PEDIATRIC DOSAGE HANDBOOK with INTERNATIONAL TRADE NAMES INDEX

Including Neonatal Dosing, Drug Administration, & Extemporaneous Preparations

Carol K. Taketomo, PharmD
Pharmacy Manager
Children's Hospital Los Angeles
Los Angeles, California

Jane Hurlburt Hodding, PharmD
Director, Pharmacy Services
Miller Children's Hospital
Long Beach, California

Donna M. Kraus, PharmD, FAPhA
Associate Professor of Pharmacy Practice
Departments of Pharmacy Practice and Pediatrics
Pediatric Clinical Pharmacist
University of Illinois at Chicago
Chicago, Illinois

LEXI-COMP

APhA

This data is intended to serve the user as a handy reference and not as a complete drug information resource. It does not include information on every therapeutic agent available. The publication covers 821 commonly used drugs and is specifically designed to present important aspects of drug data in a more concise format than is typically found in medical literature or product material supplied by manufacturers.

The nature of drug information is that it is constantly evolving because of ongoing research and clinical experience and is often subject to interpretation. While great care has been taken to ensure the accuracy of the information presented, the reader is advised that the authors, editors, reviewers, contributors, and publishers cannot be responsible for the continued currency of the information or for any errors, omissions, or the application of this information, or for any consequences arising therefrom. Therefore, the author(s) and/or the publisher shall have no liability to any person or entity with regard to claims, loss, or damage caused, or alleged to be caused, directly or indirectly, by the use of information contained herein. Because of the dynamic nature of drug information, readers are advised that decisions regarding drug therapy must be based on the independent judgment of the clinician, changing information about a drug (eg, as reflected in the literature and manufacturer's most current product information), and changing medical practices. Therefore, this data is designed to be used in conjunction with other necessary information and is not designed to be solely relied upon by any user. The user of this data hereby and forever releases the authors of this data for any and all liability of any kind that might arise out of the use of this data. The editors are not responsible for any inaccuracy of quotation or for any false or misleading implication that may arise due to the text or formulas as used or due to the quotation of revisions no longer official.

The authors, editors, and contributors have written this book in their private capacities. No official support or endorsement by any federal or state agency or pharmaceutical company is intended or inferred.

The publishers have made every effort to trace the copyright holders for borrowed material. If they have inadvertently overlooked any, they will be pleased to make the necessary arrangements at the first opportunity.

If you have any suggestions or questions regarding any information presented in this data, please contact our drug information pharmacist at (330) 650-6506.

This manual was produced using Lexi-Comp's Information Management System™ (LIMS) — a complete publishing service of Lexi-Comp Inc.

LEXI-COMP
1100 Terex Road
Hudson, Ohio 44236
(330) 650-6506

ISBN 978-1-59195-215-2 (Domestic Edition)

ISBN 978-1-59195-216-9 (International Edition)

TABLE OF CONTENTS

PREFACE

This fourteenth edition of the *Pediatric Dosage Handbook* is designed to be a practical and convenient guide to the dosing and usage of medications in children. The pediatric population is a dynamic group, with major changes in pharmacokinetics and pharmacodynamics taking place throughout infancy and childhood. Therefore, the need for the evaluation and establishment of medication dosing regimens in children of different ages is great.

Special considerations must be taken into account when dosing medications in pediatric patients. Unfortunately, due to a lack of appropriate studies, most medications commonly used in children do not have FDA approved labeling for use in pediatric patients. Only 30% of drugs used in children in a 1988 survey carried FDA approval in their labeling. Seventy-five percent of medications listed in the *1990 Physicians Desk Reference* carry some type of precaution or disclaimer statement for use in children.[1]

The FDA Modernization Act of 1997, the Children's Health Act of 2000, the Best Pharmaceuticals for Children Act of 2002, and the Pediatric Research Equity Act of 2003 will help to increase pediatric drug studies. The FDA Modernization Act of 1997 (Section 111, Public Law 105-115, 105th Congress) **encourages** pharmaceutical companies to conduct pediatric drug studies by allowing 6 months of market exclusivity to certain designated drugs. A list of drugs, for which additional pediatric information may produce pediatric healthcare benefits, was required by this law to be developed by the U.S. Department of Health and Human Services (HHS), with input from the American Academy of Pediatrics, the Pediatric Pharmacology Research Unit Network,[2] and the U.S. Pharmacopoeia. To date, the FDA has received 504 proposals from pharmaceutical companies to conduct pediatric drug studies under this Act and has issued 341 written requests for studies. If these pediatric studies are completed as the FDA has specified, then these medications will qualify for the 6 month patent extension or additional market exclusivity. One-hundred thirty-six products have already had their marketing patents extended by this law and pediatric labeling changes have occurred for 129 of these products[3]. The FDA submitted a required report on the Pediatric Exclusivity Provision to Congress in January 2001[4]. This report described the effectiveness, short comings, and economic impact of the Pediatric Exclusivity Provision. It also gave suggestions for modifications and ways to address gaps in the statute.

The pediatric section of the FDA Modernization Act was renewed by Congress and signed into law January 4, 2002. This new law, called the Best Pharmaceuticals for Children Act, reauthorizes the use of the 6-month patent extension to **encourage** pharmaceutical companies to conduct pediatric drug research. This law, which remains in effect until October 2007, calls for the establishment of an Office of Pediatric Therapeutics within the FDA and establishes an FDA Pediatric Pharmacology Advisory Committee and a Pediatric Subcommittee of the Oncologic Drugs Advisory Committee. It also creates a research fund for pediatric studies of drugs that are off patent, grants a special "priority status" to pediatric labeling changes, requires the Department of Health and Human Services (along with the Institute of Medicine) to conduct a study to assess federally funded pediatric research and calls for the development of a Final Rule that will require drug labeling to include a toll-free number to report adverse events[5].

The 1998 Pediatric Final Rule was an FDA regulation, titled "Regulations Requiring Manufacturers to Assess the Safety and Effectiveness of New Drugs and Biological Products in Pediatric Patients; Final Rule"[6]. This important regulation **required** that manufacturers conduct pediatric studies for certain new and marketed drugs and biological products. This requirement was mandatory, and its scope included new drugs (ie, new chemical entities, new dosage forms, new indications, new routes of administration, and new dosing regimens) and certain marketed drugs (ie, where the drug product offered meaningful therapeutic benefit or had substantial use in pediatric patients, AND the absence of pediatric labeling posed a risk). This FDA regulation became effective April 1, 1999, but studies mandated under this rule were not required to be submitted to the FDA before December 2, 2000. The 1998 Pediatric Final Rule and the authority of the FDA to

require manufacturers to conduct pediatric studies was challenged with a law suit. In March 2002, the FDA requested a 2-month stay on the lawsuit, so it could publish a notice and suspend the 1998 Pediatric Final Rule for 2 years. During the 2 year suspension of the Rule, the FDA planned to study whether the Best Pharmaceuticals for Children Act of 2002 made the 1998 Final Rule unnecessary. After multiple organizations lobbied Congress and the president, the Secretary of Health and Human Services announced in April 2002, that the FDA would continue to defend the Pediatric Final Rule of 1998 in court. However, on October 17, 2002, the U.S. District Court for the District of Columbia barred the FDA from enforcing the Pediatric Final Rule. Fortunately, Congress passed the Pediatric Research Equity Act of 2003 (Public Law S.650, 108th Congress). This law essentially reinstates the Pediatric Final Rule and authorizes the FDA to **require** pharmaceutical manufacturers to conduct pediatric studies of certain drugs and biological products. It also establishes an FDA Pediatric Advisory Committee.

The Children's Health Act of 2000 was signed into law on October 17, 2000. This important law establishes a Pediatric Research Initiative (headed by the Director of the NIH) and provides funds to increase support for pediatric clinical research. These three important laws, plus other FDA regulations, such as the FDA labeling changes[7] that required expanded information in the Pediatric Use section of the package insert for all prescription drugs, will certainly help to increase and disseminate pediatric drug information.

Currently, however, most commonly used pharmacy references do not include information regarding pediatric dosing, drug administration, or special pediatric concerns. It is, therefore, not surprising that in order to obtain pediatric dosing information, oftentimes the pediatric clinician is faced with extensive literature searches to arrive at a logical dose. This handbook was developed with the intent to serve as a compilation of recommended pediatric doses found in the literature and to provide relevant clinical information regarding the use of drugs in children.

New in This Edition

This new edition incorporates additions and revisions in a format that we hope the user will find beneficial. The Synonyms and Available Salts fields have been replaced with an Index Terms field which lists other names, accepted abbreviations, and various salt forms for the generic drug.

As with each edition, drug monographs have been updated and revised. Forty-seven new monographs have been added. Two monographs have been deleted because the drugs are no longer available in the U.S.: Kaolin and Pectin; Nalidixic Acid. Two monographs (Phosphate Supplements and Potassium Supplements) have been divided into separate individual monographs. This brings the total number of drug monographs to 821. The 47 new monographs added to this edition include: Abacavir and Lamivudine; Alclometasone; Antihemophilic Factor/von Willebrand Factor Complex (Human); Bromocriptine; Calcium Acetate; Calcium Carbonate; Calcium Chloride; Calcium Citrate; Calcium Glubionate; Calcium Gluconate; Calcium Lactate; Calcium Phosphate, Tribasic; Chloroprocaine; Citalopram; Fluvoxamine; Iodixanol; Magnesium Chloride; Magnesium Citrate; Magnesium Gluconate; Magnesium Hydroxide; Magnesium L-Aspartate Hydrochloride; Magnesium Oxide; Magnesium Sulfate; Measles, Mumps, Rubella, and Varicella Virus Vaccine; Mefloquine; Mepivacaine; Nabilone; Nelarabine; Nandrolone; Oxaliplatin; Papillomavirus (Types 6, 11, 16, 18) Recombinant Vaccine; Paricalcitol; Potassium Acetate; Potassium Bicarbonate; Potassium Bicarbonate and Potassium Chloride; Potassium Bicarbonate and Potassium Citrate; Potassium Chloride; Potassium Gluconate; Potassium Iodide and Iodine; Potassium Phosphate; Potassium Phosphate and Sodium Phosphate; Posaconazole; Procaine; Sodium Phosphate; Stanozolol; Teniposide; and Yellow Fever Vaccine.

In addition, a few new extemporaneous preparations have been added to this edition. This brings the total number of drug monographs with extemporaneous preparations to 89.

One new appendix piece has been added to this edition: Management of Healthcare Worker Exposures to HBV, HCV, and HIV. Appendix material has been updated to include the 2007 Childhood and Adolescent Immunization Schedule

PREFACE *(Continued)*

and the following tables were updated or revised: Antihypertensive Agents by Class; Corticosteroids, Systemic; Corticosteroids, Topical: Guidelines for Selection and Use; Multivitamin Products; OTC Cough and Cold Preparations, Pediatric; Cytochrome P450 Enzymes: Substrates, Inhibitors, and Inducers; Oral Contraceptives; Fluids, Electrolytes, and Nutrition; Endocarditis Prophylaxis; HIV Treatment Guidelines; Immunization Guidelines; Malaria; Sugar-Free Liquid Pharmaceuticals; and Carbohydrate Content of Medications.

We hope this edition continues to be a valuable and practical source of clinical drug information for the pediatric healthcare professional. We welcome comments to further improve future editions.

Footnotes

1. Food and Drug Letter, Washington Business Information, Inc. November 23, 1990.
2. "NIH Funds Network of Centers for Pediatric Drug Research," *Am J Hosp Pharm*, 1994, 51:2546.
3. http://www.fda.gov/cder/pediatric.
4. Department of Health and Human Services, U.S. Food and Drug Administration, "The Pediatric Exclusivity Provision, January 2001: Status Report to Congress," http://www.fda.gov/cder/pediatric/reportcong01.pdf.
5. Birenbaum D, "Pediatric Initiatives: A Regulatory Perspective of the U.S. Experience," June 17, 2002, http://www.fda.gov/cder/pediatric/presentation/Ped Init 2002 DB/index.htm.
6. Department of Health and Human Services, Food and Drug Administration, 21CFR Parts 201, 312, 314, and 601, Regulations Requiring Manufacturers to Assess the Safety and Effectiveness of New Drugs and Biological Products in Pediatric Patients; Final Rule," *Fed Regist*, 1998, 63(231):66631-72.
7. "Pediatric Use Drug Labeling NDA Supplements Due by December 1996 - FDA Final Rule; Agency Establishing Pediatric Subcommittee to Track Implementation," *F-D-C Reports - The Pink Sheet*, Wallace Werble Jr, Publisher, December 19, 1994.

ACKNOWLEDGMENTS

The *Pediatric Dosage Handbook* exists in its present form as the result of the concerted efforts of the following individuals: Robert D. Kerscher, publisher and chief executive officer of Lexi-Comp Inc; Steven Kerscher, president and chief operating officer; Mark Bonfiglio, BS, PharmD, RPh, chief content officer; Stacy S. Robinson, editorial manager; Joni L. Stahura, BS, PharmD, pharmacotherapy specialist; Matthew Fuller, PharmD, clinical pharmacy specialist, psychiatry (VA Medical Center, Brecksville, OH); David C. Marcus, chief information officer; Tracey Henterly, senior graphic designer; Alexandra Hart, composition specialist; and Julian I. Graubart, American Pharmacists Association (APhA), Director of Books and Electronic Products.

Special acknowledgment goes to all Lexi-Comp staff for their contributions to this handbook.

Special thanks goes to Chris Lomax, PharmD, director of pharmacy, Children's Hospital, Los Angeles, who played a significant role in bringing APhA and Lexi-Comp together.

Some of the material contained in the book was a result of pediatric pharmacy contributors throughout the United States and Canada. Lexi-Comp has assisted many pediatric medical institutions to develop hospital-specific formulary manuals that contain clinical drug information as well as dosing. Working with these pediatric clinical pharmacists, pediatric hospital pharmacy and therapeutics committees, and hospital drug information centers, Lexi-Comp has developed an evolutionary drug database that reflects the practice of pediatric pharmacy in these major pediatric institutions.

The authors wish to thank their families, friends, and colleagues who supported them in their efforts to complete this handbook.

In addition, Dr Taketomo would like to thank Robert Taketomo, PharmD, MBA and Chris Lomax, PharmD for their professional guidance and continued support, and the pharmacy staff at Childrens Hospital, Los Angeles for their assistance.

Dr Kraus would like to especially thank Keith A. Rodvold, PharmD, for his ongoing professional and personal support.

Dr Hodding would like to thank Glenn Hodding, PharmD, Carl Kildoo, PharmD, and the pediatric pharmacists at Miller Children's Hospital for their continued professional and personal support.

EDITORIAL ADVISORY PANEL

Judith A. Aberg, MD
Principal Investigator, AIDS Clinical Trials Unit
Director of HIV
Bellevue Hospital Center
Associate Professor of Medicine
New York University
New York, New York

Lora Armstrong, RPh, PharmD, BCPS
Vice President, Clinical Affairs
Pharmacy & Therapeutics Committee Formulary Process
Clinical Program Oversight
CaremarkRx
Northbrook, Illinois

William Alvarez Jr., PharmD
Clinical Specialist, Cardiology
Johns Hopkins Hospital
Baltimore, Maryland

David Au, MD
Assistant Professor of Medicine
University of Washington
Seattle, Washington

Kenneth A. Bachmann, PhD, FCP
Distinguished University Professor of Pharmacology
Codirector, Center for Applied Pharmacology
University of Toledo
Toledo, Ohio

Verna L. Baughman, MD
Professor
Anesthesiology and Neurosurgery
University of Illinois
Chicago, Illinois

Judith L. Beizer, PharmD, CGP, FASCP
Clinical Professor
Department of Clinical Pharmacy Practice
St John's University College of Pharmacy and Allied Health Professions
Jamaica, New York

Mark F. Bonfiglio, BS, PharmD, RPh
Chief Content Officer
Lexi-Comp, Inc
Hudson, Ohio

Diedra L. Bragalone, BSPharm, BCOP
Pharmacotherapy Specialist
Lexi-Comp, Inc
Hudson, Ohio

Larisa H. Cavallari, PharmD, BCPS
Assistant Professor, Section of Cardiology
University of Illinois
Chicago, Illinois

Irene H. Chenowith, MD, FACP
Medical Director of Professional Affairs
Akron General Medical Center
Akron, Ohio
Associate Professor of Internal Medicine
Northeastern Ohio Universities
College of Medicine
Rootstown, Ohio

Matthew M. Cooney, MD
Hematology/Oncology
University Hospitals of Cleveland
Cleveland, Ohio

Harold L. Crossley, DDS, PhD
Associate Professor of Pharmacology
Baltimore College of Dental Surgery
Dental School
University of Maryland Baltimore
Baltimore, Maryland

Laura Cummings, PharmD, BCPS
Clinical Pharmacy Specialist, Pediatrics
The Children's Hospital at MetroHealth
Cleveland, Ohio

Andrew J. Donnelly, PharmD, MBA
Director of Pharmacy
and
Clinical Professor of Pharmacy Practice
University of Illinois Medical Center at Chicago
Chicago, Illinois

Julie A. Dopheide, PharmD, BCPP
Associate Professor of Clinical Pharmacy,
Psychiatry and the Behavioral Sciences
University of Southern California
Schools of Pharmacy and Medicine
Los Angeles, California

Michael S. Edwards, PharmD, MBA
Assistant Director, Weinberg Pharmacy
Johns Hopkins Hospital
Baltimore, Maryland

Vicki L. Ellingrod, PharmD, BCPP
Associate Professor
University of Iowa
Iowa City, Iowa

Kelley K. Engle, BSPharm
Pharmacotherapy Specialist
Lexi-Comp, Inc
Hudson, Ohio

Margaret A. Fitzgerald, MS, APRN, BC, NP-C, FAANP
President
Fitzgerald Health Education Associates, Inc.
North Andover, Massachusetts
Family Nurse Practitioner
Greater Lawrence Family Health Center
Lawrence, Massachusetts

Lawrence A. Frazee, PharmD
Pharmacotherapy Specialist in Internal Medicine
Akron General Medical Center
Akron, Ohio

Matthew A. Fuller, PharmD, BCPS, BCPP, FASHP
Clinical Pharmacy Specialist, Psychiatry
Cleveland Department of Veterans Affairs Medical Center
Brecksville, Ohio
Associate Clinical Professor of Psychiatry
Clinical Instructor of Psychology
Case Western Reserve University
Cleveland, Ohio
Adjunct Associate Professor of Clinical Pharmacy
University of Toledo
Toledo, Ohio

EDITORIAL ADVISORY PANEL *(Continued)*

EDITORIAL ADVISORY PANEL *(Continued)*

EDITORIAL ADVISORY PANEL *(Continued)*

ABOUT THE AUTHORS

Carol K. Taketomo, PharmD

Dr Taketomo received her doctorate from the University of Southern California School of Pharmacy. Subsequently, she completed a clinical pharmacy residency at the University of California Medical Center in San Diego. With over 28 years of clinical experience at one of the largest pediatric teaching hospitals in the nation, she is an acknowledged expert in the practical aspects of pediatric drug distribution and clinical pharmacy practice. She currently holds the appointment of Adjunct Assistant Professor of Pharmacy Practice at the University of Southern California School of Pharmacy.

In her current capacity as Pharmacy Manager at Children's Hospital of Los Angeles, Dr Taketomo plays an active role in the education and training of the medical, pharmacy, and nursing staff. She coordinates the Pharmacy Department's quality assurance and drug use evaluation programs; maintains the hospital's strict formulary program; and is the editor of the house staff manual. Her particular interests are strategies to influence physician prescribing patterns and methods to decrease medication errors in the pediatric setting. She has been the author of numerous publications, and is an active presenter at professional meetings.

Dr Taketomo is a member of the American Pharmacists Association (APhA), American Society of Health-System Pharmacists (ASHP), California Society of Hospital Pharmacists (CSHP), and Southern California Pediatric Pharmacy Group.

Jane Hurlburt Hodding, PharmD

Dr Hodding earned a doctorate and completed her pharmacy residency at the University of California School of Pharmacy in San Francisco. She has held teaching positions as Assistant Clinical Professor of Pharmacy at UCSF as well as Assistant Clinical Professor of Pharmacy Practice at the University of Southern California in Los Angeles. Currently, Dr Hodding is the Director, Pharmacy Services at Miller Children's Hospital in Long Beach, California.

Throughout her 29 years of pediatric pharmacy practice, Dr Hodding has actively pursued methods to improve the safety of medication use in neonates, children, and adolescents. She has actively practiced as a clinical pharmacy specialist in neonatal intensive care, pediatric intensive care, and pediatric hematology/oncology. Parenteral nutrition is another area of focus. She has published numerous articles covering neonatal medication administration and aminoglycoside and theophylline clearance in premature infants.

Dr Hodding is a member of the American Pharmacists Association (APhA), American Society of Health-System Pharmacists (ASHP), California Society of Hospital Pharmacists (CSHP), Pediatric Pharmacy Advocacy Group (PPAG), Children's Oncology Group, and Southern California Pediatric Pharmacy Group. She is frequently an invited speaker on the topics of Medication Safety in Children, A Multidisciplinary Approach; Monitoring Drug Therapy in the NICU; Fluid and Electrolyte Therapy in Children; Drug Therapy Considerations in Children; and Parenteral Nutrition in the Premature Infant.

Donna M. Kraus, PharmD

Dr Kraus received her Bachelor of Science in Pharmacy from the University of Illinois at Chicago (UIC). She worked for several years as a hospital pediatric/obstetric satellite pharmacist before earning her doctorate degree at the UIC. Dr Kraus then completed a postdoctoral pediatric specialty residency at the University of Texas Health Science Center in San Antonio. She served as a pediatric intensive care clinical pharmacist for 15 years and for the past 9 years has been an ambulatory care pediatric clinical pharmacist, specializing in pediatric HIV pharmacotherapy and patient/parent medication adherence. Dr Kraus has also served as a clinical pharmacist consultant to a pediatric long-term care facility for

ABOUT THE AUTHORS *(Continued)*

over 21 years. She currently holds the appointment of Associate Professor of Pharmacy Practice in both the Departments of Pharmacy Practice and Pediatrics at the University of Illinois in Chicago.

In her 30 years of active pharmacy experience, Dr Kraus has dealt with pediatric pharmacy issues and pharmacotherapy problems. She is an active educator and has been a guest lecturer in China, Thailand, and Hong Kong. Dr Kraus has played a leading role in the advanced training of postgraduate pharmacists and has been the Director of the UIC (ASHP accredited) Pediatric Residency and Fellowship Program for 20 years. Dr Kraus' research areas include pediatric drug dosing and developmental pharmacokinetics and pharmacodynamics. She has published a number of articles on various issues of pediatric pharmacy and pharmacotherapy.

Dr Kraus has been an active member of numerous professional associations including the American Pharmacists Association (APhA), American Society of Health-System Pharmacists (ASHP), Illinois Pharmacists Association (IPhA), American College of Clinical Pharmacy (ACCP), Illinois College of Clinical Pharmacy (ICCP), and the Pediatric Pharmacy Advocacy Group (PPAG). She has served as Chairperson of the ASHP Commission on Therapeutics, member of the Board of Directors of Pediatric Pharmacy Advocacy Group (PPAG), and APhA, Academy of Pharmaceutical Research and Science, Member-at-Large. Dr. Kraus also served as an Editorial Board member of the *American Journal of Health-System Pharmacy* and the *Journal of Pediatric Pharmacy Practice.* Currently, she serves as an Editorial Board member of *The Journal of Pediatric Pharmacology and Therapeutics.* Dr. Kraus was awarded Fellow status by the American Pharmaceutical Association and is the APhA designated author for this handbook.

DESCRIPTION OF SECTIONS AND FIELDS USED IN THIS HANDBOOK

The *Pediatric Dosage Handbook, 14th Edition* is organized into a drug information section, an appendix, a therapeutic category & key word index, and an international trade names index.

Drug information is presented in a consistent format and provides the following:

Generic Name	U.S. adopted name. "Tall Man" lettering appears for look-alike generic drug names as recommended by the FDA. See "FDA Differentiation Project: The Use of "Tall Man" Letters" on page 27. The symbol [DSC] appears after the generic name of drugs that have been recently discontinued.
Pronunciation Guide	Phonetic listing of generic name
Medication Safety Issues	Highlights safety concerns which apply to a particular drug with a focus on name confusion, ie, drug or brand names with the potential to sound or look similar to another drug or brand name
Related Information	Cross-reference to other pertinent drug information found in the Appendix
U.S. Brand Names	Common trade names used in the U.S. The symbol [DSC] appears after trade names that have been recently discontinued.
Canadian Brand Names	Common trade names used in Canada
Index Terms	Other names, accepted abbreviations, or various salt forms for the generic drug
Therapeutic Category	Unique systematic classification of medications
Generic Available	Indicated by a "Yes" or "No" as to whether a generic form of the drug is available. Specific generic dosage forms (or exceptions) are listed in parentheses.
Use	Information pertaining to appropriate indications or use of the drug
Restrictions	Drug Enforcement Agency (DEA) classification for federally scheduled controlled substances
Medication Guide	Information regarding the FDA-required distribution of patient Medication Guides for select drugs
Pregnancy Risk Factor	Five categories established by the FDA to indicate the potential of a systemically absorbed drug for causing birth defects
Lactation	Information regarding the excretion of the drug in breast milk and whether breast-feeding is recommended or not; a notation is made when recommendations differ from the American Academy of Pediatrics
Contraindications	Information pertaining to inappropriate use of the drug, or disease states and patient populations in which the drug should not be used
Warnings	Hazardous conditions related to use of the drug
Precautions	Disease states or patient populations in which the drug should be cautiously used
Adverse Reactions	Side effects are grouped by body system and include a listing of the more common and/or serious side effects. Due to space limitations, every reported side effect is not listed.
Drug Interactions	For select drugs that have demonstrated involvement with cytochrome P450 enzymes, the initial line of this field identifies the drug as a substrate, inducer, or inhibitor of specific isoenzymes (eg, CYP1A2). A summary of this information can also be found in a tabular format within the appendix. The remainder of the field presents a description of common or significant interactions between the drug listed in the monograph and other drugs or drug classes that are commonly used in pediatric patients. Due to space limitations, the reader is advised to read the drug interaction field of both drugs involved in the interaction.
Food Interactions	Possible interactions between the drug listed in the monograph and certain foods and/or nutritional substances
Stability	Storage, refrigeration, and compatibility information
Mechanism of Action	How the drug works in the body to elicit a response
Pharmacodynamics	Dose-response relationships including onset of action, time of peak action, and duration of action

DESCRIPTION OF SECTIONS AND FIELDS USED IN THIS HANDBOOK *(Continued)*

Pharmacokinetics	Drug movement through the body over time. Pharmacokinetics deals with absorption, distribution, protein binding, metabolism, bioavailability, half-life, time to peak concentration, elimination, and clearance of drugs. Pharmacokinetic parameters help predict drug concentration and dosage requirements.
Usual Dosage	The amount of the drug to be typically given or taken during therapy Please note that doses for neonates are often listed by postnatal age (PNA) (eg, PNA ≤7 days) and/or by body weight (eg, 1200-2000 g) When both milligram and milligram per kilogram doses are listed, the milligram per kilogram dosing method is preferred. If using a milligram dosing guideline according to age, special care and lower doses should be used in children who have a low weight for their age. When ranges of doses are listed, initiate therapy at the lower end of the range and titrate the dose accordingly. References are listed at the end of drug monographs to support doses listed when little dosing information exists. For select drugs, the dosing adjustment in renal impairment or dosing interval in renal impairment is given according to creatinine clearance (Cl_{cr}). Since most studies that recommend dosing guidelines in renal dysfunction are conducted in adult patients, Cl_{cr} is usually expressed in units of mL/minute. However, in order to extrapolate the adult information to the pediatric population, one must assume that the adults studied were of standard surface area (ie, 1.73 m^2). Therefore, although the value of Cl_{cr} listed for dosing adjustment in renal impairment or dosing interval in renal impairment may be expressed in mL/minute, it is assumed to be equal to the same value in mL/minute/1.73 m^2. To calculate the dose in a pediatric patient with renal dysfunction, first calculate the normal dose (ie, the dose for a patient without renal dysfunction), then use the guidelines to adjust the dose. For example, the normal piperacillin dose for a 20 kg child is 200-300 mg/kg/day divided every 4-6 hours. If one selected 300 mg/kg/day divided every 6 hours, the dose would be 1.5 g every 6 hours in normal renal function. If Cl_{cr} was 20-40 mL/minute/1.73 m^2, the dose would be 1.5 g every 8 hours and if Cl_{cr} was <20 mL/minute/1.73 m^2, the dose would be 1.5 g every 12 hours.
Administration	Information regarding the recommended final concentrations and rates for administration of parenteral drugs are listed when appropriate, along with pertinent oral, ophthalmic, and topical administration information.
Monitoring Parameters	Laboratory tests and patient physical parameters that should be monitored for safety and efficacy of drug therapy are listed when appropriate.
Reference Range	Therapeutic and toxic serum concentrations are listed when appropriate
Test Interactions	Listing of assay interferences when relevant; (S) = Serum; (U) = Urine
Patient Information	Advice, warnings, precautions, and other information of which the patient should be informed
Nursing Implications	Comments regarding nursing care of the patient are offered when appropriate
Additional Information	Other data and facts about the drug are offered when appropriate

Dosage Forms	Information with regard to form, strength, and availability of the drug. **Note:** Additional formulation information (eg, excipients, preservatives) is included when available. Please consult product labeling for further information. The symbol [DSC] appears after dosage forms that have been recently discontinued. U.S. brand names appear in this field when more than one brand name exists for a medication. For dosage forms that are available as generic products and multiple brand names, the generic dosage forms are listed first, followed by the U.S. brand names and dosage form descriptions. Important information about ingredients found in specific dosage forms appears in brackets at the end of the dosage form entry.
Extemporaneous Preparations	Directions for preparing liquid formulations from solid drug products. May include stability information and references (listed when appropriate).
References	Bibliographic information referring to specific pediatric literature findings, especially doses

Appendix

The appendix offers a compilation of tables, guidelines, and conversion information which can often be helpful when considering patient care. This section is broken down into various sections for ease of use.

Therapeutic Category & Key Word Index

This index provides a useful listing by an easy-to-use therapeutic classification system. Also listed are controlled substances, preservative free, sugar free, and alcohol free medications.

International Trade Names Index

Alphabetical listing of international trade names covering 125 countries.

DEFINITION OF AGE GROUP TERMINOLOGY

Information in this handbook is listed according to specific age or by age group. The following are definitions of age groups and age-related terminologies. These definitions should be used unless otherwise specified in the monograph.

Gestational age (GA)	The time from conception until birth. More specifically, gestational age is defined as the number of weeks from the first day of the mother's last menstrual period (LMP) until the birth of the baby. Gestational age at birth is assessed by the date of the LMP and by physical exam (Dubowitz score).
Postnatal age (PNA)	Chronological age since birth
Postconceptional age (PCA)	Age since conception. Postconceptional age is calculated as gestational age plus postnatal age (PCA = GA + PNA).
Neonate	A full-term newborn 0-4 weeks postnatal age. This term may also be applied to a premature neonate whose postconceptional age (PCA) is 42-46 weeks.
Premature neonate	Neonate born at <38 weeks gestational age
Full-term neonate	Neonate born at 38-42 weeks (average ~40 weeks) gestational age
Infant	1 month to 1 year of age
Child/Children	1-12 years of age
Adolescent	13-18 years of age
Adult	>18 years of age

FDA PREGNANCY CATEGORIES

Throughout this book there is a field labeled Pregnancy Risk Factor and the letter A, B, C, D, or X immediately following which signifies a category. The FDA has established these five categories to indicate the potential of a systemically absorbed drug for causing birth defects. The key differentiation among the categories rests upon the reliability of documentation and the risk:benefit ratio. Pregnancy Category X is particularly notable in that if any data exists that may implicate a drug as a teratogen and the risk:benefit ratio is clearly negative, the drug is contraindicated during pregnancy.

These categories are summarized as follows:

A — Controlled studies in pregnant women fail to demonstrate a risk to the fetus in the first trimester with no evidence of risk in later trimesters. The possibility of fetal harm appears remote.

B — Either animal-reproduction studies have not demonstrated a fetal risk but there are no controlled studies in pregnant women, or animal-reproduction studies have shown an adverse effect (other than a decrease in fertility) that was not confirmed in controlled studies in women in the first trimester and there is no evidence of a risk in later trimesters.

C — Either studies in animals have revealed adverse effects on the fetus (teratogenic or embryocidal effects or other) and there are no controlled studies in women, or studies in women and animals are not available. Drugs should be given only if the potential benefits justify the potential risk to the fetus.

D — There is positive evidence of human fetal risk, but the benefits from use in pregnant women may be acceptable despite the risk (eg, if the drug is needed in a life-threatening situation or for a serious disease for which safer drugs cannot be used or are ineffective).

X — Studies in animals or human beings have demonstrated fetal abnormalities or there is evidence of fetal risk based on human experience, or both, and the risk of the use of the drug in pregnant women clearly outweighs any possible benefit. The drug is contraindicated in women who are or may become pregnant.

SYMBOLS & ABBREVIATIONS USED IN THIS HANDBOOK*

°C	degrees Celsius (Centigrade)
<	less than
>	greater than
≤	less than or equal to
≥	greater than or equal to
AAP	American Academy of Pediatrics
AAPC	antibiotic associated pseudomembranous colitis
ABG	arterial blood gas
ABMT	autologous bone marrow transplant
ACE	angiotensin-converting enzyme
ACLS	advanced cardiac life support
ADH	antidiuretic hormone
AED	antiepileptic drug
AHCPR	Agency for Health Care Policy and Research
AIDS	acquired immunodeficiency syndrome
ALL	acute lymphoblastic leukemia
ALT	alanine aminotransferase (formerly called SGPT)
AML	acute myeloblastic leukemia
ANA	antinuclear antibodies
ANC	absolute neutrophil count
ANLL	acute nonlymphoblastic leukemia
APTT	activated partial thromboplastin time
ARDS	adult respiratory distress syndrome
ASA (class I-IV)	American Society of Anesthesiology physical status classification of surgical patients according to their baseline health ASA I: Normal healthy patients ASA II: Patients having controlled disease states (eg, controlled hypertension) ASA III: Patients having a disease which compromises their organ function (eg, decompensated CHF, end stage renal failure) ASA IV: Patients who are extremely critically ill
AST	aspartate aminotransferase (formerly called SGOT)
ATP	adenosine triphosphate
AUC	area under the curve (area under the serum concentration-time curve)
A-V	atrial-ventricular
BMT	bone marrow transplant
BPD	bronchopulmonary disease
BSA	body surface area
BUN	blood urea nitrogen
CAD	coronary artery disease
CADD	computer ambulatory drug delivery
cAMP	cyclic adenosine monophosphate
CBC	complete blood count
CDC	Center for Disease Control and Prevention
CF	cystic fibrosis
CFC	chlorofluorocarbons
CHF	congestive heart failure
CI	cardiac index
Cl_{cr}	creatinine clearance
CLL	chronic lymphocytic leukemia
CML	chronic myelogenous leukemia
CMV	cytomegalovirus
CNS	central nervous system
COPD	chronic obstructive pulmonary disease
CPK	creatine phosphokinase
CPR	cardiopulmonary resuscitation

(continued)

CRF	chronic renal failure
CSF	cerebrospinal fluid
CT	computed tomography
CVA	cerebral vascular accident
CVP	central venous pressure
CYP	cytochrome
d	day
D_5/LR	dextrose 5% in lactated Ringer's
D_5/NS	dextrose 5% in sodium chloride 0.9%
D_5W	dextrose 5% in water
D_5/¼ NS	dextrose 5% in sodium chloride 0.2%
D_5/½ NS	dextrose 5% in sodium chloride 0.45%
D_{10}W	dextrose 10% in water
DIC	disseminated intravascular coagulation
DL_{co}	pulmonary diffusion capacity for carbon monoxide
DNA	deoxyribonucleic acid
[DSC]	discontinued
DVT	deep vein thrombosis
ECG	electrocardiogram
ECHO	echocardiogram
ECMO	extracorporeal membrane oxygenation
EEG	electroencephalogram
EKG	electrocardiogram
ESR	erythrocyte sedimentation rate
ESRD	end stage renal disease
E.T.	endotracheal
FDA	Food and Drug Administration (United States)
FEV_1	forced expiratory volume exhaled after 1 second
FSH	follicle-stimulating hormone
FVC	forced vital capacity
g	gram
G-6-PD	glucose-6-phosphate dehydrogenase
GA	gestational age
GABA	gamma-aminobutyric acid
GE	gastroesophageal
GERD	gastroesophageal reflux disease
GFR	glomerular filtration rate
GI	gastrointestinal
GVHD	graft versus host disease
GU	genitourinary
h	hour
Hct	hematocrit
HDL-C	high density lipoprotein cholesterol
Hgb	hemoglobin
HFA	hydrofluoroalkane
HIV	human immunodeficiency virus
HMG-CoA	hydroxymethyl glutaryl coenzyme A
HPA	hypothalamic-pituitary-adrenal
HPLC	high performance liquid chromatography
HSV	herpes simplex virus
ICP	intracranial pressure
IDDM	insulin-dependent diabetes mellitus
IgG	immune globulin G
I.M.	intramuscular
INR	international normalized ratio
ILCOR	International Liaison Committee on Resuscitation
I.O.	intraosseous
I & O	input and output
IOP	intraocular pressure

SYMBOLS & ABBREVIATIONS USED IN THIS HANDBOOK* *(Continued)*

IQ	intelligence quotient
I.T.	intrathecal
ITP	idiopathic thrombocytopenic purpura
I.V.	intravenous
IVH	intraventricular hemorrhage
IVP	intravenous push
JRA	juvenile rheumatoid arthritis
kg	kilogram
KOH	potassium hydroxide
L	liter
LDH	lactate dehydrogenase
LDL-C	low density lipoprotein cholesterol
LE	lupus erythematosus
LH	luteinizing hormone
LP	lumbar puncture
LR	lactated Ringer's
M	molar
MAC	*Mycobacterium avium* complex
MAO	monoamine oxidase
MAP	mean arterial pressure
mcg	microgram
mg	milligram
MI	myocardial infarction
min	minute
mL	milliliter
mM	millimole
mo	month
MOPP	mustargen (mechlorethamine), Oncovin® (vincristine), procarbazine, and prednisone
mOsm	milliosmoles
MRI	magnetic resonance image
MRSA	methicillin-resistant *Staphylococcus aureus*
NAEPP	National Asthma Education and Prevention Program
NCI	National Cancer Institute
ND	nasoduodenal
ng	nanogram
NG	nasogastric
NIDDM	noninsulin-dependent diabetes mellitus
NMDA	n-methyl-d-aspartate
nmol	nanomole
NMS	neuroleptic malignant syndrome
NPO	nothing per os (nothing by mouth)
NS	normal saline (0.9% sodium chloride)
½NS	0.45% sodium chloride
NSAID	nonsteroidal anti-inflammatory drug
NYHA	New York Heart Association
O.R.	operating room
OTC	over-the-counter (nonprescription)
PABA	para-aminobenzoic acid
PALS	pediatric advanced life support
PCA	postconceptional age
PCP	*Pneumocystis jiroveci* pneumonia (also called *Pneumocystis carinii* pneumonia)
PCWP	pulmonary capillary wedge pressure
PDA	patent ductus arteriosus
PE	pulmonary embolism
PICU	Pediatric Intensive Care Unit

(continued)

PIP	peak inspiratory pressure
PNA	postnatal age
prn	as needed
PSVT	paroxysmal supraventricular tachycardia
PT	prothrombin time
PTH	parathyroid hormone
PTT	partial thromboplastin time
PUD	peptic ulcer disease
PVC	premature ventricular contraction
PVR	peripheral vascular resistance
qsad	add an amount sufficient to equal
RAP	right arterial pressure
RDA	recommended daily allowance
RIA	radioimmunoassay
RNA	ribonucleic acid
RSV	respiratory syncytial virus
S-A	sino-atrial
S_{cr}	serum creatinine
SIADH	syndrome of inappropriate antidiuretic hormone
S.L.	sublingual
SLE	systemic lupus erythematosus
SSRI	selective serotonin reuptake inhibitor
STD	sexually-transmitted disease
SubQ	subcutaneous
SVR	systemic vascular resistance
SVT	supraventricular tachycardia
SWI	sterile water for injection
T_3	triiodothyronine
T_4	thyroxine
TCA	tricyclic antidepressant
TIA	transient ischemic attack
TIBC	total iron binding capacity
TNF	tissue necrosis factor
TPN	total parenteral nutrition
TSH	thyroid stimulating hormone
TT	thrombin time
UA	urine analysis
UTI	urinary tract infection
V_d	volume of distribution
V_{dss}	volume of distribution at steady-state
VF	ventricular fibrillation
VMA	vanillylmandelic acid
VT	ventricular tachycardia
VZV	varicella zoster virus
w/v	weight for volume
w/w	weight for weight
y	year

*Other than drug synonyms

SAFE WRITING

Health professionals and their support personnel frequently produce handwritten copies of information they see in print; therefore, such information is subjected to even greater possibilities for error or misinterpretation on the part of others. Thus, particular care must be given to how drug names and strengths are expressed when creating written health-care documents.

The following are a few examples of safe writing rules suggested by the Institute for Safe Medication Practices, Inc.[1]

1. There should be a space between a number and its units as it is easier to read. There should be no periods after the abbreviations mg or mL.

Correct	**Incorrect**
10 mg	10mg
100 mg	100mg

2. Never place a decimal and a zero after a whole number (2 mg is correct and 2.0 mg is **Incorrect**). If the decimal point is not seen because it falls on a line or because individuals are working from copies where the decimal point is not seen, this causes a tenfold overdose.
3. Just the opposite is true for numbers less than one. Always place a zero before a naked decimal (0.5 mL is correct, .5 mL is **Incorrect**).
4. Never abbreviate the word unit. The handwritten U or u, looks like a 0 (zero), and may cause a tenfold overdose error to be made.
5. IU is not a safe abbreviation for international units. The handwritten IU looks like IV. Write out international units or use int. units.
6. Q.D. is not a safe abbreviation for once daily, as when the Q is followed by a sloppy dot, it looks like QID which means four times daily.
7. O.D. is not a safe abbreviation for once daily, as it is properly interpreted as meaning "right eye" and has caused liquid medications such as saturated solution of potassium iodide and Lugol's solution to be administered incorrectly. There is no safe abbreviation for once daily. It must be written out in full.
8. Do not use chemical names such as 6-mercaptopurine or 6-thioguanine, as sixfold overdoses have been given when these were not recognized as chemical names. The proper names of these drugs are mercaptopurine or thioguanine.
9. Do not abbreviate drug names (5FC, 6MP, 5-ASA, MTX, HCTZ, CPZ, PBZ, etc) as they are misinterpreted and cause error.
10. Do not use the apothecary system or symbols.
11. Do not abbreviate microgram as μg; instead use mcg as there is less likelihood of misinterpretation.
12. When writing an outpatient prescription, write a complete prescription. A complete prescription can prevent the prescriber, the pharmacist, and/or the patient from making a mistake and can eliminate the need for further clarification. The legible prescriptions should contain:
    a. patient's full name
    b. for pediatric or geriatric patients: their age (or weight where applicable)
    c. drug name, dosage form and strength; if a drug is new or rarely prescribed, print this information
    d. number or amount to be dispensed
    e. complete instructions for the patient, including the purpose of the medication
    f. when there are recognized contraindications for a prescribed drug, indicate to the pharmacist that you are aware of this fact (ie, when prescribing a potassium salt for a patient receiving an ACE inhibitor, write "K serum leveling being monitored")

[1]From "Safe Writing" by Davis NM, PharmD and Cohen MR, MS, Lecturers and Consultants for Safe Medication Practices, 1143 Wright Drive, Huntington Valley, PA 19006. Phone: (215) 947-7566.

FDA NAME DIFFERENTIATION PROJECT: THE USE OF "TALL MAN" LETTERS

Confusion between similar drug names is a frequent cause of medication errors. For years, The Institute For Safe Medication Practices (ISMP), has urged generic manufacturers to use a combination of capital and lower case letters (eg, chlorproMAZINE and chlorproPAMIDE) to help distinguish drugs with look-alike names, especially when they share similar strengths. The FDA's Office of Generic Drugs has acted upon this suggestion and initiated the "Name Differentiation Project," to help decrease medication errors that result from look-alike drug names. From March to May 2001, the Office of Generic Drugs issued 142 letters encouraging manufacturers to revise product labeling and labels to visually differentiate the established drug name with the use of "Tall Man" letters.

The ISMP recommends that hospitals follow suit by making similar changes in their pharmacy-prepared labels, preprinted order forms, pharmacy and physician order entry systems, computer-generated medication administration records, drug storage location labels, and other print or electronic use of the drug name.

Lexi-Comp Medical Publishing will begin using these "Tall Man" letters for the drugs suggested by the FDA. The "Tall Man" lettering will appear in the generic name field of the monograph.

The following is a list of product names and recommended FDA revisions.

Drug Product	Recommended Revision
acetazolamide	aceta**ZOLAMIDE**
acetohexamide	aceto**HEXAMIDE**
bupropion	bu**PROP**ion
buspirone	bus**PIR**one
chlorpromazine	chlorpro**MAZINE**
chlorpropamide	chlorpro**PAMIDE**
clomiphene	clomi**PHENE**
clomipramine	clomi**PRAMINE**
cycloserine	cyclo**SERINE**
cyclosporine	cyclo**SPORINE**
daunorubicin	**DAUNO**rubicin
dimenhydrinate	dimenhy**DRINATE**
diphenhydramine	diphenhydr**AMINE**
dobutamine	**DOBUT**amine
dopamine	**DOP**amine
doxorubicin	**DOXO**rubicin
glipizide	glipi**ZIDE**
glyburide	gly**BURIDE**
hydralazine	hydr**ALAZINE**
hydroxyzine	hydr**OXY**zine
medroxyprogesterone	medroxy**PROGESTER**one
methylprednisolone	methyl**PREDNIS**olone
methyltestosterone	methyl**TESTOSTER**one
nicardipine	ni**CAR**dipine
nifedipine	**NIFE**dipine
prednisolone	predniso**LONE**
prednisone	predni**SONE**
sulfadiazine	sulfa**DIAZINE**

FDA NAME DIFFERENTIATION PROJECT: THE USE OF "TALL MAN" LETTERS *(Continued)*

Drug Product	**Recommended Revision**
sulfisoxazole	sulfi**SOXAZOLE**
tolazamide	**TOLAZ**amide
tolbutamide	**TOLBUT**amide
vinblastine	vin**BLAS**tine
vincristine	vin**CRIS**tine

References

FDA, "Name Differentiation Project." Available at http://www.fda.gov/cder/drug/MedErrors/nameDiff.htm.

Institute for Safe Medication Practices. "New Tall-Man Lettering Will Reduce Mix-Ups Due to Generic Drug Name Confusion," *ISMP Medication Safety Alert*, September 19, 2001. Available at: http://www.ismp.org.

Institute for Safe Medication Practices. "Prescription Mapping, Can Improve Efficiency While Minimizing Errors With Look-Alike Products," *ISMP Medication Safety Alert*, October 6, 1999. Available at: http://www.ismp.org.

U.S. Pharmacopeia, "USP Quality Review: Use Caution-Avoid Confusion," March 2001, No. 76. Available at: http://www.usp.org.

SELECTED REFERENCES

AHFS Drug Information, McEvoy GK, ed, Bethesda, MD: American Society of Health-System Pharmacists, 2007.

Dorr RT and Von Hoff DD, *Cancer Chemotherapy Handbook*, 2nd ed, Norwalk, CT: Appleton & Lange, 1994.

Drug Facts and Comparisons, St Louis, MO: J.B. Facts and Comparisons part of Wolters Kluwer Health, Inc, 2007.

Drug Interaction Facts, Tatro DS, ed, St Louis, MO: J.B. Lippincott Co (Facts and Comparisons Division), 2007.

Hale T, *Medications and Mother's Milk*, 9th ed, Amarillo, TX: Pharmasoft Medical Publishing, 2004.

Handbook on Extemporaneous Formulations, Bethesda, MD: American Society of Health-System Pharmacists, 1987.

Handbook of Nonprescription Drugs, 15th ed, Washington, DC: American Pharmacists Association, 2006.

Jacobs DS, DeMott WR, Grady HJ, et al, *Laboratory Test Handbook with Key Word Index*, 5th ed, Hudson, OH: Lexi-Comp Inc, 2001.

Jenson HB and Baltimore RS, *Pediatric Infectious Diseases - Principles and Practice*, 2nd ed, Philadelphia, PA: Saunders, 2002.

Lacy CF, Armstrong LL, Goldman MP, et al, *Drug Information Handbook*, 15th ed, Hudson, OH: Lexi-Comp, Inc, 2007.

Mandell GL, Bennett JE, and Dolin R, *Principles and Practice of Infectious Diseases*, 6th ed, Philadelphia, PA: Churchill Livingstone, 2004.

Nahata MC, *Pediatric Drug Formulations,* 5th ed, Cincinnati, OH: Harvey Whitney Books Company, 2003.

Nelson JD and Bradley JS, *Nelson's Pocket Book of Pediatric Antimicrobial Therapy*, 16th ed, Philadelphia, PA: Lippincott Williams & Wilkins, 2006.

PDR® Generics™, 4th ed, Montvale, New Jersey: Medical Economics Co, 1998.

Phelps SJ, Hak EB, and Crill CM, *Teddy Bear Book: Pediatric Injectable Drugs,* 8th ed, Bethesda, MD: American Society of Health-System Pharmacists, 2007.

Physician's Desk Reference, 61st, Montvale, NJ: Thomson PDR, 2007.

Pickering LK, ed, *2006 Red Book, Report of the Committee on Infectious Diseases*, 27th ed, Elk Grove Village, IL: American Academy of Pediatrics, 2006.

Piscitelli SC and Rodvold KA, eds, *Drug Interactions in Infectious Diseases*, 2nd ed, Totowa, NJ: Humana Press Inc, 2005.

Pizzo PA and Poplack DG, *Principles and Practice of Pediatric Oncology*, 4th ed, Philadelphia, PA: Lippincott Raven Publishers, 2001.

Pronsky ZM, *Powers and Moore's Food Medication Interactions*, 11th ed, Pottstown, PA: Food Medication Interactions, 2000.

Radde IC and MacLead SM, *Pediatric Pharmacology and Therapeutics*, St. Louis, MO: Mosby, 1993.

Rogers MC and Helfaer MA, *Handbook of Pediatric Intensive Care*, 3rd ed, Baltimore, MD: Lippincott Williams & Wilkins, 1998.

Rogers MC and Nichols DG, *Textbook of Pediatric Intensive Care*, 3rd ed, Baltimore, MD: Williams & Wilkins, 1996.

Rudolph AM, *Rudolph's Pediatrics*, 21st ed, Norwalk, CT: Appleton & Lange, 2002.

Textbook of Pediatric Infectious Diseases, 5th ed, Feigin RD, Cherry JD, and Buck CJ, eds, Philadelphia, PA: WB Saunders Company, 2004

Toro-Figueroa LO, Levin DL, and Morriss FC, *Essentials of Pediatric Intensive Care Manual*, St Louis, MO: Quality Medical Pub, Inc, 1992.

Trissel L, *Handbook of Injectable Drugs*, 14th ed, Bethesda, MD: American Society of Health-System Pharmacists, 2007.

Trissel LA, *Trissel's Stability of Compounded Formulations*, 3rd ed, Washington, DC: American Pharmaceutical Association, 2005.

United States Pharmacopeia Drug Information (USP DI), 27th ed, Greenwood Village, CO: Thompson Micromedex, Inc, 2007.

Yaffe SJ and Aranda JV, *Neonatal and Pediatric Pharmacology: Therapeutic Principles in Practice,* 3rd ed, Baltimore, MD: Lippincott Williams & Wilkins, 2004.

ALPHABETICAL LISTING OF DRUGS

♦ **A200® Lice [OTC]** *see* Permethrin *on page 1243*
♦ **A-ase** *see* Asparaginase *on page 161*

Abacavir (uh BACK ah veer)

Related Information
Adult and Adolescent HIV *on page 1821*
Assessment of Liver Function *on page 1810*
Pediatric HIV *on page 1816*
Perinatal HIV *on page 1831*

U.S. Brand Names Ziagen®

Canadian Brand Names Ziagen®

Index Terms Abacavir Sulfate; ABC

Therapeutic Category Antiretroviral Agent; HIV Agents (Anti-HIV Agents); Nucleoside Reverse Transcriptase Inhibitor (NRTI)

Generic Available No

Use Treatment of HIV-1 infection in combination with other antiretroviral agents. (**Note:** HIV regimens consisting of **three** antiretroviral agents are strongly recommended)

Medication Guide An FDA-approved patient medication guide, which is available with the product information and at http://www.fda.gov/cder/Offices/ODS/medication_guides.htm, must be dispensed with this medication for each new outpatient prescription and refill. A Warning Card (summarizing symptoms of hypersensitivity), which is available with the product information, must also be dispensed with this medication for each new outpatient prescription and refill.

Pregnancy Risk Factor C

Lactation Excretion in breast milk unknown/contraindicated

Contraindications Hypersensitivity to abacavir or any component [**do not rechallenge** patients who have experienced hypersensitivity reactions to abacavir, potentially fatal hypersensitivity reactions may occur (see Warnings)]; moderate or severe hepatic dysfunction

Warnings Serious and sometimes fatal hypersensitivity reactions may occur; discontinue therapy immediately in patients who show signs or symptoms of 2 or more of the following: Fever, skin rash, respiratory symptoms (including cough, dyspnea, or pharyngitis), GI symptoms (including nausea, vomiting, diarrhea, or abdominal pain), and constitutional symptoms (including fatigue, malaise, or achiness). Carefully consider the diagnosis of hypersensitivity reaction in patients who present with acute onset respiratory symptoms, even if other diagnoses, such as bronchitis, flu-like illness, pharyngitis, or pneumonia, are possible. Permanently discontinue abacavir if hypersensitivity reaction cannot be ruled out, even when other diagnoses are possible. Skin rash may be maculopapular or urticarial, but can be variable in appearance; erythema multiforme has been reported; hypersensitivity reaction may occur without a rash. Other symptoms may include edema, lethargy, myolysis, paresthesia, shortness of breath, mouth ulcerations, conjunctivitis, lymphadenopathy, and abnormal findings on chest x-ray (ie, infiltrates that can be localized). Anaphylaxis, renal failure, hepatic failure, respiratory failure, ARDS, hypotension, and death may also occur in association with hypersensitivity reactions. Laboratory abnormalities include increases in liver function tests, elevated CPK or serum creatinine, and lymphopenia.

Do not restart abacavir or any other abacavir-containing product after a hypersensitivity reaction occurs; more severe symptoms can recur within hours and may include life-threatening hypotension and death. Fatal hypersensitivity reactions have occurred following the reintroduction of abacavir in patients whose therapy was interrupted for other reasons. These patients had no identified history or had unrecognized symptoms of abacavir hypersensitivity. Reactions occurred within hours. In some cases, signs of a hypersensitivity reaction may have been previously present, but attributed to other medical conditions (acute onset respiratory diseases, gastroenteritis, reactions to other medications). If abacavir or any other abacavir-containing product is to be restarted following an interruption in therapy, the patient must first be evaluated for previously unsuspected symptoms of hypersensitivity. **Do not restart** abacavir or any other abacavir-containing product, if hypersensitivity is suspected or cannot be ruled out. Hypersensitivity reactions occur in ~8% of adult and pediatric patients; most hypersensitivity reactions occur within the first 6 weeks of therapy, but can occur at any time; one study reported a higher incidence of severe hypersensitivity reactions with once daily dosing compared with twice daily dosing (see product information); call the Abacavir Hypersensitivity Reaction Registry at 1-800-270-0425 to facilitate reporting and collection of information on patients experiencing abacavir hypersensitivity reactions (see Additional Information)

Cases of lactic acidosis, severe hepatomegaly with steatosis and death have been reported with the use of abacavir and other NRTIs; most of these cases have been in women; prolonged nucleoside use, obesity, and prior liver disease may be risk factors; use with extreme caution in patients with other risk factors for liver disease; discontinue abacavir in patients who develop laboratory or clinical evidence of lactic acidosis or pronounced hepatotoxicity

Precautions Use with caution and decrease the dose in patients with mild hepatic dysfunction (see Contraindications). Fat redistribution and accumulation [ie, central obesity, peripheral wasting, facial wasting, breast enlargement, dorsocervical fat enlargement (buffalo hump), and cushingoid appearance] have been observed in patients receiving antiretroviral agents (causal relationship not established). Always use abacavir in combination with other antiretroviral agents; do not add abacavir as a single agent to antiretroviral regimens that are failing; resistance to abacavir develops relatively slowly, but cross resistance between abacavir and other nucleoside reverse transcriptase inhibitors (NRTIs) may occur; limited response may be seen in patients with HIV isolates containing multiple mutations conferring resistance to NRTIs or in patients with a prolonged prior NRTI exposure (see Additional Information)

Immune reconstitution syndrome (an acute inflammatory response to residual or indolent opportunistic infections) may occur in HIV patients during initial treatment with combination antiretroviral agents, including abacavir; this syndrome may require further patient assessment and therapy. Systemic exposure of abacavir at 6-32 times the normal human exposure, increased the incidence of tumors (malignant and nonmalignant) in mice and rats; myocardial degeneration was seen in mice and rats receiving abacavir for 2 years at 7-24 times the expected human exposure; the clinical relevance of these findings is currently unknown

Adverse Reactions

Central nervous system: Insomnia, fever, headache, malaise, fatigue, anxiety

Dermatologic: Rash (see Warnings); erythema multiforme. **Note:** Suspected toxic epidermal necrolysis and Stevens-Johnson syndrome have been reported but patients also received medications known to be associated with these rashes; due to the similarities between these rashes and abacavir hypersensitivity reactions, abacavir should be discontinued and never restarted in such patients.

Endocrine & metabolic: Mild elevations of blood glucose (may be more frequent in pediatric patients), hypertriglyceridemia, lactic acidosis, fat redistribution and accumulation (see Precautions)

Gastrointestinal: Nausea, vomiting, diarrhea, anorexia; pancreatitis (rare); **Note:** Severe diarrhea may occur at a higher incidence in patients receiving once daily dosing

Hepatic: Hepatomegaly with steatosis; elevated liver enzymes

Neuromuscular & skeletal: Asthenia, musculoskeletal pain

Respiratory: Cough

Miscellaneous: Hypersensitivity reaction (see Warnings); immune reconstitution syndrome

Drug Interactions Use with ethanol increases abacavir AUC by 41% and prolongs half-life by 26%; abacavir may increase the clearance of methadone by 22% (a small number of patients may require an increase in methadone dosage)

Food Interactions Food does not significantly affect AUC.

Stability Store tablets and oral solution at room temperature; oral solution may be refrigerated; do not freeze

Mechanism of Action A carbocyclic analogue that is converted within cells to the active metabolite carbovir triphosphate; carbovir triphosphate serves as an alternative substrate to deoxyguanosine-5'-triphosphate (dGTP), a natural substrate for cellular DNA polymerase and reverse transcriptase; carbovir triphosphate inhibits HIV viral reverse transcriptase by competing with natural dGTP and by becoming incorporated into viral DNA causing chain termination. Abacavir is also a weak inhibitor of cellular DNA polymerases (alpha, beta, and gamma).

Pharmacokinetics

Absorption: Rapid and extensive

Distribution: Apparent V_d: Adults: 0.86 ± 0.15 L/kg

CSF to plasma AUC ratio: 27% to 33%

Protein binding: 50%

Metabolism: In the liver by alcohol dehydrogenase and glucuronyl transferase to inactive carboxylate and glucuronide metabolites; not significantly metabolized by cytochrome P450 enzymes

Bioavailability: Tablet: 83%; solution and tablet provide comparable AUCs

Half-life:

Infants ≥3 months and Children ≤13 years: 1-1.5 hours

Adults: 1.54 ± 0.63 hours

Hepatic impairment: Increases half-life by 58%

Time to peak serum concentration: Infants ≥3 months and Children ≤13 years: Within 1.5 hours

(Continued)

Abacavir *(Continued)*

Elimination: ~83% of dose excreted in the urine (1.2% as unchanged drug, 30% as 5'-carboxylic acid metabolite, 36% as the glucuronide, and 15% as other metabolites); 16% eliminated in feces

Clearance (apparent): Single dose 8 mg/kg:

Infants ≥3 months and Children ≤13 years: 17.84 mL/minute/kg

Adults: 10.14 mL/minute/kg

Usual Dosage Oral (use in combination with other antiretroviral agents):

Neonates and Infants <3 months: Not approved for use

Infants ≥3 months, Children, and Adolescents: 8 mg/kg twice daily (maximum: 300 mg twice daily); **Note:** Safety and efficacy of once daily dosing have not been established in pediatric patients

Adults: 300 mg twice daily or 600 mg once daily

Dosing adjustment in hepatic impairment:

Mild hepatic impairment (Child-Pugh score 5-6): Adults: 200 mg twice daily (using oral solution)

Moderate to severe hepatic impairment: Drug is contraindicated

Administration Oral: May be administered without regard to food

Monitoring Parameters Signs and symptoms of hypersensitivity reaction; serum glucose and triglycerides, viral load, CD4 counts

Patient Information Abacavir is not a cure for HIV. Take abacavir everyday as prescribed; do not change dose or discontinue without physician's advice. If abacavir is stopped for any reason, notify physician before restarting therapy. If a dose is missed, take it as soon as possible, then return to normal dosing schedule; if a dose is skipped, do **not** double the next dose

Serious and sometimes fatal allergic reactions may occur. Read the patient Medication Guide that you receive with each prescription and refill of abacavir; carry the Warning Card with you. Stop taking abacavir and notify physician immediately if 2 or more of the following sets of symptoms occur: Fever, rash, GI symptoms (nausea, vomiting, diarrhea or abdominal pain), flu-like symptoms (severe tiredness, achiness, or generally ill feeling), or respiratory symptoms (sore throat, shortness of breath, cough). If you experience an allergic (hypersensitivity) reaction to abacavir (or Ziagen®, Trizivir®, or Epzicom™), **never** take abacavir, Ziagen®, Trizivir®, or Epzicom™ again. If you take an abacavir-containing medication after having an allergic reaction, you may get life-threatening symptoms including very low blood pressure or death within hours.

HIV medications may cause changes in body fat, including an increase in fat in the upper back and neck, breasts, and trunk; a loss of fat from the face, arms, and legs may also occur. Some HIV medications (including abacavir) may cause a serious, but rare, condition called lactic acidosis with an increase in liver size (hepatomegaly). Before starting abacavir, inform your physician about your medical conditions, including any liver problems. Do not take Ziagen® with other abacavir-containing medications (eg, Epzicom® or Trizivir®).

Nursing Implications Inform patients of the possibility of a fatal hypersensitivity reaction and the signs and symptoms (see Warnings)

Additional Information The patient Medication Guide, which includes written manufacturer information, should be dispensed to the patient with each new prescription and refill; the Warning Card describing the hypersensitivity reaction should be given to the patient to carry with them. A familial predisposition to the abacavir hypersensitivity reaction has been reported; use abacavir with great caution in children of parents who experience a hypersensitivity reaction to abacavir (see Peyriére, 2001). Recent studies have identified genetic markers which may help predict which patients are at risk for developing the abacavir hypersensitivity reaction; further studies are needed (see Hetherington, 2002 and Mallal, 2002).

Reverse transcriptase mutations of K65R, L74V, Y115F, and M184V have been associated with abacavir resistance; at least 2-3 mutations are needed to decrease HIV susceptibility by 10-fold. The presence of a multiple number of these abacavir resistance-associated mutations, may confer cross-resistance for other nucleoside or nucleotide reverse transcriptase inhibitors (eg, didanosine, emtricitabine, lamivudine, zalcitabine, or tenofovir). A progressive decrease in abacavir susceptibility is associated with an increasing number of thymidine analogue mutations (TAMs; M41L, D67N, K70R, L210W, T215Y/F, K219E/R/H/Q/N).

A recent multicenter study, conducted in previously untreated HIV-infected children (median age: 5.3 years; range: 0.3-16.7 years), demonstrated that abacavir-containing antiretroviral regimens were more effective than regimens containing the NRTI combination of zidovudine and lamivudine; after adjusting for use of nelfinavir and controlling for baseline factors, the NRTI combination of abacavir and lamivudine showed the largest and most durable reduction in viral load, compared to the combination of zidovudine and lamivudine or zidovudine and abacavir; further studies are needed.

A high rate of early virologic failure in therapy-naive adult HIV patients has been observed with the once daily three-drug combination therapy of abacavir, lamivudine, and tenofovir. This combination should not be used as a new treatment regimen for naive or pretreated patients. Any patient currently receiving this regimen should be closely monitored and considered for regimen modification.

Dosage Forms Excipient information presented when available (limited, particularly for generics); consult specific product labeling. Available as abacavir sulfate; mg strength refers to abacavir.

Solution, oral:

Ziagen®: 20 mg/mL (240 mL) [strawberry-banana flavor]

Tablet:

300 mg

References

Briars LA, Hilao JJ, and Kraus DM, "A Review of Pediatric Human Immunodeficiency Virus Infection," *Journal of Pharmacy Practice*, 2004, 17(6):407-31.

Center for Disease Control and Prevention, "Guidelines for Using Antiretroviral Agents Among HIV-Infected Adults and Adolescents. Recommendations of the Panel on Clinical Practices for Treatment of HIV," *MMWR*, 2002, 51(RR-7):1-55.

Collura JM and Kraus DM, "New Pediatric Antiretroviral Agents," *J Pediatr Health Care*, 2000, 14(4):183-90.

Foster RH and Faulds D, "Abacavir," *Drugs*, 1998, 55(5):729-36.

Hetherington S, Hughes AR, Mosteller M, et al, "Genetic Variations in HLA-B Region and Hypersensitivity Reactions to Abacavir," *Lancet*, 2002, 359(9312):1121-2.

Hughes W, McDowell JA, Shenep J, et al, "Safety and Single-Dose Pharmacokinetics of Abacavir (1592U89) in Human Immunodeficiency Virus Type 1-Infected Children," *Antimicrob Agents Chemother*, 1999, 43(3):609-15.

Kline MW, Blanchard S, Fletcher CV, et al, "A Phase I Study of Abacavir (1592U89) Alone and in Combination With Other Antiretroviral Agents in Infants and Children With Human Immunodeficiency Virus Infection," *Pediatrics*, 1999, 103(4):e47; http://www.pediatrics.org/cgi/content/full/103/4/e47.

Mallal S, Nolan D, Witt C, et al, "Association Between Presence of HLA-B•5701, HLA-DR7, and HLA-DQ3 and Hypersensitivity to HIV-1 Reverse-Transcriptase Inhibitor Abacavir," *Lancet*, 2002, 359(9308):727-32.

Paediatric European Network for Treatment of AIDS (PENTA), "Comparison of Dual Nucleoside-Analogue Reverse-Transcriptase Inhibitor Regimens With and Without Nelfinavir in Children with HIV-1 Who Have Not Previously Been Treated: The PENTA 5 Randomised Trial," *Lancet*, 2002, 359(9308):733-40.

Panel on Clinical Practices for Treatment of HIV Infection, "Guidelines for the Use of Antiretroviral Agents in HIV-Infected Adults and Adolescents," October 10, 2006, http://www.aidsinfo.nih.gov.

Peyriére H, Nicolas J, Siffert M, et al, "Hypersensitivity Related to Abacavir in Two Members of a Family," *Ann Pharmacother*, 2001, 35(10):1291-2.

Working Group on Antiretroviral Therapy and Medical Management of HIV-Infected Children, "Guidelines for the Use of Antiretroviral Agents in Pediatric HIV Infection," October 26, 2006, http://www.aidsinfo.nih.gov.

Working Group on Antiretroviral Therapy and Medical Management of HIV-Infected Children, "Guidelines for the Use of Antiretroviral Agents in Pediatric HIV Infection. Supplement I: Pediatric Antiretroviral Drug Information," October 26, 2006, http://www.aidsinfo.nih.gov.

♦ **Abacavir, 3TC, and AZT** *see* Abacavir, Lamivudine, and Zidovudine *on page 38*

♦ **Abacavir, 3TC, and ZDV** *see* Abacavir, Lamivudine, and Zidovudine *on page 38*

♦ **Abacavir and 3TC** *see* Abacavir and Lamivudine *on page 35*

Abacavir and Lamivudine (a BAK a veer & la MI vyoo deen)

U.S. Brand Names Epzicom™

Canadian Brand Names Kivexa™

Index Terms Abacavir and 3TC; Abacavir Sulfate and Lamivudine; ABC and 3TC; Lamivudine and Abacavir; 3TC and Abacavir; 3TC and ABC

Therapeutic Category Antiretroviral Agent; HIV Agents (Anti-HIV Agents); Nucleoside Analog Reverse Transcriptase Inhibitor (NRTI)

Generic Available No

Use Treatment of HIV-1 infection (either alone or in combination with other antiretroviral agents) (**Note:** HIV regimens consisting of **three** antiretroviral agents are strongly recommended)

Medication Guide An FDA-approved patient medication guide, which is available with the product information and at http://www.fda.gov/cder/Offices/ODS/medication_guides.htm, must be dispensed with this medication for each new outpatient prescription and refill. A Warning Card (summarizing symptoms of hypersensitivity), which is available with the product information, must also be dispensed with this medication for each new outpatient prescription and refill.

Pregnancy Risk Factor C

Lactation See individual agents.

Contraindications Hypersensitivity to abacavir, lamivudine, or any component; hepatic impairment. **Do not rechallenge** patients who have experienced hypersensitivity reactions to abacavir; potentially fatal hypersensitivity reactions may occur (see Warnings).

(Continued)

Abacavir and Lamivudine *(Continued)*

Warnings Serious and sometimes fatal hypersensitivity reactions to abacavir may occur; discontinue therapy immediately in patients who show signs or symptoms of 2 or more of the following: Fever, skin rash, respiratory symptoms (including cough, dyspnea, or pharyngitis), GI symptoms (including nausea, vomiting, diarrhea, or abdominal pain), and constitutional symptoms (including fatigue, malaise, or achiness). Carefully consider the diagnosis of hypersensitivity reaction in patients who present with acute onset respiratory symptoms, even if other diagnoses, such as bronchitis, flu-like illness, pharyngitis, or pneumonia, are possible. Permanently discontinue abacavir-containing medications if hypersensitivity reaction cannot be ruled out, even when other diagnoses are possible. Skin rash may be maculopapular or urticarial, but can be variable in appearance; erythema multiforme has been reported; hypersensitivity reaction may occur without a rash. Other symptoms may include edema, lethargy, myolysis, paresthesia, shortness of breath, mouth ulcerations, conjunctivitis, lymphadenopathy, and abnormal findings on chest x-ray (ie, infiltrates that can be localized). Anaphylaxis, renal failure, hepatic failure, respiratory failure, ARDS, hypotension, and death may also occur in association with hypersensitivity reactions. Laboratory abnormalities include increases in liver function tests, elevated CPK or serum creatinine, and lymphopenia.

Do not restart abacavir, Epzicom™, or any other abacavir-containing product after a hypersensitivity reaction occurs; more severe symptoms can recur within hours and may include life-threatening hypotension and death. Fatal hypersensitivity reactions have occurred following the reintroduction of abacavir in patients whose therapy was interrupted for other reasons. These patients had no identified history or had unrecognized symptoms of abacavir hypersensitivity. Reactions occurred within hours. In some cases, signs of a hypersensitivity reaction may have been previously present, but attributed to other medical conditions (acute onset respiratory diseases, gastroenteritis, or reactions to other medications). If abacavir, Epzicom™ or any other abacavir-containing product is to be restarted following an interruption in therapy, the patient must first be evaluated for previously unsuspected symptoms of hypersensitivity. **Do not restart** abacavir, Epzicom™, or any other abacavir-containing product if hypersensitivity is suspected or cannot be ruled out. Hypersensitivity reactions occur in ~8% of adult and pediatric patients; most hypersensitivity reactions occur within the first 6 weeks of therapy, but can occur at any time; call the Abacavir Hypersensitivity Reaction Registry at 1-800-270-0425 to facilitate reporting and collection of information on patients experiencing abacavir hypersensitivity reactions (see Additional Information).

Cases of lactic acidosis, severe hepatomegaly with steatosis, and death have been reported in patients receiving nucleoside analogues; most of these cases have been in women; prolonged nucleoside use, obesity, and prior liver disease may be risk factors; use with extreme caution in patients with other risk factors for liver disease; discontinue Epzicom™ in patients who develop laboratory or clinical evidence of lactic acidosis or pronounced hepatotoxicity.

The major clinical toxicity of lamivudine in pediatric patients is pancreatitis; discontinue therapy if clinical signs, symptoms, or laboratory abnormalities suggestive of pancreatitis occur. HIV-infected patients who are coinfected with hepatitis B may experience clinical symptoms or laboratory evidence of hepatitis when a lamivudine-containing medication is discontinued; most cases are self-limited; but fatalities have been reported; monitor patients closely for at least several months after discontinuation of abacavir and lamivudine. Concomitant use of combination antiretroviral therapy with interferon alfa (with or without ribavirin) has resulted in hepatic decompensation (with some fatalities) in patients coinfected with HIV and HCV; monitor patients closely, especially for hepatic decompensation; consider discontinuation of abacavir and lamivudine if needed; consider dose reduction or discontinuation of interferon alfa, ribavirin, or both if clinical toxicities, including hepatic decompensation, worsen.

Epzicom™ contains abacavir and lamivudine as a fixed-dose combination; do not use in patients with renal dysfunction (Cl_{cr} ≤50 mL/minute) who require lamivudine dosage adjustment or in patients with hepatic dysfunction (**Note:** Abacavir is contraindicated in patients with moderate to severe hepatic dysfunction; patients with mild hepatic impairment require abacavir dosage reduction). Do not administer Epzicom™ with abacavir, lamivudine, or emtricitabine-containing products.

Precautions Fat redistribution and accumulation [ie, central obesity, peripheral wasting, facial wasting, breast enlargement, dorsocervical fat enlargement (buffalo hump), and cushingoid appearance] have been observed in patients receiving antiretroviral agents (causal relationship not established). Resistance to abacavir develops relatively slowly, but cross resistance between abacavir and other nucleoside reverse transcriptase inhibitors (NRTIs) may occur; limited response may be seen in patients with HIV isolates containing multiple mutations conferring resistance to NRTIs or in patients with a prolonged prior NRTI exposure.

Immune reconstitution syndrome (an acute inflammatory response to residual or indolent opportunistic infections) may occur in HIV patients during initial treatment with combination antiretroviral agents, including abacavir and lamivudine; this syndrome may require further patient assessment and therapy. Systemic exposure of abacavir at 6-32 times the normal human exposure, increased the incidence of tumors (malignant and nonmalignant) in mice and rats; myocardial degeneration was seen in mice and rats receiving abacavir for 2 years at 7-24 times the expected human exposure; the clinical relevance of these findings is currently unknown

Adverse Reactions See Abacavir *on page 32* and Lamivudine *on page 901*

Drug Interactions See Abacavir *on page 32* and Lamivudine *on page 901*

Food Interactions Food decreases the rate, but not the extent of absorption; in a single dose study, a high-fat meal did not change bioavailability or peak concentrations.

Stability Store at room temperature 25°C (77°F).

Mechanism of Action See Abacavir *on page 32* and Lamivudine *on page 901*

Pharmacokinetics One Epzicom™ tablet is bioequivalent, in the extent (AUC) of absorption and peak concentration, to two abacavir 300 mg tablets and two lamivudine 150 mg tablets; see Abacavir *on page 32* and Lamivudine *on page 901*

Usual Dosage Oral:

Children and Adolescents <18 years of age: Not intended for pediatric use; product is a fixed-dose combination; safety and efficacy has not been established in pediatric patients

Adolescents ≥18 years of age and Adults: 1 tablet daily

Dosage adjustment in hepatic impairment: Use is contraindicated (use individual antiretroviral agents to reduce dosage)

Dosage adjustment in renal impairment: Cl_{cr} ≤50 mL/minute: Not recommended (use individual antiretroviral agents to reduce dosage)

Administration May be administered without regards to meals.

Monitoring Parameters Signs and symptoms of abacavir hypersensitivity reaction, lactic acidosis, pronounced hepatotoxicity, and pancreatitis; serum glucose and triglycerides, viral load, CD4 counts, CBC with differential, hemoglobin, liver enzymes, serum amylase, bilirubin, renal and hepatic function tests; HIV patients should be screened for hepatitis B before starting lamivudine (see Warnings)

Patient Information Epzicom™ is not a cure for HIV. Take Epzicom™ every day as prescribed; do not change dose or discontinue without physician's advice. If Epzicom™ is stopped for any reason, notify physician before restarting therapy. If a dose is missed, take it as soon as possible, then return to normal dosing schedule; if a dose is skipped, do **not** double the next dose. Avoid alcohol. Notify physician if persistent severe abdominal pain, nausea, or vomiting occurs.

Epzicom™ contains abacavir (also called Ziagen®). Abacavir may cause serious and sometimes fatal allergic (hypersensitivity) reactions. Read the Patient Medication Guide that you receive with each prescription and refill of abacavir and lamivudine. Stop taking Epzicom™ and notify physician immediately if 2 or more of the following sets of symptoms occur: Fever, rash, GI symptoms (nausea, vomiting, diarrhea, or abdominal pain); flu-like symptoms (severe tiredness, achiness, or generally ill feeling), or respiratory symptoms (sore throat, shortness of breath, cough). If you experience an allergic (hypersensitivity) reaction to Epzicom™ (or abacavir, Ziagen®, or Trizivir®), **never** take Epzicom™, abacavir, Ziagen®, or Trizivir® again.

HIV medications may cause changes in body fat, including an increase in fat in the upper back and neck, breasts, and trunk; a loss of fat from the face, arms, and legs may also occur. Some HIV medications (including abacavir and lamivudine) may cause a serious, but rare, condition called lactic acidosis with an increase in liver size (hepatomegaly). Before starting Epzicom™, inform your physician about your medical conditions, including any kidney or liver problems (including hepatitis B infection). Do not take Epzicom™ with Combivir®, Emtriva™, Epivir®, Epivir-HBV®, Trizivir®, Truvada®, or Ziagen®.

Nursing Implications Inform patients of the possibility of a fatal abacavir hypersensitivity reaction and the signs and symptoms (see Warnings and Patient Information)

Additional Information The Patient Medication Guide, which includes written manufacturer information, should be dispensed to the patient with each new prescription and refill; a Warning Card describing the hypersensitivity reaction should be given to the patient to carry with them.

A high rate of early virologic failure in therapy-naive adult HIV patients has been observed with the once-daily three-drug combination therapy of abacavir, lamivudine, and tenofovir; this antiretroviral regimen is currently **not** recommended; any patient

(Continued)

Abacavir and Lamivudine *(Continued)*

currently receiving this regimen should be closely monitored for virologic failure and considered for treatment modification

Dosage Forms Excipient information presented when available (limited, particularly for generics); consult specific product labeling. Abacavir component is available as abacavir sulfate; mg strength refers to abacavir.

Tablet:

Epzicom™: Abacavir 600 mg and lamivudine 300 mg

References

Panel on Clinical Practices for Treatment of HIV Infection,"Guidelines for the Use of Antiretroviral Agents in HIV-infected Adults and Adolescents," October 10, 2006, http://www.aidsinfo.nih.gov.

♦ **Abacavir, Lamivudine, and Azidothymidine** *see* Abacavir, Lamivudine, and Zidovudine *on page 38*

Abacavir, Lamivudine, and Zidovudine

(uh BACK ah veer, la MI vyoo deen, & zye DOE vyoo deen)

U.S. Brand Names Trizivir®

Index Terms Abacavir, 3TC, and AZT; Abacavir, 3TC, and ZDV; Abacavir, Lamivudine, and Azidothymidine; Abacavir, Zidovudine, and Lamivudine; ABC, 3TC, and AZT; ABC, 3TC, and ZDV; Azidothymidine, Abacavir, and Lamivudine; Azidothymidine, Lamivudine and Abacavir; AZT, Abacavir, and 3TC; AZT, Abacavir, and Lamivudine; AZT, ABC, and 3TC; Compound S, Abacavir, and 3TC; Compound S, Abacavir, and Lamivudine; Compound S, ABC, and 3TC; Lamivudine, Abacavir, and Zidovudine; Lamivudine, Zidovudine, and Abacavir; 3TC, Abacavir, and AZT; 3TC, Abacavir, and ZDV; 3TC, Abacavir, and Zidovudine; 3TC, ABC, and AZT; 3TC, ABC, and ZDV; ZDV, Abacavir, and 3TC; ZDV, Abacavir, and Lamivudine; ZDV, ABC, and 3TC; Zidovudine, Abacavir, and Lamivudine

Therapeutic Category Antiretroviral Agent; HIV Agents (Anti-HIV Agents); Nucleoside Analog Reverse Transcriptase Inhibitor (NRTI)

Generic Available No

Use Treatment of HIV-1 infection (either alone or in combination with other antiretroviral agents) (**Note:** HIV regimens consisting of **three** antiretroviral agents are strongly recommended; data on the use of this triple NRTI combination regimen in patients with baseline viral loads >100,000 copies/mL is limited)

Medication Guide An FDA-approved patient medication guide, which is available with the product information and at http://www.fda.gov/cder/Offices/ODS/medication_guides.htm, must be dispensed with this medication for each new outpatient prescription and refill. A Warning Card (summarizing symptoms of hypersensitivity), which is available with the product information, must also be dispensed with this medication for each new outpatient prescription and refill.

Pregnancy Risk Factor C

Lactation See individual agents.

Contraindications Hypersensitivity to abacavir, lamivudine, zidovudine, or any component; hepatic impairment. **Do not rechallenge** patients who have experienced hypersensitivity reactions to abacavir, potentially fatal hypersensitivity reactions may occur (see Warnings)

Warnings Serious and sometimes fatal hypersensitivity reactions to abacavir may occur; discontinue therapy immediately in patients who show signs or symptoms of 2 or more of the following: Fever, skin rash, respiratory symptoms (including cough, dyspnea, or pharyngitis) and GI symptoms (including nausea, vomiting, diarrhea, or abdominal pain), and constitutional symptoms (including fatigue, malaise, or achiness). Carefully consider the diagnosis of hypersensitivity reaction in patients who present with acute onset respiratory symptoms, even if other diagnoses, such as bronchitis, flu-like illness, pharyngitis, or pneumonia, are possible. Permanently discontinue abacavir-containing medications if hypersensitivity reaction cannot be ruled out, even when other diagnoses are possible. Skin rash may be maculopapular or urticarial, but can be variable in appearance; erythema multiforme has been reported; hypersensitivity reaction may occur without a rash. Other symptoms may include edema, lethargy, myolysis, paresthesia, shortness of breath, mouth ulcerations, conjunctivitis, lymphadenopathy, and abnormal findings on chest x-ray (ie, infiltrates that can be localized). Anaphylaxis, renal failure, hepatic failure, respiratory failure, ARDS, hypotension, and death may also occur in association with hypersensitivity reactions. Laboratory abnormalities include increases in liver function tests, elevated CPK or serum creatinine, and lymphopenia.

Do not restart abacavir, Trizivir®, or any other abacavir-containing product after a hypersensitivity reaction occurs; more severe symptoms can recur within hours and may include life-threatening hypotension and death. Fatal hypersensitivity reactions have occurred following the reintroduction of abacavir in patients whose therapy was interrupted for other reasons. These patients had no identified history or had unrecognized symptoms of abacavir hypersensitivity. Reactions occurred within hours. In some cases, signs of a hypersensitivity reaction may have been previously present, but attributed to other medical conditions (acute onset respiratory diseases, gastroenteritis, reactions to other medications). If abacavir, Trizivir®, or any other abacavir-containing product is to be restarted following an interruption in therapy, the patient must first be evaluated for previously unsuspected symptoms of hypersensitivity. **Do not restart** abacavir, Trizivir®, or any other abacavir-containing product if hypersensitivity is suspected or cannot be ruled out. Hypersensitivity reactions occur in ~8% of adult and pediatric patients; most hypersensitivity reactions occur within the first 6 weeks of therapy, but can occur at any time; call the Abacavir Hypersensitivity Reaction Registry at 1-800-270-0425 to facilitate reporting and collection of information on patients experiencing abacavir hypersensitivity reactions (see Additional Information).

Cases of lactic acidosis, severe hepatomegaly with steatosis, and death have been reported in patients receiving nucleoside analogues; most of these cases have been in women; prolonged nucleoside use, obesity, and prior liver disease may be risk factors; use with extreme caution in patients with other risk factors for liver disease; discontinue Trizivir® in patients who develop laboratory or clinical evidence of lactic acidosis or pronounced hepatotoxicity.

The major clinical toxicity of lamivudine in pediatric patients is pancreatitis; discontinue therapy if clinical signs, symptoms, or laboratory abnormalities suggestive of pancreatitis occur. HIV-infected patients who are coinfected with hepatitis B may experience clinical symptoms or laboratory evidence of hepatitis when a lamivudine-containing medication is discontinued; most cases are self-limited, but fatalities have been reported; monitor patients closely for at least several months after discontinuation of abacavir, lamivudine, and zidovudine. Concomitant use of combination antiretroviral therapy with interferon alfa (with or without ribavirin) has resulted in hepatic decompensation (with some fatalities) in patients coinfected with HIV and HCV; monitor patients closely, especially for hepatic decompensation, neutropenia, and anemia; consider discontinuation of abacavir, lamivudine, and zidovudine if needed; consider dose reduction or discontinuation of interferon alfa, ribavirin, or both if clinical toxicities, including hepatic decompensation, worsen.

Zidovudine is associated with hematologic toxicity including granulocytopenia and severe anemia requiring transfusions; use with caution in patients with ANC <1000 cells/mm^3 or hemoglobin <9.5 g/dL; discontinue treatment in children with an ANC <500 cells/mm^3 until marrow recovery is observed; use of erythropoietin, or filgrastim may be necessary in some patients; prolonged use of zidovudine may cause myositis and myopathy; zidovudine has been shown to be carcinogenic in rats and mice.

Trizivir® contains abacavir, lamivudine, and zidovudine as a fixed-dose combination; do not use in patients weighing <40 kg, in patients with renal dysfunction (Cl_{cr} ≤50 mL/minute) who require lamivudine and zidovudine dosage adjustment, or in patients with hepatic dysfunction (**Note:** Patients with mild to moderate hepatic dysfunction or liver cirrhosis require zidovudine dosage adjustment; abacavir is contraindicated in patients with moderate to severe hepatic dysfunction; patients with mild hepatic impairment require abacavir dosage reduction). Do not administer Trizivir® with abacavir, lamivudine, emtricitabine, or zidovudine-containing products.

Precautions Fat redistribution and accumulation [ie, central obesity, peripheral wasting, facial wasting, breast enlargement, dorsocervical fat enlargement (buffalo hump), and cushingoid appearance] have been observed in patients receiving antiretroviral agents (causal relationship not established). Resistance to abacavir develops relatively slowly, but cross resistance between abacavir and other nucleoside reverse transcriptase inhibitors (NRTIs) may occur; limited response may be seen in patients with HIV isolates containing multiple mutations conferring resistance to NRTIs or in patients with a prolonged prior NRTI exposure.

Immune reconstitution syndrome (an acute inflammatory response to residual or indolent opportunistic infections) may occur in HIV patients during initial treatment with combination antiretroviral agents, including abacavir, lamivudine, and zidovudine; this syndrome may require further patient assessment and therapy. Systemic exposure of abacavir at 6-32 times the normal human exposure, increased the incidence of tumors (malignant and nonmalignant) in mice and rats; myocardial degeneration was seen in mice and rats receiving abacavir for 2 years at 7-24 times the expected human exposure; the clinical relevance of these findings is currently unknown

Adverse Reactions See Abacavir *on page 32*, Lamivudine *on page 901*, and Zidovudine *on page 1637*

Drug Interactions See Abacavir *on page 32*, Lamivudine *on page 901*, and Zidovudine *on page 1637*

(Continued)

Abacavir, Lamivudine, and Zidovudine *(Continued)*

Food Interactions Food decreases the rate, but not the extent of absorption (see Yuen, 2001).

Stability Store at room temperature 25°C (77°F)

Mechanism of Action See Abacavir *on page 32*, Lamivudine *on page 901*, and Zidovudine *on page 1637*

Pharmacokinetics One Trizivir® tablet is bioequivalent, in the extent (AUC) and rate of absorption (peak concentration and time to peak concentration), to one abacavir 300 mg tablet, one lamivudine 150 mg tablet, plus one zidovudine 300 mg tablet; See Abacavir *on page 32*, Lamivudine *on page 901*, and Zidovudine *on page 1637*

Usual Dosage Oral:

Children: Not intended for pediatric use; product is a fixed-dose combination

Adolescents <40 kg: Not recommended; product is a fixed-dose combination

Adolescents ≥40 kg and Adults: 1 tablet twice daily

Dosage adjustment in hepatic impairment: Use is contraindicated (use individual antiretroviral agents to reduce dosage)

Dosage adjustment in renal impairment: Cl_{cr} ≤50 mL/minute: Not recommended (use individual antiretroviral agents to reduce dosage)

Administration May be administered without regard to meals

Monitoring Parameters Signs and symptoms of abacavir hypersensitivity reaction, lactic acidosis, pronounced hepatotoxicity, anemia, bone marrow suppression, and pancreatitis; serum glucose and triglycerides, viral load, CD4 counts, CBC with differential, platelets, hemoglobin, MCV, reticulocyte count, liver enzymes, serum amylase, bilirubin, renal and hepatic function tests. HIV patients should be screened for hepatitis B infection before starting lamivudine (see Warnings).

Patient Information Trizivir® is not a cure for HIV. Take Trizivir® every day as prescribed; do not change dose or discontinue without physician's advice. If Trizivir® is stopped for any reason, notify physician before restarting therapy. If a dose is missed, take it as soon as possible, then return to normal dosing schedule; if a dose is skipped, do **not** double the next dose. Avoid alcohol. Notify physician if persistent severe abdominal pain, nausea, or vomiting occurs.

Trizivir® contains abacavir (also called Ziagen®). Abacavir may cause serious and sometimes fatal allergic (hypersensitivity) reaction. Read the Patient Medication Guide that you receive with each prescription and refill of abacavir, lamivudine, and zidovudine. Stop taking Trizivir® and notify physician immediately if 2 or more of the following sets of symptoms occur: Fever, rash, GI symptoms (nausea, vomiting, diarrhea, or abdominal pain), flu-like symptoms (severe tiredness, achiness, or generally ill feeling), or respiratory symptoms (sore throat, shortness of breath, cough). If you experience an allergic (hypersensitivity) reaction to Trizivir® (or abacavir, Ziagen®, or Epzicom™), **never** take Trizivir®, abacavir, Ziagen®, or Epzicom™ again.

Trizivir® contains zidovudine which may cause a decrease in white blood cells or red blood cells (anemia); routine blood tests can help detect these blood problems. Zidovudine may also cause muscle weakness with prolonged use, which may be a serious problem; notify physician if muscle weakness occurs.

HIV medications may cause changes in body fat, including an increase in fat in the upper back and neck, breasts, and trunk; a loss of fat from the face, arms, and legs may also occur. Some HIV medications (including abacavir, lamivudine, and zidovudine) may cause a serious, but rare, condition called lactic acidosis with an increase in liver size (hepatomegaly). Before starting Trizivir®, inform your physician about your medical conditions, including any blood, kidney, or liver problems (including hepatitis B infection). Do not take Trizivir® with Combivir®, Emtriva™, Epivir®, Epivir-HBV®, Epzicom®, Retrovir®, Truvada®, or Ziagen®.

Nursing Implications Inform patients of the possibility of a fatal abacavir hypersensitivity reaction and the signs and symptoms (see Warnings and Patient Information)

Additional Information The Patient Medication Guide, which includes written manufacturer information, should be dispensed to the patient with each new prescription and refill; a Warning Card describing the hypersensitivity reaction should be given to the patient to carry with them

Dosage Forms Excipient information presented when available (limited, particularly for generics); consult specific product labeling. Abacavir component is available as abacavir sulfate; mg strength refers to abacavir.

Tablet:

Trizivir®: Abacavir 300 mg, lamivudine 150 mg, and zidovudine 300 mg

References

Briars LA, Hilao JJ, and Kraus DM, "A Review of Pediatric Human Immunodeficiency Virus Infection," *Journal of Pharmacy Practice*, 2004, 17(6):407-31.

Center for Disease Control and Prevention, "Guidelines for Using Antiretroviral Agents Among HIV-Infected Adults and Adolescents. Recommendations of the Panel on Clinical Practices for Treatment of HIV," *MMWR*, 2002, 51(RR-7):1-55.

Panel on Clinical Practices for Treatment of HIV Infection, "Guidelines for the Use of Antiretroviral Agents in HIV-Infected Adults and Adolescents," October 10, 2006, http://www.aidsinfo.nih.gov.

Saez-Llorens X, Nelson RP, Emmanuel P, et al, "A Randomized, Double-Blind Study of Triple Nucleoside Therapy of Abacavir, Lamivudine, and Zidovudine Versus Lamivudine and Zidovudine in Previously Treated Human Immunodeficiency Virus Type 1-Infected Children," *Pediatrics*, 2001, 107(1), URL: http://www.pediatrics.org/cgi/content/full/107/1/e4.

Yuen GJ, Lou Y, Thompson NF, et al, "Abacavir/Lamivudine/Zidovudine as a Combined Formulation Tablet: Bioequivalence Compared With Each Component Administered Concurrently and the Effect of Food on Absorption," *J Clin Pharmacol*, 2001, 41(3):277-88.

- **Abacavir Sulfate** *see* Abacavir *on page 32*
- **Abacavir Sulfate and Lamivudine** *see* Abacavir and Lamivudine *on page 35*
- **Abacavir, Zidovudine, and Lamivudine** *see* Abacavir, Lamivudine, and Zidovudine *on page 38*
- **Abbott-43818** *see* Leuprolide *on page 918*
- **ABC** *see* Abacavir *on page 32*
- **ABC, 3TC, and AZT** *see* Abacavir, Lamivudine, and Zidovudine *on page 38*
- **ABC, 3TC, and ZDV** *see* Abacavir, Lamivudine, and Zidovudine *on page 38*
- **ABC and 3TC** *see* Abacavir and Lamivudine *on page 35*
- **Abelcet®** *see* Amphotericin B Lipid Complex *on page 120*
- **Abenol® (Can)** *see* Acetaminophen *on page 42*
- **ABLC** *see* Amphotericin B Lipid Complex *on page 120*
- **A/B Otic** *see* Antipyrine and Benzocaine *on page 145*
- **ABT-378/Ritonavir** *see* Lopinavir and Ritonavir *on page 954*

Acarbose (AY car bose)

Medication Safety Issues

Sound-alike/look-alike issues:

Precose® may be confused with PreCare®

International issues:

Precose® may be confused with Precosa® which is a brand name for *Saccharomyces boulardii* in Denmark, Finland, Norway, and Sweden

U.S. Brand Names Precose®

Canadian Brand Names Prandase®

Therapeutic Category Antidiabetic Agent, Alpha-glucosidase Inhibitor; Antidiabetic Agent, Oral

Generic Available No

Use Management of type II diabetes mellitus (noninsulin-dependent, NIDDM) when hyperglycemia cannot be managed by diet alone; may be used concomitantly with metformin, a sulfonylurea, or insulin to improve glycemic control

Pregnancy Risk Factor B

Lactation Excretion in breast milk unknown/use caution

Contraindications Hypersensitivity to acarbose or any component; diabetic ketoacidosis; cirrhosis; patients with inflammatory bowel disease, colonic ulceration, partial intestinal obstruction, or patients predisposed to intestinal obstruction; patients who have chronic intestinal diseases associated with marked disorders of digestion or absorption; patients who have conditions that may deteriorate as a result of increased gas formation in the intestine

Warnings Dose-related elevations in serum transaminases occurred in 15% of acarbose-treated patients in long-term studies; these elevations were asymptomatic, reversible, more common in females, and not associated with other evidence of liver dysfunction; acarbose serum levels are proportionately higher in patients with renal dysfunction (S_{cr} >2 mg/dL); until long term clinical studies are completed, use in renally-compromised patients is not recommended

Precautions Hypoglycemia may occur when used in combination with sulfonylureas or insulin; oral glucose (absorption is not affected by acarbose) should be used instead of sucrose (table sugar) for the treatment of mild to moderate hypoglycemia

Adverse Reactions

Central nervous system: Headache, vertigo, drowsiness

Dermatologic: Urticaria, erythema

Endocrine & metabolic: Hypoglycemia

Gastrointestinal: Abdominal pain, diarrhea, flatulence

Hepatic: Elevated liver enzymes

Neuromuscular & skeletal: Weakness

Drug Interactions Drugs that produce hyperglycemia (eg, diuretics, corticosteroids, phenothiazines, thyroid products, estrogens, oral contraceptives, phenytoin, nicotinic acid, sympathomimetics, calcium channel blocking drugs, rifampin, and isoniazid) may lead to a loss of glycemic control; intestinal adsorbents; digestive enzyme preparations; decreases bioavailability of digoxin resulting in decreased serum levels

(Continued)

Acarbose *(Continued)*

Mechanism of Action Competitive inhibitor of pancreatic α-glucosidases, resulting in delayed hydrolysis of ingested complex carbohydrates and disaccharides and absorption of glucose; dose-dependent reduction in postprandial serum insulin and glucose peaks; inhibits the metabolism of sucrose to glucose and fructose

Pharmacodynamics Average decrease in fasting blood sugar: 20-30 mg/dL

Pharmacokinetics

Absorption: <2% absorbed as active drug

Metabolism: Metabolized exclusively within the GI tract, principally by intestinal bacteria and by digestive enzymes; 13 metabolites have been identified

Bioavailability: Low systemic bioavailability of parent compound

Elimination: Fraction absorbed as intact drug is almost completely excreted in urine

Usual Dosage Oral:

Adolescents and Adults: Dosage must be individualized on the basis of effectiveness and tolerance; do not exceed the maximum recommended dose (use slow titration to prevent or minimize GI effects):

Initial: 25 mg 3 times/day; increase in 25 mg/day increments in 2-4 week intervals to maximum dose

Maximum dose:

Patients ≤60 kg: 50 mg 3 times/day

Patients >60 kg: 100 mg 3 times/day

Dosing adjustment in renal impairment: See Warnings

Administration Oral: Administer with first bite of each main meal

Monitoring Parameters Fasting blood glucose; hemoglobin A_{1c}; liver enzymes every 3 months for the first year of therapy and periodically thereafter

Reference Range Target range:

Blood glucose: Fasting and preprandial: 80-120 mg/dL; bedtime: 100-140 mg/dL

Glycosylated hemoglobin (hemoglobin A_{1c}): <7%

Additional Information Acarbose has been used successfully to treat postprandial hypoglycemia in children with Nissen fundoplications. Six children (4-25 months) initially received 12.5 mg before each bolus feeding of formula containing complex carbohydrates. The dosage was increased in 12.5 mg increments (dosage range: 12.5-50 mg per dose) until postprandial serum glucose was stable ≥60 mg/dL. Most commonly reported side effects were flatulence, abdominal distension, and diarrhea (Ng, 2001).

Dosage Forms Excipient information presented when available (limited, particularly for generics); consult specific product labeling.

Tablet: 25 mg, 50 mg, 100 mg

References

DeFronzo RA, "Pharmacologic Therapy for Type 2 Diabetes Mellitus," *Ann Intern Med*, 1999, 131(4):281-303.

Ng DD, Ferry RJ Jr, Kelly A, et al, "Acarbose Treatment of Postprandial Hypoglycemia in Children After Nissen Fundoplication," *J Pediatr*, 2001, 139(6):877-9.

- **Accolate®** *see* Zafirlukast *on page 1632*
- **AccuHist®** *see* Brompheniramine and Pseudoephedrine *on page 235*
- **AccuNeb®** *see* Albuterol *on page 66*
- **Accutane®** *see* Isotretinoin *on page 876*
- **ACE** *see* Captopril *on page 277*
- **Acephen™ [OTC]** *see* Acetaminophen *on page 42*
- **Acerola [OTC]** *see* Ascorbic Acid *on page 159*
- **Acetadote®** *see* Acetylcysteine *on page 51*

Acetaminophen (a seet a MIN oh fen)

Medication Safety Issues

Sound-alike/look-alike issues:

Acephen® may be confused with AcipHex®

FeverALL® may be confused with Fiberall®

Tylenol® may be confused with atenolol, timolol, Tuinal®, Tylox®

International issues:

Paralen® [Czech Republic] may be confused with Aralen® which is a brand name for chloroquine in the U.S.

Duorol® may be confused with Diuril® which is a brand name for chlorothiazide in the U.S.

Related Information

Acetaminophen Serum Level Nomogram *on page 1931*

Commonly Used Antidotes for Acute Overdoses *on page 1920*

Overdose and Toxicology *on page 1916*

U.S. Brand Names Acephen™ [OTC]; Apra Children's [OTC]; Aspirin Free Anacin® Maximum Strength [OTC]; Cetafen® [OTC]; Cetafen Extra® [OTC]; Comtrex® Sore Throat Maximum Strength [OTC]; FeverALL® [OTC]; Genapap™ [OTC]; Genapap™ Children [OTC]; Genapap™ Extra Strength [OTC]; Genapap™ Infant [OTC]; Genebs [OTC]; Genebs Extra Strength [OTC]; Infantaire [OTC]; Mapap [OTC]; Mapap Children's [OTC]; Mapap Extra Strength [OTC]; Mapap Infants [OTC]; Nortemp Children's [OTC]; Pain Eze [OTC]; Silapap® Children's [OTC]; Silapap® Infants [OTC]; Tycolene [OTC]; Tycolene Maximum Strength [OTC]; Tylenol® [OTC]; Tylenol® 8 Hour [OTC]; Tylenol® Arthritis Pain [OTC]; Tylenol® Children's [OTC]; Tylenol® Children's with Flavor Creator [OTC]; Tylenol® Extra Strength [OTC]; Tylenol® Infants [OTC]; Tylenol® Junior [OTC]; Valorin [OTC]; Valorin Extra [OTC]

Canadian Brand Names Abenol®; Apo-Acetaminophen®; Atasol®; Novo-Gesic; Pediatrix; Tempra®; Tylenol®

Index Terms APAP; N-Acetyl-P-Aminophenol; Paracetamol

Therapeutic Category Analgesic, Non-narcotic; Antipyretic

Generic Available Yes: Excludes extended release products

Use Treatment of mild to moderate pain and fever; does not have antirheumatic or systemic anti-inflammatory effects

Pregnancy Risk Factor B

Lactation Enters breast milk/compatible

Contraindications Hypersensitivity to acetaminophen or any component

Warnings May cause severe hepatic toxicity with overdose. Use with caution in patients with alcoholic liver disease. Chronic daily dosing in adults of 5-8 g of acetaminophen over several weeks or 3-4 g/day for 1 year have resulted in liver damage. Do not exceed maximum daily doses; consider acetaminophen content of combination products when evaluating the dose of acetaminophen.

Some elixir preparations contain benzoic acid; liquid preparations (ie, elixir, liquid, suspension, and drops) may contain sodium benzoate (see Dosage Forms); benzoic acid (benzoate) is a metabolite of benzyl alcohol; large amounts of benzyl alcohol (≥99 mg/kg/day) have been associated with a potentially fatal toxicity ("gasping syndrome") in neonates; the "gasping syndrome" consists of metabolic acidosis, respiratory distress, gasping respirations, CNS dysfunction (including convulsions, intracranial hemorrhage), hypotension and cardiovascular collapse; avoid use of acetaminophen products containing sodium benzoate in neonates; *in vitro* and animal studies have shown that benzoate displaces bilirubin from protein binding sites

Precautions Some products (eg, chewable tablets) contain aspartame which is metabolized to phenylalanine and must be avoided (or used with caution) in patients with phenylketonuria.

G-6-PD deficiency: Although several case reports of acetaminophen-associated hemolytic anemia have been reported in patients with G-6-PD deficiency, a direct cause and effect relationship has not been well established (concurrent illnesses such as fever or infection may precipitate hemolytic anemia in patients with G-6-PD deficiency); therefore, acetaminophen is generally thought to be safe when given in therapeutic doses to patients with G-6-PD deficiency.

Adverse Reactions

Dermatologic: Rash

Hematologic: Blood dyscrasias (neutropenia, pancytopenia, leukopenia)

Hepatic: Hepatic necrosis with overdose

Renal: Renal injury with chronic use

Miscellaneous: Hypersensitivity reactions (rare)

Drug Interactions Cytochrome P450 isoenzyme CYP1A2 substrate (minor), CYP2A6, CYP2C9, CYP2D6, CYP2E1 and CYP3A3/4 isoenzyme substrate

Enzyme inducers (barbiturates, carbamazepine, phenytoin, rifampin), carmustine (with high dose acetaminophen), isoniazid, alcohol (especially chronic use) can increase hepatotoxicity; rifampin may decrease acetaminophen's therapeutic effect; anticholinergic agents (scopolamine) may effect GI absorption; acetaminophen may increase the clearance of lamotrigine; acetaminophen may increase zidovudine concentration and toxicity

Food Interactions Rate of absorption may be decreased when given with food high in carbohydrates.

Mechanism of Action Inhibits the synthesis of prostaglandins in the CNS and peripherally blocks pain impulse generation; produces antipyresis from inhibition of hypothalamic heat-regulating center

Pharmacokinetics

Protein binding: 20% to 50%

Metabolism: At normal therapeutic dosages the parent compound is metabolized in the liver to sulfate and glucuronide metabolites, while a small amount is metabolized by microsomal mixed function oxidases to a highly reactive intermediate (N-acetyl-imidoquinone) which is conjugated with glutathione and inactivated; at

(Continued)

Acetaminophen *(Continued)*

toxic doses (as little as 4 g in a single day) glutathione can become depleted, and conjugation becomes insufficient to meet the metabolic demand causing an increase in N-acetyl-imidoquinone concentration, which is thought to cause hepatic cell necrosis.

Half-life:

Neonates: 2-5 hours

Adults: 1-3 hours

Time to peak serum concentration: 10-60 minutes after normal oral doses, but may be delayed in acute overdoses

Usual Dosage

Neonates: Oral, rectal: 10-15 mg/kg/dose every 6-8 hours as needed

International Evidence-Based Group for Neonatal Pain recommendations (Anand, 2001; Anand, 2002):

Preterm infants 28-32 weeks:

Oral: 10-12 mg/kg/dose every 6-8 hours; maximum daily dose: 40 mg/kg/day

Rectal: 20 mg/kg/dose every 12 hours; maximum daily dose: 40 mg/kg/day

Preterm infants 32-36 weeks and term infants <10 days:

Oral: 10-15 mg/kg/dose every 6 hours; maximum daily dose: 60 mg/kg/day

Rectal: Loading dose: 30 mg/kg; then 15 mg/kg/dose every 8 hours; maximum daily dose: 60 mg/kg/day

Term infants ≥10 days:

Oral: 10-15 mg/kg/dose every 4-6 hours; maximum daily dose: 90 mg/kg/day

Rectal: Loading dose: 30 mg/kg; then 20 mg/kg/dose every 6-8 hours; maximum daily dose: 90 mg/kg/day

Infants and Children:

Oral: 10-15 mg/kg/dose every 4-6 hours as needed; do **not** exceed 5 doses in 24 hours; alternatively, the following doses may be used. See table.

Acetaminophen Dosing (Oral)[1]

Weight (lbs)	Age	Dosage (mg)
6-11	0-3 mo	40
12-17	4-11 mo	80
18-23	1-2 y	120
24-35	2-3 y	160
36-47	4-5 y	240
48-59	6-8 y	320
60-71	9-10 y	400
72-95	11 y	480

[1]Manufacturer's recommendations; use of weight to select dose is preferred; if weight is not available, then use age

Rectal: 10-20 mg/kg/dose every 4-6 hours as needed. **Note:** Although the perioperative use of high-dose rectal acetaminophen (eg, 25-45 mg/kg/dose) has been investigated in several studies, its routine use remains controversial; optimal doses and dosing frequency to ensure efficacy and safety have not yet been established; further studies are needed (see Buck, 2001).

Children ≥12 years and Adults: Oral, rectal: 325-650 mg every 4-6 hours or 1000 mg 3-4 times/day; do **not** exceed 4 g/day

Administration Oral: Administer with food to decrease GI upset; shake suspension well before use; do not crush or chew extended release products

Reference Range Acute ingestions: Toxic concentration with probable hepatotoxicity: >200 mcg/mL at 4 hours or 50 mcg/mL at 12 hours after ingestion of overdose

Patient Information Avoid alcohol; do not take longer than 10 days without physician's advice

Additional Information Drops may contain saccharin.

Acetaminophen (15 mg/kg/dose given orally every 6 hours for 24 hours) did **not** relieve the intraoperative or the immediate postoperative pain associated with neonatal circumcision; some benefit was seen 6 hours after circumcision (see Howard, 1994).

There is currently no scientific evidence to support alternating acetaminophen with ibuprofen in the treatment of fever (see Mayoral, 2000).

Dosage Forms Excipient information presented when available (limited, particularly for generics); consult specific product labeling. [DSC] = Discontinued product

Caplet: 500 mg

Cetafen Extra® Strength, Genapap™ Extra Strength, Genebs Extra Strength, Mapap Extra Strength, Tycolene Maximum Strength, Tylenol® Extra Strength: 500 mg

Caplet, extended release:

Tylenol® 8 Hour, Tylenol® Arthritis Pain: 650 mg

Capsule: 500 mg

Elixir: 160 mg/5 mL (120 mL, 480 mL, 3780 mL)

Apra Children's: 160 mg/5 mL (120 mL, 480 mL, 3780 mL) [alcohol free; contains benzoic acid; cherry and grape flavors]

Mapap Children's: 160 mg/5 mL (120 mL) [alcohol free; contains benzoic acid and sodium benzoate; cherry flavor]

Gelcap:

Mapap Extra Strength, Tylenol® Extra Strength: 500 mg

Geltab:

Tylenol® Extra Strength: 500 mg

Geltab, extended release:

Tylenol® 8 Hour: 650 mg [DSC]

Liquid, oral: 500 mg/15 mL (240 mL)

Comtrex® Sore Throat Maximum Strength: 500 mg/15 mL (240 mL) [contains sodium benzoate; honey lemon flavor]

Genapap™ Children: 160 mg/5 mL (120 mL) [contains sodium benzoate; cherry and grape flavors]

Silapap®: 160 mg/5 mL (120 mL, 240 mL, 480 mL) [sugar free; contains sodium benzoate; cherry flavor]

Tylenol® Extra Strength: 500 mg/15 mL (240 mL) [contains sodium benzoate; cherry flavor]

Solution, oral: 160 mg/5 mL (120 mL, 480 mL)

Solution, oral [drops]: 80 mg/0.8 mL (15 mL) [droppers are marked at 0.4 mL (40 mg) and at 0.8 mL (80 mg)]

Genapap™ Infant: 80 mg/0.8 mL (15 mL) [fruit flavor]

Infantaire: 80 mg/0.8mL (15 mL, 30 mL)

Silapap® Infant's: 80 mg/0.8 mL (15 mL, 30 mL) [contains sodium benzoate; cherry flavor]

Suppository, rectal: 120 mg, 325 mg, 650 mg

Acephen™: 120 mg, 325 mg, 650 mg

FeverALL®: 80 mg, 120 mg, 325 mg, 650 mg

Mapap: 125 mg, 650 mg

Suspension, oral:

Mapap Children's: 160 mg/5 mL (120 mL) [contains sodium benzoate; cherry flavor]

Nortemp Children's: 160 mg/5 mL (120 mL) [alcohol free; contains sodium benzoate; cotton candy flavor]

Tylenol® Children's: 160 mg/5 mL (120 mL, 240 mL) [contains sodium benzoate; bubble gum yum, cherry blast, dye free cherry, grape splash, and very berry strawberry flavors]

Tylenol® Children's with Flavor Creator: 160 mg/5 mL (120 mL) [contains sodium 2 mg/5 mL and sodium benzoate; cherry blast flavor; packaged with apple (4), bubblegum (8), chocolate (4), & strawberry (4) sugar free flavor packets]

Suspension, oral [drops]:

Mapap Infants: 80 mg/0.8 mL (15 mL, 30 mL) [contains sodium benzoate; cherry flavor]

Tylenol® Infants: 80 mg/0.8 mL (15 mL, 30 mL) [contains sodium benzoate; cherry, dye free cherry, and grape flavors]

Tablet: 325 mg, 500 mg

Aspirin Free Anacin® Extra Strength, Genapap™ Extra Strength, Genebs Extra Strength, Mapap Extra Strength, Pain Eze, Tylenol® Extra Strength, Valorin Extra: 500 mg

Cetafen®, Genapap™, Genebs, Mapap, Tycolene, Tylenol®, Valorin: 325 mg

Tablet, chewable: 80 mg

Genapap™ Children: 80 mg [contains phenylalanine 6 mg/tablet; fruit and grape flavors]

Mapap Children's: 80 mg [contains phenylalanine 3 mg/tablet; bubble gum, fruit, and grape flavors]

Mapap Junior Strength: 160 mg [contains phenylalanine 12 mg/tablet; grape flavor]

Tablet, orally disintegrating: 80 mg, 160 mg

Tylenol® Children's Meltaways: 80 mg [bubble gum, grape, and watermelon flavors]

Tylenol® Junior Meltaways: 160 mg [bubble gum and grape flavors]

References

American Academy of Pediatrics: Committee on Drugs, "Acetaminophen Toxicity in Children," *Pediatrics*, 2001, 108(4):1020-4.

Anand KJ and International Evidence-Based Group for Neonatal Pain, "Consensus Statement for the Prevention and Management of Pain in the Newborn," *Arch Pediatr Adolesc Med*, 2001, 155(2):173-80.

(Continued)

Acetaminophen *(Continued)*

Anand KJ, Chair, International Evidence-Based Group for Neonatal Pain, personal correspondence, April 2002.

Buck ML, "Perioperative Use of High-Dose Rectal Acetaminophen," *Pediatr Pharm*, 2001, 7(9), http://www.medscape.com/viewarticle/415082.

Howard CR, Howard FM, and Weitzman ML, "Acetaminophen Analgesia in Neonatal Circumcision: The Effect on Pain," *Pediatrics*, 1994, 93(4):641-646.

Mayoral CE, Marino RV, Rosenfeld W, et al, "Alternating Antipyretics: Is This An Alternative?" *Pediatrics*, 2000, 105(5):1009-12.

Acetaminophen and Codeine (a seet a MIN oh fen & KOE deen)

Medication Safety Issues

Sound-alike/look-alike issues:

Capital® may be confused with Capitrol®

Tylenol® may be confused with atenolol, timolol, Tuinal®, Tylox®

T3 is an error-prone abbreviation (mistaken as liothyronine)

U.S. Brand Names Capital® and Codeine; Tylenol® With Codeine

Canadian Brand Names ratio-Emtec; ratio-Lenoltec; Triatec-8; Triatec-8 Strong; Triatec-30; Tylenol Elixir with Codeine; Tylenol No. 1; Tylenol No. 1 Forte; Tylenol No. 2 with Codeine; Tylenol No. 3 with Codeine; Tylenol No. 4 with Codeine

Index Terms Codeine and Acetaminophen

Therapeutic Category Analgesic, Narcotic

Generic Available Yes

Use Relief of mild to moderate pain

Restrictions C-III; C-V

Pregnancy Risk Factor C

Lactation Enters breast milk/use caution

Contraindications Hypersensitivity to acetaminophen, codeine phosphate, or any component (see Warnings)

Warnings Some tablets contain metabisulfite which may cause allergic reactions in susceptible individuals. Elixir may contain sodium benzoate; benzoic acid (benzoate) is a metabolite of benzyl alcohol; large amounts of benzyl alcohol (≥99 mg/kg/day) have been associated with a potentially fatal toxicity ("gasping syndrome") in neonates; the "gasping syndrome" consists of metabolic acidosis, respiratory distress, gasping respirations, CNS dysfunction (including convulsions, intracranial hemorrhage), hypotension and cardiovascular collapse; avoid use of acetaminophen and codeine products containing sodium benzoate in neonates; *in vitro* and animal studies have shown that benzoate displaces bilirubin from protein binding sites

Precautions Use with caution in patients with hypersensitivity reactions to other phenanthrene derivative opioid agonists (morphine, hydrocodone, hydromorphone, levorphanol, oxycodone, oxymorphone) or respiratory disease/compromise.

G-6-PD deficiency: Although several case reports of acetaminophen-associated hemolytic anemia have been reported in patients with G-6-PD deficiency, a direct cause and effect relationship has not been well established (concurrent illnesses such as fever or infection may precipitate hemolytic anemia in patients with G-6-PD deficiency); therefore, acetaminophen is generally thought to be safe when given in therapeutic doses to patients with G-6-PD deficiency.

Adverse Reactions

Acetaminophen:

- Dermatologic: Rash
- Hematologic: Blood dyscrasias (neutropenia, pancytopenia, leukopenia)
- Hepatic: Hepatic necrosis with overdose
- Renal: Renal injury with chronic use
- Miscellaneous: Hypersensitivity reactions (rare)

Codeine:

- Cardiovascular: Palpitations, hypotension, bradycardia, peripheral vasodilation
- Central nervous system: CNS depression, dizziness, drowsiness, sedation, elevated intracranial pressure
- Dermatologic: Pruritus
- Endocrine & metabolic: Antidiuretic hormone release
- Gastrointestinal: Nausea, vomiting, constipation, biliary tract spasm
- Genitourinary: Urinary retention
- Ocular: Miosis
- Respiratory: Respiratory depression
- Miscellaneous: Histamine release, physical and psychological dependence with prolonged use

Drug Interactions See Acetaminophen *on page 42* and Codeine *on page 397*

Food Interactions Rate of absorption of acetaminophen may be decreased when given with food high in carbohydrates

Mechanism of Action See individual monographs for Acetaminophen *on page 42* and Codeine *on page 397*

Pharmacokinetics See individual monographs for Acetaminophen *on page 42* and Codeine *on page 397*

Usual Dosage Oral (doses should be titrated to appropriate analgesic effect):
- Children: Analgesic: 0.5-1 mg codeine/kg/dose every 4-6 hours
  - 3-6 years: 5 mL 3-4 times/day as needed
  - 7-12 years: 10 mL 3-4 times/day as needed
  - >12 years: 15 mL every 4 hours as needed
- Adults: 1-2 tablets every 4 hours; maximum dose: 12 tablets/24 hours

Administration Oral: Administer with food to decrease GI upset; shake suspension well before use

Patient Information Codeine may be habit-forming; avoid abrupt discontinuation after prolonged use; may cause drowsiness and impair ability to perform activities requiring mental alertness or physical coordination; avoid alcohol

Nursing Implications Observe patient for excessive sedation, respiratory depression

Additional Information Tylenol® With Codeine elixir contains saccharin

Dosage Forms Excipient information presented when available (limited, particularly for generics); consult specific product labeling. [DSC] = Discontinued product; [CAN] = Canadian brand name

Caplet:
- ratio-Lenoltec No. 1 [CAN], Tylenol No. 1 [CAN]: Acetaminophen 300 mg, codeine phosphate 8 mg, and caffeine 15 mg [not available in the U.S.]
- Tylenol No. 1 Forte [CAN]: Acetaminophen 500 mg, codeine phosphate 8 mg, and caffeine 15 mg [not available in the U.S.]

Elixir, oral [C-V]: Acetaminophen 120 mg and codeine phosphate 12 mg per 5 mL (5 mL, 10 mL, 12.5 mL, 15 mL, 120 mL, 480 mL) [contains alcohol 7%]
- Tylenol® with Codeine [DSC]: Acetaminophen 120 mg and codeine phosphate 12 mg per 5 mL (480 mL) [contains alcohol 7%; cherry flavor]
- Tylenol Elixir with Codeine [CAN]: Acetaminophen 160 mg and codeine phosphate 8 mg per 5 mL (500 mL) [contains alcohol 7%, sucrose 31%; cherry flavor; not available in the U.S.]

Suspension, oral [C-V] (Capital® and Codeine): Acetaminophen 120 mg and codeine phosphate 12 mg per 5 mL (480 mL) [alcohol free; fruit punch flavor]

Tablet [C-III]: Acetaminophen 300 mg and codeine phosphate 15 mg; acetaminophen 300 mg and codeine phosphate 30 mg; acetaminophen 300 mg and codeine phosphate 60 mg
- ratio-Emtec [CAN], Triatec-30 [CAN]: Acetaminophen 300 mg and codeine phosphate 30 mg [not available in the U.S.]
- ratio-Lenoltec No. 1 [CAN]: Acetaminophen 300 mg, codeine phosphate 8 mg, and caffeine 15 mg [not available in the U.S.]
- ratio-Lenoltec No. 2 [CAN], Tylenol No. 2 with Codeine [CAN]: Acetaminophen 300 mg, codeine phosphate 15 mg, and caffeine 15 mg [not available in the U.S.]
- ratio-Lenoltec No. 3 [CAN], Tylenol No. 3 with Codeine [CAN]: Acetaminophen 300 mg, codeine phosphate 30 mg, and caffeine 15 mg [not available in the U.S.]
- ratio-Lenoltec No. 4 [CAN], Tylenol No. 4 with Codeine [CAN]: Acetaminophen 300 mg and codeine phosphate 60 mg [not available in the U.S.]
- Triatec-8 [CAN]: Acetaminophen 325 mg, codeine phosphate 8 mg, and caffeine 30 mg [not available in the U.S.]
- Triatec-8 Strong [CAN]: Acetaminophen 500 mg, codeine phosphate 8 mg, and caffeine 30 mg [not available in the U.S.]
- Tylenol® with Codeine No. 3: Acetaminophen 300 mg and codeine phosphate 30 mg [contains sodium metabisulfite]
- Tylenol® with Codeine No. 4: Acetaminophen 300 mg and codeine phosphate 60 mg [contains sodium metabisulfite]

◆ **Acetaminophen and Hydrocodone** *see* Hydrocodone and Acetaminophen *on page 779*

◆ **Acetaminophen and Oxycodone** *see* Oxycodone and Acetaminophen *on page 1191*

◆ **Acetaminophen and Propoxyphene** *see* Propoxyphene and Acetaminophen *on page 1336*

AcetaZOLAMIDE (a set a ZOLE a mide)

Medication Safety Issues

Sound-alike/look-alike issues:
- AcetaZOLAMIDE may be confused with acetoHEXAMIDE
- Diamox® Sequels® may be confused with Diabinese®, Dobutrex®, Trimox®

Related Information

Antiepileptic Drugs *on page 1902*

(Continued)

AcetaZOLAMIDE *(Continued)*

U.S. Brand Names Diamox® Sequels®

Canadian Brand Names Apo-Acetazolamide®; Diamox®

Therapeutic Category Anticonvulsant, Miscellaneous; Carbonic Anhydrase Inhibitor; Diuretic, Carbonic Anhydrase Inhibitor

Generic Available Yes: Injection, tablet

Use Reduce elevated intraocular pressure in glaucoma; diuretic; adjunct to the treatment of refractory seizures; prevent acute altitude sickness; treatment of centrencephalic epilepsies; reduce CSF production in hydrocephalus

Pregnancy Risk Factor C

Lactation Enters breast milk/not recommended (AAP rates "compatible")

Contraindications Hypersensitivity to acetazolamide, any component, or other sulfonamides; patients with hepatic disease or insufficiency; decreased serum sodium and/or potassium; adrenocortical insufficiency; hyperchloremic acidosis; or severe renal disease; long-term administration in patients with chronic noncongestive angle-closure glaucoma

Warnings Fatalities associated with sulfonamides, although rare, have occurred due to severe reactions including Stevens-Johnson syndrome, toxic epidermal necrolysis, hepatic necrosis, agranulocytosis, aplastic anemia, and other blood dyscrasias; discontinue use at first sign of rash or any sign of adverse reaction. Anorexia, tachypnea, lethargy, metabolic acidosis, and death have been reported in patients receiving acetazolamide and high-dose aspirin concomittantly. Tolerance to antiepileptic effects may require dosage adjustment.

Precautions Use with caution in patients with respiratory acidosis, COPD, diabetes mellitus, and gout; reduce dosage in patients with renal impairment; growth retardation has been reported in children receiving chronic therapy (possibly due to chronic acidosis)

Adverse Reactions

Cardiovascular: Cyanosis

Central nervous system: Drowsiness, ataxia, confusion, fatigue, vertigo, fever, seizures, dizziness, depression, malaise, headache, excitement

Dermatologic: Rash, erythema multiforme, photosensitivity, Stevens-Johnson syndrome (see Warnings), urticaria, toxic epidermal necrolysis

Endocrine & metabolic: Hypokalemia, hyperchloremic metabolic acidosis, hyperglycemia, hypoglycemia, growth retardation

Gastrointestinal: GI irritation, anorexia, nausea, vomiting, xerostomia, melena, dysgeusia, metallic taste, black stools

Genitourinary: Dysuria, polyuria

Hematologic: Bone marrow suppression, thrombocytopenia, hemolytic anemia, pancytopenia, agranulocytosis, leukopenia

Hepatic: Hepatic insufficiency, cholestatic jaundice, hepatic necrosis

Local: Pain at injection site

Neuromuscular & skeletal: Paresthesia, muscle weakness

Ocular: Myopia (transient)

Otic: Tinnitus

Renal: Renal calculi, phosphaturia, renal colic, hematuria, renal failure, polyuria

Respiratory: Hyperpnea

Drug Interactions Cytochrome P450 isoenzyme CYP3A4 inhibitor (weak)

Increases lithium excretion; may decrease the rate of excretion of other drugs such as procainamide, flecainide, quinidine, and tricyclic antidepressants; may increase the excretion of salicylates, amphetamine, and phenobarbital; may inactivate methenamine in the urine; may increase cyclosporine levels; may increase the risk of developing osteomalacia in patients receiving phenytoin or phenobarbital; topiramate may increase risk of nephrolithiasis and paresthesia; salicylates increase acetazolamide serum levels resulting in CNS toxicity; "high-dose" aspirin (see Warnings); ammonium chloride increases plasma concentration of nonionized acetazolamide; increased toxicity with propofol (cardiorespiratory instability); may increase effects of other folic acid antagonists

Food Interactions Avoid natural licorice (causes sodium and water retention and increases potassium loss)

Stability Store tablets and capsules at room temperature; after reconstitution, acetazolamide injection is stable for 12 hours at room temperature and for 1 week when refrigerated; physically incompatible with parenteral multivitamins

Mechanism of Action Competitive, reversible inhibition of the enzyme carbonic anhydrase resulting in increased renal excretion of sodium, potassium, bicarbonate, and water and decreased formation of aqueous humor; also inhibits carbonic anhydrase in CNS to retard abnormal and excessive discharge from CNS neurons

Pharmacodynamics

Onset of action:

Capsule, extended release: 2 hours

Tablet: 1-1.5 hours

I.V.: 2 minutes

Maximum effect:

Capsule, extended release: 3-6 hours

Tablet: 1-4 hours

I.V.: 15 minutes

Duration:

Capsule, extended release: 18-24 hours

Tablet: 8-12 hours

I.V.: 4-5 hours

Pharmacokinetics

Absorption: Appears to be dose dependent; erratic with daily doses >10 mg/kg

Distribution: Into erythrocytes, kidneys, and breast milk (breast milk to plasma ratio of 0.25 has been reported); crosses the blood-brain barrier and the placenta

Protein binding: 95%

Half-life: 2.4-5.8 hours

Time to peak serum concentration: Tablet: 2-4 hours

Elimination: 70% to 100% of an I.V. or tablet dose and 47% of an extended release capsule excreted unchanged in urine within 24 hours

Dialysis: 20% to 50% removed by hemodialysis

Usual Dosage

Children:

Glaucoma:

Oral: 8-30 mg/kg/day or 300-900 mg/m²/day divided every 8 hours

I.V.: 20-40 mg/kg/day divided every 6 hours, not to exceed 1 g/day

Edema: Oral, I.V.: 5 mg/kg/dose or 150 mg/m²/dose once daily

Epilepsy: Oral: 4-16 mg/kg/day in 1-4 divided doses, not to exceed 30 mg/kg/day or 1 g/day; **extended release capsule is not recommended for treatment of epilepsy**

Adults:

Glaucoma:

Chronic simple (open-angle): Oral: 250 mg 1-4 times/day or 500 mg once followed by 125-250 mg every 4 hours, or 500 mg sustained release capsule twice daily

Secondary, acute (closed-angle): I.V.: 250-500 mg, may repeat in 2-4 hours to a maximum of 1 g/day

Edema: Oral, I.V.: 250-375 mg/day

Epilepsy: Oral: 4-16 mg/kg/day in 1-4 divided doses, not to exceed 30 mg/kg/day or 1 g/day; **extended release capsule is not recommended for treatment of epilepsy**

Altitude sickness: Oral: 500-1000 mg daily in divided doses such as 250 mg every 8-12 hours or 500 mg extended release capsules every 12-24 hours; therapy should begin 24-48 hours before and continued during ascent and for at least 48 hours after arrival at the high altitude

Urine alkalinization: Oral: 5 mg/kg/dose repeated 2-3 times over 24 hours

Dosing interval in renal impairment: Children and Adults:

Cl_{cr} 10-50 mL/minute: Administer every 12 hours

Cl_{cr} <10 mL/minute: Avoid use

Administration

Oral: Administer with food to decrease GI upset; tablet may be crushed and suspended in cherry or chocolate syrup to disguise the bitter taste of the drug (See Extemporaneous Preparations)

Parenteral:

I.V.: Reconstitute with at least 5 mL SWI to provide a solution containing not more than 100 mg/mL; maximum concentration: 100 mg/mL; maximum rate of I.V. infusion: 500 mg/minute

I.M.: Not generally recommended as the drug's alkaline pH makes it very painful

Monitoring Parameters Serum electrolytes, CBC and platelet counts

Test Interactions May cause false-positive results for urinary protein with Albustix®, Labstix®, Albutest®, Bumintest®; interferes with HPLC method for assaying theophylline

Patient Information Do not crush or chew long-acting capsule; may cause dry mouth. May rarely cause photosensitivity reactions (eg, exposure to sunlight may cause severe sunburn, skin rash, redness, or itching); avoid direct exposure to sunlight; may cause drowsiness and impair ability to perform activities requiring mental alertness or physical coordination

Additional Information Sodium content of 500 mg injection: 2.049 mEq

(Continued)

AcetaZOLAMIDE *(Continued)*

Extended release capsules are indicated only for use for the adjunctive treatment of open-angle or secondary glaucoma and the prevention of high altitude sickness; avoid using extended release capsules for anticonvulsant or diuretic therapy

Acetazolamide has been used with questionable efficacy to slow the progression of hydrocephalus in neonates and infants who may not be good candidates for surgery. I.V. or oral doses of 5 mg/kg/dose every 6 hours increased by 25 mg/kg/day to a maximum of 100 mg/kg/day, if tolerated, have been used. Furosemide was used in combination with acetazolamide (Libenson, 1999).

Dosage Forms Excipient information presented when available (limited, particularly for generics); consult specific product labeling.

Capsule, extended release:

Diamox® Sequels®: 500 mg

Injection, powder for reconstitution: 500 mg

Tablet: 125 mg, 250 mg

Extemporaneous Preparations

A 25 mg/mL suspension may be made by crushing twelve 250 mg tablets and mixing with 120 mL of a 1:1 mixture of Ora-Sweet® and Ora-Plus® or a 1:1 mixture of Ora-Sweet® SF and Ora-Plus®. The resulting suspension is stable for 60 days refrigerated (Allen, 1996). When diluted in 120 mL solution of cherry syrup concentrate diluted 1:4 with simple syrup, NF, it is stable 60 days refrigerated (preferred) or at room temperature (Nahata, 2004).

A 25 mg/mL suspension may be made by crushing one hundred 250 mg tablets; add 100 mL flavor/purified water; add a mixture of 10 g Veegum (already mixed with 200 mL purified water), 300 mL 1% methylcellulose and 300 mL syrup; qsad to 1000 mL with flavor/purified water and 10 mL paraben concentrate (methylparaben 120 mg, propylparaben 12 mg, propylene glycol qsad to 100 mL); stable 79 days refrigerated (Alexander, 1991).

Allen LV and Erickson MA, "Stability of Acetazolamide, Allopurinol, Azathioprine, Clonazepam, and Flucytosine in Extemporaneously Compounded Oral Liquids," *Am J Health Sys Pharm*, 1996, 53:1944-9.

Alexander KS, Haribhakti RP, and Parker GA, "Stability of Acetazolamide in Suspension Compounded From Tablets," *Am J Hosp Pharm*, 1991, 48(6):1241-4.

Nahata, MC, Pai VB, and Hipple TF, *Pediatric Drug Formulations*, 5th ed, Cincinnati, OH: Harvey Whitney Books Co, 2004.

References

Libenson MH, Kaye EM, Rosman NP, et al, "Acetazolamide and Furosemide for Posthemorrhagic Hydrocephalus of the Newborn," *Pediatr Neurol*, 1999, 20(3):185-91.

Reiss WG and Oles KS, "Acetazolamide in the Treatment of Seizures," *Ann Pharmacother*, 1996, 30(5):514-9.

Shinnar S, Gammon K, Bergman EW Jr, et al, "Management of Hydrocephalus in Infancy: Use of Acetazolamide and Furosemide to Avoid Cerebrospinal Fluid Shunts," *J Pediatr*, 1985, 107(1):31-7.

♦ **Acetoxyl® (Can)** *see* Benzoyl Peroxide *on page 207*

♦ **Acetoxymethylprogesterone** *see* MedroxyPROGESTERone *on page 991*

Acetylcholine (a se teel KOE leen)

Medication Safety Issues

Sound-alike/look-alike issues:

Acetylcholine may be confused with acetylcysteine

U.S. Brand Names Miochol®-E

Canadian Brand Names Miochol®-E

Index Terms Acetylcholine Chloride

Therapeutic Category Cholinergic Agent, Ophthalmic; Ophthalmic Agent, Miotic

Generic Available No

Use Produces complete miosis in cataract surgery, keratoplasty, iridectomy and other anterior segment surgery where rapid miosis is required

Pregnancy Risk Factor C

Contraindications Hypersensitivity to acetylcholine chloride or any component; acute iritis and acute inflammatory disease of the anterior chamber

Warnings Open under aseptic conditions only

Precautions Systemic effects rarely occur, but can cause problems for patients with acute CHF, bronchial asthma, peptic ulcer, hyperthyroidism, GI spasm, and urinary tract obstruction

Adverse Reactions

Cardiovascular: Transient bradycardia and hypotension

Central nervous system: Headache

Ocular: Iris atrophy, temporary lens opacities (attributed to osmotic effect of 5% mannitol present in preparation)

Respiratory: Dyspnea

Miscellaneous: Diaphoresis

Drug Interactions Flurbiprofen decreases effectiveness; sodium nitrate antagonizes acetylcholine's effects

Stability Prepare solution immediately before use; do not use solution which is not clear and colorless

Mechanism of Action Causes contraction of the sphincter muscles of the iris, resulting in miosis and contraction of the ciliary muscle, leading to accommodation

Pharmacodynamics

Onset of action: Miosis occurs promptly

Duration: ~10-20 minutes

Usual Dosage Ophthalmic: Adults: Instill 0.5-2 mL of 1% injection (5-20 mg)

Administration Ophthalmic: Instill into anterior chamber before or after securing one or more sutures; instillation should be gentle and parallel to the iris face and tangential to the pupil border; in cataract surgery, acetylcholine should be used only after delivery of the lens

Dosage Forms Excipient information presented when available (limited, particularly for generics); consult specific product labeling.

Powder for solution, intraocular, as chloride:

Miochol®-E: 1:100 [20 mg; packaged with diluent (2 mL)]

♦ **Acetylcholine Chloride** *see* Acetylcholine *on page 50*

Acetylcysteine (a se teel SIS teen)

Medication Safety Issues

Sound-alike/look-alike issues:

Acetylcysteine may be confused with acetylcholine

Mucomyst® may be confused with Mucinex®

Related Information

Commonly Used Antidotes for Acute Overdoses *on page 1920*

Overdose and Toxicology *on page 1916*

U.S. Brand Names Acetadote®

Canadian Brand Names Acetylcysteine Solution; Mucomyst®; Parvolex®

Index Terms Acetylcysteine Sodium; Mercapturic Acid; Mucomyst; NAC; *N*-Acetylcysteine; *N*-Acetyl-L-cysteine

Therapeutic Category Antidote, Acetaminophen; Mucolytic Agent

Generic Available Yes: Solution for inhalation

Use

Inhalation: Adjunctive therapy in patients with abnormal or viscid mucous secretions in bronchopulmonary diseases, pulmonary complications of surgery, and cystic fibrosis; diagnostic bronchial studies

Injection, Oral: Antidote for acute acetaminophen toxicity; prevention of radiocontrast-induced renal dysfunction

Oral, rectal: Treatment of distal intestinal obstruction syndrome (previously known as "meconium ileus or its equivalent")

Pregnancy Risk Factor B

Lactation Excretion in breast milk unknown/use caution

Contraindications Hypersensitivity to acetylcysteine or any component

Warnings Serious anaphylactoid reactions including death in a patient with asthma have been reported after I.V. use; acute flushing and erythema may occur 30-60 minutes into an I.V. infusion, resolving spontaneously; the infusion may be interrupted until treatment of allergic symptoms is initiated; if acute hypersensitivity reactions occur which do not respond to medical management (eg, antihistamines, H_2 blockers) or temporarily halting infusion, discontinue use and pursue alternative management. Since increased bronchial secretions may develop after inhalation, percussion, postural drainage, and suctioning should follow.

Acetaminophen overdose: The modified Rumack-Matthew nomogram allows for stratification of patients into risk categories based on the relationship between the serum acetaminophen level and time after ingestion. There are several situations where the nomogram is of limited use. Serum acetaminophen levels obtained prior to 4-hour postingestion are not interpretable; patients presenting late may have undetectable serum concentrations, but have received a lethal dose. The nomogram is less predictive in a chronic ingestion or in an overdose with an extended release product. Acetylcysteine should be administered for any signs of hepatotoxicity even if acetaminophen serum level is low or undetectable. The nomogram also does not take into

(Continued)

Acetylcysteine *(Continued)*

account patients at higher risk of acetaminophen toxicity (eg, alcoholics, malnourished patients) or individuals ingesting higher than recommended acetaminophen doses for extended periods of time (repeated supratherapeutic ingestion).

Precautions Use with caution in patients with asthma or previous history of bronchospasm

Adverse Reactions

Cardiovascular: Tachycardia, hypotension, syncope, chest tightness, vasodilation, hypertension (after large oral doses)

Central nervous system: Drowsiness, chills, dysphoria

Dermatologic: Generalized urticaria, rash, pruritus, erythema, angioedema

Gastrointestinal: Stomatitis, nausea, vomiting, dyspepsia, hemoptysis

Hepatic: Mild elevations in liver function tests have occurred after oral therapy

Ocular: Eye pain

Respiratory: Bronchospasm, rhinorrhea, cough

Miscellaneous: Anaphylactoid reactions (I.V. use; 17% in an open label study; 1% reported as severe or moderate in 10% of patients within 15 minutes of the first infusion; severe in 1% or mild to moderate in 6% to 7% of patients after the 60 minute infusion); diaphoresis, unpleasant odor during administration

Drug Interactions May potentiate the hemodynamic effects of nitroglycerin; acetylcysteine is adsorbed by activated charcoal

Stability Store at room temperature; I.V. formulation is preservative free and stable 24 hours after dilution at room temperature; opened inhalation solution vials may be stored in the refrigerator; use within 96 hours; contact with rubber, copper, iron, and cork may inactivate the drug; the light purple color of solution does **not** affect its activity. I.V. acetylcysteine is hyperosmolar (2600 mOsm/L) and is compatible with 5% dextrose, 0.45% sodium chloride, and SWI.

Mechanism of Action Exerts mucolytic action through its free sulfhydryl group which opens up the disulfide bonds in the mucoproteins thus lowering the viscosity. The exact mechanism of action in acetaminophen toxicity is unknown. It may act by maintaining or restoring glutathione levels or by acting as an alternative substrate for conjugation with the acetaminophen's toxic metabolite.

Pharmacodynamics

Onset of action: Upon inhalation, mucus liquefaction occurs maximally within 5-10 minutes

Duration of mucus liquefaction: More than 1 hour

Pharmacokinetics

Distribution: V_d: 0.47 L/kg

Protein binding: 83%

Half-life:

- Reduced acetylcysteine: 2 hours
- Total acetylcysteine:
  - Newborns: 11 hours
  - Adults: 5.6 hours

Time to peak serum concentration: Oral: 1-2 hours

Elimination: Clearance: Adults: 0.11 L/hour/kg

Usual Dosage

Acetaminophen poisoning: Children and Adults: Begin treatment within 8 hours of ingestion to optimize therapy in patients whose serum acetaminophen levels fall above the "possible" toxicity line on the Rumack-Matthew nomogram; (see Acetaminophen Serum Level Nomogram *on page 1931* in the appendix). Treatment is also indicated in patients with a history of known or suspected acute acetaminophen ingestion of >150 mg/kg (child) or >7.5 g (adolescent or adult) total dose when plasma levels are not available within 8-10 hours of ingestion or in patients presenting >24 hours after acute ingestion who have a measurable acetaminophen level. See Warnings.

I.V.: 150 mg/kg infused over 60 minutes; followed by a 4-hour infusion of 50 mg/kg; followed by a 16-hour infusion of 100 mg/kg; equivalent to a total dose of 300 mg/kg infused over 21 hours

Oral: 140 mg/kg; followed by 17 doses of 70 mg/kg every 4 hours; repeat dose if emesis occurs within 1 hour of administration; therapy should continue until all doses are administered even though the acetaminophen plasma level has dropped below the toxic range

Nebulized inhalation:

- Infants: 1-2 mL of 20% solution or 2-4 mL of 10% solution until nebulized, given 3-4 times/day
- Children: 3-5 mL of 20% solution or 6-10 mL of 10% solution until nebulized, given 3-4 times/day
- Adolescents: 5-10 mL of 10% to 20% solution until nebulized, given 3-4 times/day

Note: Patients should receive an aerosolized bronchodilator 10-15 minutes prior to acetylcysteine

Intratracheal: Children and Adults: 1-2 mL of 10% to 20% solution every 1-4 hours as needed

Distal intestinal obstruction syndrome (previously known as meconium ileus equivalent): Varying regimens have been reported (polyethylene glycol has become more widely used for this indication):

Oral:

Children <10 years: 30 mL of 10% solution diluted in 30 mL juice or soda 3 times/day for 24 hours

Children 10 years and Adults: 60 mL of 10% solution diluted in 60 mL juice or soda 3 times/day for 24 hours

Note: Prior to treatment, administer a phosphosoda enema. A clear liquid diet should be used during the 24-hour acetylcysteine treatment

Rectal enema: Children: Varying dosages; 100-300 mL of 4% to 6% solution 2-4 times/day; 50 mL of 20% solution 1-4 times/day and 5-30 mL of 10% to 20% solution 3-4 times/day have been used; rectal enemas appear to have less favorable results than oral administration (Mascarenhas, 2003)

Prevention of radiocontrast-induced renal dysfunction (unlabeled use): Adults: Oral: 600 mg twice daily for 2 days (beginning the day before the procedure); hydrate patient concurrently

Administration

Parenteral: I.V.: Three infusions (See Usual Dosage) of different lengths: Dilute first dose (150 mg/kg) in 200 mL D_5W and infuse over 60 minutes; dilute second dose (50 mg/kg) in 500 mL D_5W and infuse over 4 hours; dilute third dose (100 mg/kg) in 1000 mL D_5W and infuse over 16 hours; for children <40 kg and patients who are fluid restricted, the manufacturer recommends reducing the diluent to a "proportional" amount. See table for manufacturer's recommended infusion guideline for patients <40 kg. Or as an alternative to proportionally lower the diluent volume, a reasonable approach might be to utilize the concentrations resulting from using the recommended dilution for the dosage in a 50 kg patient. The calculated concentration would range between 5 mg/mL (maintenance infusion) to 37.5 mg/mL (loading dose).

Infusion Guide by Weight for Patients <40 kg

Body Weight (kg)	LOADING Dose 150 mg/kg over 60 minutes		SECOND Dose 50 mg/kg over 4 hours		THIRD Dose 100 mg/kg over 16 hours	
	Acetylcysteine Dose mg (mL)	5% Dextrose (mL)	Acetylcysteine Dose mg (mL)	5% Dextrose (mL)	Acetylcysteine dose mg (mL)	5% Dextrose (mL)
10	1500 (7.5)	30	500 (2.5)	70	1000 (5)	140
15	2250 (11.25)	45	750 (3.75)	105	1500 (7.5)	210
20	3000 (15)	60	1000 (5)	140	2000 (10)	280
25	3750 (18.75)	100	1250 (6.25)	250	2500 (12.5)	500
30	4500 (22.5)	100	1500 (7.5)	250	3000 (15)	500

Oral: For treatment of acetaminophen overdosage, administer as a 5% solution; dilute the 20% solution (inhalation formulation) 1:3 with a cola, orange juice, or other soft drink; use within 1 hour of preparation

Oral inhalation: May be administered by nebulization either undiluted (both 10% and 20%) or diluted in NS

Rectal: Dilute the inhalation solution in NS to the desired final concentration and administer rectally

Monitoring Parameters When used in acetaminophen overdose, determine acetaminophen level as soon as possible, but no sooner than 4 hours after ingestion of immediate release formulations or 2 hours after ingestion of liquid formulations (to ensure peak levels have been obtained) (see Acetaminophen Serum Level Nomogram *on page 1931* in the appendix); coingestion of acetaminophen with other medications which may delay GI peristalsis eg, antihistamines, opioids, may require repeated serum levels to determine the peak serum level; liver function tests

Patient Information Clear airway by coughing deeply before aerosol treatment

Nursing Implications Anaphylactoid reactions following I.V. administration have been reported; have emergency treatments such as antihistamines and H_2 blockers readily available for potential adverse effects; assess patient for nausea, vomiting, and skin rash following oral administration for treatment of acetaminophen poisoning; intermittent aerosol treatments are commonly given when patient arises, before meals, and just before retiring at bedtime

(Continued)

Acetylcysteine *(Continued)*

Dosage Forms Excipient information presented when available (limited, particularly for generics); consult specific product labeling.

Injection, solution:

Acetadote®: 20% [200 mg/mL] (30 mL) [contains disodium edetate]

Solution, inhalation/oral: 10% [100 mg/mL] (4 mL, 10 mL, 30 mL); 20% [200 mg/mL] (4 mL, 10 mL, 30 mL)

References

Hanly JG and Fitzgerald MX, "Meconium Ileus Equivalent in Older Patients With Cystic Fibrosis," *Br Med J (Clin Res Ed)*, 1983, 286(6375):1411-3.

Mascarenhas MR, "Treatment of Gastrointestinal Problems in Cystic Fibrosis," *Curr Treat Options Gastroenterol*, 2003, 6(5):427-441.

Rashid ST, Salman M, Myint F, et al, "Prevention of Contrast-Induced Nephropathy in Vascular Patients Undergoing Angiography: A Randomized Controlled Trial of Intravenous N-Acetylcysteine," *J Vasc Surg*, 2004, 40(6):1136-41.

Tepel M, van der Giet M, Schwarzfeld C, et al, "Prevention of Radiographic-Contrast-Agent-Induced Reductions in Renal Function by Acetylcysteine," *N Engl J Med*, 2000, 343(3):180-4.

Walson PD and Groth JF Jr, "Acetaminophen Hepatotoxicity After Prolonged Ingestion," *Pediatrics*, 1993, 91(5):1021-2.

- **Acetylcysteine Sodium** *see* Acetylcysteine *on page 51*
- **Acetylcysteine Solution (Can)** *see* Acetylcysteine *on page 51*
- **Acetylsalicylic Acid** *see* Aspirin *on page 163*
- **Achromycin** *see* Tetracycline *on page 1518*
- **Aciclovir** *see* Acyclovir *on page 54*
- **Acidulated Phosphate Fluoride** *see* Fluoride *on page 675*
- **Acilac (Can)** *see* Lactulose *on page 900*
- **AcipHex®** *see* Rabeprazole *on page 1362*
- **Aclovate®** *see* Alclometasone *on page 69*
- **ACT** *see* Dactinomycin *on page 435*
- **ACT® [OTC]** *see* Fluoride *on page 675*
- **Act-D** *see* Dactinomycin *on page 435*
- **ACTH** *see* Corticotropin *on page 402*
- **ActHIB®** *see Haemophilus* b Conjugate Vaccine *on page 751*
- **Acticin®** *see* Permethrin *on page 1243*
- **Actidose-Aqua® [OTC]** *see* Charcoal, Activated *on page 328*
- **Actidose® with Sorbitol [OTC]** *see* Charcoal, Activated *on page 328*
- **Actifed® (Can)** *see* Triprolidine and Pseudoephedrine *on page 1580*
- **Actifed® Cold and Allergy [OTC] [DSC]** *see* Triprolidine and Pseudoephedrine *on page 1580*
- **Actigall®** *see* Ursodiol *on page 1586*
- **Actinomycin** *see* Dactinomycin *on page 435*
- **Actinomycin D** *see* Dactinomycin *on page 435*
- **Actinomycin CI** *see* Dactinomycin *on page 435*
- **Actiq®** *see* Fentanyl *on page 644*
- **Activase®** *see* Alteplase *on page 83*
- **Activase® rt-PA (Can)** *see* Alteplase *on page 83*
- **Activated Carbon** *see* Charcoal, Activated *on page 328*
- **Activated Charcoal** *see* Charcoal, Activated *on page 328*
- **Activated Dimethicone** *see* Simethicone *on page 1440*
- **Activated Ergosterol** *see* Ergocalciferol *on page 588*
- **Activated Methylpolysiloxane** *see* Simethicone *on page 1440*
- **Activated Protein C, Human, Recombinant** *see* Drotrecogin Alfa (Activated) *on page 549*
- **ACT® Plus [OTC]** *see* Fluoride *on page 675*
- **ACT® x2™ [OTC]** *see* Fluoride *on page 675*
- **Acular®** *see* Ketorolac *on page 889*
- **Acular LS™** *see* Ketorolac *on page 889*
- **Acular® PF** *see* Ketorolac *on page 889*
- **ACV** *see* Acyclovir *on page 54*
- **Acycloguanosine** *see* Acyclovir *on page 54*

Acyclovir (ay SYE kloe veer)

Medication Safety Issues

Sound-alike/look-alike issues:

Zovirax® may be confused with Zostrix®, Zyvox®

International issues:

Opthavir® [Mexico] may be confused with Optivar® which is a brand name for azelastine in the U.S.

U.S. Brand Names Zovirax®

Canadian Brand Names Apo-Acyclovir®; Gen-Acyclovir; Nu-Acyclovir; ratio-Acyclovir; Zovirax®

Index Terms Aciclovir; ACV; Acycloguanosine

Therapeutic Category Antiviral Agent, Oral; Antiviral Agent, Parenteral; Antiviral Agent, Topical

Generic Available Yes: Excludes cream, ointment

Use Treatment of initial and prophylaxis of recurrent mucosal and cutaneous herpes simplex (HSV 1 and HSV 2) infections; herpes simplex encephalitis; herpes zoster infections; varicella-zoster infections in healthy, nonpregnant persons >13 years of age, children >12 months of age who have a chronic skin or lung disorder or are receiving long-term aspirin therapy, and immunocompromised patients

Pregnancy Risk Factor C

Lactation Enters breast milk/use with caution (AAP rates "compatible")

Contraindications Hypersensitivity to acyclovir, valacyclovir, or any component

Warnings HSV and VZV with reduced susceptibility to acyclovir have been isolated from immunocompromised patients, especially with advanced HIV infection; renal failure, in some cases resulting in death, has occurred with acyclovir

Precautions Use with caution in patients with renal disease, dehydration, underlying neurologic disease, and in patients with hypoxia, hepatic, or electrolyte abnormalities; dosage should be reduced in patients with renal impairment

Adverse Reactions

Central nervous system: Headache, lethargy, delirium, coma, dizziness, seizures, pain, insomnia, fever, hallucinations, aggressive behavior, ataxia

Dermatologic: Skin rash, pruritus, alopecia, erythema multiforme, urticaria, photosensitivity, Stevens-Johnson syndrome, angioedema

Gastrointestinal: Nausea, vomiting, diarrhea

Hematologic: Bone marrow suppression, neutropenia, thrombotic thrombocytopenic purpura/hemolytic uremic syndrome

Hepatic: Elevated liver enzymes, hepatitis, jaundice, hyperbilirubinemia

Local: Phlebitis at injection site, tissue necrosis upon extravasation, local pain and stinging with topical use

Neuromuscular & skeletal: Tremulousness, myalgia, paresthesia

Renal: Nephrotoxicity, hematuria, elevated BUN and serum creatinine

Respiratory: Sore throat

Miscellaneous: Diaphoresis, anaphylaxis

Drug Interactions Zidovudine (neurotoxicity); probenecid decreases renal clearance of acyclovir

Food Interactions Food does not appear to affect absorption

Stability Incompatible with blood products and protein-containing solutions; reconstituted 50 mg/mL solution should be used within 12 hours; do not refrigerate reconstituted solutions as they may precipitate

Mechanism of Action Inhibits DNA synthesis and viral replication by competing with deoxyguanosine triphosphate for viral DNA polymerase and by incorporation into viral DNA

Pharmacokinetics

Absorption: Oral: 15% to 30%

Distribution: Widely distributed throughout the body including brain, kidney, lungs, liver, spleen, muscle, uterus, vagina, and the CSF; CSF acyclovir concentration is 50% of serum concentration; crosses the placenta; excreted into breast milk; V_d:

Neonates to 3 months of age: 28.8 L/1.73 m^2

Children 1-2 years: 31.6 L/1.73 m^2

Children 2-7 years: 42 L/1.73 m^2

Protein binding: <30%

Half-life, terminal phase:

Neonates: 4 hours

Children 1-12 years: 2-3 hours

Adults: 2-3.5 hours (with normal renal function)

Time to peak serum concentration: Oral: Within 1.5-2 hours

Elimination: Primary route is the kidney with 30% to 90% of a dose excreted unchanged in the urine; requires dosage adjustment with renal impairment; hemodialysis removes ~60% of a dose while removal by peritoneal dialysis is to a much lesser extent; supplemental dose recommended after hemodialysis

(Continued)

Acyclovir *(Continued)*

Usual Dosage

Genital herpes simplex virus (HSV): First infection:

Oral:

Children: 40-80 mg/kg/day in 3-4 divided doses for 5-10 days; maximum dose: 1 g/day

Adolescents and Adults: 200 mg 5 times/day or 400 mg 3 times/day for 5-10 days

I.V.: Children and Adults: 5 mg/kg/dose every 8 hours for 5-7 days

Genital HSV infection: Recurrence: Oral: Adolescents and Adults: 200 mg 5 times/day or 400 mg 3 times/day for 5 days

Recurrent genital and cutaneous (ocular) HSV episodes in a patient with frequent recurrences, chronic suppressive therapy: Oral:

Children: 40-80 mg/kg/day in 3 divided doses for up to 12 months; maximum dose: 1 g/day; re-evaluate after 12 months of treatment

Adolescents and Adults: 400 mg twice daily or 400 mg 3 times/day or 200 mg 3 times/day for as long as 12 continuous months; re-evaluate after 12 months of treatment

HSV in immunocompromised host:

Oral:

Children:1000 mg/day in 3-5 divided doses for 7-14 days; maximum dose: 80 mg/kg/day not to exceed 1 g/day

Adults: 400 mg 5 times/day for 7-14 days

I.V.:

Children <12 years: 10 mg/kg/dose every 8 hours for 7-14 days

Children ≥12 years and Adults: 5 mg/kg/dose every 8 hours for 7-14 days

Prophylaxis of HSV in immunocompromised host: Oral: Children and Adults: 600-1000 mg/day in 3-5 divided doses during period of risk; maximum dose in children: 80 mg/kg/day not to exceed 1 g/day

HSV encephalitis: I.V.:

Children 3 months to 12 years: 20 mg/kg/dose every 8 hours; some clinicians recommend 500 mg/m^2/dose every 8 hours for 14-21 days

Children >12 years and Adults: 10-15 mg/kg/dose every 8 hours for 14-21 days

Neonatal HSV: I.V.: 20 mg/kg/dose every 8 hours for 14-21 days

Varicella-zoster in immunocompromised host: I.V.:

Infants <1 year: 10 mg/kg/dose every 8 hours for 7-10 days

Children ≥1 year: 500 mg/m^2/dose every 8 hours for 7-10 days or 10 mg/kg/dose every 8 hours for 7-10 days

Varicella in immunocompetent host: Oral (initiate treatment within the first 24 hours of rash onset):

Children ≥2 years and ≤40 kg: 20 mg/kg/dose 4 times/day for 5 days; maximum dose: 3200 mg/day

Children >40 kg and Adults: 800 mg 4 times/day for 5 days

Zoster in immunocompetent host: Oral (initiate treatment within 48 hours of rash onset): Children ≥12 years and Adults: 800 mg 5 times/day for 7-10 days

Prophylaxis in bone marrow transplant recipients: I.V.:

Autologous patients who are HSV-seropositive: 250 mg/m^2/dose every 8 hours

Autologous patients who are CMV seropositive: 500 mg/m^2/dose every 8 hours; for clinically symptomatic CMV infection, consider replacing acyclovir with ganciclovir

Children and Adults: Topical: Apply ½" ribbon of ointment for a 4" square surface area every 3 hours (6 times/day) for 7 days

Dosing interval in renal impairment:

Neonates: I.V.:

S_{cr} 0.8-1.1 mg/dL: Administer 20 mg/kg/dose every 12 hours

S_{cr} 1.2-1.5 mg/dL: Administer 20 mg/kg/dose every 24 hours

S_{cr} >1.5 mg/dL: Administer 10 mg/kg/dose every 24 hours

Children ≥6 months and Adults:

Oral: See table.

Usual Dose	Creatinine Clearance	Adjusted Dose
200 mg 5 times/day	Cl_{cr} <10 mL/minute	Administer 200 mg q12h
800 mg 5 times/day	Cl_{cr} 10-25 mL/minute	Administer 800 mg q8h
	Cl_{cr} <10 mL/minute	Administer 800 mg q12h

I.V.:

Cl_{cr} 25-50 mL/minute: Administer normal dose every 12 hours

Cl_{cr} 10-25 mL/minute: Administer normal dose every 24 hours

Cl_{cr} <10 mL/minute: 50% decrease in dose, administer every 24 hours

Hemodialysis: Administer dose after dialysis

CVVHD/CVVH: Adjust dose based upon Cl_{cr} 30 mL/minute

Administration

Oral: May administer with food; shake suspension well before use

Parenteral: Reconstitute vial for injection with paraben-free SWI; administer by slow I.V. infusion over at least 1 hour at a final concentration not to exceed 7 mg/mL since rapid infusions can cause nephrotoxicity with crystalluria and renal tubular damage; in patients who require fluid restriction, a concentration of up to 10 mg/mL has been infused; concentration >10 mg/mL increases the risk of phlebitis

Monitoring Parameters Urinalysis, BUN, serum creatinine, I & O; liver enzymes, CBC; neutrophil count at least twice weekly in neonates receiving acyclovir 60 mg/kg/day I.V.

Nursing Implications Maintain adequate hydration and urine output the first 2 hours after I.V. infusion to decrease the risk of nephrotoxicity; check infusion site for phlebitis; avoid extravasation

Additional Information Sodium content of 1 g: 4.2 mEq

Dosage Forms Excipient information presented when available (limited, particularly for generics); consult specific product labeling. [DSC] = Discontinued product

Capsule: 200 mg
- Zovirax®: 200 mg

Cream, topical:
- Zovirax®: 5% (2 g, 5 g)

Injection, powder for reconstitution, as sodium: 500 mg, 1000 mg
- Zovirax®: 500 mg [DSC]

Injection, solution, as sodium [preservative free]: 25 mg/mL (20 mL, 40 mL); 50 mg/mL (10 mL, 20 mL)

Ointment, topical:
- Zovirax®: 5% (15 g)

Suspension, oral: 200 mg/5 mL (480 mL)
- Zovirax®: 200 mg/5 mL (480 mL) [banana flavor]

Tablet: 400 mg, 800 mg
- Zovirax®: 400 mg, 800 mg

References

American Academy of Pediatrics Committee on Infectious Diseases, "The Use of Oral Acyclovir in Otherwise Healthy Children With Varicella," *Pediatrics*, 1993, 91(3):674-6.

American Academy of Pediatrics, "Report of the Committee on Infectious Diseases," *2003 Red Book®*, 26th ed, 729-30.

Desparmet J, Meistelman C, Barre J, et al, "Continuous Epidural Infusion of Bupivacaine for Postoperative Pain Relief in Children," *Anesthesiology*, 1987, 67(1):108-10.

Dunkle LM, Arvin AM, Whitley RJ, et al, "A Controlled Trial of Acyclovir for Chickenpox in Normal Children," *N Engl J Med*, 1991, 325(22):1539-44.

Englund JA, Fletcher CV, and Balfour HH Jr, "Acyclovir Therapy in Neonates," *J Pediatr*, 1991, 119(1 Pt 1):129-35.

Kimberlin DW, Lin CY, Jacobs RF, et al, "Safety and Efficacy of High-Dose Intravenous Acyclovir in the Management of Neonatal Herpes Simplex Virus Infections," *Pediatrics*, 2001, 108(2):230-8.

Meyers JD, Reed EC, Shepp DH, et al, "Acyclovir for Prevention of Cytomegalovirus Infection and Disease After Allogenic Marrow Transplantation," *N Engl J Med*, 1988, 318(2):70-5.

Novelli VM, Marshall WC, Yeo J, et al, "High-Dose Oral Acyclovir for Children at Risk of Disseminated Herpes Virus Infections," *J Infect Dis*, 1985, 151(2):372.

- **Aczone™** *see* Dapsone *on page 441*
- **Adacel™** *see* Diphtheria, Tetanus Toxoids, and Acellular Pertussis Vaccine *on page 517*
- **Adalat® XL® (Can)** *see* NIFEdipine *on page 1134*
- **Adalat® CC** *see* NIFEdipine *on page 1134*
- **Adamantanamine Hydrochloride** *see* Amantadine *on page 89*

Adapalene (a DAP a leen)

U.S. Brand Names Differin®

Canadian Brand Names Differin®; Differin® XP

Index Terms CD271

Therapeutic Category Acne Products

Generic Available No

Use Topical treatment of acne vulgaris

Pregnancy Risk Factor C

Lactation Excretion in breast milk unknown/use caution

Contraindications Hypersensitivity to adapalene or any component; sunburn

Warnings Avoid excessive exposure to sunlight and sunlamps; avoid contact with abraded skin, mucous membranes, eyes, mouth, or angles of the nose

Precautions Use with caution in patients with eczema

Adverse Reactions

Dermatologic: Erythema, scaling, dry skin, skin irritation, pruritus, acne flares, photosensitivity, sunburn, skin discoloration

Local: Pruritus or burning immediately after application

(Continued)

Adapalene *(Continued)*

Ophthalmic: Eyelid edema, conjunctivitis

Drug Interactions Topical sulfur, benzoyl peroxide, salicylic acid, and resorcinol potentiate adverse reactions seen with adapalene; other topical products containing alcohol, astringents, or lime may increase drying effects

Stability Store at controlled room temperature

Mechanism of Action Retinoid-like compound which is a modulator of cellular differentiation, keratinization, and inflammatory processes, all of which represent important features in the pathology of acne vulgaris

Pharmacodynamics Onset of action: 8-12 weeks

Pharmacokinetics

Absorption: Absorption through the skin is very low; only trace amounts have been measured in serum after chronic application

Elimination: Primarily in bile

Usual Dosage Topical: Children >12 years and Adults: Apply topically once daily in the evening

Administration Topical: After cleansing the affected area with mild or soapless cleanser, using gloves, apply a thin film of medication (cream or gel) before retiring in the evening. Avoid contact with eyes, angles of the nose, lips, and mucous membranes.

Monitoring Parameters Reduction in lesion size and/or inflammation; reduction in the number of lesions

Patient Information For external use only; apply using gloves; avoid contact with eyes, mouth, mucous membranes, or open wounds. Do not apply occlusive dressing. Moisturizers may be used if necessary; however, products containing alpha hydroxy or glycolic acids should be avoided. Wax epilation should not be performed on treated skin due to the potential for skin erosions. Transient burning or stinging immediately after applying may occur. Mild to moderate redness, dryness, scaling, burning or itching are likely to occur during the first 2-4 weeks and will usually lessen with continued use; report worsening of condition or skin redness, dryness, peeling, or burning that persists between applications to the healthcare provider. May cause photosensitivity reactions (eg, exposure to sunlight may cause severe sunburn, skin rash, redness, or itching); avoid exposure to sunlight and artificial light sources (sunlamps, tanning booth/bed); wear protective clothing, wide-brimmed hats, sunglasses, and lip sunscreen (SPF ≥15); use a sunscreen [broad-spectrum sunscreen or physical sunscreen(preferred) or sunblock with SPF ≥15]; contact physician if reaction occurs.

Dosage Forms Excipient information presented when available (limited, particularly for generics); consult specific product labeling. [DSC] = Discontinued product

Cream, topical: 0.1% (15 g, 45 g)
Gel, topical: 0.1% (15 g, 45 g) [alcohol free]
Pledget, topical: 0.1% (60s) [DSC]
Solution, topical: 0.1% (30 mL) [DSC]

- ♦ **Adderall®** *see* Dextroamphetamine and Amphetamine *on page 472*
- ♦ **Adderall XR®** *see* Dextroamphetamine and Amphetamine *on page 472*
- ♦ **Adenocard®** *see* Adenosine *on page 58*
- ♦ **Adenoscan®** *see* Adenosine *on page 58*

Adenosine (a DEN oh seen)

Related Information

Adult ACLS Algorithms *on page 1660*
CPR Pediatric Drug Dosages *on page 1650*
Pediatric ALS Algorithms *on page 1657*

U.S. Brand Names Adenocard®; Adenoscan®

Canadian Brand Names Adenocard®; Adenoscan®; Adenosine Injection, USP

Index Terms 9-Beta-D-Ribofuranosyladenine

Therapeutic Category Antiarrhythmic Agent, Miscellaneous

Generic Available Yes

Use Treatment of paroxysmal supraventricular tachycardia (PSVT); used in adult ACLS algorithms for narrow-complex tachycardias, stable narrow-complex supraventricular tachycardias, and wide-complex tachycardias that are supraventricular in origin; used in PALS algorithms for probable supraventricular tachycardia; investigationally used as a continuous infusion for the treatment of primary pulmonary hypertension in adults and persistent pulmonary hypertension of the newborn (PPHN) (see Additional Information)

Pregnancy Risk Factor C

Lactation Excretion in breast milk unknown

Contraindications Hypersensitivity to adenosine or any component; second and third degree A-V block or sick sinus syndrome unless pacemaker placed

Warnings Heart block, including transient or prolonged asystole may occur as well as other arrhythmias; episodes of asystole or other arrhythmias may be fatal; if arrhythmia is not due to re-entry pathway through A-V node or sinus node (ie, atrial fibrillation, flutter, or tachycardia or ventricular tachycardia), adenosine will not terminate the arrhythmia but can produce transient ventriculoatrial or A-V block; possible mutagenic effects

Precautions Bronchoconstriction may occur in asthmatics (avoid use in patients with bronchospasm or bronchoconstriction); use with caution in patients with underlying dysfunction of sinus or A-V node, obstructive lung disease, and those taking digoxin or verapamil; initial adenosine dose should be significantly decreased in patients receiving dipyridamole

Adverse Reactions

Cardiovascular: Flushing, arrhythmias, palpitations, chest pain, bradycardia, heart block, minimal hemodynamic disturbances, hypotension (<1%)

Central nervous system: Irritability, headaches, lightheadedness, dizziness

Gastrointestinal: Nausea, metallic taste

Respiratory: Dyspnea, hyperventilation, bronchoconstriction in asthmatics

Drug Interactions Dipyridamole potentiates effects of adenosine (dose of adenosine should be significantly reduced); methylxanthines (aminophylline, theophylline, caffeine) antagonize adenosine's effects so that larger doses of adenosine or an alternative agent may be required; carbamazepine may increase heart block; digoxin and verapamil may cause ventricular fibrillation (rare cases reported)

Stability Do **not** refrigerate, precipitation may occur; contains no preservatives, discard unused portion

Mechanism of Action Slows conduction time through the A-V node, interrupting the re-entry pathways through the A-V node, restoring normal sinus rhythm

Pharmacodynamics

Onset of action: Rapid

Duration: Very brief

Pharmacokinetics

Metabolism: Removed from systemic circulation primarily by vascular endothelial cells and erythrocytes (by cellular uptake); rapidly metabolized intracellularly; phosphorylated by adenosine kinase to adenosine monophosphate (AMP) which is then incorporated into high-energy pool; intracellular adenosine is also deaminated by adenosine deaminase to inosine; inosine can be metabolized to hypoxanthine, then xanthine and finally to uric acid.

Half-life: <10 seconds

Usual Dosage Note: Adequate controlled studies in pediatric patients have not been conducted.

Manufacturer's recommendations: Rapid I.V.:

Neonates, Infants, Children, and Adolescents weighing <50 kg: Initial dose: 0.05-0.1 mg/kg; if not effective within 1-2 minutes, increase dose by 0.05-0.1 mg/kg increments every 1-2 minutes to a maximum single dose of 0.3 mg/kg or until termination of PSVT

Children and Adolescents weighing ≥50 kg and Adults: 6 mg, if not effective within 1-2 minutes, 12 mg may be given; may repeat 12 mg bolus if needed

Alternative pediatric dosing:

Neonates: Rapid I.V.: Initial dose: 0.05 mg/kg; if not effective within 2 minutes, increase dose by 0.05 mg/kg increments every 2 minutes to a maximum dose of 0.25 mg/kg or until termination of PSVT

Infants and Children: **PALS dose for treatment of SVT**: Rapid I.V.; I.O.: Initial: 0.1 mg/kg (maximum: 6 mg); if not effective, give 0.2 mg/kg (maximum: 12 mg)

Administration Parenteral: For rapid bolus I.V. use, administer over 1-2 seconds at peripheral I.V. site closest to patient's heart (I.V. administration into lower extremities may result in therapeutic failure or requirement of higher doses); follow each bolus with NS flush (infants and children: 5-10 mL; adults: 20 mL); if given peripherally in adults, elevate the extremity for 10-20 seconds after the NS flush. To administer doses <600 mcg (0.2 mL of commercial product), a dilution with NS (final concentration: 300 mcg/mL) may be made. **Note:** Preliminary results in adults suggest adenosine may be administered via a **central line** at lower doses (eg, Adults: Initial dose: 3 mg); FDA approved labeling for pediatric patients weighing <50 kg states that doses listed may be administered either peripherally or centrally (further studies are needed)

Monitoring Parameters Continuous EKG, heart rate, blood pressure, respirations

Nursing Implications Be alert for dyspnea, shortness of breath, and possible exacerbation of asthma

Additional Information Not effective in atrial flutter, atrial fibrillation, or ventricular tachycardia; short duration of action is an advantage as adverse effects are usually

(Continued)

Adenosine *(Continued)*

rapidly self-limiting; effects may be prolonged in patients with denervated transplanted hearts. Individualize treatment of prolonged adverse effects: Give I.V. fluids for hypotension, aminophylline/theophylline may antagonize effects.

Limited information is available regarding the use of adenosine for the treatment of persistent pulmonary hypertension of the newborn (PPHN); efficacy, optimal dose, and duration of therapy is not established; a randomized, masked, placebo-controlled pilot study of 18 term infants with PPHN used initial doses of 25 mcg/kg/minute (n=9); after 30 minutes, doses were increased to 50 mcg/kg/minute if no improvement in PaO_2 was observed; all patients received study drug via central line into the right atrium (inserted via the umbilical vein); significant improvement in oxygenation was observed in 4 of 9 newborns receiving 50 mcg/kg/minute; hypotension or tachycardia were not observed; further studies are needed (Kondur, 1996).

Adenosine is also available as Adenoscan®, which is used in adults as an adjunct to thallium-201 myocardial perfusion scintigraphy; see package insert for further information on this use.

Dosage Forms Excipient information presented when available (limited, particularly for generics); consult specific product labeling.

Injection, solution [preservative free]: 3 mg/mL (2 mL, 4 mL)
- Adenocard®: 3 mg/mL (2 mL, 4 mL)
- Adenoscan®: 3 mg/mL (20 mL, 30 mL)

References

Eubanks AP and Artman M, "Administration of Adenosine to a Newborn of 26 Weeks' Gestation," *Pediatr Cardiol*, 1994, 15(3):157-8.

"Guidelines 2000 for Cardiopulmonary Resuscitation and Emergency Cardiovascular Care, Part 6: Advanced Cardiovascular Life Support, The American Heart Association in Collaboration With the International Liaison Committee on Resuscitation," *Circulation*, 2000, 102(8 Suppl):I86-171.

"Guidelines 2000 for Cardiopulmonary Resuscitation and Emergency Cardiovascular Care, Part 10: Pediatric Advanced Life Support, The American Heart Association in Collaboration With the International Liaison Committee on Resuscitation," *Circulation*, 2000, 102(8 Suppl): I291-342.

Konduri GG, Garcia DC, Kazzi NJ, et al, "Adenosine Infusion Improves Oxygenation in Term Infants With Respiratory Failure," *Pediatrics*, 1996, 97(3):295-300.

McIntosh-Yellin NL, Drew BJ, and Scheinman MM, "Safety and Efficacy of Central Intravenous Bolus Administration of Adenosine for Termination of Supraventricular Tachycardia," *J Am Coll Cardiol*, 1993, 22(3):741-5.

Paul T and Pfammatter JP, "Adenosine: An Effective and Safe Antiarrhythmic Drug in Pediatrics," *Pediatr Cardiol*, 1997, 18(2):118-26.

Sherwood MC, Lau KC, and Sholler GF, "Adenosine in the Management of Supraventricular Tachycardia in Children," *J Paediatr Child Health*, 1998, 34(1):53-6.

Till J, Shinebourne EA, Rigby ML, et al, "Efficacy and Safety in the Treatment of Supraventricular Tachycardia in Infants and Children," *Br Heart J*, 1989, 62(3):204-11.

Zeigler V, "Adenosine in the Pediatric Population: Nursing Implications," *Pediatr Nurs*, 1991, 17(6):600-2.

- ♦ **Adenosine Injection, USP (Can)** *see* Adenosine *on page 58*
- ♦ **ADH** *see* Vasopressin *on page 1602*
- ♦ **Adoxa®** *see* Doxycycline *on page 543*
- ♦ **Adrenalin®** *see* Epinephrine *on page 577*
- ♦ **Adrenaline** *see* Epinephrine *on page 577*
- ♦ **Adrenocorticotropic Hormone** *see* Corticotropin *on page 402*
- ♦ **ADR (error-prone abbreviation)** *see* DOXOrubicin *on page 540*
- ♦ **Adria** *see* DOXOrubicin *on page 540*
- ♦ **Adriamycin®** *see* DOXOrubicin *on page 540*
- ♦ **Adrucil®** *see* Fluorouracil *on page 678*
- ♦ **Adsorbent Charcoal** *see* Charcoal, Activated *on page 328*
- ♦ **Advair Diskus®** *see* Fluticasone and Salmeterol *on page 694*
- ♦ **Advair® HFA** *see* Fluticasone and Salmeterol *on page 694*
- ♦ **Advate** *see* Antihemophilic Factor (Recombinant) *on page 138*
- ♦ **Advil® [OTC]** *see* Ibuprofen *on page 802*
- ♦ **Advil® (Can)** *see* Ibuprofen *on page 802*
- ♦ **Advil® Children's [OTC]** *see* Ibuprofen *on page 802*
- ♦ **Advil® Cold, Children's [OTC]** *see* Pseudoephedrine and Ibuprofen *on page 1346*
- ♦ **Advil® Cold & Sinus [OTC]** *see* Pseudoephedrine and Ibuprofen *on page 1346*
- ♦ **Advil® Cold & Sinus (Can)** *see* Pseudoephedrine and Ibuprofen *on page 1346*
- ♦ **Advil® Infants' [OTC]** *see* Ibuprofen *on page 802*
- ♦ **Advil® Junior [OTC]** *see* Ibuprofen *on page 802*
- ♦ **Advil® Migraine [OTC]** *see* Ibuprofen *on page 802*
- ♦ **Aerius® (Can)** *see* Desloratadine *on page 458*
- ♦ **AeroBid®** *see* Flunisolide *on page 669*
- ♦ **AeroBid®-M** *see* Flunisolide *on page 669*
- ♦ **Aerospan™** *see* Flunisolide *on page 669*

- **Afeditab™ CR** *see* NIFEdipine *on page 1134*
- **Afrin® Extra Moisturizing [OTC]** *see* Oxymetazoline *on page 1194*
- **Afrin® Original [OTC]** *see* Oxymetazoline *on page 1194*
- **Afrin® Severe Congestion [OTC]** *see* Oxymetazoline *on page 1194*
- **Afrin® Sinus [OTC]** *see* Oxymetazoline *on page 1194*

Agalsidase Beta (aye GAL si days BAY ta)

Medication Safety Issues

Sound-alike/look-alike issues:

Agalsidase beta may be confused with agalsidase alfa, alglucerase, alglucosidase alfa

International issues:

Agalsidase beta may be confused with agalsidase alfa, which is available in international markets

U.S. Brand Names Fabrazyme®

Canadian Brand Names Fabrazyme®

Index Terms Alpha-Galactosidase-A (Recombinant); r-h α-GAL

Therapeutic Category Enzyme, α-galactosidase A; Fabry's Disease, Treatment Agent

Generic Available No

Use Treatment of Fabry's disease

Pregnancy Risk Factor B

Lactation Excretion in breast milk unknown/use caution

Contraindications Hypersensitivity to agalsidase beta or any component

Warnings Infusion-related reactions (ranging from mild to severe) including fever, rigors, chest tightness, hypertension, hypotension, pruritus, myalgia, dyspnea, urticaria, abdominal pain, and headache have been reported; these reactions may be minimized by pretreatment with acetaminophen and an antihistamine; if an infusion related reaction occurs, regardless of pretreatment, decreasing the infusion rate, temporarily stopping the infusion, and/or additional administration of analgesics, antihistamines, or corticosteroids may ameliorate the reaction.

Precautions Use with caution in patients with compromised cardiac function (seen in advanced Fabry's disease) due to an increased potential for severe infusion related reactions; monitor these patients closely; patients may develop IgG antibodies to agalsidase beta

Adverse Reactions

Cardiovascular: Tachycardia, hypertension, hypotension, chest pain, chest tightness, bradycardia, arrhythmias, cardiac arrest, edema, pallor

Central nervous system: Headache, dizziness, fever, anxiety, depression, chills, rigors, vertigo

Dermatologic: Pruritus, urticaria

Gastrointestinal: Dyspepsia, nausea, abdominal pain, vomiting

Genitourinary: Testicular pain

Neuromuscular & skeletal: Arthrosis, skeletal pain, myalgia

Otic: Hypoacousia

Respiratory: Bronchitis, bronchospasm, laryngitis, pharyngitis, sinusitis, rhinitis, dyspnea

Miscellaneous: Hypersensitivity reactions

Drug Interactions None as yet have been identified

Stability Store in refrigerator 2°C to 8°C (36°F to 46°F); reconstituted solution is stable for 24 hours refrigerated

Mechanism of Action Agalsidase beta is a recombinant human α-galactosidase A enzyme with the same amino acid sequence as the naturally-occurring enzyme. Fabry's disease is an X-linked genetic disorder occurring in 1 in 50,000 male births, which results in a deficiency of α-galactosidase A. Lack of this enzyme leads to a progressive accumulation of glycosphingolipids, predominantly GL-3, in the vascular endothelium, leading to ischemia and infarction, especially in the kidney, heart, and brain. Clinical manifestations of Fabry's disease in childhood include intermittent severe pain in the extremities, characteristic vascular skin lesions (angiokeratomas), corneal and lenticular opacities that do not affect vision, decreased ability to sweat, intolerance to heat, cold, and exercise, mild proteinuria, and GI problems. By adulthood, this progresses to renal failure, cardiomyopathy, and cerebrovascular accidents.

Pharmacokinetics

Distribution: V_d: Adults: 80-330 mL/kg

Half-life: Adults: 45-102 minutes (dose dependent)

Usual Dosage I.V.: Children and Adults: 1 mg/kg/dose every two weeks

(Continued)

Agalsidase Beta *(Continued)*

Administration I.V.: Reconstitute vial with 7.2 mL SWI to result in 5 mg/mL concentration; swirl to dissolve; do not shake; further dilute dosage in 500 mL NS*. Initial infusion not to exceed 15 mg/hour (0.25 mg/minute); after patient tolerance to initial infusion rate is established, the infusion rate may be increased in increments of 3-5 mg/hour (0.05-0.08 mg/minute) with subsequent infusions. In clinical studies, patients have tolerated infusion rates ≥33 mg/hour. Pretreatment with acetaminophen and an antihistamine is recommended to reduce infusion related side effects (See Warnings)

*Agalsidase beta stability when diluted in NS at a concentration of 2.55 mg/mL has been demonstrated by the manufacturer. Infusion volumes as low as 100 mL were used in phase I/II clinical trials. (Personal communication, Genzyme Corporation, 2003)

Monitoring Parameters Vital signs during infusion; globotriaosylceramide (GL3) plasma levels; improvement in symptomatology

Reference Range Normal endogenous activity of alpha-galactosidase A in plasma is approximately 170 nmol/hour/mL; in patients with Fabry's disease this activity is <1.5 nmol/hour/mL

Normal (goal) globotriaosylceramide (GL3) <1.2 ng/microliter

Additional Information Agalsidase beta is an orphan drug; a Fabry Patient Support Group (800-745-4447) is available to assist patients in obtaining reimbursement from private insurers, Medicare, and Medicaid, and a Charitable Access Program sponsored by Genzyme provides the drug gratis to those patients in need. Detailed information regarding organizations and websites is also available in the Expert Panel Recommendations (Desnick, 2003)

Dosage Forms Excipient information presented when available (limited, particularly for generics); consult specific product labeling.

Injection, powder for reconstitution:

Fabrazyme®: 5 mg [contains mannitol 33 mg; derived from Chinese hamster cells]; 35 mg [contains mannitol 222 mg; derived from Chinese hamster cells]

References

Desnick RJ, Brady R, Barranger J, et al, "Fabry Disease, an Under-Recognized Multisystemic Disorder: Expert Recommendations for Diagnosis, Management, and Enzyme Replacement Therapy," *Ann Intern Med*, 2003, 138(4):338-46.

- **Agenerase®** *see* Amprenavir *on page 127*
- **$AgNO_3$** *see* Silver Nitrate *on page 1439*
- **Ah-Chew D®** *see* Phenylephrine *on page 1250*
- **AHF** *see* Antihemophilic Factor (Human) *on page 134*
- **AHF (Human)** *see* Antihemophilic Factor/von Willebrand Factor Complex (Human) *on page 141*
- **AHF (Recombinant)** *see* Antihemophilic Factor (Recombinant) *on page 138*
- **AHG** *see* Antihemophilic Factor (Human) *on page 134*
- **Ahist™** *see* Chlorpheniramine *on page 344*
- **A-hydroCort** *see* Hydrocortisone *on page 781*
- **AICC** *see* Anti-inhibitor Coagulant Complex *on page 144*
- **Airomir (Can)** *see* Albuterol *on page 66*
- **AK-Con™** *see* Naphazoline *on page 1106*
- **AK-Dilate®** *see* Phenylephrine *on page 1250*
- **Akne-Mycin®** *see* Erythromycin *on page 595*
- **AK-Pentolate® [DSC]** *see* Cyclopentolate *on page 417*
- **AK-Poly-Bac™** *see* Bacitracin and Polymyxin B *on page 196*
- **AKTob®** *see* Tobramycin *on page 1545*
- **AK-Tracin® [DSC]** *see* Bacitracin *on page 195*
- **AK-Trol® [DSC]** *see* Dexamethasone, Neomycin, and Polymyxin B *on page 464*
- **Alamag [OTC]** *see* Antacid Preparations *on page 132*
- **Alamag Plus [OTC]** *see* Antacid Preparations *on page 132*
- **Alamast®** *see* Pemirolast *on page 1226*
- **Alavert® [OTC]** *see* Loratadine *on page 959*
- **Alavert™ Allergy and Sinus [OTC]** *see* Loratadine and Pseudoephedrine *on page 961*
- **Alaway™ [OTC]** *see* Ketotifen *on page 893*
- **Albalon®** *see* Naphazoline *on page 1106*

Albendazole (al BEN da zole)

Medication Safety Issues

International issues:

Albenza® may be confused with Avanza® which is a brand name for mirtazapine in Australia

U.S. Brand Names Albenza®

Therapeutic Category Anthelmintic

Generic Available No

Use Treatment of parenchymal neurocysticercosis due to active lesions caused by larval forms of *Taenia solium*; treatment of cystic hydatid disease of the liver, lung, and peritoneum caused by the larval form of *Echinococcus granulosus*; active against *Ascaris lumbricoides* (roundworm), *Ancylostoma duodenale* and *Necator americanus* (hookworm), *Enterobius vermicularis* (pinworm), *Clonorchis sinensis* (Chinese liver fluke), *Trichuris trichiura* (whipworm), and *Capillaria philippinensis*

Pregnancy Risk Factor C

Lactation Excretion in breast milk unknown/not recommended

Contraindications Hypersensitivity to albendazole, any component, or the benzimidazole class of compounds

Warnings Fatalities due to granulocytopenia or pancytopenia associated with the use of albendazole have been reported; women of childbearing age should only begin treatment after a negative pregnancy test and should be cautioned against becoming pregnant during and for at least one month after treatment cessation with albendazole since it may cause harm to fetus.

Precautions Use with caution in patients with hepatic impairment or decreased total leukocyte count; discontinue albendazole if significant elevation of liver enzymes occur; may restart therapy when liver enzymes decrease to pretreatment values; corticosteroids should be administered 1-2 days before initiating albendazole therapy in patients with neurocysticercosis to minimize inflammatory reactions and should be followed by concurrent steroid and anticonvulsant therapy for the first week of therapy to prevent cerebral hypertension. Albendazole may induce further retinal damage in patients having retinal lesions with neurocysticercosis.

Adverse Reactions

Central nervous system: Headache, dizziness, vertigo, elevated intracranial pressure, meningeal signs, fever, seizures

Dermatologic: Rash, urticaria, alopecia

Gastrointestinal: Abdominal pain, nausea, vomiting

Hematologic: Leukopenia, pancytopenia, thrombocytopenia, granulocytopenia, agranulocytosis

Hepatic: Elevated liver enzymes, hepatotoxicity

Renal: Acute renal failure

Miscellaneous: Hypersensitivity reactions, migration of *Ascaris* through mouth and nose

Drug Interactions Cytochrome P450 isoenzyme CYP1A2 inducer; isoenzyme CYP1A2 substrate (minor) and CYP3A4 substrate (major)

Dexamethasone, cimetidine, and praziquantel increase albendazole sulfoxide (active metabolite) concentration

Food Interactions Bioavailability is increased when taken with a fatty meal

Stability Store at room temperature

Mechanism of Action Binds to β-tubulin in parasite cells inhibiting tubulin polymerization which results in the loss of cytoplasmic microtubules and inhibition of glucose uptake

Pharmacokinetics

Absorption: Poorly absorbed from the GI tract

Distribution: Widely distributed throughout the body including urine, bile, liver, cyst wall, cyst fluid, and CSF

Protein binding: 70%

Metabolism: Extensive first-pass metabolism; hepatic metabolism to albendazole sulfoxide, an active metabolite

Half-life: Albendazole sulfoxide: 8-12 hours

Time to peak serum concentration: 2-5 hours for the metabolite

Elimination: Biliary

Usual Dosage Children and Adults: Oral:

Neurocysticercosis: (patients should receive appropriate corticosteroid and anticonvulsant therapy as required):

<60 kg: 15 mg/kg/day in 2 divided doses (maximum: 800 mg/day) for 8-30 days

≥60 kg: 400 mg twice daily for 8-30 days

Hydatid disease:

<60 kg: 15 mg/kg/day in 2 divided doses (maximum: 800 mg/day) for 1-6 months

(Continued)

Albendazole *(Continued)*

≥60 kg: 400 mg twice daily for 1-6 months

Ancylostoma caninum, ascariasis (roundworm), hookworm, trichuriasis (whipworm): 400 mg as a single dose

Capillariasis: 400 mg once daily for 10 days

Clonorchis sinensis (Chinese liver fluke): 10 mg/kg/day once daily for 7 days

Cutaneous larva migrans: 400 mg once daily for 3 days

Enterobius vermicularis (pinworm): 400 mg as a single dose; repeat in 2 weeks

Filariasis (*Mansonella perstans*): 400 mg twice daily for 10 days

Trichinosis (*Trichinella spiralis*): 400 mg twice daily for 8-14 days

Visceral larva migrans: 400 mg twice daily for 5 days

Administration Oral: Administer with food

Monitoring Parameters Monitor liver function tests, CBC at start of each cycle and every 2 weeks during therapy

Dosage Forms Excipient information presented when available (limited, particularly for generics); consult specific product labeling.

Tablet: 200 mg

References

Baranwal AK, Singhi PD, Khandelwal N, et al, "Albendazole Therapy in Children With Focal Seizures and Single Small Enhancing Computerized Tomographic Lesions: A Randomized, Placebo-Controlled, Double Blind Trial," *Pediatr Infect Dis J*, 1998, 17(8):696-700.

Jung H, Sanchez M, Gonzalez-Astiazaran A, et al, "Clinical Pharmacokinetics of Albendazole in Children With Neurocysticercosis," *Am J Ther*, 1997, 4(1):23-6.

Paul I, Gnanamani G, and Nallam NR, "Intestinal Helminth Infections Among School Children in Visakhapatnam," *Indian J Pediatr*, 1999, 66(5):669-73.

Pengsaa K, Sirivichayakul C, Pojjaroen-anant C, et al, "Albendazole Treatment for *Giardia intestinalis* Infections in School Children," *Southeast Asian J Trop Med Public Health*, 1999, 30(1):78-83.

♦ **Albenza®** *see* Albendazole *on page 63*

♦ **Albert® Glyburide (Can)** *see* GlyBURIDE *on page 734*

♦ **Albert® Pentoxifylline (Can)** *see* Pentoxifylline *on page 1241*

♦ **Albumarc®** *see* Albumin *on page 64*

Albumin (al BYOO min)

Medication Safety Issues

Sound-alike/look-alike issues:

Albutein® may be confused with albuterol

Buminate® may be confused with bumetanide

U.S. Brand Names Albumarc®; Albuminar®; AlbuRx™; Albutein®; Buminate®; Flexbumin; Plasbumin®

Canadian Brand Names Plasbumin®-5; Plasbumin®-25

Index Terms Albumin (Human); Normal Human Serum Albumin; Normal Serum Albumin (Human); Salt Poor Albumin; SPA

Therapeutic Category Blood Product Derivative; Plasma Volume Expander

Generic Available Yes

Use Treatment of hypovolemia; plasma volume expansion and maintenance of cardiac output in the treatment of certain types of shock or impending shock; hypoproteinemia resulting in generalized edema or decreased intravascular volume (eg, hypoproteinemia associated with acute nephrotic syndrome, premature neonates)

Note: PALS and Neonatal Resuscitation 2000 Guidelines recommend isotonic crystalloid solutions (eg, NS or LR) as initial volume expansion; albumin is used less frequently due to limited supply, potential risk of infections, and an association with an increase in mortality (identified by meta-analyses); few studies in these analyses included children, so no firm conclusions in pediatric patients can be made

Pregnancy Risk Factor C

Lactation Excretion in breast milk unknown/compatible

Contraindications Hypersensitivity to albumin or any component; patients with severe anemia or cardiac failure

Warnings Use 25% concentration with extreme caution and infuse slowly in preterm neonates, due to increased risk of IVH (from rapid expansion of intravascular volume). Some products (eg, Albuminar®, Buminate®) contain natural rubber latex (in certain components of the product packaging) which may cause allergic reactions in susceptible individuals; avoid use in patients with allergy to latex

Precautions Rapid infusion of albumin solutions may cause vascular overload. Do not administer albumin to burn patients for the first 24 hours after the burn (capillary exudation of albumin will occur); use with caution in patients with hepatic or renal failure (added protein load) and in patients who require sodium restriction; monitor for signs of hypervolemia

Due to the occasional shortage of 5% human albumin, 5% solutions may at times be prepared by diluting 25% human albumin with NS or with D_5W (if sodium load is a concern); however, **do not use sterile water** to dilute albumin solutions, as this may result in hypotonic-associated hemolysis which can be fatal

Adverse Reactions

Cardiovascular: Precipitation of CHF or pulmonary edema, hypertension, tachycardia, hypervolemia, hypotension due to hypersensitivity reaction

Central nervous system: Fever, chills

Dermatologic: Rash

Gastrointestinal: Nausea, vomiting

Stability Use within 4 hours after opening vial, do not use if turbid or contains a deposit; do not use SWI to dilute albumin (see Precautions)

Mechanism of Action Provides increase in intravascular oncotic pressure and causes mobilization of fluids from interstitial into intravascular space

Pharmacodynamics Duration of volume expansion: ~24 hours

Pharmacokinetics Half-life: 21 days

Usual Dosage Albumin **5%** should be used in hypovolemic or intravascularly depleted patients; albumin **25%** should be used in patients with fluid or sodium restrictions (eg, patients with hypoproteinemia and generalized edema, or nephrotic syndrome) (see Additional Information). Dose depends on condition of patient: I.V.:

Hypoproteinemia: Neonates, Infants, and Children: 0.5-1 g/kg/dose of 25% albumin; may repeat every 1-2 days; up to 1.5 g/kg/day has been added to hyperalimentation solutions; see Administration

Hypovolemia:

- Neonates: Usual dose: 0.5 g/kg/dose (10 mL/kg/dose of 5% albumin); range: 0.25-0.5 g/kg/dose (5-10 mL/kg/dose of 5% albumin)
- Infants and Children: 0.5-1 g/kg/dose (10-20 mL/kg/dose of 5% albumin); may repeat as needed; maximum dose: 6 g/kg/day (120 mL/kg/day of 5% albumin); see Administration

Nephrotic syndrome: Infants and Children: 0.25-1 g/kg/dose of 25% albumin

Adults: 25 g; no more than 250 g should be administered within 48 hours

- Nephrotic syndrome: 12.5-50 g/day in 3-4 divided doses; daily dose has also been added to hyperalimentation solution; see Administration

Administration Parenteral: I.V.: Too rapid infusion may result in vascular overload

Albuminar®: May administer via the administration set provided (in-line 60 micron filter) or via any administration set; use of filter is optional; size of filter may vary according to institutional policy. Method of filter sterilization used by manufacturer includes 0.2 micron filter; however, aggregates may form under storage, shipping, and handling. Administration via very small filter will not damage product, but will slow flow rate.

Albutein®: May administer via the administration set provided (in-line 50 micron filter) or via any administration set; use of filter is optional; size of filter may vary according to institutional policy. Method of production includes passage through 0.22 micron filter. May administer via filter as small as 0.22 microns.

Buminate®: Administer via the administration set provided (in-line 15 micron filter) or via any filtered administration set; use ≥5 micron filter to ensure adequate flow rate

Plasbumin®: May administer with or without an I.V. filter; filter as small as 0.22 microns may be used

Hypoproteinemia: Infuse over 2-4 hours; for neonates, dose may be added to hyperalimentation fluid and infused over 24 hours; **Note:** Hyperalimentation fluid containing >25 g/L of albumin is more likely to occlude 0.22 micron in-line filters; but hyperalimentation solutions containing albumin in concentrations as low as 10.8 g/L have also occluded 0.22 micron filters; use ≥5 micron filter to ensure adequate flow rate; addition of albumin to hyperalimentation solutions may increase potential for growth of bacteria or fungi.

Hypovolemia: Rate of infusion depends on severity of hypovolemia and patient's symptoms; usually infuse dose over 30-60 minutes (faster infusion rates may be clinically necessary)

Maximum rates of I.V. infusion after initial volume replacement:

- 5%: 2-4 mL/minute
- 25%: 1 mL/minute

To prepare 5% albumin from 25%, see Precautions.

Monitoring Parameters Observe for signs of hypervolemia, pulmonary edema, cardiac failure, vital signs, I & O, Hgb, Hct, urine specific gravity

Nursing Implications Albumin administration must be completed within 6 hours after entering container, provided that administration is begun within 4 hours of entering the container

Additional Information In certain conditions (eg, hypoproteinemia with generalized edema, nephrotic syndrome), doses of albumin may be followed with I.V. furosemide: 0.5-1 mg/kg/dose.

(Continued)

Albumin *(Continued)*

Both albumin 5% and 25% contain 130-160 mEq/L of sodium; albumin 5% is osmotically equivalent to an equal volume of plasma; albumin 25% is osmotically equivalent to 5 times its volume of plasma.

Dosage Forms Excipient information presented when available (limited, particularly for generics); consult specific product labeling.

Injection, solution [preservative free; human]:

Albuminar®: 5% [50 mg/mL] (50 mL, 250 mL, 500 mL) [contains sodium 130-160 mEq/L and potassium ≤1 mEq/L; packaging contains dry natural rubber]; 25% [250 mg/mL] (20 mL, 50 mL, 100 mL) [contains sodium 130-160 mEq/L and potassium ≤1 mEq/L; packaging contains dry natural rubber]

AlbuRx™: 5% [50 mg/mL] (250 mL, 500 mL) [contains sodium 130-160 mEq/L and potassium ≤2 mEq/L]; 25% [250 mg/mL] (50 mL, 100 mL) [contains sodium 130-160 mEq/L and potassium ≤2 mEq/L]

Albutein®: 5% [50 mg/mL] (250 mL, 500 mL) [contains sodium 130-160 mEq/L and potassium ≤2 mEq/L]; 25% [250 mg/mL] (50 mL, 100 mL) [contains sodium 130-160 mEq/L and potassium ≤2 mEq/L]

Buminate®: 5% [50 mg/mL] (250 mL, 500 mL) [contains sodium 130-160 mEq/L and potassium ≤2 mEq/L; packaging contains dry natural rubber]; 25% [250 mg/mL] (20 mL, 50 mL, 100 mL) [contains sodium 130-160 mEq/L and potassium ≤2 mEq/L; packaging contains dry natural rubber]

Flexbumin: 25% [250 mg/mL] (50 mL, 100 mL) [contains sodium 130-160 and potassium ≤2 mEq/L]

Human Albumin Grifols®: 25% [250 mg/mL] (50 mL, 100 mL) [contains sodium 130-160 mEq/L and potassium ≤2 mEq/L]

Plasbumin®: 5% [50 mg/mL] (50 mL, 250 mL) [contains sodium ~145 mEq/L and potassium ≤2 mEq/L]; 25% [250 mg/mL] (20 mL, 50 mL, 100 mL) [contains sodium ~145 mEq/L and potassium ≤2 mEq/L]

References

"Guidelines 2000 for Cardiopulmonary Resuscitation and Emergency Cardiovascular Care, Part 10: Pediatric Advanced Life Support, The American Heart Association in Collaboration With the International Liaison Committee on Resuscitation," *Circulation*, 2000, 102(8 Suppl):I306.

"Guidelines 2000 for Cardiopulmonary Resuscitation and Emergency Cardiovascular Care, Part 11: Neonatal Resuscitation, The American Heart Association in Collaboration With the International Liaison Committee on Resuscitation," *Circulation*, 2000, 102(8 Suppl):I352.

"Hemolysis Associated With 25% Human Albumin Diluted With Sterile Water - United States, 1994-1998," *MMWR Morb Mortal Wkly Rep*, 1999, 48(8):157-9.

◆ **Albuminar®** *see* Albumin *on page 64*
◆ **Albumin (Human)** *see* Albumin *on page 64*
◆ **AlbuRx™** *see* Albumin *on page 64*
◆ **Albutein®** *see* Albumin *on page 64*

Albuterol (al BYOO ter ole)

Medication Safety Issues

Sound-alike/look-alike issues:

Albuterol may be confused with Albutein®, atenolol
Proventil® may be confused with Bentyl®, Prilosec® Prinivil®
Salbutamol may be confused with salmeterol
Ventolin® may be confused with phentolamine, Benylin®, Vantin®
Volmax® may be confused with Flomax®

Related Information

Asthma *on page 1904*

U.S. Brand Names AccuNeb®; ProAir™ HFA; Proventil®; Proventil® HFA; Ventolin® HFA; VoSpire ER®

Canadian Brand Names Airomir; Alti-Salbutamol; Apo-Salvent®; Apo-Salvent® CFC Free; Apo-Salvent® Respirator Solution; Apo-Salvent® Sterules; Gen-Salbutamol; PMS-Salbutamol; ratio-Inspra-Sal; ratio-Salbutamol; Rhoxal-salbutamol; Salbu-2; Salbu-4; Ventolin®; Ventolin® Diskus; Ventolin® HFA; Ventrodisk

Index Terms Albuterol Sulfate; Salbutamol

Therapeutic Category Adrenergic Agonist Agent; Antiasthmatic; Beta$_2$-Adrenergic Agonist Agent; Bronchodilator; Sympathomimetic

Generic Available Yes

Use Prevention and relief of bronchospasm in patients with reversible airway obstruction due to asthma or COPD; prevention of exercise-induced bronchospasm

Pregnancy Risk Factor C

Lactation Excretion in breast milk unknown/use caution

Contraindications Hypersensitivity to albuterol, any component, or adrenergic amine

Warnings Inhaled albuterol can produce paradoxical bronchospasm; discontinue therapy immediately if this occurs. Excessive or prolonged use can lead to tolerance;

excessive use has also been associated with deaths, possibly due to cardiac arrest. Outbreaks of lower respiratory tract colonization and infection have been attributed to contaminated multidose albuterol bottles (see Administration).

Precautions Use with caution in patients with hyperthyroidism, seizure disorders, diabetes mellitus; cardiovascular disorders including coronary insufficiency, hypertension, or arrhythmia

Adverse Reactions

Cardiovascular: Tachycardia, palpitations, hypertension, chest pain

Central nervous system: Nervousness, CNS stimulation, hyperactivity and insomnia occur more frequently in younger children than adults; dizziness, lightheadedness, drowsiness, headache

Dermatologic: Angioedema, urticaria

Endocrine & metabolic: Hypokalemia

Gastrointestinal: GI upset, xerostomia, heartburn, vomiting, nausea, unusual taste, hoarseness (inhalation only)

Genitourinary: Dysuria

Neuromuscular & skeletal: Tremor, weakness, muscle cramping

Respiratory: Irritation of oropharynx, coughing, paradoxical bronchospasm (oral inhalation only)

Miscellaneous: Diaphoresis (increased)

Drug Interactions Action of albuterol is antagonized by beta-adrenergic blocking agents such as propranolol; cardiovascular effects are potentiated in patients also receiving MAO inhibitors or tricyclic antidepressants; concomitant administration of sympathomimetics may result in enhanced cardiovascular effects; may decrease digoxin serum levels

Food Interactions Caffeinated beverages may increase side effects of albuterol.

Stability Liquid, tablets, MDIs, and oral inhalation solutions are stable at room temperature; discard Ventolin® HFA MDI canister after 200 actuations or 3 months after removal from moisture protective pouch; discard AccuNeb™ vial 1 week after removal from foil pouch or if solution is not colorless; oral inhalation solution compatible with cromolyn and ipratropium nebulizer solutions

Mechanism of Action Relaxes bronchial smooth muscle by action on beta$_2$-receptors with little effect on heart rate

Pharmacodynamics

Nebulization/oral inhalation:
- Peak bronchodilation: Within 0.5-2 hours nebulization
- Duration: 2-5 hours

Oral:
- Peak bronchodilatation: 2-3 hours
- Duration: 4-6 hours

Extended release tablets: Duration: Up to 12 hours

Pharmacokinetics

Metabolism: By the liver to an inactive sulfate

Half-life:
- Oral: 2.7-5 hours
- Inhalation: 3.8 hours

Elimination: 30% appears in urine as unchanged drug

Usual Dosage

Acute asthma exacerbation (NIH guidelines):

Nebulization:

Children: 0.15 mg/kg (minimum dose: 2.5 mg) every 20 minutes for 3 doses then 0.15-0.3 mg/kg (not to exceed 10 mg) every 1-4 hours as needed or 0.5 mg/kg/hour by continuous infusion

Note: Continuous nebulized albuterol at 0.3 mg/kg/hour has also been used safely in the treatment of severe status asthmaticus in children; continuous nebulized doses of 3 mg/kg/hour ± 2.2 mg/kg/hour (Katz, 1993) in children whose mean age was 20.7 months resulted in no cardiotoxicity; the optimal dosage for continuous nebulization remains to be determined

Adults: 2.5-5 mg every 20 minutes for 3 doses then 2.5-10 mg every 1-4 hours as needed or 10-15 mg/hour by continuous infusion

Inhalation: MDI: 90 mcg/spray:

Children: 4-8 puffs every 20 minutes for 3 doses then every 1-4 hours

Adults: 4-8 puffs every 20 minutes for up to 4 hours then every 1-4 hours as needed

Maintenance therapy (nonacute) (NIH guidelines):

Oral:

Immediate release formulation:

Children 2-6 years: 0.1-0.2 mg/kg/dose 3 times/day; maximum dose not to exceed 4 mg 3 times/day

Children 6-12 years: 2 mg/dose 3-4 times/day

(Continued)

Albuterol *(Continued)*

Children >12 years to Adults: 2-4 mg/dose 3-4 times/day
Sustained release formulation:
Children: 0.3-0.6 mg/kg/day in 2 divided doses; not to exceed 8 mg/day
Children >12 years to Adults: 4 mg 2 times/day; may increase to 8 mg 2 times/day
Inhalation: MDI: 90 mcg/spray:
Children ≥4 years to Adults: 1-2 inhalations every 4-6 hours; maximum 12 inhalations/day
Exercise-induced bronchospasm: Children ≥4 years to Adults: 2 inhalations 5-30 minutes before exercising
Inhalation: Children and Adults: Nebulization: See dosage table

Albuterol Nebulization Dosage (Maintenance Therapy - Non-Acute)

Age	Dose (by weight)	0.5% Solution (mL/kg)	0.083% Solution (mL/kg)	Frequency
Children <12 y	0.15-0.25 mg/kg (minimum: 1.25 mg; maximum: 5 mg)[1]	0.01-0.05 (minimum: 0.25 mL; maximum: 1 mL)[1]	0.06-0.3 (minimum: 1.5 mL; maximum: 6 mL)[1]	Every 4-6 hours
Children 12 y - Adults	1.25-5 mg	0.25-1 mL	1.5-6 mL	Every 4-8 hours

[1]Doses >2.5 mg have been associated with a higher frequency of adverse systemic effects.

or as an alternative (manufacturer's recommendation):
Children:
10-15 kg: 1.25 mg 3-4 times/day
>15 kg: 2.5 mg 3-4 times/day
AccuNeb™:
Children <12 years: 0.75-1.5 mg 3-4 times/day
Children ≥12 years to Adults: 1.5 mg 3-4 times/day
AccuNeb™ has not been studied in the treatment of acute bronchospasm; a more concentrated form may be necessary for treatment in acute bronchospasm especially in children ≥6 years.

Administration
Inhalation: Nebulization: Using 0.5% solution, dilute dosage in 1-2 mL NS (0.083% solution and AccuNeb™ do not require further dilution); adjust nebulizer flow to deliver dosage over 5-15 minutes; avoid contact of the dropper tip (multidose bottle) with any surface, including the nebulizer reservoir and associated ventilator equipment (see Warnings)
Oral: Administer with food; do not crush or chew extended release tablets (Repetabs® or Volmax®)
Oral inhalation: Prime the inhaler (before first use or if it has not been used for more than 2 weeks) by releasing 4 test sprays into the air away from the face; shake well before use; use spacer for children <8 years of age

Monitoring Parameters Serum potassium, heart rate, pulmonary function tests, respiratory rate; arterial or capillary blood gases (if patient's condition warrants)

Patient Information Do not exceed recommended dosage; may cause dry mouth; rinse mouth with water following each inhalation to help with dry throat and mouth; if more than one inhalation is necessary, wait at least 1 full minute between inhalations; notify physician if palpitations, tachycardia, chest pain, muscle tremors, dizziness, headache, flushing, or if breathing difficulty persists; limit caffeinated beverages; to prevent medication build-up or blockage in the inhaler, the actuator, with the canister removed, should be washed and air-dried once weekly

Dosage Forms Excipient information presented when available (limited, particularly for generics); consult specific product labeling.
Aerosol, for oral inhalation: 90 mcg/metered inhalation (17 g) [200 metered inhalations; contains chlorofluorocarbons]
Proventil®: 90 mcg/metered inhalation (17 g) [200 metered inhalations; contains chlorofluorocarbons]
Aerosol, for oral inhalation:
ProAir™ HFA: 90 mcg/metered inhalation (8.5 g) [200 metered inhalations; chlorofluorocarbon free]
Proventil® HFA: 90 mcg/metered inhalation (6.7 g) [200 metered inhalations; chlorofluorocarbon free]
Ventolin® HFA: 90 mcg/metered inhalation (18 g) [200 metered inhalations; chlorofluorocarbon free]
Solution for nebulization: 0.042% (3 mL); 0.083% (3 mL); 0.5% (0.5 mL, 20 mL)

AccuNeb® [preservative free]: 0.63 mg/3 mL (3 mL) [0.021%]; 1.25 mg/3 mL (3 mL) [0.042%]

Proventil®: 0.083% (3 mL) [preservative free]; 0.5% (20 mL) [contains benzalkonium chloride]

Syrup, as sulfate: 2 mg/5 mL (480 mL)

Tablet: 2 mg, 4 mg

Tablet, extended release: 4 mg, 8 mg

VoSpire ER®: 4 mg, 8 mg

References

"Guidelines for the Diagnosis and Management of Asthma. NAEPP Expert Panel Report 2," July 1997, www.nhlbi.nih.gov/guidelines/asthma/asthgdln.pdf.

Katz RW, Kelly HW, Crowley MR, et al, "Safety of Continuous Nebulized Albuterol for Bronchospasm in Infants and Children," *Pediatrics*, 1993, 92(5):666-69.

"National Asthma Education and Prevention Program. Expert Panel Report: Guidelines for the Diagnosis and Management of Asthma Update on Selected Topics--2002," *J Allergy Clin Immunol*, 2002, 110(5 Suppl):S141-219.

O'Callaghan C, Milner AD, and Swarbrick A, "Nebulized Salbutamol Does Have a Protective Effect on Airways in Children Under One Year Old," *Arch Dis Child*, 1988, 63(5):479-83.

Papo MC, Frank J, and Thompson AE, "A Prospective, Randomized Study of Continuous Versus Intermittent Nebulized Albuterol for Severe Status Asthmaticus in Children," *Crit Care Med*, 1993, 21(10):1479-86.

Rachelefsky GS and Siegel SC, "Asthma in Infants and Children - Treatment of Childhood Asthma: Part II," *J Allergy Clin Immunol*, 1985, 76(3):409-25.

Schuh S, Parkin P, Rajan A, et al, "High- Versus Low-Dose, Frequently Administered, Nebulized Albuterol in Children With Severe, Acute Asthma," *Pediatrics*, 1989, 83(4):513-8.

Schuh S, Reider MJ, Canny G, et al, "Nebulized Albuterol in Acute Childhood Asthma: Comparison of Two Doses," *Pediatrics*, 1990, 86(4):509-13.

♦ **Albuterol Sulfate** *see* Albuterol *on page 66*
♦ **Alcaine®** *see* Proparacaine *on page 1331*
♦ **Alcalak [OTC]** *see* Calcium Carbonate *on page 264*
♦ **Alcalak [OTC]** *see* Calcium Supplements *on page 272*

Alclometasone (al kloe MET a sone)

Medication Safety Issues

Sound-alike/look-alike issues:

Aclovate® may be confused with Accolate®

U.S. Brand Names Aclovate®

Index Terms Alclometasone Dipropionate

Therapeutic Category Adrenal Corticosteroid; Anti-inflammatory Agent; Corticosteroid, Topical; Glucocorticoid

Generic Available Yes

Use Treatment of inflammation of corticosteroid-responsive dermatosis (mild to moderate potency topical corticosteroid)

Pregnancy Risk Factor C

Contraindications Hypersensitivity to alclometasone or any component; viral, fungal, or tubercular skin lesions; herpes (including varicella)

Warnings Infants and small children, due to larger surface area to body weight ratio and particularly if applying to >20% of body surface area, may be more susceptible to adrenal axis suppression from topical corticosteroid therapy; systemic effects may occur when used on large areas of the body, denuded areas, for prolonged periods of time, or with an occlusive dressing. Hypothalamic pituitary adrenal (HPA) axis suppression may occur; acute adrenal insufficiency may occur with abrupt withdrawal after long term use or with stress; withdrawal or discontinuation should be done carefully; patients with HPA axis suppression may require doses of systemic glucocorticosteroids prior to, during, and after unusual stress (eg, surgery).

Precautions Safety and efficacy have not been established in children <1 year of age; not for use in treatment of diaper dermatitis; generally not for routine use on the face, underarms, or groin areas

Adverse Reactions

Dermatologic: Acne, allergic dermatitis, hypopigmentation, maceration of the skin, skin atrophy, striae, miliaria, telangiectasia

Endocrine & metabolic: HPA suppression, Cushing's syndrome, growth retardation

Local: Burning, erythema, itching, irritation, dryness, folliculitis, hypertrichosis

Systemic: HPA axis suppression, Cushing's syndrome, hyperglycemia; these reactions occur more frequently with occlusive dressings

Miscellaneous: Secondary infection

Drug Interactions No data reported

Stability Store between 2°C and 30°C (36°F and 86°F)

Mechanism of Action Possesses anti-inflammatory, antiproliferative, and immunosuppressive properties

(Continued)

Alclometasone *(Continued)*

Pharmacodynamics
Initial response:
Eczema: 5.3 days
Psoriasis: 6.7 days
Peak response:
Eczema: 13.9 days
Psoriasis: 14.8 days

Pharmacokinetics
Absorption: Topical: 3% (when left on intact skin without an occlusive dressing for 8 hours); large variation in absorption depending upon anatomical sites: Forearm 1%; scalp 4%; scrotum 36%
Metabolism: Liver, extensive

Usual Dosage Topical: Children and Adults: Apply to affected area 2-3 times/day. Therapy should be discontinued when control is achieved; if no improvement is seen, reassessment of diagnosis may be necessary. Not recommended for use >3 weeks in children. Occlusive dressings may be used when treating refractory lesions of psoriasis and other deep-seated dermatoses such as localized neurodermatitis (lichen simplex chronicus); see Warnings

Administration Topical: Apply sparingly in a thin film; rub in lightly; for external use only; avoid contact with the eyes. Do not use on open wounds or weeping lesions. Apply sparingly to occlusive dressings.

Monitoring Parameters Clinical signs and symptoms of improvement in condition; assessment of HPA suppression if treatment for prolonged periods

Patient Information Before applying, gently wash area to reduce risk of infection. Apply a thin film to cleansed area and rub in gently and thoroughly until medication vanishes. Do not use for longer than directed; notify physician if condition being treated persists or worsens.

Dosage Forms Excipient information presented when available (limited, particularly for generics); consult specific product labeling.
Cream, as dipropionate: 0.05% (15 g, 45 g, 60 g)
Ointment, as dipropionate: 0.05% (15 g, 45 g, 60 g)

- **Alclometasone Dipropionate** *see* Alclometasone *on page 69*
- **Alcohol, Absolute** *see* Ethyl Alcohol *on page 619*
- **Alcohol, Dehydrated** *see* Ethyl Alcohol *on page 619*
- **Alcomicin® (Can)** *see* Gentamicin *on page 726*
- **Aldactazide®** *see* Hydrochlorothiazide and Spironolactone *on page 778*
- **Aldactazide 25® (Can)** *see* Hydrochlorothiazide and Spironolactone *on page 778*
- **Aldactazide 50® (Can)** *see* Hydrochlorothiazide and Spironolactone *on page 778*
- **Aldactone®** *see* Spironolactone *on page 1469*

Aldesleukin (al des LOO kin)

Medication Safety Issues
Sound-alike/look-alike issues:
Aldesleukin may be confused with oprelvekin
Proleukin® may be confused with oprelvekin

High alert medication: The Institute for Safe Medication Practices (ISMP) includes this medication among its list of drugs which have a heightened risk of causing significant patient harm when used in error.

Related Information
Compatibility of Chemotherapy and Related Supportive Care Medications *on page 1777*

U.S. Brand Names Proleukin®

Canadian Brand Names Proleukin®

Index Terms Epidermal Thymocyte Activating Factor; ETAF; IL-2; Interleukin-2; Lymphocyte Mitogenic Factor; NSC-373364; T-Cell Growth Factor; TCGF; Thymocyte Stimulating Factor

Therapeutic Category Antineoplastic Agent, Miscellaneous; Biological Response Modulator

Generic Available No

Use Treatment of metastatic renal cell carcinoma and metastatic melanoma; for investigational use in tumors known to have a response to immunotherapy such as colorectal cancer and non-Hodgkin's lymphoma (alone or in combination with lymphokine-activated killer cells); investigational treatment of Kaposi's sarcoma in combination with zidovudine and acute myelogenous leukemia (AML)

Pregnancy Risk Factor C

Lactation Enters breast milk/contraindicated

Contraindications Hypersensitivity to aldesleukin or any component; abnormal thallium stress test or pulmonary function tests; organ allografts (due to increased risk of rejection); **retreatment** in patients who have experienced sustained ventricular tachycardia (≥5 beats), cardiac rhythm disturbances not controlled or unresponsive to management, recurrent chest pain with EKG changes (consistent with angina or MI), intubation required >72 hours, pericardial tamponade; renal dysfunction requiring dialysis >72 hours, coma or toxic psychosis lasting >48 hours, repetitive or difficult to control seizures, bowel ischemia/perforation, and GI bleeding requiring surgery

Warnings High-dose aldesleukin therapy is associated with capillary leak syndrome (CLS) resulting in hypotension and reduced organ perfusion (occurring within 2-12 hours after start of treatment) which may be severe and fatal; CLS may be associated with cardiac arrhythmias, angina, MI, respiratory insufficiency requiring intubation, GI bleeding or infarction, renal insufficiency, edema, and mental status changes; therapy should be restricted to patients with normal cardiac and pulmonary functions as defined by thallium stress and formal pulmonary function testing; hold aldesleukin administration in patients developing moderate to severe lethargy or somnolence as continued administration may result in coma; may exacerbate disease symptoms in patients with clinically unrecognized or untreated CNS metastases; thoroughly evaluate and treat all patients with CNS metastases prior to therapy

Precautions Use with extreme caution in patients with normal thallium stress tests and pulmonary functions tests who have a history of prior cardiac or pulmonary disease; intensive aldesleukin treatment is associated with impaired neutrophil function (reduced chemotaxis) and with an increased risk of disseminated infection (particularly with *Staphylococcus aureus*) including sepsis and bacterial endocarditis; patients with indwelling central lines are particularly at increased risk of infection; treat pre-existing bacterial infections prior to initiation of aldesleukin therapy; standard supportive care during high-dose aldesleukin treatment includes acetaminophen to relieve fever and chills and an H_2 antagonist to reduce the risk of GI ulceration and/or bleeding; aldesleukin may exacerbate autoimmune disease; closely monitor for thyroid abnormalities or other potentially autoimmune phenomena; use with caution in patients with known seizure disorders

Adverse Reactions Many adverse effects of aldesleukin are dosage and schedule dependent; greater toxicity occurs with high dose, bolus administration and the least toxicity with low dose, subcutaneous administration

Cardiovascular: Hypotension (dose-limiting, possibly fatal), sinus tachycardia, arrhythmias, edema, angina, MI, CHF, capillary leak syndrome

Central nervous system: Confusion, drowsiness, transient memory loss, dizziness, cognitive changes, fatigue, chills, malaise, somnolence, disorientation, headaches, insomnia, paranoid delusion, seizures, coma, fever, pain

Dermatologic: Macular erythematous rash, pruritus, erythema, exfoliative dermatitis, dry skin, alopecia, petechiae, purpura, vitiligo

Endocrine & metabolic: Hypomagnesemia, hypocalcemia, hypokalemia, hypophosphatemia, hyponatremia, hypoglycemia, hyperglycemia, hypermagnesemia, hypercalcemia, hyperkalemia, hyperphosphatemia, hypernatremia, thyroid dysfunction, weight gain

Gastrointestinal: Nausea, vomiting, diarrhea, stomatitis, GI bleeding, anorexia, pancreatitis

Hematologic: Anemia, thrombocytopenia, leukopenia, eosinophilia

Hepatic: Transient elevations of bilirubin and liver enzymes, jaundice, ascites, decreased clotting factors

Neuromuscular & skeletal: Weakness, rigors, arthralgia, myalgia

Renal: Oliguria, proteinuria, transient elevation in BUN, hematuria

Respiratory: Congestion, dyspnea, pleural effusion, pulmonary edema

Miscellaneous: Allergic reactions

Drug Interactions Corticosteroids may decrease efficacy; increased CNS depression when administered concomitantly with other sedating agents; increased toxicity when administered concomitantly with other potentially nephrotoxic, myelotoxic, cardiotoxic, or hepatotoxic agents; increased hypotensive effects with antihypertensives or beta-blocking agents; acute reactions including fever, chills, nausea, vomiting, pruritus, rash, diarrhea, hypotension, edema, and oliguria with iodinated contrast media (may occur within 4 weeks to several months after aldesleukin administration); hypersensitivity reactions have been reported when combined with dacarbazine, cis-platinum, tamoxifen, and interferon-alfa; exacerbation of autoimmune and inflammatory disorders and myocardial injury when used in combination with interferon-alfa

Stability Store in refrigerator; do not freeze; reconstituted solution is stable 48 hours in refrigerator or at room temperature; since aldesleukin contains no preservatives, refrigerated storage of the reconstituted solution is preferred; reconstituted solution packaged in tuberculin syringes for SubQ administration are stable 14 days refrigerated and 6 hours at room temperature; compatible **only** with D_5W; incompatible with sodium chloride solutions; do not mix with other medications

(Continued)

Aldesleukin *(Continued)*

Stability of Aldesleukin Related to Final Concentration

Infusion Duration	Final Concentration of Aldesleukin (mcg/mL)				Stability at Room Temperature (h)
	1-30	31-69	70-100	>100	
Short I.V. infusion (15 minutes)	Add albumin[1]	Not necessary to add albumin	Due to poor stability; **AVOID** use at this concentration	Not necessary to add albumin	48 h
Continuous I.V. infusion (24 h) at room temperature	Add albumin[1]	Not necessary to add albumin	Due to poor stability; **AVOID** use at this concentration	Not necessary to add albumin	48 h
Continuous I.V. infusion via CADD pump[2]	Add albumin[1]	Add albumin[1]	Due to poor stability; **AVOID** use at this concentration	Not necessary to add albumin	6 d[2]

[1]To improve stability, albumin must be added to a final concentration of 0.1% (1 mg/mL); albumin must be added first to D_5W followed by the reconstituted aldesleukin solution

[2]Continuous infusion via CADD pump or similar infusion device raises aldesleukin temperature to ≥32°C (89°F)

Mechanism of Action Aldesleukin, a human recombinant interleukin-2 product, promotes proliferation, differentiation, and recruitment of T and B cells, natural killer cells, and thymocytes; also causes cytolytic activity in some lymphocytes and subsequent interactions between lymphokine-activated killer cells and tumor-infiltrating lymphocytes; causes multiple immunological effects including activation of cellular immunity with lymphocytosis, eosinophilia, and thrombocytopenia; production of cytokines (including tumor necrosis factor, interleukin-1), and inhibition of tumor growth

Pharmacokinetics

Absorption: Oral: Not absorbed

Distribution: Primarily into plasma, lymphocytes, lungs, liver, kidney, and spleen

V_d: Adults: 4-7 L

Metabolism: Metabolized to amino acids in the cells lining the proximal convoluted tubules of the kidney

Bioavailability: I.M.: 30% to 37%

Half-life:

Children:

Distribution: 14 ± 6 minutes

Elimination: 51 ± 11 minutes

Adults:

Distribution: 6-27 minutes

Elimination: 85 minutes

Time to peak serum concentration: SubQ: 2-3 hours

Clearance: Adults: 7.2-16.1 L/hour

Usual Dosage A wide variety of dosages have been or are currently under investigation (refer to individual protocols):

AML: Children: (Investigational use only, Sievers, 1998): Continuous I.V. infusion: 9 million international units (9×10^6 international units) daily for 4 days; repeat 4 days later with 1.6 million international units (1.6×10^6 international units) daily for 10 days

Metastatic renal cell carcinoma and metastatic melanoma: Adults:

I.V.:

Initial: Treatment consists of two 5-day treatment cycles separated by a rest period: 600,000 international units/kg (0.037 mg/kg) every 8 hours for a total of 14 doses; followed by a rest period of 9 days, then repeat the 14-dose regimen; these two cycles constitute one course of therapy

Retreatment: Each treatment course should be separated by a rest period of at least 7 weeks from the date of completion; patients should be evaluated for response approximately 4 weeks after completion of a course of therapy and again immediately prior to the scheduled start of the next treatment course

SubQ: (Investigational): 11 million international units (11×10^6 international units) daily for 4 days per week for 4 consecutive weeks; repeat every 6 weeks, or alternatively, 18 million international units (18×10^6 international units) daily for 5 days followed by a 2-day rest period, then 9 million international units (9×10^6 international units) for 2 days, followed by 18 million international units (18×10^6 international units) daily for 3 days

Dosage modification for toxicity: In high-dose therapy, see manufacturer's guidelines (or refer to specific protocol for recommendations) for holding and restarting therapy; hold or interrupt a dose, **do not dose reduce**

Administration Parenteral:

I.V.: Reconstitute with 1.2 mL SWI (swirl, do not shake); resulting concentration is 1.1 mg/mL [18 million (18 x 10^6) international units/mL]; further dilute dosage in D_5W to a final concentration between 30-70 mcg/mL (0.49-1.1 million international units/mL) and infuse over 15 minutes; for continuous infusions, dilute in D_5W maintaining the same final concentration; final dilutions <30 mcg/mL or >70 mcg/mL have shown increased variability in drug stability and bioactivity; addition of albumin has been used to improve stability if final dilution concentrations <30 mcg/mL are necessary; when continuous infusion is via devices which expose aldesleukin to temperatures higher than room temperature (≥32°C/89.6°F) (eg, CADD pump or similar infusion device), drug stability is also altered; see Stability for more detailed information; do not use in-line filter when administering

SubQ: Reconstituted solution may be administered subcutaneously without further dilution (**Note**: Subcutaneous administration is a non-FDA approved route)

Monitoring Parameters Baseline chest x-ray, pulmonary function tests and thallium stress study; CBC with differential, platelet counts, electrolytes, BUN, serum creatinine, hepatic enzymes, vital signs, weight, pulse oximetry, arterial blood gases (if pulmonary symptoms), fluid intake and output

Nursing Implications See Warnings and Precautions

Additional Information

1 Cetus Unit = 6 international units

1 Roche Unit (Teceleukin) = 3 international units

1.1 mg = 18 x 10^6 international units or 3 x 10^6 Cetus units

Dosage Forms Excipient information presented when available (limited, particularly for generics); consult specific product labeling.

Injection, powder for reconstitution: 22 x 10^6 int. units [18 million int. units/mL = 1.1 mg/mL when reconstituted]

References

Sievers EL, Lange BJ, Sondel PM, et al, "Feasibility, Toxicity, and Biologic Response of Interleukin-2 After Consolidation Chemotherapy for Acute Myelogenous Leukemia: A Report From the Children's Cancer Group," *J Clin Oncol*, 1998, 16(3):914-9.

Whittington R and Faulds D, "Interleukin-2: A Review of Its Pharmacological Properties and Therapeutic Use in Patients With Cancer," *Drugs*, 1993, 46(3):446-514.

♦ **Aldomet** *see* Methyldopa *on page 1031*

♦ **Aldroxicon I [OTC]** *see* Antacid Preparations *on page 132*

♦ **Aldroxicon II [OTC]** *see* Antacid Preparations *on page 132*

♦ **Aldurazyme®** *see* Laronidase *on page 914*

♦ **Alenic Alka Tablet [OTC]** *see* Antacid Preparations *on page 132*

♦ **Aler-Cap [OTC]** *see* DiphenhydrAMINE *on page 509*

♦ **Aler-Dryl [OTC]** *see* DiphenhydrAMINE *on page 509*

♦ **Aler-Tab [OTC]** *see* DiphenhydrAMINE *on page 509*

♦ **Aleve® [OTC]** *see* Naproxen *on page 1108*

♦ **Alfenta®** *see* Alfentanil *on page 73*

Alfentanil (al FEN ta nil)

Medication Safety Issues

Sound-alike/look-alike issues:

Alfentanil may be confused with Anafranil®, fentanyl, remifentanil, sufentanil

Alfenta® may be confused with Sufenta®

Related Information

Narcotic Analgesics Comparison *on page 1705*

Overdose and Toxicology *on page 1916*

U.S. Brand Names Alfenta®

Canadian Brand Names Alfenta®; Alfentanil Injection, USP

Index Terms Alfentanil Hydrochloride

Therapeutic Category Analgesic, Narcotic; General Anesthetic

Generic Available Yes

Use Analgesia; analgesia adjunct; anesthetic agent

Restrictions C-II

Pregnancy Risk Factor C (D if used for prolonged periods or high doses at term)

Contraindications Hypersensitivity to alfentanil hydrochloride or any component; increased intracranial pressure; severe respiratory depression

Warnings Rapid I.V. infusion may result in skeletal muscle and chest wall rigidity → impaired ventilation → respiratory distress/arrest; inject slowly over 3-5 minutes; nondepolarizing skeletal muscle relaxant may be required

Precautions Use with caution in patients with bradycardia

Adverse Reactions

Cardiovascular: Bradycardia, peripheral vasodilation, hypotension

(Continued)

Alfentanil *(Continued)*

Central nervous system: Drowsiness, dizziness, sedation, CNS depression, elevated intracranial pressure
Dermatologic: Pruritus
Endocrine & metabolic: Antidiuretic hormone release
Gastrointestinal: Nausea, vomiting, constipation, biliary tract spasm
Genitourinary: Urinary tract spasm
Neuromuscular & skeletal: Skeletal muscle and chest wall rigidity especially following rapid I.V. administration
Ocular: Miosis
Respiratory: Respiratory depression, apnea, respiratory arrest
Miscellaneous: Histamine release, physical and psychological dependence with prolonged use

Drug Interactions Cytochrome P450 isoenzyme CYP3A3/4 substrate

CNS depressants, phenothiazines, tricyclic antidepressants may potentiate the adverse effects of opiate agonists; use with benzodiazepines may cause vasodilation, hypotension, and delay recovery; cimetidine may decrease and erythromycin may significantly decrease alfentanil clearance; chronic beta-blocker therapy may potentiate alfentanil-induced bradycardia; propofol may increase serum concentrations of alfentanil

Mechanism of Action Binds with stereospecific receptors at many sites within the CNS, increases pain threshold, alters pain reception, inhibits ascending pain pathways

Pharmacodynamics

Onset of action: Within 5 minutes
Duration: <15-20 minutes

Pharmacokinetics

Distribution: V_d beta:
- Newborns, premature: 1 L/kg
- Children: 0.163-0.48 L/kg
- Adults: 0.46 L/kg

Protein binding:
- Neonates: 67%
- Adults: 88% to 92%
- Bound to $alpha_1$-acid glycoprotein

Metabolism: Hepatic

Half-life, elimination:
- Newborns, premature: 320-525 minutes
- Children: 40-60 minutes
- Adults: 83-97 minutes

Usual Dosage Doses should be titrated to appropriate effects; wide range of doses is dependent upon desired degree of analgesia/anesthesia

Alfentanil: Adult Dosing

Indication	Approximate Duration of Anesthesia (min)	Induction Period (Initial Dose) (mcg/kg)	Maintenance Period (Increments/ Infusion)	Total Dose (mcg/kg)	Effects
Incremental injection	≤30	8-20	3-5 mcg/kg or 0.5-1 mcg/kg/min	8-40	Spontaneously breathing or assisted ventilation when required.
	30-60	20-50	5-15 mcg/kg	Up to 75	Assisted or controlled ventilation required. Attenuation of response to laryngoscopy and intubation.
Continuous infusion	>45	50-75	0.5-3 mcg/kg/min; average infusion rate: 1-1.5 mcg/kg/min	Dependent on duration of procedure	Assisted or controlled ventilation required. Some attenuation of response to intubation and incision, with intraoperative stability.
Anesthetic induction	>45	130-245	0.5-1.5 mcg/kg/min or general anesthetic	Dependent on duration of procedure	Assisted or controlled ventilation required. Administer slowly (over 3 minutes). Concentration of inhalation agents reduced by 30% to 50% for initial hour.

Neonates, Infants, and Children <12 years: Dose not established; A high percent of newborn infants receiving alfentanil (prior to procedures) at doses of 9-15 mcg/kg (mean dose: 11.7 mcg/kg) developed chest wall rigidity; 9 out of 20 newborns (45%) developed mild or moderate rigidity that did not affect ventilation, while 4 out of 20 (20%) had severe rigidity interfering with respiration for ~5-10 minutes; use of a skeletal muscle relaxant to prevent chest wall rigidity is recommended; however, smaller alfentanil doses may be required in newborns. Further studies are needed to determine appropriate doses of alfentanil in pediatric patients.

Adults: Use lean body weight for patients who weigh >20% over ideal body weight; see table on previous page.

Administration Parenteral: I.V.: Inject slowly over 3-5 minutes or by I.V. continuous infusion; maximum concentration: 80 mcg/mL

Monitoring Parameters Respiratory rate, blood pressure, heart rate, neurological status (for degree of analgesia/anesthesia)

Nursing Implications Alfentanil may produce more hypotension compared to fentanyl, therefore, be sure to administer slowly and ensure patient has adequate hydration; may be habit-forming; avoid abrupt discontinuation after prolonged use

Dosage Forms Excipient information presented when available (limited, particularly for generics); consult specific product labeling. Available as alfentanil hydrochloride; mg strength refers to alfentanil.

Injection, solution [preservative free]: 500 mcg/mL (2 mL, 5 mL, 10 mL)

Alfenta®: 500 mcg/mL (2 mL, 5 mL, 10 mL, 20 mL)

References

Davis PJ, Killian A, Stiller RL, et al, "Pharmacokinetics of Alfentanil in Newborn Premature Infants and Older Children," *Dev Pharmacol Ther*, 1989, 13(1):21-7.

Marlow N, Weindling AM, Van Peer A, et al, "Alfentanil Pharmacokinetics in Preterm Infants," *Arch Dis Child*, 1990, 65(4 Spec No):349-51.

Meistelman C, Saint-Maurice C, Lepaul M, et al, "A Comparison of Alfentanil Pharmacokinetics in Children and Adults," *Anesthesiology*, 1987, 66(1):13-6.

Pokela ML, Ryhanen PT, Koivisto ME, et al, "Alfentanil-Induced Rigidity in Newborn Infants," *Anesth Analg*, 1992, 75(2):252-7.

♦ **Alfentanil Hydrochloride** *see* Alfentanil *on page 73*

♦ **Alfentanil Injection, USP (Can)** *see* Alfentanil *on page 73*

Alglucerase (al GLOO ser ase)

Medication Safety Issues

Sound-alike/look-alike issues:

Alglucerase may be confused with agalsidase alfa, agalsidase beta, alglucosidase alfa

Ceredase® may be confused with Cerezyme®

U.S. Brand Names Ceredase®

Index Terms Glucocerebrosidase

Therapeutic Category Enzyme, Glucocerebrosidase; Gaucher's Disease, Treatment Agent

Generic Available No

Use Long-term enzyme replacement in patients with confirmed Type I Gaucher disease who exhibit one or more of the following conditions: Moderate to severe anemia; thrombocytopenia and bleeding tendencies; bone disease; hepatomegaly or splenomegaly; growth retardation related to Gaucher disease

Pregnancy Risk Factor C

Lactation Excretion in breast milk unknown/use caution

Contraindications Hypersensitivity to alglucerase or any component

Precautions Alglucerase is prepared from pooled human placental tissue that may contain the causative agents of some viral diseases; the risk of contamination from slowly active or latent viruses is believed to be remote due to steps taken in the manufacturing process; observe for signs of early virilization in males <10 years of age

Adverse Reactions

Central nervous system: Fever, chills, fatigue

Endocrine & metabolic: Early virilization (males <10 years)

Gastrointestinal: Abdominal discomfort, nausea, vomiting, diarrhea, oral ulcerations

Local: Discomfort, burning, and edema at the site of injection

Neuromuscular: Weakness, backache

Miscellaneous: Hypersensitivity reactions

Drug Interactions No information available at this time

Stability When diluted to 100-200 mL with NS, resultant solution is stable up to 18 hours when stored at 2°C to 8°C

Mechanism of Action Glucocerebrosidase is an enzyme prepared from human placental tissue. Gaucher's disease is an inherited metabolic disorder caused by the

(Continued)

Alglucerase *(Continued)*

defective activity of beta-glucosidase and the resultant accumulation of glucosyl ceramide laden macrophages in the liver, bone, and spleen. Alglucerase acts by replacing the missing enzyme associated with Gaucher's disease.

Pharmacodynamics

Onset of significant improvement in symptoms:

Hepatosplenomegaly and hematologic abnormalities: Occurs within 6 months

Improvement in bone mineralization: Noted at 80-104 weeks of therapy

Pharmacokinetics

Distribution: V_d: 0.05-0.28 L/kg

Half-life, elimination: ~4-10 minutes

Usual Dosage I.V. Infusion: Children, Adolescents, and Adults: 30-60 units/kg every 2 weeks; range in dosage: 2.5 units/kg 3 times/week to 60 units/kg once weekly to every 4 weeks. Initial dose should be based on disease severity and rate of progression. Children at high risk for complications from Gaucher's disease (one or more of the following: symptomatic disease including manifestations of abdominal or bone pain, fatigue, exertional limitations, weakness, and cachexia; growth failure; evidence of skeletal involvement; platelet count ≤60,000 mm^3 and/or documented abnormal bleeding episode(s); Hgb ≥2.0 g/dL below lower limit for age and sex; impaired quality of life) should receive an initial dose of 60 units/kg; failure to respond to treatment within 6 months indicates the need for a higher dosage.

Maintenance: After patient response is well established a reduction in dosage may be attempted; progressive reductions may be made at intervals of 3-6 months; assess dosage frequently to maintain consistent dosage per kg body weight

Administration Parenteral: Dilute to a final volume of 100-200 mL NS and infuse I.V. over 1-2 hours; an in-line filter should be used; do not shake solution as it denatures the enzyme

Monitoring Parameters CBC, platelets, liver function tests, MRI or CT scan (spleen and liver volume), skeletal x-rays

Dosage Forms Excipient information presented when available (limited, particularly for generics); consult specific product labeling.

Injection, solution [preservative free]:

Ceredase®: 80 units/mL (5 mL) [contains human albumin 1%]

References

Barton NW, Brady RO, Dambrosia JM, et al, "Replacement Therapy for Inherited Enzyme Deficiency - Macrophage-Targeted Glucocerebrosidase for Gaucher's Disease," *N Engl J Med*, 1991, 324(21):1464-70.

Charrow J, Andersson HC, Kaplan P, et al, "Enzyme Replacement Therapy and Monitoring for Children With Type 1 Gaucher Disease: Consensus Recommendations," *J Pediatr*, 2004, 144(1):112-20.

- **Alinia®** *see* Nitazoxanide *on page 1137*
- **Alka-Mints® [OTC]** *see* Calcium Carbonate *on page 264*
- **Alka-Mints® [OTC]** *see* Calcium Supplements *on page 272*
- **Alkeran®** *see* Melphalan *on page 997*
- **Allegra®** *see* Fexofenadine *on page 653*
- **Aller-Chlor® [OTC]** *see* Chlorpheniramine *on page 344*
- **Allerdryl® (Can)** *see* DiphenhydrAMINE *on page 509*
- **Allerfrim® [OTC]** *see* Triprolidine and Pseudoephedrine *on page 1580*
- **Allergen®** *see* Antipyrine and Benzocaine *on page 145*
- **AllerMax® [OTC]** *see* DiphenhydrAMINE *on page 509*
- **Allernix (Can)** *see* DiphenhydrAMINE *on page 509*
- **Allfen-DM** *see* Guaifenesin and Dextromethorphan *on page 748*
- **Allfen Jr** *see* Guaifenesin *on page 745*
- **Alloprin® (Can)** *see* Allopurinol *on page 76*

Allopurinol (al oh PURE i nole)

Medication Safety Issues

Sound-alike/look-alike issues:

Allopurinol may be confused with Apresoline

Zyloprim® may be confused with Xylo-Pfan®, ZORprin®

Related Information

Tumor Lysis Syndrome, Management *on page 1803*

U.S. Brand Names Aloprim™; Zyloprim®

Canadian Brand Names Alloprin®; Apo-Allopurinol®; Novo-Purol; Zyloprim®

Index Terms Allopurinol Sodium

Therapeutic Category Antigout Agent; Uric Acid Lowering Agent

Generic Available Yes

Use Prevention of attacks of gouty arthritis and nephropathy; also used in treatment of secondary hyperuricemia which may occur during treatment of tumors or leukemia; prevention of recurrent calcium oxalate calculi

Pregnancy Risk Factor C

Lactation Enters breast milk/use caution (AAP rates "compatible")

Contraindications Hypersensitivity to allopurinol or any component

Warnings Do not use to treat asymptomatic hyperuricemia; monitor liver function and complete blood counts before initiating therapy and periodically

Precautions Reduce dosage in renal impairment; discontinue drug at the first sign of rash; risk of skin rash may be increased in patients receiving amoxicillin or ampicillin; risk of hypersensitivity may be increased in patients receiving thiazides and possibly ACE inhibitors

Adverse Reactions

Cardiovascular: (reported with I.V. administration) Hypotension, flushing, hypertension, bradycardia, heart failure

Central nervous system: Drowsiness, fever, headache, chills, somnolence, agitation

Dermatologic: Pruritic maculopapular rash, exfoliative dermatitis, erythema multiforme, alopecia

Gastrointestinal: GI irritation, dyspepsia, nausea, vomiting, diarrhea, abdominal pain, gastritis

Genitourinary: Hematuria

Hematologic: Leukocytosis, leukopenia, thrombocytopenia, eosinophilia, bone marrow suppression

Hepatic: Hepatitis, elevated liver enzymes, hepatomegaly, hyperbilirubinemia, jaundice

Local: Local injection site reaction

Neuromuscular & skeletal: Peripheral neuropathy, paresthesia, neuritis, arthralgia, myoclonus

Ocular: Cataracts, optic neuritis

Renal: Renal impairment

Respiratory: Epistaxis; (reported with I.V. administration) apnea, hyperpnea, ARDS

Vascular: Necrotizing angiitis, vasculitis

Drug Interactions Inhibits metabolism of azathioprine and mercaptopurine; use with ampicillin or amoxicillin may increase the incidence of skin rash; may increase myelosuppressive effects of cyclophosphamide; large doses may decrease theophylline clearance; increased risk of hypersensitivity reactions when coadministered with ACE inhibitors and thiazide diuretics; decreased allopurinol effectiveness when coadministered with uricosuric agents; increases kidney stone formation when taken with large doses of vitamin C; aluminum hydroxide antacids decrease allopurinol's absorption; increases chlorpropamide effects; may increase risk of osteomalacia in patients receiving phenytoin or phenobarbital; prolongs the half-life of oral anticoagulants; may increase cyclosporine serum levels

Stability Reconstituted parenteral solution should be stored at room temperature; do not refrigerate; use within 10 hours of preparation; physically **incompatible** when mixed with or infused through the same line with the following: Amikacin, amphotericin B, carmustine, cefotaxime, chlorpromazine, cimetidine, clindamycin, cytarabine, dacarbazine, daunorubicin, diphenhydramine, doxorubicin, doxycycline, droperidol, floxuridine, gentamicin, haloperidol, hydroxyzine, idarubicin, imipenem-cilastatin, mechlorethamine, meperidine, metoclopramide, methylprednisolone sodium succinate, minocycline, nalbuphine, netilmicin, ondansetron, prochlorperazine, promethazine, sodium bicarbonate, streptozocin, tobramycin, vinorelbine

Mechanism of Action Decreases the production of uric acid by inhibiting the action of xanthine oxidase, an enzyme that converts hypoxanthine to xanthine and xanthine to uric acid

Pharmacodynamics Decrease in serum uric acid occurs in 1-2 days with a nadir achieved in 1-3 weeks

Pharmacokinetics

Absorption: Oral: ~80% from the GI tract

Distribution: Into breast milk; breast milk to plasma ratio: 0.9-1.4

Protein binding: <1%

Metabolism: ~75% of drug metabolized to active metabolites, chiefly oxypurinol

Half-life:

- Parent: 1-3 hours
- Oxypurinol metabolite: 18-30 hours in patients with normal renal function

Time to peak serum concentration: Within 2-6 hours

Dialysis: Allopurinol and oxypurinol are dialyzable

(Continued)

Allopurinol *(Continued)*

Usual Dosage

Prevention of acute uric acid nephropathy in myeloproliferative neoplastic disorders (beginning 1-2 days before chemotherapy): Daily doses >300 mg should be administered in divided doses:

Children ≤10 years:

I.V.: 200 mg/m²/day in 1-3 divided doses; maximum dose: 600 mg/day

Oral: 10 mg/kg/day in 2-3 divided doses or 200-300 mg/m²/day in 2-4 divided doses; maximum dose: 800 mg/day

Alternative:

<6 years: 150 mg/day in 3 divided doses

6-10 years: 300 mg/day in 2-3 divided doses

Children >10 years and Adults:

I.V.: 200-400 mg/m²/day in 1-3 divided doses; maximum: 600 mg/day

Oral: 600-800 mg/day in 2-3 divided doses

Gout: Children >10 years and Adults: Oral:

Mild: 200-300 mg/day

Severe: 400-600 mg/day

Recurrent calcium oxalate stones: Children >10 years and Adults: Oral: 200-300 mg daily in divided or single daily dosage

Dosing adjustment in renal impairment:

Cl_{cr} >50 mL/minute: No dosage change

Cl_{cr} 10-50 mL/minute: Reduce dosage to 50% of recommended

Cl_{cr} <10 mL/minute: Reduce dosage to 30% of recommended

Administration

Oral: Administer after meals with plenty of fluid

Parenteral: Reconstitute 500 mg vial with 25 mL SWI; prior to administration, further dilute with D_5W or NS to a maximum concentration of 6 mg/mL; rate of infusion is dependent upon the volume of infusate (in research studies, 100-300 mg doses were infused over 30 minutes)

Monitoring Parameters CBC, liver function tests, renal function, serum uric acid; 24-hour urinary urate (when treating calcium oxalate stones)

Reference Range

Uric acid: Male: 3.0-7.0 mg/dL; Female: 2.0-6.0 mg/dL

Urinary urate excretion: Male: <800 mg/day; Female: <750 mg/day

Patient Information Report any skin rash, painful urination, blood in urine, irritation of the eyes, or swelling of lips or mouth; avoid alcohol; drink plenty of fluids; may cause drowsiness and impair ability to perform activities requiring mental alertness or physical coordination

Dosage Forms Excipient information presented when available (limited, particularly for generics); consult specific product labeling.

Injection, powder for reconstitution, as sodium (Aloprim™): 500 mg

Tablet (Zyloprim®): 100 mg, 300 mg

Extemporaneous Preparations

A 20 mg/mL suspension may be made by crushing eight 300 mg tablets and mixing with 120 mL of either a 1:1 mixture of Ora-Sweet® and Ora-Plus® or a 1:1 mixture of Ora-Sweet® SF and Ora-Plus® or a 1:4 mixture of cherry syrup concentrate and simple syrup, NF. The resulting suspension is stable for 60 days refrigerated or at room temperature (Allen, 1996; Nahata, 2004).

A 20 mg/mL suspension may be made by crushing one 100 mg tablet; wet crushed tablet with small amount of 1% methylcellulose then add syrup NF to a final volume of 5 mL; stable 56 days refrigerated or at room temperature (Dressman, 1983; Nahata, 2004).

Allen LV and Erickson MA, "Stability of Acetazolamide, Allopurinol, Azathioprine, Clonazepam, and Flucytosine in Extemporaneously Compounded Oral Liquids," *Am J Health Sys Pharm*, 1996, 53:1944-9.

Dressman JB and Poust RI, "Stability of Allopurinol and of Five Antineoplastics in Suspension," *Am J Hosp Pharm*, 1983, 40(4):616-8.

Nahata, MC, Pai VB, and Hipple TF, *Pediatric Drug Formulations*, 5th ed, Cincinnati, OH: Harvey Whitney Books Co, 2004.

References

Bennett WM, Aronoff GR, Golper TA, et al, *Drug Prescribing in Renal Failure*, Philadelphia, PA: American College of Physicians, 1987.

Krakoff IH and Murphy ML, "Hyperuricemia in Neoplastic Disease in Children: Prevention With Allopurinol, A Xanthine Oxidase Inhibitor" *Pediatrics*, 1968, 41(1):52-6.

♦ **Allopurinol Sodium** *see* Allopurinol *on page 76*
♦ **Almacone® [OTC]** *see* Antacid Preparations *on page 132*
♦ **Almacone Double Strength® [OTC]** *see* Antacid Preparations *on page 132*
♦ **Almora® [OTC]** *see* Magnesium Gluconate *on page 971*
♦ **Almora® [OTC]** *see* Magnesium Supplements *on page 976*

- **Alocril®** *see* Nedocromil *on page 1112*
- **Aloe Vesta® 2-n-1 Antifungal [OTC]** *see* Miconazole *on page 1056*
- **Alophen® [OTC]** *see* Bisacodyl *on page 217*
- **Aloprim™** *see* Allopurinol *on page 76*
- **Alora®** *see* Estradiol *on page 605*
- **Aloxi®** *see* Palonosetron *on page 1199*
- **Alpha-Galactosidase-A (Recombinant)** *see* Agalsidase Beta *on page 61*
- **Alphagan® (Can)** *see* Brimonidine *on page 231*
- **Alphagan® P** *see* Brimonidine *on page 231*
- **Alphanate®** *see* Antihemophilic Factor (Human) *on page 134*
- **AlphaNine® SD** *see* Factor IX *on page 633*
- **Alph-E [OTC]** *see* Vitamin E *on page 1620*
- **Alph-E-Mixed [OTC]** *see* Vitamin E *on page 1620*

Alprazolam (al PRAY zoe lam)

Medication Safety Issues

Sound-alike/look-alike issues:

Alprazolam may be confused with alprostadil, lorazepam, triazolam

Xanax® may be confused with Lanoxin®, Tenex®, Tylox®, Xopenex®, Zantac®, Zyrtec®

Related Information

Overdose and Toxicology *on page 1916*

Serotonin Syndrome *on page 1955*

U.S. Brand Names Alprazolam Intensol®; Niravam™; Xanax®; Xanax XR®

Canadian Brand Names Alti-Alprazolam; Apo-Alpraz®; Apo-Alpraz® TS; Gen-Alprazolam; Novo-Alprazol; Nu-Alprax; Xanax®; Xanax TS™

Therapeutic Category Antianxiety Agent; Benzodiazepine

Generic Available Yes: Extended release tablet, immediate release tablet

Use Treatment of generalized anxiety disorder (GAD); symptoms of anxiety (short-term treatment); anxiety associated with depression; management of panic disorder, with or without agoraphobia

Restrictions C-IV

Pregnancy Risk Factor D

Lactation Enters breast milk/not recommended (AAP rates "of concern")

Contraindications Hypersensitivity to alprazolam, any component, or other benzodiazepines; severe uncontrolled pain, narrow-angle glaucoma, severe respiratory depression, pre-existing CNS depression; not to be used in pregnancy or lactation or in patients taking certain medications (see Drug Interactions)

Warnings Withdrawal symptoms including seizures have occurred 18 hours to 3 days after abrupt discontinuation; when discontinuing therapy, decrease daily dose by no more than 0.5 mg every 3 days; reduce dose in patients with significant hepatic disease

Precautions Safety and effectiveness have not been established in children <18 years of age

Adverse Reactions

Central nervous system: Drowsiness, dizziness, confusion, sedation, fatigue, headache, ataxia, abnormal coordination, somnolence, dysarthria, memory impairment, depression

Endocrine & metabolic: Weight gain or weight loss

Gastrointestinal: Xerostomia, constipation, diarrhea, nausea, vomiting, appetite increased or decreased

Ocular: Blurred vision

Miscellaneous: Physical and psychological dependence with prolonged use

Drug Interactions Cytochrome P450 isoenzyme CYP3A3/4 substrate

Enzyme inducers may increase metabolism of alprazolam; CNS depressants including alcohol may enhance CNS effects; cimetidine, clarithromycin, diltiazem, erythromycin, fluvoxamine, fluoxetine, isoniazid, nefazodone, propoxyphene, and oral contraceptives may decrease the metabolism of alprazolam (use with caution; monitor for increased adverse effects). Delavirdine, ritonavir, ketoconazole, or itraconazole may decrease the metabolism of alprazolam and significantly increase alprazolam levels; concurrent use of delavirdine or ritonavir with alprazolam is not recommended; concurrent use of ketoconazole or itraconazole is contraindicated. Alprazolam may increase plasma concentrations of imipramine (by 31%) and desipramine (by 20%); clinical significance not known, monitor patients. *In vitro* studies suggest possible interactions of alprazolam with sertraline, paroxetine, ergotamine, cyclosporine, amiodarone, nicardipine, and nifedipine (use with caution; monitor for adverse effects).

(Continued)

Alprazolam *(Continued)*

Medications that cause dry mouth or increase stomach pH may slow the disintegration or dissolution of orally-disintegrating tablets and result in slowed or decreased absorption.

Food Interactions

Extended release tablet: A high-fat meal eaten ≤2 hours before the dose may increase peak concentrations by ~25%. A high-fat meal eaten immediately before the dose may decrease the time to peak concentrations by about 33%. A high-fat meal eaten ≥1 hour after the dose may increase the time to peak concentrations by about 33%. The extent of absorption (AUC) is not affected by food.

Orally-disintegrating tablet: A high-fat meal may decrease peak concentrations by 25% and delay the time to peak concentrations by 2 hours. The AUC is not affected by food.

Stability Orally-disintegrating tablet: Store at room temperature of 20°C to 25°C (68°F to 77°F). Protect from moisture. Discard any cotton packaged inside bottle; reseal bottle tightly.

Mechanism of Action Depresses all levels of the CNS, including the limbic and reticular formation, by binding to the benzodiazepine site on the gamma-aminobutyric acid (GABA) receptor complex and modulating GABA, which is a major inhibitory neurotransmitter in the brain

Pharmacokinetics

Absorption: Oral:

Immediate release tablet: Rapidly and well absorbed

Extended release tablet: Rate of absorption is increased following night time dosing (versus morning dosing)

Distribution: 0.9-1.2 L/kg; distributes into breast milk

Protein binding: 80%

Metabolism: Extensive in the liver, primarily via cytochrome P450 isoenzyme CYP3A; major metabolites: alpha-hydroxy-alprazolam (about half as active as alprazolam), 4-hydroxyalprazolam (active), and a benzophenone metabolite (inactive). **Note:** Active metabolites are not likely to contribute to pharmacologic effects due to low levels of activity and low concentrations.

Bioavailability: Similar for extended and immediate release tablets (~90%)

Half-life: Adults: 6.3-26.9 hours; mean: 11.2 hours; **Note:** Half-life may be 25% longer in Asians compared to Caucasians.

Time to peak serum concentration:

Immediate release tablet: Within 1-2 hours

Orally-disintegrating tablet: 1.5-2 hours (if given with or without water); **Note:** Time to peak serum concentration occurs ~15 minutes earlier when taken with water (versus without)

Elimination: Excretion of metabolites and parent compound in urine

Usual Dosage Oral: **Note:** Titrate dose to effect; use lowest effective dose

Children <18 years: Immediate release: Dose not established; investigationally in children 7-16 years of age (n=13), initial doses of 0.005 mg/kg or 0.125 mg/dose were given 3 times/day for situational anxiety and increments of 0.125-0.25 mg/dose were used to increase doses to maximum of 0.02 mg/kg/dose or 0.06 mg/kg/day; a range of 0.375-3 mg/day was needed (see Pfefferbaum, 1987). **Note:** A more recent study in 17 children (8-17 years of age) with overanxious disorder or avoidant disorders used initial daily doses of 0.25 mg for children <40 kg and 0.5 mg for those >40 kg. The dose was titrated at 2-day intervals to a maximum of 0.04 mg/kg/day. Required doses ranged from 0.5-3.5 mg/day with a mean of 1.6 mg/day. Based on clinical global ratings, alprazolam appeared to be better than placebo, however, this difference was **not** statistically significant (see Simeon, 1992); further studies are needed.

Adults:

Anxiety: Immediate release: Initial: 0.25-0.5 mg 3 times/day; titrate dose upward as needed every 3-4 days; maximum dose: 4 mg/day given in divided doses

Panic disorder:

Immediate release: Initial: 0.5 mg 3 times/day; titrate dose upward as needed every 3-4 days in increments ≤1 mg/day; mean dose used in controlled trials: 5-6 mg/day; maximum dose: 10 mg/day (rarely required)

Extended release: Initial: 0.5-1 mg once daily; titrate dose upward as needed every 3-4 days in increments ≤1 mg/day; usual dose: 3-6 mg/day; maximum dose: 10 mg/day (rarely required)

Switching from immediate release to extended release: Administer the same total daily dose, but give once daily; if effect is not adequate, titrate dose as above

Administration Oral:

Immediate release tablet: Administer with food to decrease GI upset

Extended release tablet: Administer once daily, preferably in the morning; do not crush, chew, or break; swallow whole

Orally-disintegrating tablet: Do not remove tablets from bottle until right before dose; using dry hands, place tablet on top of tongue. If using one-half of tablet, immediately discard remaining half (half tablet may not remain stable). Administration with water is not necessary (water is not required to aid dissolution or swallowing)

Monitoring Parameters CNS status, respiratory rate

Patient Information May cause drowsiness and impair ability to perform activities requiring mental alertness or physical coordination; may be habit-forming; avoid abrupt discontinuation after prolonged use; avoid alcohol; limit caffeine; may cause dry mouth

Nursing Implications Assist with ambulation during beginning of therapy; allow patient to rise slowly to avoid fainting

Additional Information If used for an extended period of time, long-term usefulness of alprazolam should be periodically re-evaluated for an individual patient.

Dosage Forms Excipient information presented when available (limited, particularly for generics); consult specific product labeling.

Solution, oral [concentrate]:
Alprazolam Intensol®: 1 mg/mL (30 mL)

Tablet: 0.25 mg, 0.5 mg, 1 mg, 2 mg
Xanax®: 0.25 mg, 0.5 mg, 1 mg, 2 mg

Tablet, extended release: 0.5 mg, 1 mg, 2 mg, 3 mg
Xanax XR®: 0.5 mg, 1 mg, 2 mg, 3 mg

Tablet, orally disintegrating [scored]:
Niravam™: 0.25 mg, 0.5 mg, 1 mg, 2 mg [orange flavor]

References

Bernstein GA, Garfinkel BD, and Borchardt CM, "Comparative Studies of Pharmacotherapy for School Refusal," *J Am Acad Child Adolesc Psychiatry*, 1990, 29(5):773-81.

DeVane CL, Hill M, and Antal EJ, "Therapeutic Drug Monitoring of Alprazolam in Adolescents With Asthma," *Ther Drug Monit*, 1998, 20(3):257-60.

Pfefferbaum B, Overall JE, Boren HA, et al, "Alprazolam in the Treatment of Anticipatory and Acute Situational Anxiety in Children With Cancer," *J Am Acad Child Adolesc Psychiatry*, 1987, 26(4):532-5.

Simeon JG and Ferguson HB, "Alprazolam Effects in Children With Anxiety Disorders," *Can J Psychiatry*, 1987, 32(7):570-4.

Simeon JG, Ferguson HB, Knott V, et al, "Clinical, Cognitive, and Neurophysiological Effects of Alprazolam in Children and Adolescents With Overanxious and Avoidant Disorders," *J Am Acad Child Adolesc Psychiatry*, 1992, 31(1):29-33.

♦ **Alprazolam Intensol®** *see* Alprazolam *on page 79*

Alprostadil (al PROS ta dill)

Medication Safety Issues

Sound-alike/look-alike issues:
Alprostadil may be confused with alprazolam

U.S. Brand Names Caverject®; Caverject Impulse®; Edex®; Muse®; Prostin VR Pediatric®

Canadian Brand Names Caverject®; Muse® Pellet; Prostin® VR

Index Terms PGE_1; Prostaglandin E_1

Therapeutic Category Prostaglandin

Generic Available Yes: Solution for injection

Use Temporary maintenance of patency of ductus arteriosus in neonates with ductal-dependent congenital heart disease until surgery can be performed. These defects include cyanotic (eg, pulmonary atresia, pulmonary stenosis, tricuspid atresia, Fallot's tetralogy, transposition of the great vessels) and acyanotic (eg, interruption of aortic arch, coarctation of aorta, hypoplastic left ventricle) heart disease.

Investigationally used for the treatment of pulmonary hypertension in infants and children with congenital heart defects with left-to-right shunts

Adult males: Diagnosis and treatment of erectile dysfunction (see Additional Information)

Pregnancy Risk Factor X

Lactation Not indicated for use in women

Contraindications Hypersensitivity to alprostadil or any component; respiratory distress syndrome or persistent fetal circulation

Warnings Apnea occurs in 10% to 12% of neonates with congenital heart defects (especially in those weighing <2 kg at birth) and usually appears during the first hour of drug infusion

Precautions Use cautiously in neonates with bleeding tendencies; if hypotension or pyrexia occurs, the infusion rate should be reduced until symptoms subside; severe hypotension, apnea, or bradycardia requires drug discontinuation with cautious reinstitution at a lower dose; tissue necrosis may occur with extravasation of concentrated solutions (due to high osmolality)

(Continued)

Alprostadil *(Continued)*

Adverse Reactions

Cardiovascular: Systemic hypotension, flushing, bradycardia, rhythm disturbances, tachycardia, edema

Central nervous system: Seizure-like activity, fever

Endocrine & metabolic: Hypocalcemia, hypoglycemia, hypokalemia, hyperkalemia

Gastrointestinal: Diarrhea, gastric-outlet obstruction secondary to antral hyperplasia (occurrence related to duration of therapy and cumulative dose)

Hematologic: Inhibition of platelet aggregation

Neuromuscular & skeletal: Cortical proliferation of long bones (cortical hyperostosis) has been seen with long-term infusions (incidence and severity are related to duration of therapy and cumulative dose); **Note:** Cortical hyperostosis may present with clinical symptoms that mimic cellulitis or osteomyelitis (eg, symptomatic bone tenderness, soft tissue swelling)

Respiratory: Respiratory depression, apnea

Miscellaneous: Pretibial and soft tissue swelling, swelling of upper and lower extremities

Stability Compatible in D_5W, $D_{10}W$, and saline solutions; refrigerate ampuls at 2°C to 8°C. Avoid direct contact of undiluted alprostadil with the plastic walls of volumetric infusion chambers because the drug will interact with the plastic and create a hazy solution; discard solution and volumetric chamber if this occurs.

Mechanism of Action Causes vasodilation by means of direct effect on vascular and ductus arteriosus smooth muscle

Pharmacodynamics

Maximum effect:

Acyanotic congenital heart disease: Usual: 1.5-3 hours; range: 15 minutes to 11 hours

Cyanotic congenital heart disease: Usual: ~30 minutes

Duration: Ductus arteriosus will begin to close within 1-2 hours after drug is stopped

Pharmacokinetics

Metabolism: ~70% to 80% metabolized by oxidation during a single pass through the lungs; metabolite (13,14 dihydro-PGE_1) is active and has been identified in neonates

Half-life: 5-10 minutes; since the half-life is so short, the drug must be administered by continuous infusion

Elimination: Metabolites excreted in urine

Usual Dosage Neonates and Infants: 0.05-0.1 mcg/kg/minute; with therapeutic response, rate is reduced to lowest effective dosage; with unsatisfactory response, rate is increased gradually; maintenance: 0.01-0.4 mcg/kg/minute

PGE_1 is usually given at an infusion rate of 0.1 mcg/kg/minute; but it is often possible to reduce the dosage to ½ or even 1/10 without losing the therapeutic effect. The mixing schedule is shown in the table.

Add 1 Ampul (500 mcg) to:	Concentration (mcg/mL)	Infusion Rate to Deliver 0.1 mcg/kg/min		
		mL/kg/min	mL/kg/h	mL/kg/24 h
250 mL	2	0.05	3	72
100 mL	5	0.02	1.2	28.8
50 mL	10	0.01	0.6	14.4
25 mL	20	0.005	0.3	7.2

Administration Parenteral: I.V. continuous infusion into a large vein or alternatively through an umbilical artery catheter placed at the ductal opening; maximum concentration listed (per package insert) for I.V. infusion: 20 mcg/mL; has also been administered via continuous infusion into the right pulmonary artery for investigational treatment of pulmonary hypertension in infants and children with congenital heart defects with left-to-right shunts; rate of infusion (mL/hour) = dose (mcg/kg/minute) x weight (kg) x 60 minutes/hour divided by the concentration (mcg/mL)

Monitoring Parameters Arterial pressure, respiratory rate, heart rate, temperature, pO_2; monitor for gastric obstruction in patients receiving PGE_1 for longer than 120 hours; x-rays may be needed to assess cortical hyperostosis in patients receiving prolonged PGE_1 therapy

Nursing Implications Prepare fresh solution every 24 hours; flushing of arm or face may indicate misplacement of intra-arterial catheter and infusion of drug into subclavian or carotid artery; reposition catheter

Additional Information Therapeutic response is indicated by an increase in systemic blood pressure and pH in those with restricted systemic blood flow and acidosis, or by an increase in oxygenation (pO_2) in those with restricted pulmonary blood flow. Most cases of bone changes occurred 4-6 weeks after starting alprostadil, but it has occurred as early as 9 days; cortical hyperostosis usually resolves over 6-12 months after stopping PGE_1 therapy

Other dosage forms of alprostadil [Caverject® injection, Caverject® Impulse™ injection, Edex® injection, and Muse® Pellet (urethral)] are indicated for the diagnosis and treatment of erectile dysfunction in adult males; see package inserts for further information for this use.

Dosage Forms Excipient information presented when available (limited, particularly for generics); consult specific product labeling.

Injection, powder for reconstitution:

Caverject®: 20 mcg, 40 mcg [contains lactose; diluent contains benzyl alcohol]

Caverject Impulse®: 10 mcg, 20 mcg [prefilled injection system; contains lactose; diluent contains benzyl alcohol]

Edex®: 10 mcg, 20 mcg, 40 mcg [contains lactose; packaged in kits containing diluent, syringe, and alcohol swab]

Injection, solution: 500 mcg/mL (1 mL)

Prostin VR Pediatric®: 500 mcg/mL (1 mL) [contains dehydrated alcohol]

Pellet, urethral (Muse®): 125 mcg (6s), 250 mcg (6s), 500 mcg (6s), 1000 mcg (6s)

References

Kaufman MB and El-Chaar GM, "Bone and Tissue Changes Following Prostaglandin Therapy in Neonates," *Ann Pharmacother*, 1996, 30(3):269-74, 277.

Lewis AB, Freed MD, Heymann MA, et al, "Side Effects of Therapy With Prostaglandin E_1 in Infants With Critical Congenital Heart Disease," *Circulation*, 1981, 64(5):893-8.

Peled N, Dagan O, Babyn P, et al, "Gastric-Outlet Obstruction Induced by Prostaglandin Therapy in Neonates," *N Engl J Med*, 1992, 327(8):505-10.

Weesner KM, "Hemodynamic Effects of Prostaglandin E_1 in Patients With Congenital Heart Disease and Pulmonary Hypertension," *Cathet Cardiovasc Diagn*, 1991, 24(1):10-5.

Woo K, Emery J, and Peabody J, "Cortical Hyperostosis: A Complication of Prolonged Prostaglandin Infusion in Infants Awaiting Cardiac Transplantation," *Pediatrics*, 1994, 93(3):417-20.

- **Altachlore [OTC]** *see* Sodium Chloride *on page 1450*
- **Altafrin** *see* Phenylephrine *on page 1250*
- **Altamist [OTC]** *see* Sodium Chloride *on page 1450*
- **Altarussin DM [OTC]** *see* Guaifenesin and Dextromethorphan *on page 748*
- **Altaryl [OTC]** *see* DiphenhydrAMINE *on page 509*

Alteplase (AL te plase)

Medication Safety Issues

Sound-alike/look-alike issues:

Alteplase may be confused with Altace®

"tPA" abbreviation should not be used when writing orders for this medication; has been misread as TNKase (tenecteplase)

High alert medication: The Institute for Safe Medication Practices (ISMP) includes this medication (I.V.) among its list of drugs which have a heightened risk of causing significant patient harm when used in error.

Related Information

Antithrombotic Therapy in Children *on page 1804*

U.S. Brand Names Activase®; Cathflo® Activase®

Canadian Brand Names Activase® rt-PA; Cathflo® Activase®

Index Terms Alteplase, Recombinant; Alteplase, Tissue Plasminogen Activator, Recombinant; tPA

Therapeutic Category Thrombolytic Agent; Thrombotic Occlusion (Central Venous Catheter), Treatment Agent

Generic Available No

Use

Activase®: Thrombolytic agent used in treatment of acute MI, acute ischemic stroke, and acute massive pulmonary embolism

CathFlo® Activase®: Treatment of occluded central venous catheters

Pregnancy Risk Factor C

Lactation Excretion in breast milk unknown/use caution

Contraindications Hypersensitivity to alteplase or any component (see Additional Information)

Contraindications for use in the treatment of acute MI or pulmonary embolism: Active internal bleeding; known bleeding diathesis; history of CVA; intracranial neoplasm, arteriovenous malformation, or aneurysm; recent intracranial or intraspinal surgery or trauma; severe uncontrolled hypertension

Contraindications for use in the treatment of acute ischemic stroke: Active internal bleeding; known bleeding diathesis (including but not limited to: Current use of oral anticoagulants or an INR >1.7 or PT >15 seconds, use of heparin within 48 hours before the onset of stroke and an elevated aPTT at presentation, platelet count

(Continued)

Alteplase *(Continued)*

<100,000/mm^3); evidence of intracranial hemorrhage on pretreatment evaluation; history of intracranial hemorrhage; suspicion of subarachnoid hemorrhage; recent (within 3 months) intracranial or intraspinal surgery, serious head trauma, or previous stroke; intracranial neoplasm, arteriovenous malformation, or aneurysm; seizure at the onset of stroke; uncontrolled hypertension at time of treatment (eg, adults with blood pressures of >185 mm Hg systolic or >110 mm Hg diastolic)

Warnings Activase®: May cause bleeding (internal, superficial, or surface bleeding); concurrent use of heparin anticoagulation may increase bleeding; monitor all potential bleeding sites. Avoid I.M. injections and nonessential handling of patient; carefully perform venipunctures and only when necessary. If an arterial puncture is required, use vessel in an upper extremity that can be manually compressed. Stop alteplase (and heparin) if serious bleeding occurs (effects of heparin can be reversed by protamine). Do not exceed recommended doses; do not use doses of 150 mg to treat acute MI as this dose has been associated with an increase in intracranial hemorrhage.

Risks from alteplase may be increased in the following conditions (risks versus benefits should be weighed carefully before use): Recent major surgery (eg, organ biopsy, previous puncture of noncompressible vessels, coronary artery bypass graft, obstetrical delivery), recent trauma, recent GI or GU bleeding, current use of oral anticoagulants, cerebrovascular disease, diabetic hemorrhagic retinopathy or other hemorrhagic ophthalmic conditions, hypertension (eg, adults with systolic BP ≥175 mm Hg and/or diastolic BP ≥110 mm Hg), patients with an increased risk of left heart thrombus (eg, mitral stenosis with atrial fibrillation), acute pericarditis, subacute bacterial endocarditis, hemostatic defects including ones caused by severe renal or hepatic dysfunction, significant hepatic dysfunction, pregnancy, septic thrombophlebitis or occluded AV cannula at seriously infected site, advanced age (eg, >75 years old), any other condition in which bleeding would be a significant risk or would be especially difficult to manage due to its location.

Cholesterol embolism may occur (rare). Risk of stroke in acute MI patients who are at low risk for death from cardiac causes and who present with high blood pressure, may be greater than the survival benefit from thrombolytic therapy. Reperfusion arrhythmias may occur following coronary thrombolysis. In patients with pulmonary embolism, alteplase has not been proven to adequately treat underlying DVT; possible re-embolization from DVT may occur.

Acute ischemic stroke: Risks of alteplase therapy may be increased in patients with major early signs of infarct on CT and in those with severe neurological deficit at presentation (risks versus benefits should be weighed carefully); treatment of patients >3 hours after onset of symptoms and those with rapidly improving symptoms or minor neurological deficit is not recommended.

Precautions

Activase®: Use with caution if drug is readministered; discontinue immediately if anaphylactoid reaction occurs. For treatment of acute ischemic stroke, frequent monitoring and control of blood pressure during and after alteplase administration is recommended. For systemic use, pretreatment lab studies should include platelet count, PT/PTT, fibrinogen, fibrin degradation products, plasminogen, antithrombin III, protein S, protein C.

CathFlo® Activase®: Consider other causes of central venous catheter occlusion (eg, mechanical failure, constriction by a suture, catheter malposition, and drug precipitates or lipid deposits within the lumen of the catheter) before use; do not use vigorous suction when determining catheter occlusion (vascular wall damage or collapse of soft-walled catheters may occur); avoid excessive pressure when instilling alteplase into an occluded catheter (catheter may rupture or clot may become dislodged and enter the circulation). The use of CathFlo® Activase® has not been evaluated in patients who are at risk for bleeding; use with caution in patients with active internal bleeding or those who have had any of the following within 48 hours: Surgery, puncture of noncompressible vessels, obstetrical delivery, or percutaneous biopsy of viscera or deep tissues; use with caution in patients with thrombocytopenia, hemostatic defects including ones caused by severe renal or hepatic dysfunction, any condition in which bleeding would be a significant risk or would be especially difficult to manage due to its location, or those who are at a high risk for embolic complications (eg, venous thrombosis in the region of the catheter). Discontinue CathFlo® Activase® and withdraw from catheter if serious bleeding in a critical location occurs. Use with caution in patients with known or suspected catheter infection (use of CathFlo® Activase® in these patients may release a localized infection in the catheter into the systemic circulation). Use of >2 doses of CathFlo® Activase® has not been studied.

Adverse Reactions Note: Adverse reactions listed below have been reported with systemic use. Major adverse events after intracatheter use include: Sepsis, GI bleeding, and venous thrombosis; injection site hemorrhage in a patient with pre-existing thrombocytopenia and rupture of the catheter have also been reported.

Cardiovascular: Hypotension; reperfusion arrhythmias (following coronary thrombolysis)

Central nervous system: Fever, intracranial hemorrhage, cerebral hemorrhage

Dermatologic: Bruising (1%), rash, urticaria (rare)

Gastrointestinal: GI bleeding (5%), nausea, vomiting

Genitourinary: GU bleeding (4%)

Hematologic: Surface bleeding, internal bleeding

Local: Bleeding at catheter puncture site; bruising and inflammation with extravasation

Respiratory: Epistaxis (<1%), laryngeal edema (rare)

Miscellaneous: Anaphylactoid reaction (rare)

Drug Interactions Anticoagulants (warfarin, heparin) and drugs that affect platelet function (aspirin, NSAIDs, dipyridamole, abciximab) may increase the risk of bleeding. Aspirin and heparin have been given concurrently with and after alteplase infusions in patients with acute MI or pulmonary embolism (careful monitoring for bleeding is recommended). However, the concurrent use of aspirin or heparin with alteplase within the first 24 hours after the onset of symptoms of stroke was prohibited in the major stroke trial; therefore, safety of the use of these agents with alteplase in patients with acute ischemic stroke is unknown. Antifibrinolytic agents (aminocaproic acid) may decrease effectiveness.

Stability

Activase®: Store lyophilized product at room temperature [not to exceed 86°F (30°C)] or under refrigeration; protect from excessive light exposure during extended storage. Reconstituted solution (1 mg/mL) must be used within 8 hours (manufacturer's recommendations).

The 1 mg/mL solution may be diluted further (immediately before use) with an equal volume of NS or D_5W to yield a final concentration of 0.5 mg/mL; swirl gently, do not shake to dilute; diluted solutions are stable for 8 hours at room temperature. Dilutions to concentrations <0.5 mg/mL are not recommended for routine clinical use; dilutions <0.5 mg/mL using D_5W or SWI will result in a precipitate; an immediate formation of a precipitate following dilution of alteplase with D_5W to 0.16 mg/mL has been reported (Frazin, 1990); after reconstitution to 1 mg/mL, alteplase may be further diluted with NS to concentrations as low as 0.2 mg/mL without precipitation (Frazin, 1990); do not dilute <0.2 mg/mL; after reconstitution to 1 mg/mL, further dilution with NS to target concentrations of 0.05 mg/mL, 0.025 mg/mL, and 0.01 mg/mL resulted in <90% recovery of active alteplase (data on file at Genetech).

Solutions of 0.5 mg/mL, 1 mg/mL, and 2 mg/mL in SWI retained ≥94% of fibrinolytic activity at 48 hours when stored at 2°C in plastic syringes; these solutions retained ≥90% of fibrinolytic activity when stored in plastic syringes at -25°C or -70°C for 7 or 14 days, thawed at room temperature and then stored at 2°C for 48 hours (see Davis, 2000). Solutions of 1 mg/mL in SWI were stable for 22 weeks in plastic syringes when stored at -30°C and for ~1 month in glass vials when stored at -20°C; bioactivity remained unchanged for 6 months in propylene containers when stored at -20°C and for 2 weeks in glass vials when stored at -70°C (see review by Generali, 2001).

Do not add other medications to alteplase solutions. Alteplase is incompatible with bacteriostatic water, dobutamine, dopamine, heparin, morphine, and nitroglycerin infusions; physically compatible with lidocaine, metoprolol, and propranolol when administered via Y site.

CathFlo® Activase®: Store lyophilized product at refrigerated temperature [2°C to 8°C (36°F to 46°C)]; protect from excessive light exposure during extended storage. Reconstituted solution (1 mg/mL) must be used within 8 hours when stored at 2°C to 30°C (36°F to 81°F); do not add other medications to CathFlo® Activase® solutions

Mechanism of Action A naturally-occurring serine protease (enzyme) that initiates local fibrinolysis by binding to fibrin in a thrombus (clot) and directly activating entrapped plasminogen to plasmin; plasmin degrades fibrin, fibrinogen, and other procoagulant proteins into soluble fragments

Pharmacokinetics

Distribution: Initial: Approximates plasma volume; distribution into breast milk is unknown

Metabolism: In the liver

Half-life: Adults:

- Initial: <5 minutes
- Terminal: 72 minutes

Clearance: Plasma: Adults: 380-570 mL/minute

(Continued)

Alteplase *(Continued)*

Usual Dosage

Neonates, Infants, and Children:

Occluded I.V. catheters: Intracatheter:

Chest, 2001 and *Chest*, 2004 dosing recommendations:

Central venous catheter: **Dose listed is per lumen; for multilumen catheters, treat one lumen at a time:** [**Note:** Some institutions use lower doses (eg, 0.25 mg/0.5 mL) in neonates and infants <3 months]

Patients ≤10 kg: 0.5 mg diluted in NS to a volume equal to the internal volume of the lumen; instill in each lumen over 1-2 minutes; leave in lumen for 1-2 hours, then **aspirate out of catheter, do not infuse into patient**; flush catheter with NS

Patients >10 kg: 1 mg in 1 mL of NS; use a volume equal to the internal volume of the lumen; maximum: 2 mg in 2 mL per lumen; instill in each lumen over 1-2 minutes; leave in lumen for 1-2 hours; then **aspirate out of catheter, do not infuse into patient**; flush catheter with NS

SubQ port:

Patients ≤10 kg: 0.5 mg diluted with NS to 3 mL

Patients >10 kg: 2 mg diluted with NS to 3 mL

Manufacturer's recommendations (CathFlo® Activase®):

Central venous catheter:

Patients <30 kg: Use a 1 mg/mL concentration; instill a volume equal to 110% of the internal lumen volume of the catheter; do not exceed 2 mg in 2 mL; may instill a second dose if catheter remains occluded after 2-hour dwell time (see Administration)

Patients ≥30 kg: 2 mg in 2 mL; may instill second dose if catheter remains occluded ofter 2-hour dwell time (see Administration)

Systemic thromboses: I.V. (**Note:** Dose must be titrated to effect): *Chest*, 2004 recommendations: 0.1-0.6 mg/kg/hour for 6 hours (some patients may require longer or shorter duration of therapy). **Note:** The optimal dose for various thrombotic conditions is not established in pediatric patients; most published papers consist of case reports; few prospective pediatric studies have been conducted; several studies have used the following doses (see Levy, 1991 and Weiner, 1998). **Note:** Bleeding complications were associated with doses in the higher range.

Initial: 0.1 mg/kg/hour for 6 hours; monitor patient closely for bleeding, monitor fibrinogen levels; if no response after 6 hours, increase infusion by 0.1 mg/kg/hour at 6-hour intervals to a maximum of 0.5 mg/kg/hour; maintain fibrinogen >100 mg/dL (**Note:** Some centers maintain fibrinogen >150 mg/dL in newborns); duration of therapy is based on clinical response

Low-dose (local) infusion for occluded catheters: Note: No pediatric studies have compared local to systemic thrombolytic therapy; therefore, there is no evidence to suggest that local infusions are superior. The pediatric patients' small vessel size may increase the chance of local damage to blood vessels and formation of a new thrombus; however, local infusion may be appropriate for catheter related thromboses if the catheter is already in place (See *Chest*, 2004). Various "low-dose" regimens have been used; the following dosing recommendations are based on Doyle, 1992 and Anderson, 1991:

Initial: 0.01 mg/kg/hour for 6 hours; if no response after 6 hours, increase infusion by 0.01 mg/kg/hour at 6-hour intervals to a maximum of 0.05 mg/kg/hour; monitor patient closely; systemic fibrinolysis (decreased plasma fibrinogen levels) or bleeding has been reported in some neonates and infants receiving 0.05 mg/kg/hour; duration of therapy is based on clinical response

Adults:

Acute MI: I.V. (**Note:** Alteplase should be administered as soon as possible after symptom onset):

Accelerated infusion:

Patients >67 kg: Total dose: 100 mg given in 3 divided doses as follows: Infuse 15 mg I.V. bolus over 1-2 minutes, then infuse 50 mg over the next 30 minutes, then 35 mg over the next 60 minutes. Maximum total dose: 100 mg

Patients ≤67 kg: Infuse 15 mg I.V. bolus over 1-2 minutes, then infuse 0.75 mg/kg (maximum: 50 mg) over the next 30 minutes, then 0.5 mg/kg (maximum 35 mg) over the next 60 minutes. Maximum total dose: 100 mg

3-hour infusion:

Patients ≥65 kg: Total dose: 100 mg given as follows: Infuse 60 mg over the first hour with 6-10 mg given as an I.V. bolus, then infuse 20 mg/hour for 2 hours

Patients <65 kg: Total dose: 1.25 mg/kg given over 3 hours as described above

Acute ischemic stroke: I.V. (**Note:** Alteplase therapy should only be started within 3 hours after the onset of symptoms of stroke and after exclusion of intracranial hemorrhage by CT scan or other sensitive diagnostic imaging method): Total dose: 0.9 mg/kg (maximum: 90 mg) given over 1 hour as follows: Infuse 10% of total dose (0.09 mg/kg) I.V. bolus over 1 minute, then infuse the rest of the total dose (0.81 mg/kg) over 60 minutes

Pulmonary embolism: I.V.: 100 mg infused over 2 hours

Occluded central venous catheter: Intracatheter: Manufacturer's recommendations (CathFlo® Activase®): Patients ≥30 kg: 2 mg in 2 mL; may instill second dose if catheter remains occluded after 2-hour dwell time (see Administration); **Note:** A recent study using escalating doses of 0.5 mg, 1 mg, and 2 mg (60 minute dwell time) found that 86.2% of catheters were cleared with the 0.5 mg dose (see Davis, 2000).

Administration

Parenteral: Activase®: Reconstitute vials with supplied diluent (SWI); do not reconstitute with bacteriostatic water for injection; use large bore needle and syringe to reconstitute 50 mg vial and accompanying transfer device to reconstitute 100 mg vial (100 mg vial does not contain vacuum); swirl gently, do not shake; final concentration after reconstitution: 1 mg/mL

I.V.: May administer at a final concentration of 1 mg/mL or may dilute and administer as 0.5 mg/mL (see Stability). Prepare bolus dose using one of the following methods: 1) Remove bolus dose from reconstituted vial using syringe and needle; for 50 mg vial: do not prime syringe with air, insert needle into vial stopper; for 100 mg vial, insert needle away from puncture mark created by transfer device; 2) Remove bolus dose from a port on the infusion line after priming; 3) Program an infusion pump to deliver the bolus at the beginning of the infusion. Administer the remaining dose as follows: From 50 mg vial: Use polyvinyl chloride I.V. bag or glass vial and infusion set; from 100 mg vial: Use same puncture site made by transfer device to insert spike end of infusion set and infuse from vial.

CathFlo® Activase®: Reconstitute vial with 2.2 mL of SWI; do not reconstitute with bacteriostatic water for injection; allow vial to stand undisturbed so large bubbles may dissipate; swirl gently, do not shake; complete dissolution occurs within 3 minutes; final concentration after reconstitution: 1 mg/mL. Discard any unused solution (solution does not contain preservatives) (see Stability).

Intracatheter: Instill the appropriate dose into the occluded catheter (see Usual Dosage); leave in lumen; evaluate catheter function (by attempting to aspirate blood) after 30 minutes; if catheter is functional, aspirate 4-5 mL of blood out of catheter in patients ≥10 kg or 3 mL in patients <10 kg to remove drug and residual clot, then gently flush catheter with NS; if catheter is still occluded, leave alteplase in lumen and evaluate catheter function after 120 minutes of dwell time; if catheter is functional, aspirate 4-5 mL of blood out of catheter in patients ≥10 kg or 3 mL in patients <10 kg and gently flush with NS; if catheter remains occluded after 120 minutes of dwell time, a second dose may be instilled by repeating the above administration procedure.

Monitoring Parameters

Systemic use: Blood pressure; temperature; CBC, reticulocyte, platelet count; fibrinogen level, plasminogen, fibrin/fibrinogen degradation products, D-dimer, PT, PTT, antithrombin III, protein C; urinalysis, signs of bleeding

Intracatheter use: Catheter function (by attempting to aspirate blood); temperature, signs of sepsis, GI bleeding, bleeding at injection site, and venous thrombosis

Nursing Implications Extravasation may cause bruising or inflammation; monitor infusion site for patency of I.V.; if extravasation occurs, discontinue infusion at site of extravasation and apply local treatment; avoid I.M. injections; assess patient for bleeding

Additional Information Activase® and CathFlo® Activase® also contain L-arginine, polysorbate 80, and phosphoric acid (for pH adjustment).

Advantages of alteplase include: Low immunogenicity, short half-life, direct activation of plasminogen, and a strong and specific affinity for fibrin. Failure of thrombolytic agents in newborns/neonates may occur due to the low plasminogen concentrations (~50% to 70% of adult levels); supplementing plasminogen (via administration of fresh frozen plasma) may possibly help. Osmolality of 1 mg/mL solution is ~215 mOsm/kg.

Appropriate intracatheter use of alteplase for the treatment of occluded central venous catheters is not expected to cause systemic pharmacologic effects; in adults, if a 2 mg dose is administered I.V. (instead of being instilled into the catheter), the serum concentration of alteplase would be expected to return to normal endogenous levels within 30 minutes.

An open-label, single-arm trial of CathFlo® Activase® in pediatric patients, 2 weeks to 17 years of age (n = 310), was conducted using the manufacturer's recommended doses (see Usual Dosage); catheter function was restored in 83% of patients (similar

(Continued)

Alteplase *(Continued)*

to adults); rates of serious adverse events were also similar to adults (see CathFlo® Activase® package insert, 2005).

Dosage Forms Excipient information presented when available (limited, particularly for generics); consult specific product labeling.

Injection, powder for reconstitution, recombinant:

Activase®: 50 mg [29 million int. units; contains polysorbate 80; packaged with diluent]; 100 mg [58 million int. units; contains polysorbate 80; packaged with diluent and transfer device]

Cathflo® Activase®: 2 mg [contains polysorbate 80]

References

Anderson BJ, Keeley SR, and Johnson ND, "Caval Thrombolysis in Neonates Using Low Doses of Recombinant Human Tissue-Type Plasminogen Activator," *Anaesth Intensive Care*, 1991, 19(1):22-7.

Andrew M, Brooker L, Leaker M, et al, "Fibrin Clot Lysis by Thrombolytic Agents is Impaired in Newborns Due to a Low Plasminogen Concentration," *Thromb Haemost*, 1992, 68(3):325-30.

Cada DJ, Levien T, and Baker DE, "Alteplase," *Hospital Pharmacy*, 2002, 37(2): 148-54.

Choi M, Massicotte MP, Marzinotto V, et al, "The Use of Alteplase to Restore Patency of Central Venous Lines in Pediatric Patients: A Cohort Study," *J Pediatr*, 2001, 139(1):152-6.

Davis SN, Vermeulen L, Banton J, et al, "Activity and Dosage of Alteplase Dilution for Clearing Occlusions of Venous-Access Devices," *Am J Health Syst Pharm*, 2000, 57(11):1039-45.

Doyle E, Britto J, Freeman J, et al, "Thrombolysis With Low Dose Tissue Plasminogen Activator," *Arch Dis Child*, 1992, 67(12):1483-4.

Farnoux C, Camard O, Pinquier D, et al, "Recombinant Tissue-Type Plasminogen Activator Therapy of Thrombosis in 16 Neonates," *J Pediatr*, 1998, 133(1):137-40.

Frazin BS, "Maximal Dilution of Activase," *Am J Hosp Pharm*, 1990, 47(5):1016.

Generali J and Cada DJ, "Alteplase (t-PA) Bolus: Occluded Catheters," *Hospital Pharmacy*, 2001, 36(1):93-103.

Kothari SS, Varma S, and Wasir S, "Thrombolytic Therapy in Infants and Children," *Am Heart J*, 1994, 127(3):651-7.

Levy M, Benson LN, Burrows PE, et al, "Tissue Plasminogen Activator for the Treatment of Thromboembolism in Infants and Children," *J Pediatr*, 1991, 118(3):467-72.

Monagle P, Chan A, Massicotte P, et al, "Antithrombotic Therapy in Children: The Seventh ACCP Conference on Antithrombotic and Thrombolytic Therapy," *Chest*, 2004, 126(3 Suppl):645S-687S.

Monagle P, Michelson AD, Bovill E, et al, "Antithrombotic Therapy in Children," *Chest*, 2001, 119(1 Suppl):344S-370S.

Nowak-Gottl U, Auberger K, Halimeh S, et al, "Thrombolysis in Newborns and Infants," *Thromb Haemost*, 1999, 82 (Suppl 1):112-6.

Ponec D, Irwin D, Haire WD, et al, "Recombinant Tissue Plasminogen Activator (Alteplase) for Restoration of Flow in Occluded Central Venous Access Devices: A Double-Blind Placebo-Controlled Trial - The Cardiovascular Thrombolytic to Open Occluded Lines (COOL) Efficacy Trial," *J Vasc Interv Radiol*, 2001, 12(8):951-5.

Weiner GM, Castle VP, DiPietro MA, et al, "Successful Treatment of Neonatal Arterial Thromboses With Recombinant Tissue Plasminogen Activator," *J Pediatr*, 1998, 133(1):133-6.

♦ **Alti-Trazodone (Can)** *see* Trazodone *on page 1564*
♦ **Alti-Verapamil (Can)** *see* Verapamil *on page 1611*
♦ **Altoprev®** *see* Lovastatin *on page 964*

Aluminum Acetate (a LOO mi num AS e tate)

U.S. Brand Names Domeboro®
Index Terms Burow's Solution
Therapeutic Category Topical Skin Product
Use Astringent wet dressing for relief of inflammatory conditions of the skin and to reduce weeping that may occur in dermatitis; relieve minor skin irritations due to poison ivy, poison oak, poison sumac, insect bites, athlete's foot, and rashes caused by soaps, detergents, cosmetics, or jewelry
Pregnancy Risk Factor C
Contraindications Use with topical collagenase
Precautions Do not use plastic or other impervious material to prevent evaporation
Adverse Reactions Local: Irritation
Usual Dosage Children and Adults: Topical: Soak the affected area in the solution 2-4 times/day for 15-30 minutes or apply wet dressing soaked in the solution 2-4 times/day for 30-minute treatment periods; rewet dressing with solution every few minutes to keep it moist
Administration Topical: Keep away from eyes, external use only; one powder packet dissolved in 16 oz of water makes a modified Burow's solution equivalent to a 1:40 dilution, 2 packets: 1:20 dilution, 3 packets: 1:13 dilution. When used as a compress or wet dressing, soak a clean soft cloth in the solution. Apply cloth loosely to affected area for 15-30 minutes.
Dosage Forms Excipient information presented when available (limited, particularly for generics); consult specific product labeling.
Powder, for topical solution:
Domeboro®: Aluminum sulfate 1191 mg and calcium acetate 938 mg per packet (12s, 100s) [when powder packet is mixed with water, provides active ingredient aluminum acetate]

♦ **Aluminum and Magnesium Hydroxide** *see* Antacid Preparations *on page 132*
♦ **Aluminum Hydroxide** *see* Antacid Preparations *on page 132*
♦ **Aluminum Hydroxide and Magnesium Carbonate** *see* Antacid Preparations *on page 132*
♦ **Aluminum Hydroxide and Magnesium Hydroxide** *see* Antacid Preparations *on page 132*
♦ **Aluminum Hydroxide and Magnesium Trisilicate** *see* Antacid Preparations *on page 132*
♦ **Aluminum Hydroxide, Magnesium Hydroxide, and Simethicone** *see* Antacid Preparations *on page 132*
♦ **Aluminum Sucrose Sulfate, Basic** *see* Sucralfate *on page 1480*
♦ **Alupent®** *see* Metaproterenol *on page 1014*

Amantadine (a MAN ta deen)

Medication Safety Issues
Sound-alike/look-alike issues:
Amantadine may be confused with ranitidine, rimantadine
Symmetrel® may be confused with Synthroid®
International issues:
Symmetrel® may be confused with Somatrel® which is a brand name for somatorelin in Denmark
U.S. Brand Names Symmetrel®
Canadian Brand Names Endantadine®; PMS-Amantadine; Symmetrel®
Index Terms Adamantanamine Hydrochloride; Amantadine Hydrochloride
Therapeutic Category Anti-Parkinson's Agent; Antiviral Agent, Oral
Generic Available Yes
Use Prophylaxis and treatment of influenza A viral infection; symptomatic and adjunct treatment of parkinsonism
Pregnancy Risk Factor C
Lactation Enters breast milk/not recommended
Contraindications Hypersensitivity to amantadine hydrochloride or any component
Warnings Deaths due to amantadine overdose have been reported with the lowest lethal dose being 1 gram. Drug overdose has resulted in cardiac (ie, arrhythmia, tachycardia, hypertension), respiratory, renal, or central nervous system toxicity.
(Continued)

Amantadine *(Continued)*

Precautions Use with caution in patients with liver disease, epilepsy, history of recurrent eczematoid dermatitis, uncontrolled psychosis, and in patients receiving CNS stimulant drugs; may increase seizure activity or EEG disturbances in patients with pre-existing seizure disorders; neuroleptic malignant syndrome has been reported in patients undergoing dosage reduction or withdrawal of amantadine; modify dosage in patients with renal impairment; may need to modify dose in patients with active seizure disorders, CHF, peripheral edema, and orthostatic hypotension

Adverse Reactions

Cardiovascular: Orthostatic hypotension, edema

Central nervous system: Dizziness, confusion, headache, insomnia, difficulty in concentrating, anxiety, restlessness, irritability, hallucinations, seizures, suicide ideation, neuroleptic malignant syndrome

Dermatologic: Livedo reticularis

Gastrointestinal: Nausea, vomiting, xerostomia, anorexia, constipation

Genitourinary: Urinary retention

Drug Interactions Additive anticholinergic effects in patients receiving drugs with anticholinergic activity; additive CNS stimulant effect with CNS stimulants

Mechanism of Action As an antiviral, blocks the uncoating of influenza A virus preventing penetration of virus into host and inhibits M_2 protein in the assembly of progeny virions; antiparkinsonian activity may be due to its blocking the reuptake of dopamine into presynaptic neurons and causing direct stimulation of postsynaptic receptors

Pharmacokinetics

Absorption: Well absorbed from the GI tract

Half-life, patients with normal renal function: 10-28 hours

Time to peak serum concentration: 1-4 hours

Elimination: 80% to 90% excreted unchanged in the urine by glomerular filtration and tubular secretion

Dialysis: 0% to 5% removed by hemodialysis; no supplemental dose needed after hemodialysis or peritoneal dialysis

Usual Dosage Oral:

Children: Influenza A prophylaxis and treatment:

1-9 years: 5 mg/kg/day in 1-2 divided doses; maximum dose: 150 mg/day

≥10-12 years: 5 mg/kg/day in 1-2 divided doses; maximum dose: 200 mg/day

Note: After first influenza A virus vaccine dose, amantadine prophylaxis may be administered for up to 6 weeks, or until 2 weeks after the second dose of vaccine; administer a 10-day course of therapy following exposure; for symptomatic treatment, administer within 24-48 hours of symptom onset with usual duration of therapy between 2-5 days or for 24-48 hours after patient becomes asymptomatic

Alternative dosage for influenza A prophylaxis: Children >20 kg and Adults: 100 mg/day in 1-2 divided doses

Adults:

Parkinson's disease: 100 mg twice daily

Influenza A viral infection: 200 mg/day in 1-2 divided doses

Prophylaxis: Minimum 10-day course of therapy following exposure, or continue for 2-3 weeks after influenza A virus vaccine is given

Dosing interval in renal impairment: Adults:

Cl_{cr} 30-50 mL/minute: Administer 100 mg/day

Cl_{cr} 15-29 mL/minute: Administer 100 mg every other day

Cl_{cr} <15 mL/minute: Administer 200 mg every 7 days

Monitoring Parameters Renal function; monitor for signs of neurotoxicity

Patient Information May cause drowsiness and impair ability to perform activities requiring mental alertness or physical coordination; do not abruptly discontinue therapy, may precipitate a parkinsonian crisis; avoid alcohol; may cause dry mouth

Nursing Implications If insomnia occurs, the last daily dose should be taken several hours before retiring

Dosage Forms Excipient information presented when available (limited, particularly for generics); consult specific product labeling.

Capsule, as hydrochloride: 100 mg

Syrup, as hydrochloride: 50 mg/5 mL (480 mL)

Tablet, as hydrochloride: 100 mg

Symmetrel®: 100 mg

References

Strong DK, Eisenstat DD, Bryson SM, et al, "Amantadine Neurotoxicity in a Pediatric Patient With Renal Insufficiency," *DICP*, 1991, 25(11):1175-7.

♦ **Amantadine Hydrochloride** *see* Amantadine *on page 89*

♦ **AmBisome®** *see* Amphotericin B Liposome *on page 122*

- **AMCA** *see* Tranexamic Acid *on page 1563*
- **Americaine® [OTC]** *see* Benzocaine *on page 204*
- **Americaine® Hemorrhoidal [OTC]** *see* Benzocaine *on page 204*
- **A-Methapred** *see* MethylPREDNISolone *on page 1039*
- **Amethocaine Hydrochloride** *see* Tetracaine *on page 1517*
- **Amethopterin** *see* Methotrexate *on page 1027*
- **Ametop™ (Can)** *see* Tetracaine *on page 1517*
- **Amibid DM [DSC]** *see* Guaifenesin and Dextromethorphan *on page 748*
- **Amicar®** *see* Aminocaproic Acid *on page 96*
- **Amidate®** *see* Etomidate *on page 624*

Amifostine (am i FOS teen)

Medication Safety Issues

Sound-alike/look-alike issues:

Ethyol® may be confused with ethanol

Related Information

Compatibility of Chemotherapy and Related Supportive Care Medications *on page 1777*

U.S. Brand Names Ethyol®

Canadian Brand Names Ethyol®

Index Terms Ethiofos; Gammaphos; WR-2721; YM-08310

Therapeutic Category Antidote, Cisplatin; Cytoprotective Agent

Generic Available No

Use Cytoprotective agent which scavenges free radicals and binds to reactive drug derivatives due to radiation therapy, cisplatin, carboplatin, cyclophosphamide, ifosfamide, carmustine, melphalan, and mechlorethamine to selectively protect normal tissues against toxicity due to these agents; reduction of moderate to severe xerostomia from radiation treatment of the head and neck where the radiation port includes a substantial portion of the parotid glands

Pregnancy Risk Factor C

Lactation Excretion in breast milk unknown/not recommended

Contraindications Hypersensitivity to amifostine, aminothiol compounds, or any component; patients who are hypotensive or dehydrated

Warnings Due to limited experience and the possibility of amifostine interference with antineoplastic efficacy, amifostine should not be administered to patients in settings where chemotherapy can produce a significant survival benefit or cure, except in the context of a clinical study. Monitor serum calcium levels in patients at risk of hypocalcemia (eg, those patients receiving multiple doses of amifostine, patients with nephrotic syndrome).

Precautions Use with caution in patients with pre-existing cardiovascular or cerebrovascular conditions such as ischemic heart disease, arrhythmias, CHF, history of stroke or transient ischemic attacks; may cause hypotension; use special caution in situations where concomitant antihypertensive therapy cannot be interrupted 24 hours prior to starting amifostine or in patients in whom the adverse effects of nausea/vomiting may be more likely to have serious consequences

Adverse Reactions

Cardiovascular: Transient hypotension (62%; incidence is higher in patients with head and neck cancer, esophageal cancer, nonsmall cell lung cancer, prior neck irradiation, or hypercalcemia), flushing, warm sensation

Central nervous system: Chills, fever, dizziness, somnolence, hiccups, anxiety, malaise

Dermatologic: Rash

Endocrine & metabolic: Hypocalcemia, hypomagnesemia

Gastrointestinal: Nausea, vomiting, metallic taste in mouth

Genitourinary: Urinary retention (reversible)

Respiratory: Sneezing

Drug Interactions Antihypertensive agents may potentiate the hypotensive effects of amifostine

Stability When 500 mg amifostine is reconstituted with 9.7 mL of NS, the resultant solution is stable for 5 hours at room temperature or up to 24 hours if refrigerated; amifostine solutions diluted to 5-40 mg/mL in NS are chemically stable for 5 hours at room temperature or 24 hours if refrigerated; decreased stability in low pH conditions; incompatible with acyclovir, amphotericin B, chlorpromazine, cisplatin, ganciclovir, hydroxyzine, prochlorperazine

Mechanism of Action Amifostine is a prodrug that is converted by the plasma membrane-bound enzyme alkaline phosphatase to the active free sulfhydryl compound WR-1065, which is further oxidized to a symmetrical disulfide (WR-33278) or to mixed disulfides. The active drug scavenges free radicals, donates hydrogen

(Continued)

Amifostine *(Continued)*

ions to free radicals, and binds to active derivatives of antineoplastic agents, thus preventing the alkylation of nucleic acid. Selective protection of normal tissue is demonstrated by:

1) decreased alkaline phosphatase activity in tumor cells,
2) decreased vascularity of tumors, and
3) lower pH in tumor tissues due to the predominance of anaerobic metabolism (WR-1065 requires a pH in the range of 6.6-8.2 for uptake into tissues)

Pharmacokinetics

Distribution: V_d: Adults: 6.4 L; unmetabolized prodrug is largely confined to the intravascular compartment; active metabolite is distributed into normal tissues with high concentrations in bone marrow, GI mucosa, skin, liver, and salivary glands

Protein binding: 4%

Metabolism: Amifostine (phosphorylated prodrug) is hydrolyzed by alkaline phosphatase to an active free sulfhydryl compound (WR-1065)

Half-life:

Children: 9.3 minutes

Adults: 8 minutes

Elimination: Metabolites excreted in urine

Usual Dosage I.V. (refer to individual protocols):

Children: Limited data available on use in pediatric patients; dosing based on a prior clinical phase I trial and single case reports: 740 mg/m² once daily administered 30 minutes prior to chemotherapy; doses as high as 600 mg/m²/dose administered 15 minutes prior to and 2 hours after chemotherapy (total of 1200 mg/m²/day) have been used in phase I trials in patients treated with ifosfamide, carboplatin, and etoposide chemotherapy; repeat amifostine doses may be required when using a cytotoxic agent with a long half-life or long infusion time

Adults: 910 mg/m² once daily administered 30 minutes prior to chemotherapy; reduce dose to 740 mg/m² in patients who have a higher incidence of hypotension

Reduction of moderate to severe xerostomia from radiation of the head and neck: 200 mg/m² once daily starting 15-30 minutes prior to standard fraction radiation therapy

Administration Parenteral: I.V.: Reconstituted amifostine dose must be further diluted with NS to a final volume of 50 mL (adults) or a final concentration of 5-40 mg/mL (children). Administer amifostine doses >740 mg/m² as an I.V. intermittent infusion over 15 minutes since the 15-minute infusion is better tolerated than a more prolonged infusion. Administer 200 mg/m² dose as a 3-minute infusion. Amifostine should be interrupted if the blood pressure decreases significantly from baseline or if the patient develops symptoms related to decreased cerebral or cardiovascular perfusion. Patients experiencing decreased blood pressure should receive a rapid infusion of NS and be kept supine or placed in the Trendelenburg position. Amifostine can be restarted if the blood pressure returns to the baseline level.

Monitoring Parameters Baseline blood pressure followed by a blood pressure reading every 3-5 minutes during the 15-minute infusion; monitor electrolytes, urinalysis, serum calcium, serum magnesium; monitor I & O

Nursing Implications Pretreat patient with antiemetics; patients should be well hydrated prior to amifostine infusion; patients taking antihypertensive medications should discontinue therapy 24 hours before administration of amifostine; begin chemotherapy or radiation therapy 15 minutes after completion of amifostine

Dosage Forms Excipient information presented when available (limited, particularly for generics); consult specific product labeling.

Injection, powder for reconstitution:

Ethyol®: 500 mg

References

Adamson PC, Balis FM, Belasco JE, et al, "A Phase I Trial of Amifostine (WR-2721) and Melphalan in Children With Refractory Cancer," *Cancer Res*, 1995, 55(18): 4069-72.

Fouladi M, Stempak D, Gammon J, et al, "Phase I Trial of a Twice-Daily Regimen of Amifostine With Ifosfamide, Carboplatin, and Etoposide Chemotherapy in Children With Refractory Carcinoma," *Cancer*, 2001, 92(4):914-23.

Schuchter LM, "Guidelines for the Administration of Amifostine," *Semin Oncol*, 1996, 23(4 Suppl 8):40-3.

Shaw LM, Bonner H, and Lieberman R, "Pharmacokinetic Profile of Amifostine," *Semin Oncol*, 1996, 23(4 Suppl 8):18-22.

Amikacin (am i KAY sin)

Medication Safety Issues

Sound-alike/look-alike issues:

Amikacin may be confused with Amicar®, anakinra

Amikin® may be confused with Amicar®

Related Information

Blood Level Sampling Time Guidelines *on page 1914*

Overdose and Toxicology *on page 1916*

U.S. Brand Names Amikin®

Canadian Brand Names Amikacin Sulfate Injection, USP; Amikin®

Index Terms Amikacin Sulfate

Therapeutic Category Antibiotic, Aminoglycoside

Generic Available Yes

Use Treatment of documented gram-negative enteric infection resistant to gentamicin and tobramycin; amikacin is usually effective against *Pseudomonas, Klebsiella, Enterobacter, Serratia, Proteus,* and *E. coli*; documented infection of mycobacterial organisms susceptible to amikacin

Pregnancy Risk Factor D

Lactation Enters breast milk/compatible

Contraindications Hypersensitivity to amikacin sulfate or any component (see Warnings); cross-sensitivity may exist with other aminoglycosides

Warnings Aminoglycosides are associated with significant nephrotoxicity or ototoxicity; the ototoxicity is directly proportional to the amount of drug given and the duration of treatment. Tinnitus or vertigo are indications of vestibular injury and impending bilateral irreversible deafness. Risk of nephrotoxicity increases when used concurrently with other potentially nephrotoxic drugs; renal damage is usually reversible. Aminoglycosides can cause fetal harm when administered to a pregnant woman, and have been associated with several reports of total irreversible bilateral congenital deafness in pediatric patients exposed *in utero*. Some products contain sulfites which may cause allergic reactions in susceptible individuals.

Precautions Use with caution in neonates (due to renal immaturity that results in a prolonged half-life); patients with pre-existing renal impairment, auditory or vestibular impairment, hypocalcemia, myasthenia gravis, and in conditions which depress neuromuscular transmission; dose and/or frequency of administration must be modified in patients with renal impairment

Adverse Reactions

Central nervous system: Fever, headache, dizziness, drowsiness, ataxia, vertigo

Dermatologic: Rash

Gastrointestinal: Nausea, vomiting

Hematologic: Eosinophilia, anemia, leukopenia

Neuromuscular & skeletal: Neuromuscular blockade, tremor, paresthesia, weakness, gait instability

Otic: Ototoxicity

Renal: Nephrotoxicity

Drug Interactions Extended-spectrum penicillins (decrease serum amikacin concentration in patients with renal failure); loop diuretics may potentiate the ototoxicity of the aminoglycosides; amphotericin, vancomycin, acyclovir, cisplatin, or cephalosporins may increase nephrotoxicity; may potentiate the effects of neuromuscular blocking agents and general anesthetics; indomethacin may increase serum amikacin concentrations

Mechanism of Action Inhibits protein synthesis in susceptible bacteria by binding to ribosomal subunits

Pharmacokinetics

Distribution: Primarily into extracellular fluid (highly hydrophilic); 12% of serum concentration penetrates into bronchial secretions; poor penetration into the blood-brain barrier even when meninges are inflamed; V_d is increased in neonates and patients with edema, ascites, fluid overload; V_d is decreased in patients with dehydration; crosses the placenta

Half-life:

- Infants:
  - Low birth weight, 1-3 days of age: 7 hours
  - Full-term >7 days: 4-5 hours
- Children: 1.6-2.5 hours
- Adolescents: 1.5 ± 1 hour
- Adults: 2-3 hours
- Anuria: 28-86 hours; half-life and clearance are dependent on renal function

Time to peak serum concentration:

- I.M.: Within 45-120 minutes
- I.V.: Within 30 minutes following a 30-minute infusion

Elimination: 94% to 98% is excreted unchanged in the urine via glomerular filtration within 24 hours

Dialysis: Dialyzable (50% to 100%); supplemental dose recommended after hemodialysis or peritoneal dialysis

Usual Dosage I.M., I.V. (dosage should be based on an estimate of ideal body weight except in neonates; neonatal dosage should be based on actual weight unless the patient has hydrocephalus or hydrops fetalis):

(Continued)

Amikacin *(Continued)*

Neonates:

0-4 weeks, <1200 g: 7.5 mg/kg/dose every 18-24 hours

Postnatal age ≤7 days:

1200-2000 g: 7.5 mg/kg/dose every 12 hours

>2000 g: 7.5-10 mg/kg/dose every 12 hours

Postnatal age >7 days:

1200-2000 g: 7.5-10 mg/kg/dose every 8-12 hours

>2000 g: 10 mg/kg/dose every 8 hours

Infants and Children: 15-22.5 mg/kg/day divided every 8 hours; some consultants recommend initial doses of 30 mg/kg/day divided every 8 hours in patients who may require larger doses; see **Note**

Treatment for nontuberculous mycobacterial infection: 15-30 mg/kg/day divided every 12-24 hours as part of a multiple drug regimen; maximum dose: 1.5 g/day

Adults: 15 mg/kg/day divided every 8-12 hours; maximum: 1.5 g/day

Treatment of *M. avium* complex infection: 7.5-15 mg/kg/day divided every 12-24 hours as part of a multiple drug regimen

Dosing Interval in renal impairment: Loading dose: 5-7.5 mg/kg; subsequent dosages and frequency of administration are best determined by measurement of serum levels and assessment of renal insufficiency

Note: Some patients may require larger or more frequent doses if serum levels document the need (ie, cystic fibrosis or febrile granulocytopenic patients).

Administration Parenteral: Administer by I.M. or slow intermittent I.V. infusion over 30 minutes at a final concentration not to exceed 10 mg amikacin/mL. Administer other antibiotics such as penicillins and cephalosporins at least 1 hour before or after an amikacin dose.

Monitoring Parameters Urinalysis, urine output, BUN, serum creatinine, peak and trough serum amikacin concentrations; be alert to ototoxicity

Not all infants and children who receive aminoglycosides require monitoring of serum aminoglycoside concentrations. Indications for use of aminoglycoside serum concentration monitoring include:

- treatment course >5 days
- patients with decreased or changing renal function
- patients with poor therapeutic response
- infants <3 months of age
- atypical body constituency (obesity, expanded extracellular fluid volume)
- clinical need for higher doses or shorter intervals (eg, cystic fibrosis, burns, endocarditis, meningitis, critically ill patients, relatively resistant organisms)
- patients on hemodialysis or chronic ambulatory peritoneal dialysis
- signs of nephrotoxicity or ototoxicity
- concomitant use of other nephrotoxic agents

Reference Range

Peak: 20-30 mcg/mL

Trough: <10 mcg/mL

Patient Information Report loss of hearing, ringing or roaring in the ears, or feeling of fullness in head

Nursing Implications Aminoglycoside levels measured from blood taken from Silastic® central catheters can sometimes give falsely elevated readings; peak serum levels should be drawn 30 minutes after the end of a 30-minute infusion; trough levels are drawn within 30 minutes before the next dose; provide optimal patient hydration

Dosage Forms Excipient information presented when available (limited, particularly for generics); consult specific product labeling. [DSC] = Discontinued product

Injection, solution, as sulfate: 50 mg/mL (2 mL, 4 mL); 62.5 mg/mL (8 mL) [DSC]; 250 mg/mL (2 mL, 4 mL)

Amikin®: 50 mg/mL (2 mL); 250 mg/mL (2 mL, 4 mL) [contains metabisulfite]

References

Kenyon CF, Knoppert DC, Lee SK, et al, "Amikacin Pharmacokinetics and Suggested Dosage Modifications for the Preterm Infant," *Antimicrob Agents Chemother*, 1990, 34(2):265-8.

Public Health Service Task Force on Prophylaxis and Therapy for *Mycobacterium avium* Complex, "Recommendations on Prophylaxis and Therapy for Disseminated *Mycobacterium avium* Complex Disease in Patients Infected With the Human Immunodeficiency Virus," *N Engl J Med*, 1993, 329(12):898-904.

Starke JR and Correa AG, "Management of Mycobacterial Infection and Disease in Children," *Pediatr Infect Dis J*, 1995, 14(6):455-69.

Vogelstein B, Kowarski A, and Lietman PS, "The Pharmacokinetics of Amikacin in Children," *J Pediatr*, 1977, 91(2):333-9.

♦ **Amikacin Sulfate** *see* Amikacin *on page 92*

♦ **Amikacin Sulfate Injection, USP (Can)** *see* Amikacin *on page 92*

♦ **Amikin®** *see* Amikacin *on page 92*

Amiloride (a MIL oh ride)

Medication Safety Issues
Sound-alike/look-alike issues:
Amiloride may be confused with amiodarone, amlodipine, amrinone

Related Information
Antihypertensive Agents by Class *on page 1678*

U.S. Brand Names Midamor® [DSC]

Canadian Brand Names Apo-Amiloride®

Index Terms Amiloride Hydrochloride

Therapeutic Category Antihypertensive Agent; Diuretic, Potassium Sparing

Generic Available Yes

Use Management of edema associated with CHF, hepatic cirrhosis, and hyperaldosteronism; hypertension; primary hyperaldosteronism; hypokalemia induced by kaliuretic diuretics

Pregnancy Risk Factor B

Lactation Excretion in breast milk unknown/contraindicated

Contraindications Hypersensitivity to amiloride or any component; hyperkalemia; anuria

Warnings Due to potential severe hyperkalemia, amiloride should be discontinued in diabetic patients for at least 3 days prior to glucose tolerance testing; discontinue if serum potassium >5.5 mEq/L

Precautions Use with caution in patients with dehydration, electrolyte imbalance, metabolic or respiratory acidosis, diabetes (particularly those with nephropathy), hyponatremia, impaired renal function, or hepatic dysfunction; patients receiving potassium or other potassium-sparing diuretics; use with caution and modify dosage in patients with decreased renal function

Adverse Reactions
Cardiovascular: Angina, orthostatic hypotension, arrhythmia, palpitations
Central nervous system: Headache, dizziness, encephalopathy, vertigo, nervousness, mental confusion, insomnia, depression, somnolence
Dermatologic: Skin rash, pruritus, alopecia
Endocrine & metabolic: Hyperkalemia, hyperchloremic metabolic acidosis, dehydration, hyponatremia, gynecomastia
Gastrointestinal: Nausea, anorexia, diarrhea, vomiting, abdominal pain, appetite changes, constipation, GI bleeding, xerostomia, heartburn, flatulence, dyspepsia
Genitourinary: Impotence, dysuria, urinary frequency, bladder spasms
Hematologic: Aplastic anemia, neutropenia
Hepatic: Abnormal liver function
Neuromuscular & skeletal: Weakness, muscle cramps, joint and back pain, paresthesia, tremors
Ocular: Visual disturbances, elevated intraocular pressure
Otic: Tinnitus
Renal: Polyuria
Respiratory: Cough, dyspnea, nasal congestion, shortness of breath

Drug Interactions Potassium, other potassium-sparing diuretics, cyclosporine, tacrolimus, ACE inhibitors (eg, captopril), and angiotensin II receptor antagonists (eg, losartan) may additively increase the serum potassium; may decrease digoxin clearance and attenuate its inotropic effect; decreases lithium clearance; decreased diuresis and antihypertensive effects with concomitant NSAID use

Food Interactions Avoid natural licorice (causes sodium and water retention and increases potassium loss) and salt substitutes; food decreases absorption to ~30%

Mechanism of Action Acts directly on the distal renal tubule to inhibit sodium-potassium ion exchange; decreases sodium reabsorption in the distal tubule by inhibiting cellular sodium transport mechanisms such as the conductive sodium influx pathway and possibly the sodium-hydrogen ion exchange system; also inhibits hydrogen ion secretion; its diuretic activity is **independent** of aldosterone.

Pharmacodynamics
Onset of action: 2 hours
Maximum effect: 6-10 hours
Duration: 24 hours

Pharmacokinetics
Absorption: 50%
Distribution: Adults: V_d: 350-380 L
Metabolism: No active metabolites
Half-life: Adults:
Normal renal function: 6-9 hours
End-stage renal disease: 21-144 hours
Elimination: Unchanged drug, equally in urine and feces
(Continued)

Amiloride *(Continued)*

Usual Dosage Oral:

Hypertension:

Children: 0.4-0.625 mg/kg/day; maximum dose: 20 mg/day

Adults: 5-10 mg/day in 1-2 divided doses (JNC 7)

Edema:

Children 6-20 kg: 0.625 mg/kg/day in 1-2 divided doses; maximum dose: 10 mg/day

Children >20 kg and Adults: 5-10 mg/day in 1-2 divided doses; maximum dose: 20 mg/day

Dosing adjustment in renal impairment:

Cl_{cr} 10-50 mL/minute: Administer at 50% of normal dose

Cl_{cr} <10 mL/minute: Avoid use

Administration Oral: Administer with food or milk

Monitoring Parameters Serum potassium, sodium, creatinine, BUN, blood pressure, fluid balance

Test Interactions May falsely elevate serum digoxin levels done by radioimmunoassay

Patient Information Report to your physician any muscle cramps, weakness, nausea, or dizziness; may cause drowsiness and impair ability to perform activities requiring mental alertness or physical coordination; may cause dry mouth

Additional Information Studies utilizing aerosolized amiloride (5 mmol/L in 0.3% saline) in adult cystic fibrosis patients (Tomkiewicz, 1993) have suggested that inhaled amiloride is capable of improving the rheologic properties of the abnormally thickened mucus by increasing mucus sodium content

Dosage Forms Excipient information presented when available (limited, particularly for generics); consult specific product labeling.

Tablet, as hydrochloride: 5 mg

Extemporaneous Preparations A 1 mg/mL oral liquid may be prepared from crushed tablets added to a small quantity of sterile water to which glycerin (final concentration of 40% w/v) is added; sterile water is then added in sufficient quantity to make the desired volume; stable 21 days when refrigerated

Fawcett JP, Woods DJ, Ferry DG, et al, "Stability of Amiloride Hydrochloride Oral Liquids Prepared From Tablets and Powder," *Aust J Hosp Pharm*, 1995, 25:10-23.

References

Chobanian AV, Bakris GL, Black HR, et al, "The Seventh Report of the Joint National Committee on Prevention, Detection, Evaluation, and Treatment of High Blood Pressure: The JNC 7 Report," *JAMA*, 2003, 289(19):2560-72.

National High Blood Pressure Education Program Working Group on High Blood Pressure in Children and Adolescents, "The Fourth Report on the Diagnosis, Evaluation, and Treatment of High Blood Pressure in Children and Adolescents," *Pediatrics*, 2004, 114(2 Suppl):555-76.

Tomkiewicz RP, App, EM, Zayas JG, et al, "Amiloride Inhalation Therapy in Cystic Fibrosis. Influence on Ion Content, Hydration, and Rheology of Sputum," *Am Rev Resp Dis*, 1993, 148:1002-7.

van der Vorst MM, Kist JE, van der Heijden AJ, et al, "Diuretics in Pediatrics: Current Knowledge and Future Prospects," *Paediatr Drugs*, 2006, 8(4):245-64.

- ♦ **Amiloride Hydrochloride** *see* Amiloride *on page 95*
- ♦ **2-Amino-6-Mercaptopurine** *see* Thioguanine *on page 1527*
- ♦ **2-Amino-6-Methoxypurine Arabinoside** *see* Nelarabine *on page 1113*
- ♦ **Aminobenzylpenicillin** *see* Ampicillin *on page 123*

Aminocaproic Acid (a mee noe ka PROE ik AS id)

Medication Safety Issues

Sound-alike/look-alike issues:

Amicar® may be confused with amikacin, Amikin®, Omacor®

U.S. Brand Names Amicar®

Index Terms Epsilon Aminocaproic Acid

Therapeutic Category Hemostatic Agent

Generic Available Yes

Use Treatment of excessive bleeding resulting from systemic hyperfibrinolysis, urinary fibrinolysis, or traumatic ocular hyphema

Pregnancy Risk Factor C

Lactation Excretion in breast milk unknown/use caution

Contraindications Hypersensitivity to aminocaproic acid or any component (see Warnings); disseminated intravascular coagulation; evidence of an intravascular clotting process; use of factor IX concentrate or anti-inhibitor coagulant concentrate

Warnings Aminocaproic acid may accumulate in patients with decreased renal function; intrarenal obstruction may occur secondary to glomerular capillary thrombosis or clots in the renal pelvis and ureters; do not use in hematuria of upper urinary tract origin unless benefits outweigh potential risks; inhibition of fibrinolysis may promote clotting or thrombosis.

Injection contains benzyl alcohol which may cause allergic reactions in susceptible individuals; large amounts of benzyl alcohol (≥99 mg/kg/day) have been associated with a potentially fatal toxicity ("gasping syndrome") in neonates; the "gasping syndrome" consists of metabolic acidosis, respiratory distress, gasping respirations, CNS dysfunction (including convulsions, intracranial hemorrhage), hypotension and cardiovascular collapse; avoid use of injection in neonates; *in vitro* and animal studies have shown that benzoate, a metabolite of benzyl alcohol, displaces bilirubin from protein-binding sites

Precautions Use with caution in patients with cardiac, renal or hepatic disease; adjust dosage in patients with oliguria or end-stage renal disease; use with caution in patients at risk for veno-occlusive disease of the liver

Adverse Reactions

Cardiovascular: Hypotension, bradycardia and arrhythmias (following rapid I.V. administration), peripheral ischemia, thrombosis, stroke, syncope

Central nervous system: Dizziness, headache, malaise, seizures, confusion, delirium, hallucinations

Dermatologic: Rash, pruritus

Endocrine & metabolic: Hyperkalemia

Gastrointestinal: GI irritation, nausea, cramps, diarrhea, vomiting, abdominal pain

Genitourinary: Dry ejaculation

Hematologic: Decreased platelet function, agranulocytosis, leukopenia

Neuromuscular & skeletal: Myopathy, acute rhabdomyolysis, weakness, myalgia, elevated CPK

Ocular: Glaucoma, watery eyes

Otic: Tinnitus, deafness

Renal: Renal failure, elevated BUN

Respiratory: Nasal congestion, dyspnea, pulmonary embolism

Drug Interactions Increased risk of thrombosis with oral contraceptives, estrogens, and factor IX

Mechanism of Action Competitively inhibits activation of plasminogen thereby reducing fibrinolysin, without inhibiting lysis of clot

Pharmacodynamics Onset of action: Inhibition of fibrinolysis: Within 1-72 hours (onset shortened substantially if loading dose is used)

Pharmacokinetics

Distribution: Widely distributes through intravascular and extravascular compartments

Metabolism: Hepatic metabolism is minimal

Bioavailability: Oral: 100%

Half-life: 1-2 hours

Elimination: 40% to 60% excreted as unchanged drug in the urine within 12 hours

Usual Dosage

Children:

Oral, I.V.: Loading dose: 100-200 mg/kg; maintenance: 100 mg/kg/dose every 6 hours; maximum daily dose: 30 g

or as an alternative: I.V. loading dose: 100 mg/kg or 3 g/m^2 followed by a continuous infusion of 33.3 mg/kg/hour or 1 g/m^2/hour; total dosage should not exceed 18 g/m^2/day

Traumatic hyphema: Oral, I.V.: 100 mg/kg/dose every 4 hours (maximum dose: 5 g/dose; maximum daily dose: 30 g/day)

Adults:

Oral: For the treatment of acute bleeding syndromes due to elevated fibrinolytic activity, give 5 g during first hour, followed by 1-1.25 g/hour for about 8 hours or until bleeding stops; daily dose should not exceed 30 g

I.V.: Give 4-5 g during first hour followed by continuous infusion at the rate of 1-1.25 g/hour, continue for 8 hours or until bleeding stops

Dosing adjustment in renal impairment: Oliguria or ESRD: Reduce dose to 25% of normal

Administration

Oral: May administer without regard to food

Parenteral: Maximum concentration for I.V. administration: 20 mg/mL; administer single doses over at least 1 hour

Monitoring Parameters Fibrinogen, fibrin split products, serum creatinine kinase (long-term therapy); serum potassium (may be elevated by aminocaproic acid, especially if the patient has impaired renal function)

Reference Range Therapeutic concentration: >130 mcg/mL (concentration necessary for inhibition of fibrinolysis)

Nursing Implications Rapid I.V. injection (IVP) should be avoided since hypotension, bradycardia, and arrhythmias may result

(Continued)

Aminocaproic Acid *(Continued)*

Dosage Forms Excipient information presented when available (limited, particularly for generics); consult specific product labeling.
Injection, solution: 250 mg/mL (20 mL)
Amicar®: 250 mg/mL (20 mL) [contains benzyl alcohol]
Solution, oral: 1.25 g/5 mL (240 mL, 480 mL)
Syrup:
Amicar®: 1.25 g/5 mL (480 mL) [raspberry flavor]
Tablet [scored]: 500 mg, 1000 mg
Amicar®: 500 mg, 1000 mg

References

McGetrick JJ, Jampol LM, Goldberg MP, et al, "Aminocaproic Acid Decreases Secondary Hemorrhage After Traumatic Hyphema," *Arch Ophthalmol*, 1983, 101(7):1031-3.

Aminophylline (am in OFF i lin)

Medication Safety Issues
Sound-alike/look-alike issues:
Aminophylline may be confused with amitriptyline, ampicillin

Related Information
Asthma *on page 1904*
Overdose and Toxicology *on page 1916*
Theophylline *on page 1520*

Canadian Brand Names Phyllocontin®; Phyllocontin®-350

Index Terms Theophylline Ethylenediamine

Therapeutic Category Antiasthmatic; Bronchodilator; Respiratory Stimulant; Theophylline Derivative

Generic Available Yes

Use Bronchodilator in reversible airway obstruction due to asthma or COPD; increase diaphragmatic contractility; neonatal idiopathic apnea of prematurity

Pregnancy Risk Factor C

Lactation Enters breast milk/compatible (AAP rates "compatible")

Contraindications Hypersensitivity to aminophylline or any component; uncontrolled arrhythmias

Adverse Reactions See Theophylline *on page 1520*

Medications Affecting Theophylline Clearance Resulting in Either Increased or Decreased Serum Levels

Decreased Theophylline Level	Increased Theophylline Level
Aminoglutethimide	Alcohol
Carbamazepine	Allopurinol (>600 mg/day)
Isoproterenol (I.V.)	Beta-blockers
Isoniazid[1]	Calcium channel blockers
Ketoconazole	Cimetidine
Loop diuretics[1]	Ciprofloxacin
Nevirapine	Clarithromycin
Phenobarbital	Corticosteroids
Phenytoin	Disulfiram
Rifampin	Ephedrine
Ritonavir	Erythromycin
Sulfinpyrazone	Esmolol
Sympathomimetics	Influenza virus vaccine
	Interferon, human recombinant alpha 2-a and 2-b
	Isoniazid[1]
	Loop diuretics[1]
	Methotrexate
	Mexiletine
	Oral contraceptives
	Propafenone
	Propranolol
	Tacrine
	Thiabendazole
	Thyroid hormones
	Troleandomycin (TAO®)
	Verapamil
	Zileuton

[1]Both increased and decreased theophylline levels have been reported.

Drug Interactions Cytochrome P450 isoenzyme CYP1A2, CYP2E1 (minor), and CYP3A3/4 substrate

Decreases adenosine, benzodiazepines, and pancuronium effects; decreases zafirlukast serum levels; increases lithium clearance; increases CNS side effects with ephedrine; increases risk of cardiac arrhythmias with halothane; for medications which change aminophylline (theophylline) clearance, see tables.

Clinical Factors Reported to Affect Theophylline Clearance

Decreased Theophylline Level	Increased Theophylline Level
Smoking (cigarettes, marijuana)	Acute pulmonary edema
High protein/low carbohydrate diet	Cessation of smoking (after chronic use)
Charcoal broiled beef	Cor pulmonale
	Congestive heart failure
	Hypothyroidism
	Fever (≥102° for 24 hours or more, or lesser temperature elevations for longer periods)
	Hepatic cirrhosis/acute hepatitis
	Renal failure in infants <3 mo of age
	Sepsis with multisystem organ failure
	Shock
	Viral illness

Food Interactions Food does not appreciably affect absorption; avoid extremes of dietary protein and carbohydrate intake; limit charcoal-broiled foods and caffeinated beverages

Mechanism of Action See Theophylline *on page 1520*

Pharmacokinetics Aminophylline is the ethylenediamine salt of theophylline, pharmacokinetic parameters are those of **theophylline**; fraction available: 80% (eg, 100 mg aminophylline = 80 mg theophylline); see Theophylline *on page 1520*

Usual Dosage All dosages based upon **aminophylline**; dose should be based on ideal body weight

Neonates:

Apnea of prematurity: Oral, I.V.:

Loading dose: 5 mg/kg

Maintenance: Initial: 5 mg/kg/day every 12 hours; increased dosages may be indicated as liver metabolism matures (usually >30 days of life); monitor serum levels to determine appropriate dosages

Theophylline levels should be initially drawn after 3 days of therapy; repeat levels are indicated 3 days after each increase in dosage or weekly if on a stabilized dosage

Infants, Children, and Adults: Treatment of acute bronchospasm: I.V.: Loading dose (in patients not currently receiving aminophylline or theophylline): 6 mg/kg (based on aminophylline) given I.V. over 20-30 minutes

Guidelines for Drawing Theophylline Serum Levels

Dosage Form	Time to Draw Level[1]
I.V. bolus	30 min after end of 30-min infusion
I.V. continuous infusion	12-24 h after initiation of infusion
P.O. liquid, fast-release formulation	Peak: 1 h postdose after at least 1 day of therapy Trough: Just before a dose after at least 1 day of therapy

[1]The time to achieve steady-state serum levels is prolonged in patients with longer half-lives (eg, premature neonates, infants, and adults with cardiac or liver failure (see theophylline half-life table). In these patients, serum theophylline levels should be drawn after 48-72 hours of therapy; serum levels may need to be done prior to steady-state to assess the patient's current progress or evaluate potential toxicity.

Approximate I.V. maintenance dosages are based upon **continuous infusions**; intermittent dosing (often used in children <6 months of age) may be determined by multiplying the hourly infusion rate by 24 hours and dividing by the desired number of doses/day (usually in 3-4 doses/day)

6 weeks to 6 months: 0.5 mg/kg/hour

6 months to 1 year: 0.6-0.7 mg/kg/hour

1-9 years: 1-1.2 mg/kg/hour

9-12 years and young adult smokers: 0.9 mg/kg/hour

(Continued)

Aminophylline *(Continued)*

12-16 years: 0.7 mg/kg/hour

Adults (healthy, nonsmoking): 0.7 mg/kg/hour

Older patients and patients with cor pulmonale, patients with CHF or liver failure: 0.25 mg/kg/hour

Oral dose: See Theophylline *on page 1520*, (consider mg theophylline available when using aminophylline products)

Dosage should be adjusted according to serum level measurements during the first 12- to 24-hour period. See table on previous page.

Administration

Oral: May be administered without regard to meals

Parenteral: Do not administer I.M. (I.M. administration causes intense pain); dilute with I.V. fluid to a concentration of 1 mg/mL and infuse over 20-30 minutes; maximum concentration: 25 mg/mL; maximum rate of infusion: 0.36 mg/kg/minute, and not to exceed 25 mg/minute

Monitoring Parameters Serum theophylline levels, heart rate, respiratory rate, number and severity of apnea spells (when used for apnea of prematurity); arterial or capillary blood gases (if applicable); pulmonary function tests

Reference Range Therapeutic: For asthma 10-20 mcg/mL; for neonatal apnea 6-13 mcg/mL (serum levels are reduced for neonatal apnea due to decreased binding of theophylline to fetal albumin resulting in a greater amount of free "active" theophylline)

Dosage Forms Excipient information presented when available (limited, particularly for generics); consult specific product labeling.

Injection, solution, as dihydrate: 25 mg/mL (10 mL, 20 mL)

Tablet, as dihydrate: 100 mg, 200 mg

References

Bhatt-Mehta V and Schumacher RE, "Treatment of Apnea of Prematurity," *Paediatr Drugs*, 2003, 5(3):195-210.

"National Asthma Education and Prevention Program. Expert Panel Report: Guidelines for the Diagnosis and Management of Asthma Update on Selected Topics--2002," *J Allergy Clin Immunol*, 2002, 110(5 Suppl):S141-219.

◆ **5-Aminosalicylic Acid** *see* Mesalamine *on page 1011*

◆ **Aminoxin® [OTC]** *see* Pyridoxine *on page 1353*

Amiodarone (a MEE oh da rone)

Medication Safety Issues

Sound-alike/look-alike issues:

Amiodarone may be confused with amiloride, amrinone

Cordarone® may be confused with Cardura®, Cordran®

High alert medication: The Institute for Safe Medication Practices (ISMP) includes this medication among its list of drugs which have a heightened risk of causing significant patient harm when used in error.

Related Information

CPR Pediatric Drug Dosages *on page 1650*

Pediatric ALS Algorithms *on page 1657*

U.S. Brand Names Cordarone®; Pacerone®

Canadian Brand Names Alti-Amiodarone; Amiodarone Hydrochloride for Injection®; Apo-Amiodarone®; Cordarone®; Gen-Amiodarone; Novo-Amiodarone; PMS-Amiodarone; Rhoxal-amiodarone; Sandoz-Amiodarone

Index Terms Amiodarone Hydrochloride

Therapeutic Category Antiarrhythmic Agent, Class III

Generic Available Yes

Use

Oral: Management of life-threatening recurrent ventricular arrhythmias [eg, recurrent ventricular fibrillation (VF) or recurrent hemodynamically unstable ventricular tachycardia (VT)] unresponsive to other therapy or in patients intolerant to other therapy

I.V.: Initiation of management and prophylaxis of frequently recurrent VF and hemodynamically unstable VT unresponsive to other therapy; VF and VT in patients requiring amiodarone who are not able to take oral therapy

Note: Also has been used to treat supraventricular arrhythmias unresponsive to other therapy. Amiodarone is recommended in the PALS guidelines for SVT (unresponsive to vagal maneuvers and adenosine). It is recommended in both the PALS and ACLS guidelines for cardiac arrest with pulseless VT or VF (unresponsive to defibrillation, CPR, and vasopressor administration) and control of hemodynamically-stable VT or wide-complex tachycardia of uncertain origin. The drug is also recommended in the ACLS guidelines for re-entry SVT (unresponsive to vagal maneuvers and adenosine); control of rapid ventricular rate due to conduction via an accessory pathway in pre-excited atrial arrhythmias; and control of polymorphic VT with a normal QT interval. A benzyl alcohol free and polysorbate free injectable product is currently under development.

Medication Guide An FDA-approved patient medication guide, which is available with the product information and at http://www.fda.gov/cder/Offices/ODS/medication_guides.htm, must be dispensed with this medication for each new outpatient prescription and refill for oral administration.

Pregnancy Risk Factor D

Lactation Enters breast milk/not recommended (AAP rates "of concern")

Contraindications Hypersensitivity to amiodarone, iodine, or any component (see Warnings); severe sinus node dysfunction; marked sinus bradycardia, second or third degree A-V block; cardiogenic shock; bradycardia-induced syncope, except if pacemaker is placed

Warnings Not considered first-line antiarrhythmic due to high incidence of toxicity; 75% of patients experience adverse effects with large doses. Discontinuation is required in 5% to 20% of patients. Pulmonary and hepatic toxicities may be fatal (see Adverse Reactions); reserve for use in life-threatening arrhythmias refractory to other therapy. Amiodarone may worsen or precipitate arrhythmias, including torsade de pointes; when possible, hypokalemia and hypomagnesemia should be corrected prior to I.V. amiodarone use due to increased risk for torsade de pointes. Amiodarone is a potent inhibitor of cytochrome P450 enzymes and p-glycoprotein; serious drug interactions may occur (see Drug Interactions); prolongation of the QT interval, with or without torsade de pointes, has been reported in patients receiving amiodarone concomitantly with macrolide antibiotics, azoles, or fluroquinolones. Hypotension with I.V. product occurs in about 16% of patients, may be associated with infusion rate, and may be fatal. Bradycardia and AV block may occur; temporary pacemaker should be available when I.V. product is used in patients with known predisposition to bradycardia or AV block. Patients should be hospitalized for initiation of therapy and loading dose administration. Optic neuropathy and/or optic neuritis resulting in visual impairment may occur at any time and can progress to permanent blindness; prompt ophthalmic exam is recommended if visual impairment occurs; re-evaluate amiodarone therapy if optic neuropathy or neuritis occurs. Corneal refractive laser surgery is generally contraindicated in patients receiving amiodarone (per manufacturers of the laser surgery devices).

Injectable products (Cordarone® and generic) contain polysorbate (Tween®) 80 and benzyl alcohol; benzyl alcohol may cause allergic reactions in susceptible individuals; large amounts of benzyl alcohol (≥99 mg/kg/day) have been associated with a potentially fatal toxicity ("gasping syndrome") in neonates; the "gasping syndrome" consists of metabolic acidosis, respiratory distress, gasping respirations, CNS dysfunction (including convulsions, intracranial hemorrhage), hypotension and cardiovascular collapse; use amiodarone products containing benzyl alcohol with caution in neonates (see also Precautions); a benzyl alcohol free and polysorbate free injection is currently under development; *in vitro* and animal studies have shown that benzoate, a metabolite of benzyl alcohol, displaces bilirubin from protein binding sites

Precautions Amiodarone HCl contains 37% iodine by weight; avoid use during pregnancy and while breast-feeding (fetal/neonatal goiters, hypothyroidism, and possible cerebral damage may occur); amiodarone may cause hypothyroidism or hyperthyroidism; hyperthyroidism may result in potentially fatal thyrotoxicosis or breakthrough or aggravation of potentially fatal arrhythmias; consider the possibility of hyperthyroidism if any new signs of arrhythmia appear; use with caution and monitor thyroid function closely in patients with thyroid disease (**Note:** Oral amiodarone has caused dose-related thyroid tumors in rats; cases of thyroid nodules/thyroid cancer have been reported in patients treated with amiodarone; hyperthyroidism was also present in some of these patients).

Safety and efficacy of amiodarone have not been established in pediatric patients. I.V. amiodarone has been shown to leach out plasticizers [eg, DEHP or di-(2-ethylhexyl)phthalate] from I.V. tubing, including polyvinyl chloride tubing. Polysorbate (Tween®) 80, an ingredient found in I.V. amiodarone, is also known to leach DEHP from polyvinyl chloride tubing. In immature animals, exposure to DEHP may adversely affect the development of the male reproductive tract. In order to decrease the potential exposure of infants to plasticizers, consider the use of bolus dosing in 1 mg/kg aliquots as described by Perry, 1996; see Usual Dosage. See also http://www.fda.gov/medwatch/safety/2001/safety01.htm#cordar.

Adverse Reactions

Cardiovascular: Proarrhythmia (including torsade de pointes), atropine-resistant bradycardia, heart block, sinus arrest, myocardial depression, CHF, paroxysmal ventricular tachycardia, cardiogenic shock, hypotension [**Note:** Hypotension may be potentially fatal with I.V. use; in adults, I.V. daily doses >2100 mg are associated with a greater risk of hypotension; in pediatric patients 30 days-15 years of age (n=61), dose-related cardiovascular adverse reactions were common (hypotension

(Continued)

Amiodarone *(Continued)*

36%, bradycardia 20%, and AV block 15%) and in some cases severe or life-threatening]

Central nervous system (20% to 40% incidence): Lack of coordination, fatigue, malaise, abnormal gait, dizziness, headache, insomnia, nightmares, ataxia, behavioral changes, fever

Dermatologic: Discoloration of skin (slate blue), photosensitivity, rash, angioedema, pruritus; skin cancer (postmarketing reports)

Endocrine & metabolic: Hypothyroidism (or less commonly hyperthyroidism, see Additional Information), hyperglycemia, elevated triglycerides, SIADH

Gastrointestinal: Nausea, vomiting, anorexia, constipation

Genitourinary: Sterile epididymitis

Hematologic: Coagulation abnormalities, thrombocytopenia; neutropenia, pancytopenia, hemolytic anemia, aplastic anemia

Hepatic: Elevated liver enzymes, elevated bilirubin, elevated serum ammonia, severe hepatic toxicity (potentially fatal); **Note:** Hepatocellular necrosis, hepatic coma, acute renal failure, and death have been associated with I.V. loading doses at much higher concentrations and I.V. rates of infusion much faster than recommended

Local: Injection site reactions (25% of pediatric patients); phlebitis (with I.V. formulation; concentration dependent)

Neuromuscular & skeletal: Paresthesia, tremor, peripheral neuropathy (rare), muscle weakness, rhabdomyolysis

Ocular: Corneal microdeposits, halos or blurred vision (10% incidence), photophobia, optic neuropathy, optic neuritis, visual impairment, permanent blindness (**Note:** Asymptomatic corneal microdeposits alone do not require dose reduction or discontinuation)

Renal: Renal impairment (postmarketing reports)

Respiratory (potentially fatal): Interstitial pneumonitis, hypersensitivity pneumonitis, pulmonary fibrosis [may present with cough, fever, dyspnea, malaise, chest x-ray changes (pulmonary infiltrates and/or mass)]; adult respiratory distress syndrome; **Note:** Use of lower amiodarone doses (loading and maintenance) may be associated with a lower incidence of pulmonary toxicity. Early onset pulmonary toxicity (ie, occurring over days to weeks) has been reported with oral amiodarone (with or without initial I.V. use) and may progress to respiratory failure or death.

Miscellaneous: Anaphylaxis, anaphylactoid reactions (including shock); thyroid nodules/thyroid cancer (postmarketing reports)

Drug Interactions Cytochrome P450 isoenzyme CYP3A3/4 and CYP2C8 substrate; isoenzyme CYP1A2, CYP2C9, CYP2D6, and CYP3A3/4 inhibitor; p-glycoprotein inhibitor

Amiodarone inhibits certain P450 enzymes and p-glycoprotein and may increase plasma concentrations of digoxin, cyclosporine, flecainide, lidocaine, methotrexate, theophylline, procainamide, quinidine, warfarin, and phenytoin resulting in toxicities. **Note:** Dosage reduction of these agents and follow-up serum concentration monitoring are recommended (eg, a 50% dosage reduction in digoxin, 30% dosage reduction in flecainide, and a 30% to 50% dosage reduction in warfarin have been recommended).

Combined use of amiodarone with beta-blockers, digitalis glycosides, or calcium channel blockers may result in bradycardia, sinus arrest and heart block; use with class I antiarrhythmics may cause ventricular arrhythmias; amiodarone and general anesthetics may result in bradycardia, hypotension, heart block; use with fentanyl may cause bradycardia, hypotension, decreased cardiac output; combined use of amiodarone with lovastatin or simvastatin may result in an increased risk of myopathy or rhabdomyolysis (dosage reduction of lovastatin or simvastatin is recommended); amiodarone may inhibit the metabolism of dextromethorphan; use of amiodarone with fluindione (an oral vitamin K antagonist) may result in increased bleeding; amiodarone may decrease the metabolism of clopidogrel to its active metabolite and result in ineffective inhibition of platelet aggregation. Phenytoin, rifampin and cholestyramine may decrease and cimetidine may increase amiodarone serum levels. Protease inhibitors may increase the serum concentration of amiodarone; monitor patients receiving concomitant indinavir closely; concurrent use of amiodarone with ritonavir or nelfinavir is not recommended.

The herbal medicine St John's wort (*Hypericum perforatum*) may significantly decrease concentrations of amiodarone and is **not** recommended for concurrent use. Concomitant use with antiarrhythmic agents or other drugs that prolong the QT interval may cause arrhythmias, including torsade de pointes; reserve the combined use of amiodarone with other antiarrhythmic agents for life-threatening ventricular arrhythmias in patients who do not completely respond to a single agent; carefully evaluate the risks and benefits of concurrent use of any drug known to prolong the QT interval (including macrolide antibiotics, azoles, and fluroquinolones), see Warnings; QT prolongation and torsade de pointes have been reported with the concurrent use of amiodarone and loratadine or trazodone. **Note:** Due to the long half-life of amiodarone, drug interactions may potentially occur even after discontinuation of amiodarone.

Food Interactions Food increases rate and extent of oral absorption (high fat meal increased AUC by a mean of 2.3 times). Grapefruit juice increases oral amiodarone AUC by 50% and peak serum concentrations by 84%; avoid grapefruit juice during amiodarone therapy.

Stability

Storage:

Tablets: Store at controlled room temperature; protect from light; dispense in a light-resistant, tightly closed container

Injection: Store at controlled room temperature; protect from light during storage; protect from excessive heat; there is no need to protect diluted solutions from light during I.V. administration

Compatibility: Injection is compatible in D_5W at concentrations of 1-6 mg/mL for 24 hours in glass or polyolefin bottles and for 2 hours in polyvinyl chloride bags; although amiodarone adsorbs to polyvinyl chloride tubing, all clinical studies used polyvinyl chloride tubing and the recommended doses take adsorption into account, therefore, in adults, polyvinyl chloride tubing is recommended; amiodarone I.V. in D_5W is **not** compatible with aminophylline, cefamandole, cefazolin, mezlocillin, heparin, or sodium bicarbonate when administered together at the Y-site (a precipitate will occur)

Mechanism of Action A class III antiarrhythmic agent which inhibits adrenergic stimulation (possesses alpha- and beta-adrenergic-blocking properties); affects sodium, potassium, and calcium channels; prolongs the action potential and refractory period in myocardial tissue; decreases A-V conduction and sinus node function; possesses vasodilatory and negative inotropic effects

Pharmacodynamics

Onset of action: Oral: 2-3 days to 1-3 weeks after starting therapy; I.V.: (electrophysiologic effects) within hours; antiarrhythmic effects: 2-3 days to 1-3 weeks; mean onset of effect may be shorter in children vs adults and in patients receiving I.V. loading doses

Maximum effect: Oral: 1 week to 5 months

Duration of effects after discontinuation of oral therapy: Variable, 2 weeks to months: Children: less than a few weeks; adults: several months

Pharmacokinetics

Absorption: Oral: Slow and incomplete

Distribution: Amiodarone and its active metabolite cross the placenta; both distribute to breast milk in concentrations higher than maternal plasma concentrations

I.V.: Rapid redistribution with a decrease to 10% of peak values within 30-45 minutes after completion of infusion

V_{dss}: I.V. single dose in adults: Mean range: 40-84 L/kg

V_d: Oral dose in adults: 66 L/kg: range: 18-148 L/kg

Protein binding: >96%

Metabolism: In the liver and possibly the GI tract via cytochrome P450 enzymes; the major metabolite N-desethylamiodarone is active

Bioavailability: Oral: ~50% (range: 35% to 65%)

Half-life:

Amiodarone:

Single dose in adults: Mean: 58 days (range 15-142 days)

Oral chronic therapy in adults: Mean range: 40-55 days (range: 26-107 days)

I.V. single dose in adults: Mean range: 20-47 days

Half-life is shortened in children vs adults

N-desethylamiodarone (active metabolite):

Single dose in adults: Mean: 36 days (range 14-75 days)

Oral chronic therapy in adults: Mean: 61 days

Elimination: Via biliary excretion; possible enterohepatic recirculation; <1% excreted unchanged in urine

Dialysis: Nondialyzable (parent and metabolite)

Usual Dosage

Infants and Children:

Oral: **Note:** Calculate dose using body surface area for children <1 year of age: Loading dose: 10-15 mg/kg/day or 600-800 mg/1.73 m^2/day in 1-2 divided doses/day for 4-14 days or until adequate control of arrhythmia or prominent adverse effects occur; dosage should then be reduced to 5 mg/kg/day or 200-400 mg/1.73 m^2/day given once daily for several weeks; if arrhythmia does not recur, reduce to lowest effective dosage possible; usual daily minimal dose: 2.5 mg/kg; maintenance doses may be given for 5 of 7 days/week.

(Continued)

Amiodarone *(Continued)*

Note: A more aggressive dosing regimen was used in neonates and infants (n=50; (mean age: 1 ± 1.5 months) <9 months of age, treated for various types of SVT; 90% of patients at discharge and 100% of patients within 3 months of discharge were free of tachycardia; however, patients who received a higher loading dose (20 mg/kg/day in 2 divided doses) were more likely to have a prolongation of the corrected QT interval (see Etheridge, 2001); further studies are needed.

I.V., I.O.: **Note:** Use with caution when administering amiodarone with other drugs that prolong the QT interval (consider consulting expert)

PALS dose for treatment of pulseless VT or VF: 5 mg/kg rapid I.V. bolus or I.O.; may repeat up to 15 mg/kg; maximum: 300 mg

PALS dose for treatment of perfusing tachycardias: 5 mg/kg I.V. given over 20-60 minutes or I.O.; may repeat up to 15 mg/kg; maximum: 300 mg

I.V.: Limited data is available. Four retrospective studies (Figa, 1994; Raja, 1994; Soult, 1995; Celiker, 1998) used I.V. loading doses of 5 mg/kg. Loading doses were administered over 1 hour in three of these studies to treat various life-threatening tachyarrhythmias including junctional ectopic tachycardia after cardiac surgery (in conjunction with atrial pacing). Soult 1995 used I.V. amiodarone for short-term treatment of paroxysmal supraventricular tachycardia (PSVT) and administered the loading dose via slow I.V. bolus over 5 minutes. For continuous infusion, Figa 1994 and Celiker 1998, used initial maintenance doses of 5 mcg/kg/minute (7.2 mg/kg/day) which was increased incrementally until the desired effect was seen or a maximum dose of 15 mcg/kg/minute (21.6 mg/kg/day) was reached. The mean effective dose in the study by Figa 1994 (n=30) was 9.5 mcg/kg/minute (13.7 mg/kg/day) and in Celiker 1998 (n=12) was 10 ± 4.7 mcg/kg/minute (range: 5-15 mcg/kg/minute).

A multicenter study (Perry, 1996; n=40; mean age 5.4 years with 24 of 40 children <2 years of age) used an I.V. loading dose of 5 mg/kg that was divided into five 1 mg/kg aliquots, with each aliquot given over 5-10 minutes. Additional 1-5 mg/kg doses could be administered 30 minutes later in a similar fashion if needed. The mean loading dose was 6.3 mg/kg. A maintenance dose (continuous infusion of 10-15 mg/kg/day) was administered to 21 of the 40 patients. Further studies are needed.

Adults:

ACLS dose for cardiac arrest due to pulseless VT or VF: I.V., I.O.: Initial: 300 mg diluted in 20-30 mL D_5W or NS given rapid I.V. push or given I.O.; one supplemental bolus dose of 150 mg given by rapid I.V. infusion or I.O. may be given for recurring VF or pulseless VT

ACLS doses for perfusing tachycardias: I.V.: See manufacturer's recommendations below for ventricular arrhythmias, for loading dose and continuous infusion; ACLS also recommends: Bolus doses for hemodynamically stable VT or wide QRS tachycardia of uncertain origin (regular rhythm): 150 mg given over 10 minutes; may repeat as needed to a maximum of 2.2 g/24 hours; for pre-excited atrial fibrillation: Consider 150 mg I.V. over 10 minutes

Ventricular arrhythmias (manufacturer's recommendations):

Oral: Loading dose: 800-1600 mg/day divided in 1-2 doses/day for 1-3 weeks, then 600-800 mg/day in 1-2 doses/day for 1 month; maintenance: 400 mg/day; lower doses are recommended for supraventricular arrhythmias.

I.V.: Loading dose: 1050 mg delivered over 24 hours as follows: 150 mg given over 10 minutes (at a rate of 15 mg/minute) followed by 360 mg given over 6 hours (at a rate of 1 mg/minute); follow with maintenance dose: 540 mg given over the next 18 hours (at a rate of 0.5 mg/minute); after the first 24 hours the maintenance dose is continued at 0.5 mg/minute; additional supplemental bolus doses of 150 mg infused over 10 minutes may be given for breakthrough VF or hemodynamically unstable VT; maintenance dose infusion may be increased to control arrhythmia; maximum daily dose: 2.1 g

Atrial fibrillation (see Goldschlager, 2000):

Oral: Loading dose: 600-800 mg/day divided in 2 doses/day for 2-4 weeks, then 400 mg/day; at 3-6 months, dose may be reduced further to 100-300 mg/day based on clinical efficacy and adverse effects; usual maintenance: 200 mg/day; **Note:** some patients may require higher maintenance doses or increased maintenance doses for short periods of time for breakthrough arrhythmias; some patients can be maintained with 200 mg/day given for 5 of 7 days/week

Transition from I.V. to oral therapy: Optimal initial daily dose depends on I.V. dose administered and oral bioavailability; use the following as a guide for an initial daily dose, assuming patient received 0.5 mg/minute for the listed duration of I.V. infusion:

<1 week infusion: 800-1600 mg/day

1-3 week infusion: 600-800 mg/day

>3 week infusion: 400 mg/day

Dosing adjustment in renal impairment: No adjustment necessary

Administration

Oral: Administer at same time in relation to meals; do not administer with grapefruit juice

I.V.: Adjust administration rate to patient's clinical condition and urgency; give slowly to patients who have a pulse (ie, perfusing arrhythmia); may be given rapidly to patients with ventricular fibrillation or in cardiac arrest. Do not exceed recommended I.V. concentrations or rates of infusion (severe hepatic toxicity may occur; see Adverse Reactions). Slow the infusion rate if hypotension or bradycardia develops. Injection must be diluted before I.V. use. Adults: Usual dilutions: First loading infusion: 150 mg in 100 mL D_5W (1.5 mg/mL) for infusion over 10 minutes; then 900 mg in 500 mL D_5W (1.8 mg/mL) to deliver rest of dose. Administer via central venous catheter, if possible; increased phlebitis may occur with peripheral infusions >3 mg/mL in D_5W, but concentrations ≤2.5 mg/mL may be less irritating; the use of a central venous catheter with concentrations >2 mg/mL for infusions >1 hour is recommended. Maximum concentration for infusion: 6 mg/mL. Use glass or polyolefin bottles for infusions >2 hours; the use of polyvinyl chloride tubing is recommended in adults (see Stability). Must be infused via volumetric infusion device; drop size of I.V. solution may be reduced and underdosage may occur if drop counter infusion sets are used. Use in-line filter during administration. Adults: Do not exceed 30 mg/minute initial infusion rate; infants and children: See Usual Dosage I.V. and Precautions

Monitoring Parameters Heart rate and rhythm, blood pressure, EKG, chest x-ray, pulmonary function tests, thyroid function tests (see Additional Information); serum glucose, electrolytes (especially potassium and magnesium), triglycerides, liver enzymes; ophthalmologic exams including fundoscopy and slit-lamp examinations, physical signs and symptoms of thyroid dysfunction (lethargy, edema of hands and feet, weight gain or loss), and pulmonary toxicity (dyspnea, cough; oxygen saturation, blood gases)

Reference Range Therapeutic: Chronic oral dosing: 1-2.5 mg/L (SI: 2-4 micromoles/L) (parent); desethyl metabolite (active) is present in equal concentration to parent drug; serum levels may not be of great value for predicting toxicity and efficacy; toxicity may occur even at therapeutic concentrations

Patient Information Read the patient Medication Guide that you receive with each prescription and refill of amiodarone. Report the use of other medications, nonprescription medications, and herbal or natural products to your physician and pharmacist. Avoid grapefruit juice and the herbal medicine, St John's wort. Notify physician or get medical help immediately if shortness of breath, wheezing, chest pain, spitting up of blood, yellow eyes, brown or dark-colored urine, heart pounding, lightheadedness, fainting, weakness, heat or cold intolerance, weight gain or loss, sweating, thinning of hair, changes in menses, swelling of neck (goiter), nervousness, irritability, restlessness, decreased concentration, depression, or tremor occurs. Notify physician if persistent dry cough or decreased vision occurs. May discolor skin to a slate blue color. May cause photosensitivity reactions (eg, exposure to sunlight may cause severe sunburn, skin rash, redness, or itching); avoid exposure to sunlight and artificial light sources (sunlamps, tanning booth/bed); wear protective clothing, wide-brimmed hats, sunglasses, and lip sunscreen (SPF ≥15); use a sunscreen [broad-spectrum sunscreen or physical sunscreen (preferred) or sunblock with SPF ≥15]; contact physician if reaction occurs.

Nursing Implications Ambulation of patient may be impaired due to adverse effects; due to possible infusion rate-related hypotension, the I.V. infusion rate should be carefully monitored

Additional Information Intoxication with amiodarone necessitates EKG monitoring; bradycardia may be atropine resistant, I.V. isoproterenol or cardiac pacemaker may be required; hypotension, cardiogenic shock, heart block, QT prolongation and hepatotoxicity may also be seen; patients should be monitored for several days following overdose due to long half-life

I.V. product is used for acute treatment; the duration of I.V. treatment is usually 48-96 hours, however, in adults, infusions may be used cautiously for 2-3 weeks; there is limited experience with administering infusions for >3 weeks

Use of amiodarone 300 mg I.V. in adults with cardiac arrest (out-of-hospital) due to refractory ventricular arrhythmias improved the rate of survival to hospital admission (see Kudenchuk, 1999). In a randomized, double blind, placebo controlled trial in adults with shock-resistant ventricular fibrillation (out-of-hospital), I.V. amiodarone [initial dose: 5 mg/kg; second dose (if needed): 2.5 mg/kg] resulted in higher rates of survival to hospital admission as compared to I.V. lidocaine [initial dose: 1.5 mg/kg; second dose (if needed): 1.5 mg/kg] (see Dorian, 2002).

(Continued)

Amiodarone *(Continued)*

Thyroid function tests: Amiodarone partially inhibits the peripheral conversion of thyroxine (T_4) to triiodothyronine (T_3); serum T_4 and reverse triiodothyronine (RT_3) concentrations may be increased and serum T_3 may be decreased; most patients remain clinically euthyroid, however, clinical hypothyroidism or hyperthyroidism may occur. **Note:** Amiodarone HCl contains 37% iodine by weight and is a potential source of large amounts of iodine; ~3 mg of inorganic iodine per 100 mg of amiodarone is released into the systemic circulation (RDA for iodine in Adults is 150 mcg).

Dosage Forms Excipient information presented when available (limited, particularly for generics); consult specific product labeling. [DSC] = Discontinued product

Injection, solution, as hydrochloride: 50 mg/mL (3 mL, 9 mL, 18 mL) [contains benzyl alcohol and polysorbate (Tween®) 80] [DSC]

Cordarone®: 50 mg/mL (3 mL) [contains benzyl alcohol and polysorbate (Tween®) 80]

Tablet, as hydrochloride [scored]: 200 mg, 400 mg

Cordarone®: 200 mg

Pacerone®: 100 mg [not scored], 200 mg, 300 mg [DSC], 400 mg

Extemporaneous Preparations

A 5 mg/mL oral suspension can be made from tablets; two stability studies using different vehicles exist; a 5 mg/mL oral suspension made with simple syrup NF containing methylcellulose 1% (50:50, v/v) was stable for 42 days at room temperature (25°C) and 91 days under refrigeration (4°C) in both glass and plastic prescription bottles (Nahata, 1997); label "shake well" and "protect from light"

Five 200 mg tablets were crushed in a mortar; the vehicle (either a 1:1 mixture of Ora-Sweet® and Ora-Plus® or a 1:1 mixture of Ora-Sweet® SF and Ora-Plus®) was adjusted to a pH between 6-7 using a sodium bicarbonate solution (5 g/100 mL of distilled water). A small amount of the vehicle was added to the mortar to make a uniform paste; geometric amounts of the vehicle were added while mixing to **almost** the desired volume; suspension was transferred to a graduate and qsad to 200 mL while mixing. Suspensions prepared in both vehicles were stable for 42 days at room temperature (25°C) and 91 days under refrigeration (4°C) in plastic prescription bottles (Nahata 1999); label "shake well" and "protect from light"

Neither of these 2 studies determined microbial growth; extended storage under refrigeration is recommended

Nahata MC, "Stability of Amiodarone in an Oral Suspension Stored Under Refrigeration and at Room Temperature," *Ann Pharmacother*, 1997, 31(7-8):851-2.

Nahata MC, Morosco RS, and Hipple TF, "Stability of Amiodarone in Extemporaneous Oral Suspensions Prepared From Commercially Available Vehicles," *J Ped Pharmacy Practice*, 1999, 4(4):186-9.

References

American Heart Association Emergency Cardiovascular Care Committee, " 2005 American Heart Association (AHA) Guidelines for Cardiopulmonary Resuscitation (CPR) and Emergency Cardiovascular Care (ECC), Part 7.2: Management of Cardiac Arrest, Part 7.3: Management of Symptomatic Bradycardia and Tachycardia, and Part 12: Pediatric Advanced Life Support," *Circulation*, 2005, 112(24 Suppl):IV58-77,167-87.

Celiker A, Ceviz N, and Ozme S, "Effectiveness and Safety of Intravenous Amiodarone in Drug-Resistant Tachyarrhythmias of Children," *Acta Paediatr Jpn*, 1998, 40(6):567-72.

Coumel P and Fidelle J, "Amiodarone in the Treatment of Cardiac Arrhythmias in Children: One Hundred Thirty-Five Cases," *Am Heart J*, 1980, 100(6 Pt 2):1063-9.

Dorian P, Cass D, Schwartz B, et al, "Amiodarone as Compared With Lidocaine for Shock-Resistant Ventricular Fibrillation," *N Engl J Med*, 2002, 346(12):884-90.

Drago F, Mazza A, Guccione P, et al, "Amiodarone Used Alone or in Combination With Propranolol: A Very Effective Therapy for Tachyarrhythmias in Infants and Children," *Pediatr Cardiol*, 1998, 19(6):445-9.

Etheridge SP, Craig JE, and Compton SJ, "Amiodarone is Safe and Highly Effective Therapy for Supraventricular Tachycardia in Infants," *Am Heart J*, 2001, 141(1):105-10.

Figa FH, Gow RM, Hamilton RM, et al, "Clinical Efficacy and Safety of Intravenous Amiodarone in Infants and Children," *Am J Cardiol*, 1994, 74(6):573-7.

Garson A Jr, Gillette PC, McVey P, et al, "Amiodarone Treatment of Critical Arrhythmias in Children and Young Adults," *J Am Coll Cardiol*, 1984, 4(4):749-55.

Goldschlager N, Epstein AE, Naccarelli G, et al, "Practical Guidelines for Clinicians Who Treat Patients With Amiodarone," *Arch Intern Med*, 2000, 160(12):1741-8.

Kudenchuk PJ, Cobb LA, Copass MK, et al, "Amiodarone for Resuscitation After Out-of-Hospital Cardiac Arrest Due to Ventricular Fibrillation," *N Engl J Med*, 1999, 341(12):871-8.

Paul T and Guccione P, "New Antiarrhythmic Drugs in Pediatric Use: Amiodarone," *Pediatr Cardiol*, 1994, 15(3):132-8.

Perry JC, Fenrich AL, Hulse JE, et al, "Pediatric Use of Intravenous Amiodarone: Efficacy and Safety in Critically Ill Patients From a Multicenter Protocol," *J Am Coll Cardiol*, 1996, 27(5):1246-50.

Raja P, Hawker RE, Chaikitpinyo A, et al, "Amiodarone Management of Junctional Ectopic Tachycardia After Cardiac Surgery in Children," *Br Heart J*, 1994, 72(3):261-5.

Shahar E, Barzilay Z, Frand M, et al, "Amiodarone in Control of Sustained Tachyarrhythmias in Children With Wolff-Parkinson-White Syndrome," *Pediatrics*, 1983, 72(6):813-6.

Shuler CO, Case CL, and Gillette PC, "Efficacy and Safety of Amiodarone in Infants," *Am Heart J*, 1993, 125(5 Pt 1):1430-2.

Soult JA, Munoz M, Lopez JD, et al, "Efficacy and Safety of Intravenous Amiodarone for Short-Term Treatment of Paroxysmal Supraventricular Tachycardia in Children," *Pediatr Cardiol*, 1995, 16(1):16-9.

♦ **Amiodarone Hydrochloride** *see* Amiodarone *on page 100*

- **Amiodarone Hydrochloride for Injection® (Can)** *see* Amiodarone *on page 100*
- **Amitone® [OTC] [DSC]** *see* Calcium Supplements *on page 272*

Amitriptyline (a mee TRIP ti leen)

Medication Safety Issues
Sound-alike/look-alike issues:
Amitriptyline may be confused with aminophylline, imipramine, nortriptyline
Elavil® may be confused with Aldoril®, Eldepryl®, enalapril, Equanil®, Mellaril®, Oruvail®, Plavix®

Related Information
Antidepressant Agents *on page 1681*
Medications for Which A Single Dose May Be Fatal When Ingested By A Toddler *on page 1932*
Overdose and Toxicology *on page 1916*
Serotonin Syndrome *on page 1955*

Canadian Brand Names Apo-Amitriptyline®; Levate®; Novo-Triptyn; PMS-Amitriptyline

Index Terms Amitriptyline Hydrochloride; Elavil

Therapeutic Category Antidepressant, Tricyclic; Antimigraine Agent

Generic Available Yes

Use Treatment of various forms of depression, often in conjunction with psychotherapy; analgesic for certain chronic and neuropathic pain; migraine prophylaxis

Medication Guide An FDA-approved patient medication guide, which is available with the product information and at http://www.fda.gov/cder/Offices/ODS/medication_guides.htm, must be dispensed with this medication for each new outpatient prescription and refill.

Pregnancy Risk Factor C

Lactation Enters breast milk/not recommended (AAP rates "of concern")

Contraindications Hypersensitivity to amitriptyline (cross-sensitivity with other tricyclics may occur) or any component; narrow-angle glaucoma; use of MAO inhibitors within 14 days (potentially fatal reactions may occur, see Drug Interactions); concurrent use of cisapride; use during acute recovery phase after MI

Warnings Amitriptyline is not approved for use in pediatric patients. Clinical worsening of depression or suicidal ideation and behavior may occur in children and adults with major depressive disorder. In clinical trials, antidepressants increased the risk of suicidal thinking and behavior (suicidality) in children, adolescents, and young adults (18-24 years of age) with major depressive disorder and other psychiatric disorders. This risk must be considered before prescribing antidepressants for any clinical use. Short-term studies did **not** show an increased risk of suicidality with antidepressant use in patients >24 years of age and showed a decreased risk in patients ≥65 years.

Patients of all ages who are treated with antidepressants for any indication require appropriate monitoring and close observation for clinical worsening of depression, suicidality, and unusual changes in behavior, especially during the first few months after antidepressant initiation or when the dose is adjusted. Family members and caregivers should be instructed to closely observe the patient (ie, daily) and communicate condition with healthcare provider. Patients should also be monitored for associated behaviors (eg, anxiety, agitation, panic attacks, insomnia, irritability, hostility, aggressiveness, impulsivity, akathisia, hypomania, mania) which may increase the risk for worsening depression or suicidality. Worsening depression or emergence of suicidality (or associated behaviors listed above) that is abrupt in onset, severe, or not part of the presenting symptoms, may require discontinuation or modification of drug therapy.

Do not discontinue abruptly in patients receiving high doses chronically (withdrawal symptoms may occur; see Adverse Reactions). To reduce risk of intentional overdose, write prescriptions for the smallest quantity consistent with good patient care. Screen individuals for bipolar disorder prior to treatment (using antidepressants alone may induce manic episodes in patients with this condition). May worsen psychosis in some patients.

Precautions Use with caution in patients with cardiac conduction disturbances, cardiovascular disease, seizure disorders, diabetes mellitus, narrow-angle glaucoma, increased intraocular pressure, history of urinary retention or bowel obstruction, hepatic or renal dysfunction, hyperthyroidism or those receiving thyroid hormone replacement; degree of sedation, anticholinergic effects, and risk of orthostatic hypotension are very high relative to other antidepressants; manufacturer does not recommend use in children <12 years of age

Adverse Reactions Anticholinergic effects may be pronounced; moderate to marked sedation can occur (tolerance to these effects usually occurs)
(Continued)

Amitriptyline *(Continued)*

Cardiovascular: Postural hypotension, arrhythmias, tachycardia, sudden death, cardiomyopathy (very rare)

Central nervous system: Sedation, fatigue, anxiety, confusion, insomnia, impaired cognitive function, seizures; extrapyramidal symptoms are possible; suicidal thinking and behavior (see Warnings)

Dermatologic: Photosensitivity, urticaria, rash

Endocrine & metabolic: SIADH (rare), weight gain, hyperglycemia, hypoglycemia

Gastrointestinal: Xerostomia, constipation, decrease of lower esophageal sphincter tone, GE reflux, increased appetite

Genitourinary: Urinary retention, discoloration of urine (blue-green)

Hematologic: Rarely agranulocytosis, leukopenia, eosinophilia

Hepatic: Elevated liver enzymes, cholestatic jaundice

Neuromuscular & skeletal: Tremor, weakness

Ocular: Blurred vision, increased intraocular pressure

Miscellaneous: Allergic reactions; withdrawal symptoms following abrupt discontinuation (headache, nausea, malaise)

Drug Interactions Cytochrome P450 isoenzyme CYP1A2, CYP2C9, CYP2C19, CYP2D6 and CYP3A3/4 substrate

Amitriptyline may decrease the effects of clonidine and guanethidine; with clonidine, hypertensive crisis may occur following discontinuation of clonidine; amitriptyline may increase the effects of CNS depressants (including alcohol), adrenergic agents (epinephrine, isoproterenol), anticholinergic agents and warfarin. With MAO inhibitors, hyperpyrexia, tachycardia, hypertension, confusion, seizures, and death have been reported. The herbal medicine St John's wort (*Hypericum perforatum*) may increase serious side effects; its use is **not** recommended. Cimetidine, fluoxetine, quinidine, propafenone, flecainide, paroxetine, and methylphenidate may decrease the metabolism and phenobarbital, carbamazepine, and rifampin may increase the metabolism of amitriptyline; amitriptyline may potentiate the cardiac effects of cisapride (do not administer concurrently); concurrent use of high-dose TCAs and ritonavir may cause the serotonin syndrome; concomitant use with disulfiram may cause delirium

Food Interactions Riboflavin dietary requirements may be increased; increased dietary fiber may decrease drug effect

Mechanism of Action Increases the synaptic concentration of serotonin and/or norepinephrine in the CNS by inhibition of their reuptake by the presynaptic neuronal membrane

Pharmacodynamics Onset of action: Therapeutic antidepressant effects begin in 7-21 days; maximum effects may not occur for ≥2 weeks and as long as 4-6 weeks

Pharmacokinetics

Absorption: Oral: Rapid, well absorbed

Distribution: Crosses placenta; enters breast milk

Protein binding: >90%

Metabolism: In the liver to nortriptyline (active), hydroxy derivatives and conjugated derivatives

Half-life, adults: 9-25 hours (15-hour average)

Time to peak serum concentration: Within 4 hours

Elimination: Renal excretion of 18% as unchanged drug; small amounts eliminated in feces by bile

Dialysis: Nondialyzable

Usual Dosage Oral:

Chronic pain management: Children: Initial: 0.1 mg/kg at bedtime, may advance as tolerated over 2-3 weeks to 0.5-2 mg/kg at bedtime

Depressive disorders: **Note:** Not FDA approved for use in pediatric patients; controlled clinical trials have not shown tricyclic antidepressants to be superior to placebo for the treatment of depression in children and adolescents (see Dopheide, 2006 and Wagner, 2005).

Children: Investigationally initial doses of 1 mg/kg/day given in 3 divided doses with increases to 1.5 mg/kg/day have been reported in a small number of children (n=9) 9-12 years of age; clinically, doses up to 3 mg/kg/day (5 mg/kg/day if monitored closely) have been proposed

Adolescents: Initial: 25-50 mg/day; may give in divided doses; increase gradually to 100 mg/day in divided doses; maximum dose: 200 mg/day

Migraine prophylaxis: Children: Limited studies exist; one small study (n=24; mean age: 8 years; range: 6-12 years) used increasing doses over 5 days to reach a final dose of 1.5 mg/kg/day; effectiveness was seen in 19 of 24 patients, but 5 children dropped out of the trial due to adverse effects (see Sorge, 1982). A recent large open-label trial in 192 children (mean age 12 ± 3 years) with >3 headaches/month (61% with migraine, 8% with migraine with aura, and 10% with tension-type headaches) used an initial dose of 0.25 mg/kg/day given before bedtime; doses were increased every 2 weeks by 0.25 mg/kg/day to a final dose of 1 mg/kg/day; patients also used appropriate abortive medications and lifestyle adjustments; at initial re-evaluation (mean: 67 days after initiation of therapy), the mean number of headaches per month significantly decreased from 17.1 to 9.2; the mean duration of headaches decreased from 11.5 to 6.3 hours; continued improvement was observed at follow-up visits; minimal adverse effects were reported. **Note:** Mean final dose was 0.99 ± 0.23 mg/kg; range: 0.16-1.7 mg/kg/day; EKGs were obtained on children receiving >1 mg/kg/day or in those describing a cardiac side effect (see Hershey, 2000). Further studies are needed.

Depression: Adults: Initial: 50-100 mg/day single dose at bedtime or in divided doses; dose may be gradually increased up to 300 mg/day; once symptoms are controlled, decrease gradually to lowest effective dose

Administration Oral: May administer with food to decrease GI upset

Monitoring Parameters Heart rate, blood pressure, mental status, weight. Monitor patient periodically for symptom resolution; monitor for worsening depression, suicidality, and associated behaviors (especially at the beginning of therapy or when doses are increased or decreased; see Warnings).

Reference Range Note: Plasma levels do not always correlate with clinical effectiveness

Therapeutic:

Amitriptyline plus nortriptyline (active metabolite): 100-250 ng/mL (SI: 360-900 nmol/L)

Nortriptyline 50-150 ng/mL (SI: 190-570 nmol/L)

Toxic: >500 ng/mL (SI: >1800 nmol/L)

Patient Information Read the patient Medication Guide that you receive with each prescription and refill of amitriptyline. An increased risk of suicidal thinking and behavior has been reported with the use of antidepressants in children, adolescents, and young adults (18-24 years of age). Notify physician if you feel more depressed, have thoughts of suicide, or become more agitated or irritable (see Warnings). Avoid alcohol and the herbal medicine St John's wort; limit caffeine intake; may cause drowsiness and impair ability to perform activities requiring mental alertness or physical coordination; may cause dry mouth; do not discontinue abruptly; may discolor urine to a blue-green color. May cause photosensitivity reactions (eg, exposure to sunlight may cause severe sunburn, skin rash, redness, or itching); avoid exposure to sunlight and artificial light sources (sunlamps, tanning booth/bed); wear protective clothing, wide-brimmed hats, sunglasses, and lip sunscreen (SPF ≥15); use a sunscreen [broad-spectrum sunscreen or physical sunscreen (preferred) or sunblock with SPF ≥15]; contact physician if reaction occurs.

Additional Information Due to promotion of weight gain with amitriptyline, other antidepressants (ie, imipramine or desipramine) may be preferred in heavy or obese children and adolescents

Dosage Forms Excipient information presented when available (limited, particularly for generics); consult specific product labeling.

Tablet, as hydrochloride: 10 mg, 25 mg, 50 mg, 75 mg, 100 mg, 150 mg

References

Dopheide JA, "Recognizing and Treating Depression in Children and Adolescents," *Am J Health Syst Pharm*, 2006, 63(3):233-43.

Elser JM and Woody RC, "Migraine Headache in the Infant and Young Child," *Headache*, 1990, 30(6):366-8.

Hershey AD, Powers SW, Bentti AL, et al, "Effectiveness of Amitriptyline in the Prophylactic Management of Childhood Headaches," *Headache*, 2000, 40(7):539-49.

Kashani JH, Shekim WO, and Reid JC, "Amitriptyline in Children With Major Depressive Disorder: A Double-Blind Crossover Pilot Study," *J Am Acad Child Psychiatry*, 1984, 23(3):348-51.

Levy HB, Harper CR, and Weinberg WA, "A Practical Approach to Children Failing in School," *Pediatr Clin North Am*, 1992, 39(4):895-928.

Sorge F, Barone P, Steardo L, et al, "Amitriptyline as a Prophylactic for Migraine in Children," *Acta Neurol (Napoli)*, 1982, 4(5):362-7.

Wagner KD, "Pharmacotherapy for Major Depression in Children and Adolescents," *Prog Neuropsychopharmacol Biol Psychiatry*, 2005, 29(5):819-26.

♦ **Amitriptyline Hydrochloride** *see* Amitriptyline *on page 107*

♦ **AmLactin® [OTC]** *see* Lactic Acid and Ammonium Hydroxide *on page 898*

Amlodipine (am LOE di peen)

Medication Safety Issues

Sound-alike/look-alike issues:

Amlodipine may be confused with amiloride

Norvasc® may be confused with Navane®, Norvir®, Vascor®

Related Information

Antihypertensive Agents by Class *on page 1678*

(Continued)

Amlodipine *(Continued)*

U.S. Brand Names Norvasc®

Canadian Brand Names Norvasc®

Index Terms Amlodipine Besylate

Therapeutic Category Antianginal Agent; Antihypertensive Agent; Calcium Channel Blocker

Generic Available Yes

Use Treatment of hypertension; chronic stable angina; vasospastic (Prinzmetal's) angina; angiographically documented CAD [to decrease risk of hospitalization (due to angina) and coronary revascularization procedure]

Pregnancy Risk Factor C

Lactation Excretion in breast milk unknown/not recommended

Contraindications Hypersensitivity to amlodipine or any component

Warnings May increase frequency, duration, and severity of angina or precipitate acute MI during initiation of therapy or dosage increase (particularly in patients with severe obstructive coronary artery disease)

Precautions Use with caution in patients with CHF or severe aortic stenosis; use with caution and reduce the dose in patients with severe hepatic impairment; acute hypotension may rarely occur

Adverse Reactions

Cardiovascular system: Peripheral edema, flushing, palpitations; rarely: hypotension, arrhythmia, chest pain, syncope, peripheral ischemia, vasculitis; MI (rare)

Central nervous system: Headache, dizziness, somnolence, fatigue; less common: vertigo, insomnia, abnormal dreams, nervousness, depression, anxiety

Dermatologic: Rash, pruritus, erythema multiforme, angioedema

Endocrine & Metabolic: Sexual dysfunction, gynecomastia, hyperglycemia, weight gain, weight loss

Gastrointestinal: Nausea, abdominal pain, dyspepsia, anorexia, constipation, diarrhea, dysphagia, pancreatitis, vomiting, xerostomia; gingival hyperplasia (may be less than with nifedipine)

Hematologic: Thrombocytopenia, leukopenia, purpura

Hepatic: Jaundice, elevated liver enzymes

Neuromuscular & skeletal: Muscle cramps, asthenia, arthralgia, myalgia, paresthesia, peripheral neuropathy, hypoesthesia, tremor

Ocular: Diplopia, abnormal vision, eye pain, conjunctivitis

Otic: Tinnitus

Respiratory: Dyspnea, epistaxis

Miscellaneous: Diaphoresis, hypersensitivity reactions, thirst

Drug Interactions Cytochrome P450 isoenzyme CYP3A4 substrate

Azole antifungal agents may inhibit the metabolism of amlodipine and result in an increase in amlodipine serum concentrations or effect; calcium may decrease the pharmacologic effect of calcium channel blockers; rifampin may decrease amlodipine serum concentrations; amlodipine may (or may not) increase cyclosporine serum concentrations (conflicting studies exist)

Food Interactions Food does not affect the bioavailability of amlodipine. Grapefruit juice increased amlodipine peak serum concentrations by 15% and AUC by 16% in one single dose study (Josefsson, 1996); however, repeated daily ingestion of grapefruit juice did **not** affect amlodipine pharmacokinetics in another single-dose amlodipine study (Vincent, 2000); multiple dose amlodipine-grapefruit juice interaction studies are needed. Avoid natural licorice (causes sodium and water retention and increases potassium loss)

Stability Store at room temperature of 15°C to 30°C (59°F to 86°F); dispense in tightly-closed, light-resistant container

Mechanism of Action Inhibits calcium ions from entering the "slow channels" or select voltage-sensitive areas of vascular smooth muscle and myocardium during depolarization; produces a relaxation of coronary vascular smooth muscle and coronary vasodilation; increases myocardial oxygen delivery in patients with vasospastic angina

Pharmacodynamics Antihypertensive effects: Duration: ≥24 hours with chronic daily dosing

Pharmacokinetics

Absorption: Oral: Well absorbed

Distribution: Distribution into breast milk is unknown

Mean V_d:

Children >6 years: Similar to adults on a per kg basis

Adults: 21 L/kg

Protein binding: 93%

Metabolism: In the liver with 90% metabolized to inactive metabolites

Bioavailability: 64% to 90%

Half-life: Terminal: 30-50 hours
Time to peak serum concentrations: 6-12 hours
Elimination: 10% of unchanged drug and 60% of metabolites are excreted in the urine
Clearance: May be decreased in patients with hepatic insufficiency or moderate to severe heart failure; weight-adjusted clearance in children >6 years of age is similar to adults
Dialysis: Not dialyzable

Usual Dosage Oral:
Children: Hypertension: Manufacturer recommendations: Children 6-17 years: 2.5-5 mg once daily; doses >5 mg daily have not been fully studied
Limited information exists in the literature. In one prospective study, 21 hypertensive children (mean age: 13.1 years; range: 6-17 years) received the following initial daily doses of amlodipine based on weight groups: Children <50 kg: 0.05 mg/kg/day; children 50-70 kg: 2.5 mg daily; children >70 kg: 5 mg daily; mean initial dose: 0.07 ± 0.04 mg/kg/day; doses were increased by 25% to 50% (rounded to the nearest 2.5 mg) every 5-7 days to a maximum of 0.5 mg/kg/day, as needed to control blood pressure; the mean required dose was almost twice as high for children <13 years of age (0.29 ± 0.13 mg/kg/day) compared to children ≥13 years of age (0.16 ± 0.11 mg/kg/day) (see Tallian, 1999).
In a small randomized crossover trial, amlodipine was compared to nifedipine or felodipine in 11 hypertensive children (mean age: 16 years; range: 9-17 years); amlodipine was administered once daily as a liquid preparation (tablets dissolved in water immediately prior to administration); an initial daily dose of 0.1 mg/kg/day (maximum: 5 mg daily) was increased by 50% to 100% after 1 week to a maximum of 10 mg/day, as needed for blood pressure control; mean initial dose: 0.09 ± 0.01 mg/kg/day; mean required dose: 0.12 mg/kg/day (Rogan, 2000). A third prospective study used fixed mg doses, rather than dosing on a mg/kg basis (Pfammatter, 1998).
Four retrospective studies used a variety of initial amlodipine doses ranging from 0.05-0.13 mg/kg/day; mean required dose after dosage titration (for all aged patients) ranged from 0.15-0.17 mg/kg/day (Khattak, 1998; Silverstein, 1999; Flynn, 2000a; Parker 2002). Two of these studies noted a relationship between dose and age, with younger patients requiring higher mg/kg/day doses. Several retrospective studies used twice daily dosing in younger children, but it is unknown whether this reflects altered pharmacokinetics or physician prescribing habits. Further pediatric studies are needed.
Adults:
Hypertension: Initial: 2.5-5 mg once daily; use initial dose of 2.5 mg once daily in patients who are small, fragile, or elderly, and when adding amlodipine to other antihypertensive therapy; in general, titrate dose over 7-14 days to fully assess effects; usual dose: 5 mg once daily; maximum dose: 10 mg once daily; usual dosage range (JNC 7): 2.5-10 mg once daily
Angina or CAD: 5-10 mg once daily; use lower dose for patients with hepatic impairment and in the elderly; most patients with CAD require 10 mg once daily
Dosing adjustment in renal impairment: Not needed; patients may receive the usual initial dose
Dosing adjustment in hepatic impairment: Adults: Initial: 2.5 mg once daily

Administration Oral: May be administered without regard to food; use caution if administered with grapefruit juice (see Food Interactions)

Monitoring Parameters Blood pressure, liver enzymes

Patient Information Do not discontinue abruptly; report unrelieved headache, vomiting, palpitations, peripheral or facial swelling, weight gain, or respiratory changes; may cause dizziness or drowsiness and impair ability to perform activities requiring mental alertness or physical coordination; may cause dry mouth

Dosage Forms Excipient information presented when available (limited, particularly for generics); consult specific product labeling. Available as amlodipine besylate; mg strength refers to amlodipine.
Tablet: 2.5 mg, 5 mg, 10 mg
Norvasc®: 2.5 mg, 5 mg, 10 mg

Extemporaneous Preparations A 1 mg/mL oral suspension made from tablets and two different vehicles (a 1:1 mixture of simple syrup and 1% methylcellulose or a 1:1 mixture of OraPlus® and OraSweet®) was stable for 56 days at room temperature (25°C) and 91 days under refrigeration (4°C) when stored in amber plastic prescription bottles; grind fifty 5 mg tablets in a mortar into a fine powder; add a small amount of the vehicle and mix well to form a uniform paste; mix while adding the vehicle in geometric proportions to **almost** 250 mL; transfer to a calibrated bottle and qsad with vehicle to 250 mL. Microbial growth was not determined in this study; extended storage under refrigeration is recommended to minimize microbial contamination. Label "shake well" and "refrigerate"
Nahata MC, Morosco RS, and Hipple TF, "Stability of Amlodipine Besylate in Two Liquid Dosage Forms," *J Am Pharm Assoc*, 1999, 39(3):375-7.
(Continued)

Amlodipine *(Continued)*

References

Chobanian AV, Bakris GL, Black HR, et al, "The Seventh Report of the Joint National Committee on Prevention, Detection, Evaluation, and Treatment of High Blood Pressure: The JNC 7 report," *JAMA*, 2003, 289(19):2560-72.

Flynn JT and Pasko DA, "Calcium Channel Blockers: Pharmacology and Place in Therapy of Pediatric Hypertension," *Pediatr Nephrol*, 2000, 15(3-4):302-16.

Flynn JT, Smoyer WE, and Bunchman TE, "Treatment of Hypertensive Children With Amlodipine," *Am J Hypertens*, 2000a, 13(10):1061-6.

Josefsson M, Zackrisson AL, and Ahlner J, "Effect of Grapefruit Juice on the Pharmacokinetics of Amlodipine in Healthy Volunteers," *Eur J Clin Pharmacol*, 1996, 51(2):189-93.

Khattak S, Rogan JW, Saunders EF, et al, "Efficacy of Amlodipine in Pediatric Bone Marrow Transplant Patients," *Clin Pediatr (Phila)*, 1998, 37(1):31-5.

Parker ML, Robinson RF, and Nahata MC, "Amlodipine Therapy in Pediatric Patients With Hypertension," *J Am Pharm Assoc*, 2002, 42(1):114-7.

Pfammatter JP, Clericetti-Affolter C, Truttmann AC, et al, "Amlodipine Once-Daily in Systemic Hypertension," *Eur J Pediatr*, 1998, 157(8):618-21.

Rogan JW, Lyszkiewicz DA, Blowey D, et al, "A Randomized Prospective Crossover Trial of Amlodipine in Pediatric Hypertension," *Pediatr Nephrol*, 2000, 14(12):1083-7.

Silverstein DM, Palmer J, Baluarte HJ, et al, "Use of Calcium-Channel Blockers in Pediatric Renal Transplant Recipients," *Pediatr Transplant*, 1999, 3(4):288-92.

Tallian KB, Nahata MC, Turman MA, et al, "Efficacy of Amlodipine in Pediatric Patients With Hypertension," *Pediatr Nephrol*, 1999, 13(4):304-10.

Vincent J, Harris SI, Foulds G, et al, "Lack of Effect of Grapefruit Juice on the Pharmacokinetics and Pharmacodynamics of Amlodipine," *Br J Clin Pharmacol*, 2000, 50(5):455-63.

♦ **Amlodipine Besylate** *see* Amlodipine *on page 109*

♦ **Ammens® Medicated Deodorant [OTC]** *see* Zinc Oxide *on page 1640*

♦ **Ammonapse** *see* Sodium Phenylbutyrate *on page 1455*

Ammonium Chloride (a MOE nee um KLOR ide)

Index Terms NH_4Cl

Therapeutic Category Metabolic Alkalosis Agent; Urinary Acidifying Agent

Generic Available Yes

Use Diuretic or systemic and urinary acidifying agent; treatment of hypochloremia

Pregnancy Risk Factor C

Contraindications Hypersensitivity to ammonium chloride or any component; severe hepatic and renal dysfunction; patients with primary respiratory acidosis

Adverse Reactions

Cardiovascular: Bradycardia
Central nervous system: Mental confusion, coma, headache
Dermatologic: Rash
Endocrine & metabolic: Metabolic acidosis secondary to hyperchloremia
Gastrointestinal: GI irritation
Local: Pain at site of injection
Respiratory: Hyperventilation

Drug Interactions Chlorpropamide's effects may be enhanced due to decreased urinary excretion; may decrease flecainide levels due to increased urinary excretion; systemic acidosis may occur when used with spironolactone

Mechanism of Action Its dissociation to ammonium and chloride ions increases acidity by increasing free hydrogen ion concentration which combines with bicarbonate ion to form CO_2 and water; the net result is the replacement of bicarbonate ions by chloride ions

Pharmacokinetics

Metabolism: In the liver
Elimination: In urine

Usual Dosage

The following equations represent different methods of chloride or alkalosis correction utilizing either the serum HCO_3^-, the serum Cl^- or the base excess: Children and Adults: I.V. (**Note:** Ammonium chloride is an alternative treatment and should be used only after sodium and potassium chloride supplementation has been optimized.):

Correction of refractory hypochloremic metabolic alkalosis: mEq NH_4Cl = 0.5 L/kg x wt in kg x [serum HCO_3^- - 24] mEq/L; give 1/2 to 2/3 of the calculated dose, then re-evaluate

Correction of hypochloremia: mEq NH_4Cl = 0.2 L/kg x wt in kg x [103 - serum Cl^-] mEq/L, give 1/2 to 2/3 of calculated dose, then re-evaluate

Correction of alkalosis via base excess method: mEq NH_4Cl = 0.3 L/kg x wt in kg x base excess (mEq/L), give 1/2 to 2/3 of calculated dose, then re-evaluate

Children: I.V.: 75 mg/kg/day in 4 divided doses for urinary acidification; maximum daily dose: 6 g

Adults: I.V.: 1.5 g/dose every 6 hours

Administration

Parenteral: Dilute to 0.2 mEq/mL and infuse I.V. over 3 hours; maximum concentration: 0.4 mEq/mL; maximum rate of infusion: 1 mEq/kg/hour

Monitoring Parameters Serum electrolytes, serum ammonia

Nursing Implications Rapid I.V. injection may increase the likelihood of ammonia toxicity

Dosage Forms Excipient information presented when available (limited, particularly for generics); consult specific product labeling.

Injection, solution: Ammonium 5 mEq/mL and chloride 5 mEq/mL (20 mL) [equivalent to ammonium chloride 267.5 mg/mL]

- ♦ **Ammonium Lactate** *see* Lactic Acid and Ammonium Hydroxide *on page 898*
- ♦ **Ammonium Molybdate** *see* Trace Metals *on page 1558*
- ♦ **Ammonul®** *see* Sodium Phenylacetate and Sodium Benzoate *on page 1453*
- ♦ **Amnesteem™** *see* Isotretinoin *on page 876*
- ♦ **Amoclan** *see* Amoxicillin and Clavulanic Acid *on page 115*

Amoxicillin (a moks i SIL in)

Medication Safety Issues

Sound-alike/look-alike issues:

Amoxicillin may be confused with amoxapine, Amoxil®, Atarax®

Amoxil® may be confused with amoxapine, amoxicillin

International issues:

Fisamox® [Australia] may be confused with Fosamax® which is a brand name for alendronate in the U.S.

Fisamox® [Australia] may be confused with Vigamox™ which is a brand name for moxifloxacin in the U.S.

Related Information

Endocarditis Prophylaxis *on page 1812*

U.S. Brand Names Amoxil®

Canadian Brand Names Apo-Amoxi®; Gen-Amoxicillin; Lin-Amox; Novamoxin®; Nu-Amoxi; PHL-Amoxicillin; PMS-Amoxicillin

Index Terms Amoxicillin Trihydrate; Amoxycillin; *p*-Hydroxyampicillin

Therapeutic Category Antibiotic, Penicillin

Generic Available Yes: Excludes drops

Use Treatment of otitis media, sinusitis, and infections involving the respiratory tract, skin, and urinary tract due to susceptible *H. influenzae*, *N. gonorrhoeae*, *E. coli*, *P. mirabilis*, *E. faecalis*, streptococci, and nonpenicillinase-producing staphylococci; treatment of Lyme disease in children <8 years of age; prophylaxis of bacterial endocarditis; prophylaxis of postexposure inhalational anthrax; *H. pylori* eradication to reduce the risk of duodenal ulcer recurrence

Pregnancy Risk Factor B

Lactation Enters breast milk/compatible

Contraindications Hypersensitivity to amoxicillin, penicillin, or any component

Warnings Epstein-Barr virus infection, acute lymphocytic leukemia or cytomegalovirus infection increases risk for amoxicillin-induced maculopapular rash; some oral suspensions may contain sodium benzoate; benzoic acid (benzoate) is a metabolite of benzyl alcohol; large amounts of benzyl alcohol (≥99 mg/kg/day) have been associated with a potentially fatal toxicity ("gasping syndrome") in neonates; the "gasping syndrome" consists of metabolic acidosis, respiratory distress, gasping respirations, CNS dysfunction (including convulsions, intracranial hemorrhage), hypotension and cardiovascular collapse; avoid use of amoxicillin products containing sodium benzoate in neonates; *in vitro* and animal studies have shown that benzoate displaces bilirubin from protein binding sites

Precautions In patients with renal dysfunction, doses and/or frequency of administration should be modified in response to the degree of renal impairment; use with caution in patients with history of cephalosporin allergy; chewable tablets contain aspartame which is metabolized to phenylalanine and must be used with caution in patients with phenylketonuria

Adverse Reactions

Central nervous system: Fever, hyperactivity, agitation, seizures

Dermatologic: Rash, exfoliative dermatitis, Stevens-Johnson syndrome, erythema multiforme, acute generalized exanthematous pustulosis, urticaria

Gastrointestinal: Diarrhea, nausea, vomiting, pseudomembranous colitis

Hematologic: Anemia, leukopenia, neutropenia, eosinophilia, thrombocytopenia, prolongation of bleeding time, hemolytic anemia

Hepatic: Elevated AST and ALT, cholestatic jaundice, acute cytolytic hepatitis

Miscellaneous: Superinfection, hypersensitivity reactions, serum sickness, vasculitis, anaphylaxis; rare: Tooth discoloration (brown, yellow, or gray)

(Continued)

Amoxicillin *(Continued)*

Drug Interactions Probenecid (increases serum amoxicillin concentration); allopurinol may increase frequency for amoxicillin rash; decreases oral contraceptive efficacy

Food Interactions Food does not interfere with absorption

Stability Suspensions are stable for 14 days at room temperature or if refrigerated; refrigeration is preferred

Mechanism of Action Interferes with bacterial cell wall synthesis during active multiplication by binding to one or more of the penicillin-binding proteins, causing cell wall death and resultant bactericidal activity against susceptible bacteria

Pharmacokinetics

Absorption: Oral: Rapid and nearly complete (74% to 92% of a single dose is absorbed)

Distribution: Into liver, lungs, prostate, muscle, middle ear effusions, maxillary sinus secretions, bile, and into ascitic and synovial fluids; excreted into breast milk

Protein binding: 17% to 20%, lower in neonates

Metabolism: Partial

Half-life:

- Neonates, full-term: 3.7 hours
- Infants and children: 1-2 hours
- Adults with normal renal function: 0.7-1.4 hours
- Patients with Cl_{cr} <10 mL/minute: 7-21 hours

Time to peak serum concentration:

- Capsule: Within 2 hours
- Suspension: Neonates: 3-4.5 hours; children: 1 hour

Elimination: Renal excretion (80% unchanged drug)

Dialysis: Moderately dialyzable (20% to 50%); ~30% removed by 3-hour hemodialysis; supplemental dose is recommended after hemodialysis

Usual Dosage Oral:

Neonates and Infants: ≤3 months: 20-30 mg/kg/day in divided doses every 12 hours

Infants >3 months and Children: 25-50 mg/kg/day in divided doses every 8 hours or 25-50 mg/kg/day in divided doses every 12 hours

- Acute otitis media due to highly resistant strains of *S. pneumoniae*: 80-90 mg/kg/day divided every 12 hours
- Uncomplicated gonorrhea:
  - <2 years, probenecid is contraindicated in this age group
  - ≥2 years: 50 mg/kg plus probenecid 25 mg/kg as a single dose
- Endocarditis prophylaxis: 50 mg/kg 1 hour before procedure, not to exceed adult dose
- Postexposure inhalational anthrax prophylaxis:
  - <40 kg: 45 mg/kg/day in divided doses every 8 hours
  - ≥40 kg: 500 mg every 8 hours

Adults: 250-500 mg every 8 hours or 500-875 mg tablets twice daily; maximum dose: 2-3 g/day

- Uncomplicated gonorrhea: 3 g plus probenecid 1 g as a single dose
- Endocarditis prophylaxis: 2 g 1 hour before procedure
- *H. pylori* eradication: 1 g twice daily for 14 days in combination with a proton pump inhibitor and at least one other antibiotic (clarithromycin)

Dosing interval in renal impairment: Note: The 875 mg tablet should not be used in patients with a Cl_{cr} <30 mL/minute

- Cl_{cr} 10-30 mL/minute: Administer every 12 hours
- Cl_{cr} <10 mL/minute: Administer every 24 hours

Administration Oral: May be administered on an empty or full stomach; may be mixed with formula, milk, cold drink, or juice; administer dose immediately after mixing; shake suspension well before use

Monitoring Parameters With prolonged therapy, monitor renal, hepatic, and hematologic function periodically; monitor for diarrhea

Patient Information May cause tooth discoloration (most reports occurred in pediatric patients); tooth brushing or dental cleaning will reduce or eliminate discoloration.

Additional Information Appearance of a rash should be carefully evaluated to differentiate a nonallergic amoxicillin rash from a hypersensitivity reaction. Amoxicillin rash occurs in 5% to 10% of children receiving amoxicillin and is a generalized dull, red, maculopapular rash, generally appearing 3-14 days after the start of therapy. It normally begins on the trunk and spreads over most of the body. It may be most intense at pressure areas, elbows, and knees. Incidence of amoxicillin rash is higher in patients with viral infections, cytomegalovirus infections, infectious mononucleosis, lymphocytic leukemia, or patients with hyperuricemia who are receiving allopurinol.

Dosage Forms Excipient information presented when available (limited, particularly for generics); consult specific product labeling.

Capsule: 250 mg, 500 mg

Amoxil®: 500 mg

Powder for oral suspension: 125 mg/5 mL (80 mL, 100 mL, 150 mL); 200 mg/5 mL (50 mL, 75 mL, 100 mL); 250 mg/5 mL (80 mL, 100 mL, 150 mL); 400 mg/5 mL (50 mL, 75 mL, 100 mL)

Amoxil®: 200 mg/5 mL (50 mL, 75 mL, 100 mL) [contains sodium benzoate; bubble gum flavor]; 250 mg/5 mL (100 mL, 150 mL) [contains sodium benzoate; bubble gum flavor]; 400 mg/5 mL (5 mL, 50 mL, 75 mL, 100 mL) [contains sodium benzoate; bubble gum flavor]

Powder for oral suspension [drops]:

Amoxil®: 50 mg/mL (30 mL) [contains sodium benzoate; bubble gum flavor]

Tablet: 500 mg, 875 mg

Amoxil®: 500 mg, 875 mg

Tablet, chewable: 125 mg, 200 mg, 250 mg, 400 mg

Amoxil®: 200 mg [contains phenylalanine 1.82 mg/tablet; cherry banana peppermint flavor]; 400 mg [contains phenylalanine 3.64 mg/tablet; cherry banana peppermint flavor]

References

Bogunlewlcz M and Leung DY, "Hypersensitivity Reactions to Antibiotics Commonly Used in Children," *Pediatr Infect Dis J*, 1995, 14(3):221-31.

Canafax, DM, Yuan Z, Chonmaitree T, et al, "Amoxicillin Middle Ear Fluid Penetration and Pharmacokinetics in Children with Acute Otitis Media," *Pediatr Infect Dis J*, 1998, 17(2):149-56.

CDC and Johns Hopkins Working Group on Civilian Biodefense, "Commentary on Non-Labeled Dosing of Oral Amoxicillin in Adults and Pediatrics for Post-Exposure Inhalational Anthrax," December 10, 2001, http://www.fda.gov/cder/drugprepare/amox-anthrax.htm.

Dajani AS, Taubert KA, Wilson WW, et al, "Prevention of Bacterial Endocarditis. Recommendations by the American Heart Association," *JAMA*, 1997, 277(22):1794-1801.

Amoxicillin and Clavulanic Acid

(a moks i SIL in & klav yoo LAN ic AS id)

Medication Safety Issues

Sound-alike/look-alike issues:

Augmentin® may be confused with Azulfidine®

U.S. Brand Names Amoclan; Augmentin®; Augmentin ES-600®; Augmentin XR®

Canadian Brand Names Alti-Amoxi-Clav; Apo-Amoxi-Clav®; Augmentin®; Clavulin®; Novo-Clavamoxin; ratio-Aclavulanate

Index Terms Clavulanic Acid and Amoxicillin

Therapeutic Category Antibiotic, Beta-lactam and Beta-lactamase Combination; Antibiotic, Penicillin

Generic Available Yes: Excludes extended release

Use Infections caused by susceptible organisms involving the lower respiratory tract, otitis media, sinusitis, skin and skin structure, and urinary tract; spectrum same as amoxicillin in addition to beta-lactamase producing *M. catarrhalis*, *H. influenzae*, *N. gonorrhoeae*, and *S. aureus* (not MRSA)

Pregnancy Risk Factor B

Lactation Enters breast milk/use caution (AAP rates "compatible")

Contraindications Hypersensitivity to amoxicillin, clavulanic acid, penicillins, or any component; history of amoxicillin/clavulanic acid-associated cholestatic jaundice or hepatic dysfunction

Warnings Epstein-Barr virus infection, acute lymphocytic leukemia or cytomegalovirus infection increase the risk for amoxicillin-induced maculopapular rash. Pseudomembranous colitis has been reported; prolonged use may result in superinfection

Precautions Use with caution in patients with history of cephalosporin hypersensitivity; in patients with renal dysfunction, doses and/or frequency of administration should be modified in response to the degree of renal impairment. The "BID" formulation may contain aspartame which is metabolized to phenylalanine and must be avoided or used with caution in patients with phenylketonuria.

Adverse Reactions

Central nervous system: Headache, agitation

Dermatologic: Rash, urticaria, exfoliative dermatitis, Stevens-Johnson syndrome

Gastrointestinal: Nausea, vomiting, abdominal pain, pseudomembranous colitis; incidence of diarrhea (9%) is higher than with amoxicillin alone

Genitourinary: Vaginal candidiasis

Hepatic: Elevated AST, ALT, alkaline phosphatase, and bilirubin

Miscellaneous: Superinfection, hypersensitivity reactions, serum sickness, vasculitis, anaphylaxis

Drug Interactions Probenecid (increases serum amoxicillin concentration), allopurinol (may increase incidence of rash); amoxicillin and clavulanic acid may reduce the efficacy of oral contraceptives

(Continued)

Amoxicillin and Clavulanic Acid *(Continued)*

Stability Reconstituted oral suspension should be refrigerated; discard unused suspension after 10 days; store tablets, chewable tablets, and powder for oral suspension at room temperature

Mechanism of Action Clavulanic acid binds and inhibits beta-lactamases that inactivate amoxicillin resulting in amoxicillin having an expanded spectrum of activity; amoxicillin interferes with bacterial cell wall synthesis by binding to one or more of the penicillin-binding proteins and causing cell wall death

Pharmacokinetics

Absorption: Both amoxicillin and clavulanate are well absorbed

Distribution: Both widely distributed into lungs, pleural, peritoneal, synovial, and ascitic fluid as well as bone, gynecologic tissue, and middle ear fluid; crosses the placenta; excreted in breast milk

Protein binding:

Amoxicillin: 17% to 20%

Clavulanate: 25%

Metabolism: Clavulanic acid: Metabolized in the liver

Half-life of both agents in adults with normal renal function: ~1 hour; amoxicillin pharmacokinetics are not affected by clavulanic acid

Time to peak serum concentration: Within 2 hours

Elimination: Amoxicillin: 60% to 80%; excreted unchanged in the urine

Dialysis: ~30% of amoxicillin removed by 3-hour hemodialysis; supplemental dose recommended after hemodialysis (do **not** use extended release tablets)

Usual Dosage Oral (dosing based on amoxicillin component):

Neonates and Infants <3 months: 30 mg/kg/day divided every 12 hours using the 125 mg/5 mL suspension

Children <40 kg: 20-40 mg (amoxicillin component)/kg/day in divided doses every 8 hours **or** 25-45 mg (amoxicillin component)/kg/day divided every 12 hours using either 200 mg/5 mL or 400 mg/5 mL suspension, or 200 mg, 400 mg chewable tablet formulation

Multidrug-resistant pneumococcal otitis media: 80-90 mg/kg/day divided every 12 hours (use a 7:1 "BID" formulation or Augmentin ES-600®)

Note: Children <40 kg should not receive the 250 mg film-coated tablets which contain a higher dose of clavulanic acid than the 250 mg chewable tablets.

Children ≥16 years and Adults:

Acute bacterial sinusitis: Extended release tablet: 2000 mg every 12 hours for 10 days

Community-acquired pneumonia: Extended release tablet: 2000 mg every 12 hours for 7-10 days

Adults:

Less severe infection: 250 mg every 8 hours or 500 mg every 12 hours

More severe infections and respiratory tract infections: 500 mg every 8 hours or 875 mg every 12 hours

Dosing interval in renal impairment:

Cl_{cr} <30 mL/minute: Do not use 875 mg tablet or extended release tablet

Cl_{cr} 10-30 mL/minute: Administer 250-500 mg every 12 hours

Cl_{cr} <10 mL/minute: Administer 250-500 mg every 24 hours

Administration Oral: Administer at the start of a meal to decrease the frequency or severity of GI side effects; do not administer with a high fat meal (clavulanate absorption is decreased); may mix with milk, formula, or juice; shake suspension well before use

Monitoring Parameters With prolonged therapy, monitor renal, hepatic, and hematologic function periodically

Test Interactions May interfere with urinary glucose determinations using Clinitest®

Patient Information Adverse GI effects may occur less frequently if taken with food. Report persistent diarrhea to physician.

Additional Information Since both the 250 mg and 500 mg tablets contain the same amount of clavulanic acid, two 250 mg tablets are not equivalent to one 500 mg tablet. Four 250 mg tablets or two 500 mg tablets are **not** equivalent to a single 1000 mg extended release tablet.

Appearance of a rash should be carefully evaluated to differentiate a nonallergic amoxicillin rash from a hypersensitivity reaction. Amoxicillin rash occurs in 5% to 10% of children receiving amoxicillin and is a generalized dull, red, maculopapular rash, generally appearing 3-14 days after the start of therapy. It normally begins on the trunk and spreads over most of the body. It may be most intense at pressure areas, elbows, and knees. Incidence of amoxicillin rash is higher in patients with viral infections, *Salmonella* infections, lymphocytic leukemia, or patients with hyperuricemia who are receiving allopurinol.

Dosage Forms Excipient information presented when available (limited, particularly for generics); consult specific product labeling. [DSC] = Discontinued product

Powder for oral suspension: 200: Amoxicillin 200 mg and clavulanate potassium 28.5 mg per 5 mL (50 mL, 75 mL, 100 mL) [contains phenylalanine]; 400: Amoxicillin 400 mg and clavulanate potassium 57 mg per 5 mL (50 mL, 75 mL, 100 mL) [contains phenylalanine]; 600: Amoxicillin 600 mg and clavulanic potassium 42.9 mg per 5 mL (75 mL, 125 mL, 200 mL) [contains phenylalanine]

Amoclan:

200: Amoxicillin 200 mg and clavulanate potassium 28.5 mg per 5 mL (50 mL, 75 mL, 100 mL) [contains phenylalanine 7 mg/5 mL and potassium 0.14 mEq/5 mL; fruit flavor]

400: Amoxicillin 400 mg and clavulanate potassium 57 mg per 5 mL (50 mL, 75 mL, 100 mL) [contains phenylalanine 7 mg/5 mL and potassium 0.29 mEq/5 mL; fruit flavor]

Augmentin®:

125: Amoxicillin 125 mg and clavulanate potassium 31.25 mg per 5 mL (75 mL, 100 mL, 150 mL) [contains potassium 0.16 mEq/5 mL; banana flavor]

200: Amoxicillin 200 mg and clavulanate potassium 28.5 mg per 5 mL (50 mL, 75 mL, 100 mL) [contains phenylalanine 7 mg/5 mL and potassium 0.14 mEq/5 mL; orange flavor]

250: Amoxicillin 250 mg and clavulanate potassium 62.5 mg per 5 mL (75 mL, 100 mL, 150 mL) [contains potassium 0.32 mEq/5 mL; orange flavor]

400: Amoxicillin 400 mg and clavulanate potassium 57 mg per 5 mL (50 mL, 75 mL, 100 mL) [contains phenylalanine 7 mg/5 mL and potassium 0.29 mEq/5 mL; orange flavor]

Augmentin ES-600®: Amoxicillin 600 mg and clavulanic potassium 42.9 mg per 5 mL (75 mL, 125 mL, 200 mL) [contains phenylalanine 7 mg/5 mL and potassium 0.23 mEq/5 mL; strawberry cream flavor]

Tablet: 250: Amoxicillin 250 mg and clavulanate potassium 125 mg; 500: Amoxicillin 500 mg and clavulanate potassium 125 mg; 875: Amoxicillin 875 mg and clavulanate potassium 125 mg

Augmentin®:

250: Amoxicillin 250 mg and clavulanate potassium 125 mg [contains potassium 0.63 mEq/tablet]

500: Amoxicillin 500 mg and clavulanate potassium 125 mg [contains potassium 0.63 mEq/tablet]

875: Amoxicillin 875 mg and clavulanate potassium 125 mg [contains potassium 0.63 mEq/tablet]

Tablet, chewable: 200: Amoxicillin 200 mg and clavulanate potassium 28.5 mg [contains phenylalanine]; 400: Amoxicillin 400 mg and clavulanate potassium 57 mg [contains phenylalanine]

Augmentin®:

125: Amoxicillin 125 mg and clavulanate potassium 31.25 mg [contains potassium 0.16 mEq/tablet; lemon-lime flavor] [DSC]

200: Amoxicillin 200 mg and clavulanate potassium 28.5 mg [contains phenylalanine 2.1 mg/tablet and potassium 0.14 mEq/tablet; cherry-banana flavor]

250: Amoxicillin 250 mg and clavulanate potassium 62.5 mg [contains potassium 0.32 mEq/tablet; lemon-lime flavor]

400: Amoxicillin 400 mg and clavulanate potassium 57 mg [contains phenylalanine 4.2 mg/tablet and potassium 0.29 mEq/tablet; cherry-banana flavor]

Tablet, extended release:

Augmentin XR®: Amoxicillin 1000 mg and clavulanic acid 62.5 mg [contains potassium 29.3 mg (1.27 mEq) and sodium 12.6 mg (0.32 mEq) per tablet; packaged in either a 7-day or 10-day package]

References

Gan VN, Kusmiesz H, Shelton S, et al, "Comparative Evaluation of Loracarbef and Amoxicillin-Clavulanate for Acute Otitis Media," *Antimicrob Agents Chemother*, 1991, 35(5):967-71.

Hoberman A, Paradise JL, Burch DJ, et al, "Equivalent Efficiency and Reduced Occurrence of Diarrhea From a New Formulation of Amoxicillin/Clavulanate Potassium (Augmentin®) for Treatment of Acute Otitis Media in Children," *Pediatr Infect Dis J*, 1997, 16(5):463-70.

Reed MD, "Clinical Pharmacokinetics of Amoxicillin and Clavulanate," *Pediatr Infect Dis J*, 1996, 15(10):949-54.

Thoene DE and Johnson CE, "Pharmacotherapy of Otitis Media," *Pharmacotherapy*, 1991, 11(3):212-21.

Todd PA and Benfield P, "Amoxicillin/Clavulanic Acid. An Update of Its Antibacterial Activity, Pharmacokinetic Properties and Therapeutic Use," *Drugs*, 1990, 39(2):264-307.

♦ **Amoxicillin Trihydrate** *see* Amoxicillin *on page 113*

♦ **Amoxil®** *see* Amoxicillin *on page 113*

♦ **Amoxycillin** *see* Amoxicillin *on page 113*

♦ **Amphadase™** *see* Hyaluronidase *on page 774*

♦ **Amphetamine and Dextroamphetamine** *see* Dextroamphetamine and Amphetamine *on page 472*

♦ **Amphocin® [DSC]** *see* Amphotericin B (Conventional) *on page 118*

♦ **Amphotec® (Can)** *see* Amphotericin B Lipid Complex *on page 120*

Amphotericin B (Conventional)

(am foe TER i sin bee con VEN sha nal)

Medication Safety Issues

Safety issues:

Conventional amphotericin formulations (Amphocin®, Fungizone®) may be confused with lipid-based formulations (AmBisome®, Abelcet®, Amphotec®).

Large overdoses have occurred when conventional formulations were dispensed inadvertently for lipid-based products. Single daily doses of conventional amphotericin formulation never exceed 1.5 mg/kg.

U.S. Brand Names Amphocin® [DSC]

Canadian Brand Names Fungizone®

Index Terms Amphotericin B Desoxycholate

Therapeutic Category Antifungal Agent, Systemic; Antifungal Agent, Topical

Generic Available Yes

Use Treatment of severe systemic infections and meningitis caused by susceptible fungi such as *Candida* species, *Histoplasma capsulatum, Cryptococcus neoformans, Aspergillus* species, *Mucor* species, *Blastomyces dermatitidis, Torulopsis glabrata, Sporothrix schenckii, Paracoccidioides brasiliensis*, and *Coccidioides immitis*; fungal peritonitis; irrigant for bladder fungal infections; treatment of amebic meningoencephalitis caused by *Naegleria fowleri*

Pregnancy Risk Factor B

Lactation Excretion in breast milk unknown/contraindicated

Contraindications Hypersensitivity to amphotericin or any component

Warnings I.V. amphotericin is used primarily for the treatment of patients with progressive and potentially fatal fungal infections; not to be used for common clinically inapparent forms of fungal disease; anaphylaxis has been reported with amphotericin B-containing drugs; facilities for cardiopulmonary resuscitation should be available during administration due to the possibility of anaphylactic reaction

Precautions Due to the nephrotoxic potential of amphotericin, other nephrotoxic drugs should be avoided. Acute pulmonary reactions have been reported in patients simultaneously receiving intravenous amphotericin B and leukocyte transfusions; separate these infusions temporally as much as possible and monitor pulmonary function.

Adverse Reactions

Cardiovascular: Hypotension, hypertension, cardiac arrhythmias, shock, flushing

Central nervous system: Fever, chills, and headache are the most common adverse effects reported with amphotericin B infusion; delirium, seizures, malaise

Dermatologic: Rash, pruritus, urticaria

Endocrine & metabolic: Hypokalemia, hypomagnesemia, weight loss

Gastrointestinal: Anorexia, nausea, vomiting, steatorrhea

Hematologic: Anemia, leukopenia, thrombocytopenia

Hepatic: Acute hepatic failure, jaundice; elevated AST, ALT, and bilirubin

Local: Phlebitis

Renal: Renal tubular acidosis, renal failure (oliguria, azotemia, elevated serum creatinine)

Respiratory: Wheezing, hypoxemia, bronchospasm

Miscellaneous: Anaphylactoid reaction

Adverse effects due to intrathecal amphotericin:

Central nervous system: Headache, pain along lumbar nerves, arachnoiditis

Gastrointestinal: Nausea, vomiting

Genitourinary: Urinary retention

Neuromuscular & skeletal: Paresthesia, leg and back pain, foot drop

Ocular: Vision changes

Drug Interactions Nephrotoxic drugs may cause additive toxic effects; corticosteroids may increase potassium depletion caused by amphotericin; may predispose patients receiving cardiac glycosides or skeletal muscle relaxants to toxicity secondary to hypokalemia; imidazole derivatives (eg, miconazole, fluconazole, ketoconazole) may antagonize the effect and induce fungal resistance to amphotericin; may increase toxicity of flucytosine by increasing cellular uptake and/or impairing its renal excretion; may potentiate renal toxicity, bronchospasm, and hypotension of antineoplastic agents

Stability Reconstitute only with SWI without preservatives, not bacteriostatic water; benzyl alcohol, sodium chloride, or other electrolyte solutions may cause precipitation; can be diluted in D_5W, $D_{10}W$, up to $D_{20}W$; for I.V. infusion, an in-line filter (>1 micron mean pore diameter) may be used; irrigating solutions should be diluted in sterile water; short-term exposure (<24 hours) to light during I.V. infusion does **not** appreciably affect potency

Mechanism of Action Binds to ergosterol altering cell membrane permeability in susceptible fungi and causing leakage of cell components with subsequent cell death

Pharmacokinetics

Absorption: Poor oral absorption

Distribution: Minimal amounts enter the aqueous humor, bile, amniotic fluid, pericardial fluid, pleural fluid, and synovial fluid; poor CSF penetration

Protein binding: 90%

Half-life: Increased in small neonates and young infants

Initial: 15-48 hours

Terminal phase: 15 days

Elimination: 2% to 4% of dose eliminated in urine unchanged; ~40% eliminated over 7-day period and may be detected in urine for up to 8 weeks after discontinued use

Dialysis: Poorly dialyzed

Usual Dosage Medication errors, including deaths, have resulted from confusion between lipid-based forms of amphotericin (Abelcet®, Amphotec®, AmBisome®) and conventional amphotericin B for injection; conventional amphotericin B for injection doses should not exceed 1.5 mg/kg/day

Neonates, Infants, and Children:

I.V.: Test dose: 0.1 mg/kg/dose to a maximum of 1 mg; infuse over 20-60 minutes; an alternative method to the 0.1 mg/kg test dose is to initiate therapy with 0.25 mg/kg amphotericin administered over 6 hours; frequent observation of the patient and assessment of vital signs during the first several hours of the infusion is recommended

Initial therapeutic dose: If the 0.1 mg/kg test dose is tolerated without the occurrence of serious adverse effects, a therapeutic dose of 0.4 mg/kg can be given the same day as the test dose

The daily dose can then be gradually increased, usually in 0.25 mg/kg increments on each subsequent day until the desired daily dose is reached; in critically ill patients, more rapid dosage acceleration (up to 0.5 mg/kg increments on each subsequent day) may be warranted

Maintenance dose: 0.25-1 mg/kg/day given once daily; infuse over 2-6 hours; rapidly progressing disease may require short-term use of doses to 1.5 mg/kg/day; once therapy has been established, amphotericin B can be administered on an every-other-day basis at 1-1.5 mg/kg/dose

Intrathecal, intraventricular, or intracisternal (preferably into the lateral ventricles through a cisternal Ommaya reservoir): 25-100 mcg every 48-72 hours; increase to 500 mcg as tolerated

Adults:

I.V.: Test dose: 1 mg infused over 20-30 minutes

Initial therapeutic dose (if the test dose is tolerated): 0.25 mg/kg

The daily dose can then be gradually increased, usually in 0.25 mg/kg increments on each subsequent day until the desired daily dose is reached

Maintenance dose: 0.25-1 mg/kg/day once daily, infuse over 2-6 hours; or 1-1.5 mg/kg/dose every other day; do not exceed 1.5 mg/kg/day

Intrathecal, intraventricular, or intracisternal (preferably into the lateral ventricles through a cisternal Ommaya reservoir): 25-100 mcg every 48-72 hours; increase to 500 mcg as tolerated

Children and Adults:

Bladder irrigation: 5-15 mg amphotericin/100 mL of sterile water irrigation solution at 100-300 mL/day. Fluid is instilled into the bladder; the catheter is clamped for 60-120 minutes and the bladder drained. Perform irrigation 3-4 times/day for 2-5 days.

Dialysate: 1-4 mg/L of peritoneal dialysis fluid either with or without low-dose I.V. amphotericin B therapy

Note: Amphotericin B has been administered intranasally to reduce the frequency of invasive aspergillosis in neutropenic patients; 7 mg amphotericin B in 7 mL sterile water was placed in a De Vilbiss atomizer and the aerosolized solution was instilled intranasally to each nostril 4 times/day delivering an average of 5 mg amphotericin/day

Dosing adjustment in renal impairment: Dosage adjustments are not necessary with pre-existing renal impairment; if decreased renal function is due to amphotericin, the daily dose can be decreased by 50% or the dose can be given every other day. Therapy may be held until serum creatinine concentrations begin to decline.

Administration Parenteral: Amphotericin is administered by I.V. infusion over 2-3 hours (range: 1-6 hours) at a final concentration not to exceed 0.1 mg/mL through a peripheral venous catheter; in patients unable to tolerate a large fluid volume, amphotericin B at a final concentration not to exceed 0.5 mg/mL in D_5W or $D_{10}W$ may be administered through a central venous catheter

Monitoring Parameters BUN and serum creatinine levels should be determined every other day while therapy is increased and at least weekly thereafter; serum

(Continued)

Amphotericin B (Conventional) *(Continued)*

potassium and magnesium should be monitored closely; monitor electrolytes, liver function, hematocrit, CBC regularly; monitor I & O; monitor for signs of hypokalemia (muscle weakness, cramping, drowsiness, EKG changes, etc); blood pressure, temperature, pulse, respiration

Nursing Implications Cardiovascular collapse has been reported after rapid amphotericin injection; may premedicate patients who experience mild adverse reactions with acetaminophen and diphenhydramine 30 minutes prior to the amphotericin infusion. Meperidine and ibuprofen may help to reduce fevers and chills. Hydrocortisone can be added to the infusion solution to reduce febrile and other systemic reactions. Heparin 1 unit per 1 mL of infusion solution can be added to reduce phlebitis.

Additional Information A study by Harbarth, et al, reported that 29% of patients who experienced moderate to severe nephrotoxicity during conventional amphotericin B treatment had 3 or more risk factors which included body weight ≥90 kg, male sex, mean daily amphotericin B dosage ≥35 mg, chronic kidney disease, or concomitant use of amikacin or cyclosporine. Amphotericin B-induced nephrotoxicity may be minimized by sodium loading with 10-15 mL/kg of NS infused prior to each amphotericin B dose or pentoxifylline, and avoiding use of other nephrotoxic agents

Dosage Forms Excipient information presented when available (limited, particularly for generics); consult specific product labeling. [DSC] = Discontinued product

Injection, powder for reconstitution, as desoxycholate: 50 mg

Amphocin®: 50 mg [DSC]

References

The Ad Hoc Advisory Panel on Peritonitis Management. "Continuous Ambulatory Peritoneal Dialysis (CAPD) Peritonitis Treatment Recommendations: 1989 Update," *Perit Dial Int*, 1989, 9(4):247-56.

Benson JM and Nahata MC, "Pharmacokinetics of Amphotericin B in Children," *Antimicrob Agents Chemother*, 1989, 33(11):1989-93.

Bianco JA, Almgren J, Kern DL, et al, "Evidence That Oral Pentoxifylline Reverses Acute Renal Dysfunction in Bone Marrow Transplant Recipients Receiving Amphotericin B and Cyclosporine," *Transplantation*, 1991, 51(4):925-7.

Branch RA, "Prevention of Amphotericin B-Induced Renal Impairment. A Review on the Use of Sodium Supplementation," *Arch Intern Med*, 1988, 148(11):2389-94.

Harbarth S, Pestotnik SL, Lloyd JF, et al, "The Epidemiology of Nephrotoxicity Associated With Conventional Amphotericin B Therapy," *Am J Med*, 2001, 111(7):528-34.

Jeffery GM, Beard ME, Ikram RB, et al, "Intranasal Amphotericin B Reduces the Frequency of Invasive Aspergillosis in Neutropenic Patients," *Am J Med*, 1991, 90(6):685-92.

Kintzel PE and Smith GH, "Practical Guidelines for Preparing and Administering Amphotericin B," *Am J Hosp Pharm*, 1992, 49(5):1156-64.

Koren G, Lau A, Klein J, et al, "Pharmacokinetics and Adverse Effects of Amphotericin B in Infants and Children," *J Pediatr*, 1988, 113(3):559-63.

♦ **Amphotericin B Desoxycholate** *see* Amphotericin B (Conventional) *on page 118*

Amphotericin B Lipid Complex

(am foe TER i sin bee LIP id KOM pleks)

Medication Safety Issues

Safety issues:

Lipid-based amphotericin formulations (Abelcet®) may be confused with conventional formulations (Amphocin®, Fungizone®)

Large overdoses have occurred when conventional formulations were dispensed inadvertently for lipid-based products. Single daily doses of conventional amphotericin formulation never exceed 1.5 mg/kg.

U.S. Brand Names Abelcet®

Canadian Brand Names Abelcet®; Amphotec®

Index Terms ABLC

Therapeutic Category Antifungal Agent, Systemic

Generic Available No

Use Treatment of aspergillosis or invasive fungal infections in patients who are refractory to or intolerant of conventional amphotericin B therapy (refractory to or intolerant is defined as renal dysfunction with a serum creatinine ≥1.5 mg/dL that develops during therapy, or disease progression after a total dose of conventional amphotericin B of at least 10 mg/kg). This indication is primarily based on results of emergency studies for the treatment of aspergillosis; may be useful in the treatment of hepatosplenic candidiasis and cryptococcal meningitis.

Pregnancy Risk Factor B

Lactation Enters breast milk/contraindicated

Contraindications Hypersensitivity to amphotericin B, dimyristoylphosphatidylcholine (DMPC) and dimyristoylphosphatidylglycerol (DMPG) which are two phospholipids in the formulation, or any component

Warnings Anaphylaxis has been reported with amphotericin B-containing drugs; facilities for cardiopulmonary resuscitation should be available during administration due to the possibility of anaphylactic reaction

Precautions Due to the nephrotoxic potential of amphotericin B, other nephrotoxic drugs should be avoided. Acute pulmonary reactions have been reported in patients simultaneously receiving intravenous amphotericin B and leukocyte transfusions; separate these infusions temporally as much as possible and monitor pulmonary function.

Adverse Reactions

Cardiovascular: Hypotension, cardiac arrest, arrhythmias, flushing

Central nervous system: Headache; transient chills and fever and during infusion of the drug are the most common effects reported with ABLC

Dermatologic: Rash, pruritus

Endocrine & metabolic: Hypokalemia, bilirubinemia, hypomagnesemia

Gastrointestinal: Diarrhea, abdominal pain

Hematologic: Thrombocytopenia, leukopenia, anemia

Renal: Renal tubular acidosis, elevated serum creatinine (occurs to a lesser degree than with conventional amphotericin B), azotemia, oliguria

Respiratory: Dyspnea, respiratory failure

Miscellaneous: Anaphylactoid and other allergic reactions

Drug Interactions Nephrotoxic drugs may cause additive nephrotoxic effects; corticosteroids may increase potassium depletion caused by amphotericin; may predispose patients receiving cardiac glycosides or skeletal muscle relaxants to toxicity secondary to hypokalemia; may increase myelotoxicity and nephrotoxicity of zidovudine; imidazole derivatives (eg, miconazole, fluconazole, ketoconazole) may antagonize the effect and induce fungal resistance to amphotericin; may increase toxicity of flucytosine by increasing cellular uptake and/or impairing its renal excretion; may potentiate renal toxicity, bronchospasm, and hypotension of antineoplastic agents

Stability Prior to admixture, refrigerate vial and protect from light; diluted ABLC infusion solution in D_5W is stable up to 48 hours refrigerated and an additional 6 hours at room temperature. Do not freeze. Do not dilute with saline solutions or mix with other drugs or electrolytes.

Mechanism of Action Binds to ergosterol altering cell membrane permeability in susceptible fungi and causing leakage of cell components with subsequent cell death

Pharmacokinetics Exhibits nonlinear kinetics; volume of distribution and clearance from blood increases with increasing dose

Distribution: High tissue concentration found in the liver, spleen, and lung

Half-life, terminal: 173 hours

Elimination: 0.9% of dose excreted in urine over 24 hours; effects of hepatic and renal impairment on drug disposition are unknown

Dialysis: ABLC is not hemodialyzable

Usual Dosage Children and Adults: I.V.: 2.5-5 mg/kg given as a once daily infusion

Dosing adjustment in renal failure: Renal toxicity is dose dependent; there are no firm guidelines for dose adjustment based on lab test results (serum creatinine levels).

Administration Parenteral: I.V.: Prior to administration, amphotericin B lipid complex 5 mg/mL concentrated suspension must be diluted in D_5W by gently shaking the vial until solution contains no sediment; the appropriate dose is drawn into one or more sterile 20 mL syringes using an 18 gauge needle. The needle is removed and replaced with a 5 micrometer filter needle which can be used to filter the contents of up to 4 vials of drug. Contents of the syringe are injected via the filter needle into the I.V. container of D_5W diluting amphotericin B lipid complex to a final concentration of 1 mg/mL; a maximum concentration of 2 mg/mL may be used in fluid-restricted patients. Shake the I.V. container of diluted drug to insure that contents are thoroughly mixed then administer at a rate of 2.5 mg/kg/hour (over 2 hours). The manufacturer recommends that an in-line filter should NOT be used during administration of amphotericin B lipid complex.

Monitoring Parameters BUN, serum creatinine, liver function tests, serum electrolytes, CBC; vital signs, I & O; monitor for signs of hypokalemia (muscle weakness, cramping, drowsiness, EKG changes, etc)

Nursing Implications If infusion time exceeds 2 hours, mix the contents by gently rotating the infusion bag every 2 hours.

Additional Information Management of side effects is similar to conventional amphotericin B. [See Amphotericin B (Conventional) *on page 118* for suggested management guidelines of side effects.]

Dosage Forms Excipient information presented when available (limited, particularly for generics); consult specific product labeling.

Injection, suspension [preservative free]: 5 mg/mL (20 mL)

References

De Marie S, "Clinical Use of Liposomal and Lipid-Complexed Amphotericin B," *J Antimicrob Chemother*, 1994, 33(5):907-16.

Kline S, Larsen TA, Fieber L, et al, "Limited Toxicity of Prolonged Therapy With High Doses of Amphotericin B Lipid Complex," *Clin Infect Dis*, 1995, 21(5):1154-8.

Amphotericin B Liposome (am foe TER i sin bee LYE po som)

Medication Safety Issues

Safety issues:

Lipid-based amphotericin formulations (AmBisome®) may be confused with conventional formulations (Amphocin®, Fungizone®)

Large overdoses have occurred when conventional formulations were dispensed inadvertently for lipid-based products. Single daily doses of conventional amphotericin formulation never exceed 1.5 mg/kg.

U.S. Brand Names AmBisome®

Canadian Brand Names AmBisome®

Index Terms L-AmB

Therapeutic Category Antifungal Agent, Systemic

Generic Available No

Use Treatment of aspergillosis, candidiasis, or cryptococcosis in patients who are refractory to or intolerant of conventional amphotericin B therapy (refractory to or intolerant is defined as renal dysfunction with a serum creatinine ≥1.5 mg/dL that develops during therapy, or disease progression after a total dose of conventional amphotericin B of at least 10 mg/kg); empiric therapy for presumed fungal infection in febrile, neutropenic bone marrow transplant patients or febrile, neutropenic acute nonlymphocytic leukemia patients after an unsuccessful trial of antibiotics; treatment of cryptococcal meningitis in HIV infected patients; treatment of visceral leishmaniasis; treatment of suspected or proven fungal infections in patients with renal impairment

Pregnancy Risk Factor B

Lactation Excretion in breast milk unknown/contraindicated

Contraindications Hypersensitivity to amphotericin B or any component

Warnings Anaphylaxis has been reported with amphotericin B-containing drugs; if a severe anaphylactic reaction occurs, discontinue infusion immediately; patient should not receive further infusions of amphotericin B liposome; facilities for cardiopulmonary resuscitation should be available during administration due to the possibility of anaphylactic reaction

Precautions Due to the nephrotoxic potential of amphotericin B, other nephrotoxic drugs should be avoided. Acute pulmonary reactions have been reported in patients simultaneously receiving intravenous amphotericin B and leukocyte transfusions; separate these infusions temporally as much as possible and monitor pulmonary function.

Adverse Reactions

Cardiovascular: Hypotension, arrhythmias, chest pain, cardiac arrest, vasodilatation, hypertension, tachycardia

Central nervous system: Headache, transient chills or rigors (18%), fever (17%), anxiety, insomnia, dizziness, hallucinations, asthenia

Dermatologic: Pruritus, rash, diaphoresis

Endocrine & metabolic: Hypokalemia, bilirubinemia, hypomagnesemia, hyperglycemia, hypocalcemia, hyperphosphatemia

Gastrointestinal: Diarrhea, nausea, vomiting, abdominal pain

Hematologic: Anemia, thrombocytopenia, leukopenia

Hepatic: Elevated ALT, AST, and alkaline phosphatase

Renal: Renal tubular acidosis, elevated serum creatinine and BUN (19%; occurs to a lesser degree than with conventional amphotericin B), oliguria, hematuria

Respiratory: Dyspnea, respiratory failure, cough, epistaxis

Miscellaneous: Anaphylactoid and other allergic reactions

Drug Interactions Nephrotoxic drugs may cause additive nephrotoxic effects; corticosteroids may increase potassium depletion caused by amphotericin; may predispose patients receiving cardiac glycosides or skeletal muscle relaxants to toxicity secondary to hypokalemia; may result in acute pulmonary toxicity in patients simultaneously receiving leukocyte transfusions; ketoconazole, fluconazole may induce fungal resistance to amphotericin B; may increase toxicity of flucytosine by increasing cellular uptake and/or impairing its renal excretion; may potentiate renal toxicity, bronchospasm and hypotension of antineoplastic agents

Stability Store unopened vials at temperatures ≤25°C (77°F); reconstituted drug is stable for 24 hours under refrigeration. Do not dilute with saline solutions or mix with other drugs or electrolytes since this may cause precipitation of AmBisome®. AmBisome® is stable when further diluted to a concentration of 0.2-2 mg/mL in D_5W and $D_{10}W$ or 2 mg/mL in $D_{20}W$ and $D_{25}W$ (see table on next page).

Mechanism of Action Binds to ergosterol altering cell membrane permeability in susceptible fungi and causing leakage of cell components with subsequent cell death

Pharmacokinetics Exhibits nonlinear kinetics (greater than proportional increase in serum concentration with an increase in dose)

Distribution: V_d: 0.1-0.16 L/kg
Half-life (terminal): 100-153 hours

AmBisome® Stability

	Solution	Temperature	Stability
D_5W	2 mg/mL	2°C to 8°C	14 days
	0.2 mg/mL	2°C to 8°C	11 days
	0.2-2 mg/mL	23°C to 27°C	24 hours
$D_{10}W$	0.2-2 mg/mL	2°C to 8°C	48 hours
$D_{20}W$	2 mg/mL	2°C to 8°C	48 hours
$D_{25}W$	2 mg/mL	2°C to 8°C	48 hours

Usual Dosage Infants ≥1 month, Children, and Adults: I.V.:
Empiric therapy: 3 mg/kg/day given as a once daily infusion
Systemic fungal infections: 3-5 mg/kg/day given as a once daily infusion; doses as high as 10 mg/kg/day have been used in patients with documented *Aspergillus* infection
Cryptococcal meningitis in HIV infected patients: 6 mg/kg/day given as a once daily infusion
Visceral leishmaniasis:
Immunocompetent patients:
Days 1-5: 3 mg/kg/day once daily
Days 14 and 21: 3 mg/kg/dose
Note: Repeat course may be given to patients who do not achieve parasitic clearance
Immunocompromised patients:
Days 1-5: 4 mg/kg/day once daily
Days 10, 17, 24, 31, 38: 4 mg/kg/dose

Administration Parenteral: I.V.: Do not use in-line filter less than 1 micron to administer AmBisome®. Flush line with D_5W prior to infusion; infusion of diluted AmBisome® should start within 6 hours of preparation; infuse over 2 hours; infusion time may be reduced to 1 hour in patients who tolerate the treatment; AmBisome® may be diluted with D_5W, $D_{10}W$, or $D_{20}W$ to a final concentration of 1-2 mg/mL; lower concentrations (0.2-0.5 mg/mL) may be administered to infants and small children to provide sufficient volume for infusion

Monitoring Parameters BUN, serum creatinine, liver function tests, serum electrolytes, CBC, vital signs, I & O; monitor for signs of hypokalemia (muscle weakness, cramping, drowsiness, EKG changes)

Nursing Implications Management of side effects is similar to conventional amphotericin B. [See Amphotericin B (Conventional) *on page 118* for suggested management guidelines of side effects.]

Dosage Forms Excipient information presented when available (limited, particularly for generics); consult specific product labeling.
Injection, powder for reconstitution:
AmBisome®: 50 mg [contains soy and sucrose]

References

Emminger W, Graninger W, Emminger-Schmidmeir W, et al, "Tolerance of High Doses of Amphotericin B by Infusion of a Liposomal Formulation in Children With Cancer," *Ann Hematol*, 1994, 68:27-31.
Ringden O, Andstrom E, Remberger M, et al, "Safety of Liposomal Amphotericin B (AmBisome®) In 187 Transplant Recipients Treated With Cyclosporin," *Bone Marrow Transplant*, 1994, 14 Suppl 5:S10-4.
Walsh TJ, Goodman JL, Pappas P, et al, "Safety, Tolerance, and Pharmacokinetics of High-Dose Liposomal Amphotericin B (AmBisome®) in Patients Infected With Aspergillus Species and Other Filamentous Fungi: Maximum Tolerated Dose Study," *Antimicrob Agents Chemother*, 2001, 45(12):3487-96.
Walsh TJ, Finberg RW, Arndt C, et al, "Liposomal Amphotericin B for Empirical Therapy in Patients With Persistent Fever and Neutropenia," *N Engl J Med*, 1999, 340:764-71.

Ampicillin (am pi SIL in)

Medication Safety Issues
Sound-alike/look-alike issues:
Ampicillin may be confused with aminophylline

Related Information
Endocarditis Prophylaxis *on page 1812*

Canadian Brand Names Apo-Ampi®; Novo-Ampicillin; Nu-Ampi

Index Terms Aminobenzylpenicillin; Ampicillin Sodium; Ampicillin Trihydrate

Therapeutic Category Antibiotic, Penicillin

Generic Available Yes

Use Treatment of susceptible bacterial infections caused by streptococci, pneumococci, enterococci, nonpenicillinase-producing staphylococci, *Listeria*, meningococci; some strains of *H. influenzae, P. mirabilis, Salmonella, Shigella, E. coli, Enterobacter*,
(Continued)

Ampicillin *(Continued)*

and *Klebsiella*; initial empiric treatment of neonates with suspected bacterial sepsis or meningitis used in combination with an aminoglycoside or cefotaxime; endocarditis prophylaxis

Pregnancy Risk Factor B

Lactation Enters breast milk/use caution

Contraindications Hypersensitivity to ampicillin (penicillins) or any component

Warnings Epstein-Barr virus infection, acute lymphocytic leukemia or cytomegalovirus infection increases risk for ampicillin-induced maculopapular rash

Precautions Dosage adjustment may be necessary in patients with renal impairment (Cl_{cr} <10-15 mL/minute); use with caution in patients allergic to cephalosporins

Adverse Reactions

Central nervous system: Seizures, headache, dizziness, drug fever

Dermatologic: Rash, urticaria, exfoliative dermatitis, Stevens-Johnson syndrome

Gastrointestinal: Diarrhea (20%), nausea, vomiting, glossitis, pseudomembranous enterocolitis, oral candidiasis

Hematologic: Eosinophilia, hemolytic anemia, thrombocytopenia, neutropenia, prolongation of bleeding time

Renal: Interstitial nephritis

Miscellaneous: Anaphylaxis, hypersensitivity reactions, serum sickness, vasculitis, superinfection

Drug Interactions Estrogen-containing oral contraceptives (decreases contraceptive effectiveness), aminoglycosides, probenecid (increases ampicillin serum levels), chloroquine (decreases bioavailability of ampicillin), allopurinol (possible increased frequency of ampicillin rash)

Food Interactions Food decreases rate and extent of absorption

Stability Oral suspension is stable for 14 days under refrigeration; reconstituted solutions for I.M. or direct I.V. should be used within 1 hour; solutions for I.V. infusion will be inactivated by dextrose at room temperature; if dextrose-containing solutions are to be used as a diluent, the resultant solution will only be stable for 2 hours vs 8 hours in solutions containing NS

Mechanism of Action Interferes with bacterial cell wall synthesis by binding to one or more penicillin-binding proteins during active multiplication; inhibits the final transpeptidation step of peptidoglycan synthesis causing cell wall death and resultant bactericidal activity against susceptible bacteria

Pharmacokinetics

Absorption: Oral: 50%

Distribution: Into bile; penetration into CSF occurs with inflamed meninges only; low excretion into breast milk

Protein binding:
- Neonates: 10%
- Adults: 15% to 18%

Half-life:
- Neonates:
  - 2-7 days: 4 hours
  - 8-14 days: 2.8 hours
  - 15-30 days: 1.7 hours
- Children and Adults: 1-1.8 hours
- Anuric patients: 8-20 hours

Time to peak serum concentration: Oral: Within 1-2 hours

Elimination: ~90% of drug excreted unchanged in urine within 24 hours; excreted in bile

Dialysis: ~40% is removed by hemodialysis

Usual Dosage

Children: Oral: 50-100 mg/kg/day divided every 6 hours; maximum dose: 2-3 g/day

Adults: Oral: 250-500 mg every 6 hours

Neonates: I.M., I.V.:
- Postnatal age ≤7 days:
  - ≤2000 g: 50 mg/kg/day divided every 12 hours; meningitis: 100 mg/kg/day divided every 12 hours
  - >2000 g: 75 mg/kg/day divided every 8 hours; meningitis: 150 mg/kg/day divided every 8 hours
  - Group B streptococcal meningitis: 200 mg/kg/day divided every 8 hours
- Postnatal age >7 days:
  - <1200 g: 50 mg/kg/day divided every 12 hours; meningitis: 100 mg/kg/day divided every 12 hours
  - 1200-2000 g: 75 mg/kg/day divided every 8 hours; meningitis: 150 mg/kg/day divided every 8 hours
  - >2000 g: 100 mg/kg/day divided every 6 hours; meningitis: 200 mg/kg/day divided every 6 hours

Group B streptococcal meningitis: 300 mg/kg/day divided every 6 hours

Infants and Children: I.M., I.V.: 100-200 mg/kg/day divided every 6 hours; meningitis: 200-400 mg/kg/day divided every 6 hours; maximum dose: 12 g/day

Endocarditis prophylaxis:

50 mg/kg within 30 minutes before procedure (dental, oral, respiratory tract, or esophageal procedures); maximum dose: 2 g

50 mg/kg (maximum dose: 2 g) plus gentamicin 1.5 mg/kg (maximum dose: 120 mg) within 30 minutes of starting the procedure; 25 mg/kg 6 hours later (for high-risk patients undergoing genitourinary and GI tract procedures)

Adults: I.M., I.V.: 500 mg to 3 g every 6 hours; maximum dose: 14 g/day

Endocarditis prophylaxis:

2 g within 30 minutes before procedure (dental, oral, respiratory tract, or esophageal procedures)

2 g plus gentamicin 1.5 mg/kg (maximum dose: 120 mg) within 30 minutes of starting the procedure; 1 g 6 hours later (for high-risk patients undergoing genitourinary and GI tract procedures)

Dosing interval in renal impairment: Adults:

Cl_{cr} 10-30 mL/minute: Administer every 6-12 hours

Cl_{cr} <10 mL/minute: Administer every 12 hours

Administration

Oral: Administer with water 1-2 hours prior to food on an empty stomach; shake suspension well before using

Parenteral: Ampicillin may be administered IVP over 3-5 minutes at a rate not to exceed 100 mg/minute or I.V. intermittent infusion over 15-30 minutes; final concentration for I.V. administration should not exceed 100 mg/mL (IVP) or 30 mg/mL (I.V. intermittent infusion)

Monitoring Parameters With prolonged therapy monitor renal, hepatic, and hematologic function periodically; observe for change in bowel frequency

Test Interactions False-positive urinary glucose (Benedict's solution, Clinitest®); + Coombs' [direct]

Nursing Implications Ampicillin and gentamicin should not be mixed in the same I.V. tubing or administered concurrently

Additional Information Appearance of a rash should be carefully evaluated to differentiate a nonallergic ampicillin rash from a hypersensitivity reaction. Ampicillin rash occurs in 5% to 10% of children receiving ampicillin and is a generalized dull red, maculopapular rash, generally appearing 3-14 days after the start of therapy. It normally begins on the trunk and spreads over most of the body. It may be most intense at pressure areas, elbows, and knees. Incidence of ampicillin rash is higher in patients with viral infections, infectious mononucleosis, lymphocytic leukemia, or patients with hyperuricemia who are receiving allopurinol.

Sodium content of suspension (250 mg/5 mL, 5 mL): 10 mg (0.4 mEq)

Sodium content of 1 g: 66.7 mg (3 mEq)

Dosage Forms Excipient information presented when available (limited, particularly for generics); consult specific product labeling.

Capsule: 250 mg, 500 mg

Injection, powder for reconstitution, as sodium: 125 mg, 250 mg, 500 mg, 1 g, 2 g, 10 g

Powder for oral suspension: 125 mg/5 mL (100 mL, 200 mL); 250 mg/5 mL (100 mL, 200 mL)

References

Boguniewicz M and Leung DY, "Hypersensitivity Reactions to Antibiotics Commonly Used in Children," *Pediatr Infect Dis J*, 1995, 14(3):221-31.

Brown RD, Campoli-Richards DM, "Antimicrobial Therapy in Neonates, Infants, and Children," *Clin Pharmacokinet*, 1989, 17(Suppl 1):105-15.

Ampicillin and Sulbactam (am pi SIL in & SUL bak tam)

U.S. Brand Names Unasyn®

Canadian Brand Names Unasyn®

Index Terms Sulbactam and Ampicillin

Therapeutic Category Antibiotic, Beta-lactam and Beta-lactamase Combination; Antibiotic, Penicillin

Generic Available Yes

Use Treatment of susceptible bacterial infections involved with skin and skin structure, intra-abdominal infections, gynecological infections; spectrum is that of ampicillin plus organisms producing beta-lactamases such as *S. aureus*, *H. influenzae*, *E. coli*, *Klebsiella*, *Acinetobacter*, *Enterobacter*, and anaerobes

Pregnancy Risk Factor B

Lactation Enters breast milk/use caution

(Continued)

Ampicillin and Sulbactam *(Continued)*

Contraindications Hypersensitivity to ampicillin, sulbactam, any component, or penicillins

Warnings Epstein-Barr virus infection, acute lymphocytic leukemia or cytomegalovirus infection increases risk for ampicillin-induced maculopapular rash; not FDA approved for children <12 years of age

Precautions Modify dosage in patients with renal impairment; use with caution in patients allergic to cephalosporins

Adverse Reactions

Cardiovascular: Chest pain

Central nervous system: Fatigue, malaise, headache, chills, dizziness, seizures

Dermatologic: Rash (2%), itching, urticaria, exfoliative dermatitis, Stevens-Johnson syndrome

Gastrointestinal: Diarrhea (3%), nausea, vomiting, candidiasis, flatulence, pseudomembranous colitis, hairy tongue

Genitourinary: Dysuria, hematuria

Hematologic: Decreased WBC, neutrophils, platelets, hemoglobin, and hematocrit

Hepatic: Elevated liver enzymes

Local: Pain at injection site (I.M.: 16%, I.V.: 3%), thrombophlebitis (3%)

Renal: Elevated BUN, elevated serum creatinine

Miscellaneous: Hypersensitivity reactions, anaphylaxis, serum sickness, vasculitis, superinfection

Drug Interactions Probenecid (decreased elimination of ampicillin and sulbactam); allopurinol (possible increased frequency of ampicillin rash); efficacy of oral contraceptives may be reduced

Stability Ampicillin/sulbactam infusion solution is stable for 8 hours in NS at room temperature; incompatible when mixed with aminoglycosides

Mechanism of Action Sulbactam has very little antibacterial activity by itself. The addition of sulbactam, a beta-lactamase inhibitor, to ampicillin extends the spectrum of ampicillin to include beta-lactamase producing organisms; ampicillin acts by inhibiting bacterial cell wall synthesis during the stage of active multiplication

Pharmacokinetics

Distribution: Into bile, blister and tissue fluids; poor penetration into CSF with uninflamed meninges; higher concentrations attained with inflamed meninges

Protein binding:

- Ampicillin: 28%
- Sulbactam: 38%

Half-life: Ampicillin and sulbactam are similar: 1-1.8 hours and 1-1.3 hours, respectively in patients with normal renal function

Elimination: ~75% to 85% of both drugs are excreted unchanged in urine within 8 hours following administration

Usual Dosage Unasyn® (ampicillin/sulbactam) is a combination product; each 3 g vial contains 2 g of ampicillin and 1 g of sulbactam. Dosage recommendations are based on the **ampicillin** component.

I.M., I.V.:

- Infants ≥1 month: 100-150 mg ampicillin/kg/day divided every 6 hours
  - Meningitis: 200-300 mg ampicillin/kg/day divided every 6 hours
- Children: 100-200 mg ampicillin/kg/day divided every 6 hours
  - Meningitis: 200-400 mg ampicillin/kg/day divided every 6 hours; maximum dose: 8 g ampicillin/day
- Adults: 1-2 g ampicillin every 6-8 hours; maximum dose: 12 g ampicillin/day

Dosing interval in renal impairment:

- Cl_{cr} 15-29 mL/minute: Administer every 12 hours
- Cl_{cr} 5-14 mL/minute: Administer every 24 hours

Administration Parenteral: May be administered by slow I.V. injection over 10-15 minutes at a final concentration for administration not to exceed 45 mg Unasyn® (30 mg ampicillin and 15 mg sulbactam)/mL or by intermittent infusion over 15-30 minutes

Monitoring Parameters With prolonged therapy monitor hematologic, renal, and hepatic function; observe for change in bowel frequency

Test Interactions False-positive urinary glucose levels (Benedict's solution, Clinitest®); positive Coombs' [direct]

Additional Information Sodium content of 1.5 g (1 g ampicillin plus 0.5 g sulbactam): 5 mEq

Dosage Forms Excipient information presented when available (limited, particularly for generics); consult specific product labeling.

Injection, powder for reconstitution: 1.5 g: Ampicillin 1 g and sulbactam 0.5 g [contains sodium 115 mg (5 mEq)/1.5 g)]; 3 g: Ampicillin 2 g and sulbactam 1 g [contains sodium 115 mg (5 mEq)/1.5 g)]; 15 g: Ampicillin 10 g and sulbactam 5 g [bulk package; contains sodium 115 mg (5 mEq)/1.5 g)]

Unasyn®:

1.5 g: Ampicillin 1 g and sulbactam 0.5 g [contains sodium 115 mg (5 mEq)/1.5 g]

3 g: Ampicillin 2 g and sulbactam 1 g [contains sodium 115 mg (5 mEq)/1.5 g)]

15 g: Ampicillin 10 g and sulbactam 5 g [bulk package; contains sodium 115 mg (5 mEq)/1.5 g)]

References

Dajani AS, "Sulbactam/Ampicillin in Pediatric Infections," *Drugs*, 1988, 35(Suppl 7):35-8.

Goldfarb J, Aronoff SC, Jaffé A, et al, "Sultamicillin in the Treatment of Superficial Skin and Soft Tissue Infections in Children," *Antimicrob Agents Chemother*, 1987, 31(4):663-4.

Kulhanjian J, Dunphy MG, Hamstra S, et al, "Randomized Comparative Study of Ampicillin/Sulbactam vs Ceftriaxone for Treatment of Soft Tissue and Skeletal Infections in Children," *Pediatr Infect Dis J*, 1989, 8(9):605-10.

Syriopoulou V, Bitsi M, Theodoridis C, et al, "Clinical Efficacy of Sulbactam/Ampicillin in Pediatric Infections Caused by Ampicillin-Resistant or Penicillin-Resistant Organisms," *Rev Infect Dis*, 1986, 8(Suppl 5):S630-3.

♦ **Ampicillin Sodium** *see* Ampicillin *on page 123*

♦ **Ampicillin Trihydrate** *see* Ampicillin *on page 123*

Amprenavir (am PRE na veer)

Related Information

Adult and Adolescent HIV *on page 1821*
Assessment of Liver Function *on page 1810*
Pediatric HIV *on page 1816*
Perinatal HIV *on page 1831*

U.S. Brand Names Agenerase®

Canadian Brand Names Agenerase®

Therapeutic Category Antiretroviral Agent; HIV Agents (Anti-HIV Agents); Protease Inhibitor

Generic Available No

Use Treatment of HIV infection in combination with other antiretroviral agents (Note: HIV regimens consisting of **three** antiretroviral agents are strongly recommended)

Pregnancy Risk Factor C

Lactation Excretion in breast milk unknown/contraindicated

Contraindications Hypersensitivity to amprenavir or any component; concurrent therapy with astemizole, cisapride, dihydroergotamine, ergonovine, ergotamine, methylergonovine, pimozide, midazolam, or triazolam; due to the high amount of propylene glycol, amprenavir oral **solution** is contraindicated in infants and children <4 years, pregnancy, renal or hepatic failure, and in patients receiving disulfiram or metronidazole

Warnings Amprenavir is a potent CYP3A4 isoenzyme inhibitor that interacts with numerous drugs. Due to potential serious and/or life-threatening drug interactions, some drugs are contraindicated (see Contraindications and Drug interactions) and the following drugs require concentration monitoring if coadministered with amprenavir: amiodarone, systemic lidocaine, tricyclic antidepressants, and quinidine. Concurrent use with rifampin, hormonal contraceptives, or certain cholesterol-lowering agents (lovastatin, simvastatin) is **not** recommended.

Amprenavir oral solution contains a high amount of propylene glycol and should only be used when the capsules or other protease inhibitors are not options; women and certain ethnic groups (Native Americans, Eskimos, Asians) may have a decreased capacity to metabolize propylene glycol and therefore, may be at a higher risk for adverse effects of propylene glycol; patients with renal or hepatic impairment are also at higher risk for adverse effects of propylene glycol (use oral solution with caution); when using the oral solution, monitor patients for propylene glycol adverse effects (see Monitoring Parameters); change patient to capsule formulation as soon as patient is able to take capsules.

Severe and life-threatening skin reactions (eg, Stevens-Johnson syndrome) may occur; discontinue amprenavir in patients who develop severe or life-threatening rashes or in patients with moderate rashes and systemic symptoms. Spontaneous bleeding episodes have been reported in patients with hemophilia type A and B receiving protease inhibitors. New onset diabetes mellitus, exacerbations of diabetes, and hyperglycemia have been reported in HIV-infected patients receiving protease inhibitors. Acute hemolytic anemia has been reported.

Precautions Use with caution in patients with diabetes mellitus, sulfonamide allergy (amprenavir is a sulfonamide), or hemophilia. Use with caution and decrease the dose in patients with hepatic impairment. Capsules and oral solution contain high amounts of vitamin E; additional supplements of vitamin E should be avoided. Fat redistribution and accumulation [ie, central obesity, peripheral wasting, facial wasting, breast enlargement, dorsocervical fat enlargement (buffalo hump), and cushingoid

(Continued)

Amprenavir *(Continued)*

appearance] have been observed in patients receiving antiretroviral agents (causal relationship not established). Immune reconstitution syndrome (an acute inflammatory response to residual or indolent opportunistic infections) may occur in HIV patients during initial treatment with combination antiretroviral agents, including amprenavir; this syndrome may require further patient assessment and therapy.

Adverse Reactions Note: Percent incidence of adverse reactions are similar in adult and pediatric patients; percent incidence listed reflects combination antiretroviral therapy (but not concurrent therapy with ritonavir; see package insert)

Central nervous system: Depression or mood disorders (9% to 16%), headache, fatigue

Dermatologic: Rash (22% incidence; usually mild to moderate, maculopapular, some pruritic; median onset: 11 days, range: 7-73 days); severe or life-threatening rash, including Stevens-Johnson syndrome (1% of patients, 4% of patients who develop a rash)

Endocrine & metabolic: Hyperglycemia (>116 mg/dL: 45% to 53%), hypertriglyceridemia (>213 mg/dL: 41% to 56%), hypercholesterolemia (>283 mg/dL: 7% to 13%), new onset diabetes, exacerbation of diabetes mellitus, ketoacidosis, elevated serum creatine phosphokinase, fat redistribution and accumulation (see Precautions)

Gastrointestinal: Nausea (43% to 74%), vomiting (24% to 34%), diarrhea (39% to 60%), taste disorders (2% to 10%)

Hematologic: Acute hemolytic anemia (rare, one case reported), spontaneous bleeding in hemophiliacs, neutropenia

Hepatic: Elevated liver enzymes

Neuromuscular & skeletal: Paresthesia [perioral (26% to 31%) or peripheral (10% to 14%)]

Miscellaneous: Immune reconstitution syndrome

Drug Interactions Cytochrome P450 isoenzyme CYP2C9 (minor), CYP3A4 (major), CYP3A5 (minor) substrate; isoenzyme CYP2C19 (weak) and CYP3A4 (strong) inhibitor

Amprenavir may inhibit the metabolism of the following drugs and cause serious or life-threatening adverse effects: Astemizole, cisapride, dihydroergotamine, ergotamine, midazolam, and triazolam (concurrent therapy with these drugs and amprenavir is contraindicated); **Note:** If amprenavir and ritonavir capsules are used concurrently, flecainide and propafenone are also contraindicated; amprenavir may increase the toxic effects of amiodarone, lidocaine, quinidine, warfarin, cyclosporine, tacrolimus, rapamycin, and tricyclic antidepressants (serum concentration monitoring of these drugs is necessary); amprenavir may increase the serum concentration of bepridil and result in life-threatening cardiac arrhythmias (use with caution; monitor closely); amprenavir significantly increases the AUC of rifabutin by 193% (rifabutin dose should be decreased by at least ½ the recommended dose when used in combination with amprenavir); amprenavir may increase the AUC of ketoconazole and zidovudine and decrease the AUC of indinavir and saquinavir; amprenavir may increase serum concentrations or toxicity of diltiazem, nifedipine, alprazolam, clorazepate, diazepam, flurazepam, itraconazole, dapsone, erythromycin, loratadine, sildenafil, carbamazepine, pimozide, trazodone, and cholesterol-lowering agents (concurrent use of lovastatin or simvastatin is **not** recommended; concurrent use of atorvastatin may increase risk of myopathy and rhabdomyolysis; use lowest possible dose of atorvastatin and carefully monitor patient; consider use of pravastatin or fluvastatin for concurrent use with amprenavir). Ritonavir significantly increases fluticasone serum concentrations and may result in systemic corticosteroid effects (eg, Cushing's syndrome and adrenal suppression); amprenavir plus ritonavir use with fluticasone is expected to have the same effect; concurrent use of amprenavir plus ritonavir with fluticasone is **not** recommended unless benefits outweigh risks; use of amprenavir without ritonavir may increase fluticasone serum concentrations (use with caution; consider alternative agent, especially with long-term use).

Rifampin significantly reduces amprenavir plasma concentrations (AUC of amprenavir is decreased by about 90%) and should **not** be used concurrently; hormonal contraceptives (eg, ethinyl estradiol/norethindrone) decrease amprenavir serum concentrations and should **not** be used concurrently (nonhormonal contraception is recommended); methadone may decrease the serum concentrations of amprenavir (consider alternative antiretroviral agent); amprenavir may decrease plasma concentrations of methadone (increase in methadone dosage may be required); amprenavir may decrease serum concentrations of delavirdine and result in a loss of virological response and possible delavirdine resistance (concomitant use of amprenavir and delavirdine is **not** recommended); the herbal medicine St John's wort (*Hypericum perforatum*) may significantly decrease concentrations of amprenavir and is **not** recommended for concurrent use; efavirenz decreases amprenavir concentrations by 39%; saquinavir decreases amprenavir AUC by 32%; dexamethasone may decrease amprenavir serum concentrations (use with caution); nevirapine, phenobarbital, phenytoin, or carbamazepine may decrease amprenavir concentrations; abacavir, clarithromycin, indinavir, ketoconazole, or zidovudine may increase the AUC of amprenavir; nelfinavir may increase the trough concentrations of amprenavir; cimetidine, lopinavir/ritonavir, or ritonavir may increase amprenavir concentrations [**Note:** Amprenavir dose of capsules should be decreased when used in combination with ritonavir capsules (see Usual Dosage)]; use of amprenavir oral solution with ritonavir oral solution is not recommended (see paragraph below)

Antacids or didanosine (buffered formulations) should be given at least 1 hour before or after amprenavir; vitamin E supplements should be avoided (amprenavir products contain high amounts of vitamin E); alcohol may interact with the high amount of propylene glycol in the oral solution and should be avoided; concomitant use of ritonavir oral solution with amprenavir oral solution is not recommended due to the large amounts of propylene glycol in amprenavir oral solution and ethanol in ritonavir oral solution [**Note:** Propylene glycol and ethanol (alcohol) may compete for the same metabolic pathway]

Food Interactions A high fat meal may decrease mean AUC by 14%

Stability Capsules and solution: Store at room temperature; do not refrigerate

Mechanism of Action A protease inhibitor which acts on an enzyme (protease) late in the HIV replication process after the virus has entered into the cell's nucleus; amprenavir binds to the protease activity site and inhibits the activity of the enzyme, thus preventing cleavage of viral polyprotein precursors (gag-pol protein precursors) into individual functional proteins found in infectious HIV; this results in the formation of immature, noninfectious viral particles

Pharmacokinetics

Distribution: V_d (apparent): Adults: 430 L

Protein binding: 90%; high affinity binding protein: alpha$_1$ acid glycoprotein; also binds to albumin (but to a lesser extent)

Metabolism: In the liver primarily via cytochrome P450 CYP3A4 isoenzyme system; glucuronide conjugation of oxidized metabolites also occurs

Bioavailability: Absolute bioavailability not established; oral solution is 14% less bioavailable than capsules (do not interchange on a mg per mg basis)

Half-life: Adults: 7.1-10.6 hours

Time to peak serum concentration (single dose): 1-2 hours

Elimination: Minimal excretion of unchanged drug in urine (<3%) and feces; 75% of dose excreted as metabolites via biliary tract into feces and 14% excreted as metabolites in urine

Usual Dosage Oral (use in combination with other antiretroviral agents): **Note:** Due to differences in bioavailability, capsules and solution are **not** interchangeable on a mg per mg basis; **Note:** Amprenavir 150 mg capsules have been discontinued; consider use of fosamprenavir in appropriate patients (see Fosamprenavir monograph):

Neonates, Infants, and Children <4 years:

Capsules: Not approved for use

Solution: Contraindicated due to potential toxicity from propylene glycol

Children 4-12 years and Adolescents 13-16 years with a body weight <50 kg:

Capsules: 20 mg/kg twice daily or 15 mg/kg 3 times/day; maximum: 2400 mg/day

Solution: 22.5 mg/kg (1.5 mL/kg) twice daily or 17 mg/kg (1.1 mL/kg) 3 times/day; maximum: 2800 mg/day

Note: Concomitant therapy of amprenavir oral solution with ritonavir oral solution is not recommended (see Drug Interactions)

Adolescents 13-16 years with a body weight ≥50 kg and Adults:

Capsules: 1200 mg twice daily

Solution: 1400 mg twice daily

Adults:

Concomitant therapy with ritonavir: Capsules: Amprenavir 1200 mg (with ritonavir 200 mg) once daily or amprenavir 600 mg (with ritonavir 100 mg) twice daily

Concomitant therapy with efavirenz: Capsules: Amprenavir 1200 mg (with ritonavir 200 mg) twice daily plus efavirenz 600 mg once daily. **Note:** Ritonavir boosting of amprenavir should always be used when regimen includes efavirenz

Dosing adjustment in hepatic impairment: Adults:

Capsules:

Child-Pugh score 5-8: 450 mg twice daily

Child-Pugh score 9-12: 300 mg twice daily

Solution:

Child-Pugh score 5-8: 513 mg (34 mL) twice daily

Child-Pugh score 9-12: 342 mg (23 mL) twice daily

Administration May be administered without regard to meals; avoid administration with high fat meals; do not administer concurrently with antacids

(Continued)

Amprenavir *(Continued)*

Monitoring Parameters Signs and symptoms of rash or adverse effects; serum glucose, triglycerides, cholesterol, liver enzymes, CBC with differential, CD4 cell count, viral load; patients treated with amprenavir oral solution need to be monitored for adverse effects of propylene glycol, such as hyperosmolality, lactic acidosis, seizures, stupor, tachycardia, renal toxicity, and hemolysis

Patient Information Inform your physician if you have a sulfa allergy; amprenavir is not a cure for HIV; notify physician immediately if rash develops; some medicines should not be taken with amprenavir; report the use of other medications, nonprescription medications, and herbal or natural products to your physician and pharmacist; avoid the herbal medicine St John's wort and vitamin E supplements; take amprenavir every day as prescribed; do not change dose or discontinue without physician's advice; if a dose is missed, take it as soon as possible, then return to normal dosing schedule; if a dose is skipped, do not double the next dose; avoid alcohol and ritonavir oral solution if taking amprenavir oral solution

HIV medications may cause changes in body fat, including an increase in fat in the upper back and neck, breasts, and trunk; a loss of fat from the face, arms, and legs may also occur.

Additional Information To increase amprenavir solubility, propylene glycol has been added to the oral solution. **Note:** The recommended pediatric (twice daily) dose of the oral solution delivers 1650 mg/kg/day of propylene glycol; the acceptable amount of propylene glycol (when used as an excipient) is not known; however, the amount of propylene glycol found in amprenavir oral solution exceeds the WHO standards (25 mg/kg/day) for use as a food additive in infants. Treatment of overdose of the oral solution should include monitoring and management of propylene glycol adverse effects including acid-base abnormalities (see Monitoring Parameters); hemodialysis for removal of propylene glycol may be needed.

To increase amprenavir bioavailability, *d*-alpha tocopherol polyethylene glycol 1000 succinate (TPGS; a form of vitamin E) has been added in significant concentrations to the product formulations (see Dosage Forms). **Note:** The recommended pediatric dose of the oral solution delivers 138 international units/kg/day of vitamin E; this significantly exceeds the pediatric RDA of 10 international units. The recommended adult dose in capsule form delivers 1744 international units/day of vitamin E; this significantly exceeds the adult RDA of 30 international units. Long-term effects of high dose vitamin E are not well defined; high doses of vitamin E may worsen blood coagulation defects of vitamin K deficiency that are caused by malabsorption or from anticoagulant therapy.

Dosage Forms Excipient information presented when available (limited, particularly for generics); consult specific product labeling.

Capsule:
- Agenerase®: 50 mg [contains vitamin E 36.3 int. units (as TPGS)]

Solution, oral:
- Agenerase®: 15 mg/mL (240 mL) [contains propylene glycol 550 mg/mL and vitamin E 46 int. units/mL; grape-bubble gum-peppermint flavor]

References

Adkins JC and Faulds D, "Amprenavir," *Drugs*, 1998, 55(6):837-42.

Briars LA, Hilao JJ, and Kraus DM, "A Review of Pediatric Human Immunodeficiency Virus Infection," *Journal of Pharmacy Practice*, 2004, 17(6):407-31.

Center for Disease Control and Prevention, "Guidelines for Using Antiretroviral Agents Among HIV-Infected Adults and Adolescents. Recommendations of the Panel on Clinical Practices for Treatment of HIV," *MMWR*, 2002, 51(RR-7):1-55.

Collura JM and Kraus DM, "New Pediatric Antiretroviral Agents," *J Pediatr Health Care*, 2000, 14(4):183-90.

Panel on Clinical Practices for Treatment of HIV Infection, "Guidelines for the Use of Antiretroviral Agents in HIV-Infected Adults and Adolescents," October 10, 2006, http://www.aidsinfo.nih.gov.

Piscitelli SC, Burstein AH, Chaitt D, et al, "Indinavir Concentrations and St. John's Wort," *Lancet*, 2000, 355(9203):547-8.

Sadler BM, Hanson CD, Chittick GE, et al, "Safety and Pharmacokinetics of Amprenavir (141W94), a Human Immunodeficiency Virus (HIV) Type 1 Protease Inhibitor, Following Oral Administration of Single Doses to HIV-Infected Adults," *Antimicrob Agents Chemother*, 1999, 43(7):1686-92.

Working Group on Antiretroviral Therapy and Medical Management of HIV-Infected Children, "Guidelines for the Use of Antiretroviral Agents in Pediatric HIV Infection," October 26, 2006, http://www.aidsinfo.nih.gov.

Working Group on Antiretroviral Therapy and Medical Management of HIV-Infected Children, "Guidelines for the Use of Antiretroviral Agents in Pediatric HIV Infection. Supplement I: Pediatric Antiretroviral Drug Information," October 26, 2006, http://www.aidsinfo.nih.gov.

♦ **Amrinone Lactate** *see* Inamrinone *on page 822*

Amyl Nitrite (AM il NYE trite)

Index Terms Isoamyl Nitrite

Therapeutic Category Antidote, Cyanide; Vasodilator, Coronary

Generic Available Yes

Use Coronary vasodilator in angina pectoris; an adjunct in treatment of cyanide poisoning

Pregnancy Risk Factor C

Lactation Excretion in breast milk unknown/not recommended

Contraindications Hypersensitivity to nitrates or any component; severe anemia; recent head trauma or cerebral hemorrhage; glaucoma; hyperthyroidism; recent MI

Warnings Postural hypotension with episodes of dizziness, weakness, or syncope may occur after inhalation; may cause harm to the fetus if administered to a pregnant woman (may significantly decrease systemic blood pressure and blood flow)

Precautions Use with great caution in patients with increased intracranial pressure or low systolic blood pressure; tolerance to coronary vasodilator effects may occur (to minimize tolerance, use lowest effective initial dose and alternate with another coronary vasodilator); high doses of nitrates may cause methemoglobinemia (especially in patients with methemoglobin reductase deficiency or other metabolic abnormalities)

Adverse Reactions

Cardiovascular: Postural hypotension; cutaneous flushing of head, neck, and clavicular area; tachycardia; palpitations; vasodilation; syncope

Central nervous system: Headache, dizziness, restlessness

Dermatologic: Skin rash (contact dermatitis)

Gastrointestinal: Nausea, vomiting

Hematologic: Hemolytic anemia

Neuromuscular & skeletal: Weakness

Ocular: Elevated intraocular pressure

Miscellaneous: Tolerance to coronary vasodilator effects may occur

Drug Interactions Alcohol (may increase side effects and cause severe hypotension or cardiovascular collapse); medications that cause hypotension may increase the postural hypotensive effects of amyl nitrite

Stability Store in cool place, protect from light; flammable, avoid exposure to heat or flame

Mechanism of Action Vasodilator (vascular smooth muscle relaxant) which decreases afterload and improves myocardial blood supply via coronary artery vasodilation; antidote for cyanide poisoning: promotes formation of methemoglobin which combines with cyanide molecule to form cyanmethemoglobin (nontoxic)

Pharmacodynamics

Onset of action: Within 30 seconds

Duration: 3-5 minutes

Pharmacokinetics

Absorption: Inhalation: Readily absorbed through respiratory tract

Metabolism: In the liver to form inorganic nitrates (less potent)

Half-life:

Amyl nitrite: <1 hour

Methemoglobin: 1 hour

Elimination: Renal; ~33%

Usual Dosage Nasal inhalation:

Children and Adults: Cyanide poisoning: Inhale the vapor from a 0.3 mL crushed ampul every minute for 15-30 seconds until I.V. sodium nitrite infusion is available

Adults: Angina: 1-6 inhalations from 1 crushed ampul; may repeat in 3-5 minutes

Administration Give by nasal inhalation with patient in recumbent or seated position; crush ampul in woven covering between finger and hold under patient's nostrils

Monitoring Parameters Blood pressure; with treatment for cyanide poisoning: methemoglobin levels, arterial blood gas

Patient Information Remain seated or lying down during administration because of possible hypotension and dizziness; do not get up suddenly after use; avoid alcohol; if angina pain is not relieved after 2 doses, seek immediate medical attention

Nursing Implications To facilitate recovery from symptoms of postural hypotension, place patient in head-down position; may also use measures such as deep breathing and movement of extremities

Additional Information Amyl nitrite has been used to treat penile erections after urological surgery (eg, circumcisions in adults) and has been used to change the intensity of heart murmurs to aid in their diagnosis

Dosage Forms Excipient information presented when available (limited, particularly for generics); consult specific product labeling.

Vapor for inhalation [crushable covered glass capsules]: Amyl nitrite USP (0.3 mL)

♦ **Amyl Nitrite,Sodium Thiosulfate, and Sodium Nitrite** *see* Sodium Nitrite, Sodium Thiosulfate, and Amyl Nitrite *on page 1452*

♦ **Anaprox®** *see* Naproxen *on page 1108*

♦ **Anaprox® DS** *see* Naproxen *on page 1108*

♦ **Anaspaz®** *see* Hyoscyamine *on page 798*

♦ **Anbesol® [OTC]** *see* Benzocaine *on page 204*

- **Anbesol® Baby [OTC]** *see* Benzocaine *on page 204*
- **Anbesol® Baby (Can)** *see* Benzocaine *on page 204*
- **Anbesol® Cold Sore Therapy [OTC]** *see* Benzocaine *on page 204*
- **Anbesol® Jr. [OTC]** *see* Benzocaine *on page 204*
- **Anbesol® Maximum Strength [OTC]** *see* Benzocaine *on page 204*
- **Ancholc Acid** *see* Azelaic Acid *on page 188*
- **Ancobon®** *see* Flucytosine *on page 662*
- **Andehist NR Drops [DSC]** *see* Carbinoxamine and Pseudoephedrine *on page 286*
- **Andehist NR Syrup** *see* Brompheniramine and Pseudoephedrine *on page 235*
- **Andriol® (Can)** *see* Testosterone *on page 1511*
- **Androderm®** *see* Testosterone *on page 1511*
- **AndroGel®** *see* Testosterone *on page 1511*
- **Andropository (Can)** *see* Testosterone *on page 1511*
- **Androstanazole** *see* Stanozolol *on page 1471*
- **Anestacon®** *see* Lidocaine *on page 933*
- **Aneurine Hydrochloride** *see* Thiamine *on page 1526*
- **Anexate® (Can)** *see* Flumazenil *on page 667*
- **Anexsia®** *see* Hydrocodone and Acetaminophen *on page 779*
- **Anhydrous Glucose** *see* Dextrose *on page 479*
- **Ansaid® [DSC]** *see* Flurbiprofen *on page 688*
- **Ansaid® (Can)** *see* Flurbiprofen *on page 688*
- **Ansamycin** *see* Rifabutin *on page 1382*

Antacid Preparations (ant AS id prep a RAE shuns)

Related Information

Calcium Supplements *on page 272*
Magnesium Supplements *on page 976*

U.S. Brand Names Alamag [OTC]; Alamag Plus [OTC]; Aldroxicon I [OTC]; Aldroxicon II [OTC]; Alenic Alka Tablet [OTC]; Almacone® [OTC]; Almacone Double Strength® [OTC]; ALternaGel® [OTC]; Dermagran® [OTC]; Gaviscon® Tablet [OTC]; Gelusil® [OTC]; Genaton Tablet [OTC]; Maalox® [OTC]; Maalox® Max [OTC]; Mi-Acid [OTC]; Mi-Acid Maximum Strength [OTC]; Mintox Extra Strength [OTC]; Mintox Plus [OTC]; Mylanta® Liquid [OTC]; Mylanta® Maximum Strength Liquid [OTC]; Rulox [OTC]; Rulox No. 1 [DSC]

Index Terms Aluminum and Magnesium Hydroxide; Aluminum Hydroxide; Aluminum Hydroxide and Magnesium Carbonate; Aluminum Hydroxide and Magnesium Hydroxide; Aluminum Hydroxide and Magnesium Trisilicate; Aluminum Hydroxide, Magnesium Hydroxide, and Simethicone; Magaldrate

Therapeutic Category Antacid; Gastrointestinal Agent, Gastric or Duodenal Ulcer Treatment

Generic Available Yes

Use Adjunct for the relief of peptic ulcer pain and to promote healing of peptic ulcers; relief of stomach upset associated with hyperacidity; prevention of stress ulcer bleeding; treatment of duodenal ulcer and gastroesophageal reflux disease. Aluminum hydroxide is also used to reduce phosphate absorption in hyperphosphatemia; calcium carbonate is used to treat calcium deficiency and to bind phosphate; magnesium oxide is used to treat hypomagnesemia.

Contraindications Magnesium-containing antacids should not be used in patients with a creatinine clearance <30 mL/minute

Warnings Use aluminum-containing antacids with caution in patients with: Decreased bowel motility and dehydration, gastric outlet obstruction, renal failure, and in patients who have an upper GI hemorrhage; use magnesium-containing products with caution in patients with renal impairment; use sodium-containing antacids with caution in patients on low-sodium diets, and in patients with CHF, edema, renal failure, or hepatic failure; some tablets contain tartrazine which may cause allergic reactions in susceptible individuals

Precautions Maalox® Quick Dissolve tablets contain aspartame which is metabolized to phenylalanine and must be avoided or used with caution in patients with phenylketonuria.

Adverse Reactions

Aluminum-containing antacids:

Central nervous system: Dementia, encephalopathy, malaise, seizures, confusion, coma

Endocrine & metabolic: Hypophosphatemia, hyperaluminemia, osteoporosis

Gastrointestinal: Constipation, anorexia

Genitourinary: Urinary calculi
Neuromuscular & skeletal: Muscle weakness, osteomalacia

Calcium-containing antacids:
Endocrine & metabolic: Milk-alkali syndrome (hypercalcemia, metabolic alkalosis), hypophosphatemia
Gastrointestinal: Constipation, flatulence, nausea

Magnesium-containing antacids:
Endocrine & metabolic: Hypermagnesemia, fluid and electrolyte imbalance
Gastrointestinal: Laxative effects, diarrhea

Sodium-containing antacids:
Cardiovascular: Fluid retention
Endocrine & metabolic: Metabolic alkalosis, sodium overload
Gastrointestinal: Flatulence

Drug Interactions Aluminum-, calcium-, or magnesium-containing antacids (decrease tetracycline and quinolone absorption); antacids decrease absorption of delavirdine, itraconazole, ketoconazole, iron, digoxin, phenytoin, indomethacin, chlorpromazine; increased absorption of buffered or enteric-coated aspirin; aluminum hydroxide (decreased absorption of isoniazid); sucralfate antacids (may impair binding of sucralfate to ulcerated mucosa)

Food Interactions Aluminum-containing antacids (except aluminum phosphate) form insoluble salts with dietary phosphorus decreasing phosphorus absorption

Stability Avoid freezing aluminum hydroxide and magnesium hydroxide

Mechanism of Action Neutralizes gastric acidity increasing gastric pH; inhibits proteolytic activity of pepsin when gastric pH is increased >4; binds bile salts

Pharmacodynamics
Duration: Dependent on gastric emptying time
Fasting state: 20-60 minutes
1 hour after meals: May be up to 3 hours

Usual Dosage Oral: Aluminum/magnesium hydroxide combination (for extra strength or concentrated suspension, use half the volume of the stated dose):

Peptic ulcer disease:
Infants: 1-2 mL/kg/dose 1-3 hours after meals and at bedtime
Children: 5-15 mL/dose every 3-6 hours or 1-3 hours after meals and at bedtime
Adults: 15-45 mL every 3-6 hours or 1-3 hours after meals and at bedtime

Prophylaxis against GI bleeding:
Neonates: 1 mL/kg every 4 hours as needed
Infants: 2-5 mL/dose every 1-2 hours, titrate to gastric pH >3.5
Children: 5-15 mL/dose every 1-2 hours, titrate to gastric pH >3.5
Adults: 30-60 mL every 1-2 hours, titrate to gastric pH >3.5

Hyperphosphatemia:
Children: Use $Al(OH)_3$ or aluminum carbonate gel product only: 50-150 mg/kg/day (as aluminum hydroxide gel) divided every 4-6 hours; titrate to normal serum phosphorus level
Adults: 30-40 mL of $Al(OH)_3$ 3-4 times/day between meals and at bedtime

Administration Oral: Thoroughly chew tablets before swallowing; shake suspensions well before use; administer prior to meals when stomach acidity is highest

Monitoring Parameters GI complaints, stool frequency; serum phosphate concentrations in patients on hemodialysis receiving chronic aluminum-containing antacid therapy; serum calcium, phosphate, and bicarbonate in patients receiving large doses of calcium carbonate; serum electrolytes in patients with renal impairment receiving magnesium-containing antacids

Patient Information Antacids may impair or increase absorption of many drugs, do not take oral medications within 1-2 hours of an antacid dose unless specifically instructed to do so

Additional Information Antacid products containing alginic acid form a viscous solution that serves as a protective barrier for the esophagus against reflux of gastric contents.

Dosage Forms Excipient information presented when available (limited, particularly for generics); consult specific product labeling; [DSC] = Discontinued product

Aluminum hydroxide:
Ointment (Dermagran®): 0.275% (120 g)
Suspension, oral: 320 mg/5 mL (473 mL)
ALternaGel®: 600 mg/5 mL (360 mL)

Aluminum hydroxide and magnesium hydroxide:
Suspension: Aluminum hydroxide 225 mg and magnesium hydroxide 200 mg per 5 mL (360 mL)
Alamag, Rulox: Aluminum hydroxide 225 mg and magnesium hydroxide 200 mg per 5 mL (360 mL)
Tablet, chewable:
Alamag: Aluminum hydroxide 300 mg and magnesium hydroxide 150 mg

(Continued)

Antacid Preparations *(Continued)*

Rulox No. 1: Aluminum hydroxide 200 mg and magnesium hydroxide 200 mg [DSC]

Aluminum hydroxide and magnesium trisilicate:

Tablet, chewable: Aluminum hydroxide 80 mg and magnesium trisilicate 20 mg

Alenic Alka: Aluminum hydroxide 80 mg and magnesium trisilicate 20 mg [butterscotch flavor]

Gaviscon®: Aluminum hydroxide 80 mg and magnesium trisilicate 20 mg [contains sodium 0.8 mEq/tablet; butterscotch flavor]

Genaton: Aluminum hydroxide 80 mg and magnesium trisilicate 20 mg

Aluminum hydroxide, magnesium hydroxide, and simethicone:

Liquid: Aluminum hydroxide 200 mg, magnesium hydroxide 200 mg, and simethicone 20 mg per 5 mL (360 mL); aluminum hydroxide 400 mg, magnesium hydroxide 400 mg, and simethicone 40 mg per 5 mL (360 mL)

Aldroxicon I: Aluminum hydroxide 200 mg, magnesium hydroxide 200 mg, and simethicone 20 mg per 5 mL (30 mL)

Aldroxicon II: Aluminum hydroxide 400 mg, magnesium hydroxide 400 mg, and simethicone 40 mg per 5 mL (30 mL)

Almacone®: Aluminum hydroxide 200 mg, magnesium hydroxide 200 mg, and simethicone 20 mg per 5 mL (360 mL)

Almacone Double Strength®: Aluminum hydroxide 400 mg, magnesium hydroxide 400 mg, and simethicone 40 mg per 5 mL (360 mL)

Maalox®: Aluminum hydroxide 200 mg, magnesium hydroxide 200 mg, and simethicone 20 mg per 5 mL (360 mL, 770 mL) [lemon and mint flavors]

Maalox® Max: Aluminum hydroxide 400 mg, magnesium hydroxide 400 mg, and simethicone 40 mg per 5 mL (360 mL, 770 mL) [cherry, vanilla creme, and wild berry flavors]

Mi-Acid: Aluminum hydroxide 200 mg, magnesium hydroxide 200 mg, and simethicone 20 mg per 5 mL (360 mL)

Mi-Acid Maximum Strength: Aluminum hydroxide 400 mg, magnesium hydroxide 400 mg, and simethicone 40 mg per 5 mL (360 mL)

Mintox Extra Strength: Aluminum hydroxide 500 mg, magnesium hydroxide 450 mg, and simethicone 40 mg per 5 mL (360 mL) [lemon creme flavor]

Mylanta®: Aluminum hydroxide 200 mg, magnesium hydroxide 200 mg, and simethicone 20 mg per 5 mL (180 mL, 360 mL, 720 mL) [original, cherry, and mint flavors]

Mylanta® Maximum Strength: Aluminum hydroxide 400 mg, magnesium hydroxide 400 mg, and simethicone 40 mg per 5 mL (180 mL, 360 mL, 720 mL) [original, cherry, orange creme, and mint flavors]

Suspension (Alamag Plus): Aluminum hydroxide 225 mg, magnesium hydroxide 200 mg, and simethicone 25 mg per 5 mL (360 mL)

Tablet, chewable: Aluminum hydroxide 200 mg, magnesium hydroxide 200 mg, and simethicone 25 mg

Alamag Plus: Aluminum hydroxide 200 mg, magnesium hydroxide 200 mg, and simethicone 25 mg [cherry flavor]

Almacone®: Aluminum hydroxide 200 mg, magnesium hydroxide 200 mg, and simethicone 20 mg [peppermint flavor]

Gelusil®: Aluminum hydroxide 200 mg, magnesium hydroxide 200 mg, and simethicone 25 mg [peppermint flavor]

Mintox Plus: Aluminum hydroxide 200 mg, magnesium hydroxide 200 mg, and simethicone 25 mg

References

Nord KS, "Peptic Ulcer Disease in the Pediatric Population," *Pediatr Clin North Am*, 1988, 35(1):117-140.

♦ **Anti-CD20 Monoclonal Antibody** *see* Rituximab *on page 1398*

♦ **Antidigoxin Fab Fragments, Ovine** *see* Digoxin Immune Fab *on page 498*

♦ **Antidiuretic Hormone** *see* Vasopressin *on page 1602*

Antihemophilic Factor (Human)

(an tee hee moe FIL ik FAK tor HYU man)

U.S. Brand Names Alphanate®; Hemofil M; Koāte®-DVI; Monarc-M™; Monoclate-P®

Canadian Brand Names Hemofil M

Index Terms AHF; AHG; Factor VIII

Therapeutic Category Antihemophilic Agent; Blood Product Derivative

Generic Available Yes

Use Prevention and treatment of hemorrhagic episodes in patients with hemophilia A (classical hemophilia); perioperative management of patients with hemophilia A; can provide therapeutic effects in patients with acquired factor VIII inhibitors <10 Bethesda units/mL

Pregnancy Risk Factor C

Lactation Excretion in breast milk unknown/use caution

Contraindications

All products: Hypersensitivity to any component (see Warnings and table)

Antihemophilic factor, human (Method M, monoclonal purified); Hemofil® M; Monarc® M; Monoclate-P®: Hypersensitivity to mouse protein

Antihemophilic Factor (Human) Products

Note: Source of all products is pooled human plasma

Product	Preparation and Purification Methods	Viral Inactivation	Stabilizers and Excipients
Alphanate®	• Cryoprecipitation • Fractional solubilization • Affinity chromatography (heparin/argose)	• Organic solvent/ detergent treatment • Heat treatment (dry; 80°C x 72 hours)	• Albumin (human)[1] • Calcium • Glycine • Heparin • Histidine • Imidazole • Arginine • Polyethylene glycol • Polysorbate 80 • Sodium • Tri-n-butyl phosphate
Hemofil® M	• Method M process • Immunoaffinity chromatography using murine monoclonal antibody • Ion exchange chromatography	• Organic solvent/ detergent treatment	• Albumin (human)[1] • Polyethylene glycol[1] • Histidine[1] • Glycine[1] • Mouse protein • Tri-n-butyl phosphate • Octoxynol 9
Koāte®-DVI	• Purified from cold insoluble fraction of fresh-frozen plasma • Gel permeation chromatography	• Organic solvent/ detergent treatment • Heat treatment (dry; in lyophilized form in final container; 80°C x 72 hours)	• Albumin (human) • Polyethylene glycol • Glycine • Polysorbate 80 • Tri-n-butyl phosphate • Calcium • Aluminum • Histidine
Monarc® M	• Method M process • Immunoaffinity chromatography using murine monoclonal antibody • Ion exchange chromatography	• Organic solvent/ detergent treatment	• Albumin (human)[1] • Polyethylene glycol[1] • Histidine[1] • Glycine[1] • Mouse protein • Tri-n-butyl phosphate • Octoxynol 9
Monoclate-P®	• Immunoaffinity chromatography using murine monoclonal antibody	• Heat treatment in aqueous solution (pasteurization; 60°C x 10 hours)	• Albumin (human)[1] • Sodium (300-450 millimoles/L) • Calcium chloride • Mannitol • Histidine • Hydrochloric acid and/or sodium hydroxide (pH adjustment) • Mouse protein

[1]Listed as a stabilizer in the product's package insert

Warnings Hemofil® M and Monarc® M contain natural rubber latex (in certain components of the product packaging) which may cause allergic reactions in susceptible individuals; avoid use in patients with allergy to latex

Precautions Human antihemophilic factor is prepared from pooled plasma and even with heat treated or other viral attenuated processes, the risk of viral transmission (ie, viral hepatitis, HIV, parvovirus B19, and theoretically, Creutzfeldt-Jacob disease agent) is not totally eradicated. Hepatitis B vaccination is recommended for all patients receiving human antihemophilic factor and hepatitis A vaccination is recommended for seronegative patients. [**Note:** The use of recombinant antihemophilic factor products (such as Advate, Helixate® FS, Kogenate® FS, Recombinate™, or ReFacto®) substantially decreases the risk of viral transmission because these products are biosynthetically prepared.] Progressive anemia and hemolysis may occur in individuals with blood groups A, B, and AB who receive large or frequent doses of human antihemophilic factor due to trace amounts of blood group A and B isohemagglutinins (see Monitoring Parameters).

Formation of factor VIII inhibitors (neutralizing antibodies to AHF human) may occur (see Adverse Reactions); monitor patients appropriately (see Monitoring Parameters). Allergic-type hypersensitivity reactions are possible; discontinue therapy immediately if urticaria, hives, hypotension, tightness of the chest, wheezing, dyspnea, faintness, or anaphylaxis develop. Products vary by preparation method (see table); final formulations contain human albumin

Adverse Reactions

Cardiovascular: Flushing, tachycardia, fever, chills, chest tightness

Central nervous system: Headache, lethargy, somnolence, dizziness, nervousness

Dermatologic: Urticaria, rash, pruritus

(Continued)

Antihemophilic Factor (Human) *(Continued)*

Gastrointestinal: Nausea, vomiting, GI upset; unusual taste (one patient)

Local: Injection site reactions, stinging; phlebitis

Neuromuscular & skeletal: Paresthesia

Ocular: Blurred vision

Miscellaneous: Hypersensitivity reactions, anaphylaxis (see Precautions); allergic vasomotor reactions, edema, development of inhibitor antibodies (3% to 52%); inhibitor antibodies are IgG immunoglobulins that neutralize the activity of factor VIII; an increase of inhibitor antibody concentration is seen at 2-7 days, with peak concentrations at 1-3 weeks after therapy. Children <5 years of age are at greatest risk; higher doses of AHF may be needed if antibody is present; if antibody concentration is >10 Bethesda units/mL, patients may not respond to larger doses and alternative treatment modalities may be needed (see Additional Information).

Stability

Storage: Store unopened vials under refrigeration 2°C to 8°C (36°F to 46°F); avoid freezing (to prevent damage to diluent vial)

Alphanate®: May also be stored at room temperature (≤30°C or 86°F) for up to 2 months

Hemofil® M: May also be stored at room temperature (≤30°C or 86°F)

Koate®-DVI: May also be stored at room temperature (≤25°C or 77°F) for up to 6 months

Monarc® M: May also be stored at room temperature (≤30°C or 86°F) for up to 12 months

Monoclate-P®: May also be stored at room temperature (≤30°C or 86°F) for up to 6 months

Reconstitution: If refrigerated, the dried concentrate and diluent should be warmed to room temperature before reconstitution; see individual product labeling for specific reconstitution guidelines; gently agitate or rotate vial after adding diluent, do not shake vigorously (**Note:** For Koate®-DVI: Swirl vigorously without creating excessive foaming); use filter needle provided by manufacturer to draw product into syringe; use one filter needle per vial; do **not** refrigerate after reconstitution (precipitation may occur); administer within 3 hours after reconstitution; **Note:** Use plastic syringes, since AHF may stick to the surface of glass syringes

Mechanism of Action Factor VIII is a protein in normal plasma which is necessary for clot formation and maintenance of hemostasis; it activates factor X in conjunction with activated factor IX; activated factor X converts prothrombin to thrombin, which converts fibrinogen to fibrin and with factor XIII forms a stable clot

Pharmacodynamics Maximum effect: 1-2 hours

Pharmacokinetics

Distribution: Does not readily cross the placenta

Half-life: 4-24 hours; mean = 12 hours (biphasic)

Usual Dosage Children and Adults: I.V.: Individualize dosage based on coagulation studies performed prior to and during treatment at regular intervals:

Hemophilia A: For every 1 international unit per kg body weight of AHF (human) administered, factor VIII level should increase by 2%; calculated dosage should be adjusted to the actual vial size

Formula to calculate dosage required, based on desired increase in factor VIII (% of normal) (**Note:** This formula assumes that the patient's baseline AHF level is <1%): International units required = Body weight (kg) x 0.5 x desired increase in factor VIII (international units/dL or % of normal)

Hospitalized patients: 20-50 units/kg/dose; may be higher for special circumstances. Dose can be given every 12-24 hours and more frequently in special circumstances.

Hemophilia A with high titer of inhibitor antibody: 50-75 units/kg/hour has been given

General dosing guidelines (consult individual product labeling for specific dosage recommendations):

Minor hemorrhage (required peak postinfusion AHF level: 20% to 40%): 10-20 international units/kg; repeat every 12-24 hours for 1-3 days until bleeding is resolved or healing achieved; mild superficial or early hemorrhages may respond to a single dose

Moderate hemorrhage (required peak postinfusion AHF level: 30% to 60%): 15-30 international units/kg; repeat every 12-24 hours for ≥3 days until pain and disability are resolved

Alternatively (to achieve peak postinfusion AHF level: 50%) Initial: 25 international units/kg; maintenance: 10-15 international units/kg every 8-12 hours

Severe/life-threatening hemorrhage (required peak postinfusion AHF level: 60% to 100%): 30-50 international units/kg; repeat every 8-24 hours until threat is resolved

Alternatively (to achieve peak postinfusion AHF level: 80% to 100%): 40-50 international units/kg; maintenance: 20-25 international units/kg every 8-12 hours

Minor surgery (required peak postinfusion AHF level: Range 30% to 80%): 15-40 international units/kg; dose is highly dependent upon procedure and specific product recommendations; for some procedures, a single dose plus oral antifibrinolytic therapy within 1 hour is sufficient; in other procedures, may repeat dose every 12-24 hours as needed

Major surgery (required peak pre- and postsurgery AHF level: 80% to 100%): 40-50 international units/kg; repeat every 8-24 hours depending on state of healing

Prophylaxis: May also be given on a regular schedule to prevent bleeding

Administration Parenteral: I.V. administration only; see Stability for reconstitution and dosage preparation; administer through a separate line, do not mix with drugs or other I.V. fluids.

Maximum rate of administration is product dependent:

Alphanate®, Hemofil® M, Monarc® M: 10 mL/minute

Monoclate-P®: 2 mL/minute

Koate®-DVI: Total dose may be given over 5-10 minutes; adjust administration rate based on patient response

Monitoring Parameters Bleeding; heart rate and blood pressure (before and during I.V. administration); AHF levels prior to and during treatment; monitor for development of inhibitor antibodies by clinical observation (eg, inadequate control of bleeding with adequate doses) and laboratory tests (eg, inhibitor level, Bethesda assay); in patients with blood groups A, B, or AB who receive large or frequent doses, monitor Hct, direct Coombs' test, and signs of intravascular hemolysis

Reference Range

Plasma antihemophilic factor level:

Normal range: 50% to 150%

Level to prevent spontaneous hemorrhage: 5%

Required peak postinfusion AHF activity in blood (as % of normal or units/dL plasma):

Early hemarthrosis, muscle bleed, or oral bleed: 20% to 40%

More extensive hemarthrosis, muscle bleed, or hematoma: 30% to 60%

Life-threatening bleeds (such as head injury, throat bleed, severe abdominal pain): 80% to 100%

Minor surgery, including tooth extraction: 60% to 80%

Major surgery: 80% to 100% (pre- and postoperative)

Patient Information This medication can only be given intravenously. Stop taking antihemophilic factor human and notify physician immediately if any of the following signs or symptoms of an allergic (hypersensitivity) reaction occur: Itching, hives, low blood pressure, tightness in chest, wheezing, or anaphylaxis. Wear identification indicating that you have a hemophilic condition.

Nursing Implications Reduce rate of administration or temporarily discontinue if patient experiences tachycardia or any other adverse reaction; hypersensitivity reactions (eg, hives, chest tightness, itching, wheezing, dyspnea, faintness, hypotension, anaphylaxis) may occur (see Precautions)

Additional Information One international unit of AHF is equal to the factor VIII activity present in 1 mL of normal human plasma. If bleeding is not controlled with adequate dose, test for the presence of factor VIII inhibitor; larger doses of AHF may be therapeutic with inhibitor titers <10 Bethesda units/mL; it may not be possible or practical to control bleeding if inhibitor titers >10 Bethesda units/mL (due to the very large AHF doses required); other treatments [eg, antihemophilic factor (porcine), factor IX complex concentrates, recombinant factor VIIa, or anti-inhibitor coagulant complex] may be needed in patients with inhibitor titers >10 Bethesda units/mL.

Dosage Forms

Injection, powder for reconstitution:

Alphanate®: Vial labeled with international units [contains sodium ≤10 mEq/vial and albumin]

Hemofil M: Vial labeled with international units [contains albumin; derived from mouse proteins; packaging may contain natural rubber latex]

Koate®-DVI: ~250 int. units, ~500 int. units, ~1000 int. units [contains albumin]

Monarc-M™: Vial labeled with international units [contains albumin; derived from mouse proteins; packaging may contain natural rubber latex]

Monoclate-P®: ~250 int. units, ~500 int. units, ~1000 int. units, ~1500 int. units [contains albumin; derived from mouse proteins]

References

Liesner RJ, "Prophylaxis in Haemophilic Children," *Blood Coagul Fibrinolysis*, 1997, 8(Suppl 1):S7-10.

Scharrer I, Bray GL, and Neutzling O, "Incidence of Inhibitors in Haemophilia A Patients--A Review of Recent Studies of Recombinant and Plasma-Derived Factor VIII Concentrates," *Haemophilia*, 1999, 5(3):145-54.

Shord SS and Lindley CM, "Coagulation Products and Their Uses," *Am J Health Syst Pharm*, 2000, 57(15):1403-20.

Antihemophilic Factor (Recombinant)

(an tee hee moe FIL ik FAK tor ree KOM be nant)

U.S. Brand Names Advate; Helixate® FS; Kogenate® FS; Recombinate; ReFacto®

Canadian Brand Names Helixate® FS; Kogenate®; Kogenate® FS; Recombinate; ReFacto®

Index Terms AHF (Recombinant); Factor VIII (Recombinant); rAHF

Therapeutic Category Antihemophilic Agent

Generic Available No

Use Prevention and control of hemorrhagic episodes in patients with hemophilia A in whom a deficiency of activity in factor VIII has been demonstrated; perioperative management of patients with hemophilia A; can provide therapeutic effects in patients with acquired factor VIII inhibitors <10 Bethesda units/mL; **Note:** AHF recombinant is not indicated for the treatment of von Willebrand disease

Pregnancy Risk Factor C

Lactation Excretion in breast milk unknown/use caution

Contraindications

All products: Hypersensitivity or intolerance to any component (see Warnings and table)

Advate; Helixate® FS; Kogenate® FS: Hypersensitivity to mouse or hamster protein

Recombinate™; ReFacto®: Hypersensitivity to mouse, hamster, or bovine protein

Antihemophilic Factor (Recombinant) Products

Product	Synthesis	Purification Methods	Stabilizers and Excipients
Advate	• Recombinant DNA technology • Chinese Hamster Ovary (CHO) cell line • Plasma/Albumin " free method	• Solvent/detergent virus inactivation • Column chromatography • Monoclonal antibody immunoaffinity chromatography	• Mannitol[1] • Trehalose[1] • Sodium[1] • Histidine[1] • Tris[1] • Calcium[1] • Polysorbate-80[1] • Glutathione[1] • von Willebrand factor (insignificant amounts)[1]
Helixate® FS	• Recombinant DNA technology • Baby Hamster Kidney (BHK) cells • Human Plasma Protein Solution (HPPS) and recombinant insulin in cell culture medium	• Solvent/detergent virus inactivation • Ion exchange chromatography • Monoclonal antibody immunoaffinity chromatography • Other chromatographic steps	• Sucrose[1] • Glycine[1] • Histidine[1] • Calcium chloride • Sodium • Chloride • Polysorbate-80 • Imidazole • Tri-n-butyl phosphate • Copper
Kogenate® FS	• Recombinant DNA technology • Baby Hamster Kidney (BHK) cells • Human Plasma Protein Solution (HPPS) and recombinant insulin in cell culture medium	• Solvent/detergent virus inactivation • Ion exchange chromatography • Monoclonal antibody immunoaffinity chromatography • Other chromatographic steps	• Sucrose[1] • Glycine[1] • Histidine[1] • Calcium chloride • Sodium • Chloride • Polysorbate-80 • Imidazole • Tri-n-butyl phosphate • Copper
Recombinate™	• Recombinant DNA technology • Chinese Hamster Ovary (CHO) cell line	• Column chromatography • Monoclonal antibody immunoaffinity chromatography	• Albumin (human)[1] • Calcium[1] • Polyethylene glycol[1] • Sodium[1] • Histidine[1] • Polysorbate-80[1] • von Willebrand factor[1] (insignificant amounts)
ReFacto®	• Recombinant DNA technology • Chinese Hamster Ovary (CHO) cell line • Human Serum Albumin and recombinant insulin in cell culture medium	• Chromatography	• Sodium chloride • Sucrose • L-histadine • Calcium chloride • Polysorbate-80

[1]Listed as a stabilizer in the product's package insert

Warnings Recombinate™ contains natural rubber latex (in certain components of the product packaging) which may cause allergic reactions in susceptible individuals; avoid use in patients with allergy to latex.

Precautions Formation of factor VIII inhibitors (neutralizing antibodies to AHF recombinant) may occur; antibody formation may occur at any time, but is more common in young children with severe hemophilia during the first years of therapy, or in patients at any age who received little prior therapy with factor VIII; monitor patients appropriately (see Monitoring Parameters). Although remote, formation of antibodies to mouse, hamster, or bovine protein may occur (products may contain trace amounts of these proteins). Allergic type hypersensitivity reactions are theoretically possible;

discontinue therapy immediately if urticaria, hives, hypotension, tightness of the chest, wheezing or anaphylaxis develop; emergency treatment and resuscitative measures (eg, epinephrine, oxygen) may be needed. Products vary by preparation method (see table). Recombinate™ formulation is stabilized using human albumin; Helixate® FS, Kogenate® FS, and ReFacto® formulations are stabilized using sucrose

Adverse Reactions

Cardiovascular: Flushing, vasodilation, fever, chills, chest discomfort, hypotension (slight), mildly elevated blood pressure, angina pectoris, tachycardia

Central nervous system: Mild fatigue, dizziness, headache, lethargy, asthenia, somnolence, depersonalization

Dermatologic: Urticaria, rash, pruritus

Gastrointestinal: Nausea, vomiting, diarrhea, sore throat, unusual taste, constipation, anorexia

Hepatic: Elevated aminotransferase, elevated bilirubin

Local: Injection site reactions (burning, pruritus, erythema)

Neuromuscular & skeletal: Muscle weakness

Ocular: Abnormal vision

Respiratory: Epistaxis, rhinitis, dyspnea, cough

Miscellaneous: Cold feet, adenopathy, allergic reactions, anaphylaxis, permanent venous catheter access complications, diaphoresis, elevated CPK, development of inhibitor antibodies; inhibitor antibodies are IgG immunoglobulins that neutralize the activity of factor VIII; higher doses of AHF recombinant may be needed if antibody is present; if antibody concentration is >10 Bethesda units/mL, patients may not respond to larger doses and alternative treatment modalities may be needed (see Additional Information)

Stability

Storage: Store unopened vials under refrigeration 2°C to 8°C (36°F to 46°F); avoid freezing

Advate: May also be stored at room temperature [22°C to 28°C (72°F to 82°F)] for up to 6 months

Helixate® FS, Kogenate® FS, ReFacto®: May also be stored at room temperature (≤25°C or 77°F) for up to 3 months. Avoid extreme or prolonged exposure to light during storage (store drug in carton before use)

Recombinate™: May also be stored at room temperature (≤30°C or 86°F)

Mechanism of Action Antihemophilic factor (recombinant) has the same biological activity as AHF (factor VIII) derived from human plasma; factor VIII is a protein in normal plasma which is necessary for clot formation and maintenance of hemostasis; factor VIII activates factor X in conjunction with activated factor IX; activated factor X converts prothrombin to thrombin, which converts fibrinogen to fibrin, and with factor XIII forms a stable clot

Pharmacokinetics Half-life: Mean: 11-16 hours

Usual Dosage Neonates, Infants, Children, and Adults: I.V.: **Individualize dosage based on coagulation studies performed prior to treatment and at regular intervals during treatment;** for every 1 international unit per kg body weight of rAHF administered, factor VIII level should increase by 2%; calculated dosage should be adjusted to the actual vial size

Formula to calculate dosage required, based on desired increase in factor VIII (% of normal) (**Note:** This formula assumes that the patient's baseline AHF level is <1%): International units required = body weight (kg) x 0.5 x desired increase in factor VIII (international units/dL or % of normal)

General dosing guidelines (consult individual product labeling for specific dosage recommendations):

Minor hemorrhage (required peak postinfusion AHF level: 20% to 40%): 10-20 international units/kg; repeat every 12-24 hours for 1-3 days until bleeding is resolved or healing achieved; mild, superficial, or early hemorrhages may respond to a single dose

Moderate hemorrhage (required peak post-infusion AHF level: 30% to 60%): 15-30 international units/kg, repeat every 12-24 hours for 3-4 days until pain and disability are resolved

Severe/life-threatening hemorrhage:

Helixate® FS, Kogenate® FS (required peak post-infusion AHF level: 80% to 100%): Initial: 40-50 international units/kg; maintenance: 20-25 international units/kg every 8-12 hours

Advate, Recombinate™, ReFacto® (required peak post-infusion AHF level: 60% to 100%): 30-50 international units/kg; repeat every 8-24 hours until threat is resolved

Minor surgery (required peak post-infusion AHF level: range: 30% to 80%): 15-40 international units/kg; dose is highly dependent upon procedure and specific

(Continued)

Antihemophilic Factor (Recombinant) *(Continued)*

product recommendations; for some procedures, a single dose plus oral antifibrinolytic therapy within 1 hour is sufficient; in other procedures, may repeat dose in 12-24 hours as needed

Major surgery:

Advate (required peak pre- and post-surgery AHF level: 80% to 120%): 40-60 international units/kg; repeat every 8-24 hours depending on state of healing

Helixate® FS, Kogenate® FS (required peak pre- and post-surgery AHF level: 100%): 50 international units/kg; may repeat every 6-12 hours initially and until healing complete (10-14 days); intensity of regimen is dependent on type of surgery and postoperative care

Recombinate™, ReFacto® (required peak pre- and post-surgery AHF level: 80% to 100%): 40-50 international units/kg; repeat every 8-24 hours depending on state of healing

Prophylaxis: May also be given on a regular schedule to prevent bleeding

Administration

Reconstitution: If refrigerated, the dried concentrate and diluent should be warmed to room temperature before reconstitution; see individual product labeling for specific reconstitution guidelines; gently agitate or rotate vial after adding diluent, do not shake vigorously; use filter needle provided by manufacturer to draw product into syringe; do **not** refrigerate after reconstitution; administer within 3 hours after reconstitution; **Note:** Use plastic syringes, since rAHF may stick to the surface of glass syringes

Parenteral: I.V. administration only; total dose may be administered over 5-10 minutes; Advate may be administered over ≤5 minutes; maximum rate of infusion (all products): 10 mL/minute; adjust administration rate based on patient response; for Advate, Helixate® FS, Kogenate® FS, and ReFacto®, use sterile administration set provided by manufacturer

Monitoring Parameters Bleeding; heart rate and blood pressure (before and during I.V. administration); AHF levels prior to and during treatment; monitor for the development of inhibitor antibodies by clinical observations (eg, inadequate control of bleeding with adequate doses) and laboratory tests (eg, inhibitor level, Bethesda assay)

Reference Range

Plasma antihemophilic factor level:

Normal range: 50% to 150%

Level to prevent spontaneous hemorrhage: 5%

Required peak post-infusion AHF activity in blood (as % of normal or units/dL plasma):

Early hemarthrosis, muscle bleed, or oral bleed: 20% to 40%

More extensive hemarthrosis, muscle bleed, or hematoma: 30% to 60%

Life-threatening bleeds (such as head injury, throat bleed, severe abdominal pain): 80% to 100%

Minor surgery, including tooth extraction: 60% to 80%

Major surgery: 80% to 100% (pre- and postoperative)

Patient Information This medication can only be given intravenously. Stop taking antihemophilic factor recombinant and notify physician immediately if any of the following signs or symptoms of an allergic (hypersensitivity) reaction occur: Itching, hives, low blood pressure, tightness of the chest, wheezing, or anaphylaxis. Wear identification indicating that you have a hemophilic condition.

Nursing Implications Reduce rate of administration, or temporarily discontinue, if patient experiences any adverse reactions; hypersensitivity reactions (eg, hives, chest tightness, itching, wheezing, hypotension) are possible

Additional Information One international unit of rAHF is equal to the factor VIII activity present in 1 mL of fresh pooled human plasma. If bleeding is not controlled with adequate dose, test for the presence of factor VIII inhibitor; larger doses of rAHF may be therapeutic with inhibitor titers <10 Bethesda units/mL; it may not be possible or practical to control bleeding if inhibitor titers >10 Bethesda units/mL (due to the very large rAHF doses required); other treatments [eg, antihemophilic factor (porcine), factor IX complex concentrates, recombinant factor VIIa, or anti-inhibitor coagulant complex] may be needed in patients with inhibitor titers >10 Bethesda units/mL

Dosage Forms Excipient information presented when available (limited, particularly for generics); consult specific product labeling.

Injection, powder for reconstitution, recombinant [preservative free]:

Advate: 250 int. units, 500 int. units, 1000 int. units, 1500 int. units, 2000 int. units [plasma/albumin free; contains sodium 108 mEq/L, mannitol; derived from hamster or mouse proteins]

Helixate® FS, Kogenate® FS: 250 int. units, 500 int. units, 1000 int. units [albumin free; contains sucrose 28 mg/vial, sodium 27-36 mEq/L; derived from hamster or mouse protein]

Recombinate: 250 int. units, 500 units, 1000 int. units [contains human albumin, sodium 180 mEq/L; derived from bovine, hamster or mouse proteins; packaging contains natural rubber latex]

ReFacto®: 250 int. units, 500 units, 1000 int. units, 2000 int. units [contains sucrose; derived from hamster or mouse proteins]

References

Abshire TC, Brackmann HH, Scharrer I, et al, "Sucrose Formulated Recombinant Human Antihemophilic Factor VIII is Safe and Efficacious for Treatment of Hemophilia A in Home Therapy. International Kogenate-FS Study Group," *Thromb Haemost*, 2000, 83(6):811-6.

Bray GL, Gomperts ED, Courter S, et al, "A Multicenter Study of Recombinant Factor VIII (Recombinate): Safety, Efficacy, and Inhibitor Risk in Previously Untreated Patients With Hemophilia A. The Recombinate Study Group," *Blood*, 1994, 83(9):2428-35.

Kelly KM, Butler RB, Farace L, et al, "Superior In Vivo Response of Recombinant Factor VIII Concentrate in Children With Hemophilia A," *J Pediatr*, 1997, 130(4):537-40.

Liesner RJ, "Prophylaxis in Haemophilic Children," *Blood Coagul Fibrinolysis*, 1997, 8(Suppl 1):S7-10.

Scharrer I, Bray GL, and Neutzling O, "Incidence of Inhibitors in Haemophilia A Patients - A Review of Recent Studies of Recombinant and Plasma-Derived Factor VIII Concentrates," *Haemophilia*, 1999, 5(3):145-54.

Shord SS and Lindley CM, "Coagulation Products and Their Uses," *Am J Health Syst Pharm*, 2000, 57(15):1403-20.

Schwartz RS, Abildgaard CF, Aledort LM, et al, "Human Recombinant DNA-Derived Antihemophilic Factor (Factor VIII) in the Treatment of Hemophilia A. Recombinant Factor VIII Study Group," *N Engl J Med*, 1990, 323(26):1800-5.

Antihemophilic Factor/von Willebrand Factor Complex (Human)

(an tee hee moe FIL ik FAK tor von WILL le brand FAK tor KOM plex HYU man)

U.S. Brand Names Humate-P®

Canadian Brand Names Humate-P®

Index Terms AHF (Human); Factor VIII (Human); FVIII/vWF

Therapeutic Category Antihemophilic Agent; Blood Product Derivative

Generic Available No

Use

Hemophilia A: Prevention and treatment of hemorrhagic episodes

Von Willebrand disease (including severe disease and mild-to-moderate disease where the use of desmopressin is suspected or known to be inadequate): Treatment of spontaneous and trauma-induced hemorrhagic episodes; prevention of excessive perioperative bleeding

Pregnancy Risk Factor C

Lactation Excretion in breast milk unknown/use caution

Contraindications History of anaphylactic or severe systemic response to antihemophilic factor or von Willebrand factor products; hypersensitivity to any component; see table

Antihemophilic Factor/von Willebrand Factor Complex (Human) Product

Note: Source is pooled human plasma

Product	Preparation and Purification Methods	Viral Inactivation	Stabilizers and Excipients
Humate-P®	• Purified from cold insoluble fraction of fresh-frozen plasma	• Cryoprecipitation • Aluminum hydroxide adsorption, glycine precipitation and sodium chloride precipitation • Heat treatment in aqueous solution (pasteurization; 60°C x 10 hours)	• Glycine • Sodium citrate • Sodium chloride • Albumin (human) • Other proteins • Fibrinogen (<0.2 mg/mL)

Warnings Thromboembolic events in patients with von Willebrand disease receiving antihemophilic factor/von Willebrand factor complex have been reported; risk of these events may be higher in patients with other risk factors for thrombosis and in females; use antihemophilic factor/von Willebrand factor complex with caution in these patients; consider antithrombotic measures

Precautions Human antihemophilic factor/von Willebrand factor complex is prepared from pooled plasma; even with heat treated or other viral attenuated processes, the risk of viral transmission (ie, viral hepatitis, HIV, parvovirus B19, and theoretically, Creutzfeldt-Jacob disease agent) is not totally eradicated. Hepatitis B vaccination is recommended for all patients receiving human antihemophilic factor/von Willebrand factor complex and hepatitis A vaccination is recommended for seronegative patients. Progressive anemia and hemolysis may occur in individuals with blood groups A, B, and AB who receive large or frequent doses of human antihemophilic

(Continued)

Antihemophilic Factor/von Willebrand Factor Complex (Human) *(Continued)*

factor/von Willebrand factor complex due to trace amounts of blood group A and B isohemagglutinins (see Monitoring Parameters).

Formation of factor VIII inhibitors (neutralizing antibodies to AHF human) may occur (see Adverse Reactions); monitor patients appropriately (see Monitoring Parameters); optimal dosage should be determined by clinical response. Allergic-type hypersensitivity reactions are possible; discontinue therapy immediately if urticaria, hives, hypotension, tightness of the chest, wheezing, dyspnea, faintness, or anaphylaxis develop.

Adverse Reactions

Cardiovascular: Edema, chest tightness, thromboembolic events, vasodilation, hypervolemia

Central nervous system: Fever, chills, headache, dizziness

Dermatologic: Urticaria, rash, pruritus

Gastrointestinal: Nausea, vomiting

Hematologic: Pseudothrombocytopenia (platelet clumping with a false low reading)

Hepatic: Elevated SGPT (one possible case reported)

Local: Phlebitis

Neuromuscular & skeletal: Paresthesia, extremity pain

Ocular: Blurred vision

Miscellaneous: Hypersensitivity reactions, anaphylaxis (see Precautions); development of inhibitor antibodies to Factor VIII; inhibitor antibodies are IgG immunoglobulins that neutralize the activity of factor VIII; an increase of inhibitor antibody concentration is seen at 2-7 days, with peak concentrations at 1-3 weeks after therapy. Children <5 years of age are at greatest risk; higher doses of AHF may be needed if antibody is present; if antibody concentration is >10 Bethesda units/mL, patients may not respond to larger doses and alternative treatment modalities may be needed (see Additional Information).

Stability Store unopened vials under refrigeration 2°C to 8°C (36°F to 46°F); may also be stored at room temperature (≤30°C or 86°F) for up to 6 months; avoid freezing (to prevent damage to diluent vial). If refrigerated, the dried concentrate and diluent should be warmed to room temperature before reconstitution; see product labeling for specific reconstitution guidelines; gently agitate or rotate vial after adding diluent, do not shake vigorously; administer within 3 hours after reconstitution; do not refrigerate after reconstitution, precipitation may occur; **Note:** Use plastic syringes, since AHF may stick to the surface of glass syringes

Mechanism of Action Factor VIII and von Willebrand factor (vWF), obtained from pooled human plasma, are used to replace endogenous factor VIII and vWF in patients with hemophilia or vWD. Factor VIII is a protein in normal plasma which is necessary for clot formation and maintenance of hemostasis; it activates factor X in conjunction with activated factor IX; activated factor X converts prothrombin to thrombin, which converts fibrinogen to fibrin and with factor XIII forms a stable clot. vWF promotes platelet aggregation and adhesion to damaged vascular endothelium and acts as a stabilizing carrier protein for factor VIII. [Circulating levels of functional vWF are measured as ristocetin cofactor activity (vWF:RCo)]

Pharmacodynamics Maximum effect: 1-2 hours

Pharmacokinetics Half-life, elimination:

FVIII:C: 8-17 hours (mean: 12 hours) in patients with hemophilia

VWF:RCo: 3-34 hours (median: 10 hours) in patients with vWD

Usual Dosage Children and Adults: I.V.: Individualize dosage based on coagulation studies performed prior to and during treatment at regular intervals:

Hemophilia A: For every 1 international unit per kg body weight of Factor VIII activity (FVIII) administered, factor VIII level should increase by 2 international units/dL (or 2%); calculated dosage should be adjusted to the actual vial size

Formula to calculate dosage required, based on desired increase in factor VIII (% of normal) (**Note:** This formula assumes that the patient's baseline AHF level is <1%): International units required = Body weight (kg) x 0.5 x desired increase in factor VIII (international units/dL or % of normal)

General dosing guidelines:

Minor hemorrhage: Loading dose: FVIII:C 15 international units/kg to achieve FVIII:C plasma level ~30% of normal. One infusion may be adequate. If second infusion is needed, half the loading dose may be given once or twice daily for 1-2 days.

Moderate hemorrhage: Loading dose: FVIII:C 25 international units/kg to achieve FVIII:C plasma level ~50% of normal. Maintenance: FVIII:C 15 international units/kg every 8-12 hours for 1-2 days in order to maintain FVIII:C plasma levels at 30% of normal. Repeat the same dose once or twice daily for up to 7 days or until adequate wound healing.

Life-threatening hemorrhage: Loading dose: FVIII:C 40-50 international units/kg. Maintenance: FVIII:C 20-25 international units/kg every 8 hours to maintain FVIII:C plasma levels at 80% to 100% of normal for 7 days. Continue same dose once or twice daily for another 7 days in order to maintain FVIII:C levels at 30% to 50% of normal.

von Willebrand disease: For every 1 international unit per kg body weight of factor VIII administered, von Willebrand factor: ristocetin cofactor (vWF:RCo) level should increase by approximately 5 international units/dL

Treatment:

Type 1, mild (if desmopressin is not appropriate; baseline vWF:RCo activity usually >30%): Major hemorrhage:

Loading dose: 40-60 international units/kg

Maintenance dose: 40-50 international units/kg every 8-12 hours for 3 days, keeping vWF:RCo trough level >50%; follow with 40-50 international units/kg daily for up to 7 days

Type 1, moderate or severe (baseline vWF:RCo activity usually <30%):

Minor hemorrhage: 40-50 international units/kg for 1-2 doses

Major hemorrhage:

Loading dose: 50-75 international units/kg

Maintenance dose: 40-60 international units/kg every 8-12 hours for 3 days keeping vWF:RCo trough level >50%; follow with 40-60 international units/kg daily for up to 7 days

Types 2 (all variants) and 3:

Minor hemorrhage: 40-50 international units/kg for 1-2 doses

Major hemorrhage:

Loading dose: 60-80 international units/kg

Maintenance dose: 40-60 international units/kg every 8-12 hours for 3 days, keeping vWF:RCo trough level >50%; follow with 40-60 international units/kg daily for up to 7 days

Administration Parenteral: I.V. administration only; see Stability for reconstitution and dosage preparation; administer through a separate line, do not mix with drugs or other I.V. fluids. Maximum rate of administration: 4 mL/minute

Monitoring Parameters Bleeding; heart rate and blood pressure (before and during I.V. administration). AHF levels prior to and during treatment. Monitor for development of inhibitor antibodies by clinical observation (eg, inadequate control of bleeding with adequate doses) and laboratory tests (eg, inhibitor level, Bethesda assay). In patients with blood groups A, B, or AB who receive large or frequent doses, monitor Hct, direct Coombs' test, and signs of intravascular hemolysis. vWF activity [circulating levels of functional vWF are measured as ristocetin cofactor activity (vWF:RCo)]

Reference Range

Hemophilia: Classification of hemophilia; normal is defined as 1 international unit/mL of factor VII:C:

Severe: Factor level <1% of normal

Moderate: Factor level 1% to 5% of normal

Mild: Factor level >5% to <40% of normal

Plasma antihemophilic factor level:

Normal range: 50% to 150%

Level to prevent spontaneous hemorrhage: 5%

Required peak postinfusion AHF activity in blood (as % of normal or units/dL plasma):

Early hemarthrosis, muscle bleed, or oral bleed: 20% to 40%

More extensive hemarthrosis, muscle bleed, or hematoma: 30% to 60%

Life-threatening bleeds (such as head injury, throat bleed, severe abdominal pain): 80% to 100%

Minor surgery, including tooth extraction: 60% to 80%

Major surgery: 80% to 100% (pre- and postoperative)

Von Willebrand disease: Classification of von Willebrand disease:

Severe forms: vWF:RCo <10 units/dL and factor VIII:C <20 units/dL

Moderate forms: vWF:RCo 10-30 units/dL and factor VIII:C 20-40 units/dL

Mild forms: vWF:RCo 30-50 units/dL and factor VIII:C 40-60 units/dL

Note: Circulating levels of functional VWF are measured as ristocetin cofactor activity (vWF:RCo)]

Patient Information This medication can only be given intravenously. Stop taking this medication and notify physician immediately if any of the following signs or symptoms of an allergic (hypersensitivity) reaction occur: Itching, hives, low blood pressure, tightness in chest, wheezing, or anaphylaxis. Report immediately any sudden-onset headache, chest or back pain, low-grade fever, stomach pain, or nausea/vomiting to prescriber. Wear identification indicating that you have a hemophilic condition.

Nursing Implications Assess potential for interactions with other pharmacological agents patient may be taking that may affect coagulation or platelet function. Hypersensitivity reactions (eg, hives, chest tightness, itching, wheezing, dyspnea, chills,

(Continued)

Antihemophilic Factor/von Willebrand Factor Complex (Human) *(Continued)*

fever, faintness, hypotension, anaphylaxis) may occur (see Precautions). Reduce rate of administration or temporarily discontinue if patient experiences tachycardia or any other adverse reaction. Patient should be monitored closely during and after infusion for any change in vital signs, cardiac and CNS status, or hypersensitivity reactions. Assess response [eg, results of laboratory tests (hematocrit and coagulation studies)], therapeutic effectiveness (bleeding and coagulation status), and adverse reactions (eg, bleeding or anemia).

Additional Information One international unit of AHF is equal to the factor VIII activity present in 1 mL of normal human plasma. If bleeding is not controlled with adequate dose, test for the presence of factor VIII inhibitor; larger doses of AHF may be therapeutic with inhibitor titers <10 Bethesda units/mL; it may not be possible or practical to control bleeding if inhibitor titers >10 Bethesda units/mL (due to the very large AHF doses required); other treatments [eg, antihemophilic factor (porcine), factor IX complex concentrates, recombinant factor VIIa, or anti-inhibitor coagulant complex] may be needed in patients with inhibitor titers >10 Bethesda units/mL.

Dosage Forms Excipient information presented when available (limited, particularly for generics); consult specific product labeling.

Injection, powder for reconstitution:

Humate-P®: FVIII 250 int. units and vWF:RCo 600 int. units [human derived; contains albumin; packaged with diluent]; FVIII 500 int. units and vWF:RCo 1200 int. units [human derived; contains albumin; packed with diluent]; FVIII 1000 int. units and vWF:RCo 2400 int. units [human derived; contains albumin; packaged with diluent]

Anti-inhibitor Coagulant Complex

(an tee-in HI bi tor coe AG yoo lant KOM pleks)

U.S. Brand Names Autoplex® T [DSC]; Feiba VH

Canadian Brand Names Feiba VH Immuno

Index Terms AICC; Coagulant Complex Inhibitor

Therapeutic Category Antihemophilic Agent; Blood Product Derivative

Generic Available No

Use Control of spontaneous bleeding episodes or to cover surgical interventions in hemophilia A and hemophilia B patients with factor VIII inhibitors

Pregnancy Risk Factor C

Lactation Excretion in breast milk unknown/use caution

Contraindications Hypersensitivity to anti-inhibitor coagulant complex or any component; disseminated intravascular coagulation (DIC); fibrinolysis; patients with a normal coagulation mechanism

Warnings Not for use in patients with bleeding episodes resulting from coagulation factor deficiencies without circulating inhibitors. Products are prepared from pooled human plasma; such plasma may contain the causative agents of viral diseases; risk of transmission is extremely rare. Reserve use for patients with circulating inhibitors to Factor VIII only. aPTT, WBCT, and TEG tests do not correlate with clinical efficacy; dosing to normalize these values may result in DIC. Discontinue immediately if symptoms of DIC occur. Thromboembolic events may occur, particularly following administration of high doses and/or in patients with thrombotic risk factors. Patients receiving single doses >100 units/kg or daily doses >200 units/kg must be monitored for the development of DIC and/or symptoms of acute coronary ischemia. Anamnestic rises in inhibitor (antibody) levels have been observed in 20% of the patients which may result in prolonged refractoriness to subsequent therapy. Transient hypofibrinogenemia has been reported in a few pediatric patients; all patients responded favorably to cryoprecipitate and did not develop DIC; measure fibrinogen levels in pediatric patients prior to initiation of therapy

Precautions Use with extreme caution in patients with thrombotic risk factors; hypotension may be more prevalent if administered more than one hour after reconstitution of anti-inhibitor coagulant complex due to increased prekallikrein activator activity; if infusion-related side effects occur (eg, headache, heart rate changes, hypotension or flushing), temporarily discontinue the infusion until the symptoms disappear and resume at a slower rate

Adverse Reactions

Cardiovascular: Hypotension, flushing, and tachycardia (related to the rate of infusion), chest pain, MI

Central nervous system: Fever, chills, headache, dizziness, drowsiness

Dermatologic: Rash, urticaria

Gastrointestinal: Nausea, abdominal pain

Hematologic: DIC, thromboembolic events

Miscellaneous: Anaphylaxis

Drug Interactions Increased thrombosis with aminocaproic acid and tranexamic acid; consider separating therapy from anti-inhibitor coagulant complex by at least 12 hours

Stability Refrigerate freeze-dried powder at 2°C to 8°C (36°F to 46°F); avoid freezing; do not refrigerate after reconstitution; Feiba VH® is stable at room temperature for up to 6 months

Mechanism of Action Anti-inhibitor coagulant complex contains varying amounts of factors II (prothrombin), VII (proconvertin or serum prothrombin conversion accelerator), IX (Christmas factor or plasma thromboplastin component), and X (Stuart-Prower factor) prepared from pooled human plasma. Factors VII and X may be activated or partially-activated forms. The exact mechanism of action is not completely known but has been described as "inhibitor bypassing activity".

Usual Dosage Dosage is dependent upon the severity and location of bleeding, type and level of inhibitors, and whether the patient has a history of an anamnestic increase in antihemophilic inhibitor levels following use of preparations containing antihemophilic factor. The two formulations listed below differ from each other in the amounts of their individual components but the clinical significance related to efficacy and/or adverse effects is unknown. In addition, each formulation uses a different method of standardization, so recommended dosages are not considered equivalent. The dosage recommendations below reflect the manufacturer's recommendations with duration of use dependent upon the patient's response.

Children and Adults: I.V.:

Feiba VH®: 50-100 Feiba VH® immuno units/kg; not to exceed 200 Feiba VH® immuno units/kg/day; dosage may vary with the bleeding site and severity:

Joint hemorrhage: 50 Feiba VH® immuno units/kg every 12 hours; may increase to 100 Feiba VH® immuno units/kg

Mucous membrane bleeding: 50 Feiba VH® immuno units/kg every 6 hours; may increase to 100 Feiba VH® immuno units/kg every 6 hours for only two doses; not to exceed 200 Feiba VH immuno units/kg/day

Soft tissue hemorrhage: 100 Feiba VH® immuno units/kg every 12 hours

Other severe hemorrhages: 100 Feiba VH® immuno units/kg every 6-12 hours

Autoplex® T: 25-100 antihemophilic factor correctional units/kg every 6 hours

Administration I.V.: Reconstitute with provided diluent; swirl gently; do not shake; use within 3 hours of reconstitution; administer without further dilution; Feiba VH®: Maximum rate: 2 units/kg/minute; Autoplex® T: Initial rate of 2 mL/minute with a gradual increase to a maximum of 10 mL/minute

Monitoring Parameters Hemoglobin, hematocrit, bleeding at site, PTT, fibrinogen, platelets, fibrin split products, Factor VIII inhibitor levels

Reference Range Factor VIII inhibitor levels: <2 Bethesda Units (B.U.) antihemophilic factor is the preferred treatment agent; 2-10 B.U. either anti-inhibitor coagulant complex or antihemophilic factor may be used; >10 B.U. anti-inhibitor coagulant complex is the preferred treatment agent

Patient Information Report sudden onset headache, rash, chest or back pain, wheezing or respiratory difficulties, hives, itching, or acute feelings of anxiety. Wear identification indicating that you have a hemophilic condition.

Dosage Forms Excipient information presented when available (limited, particularly for generics); consult specific product labeling.

Injection, powder for reconstitution:

Autoplex® T: Each bottle is labeled with correctional units of factor VIII [contains heparin 2 units/mL and sodium 162-192 mEq/L; packaging contains natural rubber latex] [DSC]

Feiba VH: Each bottle is labeled with Immuno units of factor VIII [heparin free; contains sodium 8 mg/mL; packaging contains natural rubber latex]

Antipyrine and Benzocaine (an tee PYE reen & BEN zoe kane)

Medication Safety Issues

Sound-alike/look-alike issues:

Auralgan® may be confused with Ophthalgan®

U.S. Brand Names A/B Otic; Allergen®; Aurodex

Canadian Brand Names Auralgan®

Index Terms Benzocaine and Antipyrine

Therapeutic Category Otic Agent, Analgesic; Otic Agent, Cerumenolytic

Generic Available Yes

Use Temporary relief of pain and reduction of inflammation associated with acute congestive and serous otitis media, swimmer's ear, otitis externa; facilitates ear wax removal

Pregnancy Risk Factor C

(Continued)

Antipyrine and Benzocaine *(Continued)*

Contraindications Hypersensitivity to antipyrine, benzocaine, or any component; perforated tympanic membrane

Warnings Use of otic anesthetics may mask symptoms of a fulminating middle ear infection (acute otitis media); not intended for prolonged use

Adverse Reactions

Hematologic: Methemoglobinemia
Local: Burning, stinging, tenderness, edema
Miscellaneous: Hypersensitivity reactions

Usual Dosage Infants, Children, and Adults: Otic: Fill ear canal; moisten cotton pledget, place in external ear, repeat every 1-2 hours until pain and congestion is relieved; for ear wax removal instill drops 3-4 times/day for 2-3 days

Dosage Forms Excipient information presented when available (limited, particularly for generics); consult specific product labeling.

Solution, otic [drops]: Antipyrine 5.4% and benzocaine 1.4% (10 mL)
A/B Otic, Allergen®, Aurodex: Antipyrine 5.4% and benzocaine 1.4% (15 mL)

References

Rodriguez LF, Smolik LM, and Zbehlik AJ, "Benzocaine-Induced Methemoglobinemia: Report of a Severe Reaction and Review of the Literature," *Ann Pharmacother*, 1994, 28(5):643-9.

Antithymocyte Globulin (Equine)

(LIM foe site i MYUN GLOB yoo lin E kwine)

Medication Safety Issues

Sound-alike/look-alike issues:
Atgam® may be confused with Ativan®

U.S. Brand Names Atgam®

Canadian Brand Names Atgam®

Index Terms Antithymocyte Immunoglobulin; ATG; Horse Antihuman Thymocyte Gamma Globulin; Lymphocyte Immune Globulin

Therapeutic Category Immunosuppressant Agent

Generic Available No

Use Prevention and/or treatment of allograft rejection; treatment of moderate to severe aplastic anemia in patients not considered suitable candidates for bone marrow transplantation; prevention of graft-vs-host disease following bone marrow transplantation

Pregnancy Risk Factor C

Lactation Excretion in breast milk unknown/use caution

Contraindications Hypersensitivity to ATG, any component, or other equine gamma globulins; severe, unremitting leukopenia and/or thrombocytopenia

Warnings Should only be used by physicians experienced in immunosuppressive therapy or management of renal transplant patients; adequate laboratory and supportive medical resources must be readily available in the facility for patient management. Anaphylaxis (symptoms can include hypotension, respiratory distress, pain in the chest, rash, and tachycardia) may occur at any time during ATG therapy. Epinephrine and oxygen should be readily available to treat anaphylaxis.

Adverse Reactions

Cardiovascular: Hypotension, hypertension, tachycardia, edema
Central nervous system: Seizures, fever, headache, chills
Dermatologic: Rash, pruritus, urticaria
Gastrointestinal: Diarrhea, nausea, stomatitis
Hematologic: Leukopenia, thrombocytopenia, hemolysis, anemia
Local: Thrombophlebitis
Neuromuscular & skeletal: Arthralgia; pain in the chest, flank, or back; weakness
Renal: Acute renal failure
Respiratory: Dyspnea
Miscellaneous: Lymphadenopathy, serum sickness, night sweats; anaphylaxis may be indicated by hypotension or respiratory distress

Stability Store in refrigerator; dilute in ½NS or NS; when diluted to concentrations up to 4 mg/mL, ATG infusion solution is stable for 24 hours; use of dextrose solutions is not recommended; precipitation can occur in solutions with a low salt concentration (ie, D_5W)

Mechanism of Action May involve elimination of antigen-reactive T-lymphocytes (killer cells) in peripheral blood or alteration of T-cell function

Pharmacokinetics

Distribution: Poor into lymphoid tissues; binds to circulating lymphocytes, granulocytes, platelets, bone marrow cells
Half-life, plasma: 1.5-12 days
Elimination: ~1% of dose excreted in urine

Usual Dosage Intradermal skin test is recommended prior to administration of the initial dose of ATG; use 0.1 mL of a 1:1000 dilution of ATG in NS; observe the skin test every 15 minutes for 1 hour; a local reaction ≥10 mm diameter with a wheal or erythema or both should be considered a positive skin test

I.V.:

Children:

Aplastic anemia protocol: 10-20 mg/kg/day for 8-14 days, or 40 mg/kg/day once daily over 4 hours for 4 days; then give 10-30 mg/kg/dose every other day for 7 more doses

Cardiac allograft: 10 mg/kg/day for 7 days or as per protocol

Renal allograft: 5-25 mg/kg/day or as per protocol

Children and Adults:

Rejection prevention: 15 mg/kg/day for 14 days, then give every other day for 7 more doses; initial dose should be administered within 24 hours before or after transplantation

Rejection treatment: 10-15 mg/kg/day for 14 days, then give every other day for 7 more doses

Administration Parenteral: Administer via central line; use of high flow veins will minimize the occurrence of phlebitis and thrombosis; administer by slow I.V. infusion through a 0.2-1 micron in-line filter over 4-8 hours at a final concentration not to exceed 4 mg ATG/mL

Monitoring Parameters Lymphocyte profile; CBC with differential and platelet count, vital signs during administration, renal function test

Nursing Implications Patient may need to be pretreated with an antipyretic, antihistamine, and/or corticosteroid to prevent chills, fever, itching, and erythema

Dosage Forms Excipient information presented when available (limited, particularly for generics); consult specific product labeling.

Injection, solution:

Atgam®: 50 mg/mL (5 mL)

References

Rosenfeld SJ, Kimball J, Vining D, et al, "Intensive Immunosuppression With Antithymocyte Globulin and Cyclosporine as Treatment for Severe Acquired Aplastic Anemia," *Blood*, 1995, 85(11):3058-65.

Whitehead B, James I, Helms P, et al, "Intensive Care Management of Children Following Heart and Heart-Lung Transplantation," *Intensive Care Med*, 1990, 16(7):426-30.

Antithymocyte Globulin (Rabbit)

(an te THY moe site GLOB yu lin (RAB bit)

U.S. Brand Names Thymoglobulin®

Index Terms Antithymocyte Immunoglobulin; rATG

Therapeutic Category Immunosuppressant Agent

Generic Available No

Use Prevention and/or treatment of acute rejection after renal, bone marrow, heart/lung, liver, intestinal, or multivisceral transplantation in conjunction with other immunosuppressive agents. Treatment of aplastic anemia in patients who failed to respond to antithymocyte immunoglobulin (equine).

Pregnancy Risk Factor C

Lactation Excretion in breast milk unknown/use caution

Contraindications Hypersensitivity to antithymocyte globulin, rabbit proteins, or any component; acute viral illness

Warnings Should only be used by physicians experienced in immunosuppressive therapy for the treatment of transplant patients; adequate laboratory and supportive medical resources must be readily available in the facility for patient management. Anaphylaxis has been reported with the use of antithymocyte globulin (rabbit). Epinephrine, oxygen, and resuscitative equipment should be readily available to treat anaphylaxis. Thrombocytopenia or neutropenia may result from cross-reactive antibodies and is reversible following dose reduction or discontinuation.

Precautions Infusion may cause fever and chills. Infuse first dose slowly over a minimum of 6 hours into a high flow vein; 1 hour prior to infusion, premedicate with corticosteroids, acetaminophen, and/or an antihistamine to reduce incidence of side effects during infusion. Reduce dose in patients with WBC between 2000-3000 cells/mm^3 or if the platelet count is between 50,000-75,000 cells/mm^3. Consider discontinuing antithymocyte globulin (rabbit) if WBC <2000 cells/mm^3 or platelets <50,000 cells/mm^3.

Adverse Reactions

Cardiovascular: Hypotension or hypertension, tachycardia, peripheral edema

Central nervous system: Fever, chills, headache, malaise, dizziness, asthenia

Endocrine & metabolic: Hyperkalemia

Gastrointestinal: Abdominal pain, diarrhea, nausea, vomiting

Hematologic: Thrombocytopenia, neutropenia, leukopenia

(Continued)

Antithymocyte Globulin (Rabbit) *(Continued)*

Respiratory: Dyspnea

Miscellaneous: Increased risk of infection, lymphoma, post-transplant lymphoproliferative disease; anaphylaxis; diaphoresis

Drug Interactions Immunosuppressants (additive immunosuppressive effects or over-immunosuppression)

Stability Store intact vial in refrigerator; protect from light; do not freeze. Allow diluent and contents of vial to reach room temperature prior to reconstitution; use within 4 hours of reconstitution if stored at room temperature; compatible with D_5W or NS; Y-site injection compatible with hydrocortisone sodium succinate and heparin 100 units/mL in D_5W or NS; incompatible with heparin 2 units/mL in D_5W

Mechanism of Action Possible mechanism may involve elimination of antigen-reactive T-lymphocytes (killer cells) in peripheral blood or alteration of T-cell function

Pharmacodynamics Onset of action (T-cell depletion): Within one day

Pharmacokinetics Half-life: 2-3 days

Usual Dosage IV: (refer to individual protocols):

Children:

Bone marrow transplantation: 1.5-3 mg/kg/day once daily for 4 consecutive days before transplantation

Treatment of graft-versus-host disease: 1.5 mg/kg/dose once daily or every other day

Renal transplantation:

Induction: 1-2 mg/kg/day once daily for 4-5 days initiated at time of transplant

Acute rejection: 1.5mg/kg/day once daily for 7-14 days

Heart/lung transplantation:

Induction: 1-2 mg/kg/day depending on baseline platelet count once daily for 5 days

Rejection: 2 mg/kg/day once daily for 5 days

Liver, intestinal, or multivisceral transplant:

Preconditioning/induction: Pretransplant: 2 mg/kg; postop day 1: 3 mg/kg

Rejection: 1.5 mg/kg/day once daily for 7-14 days based upon biopsy results; maximum dose: 2 mg/kg/dose

Adults:

Acute renal transplant rejection: 1.5 mg/kg/day once daily for 7-14 days

Aplastic Anemia: 3.5 mg/kg/day once daily for 5 days

Administration Parenteral: Administer by slow I.V. infusion over 6-12 hours for the preconditioning/induction dose or over 6 hours for the initial acute rejection treatment dose; infuse over 4 hours for subsequent doses if first dose tolerated. Administer through an in-line filter with pore size of 0.22 microns via central line or high flow vein at a final concentration of 0.5 to 2 mg/mL in NS or D_5W.

Monitoring Parameters Platelet count, CBC with differential, lymphocyte count, vital signs during infusion

Test Interactions Potential interference with rabbit antibody-based immunoassays

Nursing Implications Patient may need to be pretreated with an antipyretic, antihistamine, and corticosteroid 1 hour prior to each dose of antithymocyte globulin (rabbit). Mild itching and erythema can be treated with an antihistamine. Chills and fever can be treated by slowing the infusion rate or administering an additional dose of corticosteroid. If anaphylaxis occurs, terminate infusion immediately.

Additional Information Antiviral therapy should be given prophylactically during antithymocyte globulin (rabbit) use.

Dosage Forms Excipient information presented when available (limited, particularly for generics); consult specific product labeling.

Injection, powder for reconstitution:

Thymoglobulin®: 25 mg

References

Di Filippo S, Boissonnat P, Sassolas F, et al, "Rabbit Antithymocyte Globulin as Induction Immunotherapy in Pediatric Heart Transplantation," *Transplantation*, 2003, 75(3):354-8.

Horan JT, Liesveld JL, Fenton P, et al, "Hematopoietic Stem Cell Transplantation for Multiply Transfused Patients With Sickle Cell Disease and Thalassemia After Low-Dose Total Body Irradiation, Fludarabine, and Rabbit Anti-thymocyte Globulin," *Bone Marrow Transplant*, 2005, 35(2):171-7.

Starzl TE, Murase N, Abu-Elmagd K, et al, "Tolerogenic Immunosuppression for Organ Transplantation," *Lancet*, 2003, 361(9368):1502-10.

Trissel LA and Saenz CA, "Physical Compatibility of Antithymocyte Globulin (Rabbit) With Heparin Sodium and Hydrocortisone Sodium Succinate," *Am J Health Syst Pharm*, 2003, 60(16):1650-2.

♦ **Antithymocyte Immunoglobulin** *see* Antithymocyte Globulin (Equine) *on page 146*

♦ **Antithymocyte Immunoglobulin** *see* Antithymocyte Globulin (Rabbit) *on page 147*

♦ **Antitumor Necrosis Factor-Alpha** *see* Infliximab *on page 830*

Antivenin (*Latrodectus mactans*)

(an tee VEN in lak tro DUK tus MAK tans)

Index Terms Black Widow Spider Species Antivenin (*Latrodectus mactans*)

Therapeutic Category Antivenin

Generic Available No

Use Treatment of severe systemic symptoms refractory to supportive measures due to black widow spider bites.

Pregnancy Risk Factor C

Lactation Excretion in breast milk unknown/use caution

Warnings Anaphylaxis and serum sickness have been reported in patients who received *Latrodectus mactans* antivenin. Patients with atopic sensitivity to horses may have an increased risk of experiencing an immediate sensitivity reaction to the antivenin. Desensitization may need to be performed on patients with positive skin or conjunctival test reaction or history of sensitivity to equine serum; epinephrine and oxygen should be readily available to treat anaphylaxis. *Latrodectus mactans* antivenin contains thimerosal which has been associated with neurologic and renal toxicities.

Adverse Reactions

Cardiovascular: Shock, flushing, hypotension, edema of face, tongue and throat

Dermatologic: Pruritus, urticaria

Gastrointestinal: Vomiting

Respiratory: Cough, dyspnea, bronchospasm

Miscellaneous: Anaphylaxis, serum sickness (occurs 7-14 days after antivenin administration in 75% of patients)

Stability Refrigerate; do not freeze

Mechanism of Action Neutralizes the venom of black widow spiders

Pharmacodynamics Onset of action: Within 30 minutes with symptoms subsiding after 1-3 hours

Pharmacokinetics Data in humans is not available.

Usual Dosage The initial dose of antivenin should be administered as soon as possible for prompt relief of symptoms. Delayed antivenin administration (up to 90 hours after bite) may still be effective in treating patients with prolonged or refractory symptoms resulting from black widow spider bites.

Sensitivity testing: Intradermal skin test or conjunctival test must be performed prior to antivenin administration:

Intradermal skin test: Use 0.02 mL of a 1:10 dilution of normal horse serum in NS. An intradermal control of 0.02 mL NS should also be administered. Read skin test after 10 minutes. Positive reaction consists of an urticarial wheal surrounded by a zone of erythema.

Conjunctival test: Positive reaction consists of reddening of the conjunctiva and itching of the eye 10 minutes following test.

Children: Instill one drop of 1:100 dilution of horse serum into conjunctival sac.

Adults: Instill one drop of 1:10 dilution of horse serum into the conjunctival sac.

Desensitization: (Desensitization is only utilized when antivenin is considered a necessary lifesaving treatment in patients with history of allergy or with mildly positive sensitivity tests): SubQ: Inject 0.1 mL, followed by 0.2 mL and 0.5 mL of a 1:100 antivenin dilution administered in 15- to 30-minute intervals (30 minutes preferably); repeat procedure with a 1:10 dilution of antivenin; then repeat procedure with undiluted antivenin. If a reaction occurs after a desensitization injection, apply tourniquet proximal to the injection site and administer epinephrine proximal to the tourniquet or into another extremity. After 30 minutes, continue desensitization procedure by injecting the last dose that did not evoke a reaction. If no reaction occurs after 0.5 mL of undiluted antivenin is administered, continue to administer 0.5 mL of undiluted antivenin at 15-minute intervals until the entire dose (2.5 mL) has been injected.

If sensitivity test is negative, antivenin may be administered:

Children <12 years: I.V.: Entire contents of a reconstituted vial (2.5 mL); second dose may be needed in some cases

Adults: I.M., I.V.: Entire contents of a reconstituted vial (2.5 mL); administer I.V. to patients in shock or for management of severe cases; second dose may be needed in some cases

Administration Parenteral: Reconstitute vial containing 6000 units of antivenin with 2.5 mL SWI; shake vial (with the needle still in the rubber stopper) to dissolve powder. Visually inspect vial for particulate matter.

I.M.: Administer into the anterolateral thigh. Apply tourniquet if an adverse reaction occurs.

(Continued)

Antivenin (*Latrodectus mactans*) *(Continued)*

I.V.: Dilute reconstituted antivenin with 10-50 mL of NS; infuse over 15 minutes. If an immediate hypersensitivity reaction occurs, immediately interrupt antivenin infusion and provide appropriate supportive therapy. If administration of antivenin can be resumed after control of the reaction, reinitiate at a slower infusion rate.

Monitoring Parameters Vital signs; signs and symptoms of allergy, anaphylaxis, and serum sickness

Additional Information The venom of the black widow spider is a neurotoxin that causes release of a presynaptic neurotransmitter. Within 1 hour of the bite, clinical effects such as sharp pain, muscle spasm, weakness, tremor, severe abdominal pain with rigidity, hypertension, respiratory distress, diaphoresis, and facial swelling may be seen.

Dosage Forms Excipient information presented when available (limited, particularly for generics); consult specific product labeling.

Injection, powder for reconstitution: 6000 antivenin units [equine origin; contains thimerosal; packaged with diluent and normal horse serum for sensitivity testing]

References

Saucier JR, "Arachnid Envenomation," *Emerg Med Clin North Am*, 2004, 22(2):405-22

- ♦ **Antivenin Polyvalent [Equine]** *see Crotalidae* Polyvalent Antivenin (Equine) *on page 409*
- ♦ **Antivert®** *see* Meclizine *on page 988*
- ♦ **Antizol®** *see* Fomepizole *on page 702*
- ♦ **Anucort-HC®** *see* Hydrocortisone *on page 781*
- ♦ **Anu-Med [OTC]** *see* Phenylephrine *on page 1250*
- ♦ **Anusol-HC®** *see* Hydrocortisone *on page 781*
- ♦ **Anusol® HC-1 [OTC]** *see* Hydrocortisone *on page 781*
- ♦ **Anzemet®** *see* Dolasetron *on page 528*
- ♦ **APAP** *see* Acetaminophen *on page 42*
- ♦ **Apidra®** *see* Insulin Glulisine *on page 841*
- ♦ **Apo-Acetaminophen® (Can)** *see* Acetaminophen *on page 42*
- ♦ **Apo-Acetazolamide® (Can)** *see* AcetaZOLAMIDE *on page 47*
- ♦ **Apo-Acyclovir® (Can)** *see* Acyclovir *on page 54*
- ♦ **Apo-Allopurinol® (Can)** *see* Allopurinol *on page 76*
- ♦ **Apo-Alpraz® (Can)** *see* Alprazolam *on page 79*
- ♦ **Apo-Alpraz® TS (Can)** *see* Alprazolam *on page 79*
- ♦ **Apo-Amiloride® (Can)** *see* Amiloride *on page 95*
- ♦ **Apo-Amiodarone® (Can)** *see* Amiodarone *on page 100*
- ♦ **Apo-Amitriptyline® (Can)** *see* Amitriptyline *on page 107*
- ♦ **Apo-Amoxi® (Can)** *see* Amoxicillin *on page 113*
- ♦ **Apo-Amoxi-Clav® (Can)** *see* Amoxicillin and Clavulanic Acid *on page 115*
- ♦ **Apo-Ampi® (Can)** *see* Ampicillin *on page 123*
- ♦ **Apo-Atenol® (Can)** *see* Atenolol *on page 170*
- ♦ **Apo-Azathioprine® (Can)** *see* Azathioprine *on page 187*
- ♦ **Apo-Azithromycin® (Can)** *see* Azithromycin *on page 191*
- ♦ **Apo-Baclofen® (Can)** *see* Baclofen *on page 197*
- ♦ **Apo-Beclomethasone® (Can)** *see* Beclomethasone *on page 200*
- ♦ **Apo-Benztropine® (Can)** *see* Benztropine *on page 208*
- ♦ **Apo-Bisacodyl® (Can)** *see* Bisacodyl *on page 217*
- ♦ **Apo-Brimonidine® (Can)** *see* Brimonidine *on page 231*
- ♦ **Apo-Bromocriptine® (Can)** *see* Bromocriptine *on page 232*
- ♦ **Apo-Buspirone® (Can)** *see* BusPIRone *on page 250*
- ♦ **Apo-Cal® (Can)** *see* Calcium Carbonate *on page 264*
- ♦ **Apo-Calcitonin® (Can)** *see* Calcitonin *on page 258*
- ♦ **Apo-Capto® (Can)** *see* Captopril *on page 277*
- ♦ **Apo-Carbamazepine® (Can)** *see* Carbamazepine *on page 279*
- ♦ **Apo-Carvedilol® (Can)** *see* Carvedilol *on page 293*
- ♦ **Apo-Cefaclor® (Can)** *see* Cefaclor *on page 301*
- ♦ **Apo-Cefadroxil® (Can)** *see* Cefadroxil *on page 302*
- ♦ **Apo-Cefoxitin® (Can)** *see* Cefoxitin *on page 313*
- ♦ **Apo-Cefprozil® (Can)** *see* Cefprozil *on page 316*
- ♦ **Apo-Cefuroxime® (Can)** *see* Cefuroxime *on page 322*
- ♦ **Apo-Cephalex® (Can)** *see* Cephalexin *on page 324*
- ♦ **Apo-Cetirizine® (Can)** *see* Cetirizine *on page 327*
- ♦ **Apo-Cimetidine® (Can)** *see* Cimetidine *on page 355*

- ♦ **Apo-Salvent® Respirator Solution (Can)** *see* Albuterol *on page 66*
- ♦ **Apo-Salvent® Sterules (Can)** *see* Albuterol *on page 66*
- ♦ **Apo-Sertraline® (Can)** *see* Sertraline *on page 1429*
- ♦ **Apo-Simvastatin® (Can)** *see* Simvastatin *on page 1441*
- ♦ **Apo-Sotalol® (Can)** *see* Sotalol *on page 1463*
- ♦ **Apo-Sulfatrim® (Can)** *see* Sulfamethoxazole and Trimethoprim *on page 1487*
- ♦ **Apo-Sulfatrim® DS (Can)** *see* Sulfamethoxazole and Trimethoprim *on page 1487*
- ♦ **Apo-Sulfatrim® Pediatric (Can)** *see* Sulfamethoxazole and Trimethoprim *on page 1487*
- ♦ **Apo-Sulin® (Can)** *see* Sulindac *on page 1493*
- ♦ **Apo-Sumatriptan® (Can)** *see* Sumatriptan *on page 1495*
- ♦ **Apo-Tetra® (Can)** *see* Tetracycline *on page 1518*
- ♦ **Apo-Theo LA® (Can)** *see* Theophylline *on page 1520*
- ♦ **Apo-Timol® (Can)** *see* Timolol *on page 1542*
- ♦ **Apo-Timop® (Can)** *see* Timolol *on page 1542*
- ♦ **Apo-Trazodone® (Can)** *see* Trazodone *on page 1564*
- ♦ **Apo-Trazodone D® (Can)** *see* Trazodone *on page 1564*
- ♦ **Apo-Triazo® (Can)** *see* Triazolam *on page 1572*
- ♦ **Apo-Trihex® (Can)** *see* Trihexyphenidyl *on page 1575*
- ♦ **Apo-Trimethoprim® (Can)** *see* Trimethoprim *on page 1578*
- ♦ **Apo-Valproic® (Can)** *see* Valproic Acid and Derivatives *on page 1592*
- ♦ **Apo-Verap® (Can)** *see* Verapamil *on page 1611*
- ♦ **Apo-Verap® SR (Can)** *see* Verapamil *on page 1611*
- ♦ **Apo-Warfarin® (Can)** *see* Warfarin *on page 1626*
- ♦ **Apo-Zidovudine® (Can)** *see* Zidovudine *on page 1637*
- ♦ **APPG** *see* Penicillin G Procaine *on page 1233*
- ♦ **Apra Children's [OTC]** *see* Acetaminophen *on page 42*

Aprepitant (ap RE pi tant)

Related Information
Assessment of Liver Function *on page 1810*

U.S. Brand Names Emend®

Index Terms L 754030; MK 869

Therapeutic Category Antiemetic; Substance P/Neurokinin 1 (NK_1) Receptor Antagonist

Generic Available No

Use Prevention of acute and delayed chemotherapy-induced emesis when used as an adjunctive agent with a 5-HT_3 antagonist and a corticosteroid; prevention of postoperative nausea and vomiting

Pregnancy Risk Factor B

Lactation Excretion in breast milk unknown/not recommended

Contraindications Hypersensitivity to aprepitant or any component; concurrent use with pimozide, terfenadine, astemizole, or cisapride

Warnings Aprepitant has a potential to significantly interact with many medications (see Drug Interactions); potential increased serum levels of pimozide, terfenadine, astemizole, or cisapride could result in serious or life-threatening adverse effects; concomitant use with warfarin may result in clinically significant decrease in INR; patients on warfarin should have INR monitored closely, particularly at 7-10 days following initiation of 3-day aprepitant therapy. The efficacy of oral contraceptives may also be reduced during treatment with aprepitant; alternative methods of birth control should be used during aprepitant therapy.

Precautions Aprepitant is a moderate cytochrome P450 isoenzyme CYP3A4 inhibitor; use with caution in patients receiving medications metabolized by CYP3A4 as a reduction in metabolism and consequent elevation of serum levels may occur; the effect of aprepitant on the pharmacokinetics of orally administered CYP3A4 substrates may be greater than that seen with I.V. administered CYP3A4 substrates. Use with caution and monitor use closely in patients receiving docetaxel, paclitaxel, etoposide, irinotecan, ifosfamide, imatinib, vinorelbine, vinblastine, and vincristine as they are known to be metabolized by CYP3A4 isoenzymes

Adverse Reactions
Cardiovascular: Hypertension, hypotension, MI, tachycardia, bradycardia
Central nervous system: Confusion, depression, anxiety, headache, insomnia, dizziness, fatigue (18% to 22%), fever
Dermatologic: Rash, alopecia, urticaria, angioedema, Stevens-Johnson syndrome (rare)
(Continued)

Aprepitant *(Continued)*

Endocrine & metabolic: Anorexia, hyperglycemia, hypokalemia, weight loss, hyponatremia

Gastrointestinal: Abdominal pain, constipation (9% to 12%), diarrhea, epigastric discomfort, gastritis, heartburn, nausea (7% to 13%), vomiting, dysgeusia, dyspepsia, dysphagia, flatulence, taste disturbance, vocal disturbance, pharyngitis, increased salivation, hiccups

Genitourinary: Dysuria

Hematologic: Anemia, thrombocytopenia, neutropenia

Hepatic: Elevated serum transaminases

Neuromuscular & skeletal: Weakness (3% to 18%), myalgia, muscle pain

Otic: Tinnitus

Renal: Renal insufficiency, elevated serum creatinine, proteinuria

Respiratory: Hiccups (11%), cough, dyspnea, pneumonitis, respiratory insufficiency

Drug Interactions Cytochrome P450 isoenzyme CYP3A4 substrate, moderate inhibitor, and inducer; CYP2C9 inducer

Aprepitant induces the metabolism of warfarin (monitor INR closely, particularly in the 7- to 10-day period post-aprepitant therapy), tolbutamide, and other drugs known to be metabolized by CYP2C9; decreases AUC of oral contraceptives which may result in reduced efficacy; increases serum levels of medications primarily metabolized by CYP3A4 such as pimozide, terfenadine, astemizole, cisapride, docetaxel, paclitaxel, etoposide, irinotecan, ifosfamide, imatinib, vinorelbine, vinblastine, and vincristine; increases serum levels of pimozide, terfenadine, astemizole, and cisapride (see Contraindications); increases AUC for corticosteroids (reduce the oral dexamethasone dose by 50%, I.V. methylprednisolone dose by 25%, and oral methylprednisolone dose by 50%); increases serum level of midazolam and potentially other benzodiazepines; CYP3A4 inhibitors (ketoconazole, itraconazole, nefazodone, troleandomycin, clarithromycin, ritonavir, nelfinavir) may significantly increase aprepitant serum levels; CYP3A4 inducers (rifampin, carbamazepine, and phenytoin) may reduce aprepitant serum levels; diltiazem increases aprepitant serum levels; when concomitantly used with paroxetine, serum levels of both agents are reduced

Stability Store capsules at room temperature.

Mechanism of Action Aprepitant is a selective high-affinity antagonist of human substance P/neurokinin 1 receptors. Antiemetic activity is via central action with little or no affinity for serotonin, dopamine, and corticosteroid receptors.

Pharmacokinetics

Distribution: V_d: Adults: 70 L

Protein binding: >95%

Metabolism: Extensive hepatic metabolism primarily by CYP3A4 with minor metabolism by CYP1A2 and CYP2C19

Bioavailability: 60% to 65%

Half-life: Adults: 9-13 hours

Time to peak serum concentration: 3-4 hours

Elimination:

Clearance: Adults: 62-90 mL/minute

Usual Dosage Oral: **Note:** Aprepitant has not been studied for chronic continuous therapy and its use for chronic therapy is not recommended.

Prevention of chemotherapy-induced emesis: Adults: 125 mg one hour prior to chemotherapy followed by 80 mg once daily for the next two days. Use in combination with a 5-HT_3 antagonist and a corticosteroid.

Note: Aprepitant has only been studied in a three-day regimen combined with a corticosteroid and 5-HT_3 antagonist. Efficacy as a single agent or for prolonged treatment has not been demonstrated.

Prevention of postoperative nausea and vomiting: Adults: 40 mg within 3 hours prior to induction of anesthesia

Dosage adjustment in renal impairment: No dosage adjustment needed

Dosage adjustment in hepatic impairment: No dosage adjustment needed in mild to moderate hepatic insufficiency; the pharmacokinetic profile of aprepitant in severe hepatic insufficiency (Child-Pugh score >9) has not be studied

Administration Oral: May be administered without regard to food, one hour prior to chemotherapy on the first day of treatment and in the morning on the subsequent next two days or within 3 hours prior to induction of anesthesia

Patient Information Aprepitant may react with many other medications; report all medication use including OTC and herbal products to your physician; due to potential decrease effectiveness of oral contraceptives, alternative contraceptive methods should be used during therapy

Dosage Forms Excipient information presented when available (limited, particularly for generics); consult specific product labeling.

Capsule:
Emend®: 40 mg, 80 mg, 125 mg
Combination package: Capsule 80 mg (2s), capsule 125 mg (1s)

- **Apresoline [DSC]** *see* HydrALAZINE *on page 775*
- **Apresoline® (Can)** *see* HydrALAZINE *on page 775*
- **Aprodine® [OTC]** *see* Triprolidine and Pseudoephedrine *on page 1580*

Aprotinin (a proe TYE nin)

U.S. Brand Names Trasylol®

Canadian Brand Names Trasylol®

Therapeutic Category Hemostatic Agent

Generic Available No

Use Prophylactic use to reduce perioperative blood loss and the need for blood transfusion in patients undergoing cardiopulmonary bypass in the course of coronary artery bypass graft surgery (CABG); in selected repeat cases of primary CABG surgery where the risk of bleeding is especially high or where transfusion is unavailable or unacceptable

Pregnancy Risk Factor B

Lactation Excretion in breast milk unknown/use caution

Contraindications Hypersensitivity to aprotinin or any component

Warnings Patients with a provious exposure to aprotinin (particularly when re-exposure is within 6 months) are at an increased risk for hypersensitivity reactions including anaphylactic or anaphylactoid reactions; emergency medications to treat severe hypersensitivity reactions should be readily available; pretreatment with an antihistamine and H_2 blocker before administration of the loading dose is recommended in these patients; delay the addition of aprotinin into the pump prime solution until the loading dose has safely been administered.

The FDA has issued a Public Health Advisory alerting physicians who perform heart bypass surgery and their patients that aprotinin has been linked to an increased risk of death, serious kidney damage, CHF, and stroke in observational studies. The FDA is advising healthcare providers to limit the use of aprotinin to patients where benefit of reducing blood loss is essential to management (outweighs the risks), to carefully monitor patients for the occurrence of toxicity, and to report adverse events associated with its use to the FDA. Safety and efficacy in children have not been established.

Precautions All patients treated with aprotinin should first receive a test dose at least 10 minutes before the loading dose to assess the potential for allergic reactions

Adverse Reactions

Cardiovascular: Atrial fibrillation, MI, CHF, atrial flutter, ventricular tachycardia, ventricular extrasystoles, supraventricular tachycardia, stroke, chest pain, hypotension, pericardial effusion, pulmonary hypertension, pericarditis

Central nervous system: Fever, mental confusion, seizures, agitation, dizziness, anxiety, insomnia

Endocrine & metabolic: Hyperglycemia, hypokalemia, acidosis

Gastrointestinal: Nausea, vomiting, constipation, diarrhea, GI hemorrhage

Hematologic: Hemolysis, anemia, thrombosis, increased CPK

Hepatic: Liver damage, jaundice

Local: Phlebitis

Neuromuscular & skeletal: Arthralgia

Renal: Decreased renal function, renal failure, renal tubular acidosis

Respiratory: Dyspnea, bronchoconstriction, pulmonary edema, apnea, increased cough

Miscellaneous: Anaphylaxis (see Warnings)

Drug Interactions Decreases effects of fibrinolytic agents such as streptokinase or anistreplase; decreases effects of captopril; prolonged activated clotting time when used with heparin

Stability Store between 2°C to 25°C (36°F to 77°F); do not freeze; do not mix with other medications; incompatible with corticosteroids, heparin (see Administration), amino acids, and fat emulsion

Mechanism of Action Aprotinin, a serine protease inhibitor, modulates the systemic inflammatory response associated with cardiopulmonary bypass surgery; inhibits plasmin, kallikrein, and platelet activation producing antifibrinolytic effects; is a weak inhibitor of plasma pseudocholinesterase; inhibits the contact phase activation of coagulation and preserves adhesive platelet glycoproteins making them resistant to damage from increased circulating plasmin or mechanical injury occurring during cardiopulmonary bypass

Pharmacokinetics

Metabolism: Slowly degraded by lysosomal enzymes

(Continued)

Aprotinin *(Continued)*

Half-life, elimination: 150 minutes; terminal elimination: 10 hours

Elimination: <10% excreted unchanged in the urine

Usual Dosage I.V.: Test dose: All patients should receive a test dose at least 10 minutes prior to the loading dose to assess the potential for allergic reactions

Infants and Children: No conclusive dosage regimen has been established; variable dosage recommendations in the literature. Test dose: (dosage not well documented in studies) 0.1 mg/kg (maximum: 1.4 mg) has been used. The following dosage ranges have been reported in the literature:

10,000-35,000 Kallikrein inhibitor units/kg (1.4-4.9 mg/kg) loading dose

10,000-35,000 Kallikrein inhibitor units/kg (1.4-4.9 mg/kg) into pump prime volume

10,000-35,000 Kallikrein inhibitor units/kg/hour (1.4-4.2 mg/kg/hour) continuous infusion

Alternative (based upon surface area):

120-240 mg/m^2 (857,142-1,714,284 Kallikrein inhibitor units/ m^2) loading dose

120-240 mg/m^2 (857,142-1,714,284 Kallikrein inhibitor units/m^2) into pump prime volume

28-56 mg/m^2/hour (200,000-400,000 Kallikrein inhibitor units/ m^2/hour) continuous infusion

Adults: Test dose: 1 mL (1.4 mg)

Regimen A (standard dose):

2 million Kallikrein inhibitor units (280 mg) loading dose

2 million Kallikrein inhibitor units (280 mg) into pump prime volume

500,000 Kallikrein inhibitor units/hour (70 mg/hour) continuous infusion during surgery

Regimen B (low dose):

1 million Kallikrein inhibitor units (140 mg) loading dose

1 million Kallikrein inhibitor units (140 mg) into pump prime volume

250,000 Kallikrein inhibitor units/hour (35 mg/hour) continuous infusion during surgery

Dosage adjustment in renal impairment: No adjustment required

Dosage adjustment in hepatic impairment: No information available

Administration Parenteral: For I.V. use only; all I.V. doses should be administered through a central line; infuse test dose over at least 10 minutes; infuse loading dose over 20-30 minutes with patient in the supine position; add pump priming dose while recirculating the priming fluid of the cardiopulmonary bypass circuit. To avoid physical incompatibility with heparin when adding to pump-prime solution, each agent should be added during recirculation to assure adequate dilution.

Monitoring Parameters Bleeding times, prothrombin time (PT), activated clotting time (ACT), platelet count, CBC, Hct, Hgb, and fibrinogen degradation products; for toxicity also include renal function tests and blood pressure

Because aPPT and ACT are difficult to interpret with aprotinin use, the manufacturer recommends two different ways to administer heparin:

1) Fixed heparin dosing where a standard loading dose of heparin plus the quantity of heparin added to the prime volume of the cardiopulmonary bypass (CPB) circuit should total at least 350 units/kg; additional heparin should be administered based upon the patient's weight and duration of CPB.

2) Heparin dosing based upon a protamine titration method. A heparin dose response, assessed by protamine titration, should be performed prior to administration of aprotinin to determine the heparin loading dose. Additional heparin should be administered on the basis of heparin levels measured by protamine titration. Heparin levels during bypass should not be allowed to drop below 2.7 units/mL (2 mg/kg) or below the level indicated by heparin dose response testing.

Reference Range Antiplasmin effects occur when plasma aprotinin concentrations are 125 kallikrein inhibitor units/mL and antikallikrein effects occur when plasma levels are 250-500 kallikrein inhibitor units/mL; it remains unknown if these plasma concentrations are required for clinical benefits to occur during cardiopulmonary bypass.

While institutional protocols may vary, a minimal celite ACT of 750 seconds or kaolin-ACT of 480 seconds is recommended in the presence of aprotinin. Consult the manufacturer's information on specific ACT test interpretation in the presence of aprotinin.

Test Interactions Aprotinin prolongs whole blood clotting time of heparinized blood as determined by the Hemochrom® method or similar surface activation methods; patients may require additional heparin even in the presence of activated clotting time levels that appear to represent adequate anticoagulation

Additional Information Due to interference with aprotinin and ACT, the amount of protamine administered to reverse heparin activity should be based upon the amount of heparin administered and not the ACT value.

Dosage Forms Excipient information presented when available (limited, particularly for generics); consult specific product labeling.

Injection, solution:

Trasylol®: 1.4 mg/mL [10,000 KIU/mL] (100 mL, 200 mL) [bovine derived]

References

Arnold DM, Fergusson DA, Chan AK, et al, "Avoiding Transfusions in Children Undergoing Cardiac Surgery: A Meta-Analysis of Randomized Trials of Aprotinin," *Anesth Analg*, 2006, 102(3):731-7.

Boldt J, "Endothelial-Related Coagulation in Pediatric Surgery," *Ann Thorac Surg*, 1998, 65(6 Suppl):S56-9.

Carrel TP, Schwanda M, Vogt P, et al, "Aprotinin in Pediatric Cardiac Operations: A Benefit in Complex Malformations and With High-Dose Regimen Only," *Ann Thorac Surg*, 1998, 66(1):153-8.

Miller BE, Tosone SR, Tam VK, et al, "Hematologic and Economic Impact of Aprotinin in Reoperative Pediatric Cardiac Operations," *Ann Thorac Surg*, 1998, 66(2):535-41.

Penkoske P, Entwistle LM, Marchak BE, et al, "Aprotinin in Children Undergoing Repair of Congenital Heart Defects," *Ann Thorac Surg*, 1995, 60(6 Suppl):S529-32.

Spray TL, "Use of Aprotinin in Pediatric Organ Transplantation," *Ann Thorac Surg*, 1998, 65(6 Suppl):S71-3.

♦ **Aquachloral® Supprettes®** *see* Chloral Hydrate *on page 331*
♦ **Aquacort® (Can)** *see* Hydrocortisone *on page 781*
♦ **AquaMEPHYTON® (Can)** *see* Phytonadione *on page 1258*
♦ **Aquanil™ HC [OTC]** *see* Hydrocortisone *on page 781*
♦ **Aquasol A®** *see* Vitamin A *on page 1619*
♦ **Aquasol E® [OTC]** *see* Vitamin E *on page 1620*
♦ **Aquavit-E [OTC]** *see* Vitamin E *on page 1620*
♦ **Aqueous Procaine Penicillin G** *see* Penicillin G Procaine *on page 1233*
♦ **Ara-C** *see* Cytarabine *on page 429*
♦ **Arabinosylcytosine** *see* Cytarabine *on page 429*
♦ **Aralen®** *see* Chloroquine *on page 340*
♦ **Aranesp®** *see* Darbepoetin Alfa *on page 444*
♦ **Aredia®** *see* Pamidronate *on page 1200*

Arginine (AR ji neen)

U.S. Brand Names R-Gene®

Index Terms Arginine Hydrochloride

Therapeutic Category Diagnostic Agent, Growth Hormone Function; Metabolic Alkalosis Agent; Urea Cycle Disorder (UCD) Treatment Agent

Generic Available No

Use Pituitary function test (stimulant for the release of growth hormone); management of severe, uncompensated, metabolic alkalosis (pH ≥7.55) **after** optimizing therapy with sodium or potassium chloride supplements; treatment agent for urea cycle disorders

Pregnancy Risk Factor B

Lactation Enters breast milk/use caution

Contraindications Hypersensitivity to arginine or any component; renal or hepatic failure

Warnings Use extreme caution when administering to neonates and children as overdosage has resulted in hyperchloremic metabolic acidosis, cerebral edema, or possibly death.

Precautions Arginine hydrochloride is metabolized to nitrogen-containing products for excretion; the temporary effect of a high nitrogen load on the kidneys should be evaluated; accumulation of excess arginine may result in an overproduction of nitric oxide, leading to vasodilation and hypotension; each 1 mEq chloride delivers 1 mEq hydrogen; monitor acid base balance closely, particularly in neonates

Adverse Reactions

Cardiovascular: Flushing (after rapid I.V. administration), hypotension
Central nervous system: Headache (after rapid I.V. administration)
Dermatologic: Rash
Endocrine & metabolic: Hyperglycemia, hyperkalemia, metabolic acidosis
Gastrointestinal: Nausea, vomiting, abdominal pain, bloating
Hematologic: Thrombocytopenia (rare)
Local: Venous irritation, severe tissue necrosis with extravasation
Miscellaneous: Elevated serum gastrin concentration

Drug Interactions Estrogen-progesterone combinations, spironolactone (potentially fatal hyperkalemia has been reported in patients with hepatic disease)

Mechanism of Action Stimulates pituitary release of growth hormone and prolactin and pancreatic release of glucagon and insulin; patients with impaired pituitary function have lower or no increase in plasma concentrations of growth hormone after administration of arginine. Arginine hydrochloride has been used for treatment of

(Continued)

Arginine *(Continued)*

hypochloremic metabolic alkalosis due to its high chloride content. Arginine becomes an essential amino acid in ASL deficiency due to a decrease in the conversion of argininosuccinate to arginine; in other urea cycle disorders, arginine is used not only to increase its serum concentration but also to prevent the breakdown of endogenous protein.

Pharmacokinetics

Absorption: Oral: Well absorbed

Time to peak serum concentration: Within 2 hours

Usual Dosage I.V.:

Growth hormone reserve test:

Children: 500 mg/kg over 30 minutes

Adults: 300 mL over 30 minutes

Treatment of urea cycle disorders: Neonates, Infants, Children, and Adults:

Argininosuccinic acid lyase (ASL) or argininosuccinic acid synthetase (ASS) disorders or pending definitive diagnosis: 600 mg/kg as a loading dose followed by 600 mg/kg/day as a continuous infusion

Carbamyl phosphate synthetase (CPS) or ornithine transcarbamylase (OTC) disorder: 200 mg/kg as a loading dose followed by 200 mg/kg/day as a continuous infusion

Intermittent hyperammonemic crisis in patients with urea cycle disorders: Neonates, Infants, Children, and Adults:

ASL or ASS: 0.6 g/kg or 12 g/m^2 loading dose followed by 0.6 g/kg/day or 12 g/m^2/day continuous infusion

CPS or OTC: 0.2 g/kg or 4 g/m^2 loading dose followed by 0.2 g/kg/day or 4 g/m^2/day continuous infusion

Metabolic alkalosis: Infants, Children, and Adults: Arginine hydrochloride dose (g) = weight (kg) x 0.1 x [HCO_3^- - 24] where HCO_3^- = the patient's serum bicarbonate concentration in mEq/L; give $\frac{1}{2}$ to $\frac{2}{3}$ of calculated dose and re-evaluate

Note: Arginine hydrochloride is an alternative treatment for uncompensated metabolic alkalosis after sodium chloride and potassium chloride supplementation have been optimized

To correct hypochloremia: Infants, Children, and Adults: Arginine hydrochloride dose (mEq) = 0.2 x weight (kg) x [103 - Cl^-] where Cl^- = the patient's serum chloride concentration in mEq/L; give $\frac{1}{2}$ to $\frac{2}{3}$ of calculated dose and re-evaluate

Note: Arginine hydrochloride should never be used as initial therapy for chloride supplementation but as an alternative in the patient who is unresponsive to sodium chloride or potassium chloride supplementation.

Administration Parenteral: May be infused without further dilution (however, very irritating to tissues, dilution is recommended); administration through a central line is recommended; maximum rate of I.V. infusion: 1 g/kg/hour (4.75 mEq/kg/hour) (maximum dose: 60 g/hour = 285 mEq over 1 hour); infuse loading doses for urea cycle disorders over 90 minutes

Monitoring Parameters Acid-base status (arterial or capillary blood gases), serum electrolytes, BUN, glucose, plasma growth hormone concentrations (when evaluating growth hormone reserve), plasma ammonia and amino acids (when treating urea cycle disorders)

Reference Range If intact pituitary function, human growth hormone levels should rise after arginine administration to 10-30 ng/mL (control range: 0-6 ng/mL)

Nursing Implications I.V. infiltration of arginine hydrochloride may cause necrosis and phlebitis; prolongation of the infusion may diminish the stimulus to the pituitary gland and nullify the test

Additional Information When treating urea cycle disorders, sodium bicarbonate use may be necessary to neutralize the acidifying effects of arginine HCl.

Dosage Forms Excipient information presented when available (limited, particularly for generics); consult specific product labeling.

Injection, solution, as hydrochloride: 10% [100 mg/mL = 950 mOsm/L] (300 mL) [contains chloride 0.475 mEq/mL]

References

Batshaw ML, MacArthur RB, and Tuchman M, "Alternative Pathway Therapy for Urea Cycle Disorders: Twenty Years Later," *J Pediatr*, 2001, 138(1 Suppl):S46-54.

Bushinsky DA and Gennari FJ, "Life-Threatening Hyperkalemia Induced by Arginine," *Ann Intern Med*, 1978, 89(5 Pt 1):632-4.

Summar M, "Current Strategies for the Management of Neonatal Urea Cycle Disorders," *J Pediatr*, 2001, 138(1 Suppl):S30-9.

♦ **Arginine Hydrochloride** *see* Arginine *on page 157*

♦ **8-Arginine Vasopressin** *see* Vasopressin *on page 1602*

♦ **Aristocort® [DSC]** *see* Triamcinolone *on page 1568*

♦ **Aristocort® A [DSC]** *see* Triamcinolone *on page 1568*

♦ **Aristospan®** *see* Triamcinolone *on page 1568*

Ascorbic Acid (a SKOR bik AS id)

Medication Safety Issues

International issues:

Rubex® [Ireland] may be confused with Revex® which is a brand name for nalmefene in the U.S.

Rubex® [Ireland]: Brand name for doxurbicin in the U.S.

U.S. Brand Names Acerola [OTC]; Asco-Caps [OTC]; Ascocid® [OTC]; Asco-Tabs [OTC]; Cecon® [OTC]; Cemill [OTC]; Cenolate®; C-Gel [OTC]; C-Gram [OTC]; Chew-C [OTC]; C-Time [OTC]; Dull-C® [OTC]; Mild-C® [OTC]; One Gram C [OTC]; Time-C [OTC]; Time-C-Bio [OTC]; Vicks® Vitamin C [OTC]; Vita-C® [OTC]

Canadian Brand Names Proflavanol C™; Revitalose C-1000®

Index Terms Vitamin C

Therapeutic Category Nutritional Supplement; Urinary Acidifying Agent; Vitamin, Water Soluble

Generic Available Yes

Use Prevention and treatment of scurvy; urinary acidification; dietary supplementation; prevention and reduction in the severity of colds

Pregnancy Risk Factor A (C if used in doses above RDA recommendation)

Lactation Enters breast milk/compatible

Contraindications Hypersensitivity to ascorbic acid or any component (see Warnings); large doses during pregnancy

Warnings Cenolate® injection contains sulfites which may cause allergic reactions in susceptible individuals

Precautions Some products contain aspartame which is metabolized to phenylalanine and must be avoided (or used with caution) in patients with phenylketonuria.

Adverse Reactions

Cardiovascular: Flushing

Central nervous system: Faintness, dizziness, headache, fatigue

Gastrointestinal: Nausea, vomiting, heartburn, diarrhea

Renal: Hyperoxaluria

Drug Interactions Aspirin, iron, oral contraceptives (increases estrogen levels), decreased warfarin effect

Stability Injectable form should be stored under refrigeration (2°C to 8°C); protect oral dosage forms from light; ascorbic acid solution is rapidly oxidized

Mechanism of Action Necessary for collagen formation and tissue repair in the body; involved in some oxidation-reduction reactions as well as many other metabolic reactions

Pharmacodynamics Reversal of scurvy symptoms: 2 days to 3 weeks

Pharmacokinetics

Absorption: Oral: Readily absorbed; absorption is an active process and is thought to be dose-dependent

Distribution: Widely distributed

Protein binding: 25%

Metabolism: In the liver by oxidation and sulfation

Elimination: In urine; there is an individual specific renal threshold for ascorbic acid; when blood levels are high, ascorbic acid is excreted in urine, whereas when the levels are subthreshold very little if any ascorbic acid is excreted into urine

Usual Dosage Oral, I.M., I.V., SubQ:

Recommended adequate intake (AI):

0-6 months: 40 mg

6-12 months: 50 mg

(Continued)

Ascorbic Acid *(Continued)*

Recommended daily allowance (RDA):
- 1-3 years: 15 mg
- 4-8 years: 25 mg
- 9-13 years: 45 mg
- 14-18 years: Males: 75 mg, females: 65 mg
- 19 years to Adults: Males: 90 mg, females: 75 mg

Children:
- Scurvy: 100-300 mg/day in divided doses
- Urinary acidification: 500 mg every 6-8 hours
- Dietary supplement (variable): 35-100 mg/day

Adults:
- Scurvy: 100-250 mg 1-2 times/day
- Urinary acidification: 4-12 g/day in 3-4 divided doses
- Dietary supplement (variable): 50-200 mg/day
- Prevention and treatment of cold: 1-3 g/day

Children and Adults: To increase iron excretion during deferoxamine administration: 100-200 mg/day during deferoxamine therapy

Administration

Oral: May be administered without regard to meals

Parenteral: Use only in circumstances when the oral route is not possible; I.M. preferred parenteral route due to improved utilization; for I.V. use dilute in equal volume D_5W or NS, and infuse over at least 10 minutes

Reference Range

Normal levels: 10-20 mcg/mL

Scurvy: <1-1.5 mcg/mL

Test Interactions False-positive urinary glucose with cupric sulfate reagent, false-negative urinary glucose with glucose oxidase method, false-negative amine-dependent stool occult blood test

Additional Information Sodium content of 1 g: ~5 mEq

Dosage Forms Excipient information presented when available (limited, particularly for generics); consult specific product labeling.

Caplet: 1000 mg

Caplet, timed release: 500 mg, 1000 mg

Capsule:
- Mild-C®: 500 mg

Capsule, softgel:
- C-Gel: 1000 mg

Capsule, sustained release:
- C-Time: 500 mg

Capsule, timed release: 500 mg
- Asco-Caps: 500 mg, 1000 mg [sugar free]
- Time-C®: 500 mg

Crystals for solution, oral: 4 g/teaspoonful (170 g, 1000 g)
- Mild-C®: 3600 mg/teaspoonful [contains calcium 400 mg/teaspoonful]
- Vita-C®: 4 g/teaspoonful (100 g, 454 g)

Injection, solution: 500 mg/mL (50 mL)
- Cenolate®: 500 mg/mL (1 mL, 2 mL) [contains sodium hydrosulfite]

Liquid, oral: 500 mg/5 mL

Lozenge:
- Vicks® Vitamin C: 25 mg [contains sodium 5 mg; orange flavor]

Powder, for solution, oral:
- Ascocid®: 4000 mg/5 mL (227 g); 4300 mg/5 mL (227 g, 454 g); 5000 mg/5 mL (227 g, 454 g)
- Dull-C®: 4 g/teaspoonful

Solution, oral:
- Cecon®: 90 mg/mL

Tablet: 100 mg, 250 mg, 500 mg, 1000 mg
- Asco-Tabs: 1000 mg [sugar free]
- Ascocid®: 500 mg [sugar free]
- C-Gram, One Gram C: 1000 mg

Tablet, chewable: 250 mg, 500 mg
- Acerola: 500 mg [cherry flavor]
- Chew-C: 500 mg [orange flavor]
- Mild-C®: 250 mg

Tablet, timed release: 500 mg, 1000 mg
- Cemill: 500 mg, 1000 mg
- Mild-C®: 1000 mg
- Time-C-Bio: 500 mg

References

"Dietary Reference Intakes for Vitamin C, Vitamin E, Selenium, and Carotenoids. A Report of the Panel on Dietary Antioxidants and Related Compounds Food and Nutrition Board, Institute of Medicine," National Academy of Sciences, Washington, DC: National Academy Press, 2000.

- **Asco-Tabs [OTC]** *see* Ascorbic Acid *on page 159*
- **Ascriptin® [OTC]** *see* Aspirin *on page 163*
- **Ascriptin® Maximum Strength [OTC]** *see* Aspirin *on page 163*
- **Asmanex® Twisthaler®** *see* Mometasone Furoate *on page 1076*
- **ASN-ase** *see* Asparaginase *on page 161*

Asparaginase (a SPIR a ji nase)

Medication Safety Issues

Sound-alike/look-alike issues:

Asparaginase may be confused with pegaspargase

Elspar® may be confused with Elaprase™

High alert medication: The Institute for Safe Medication Practices (ISMP) includes this medication among its list of drugs which have a heightened risk of causing significant patient harm when used in error.

Related Information

Compatibility of Chemotherapy and Related Supportive Care Medications *on page 1777*

Emetogenic Potential of Single Chemotherapeutic Agents *on page 1776*

U.S. Brand Names Elspar®

Canadian Brand Names Elspar®; Kidrolase®

Index Terms A-ase; ASN-ase; *E. coli* Asparaginase; LASP; L-asparaginase; NSC-109229 (*E. coli*)

Therapeutic Category Antineoplastic Agent, Miscellaneous

Generic Available No

Use In combination therapy for the treatment of acute lymphocytic leukemia; treatment of lymphoma

Pregnancy Risk Factor C

Lactation Excretion in breast milk unknown/not recommended

Contraindications Hypersensitivity to *E. coli*, asparaginase, or any component (if a reaction to Elspar® occurs, obtain investigational *Erwinia* preparation from Opi SA, Pharmaceuticals for Rare Diseases, Les Jardins d'Eole, France or pegaspargase is another alternative - use with caution); pancreatitis

Warnings The FDA currently recommends that procedures for proper handling and disposal of antineoplastic agents be considered; asparaginase should be administered under the supervision of a physician experienced in the use of cancer chemotherapy agents; allergic reactions to asparaginase are frequent; be prepared to treat anaphylaxis at each administration

Precautions Use with caution in patients with an underlying coagulopathy, impaired renal function, or in patients with pre-existing liver impairment; discontinue asparaginase at the first sign of renal failure or pancreatitis. Appropriate measures should be taken to prevent hyperuricemia and uric acid nephropathy (consider allopurinol, hydration, and urinary alkalinization).

Adverse Reactions

Cardiovascular: Hypotension, edema

Central nervous system: Fever, drowsiness, seizures, chills, malaise, lethargy, coma, agitation, headache, stroke, confusion, dizziness, hallucinations, depression

Dermatologic: Rash, pruritus, urticaria, angioedema

Endocrine & metabolic: Hyperglycemia, transient diabetes mellitus, hyperammonemia, hyperuricemia, hypoalbuminemia; decreased thyroxine and thyroxine-binding globulin concentration

Gastrointestinal: Vomiting, pancreatitis, nausea, anorexia, abdominal cramps

Hematologic: Leukopenia, coagulation abnormalities (prolonged thrombin, PT, and partial prothrombin times), reduced fibrinogen

Hepatic: Hepatotoxicity (elevated liver enzymes and alkaline phosphatase, hypoalbuminemia, hyperbilirubinemia), hepatic failure

Neuromuscular & skeletal: Arthralgia

Renal: Azotemia, acute renal failure

Respiratory: Coughing, laryngeal edema, bronchospasm

Miscellaneous: Hypersensitivity reactions (incidence in children is 20% with *E. coli* asparaginase and <5% with *Erwinia* asparaginase); anaphylaxis

Drug Interactions Methotrexate (decreased antineoplastic effect if given prior to methotrexate); vincristine (increases toxicity if given concomitantly); prednisone (increases hyperglycemic effect)

(Continued)

Asparaginase *(Continued)*

Stability Refrigerate; no loss in potency was noted after storage for 1 week at room temperature, however, the manufacturer recommends that reconstituted solutions should be discarded after 8 hours since there is no preservative; discard immediately if solution becomes cloudy; use of a 0.2 micron filter may result in some loss of potency

Mechanism of Action Inhibits protein synthesis by deaminating asparagine and depriving tumor cells of this essential amino acid

Pharmacokinetics

Absorption: Not absorbed from GI tract, therefore requires parenteral administration

Distribution: Asparaginase not detected in CSF but CSF asparagine is depleted; asparaginase is detected in lymph

V_d: 4-5 L/kg (~70% to 80% of plasma volume)

Half-life:

E. coli L-asparaginase: 24-36 hours

Patients who have had a hypersensitivity reaction to asparaginase have a decreased half-life

Note: *Erwinia* L-asparaginase: Significantly shorter than for the *E. coli*-derived product; mean half-life *Erwinia* L-asparaginase: 10-15 hours

Time to peak plasma levels: I.M.: 14-24 hours

Elimination: Clearance is unaffected by age, renal function, or hepatic function; only trace amounts appear in the urine

Usual Dosage Children and Adults: Refer to individual protocols

Perform intradermal sensitivity testing with 2 units of asparaginase before the initial dose and when a week or more has elapsed between doses (**Note:** False-negative rates of up to 80% to test doses of 2-5 units have been reported):

I.M. (preferred): 6000-10,000 units/m^2/dose 3 times/week for 3 weeks for combination therapy; high-dose I.M. regimen of 25,000 units/m^2/dose once weekly for 9 doses has also been used

I.V.: 1000 units/kg/day for 10 days for combination therapy or 200 units/kg/day for 28 days if combination therapy is inappropriate

Administration

I.M.: Reconstitute vial with NS. Maximum 2 mL volume is recommended for I.M. injections; if the volume to be administered is >2 mL, use multiple injection sites

I.V.: Must be infused over a minimum of 30 minutes; dilute dose in 50-250 mL of D_5W or NS

Monitoring Parameters Vital signs during administration, CBC, urinalysis, amylase, liver enzymes, bilirubin, prothrombin time, renal function tests, urine glucose, blood glucose, uric acid

Patient Information Notify physician if fever, sore throat, painful/burning urination, bruising, bleeding, or shortness of breath occurs

Nursing Implications I.M. route is associated with a more delayed, less severe anaphylactoid reaction compared to the I.V. route; patients should be observed for one hour following an I.M. injection for signs of severe hypersensitivity; appropriate agents for maintenance of an adequate airway and treatment of a hypersensitivity reaction (antihistamine, epinephrine, oxygen, I.V. corticosteroids) should be readily available. Asparaginase is irritating to eyes, skin, and the upper respiratory tract; avoid inhalation of aerosols or contact with skin, eyes, or mucous membranes.

Dosage Forms Excipient information presented when available (limited, particularly for generics); consult specific product labeling.

Injection, powder for reconstitution:

Elspar®: 10,000 units

References

Asselin BL, Whitin JC, Coppola DJ, et al, "Comparative Pharmacokinetic Studies of Three Asparaginase Preparations," *J Clin Oncol*, 1993, 11(9):1780-6.

Avramis VI, Sencer S, Periclou AP, et al, "A Randomized Comparison of Native *Escherichia coli* Asparaginase and Polyethylene Glycol Conjugated Asparaginase for Treatment of Children With Newly Diagnosed Standard-Risk Acute Lymphoblastic Leukemia: A Children's Cancer Group Study," *Blood*, 2002, 99(6):1986-94.

Clavell LA, Gelber RD, Cohen HJ, et al, "Four-Agent Induction and Intensive Asparaginase Therapy for Treatment of Childhood Acute Lymphoblastic Leukemia," *N Engl J Med*, 1986, 315(11):657-63.

Nesbit M, Chard R, Evans A, et al, "Evaluation of Intramuscular Versus Intravenous Administration of L-Asparaginase in Childhood Leukemia," *Am J Pediatr Hematol Oncol*, 1979, 1(1):9-13.

Ortega JA, Nesbit ME Jr, and Donaldson MH, "L-Asparaginase, Vincristine, and Prednisone for Induction of First Remission in Acute Lymphocytic Leukemia," *Cancer Res*, 1977, 37(2):535-40.

♦ **Aspart Insulin** *see* Insulin Aspart *on page 836*

♦ **Aspercin [OTC]** *see* Aspirin *on page 163*

♦ **Aspergum® [OTC]** *see* Aspirin *on page 163*

Aspirin (AS pir in)

Medication Safety Issues

Sound-alike/look-alike issues:

Aspirin may be confused with Afrin®, Asendin®

Ascriptin® may be confused with Aricept®

Ecotrin® may be confused with Akineton®, Edecrin®, Epogen®

Halfprin® may be confused with Halfan®, Haltran®

ZORprin® may be confused with Zyloprim®

International issues:

Cartia® [multiple international markets] may be confused with Cartia XT™ which is a brand name for diltiazem in the U.S.

Related Information

Antithrombotic Therapy in Children *on page 1804*

Overdose and Toxicology *on page 1916*

U.S. Brand Names Ascriptin® [OTC]; Ascriptin® Maximum Strength [OTC]; Aspercin [OTC]; Aspergum® [OTC]; Aspirtab [OTC]; Bayer® Aspirin Extra Strength [OTC]; Bayer® Aspirin Regimen Adult Low Dose [OTC]; Bayer® Aspirin Regimen Children's [OTC]; Bayer® Aspirin Regimen Regular Strength [OTC]; Bayer® Genuine Aspirin [OTC]; Bayer® Plus Extra Strength [OTC]; Bayer® Women's Aspirin Plus Calcium [OTC]; Buffasal [OTC]; Bufferin® [OTC]; Bufferin® Extra Strength [OTC]; Buffinol [OTC]; Easprin®; Ecotrin® [OTC]; Ecotrin® Low Strength [OTC]; Ecotrin® Maximum Strength [OTC]; Genacote™ [OTC]; Halfprin® [OTC]; St. Joseph® Adult Aspirin [OTC]; ZORprin®

Canadian Brand Names Asaphen; Asaphen E.C.; Entrophen®; Novasen

Index Terms Acetylsalicylic Acid; ASA

Therapeutic Category Analgesic, Non-narcotic; Anti-inflammatory Agent; Antiplatelet Agent; Antipyretic; Nonsteroidal Anti-inflammatory Drug (NSAID), Oral; Salicylate

Generic Available Yes: Excludes gum

Use Treatment of mild to moderate pain, inflammation and fever; adjunctive treatment of Kawasaki disease; prevention of vascular mortality during suspected acute MI; prevention of recurrent MI; prevention of MI in patients with angina; prevention of recurrent stroke and mortality following TIA or stroke; management of rheumatoid arthritis, rheumatic fever, osteoarthritis, and gout (high dose); adjunctive therapy in revascularization procedures (coronary artery bypass graft, percutaneous transluminal coronary angioplasty, carotid endarterectomy)

Pregnancy Risk Factor C (D if full-dose aspirin in 3rd trimester)

Lactation Enters breast milk/use caution

Contraindications Hypersensitivity to salicylates, any component, or other NSAIDs; bleeding disorders; hepatic failure

Warnings Do not use aspirin in children and teenagers who have or who are recovering from chickenpox or flu symptoms (due to the association with Reye's syndrome); when using aspirin, changes in behavior (along with nausea and vomiting) may be an early sign of Reye's syndrome; instruct patients and caregivers to contact their healthcare provider if these symptoms occur.

Precautions Use with caution in patients with impaired renal function, erosive gastritis, peptic ulcer, gout, platelet and bleeding disorders

Adverse Reactions

Dermatologic: Rash, urticaria

Gastrointestinal: Nausea, vomiting, GI distress, GI bleeding, ulcers

Hematologic: Inhibition of platelet aggregation

Hepatic: Hepatotoxicity

Otic: Tinnitus

Renal: Interstitial nephritis, renal papillary necrosis

Respiratory: Bronchospasm

Drug Interactions Aspirin may increase methotrexate serum levels and may displace valproic acid from binding sites which can result in toxicity. Aspirin may increase free (unbound) buspirone concentrations. Use of warfarin, heparin, low molecular weight heparins, urokinase, streptokinase, alteplase, and platelet inhibitors (eg, dipyridamole) with aspirin may cause an increase in bleeding.

Use of NSAIDs with aspirin may cause an increase in GI adverse effects and a possible decrease in serum concentration of NSAIDs. Ibuprofen and other COX-1 inhibitors may reduce the cardioprotective (antiplatelet effect) of aspirin depending upon when it is administered. Avoid giving these agents on a regular basis in patients requiring the antiplatelet effect of aspirin. If used occasionally, a single dose of ibuprofen should be taken 30-120 minutes after aspirin (immediate release; not enteric coated) ingestion or at least 8 hours should elapse after ibuprofen dosing before giving aspirin (see Catella-Lawson, 2001).

(Continued)

Aspirin *(Continued)*

Aspirin may antagonize effects of probenecid. Aspirin, especially high doses, may decrease the antihypertensive effects of ACE inhibitors. Buffered preparations may decrease the oral absorption of tetracycline or ketoconazole, therefore, administer 3-4 hours apart. Use with alcohol may increase damage to gastric mucosa.

Food Interactions Aspirin may increase the renal excretion of vitamin C and may decrease serum folate levels; some suggest increasing the dietary intake of foods that are high in vitamin C and folic acid

Stability Keep suppositories in refrigerator, do not freeze; hydrolysis of aspirin occurs upon exposure to water or moist air, resulting in salicylate and acetate; acetate possesses a vinegar-like odor; do not use if a strong odor is present

Mechanism of Action Inhibits prostaglandin synthesis, acts on the hypothalamus heat-regulating center to reduce fever, blocks prostaglandin synthetase action which prevents formation of the platelet-aggregating substance thromboxane A_2

Pharmacokinetics

Absorption: From the stomach and small intestine

Distribution: Readily distributes into most body fluids and tissues; hydrolyzed to salicylate (active) by esterases in the GI mucosa, red blood cells, synovial fluid and blood

Metabolism: Primarily by hepatic microsomal enzymes

Half-life: 15-20 minutes; metabolic pathways are saturable such that salicylate half-life is dose-dependent ranging from 3 hours at lower doses (300-600 mg), 5-6 hours (after 1 g) and 10 hours with higher doses

Time to peak serum concentration: Salicylate: ~1-2 hours; may be delayed with controlled or timed-release preparations

Elimination: Renal as salicylate and conjugated metabolites

Dialysis: Dialyzable: 50% to 100%

Usual Dosage

Children:

Analgesic and antipyretic: Oral, rectal: 10-15 mg/kg/dose every 4-6 hours; maximum dose: 4 g/day

Anti-inflammatory: Oral: Initial: 60-90 mg/kg/day in divided doses; usual maintenance: 80-100 mg/kg/day divided every 6-8 hours; monitor serum concentrations

Antiplatelet effects: Adequate pediatric studies have not been performed; pediatric dosage is derived from adult studies and clinical experience and is not well established; suggested doses have ranged from 3-5 mg/kg/day to 5-10 mg/kg/day given as a single daily dose. Doses are rounded to a convenient amount (eg, ½ of 81 mg tablet).

Mechanical prosthetic heart valves: 6-20 mg/kg/day given as a single daily dose (used in combination with an oral anticoagulant in children who have systemic embolism despite adequate oral anticoagulation therapy and used in combination with low-dose anticoagulation when full-dose oral anticoagulation is contraindicated; see Monagle, 2004)

Blalock-Taussig shunts, primary prophylaxis: 5 mg/kg/day given as a single daily dose

Patients following Fontan surgery, primary prophylaxis: 5 mg/kg/day given as a single daily dose

Arterial ischemic stroke: 2-5 mg/kg/day given as single daily dose after anticoagulation therapy has been discontinued

Kawasaki disease: Oral: 80-100 mg/kg/day divided every 6 hours for up to 14 days; monitor serum concentrations; after fever resolves: 3-5 mg/kg/day once daily. In patients without coronary artery abnormalities, give lower dose for >7 weeks or until ESR and platelet count are normal. In patients with coronary artery abnormalities, low-dose aspirin should be continued indefinitely (in addition to therapy with warfarin; see Monagle, 2004)

Adults:

Analgesic and antipyretic: Oral, rectal: 325-1000 mg every 4-6 hours up to 4 g/day

Anti-inflammatory: Oral: Initial: 2.4-3.6 g/day in divided doses; usual maintenance: 3.6-5.4 g/day; monitor serum concentrations

Suspected acute MI: Oral: Initial: 160-162.5 mg as soon as MI is suspected; then 160-162.5 mg once daily for 30 days post MI; then consider further aspirin treatment

MI prophylaxis: Oral: 75-325 mg once daily (continue indefinitely)

Prevention of stroke following ischemic stroke or TIA: Oral: 50-325 mg once daily (continue indefinitely)

Administration Oral: Administer with water, food, or milk to decrease GI upset. Do not crush or chew controlled release, timed release, or enteric coated tablets; these preparations should be swallowed whole

Monitoring Parameters Serum salicylate concentration with chronic use

Reference Range

Therapeutic levels:

Anti-inflammatory effect: 150-300 mcg/mL

Analgesic and antipyretic effect: 30-50 mcg/mL

Timing of serum samples: Peak levels usually occur 2 hours after normal doses but may occur 6-24 hours after acute toxic ingestion.

Salicylate serum concentrations correlate with the pharmacological actions and adverse effects observed. See table.

Serum Salicylate: Clinical Correlations

Serum Salicylate Concentration (micrograms/mL)	Desired Effects	Adverse Effects/Intoxication
~100	Antiplatelet Antipyresis Analgesia	GI intolerance and bleeding, hypersensitivity, hemostatic defects
150-300	Anti-inflammatory	Mild salicylism
250-400	Treatment of rheumatic fever	Nausea/vomiting, hyperventilation, salicylism, flushing, sweating, thirst, headache, diarrhea, and tachycardia
>400-500		Respiratory alkalosis, hemorrhage, excitement, confusion, asterixis, pulmonary edema, convulsions, tetany, metabolic acidosis, fever, coma, cardiovascular collapse, renal and respiratory failure

Test Interactions False-negative results for glucose oxidase urinary glucose tests (Clinistix®); false-positives using the cupric sulfate method (Clinitest®); interferes with Gerhardt test, VMA determination; 5-HIAA, xylose tolerance test and T_3 and T_4

Patient Information Avoid alcohol; watch for bleeding gums or signs of GI bleeding, (bright red blood in emesis or stool, coffee ground-like emesis, black tarry stools); notify physician if ringing in the ears, persistent GI pain, GI bleeding, or changes in behavior (along with nausea and vomiting) occur (see Warnings)

Dosage Forms Excipient information presented when available (limited, particularly for generics); consult specific product labeling. [DSC] = Discontinued product

Caplet:

Bayer® Aspirin Extra Strength: 500 mg

Bayer® Aspirin Regimen Regular Strength: 325 mg

Bayer® Genuine Aspirin: 325 mg

Bayer® Plus Extra Strength: 500 mg [contains calcium carbonate]

Bayer® Women's Aspirin Plus Calcium: 81 mg [contains elemental calcium 300 mg]

Caplet, buffered:

Ascriptin® Maximum Strength: 500 mg [contains aluminum hydroxide, calcium carbonate, and magnesium hydroxide]

Gelcap:

Bayer® Aspirin Extra Strength: 500 mg [DSC]

Gum:

Aspergum®: 227 mg [cherry or orange flavor]

Suppository, rectal: 300 mg, 600 mg

Tablet: 325 mg

Aspercin, Aspirtab: 325 mg

Bayer® Genuine Aspirin: 325 mg

Tablet, buffered: 325 mg

Ascriptin®: 325 mg [contains aluminum hydroxide, calcium carbonate, and magnesium hydroxide]

Buffasal: 325 mg [contains magnesium oxide]

Bufferin®: 325 mg [contains calcium carbonate, magnesium oxide, and magnesium carbonate; contains calcium 65 mg/tablet, magnesium 50 mg/tablet]

Bufferin® Extra Strength: 500 mg [contains calcium carbonate, magnesium oxide, and magnesium carbonate; contains calcium 90 mg/tablet, magnesium 70 mg/tablet]

Buffinol: 325 mg [contains magnesium oxide]

Tablet, chewable: 81 mg

Bayer® Aspirin Regimen Children's: 81 mg [cherry or orange flavor]

St. Joseph® Adult Aspirin: 81 mg [orange flavor]

Tablet, controlled release (ZORprin®): 800 mg

Tablet, enteric coated: 81 mg, 325 mg, 500 mg, 650 mg, 975 mg

Bayer® Aspirin Regimen Adult Low Dose, Ecotrin® Low Strength, St. Joseph Adult Aspirin: 81 mg

(Continued)

Aspirin *(Continued)*

Easprin®: 975 mg
Ecotrin®, Genacote™: 325 mg
Ecotrin® Maximum Strength: 500 mg
Halfprin®: 81 mg, 162 mg

References

Capone ML, Sciulli MG, Tacconelli S, et al, "Pharmacodynamic Interaction of Naproxen With Low-Dose Aspirin in Healthy Subjects," *J Am Coll Cardiol*, 2005, 45(8):1295-1301.

Catella-Lawson F, Reilly MP, Kapoor SC, et al, "Cyclooxygenase Inhibitors and the Antiplatelet Effects of Aspirin," *N Engl J Med*, 2001, 345(25):1809-17.

Cryer B, Verlin RG, Cooper SA, et al, "Double-Blind, Randomized, Parallel, Placebo-Controlled Study Of Ibuprofen Effects On Thromboxane B2 Concentrations In Aspirin-Treated Healthy Adult Volunteers," *Clin Ther*, 2005, 27 (2):185-191.

Hathaway WE, "Use of Antiplatelet Agents in Pediatric Hypercoagulable States," *Am J Dis Child*, 1984, 138(3):301-4.

Monagle P, Chan A, Massicotte P, et al, "Antithrombotic Therapy in Children: The Seventh ACCP Conference on Antithrombotic and Thrombolytic Therapy," *Chest*, 2004, 126(3 Suppl):645S-687S.

Monagle P, Michelson AD, Bovill E, et al, "Antithrombotic Therapy in Children," *Chest*, 2001, 119(1 Suppl):344S-370S.

Pickering LK, ed, *2000 Red Book, Report of the Committee on Infectious Diseases*, 25th ed, Elk Grove Village IL: American Academy of Pediatrics, 2000, 360-3.

♦ **Aspirin and Oxycodone** *see* Oxycodone and Aspirin *on page 1193*
♦ **Aspirin Free Anacin® Maximum Strength [OTC]** *see* Acetaminophen *on page 42*
♦ **Aspirtab [OTC]** *see* Aspirin *on page 163*
♦ **Astelin®** *see* Azelastine *on page 189*
♦ **Astramorph/PF™** *see* Morphine Sulfate *on page 1082*
♦ **Atarax® (Can)** *see* HydrOXYzine *on page 796*
♦ **Atasol® (Can)** *see* Acetaminophen *on page 42*

Atazanavir (at a za NA veer)

Related Information

Adult and Adolescent HIV *on page 1821*
Assessment of Liver Function *on page 1810*
Pediatric HIV *on page 1816*
Perinatal HIV *on page 1831*

U.S. Brand Names Reyataz®

Canadian Brand Names Reyataz®

Index Terms Atazanavir Sulfate; BMS-232632

Therapeutic Category Antiretroviral Agent; HIV Agents (Anti-HIV Agents); Protease Inhibitor

Generic Available No

Use Treatment of HIV infection in combination with other antiretroviral agents [**Note:** HIV regimens consisting of **three** antiretroviral agents are strongly recommended; low-dose ritonavir (booster dose) is recommended in combination with atazanavir in antiretroviral-experienced patients with prior virologic failure; see Usual Dosage]

Pregnancy Risk Factor B

Lactation Excretion in breast milk unknown/contraindicated

Contraindications Hypersensitivity to atazanavir or any component; concurrent therapy with medications that largely rely on cytochrome P450 isoenzyme CYP3A for clearance and that have an association between increased plasma concentrations and serious or life-threatening effects (eg, cisapride, dihydroergotamine, ergotamine, ergonovine, methylergonovine, midazolam, pimozide, triazolam)

Warnings Atazanavir is an inhibitor of cytochrome P450 isoenzyme CYP3A and uridine diphosphate glucuronosyl transferase (UGT1A1; a glucuronidation enzyme). Administration of atazanavir with drugs that are primarily metabolized by CYP3A or UGT1A1 may result in increased serum concentrations of the other drug and lead to an increase or prolongation of adverse effects. Due to potential serious and/or life-threatening drug interactions, some drugs are contraindicated or not recommended for concurrent use; other drug interactions require dosage or regimen adjustment or monitoring of serum concentrations of drugs coadministered with atazanavir (see Contraindications and Drug Interactions).

Asymptomatic elevations in unconjugated (indirect) bilirubin occur commonly during therapy with atazanavir; this reversible hyperbilirubinemia is related to inhibition of uridine diphosphate glucuronosyl transferase; consider alternative therapy if bilirubin is >5 times upper limits of normal (long-term safety data is not available for such patients) or if jaundice or scleral icterus become a cosmetic concern for the patient; evaluate alternative etiologies if elevated transaminase also occur. Optimal dosing of atazanavir in pediatric patients has not been established; do not use in infants <3 months of age due to potential risk of kernicterus.

Skin rash may occur with atazanavir use (median onset 8 weeks); treatment may be continued if rash is mild to moderate (rash may resolve; median duration 1.3 weeks); discontinue therapy in cases of severe rash.

Precautions Atazanavir may prolong the P-R interval; rare cases of second-degree AV block and other conduction abnormalities have also been reported; use with caution in patients with pre-existing conduction abnormalities or with medications which prolong A-V conduction (dosage adjustment is required with some agents; see Drug Interactions). Hyperglycemia, changes in glucose tolerance, exacerbation of diabetes, DKA, and new-onset diabetes mellitus have been reported in patients receiving protease inhibitors (use with caution in patients with diabetes mellitus).

Use with caution in patients with mild to moderate hepatic impairment; consider dosage adjustment in patients with moderate hepatic dysfunction; atazanavir is not recommended for use in patients with severe hepatic impairment. Atazanavir may exacerbate pre-existing hepatic dysfunction; use with caution in patients with hepatitis B or C or in patients with marked elevations in hepatic transaminases. Use with caution in patients with hemophilia; spontaneous bleeding episodes have been reported in patients with hemophilia type A and B receiving protease inhibitors. Fat redistribution and accumulation [ie, central obesity, peripheral wasting, facial wasting, breast enlargement, dorsocervical fat enlargement (buffalo hump), and cushingoid appearance] have been observed in patients receiving antiretroviral agents (causal relationship not established). Immune reconstitution syndrome (an acute inflammatory response to residual or indolent opportunistic infections) may occur in HIV patients during initial treatment with combination antiretroviral agents, including atazanavir; this syndrome may require further patient assessment and therapy.

Adverse Reactions

Cardiovascular: Prolongation of the P-R interval (concentration and dose dependent); rarely: second-degree AV block, other conduction abnormalities

Central nervous system: Headache, fever, depression, insomnia, dizziness, fatigue, pain

Dermatologic: Rash (incidence 21%; usually mild to moderate; maculopapular; see Warnings); erythema multiforme, Stevens-Johnson syndrome

Endocrine & metabolic: Hyperglycemia, new-onset diabetes, exacerbation of diabetes mellitus; hypertriglyceridemia, hypercholesterolemia (less common than with other protease inhibitors); fat redistribution and accumulation (see Precautions)

Gastrointestinal: Nausea, abdominal pain, vomiting, diarrhea

Hepatic: Unconjugated hyperbilirubinemia (incidence: 35% to 49%), jaundice (7% to 9%), elevated liver enzymes, elevated amylase

Neuromuscular & skeletal: Peripheral neuropathy, back pain, arthralgia

Ocular: Scleral icterus

Respiratory: Increased cough

Miscellaneous: Immune reconstitution syndrome (see Precautions)

Drug Interactions Cytochrome P450 isoenzyme CYP3A4 substrate; isoenzyme CYP1A2 (weak), CYP2C8 (strong), CYP2C9 (weak), and CYP3A4 (strong) inhibitor; uridine diphosphate glucuronosyl transferase (UGT1A1) inhibitor

Atazanavir may inhibit the metabolism of the following drugs and cause serious or life-threatening adverse effects: Cisapride, dihydroergotamine, ergotamine, ergonovine, methylergonovine, midazolam, pimozide, triazolam (concurrent therapy with these drugs and atazanavir is contraindicated). Atazanavir significantly increases the AUC of rifabutin by >200% (rifabutin dose should be decreased by up to 75% of the normal dose when used in combination with amprenavir). Atazanavir may increase serum concentrations or serious toxicities of irinotecan (concurrent use is **not** recommended); amiodarone, bepridil, lidocaine, quinidine, tricyclic antidepressants (use with caution; serum concentration monitoring of these drugs is necessary); warfarin (monitor INR); diltiazem (consider a 50% dosage reduction in diltiazem; monitor EKG); nifedipine, felodipine, nicardipine, verapamil (consider dosage titration of calcium channel blocker; monitor EKG); sildenafil or other phosphodiesterase-5 (PDE-5) enzyme inhibitors (use decreased dose of sildenafil or other PDE-5 enzyme inhibitor); cholesterol-lowering agents (concurrent use of lovastatin or simvastatin is **not** recommended; use atorvastatin with caution); cyclosporine, sirolimus, tacrolimus (monitor immunosuppressant serum concentrations); clarithromycin (consider a 50% dosage reduction in clarithromycin; consider alternative antibiotic for non-MAC infections); ethinyl estradiol and norethindrone oral contraceptive agents or contraceptive patch (alternative, nonhormonal methods of contraception are recommended); trazodone (use with caution and consider dosage reduction of trazodone). Atazanavir increases serum concentrations of saquinavir (appropriate concurrent doses have not been established). Ritonavir significantly increases fluticasone serum concentrations and may result in systemic corticosteroid effects (eg, Cushing's syndrome and adrenal suppression); atazanavir plus ritonavir use with fluticasone is expected to have the same effect; concurrent use of atazanavir plus ritonavir with fluticasone is

(Continued)

Atazanavir *(Continued)*

not recommended unless benefits outweigh risks; use of atazanavir without ritonavir may increase fluticasone serum concentrations (use with caution; consider alternative agent, especially with long-term use).

Ritonavir increases serum concentrations of atazanavir (dosage adjustment is required; see Usual Dosage). Voriconazole may increase atazanavir concentrations. Efavirenz significantly decreases atazanavir serum concentrations and may result in a loss or lack of virologic response and possible resistance to atazanavir (booster doses of ritonavir are required for patients receiving atazanavir and efavirenz; see Usual Dosage). Nevirapine may decrease atazanavir serum concentrations (due to lack of studies, concurrent use is **not** recommended). Tenofovir significantly decreases atazanavir serum concentrations and may result in a loss or lack of virologic response and possible resistance to atazanavir (booster doses of ritonavir are required for patients receiving atazanavir and tenofovir; see Usual Dosage). Atazanavir may increase tenofovir serum concentrations and adverse effects (monitor patients). Rifampin significantly reduces plasma concentrations of protease inhibitors (concurrent use of rifampin and atazanavir is **not** recommended). Other enzyme inducers (eg, carbamazepine, phenobarbital) may decrease atazanavir serum concentrations. The herbal medicine St John's wort (*Hypericum perforatum*) may significantly decrease concentrations of atazanavir and is **not** recommended for concurrent use.

Medications that increase gastrointestinal pH may decrease the solubility of atazanavir and significantly decrease atazanavir plasma concentrations; concurrent use of proton pump inhibitors and atazanavir (with or without ritonavir) is **not** recommended (**Note:** Omeprazole significantly decreased atazanavir plasma concentrations even though atazanavir was given with booster doses of ritonavir); atazanavir should be administered at least 2 hours before and at least 10 hours after H_2-receptor antagonists (see Usual Dosage); atazanavir should be administered 2 hours before or 1 hour after antacids or buffered medications, including didanosine buffered formulations. Concurrent administration of didanosine enteric-coated capsules and atazanavir with food resulted in a decrease in didanosine AUC; atazanavir should be administered 2 hours before or 1 hour after didanosine enteric-coated capsules. Use of atazanavir with indinavir may increase the risk of hyperbilirubinemia (concurrent use is **not** recommended).

Food Interactions Food increases oral bioavailability and decreases interpatient pharmacokinetic variability.

Stability Store at room temperature.

Mechanism of Action An azapeptide protease inhibitor which acts on an enzyme (protease) late in the HIV replication process after the virus has entered into the cell's nucleus. Atazanavir binds to the protease activity site and inhibits the activity of the enzyme, thus preventing cleavage of viral polyprotein precursors (gag-pol protein precursors) into individual functional proteins found in infectious HIV. This results in the formation of immature, noninfectious viral particles.

Pharmacokinetics

Distribution: CSF: Plasma concentration ratio (range): 0.0021-0.226

Protein binding: 86%; binds to both alpha$_1$-acid glycoprotein and albumin (similar affinity)

Metabolism: Extensively metabolized in the liver, primarily by cytochrome P450 isoenzyme CYP3A; also undergoes biliary elimination; major biotransformation pathways include mono-oxygenation and dioxygenation; minor pathways for parent drug or metabolites include glucuronidation, N-dealkylation, hydrolysis and oxygenation with dehydrogenation; 3 minor inactive metabolites have been identified

Half-life:

- Adults: 6.5 hours
- Adults with hepatic impairment: 12 hours

Time to peak serum concentration: 2 hours

Elimination: 13% of the dose is excreted in the urine (7% as unchanged drug); 79% of the dose is excreted in feces (20% as unchanged drug)

Dialysis: Not likely to remove significant amounts of atazanavir (due to high protein binding and extensive hepatic metabolism)

Usual Dosage Oral (use in combination with other antiretroviral agents):

Neonates and Infants <3 months: Not recommended due to risk of kernicterus

Infants ≥3 months and Children <16 years: Not approved for use (see Additional Information)

Adolescents ≥16 years and Adults:

- Antiretroviral-naive patients: 400 mg once daily (**Note:** No information exists regarding the coadministration of atazanavir plus ritonavir in antiretroviral-naive patients)

Antiretroviral-experienced patients: 300 mg once daily **plus** ritonavir 100 mg once daily (**Note:** Atazanavir **without** ritonavir is **not** recommended in antiretroviral-experienced patients with prior virologic failure)

Coadministration with efavirenz:

Antiretroviral-naive patients: Atazanavir 300 mg **plus** ritonavir 100 mg is recommended to be given with efavirenz 600 mg (all as a single daily dose); administer with food; do **not** use efavirenz and atazanavir without booster doses of ritonavir (see Drug Interactions)

Antiretroviral-experienced patients: Dosing recommendations not established

Coadministration with tenofovir: Atazanavir 300 mg **plus** ritonavir 100 mg is recommended to be given with tenofovir 300 mg (all as a single daily dose); administer with food; do **not** use tenofovir and atazanavir without booster doses of ritonavir (see Drug Interactions)

Coadministration with H_2-receptor antagonists:

Antiretroviral-naive patients: Atazanavir 400 mg once daily (with food) at least 2 hours before and at least 10 hours after the H_2-blocker **OR** atazanavir 300 mg **plus** ritonavir 100 mg once daily administered with food (and no need to separate from administration of H_2-blocker)

Antiretroviral-experienced patients: Atazanavir 300 mg **plus** ritonavir 100 mg once daily (with food) at least 2 hours before and at least 10 hours after the H_2-blocker

Dosage adjustment in renal impairment: No recommendations available

Dosage adjustment in hepatic impairment: Adolescents ≥16 years and Adults:

Moderate hepatic impairment (Child-Pugh Class B): Patients without prior virologic failure: Reduce dose to 300 mg once daily

Severe hepatic impairment (Child-Pugh Class C): Do not use

Note: The pharmacokinetics of atazanavir plus ritonavir have not been assessed in patients with hepatic impairment; concurrent use is not recommended

Administration Administer with food to enhance absorption; swallow capsules whole, do not open; administer atazanavir 2 hours before or 1 hour after didanosine buffered formulations, didanosine enteric-coated capsules, other buffered medications, or antacids; administer atazanavir at least 2 hours before and at least 10 hours after H_2-receptor antagonists (see Usual Dosage)

Monitoring Parameters CD4 cell count, viral load, serum glucose, bilirubin, triglycerides, cholesterol, liver enzyme tests (especially in patients with a history of hepatitis B or C)

Patient Information Atazanavir may cause changes in the EKG (notify physician if dizziness or lightheadedness occur); atazanavir may cause elevated bilirubin levels and yellowing of the skin or whites of the eye (other medication can be used if these side effects are of concern); atazanavir may cause a skin rash that will usually go away with continued use of the drug (notify healthcare provider if skin rash occurs). Some medicines should not be taken with atazanavir; report the use of other medications, nonprescription medications and herbal or natural products to your physician and pharmacist; avoid the herbal medicine St John's wort. Atazanavir is not a cure for HIV; take atazanavir everyday as prescribed; do not change dose or discontinue without physician's advice; if a dose is missed, take it as soon as possible, then return to normal dosing schedule; if it is within 6 hours of your next dose, do not take the missed dose; if a dose is skipped, do not double the next dose.

HIV medications may cause changes in body fat, including an increase in fat in the upper back and neck, breasts, and trunk; a loss of fat from the face, arms, and legs may also occur.

Additional Information Preliminary pediatric studies have shown that appropriate atazanavir serum concentrations are difficult to achieve in children even with higher doses; optimal dosing in children is being investigated; the addition of low-dose ritonavir (booster doses) to increase atazanavir serum concentrations may be required and is currently being evaluated. A powder formulation is also being studied in pediatric patients (Working Group, 2005).

Dosage Forms Excipient information presented when available (limited, particularly for generics); consult specific product labeling.

Capsule, as sulfate:

Reyataz®: 100 mg, 150 mg, 200 mg, 300 mg

References

Briars LA, Hilao JJ, and Kraus DM, "A Review of Pediatric Human Immunodeficiency Virus Infection," *Journal of Pharmacy Practice*, 2004, 17(6):407-31.

Goldsmith DR and Perry CM, "Atazanavir," *Drugs*, 2003, 63(16):1679-93.

Morris JL and Kraus DM, "New Antiretroviral Therapies for Pediatric HIV Infection," *J Pediatr Pharmacol Ther*, 2005, 10:215-47.

Musial BL, Chojnacki JK, and Coleman CI, "Atazanavir: A New Protease Inhibitor to Treat HIV Infection," *Am J Health Syst Pharm*, 2004, 61(13):1365-74.

Panel on Clinical Practices for Treatment of HIV Infection, "Guidelines for the Use of Antiretroviral Agents in HIV-Infected Adults and Adolescents," October 10, 2006, http://www.aidsinfo.nih.gov.

(Continued)

Atazanavir *(Continued)*

Working Group on Antiretroviral Therapy and Medical Management of HIV-Infected Children, "Guidelines for the Use of Antiretroviral Agents in Pediatric HIV Infection," October 26, 2006, http://www.aidsinfo.nih.gov.

♦ **Atazanavir Sulfate** *see* Atazanavir *on page 166*

Atenolol (a TEN oh lole)

Medication Safety Issues

Sound-alike/look-alike issues:

Atenolol may be confused with albuterol, Altenol®, timolol, Tylenol®

Tenormin® may be confused with Imuran®, Norpramin®, thiamine, Trovan®

International issues:

Betanol® [Bangladesh] may be confused with Patanol® which is a brand name for olopatadine in the U.S.

Related Information

Antihypertensive Agents by Class *on page 1678*

Overdose and Toxicology *on page 1916*

U.S. Brand Names Tenormin®

Canadian Brand Names Apo-Atenol®; Gen-Atenolol; Novo-Atenol; Nu-Atenol; PMS-Atenolol; RAN™-Atenolol; Rhoxal-atenolol; Riva-Atenolol; Sandoz-Atenolol; Tenolin; Tenormin®

Therapeutic Category Antianginal Agent; Antihypertensive Agent; Beta-Adrenergic Blocker

Generic Available Yes: Tablet

Use Treatment of hypertension, alone or in combination with other agents; management of angina pectoris; antiarrhythmic; post-MI patients; acute alcohol withdrawal

Pregnancy Risk Factor D

Lactation Enters breast milk/use caution

Contraindications Hypersensitivity to atenolol or any component; pulmonary edema, cardiogenic shock, bradycardia, heart block, or uncompensated CHF

Warnings Abrupt withdrawal of the drug should be avoided; drug should be discontinued over 1-2 weeks. Atenolol should not be administered to patients with untreated pheochromocytoma. Atenolol may mask clinical signs of hyperthyroidism (exacerbation of symptoms of hyperthyroidism, including thyroid storm, may occur following abrupt discontinuation).

Precautions Use with caution and modify dosage in patients with renal impairment; use with caution in patients with CHF, bronchospastic disease, diabetes mellitus, and hyperthyroidism. Use with caution in nursing women; clinically significant bradycardia may occur in breast-fed infants; infants with renal dysfunction and premature infants may be at higher risk for adverse effects; breast-fed infants and neonates born to mothers receiving atenolol may be at increased risk for hypoglycemia. Patients who have a history of anaphylactic hypersensitivity reactions to various substances may be more reactive while receiving beta-blockers; these patients may not be responsive to the normal doses of epinephrine used to treat hypersensitivity reactions.

Adverse Reactions

Cardiovascular: Bradycardia, hypotension, second or third degree A-V block, CHF, chest pain, edema, Raynaud's phenomenon

Central nervous system: Dizziness, fatigue, lethargy, headache, nightmares, insomnia, confusion, mental impairment

Gastrointestinal: Constipation, nausea, diarrhea

Respiratory: Wheezing and dyspnea have occurred with higher doses (eg, >100 mg/day in adults)

Drug Interactions Catecholamine-depleting drugs, such as reserpine, may have additive effects (hypotension, bradycardia); hypotensive agents, diuretics, cardiac glycosides, amiodarone, calcium channel blockers, agents that slow AV conduction, and myocardial depressant general anesthetics may have additive effects with beta-blockers; abrupt withdrawal of clonidine while receiving beta-blockers may result in an exaggerated hypertensive crisis; NSAIDs and indomethacin may decrease the antihypertensive effects of beta-blockers; atenolol (especially at higher doses) may reverse the therapeutic effects of theophylline

Mechanism of Action Competitively blocks response to beta-adrenergic stimulation; selectively blocks $beta_1$-receptors with little or no effect on $beta_2$-receptors except at high doses; does not possess membrane stabilizing or intrinsic sympathomimetic (partial agonist) activities

Pharmacodynamics

Beta-blocking effect:

Onset of action: Oral: ≤1 hour

Maximum effect:
Oral: 2-4 hours
I.V.: ≤5 minutes
Duration:
Oral: ≥24 hours
I.V.: 12 hours
Antihypertensive effect:
Duration: Oral: 24 hours

Pharmacokinetics

Absorption: Incomplete from the GI tract; ~50% absorbed

Distribution: Does not cross the blood-brain barrier; low lipophilicity; distributes into breast milk at a concentration 1.5-6.8 times the maternal plasma concentration (see Precautions)

Protein binding: Low (6% to 16%)

Half-life, beta:
Neonates: Mean: 16 hours, up to 35 hours
Children 5-16 years of age: Mean: 4.6 hours; range: 3.5-7 hours; children >10 years of age may have longer half-life (>5 hours) compared to children 5-10 years of age (<5 hours)
Adults: 6-7 hours
Prolonged half-life with renal dysfunction

Time to peak serum concentration: Oral: Within 2-4 hours

Elimination: 40% as unchanged drug in urine, 50% in feces

Dialysis: Moderately dialyzable (20% to 50%)

Usual Dosage

Oral:
Children: Initial: 0.8-1 mg/kg/dose given daily; range: 0.8-1.5 mg/kg/day; maximum dose: 2 mg/kg/day; do not exceed adult maximum dose of 100 mg/day
Adults:
Initial: 25-50 mg/dose given daily; usual dose: 50-100 mg/dose given daily; usual dosage range for hypertension (JNC 7): 25-100 mg once daily
Maximum dose: Hypertension: 100 mg given daily; angina: 200 mg given daily
Dosing interval in renal impairment: See table

Creatinine Clearance	Maximum Oral Dose	Frequency of Administration
15-35 mL/min	50 mg or 1 mg/kg/dose	Daily
<15 mL/min	50 mg or 1 mg/kg/dose	Every other day

I.V.: Adults: For early treatment of MI: 5 mg slow I.V. over 5 minutes; may repeat in 10 minutes; if both doses are tolerated, may start oral atenolol 50 mg every 12 hours for 6-9 days post MI

Administration

Oral: May be administered without regard to food

Parenteral: Administer by slow I.V. injection at a rate not to exceed 1 mg/minute; the injection can be administered undiluted or diluted with a compatible I.V. solution

Monitoring Parameters Blood pressure, heart rate, EKG, fluid intake and output, daily weight, respiratory rate

Patient Information Abrupt withdrawal of the drug should be avoided

Additional Information In diabetic patients, atenolol may potentiate hypoglycemia and mask signs and symptoms of hypoglycemia; limited data suggests that atenolol may have a shorter half-life and faster clearance in patients with Marfan syndrome. Higher doses (2 mg/kg/day divided every 12 hours) have been used in patients with Marfan syndrome (6-22 years of age) to decrease aortic root growth rate and prevent aortic dissection or rupture; further studies are needed.

Dosage Forms Excipient information presented when available (limited, particularly for generics); consult specific product labeling.

Injection, solution: 0.5 mg/mL (10 mL)

Tablet: 25 mg, 50 mg, 100 mg

Extemporaneous Preparations

A 2 mg/mL atenolol oral liquid compounded from tablets and a commercially available oral diluent was found to be stable for up to 40 days when stored at 5°C or 25°C (Garner, 1994)

Stability of a 2 mg/mL atenolol oral liquid compounded from tablets and several different vehicles was studied at room temperature in amber prescription bottles. The 2 mg/mL atenolol oral liquid in Ora-Sweet® SF was stable for 90 days; in a vehicle of simple syrup, the preparation was stable for approximately 3 weeks; when formulated in Ora-Sweet® however, the preparation was stable for <1 week (Patel, 1997)

(Continued)

Atenolol *(Continued)*

Garner SS, Wiest DB, and Reynolds ER, "Stability of Atenolol in an Extemporaneously Compounded Oral Liquid," *Am J Hosp Pharm*, 1994, 51(4):508-11.

Patel D, Doski DH, and Desai A, "Short-Term Stability of Atenolol in Oral Liquid Formulations," *Int J Pharmaceut Compd*, 1997, 1:437-9.

References

Buck ML, Wiest D, Gillette PC, et al, "Pharmacokinetics and Pharmacodynamics of Atenolol in Children," *Clin Pharmacol Ther*, 1989, 46(6):629-33.

Case CL, Trippel DL, and Gillette PC, "New Antiarrhythmic Agents in Pediatrics," *Pediatr Clin North Am*, 1989, 36(5):1293-320.

Chobanian AV, Bakris GL, Black HR, et al, "The Seventh Report of the Joint National Committee on Prevention, Detection, Evaluation, and Treatment of High Blood Pressure: The JNC 7 report," *JAMA*, 2003, 289(19):2560-72.

Trippel DL and Gillette PC, "Atenolol in Children With Supraventricular Tachycardia," *Am J Cardiol*, 1989, 64(3):233-6.

Trippel DL and Gillette PC, "Atenolol in Children With Ventricular Arrhythmias," *Am Heart J*, 1990, 119(6):1312-6.

♦ **ATG** *see* Antithymocyte Globulin (Equine) *on page 146*

♦ **Atgam®** *see* Antithymocyte Globulin (Equine) *on page 146*

♦ **Ativan®** *see* Lorazepam *on page 962*

Atomoxetine (AT oh mox e teen)

Related Information

Assessment of Liver Function *on page 1810*

U.S. Brand Names Strattera®

Canadian Brand Names Strattera®

Index Terms Atomoxetine Hydrochloride; LY139603; Methylphenoxy-Benzene Propanamine; Tomoxetine

Therapeutic Category Norepinephrine Reuptake Inhibitor, Selective

Generic Available No

Use Treatment of attention deficit/hyperactivity disorder (ADHD); has been used investigationally to treat depression

Medication Guide An FDA-approved patient medication guide, which is available with the product information and at http://www.fda.gov/cder/Offices/ODS/medication_guides.htm, must be dispensed with this medication for each new outpatient prescription and refill.

Pregnancy Risk Factor C

Lactation Excretion in breast milk unknown/use caution

Contraindications Hypersensitivity to atomoxetine or any component; concurrent use or use within 14 days of MAO inhibitors; narrow-angle glaucoma

Warnings Atomoxetine has been associated with an increased risk of suicidal thinking in children and adolescents with ADHD. This risk must be considered before prescribing atomoxetine in pediatric patients. Children and adolescents who start treatment with atomoxetine require close monitoring for suicidal thinking and behavior (ie, suicidality), unusual changes in behavior, or clinical worsening, especially during the first few months after initiation of a course of therapy or when the dosage is changed. Family members and caregivers should be instructed to closely observe the patient and communicate their condition with the healthcare provider. Recommended monitoring includes daily observation by family members and caregivers, at least weekly face-to-face visits with patients or their family members or caregivers during the first 4 weeks of treatment, then every other week visits for the next 4 weeks, then at 12 weeks, and then as clinically indicated beyond 12 weeks. In addition, contact by phone may be appropriate between visits. Patients should also be monitored for associated behaviors (eg, agitation, irritability, anxiety, akathisia, aggressiveness, insomnia, hostility, impulsivity, panic attacks, hypomania, mania) which may be precursors to emerging suicidality. Emergence of suicidality or associated behaviors listed above, that is abrupt in onset, severe, or not part of the presenting symptoms, may require discontinuation or modification of drug therapy.

Screen individuals for bipolar disorder prior to treatment (atomoxetine may induce mixed/manic episodes in patients at risk for bipolar disorder). Although rare, severe liver injury has been reported and may progress to liver failure, death, or the need for liver transplantation; discontinue atomoxetine and do not restart in patients who develop jaundice or laboratory evidence of liver injury; obtain liver enzyme levels if patient develops signs of liver dysfunction (eg, dark urine, jaundice, pruritus, right upper quadrant tenderness, or unexplained flu-like symptoms). Allergic reactions (including rash, urticaria, and angioneurotic edema) may occur. Suppression of growth may occur with long-term use in children (monitor carefully; consider interruption of therapy in children who are not growing or gaining weight appropriately).

Aggressive behavior or hostility has been observed in patients receiving atomoxetine (causal relationship not established).

Precautions May cause increased heart rate or blood pressure, use with caution in patients with hypertension, tachycardia, or other cardiovascular or cerebrovascular disease; may cause orthostatic hypotension, use with caution in patients with conditions that predispose to hypotension; may cause urinary retention or hesitancy, use with caution in patients with a history of urinary retention or bladder outlet obstruction; use with caution and reduce the dose in patients with hepatic dysfunction; use with caution in patients who are cytochrome P450 CYP2D6 poor metabolizers; use with caution and modify dose in patients receiving strong CYP2D6 inhibitors (see Drug Interactions and Usual Dosage). Safety and efficacy have not been established in children <6 years of age; safety and efficacy of long-term use have not been established.

Adverse Reactions **Note:** Adverse reactions reported to be increased in poor metabolizers of CYP2D6 substrates include: Decreased appetite, insomnia, sedation, depression, tremor, early morning awakening, pruritus, and mydriasis

Cardiovascular: Palpitations, tachycardia, hypertension, orthostatic hypotension, chest pain

Central nervous system: Headache, insomnia, fatigue, lethargy, irritability, somnolence, dizziness, mood swings, abnormal dreams, sleep disorder, pyrexia, rigors, crying, aggression, sedation, depression, early morning awakening; suicidal thinking and behavior (0.4%; see Warnings)

Dermatologic: Dermatitis, pruritus

Endocrine & metabolic: Weight loss, dysmenorrhea, decreased libido, menstruation disorders, hot flashes

Gastrointestinal: Xerostomia, abdominal pain, vomiting, decreased appetite, dyspepsia, diarrhea, flatulence, constipation, nausea

Genitourinary: Sexual dysfunction

Hepatic: Rare: Severe liver injury including elevated liver enzymes, hyperbilirubinemia, jaundice (**Note:** Liver injury may rarely progress to liver failure or death; see Warnings)

Neuromuscular & skeletal: Paresthesia, myalgia, tremor

Ocular: Mydriasis

Renal: Urinary retention, urinary hesitation, difficulty in micturition

Respiratory: Cough, rhinorrhea, sinus headache

Miscellaneous: Increased diaphoresis, sinusitis, ear infection, influenza, hypersensitivity reactions, urticaria, angioedema

Drug Interactions Cytochrome P450 isoenzyme CYP2D6 and CYP2C19 (minor) substrate

Concurrent use or use within 2 weeks of MAO inhibitors may cause serious and potentially fatal reactions, eg, hyperthermia, rigidity, myoclonus, mental status changes, autonomic instability, neuroleptic malignant syndrome (combined use is contraindicated). Atomoxetine may potentiate cardiovascular effects of albuterol and sympathomimetic or pressor agents (use atomoxetine with caution and monitor patients closely); atomoxetine may increase midazolam serum concentrations (monitor patients). Cytochrome P450 CYP2D6 inhibitors (eg, paroxetine, fluoxetine, quinidine) may increase atomoxetine concentrations in extensive metabolizers (atomoxetine dosage reduction may be needed; see Usual Dosage).

Food Interactions A high fat meal decreases the rate, but not the extent of absorption.

Stability Store at room temperature of 25°C (77°F).

Mechanism of Action Enhances norepinephrine activity by selectively inhibiting norepinephrine reuptake; little to no activity at other neuronal reuptake pumps or receptor sites

Pharmacokinetics

Absorption: Oral: Rapid

Distribution: V_d: Adults: I.V.: 0.85 L/kg

Protein binding: 98%, primarily albumin

Metabolism: Extensive in the liver, primarily by oxidative metabolism via cytochrome P450 CYP2D6 to 4-hydroxyatomoxetine (major metabolite regardless of CYP2D6 status, active, equipotent to atomoxetine) with subsequent glucuronidation; also metabolized via CYP2C19 to N-desmethlyatomoxetine (active, minimal activity); **Note:** CYP2D6 poor metabolizers have atomoxetine AUCs that are ~10-fold higher and peak concentrations that are ~5-fold greater than extensive metabolizers; 4-hyroxyatomoxetine plasma concentrations are very low (extensive metabolizers: 1% of atomoxetine concentrations; poor metabolizers: 0.1% of atomoxetine concentrations)

Bioavailability: Extensive metabolizers: 63%; poor metabolizers: 94%

Half-life: Adults:

Atomoxetine: Extensive metabolizers: 5.2 hours; poor metabolizers: 21.6 hours

4-hydroxyatomoxetine: Extensive metabolizers: 6-8 hours

(Continued)

Atomoxetine *(Continued)*

N-desmethlyatomoxetine: Extensive metabolizers: 6-8 hours; poor metabolizers: 34-40 hours

Elimination: Urine: <3% is excreted unchanged; 80% excreted as 4-hydroxyatomoxetine glucuronide; feces: <17%

Usual Dosage Oral:

Children and Adolescents ≤70 kg: Initial: 0.5 mg/kg/day; increase after a minimum of 3 days to approximately 1.2 mg/kg/day; may administer once daily in the morning or divide into two doses and administer in the morning and late afternoon/early evening. Maximum daily dose: 1.4 mg/kg/day or 100 mg/day, whichever is less.

Note: Doses >1.2 mg/kg/day have not been shown to provide additional benefit.

Note: In patients receiving strong CYP2D6 inhibitors (eg, paroxetine, fluoxetine, quinidine), maintain the above listed initial dose for 4 weeks; increase dose to 1.2 mg/kg/day only if clinically needed and the initial dose is well tolerated; do not exceed 1.2 mg/kg/day

Children and Adolescents >70 kg and Adults: Initial: 40 mg/day; increase after a minimum of 3 days to approximately 80 mg/day; may administer once daily in the morning or divide into two doses and administer in morning and late afternoon/early evening. May increase (if needed) to 100 mg/day in 2-4 additional weeks

Note: In patients receiving strong CYP2D6 inhibitors (eg, paroxetine, fluoxetine, quinidine), maintain the above listed initial dose for 4 weeks; increase dose to 80 mg/day only if clinically needed and the initial dose is well tolerated; do not exceed 80 mg/day

Dosage adjustment in renal impairment: No adjustment needed

Dosage adjustment in hepatic impairment:

Moderate hepatic impairment (Child-Pugh class B): All doses should be reduced to 50% of normal

Severe hepatic impairment (Child-Pugh class C): All doses should be reduced to 25% of normal

Administration Oral: May be administered without regard to food. Do not open capsule; swallow whole (atomoxetine is an ocular irritant; see Additional Information).

Monitoring Parameters Weight, height (in children); blood pressure, heart rate; liver enzymes in patients with symptoms of liver dysfunction; monitor for suicidality and associated behaviors (see Warnings)

Patient Information An increased risk of suicidal thinking and behavior has been reported with the use of atomoxetine in children and adolescents; notify physician if you feel depressed, have thoughts of suicide, or become more agitated or irritable (see Warnings). Read the patient Medication Guide that you receive with each prescription and refill of atomoxetine. Inform physician if you have allergies, narrow-angle glaucoma, current or past liver problems, or high or low blood pressure; notify physician if you experience problems with rapid or irregular heartbeats, dark urine, yellow skin or eyes, abdominal pain, itching, unexplained flu-like symptoms, or an increase in aggression or hostility. Some medicines should not be taken with atomoxetine; report the use of other medications, nonprescription medications, and herbal or natural products to your physician and pharmacist. If a dose is missed, take it as soon as possible, but do not take more than the prescribed total daily amount in any 24-hour period. May cause dizziness and impair ability to perform activities requiring mental alertness or physical coordination; may cause weight loss; may cause decreased growth in children; may make it difficult to urinate; may cause dry mouth

Additional Information Atomoxetine hydrochloride is the R(-) isomer. Therapy may be discontinued without being tapered. Total daily doses >150 mg/day and single doses >120 mg/dose have not been systematically evaluated. Medications used to treat ADHD should be part of a total treatment program that may include other components such as psychological, educational, and social measures. If used for an extended period of time, long-term usefulness of atomoxetine should be periodically re-evaluated for the individual patient.

Atomoxetine is an ocular irritant; avoid contact with eye; if capsule contents come into contact with eye, flush eye immediately with water and obtain medical advice; wash hands and any potentially contaminated surface as soon as possible

Dosage Forms Excipient information presented when available (limited, particularly for generics); consult specific product labeling. Available as atomoxetine hydrochloride; mg strength refers to atomoxetine

Capsule:

Strattera®: 10 mg, 18 mg, 25 mg, 40 mg, 60 mg, 80 mg, 100 mg

References

Biderman J, Heiligenstein JH, Faries DE, at al, "Efficacy of Atomoxetine Versus Placebo in School-Age Girls With Attention-Deficit/Hyperactivity Disorder," *Pediatrics*, 2002, 110(6), http://www.pediatrics.org/cgi/content/full/110/6/e75.

Kratochvil CJ, Heiligenstein JH, Dittmann R, et al, "Atomoxetine and Methylphenidate Treatment in Children With ADHD: A Prospective, Randomized, Open-Label trial," *J Am Acad Child Adolesc Psychiatry*, 2002, 41(7):776-84.

Michelson D, Allen AJ, Busner J, et al, "Once-Daily Atomoxetine Treatment for Children and Adolescents With Attention Deficit Hyperactivity Disorder: A Randomized, Placebo-Controlled Study," *Am J Psychiatry*, 2002, 159(11):1896-901.

Michelson D, Faries D, Wernicke J, et al, "Atomoxetine in the Treatment of Children and Adolescents With Attention-Deficit/Hyperactivity Disorder: A Ramdomized, Placebo-Controlled, Dose-Response Study," *Pediatrics*, 2001, 108(5), http://www.pediatrics.org/cgi/content/full/108/5/e83.

Spencer T, Heiligenstein JH, Biederman J, et al, "Results From 2 Proof-of-Concept, Placebo-Controlled Studies of Atomoxetine in Children With Attention-Deficit/Hyperactivity Disorder," *J Clin Psychiatry*, 2002, 63(12):1140-7.

Wernicke JF and Kratochvil CJ, "Safety Profile of Atomoxetine in the Treatment of Children and Adolescents With ADHD," *J Clin Psychiatry*, 2002, 63(Suppl 12):50-5.

♦ **Atomoxetine Hydrochloride** *see* Atomoxetine *on page 172*

Atorvastatin (a TORE va sta tin)

Medication Safety Issues

Sound-alike/look-alike issues:

Lipitor® may be confused with Levatol®

U.S. Brand Names Lipitor®

Canadian Brand Names Lipitor®

Therapeutic Category Antilipemic Agent; HMG-CoA Reductase Inhibitor

Generic Available No

Use Hyperlipidemia: Adjunct to dietary therapy to decrease elevated serum total and low density lipoprotein cholesterol (LDL-C), apolipoprotein B (apo-B), and triglyceride levels, and to increase high density lipoprotein cholesterol (HDL-C) in patients with primary hypercholesterolemia (heterozygous, familial and nonfamilial) and mixed dyslipidemia (Fredrickson types IIa and IIb); treatment of homozygous familial hypercholesterolemia; treatment of isolated hypertriglyceridemia (Fredrickson type IV) and type III hyperlipoproteinemia; treatment of primary dysbetalipoproteinemia (Fredrickson Type III)

Primary prevention of cardiovascular disease in high risk patients; risk factors include: Age ≥55 years, smoking, hypertension, low HDL-C or family history of early coronary heart disease; secondary prevention of cardiovascular disease to reduce the risk of MI, stroke, revascularization procedures, and angina in patients with evidence of heart disease and to reduce the risk of hospitalization for heart failure

Pregnancy Risk Factor X

Lactation Enters breast milk/contraindicated

Contraindications Hypersensitivity to atorvastatin or any component; active liver disease; unexplained persistent elevations of serum transaminases; pregnancy

Warnings Rhabdomyolysis with or without acute renal failure secondary to myoglobinuria has occurred rarely. Risk is increased with concurrent use of amiodarone, clarithromycin, danazol, diltiazem, fluvoxamine, amprenavir, delavirdine, indinavir, nefazodone, nelfinavir, ritonavir, verapamil, troleandomycin, cyclosporine, fibric acid derivatives, erythromycin, niacin, or azole antifungals. Assess the risk versus benefit before combining any of these medications with atorvastatin. Temporarily discontinue atorvastatin in any patient experiencing an acute or serious condition predisposing to renal failure secondary to rhabdomyolysis. Patients with a history of hemorrhagic stroke may be at increased risk for another when taking atorvastatin.

Precautions Persistent increases in serum transaminases have occurred (incidence in clinical trials 0.7% overall and highest with the 80 mg dose, 2.3%); liver function tests must be monitored at the initiation of therapy and 12 weeks following initiation of therapy or increase in dosage, and then periodically eg, semiannually, thereafter. Liver enzyme changes generally occur in the first 3 months of treatment. Use with caution in patients who consume substantial quantities of alcohol or have a previous history of liver disease.

Adverse Reactions

Cardiovascular: Angina, postural hypotension, palpitations, hypertension, phlebitis, arrhythmia, vasodilatation, chest pain, edema, sweating, angioneurotic edema

Central nervous system: Dizziness, headache, somnolence, fatigue, insomnia, depression, amnesia, abnormal dreams, emotional lability, migraine, decreased libido

Dermatologic: Eczema, pruritus, rash, photosensitivity, alopecia, dry skin, acne, seborrhea, skin ulcer, erythema multiforme, Stevens-Johnson syndrome, toxic epidermal necrolysis

Endocrine & metabolic: Hyperglycemia, gout, hypoglycemia

Gastrointestinal: Constipation, dyspepsia, flatulence, abdominal pain, diarrhea, nausea, pancreatitis, gastroenteritis, gastritis, vomiting, xerostomia, rectal hemorrhage, esophagitis, eructation, glossitis, mouth ulceration, anorexia, increased appetite, stomatitis, biliary pain, cheilitis, duodenal ulcer, dysphagia, enteritis,

(Continued)

Atorvastatin *(Continued)*

melena, gum hemorrhage, stomach ulcer, tenesmus, ulcerative stomatitis, taste perversion, taste loss

Genitourinary: Urinary frequency, cystitis, hematuria, impotence, dysuria, kidney calculus, nocturia, epididymitis, vaginal hemorrhage, albuminuria, metrorrhagia, urinary retention, urinary incontinence, abnormal ejaculation, uterine hemorrhage, UTI

Hematologic: Thrombocytopenia, anemia

Hepatic: Elevated serum transaminases, hepatitis, cholestatic jaundice

Neuromuscular & skeletal: Elevated CPK, myalgia, muscle cramps, myopathy, bursitis, tenosynovitis, myasthenia, tendinous contracture, myositis, hypertonia, peripheral neuropathy, torticollis, facial paralysis, paresthesias, rhabdomyolysis, arthralgias, hyperkinesias, neck rigidity, tendon rupture

Ocular: Dry eyes, amblyopia, refraction disorder, eye hemorrhage, glaucoma, diplopia

Otic: Tinnitus, deafness

Renal: Nephritis

Respiratory: Sinusitis, pharyngitis, bronchitis, rhinitis, dyspnea, asthma, pneumonia

Miscellaneous: Hypersensitivity reactions including anaphylaxis

Drug Interactions Cytochrome P450 isoenzyme CYP3A3/4 enzyme substrate; isoenzyme CYP3A4 inhibitor

Plasma concentrations may be decreased when given with magnesium-aluminum hydroxide-containing antacids; cholestyramine and colestipol reduce absorption; clofibrate, fenofibrate, gemfibrozil, niacin (≥1 g/day), amiodarone, and cyclosporine may increase the risk of myopathy and rhabdomyolysis (see Warnings); CYP3A3/4 inhibitors (clarithromycin, cyclosporine, danazol, diltiazem, fluconazole, fluvoxamine, erythromycin, delavirdine, amprenavir, indinavir, itraconazole, ketoconazole, miconazole, nefazodone, nelfinavir, ritonavir, saquinavir, troleandomycin, and verapamil) increase atorvastatin blood levels and may increase the risk of atorvastatin-induced myopathy and rhabdomyolysis (see Warnings); bosentan may decrease atorvastatin serum level; atorvastatin may increase digoxin serum level; increased AUC values for oral contraceptives (norethindrone 30% and ethinyl estradiol 20%) occur when coadministered with atorvastatin; atorvastatin may decrease antiplatelet activity of clopidogrel; the herbal medicine St John's wort (*Hypericum perforatum*) may decrease atorvastatin serum levels

Food Interactions Atorvastatin serum concentration may be increased when taken with large quantities (>1 quart/day) of grapefruit juice; avoid concurrent use

Stability Tablets should be stored in well closed container at controlled room temperature between 20°C to 25°C (68°F to 77°F)

Mechanism of Action Atorvastatin is a selective, competitive inhibitor of 3-hydroxy-3-methylglutaryl-coenzyme A (HMG-CoA) reductase, the enzyme that catalyzes the rate-limiting step in cholesterol biosynthesis

Pharmacodynamics

Onset of action: Within 2 weeks

Maximum effect: After 4 weeks

LDL reduction: 10 mg/day: 39% (for each doubling of this dose, LDL is lowered approximately 6%)

Pharmacokinetics

Absorption: Oral: Rapidly absorbed; extensive first-pass metabolism in GI mucosa and liver

Distribution: V_d: Adults: 381 L

Protein binding: >98%

Metabolism: Extensive metabolism to ortho- and parahydroxylated derivatives and various beta-oxidation products with equivalent *in vitro* activity to atorvastatin

Bioavailability: Absolute: 14%

Half-life: Adults: 14 hours (half-life of inhibitory activity due to active metabolites is 20-30 hours)

Time to peak serum concentration: 1-2 hours

Elimination: Primarily in bile following hepatic and/or extra-hepatic metabolism; does not appear to undergo enterohepatic recirculation; <2% excreted in urine

Usual Dosage Oral: Dosage should be individualized according to the baseline LDL-C level, the recommended goal of therapy, and patient response; adjustments should be made at intervals of 2-4 weeks

Hyperlipidemia:

Children 10-17 years: 10 mg once daily; may increase to 20 mg once daily; doses >20 mg have not been studied

Adolescents >17 years and Adults:

Initial: 10-20 mg once daily; patients who require a reduction of >45% in LDL-C may be started at 40 mg once daily

Maintenance: Recommended dosage range: 10-80 mg/day

Heterozygous familial and nonfamilial hypercholesterolemia:

Adolescents 10-17 years: 10 mg once daily; may increase to a maximum of 20 mg/day

Adults: 10-20 mg once daily; may increase to a maximum of 80 mg/day

Homozygous familial hypercholesterolemia: Adults: 10-80 mg/day

Primary prevention of cardiovascular disease: Adults: 10 mg once daily

Dosing adjustment in renal impairment: Adults: Because atorvastatin does not undergo significant renal excretion, dose modification is not necessary

Dosing adjustment in hepatic impairment: Avoid use in active liver disease

Administration Oral: May be taken without regard to meals or time of day

Monitoring Parameters Serum cholesterol (total and fractionated), CPK; liver function tests (see Precautions)

Reference Range Hypercholesterolemia as defined by serum cholesterol, LDL-C, TG concentration: See table below; desired: HDL-C <40 mg/dL

Classification of Blood Cholesterol, LDL-C, and Triglyceride Concentrations[1]

Classification	Cholesterol (mg/dL)		LDL-C (mg/dL)		Triglycerides (mg/dL)
	Children	Adults	Children	Adults	Adults
Acceptable/optimal	<170	<200	<110	<100	<150
Above optimal	†	†	†	100 120	†
Borderline high	170-199	200-239	110-129	130-159	150-199
High	≥200	≥240	≥130	160-189	200-499
Very high	†	†	†	≥190	≥500

[1]Adapted from American Academy of Pediatrics Committee on Nutrition, "Cholesterol in Childhood," *Pediatrics*, 1998, 101(1 Pt 1):141-7 and "Third Report of the National Cholesterol Education Program Expert Panel on Detection, Evaluation, and Treatment of High Blood Cholesterol in Adults (Adult Treatment Panel III)," May 2001, www.nhlbi.nih.gov/guidelines/cholesterol.

†Lack of specific type of classification in either pediatric or adult recommendations.

Patient Information May rarely cause photosensitivity reactions (eg, exposure to sunlight may cause severe sunburn, skin rash, redness, or itching); avoid direct exposure to sunlight. Report severe and unresolved gastric upset, any vision changes, muscle pain and weakness, changes in color of urine or stool, yellowing of skin or eyes, and any unusual bruising. Female patients of childbearing age must be counseled to use 2 effective forms of contraception simultaneously, unless absolute abstinence is the chosen method; this drug may cause severe fetal defects. May cause dry mouth.

Additional Information The current recommendation for treatment of hypercholesterolemia in children is limited to children ≥10 years of age who, after a 6-month to 1-year trial of diet therapy, continue to have LDL-C concentrations ≥190 mg/dL alone, or LDL-C concentrations ≥160 mg/dL and a family history of premature coronary artery disease or two or more other coronary artery disease risk factors (AAP Committee on Nutrition, 1998). For each 1% lowering in LDL-C, the relative risk for major cardiovascular events is reduced by approximately 1%. For more specific risk assessment and treatment recommendations for adults, see NCEP ATPIII, 2004.

Dosage Forms Excipient information presented when available (limited, particularly for generics); consult specific product labeling.

Tablet:

Lipitor®: 10 mg, 20 mg, 40 mg, 80 mg

References

American Academy of Pediatrics Committee on Nutrition, "Cholesterol in Childhood," *Pediatrics*, 1998, 101(1 Pt 1):141-7.

American Academy of Pediatrics, "National Cholesterol Education Program: Report of the Expert Panel on Blood Cholesterol Levels in Children and Adolescents," *Pediatrics*, 1992, 89(3 Pt 2):525-84.

Argent E, Kainer G, Aitken M, et al, "Atorvastatin Treatment for Hyperlipidemia in Pediatric Renal Transplant Recipients," *Pediatr Transplant*, 2003, 7(1):38-42.

Belay B, Belamarich PF, and Tom-Revzon C, "The Use of Statins in Pediatrics: Knowledge Base, Limitations, and Future Directions," *Pediatrics*, 2007, 119(2):370-80.

Duplaga BA, "Treatment of Childhood Hypercholesterolemia With HMG-CoA Reductase Inhibitors," *Ann Pharmacother*, 1999, 33(11):1224-7.

Grundy SM, Cleeman JI, Merz CN, et al, "Implications of Recent Clinical Trials for the National Cholesterol Education Program Adult Treatment Panel III Guidelines," *Circulation*, 2004, 110(2):227-39.

McCrindle BW, Ose L, and Marais AD, "Efficacy and Safety of Atorvastatin in Children and Adolescents With Familial Hypercholesterolemia or Severe Hyperlipidemia: A Multicenter, Randomized, Placebo-Controlled Trial," *J Pediatr*, 2003, 143(1):74-80.

"Third Report of the National Cholesterol Education Program Expert Panel on Detection, Evaluation, and Treatment of High Blood Cholesterol in Adults (Adult Treatment Panel III)," May 2001, www.nhlbi.nih.gov/guidelines/cholesterol.

Atovaquone (a TOE va kwone)

U.S. Brand Names Mepron®
Canadian Brand Names Mepron®
Index Terms Hydroxy-1,4-naphthoquinone
Therapeutic Category Antiprotozoal
Generic Available No
Use Second-line treatment of mild to moderate *Pneumocystis carinii* pneumonia (PCP) in patients intolerant of trimethoprim/sulfamethoxazole (TMP/SMX); mild to moderate PCP is defined as an alveolar-arterial oxygen diffusion gradient ≤45 mm Hg and PaO_2 ≥60 mm Hg on room air; patients intolerant of TMP/SMX are defined as having a significant rash (ie, Stevens-Johnson-like syndrome), neutropenia, or hemolysis; prevention of PCP in patients who are intolerant to TMP/SMX; treatment of babesiosis
Pregnancy Risk Factor C
Lactation Excretion in breast milk unknown/use caution
Contraindications Hypersensitivity to atovaquone or any component (see Warnings)
Warnings Clinical experience with atovaquone has been limited to patients with mild to moderate PCP; treatment of more severe episodes of PCP has not been systematically studied

Suspension contains benzyl alcohol which may cause allergic reactions in susceptible individuals; large amounts of benzyl alcohol (≥99 mg/kg/day) have been associated with a potentially fatal toxicity ("gasping syndrome") in neonates; the "gasping syndrome" consists of metabolic acidosis, respiratory distress, gasping respirations, CNS dysfunction (including convulsions, intracranial hemorrhage), hypotension and cardiovascular collapse; avoid use in neonates; *in vitro* and animal studies have shown that benzoate, a metabolite of benzyl alcohol, displaces bilirubin from protein binding sites

Precautions For patients who have difficulty taking atovaquone with food or who have chronic diarrhea, stomach or intestinal problems which may result in drug malabsorption, parenteral therapy with other agents should be considered since a low serum atovaquone concentration could lead to treatment failure
Adverse Reactions
Central nervous system: Fever, headache, insomnia, dizziness, pain
Dermatologic: Maculopapular rash, erythema multiforme, pruritus
Endocrine & metabolic: Hyponatremia
Gastrointestinal: Nausea, vomiting, diarrhea, abdominal pain, constipation, anorexia, elevated amylase
Hematologic: Rare: Neutropenia, anemia
Hepatic: Elevated hepatic enzymes, cholestasis
Respiratory: Cough, sinusitis
Miscellaneous: Diaphoresis
Drug Interactions Rifampin may decrease plasma atovaquone concentration; since atovaquone is highly protein bound, it may compete for protein binding sites with other highly protein-bound agents like warfarin (however, there have been no drug-drug interactions of this type reported to date)
Food Interactions Administration with food increases bioavailability of atovaquone suspension 1.4-fold over that achieved in a fasting state or up to 3-fold with a high fat meal
Stability Store at room temperature; do not freeze
Mechanism of Action The mechanism of action against *Pneumocystis carinii* has not been fully elucidated; in *Plasmodium* species, atovaquone selectively inhibits the mitochondrial electron-transport system at the cytochrome bc_1 complex resulting in depletion of dihydroorotate dehydrogenase and ultimately resulting in the inhibition of nucleic acid and adenosine triphosphate synthesis
Pharmacokinetics
Absorption: Oral:
Infants and Children <2 years of age: Decreased absorption
Adults: Oral suspension: Absorption is enhanced 1.4-fold with food; decreased absorption with single doses exceeding 750 mg
Distribution: V_{dss}: 0.6 L/kg; CSF concentration is <1% of the plasma concentration
Protein binding: >99%
Bioavailability: Suspension (administered with food): 47%
Half-life, elimination:
Children (4 months to 12 years): 60 hours (range: 31-163 hours)
Adults: 2.9 days
Adults with AIDS: 2.2 days
Time to peak serum concentration: Dual peak serum concentrations at 1 to 8 hours and at 24 to 96 hours after dose due to enterohepatic cycling

Elimination: ~94% is recovered as unchanged drug in feces; 0.6% excreted in urine

Usual Dosage Oral:

Children:

Treatment: Dose of 40 mg/kg/day divided twice daily (maximum dose: 1500 mg/day) may be necessary to attain comparable plasma concentrations associated with the successful treatment of PCP as seen in adults.

Prophylaxis of *Pneumocystis carinii* pneumonia:

1-3 months of age and >24 months of age: 30 mg/kg/day once daily (maximum dose: 1500 mg/day)

4-24 months of age: 45 mg/kg/day once daily (maximum dose: 1500 mg/day)

Babesiosis: 40 mg/kg/day divided twice daily (maximum dose: 1500 mg/day) with azithromycin 12 mg/kg/day once daily for 7-10 days

Adolescents 13-16 years and Adults:

Treatment: 750 mg/dose twice daily for 21 days

Prophylaxis of *Pneumocystis carinii* pneumonia: 1500 mg once daily

Babesiosis: 750 mg/dose twice daily for 7-10 days with azithromycin 1000 mg once daily for 3 days then 500 mg once daily for 7 days

Administration Oral: Administer with food or a high-fat meal; shake suspension well before using

Monitoring Parameters CBC with differential, liver enzymes, serum chemistries, serum amylase

Additional Information The suspension contains the inactive ingredient poloxamer 188

Dosage Forms Excipient information presented when available (limited, particularly for generics); consult specific product labeling.

Suspension, oral: 750 mg/5 mL (5 mL, 210 mL) [contains benzyl alcohol; citrus flavor]

References

Centers for Disease Control and Prevention, "2001 USPHS/IDSA Guidelines for the Prevention of Opportunistic Infections in Persons Infected With Human Immunodeficiency Virus," November 28, 2001, http://www.aidsinfo.nih.gov

Haile LG and Flaherty JF, "Atovaquone: A Review," *Ann Pharmacother*, 1993, 27(12):1488-94.

Hughes W, Dorenbaum A, Yogev R, et al, "Phase I Safety and Pharmacokinetics Study of Micronized Atovaquone Human Immunodeficiency Virus-Infected Infants and Children. Pediatric AIDS Clinical Trials Group," *Antimicrob Agents Chemother*, 1998, 42(6):1315-8.

Hughes W, Leoung G, Kramer F, et al, "Comparison of Atovaquone (566C80) With Trimethoprim-Sulfamethoxazole to Treat *Pneumocystis carinii* Pneumonia in Patients With AIDS," *N Engl J Med*, 1993, 328(21):1521-7.

Atracurium (a tra KYOO ree um)

Medication Safety Issues

High alert medication: The Institute for Safe Medication Practices (ISMP) includes this medication among its list of drugs which have a heightened risk of causing significant patient harm when used in error.

Canadian Brand Names Atracurium Besylate Injection

Index Terms Atracurium Besylate

Therapeutic Category Neuromuscular Blocker Agent, Nondepolarizing; Skeletal Muscle Relaxant, Paralytic

Generic Available Yes

Use Eases endotracheal intubation as an adjunct to general anesthesia and relaxes skeletal muscle during surgery or mechanical ventilation

Pregnancy Risk Factor C

Lactation Excretion in breast milk unknown/use caution

Contraindications Hypersensitivity to atracurium besylate or any component

Warnings Reduce initial dosage and inject slowly (over 1-2 minutes) in patients in whom substantial histamine release would be potentially hazardous (eg, patients with clinically important cardiovascular disease); maintenance of an adequate airway and respiratory support is critical; formulation with preservative contains benzyl alcohol which may cause allergic reactions in susceptible individuals; large amounts of benzyl alcohol (≥99 mg/kg/day) have been associated with a potentially fatal toxicity ("gasping syndrome") in neonates; the "gasping syndrome" consists of metabolic acidosis, respiratory distress, gasping respirations, CNS dysfunction (including convulsions, intracranial hemorrhage), hypotension and cardiovascular collapse; avoid use of atracurium products containing benzyl alcohol in neonates; use preservative free product; *in vitro* and animal studies have shown that benzoate, a metabolite of benzyl alcohol, displaces bilirubin from protein binding sites; avoid use of preservative-containing formulation in neonates

Certain clinical conditions may result in potentiation or antagonism of neuromuscular blockade, see table on next page. Increased sensitivity in patients with myasthenia gravis, Eaton-Lambert syndrome; resistance to neuromuscular blockade in burn patients (>30% of body) for period of 5-70 days postinjury; resistance in patients with muscle

(Continued)

Atracurium *(Continued)*

trauma, denervation, immobilization, infection, chronic treatment with atracurium. When used in conjunction with anesthetics, bradycardia may be more common with atracurium than with other neuromuscular blocking agents; it has no clinically significant effects on heart rate to counteract the bradycardia produced by anesthetics.

Clinical Conditions Affecting Neuromuscular Blockade

Potentiation	Antagonism
Electrolyte abnormalities	Alkalosis
Severe hyponatremia	Hypercalcemia
Severe hypocalcemia	Demyelinating lesions
Severe hypokalemia	Peripheral neuropathies
Hypermagnesemia	Diabetes mellitus
Neuromuscular diseases	
Acidosis	
Acute intermittent porphyria	
Renal failure	
Hepatic failure	

Precautions Due to potential histamine release, use with caution in patients in whom histamine release may be hazardous (eg, cardiovascular disease, asthma); patients with severe electrolyte disorders; patients with myasthenia gravis

Adverse Reactions

Cardiovascular: Effects are minimal and transient

Dermatologic: Erythema, itching, urticaria

Respiratory: Wheezing, bronchial secretions (increased)

Drug Interactions See table.

Potential Drug Interactions

Potentiation	Antagonism
Inhalation anesthetics	Calcium
Desflurane, sevoflurane, enflurane and isoflurane > halothane > nitrous oxide	Carbamazepine
	Phenytoin
	Steroids (chronic administration)
Antibiotics	Theophylline
Aminoglycosides, polymyxins, clindamycin, vancomycin, tetracycline	Anticholinesterases[1]
	Neostigmine, pyridostigmine, edrophonium, echothiophate ophthalmic solution
Magnesium	
Antiarrhythmics	
Quinidine, procainamide, bretylium, and possibly lidocaine	Caffeine
	Azathioprine
Diuretics	
Furosemide, mannitol, thiazides	
Amphotericin B (secondary to hypokalemia)	
Local anesthetics	
Dantrolene (directly depresses skeletal muscle)	
Beta blockers	
Calcium channel blockers	
Ketamine	
Lithium	
Succinylcholine (when administered prior to nondepolarizing neuromuscular-blocking agent)	
Cyclosporine	

[1]Can prolong the effects of acetylcholine

Stability Refrigerate; stable at room temperature for 14 days; unstable in alkaline solutions; compatible with D_5W, D_5NS, and NS; do not dilute in LR

Mechanism of Action Blocks neural transmission at the myoneural junction by binding with cholinergic receptor sites

Pharmacodynamics

Onset of action: I.V.: 1-4 minutes

Maximum effect: Within 3-5 minutes
Duration: Recovery begins in 20-35 minutes when anesthesia is balanced

Pharmacokinetics
Distribution: V_d:
Infants: 0.21 L/kg
Children: 0.13 L/kg
Adults: 0.1 L/kg
Metabolism: Some metabolites are active; undergoes rapid nonenzymatic degradation (Hofmann elimination) in the bloodstream; additional metabolism occurs via ester hydrolysis
Half-life: Elimination:
Infants: 20 minutes
Children: 17 minutes
Adults: 16 minutes
Elimination: Clearance:
Infants: 7.9 mL/kg/minute
Children: 6.8 mL/kg/minute
Adults: 5.3 mL/kg/minute

Usual Dosage I.V.:
Neonates, Infants, and Children ≤2 years:
0.3-0.4 mg/kg initially followed by maintenance doses of 0.3-0.4 mg/kg as needed to maintain neuromuscular blockade
or
Continuous infusion: 0.6-1.2 mg/kg/hour or 10-20 mcg/kg/minute
Children >2 years to Adults:
0.4-0.5 mg/kg then 0.08-0.1 mg/kg 20-45 minutes after initial dose to maintain neuromuscular block
or
Continuous infusion: 0.4-0.8 mg/kg/hour or 6.7-13 mcg/kg/minute (range: 2-15 mcg/kg/minute)
Dosage adjustment in hepatic or renal impairment: Not necessary
Dosage adjustment with enflurane or isoflurane: Reduce dosage by 33%
Dosage adjustment with induced hypothermia (cardio-bypass surgery): Reduce dosage by 50%

Administration Parenteral: May be administered without further dilution by rapid I.V. injection; for continuous infusions, dilute to a maximum concentration of 0.5 mg/mL (more concentrated solutions have reduced stability, ie, <24 hours at room temperature); not for I.M. injection due to tissue irritation

Monitoring Parameters Muscle twitch response to peripheral nerve stimulation, heart rate, blood pressure

Additional Information Neuromuscular blockade may be reversed with neostigmine; atropine or glycopyrrolate should be available to treat excessive cholinergic effects from neostigmine

Dosage Forms Excipient information presented when available (limited, particularly for generics); consult specific product labeling.
Injection, as besylate: 10 mg/mL (10 mL) [contains benzyl alcohol]
Injection, as besylate [preservative free]: 10 mg/mL (5 mL)

References
Martin LD, Bratton SL, and O'Rourke PP, "Clinical Uses and Controversies of Neuromuscular Blocking Agents in Infants and Children," *Crit Care Med*, 1999, 27(7):1358-68.

♦ **Atracurium Besylate** *see* Atracurium *on page 179*
♦ **Atracurium Besylate Injection (Can)** *see* Atracurium *on page 179*
♦ **AtroPen®** *see* Atropine *on page 181*

Atropine (A troe peen)

Medication Safety Issues
International issues:
Genatropine® [France] may be confused with Genotropin®

Related Information
Asthma *on page 1904*
Commonly Used Antidotes for Acute Overdoses *on page 1920*
Compatibility of Medications Mixed in A Syringe *on page 1941*
CPR Pediatric Drug Dosages *on page 1650*
Overdose and Toxicology *on page 1916*
(Continued)

Atropine *(Continued)*

U.S. Brand Names AtroPen®; Atropine-Care®; Isopto® Atropine; Sal-Tropine™

Canadian Brand Names Dioptic's Atropine Solution; Isopto® Atropine

Index Terms Atropine Sulfate

Therapeutic Category Antiasthmatic; Anticholinergic Agent; Anticholinergic Agent, Ophthalmic; Antidote, Organophosphate Poisoning; Antispasmodic Agent, Gastrointestinal; Bronchodilator; Ophthalmic Agent, Mydriatic

Generic Available Yes: Excludes tablet

Use Preoperative medication to inhibit salivation and secretions; treatment of sinus bradycardia; treatment of asystole and pulseless electrical activity (adults); management of peptic ulcer; reversal of the muscarinic effects of cholinergic agents such as neostigmine and pyridostigmine; treatment of exercise-induced bronchospasm; antidote for organophosphate or carbamate pesticide poisoning; used to produce mydriasis and cycloplegia for examination of the retina and optic disk and accurate measurement of refractive errors; treatment of uveitis

Pregnancy Risk Factor C

Lactation Enters breast milk (trace amounts)/use caution (AAP rates "compatible")

Contraindications Hypersensitivity to atropine sulfate or any component; narrow-angle glaucoma; tachycardia; thyrotoxicosis; obstructive disease of the GI tract; obstructive uropathy

Warnings The AtroPen® formulation is available for use primarily by the Department of Defense as an initial treatment of the muscarinic symptoms of insecticide or nerve agent poisoning; its use should be reserved for individuals who have had adequate training in the recognition and treatment of this type of intoxication.

Precautions Use with caution in children with spastic paralysis or brain damage; children are at increased risk for rapid rise in body temperature due to suppression of sweat gland activity; paradoxical hyperexcitability may occur in children given large doses; infants with Down's syndrome have both increased sensitivity to cardiac effects and mydriasis

Adverse Reactions

Cardiovascular: Tachycardia, palpitations, flushing, arrhythmias

Central nervous system: Fatigue, delirium, headache, restlessness, ataxia, confusion, dizziness, hyperpyrexia

Dermatologic: Dry hot skin, dry mucous membranes, rash

Gastrointestinal: Impaired GI motility, xerostomia, constipation, abdominal distension, nausea, vomiting, loss of libido

Genitourinary: Urinary retention, impotency

Local: Pain at injection site

Neuromuscular & skeletal: Tremor, hypertonia

Ocular: Blurred vision, photophobia, mydriasis, dry eyes

Respiratory: Tachypnea, shallow respirations, stridor, laryngitis, pulmonary edema, respiratory failure

Drug Interactions Additive effects when administered with other anticholinergic agents; may alter response to beta-adrenergic blockers

Stability Store at controlled room temperature; protect AtroPen® from light

Mechanism of Action Blocks the action of acetylcholine at parasympathetic sites in smooth muscle, secretory glands, and the CNS; increases cardiac output, dries secretions, antagonizes histamine and serotonin

Pharmacodynamics

Inhibition of salivation:
- Onset of action:
  - Oral: 30-60 minutes
  - I.M.: 30 minutes
- Maximum effect:
  - Oral: 2 hours
  - I.M.: 1-1.6 hours
- Duration: Oral, I.M.: Up to 4 hours

Increased heart rate:
- Onset of action:
  - Oral: 30 minutes to 2 hours
  - I.M.: 5-40 minutes
- Maximum effect:
  - Oral: 1-2 hours
  - I.M.: 20 minutes to 1 hour
  - I.V.: 2-4 minutes

Bronchodilation: Oral Inhalation:
- Onset of action: 15 minutes
- Maximum effect: 15 minutes to 1.5 hours

Pharmacokinetics

Absorption: Well absorbed from all dosage forms

Distribution: Widely distributes throughout the body; crosses the placenta; trace amounts appear in breast milk; crosses the blood-brain barrier

Protein binding: 14% to 22%

Metabolism: In the liver

Half-life:

Children <2 years: 6.9 ± 3 hours

Children >2 years: 2.5 ± 1.2 hours

Adults: 3 ± 0.9 hours

Elimination: Both metabolites and unchanged drug (13% to 50%) are excreted into urine

Usual Dosage Note: Doses <0.1 mg have been associated with paradoxical bradycardia

Neonates, Infants and Children:

Preanesthetic: Oral, I.M., I.V., SubQ:

<5 kg: 0.02 mg/kg/dose 30-60 minutes preop then every 4-6 hours as needed; use of a minimum dosage of 0.1 mg in neonates <5 kg will result in dosages >0.02 mg/kg; there is no documented minimum dosage in this age group

>5 kg: 0.01-0.02 mg/kg/dose to a maximum 0.4 mg/dose 30-60 minutes preop; minimum dose: 0.1 mg

Bradycardia: I.V., intratracheal, I.O.: 0.02 mg/kg, minimum dose 0.1 mg, maximum single dose: 0.5 mg in children and 1 mg in adolescents; may repeat in 5 minutes; maximum total dose of 1 mg in children or 2 mg in adolescents. (**Note:** For intratracheal administration, must be diluted; see Administration.) When treating bradycardia in neonates, reserve use for those patients unresponsive to improved oxygenation and epinephrine.

Children:

Bronchospasm: Inhalation: 0.03-0.05 mg/kg/dose 3-4 times/day; maximum: 2.5 mg/dose

Refraction: Ophthalmic:

Infants <1 year: Instill 1 drop of 0.25% solution 3 times/day for 3 days before the procedure

Children: 1-5 years: Instill 1 drop of 0.5% solution 3 times/day for 3 days before the procedure

Children >5 years or Children with dark irides: Instill 1 drop of 1% solution 3 times/day for 3 days before the procedure

Organophosphate or carbamate poisoning:

I.V.: 0.02-0.05 mg/kg every 10-20 minutes until atropine effect (dry flushed skin, tachycardia, mydriasis, fever) is observed then every 1-4 hours for at least 24 hours

I.M.: AtroPen®:

Children 6 months to 4 years (15-40 lbs): 0.5 mg (blue pen)

Children 4-10 years (40-90 lbs): 1 mg (dark red pen)

Children >10 years (>90 lbs): 2 mg (green pen)

Mild symptoms: 1 injection as soon as exposure is known or suspected

Severe symptoms: 2 additional injections (3 total) given in rapid succession 10 minutes after receiving the first injection

Uveitis: Ophthalmic: Instill 1 drop of 0.5% solution 1-3 times daily

Adults (doses <0.5 mg have been associated with paradoxical bradycardia):

Asystole and slow pulseless electrical activity: I.V.: 1 mg; may repeat every 3-5 minutes as needed to a total dose of 0.04 mg/kg

Preanesthetic: Oral, I.M., I.V., SubQ: 0.4-0.6 mg 30-60 minutes preop

Bradycardia: I.V.: 0.5-1 mg every 5 minutes, not to exceed a total of 2 mg or 0.04 mg/kg

Bronchospasm: Inhalation: 0.025-0.05 mg/kg/dose every 4-6 hours as needed; maximum: 2.5 mg/dose

Organophosphate or carbamate poisoning:

I.V.: 1-2 mg/dose every 10-20 minutes until atropine effect (dry flushed skin, tachycardia, mydriasis, fever) is observed then every 1-4 hours for at least 24 hours; up to 50 mg in first 24 hours and 2 g over several days may be given in cases of severe intoxication

I.M.: AtroPen®: 2 mg (green pen) administered as soon as exposure is known or suspected; if severe symptoms, administer 2 additional injections (3 total) in rapid succession 10 minutes after receiving the first injection

Refraction: Ophthalmic: Instill 1-2 drops of 1% solution before the procedure

Uveitis: Ophthalmic: Instill 1-2 drops of 1% solution up to 4 times/day

Administration

Intratracheal: Administer and flush with 5 mL NS followed by 5 manual ventilations

(Continued)

Atropine *(Continued)*

Parenteral:

I.V.: Administer undiluted by rapid I.V. injection; slow injection may result in paradoxical bradycardia

I.M.: AtroPen®: Administer to outer thigh. May be given through clothing as long as pockets at the injection site are empty. Hold autoinjector in place for 10 seconds following injection; massage the injection site.

Oral: Administer without regard to food

Ophthalmic: Due to the discontinuance of 0.5% ophthalmic solutions commercially, 0.5% and 0.25% solutions may be prepared by dilution of 1% atropine ophthalmic solution with artificial tears; a 1:1 dilution for 0.5% and a 1:4 dilution for 0.25%; instill solution into conjunctival sac of affected eye(s); avoid contact of bottle tip with eye or skin

Monitoring Parameters Heart rate; organophosphate or carbamate poisoning symptomatology

Patient Information May cause dry mouth

Dosage Forms Excipient information presented when available (limited, particularly for generics); consult specific product labeling.

Injection, solution, as sulfate: 0.05 mg/mL (5 mL); 0.1 mg/mL (5 mL, 10 mL); 0.4 mg/0.5 mL (0.5 mL); 0.4 mg/mL (0.5 mL, 1 mL, 20 mL); 1 mg/mL (1 mL)

AtroPen® [prefilled autoinjector]: 0.5 mg/0.7 mL (0.7 mL); 1 mg/0.7 mL (0.7 mL); 2 mg/0.7 mL (0.7 mL)

Ointment, ophthalmic, as sulfate: 1% (3.5 g)

Solution, ophthalmic, as sulfate: 1% (2 mL, 5 mL, 15 mL)

Atropine-Care®: 1% (2 mL) [contains benzalkonium chloride]

Isopto® Atropine: 1% (5 mL, 15 mL) [contains benzalkonium chloride]

Tablet, as sulfate (Sal-Tropine™): 0.4 mg

References

"2005 American Heart Association (AHA) Guidelines for Cardiopulmonary Resuscitation (CPR) and Emergency Cardiovascular Care (ECC) of Pediatric and Neonatal Patients: Pediatric Advanced Life Support," *Pediatrics*, 2006, 117(5):1005-28.

♦ **Atropine and Diphenoxylate** *see* Diphenoxylate and Atropine *on page 512*

♦ **Atropine-Care®** *see* Atropine *on page 181*

♦ **Atropine, Hyoscyamine, Scopolamine, and Phenobarbital** *see* Hyoscyamine, Atropine, Scopolamine, and Phenobarbital *on page 800*

♦ **Atropine Sulfate** *see* Atropine *on page 181*

♦ **Atrovent®** *see* Ipratropium *on page 863*

♦ **Atrovent® HFA** *see* Ipratropium *on page 863*

Attapulgite (at a PULL gite)

Medication Safety Issues

Sound-alike/look-alike issues:

Kaopectate® may be confused with Kayexalate®

International issues:

Diasorb®: Brand name for loperamide in Great Britain

U.S. Brand Names Children's Kaopectate® [OTC] [DSC]; Diasorb® [OTC]; Kaopectate® Advanced Formula [OTC] [DSC]; Kaopectate® Maximum Strength Caplets [OTC] [DSC]

Canadian Brand Names Kaopectate®

Therapeutic Category Antidiarrheal

Generic Available Yes

Use Treatment of uncomplicated diarrhea

Pregnancy Risk Factor B

Contraindications Hypersensitivity to attapulgite or any component

Warnings Not to be used for self-medication for diarrhea >48 hours or in the presence of high fever in infants and children <3 years of age; do not use for diarrhea associated with pseudomembranous enterocolitis or in diarrhea caused by toxigenic bacteria

Adverse Reactions

Gastrointestinal: Constipation

Respiratory: Pneumoconiosis (from inhalation of the powder chronically as it contains large amounts of silica)

Drug Interactions May inhibit GI absorption of promazine, digoxin, clindamycin, tetracycline, and penicillamine

Mechanism of Action Controls diarrhea because of its absorbent action

Usual Dosage Adequate controlled clinical studies documenting the efficacy of attapulgite are lacking; its usage and dosage has been primarily empiric; the following are manufacturer's recommended dosages

Oral: Give after each bowel movement

Children:

3-6 years: 300-750 mg/dose; maximum dose: 7 doses/day or 2250 mg/day

6-12 years: 600-1500 mg/dose; maximum dose: 7 doses/day or 4500 mg/day

Children >12 years and Adults: 1200-3000 mg/dose; maximum dose: 8 doses/day or 9000 mg/day

Administration May be administered without regard to meals; shake liquid preparation well before use

Patient Information Do not exceed maximum number of doses per day; drink plenty of fluids; contact your physician if diarrhea persists more than 48 hours or if fever develops in children <3 years of age

Additional Information Kaopectate®, Kaopectate® Advanced Formula, Children's Kaopectate®, and Kaopectate® Maximum Strength have been reformulated. Previously, Kaopectate® contained attapulgite. The new formulation contains only bismuth subsalicylate. Bismuth salicylate has significant contraindications, particularly in children with influenza and chickenpox. Please refer to bismuth monograph for product information. During the transition period, the older formulation may still be available, read product label closely.

Dosage Forms Excipient information presented when available (limited, particularly for generics); consult specific product labeling. [DSC] = Discontinued product

Caplet (Kaopectate® Maximum Strength [DSC]): 750 mg

Liquid, oral concentrate: Activated attapulgite 600 mg/15 mL (120 mL, 180 mL, 240 mL); activated attapulgite 750 mg/15 mL (120 mL, 360 mL)

Children's Kaopectate® [DSC]: Activated attapulgite 300 mg/7.5 mL (180 mL) [cherry flavor]

Diasorb®: Activated attapulgite 750 mg/5 mL (120 mL) [cola flavor; sugar free]

Kaopectate® Advanced Formula [DSC]: Activated attapulgite 750 mg/15 mL (90 mL, 240 mL, 360 mL) [peppermint flavor]

♦ **Attenuvax®** *see* Measles Virus Vaccine (Live) *on page 984*

♦ **Augmentin®** *see* Amoxicillin and Clavulanic Acid *on page 115*

♦ **Augmentin ES-600®** *see* Amoxicillin and Clavulanic Acid *on page 115*

♦ **Augmentin XR®** *see* Amoxicillin and Clavulanic Acid *on page 115*

♦ **Auralgan® (Can)** *see* Antipyrine and Benzocaine *on page 145*

Auranofin (au RANE oh fin)

Medication Safety Issues

Sound-alike/look-alike issues:

Ridaura® may be confused with Cardura®

U.S. Brand Names Ridaura®

Canadian Brand Names Ridaura®

Therapeutic Category Gold Compound

Generic Available No

Use Management of active stage of classic or definite rheumatoid or psoriatic arthritis in patients who do not respond to or tolerate other agents; adjunctive or alternative therapy for pemphigus

Pregnancy Risk Factor C

Lactation Enters breast milk/contraindicated

Contraindications Hypersensitivity to auranofin or any component; renal disease; history of blood dyscrasias; CHF; exfoliative dermatitis; necrotizing enterocolitis; urticaria, eczema, SLE, bone marrow aplasia, pulmonary fibrosis; history of severe toxicity resulting from previous exposure to other heavy metals; patients who have recently received radiation therapy

Warnings Explain the possibility of adverse reactions before initiating therapy; signs of gold toxicity include decrease in hemoglobin, leukocytes, granulocytes and platelets, proteinuria, hematuria, pruritus, stomatitis or persistent diarrhea; advise patients to report any symptoms of toxicity; therapy should be discontinued if platelet count falls to <100,000/mm^3

Precautions Use with caution and modify dose in patients with renal impairment

Adverse Reactions

Central nervous system: Confusion, hallucinations, seizures

Dermatologic: Dermatitis, pruritus, alopecia, chrysiasis, rash, angioedema, photosensitivity

Gastrointestinal: Diarrhea, loose stools, stomatitis, abdominal cramping, metallic taste, glossitis, ulcerative enterocolitis, GI hemorrhage, gingivitis, dysphagia

(Continued)

Auranofin *(Continued)*

Hematologic: Thrombocytopenia, aplastic anemia, eosinophilia, leukopenia
Hepatic: Elevated liver enzymes, jaundice, hepatitis
Neuromuscular & skeletal: Peripheral neuropathy
Ocular: Conjunctivitis, iritis, corneal ulcers
Renal: Proteinuria, hematuria, nephrotic syndrome
Respiratory: Interstitial pneumonitis, fibrosis, gold bronchitis

Drug Interactions Possible increase of phenytoin serum levels (1 case reported); penicillamine, antimalarials, hydroxychloroquine, cytotoxic drugs, or immunosuppressive agents

Mechanism of Action Unknown, acts principally via immunomodulating effects and by decreasing lysosomal enzyme release; may alter cellular mechanisms by inhibiting sulfhydryl systems

Pharmacodynamics Onset of action: Therapeutic response may not be seen for 3-4 months after start of therapy

Pharmacokinetics

Absorption: Oral: Only about 20% to 25% of gold in a dose is absorbed
Protein binding: 60%
Half-life: 21-31 days (half-life dependent upon single or multiple dosing)
Time to peak serum concentration: Within 2 hours
Elimination: 60% of absorbed gold is eliminated in urine while the remainder is eliminated in feces

Usual Dosage Oral:

Children: Initial: 0.1 mg/kg/day in 1-2 divided doses; usual maintenance: 0.15 mg/kg/day in 1-2 divided doses; maximum dose: 0.2 mg/kg/day in 1-2 divided doses

Adults: 6 mg/day in 1-2 divided doses; after 3 months may be increased to 9 mg/day in 3 divided doses; if still no response after 3 months at 9 mg/day, discontinue drug

Dosing adjustment in renal impairment:

Cl_{cr} 50-80 mL/minute: Reduce dose to 50%
Cl_{cr} <50 mL/minute: Avoid use

Monitoring Parameters CBC with differential, platelet count, urinalysis, baseline renal and liver function tests

Reference Range Gold: Normal: 0-0.1 mcg/mL (SI: 0-0.0064 micromoles/L); Therapeutic: 1-3 mcg/mL (SI: 0.06-0.18 micromoles/L); Urine <0.1 mcg/24 hours

Test Interactions May enhance the response to a tuberculin skin test

Patient Information Notify your physician of pruritus, sore mouth, indigestion, metallic taste; observe careful oral hygiene. May cause photosensitivity reactions (eg, exposure to sunlight may cause severe sunburn, skin rash, redness, or itching); avoid exposure to sunlight and artificial light sources (sunlamps, tanning booth/bed); wear protective clothing, wide-brimmed hats, sunglasses, and lip sunscreen (SPF ≥15); use a sunscreen [broad-spectrum sunscreen or physical sunscreen (preferred) or sunblock with SPF ≥15]; contact physician if reaction occurs.

Additional Information Metallic taste may indicate stomatitis

Dosage Forms Excipient information presented when available (limited, particularly for generics); consult specific product labeling.

Capsule: 3 mg [29% gold]

- **Aurodex** *see* Antipyrine and Benzocaine *on page 145*
- **Aurolate®** *see* Gold Sodium Thiomalate *on page 739*
- **Autoplex® T [DSC]** *see* Anti-inhibitor Coagulant Complex *on page 144*
- **Avagard™ [OTC]** *see* Chlorhexidine Gluconate *on page 337*
- **Avage™** *see* Tazarotene *on page 1501*
- **Avandia®** *see* Rosiglitazone *on page 1406*
- **Avaxim® (Can)** *see* Hepatitis A Vaccine *on page 761*
- **Avaxim®-Pediatric (Can)** *see* Hepatitis A Vaccine *on page 761*
- **Aventyl® (Can)** *see* Nortriptyline *on page 1149*
- **Avinza®** *see* Morphine Sulfate *on page 1082*
- **Avita®** *see* Tretinoin *on page 1567*
- **Axid®** *see* Nizatidine *on page 1145*
- **Axid® AR [OTC]** *see* Nizatidine *on page 1145*
- **Aygestin®** *see* Norethindrone *on page 1148*
- **Ayr® Baby Saline [OTC]** *see* Sodium Chloride *on page 1450*
- **Ayr® Saline [OTC]** *see* Sodium Chloride *on page 1450*
- **Ayr® Saline No-Drip [OTC]** *see* Sodium Chloride *on page 1450*
- **Azactam®** *see* Aztreonam *on page 194*
- **Azasan®** *see* Azathioprine *on page 187*

Azathioprine (ay za THYE oh preen)

Medication Safety Issues

Sound-alike/look-alike issues:

Azathioprine may be confused with azatadine, azidothymidine, Azulfidine®

Imuran® may be confused with Elmiron®, Enduron®, Imdur®, Inderal®, Tenormin®

Azathioprine is metabolized to mercaptopurine; concurrent use of these commercially-available products has resulted in profound myelosuppression.

U.S. Brand Names Azasan®; Imuran®

Canadian Brand Names Alti-Azathioprine; Apo-Azathioprine®; Gen-Azathioprine; Imuran®; Novo-Azathioprine

Index Terms Azathioprine Sodium

Therapeutic Category Antineoplastic Agent, Adjuvant; Immunosuppressant Agent

Generic Available Yes

Use Adjunct with other agents in prevention of transplant rejection; used as an immunosuppressant in a variety of autoimmune diseases such as SLE, severe rheumatoid arthritis unresponsive to other agents, and nephrotic syndrome

Pregnancy Risk Factor D

Lactation Enters breast milk/not recommended

Contraindications Hypersensitivity to azathioprine or any component; pregnancy and lactation

Warnings Chronic immunosuppression increases the risk of neoplasia, particularly lymphoma and skin cancers; mutagenic potential in both men and women; may cause irreversible bone marrow suppression

Precautions Use with caution in patients with liver disease, renal impairment, and those with cadaveric kidneys; modify dosage in patients with renal impairment; reduce dosage to 25% to 33% of usual dosage in patients receiving allopurinol and azathioprine concurrently; discontinue azathioprine therapy in patients with hepatic veno-occlusive disease

Adverse Reactions

Central nervous system: Fever, chills

Dermatologic: Alopecia, erythematous or maculopapular rash

Gastrointestinal: Nausea, vomiting, anorexia, diarrhea, aphthous stomatitis, pancreatitis

Hematologic: Bone marrow depression (leukopenia, thrombocytopenia, anemia)

Hepatic: Hepatotoxicity, jaundice, hepatic veno-occlusive disease

Neuromuscular & skeletal: Arthralgias

Ocular: Retinopathy

Miscellaneous: Rare hypersensitivity reactions which include myalgias, rigors, dyspnea, hypotension, serum sickness, rash

Drug Interactions Allopurinol inhibits the metabolic pathway of azathioprine by inhibiting xanthine oxidase and blocking the conversion of mercaptopurine to inactive products which increases azathioprine's effects; nondepolarizing neuromuscular blockers (decreased blockade); captopril or enalapril in combination with azathioprine has resulted in severe anemia

Stability Reconstituted 10 mg/mL injection is stable for 24 hours at room temperature; stable in neutral or acid solutions, but is hydrolyzed to mercaptopurine in alkaline solutions

Mechanism of Action Antagonizes purine metabolism and may inhibit synthesis of DNA, RNA, and proteins; may also interfere with cellular metabolism and inhibit mitosis

Pharmacokinetics

Distribution: Crosses the placenta

Protein binding: ~30%

Metabolism: Extensive by hepatic xanthine oxidase to 6-mercaptopurine (active)

Bioavailability: ~50%

Half-life:

Parent: 12 minutes

6-mercaptopurine: 0.7-3 hours; with anuria: 50 hours

Elimination: Small amount eliminated as unchanged drug; metabolites eliminated eventually in the urine

Dialysis: Slightly dialyzable (5% to 20%)

Usual Dosage Children and Adults:

Transplantation: Oral, I.V.: Initial: 2-5 mg/kg/dose once daily; maintenance: 1-3 mg/kg/dose once daily

Lupus nephritis: Oral: 2-3 mg/kg/dose once daily

Rheumatoid arthritis: Oral: 1 mg/kg/dose once daily for 6-8 weeks; increase by 0.5 mg/kg every 4 weeks until response or up to 2.5 mg/kg/day

(Continued)

Azathioprine *(Continued)*

Dosing interval in renal impairment:

Cl_{cr} 10-50 mL/minute: Administer every 36 hours or administer 75% of dose once daily

Cl_{cr} <10 mL/minute: Administer every 48 hours or administer 50% of dose once daily

Administration

Oral: Administer with food to decrease GI upset

Parenteral: Administer IVP over 5 minutes at a concentration not to exceed 10 mg/mL; or may be further diluted with NS or D_5W and administered by intermittent infusion over 15-60 minutes

Monitoring Parameters CBC, platelet counts, creatinine, total bilirubin, alkaline phosphatase, liver function tests

Patient Information Response in rheumatoid arthritis may not occur for up to 2-3 months; inform physician of persistent sore throat, unusual bleeding or bruising, or fatigue

Dosage Forms Excipient information presented when available (limited, particularly for generics); consult specific product labeling.

Injection, powder for reconstitution: 100 mg

Tablet [scored]: 50 mg

Azasan®: 75 mg, 100 mg

Imuran®: 50 mg

Extemporaneous Preparations A 50 mg/mL suspension compounded from one-hundred twenty 50 mg tablets comminuted to a fine powder in a mortar with 40 mL of a 1:1 mixture of Ora-Sweet® and Ora-Plus® added and mixed to a fine paste, and then adding the 1:1 mixture of Ora-Sweet® and Ora-Plus® to a total volume of 120 mL, was stable for 60 days at 5°C and 25°C when protected from light. Label "shake well before using" and "protect from light."

Allen LV Jr and Erickson MA, "Stability of Acetazolamide, Allopurinol, Azathioprine, Clonazepam, and Flucytosine in Extemporaneously Compounded Oral Liquids," *Am J Health Syst Pharm*, 1996, 53(16):1944-9.

References

American College of Rheumatology Ad Hoc Committee on Clinical Guidelines, "Guidelines for Monitoring Drug Therapy in Rheumatoid Arthritis," *Arthritis Rheum*, 1996, 39(5):723-31.

Baum D, Bernstein D, Starnes VA, et al, "Pediatric Heart Transplantation at Stanford: Results of a 15-Year Experience," *Pediatrics*, 1991, 88(2):203-14.

Leichter HE, Sheth KJ, Gerlach MJ, et al, "Outcome of Renal Transplantation in Children Aged 1-5 and 6-18 Years," *Child Nephrol Urol*, 1992, 12(1):1-5.

♦ **Azathioprine Sodium** *see* Azathioprine *on page 187*

Azelaic Acid (a zeh LAY ik AS id)

U.S. Brand Names Azelex®; Finacea®

Canadian Brand Names Finacea®

Index Terms Anchoic Acid; Lepargylic Acid

Therapeutic Category Acne Products

Generic Available No

Use Topical treatment of mild to moderate acne vulgaris; treatment of inflammatory papules and pustules of mild to moderate rosacea

Pregnancy Risk Factor B

Lactation Enters breast milk/use caution

Contraindications Hypersensitivity to azelaic acid, propylene glycol, or any component

Warnings Cream and gel contain benzoic acid; benzoic acid (benzoate) is a metabolite of benzyl alcohol; large amounts of benzyl alcohol (≥99 mg/kg/day) have been associated with a potentially fatal toxicity ("gasping syndrome") in neonates; do not use in neonates; *in vitro* and animal studies have shown that benzoate displaces bilirubin from protein binding sites

Precautions Due to isolated reports of hypopigmentation, use cautiously in patients with dark complexions; for topical use only; avoid contact with eyes, mouth, mucous membranes, or open wounds

Adverse Reactions

Dermatologic: Pruritus, erythema, dry skin, rash, peeling, dermatitis, hypopigmentation (vitiligo depigmentation and small depigmented spots), hypertrichosis

Local: Burning, tingling

Respiratory: Worsening of asthma

Miscellaneous: Exacerbation of recurrent herpes labialis

Drug Interactions None known

Stability Store at controlled room temperature.

Mechanism of Action Azelaic acid is a dietary constituent of whole grain cereals and animal products; its exact mechanism of action has not been determined; azelaic acid possesses antimicrobial activity against *Propionibacterium acnes* and *Staphylococcus epidermidis*; normalization of keratinization leading to an anticomedonal effect may also contribute to its clinical activity

Pharmacodynamics

Onset of action: Within 4 weeks

Maximum effect: 1-4 months

Pharmacokinetics

Absorption: ~3% to 5% penetrates stratum corneum; up to 10% found in epidermis and dermis; 4% systemic absorption

Half-life: Adults: 12 hours

Excretion: Primarily unchanged in the urine

Usual Dosage Topical:

Acne vulgaris: Children >12 years and Adults: Apply 20% azelaic acid twice daily in the morning and evening; may reduce to once daily if persistent skin irritation occurs

Rosacea: Adults: Apply 15% azelaic acid gel to affected areas of the face twice daily in the morning and evening

Administration Topical: After skin is thoroughly washed with a mild soap or a soapless cleansing lotion and patted dry, apply a thin film and massage into the affected area. Wash hands following application.

Monitoring Parameters Reduction in lesion size and/or inflammation; reduction in the number of lesions

Patient Information For external use only; avoid contact with eyes, mouth, mucous membranes, or open wounds. Avoid use of alcoholic skin cleansers, tinctures, and astringents, abrasives and peeling agents. Do not apply occlusive dressings; temporary skin irritation may occur when applied to broken or inflamed skin, usually at the start of treatment; report abnormal changes in skin color or persistent skin irritation to the healthcare provider. Gel: Avoid spicy foods, thermally hot foods and drinks, and alcoholic beverages that might cause erythema, flushing, or blushing.

Dosage Forms Excipient information presented when available (limited, particularly for generics); consult specific product labeling.

Cream:

Azelex®: 20% (30 g, 50 g) [contains benzoic acid and propylene glycol]

Gel:

Finacea®: 15% (30 g) [contains benzoic acid and propylene glycol]

Azelastine (a ZEL as teen)

Medication Safety Issues

Sound-alike/look-alike issues:

Optivar® may be confused with Optiray®

International issues:

Optivar® may be confused with Opthavir® which is a brand name for acyclovir in Mexico

U.S. Brand Names Astelin®; Optivar®

Canadian Brand Names Astelin®

Index Terms Azelastine Hydrochloride

Therapeutic Category Antiallergic, Ophthalmic; Antihistamine, Nasal

Generic Available No

Use

Nasal: Treatment of the symptoms of seasonal allergic rhinitis (SAR) and vasomotor rhinitis

Ophthalmic: Treatment of itching of the eye associated with allergic conjunctivitis

Pregnancy Risk Factor C

Lactation Excretion in breast milk unknown/use caution

Contraindications Hypersensitivity to azelastine or any component

Warnings Ophthalmic solution not for use in contact lens-related irritation; preservative in ophthalmic solution may be absorbed by soft contact lenses; wait at least 10 minutes after instillation before inserting soft contact lenses

Precautions Use with caution in asthmatics; patients with hepatic or renal dysfunction may require lower doses

Adverse Reactions

Cardiovascular: Flushing, hypertension, tachycardia

Central nervous system: Drowsiness, headache, somnolence, fatigue, vertigo, depression, nervousness, hypoesthesia

Dermatologic: Contact dermatitis, eczema, hair and follicle infection, furunculosis

Endocrine & metabolic: Weight gain

(Continued)

Azelastine *(Continued)*

Gastrointestinal: Nausea, xerostomia, bitter taste, glossitis, ulcerative stomatitis, aphthous stomatitis, constipation, abdominal pain

Genitourinary: Urinary frequency, hematuria

Neuromuscular & skeletal: Myalgia, hyperkinesia

Ocular: Conjunctivitis, watery eyes, eye pain, transient eye burning/stinging (ophthalmic use)

Respiratory: Nasal burning, paroxysmal sneezing, rhinitis, epistaxis, bronchospasm, coughing, throat burning, laryngitis (nasal use)

Drug Interactions Cytochrome P450 isoenzyme CYP1A2, CYP2C19, CYP2D6, and CYP3A4 substrate (minor); CYP2B6 (weak), CYP2C9 (weak), CYP2C19 (weak), CYP2D6 (weak), and CYP3A4 (weak) inhibitor

May cause additive sedation when concomitantly administered with other CNS depressant medications; may enhance adverse/toxic effects of other anticholinergics; cimetidine may increase serum levels/toxicity

Stability Stable 3 months after opening

Mechanism of Action Competes with histamine for H_1-receptor sites on effector cells in the blood vessels and respiratory tract; reduces hyper-reactivity of the airways; increases the motility of bronchial epithelial cilia, improving mucociliary transport

Pharmacodynamics

Onset of action: 30 minutes to 1 hour

Maximum effect: 3 hours

Duration: 12 hours

Pharmacokinetics

Protein binding: 88%

Metabolism: Metabolized by cytochrome P450 enzyme system; active metabolite desmethylazelastine

Bioavailability: After intranasal administration: 40%

Half-life, elimination: 22 hours

Time to peak serum concentration: 2-3 hours

Elimination: Clearance: 0.5 L/hour/kg

Usual Dosage

Intranasal:

Children 5-12 years: 1 spray each nostril twice daily

Children ≥12 years and Adults: 2 sprays each nostril twice daily

Ophthalmic: Children ≥3 years and Adults: Instill 1 drop into each affected eye twice daily

Administration

Intranasal: Before use, the child-resistant screw cap on the bottle should be replaced with the pump unit and the delivery system should be primed with 4 sprays or until a fine mist appears; when 3 or more days have elapsed since the last use, the pump should be reprimed with 2 sprays or until a fine mist appears

Ophthalmic: Apply finger pressure to lacrimal sac during and for 1-2 minutes after instillation to decrease risk of systemic effects; avoid contact of bottle tip with skin or eye

Patient Information May cause drowsiness and impair ability to perform activities requiring mental alertness or physical coordination; may cause dry mouth

Dosage Forms Excipient information presented when available (limited, particularly for generics); consult specific product labeling.

Solution, intranasal, as hydrochloride [spray]:

Astelin®: 1 mg/mL(30 mL) [contains benzalkonium chloride; 137 mcg/spray; 200 metered sprays]

Solution, ophthalmic, as hydrochloride:

Optivar®: 0.05% (6 mL) [contains benzalkonium chloride]

References

McNeely W and Wiseman LR, "Intranasal Azelastine. A Review of Its Efficacy in the Management of Allergic Rhinitis," *Drugs*, 1988, 56(1):91-114.

♦ **Azelastine Hydrochloride** *see* Azelastine *on page 189*

♦ **Azelex**® *see* Azelaic Acid *on page 188*

♦ **Azidothymidine** *see* Zidovudine *on page 1637*

♦ **Azidothymidine, Abacavir, and Lamivudine** *see* Abacavir, Lamivudine, and Zidovudine *on page 38*

♦ **Azidothymidine, Lamivudine and Abacavir** *see* Abacavir, Lamivudine, and Zidovudine *on page 38*

Azithromycin (az ith roe MYE sin)

Medication Safety Issues
Sound-alike/look-alike issues:
Azithromycin may be confused with erythromycin
Zithromax® may be confused with Zinacef®

Related Information
Endocarditis Prophylaxis *on page 1812*

U.S. Brand Names Zithromax®; Zmax™

Canadian Brand Names Apo-Azithromycin®; CO Azithromycin; Dom-Azithromycin; GMD-Azithromycin; Novo-Azithromycin; PHL-Azithromycin; PMS-Azithromycin; ratio-Azithromycin; Sandoz-Azithromycin; Zithromax®

Index Terms Azithromycin Dihydrate; Zithromax® TRI-PAK™; Zithromax® Z-PAK®

Therapeutic Category Antibiotic, Macrolide

Generic Available Yes: Injection, powder for oral suspension, tablet

Use Treatment of mild to moderate upper and lower respiratory tract infections, community-acquired pneumonia, infections of the skin and skin structure, acute otitis media, and urethritis and cervicitis due to susceptible strains of *C. trachomatis, N. gonorrhoeae, M. catarrhalis, H. influenzae, S. aureus, S. pneumoniae, Mycoplasma pneumoniae, M. avium* complex, *C. psittaci*, and *C. pneumoniae*; treatment of babesiosis; pertussis; endocarditis prophylaxis; treatment of CF lung disease

Pregnancy Risk Factor B

Lactation Enters breast milk/use caution

Contraindications Hypersensitivity to azithromycin, erythromycin, any component, or macrolide antibiotics

Warnings Oral azithromycin should not be used to treat pneumonia that is considered inappropriate for outpatient oral therapy; may mask or delay symptoms of incubating gonorrhea or syphilis so appropriate culture and susceptibility tests should be performed prior to initiating azithromycin; pseudomembranous colitis has been reported with use of macrolide antibiotics; patients who experience allergic reactions to azithromycin may require prolonged periods of observation and symptomatic treatment possibly due to the drug's long tissue half-life

Precautions Use with caution in patients with impaired hepatic function and patients with severe renal impairment (Cl_{cr} <10 mL/minute)

Adverse Reactions
Cardiovascular: Palpitations, chest pain, ventricular arrhythmias, hypotension
Central nervous system: Headache, dizziness, agitation, nervousness, insomnia, fever, fatigue, seizures
Dermatologic: Rash, pruritus, angioedema, photosensitivity, Stevens-Johnson syndrome, toxic epidermal necrolysis
Gastrointestinal: Diarrhea (6%), nausea (2%), abdominal pain (2.5%), vomiting, anorexia, pseudomembranous colitis, pancreatitis, oral candidiasis
Genitourinary: Vaginitis
Hematologic: Anemia, leukopenia, thrombocytopenia
Hepatic: Elevated hepatic enzymes, cholestatic jaundice
Local: Pain at injection site, inflammation
Otic: Ototoxicity
Renal: Nephritis, acute renal failure
Miscellaneous: Anaphylaxis

Drug Interactions Cytochrome P450 isoenzyme CYP3A3/4 substrate; CYP3A3/4 isoenzyme inhibitor (mild)
Aluminum- and magnesium-containing antacids decrease azithromycin peak serum levels by 24%; monitor patients receiving azithromycin and drugs known to interact with erythromycin (ie, theophylline, cisapride, anticoagulants) since there are still very few studies examining drug-drug interactions with azithromycin; azithromycin may increase levels of tacrolimus, phenytoin, ergot alkaloids, alfentanil, astemizole, terfenadine, bromocriptine, carbamazepine, cyclosporine, digoxin, disopyramide, and triazolam; avoid use with pimozide due to risk of cardiotoxicity; nelfinavir may increase azithromycin serum levels (monitor for azithromycin side effects)

Food Interactions Presence of food does not affect bioavailability of the tablet formulation, oral suspension, or the 1 g suspension regimen

Stability Store intact vials of injection, dry powder for oral suspension, and tablets at room temperature.
Oral suspension: After reconstitution, multiple dose oral suspension may be stored for 10 days at room temperature or in the refrigerator.
Injection: After reconstituting 500 mg vial at a concentration of 100 mg/mL, solution is stable for 24 hours at room temperature. If solution is further diluted with a compatible diluent to a 1-2 mg/mL concentration, this solution is stable for 24 hours at room temperature or 7 days if refrigerated.
(Continued)

Azithromycin *(Continued)*

Mechanism of Action Inhibits bacterial RNA-dependent protein synthesis by binding to the 50S ribosomal subunit which results in the blockage of transpeptidation

Pharmacokinetics

Absorption: Oral: Rapid from the GI tract

Distribution: Extensive tissue distribution into skin, lungs, bone, prostate, cervix; CSF concentrations are low; crosses the placenta

Protein binding: 7% to 50% (concentration-dependent and dependent on $alpha_1$-acid glycoprotein levels)

Metabolism: In the liver to inactive metabolites

Bioavailability: Capsule, tablet, oral suspension: 34% to 52%

Half-life, terminal: 68 hours

Time to peak serum concentration: Oral: 2-3 hours

Elimination: 50% of dose is excreted unchanged in bile; 6% of dose is excreted unchanged in urine

Usual Dosage

Oral:

Infants <6 months: Pertussis: 10 mg/kg/dose once daily for 5 days

Children ≥6 months:

Respiratory tract infections: 10 mg/kg on day 1 (maximum dose: 500 mg/day) followed by 5 mg/kg/day once daily on days 2-5 (maximum dose: 250 mg/day)

Otitis media:

Single dose regimen: 30 mg/kg as a single dose (maximum dose: 1500 mg)

Three-day regimen: 10 mg/kg once daily for 3 days (maximum dose: 500 mg/day)

Five-day regimen: 10 mg/kg on day 1 (maximum dose: 500 mg), followed by 5 mg/kg once daily on days 2-5 (maximum dose: 250 mg/day)

Pertussis: 10 mg/kg on day 1 (maximum dose: 500 mg), followed by 5 mg/kg/day once daily on days 2-5 (maximum dose: 250 mg/day)

Children ≥2 years: Pharyngitis, tonsillitis: 12 mg/kg/day once daily for 5 days (maximum dose: 500 mg/day)

Children:

Chancroid: Single 20 mg/kg dose (maximum dose: 1 g)

Uncomplicated chlamydial urethritis or cervicitis:

Children <8 years and ≥45 kg: Single 1 g dose

Children ≥8 years: Single 1 g dose

Primary prevention of disseminated MAC: 5 mg/kg/day once daily (maximum dose: 250 mg/day) or 20 mg/kg (maximum dose: 1200 mg) once weekly given alone or in combination with rifabutin

Treatment and secondary prevention of disseminated MAC: 5 mg/kg/day once daily (maximum dose: 250 mg/day) in combination with ethambutol, with or without rifabutin

Babesiosis: 12 mg/kg/day once daily for 7-10 days with oral atovaquone 40 mg/kg/day divided twice daily

Endocarditis prophylaxis: 15 mg/kg/dose 1 hour before procedure

Children ≥6 years, weight ≥25 kg and Adolescents: CF patients with chronic *Pseudomonas aeruginosa* infection:

≥25 kg to <40 kg: 250 mg on Mondays, Wednesdays, Fridays (MWF). If intolerable side effects occur, decrease dose to twice a week, or if necessary, once weekly.

≥40 kg: 500 mg on Mondays, Wednesdays, Fridays (MWF). If intolerable side effects occur, decrease dose to twice a week, or if necessary, once weekly.

Adolescents ≥16 years and Adults:

Respiratory tract, skin and soft tissue infections: 500 mg on day 1 followed by 250 mg/day once daily on days 2-5

Alternative regimen for bacterial exacerbation of COPD: 500 mg once daily for 3 days

Chancroid or nongonococcal urethritis and cervicitis due to *C. trachomatis*: Single 1 g dose

Urethritis and cervicitis due to *N. gonorrhoeae*: Single 2 g dose

Prevention of disseminated MAC: 1200 mg once weekly alone or in combination with rifabutin

Treatment and secondary prevention of disseminated MAC: 500 mg once daily in combination with ethambutol, with or without rifabutin

Pertussis: 500 mg on day 1 followed by 250 mg once daily on days 2-5

I.V.: Adolescents ≥16 years and Adults: 500 mg once daily for 2 days followed by a switch to oral azithromycin therapy

Administration

Oral: Shake suspension well before use; oral suspension, tablet, or the 1 g suspension regimen formulation may be administered with or without food; do not administer with antacids that contain aluminum or magnesium; azithromycin 1 g oral suspension for a single dose regimen should be prepared by mixing contents of 1 packet with approximately 60 mL of water. Have the patient drink the entire contents immediately; add an additional 60 mL of water, mix, and drink.

Parenteral: Administer infusion at a final concentration of 1 mg/mL over 3 hours; for a 2 mg/mL concentration, infuse over 1 hour; do not infuse over a period of less than 60 minutes

Monitoring Parameters Liver function tests, WBC with differential; monitor patients receiving azithromycin and drugs known to interact with erythromycin (ie, theophylline, digoxin, anticoagulants, triazolam) since there are still very few studies examining drug-drug interactions with azithromycin

Patient Information Report any symptoms of chest pain, heart palpitations, and yellowing of skin or eyes. May cause photosensitivity reactions (eg, exposure to sunlight may cause severe sunburn, skin rash, redness, or itching); avoid exposure to sunlight and artificial light sources (sunlamps, tanning booth/bed); wear protective clothing, wide-brimmed hats, sunglasses, and lip sunscreen (SPF ≥15); use a sunscreen [broad-spectrum sunscreen or physical sunscreen (preferred) or sunblock with SPF ≥15]; contact physician if reaction occurs.

Dosage Forms Excipient information presented when available (limited, particularly for generics); consult specific product labeling.

Note: Strength expressed as base

Injection, powder for reconstitution, as dihydrate: 500 mg

Zithromax®: 500 mg [contains sodium 114 mg (4.96 mEq) per vial]

Injection, powder for reconstitution, as monohydrate: 500 mg

Microspheres for oral suspension, extended release, as dihydrate:

Zmax™: 2 g [single-dose bottle; contains sodium 148 mg per bottle; cherry and banana flavor]

Injection, powder for reconstitution, as monohydrate: 500 mg

Powder for oral suspension, as monohydrate: 100 mg/5 mL (15 mL); 200 mg/5 mL (15 mL, 22.5 mL, 30 mL)

Powder for oral suspension, immediate release, as dihydrate:

Zithromax®: 100 mg/5 mL (15 mL) [contains sodium 3.7 mg/ 5 mL; cherry creme de vanilla and banana flavor]; 200 mg/5 mL (15 mL, 22.5 mL, 30 mL) [contains sodium 7.4 mg/5 mL; cherry creme de vanilla and banana flavor]; 1 g [single-dose packet; contains sodium 37 mg per packet; cherry creme de vanilla and banana flavor]

Tablet, as dihydrate:

Zithromax®: 250 mg [contains sodium 0.9 mg per tablet]; 500 mg [contains sodium 1.8 mg per tablet]; 600 mg [contains sodium 2.1 mg per tablet]

Zithromax® TRI-PAK™ [unit-dose pack]: 500 mg (3s) [contains sodium 1.8 mg per tablet]

Zithromax® Z-PAK® [unit-dose pack]: 250 mg (6s) [contains sodium 0.9 mg per tablet]

Tablet, as monohydrate: 250 mg, 500 mg, 600 mg

References

Drew RH and Gallis HA, "Azithromycin-Spectrum of Activity, Pharmacokinetics, and Clinical Applications," *Pharmacotherapy*, 1992, 12(3):161-73.

Foulds G, Shepard RM, and Johnson RB, "The Pharmacokinetics of Azithromycin in Human Serum and Tissues," *J Antimicrob Chemother*, 1990, 25(Suppl A):73-82.

Nahata MC, Koranyi KI, Gadgil SD, et al, "Pharmacokinetics of Azithromycin After Oral Administration of Multiple Doses of Suspension," *Antimicrob Agents Chemother*, 1993, 37(2):314-16.

Saiman L, Marshall BC, Mayer-Hamblett N, et al, "Azithromycin in Patients With Cystic Fibrosis Chronically Infected With *Pseudomonas aeruginosa*: A Randomized Controlled Trial," *JAMA*, 2003, 290(13):1749-56.

Starke JR and Correa AG, "Management of Mycobacterial Infection and Disease in Children," *Pediatr Infect Dis J*, 1995, 14(6):455-69.

Tiwari T, Murphy TV, and Moran J, "Recommended Antimicrobial Agents for the Treatment and Postexposure Prophylaxis of Pertussis: 2005 CDC Guidelines," *MMWR*, 2005, 54(RR-14):1-16.

"2001 USPHS/IDSA Guidelines for the Prevention of Opportunistic Infections in Persons Infected With Human Immunodeficiency Virus. USPHS/IDSA Prevention of Opportunistic Working Group," November 28, 2001, http://http://www.aidsinfo.nih.gov.

Workowski KA and Levine WC, "Sexually Transmitted Diseases - Treatment Guidelines - 2002," *MMWR*, 2002, 51:1-80.

- ♦ **Azithromycin Dihydrate** *see* Azithromycin *on page 191*
- ♦ **Azmacort®** *see* Triamcinolone *on page 1568*
- ♦ **AZO-Gesic® [OTC]** *see* Phenazopyridine *on page 1244*
- ♦ **AZO-Standard® [OTC]** *see* Phenazopyridine *on page 1244*
- ♦ **AZT™ (Can)** *see* Zidovudine *on page 1637*
- ♦ **AZT, Abacavir, and 3TC** *see* Abacavir, Lamivudine, and Zidovudine *on page 38*
- ♦ **AZT, Abacavir, and Lamivudine** *see* Abacavir, Lamivudine, and Zidovudine *on page 38*

◆ **AZT, ABC, and 3TC** *see* Abacavir, Lamivudine, and Zidovudine *on page 38*
◆ **AZT and 3TC** *see* Lamivudine and Zidovudine *on page 904*
◆ **AZT (error-prone abbreviation)** *see* Zidovudine *on page 1637*
◆ **Azthreonam** *see* Aztreonam *on page 194*

Aztreonam (AZ tree oh nam)

Medication Safety Issues
Sound-alike/look-alike issues:
Aztreonam may be confused with azidothymidine

U.S. Brand Names Azactam®

Canadian Brand Names Azactam®

Index Terms Azthreonam

Therapeutic Category Antibiotic, Miscellaneous

Generic Available No

Use Treatment of patients with documented multidrug resistant aerobic gram-negative infection in which beta-lactam therapy is contraindicated; used for UTI, lower respiratory tract infections, septicemia, skin/skin structure infections, intra-abdominal infections and gynecological infections caused by susceptible *Enterobacteriaceae*, *E. coli*, *K. pneumoniae*, *P. mirabilis*, *S. marcescens*, *Citrobacter* species, *H. influenzae*, and *P. aeruginosa*

Pregnancy Risk Factor B

Lactation Enters breast milk/not recommended (AAP rates "compatible")

Contraindications Hypersensitivity to aztreonam or any component

Warnings Check for hypersensitivity to other beta-lactams (hypersensitivity reactions to aztreonam have occurred rarely in patients with a history of penicillin or cephalosporin hypersensitivity); prolonged use may result in superinfection

Precautions Use with caution and reduce dose in patients with renal impairment

Adverse Reactions
Cardiovascular: Hypotension, transient EKG changes
Central nervous system: Seizures, confusion, fever
Dermatologic: Rash, toxic epidermal necrolysis, urticaria, pruritus
Gastrointestinal: Diarrhea, nausea, vomiting, abdominal pain, pseudomembranous colitis
Hematologic: Eosinophilia, leukopenia, neutropenia, thrombocytopenia, anemia
Hepatic: Elevated liver enzymes, hepatitis, jaundice
Local: Pain at injection site, thrombophlebitis, swelling at injection site
Renal: Elevated BUN and serum creatinine
Miscellaneous: Anaphylaxis

Drug Interactions Avoid antibiotics that induce beta-lactamase production (cefoxitin, imipenem); probenecid and furosemide increases aztreonam serum levels

Stability Reconstituted solution is stable 48 hours at room temperature and 7 days when refrigerated; incompatible when mixed with nafcillin, metronidazole, or cephradine

Mechanism of Action Binds to penicillin-binding protein 3 which produces filamentation of the bacterium inhibiting bacterial cell wall synthesis and causing cell wall destruction

Pharmacokinetics
Absorption: I.M.: Well absorbed
Distribution: Widely distributed into body tissues, cerebrospinal fluid, bronchial secretions, peritoneal fluid, bone, and breast milk; crosses the placenta
V_d:
Neonates: 0.26-0.36 L/kg
Children: 0.2-0.29 L/kg
Adults: 0.2 L/kg
Protein binding: 56%
Half-life:
Neonates:
<7 days, ≤2.5 kg: 5.5-9.9 hours
<7 days, >2.5 kg: 2.6 hours
1 week to 1 month: 2.4 hours
Children 2 months to 12 years: 1.7 hours
Children with cystic fibrosis: 1.3 hours
Adults: 1.3-2.2 hours (half-life prolonged in renal failure)
Time to peak serum concentration: Within 60 minutes after an I.M. dose
Elimination: 60% to 70% excreted unchanged in the urine and partially excreted in feces
Dialysis: Moderately dialyzable
Hemodialysis: 27% to 58% in 4 hours

Peritoneal dialysis: 10% with a 6-hour dwell time

Usual Dosage I.M., I.V.:

Neonates:

Postnatal age ≤7 days:

≤2000 g: 60 mg/kg/day divided every 12 hours

>2000 g: 90 mg/kg/day divided every 8 hours

Postnatal age >7 days:

<1200 g: 60 mg/kg/day divided every 12 hours

1200-2000 g: 90 mg/kg/day divided every 8 hours

>2000 g: 120 mg/kg/day divided every 6 hours

Children >1 month: 90-120 mg/kg/day divided every 6-8 hours

Cystic fibrosis: 50 mg/kg/dose every 6-8 hours (ie, up to 200 mg/kg/day); maximum dose: 8 g/day

Adults:

Urinary tract infection: 500 mg to 1 g every 8-12 hours

Moderately severe systemic infections: 1 g I.V. or I.M. or 2 g I.V. every 8-12 hours

Severe systemic or life-threatening infections (especially if caused by *Pseudomonas aeruginosa*): I.V.: 2 g every 6-8 hours; maximum dose: 8 g/day

Dosing adjustment in renal impairment:

Cl_{cr} 10-30 mL/minute: Reduce dose by 50%; give at the usual interval

Cl_{cr} <10 mL/minute: Reduce dose by 75%; give at the usual interval

Administration Parenteral:

I.V.: Administer by IVP over 3-5 minutes at a maximum concentration of 66 mg/mL or by intermittent infusion over 20-60 minutes at a final concentration not to exceed 20 mg/mL

I.M.: Deep I.M. injection into a large muscle mass such as the upper outer quadrant of the gluteus maximus or lateral part of the thigh

Monitoring Parameters Periodic liver function test

Test Interactions False positive urine glucose (Clinitest®), positive Coombs' test

Dosage Forms Excipient information presented when available (limited, particularly for generics); consult specific product labeling.

Infusion [premixed]: 1 g (50 mL); 2 g (50 mL)

Injection, powder for reconstitution: 500 mg, 1 g, 2 g

References

Bosso JA and Black PG, "The Use of Aztreonam in Pediatric Patients: A Review," *Pharmacotherapy*, 1991, 11(1):20-5.

Stutman HR, Chartrand SA, Tolentino T, et al, "Aztreonam Therapy for Serious Gram-Negative Infections in Children," *Am J Dis Child*, 1986, 140(11):1147-51.

♦ **Azulfidine®** *see* Sulfasalazine *on page 1490*

♦ **Azulfidine® EN-tabs®** *see* Sulfasalazine *on page 1490*

♦ **Babee® Cof Syrup [OTC]** *see* Dextromethorphan *on page 477*

♦ **BabyBIG®** *see* Botulism Immune Globulin (Intravenous-Human) *on page 230*

♦ **Bacid® [OTC]** *see Lactobacillus acidophilus* and *Lactobacillus bulgaricus on page 898*

♦ **Bacid® (Can)** *see Lactobacillus acidophilus* and *Lactobacillus bulgaricus on page 898*

♦ **Baciguent® [OTC]** *see* Bacitracin *on page 195*

♦ **Baciguent® (Can)** *see* Bacitracin *on page 195*

♦ **BaciiM®** *see* Bacitracin *on page 195*

♦ **Baciject® (Can)** *see* Bacitracin *on page 195*

Bacitracin (bas i TRAY sin)

Medication Safety Issues

Sound-alike/look-alike issues:

Bacitracin may be confused with Bactrim®, Bactroban®

U.S. Brand Names AK-Tracin® [DSC]; Baciguent® [OTC]; BaciiM®

Canadian Brand Names Baciguent®; Baciject®

Therapeutic Category Antibiotic, Miscellaneous; Antibiotic, Topical

Generic Available Yes

Use Treatment of pneumonia and empyema caused by susceptible staphylococci; prevention or treatment of superficial skin infections; due to its toxicity, use of bacitracin systemically or as an irrigant should be limited to situations where less toxic alternatives would not be effective; treatment of antibiotic-associated colitis

Pregnancy Risk Factor C

Lactation Excretion in breast milk unknown/use caution

Contraindications Hypersensitivity to bacitracin or any component; I.M. use is contraindicated in patients with renal impairment

Warnings I.M. use may cause renal failure due to tubular and glomerular necrosis; do **not** administer intravenously because severe thrombophlebitis occurs; bacitracin may be absorbed from denuded areas and irrigation sites

(Continued)

Bacitracin *(Continued)*

Precautions Prolonged use may result in overgrowth of nonsusceptible organisms

Adverse Reactions

Cardiovascular: Hypotension, tightness of chest
Central nervous system: Pain
Dermatologic: Rash, itching
Gastrointestinal: Anorexia, nausea, vomiting, diarrhea, rectal itching and burning
Hematologic: Blood dyscrasias
Renal: With I.M. use: Renal tubular and glomerular necrosis, azotemia, renal failure
Miscellaneous: Diaphoresis, edema of lips and face

Drug Interactions Nephrotoxic drugs (increase toxicity), neuromuscular blocking agents and anesthetics (increase neuromuscular blockade)

Stability Sterile powder should be stored in the refrigerator; once reconstituted, bacitracin is stable for 1 week under refrigeration (2°C to 8°C); incompatible with diluents containing parabens

Mechanism of Action Inhibits bacterial cell wall synthesis by preventing transfer of mucopeptides into the growing cell wall

Pharmacokinetics

Absorption: Poor from mucous membranes and intact skin; rapid following I.M. administration
Protein binding: Minimally bound to plasma proteins
Time to peak serum concentration: I.M.: Within 1-2 hours
Elimination: Slow elimination into the urine with 10% to 40% of a dose excreted within 24 hours

Usual Dosage

I.M. (not recommended):
Infants:
≤2.5 kg: 900 units/kg/day in 2-3 divided doses
>2.5 kg: 1000 units/kg/day in 2-3 divided doses
Children: 800-1200 units/kg/day divided every 8 hours
Adults: 10,000-25,000 units/dose every 6 hours; not to exceed 100,000 units/day
Children and Adults:
Topical: Apply 1-5 times/day
Irrigation, solution: 50-100 units/mL in NS, LR, or sterile water for irrigation; soak sponges in solution for topical compresses 1-5 times/day or as needed during surgical procedures
Antibiotic-associated colitis: Adults: Oral: 25,000 units every 6 hours for 7-10 days

Administration

Parenteral: For I.M. administration, pH of urine should be kept above 6 by using sodium bicarbonate; bacitracin sterile powder should be dissolved in NS injection containing 2% procaine hydrochloride; administer I.M. injection into the upper outer quadrant of the buttocks; alternate injection sites
Topical: Apply thin layer to the cleansed affected area. May cover with a sterile bandage. For external use only. Do not use topical ointment in the eyes.

Monitoring Parameters I.M.: Urinalysis, renal function tests

Patient Information Topical bacitracin should not be used for longer than 1 week unless directed by a physician

Dosage Forms Excipient information presented when available (limited, particularly for generics); consult specific product labeling. [DSC] = Discontinued product
Injection, powder for reconstitution (BaciiM®): 50,000 units
Ointment, ophthalmic (AK-Tracin® [DSC]): 500 units/g (3.5 g)
Ointment, topical: 500 units/g (0.9 g, 15 g, 30 g, 120 g, 454 g)
Baciguent®: 500 units/g (15 g, 30 g)

References

Kelly CP, Pothoulakis C, and LaMont JT, "*Clostridium difficile* Colitis," *N Engl J Med*, 1994, 330(4):257-62.

Bacitracin and Polymyxin B (bas i TRAY sin & pol i MIKS in bee)

Medication Safety Issues

Sound-alike/look-alike issues:
Betadine® may be confused with Betagan®, betaine

U.S. Brand Names AK-Poly-Bac™; Betadine® First Aid Antibiotics + Moisturizer [OTC] [DSC]; Polysporin® [OTC]

Canadian Brand Names LID-Pack®; Optimyxin®

Index Terms Polymyxin B and Bacitracin

Therapeutic Category Antibiotic, Ophthalmic; Antibiotic, Topical

Generic Available Yes

Use Treatment of superficial infections involving the conjunctiva and/or cornea caused by susceptible organisms; prevent infection in minor cuts, scrapes and burns

Pregnancy Risk Factor C

Lactation Excretion in breast milk unknown/use caution

Contraindications Hypersensitivity to polymyxin, bacitracin, or any component

Precautions Prolonged use may result in overgrowth of nonsusceptible organisms

Adverse Reactions

Local: Rash, itching, burning, edema

Ocular: Conjunctival erythema

Miscellaneous: Anaphylactoid reactions

Pharmacokinetics Absorption: Insignificant from intact skin or mucous membrane

Usual Dosage Children and Adults:

Ophthalmic: Instill 1/4" to 1/2" directly into conjunctival sac(s) every 3-4 hours depending on severity of the infection

Topical: Apply a small amount of ointment or dusting of powder to the affected area 1-3 times/day

Administration Ophthalmic: Do not use topical ointment in the eyes; avoid contact of tube tip with skin or eye

Patient Information Do not use longer than 1 week unless directed by physician; ophthalmic ointment may cause blurred vision

Dosage Forms Excipient information presented when available (limited, particularly for generics); consult specific product labeling. [DSC] = Discontinued product

Ointment, ophthalmic: Bacitracin 500 units and polymyxin B 10,000 units per g (3.5 g)

AK-Poly-Bac™: Bacitracin 500 units and polymyxin 10,000 units per g (3.5 g)

Ointment, topical: Bacitracin 500 units and polymyxin B 10,000 units per g in white petrolatum (15 g, 30 g)

Betadine® First Aid Antibiotics + Moisturizer: Bacitracin 500 units and polymyxin B 10,000 units per g (14 g) [DSC]

Polysporin®: Bacitracin 500 units and polymyxin B 10,000 units per g (0.9 g, 15 g, 30 g)

Powder, topical:

Polysporin®: Bacitracin 500 units and polymyxin B 10,000 units per g (10 g)

Baclofen (BAK loe fen)

Medication Safety Issues

Sound-alike/look-alike issues:

Baclofen may be confused with Bactroban®

Lioresal® may be confused with lisinopril, Lotensin®

Related Information

Commonly Used Antidotes for Acute Overdoses *on page 1920*

U.S. Brand Names Lioresal®

Canadian Brand Names Apo-Baclofen®; Gen-Baclofen; Lioresal®; Liotec; Nu-Baclo; PMS-Baclofen

Therapeutic Category Skeletal Muscle Relaxant, Nonparalytic

Generic Available Yes: Tablets only

Use Treatment of cerebral spasticity, reversible spasticity associated with multiple sclerosis or spinal cord lesions; intrathecal use for the management of spasticity in patients who are unresponsive to oral baclofen or experience intolerable CNS side effects; treatment of trigeminal neuralgia; adjunctive treatment of tardive dyskinesia

Pregnancy Risk Factor C

Lactation Enters breast milk (small amounts)/compatible

Contraindications Hypersensitivity to baclofen or any component

Warnings Should not be used when spasticity is used to maintain posture or balance; due to the life-threatening complications of intrathecal use, physicians must be adequately trained in its use; physostigmine should be available to reverse life-threatening central nervous side effects (eg, respiratory depression); injection for intrathecal use is not recommended or intended for I.V., I.M., SubQ or epidural administration; abrupt withdrawal of oral baclofen has been reported to precipitate hallucinations and/or seizures. Abrupt discontinuation of intrathecal baclofen regardless of the cause, has resulted in sequelae that include high fever, altered mental status, exaggerated rebound spasticity, and muscle rigidity, that in rare cases, has advanced to rhabdomyolysis, multiple organ system failure, and death. Early symptoms of withdrawal include: Return of baseline spasticity, pruritus, hypotension, and paresthesias. Clinical characteristics of advanced withdrawal may resemble autonomic dysreflexia, sepsis, malignant hyperthermia, neuroleptic-malignant syndrome, and other conditions associated with hypermetabolic state or widespread rhabdomyolysis. Patients at increased risk include spinal cord injuries at T-6 or above, patients with communication difficulties, and history of withdrawal symptoms from oral baclofen. If restoration of intrathecal baclofen is delayed, oral baclofen or benzodiazepine treatment may be used as a temporary measure.

(Continued)

Baclofen *(Continued)*

Precautions Use with caution in patients with seizure disorder, impaired renal function, peptic ulcer disease, stroke, ovarian cysts, psychotic disorders, autonomic dysreflexia (intrathecal therapy)

Adverse Reactions

Cardiovascular: Hypotension, cardiovascular collapse (with intrathecal therapy), chest pain, palpitations

Central nervous system: Drowsiness, fatigue, vertigo, dizziness, psychiatric disturbances, insomnia, slurred speech, headache, hypotonia, ataxia, life-threatening CNS depression (with intrathecal use)

Dermatologic: Rash, pruritus

Gastrointestinal: Nausea, constipation, anorexia, dysgeusia, diarrhea, abdominal pain, xerostomia

Genitourinary: Impotence, urinary frequency, nocturia

Renal: Hematuria

Respiratory: Respiratory failure (with intrathecal administration), dyspnea

Miscellaneous: Diaphoresis

Drug Interactions Increased CNS depression when administered with other CNS depressants (eg, opiates, alcohol, benzodiazepines), tricyclic antidepressants; MAO inhibitors; baclofen may decrease lithium's effect

Mechanism of Action Inhibits the transmission of both monosynaptic and polysynaptic reflexes at the spinal cord level, possibly by hyperpolarization of primary afferent fiber terminals, with resultant relief of muscle spasticity

Pharmacodynamics

Oral: Muscle relaxation effects require 3-4 days and maximal clinical effects are not seen for 5-10 days

Intrathecal:

- Bolus:
  - Onset of action: 30 minutes to 1 hour
  - Maximum effect: 4 hours
  - Duration: 4-8 hours
- Continuous intrathecal infusion:
  - Onset of action: 6-8 hours
  - Maximum activity: 24-48 hours

Pharmacokinetics

Oral:

- Absorption: Rapid; absorption from the GI tract is thought to be dose dependent
- Protein binding: 30%
- Metabolism: Minimal in the liver (15%)
- Half-life: 2.5-4 hours
- Time to peak serum concentration: Oral: Within 2-3 hours
- Elimination: 85% of dose excreted in urine and feces as unchanged drug

Intrathecal:

- Half-life, CSF elimination: 1.5 hours
- Clearance, CSF: 30 mL/hour

Usual Dosage

Oral:

- Children:
  - 2-7 years: Initial: 10-15 mg/day divided every 8 hours; titrate dose every 3 days in increments of 5-15 mg/day to a maximum of 40 mg/day
  - ≥8 years: Titrate dosage as above to a maximum of 60 mg/day
- Adults: 5 mg 3 times/day, may increase 5 mg/dose every 3 days to a maximum of 80 mg/day

Intrathecal: Children and Adults:

- Screening dosage: 50 mcg for 1 dose and observe for 4-8 hours; very small children may receive 25 mcg; if ineffective, a repeat dosage increased by 50% (eg, 75 mcg) may be repeated in 24 hours; if still suboptimal, a third dose increased by 33% (eg, 100 mcg) may be repeated in 24 hours; patients who do not respond to 100 mcg intrathecally should not be considered for continuous chronic administration via an implantable pump
- Maintenance dose: Continuous infusion: Initial: Depending upon the screening dosage and its duration:
  - If the screening dose duration >8 hours: Daily dose = effective screening dose
  - If the screening dose duration <8 hours: Daily dose = **twice** effective screening dose
  - Continuous infusion dose mcg/hour = daily dose divided by 24 hours
  - **Note:** Further adjustments in infusion rate may be done every 24 hours as needed; for spinal cord-related spasticity, increase in 10% to 30% increments/24 hours; for spasticity of cerebral origin, increase in 5% to 10% increments/24 hours

Average daily dose:

Children ≤12 years: 100-300 mcg/day (4.2-12.5 mcg/hour); doses as high as 1000 mcg/day have been used

Children >12 years and Adults: 300-800 mcg/day (12.5-33 mcg/hour); doses as high as 2000 mcg/day have been used

Administration

Oral: Administer with food or milk

Parenteral: Intrathecal: Test dosage: Use dilute concentration (50 mcg/mL) and inject over at least 1 minute; for maintenance infusion via implantable infusion pump, concentrations of 500-2000 mcg/mL may be used; do not abruptly discontinue intrathecal baclofen administration (see Warnings)

Monitoring Parameters Muscle rigidity, spasticity (decrease in number and severity of spasms), modified Ashworth score

Patient Information Avoid alcohol and other CNS depressants; may cause drowsiness and impair ability to perform activities requiring mental alertness or physical coordination; may cause dry mouth; do not abruptly discontinue therapy

Dosage Forms Excipient information presented when available (limited, particularly for generics); consult specific product labeling.

Injection, solution, intrathecal [preservative free]:

Lioresal®: 50 mcg/mL (1 mL); 500 mcg/mL (20 mL); 2000 mcg/mL (5 mL, 20 mL)

Tablet: 10 mg, 20 mg

Extemporaneous Preparations

A 5 mg/mL suspension may be made by crushing thirty 20 mg tablets; levigate with a small amount of glycerin to form a paste. Add simple syrup incrementally to a total volume of 120 mL; shake well; refrigerate; stable 35 days (Johnson, 1993)

A 10 mg/mL oral suspension may be made by crushing one hundred twenty 10 mg tablets; gradually add 60 mL Ora-Sweet® or Ora-Plus® and mix until a uniform paste, then add more vehicle to make a total volume of 120 mL; refrigerate; shake well; stable 60 days (Allen, 1996)

Allen LV Jr and Erickson MA 3rd, "Stability of Baclofen, Captopril, Diltiazem Hydrochloride, Dipyridamole, and Flecainide Acetate in Extemporaneously Compounded Oral Liquids," *Am J Health Syst Pharm*, 1996, 53(18):2179-84.

Johnson CE and Hart SM, "Stability of an Extemporaneously Compounded Baclofen Oral Liquid," *Am J Hosp Pharm*, 1993, 50(11):2353-5.

♦ **BactoShield® CHG [OTC]** *see* Chlorhexidine Gluconate *on page 337*
♦ **Bactrim™** *see* Sulfamethoxazole and Trimethoprim *on page 1487*
♦ **Bactrim™ DS** *see* Sulfamethoxazole and Trimethoprim *on page 1487*
♦ **Bactroban®** *see* Mupirocin *on page 1091*
♦ **Bactroban® Nasal** *see* Mupirocin *on page 1091*
♦ **Baking Soda** *see* Sodium Bicarbonate *on page 1448*
♦ **BAL** *see* Dimercaprol *on page 508*
♦ **Balacet 325™** *see* Propoxyphene and Acetaminophen *on page 1336*
♦ **BAL in Oil®** *see* Dimercaprol *on page 508*
♦ **Balmex® [OTC]** *see* Zinc Oxide *on page 1640*
♦ **Balminil Decongestant (Can)** *see* Pseudoephedrine *on page 1344*
♦ **Balminil DM E (Can)** *see* Guaifenesin and Dextromethorphan *on page 748*
♦ **Balminil Expectorant (Can)** *see* Guaifenesin *on page 745*
♦ **Balnetar® [OTC]** *see* Coal Tar *on page 394*
♦ **Balnetar® (Can)** *see* Coal Tar *on page 394*
♦ **Band-Aid® Hurt-Free™ Antiseptic Wash [OTC]** *see* Lidocaine *on page 933*
♦ **Banophen® [OTC]** *see* DiphenhydrAMINE *on page 509*
♦ **Banophen® Anti-Itch [OTC]** *see* DiphenhydrAMINE *on page 509*
♦ **Baridium® [OTC]** *see* Phenazopyridine *on page 1244*
♦ **Base Ointment** *see* Zinc Oxide *on page 1640*
♦ **Bausch & Lomb® Computer Eye Drops [OTC]** *see* Glycerin *on page 736*
♦ **Bayer® Aspirin Extra Strength [OTC]** *see* Aspirin *on page 163*
♦ **Bayer® Aspirin Regimen Adult Low Dose [OTC]** *see* Aspirin *on page 163*
♦ **Bayer® Aspirin Regimen Children's [OTC]** *see* Aspirin *on page 163*
♦ **Bayer® Aspirin Regimen Regular Strength [OTC]** *see* Aspirin *on page 163*
♦ **Bayer® Genuine Aspirin [OTC]** *see* Aspirin *on page 163*
♦ **Bayer® Plus Extra Strength [OTC]** *see* Aspirin *on page 163*
♦ **Bayer® Women's Aspirin Plus Calcium [OTC]** *see* Aspirin *on page 163*
♦ **BayGam® [DSC]** *see* Immune Globulin (Intramuscular) *on page 817*
♦ **BayGam® (Can)** *see* Immune Globulin (Intramuscular) *on page 817*
♦ **Baza® Antifungal [OTC]** *see* Miconazole *on page 1056*
♦ **BCI-Fluoxetine (Can)** *see* Fluoxetine *on page 681*

♦ **BCI-Gabapentin (Can)** *see* Gabapentin *on page 716*
♦ **BCI-Metformin (Can)** *see* Metformin *on page 1016*
♦ **BCI-Ranitidine (Can)** *see* Ranitidine *on page 1366*
♦ **BCI-Simvastatin (Can)** *see* Simvastatin *on page 1441*
♦ **BCNU** *see* Carmustine *on page 290*
♦ **Bebulin® VH** *see* Factor IX Complex (Human) *on page 635*

Beclomethasone (be kloe METH a sone)

Medication Safety Issues

Sound-alike/look-alike issues:

Vanceril® may be confused with Vancenase®

Related Information

Asthma *on page 1904*

U.S. Brand Names Beconase® AQ; QVAR®

Canadian Brand Names Apo-Beclomethasone®; Gen-Beclo; Nu-Beclomethasone; Propaderm®; QVAR®; Rivanase AQ; Vanceril® AEM

Index Terms Beclomethasone Dipropionate

Therapeutic Category Adrenal Corticosteroid; Anti-inflammatory Agent; Antiasthmatic; Corticosteroid, Inhalant (Oral); Corticosteroid, Intranasal; Glucocorticoid

Generic Available No

Use

Oral inhalation: Long-term (chronic) control of persistent bronchial asthma; **NOT** indicated for the relief of acute bronchospasm. Also used to help reduce or discontinue oral corticosteroid therapy for asthma.

Intranasal: Management of seasonal or perennial rhinitis and nasal polyposis

Pregnancy Risk Factor C

Lactation Excretion in breast milk unknown/use caution

Contraindications Hypersensitivity to beclomethasone or any component; primary treatment of status asthmaticus or other acute episodes of bronchial asthma where intensive treatment is needed

Warnings Fatalities have occurred due to adrenal insufficiency in asthmatic patients during and after switching from systemic corticosteroids to aerosol steroids; several months may be required for full recovery of hypothalamic-pituitary-adrenal (HPA) function; patients receiving higher doses of systemic corticosteroids (eg, adults receiving ≥20 mg of prednisone per day) may be at greater risk; during this period of HPA suppression, aerosol steroids do **not** provide the systemic glucocorticoid or mineralocorticoid activity needed to treat patients requiring stress doses (ie, patients with major stress such as trauma, surgery, or infections, or other conditions associated with severe electrolyte loss). When used at high doses or for a prolonged time, hypercorticism and HPA suppression (including adrenal crisis) may occur; use with inhaled or systemic corticosteroids (even alternate-day dosing) may increase risk of HPA suppression. Acute adrenal insufficiency may occur with abrupt withdrawal after long-term use or with stress; withdrawal and discontinuation of corticosteroids should be done carefully; patients with HPA axis suppression may require doses of systemic glucocorticosteroids prior to, during, and after unusual stress (eg, surgery). Immunosuppression may occur; patients may be more susceptible to infections; avoid exposure to chickenpox and measles. Switching from systemic corticosteroids to inhalation may unmask allergic conditions (such as eczema, conjunctivitis, and rhinitis) that were previously suppressed by systemic steroids. Bronchospasm may occur after use of inhaled asthma medications (see Additional Information).

Precautions Avoid using higher than recommended dosages; suppression of HPA function, suppression of linear growth (ie, reduction of growth velocity), reduced bone mineral density, hypercorticism (Cushing's syndrome), hyperglycemia, or glucosuria may occur. Use with extreme caution in patients with respiratory tuberculosis, untreated systemic infections, or ocular herpes simplex. Use with caution and monitor patients closely with hepatic dysfunction. Rare cases of increased IOP, glaucoma, or cataracts may occur.

Adverse Reactions

Central nervous system: Headache, dizziness, malaise, fatigue, insomnia

Endocrine & metabolic: HPA suppression, Cushing's syndrome, growth suppression, hyperglycemia, dysmenorrhea

Gastrointestinal: Xerostomia, sore throat, pharyngitis, nausea, vomiting, diarrhea, dyspepsia

Local: Growth of *Candida* in the mouth, throat, or nares

Neuromuscular & skeletal: Growth velocity suppression (reported in asthmatic children receiving oral inhalation 2 puffs 4 times/day); muscular soreness, osteoporosis, decreased bone mineral density

Ocular: Cataracts, increased IOP, glaucoma

Respiratory: Cough, sneezing, hoarseness; irritation and burning of the nasal mucosa, nasal ulceration, epistaxis, rhinorrhea, nasal congestion (intranasal use)
Miscellaneous: Immunosuppression, anaphylactoid reactions (rare)

Drug Interactions Cytochrome P450 isoenzyme CYP3A substrate
Interactions similar to other corticosteroids may potentially occur

Stability Do not store near heat or open flame; store QVAR® so inhaler rests on concave end of canister (with plastic actuator on top); use Vanceril® within 6 months after removal from moisture protective package

Mechanism of Action Controls the rate of protein synthesis, depresses the migration of polymorphonuclear leukocytes and fibroblasts, reverses capillary permeability, and stabilizes lysosomal membranes at the cellular level to prevent or control inflammation

Pharmacodynamics
Onset of action:
Oral inhalation: Within 1-2 days in some patients; usually within 1-2 weeks
Nasal inhalation: Within a few days up to 2 weeks
Maximum effect: Oral inhalation: 3-4 weeks

Pharmacokinetics
Absorption: Inhalation: Readily absorbed; quickly hydrolyzed by pulmonary esterases prior to absorption; oral: 90%
Distribution: 10% to 25% of inhaled dose reaches respiratory tract (50% with QVAR®); secreted into breast milk
Protein binding: 87%
Metabolism: In the liver via cytochrome P450 isoenzyme CYP3A to 3 major metabolites: Beclomethasone-17-monopropionate (17-BMP), beclomethasone-21-monopropionate (21-BMP), and beclomethasone (BOH); most active metabolite is 17-BMP
Half-life: Biphasic: Initial 3 hours; terminal: 15 hours
Elimination: Primary route of excretion is via feces; 12% to 15% of oral dose excreted in urine as metabolites

Usual Dosage
Aqueous inhalation, nasal:
Beconase® AQ:
Children 6-12 years: Initial: 1 inhalation in each nostril twice daily; may increase if needed to 2 inhalations in each nostril twice daily; once symptoms are adequately controlled, decrease dose to 1 inhalation in each nostril twice daily
Children ≥12 years and Adults: 1-2 inhalations in each nostril twice daily
Oral inhalation (doses should be titrated to the lowest effective dose once asthma is controlled):
QVAR®:
Children 5-11 years: Initial: 40 mcg twice daily; maximum dose: 80 mcg twice daily
Children ≥12 years and Adults:
No previous inhaled corticosteroids: Initial: 40-80 mcg twice daily; maximum dose: 320 mcg twice daily
Previous inhaled corticosteroid use: Initial: 40-160 mcg twice daily; maximum dose: 320 mcg twice daily
Note: Therapeutic ratio between QVAR® and other beclomethasone inhalers has not been established; when switching to QVAR®, monitor patients for efficacy and adverse effects (see Additional Information)
NIH Asthma Guidelines (NAEPP, 2002; NIH, 1997) [give in divided doses]:
HFA formulation (eg, QVAR®):
Children ≤12 years:
"Low" dose: 80-160 mcg/day (40 mcg/puff: 2-4 puffs/day or 80 mcg/puff: 1-2 puffs/day)
"Medium" dose: 160-320 mcg/day (40 mcg/puff: 4-8 puffs/day or 80 mcg/puff: 2-4 puffs/day)
"High" dose: >320 mcg/day (40 mcg/puff: >8 puffs/day or 80 mcg/puff: >4 puff/day)
Children >12 years and Adults:
"Low" dose: 80-240 mcg/day (40 mcg/puff: 2-6 puffs/day or 80 mcg/puff: 1-3 puffs/day)
"Medium" dose: 240-480 mcg/day (40 mcg/puff: 6-12 puffs/day or 80 mcg/puff: 3-6 puffs/day)
"High" dose: >480 mcg/day (40 mcg/puff: >12 puffs/day or 80 mcg/puff: 6 puffs/day)

Administration
Nasal inhalation: Shake container well before use; gently blow nose to clear nasal passages before administration; occlude one nostril with finger while carefully inserting nasal applicator into other nostril to administer dose
(Continued)

Beclomethasone *(Continued)*

Oral inhalation: Prime canister before use; use a spacer device for children <8 years of age; rinse mouth after use to prevent *Candida* infection. Do not wash or put inhaler in water; mouthpiece may be cleaned with a dry tissue or cloth.

Monitoring Parameters Check mucous membranes for signs of fungal infection. Monitor growth in pediatric patient. Monitor IOP with therapy >6 weeks

Patient Information Notify physician if condition being treated persists or worsens; do not decrease dose or discontinue without physician approval; may cause dry mouth; avoid spraying in eyes; avoid exposure to chicken pox or measles; if exposed, seek medical advice without delay; discard canister when labeled number of metered doses (sprays) have been used. QVAR® may taste differently and have a different feeling during inhalation compared to other inhalers containing chlorofluorocarbons (CFCs).

Oral inhalant: Rinse mouth after inhalation to decrease chance of oral candidiasis; report sore mouth or mouth lesions to physician

Additional Information

Oral inhalation: If bronchospasm with wheezing occurs after use, a fast-acting bronchodilator may be used; discontinue orally inhaled corticosteroid and initiate alternative chronic therapy.

QVAR®: Does not contain chlorofluorocarbons (CFCs), uses hydrofluoroalkane (HFA) as the propellant; is a solution formulation (other beclomethasone inhalers are suspension aerosols); uses smaller-size particles which results in a higher percent of drug delivered to the respiratory tract and lower recommended doses than other products. An open-label, randomized, multicenter, 12-month study in 300 asthmatic children 5-11 years of age indicated that QVAR® provided long-term control of asthma at approximately half the dose compared with a CFC propelled beclomethasone MDI and spacer (see Pederson, 2002). Further studies are needed to define therapeutic ratio between QVAR® and other beclomethasone inhalers.

Aqueous beclomethasone nasal spray (42 mcg/inhalation; 2 sprays in each nostril twice daily for 4 weeks, followed by 1 spray in each nostril twice daily) may be useful in reducing adenoidal hypertrophy and nasal airway obstruction in children 5-11 years of age (Demain, 1995)

Dosage Forms Excipient information presented when available (limited, particularly for generics); consult specific product labeling.

Aerosol for oral inhalation, as dipropionate:

QVAR®: 40 mcg/inhalation [100 metered actuations] (7.3 g); 80 mcg/inhalation [100 metered actuations] (7.3 g)

Suspension, intranasal, as dipropionate [aqueous spray]:

Beconase® AQ: 42 mcg/inhalation [180 metered sprays (25 g)

References

Demain JG and Goetz DW, "Pediatric Adenoidal Hypertrophy and Nasal Airway Obstruction: Reduction With Aqueous Nasal Beclomethasone," *Pediatrics*, 1995, 95(3):355-64.

Expert Panel Report 2, "Guidelines for the Diagnosis and Management of Asthma," *Clinical Practice Guidelines*, National Institutes of Health, National Heart, Lung, and Blood Institute, NIH Publication No. 94-4051, April, 1997.

Kobayashi RH, Tinkelman DG, Reese ME, et al, "Beclomethasone Dipropionate Aqueous Nasal Spray for Seasonal Allergic Rhinitis in Children," *Ann Allergy*, 1989, 62(3):205-8.

"National Asthma Education and Prevention Program. Expert Panel Report: Guidelines for the Diagnosis and Management of Asthma Update on Selected Topics--2002," *J Allergy Clin Immunol*, 2002, 110(5 Suppl):S141-219.

Pedersen S, Warner J, Wahn U, et al, "Growth, Systemic Safety, and Efficacy During 1 Year of Asthma Treatment With Different Beclomethasone Dipropionate Formulations: An Open-Label, Randomized Comparison of Extra Fine and Conventional Aerosols in Children," *Pediatrics*, 2002, 109(6), http://www.pediatrics.org/cgi/content/full/109/6/e92.

Tinkelman DG, Reed CE, Nelson HS, et al, "Aerosol Beclomethasone Dipropionate Compared With Theophylline as Primary Treatment of Chronic, Mild to Moderately Severe Asthma in Children," *Pediatrics*, 1993, 92(1):64-77.

Wyatt R, Waschek J, Weinberger M, et al, "Effects of Inhaled Beclomethasone Dipropionate and Alternate-Day Prednisone on Pituitary-Adrenal Function in Children With Chronic Asthma," *N Engl J Med*, 1978, 299(25):1387-92.

♦ **Beclomethasone Dipropionate** *see* Beclomethasone *on page 200*

♦ **Beconase® AQ** *see* Beclomethasone *on page 200*

♦ **Belladonna Alkaloids With Phenobarbital** *see* Hyoscyamine, Atropine, Scopolamine, and Phenobarbital *on page 800*

Belladonna and Opium (bel a DON a & OH pee um)

U.S. Brand Names B&O Supprettes®

Index Terms Opium and Belladonna

Therapeutic Category Analgesic, Narcotic; Antispasmodic Agent, Urinary

Generic Available Yes

Use Relief of moderate to severe pain associated with rectal or bladder tenesmus that may occur in postoperative states and neoplastic situations; relief of pain associated with ureteral spasms not responsive to non-narcotic analgesics and to space intervals between injections of opiates

Restrictions C-II

Pregnancy Risk Factor C

Lactation Excretion in breast milk unknown/use caution

Contraindications Hypersensitivity to belladonna, atropine, opium alkaloids, morphine, or any component; glaucoma; severe renal or hepatic disease; obstructive uropathy; obstructive disease of the GI tract; severe respiratory depression; convulsive disorders; acute alcoholism; premature labor

Warnings Opium shares the toxic potential of opiate agonists; usual precautions of opiate agonist therapy should be observed; not recommended for use in children <12 years

Precautions Use with caution in patients with cardiac, respiratory, hepatic, or renal dysfunction, severe prostatic hypertrophy, or history of narcotic abuse; use with caution in patients with increased intracranial pressure

Adverse Reactions

Cardiovascular: Orthostatic hypotension, ventricular fibrillation, tachycardia, palpitations

Central nervous system: Confusion, drowsiness, headache, loss of memory, fatigue, ataxia, CNS depression, physical and psychological dependence

Dermatologic: Dry skin, increased sensitivity to light, rash, pruritus, urticaria

Endocrine & metabolic: Decreased flow of breast milk, antidiuretic hormone release

Gastrointestinal: Constipation, dry throat, xerostomia, dysphagia, bloated feeling, nausea, vomiting, constipation, biliary tract spasm

Genitourinary: Dysuria, urinary retention, urinary tract spasm

Neuromuscular & skeletal: Weakness

Ocular: Intraocular pain, blurred vision, photophobia

Respiratory: Dry nose, respiratory depression

Miscellaneous: Diaphoresis (decreased), histamine release

Drug Interactions CNS depressants (eg, alcohol, narcotics, benzodiazepines, tricyclic antidepressants, MAO inhibitors, phenothiazines) may increase effects/toxicity; additive effects with other anticholinergic agents

Food Interactions Avoid ethanol (may increase sedation).

Stability Store at room temperature; avoid freezing

Mechanism of Action Anticholinergic alkaloids act primarily by competitive inhibition of the muscarinic actions of acetylcholine on structures innervated by postganglionic cholinergic neurons and on smooth muscle; resulting effects include antisecretory activity on exocrine glands and intestinal mucosa and smooth muscle relaxation. Contains many narcotic alkaloids including morphine; its mechanism for gastric motility inhibition is primarily due to this morphine content; it results in a decrease in digestive secretions, an increase in GI muscle tone, and therefore a reduction in GI propulsion.

Pharmacodynamics Opium: Onset of action: Within 30 minutes

Pharmacokinetics Metabolism: Hepatic

Usual Dosage Rectal: Adults: 1 suppository 1-2 times/day, up to 4 doses/day

Administration Rectal: Remove from foil; moisten finger and suppository; insert rectally

Patient Information Drug may cause physical and/or psychological dependence; avoid abrupt discontinuation after prolonged use. Avoid alcohol; may cause drowsiness and impair ability to perform activities requiring mental alertness or physical coordination; may cause dry mouth

Dosage Forms Excipient information presented when available (limited, particularly for generics); consult specific product labeling.

Suppository: Belladonna extract 16.2 mg and opium 30 mg; belladonna extract 16.2 mg and opium 60 mg

B&O Supprettes® #15 A: Belladonna extract 16.2 mg and opium 30 mg

B&O Supprettes® #16 A: Belladonna extract 16.2 mg and opium 60 mg

- **Benadryl® (Can)** *see* DiphenhydrAMINE *on page 509*
- **Benadryl® Allergy [OTC]** *see* DiphenhydrAMINE *on page 509*
- **Benadryl® Children's Allergy [OTC]** *see* DiphenhydrAMINE *on page 509*
- **Benadryl® Children's Allergy Fastmelt® [OTC]** *see* DiphenhydrAMINE *on page 509*
- **Benadryl® Children's Dye-Free Allergy [OTC]** *see* DiphenhydrAMINE *on page 509*
- **Benadryl® Injection** *see* DiphenhydrAMINE *on page 509*
- **Benadryl® Itch Stopping [OTC]** *see* DiphenhydrAMINE *on page 509*

- ♦ **Benadryl® Itch Stopping Extra Strength [OTC]** *see* DiphenhydrAMINE *on page 509*
- ♦ **BeneFix®** *see* Factor IX *on page 633*
- ♦ **Beneflur® (Can)** *see* Fludarabine *on page 664*
- ♦ **Benemid [DSC]** *see* Probenecid *on page 1313*
- ♦ **Benoxyl® (Can)** *see* Benzoyl Peroxide *on page 207*
- ♦ **Ben-Tann** *see* DiphenhydrAMINE *on page 509*
- ♦ **Bentyl®** *see* Dicyclomine *on page 490*
- ♦ **Bentylol® (Can)** *see* Dicyclomine *on page 490*
- ♦ **Benuryl™ (Can)** *see* Probenecid *on page 1313*
- ♦ **Benylin® D for Infants (Can)** *see* Pseudoephedrine *on page 1344*
- ♦ **Benylin® DM-E (Can)** *see* Guaifenesin and Dextromethorphan *on page 748*
- ♦ **Benylin® E Extra Strength (Can)** *see* Guaifenesin *on page 745*
- ♦ **Benzac® AC** *see* Benzoyl Peroxide *on page 207*
- ♦ **Benzac AC® (Can)** *see* Benzoyl Peroxide *on page 207*
- ♦ **Benzac® AC Wash** *see* Benzoyl Peroxide *on page 207*
- ♦ **BenzaClin®** *see* Clindamycin and Benzoyl Peroxide *on page 382*
- ♦ **Benzac® W [DSC]** *see* Benzoyl Peroxide *on page 207*
- ♦ **Benzac W® Gel (Can)** *see* Benzoyl Peroxide *on page 207*
- ♦ **Benzac® W Wash** *see* Benzoyl Peroxide *on page 207*
- ♦ **Benzac W® Wash (Can)** *see* Benzoyl Peroxide *on page 207*
- ♦ **Benzagel®** *see* Benzoyl Peroxide *on page 207*
- ♦ **Benzagel® Wash [DSC]** *see* Benzoyl Peroxide *on page 207*
- ♦ **BenzaShave®** *see* Benzoyl Peroxide *on page 207*
- ♦ **Benzathine Benzylpenicillin** *see* Penicillin G Benzathine *on page 1230*
- ♦ **Benzathine Penicillin G** *see* Penicillin G Benzathine *on page 1230*
- ♦ **Benzene Hexachloride** *see* Lindane *on page 939*
- ♦ **Benzhexol Hydrochloride** *see* Trihexyphenidyl *on page 1575*
- ♦ **Benziq™** *see* Benzoyl Peroxide *on page 207*
- ♦ **Benziq™ LS** *see* Benzoyl Peroxide *on page 207*
- ♦ **Benzmethyzin** *see* Procarbazine *on page 1320*

Benzocaine (BEN zoe kane)

Medication Safety Issues
Sound-alike/look-alike issues:
Orabase®-B may be confused with Orinase®

U.S. Brand Names Americaine® [OTC]; Americaine® Hemorrhoidal [OTC]; Anbesol® [OTC]; Anbesol® Baby [OTC]; Anbesol® Cold Sore Therapy [OTC]; Anbesol® Jr. [OTC]; Anbesol® Maximum Strength [OTC]; Benzodent® [OTC]; Cepacol® Sore Throat [OTC]; Chiggerex® [OTC]; Chiggertox® [OTC]; Cylex® [OTC]; Dentapaine [OTC]; Dent's Extra Strength Toothache [OTC]; Dent's Maxi-Strength Toothache [OTC]; Dermoplast® Antibacterial [OTC]; Dermoplast® Pain Relieving [OTC]; Detane® [OTC]; Foille® [OTC]; HDA® Toothache [OTC]; Hurricaine® [OTC]; Ivy-Rid® [OTC]; Kanka® Soft Brush™ [OTC]; Lanacane® [OTC]; Lanacane® Maximum Strength [OTC]; Mycinettes® [OTC]; Orabase® with Benzocaine [OTC]; Orajel® Baby Daytime and Nighttime [OTC]; Orajel® Baby Teething [OTC]; Orajel® Baby Teething Nighttime [OTC]; Orajel® Denture Plus [OTC]; Orajel® Maximum Strength [OTC]; Orajel® Medicated Toothache [OTC]; Orajel® Mouth Sore [OTC]; Orajel® Multi-Action Cold Sore [OTC]; Orajel PM® [OTC]; Orajel® Ultra Mouth Sore [OTC]; Oticaine; Otocaine™; Outgro® [OTC]; Red Cross™ Canker Sore [OTC]; Rid-A-Pain Dental Drops [OTC]; Skeeter Stik [OTC]; Sting-Kill [OTC]; Tanac® [OTC]; Thorets [OTC]; Trocaine® [OTC]; Zilactin®-B [OTC]; Zilactin Toothache and Gum Pain® [OTC]

Canadian Brand Names Anbesol® Baby; Zilactin-B®; Zilactin Baby®

Index Terms Ethyl Aminobenzoate

Therapeutic Category Analgesic, Topical; Local Anesthetic, Oral; Local Anesthetic, Topical

Generic Available Yes: Lozenge, otic drops

Use Temporary relief of pain associated with pruritic dermatosis, pruritus, minor burns, toothache, minor sore throat pain, canker sores, hemorrhoids, rectal fissures; anesthetic lubricant for passage of catheters and endoscopic tubes

Pregnancy Risk Factor C

Lactation Excretion in breast milk unknown/use caution

Contraindications Hypersensitivity to benzocaine, other ester-type local anesthetics, or any component (see Warnings); secondary bacterial infection of area; perforated tympanic membrane (otic formulations only)

Warnings Benzocaine sprays used in the mouth, throat, and other mucous membranes, particularly when using higher concentrations (14% to 25%), have been associated with an increased risk for developing methemoglobinemia; patients with asthma, bronchitis, emphysema, mucosal damage or inflammation at the application site, heart disease, malnutrition, and children <4 months of age may be at greater risk for developing methemoglobinemia; use cautiously or select another product for these patients. Patients with a greater tendency for elevated levels of methemoglobin, eg, G6PD deficiency, hemoglobin-M disease, NADH-methemoglobin reductase deficiency, and pyruvate-kinase deficiency may benefit from products with an alternative anesthetic (eg, lidocaine). Monitor for signs and symptoms of methemoglobinemia including pale, gray, or blue colored skin, headache, lightheadedness, shortness of breath, anxiety, fatigue, and tachycardia. The classical clinical finding of methemoglobinemia is chocolate brown-colored arterial blood. However, suspected cases should be confirmed by co-oximetry, which yields a direct and accurate measure of methemoglobin levels (standard pulse oximetry readings or arterial blood gas values are not reliable). Clinically significant methemoglobinemia requires immediate treatment.

Topical use prior to cosmetic procedures can result in high systemic levels and lead to toxic effects (eg arrhythmias, seizures, coma, respiratory depression, and death), particularly when applied in large amounts to cover large areas and/or left on for long periods of time or used with materials, wraps, or dressings to cover the skin after anesthetic application. These practices may increase the degree of systemic absorption and should be avoided. The FDA is recommending consumers consult their healthcare provider for instructions on safe use prior to applying topical anesthetics for medical or cosmetic purposes. Use of products with the lowest amount of anesthetic with the least amount of application possible to relieve pain is also recommended.

Some products contain tartrazine and benzyl alcohol which may cause allergic reactions in susceptible individuals; large amounts of benzyl alcohol (≥99 mg/kg/day) have been associated with a potentially fatal toxicity ("gasping syndrome") in neonates; the "gasping syndrome" consists of metabolic acidosis, respiratory distress, gasping respirations, CNS dysfunction (including convulsions, intracranial hemorrhage), hypotension and cardiovascular collapse; avoid use of injection in neonates. *In vitro* and animal studies have shown that benzoate, a metabolite of benzyl alcohol, displaces bilirubin from protein-binding sites.

Adverse Reactions

Cardiovascular: Edema, arrhythmias (see Warnings)
Central nervous system: Seizures (see Warnings)
Dermatologic: Angioedema, urticaria
Genitourinary: Urethritis
Hematologic: Methemoglobinemia in infants
Local: Contact dermatitis, burning, stinging, tenderness

Drug Interactions May antagonize actions of sulfonamides

Stability Store at room temperature.

Mechanism of Action Blocks both the initiation and conduction of nerve impulses from sensory nerves by decreasing the neuronal membrane's permeability to sodium ions, which results in inhibition of depolarization with resultant blockade of conduction

Pharmacokinetics

Absorption: Poor after topical administration to intact skin, but well absorbed from mucous membranes and traumatized skin
Metabolism: Hydrolyzed in plasma and to a lesser extent in the liver by cholinesterase
Elimination: Excretion of the metabolites in urine

Usual Dosage Children and Adults:

Mucous membranes: Dosage varies depending on area to be anesthetized and vascularity of tissues
Oral mouth/throat preparations: Do not administer for >2 days or in children <2 years of age, unless directed by a physician; refer to specific package labeling
Otic: 4-5 drops into ear canal; may repeat every 1-2 hours as needed
Topical: Apply to affected area as needed

Administration

Mucous membranes: Apply to mucous membrane; do not eat for 1 hour after application to oral mucosa
Otic: After instilling into external ear canal, insert cotton pledget into ear canal
Topical: Apply evenly; do not apply to deep or puncture wounds or to serious burns

Monitoring Parameters Monitor patients for signs and symptoms of methemoglobinemia such as pallor, cyanosis, nausea, muscle weakness, dizziness, confusion, agitation, dyspnea, and tachycardia; co-oximetry (see Warnings)

Patient Information Consult healthcare provider for safe application practice prior to application; do not eat for 1 hour after application to oral mucosa; do not chew gum while mouth or throat is anesthetized due to potential biting trauma; do not overuse; do not apply to infected areas or to large areas of broken skin
(Continued)

Benzocaine *(Continued)*

Dosage Forms Excipient information presented when available (limited, particularly for generics); consult specific product labeling.

Aerosol, oral spray (Hurricaine®): 20% (60 mL) [dye free; cherry flavor]

Aerosol, topical spray:
- Americaine®: 20% (60 mL)
- Dermoplast® Antibacterial: 20% (83 mL) [contains aloe vera, benzethonium chloride, menthol]
- Dermoplast® Pain Relieving: 20% (60 mL, 83 mL) [contains menthol]
- Foille®: 5% (92 g) [contains chloroxylenol 0.63% and corn oil]
- Ivy-Rid®: 2% (83 mL)
- Lanacane® Maximum Strength: 20% (120 mL) [contains alcohol]
- Solarcaine®: 20% (120 mL) [contains triclosan 0.13%, alcohol 35%]

Combination package (Orajel® Baby Daytime and Nighttime):
- Gel, oral [Daytime Regular Formula]: 7.5% (5.3 g)
- Gel, oral [Nighttime Formula]: 10% (5.3 g)

Cream, oral:
- Benzodent®: 20% (7.5 g, 30 g)
- Orajel PM®: 20% (5.3 g, 7 g)

Cream, topical:
- Lanacane®: 6% (30 g, 60 g)
- Lanacane® Maximum Strength: 20% (30 g)

Gel, oral:
- Anbesol®: 10% (7.5 g) [contains benzyl alcohol; cool mint flavor]
- Anbesol® Baby: 7.5% (7.5 g) [contains benzoic acid; grape flavor]
- Anbesol® Jr.: 10% (7 g) [contains benzyl alcohol; bubble gum flavor]
- Anbesol® Maximum Strength: 20% (7.5 g, 10 g) [contains benzyl alcohol]
- Dentapaine: 20% (11 g) [contains clove oil]
- HDA® Toothache: 6.5% (15 mL) [contains benzyl alcohol]
- Hurricaine®: 20% (5 g) [dye free; wild cherry flavor]; (30 g) [dye free; mint, pina colada, watermelon, and wild cherry flavors]
- Kanka® Soft Brush™: 20% (2 mL) [packaged in applicator with brush tip]
- Orabase® with Benzocaine®: 20% (7 g) [contains ethyl alcohol 48%; mild mint flavor]
- Orajel®: 10% (5.3 g, 7 g, 9.4 g)
- Orajel® Baby Teething: 7.5% (9.4 g, 11.9 g) [cherry flavor]
- Orajel® Baby Teething Nighttime: 10% (5.3 g)
- Orajel® Denture Plus: 15% (9 g) [contains menthol 2%, ethyl alcohol 66.7%]
- Orajel® Maximum Strength: 20% (5.3 g, 7 g, 9.4 g, 11.9 g)
- Orajel® Mouth Sore: 20% (5.3 g, 9.4 g, 11.9 g) [contains benzalkonium chloride 0.02%, zinc chloride 0.1%]
- Orajel® Multi-Action Cold Sore: 20% (9.4 g) [contains allantoin 0.5%, camphor 3%, dimethicone 2%]
- Orajel® Ultra Mouth Sore: 15% (9.4 g) [contains ethyl alcohol 66.7%, menthol 2%]
- Zilactin®-B: 10% (7.5 g)

Gel, topical (Detane®): 7.5% (15 g)

Liquid, oral:
- Anbesol®: 10% (9 mL) [cool mint flavor]
- Anbesol® Maximum Strength: 20% (9 mL) [contains benzyl alcohol]
- Hurricaine®: 20% (30 mL) [pina colada and wild cherry flavors]
- Orajel® Baby Teething: 7.5% (13 mL) [very berry flavor]
- Orajel® Maximum Strength: 20% (13 mL) [contains ethyl alcohol 44%, tartrazine]

Liquid, oral drop:
- Dent's Maxi-Strength Toothache: 20% (3.7 mL) [contains alcohol 74%]
- Rid-A-Pain Dental Drops: 6.3% (30 mL) [contains alcohol 70%]

Liquid, topical:
- Chiggertox®: 2% (30 mL)
- Outgro®: 20% (9 mL)
- Skeeter Stik: 5% (14 mL) [contains menthol]
- Tanac®: 10% (13 mL) [contains benzalkonium chloride]

Lozenge: 6 mg (18s) [contains menthol]; 15 mg (10s)
- Cepacol® Sore Throat: 10 mg (18s) [contains cetylpyridinium, menthol; cherry, citrus, honey lemon, and menthol flavors]
- Cepacol® Sore Throat: 10 mg (16s) [sugar free; contains cetylpyridinium, menthol; cherry and menthol flavors]
- Cylex®: 15 mg [sugar free; contains cetylpyridinium chloride 5 mg; cherry flavor]
- Mycinettes®: 15 mg (12s) [sugar free; contains sodium 9 mg; cherry or regular flavor]
- Thorets: 18 mg (500s) [sugar free]
- Trocaine®: 10 mg (40s, 400s)

Ointment, oral:
Anbesol® Cold Sore Therapy: 20% (7.1 g) [contains benzyl alcohol, allantoin, aloe, camphor, menthol, vitamin E]
Red Cross™ Canker Sore: 20% (7.5 g) [contains coconut oil]
Ointment, rectal (Americaine® Hemorrhoidal): 20% (30 g)
Ointment, topical:
Chiggerex®: 2% (50 g) [contains aloe vera]
Foille®: 5% (3.5 g, 14 g, 28 g) [contains chloroxylenol 0.1%, benzyl alcohol; corn oil base]
Pads, topical (Sting-Kill): 20% (8s) [contains menthol and tartrazine]
Paste, oral (Orabase® with Benzocaine): 20% (6 g)
Solution, otic drops (Oticaine, Otocaine™): 20% (15 mL)
Swabs, oral:
Hurricaine®: 20% (6s, 100s) [dye free; wild cherry flavor]
Orajel® Baby Teething: 7.5% (12s) [berry flavor]
Orajel® Medicated Mouth Sore, Orajel® Medicated Toothache: 20% (8s, 12s) [contains tartrazine]
Zilactin® Toothache and Gum Pain: 20% (8s) [grape flavor]
Swabs, topical (Sting-Kill): 20% (5s) [contains menthol and tartrazine]
Wax, oral (Dent's Extra Strength Toothache Gum): 20% (1 g)

- **Benzocaine and Antipyrine** *see* Antipyrine and Benzocaine *on page 145*
- **Benzodent® [OTC]** *see* Benzocaine *on page 201*

Benzoyl Peroxide (BEN zoe il peer OKS ide)

Medication Safety Issues
Sound-alike/look-alike issues:
Benoxyl® may be confused with Brevoxyl®, Peroxyl®
Benzac® may be confused with Benza®
Brevoxyl® may be confused with Benoxyl®
Fostex® may be confused with pHisoHex®

U.S. Brand Names Benzac® AC; Benzac® AC Wash; Benzac® W [DSC]; Benzac® W Wash; Benzagel®; Benzagel® Wash [DSC]; BenzaShave®; Benziq™; Benziq™ LS; Brevoxyl®; Brevoxyl® Cleansing; Brevoxyl® Wash; Clearplex [OTC]; Clinac™ BPO; Del Aqua®; Desquam-E™; Desquam-X®; Exact® Acne Medication [OTC]; Fostex® 10% BPO [OTC]; Loroxide® [OTC]; Neutrogena® Acne Mask [OTC]; Neutrogena® On The Spot® Acne Treatment [OTC]; Oxy 10® Balanced Medicated Face Wash [OTC]; Oxy 10® Balance Spot Treatment [OTC]; Palmer's® Skin Success Acne [OTC]; PanOxyl®; PanOxyl®-AQ; PanOxyl® Aqua Gel; PanOxyl® Bar [OTC]; Seba-Gel™; Triaz®; Triaz® Cleanser; Zapzyt® [OTC]; Zoderm®

Canadian Brand Names Acetoxyl®; Benoxyl®; Benzac AC®; Benzac W® Gel; Benzac W® Wash; Desquam-X®; Oxyderm™; PanOxyl®; Solugel®

Therapeutic Category Acne Products; Topical Skin Product

Generic Available Yes: Excludes cream, pads, and soap

Use Adjunctive treatment of mild to moderate acne vulgaris

Pregnancy Risk Factor C

Contraindications Hypersensitivity to benzoyl peroxide, benzoic acid, or any component

Warnings Discontinue if burning, swelling, or undue dryness occurs

Precautions For external use only; may bleach colored fabrics; avoid contact with eyes, eyelids, lips, mucous membranes, and highly inflamed or denuded skin

Adverse Reactions
Dermatologic: Contact dermatitis
Local: Irritation, stinging, dryness, peeling, erythema

Mechanism of Action Releases free-radical oxygen which oxidizes bacterial proteins in the sebaceous follicles decreasing the number of anaerobic bacteria and irritating free fatty acids; exerts a keratolytic activity and a comedolytic effect

Pharmacokinetics
Absorption: ~5% through the skin
Metabolism: Major metabolite is benzoic acid
Elimination: In the urine as benzoate

Usual Dosage Children and Adults: Topical: Apply sparingly 1-3 times/day; initially apply for 15 minutes; length of exposure, strength, and frequency of application are increased as tolerated

Administration Topical: Shake lotion before using; cleanse skin before applying; for external use only; avoid contact with eyes and mucous membranes

Additional Information Granulation may indicate effectiveness; gels are more penetrating than creams and last longer than creams or lotions
(Continued)

Benzoyl Peroxide *(Continued)*

Dosage Forms Excipient information presented when available (limited, particularly for generics); consult specific product labeling. [DSC] = Discontinued product

Cream, topical:

BenzaShave®: 5% (120 g); 10% (120 g) [contains sodium coconut sulfate and coconut acid]

Exact® Acne Medication: 5% (18 g)

Neutrogena® Acne Mask: 5% (60 g)

Neutrogena® On The Spot® Acne Treatment: 2.5% (22.5 g)

Zoderm®: 4.5% (125 mL) [contains urea 10%]; 6.5% (125 mL) [contains urea 10%]; 8.5% (125 mL) [contains urea 10%]

Emulsion, topical [cleanser]:

Zoderm®: 4.5% (400 mL) [contains urea 10%]; 6.5% (400 mL) [contains urea 10%]; 8.5% (400 mL) [contains urea 10%]

Gel, topical: 2.5% (60 g); 5% (45 g, 60 g, 90 g); 10% (45 g, 60 g, 90 g)

Benzac® AC [water based]: 5% (60 g); 10% (60 g)

Benzac® W [water based]: 2.5% (60 g); 5% (60 g); 10% (60 g) [DSC]

Benzagel®: 5% (45 g); 10% (45 g)

Benzagel® Wash [water based]: 10% (60 g) [DSC]

Benziq™: 5.25% (50 g)

Benziq™ LS: 2.75% (50 g)

Brevoxyl®: 4% (43 g, 90 g); 8% (43 g, 90 g)

Clearplex: 5% (45 g); 10% (45 g)

Clinac™ BPO: 7% (45 g)

Desquam-E™ [water based]: 2.5% (42.5 g); 5% (42.5 g) [emollient gel]

Desquam-X®: 5% (42.5 g, 90 g); 10% (42.5 g, 90 g)

Fostex® 10% BPO: 10% (45 g)

Oxy 10® Balance Spot Treatment: 5% (30 g); 10% (30 g)

PanOxyl® [alcohol based]: 5% (57 g, 113 g); 10% (57 g, 113 g)

PanOxyl® AQ [water based]: 2.5% (57 g, 113 g); 5% (57 g, 113 g); 10% (57 g, 113 g)

PanOxyl® Aqua Gel [water based]: 10% (42.5 g)

Seba-Gel™: 5% (90 g); 10% (90 g)

Triaz®: 3% (42.5 g) [DSC]; 6% (42.5 g) [DSC]

Triaz® Cleanser: 3% (170 g, 340 g); 6% (170 g, 340 g); 10% (170 g, 340 g)

Zapzyt®: 10% (30 g)

Zoderm®: 4.5% (125 mL) [contains urea 10%]; 6.5% (125 mL) [contains urea 10%]; 8.5% (125 mL) [contains urea 10%]

Liquid, topical: 2.5% (240 mL); 5% (120 mL, 150 mL, 240 mL); 10% (150 mL, 240 mL)

Benzac® AC Wash [water based]: 5% (240 mL); 10% (240 mL)

Benzac® W Wash [water based]: 5% (240 mL)

Benziq™ [wash]: 5.25% (175 g)

Del-Aqua®: 5% (45 mL); 10% (45 mL)

Desquam-X®: 5% (150 mL)

Oxy-10® Balance Medicated Face Wash: 10% (240 mL)

Lotion, topical: 5% (30 mL); 10% (30 mL)

Brevoxyl® Cleansing: 4% (297 g); 8% (297 g) [in a lathering vehicle]

Brevoxyl® Wash: 4% (170 g); 8% (170 g) [in a lathering vehicle]

Fostex® 10% BPO: 10% (150 mL)

Loroxide®: 5.5% (26 mL)

Palmer's® Skin Success Acne: 10% (30 mL) [contains vitamin E and aloe]

Pad, topical:

Triaz®: 3% (30s, 60s); 6% (30s, 60s); 9% (30s)

Zoderm®: 4.5% (30s); 6.5% (30s); 8.5% (30s)

Soap, topical [bar]:

Fostex® 10% BPO: 10% (113 g)

PanOxyl® Bar: 5% (113 g); 10% (113 g)

References

Winston MH and Shalita AR, "Acne Vulgaris: Pathogenesis and Treatment," *Pediatr Clin North Am*, 1991, 38(4):889-903.

♦ **Benzoyl Peroxide and Clindamycin** *see* Clindamycin and Benzoyl Peroxide *on page 382*

Benztropine (BENZ troe peen)

Medication Safety Issues

Sound-alike/look-alike issues:

Benztropine may be confused with bromocriptine

Related Information

Acute Dystonic Reactions, Management *on page 1894*

Commonly Used Antidotes for Acute Overdoses *on page 1920*
Overdose and Toxicology *on page 1916*

U.S. Brand Names Cogentin®

Canadian Brand Names Apo-Benztropine®

Index Terms Benztropine Mesylate

Therapeutic Category Anti-Parkinson's Agent; Anticholinergic Agent; Antidote, Drug-induced Dystonic Reactions

Generic Available Yes: Tablet

Use Adjunctive treatment of parkinsonism; also used in treatment of drug-induced extrapyramidal effects (except tardive dyskinesia) and acute dystonic reactions

Pregnancy Risk Factor C

Lactation Excretion in breast milk unknown/use caution

Contraindications Hypersensitivity to benztropine mesylate or any component; children <3 years of age; patients with narrow-angle glaucoma, pyloric or duodenal obstruction, stenosing peptic ulcers; bladder neck obstructions; achalasia; myasthenia gravis

Precautions Use with caution in hot weather or during exercise; may cause anhydrosis and hyperthermia; increased risk of hyperthermia in alcoholics, patients with CNS disease, and with prolonged outdoor exposure

Adverse Reactions

Cardiovascular: Tachycardia, orthostatic hypotension, ventricular fibrillation, palpitations

Central nervous system: Drowsiness, nervousness, hallucinations, coma

Dermatologic: Dry skin

Endocrine & metabolic: Decreased flow of breast milk

Gastrointestinal: Nausea, vomiting, xerostomia, constipation, dry throat, dysphagia

Neuromuscular & skeletal: Weakness

Ocular: Blurred vision, mydriasis, elevated intraocular pressure, pain

Respiratory: Dry nose

Miscellaneous: Diaphoresis (decreased)

Drug Interactions As an anticholinergic, benztropine may potentiate the CNS depressant effects of CNS depressants; may inhibit the therapeutic response to neuroleptics; central and/or peripheral anticholinergic syndrome can occur when administered with amantadine, rimantadine, narcotic analgesics, phenothiazides, TCAs, quinidine, and antihistamines

Mechanism of Action Thought to partially block striatal cholinergic receptors to help balance cholinergic and dopaminergic activity

Pharmacodynamics

Onset of action:

Oral: Within 1 hour

Parenteral: Within 15 minutes

Duration: 6-48 hours

Usual Dosage

Drug-induced extrapyramidal reaction: Oral, I.M., I.V.:

Children >3 years: 0.02-0.05 mg/kg/dose 1-2 times/day; use in children <3 years should be reserved for life-threatening emergencies

Adults: 1-4 mg/dose 1-2 times/day

Acute dystonia: Adults: I.M., I.V.: 1-2 mg as a single dose

Parkinsonism: Adults: Oral: 0.5-6 mg/day in 1-2 divided doses; begin with 0.5 mg/day; increase in 0.5 mg increments at 5- to 6-day intervals to achieve the desired effect

Administration

Oral: Administer with food to decrease GI upset

Parenteral: I.V. route should be reserved for situations when oral or I.M. are not appropriate

Patient Information May causes drowsiness and impair ability to perform activities requiring mental alertness or physical coordination; may cause dry mouth.

Dosage Forms Excipient information presented when available (limited, particularly for generics); consult specific product labeling.

Injection, solution, as mesylate (Cogentin®): 1 mg/mL (2 mL)

Tablet, as mesylate: 0.5 mg, 1 mg, 2 mg

♦ **Benztropine Mesylate** *see* Benztropine *on page 208*

♦ **Benzylpenicillin Benzathine** *see* Penicillin G Benzathine *on page 1230*

♦ **Benzylpenicillin Potassium** *see* Penicillin G (Parenteral/Aqueous) *on page 1231*

♦ **Benzylpenicillin Sodium** *see* Penicillin G (Parenteral/Aqueous) *on page 1231*

Benzylpenicilloyl-polylysine [DSC]
(BEN zil pen i SIL oyl pol i LIE seen)

U.S. Brand Names Pre-Pen® [DSC]
Index Terms Penicilloyl-polylysine; PPL
Therapeutic Category Diagnostic Agent, Penicillin Allergy Skin Test
Generic Available No
Use Adjunct in assessing the risk of administering penicillin (penicillin or benzylpenicillin) in patients with a history of clinical penicillin hypersensitivity
Pregnancy Risk Factor C
Contraindications Patients known to be extremely hypersensitive to penicillin
Warnings PPL test alone has a sensitivity rate of 76% and does not identify those patients who react to a minor antigenic determinant; does not appear to reliably predict the occurrence of late reactions and patients at risk for anaphylaxis can be missed; PPL test alone is estimated to miss 3% to 6% of penicillin-allergic patients who are at risk for serious or fatal reactions
Adverse Reactions
Dermatologic: Erythema, urticaria
Local: Pruritus, wheal, edema
Miscellaneous: Systemic allergic reactions occur rarely
Drug Interactions Antihistamines, tricyclic antidepressants, and sympathomimetic agents may affect skin response
Stability Store in refrigerator; discard if left at room temperature for longer than 1 day
Mechanism of Action Elicits IgE antibodies which produce type I accelerated urticarial reactions to penicillins
Usual Dosage Children and Adults:
Scratch test: Use scratch technique with a 20-gauge needle to make 3-5 mm nonbleeding scratch on epidermis, apply a small drop of solution to scratch, rub in gently with applicator or toothpick. A positive reaction consists of a pale wheal surrounding the scratch site which develops within 10 minutes and ranges from 5-15 mm or more in diameter.
Intradermal test: Use intradermal test with a tuberculin syringe with a 26- to 30-gauge short bevel needle; a dose of 0.01-0.02 mL is injected intradermally. A control of NS should be injected at least 1½" from the PPL test site. Most skin responses to the intradermal test will develop within 5-15 minutes.

Interpretation:
(-) Negative: No reaction
(+/-) Equivocal: Wheal only slightly larger than original bleb with or without erythematous flare and larger than control site
(+) Positive: Itching and marked increase in size of original bleb
Control site should not exhibit any reaction
Administration Parenteral: PPL is administered by a scratch technique or by intradermal injection. For initial testing, PPL should always be applied via the scratch technique on the inner volar surface of the forearm. Do not administer intradermally to patients who have positive reactions to a scratch test.
Intradermal test: Administer on the upper, outer arm at least several inches below the deltoid muscle
Nursing Implications Always use scratch test for initial testing
Additional Information Hydroxyzine and diphenhydramine should be discontinued for at least 4 days and astemizole for 6-8 weeks before skin testing
Dosage Forms Excipient information presented when available (limited, particularly for generics); consult specific product labeling. [DSC] = Discontinued product
Injection, solution: 6 x 10^{-5} M (0.25 mL) [DSC]
References
Boguniewicz M and Leung DYM, "Hypersensitivity Reactions to Antibiotics Commonly Used in Children," *Pediatr Infect Dis J*, 1995, 14(3):221-31.

Beractant (ber AKT ant)

Medication Safety Issues
Sound-alike/look-alike issues:
Survanta® may be confused with Sufenta®
U.S. Brand Names Survanta®
Canadian Brand Names Survanta®
Index Terms Bovine Lung Surfactant; Natural Lung Surfactant
Therapeutic Category Lung Surfactant
Generic Available No

Use Prevention and treatment of respiratory distress syndrome (RDS) in premature infants

Prophylactic therapy: Infants with body weight <1250 g who are at risk for developing or with evidence of surfactant deficiency

Rescue therapy: Treatment of infants with RDS confirmed by x-ray and requiring mechanical ventilation

Warnings Rapidly affects oxygenation and lung compliance and should be restricted to a highly supervised use in a clinical setting with immediate availability of clinicians experienced with intubation and ventilatory management of premature infants. If transient episodes of bradycardia and decreased oxygen saturation occur, discontinue the dosing procedure and initiate measures to alleviate the condition; produces rapid improvements in lung oxygenation and compliance that may require immediate reductions in ventilator settings and FiO_2.

Precautions Use of beractant in infants <600 g birth weight or >1750 g birth weight has not been evaluated

Adverse Reactions During the dosing procedure:

Cardiovascular: Transient bradycardia, vasoconstriction, hypotension, hypertension, pallor

Respiratory: Oxygen desaturation, endotracheal tube blockage, hypocarbia, hypercarbia, apnea, pulmonary air leaks, pulmonary interstitial emphysema, pulmonary hemorrhage

Miscellaneous: Increased probability of post-treatment nosocomial sepsis

Stability Refrigerate; protect from light; prior to administration warm by standing at room temperature for 20 minutes or hold in hand for 8 minutes; artificial warming methods should **not** be used; unused, unopened vials warmed to room temperature may be returned to the refrigerator within 8 hours of warming only once

Mechanism of Action Replaces deficient or ineffective endogenous lung surfactant in neonates with respiratory distress syndrome (RDS) or in neonates at risk of developing RDS. Surfactant prevents the alveoli from collapsing during expiration by lowering surface tension between air and alveolar surfaces.

Usual Dosage Intratracheal: Neonates:

Prophylactic treatment: Give 4 mL/kg as soon as possible; as many as 4 doses may be administered during the first 48 hours of life, no more frequently than 6 hours apart. The need for additional doses is determined by evidence of continuing respiratory distress or if the infant is still intubated and requiring at least 30% inspired oxygen to maintain a $PaO_2 \leq 80$ torr.

Rescue treatment: Give 4 mL/kg as soon as the diagnosis of RDS is made; may repeat if needed, no more frequently than every 6 hours to a maximum of 4 doses

Administration Intratracheal: For intratracheal administration only. Do not shake; if settling occurs during storage, gently swirl. Suction infant prior to administration; inspect solution to verify complete mixing of the suspension. Administer intratracheally by instillation through a 5-French end-hole catheter inserted into the infant's endotracheal tube. Administer the dose in four 1 mL/kg aliquots. Each quarter-dose is instilled over 2-3 seconds; each quarter-dose is administered with the infant in a different position; slightly downward inclination with head turned to the right, then repeat with head turned to the left; then slightly upward inclination with head turned to the right, then repeat with head turned to the left.

Monitoring Parameters Continuous heart rate and transcutaneous O_2 saturation should be monitored during administration; frequent ABG sampling is necessary to prevent postdosing hyperoxia and hypocarbia.

Dosage Forms Excipient information presented when available (limited, particularly for generics); consult specific product labeling.

Suspension, intratracheal [preservative free; bovine derived]:

Survanta®: 25 mg/mL (4 mL, 8 mL)

- **9-Beta-D-Ribofuranosyladenine** *see* Adenosine *on page 58*
- **Betacaine® (Can)** *see* Lidocaine *on page 933*
- **Betaderm (Can)** *see* Betamethasone *on page 212*
- **Betadine® First Aid Antibiotics + Moisturizer [OTC] [DSC]** *see* Bacitracin and Polymyxin B *on page 196*
- **Betagan®** *see* Levobunolol *on page 925*
- **Beta-HC®** *see* Hydrocortisone *on page 781*

Betaine (BAY tayne)

Medication Safety Issues

Sound-alike/look-alike issues:

Betaine may be confused with Betadine®

Cystadane® may be confused with cysteamine, cysteine

(Continued)

Betaine *(Continued)*

U.S. Brand Names Cystadane®
Canadian Brand Names Cystadane®
Index Terms Betaine Anhydrous
Therapeutic Category Homocystinuria, Treatment Agent
Generic Available No
Use Treatment agent to reduce elevated homocysteine blood levels in homocystinuria; homocystinuria includes deficiencies or defects in cystathionine beta-synthase (CBS), 5,10-methylenetetrahydrofolate reductase (MTHFR), and cobalamin cofactor metabolism (cbl)
Pregnancy Risk Factor C
Lactation Excretion in breast milk unknown/use caution
Contraindications Hypersensitivity to betaine or any component
Warnings Cerebral edema has been reported in patients with hypermethioninemia, including a few patients treated with betaine. Treatment of CBS with betaine may further increase methionine serum levels (due to remethylation of homocysteine to methionine); monitor methionine serum levels in patients with CBS deficiency; maintain methionine levels <1,000 micromol/L.
Adverse Reactions Gastrointestinal: Nausea, vomiting, diarrhea, GI distress
Stability Store at room temperature; protect from moisture
Mechanism of Action Betaine reduces homocysteine blood concentrations by acting as a methyl group donor in the remethylation of homocysteine to methionine
Usual Dosage Oral:

Children <3 years: 100 mg/kg/day divided into 2 doses; increase at weekly intervals in 50 mg/kg/day increments

Children ≥3 years and Adults: 3 g twice daily; doses up to 20 g/day have been needed to control homocysteine plasma concentrations in some patients

Note: Minimal benefit has been shown in patients treated with >150 mg/kg/day or >20 g/day

Administration Oral: Shake bottle lightly before opening; measure prescribed amount with provided measuring scoop and dissolve in 4-6 ounces of water, juice, milk, or formula; administer immediately; do not use if powder does not completely dissolve or gives a colored solution
Monitoring Parameters Plasma homocysteine concentration (should be low or undetectable); plasma methionine (CBS patients)
Additional Information Orphan drug; may only be obtained by contacting Chronimed Inc at 1-800-900-4267; vitamin B_6, vitamin B_{12}, and folate have been helpful in the management of homocystinuria and are often used in conjunction
Dosage Forms Excipient information presented when available (limited, particularly for generics); consult specific product labeling.

Powder for oral solution, anhydrous:

Cystadane®: 1 g/scoop (180 g) [1 scoop = 1.7 mL]

References

Burns SP, Iles RA, Ryalls M, et al "Methylgenesis From Betaine in Cystathionine-Beta-Synthase Deficiency," *Biochem Soc Trans*, 1993, 21:455S.
Devlin AM, Hajipour L, Gholkar A, "Cerebral Edema Associated With Betaine Treatment in Classical Homocystinuria," *J Pediatr*, 2001,144(4):545-8.
Kishi T, Kawamura I, Harada Y, et al, "Effect of Betaine on S-Adenosylmethionine Levels in the Cerebrospinal Fluid in a Patient With Methylenetetrahydrofolate Reductase Deficiency and Peripheral Neuropathy," *J Inherit Metab Dis*, 1994, 17(5):560-5.
Lawson-Yuen A and Levy, HL, "The Use of Betaine in the Treatment of Elevated Homocysteine," *Mol Genet Metab*, 2006, 88(3):201-7.
Matthews A, Johnson TN, Rostami-Hodjegan A, et al, "An Indirect Response Model of Homocysteine Suppression by Betaine: Optimising the Dosage Regimen of Betaine in Homocystinuria," *Br J Clin Pharmacol*, 2002, 54(2):140-6.
Smolin LA, Benevenga NJ, and Berlow S, "The Use of Betaine for the Treatment of Homocystinuria," *J Pediatr*, 1981, 99:467-72.

♦ **Betaine Anhydrous** *see* Betaine *on page 211*
♦ **Betaject™ (Can)** *see* Betamethasone *on page 212*
♦ **Betaloc® (Can)** *see* Metoprolol *on page 1046*
♦ **Betaloc® Durules® (Can)** *see* Metoprolol *on page 1046*

Betamethasone (bay ta METH a sone)

Medication Safety Issues

Sound-alike/look-alike issues:

Luxiq® may be confused with Lasix®

International issues:

Beta-Val® may be confused with Betanol® which is a brand name for metipranolol in Monaco

Related Information

Corticosteroids, Topical: Guidelines for Selection and Use *on page 1686*

U.S. Brand Names Beta-Val®; Celestone®; Celestone® Soluspan®; Diprolene®; Diprolene® AF; Luxiq®

Canadian Brand Names Betaderm; Betaject™; Betnesol®; Betnovate®; Celestone® Soluspan®; Diprolene® Glycol; Diprosone®; Ectosone; Prevex® B; Taro-Sone®; Topilene®; Topisone®; Valisone® Scalp Lotion

Index Terms Betamethasone Dipropionate; Betamethasone Dipropionate, Augmented; Betamethasone Sodium Phosphate; Betamethasone Valerate; Flubenisolone

Therapeutic Category Adrenal Corticosteroid; Anti-inflammatory Agent; Corticosteroid, Systemic; Corticosteroid, Topical; Glucocorticoid

Generic Available Yes: Excludes aerosol, injection, solution

Use Anti-inflammatory; immunosuppressant agent; corticosteroid replacement therapy

Topical: Inflammatory dermatoses such as psoriasis, seborrheic or atopic dermatitis, neurodermatitis, inflammatory phase of xerosis, late phase of allergic dermatitis or irritant dermatitis; Foam: Inflammatory and pruritic symptoms of scalp dermatoses responsive to corticosteroids

Pregnancy Risk Factor C

Lactation Excretion in breast milk unknown/use caution

Contraindications Hypersensitivity to betamethasone or any component; systemic fungal infections

Warnings Hypothalamic-pituitary-adrenal (HPA) axis suppression may occur; acute adrenal insufficiency (adrenal crisis) may occur with abrupt withdrawal after long-term use or with stress; withdrawal or discontinuation of corticosteroids should be done carefully; patients with HPA axis suppression may require increased doses of systemic glucocorticosteroids prior to, during, and after unusual stress (eg, surgery). Immunosuppression may occur; patients may be more susceptible to infection; avoid exposure to chicken pox and measles. Corticosteroids may mask signs of infection. Corticosteroids may activate latent opportunistic infections or exacerbate systemic fungal infections. May cause osteoporosis (at any age) or inhibition of bone growth in pediatric patients. Acute myopathy may occur with high doses, elevated IOP may occur (especially with prolonged use), CNS effects (ranging from euphoria to psychosis) may occur. Rare cases of anaphylactoid reactions have been reported with corticosteroids.

Topical: Infants and small children may be more susceptible to HPA axis suppression from topical corticosteroid therapy; systemic effects may occur when used on large areas of the body, denuded areas, for prolonged periods of time, or with an occlusive dressing; do not use in diaper area or with occlusive dressings, especially on weeping or exudative lesions; discontinue if skin irritation or contact dermatitis occurs; do not use very high potency topical products for the treatment of rosacea or perioral dermatitis (see Additional Information).

Oral solution contains propylene glycol and sodium benzoate; benzoic acid (benzoate) is a metabolite of benzyl alcohol; large amounts of benzyl alcohol (≥99 mg/kg/day) have been associated with a potentially fatal toxicity ("gasping syndrome") in neonates; the "gasping syndrome" consists of metabolic acidosis, respiratory distress, gasping respirations, CNS dysfunction (including convulsions, intracranial hemorrhage), hypotension and cardiovascular collapse; avoid use of betamethasone products containing sodium benzoate in neonates; *in vitro* and animal studies have shown that benzoate displaces bilirubin from protein binding sites

Precautions Avoid using higher than recommended doses; suppression of HPA axis, suppression of linear growth (ie, reduction of growth velocity), reduced bone mineral density, hypercorticism (Cushing's syndrome), hyperglycemia, or glucosuria may occur; titrate to lowest effective dose. Reduction in growth velocity may occur when corticosteroids are administered to pediatric patients by any route (monitor growth). Use with extreme caution in patients with respiratory tuberculosis, untreated systemic infections, or ocular herpes simplex; use with caution in patients with thyroid dysfunction, cirrhosis, nonspecific ulcerative colitis, hypertension, renal impairment, osteoporosis, thromboembolic tendencies, CHF, recent MI, convulsive disorders, myasthenia gravis, thrombophlebitis, peptic ulcer, diabetes, glaucoma, cataracts, or hepatic impairment. Prolonged use may result in cataracts or glaucoma.

Use topical products sparingly in children, systemic effects may be seen; **Note:** Due to the high incidence of developing adrenal suppression, augmented topical products (eg, Diprolene® AF cream, Diprolene® lotion) are not recommended for use in children ≤12 years of age (see Additional Information). Foam is not recommended for children <16 years.

Adverse Reactions

Cardiovascular: Edema, hypertension, CHF

(Continued)

Betamethasone *(Continued)*

Central nervous system: Convulsions, vertigo, confusion, headache, psychoses, pseudotumor cerebri, euphoria, insomnia, intracranial hypertension, nervousness

Dermatologic: Thin fragile skin, hyperpigmentation or hypopigmentation, acne, impaired wound healing, skin atrophy (bruising, shininess, telangiectasia, thinness, loss of skin markings), erythema, rash, dry skin

Endocrine & metabolic: HPA suppression, Cushingoid state, sodium and water retention, growth suppression, glucose intolerance, hypokalemia

Gastrointestinal: Peptic ulcer, nausea, vomiting

Local: Burning, itching, stinging, sterile abscess, irritation, erythema, folliculitis, vesiculation, acneform eruptions, contact dermatitis

Neuromuscular & skeletal: Muscle weakness, decreased bone mineral density, osteoporosis, fractures

Ocular: Cataracts, elevated IOP, glaucoma

Miscellaneous: Immunosuppression, anaphylactoid reactions (rare)

Drug Interactions Cytochrome P450 isoenzyme CYP3A substrate

Barbiturates, phenytoin and rifampin will decrease corticosteroid effects; salicylates; NSAIDs; diuretics (potassium depleting); caffeine and alcohol may increase risk for GI ulcer; with systemic use: Live virus vaccines (increase risk of viral infection), vaccines may have decreased effects

Food Interactions Systemic use of corticosteroids may require a diet with increased potassium, vitamins A, B_6, C, D, folate, calcium, zinc, and phosphorus and decreased sodium

Stability Store at controlled room temperature; foam canister is flammable; avoid fire, flame, heat; do not store at >120°F (49°C)

Mechanism of Action Controls the rate of protein synthesis, depresses the migration of polymorphonuclear leukocytes and fibroblasts, reverses capillary permeability, and causes lysosomal stabilization at the cellular level to prevent or control inflammation

Pharmacokinetics

Protein binding: 64%

Metabolism: Hepatic

Elimination: <5% of dose excreted renally as unchanged drug; small amounts eliminated via biliary tract

Usual Dosage Base dosage on severity of disease and patient response

I.M.:

Children: Use lowest dose listed as initial dose for adrenocortical insufficiency (physiologic replacement); 0.0175-0.125 mg base/kg/day divided every 6-12 hours **or** 0.5-7.5 mg base/m^2/day divided every 6-12 hours

Adolescents and Adults: 0.6-9 mg/day divided every 12-24 hours

Oral:

Children: Use lowest dose listed as initial dose for adrenocortical insufficiency (physiologic replacement); 0.0175-0.25 mg/kg/day divided every 6-8 hours **or** 0.5-7.5 mg/m^2/day divided every 6-8 hours

Adolescents and Adults: 2.4-4.8 mg/day in 2-4 doses; range: 0.6-7.2 mg/day

Topical: Use smallest amount for shortest period of time to avoid HPA suppression; discontinue use once control is achieved; reassess diagnosis if no improvement is seen within 2 weeks

Children and Adults: Apply thin film 1-2 times/day (see Precautions and Additional Information)

Adolescents ≥13 years and Adults:

Diprolene® AF cream: Apply thin film 1-2 times/day; maximum: 45 g of cream/week; do not use >2 weeks

Diprolene® Lotion: Apply a few drops once or twice daily; maximum: 50 mL/week; do not use >2 weeks

Diprolene® Gel: Apply thin film once or twice daily; maximum: 50 g/week; do not use >2 weeks

Adolescents ≥16 years and Adults: Luxiq® foam: Apply twice daily (in morning and at night)

Administration

Oral: Administer with food to decrease GI effects

Parenteral: Do not administer injectable suspension I.V.; shake injectable suspension before use

Topical: Apply sparingly, rub in gently until it disappears; do not apply to face, axillae, or inguinal areas; not for use on broken skin, in areas of infection, or in diaper area. Do not apply to wet skin unless directed; do not cover with occlusive dressing.

Foam: Invert can, dispense small amount of foam onto saucer or other cool surface; foam will melt upon contact with warm skin (do not dispense directly into hands); use fingers to apply small amounts of foam to affected scalp area; rub in gently until it disappears; avoid fire, flame, or smoking during use; contents of can are flammable and under pressure

Test Interactions Skin tests

Patient Information

Systemic use: Avoid alcohol and caffeine; do not decrease dose or discontinue without physician's approval

Topical use: Avoid contact with eyes; do not use occlusive dressings or other corticosteroid-containing products unless directed by physician

Additional Information Long-acting corticosteroid with minimal or no sodium-retaining potential. Topical products: Very high potency: Augmented betamethasone dipropionate ointment and lotion; high potency: Augmented betamethasone dipropionate cream and betamethasone dipropionate cream and ointment; intermediate potency: Betamethasone dipropionate lotion and betamethasone valerate cream. Topical products labeled as augmented use a vehicle that augments (increases) the penetration of the drug into the skin.

Several recent studies conducted in children ≤12 years of age with atopic dermatitis demonstrated a high incidence of adrenal suppression when topical betamethasone products were applied twice daily for 2-3 weeks. Adrenal suppression occurred in 19 of 60 (32%) evaluable patients (3 months to 12 years of age) using Diprolene® AF cream 0.05%. A higher percent incidence of adrenal suppression was noted in younger children and infants (see product package insert). Pediatric patients may be more susceptible to adrenal suppression and other systemic side effects of topical corticosteroids, due to their larger skin surface area to body weight ratio. The smallest effective dose of topical corticosteroids should be used in pediatric patients.

Dosage Forms Excipient information presented when available (limited, particularly for generics); consult specific product labeling.

Note: Potency expressed as betamethasone base.

Aerosol, topical, as valerate [foam]:

Luxiq®: 0.12% (50 g, 100 g, 150 g) [strength expressed as salt; contains ethanol 60.4%]

Cream, topical, as dipropionate: 0.05% (15 g, 45 g)

Cream, topical, as dipropionate augmented: 0.05% (15 g, 50 g)

Diprolene® AF: 0.05% (15 g, 50 g)

Cream, topical, as valerate (Beta-Val®): 0.1% (15 g, 45 g)

Beta-Val®: 0.1% (15 g, 45 g)

Gel, topical, as dipropionate augmented: 0.05% (15 g, 50 g)

Injection, suspension:

Celestone® Soluspan®: Betamethasone sodium phosphate 3 mg and betamethasone acetate 3 mg per 1 mL (5 mL) [6 mg/mL]

Lotion, topical, as dipropionate: 0.05% (60 mL)

Lotion, topical, as dipropionate augmented:

Diprolene®: 0.05% (30 mL, 60 mL)

Lotion, topical, as valerate: 0.1% (60 mL)

Beta-Val®: 0.1% (60 mL)

Ointment, topical, as dipropionate: 0.05% (15 g, 45 g)

Ointment, topical, as dipropionate augmented: 0.05% (15 g, 50 g)

Diprolene®: 0.05% (15 g, 50 g)

Ointment, topical, as valerate: 0.1% (15 g, 45 g)

Solution, as base:

Celestone®: 0.6 mg/5 mL (118 mL) [contains alcohol and sodium benzoate; cherry-orange flavor]

♦ **Betamethasone Dipropionate** *see* Betamethasone *on page 212*

♦ **Betamethasone Dipropionate, Augmented** *see* Betamethasone *on page 212*

♦ **Betamethasone Sodium Phosphate** *see* Betamethasone *on page 212*

♦ **Betamethasone Valerate** *see* Betamethasone *on page 212*

♦ **Betapace®** *see* Sotalol *on page 1463*

♦ **Betapace AF®** *see* Sotalol *on page 1463*

♦ **Betasept® [OTC]** *see* Chlorhexidine Gluconate *on page 337*

♦ **Betatar® Gel [OTC]** *see* Coal Tar *on page 394*

♦ **Beta-Val®** *see* Betamethasone *on page 212*

♦ **Betaxin® (Can)** *see* Thiamine *on page 1526*

Bethanechol (be THAN e kole)

Medication Safety Issues

Sound-alike/look-alike issues:

Bethanechol may be confused with betaxolol

(Continued)

Bethanechol *(Continued)*

U.S. Brand Names Urecholine®

Canadian Brand Names Duvoid®; Myotonachol®; PMS-Bethanechol

Index Terms Bethanechol Chloride

Therapeutic Category Cholinergic Agent

Generic Available Yes

Use Treatment of nonobstructive urinary retention and retention due to neurogenic bladder; gastroesophageal reflux

Pregnancy Risk Factor C

Lactation Excretion in breast milk unknown/contraindicated

Contraindications Hypersensitivity to bethanechol chloride or any component; do not use in patients with mechanical obstruction of the GI or GU tract; do not use in patients with hyperthyroidism, peptic ulcer, bronchial asthma, or cardiac disease

Adverse Reactions

Cardiovascular: Hypotension, cardiac arrest, flushed skin (vasomotor response)
Central nervous system: Headache
Gastrointestinal: Abdominal cramps, diarrhea, nausea, vomiting, salivation
Genitourinary: Urinary frequency
Hepatic: Elevated liver enzymes, elevated bilirubin
Ocular: Miosis, lacrimation
Respiratory: Bronchial constriction
Miscellaneous: Diaphoresis

Drug Interactions Ganglionic blockers may cause a critical fall in blood pressure; additive effects with other cholinergic agents; quinidine, and procainamide decrease the effects of bethanechol; anticholinergic agents (atropine, antihistamines, TCAs, phenothiazine) may decrease bethanechol's effects

Mechanism of Action Stimulates cholinergic receptors in the smooth muscle of the urinary bladder and GI tract resulting in increased peristalsis, increased GI and pancreatic secretions, bladder muscle contraction, and increased ureteral peristaltic waves

Pharmacodynamics

Onset of action: Oral: 30-90 minutes
Duration: Oral: Up to 6 hours

Pharmacokinetics

Absorption: Oral: Variable
Metabolic fate and excretion have not been determined

Usual Dosage Oral:

Children:

Abdominal distention or urinary retention: 0.6 mg/kg/day divided 3-4 times/day
Gastroesophageal reflux: 0.1-0.2 mg/kg/dose or 3 mg/m^2/dose given 30 minutes to 1 hour before each meal to a maximum of 4 times/day

Adults: 10-50 mg 2-4 times/day

Administration Oral: Administer on an empty stomach to reduce nausea and vomiting

Patient Information Dizziness, lightheadedness, or fainting may occur especially when getting up from a lying position

Dosage Forms Excipient information presented when available (limited, particularly for generics); consult specific product labeling.

Tablet, as chloride: 5 mg, 10 mg, 25 mg, 50 mg

Extemporaneous Preparations

A 1 mg/mL solution may be made by crushing twelve 10 mg tablets; add sterile water in increments to a total volume of 120 mL; shake well; refrigerate; stable for 30 days (Schlatter, 1997).

A 5 mg/mL suspension may be made by crushing twelve 50 mg tablets; add to a total volume of 120 mL of a 1:1 mixture of Ora-Plus®:Ora-Sweet® or Ora-Plus®:Ora-Sweet® SF or 1:4 concentrated cherry syrup and simple syrup, NF mixture; stable 60 days refrigerated (preferred) or at room temperature; label "shake well" and protect from light (Allen, 1998; Nahata, 2004).

Allen LV Jr and Erickson MA, "Stability of Bethanechol Chloride, Pyrazinamide, Quinidine Sulfate, Rifampin, and Tetracycline Hydrochloride in Extemporaneously Compounded Oral Liquids," *Am J Health Syst Pharm*, 1998, 55(17):1804-9.

Nahata, MC, Pai VB, and Hipple TF, *Pediatric Drug Formulations*, 5th ed, Cincinnati, OH: Harvey Whitney Books Co, 2004.

Schlatter JL and Saulnier JL, "Bethanechol Chloride Oral Solutions: Stability and Use in Infants," *Ann Pharmacother*, 1997, 31(3):294-6.

♦ **Bethanechol Chloride** *see* Bethanechol *on page 215*
♦ **Betimol®** *see* Timolol *on page 1542*
♦ **Betnesol® (Can)** *see* Betamethasone *on page 212*

♦ **Betnovate® (Can)** *see* Betamethasone *on page 212*
♦ **Biaxin®** *see* Clarithromycin *on page 375*
♦ **Biaxin® XL** *see* Clarithromycin *on page 375*
♦ **Bicillin® L-A** *see* Penicillin G Benzathine *on page 1230*
♦ **BiCNU®** *see* Carmustine *on page 290*
♦ **BIG-IV** *see* Botulism Immune Globulin (Intravenous-Human) *on page 230*
♦ **Biltricide®** *see* Praziquantel *on page 1302*
♦ **Biobase™ (Can)** *see* Ethyl Alcohol *on page 619*
♦ **Biobase-G™ (Can)** *see* Ethyl Alcohol *on page 619*
♦ **Biocef®** *see* Cephalexin *on page 324*
♦ **BioQuin® Durules™ (Can)** *see* Quinidine *on page 1356*
♦ **Bio-Statin®** *see* Nystatin *on page 1156*

Biotin (BYE oh tin)

Index Terms Coenzyme R; Vitamin Bw; Vitamin H

Therapeutic Category Biotinidase Deficiency, Treatment Agent; Nutritional Supplement; Vitamin, Water Soluble

Use Treatment of primary biotinidase deficiency; nutritional biotin deficiency; component of the vitamin B complex

Contraindications Hypersensitivity to biotin or any component

Food Interactions Large amounts of raw egg whites prevent biotin absorption

Mechanism of Action A member of the B-complex group of vitamins; biotin is required for various metabolic functions such as gluconeogenesis, lipogenesis, fatty acid biosynthesis, propionate metabolism, and the catabolism of branched-chain amino acids; there are 9 known biotin-dependent enzymes; the enzyme biotinidase regenerates biotin in the body and is also required for the release of dietary protein-bound biotin.

Biotinidase deficiency is an autosomal recessively inherited metabolic disorder characterized by deficient activity of the enzyme in serum. Children with the disorder usually exhibit seizures, hypotonia, ataxia, skin rash, alopecia, metabolic ketoacidosis, and organic aciduria.

Usual Dosage Oral:

RDA: Infants, Children, and Adults: There is no official RDA, however 100-200 mcg/day is considered adequate

Biotinidase deficiency: Neonates, Infants, Children, and Adults: 5-10 mg once daily

Biotin deficiency: Children and Adults: 5-20 mg once daily

Administration Oral: May be administered without regard to meals

Reference Range Serum biotinidase activity

Dosage Forms Capsule: 1 mg

References

McVoy JR, Levy HL, Lawler M, et al, "Partial Biotinidase Deficiency: Clinical and Biochemical Features," 1990, *J Pediatr*, 116(1):78-83.

Salbert BA, Pellock JM, and Wolf B, "Characterization of Seizures Associated With Biotinidase Deficiency," *Neurology*, 1993, 43(7):1351-5.

Wastell HJ, Bartlett K, Dale G, et al, "Biotinidase Deficiency: A Survey of 10 Cases," *Arch Dis Child*, 1988, 63(10):1244-9.

♦ **Biphentin® (Can)** *see* Methylphenidate *on page 1034*
♦ **Bisac-Evac™ [OTC]** *see* Bisacodyl *on page 217*

Bisacodyl (bis a KOE dil)

Medication Safety Issues

Sound-alike/look-alike issues:

Doxidan® may be confused with doxepin

Modane® may be confused with Matulane®, Moban®

U.S. Brand Names Alophen® [OTC]; Bisac-Evac™ [OTC]; Bisacodyl Uniserts® [OTC] [DSC]; Bisolax™ [OTC]; Correctol® Tablets [OTC]; Dacodyl™ [OTC]; Doxidan® [OTC]; Dulcolax® [OTC]; ex-lax® Ultra [OTC]; Fematrol [OTC]; Femilax™ [OTC]; Fleet® Bisacodyl [OTC]; Fleet® Stimulant Laxative [OTC]; Veracolate [OTC]

Canadian Brand Names Apo-Bisacodyl®; Carter's Little Pills®; Dulcolax®; Gentlax®

Therapeutic Category Laxative, Stimulant

Generic Available Yes: Excludes enema

Use Treatment of constipation; colonic evacuation prior to procedures or examination

Pregnancy Risk Factor C

Contraindications Hypersensitivity to bisacodyl or any component; do not use in patients with abdominal pain, appendicitis, obstruction, nausea or vomiting; not to be used during pregnancy or lactation

(Continued)

Bisacodyl *(Continued)*

Warnings Stimulant laxatives are habit-forming; long-term use may result in laxative dependence and loss of normal bowel function.

Precautions Bisacodyl tannex powder for preparation as a rectal solution should be used with caution in patients with ulceration of the colon

Adverse Reactions

Endocrine & metabolic: Electrolyte and fluid imbalance (metabolic acidosis or alkalosis, hypocalcemia)

Gastrointestinal: Abdominal cramps, nausea, vomiting, diarrhea, rectal burning, proctitis (rare)

Food Interactions Administration within 1 hour of ingesting antacids, alkaline material, milk, or dairy products will cause premature dissolution of the enteric coating and resultant gastric irritation

Stability Store enteric-coated tablets and rectal suppositories at <30°C.

Mechanism of Action Stimulates peristalsis by directly irritating the smooth muscle of the intestine, possibly the colonic intramural plexus; alters water and electrolyte secretion producing net intestinal fluid accumulation and laxation

Pharmacodynamics Onset of action:

Oral: Within 6-10 hours

Rectal: 15-60 minutes

Pharmacokinetics

Absorption: Oral, rectal: <5% absorbed systemically

Metabolism: In the liver

Elimination: Conjugated metabolites excreted in breast milk, bile, and urine

Usual Dosage

Bisacodyl (Dulcolax®) tablet: Oral:

- Children 3-12 years: 5-10 mg or 0.3 mg/kg/day as a single dose
- Children ≥12 years and Adults: 5-15 mg/day as a single dose; maximum dose: 30 mg

Bisacodyl (Dulcolax®) suppository: Rectal:

- Children:
  - <2 years: 5 mg/day as a single dose
  - 2-11 years: 5-10 mg/day as a single dose
- Children ≥12 years and Adults: 10 mg/day as a single dose

Administration Oral: Administer on an empty stomach with water; patient should swallow tablet whole; do not break or chew enteric-coated tablet; do not administer within 1 hour of ingesting antacids, alkaline material, milk, or dairy products

Patient Information Should not be used regularly for more than 1 week

Additional Information In a randomized prospective study of 70 patients, bisacodyl tablets were given orally once daily in the morning for 2 days before colonoscopy to 19 patients (dose for children <5 years: 5 mg; 5-12 years: 10 mg; >12 years: 15 mg) with a Fleet® enema given on the morning of the procedure without any dietary restriction. Results showed that bisacodyl without dietary restriction provided unsatisfactory colon cleansing.

Dosage Forms Excipient information presented when available (limited, particularly for generics); consult specific product labeling. [DSC] = Discontinued product

Solution, rectal [enema]:

- Fleet® Bisacodyl: 10 mg/30 mL (37 mL)

Suppository, rectal: 10 mg

- Bisac-Evac™, Bisacodyl Uniserts® [DSC], Bisolax™, Dulcolax®: 10 mg

Tablet [enteric coated]: 5 mg

- Alophen®, Bisac-Evac™, Correctol®, Dacodyl™, Dulcolax®, ex-lax® Ultra, Fematrol, Femilax™, Veracolate: 5 mg

Tablet, delayed release: 5 mg

- Doxidan®, Fleet® Stimulant Laxative: 5 mg

References

BaKer SS, Liptak GS, Colletti RB, et al, "Constipation in Infants and Children: Evaluation and Treatment," 2000, www.naspgn.org/constipation.

Dahshan A, Lin CH, Peters J, et al, "A Randomized, Prospective Study to Evaluate the Efficacy and Acceptance of Three Bowel Preparations for Colonoscopy in Children," *Am J Gastroenterol*, 1999, 94(12):3497-501.

◆ **Bisacodyl Uniserts® [OTC] [DSC]** *see* Bisacodyl *on page 217*

◆ **bis-chloronitrosourea** *see* Carmustine *on page 290*

◆ **Bismatrol** *see* Bismuth *on page 219*

◆ **Bismatrol [OTC]** *see* Bismuth *on page 219*

◆ **Bismatrol Maximum Strength [OTC]** *see* Bismuth *on page 219*

Bismuth (BIZ muth)

Medication Safety Issues

Sound-alike/look-alike issues:

Kaopectate® may be confused with Kayexalate®

Maalox® Total Stomach Relief® is a different formulation than Maalox®

U.S. Brand Names Bismatrol [OTC]; Bismatrol Maximum Strength [OTC]; Diotame® [OTC]; Kaopectate® [OTC]; Kaopectate® Extra Strength [OTC]; Kao-Tin [OTC]; Kapectolin [OTC]; Maalox® Total Stomach Relief® [OTC]; Pepto-Bismol® [OTC]; Pepto-Bismol® Maximum Strength [OTC]

Index Terms Bismatrol; Bismuth Subgallate; Bismuth Subsalicylate; Pink Bismuth

Therapeutic Category Antidiarrheal; Gastrointestinal Agent, Gastric or Duodenal Ulcer Treatment

Generic Available Yes

Use

Subsalicylate formulation: Symptomatic treatment of mild, nonspecific diarrhea including traveler's diarrhea; chronic infantile diarrhea; adjunctive treatment of *Helicobacter pylori*-associated antral gastritis

Subgallate formulation: An aid to reduce fecal odors from a colostomy or ileostomy

Pregnancy Risk Factor C (D in 3rd trimester)

Lactation Excretion in breast milk unknown (salicylates enter breast milk)/use caution

Contraindications Hypersensitivity to bismuth, salicylates, or any component; history of severe GI bleeding or coagulopathy

Warnings Kaopectate® has been reformulated to contain **only** bismuth subsalicylate; follow dosage recommendations closely. Do not use subsalicylate in patients with influenza or chickenpox because of the risk of Reye's syndrome; when using bismuth subsalicylate, changes in behavior (along with nausea and vomiting) may be an early sign of Reye's syndrome; instruct patients and caregivers to contact their healthcare provider if these symptoms occur; subsalicylate should be used with caution if patient is taking aspirin, due to additive toxicity; use with caution in children <3 years of age; be aware of salicylate content when prescribing for use in children

Precautions May interfere with radiologic examinations of GI tract as bismuth is radiopaque

Adverse Reactions

Central nervous system: Anxiety, confusion, slurred speech, headache, mental depression

Gastrointestinal: Impaction (infants and debilitated patients), grayish-black stools, darkened tongue

Neuromuscular & skeletal: Muscle spasms, weakness

Otic: Tinnitus, loss of hearing

Drug Interactions Decreases absorption of tetracycline; increases toxicity of aspirin (due to absorption of salicylate), warfarin, hypoglycemics

Mechanism of Action Adsorbs extra water in large intestine, as well as toxins; forms a protective coat on the intestinal mucosa; appears to have antisecretory (salicylate moiety) and antimicrobial effects (bismuth moiety) against bacterial and viral pathogens

Pharmacokinetics

Absorption: Bismuth is minimally absorbed (<1%) across the GI tract while salicylate salt is readily absorbed (80%)

Distribution: Salicylate: V_d: 170 mL/kg

Protein binding, plasma: Bismuth and salicylate: >90%

Metabolism: Bismuth salts undergo chemical dissociation after oral administration; salicylate is extensively metabolized in the liver

Half-life:

Bismuth: Terminal: 21-72 days

Salicylate: Terminal: 2-5 hours

Elimination:

Bismuth: Renal, biliary

Salicylate: Only 10% excreted unchanged in urine

Usual Dosage Oral: Bismuth subsalicylate **(bismuth subsalicylate liquid dosages expressed in mL of 262 mg/15 mL concentration):**

Nonspecific diarrhea: Children: 100 mg/kg/day divided into 5 equal doses for 5 days (maximum: 4.19 g/day) **or**

Children: Up to 8 doses/24 hours:

3-6 years: 1/3 tablet or 5 mL (87 mg)every 30 minutes to 1 hour as needed

6-9 years: 2/3 tablet or 10 mL (175 mg) every 30 minutes to 1 hour as needed

9-12 years: 1 tablet or 15 mL (262 mg) every 30 minutes to 1 hour as needed

Adults: 2 tablets or 30 mL (524 mg) every 30 minutes to 1 hour as needed up to 8 doses/24 hours

(Continued)

Bismuth *(Continued)*

Chronic infantile diarrhea:

2-24 months: 2.5 mL (44 mg) every 4 hours

24-48 months: 5 mL (87 mg) every 4 hours

48-70 months: 10 mL (175 mg) every 4 hours

Prevention of traveler's diarrhea: Adults: 2.1 g/day or 2 tablets 4 times/day before meals and at bedtime

Helicobacter pylori-associated antral gastritis: Dosage in children is not well established, the following dosages have been used [in conjunction with ampicillin and metronidazole or (in adults) tetracycline and metronidazole]:

Children ≤10 years: 15 mL (262 mg) 4 times/day for 6 weeks

Children >10 years and Adults: 30 mL (524 mg) solution or two 262 mg tablets 4 times/day for 6 weeks

Dosing adjustment in renal impairment: Avoid use in patients with renal failure

Administration Oral: Shake liquid well before using; chew tablets or allow to dissolve in mouth before swallowing

Test Interactions Bismuth absorbs x-rays and may interfere with diagnostic procedures of GI tract

Patient Information May darken stools; if diarrhea persists for more than 2 days, consult a physician; may turn tongue black; notify physician if behavioral changes along with nausea and vomiting occur (see Warnings)

Additional Information Bismuth subsalicylate: 262 mg = 130 mg nonaspirin salicylate; 525 mg = 236 mg nonaspirin salicylate

Dosage Forms Excipient information presented when available (limited, particularly for generics); consult specific product labeling.

Caplet, as subsalicylate: 262 mg

Pepto-Bismol®: 262 mg [sugar free; contains sodium 2 mg]

Liquid, as subsalicylate: 262 mg/15 mL (240 mL, 360 mL, 480 mL); 525 mg/15 mL (240 mL, 360 mL)

Bismatrol: 262 mg/15 mL (240 mL)

Bismatrol Maximum Strength: 525 mg/15 mL (240 mL)

Diotame®: 262 mg/15 mL (30 mL)

Kaopectate®: 262 mg/15 mL (180 mL, 240 mL, 360 mL) [contains sodium 10 mg/15 mL; regular and peppermint flavor]

Kaopectate® Extra Strength: 525 mg/15 mL (240 mL) [contains sodium 11 mg/15 mL; peppermint flavor]

Kaotin: 262 mg/15 mL (240 mL, 480 mL)

Maalox® Total Stomach Relief®: 525 mg/15 mL (360 mL) [contains sodium 3.3 mg/15mL; strawberry and peppermint flavor]

Pepto-Bismol®: 262 mg/15 mL (120 mL, 240 mL, 360 mL, 480 mL) [sugar free; contains sodium 6 mg/15 mL and benzoic acid; wintergreen flavor]

Pepto-Bismol® Maximum Strength: 525 mg/15 mL (120 mL, 240 mL, 360 mL) [sugar free; contains sodium 6 mg/15 mL and benzoic acid; wintergreen flavor]

Suspension:

Kapectolin: 262 mg/15 mL (480 mL) [mint flavor]

Tablet, chewable, as subsalicylate: 262 mg

Bismatrol: 262 mg

Diotame®: 262 mg

Pepto-Bismol®: 262 mg [sugar free; contains sodium <1 mg; cherry flavor]

References

Drumm B, Sherman P, Karmali M, et al, "Treatment of *Campylobacter pylori*-associated Antral Gastritis in Children With Bismuth Subsalicylate and Ampicillin," *J Pediatr*, 1988, 113(5):908-12.

Soriano-Brucher HE, Avendano P, O'Ryan M, et al, "Use of Bismuth Subsalicylate in Acute Diarrhea in Children," *Rev Infect Dis*, 1990, 12(Suppl 1):S51-5.

Walsh JH and Peterson WL, "The Treatment of *Helicobacter pylori* Infection in the Management of Peptic Ulcer Disease," *N Engl J Med*, 1995, 333(15):984-91.

♦ **Bismuth Subgallate** *see* Bismuth *on page 219*

♦ **Bismuth Subsalicylate** *see* Bismuth *on page 219*

♦ **Bisolax™ [OTC]** *see* Bisacodyl *on page 217*

♦ **Bistropamide** *see* Tropicamide *on page 1582*

♦ **Black-Draught Tablets [OTC]** *see* Senna *on page 1427*

♦ **Black Widow Spider Species Antivenin (*Latrodectus mactans*)** *see* Antivenin (*Latrodectus mactans*) *on page 149*

♦ **Blenoxane®** *see* Bleomycin *on page 221*

♦ **Bleo** *see* Bleomycin *on page 221*

Bleomycin (blee oh MYE sin)

Medication Safety Issues

Sound-alike/look-alike issues:

Bleomycin may be confused with Cleocin®

High alert medication: The Institute for Safe Medication Practices (ISMP) includes this medication among its list of drugs which have a heightened risk of causing significant patient harm when used in error.

Related Information

Compatibility of Chemotherapy and Related Supportive Care Medications *on page 1777*

Emetogenic Potential of Single Chemotherapeutic Agents *on page 1776*

U.S. Brand Names Blenoxane®

Canadian Brand Names Blenoxane®; Bleomycin Injection, USP

Index Terms Bleo; Bleomycin Sulfate; BLM; NSC-125066

Therapeutic Category Antineoplastic Agent, Antibiotic

Generic Available Yes

Use Palliative treatment of squamous cell carcinoma, testicular carcinoma, and germ cell tumors; Hodgkin's lymphoma, non-Hodgkin's lymphoma, renal carcinoma, and soft tissue sarcoma; sclerosing agent to control malignant effusions

Pregnancy Risk Factor D

Lactation Excretion in breast milk unknown/not recommended

Contraindications Hypersensitivity to bleomycin sulfate or any component

Warnings The FDA currently recommends that procedures for proper handling and disposal of antineoplastic agents be considered. Occurrence of pulmonary fibrosis is higher in elderly patients and in those receiving a total cumulative dose >400 units; pulmonary toxicity has occurred at a total dosage <200 units or 250 units/m^2 in younger patients; pulmonary irradiation and use of supplemental oxygen increase the chance for developing toxic pulmonary reactions in patients previously treated with bleomycin; a severe idiosyncratic reaction consisting of hypotension, mental confusion, fever, chills, and wheezing is possible.

Precautions Use with caution in patients with renal or pulmonary impairment; dosage modification is recommended in patients with renal impairment; dosage modification may be necessary in patients with a 20% decrease from baseline in FEV_1, FVC, or DL_{co}; administer test dose to lymphoma patients prior to starting therapy

Adverse Reactions

Cardiovascular: Cerebrovascular accident, hypotension, Raynaud's phenomenon

Central nervous system: Fever, chills, malaise

Dermatologic: Hyperpigmentation, hyperkeratosis of hands and nails, rash, alopecia, desquamation

Gastrointestinal: Stomatitis, vomiting, anorexia, mild nausea

Hematologic: Thrombocytopenia, leukopenia

Local: Phlebitis

Respiratory: Interstitial pneumonitis (10%), pulmonary fibrosis (cumulative lifetime dose should not exceed 400 units or 250 units/m^2 in younger patients), dyspnea, tachypnea, nonproductive cough, rales

Miscellaneous: Anaphylactoid reactions

Drug Interactions Phenytoin (decreases phenytoin concentrations), cisplatin (decreases bleomycin clearance), bleomycin may decrease digoxin absorption; concurrent use with amphotericin B products may increase nephrotoxicity and risk for hypotension and bronchospasm

Stability Refrigerate; intact vials are stable 28 days at room temperature; reconstituted solution is stable for 24 hours at room temperature; incompatible with amino acid solutions, ascorbic acid, cefazolin, furosemide, diazepam, hydrocortisone, mitomycin, nafcillin, penicillin G, aminophylline, copper; dilution in dextrose solutions may result in a 10% loss of activity within 24 hours

Mechanism of Action Inhibits synthesis of DNA; binds to DNA leading to single- and double-strand breaks by a Fe^{++}-O_2-catalyzed free radical reaction

Pharmacokinetics

Distribution: Into skin, lungs, kidneys, peritoneum, and lymphatics

Protein binding: <10%

Half-life: Dependent upon renal function

Children: 2.1-3.5 hours

Adults, with normal renal function: 2-3 hours

Time to peak serum concentration: I.M.: Within 30-60 minutes

Elimination: 60% to 70% of a dose excreted in the urine as active drug

Dialysis: Not removed by hemodialysis

(Continued)

Bleomycin *(Continued)*

Usual Dosage Refer to individual protocol

Children and Adults:

I.M., I.V., SubQ:

Test dose for lymphoma patients: 1-2 units of bleomycin for the first 2 doses; monitor vital signs every 15 minutes; wait a minimum of 1 hour before administering remainder of dose

Treatment: 10-20 units/m^2 (0.25-0.5 units/kg) 1-2 times/week in combination regimens or once every 2-4 weeks

Germ cell tumors: 15 units/m^2/dose once weekly for 3 weeks per regimen

Hodgkin's disease: 10 units/m^2/dose on days 1 and 15 of cycle

I.V. continuous infusion: 15-20 units/m^2/day over 24 hours for 3-5 days

Adults: Intracavitary injection for pleural effusion: 15-60 units (dose generally does not exceed 1 unit/kg); drug is diluted with 50-100 mL of NS and is instilled into the pleural cavity via a thoracostomy tube

Dosing adjustment in renal impairment:

Cl_{cr} 25-50 mL/minute: Reduce dose by 25%

Cl_{cr} <25 mL/minute: Reduce dose by 50% to 75%

Administration Parenteral:

I.V.: Administer I.V. slowly over at least 10 minutes (no greater than 1 unit/minute) at a concentration not to exceed 3 units/mL; bleomycin for I.V. continuous infusion can be further diluted in NS (preferred) or D_5W; administration by continuous infusion may produce less severe pulmonary toxicity.

I.M., SubQ: 15 units/mL concentration may be used for I.M., SubQ administration

Monitoring Parameters Pulmonary function tests (total lung volume, FEV_1, FVC, DL_{co}), renal function tests, chest x-ray; vital signs and temperature initially; CBC with differential and platelet count

Patient Information Report any coughing, shortness of breath, or wheezing to physician

Nursing Implications Fever and chills can occur 2-6 hours following parenteral administration; pretreatment with acetaminophen, antihistamine, and hydrocortisone may decrease the severity of fever and chills

Dosage Forms Excipient information presented when available (limited, particularly for generics); consult specific product labeling.

Injection, powder for reconstitution, as sulfate: 15 units, 30 units

References

Alberts DS, Chen HS, Liu R, et al, "Bleomycin Pharmacokinetics in Man. I. Intravenous Administration," *Cancer Chemother Pharmacol*, 1978, 1(3):177-81.

Berg SL, Grisell DL, Delaney TF, et al, "Principles of Treatment of Pediatric Solid Tumors," *Pediatr Clin North Am*, 1991, 38(2):249-67.

◆ **Bleomycin Injection, USP (Can)** *see* Bleomycin *on page 221*
◆ **Bleomycin Sulfate** *see* Bleomycin *on page 221*
◆ **Bleph®-10** *see* Sulfacetamide *on page 1483*
◆ **Blis-To-Sol® [OTC]** *see* Tolnaftate *on page 1550*
◆ **BLM** *see* Bleomycin *on page 221*
◆ **Blocadren®** *see* Timolol *on page 1542*
◆ **BMS-232632** *see* Atazanavir *on page 166*
◆ **Bonamine™ (Can)** *see* Meclizine *on page 988*
◆ **Bonine® [OTC]** *see* Meclizine *on page 988*
◆ **Bonine® (Can)** *see* Meclizine *on page 988*
◆ **Boostrix®** *see* Diphtheria, Tetanus Toxoids, and Acellular Pertussis Vaccine *on page 517*

Bosentan (boe SEN tan)

Related Information

World Health Organization (WHO) Functional Classification of Pulmonary Hypertension *on page 1680*

U.S. Brand Names Tracleer®

Canadian Brand Names Tracleer®

Therapeutic Category Endothelin Receptor Antagonist

Generic Available No

Use Treatment of pulmonary arterial hypertension (PAH) in patients with World Health Organization (WHO) Class III or IV symptoms to improve exercise capacity and decrease the rate of clinical deterioration

Restrictions Bosentan (Tracleer®) is available only through a limited distribution program directly from the manufacturer (Actelion Pharmaceuticals 1-866-228-3546). It is not available through wholesalers or individual pharmacies.

Medication Guide An FDA-approved patient medication guide, which is available with the product information and at http://www.fda.gov/cder/Offices/ODS/medication_guides.htm, must be dispensed with this medication for each new outpatient prescription and refill.

Pregnancy Risk Factor X

Lactation Excretion in breast milk unknown/not recommended

Contraindications Hypersensitivity to bosentan or any component; pregnancy; concurrent use of cyclosporine or glyburide

Warnings Serious hepatic injury, including rare reports of cirrhosis and liver failure may occur. Elevations in liver aminotransferases (ALT and AST) of at least 3 times the upper limit of normal may occur in 11% of patients with elevations in bilirubin in some cases. Monitor liver enzymes at baseline and monthly thereafter. Use with caution in patients with mildly impaired liver function; avoid use in moderate-to-severe hepatic impairment. Avoid use in patients with elevated serum transaminases (>3 times upper limit of normal) at baseline; adjust dosage if elevations in liver enzymes occur during therapy. Treatment should be discontinued in patients who develop elevated transaminases (ALT or AST) in combination with symptoms of hepatic injury (unusual fatigue, jaundice, nausea, vomiting, abdominal pain, and/or fever) or elevated serum bilirubin ≥2 times upper limit of normal.

Major birth defects may occur if bosentan is used during pregnancy (use in pregnancy is contraindicated). Exclude pregnancy prior to initiation of therapy; obtain monthly pregnancy tests in women of childbearing potential during therapy. Patients must be instructed to use effective, nonhormonal contraception throughout treatment. Efficacy of hormonal contraceptives may be decreased (see Drug Interactions), and should not be the sole contraceptive method in patients receiving bosentan. Women of childbearing potential should not be exposed to the drug by crushing the tablets; tablets should be dissolved in water if necessary (see Extemporaneous Preparations).

Precautions Use with caution in patients with low hemoglobin levels or ischemic cardiovascular disease. Bosentan may cause dose-related decreases in hemoglobin and hematocrit (monitoring of hemoglobin is recommended). May cause fluid retention, worsening of CHF, weight gain, and leg edema. If pulmonary edema occurs, consider the possibility of pulmonary veno-occlusive disease and discontinue bosentan. Safety and efficacy in pediatric patients have not been established.

Adverse Reactions Percent incidence is from adult studies:

- Cardiovascular: Flushing (7% to 9%), edema (lower limb: 5% to 8%; generalized: 4%), hypotension (7%), palpitation (5%); worsening of CHF
- Central nervous system: Headache (16% to 22%), fatigue (4%)
- Dermatologic: Pruritus (4%)
- Endocrine & metabolic: Fluid retention, weight gain
- Gastrointestinal: Dyspepsia (4%)
- Hematologic: Decreased hemoglobin (≥1 g/dL in up to 57% of patients, typically in first 6 weeks of therapy; markedly decreased hemoglobin may occur in up to 6% of patients), anemia (3%)
- Hepatic: Elevated liver enzymes (**Note:** Transaminases are increased >3 times the upper limit of normal in up to 11% of patients; elevations are dose-dependent, may occur at any time, usually progress slowly, typically are asymptomatic, and usually are reversible after drug interruption or discontinuation), abnormal hepatic function (6% to 8%), hepatic cirrhosis (rare; reported after prolonged use >12 months in patients receiving multiple medications), liver failure (rare), elevated bilirubin
- Respiratory: Nasopharyngitis (11%)
- Miscellaneous: Hypersensitivity, rash, angioneurotic edema (several reports)

Drug Interactions Cytochrome P450 isoenzyme CYP2C9 and CYP3A4 substrate; isoenzyme CYP2C9 and CYP3A4 inducer; possible isoenzyme CYP2C19 inducer

Cyclosporine significantly increases serum concentrations of bosentan (concurrent use of cyclosporine is contraindicated). Based on animal studies, tacrolimus may significantly increase serum concentrations of bosentan (use tacrolimus with caution; monitor patients closely). Bosentan may enhance the metabolism of cyclosporine, decreasing its serum concentrations by ~50%; effect on sirolimus and/or tacrolimus has not been specifically evaluated, but may be similar. Concurrent use with glyburide resulted in an increased risk of serum transaminase elevations (concurrent use of glyburide is contraindicated).

Cytochrome P450 CYP2C8/9 inhibitors (such as amiodarone, fluconazole, ketoconazole, nicardipine, NSAIDs, and sulfonamides) or isoenzyme CYP3A4 inhibitors (such as clarithromycin, erythromycin, isoniazid, ketoconazole, nefazodone, nicardipine, propofol, protease inhibitors, quinidine, telithromycin, and verapamil) may increase bosentan serum concentrations or effects (use with caution; monitor patients closely for increased effects). Concurrent use of bosentan with a potent CYP2C9 inhibitor

(Continued)

Bosentan *(Continued)*

plus a CYP3A4 inhibitor is **not** recommended. Cytochrome P450 CYP2C8/9 inducers (such as carbamazepine, phenobarbital, phenytoin, and rifampin) and isoenzyme CYP3A4 inducers (such as carbamazepine, nevirapine, phenobarbital, phenytoin, and rifamycins) may decrease bosentan serum concentrations or effects (use with caution; monitor patients). The herbal medicine St John's wort (*Hypericum perforatum*) may potentially decrease serum concentrations of bosentan and is **not** recommended for concurrent use.

Bosentan may decrease the serum concentrations or effects of CYP2C8/9 substrates [such as fluoxetine, glipizide, phenytoin, rosiglitazone, sertraline, and warfarin (monitor INR)] and CYP3A4 substrates (such as benzodiazepines, calcium channel blockers, ergot derivatives, nefazodone, tacrolimus, and venlafaxine). Bosentan decreased plasma concentrations of simvastatin by ~50% and may decrease plasma concentrations of lovastatin and atorvastatin (monitor cholesterol concentrations; adjustment of statin dosage may be needed). Concurrent use with sildenafil increased bosentan plasma concentrations by 50% and decreased sildenafil concentrations by 63% (dosage adjustments of either drug is **not** needed).

Bosentan significantly decreases the serum concentrations of oral hormonal contraceptives (both estrogen and progesterone); hormonal contraceptives (including oral, transdermal, injectable, and implantable dosage forms) may not be effective in patients receiving bosentan and must not be used as the sole contraceptive method; nonhormonal contraception must be used throughout treatment.

Food Interactions Food does not affect bioavailability.

Stability Store at 20°C to 25°C (68°F to 77°F).

Mechanism of Action Bosentan acts as a competitive antagonist and blocks endothelin receptors on vascular endothelium and smooth muscle. Stimulation of endothelin receptors is associated with vasoconstriction and proliferation (**Note:** Patients with PAH have elevated lung tissue and plasma concentrations of endothelin). Although bosentan blocks both ET_A and ET_B receptors, the affinity is slightly higher for the A subtype. In clinical trials, bosentan significantly increased cardiac index and decreased pulmonary artery pressure, pulmonary vascular resistance, and mean right atrial pressure. Improvement in symptoms of PAH and exercise capacity, and a decrease in the rate of clinical deterioration were observed.

Pharmacokinetics

Distribution: Unknown if distributes into breast milk; does not distribute into RBCs; V_d: Adults: 18 L

Protein binding: >98% to plasma proteins (primarily albumin)

Metabolism: Extensive in the liver via cytochrome P450 isoenzymes CYP2C9 and CYP3A4 to three metabolites (one has pharmacologic activity and may account for 10% to 20% of drug effect); steady-state plasma concentrations are 50% to 65% of those attained after single dose (most likely due to autoinduction of liver enzymes); steady-state is attained within 3-5 days

Bioavailability: 50%

Half-life: Healthy subjects: 5 hours; half-life may be prolonged in PAH, as AUC is 2-fold greater in adults with PAH versus healthy subjects

Time to peak serum concentration: Oral: Within 3-5 hours

Elimination: Biliary excretion; <3% of dose is excreted in the urine

Usual Dosage Oral:

Infants and Children: Limited information available; several pediatric studies have used the following doses based on body weight in patients as young as 9 months of age (see Barst, 2003; Rosenzweig, 2005; Ivy, 2004):

<10 kg (only 3 patients reported; see Rosenzweig, 2005): Initial: 15.6 mg daily for 4 weeks; increase to maintenance dose of 15.6 mg twice daily; **Note:** Based on an extrapolation of study doses used in Barst, 2003, the following doses are recommended for patients <10 kg: Initial: 1-2 mg/kg twice daily for 4 weeks; increase to maintenance dose of 2-4 mg/kg twice daily (Villanueva, 2006)

10-20 kg: Initial: 31.25 mg daily for 4 weeks; increase to maintenance dose of 31.25 mg twice daily

>20-40 kg: Initial: 31.25 mg twice daily for 4 weeks; increase to maintenance dose of 62.5 mg twice daily

>40 kg: Initial: 62.5 mg twice daily for 4 weeks; increase to maintenance dose of 125 mg twice daily

Note: A smaller pediatric study of 7 patients, 1.5-6.4 years of age (median: 3.8 years) used initial doses of 1.5 mg/kg/day divided into 1-3 doses/day (in capsule form) for 4 weeks; doses were increased to maintenance doses of 3 mg/kg/day (see Gilbert, 2005)

Adolescents >12 years who are <40 kg: Manufacturer's recommendations: Initial and maintenance: 62.5 mg twice daily

Adults: Initial: 62.5 mg twice daily for 4 weeks; increase to maintenance dose of 125 mg twice daily; adults <40 kg should be maintained at 62.5 mg twice daily.

Note: Doses >125 mg twice daily do not provide additional benefit sufficient to offset the increased risk of hepatic injury. When discontinuing treatment, consider a reduction in dosage to 62.5 mg twice daily for 3-7 days (to avoid clinical deterioration).

Dosage adjustment in renal impairment: No dosage adjustment required.

Dosage adjustment in hepatic impairment: Use with caution in patients with mild hepatic impairment. Avoid use in patients with moderate-to-severe hepatic insufficiency and in patients with elevated serum transaminases (>3 times upper limit of normal) at baseline

Dosage adjustment in patients who develop elevations of aminotransferases:

Adult guidelines: Note: If any elevation, regardless of degree, is accompanied by clinical symptoms of hepatic injury (unusual fatigue, nausea, vomiting, abdominal pain, fever, or jaundice) or a serum bilirubin ≥2 times the upper limit of normal, treatment should be stopped.

AST/ALT >3 times but ≤5 times upper limit of normal: Confirm elevation with additional test; if confirmed, reduce dose or interrupt treatment. Monitor transaminase levels at least every 2 weeks. May continue or reintroduce treatment, as appropriate, following return to pretreatment aminotransferase values. Begin with initial dose (above) and recheck transaminases within 3 days.

AST/ALT >5 times but ≤8 times upper limit of normal: Confirm elevation with additional test; if confirmed, stop treatment. Monitor transaminase levels at least every 2 weeks. May consider reintroduction of treatment, as appropriate, following return to pretreatment aminotransferase values.

AST/ALT >8 times upper limit of normal: Stop treatment.

Administration Oral: May be administered without regard to meals.

Monitoring Parameters Serum transaminase (AST and ALT) should be determined prior to the initiation of therapy and at monthly intervals thereafter. A woman of childbearing potential must have a negative pregnancy test prior to the initiation of therapy and monthly thereafter. Hemoglobin and hematocrit should be measured at baseline, after 1 and 3 months of treatment, and every 3 months thereafter. Monitor for clinical signs and symptoms of liver injury.

Patient Information Read the patient Medication Guide that you receive with each prescription and refill of bosentan. Some medicines should not be taken with bosentan; report the use of other medications, nonprescription medications, and herbal or natural products to your physician and pharmacist; avoid the herbal medicine St John's wort. Bosentan may cause liver damage and low red blood cell levels; blood tests to check for these side effects must be performed frequently. Notify physician if persistent headache or GI problems, swelling of extremities, or unusual weight gain, chest pain or palpitations, unusual fatigue or weakness, yellowing of skin or eyes, change in color of stool or urine, or other persistent reactions occur.

Bosentan may cause major birth defects and must not be taken by women who are pregnant or who may become pregnant; women who are able to become pregnant must use an effective birth control method while taking bosentan; bosentan may decrease the effectiveness of hormonal contraceptives, including birth control pills, skin patches, shots, and implants (talk to your doctor about using an alternative, nonhormonal, form of contraception); pregnancy tests (either urine or blood tests) must be performed every month while taking bosentan in women who are able to become pregnant; notify physician immediately if you think you might be pregnant. Do not crush tablets; women who are able to become pregnant should avoid exposure to bosentan powder (dust) from cutting tablets; tablets should be dissolved in water if necessary (see Extemporaneous Preparations).

Nursing Implications Assess results of laboratory tests, therapeutic effectiveness, and adverse reactions on a regular basis during therapy. Assess for fluid retention. Instruct patient on appropriate use, side effects/appropriate interventions, and adverse symptoms to report.

Bosentan is a teratogen (Pregnancy Risk Factor X); avoid exposure to bosentan powder (dust) when cutting the tablets (use gloves and mask); do not crush the tablets; (see Extemporaneous Preparations).

Additional Information The addition of bosentan to epoprostenol therapy in 8 children (8-18 years of age) with idiopathic PAH allowed for a reduction in the epoprostenol dose (and its associated side effects) in 7 of the 8 children. Epoprostenol was able to be discontinued in 3 of the 8 children (see Ivy, 2004).

Clinical studies in adults have shown that bosentan was **not** effective in the treatment of CHF in patients with left ventricular dysfunction; hospitalizations for CHF were more common during the first 1-2 months after initiation of the drug.

Dosage Forms Excipient information presented when available (limited, particularly for generics); consult specific product labeling.

(Continued)

Bosentan *(Continued)*

Tablet:

Tracleer®: 62.5 mg, 125 mg

Extemporaneous Preparations Note: Tablets are not scored; a commercial pill cutter should be used to prepare a 31.25 mg dose from the 62.5 mg tablet; the half-cut 62.5 mg tablets are stable for up to 4 weeks, when stored at room temperature in the high-density polyethylene plastic bottle provided by the manufacturer of the drug. Since bosentan is classified as a teratogen (Pregnancy Risk Factor X), individuals should avoid exposure to bosentan powder (dust) by taking appropriate measures (eg, using gloves and mask); women of childbearing potential should avoid all possible exposure to the dust.

Crushing of the tablets is not recommended; bosentan tablets will disintegrate rapidly (within 5 minutes) in 5-25 mL of water, to create a suspension. An appropriate aliquot of the suspension can be used to deliver the prescribed dose. The suspension is stable for up to 24 hours when stored at room temperature in a 10 mL syringe. Bosentan should not be mixed or dissolved in liquids with a low (acidic) pH (eg, fruit juices) due to poor solubility; the drug is most soluble in solutions with a pH >8.5.

Villanueva D. Medical Information Manager, Actelion, personal correspondence, March 2006.

References

Adatia I, "Improving the Outcome of Childhood Pulmonary Arterial Hypertension: The Effect of Bosentan in the Setting of a Dedicated Pulmonary Hypertension Clinic," *J Am Coll Cardiol*, 2005, 46(4):705-6.

Barst RJ, Ivy D, Dingemanse J, et al, "Pharmacokinetics, Safety, and Efficacy of Bosentan in Pediatric Patients With Pulmonary Arterial Hypertension," *Clin Pharmacol Ther*, 2003, 73(4):372-82.

Gilbert N, Luther YC, Miera O, et al, "Initial Experience With Bosentan (Tracleer®) as Treatment for Pulmonary Arterial Hypertension (PAH) Due to Congenital Heart Disease in Infants and Young Children," *Z Kardiol*, 2005, 94(9):570-4.

Ivy DD, Doran A, Claussen L, et al, "Weaning and Discontinuation of Epoprostenol in Children With Idiopathic Pulmonary Arterial Hypertension Receiving Concomitant Bosentan," *Am J Cardiol*, 2004, 93(7):943-6.

Rosenzweig EB, Ivy DD, Widlitz A, et al, "Effects of Long-Term Bosentan in Children With Pulmonary Arterial Hypertension," *J Am Coll Cardiol*, 2005, 46(4):697-704.

Villanueva D. Medical Information Manager, Actelion, personal correspondence, March 2006.

♦ **B&O Supprettes®** *see* Belladonna and Opium *on page 202*

♦ **Botox®** *see* Botulinum Toxin Type A *on page 226*

♦ **Botox® Cosmetic** *see* Botulinum Toxin Type A *on page 226*

Botulinum Toxin Type A (BOT yoo lin num TOKS in type aye)

U.S. Brand Names Botox®; Botox® Cosmetic

Canadian Brand Names Botox®; Botox® Cosmetic

Index Terms BTX-A

Therapeutic Category Muscle Contracture, Treatment; Ophthalmic Agent, Toxin

Generic Available No

Use Treatment of strabismus and blepharospasm associated with dystonia (including benign essential blepharospasm or VII nerve disorders); treatment of dynamic muscle contracture in pediatric cerebral palsy patients (orphan drug); treatment of cervical dystonia; treatment of severe primary axillary hyperhidrosis (not adequately controlled with topical treatments); temporary improvement in the appearance of lines and wrinkles of the face (moderate to severe glabellar lines associated with corrugator and/or procerus muscle activity) in adult patients ≤65 years of age

Unlabeled uses: Treatment of sialorrhea; palmar hyperhidrosis, esophageal achalasia, chronic anal fissure; migraine headache

Pregnancy Risk Factor C

Lactation Excretion in breast milk unknown/not recommended

Contraindications Hypersensitivity to botulinum A toxin or any component; infection at the site of injection

Warnings The European formulation of botulinum A toxin (Dysport®) is not equivalent in potency to Botox®; the Dysport®:Botox® equivalency ratio is ~3:1 or 4:1, respectively; patients treated for cervical dystonia may experience dysphagia which rarely may result in dyspnea, aspiration, and pneumonia; weakness of hand muscles and blepharoptosis may occur in patients who also receive treatment for palmar and facial hyperhidrosis respectively

Precautions Presence of antibodies to botulinum toxin type A may reduce the effectiveness of therapy; to minimize the development of antibodies, keep the dose of botulinum toxin type A as low as possible. Reduced blinking from botulinum toxin type A injection of the orbicularis muscle can lead to corneal exposure, persistent epithelial defect, and corneal ulceration, especially in patients with VII nerve disorders; carefully test corneal sensation in eyes previously operated upon. Avoid injection into the lower lid area to avoid ectropion, and vigorously treat any epithelial defect (this may require protective drops, ointment, therapeutic soft contact lenses, or closure of the eye by patching). Retrobulbar hemorrhages sufficient to compromise retinal circulation have occurred from needle penetrations into the orbit; have appropriate instruments to decompress the orbit accessible; ocular (globe) penetrations by needles have also occurred (an ophthalmoscope to diagnose this condition should be available).

Use with caution in patients with peripheral motor neuropathic diseases (eg, amyotrophic lateral sclerosis or motor neuropathy) or neuromuscular junction disorders (eg, myasthenia gravis or Lambert-Eaton syndrome) as these patients may be at increased risk for development of significant systemic side effects including severe dysphagia and respiratory compromise; use cautiously if there is inflammation present at the proposed injection site or when excessive weakness or atrophy is present in the target muscles

Adverse Reactions

Cardiovascular: Arrhythmia, MI (rare)

Central nervous system: Fever, anxiety, dizziness, drowsiness, speech disorder

Dermatologic: Rash, keratitis, pruritus, erythema multiforme, psoriasiform eruption, nonaxillary sweating (after primary hyperhidrosis treatment)

Gastrointestinal: Dysphagia (particularly after treatment of cervical dystonia), dyspepsia, xerostomia, pharyngitis

Local: Pain, tenderness, erythema and bruising at injection site

Neuromuscular & skeletal: Muscle weakness, temporary loss of function around injection site

Ocular: Dry eyes, lagophthalmos, ptosis, photophobia, vertical deviation, tearing, diplopia, eyelid edema, spatial disorientation, blepharospasm, ectropion, entropion, retrobulbar hemorrhage

Respiratory: Cough, rhinitis

Miscellaneous: Infection, flu-like syndrome, hypersensitivity reactions

Drug Interactions Effects of botulinum toxin may be potentiated by aminoglycoside antibiotics, or any other drug that interferes with neuromuscular transmission

Stability Store lyophilized product in refrigerator at 2°C to 8°C (36°F to 46°F); administer within 4 hours after reconstitution; reconstituted solution may be stored in the refrigerator (2°C to 8°C/36°F to 46°F) until administered; do not freeze reconstituted solution

Mechanism of Action Botulinum A toxin is a neurotoxin produced by *Clostridium botulinum*, a spore-forming anaerobic bacillus; it blocks neuromuscular conduction by binding to receptor sites on motor nerve terminals, entering the nerve terminals and inhibiting the release of acetylcholine. When injected intramuscularly at therapeutic doses, it produces a localized chemical denervation muscle paralysis. When the muscle is chemically denervated, it atrophies and may develop extrajunctional acetylcholine receptors. There is evidence that the nerve can sprout and reinnervate the muscle, with the weakness being reversible. Following several weeks of paralysis, alignment of the eye is measurably changed, despite return of innervation to the injected muscle. When injected intradermally, a temporary chemical denervation of the sweat gland reduces local sweating.

Pharmacodynamics

Strabismus:
- Onset of action: 1-2 days after injection
- Duration of paralysis: 2-6 weeks

Blepharospasm:
- Onset of action: 3 days after injection
- Maximum effect: 1-2 weeks
- Duration of paralysis: 3 months

Spasticity associated with cerebral palsy
- Onset of action: Several days
- Duration of paralysis: 3-8 months

Reduction in axillary sweat production:
- Duration of effect: 201 days (mean)

Usual Dosage I.M.:

Strabismus:

Children 2 months to 12 years:
- Horizontal or vertical deviations <20 prism diopters: 1.25 units into any one muscle
- Horizontal or vertical deviations 20-25 prism diopters: 1-2.5 units into any one muscle
- Persistent VI nerve palsy of ≥1 month duration: 1-1.25 units into the medial rectus muscle

Children ≥12 years and Adults:
- Horizontal or vertical deviations <20 prism diopters: 1.25-2.5 units into any one muscle

(Continued)

Botulinum Toxin Type A *(Continued)*

Horizontal or vertical deviations 20-50 prism diopters: 2.5-5 units into any one muscle

Persistent VI nerve palsy of ≥1 month duration: 1.25-2.5 units into the medial rectus muscle

Note: Re-examine patient 7-14 days after each injection to assess effects; dosage may be increased up to twofold of the previously administered dose; do not exceed 25 units as a single injection for any one muscle

Blepharospasm: Adults: Initial: 1.25-2.5 units injected into the medial and lateral pretarsal orbicularis oculi of the upper lid and into the lateral pretarsal orbicularis oculi of the lower lid; dose may be increased up to 2.5-5 units at repeat treatment sessions; do not exceed 5 units per injection or cumulative dose of 200 units in a 30-day period

Spasticity associated with cerebral palsy: Children >18 months to Adolescents: Small muscle: 1-2 units/kg; large muscle: 3-6 units/kg; maximum dose per injection site: 50 units; maximum dose for any one visit: 12 units/kg, up to 400 units; no more than 400 units should be administered during a 3-month period

Cervical dystonia: Adults: Initial and sequential doses should be individualized related to the patient's head and neck position, localization of pain, muscle hypertrophy, and patient response; mean dosage used in research trials: 236 units (range: 198-300 units) divided among affected muscles; limit total dose into sternocleidomastoid muscles to ≤100 units

Severe primary axillary hyperhidrosis: Adults: Intradermal: 50 units per axilla injected in 0.1-0.2 mL aliquots

Reduction of glabellar lines: Adults ≤65 years: I.M.: An effective dose is determined by gross observation of the patient's ability to activate the superficial muscles injected. The location, size and use of muscles may vary markedly among individuals. Inject 0.1 mL dose into each of five sites, two in each corrugator muscle and one in the procerus muscle (total dose 0.5 mL).

Administration Parenteral: For I.M. or intradermal administration only by individuals understanding the relevant neuromuscular and orbital anatomy and any alterations to the anatomy due to prior surgical procedures and standard electromyographic techniques; reconstitute vial with preservative-free NS to obtain an optimal injection volume of 0.1 mL; suggested diluent volumes and resulting concentrations: 1 mL (10 units/0.1 mL); 2 mL (5 units/0.1 mL), 4 mL (2.5 units/0.1 mL) or 8 mL (1.25 units/0.1 mL); gently swirl as botulinum toxin type A is denatured by violent agitation. Local site reactions may be minimized by careful injection into the target muscle, using a minimal volume, and slowing the rate of injection. Application of ice and topical anesthetics to the injection site may also be used.

Monitoring Parameters

Cervical dystonia: Toronto Western Spasmodic Torticollis Rating Scale (TWSTRS) which evaluates severity, disability, and pain

Cerebral palsy: Modified Ashworth Scale, Tardieu Scale, Gross Motor Function Measure; treatment goals include: Improved gait and balance, facilitation of patient care, increased comfort with therapy, improved tolerance of bracing, and prevention of musculoskeletal complications

Patient Information Patients with blepharospasm may have been extremely sedentary for a long time; sedentary patients should be cautioned to resume activity slowly and carefully following injection; may cause dry mouth

Dosage Forms Excipient information presented when available (limited, particularly for generics); consult specific product labeling.

Injection, powder for reconstitution [preservative free]: *Clostridium botulinum* toxin type A 100 units [contains human albumin]

References

"Botulinum Toxin," *NIH Consens Statement*, 1990, 12-14, 8(8):1-20.

Benson J and Daugherty KK, "Botulinum Toxin A in the Treatment of Sialorrhea," *Ann Pharmacother*, 2007, 41(1):79-85.

Charles PD, "Botulinum Neurotoxin Serotype A: A Clinical Update on Non-cosmetic Uses," *Am J Health Syst Pharm*, 2004, 61(22 Suppl 6):S11-23.

Cheng CM, Chen JS, and Patel RP, "Unlabeled Uses of Botulinum Toxins: A Review, Part 1," *Am J Health Syst Pharm*, 2006, 63(2):145-52.

Cheng CM, Chen JS, and Patel RP, "Unlabeled Uses of Botulinum Toxins: A Review, Part 2," *Am J Health Syst Pharm*, 2006, 63(3):225-32.

Criswell SR, Crowner BE, and Racette BA, "The Use of Botulinum Toxin Therapy for Lower-Extremity Spasticity in Children With Cerebral Palsy," *Neurosurg Focus*, 2006, 21(2):e1.

Russman BS, Tilton A, and Gormley ME Jr, "Cerebral Palsy: A Rational Approach to a Treatment Protocol, and the Role of Botulinum Toxin in Treatment," *Muscle Nerve Suppl*, 1997, 6:S181-S193.

Scott AB, Magoon EH, McNeer KW, et al, "Botulinum Treatment of Childhood Strabismus," *Ophthalmology*, 1990, 97(11):1434-8.

Botulinum Toxin Type B (BOT yoo lin num TOKS in type bee)

U.S. Brand Names Myobloc®

Index Terms *Clostridium botulinum* Toxin Type B

Therapeutic Category Muscle Contracture, Treatment

Generic Available No

Use Treatment of cervical dystonia

Pregnancy Risk Factor C

Lactation Excretion in breast milk unknown/not recommended

Contraindications Hypersensitivity to botulinum B toxin or any component

Warnings Use of botulinum B toxin should be reserved for healthcare providers familiar and experienced in the assessment and management of patients with cervical dystonia

Precautions Use with caution in patients with peripheral motor neuropathic diseases (eg, amyotrophic lateral sclerosis or motor neuropathy) or neuromuscular junction disorders (eg, myasthenia gravis or Lambert-Eaton syndrome) as these patients may be at increased risk for development of significant systemic side effects including severe dysphagia and respiratory compromise; use cautiously if there is inflammation present at the proposed injection site or when excessive weakness or atrophy is present in the target muscles

Adverse Reactions

Cardiovascular: Chest pain, vasodilation, peripheral edema

Central nervous system: Headache, fever, chills, malaise, dizziness, anxiety, somnolence, confusion

Dermatologic: Pruritus

Gastrointestinal: Dysphagia, dyspepsia, xerostomia, nausea, glossitis, stomatitis, taste perversion

Genitourinary: Urinary tract infection, cystitis, vaginal moniliasis

Local: Pain, bruising at injection site

Neuromuscular & skeletal: Weakness, neck pain, back pain, arthralgia, tremor

Ocular: Amblyopia, abnormal vision

Otic: Otitis media, tinnitus

Respiratory: Cough, rhinitis, pneumonia

Miscellaneous: Flu-like syndrome, viral infection, hypersensitivity reactions, abscess, cysts

Drug Interactions Effects of botulinum toxin may be potentiated by aminoglycoside antibiotics, or any drug that interferes with neuromuscular transmission

Stability Store solution in refrigerator at 2°C to 8°C (36°F to 46°F); stable for 4 hours at room temperature after dilution with NS

Mechanism of Action Botulinum B toxin is one of seven neurotoxins (A through G) produced by *Clostridium botulinum*, a spore-forming anaerobic bacillus; it blocks neuromuscular conduction by binding to receptor sites on motor nerve terminals, entering the nerve terminals and inhibiting the release of acetylcholine. Botulinum B also cleaves synaptic vesicle associated membrane protein (VAMP), a component of the protein complex involved in neurotransmitter release. When injected intramuscularly at therapeutic doses, it produces a localized chemical denervation muscle paralysis. When the muscle is chemically denervated, it atrophies and may develop extrajunctional acetylcholine receptors. There is evidence that the nerve can sprout and reinnervate the muscle, with the weakness being reversible.

Pharmacodynamics Duration of paralysis: 12-16 weeks

Usual Dosage I.M.: Adults: 2500-5000 units divided among affected muscles; patients without a prior history of tolerating botulinum toxin injections should receive a lower initial dose; subsequent doses should be individualized related to the patient's response; doses up to 10,000 units have been used

Administration Parenteral: For I.M. administration only by individuals understanding the relevant neuromuscular anatomy and any alterations to the anatomy due to prior surgical procedures and standard electromyographic techniques; solution may be diluted with NS prior to administration

Monitoring Parameters Toronto Western Spasmodic Torticollis Rating Scale (TWSTRS) which evaluates severity, disability, and pain

Patient Information May cause dry mouth

Dosage Forms Excipient information presented when available (limited, particularly for generics); consult specific product labeling.

Injection, solution [preservative free]:

Myobloc®: 5000 units/mL (0.5 mL, 1 mL, 2 mL) [contains albumin 0.05%]

References

"Botulinum Toxin," *NIH Consens Statement*, 1990, 12-14, 8(8):1-20.

Figgitt DP and Noble S, "Botulinum Toxin B: A Review of Its Therapeutic Potential in the Management of Cervical Dystonia," *Drugs*, 2002, 62(4):705-22.

Botulism Immune Globulin (Intravenous-Human)

(BOT yoo lism i MYUN GLOB you lin, in tra VEE nus, YU man)

U.S. Brand Names BabyBIG®

Index Terms BIG-IV

Therapeutic Category Immune Globulin

Generic Available No

Use Treatment of infant botulism caused by toxin type A or B in patients <1 year of age.

Restrictions In order to obtain this product, an invoice and purchase agreement must be completed and faxed to the Infant Botulism Treatment and Prevention Program (IBTPP) at 510-231-7609 (normal business hours) or 510-217-4449 (nights, weekends, and holidays).

After faxing the purchase agreement, the original copy of the purchase agreement must be returned to the IBTPP via overnight courier, and payment must be wired within 5 business days.

Arrange for courier pick-up of BabyBIG® from FFF Enterprises in Temecula, CA.

Pregnancy Risk Factor C

Contraindications Hypersensitivity to immune globulin or any component; IgA deficiency (BabyBIG® contains trace amounts of immunoglobulin A)

Warnings Renal dysfunction and/or acute renal failure has been reported with the administration of IVIG; 88% of the cases were associated with the administration of sucrose-containing IVIG products at doses of 400 mg/kg or greater. BabyBIG® contains sucrose as a stabilizer. BabyBIG® is made from human plasma which carries the risk of blood-borne virus transmission, including the disease-causing agent for Creutzfeldt-Jakob disease. Like any other blood product, the risks and benefits of this agent should be discussed between the patient's legal guardian and the attending physician. An aseptic meningitis syndrome has been reported to occur with high total doses of other I.V. immune globulin products (eg, 2 g/kg of IVIG). Symptoms usually present within hours to days of treatment. Signs and symptoms may include severe headache, nuchal rigidity, photophobia, nausea, vomiting, painful eye movement, and fever. Cerebrospinal fluid may be positive with pleocytosis and elevated protein levels.

Precautions Use with caution in patients at increased risk for developing acute renal failure (patients with pre-existing renal insufficiency, diabetes mellitus, volume depletion, sepsis, paraproteinemia, and concomitant nephrotoxic drugs). Assure that patients are not volume depleted prior to the initiation of BabyBIG®.

Adverse Reactions

Dermatologic: Erythematous rash

Renal: Acute renal failure, renal dysfunction, proximal tubular nephropathy, osmotic nephrosis, elevated BUN/serum creatinine

Miscellaneous: Anaphylaxis; infusion rate-related effects: Increased blood pressure, irritability, chills, muscle cramps, back pain, fever, nausea, vomiting, wheezing

Drug Interactions Vaccination with live viruses (polio, measles, mumps, rubella) should be deferred until ~5 months after administration of BabyBIG® due to the possibility of interference with the immune response. If patients are vaccinated shortly before BabyBIG® administration, revaccination may be necessary.

Stability Store between 2°C to 8°C (35.6°F to 46.4°F). Since BabyBIG® does not contain a preservative, reconstituted vials should be used within 2 hours. Do not mix with other drugs.

Mechanism of Action BabyBIG® contains antibody titers against botulinum toxin type A of at least 15 international units/mL and botulinum toxin type B of at least 4 international units/mL at levels sufficient to neutralize expected levels of circulating neurotoxin.

Pharmacodynamics Duration: ~6 months with a single infusion

Pharmacokinetics Half-life: ~28 days

Usual Dosage I.V.: Infants <1 year: Total dose is 50 mg/kg as a single I.V. infusion. Start as soon as diagnosis of infant botulism is made.

Administration Do not administer I.M. or SubQ

I.V. infusion: Add 2 mL SWI to 100 mg vial, resulting in 50 mg/mL solution; rotate vial gently to wet all the powder and avoid foaming. Do not shake vial. Allow solution to stand 30 minutes until it clears. Use within 2 hours of reconstitution. Use low volume tubing for administration via a separate line. If this is not possible, piggyback BabyBIG® into a pre-existing line containing either NS or a dextrose solution ($D_{2.5}W$, D_5W, $D_{10}W$, or $D_{20}W$) with or without added NaCl. Do not dilute more than 1:2 with any of the above solutions. Drug concentration should be no less than 25 mg/mL. Administer via an in-line 18 micron filter.

Initial: Administer slowly at 25 mg/kg/hour for the first 15 minutes; after 15 minutes, rate may be increased to the maximum infusion rate of 50 mg/kg/hour to the end of the infusion (infusion should conclude within 4 hours of reconstitution).

Monitoring Parameters Vital signs and blood pressure monitored continuously during the infusion. BUN and serum creatinine should be monitored prior to initial infusion. Periodic monitoring of renal function tests and urine output in patients at risk for developing renal failure.

Nursing Implications Appropriate agents for treatment of a hypersensitivity reaction (eg, epinephrine) should be readily available; adverse reactions may also be alleviated by decreasing the rate or the concentration of infusion, or temporarily interrupting the infusion

Dosage Forms Excipient information presented when available (limited, particularly for generics); consult specific product labeling.

Injection, powder for reconstitution [preservative free]:

BabyBIG®: ~100 mg [contains albumin and sucrose; packaged with SWFI]

References

Arnon SS, Schechter R, Maslanka SE, et al, "Human Botulism Immune Globulin for the Treatment of Infant Botulism," *N Engl J Med*, 2006, 354(5):462-71.

Infant Botulism Treatment and Prevention Program, Department of Communicable Disease Control, California Department of Health Services, http://infantbotulism.org

- **Boudreaux's® Butt Paste [OTC]** *see* Zinc Oxide *on page 1640*
- **Bovine Lung Surfactant** *see* Beractant *on page 210*
- **Bovine Lung Surfactant** *see* Calfactant *on page 275*
- **Breathe Right® Saline [OTC]** *see* Sodium Chloride *on page 1450*
- **Brethaire [DSC]** *see* Terbutaline *on page 1510*
- **Brevibloc®** *see* Esmolol *on page 601*
- **Brevital® (Can)** *see* Methohexital *on page 1025*
- **Brevital® Sodium** *see* Methohexital *on page 1025*
- **Brevoxyl®** *see* Benzoyl Peroxide *on page 207*
- **Brevoxyl® Cleansing** *see* Benzoyl Peroxide *on page 207*
- **Brevoxyl® Wash** *see* Benzoyl Peroxide *on page 207*
- **Bricanyl [DSC]** *see* Terbutaline *on page 1510*
- **Bricanyl® (Can)** *see* Terbutaline *on page 1510*

Brimonidine (bri MOE ni deen)

Medication Safety Issues

Sound-alike/look-alike issues:

Brimonidine may be confused with bromocriptine

U.S. Brand Names Alphagan® P

Canadian Brand Names Alphagan®; Apo-Brimonidine®; PMS-Brimonidine Tartrate; ratio-Brimonidine

Index Terms Brimonidine Tartrate

Therapeutic Category Alpha-Adrenergic Agonist, Ophthalmic; Glaucoma, Treatment Agent

Generic Available Yes

Use Lowering of IOP in patients with open-angle glaucoma or ocular hypertension

Pregnancy Risk Factor B

Lactation Excretion in breast milk unknown/not recommended

Contraindications Hypersensitivity to brimonidine or any component; use during or within 14 days of MAO inhibitor therapy

Warnings May cause CNS depression, particularly in young children; the most common adverse effect reported in a study of pediatric glaucoma patients was somnolence and decreased alertness (50% to 83% in children 2-6 years of age); these effects resulted in a 16% discontinuation of treatment rate; children >7 years (>20 kg) had a much lower rate of somnolence (25%); apnea, bradycardia, hypotension, hypothermia, hypotonia, and somnolence have been reported in infants receiving brimonidine; brimonidine is not approved for use in children <2 years

Precautions Use with caution in patients with severe cardiovascular disease, hepatic or renal impairment, depression, cerebral or coronary insufficiency, Raynaud's phenomenon, orthostatic hypotension, or thromboangiitis

Adverse Reactions

Cardiovascular: Hypertension, bradycardia, hypotension, tachycardia

Central nervous system: Headache, dizziness, somnolence (see Warnings), decreased alertness, insomnia, hypothermia (in infants only)

Dermatologic: Rash

Gastrointestinal: Xerostomia, taste perversion, dyspepsia, pharyngitis

Local: Stinging, burning sensation

Neuromuscular & skeletal: Hypotonia (in infants only)

Ocular: Allergic conjunctivitis, conjunctival hyperemia, eye pruritus (10% to 20%); conjunctival folliculosis, visual disturbances (5% to 9%); blepharitis, conjunctival

(Continued)

Brimonidine *(Continued)*

edema, conjunctival hemorrhage, conjunctivitis, discharge, dryness, irritation, eye pain, eyelid edema, eyelid erythema, foreign body sensation, photophobia, superficial punctate keratopathy, visual field defect, vitreous floaters, worsened visual acuity, corneal erosion (rare), iritis, miosis

Respiratory: Bronchitis, cough, dyspnea, rhinitis, sinus infection, sinusitis, nasal dryness, apnea

Miscellaneous: Flu-like syndrome, hypersensitivity reactions

Drug Interactions Additive effects with other IOP-lowering agents; additive or potentiating effects with CNS depressants; MAO inhibitors

Stability Store at controlled room temperature (59°F to 77°F)

Mechanism of Action Brimonidine is an alpha-adrenergic receptor agonist that reduces aqueous humor production and increases uveoscleral outflow

Pharmacodynamics Onset of action: Peak effect: 2 hours

Pharmacokinetics

Metabolism: Extensive in liver

Half-life: 2 hours

Time to peak serum concentration: Ophthalmic: Within 0.5-2.5 hours

Usual Dosage Ophthalmic: Children ≥2 years and Adults: Instill 1 drop into lower conjunctival sac of affected eye(s) 3 times/day (approximately every 8 hours)

Administration Ophthalmic: Instill into conjunctival sac avoiding contact of bottle tip with skin or eye; apply finger pressure to lacrimal sac during and for 1-2 minutes after instillation to decrease risk of absorption and systemic effects. Administer other topical ophthalmic medications at least 5 minutes apart; generic formulation contains benzalkonium chloride which may be absorbed by soft contact lenses; wait at least 15 minutes after administration to insert soft contact lenses.

Monitoring Parameters IOP

Patient Information Brimonidine may cause dizziness, drowsiness, visual disturbances, and impair ability to perform activities requiring mental alertness or physical coordination; may cause dry mouth

Dosage Forms Excipient information presented when available (limited, particularly for generics); consult specific product labeling.

Solution, ophthalmic, as tartrate: 0.2% (5 mL, 10 mL, 15 mL) [may contain benzalkonium chloride]

Alphagan® P: 0.1% (5 mL, 10 mL, 15 mL) [contains Purite® as preservative]; 0.15% (5 mL, 10 mL, 15 mL) [contains Purite® as preservative]

References

Berlin RJ, Lee UT, Samples JR, et al, "Ophthalmic Drops Causing Coma in an Infant," *J Pediatr*, 2001, 138(3):441-3.

Carlsen JO, Zabriskie NA, Kwon YH, et al, "Apparent Central Nervous System Depression in Infants After the Use of Topical Brimonidine," *Am J Ophthalmol*, 1999, 128(2):255-6.

Enyedi LB and Freedman SF, "Safety and Efficacy of Brimonidine in Children With Glaucoma," *J AAPOS*, 2001, 5(5):281-4.

♦ **Brimonidine Tartrate** *see* Brimonidine *on page 231*

♦ **Brioschi® [OTC]** *see* Sodium Bicarbonate *on page 1448*

♦ **British Anti-Lewisite** *see* Dimercaprol *on page 508*

♦ **BRL 43694** *see* Granisetron *on page 742*

♦ **Bromaline® [OTC]** *see* Brompheniramine and Pseudoephedrine *on page 235*

♦ **Bromaxefed RF [DSC]** *see* Brompheniramine and Pseudoephedrine *on page 235*

♦ **Bromfenex®** *see* Brompheniramine and Pseudoephedrine *on page 235*

♦ **Bromfenex® PD** *see* Brompheniramine and Pseudoephedrine *on page 235*

♦ **Bromhist-NR** *see* Brompheniramine and Pseudoephedrine *on page 235*

♦ **Bromhist Pediatric** *see* Brompheniramine and Pseudoephedrine *on page 235*

Bromocriptine (broe moe KRIP teen)

Medication Safety Issues

Sound-alike/look-alike issues:

Bromocriptine may be confused with benztropine, brimonidine

Parlodel® may be confused with pindolol, Provera®

U.S. Brand Names Parlodel®; Parlodel® SnapTabs®

Canadian Brand Names Apo-Bromocriptine®; Parlodel®; PMS-Bromocriptine

Index Terms Bromocriptine Mesylate

Therapeutic Category Anti-Parkinson's Agent, Dopamine Agonist; Ergot Derivative

Generic Available Yes

Use Treatment of dysfunctions associated with hyperprolactinemia including amenorrhea with or without galactorrhea, infertility, or hypogonadism; treatment of prolactin-secreting adenomas; treatment of acromegaly; treatment of Parkinson's disease; neuroleptic malignant syndrome (unlabeled use)

Pregnancy Risk Factor B

Lactation Enters breast milk/not recommended

Contraindications Hypersensitivity to bromocriptine, ergot alkaloids, or any component; hereditary problems of galactose intolerance, severe lactase deficiency, or glucose-galactose malabsorption; ergot alkaloids are contraindicated with potent inhibitors of CYP3A4 (includes protease inhibitors, azole antifungals, and some macrolide antibiotics); concomitant use with serotonin agonists (includes buspirone, SSRIs, TCAs, nefazodone, sumatriptan, and trazodone) and sibutramine (see Drug Interactions); uncontrolled hypertension; severe ischemic heart disease or peripheral vascular disorders; pregnancy (risk to benefit evaluation must be performed in women who become pregnant during treatment for acromegaly, prolactinoma, or Parkinson's disease); hypertensive disorders of pregnancy (including eclampsia, preeclampsia, or pregnancy-induced hypertension) are indications for withdrawing therapy in these patients unless withdrawal is considered to be medically contraindicated

Warnings Complete evaluation of pituitary function should be completed prior to initiation of treatment. Patients not seeking pregnancy or those with large adenomas should be advised to use contraception other than oral contraceptives during treatment with bromocriptine. Pregnancy testing is recommended at least every 4 weeks during the amenorrheic period and, once menses are reinitiated, every time a patient misses a menstrual period.

Symptomatic hypotension may occur in a significant number of patients especially during the first days of treatment. Ergot alkaloids and derivatives have been associated with fibrotic valve thickening (eg, aortic, mitral, tricuspid); usually associated with long-term, chronic use. Hypertension, seizures, MI, and stroke have been rarely associated with therapy. Severe headache or visual changes may precede events. The onset of reactions may be immediate or delayed (often may occur in the second week of therapy). Patients who receive bromocriptine during and immediately following pregnancy as a continuation of previous therapy (eg, acromegaly) should be closely monitored for cardiovascular effects. Prolactin-secreting adenomas may expand and compress the optic or other cranial nerves. Monitoring and careful evaluation of visual changes during the treatment of hyperprolactinemia is recommended to differentiate between tumor shrinkage and traction on the optic chiasm. Rapidly progressing visual field loss requires neurosurgical consultation. In most cases, compression resolves following delivery.

Rare cases of pleural and pericardial effusions as well as pleural and pulmonary fibrosis and constrictive pericarditis have been reported, particularly with long term and high-dose treatment. Retroperitoneal fibrosis has also been reported.

In the treatment of acromegaly, discontinuation is recommended if tumor expansion occurs during therapy. Cold sensitive digital vasospasm may occur in some patients with acromegaly and may be reversed with dosage reduction. Discontinuation of therapy in patients with macroadenomas has been associated with rapid regrowth of tumor and increased prolactin serum levels. Safety and effectiveness have not been established in children <15 years of age for pituitary adenoma. Patients treated with pituitary radiation should have an annual 4-8 week withdrawal from bromocriptine to assess both the clinical effects of radiation on the disease process as well as the effects of bromocriptine. Recurrence of signs and symptoms or increases in growth hormone indicate the need to resume treatment.

Safety has not been established for use >2 years in patients with Parkinson's disease. Concurrent use with levodopa has been associated with an increased risk of hallucinations; consider dosage reduction and/or discontinuation in patients with hallucinations. Hallucinations may require weeks to months before resolution. Bromocriptine has been associated with sudden onset of sleep during daily activities, in some cases without awareness or warning signs. A reduction in dosage or termination of therapy may be necessary.

Precautions Use with caution in patients with cardiovascular disease (myocardial infarction, arrhythmia), peptic ulcer, dementia, hepatic impairment, and psychosis. Should not be used postpartum in women with coronary artery disease or other cardiovascular disease; use to control or prevent lactation or in patients with uncontrolled hypertension is not recommended. Concurrent antihypertensives or drugs which may alter blood pressure should be used with caution.

Adverse Reactions Note: Frequency of adverse effects may vary by dose and/or indication.

Cardiovascular: Hypotension (up to 30%), orthostasis, vasospasm (cold-sensitive), exacerbation of Raynaud's syndrome, syncope, arrhythmias, bradycardia, MI, hypertension, vasovagal reaction, mottled skin, pericardial effusions, constrictive pericarditis (rare)

(Continued)

Bromocriptine *(Continued)*

Central nervous system: Headache (19%), dizziness (17%), fatigue, lightheadedness, drowsiness, hallucinations (visual), seizures, nightmares, paranoia, psychosis, vertigo, insomnia, lassitude, CSF rhinorrhea (rare when treating large prolactinomas), ataxia, psychomotor agitation

Dermatologic: Alopecia, rash

Gastrointestinal: Nausea (49%), constipation, anorexia, vomiting, abdominal cramps, diarrhea, dyspepsia, GI bleeding, xerostomia, retroperitoneal fibrosis (rare), dysphagia

Hepatic: Increased transaminases, increased CPK

Muscular & skeletal: Muscle cramps, paresthesia, tingling, dyskinesia

Ocular: Blepharospasm, visual changes

Renal: Increased BUN

Respiratory: Nasal congestion, pulmonary infiltrates, pleural effusion, pulmonary fibrosis, pleural fibrosis

Miscellaneous: Pulmonary infiltrates, pleural effusion

Withdrawal reactions: Abrupt discontinuation has resulted in rare cases of a withdrawal reaction with symptoms similar to neuroleptic malignant syndrome.

Drug Interactions Cytochrome P450 isoenzyme CYP3A4 substrate (major); CYP1A2 (weak) and CYP3A4 (weak) inhibitor

Alpha agonists/sympathomimetics may enhance the adverse/toxic effect of bromocriptine, including increased blood pressure, ventricular arrhythmias, and seizures (**Note:** The use of epinephrine in combination local anesthetics should pose no clinical concern). Alcohol may enhance the adverse effects of bromocriptine; antihypertensives may increase the risk of hypotension and/or orthostasis; antifungals, azole derivatives (itraconazole, ketoconazole) increase levels of ergot alkaloids by inhibiting CYP3A4 metabolism, resulting in toxicity; concomitant use is contraindicated.

Antipsychotics and metoclopramide may diminish the effects of bromocriptine (due to dopamine antagonism); these combinations should generally be avoided; CYP3A4 inhibitors may increase the levels/effects of bromocriptine. Example inhibitors include azole antifungals, clarithromycin, diclofenac, doxycycline, erythromycin, imatinib, isoniazid, nefazodone, nicardipine, propofol, protease inhibitors, quinidine, telithromycin, and verapamil. Levodopa may increase the risk of hallucinations; dosage reduction may be required.

Macrolide antibiotics (erythromycin, clarithromycin, telithromycin, and troleandomycin) may increase levels of ergot alkaloids by inhibiting CYP3A4 metabolism, resulting in toxicity (ischemia, vasospasm); concomitant use is contraindicated. MAO inhibitors may increase the serotonergic effects of ergot derivatives; monitor for signs and symptoms of serotonin syndrome.

Protease inhibitors (ritonavir, amprenavir, indinavir, nelfinavir, and saquinavir) increase blood levels of ergot alkaloids by inhibiting CYP3A4 metabolism; acute ergot toxicity has been reported; concomitant use is contraindicated.

Serotonin agonists (buspirone, SSRIs, TCAs, nefazodone, sumatriptan, and trazodone) and sibutramine may increase the risk of serotonin syndrome; concurrent use with ergot alkaloids is contraindicated.

Food Interactions The herbal medicine St John's wort (*Hypericum perforatum*) may decrease bromocriptine levels.

Mechanism of Action Semisynthetic ergot alkaloid derivative and a dopamine receptor agonist which activates postsynaptic dopamine receptors in the tuberoinfundibular process which results in inhibition of pituitary prolactin secretion. Stimulation of dopamine receptors in the corpus striatum is beneficial in the treatment of Parkinson's disease, a condition characterized by a progressive deficiency in dopamine synthesis.

Pharmacodynamics Reduction of prolactin levels:

Onset of action: 1-2 hours

Maximum effect: 5-10 hours

Duration: 8-12 hours

Pharmacokinetics

Bioavailability: 28%

Protein binding: 90% to 96%

Metabolism: Primarily hepatic with extensive first-pass biotransformation

Half-life: Biphasic with terminal half-life: 15 hours; range: 8-20 hours

Time to peak serum concentration: 1-2 hours

Elimination: Feces; urine (2% to 6% as unchanged drug)

Usual Dosage Oral:

Hyperprolactinemia:

Children 11-15 years (based on limited information): Initial: 1.25-2.5 mg daily; dosage may be increased as tolerated to achieve a therapeutic response (range: 2.5-10 mg daily)

Children ≥16 years and Adults: Initial: 1.25-2.5 mg/day; may be increased by 2.5 mg/day as tolerated every 2-7 days until optimal response (range: 2.5-15 mg/day)

Parkinsonism: Adults: 1.25 mg twice daily, increased by 2.5 mg/day in 2- to 4-week intervals (usual dose range is 30-90 mg/day in 3 divided doses), though elderly patients can usually be managed on lower doses

Neuroleptic malignant syndrome (unlabeled use): Adults: 2.5-5 mg 3 times/day

Acromegaly: Adults: Initial: 1.25-2.5 mg daily increasing by 1.25-2.5 mg daily as necessary every 3-7 days; usual dose: 20-30 mg/day (maximum: 100 mg/day)

Dosing adjustment in hepatic impairment: No guidelines are available; however, may be necessary

Administration Oral: May be taken with food to decrease GI distress

Monitoring Parameters Monitor blood pressure closely as well as hepatic, hematopoietic, and cardiovascular function; visual field monitoring is recommended (prolactinoma); pregnancy testing (see Warnings); growth hormone and prolactin levels

Patient Information Take exactly as directed (may be prescribed in conjunction with levodopa/carbidopa); do not change dosage or discontinue this medicine without consulting prescriber. Therapeutic effects may take several weeks or months to achieve and you may need frequent monitoring during first weeks of therapy. Take with meals if GI upset occurs, before meals if dry mouth occurs, or after eating if drooling or if nausea occurs. Take at the same time each day. Maintain adequate hydration (2-3 L/day of fluids) unless instructed to restrict fluid intake; void before taking medication. Do not use alcohol, prescription or OTC sedatives, or CNS depressants without consulting prescriber. Urine or perspiration may appear darker. You may experience drowsiness, dizziness, confusion, or vision changes (use caution when driving, climbing stairs, or engaging in tasks requiring alertness until response to drug is known); orthostatic hypotension (use caution when rising from sitting or lying position); constipation (increased exercise, fluids, fruit, or fiber may help); nasal congestion (consult prescriber for appropriate relief); or nausea, vomiting, loss of appetite, or stomach discomfort (small frequent meals, frequent mouth care, chewing gum, or sucking lozenges may help). Report unresolved constipation or vomiting; chest pain or irregular heartbeat; acute headache or dizziness; CNS changes (eg, hallucination, loss of memory, seizures, acute headache, nervousness); painful or difficult urination; increased muscle spasticity, rigidity, or involuntary movements; skin rash; or significant worsening of condition.

Additional Information Usually used with levodopa or levodopa/carbidopa to treat Parkinson's disease. When adding bromocriptine, the dose of levodopa/carbidopa can usually be decreased.

Dosage Forms Excipient information presented when available (limited, particularly for generics); consult specific product labeling.

Capsule, as mesylate: 5 mg

Parlodel®: 5 mg

Tablet, as mesylate: 2.5 mg

Parlodel® SnapTabs®: 2.5 mg

References

de Groot AN, van Dongen PW, Vree TB, et al, "Ergot Alkaloids. Current Status and Review of Clinical Pharmacology and Therapeutic Use Compared With Other Oxytocics in Obstetrics and Gynaecology," *Drugs*, 1998, 56(4):523-35.

Gillam MP, Fideleff H, Boquete HR, et al, "Prolactin Excess: Treatment and Toxicity," *Pediatr Endocrinol Rev*, 2004, 2(suppl)1:108-14.

Lejoyeux M, et al, "Serotonin Syndrome: Incidence, Symptoms, and Treatment," *CNS Drugs*, 1994, 2:132-43.

Melmed S and Braunstein GD, "Bromocriptine and Pleuropulmonary Disease," *Arch Intern Med*, 1989, 149(2):258-9.

Molitch ME, "Management of Prolactinomas During Pregnancy," *J Reprod Med*, 1999, 44(12 Suppl):1121-6.

Morgans D, "Re: Parlodel," *Aust N Z J Obstet Gynaecol*, 1995, 35(2):228-9.

Mueller PS, Vester JW, and Fermaglich J, "Neuroleptic Malignant Syndrome. Successful Treatment With Bromocriptine," *JAMA*, 1983, 249(3):386-8.

Parkes D, "Drug Therapy: Bromocriptine," *N Engl J Med*, 1979, 301(16):873-8.

♦ **Bromocriptine Mesylate** *see* Bromocriptine *on page 232*

Brompheniramine and Pseudoephedrine

(brome fen IR a meen & soo doe e FED rin)

Medication Safety Issues

Sound-alike/look-alike issues:

Bromfed® may be confused with Bromphen®

(Continued)

Brompheniramine and Pseudoephedrine *(Continued)*

Related Information
OTC Cough and Cold Preparations, Pediatric *on page 1706*

U.S. Brand Names AccuHist®; Andehist NR Syrup; Bromaline® [OTC]; Bromaxefed RF [DSC]; Bromfenex®; Bromfenex® PD; Bromhist-NR; Bromhist Pediatric; Brotapp; Brovex SR; Children's Dimetapp® Elixir Cold & Allergy [OTC] [DSC]; Dimaphen [OTC]; Histex™ SR; Lodrane®; Lodrane® 12D; Lodrane® 24D; Lodrane® D; LoHist 12D; LoHist LQ; LoHist PD; Sildec Syrup; Touro® Allergy

Index Terms Brompheniramine Maleate and Pseudoephedrine Hydrochloride; Brompheniramine Maleate and Pseudoephedrine Sulfate; Pseudoephedrine and Brompheniramine

Therapeutic Category Antihistamine/Decongestant Combination

Generic Available Yes

Use Temporary relief of nasal congestion, running nose, sneezing, and itchy, watery eyes; also promotes nasal or sinus drainage

Pregnancy Risk Factor C

Lactation Enters breast milk/not recommended

Contraindications Hypersensitivity to brompheniramine, pseudoephedrine, or any component; MAO inhibitor therapy, severe hypertension, severe coronary artery disease

Warnings Some products may contain sodium benzoate; benzoic acid (benzoate) is a metabolite of benzyl alcohol; large amounts of benzyl alcohol (≥99 mg/kg/day) have been associated with a potentially fatal toxicity ("gasping syndrome") in neonates; the "gasping syndrome" consists of metabolic acidosis, respiratory distress, gasping respirations, CNS dysfunction (including convulsions, intracranial hemorrhage), hypotension and cardiovascular collapse; avoid use in neonates; *in vitro* and animal studies have shown that benzoate displaces bilirubin from protein binding sites

Precautions Use with caution in patients with mild-moderate hypertension, heart disease, arrhythmias, diabetes mellitus, thyroid disease, asthma, glaucoma, and prostatic hypertrophy

Adverse Reactions See individual monograph for Pseudoephedrine *on page 1344*.
Brompheniramine component only:
- Cardiovascular: Palpitations
- Central nervous system: Paradoxical excitability, drowsiness, dizziness, headache, fever, nervousness, depression
- Dermatologic: Rash, photosensitivity, angioedema
- Endocrine & metabolic: Weight gain
- Gastrointestinal: Nausea, anorexia, xerostomia, appetite increase, diarrhea, abdominal pain
- Hepatic: Hepatitis
- Neuromuscular & skeletal: Myalgia, paresthesia
- Respiratory: Bronchospasm, epistaxis, thickening of bronchial secretions

Drug Interactions See individual monograph for Pseudoephedrine *on page 1344*.
Brompheniramine component only: May cause additive sedation with other CNS depressants; may cause additive anticholinergic effects with other anticholinergic agents; MAO inhibitors

Pharmacodynamics See individual monograph for Pseudoephedrine *on page 1344*.
Brompheniramine component only:
- Maximum effect: Maximal clinical effects seen within 3-9 hours
- Duration: Varies with formulation

Pharmacokinetics See individual monograph for Pseudoephedrine *on page 1344*.
Brompheniramine component only:
- Metabolism: Extensive by the liver
- Half-life: 12-34 hours
- Time to peak serum concentration: Oral: Within 2-5 hours
- Elimination: In urine as inactive metabolites

Usual Dosage Oral:
Manufacturer's recommendations:
- Children's Dimetapp® Elixir Cold & Allergy:
  - Children 6-12 years: 10 mL (pseudoephedrine 30 mg) every 4 hours
  - Children >12 years and Adults: 20 mL (pseudoephedrine 60 mg) every 4 hours
- Lodrane® D suspension:
  - Children 2-6 years: 1.25 mL (pseudoephedrine 15 mg) every 12 hours
  - Children 6-12 years: 2.5 mL (pseudoephedrine 30 mg) every 12 hours; not to exceed 2 doses/day
  - Children >12 years and Adults: 5 mL (pseudoephedrine 60 mg) every 12 hours not to exceed 2 doses/day

Lodrane® 12D:

Children 6-12 years: 1 tablet (pseudoephedrine 45 mg) every 12 hours; not to exceed 2 tablets/day

Children >12 years and Adults: 1-2 tablets (pseudoephedrine 45-90 mg) every 12 hours; not to exceed 4 tablets/day

Lodrane® 24D:

Children 6-12 years: 1 capsule (pseudoephedrine 90 mg) once daily

Children >12 years and Adults: 1-2 capsules (pseudoephedrine 90-180 mg) once daily

Alternative pediatric dosing: May dose according to the pseudoephedrine component:

Infants and Children <2 years: 4 mg/kg/day in divided doses every 6 hours

Children 2-5 years: 15 mg every 6 hours; maximum dose: 60 mg/24 hours

Children 6-12 years: 30 mg every 6 hours or extended release product 60 mg every 12 hours; maximum dose: 120 mg/24 hours

Children >12 years and Adults: 30-60 mg every 6 hours or extended release product 120 mg every 12 hours; maximum dose: 240 mg/24 hours

Administration Oral: Administer with food

Test Interactions False-positive test for amphetamines by EMIT assay

Patient Information May cause drowsiness and impair ability to perform activities requiring mental alertness or physical coordination. May cause photosensitivity reactions (eg, exposure to sunlight may cause severe sunburn, skin rash, redness, or itching); avoid direct exposure to sunlight

Dosage Forms Excipient information presented when available (limited, particularly for generics); consult specific product labeling. [DSC] = Discontinued product

Capsule, extended release:

Bromfenex®: Brompheniramine maleate 12 mg and pseudoephedrine hydrochloride 120 mg

Bromfenex® PD: Brompheniramine maleate 6 mg and pseudoephedrine hydrochloride 60 mg

Histex™ SR: Brompheniramine maleate 10 mg and pseudoephedrine hydrochloride 120 mg [DSC]

Lodrane® 24D: Brompheniramine maleate 12 mg and pseudoephedrine hydrochloride 90 mg

Capsule, sustained release:

Brovex SR: Brompheniramine maleate 9 mg and pseudoephedrine hydrochloride 90 mg

Touro® Allergy: Brompheniramine maleate 5.75 mg and pseudoephedrine hydrochloride 60 mg

Elixir:

Children's Dimetapp® Elixir Cold & Allergy: Brompheniramine maleate 1 mg and pseudoephedrine hydrochloride 15 mg per 5 mL (240 mL) [alcohol free; contains sodium benzoate; grape flavor] [DSC]

Dimaphen: Brompheniramine maleate 1 mg and pseudoephedrine hydrochloride 15 mg per 5 mL (120 mL, 480 mL)

Liquid: Brompheniramine maleate 4 mg and pseudoephedrine hydrochloride 60 mg per 5 mL (480 mL)

Brotapp: Brompheniramine maleate 1 mg and pseudoephedrine hydrochloride 15 mg per 5 mL (120 mL, 240 mL, 480 mL) [grape flavor]

Lodrane®: Brompheniramine maleate 4 mg and pseudoephedrine hydrochloride 60 mg per 5 mL (480 mL) [alcohol free, dye free, sugar free; cherry flavor]

LoHist LQ: Brompheniramine maleate 4 mg and pseudoephedrine hydrochloride 60 mg per 5 mL (480 mL) [cherry flavor]

Liquid, oral [drops]:

AccuHist®: Brompheniramine maleate 1 mg and pseudoephedrine hydrochloride 12.5 mg per 1 mL (30 mL) [sugar free; cherry flavor]

Bromhist NR: Brompheniramine maleate 1 mg and pseudoephedrine hydrochloride 12.5 mg per 1 mL (30 mL) [cherry flavor]

Bromhist Pediatric: Brompheniramine maleate 1 mg and pseudoephedrine hydrochloride 15 mg per 1 mL (30 mL) [cherry flavor]

LoHist PD: Brompheniramine maleate 1 mg and pseudoephedrine hydrochloride 12.5 mg per 1 mL (30 mL) [cherry flavor]

Solution:

Bromaline®: Brompheniramine maleate 1 mg and pseudoephedrine hydrochloride 15 mg per 5 mL (120 mL, 480 mL) [alcohol free; contains sodium benzoate; grape flavor]

Suspension:

Lodrane® D: Brompheniramine tannate 8 mg and pseudoephedrine tannate 90 mg per 5 mL (480 mL) [alcohol free, sugar free; strawberry flavor]

Syrup:

Andehist NR: Brompheniramine maleate 4 mg and pseudoephedrine sulfate 45 mg per 5 mL (473 mL) [raspberry flavor]

(Continued)

Brompheniramine and Pseudoephedrine *(Continued)*

Bromaxefed RF: Brompheniramine maleate 4 mg and pseudoephedrine hydrochloride 45 mg per 5 mL (120 mL, 480 mL) [alcohol free; cherry flavor]

Sildec: Brompheniramine maleate 4 mg and pseudoephedrine hydrochloride 45 mg per 5 mL (480 mL) [raspberry flavor]

Tablet, extended release:

Lodrane® 12D: Brompheniramine maleate 6 mg and pseudoephedrine hydrochloride 45 mg [dye free]

LoHist 12D: Brompheniramine maleate 6 mg and pseudoephedrine hydrochloride 45 mg

Tablet, sustained release: Brompheniramine maleate 6 mg and pseudoephedrine hydrochloride 45 mg

- ♦ **Brompheniramine Maleate and Pseudoephedrine Hydrochloride** *see* Brompheniramine and Pseudoephedrine *on page 235*
- ♦ **Brompheniramine Maleate and Pseudoephedrine Sulfate** *see* Brompheniramine and Pseudoephedrine *on page 235*
- ♦ **Broncho Saline® [OTC] [DSC]** *see* Sodium Chloride *on page 1450*
- ♦ **Brontex®** *see* Guaifenesin and Codeine *on page 746*
- ♦ **Brotapp** *see* Brompheniramine and Pseudoephedrine *on page 235*
- ♦ **Brovex SR** *see* Brompheniramine and Pseudoephedrine *on page 235*
- ♦ **BTX-A** *see* Botulinum Toxin Type A *on page 226*

Budesonide (byoo DES oh nide)

Related Information

Asthma *on page 1904*

U.S. Brand Names Entocort® EC; Pulmicort Flexhaler®; Pulmicort Respules®; Pulmicort Turbuhaler®; Rhinocort® Aqua®

Canadian Brand Names Entocort®; Gen-Budesonide AQ; Pulmicort®; Rhinocort® Turbuhaler®

Therapeutic Category Adrenal Corticosteroid; Anti-inflammatory Agent; Antiasthmatic; Corticosteroid, Inhalant (Oral); Corticosteroid, Intranasal; Corticosteroid, Oral; Glucocorticoid

Generic Available No

Use

Intranasal:

Children and Adults: Management of seasonal or perennial allergic rhinitis

Adults: Nonallergic perennial rhinitis

Nebulization: Children 12 months to 8 years: Maintenance therapy and prophylaxis of bronchial asthma; **not** indicated for the relief of acute bronchospasm

Oral: Treatment of mild to moderate active Crohn's disease of the ileum and/or ascending colon; maintenance of remission (for up to 3 months) of mild to moderate Crohn's disease of the ileum and/or ascending colon

Oral inhalation: Long-term (chronic) control of persistent bronchial asthma; **NOT** indicated for the relief of acute bronchospasm; also indicated in bronchial asthma patients requiring oral corticosteroids (inhalation may decrease or eliminate need for oral steroids over time)

Pregnancy Risk Factor Pulmicort® Respules® and Turbuhaler® and Rhinocort® Aqua®: B; Entocort®: C

Lactation Enters breast milk/use caution

Contraindications Hypersensitivity to budesonide or any component; Pulmicort® Respules® and Pulmicort® Turbuhaler®: Primary treatment of status asthmaticus or other acute episodes of bronchial asthma where intensive treatment is needed

Warnings

Oral inhalation and nebulization: Fatalities have occurred due to adrenal insufficiency in asthmatic patients during and after switching from systemic corticosteroids to aerosol steroids; several months may be required for full recovery of hypothalamic-pituitary-adrenal (HPA) function; patients receiving higher doses of systemic corticosteroids (eg, adults receiving ≥20 mg of prednisone per day may be at greater risk; during this period of HPA suppression, aerosol steroids do **not** provide the systemic glucocorticoid or mineral corticoid activity needed to treat patients requiring stress doses (ie, patients with major stress such as trauma, surgery, or infections, or other conditions associated with severe electrolyte loss). When used at high doses, HPA suppression may occur; use with inhaled or systemic corticosteroids (even alternate-day dosing) may increase risk of HPA suppression. Acute adrenal insufficiency may occur with abrupt withdrawal after long-term use or with stress; withdrawal and discontinuation of corticosteroids should be done carefully; patients with HPA axis suppression may require doses of systemic glucocorticosteroids prior to, during, and after unusual stress (eg, surgery). Immunosuppression may occur; patients may be more susceptible to infections; avoid exposure to chickenpox and measles. Bronchospasm may occur after use of inhaled asthma medications (see Additional Information).

Oral: HPA axis suppression may occur; adrenal suppression may occur when switching patients from systemic corticosteroids to oral budesonide (due to lower bioavailability); withdrawal and discontinuation of systemic corticosteroids should be done carefully (monitoring of adrenocorticoid function may be needed); patients with HPA axis suppression may require increased doses of systemic glucocorticosteroids prior to, during, and after unusual stress (eg, surgery). Immunosuppression may occur; patients may be more susceptible to infections; avoid exposure to chickenpox and measles.

Precautions Avoid using higher than recommended dosages; suppression of HPA function, suppression of linear growth (ie, reduction of growth velocity), reduced bone mineral density, or hypercorticism (Cushing's syndrome) may occur; titrate to lowest effective dose. Reduction in growth velocity may occur when corticosteroids are administered to pediatric patients, even at recommended doses via oral, inhaled, nebulized, or intranasal route (monitor growth). Use of oral, inhaled, nebulized, or nasal budesonide in place of systemic corticosteroids may unmask allergies (eg, eczema, rhinitis) that were previously controlled by the systemic corticosteroids. Use oral budesonide with caution in patients with hypertension, tuberculosis, osteoporosis, diabetes mellitus, peptic ulcer disease, glaucoma, cataracts, or a family history of glaucoma or diabetes mellitus; use oral budesonide with caution and consider dosage reduction in patients with hepatic cirrhosis. Use inhaled budesonide with extreme caution in patients with respiratory tuberculosis, untreated systemic infections, or ocular herpes simplex. Rare cases of increased IOP, glaucoma, or cataracts may occur with inhaled corticosteroids.

Adverse Reactions

Cardiovascular: Facial edema

Central nervous system: Nervousness, migraine, insomnia, fatigue, dizziness, headache, fever, amnesia

Dermatologic: Rash, pruritus, contact dermatitis

Endocrine & metabolic: HPA suppression, hypokalemia, Cushingoid state, weight gain

Gastrointestinal: Xerostomia, dysgeusia, GI irritation, nausea, abdominal pain, vomiting, diarrhea

Hematologic: Leukocytosis, purpura

Local: Nasal irritation, burning, or ulceration; pharyngitis; growth of *Candida* in the mouth, throat, or nares

Neuromuscular & skeletal: Growth suppression, fracture, myalgia, arthralgia, decreased bone mineral density

Ocular: Conjunctivitis

Otic: Otitis media

Respiratory: Cough, epistaxis, wheezing, decreased sense of smell, hoarseness, respiratory infection, rhinitis, sinusitis

Miscellaneous: Immunosuppression, anaphylactoid reactions (rare)

Drug Interactions Cytochrome P450 isoenzyme CYP3A4 substrate

Ketoconazole, itraconazole, cimetidine, clarithromycin, erythromycin, ritonavir, indinavir, saquinavir, or other CYP3A4 inhibitors may increase budesonide serum concentrations (use with caution with all dosage forms of budesonide; monitor for signs of hypercorticoidism; consider reduction of oral budesonide dose); interactions similar to other corticosteroids may potentially occur; since dissolution of the coating of the oral capsules is pH dependent (see Additional Information), absorption of budesonide capsules may be altered by drugs that change the gastrointestinal pH

Food Interactions A high-fat meal delays the time to peak concentration by 2.5 hours, but does not affect the extent of oral absorption; grapefruit juice significantly increases oral absorption

Stability

Capsule: Store at room temperature in a tightly closed container

Intranasal inhaler: Use within 6 months after opening; avoid storage in high humidity; do not store or use by heat or open flame

Nebulization: Store Respules® upright at room temperature (68°F to 77°F); do not refrigerate or freeze; do not mix with other medications; after foil packet has been opened, Respules® are stable for 2 weeks when protected from light; return unused Respules® to foil packet to protect from light; use opened Respules® promptly

Oral inhaler: Keep clean and dry; store at room temperature 68°F to 77°F

Mechanism of Action Controls the rate of protein synthesis, depresses the migration of polymorphonuclear leukocytes and fibroblasts, reverses capillary permeability, and

(Continued)

Budesonide *(Continued)*

stabilizes lysosomal membranes at the cellular level to prevent or control inflammation

Pharmacodynamics Clinical effects are due to direct local effect, rather than systemic absorption

Onset of action:

Oral inhalation; intranasal inhaler: Within 24 hours

Intranasal spray (Rhinocort® Aqua®): Within 10 hours

Nebulization (control of asthma symptoms): Within 2-8 days

Maximum effect:

Intranasal spray: 2 weeks

Nebulization: 4-6 weeks

Oral inhalation: 1-2 weeks or more

Duration after discontinuation: Intranasal: Several days

Pharmacokinetics

Absorption:

Intranasal spray: 34% of dose delivered reaches systemic circulation

Oral inhalation: 39% of the metered dose is systemically available

Distribution: V_d:

Children 4-6 years: 3 L/kg

Adults: ~200 L or 2.2-3.9 L/kg

Protein binding: 85% to 90%

Metabolism: Extensively metabolized by the liver via cytochrome P450 CYP3A isoenzyme to 2 major metabolites: 16α-hydroxyprednisolone and 6β-hydroxybudesonide; both are <1% as active as parent

Bioavailability:

Nebulization: Children 4-6 years: 6%; **Note:** AUC of single 1 mg dose was comparable to a single 2 mg dose in healthy adults

Oral: ~10% (large first pass effect); **Note:** Oral bioavailability is 2.5-fold higher in patients with hepatic cirrhosis

Half-life:

Children: 4-6 years: 2.3 hours (after nebulization)

Children 10-14 years: 1.5 hours

Adults: 2-3.6 hours

Time to peak serum concentration: Oral: 30-600 minutes

Elimination: 60% to 66% of dose renally excreted as metabolites; no unchanged drug found in urine

Clearance:

Children 4-6 years: 0.5 L/minute (~50% greater than healthy adults after weight adjustment)

Adults: 0.9-1.8 L/minute

Usual Dosage

Intranasal: Children ≥6 years and Adults:

Rhinocort® Aqua® (32 mcg/spray): Initial: 2 sprays (1 spray/nostril) once daily (64 mcg/day); dose may be increased if needed

Maximum dose:

Children <12 years: 4 sprays (2 sprays/nostril) once daily (128 mcg/day)

Children ≥12 years and Adults: 8 sprays (4 sprays/nostril) once daily (256 mcg/day)

Nebulization: Pulmicort® Respules®: Doses should be titrated to the lowest effective dose once asthma is controlled:

Manufacturer's recommendations: Children 12 months to 8 years:

Previously treated with bronchodilators alone: Initial: 0.25 mg twice daily or 0.5 mg once daily; maximum dose: 0.5 mg/day

Previously treated with inhaled corticosteroids: Initial: 0.25 mg twice daily or 0.5 mg once daily; maximum dose: 1 mg/day

Previously treated with oral corticosteroids: Initial: 0.5 mg twice daily or 1 mg once daily; maximum dose: 1 mg/day

Symptomatic children not responding to nonsteroidal asthma medications: Initial: 0.25 mg once daily may be considered

Oral:

Children: A retrospective study of 62 children (mean age: 14.1 ± 2.5 years; range: 9.5-18 years) used oral budesonide in doses of 0.45 mg/kg/day (maximum dose: 9 mg/day) for the treatment of mild to moderate Crohn's disease (see Levine, 2002); further studies are needed

Adults:

Active Crohn's disease (treatment): 9 mg once daily in the morning for ≤8 weeks; may repeat the 8-week course for recurring episodes of active Crohn's disease; **Note:** When switching patients from oral prednisolone to oral budesonide, do not stop prednisolone abruptly; prednisolone taper should begin at the same time that budesonide is started

Maintenance of remission: Following treatment of active disease and control of symptoms (Crohn's Disease Activity Index <150), use 6 mg once daily for up to 3 months; if symptoms are still controlled at 3 months, taper the dose to complete cessation; continuing remission dose >3 months has not been demonstrated to result in substantial benefit.

Oral inhalation: Note: Doses should be titrated to the lowest effective dose once asthma is controlled; Manufacturer's recommendations:

Children ≥6 years:

Previously treated with bronchodilators alone or with inhaled corticosteroids: Initial: 200 mcg (1 puff) twice daily; maximum dose: 400 mcg (2 puffs) twice daily

Treated with oral corticosteroids: Initial: 400 mcg (2 puffs) twice daily (maximum dose)

Adults:

Previously treated with bronchodilators alone: Initial: 200-400 mcg (1-2 puffs) twice daily; maximum dose: 400 mcg (2 puffs) twice daily

Treated with inhaled corticosteroids: Initial: 200-400 mcg (1-2 puffs) twice daily; maximum dose: 800 mcg (4 puffs) twice daily

Treated with oral corticosteroids: Initial: 400-800 mcg (2-4 puffs) twice daily; maximum dose: 800 mcg (4 puffs) twice daily

NIH Asthma Guidelines (NAEPP, 2002):

Nebulization [give once daily or in divided doses twice daily]:

Children ≤12 years:

"Low" dose: 0.5 mg/day

"Medium" dose: 1 mg/day

"High" dose: 2 mg/day daily

Oral inhalation [give in divided doses twice daily]:

Children ≤12 years:

"Low" dose: 200-400 mcg/day (1-2 inhalations/day)

"Medium" dose: 400-800 mcg/day (2-4 inhalations/day)

"High" dose: >800 mcg/day (>4 inhalations/day)

Children >12 years and Adults:

"Low" dose: 200-600 mcg/day (1-3 inhalations/day)

"Medium" dose: 600-1200 mcg/day (3-6 inhalations/day)

"High" dose: >1200 mcg/day (>6 inhalations/day)

Dosage adjustment in moderate to severe liver dysfunction: Oral: Monitor for signs and symptoms of hypercorticism; consider dosage reduction

Administration

Intranasal spray: Clear nasal passage by blowing nose prior to use; shake container gently before use

Nebulization: Shake gently with a circular motion before use. Administer only with a compressed air driven jet nebulizer; do not use an ultrasonic nebulizer; use adequate flow rates and administer via appropriate size face mask or mouthpiece; avoid exposure of nebulized medication to eyes

Oral: May be administered without regard to meals; do not chew, crush, break, or open capsule; swallow whole; do not administer with grapefruit juice

Oral inhaler: Do **not** shake inhaler; do not use inhaler with a spacer

Monitoring Parameters Monitor growth in pediatric patients; inhalation and intranasal: Check mucous membranes for signs of fungal infection

Patient Information Notify physician if condition being treated persists or worsens; do not decrease dose or discontinue without physician approval; avoid exposure to chicken pox or measles; if exposed, seek medical advice without delay; may cause dry mouth

Nebulization: Rinse mouth after treatment and wash face after using face mask to decrease chance of oral candidiasis and steroid effects on skin

Oral: Avoid grapefruit juice and grapefruit

Oral inhaler: Rinse mouth after inhalation to decrease chance of oral candidiasis; report sore mouth or mouth lesions to physician. A red mark will appear on the indicator window of the Pulmicort Turbuhaler® when 20 doses are left.

Additional Information If bronchospasm with wheezing occurs after use of oral inhaler, a fast-acting bronchodilator may be used; discontinue orally inhaled corticosteroid and initiate alternative chronic therapy. Pulmicort® Turbuhaler® delivers budesonide as a fine powder.

A 12-week study in infants (n=141; 6-12 months of age) receiving budesonide nebulizations (0.5 mg or 1 mg once daily) versus placebo demonstrated a budesonide dose-dependent suppression of linear growth; in addition, although mean changes

(Continued)

Budesonide *(Continued)*

from baseline did not indicate budesonide-induced adrenal suppression, 6 infants who received budesonide had subnormal stimulated cortisol levels at week 12. Children and adolescents (n=18; 6-15 years) receiving budesonide nebulizations of 1 and 2 mg twice daily showed a significant reduction in urinary cortisol excretion; this reduction was not seen when patients were dosed at 1 mg/day (maximum recommended dose). Long-term effects of chronic use of budesonide nebulization on immunological or developmental processes of upper airways, mouth, and lung are unknown.

Budesonide capsules (Entocort® EC) contain granules in an ethylcellulose matrix; the granules are coated with a methacrylic acid polymer to protect from dissolution in the stomach; the coating dissolves at a pH >5.5 (duodenal pH); the ethylcellulose matrix controls the release of drug in a time-dependent manner (until the drug reaches the ileum and ascending colon)

Dosage Forms Excipient information presented when available (limited, particularly for generics); consult specific product labeling. [CAN] = Canadian brand name

Capsule, enteric coated:
- Entocort® EC: 3 mg

Powder for oral inhalation:
- Pulmicort Flexhaler®: 90 mcg/inhalation (165 mg) [delivers ~80 mcg/inhalation; 60 actuations]
- Pulmicort Flexhaler®: 180 mcg/inhalation (225 mg) [delivers ~160 mcg/inhalation; 120 actuations]
- Pulmicort Turbuhaler®: 200 mcg/inhalation (104 g) [delivers ~160 mcg/inhalation; 200 metered actuations]
- Pulmicort Turbuhaler® [CAN]: 100 mcg/inhalation [delivers 200 metered actuations]; 200 mcg/inhalation [delivers 200 metered actuations]; 400 mcg/inhalation [delivers 200 metered actuations] [not available in the U.S.]

Suspension, intranasal [spray]:
- Rhinocort® Aqua®: 32 mcg/inhalation (8.6 g) [120 metered actuations]

Suspension for nebulization:
- Pulmicort Respules®: 0.25 mg/2 mL (30s), 0.5 mg/2 mL (30s)

References

"Budesonide (Entocort™ EC) for Crohn's Disease," *Med Lett Drugs Ther*, 2002, 44(1122):6-8.

Expert Panel Report 2, "Guidelines for the Diagnosis and Management of Asthma," *Clinical Practice Guidelines*, National Institutes of Health, National Heart, Lung, and Blood Institute, NIH Publication No. 94-4051, April, 1997.

Levine A, Broide E, Stein M, et al, "Evaluation of Oral Budesonide for Treatment of Mild and Moderate Exacerbations of Crohn's Disease in Children," *J Pediatr*, 2002, 140(1):75-80.

"National Asthma Education and Prevention Program. Expert Panel Report: Guidelines for the Diagnosis and Management of Asthma Update on Selected Topics--2002," *J Allergy Clin Immunol*, 2002, 110(5 Suppl):S141-219.

Szefler SJ, "A Review of Budesonide Inhalation Suspension in the Treatment of Pediatric Asthma," *Pharmacotherapy*, 2001, 21(2):195-206.

♦ **Buffasal [OTC]** *see* Aspirin *on page 163*
♦ **Bufferin® [OTC]** *see* Aspirin *on page 163*
♦ **Bufferin® Extra Strength [OTC]** *see* Aspirin *on page 163*
♦ **Buffinol [OTC]** *see* Aspirin *on page 163*

Bumetanide (byoo MET a nide)

Medication Safety Issues

Sound-alike/look-alike issues:
- Bumetanide may be confused with Buminate®
- Bumex® may be confused with Brevibloc®, Buprenex®, Permax®

Related Information

Antihypertensive Agents by Class *on page 1678*

U.S. Brand Names Bumex®

Canadian Brand Names Bumex®; Burinex®

Therapeutic Category Antihypertensive Agent; Diuretic, Loop

Generic Available Yes

Use Management of edema secondary to CHF or hepatic or renal disease including nephrotic syndrome; may also be used alone or in combination with antihypertensives in the treatment of hypertension

Pregnancy Risk Factor C

Lactation Excretion in breast milk unknown/use caution

Contraindications Hypersensitivity to bumetanide or any component; anuria or increasing azotemia; hepatic coma; severe electrolyte depletion (until condition is improved or corrected)

Warnings Loop diuretics are potent diuretics; excess amounts can lead to profound diuresis with fluid and electrolyte loss; close medical supervision and dose evaluation is required. Injection contains benzyl alcohol which may cause allergic reactions in susceptible individuals; large amounts of benzyl alcohol (≥99 mg/kg/day) have been associated with a potentially fatal toxicity ("gasping syndrome") in neonates; the "gasping syndrome" consists of metabolic acidosis, respiratory distress, gasping respirations, CNS dysfunction (including convulsions, intracranial hemorrhage), hypotension and cardiovascular collapse; *in vitro* and animal studies have shown that benzoate, a metabolite of benzyl alcohol, displaces bilirubin from protein binding sites; avoid or use injection cautiously in neonates. *In vitro* studies using pooled sera from critically ill neonates have also shown bumetanide to be a potent displacer of bilirubin; avoid use in neonates at risk for kernicterus; increased risk of ototoxicity with rapid I.V. administration, renal impairment, excessive doses, and concurrent use of other ototoxins

Precautions Use with caution in patients with cirrhosis; allergy to sulfonamides may result in cross hypersensitivity to bumetanide

Adverse Reactions

Cardiovascular: Hypotension, chest pain
Central nervous system: Dizziness, headache, encephalopathy, vertigo
Dermatologic: Rash, pruritus, urticaria
Endocrine & metabolic: Hyperglycemia, hypokalemia, hypochloremia, hypomagnesemia, hyponatremia, hyperuricemia
Gastrointestinal: Cramps, nausea, vomiting, diarrhea, abdominal pain, xerostomia
Hematologic: Thrombocytopenia (rare)
Hepatic: Elevated liver enzymes
Neuromuscular & skeletal: Weakness, muscle cramps, arthritic pain
Otic: Ototoxicity (with rapid I.V. administration)
Renal: Decreased uric acid excretion, elevated serum creatinine, azotemia

Drug Interactions Decreased blood pressure when used with other antihypertensive agents and ACE inhibitors (may need to decrease dose of one or both agents); indomethacin and probenecid may decrease bumetanide's effect; decreased lithium excretion; ototoxic drugs (aminoglycoside antibiotics, cisplatin); cholestyramine may decrease absorption

Stability Store at room temperature; light sensitive, may discolor when exposed to light

Mechanism of Action Inhibits reabsorption of sodium and chloride in the ascending loop of Henle and proximal renal tubule, interfering with the chloride-binding cotransport system, thus causing increased excretion of water, sodium, chloride, magnesium, calcium, and phosphate

Pharmacodynamics

Onset of action:
- Oral, I.M.: Within 30-60 minutes
- I.V.: Within a few minutes

Maximum effect:
- Oral, I.M.: 1-2 hours
- I.V.: 15-30 minutes

Duration:
- Oral: 4-6 hours
- I.V.: 2-3 hours

Pharmacokinetics

Distribution: V_d: Neonates and infants: 0.26-0.39 L/kg
Protein binding: 95%
- Neonates: 97%

Metabolism: Partial metabolism occurs in the liver
Bioavailability: 72% to 96%
Half-life:
- Premature and full term neonates: 6 hours (range up to 15 hours)
- Infants <2 months: 2.5 hours
- Infants 2-6 months: 1.5 hours
- Adults: 1-1.5 hours

Time to peak serum concentration: 0.5-2 hours
Elimination: Unchanged drug excreted in urine (45%); biliary/fecal (2%)
- Clearance:
  - Preterm and full term neonates: 0.2-1.1 mL/minute/kg
  - Infants <2 months: 2.17 mL/minute/kg
  - Infants 2-6 months: 3.8 mL/minute/kg
  - Adults: 2.9 ± 0.2 mL/minute/kg

Usual Dosage

Oral, I.M., I.V.:
- Neonates (see Warnings): 0.01-0.05 mg/kg/dose every 24-48 hours
- Infants and Children: 0.015-0.1 mg/kg/dose every 6-24 hours (maximum dose: 10 mg/day)

(Continued)

Bumetanide *(Continued)*

Adults:

Edema:

Oral: 0.5-2 mg/dose (maximum dose: 10 mg/day) 1-2 times/day

I.M., I.V.: 0.5-1 mg/dose; may repeat in 2-3 hours for up to 2 doses if needed (maximum dose: 10 mg/day)

Continuous I.V. infusion: 0.9-1 mg/hour

Hypertension: Oral: 0.5-2 mg divided twice daily; maximum dose: 5 mg/day

Administration

Oral: Administer with food to decrease GI irritation

Parenteral: Administer without additional dilution by direct I.V. injection over 1-2 minutes; for intermittent I.V. infusion, dilute in D_5W, LR, or NS and infuse over 5 minutes; for continuous infusion, dilute in D_5W to a final concentration of 0.024 mg/mL

Monitoring Parameters Blood pressure, serum electrolytes, renal function, urine output

Patient Information May cause dry mouth

Additional Information Patients with impaired hepatic function must be monitored carefully, often requiring reduced doses; larger doses may be necessary in patients with impaired renal function to obtain the same therapeutic response; 1 mg bumetanide approximately equivalent in potency to 40 mg furosemide

Dosage Forms Excipient information presented when available (limited, particularly for generics); consult specific product labeling.

Injection, solution: 0.25 mg/mL (2 mL, 4 mL, 10 mL) [contains benzyl alcohol]

Tablet (Bumex®): 0.5 mg, 1 mg, 2 mg

References

Chobanian AV, Bakris GL, Black HR, et al, "The Seventh Report of the Joint National Committee on Prevention, Detection, Evaluation, and Treatment of High Blood Pressure: The JNC 7 Report," *JAMA*, 2003, 289(19):2560-72.

Wells TG, "The Pharmacology and Therapeutics of Diuretics in the Pediatric Patient," *Pediatr Clin North Am*, 1990, 37(2):463-504.

♦ **Bumex®** *see* Bumetanide *on page 242*

♦ **Buminate®** *see* Albumin *on page 64*

♦ **Buphenyl®** *see* Sodium Phenylbutyrate *on page 1455*

Bupivacaine (byoo PIV a kane)

Medication Safety Issues

Sound-alike/look-alike issues:

Bupivacaine may be confused with mepivacaine, ropivacaine

Marcaine® may be confused with Narcan®

U.S. Brand Names Marcaine®; Marcaine® Spinal; Sensorcaine®; Sensorcaine®-MPF; Sensorcaine®-MPF Spinal

Canadian Brand Names Marcaine®; Sensorcaine®

Index Terms Bupivacaine Hydrochloride

Therapeutic Category Local Anesthetic, Injectable

Generic Available Yes

Use Local anesthetic (injectable) for peripheral nerve block, infiltration, sympathetic block, caudal or epidural block, retrobulbar block

Pregnancy Risk Factor C

Lactation Enters breast milk/not recommended

Contraindications Hypersensitivity to bupivacaine hydrochloride, other amide-type anesthetics, or any component (see Warnings); not recommended for I.V. regional anesthesia (Bier block); obstetrical paracervical block anesthesia (use is associated with fetal bradycardia and death); 0.75% concentration in obstetrical anesthesia

Warnings Convulsions due to systemic toxicity leading to cardiac arrest have been reported, presumably following unintentional I.V. injection; some products contain sulfites which may cause allergic reactions in susceptible individuals; **do not use solutions containing preservatives for caudal or epidural block.** Infants may be at greater risk for bupivacaine toxicity because α_1-acid-glycoprotein, the major serum protein to which bupivacaine is bound, is lower in infants compared with older children; use epidural infusions with caution in infants and monitor closely; increased toxicity may be minimized by limiting the duration of infusion to ≤48 hours (McCloskey, 1992). Reduce epidural infusion dosage in patients with seizure disorders or at increased risk for seizures (eg, electrolyte imbalance) (Berde, 1992).

Precautions Use with caution in patients with liver disease and impaired cardiovascular function; when used for epidural anesthesia, a smaller test dose is recommended to evaluate the patient's response

Adverse Reactions

Cardiovascular: Cardiac arrest, hypotension, bradycardia, palpitations
Central nervous system: Headache, restlessness, anxiety, dizziness, seizures
Dermatologic: Pruritus, angioneurotic edema
Gastrointestinal: Nausea, vomiting
Neuromuscular & skeletal: Weakness
Ocular: Blurred vision
Otic: Tinnitus
Respiratory: Apnea, sneezing
Miscellaneous: Hypersensitivity reactions

Drug Interactions Interactions relate to use in combination with epinephrine; see Epinephrine monograph

Stability Store at room temperature; solutions containing epinephrine should be protected from light; bupivacaine 0.4375 mg/mL when mixed with epinephrine 0.6875 mcg/mL and fentanyl 1.25 mcg/mL is stable refrigerated for 20 days and at room temperature for 48 hours; bupivacaine 625 mcg/mL or 1250 mcg/mL mixed with morphine sulfate 100 mcg/mL or 500 mcg/mL in NS is stable for 72 hours at room temperature

Mechanism of Action Blocks both the initiation and conduction of nerve impulses by decreasing the neuronal membrane's permeability to sodium ions, which results in inhibition of depolarization with resultant blockade of conduction

Pharmacodynamics

Onset of anesthetic action: Dependent on total dose, concentration, and route administered, but generally occurs within 4-10 minutes
Duration: 1.5-8.5 hours (depending upon route of administration)

Pharmacokinetics

Distribution: V_d:
- Infants: 3.9 ± 2 L/kg
- Children: 2.7 ± 0.2 L/kg

Protein binding: 84% to 95%
Metabolism: In the liver
Half-life (age-dependent):
- Neonates: 8.1 hours
- Adults: 2.7 hours

Time to peak serum concentration: Caudal, epidural, or peripheral nerve block: 30-45 minutes
Elimination: Small amounts (~6%) excreted in urine unchanged
Clearance:
- Infants: 7.1 ± 3.2 mL/kg/minute
- Children: 10 ± 0.7 mL/kg/minute

Usual Dosage Dose varies with procedure, depth of anesthesia, vascularity of tissues, duration of anesthesia and condition of patient

Caudal block (with or without epinephrine, **preservative free**):
- Children: 1-3.7 mg/kg
- Adults: 15-30 mL of 0.25% or 0.5%

Epidural block, **preservative free** (other than caudal block):
- Children: 1.25 mg/kg/dose
- Adults: 10-20 mL of 0.25%, 0.5%, or 0.75%

Peripheral nerve block: 5 mL dose of 0.25% or 0.5% (12.5-25 mg); maximum dose: 400 mg/day
Sympathetic nerve block: 20-50 mL of 0.25% (no epinephrine) solution
Continuous epidural (caudal or lumbar) infusion (limited information in neonates, infants, and children):
- Loading dose: 2-2.5 mg/kg (0.8-1 mL/kg of 0.25% bupivacaine)
- Infusion dose: See table

Bupivacaine Infusion Dose

Age	Dose	Dose (using 0.25% solution)	Dose (using 0.125% solution)	Dose (using 0.05% solution)
Neonates and Infants ≤4 months	0.2-0.25 mg/kg/h	0.08-0.1 mL/kg/h	0.16-0.2 mL/kg/h	0.4-0.5 mL/kg/h
Infants >4 months and Children	0.4-0.5 mg/kg/h	0.16-0.2 mL/kg/h	0.32-0.4 mL/kg/h	0.8-1 mL/kg/h
Adults	5-20 mg/h	2-8 mL/h	4-16 mL/h	10-40 mL/h

Administration Solutions containing preservatives should not be used for epidural or caudal blocks; for epidural infusion, may use undiluted or diluted with preservative free NS

(Continued)

Bupivacaine *(Continued)*

Reference Range Toxicity: 2-4 mcg/mL (however, some experts have suggested that the rate of rise of the serum level is more predictive of toxicity than the actual value; Scott, 1975)

Patient Information May experience temporary loss of sensation and motor activity, usually in the lower half of the body following caudal or lumbar epidural anesthesia

Additional Information For epidural infusion, lower dosages of bupivacaine may be effective when used in combination with narcotic analgesics

Dosage Forms Excipient information presented when available (limited, particularly for generics); consult specific product labeling.

Injection, solution, as hydrochloride [preservative free]: 0.25% [2.5 mg/mL] (10 mL, 20 mL, 30 mL, 50 mL); 0.5% [5 mg/mL] (10 mL, 20 mL, 30 mL); 0.75% [7.5 mg/mL] (10 mL, 20 mL, 30 mL)

Marcaine®: 0.25% [2.5 mg/mL] (10 mL, 30 mL); 0.5% [5 mg/mL] (10 mL, 30 mL); 0.75% [7.5 mg/mL] (10 mL, 30 mL)

Marcaine® Spinal: 0.75% [7.5 mg/mL] (2 mL) [in dextrose 8.25%]

Sensorcaine®-MPF: 0.25% [2.5 mg/mL] (10 mL, 30 mL); 0.5% [5 mg/mL] (10 mL, 30 mL); 0.75% [7.5 mg/mL] (10 mL, 30 mL)

Sensorcaine®-MPF Spinal: 0.75% [7.5 mg/mL] (2 mL) [in dextrose 8.25%]

Injection, solution, as hydrochloride:

Marcaine®, Sensorcaine®: 0.25% [2.5 mg/mL] (50 mL); 0.5% [5 mg/mL] (50 mL) [contains methylparaben]

References

Berde CB, "Convulsions Associated With Pediatric Regional Anesthesia," *Anesth Analg*, 1992, 75(2):164-6.

Desparmet J, Meistelman C, Barre J, et al, "Continuous Epidural Infusion of Bupivacaine for Postoperative Pain Relief in Children," *Anesthesiology*, 1987, 67(1):108-10.

Luz G, Innerhofer P, Bachmann B, et al, "Bupivacaine Plasma Concentrations During Continuous Epidural Anesthesia in Infants and Children," *Anesth Analg*, 1996, 82(2):231-4.

McCloskey JJ, Haun SE, and Deshpande JK, "Bupivacaine Toxicity Secondary to Continuous Caudal Epidural Infusion in Children," *Anesth Analg*, 1992, 75(2):287-90.

Scott DB, "Evaluation of Clinical Tolerance of Local Anaesthetic Agents," *Br J Anaesth*, 1975, 47:328-31.

♦ **Bupivacaine Hydrochloride** *see* Bupivacaine *on page 244*

♦ **Buprenex®** *see* Buprenorphine *on page 246*

Buprenorphine (byoo pre NOR feen)

Medication Safety Issues

Sound-alike/look-alike issues:

Buprenex® may be confused with Brevibloc®, Bumex®

U.S. Brand Names Buprenex®; Subutex®

Canadian Brand Names Buprenex®; Subutex®

Index Terms Buprenorphine Hydrochloride

Therapeutic Category Analgesic, Narcotic; Opiate Partial Agonist

Generic Available Yes: Injection

Use

Injection: Management of moderate to severe pain

Sublingual tablet: Treatment of opioid dependence

Restrictions Injection: C-V/C-III; Tablet: C-III

Pregnancy Risk Factor C

Lactation Enters breast milk/not recommended

Contraindications Hypersensitivity to buprenorphine or any component

Warnings Respiratory depression may occur; use with caution and in reduced doses in patients with pre-existing respiratory depression, decreased respiratory reserve, hypoxia, hypercapnia, significant COPD, or cor pulmonale, and in those receiving medications with CNS or respiratory depressant effects; respiratory depression may not be reversible with naloxone; mechanical ventilation may be required.

May cause CNS depression; warn patients of possible impairment of alertness or physical coordination (see Patient Information); interactions with other CNS drugs may occur (see Drug Interactions); physical and psychological dependence may occur; abrupt discontinuation after prolonged use may result in withdrawal symptoms (**Note:** Compared to full opioid agonists, withdrawal from buprenorphine may be milder and may be delayed in onset); narcotic antagonist activity of buprenorphine may precipitate acute narcotic withdrawal in opioid-dependent individuals.

Hepatitis and other hepatic events (see Adverse Reactions) have been reported in patients receiving buprenorphine for the treatment of opioid dependence; infection with viral hepatitis, concomitant use of potentially hepatotoxic drugs, pre-existing liver enzyme abnormalities, ongoing drug use may have contributed to liver abnormalities. Acute and chronic hypersensitivity reactions have also been reported. Orthostatic hypotension may occur in ambulatory patients.

Precautions Use with caution in patients with head injury; increased intracranial pressure; CNS depression; coma; toxic psychosis; seizures; acute abdominal conditions; biliary tract disease, pancreatitis; severe renal, respiratory, or hepatic insufficiency; hypothyroidism; Addison's disease; urethral stricture, prostatic hypertrophy; acute alcoholism; delirium tremens, kyphoscoliosis, and in children or debilitated patients. Safety and efficacy of injection in children <2 years of age and of sublingual tablets in children <16 years of age have not been established.

Adverse Reactions

Cardiovascular: Hypotension, bradycardia, tachycardia, hypertension, Wenckebach block, orthostatic hypotension

Central nervous system: Sedation, dizziness, vertigo, CNS depression, headache, confusion, euphoria, fatigue, nervousness, depression, slurred speech, dreaming, psychosis, anxiety, insomnia

Dermatologic: Pruritus, rash, hives

Gastrointestinal: Nausea, vomiting, constipation, xerostomia, abdominal pain, dyspepsia

Genitourinary: Urinary retention

Hepatic: Sublingual tablets: elevated liver enzymes, hepatitis with jaundice, cytolytic hepatitis, hepatic failure, hepatic necrosis, hepatorenal syndrome, hepatic encephalopathy

Local: Injection site reaction

Neuromuscular & skeletal: Weakness, paresthesia

Ocular: Miosis, diplopia, visual abnormalities, blurred vision

Otic: Tinnitus

Respiratory: Respiratory depression, hypoventilation, dyspnea, cyanosis

Miscellaneous: Physical and psychological dependence, diaphoresis; hypersensitivity reactions, angioneurotic edema, anaphylactic shock

Drug Interactions Cytochrome P450 isoenzyme CYP3A4 substrate

CNS depressants may potentiate the CNS adverse effects of buprenorphine; respiratory and cardiovascular collapse may occur with concurrent use with diazepam; I.V. misuse (self-injection of crushed buprenorphine tablets) with benzodiazepines has been associated with coma and death; use with MAO inhibitors may increase adverse effects (use with caution); CYP3A4 enzyme inhibitors, such as azole antifungal agents (eg, ketoconazole), macrolide antibiotics (eg, erythromycin), and protease inhibitors (eg, ritonavir) may increase buprenorphine serum concentrations or effect (monitor closely and adjust buprenorphine dose if needed); CYP3A4 enzyme inducers (eg, carbamazepine, phenytoin, rifampin) may decrease buprenorphine serum concentrations or effect (monitor closely and adjust buprenorphine dose if needed)

Stability

Injection: Protect from exposure to excessive heat of >40°C (>104°F) or prolonged exposure to light.

Sublingual tablet: Store at room temperature of 25°C (77°F).

Mechanism of Action Binds to opiate receptors in the CNS, causing inhibition of ascending pain pathways, altering perception of and response to pain; produces generalized CNS depression. Can be classified as a partial agonist with both agonist and antagonist activity (ie, partial agonist at the mu opioid receptor and an antagonist at the kappa opioid receptor). When used as recommended, buprenorphine acts as a classic mu receptor agonist (like morphine). *In vitro* studies demonstrate a very slow rate of dissociation from the mu receptor which may account for buprenorphine's longer duration of action (compared to morphine), unpredictability of reversal by opioid antagonists, and low level of apparent physical dependence.

Pharmacodynamics I.M.:

Onset of action: 15 minutes

Maximum effect: 1 hour

Duration: ≥6 hours

Pharmacokinetics

Distribution: Distributes into breast milk at concentrations greater than maternal plasma

V_d:

Premature neonates 27-32 weeks GA (n=11) (mean ± SD): 6.2 ± 2.1 L/kg

Children 4-7 years (n=10) (mean ± SD): 3.2 ± 2 L/kg

Protein binding: 96%, primarily to alpha and beta globulin

Metabolism: In the liver, via both N-dealkylation (to an active metabolite, norbuprenorphine) and glucuronidation; norbuprenorphine also undergoes glucuronidation; two other unidentified metabolites have been found; extensive first-pass effect

Half-life:

I.V.:

Premature neonates 27-32 weeks GA (n=11) (mean ± SD): 20 ± 8 hours

Adults: 2.2 hours

Sublingual: Adults: 37 hours

(Continued)

Buprenorphine *(Continued)*

Elimination: 30% of the dose is excreted in the urine (1% as unchanged drug; 9.4% as conjugated drug; 2.7% as norbuprenorphine; and 11% as conjugated norbuprenorphine) and 69% in feces (33% as unchanged drug; 5% as conjugated drug; 21% as norbuprenorphine; and 2% as conjugated norbuprenorphine)

Clearance: Related to hepatic blood flow

Premature neonates 27-32 weeks GA (n=11): 0.23 ± 0.07 L/hour/kg

Children 4-7 years: 3.6 ± 1.1 L/hour/kg

Adults: 0.78-1.32 L/hour/kg

Usual Dosage Dose should be titrated to appropriate effect. Use ½ of the dose listed in patients with pre-existing respiratory depression, decreased respiratory reserve, hypoxia, hypercapnia, significant COPD, or cor pulmonale, and in those receiving medications with CNS or respiratory depressant effects.

Moderate to severe pain:

Children 2-12 years: I.M., slow I.V. injection: 2-6 mcg/kg every 4-6 hours; **Note:** 3 mcg/kg/dose has been most commonly studied (see References); not all children have faster clearance rates than adults; some children may require dosing intervals of every 6-8 hours; observe clinical effects to establish the proper dosing interval

Children ≥13 years and Adults: I.M., slow I.V. injection: Initial: Opiate-naive: 0.3 mg every 6-8 hours as needed; initial dose (up to 0.3 mg) may be repeated once in 30-60 minutes if clinically needed; **Note:** In adults, single doses of up to 0.6 mg administered I.M. may occasionally be required

Opioid dependence: Note: Do not start induction with buprenorphine until objective and clear signs of withdrawal are apparent (otherwise withdrawal may be precipitated). Children ≥16 years and Adults: Sublingual:

Induction: Target range: 12-16 mg/day (doses during one induction study used 8 mg on day 1, followed by 16 mg on day 2; other studies accomplished induction over 3-4 days). Treatment should begin at least 4 hours after last use of heroin or short-acting opioid, preferably when first signs of withdrawal appear. Titrating dose to clinical effect should be done as rapidly as possible to prevent undue withdrawal symptoms.

Maintenance: **Note:** Patients should be switched to the buprenorphine/naloxone combination product for maintenance and for unsupervised therapy; initial target dose: 12-16 mg/day; then adjust dose in 2-4 mg increments/decrements to a dose that adequately suppresses opioid withdrawal; usual range: 4-24 mg/day

Administration

Oral: Sublingual: Place tablet under the tongue until dissolved; do not swallow. If 2 or more tablets are needed per dose, all tablets may be placed under the tongue at once, or 2 tablets may be placed under the tongue at a time; to ensure consistent bioavailability, subsequent doses should always be taken the same way.

Parenteral:

I.M.: Administer via deep I.M. injection

I.V.: Administer slowly, over at least 2 minutes

Monitoring Parameters Pain relief, respiratory rate, mental status, blood pressure; liver enzymes (baseline and periodic) with use of sublingual tablets

Patient Information May cause drowsiness and impair ability to perform activities requiring mental alertness or physical coordination; may cause postural hypotension (use caution when changing positions from lying or sitting to standing); avoid alcohol, sedatives, benzodiazepines, tranquilizers, and antidepressants; report the use of other prescription and nonprescription medications to your physician and pharmacist. May be habit-forming; use exactly as directed; do not increase dose or frequency; do not discontinue abruptly, dose should be tapered to prevent withdrawal. May cause dry mouth.

Additional Information Equianalgesic doses (parenteral): Buprenorphine 0.3 mg = morphine 10 mg; buprenorphine has a longer duration of action than morphine

Symptoms of overdose include CNS and respiratory depression, pinpoint pupils, hypotension, and bradycardia; treatment is supportive; naloxone may have limited effects in reversing respiratory depression; doxapram has also been used as a respiratory stimulant.

Neonatal withdrawal symptoms (including tremor, agitation, hypertonia, and myoclonus) have been reported in infants of women receiving buprenorphine sublingual tablets during pregnancy; onset of symptoms ranged from day 1 to day 8 of life, most occurring on day 1 of life; rare cases of convulsions (with one case of apnea and bradycardia) have also been reported

Dosage Forms Excipient information presented when available (limited, particularly for generics); consult specific product labeling. Available as buprenorphine hydrochloride; mg strength refers to buprenorphine

Injection, solution: 0.3 mg/mL (1 mL) [C-III]

Buprenex®: 0.3 mg/mL (1 mL) [C-V]

Tablet, sublingual:

Subutex®: 2 mg, 8 mg

References

Barrett DA, Simpson J, Rutter N, et al, "The Pharmacokinetics and Physiological Effects of Buprenorphine Infusion in Premature Neonates," *Br J Clin Pharmacol*, 1993, 36(3):215-9.

Hamunen K, Olkkola KT, and Maunuksela EL, "Comparison of the Ventilatory Effects of Morphine and Buprenorphine in Children," *Acta Anaesthesiol Scand*, 1993, 37(5):449-53.

Maunuksela EL, Korpela R, and Olkkola KT, "Comparison of Buprenorphine With Morphine in the Treatment of Postoperative Pain in Children," *Anesth Analg*, 1988, 67(3):233-9.

Maunuksela EL, Korpela R, and Olkkola KT, "Double-Blind, Multiple-Dose Comparison of Buprenorphine and Morphine in Postoperative Pain of Children," *Br J Anaesth*, 1988, 60(1):48-55.

Olkkola KT, Leijala MA, and Maunuksela EL, "Paediatric Ventilatory Effects of Morphine and Buprenorphine Revisited," *Paediatr Anaesth*, 1995, 5(5):303-5.

Olkkola KT, Maunuksela EL, and Korpela R, "Pharmacokinetics of Intravenous Buprenorphine in Children," *Br J Clin Pharmacol*, 1989, 28(2):202-4.

Buprenorphine and Naloxone (byoo pre NOR feen & nal OKS one)

U.S. Brand Names Suboxone®

Index Terms Buprenorphine Hydrochloride and Naloxone Hydrochloride Dihydrate; Naloxone and Buprenorphine; Naloxone Hydrochloride Dihydrate and Buprenorphine Hydrochloride

Therapeutic Category Analgesic, Narcotic; Opiate Partial Agonist

Generic Available No

Use Treatment of opioid dependence

Restrictions C-III

Pregnancy Risk Factor C

Lactation Buprenorphine: Enters breast milk/not recommended

Contraindications Hypersensitivity to buprenorphine, naloxone, or any component

Warnings Respiratory depression may occur; use with caution and in reduced doses in patients with pre-existing respiratory depression, decreased respiratory reserve, hypoxia, hypercapnia, significant COPD, or cor pulmonale, and in those receiving medications with CNS or respiratory depressant effects; respiratory depression may not be reversible with naloxone; mechanical ventilation may be required.

May cause CNS depression; warn patients of possible impairment of alertness or physical coordination (see Patient Information); interactions with other CNS drugs may occur (see Drug Interactions); physical and psychological dependence may occur; abrupt discontinuation after prolonged use may result in withdrawal symptoms (**Note:** Compared to full opioid agonists, withdrawal from buprenorphine may be milder and may be delayed in onset); narcotic antagonist activity of buprenorphine may precipitate acute narcotic withdrawal in opioid-dependent individuals.

Naloxone may precipitate intense withdrawal symptoms in patients addicted to opiates when administered before the opioid effects have subsided, or if misused parenterally in opioid-dependent individuals. Combination product of buprenorphine and naloxone is indicated for maintenance therapy and should not be used for induction. Oral buprenorphine is not approved for management of pain.

Hepatitis and other hepatic events (see Adverse Reactions) have been reported in patients receiving buprenorphine for the treatment of opioid dependence; infection with viral hepatitis, concomitant use of potentially hepatotoxic drugs, pre-existing liver enzyme abnormalities, ongoing drug use may have contributed to liver abnormalities. Acute and chronic hypersensitivity reactions have also been reported. Orthostatic hypotension may occur in ambulatory patients.

Precautions Use with caution in patients with head injury; increased intracranial pressure; CNS depression; coma; toxic psychosis; seizures; acute abdominal conditions; biliary tract disease, pancreatitis; severe renal, respiratory, or hepatic insufficiency; hypothyroidism; Addison's disease; urethral stricture, prostatic hypertrophy; acute alcoholism; delirium tremens, kyphoscoliosis, and in children or debilitated patients. Safety and efficacy in children <16 years of age have not been established.

Adverse Reactions See individual monographs for Buprenorphine *on page 246* and Naloxone *on page 1103*

Drug Interactions See monograph for Buprenorphine *on page 246*

Stability Store a room temperature of 25°C (77°F)

Mechanism of Action See individual monographs for Buprenorphine *on page 246* and Naloxone *on page 1103*

Pharmacokinetics See individual monographs for Buprenorphine *on page 246* and Naloxone *on page 1103*

Absorption: Absorption of the combination product is variable between patients following sublingual use, but variability within each individual patient is low.

(Continued)

Buprenorphine and Naloxone *(Continued)*

Usual Dosage Dose should be titrated to appropriate effect.

Opioid dependence: Children ≥16 years and Adults: Sublingual:

Induction: **Note:** Combination product (buprenorphine and naloxone) is not recommended for use during induction; initial treatment should begin using buprenorphine sublingual tablets (see buprenorphine monograph).

Maintenance: **Note:** Patients should be switched to the buprenorphine and naloxone combination product for maintenance and for unsupervised therapy; initial target dose: 12-16 mg/day (based on buprenorphine content); then adjust dose in 2-4 mg increments/decrements to a dose that adequately suppresses opioid withdrawal; usual range: 4-24 mg/day

Administration Oral: Sublingual: Place tablet under the tongue until dissolved; do not swallow. If 2 or more tablets are needed per dose, all tablets may be placed under the tongue at once, or 2 tablets may be placed under the tongue at a time; to ensure consistent bioavailability, subsequent doses should always be taken the same way.

Monitoring Parameters Symptoms of withdrawal, respiratory rate, mental status, blood pressure; liver enzymes (baseline and periodic)

Patient Information May cause drowsiness and impair ability to perform activities requiring mental alertness or physical coordination; may cause postural hypotension (use caution when changing positions from lying or sitting to standing); avoid alcohol, sedatives, benzodiazepines, tranquilizers, and antidepressants; report the use of other prescription and nonprescription medications to your physician and pharmacist. May be habit-forming; use exactly as directed; do not increase dose or frequency; do not discontinue abruptly, dose should be tapered to prevent withdrawal. May cause dry mouth.

Additional Information Sublingual tablets contain a free base ratio of buprenorphine to naloxone of 4 to 1. Naloxone has been added to the formulation to decrease the abuse potential of crushing and dissolving tablets in water and using as an injection (precipitation of severe withdrawal would occur in opioid dependent patients if the tablets were misused in this manner).

Symptoms of overdose include CNS and respiratory depression, pinpoint pupils, hypotension, and bradycardia; treatment is supportive; parenteral naloxone may have limited effects in reversing respiratory depression; doxapram has also been used as a respiratory stimulant.

Neonatal withdrawal symptoms (including tremor, agitation, hypertonia, and myoclonus) have been reported in infants of women receiving buprenorphine sublingual tablets during pregnancy; onset of symptoms ranged from day 1 to day 8 of life, most occurring on day 1 of life; rare cases of convulsions (with one case of apnea and bradycardia) have also been reported

Dosage Forms Excipient information presented when available (limited, particularly for generics); consult specific product labeling. Available as buprenorphine hydrochloride and naloxone hydrochloride dihydrate; mg strength refers to buprenorphine and naloxone free bases

Tablet, sublingual: Buprenorphine 2 mg and naloxone 0.5 mg; buprenorphine 8 mg and naloxone 2 mg [lemon-lime flavor]

♦ **Buprenorphine Hydrochloride** *see* Buprenorphine *on page 246*
♦ **Buprenorphine Hydrochloride and Naloxone Hydrochloride Dihydrate** *see* Buprenorphine and Naloxone *on page 249*
♦ **Burinex® (Can)** *see* Bumetanide *on page 242*
♦ **Burnamycin [OTC]** *see* Lidocaine *on page 933*
♦ **Burn Jel [OTC]** *see* Lidocaine *on page 933*
♦ **Burn-O-Jel [OTC]** *see* Lidocaine *on page 933*
♦ **Burow's Solution** *see* Aluminum Acetate *on page 89*
♦ **Buscopan® (Can)** *see* Scopolamine *on page 1421*
♦ **BuSpar®** *see* BusPIRone *on page 250*
♦ **Buspirex (Can)** *see* BusPIRone *on page 250*

BusPIRone (byoo SPYE rone)

Medication Safety Issues

Sound-alike/look-alike issues:

BusPIRone may be confused with buPROPion

Related Information

Serotonin Syndrome *on page 1955*

U.S. Brand Names BuSpar®

Canadian Brand Names Apo-Buspirone®; BuSpar®; Buspirex; Bustab®; Gen-Buspirone; Lin-Buspirone; Novo-Buspirone; Nu-Buspirone; PMS-Buspirone

Index Terms Buspirone Hydrochloride

Therapeutic Category Antianxiety Agent

Generic Available Yes

Use Management of anxiety disorders

Pregnancy Risk Factor B

Lactation Excretion in breast milk unknown/not recommended

Contraindications Hypersensitivity to buspirone or any component

Warnings Do not use concurrently with MAO inhibitors or within 10 days of MAO inhibitors as significant increases in blood pressure may occur

Precautions Use with caution in patients with hepatic or renal dysfunction; use in severe hepatic or renal impairment is not recommended; buspirone does not prevent or treat withdrawal from benzodiazepines or sedative/hypnotic drugs

Adverse Reactions

Cardiovascular: Chest pain, tachycardia

Central nervous system: Dizziness, lightheadedness, headache, fatigue, restlessness, confusion, insomnia, nightmares, sedation (about $\frac{1}{3}$ of that with benzodiazepines), disorientation, excitement, fever, drowsiness (more common with ≥20 mg/day), akathisia; possible psychotic deterioration has been reported (two pediatric cases, see Soni, 1992)

Dermatologic: Rash, urticaria

Gastrointestinal: Nausea, vomiting, diarrhea, flatulence, xerostomia

Hematologic: Rare: Leukopenia, eosinophilia, thrombocytopenia

Neuromuscular & skeletal: Muscle weakness, numbness

Ocular: Blurred vision

Otic: Tinnitus

Drug Interactions Cytochrome P450 isoenzyme CYP3A4 substrate

Use with MAO inhibitors may cause significant increases in blood pressure; alcohol or other CNS depressants may increase CNS adverse effects; buspirone may increase haloperidol levels; buspirone may displace digoxin from serum proteins; fluoxetine; use with warfarin may increase PT; erythromycin, itraconazole, ketoconazole, nefazodone, diltiazem, verapamil, or other inhibitors of CYP3A4 may increase buspirone plasma concentrations (the dose of buspirone should be reduced); when used with diazepam, buspirone may increase nordiazepam serum concentrations; aspirin may increase and flurazepam may decrease free (unbound) buspirone concentrations; rifampin, phenytoin, phenobarbital, carbamazepine, dexamethasone, or other inducers of CYP3A4 may decrease serum concentrations of buspirone (dosage adjustment of buspirone may be needed)

Food Interactions Food may delay oral absorption, decrease the first-pass metabolism effect and increase oral bioavailability; grapefruit juice may greatly increase buspirone concentrations

Stability Protect from light; store at room temperature

Mechanism of Action Decreases the spontaneous firing of serotonin-containing neurons in the CNS by selectively binding to and acting as agonist at presynaptic CNS serotonin 5-HT_1A receptors; possesses partial agonist activity (mixed agonist/antagonist) at postsynaptic 5-HT_2A receptors; does not bind to benzodiazepine-GABA receptors; binds to $dopamine_2$ receptors; may have other effects on other neurotransmitter systems; buspirone is "anxiolytic-select" and does not possess the anticonvulsant, muscle relaxant, or sedative effects of the benzodiazepines; little potential for abuse, tolerance, or withdrawal reactions

Pharmacodynamics

Onset of action: Within 2 weeks

Maximum effect: 3-4 weeks, up to 4-6 weeks

Pharmacokinetics

Absorption: Rapid and complete, but bioavailability is limited by extensive first-pass effect; only 1.5% to 13% (mean 4%) of the oral dose reaches the systemic circulation unchanged

Protein binding: 86%

Metabolism: In the liver by oxidation (by cytochrome P450 isoenzyme CYP3A4) to several metabolites including 1-pyrimidinyl piperazine (about $\frac{1}{4}$ as active as buspirone)

Half-life: Adults: Mean: 2-3 hours; increased with renal or liver dysfunction

Elimination: 29% to 63% excreted in urine (primarily as metabolites)

Usual Dosage Oral:

Children and Adolescents: Anxiety disorders: Limited information is available; dose is not well established. One pilot study of 15 children, 6-14 years of age (mean 10 years), with mixed anxiety disorders, used initial doses of 5 mg daily; doses were individualized with increases in increments of 5 mg/day every week as needed to a maximum dose of 20 mg/day divided into 2 doses; the mean dose required: 18.6 mg/day (Simeon, 1994). Some authors (Carrey, 1996 and Kutcher, 1992), based on their clinical experience, recommend higher doses (eg, 15-30 mg/day in 2

(Continued)

BusPIRone *(Continued)*

divided doses). An open-label study in 25 prepubertal inpatients (mean age: 8 ± 1.8 years; range: 5-11 years) with anxiety symptoms and moderately aggressive behavior used initial doses of 5 mg daily; doses were titrated upwards (over 3 weeks) by 5-10 mg every 3 days to a maximum dose of 50 mg/day; doses >5 mg/day were administered in 2 divided doses/day; buspirone was discontinued in 25% of the children due to increased aggression and agitation or euphoric mania; mean optimal dose (n=19): 28 mg/day; range: 10-50 mg/day; median: 30 mg/day (Pfeffer, 1997). Two placebo-controlled 6-week trials in children and adolescents (n=559; age: 6-17 years) with generalized anxiety disorder studied doses of 7.5-30 mg twice daily (15-60 mg/day); no significant differences between buspirone and placebo with respect to generalized anxiety disorder symptoms were observed (see package insert).

Adults: Initial: 7.5 mg twice daily; increase in increments of 5 mg/day every 2-3 days as needed to a maximum of 60 mg/day; usual dose: 20-30 mg/day in 2 or 3 divided doses; **Note:** For patients receiving concomitant therapy with cytochrome P450 CYP3A4 inhibitors, a lower dose of buspirone is recommended (eg, 2.5 mg twice daily for patients receiving erythromycin; 2.5 mg daily for patients receiving itraconazole or nefazodone); with further dosage adjustments based on clinical assessment

Dosing adjustment in renal impairment:

Mild to moderate renal dysfunction: Dose reductions not required

Patients with anuria: Reduce dose by 25% to 50%; further studies are needed

Administration Oral: Administer in a consistent manner in relation to food (ie, either always with food or always without food); may administer with food to decrease GI upset; use caution if administered with grapefruit juice; avoid large amounts of grapefruit juice (see Food Interactions)

Monitoring Parameters Mental status, signs and symptoms of anxiety, liver and renal function

Patient Information Avoid alcohol and large amounts of grapefruit juice; may cause drowsiness and impair ability to perform activities requiring mental alertness or physical coordination; may cause dry mouth

Additional Information Not appropriate for "as needed" (prn) use or for brief, situational anxiety; buspirone is equipotent to diazepam on a milligram to milligram basis in the treatment of anxiety; however, unlike diazepam, the onset of buspirone is delayed (see Pharmacodynamics)

Dosage Forms Excipient information presented when available (limited, particularly for generics); consult specific product labeling.

Tablet, as hydrochloride: 5 mg, 7.5 mg, 10 mg, 15 mg, 30 mg

BuSpar®: 5 mg, 10 mg, 15 mg, 30 mg

References

Carrey NJ, Wiggins DM, and Milin RP, "Pharmacological Treatment of Psychiatric Disorders in Children and Adolescents," *Drugs*, 1996, 51(5):750-9.

Hanna GL, Feibusch EL, and Albright KJ, "Buspirone Treatment of Anxiety, Associated With Pharyngeal Dysphagia in a Four-Year Old," *J Child Adolesc Psychopharmacol*, 1997, 7(2):137-43.

Kutcher SP, Reiter S, Gardner DM, et al, "The Pharmacotherapy of Anxiety Disorders in Children and Adolescents," *Psychiatr Clin North Am*, 1992, 15(1):41-67.

Pfeffer CR, Jiang H, and Domeshek LJ, "Buspirone Treatment of Psychiatrically Hospitalized Prepubertal Children With Symptoms of Anxiety and Moderately Severe Aggression," *J Child Adolesc Psychopharmacol*, 1997, 7(3):145-55.

Simeon JG, Knott VJ, DuBois C, et al, "Buspirone Therapy of Mixed Anxiety Disorders in Childhood and Adolescence: A Pilot Study," *J Child Adolesc Psychopharmacol*, 1994, 4(3):159-70.

Soni P and Weintraub AL, "Buspirone-Associated Mental Status Changes," *J Am Acad Child Adolesc Psychiatry*, 1992, 31(6):1098-9.

♦ **Buspirone Hydrochloride** *see* BusPIRone *on page 250*

♦ **Bustab® (Can)** *see* BusPIRone *on page 250*

Busulfan (byoo SUL fan)

Medication Safety Issues

Sound-alike/look-alike issues:

Busulfan may be confused with Butalan®

Myleran® may be confused with Leukeran®, melphalan, Mylicon®

High alert medication: The Institute for Safe Medication Practices (ISMP) includes this medication among its list of drugs which have a heightened risk of causing significant patient harm when used in error.

Related Information

Compatibility of Chemotherapy and Related Supportive Care Medications *on page 1777*

Emetogenic Potential of Single Chemotherapeutic Agents *on page 1776*

U.S. Brand Names Busulfex®; Myleran®

Canadian Brand Names Busulfex®; Myleran®

Index Terms 1,4-Butanediol Dimethanesulfonate; NSC-750

Therapeutic Category Antineoplastic Agent, Alkylating Agent

Generic Available No

Use Chronic myelogenous leukemia (CML); component of marrow-ablative conditioning regimen prior to bone marrow transplantation (BMT) for refractory leukemias, lymphomas, and pediatric solid tumors

Pregnancy Risk Factor D

Lactation Excretion in breast milk unknown/contraindicated

Contraindications Hypersensitivity to busulfan or any component; failure to respond to previous courses; should not be used in pregnancy or lactation

Warnings The FDA currently recommends that procedures for proper handling and disposal of antineoplastic agents be considered; discontinue busulfan if lung toxicity develops; busulfan is potentially carcinogenic; malignant tumors and acute leukemias have been reported in patients who received busulfan; busulfan is associated with ovarian failure including failure to achieve puberty in females

Profound myelosuppression with severe granulocytopenia, thrombocytopenia, and anemia are the most frequent serious adverse events occurring when high-dose busulfan is used as a conditioning regimen. Seizures have been reported in patients receiving high-dose busulfan. Prophylactic anticonvulsant therapy should be initiated prior to high-dose busulfan therapy. High busulfan AUC values (>1500 micromolar/minute) may be associated with an increased risk of developing hepatic veno-occlusive disease (HVOD). Patients who have received prior radiation therapy, ≥3 cycles of chemotherapy, or prior progenitor cell transplant may be at increased risk for developing HVOD. Of the patients who developed HVOD, it was fatal in 40% of the cases.

Precautions May induce severe bone marrow hypoplasia; reduce dosage in patients with bone marrow suppression; use with extreme caution in patients who have recently received other myelosuppressive drugs or radiation therapy; use with caution in patients with a history of seizure disorder, head trauma, or when receiving other epileptogenic drugs

Adverse Reactions

Cardiovascular: Cardiac tamponade (reported in a small number of thalassemia patients who received busulfan and cyclophosphamide as part of a BMT conditioning regimen), edema, tachycardia

Central nervous system: Dizziness, seizures, fever, chills, insomnia, confusion, hallucinations

Dermatologic: Hyperpigmentation, alopecia, rash, urticaria

Endocrine & metabolic: Addisonian-like syndrome (hyperpigmentation, wasting, hypotension), hyperuricemia, gynecomastia, testicular atrophy, amenorrhea, sterility, hyperglycemia, hypomagnesemia, hypokalemia

Gastrointestinal: Nausea, vomiting, mucositis, diarrhea, abdominal pain, constipation, ileus, anorexia, pancreatitis

Genitourinary: Hemorrhagic cystitis

Hematologic: Myelosuppression with nadirs of 14-21 days for leukopenia and thrombocytopenia; anemia, aplastic anemia, thrombosis

Hepatic: Hepatic impairment, hepatic veno-occlusive disease (7.7% to 12% with high-dose busulfan), hyperbilirubinemia, hepatocellular necrosis, ascites

Ocular: Blurred vision, subcapsular cataracts, corneal thinning

Respiratory: Pulmonary fibrosis (may occur 4 months to 10 years after initiation of therapy), dyspnea

Drug Interactions Cytochrome P450 isoenzyme CYP3A3/4 substrate

Thioguanine (may increase hepatotoxicity); itraconazole (may decrease busulfan clearance by 25% and increase busulfan toxicity); phenytoin lowers busulfan plasma AUC by 15%; acetaminophen may decrease busulfan clearance

Food Interactions No clear or firm data on the effect of food on busulfan bioavailability

Stability Store tablets at room temperature. Store intact ampuls in the refrigerator; diluted busulfan solution is stable for up to 8 hours at room temperature; infusion must be completed within that 8 hour time frame. If diluted in NS, the solution is stable for 12 hours if refrigerated, but the infusion must be completed within that 12-hour time frame.

Mechanism of Action Interferes with the normal function of DNA by alkylation of intracellular nucleophiles and cross-linking the strands of DNA

Pharmacokinetics

Absorption: Oral: 70% absorbed

Distribution: Crosses into CSF, saliva, placenta, and liver

V_d: Children: 0.64 L/kg

Protein binding: 32% to 55%

(Continued)

Busulfan *(Continued)*

Metabolism: Extensive in the liver by conjugation with glutathione
Half-life:
Children: 2.5 hours
Adults: 2.3-2.6 hours
Time to peak serum concentration: Oral: Within 1-2 hours
Elimination: 10% to 50% excreted in urine as metabolites, 1% excreted unchanged in urine within 24 hours; total plasma clearance rate is 2-4 times higher in children than in adults
Clearance:
Children: 3.37 mL/minute/kg
Adults: 2.52 mL/minute/kg (range: 1.49-4.31 mL/minute/kg)

Usual Dosage Refer to individual protocols; dose should be based on ideal body weight:

Children:

Oral:

Remission induction of CML: 0.06-0.12 mg/kg once daily **or** 1.8-4.6 mg/m^2/day once daily; titrate dose to maintain a leukocyte count >40,000/mm^3; discontinue busulfan if counts fall to ≤20,000/mm^3

BMT marrow-ablative conditioning regimen: 1 mg/kg/dose every 6 hours for 16 doses

Hematopoietic stem cell transplant regimen: Children ≤6 years: 40 mg/m^2/dose every 6 hours for 16 doses

I.V.: High-dose BMT or peripheral blood progenitor cell transplantation conditioning regimen: Dose based on actual body weight:

≤12 kg: 1.1 mg/kg/dose every 6 hours for 16 doses over 4 consecutive days

>12 kg: 0.8 mg/kg/dose every 6 hours for 16 doses over 4 consecutive days

Dosage adjustment based on therapeutic drug monitoring:

Adjusted dose (mg) = Actual dose (mg) x target AUC (micromolar•minute) / actual AUC (micromolar•minute)

Target AUC = 1125 micromolar•minute

Adults:

Oral:

Remission induction of CML: 4-8 mg/day or 0.06 mg/kg/day

Maintenance dose: Controversial; range is from 1-4 mg/day to 2 mg/week; reduce dose in proportion to the decrease in leukocyte count or discontinue busulfan when the leukocyte count falls to ≤20,000/mm^3

I.V.: High-dose BMT conditioning regimen: 0.8 mg/kg/dose every 6 hours for 16 doses over 4 consecutive days

I.V. dose for obese patients: Dose should be based on adjusted ideal body weight (AIBW)

AIBW = Ideal body weight (IBW) + 0.25 x (actual weight - IBW)

Administration

Oral: May be administered without regard to meals. To facilitate ingestion of high doses, insert multiple tablets into clear gelatin capsules for administration.

Parenteral: Filter busulfan using 5 micron syringe filter provided, using one filter per ampul. If using the syringe filter in the forward flow direction, allow for ~0.16 mL of residual busulfan to remain in the filter. Dilute busulfan injection with either NS or D_5W to a final concentration of ≥0.5 mg/mL (diluent volume should be 10 times the volume of busulfan injection); infuse over 2 hours through a central venous catheter; flush line before and after each infusion with D_5W or NS. Do **not** use polycarbonate syringes or filters.

Monitoring Parameters CBC with differential and platelet count, hemoglobin, liver function tests, bilirubin, alkaline phosphatase; monitor busulfan plasma concentration

Patient Information Report any difficulty in breathing, cough, fever, sore throat, bleeding or bruising to physician. Report any signs of abrupt weakness, fatigue, anorexia, weight loss, nausea, vomiting, and melanoderma. Female patients of childbearing potential should avoid becoming pregnant during and for one month following therapy.

Additional Information One method used to prevent seizures during high-dose busulfan (~4 mg/kg/day for 4 days) is to initiate a standard loading dose of phenytoin (15 mg/kg) 1 day prior to starting busulfan therapy followed by a maintenance dose adjusted to maintain a therapeutic phenytoin concentration until 24 hours after the final busulfan dose

"Juvenile type" chronic myelogenous leukemia which typically occurs in young children and is associated with the absence of Philadelphia chromosome responds poorly to busulfan.

Dosage Forms Excipient information presented when available (limited, particularly for generics); consult specific product labeling.

Injection, solution:

Busulfex®: 6 mg/mL (10 mL)

Tablet:

Myleran®: 2 mg

Extemporaneous Preparations A 2 mg/mL oral suspension can be prepared in a vertical flow hood using simple syrup; crush one-hundred twenty 2 mg tablets into a fine powder in a mortar; levigate with a small amount of simple syrup and mix to make a uniform paste; mix while adding simple syrup in geometric portions to almost 120 mL; pour contents into a graduated cylinder; rinse mortar and pestle with simple syrup, transfer to the graduated cylinder, and qsad with vehicle to 120 mL. Transfer contents of the graduated cylinder into an amber prescription bottle. Preparation is stable for 30 days when stored under refrigeration; label "shake well" and "caution chemotherapy"

Allen LV, "Busulfan Oral Suspension," *US Pharmacist*, 1990, 15:94-5.

References

Bolinger AM, Zangwill AB, Slattery JT, et al, "An Evaluation of Engraftment, Toxicity and Busulfan Concentration in Children Receiving Bone Marrow Transplantation for Leukemia or Genetic Disease," *Bone Marrow Transplant*, 2000, 25(9):925-30.

Heard BE and Cooke RA, "Busulphan Lung," *Thorax*, 1968, 23(2):187-93.

Ozkaynak MF, Weinberg K, Kohn D, et al, "Hepatic Veno-Occlusive Disease Post-Bone Marrow Transplantation in Children Conditioned With Busulfan and Cyclophosphamide: Incidence, Risk Factors, and Clinical Outcome," *Bone Marrow Transplant*, 1991, 7(6):467-74.

Regazzi MB, Locatelli F, Buggia I, et al, "Disposition of High Dose Busulfan in Pediatric Patients Undergoing Bone Marrow Transplantation," *Clin Pharmacol Ther*, 1993, 54(1):45-52.

Vassal G, Gouyette A, Hartmann O, et al, "Pharmacokinetics of High-Dose Busulfan in Children," *Cancer Chemother Pharmacol*, 1989, 24(6):386-90.

◆ **Busulfex®** *see* Busulfan *on page 252*

◆ **1,4-Butanediol Dimethanesulfonate** *see* Busulfan *on page 252*

◆ **BW-430C** *see* Lamotrigine *on page 906*

◆ **BW524W91** *see* Emtricitabine *on page 562*

◆ **C2B8** *see* Rituximab *on page 1398*

◆ **C2B8 Monoclonal Antibody** *see* Rituximab *on page 1398*

◆ **CaEDTA** *see* Edetate Calcium Disodium *on page 553*

◆ **Cafcit®** *see* Caffeine *on page 255*

◆ **Cafergor® (Can)** *see* Ergotamine and Caffeine *on page 592*

◆ **Cafergot®** *see* Ergotamine and Caffeine *on page 592*

Caffeine (KAF een)

Related Information

Overdose and Toxicology *on page 1916*

U.S. Brand Names Cafcit®; Enerjets [OTC]; No Doz® Maximum Strength [OTC]; Vivarin® [OTC]

Index Terms Caffeine and Sodium Benzoate; Caffeine Citrate; Sodium Benzoate and Caffeine

Therapeutic Category Central Nervous System Stimulant, Nonamphetamine; Diuretic; Respiratory Stimulant

Generic Available Yes: Tablet, caffeine and sodium benzoate injection

Use

Treatment of idiopathic apnea of prematurity **(caffeine citrate)**

Emergency stimulant in acute circulatory failure; diuretic; treatment of spinal puncture headaches **(caffeine sodium benzoate)**

Pregnancy Risk Factor C

Lactation Enters breast milk/use caution (AAP rates "compatible")

Contraindications Hypersensitivity to caffeine or any component; sodium benzoate salt form in neonates (see Warnings)

Warnings Do not interchange the caffeine citrate salt formulation with the caffeine sodium benzoate formulation; sodium benzoate has been associated with a potentially fatal toxicity ("gasping syndrome") in neonates; the "gasping syndrome" consists of metabolic acidosis, respiratory distress, gasping respirations, CNS dysfunction (including convulsions, intracranial hemorrhage), hypotension and cardiovascular collapse; *in vitro* and animal studies have shown that benzoate also displaces bilirubin from protein-binding sites; avoid use of products containing sodium benzoate in neonates. During a Cafcit® double-blind, placebo-controlled study, 6 of 85 patients developed necrotizing enterocolitis (NEC); 5 of these 6 patients had received caffeine citrate; although no causal relationship has been established, neonates who receive caffeine citrate should be closely monitored for the development of NEC. Caffeine serum levels should be closely monitored to optimize therapy and prevent serious toxicity.

(Continued)

Caffeine *(Continued)*

Precautions Use with caution in patients with a history of peptic ulcer, impaired renal or hepatic function, seizure disorders, or cardiovascular disease; avoid in patients with symptomatic cardiac arrhythmias

Adverse Reactions

Cardiovascular: Cardiac arrhythmias, tachycardia, extrasystoles

Central nervous system: Insomnia, restlessness, agitation, irritability, hyperactivity, jitteriness, headache, nervousness, anxiety

Endocrine & metabolic: Hypoglycemia, hyperglycemia

Gastrointestinal: Nausea, vomiting, gastric irritation, necrotizing enterocolitis, GI hemorrhage

Genitourinary: Increased urine output

Neuromuscular & skeletal: Muscle tremors or twitches

Drug Interactions Cytochrome P450 isoenzyme CYP1A2, CYP2E1, and CYP3A3/4 substrate

Enhances the positive cardiac inotropic and chronotropic effects of beta-adrenergic agonists; cimetidine, ketoconazole, fluconazole, mexiletine, and phenylpropanolamine may impair caffeine metabolism (increase serum levels); caffeine decreases the hemodynamic effect of adenosine; phenobarbital and phenytoin may increase caffeine elimination (lower serum levels)

Stability Caffeine citrate: Injection and oral solution contain no preservatives; injection is chemically stable for at least 24 hours at room temperature when diluted to 10 mg/mL (as caffeine citrate) with D_5W, $D_{50}W$, Intralipid® 20%, and Aminosyn® 8.5%; also compatible with dopamine (600 mcg/mL), calcium gluconate 10%, heparin (1 unit/mL), and fentanyl (10 mcg/mL) at room temperature for 24 hours

Mechanism of Action Increases levels of 3'5' cyclic AMP by inhibiting phosphodiesterase; CNS stimulant which increases medullary respiratory center sensitivity to carbon dioxide, stimulates central inspiratory drive, and improves skeletal muscle contraction (diaphragmatic contractility); prevention of apnea may occur by competitive inhibition of adenosine

Pharmacokinetics

Distribution: V_d:

- Neonates: 0.8-0.9 L/kg
- Children >9 months to Adults: 0.6 L/kg

Protein binding: 17%

Metabolism: Interconversion between caffeine and theophylline has been reported in preterm neonates (caffeine levels are ~25% of measured theophylline after theophylline administration and ~3% to 8% of caffeine would be expected to be converted to theophylline)

Half-life:

- Neonates: 72-96 hours (range: 40-230 hours)
- Infants >9 months, Children, and Adults: 5 hours

Time to peak serum concentration: Oral: Within 30 minutes to 2 hours

Elimination:

- Neonates ≤1 month: 86% excreted unchanged in urine
- Infants >1 month and Adults: Extensively liver metabolized to a series of partially demethylated xanthines and methyluric acids
- Clearance:
  - Neonates: 8.9 mL/hour/kg (range: 2.5-17)
  - Adults: 94 mL/hour/kg

Usual Dosage

Apnea of prematurity: **Caffeine citrate:** Neonates: Oral, I.V.:

Loading dose: 10-20 mg/kg as caffeine citrate (5-10 mg/kg as caffeine base). If theophylline has been administered to the patient within the previous 3 days, a full or modified loading dose (50% to 75% of a loading dose) may be given (caffeine is a significant metabolite of theophylline in the newborn; see Pharmacokinetics).

Maintenance dose: 5 mg/kg/day as caffeine citrate (2.5 mg/kg/day as caffeine base) once daily starting 24 hours after the loading dose. Maintenance dose is adjusted based on patient's response (efficacy and adverse effects), and serum caffeine concentrations.

Stimulant/diuretic: **Caffeine sodium benzoate:** Adults: I.M., I.V.: 500 mg as a single dose

Treatment of spinal puncture headache: **Caffeine sodium benzoate:** Adults: I.V.: 500 mg as a single dose; may repeat in 4 hours if headache unrelieved (see Administration)

Administration

Oral: May be administered without regard to feedings or meals; may administer injectable formulation (caffeine citrate) orally

Parenteral:

Caffeine citrate: Infuse loading dose over at least 30 minutes; maintenance dose may be infused over at least 10 minutes; may administer without dilution or diluted with D_5W to 10 mg caffeine citrate/mL

Caffeine sodium benzoate: I.V. as slow direct injection; for spinal headaches, dilute in 1000 mL NS and infuse over 1 hour; follow with 1000 mL NS, infuse over 1 hour; administer I.M. undiluted

Monitoring Parameters Heart rate, number and severity of apnea spells, serum caffeine levels

Reference Range

Therapeutic: Apnea of prematurity: 8-20 mcg/mL

Potentially toxic: >20 mcg/mL

Toxic: >50 mcg/mL

Dosage Forms Excipient information presented when available (limited, particularly for generics); consult specific product labeling.

Caplet:

NoDoz® Maximum Strength, Vivarin®: 200 mg

Injection, solution, as citrate [preservative free] (Cafcit®): 20 mg/mL (3 mL) [equivalent to 10 mg/mL caffeine base]

Injection, solution [with sodium benzoate]: Caffeine 125 mg/mL and sodium benzoate 125 mg/mL (2 mL); caffeine 121 mg/mL and sodium benzoate 129 mg/mL (2 mL)

Lozenge:

Enerjets®: 75 mg [classic coffee, hazelnut cream, or mochamint flavor]

Solution, oral, as citrate [preservative free]:

Cafcit®: 20 mg/mL (3 mL) [equivalent to 10 mg/mL caffeine base]

Tablet: 200 mg

Vivarin®: 200 mg

Extemporaneous Preparations

An oral solution of 20 mg/mL caffeine citrate, prepared from 10 g caffeine (anhydrous) combined with 10 g citric acid USP and 1000 mL SWI is stable for 3 months refrigerated (Nahata, 1987).

An oral solution 20 mg/mL caffeine citrate may be made by dissolving 5 g anhydrous caffeine and 5 g citric acid USP in 250 mL SWI. Stir solution until completely clear; add 2:1 simple syrup:cherry syrup mixture to a final volume of 500 mL; stable refrigerated 90 days (Eisenberg, 1984).

Eisenberg MG and Kang N, "Stability of Citrated Caffeine Solutions for Injectable and Enteral Use," *Am J Hosp Pharm*, 1984, 41(11):2405-6.

Nahata, MC, Pai VB, and Hipple TF, *Pediatric Drug Formulations*, 5th ed, Cincinnati, OH: Harvey Whitney Books Co, 2004.

References

Bhatt-Mehta V and Schumacher RE, "Treatment of Apnea of Prematurity," *Paediatr Drugs*, 2003, 5(3):195-210.

Erenberg A, Leff RD, Haack DG, et al, "Caffeine Citrate for the Treatment of Apnea of Prematurity: A Double-Blind, Placebo-Controlled Study," *Pharmacotherapy*, 2000, 20(6):644-52.

Kriter KE and Blanchard J, "Management of Apnea in Infants," *Clin Pharm*, 1989, 8(8):577-87.

♦ **Caffeine and Ergotamine** *see* Ergotamine and Caffeine *on page 592*

♦ **Caffeine and Sodium Benzoate** *see* Caffeine *on page 255*

♦ **Caffeine Citrate** *see* Caffeine *on page 255*

Calamine Lotion (KAL a myne loe shun)

Index Terms Lotio Calaminae

Therapeutic Category Topical Skin Product

Use Employed primarily as an astringent, protectant, and soothing agent for conditions such as poison ivy, poison oak, poison sumac, sunburn, insect bites, or minor skin irritations

Precautions For external use only

Adverse Reactions

Dermatologic: Rash

Local: Irritation

Usual Dosage Topical: Apply 1-4 times/day as needed; reapply after bathing

Administration Topical: Shake well before using; avoid contact with the eyes; do not use on open wounds or burns

Additional Information Active ingredients: Calamine, zinc oxide

Dosage Forms Excipient information presented when available (limited, particularly for generics); consult specific product labeling.

Lotion:

Topical: Calamine 8%, zinc oxide 8%, glycerin 2% and bentonite magma in calcium hydroxide solution (120 mL, 240 mL, 480 mL)

(Continued)

Calamine Lotion *(Continued)*

Topical, phenolated: Calamine 8%, zinc oxide 8%, glycerin 2%, bentonite magma, and phenol 1% in calcium hydroxide solution (120 mL, 240 mL)

- **Calan®** *see* Verapamil *on page 1611*
- **Calan® SR** *see* Verapamil *on page 1611*
- **Calcarb 600 [OTC]** *see* Calcium Carbonate *on page 264*
- **Calcarb 600 [OTC]** *see* Calcium Supplements *on page 272*
- **Calci-Chew® [OTC]** *see* Calcium Carbonate *on page 264*
- **Calci-Chew® [OTC]** *see* Calcium Supplements *on page 272*
- **Calciferol™** *see* Ergocalciferol *on page 588*
- **Calcijex®** *see* Calcitriol *on page 259*
- **Calcimar® (Can)** *see* Calcitonin *on page 258*
- **Calci-Mix® [OTC]** *see* Calcium Carbonate *on page 264*
- **Calci-Mix® [OTC]** *see* Calcium Supplements *on page 272*
- **Calcionate [OTC]** *see* Calcium Glubionate *on page 268*
- **Calcite-500 (Can)** *see* Calcium Carbonate *on page 264*

Calcitonin (kal si TOE nin)

Medication Safety Issues

Sound-alike/look-alike issues:

Calcitonin may be confused with calcitriol

Miacalcin® may be confused with Micatin®

Calcitonin nasal spray is administered as a single spray into **one** nostril daily, using alternate nostrils each day.

U.S. Brand Names Fortical®; Miacalcin®

Canadian Brand Names Apo-Calcitonin®; Calcimar®; Caltine®; Miacalcin® NS

Index Terms Calcitonin (Salmon)

Therapeutic Category Antidote, Hypercalcemia

Generic Available No

Use

Parenteral: Treatment of Paget's disease of bone and as adjunctive therapy for hypercalcemia; also used in postmenopausal osteoporosis and osteogenesis imperfecta

Intranasal: Postmenopausal osteoporosis in women >5 years postmenopause with low bone mass

Pregnancy Risk Factor C

Lactation Excretion in breast milk unknown/not recommended

Contraindications Hypersensitivity to calcitonin, salmon protein, or any component

Precautions Due to potential hypersensitivity reactions, a skin test is recommended prior to initiating parenteral therapy; the skin test is 0.1 mL of 10 unit/mL calcitonin injection in NS (must be prepared) injected intradermally; observe injection site for 15 minutes for wheal or significant erythema; when using intranasal formulation, periodic nasal examinations are recommended

Adverse Reactions

Cardiovascular: Flushing of the face, edema, hypertension, angina, tachycardia, palpitation, MI, thrombophlebitis

Central nervous system: Dizziness, headache, chills, fever, fatigue, anxiety, vertigo, migraine, neuralgia, agitation

Dermatologic: Erythematous rash, eczema, alopecia, pruritus

Endocrine & metabolic: Increase weight, goiter, hyperthyroidism

Gastrointestinal: Nausea, vomiting, diarrhea, anorexia, metallic taste, dyspepsia, constipation, abdominal pain, flatulence, gastritis, xerostomia, thirst

Genitourinary: Hematuria, renal calculus, cystitis

Hepatic: Cholelithiasis, hepatitis

Local: Injection site reactions (10%)

Neuromuscular & skeletal: Weakness, tingling of palms and soles, back and joint pain, arthralgia, polymyalgia rheumatica, stiffness, paresthesia

Ocular: Periorbital edema

Otic: Tinnitus

Renal: Diuresis, pyelonephritis

Respiratory: Shortness of breath; nasal congestion, rhinitis, epistaxis, nasal sores, and sore bridge of nose (nasal spray)

Miscellaneous: Hypersensitivity reactions, lymphadenopathy, influenza-like symptoms

Stability

Injection: Store under refrigeration; stable for up to 2 weeks at room temperature

Nasal spray: Store unopened bottle under refrigeration; do not freeze; once the pump has been activated, store at room temperature; stable at room temperature for 30 days

Mechanism of Action Calcitonin directly inhibits osteoclastic bone resorption; promotes the renal excretion of calcium, phosphate, sodium, magnesium and potassium by decreasing tubular reabsorption; increases the jejunal secretion of water, sodium, potassium, and chloride

Pharmacodynamics

Hypercalcemia:

Onset of action:

I.M., SubQ: 15 minutes

I.V.: Immediate

Maximum effect: I.M., SubQ: 4 hours

Duration:

I.M., SubQ: 8-24 hours

I.V.: 30 minutes to 12 hours

Pharmacokinetics

Absorption: Intranasal: Rapidly but highly variable and lower than I.M. administration

Metabolism: Rapidly in the kidneys, blood, and peripheral tissues

Bioavailability: Intranasal: 3%

Half-life, elimination: Intranasal: 43 minutes

Time to peak serum concentration:

Intranasal: 31-39 minutes

I.V.: 16-25 minutes

Elimination: As inactive metabolites in urine

Clearance: Salmon calcitonin: 3.1 mL/kg/minute

Usual Dosage Dosage for children not established; Adults:

Paget's disease:

I.M., SubQ: Initial: 100 international units/day; maintenance dose: 50 international units/day or 50-100 international units every 1-3 days

Intranasal: 200-400 international units (1-2 sprays) per day

Hypercalcemia: Initial: I.M., SubQ: 4 international units/kg every 12 hours; may increase up to 8 international units/kg every 12 hours to a maximum of every 6 hours

Osteogenesis imperfecta: I.M., SubQ: 2 international units/kg 3 times/week

Postmenopausal osteoporosis:

I.M., SubQ: 100 international units/day

Intranasal: 200 international units (1 spray) into **one** nostril daily

Administration

Intranasal: Spray into **one** nostril daily; alternate nostrils to reduce irritation. Before priming a new pump, allow it to reach room temperature first.

Parenteral: Do not exceed 2 mL volume per injection site; may be administered SubQ or I.M.

Monitoring Parameters Serum electrolytes and calcium; alkaline phosphatase and 24-hour urine collection for hydroxyproline excretion (Paget's disease); urinalysis (urine sediment); serum calcium; periodic nasal exams (intranasal use only)

Reference Range Therapeutic: <19 pg/mL (SI: 19 ng/L) basal, depending on the assay

Patient Information Nasal spray: Notify physician if you develop significant nasal irritation; alternate nostrils; in treatment of postmenopausal osteoporosis, maintain adequate vitamin D intake and supplemental calcium

Dosage Forms Excipient information presented when available (limited, particularly for generics); consult specific product labeling.

Injection, solution [calcitonin-salmon]:

Miacalcin®: 200 int. units/mL (2 mL)

Solution, intranasal [spray, calcitonin-salmon]:

Fortical®: 200 int. units/0.09 mL (3.7 mL) [rDNA origin; contains benzyl alcohol; delivers 30 doses, 200 units/actuation]

Miacalcin®: 200 int. units/0.09 mL (3.7 mL) [contains benzalkonium chloride; delivers 30 doses, 200 units/actuation]

♦ **Calcitonin (Salmon)** *see* Calcitonin *on page 258*

♦ **Cal-Citrate® 250 [OTC]** *see* Calcium Citrate *on page 267*

♦ **Cal-Citrate® 250 [OTC]** *see* Calcium Supplements *on page 272*

Calcitriol (kal si TRYE ole)

Medication Safety Issues

Sound-alike/look-alike issues:

Calcitriol may be confused with calcifediol, Calciferol®, calcitonin

(Continued)

Calcitriol *(Continued)*

Dosage is expressed in mcg (micrograms), **not** mg (milligrams); rare cases of acute overdose have been reported

U.S. Brand Names Calcijex®; Rocaltrol®

Canadian Brand Names Calcijex®; Rocaltrol®

Index Terms 1,25 Dihydroxycholecalciferol

Therapeutic Category Rickets, Treatment Agent; Vitamin D Analog; Vitamin, Fat Soluble

Generic Available Yes

Use Management of secondary hyperparathyroidism and resultant metabolic bone disease in patients with moderate to severe chronic renal failure not yet on dialysis; management of hypocalcemia and resultant metabolic bone disease in patients on chronic renal dialysis; management of hypocalcemia in patients with hypoparathyroidism and pseudohypoparathyroidism

Pregnancy Risk Factor C

Lactation Enters breast milk/not recommended

Contraindications Hypersensitivity to calcitriol or any component; hypercalcemia; vitamin D toxicity; abnormal sensitivity to the effects of vitamin D

Warnings Excessive administration may lead to over suppression of PTH, hypercalcemia, hypercalciuria, hyperphosphatemia, and adynamic bone disease. Acute hypercalcemia may increase risk of cardiac arrhythmias and seizures. Chronic hypercalcemia may lead to generalized vascular and other soft-tissue calcification. Phosphate and vitamin D (and its derivatives) should be withheld during therapy to avoid hypercalcemia. Monitor serum calcium levels closely; the calcitriol dosage should be adjusted accordingly; serum calcium times phosphorus product (Ca x P) should not exceed 65 mg^2/dL^2 for infants and children <12 years of age and 55 mg^2/dL^2 for adolescents and adults. Not indicated for use in patients with rapidly worsening kidney function or those who are noncompliant with medications or follow-up (K/DOQI Guidelines, 2003).

Precautions

Hypercalcemia potentiates digoxin toxicity; use concomitantly with caution

Adverse Reactions Effects primarily associated with hypercalcemia

Cardiovascular: Elevated blood pressure, cardiac arrhythmias

Central nervous system: Somnolence, headache, hyperthermia, apathy

Dermatologic: Pruritus

Endocrine & metabolic: Hypercholesterolemia, hypercalcemia, polydipsia, weight loss, hyperphosphatemia

Gastrointestinal: Nausea, vomiting, constipation, anorexia, xerostomia, pancreatitis, metallic taste

Genitourinary: Nocturia

Hepatic: Elevated liver enzymes

Neuromuscular & skeletal: Myalgia, bone pain, weakness

Ocular: Calcific conjunctivitis, photophobia

Renal: Polyuria, uremia, albuminuria, nephrocalcinosis, UTIs, hypercalciuria

Respiratory: Rhinorrhea

Miscellaneous: Hypersensitivity reactions, dehydration

Drug Interactions May antagonize the effects of calcium channel blockers by increasing serum calcium levels; may be associated with digoxin toxicity by increasing calcium levels; an additive increase in calcium levels due to decreased calcium excretion by thiazide diuretics; magnesium-containing antacids (potential development of hypermagnesemia); cholestyramine, colestipol, orlistat, and excessive use of mineral oil decrease absorption; ketoconazole may inhibit both the synthetic and catabolic enzymes of calcitriol; corticosteroids decrease calcium absorption counteracting the calcitriol function of increasing calcium absorption

Stability Store at room temperature; protect from light and heat

Mechanism of Action Calcitriol, the active form of vitamin D (1,25 hydroxyvitamin D_3), binds to and activates the vitamin D receptor in kidney, parathyroid gland, intestine, and bone, stimulating intestinal calcium transport and absorption. It reduces PTH levels and improves calcium and phosphate homeostasis by stimulating bone resorption of calcium and increasing renal tubular reabsorption of calcium. Decreased renal conversion of vitamin D to its primary active metabolite (1,25 hydroxyvitamin D) in chronic renal failure leads to reduced activation of vitamin D receptor, which subsequently removes inhibitory suppression of parathyroid hormone (PTH) release; increased serum PTH (secondary hyperparathyroidism) reduces calcium excretion and enhances bone resorption.

Pharmacodynamics Oral:

Onset of action: 2 hours

Maximum effect: 10 hours

Duration: 3-5 days

Pharmacokinetics

Distribution: Breast milk: Very low (levels 2.2 ± 0.1 pg/mL)

Protein binding: 99.9%

Metabolism: Primarily to 1,24,25-trihydroxycholecalciferol and 1,24,25-trihydroxy ergocalciferol

Half-life:

Children 1.8-16 years undergoing peritoneal dialysis: 27.4 hours

Adults without renal dysfunction: 5-8 hours

Adults with CRF: 16.2-21.9 hours

Time to peak serum concentration: Oral: 3-6 hours

Elimination: Feces 27% and urine 7% excreted unchanged in 24 hours

Clearance: Children 1.8-16 years undergoing peritoneal dialysis: 15.3 mL/hour/kg

Usual Dosage

Management of hypocalcemia in patients with chronic kidney disease (CKD): Indicated for therapy when serum levels of 25(OH)D are >30 ng/mL (75 nmol/L) and serum levels of intact parathyroid hormone (iPTH) are above the target range for the stage of CKD (see Reference Range); serum levels of corrected total calcium are <9.5-10 mg/dL (2.37 mmol/L) and serum levels of phosphorus in children are less than age-appropriate upper limits of normal or in adults <4.6 mg/dL (1.49 mmol/L) (K/DOQI Guidelines, 2005):

Children and Adolescents: CKD Stages 2-4: Oral:

<10 kg: 0.05 mcg every other day

10-20 kg: 0.1-0.15 mcg daily

>20 kg: 0.25 mcg daily

Dosage adjustment:

If iPTH decrease is <30% after 3 months of therapy and serum levels of calcium and phosphorus are within the target ranges based upon the CKD Stage (see Reference Range), increase dosage by 50%

If iPTH decrease < target range for CKD stage (see Reference Range) hold calcitriol therapy until iPTH increases to above target range; resume therapy at half the previous dosage (if dosage <0.25 mcg capsule or 0.05 mcg liquid, use every other day therapy)

If serum levels of total corrected calcium exceed 10.2 mg/dL (2.37 mmol/L) hold calcitriol therapy until serum calcium decreased to <9.8 mg/dL (2.37 mmol/L); resume therapy at half the previous dosage (if dosage <0.25 mcg capsule or 0.05 mcg liquid, use every other day therapy)

If serum levels of phosphorus increase to > age-appropriate upper limits, hold calcitriol therapy (initiate or increase phosphate binders until the levels of serum phosphorus decrease to age-appropriate limits); resume therapy at half the previous dosage

Children and Adolescents: CKD Stage 5: Oral, I.V.: Serum calcium times phosphorus product (Ca x P) should not exceed 65 mg^2/dL^2 for infants and children <12 years of age and 55 mg^2/dL^2 for adolescents, serum phosphorus should be within target (see Reference Range), serum calcium <10 mg/dL (2.37 mmol/L):

iPTH 300-500 pg/mL: 0.0075 mcg/kg per dialysis session (3 times/week); not to exceed 0.25 mcg daily

iPTH >500-1000 pg/mL: 0.015 mcg/kg per dialysis session (3 times/week); not to exceed 0.5 mcg daily

iPTH >1000 pg/mL: 0.025 mcg/kg per dialysis session (3 times/week); not to exceed 1 mcg daily

Dosage adjustment: If iPTH decrease is <30% after 3 months of therapy and serum levels of calcium and phosphorus are within the target ranges based upon the CKD Stage 5 (see Reference Range), increase dosage by 50%

Adult CKD Stages 3 or 4: Serum calcium <9.5 mg/dL (2.37 mmol/L), serum phosphorus <5.5 mg/dL (1.77 mmol/L), serum calcium times phosphorus product (Ca x P) <55 mg^2/dL^2:

iPTH 300-600 pg/mL: Oral, I.V.: 0.5-1.5 mcg per dialysis session (3 times/week)

iPTH 600-1000 pg/mL: I.V.: 1-3 mcg per dialysis session (3 times/week); Oral: 1-4 mcg per dialysis session (3 times/week)

iPTH >1000 pg/mL: I.V. 3-5 mcg per dialysis session (3 times/week); Oral: 3-7 mcg per dialysis session (3 times/week)

Dosage adjustment:

If iPTH decrease < target range for CKD stage 5 (see Reference Range) hold calcitriol therapy until iPTH increases to above target range; resume therapy at half the previous dosage (if dosage <0.25 mcg capsule or 0.05 mcg liquid, use every other day therapy)

If serum levels of total corrected calcium exceed 9.5 mg/dL (2.37 mmol/L) hold calcitriol therapy until serum calcium decreased to <9.5 mg/dL (2.37 mmol/L); resume therapy at half the previous dosage (if dosage <0.25 mcg capsule or 0.05 mcg liquid, use every other day therapy)

(Continued)

Calcitriol *(Continued)*

If serum levels of phosphorus increase to >4.6 mg/dL (1.49 mmol/L), hold calcitriol therapy (initiate or increase phosphate binders until the levels of serum phosphorus decrease to 4.6 mg/dL (1.49 mmol/L); resume therapy at prior dosage

Note: Intermittent administration of calcitriol by I.V. or oral routes is more effective than daily oral calcitriol in lowering iPTH levels.

Hypoparathyroidism/pseudohypoparathyroidism: Oral (evaluate dosage at 2- to 4-week intervals):

Children:

<1 year: 0.04-0.08 mcg/kg once daily

1-5 years: 0.25-0.75 mcg once daily

Children >6 years and Adults: 0.5-2 mcg once daily

Vitamin D-dependent rickets: Children and Adults: Oral: 1 mcg once daily

Vitamin D-resistant rickets (familial hypophosphatemia): Children and Adults: Oral: Initial: 0.015-0.02 mcg/kg once daily; maintenance: 0.03-0.06 mcg/kg once daily; maximum dose: 2 mcg once daily

Hypocalcemia in premature infants: Oral: 1 mcg once daily for the first 5 days of life

Hypocalcemic tetany in premature infants: I.V.: 0.05 mcg/kg once daily for 5-12 days

Administration

Oral: May be administered with or without meals; when administering small doses from the liquid-filled capsules, consider the following concentration for Rocaltrol®:

0.25 mcg capsule = 0.25 mcg per 0.17 mL

0.5 mcg capsule = 0.5 mcg per 0.17 mL

Parenteral: May be administered undiluted as a bolus dose I.V. through the catheter at the end of hemodialysis

Monitoring Parameters Signs and symptoms of vitamin D intoxication

Serum calcium and phosphorus:

I.V.: Twice weekly during initial phase, then at least monthly once dose established

Oral: At least every 2 weeks for 3 months or following dose adjustment, then monthly for 3 months, then every 3 months

Serum or plasma intact parathyroid hormone (iPTH): At least every 2 weeks for 3 months or following dose adjustment, then monthly for 3 months, then as per K/DOQI Guidelines below.

Per Kidney Disease Outcome Quality Initiative Practice Guidelines: Children (K/DOQI, 2005):

Stage 3 CKD: iPTH every 6 months

Stage 4 CKD: iPTH every 3 months

Stage 5 CKD: iPTH every 3 months

Per Kidney Disease Outcome Quality Initiative Practice Guidelines: Adults (K/DOQI, 2003):

Stage 3 CKD: iPTH every 12 months

Stage 4 CKD: iPTH every 3 months

Stage 5 CKD: iPTH every 3 months

Reference Range

Chronic kidney disease (CKD) is defined either as kidney damage or GFR <60 mL/minute/1.73 m^2 for ≥3 months); stages of CKD are described below:

CKD Stage 1: Kidney damage with normal or increased GFR; GFR >90 mL/minute/1.73m^2

CKD Stage 2: Kidney damage with mild decrease in GFR; GFR 60-89 mL/minute/1.73 m^2

CKD Stage 3: Moderate decrease in GFR; GFR 30-59 mL/minute/1.73 m^2

CKD Stage 4: Severe decrease in GFR; GFR 15-29 mL/minute/1.73 m^2

CKD Stage 5: Kidney failure; GFR <15 mL/minute/1.73 m^2 or dialysis

Target range for iPTH:

Stage 2 CKD: Children: 35-70 pg/mL (3.85-7.7 pmol/L)

Stage 3 CKD: Children and Adults: 35-70 pg/mL (3.85-7.7 pmol/L)

Stage 4 CKD: Children and Adults: 70-110 pg/mL (7.7-12.1 pmol/L)

Stage 5 CKD:

Children: 200-300 pg/mL (22-33 pmol/L)

Adults: 150-300 pg/mL (16.5-33 pmol/L)

Serum phosphorous:

Stages 1-4 CKD: Children: At or above the age-appropriate lower limits and no higher than age-appropriate upper limits

Stage 3 and 4 CKD: Adults: ≥2.7 to <4.6 mg/dL (≥0.87 to <1.49 mmol/L)

Stage 5 CKD:

Children 1-12 years: 4-6 mg/dL (1.29-1.94 mmol/L)

Children >12 years and Adults: 3.5-5.5 mg/dL (1.13-1.78 mmol/L)

Patient Information Take as directed; do not increase dosage without consulting healthcare provider. Adhere to diet as recommended (do not take any other phosphate or vitamin D-related compounds while taking calcitriol). You may experience nausea, vomiting, dry mouth (small frequent meals, frequent mouth care, chewing gums, or sucking lozenges may help).

Dosage Forms Excipient information presented when available (limited, particularly for generics); consult specific product labeling.

Capsule, softgel: 0.25 mcg, 0.5 mcg
- Rocaltrol®: 0.25 mcg, 0.5 mcg [each strength contains coconut oil]

Injection, solution: 1 mcg/mL (1 mL)
- Calcijex®: 1 mcg/mL (1 mL) [contains aluminum]

Solution, oral: 1 mcg/mL (15 mL)
- Rocaltrol®: 1 mcg/mL (15 mL) [contains palm seed oil]

References

"K/DOQI Clinical Practice Guidelines for Bone Metabolism and Disease in Children With Chronic Kidney Disease," *Am J Kidney Dis*, 2005, 46(4 Suppl 1):S1-121.

"K/DOQI Clinical Practice Guidelines for Bone Metabolism and Disease in Chronic Kidney Disease. Guideline 1. Evaluation of Calcium and Phosphorus Metabolism," *Am J Kidney Dis* , 2003, 42(4 Suppl 3):52-7.

"K/DOQI Clinical Practice Guidelines for Bone Metabolism and Disease in Chronic Kidney Disease. Guideline 3. Evaluation of Serum Phosphorus Levels," *Am J Kidney Dis* , 2003, 42(4 Suppl 3):62-3.

"K/DOQI Clinical Practice Guidelines for Chronic Kidney Disease: Evaluation, Classification, and Stratification, Part 4. Definition and Classification of Stages of Chronic Kidney Disease," *Am J Kidney Dis*, 2002, 39(2 Suppl 1):46-75.

Sanchez CP, "Secondary Hyperparathyroidism in Children With Chronic Renal Failure: Pathogenesis and Treatment," *Paediatr Drugs*, 2003, 5(11): 763-76.

Ziolkowska H, "Minimizing Bone Abnormalities in Children With Renal Failure," *Paediatr Drugs*, 2006, 8(4):205-22.

Calcium Acetate (KAL see um AS e tate)

Medication Safety Issues

Sound-alike/look-alike issues:
- PhosLo® may be confused with Phos-Flur®, ProSom™

U.S. Brand Names PhosLo®

Canadian Brand Names PhosLo®

Therapeutic Category Calcium Salt; Electrolyte Supplement, Parenteral

Generic Available Yes: Solution for injection

Use Treatment and prevention of calcium depletion (injection); treatment of hyperphosphatemia in end-stage renal failure

Pregnancy Risk Factor C

Contraindications See Calcium Supplements *on page 272.*

Warnings See Calcium Supplements *on page 272.* Avoid use of calcium acetate in dialysis patients with hypercalcemia or whose plasma PTH concentrations are <150 pg/mL on two consecutive measurements.

Precautions See Calcium Supplements *on page 272.*

Adverse Reactions See Calcium Supplements *on page 272.*

Drug Interactions See Calcium Supplements *on page 272.*

Food Interactions See Calcium Supplements *on page 272.*

Stability Store at room temperature; parenteral solutions are incompatible with bicarbonates, phosphates, and sulfate formulations; mixing will result in precipitation. TPN solutions containing phosphate and calcium are compatible depending upon the parenteral amino-acid formulation and its concentration.

Mechanism of Action Calcium moderates nerve and muscle performance via action potential excitation threshold regulation; it is necessary for maintaining the functional integrity of nervous, muscular, and skeletal systems and cell-membrane and capillary permeability. Calcium acetate combines with dietary phosphate to form insoluble calcium phosphate which is excreted in feces and reduces phosphate absorption.

Pharmacokinetics See Calcium Supplements *on page 272.*

Usual Dosage

Recommended daily allowance (RDA) and adequate intake: See Calcium Supplements *on page 272.*

Treatment of hyperphosphatemia in end-stage renal failure: Oral: Adults: Dose expressed in mg of **calcium acetate** (PhosLo®): 1334 mg (two 667 mg capsules) with each meal; may increase up to 2668 mg (four 667 mg capsules) with each meal

Daily maintenance calcium: I.V.:
- Neonates: 3-4 mEq/kg/day
- Infants and Children <25 kg: 1-2 mEq/kg/day
- Children 25-45 kg: 0.5-1.5 mEq/kg/day
- Children >45 kg and Adults: 0.2-0.3 mEq/kg/day or 10-20 mEq/day

Dosage adjustment in renal impairment: Cl_{cr} <25 mL/minute may require dosage adjustment depending upon serum calcium level

(Continued)

Calcium Acetate *(Continued)*

Administration

Oral: Administer with plenty of fluids with meals to optimize effectiveness

Parenteral:

I.V.: For direct I.V. injection infuse slow IVP over 3-5 minutes or at a rate not to exceed 0.7-1.8 mEq/minute

I.V. infusion: Infuse 0.6-1.2 mEq/kg over 1 hour

Do not inject calcium salts I.M. or administer SubQ since severe necrosis and sloughing may occur; extravasation of calcium can result in severe necrosis and tissue sloughing. Do not use scalp vein or small hand or foot veins for I.V. administration. Not for endotracheal administration.

Monitoring Parameters See Calcium Supplements *on page 272.*

Reference Range See Calcium Supplements *on page 272.*

Additional Information 1 g calcium acetate = 250 mg elemental calcium = 12.7 mEq calcium. Due to a poor correlation between the serum ionized calcium (free) and total serum calcium, particularly in states of low albumin or acid/base imbalances, direct measurement of ionized calcium is recommended. If ionized calcium is unavailable, in low albumin states, the corrected **total** serum calcium may be estimated by this equation (assuming a normal albumin of 4 g/dL); corrected total calcium = total serum calcium + 0.8(4 - measured serum albumin)

Dosage Forms Excipient information presented when available (limited, particularly for generics); consult specific product labeling. [DSC] = Discontinued product. **Note:** Elemental calcium listed in brackets:

Gelcap:

PhosLo®: 667 mg [169 mg]

Injection, solution: 0.5 mEq/mL (10 mL, 50 mL, 100 mL) [DSC]

Calcium Carbonate (KAL see um KAR bun ate)

Medication Safety Issues

Sound-alike/look-alike issues:

Florical® may be confused with Fiorinal®

Mylanta® may be confused with Mynatal®

Nephro-Calci® may be confused with Nephrocaps®

Os-Cal® may be confused with Asacol®

International issues:

Remegel® [Great Britain, Ireland, Italy] may be confused with Renagel® which is a brand name for sevelamer in the U.S.

U.S. Brand Names Alcalak [OTC]; Alka-Mints® [OTC]; Calcarb 600 [OTC]; Calci-Chew® [OTC]; Calci-Mix® [OTC]; Cal-Gest [OTC]; Cal-Mint [OTC]; Caltrate® 600 [OTC]; Children's Pepto [OTC]; Chooz® [OTC]; Florical® [OTC]; Maalox® Regular Chewable [OTC]; Mylanta® Children's [OTC]; Nephro-Calci® [OTC]; Nutralox® [OTC]; Os-Cal® 500 [OTC] [DSC]; Oysco 500 [OTC]; Oyst-Cal 500 [OTC]; Rolaids® Softchews [OTC]; Titralac™ [OTC]; Tums® [OTC]; Tums® E-X [OTC]; Tums® Extra Strength Sugar Free [OTC]; Tums® Smoothies™ [OTC]; Tums® Ultra [OTC]

Canadian Brand Names Apo-Cal®; Calcite-500; Caltrate®; Caltrate® Select; Os-Cal®

Therapeutic Category Antacid; Calcium Salt; Electrolyte Supplement, Oral

Generic Available Yes

Use Symptomatic relief of hyperacidity associated with peptic ulcer, gastritis, esophagitis, and hiatal hernia; treatment of hyperphosphatemia in end-stage renal failure; dietary supplement; prevention and treatment of calcium deficiency; topical treatment of hydrofluoric acid burns; adjunctive prevention and treatment of osteoporosis

Pregnancy Risk Factor C

Contraindications See Calcium Supplements *on page 272.*

Warnings See Calcium Supplements *on page 272.* Milk-Alkali syndrome (hypercalcemia, metabolic alkalosis, and rarely, renal insufficiency) has been associated with ingestion of large quantities of milk concomitantly with calcium carbonate; patients with renal impairment or dehydration and electrolyte imbalance are at increased risk for developing this syndrome; monitor calcium serum levels periodically

Precautions See Calcium Supplements *on page 272.* When used chronically as an antacid, calcium carbonate has been associated with gastric hypersecretion and acid rebound.

Adverse Reactions See Calcium Supplements *on page 272.*

Drug Interactions See Calcium Supplements *on page 272.*

Food Interactions See Calcium Supplements *on page 272.*

Stability Store at room temperature.

Mechanism of Action Calcium moderates nerve and muscle performance via action potential excitation threshold regulation; it is necessary for maintaining the functional integrity of nervous, muscular, and skeletal systems and cell-membrane and capillary permeability. Calcium carbonate combines with dietary phosphate to form insoluble calcium phosphate which is excreted in feces and reduces phosphate absorption .

Pharmacodynamics Acid neutralizing capacity: Tums® 500 mg: 10 mEq, Tums® E-X 750 mg: 15mEq; Tums® Ultra 1000 mg: 20 mEq

Pharmacokinetics See Calcium Supplements *on page 272.*

Usual Dosage Oral:

Recommended daily allowance (RDA) and adequate intake: See Calcium Supplements *on page 272.*

Antacid:

Children 2-5 years: Children's Pepto, Mylanta® Children's: 1 tablet (400 mg calcium carbonate) as symptoms occur; not to exceed 3 tablets/day

Children >5-11 years: Children's Pepto, Mylanta® Children's: 2 tablets (800 mg calcium carbonate) as symptoms occur; not to exceed 6 tablets/day

Children >11 years and Adults:

Tums®, Tums® E-X: Chew 2-4 tablets as symptoms occur; not to exceed 15 tablets (Tums®) or 10 tablets (Tums® E-X) per day

Tums® Ultra: Chew 2-3 tablets as symptoms occur; not to exceed 7 tablets per day

Hypocalcemia (dose depends on clinical condition and serum calcium level): Dose expressed in mg of **elemental calcium**:

Neonates: 50-150 mg/kg/day in 4-6 divided doses; not to exceed 1 g/day

Children: 45-65 mg/kg/day in 4 divided doses

Adults: 1-2 g or more per day in 3-4 divided doses

Treatment of hyperphosphatemia in end-stage renal failure: Children and Adults: Dose expressed in mg of **calcium carbonate**: 1 g with each meal; increase as needed; range: 4-7 g/day

Adjunctive prevention and treatment of osteoporosis: Adults: 500 mg **elemental calcium** 2-3 times/day; recommended dosage includes dietary intake and should be adjusted depending upon the patient's diet; to improve absorption do not administer more than 500 mg **elemental calcium**/dose

Hydrofluoric acid (HF) burns (HF concentration <20%): Topical: Various topical calcium preparations have been used anecdotally for treatment of dermal exposure to HF solutions; calcium carbonate at concentrations ranging from 2.5% to 33% has been used; a topical calcium carbonate preparation must be compounded (see Extemporaneous Preparations); apply topically as needed

Dosage adjustment in renal impairment: Cl_{cr} <25 mL/minute may require dosage adjustment depending upon serum calcium level

Administration

Oral: Administer with plenty of fluids with or immediately following meals; if using for phosphate-binding, administer with meals

Suspension: Shake well before administration

Chewable tablets: Thoroughly chew tablets before swallowing

Topical: Massage calcium carbonate slurry into exposed area for 15 minutes

Monitoring Parameters See Calcium Supplements *on page 272.*

Reference Range See Calcium Supplements *on page 272.*

Additional Information 1 g calcium carbonate = 400 mg elemental calcium = 20 mEq calcium. Due to a poor correlation between the serum ionized calcium (free) and total serum calcium, particularly in states of low albumin or acid/base imbalances, direct measurement of ionized calcium is recommended. If ionized calcium is unavailable, in low albumin states, the corrected **total** serum calcium may be estimated by this equation (assuming a normal albumin of 4 g/dL); corrected total calcium = total serum calcium + 0.8(4 - measured serum albumin)

Dosage Forms Excipient information presented when available (limited, particularly for generics); consult specific product labeling. [DSC] = Discontinued product

Capsule:

Calci-Mix®: 1250 mg [equivalent to elemental calcium 500 mg]

Florical®: 364 mg [equivalent to elemental calcium 145.6 mg; contains sodium fluoride 3.75 mg]

Gum, chewing: 250 mg (30s)

Chooz®: 500 mg [equivalent to elemental calcium 200 mg; mint flavor]

Powder: 4000 mg/teaspoonful (480 g) [equivalent to 1600 mg elemental calcium/teaspoonful]

Suspension, oral: 1250 mg/5 mL (5 mL, 500 mL) [equivalent to elemental calcium 500 mg/5 mL; mint flavor]

Tablet: 1250 mg [equivalent to elemental calcium 500 mg]; 1500 mg [equivalent to elemental calcium 600 mg]

Calcarb 600, Caltrate® 600, Nephro-Calci®: 1500 mg [equivalent to elemental calcium 600 mg]

Florical®: 364 mg [equivalent to elemental calcium 145.6 mg; contains sodium fluoride 8.3 mg]

(Continued)

Calcium Carbonate *(Continued)*

Os-Cal® 500: 1250 mg [equivalent to elemental calcium 500 mg; contains tartrazine] [DSC]

Oysco 500, Oyst-Cal 500: 1250 mg [equivalent to elemental calcium 500 mg]

Tablet, chewable: 500 mg [equivalent to elemental calcium 200 mg]; 650 mg [equivalent to elemental calcium 260 mg]; 750 mg [equivalent to elemental calcium 300 mg]

Alcalak: 420 mg [equivalent to elemental calcium 168 mg; mint flavor]

Alka-Mints®: 850 mg [equivalent to elemental calcium 340 mg; spearmint flavor]

Cal-Gest: 500 mg [equivalent to elemental calcium 200 mg; assorted flavors]

Calci-Chew®: 1250 mg [equivalent to elemental calcium 500 mg; cherry, lemon, and orange flavors]

Cal-Mint: 650 mg [equivalent to elemental calcium 260 mg; mint flavor]

Children's Pepto: 400 mg [equivalent to elemental calcium 161 mg; bubble gum or watermelon flavors]

Maalox® Regular: 600 mg [equivalent to elemental calcium 222 mg; contains phenylalanine 0.5 mg/tablet; lemon flavor]

Mylanta® Children's: 400 mg [equivalent to elemental calcium 160 mg; bubble gum flavor]

Nutralox®: 420 mg [equivalent to elemental calcium 168 mg; sugar free; mint flavor]

Os-Cal® 500: 1250 mg [equivalent to elemental calcium 500 mg; Bavarian cream flavor] [DSC]

Titralac™: 420 mg [equivalent to elemental calcium 168 mg; sugar free; contains sodium 1.1 mg/tablet; spearmint flavor]

Tums®: 500 mg [equivalent to elemental calcium 200 mg; contains tartrazine; assorted fruit and peppermint flavors]

Tums® E-X: 750 mg [equivalent to elemental calcium 300 mg; contains tartrazine; assorted fruit, cool relief mint, fresh blend, tropical assorted fruit, wintergreen, and assorted berry flavors]

Tums® Extra Strength Sugar Free: 750 mg [equivalent to elemental calcium 300 mg; sugar free; contains phenylalanine <1 mg/tablet; orange cream flavor]

Tums® Smoothies™: 750 mg [equivalent to elemental calcium 300 mg; contains tartrazine; assorted fruit, assorted tropical fruit, peppermint flavors]

Tums® Ultra®: 1000 mg [equivalent to elemental calcium 400 mg; contains tartrazine; assorted berry, assorted fruit, assorted tropical fruit, peppermint, and spearmint flavors]

Tablet, softchew:

Rolaids®: 1177 mg [equivalent to elemental calcium 471 mg; contains coconut oil and soy lecithin; vanilla creme and wild cherry flavors]

Extemporaneous Preparations Calcium carbonate slurry: 32.5% slurry can be prepared by triturating ten 650 mg tablets into a fine powder and adding 20 mL of water-soluble lubricant gel (eg, K-Y® Jelly)

Calcium Chloride (KAL see um KLOR ide)

Related Information

CPR Pediatric Drug Dosages *on page 1650*

Therapeutic Category Calcium Salt; Electrolyte Supplement, Parenteral

Generic Available Yes

Use Treatment and prevention of calcium depletion; treatment of hypocalcemic tetany; hypermagnesemia, cardiac disturbances of hyperkalemia, hypocalcemia, or calcium channel blocking agent toxicity

Pregnancy Risk Factor C

Contraindications See Calcium Supplements *on page 272.*

Warnings See Calcium Supplements *on page 272.*

Precautions See Calcium Supplements *on page 272.*

Adverse Reactions See Calcium Supplements *on page 272.*

Drug Interactions See Calcium Supplements *on page 272.*

Food Interactions See Calcium Supplements *on page 272.*

Stability Store at room temperature; parenteral solutions are incompatible with bicarbonates, phosphates, and sulfate formulations; mixing will result in precipitation. TPN solutions containing phosphate and calcium are compatible depending upon the parenteral amino-acid formulation and its concentration.

Mechanism of Action Calcium moderates nerve and muscle performance via action potential excitation threshold regulation; it is necessary for maintaining the functional integrity of nervous, muscular, and skeletal systems and cell-membrane and capillary permeability.

Pharmacokinetics See Calcium Supplements *on page 272.*

Usual Dosage
Hypocalcemia: I.V.: Dosage expressed in mg of **calcium chloride**:
Manufacturer's recommendations: Children: 2.7-5 mg/kg/dose every 4-6 hours
Alternative pediatric dosing: Neonates, Infants, and Children: 10-20 mg/kg/dose, repeat every 4-6 hours if needed
Adults: 500 mg to 1 g/dose every 6 hours
Cardiac arrest in the presence of hyperkalemia or hypocalcemia, magnesium toxicity, or calcium antagonist toxicity: I.V., I.O.: Dosage expressed in mg of **calcium chloride**:
Neonates, Infants, and Children: 20 mg/kg; may repeat in 10 minutes if necessary; if effective, consider I.V. infusion of 20-50 mg/kg/hour
Adults: 2-4 mg/kg; may repeat in 10 minutes if necessary
Hypocalcemia secondary to citrated blood infusion: I.V.: Give 0.45 mEq **elemental** calcium for each 100 mL citrated blood infused
Tetany: I.V.: Dose expressed in mg of **calcium chloride**:
Neonates, Infants, and Children: 10 mg/kg over 5-10 minutes; may repeat after 6 hours or follow with an infusion with a maximum dose of 200 mg/kg/day
Adults: 1 g over 10-30 minutes; may repeat after 6 hours
Dosage adjustment in renal impairment: Cl_{cr} <25 mL/minute may require dosage adjustment depending upon serum calcium level

Administration Parenteral:
I.V.: For direct I.V. injection infuse slow IVP over 3-5 minutes or at a maximum rate of 50-100 mg calcium chloride/minute; in situations of cardiac arrest, calcium chloride may be administered over 10-20 seconds
I.V. infusion: Dilute to a final concentration of 20 mg/mL; administer 45-90 mg calcium chloride/kg over 1 hour; 0.6-1.2 mEq calcium/kg over 1 hour
Do not inject calcium salts I.M. or administer SubQ since severe necrosis and sloughing may occur; extravasation of calcium can result in severe necrosis and tissue sloughing. Do not use scalp vein or small hand or foot veins for I.V. administration. Not for endotracheal administration.

Monitoring Parameters See Calcium Supplements *on page 272.*

Reference Range See Calcium Supplements *on page 272.*

Additional Information 1 g calcium chloride = 270 mg elemental calcium = 13.5 mEq calcium. Due to a poor correlation between the serum ionized calcium (free) and total serum calcium, particularly in states of low albumin or acid/base imbalances, direct measurement of ionized calcium is recommended. If ionized calcium is unavailable, in low albumin states, the corrected **total** serum calcium may be estimated by this equation (assuming a normal albumin of 4 g/dL); corrected total calcium = total serum calcium + 0.8(4 - measured serum albumin)

Dosage Forms Excipient information presented when available (limited, particularly for generics); consult specific product labeling.
Injection, solution [preservative free]: 10% (10 mL) [present as calcium chloride 100 mg (1.36 mEq)/mL; provides elemental calcium 27.2 mg/mL (1.36 mEq)/mL]
Injection, solution: 10% (10 mL) [present as calcium chloride 100 mg (1.36 mEq)/mL; provides elemental calcium 27.2 mg (1.36 mEq)/mL]

Calcium Citrate (KAL see um SIT rate)

Medication Safety Issues
Sound-alike/look-alike issues:
Citracal® may be confused with Citrucel®

U.S. Brand Names Cal-Citrate® 250 [OTC]; Citracal® [OTC]

Canadian Brand Names Osteocit®

Therapeutic Category Calcium Salt; Electrolyte Supplement, Oral

Generic Available Yes

Use Treatment of hyperphosphatemia in end-stage renal failure; dietary supplement; prevention and treatment of calcium deficiency; adjunctive prevention and treatment of osteoporosis

Pregnancy Risk Factor C

Contraindications See Calcium Supplements *on page 272.*

Warnings See Calcium Supplements *on page 272.*

Precautions See Calcium Supplements *on page 272.*

Adverse Reactions See Calcium Supplements *on page 272.*

Drug Interactions See Calcium Supplements *on page 272.*

Food Interactions See Calcium Supplements *on page 272.*

Stability Store at room temperature.

Mechanism of Action Calcium moderates nerve and muscle performance via action potential excitation threshold regulation; it is necessary for maintaining the functional integrity of nervous, muscular, and skeletal systems and cell-membrane and capillary
(Continued)

Calcium Citrate *(Continued)*

permeability. Calcium citrate combines with dietary phosphate to form insoluble calcium phosphate which is excreted in feces and reduces phosphate absorption

Pharmacokinetics See Calcium Supplements *on page 272.*

Usual Dosage Oral:

Recommended daily allowance (RDA) and adequate intake: See Calcium Supplements *on page 272.*

Hypocalcemia (dose depends on clinical condition and serum calcium level): Dose expressed in mg of **elemental calcium:**

Neonates: 50-150 mg/kg/day in 4-6 divided doses; not to exceed 1 g/day

Children: 45-65 mg/kg/day in 4 divided doses

Adults: 1-2 g or more per day in 3-4 divided doses

Dietary supplement: Adults: 500 mg to 2 g divided 2-4 times/day

Adjunctive prevention and treatment of osteoporosis: Adults: 500 mg elemental calcium 2-3 times/day; recommended dosage includes dietary intake and should be adjusted depending upon the patient's diet; to improve absorption do not administer more than 500 mg **elemental calcium**/dose

Dosage adjustment in renal impairment: Cl_{cr} <25 mL/minute may require dosage adjustment depending upon serum calcium level

Administration Oral: Administer with plenty of fluids; may administer without regard to food when using to treat/prevent deficiency conditions; administer with food when treating hyperphosphatemia or when administering granule formulation

Monitoring Parameters See Calcium Supplements *on page 272.*

Reference Range See Calcium Supplements *on page 272.*

Additional Information 1 g calcium citrate = 211mg elemental calcium = 10.6 mEq calcium. Due to a poor correlation between the serum ionized calcium (free) and total serum calcium, particularly in states of low albumin or acid/base imbalances, direct measurement of ionized calcium is recommended. If ionized calcium is unavailable, in low albumin states, the corrected **total** serum calcium may be estimated by this equation (assuming a normal albumin of 4 g/dL); corrected total calcium = total serum calcium + 0.8(4 - measured serum albumin)

Dosage Forms Excipient information presented when available (limited, particularly for generics); consult specific product labeling.

Granules: 760 mg/teaspoonful (480 g)

Tablet: Elemental calcium 200 mg, 250 mg

Cal-Citrate®: Elemental calcium 250 mg

Citracal®: 950 mg [equivalent to elemental calcium 200 mg]

♦ **Calcium Disodium Edetate** *see* Edetate Calcium Disodium *on page 553*

♦ **Calcium Disodium Versenate®** *see* Edetate Calcium Disodium *on page 553*

♦ **Calcium EDTA** *see* Edetate Calcium Disodium *on page 553*

Calcium Glubionate (KAL see um gloo BYE oh nate)

Medication Safety Issues

Sound-alike/look-alike issues:

Calcium glubionate may be confused with calcium gluconate

U.S. Brand Names Calcionate [OTC]

Therapeutic Category Calcium Salt; Electrolyte Supplement, Oral

Generic Available Yes

Use Treatment and replacement of calcium deficiency; dietary supplement; adjunctive prevention and treatment of osteoporosis

Pregnancy Risk Factor C

Contraindications See Calcium Supplements *on page 272.*

Warnings See Calcium Supplements *on page 272.*

Precautions See Calcium Supplements *on page 272.*

Adverse Reactions See Calcium Supplements *on page 272.*

Drug Interactions See Calcium Supplements *on page 272.*

Food Interactions See Calcium Supplements *on page 272.*

Stability Store at room temperature.

Mechanism of Action Calcium moderates nerve and muscle performance via action potential excitation threshold regulation; it is necessary for maintaining the functional integrity of nervous, muscular, and skeletal systems and cell-membrane and capillary permeability.

Pharmacokinetics See Calcium Supplements *on page 272.*

Usual Dosage Oral:

Recommended daily allowance (RDA) and adequate intake: See Calcium Supplements *on page 272.*

Hypocalcemia (dose depends on clinical condition and serum calcium level):
Dose expressed in mg of **elemental calcium**:
Neonates: 50-150 mg/kg/day in 4-6 divided doses; not to exceed 1 g/day
Children: 45-65 mg/kg/day in 4 divided doses
Adults: 1-2 g or more per day in 3-4 divided doses
Dose expressed in mg of **calcium glubionate**:
Neonates: 1200 mg/kg/day in 4-6 divided doses
Infants and Children: 600-2000 mg/kg/day in 4 divided doses up to a maximum of 9 g/day
Adults: 6-18 g/day in divided doses
Adjunctive prevention and treatment of osteoporosis: Adults: 500 mg **elemental calcium** 2-3 times/day; recommended dosage includes dietary intake and should be adjusted depending upon the patient's diet; to improve absorption do not administer more than 500 mg **elemental calcium**/dose
Dosage adjustment in renal impairment: Cl_{cr} <25 mL/minute may require dosage adjustment depending upon serum calcium level

Administration Oral: Administer with plenty of fluids with or following meals; for phosphate binding, administer on an empty stomach before meals to optimize effectiveness

Monitoring Parameters See Calcium Supplements *on page 272.*

Reference Range See Calcium Supplements *on page 272.*

Additional Information 1 g calcium glubionate = 64 mg elemental calcium = 3.2 mEq calcium. Due to a poor correlation between the serum ionized calcium (free) and total serum calcium, particularly in states of low albumin or acid/base imbalances, direct measurement of ionized calcium is recommended. If ionized calcium is unavailable, in low albumin states, the corrected **total** serum calcium may be estimated by this equation (assuming a normal albumin of 4 g/dL); corrected total calcium = total serum calcium + 0.8(4 - measured serum albumin)

Dosage Forms Excipient information presented when available (limited, particularly for generics); consult specific product labeling.
Syrup:
Calcionate: 1.8 g/5 mL (480 mL) [equivalent to elemental calcium 115 mg/5 mL; contains benzoic acid; caramel and orange flavor]

Calcium Gluconate (KAL see um GLOO koe nate)

Medication Safety Issues
Sound-alike/look-alike issues:
Calcium gluconate may be confused with calcium glubionate

Therapeutic Category Antidote, Hydrofluoric Acid; Calcium Salt; Electrolyte Supplement, Oral; Electrolyte Supplement, Parenteral

Generic Available Yes

Use Treatment and prevention of calcium depletion; treatment of hypocalcemic tetany; hypermagnesemia, cardiac disturbances of hyperkalemia, hypocalcemia, or calcium channel blocking agent toxicity; adjunctive prevention and treatment of osteoporosis; topical treatment of hydrofluoric acid burns

Pregnancy Risk Factor C

Lactation Enters breast milk

Contraindications See Calcium Supplements *on page 272.*

Warnings See Calcium Supplements *on page 272.*

Precautions See Calcium Supplements *on page 272.*

Adverse Reactions See Calcium Supplements *on page 272.*

Drug Interactions See Calcium Supplements *on page 272.*

Food Interactions See Calcium Supplements *on page 272.*

Stability Store at room temperature; parenteral solutions are incompatible with bicarbonates, phosphates, and sulfate formulations; mixing will result in precipitation. TPN solutions containing phosphate and calcium are compatible depending upon the parenteral amino-acid formulation and its concentration.

Mechanism of Action Calcium moderates nerve and muscle performance via action potential excitation threshold regulation; it is necessary for maintaining the functional integrity of nervous, muscular, and skeletal systems and cell-membrane and capillary permeability.

Pharmacokinetics See Calcium Supplements *on page 272.*

Usual Dosage
Recommended daily allowance (RDA) and adequate intake: See Calcium Supplements *on page 272.*
Hypocalcemia (dose depends on clinical condition and serum calcium level): Oral:
Dose expressed in mg of **elemental calcium**:
Neonates: 50-150 mg/kg/day in 4-6 divided doses; not to exceed 1 g/day
(Continued)

Calcium Gluconate *(Continued)*

Children: 45-65 mg/kg/day in 4 divided doses
Adults: 1-2 g or more per day in 3-4 divided doses
Dose expressed in mg of **calcium gluconate**:
Neonates: 500-1500 mg/kg/day in 4-6 divided doses
Infants and Children: 500-725 mg/kg/day in 3-4 divided doses
Adults: 500 mg to 2 g 2-4 times/day

Hypocalcemia (dose depends on clinical condition and serum calcium level): I.V.:
Dose expressed in mg of **calcium gluconate**:
Neonates: 200-800 mg/kg/day as a continuous infusion or in 4 divided doses
Infants and Children: 200-500 mg/kg/day as a continuous infusion or in 4 divided doses
Adults: 2-15 g/day as a continuous infusion or in divided doses

Cardiac arrest in the presence of hyperkalemia or hypocalcemia, magnesium toxicity, or calcium antagonist toxicity: I.V., I.O.: Dosage expressed in mg of **calcium gluconate**:
Neonates, Infants, and Children: 60-100 mg/kg/dose (maximum: 3 g/dose); may repeat in 10 minutes if necessary; if effective, consider I.V. infusion
Adults: 500-800 mg (maximum: 3 g/dose); may repeat in 10 minutes if necessary

Hypocalcemia secondary to citrated blood infusion: I.V.: Give 0.45 mEq **elemental calcium** for each 100 mL citrated blood infused

Tetany: I.V.: Dose expressed in mg of **calcium gluconate**:
Neonates, Infants, and Children: 100-200 mg/kg/dose; over 5-10 minutes; may repeat after 6 hours or follow with an infusion with a maximum dose of 500 mg/kg/day
Adults: 1-3 g over 10-30 minutes; may repeat after 6 hours

Daily maintenance calcium: I.V.:
Neonates: 3-4 mEq/kg/day
Infants and Children <25kg: 1-2 mEq/kg/day
Children 25-45 kg: 0.5-1.5 mEq/kg/day
Children >45 kg and Adults: 0.2-0.3 mEq/kg/day or 10-20 mEq/day

Adjunctive prevention and treatment of osteoporosis: Oral: Adults: 500 mg **elemental calcium** 2-3 times/day; recommended dosage includes dietary intake and should be adjusted depending upon the patient's diet; to improve absorption, do not administer more than 500 mg **elemental calcium**/dose

Dosage adjustment in renal impairment: Cl_{cr} <25 mL/minute may require dosage adjustment depending upon serum calcium level

Hydrofluoric acid (HF) burns (HF concentration <20%): Topical: Various topical calcium preparations have been used anecdotally for treatment of dermal exposure to HF solutions; calcium gluconate at concentrations ranging from 2.5% to 33% has been used; a topical calcium gluconate preparation must be compounded (see Extemporaneous Preparations); apply topically as needed

Administration

Oral: Administer with plenty of fluids with or following meals; for phosphate-binding, administer on an empty stomach before meals to optimize effectiveness; powder may be added to food

Parenteral:
I.V.: For direct I.V. injection, infuse slow IVP over 3-5 minutes or at a maximum rate of 50-100 mg calcium gluconate/minute; in situations of cardiac arrest, calcium gluconate may be administered over 10-20 seconds
I.V. infusion: Dilute to 50 mg/mL and infuse at 120-240 mg/kg (0.6-1.2mEq calcium/kg) over 1 hour
Do not inject calcium salts I.M. or administer SubQ since severe necrosis and sloughing may occur; extravasation of calcium can result in severe necrosis and tissue sloughing. Do not use scalp vein or small hand or foot veins for I.V. administration. Not for endotracheal administration.

Topical: Massage calcium gluconate gel into exposed area for 15 minutes

Monitoring Parameters See Calcium Supplements *on page 272.*

Reference Range See Calcium Supplements *on page 272.*

Additional Information 1 g calcium gluconate = 90 mg elemental calcium = 4.5 mEq calcium. Due to a poor correlation between the serum ionized calcium (free) and total serum calcium, particularly in states of low albumin or acid/base imbalances, direct measurement of ionized calcium is recommended. If ionized calcium is unavailable, in low albumin states, the corrected **total** serum calcium may be estimated by this equation (assuming a normal albumin of 4 g/dL); corrected total calcium = total serum calcium + 0.8(4 - measured serum albumin)

Dosage Forms Excipient information presented when available (limited, particularly for generics); consult specific product labeling.

Injection, solution [preservative free]: 10% [100 mg/mL] (10 mL, 50 mL, 100 mL, 200 mL) [equivalent to elemental calcium 9 mg/mL; calcium 0.46 mEq/mL]

Powder: 347 mg/tablespoonful (480 g)

Tablet: 500 mg [equivalent to elemental calcium 45 mg]; 650 mg [equivalent to elemental calcium 58.5 mg]; 975 mg [equivalent to elemental calcium 87.75 mg]

Extemporaneous Preparations Calcium gluconate gel: Crush 3.5 g calcium gluconate tablets into a fine powder; add to 5 oz tube of water-soluble surgical lubricant (eg, K-Y® Jelly) or add 3.5 g calcium gluconate injection to 5 oz of water-soluble surgical lubricant (calcium carbonate may be substituted; do not use calcium chloride due to potential for irritation)

Calcium Lactate (KAL see um LAK tate)

Therapeutic Category Calcium Salt; Electrolyte Supplement, Oral

Generic Available Yes

Use Prevention and treatment of calcium deficiency; dietary supplement; adjunctive prevention and treatment of osteoporosis

Pregnancy Risk Factor C

Contraindications See Calcium Supplements *on page 272.*

Warnings See Calcium Supplements *on page 272.*

Precautions See Calcium Supplements *on page 272.*

Adverse Reactions See Calcium Supplements *on page 272.*

Drug Interactions See Calcium Supplements *on page 272.*

Food Interactions See Calcium Supplements *on page 272.*

Stability Store at room temperature.

Mechanism of Action Calcium moderates nerve and muscle performance via action potential excitation threshold regulation; it is necessary for maintaining the functional integrity of nervous, muscular, and skeletal systems and cell-membrane and capillary permeability.

Pharmacokinetics See Calcium Supplements *on page 272.*

Usual Dosage Oral:

Recommended daily allowance (RDA) and Adequate Intake: See Calcium Supplements *on page 272.*

Hypocalcemia (dose depends on clinical condition and serum calcium level):

- Dose expressed in mg of **elemental calcium**:
  - Neonates: 50-150 mg/kg/day in 4-6 divided doses; not to exceed 1 g/day
  - Children: 45-65 mg/kg/day in 4 divided doses
  - Adults: 1-2 g or more per day in 3-4 divided doses
- Dose expressed in mg of **calcium lactate**:
  - Neonates and Infants: 400-500 mg/kg/day divided every 4-6 hours
  - Children: 500 mg/kg/day divided every 6-8 hours; maximum daily dose: 9 g
  - Adults: 1.5-3 g/day divided every 8 hours; maximum daily dose: 9 g

Adjunctive prevention and treatment of osteoporosis: Adults: 500 mg elemental calcium 2-3 times/day; recommended dosage includes dietary intake and should be adjusted depending upon the patient's diet; to improve absorption do not administer more than 500 mg **elemental calcium**/dose

Dosage adjustment in renal impairment: Cl_{cr} <25 mL/minute may require dosage adjustment depending upon serum calcium level

Administration Oral: Administer with plenty of fluids with or following meals

Monitoring Parameters See Calcium Supplements *on page 272.*

Reference Range See Calcium Supplements *on page 272.*

Additional Information

1 g calcium lactate = 130 mg elemental calcium = 6.5 mEq calcium. Due to a poor correlation between the serum ionized calcium (free) and total serum calcium, particularly in states of low albumin or acid/base imbalances, direct measurement of ionized calcium is recommended. If ionized calcium is unavailable, in low albumin states, the corrected **total** serum calcium may be estimated by this equation (assuming a normal albumin of 4 g/dL); corrected total calcium = total serum calcium + 0.8(4 - measured serum albumin)

Dosage Forms Excipient information presented when available (limited, particularly for generics); consult specific product labeling.

Tablet: 650 mg [equivalent to elemental calcium 84.5 mg]

◆ **Calcium Leucovorin** *see* Leucovorin *on page 916*

Calcium Phosphate, Tribasic (KAL see um FOS fate tri BAY sik)

U.S. Brand Names Posture® [OTC]

Index Terms Tricalcium Phosphate

Therapeutic Category Calcium Salt; Electrolyte Supplement, Oral

Generic Available No

(Continued)

Calcium Phosphate, Tribasic *(Continued)*

Use Prevention and treatment of calcium deficiency; dietary supplement; adjunctive prevention and treatment of osteoporosis

Pregnancy Risk Factor C

Contraindications See Calcium Supplements *on page 272.*

Warnings See Calcium Supplements *on page 272.* Avoid use of calcium phosphate, tribasic, in dialysis patients with hypercalcemia, or whose plasma PTH concentrations are <150 pg/mL on two consecutive measurements.

Precautions See Calcium Supplements *on page 272.*

Adverse Reactions See Calcium Supplements *on page 272.*

Drug Interactions See Calcium Supplements *on page 272.*

Food Interactions See Calcium Supplements *on page 272.*

Stability Store at room temperature.

Mechanism of Action Calcium moderates nerve and muscle performance via action potential excitation threshold regulation; it is necessary for maintaining the functional integrity of nervous, muscular, and skeletal systems and cell-membrane and capillary permeability.

Pharmacokinetics See Calcium Supplements *on page 272.*

Usual Dosage Oral:

Recommended daily allowance (RDA) and adequate intake: See Calcium Supplements *on page 272.*

Hypocalcemia (dose depends on clinical condition and serum calcium level): Dose expressed in mg of **elemental calcium**:

Children: 45-65 mg/kg/day in 4 divided doses

Adults: 1-2 g or more per day in 3-4 divided doses

Adjunctive prevention and treatment of osteoporosis: Adults: 500 mg **elemental calcium** 2-3 times/day; recommended dosage includes dietary intake and should be adjusted depending upon the patient's diet; to improve absorption do not administer more than 500 mg **elemental calcium**/dose

Dosage adjustment in renal impairment: Cl_{cr} <25 mL/minute may require dosage adjustment depending upon serum calcium level

Monitoring Parameters See Calcium Supplements *on page 272.*

Reference Range See Calcium Supplements *on page 272.*

Additional Information

1 g calcium phosphate, tribasic = 390 mg elemental calcium = 19.3 mEq calcium. Due to a poor correlation between the serum ionized calcium (free) and total serum calcium, particularly in states of low albumin or acid/base imbalances, direct measurement of ionized calcium is recommended. If ionized calcium is unavailable, in low albumin states, the corrected **total** serum calcium may be estimated by this equation (assuming a normal albumin of 4 g/dL); corrected total calcium = total serum calcium + 0.8(4 - measured serum albumin)

Dosage Forms Excipient information presented when available (limited, particularly for generics); consult specific product labeling.

Caplet:

Posture®: Calcium 600 mg and phosphorus 280 mg [as tricalcium phosphate]

Calcium Supplements (KAL see um SUP la ments)

Related Information

Antacid Preparations *on page 132*
Calcium Acetate *on page 263*
Calcium Carbonate *on page 264*
Calcium Chloride *on page 266*
Calcium Citrate *on page 267*
Calcium Glubionate *on page 268*
Calcium Gluconate *on page 269*
Calcium Lactate *on page 271*
Calcium Phosphate, Tribasic *on page 271*

U.S. Brand Names Alcalak [OTC]; Alka-Mints® [OTC]; Amitone® [OTC] [DSC]; Calcarb 600 [OTC]; Calci-Chew® [OTC]; Calci-Mix® [OTC]; Cal-Citrate® 250 [OTC]; Cal-Gest [OTC]; Cal-Mint [OTC]; Caltrate® 600 [OTC]; Children's Pepto [OTC]; Chooz® [OTC]; Citracal® [OTC]; Florical® [OTC]; Maalox® Quick Dissolve [OTC]; Mylanta® Children's [OTC]; Nephro-Calci® [OTC]; Nutralox® [OTC]; Os-Cal® 500 [OTC]; Oysco® 500 [OTC]; Oyst-Cal 500 [OTC]; PhosLo®; Posture®; Rolaids® Softchews [OTC]; Titralac® [OTC]; Titralac® Extra Strength [OTC]; Tums® [OTC]; Tums® E-X [OTC]; Tums® Extra Strength Sugar Free [OTC]; Tums® Smoothies™ [OTC]; Tums® Ultra® [OTC]

Therapeutic Category Antacid; Antidote, Hydrofluoric Acid; Calcium Salt; Electrolyte Supplement, Oral; Electrolyte Supplement, Parenteral

Generic Available Yes

Use

Treatment and prevention of calcium depletion:

Injection: See Calcium Acetate *on page 263*, Calcium Chloride *on page 266*, and Calcium Gluconate *on page 269*

Oral: See Calcium Glubionate *on page 268*, Calcium Citrate *on page 267*, Calcium Carbonate *on page 264*, and Calcium Lactate *on page 271*

Relief of acid indigestion, heartburn: See Calcium Carbonate *on page 264*

Treatment of hypocalcemic tetany; hypermagnesemia, cardiac disturbances of hyperkalemia, hypocalcemia, or calcium channel blocking agent toxicity: See Calcium Chloride *on page 266* and Calcium Gluconate *on page 269*

Treatment and prevention of hyperphosphatemia in chronic renal failure: See Calcium Acetate *on page 263*, Calcium Carbonate *on page 264*, and Calcium Citrate *on page 267*

Adjunctive prevention and treatment of osteoporosis: See Calcium Carbonate *on page 264*, Calcium Citrate *on page 267*, Calcium Glubionate *on page 268*, Calcium Gluconate *on page 269*, and Calcium Lactate *on page 271*

Topical treatment of hydrofluoric acid burns: See Calcium Carbonate *on page 264* and Calcium Gluconate *on page 269*

Pregnancy Risk Factor C

Contraindications Hypersensitivity to calcium formulation (see Warnings); hypercalcemia, renal calculi, ventricular fibrillation

Warnings Multiple salt forms of calcium exist; close attention must be paid to the salt form when ordering and administering calcium; incorrect selection or substitution of one salt for another without proper dosage adjustment may result in serious over- or under-dosing. Some products may contain tartrazine which may cause allergic reactions in susceptible individuals. Avoid use of calcium-containing phosphate binders (calcium acetate or phosphate) in dialysis patients with hypercalcemia or whose plasma PTH concentrations are <150 pg/mL on two consecutive measurements. Milk-Alkali syndrome (hypercalcemia, metabolic alkalosis, and rarely, renal insufficiency) has been associated with ingestion of large quantities of milk concomitantly with calcium carbonate; patients with renal impairment or dehydration and electrolyte imbalance are at increased risk for developing this syndrome; monitor calcium serum levels periodically

Precautions Use cautiously in patients with sarcoidosis, respiratory failure, acidosis, renal or cardiac disease; avoid too rapid I.V. administration; avoid extravasation; use with caution in digitalized patients; some products may contain aspartame which is metabolized to phenylalanine and must be avoided in patients with phenylketonuria

Adverse Reactions

Cardiovascular: Vasodilation, hypotension, bradycardia, cardiac arrhythmias, ventricular fibrillation, syncope

Central nervous system: Headache, mental confusion, dizziness, lethargy, coma

Dermatologic: Erythema

Endocrine & metabolic: Hypercalcemia, milk-alkali syndrome (calcium carbonate), hypophosphatemia, hypercalciuria, hypomagnesemia

Gastrointestinal: Constipation, nausea, vomiting, xerostomia, elevated serum amylase

Local: Tissue necrosis (I.V. administration)

Neuromuscular & skeletal: Muscle weakness

Drug Interactions May potentiate digoxin toxicity; may antagonize the effects of calcium channel blockers (eg, verapamil); when administered orally, calcium decreases the absorption of tetracycline, atenolol, iron, quinolone antibiotics, alendronate, sodium fluoride, and zinc; high doses of calcium with thiazide diuretics may result in milk-alkali syndrome and hypercalcemia; decreases potassium-binding ability of polystyrene sulfonate; PPIs and H_2 blockers may reduce absorption of calcium carbonate

Food Interactions Do not give orally with bran, foods high in oxalates (spinach, sweet potatoes, rhubarb, beans), or phytic acid (unleavened bread, raw beans, seeds, nuts, grains, soy isolates) which may decrease calcium absorption; minimize administration with dairy products (when treating deficiency state) as this will reduce absorption

Stability Store at room temperature; parenteral solutions are incompatible with bicarbonates, phosphates, and sulfate formulations; mixing will result in precipitation. TPN solutions containing phosphate and calcium are compatible depending upon the parenteral amino-acid formulation and its concentration.

Mechanism of Action Calcium moderates nerve and muscle performance via action potential excitation threshold regulation; it is necessary for maintaining the functional integrity of nervous, muscular, and skeletal systems and cell-membrane and capillary permeability. Calcium acetate and carbonate combines with dietary phosphate to form insoluble calcium phosphate which is excreted in feces and reduces phosphate absorption. Neutralizes acidity of stomach (carbonate salt).

(Continued)

Calcium Supplements *(Continued)*

Pharmacokinetics

Absorption: 25% to 35%; varies with age (infants 60%, prepubertal children 28%, pubertal children 34%, young adults 25%); decreased absorption occurs in patients with achlorhydria, renal osteodystrophy, steatorrhea, or uremia

Protein binding: 45%

Elimination: Primarily in the feces as unabsorbed calcium

Usual Dosage See individual calcium monographs.

Recommended daily allowance (RDA): Dosage is in terms of elemental calcium:

- <6 months: 400 mg/day
- 6-12 months: 600 mg/day
- 1-10 years: 800 mg/day
- 11-24 years: 1200 mg/day
- Adults >24 years: 800 mg/day

Adequate intake (1997 National Academy of Science Recommendations): **Dosage is in terms of elemental calcium:**

- 0-6 months: 210 mg/day
- 7-12 months: 270 mg/day
- 1-3 years: 500 mg/day
- 4-8 years: 800 mg/day
- 9-18 years: 1300 mg/day
- 19-50 years: 1000 mg/day
- >50 years: 1200 mg/day

Oral: **Note:** For comparison information of calcium salts, see table.

Elemental Calcium Content of Calcium Salts

Calcium Salt	Elemental Calcium (mg/1 g of salt form)	mEq calcium per gram	Approximate Equivalent Doses (mg of calcium salt)
Calcium acetate	250	12.7	354
Calcium carbonate	400	20	225
Calcium chloride	270	13.5	330
Calcium citrate	211	10.6	425
Calcium glubionate	64	3.2	1400
Calcium gluconate	90	4.5	1000
Calcium lactate	130	6.5	700
Calcium phosphate, tribasic	390	19.3	233

Administration

See individual calcium monographs.

Monitoring Parameters Serum calcium (ionized calcium preferred if available, see Additional Information), phosphate, magnesium, heart rate, EKG

Reference Range

Calcium: Newborns: 7.0-12.0 mg/dL; 0-2 years: 8.8-11.2 mg/dL; 2 years to adults: 9.0-11.0 mg/dL

Calcium, ionized, whole blood: 4.4-5.4 mg/dL

Patient Information May cause dry mouth

Additional Information Due to a poor correlation between the serum ionized calcium (free) and total serum calcium, particularly in states of low albumin or acid/base imbalances, direct measurement of ionized calcium is recommended. If ionized calcium is unavailable, in low albumin states, the corrected **total** serum calcium may be estimated by this equation (assuming a normal albumin of 4 g/dL); corrected total calcium = total serum calcium + 0.8(4 - measured serum albumin)

Dosage Forms See individual monographs.

Extemporaneous Preparations

Calcium gluconate gel: Crush 3.5 g calcium gluconate tablets into a fine powder; add to 5 oz tube of water-soluble surgical lubricant (eg, K-Y® Jelly) or add 3.5 g calcium gluconate injection to 5 oz of water-soluble surgical lubricant (calcium carbonate may be substituted; do not use calcium chloride due to potential for irritation)

Calcium carbonate slurry: 32.5% slurry can be prepared by triturating ten 650 mg tablets into a fine powder and adding 20 mL of water-soluble lubricant gel (eg, K-Y® Jelly)

References

"2005 American Heart Association (AHA) Guidelines for Cardiopulmonary Resuscitation (CPR) and Emergency Cardiovascular Care (ECC) of Pediatric and Neonatal Patients: Pediatric Advanced Life Support," *Pediatrics*, 2006, 117(5):1005-28.

Baker SS, Cochran WJ, Flores CA, et al, "American Academy of Pediatrics. Committee on Nutrition: Calcium Requirements of Infants, Children, and Adolescents," *Pediatrics*, 1999, 104(5):1152-7.
"Dietary Reference Intakes for Calcium, Phosphorus, Magnesium, Vitamin D, and Fluoride. Standing Committee on the Scientific Evaluation of Dietary Reference Intakes, Food and Nutrition Board, Institute of Medicine," National Academy of Sciences, Washington, DC: National Academy Press, 1997.
NIH Consensus Conference, "Optimal Calcium Intake," *JAMA*, 1994, 272(24):1942-8.

♦ **Caldecort® [OTC]** *see* Hydrocortisone *on page 781*

Calfactant (cal FAC tant)

U.S. Brand Names Infasurf®
Index Terms Bovine Lung Surfactant
Therapeutic Category Lung Surfactant
Generic Available No

Use Prevention and treatment of respiratory distress syndrome (RDS) in premature infants
Prophylactic therapy: Infants <29 weeks at significant risk for RDS
Treatment: Infants ≤72 hours of age with RDS (confirmed by clinical and radiologic findings and requiring endotracheal intubation)

Warnings Rapidly affects oxygenation and lung compliance and should be restricted to a highly supervised use in a clinical setting with immediate availability of clinicians experienced with intubation and ventilatory management of premature infants; if transient episodes of bradycardia and decreased oxygen saturation occur, discontinue the dosing procedure and initiate measures to alleviate the condition; produces rapid improvement in lung oxygenation and compliance that may require immediate reductions in ventilator settings and FiO_2; for intratracheal administration only

Precautions Transient episodes of reflux of calfactant into the endotracheal tube, cyanosis, bradycardia, or airway obstruction have occurred during dosing procedures; such episodes may require stopping administration and taking appropriate measures to alleviate the condition before resuming therapy

Adverse Reactions Most adverse reactions occur during the dosing procedure
Cardiovascular: Bradycardia, cyanosis
Respiratory: Airway obstruction, pneumothorax, pulmonary hemorrhage, apnea

Stability Refrigerate; protect from light; unopened, unused warmed vials of calfactant may be returned to refrigerator within 24 hours for future use; repeated warming to room temperature should be avoided

Mechanism of Action Replaces deficient or ineffective endogenous lung surfactant in neonates with RDS or in neonates at risk of developing RDS; surfactant prevents the alveoli from collapsing during expiration by lowering surface tension between air and alveolar surfaces

Usual Dosage Intratracheal: Neonates: 3 mL/kg every 12 hours up to a total of 3 doses; repeat doses have been administered as early as 6 hours after the previous dose for a total of up to four doses (if the infant was still intubated and required at least 30% inspired oxygen to maintain a PaO_2 ≤80 torr)

Administration Intratracheal: Gently swirl to redisperse suspension; do not shake; administer dosage divided into two aliquots of 1.5 mL/kg each into the endotracheal tube; after each instillation, reposition the infant with either the right or left side dependent; administration is made while ventilation is continued over 20-30 breaths for each aliquot, with small bursts timed only during the inspiratory cycles; a pause followed by evaluation of the respiratory status and repositioning should separate the two aliquots; calfactant dosage has also been divided into four equal aliquots and administered with repositioning in four different positions (prone, supine, right and left lateral)

Monitoring Parameters Continuous heart rate and transcutaneous O_2 saturation should be monitored during administration; frequent ABG sampling is necessary to prevent postdosing hyperoxia and hypocarbia

Dosage Forms Excipient information presented when available (limited, particularly for generics); consult specific product labeling.
Suspension, intratracheal [preservative free; calf lung derived]:
Infasurf®: 35 mg/mL (3 mL, 6 mL)

References
Hudak ML, Martin DJ, Egan EA, et al, "A Multicenter Randomized Masked Comparison Trail of Synthetic Surfactant Versus Calf Lung Surfactant Extract in the Prevention of Neonatal Respiratory Distress Syndrome," *Pediatrics*, 1997, 100(1):39-50.
Bloom BT, Kattwinkel J, Hall RT, et al, "Comparison of Infasurf® (Calf Lung Surfactant Extract) to Survanta® (Beractant) in the Treatment and Prevention of Respiratory Distress Syndrome," *Pediatrics*, 1997, 100(1):31-8.

♦ **Cal-Gest [OTC]** *see* Calcium Carbonate *on page 264*
♦ **Cal-Gest [OTC]** *see* Calcium Supplements *on page 272*
♦ **Cal-Mint [OTC]** *see* Calcium Carbonate *on page 264*
♦ **Cal-Mint [OTC]** *see* Calcium Supplements *on page 272*

- ♦ **Caltine® (Can)** *see* Calcitonin *on page 258*
- ♦ **Caltrate® (Can)** *see* Calcium Carbonate *on page 264*
- ♦ **Caltrate® 600 [OTC]** *see* Calcium Carbonate *on page 264*
- ♦ **Caltrate® 600 [OTC]** *see* Calcium Supplements *on page 272*
- ♦ **Caltrate® Select (Can)** *see* Calcium Carbonate *on page 264*
- ♦ **Camila™** *see* Norethindrone *on page 1148*
- ♦ **Camphorated Tincture of Opium (error-prone synonym)** *see* Paregoric *on page 1213*
- ♦ **Camptosar®** *see* Irinotecan *on page 865*
- ♦ **Camptothecin-11** *see* Irinotecan *on page 865*
- ♦ **Canasa™** *see* Mesalamine *on page 1011*
- ♦ **Cancidas®** *see* Caspofungin *on page 298*
- ♦ **Candistatin® (Can)** *see* Nystatin *on page 1156*
- ♦ **Canesten® Topical (Can)** *see* Clotrimazole *on page 393*
- ♦ **Canesten® Vaginal (Can)** *see* Clotrimazole *on page 393*
- ♦ **Cankaid® [OTC]** *see* Carbamide Peroxide *on page 283*
- ♦ **Capex™** *see* Fluocinolone *on page 672*
- ♦ **Capital® and Codeine** *see* Acetaminophen and Codeine *on page 46*
- ♦ **Capoten®** *see* Captopril *on page 277*
- ♦ **Capoten™ (Can)** *see* Captopril *on page 277*
- ♦ **Capsagel® [OTC]** *see* Capsaicin *on page 276*

Capsaicin (kap SAY sin)

Medication Safety Issues

Sound-alike/look-alike issues:

Zostrix® may be confused with Zestril®, Zovirax®

U.S. Brand Names ArthriCare® for Women Extra Moisturizing [OTC] [DSC]; ArthriCare® for Women Multi-Action [OTC] [DSC]; ArthriCare® for Women Silky Dry [OTC] [DSC]; ArthriCare® for Women Ultra Strength [OTC] [DSC]; Capsagel® [OTC]; Capzasin-HP® [OTC]; Capzasin-P® [OTC]; Zostrix® [OTC]; Zostrix®-HP [OTC]

Canadian Brand Names Zostrix®; Zostrix® H.P.

Therapeutic Category Analgesic, Topical; Topical Skin Product

Generic Available Yes: Cream

Use Topical treatment of pain associated with postherpetic neuralgia, rheumatoid arthritis, osteoarthritis, diabetic neuropathy, and postsurgical pain; also used for treatment of pain associated with psoriasis, chronic neuralgias unresponsive to other forms of therapy, and intractable pruritus

Contraindications Hypersensitivity to capsaicin or any component

Warnings Avoid contact with eyes, mucous membrane, or with damaged or irritated skin

Precautions Since warm water or excessive sweating may intensify the localized burning sensation after capsaicin application, the affected area should not be tightly bandaged or exposed to direct sunlight or a heat lamp

Adverse Reactions

Dermatologic: Erythema

Local: Itching, burning, or stinging sensation

Respiratory: Cough

Mechanism of Action Induces release of substance P, the principal chemomediator of pain impulses from the periphery to the CNS, from peripheral sensory neurons. After repeated application, capsaicin depletes the neuron of substance P and prevents reaccumulation.

Pharmacodynamics

Onset of action: Pain relief is usually seen within 14-28 days of regular topical application; maximal response may require 4-6 weeks of continuous therapy

Duration: Several hours

Usual Dosage Children ≥2 years and Adults: Topical: Apply to affected area at least 3-4 times/day; application frequency less than 3-4 times/day prevents the total depletion, inhibition of synthesis, and transport of substance P resulting in decreased clinical efficacy and increased local discomfort

Administration Topical: Should not be applied to wounds or damaged skin; avoid eye and mucous membrane exposure

Patient Information For external use only. Avoid washing treated areas for 30 minutes after application

Nursing Implications Wash hands with soap and water after applying to avoid spreading cream to eyes or other sensitive areas of the body

Additional Information In patients with severe and persistent local discomfort, pretreatment with topical lidocaine 5% ointment or concurrent oral analgesics for the first 2 weeks of therapy have been effective in alleviating the initial burning sensation and enabling continuation of topical capsaicin

Dosage Forms Excipient information presented when available (limited, particularly for generics); consult specific product labeling. [DSC] = Discontinued product

Cream, topical: 0.025% (60 g); 0.075% (60 g)

ArthriCare® for Women Multi-Action: 0.025% (42 g) [contains menthol] [DSC]

ArthriCare® for Women Silky Dry: 0.025% (42 g) [DSC]

ArthriCare® for Women Ultra Strength: 0.075% (42 g) [contains benzalkonium chloride and menthol] [DSC]

Capzasin-P®: 0.025% (45 g)

Capzasin-HP®: 0.075% (45 g)

Zostrix®: 0.025% (60 g)

Zostrix®-HP: 0.075% (60 g)

Gel, topical:

Capsagel®: 0.025% (60 g); 0.05% (60 g); 0.075% (30 g)

Lotion, topical:

ArthriCare® for Women Extra Moisturizing: 0.025% (120 mL, 240 mL) [DSC]

References

Bernstein JE, Korman NJ, Bickers DR, et al, "Topical Capsaicin Treatment of Chronic Postherpetic Neuralgia," *J Am Acad Dermatol*, 1989, 21(2 Pt 1):265-70.

Captopril (KAP toe pril)

Medication Safety Issues

Sound-alike/look-alike issues:

Captopril may be confused with Capitrol®, carvedilol

International issues:

Acepril® [Great Britain] may be confused with Accupril® which is a brand name for quinapril in the U.S.

Acepril®: Brand name for enalapril in Hungary and Switzerland; brand name for lisinopril in Denmark

Related Information

Antihypertensive Agents by Class *on page 1678*

U.S. Brand Names Capoten®

Canadian Brand Names Alti-Captopril; Apo-Capto®; Capoten™; Gen-Captopril; Novo-Captopril; Nu-Capto; PMS-Captopril

Index Terms ACE

Therapeutic Category Angiotensin-Converting Enzyme (ACE) Inhibitor; Antihypertensive Agent

Generic Available Yes

Use Management of hypertension; treatment of CHF; in post-MI patients, improves survival in clinically stable patients with left-ventricular dysfunction

Pregnancy Risk Factor C (1st trimester); D (may cause injury and death to the developing fetus when used during the second and third trimester of pregnancy)

Lactation Enters breast milk/not recommended (AAP rates "compatible")

Contraindications Hypersensitivity to captopril, any component, or other ACE inhibitors

Warnings Serious adverse effects including angioedema, anaphylactoid reactions, neutropenia, agranulocytosis, proteinuria, hypotension, and hepatic failure may occur (see Adverse Reactions); risk of neutropenia is increased 15 fold to 1 per 500 in patients with renal dysfunction, and increased to 3.7% in patients with both collagen vascular disease and renal dysfunction

Precautions Use with caution and modify dosage in patients with renal impairment, especially those with severe renal artery stenosis; elevated BUN and serum creatinine may occur in these patients after decrease in blood pressure with captopril; dosage reduction of captopril or discontinuation of concurrent diuretic may be needed; control of blood pressure while maintaining adequate renal perfusion may not be possible in some of these patients. Use with caution in patients with collagen vascular disease and in patients with volume depletion.

Adverse Reactions

Cardiovascular: Hypotension, tachycardia

Central nervous system: Headache, dizziness, fatigue, insomnia, fever

Dermatologic: Rash, angioedema. **Note:** The relative risk of angioedema with ACE inhibitors is higher within the first 30 days of use (compared to >1 year of use), for Black Americans (compared to Whites), for lisinopril or enalapril (compared to captopril), and for patients previously hospitalized within 30 days (Brown, 1996).

Endocrine & metabolic: Hyperkalemia

Gastrointestinal: Ageusia

(Continued)

Captopril *(Continued)*

Hematologic: Neutropenia, agranulocytosis, eosinophilia

Hepatic: Cholestatic jaundice, fulminant hepatic necrosis (rare, but potentially fatal)

Renal: Elevated BUN and serum creatinine, proteinuria, oliguria

Respiratory: Cough, dyspnea; **Note:** An isolated dry cough lasting >3 weeks was reported in 7 of 42 pediatric patients (17%) receiving ACE inhibitors (see von Vigier, 2000)

Drug Interactions Cytochrome P450 isoenzyme CYP2D6 substrate

Captopril plus potassium supplements or potassium-sparing diuretics may cause an additive hyperkalemic effect; captopril plus indomethacin or NSAIDs may result in a reduced antihypertensive response to captopril

Food Interactions Absorption of captopril may be reduced by food; long-term use of captopril may result in a zinc deficiency which can result in a decrease in taste perception; zinc supplements may be used; limit salt substitutes or potassium-rich diet; avoid natural licorice (causes sodium and water retention and increases potassium loss)

Stability Unstable in aqueous solutions

Mechanism of Action Competitive inhibitor of angiotensin-converting enzyme (ACE); prevents conversion of angiotensin I to angiotensin II, a potent vasoconstrictor; results in lower levels of angiotensin II which causes an increase in plasma renin activity and a reduction in aldosterone secretion

Pharmacodynamics

Onset of action: Decrease in blood pressure within 15 minutes

Maximum effect: 60-90 minutes; may require several weeks of therapy before full hypotensive effect is seen

Duration: Dose-related

Pharmacokinetics

Absorption: 60% to 75%

Distribution: 7 L/kg

Protein binding: 25% to 30%

Metabolism: 50% metabolized

Half-life:

- Infants with CHF: 3.3 hours; range: 1.2-12.4 hours
- Children: 1.5 hours; range: 0.98-2.3 hours
- Normal adults (dependent upon renal and cardiac function): 1.9 hours
- Adults with CHF: 2.1 hours
- Anuria: 20-40 hours

Time to peak serum concentration: Within 1-2 hours

Elimination: 95% excreted in urine in 24 hours

Usual Dosage Note: Dosage must be titrated according to patient's response; use lowest effective dose; lower doses (~½ of those listed) should be used in patients who are sodium and water depleted due to diuretic therapy; Oral:

Newborns and premature Neonates: Initial: 0.01 mg/kg/dose every 8-12 hours; titrate dose

Neonates: Initial: 0.05-0.1 mg/kg/dose every 8-24 hours; titrate dose up to 0.5 mg/kg/dose given every 6-24 hours

Infants: Initial: 0.15-0.3 mg/kg/dose; titrate dose upward to maximum of 6 mg/kg/day in 1-4 divided doses; usual required dose: 2.5-6 mg/kg/day

Children: Initial: 0.3-0.5 mg/kg/dose; titrate upward to maximum of 6 mg/kg/day in 2-4 divided doses

Older Children: Initial: 6.25-12.5 mg/dose every 12-24 hours; titrate upward to maximum of 6 mg/kg/day in 2-4 divided doses

Adolescents and Adults: Initial: 12.5-25 mg/dose given every 8-12 hours; increase by 25 mg/dose at 1-2 week intervals based on patient response; maximum dose: 450 mg/day; usual dosage range for hypertension (JNC 7): Adolescents ≥18 years and Adults: 25-100 mg/day in 2 divided doses

Dosing adjustment in renal impairment:

- Cl_{cr} 10-50 mL/minute: Administer 75% of dose
- Cl_{cr} <10 mL/minute: Administer 50% of dose

Administration Oral: Administer on an empty stomach 1 hour before meals or 2 hours after meals

Monitoring Parameters Blood pressure, BUN, serum creatinine, renal function, urine dipstick for protein, WBC with differential, serum potassium

Patient Information Limit alcohol; notify physician if swelling of face, lips, tongue, difficulty in breathing, or persistent cough occurs; do not use salt substitute (potassium-containing) without physician advice

Nursing Implications Discontinue if angioedema occurs; monitor blood pressure for hypotension within 1-3 hours after first dose or after a new higher dose

Additional Information Severe hypotension may occur in patients who are sodium and/or volume depleted

Dosage Forms Excipient information presented when available (limited, particularly for generics); consult specific product labeling.

Tablet: 12.5 mg, 25 mg, 50 mg, 100 mg

Extemporaneous Preparations

Captopril has limited stability in aqueous preparations. The addition of an antioxidant [sodium ascorbate (using an injectable product) or ascorbic acid (using tablets)] has been shown to increase the stability of captopril in solution; captopril (1 mg/mL) in syrup with methylcellulose is stable for 7 days stored either at 4°C or 22°C. Captopril (1 mg/mL) in distilled water (no additives) is stable for 14 days if stored at 4°C and 7 days if stored at 22°C; captopril (1 mg/mL) with sodium ascorbate (5 mg/mL) in distilled water is stable for 56 days at 4°C and 14 days at 22°C (Nahata, 1994); captopril (1 mg/mL) with ascorbic acid (5 mg/mL) in distilled water is stable for 56 days at 4°C and 28 days at 22°C (Nahata, 1994a); captopril (1 mg/mL) in an undiluted syrup containing preservatives is stable for 30 days at 5°C in amber glass containers (Lye, 1997).

Captopril (0.75 mg/mL) in cherry syrup is stable for only 2 days in amber clear plastic containers stored at room temperature or under refrigeration; captopril (0.75 mg/mL) in either a 1:1 mixture of Ora-Sweet® and Ora-Plus® or a 1:1 mixture of Ora-Sweet® SF and Ora-Plus® is stable for 10 days or less depending on the storage temperature (see Allen, 1996).

Powder papers can also be made; powder papers are stable for 12 weeks when stored at room temperature (Taketomo, 1990).

Allen LV and Erickson MA, "Stability of Baclofen, Captopril, Diltiazem Hydrochloride, Dipyridamole, and Flecainide Acetate in Extemporaneously Compounded Oral Liquids," *Am J Health Sys Pharm*, 1996, 53(18):2179-84.

Lye MY, Yow KL, Lim LY, et al, "Effects of Ingredients on Stability of Captopril in Extemporaneously Prepared Oral Liquids," *Am J Health Syst Pharm*, 1997, 54(21):2483-7.

Nahata MC, Morosco RS, and Hipple TF, "Stability of Captopril in Three Liquid Dosage Forms," *Am J Hosp Pharm*, 1994, 51(1):95-6.

Nahata MC, Morosco RS, and Hipple TF, "Stability of Captopril in Liquid Containing Ascorbic Acid or Sodium Ascorbate," *Am J Hosp Pharm*, 1994a, 51(13):1707-8.

Taketomo CK, Chu SA, Cheng MH, et al, "Stability of Captopril in Powder Papers Under Three Storage Conditions," *Am J Hosp Pharm*, 1990, 47(8):1799-801.

References

Brown NJ, Ray WA, Snowden M, et al, "Black Americans Have an Increased Rate of Angiotensin-Converting Enzyme Inhibitor-Associated Angioedema," *Clin Pharmacol Ther*, 1996, 60(1):8-13.

Chobanian AV, Bakris GL, Black HR, et al, "The Seventh Report of the Joint National Committee on Prevention, Detection, Evaluation, and Treatment of High Blood Pressure: The JNC 7 report," *JAMA*, 2003, 289(19):2560-72.

Friedman WF and George BL, "New Concepts and Drugs in the Treatment of Congestive Heart Failure," *Pediatr Clin North Am*, 1984, 31(6):1197-227.

Levy M, Koren G, Klein J, et al, "Captopril Pharmacokinetics, Blood Pressure Response and Plasma Renin Activity in Normotensive Children With Renal Scarring," *Dev Pharmacol Ther*, 1991, 16(4):185-93.

Mirkin BL and Newman TJ, "Efficacy and Safety of Captopril in the Treatment of Severe Childhood Hypertension: Report of the International Collaborative Study Group," *Pediatrics*, 1985, 75(6):1091-100.

Pereira CM, Tam YK, Collins-Nakai RL, "The Pharmacokinetics of Captopril in Infants With Congestive Heart Failure," *Ther Drug Monit*, 1991, 13(3):209-14.

von Vigier RO, Mozzettini S, Truttmann AC, et al, "Cough is Common in Children Prescribed Converting Enzyme Inhibitors," *Nephron*, 2000, 84(1):98.

- **Capzasin-HP® [OTC]** *see* Capsaicin *on page 276*
- **Capzasin-P® [OTC]** *see* Capsaicin *on page 276*
- **Carac™** *see* Fluorouracil *on page 678*
- **Carafate®** *see* Sucralfate *on page 1480*
- **Carapres® (Can)** *see* Clonidine *on page 389*

Carbamazepine (kar ba MAZ e peen)

Medication Safety Issues

Sound-alike/look-alike issues:

Carbatrol® may be confused with Cartrol®

Epitol® may be confused with Epinal®

Tegretol®, Tegretol®-XR may be confused with Mebaral®, Tegrin®, Toprol-XL®, Toradol®, Trental®

Related Information

Antiepileptic Drugs *on page 1902*

Blood Level Sampling Time Guidelines *on page 1914*

Overdose and Toxicology *on page 1916*

Serotonin Syndrome *on page 1955*

(Continued)

Carbamazepine *(Continued)*

U.S. Brand Names Carbatrol®; Epitol®; Equetro™; Tegretol®; Tegretol®-XR

Canadian Brand Names Apo-Carbamazepine®; Gen-Carbamazepine CR; Mapezine®; Novo-Carbamaz; Nu-Carbamazepine; PMS-Carbamazepine; Taro-Carbamazepine Chewable; Tegretol®

Index Terms CBZ; SPD417

Therapeutic Category Anticonvulsant, Miscellaneous

Generic Available Yes: Excludes capsule (extended release), tablet (extended release)

Use Treatment of generalized tonic-clonic, partial (especially complex partial), and mixed partial or generalized seizure disorder; to relieve pain in trigeminal neuralgia or diabetic neuropathy; treatment of bipolar disorders (Equetro™ is approved for this use)

Pregnancy Risk Factor D

Lactation Enters breast milk/not recommended (AAP rates "compatible")

Contraindications Hypersensitivity to carbamazepine, tricyclic antidepressants, or any component; patients with a history of bone marrow suppression; concomitant use or use within 14 days of MAO inhibitors

Warnings Potentially fatal blood cell abnormalities have been reported following treatment; history of adverse hematologic reaction to any drug may place patient at increased risk; early detection of hematologic change is important; advise patients of early signs and symptoms which are: fever, sore throat, mouth ulcers, infections, easy bruising, petechial or purpuric hemorrhage. Potentially fatal, severe dermatologic reactions (including Stevens-Johnson syndrome and toxic epidermal necrolysis) may occur; hepatic failure (rare) and multi-organ hypersensitivity reactions may occur (see Adverse Reactions); consider discontinuation of carbamazepine if any evidence of hypersensitivity occurs. Do not abruptly discontinue in patients being treated for seizures (precipitation of status epilepticus may occur). Carbamazepine may activate latent psychosis.

Substitution of Tegretol® with generic carbamazepine has resulted in decreased carbamazepine levels and increased seizure activity, as well as increased carbamazepine levels and toxicity. Monitoring of carbamazepine serum concentrations is mandatory when patients are switched from any product to another.

Precautions Use with caution and only after benefit-to-risk assessment in patients with history of cardiac disease, hepatic disease, renal failure, adverse hematologic reactions to other drugs, or history of hypersensitivity reactions to other anticonvulsants (eg, phenobarbital, phenytoin); use with caution in patients with increased IOP (carbamazepine has mild anticholinergic effects); higher peak concentrations occur with the suspension, so treatment is initiated with lower amounts per dose and increased slowly to avoid adverse effects. Long-term risks and benefits of carbamazepine in the treatment of bipolar disorder have not been evaluated; periodic assessment of risks and benefits should be conducted for individual patient.

Adverse Reactions

Cardiovascular: Edema, CHF, syncope, dysrhythmias, heart block

Central nervous system: Sedation, dizziness, drowsiness, somnolence, fatigue, slurred speech, ataxia, confusion

Dermatologic: Rash, Stevens-Johnson syndrome, toxic epidermal necrolysis, photosensitivity, pruritus

Endocrine & metabolic: SIADH, hyponatremia

Gastrointestinal: Nausea, diarrhea, vomiting, abdominal cramps, pancreatitis, xerostomia

Genitourinary: Urinary retention

Hematologic: Neutropenia (can be transient), aplastic anemia, agranulocytosis, thrombocytopenia

Hepatic: Elevated liver enzymes, jaundice, hepatitis; hepatic failure (very rare)

Ocular: Nystagmus, diplopia, blurred vision

Miscellaneous: Multi-organ hypersensitivity reactions (rare): Reactions may include vasculitis, lymphadenopathy, fever, rash, lymphoma-like symptoms, arthralgia, eosinophilia, leukopenia, elevated liver enzymes, hepato-splenomegaly

Drug Interactions Cytochrome P450 isoenzyme CYP2C8 and CYP3A3/4 substrate; isoenzyme CYP1A2, CYP2C, and CYP3A3/4 inducer

Enzyme inhibitors, such as acetazolamide, cimetidine, clarithromycin, danazol, diltiazem, erythromycin, fluoxetine, fluvoxamine, isoniazid, itraconazole, ketoconazole, loratadine, nefazodone, propoxyphene, protease inhibitors, quinine, verapamil, and zileuton may inhibit hepatic metabolism of carbamazepine with resultant increase of carbamazepine serum concentrations and toxicity. Enzyme inducers, such as rifampin, phenobarbital, phenytoin, primidone, and methsuximide may decrease serum concentration of carbamazepine. Carbamazepine may induce the metabolism of benzodiazepines, oral or subdermal contraceptives (consider alternative or back-up methods of contraception), corticosteroids, cyclosporine, delavirdine (may result in loss of virologic response), doxorubicin, doxycycline, ethosuximide, etoposide, lamotrigine, methotrexate, midazolam, phenytoin, ritonavir, saquinavir, teniposide, theophylline, thyroid hormones, tiagabine, topiramate, valproic acid, vincristine, and warfarin. Carbamazepine may increase the serum concentration of clomipramine, phenytoin, and primidone. Use with lithium may increase neurotoxic side effects. Antimalarial drugs (chloroquine, mefloquine) may antagonize the activity of carbamazepine. Use with alcohol or other CNS acting agents may potentiate adverse effects of carbamazepine. Ritonavir and cefixime may affect the metabolism of carbamazepine. Administration of Tegretol® suspension in combination with liquid chlorpromazine or thioridazine results in an orange rubbery precipitate

Food Interactions Extended release capsules (Carbatrol®, Equetro™): A high fat meal may increase the rate of absorption, reduce time to peak concentration (from 24 hours to 14 hours), and increase peak concentrations, but does not effect extent of absorption (AUC)

Grapefruit juice increases the oral bioavailability of carbamazepine by an average of 40%

Stability Store at room temperature, below 30°C (86°F).

Tablets, chewable: Protect from moisture and light; dispense in tight, light-resistant container

Tablets and extended release tablets: Protect from moisture; dispense in tightly closed container

Suspension: Dispense in tight, light-resistant container

Capsules, extended release: Protect from light

Mechanism of Action

Epilepsy: May depress activity in the nucleus ventralis of the thalamus or decrease synaptic transmission or decrease summation of temporal stimulation leading to neural discharge, by limiting influx of sodium ions across cell membrane; other unknown mechanisms.

Bipolar disorder: Mechanism of action is unknown.

Carbamazepine also stimulates the release of ADH and potentiates its action in promoting reabsorption of water; chemically related to tricyclic antidepressants; in addition to anticonvulsant effects, carbamazepine has anticholinergic, antineuralgic, antidiuretic, muscle relaxant and antiarrhythmic properties

Pharmacokinetics

Absorption: Slowly from the GI tract

Distribution: Carbamazepine and its active epoxide metabolite distribute into breast milk

V_d:
- Neonates: 1.5 L/kg
- Children: 1.9 L/kg
- Adults: 0.59-2 L/kg

Protein binding: Carbamazepine: 75% to 90%, bound to alpha$_1$-acid glycoprotein and nonspecific binding sites on albumin; protein binding may be decreased in newborns
- Epoxide metabolite: 50% protein bound

Metabolism: Induces liver enzymes to increase metabolism and shorten half-life over time; metabolized in the liver by cytochrome P450 3A4 to active epoxide metabolite; epoxide metabolite is metabolized by epoxide hydrolase to the trans-diol metabolite; ratio of serum epoxide to carbamazepine concentrations may be higher in patients receiving polytherapy (vs monotherapy) and in infants (vs older children); boys may have faster carbamazepine clearances and may, therefore, require higher mg/kg/day doses of carbamazepine compared to girls of similar age and weight

Bioavailability, oral: 75% to 85%; relative bioavailability of extended release tablet to suspension: 89%

Half-life:
- Carbamazepine:
  - Initial: 25-65 hours
  - Multiple dosing:
    - Children: 8-14 hours
    - Adults: 12-17 hours
- Epoxide metabolite: 34 ± 9 hours

Time to peak serum concentration: Unpredictable, within 4-8 hours
- Chronic administration:
  - Suspension: 1.5 hours
  - Tablet: 4-5 hours
  - Extended release tablet: 3-12 hours

Elimination: 1% to 3% excreted unchanged in urine

(Continued)

Carbamazepine *(Continued)*

Usual Dosage Dosage must be adjusted according to patient's response and serum concentrations. Administer tablets (chewable or conventional) in 2-3 divided doses daily and suspension in 4 divided doses daily. (See Additional Information for investigational oral loading dose and rectal maintenance dose information.) Oral:

Epilepsy:

Children:

<6 years: Initial: 10-20 mg/kg/day divided twice or 3 times daily as tablets or 4 times/day as suspension; increase dose every week until optimal response and therapeutic levels are achieved; maintenance dose: Divide into 3-4 doses daily (tablets or suspension); maximum recommended dose: 35 mg/kg/day

6-12 years: Initial: 100 mg twice daily (tablets or extended release tablets) or 50 mg of suspension 4 times/day (200 mg/day); increase by up to 100 mg/day at weekly intervals using a twice daily regimen of extended release tablets or 3-4 times daily regimen of other formulations until optimal response and therapeutic levels are achieved; usual maintenance: 400-800 mg/day; maximum recommended dose: 1000 mg/day

Note: Children <12 years who receive ≥400 mg/day of carbamazepine may be converted to extended release capsules (Carbatrol®) using the same total daily dosage divided twice daily

Children >12 years and Adults: Initial: 200 mg twice daily (tablets, extended release tablets, or extended release capsules) or 100 mg of suspension 4 times/day (400 mg daily); increase by up to 200 mg/day at weekly intervals using a twice daily regimen of extended release tablets or capsules, or a 3-4 times/day regimen of other formulations until optimal response and therapeutic levels are achieved; usual dose: 800-1200 mg/day

Maximum recommended doses:

Children 12-15 years: 1000 mg/day

Children >15 years: 1200 mg/day

Adults: 1600 mg/day; however, some patients have required up to 1.6-2.4 g/day

Bipolar disorder (Equetro™): Adults: Initial: 200 mg twice daily; adjust dose by 200 mg/day increments until optimal response is achieved; maximum dose: 1600 mg/day

Dosing adjustment in renal impairment: Cl_{cr} <10 mL/minute: Administer 75% of recommended dose; monitor serum levels

Administration

Oral: Administer with food to decrease GI upset; avoid administration with grapefruit juice; extended release capsules (Carbatrol®, Equetro™) may be taken without regard to meals; suspension dosage should be administered on a 3-4 times/day schedule vs tablet (conventional or chewable) which can be administered 2-4 times/day; extended release (XR) tablets should be dosed twice daily; do not crush or chew XR tablets; examine XR tablets for cracks or chips; do not use damaged XR tablets or XR tablets without a release portal; chewable tablet should be chewed well and swallowed. Swallow extended release capsules whole or open and sprinkle contents on small amount of soft food (eg, 1 teaspoonful of applesauce); swallow sprinkle/food mixture immediately; do not chew; do not store for later use; drink fluids after dose to make sure mixture is completely swallowed

Suspension: Tegretol® should not be administered with diluents or other liquid medicines due to the possibility of a component interaction (see Drug Interactions); shake suspension well before use

Monitoring Parameters CBC with platelet count, reticulocytes, serum iron, liver function tests, ophthalmic examinations (including slit-lamp, fundoscopy, and tonometry), urinalysis, BUN, lipid panel, serum drug concentrations, thyroid function tests, serum sodium; observe patient for excessive sedation especially when instituting or increasing therapy

Reference Range Therapeutic: 4-12 mcg/mL (SI: 17-51 micromoles/L). Patients who require higher levels [8-12 mcg/mL (SI: 34-51 micromoles/L)] should be carefully monitored. Side effects (especially CNS) occur commonly at higher levels. If other anticonvulsants (enzyme inducers) are given, therapeutic range is 4-8 mcg/mL (SI: 17-34 micromoles/L) due to increase in unmeasured active epoxide metabolite.

Test Interactions Carbamazepine may interfere with a serum immunoassay for tricyclic antidepressants; false-positive qualitative serum tricyclic antidepressant drug screen results have been reported in patients with carbamazepine intoxication (see Matos, 2000). Carbamazepine may interfere with some pregnancy tests.

Patient Information Avoid alcohol and grapefruit juice. May cause drowsiness and impair ability to perform activities requiring mental alertness or physical coordination. May cause dry mouth. Report fever, sore throat, infection, mouth ulcers, easy bruising, bleeding, loss of appetite, nausea, vomiting, or yellow skin or eyes to physician. Report the use of other medications, nonprescription medications, and herbal or natural products to your physician and pharmacist. The tablet coating of Tegretol®-XR tablet is not absorbed and may appear in the stool. May cause photosensitivity reactions (eg, exposure to sunlight may cause severe sunburn, skin rash, redness, or itching); avoid exposure to sunlight and artificial light sources (sunlamps, tanning booth/bed); wear protective clothing, wide-brimmed hats, sunglasses, and lip sunscreen (SPF ≥15); use a sunscreen [broad-spectrum sunscreen or physical sunscreen (preferred) or sunblock with SPF ≥15]; contact physician if reaction occurs.

Additional Information Carbamazepine is not effective in absence, myoclonic, akinetic, or febrile seizures; exacerbation of certain seizure types have been seen after initiation of carbamazepine therapy in children with mixed seizure disorders

Investigationally, loading doses of the suspension (10 mg/kg for children <12 years of age and 8 mg/kg for children >12 years) were given (via NG or ND tubes followed by 5-10 mL of water to flush through tube) to PICU patients with frequent seizures/status; 5 of 6 patients attained mean plasma concentrations of 4.3 mcg/mL and 7.3 mcg/mL at 1 and 2 hours postload; concurrent enteral feeding or ileus may delay absorption of loading dose (Miles, 1990)

Carbamazepine suspension may be administered rectally as maintenance doses, if oral therapy is not possible (**Note:** Rectally administered carbamazepine is not useful in status epilepticus due to its slow absorption); when using carbamazepine suspension rectally, administer the same total daily dose, but give in small, diluted, multiple doses; dilute the oral suspension with an equal volume of water; if defecation occurs within the first 2 hours, repeat the dose (see Graves, 1987)

Extended release capsule (Cabatrol®, Equetro™) contain three different types of beads: Immediate-, extended-, and enteric-release; the combination of the ratio of bead types allows for twice daily dosing.

A recent study (Relling, 2000) demonstrated that enzyme-inducing antiepileptic drugs (AEDs) (carbamazepine, phenobarbital, and phenytoin) increased systemic clearance of antileukemic drugs (teniposide and methotrexate) and were associated with a worse event-free survival, CNS relapse, and hematologic relapse, (ie, lower efficacy), in B-lineage ALL children receiving chemotherapy; the authors recommend using nonenzyme-inducing AEDs in patients receiving chemotherapy for ALL.

Dosage Forms Excipient information presented when available (limited, particularly for generics); consult specific product labeling.

Capsule, extended release:
  Carbatrol®, Equetro™: 100 mg, 200 mg, 300 mg
Suspension, oral: 100 mg/5 mL (10 mL, 450 mL)
  Tegretol®: 100 mg/5 mL (450 mL) [citrus vanilla flavor]
Tablet: 200 mg
  Epitol®, Tegretol®: 200 mg
Tablet, chewable: 100 mg
  Tegretol®: 100 mg
Tablet, extended release:
  Tegretol®-XR: 100 mg, 200 mg, 400 mg

References

Gilman JT, "Carbamazepine Dosing for Pediatric Seizure Disorders: The Highs and Lows," *DICP*, 1991, 25(10):1109-12.

Graves NM and Kriel RL, "Rectal Administration of Antiepileptic Drugs in Children," *Pediatr Neurol*, 1987, 3(6):321-6.

Korinthenberg R, Haug C, and Hannak D, "The Metabolization of Carbamazepine to CBZ-10,11 Epoxide in Children From the Newborn Age to Adolescence," *Neuropediatrics*, 1994, 25(4):214-6.

Liu H and Delgado MR, "Influence of Sex, Age, Weight, and Carbamazepine Dose on Serum Concentrations, Concentration Ratios, and Level/Dose Ratios of Carbamazepine and Its Metabolites," *Ther Drug Monit*, 1994, 16(5):469-76.

Matos ME, Burns MM, and Shannon MW, "False-Positive Tricyclic Antidepressant Drug Screen Results Leading to the Diagnosis of Carbamazepine Intoxication," *Pediatrics*, 2000, 105(5), http://www.pediatrics.org/cgi/content/full/105/5/e66.

Miles MV, Lawless ST, Tennison MB, et al, "Rapid Loading of Critically Ill Patients With Carbamazepine Suspension," *Pediatrics*, 1990, 86(2):263-6.

Relling MV, Pui CH, Sandlund JT, et al, "Adverse Effect of Anticonvulsants on Efficacy of Chemotherapy for Acute Lymphoblastic Leukaemia," *Lancet*, 2000, 356(9226):285-90.

Carbamide Peroxide (KAR ba mide per OKS ide)

U.S. Brand Names Cankaid® [OTC]; Debrox® [OTC]; Dent's Ear Wax [OTC]; E•R•O [OTC]; Gly-Oxide® [OTC]; Murine® Ear Wax Removal System [OTC]; Orajel® Perioseptic® Spot Treatment [OTC]

Index Terms Urea Peroxide

Therapeutic Category Otic Agent, Cerumenolytic

Generic Available Yes

Use

Oral: Relief of minor inflammation of gums, oral mucosal surfaces and lips including canker sores and dental irritation; adjunct in oral hygiene

(Continued)

Carbamide Peroxide *(Continued)*

Otic: Emulsify and disperse ear wax

Pregnancy Risk Factor C

Contraindications Hypersensitivity to carbamide peroxide or any component; otic preparation should not be used in patients with a perforated tympanic membrane or following otic surgery; ear drainage, ear pain, or rash in the ear; dizziness; oral preparation should not be used for self medication in children <3 years of age

Warnings With prolonged use of oral carbamide peroxide, there is a potential for overgrowth of opportunistic organisms, damage to periodontal tissues, delayed wound healing

Adverse Reactions

Central nervous system: Dizziness

Dermatologic: Rash

Local: Irritation, tenderness, pain, redness

Stability Protect from heat and direct light

Mechanism of Action Carbamide peroxide releases hydrogen peroxide which serves as a source of nascent oxygen upon contact with catalase; deodorant action is probably due to inhibition of odor-causing bacteria; softens impacted cerumen due to its foaming action

Pharmacodynamics Onset of action: Otic: Slight disintegration of hard ear wax in 24 hours

Usual Dosage

Oral: Children and Adults: Solution: Apply several drops undiluted to affected area of the mouth 4 times/day after meals and at bedtime for up to 7 days, expectorate after 2-3 minutes; as an adjunct to oral hygiene after brushing, swish 10 drops for 2-3 minutes, then expectorate

Otic: Solution:

Children <12 years: Individualize the dose according to patient size; 3 drops (range: 1-5 drops) twice daily for up to 4 days

Children ≥12 years and Adults: Instill 5-10 drops twice daily for up to 4 days

Administration

Oral: Apply undiluted solution with an applicator or cotton swab to the affected area after meals and at bedtime; or place drops on the tongue, mix with saliva, swish in the mouth for several minutes, then expectorate. Patient should not rinse mouth or drink fluids for 5 minutes after oral administration.

Otic: Instill drops into the external ear canal; keep drops in ear for several minutes by keeping head tilted or placing cotton in ear. Gently irrigate ear canal with warm water to remove loosened cerumen.

Patient Information Contact physician if dizziness or otic redness, rash, irritation, tenderness, pain, drainage or discharge develop; do not use in the eye

Nursing Implications Drops foam on contact with ear wax

Dosage Forms Excipient information presented when available (limited, particularly for generics); consult specific product labeling.

Solution, oral: 10% (60 mL)

Cankaid®: 10% (22 mL) [in anhydrous glycerol]

Gly-Oxide®: 10% (15 mL, 60 mL) [contains glycerin]

Orajel® Perioseptic® Spot Treatment: 15% (13.3 mL) [contains anhydrous glycerin]

Solution, otic: 6.5% (15 mL)

Debrox®: 6.5% (15 mL, 30 mL) [contains propylene glycol]

Dent's Ear Wax: 6.5% (3.7 mL) [contains glycerin]

E•R•O: 6.5% (15 mL)

Murine® Ear Wax Removal System: 6.5% (15 mL) [contains alcohol 6.3% and glycerin]

♦ **Carbatrol®** *see* Carbamazepine *on page 279*

♦ **Carbaxefed RF [DSC]** *see* Carbinoxamine and Pseudoephedrine *on page 286*

Carbenicillin (kar ben i SIL in)

U.S. Brand Names Geocillin®

Index Terms Carbenicillin Indanyl Sodium; Carindacillin

Therapeutic Category Antibiotic, Penicillin (Antipseudomonal)

Generic Available No

Use Treatment of urinary tract infections, asymptomatic bacteriuria, or prostatitis caused by susceptible strains of *Pseudomonas aeruginosa*, *E. coli*, indole-positive *Proteus*, and *Enterobacter*

Pregnancy Risk Factor B

Lactation Enters breast milk/use caution

Contraindications Hypersensitivity to carbenicillin, any component, or penicillins

Warnings Oral carbenicillin should be limited to treatment of urinary tract infections

Precautions Use with caution in patients with history of cephalosporin hypersensitivity; do not use in patients with severe renal impairment (Cl_{cr} <10 mL/minute) since drug concentration in urine is reduced and inadequate for treatment of UTIs

Adverse Reactions

Dermatologic: Rash, urticaria, pruritus

Gastrointestinal: Nausea, vomiting, diarrhea, abdominal cramps, furry tongue

Genitourinary: Vaginitis

Hematologic: Eosinophilia, hemolytic anemia, neutropenia, leukopenia, thrombocytopenia

Hepatic: Elevated liver enzymes, hepatotoxicity

Drug Interactions Probenecid, lithium

Mechanism of Action Interferes with bacterial cell wall synthesis during active multiplication

Pharmacokinetics

Absorption: Oral: 30% to 40%; in patients with normal renal function, serum concentrations of carbenicillin following oral absorption are inadequate for the treatment of systemic infections

Protein binding: 50%

Half-life:

Neonates:

<7 days, ≤2.5 kg: 4 hours

<7 days, >2.5 kg: 2.7 hours

Children: 0.8-1.8 hours

Adults: 1-1.5 hours; prolonged to 10-20 hours with renal insufficiency

Time to peak serum concentration: Within 30-120 minutes

Elimination: Carbenicillin and its metabolites are excreted in the urine; ~80% to 99% of the dose is excreted unchanged in the urine

Dialysis: Moderately dialyzable (20% to 50%)

Usual Dosage Oral:

Children: 30-50 mg/kg/day divided every 6 hours; maximum dose: 2-3 g/day

Adults:

Urinary tract infections: 1-2 tablets every 6 hours

Prostatitis: 2 tablets every 6 hours

Administration Oral: Administer with water

Monitoring Parameters Renal, hepatic, and hematologic function tests

Test Interactions False-positive urine or serum proteins; false-positive urine glucose (Clinitest®)

Patient Information Tablets have a bitter taste

Additional Information Sodium content of 382 mg tablet: 23 mg (1 mEq)

Dosage Forms Excipient information presented when available (limited, particularly for generics); consult specific product labeling.

Tablet: 382 mg [contains sodium 23 mg/tablet]

♦ **Carbenicillin Indanyl Sodium** *see* Carbenicillin *on page 284*

Carbinoxamine (kar bi NOKS a meen)

U.S. Brand Names Palgic®

Index Terms Carbinoxamine Maleate

Therapeutic Category Antihistamine

Generic Available No

Use Relief of symptoms of seasonal and perennial allergic rhinitis, vasomotor rhinitis, allergic conjunctivitis, urticaria, angioedema, and dermatographism

Pregnancy Risk Factor C

Lactation Excretion in breast milk unknown/contraindicated

Contraindications Hypersensitivity to carbinoxamine or any component of the formulation; use with or within 14 days of MAO inhibitor therapy; children <2 years of age

Warnings Due to an association with the use of carbinoxamine and increased fatalities in children <2 years of age, the FDA is not recommending the use of carbinoxamine in children <2 years of age.

Precautions Use with caution in patients with mild to moderate hypertension, cardiovascular disease, diabetes, asthma, thyroid disease, increased intraocular pressure, GU or GI obstruction or symptomatic prostatic hypertrophy

Adverse Reactions

Cardiovascular: Hypotension, palpitations, tachycardia, extrasystoles, chills

Central nervous system: Dizziness, paradoxical excitability (children), headache, nervousness, sedation, fatigue, confusion, seizures, hysteria, euphoria, insomnia, irritability, vertigo

Dermatologic: Urticaria, rash, photosensitivity

(Continued)

Carbinoxamine *(Continued)*

Gastrointestinal: Anorexia, diarrhea, heartburn, nausea, vomiting, xerostomia
Hematologic: Hemolytic anemia (rare), thrombocytopenia (rare), agranulocytosis (rare)
Neuromuscular & skeletal: Weakness, tremor, paresthesia, neuritis
Ocular: Diplopia, blurred vision
Otic: Tinnitus, acute labyrinthitis
Renal: Polyuria
Respiratory: Thickening of bronchial secretions, chest tightness, wheezing
Miscellaneous: Excessive perspiration, anaphylactic shock

Drug Interactions May produce severe hypertensive episodes when used with MAO inhibitors; additive effects with other antihistamines, anticholinergics, sedatives, alcohol, barbiturates, and other CNS depressants

Stability Store at controlled room temperature of 15°C to 30°C (59°F to 86°F).

Mechanism of Action Carbinoxamine competes with histamine for H_1-receptor sites on effector cells in the gastrointestinal tract, blood vessels, and respiratory tract.

Pharmacodynamics Duration: 3-6 hours

Pharmacokinetics Half-life: Adults: 10-20 hours

Usual Dosage Oral:

Infants and Children: 0.2-0.4 mg/kg/day divided 3-4 times/day

Alternate dosing (manufacturer's recommendation); **Note:** When using this recommendation, be sure to compare with the weight-based dosage listed above as the age-based dosage may exceed 0.4 mg/kg/day in some individuals):
Palgic®:
2-3 years: 2 mg (2.5 mL) 3-4 times/day
3-6 years: 2-4 mg (2.5-5 mL) 3-4 times/day
>6 years: 4-6 mg (5-7.5 mL) 3-4 times/day
Adults: 4-8 mg 3-4 times/day

Administration Oral: Administer without regard to food

Patient Information May cause drowsiness or impair ability to perform activities requiring mental alertness or physical coordination; may cause blurred vision; may also cause CNS excitation and difficulty sleeping; may cause dry mouth; avoid alcohol; may rarely cause photosensitivity reactions (eg, exposure to sunlight may cause severe sunburn, skin rash, redness, or itching); avoid direct exposure to sunlight

Dosage Forms Excipient information presented when available (limited, particularly for generics); consult specific product labeling.
Solution, as maleate:
Palgic®: 4 mg/5 mL (480 mL) [bubble gum flavor]
Tablet, as maleate [scored]:
Palgic®: 4 mg

Carbinoxamine and Pseudoephedrine

(kar bi NOKS a meen & soo doe e FED rin)

U.S. Brand Names Andehist NR Drops [DSC]; Carbaxefed RF [DSC]; Carboxine-PSE [DSC]; Cordron-D NR [DSC]; Hydro-Tussin™-CBX; Palgic®-D [DSC]; Palgic®-DS [DSC]; Pediatex™-D [DSC]; Sildec [DSC]

Index Terms Pseudoephedrine and Carbinoxamine

Therapeutic Category Antihistamine/Decongestant Combination

Generic Available Yes

Use Temporary relief of nasal congestion, running nose, sneezing, itching of nose or throat, and itchy, watery eyes due to the common cold, hay fever, or other respiratory allergies

Pregnancy Risk Factor C

Lactation Enters breast milk/contraindicated

Contraindications Hypersensitivity to carbinoxamine, pseudoephedrine, or any component; severe hypertension or coronary artery disease, MAO inhibitor therapy, GI or GU obstruction, narrow-angle glaucoma

Warnings Due to an association with the use of carbinoxamine and increased fatalities in children <2 years of age, the FDA is not recommending the use of carbinoxamine in children <2 years of age.

Some products contains sodium benzoate; benzoic acid (benzoate) is a metabolite of benzyl alcohol; large amounts of benzyl alcohol (≥99 mg/kg/day) have been associated with a potentially fatal toxicity ("gasping syndrome") in neonates; the "gasping syndrome" consists of metabolic acidosis, respiratory distress, gasping respirations, CNS dysfunction (including convulsions, intracranial hemorrhage), hypotension and cardiovascular collapse; avoid use in neonates; *in vitro* and animal studies have shown that benzoate displaces bilirubin from protein binding sites

Precautions Use with caution in patients with mild to moderate hypertension, heart disease, diabetes, asthma, thyroid disease, or prostatic hypertrophy

Adverse Reactions

Cardiovascular: Hypertension, tachycardia, arrhythmias, edema, palpitations

Central nervous system: Sedation, CNS stimulation, headache, seizures, drowsiness, fatigue, nervousness, depression

Dermatologic: Angioedema, photosensitivity, rash

Gastrointestinal: Nausea, vomiting, xerostomia, anorexia, diarrhea, heart burn

Genitourinary: Dysuria

Hepatic: Hepatitis

Neuromuscular & skeletal: Weakness, myalgia, paresthesia

Ocular: Diplopia

Respiratory: Bronchospasm, epistaxis

Renal: Polyuria

Drug Interactions May produce severe hypertensive episodes when used with MAO inhibitors; may inhibit hypotensive effects of beta-adrenergic blocking agents; additive effects with other sympathomimetics, sedatives, alcohol, barbiturates, and other CNS depressants

Mechanism of Action Carbinoxamine competes with histamine for H_1-receptor sites on effector cells in the GI tract, blood vessels, and respiratory tract; pseudoephedrine directly stimulates alpha-adrenergic receptors of respiratory mucosa causing vasoconstriction; directly stimulates beta-adrenergic receptors causing bronchial relaxation, increased heart rate and contractility

Usual Dosage Oral:

Children: May dose according to pseudoephedrine component: 4 mg/kg/day **or** the carbinoxamine component: 0.2-0.4 mg/kg/day

Administration Oral: Do not crush or chew extended release tablets

Patient Information May cause drowsiness or impair ability to perform activities requiring mental alertness or physical coordination; may cause blurred vision; may also cause CNS excitation and difficulty sleeping; may cause dry mouth; avoid alcohol. May rarely cause photosensitivity reactions (eg, exposure to sunlight may cause severe sunburn, skin rash, redness, or itching); avoid direct exposure to sunlight

Dosage Forms Excipient information presented when available (limited, particularly for generics); consult specific product labeling. [DSC] = Discontinued product

Liquid:

Cordron-D NR: Carbinoxamine maleate 2 mg and pseudoephedrine hydrochloride 12.5 mg per 5 mL (480 mL) [cotton candy flavor] [DSC]

Pediatex™-D: Carbinoxamine maleate 2 mg and pseudoephedrine hydrochloride 20 mg per 5 mL (480 mL) [alcohol free, dye free, sugar free; cotton candy flavor] [DSC]

Solution: Carbinoxamine maleate 2 mg and pseudoephedrine hydrochloride 25 mg per 5 mL (480 mL) [DSC]

Carboxine-PSE: Carbinoxamine maleate 2 mg and pseudoephedrine hydrochloride 20 mg per 5 mL (480 mL) [peach flavor] [DSC]

Solution, oral drops:

Andehist NR: Carbinoxamine maleate 1 mg and pseudoephedrine hydrochloride 15 mg per mL (30 mL) [alcohol and sugar free; raspberry flavor] [DSC]

Carbaxefed RF: Carbinoxamine maleate 1 mg and pseudoephedrine hydrochloride 15 mg per mL (30 mL) [alcohol free; contains sodium benzoate; cherry flavor] [DSC]

Sildec: Carbinoxamine maleate 1 mg and pseudoephedrine hydrochloride 15 mg per mL (30 mL) [raspberry flavor] [DSC]

Syrup: Carbinoxamine maleate 2 mg and pseudoephedrine hydrochloride 25 mg per 5 mL (480 mL)

Hydro-Tussin™-CBX, Palgic®-DS [DSC]: Carbinoxamine maleate 2 mg and pseudoephedrine hydrochloride 25 mg per 5 mL (480 mL) [alcohol, dye, and sugar free; strawberry/pineapple flavor]

Tablet, timed release:

Palgic®-D: Carbinoxamine maleate 8 mg and pseudoephedrine hydrochloride 80 mg [dye free] [DSC]

♦ **Carbinoxamine Maleate** *see* Carbinoxamine *on page 285*

♦ **Carbocaine®** *see* Mepivacaine *on page 1005*

♦ **Carbolith™ (Can)** *see* Lithium *on page 948*

Carboplatin (KAR boe pla tin)

Medication Safety Issues

Sound-alike/look-alike issues:

Carboplatin may be confused with cisplatin, oxaliplatin

Paraplatin® may be confused with Platinol®

High alert medication: The Institute for Safe Medication Practices (ISMP) includes this medication among its list of drugs which have a heightened risk of causing significant patient harm when used in error.

Related Information

Compatibility of Chemotherapy and Related Supportive Care Medications *on page 1777*

Emetogenic Potential of Single Chemotherapeutic Agents *on page 1776*

U.S. Brand Names Paraplatin® [DSC]

Canadian Brand Names Paraplatin-AQ

Index Terms CBDCA; NSC-241240

Therapeutic Category Antineoplastic Agent, Alkylating Agent

Generic Available Yes

Use Treatment of ovarian carcinoma; treatment of small cell lung cancer, squamous cell carcinoma of the esophagus; solid tumors of the bladder, cervix and testes; pediatric brain tumor, neuroblastoma, bony and soft tissue sarcomas, germ cell tumors, and high-dose therapy with stem cell/bone marrow transplants

Pregnancy Risk Factor D

Lactation Excretion in breast milk unknown/contraindicated

Contraindications Hypersensitivity to carboplatin, cisplatin, any component, other platinum-containing compounds, or mannitol; severe bone marrow suppression or excessive bleeding

Warnings The FDA currently recommends that procedures for proper handling and disposal of antineoplastic agents be considered. When carboplatin is dosed using AUC as the endpoint, note that the calculated dose is the dose administered, not the dose based on body surface area

Precautions Bone marrow suppression, which may be severe, and vomiting are dose-related; high doses have also resulted in severe abnormalities of liver function; reduce dosage in patients with bone marrow suppression and impaired renal function (creatinine clearance values <60 mL/minute)

Adverse Reactions

Cardiovascular: Hypotension

Central nervous system: Pain

Dermatologic: Urticaria, rash, alopecia, pruritus, erythema

Endocrine & metabolic: Electrolyte abnormalities such as hypocalcemia, hypokalemia, hypomagnesemia

Gastrointestinal: Nausea, vomiting, diarrhea, anorexia, hemorrhagic colitis, mucositis, constipation, metallic taste

Hematologic: Neutropenia, leukopenia, thrombocytopenia (platelet count reaches a nadir between 14-21 days), anemia

Hepatic: Abnormal liver function tests

Neuromuscular & skeletal: Peripheral neuropathy, weakness

Otic: Tinnitus, hearing loss at high tones

Renal: Nephrotoxicity, elevated BUN and serum creatinine, hematuria

Respiratory: Bronchospasm, interstitial pneumonia

Miscellaneous: Anaphylactic-like reactions

Drug Interactions Aminoglycosides (increased ototoxicity and nephrotoxicity); nephrotoxic drugs (increased renal toxicity); decreases phenytoin serum levels

Stability Store unopened vials at room temperature; protect from light; after reconstitution, solutions are stable for 8 hours; 2 mg/mL solutions diluted in D_5W for infusion are stable for 24 hours; 7 mg/mL solutions diluted in NS for infusion are stable for 24 hours; aluminum reacts with carboplatin resulting in a precipitate and loss of potency

Mechanism of Action Platination of DNA results in possible cross-linking and interference with the function of DNA

Pharmacokinetics

Distribution: V_d: 16 L/kg

Protein binding: 0%; however, platinum is 30% protein bound

Half-life: Patients with Cl_{cr} >60 mL/minute: 2.5-5.9 hours

Elimination: ~60% to 80% is excreted renally

Usual Dosage I.V. (refer to individual protocols):

Infants and Children <3 years or ≤12 kg: Various protocols calculate dosage on the basis of body weight rather than body surface area

Children:

Solid tumor: 560 mg/m^2 once every 4 weeks

Sarcoma (bony/soft tissue): 400 mg/m^2/day for 2 days

Brain tumor: 175 mg/m^2 once weekly for 4 weeks with a 2-week recovery period between courses; dose is then adjusted on platelet count and neutrophil count values; courses should not be repeated until the platelet count is ≥100,000/mm^3 and the neutrophil count is ≥2000/mm^3

Bone marrow transplant preparative regimen: 500 mg/m^2/day for 3 days

Retinoblastoma: Subconjunctival injection of carboplatin for intraocular retinoblastoma has been administered using 1-2 mL of a 10 mg/mL solution per dose to affected eye(s)

Alternative carboplatin dosing: Some investigators calculate pediatric carboplatin doses using a modified Calvert formula: Dosing based on target AUC (modified Calvert formula for use in children): Total dose (mg) = [Target AUC (mg/mL/minute)] x [GFR (mL/minute) + (0.36 x body weight in kilograms)]

Note: Calvert formula was based on using chromic edetate (^{51}Cr-EDTA) plasma clearance to establish GFR. Some clinicians have recommended that methods for estimating Cl_{cr} not be substituted for GFR since carboplatin dosing based on such estimates may not be predictive.

Note: The dose of carboplatin calculated is TOTAL mg DOSE not mg/m^2

Adults:

Single agent: 360 mg/m^2 once every 4 weeks; dose is then adjusted on platelet count and neutrophil count values; courses should not be repeated until the platelet count is ≥100,000/mm^3 and the neutrophil count is ≥2000/mm^3

Calvert formula: See table

Calvert Formula for Carboplatin Dosing in Adults
Total dose (mg) = Target AUC(mg/mL/minute) x (GFR + 25)

Single Agent Carboplatin/No Prior Chemotherapy	Total dose (mg): 6-8 (GFR + 25)
Single Agent Carboplatin/Prior Chemotherapy	Total dose (mg): 4-6 (GFR + 25)
Combination Chemotherapy/No Prior Chemotherapy	Total dose (mg): 4.5-6 (GFR + 25)
Combination Chemotherapy/Prior Chemotherapy	Use a target AUC value <5 for the initial cycle

Dosing adjustment in renal impairment: Adults: Calvert formula (dosing adjustment for renal impairment is implied with this formula):

Total dose (mg) = [Target AUC (mg/mL/minute)] x [GFR (mL/minute) + 25]

Note: The dose of carboplatin calculated is TOTAL mg DOSE not mg/m^2; target AUC will vary depending upon: Number of agents in the regimen and treatment status (ie, previously untreated or treated)

Administration Parenteral: Administer by I.V. intermittent infusion over 15 minutes to 1 hour, or by continuous infusion (continuous infusion regimens may be less toxic than the bolus route); reconstituted carboplatin 10 mg/mL should be further diluted to a final concentration of 0.5-2 mg/mL with D_5W or NS for administration

Monitoring Parameters CBC with differential and platelet count, serum electrolytes, urinalysis, creatinine clearance, liver function tests

Nursing Implications Needle or intravenous administration sets containing aluminum parts should not be used in the administration or preparation of carboplatin (aluminum can interact with carboplatin resulting in precipitate formation and loss of potency)

Dosage Forms Excipient information presented when available (limited, particularly for generics); consult specific product labeling. [DSC] = Discontinued product

Injection, powder for reconstitution: 50 mg, 150 mg, 450 mg

Paraplatin®: 50 mg, 150 mg, 450 mg [DSC]

Injection, solution: 10 mg/mL (5 mL, 15 mL, 45 mL, 60 mL)

Paraplatin®: 10 mg/mL (5 mL, 15 mL, 45 mL, 60 mL) [DSC]

References

Abramson DH, Frank CM, and Dunkel IJ, "A Phase I/II Study of Subconjunctival Carboplatin for Intraocular Retinoblastoma," *Ophthalmology*, 1999, 106(10):1947-50.

Cairo MS, "The Use of Ifosfamide, Carboplatin, and Etoposide in Children With Solid Tumors," *Semin Oncol*, 1995, 22(3 Suppl 7):23-7.

Lovett D, Kelsen D, Eisenberger M, et al, "A Phase II Trial of Carboplatin and Vinblastine in the Treatment of Advanced Squamous Cell Carcinoma of the Esophagus," *Cancer*, 1991, 67(2):354-6.

Newell DR, Pearson AD, Balmanno K, et al, "Carboplatin Pharmacokinetics in Children: The Development of a Pediatric Dosing Formula. The United Kingdom Children's Cancer Study Group," *J Clin Oncol*, 1993, 11(12):2314-23.

Zeltzer PM, Epport K, Nelson MD Jr, et al, "Prolonged Response to Carboplatin in an Infant With Brain Stem Glioma," *Cancer*, 1991, 67(1):43-7.

♦ **Carboxine-PSE [DSC]** *see* Carbinoxamine and Pseudoephedrine *on page 286*

♦ **Cardene®** *see* NiCARdipine *on page 1130*

Carmustine (kar MUS teen)

Medication Safety Issues

Sound-alike/look-alike issues:

Carmustine may be confused with lomustine

High alert medication: The Institute for Safe Medication Practices (ISMP) includes this medication among its list of drugs which have a heightened risk of causing significant patient harm when used in error.

Related Information

Compatibility of Chemotherapy and Related Supportive Care Medications *on page 1777*

Emetogenic Potential of Single Chemotherapeutic Agents *on page 1776*

U.S. Brand Names BiCNU®; Gliadel®

Canadian Brand Names BiCNU®; Gliadel Wafer®

Index Terms BCNU; bis-chloronitrosourea; Carmustinum; NSC-409962; WR-139021

Therapeutic Category Antineoplastic Agent, Alkylating Agent (Nitrosourea)

Generic Available No

Use

Injection: Treatment of brain tumors, multiple myeloma, Hodgkin's disease, and non-Hodgkin's lymphomas; some activity in malignant melanoma, lung and colon cancer

Wafer (implant): Adjunct to surgery in patients with high grade malignant glioma or in patients with recurrent glioblastoma multiforme

Pregnancy Risk Factor D

Lactation Excretion in breast milk unknown/not recommended

Contraindications Hypersensitivity to carmustine or any component

Warnings The FDA currently recommends that procedures for proper handling and disposal of antineoplastic agents be considered. Bone marrow suppression, notably thrombocytopenia and leukopenia, may lead to bleeding and overwhelming infection in an already compromised patient; myelosuppressive effects will last for at least 6 weeks after a dose, do not give courses more frequently than every 6 weeks because the toxicity is cumulative; pulmonary toxicity is more common in patients receiving a cumulative dose >1400 mg/m^2, patients with recent mediastinal irradiation, and in patients with a past history of lung disease; delayed-onset pulmonary fibrosis has occurred up to 17 years after carmustine treatment in children and adolescents; acute leukemia has been reported in patients receiving long-term carmustine.

Cases of intracerebral mass effect unresponsive to corticosteroids, including one case leading to brain herniation, have been reported. Monitor patients receiving Gliadel® implant for seizures, intracranial infections, abnormal wound healing, and brain edema. Carmustine injection diluent contains absolute alcohol which can cause an "alcohol flushing syndrome" in susceptible patients; use with caution in patients with aldehyde dehydrogenase-2 deficiency.

Precautions Administer with caution to patients with depressed platelet, leukocyte or erythrocyte counts and in patients with renal or hepatic impairment; dosage reduction is recommended in patients with compromised bone marrow function (decreased leukocyte and platelet counts)

Adverse Reactions

Cardiovascular: Flushing; high dose (≥300 mg/m^2) can produce hypotension, tachycardia, confusion, chest pain

Central nervous system: Ataxia, dizziness, seizures, fever, headache

Dermatologic: Dermatitis, hyperpigmentation, alopecia, rash

Gastrointestinal: Nausea, vomiting, diarrhea, esophagitis, anorexia, mucositis, metallic taste

Hematologic: Myelosuppression (leukopenia, thrombocytopenia) with nadir at 28 days, anemia

Hepatic: Hepatotoxicity, elevated liver enzymes and serum bilirubin, jaundice, veno-occlusive disease with high doses

Local: Pain and thrombophlebitis at injection site, burning sensation

Ocular: Retinitis, optic neuritis

Renal: Renal failure, azotemia

Respiratory: Pulmonary fibrosis, cough, dyspnea, tachypnea

Drug Interactions Cimetidine (potentiates myelosuppressive effects); may potentiate hepatotoxicity with high doses of acetaminophen; may decrease serum digoxin and phenytoin levels; metronidazole (disulfiram reaction)

Stability Store vial in refrigerator; protect from light and heat; discard vial if oily film is found on the bottom of the vial; reconstituted solution is stable for 8 hours at room temperature, 24 hours when refrigerated, or 48 hours when refrigerated after further dilution in D_5W or NS in a glass bottle to a concentration of 0.2 mg/mL; incompatible with sodium bicarbonate; adsorption of carmustine to plastics and polyvinyl chloride-based infusion containers has been documented. Store Gliadel® wafers at or below -20°C (-4°F).

Mechanism of Action Inhibits key enzymatic reactions involved with DNA synthesis; carbamoylation of amine groups on proteins; interferes with the normal function of DNA by alkylation and forms DNA-protein cross-links

Pharmacokinetics

Distribution: Readily crosses the blood-brain barrier since it is highly lipid soluble; CSF:plasma ratio >90%; distributes into breast milk

Protein binding: 75%

Metabolism: Denitrosation through action of microsomal enzymes; some enterohepatic circulation occurs

Half-life, terminal: 20-70 minutes (active metabolites may persist for days)

Elimination: ~60% to 70% excreted as metabolites in the urine and 6% to 10% excreted as CO_2 by the lungs

Usual Dosage

I.V. infusion (refer to individual protocols):

Children: 200-250 mg/m^2 every 4-6 weeks as a single dose; next dose is to be determined based on clinical and hematologic response to the previous dose (a repeat course should not be given until platelets are >100,000/mm^3 and leukocytes are >4000/mm^3)

BMT-conditioning agent: 300-600 mg/m^2 over at least 2 hours or may be divided into 2 doses administered 12 hours apart or 100 mg/m^2 every 12 hours for 6 doses

Adults: 150-200 mg/m^2 every 6 weeks as a single dose or divided into 75-100 mg/m^2/dose on 2 successive days; next dose is to be determined based on clinical and hematologic response to the previous dose (a repeat course should not be given until platelets are >100,000/mm^3 and leukocytes are >4000/mm^3)

Intracranial implant (wafer): Adults: Place 8 wafers (total dose: 61.6 mg) in the resection cavity; should the size and shape not accommodate 8 wafers, the maximum number of wafers as allowed should be placed

Administration Parenteral: Reconstitute 100 mg vial with 3 mL sterile dehydrated (absolute) alcohol followed by addition of 27 mL SWI. Further dilute the 3.3 mg of carmustine per mL solution with NS or D_5W in a glass or polyolefin container to a final concentration of 0.2-1 mg/mL and administer by I.V. infusion over 1-2 hours to prevent vein irritation; rapid I.V. carmustine infusion may result in flushing, hypotension, and agitation; carmustine has also been administered over 15-45 minutes diluted in 100-250 mL D_5W with monitoring for vein irritation; burning sensation and pain at I.V. site can be decreased with reduction of infusion rate and further dilution of solution or placing ice pack on I.V. site; flush line before and after carmustine administration to ensure vein patency

Monitoring Parameters CBC with differential and platelet count; pulmonary function, liver function, and renal function tests; monitor blood pressure and infusion site during administration

Patient Information Report occurrence of fever, sore throat, unusual bleeding or bruising to physician; may discolor skin brown; women of childbearing potential should avoid becoming pregnant while on carmustine therapy

Nursing Implications Must administer in glass containers; do not mix or administer with solutions containing sodium bicarbonate; accidental skin contact may cause transient burning and brown discoloration of the skin

Additional Information Myelosuppressive effects:

WBC: Moderate (nadir: 5-6 weeks)

Platelets: Severe (nadir: 4-5 weeks)

Dosage Forms Excipient information presented when available (limited, particularly for generics); consult specific product labeling.

Injection, powder for reconstitution:

BiCNU®: 100 mg [packaged with 3 mL of absolute alcohol as diluent]

Wafer, implant:

Gliadel®: 7.7 mg (8s)

(Continued)

Carmustine *(Continued)*

References

Aronin PA, Mahaley MS Jr, Rudnick SA, et al, "Prediction of BCNU Pulmonary Toxicity in Patients With Malignant Gliomas," *N Engl J Med*, 1980, 303(4):183-8.

Colvin M, Hartner J and Summerfield M, "Stability of Carmustine in the Presence of Sodium Bicarbonate," *Am J Hosp Pharm*, 1980, 37(5):677-8.

Dunkel IJ, Garvin JH Jr, Goldman S, et al, "High Dose Chemotherapy With Autologous Bone Marrow Rescue for Children With Diffuse Pontine Brain Stem Tumors. Children's Cancer Group," *J Neurooncol*, 1998, 37(1):67-73.

O'Driscoll BR, Hasleton PS, Taylor PM, et al, "Active Lung Fibrosis Up to 17 Years After Chemotherapy With Carmustine (BCNU) in Childhood," *N Engl J Med*, 1990, 323(6):378-82.

♦ **Carmustinum** *see* Carmustine *on page 290*

Carnitine (KAR ni teen)

Medication Safety Issues

Sound-alike/look-alike issues:

Levocarnitine may be confused with levocabastine

U.S. Brand Names Carnitor®; Carnitor® SF

Canadian Brand Names Carnitor®

Index Terms L-Carnitine

Therapeutic Category Nutritional Supplement

Generic Available Yes

Use Treatment of primary or secondary carnitine deficiency; prevention and treatment of carnitine deficiency (injection) in patients undergoing dialysis for end-stage renal disease (ESRD)

Pregnancy Risk Factor B

Lactation Excretion in breast milk unknown/use caution

Contraindications Hypersensitivity to carnitine or any component

Precautions Use with caution in patients with seizure disorders; both new onset seizure activity and increased frequency of seizures have been reported. Safety and efficacy of oral carnitine has not been established in ESRD. Chronic administration of high doses of oral carnitine in patients with severely compromised renal function or ESRD on dialysis may result in accumulation of potentially toxic metabolites, trimethylamine and trimethylamine-N-oxide.

Adverse Reactions

Cardiovascular: I.V. use: Hypertension (18% to 21%), chest pain (6% to 15%), tachycardia (5% to 9%), palpitation, atrial fibrillation, ECG abnormality

Central nervous system: Myasthenia (in uremic patients on D,L-carnitine not L-carnitine), dizziness, fever, depression, seizures, headache, vertigo

Dermatologic: Rash

Endocrine & metabolic: Parathyroid disorder

Gastrointestinal: Nausea, vomiting, abdominal cramps, diarrhea, gastritis, taste perversion, anorexia

Neuromuscular & skeletal: Weakness, paresthesia, myasthenia (mild)

Respiratory: Cough, rhinitis, bronchitis

Miscellaneous: Body odor (dose-related), allergic reactions

Drug Interactions D,L-carnitine sold in health food stores as vitamin B_T, competitively inhibits L-carnitine

Stability Store at room temperature; protect from light

Mechanism of Action Endogenous substance required in energy metabolism; facilitates long chain fatty acid entry into the mitochondria; modulates intracellular coenzyme A homeostasis; carnitine deficiency exists when there is insufficient carnitine to buffer toxic acyl-Co A compounds; secondary carnitine deficiency may be a consequence of inborn errors of metabolism

Pharmacokinetics

Metabolism: Major metabolites: Trimethylamine, trimethylamine-N-oxide and acylcarnitine

Half-life, terminal: Adults: 17.4 hours

Bioavailability:

Tablet: 15.1% ± 5.3%

Solution: 15.9% ± 4.9%

Time to peak serum concentration: Oral: 3.3 hours

Elimination: Renal excretion of free and conjugated metabolites (acylcarnitine)

Clearance: 4 L/hour

Excretion: Urine 76% with 4% to 9% as unchanged drug; feces <1%

Usual Dosage

Primary carnitine deficiency:

Oral:

Children: 50-100 mg/kg/day divided 2-3 times/day, maximum 3 g/day; dosage must be individualized based upon patient response; higher dosages have been used

Adults: 330-990 mg/dose 2-3 times/day; maximum: 3 g/day

I.V.: Children and Adults: 50 mg/kg as a loading dose, followed (in severe cases) by 50 mg/kg/day infusion; maintenance: 50 mg/kg/day divided every 4-6 hours, increase as needed to a maximum of 300 mg/kg/day

ESRD patients on hemodialysis: Adults: I.V.: Predialysis carnitine levels below normal (30-60 micromoles): 10-20 mg/kg after each dialysis session; maintenance doses as low as 5 mg/kg may be used after 3-4 weeks of therapy depending upon response (carnitine level); National Kidney Foundation guidelines recommend basing treatment on clinical signs and symptoms; evaluate response at 3-month intervals and discontinue if no clinical improvement noted within 9-12 months.

Supplement to parenteral nutrition: I.V.: Neonates: 10-20 mg/kg/day in parenteral nutrition solution

Administration

Oral: Dilute in beverages or liquid food; administer with meals; consume slowly

Parenteral: May be administered by direct I.V. infusion over 2-3 minutes or as a continuous infusion diluted to 0.5-8 mg/mL in LR or NS

Monitoring Parameters Serum triglycerides, fatty acids, and carnitine levels

Reference Range Plasma free carnitine level: >20 micromoles/L; plasma total carnitine level 30-60 micromoles/L; to evaluate for carnitine deficiency determine the plasma acylcarnitine/free carnitine ratio (A/F ratio)

A/F ratio = [plasma total carnitine - free carnitine] divided by free carnitine

Normal plasma A/F ratio = 0.25; in carnitine deficiency A/F ratio >0.4

Additional Information Routine prophylactic use of carnitine in children receiving valproic acid to avoid carnitine deficiency and hepatotoxicity is probably not indicated

Dosage Forms Excipient information presented when available (limited, particularly for generics); consult specific product labeling.

Capsule: 250 mg

Injection, solution: 200 mg/mL (5 mL, 12.5 mL)

Carnitor®: 200 mg/mL (5 mL)

Solution, oral: 100 mg/mL (118 mL)

Carnitor®: 100 mg/mL (118 mL) [cherry flavor]

Carnitor® SF: 100 mg/mL (118 mL) [sugar free; cherry flavor]

Tablet: 330 mg, 500 mg

Carnitor®: 330 mg

References

Bonner CM, De Brie KL, Hug G, et al, "Effects of Parenteral L-Carnitine Supplementation on Fat Metabolism and Nutrition in Premature Neonates," *J Pediatr*, 1995, 126(2):287-92.

Borum PR, "Carnitine in Neonatal Nutrition," *J Child Neurol*, 1995, 10(Suppl 2):S25-31.

Eknoyan G, Latos DL, and Lindberg J, "Practice Recommendations for the Use of L-carnitine in Dialysis-Related Carnitine Disorder. National Kidney Foundation Carnitine Consensus Conference," *Am J Kidney Dis*, 2003, 41(4):868-76.

Helms RA, Mauer EC, and Hay WW Jr, "Effect of Intravenous L-Carnitine on Growth Parameters and Fat Metabolism During Parenteral Nutrition in Neonates," *JPEN J Parenter Enteral Nutr*, 1990, 14(5):448-53.

- **Carnitor®** *see* Carnitine *on page 292*
- **Carnitor® SF** *see* Carnitine *on page 292*
- **Carrington Antifungal [OTC]** *see* Miconazole *on page 1056*
- **Carter's Little Pills® (Can)** *see* Bisacodyl *on page 217*
- **Cartia XT™** *see* Diltiazem *on page 503*

Carvedilol (KAR ve dil ole)

Medication Safety Issues

Sound-alike/look-alike issues:

Carvedilol may be confused with captopril, carteolol

International issues:

Talliton® [Hungary] may be confused with Talacen® which is a brand name for pentazocine/acetaminophen combination in the U.S.

Related Information

Antihypertensive Agents by Class *on page 1678*

U.S. Brand Names Coreg®; Coreg CR™

Canadian Brand Names Apo-Carvedilol®; Coreg®; Novo-Carvedilol; PMS-Carvedilol; RAN™-Carvedilol; ratio-Carvedilol

Therapeutic Category Antihypertensive Agent; Beta-Adrenergic Blocker, Nonselective With Alpha-Blocking Activity

Generic Available No

(Continued)

Carvedilol *(Continued)*

Use Treatment of mild to severe CHF of cardiomyopathic or ischemic origin (usually in addition to standard therapy); management of hypertension; reduction of cardiovascular mortality in patients with left ventricular dysfunction following MI

Pregnancy Risk Factor C (D in 2nd and 3rd trimesters)

Lactation Excretion in breast milk unknown/not recommended

Contraindications Hypersensitivity to carvedilol or any component; bronchial asthma or related bronchospastic conditions; sick sinus syndrome, second or third degree heart block, or severe bradycardia (except in patients with a functioning artificial pacemaker); cardiogenic shock; decompensated cardiac failure requiring intravenous inotropic therapy; severe hepatic impairment

Warnings May cause bradycardia, hypotension, postural hypotension, or syncope; to decrease risk of significant hypotension or syncope, initiate carvedilol cautiously and monitor closely while slowly titrating dose upwards; worsening of CHF or fluid retention may occur; adjustment of dose or other medications (eg, diuretics) may be required. Due to risk of syncope, avoid driving or hazardous tasks during initiation of therapy.

Beta blockers may block hypoglycemia-induced tachycardia and blood pressure changes; nonselective beta blockers may augment the insulin-induced hypoglycemia and delay the recovery of serum glucose concentrations; use with caution in patients with diabetes mellitus; worsening hyperglycemia may occur (monitor serum glucose). Use with caution in patients with peripheral vascular disease (may aggravate arterial insufficiency); use caution with anesthetic agents that decrease myocardial function. May mask signs of hyperthyroidism (eg, tachycardia); exacerbation of hyperthyroidism or thyroid storm may occur if beta blockers are abruptly discontinued. Exacerbation of angina, arrhythmias, and in some cases MI may occur following abrupt discontinuation of beta blockers; avoid abrupt discontinuation, wean carvedilol slowly over 1-2 weeks, monitor for signs and symptoms of ischemia.

Deterioration of renal function may rarely occur in patients with CHF receiving carvedilol; patients with underlying renal dysfunction, diffuse vascular disease, ischemic heart disease or low blood pressure (eg, adults with systolic blood pressure <100 mm Hg) may be at risk; monitor renal function closely in these patients; decrease carvedilol dose or discontinue drug if renal function worsens.

Precautions Use with caution in patients with pheochromocytoma or Prinzmetal's variant angina. Beta blockers should be avoided in patients with bronchospastic disease (see Contraindications); if administered to patients, use the lowest possible dose and monitor patients carefully. Patients who have a history of severe anaphylactic hypersensitivity reactions to various substances may be more reactive while receiving beta blockers; these patients may not be responsive to the normal doses of epinephrine used to treat hypersensitivity reactions. Use caution with concurrent use of verapamil or diltiazem (bradycardia or heart block can occur). Safety and efficacy in children <18 years of age have not been established.

Adverse Reactions

Cardiovascular: Hypotension, bradycardia, syncope, postural hypotension, edema, hypertension, AV block, angina, palpitations

Central nervous system: Dizziness, fatigue, headache, fever, paresthesia, somnolence, insomnia, malaise

Endocrine & metabolic: Hyperglycemia, weight gain, hypercholesterolemia, hypertriglyceridemia

Gastrointestinal: Diarrhea, nausea, vomiting

Hematologic: Thrombocytopenia

Hepatic: Elevated liver enzymes

Neuromuscular & skeletal: Asthenia, arthralgia, paresthesia

Ocular: Blurred vision

Renal: Elevated BUN, decreased renal function (rare; see Warnings)

Respiratory: Increased cough, nasopharyngitis, rhinitis, nasal congestion, sinus congestion

Drug Interactions Cytochrome P450 isoenzyme CYP 1A2 (minor), CYP2C19 (minor), CYP2C9 (major), CYP2D6 (major), CYP2E1 (minor) and CYP3A4 (minor) substrate

Carvedilol may increase serum concentrations of cyclosporine or digoxin (monitor serum concentrations and adjust dosage as needed); cimetidine and other enzyme inhibitors may increase carvedilol serum concentrations; although not studied, inhibitors of CYP2D6 (eg, fluoxetine, paroxetine, propafenone, quinidine) may increase the serum concentrations of R(+) carvedilol; rifampin and other enzyme inducers may significantly decrease serum carvedilol concentrations; concurrent use with catecholamine-depleting agents (eg, reserpine or MAO inhibitors) may increase risk of hypotension or severe bradycardia (monitor closely); use with clonidine may potentiate effects (hypotension, bradycardia); abrupt withdrawal of clonidine while receiving beta blockers may result in an exaggerated hypertensive crisis; concurrent use with verapamil, diltiazem, or similar calcium channel blockers may result in conduction disturbances or hypotension (monitor closely); beta blockers may enhance the effects of insulin and oral hypoglycemic agents in reducing blood sugar and may mask symptoms of hypoglycemia (monitor blood glucose closely). Ethanol may affect the release properties of the extended release capsule and cause a faster rate of release (separate administration by at least 2 hours).

Food Interactions

Immediate release tablets: Food decreases the rate, but not the extent of absorption.

Extended release capsules: Compared with a standard meal, a high fat meal increases AUC and peak serum concentrations by ~20%; administration on an empty stomach decreases AUC by 27% and peak serum concentrations by 43%. In adults, administration of capsule contents on applesauce decreases the rate, but not the extent of absorption.

Stability

Immediate release tablets: Store below 30°C (86°F); protect from moisture; dispense in tightly closed, light resistant container

Extended release capsules: Store at controlled room temperature; dispense in tightly closed, light resistant container

Mechanism of Action Nonselective beta-adrenergic blocker with alpha-adrenergic blocking activity. Available as a racemic mixture; the S(-) enantiomer possesses the nonselective beta-adrenoreceptor blocking activity, while the alpha-adrenergic blocking activity is present in both R(+) and S(-) enantiomers at equal potency. Does not possess intrinsic sympathomimetic activity.

Associated effects in hypertensive patients include reduction of cardiac output, reduction of exercise- or beta agonist-induced tachycardia, reduction of reflex orthostatic tachycardia, vasodilation, decreased peripheral vascular resistance (especially in standing position), decreased renal vascular resistance, reduced plasma renin activity, and increased levels of atrial natriuretic peptide. In CHF patient, associated effects include decreased systemic blood pressure, decreased pulmonary capillary wedge pressure, decreased pulmonary artery pressure, decreased heart rate, decreased systemic vascular resistance, decreased right arterial pressure, increased stroke volume index, and increased left ventricular ejection fraction.

Pharmacodynamics Oral:

Onset of action:
- Alpha-blockade: Within 30 minutes
- Beta-blockade: Within 1 hour

Maximum effect: Antihypertensive effect, multiple dosing: 7-14 days

Pharmacokinetics

Absorption: Oral: Rapid and extensive, but with large first pass effect; first pass effect is stereoselective with R(+) enantiomer achieving plasma concentrations 2-3 times higher than S(-) enantiomer

Distribution: Distributes into extravascular tissues
- V_d: Adults: 115 L

Protein binding: >98%, primarily to albumin

Metabolism: Extensively metabolized in the liver, primarily via cytochrome P450 isoenzymes CYP2D6 and CYP2C9 and to a lesser extent via CYP3A4, CYP2C19, CYP1A2 and CYP2E1; metabolized predominantly by aromatic ring oxidation and glucuronidation; oxidative metabolites undergo conjugation via glucuronidation and sulfation; three active metabolites (4′-hydroxyphenyl metabolite is 13 times more potent than parent drug for beta blocking activity; however, active metabolites achieve plasma concentrations of only 1/10 of those for carvedilol). Metabolism is subject to genetic polymorphism; CYP2D6 poor metabolizers have a 2-3 fold higher plasma concentration of the R(+) enantiomer and a 20% to 25% increase in the S(-) enantiomer compared to extensive metabolizers.

Bioavailability: Immediate release tablets: 25% to 35%; extended release capsules: 85% of immediate release; bioavailability is increased in patients with CHF

Half-life:
- (Laer, 2002):
  - Infants and children 6 weeks of age to 3.5 years (n = 8): 2.2 hours
  - Children 5.5-19 years (n = 7): 3.6 hours
  - Adults 24-37 years (n = 9): 5.2 hours
- (Manufacturer):
  - Adults (in general): 7-10 hours
  - R(+)-carvedilol: 5-9 hours
  - S(-)-carvedilol: 7-11 hours

Time to peak serum concentration: Extended release capsules: 5 hours

Elimination: <2% excreted unchanged in urine; metabolites are excreted via bile, into the feces

Dialysis: Hemodialysis does not significantly clear carvedilol

(Continued)

Carvedilol *(Continued)*

Usual Dosage Oral: **Note:** Individualize dosage for each patient; monitor patients closely during initiation and upwards titration of dose; reduce dosage if bradycardia or hypotension occurs

Infants and Children: **Heart Failure:** Immediate release tablets: Dose not established. Several case series and smaller studies have used a wide range of initial and target maintenance doses.

Although retrospective, the largest pediatric study to date (n = 46; age range 3 months to 19 years) used mean initial doses of 0.08 mg/kg/dose given twice daily. Doses were increased as tolerated by doubling the dose every 2 weeks. The dose was increased over a mean of 11 weeks to a mean maintenance dose of 0.46 mg/kg/dose given twice daily (see Bruns, 2001). Another retrospective study of 24 patients (mean age: 7.2 ± 6.4 years) used mean initial doses of 0.075 mg/kg/dose given twice daily. Doses were increased by 50% to 100% every 1-2 weeks with a target dose of 0.5 mg/kg/dose given twice daily. The mean maintenance dose achieved (after a median of 14 weeks of titration) was 0.98 mg/kg/day given in 2 divided doses per day (see Rusconi, 2004).

A large prospective randomized placebo controlled trial of 150 pediatric patients ranging in age from birth to 17 years will compare two doses of carvedilol. The following doses will be used. Initial: 0.05 mg/kg/dose given twice daily; maximum initial dose: 3.125 mg twice daily. Doses will be increased as tolerated by doubling the dose every 2 weeks until the target dose is attained. The "low dose" target dose will be 0.2 mg/kg/dose given twice daily; maximum: 12.5 mg twice daily. The "high dose" target dose will be 0.4 mg/kg/dose given twice daily; maximum: 25 mg twice daily (See Shady, 2002).

Note: Due to faster carvedilol elimination, 3 times daily dosing and a higher target dose per kg may be needed in young children (eg, <3.5 years) (see Laer, 2002). Further studies are needed to establish the optimal pediatric dose.

Adults:

CHF: Note: Prior to initiating therapy, other CHF medications should be stabilized and fluid retention minimized.

Immediate release tablets: Initial: 3.125 mg twice daily for 2 weeks; if tolerated, may increase to 6.25 mg twice daily. May double the dose every 2 weeks to the highest dose tolerated by patient.

Maximum recommended dose:

Mild to moderate heart failure:

<85 kg: 25 mg twice daily

>85 kg: 50 mg twice daily

Severe heart failure: 25 mg twice daily

Extended release capsules: Initial: 10 mg once daily for 2 weeks; if tolerated, may double the dose every 2 weeks up to 80 mg once daily; maintain on lower dose if higher dose is not tolerated.

Hypertension: Note: Use standing systolic blood pressure measured ~1 hour after dose as a guide for tolerance and trough blood pressure as a guide for efficacy.

Immediate release tablets: Initial: 6.25 mg twice daily; if tolerated, dose should be maintained for 1-2 weeks, then increased to 12.5 mg twice daily as needed. Dosage may be increased after 1-2 weeks if tolerated, to a maximum of 25 mg twice daily; maximum dose: 50 mg/day

Extended release capsules: Initial: 20 mg once daily; if tolerated, dose should be maintained for 1-2 weeks, then increased to 40 mg once daily as needed. Dosage may be increased after 1-2 weeks if tolerated, to 80 mg once daily; maximum dose: 80 mg once daily.

Left ventricular dysfunction following MI: Note: Initiate only after patient is hemodynamically stable and fluid retention has been minimized.

Immediate release tablets: Initial: 3.125-6.25 mg twice daily; use lower dose listed in patients with low blood pressure, low heart rate, or fluid retention; increase dosage incrementally (eg, from 6.25 to 12.5 mg twice daily) at intervals of 3-10 days, as tolerated, to a target dose of 25 mg twice daily.

Extended release capsules: Initial: 20 mg once daily; increase dosage incrementally (eg, from 20 mg to 40 mg once daily) at intervals of 3-10 days, as tolerated, to a target dose of 80 mg once daily; maintain on lower dose if higher dose is not tolerated.

Dosing adjustment in renal impairment: None recommended. **Note:** Mean AUCs were 40% to 50% higher in patients with moderate to severe renal dysfunction who received immediate release carvedilol, but the ranges of AUCs were similar to patients with normal renal function

Dosing adjustment in hepatic impairment: Use is contraindicated in patients with severe liver dysfunction, as drug is extensively metabolized by the liver. **Note:** Patients with cirrhotic liver disease achieved carvedilol serum concentrations 4-7

fold higher than normal patients following a single dose of immediate release carvedilol

Administration

Immediate release tablets: Administer with food to decrease the risk of orthostatic hypotension.

Extended release capsules: Administer with food, preferably in the morning; do not crush or chew capsule, swallow whole. Capsule may be opened and contents sprinkled on a spoonful of applesauce; swallow applesauce/medication mixture immediately; do not chew; do not store for later use; do not use warm applesauce; drink fluids after dose to make sure mixture is completely swallowed. Separate administration from alcohol consumption (including alcohol containing prescription and nonprescription medications) by at least 2 hours.

Monitoring Parameters Heart rate, blood pressure (seated and standing base); weight, BUN, serum creatinine, liver function, serum glucose, cholesterol, and triglycerides

Patient Information May cause fatigue, dizziness, low blood pressure (especially when standing), or fainting; rise slowly from sitting or lying position; may impair ability to perform activities requiring mental alertness or physical coordination; report unresolved swelling of extremities, weight gain, dizziness, fatigue, or fainting to healthcare provider; if diabetic, monitor serum glucose closely (drug may alter glucose tolerance or mask signs of hypoglycemia). Do not drink alcohol, or take prescription or nonprescription medications containing alcohol, 2 hours before or after taking the controlled release capsule (Coreg CR™); serious adverse effects may occur.

Nursing Implications Due to its alpha-blocking effects, carvedilol decreases blood pressure more in the standing position than in the supine position; be aware that postural hypotension and syncope may occur (see Warnings)

Additional Information Cytochrome P450 isoenzyme CYP2D6 poor metabolizers may have a higher rate of dizziness during initiation and upwards titration of carvedilol, perhaps due to the higher serum concentrations of the alpha blocking R(+) enantiomer and resulting vasodilation.

CHF: Carvedilol is a nonselective beta blocker with alpha-blocking and antioxidant properties. It is the only beta blocker approved in adults for the treatment of heart failure. Beta blocker therapy, without intrinsic sympathomimetic activity, should be initiated in adult patients with **stable** CHF (NYHA Class II-IV). To date, carvedilol, sustained release metoprolol, and bisoprolol have demonstrated a beneficial effect on morbidity and mortality. It is important that beta blocker therapy be instituted initially at very low doses with gradual and very careful titration. Because carvedilol has alpha-adrenergic blocking effects, it may lower blood pressure to a greater extent. The definitive clinical benefits of the antioxidant property are not known at this time.

Coreg CR™ extended release capsules are hard gelatin capsules filled with immediate-release and controlled-release microparticles containing carvedilol phosphate; the microparticles are drug-layered and coated with methacrylic acid copolymers.

Dosage Forms Excipient information presented when available (limited, particularly for generics); consult specific product labeling.

Capsule, extended release; as phosphate:
- Coreg CR™: 10 mg, 20 mg, 40 mg, 80 mg

Tablet:
- Coreg®: 3.125 mg, 6.25 mg, 12.5 mg, 25 mg

Extemporaneous Preparations Stability information of liquid carvedilol preparations has not been published, but is available from the manufacturer (see below). Two studies have used aqueous preparations. One study used a liquid suspension by dissolving one 3.125 mg tablet in 3 mL of water (see Bruns, 2001). A second study briefly mentions making a 1 mg/mL solution in water, details were not provided (see Rusconi, 2004).

Carvedilol oral liquid suspensions (0.1 mg/mL and 1.67 mg/mL) made from tablets, water, Ora-Plus®, and Ora-Sweet® were stable for 12 weeks when stored in glass amber bottles at room temperature (25°C); use one 3.125 mg tablet for the 0.1 mg/mL suspension or two 25 mg tablets for the 1.67 mg/mL suspension; grind the tablet(s) and compound a mixture with 5 mL of water, 15 mL Ora-Plus®, and 10 mL Ora-Sweet®; final volume of each suspension: 30 mL; label "shake well"; microbial testing at 5 and 12 weeks showed <10 colony forming units/mL for both aerobic count and the total combined mold and yeast count (data on file, GlaxoSmithKline, Philadelphia, PA: DOF #132).

References

Azeka E, Franchini Ramires JA, Valler C, et al, "Delisting of Infants and Children From the Heart Transplantation Waiting List After Carvedilol Treatment," *J Am Coll Cardiol*, 2002, 40(11):2034-8.

Bruns LA and Canter CE, "Should Beta-Blockers be Used for the Treatment of Pediatric Patients With Chronic Heart Failure?" *Paediatr Drugs*, 2002, 4(12):771-8.

Bruns LA, Chrisant MK, Lamour JM, et al, "Carvedilol as Therapy in Pediatric Heart Failure: An Initial Multicenter Experience," *J Pediatr*, 2001, 138(4):505-11.

(Continued)

Carvedilol *(Continued)*

Gachara N, Prabhakaran S, Srinivas S, et al, "Efficacy and Safety of Carvedilol in Infants With Dilated Cardiomyopathy: A Preliminary Report," *Indian Heart J*, 2001, 53(1):74-8.
Giardini A, Formigari R, Bronzetti G, et al, "Modulation of Neurohormonal Activity After Treatment of Children in Heart Failure With Carvedilol," *Cardiol Young*, 2003, 13(4):333-6.
Laer S, Mir TS, Behn F, et al, "Carvedilol Therapy in Pediatric Patients With Congestive Heart Failure: A Study Investigating Clinical and Pharmacokinetic Parameters," *Am Heart J*, 2002, 143(5):916-22.
Ratnapalan S, Griffiths K, Costei AM, et al, "Digoxin-Carvedilol Interactions in Children," *J Pediatr*, 2003, 142(5):572-4.
Rusconi P, Gomez-Marin O, Rossique-Gonzalez M, et al, "Carvedilol in Children With Cardiomyopathy: 3-Year Experience at a Single Institution," *J Heart Lung Transplant*, 2004, 23(7):832-8.
Shaddy RE, Curtin EL, Sower B, et al, "The Pediatric Randomized Carvedilol Trial in Children With Heart Failure: Rationale and Design," *Am Heart J*, 2002, 144(3):383-9.

Cascara (kas KAR a)

Index Terms Cascara Sagrada
Therapeutic Category Laxative, Stimulant
Generic Available Yes
Use Temporary relief of constipation; sometimes used with milk of magnesia ("black and white" mixture)
Pregnancy Risk Factor C
Contraindications Nausea, vomiting, abdominal pain, fecal impaction, intestinal obstruction, GI bleeding, appendicitis, CHF
Warnings Long-term use may result in laxative dependence
Adverse Reactions
Cardiovascular: Faintness
Endocrine & metabolic: Electrolyte and fluid imbalance
Gastrointestinal: Abdominal cramps, nausea, diarrhea, benign pigmentation of the colonic mucosa (with prolonged use)
Genitourinary: Discoloration of urine (reddish, pink, or brown)
Stability Protect from light and heat
Mechanism of Action Direct chemical irritation of the intestinal mucosa resulting in an increased rate of colonic motility and change in fluid and electrolyte secretion
Pharmacodynamics Onset of action: 6-10 hours
Pharmacokinetics
Absorption: Oral: Small amount from small intestine
Metabolism: In the liver
Usual Dosage Oral (**aromatic** fluid extract):
Infants: 1.25 mL/day as a single dose (range: 0.5-2 mL) as needed
Children 2-11 years: 2.5 mL/day as a single dose (range: 1-3 mL) as needed
Children ≥12 years and Adults: 5 mL/day (range: 2-6 mL) as needed at bedtime
Administration Oral: Administer on an empty stomach at bedtime; drink plenty of fluids
Patient Information Should not be used regularly for more than 1 week; may discolor urine reddish, pink, or brown
Additional Information Cascara sagrada fluid extract is 5 times more potent than cascara sagrada aromatic fluid extract
Dosage Forms Excipient information presented when available (limited, particularly for generics); consult specific product labeling.
Aromatic fluid extract: 120 mL, 473 mL
Tablet: 325 mg

♦ **Cascara Sagrada** *see* Cascara *on page 298*

Caspofungin (kas poe FUN jin)

Related Information
Assessment of Liver Function *on page 1810*
U.S. Brand Names Cancidas®
Canadian Brand Names Cancidas®
Index Terms Caspofungin Acetate
Therapeutic Category Antifungal Agent, Echinocandin; Antifungal Agent, Systemic
Generic Available No
Use Treatment of invasive aspergillosis in patients who are refractory to or intolerant of other therapies (ie, amphotericin B, lipid formulations of amphotericin B, and/or itraconazole); candidemia, intra-abdominal abscess, peritonitis, and pleural space infection caused by susceptible *Candida* species; esophageal candidiasis; empiric therapy of presumed fungal infection in febrile neutropenic patients
Pregnancy Risk Factor C
Lactation Excretion in breast milk unknown/use caution

Contraindications Hypersensitivity to caspofungin or any component

Warnings Transient elevations of alanine transaminase (ALT) and aspartate transaminase (AST) have been reported with concomitant use of caspofungin and cyclosporine (avoid concurrent use of cyclosporine).

Precautions Use with caution and modify dose in patients with moderate hepatic impairment; use with caution and modify dose in patients on concurrent drugs which induce drug clearance such as efavirenz, nevirapine, phenytoin, dexamethasone, carbamazepine, or rifampin (see Drug Interactions)

Adverse Reactions

Cardiovascular: Facial swelling, peripheral edema, flushing

Central nervous system: Chills, fever, headache, insomnia

Dermatologic: Rash, pruritus, erythema

Endocrine & metabolic: Hypokalemia, hypercalcemia, hypomagnesemia

Gastrointestinal: Diarrhea, vomiting, nausea, abdominal pain

Hematologic: Eosinophilia, anemia, decreased hemoglobin, neutropenia, thrombocytopenia, leukopenia

Hepatic: Elevated alkaline phosphatase, ALT, AST, serum bilirubin; hepatic impairment

Local: Phlebitis, thrombophlebitis

Neuromuscular & skeletal: Tremor, paresthesia, myalgia

Renal: Elevated creatinine, proteinuria, hematuria

Respiratory: Bronchospasm, dyspnea

Miscellaneous: Anaphylaxis, flu-like syndrome, ARDS, diaphoresis

Drug Interactions Decreases blood concentration of tacrolimus (monitor tacrolimus blood concentrations); cyclosporine may increase caspofungin concentrations and AUC by 35% (see Warnings); rifampin may decrease caspofungin trough concentrations by 30% (adjust caspofungin daily dose; eg, in adults, increase caspofungin dose to 70 mg/day); efavirenz, nevirapine, phenytoin, dexamethasone, or carbamazepine may decrease caspofungin concentration (adjust caspofungin daily dose)

Stability Store lyophilized vial in refrigerator at 2°C to 8°C (36°F to 46°F); reconstitute 50 mg or 70 mg vial with the appropriate volume of NS (consult manufacturer's prescribing information for details); reconstituted solution may be stored in the refrigerator for 1 hour prior to preparation of the infusion solution; final infusion solution may be stored at room temperature (≤25°C or ≤77°F) for 24 hours or for 48 hours in the refrigerator; caspofungin is not stable in dextrose-containing solutions

Mechanism of Action Inhibits synthesis of beta (1,3)-D-glucan, an essential cell wall component of susceptible fungi

Pharmacokinetics

Protein binding: 97% to albumin

Metabolism: Via hydrolysis and N-acetylation in the liver; undergoes spontaneous chemical degradation to an open-ring peptide and hydrolysis to amino acids

Half-life: Adults: Beta (distribution): 9-11 hours; terminal: 40-50 hours; beta phase half-life is 32% to 43% lower in pediatric patients than in adult patients

Elimination: 35% of dose excreted in feces, 41% of dose excreted in urine; 1.4% of dose excreted unchanged in urine

Dialysis: Not dialyzable

Usual Dosage I.V.: Safety and efficacy in pediatric patients has not been established

Note: Caspofungin treatment duration should be based on patient status and clinical response. Empiric therapy should be given until neutropenia resolves. In neutropenic patients, continue treatment for at least 7 days after both signs and symptoms of infection and neutropenia resolve. In patients with positive cultures, continue treatment for at least 14 days after the last positive culture.

Children 2-11 years: Loading dose: 70 mg/m²/day on day 1, maximum dose: 70 mg; followed by 50 mg/m²/day, maximum dose: 50 mg, once daily thereafter

Children >12 years, Adolescents, and Adults: Loading dose: 70 mg on day 1, followed by 50 mg once daily thereafter; 70 mg daily dose has been administered and well tolerated in patients not clinically responding to the daily 50 mg dose; may need to adjust dose in patients receiving a concomitant enzyme inducer

Esophageal candidiasis: 50 mg once daily

Patients receiving concomitant enzyme inducer:

Patients receiving rifampin: 70 mg caspofungin once daily

Patients receiving carbamazepine, dexamethasone, phenytoin, nevirapine, or efavirenz: May require an increase in caspofungin dose to 70 mg once daily

Dosing adjustment in renal impairment: No adjustment needed

Dosing adjustment in hepatic impairment:

Mild hepatic impairment (Child-Pugh score 5 to 6): No dosage adjustment necessary

Moderate hepatic impairment (Child-Pugh score 7 to 9): Decrease daily dose by 30%

(Continued)

Caspofungin *(Continued)*

Administration Parenteral: I.V.: Administer by slow I.V. infusion over 1 hour at a maximum concentration of 0.47 mg/mL diluted in NS, LR, 0.45% sodium chloride, or 0.225% sodium chloride injection. Do not mix or coinfuse with other medications. **Do not use** diluents containing dextrose.

Monitoring Parameters Periodic liver function tests, serum potassium, CBC, hemoglobin

Nursing Implications Infuse slowly over 1 hour; possible histamine-related reactions have been reported (monitor during infusion)

Dosage Forms Excipient information presented when available (limited, particularly for generics); consult specific product labeling.

Injection, powder for reconstitution, as acetate: 50 mg [contains sucrose 39 mg], 70 mg [contains sucrose 54 mg]

References

Walsh TJ, Adamson PC, Seibel NL, et al, "Pharmacokinetics (PK) of Caspofungin (CAS) in Pediatric Patients (#M-896)," 42nd Interscience Conference on Antimicrobial Agents and Chemotherapy, San Diego, CA, Sept 27-30, 2002.

Walsh TJ, Adamson PC, Seibel NL, et al, "Pharmacokinetics, Safety, and Tolerability of Caspofungin in Children and Adolescents," *Antimicrob Agents Chemother*, 2005, 49(11):4536-45.

Walsh TJ, Teppler H, Donowitz GR, et al, "Caspofungin Versus Liposomal Amphotericin B for Empirical Antifungal Therapy in Patients With Persistent Fever and Neutropenia," *N Engl J Med*, 2004, 351(14):1391-402.

♦ **Caspofungin Acetate** *see* Caspofungin *on page 298*

Castor Oil (KAS tor oyl)

Index Terms Oleum Ricini

Therapeutic Category Laxative, Stimulant

Generic Available Yes: Oil

Use Preparation for rectal or bowel examination or surgery; rarely used to relieve constipation; also applied to skin as emollient and protectant

Pregnancy Risk Factor X

Contraindications Hypersensitivity to castor oil; nausea, vomiting, abdominal pain, fecal impaction, GI bleeding, appendicitis, CHF, menstruation, dehydration

Warnings Long-term use may result in laxative dependence

Adverse Reactions

Central nervous system: Dizziness

Endocrine & metabolic: Electrolyte disturbance, dehydration

Gastrointestinal: Abdominal cramps, nausea, diarrhea

Stability Protect from heat (emulsion should be protected from freezing)

Mechanism of Action Acts primarily in the small intestine; hydrolyzed to ricinoleic acid which reduces net absorption of fluid and electrolytes and stimulates peristalsis

Pharmacodynamics Onset of action: Oral: Within 2-6 hours

Usual Dosage Oral:

Castor oil:

- Infants <2 years: 1-5 mL or 15 mL/m^2/dose as a single dose
- Children 2-11 years: 5-15 mL as a single dose
- Children ≥12 years and Adults: 15-60 mL as a single dose

Emulsified castor oil:

- Infants: 2.5-7.5 mL/dose
- Children:
  - <2 years: 5-15 mL/dose
  - 2-11 years: 7.5-30 mL/dose
- Children ≥12 years and Adults: 30-60 mL/dose

Administration Oral: Do not administer at bedtime because of rapid onset of action; chill or administer with milk, juice or carbonated beverage to improve palatability; administer on an empty stomach; castor oil emulsions should be shaken well before use

Monitoring Parameters I & O, serum electrolytes, stool frequency

Dosage Forms Excipient information presented when available (limited, particularly for generics); consult specific product labeling.

Oil, oral: 100% (60 mL, 120 mL, 180 mL, 480 mL, 3840 mL)

♦ **Cataflam®** *see* Diclofenac *on page 486*
♦ **Catapres®** *see* Clonidine *on page 389*
♦ **Catapres-TTS®** *see* Clonidine *on page 389*
♦ **Cathflo® Activase®** *see* Alteplase *on page 83*
♦ **Caverject®** *see* Alprostadil *on page 81*
♦ **Caverject Impulse®** *see* Alprostadil *on page 81*
♦ **CaviRinse™** *see* Fluoride *on page 675*

- **CB-1348** *see* Chloramubucil *on page 333*
- **CBDCA** *see* Carboplatin *on page 288*
- **CBZ** *see* Carbamazepine *on page 279*
- **CCNU** *see* Lomustine *on page 951*
- **CD271** *see* Adapalene *on page 57*
- **2-CdA** *see* Cladribine *on page 373*
- **CDDP** *see* Cisplatin *on page 366*
- **Ceclor® (Can)** *see* Cefaclor *on page 301*
- **Cecon® [OTC]** *see* Ascorbic Acid *on page 159*
- **CEE** *see* Estrogens (Conjugated/Equine) *on page 610*
- **CeeNU®** *see* Lomustine *on page 951*

Cefaclor (SEF a klor)

Medication Safety Issues
Sound-alike/look-alike issues:
Cefaclor may be confused with cephalexin

U.S. Brand Names Raniclor™

Canadian Brand Names Apo-Cefaclor®; Ceclor®; Novo-Cefaclor; Nu-Cefaclor; PMS-Cefaclor

Therapeutic Category Antibiotic, Cephalosporin (Second Generation)

Generic Available Yes: Excludes chewable tablet

Use Infections caused by susceptible bacteria including *Staph aureus*, *S. pneumoniae*, *S. pyogenes*, and *H. influenzae* (excluding β-lactamase negative, ampicillin-resistant strains); treatment of otitis media, sinusitis, and infections involving the respiratory tract, skin and skin structure, bone and joint; treatment of urinary tract infections caused by *E. coli*, *Klebsiella*, and *Proteus mirabilis*

Pregnancy Risk Factor B

Lactation Enters breast milk/use caution

Contraindications Hypersensitivity to cefaclor, any component, or cephalosporins

Warnings Prolonged use may result in superinfection; do not use in patients with immediate-type hypersensitivity reactions to penicillin

Precautions Use with caution in patients with impaired renal function, history of colitis, or history of penicillin hypersensitivity; modify dosage in patients with severe renal impairment. Chewable tablets contain aspartame which is metabolized to phenylalanine and must be avoided (or used with caution) in patients with phenylketonuria.

Adverse Reactions
Central nervous system: Dizziness, agitation, insomnia, confusion, fever
Dermatologic: Rash, urticaria, pruritus, erythema multiforme, Stevens-Johnson syndrome, toxic epidermal necrolysis, angioedema
Gastrointestinal: Nausea, vomiting, diarrhea, pseudomembranous colitis
Genitourinary: Genital moniliasis, vaginitis
Hematologic: Eosinophilia, neutropenia, aplastic anemia, agranulocytosis, thrombocytopenia
Hepatic: Elevated liver enzymes, cholestatic jaundice
Renal: Interstitial nephritis
Miscellaneous: Anaphylaxis (rare); serum sickness-like reaction (estimated incidence ranges from 0.024% to 0.2% per drug course); majority of reactions have occurred in children <5 years of age with symptoms of fever, rash, erythema multiforme, and arthralgia, often occurring during the second or third exposure

Drug Interactions Probenecid (increased cefaclor concentration)

Food Interactions Capsules and suspension: Food or milk delays and decreases peak concentration

Stability Store capsule, chewable tablet, and unreconstituted powder for oral suspension at room temperature. Refrigerate suspension after reconstitution; discard after 14 days.

Mechanism of Action Inhibits bacterial cell wall synthesis by binding to one or more of the penicillin-binding proteins and interfering with the final transpeptidation step of peptidoglycan synthesis resulting in cell wall death

Pharmacokinetics
Absorption: Oral: Well absorbed; acid stable
Distribution: Distributes into tissues and fluids including bone, pleural and synovial fluid; crosses the placenta; appears in breast milk
Protein binding: 25%
Half-life: 30-60 minutes (prolonged with renal impairment)
Time to peak serum concentration:
Capsule: 60 minutes
Suspension and chewable tablet: 45-60 minutes

(Continued)

Cefaclor *(Continued)*

Elimination: Most of dose (80%) excreted unchanged in urine by glomerular filtration and tubular secretion

Dialysis: Moderately dialyzable (20% to 50%)

Usual Dosage Oral:

Children >1 month: 20-40 mg/kg/day divided every 8-12 hours; maximum dose: 2 g/day (twice daily option is for treatment of otitis media or pharyngitis)

Otitis media: 40 mg/kg/day divided every 12 hours

Pharyngitis: 20 mg/kg/day divided every 12 hours

Adults: 250-500 mg every 8 hours

Dosing adjustment in renal impairment: Cl_{cr} <10 mL/minute: Administer 50% of dose

Administration Oral:

Capsule, suspension: Administer 1 hour before or 2 hours after a meal; shake suspension well before use

Tablet, chewable: Administer 1 hour before or 2 hours after a meal; chew tablet before swallowing

Monitoring Parameters With prolonged therapy, monitor CBC and stool frequency periodically

Test Interactions Positive Coombs' [direct], false-positive urine glucose (Clinitest®), false ↑ of serum or urine creatinine

Patient Information Counsel patient that cefaclor should only be used to treat bacterial infections. Entire course of medication should be taken even if patient feels better early in the course. Report persistent diarrhea to physician.

Dosage Forms Excipient information presented when available (limited, particularly for generics); consult specific product labeling.

Capsule: 250 mg, 500 mg

Powder for oral suspension: 125 mg/5 mL (75 mL, 150 mL); 250 mg/5 mL (75 mL, 150 mL); 375 mg/5 mL (50 mL, 100 mL)

Tablet, chewable:

Raniclor™: 250 mg [contains phenylalanine 5.6 mg/tablet and tartrazine; fruity flavor]; 375 mg [contains phenylalanine 8.4 mg/tablet and tartrazine; fruity flavor]

Tablet, extended release: 500 mg

References

Boguniewicz M and Leung DYM, "Hypersensitivity Reactions to Antibiotics Commonly Used in Children," *Pediatr Infect Dis J*, 1995, 14(3):221-31.

Hyslop DL, "Cefaclor Safety Profile: A Ten Year Review," *Clin Ther*, 1988, 11(Suppl A):83-94.

Levine LR, "Quantitative Comparison of Adverse Reactions to Cefaclor vs Amoxicillin in a Surveillance Study," *Pediatr Infect Dis*, 1985, 4(4):358-61.

Cefadroxil (sef a DROKS il mon o HYE drate)

U.S. Brand Names Duricef®

Canadian Brand Names Apo-Cefadroxil®; Duricef®; Novo-Cefadroxil

Index Terms Cefadroxil Monohydrate

Therapeutic Category Antibiotic, Cephalosporin (First Generation)

Generic Available Yes

Use Treatment of susceptible bacterial infections including group A beta-hemolytic streptococcal pharyngitis or tonsillitis; skin and soft tissue infections caused by streptococci or staphylococci; urinary tract infections caused by *Klebsiella*, *E. coli*, and *Proteus mirabilis*

Pregnancy Risk Factor B

Lactation Enters breast milk (small amounts)/use caution (AAP rates "compatible")

Contraindications Hypersensitivity to cefadroxil, any component, or cephalosporins

Warnings Prolonged use may result in superinfection; do not use in patients with immediate-type hypersensitivity reaction to penicillin

Oral suspension contains sodium benzoate; benzoic acid (benzoate) is a metabolite of benzyl alcohol; large amounts of benzyl alcohol (≥99 mg/kg/day) have been associated with a potentially fatal toxicity ("gasping syndrome") in neonates; the "gasping syndrome" consists of metabolic acidosis, respiratory distress, gasping respirations, CNS dysfunction (including convulsions, intracranial hemorrhage), hypotension and cardiovascular collapse; use cefadroxil oral suspensions containing sodium benzoate with caution in neonates; *in vitro* and animal studies have shown that benzoate displaces bilirubin from protein binding sites

Precautions Use with caution in patients who are hypersensitive to penicillin; modify dosage in patients with renal impairment

Adverse Reactions

Dermatologic: Rash

Gastrointestinal: Nausea, vomiting, diarrhea, pseudomembranous colitis

Genitourinary: Vaginitis
Hematologic: Transient neutropenia

Drug Interactions Probenecid may decrease renal tubular secretion and increase cefadroxil serum concentrations

Food Interactions Concomitant administration with food, infant formula, or cow's milk does **not** significantly affect absorption

Stability Refrigerate suspension after reconstitution; discard after 14 days

Mechanism of Action Interferes with bacterial cell wall synthesis during active replication, causing cell wall death and resultant bactericidal activity against susceptible bacteria

Pharmacokinetics

Absorption: Oral: Rapid; well absorbed from GI tract
Distribution: V_d: 0.31 L/kg; crosses the placenta; appears in breast milk
Protein binding: 20%
Half-life: 1-2 hours; 20-24 hours in renal failure
Time to peak serum concentration: Within 70-90 minutes
Elimination: >90% of dose excreted unchanged in urine within 24 hours

Usual Dosage Oral:

Infants and Children: 30 mg/kg/day divided twice daily up to a maximum of 2 g/day
Adolescents and Adults: 1-2 g/day in 1-2 divided doses; maximum dose for adults: 4 g/day

Dosing interval in renal impairment:

Cl_{cr} 10-25 mL/minute: Administer every 24 hours
Cl_{cr} <10 mL/minute: Administer every 36 hours

Administration Oral: May be administered without regard to food; administration with food may decrease nausea or vomiting; shake suspension well before use

Monitoring Parameters Stool frequency, resolution of infection

Test Interactions Positive Coombs' [direct], false-positive with urinary glucose tests using cupric sulfate (Clinitest®, Benedict's solution)

Patient Information Report persistent diarrhea; entire course of medication (eg, 10-14 days) should be taken to ensure eradication of organism

Dosage Forms Excipient information presented when available (limited, particularly for generics); consult specific product labeling. [DSC] = Discontinued product

Capsule, as monohydrate: 500 mg
Duricef®: 500 mg [DSC]

Powder for oral suspension, as monohydrate: 250 mg/5 mL (50 mL, 100 mL); 500 mg/5 mL (75 mL, 100 mL)
Duricef®: 250 mg/5 mL (50 mL, 100 mL); 500 mg/5 mL (75 mL, 100 mL) [contains sodium benzoate; orange-pineapple flavor]

Tablet, as monohydrate: 1 g
Duricef®: 1 g [DSC]

♦ **Cefadroxil Monohydrate** *see* Cefadroxil *on page 302*

Cefazolin (sef A zoe lin)

Medication Safety Issues

Sound-alike/look-alike issues:
Cefazolin may be confused with cefprozil, cephalexin, cephalothin
Kefzol® may be confused with Cefzil®

Related Information

Endocarditis Prophylaxis *on page 1812*

Index Terms Cefazolin Sodium

Therapeutic Category Antibiotic, Cephalosporin (First Generation)

Generic Available Yes

Use Treatment of respiratory tract, skin and skin structure, urinary tract, biliary tract, bone and joint infections and septicemia due to susceptible gram-positive cocci (except enterococcus); some gram-negative bacilli including *E. coli*, *Proteus*, and *Klebsiella* may be susceptible; perioperative prophylaxis; bacterial endocarditis prophylaxis for dental and upper respiratory procedures

Pregnancy Risk Factor B

Lactation Enters breast milk (small amounts)/use caution (AAP rates "compatible")

Contraindications Hypersensitivity to cefazolin sodium, any component, or cephalosporins

Warnings Prolonged use may result in superinfection; do not use in patients with immediate-type hypersensitivity reactions to penicillin

Precautions Use with caution in patients with a history of colitis, renal or hepatic impairment, poor nutritional state, patients previously stabilized on anticoagulant therapy, or in patients with a history of hypersensitivity to penicillins; modify dosage in patients with renal impairment

(Continued)

Cefazolin *(Continued)*

Adverse Reactions

Central nervous system: Fever, CNS irritation, seizures

Dermatologic: Rash, urticaria, pruritus, Stevens-Johnson syndrome

Gastrointestinal: Nausea, vomiting, diarrhea, pseudomembranous colitis, oral candidiasis

Hematologic: Leukopenia, thrombocytopenia, eosinophilia, neutropenia

Hepatic: Transient elevation of liver enzymes, hepatitis

Local: Thrombophlebitis, pain at injection site

Renal: Elevated BUN and serum creatinine; renal failure

Miscellaneous: Anaphylaxis

Drug Interactions Probenecid may decrease renal tubular secretion and increase cefazolin serum concentrations; nephrotoxic agents

Stability Store intact vials at room temperature; protect from light. Reconstituted solution is stable for 24 hours at room temperature or 10 days when refrigerated; thawed solutions of the commercially available frozen cefazolin injections are stable for 48 hours at room temperature or 10 days when refrigerated

Mechanism of Action Inhibits bacterial cell wall synthesis by binding to one or more of the penicillin-binding proteins and interfering with the final transpeptidation step of peptidoglycan synthesis resulting in cell wall death

Pharmacokinetics

Distribution: Crosses the placenta; small amounts appear in breast milk; CSF penetration is poor; penetrates bone and synovial fluid well; distributes into bile

Protein binding: 74% to 86%

Metabolism: Hepatic is minimal

Half-life:

- Neonates: 3-5 hours
- Adults: 90-150 minutes (prolonged with renal impairment)

Time to peak serum concentration:

- I.M.: Within 0.5-2 hours
- I.V.: Within 5 minutes

Elimination: 80% to 100% excreted unchanged in urine

Dialysis: Moderately dialyzable (20% to 50%)

Usual Dosage I.M., I.V.:

Neonates:

- Postnatal age ≤7 days: 40 mg/kg/day divided every 12 hours
- Postnatal age >7 days:
  - ≤2000 g: 40 mg/kg/day divided every 12 hours
  - >2000 g: 60 mg/kg/day divided every 8 hours

Infants and Children: 50-100 mg/kg/day divided every 8 hours; maximum dose: 6 g/day

- Bacterial endocarditis prophylaxis for dental and upper respiratory procedures in penicillin allergic patients (see Precautions): 25 mg/kg 30 minutes before procedure; maximum dose: 1 g

Adults: 0.5-2 g every 6-8 hours; maximum dose: 12 g/day

- UTI: 1 g every 12 hours
- Bacterial endocarditis prophylaxis for dental and upper respiratory procedures in penicillin allergic patients (see Precautions): 1 g 30 minutes before procedure
- Perioperative prophylaxis: 1 g 30-60 minutes prior to surgery; 0.5-1 g every 8 hours for 24 hours postoperatively depending on the procedure

Dosing interval in renal impairment:

- Cl_{cr} 10-30 mL/minute: Administer every 12 hours
- Cl_{cr} <10 mL/minute: Administer every 24 hours

Administration Parenteral:

I.V.: Cefazolin may be administered IVP over 3-5 minutes at a maximum concentration of 100 mg/mL or I.V. intermittent infusion over 10-60 minutes at a final concentration for I.V. administration of 20 mg/mL. In fluid-restricted patients, a concentration of 138 mg/mL has been administered IVP.

I.M.: Deep I.M. injection into a large muscle mass. May dilute vial using SWI to a final concentration between 225-330 mg/mL (see package insert). Shake well before use.

Monitoring Parameters Renal function periodically when used in combination with other nephrotoxic drugs, hepatic function tests, and CBC; prothrombin time in patients at risk

Test Interactions False-positive urine glucose using Clinitest®, positive Coombs' [direct], false ↑ serum or urine creatinine

Additional Information Sodium content of 1 g: 2 mEq

Dosage Forms Excipient information presented when available (limited, particularly for generics); consult specific product labeling.

Infusion [premixed in D_5W]: 1 g (50 mL)

Injection, powder for reconstitution: 500 mg, 1 g, 10 g, 20 g

References

Dajani AS, Taubert KA, Wilson WW, et al, "Prevention of Bacterial Endocarditis. Recommendations by the American Heart Association," *JAMA*, 1997, 277(22):1794-801.

Pickering LK, O'Connor DM, Anderson D, et al, "Clinical and Pharmacologic Evaluation of Cefazolin in Children," *J Infect Dis* 1973, 128(Suppl):S407-1.

Robinson DC, Cookson TL, and Grisafe JA, "Concentration Guidelines for Parenteral Antibiotics in Fluid-Restricted Patients," *Drug Intell Clin Pharm*, 1987, 21(12):985-9.

♦ **Cefazolin Sodium** *see* Cefazolin *on page 303*

Cefdinir (SEF di ner)

U.S. Brand Names Omnicef®

Canadian Brand Names Omnicef®

Index Terms CFDN

Therapeutic Category Antibiotic, Cephalosporin (Third Generation)

Generic Available No

Use Infections caused by susceptible organisms including *S. pneumoniae* (penicillin-susceptible strains only; inadequate activity against resistant pneumococcus), *H. influenzae* (including beta-lactamase-producing strains), *H. parainfluenzae* (including beta-lactamase-producing strains), *M. catarrhalis* (including beta-lactamase-producing strains), *S. aureus* (inactive against methicillin-resistant staphylococci), and *S. pyogenes*; treatment of infections involving the respiratory tract, skin and skin structure, and otitis media

Pregnancy Risk Factor B

Lactation Excretion in breast milk unknown/use caution

Contraindications Hypersensitivity to cefdinir, any component, or cephalosporins

Warnings Pseudomembranous colitis has been reported with cefdinir; prolonged use may result in superinfection; serum sickness-like reactions have been reported with signs and symptoms occurring after a few days of therapy and resolving a few days after drug discontinuation. Discontinue cefdinir if an allergic reaction occurs. Powder for oral suspension contains sodium benzoate; benzoic acid (benzoate) is a metabolite of benzyl alcohol; large amounts of benzyl alcohol (≥99 mg/kg/day) have been associated with a potentially fatal toxicity ("gasping syndrome") in neonates; avoid use of cefdinir products containing sodium benzoate in neonates; *in vitro* and animal studies have shown that benzoate displaces bilirubin from protein binding sites

Precautions Use with caution in patients with impaired renal function, history of colitis, or in penicillin-sensitive patients; modify dosage in patients with severe renal impairment

Adverse Reactions

Central nervous system: Headache, hyperactivity, insomnia, somnolence, seizures, dizziness

Dermatologic: Rash, pruritus, diaper rash, Stevens-Johnson syndrome, erythema multiforme, toxic epidermal necrolysis

Gastrointestinal: Diarrhea, nausea, vomiting, abdominal pain, pseudomembranous colitis, dyspepsia

Genitourinary: Vaginitis, microhematuria, vaginal moniliasis

Hematologic: Leukopenia, neutropenia, hemolytic anemia, eosinophilia, thrombocytopenia

Hepatic: Elevated AST, ALT, alkaline phosphatase; cholestatic jaundice, prolonged PT, hepatitis

Renal: Elevated BUN/serum creatinine, acute renal failure

Miscellaneous: Serum sickness-like reactions, anaphylaxis

Drug Interactions Probenecid increases cefdinir serum levels; aluminum- or magnesium-containing antacids decrease cefdinir absorption by 40%; iron decreases cefdinir absorption by 80%

Food Interactions Total absorption is not affected by food. Iron-fortified infant formula has no significant effect on cefdinir absorption (cefdinir can be administered with iron-fortified infant formula)

Stability Store at room temperature; reconstituted suspension stable for 10 days at room temperature

Mechanism of Action Inhibits bacterial cell wall synthesis by binding to one or more of the penicillin-binding proteins resulting in disruption of cell wall synthesis and cell lysis

Pharmacokinetics

Absorption: High-fat meal decreases extent of absorption by 10%

Distribution: Penetrates into blister fluid, middle ear fluid, tonsils, sinus, and lung tissues

V_d:

Children 6 months to 12 years: 0.67 L/kg

(Continued)

Cefdinir *(Continued)*

Adults: 0.35 L/kg
Protein binding: 60% to 70%
Bioavailability:
Capsules: 16% to 21%
Suspension: 25%
Half-life, elimination: 1.7 (± 0.6) hours with normal renal function
Time to peak serum concentration: 2-4 hours
Elimination: 11.6% to 18.4% of a dose is excreted unchanged in urine
Dialysis: ~63% is removed by hemodialysis (4 hours duration)

Usual Dosage Oral:

Infants and Children (≥6 months to 12 years):
- Otitis media or pharyngitis/tonsillitis: 14 mg/kg/day divided every 12 hours for 5-10 days or 14 mg/kg/day once daily for 10 days; maximum: 600 mg/day
- Skin and skin structure infection: 14 mg/kg/day divided twice daily for 10 days; maximum: 600 mg/day
- Acute maxillary sinusitis: 14 mg/kg/day divided every 12 hours for 10 days or 14 mg/kg/day once daily for 10 days; maximum: 600 mg/day

Children >12 years and Adults:
- Acute exacerbations of chronic bronchitis or pharyngitis/tonsillitis: 600 mg once daily for 10 days or 300 mg every 12 hours for 5-10 days
- Skin and skin structure infection or community-acquired pneumonia: 300 mg every 12 hours for 10 days
- Acute maxillary sinusitis: 600 mg once daily for 10 days or 300 mg every 12 hours for 10 days

Dosing adjustment in renal impairment: Cl_{cr} <30 mL/minute:
- Children ≥6 months to 12 years: 7 mg/kg/dose once daily
- Adults: 300 mg once daily
- Patients receiving hemodialysis: 300 mg or 7 mg/kg/dose starting at the conclusion of each hemodialysis session with subsequent doses every other day

Administration Oral: May administer with or without food; administer with food if stomach upset occurs; administer cefdinir at least 2 hours before or after antacids or iron supplements; shake suspension well before use

Monitoring Parameters Evaluate renal function before and during therapy; with prolonged therapy, monitor coagulation tests, CBC, and liver function test periodically

Test Interactions Positive Coombs' [direct]; may produce false-positive reaction to urine glucose with Clinitest®; may produce false-positive reaction for ketones in the urine with tests using nitroprusside

Patient Information Report persistent diarrhea to physician; may discolor stools red if taken with iron

Additional Information Oral suspension contains 2.86 g of sucrose per teaspoon.

Dosage Forms Excipient information presented when available (limited, particularly for generics); consult specific product labeling.

Capsule: 300 mg
Powder for oral suspension: 125 mg/5 mL (60 mL, 100 mL) [contains sodium benzoate and sucrose 2.86 g/5 mL; strawberry flavor]; 250 mg/5 mL (60 mL, 100 mL) [contains sodium benzoate and sucrose 2.86 g/5 mL; strawberry flavor]

References

Klein JO and McCracken GH Jr, "Summary: Role of a New Oral Cephalosporin, Cefdinir, for Therapy of Infections of Infants and Children," *Pediatr Infect Dis J*, 2000, 19(12 Suppl):S181-3.
Perry CM and Scott LJ, "Cefdinir: A Review of Its Use in the Management of Mild-to-Moderate Bacterial Infections," *Drugs*, 2004, 64(13):1433-64.

Cefepime (SEF e pim)

U.S. Brand Names Maxipime®

Canadian Brand Names Maxipime®

Index Terms Cefepime Hydrochloride

Therapeutic Category Antibiotic, Cephalosporin (Fourth Generation)

Generic Available No

Use Treatment of lower respiratory tract infections, cellulitis, other skin and soft tissue infections, and urinary tract infections; empiric monotherapy in febrile neutropenia; considered a fourth generation cephalosporin because it is active against aerobic gram-negative bacteria, including *Pseudomonas aeruginosa*, active against some gram-negative bacteria that are resistant to third-generation cephalosporins, and more active than third-generation cephalosporins against gram-positive bacteria such as *Staphylococcus aureus*

Pregnancy Risk Factor B

Lactation Enters breast milk/use caution

Contraindications Hypersensitivity to cefepime, any component, or cephalosporins

Warnings Modify dosage in patients with severe renal impairment; prolonged use may result in superinfection; use with caution in patients with penicillin hypersensitivity; do not use in patients with immediate-type hypersensitivity reactions to penicillin

Adverse Reactions

Central nervous system: Headache, lightheadedness, fever, encephalopathy
Dermatologic: Maculopapular rash, pruritus, urticaria
Gastrointestinal: Dyspepsia, diarrhea, nausea, vomiting, pseudomembranous colitis
Hematologic: Neutropenia after extended therapy, transient leukopenia and thrombocytopenia, agranulocytosis, eosinophilia, anemia
Hepatic: Transient elevations in LFTs
Local: Phlebitis
Ocular: Blurred vision
Renal: Elevated BUN, elevated serum creatinine
Miscellaneous: Anaphylaxis including anaphylactic shock

Drug Interactions Probenecid decreases the clearance of cefepime; aminoglycosides increase nephrotoxic potential

Stability Store vial at room temperature and protect from light; incompatible with metronidazole, vancomycin, aminoglycosides, and aminophylline

Mechanism of Action Inhibits bacterial cell wall synthesis by binding to one or more of the penicillin-binding proteins; inhibits the final transpeptidation step of peptidoglycan synthesis in bacterial cell walls

Pharmacokinetics

Distribution: V_d:
- Infants (PCA <30 weeks): 0.51 L/kg
- Children (2 months to 6 years): 0.32-0.35 L/kg
- Adults: 14-20 L; penetrates into inflammatory fluid at concentrations ~80% of serum levels and into bronchial mucosa at levels ~60% of plasma levels; excreted in breast milk at very low concentrations

Protein binding: 16% to 19%
Metabolism: Very little
Half-life:
- Children 2 months to 6 years: 1.77-1.96 hours
- Adults: 2 hours

Elimination: At least 85% eliminated as unchanged drug in urine
Dialysis: 45% to 68% removed by hemodialysis

Usual Dosage I.M., I.V.:

Neonates <14 days of age: 30 mg/kg/dose every 12 hours should provide antibiotic exposure equivalent to or greater than 50 mg/kg/dose every 8 hours used in older infants and children

Children 2 months to 16 years, ≤40 kg in weight: 50 mg/kg/dose every 12 hours
- Febrile neutropenic patients: 50 mg/kg/dose every 8 hours
- Cefepime has been studied in 12 cystic fibrosis patients (ages 4-41 years) with bronchopulmonary infection at a dose of 50 mg/kg/dose every 8 hours (maximum dose: 2 g/dose every 8 hours); cefepime was as effective as cefotaxime in 90 children <15 years of age who were randomized to receive cefepime 50 mg/kg/dose every 8 hours (n=43) or cefotaxime 50 mg/kg/dose every 6 hours (n=47) for the treatment of bacterial meningitis

Adults: 1-2 g every 12 hours; high doses or more frequent administration may be required in pseudomonal infections
- UTIs: 500 mg every 12 hours
- Empiric monotherapy in febrile neutropenia: 2 g every 8 hours

Dosing Adjustment in Renal Impairment, Adults

Cl_{cr} (mL/min)	Infection		
	Mild to Moderate	Moderate to Severe	Severe
30-60	0.5-1 g I.M./I.V. every 24 hours	1-2 g I.V. every 24 hours	2 g I.V. every 24 hours
11-29	0.5 g I.M./I.V. every 24 hours	0.5-1 g I.V. every 24 hours	1 g I.V. every 24 hours
≤10	0.25 g I.M./I.V. every 24 hours	0.25-0.5 g I.V. every 24 hours	0.5 g I.V. every 24 hours

Administration Parenteral:

I.V.: Cefepime may be administered by I.V. intermittent infusion over 20-30 minutes; final concentration for I.V. administration should not exceed 40 mg/mL in D_5W, NS, $D_{10}W$, D_5/NS, or D_5/LR; in clinical trials, cefepime was administered by direct I.V. injection over 3-5 minutes at a final concentration of 100 mg/mL for mild to moderate infections

(Continued)

Cefepime *(Continued)*

I.M.: Deep I.M. injection. May dilute vial using SWI, NS, D_5W, or 0.5% or 1% lidocaine to a final concentration of 280 mg/mL (see package insert)

Monitoring Parameters With prolonged therapy, monitor renal and hepatic function periodically; number and type of stools/day for diarrhea; CBC with differential

Test Interactions Positive Coombs' [direct]; may falsely elevate creatinine values when Jaffé reaction is used; may cause false-positive results in urine glucose tests when using Clinitest®; false-positive urinary proteins and steroids

Patient Information Report side effects such as diarrhea, dyspepsia, headache, blurred vision, and lightheadedness to your physician

Nursing Implications Do not admix with aminoglycosides

Dosage Forms Excipient information presented when available (limited, particularly for generics); consult specific product labeling.

Injection, powder for reconstitution, as hydrochloride: 500 mg, 1 g, 2 g

References

Arguedas AG, Stutman HR, Zaleska M, et al, "Cefepime. Pharmacokinetics and Clinical Response in Patients With Cystic Fibrosis," *Am J Dis Child*, 1992, 146(7):797-802.

Blumer JL, Reed MD, Lemon E, et al, "Pharmacokinetics (PK) of Cefepime in Pediatric Patients Administered Single and Multiple 50 mg/kg Doses Every 8 Hours by the Intravenous (I.V.) or Intramuscular (I.M.) Route," 34th Interscience Conference on Antimicrobial Agents and Chemotherapy, 1994, Orlando, Fl. Abs. A69.

Capparelli E, Hochwald C, Rasmussen M, et al, "Population Pharmacokinetics of Cefepime in the Neonate," *Antimicrob Agents Chemother*, 2005, 49(7):2760-6.

Saez-Llorens X, Castano E, Garcia R, et al, "Prospective Randomized Comparison of Cefepime and Cefotaxime for Treatment of Bacterial Meningitis in Infants and Children", *Antimicrob Agents Chemother*, 1995, 39(4):937-40.

Wynd MA and Paladino JA, "Cefepime: A Fourth-Generation Parenteral Cephalosporin," *Ann Pharmacother*, 1996, 30(12):1414-24.

♦ **Cefepime Hydrochloride** *see* Cefepime *on page 306*

Cefixime (sef IKS eem)

Medication Safety Issues

Sound-alike/look-alike issues:

Suprax® may be confused with Sporanox®, Surbex®

International issues:

Cefiton® [Portugal] may be confused with Cefotan® which is a brand name for cefotetan in the U.S.

Cefiton® [Portugal] may be confused with Ceftim® which is a brand name for ceftazidime in Italy

Cefiton® [Portugal] may be confused with Ceftin® which is a brand name for cefuroxime in the U.S.

Cefiton® [Portugal] may be confused with Lexotan® which is a brand name for bromazepam in multiple international markets

U.S. Brand Names Suprax®

Canadian Brand Names Suprax®

Index Terms Cefixime Trihydrate

Therapeutic Category Antibiotic, Cephalosporin (Third Generation)

Generic Available No

Use Treatment of urinary tract infections, otitis media, respiratory infections due to susceptible organisms including *S. pneumoniae* and *pyogenes*, *H. influenzae*, *M. catarrhalis*, and many *Enterobacteriaceae*; documented poor compliance with other oral antimicrobials; outpatient therapy of serious soft tissue or skeletal infections due to susceptible organisms; single-dose oral treatment of uncomplicated cervical/urethral gonorrhea due to *N. gonorrhoeae*; treatment of shigellosis in areas with a high rate of resistance to TMP-SMX

Pregnancy Risk Factor B

Lactation Excretion in breast milk unknown/use caution

Contraindications Hypersensitivity to cefixime, any component, or cephalosporins

Warnings Prolonged use may result in superinfection; do not use in patients with immediate-type hypersensitivity reactions to penicillin

Suspension contains sodium benzoate; benzoic acid (benzoate) is a metabolite of benzyl alcohol; large amounts of benzyl alcohol (≥99 mg/kg/day) have been associated with a potentially fatal toxicity ("gasping syndrome") in neonates; the "gasping syndrome" consists of metabolic acidosis, respiratory distress, gasping respirations, CNS dysfunction (including convulsions, intracranial hemorrhage), hypotension and cardiovascular collapse; use suspension containing sodium benzoate with caution in neonates; *in vitro* and animal studies have shown that benzoate displaces bilirubin from protein binding sites

Precautions Use with caution in patients hypersensitive to penicillin, patients with impaired renal function, and patients with a history of colitis; modify dosage in patients with renal impairment

Adverse Reactions

Central nervous system: Headache, fever, dizziness, fatigue, nervousness, insomnia, seizures, somnolence

Dermatologic: Skin rash, urticaria, pruritus, angioedema, Stevens-Johnson syndrome, erythema multiforme, toxic epidermal necrolysis

Gastrointestinal: Nausea, diarrhea (up to 15% of children), abdominal pain, pseudomembranous colitis

Genitourinary: Vaginitis, dysuria

Hematologic: Eosinophilia, thrombocytopenia, leukopenia

Hepatic: Transient elevation of liver enzymes, hepatitis, jaundice

Neuromuscular & skeletal: Arthralgia

Renal: Transient elevation of BUN and serum creatinine, acute renal failure

Miscellaneous: Anaphylaxis

Drug Interactions Probenecid (increases cefixime concentration); cefixime may increase carbamazepine serum concentrations; warfarin (increased prothrombin time)

Food Interactions Food delays the time to reach peak concentrations

Stability After reconstitution, suspension may be stored for 14 days at room temperature or under refrigeration

Mechanism of Action Inhibits bacterial cell wall synthesis by binding to one or more of the penicillin-binding proteins; inhibits the final transpeptidation step of peptidoglycan synthesis resulting in cell wall death

Pharmacokinetics

Absorption: Oral: 40% to 50%

Distribution: Into bile, sputum, middle ear fluid; crosses the placenta

Protein binding: 65%

Half-life:

- Normal renal function: 3-4 hours
- Renal failure: Up to 11.5 hours

Time to peak serum concentration: Within 2-6 hours; peak serum concentrations are 25% to 50% higher for the oral suspension versus tablets (tablets are no longer commercially available in the U.S.)

Elimination: 50% of absorbed dose excreted as active drug in urine and 10% in bile

Dialysis: 10% removed by hemodialysis

Usual Dosage Oral:

Infants and Children: 8 mg/kg/day divided every 12-24 hours; maximum dose: 400 mg/day

- Treatment of acute UTI: 16 mg/kg/day divided every 12 hours on day 1, then 8 mg/kg/day every 24 hours for 13 days
- Prophylaxis after sexual victimization: 8 mg/kg in a single dose (maximum dose: 400 mg) **plus** azithromycin 20 mg/kg in a single dose (maximum dose: 1 g); also begin or complete hepatitis B virus immunization and consider prophylaxis for trichomoniasis and bacterial vaginosis

Adolescents and Adults: 400 mg/day divided every 12-24 hours

- Uncomplicated cervical/urethral gonorrhea due to *N. gonorrhoeae*: 400 mg as a single dose plus azithromycin 1 g orally in a single dose **or** doxycycline 100 mg orally twice daily for 7 days
- Prophylaxis after sexual victimization: 400 mg in a single dose **plus** azithromycin 1 g orally in a single dose **or** doxycycline 100 mg orally twice daily for 7 days **plus** metronidazole 2 g orally in a single dose **plus** hepatitis B virus immunization if not fully immunized plus consider prophylaxis for HIV depending on circumstances

Dosing adjustment in renal impairment:

- Cl_{cr} 21-60 mL/minute: Administer 75% of the standard dose
- Cl_{cr} <20 mL/minute: Administer 50% of the standard dose

Administration Oral: May be administered with or without food; administer with food to decrease GI distress; shake suspension well before use

Monitoring Parameters With prolonged therapy, monitor renal and hepatic function periodically; number and type of stools/day for diarrhea

Test Interactions False-positive reaction for urine glucose using Clinitest®; false-positive urine ketones using tests with nitroprusside

Patient Information Report problems with diarrhea

Dosage Forms Excipient information presented when available (limited, particularly for generics); consult specific product labeling.

Powder for oral suspension, as trihydrate:

- Suprax®: 100 mg/5 mL (50 mL, 75 mL, 100 mL) [contains sodium benzoate; strawberry flavor]

(Continued)

Cefixime *(Continued)*

References

Ashkenazi S, Amir J, Waisman Y, et al, "A Randomized, Double-Blind Study Comparing Cefixime and Trimethoprim-Sulfamethoxazole in the Treatment of Childhood Shigellosis," *J Pediatr*, 1993, 123(5):817-21.

"2002 Guidelines for the Treatment of Sexually Transmitted Diseases. Centers for Disease Control and Prevention," *MMWR Morb Mortal Wkly Rep*, 2002, 51(RR-6):1-80.

Hoberman A, Wald ER, Hickey RW, et al, "Oral Versus Initial Intravenous Therapy for Urinary Tract Infections in Young Febrile Children," *Pediatrics*, 1999, 104(1 Pt 1):79-86.

Johnson CE, Carlin SA, Super DM, et al, "Cefixime Compared With Amoxicillin for Treatment of Acute Otitis Media," *J Pediatr*, 1991, 119(1):117-22.

♦ **Cefixime Trihydrate** *see* Cefixime *on page 308*
♦ **Cefizox®** *see* Ceftizoxime *on page 318*
♦ **Cefotan® [DSC]** *see* Cefotetan *on page 311*
♦ **Cefotan® (Can)** *see* Cefotetan *on page 311*

Cefotaxime (sef oh TAKS eem)

Medication Safety Issues

Sound-alike/look-alike issues:

Cefotaxime may be confused with cefoxitin, ceftizoxime, cefuroxime

International issues:

Spectrocef® [Italy] may be confused with Spectracef™ which is a brand name for cefditoren in the U.S.

U.S. Brand Names Claforan®

Canadian Brand Names Claforan®

Index Terms Cefotaxime Sodium

Therapeutic Category Antibiotic, Cephalosporin (Third Generation)

Generic Available Yes: Powder

Use Treatment of susceptible lower respiratory tract, skin and skin structure, bone and joint, intra-abdominal and genitourinary tract infections; treatment of a documented or suspected meningitis due to susceptible organisms such as *H. influenzae* and *N. meningitidis*; indicated for *Neisseria gonorrhoeae* infections (including uncomplicated cervical and urethral gonorrhea and gonorrhea pelvic inflammatory disease); nonpseudomonal gram-negative rod infection in a patient at risk of developing aminoglycoside-induced nephrotoxicity and/or ototoxicity; infection due to an organism whose susceptibilities clearly favor cefotaxime over cefuroxime or an aminoglycoside

Pregnancy Risk Factor B

Lactation Enters breast milk/use caution (AAP rates "compatible")

Contraindications Hypersensitivity to cefotaxime, any component, or cephalosporins

Warnings Prolonged use may result in superinfection; do not use in patients with immediate-type hypersensitivity reactions to penicillin; cefotaxime rapid bolus injection (over <1 minute through a central venous catheter) has been associated with potentially life-threatening arrhythmias

Precautions Use with caution in patients with history of penicillin hypersensitivity, impaired renal function, or history of colitis; modify dosage in patients with Cl_{cr} <20 mL/minute

Adverse Reactions

Cardiovascular: Arrhythmias
Central nervous system: Fever, headache
Dermatologic: Rash, pruritus
Gastrointestinal: Antibiotic-associated pseudomembranous colitis, diarrhea, nausea, vomiting
Hematologic: Transient neutropenia, thrombocytopenia, eosinophilia, leukopenia
Hepatic: Transient elevation of liver enzymes
Local: Phlebitis, pain at injection site
Renal: Transient elevation of BUN and serum creatinine

Drug Interactions Probenecid (increases cefotaxime concentration)

Stability Reconstituted solution is stable for 24 hours at room temperature and 10 days when refrigerated

Mechanism of Action Inhibits bacterial cell wall synthesis by binding to one or more of the penicillin-binding proteins; inhibits the final transpeptidation step of peptidoglycan synthesis resulting in cell wall death

Pharmacokinetics

Distribution: Into bronchial secretions, middle ear effusions, bone, bile; penetration into CSF when meninges are inflamed; crosses the placenta; appears in breast milk
Protein binding: 31% to 50%
Metabolism: Partially metabolized in the liver to active metabolite, desacetylcefotaxime

Half-life:

Cefotaxime:

Neonates, premature: <1 week: 5-6 hours

Neonates, full-term: <1 week: 2-3.4 hours; 1-4 weeks: 2 hours

Children: 1.5 hours

Adults: 1-1.5 hours (prolonged with renal and/or hepatic impairment)

Desacetylcefotaxime: Adults: 1.5-1.9 hours (prolonged with renal impairment)

Time to peak serum concentration: I.M.: Within 30 minutes

Elimination: 40% to 60% of a dose excreted as unchanged drug and 24% excreted as desacetylcefotaxime in the urine

Dialysis: Moderately dialyzable (20% to 50%)

Usual Dosage I.M., I.V.:

Neonates: 0-4 weeks: <1200 g: 100 mg/kg/day divided every 12 hours

Postnatal age ≤7 days:

1200-2000 g: 100 mg/kg/day divided every 12 hours

>2000 g: 100-150 mg/kg/day divided every 8-12 hours

Postnatal age >7 days:

1200-2000 g: 150 mg/kg/day divided every 8 hours

>2000 g: 150-200 mg/kg/day divided every 6-8 hours

Infants and Children 1 month to 12 years:

<50 kg: 100-200 mg/kg/day divided every 6-8 hours

Meningitis: 200 mg/kg/day divided every 6 hours; 225-300 mg/kg/day divided every 6-8 hours has been used to treat invasive pneumococcal meningitis

≥50 kg: Moderate to severe infection: 1-2 g every 6-8 hours; life-threatening infection: 2 g/dose every 4 hours; maximum dose: 12 g/day

Children >12 years and Adults: 1-2 g every 6-8 hours (up to 12 g/day)

Dosing adjustment in renal impairment: Cl_{cr} <20 mL/minute: Reduce dose by 50%

Administration Parenteral:

I.V.: Cefotaxime may be administered IVP over 3-5 minutes at a maximum concentration of 100 mg/mL or I.V. intermittent infusion over 15-30 minutes at a final concentration of 20-60 mg/mL; in fluid-restricted patients, a concentration of 150 mg/mL may be administered IVP; rapid IVP over <1 minute may cause arrhythmias (see Warnings)

I.M.: Deep I.M. injection into a large muscle mass such as the upper outer quadrant of the gluteus maximus. Doses as large as 2 g should be divided and administered at 2 different sites. May dilute vial using SWI to a final concentration between 230-330 mg/mL (see package insert).

Monitoring Parameters With prolonged therapy, monitor renal, hepatic, and hematologic function periodically; number and type of stools/day for diarrhea

Test Interactions Positive Coombs' [direct]

Additional Information Sodium content of 1 g: 2.2 mEq

Dosage Forms Excipient information presented when available (limited, particularly for generics); consult specific product labeling.

Infusion, as sodium [premixed iso-osmotic solution]:

Claforan®: 1 g (50 mL); 2 g (50 mL) [contains sodium 50.5 mg (2.2 mEq) per cefotaxime 1 g]

Injection, powder for reconstitution, as sodium: 500 mg, 1 g, 2 g, 10 g, 20 g

Claforan®: 500 mg, 1 g, 2 g, 10 g [contains sodium 50.5 mg (2.2 mEq) per cefotaxime 1 g]

References

Spritzer R, Kamp HJ, Dzoljic G, et al, "Five Years of Cefotaxime Use in a Neonatal Intensive Care Unit," *Pediatr Infect Dis J*, 1990, 9(2):92-6.

♦ **Cefotaxime Sodium** *see* Cefotaxime *on page 310*

Cefotetan (SEF oh tee tan)

Medication Safety Issues

Sound-alike/look-alike issues:

Cefotetan may be confused with cefoxitin, Ceftin®

Cefotan® may be confused with Ceftin®

International issues:

Cefotan® may be confused with Lexotan® which is a brand name for bromazepam in multiple international markets

Cefotan® may be confused with Cefiton® which is a brand name for cefixime in Portugal

U.S. Brand Names Cefotan® [DSC]

Canadian Brand Names Cefotan®

Index Terms Cefotetan Disodium

Therapeutic Category Antibiotic, Cephalosporin (Second Generation)

Generic Available No

(Continued)

Cefotetan *(Continued)*

Use Treatment of susceptible lower respiratory tract, skin and skin structure, bone and joint, urinary tract, sepsis, gynecologic, and intra-abdominal infections; active against anaerobes including *Bacteroides* species of GI tract, gram-negative enteric bacilli including *E. coli*, *Klebsiella*, and *Proteus*; active against many strains of *N. gonorrhoeae*; inactive against *Enterobacter* sp.; less active against staphylococci and streptococci than first generation cephalosporins; preoperative prophylaxis

Pregnancy Risk Factor B

Lactation Enters breast milk (small amounts)/use caution

Contraindications Hypersensitivity to cefotetan, cephalosporins, any component, or patients who have experienced a cephalosporin-associated hemolytic anemia

Warnings Prolonged use may result in superinfection; do not use in patients with immediate-type hypersensitivity reactions to penicillin. May cause pseudomembranous colitis or secondary antibiotic-associated colitis. Severe cases of immune mediated hemolytic anemia have been reported with cefotetan administration. Risk of developing cefotetan-induced hemolytic anemia is 3-fold higher relative to other cephalosporins. Monitor hematologic parameters; blood transfusion may be needed.

Precautions Use with caution and modify dosage in patients with renal impairment; use with caution in patients with history of colitis or penicillin hypersensitivity

Adverse Reactions

Central nervous system: Seizures, fever

Dermatologic: Rash, pruritus, urticaria

Gastrointestinal: Diarrhea, nausea, vomiting, pseudomembranous colitis

Hematologic: Neutropenia, leukopenia, thrombocytopenia, eosinophilia, hemolytic anemia, bleeding, prolongation of PT

Hepatic: Elevated serum AST, ALT, alkaline phosphatase, LDH

Local: Phlebitis, pain at the injection site, edema

Renal: Elevated BUN, elevated serum creatinine, nephrotoxicity (rare)

Miscellaneous: Anaphylaxis

Drug Interactions Alcohol (disulfiram-like reaction which includes flushing, sweating, headache, and tachycardia), anticoagulants (may increase the risk of hemorrhage), aminoglycosides (additive nephrotoxicity)

Stability Thawed solutions of the commercially available frozen cefotetan injections are stable for 48 hours at room temperature or 21 days when refrigerated; do not refreeze; incompatible with aminoglycosides, heparin, and tetracycline

Mechanism of Action Inhibits bacterial cell wall synthesis by binding to one or more of the penicillin-binding proteins; inhibits the final transpeptidation step of peptidoglycan synthesis resulting in cell wall death

Pharmacokinetics

Absorption: I.M.: Completely absorbed

Distribution: Distributes into tissues and fluids including gallbladder, kidney, skin, tonsils, uterus, sputum, prostatic and peritoneal fluids; poor penetration into CSF; crosses the placenta; small amounts appear in breast milk

Protein binding: 76% to 91%

Half-life: Adults: 3.5 hours, prolonged in patients with impaired renal function (up to 10 hours)

Time to peak serum concentration: I.M.: Within 1.5-3 hours

Elimination: 49% to 81% excreted as unchanged drug in urine, 20% of dose is excreted in bile

Dialysis: <10% removed by hemodialysis

Usual Dosage I.V.: Safety and efficacy in children have not been established

Children: 40-80 mg/kg/day divided every 12 hours; maximum dose: 6 g/day

Preoperative prophylaxis: 40 mg/kg 30-60 minutes prior to procedure; **Note:** May add gentamicin 2 mg/kg for cases of ruptured viscus

Adolescents and Adults: 2-4 g/day divided every 12 hours; maximum dose: 6 g/day

Urinary tract infections: 1-2 g/day divided every 12-24 hours

Preoperative prophylaxis: 1-2 g 30-60 minutes prior to procedure

Pelvic inflammatory disease: 2 g every 12 hours continued for 24-48 hours after significant clinical improvement is demonstrated **plus** doxycycline 100 mg I.V. or orally every 12 hours for 14 days

Dosing interval in renal impairment:

Cl_{cr} 10-30 mL/minute: Administer every 24 hours

Cl_{cr} <10 mL/minute: Administer every 48 hours

Administration Parenteral: I.V. intermittent: Infuse over 20-60 minutes at a concentration of 10-40 mg/mL

Monitoring Parameters CBC, prothrombin time, renal function tests; number and type of stools/day for diarrhea; signs and symptoms of hemolytic anemia

Test Interactions Positive Coombs' [direct], false-positive urine glucose (Clinitest®), falsely elevated serum or urinary creatinine (Jaffé reaction)

Patient Information Avoid alcohol during and for at least 72 hours after the last cefotetan dose.

Additional Information Sodium content of 1 g: 3.5 mEq; chemical structure contains a methyltetrazolethiol side chain which may be responsible for the disulfiram-like reaction with alcohol and increased risk of bleeding

Dosage Forms Excipient information presented when available (limited, particularly for generics); consult specific product labeling. [DSC] = Discontinued product

Infusion [premixed iso-osmotic solution]: 1 g (50 mL); 2 g (50 mL) [contains sodium 80 mg/g (3.5 mEq/g)] [DSC]

Injection, powder for reconstitution: 1 g, 2 g [contains sodium 80 mg/g (3.5 mEq/g)] [DSC]

References

Martin C, Thomachot L, and Albanese J, "Clinical Pharmacokinetics of Cefotetan," *Clin Pharmacokinet*, 1994, 26(4):248-58.

♦ **Cefotetan Disodium** *see* Cefotetan *on page 311*

Cefoxitin (se FOKS i tin)

Medication Safety Issues

Sound-alike/look-alike issues:

Cefoxitin may be confused with cefotaxime, cefotetan, Cytoxan®

Mefoxin® may be confused with Lanoxin®

U.S. Brand Names Mefoxin®

Canadian Brand Names Apo-Cefoxitin®

Index Terms Cefoxitin Sodium

Therapeutic Category Antibiotic, Cephalosporin (Second Generation)

Generic Available Yes: Powder for injection

Use Treatment of susceptible lower respiratory tract, skin and skin structure, bone and joint, genitourinary tract, sepsis, gynecologic, and intra-abdominal infections; active against anaerobes including *Bacteroides* species of the GI tract, gram-negative enteric bacilli including *E. coli*, *Klebsiella*, and *Proteus*; active against many strains of *N. gonorrhoeae*; inactive against *Enterobacter* sp.; perioperative prophylaxis

Pregnancy Risk Factor B

Lactation Enters breast milk (small amounts)/use caution (AAP rates "compatible")

Contraindications Hypersensitivity to cefoxitin, any component, or cephalosporins

Warnings Prolonged use may result in superinfection; high doses in children have been associated with an increased incidence of eosinophilia and elevation of serum AST; safety and efficacy in infants <3 months have not been established; do not use in patients with immediate-type hypersensitivity reactions to penicillin

Precautions Use with caution and modify dosage in patients with renal impairment; use with caution in patients with history of colitis or penicillin hypersensitivity

Adverse Reactions

Central nervous system: Fever, headache

Dermatologic: Rash, pruritus, exfoliative dermatitis

Gastrointestinal: Pseudomembranous colitis, diarrhea, nausea, vomiting

Hematologic: Transient leukopenia, thrombocytopenia, neutropenia, anemia, eosinophilia

Hepatic: Transient elevation of liver enzymes, AST, ALT, and alkaline phosphatase

Local: Thrombophlebitis, pain at injection site

Renal: Transient elevation of BUN and serum creatinine

Drug Interactions Probenecid (increases serum concentration of cefoxitin)

Stability Reconstituted solution is stable for 24 hours at room temperature and for 1 week under refrigeration; thawed solutions of the commercially available frozen cefoxitin injections are stable for 24 hours at room temperature or 5 days when refrigerated

Mechanism of Action Inhibits bacterial cell wall synthesis by binding to one or more of the penicillin-binding proteins; inhibits the final transpeptidation step of peptidoglycan synthesis resulting in cell wall death

Pharmacokinetics

Distribution: Distributes into tissues and fluids including ascitic, pleural, bile, and synovial fluids; poor penetration into CSF even with inflamed meninges; crosses the placenta; small amounts appear in breast milk

Protein binding: 65% to 79%

Half-life:

Infants (10-53 days of age): 1.4 hours

Adults: 45-60 minutes, increases significantly with renal insufficiency

Time to peak serum concentration: I.M.: Within 20-30 minutes

Elimination: Rapidly excreted as unchanged drug (85%) in the urine

Dialysis: Moderately dialyzable (20% to 50%)

(Continued)

Cefoxitin *(Continued)*

Usual Dosage I.M., I.V.:

Neonates: 90-100 mg/kg/day divided every 8 hours

Infants ≥3 months and Children:

Mild-moderate infection: 80-100 mg/kg/day divided every 6-8 hours

Severe infection: 100-160 mg/kg/day divided every 4-6 hours; maximum dose: 12 g/day

Perioperative prophylaxis: 30-40 mg/kg 30-60 minutes prior to surgery followed by 30-40 mg/kg/dose every 6 hours for no more than 24 hours after surgery depending on the procedure

Adolescents and Adults: 1-2 g every 6-8 hours (I.M. injection is painful); maximum dose: 12 g/day

Pelvic inflammatory disease: I.V.: 2 g every 6 hours continued for 24-48 hours after significant clinical improvement is demonstrated **plus** doxycycline 100 mg I.V. or orally every 12 hours for 14 days

Perioperative prophylaxis: 1-2 g 30-60 minutes prior to surgery followed by 1-2 g every 6-8 hours for no more than 24 hours after surgery depending on the procedure

Dosing interval in renal impairment:

Cl_{cr} 30-50 mL/minute: Administer every 8-12 hours

Cl_{cr} 10-30 mL/minute: Administer every 12-24 hours

Cl_{cr} <10 mL/minute: Administer every 24-48 hours

Administration Parenteral:

IVP: Administer over 3-5 minutes at a maximum concentration of 200 mg/mL

I.V. intermittent infusion: Administer over 10-60 minutes at a final concentration not to exceed 40 mg/mL

I.M.: Deep I.M. injection into a large muscle mass such as the upper outer quadrant of the gluteus maximus. May dilute vial using SWI or 0.5% or 1% lidocaine to a final concentration of 400 mg/mL (see package insert)

Monitoring Parameters Renal function periodically when used in combination with other nephrotoxic drugs; liver function and hematologic function tests; number and type of stools/day for diarrhea

Test Interactions Positive Coombs' [direct]; false-positive urine glucose (Clinitest®), false ↑ in serum or urine creatinine

Additional Information Sodium content of 1 g: 53 mg (2.3 mEq)

Dosage Forms Excipient information presented when available (limited, particularly for generics); consult specific product labeling.

Infusion, as sodium [premixed iso-osmotic solution]: 1 g (50 mL); 2 g (50 mL) [contains sodium 53.8 mg/g (2.3 mEq/g)]

Injection, powder for reconstitution, as sodium: 1 g, 2 g, 10 g [contains sodium 53.8 mg/g (2.3 mEq/g)]

References

Feldman WE, Moffitt S, and Sprow N, "Clinical and Pharmacokinetic Evaluation of Parenteral Cefoxitin in Infants and Children," *Antimicrob Agents Chemother*, 1980, 17(4):669-74.

Regazzi MB, Chirico G, Cristiani D, et al, "Cefoxitin in Newborn Infants. A Clinical and Pharmacokinetic Study," *Eur J Clin Pharmacol*, 1983, 25(4):507-9.

♦ **Cefoxitin Sodium** *see* Cefoxitin *on page 313*

Cefpodoxime (sef pode OKS eem)

Medication Safety Issues

Sound-alike/look-alike issues:

Vantin® may be confused with Ventolin®

U.S. Brand Names Vantin®

Canadian Brand Names Vantin®

Index Terms Cefpodoxime Proxetil

Therapeutic Category Antibiotic, Cephalosporin (Third Generation)

Generic Available Yes: Tablet

Use Treatment of susceptible acute, community-acquired pneumonia caused by *S. pneumoniae* or nonbeta-lactamase producing *H. influenzae*; alternative regimen for acute uncomplicated gonorrhea caused by *N. gonorrhoeae*; uncomplicated skin and skin structure infections caused by *S. aureus* or *S. pyogenes*; acute otitis media caused by *S. pneumoniae, H. influenzae*, or *M. catarrhalis*; pharyngitis or tonsillitis; and uncomplicated urinary tract infections caused by *E. coli*, *Klebsiella*, and *Proteus*; inactive against *Pseudomonas* and *Enterobacter* spp.

Pregnancy Risk Factor B

Lactation Enters breast milk (small amounts)/use caution

Contraindications Hypersensitivity to cefpodoxime, any component, or cephalosporins

Warnings Prolonged use may result in superinfection; do not use in patients wi immediate-type hypersensitivity reactions to penicillin

Suspension contains sodium benzoate; benzoic acid (benzoate) is a metabolite of benzyl alcohol; large amounts of benzyl alcohol (≥99 mg/kg/day) have been associated with a potentially fatal toxicity ("gasping syndrome") in neonates; the "gasping syndrome" consists of metabolic acidosis, respiratory distress, gasping respirations, CNS dysfunction (including convulsions, intracranial hemorrhage), hypotension and cardiovascular collapse; use suspension containing sodium benzoate with caution in neonates; *in vitro* and animal studies have shown that benzoate displaces bilirubin from protein binding sites

Precautions Use with caution in patients with history of penicillin hypersensitivity, impaired renal function, and patients with a history of colitis; modify dosage in patients with renal impairment

Adverse Reactions

Central nervous system: Headache

Dermatologic: Rash

Gastrointestinal: Nausea (3.8%), vomiting, abdominal pain, diarrhea (7.1%), pseudomembranous colitis

Genitourinary: Vaginal fungal infections (3.3%)

Hematologic: Eosinophilia, leukocytosis, thrombocytosis, decrease in hemoglobin or hematocrit, leukopenia, prolonged PT and PTT

Hepatic: Transient elevation in AST, ALT, bilirubin

Renal: Elevated BUN, elevated serum creatinine

Drug Interactions Antacids and H_2-receptor antagonists (reduce absorption and serum concentration of cefpodoxime); probenecid (inhibits renal excretion of cefpodoxime)

Food Interactions Food increases oral bioavailability

Stability After reconstitution, suspension may be stored in refrigerator for 14 days

Mechanism of Action Inhibits bacterial cell wall synthesis by binding to one or more of the penicillin-binding proteins; inhibits the final transpeptidation step of peptidoglycan synthesis resulting in cell wall death

Pharmacokinetics

Absorption: Enhanced in the presence of food or low gastric pH

Distribution: Good tissue penetration, including lung and tonsils; penetrates into pleural fluid; poor penetration into CSF; small amounts appear in breast milk

Protein binding: 18% to 23%

Metabolism: Following oral administration, cefpodoxime proxetil is de-esterified in the GI tract to the active metabolite, cefpodoxime

Bioavailability: Oral: 50%

Half-life: 2.2 hours (prolonged with renal impairment)

Time to peak serum concentration: Within 2-3 hours

Elimination: Primarily by the kidney with 80% of absorbed dose excreted unchanged in urine in 24 hours

Usual Dosage Oral:

Infants >6 months and Children to 12 years: 10 mg/kg/day divided every 12 hours; maximum dose: 800 mg/day

Adolescents and Adults: 100-400 mg/dose every 12 hours

Uncomplicated gonorrhea: 200 mg as a single dose

Dosing adjustment in renal impairment: Cl_{cr} <30 mL/minute: Administer every 24 hours; patients on hemodialysis, administer dose 3 times/week

Dosing adjustment in hepatic impairment: Not necessary in patient with cirrhosis

Administration Oral:

Tablet: Administer with food

Suspension: May administer with or without food; shake suspension well before use

Monitoring Parameters Observe patient for diarrhea; with prolonged therapy, monitor renal function periodically

Test Interactions Positive Coombs' [direct]

Dosage Forms Excipient information presented when available (limited, particularly for generics); consult specific product labeling.

Granules for oral suspension: 50 mg/5 mL (50 mL, 75 mL, 100 mL); 100 mg/5 mL (50 mL, 75 mL, 100 mL) [contains sodium benzoate; lemon creme flavor]

Tablet: 100 mg, 200 mg

References

Borin MT, "A Review of the Pharmacokinetics of Cefpodoxime Proxetil," *Drugs*, 1991, 42(Suppl 3):13-21.

Fujii R, "Clinical Trials of Cefpodoxime Proxetil Suspension in Pediatrics," *Drugs*, 1991, 42(Suppl 3):57-60.

Mendelman PM, Del-Beccaro MA, McLinn SE, et al, "Cefpodoxime Proxetil Compared With Amoxicillin-Clavulanate for the Treatment of Otitis Media," *J Pediatr*, 1992, 121(3):459-65.

♦ **Cefpodoxime Proxetil** *see* Cefpodoxime *on page 314*

Cefprozil (sef PROE zil)

Medication Safety Issues

Sound-alike/look-alike issues:

Cefprozil may be confused with cefazolin, cefuroxime

Cefzil® may be confused with Cefol®, Ceftin®, Kefzol®

U.S. Brand Names Cefzil®

Canadian Brand Names Apo-Cefprozil®; Cefzil®

Therapeutic Category Antibiotic, Cephalosporin (Second Generation)

Generic Available Yes

Use Infections caused by susceptible organisms including *S. pneumoniae*, *H. influenzae*, *M. catarrhalis*, *S. aureus*, *S. pyogenes*; treatment of infections involving the respiratory tract, skin and skin structure, and otitis media

Pregnancy Risk Factor B

Lactation Enters breast milk/use caution (AAP rates "compatible")

Contraindications Hypersensitivity to cefprozil, any component, or cephalosporins

Warnings Prolonged use may result in superinfection; do not use in patients with immediate-type hypersensitivity reactions to penicillin

Oral suspension contains sodium benzoate; benzoic acid (benzoate) is a metabolite of benzyl alcohol; large amounts of benzyl alcohol (≥99 mg/kg/day) have been associated with a potentially fatal toxicity ("gasping syndrome") in neonates; the "gasping syndrome" consists of metabolic acidosis, respiratory distress, gasping respirations, CNS dysfunction (including convulsions, intracranial hemorrhage), hypotension and cardiovascular collapse; use oral suspension containing sodium benzoate with caution in neonates; *in vitro* and animal studies have shown that benzoate displaces bilirubin from protein binding sites

Precautions Use with caution in patients with impaired renal function, history of colitis, or in penicillin-sensitive patients; modify dosage in patients with severe renal impairment; some products (eg, oral suspension) contain aspartame which is metabolized to phenylalanine and must be used with caution in patients with phenylketonuria.

Adverse Reactions

Central nervous system: Headache, hyperactivity, insomnia, confusion, dizziness

Dermatologic: Rash, pruritus, diaper rash

Gastrointestinal: Diarrhea, nausea, vomiting, abdominal pain

Genitourinary: Vaginitis

Hematologic: Decrease in leukocyte and platelet count, eosinophilia

Hepatic: Elevated AST, ALT, and alkaline phosphatase; cholestatic jaundice; prolonged PT

Renal: Elevated BUN and serum creatinine

Miscellaneous: Serum sickness-like reactions

Drug Interactions Probenecid increases cefprozil serum levels

Food Interactions Total absorption is not affected by food

Stability Refrigerate suspension after reconstitution; discard after 14 days

Mechanism of Action Inhibits bacterial cell wall synthesis by binding to one or more of the penicillin-binding proteins resulting in disruption of cell wall synthesis and cell lysis

Pharmacokinetics

Absorption: Oral: Well absorbed (95%)

Distribution: Low excretion into breast milk

Protein binding: 35% to 45%

Bioavailability: 94%

Half-life, elimination: 1.3 hours (normal renal function)

Time to peak serum concentration: 1.5 hours (fasting state)

Elimination: 61% excreted unchanged in urine

Dialysis: ~55% is removed by hemodialysis

Usual Dosage Oral:

Infants >6 months and Children to 12 years:

Otitis media: 30 mg/kg/day divided every 12 hours; maximum dose: 1 g/day

Children 2-12 years:

Pharyngitis/tonsillitis: 15 mg/kg/day divided every 12 hours; maximum dose: 1 g/day

Skin and skin structure infection: 20 mg/kg once daily

Children >12 years and Adults: 250-500 mg every 12 hours or 500 mg every 24 hours

Dosing adjustment in renal impairment: Cl_{cr} <30 mL/minute: Reduce dose by 50%

Administration Oral: May administer with or without food; administer with food if stomach upset occurs; chilling improves flavor of suspension (do not freeze); shake suspension well before use

Monitoring Parameters Evaluate renal function before and during therapy; with prolonged therapy, monitor coagulation tests, CBC, and liver function tests periodically

Test Interactions Positive Coombs' [direct]; may produce false-positive reaction for urine glucose with Clinitest®

Patient Information Report persistent diarrhea to physician

Additional Information Suspension also contains FD&C red No. 3, glycine, carboxymethylcellulose, and sucrose

Dosage Forms Excipient information presented when available (limited, particularly for generics); consult specific product labeling.

Powder for oral suspension, as anhydrous: 125 mg/5 mL (50 mL, 75 mL, 100 mL); 250 mg/5 mL (50 mL, 75 mL, 100 mL)

Cefzil®: 125 mg/5 mL (50 mL, 75 mL, 100 mL) [contains phenylalanine 28 mg/5 mL and sodium benzoate; bubble gum flavor]; 250 mg/5 mL (50 mL, 75 mL, 100 mL) [contains phenylalanine 28 mg/5 mL and sodium benzoate; bubble gum flavor]

Tablet, as anhydrous: 250 mg, 500 mg

Cefzil®: 250 mg, 500 mg

References

Arguedas AG, Zaleska M, Stutman HR, et al, "Comparative Trial of Cefprozil vs Amoxicillin Clavulanate Potassium in the Treatment of Children With Acute Otitis Media With Effusion," *Pediatr Infect Dis J*, 1991, 10(5):375-80.

Barriere SL, "Review of *In Vitro* Activity, Pharmacokinetic Characteristics, Safety, and Clinical Efficacy of Cefprozil, a New Oral Cephalosporin," *Ann Pharmacother*, 1993, 27(9):1082-9.

Lowery N, Kearns GL, Young RA, et al, "Serum Sickness-Like Reactions Associated With Cefprozil Therapy," *J Pediatr*, 1994, 125(2):325-8.

Ceftazidime (SEF tay zi deem)

Medication Safety Issues

Sound-alike/look-alike issues:

Ceftazidime may be confused with ceftizoxime

Ceptaz® may be confused with Septra®

Tazicef® may be confused with Tazidime®

Tazidime® may be confused with Tazicef®

International issues:

Ceftim® [Italy] may be confused with Ceftin® which is a brand name for cefuroxime in the U.S.

Ceftim® [Italy] may be confused with Cefiton® which is a brand name for cefixime in Portugal

Ceftim® [Italy] may be confused with Ceftina® which is a brand name for cefalotin in Mexico

U.S. Brand Names Fortaz®; Tazicef®

Canadian Brand Names Fortaz®

Therapeutic Category Antibiotic, Cephalosporin (Third Generation)

Generic Available No

Use Treatment of infections of the respiratory tract, urinary tract, skin and skin structure, intra-abdominal, osteomyelitis, sepsis, and meningitis caused by susceptible gram-negative aerobic organisms such as Enterobacteriaceae and *Pseudomonas*; pseudomonal infection in patient at risk of developing aminoglycoside-induced nephrotoxicity and/or ototoxicity; empiric therapy for febrile, granulocytopenic patients

Pregnancy Risk Factor B

Lactation Enters breast milk (small amounts)/use caution (AAP rates "compatible")

Contraindications Hypersensitivity to ceftazidime, any component, or cephalosporins

Warnings Prolonged use may result in superinfection; do not use in patients with immediate-type hypersensitivity reactions to penicillin

Precautions Use with caution and modify dosage in patients with impaired renal function; use with caution in patients with history of colitis or patients with penicillin hypersensitivity

Adverse Reactions

Central nervous system: Fever, headache, dizziness, coma

Dermatologic: Rash, pruritus, urticaria

Gastrointestinal: Pseudomembranous colitis, diarrhea, nausea, vomiting, candidiasis

Hematologic: Transient leukopenia, thrombocytopenia, eosinophilia, thrombocytosis, hemolytic anemia

Hepatic: Transient elevation of liver enzymes, jaundice, hyperbilirubinemia

Local: Phlebitis, pain at injection site

Neuromuscular & skeletal: Myoclonia

Renal: Transient elevation of BUN and serum creatinine, renal impairment

Miscellaneous: Anaphylaxis

Drug Interactions Probenecid decreases renal clearance of ceftazidime; aminoglycosides may increase risk of nephrotoxicity

(Continued)

Ceftazidime *(Continued)*

Stability Reconstituted solution is stable for 24 hours at room temperature and 10 days when refrigerated; incompatible with sodium bicarbonate; potentially incompatible with aminoglycosides

Mechanism of Action Bactericidal antibiotic with a mechanism similar to that of penicillins by binding to one or more of the penicillin-binding proteins; inhibits mucopeptide synthesis in the bacterial cell wall

Pharmacokinetics

Distribution: Widely distributed throughout the body including bone, bile, skin, CSF (diffuses into CSF at higher concentrations when the meninges are inflamed), endometrium, heart, pleural and lymphatic fluids; distributes into breast milk

Protein binding: 17%

Half-life:

- Neonates <23 days: 2.2-4.7 hours
- Adults: 1-2 hours (prolonged with renal impairment)

Time to peak serum concentration: I.M.: Within 60 minutes

Elimination: By glomerular filtration with 80% to 90% of the dose excreted as unchanged drug in urine within 24 hours

Dialysis: Dialyzable (50% to 100%)

Usual Dosage I.M., I.V.:

Neonates: 0-4 weeks: <1200 g: 100 mg/kg/day divided every 12 hours

- Postnatal age ≤7 days:
  - 1200-2000 g: 100 mg/kg/day divided every 12 hours
  - >2000 g: 100-150 mg/kg/day divided every 8-12 hours
- Postnatal age >7 days: ≥1200 g: 150 mg/kg/day divided every 8 hours

Infants and Children 1 month to 12 years: 100-150 mg/kg/day divided every 8 hours; maximum dose: 6 g/day

- Meningitis: 150 mg/kg/day divided every 8 hours; maximum dose: 6 g/day

Adults: 1-2 g every 8-12 hours

- Urinary tract infections: 250-500 mg every 12 hours

Dosing interval in renal impairment:

- Cl_{cr} 30-50 mL/minute: Administer every 12 hours
- Cl_{cr} 10-30 mL/minute: Administer every 24 hours
- Cl_{cr} <10 mL/minute: Administer every 24-48 hours

Administration Parenteral: Any carbon dioxide bubbles that may be present in the withdrawn solution should be expelled prior to injection

IVP: Administer over 3-5 minutes at a maximum concentration of 180 mg/mL

I.V. intermittent infusion: Administer over 15-30 minutes at a final concentration ≤40 mg/mL

I.M.: Deep I.M. injection into a large muscle mass such as the upper outer quadrant of the gluteus maximus or lateral part of the thigh. May dilute vial using SWI or 0.5% or 1% lidocaine to a final concentration of 280 mg/mL (see package insert)

Monitoring Parameters Renal function periodically when used in combination with aminoglycosides; with prolonged therapy also monitor hepatic and hematologic function periodically; number and type of stools/day for diarrhea

Test Interactions Positive Coombs' [direct], false-positive urine glucose (Clinitest®)

Additional Information Sodium content of 1 g: 2.3 mEq

Dosage Forms Excipient information presented when available (limited, particularly for generics); consult specific product labeling.

Infusion, as sodium [premixed iso-osmotic solution]:

- Fortaz®: 1 g (50 mL); 2 g (50 mL)

Injection, powder for reconstitution:

- Fortaz®: 500 mg, 1 g, 2 g, 6 g [contains sodium carbonate]
- Tazicef®: 1 g, 2 g, 6 g [contains sodium carbonate]

References

McCracken GH Jr, Threlkeld N, and Thomas ML, "Pharmacokinetics of Ceftazidime in Newborn Infants," *Antimicrob Agents Chemother*, 1984, 26(4):583-4.

Robinson DG, Cookson TL, and Frisafe JA, "Concentration Guidelines for Parenteral Antibiotics in Fluid-Restricted Patients," *Drug Intell Clin Pharm*, 1987, 21(12):985-9.

♦ **Ceftin®** *see* Cefuroxime *on page 322*

Ceftizoxime (sef ti ZOKS eem)

Medication Safety Issues

Sound-alike/look-alike issues:

- Ceftizoxime may be confused with cefotaxime, ceftazidime, cefuroxime

U.S. Brand Names Cefizox®

Canadian Brand Names Cefizox®

Index Terms Ceftizoxime Sodium

Therapeutic Category Antibiotic, Cephalosporin (Third Generation)

Generic Available No

Use Treatment of susceptible bacterial infections, mainly respiratory tract, skin and skin structure, bone and joint, urinary tract and sepsis; as a third generation cephalosporin, ceftizoxime has activity against gram-negative enteric bacilli (eg, *E. coli*, *Klebsiella*), and cocci (eg, *Neisseria*), and variable activity against gram-positive cocci (*Staphylococcus* and *Streptococcus*); ceftizoxime has some anaerobic coverage but is less active against *B. fragilis* than cefoxitin; also indicated for *Neisseria gonorrhoeae* infections (including uncomplicated cervical and urethral gonorrhea and gonorrhea pelvic inflammatory disease), and *Haemophilus influenzae* meningitis

Pregnancy Risk Factor B

Lactation Enters breast milk (small amounts)/use caution

Contraindications Hypersensitivity to ceftizoxime, any component, or cephalosporins

Warnings Prolonged use may result in superinfection; do not use in patients with immediate-type hypersensitivity reaction to penicillin

Precautions Use with caution in patients who are hypersensitive to penicillins; use with caution and modify dosage in patients with renal impairment

Adverse Reactions

Central nervous system: Fever

Dermatologic: Rash, pruritus

Gastrointestinal: Diarrhea, occasionally nausea and vomiting

Genitourinary: Vaginitis (rare)

Hematologic: Positive Coombs' test, eosinophilia, thrombocytosis (transient); rarely: anemia, leukopenia, neutropenia, thrombocytopenia

Hepatic: Elevated bilirubin; transient elevation of AST, ALT, alkaline phosphatase

Local: Pain, burning at injection site

Neuromuscular & skeletal: Numbness

Renal: Transient elevations of BUN and serum creatinine

Drug Interactions Probenecid may decrease renal tubular secretion and increase ceftizoxime serum concentrations

Stability Reconstituted solution is stable for 24 hours at room temperature and 96 hours when refrigerated; for I.V. infusion in NS or D_5W solution is stable for 24 hours at room temperature, 96 hours when refrigerated or 12 weeks when frozen; after freezing, thawed solution is stable for 24 hours at room temperature or 10 days when refrigerated; do not refreeze; do not mix with aminoglycosides

Mechanism of Action Interferes with bacterial cell wall synthesis during active replication, causing cell wall death and resultant bactericidal activity against susceptible bacteria

Pharmacokinetics

Distribution: V_d: 0.35-0.5 L/kg; penetrates CSF

Protein binding: 30%

Half-life: 1.6 hours, increases to 25 hours when Cl_{cr} falls to <10 mL/minute

Time to peak serum concentration: I.M.: Within 0.5-1 hour

Elimination: Excreted unchanged in urine

Dialysis: Moderately dialyzable (20% to 50%)

Usual Dosage I.M., I.V.:

Infants ≥6 months and Children: 150-200 mg/kg/day divided every 6-8 hours; maximum dose: 12 g/24 hours

Adults: 1-2 g every 8-12 hours

Life-threatening infections: Up to 2 g every 4 hours or 4 g every 8 hours

Uncomplicated gonorrhea: I.M.: 1 g (single dose)

Dosing interval in renal impairment:

Cl_{cr} 50-80 mL/minute: Administer every 8-12 hours

Cl_{cr} 10-50 mL/minute: Administer every 36-48 hours

Cl_{cr} <10 mL/minute: Administer every 48-72 hours

Administration Parenteral:

I.V. intermittent infusion: Administer over 30 minutes; usual dilution: 1 g/50 mL, doses >1 g are usually diluted to 100 mL

I.V. direct (bolus) injection: Administer slowly over 3-5 minutes at a concentration of 95 mg/mL

Test Interactions May falsely elevate creatine values when Jaffé reaction is used; may cause false-positive urinary glucose tests using cupric sulfate (Clinitest®, Benedict's solution)

Additional Information Sodium content of 1 g ceftizoxime: 60 mg (2.6 mEq); ceftizoxime does not cover *Chlamydia trachomatis* infections and must, therefore, be used with appropriate antichlamydial agents when treating pelvic inflammatory disease if *C. trachomatis* is suspected

(Continued)

Ceftizoxime *(Continued)*

Dosage Forms Available as sodium ceftizoxime; mg strength refers to ceftizoxime; [DSC] = Discontinued product
Infusion [premixed iso-osmotic solution]:
Cefizox®: 1 g (50 mL); 2 g (50 mL)
Injection, powder for reconstitution:
Cefizox®: 1 g, 2 g, 10 g [DSC]

♦ **Ceftizoxime Sodium** *see* Ceftizoxime *on page 318*

Ceftriaxone (sef trye AKS one)

Medication Safety Issues
Sound-alike/look-alike issues:
Rocephin® may be confused with Roferon®

Related Information
Endocarditis Prophylaxis *on page 1812*

U.S. Brand Names Rocephin®

Canadian Brand Names Rocephin®

Index Terms Ceftriaxone Sodium

Therapeutic Category Antibiotic, Cephalosporin (Third Generation)

Generic Available Yes

Use Treatment of sepsis, meningitis, infections of the lower respiratory tract, skin and skin structure, bone and joint, intra-abdominal and urinary tract due to susceptible organisms; as a third generation cephalosporin, ceftriaxone has activity against gram-negative aerobic bacteria (ie, *H. influenzae*, Enterobacteriaceae, *Neisseria*), and variable activity against gram-positive cocci; considered inactive against *Pseudomonas aeruginosa* and *C. trachomatis*; documented or suspected infection due to susceptible organisms in home care patients and patients without I.V. line access; treatment of documented or suspected gonococcal infection or chancroid; emergency room management of patients at high risk for bacteremia, periorbital or buccal cellulitis, salmonellosis or shigellosis and pneumonia of unestablished etiology (<5 years of age); treatment of resistant acute otitis media; in children with acute otitis media who are unable to take oral antibiotics

Pregnancy Risk Factor B

Lactation Enters breast milk/use caution (AAP rates "compatible")

Contraindications Hypersensitivity to ceftriaxone sodium, any component, or cephalosporins; do not use in hyperbilirubinemic neonates, particularly those who are premature since ceftriaxone is reported to displace bilirubin from albumin binding sites increasing the risk for kernicterus

Warnings Prolonged use may result in superinfection with yeasts, enterococci, *B. fragilis*, or *P. aeruginosa*; do not use in patients with immediate-type hypersensitivity reactions to penicillin

Precautions Use with caution in patients with gallbladder, biliary tract, liver, or pancreatic disease; or in patients with history of colitis or penicillin hypersensitivity

Adverse Reactions
Central nervous system: Fever, chills, headache, dizziness
Dermatologic: Rash, pruritus
Gastrointestinal: Diarrhea, nausea, vomiting, sludging in the gallbladder, cholelithiasis, pseudomembranous colitis
Genitourinary: Vaginitis, casts in urine
Hematologic: Eosinophilia, leukopenia, anemia, thrombocytopenia, thrombocytosis, bleeding, neutropenia
Hepatic: Transient elevation in liver enzymes, jaundice, elevation in serum bilirubin
Local: Pain at injection site
Renal: Elevated BUN and serum creatinine

Drug Interactions High-dose probenecid (decreases elimination half-life of ceftriaxone); aminoglycosides may increase risk of nephrotoxicity

Stability Reconstituted solution (100 mg/mL) is stable for 3 days at room temperature and 10 days when refrigerated; reconstituted solution (250 mg/mL) is stable for 24 hours at room temperature and 3 days when refrigerated

Mechanism of Action Inhibits bacterial cell wall synthesis by binding to one or more of the penicillin-binding proteins; inhibits the final transpeptidation step of peptidoglycan synthesis resulting in cell wall death

Pharmacokinetics
Distribution: Widely distributed throughout the body including gallbladder, lungs, bone, bile, CSF (diffuses into the CSF at higher concentrations when the meninges are inflamed); crosses the placenta
Protein binding: 85% to 95%

Half-life:
Neonates:
1-4 days: 16 hours
9-30 days: 9 hours
Adults: 5-9 hours (with normal renal and hepatic function)
Time to peak serum concentration: I.M.: Within 1-2 hours
Elimination: Unchanged in the urine (33% to 65%) by glomerular filtration and in feces via bile
Dialysis: Not dialyzable (0% to 5%)

Usual Dosage I.M., I.V.:
Neonates:
Postnatal age ≤7 days: 50 mg/kg/day given every 24 hours
Postnatal age >7 days:
≤2000 g: 50 mg/kg/day given every 24 hours
>2000 g: 50-75 mg/kg/day given every 24 hours
Gonococcal prophylaxis: 25-50 mg/kg as a single dose (dose not to exceed 125 mg)
Gonococcal infection: 25-50 mg/kg/day (maximum dose: 125 mg) given every 24 hours for 7 days, up to 10-14 days if meningitis is documented
Note: Use cefotaxime in place of ceftriaxone in hyperbilirubinemic neonates
Infants and Children: 50-75 mg/kg/day divided every 12-24 hours
Meningitis: 80-100 mg/kg/day divided every 12-24 hours; loading dose of 75 mg/kg may be administered at the start of therapy; maximum dose: 4 g/day
Chemoprophylaxis for high-risk contacts of patients with invasive meningococcal disease:
≤12 years: I.M.: 125 mg in a single dose
>12 years: I.M.: 250 mg in a single dose
Uncomplicated gonococcal infections, sexual assault, and STD prophylaxis: I.M.: 125 mg in a single dose
Complicated gonococcal infections: I.M., I.V.:
<45 kg:
Peritonitis, arthritis, or bacteremia: 50 mg/kg/day once daily for 7 days; maximum dose: 1 g/day
Conjunctivitis: 50 mg/kg (maximum dose: 1 g) in a single dose
Meningitis or endocarditis: 50 mg/kg/day divided every 12 hours for 10-14 days (meningitis), for 28 days (endocarditis); maximum dose: 2 g/day
>45 kg:
Disseminated gonococcal infections: 1 g/day once daily for 7 days
Meningitis: 1-2 g/dose every 12 hours for 10-14 days
Endocarditis: 1-2 g/dose every 12 hours for 28 days
Conjunctivitis: I.M.: 1 g in a single dose
Chancroid: I.M.: 50 mg/kg as a single dose (maximum dose: 250 mg)
Acute epididymitis: I.M.: 250 mg in a single dose
Acute otitis media: 50 mg/kg in a single dose (maximum dose: 1 g)
Persistent or relapsing acute otitis media: 50 mg/kg once daily for 3 days (maximum dose: 1 g/day)
Adults: 1-2 g every 12-24 hours depending on the type and severity of the infection; maximum dose: 4 g/day
Dosing interval in renal impairment: No change necessary with dose ≤2 g/day

Administration Parenteral:
IVP: Administer over 2-4 minutes at a maximum concentration of 40 mg/mL. Rapid IVP injection over 5 minutes of a 2 g dose resulted in tachycardia, restlessness, diaphoresis, and palpitations in an adult patient
I.V. intermittent infusion: Administer over 10-30 minutes; final concentration for I.V. administration should not exceed 40 mg/mL
I.M. injection: May be diluted with SWI or 1% lidocaine to a final concentration of 250 mg/mL or may be concentrated by using the manufacturer's recommended diluent volume of 1% lidocaine with a resultant concentration of 350 mg/mL; administer I.M. injections deep into a large muscle mass

Monitoring Parameters CBC with differential, platelet count, PT, renal and hepatic function tests periodically; number and type of stools/day for diarrhea

Test Interactions False-positive urine glucose with Clinitest®; may falsely elevate serum or urinary creatinine values when a manual Jaffé method is used

Additional Information Sodium content of 1 g: 3.6 mEq

Dosage Forms Excipient information presented when available (limited, particularly for generics); consult specific product labeling.
Note: Contains sodium 83 mg (3.6 mEq) per ceftriaxone 1 g
Infusion [premixed in dextrose]: 1 g (50 mL); 2 g (50 mL)
Injection, powder for reconstitution: 250 mg, 500 mg, 1 g, 2 g, 10 g
(Continued)

Ceftriaxone *(Continued)*

References

Bradley JS, Compogiannis LS, Murray WE, et al, "Pharmacokinetics and Safety of Intramuscular Injection of Concentrated Ceftriaxone in Children," *Clin Pharm*, 1992, 11(11):961-4.

Centers for Disease Control and Prevention, "2002 Guidelines for Treatment of Sexually Transmitted Diseases," *MMWR Morb Mortal Wkly Rep*, 2002, 51(RR-6):1-80.

Committee on Adolescence, American Academy of Pediatrics, "Sexual Assault and the Adolescent," *Pediatrics*, 1994, 94(5):761-5.

Dowell SF, Butler JC, Giebink GS, et al, "Acute Otitis Media: Management and Surveillance in an era of Pneumococcal Resistance--A Report From the Drug-Resistant *Streptococcus pneumoniae* Therapeutic Working Group," *Pediatr Infect Dis J*, 1999, 18(1):1-9.

Richards DM, Heel RC, Brogden RN, et al, "Ceftriaxone: A Review of Its Antibacterial Activity, Pharmacological Properties and Therapeutic Use," *Drugs*, 1984, 27(6):469-527.

♦ **Ceftriaxone Sodium** *see* Ceftriaxone *on page 320*

Cefuroxime (se fyoor OKS eem)

Medication Safety Issues

Sound-alike/look-alike issues:

Cefuroxime may be confused with cefotaxime, cefprozil, ceftizoxime, deferoxamine

Ceftin® may be confused with Cefotan®, cefotetan, Cefzil®, Cipro®

Zinacef® may be confused with Zithromax®

International issues:

Ceftin® may be confused with Cefiton® which is a brand name for cefixime in Portugal

Ceftin® may be confused with Ceftina® which is a brand name for cefalotin in Mexico

Ceftin® may be confused with Ceftim® which is a brand name for ceftazidime in Italy

U.S. Brand Names Ceftin®; Zinacef®

Canadian Brand Names Apo-Cefuroxime®; Ceftin®; ratio-Cefuroxime; Zinacef®

Index Terms Cefuroxime Axetil; Cefuroxime Sodium

Therapeutic Category Antibiotic, Cephalosporin (Second Generation)

Generic Available Yes: Excludes powder for oral suspension

Use A second generation cephalosporin useful in infections caused by susceptible staphylococci, group B streptococci, pneumococci, *H. influenzae* (type A and B), *E. coli*, *Enterobacter*, and *Klebsiella*; treatment of susceptible infections of the upper and lower respiratory tract, otitis media, acute bacterial maxillary sinusitis, urinary tract, skin and soft tissue, bone and joint, and sepsis

Pregnancy Risk Factor B

Lactation Enters breast milk/use caution

Contraindications Hypersensitivity to cefuroxime, any component, or cephalosporins

Warnings Prolonged use may result in superinfection; patients with renal or hepatic impairment, poor nutritional state, patients previously stabilized on anticoagulant therapy, or who have received a prolonged course of antimicrobial therapy are at risk for developing a fall in prothrombin activity. Monitor prothrombin time and consider administering vitamin K if indicated. Safety and efficacy in infants <3 months of age have not been established; do not use in patients with immediate-type hypersensitivity reactions to penicillin

Precautions Use with caution and modify dosage in patients with renal impairment; use with caution in patients with history of colitis or history of penicillin hypersensitivity

Adverse Reactions

Central nervous system: Fever, headache, dizziness, vertigo, seizures

Dermatologic: Rash, pruritus, erythema multiforme, diaper rash, urticaria

Gastrointestinal: Nausea, vomiting, diarrhea, stomach cramps, GI bleeding, antibiotic-associated colitis, stomatitis

Genitourinary: Vaginitis

Hematologic: Hemolytic anemia, transient neutropenia and leukopenia, decreased hemoglobin and hematocrit, eosinophilia, increased prothrombin time

Hepatic: Transient elevation in liver enzymes, hepatitis, cholestasis

Local: Pain at injection site, thrombophlebitis

Renal: Elevated BUN and serum creatinine

Miscellaneous: Anaphylaxis

Drug Interactions Probenecid (increases serum cefuroxime concentration); aminoglycosides may increase risk of nephrotoxicity

Food Interactions Food and milk increase bioavailability and peak levels

Stability Reconstituted injectable solution (100 mg/mL) or injectable suspension (200-220 mg/mL) is stable for 24 hours at room temperature or 48 hours when refrigerated; reconstituted oral suspension can be stored in the refrigerator or at room temperature; discard after 10 days

Mechanism of Action Inhibits bacterial cell wall synthesis by binding to one or mc of the penicillin-binding proteins; inhibits the final transpeptidation step of peptid glycan synthesis resulting in cell wall death

Pharmacokinetics

Absorption: Oral: Increased when given with or shortly after food or infant formula

Distribution: Into bronchial secretions, synovial and pericardial fluid, kidneys, heart, liver, bone and bile; penetrates into CSF with inflamed meninges; crosses the placenta; excreted into breast milk

Protein binding: 33% to 50%

Bioavailability: Oral cefuroxime axetil tablets: 37% to 52%; cefuroxime axetil suspension is less bioavailable than the tablet (91% of the AUC for tablets)

Half-life:

Neonates:

≤3 days: 5.1-5.8 hours

6-14 days: 2-4.2 hours

3-4 weeks: 1-1.5 hours

Adults: 1-2 hours (prolonged in renal impairment)

Time to peak serum concentration:

Oral: 2-3 hours

I.M.: Within 15-60 minutes

Elimination: Primarily 66% to 100% as unchanged drug in urine by both glomerular filtration and tubular secretion

Dialysis: Dialyzable

Usual Dosage

I.M., I.V.:

Neonates: 50-100 mg/kg/day divided every 12 hours

Children: 75-150 mg/kg/day divided every 8 hours; maximum dose: 6 g/day

Meningitis: Not recommended due to reports of treatment failures and slower bacteriologic response time (doses of 200-240 mg/kg/day divided every 6-8 hours have been used); maximum dose: 9 g/day

Adults: 750 mg to 1.5 g/dose every 8 hours

Oral: **Cefuroxime axetil film-coated tablets and oral suspension are not bioequivalent and are not substitutable on a mg/mg basis**

Infants ≥3 months to Children 12 years:

Pharyngitis, tonsillitis: Suspension: 20 mg/kg/day (maximum dose: 500 mg/day) in 2 divided doses

Acute otitis media, acute bacterial maxillary sinusitis, impetigo:

Suspension: 30 mg/kg/day (maximum dose: 1 g/day) in 2 divided doses

Tablet: 250 mg every 12 hours

Adolescents and Adults: 250-500 mg twice daily

Uncomplicated urinary tract infection: 125-250 mg every 12 hours

Uncomplicated gonorrhea: Single 1 g dose

Early Lyme disease: 500 mg twice daily for 20 days

Dosing interval in renal impairment:

Cl_{cr} 10-20 mL/minute: Administer every 12 hours

Cl_{cr} <10 mL/minute: Administer every 24 hours

Administration

Oral: Cefuroxime axetil suspension must be administered with food; shake suspension well before use; tablets may be administered with or without food; administer with food to decrease GI upset; avoid crushing the tablet due to its bitter taste

Parenteral:

IVP: Administer over 3-5 minutes at a maximum concentration of 100 mg/mL

I.V. intermittent infusion: Administer over 15-30 minutes at a final concentration for administration ≤30 mg/mL; in fluid restricted patients, a concentration of 137 mg/mL may be administered

I.M.: I.M. injection is less painful when administered as an injectable suspension rather than a solution (see Stability), and is less painful when administered into the buttock rather than the thigh

Monitoring Parameters With prolonged therapy, monitor renal, hepatic, and hematologic function periodically; number and type of stools/day for diarrhea; and prothrombin time

Test Interactions Positive Coombs' [direct]; false-positive urine glucose with Clinitest®

Dosage Forms Excipient information presented when available (limited, particularly for generics); consult specific product labeling.

Note: Strength expressed as base

Infusion, as sodium [premixed]: 750 mg (50 mL); 1.5 g (50 mL)

Zinacef®: 750 mg (50 mL); 1.5 g (50 mL) [contains sodium 4.8 mEq (111 mg) per 750 mg]

Injection, powder for reconstitution, as sodium: 750 mg, 1.5 g, 7.5 g

Zinacef®: 750 mg, 1.5 g, 7.5 g [contains sodium 1.8 mEq (41 mg) per 750 mg]

(Continued)

efuroxime *(Continued)*

Powder for oral suspension, as axetil:

Ceftin®: 125 mg/5 mL (100 mL) [contains phenylalanine 11.8 mg/5 mL; tutti-frutti flavor]; 250 mg/5 mL (50 mL, 100 mL) [contains phenylalanine 25.2 mg/5 mL; tutti-frutti flavor]

Tablet, as axetil: 250 mg, 500 mg

Ceftin®: 250 mg, 500 mg

References

de Louvois J, Mulhall A, and Hurley R, "Cefuroxime in the Treatment of Neonates," *Arch Dis Child*, 1982, 57(1):59-62.

Gooch WM 3rd, Blair E, Puopolo A, et al, "Effectiveness of Five Days of Therapy With Cefuroxime Axetil Suspension for Treatment of Acute Otitis Media," *Pediatr Infect Dis J*, 1996, 15(2):157-64.

Nelson JD, "Cefuroxime: A Cephalosporin With Unique Applicability to Pediatric Practice," *Pediatr Infect Dis*, 1983, 2(5):394-6.

Thoene DE and Johnson CE, "Pharmacotherapy of Otitis Media," *Pharmacotherapy*, 1991, 11(3):212-21.

♦ **Cefuroxime Axetil** *see* Cefuroxime *on page 322*
♦ **Cefuroxime Sodium** *see* Cefuroxime *on page 322*
♦ **Cefzil®** *see* Cefprozil *on page 316*
♦ **Celestone®** *see* Betamethasone *on page 212*
♦ **Celestone® Soluspan®** *see* Betamethasone *on page 212*
♦ **Celexa®** *see* Citalopram *on page 368*
♦ **CellCept®** *see* Mycophenolate *on page 1093*
♦ **Celontin®** *see* Methsuximide *on page 1030*
♦ **Cemill [OTC]** *see* Ascorbic Acid *on page 159*
♦ **Cenolate®** *see* Ascorbic Acid *on page 159*
♦ **Centany™** *see* Mupirocin *on page 1091*
♦ **Cepacol® Sore Throat [OTC]** *see* Benzocaine *on page 204*

Cephalexin (sef a LEKS in)

Medication Safety Issues

Sound-alike/look-alike issues:

Cephalexin may be confused with cefaclor, cefazolin, cephalothin, ciprofloxacin

Related Information

Endocarditis Prophylaxis *on page 1812*

U.S. Brand Names Biocef®; Keflex®; Panixine DisperDose™ [DSC]

Canadian Brand Names Apo-Cephalex®; Keftab®; Novo-Lexin; Nu-Cephalex

Index Terms Cephalexin Monohydrate

Therapeutic Category Antibiotic, Cephalosporin (First Generation)

Generic Available Yes: Excludes tablet for oral suspension

Use Treatment of susceptible bacterial infections, including those caused by group A beta-hemolytic *Streptococcus*, *Staphylococcus*, *Klebsiella pneumoniae*, *E. coli*, and *Proteus mirabilis*; not active against enterococci or methicillin-resistant staphylococci; used to treat susceptible infections of the respiratory tract, skin and skin structure, bone, genitourinary tract, and otitis media; alternative therapy for endocarditis prophylaxis

Pregnancy Risk Factor B

Lactation Enters breast milk (small amounts)/use caution

Contraindications Hypersensitivity to cephalexin, any component, or cephalosporins

Warnings Prolonged use may result in GI or genitourinary superinfection; do not use in patients with immediate-type hypersensitivity reactions to penicillin

Precautions Use with caution and modify dosage in patients with renal impairment; use with caution in patients with history of colitis or history of penicillin hypersensitivity. Tablets for oral suspension contain aspartame which is metabolized to phenylalanine and must be avoided (or used with caution) in patients with phenylketonuria.

Adverse Reactions

Central nervous system: Dizziness, headache, fatigue, fever, confusion

Dermatologic: Rash, urticaria, angioedema; erythema multiforme, Stevens-Johnson syndrome, toxic epidermal necrolysis (rare)

Gastrointestinal: Nausea, vomiting, pseudomembranous colitis, diarrhea, cramps, gastritis

Genitourinary: Vaginal moniliasis, vaginitis

Hematologic: Transient neutropenia, thrombocytopenia, anemia, eosinophilia

Hepatic: Transient elevation in liver enzymes, hepatitis, cholestatic jaundice

Neuromuscular & skeletal: Arthralgia, arthritis

Renal: Interstitial nephritis (rare)

Miscellaneous: Anaphylaxis

Drug Interactions Probenecid increases serum concentration of cephalexin

Food Interactions Food may delay absorption

Stability Refrigerate suspension after reconstitution; discard after 14 days; tablets for oral suspension should be used immediately after dissolving

Mechanism of Action Inhibits bacterial cell wall synthesis by binding to one or more of the penicillin-binding proteins; inhibits the final transpeptidation step of peptidoglycan synthesis resulting in cell wall death

Pharmacokinetics

Absorption: Delayed in young children and may be decreased up to 50% in neonates

Distribution: Into tissues and fluids including bone, pleural and synovial fluid; crosses the placenta; appears in breast milk

Protein binding: 6% to 15%

Half-life:

- Neonates: 5 hours
- Children 3-12 months: 2.5 hours
- Adults: 0.5-1.2 hours (prolonged with renal impairment)

Time to peak serum concentration: Oral: Within 60 minutes

Elimination: 80% to 100% of dose excreted as unchanged drug in urine within 8 hours

Dialysis: Moderately dialyzable (20% to 50%)

Usual Dosage Oral:

Children: 25-50 mg/kg/day divided every 6-8 hours; severe infections: 50-100 mg/kg/day divided every 6-8 hours; maximum dose: 4 g/day

- Otitis media: 75-100 mg/kg/day divided every 6 hours
- Streptococcal pharyngitis, skin and skin structure infections: 25-50 mg/kg/day divided every 12 hours
- Endocarditis prophylaxis: 50 mg/kg 1 hour prior to procedure (maximum: 2 g)
- Uncomplicated cystitis: Children >15 years: 500 mg every 12 hours for 7-14 days

Adults: 250-500 mg every 6 hours; maximum dose: 4 g/day

- Streptococcal pharyngitis, skin and skin structure infections: 500 mg every 12 hours
- Endocarditis prophylaxis: 2 g 1 hour prior to procedure
- Uncomplicated cystitis: 500 mg every 12 hours for 7-14 days

Dosing interval in renal impairment:

- Cl_{cr} 10-40 mL/minute: Administer every 8-12 hours
- Cl_{cr} <10 mL/minute: Administer every 12-24 hours

Administration Oral: Administer on an empty stomach (ie, 1 hour prior to, or 2 hours after meals); administer with food if GI upset occurs; shake suspension well before use

Tablet for oral suspension: Mix tablet in a small amount of water (~10 mL); stir until thoroughly mixed; entire mixture should be administered immediately after mixing; rinse container with an additional small amount of water and drink contents to assure the whole dose is taken. **Do not** chew or swallow tablets. **Do not** mix with liquids other than water.

Monitoring Parameters With prolonged therapy, monitor renal, hepatic, and hematologic function periodically; number and type of stools/day for diarrhea

Test Interactions False-positive urine glucose with Clinitest®; positive Coombs' [direct]; false ↑ serum or urine creatinine

Patient Information Counsel patient that cephalexin should only be used to treat bacterial infections. Entire course of medication should be taken even if patient feels better early in the course. Report prolonged diarrhea.

Dosage Forms Excipient information presented when available (limited, particularly for generics); consult specific product labeling. [DSC] = Discontinued product

Capsule: 250 mg, 500 mg

- Biocef®: 500 mg
- Keflex®: 250 mg, 333 mg [DSC], 500 mg, 750 mg

Powder for oral suspension: 125 mg/5 mL (100 mL, 200 mL); 250 mg/5 mL (100 mL, 200 mL)

- Biocef®: 125 mg/5 mL (100 mL); 250 mg/5 mL (100 mL)
- Keflex®: 125 mg/5 mL (100 mL, 200 mL); 250 mg/5 mL (100 mL, 200 mL)

Tablet, for oral suspension (Panixine DisperDose™): 125 mg [contains phenylalanine 2.8 mg; peppermint flavor], 250 mg [contains phenylalanine 5.6 mg; peppermint flavor] [DSC]

♦ **Cephalexin Monohydrate** *see* Cephalexin *on page 324*

Cephradine (SEF ra deen)

Medication Safety Issues

Sound-alike/look-alike issues:

- Cephradine may be confused with cephapirin
- Velosef® may be confused with Vasosulf®

(Continued)

Cephradine *(Continued)*

U.S. Brand Names Velosef®

Therapeutic Category Antibiotic, Cephalosporin (First Generation)

Generic Available No

Use Treatment of susceptible bacterial infections, including skin and skin structure infections caused by *Streptococcus* or *Staphylococcus*; urinary tract infections caused by *Klebsiella, E. coli*, and *Proteus mirabilis*; respiratory tract infections caused by group A beta-hemolytic streptococci and *Streptococcus pneumoniae*; otitis media caused by group A beta-hemolytic streptococci, *Streptococcus pneumoniae*, or *H. influenzae*

Pregnancy Risk Factor B

Lactation Enters breast milk/use caution

Contraindications Hypersensitivity to cephradine, any component, or cephalosporins

Warnings Prolonged use may result in superinfection; do not use in patients with immediate-type hypersensitivity reaction to penicillin

Precautions Use with caution in patients with a history of penicillin hypersensitivity; reduce dose in patients with renal impairment

Adverse Reactions

Dermatologic: Rash

Gastrointestinal: Diarrhea, nausea, vomiting, pseudomembranous colitis

Genitourinary: Vaginitis

Hematologic: Transient neutropenia, eosinophilia, leukopenia

Hepatic: Elevated liver enzymes, elevated bilirubin

Neuromuscular & skeletal: Arthralgia

Renal: Elevated BUN and serum creatinine

Drug Interactions Probenecid may decrease renal tubular secretion and increase cephradine serum concentrations

Food Interactions Food will decrease the rate, but not the extent of oral absorption

Stability Oral suspension: Stable for 7 days at room temperature, or 14 days at 2°C to 8°C after reconstitution

Mechanism of Action Interferes with bacterial cell wall synthesis during active replication, causing cell wall death and resultant bactericidal activity against susceptible bacteria

Pharmacokinetics

Absorption: Well absorbed from GI tract

Distribution: V_d: 0.25 L/kg; crosses the placenta; appears in breast milk

Protein binding: 6% to 20%

Half-life: Adults: 0.7-2 hours; Children: 1 hour; half-life increases with renal dysfunction

Time to peak serum concentration: Oral: Within 1-2 hours

Elimination: Excreted unchanged in the urine (80% to 90%) via glomerular filtration and tubular secretion

Usual Dosage Oral:

Infants ≥9 months and Children:

- Usual: 25-50 mg/kg/day in divided doses every 6-12 hours
- Otitis media: 75-100 mg/kg/day in divided doses every 6-12 hours
- Maximum dose: 4 g/day

Adults: Oral: 250-500 mg every 6-12 hours

Dosing adjustment in renal impairment:

- Cl_{cr} 10-50 mL/minute: Administer 50% of dose given at normal interval
- Cl_{cr} <10 mL/minute: Administer 25% of dose given at normal interval

or

- Cl_{cr} 25-50 mL/minute: Administer normal dose every 12 hours
- Cl_{cr} 10-25 mL/minute: Administer normal dose every 24 hours
- Cl_{cr} <10 mL/minute: Administer normal dose every 36 hours

Administration Oral: May be administered without regard to food; shake suspension well before use

Monitoring Parameters Periodic renal and hepatic function tests; number and type of stools/day for diarrhea; resolution of infection

Test Interactions False-positive Coombs' test; may falsely elevate creatinine values when Jaffé reaction is used; may cause false-positive results in urine glucose tests using cupric sulfate (Benedict's solution, Clinitest®)

Patient Information Report persistent diarrhea; entire course of medication (eg, 10-14 days) should be taken to ensure eradication of organism

Additional Information Efficacy not established for twice daily dosing in infants <9 months of age; parenteral product no longer available in the United States

Dosage Forms Excipient information presented when available (limited, particularly for generics); consult specific product labeling. [DSC] = Discontinued product

Capsule: 250 mg, 500 mg [DSC]

Powder for oral suspension: 250 mg/5 mL (100 mL) [fruit flavor]

References

Donowitz GR and Mandell GL, "Drug Therapy. Beta-Lactam Antibiotics (1)," *N Engl J Med*, 318(7):419-26.

Donowitz GR and Mandell GL, "Drug Therapy. Beta-Lactam Antibiotics (2)," *N Engl J Med*, 1 318(8):490-500.

Gustaferro CA and Steckelberg JM, "Cephalosporin Antimicrobial Agents and Related Compounds," *Ma Clin Proc*, 1991, 66(10):1064-73.

Smith GH, "Oral Cephalosporins in Perspective," *DICP*, 1990, 24(1):45-51.

- **Cerebyx®** *see* Fosphenytoin *on page 711*
- **Ceredase®** *see* Alglucerase *on page 75*
- **Cerezyme®** *see* Imiglucerase *on page 811*
- **Cerubidine®** *see* DAUNOrubicin *on page 447*
- **Cerumenex® [DSC]** *see* Triethanolamine Polypeptide Oleate-Condensate *on page 1574*
- **Cerumenex® (Can)** *see* Triethanolamine Polypeptide Oleate-Condensate *on page 1574*
- **C.E.S.** *see* Estrogens (Conjugated/Equine) *on page 610*
- **C.E.S.® (Can)** *see* Estrogens (Conjugated/Equine) *on page 610*
- **Cesamet™** *see* Nabilone *on page 1097*
- **Cetacort®** *see* Hydrocortisone *on page 781*
- **Cetafen® [OTC]** *see* Acetaminophen *on page 42*
- **Cetafen Extra® [OTC]** *see* Acetaminophen *on page 42*
- **Cetamide™ (Can)** *see* Sulfacetamide *on page 1483*
- **Ceta-Plus®** *see* Hydrocodone and Acetaminophen *on page 779*

Cetirizine (se TI ra zeen)

Medication Safety Issues

Sound-alike/look-alike issues:

Zyrtec® may be confused with Serax®, Xanax®, Zantac®, Zyprexa®

U.S. Brand Names Zyrtec®

Canadian Brand Names Apo-Cetirizine®; Reactine™

Index Terms Cetirizine Hydrochloride; P-071; UCB-P071

Therapeutic Category Antihistamine

Generic Available No

Use Relief of symptoms associated with perennial and seasonal allergic rhinitis; treatment of the uncomplicated skin manifestations of chronic idiopathic urticaria

Pregnancy Risk Factor B

Lactation Enters breast milk/not recommended

Contraindications Hypersensitivity to cetirizine, hydroxyzine, or any component

Warnings Doses >10 mg/day may cause significant drowsiness

Precautions Use with caution in patients with hepatic or renal dysfunction

Adverse Reactions

Cardiovascular: Palpitations, tachycardia, hypertension, hypotension

Central nervous system: Headache, drowsiness, somnolence, fatigue, dizziness, depression, confusion, vertigo, ataxia, syncope, hallucinations, convulsions (rare), aggressive reactions (rare), suicidal ideation (rare)

Dermatologic: Rash, photosensitivity, pruritus

Gastrointestinal: Diarrhea, flatulence, constipation, xerostomia, dyspepsia, abdominal pain, pharyngitis, taste loss, taste perversion, anorexia

Genitourinary: Dysuria, cystitis, polyuria, urinary incontinence, dysmenorrhea, vaginitis

Hematologic: Hemolytic anemia (rare), thrombocytopenia (rare)

Hepatic: Transient hepatic enzyme elevation, cholestasis, hepatitis (rare)

Neuromuscular & skeletal: Paresthesias, hyperkinesia, hypertonia, tremor, leg cramps

Otic: Tinnitus, ototoxicity, earache (<2%)

Renal: Glomerulonephritis (rare)

Respiratory: Cough, epistaxis, bronchospasm

Miscellaneous: Anaphylaxis (rare)

Drug Interactions Cytochrome P450 isoenzyme CYP3A4 substrate

Increased cetirizine toxicity: CNS depressants, anticholinergics; theophylline may decrease cetirizine clearance with potential increased toxicity

Stability Store at room temperature; protect syrup from light

Mechanism of Action Cetirizine, a metabolite of hydroxyzine, competes with histamine for H_1-receptor sites on effector cells in the GI tract, blood vessels, and respiratory tract

(Continued)

izine *(Continued)*

armacodynamics
Onset of action: 20-60 minutes
Duration: 24 hours

Pharmacokinetics
Absorption: Well absorbed from the GI tract
Distribution: V_d:
Children: 0.7 L/kg
Adults: 0.5-0.8 L/kg
Protein binding: 93%
Metabolism: Exact fate is unknown, limited hepatic metabolism
Half-life:
Children: 6.2 hours
Adults: 7.4-9 hours
Adults with mild-moderate renal failure: 19-21 hours
Time to peak serum concentration: 1 hour
Elimination: 60% to 70% excreted unchanged in urine
Dialysis: <10% removed during hemodialysis

Usual Dosage Oral:
Children 6-12 months: 2.5 mg once daily
Children 12-23 months: Initial: 2.5 mg once daily; dosage may be increased to 2.5 mg twice daily
Children 2-5 years: 2.5 mg/day; may be increased to a maximum of 5 mg/day given either as a single dose or divided into 2 doses
Children ≥6 years to Adults: 5-10 mg/day as a single dose or divided into 2 doses
Dosage adjustment in renal or hepatic impairment:
Children <6 years: Cetirizine use not recommended
Children 6-11 years: <2.5 mg once daily
Children ≥12 and Adults:
Cl_{cr} 11-31 mL/minute, hemodialysis, or hepatic impairment: 5 mg once daily
Cl_{cr} <11 mL/minute, not on dialysis: Cetirizine use not recommended

Administration Oral: Administer without regard to food

Patient Information May cause drowsiness and impair ability to perform activities requiring mental alertness or physical coordination; may cause dry mouth. May cause photosensitivity reactions (eg, exposure to sunlight may cause severe sunburn, skin rash, redness, or itching); avoid exposure to sunlight and artificial light sources (sunlamps, tanning booth/bed); wear protective clothing, wide-brimmed hats, sunglasses, and lip sunscreen (SPF ≥15); use a sunscreen [broad-spectrum sunscreen or physical sunscreen (preferred) or sunblock with SPF ≥15]; contact physician if reaction occurs.

Dosage Forms Excipient information presented when available (limited, particularly for generics); consult specific product labeling.
Syrup, as hydrochloride: 5 mg/5 mL (120 mL, 480 mL) [banana-grape flavor]
Tablet, as hydrochloride: 5 mg, 10 mg
Tablet, chewable, as hydrochloride: 5 mg, 10 mg [grape flavor]

- ♦ **Cetirizine Hydrochloride** *see* Cetirizine *on page 327*
- ♦ **CFDN** *see* Cefdinir *on page 305*
- ♦ **CG** *see* Chorionic Gonadotropin *on page 351*
- ♦ **C-Gel [OTC]** *see* Ascorbic Acid *on page 159*
- ♦ **C-Gram [OTC]** *see* Ascorbic Acid *on page 159*
- ♦ **Charcadole® (Can)** *see* Charcoal, Activated *on page 328*
- ♦ **Charcadole®, Aqueous (Can)** *see* Charcoal, Activated *on page 328*
- ♦ **Charcadole® TFS (Can)** *see* Charcoal, Activated *on page 328*
- ♦ **Char-Caps [OTC]** *see* Charcoal, Activated *on page 328*

Charcoal, Activated (CHAR kole AK tiv ay ted)

Medication Safety Issues
Sound-alike/look-alike issues:
Actidose® may be confused with Actos®

U.S. Brand Names Actidose-Aqua® [OTC]; Actidose® with Sorbitol [OTC]; Char-Caps [OTC]; Charcoal Plus® DS [OTC]; Charcocaps® [OTC]; EZ-Char™ [OTC]; Kerr Insta-Char® [OTC]

Canadian Brand Names Charcadole®; Charcadole®, Aqueous; Charcadole® TFS

Index Terms Activated Carbon; Activated Charcoal; Adsorbent Charcoal; Liquid Antidote; Medicinal Carbon; Medicinal Charcoal

Therapeutic Category Antidiarrheal; Antidote, Adsorbent; Antiflatulent

Generic Available Yes: Powder

Use Emergency treatment in poisoning by drugs and chemicals (see Additional Information); repetitive doses for GI dialysis in drug overdose to enhance the elimination of certain drugs (eg, theophylline, phenobarbital, carbamazepine, dapsone, quinine) and in uremia to adsorb various waste products

Pregnancy Risk Factor C

Lactation Does not enter breast milk/compatible

Contraindications Patients with an unprotected airway (eg, depressed CNS state without endotracheal intubation); patients at increased risk and severity of aspiration (eg, ingestion of hydrocarbon with a high potential for aspiration); patients at risk of GI perforation or hemorrhage due to medical conditions, recent surgery, or other pathology; **Note**: Ingestion of a corrosive (caustic) substance is **not** a contraindication if charcoal is used for coingested systemic toxin. Charcoal is not effective for cyanide, mineral acids, caustic alkalis, organic solvents, iron, ethanol, methanol or lithium poisonings; do not use charcoal with sorbitol in patients with fructose intolerance; charcoal with sorbitol is not recommended in children <1 year of age

Warnings If charcoal in sorbitol is administered, doses should be limited to prevent excessive fluid and electrolyte losses

Precautions When using ipecac with charcoal, induce vomiting with ipecac before administering activated charcoal since charcoal adsorbs ipecac syrup; charcoal may cause vomiting which is hazardous in petroleum distillate and caustic ingestions; charcoal (especially in multiple doses) may adsorb maintenance medications and place the patient at risk for exacerbation of concomitant disorders

Adverse Reactions

Gastrointestinal: Vomiting (**Note:** Use of charcoal with sorbitol may increase rate of emesis), constipation, intestinal obstruction, black stools; diarrhea if product contains sorbitol

Ocular: Corneal abrasions if spilled into eyes

Miscellaneous: Aspiration may cause tracheal obstruction in infants, but usually not a major problem in adults; aspiration pneumonitis, bronchiolitis obliterans, and ARDS have been reported following aspiration of charcoal; however, these problems may be due to the aspiration of gastric contents and not charcoal per se

Food Interactions Milk, ice cream, sherbet, or marmalade may reduce charcoal's effectiveness; chocolate or fruit syrup do not appear to reduce efficacy

Stability Adsorbs gases from air; store in closed container

Mechanism of Action Adsorbs toxic substances or irritants, thus inhibiting GI absorption; for select drugs, increases drug clearance by interfering with enterohepatic recycling or causing dialysis across intestinal membrane; adsorbs intestinal gas; the addition of sorbitol results in hyperosmotic laxative action causing catharsis

Pharmacodynamics In studies using adult human volunteers: Mean **reduction** in drug absorption following a single dose of activated charcoal:

All size doses of activated charcoal:

- Given within 30 minutes after ingestion: 69.1% reduction
- Given at 60 minutes after ingestion: 34.4% reduction

50 g activated charcoal:

- Given within 30 minutes after ingestion: 88.6% reduction
- Given at 60 minutes after ingestion: 37.3% reduction

Pharmacokinetics

Absorption: Not absorbed from the GI tract

Metabolism: Not metabolized

Elimination: Excreted as charcoal in feces

Usual Dosage Oral:

Acute poisoning:

Single dose: Charcoal with sorbitol (**Note:** The use of repeated oral charcoal with sorbitol doses is not recommended):

- Infants <1 year: Not recommended
- Children 1-12 years: 1-2 g/kg or 25-50 g or approximately 5-10 times the weight of the ingested poison on a gram-to-gram basis; 1 g adsorbs 100-1000 mg of poison; in young children sorbitol should be repeated **no more** than 1-2 times/day
- Adolescents and Adults: 30-100 g

Single dose: Charcoal in water (a cathartic such as sorbitol should be added in appropriate doses):

- Infants <1 year: 1 g/kg
- Children 1-12 years: 1-2 g/kg or 25-50 g
- Adolescents and Adults: 30-100 g or 1-2 g/kg

Multiple dose: Charcoal in water (doses are repeated until clinical observations of toxicity subside and serum drug concentrations have returned to a subtherapeutic range or until the development of absent bowel sounds or ileus; use only one dose of cathartic daily):

- Infants <1 year: 1 g/kg every 4-6 hours

(Continued)

Charcoal, Activated *(Continued)*

Children 1-12 years: 1-2 g/kg or 15-30 g every 2-6 hours
Adolescents and Adults: 25-60 g or 1-2 g/kg every 2-6 hours
Gastric dialysis: Adults: 20-50 g every 6 hours for 1-2 days

Administration Oral: Administer as soon as possible after ingestion, preferably within 1 hour for greatest effect; shake well before use; do not mix with milk, ice cream, sherbet, or marmalade; may be mixed with chocolate or fruit syrup to increase palatability; instruct patient to drink slowly, rapid administration may increase frequency of vomiting; if patient has persistent vomiting, multiple doses may be administered as a continuous enteral infusion

Monitoring Parameters Fluid status, sorbitol intake, number of stools, electrolytes if increase in stools or diarrhea occurs; continually assess for active bowel sounds in patients receiving multiple dose activated charcoal

Patient Information Charcoal causes the stools to turn black

Nursing Implications Charcoal slurries that are too concentrated may clog airways, if aspirated

Additional Information 5-6 tablespoonfuls of activated charcoal powder is approximately equal to 30 g; minimum dilution of 240 mL water per 20-30 g activated charcoal should be mixed as an aqueous slurry; multiple dose activated charcoal has been shown to be effective in increasing the elimination of certain drugs (carbamazepine, theophylline, phenobarbital) even after these drugs have been absorbed

The Position Statement on single-dose activated charcoal by The American Academy of Clinical Toxicology and The European Association of Poisons Centres and Clinical Toxicologists (AACT and EAPCCT, 1997) does not advocate **routine** use of single dose activated charcoal in the treatment of poisoned patients; scientific literature supports the use of activated charcoal within 1 hour of toxin ingestion, when it will be more likely to produce benefit. Therefore, this publication states that activated charcoal may be considered up to 1 hour following ingestion of a potentially toxic amount of poison; the use of activated charcoal may be considered greater than 1 hour following ingestion, but there are no studies to support or exclude its use. Furthermore, based on current literature, the routine administration of a cathartic with activated charcoal is not recommended; when cathartics are used, only a single dose should be administered so as to decrease adverse effects (AACT and EAPCCT, 1997a).

A recent policy statement by the American Academy of Pediatrics states that it is currently premature to recommend the **routine** administration of activated charcoal as a home treatment strategy for poisonings (see AAP, 2003).

Dosage Forms Excipient information presented when available (limited, particularly for generics); consult specific product labeling.

Capsule:
- Char-Caps, Charcocaps®: 260 mg

Liquid:
- Actidose-Aqua®: 15 g (72 mL); 25 g (120 mL); 50 g (240 mL)
- Kerr Insta-Char®: 25 g (120 mL) [cherry flavor]; 50 g (240 mL) [unflavored or cherry flavor]

Liquid [with sorbitol]:
- Actidose® with Sorbitol: 25 g (120 mL); 50 g (240 mL)
- Kerr Insta-Char®: 25 g (120 mL); 50 g (240 mL) [cherry flavor]

Pellet:
- EZ-Char™: 25 g

Powder for suspension: 30 g, 240 g

Tablet:
- Charcoal Plus® DS: 250 mg

References

American Academy of Pediatrics Committee on Injury, Violence, and Poison Prevention, "Poison Treatment in the Home," *Pediatrics*, 2003, 112(5):1182-5.

Burns MM, "Activated Charcoal as the Sole Intervention for Treatment After Childhood Poisoning," *Curr Opin Pediatr*, 2000, 12(2):166-71.

Farley TA, "Severe Hypernatremic Dehydration After Use of an Activated Charcoal-Sorbitol Suspension," *J Pediatr*, 1986, 109(4):719-22.

"Position Statement and Practice Guidelines on the Use of Multi-dose Activated Charcoal in the Treatment of Acute Poisoning. American Academy of Clinical Toxicology; European Association of Poisons Centres and Clinical Toxicologists," *J Toxicol Clin Toxicol*, 1999, 37(6):731-51.

"Position Statement: Cathartics. American Academy of Clinical Toxicology; European Association of Poisons Centres and Clinical Toxicologists," *J Toxicol Clin Toxicol*, 1997a, 35(7):743-52.

"Position Statement: Single-Dose Activated Charcoal. American Academy of Clinical Toxicology; European Association of Poisons Centres and Clinical Toxicologists," *J Toxicol Clin Toxicol*, 1997, 35(7):721-41.

Shannon M, "Ingestion of Toxic Substances by Children," *N Engl J Med*, 2000, 342(3):186-91.

♦ **Charcoal Plus® DS [OTC]** *see* Charcoal, Activated *on page 328*
♦ **Charcocaps® [OTC]** *see* Charcoal, Activated *on page 328*
♦ **Chemet®** *see* Succimer *on page 1477*

- **Cheracol®** *see* Guaifenesin and Codeine *on page 746*
- **Cheracol® D [OTC]** *see* Guaifenesin and Dextromethorphan *on page 748*
- **Cheracol® Plus [OTC]** *see* Guaifenesin and Dextromethorphan *on page 748*
- **Chew-C [OTC]** *see* Ascorbic Acid *on page 159*
- **CHG** *see* Chlorhexidine Gluconate *on page 337*
- **Chickenpox Vaccine** *see* Varicella Virus Vaccine *on page 1599*
- **Chiggerex® [OTC]** *see* Benzocaine *on page 204*
- **Chiggertox® [OTC]** *see* Benzocaine *on page 204*
- **Children's Advil® Cold (Can)** *see* Pseudoephedrine and Ibuprofen *on page 1346*
- **Children's Dimetapp® Elixir Cold & Allergy [OTC] [DSC]** *see* Brompheniramine and Pseudoephedrine *on page 235*
- **Children's Kaopectate® [OTC] [DSC]** *see* Attapulgite *on page 184*
- **Children's Pepto [OTC]** *see* Calcium Carbonate *on page 264*
- **Children's Pepto [OTC]** *see* Calcium Supplements *on page 272*
- **Children's Motion Sickness Liquid (Can)** *see* DimenhyDRINATE *on page 507*
- **ChiRhoStim™** *see* Secretin *on page 1425*
- **Chloral** *see* Chloral Hydrate *on page 331*

Chloral Hydrate (KLOR al HYE drate)

Related Information

Preprocedure Sedatives in Children *on page 1895*

U.S. Brand Names Aquachloral® Supprettes®; Somnote™

Canadian Brand Names PMS-Chloral Hydrate

Index Terms Chloral; Hydrated Chloral; Trichloroacetaldehyde Monohydrate

Therapeutic Category Hypnotic; Sedative

Generic Available Yes: Syrup

Use Short-term sedative and hypnotic (<2 weeks), sedative/hypnotic prior to nonpainful therapeutic or diagnostic procedures (eg, EEG, CT scan, MRI, ophthalmic exam, dental procedure)

Restrictions C-IV

Pregnancy Risk Factor C

Lactation Enters breast milk/compatible

Contraindications Hypersensitivity to chloral hydrate or any component (see Warnings); hepatic or renal impairment; severe cardiac disease. Oral forms are also contraindicated in patients with gastritis, esophagitis, or gastric or duodenal ulcers.

Warnings Deaths and permanent neurologic injury from respiratory compromise have been reported in children sedated with chloral hydrate; respiratory obstruction may occur in children with tonsillar and adenoidal hypertrophy, obstructive sleep apnea, and Leigh's encephalopathy, and in ASA class III children; depressed levels of consciousness may occur; chloral hydrate should **not** be administered for sedation by nonmedical personnel or in a nonsupervised medical environment; sedation with chloral hydrate requires careful patient monitoring (see Monitoring Parameters) (Cote, 2000); animal studies suggest that chloral hydrate may depress the genioglossus muscle and other airway-maintaining muscles in patients who are already at risk for life-threatening airway obstruction (eg, obstructive sleep apnea); alternative sedative agents should be considered for these patients (see Hershenson, 1984).

Trichloroethanol (TCE), an active metabolite of chloral hydrate, is a carcinogen in mice; there is no data in humans. The 325 mg suppositories contain tartrazine which may cause allergic reactions in susceptible individuals. Syrup contains sodium benzoate; benzoic acid (benzoate) is a metabolite of benzyl alcohol; large amounts of benzyl alcohol (≥99 mg/kg/day) have been associated with a potentially fatal toxicity ("gasping syndrome") in neonates; the "gasping syndrome" consists of metabolic acidosis, respiratory distress, gasping respirations, CNS dysfunction (including convulsions, intracranial hemorrhage), hypotension and cardiovascular collapse; use chloral hydrate products containing sodium benzoate with caution in neonates; *in vitro* and animal studies have shown that benzoate displaces bilirubin from protein binding sites

Precautions Use with caution in neonates, drug and metabolites may accumulate with repeated use; prolonged use in neonates is associated with direct hyperbilirubinemia [active metabolite (TCE) competes with bilirubin for glucuronide conjugation in the liver]; use with caution in patients with porphyria. Tolerance to hypnotic effect develops, therefore, not recommended for use >2 weeks; taper dosage to avoid withdrawal with prolonged use. Avoid use in patients with moderate to severe renal failure (Cl_{cr} <50 mL/minute).

(Continued)

Chloral Hydrate *(Continued)*

Adverse Reactions

Central nervous system: Disorientation, sedation, excitement (paradoxical), dizziness, fever, headache, ataxia

Dermatologic: Rash, urticaria

Gastrointestinal: Gastric irritation, nausea, vomiting, diarrhea, flatulence

Hematologic: Leukopenia, eosinophilia

Respiratory: Respiratory depression when combined with other sedatives or narcotics

Miscellaneous: Physical and psychological dependence with prolonged use

Drug Interactions May potentiate effects of warfarin, CNS depressants, alcohol; vasodilation reaction (flushing, tachycardia, etc) may occur with concurrent use of alcohol; concomitant use of furosemide (I.V.) may result in flushing, sweating, and blood pressure changes; chloral hydrate may increase the conversion of cyclophosphamide and ifosfamide to active metabolites and may increase toxicity

Stability Sensitive to light; exposure to air causes volatilization; store in light-resistant, airtight container at room temperature; do not refrigerate

Mechanism of Action Central nervous system depressant effects are primarily due to its active metabolite trichloroethanol, mechanism unknown; in neonates, chloral hydrate itself may play a role in the immediate sedative effects; **Note:** Chloral hydrate does not interfere with EEG results (unlike barbiturates and benzodiazepines)

Pharmacodynamics

Onset of action: 10-20 minutes

Maximum effect: Within 30-60 minutes

Duration: 4-8 hours

Pharmacokinetics

Absorption: Oral, rectal: Well absorbed

Distribution: Crosses the placenta; distributes to breast milk

Protein binding: Trichloroethanol: 35% to 40%; trichloroacetic acid: ~94% (may compete with bilirubin for albumin binding sites)

Metabolism: Rapidly metabolized by alcohol dehydrogenase to trichloroethanol (active metabolite); trichloroethanol undergoes glucuronidation in the liver; variable amounts of chloral hydrate and trichloroethanol are metabolized in liver and kidney to trichloroacetic acid (inactive)

Half-life:

- Chloral hydrate: Infants: 1 hour
- Trichloroethanol (active metabolite):
  - Neonates: Range: 8.5-66 hours
  - Half-life decreases with increasing postconceptional age (PCA):
    - Preterm infants (PCA 31-37 weeks): Mean half-life: 40 hours
    - Term infants (PCA 38-42 weeks): Mean half-life: 28 hours
    - Older children (PCA 57-708 weeks): Mean half-life: 10 hours
  - Adults: 8-11 hours
- Trichloroacetic acid: Adults: 67.2 hours

Elimination: Metabolites excreted in urine; small amounts excreted in feces via bile

Dialysis: Dialyzable (50% to 100%)

Usual Dosage Oral, rectal:

Neonates: 25 mg/kg/dose for sedation prior to a procedure; **Note:** Repeat doses should be used with great caution, as drug and metabolites accumulate with repeated use; toxicity has been reported after 3 days in a preterm neonate and after 7 days in a term neonate receiving chloral hydrate 40-50 mg/kg every 6 hours

Infants and Children:

- Sedation, anxiety: 25-50 mg/kg/day divided every 6-8 hours, maximum dose: 500 mg/dose
- Prior to EEG: 25-50 mg/kg/dose 30-60 minutes prior to EEG; may repeat in 30 minutes to a total maximum of 100 mg/kg or 1 g total for infants and 2 g total for children
- Hypnotic: 50 mg/kg; maximum dose: 2 g/dose/day
- Sedation, nonpainful procedure: 50-75 mg/kg/dose 30-60 minutes prior to procedure; may repeat 30 minutes after initial dose if needed, to a total maximum dose of 120 mg/kg or 1 g total for infants and 2 g total for children

Adults:

- Sedation, anxiety: 250 mg 3 times/day
- Hypnotic: 500-1000 mg at bedtime or 30 minutes prior to procedure, not to exceed 2 g/24 hours

Dosing adjustment in renal impairment:

- Cl_{cr} ≥50 mL/minute: No dosage adjustment needed
- Cl_{cr} <50 mL/minute: Avoid use

Administration Oral: Minimize unpleasant taste and gastric irritation by administering with water, infant formula, fruit juice, or ginger ale; do not crush capsule, contains drug in liquid form with unpleasant taste

Monitoring Parameters Level of sedation; vital signs and O_2 saturation with doses used for sedation prior to procedure

Test Interactions False-positive urine glucose using Clinitest® method; may interfere with fluorometric urine catecholamine and urinary 17-hydroxycorticosteroid tests

Patient Information May cause drowsiness and impair ability to perform activities requiring mental alertness or physical coordination; avoid alcohol and other CNS depressants; may be habit-forming; avoid abrupt discontinuation after prolonged use

Nursing Implications May cause irritation of skin and mucous membranes

Additional Information Not an analgesic; osmolality of 500 mg/5 mL syrup is approximately 3500 mOsm/kg

Dosage Forms Excipient information presented when available (limited, particularly for generics); consult specific product labeling.

Capsule (Somnote™): 500 mg

Suppository, rectal (Aquachloral® Supprettes®): 325 mg [contains tartrazine], 650 mg

Syrup: 500 mg/5 mL (480 mL) [contains sodium benzoate]

References

American Academy of Pediatrics, Committee on Drugs and Committee on Environmental Health, "Use of Chloral Hydrate for Sedation in Children," *Pediatrics*, 1993, 92(3):471-3.

Buck ML, "Chloral Hydrate Use During Infancy," *Neonatal Pharmacology Quarterly*, 1992, 1(1):31-7.

Cote CJ, Karl HW, Notterman DA, et al, "Adverse Sedation Events in Pediatrics: Analysis of Medications Used for Sedation," *Pediatrics*, 2000, 106(4):633-44.

Hershenson M, Brouillette RT, Olsen E, et al, "The Effect of Chloral Hydrate on Genioglossus and Diaphragmatic Activity," *Pediatr Res*, 1984, 18(6):516-9.

Mayers DJ, Hindmarsh KW, Gorecki DK, et al, "Sedative/Hypnotic Effects of Chloral Hydrate in the Neonate: Trichloroethanol or Parent Drug?" *Dev Pharmacol Ther*, 1992, 19(2-3):141-6.

Mayers DJ, Hindmarsh KW, Sankaran K, et al, "Chloral Hydrate Disposition Following Single-Dose Administration to Critically Ill Neonates and Children," *Dev Pharmacol Ther*, 1991, 16(2):71-7.

Steinberg AD, "Should Chloral Hydrate be Banned?" *Pediatrics*, 1993, 92(3)442-6.

Chlorambucil (klor AM byoo sil)

Medication Safety Issues

Sound-alike/look-alike issues:

Chlorambucil may be confused with Chloromycetin®

Leukeran® may be confused with Alkeran®, leucovorin, Leukine®, Myleran®

High alert medication: The Institute for Safe Medication Practices (ISMP) includes this medication among its list of drugs which have a heightened risk of causing significant patient harm when used in error.

Related Information

Emetogenic Potential of Single Chemotherapeutic Agents *on page 1776*

U.S. Brand Names Leukeran®

Canadian Brand Names Leukeran®

Index Terms CB-1348; Chlorambucilum; Chloraminophene; Chlorbutinum; NSC-3088; WR-139013

Therapeutic Category Antineoplastic Agent, Alkylating Agent (Nitrogen Mustard)

Generic Available No

Use Treatment of chronic lymphocytic leukemia (CLL), Hodgkin's and non-Hodgkin's lymphoma; breast and ovarian carcinoma, testicular carcinoma, choriocarcinoma; Waldenström's macroglobulinemia, and nephrotic syndrome unresponsive to conventional therapy

Pregnancy Risk Factor D

Lactation Excretion in breast milk unknown/not recommended

Contraindications Hypersensitivity to chlorambucil or any component; cross hypersensitivity (skin rash) may occur with other alkylating agents; previous resistance

Warnings The FDA currently recommends that procedures for proper handling and disposal of antineoplastic agents be considered. Chlorambucil can severely suppress bone marrow function; affects human fertility; carcinogenic in humans and probably mutagenic and teratogenic as well; chromosomal damage has been documented; secondary AML may be associated with chronic therapy and large cumulative doses. Severe skin reactions (eg, erythema multiforme, Stevens-Johnson syndrome and toxic epidermal necrolysis) have been reported.

Precautions Use with caution in patients with seizure disorder, head trauma, patients receiving epileptogenic drugs, and in patients with bone marrow suppression; avoid administration of live vaccines to immunocompromised patients; children with nephrotic syndrome may have an increased risk of seizures; reduce initial dosage if patient has received radiation therapy, myelosuppressive drugs, or has a depressed baseline leukocyte or platelet count within the previous 4 weeks.

Adverse Reactions

Central nervous system: Seizures, fever, agitation, irritability, hyperactivity, confusion, ataxia, hallucinations

(Continued)

Chlorambucil *(Continued)*

Dermatologic: Rash, pruritus, erythema multiforme, toxic epidermal necrolysis, urticaria, angioneurotic edema, Stevens-Johnson syndrome
Endocrine & metabolic: Hyperuricemia, menstrual cramps, amenorrhea, infertility
Gastrointestinal: Nausea, vomiting, abdominal pain, stomatitis, diarrhea
Genitourinary: Oligospermia, azoospermia
Hematologic: Leukopenia, thrombocytopenia, anemia, lymphocytopenia, neutropenia (risk of irreversible bone marrow damage occurs as total chlorambucil dose approaches 6.5 mg/kg)
Hepatic: Hepatotoxicity, jaundice
Neuromuscular & skeletal: Tremor, muscular twitching, weakness, myoclonia, peripheral neuropathy
Respiratory: Pulmonary fibrosis, interstitial pneumonia
Miscellaneous: Secondary malignancies

Drug Interactions Phenobarbital (possible increased chlorambucil toxicity); live vaccines (unknown whether secondary transmission of infection from live vaccines can occur)

Food Interactions Avoid acidic foods, hot foods, and spices; delayed absorption when administered with food

Stability Store in refrigerator; protect from light

Mechanism of Action Interferes with DNA replication and RNA transcription by alkylation and cross-linking the strands of DNA; immunosuppressive activity due to suppression of lymphocytes

Pharmacokinetics
Absorption: Oral: Rapid and almost completely absorbed from GI tract
Distribution: To liver, ascitic fluid, fat; extensively bound to plasma and tissue proteins; crosses the placenta
Protein binding: ~99%
Metabolism: In the liver to an active metabolite, phenylacetic acid mustard
Bioavailability: 56% to 100%
Half-life: Chlorambucil: 1.5 hours; phenylacetic acid mustard: 2.5 hours
Time to peak serum concentration: Chlorambucil: Within 1 hour; phenylacetic acid mustard: Within 2-4 hours
Elimination: 60% excreted in urine within 24 hours principally as metabolites; <1% excreted as unchanged drug or phenylacetic acid mustard in urine
Dialysis: Probably not dialyzable

Usual Dosage Oral (refer to individual protocols):
Children:
General short courses: 0.1-0.2 mg/kg/day or 4.5 mg/m^2/day once daily for 3-6 weeks for remission induction (usual: 4-10 mg/day); maintenance therapy: 0.03-0.1 mg/kg/day (usual: 2-4 mg/day)
Relapsing steroid-sensitive nephrotic syndrome: 0.2 mg/kg/day once daily for 8 weeks
CLL:
Biweekly regimen: Initial: 0.4 mg/kg/dose every 2 weeks; increase dose by 0.1 mg/kg every 2 weeks until a response occurs and/or myelosuppression occurs
Monthly regimen: Initial: 0.4 mg/kg every 4 weeks, increase dose by 0.2 mg/kg every 4 weeks until a response occurs and/or myelosuppression occurs
Malignant lymphomas:
Non-Hodgkin's lymphoma: 0.1 mg/kg/day
Hodgkin's: 0.2 mg/kg/day
Adults: 0.1-0.2 mg/kg/day or 3-6 mg/m^2/day once daily for 3-6 weeks, then adjust dose on basis of blood counts

Administration Oral: Administer 30-60 minutes before food; do not administer with acidic foods, hot foods, and spices

Monitoring Parameters Liver function tests, CBC with differential, hemoglobin, leukocyte and platelet counts, serum uric acid

Patient Information Notify physician if fever, sore throat, persistent cough, skin rash, seizures, amenorrhea, unusual lumps/masses, or bleeding occurs; avoid acidic foods, hot foods, and spices. Discontinue chlorambucil if skin reaction occurs. Women of childbearing potential should avoid becoming pregnant while on chlorambucil.

Additional Information Myelosuppressive effects:
WBC: Moderate
Platelets: Moderate
Onset (days): 7
Nadir (days): 14-21

Dosage Forms Excipient information presented when available (limited, particularly for generics); consult specific product labeling.

Tablet:

Leukeran®: 2 mg

Extemporaneous Preparations A 2 mg/mL suspension was stable for 7 days when refrigerated and compounded as follows: Pulverize sixty 2 mg tablets; levigate with a small amount of glycerin; add 20 mL Cologel® [DSC] and levigate until a uniform mixture is obtained; add a 2:1 simple syrup/cherry syrup mixture to make a total volume of 60 mL; label "refrigerate" and "shake well before use"

Dressman JB and Poust RI, "Stability of Allopurinol and of Five Antineoplastics in Suspension," *Am J Hosp Pharm*, 1983, 40(4):616-8.

References

Baluarte HJ, Hiner L, and Gruskin AB, "Chlorambucil Dosage in Frequently Relapsing Nephrotic Syndrome: A Controlled Clinical Trial," *J Pediatr*, 1978, 92(2):295-8.

Durkan A, Hodson EM, Willis NS, et al, "Non-corticosteroid Treatment for Nephrotic Syndrome in Children," *Cochrane Database Syst Rev*, 2005, 18(2):CD002290.

Singh BN and Malhotra BK, "Effects of Food on the Clinical Pharmacokinetics of Anticancer Agents: Underlying Mechanisms and Implications for Oral Chemotherapy," *Clin Pharmacokinet*, 2004, 43(15):1127-56.

Williams SA, Makker SP, and Grupe WE, "Seizures: A Significant Side Effect of Chlorambucil Therapy in Children," *J Pediatr*, 1978, 93(3):516-8.

♦ **Chlorambucilum** *see* Chlorambucil *on page 333*

♦ **Chloraminophene** *see* Chlorambucil *on page 333*

Chloramphenicol (klor am FEN i kole)

Medication Safety Issues

Sound-alike/look-alike issues:

Chloromycetin® may be confused with chlorambucil, Chlor-Trimeton®

Related Information

Blood Level Sampling Time Guidelines *on page 1914*

U.S. Brand Names Chloromycetin® Sodium Succinate

Canadian Brand Names Chloromycetin®; Chloromycetin® Succinate; Diochloram®; Pentamycetin®

Therapeutic Category Antibiotic, Miscellaneous

Generic Available Yes

Use Treatment of serious infections due to organisms resistant to other less toxic antibiotics or when its penetrability into the site of infection is clinically superior to other antibiotics to which the organism is sensitive; useful in infections caused by *Bacteroides, H. influenzae, Neisseria meningitidis, S. pneumoniae, Salmonella,* and *Rickettsia*

Pregnancy Risk Factor C

Lactation Enters breast milk/not recommended (AAP rates "of concern")

Contraindications Hypersensitivity to chloramphenicol or any component

Warnings Serious and fatal blood dyscrasias have occurred after both short-term and prolonged therapy; should not be used when less potentially toxic agents are effective; prolonged use may result in superinfection; breast-feeding is not recommended

Precautions Use with caution in patients with G-6-PD deficiency, impaired renal or hepatic function and in neonates; monitor serum concentrations and CBC in all patients; reduce dose in patients with hepatic and renal impairment

Adverse Reactions

Cardiovascular: Cardiotoxicity (left ventricular dysfunction), gray baby syndrome (see Additional Information)

Central nervous system: Nightmares, headache

Dermatologic: Rash

Gastrointestinal: Diarrhea, stomatitis, enterocolitis, vomiting, nausea

Hematologic: Bone marrow suppression, aplastic anemia, neutropenia, thrombocytopenia, hemolysis in patients with G-6-PD deficiency, anemia (see Additional Information)

Hepatic: Hepatitis-pancytopenia syndrome

Neuromuscular & skeletal: Peripheral neuropathy

Ocular: Optic neuritis

Miscellaneous: Anaphylaxis

Drug Interactions Cytochrome P450 isoenzyme CYP2C9 inhibitor

Chloramphenicol inhibits the metabolism of chlorpropamide, phenytoin, cyclosporine, tacrolimus, oral anticoagulants; phenobarbital and rifampin may decrease concentration of chloramphenicol; phenytoin may increase chloramphenicol concentration

Food Interactions May decrease intestinal absorption of vitamin B_{12}; may have increased dietary need for riboflavin, pyridoxine, and vitamin B_{12}

Stability Reconstituted parenteral solution (100 mg/mL) is stable for 30 days at room temperature

(Continued)

Chloramphenicol *(Continued)*

Mechanism of Action Reversibly binds to 50S ribosomal subunits of susceptible organisms preventing amino acids from being transferred to growing peptide chains thus inhibiting protein synthesis

Pharmacokinetics

Distribution: Readily crosses the placenta; appears in breast milk; distributes to most tissues and body fluids; good CSF and brain penetration

CSF concentration with uninflamed meninges: 21% to 50% of plasma concentration

CSF concentration with inflamed meninges: 45% to 89% of plasma concentration

Protein binding: 60%

Metabolism: Extensive in the liver (90%) to inactive metabolites, principally by glucuronidation; chloramphenicol sodium succinate must be hydrolyzed by esterases to active base.

Half-life:

Neonates:

1-2 days: 24 hours

10-16 days: 10 hours

Adults: 1.6-3.3 hours (prolonged with hepatic insufficiency)

Elimination: 5% to 15% excreted as unchanged drug in urine and 4% excreted in bile; in neonates, 6% to 80% of the dose may be excreted unchanged in urine

Dialysis: Slightly dialyzable (5% to 20%)

Usual Dosage

Neonates: Initial loading dose: I.V. (I.M. administration is not recommended): 20 mg/kg (the first maintenance dose should be given 12 hours after the loading dose)

Maintenance dose: Postnatal age:

≤7 days: 25 mg/kg/day once every 24 hours

>7 days, ≤2000 g: 25 mg/kg/day once every 24 hours

>7 days, >2000 g: 50 mg/kg/day divided every 12 hours

Meningitis: I.V.: Infants and Children: Maintenance dose: 75-100 mg/kg/day divided every 6 hours

Other infections: I.V.:

Infants and Children: 50-75 mg/kg/day divided every 6 hours; maximum daily dose: 4 g/day

Adults: 50 mg/kg/day in divided doses every 6 hours; maximum daily dose: 4 g/day

Dosing adjustment in renal and/or hepatic impairment: Dose reduction should be based upon serum chloramphenicol concentrations

Administration Parenteral:

IVP: Administer over 5 minutes at a maximum concentration of 100 mg/mL

I.V. intermittent infusion: Administer over 15-30 minutes at a final concentration for administration ≤20 mg/mL

Monitoring Parameters CBC with reticulocyte and platelet counts, hematocrit, serum iron level, iron-binding capacity, periodic liver and renal function tests, serum drug concentration

Reference Range

Meningitis:

Peak: 15-25 mcg/mL

Trough: 5-15 mcg/mL

Other infections:

Peak: 10-20 mcg/mL

Trough: 5-10 mcg/mL

Nursing Implications Draw peak levels 90 minutes after the end of a 30-minute infusion; trough levels should be drawn just prior to the next dose

Additional Information Sodium content of 1 g injection: 2.25 mEq

Three major toxicities associated with chloramphenicol include:

Aplastic anemia, an idiosyncratic reaction which can occur with any route of administration; usually occurs 3 weeks to 12 months after initial exposure to chloramphenicol; incidence: 1 in 40,000 cases

Bone marrow suppression is thought to be dose-related with serum concentrations >25 mcg/mL and reversible once chloramphenicol is discontinued; anemia and neutropenia may occur during the first week of therapy

Gray baby syndrome is characterized by circulatory collapse, hypothermia, cyanosis, acidosis, abdominal distention, myocardial depression, coma, and death; reaction appears to be associated with serum levels ≥50 mcg/mL; may result from drug accumulation in patients with impaired hepatic or renal function; may occur after 3-4 days of therapy or within hours of initiating therapy

Dosage Forms Excipient information presented when available (limited, particularly for generics); consult specific product labeling.

Injection, powder for reconstitution: 1 g [contains sodium ~52 mg/g (2.25 mEq/g)]

References

Nahata MC and Powell DA, "Bioavailability and Clearance of Chloramphenicol After Intravenous Chloramphenicol Succinate," *Clin Pharmacol Ther*, 1981, 30(3):368-72.

♦ **ChloraPrep® [OTC]** *see* Chlorhexidine Gluconate *on page 337*
♦ **Chlorbutinum** *see* Chlorambucil *on page 333*
♦ **Chlorethazine** *see* Mechlorethamine *on page 987*
♦ **Chlorethazine Mustard** *see* Mechlorethamine *on page 987*

Chlorhexidine Gluconate (klor HEKS i deen GLOO koe nate)

Medication Safety Issues

Sound-alike/look-alike issues:

Peridex® may be confused with Precedex™

U.S. Brand Names Avagard™ [OTC]; BactoShield® CHG [OTC]; Betasept® [OTC]; ChloraPrep® [OTC]; Dyna-Hex® [OTC]; Hibiclens® [OTC]; Hibistat® [OTC]; Operand® Chlorhexidine Gluconate [OTC]; Peridex®; PerioChip®; PerioGard®

Canadian Brand Names Hibidil® 1:2000; ORO-Clense

Index Terms CHG; 3M™ Avagard™ [OTC]

Therapeutic Category Antibacterial, Topical; Antibiotic, Oral Rinse

Generic Available Yes: Oral liquid

Use Skin cleanser for surgical scrub; cleanser for skin wounds; germicidal hand rinse; antibacterial dental rinse to reduce plaque formation and control gingivitis; prophylactic dental rinse to prevent oral infections in immunocompromised patients, particularly bone marrow transplant patients receiving cytotoxic therapy; and short-term substitute for toothbrushing in situations where the patient is unable to tolerate mechanical stimulation of the gums

Pregnancy Risk Factor B

Contraindications Hypersensitivity to chlorhexidine gluconate or any component; do not use as a preoperative skin preparation of the face or head (except Hibiclens® liquid) as serious, permanent eye injury has occurred when chlorhexidine gluconate enters and remains in the eye during surgery.

Warnings For topical use only; there have been several case reports of anaphylaxis following disinfection with chlorhexidine; a case of bradycardic episodes after breast-feeding in a 2 day old infant whose mother used chlorhexidine gluconate topically on her breasts to prevent mastitis has been reported

Precautions Staining of oral surfaces, teeth, restorations, and dorsum of tongue may occur and may be visible as soon as 1 week after therapy begins; staining is more pronounced when there is a heavy accumulation of unremoved plaque and when teeth fillings have rough surfaces; stain does not have clinically adverse effect, but because removal may not be possible, patients with frontal restoration should be advised of the potential permanency of the stain; avoid contact with meninges; corneal injury has been associated with direct eye contact (see Contraindications); deafness has been associated with direct instillation into the middle ear through a perforated eardrum

Adverse Reactions

Dermatologic: Skin irritation

Gastrointestinal: Tongue irritation, minor irritation and superficial desquamation of oral mucosa (particularly among children), increased tartar on teeth, staining of oral surfaces (mucosa, teeth, and dorsum of tongue; see Warnings), dysgeusia, transient parotiditis; toothache (chip)

Ocular: Corneal damage (see Precautions)

Otic: Deafness (see Precautions)

Respiratory: Nasal congestion, shortness of breath

Miscellaneous: Edema of face, anaphylactoid reactions

Drug Interactions When combined with nystatin, *in vitro*, the minimum inhibitory concentrations (MIC) of susceptible organisms, were increased to both agents.

Stability Store away from heat and direct light; do not freeze

Mechanism of Action The bactericidal effect of chlorhexidine is a result of the binding of this cationic molecule to negatively charged bacterial cell walls and extramicrobial complexes. At low concentrations, this causes an alteration of bacterial cell osmotic equilibrium and leakage of potassium and phosphorous resulting in a bacteriostatic effect. At high concentrations of chlorhexidine, the cytoplasmic contents of the bacterial cell precipitate and result in cell death. Chlorhexidine is active against gram-positive and gram-negative organisms, facultative anaerobes, anaerobes, and yeast.

Pharmacokinetics

Absorption: ~30% of chlorhexidine is retained in the oral cavity following rinsing and is slowly released into the oral fluids; chlorhexidine is poorly absorbed from the GI tract and is not absorbed topically through intact skin

(Continued)

Chlorhexidine Gluconate *(Continued)*

Serum concentrations: Detectable levels are not present in the plasma 12 hours after administration

Elimination: Primarily through the feces (~90%); <1% excreted in the urine

Usual Dosage

Oral rinse (Peridex® or PerioGard®) (see Administration: Oral):

Children and Adults: 15 mL twice daily

Immunocompromised patient: 10-15 mL, 2-3 times/day

Cleanser: Children and Adults: Apply 5 mL per scrub or hand wash; apply 25 mL per body wash or hair wash

Administration

Oral rinse: Precede use of solution by flossing and brushing teeth, completely rinse toothpaste from mouth; swish undiluted oral rinse around in mouth for 30 seconds, then expectorate; caution patient not to swallow the medicine; avoid eating for 2-3 hours after treatment.

Topical:

Surgical scrub: Scrub 3 minutes and rinse thoroughly, wash for an additional 3 minutes

Hand wash: Wash for 15 seconds and rinse

Hand rinse: Rub vigorously for 15 seconds

Body wash: Wet body and/or hair, apply, rinse thoroughly, repeat.

Monitoring Parameters Improvement in gingival inflammation and bleeding; development of teeth or denture discoloration; dental prophylaxis to remove stains at regular intervals of no greater than 6 months.

Test Interactions If chlorhexidine is used as a disinfectant before midstream urine collection, a false-positive urine protein may result (when using dipstick method based upon a pH indicator color change).

Patient Information

Oral rinse: Use after tooth brushing; do not swallow, do not rinse after use; may cause reduced taste perception which is reversible; may cause discoloration of teeth which may be removed with professional dental cleaning; notify dentist or physician if difficulty breathing or flushing or swelling of face occurs

Topical administration is for external use only; if accidentally enters eyes or ears, rinse out promptly and thoroughly with water

Dosage Forms Excipient information presented when available (limited, particularly for generics); consult specific product labeling.

Chip, for periodontal pocket insertion:

PerioChip®: 2.5 mg

Liquid, topical [surgical scrub]:

Avagard™: 1% (500 mL) [contains ethyl alcohol and moisturizers]

BactoShield® CHG: 2% (120 mL, 480 mL, 750 mL, 1000 mL, 3800 mL); 4% (120 mL, 480 mL, 750 mL, 1000 mL, 3800 mL) [contains isopropyl alcohol]

Betasept®: 4% (120 mL, 240 mL, 480 mL, 960 mL, 3840 mL) [contains isopropyl alcohol]

ChloraPrep®: 2% (0.67 mL, 1.5 mL, 3 mL, 10.5 mL) [contains isopropyl alcohol 70%; prefilled applicator]

Dyna-Hex®: 2% (120 mL, 960 mL, 3840 mL); 4% (120 mL, 960 mL, 3840 mL)

Hibiclens®: 4% (15 mL, 120 mL, 240 mL, 480 mL, 960 mL, 3840 mL) [contains isopropyl alcohol]

Operand® Chlorhexidine Gluconate: 2% (120 mL); 4% (120 mL, 240 mL, 480 mL, 960 mL, 3840 mL) [contains isopropyl alcohol]

Liquid, oral rinse: 0.12% (480 mL)

Peridex®: 0.12% (480 mL) [contains alcohol 11.6%]

PerioGard®: 0.12% (480 mL) [contains alcohol 11.6%; mint flavor]

Pad [prep pad] (Hibistat®): 0.5% (50s) [contains isopropyl alcohol]

Sponge/Brush (BactoShield® CHG): 4% per sponge/brush [contains isopropyl alcohol]

References

Quinn MW and Bini RM, "Bradycardia Associated With Chlorhexidine Spray," *Arch Dis Child*, 1989, 64(6):892-3.

Yong D, Parker FC, and Foran SM, "Severe Allergic Reactions and Intra-Urethral Chlorhexidine Gluconate," *Med J Aust*, 1995, 162(5):257-8.

♦ **Chlormeprazine** *see* Prochlorperazine *on page 1321*

♦ **2-Chlorodeoxyadenosine** *see* Cladribine *on page 373*

♦ **Chloromag®** *see* Magnesium Chloride *on page 969*

♦ **Chloromag®** *see* Magnesium Supplements *on page 976*

♦ **Chloromycetin® (Can)** *see* Chloramphenicol *on page 335*

♦ **Chloromycetin® Sodium Succinate** *see* Chloramphenicol *on page 335*

♦ **Chloromycetin® Succinate (Can)** *see* Chloramphenicol *on page 335*

Chloroprocaine (klor oh PROE kane)

Medication Safety Issues

Sound-alike/look-alike issues:

Nesacaine® may be confused with Neptazane®

U.S. Brand Names Nesacaine®; Nesacaine®-MPF

Canadian Brand Names Nesacaine®-CE

Index Terms Chloroprocaine Hydrochloride

Therapeutic Category Local Anesthetic, Injectable

Generic Available Yes

Use Production of local or regional analgesia and anesthesia by local infiltration and peripheral nerve block techniques

Pregnancy Risk Factor C

Lactation Excretion in breast milk unknown/use caution

Contraindications Hypersensitivity to chloroprocaine, PABA, any anesthetic of the ester type, or any component of the formulation; cerebrospinal diseases such as meningitis or syphilis, and septicemia (spinal anesthetic use)

Warnings Convulsions and cardiac arrhythmias resulting in cardiac arrest have been reported, presumably due to systemic toxicity following unintentional I.V. injection; should be administered in small incremental doses. Chloroprocaine solutions containing preservatives (methylparaben) are not to be used for lumbar or caudal anesthesia. When using for obstetrical anesthesia, 5% to 10% of cases where initial total doses of 120-400 mg were administered, have been associated with fetal bradycardia.

Precautions Use with extreme caution as lumbar or caudal anesthesia in patients with existing neurologic disease, spinal deformities, or severe hypertension; use with caution in patients with hypotension, cardiac disease, and hepatic or renal disease. Use caution in debilitated, elderly, or acutely-ill patients; dose reduction may be required.

Adverse Reactions Degree of adverse effects in the CNS and cardiovascular system is directly related to the blood level of procaine, route of administration, and physical status of the patient. The effects below are more likely to occur after systemic administration rather than infiltration.

Cardiovascular: Bradycardia, cardiac arrest, decreased cardiac output, heart block, hypertension, hypotension, myocardial depression, syncope, tachycardia, ventricular arrhythmias

Central nervous system: Anxiety, chills, seizures, depression, dizziness, excitation, restlessness, tremors, fever, headache

Dermatologic: Angioneurotic edema, erythema, pruritus, urticaria

Gastrointestinal: Fecal incontinence, nausea, vomiting

Genitourinary: Incontinence, urinary retention

Neuromuscular & skeletal: Paralysis, tremors, paresthesia, weakness

Ocular: Blurred vision, pupil constriction

Otic: Tinnitus

Respiratory: Apnea, hypoventilation, sneezing, laryngeal edema

Miscellaneous: Allergic reaction, anaphylactoid reaction, diaphoresis

Drug Interactions Decreased effect of sulfonamides with the aminobenzoic metabolite of procaine

Stability Store at controlled room temperature of 15°C to 30°C (59°F to 86°F); protect from light. Solutions may not be resterilized by autoclaving.

Mechanism of Action Blocks both the initiation and conduction of nerve impulses by decreasing the neuronal membrane's permeability to sodium ions, which results in inhibition of depolarization with resultant blockade of conduction

Pharmacodynamics

Onset of action: 6-12 minutes

Duration (patient, type of block, concentration, and method of anesthesia dependent): Up to 1 hour

Pharmacokinetics

Metabolism: Rapidly hydrolyzed by plasma enzymes to 2-chloro-4-aminobenzoic acid and 8-diethylaminoethanol (80% conjugated before elimination)

Half-life (*in vitro*):

Neonates: 43 ± 2 seconds

Adult males: 21 ± 2 seconds

Adult females: 25 ± 1 second

Elimination: Very little excreted as unchanged drug in urine; metabolites: Cloro-aminobenzoic acid and diethylaminoethanol primarily excreted unchanged in urine

Usual Dosage Dose varies with procedure, desired depth, and duration of anesthesia, desired muscle relaxation, vascularity of tissues, physical condition, and age of

(Continued)

Chloroprocaine *(Continued)*

patient. The smallest dose and concentration required to produce the desired effect should be used.

Children >3 years: Maximum dose without epinephrine: 11 mg/kg

Adults: Maximum dose: 11 mg/kg; not to exceed 800 mg per treatment; with epinephrine: 14 mg/kg; not to exceed 1000 mg per treatment

Infiltration and peripheral nerve block:

- Mandibular: 2-3 mL (40-60 mg) using 2%
- Infraorbital: 0.5-1 mL (10-20 mg) using 2%
- Brachial plexus: 30-40 mL (600-800 mg) using 2%
- Digital (without epinephrine): 3-4 mL (30-40 mg) using 1%
- Pudendal: 10 mL (200 mg) into each side (2 sites) using 2%
- Paracervical: 3 mL (30 mg) per each of four sites using 1%

Caudal and lumbar epidural block:

- Caudal: 15-25 mL using 2% to 3% solution; may repeat dose at 40- to 60-minute intervals
- Lumbar: 2-2.5 mL per segment using 2% to 3% solution; usual total volume 15-25 mL; repeated doses 2-6 mL less than the original dose may be given at 40- to 50-minutes intervals

Administration Parenteral: Administer in small incremental doses; when using continuous intermittent catheter techniques, use frequent aspirations before and during the injection to avoid intravascular injection

Monitoring Parameters Blood pressure, heart rate, respiration, signs of CNS toxicity (lightheadedness, dizziness, tinnitus, restlessness, tremors, twitching, drowsiness, circumoral paresthesia)

Patient Information You will experience decreased sensation to pain, heat, or cold in the area and/or decreased muscle strength (depending on area of application) until effects wear off; use necessary caution to reduce incidence of possible injury until full sensation returns. Report irritation, pain, burning at injection site; chest pain or palpitations; or respiratory difficulty.

Dosage Forms Excipient information presented when available (limited, particularly for generics); consult specific product labeling.

Injection, solution, as hydrochloride (Nesacaine®): 1% (30 mL); 2% (30 mL) [contains disodium EDTA and methylparaben]

Injection, solution, as hydrochloride [preservative free] (Nesacaine®-MPF): 2% (20 mL); 3% (20 mL)

♦ **Chloroprocaine Hydrochloride** *see* Chloroprocaine *on page 339*

Chloroquine (KLOR oh kwin)

Medication Safety Issues

International issues:

- Aralen® may be confused with Oralon® which is a brand name for povidone-iodine in Japan
- Aralen® may be confused with Paralen® which is a brand name for acetaminophen in the Czech Republic

Related Information

Malaria *on page 1855*

Medications for Which A Single Dose May Be Fatal When Ingested By A Toddler *on page 1932*

U.S. Brand Names Aralen®

Canadian Brand Names Aralen®; Novo-Chloroquine

Index Terms Chloroquine Phosphate

Therapeutic Category Amebicide; Antimalarial Agent

Generic Available Yes

Use Suppression or chemoprophylaxis of malaria in chloroquine-sensitive areas; treatment of uncomplicated or mild-moderate malaria due to susceptible *Plasmodium* species, except chloroquine-resistant *Plasmodium falciparum*; extraintestinal amebiasis; rheumatoid arthritis; discoid lupus erythematosus, scleroderma, pemphigus

Pregnancy Risk Factor C

Lactation Enters breast milk/not recommended (AAP considers "compatible")

Contraindications Hypersensitivity to chloroquine or any component; retinal or visual field changes; patients with psoriasis. Avoid use in pregnancy except in the suppression or treatment of malaria when in the judgment of the physician, benefit outweighs potential risk to the fetus.

Warnings Resistance of *Plasmodium falciparum* to chloroquine is widespread (includes areas like sub-Saharan Africa, Southeast Asia, Indian subcontinent, and large portions of South America); cases of *Plasmodium vivax* resistance have been reported. Sudden deaths have been reported after overdose of parenteral chloroquine in children. In no instance should the single dose of parenteral chloroquine administered to infants or children exceed 5 mg base/kg.

Precautions Use with caution in patients with liver disease, G-6-PD deficiency, seizure disorders, pre-existing auditory damage, or in conjunction with hepatotoxic drugs

Adverse Reactions

Cardiovascular: Hypotension, EKG changes (inversion or depression of T-wave with widening of the QRS complex), cardiomyopathy

Central nervous system: Fatigue, personality changes, headache, delirium, depression, confusion, agitation, psychotic episodes, seizures

Dermatologic: Pruritus, hair bleaching, skin eruptions, exfoliative dermatitis, photosensitivity, hair loss

Endocrine & metabolic: Weight loss

Gastrointestinal: Anorexia, nausea, vomiting, diarrhea, stomatitis, abdominal cramps

Hematologic: Blood dyscrasias (neutropenia, aplastic anemia, thrombocytopenia)

Neuromuscular & skeletal: Peripheral neuropathy, neuromyopathy, weakness, myalgia, depression of tendon reflexes

Ocular: Retinopathy, blurred vision, corneal opacity, photophobia, blindness

Otic: Tinnitus, deafness, reduced hearing

Drug Interactions Cytochrome P450 isoenzyme CYP2D6 and CYP3A4 substrate; isoenzyme CYP2D6 inhibitor

Intradermally administered rabies vaccine; cimetidine increases levels of chloroquine; urinary acidifiers increase the elimination of chloroquine; antacids and kaolin decrease absorption of chloroquine; chloroquine may increase cyclosporine levels (monitor serum cyclosporine levels); chloroquine may decrease the absorption of ampicillin

Stability Protect from light

Mechanism of Action Binds to and inhibits DNA and RNA polymerase; interferes with metabolism and hemoglobin utilization by parasites; inhibits prostaglandin effects

Pharmacokinetics

Absorption: Oral: Rapid

Distribution: Widely distributed in body tissues including eyes, heart, kidneys, liver, and lungs where retention is prolonged; crosses the placenta; appears in breast milk

Protein binding: 50% to 65%

Metabolism: Partial hepatic

Half-life: 3-5 days

Time to peak serum concentration: Oral: Within 1-2 hours

Elimination: ~70% of dose excreted unchanged in urine; acidification of the urine increases elimination of drug; small amounts of drug may be present in urine months following discontinuation of therapy

Dialysis: Minimally removed by hemodialysis

Usual Dosage (Dosage expressed in terms of base):

Oral:

Suppression or prophylaxis of malaria:

Children: Administer 5 mg base/kg/week on the same day each week (not to exceed 300 mg base/dose); begin 1-2 weeks prior to exposure; continue for 4 weeks after leaving endemic area; if suppressive therapy is not begun prior to exposure, double the initial loading dose to 10 mg base/kg and give in 2 divided doses 6 hours apart, followed by the usual dosage regimen

Adults: 300 mg/week (base) on the same day each week; begin 1-2 weeks prior to exposure; continue for 4 weeks after leaving endemic area; if suppressive therapy is not begun prior to exposure, double the initial loading dose to 600 mg base and give in 2 divided doses 6 hours apart, followed by the usual dosage regimen

Acute attack:

Children: 10 mg base/kg (maximum dose: 600 mg base) stat, then 5 mg base/kg (maximum dose: 300 mg base) 6 hours later and then 5 mg base/kg/day (maximum daily dose: 300 mg base) once daily for 2 days

Adults: 600 mg base/dose one time, then 300 mg base/dose 6 hours later, and then 300 mg base/dose once daily for 2 days

Extraintestinal amebiasis:

Children: 10 mg base/kg once daily for 2-3 weeks (up to 300 mg base/day)

Adults: 600 mg base/day for 2 days followed by 300 mg base/day for at least 2-3 weeks

Rheumatoid arthritis: Adults: 150 mg base once daily

I.M.:

Severe malaria when oral therapy is not feasible:

Children: 5 mg base/kg (maximum dose: 200 mg base); dose may be repeated in 6 hours; maximum dose: 10 mg base/kg in a 24-hour period

(Continued)

Chloroquine *(Continued)*

Adults: Initial: 160-200 mg base, may repeat in 6 hours if needed; maximum: 800 mg base in the first 24 hours. Convert to oral dosing as soon as possible and continue for 3 days until 1.5 g base has been given.

Dosing adjustment in renal impairment: Cl_{cr} <10 mL/minute: Administer 50% of dose

Administration

Oral: Administer with meals to decrease GI upset; chloroquine phosphate tablets have also been mixed with chocolate syrup or enclosed in gelatin capsules to mask the bitter taste

Parenteral: Cautious administration of frequent small doses by I.M. or SubQ injection in children with severe malaria may reduce risk of severe adverse effects (eg, 2.5 mg base/kg every 4 hours not to exceed 10 mg base/kg in a 24-hour period)

Monitoring Parameters Periodic CBC, examination for muscular weakness and ophthalmologic examination in patients receiving prolonged therapy

Patient Information Report any visual disturbances, muscular weakness, or difficulty in hearing or ringing in the ears; tablets are bitter tasting. May cause photosensitivity reactions (eg, exposure to sunlight may cause severe sunburn, skin rash, redness, or itching); avoid exposure to sunlight and artificial light sources (sunlamps, tanning booth/bed); wear protective clothing, wide-brimmed hats, sunglasses, and lip sunscreen (SPF ≥15); use a sunscreen [broad-spectrum sunscreen or physical sunscreen (preferred) or sunblock with SPF ≥15]; contact physician if reaction occurs.

Dosage Forms Excipient information presented when available (limited, particularly for generics); consult specific product labeling.

Tablet, as phosphate: 250 mg [equivalent to 150 mg base]; 500 mg [equivalent to 300 mg base]

Aralen®: 500 mg [equivalent to 300 mg base]

Extemporaneous Preparations A 15 mg chloroquine phosphate/mL suspension (equivalent to 9 mg chloroquine base/mL) is made by pulverizing three Aralen® 500 mg phosphate = 300 mg base/tablet, levigating with 15 mL of a 1:1 vehicle of Ora-Sweet® and Ora-Plus®, and adding vehicle by geometric proportion, levigating until a uniform mixture is obtained; qsad to 100 mL with vehicle, stable for up to 60 days when stored at 5°C or 25°C and protected from light. Label "shake well before using" and "protect from light."

Allen LV Jr and Erickson MA, "Stability of Alprazolam, Chloroquine Phosphate, Cisapride, Enalapril Maleate, and Hydralazine Hydrochloride in Extemporaneously Compounded Oral Liquids," *Am J Health Syst Pharm*, 1998, 55(18):1915-20.

References

Wyler DJ, "Malaria Chemoprophylaxis for the Traveler," *N Engl J Med*, 1993, 329(1):31-7.

♦ **Chloroquine Phosphate** *see* Chloroquine *on page 340*

Chlorothiazide (klor oh THYE a zide)

Medication Safety Issues

International issues:

Diuril® may be confused with Duorol® which is a brand name for acetaminophen in Spain

Related Information

Antihypertensive Agents by Class *on page 1678*

U.S. Brand Names Diuril®

Canadian Brand Names Diuril®

Therapeutic Category Antihypertensive Agent; Diuretic, Thiazide

Generic Available Yes: Tablet

Use Management of mild to moderate hypertension; edema associated with CHF, pregnancy, or nephrotic syndrome

Pregnancy Risk Factor C

Lactation Enters breast milk/use caution (AAP rates "compatible")

Contraindications Hypersensitivity to chlorothiazide or any component; cross-sensitivity with other thiazides or sulfonamides; do not use in anuric patients

Warnings The injection must not be administered subcutaneously or I.M.

Precautions Use with caution in patients with severe renal disease, impaired hepatic function, moderate-high cholesterol concentrations, and in patients with high triglycerides

Adverse Reactions

Cardiovascular: Hypotension, arrhythmia, weak pulse

Central nervous system: Dizziness, vertigo, headache, fever

Dermatologic: Rash, photosensitivity

Endocrine & metabolic: Hypokalemia, hypochloremic alkalosis, hyperglycemia, hyperlipidemia, hyperuricemia
Gastrointestinal: Anorexia, nausea, vomiting, cramping, diarrhea, pancreatitis, constipation
Hematologic: Rarely blood dyscrasias, thrombocytopenia
Hepatic: Intrahepatic cholestasis
Neuromuscular & skeletal: Muscle weakness, paresthesia
Ocular: Blurred vision
Renal: Prerenal azotemia, hematuria

Drug Interactions NSAIDs with chlorothiazide may result in decreased antihypertensive effect; additive potassium losses with steroids, loop diuretics and amphotericin B; decreases lithium clearance; increases hypersensitivity reactions to allopurinol; increases hyperglycemia with diazoxide; decreased absorption of chlorothiazide when administered with cholestyramine; milk-alkali syndrome with high calcium dosages

Food Interactions Avoid natural licorice (causes sodium and water retention and increases potassium loss); may need to decrease sodium and calcium, may need to increase potassium, zinc, magnesium, and riboflavin in diet

Stability Reconstituted injection is stable for 24 hours at room temperature

Mechanism of Action Inhibits sodium reabsorption in the distal tubules causing increased excretion of sodium, chloride, potassium, bicarbonate, magnesium, phosphate, calcium (transiently) and water

Pharmacodynamics
Diuresis: Onset of action: Oral: Within 2 hours
Duration:
Oral: ~6-12 hours
I.V.: 2 hours

Pharmacokinetics
Absorption: Oral: Poor (~10% to 20%); dose dependent
Distribution: Breast milk to plasma ratio: 0.05
Half-life: Adults: 45-120 minutes
Time to peak serum concentration: Within 4 hours
Elimination: Excreted unchanged in urine

Usual Dosage I.V. dosage in infants and children has not been established. The following I.V. dosages in infants and children are based upon anecdotal reports. Lower dosing regimens have been extrapolated from oral dosing recommendations as 10% to 20% of an oral dose is absorbed.

Neonates and Infants <6 months:
Oral: 20-40 mg/kg/day in 2 divided doses; maximum: 375 mg/day
I.V.: 2-8 mg/kg/day in 2 divided doses; doses up to 20 mg/kg/day have been used
Infants >6 months and Children:
Oral: 20 mg/kg/day in 2 divided doses; maximum: 1 g/day
I.V.: 4 mg/kg/day divided in 1-2 doses; doses up to 20 mg/kg/day have been used
Adults:
Hypertension: Oral: 125-500 mg once daily
Edema:
Oral: 500 mg to 2 g/day divided in 1-2 doses
I.V.:100-500 mg/day divided in 1-2 doses

Administration
Oral: Administer with food; shake suspension well before use
Parenteral: Dilute 500 mg vial with 18 mL SWI (resulting in 27.8 mg/mL concentration); administer by direct I.V. infusion over 3-5 minutes or infusion over 30 minutes in dextrose or NS; avoid extravasation of parenteral solution since it is extremely irritating to tissues

Monitoring Parameters Serum electrolytes (sodium, potassium, chloride, and bicarbonate), glucose, uric acid, triglycerides; body weight; blood pressure

Patient Information May cause photosensitivity reactions (eg, exposure to sunlight may cause severe sunburn, skin rash, redness, or itching); avoid exposure to sunlight and artificial light sources (sunlamps, tanning booth/bed); wear protective clothing, wide-brimmed hats, sunglasses, and lip sunscreen (SPF ≥15); use a sunscreen [broad-spectrum sunscreen or physical sunscreen (preferred) or sunblock with SPF ≥15]; contact physician if reaction occurs.

Dosage Forms Excipient information presented when available (limited, particularly for generics); consult specific product labeling.
Injection, powder for reconstitution, as sodium: 500 mg
Suspension, oral: 250 mg/5 mL (237 mL) [contains alcohol 0.5% and benzoic acid]
Tablet: 250 mg, 500 mg

Extemporaneous Preparations A 50 mg/mL oral suspension may be made by crushing ten 500 mg chlorothiazide tablets; levigate with glycerin to form a uniform paste. Add 2 grams carboxymethylcellulose gel (2 g carboxymethylcellulose is mixed
(Continued)

Chlorothiazide *(Continued)*

with 5-10 mL water to form paste, additional 40 mL water is added and heated to 60°C with moderate stirring until dissolution occurs; this is cooled and allowed to stand for 1-2 hours to form a clear gel). Dissolve 500 mg citric acid in 5 mL water; add to chlorothiazide carboxymethylcellulose mixture with 0.1% parabens; qs to 100 mL with water (Nahata, 2004).

Nahata, MC, Pai VB, and Hipple TF, *Pediatric Drug Formulations*, 5th ed, Cincinnati, OH: Harvey Whitney Books Co, 2004.

References

Chobanian AV, Bakris GL, Black HR, et al, "The Seventh Report of the Joint National Committee on Prevention, Detection, Evaluation, and Treatment of High Blood Pressure: The JNC 7 Report," *JAMA*, 2003, 289(19):2560-72.

♦ **Chlorphen [OTC]** *see* Chlorpheniramine *on page 344*

Chlorpheniramine (klor fen IR a meen)

Medication Safety Issues
Sound-alike/look-alike issues:
Chlor-Trimeton® may be confused with Chloromycetin®

Related Information
OTC Cough and Cold Preparations, Pediatric *on page 1706*
Overdose and Toxicology *on page 1916*

U.S. Brand Names Ahist™; Aller-Chlor® [OTC]; Chlorphen [OTC]; Chlor-Trimeton® [OTC]; Diabetic Tussin® Allergy Relief [OTC]; PediaTan™; QDALL® AR; Teldrin® HBP [OTC]

Canadian Brand Names Chlor-Tripolon®; Novo-Pheniram

Index Terms Chlorpheniramine Maleate; CTM

Therapeutic Category Antihistamine

Generic Available Yes: Syrup, tablet

Use Perennial and seasonal allergic rhinitis and other allergic symptoms including urticaria

Pregnancy Risk Factor B

Contraindications Hypersensitivity to chlorpheniramine maleate or any component; narrow-angle glaucoma, bladder neck obstruction, symptomatic prostatic hypertrophy, stenosing peptic ulcer, pyloroduodenal obstruction

Precautions Use with caution in patients with asthma; young children may be more susceptible to side effects and CNS stimulation

Adverse Reactions
Cardiovascular: Palpitations
Central nervous system: Drowsiness, vertigo, headache, excitability (children may be at increased risk for developing CNS stimulation), nervousness, fatigue, dizziness, depression
Dermatologic: Dermatitis, photosensitivity, angioedema
Endocrine & metabolic: Weight gain
Gastrointestinal: Nausea, xerostomia, diarrhea, abdominal pain, appetite increase
Genitourinary: Urinary retention
Neuromuscular & skeletal: Weakness, arthralgia, paresthesia
Ocular: Diplopia, blurred vision
Renal: Polyuria
Respiratory: Thickening of bronchial secretions, pharyngitis, epistaxis

Drug Interactions Cytochrome P450 isoenzyme CYP2D6 substrate
May cause additive sedation when concomitantly administered with other CNS depressant medications

Mechanism of Action Competes with histamine for H_1-receptor sites on effector cells in the GI tract, blood vessels, and respiratory tract

Pharmacodynamics
Onset of action: Oral: 6 hours
Duration: Oral: 24 hours

Pharmacokinetics (Data from chlorpheniramine maleate)
Distribution: V_d:
Children: 3.8 L/kg
Adults: 2.5-3.2 L/kg
Protein binding: 69% to 72%
Metabolism: Substantial metabolism in GI mucosa and on first pass through liver
Bioavailability: Chlorpheniramine:
Solution: 35% to 60%
Tablet: 25% to 45%
Half-life:
Children: Average: 9.6-13.1 hours (range: 5.2-23.1 hours)

Adults: 12-43 hours

Time to peak serum concentration: Oral (solution and conventional tablets): 2-6 hours

Elimination: 35% excreted in 48 hours

Usual Dosage

Chlorpheniramine maleate: Oral:

Children <12 years: Oral: 0.35 mg/kg/day in divided doses every 4-6 hours or as an alternative

2-5 years: 1 mg every 4-6 hours

6-11 years: 2 mg every 4-6 hours, not to exceed 12 mg/day or timed release 8 mg every 12 hours

Children ≥12 years and Adults: 4 mg every 4-6 hours, not to exceed 24 mg/day or timed release 8-12 mg every 12 hours

Dexchlorpheniramine maleate: Oral:

Children 2-5 years: 0.5 mg every 4-6 hours, not to exceed 3 mg/day

Children 6-11 years: 1 mg every 4-6 hours, not to exceed 6 mg/day

Children ≥12 years and Adults: 2 mg every 4-6 hours; not to exceed 12 mg/day

Administration Oral: Administer with food to decrease GI distress; do not crush or chew timed release tablets

Patient Information May cause drowsiness and impair ability to perform activities requiring mental alertness or physical coordination; may cause dry mouth. May cause photosensitivity reactions (eg, exposure to sunlight may cause severe sunburn, skin rash, redness, or itching); avoid direct exposure to sunlight

Dosage Forms Excipient information presented when available (limited, particularly for generics); consult specific product labeling.

Capsule, variable release, as maleate:

QDALL® AR: Chlorpheniramine 12 mg [immediate release and sustained release]

Suspension, as tannate:

PediaTan™: 8 mg/5 mL (480 mL) [sugar free; contains sodium benzoate; bubble gum flavor]

Syrup, as maleate:

Aller-Chlor®: 2 mg/5 mL (120 mL) [contains alcohol 5%]

Diabetic Tussin® Allergy Relief: 2 mg/5 mL (120 mL) [alcohol free, dye free, sugar free]

Tablet, as maleate: 4 mg

Aller-Chlor®, Chlor-Trimeton®, Chlorphen, Teldrin® HBP: 4 mg

Tablet, extended release, as maleate:

Chlor-Trimeton®: 12 mg

Tablet, long acting, as tannate [scored]:

Ahist™: 12 mg

◆ **Chlorpheniramine Maleate** *see* Chlorpheniramine *on page 344*

ChlorproMAZINE (klor PROE ma zeen)

Medication Safety Issues

Sound-alike/look-alike issues:

ChlorproMAZINE may be confused with chlorproPAMIDE, clomiPRAMINE, prochlorperazine, promethazine

Thorazine® may be confused with thiamine, thioridazine

Related Information

Compatibility of Medications Mixed in A Syringe *on page 1941*

Medications for Which A Single Dose May Be Fatal When Ingested By A Toddler *on page 1932*

Overdose and Toxicology *on page 1916*

Prochlorperazine *on page 1321*

Canadian Brand Names Largactil®; Novo-Chlorpromazine

Index Terms Chlorpromazine Hydrochloride; CPZ

Therapeutic Category Antiemetic; Antipsychotic Agent; Phenothiazine Derivative

Generic Available Yes

Use Treatment of nausea and vomiting, schizophrenia, Tourette's syndrome, mania, acute intermittent porphyria, restlessness and apprehension prior to surgery, intractable hiccups (adults), severe behavioral problems (children); used as an adjunct in the treatment of tetanus

Pregnancy Risk Factor C

Lactation Enters breast milk/not recommended (AAP rates "of concern")

Contraindications Hypersensitivity to chlorpromazine hydrochloride or any component (see Warnings); cross-sensitivity with other phenothiazines may exist; avoid use in patients with narrow-angle glaucoma, bone marrow suppression, severe liver or cardiac disease

Warnings Significant hypotension may occur, particularly with parenteral administration.

(Continued)

ChlorproMAZINE *(Continued)*

Tablets may contain benzoic acid; benzoic acid (benzoate) is a metabolite of benzyl alcohol; large amounts of benzyl alcohol (≥99 mg/kg/day) have been associated with a potentially fatal toxicity ("gasping syndrome") in neonates; the "gasping syndrome" consists of metabolic acidosis, respiratory distress, gasping respirations, CNS dysfunction (including convulsions, intracranial hemorrhage), hypotension and cardiovascular collapse; use chlorpromazine products containing benzoic acid with caution in neonates; *in vitro* and animal studies have shown that benzoate displaces bilirubin from protein binding sites

Precautions Use with caution in patients with cardiovascular, renal, or hepatic disease; chronic respiratory diseases (especially in children); seizures; significant medical disorders or children with acute illnesses

Adverse Reactions

Cardiovascular: Hypotension (especially with I.V. use), orthostatic hypotension, tachycardia, arrhythmias

Central nervous system: Sedation, drowsiness, restlessness, anxiety, extrapyramidal reactions, pseudoparkinsonian signs and symptoms, tardive dyskinesia, neuroleptic malignant syndrome, seizures, altered central temperature regulation

Dermatologic: Hyperpigmentation, pruritus, rash, photosensitivity; oral solution or injection may cause contact dermatitis (avoid contact with skin)

Endocrine & metabolic: Amenorrhea, galactorrhea, gynecomastia, weight gain

Gastrointestinal: Xerostomia, constipation, GI upset

Genitourinary: Impotence, urinary retention

Hematologic: Agranulocytosis, leukopenia (usually in patients with large doses for prolonged periods), thrombocytopenia, hemolytic anemia, eosinophilia

Hepatic: Cholestatic jaundice (rare)

Local: Thrombophlebitis

Ocular: Retinal pigmentation, blurred vision

Miscellaneous: Anaphylactoid reactions

Drug Interactions Cytochrome P450 isoenzyme CYP1A2, CYP2D6, and CYP3A3/4 substrate; isoenzyme CYP2D6 inhibitor

Additive effects with other CNS depressants; epinephrine may cause hypotension in patients receiving chlorpromazine due to phenothiazine-induced alpha-adrenergic blockade and unopposed epinephrine $beta_2$ action; thiazide diuretics may increase the orthostatic hypotension of phenothiazines; chlorpromazine may increase valproic acid, phenytoin, and haloperidol serum concentrations; use with propranolol will result in an increase in plasma concentrations of both chlorpromazine and propranolol; chlorpromazine may decrease the effects of oral anticoagulants; absorption of chlorpromazine may be decreased if administered concomitantly with aluminum- or magnesium-containing antacids; liquid preparations of chlorpromazine will form an orange rubbery precipitate if mixed with or administered simultaneously with carbamazepine suspension; may interact with metyrapone and reduce test effectiveness; may interact with tranexamic acid

Food Interactions Increases riboflavin elimination and may induce depletion; some may recommend increasing riboflavin in diet; may also decrease absorption of vitamin B_{12}; brown precipitate may occur when chlorpromazine is mixed with caffeine-containing liquids

Stability Protect oral dosage forms from light; diluted injection (1 mg/mL) with NS stored in 5 mL vials remains stable for 30 days

Mechanism of Action Blocks postsynaptic mesolimbic dopaminergic receptors in the brain; exhibits a strong alpha-adrenergic blocking effect and depresses the release of hypothalamic and hypophyseal hormones

Pharmacodynamics

Onset of action:

- Oral: 30-60 minutes
- Antipsychotic effects: Gradual, may take up to several weeks

Maximum antipsychotic effect: 6 weeks to 6 months

Duration: Oral: 4-6 hours

Pharmacokinetics

Absorption: Oral: Rapid and virtually complete; large first-pass effect due to metabolism during absorption in the GI mucosa

Distribution: Widely distributed into most body tissues and fluids; crosses blood-brain barrier and placenta; appears in breast milk; V_d: 8-160 L/kg (adults)

Protein binding: 90% to 99%

Metabolism: Extensively in the liver by demethylation (followed by glucuronide conjugation) and amine oxidation

Bioavailability: Oral: ~32%

Half-life, biphasic:

- Initial:
  - Children: 1.1 hours

Adults: ~2 hours
Terminal:
Children: 7.7 hours
Adults: ~30 hours
Elimination: <1% excreted in urine as unchanged drug within 24 hours
Dialysis: Not dialyzable (0% to 5%)

Usual Dosage

Neonates: Neonatal abstinence syndrome (withdrawal from maternal narcotic use):
I.M. and Oral: Initial: I.M.: 0.5-0.7 mg/kg/dose given every 6 hours; change to oral after ~4 days, decrease dose gradually over 2-3 weeks. **Note:** Chlorpromazine is rarely used for neonatal abstinence syndrome due to adverse effects such as hypothermia and eosinophilia. Other agents (eg, phenobarbital or a 25-fold dilution of tincture of opium) are preferred.

Infants ≥6 months and Children:
Schizophrenia/psychoses:
Oral: 0.5-1 mg/kg/dose every 4-6 hours; older children may require 200 mg/day or higher
I.M., I.V.: 0.5-1 mg/kg/dose every 6-8 hours
Maximum recommended doses:
Children <5 years (<22.7 kg): 40 mg/day
Children 5-12 years (22.7-45.5 kg): 75 mg/day
Nausea and vomiting:
Oral: 0.5-1 mg/kg/dose every 4-6 hours as needed
I.M., I.V.: 0.5-1 mg/kg/dose every 6-8 hours; maximum recommended doses:
Children <5 years (<22.7 kg): 40 mg/day
Children 5-12 years (22.7-45.5 kg): 75 mg/day

Adults:
Schizophrenia/psychoses:
Oral: Range: 30-800 mg/day in 1-4 divided doses, initiate at lower doses and titrate as needed; usual dose is 200 mg/day; some patients may require 1-2 g/day
I.M., I.V.: 25 mg initially, may repeat (25-50 mg) in 1-4 hours, gradually increase to a maximum of 400 mg/dose every 4-6 hours until patient controlled; usual dose 300-800 mg/day
Nausea and vomiting:
Oral: 10-25 mg every 4-6 hours
I.M., I.V.: 25-50 mg every 4-6 hours

Administration

Oral: Administer with water, food, or milk to decrease GI upset. Do not administer chlorpromazine liquid preparations simultaneously with carbamazepine suspension (see Drug Interactions).

Parenteral: Do not administer SubQ (tissue damage and irritation may occur); for direct I.V. injection: Dilute with NS to a maximum concentration of 1 mg/mL, administer slow I.V. at a rate not to exceed 0.5 mg/minute in children and 1 mg/minute in adults

Monitoring Parameters Periodic eye exam with prolonged therapy; blood pressure with parenteral administration; CBC with differential

Reference Range Relationship of plasma concentration to clinical response is not well established
Therapeutic: 50-300 ng/mL (SI: 157-942 nmol/L)
Toxic: >750 ng/mL (SI: >2355 nmol/L)

Test Interactions False-positives for phenylketonuria, amylase, uroporphyrins, urobilinogen; possible false-negative pregnancy urinary test

Patient Information May cause drowsiness and impair ability to perform activities requiring mental alertness or physical coordination; may cause dry mouth; avoid alcohol. May cause photosensitivity reactions (eg, exposure to sunlight may cause severe sunburn, skin rash, redness, or itching); avoid exposure to sunlight and artificial light sources (sunlamps, tanning booth/bed); wear protective clothing, wide-brimmed hats, sunglasses, and lip sunscreen (SPF ≥15); use a sunscreen [broad-spectrum sunscreen or physical sunscreen (preferred) or sunblock with SPF ≥15]; contact physician if reaction occurs.

Nursing Implications Avoid contact of injection with skin (may cause contact dermatitis; use of rubber gloves is recommended)

Additional Information Although chlorpromazine has been used in combination with meperidine and promethazine as a premedication ("lytic cocktail"), this combination may have a higher rate of adverse effects compared to alternative sedatives/analgesics (see AAP, 1995). Use decreased doses in elderly or debilitated patients; dystonic reactions may be more common in patients with hypocalcemia; extrapyramidal reactions may be more common in pediatric patients, especially those with dehydration or acute illnesses (viral or CNS infections).

(Continued)

ChlorproMAZINE *(Continued)*

Dosage Forms Excipient information presented when available (limited, particularly for generics); consult specific product labeling.

Injection, solution, as hydrochloride: 25 mg/mL (1 mL, 2 mL)

Tablet, as hydrochloride: 10 mg, 25 mg, 50 mg, 100 mg, 200 mg

References

American Academy of Pediatrics Committee on Drugs, "Reappraisal of Lytic Cocktail/Demerol®, Phenergan®, and Thorazine® (DPT) for the Sedation of Children," *Pediatrics*, 1995, 95(4):598-602.

Furlanut M, Benetello P, Baraldo M, et al, "Chlorpromazine Disposition in Relation to Age in Children," *Clin Pharmacokinet*, 1990, 18(4):329-31.

♦ **Chlorpromazine Hydrochloride** *see* ChlorproMAZINE *on page 345*
♦ **Chlor-Trimeton® [OTC]** *see* Chlorpheniramine *on page 344*
♦ **Chlor-Tripolon® (Can)** *see* Chlorpheniramine *on page 344*
♦ **Chlor-Tripolon ND® (Can)** *see* Loratadine and Pseudoephedrine *on page 961*

Chlorzoxazone (klor ZOKS a zone)

Medication Safety Issues

Sound-alike/look-alike issues:

Parafon Forte® may be confused with Fam-Pren Forte

U.S. Brand Names Parafon Forte® DSC

Canadian Brand Names Parafon Forte®; Strifon Forte®

Therapeutic Category Skeletal Muscle Relaxant, Nonparalytic

Generic Available Yes

Use Symptomatic treatment of muscle spasm and pain associated with acute musculoskeletal conditions

Pregnancy Risk Factor C

Lactation Excretion in breast milk unknown/not recommended

Contraindications Hypersensitivity to chlorzoxazone or any component; impaired liver function

Warnings Serious (including fatal) hepatocellular toxicity has been reported rarely

Adverse Reactions

Cardiovascular: Tachycardia, tightness in chest, flushing of face, syncope

Central nervous system: Drowsiness, dizziness, lightheadedness, headache, paradoxical stimulation, ataxia

Dermatologic: Rash, urticaria, petechiae, angioneurotic edema, erythema multiforme

Gastrointestinal: Nausea, vomiting, diarrhea, GI bleeding (rare), stomach cramps

Genitourinary: Discoloration of urine (orange or purple-red)

Hematologic: Anemia, granulocytopenia, eosinophilia

Hepatic: Hepatitis

Neuromuscular & skeletal: Paresthesia, trembling

Ocular: Burning of eyes

Respiratory: Shortness of breath

Miscellaneous: Hiccups

Drug Interactions Cytochrome P450 isoenzyme CYP2E1 substrate

May cause additive sedation when concomitantly administered with other CNS depressant medications

Food Interactions Watercress may decrease chlorzoxazone clearance

Mechanism of Action Acts on the spinal cord and subcortical levels of the brain to inhibit multisynaptic reflex arcs involved in producing and maintaining skeletal muscle spasms

Pharmacodynamics

Onset of action: Within 60 minutes

Duration: 3-4 hours

Pharmacokinetics

Absorption: Oral: Readily

Metabolism: Extensive in the liver by glucuronidation

Half-life: ~60 minutes

Time to peak serum concentration: Adults: 1-2 hours

Elimination: In urine as conjugates; <1% excreted unchanged in urine

Usual Dosage Oral:

Children: 20 mg/kg/day or 600 mg/m^2/day in 3-4 divided doses

Adults: 250-750 mg 3-4 times/day

Administration Oral: Administer with food

Monitoring Parameters Periodic liver function tests

Patient Information May color urine orange or purple-red; may cause drowsiness and impair ability to perform activities requiring mental alertness or physical coordination; notify physician if experiencing fever, rash, anorexia, right upper quadrant pain, dark urine, or jaundice

Dosage Forms Excipient information presented when available (limited, particularly for generics); consult specific product labeling.
Caplet (Parafon Forte® DSC): 500 mg
Tablet: 250 mg, 500 mg

Cholestyramine Resin (koe LES tir a meen REZ in)

U.S. Brand Names Prevalite®; Questran®; Questran® Light

Canadian Brand Names Novo-Cholamine; Novo-Cholamine Light; PMS-Cholestyramine; Questran®; Questran® Light Sugar Free

Therapeutic Category Antilipemic Agent

Generic Available Yes

Use Adjunct in the management of primary hypercholesterolemia; pruritus associated with elevated levels of bile acids; diarrhea associated with excess fecal bile acids; pseudomembraneous colitis

Pregnancy Risk Factor C

Lactation Does not enter breast milk/use caution

Contraindications Hypersensitivity to cholestyramine or any component; avoid using in complete biliary obstruction or biliary atresia

Precautions Use with caution in patients with constipation or recent abdominal surgery (see Additional Information); some products (eg, Prevalite® and Questran® Light) contain aspartame which is metabolized to phenylalanine and must be avoided (or used with caution) in patients with phenylketonuria.

Adverse Reactions
Dermatologic: Rash
Endocrine & metabolic: Hyperchloremic acidosis
Gastrointestinal: Constipation, nausea, vomiting, abdominal distention and pain, steatorrhea, malabsorption of fat-soluble vitamins
Genitourinary: Increased urinary calcium excretion
Hematologic: Hypoprothrombinemia
Local: Irritation of perianal area, skin, or tongue

Drug Interactions May decrease oral absorption of digitalis glycosides, warfarin, thyroid hormones, thiazide diuretics, propranolol, phenobarbital, amiodarone, methotrexate, NSAIDs, and other drugs by binding to the drug in the intestine (administer medications at least 1 hour before or at least 4-6 hours after cholestyramine)

Food Interactions Cholestyramine (especially high doses or long-term therapy) may decrease the absorption of fat-soluble vitamins (vitamins A, D, E, and K), folic acid, calcium, iron, zinc, and magnesium; deficiencies may occur including hypoprothrombinemia and increased bleeding from vitamin K deficiency; supplementation of vitamins A, D, E, and K, folic acid, and iron may be required with high-dose, long-term therapy (administer vitamins or mineral supplements at least 1 hour before or at least 4-6 hours after cholestyramine)

Mechanism of Action Forms a nonabsorbable complex with bile acids in the intestine, releasing chloride ions in the process; inhibits enterohepatic reuptake of intestinal bile salts and thereby increases the fecal loss of bile salt-bound low density lipoprotein cholesterol

Pharmacodynamics
Maximum effect on serum cholesterol levels: Within 4 weeks

Pharmacokinetics
Absorption: Not absorbed from the GI tract
Elimination: Forms an insoluble complex with bile acids which is excreted in feces

Usual Dosage Oral (dosages are expressed in terms of anhydrous resin):
Children: 240 mg/kg/day in 3 divided doses; need to titrate dose depending on indication
Hypercholesterolemia (**Note:** Doses >8 g/day may not provide additional significant cholesterol-lowering effects, but may increase adverse effects): Some centers use the following doses (see Sprecher, 1996):
Children ≤10 years: Initial: 2 g/day; titrate dose based on efficacy and tolerance; range: 1-4 g/day
Children >10 years and Adolescents: Initial: 2 g/day; titrate dose based on efficacy and tolerance, up to 8 g/day
Note: Lipid-lowering effects are better if dose is administered as a single daily dose with the evening meal (single daily morning doses are less effective); if patients cannot tolerate once daily dosing, the dose/day may be divided into 2 doses and administered with the morning and evening meals; may also be administered in 3 divided doses/day (Daniels, 2002)
Adults: 3-4 g 3-4 times/day to a maximum of 16-32 g/day in 2-4 divided doses

Administration Oral: Administer at mealtime; do not administer the powder in its dry form; just prior to administration, mix with 2-6 ounces of water, noncarbonated liquid, or applesauce; to minimize binding of concomitant medications, administer other
(Continued)

Cholestyramine Resin *(Continued)*

drugs including vitamins or mineral supplements at least 1 hour before or at least 4-6 hours after cholestyramine

Monitoring Parameters Serum cholesterol, serum triglycerides; with prolonged use, prothrombin time, liver enzymes, CBC, electrolytes; number of stools/day

Nursing Implications Maintain adequate oral fluid intake to avoid constipation; with high-dose, long-term therapy, use of daily multivitamin with iron and folic acid is recommended

Additional Information Overdose may result in GI obstruction; intestinal obstruction has been reported in patients with recent abdominal surgery (see Tonstad, 1996)

Dosage Forms Excipient information presented when available (limited, particularly for generics); consult specific product labeling.

Powder for oral suspension: 4 g of resin/5 g of powder (5 g packets, 210 g can) [contains phenylalanine 14 mg/5 g]; 4 g of resin/5.7 g of powder (5.7 g packets, 240 g can) [light formulation]; 4 g of resin/9 g of powder (9 g packets, 378 g can)

Prevalite®: 4 g of resin/5.5 g of powder (5.5 g packets, 231 g can) [contains phenylalanine 14.1 mg/5.5 g; orange flavor]

Questran®: 4 g of resin/9 g of powder (9 g packets, 378 g can)

Questran® Light: 4 g of resin/6.4 g of powder (5 g packets, 268 g can) [contains phenylalanine 28.1 g/6.4 g]

References

Daniels SR, personal communication, May 2002.

McCrindle BW, O'Neill MB, Cullen-Dean G, et al, "Acceptability and Compliance With Two Forms of Cholestyramine in the Treatment of Hypercholesterolemia in Children: A Randomized, Crossover Trial," *J Pediatr*, 1997, 130(2):266-73.

Sprecher DL and Daniels SR, "Rational Approach to Pharmacologic Reduction of Cholesterol Levels in Children," *J Pediatr*, 1996, 129(1):4-7.

Tonstad S, Knudtzon J, Sivertsen M, et al, "Efficacy and Safety of Cholestyramine Therapy in Peripubertal and Prepubertal Children With Familial Hypercholesterolemia," *J Pediatr*, 1996, 129(1):42-9.

Choline Magnesium Trisalicylate

(KOE leen mag NEE zhum trye sa LIS i late)

Related Information

Overdose and Toxicology *on page 1916*

U.S. Brand Names Trilisate® [DSC]

Index Terms Tricosal

Therapeutic Category Analgesic, Non-narcotic; Anti-inflammatory Agent; Antipyretic; Nonsteroidal Anti-inflammatory Drug (NSAID), Oral; Salicylate

Generic Available Yes

Use Management of osteoarthritis, rheumatoid arthritis, and other arthritides; treatment of acute painful shoulder, mild to moderate pain, and fever

Pregnancy Risk Factor C (D in 3rd trimester)

Lactation Enters breast milk/use caution

Contraindications Hypersensitivity to salicylates, any component, or other nonacetylated salicylates

Warnings Do not use salicylates in children and teenagers who have or who are recovering from chickenpox or flu symptoms (due to the association with Reye's syndrome); when using salicylates, changes in behavior (along with nausea and vomiting) may be an early sign of Reye's syndrome; instruct patients and caregivers to contact their healthcare provider if these symptoms occur.

Precautions Use with extreme caution in patients with impaired renal function, erosive gastritis or peptic ulcer

Adverse Reactions

Dermatologic: Rash, pruritus, urticaria

Gastrointestinal: Nausea, vomiting, GI distress, ulceration

Hepatic: Hepatotoxicity

Otic: Tinnitus

Respiratory: Pulmonary edema

Drug Interactions Antacids may decrease salicylate concentration; salicylates may increase hypoprothrombinemic effect of warfarin

Mechanism of Action Inhibits prostaglandin synthesis; acts on the hypothalamus heat-regulating center to reduce fever; blocks the generation of pain impulses

Pharmacokinetics

Absorption: From stomach and small intestine

Distribution: Readily distributes into most body fluids and tissues; crosses the placenta; appears in breast milk

Protein binding: 90% to 95%

Metabolism: Hepatic microsomal enzyme system

Half-life: Dose-dependent, ranging from 2-3 hours at low doses to 30 hours at high doses
Time to peak serum concentration:
Solution: 20-35 minutes
Tablet: Within ~2 hours
Elimination: 10% excreted as unchanged drug

Usual Dosage Oral (based on **total salicylate content**):
Children: 30-60 mg/kg/day given in 3-4 divided doses
Adults: 500 mg to 1.5 g 1-3 times/day

Administration Oral: Administer with food or milk to decrease GI upset; liquid may be mixed with fruit juice just before drinking; do not administer with antacids

Monitoring Parameters Serum salicylate levels; serum magnesium with high doses or in patients with decreased renal function

Reference Range
Salicylate blood levels for anti-inflammatory effect: 150-300 mcg/mL
Analgesia and antipyretic effect: 30-50 mcg/mL

Test Interactions False-negative results for Clinistix® urine test; false-positive results with Clinitest®

Patient Information Avoid alcohol; notify physician if ringing in ears, persistent GI pain, GI bleeding, or changes in behavior (along with nausea and vomiting) occur (see Warnings)

Additional Information Salicylate salts do not inhibit platelet aggregation and, therefore, should not be substituted for aspirin in the prophylaxis of thrombosis (ie, for aspirin's antiplatelet effects)

Dosage Forms Excipient information presented when available (limited, particularly for generics); consult specific product labeling.
Liquid: 500 mg/5 mL (240 mL) [choline salicylate 293 mg and magnesium salicylate 362 mg per 5 mL; cherry cordial flavor]
Tablet: 500 mg [choline salicylate 293 mg and magnesium salicylate 362 mg]; 750 mg [choline salicylate 440 mg and magnesium salicylate 544 mg]; 1000 mg [choline salicylate 587 mg and magnesium salicylate 725 mg]

References
Berde C, Ablin A, Glazer J, et al, "American Academy of Pediatrics Report of the Subcommittee on Disease-Related Pain in Childhood Cancer," *Pediatrics*, 1990, 86(5 Pt 2):818-25.

♦ **Chooz® [OTC]** *see* Calcium Carbonate *on page 264*
♦ **Chooz® [OTC]** *see* Calcium Supplements *on page 272*

Chorionic Gonadotropin (kor ee ON ik goe NAD oh troe pin)

U.S. Brand Names Novarel®; Pregnyl®
Canadian Brand Names Humegon®; Pregnyl®; Profasi® HP
Index Terms CG; hCG
Therapeutic Category Gonadotropin; Ovulation Stimulator
Generic Available Yes
Use Treatment of hypogonadotropic hypogonadism, prepubertal cryptorchidism; induce ovulation and pregnancy in anovulatory, infertile women
Pregnancy Risk Factor X
Lactation Excretion in breast milk unknown/use caution
Contraindications Hypersensitivity to chorionic gonadotropin or any component (see Warnings); precocious puberty, prostatic carcinoma or other androgen-dependent neoplasms; pregnancy

Warnings hCG is **not** effective in the treatment of obesity. hCG should only be used by clinicians who are experienced in the management of fertility disorders. May cause ovarian hyperstimulation syndrome (OHSS); if severe, treatment should be discontinued and patient should be hospitalized. OHSS results in a rapid (<24 hours to 7 days) accumulation of fluid in the peritoneal cavity, thorax, and possibly, the pericardium, which may become more severe if pregnancy occurs; monitor for ovarian enlargement. Use may lead to multiple births, arterial thromboembolism, enlargement or rupture of pre-existing ovarian cysts with resultant hemoperitoneum.

Pregnyl® contains benzyl alcohol which may cause allergic reactions in susceptible individuals; large amounts of benzyl alcohol (≥99 mg/kg/day) have been associated with a potentially fatal toxicity ("gasping syndrome") in neonates; the "gasping syndrome" consists of metabolic acidosis, respiratory distress, gasping respirations, CNS dysfunction (including convulsions, intracranial hemorrhage), hypotension and cardiovascular collapse; avoid use of Pregnyl® in neonates. *In vitro* and animal studies have shown that benzoate, a metabolite of benzyl alcohol, displaces bilirubin from protein-binding sites.

Precautions Use with caution in patients with asthma, seizure disorders, migraine, cardiac or renal disease; may induce precocious puberty in children being treated for

(Continued)

Chorionic Gonadotropin *(Continued)*

cryptorchidism; discontinue if signs of precocious puberty occur; safety and efficacy in children <4 years of age has not been established

Adverse Reactions

Cardiovascular: Edema, arterial thromboembolism

Central nervous system: Irritability, restlessness, depression, fatigue, headache, aggressive behavior

Endocrine & metabolic: Gynecomastia, precocious puberty, ovarian hyperstimulation (see Warnings), enlargement of preexisting ovarian cysts or rupture of ovarian cysts

Local: Pain at the injection site

Neuromuscular & skeletal: Premature closure of epiphyses

Respiratory: Shortness of breath, dyspnea

Miscellaneous: Hypersensitivity reactions

Stability Following reconstitution with provided diluent, stable for 30-90 days (depending upon preparation) when stored at 2°C to 15°C

Mechanism of Action Stimulates production of gonadal steroid hormones by causing production of androgen by the testis; as a substitute for luteinizing hormone (LH) to stimulate ovulation

Pharmacokinetics

Distribution: Distributes mainly into the testes in males and into the ovaries in females

Half-life, biphasic:

Initial: 11 hours

Terminal: 23 hours

Time to peak serum concentration: 6 hours

Elimination: Approximately 10% to 12% excreted unchanged in urine within 24 hours; detectable amounts may continue to be excreted in the urine for up to 3-4 days

Usual Dosage

Children: I.M. (many regimens have been described):

Prepubertal cryptorchidism:

1000-2000 units/m^2/dose 3 times/week for 3 weeks or 4000 units 3 times/week for 3 weeks

or

5000 units every second day for 4 injections

or

500 units 3 times/week for 4-6 weeks

Hypogonadotropic hypogonadism:

500-1000 units 3 times/week for 3 weeks, followed by the same dose twice weekly for 3 weeks

or

1000-2000 units 3 times/week

or

4000 units 3 times/week for 6-9 months; reduce dosage to 2000 units 3 times/week for additional 3 months

Adults:

Induction of ovulation: Females: 5000-10,000 units the day following the last dose of menotropins

Spermatogenesis induction associated with hypogonadotropic hypogonadism: Male: Treatment regimens vary (range: 1000-2000 units 2-3 times a week). Administer hCG until serum testosterone levels are normal (may require 2-3 months of therapy), then may add follitropin alfa or menopausal gonadotropin if needed to induce spermatogenesis; continue hCG at the dose required to maintain testosterone levels.

Administration Parenteral: Administer I.M. only

Monitoring Parameters

Male: Serum testosterone levels, semen analysis

Female: Ultrasound and/or estradiol levels to assess follicle development; ultrasound to assess number and size of follicles; ovulation (basal body temperature, serum progestin level, menstruation, sonography)

Reference Range Depends on application and methodology; <3 milli international units/mL (SI: <3 units/L) usually normal (nonpregnant)

Test Interactions Cross reacts with radioimmunoassay of gonadotropins, especially LH

Dosage Forms Excipient information presented when available (limited, particularly for generics); consult specific product labeling.

Injection, powder for reconstitution: 10,000 units [packaged with diluent; diluent contains benzyl alcohol and mannitol]

Novarel®: 10,000 units [packaged with diluent; diluent contains benzyl alcohol and mannitol]

Pregnyl®: 10,000 units [packaged with diluent; diluent contains benzyl alcohol]

- **Chromium Chloride** *see* Trace Metals *on page 1558*
- **Chronovera® (Can)** *see* Verapamil *on page 1611*

Cidofovir (si DOF o veer)

U.S. Brand Names Vistide®

Index Terms HPMPC

Therapeutic Category Antiviral Agent, Parenteral

Generic Available No

Use Treatment of cytomegalovirus (CMV) retinitis in patients with acquired immunodeficiency syndrome; antiviral agent with activity against ganciclovir-resistant CMV, foscarnet-resistant CMV, acyclovir-resistant HSV or VZV, and adenovirus; treatment of recurrent respiratory papillomatosis

Pregnancy Risk Factor C

Lactation Excretion in breast milk unknown/contraindicated

Contraindications Hypersensitivity to cidofovir or any component; history of clinically severe hypersensitivity to probenecid or other sulfa-containing medications; patients with a serum creatinine >1.5 mg/dL, creatinine clearance ≤55 mL/minute, urine protein ≥100 mg/dL (≥2 plus proteinuria); patients who are receiving other nephrotoxic agents; direct intraocular injection

Warnings Safety and efficacy have not been established in children; due to risk of long-term carcinogenicity and reproductive toxicity, administration of cidofovir to children warrants extreme caution. Prepare admixture in a Class II laminar flow hood; administer and dispose according to guidelines issued for cytotoxic drugs. Acute renal failure resulting in dialysis and/or contributing to death has been reported to occur after as few as one or two cidofovir doses; neutropenia and ocular hypotony have been reported in association with cidofovir treatment.

Precautions Modify dose in patients with changing renal function due to dose-dependent nephrotoxicity. Cidofovir administration must be accompanied by oral probenecid and NS I.V. prehydration to reduce possible nephrotoxicity.

Adverse Reactions

Cardiovascular: Hypotension, pallor, syncope, tachycardia, cardiomyopathy, edema, hypertension

Central nervous system: Headache, agitation, dizziness, fever, chills, amnesia, confusion, seizures, insomnia, personality/mood disorder, hallucinations, anxiety, somnolence, malaise

Dermatologic: Alopecia, rash, acne, skin discoloration, pruritus, urticaria

Endocrine & metabolic: Metabolic acidosis, hyperglycemia, hyperlipidemia, hypocalcemia, hypokalemia, dehydration, hypomagnesemia, hyponatremia, hypophosphatemia

Gastrointestinal: Nausea, vomiting, diarrhea, anorexia, abdominal pain, constipation, dyspepsia, gastritis, abnormal taste, stomatitis, colitis, cholangitis, pancreatitis, dysphagia

Genitourinary: Glycosuria, urinary incontinence, hematuria, proteinuria

Hematologic: Neutropenia (not dose-related; occurs in up to 24% of AIDS patients), thrombocytopenia, anemia

Hepatic: Hepatomegaly, elevated SGOT and SGPT

Neuromuscular & skeletal: Weakness, paresthesia, skeletal pain, peripheral neuropathy

Ocular: Amblyopia, conjunctivitis, iritis, uveitis, decreased intraocular pressure, ocular hypotony, retinal detachment

Renal: Tubular damage (dose-dependent), elevated BUN and serum creatinine, Fanconi-like syndrome

Respiratory: Asthma, bronchitis, coughing, dyspnea, pharyngitis, pneumonia, rhinitis, sinusitis

Miscellaneous: Diaphoresis, allergic reactions

Drug Interactions Aminoglycosides, amphotericin B, foscarnet, vancomycin, I.V. pentamidine and NSAIDs increase nephrotoxicity (cidofovir is contraindicated in patients who are receiving other nephrotoxic drugs); probenecid may decrease zidovudine clearance (temporarily discontinue zidovudine or decrease its dose by 50% on the days of cidofovir administration only); probenecid reduces the risk of cidofovir-induced nephrotoxicity by decreasing its concentration in proximal tubular cells; ganciclovir ocular implant (increased toxicity)

Stability Store vials at room temperature; cidofovir admixture is stable for 24 hours under refrigeration.

Mechanism of Action Cidofovir is converted to cidofovir diphosphate which is the active intracellular metabolite; suppresses CMV replication by selective inhibition of viral DNA polymerase; incorporation of cidofovir into the growing viral DNA chain results in reduction in the rate of viral DNA synthesis

(Continued)

Cidofovir *(Continued)*

Pharmacokinetics

Distribution: V_d: 0.54 L/kg; does not cross significantly into the CSF

Protein binding: <6%

Metabolism: Cidofovir is phosphorylated intracellularly to the active metabolite cidofovir diphosphate

Half-life: ~2.6 hours (cidofovir); 17 hours (cidofovir diphosphate)

Elimination: Renal tubular secretion and glomerular filtration

Renal clearance without probenecid: 130-170 mL/minute/1.73 m^2

Renal clearance with probenecid: 70-125 mL/minute/1.73 m^2

Usual Dosage

I.V.: Administration of cidofovir must be accompanied by concomitant oral probenecid and I.V. NS hydration

Children:

Adenovirus: **Note:** Limited information regarding cidofovir use in pediatric patients is currently available in the literature; some centers have used doses of 1 mg/kg/dose 3 times/week or 5 mg/kg/dose once weekly for 3 weeks then every 2 weeks for the treatment of adenovirus infection after bone marrow transplantation. Oral probenecid 1.25 g/m^2/dose is administered 3 hours prior to and 1 hour and 8 hours after completion of each 1-hour cidofovir infusion. NS bolus equal to 3 times the maintenance fluid is administered for 1 hour before cidofovir infusion and 1 hour after, then decrease to 2 times the maintenance fluid for the subsequent 2 hours.

Cytomegalovirus (CMV) retinitis:

Induction: 5 mg/kg/dose one time with probenecid and hydration

Maintenance: 3 mg/kg/dose once weekly with probenecid and hydration

Adults: Cytomegalovirus (CMV) retinitis: Administer 2 g probenecid orally 3 hours prior to each cidofovir dose and 1 g at 2 and 8 hours after completion of the cidofovir infusion (total probenecid dose: 4 g); infuse one liter NS over 1-2 hours prior to the cidofovir infusion; may administer second liter of NS over 1-3 hours with or immediately after the cidofovir infusion if tolerated

Induction: 5 mg/kg/dose once weekly for 2 consecutive weeks

Maintenance: 5 mg/kg/dose once every other week

Intralesional: Children and Adults: Recurrent respiratory papillomatosis: Injection volume is adapted case by case according to lesion extension and so not to cause airway obstruction. Injection is administered once monthly for 3-4 doses (see Naiman, 2003).

Dosing adjustment in renal impairment: If the serum creatinine increases by 0.3-0.4 mg/dL above baseline, reduce the cidofovir dose to 3 mg/kg; discontinue cidofovir therapy for increases ≥0.5 mg/dL above baseline or development of ≥3+ proteinuria.

Administration Do **not** administer by direct intraocular injection due to risk of iritis, ocular hypotony, and permanent visual impairment.

Parenteral: Administer by I.V. infusion over 1 hour. Dilute in 100 mL NS or D_5W or to a final concentration not to exceed 8 mg/mL.

Intralesional: May administer a solution with final concentration of 5-10 mg/mL

Monitoring Parameters Monitor renal function (BUN, serum creatinine), urinalysis (urine glucose and protein), CBC with differential (neutrophil count), electrolytes (calcium, magnesium, phosphorus, uric acid), liver function tests (SGOT/SGPT), intraocular pressure and visual acuity

Patient Information Cidofovir is not a cure for CMV retinitis; regular follow-up ophthalmologic exams and careful monitoring of renal function are necessary; report any rash immediately to your physician; use contraception during and for 3 months following treatment

Nursing Implications Administration of probenecid with a meal may decrease associated nausea; acetaminophen and antihistamines may ameliorate hypersensitivity reactions. Handle and dispose of cidofovir according to guidelines issued for cytotoxic drugs. Maintain adequate patient hydration.

Dosage Forms Excipient information presented when available (limited, particularly for generics); consult specific product labeling.

Injection, solution [preservative free]: 75 mg/mL (5 mL)

References

Cesaro S, Zhou X, Manzardo C, et al, "Cidofovir for Cytomegalovirus Reactivation in Pediatric Patients After Hematopoietic Stem Cell Transplantation," *J Clin Virol*, 2005, 34(2):129-32.

Izadifar-legrand F, Berrebi D, Faye A, et al, "Early Diagnosis of Adenovirus Infection and Treatment With Cidofovir After Bone Marrow Transplantation in Children," *Blood*, 1999, 94:341a.

Lalezari JP, Holland GN, Kramer F, et al, "Randomized, Controlled Study of the Safety and Efficacy of Intravenous Cidofovir for the Treatment of Relapsing Cytomegalovirus Retinitis in Patients With AIDS," *J Acquir Immune Defic Syndr Hum Retrovirol*, 1998, 17(4):339-44.

Legrand F, Berrebi D, Houhou N, et al, "Early Diagnosis of Adenovirus Infection and Treatment With Cidofovir After Bone Marrow Transplantation in Children," *Bone Marrow Transplant*, 2001, 27(6):621-6.

Naiman AN, Ceruse P, Coulombeau B, et al, "Intralesional Cidofovir and Surgical Excision for Laryngeal Papillomatosis," *Laryngoscope*, 2003, 113(12):2174-81.
Ribaud P, Scieux C, Freymuth F, et al, "Successful Treatment of Adenovirus Disease With Intravenous Cidofovir in an Unrelated Stem-Cell Transplant Recipient," *Clinical Infectious Diseases*, 1999, 28(3):690-1.

- **Cilastatin and Imipenem** *see* Imipenem and Cilastatin *on page 813*
- **Ciloxan®** *see* Ciprofloxacin *on page 357*

Cimetidine (sye MET i deen)

Medication Safety Issues
Sound-alike/look-alike issues:
Cimetidine may be confused with simethicone

U.S. Brand Names Tagamet® [DSC]; Tagamet® HB 200 [OTC]

Canadian Brand Names Apo-Cimetidine®; Gen-Cimetidine; Novo-Cimetidine; Nu-Cimet; PMS-Cimetidine; Tagamet® HB

Therapeutic Category Gastrointestinal Agent, Gastric or Duodenal Ulcer Treatment; Histamine H_2 Antagonist

Generic Available Yes

Use Short-term treatment of active duodenal ulcers and benign gastric ulcers; long-term prophylaxis of duodenal ulcer; gastric hypersecretory states; gastroesophageal reflux (GERD); prevention of upper GI bleeding in critically ill patients; over-the-counter (OTC) formulation for relief of acid indigestion, heartburn, or sour stomach

Pregnancy Risk Factor B

Lactation Enters breast milk/not recommended

Contraindications Hypersensitivity to cimetidine or any component (see Warnings)

Warnings Rapid I.V. administration may cause hypotension or cardiac arrhythmias. Use of gastric acid inhibitors including proton pump inhibitors and H_2 blockers has been associated with an increased risk for development of acute gastroenteritis and community-acquired pneumonia (Canani, 2006). A large epidemiological study has suggested an increased risk for developing pneumonia in patients receiving H_2 receptor antagonists; however, a causal relationship with cimetidine has not been demonstrated.

Injection (8 mL vial) contains benzyl alcohol which may cause allergic reactions in susceptible individuals; large amounts of benzyl alcohol (≥99 mg/kg/day) have been associated with a potentially fatal toxicity ("gasping syndrome") in neonates; the "gasping syndrome" consists of metabolic acidosis, respiratory distress, gasping respirations, CNS dysfunction (including convulsions, intracranial hemorrhage), hypotension and cardiovascular collapse; avoid use of injection containing benzyl alcohol in neonates. *In vitro* and animal studies have shown that benzoate, a metabolite of benzyl alcohol, displaces bilirubin from protein-binding sites.

Precautions Modify dosage in patients with renal and/or hepatic impairment; multiple drug interactions exist requiring dose modifications of other medications or cimetidine (see Drug Interactions)

Adverse Reactions
Cardiovascular: Bradycardia, hypotension, cardiac arrhythmias (after rapid I.V. administration), tachycardia
Central nervous system: Dizziness, mental confusion, agitation, headache, psychosis, drowsiness, fever
Dermatologic: Rash
Endocrine & metabolic: Gynecomastia
Gastrointestinal: Mild diarrhea, nausea, vomiting
Hematologic: Neutropenia, agranulocytosis, thrombocytopenia
Hepatic: Elevated AST and ALT
Neuromuscular & skeletal: Myalgia
Renal: Elevated serum creatinine
Respiratory: Pneumonia (causal relationship has not been established; see Warnings)

Drug Interactions Cytochrome P450 isoenzyme CYP1A2, CYP2C9, CYP2C19, CYP2D6, CYP3A3/4, and CYP2C18 inhibitor; isoenzyme CYP3A3/4 substrate
Cimetidine reduces the hepatic metabolism of drugs metabolized by the cytochrome P450 pathway which may result in decreased elimination of lidocaine, diazepam, theophylline, phenytoin, gabapentin, metronidazole, triamterene, procainamide, quinidine, propranolol, carbamazepine, chloroquine, lomustine, warfarin, flecainide, and tricyclic antidepressants; antacids, metoclopramide, and anticholinergics may reduce the absorption of cimetidine; cimetidine may decrease the absorption of iron, melphalan, indomethacin, ketoconazole, tetracyclines, delavirdine, and possibly fluconazole; cimetidine may decrease digoxin serum levels; may increase diltiazem, flecainide, praziquantel, tacrolimus, cyclosporin, nevirapine, mexiletine,
(Continued)

Cimetidine *(Continued)*

and pentoxifylline serum levels; cimetidine decreases the renal clearance of zalcitabine and zidovudine; potentiates myelosuppressive effects of carmustine; may increase didanosine absorption

Food Interactions Limit xanthine-containing foods and beverages

Stability Protect from light; store at room temperature; do not refrigerate the injection since precipitation may occur (can be redissolved by warming without degradation); stable in parenteral nutrition solutions for up to 7 days when protected from light

Mechanism of Action Competitive inhibition of histamine at H_2-receptors of the gastric parietal cells resulting in reduced gastric acid secretion

Pharmacokinetics

Distribution: Crosses the placenta; breast milk to plasma ratio: 4.6-11.76
Protein binding: 13% to 25%
Metabolism: Hepatic with a sulfoxide as the major metabolite
Bioavailability: 60% to 70%
Half-life:
- Neonates: 3.6 hours
- Children: 1.4 hours
- Adults with normal renal function: 2 hours

Time to peak serum concentration: Oral: 45-90 minutes
Elimination: Primarily in urine (48% unchanged drug); some excretion in bile and feces

Usual Dosage

Neonates: Oral, I.M., I.V.: 5-10 mg/kg/day in divided doses every 8-12 hours
Infants: Oral, I.M., I.V.: 10-20 mg/kg/day divided every 6-12 hours
Children: Oral, I.M., I.V.: 20-40 mg/kg/day in divided doses every 6 hours
Adults:
- Short-term treatment of active ulcers:
  - Oral: 300 mg 4 times/day or 800 mg at bedtime or 400 mg twice daily for up to 8 weeks
  - I.M., I.V.: 300 mg every 6 hours or 150 mg single dose followed by 37.5 mg/hour by continuous infusion; adjust dosage to maintain an intragastric pH ≥5 or acid secretory rate of <10 mEq/hour; (average dose 160 mg/hour; range: 40-600 mg/hour)
- Duodenal ulcer prophylaxis: Oral: 400-800 mg at bedtime
- Gastric hypersecretory conditions: Oral, I.M., I.V.: 300-600 mg every 6 hours; dosage not to exceed 2.4 g/day
- GERD: Oral: 800 mg twice daily or 400 mg 4 times/day for 12 weeks
- Acid indigestion, heartburn, sour stomach relief (OTC use): Oral: 100 mg right before or up to 30 minutes before a meal; no more than 2 tablets per day
- Prevention of upper GI bleeding: Continuous I.V. infusion of 50 mg/hour

Dosing interval in renal impairment using 5-10 mg/kg/dose in children or 300 mg in adults (titrate dose to gastric pH and Cl_{cr}):
- Cl_{cr} >40 mL/minute: Administer every 6 hours
- Cl_{cr} 20-40 mL/minute: Administer every 8 hours or reduce dose by 25%
- Cl_{cr} <20 mL/minute: Administer every 12 hours or reduce dose by 50%

Hemodialysis: Administer after dialysis and every 12 hours during the interdialysis period

Dosing adjustment in hepatic impairment: Reduce dosage in severe liver disease

Administration

Oral: Administer with food; do not administer with antacids
Parenteral: Can be administered as a slow I.V. push over 15 minutes (minimum 5 minutes; rapid administration has been associated with hypotension and cardiac arrhythmias) at a concentration not to exceed 15 mg/mL; or preferably as an I.V. intermittent or I.V. continuous infusion. Intermittent infusions are administered over 15-30 minutes at a final concentration not to exceed 6 mg/mL; for patients with an active bleed, preferred method of administration is continuous infusion; may be administered intramuscularly

Monitoring Parameters Blood pressure and heart rate with I.V. push administration; CBC; gastric pH

Patient Information Avoid excessive amount of coffee and aspirin; when self medicating, if symptoms of heartburn, acid indigestion, or sour stomach persist after 2 weeks of continuous use of the drug, consult a clinician; notify your physician if taking other medications (multiple drug interactions exist)

Dosage Forms Excipient information presented when available (limited, particularly for generics); consult specific product labeling. [DSC] = Discontinued product
Infusion, as hydrochloride [premixed in NS]: 300 mg (50 mL)
Injection, solution, as hydrochloride: 150 mg/mL (2 mL, 8 mL) [8 mL size contains benzyl alcohol]

Liquid, oral, as hydrochloride: 300 mg/5 mL (240 mL, 480 mL) [contains alcohol 2.8%; mint-peach flavor]

Tablet: 200 mg [OTC], 300 mg, 400 mg, 800 mg

Tagamet®: 300 mg, 400 mg [DSC]

Tagamet® HB 200: 200 mg

References

Canani RB, Cirillo P, Roggero P, et al, "Therapy With Gastric Acidity Inhibitors Increases the Risk of Acute Gastroenteritis and Community-Acquired Pneumonia in Children," *Pediatrics*, 2006, 117(5):e817-20.

Lambert J, Mobassaleh M, and Grand RJ, "Efficacy of Cimetidine for Gastric Acid Suppression in Pediatric Patients," *J Pediatr*, 1992, 120(3):474-8.

Lloyd CW, Martin WJ, Taylor BD, et al, "Pharmacokinetics and Pharmacodynamics of Cimetidine and Metabolites in Critically Ill Children," *J Pediatr*, 1985, 107(2):295-300.

Lloyd CW, Martin WJ, and Taylor BD, "The Pharmacokinetics of Cimetidine and Metabolites in a Neonate," *Drug Intell Clin Pharm*, 1985, 19(3):203-5.

Somogyi A and Gugler R, "Clinical Pharmacokinetics of Cimetidine," *Clin Pharmacokinet*, 1983, 8(6):463-95.

♦ **Cipro®** *see* Ciprofloxacin *on page 357*

♦ **Cipro® XL (Can)** *see* Ciprofloxacin *on page 357*

♦ **Ciprodex®** *see* Ciprofloxacin and Dexamethasone *on page 361*

Ciprofloxacin (sip roe FLOKS a sin)

Medication Safety Issues

Sound-alike/look-alike issues:

Ciprofloxacin may be confused with cephalexin

Ciloxan® may be confused with cinoxacin, Cytoxan®

Cipro® may be confused with Ceftin®

U.S. Brand Names Ciloxan®; Cipro®; Cipro® XR; Proquin® XR

Canadian Brand Names Apo-Ciproflox®; Ciloxan®; Cipro®; Cipro® XL; CO Ciprofloxacin; Gen-Ciprofloxacin; Novo-Ciprofloxacin; PMS-Ciprofloxacin; RAN™-Ciprofloxacin; ratio-Ciprofloxacin; Rhoxal-ciprofloxacin; Sandoz-Ciprofloxacin; Taro-Ciprofloxacin

Index Terms Ciprofloxacin Hydrochloride

Therapeutic Category Antibiotic, Ophthalmic; Antibiotic, Quinolone

Generic Available Yes: Excludes infusion, suspension, ointment

Use Treatment of documented or suspected pseudomonal infection of the respiratory or urinary tract, skin and soft tissue, bone and joint, eye and ear; treatment of complicated UTIs and pyelonephritis in children 1-17 years of age due to *E. coli*; documented multidrug-resistant, aerobic gram-negative bacilli, some gram-positive staphylococci, and *Mycobacterium tuberculosis*; documented infectious diarrhea due to *Campylobacter jejuni*, *Shigella*, or *E. coli*; typhoid fever caused by *Salmonella typhi*; osteomyelitis caused by susceptible organisms in which parenteral therapy is not feasible; uncomplicated cervical and urethral gonorrhea due to *N. gonorrhoeae*; chronic bacterial prostatitis caused by *E. coli* or *Proteus mirabilis*; pulmonary exacerbation of cystic fibrosis; empiric therapy for febrile neutropenia in combination with piperacillin; initial therapy or postexposure prophylaxis for inhalational anthrax; used ophthalmically for treatment of corneal ulcers and conjunctivitis due to susceptible organisms; extended release tablet is used for the treatment of UTI and acute uncomplicated pyelonephritis caused by susceptible *E. coli* and *Klebsiella pneumoniae*

Pregnancy Risk Factor C

Lactation Enters breast milk/not recommended (AAP rates "compatible")

Contraindications Hypersensitivity to ciprofloxacin, any component, or other quinolones; concomitant administration with tizanidine; not recommended for use in pregnant women or during breast-feeding

Warnings Ciprofloxacin is not a drug of first choice in the pediatric population due to reported adverse events related to joints and/or surrounding tissues. Ciprofloxacin has caused arthropathy with erosions of the cartilage in weight bearing joints of immature animals; green discoloration of teeth in newborns has been reported; Achilles tendonitis and tendon rupture have been reported with fluoroquinolones with risk increased in patients taking concomitant corticosteroids; if patient experiences pain, inflammation, or tendon rupture, discontinue ciprofloxacin. Prolonged use may result in superinfection; CNS stimulation, increased intracranial pressure, and toxic psychosis may occur resulting in tremors, restlessness, confusion, and very rarely hallucinations, depression, nightmares, suicidal ideation, or convulsive seizures. If these reactions occur, discontinue ciprofloxacin. Rare cases of polyneuropathy affecting small and/or large axons resulting in paresthesias, hypoesthesias, dysesthesias, and weakness have been reported in patients receiving ciprofloxacin. Discontinue ciprofloxacin if patient experiences pain, burning, tingling, numbness, weakness, or is found to have deficits in light touch, pain, temperature, position sense, vibrating sensation, or motor strength.

(Continued)

Ciprofloxacin *(Continued)*

Coadministration of ciprofloxacin with drugs metabolized by CYP1A2 (eg, theophylline, caffeine, tizanidine) may result in increased plasma concentrations of the coadministered drug with corresponding side effects. Serious and fatal reactions including cardiac arrest, seizure, status epilepticus, and respiratory failure have been reported in patients receiving ciprofloxacin and theophylline concurrently. Serum theophylline levels should be monitored and dosage adjustments made when concomitant use cannot be avoided. Hypotension and oversedation have been reported when ciprofloxacin and tizanidine were given concomitantly (concomitant administration of tizanidine and ciprofloxacin is contraindicated). Severe hypersensitivity reactions, including life-threatening anaphylactic shock, have been reported in patients receiving quinolones. If an allergic reaction occurs, discontinue drug immediately.

Precautions Use with caution in patients with known or suspected CNS disorders, seizure disorders, severe cerebral arteriosclerosis, or renal impairment; modify dosage in patients with renal impairment

Adverse Reactions

Cardiovascular: Torsade de pointes, syncope, hypertension, hypotension, arrhythmia, angina pectoris, tachycardia, flushing, vasculitis, migraine, palpitation, atrial flutter

Central nervous system: Headache, restlessness, dizziness, confusion, seizures, insomnia, nervousness, hallucinations, agitation, somnolence, fever, nightmares, depression, paranoia

Dermatologic: Rash, photosensitivity, pruritus, urticaria, erythema multiforme, Stevens-Johnson syndrome, angioedema, exfoliative dermatitis, Lyell's syndrome

Endocrine & metabolic: Elevated serum triglyceride, cholesterol, and lipase; hyperglycemia

Gastrointestinal: Nausea, diarrhea, vomiting, GI bleeding, abdominal pain, constipation, pseudomembranous colitis, pancreatitis, anorexia

Genitourinary: Crystalluria

Hematologic: Anemia, eosinophilia, neutropenia, agranulocytosis

Hepatic: Elevated liver enzymes, cholestatic jaundice, hepatitis

Local: With I.V.: Phlebitis, burning, pain, erythema, and swelling (occurs more frequently with infusion time <30 minutes)

Neuromuscular & skeletal: Arthralgia, joint and back pain, tremor, joint stiffness, arthritis, myoclonus, tendonitis, tendon rupture, peripheral neuropathy, myalgia, paresthesias, hypoesthesias, dysesthesias, weakness

Ocular: Nystagmus, blurred vision; ophthalmic ointment: Visual blurring, retardation of corneal healing, dry eye, eye pain, keratoconjunctivitis, photophobia

Otic: Hearing loss

Renal: Elevated BUN and serum creatinine, acute renal failure, interstitial nephritis, hematuria

Respiratory: Dyspnea, bronchospasm, pulmonary edema

Miscellaneous: Anaphylaxis, serum sickness, diaphoresis

Drug Interactions Cytochrome P450 isoenzyme CYP1A2 inhibitor

Magnesium-, aluminum- or calcium-containing antacids, sucralfate, and sevelamer decrease ciprofloxacin absorption by up to 90% if given at the same time; antacids in didanosine formulation chelate ciprofloxacin and decrease its absorption (administer ciprofloxacin 2 hours before or 6 hours after antacids, calcium, zinc, sucralfate, highly-buffered drugs, and didanosine); probenecid decreases renal clearance of ciprofloxacin and can increase ciprofloxacin concentrations by 50%; ciprofloxacin decreases theophylline, caffeine, tizanidine, warfarin, ropivacaine, clozapine, diazepam, methadone, olanzapine, and cyclosporine clearance; NSAID (increase CNS stimulation and may provoke seizures); may enhance hypoprothrombinemic effect of warfarin (monitor INR or prothrombin time); ciprofloxacin inhibits renal tubular transport of methotrexate increasing plasma methotrexate levels (monitor); may decrease serum levels of phenytoin; concomitant administration with glyburide may result in severe hypoglycemia; foscarnet (increased risk of seizures); ziprasidone (additive cardiotoxicity)

Food Interactions Dairy foods (milk, yogurt) and mineral supplements decrease ciprofloxacin concentrations; avoid concomitant administration with dairy products, enteral feedings (enteral feeds need to be discontinued for 1-2 hours prior to and after ciprofloxacin administration), mineral supplements, iron, zinc, or with calcium-fortified juices; ciprofloxacin increases caffeine concentrations; use caution with xanthine-containing foods and beverages

Stability Premixed bags: Out of overwrap stability: 14 days at room temperature; reconstituted oral suspension: Stable for 14 days when stored at room temperature or refrigerated; store tablets, intact injection vial, ophthalmic solution/ointment, and oral suspension prior to reconstitution at room temperature; protect from intense light; protect from freezing

Mechanism of Action Inhibits DNA-gyrase and topoisomerase IV in susceptible organisms; inhibits relaxation of supercoiled DNA and promotes breakage of double-stranded DNA

Pharmacokinetics

Absorption: Oral: Well absorbed. 500 mg orally every 12 hours produces an equivalent AUC to that produced by 400 mg I.V. over 60 minutes every 12 hours.

Distribution: Widely distributed into body tissues and fluids with high concentration in bile, saliva, urine, sputum, stool, lungs, liver, skin, muscle, prostate, genital tissue, and bone; low concentration in CSF; crosses the placenta; appears in breast milk

Protein binding: 16% to 43%

Metabolism: Partially in the liver to four active metabolites

Bioavailability: Oral: 50% to 85%; younger CF patients have a lower bioavailability of 68% versus CF patients >13 years of age with bioavailability of 95%

Half-life:
- Children: 4-5 hours
- Adults with normal renal function: 3-5 hours

Time to peak serum concentration: Oral: Immediate release tablet: Within 0.5-2 hours; Extended release tablet: Cipro® XR: 1-4 hours; Proquin® XR: 3.5-8.7 hours

Elimination: 30% to 50% excreted as unchanged drug in urine via glomerular filtration and active tubular secretion; 20% to 40% excreted in feces primarily from biliary excretion; <1% excreted in bile as unchanged drug
- Clearance: After I.V.:
  - CF child: 0.84 L/hour/kg
  - Adult: 0.5-0.6 L/hour/kg

Dialysis: Only small amounts of ciprofloxacin are removed by dialysis (<10%)

Usual Dosage Note: Extended release tablets and immediate release formulations are not interchangeable. Unless otherwise specified, oral dosing reflects the use of immediate release formulation.

Neonates: I.V. ciprofloxacin has been used in 23 neonates at doses ranging from 7-40 mg/kg/day divided every 12 hours (Schaad, 1995)

Children:
- Oral: 20-30 mg/kg/day in 2 divided doses; maximum dose: 1.5 g/day
- I.V.: 20-30 mg/kg/day divided every 12 hours; maximum dose: 800 mg/day
- Inhalational anthrax (postexposure): Initial treatment:
  - I.V.: 20 mg/kg/day divided every 12 hours for 60 days; maximum dose: 800 mg/day (substitute oral antibiotics for I.V. antibiotics as soon as clinical condition improves)
  - Oral: 30 mg/kg/day divided every 12 hours for 60 days; maximum dose: 1000 mg/day
- Complicated UTI or pyelonephritis:
  - I.V.: 18-30 mg/kg/day divided every 8 hours for 10-21 days; maximum dose: 1200 mg/day
  - Oral: 20-40 mg/kg/day divided every 12 hours for 10-21 days; maximum dose: 1500 mg/day
- Cystic fibrosis:
  - Oral: 40 mg/kg/day divided every 12 hours; maximum dose: 2 g/day
  - I.V.: 30 mg/kg/day divided every 8-12 hours; maximum dose: 1.2 g/day

Adults:
- Oral: 250-750 mg every 12 hours, depending on severity of infection and susceptibility
  - Acute sinusitis: Mild/moderate: 500 mg every 12 hours for 10 days
  - Uncomplicated UTI/acute cystitis:
    - Extended release tablet: 500 mg every 24 hours for 3 days
    - Immediate release formulation: Acute uncomplicated: 250 mg every 12 hours for 3 days; 250 mg every 12 hours for 7-14 days for mild to moderate UTI
  - Complicated UTI or acute uncomplicated pyelonephritis:
    - Extended release tablet: 1000 mg every 24 hours for 7-14 days
    - Immediate release formulation: 500 mg every 12 hours for 7-14 days
  - Bone and joint infections:
    - Mild/moderate: 500 mg every 12 hours for ≥4 to 6 weeks
    - Severe/complicated: 750 mg every 12 hours for ≥4 to 6 weeks
  - Chemoprophylaxis regimen for high-risk contacts of invasive meningococcal disease: 500 mg as a single dose
  - Chronic bacterial prostatitis: 500 mg every 12 hours for 28 days
  - Infectious diarrhea: 500 mg every 12 hours for 5-7 days
  - Skin and skin structure infections:
    - Mild/moderate: 500 mg every 12 hours for 7-14 days
    - Severe/complicated: 750 mg every 12 hours for 7-14 days
  - Uncomplicated gonorrhea: 500 mg as a single dose
  - Chancroid: 500 mg twice daily for 3 days

(Continued)

Ciprofloxacin *(Continued)*

Lower respiratory tract infection:
Mild/moderate: 500 mg every 12 hours for 7-14 days
Severe/complicated: 750 mg every 12 hours for 7-14 days
Typhoid fever: 500 mg every 12 hours for 10 days
Inhalational anthrax (postexposure prophylaxis): 500 mg every 12 hours for 60 days
I.V.: 200-400 mg every 8-12 hours depending on severity of infection
Lower respiratory tract, skin and skin structure infection:
Mild/moderate: 400 mg every 12 hours for 7-14 days
Severe/complicated: 400 mg every 8 hours for 7-14 days
Treatment of anthrax infection: 400 mg every 12 hours for 60 days (substitute oral antibiotics for I.V. antibiotics as soon as clinical condition improves)
Empiric therapy in febrile neutropenic patients: 400 mg every 8 hours in combination with piperacillin for 7-14 days
Ophthalmic:
Children ≥1 year and Adults: Solution: Instill 1-2 drops into the affected eye(s) every 2 hours while awake for 2 days, then 1-2 drops every 4 hours while awake for the next 5 days
Treatment of corneal ulcers: Instill 2 drops every 15 minutes for the first 6 hours, then 2 drops every 30 minutes for the remainder of the first day; on the second day, 2 drops every hour; then 2 drops every 4 hours thereafter
Children ≥2 years and Adults: Ointment: Instill ½" ointment ribbon 3 times/day for 2 days, then twice daily for the next 5 days

Dosing interval in renal impairment: Adults:
Cl_{cr} 30-50 mL/minute: Oral: 250-500 mg every 12 hours
Cl_{cr} <30 mL/minute:
Immediate release formulations: 250-500 mg every 18 hours
Extended release tablet: Complicated UTI or acute uncomplicated pyelonephritis: 500 mg every 24 hours
Patients on hemodialysis or peritoneal dialysis: Immediate release formulations: 250-500 mg every 24 hours after dialysis

Administration
Oral: Administer immediate release tablets 2 hours after a meal; may administer with food to minimize GI upset; extended release tablet and oral suspension may be administered with or without food; Proquin® XR should be administered with a main meal (evening meal preferred); do not administer oral suspension through a feeding tube (suspension will adhere to the feeding tube); to prepare oral suspension, pour the microcapsules (small bottle) completely into the large bottle of diluent - DO NOT ADD WATER TO THE SUSPENSION. Shake suspension vigorously for 15 seconds before use. Avoid antacid use. Drink plenty of fluids to maintain proper hydration and urine output
Nasogastric/orogastric tube: Crush immediate release tablet and mix with water. Flush feeding tube before and after ciprofloxacin administration with water. Hold tube feeding at least 1 hour before and 2 hours after administration.
Parenteral: Administer by slow I.V. infusion over 60 minutes to reduce the risk of venous irritation (burning, pain, erythema, and swelling); final concentration for administration should not exceed 2 mg/mL
Ophthalmic: For topical ophthalmic use only. Avoid contacting tip with skin or eye.
Ointment: Instill ointment in the lower conjunctival sac
Solution: Apply finger pressure to lacrimal sac during and for 1-2 minutes after instillation to decrease risk of absorption and systemic effects

Monitoring Parameters Monitor renal, hepatic, and hematopoietic function periodically; number and type of stools/day for diarrhea. Patients receiving concurrent ciprofloxacin and theophylline should have serum levels of theophylline monitored; monitor INR in patients receiving warfarin; patients receiving concurrent ciprofloxacin and cyclosporine should have cyclosporine levels monitored

Reference Range Avoid peak serum concentrations >5 mcg/mL

Patient Information Do not chew microcapsules of the oral suspension; do not split, crush, or chew extended release tablet; avoid caffeine; may cause dizziness or lightheadedness and impair ability to perform activities requiring mental alertness or physical coordination. Notify physician if tendon pain or swelling occurs, signs of allergy; burning, tingling, numbness, or weakness develops or persistent diarrhea occurs. Remove contact lenses prior to administration of ophthalmic solution and ointment. May cause photosensitivity reactions (eg, exposure to sunlight may cause severe sunburn, skin rash, redness, or itching); avoid exposure to sunlight and artificial light sources (sunlamps, tanning booth/bed); wear protective clothing, wide-brimmed hats, sunglasses, and lip sunscreen (SPF ≥15); use a sunscreen [broad-spectrum sunscreen or physical sunscreen (preferred) or sunblock with SPF ≥15]; contact physician if reaction occurs.

Nursing Implications Administer immediate release ciprofloxacin and Cipro® XR at least 2 hours before or 6 hours after, and Proquin® XR at least 4 hours before or 2 hours after antacids or other products containing calcium, iron, or zinc (including dairy products or calcium-fortified juices), sucralfate, or highly buffered drugs; ensure adequate patient hydration to prevent crystalluria. Cipro® XR and Proquin® XR are not interchangeable with ciprofloxacin immediate-release tablets.

Additional Information Although fluoroquinolones are only FDA approved for use in children for complicated UTI, pyelonephritis, and postexposure treatment for inhalational anthrax, the AAP has provided a list of other possible uses for fluoroquinolones once risks and benefits have been assessed to justify its use:

- UTI caused by *Pseudomonas aeruginosa* or other multidrug-resistant, gram-negative bacteria susceptible to fluoroquinolones
- Chronic suppurative otitis media or otitis externa caused by *P. aeruginosa*
- Chronic or acute osteomyelitis or osteochondritis caused by *P. aeruginosa*
- Mycobacterial infections caused by isolates sensitive to fluoroquinolones
- Gram-negative bacterial infections in immunocompromised hosts in which oral therapy is desired or resistance to alternative agents is present

Dosage Forms Excipient information presented when available (limited, particularly for generics); consult specific product labeling.

Infusion [premixed in D_5W]:
Cipro®: 200 mg (100 mL); 400 mg (200 mL) [latex free]
Injection, solution: 10 mg/mL (20 mL, 40 mL)
Cipro®: 10 mg/mL (20 mL, 40 mL)
Microcapsules for suspension, oral:
Cipro®: 250 mg/5 mL (100 mL); 500 mg/5 mL (100 mL) [strawberry flavor]
Ointment, ophthalmic, as hydrochloride:
Ciloxan®: 3.33 mg/g [0.3% base] (3.5 g)
Solution, ophthalmic, as hydrochloride: 3.5 mg/mL (2.5 mL, 5mL, 10 mL) [0.3% base]
Ciloxin®: 3.5 mg/mL (2.5 mL, 5mL, 10 mL) [0.3% base; contains benzalkonium chloride]
Tablet: 250 mg, 500 mg, 750 mg
Cipro®: 250 mg, 500 mg, 750 mg
Tablet, extended release: 500 mg, 1000 mg
Cipro® XR: 500 mg [equivalent to ciprofloxacin hydrochloride 287.5 mg and ciprofloxacin base 212.6 mg]; 1000 mg [equivalent to ciprofloxacin hydrochloride 574.9 mg and ciprofloxacin base 425.2 mg]
Proquin® XR: 500 mg
Tablet, extended release [dose pack]:
Proquin® XR: 500 mg (3s)

References

Campoli-Richards DM, Monk JP, Price A, et al, "Ciprofloxacin: A Review of Its Antibacterial Activity, Pharmacokinetic Properties and Therapeutic Use," *Drugs*, 1988, 35(4):373-447.
Inglesby TV, Henderson DA, Bartlett JG, et al, "Anthrax as a Biological Weapon: Medical and Public Health Management. Working Group on Civilian Biodefense," *JAMA*, 1999, 281(18):1735-45.
Rodriguez WJ, and Wiedermann BL, "The Role of Newer Oral Cephalosporins, Fluoroquinolones, and Macrolides in the Treatment of Pediatric Infections," *Adv Pediatr Infect Dis*, 1994, 9:125-59.
Rubio TT, Miles MV, Lettieri JT, et al, "Pharmacokinetic Disposition of Sequential Intravenous/Oral Ciprofloxacin in Pediatric Cystic Fibrosis Patients with Acute Pulmonary Exacerbation," *Pediatr Infect Dis J*, 1997, 16:112-7
Schaad UB, abdus Salam M, Aujard Y, et al, "Use of Fluoroquinolones in Pediatrics: Consensus Report of an International Society of Chemotherapy Commission," *Pediatr Infect Dis J*, 1995, 14(1):1-9.

Ciprofloxacin and Dexamethasone

(sip roe FLOKS a sin & deks a METH a sone)

U.S. Brand Names Ciprodex®

Canadian Brand Names Ciprodex®

Index Terms Ciprofloxacin Hydrochloride and Dexamethasone; Dexamethasone and Ciprofloxacin

Therapeutic Category Antibiotic/Corticosteroid, Otic

Generic Available No

Use Treatment of acute otitis media in pediatric patients with tympanostomy tubes due to *S. aureus, S. pneumoniae, H. influenzae, M. catarrhalis*, or *P. aeruginosa*; acute otitis externa in children and adults due to *S. aureus* or *P. aeruginosa*

Pregnancy Risk Factor C

Lactation Excretion in breast milk unknown/not recommended

Contraindications Hypersensitivity to ciprofloxacin, other quinolones, dexamethasone, or any component; herpes simplex or other viral infections of the external ear canal

Warnings For otic use only; do not administer parenterally or ophthalmically

Adverse Reactions

Central nervous system: Irritability, dizziness
(Continued)

Ciprofloxacin and Dexamethasone *(Continued)*

Dermatologic: Rash
Gastrointestinal: Taste perversion
Otic: Ear discomfort (3%), ear pain (2.3%), ear precipitate (residue) (0.5%), tinnitus, ear pruritus and erythema

Stability Store at room temperature; avoid freezing; protect from light

Pharmacokinetics Time to peak serum concentration: 15 minutes to 2 hours post dose application

Usual Dosage Otic: Children ≥6 months and Adults: Acute otitis media in patients with tympanostomy tubes or acute otitis externa: Instill 4 drops into affected ear(s) twice daily for 7 days

Administration To avoid dizziness which may result from the instillation of a cold solution, warm bottle in hand for 1-2 minutes. Shake suspension well before using; avoid contamination of the tip of the bottle to fingers, ear, or any surfaces. Patient should lie with affected ear upward and maintain position for 60 seconds after suspension is instilled.

Acute otitis media with tympanostomy tubes: Instill drops then gently press the tragus 5 times in a pumping motion to allow the drops to pass through the tube into the middle ear.

Acute otitis externa: Gently pull the outer ear lobe upward and backward to allow the drops to flow down into the ear canal.

Patient Information Keep infected ear(s) clean and dry. Avoid swimming unless otherwise instructed by physician. Discontinue otic suspension and notify physician immediately if rash or an allergic reaction occurs.

Dosage Forms Excipient information presented when available (limited, particularly for generics); consult specific product labeling.

Suspension, otic: Ciprofloxacin 0.3% and dexamethasone 0.1% (7.5 mL) [contains benzalkonium chloride]

References

Roland PS, Dohar JE, Lanier BJ, et al, "Topical Ciprofloxacin/Dexamethasone Otic Suspension is Superior to Ofloxacin Otic Solution in the Treatment of Granulation Tissue in Children With Acute Otitis Media With Otorrhea Through Tympanostomy Tubes," *Otolaryngol Head Neck Surg*, 2004, 130(6):736-41.

Ciprofloxacin and Hydrocortisone

(sip roe FLOKS a sin & hye droe KOR ti sone)

Related Information

Ciprofloxacin *on page 357*
Hydrocortisone *on page 781*

U.S. Brand Names Cipro® HC

Canadian Brand Names Cipro® HC

Index Terms Ciprofloxacin Hydrochloride and Hydrocortisone; Hydrocortisone and Ciprofloxacin

Therapeutic Category Antibiotic/Corticosteroid, Otic

Generic Available No

Use Treatment of acute bacterial otitis externa due to susceptible strains of *S. aureus*, *P. aeruginosa*, or *Proteus mirabilis*

Pregnancy Risk Factor C

Contraindications Hypersensitivity to ciprofloxacin, hydrocortisone, any component, or other quinolones; patients with perforated tympanic membrane; patients with viral infections of the external ear canal

Adverse Reactions

Central nervous system: Headache
Dermatologic: Pruritus, fungal dermatitis, rash, urticaria, alopecia
Neuromuscular & skeletal: Paresthesia, hypoesthesia
Respiratory: Cough

Usual Dosage Children ≥1 year and Adults: Otic: Instill 3 drops into the affected ear(s) twice daily for 7 days

Administration Otic: Warm suspension by holding bottle in hand prior to instillation; shake well before use; patient should lie with affected ear upward and maintain position for 30-60 seconds after suspension is instilled into the ear canal

Dosage Forms Excipient information presented when available (limited, particularly for generics); consult specific product labeling.

Suspension, otic: Ciprofloxacin hydrochloride 0.2% and hydrocortisone 1% (10 mL) [contains benzyl alcohol]

♦ **Ciprofloxacin Hydrochloride** *see* Ciprofloxacin *on page 357*

♦ **Ciprofloxacin Hydrochloride and Dexamethasone** *see* Ciprofloxacin and Dexamethasone *on page 361*

- **Ciprofloxacin Hydrochloride and Hydrocortisone** *see* Ciprofloxacin and Hydrocortisone *on page 362*
- **Cipro® HC** *see* Ciprofloxacin and Hydrocortisone *on page 362*
- **Cipro® XR** *see* Ciprofloxacin *on page 357*

Cisapride *U.S. - Available Via Limited-Access Protocol Only* (SIS a pride)

Medication Safety Issues
Sound-alike/look-alike issues:
Propulsid® may be confused with propranolol

U.S. Brand Names Propulsid®

Therapeutic Category Gastrointestinal Agent, Prokinetic

Generic Available No

Use Treatment of nocturnal symptoms of gastroesophageal reflux disease (GERD), also demonstrated effectiveness for gastroparesis, refractory constipation, and nonulcer dyspepsia in patients failing other therapies (see Warnings)

Pregnancy Risk Factor C

Lactation Enters breast milk/use caution (AAP rates "compatible")

Contraindications Hypersensitivity to cisapride or any component; GI hemorrhage, mechanical obstruction, GI perforation, or other situations when GI motility stimulation is dangerous; patients with CHF, renal failure, multisystem organ failure, and COPD; patients at risk for developing or who have hypokalemia, hypocalcemia, or hypomagnesemia (eg, severe dehydration, vomiting, diarrhea, malnutrition, or receiving chronic diuretic therapy); patients with a known family history of congenital long-QT syndrome; prolonged QT intervals (QT_c >450), ventricular arrhythmias, ischemic heart disease, sinus node dysfunction, clinically significant bradycardia, and second or third degree AV block; patients receiving medications known to prolong the QT interval such as quinidine, procainamide, sotalol, amitriptyline (and other tricyclic antidepressants), maprotiline, phenothiazines, sertindole, astemizole, bepridil, or sparfloxacin, (see Warnings and Drug Interactions); serious cardiac arrhythmias including ventricular tachycardia, ventricular fibrillation, torsade de pointes, and QT prolongations have been reported in patients taking medications which inhibit cytochrome P450 3A4; some of these events have been fatal; do not coadminister with ketoconazole, itraconazole, fluconazole, miconazole, erythromycin, clarithromycin, nefazodone, delavirdine, indinavir, nelfinavir, ritonavir, saquinavir, or troleandomycin; do not coadminister with grapefruit juice

Warnings Serious cardiac arrhythmias including ventricular tachycardia, ventricular fibrillation, torsade de pointes, and QT prolongation have been reported in patients receiving cisapride; more than 270 cases have been reported including 70 fatalities; 85% of these cases occurred in patients with known risk factors (see Contraindications); for this reason, cisapride is available only for use in patients with severely debilitating conditions who meet specific criteria for a limited-access program directly through PRA International; for more information contact them at 877-795-4247

Precautions Use with caution in neonates, particularly if premature due to a potential increased risk of serious cardiac arrhythmias; decreased cisapride clearance found in neonates may result in increased serum levels; a 12-lead EKG (measuring QT intervals) should be done in all patients before beginning therapy

Adverse Reactions
Cardiovascular: Sinus tachycardia, QT interval prolongation, serious cardiac arrhythmias (see Warnings and Contraindications)
Central nervous system: Headache, insomnia, anxiety, nervousness, confusion
Dermatologic: Rash, pruritus
Endocrine & metabolic: Hypoglycemia with acidosis, hyperglycemia
Gastrointestinal: Diarrhea, abdominal pain, nausea, flatulence, dyspepsia, constipation, xerostomia
Genitourinary: Vaginitis (rare), urinary frequency
Hematologic: Thrombocytopenia, leukopenia, aplastic anemia, pancytopenia, hemolytic anemia, methemoglobinemia
Hepatic: Hepatitis, elevated liver enzymes
Neuromuscular & skeletal: Arthralgia, tremor
Respiratory: Rhinitis, sinusitis, cough, apnea
Miscellaneous: Positive ANA

Drug Interactions Cytochrome P450 isoenzyme CYP3A3/4 substrate
Decreased absorption of digoxin; decreased effect with atropine
Increased effect/toxicity of warfarin, diazepam (increased levels); increased bioavailability of cisapride with cimetidine and ranitidine use
Concomitant administration with ketoconazole has resulted in markedly elevated cisapride plasma concentrations and prolonged QT intervals on the EKG. These

(Continued)

Cisapride *U.S. - Available Via Limited-Access Protocol Only (Continued)*

prolonged intervals have rarely been associated with serious ventricular arrhythmias and torsade de pointes; some of these adverse reactions have been fatal. Since the interaction is due to a decrease in cytochrome P450 metabolism induced by ketoconazole, it is expected that similar reactions would occur with itraconazole, miconazole, fluconazole, troleandomycin, delavirdine, indinavir, erythromycin, clarithromycin, nefazodone, nelfinavir, amprenavir, ritonavir, and saquinavir; see Contraindications and Food Interactions

Food Interactions Do not use grapefruit juice which increases cisapride bioavailability

Mechanism of Action A GI prokinetic agent which enhances the release of acetylcholine at the myenteric plexus. *In vitro* studies have shown cisapride to have serotonin-4 receptor agonistic properties; it has no dopamine receptor blocking activity and, therefore, no extrapyramidal side effects or central antiemetic activity. It increases lower esophageal sphincter pressure, increases the amplitude of peristalsis, accelerates gastric emptying, improves antroduodenal coordination, increases colonic motility, and enhances cecal and ascending colonic emptying.

Pharmacodynamics Onset of action: 0.5-1 hour

Pharmacokinetics

Distribution: Breast milk to plasma ratio: 0.045

Protein binding: 98%

Metabolism: Extensive in liver via cytochrome P450 isoenzyme CYP 3A3/4 to norcisapride, which is eliminated in urine and feces

Bioavailability: 40% to 50%

Half-life: 7-10 hours

Elimination: <10% of dose excreted into feces and urine

Usual Dosage Oral:

Neonates: 0.15-0.2 mg/kg/dose 3-4 times/day; maximum dose: 0.8 mg/kg/day

Infants and Children: 0.15-0.3 mg/kg/dose 3-4 times/day; maximum dose: 10 mg/dose

Adults: Initial: 10 mg 4 times/day at least 15 minutes before meals and at bedtime; in some patients the dosage will need to be increased to 20 mg to obtain a satisfactory result

Dosage adjustment in liver dysfunction: Reduce daily dosage by 50%

Administration Oral: Administer 15 minutes before meals or feeding

Monitoring Parameters EKG (prior to beginning therapy), serum electrolytes in patients on diuretic therapy (prior to beginning therapy and periodically thereafter); see Contraindications

Patient Information May cause dry mouth.

References

Cucchiara S, Staiano A, Boccieri A, et al, "Effects of Cisapride on Parameters of Oesophageal Motility and on the Prolonged Intraoesophageal pH Test in Infants With Gastro-Oesophageal Reflux Disease," *Gut*, 1990, 31(1):21-5.

Hill SL, Evangelista KJ, Pizzi AM, et al, "Proarrhythmia Associated With Cisapride in Children," *Pediatrics*, 1998, 101(6):1053-6.

Khongphatthanayothin A, Lane J, Thomas D, et al, "Effects of Cisapride on QT Interval in Children," *J Pediatr*, 1998, 133(1):51-6.

Lander A, "The Risks and Benefits of Cisapride in Premature Neonates, Infants and Children," *Arch Dis Child*, 1998, 79:469-71.

Lewin MB, Bryant RM, Fenrich AL, et al, "Cisapride-Induced QT Interval," *J Pediatr*, 1996, 128(2):279-81.

Tolia V, "Long-Term Use of Cisapride in Premature Neonates of <34 Weeks Gestational Age," *J Pediatr Gastroenterol Nutr*, 1990, 11:420-2.

Van Eygen M and Van Ravensteyn H, "Effect of Cisapride on Excessive Regurgitation in Infants," *Clin Ther*, 1989, 11(5):669-77.

Cisatracurium (sis a tra KYOO ree um)

Medication Safety Issues

Sound-alike/look-alike issues:

Nimbex® may be confused with Revex®

High alert medication: The Institute for Safe Medication Practices (ISMP) includes this medication among its list of drugs which have a heightened risk of causing significant patient harm when used in error.

U.S. Brand Names Nimbex®

Canadian Brand Names Nimbex®

Index Terms Cisatracurium Besylate

Therapeutic Category Neuromuscular Blocker Agent, Nondepolarizing; Skeletal Muscle Relaxant, Paralytic

Generic Available No

Use Eases endotracheal intubation as an adjunct to general anesthesia and relaxes skeletal muscle during surgery or mechanical ventilation

Pregnancy Risk Factor B

Lactation Excretion in breast milk unknown/use caution

Contraindications Hypersensitivity to cisatracurium or any component (see Warnings)

Warnings Maintenance of an adequate airway and respiratory support is critical. Due to its intermediate onset of action, cisatracurium is not recommended for rapid sequence intubation; certain clinical conditions may result in potentiation or antagonism of neuromuscular blockade, see table on next page.

10 mL multiple use vials contain benzyl alcohol as a preservative; benzyl alcohol may cause allergic reactions in susceptible individuals; large amounts of benzyl alcohol (≥99 mg/kg/day) have been associated with a potentially fatal toxicity ("gasping syndrome") in neonates; the "gasping syndrome" consists of metabolic acidosis, respiratory distress, gasping respirations, CNS dysfunction (including convulsions, intracranial hemorrhage), hypotension and cardiovascular collapse; avoid use of vials containing benzyl alcohol in neonates; *in vitro* and animal studies have shown that benzoate, a metabolite of benzyl alcohol, displaces bilirubin from protein-binding sites

Increased sensitivity in patients with myasthenia gravis, Eaton-Lambert syndrome, resistance to neuromuscular blockade in burn patients (>30% of body) for period of 5-70 days postinjury; resistance to neuromuscular blockade in patients with muscle trauma, denervation, immobilization, infection

Precautions Certain clinical conditions may result in potentiation or antagonism of neuromuscular blockade, see table on next page.

Adverse Reactions

Cardiovascular: Rarely mild histamine release, cardiovascular effects are minimal and transient

Dermatologic: Rash, pruritus

Respiratory: Wheezing, bronchospasm, laryngospasm (rare)

Miscellaneous: Hypersensitivity reactions including anaphylaxis

Drug Interactions See table below.

Stability Protect from light; refrigerate; once removed from refrigerator, stable 21 days even if re-refrigerated; unstable in alkaline solutions; **compatible** with D_5W, D_5NS, and NS; do not dilute in LR; **incompatible** for Y-site administration with propofol or ketorolac; **compatible** for Y-site administration with sufentanil, alfentanil, fentanyl, midazolam, and droperidol.

Potential Drug Interactions

Potentiation	Antagonism
Inhalation anesthetics	Calcium
Desflurane, sevoflurane, enflurane and isoflurane > halothane > nitrous oxide	Carbamazepine
	Phenytoin
	Steroids (chronic administration)
Antibiotics	Theophylline
Aminoglycosides, polymyxins, clindamycin, vancomycin, tetracycline	Anticholinesterases[1]
	Neostigmine, pyridostigmine, edrophonium, echothiophate ophthalmic solution
Magnesium	
Antiarrhythmics	
Quinidine, procainamide, bretylium, and possibly lidocaine	Caffeine
	Azathioprine
Diuretics	
Furosemide, mannitol, thiazides	
Amphotericin B (secondary to hypokalemia)	
Local anesthetics	
Dantrolene (directly depresses skeletal muscle)	
Beta blockers	
Calcium channel blockers	
Ketamine	
Lithium	
Succinylcholine (when administered prior to nondepolarizing neuromuscular-blocking agent)	
Cyclosporine	

[1]Can prolong the effects of acetylcholine

(Continued)

Cisatracurium *(Continued)*

Clinical Conditions Affecting Neuromuscular Blockade

Potentiation	Antagonism
Electrolyte abnormalities	Alkalosis
Severe hyponatremia	Hypercalcemia
Severe hypocalcemia	Demyelinating lesions
Severe hypokalemia	Peripheral neuropathies
Hypermagnesemia	Diabetes mellitus
Neuromuscular diseases	
Acidosis	
Acute intermittent porphyria	
Renal failure	
Hepatic failure	

Mechanism of Action Blocks neural transmission at the myoneural junction by binding with cholinergic receptor sites

Pharmacodynamics

Onset of action: I.V.: Within 2-3 minutes

Maximum effect: Within 3-5 minutes

Duration: Dose dependent, 35-45 minutes after a single 0.1 mg/kg dose; recovery begins in 20-35 minutes when anesthesia is balanced; recovery is attained in 90% of patients in 25-93 minutes

Pharmacokinetics

Distribution: V_d: Adults: 0.16 L/kg

Metabolism: Some metabolites are active; 80% of drug clearance is via a rapid nonenzymatic degradation (Hofmann elimination) in the bloodstream; additional metabolism occurs via ester hydrolysis

Half-life: 22-31 minutes

Elimination: <10% of dose excreted as unchanged drug in urine

Clearance:

Children: 5.9 mL/kg/minute

Adults: 5.1 mL/kg/minute

Usual Dosage I.V.:

Children 2-12 years: Initial: 0.1 mg/kg followed by maintenance dose of 0.03 mg/kg as needed to maintain neuromuscular blockade

Children >12 years to Adults: Initial: 0.15-0.2 mg/kg followed by maintenance dose of 0.03 mg/kg 40-65 minutes later or as needed to maintain neuromuscular blockade

Continuous infusion:

Children ≥2 years: 1-4 mcg/kg/minute

Adults: 1-3 mcg/kg/minute

Note: There may be wide interpatient variability in dosage (range 0.5-10 mcg/kg/minute in adults) which may increase and decrease over time; optimize patient dosage by utilizing a peripheral nerve stimulator

Administration Parenteral: May be administered without further dilution by rapid I.V. injection over 5-10 seconds; for continuous infusions, dilute to a concentration of 0.1-0.4 mg/mL in D_5W or NS; not for I.M. injection due to tissue irritation

Monitoring Parameters Muscle twitch response to peripheral nerve stimulation, heart rate, blood pressure

Additional Information Neuromuscular blocking potency is 3 times that of atracurium; maximum block is up to 2 minutes longer than for equipotent doses of atracurium; laudanosine, a metabolite without neuromuscular blocking activity has been associated with hypotension and seizure activity in animal studies.

Dosage Forms Excipient information presented when available (limited, particularly for generics); consult specific product labeling.

Injection, solution: 2 mg/mL (5 mL); 10 mg/mL (20 mL)

Injection, solution: 2 mg/mL (10 mL) [contains benzyl alcohol]

References

Martin LD, Bratton SL, and O'Rourke PP, "Clinical Uses and Controversies of Neuromuscular Blocking Agents in Infants and Children," *Crit Care Med*, 1999, 27(7):1358-68.

♦ **Cisatracurium Besylate** *see* Cisatracurium *on page 364*

Cisplatin (SIS pla tin)

Medication Safety Issues

Sound-alike/look-alike issues:

Cisplatin may be confused with carboplatin

Platinol®-AQ may be confused with Paraplatin®, Patanol®, Plaquenil®

High alert medication: The Institute for Safe Medication Practices (ISMP) includes this medication among its list of drugs which have a heightened risk of causing significant patient harm when used in error.

Doses >100 mg/m^2 once every 3-4 weeks are rarely used and should be verified with the prescriber.

Related Information

Compatibility of Chemotherapy and Related Supportive Care Medications *on page 1777*
Emetogenic Potential of Single Chemotherapeutic Agents *on page 1776*
Extravasation Treatment *on page 1726*

U.S. Brand Names Platinol®-AQ [DSC]

Index Terms CDDP

Therapeutic Category Antineoplastic Agent, Alkylating Agent

Generic Available Yes

Use Treatment of testicular, ovarian, and breast cancer; advanced bladder cancer, osteosarcoma, Hodgkin's and non-Hodgkin's lymphoma, head or neck cancer, cervical cancer, lung cancer, brain tumors, neuroblastoma; used alone or in combination with other agents

Pregnancy Risk Factor D

Lactation Enters breast milk/contraindicated

Contraindications Hypersensitivity to cisplatin, platinum-containing agents, or any component; pre-existing renal impairment, hearing impairment, and myelosuppression; pregnancy

Warnings The FDA currently recommends that procedures for proper handling and disposal of antineoplastic agents be considered. Cumulative renal toxicity may be severe; dose-related toxicities include myelosuppression, nausea and vomiting; ototoxicity, especially pronounced in children, is manifested by tinnitus or loss of high frequency hearing and occasionally, deafness

Precautions All patients should receive adequate hydration prior to and for 24 hours after cisplatin administration with a sodium chloride-containing I.V. solution to promote chloruresis, with or without mannitol and/or furosemide, to ensure good urine output and decrease the chance of nephrotoxicity; reduce dosage in renal impairment and in infants <6 months of age due to their decreased renal function and renal tubular secretion; serum magnesium, as well as electrolytes, should be monitored before and within 48 hours after cisplatin therapy. Patients who are magnesium-depleted should receive replacement therapy before the start of cisplatin.

Adverse Reactions

Cardiovascular: Bradycardia, arrhythmias, Raynaud's phenomenon

Central nervous system: Seizures, encephalopathy

Dermatologic: Mild alopecia

Endocrine & metabolic: Hypomagnesemia, hypocalcemia, hypokalemia, hypophosphatemia, hyperuricemia

Gastrointestinal: Nausea and vomiting occur in 76% to 100% of patients and is dose-related

Hematologic: Myelosuppression

Hepatic: Elevated liver enzymes

Local: Phlebitis, tissue sloughing and necrosis if infiltrated

Neuromuscular & skeletal: Peripheral neuropathy (related to cumulative doses >200 mg/m^2)

Ocular: Papilledema, optic neuritis

Otic: Ototoxicity (especially pronounced in children; hearing loss in the high-frequency range is related to a cumulative dose of cisplatin >400 mg/m^2)

Renal: Nephrotoxicity (damage to the proximal tubules), azotemia, elevated BUN and serum creatinine

Miscellaneous: Anaphylactoid reactions (bronchoconstriction, tachycardia, hypotension, facial edema)

Drug Interactions Aminoglycosides, amphotericin B, and other nephrotoxic drugs (increase risk of nephrotoxicity); loop diuretics, aminoglycosides (potentiate ototoxicity); synergistic antineoplastic activity with cytarabine, 5-fluorouracil, etoposide; reduces renal elimination of methotrexate

Stability Reconstituted powder for injection is stable for 20 hours at room temperature; do not refrigerate reconstituted solution since precipitation may occur; protect from light; incompatible with sodium bicarbonate; do not infuse in solutions containing <0.2% sodium chloride; stable when combined with mannitol (12.5-50 g mannitol/L)

Mechanism of Action Platination of DNA leads to reactive intermediates that bind to DNA and form intrastrand and interstrand DNA cross-links

(Continued)

Cisplatin *(Continued)*

Pharmacokinetics

Distribution: I.V.: Rapid tissue distribution; CSF unbound platinum concentration: 40% of the plasma concentration

Protein binding: >90%; only the free (unbound) platinum and parent drug are cytotoxic

Metabolism: Undergoes nonenzymatic metabolism

Half-life, terminal: Children:

Free drug: 1.3 hours

Total platinum: 44 hours

Elimination: ~50% of dose excreted in urine within 5 days in an inactive form

Dialysis: Minimally removed by hemodialysis

Usual Dosage Children and Adults: I.V. (refer to individual protocols): **TO PREVENT POSSIBLE OVERDOSE, VERIFY ANY CISPLATIN DOSE EXCEEDING 120 mg/m² PER COURSE**:

Intermittent dosing schedule: 37-75 mg/m² once every 2-3 weeks or 50-100 mg/m² over 4-6 hours, once every 21-28 days

Daily dosing schedule: 15-20 mg/m²/day for 5 days every 3-4 weeks

Osteogenic sarcoma or neuroblastoma: 60-100 mg/m² on day 1 every 3-4 weeks

Recurrent brain tumors: 60 mg/m² once daily for 2 consecutive days every 3-4 weeks

Bone marrow/blood cell transplantation: Continuous infusion: High dose: 55 mg/m²/day for 72 hours; total dose = 165 mg/m²

Dosing adjustment in renal impairment:

Cl_{cr} 10-50 mL/minute: Administer 75% of dose

Cl_{cr} <10 mL/minute: Administer 50% of dose

Administration Parenteral: I.V.: Administer according to protocol; rate of administration has varied from a 15- to 20-minute infusion, 1 mg/minute infusion, 6- to 8-hour infusion or 24-hour infusion; rapid I.V. injection may be associated with increased nephrotoxicity or ototoxicity compared to a slower I.V. infusion

Monitoring Parameters Renal function tests (serum creatinine, BUN, Cl_{cr}), electrolytes (particularly magnesium, calcium, potassium), hearing test, neurologic exam (with high dose), liver function tests periodically, CBC with differential and platelet count, urine output, urinalysis

Nursing Implications Needles, syringes, catheters, or I.V. administration sets that contain aluminum parts should not be used for administration of drug; methods to prevent nephrotoxicity include prehydration, diuresis with mannitol, and administration of sodium chloride containing I.V. solutions to promote chloruresis. Adequate hydration and urinary output should be maintained for 24 hours after administration. Extravasation may cause tissue sloughing and necrosis; care should be taken to avoid extravasation. Infiltration of cisplatin infusions with concentrations >0.5 mg/mL may result in a more severe tissue toxicity.

Additional Information Myelosuppressive effects:

WBC: Mild

Platelets: Mild

Onset (days): 10

Nadir (days): 18-23

Recovery (days): 21-40

Dosage Forms Excipient information presented when available (limited, particularly for generics); consult specific product labeling. [DSC] = Discontinued product

Injection, solution: 1 mg/mL (50 mL, 100 mL, 200 mL)

Platinol®-AQ: 1 mg/mL (50 mL, 100 mL) [contains sodium 9 mg/mL] [DSC]

References

Costello MA, Dominick C, and Clerico A, "A Pilot Study of 5-Day Continuous Infusion of High-Dose Cisplatin and Pulsed Etoposide in Childhood Solid Tumors," *Am J Pediatr Hematol Oncol*, 1988, 10:103-8.

Reece PA, Stafford I, Abbott RL, et al, "Two-Versus 24-Hour Infusion of Cisplatin: Pharmacokinetic Considerations," *J Clin Oncol*, 1989, 7(2):270-5.

♦ **13-*cis*-Retinoic Acid** *see* Isotretinoin *on page 876*

Citalopram (sye TAL oh pram)

Medication Safety Issues

Sound-alike/look-alike issues:

Celexa® may be confused with Celebrex®, Cerebra®, Cerebyx®, Ranexa™, Zyprexa®

Related Information

Antidepressant Agents *on page 1681*

U.S. Brand Names Celexa®

Canadian Brand Names Apo-Citalopram®; Celexa®; CO Citalopram; Dom-Citalopram; Gen-Citalopram; Novo-Citalopram; PHL-Citalopram;

PMS-Citalopram; RAN™-Citalopram; ratio-Citalopram; Rhoxal-citalopram; Sandoz-Citalopram

Index Terms Citalopram Hydrobromide; Nitalapram

Therapeutic Category Antidepressant, Selective Serotonin Reuptake Inhibitor (SSRI)

Generic Available Yes

Use Treatment of depression; obsessive-compulsive disorder (OCD) in children

Medication Guide An FDA-approved patient medication guide, which is available with the product information and at http://www.fda.gov/cder/Offices/ODS/medication_guides.htm, must be dispensed with this medication for each new outpatient prescription and refill.

Pregnancy Risk Factor C

Lactation Enters breast milk/not recommended

Contraindications Hypersensitivity to citalopram or any component; use with MAO inhibitors within 14 days (potentially fatal reactions may occur, see Drug Interactions); concurrent use of pimozide

Warnings Citalopram is not approved for use in pediatric patients. Clinical worsening of depression or suicidal ideation and behavior may occur in children and adults with major depressive disorder. In clinical trials, antidepressants increased the risk of suicidal thinking and behavior (suicidality) in children, adolescents, and young adults (18-24 years of age) with major depressive disorder and other psychiatric disorders. This risk must be considered before prescribing antidepressants for any clinical use. Short-term studies did **not** show an increased risk of suicidality with antidepressant use in patients >24 years of age and showed a decreased risk in patients ≥65 years.

Patients of all ages who are treated with antidepressants for any indication require appropriate monitoring and close observation for clinical worsening of depression, suicidality, and unusual changes in behavior, especially during the first few months after antidepressant initiation or when the dose is adjusted. Family members and caregivers should be instructed to closely observe the patient (ie, daily) and communicate condition with healthcare provider. Patients should also be monitored for associated behaviors (eg, anxiety, agitation, panic attacks, insomnia, irritability, hostility, aggressiveness, impulsivity, akathisia, hypomania, mania) which may increase the risk for worsening depression or suicidality. Worsening depression or emergence of suicidality (or associated behaviors listed above) that is abrupt in onset, severe, or not part of the presenting symptoms, may require discontinuation or modification of drug therapy.

Avoid abrupt discontinuation; withdrawal syndrome with discontinuation symptoms (including agitation, dysphoria, anxiety, confusion, dizziness, hypomania, nightmares, irritability, sensory disturbances, headache, lethargy, emotional lability, insomnia, tinnitus, and seizures) may occur if therapy is abruptly discontinued or dose reduced; taper the dose to minimize risks of discontinuation symptoms. If intolerable symptoms occur following a decrease in dosage or upon discontinuation of therapy, consider resuming the previous dose with a more gradual taper. To reduce risk of intentional overdose, write prescriptions for the smallest quantity consistent with good patient care.

May worsen psychosis in some patients or precipitate a shift to mania or hypomania in patients with bipolar disorder. Monotherapy in patients with bipolar disorder should be avoided. Patients presenting with depressive symptoms should be screened for bipolar disorder. Citalopram is not FDA approved for the treatment of bipolar depression.

Potentially fatal serotonin syndrome may occur when SSRIs are used in combination with serotonergic drugs (eg, triptans) or drugs that impair the metabolism of serotonin (eg, MAO inhibitors); see Drug Interactions

Precautions Citalopram may cause abnormal bleeding (eg, ecchymosis, purpura, upper GI bleeding); use with caution in patients with impaired platelet aggregation and with concurrent use of aspirin, NSAIDs, or other drugs that affect coagulation. May impair cognitive or motor performance. Use with caution in patients with seizure disorders, concomitant illnesses that may effect hepatic metabolism or hemodynamic responses (eg, unstable cardiac disease, recent MI), and in suicidal patients; use with caution and decrease dose in patients with hepatic dysfunction; use with caution in patients with severe renal impairment.

Use with caution during third trimester of pregnancy [newborns may experience adverse effects or withdrawal symptoms (consider risk and benefits), see Additional Information; exposure to SSRIs late in pregnancy may also be associated with an increased risk for persistent pulmonary hypertension of the newborn (see Chambers, 2006)]; high doses of citalopram have been associated with teratogenicity in animals. Use with caution in patients receiving diuretics or those who are volume depleted (may cause hyponatremia or SIADH). No clinical studies have assessed the

(Continued)

Citalopram *(Continued)*

combined use of citalopram and electroconvulsive therapy; however, use with caution in patients receiving electroconvulsive therapy; may increase the risks associated with electroconvulsive therapy, consider discontinuing, when possible, prior to electroconvulsive therapy treatment.

Adverse Reactions Predominant adverse effects are CNS and GI.

Central nervous system: Somnolence, dizziness, insomnia, anxiety, anorexia, agitation, yawning, apathy, fatigue, fever; suicidal thinking and behavior (see Warnings)

Note: SSRI-associated behavioral activation (ie, restlessness, hyperkinesis, hyperactivity, agitation) is 2- to 3-fold more prevalent in children compared to adolescents; it is more prevalent in adolescents compared to adults. Somnolence (including sedation and drowsiness) is more common in adults compared to children and adolescents (see Safer, 2006).

Dermatologic: Rash, pruritus

Endocrine & metabolic: Hyponatremia, SIADH (usually in volume-depleted patients); sexual dysfunction

Gastrointestinal: Nausea, xerostomia, diarrhea, dyspepsia, vomiting, abdominal pain, weight loss

Note: SSRI-associated vomiting is 2- to 3-fold more prevalent in children compared to adolescents; it is more prevalent in adolescents compared to adults.

Hematologic: Altered platelet function (rare), increased bleeding, bruising

Neuromuscular & skeletal: Tremor, arthralgia, myalgia, asthenia

Respiratory: Cough, rhinitis, sinusitis

Miscellaneous: Diaphoresis; withdrawal symptoms following abrupt discontinuation (see Warnings)

Drug Interactions Cytochrome P450 isoenzyme CYP2C19 (major), 2D6 (minor), 3A4 (major) substrate; CYP1A2 (weak), 2B6 (weak), 2C19 (weak), 2D6 (weak) inhibitor

With MAO inhibitors, fever, tremors, seizures, delirium, coma may occur (use of MAO inhibitors within 14 days of citalopram use is contraindicated). Tryptophan (which can be metabolized to serotonin) and the herbal medicine St John's wort (*Hypericum perforatum*) may increase serious side effects (the use of these agents is not recommended). Concurrent selegiline has been associated with mania, hypertension, and serotonin syndrome.

Combined use of SSRIs and amphetamine, buspirone, meperidine, nefazodone, serotonin agonists, sibutramine, other SSRIs, sympathomimetics, ritonavir, linezolid, lithium, tramadol, and venlafaxine may increase the risk of serotonin syndrome. Use of SSRIs with sumatriptan may cause weakness, incoordination, hyper-reflexia and an increased risk of serotonin syndrome; use triptans with caution in patients receiving SSRIs; monitor carefully, especially during initiation of treatment and dosage increases.

Risk of hyponatremia may increase with concurrent use of loop diuretics. Citalopram may increase the hypoprothrombinemic response to warfarin. Concomitant use of citalopram with NSAIDs, aspirin, or other drugs affecting coagulation has been associated with an increased risk of bleeding. Alcohol and other CNS depressants may increase CNS adverse effects.

Citalopram increased metoprolol serum concentrations by two-fold (effects on blood pressure and heart rate were not clinically significant). Cimetidine increases citalopram AUC by 43% and peak serum concentrations by 39% (clinical significance unknown). Cytochrome P450 isoenzyme CYP2C19 and CYP3A4 inducers may decrease the levels/effects of citalopram (**Note:** Ketoconazole did not significantly affect citalopram pharmacokinetics)

Food Interactions Absorption is not affected by food.

Tryptophan supplements may increase serious side effects; its use is **not recommended**

Stability Store at 25°C (77°F); excursions permitted to 15°C to 30°C (59°F to 86°F).

Mechanism of Action A bicyclic phthalane derivative, citalopram selectively inhibits serotonin reuptake in the presynaptic neurons; minimal or no effect on reuptake of norepinephrine or dopamine; does not significantly bind to alpha-adrenergic, histamine or cholinergic receptors; may therefore be useful in patients at risk from sedation, hypotension, and anticholinergic effects of tricyclic antidepressants. Citalopram is a racemic mixture; activity is primarily due to S enantiomer.

Pharmacodynamics

Onset of action: 1-2 weeks

Maximum effect: 8-12 weeks

Duration: 1-2 days

Pharmacokinetics

Distribution: V_d: Adults: 12 L/kg

Protein binding, plasma: ~80%

Metabolism: Extensively hepatic, primarily via CYP3A4 and CYP2C19; metabolized to N-demethylated, N-oxide, and deaminated metabolites

Bioavailability: 80%; tablets and oral solution are bioequivalent

Half-life elimination: Adults: Range: 24-48 hours; mean: 35 hours (doubled with hepatic impairment)

Time to peak serum concentration: 1 to 6 hours, average within 4 hours

Elimination: Urine (10% as unchanged drug)

Clearance: Hepatic impairment: Decreased by 37%; Mild to moderate renal impairment: Decreased by 17%; Severe renal impairment (Cl_{cr} <20 mL/minute): No information available

Usual Dosage

Children and Adolescents: **Note:** Slower titration of dose every 2-4 weeks may minimize risk of SSRI associated behavioral activation, which has been shown to increase risk of suicidal behavior.

Depression: **Note:** Not FDA approved; see Warnings. Limited information is available; only one randomized, placebo controlled trial has shown citalopram to be effective for the treatment of depression in pediatric patients (see Wagner, 2004); other controlled unpublished pediatric trials have **not** shown benefit (see Sharp, 2006 and Wagner, 2005). Some experts recommend the following doses (see Dopheide, 2006):

Children ≤11 years: Initial: 10 mg/day given once daily; increase dose slowly by 5 mg/day every 2 weeks as clinically needed; dosage range: 20-60 mg/day

Children and Adolescents ≥12 years: Initial: 20 mg/day given once daily; increase dose slowly by 10 mg/day every 2 weeks as clinically needed; dosage range: 20"60 mg/day

Obsessive-compulsive disorder: **Note:** Not FDA approved; see Warnings. Limited information is available; several open label trials have been published (see Thomsen, 1997; Thomsen, 2001; Mukaddes, 2003). Some experts recommend the following doses:

Children ≤11 years: Initial: 5-10 mg/day given once daily; increase dose slowly by 5 mg/day every 2 weeks as clinically needed; dosage range: 10-40 mg/day.

Children and Adolescents ≥12 years: Initial: 10-20 mg/day given once daily; increase dose slowly by 10 mg/day every 2 weeks as clinically needed; dosage range: 10-40 mg/day.

Note: Higher mg/kg doses are needed in children compared to adolescents.

Adults: Depression: Initial: 20 mg/day given once daily; may increase daily dose in 20 mg increments at intervals of ≥1 week; usual dose: 40 mg/day; doses >40 mg are not usually necessary and may not increase effectiveness; maximum dose: 60 mg/day

Dosage adjustment in hepatic impairment: Initial: 20 mg/day; usual dose: 20 mg/day; in nonresponsive patients, may titrate to maximum dose of 40 mg/day

Dosage adjustment in renal impairment: Mild or moderate renal impairment: No dosage adjustment needed; Severe renal impairment: Use with caution

Administration May be administered without regard to meals

Monitoring Parameters Monitor patient periodically for symptom resolution; monitor for worsening depression, suicidality, and associated behaviors (especially at the beginning of therapy or when doses are increased or decreased; see Warnings). Monitor for anxiety, social functioning, mania, panic attacks; akathisia

Patient Information Read the patient Medication Guide that you receive with each prescription and refill of citalopram. An increased risk of suicidal thinking and behavior has been reported with the use of antidepressants in children, adolescents, and young adults (18-24 years of age). Notify physician if you feel more depressed, have thoughts of suicide, or become more agitated or irritable (see Warnings). Avoid alcohol, caffeine, CNS stimulants, tryptophan supplements, and the herbal medicine St John's wort; avoid aspirin, NSAIDs, or other drugs that affect coagulation (may increase risks of bleeding); may cause dizziness or drowsiness and impair ability to perform activities requiring mental alertness or physical coordination; may cause dry mouth. Some medicines should not be taken with citalopram or should not be taken for a while after citalopram has been discontinued; report the use of other medications, nonprescription medications, and herbal or natural products to your physician and pharmacist. It may take up to 4 weeks to see therapeutic effects from this medication. Take as directed; do not alter dose or frequency without consulting prescriber; avoid abrupt discontinuation.

Nursing Implications Assess other medications patient may be taking for possible interaction (especially MAO inhibitors, P450 inhibitors, and other CNS active agents). Assess mental status for depression, suicidal ideation, anxiety, social functioning, mania, or panic attack.

Additional Information If used for an extended period of time, long-term usefulness of citalopram should be periodically re-evaluated for the individual patient. A recent report describes 5 children (age: 8-15 years) who developed epistaxis (n=4) or bruising (n=1) while receiving SSRI therapy (sertraline) (Lake, 2000).

(Continued)

Citalopram *(Continued)*

Neonates born to women receiving SSRIs later during the third trimester may experience respiratory distress, apnea, cyanosis, temperature instability, vomiting, feeding difficulty, hypoglycemia, constant crying, irritability, hypotonia, hypertonia, hyper-reflexia, tremor, jitteriness, and seizures; these symptoms may be due to a direct toxic effect, withdrawal syndrome, or (in some cases) serotonin syndrome. Withdrawal symptoms occur in 30% of neonates exposed to SSRIs *in utero*; monitor newborns for at least 48 hours after birth; long-term effects of *in utero* exposure to SSRIs are unknown (see Levinson-Castiel, 2006).

Dosage Forms Excipient information presented when available (limited, particularly for generics); consult specific product labeling.

Solution, oral: 10 mg/5 mL (240 mL)

Celexa®: 10 mg/5 mL (240 mL) [alcohol free, sugar free; peppermint flavor]

Tablet: 10 mg, 20 mg, 40 mg

Celexa®: 10 mg, 20 mg, 40 mg

References

Bernard L, Stern R, Lew D, et al, "Serotonin Syndrome After Concomitant Treatment With Linezolid and Citalopram," *Clin Infect Dis*, 2003, 36(9):1197.

Chambers CD, Hernandez-Diaz S, Van Marter LJ, et al, "Selective Serotonin-Reuptake Inhibitors and Risk of Persistent Pulmonary Hypertension of the Newborn," *N Engl J Med*, 2006, 354(6):579-87.

Dopheide JA, "Recognizing and Treating Depression in Children and Adolescents," *Am J Health Syst Pharm*, 2006, 63(3):233-43.

Lake MB, Birmaher B, Wassick S, et al, "Bleeding and Selective Serotonin Reuptake Inhibitors in Childhood and Adolescence," *J Child Adolesc Psychopharmacol*, 2000, 10(1):35-8.

Levinson-Castiel R, Merlob P, Linder N, et al, "Neonatal Abstinence Syndrome After *in utero* Exposure to Selective Serotonin Reuptake Inhibitors in Term Infants," *Arch Pediatr Adolesc Med*, 2006, 160(2):173-6.

Mahlberg R, Kunz D, Sasse J, et al, "Serotonin Syndrome With Tramadol and Citalopram," *Am J Psychiatry*, 2004, 161(6):1129.

Mukaddes NM, Abali O, and Kaynak N, "Citalopram Treatment of Children and Adolescents With Obsessive-Compulsive Disorder: A Preliminary Report," *Psychiatry Clin Neurosci*, 2003, 57(4):405-8

Pass SE and Simpson RW, "Discontinuation and Reinstitution of Medications During the Perioperative Period," *Am J Health Syst Pharm*, 2004, 61(9):899-912.

Reinblatt SP and Riddle MA, "Selective Serotonin Reuptake Inhibitors-Induced Apathy: A Pediatric Case Series," *J Child Adolesc Psychopharmacol*, 2006, 6(1/2):227-33.

Safer DJ and Zito JM, "Treatment Emergent Adverse Effects of Selective Serotonin Reuptake Inhibitors by Age Group: Children vs. Adolescents," *J Child Adolesc Psychopharmacol*, 2006, 16(1/2):159-69.

Sharp SC and Hellings JA, "Efficacy and Safety of Selective Serotonin Reuptake Inhibitors in the Treatment of Depression in Children and Adolescents: Practitioner Review," *Clin Drug Investig*, 2006, 26(5):247-55.

Tahir N, "Serotonin Syndrome as a Consequence of Drug-Resistant Infections: An Interaction Between Linezolid and Citalopram," *J Am Med Dir Assoc*, 2004, 5(2):111-3.

Thomsen PH, "Child and Adolescent Obsessive-Compulsive Disorder Treated With Citalopram: Findings From an Open Trial of 23 Cases," *J Child Adolesc Psychopharmacol*, 1997, 7(3):157-66.

Thomsen PH, Ebbesen C, and Persson C, "Long-Term Experience With Citalopram in the Treatment of Adolescent OCD," *J Am Acad Child Adolesc Psychiatry*, 2001, 40(8):895-902.

Wagner KD, "Pharmacotherapy for Major Depression in Children and Adolescents," *Prog Neuropsychopharmacol Biol Psychiatry*, 2005, 29(5):819-26.

Wagner KD, Robb AS, Findling RL, et al, "A Randomized, Placebo-Controlled Trial of Citalopram for the Treatment of Major Depression in Children and Adolescents," *Am J Psych*, 2004, 161(6):1079-83.

♦ **Citalopram Hydrobromide** *see* Citalopram *on page 368*

♦ **Citracal® [OTC]** *see* Calcium Citrate *on page 267*

♦ **Citracal® [OTC]** *see* Calcium Supplements *on page 272*

Citrate and Citric Acid (SIT rate & SIT rik AS id)

Index Terms Shohl's Solution, Modified

Therapeutic Category Alkalinizing Agent, Oral

Use Treatment of metabolic acidosis; alkalinizing agent in conditions where long-term maintenance of an alkaline urine is desirable

Potassium citrate: Prevention of uric acid nephrolithiasis, prevention of calcium renal stones in patients with hypocitraturia; urinary alkalizer when sodium citrate is contraindicated

Pregnancy Risk Factor C

Contraindications Hypersensitivity to citrate, citric acid, or any component; patients receiving sodium-restricted diet (sodium salts); severe renal impairment with oliguria, azotemia, or anuria; untreated Addison's disease, acute dehydration, heat cramps, severe myocardial damage, hyperkalemia (potassium salts); Urocit®-K (wax matrix tablet) is contraindicated in patients with delayed gastric emptying, intestinal obstruction, or stricture, patients receiving anticholinergic medications and in patients with peptic ulcer disease

Warnings Conversion to bicarbonate may be impaired in patients with hepatic failure, in shock, or who are severely ill. Some products contain sodium benzoate; benzoic acid (benzoate) is a metabolite of benzyl alcohol; large amounts of benzyl alcohol (≥99 mg/kg/day) have been associated with a potentially fatal toxicity ("gasping syndrome") in neonates; the "gasping syndrome" consists of metabolic acidosis, respiratory distress, gasping respirations, CNS dysfunction (including convulsions, intracranial hemorrhage), hypotension and cardiovascular collapse; avoid use of sodium benzoate containing products in neonates; *in vitro* and animal studies have shown that benzoate displaces bilirubin from protein binding sites

Precautions Use sodium salts with caution in patients with CHF, hypertension, pulmonary edema; may predispose patient to urolithiasis

Adverse Reactions

Central nervous system: Tetany

Endocrine & metabolic: Metabolic alkalosis, hypernatremia (if sodium salt used), hypocalcemia, hyperkalemia (if potassium salt used)

Gastrointestinal: Diarrhea, nausea, vomiting, stenotic or ulcerative lesions (wax matrix tablets)

Drug Interactions

Decreased effect/levels of chlorpropamide, lithium, methenamine, methotrexate, salicylates, and tetracycline due to urinary alkalinization

Increased toxicity/levels of amphetamines, flecainide, ephedrine, pseudoephedrine, quinidine, and quinine due to urinary alkalinization

Potassium-sparing diuretics, salt substitutes, captopril, and enalapril may result in increased serum potassium (potassium-containing salt forms only)

Mechanism of Action Citrate salts are oxidized in the body to form bicarbonate

Usual Dosage Oral (dilute in water or juice):

Infants and Children: 2-3 mEq/kg/day in divided doses 3-4 times/day **or** 5-15 mL with water after meals and at bedtime

Adults:

Solution: 15-30 mL with water after meals and at bedtime

Wax matrix tablet (Urocit®-K): 30-60 mEq/day in divided doses 3-4 times/day

Administration Oral: Dilute with water or juice and administer after meals; do not crush or chew wax matrix tablets (Urocit®-K)

Monitoring Parameters Serum sodium, bicarbonate, potassium, urine pH

Dosage Forms

Crystals (Polycitra®-K): Potassium citrate monohydrate 1100 mg and citric acid monohydrate 334 mg per 5 mL when reconstituted [potassium 2 mEq and is equivalent to bicarbonate 2 mEq per mL] (unit dose packets)

Solution, oral:

Modified Shohl's, Bicitra® (alcohol free): Sodium citrate dihydrate 500 mg and citric acid monohydrate 334 mg per 5 mL [sodium 1 mEq and is equivalent to bicarbonate 1 mEq per mL] (15 mL, 30 mL, 120 mL, 473 mL)

Oracit®: Sodium citrate 490 mg and citric acid 640 mg per 5 mL [sodium 1 mEq and is equivalent to bicarbonate 1 mEq per mL] (15 mL, 30 mL, 500 mL)

Polycitra®-K (alcohol free): Potassium citrate monohydrate 1100 mg and citric acid monohydrate 334 mg per 5 mL [potassium 2 mEq, and is equivalent to bicarbonate 2 mEq per mL] (473 mL)

Syrup, alcohol and sugar free (Polycitra®-LC): Potassium citrate monohydrate 550 mg, sodium citrate dihydrate 500 mg, and citric acid monohydrate 334 mg per 5 mL [potassium 1 mEq, sodium 1 mEq, and is equivalent to bicarbonate 2 mEq per mL] (473 mL)

Syrup, alcohol free (Polycitra®): Potassium citrate monohydrate 550 mg, sodium citrate dihydrate 500 mg, and citric acid monohydrate 334 mg per 5 mL [potassium 1 mEq, sodium 1 mEq, and is equivalent to bicarbonate 2 mEq per mL] (473 mL)

◆ **Citrate of Magnesia** *see* Magnesium Citrate *on page 970*
◆ **Citrate of Magnesia (Magnesium Citrate)** *see* Magnesium Supplements *on page 976*
◆ **Citroma® [OTC]** *see* Magnesium Citrate *on page 970*
◆ **Citro-Mag® (Can)** *see* Magnesium Citrate *on page 970*
◆ **Citrovorum Factor** *see* Leucovorin *on page 916*
◆ **CL-65336** *see* Tranexamic Acid *on page 1563*

Cladribine (KLA dri been)

Medication Safety Issues

Sound-alike/look-alike issues:

Cladribine may be confused with clofarabine

Leustatin® may be confused with lovastatin

High alert medication: The Institute for Safe Medication Practices (ISMP) includes this medication among its list of drugs which have a heightened risk of causing significant patient harm when used in error.

Related Information

Compatibility of Chemotherapy and Related Supportive Care Medications *on page 1777*

(Continued)

Cladribine *(Continued)*

U.S. Brand Names Leustatin®

Canadian Brand Names Leustatin®

Index Terms 2-CdA; 2-Chlorodeoxyadenosine; NSC-105014

Therapeutic Category Antineoplastic Agent, Antimetabolite (Purine)

Generic Available Yes

Use Treatment of hairy cell leukemia, chronic myeloid leukemia, and chronic lymphocytic leukemia; cladribine has activity in the treatment of Langerhans cell histiocytosis (LCH), non-Hodgkin's lymphomas, T-cell lymphomas, relapsed acute lymphocytic leukemia and relapsed acute myeloid leukemia

Pregnancy Risk Factor D

Lactation Excretion in breast milk unknown/not recommended

Contraindications Hypersensitivity to cladribine or any component

Warnings The FDA currently recommends that procedures for proper handling and disposal of antineoplastic agents be considered. Serious neurological toxicity has been reported in patients who received cladribine by continuous infusion at high doses (0.4-0.8 mg/kg/day or >16 mg/m^2/day); neurologic toxicity appears to be dose-related. Severe neurologic toxicity has been reported rarely with standard dosing regimens. Acute nephrotoxicity has been observed with cladribine doses of 0.4-0.8 mg/kg/day, especially in patients concurrently receiving other nephrotoxic agents.

Precautions Dose-limiting toxicity is myelosuppression; use with caution in patients with pre-existing hematologic or immunologic abnormalities; prophylactic administration of allopurinol should be considered in patients receiving cladribine due to the potential for hyperuricemia secondary to tumor lysis; appropriate antibiotic therapy should be administered promptly in patients exhibiting signs and symptoms of neutropenia and infection.

Adverse Reactions

Cardiovascular: Edema, tachycardia

Central nervous system: Fever (69%), fatigue (45%), headache, dizziness, insomnia, malaise, irreversible neurologic toxicity (paraparesis/quadriparesis) at high doses (0.4-0.8 mg/kg/day or >16 mg/m^2/day)

Dermatologic: Pruritus, erythema, rash

Gastrointestinal: Constipation, abdominal pain, nausea, vomiting, decreased appetite, diarrhea

Hematologic: Myelosuppression (prolonged pancytopenia), thrombocytopenia, aplastic anemia, hemolytic anemia

Hepatic: Reversible, mild elevations of bilirubin and transaminase levels

Local: Injection site reactions, pain

Neuromuscular & skeletal: Myalgia, trunk pain

Renal: Acute nephrotoxicity reported at high doses (rare)

Respiratory: Abnormal breath sounds, cough, shortness of breath

Stability Refrigerate unopened vials (2°C to 8°C/36°F to 46°F); protect from light. Solutions should be administered immediately after the initial dilution or stored in the refrigerator (2°C to 8°C) for ≤8 hours. **The use of D_5W as a diluent is not recommended due to increased degradation of cladribine;** should not be mixed with other intravenous drugs or additives or infused simultaneously via a common intravenous line. Diluted solution of cladribine in NS is stable for 24 hours at room temperature under normal room light in polyvinyl chloride infusion containers.

Mechanism of Action A purine nucleoside analogue; prodrug which enters the cells through a transport system and is activated via phosphorylation by deoxycytidine kinase to a 5'-triphosphate derivative. This active form incorporates into DNA resulting in inhibition of DNA synthesis and early chain termination. The induction of strand breaks results in a drop in the cofactor nicotinamide adenine dinucleotide and disruption of cell metabolism. ATP is depleted to deprive cells of an important source of energy. Cladribine kills both resting as well as dividing cells.

Pharmacokinetics

Distribution: V_d:

Children: 305 L/m^2

Adults: 0.5-9 L/kg (53-160 L/m^2)

CSF: Plasma concentration ratio: 18.2%

Protein binding: 20%

Bioavailability: SubQ: 100%

Half-life: 19.7 hours ± 3.4 hours

Elimination: 21% to 44% renally excreted

Usual Dosage I.V.: (refer to individual protocols):

Children:

Hairy cell leukemia: 0.09 mg/kg/day continuous infusion for 7 days

AML:

<3 years: 0.3 mg/kg/day over 2 hours daily for 5 days

≥3 years: 9 mg/m^2/day over 2 hours daily for 5 days or 8.9 mg/m^2/day over 24 hours for 5 days

Langerhans cell histiocytosis: 5-7 mg/m^2/day for 5 days; repeat every 21-28 days; do not administer if platelet count <100,000

Adults: 0.09-0.1 mg/kg/day continuous infusion for 7 consecutive days

Administration Parenteral: I.V.: **Single daily infusion:** May administer diluted in NS as an intermittent infusion or continuous infusion; administer through a 0.22 micron in-line filter

Monitoring Parameters CBC with differential and platelet count; creatinine clearance before initial dose; periodic renal and hepatic function tests

Nursing Implications Cladribine I.V. solution for administration should be inspected visually for particulates. A precipitate may occur at low temperatures and may be resolubilized at room temperature or by shaking the solution vigorously.

Dosage Forms Excipient information presented when available (limited, particularly for generics); consult specific product labeling.

Injection, solution [preservative free]: 1 mg/mL (10 mL)

References

Kearns CM, Blakley RL, Santane VM, et al, "Pharmacokinetics of Cladribine (2-Chlorodeoxyadenosine) in Children with Acute Leukemia," *Cancer Research*, 1994, 54:1235-39.

Larson RA, et al, "Dose Escalation Trial of Cladribine Using 5 Daily I.V. Infusions in Patients with Advanced Hematologic Malignancies," *J Clin Oncol*, 1996, 14(1):188-95.

Liliemark J, "The Clinical Pharmacokinetics of Cladribine," *Clin Pharmacokinet*, 1997, 32:120-131.

Rodriguez-Galindo C, Kelly P, Jeng M, et al, "Treatment of Children With Langerhans Cell Histiocytosis With 2-Chlorodeoxyadenosine," *Am J Hematol*, 2002, 69(3):179-84.

Stine KC, Saylors RL, Williams LL, et al, "2-Chlorodeoxyadenosine (2-CDA) for the Treatment of Refractory or Recurrent Langerhans Cell Histiocytosis (LCH) in Pediatric Patients," *Med Pediatr Oncol*, 1997, 29:288-92.

♦ **Claforan®** *see* Cefotaxime *on page 310*

♦ **Claravis™** *see* Isotretinoin *on page 876*

♦ **Clarinex®** *see* Desloratadine *on page 458*

Clarithromycin (kla RITH roe mye sin)

Medication Safety Issues

Sound-alike/look-alike issues:

Clarithromycin may be confused with erythromycin

Related Information

Endocarditis Prophylaxis *on page 1812*

U.S. Brand Names Biaxin®; Biaxin® XL

Canadian Brand Names Biaxin®; Biaxin® XL; ratio-Clarithromycin

Therapeutic Category Antibiotic, Macrolide

Generic Available Yes: Tablet

Use Treatment of upper and lower respiratory tract infections, community-acquired pneumonia, acute otitis media, and infections of the skin and skin structure due to susceptible strains of *S. aureus*, *S. pyogenes*, *S. pneumoniae*, *H. influenzae*, *M. catarrhalis*, *Mycoplasma pneumoniae*, *C. trachomatis*, and *Legionella* species; prophylaxis and treatment of *Mycobacterium avium* complex (MAC) disease in patients with advanced HIV infection; treatment of *Helicobacter pylori* infection; infective endocarditis prophylaxis for dental procedures in penicillin-allergic patients; postexposure prophylaxis and treatment of pertussis

Pregnancy Risk Factor C

Lactation Excretion in breast milk unknown/use caution

Contraindications Hypersensitivity to clarithromycin, any component, erythromycin, or any macrolide antibiotics; concomitant administration of terfenadine, astemizole, pimozide, or cisapride with clarithromycin may result in QT interval prolongation, ventricular tachycardia, ventricular fibrillation, hypotension, palpitations, cardiac arrest, and death; coadministration of clarithromycin with ergot derivatives

Warnings Safety and efficacy of clarithromycin have not been established in children <6 months of age; pseudomembranous colitis has been reported with use of clarithromycin. Colchicine toxicity with death has been reported with concomitant use of clarithromycin (some events occurred in patients with renal impairment).

Precautions Use with caution in patients with hepatic or renal impairment; reduce dosage or prolong dosing interval in patients with severe renal impairment with or without coexisting hepatic impairment. When clarithromycin and colchicine are coadministered together, inhibition of CYP3A and p-glycoprotein may lead to increased exposure to colchicine (monitor for symptoms of colchicine toxicity).

Adverse Reactions

Cardiovascular: QT prolongation, ventricular tachycardia

(Continued)

Clarithromycin *(Continued)*

Central nervous system: Headache, hallucinations, anxiety, confusion, convulsions, insomnia, vertigo, nightmares, psychosis

Dermatologic: Pruritus, rash, Stevens-Johnson syndrome, urticaria, toxic epidermal necrolysis

Gastrointestinal: Diarrhea, nausea, vomiting, abdominal pain, pseudomembranous colitis, pancreatitis, dysgeusia, tooth discoloration (reversible with dental cleaning), stomatitis; incidence of adverse GI effects (diarrhea, nausea, vomiting, dyspepsia, abdominal pain) is lower (13%) compared to erythromycin treated patients (32%)

Hematologic: Elevated prothrombin time, decreased WBC, thrombocytopenia

Hepatic: Elevated liver enzymes, hyperbilirubinemia, hepatitis, jaundice

Otic: Hearing loss, tinnitus

Renal: Elevated BUN and serum creatinine

Miscellaneous: Anaphylaxis (rare)

Drug Interactions Cytochrome P450 isoenzyme CYP3A3/4 substrate; CYP1A2 and CYP3A3/4 isoenzyme inhibitor

Clarithromycin has been shown to increase serum **theophylline** levels by as much as 20%; **carbamazepine** levels have been shown to increase after a single dose of clarithromycin; hepatic metabolism of terfenadine, astemizole, pimozide, and cisapride are reduced by clarithromycin (see Contraindications); increases serum level of digoxin, cyclosporine, sildenafil, quinidine, sirolimus, disopyramide, tacrolimus, ergot alkaloids, omeprazole, lovastatin, simvastatin, and triazolam; potentiates the effects of warfarin; fluconazole and ritonavir increase serum level of clarithromycin; efavirenz decreases clarithromycin levels while increasing the levels of its metabolite

Food Interactions

Immediate release formulations: Food may delay the rate but not the extent of oral absorption

Extended release formulations: Food increases AUC by 30% relative to fasting conditions

Stability Reconstituted oral suspension should **not** be refrigerated because it might gel; microencapsulated particles of clarithromycin in suspension are stable for 14 days when stored at room temperature

Mechanism of Action Inhibits bacterial RNA-dependent protein synthesis by binding to the 50S ribosomal subunit; the 14-hydroxy metabolite of clarithromycin is twice as active as the parent compound

Pharmacokinetics

Absorption: Rapid from the GI tract; food delays onset of absorption and formation of active metabolite, but does not affect the extent of tablet absorption; in pediatric patients, coadministration of the suspension with food did not significantly alter the extent of clarithromycin absorption or formation of the 14-OH metabolite (active)

Distribution: Widely distributed throughout the body with tissue concentrations higher than serum concentrations

Protein binding: 65% to 70%

Metabolism: In the liver to active and inactive metabolites; undergoes extensive first-pass metabolism

Bioavailability: 50% to 68%

Half-life: Dose-dependent, prolonged with renal dysfunction

- Clarithromycin:
  - 250 mg dose: 3-4 hours
  - 500 mg dose: 5-7 hours
- 14-hydroxy metabolite:
  - 250 mg dose: 5-6 hours
  - 500 mg dose: 7-9 hours

Time to peak serum concentration: Immediate release formulations: 2-3 hours

Elimination: After a 250 mg dose, 20% is excreted unchanged in urine, 10% to 15% is excreted as active metabolite 14-OH clarithromycin, and 4% is excreted in feces

Usual Dosage Oral:

Infants and Children:

- Acute otitis media: 15 mg/kg/day divided every 12 hours for 10 days
- Respiratory, skin and skin structure infections: 15 mg/kg/day divided every 12 hours for 7-14 days
- Infective endocarditis prophylaxis for dental procedures in patients allergic to penicillins or ampicillin: 15 mg/kg 30-60 minutes before procedure; maximum dose: 500 mg
- Prophylaxis for first episode of MAC with the following CD4$^+$ T-lymphocyte counts (see below): 15 mg/kg/day divided every 12 hours; maximum dose: 1 g/day
  - Children <12 months: <750 cells/microliter
  - 1-2 years: <500 cells/microliter
  - 2-6 years: <75 cells/microliter

≥6 years: <50 cells/microliter

Prophylaxis for recurrence of MAC: 15 mg/kg/day divided every 12 hours; maximum dose: 1 g/day (use in combination with ethambutol and with or without rifabutin)

Pertussis: Infants and Children ≥1 month: 15 mg/kg/day divided every 12 hours for 7 days; maximum dose: 1 g/day; **Note:** Use azithromycin in infants <1 month

Adolescents and Adults: Immediate-release tablet: 250 mg every 12 hours for 7-14 days for all indications except sinusitis and chronic bronchitis due to *H. influenzae*; for these indications, 500 mg every 12 hours for 7-14 days

Infective endocarditis prophylaxis for dental procedures in patients allergic to penicillins or ampicillin: 500 mg 30-60 minutes before procedure

Prophylaxis for first episode of MAC in patients with CD4+ T-lymphocyte count <50 cells/microliter: 500 mg twice daily

Prophylaxis for recurrence of MAC: 500 mg twice daily in combination with ethambutol and with or without rifabutin

Helicobacter pylori (combination therapy with omeprazole or with bismuth subsalicylate, tetracycline, and an H_2-receptor antagonist): 250 mg twice daily up to 500 mg 3 times/day

Pertussis: 500 mg twice daily for 7 days

Adolescents and Adults: Extended-release tablet: Two 500 mg tablets every 24 hours for 7 days for chronic bronchitis and community-acquired pneumonia; two 500 mg tablets every 24 hours for 14 days for sinusitis

Dosing adjustment in renal impairment: Cl_{cr} <30 mL/minute: Decrease dose by 50% and administer once or twice daily

Administration Oral: May administer immediate-release tablet or oral suspension with or without meals; extended-release tablet must be administered with food; do not crush or chew extended-release tablet; may administer with milk; shake suspension well before use

Monitoring Parameters Monitor serum concentration of drugs whose concentrations may be affected in patients receiving concomitant clarithromycin (ie, theophylline, carbamazepine, quinidine, digoxin, anticoagulants, triazolam); liver function tests; hearing (in patients receiving long-term treatment with clarithromycin); observe for changes in bowel frequency

Dosage Forms Excipient information presented when available (limited, particularly for generics); consult specific product labeling.

Granules for oral suspension:

Biaxin®: 125 mg/5 mL (50 mL, 100 mL); 250 mg/5 mL (50 mL, 100 mL) [fruit punch flavor]

Tablet: 250 mg, 500 mg

Biaxin®: 250 mg, 500 mg

Tablet, extended release: 500 mg

Biaxin® XL: 500 mg

References

Aspin MM, Hoberman A, McCarty J, et al, "Comparative Study of the Safety and Efficacy of Clarithromycin and Amoxicillin-Clavulanate in the Treatment of Acute Otitis Media in Children," *J Pediatr*, 1994, 125(1):136-41.

Guay DR and Craft JC, "Overview of the Pharmacology of Clarithromycin Suspension in Children and a Comparison With That in Adults," *Pediatr Infect Dis J*, 1993, 12(12 Suppl 3):S106-11.

Husson RN, Ross LA, Sandelli S, et al, "Orally Administered Clarithromycin for the Treatment of Systemic *Mycobacterium avium* Complex Infection in Children With Acquired Immunodeficiency Syndrome," *J Pediatr*, 1994, 124(5 Pt 1):807-14.

Kaplan JE, Masur H, and Holmes KK, "Guidelines for Preventing Opportunistic Infections Among HIV-Infected Persons - 2002 Recommendations of the USPHS and IDSA," *MMWR*, 2002, 51(RR-8):1-46.

Neu HC, "The Development of Macrolides: Clarithromycin in Perspective," *J Antimicrob Chemother*, 1991, 27(Suppl A):1-9.

Tiwari T, Murphy TV, and Moran J, "Recommended Antimicrobial Agents for the Treatment and Postexposure Prophylaxis of Pertussis: 2005 CDC Guidelines," *MMWR Recomm Rep*, 2005, 54(RR-14):1-16.

Wilson W, Taubert KA, Gewitz M, et al, "Prevention of Infective Endocarditis. Guidelines From the American Heart Association, " *Circulation*, 2007, 115:1-20.

♦ **Claritin® (Can)** *see* Loratadine *on page 959*

♦ **Claritin® 24 Hour Allergy [OTC]** *see* Loratadine *on page 959*

♦ **Claritin-D® 12-Hour [OTC]** *see* Loratadine and Pseudoephedrine *on page 961*

♦ **Claritin-D® 24-Hour [OTC]** *see* Loratadine and Pseudoephedrine *on page 961*

♦ **Claritin® Allergic Decongestant (Can)** *see* Oxymetazoline *on page 1194*

♦ **Claritin® Extra (Can)** *see* Loratadine and Pseudoephedrine *on page 961*

♦ **Claritin® Hives Relief [OTC]** *see* Loratadine *on page 959*

♦ **Claritin® Kids (Can)** *see* Loratadine *on page 959*

♦ **Claritin® Liberator (Can)** *see* Loratadine and Pseudoephedrine *on page 961*

♦ **Clarus™ (Can)** *see* Isotretinoin *on page 876*

♦ **Clavulanic Acid and Amoxicillin** *see* Amoxicillin and Clavulanic Acid *on page 115*

♦ **Clavulin® (Can)** *see* Amoxicillin and Clavulanic Acid *on page 115*

♦ **Clear eyes® for Dry Eyes and ACR Relief [OTC]** *see* Naphazoline *on page 1106*
♦ **Clear eyes® for Dry Eyes and Redness Relief [OTC]** *see* Naphazoline *on page 1106*
♦ **Clear eyes® Redness Relief [OTC]** *see* Naphazoline *on page 1106*
♦ **Clear eyes® Seasonal Relief [OTC]** *see* Naphazoline *on page 1106*
♦ **Clearplex [OTC]** *see* Benzoyl Peroxide *on page 207*

Clemastine (KLEM as teen)

U.S. Brand Names Dayhist® Allergy [OTC]; Tavist® Allergy [OTC]

Index Terms Clemastine Fumarate

Therapeutic Category Antihistamine

Generic Available Yes

Use Perennial and seasonal allergic rhinitis and other allergic symptoms including urticaria

Pregnancy Risk Factor C

Lactation Enters breast milk/not recommended

Contraindications Hypersensitivity to clemastine or any component; narrow-angle glaucoma; patients receiving MAO inhibitors

Precautions Use with caution in patients with stenosing peptic ulcer, GI or GU obstruction, asthma, or prostatic hypertrophy

Adverse Reactions

Cardiovascular: Bradycardia, edema, palpitations

Central nervous system: Drowsiness, fatigue, headache, dizziness, vertigo, ataxia, CNS stimulation (more common in children)

Dermatologic: Rash, angioedema, photosensitivity

Endocrine & metabolic: Weight gain

Gastrointestinal: Nausea, vomiting, xerostomia, gastritis, appetite increase, diarrhea, abdominal pain

Hepatic: Hepatitis

Neuromuscular & skeletal: Arthralgia, myalgia, paresthesia

Respiratory: Shortness of breath, pharyngitis, bronchospasm, epistaxis

Drug Interactions Increased toxicity (CNS depression or excessive anticholinergic activity): CNS depressants, MAO inhibitors, tricyclic antidepressants, phenothiazines

Mechanism of Action Competes with histamine for H_1-receptor sites on effector cells in the GI tract, blood vessels, and respiratory tract

Pharmacodynamics

Onset of action: 2 hours after administration

Maximum effect: 5-7 hours

Duration: 10-12 hours

Pharmacokinetics

Absorption: Oral: Well absorbed

Distribution: Breast milk to plasma ratio: 0.25-0.5

Metabolism: In the liver

Time to peak serum concentration: 2-4 hours

Elimination: Majority of an oral dose eliminated in the urine

Usual Dosage Oral:

Infants and Children <6 years: 0.05 mg/kg/day as **clemastine base** or 0.335-0.67 mg/day clemastine fumarate (0.25-0.5 mg base/day) divided into 2 or 3 doses; maximum daily dosage: 1.34 mg (1 mg base)

Children 6-12 years: 0.67-1.34 mg clemastine fumarate (0.5-1 mg base) twice daily; do not exceed 4.02 mg/day (3 mg/day base)

Children ≥12 years and Adults: 1.34 mg clemastine fumarate (1 mg base) twice daily to 2.68 mg (2 mg base) 3 times/day; do not exceed 8.04 mg/day (6 mg base)

Administration Oral: Administer with food

Monitoring Parameters Look for a reduction of rhinitis, urticaria, eczema, pruritus, or other allergic symptoms

Patient Information Avoid alcohol; may cause drowsiness and impair ability to perform activities requiring mental alertness or physical coordination; may cause dry mouth. May rarely cause photosensitivity reactions (eg, exposure to sunlight may cause severe sunburn, skin rash, redness, or itching); avoid direct exposure to sunlight

Dosage Forms Excipient information presented when available (limited, particularly for generics); consult specific product labeling.

Syrup, as fumarate [prescription formulation]: 0.67 mg/5 mL (120 mL) [0.5 mg base/5 mL; contains alcohol 5.5%; citrus flavor]

Tablet, as fumarate: 1.34 mg [1 mg base; OTC], 2.68 mg [2 mg base; prescription formulation]

Dayhist® Allergy, Tavist® Allergy: 1.34 mg [1 mg base]

- ♦ **Clemastine Fumarate** *see* Clemastine *on page 378*
- ♦ **Cleocin®** *see* Clindamycin *on page 379*
- ♦ **Cleocin HCl®** *see* Clindamycin *on page 379*
- ♦ **Cleocin Pediatric®** *see* Clindamycin *on page 379*
- ♦ **Cleocin Phosphate®** *see* Clindamycin *on page 379*
- ♦ **Cleocin T®** *see* Clindamycin *on page 379*
- ♦ **Cleocin® Vaginal Ovule** *see* Clindamycin *on page 379*
- ♦ **Climara®** *see* Estradiol *on page 605*
- ♦ **Clinac™ BPO** *see* Benzoyl Peroxide *on page 207*
- ♦ **Clindagel®** *see* Clindamycin *on page 379*
- ♦ **ClindaMax™** *see* Clindamycin *on page 379*

Clindamycin (klin da MYE sin)

Medication Safety Issues

Sound-alike/look-alike issues:

Cleocin® may be confused with bleomycin, Clinoril®, Lincocin®

Related Information

Endocarditis Prophylaxis *on page 1812*

Malaria *on page 1855*

U.S. Brand Names Cleocin®; Cleocin HCl®; Cleocin Pediatric®; Cleocin Phosphate®; Cleocin T®; Cleocin® Vaginal Ovule; Clindagel®; ClindaMax™; Clindesse™; Clindets® [DSC]; Evoclin™

Canadian Brand Names Alti-Clindamycin; Apo-Clindamycin®; Clindamycin Injection, USP; Clindoxyl®; Dalacin® C; Dalacin® T; Dalacin® Vaginal; Novo-Clindamycin; Riva-Clindamycin; Taro-Clindamycin

Index Terms Clindamycin Hydrochloride; Clindamycin Palmitate; Clindamycin Phosphate

Therapeutic Category Acne Products; Antibiotic, Anaerobic; Antibiotic, Miscellaneous

Generic Available Yes: Excludes foam, granules, vaginal suppositories, vaginal cream

Use Useful agent against most aerobic gram-positive staphylococci and streptococci (except enterococci); useful against *Fusobacterium, Bacteroides* species and *Actinomyces* for treatment of respiratory tract infections, skin and soft tissue infections, sepsis, intra-abdominal infections, and infections of the female pelvis and genital tract; bacterial endocarditis prophylaxis for dental and upper respiratory procedures in penicillin-allergic patients; perioperative prophylaxis for head and neck surgery (incision through oral mucosa), colorectal surgery, appendectomy, or surgery for ruptured viscus; treatment of babesiosis; used topically in treatment of acne vulgaris; used intravaginally for treatment of bacterial vaginosis

Pregnancy Risk Factor B

Lactation Enters breast milk/compatible

Contraindications Hypersensitivity to clindamycin, lincomycin, or any component (see Warnings); previous pseudomembranous colitis, hepatic impairment, regional enteritis or ulcerative colitis

Warnings Use of topical and systemic clindamycin can cause severe and possibly fatal colitis characterized by severe persistent diarrhea, severe abdominal cramps and possibly, the passage of blood and mucus; discontinue drug if significant diarrhea occurs. Antiperistaltic agents such as opiates or diphenoxylate with atropine may prolong and worsen the condition.

Capsule contains tartrazine which may cause allergic reactions in susceptible individuals. Injection contains benzyl alcohol which may cause allergic reactions in susceptible individuals; large amounts of benzyl alcohol (≥99 mg/kg/day) have been associated with a potentially fatal toxicity ("gasping syndrome") in neonates; the "gasping syndrome" consists of metabolic acidosis, respiratory distress, gasping respirations, CNS dysfunction (including convulsions, intracranial hemorrhage), hypotension and cardiovascular collapse; use clindamycin injection products containing benzyl alcohol with caution in neonates; *in vitro* and animal studies have shown that benzoate, a metabolite of benzyl alcohol, displaces bilirubin from protein binding sites

Precautions Use with caution and modify dosage in patients with severe renal and/or hepatic impairment; use with caution in atopic patients

Adverse Reactions

Cardiovascular: Hypotension, cardiac arrest (with rapid I.V. administration); arrhythmia due to QT_c prolongation

Central nervous system: Dizziness, headache

Dermatologic: Urticaria, rash, Stevens-Johnson syndrome, dry skin, erythema, pruritus

(Continued)

Clindamycin *(Continued)*

Gastrointestinal: Diarrhea, nausea, vomiting, pseudomembranous colitis, esophagitis, abdominal pain
Genitourinary: Vaginal candidiasis, vaginitis
Hematologic: Eosinophilia, granulocytopenia, thrombocytopenia, neutropenia
Hepatic: Elevated liver enzymes
Local: Sterile abscess at I.M. injection site; thrombophlebitis, erythema, pain, swelling; application site burning, pruritus, dryness
Neuromuscular & skeletal: Polyarthritis (rare)
Renal: Rare: Renal dysfunction
Miscellaneous: Hypersensitivity reactions

Drug Interactions Cytochrome P450 isoenzyme CYP3A3/4 substrate
Clindamycin may increase the neuromuscular blocking action of tubocurarine, pancuronium

Stability Store foam at room temperature (Flammable: Do not expose to heat, fire, or flame). Do **not** refrigerate the reconstituted oral solution because it will thicken; oral solution stable for 2 weeks at room temperature following reconstitution; I.V. clindamycin is incompatible with aminophylline, tobramycin

Mechanism of Action Reversibly binds to 50S ribosomal subunits preventing peptide bond formation thus inhibiting bacterial protein synthesis; bacteriostatic or bactericidal depending on drug concentration, infection site, and organism

Pharmacokinetics
Absorption:
Oral: 90% of clindamycin hydrochloride is rapidly absorbed; clindamycin palmitate must be hydrolyzed in the GI tract before it is active
Topical: ~10% absorbed systemically
Distribution: No significant levels are seen in CSF, even with inflamed meninges; crosses the placenta; distributes into breast milk, saliva, ascites fluid, pleural fluid, bone, and bile
Protein binding: 94%
Bioavailability: Oral: ~90%
Half-life:
Neonates:
Premature: 8.7 hours
Full-term: 3.6 hours
Infants 1 month to 1 year: 3 hours
Children and Adults with normal renal function: 2-3 hours
Time to peak serum concentration:
Oral: Within 60 minutes
I.M.: Within 1-3 hours
Elimination: Most of the drug is eliminated by hepatic metabolism; 10% of an oral dose excreted in urine and 3.6% excreted in feces as active drug and metabolites
Dialysis: Not dialyzable (0% to 5%)

Usual Dosage
Neonates: I.M., I.V.:
Postnatal age ≤7 days:
≤2000 g: 10 mg/kg/day divided every 12 hours
>2000 g: 15 mg/kg/day divided every 8 hours
Postnatal age >7 days:
<1200 g: 10 mg/kg/day divided every 12 hours
1200-2000 g: 15 mg/kg/day divided every 8 hours
>2000 g: 20-30 mg/kg/day divided every 6-8 hours
Infants and Children:
Oral: 10-30 mg/kg/day divided every 6-8 hours; maximum dose: 1.8 g/day
I.M., I.V.: 25-40 mg/kg/day divided every 6-8 hours; doses as high as 4.8 g/day have been given I.V. in life-threatening situations
Bacterial endocarditis prophylaxis for dental and upper respiratory procedures in penicillin allergic patients:
Oral: 20 mg/kg 1 hour before procedure **or** I.V.: 20 mg/kg 30 minutes before procedure; maximum dose: 600 mg
Perioperative prophylaxis: I.V.: 10 mg/kg (maximum: 600 mg) plus gentamicin 2 mg/kg (maximum: 120 mg) 30 minutes prior to the procedure
Babesiosis: Oral: 20-40 mg/kg/day divided every 8 hours for 7 days plus quinine
Children and Adults: Topical:
Gel, pledget, lotion, solution: Apply a thin film twice daily
Foam: Apply once daily in an amount that will cover the affected area
Adolescents and Adults:
Oral: 150-450 mg/dose every 6-8 hours; maximum dose: 1.8 g/day
I.M., I.V.: 1.2-2.7 g/day in 2-4 divided doses; doses as high as 4.8 g/day have been given I.V. in life-threatening situations

Vaginal:

Cream: One full applicator (100 mg) inserted intravaginally once daily before bedtime for 3 or 7 consecutive days

Suppository: Insert one ovule (100 mg) intravaginally once daily before bedtime for 3 days

Bacterial endocarditis prophylaxis for dental and upper respiratory procedures in penicillin allergic patients:

Oral: 600 mg 1 hour before procedure **or** I.V.: 600 mg 30 minutes before procedure

Perioperative prophylaxis: I.V.: 600 mg plus gentamicin 1.5 mg/kg (maximum: 120 mg) 30 minutes prior to the procedure

Pelvic inflammatory disease: 900 mg I.V. every 8 hours for 24-48 hours after significant clinical improvement, followed by 600 mg orally 3 times/day to complete a 14-day course

Babesiosis:

I.V.: 1.2 g twice daily plus quinine

or

Oral: 600 mg 3 times/day for 7 days plus quinine

Dosing interval in renal/hepatic impairment: Reduce dosage in patients with severe renal or hepatic impairment

Administration

Intravaginal: Do not use for topical therapy, instillation in the eye, or oral administration. Wash hands; insert applicator into vagina and expel suppository or cream. Remain lying down for 30 minutes following administration. Wash applicator with soap and water following suppository use; if administering the cream, use each disposable applicator only once

Oral: Capsule should be taken with a full glass of water to avoid esophageal irritation; shake oral solution well before use; may administer with or without meals

Parenteral: Administer by I.V. intermittent infusion over at least 10-60 minutes, at a rate **not** to exceed 30 mg/minute; hypotension and cardiopulmonary arrest have been reported following rapid I.V. administration; final concentration for administration should not exceed 18 mg/mL

Topical: Do not use intravaginally, instill in the eye, or administer orally

Foam: Before applying foam, wash affected area with mild soap, then dry. Do not dispense foam directly onto hands or face. Remove cap, hold can at an upright angle and dispense foam directly into the cap or onto a cool surface. If can is warm or foam is runny, run can under cold water. Use fingertips to pick up small amounts of foam and gently massage into affected area until foam disappears. Avoid fire, flame, or smoking during or immediately following application.

Lotion: Shake well before use

Monitoring Parameters Observe for changes in bowel frequency; during prolonged therapy monitor CBC with differential, platelet count, hepatic and renal function tests periodically

Patient Information Report any severe diarrhea immediately; clindamycin vaginal cream (oil-based) may weaken latex condoms for up to 72 hours after completing therapy

Dosage Forms Excipient information presented when available (limited, particularly for generics); consult specific product labeling. [DSC] = Discontinued product

Note: Strength is expressed as base

Capsule, as hydrochloride: 150 mg, 300 mg

Cleocin HCl®: 75 mg [contains tartrazine], 150 mg [contains tartrazine], 300 mg

Cream, vaginal, as phosphate:

Cleocin®: 2% (40 g) [contains benzyl alcohol and mineral oil; packaged with 7 disposable applicators]

Clindesse™: 2% (5 g) [contains mineral oil; prefilled single disposable applicator]

Foam, topical, as phosphate:

Evoclin™: 1% (50 g, 100 g) [contains ethanol 58%]

Gel, topical, as phosphate: 1% (30 g, 60 g)

Cleocin T®: 1% (30 g, 60 g)

Clindagel®: 1% (40 mL, 75 mL)

ClindaMax™: 1% (30 g, 60 g)

Granules for oral solution, as palmitate:

Cleocin Pediatric®: 75 mg/5 mL (100 mL) [cherry flavor]

Infusion, as phosphate [premixed in D_5W]:

Cleocin Phosphate®: 300 mg (50 mL); 600 mg (50 mL); 900 mg (50 mL)

Injection, solution, as phosphate: 150 mg/mL (2 mL, 4 mL, 6 mL, 60 mL)

Cleocin Phosphate®: 150 mg/mL (2 mL, 4 mL, 6 mL, 60 mL) [contains benzyl alcohol and disodium edetate 0.5 mg]

Lotion, as phosphate: 1% (60 mL)

Cleocin T®, ClindaMax™: 1% (60 mL)

Pledgets, topical: 1% (60s) [contains alcohol]

(Continued)

Clindamycin *(Continued)*

Cleocin T®: 1% (60s) [contains isopropyl alcohol 50%]
Clindets®: 1% (69s) [contains isopropyl alcohol 52%] [DSC]
Solution, topical, as phosphate: 1% (30 mL, 60 mL)
Cleocin T®: 1% (30 mL, 60 mL) [contains isopropyl alcohol 50%]
Suppository, vaginal, as phosphate:
Cleocin® Vaginal Ovule: 100 mg (3s) [contains oleaginous base; single reusable applicator]

References

Dajani AS, Taubert KA, Wilson W, et al, "Prevention of Bacterial Endocarditis. Recommendations by the American Heart Association," *JAMA*, 1997, 277(22):1794-801.

Clindamycin and Benzoyl Peroxide

(klin da MYE sin & BEN zoe il peer OKS ide)

U.S. Brand Names BenzaClin®; Duac™

Canadian Brand Names BenzaClin®

Index Terms Benzoyl Peroxide and Clindamycin; Clindamycin Phosphate and Benzoyl Peroxide

Therapeutic Category Acne Products; Topical Skin Product

Generic Available No

Use Topical treatment of acne vulgaris

Pregnancy Risk Factor C

Lactation Excretion in breast milk unknown/not recommended

Contraindications Hypersensitivity to benzoyl peroxide, clindamycin, lincomycin, or any component; history of regional enteritis, ulcerative colitis, or antibiotic-associated colitis; concurrent use with erythromycin

Warnings Use of topical clindamycin results in absorption from the skin surface; diarrhea, bloody diarrhea, and colitis (including pseudomembranous colitis) have been reported with the use of topical and systemic clindamycin; the colitis is usually characterized by severe persistent diarrhea and severe abdominal cramps and may be associated with the passage of blood and mucus; discontinue drug if significant diarrhea occurs. Antiperistaltic agents such as opiates or diphenoxylate with atropine may prolong and worsen the condition. May bleach hair or clothing.

Precautions Avoid contact with eyes and mucous membranes; use of antibiotic agents may be associated with the overgrowth of nonsusceptible organisms including fungi; if this occurs, discontinue use; concomitant topical acne therapy should be used with caution because a possible cumulative irritancy effect may occur, especially with the use of peeling, desquamating, or abrasive agents

Adverse Reactions

Dermatologic: Dry skin, pruritus, peeling, erythema, photosensitivity
Gastrointestinal: Colitis, diarrhea, AAPC

Drug Interactions Use with erythromycin may lead to antagonism of antimicrobial effects; increased topical adverse effects with tretinoin

Stability

BenzaClin®: Store at room temperature; stable at room temperature after reconstitution with purified water for 10 weeks
Duac™: Store in refrigerator until dispensed; stable at room temperature for 60 days

Mechanism of Action Clindamycin and benzoyl peroxide have activity against *Propionibacterium acnesin vitro*. This organism has been associated with acne vulgaris. Benzoyl peroxide releases free-radical oxygen which oxidizes bacterial proteins in the sebaceous follicles decreasing the number of anaerobic bacteria and decreasing irritating-type free fatty acids. Clindamycin reversibly binds to 50S ribosomal subunits preventing peptide bond formation thus inhibiting bacterial protein synthesis; bacteriostatic or bactericidal depending on the drug concentration, infection site, and organism.

Pharmacodynamics See individual agents

Pharmacokinetics See individual agents

Usual Dosage Topical: Children ≥12 years and Adults:
BenzaClin®: Apply twice daily (morning and evening)
Duac™: Apply once daily in the evening

Administration Topical: Skin should be clean and dry before applying. Apply to affected areas avoiding contact with eyes, inside of nose, mouth, and all mucous membranes.

Patient Information Avoid contact with eyes, inside of nose, mouth, and all mucous membranes; may bleach hair and clothing; notify physician if severe diarrhea, dryness, redness or peeling occurs. May cause photosensitivity reactions (eg, exposure to sunlight may cause severe sunburn, skin rash, redness, or itching); avoid exposure to sunlight and artificial light sources (sunlamps, tanning booth/bed); wear protective clothing, wide-brimmed hats, sunglasses, and lip sunscreen (SPF ≥15); use a sunscreen [broad-spectrum sunscreen or physical sunscreen(preferred) or sunblock with SPF ≥15]; contact physician if reaction occurs.

Dosage Forms Excipient information presented when available (limited, particularly for generics); consult specific product labeling.

Gel, topical:

BenzaClin®: Clindamycin phosphate 1% and benzoyl peroxide 5% (25 g, 50 g)

Duac™: Clindamycin phosphate 1% and benzoyl peroxide 5% (45 g)

- ♦ **Clindamycin Hydrochloride** *see* Clindamycin *on page 379*
- ♦ **Clindamycin Injection, USP (Can)** *see* Clindamycin *on page 379*
- ♦ **Clindamycin Palmitate** *see* Clindamycin *on page 379*
- ♦ **Clindamycin Phosphate** *see* Clindamycin *on page 379*
- ♦ **Clindamycin Phosphate and Benzoyl Peroxide** *see* Clindamycin and Benzoyl Peroxide *on page 382*
- ♦ **Clindesse™** *see* Clindamycin *on page 379*
- ♦ **Clindets® [DSC]** *see* Clindamycin *on page 379*
- ♦ **Clindoxyl® (Can)** *see* Clindamycin *on page 379*
- ♦ **Clinoril®** *see* Sulindac *on page 1493*

Clobetasol (kloe BAY ta sol)

Medication Safety Issues

International issues:

Clobex® may be confused with Codex® which is a brand name for *Saccharomyces boulardii* in Italy

Related Information

Corticosteroids, Topical: Guidelines for Selection and Use *on page 1686*

U.S. Brand Names Clobevate®; Clobex®; Cormax®; Olux®; Olux-E™; Temovate®; Temovate E®

Canadian Brand Names Clobex®; Dermovate®; Gen-Clobetasol; Novo-Clobetasol; Taro-Clobetasol

Index Terms Clobetasol Propionate

Therapeutic Category Adrenal Corticosteroid; Anti-inflammatory Agent; Corticosteroid, Topical; Glucocorticoid

Generic Available Yes: Excludes foam, lotion, shampoo, spray

Use Short-term relief of inflammation and pruritus associated with corticosteroid-responsive dermatoses

Pregnancy Risk Factor C

Lactation Excretion in breast milk unknown/use caution

Contraindications Hypersensitivity to clobetasol propionate, other corticosteroids, or any component; the solution for scalp application is also contraindicated for use in patients with primary scalp infections

Warnings Hypothalamic-pituitary-adrenal (HPA) axis suppression may occur with topical clobetasol use, even at low doses; acute adrenal insufficiency may occur with abrupt withdrawal after long-term use or with stress; withdrawal or discontinuation should be done carefully; patients with HPA axis suppression may require increased doses of systemic glucocorticosteroids prior to, during, and after unusual stress (eg, surgery). Adverse systemic effects (including HPA axis suppression) may occur when topical steroids are used on large areas of the body, denuded areas, for prolonged periods of time, with an occlusive dressing, and/or in pediatric patients; infants and small children may be more susceptible to HPA axis suppression or other systemic toxicities due to a larger skin surface area to body mass ratio; use with caution in pediatric patients; due to the increased risk of HPA axis suppression and other systemic toxicities, the use of any clobetasol product for the treatment of steroid-responsive dermatoses is not recommended in children <12 years of age; use of clobetasol lotion or spray for moderate to severe plaque-type psoriasis in children <18 years is not recommended.

Do not use topical clobetasol for the treatment of rosacea or perioral dermatitis; do not apply to the face, groin, or axillae. Do not exceed maximum recommended dose or duration of therapy due to the potential development of HPA axis suppression.

Precautions Avoid using higher than recommended doses; suppression of HPA axis, suppression of linear growth (ie, reduction of growth velocity), reduced bone mineral, or hypercorticism (Cushing's syndrome) may occur. Discontinue treatment if local irritation develops. Use appropriate antibacterial or antifungal agents to treat concomitant skin infections; discontinue clobetasol treatment if infection does not resolve promptly.

(Continued)

Clobetasol *(Continued)*

Adverse Reactions

Central nervous system: Intracranial hypertension (systemic effect reported in children treated with topical corticosteroids); headache (with scalp application)

Dermatologic: Burning, stinging, cracking and fissuring of the skin, local pain, pigmentation change, dryness, erythema, folliculitis, irritation, pruritus, skin atrophy, telangiectasia. **Note:** Other dermatologic effects reported with scalp application: Scalp pustules, tightness of the scalp, dermatitis, tenderness, and hair loss. Other effects reported with other high-potency topical steroids: Acne eruptions, allergic contact dermatitis, hypertrichosis, hypopigmentation, maceration of the skin, miliaria, striae, perioral dermatitis, secondary infection.

Endocrine & metabolic: Hyperglycemia, HPA axis suppression, Cushing's syndrome, growth retardation

Neuromuscular & skeletal: Numbness of the fingers

Ocular: Eye irritation (with scalp application)

Renal: Glycosuria

Drug Interactions None identified

Stability

Cream, emollient cream, ointment: Store at room temperature, between 15°C to 30°C (59°F to 86°F). Do not refrigerate.

Foam: Store at room temperature of 20°C to 25°C (68°F to 77°F); do not expose to heat or temperatures >49°C (120°F). Can is pressurized; do not puncture or incinerate. Contents are flammable; avoid flame, fire, or smoking during and immediately after application.

Gel: Store between 2°C to 30°C (36°F to 86°F)

Lotion: Store at room temperature of 20°C to 25°C (68°F to 77°F). Do not freeze.

Solution: Do not use near open flame.

Cormax® scalp application: Store at room temperature between 15°C to 30°C (59°F to 86°F); do not refrigerate.

Temovate® scalp application: Store between 4°C to 25°C (39°F to 77°F).

Spray: Store at controlled room temperature; do not refrigerate or freeze; do not store at >30°C; spray is flammable; avoid heat, do not use near open flame

Mechanism of Action Not well defined topically; possesses anti-inflammatory, antipruritic, antiproliferative, vasoconstrictive, and immunosuppressive properties

Pharmacokinetics

Absorption: Percutaneous absorption varies and depends on many factors including vehicle used, integrity of epidermis, dose, and use of occlusive dressing; absorption is increased by occlusive dressings or with decreased integrity of skin (eg, inflammation or skin disease); gel has greater absorption than cream

Metabolism: Hepatic

Elimination: Drug and metabolites are excreted in urine and bile

Usual Dosage Topical: Use the smallest amount for the shortest period of time to avoid HPA suppression; discontinue therapy when control is achieved; reassess diagnosis if no improvement is seen within 2 weeks.

Children <12 years: Use not recommended (high risk of systemic adverse effects, eg, HPA axis suppression, Cushing's syndrome)

Children ≥12 years and Adults:

Steroid-responsive dermatoses:

Cream, emollient cream, gel, lotion, ointment: Apply sparingly twice daily for up to 2 weeks; maximum dose: 50 g/week or 50 mL/week

Foam, solution: Apply sparingly to affected area of scalp twice daily for up to 2 weeks; maximum dose: 50 g/week or 50 mL/week

Mild to moderate plaque-type psoriasis of nonscalp areas: Foam: Apply sparingly to affected area twice daily for up to 2 weeks; maximum dose: 50 g/week; do not apply to face or intertriginous areas

Moderate to severe plaque-type psoriasis: Emollient cream: Apply sparingly twice daily for up to 2 weeks; if response is not adequate, may be used for up to 2 more weeks if application is <10% of body surface area; use with caution; maximum dose: 50 g/week

Children ≥18 years and Adults: Moderate to severe plaque-type psoriasis:

Lotion: Apply sparingly twice daily for up to 2 weeks; if response is not adequate, may be used for up to 2 more weeks if application is <10% of body surface area; use with caution; maximum dose: 50 mL/week (see Additional Information)

Spray: Apply sparingly twice daily for up to 2 weeks; if response is not adequate, may be used for up to 2 more weeks, but use should be limited to skin lesions that have not sufficiently improved; maximum dose: 50 g (59 mL) per week

Administration

Topical: All products: Apply sparingly to clean dry skin of affected area, gently rub in until disappears; do not use on open skin; do not apply to face, underarms, or groin area; avoid contact with eyes and lips; do not occlude affected area; wash hands after applying

Foam: Turn can upside down and spray a small amount (maximum: 1 ½ capful or about the size of a golf ball) of foam into the cap, other cool surface, or to affected area. If the can is warm or foam is runny, place can under cold, running water. If fingers are warm, rinse with cool water and dry prior to handling (foam will melt on contact with warm skin). Massage foam into affected area.

Monitoring Parameters Assess HPA axis suppression in patients using potent topical steroids applied to a large surface area or to areas under occlusion (eg, ACTH stimulation test, morning plasma cortisol test, urinary free cortisol test)

Patient Information Avoid contact with eyes and lips; do not apply to face, underarms, or groin area; do not bandage, cover, or wrap affected area unless directed by physician; wash hands after applying. Use only as prescribed and for the minimum amount of time required; do not use for longer than directed; notify physician if condition being treated persists or worsens; inform physician of use if surgery is to be considered.

Additional Information Considered to be a super high potency topical corticosteroid; clobetasol is a prednisolone analog with a high level of glucocorticoid activity and slight degree of mineralocorticoid activity. Nine of 14 pediatric patients (12-17 years of age) with moderate to severe atopic dermatitis (involving ≥20% BSA), who were treated with clobetasol lotion 0.05% twice daily for 2 weeks, developed adrenal suppression (versus 2 of 10 patients treated with the cream). Due to this high incidence of adrenal suppression, the lotion is not approved for this indication in children <18 years of age.

Dosage Forms Excipient information presented when available (limited, particularly for generics); consult specific product labeling.

Cream, as propionate: 0.05% (15 g, 30 g, 45 g, 60 g)
- Cormax®: 0.05% (30 g)
- Temovate®: 0.05% (30 g, 60 g)

Cream, as propionate [in emollient base]: 0.05% (15 g, 30 g, 60 g)
- Temovate E®: 0.05% (60 g)

Foam, topical, as propionate:
- Olux®: 0.05% (50 g, 100 g) [contains ethanol 60%]
- Olux-E™: 0.05% (50 g, 100 g)

Gel, as propionate: 0.05% (15 g, 30 g, 60 g)
- Clobevate®: 0.05% (45 g)
- Temovate®: 0.05% (60 g)

Lotion, as propionate:
- Clobex®: 0.05% (30 mL, 59 mL)

Ointment, as propionate: 0.05% (15 g, 30 g, 45 g, 60 g)
- Cormax®: 0.05% (15 g, 45 g)
- Temovate®: 0.05% (15 g, 30 g)

Shampoo, as propionate:
- Clobex®: 0.05% (120 mL) [contains alcohol]

Solution, topical, as propionate [for scalp application]: 0.05% (25 mL, 50 mL)
- Cormax®: 0.05% (25 mL, 50 mL) [contains isopropyl alcohol 40%]
- Temovate®: 0.05% (50 mL) [contains isopropyl alcohol 40%]

Solution, topical, as propionate [spray]:
- Clobex®: 0.05% (60 mL, 125 mL) [contains alcohol]

♦ **Clobetasol Propionate** *see* Clobetasol *on page 383*
♦ **Clobevate®** *see* Clobetasol *on page 383*
♦ **Clobex®** *see* Clobetasol *on page 383*

Clofarabine (klo FARE a been)

Medication Safety Issues

High alert medication: The Institute for Safe Medication Practices (ISMP) includes this medication among its list of drugs which have a heightened risk of causing significant patient harm when used in error.

U.S. Brand Names Clolar™

Index Terms Clofarex; NSC606869

Therapeutic Category Antineoplastic Agent, Antimetabolite (Purine Antagonist)

Generic Available No

Use Treatment of pediatric patients (1-21 years of age) with relapsed or refractory acute lymphoblastic leukemia after at least two prior treatment regimens

Pregnancy Risk Factor D

Lactation Excretion in breast milk unknown/not recommended

Contraindications Hypersensitivity to clofarabine or any component

(Continued)

Clofarabine *(Continued)*

Warnings The FDA currently recommends that procedures for proper handling and disposal of antineoplastic agents be considered. May cause fetal harm when administered to a pregnant woman (women of childbearing potential should be advised to avoid becoming pregnant while on clofarabine). Bone marrow suppression (appears to be dose dependent and reversible) increases the risk of infection. Tumor lysis syndrome and cytokine release may develop into systemic inflammatory response syndrome (SIRS)/capillary leak syndrome, and organ dysfunction. Discontinue clofarabine if SIRS, capillary leak syndrome, or hypotension occurs. If hypotension resolves without pharmacological intervention, clofarabine can be restarted at a lower dose.

I.V. fluids should be administered throughout the 5 days of clofarabine administration; administer allopurinol if hyperuricemia is expected.

Precautions Safety and efficacy have not been established with renal or hepatic impairment; use with caution. Avoid concomitant use of nephrotoxic or hepatotoxic drugs.

Adverse Reactions

Cardiovascular: Hypotension, capillary leak syndrome, tachycardia, flushing, pericardial effusion

Central nervous system: Dizziness, lightheadedness, fainting spells, fatigue, fever, headache

Dermatologic: Rash, erythema, pruritus, palmar-plantar erythrodysesthesia syndrome

Endocrine & metabolic: Tumor lysis syndrome, hyperuricemia

Gastrointestinal: Vomiting, diarrhea, nausea, abdominal pain, anorexia

Hematologic: Neutropenia, anemia, thrombocytopenia, leukopenia

Hepatic: Hyperbilirubinemia, elevated liver enzymes, jaundice, hepatomegaly

Renal: Hematuria, elevated serum creatinine

Respiratory: Tachypnea, respiratory distress, pulmonary edema, cough

Miscellaneous: Sepsis, systemic inflammatory response syndrome

Stability Store undiluted drug at room temperature; diluted solution is stable for 24 hours at room temperature. To prevent drug incompatibilities, do not mix with other medications.

Mechanism of Action Clofarabine, a purine nucleoside analog is metabolized to clofarabine 5'-triphosphate which competes with deoxyadenosine triphosphate for binding to ribonucleotide reductase and DNA polymerase. Clofarabine inhibits DNA synthesis, terminates DNA chain elongation, and inhibits DNA repair resulting in decreased cell replication and repair. Clofarabine disrupts the mitochondrial membrane which results in the release of proteins, cytochrome C and apoptosis-inducing factor leading to cell death.

Pharmacokinetics

Distribution: V_d: 172 L/m^2

Protein binding: 47%

Metabolism: Intracellularly by deoxycytidine kinase and mono- and di-phosphokinases to active metabolite clofarabine 5'-triphosphate

Half-life: 5.2 hours

Elimination: 49% to 60% excreted in urine as unchanged drug

Clearance: 28.8 L/hour/m^2

Usual Dosage I.V. infusion:

Children 1-21 years of age: 52 mg/m^2/day once daily for 5 days; repeat dosing schedule every 2-6 weeks following recovery or return to baseline organ function

Adults: Refractory and/or relapsed hematologic malignancy: 40 mg/m^2/day for 5 days every 28 days

Administration Parenteral: I.V. infusion: Filter clofarabine through a 0.2 µm syringe filter and then further dilute dose with D_5W or NS; administer by I.V. infusion over 2 hours

Monitoring Parameters Renal and hepatic function tests, blood pressure, cardiac function, respiratory status, CBC with differential, platelet count, urine output

Patient Information Female patients of childbearing potential should avoid pregnancy during clofarabine therapy by using effective forms of contraception; avoid breast-feeding during treatment

Nursing Implications Ensure adequate hydration by giving continuous I.V. fluids throughout the 5 days of clofarabine administration to prevent tumor lysis and other adverse effects.

Additional Information Use of prophylactic steroids (eg, hydrocortisone 100 mg/m^2 on days 1 through 3 of each cycle) may prevent signs or symptoms of SIRS or capillary leak syndrome.

Dosage Forms Excipient information presented when available (limited, particularly for generics); consult specific product labeling.

Injection, solution [preservative free]: 1 mg/mL (20 mL)

References

Jeha S, Gandhi V, Chan KW, et al, "Clofarabine, a Novel Nucleoside Analog, Is Active in Pediatric Patients With Advanced Leukemia," *Blood*, 2004, 103(3):784-9.

- **Clofarex** *see* Clofarabine *on page 385*
- **Clolar™** *see* Clofarabine *on page 385*
- **Clonapam (Can)** *see* Clonazepam *on page 387*

Clonazepam (kloe NA ze pam)

Medication Safety Issues

Sound-alike/look-alike issues:

Clonazepam may be confused with clofazimine, clonidine, clorazepate, clozapine, lorazepam

Klonopin® may be confused with clofazimine, clonidine, clorazepate, clozapine, lorazepam

Related Information

Antiepileptic Drugs *on page 1902*

Overdose and Toxicology *on page 1916*

U.S. Brand Names Klonopin®

Canadian Brand Names Alti-Clonazepam; Apo-Clonazepam®; Clonapam; CO Clonazepam; Gen-Clonazepam; Klonopin®; Novo-Clonazepam; Nu-Clonazepam; PMS-Clonazepam; Rho®-Clonazepam; Rivotril®; Sandoz-Clonazepam

Therapeutic Category Anticonvulsant, Benzodiazepine; Benzodiazepine

Generic Available Yes

Use Alone or as an adjunct in the treatment of absence (petit mal), petit mal variant (Lennox-Gastaut), infantile spasms, akinetic, and myoclonic seizures; panic disorder with or without agoraphobia

Restrictions C-IV

Pregnancy Risk Factor D

Lactation Enters breast milk/not recommended

Contraindications Hypersensitivity to clonazepam, any component, or other benzodiazepines; severe liver disease, acute narrow-angle glaucoma

Precautions Use with caution in patients with chronic respiratory disease, hepatic disease, or impaired renal function; abrupt discontinuance may precipitate withdrawal symptoms, status epilepticus or seizures (withdraw gradually when discontinuing therapy; see Additional Information); worsening of seizures may occur when clonazepam is added to patients with multiple seizure types

Adverse Reactions

Cardiovascular: Hypotension

Central nervous system: Drowsiness, changes in behavior or personality, aggression, vertigo, confusion, depression, memory impairment, decreased concentration, headache, ataxia, hypotonia

Dermatologic: Rash

Gastrointestinal: Nausea, xerostomia, vomiting, diarrhea, constipation, anorexia, hypersalivation

Hematologic: Thrombocytopenia, anemia, leukopenia, eosinophilia

Neuromuscular & skeletal: Tremor, choreiform movements

Ocular: Nystagmus, blurred vision

Respiratory: Bronchial hypersecretion, respiratory depression

Miscellaneous: Physical and psychological dependence

Drug Interactions Cytochrome P450 isoenzyme CYP3A3/4 substrate

CNS depressants or alcohol increase sedation; phenytoin, carbamazepine, rifampin, or barbiturates increase clonazepam clearance; drugs that inhibit cytochrome P450 isoenzyme CYP3A3/4 may increase levels and effects of clonazepam (monitor for altered benzodiazepine response); concurrent use with valproic acid may result in absence status; propantheline may decrease clonazepam serum concentrations

Stability Store at 25°C (77°F); excursions permitted to 15°C to 30°C (59°F to 80°F)

Mechanism of Action Suppresses the spike-and-wave discharge in absence seizures by depressing nerve transmission in the motor cortex; depresses all levels of the CNS, including the limbic and reticular formation, by binding to the benzodiazepine site on the gamma-aminobutyric acid (GABA) receptor complex and modulating GABA, which is a major inhibitory neurotransmitter in the brain

Pharmacodynamics

Onset of action: 20-60 minutes

Duration:

Infants and young children: Up to 6-8 hours

Adults: Up to 12 hours

Pharmacokinetics

Absorption: Oral: Well absorbed

(Continued)

Clonazepam *(Continued)*

Distribution: V_d: Adults: 1.5-4.4 L/kg
Protein binding: 85%
Metabolism: Extensively metabolized in the liver; undergoes nitroreduction to 7-aminoclonazepam, followed by acetylation to 7-acetamidoclonazepam; nitroreduction and acetylation are via cytochrome P450 enzyme system; metabolites undergo glucuronide and sulfate conjugation
Bioavailability: 90%
Half-life:
Children: 22-33 hours
Adults: Usual: 30-40 hours; range: 19-50 hours
Elimination: Metabolites excreted as glucuronide or sulfate conjugates; <2% excreted unchanged in urine

Usual Dosage Oral:
Seizure disorders:
Infants and Children <10 years or 30 kg:
Initial daily dose: 0.01-0.03 mg/kg/day (maximum initial dose: 0.05 mg/kg/day) given in 2-3 divided doses; increase by no more than 0.5 mg every third day until seizures are controlled or adverse effects seen
Maintenance dose: 0.1-0.2 mg/kg/day divided 3 times/day; not to exceed 0.2 mg/kg/day
Children ≥10 years (>30 kg) and Adults:
Initial daily dose not to exceed 1.5 mg given in 3 divided doses; may increase by 0.5-1 mg every third day until seizures are controlled or adverse effects seen
Maintenance dose: 0.05-0.2 mg/kg/day; do not exceed 20 mg/day
Panic disorder: Adolescents ≥18 years and Adults: Initial: 0.25 mg twice daily; increase in increments of 0.125-0.25 mg twice daily every 3 days; target dose: 1 mg/day; maximum dose: 4 mg/day

Administration
Oral: May administer with food or water to decrease GI distress
Orally-disintegrating tablet: Open pouch and peel back foil on the blister; do not push tablet through foil. Use dry hands to remove tablet and place in mouth. May be swallowed with or without water. Use immediately after removing from package.

Monitoring Parameters Long-term use: CBC with differential, platelets, liver enzymes

Reference Range Relationship between serum concentration and seizure control is not well established; measurement at random times postdose may contribute to this problem; predose concentrations are recommended
Proposed therapeutic levels: 20-80 ng/mL
Potentially toxic concentration: >80 ng/mL

Patient Information Avoid alcohol; limit caffeine; may cause drowsiness and impair ability to perform activities requiring mental alertness or physical coordination; may be habit-forming; avoid abrupt discontinuation after prolonged use; may cause dry mouth

Additional Information Ethosuximide or valproic acid may be preferred for treatment of absence (petit mal) seizures. Clonazepam-induced behavioral disturbances may be more frequent in mentally handicapped patients. When discontinuing therapy in children, the clonazepam dose may be safely reduced by ≤0.04 mg/kg/week and discontinued when the daily dose is ≤0.04 mg/kg/day. When discontinuing therapy in adults treated for panic disorder, the clonazepam dose may be decreased by 0.125 mg twice daily every 3 days, until the drug is completely withdrawn. Treatment of panic disorder for >9 weeks has not been studied; long-term usefulness of clonazepam for the treatment of panic disorder should be re-evaluated periodically.

Dosage Forms Excipient information presented when available (limited, particularly for generics); consult specific product labeling.
Tablet: 0.5 mg, 1 mg, 2 mg
Tablet, orally disintegrating [wafer]: 0.125 mg, 0.25 mg, 0.5 mg, 1 mg, 2 mg

Extemporaneous Preparations A 0.1 mg/mL oral liquid can be made using 3 different vehicles (cherry syrup; a 1:1 mixture of Ora-Sweet® and Ora-Plus®; or a 1:1 mixture of Ora-Sweet® SF and Ora-Plus®); crush six 2 mg tablets into a fine powder in a mortar; add 10 mL of the vehicle and mix to make a uniform paste; mix while adding the vehicle in geometric portions to **almost** 120 mL; transfer to a calibrated bottle and qsad with vehicle to 120 mL; preparation is stable for 60 days when stored in amber prescription bottles in the dark at room temperature (25°C) or under refrigeration (5°C); label "shake well" and "protect from light"

Allen LV and Erickson MA, "Stability of Acetazolamide, Allopurinol, Azathioprine, Clonazepam, and Flucytosine in Extemporaneously Compounded Oral Liquids," *Am J Health Syst Pharm*, 1996, 53(16):1944-9.

References

Sugai K, "Seizures With Clonazepam: Discontinuation and Suggestions for Safe Discontinuation Rates in Children," *Epilepsia*, 1993, 34(6):1089-97.
Walson PD and Edge JH, "Clonazepam Disposition in Pediatric Patients," *Ther Drug Monit*, 1996, 18(1):1-5.

Clonidine (KLOE ni deen)

Medication Safety Issues

Sound-alike/look-alike issues:

Clonidine may be confused with Clomid®, clomiPHENE, clonazepam, clozapine, Klonopin™, quinidine

Catapres® may be confused with Cataflam®, Cetapred®, Combipres®

Transdermal patch may contain conducting metal (eg, aluminum); remove patch prior to MRI.

Related Information

Antihypertensive Agents by Class *on page 1678*

U.S. Brand Names Catapres®; Catapres-TTS®; Duraclon™

Canadian Brand Names Apo-Clonidine®; Carapres®; Dixarit®; Novo-Clonidine; Nu-Clonidine

Index Terms Clonidine Hydrochloride

Therapeutic Category Adrenergic Agonist Agent; Alpha-Adrenergic Agonist; Analgesic, Non-narcotic (Epidural); Antihypertensive Agent

Generic Available Yes: Tablet

Use Management of hypertension; aid in the diagnosis of pheochromocytoma and growth hormone deficiency; used for heroin withdrawal and smoking cessation therapy in adults; alternate agent for the treatment of attention-deficit/hyperactivity disorder (ADHD); adjunct in the treatment of neuropathic pain; epidural form is used in combination with opiates for relief of severe pain in cancer patients whose pain was not relieved by opiates alone

Pregnancy Risk Factor C

Lactation Enters breast milk/not recommended

Contraindications Hypersensitivity to clonidine hydrochloride or any component; epidural injection is contraindicated in patients receiving anticoagulation therapy and in patients with a bleeding diathesis or an infection at the injection site. Administration of epidural clonidine above the C_4 dermatome is contraindicated.

Warnings Do not abruptly discontinue as rapid increase in blood pressure and symptoms of sympathetic overactivity (such as increased heart rate, tremors, agitation, anxiety, insomnia, sweating, palpitations) may occur; if need to discontinue, taper dose gradually over more than 1 week. EKG abnormalities and 4 cases of sudden cardiac death have been reported in children receiving clonidine with methylphenidate; reduce dose of methylphenidate by 40% when used concurrently with clonidine; consider EKG monitoring. Epidural clonidine is not recommended for perioperative, obstetrical, or postpartum pain [due to the risk of hemodynamic instability (hypotension, bradycardia)], in patients with severe cardiovascular disease, or those who are hemodynamically unstable.

Precautions Dosage modification is required in patients with renal impairment; use with caution in cerebrovascular disease, coronary insufficiency, renal impairment, sinus node dysfunction; monitor patients for signs of depression (especially those with a history of affective disorders)

Adverse Reactions

Cardiovascular: Raynaud's phenomenon, hypotension, bradycardia, palpitations, tachycardia, CHF, rebound hypertension if discontinued abruptly

Central nervous system: Drowsiness, sedation, headache, dizziness, fatigue, insomnia, anxiety, depression

Dermatologic: Rash, local skin reactions with patch

Endocrine & metabolic: Sodium and water retention, parotid pain

Gastrointestinal: Constipation, anorexia, xerostomia

Respiratory: Respiratory depression and ventilatory abnormalities with high epidural doses

Drug Interactions Use with methylphenidate may potentially increase EKG effects (see Warnings); tricyclic antidepressants antagonize hypotensive effects of clonidine; beta-blockers may potentiate bradycardia in patients receiving clonidine and may increase the rebound hypertension seen with clonidine withdrawal; discontinue beta-blocker several days before clonidine is tapered off; CNS depressants and alcohol may increase sedative effects; use with opiates may increase hypotension; epidural clonidine may prolong the effects of epidural local anesthetics

Food Interactions Avoid natural licorice (causes sodium and water retention and increases potassium loss)

Stability Epidural injection: Discard unused portion of vial (injection is preservative free); do not use with preservative

(Continued)

Clonidine *(Continued)*

Mechanism of Action Stimulates $alpha_2$-adrenoreceptors in the brain stem, thus activating an inhibitory neuron, resulting in reduced sympathetic outflow, producing a decrease in vasomotor tone and heart rate

Epidural use: Prevents pain signal transmission to the brain and produces analgesia at presynaptic and postjunctional $alpha_2$-adrenoreceptors in the spinal cord

Pharmacodynamics Antihypertensive effects: Oral:
Onset of action: 30-60 minutes
Maximum effect: Within 2-4 hours
Duration: 6-10 hours

Pharmacokinetics
Distribution: V_d: Adults: 2.1 L/kg
Protein binding: 20% to 40%
Metabolism: Hepatic to inactive metabolites
Bioavailability, oral: 75% to 95%
Half-life, serum:
Neonates: 44-72 hours
Children: 8-12 hours
Adults:
Normal renal function: 6-20 hours
Renal impairment: 18-41 hours
Half-life, CSF: Adults: 1.3 ± 0.5 hours
Elimination: 65% excreted in urine (32% unchanged) and 22% excreted in feces via enterohepatic recirculation
Dialysis: Not dialyzable (0% to 5%)

Usual Dosage
Children:
Hypertension: Oral: Initial: 5-10 mcg/kg/day in divided doses every 8-12 hours; increase gradually, if needed, to 5-25 mcg/kg/day in divided doses every 6 hours; maximum dose: 0.9 mg/day
ADHD: Oral: Initial: 0.05 mg/day, increase every 3-7 days by 0.05 mg/day to 3-5 mcg/kg/day given in divided doses 3-4 times/day; usual maximum dose: 0.3-0.4 mg/day. **Note:** Some centers use doses as high as 8 mcg/kg/day or 0.5 mg/day (see Hunt, 1990).
Clonidine tolerance test (test of growth hormone release from the pituitary): Oral: 0.15 mg/m^2 or 4 mcg/kg as a single dose
Analgesia: Epidural (continuous infusion): Reserved for cancer patients with severe intractable pain, unresponsive to other analgesics or epidural or spinal opiates: Initial: 0.5 mcg/kg/hour; adjust with caution, based on clinical effect; usual range: 0.5-2 mcg/kg/hour; do not exceed adult doses
Neuropathic pain: Oral: Some centers use the following doses (see Galloway, 2000): Initial: 2 mcg/kg/dose every 4-6 hours; increase incrementally over several days; range: 2-4 mcg/kg/dose every 4-6 hours; may also be given as transdermal (see Transdermal)
Transdermal: Children may be switched to the transdermal delivery system after oral therapy is titrated to an optimal and stable dose; a transdermal dose approximately equivalent to the total oral daily dose may be used (see Hunt, 1990; see Administration)

Adults:
Hypertension:
Oral: Initial dose: 0.1 mg twice daily, usual maintenance dose: 0.2-1.2 mg/day in 2-4 divided doses; maximum recommended dose: 2.4 mg/day; usual dosage range (JNC 7): 0.1-0.8 mg/day in 2 divided doses
Transdermal: Applied once weekly as transdermal delivery system; begin therapy with 0.1 mg/day patch applied once every 7 days; increase by 0.1 mg/day at 1-2 week intervals based on response; hypotensive action may not begin until 2-3 days after initial application; doses >0.6 mg/day do not improve efficacy; usual dosage range (JNC 7): 0.1-0.3 mg/day patch applied once weekly
Analgesia: Epidural (continuous infusion): Initial: 30 mcg/hour; titrate to clinical effect; usual maximum dose: 40 mcg/hour

Administration
Epidural: Dilute the 500 mcg/mL product with preservative free NS to a final concentration of 100 mcg/mL prior to use; visually inspect for particulate matter and discoloration prior to administration (whenever permitted by container and solution)
Oral: May be administered without regard to meals
Transdermal: Patches should be applied at bedtime to a clean, hairless area of the upper arm or chest; rotate patch sites weekly in adults; in children, the patch may need to be changed more frequently (eg, every 3-5 days); **Note:** Transdermal patch is a membrane-controlled system; do **not** cut the patch to deliver partial doses; rate of drug delivery, reservoir contents, and adhesion may be affected if cut; if partial

dose is needed, surface area of patch can be blocked proportionally using adhesive bandage (see Lee, 1997)

Monitoring Parameters Blood pressure, heart rate; consider EKG monitoring in patients with history of heart disease or concurrent use of medications affecting cardiac conduction; with epidural administration: Blood pressure, heart rate; pulse oximetry with large bolus doses; monitor infusion pump and catheter tubing for obstruction or dislodgment throughout the course of therapy to decrease risk of inadvertent abrupt discontinuation

Patient Information Avoid alcohol; may cause drowsiness and impair ability to perform activities requiring mental alertness or physical coordination; do not stop drug abruptly; may cause dry mouth

Nursing Implications Counsel patient/parent about compliance and danger of withdrawal reaction if doses are missed or drug is discontinued

Additional Information Epidural clonidine may be more effective in the treatment of neuropathic pain compared to somatic or visceral pain; clonidine-induced symptomatic bradycardia may be treated with atropine

Dosage Forms Excipient information presented when available (limited, particularly for generics); consult specific product labeling.

Injection, epidural solution, as hydrochloride [preservative free] (Duraclon™): 100 mcg/mL (10 mL); 500 mcg/mL (10 mL)

Patch, transdermal [once-weekly patch]:

Catapres-TTS®-1: 0.1 mg/24 hours (4s)

Catapres-TTS®-2: 0.2 mg/24 hours (4s)

Catapres-TTS®-3: 0.3 mg/24 hours (4s)

Tablet, as hydrochloride (Catapres®): 0.1 mg, 0.2 mg, 0.3 mg

Extemporaneous Preparations A 0.1 mg/mL oral suspension compounded from tablets is stable for 28 days when stored in amber glass bottles and refrigerated (4°C); thirty 0.2 mg tablets are crushed in a glass mortar and ground to a fine powder; 2 mL Purified Water USP is slowly added, and triturated to make a fine paste; Simple Syrup, NF is slowly added in 15 mL increments and triturated; qsad 60 mL; shake well before use

Levinson ML and Johnson CE, "Stability of an Extemporaneously Compounded Clonidine Hydrochloride Oral Liquid," *Am J Hosp Pharm*, 1992, 49(1):122-5.

References

Chobanian AV, Bakris GL, Black HR, et al, "The Seventh Report of the Joint National Committee on Prevention, Detection, Evaluation, and Treatment of High Blood Pressure: The JNC 7 report," *JAMA*, 2003, 289(19):2560-72.

Chafin CC, Hovinga CA,and Phelps SJ, "Clonidine in the Treatment of Attention Deficit Hyperactivity Disorder," *Journal of Pediatric Pharmacy Practice*, 1999, 4(6):308-15.

Galloway KS and Yaster M, "Pain and Symptom Control in Terminally Ill Children," *Pediatr Clin North Am*, 2000, 47(3):711-46.

Hart-Santora D and Hart LL, "Clonidine in Attention Deficit Hyperactivity Disorder," *Ann Pharmacother*, 1992, 26(1):37-9.

Hunt RD, Capper L, and O'Connell P, "Clonidine in Child and Adolescent Psychiatry," *J Child Adol Psychpharm*, 1990, 1(1):87-102.

Hunt RD, Minderaa RB, and Cohen DJ, "The Therapeutic Effect of Clonidine in Attention Deficit Disorder With Hyperactivity: A Comparison With Placebo and Methylphenidate," *Psychopharmacol Bull*, 1986, 22(1):229-35.

Lee NA and Anderson PO, "Giving Partial Doses of Transdermal Patches," *Am J Health Syst Pharm*, 1997, 54(15):1759-60.

Rocchini AP, "Childhood Hypertension: Etiology, Diagnosis, and Treatment," *Pediatr Clin North Am*, 1984, 31(6):1259-73.

Sinaiko AR, "Pharmacologic Management of Childhood Hypertension," *Pediatr Clin North Am*, 1993, 40(1):195-212.

♦ **Clonidine Hydrochloride** *see* Clonidine *on page 389*

Clorazepate (klor AZ e pate)

Medication Safety Issues

Sound-alike/look-alike issues:

Clorazepate may be confused with clofibrate, clonazepam

Related Information

Overdose and Toxicology *on page 1916*

U.S. Brand Names Tranxene® SD™; Tranxene® SD™-Half Strength; Tranxene® T-Tab®

Canadian Brand Names Apo-Clorazepate®; Novo-Clopate

Index Terms Clorazepate Dipotassium; Tranxene T-Tab®

Therapeutic Category Anticonvulsant, Benzodiazepine; Benzodiazepine; Sedative

Generic Available Yes

Use Treatment of generalized anxiety and panic disorders; management of alcohol withdrawal; adjunct anticonvulsant in management of partial seizures

Restrictions C-IV

Pregnancy Risk Factor D

(Continued)

Clorazepate *(Continued)*

Lactation Excretion in breast milk unknown/not recommended

Contraindications Hypersensitivity to clorazepate dipotassium or any component; cross-sensitivity with other benzodiazepines may exist; avoid using in patients with pre-existing CNS depression, severe uncontrolled pain, or narrow-angle glaucoma

Warnings Abrupt discontinuation may cause withdrawal symptoms or seizures

Precautions Use with caution in patients with hepatic or renal disease

Adverse Reactions

Cardiovascular: Hypotension

Central nervous system: Drowsiness, dizziness, confusion, amnesia, nervousness, headache, depression, ataxia, insomnia, fatigue, irritability, slurred speech

Dermatologic: Rash

Gastrointestinal: Nausea, xerostomia

Hematologic: Reduced hematocrit (with long-term use)

Neuromuscular & skeletal: Tremor

Ocular: Blurred vision, diplopia

Miscellaneous: Physical and psychological dependence with long-term use; long-term use may also be associated with renal or hepatic injury

Drug Interactions Cytochrome P450 isoenzyme CYP3A3/4 substrate

Cimetidine or other hepatic enzyme inhibitors may decrease hepatic clearance, monitor for altered benzodiazepine response; concurrent use of clorazepate with ritonavir is not recommended

Stability Unstable in water

Mechanism of Action Depresses all levels of the CNS, including the limbic and reticular formation, by binding to the benzodiazepine site on the gamma-aminobutyric acid (GABA) receptor complex and modulating GABA, which is a major inhibitory neurotransmitter in the brain

Pharmacokinetics

Absorption: Rapidly decarboxylated to desmethyldiazepam (active) in acidic stomach prior to absorption

Distribution: Crosses the placenta

Metabolism: In the liver to oxazepam (active)

Half-life, adults:

Desmethyldiazepam: 48-96 hours

Oxazepam: 6-8 hours

Time to peak serum concentration: Oral: Within 1 hour

Elimination: Primarily in urine

Usual Dosage Oral:

Anticonvulsant:

Children: Initial dose: 0.3 mg/kg/day; maintenance dose: 0.5-3 mg/kg/day divided 2-4 times/day

or

Children 9-12 years: Initial: 3.75-7.5 mg/dose twice daily; increase dose by 3.75 mg at weekly intervals, not to exceed 60 mg/day in 2-3 divided doses

Children >12 years and Adults: Initial: Up to 7.5 mg/dose 2-3 times/day; increase dose by 7.5 mg at weekly intervals; usual dose: 0.5-1 mg/kg/day; not to exceed 90 mg/day

Anxiety: Adults: 7.5-15 mg 2-4 times/day, or given as single dose of 15-22.5 mg at bedtime

Alcohol withdrawal: Adults: Initial: 30 mg, then 15 mg 2-4 times/day on first day; maximum daily dose: 90 mg; gradually decrease dose over subsequent days

Administration Oral: May administer with food or water to decrease GI upset

Monitoring Parameters Excessive CNS depression, respiratory rate, and cardiovascular status; with prolonged use: CBC, liver enzymes, renal function

Reference Range Therapeutic: 0.12-1 mcg/mL (SI: 0.36-3.01 micromoles/L)

Patient Information Avoid alcohol; may cause drowsiness and impair ability to perform activities requiring mental alertness or physical coordination; may be habit-forming; avoid abrupt discontinuation after prolonged use; may cause dry mouth

Dosage Forms Excipient information presented when available (limited, particularly for generics); consult specific product labeling.

Tablet, as dipotassium: 3.75 mg, 7.5 mg, 15 mg

Tranxene® SD™: 22.5 mg [once daily]

Tranxene® SD™-Half Strength: 11.25 mg [once daily]

Tranxene® T-Tab®: 3.75 mg, 7.5 mg, 15 mg

References

Fenichel GM, *Clinical Pediatric Neurology: A Signs and Symptoms Approach*, 2nd ed, Philadelphia, PA: WB Saunders Co, 1993.

Fujii T, Okuno T, Go T, et al, "Clorazepate Therapy for Intractable Epilepsy," *Brain Dev*, 1987, 9(3):288-91.

Mimaki T, Tagawa T, Ono J, et al, "Antiepileptic Effect and Serum Levels of Clorazepate on Children With Refractory Seizures," *Brain Dev*, 1984, 6(6):539-44.

♦ **Clorazepate Dipotassium** *see* Clorazepate *on page 391*
♦ ***Clostridium botulinum* Toxin Type B** *see* Botulinum Toxin Type B *on page 229*
♦ **Clotrimaderm (Can)** *see* Clotrimazole *on page 393*

Clotrimazole (kloe TRIM a zole)

Medication Safety Issues

Sound-alike/look-alike issues:

Clotrimazole may be confused with co-trimoxazole
Lotrimin® may be confused with Lotrisone®, Otrivin®
Mycelex® may be confused with Myoflex®

International issues:

Cloderm®: Brand name for clocortolone in the United States
Canesten® [multiple international markets] may be confused with Cenestin® which is a brand name for estrogens (conjugated a/synthetic) in the U.S.
Canesten® [multiple international markets]: Brand name for fluconazole in Great Britain
Mycelex® may be confused with Mucolex® which is a brand name for carbocysteine in Ireland, Portugal, and Thailand; a brand name for guaifenesin in Hong Kong

U.S. Brand Names Cruex® Cream [OTC]; Gyne-Lotrimin® 3 [OTC]; Lotrimin® AF Athlete's Foot Cream [OTC]; Lotrimin® AF Athlete's Foot Solution [OTC]; Lotrimin® AF Jock Itch Cream [OTC]; Mycelex®; Mycelex®-7 [OTC]; Mycelex® Twin Pack [OTC]

Canadian Brand Names Canesten® Topical; Canesten® Vaginal; Clotrimaderm; Trivagizole-3®

Therapeutic Category Antifungal Agent, Oral Nonabsorbed; Antifungal Agent, Topical; Antifungal Agent, Vaginal

Generic Available Yes: Cream, solution, troche

Use Treatment of susceptible fungal infections, including oropharyngeal candidiasis, dermatophytoses, superficial mycoses, cutaneous candidiasis, as well as vulvovaginal candidiasis; limited data suggests that the use of clotrimazole troches may be effective for prophylaxis against oropharyngeal candidiasis in neutropenic patients

Pregnancy Risk Factor B (topical); C (troches)

Lactation Excretion in breast milk unknown

Contraindications Hypersensitivity to clotrimazole or any component

Warnings Clotrimazole troches should not be used for treatment of systemic fungal infection

Precautions Safety and effectiveness of clotrimazole lozenges (troches) in children <3 years of age have not been established

Adverse Reactions

Dermatologic: Erythema, pruritus, urticaria, skin fissures, blistering
Gastrointestinal: Nausea and vomiting may occur in patients on clotrimazole troches; lower abdominal cramps may occur in patients receiving clotrimazole vaginal tablets
Hepatic: Abnormal liver function tests (causal relationship between troches and elevated LFTs not clearly established)
Local: Mild burning, irritation, stinging of skin or vaginal area

Mechanism of Action Binds to phospholipids in the fungal cell membrane altering cell wall permeability resulting in loss of essential intracellular elements

Pharmacokinetics

Absorption: Negligible through intact skin when administered topically; 3% to 10% of an intravaginal dose is absorbed
Distribution: Following oral/topical administration, clotrimazole is present in saliva for up to 3 hours following 30 minutes of dissolution time in the mouth

Usual Dosage

Children >3 years and Adults:
Topical/Oral: 10 mg troche dissolved slowly 5 times/day
Topical: Apply twice daily

Children >12 years and Adults: Vaginal: 100 mg/day at bedtime for 7 days or 200 mg/day at bedtime for 3 days or 500 mg single dose; or 5 g (= 1 applicatorful) of 1% vaginal cream daily at bedtime for 7-14 days

Administration

Oral: Dissolve lozenge (troche) in mouth over 15-30 minutes
Topical: Apply sparingly and rub gently into the cleansed, affected area and surrounding skin; do not apply to the eye
Vaginal: Wash hands before using. Insert full applicator into vagina gently and expel cream, or insert tablet into vagina. Wash applicator with soap and water following use. Remain lying down for 30 minutes following administration.

Monitoring Parameters Periodic liver function tests during oral therapy with clotrimazole lozenges

(Continued)

Clotrimazole *(Continued)*

Patient Information Vaginal cream and tablet are oil-based and may weaken latex condoms and diaphragms; avoid intercourse during therapy. Do not use tampons until therapy is complete.

Dosage Forms Excipient information presented when available (limited, particularly for generics); consult specific product labeling.

Combination pack (Mycelex®-7): Vaginal tablet 100 mg (7s) and vaginal cream 1% (7 g)

Cream, topical: 1% (15 g, 30 g, 45 g)

Cruex®: 1% (15 g)

Lotrimin® AF Athlete's Foot: 1% (12 g, 24 g)

Lotrimin® AF Jock Itch: 1% (12 g)

Cream, vaginal: 2% (21 g)

Mycelex®-7: 1% (45 g)

Solution, topical: 1% (10 mL, 30 mL)

Lotrimin® AF Athlete's Foot: 1% (10 mL)

Tablet, vaginal (Gyne-Lotrimin® 3): 200 mg (3s)

Troche (Mycelex®): 10 mg

♦ **CMA-676** *see* Gemtuzumab Ozogamicin *on page 723*

♦ **CMV-IGIV** *see* Cytomegalovirus Immune Globulin (Intravenous-Human) *on page 431*

♦ **Coagulant Complex Inhibitor** *see* Anti-inhibitor Coagulant Complex *on page 144*

♦ **Coagulation Factor VIIa** *see* Factor VIIa (Recombinant) *on page 631*

Coal Tar (KOLE tar)

Medication Safety Issues

Sound-alike/look-alike issues:

Pentrax® may be confused with Permax®

Tegrin® may be confused with Tegretol®

U.S. Brand Names Balnetar® [OTC]; Betatar® Gel [OTC]; Cutar® [OTC]; Denorex® Original Therapeutic Strength [OTC]; DHS™ Tar [OTC]; DHS™ Targel [OTC]; Doak® Tar [OTC]; Exorex®; Fototar® [OTC]; Ionil T® [OTC]; Ionil T® Plus [OTC]; MG 217® [OTC]; MG 217® Medicated Tar [OTC]; Neutrogena® T/Gel [OTC]; Neutrogena® T/Gel Extra Strength [OTC]; Neutrogena® T/Gel Stubborn Itch Control [OTC]; Oxipor® VHC [OTC]; Polytar® [OTC]; PsoriGel® [OTC] [DSC]; Reme-T™ [OTC]; Tera-Gel™ [OTC]; Zetar® [OTC]

Canadian Brand Names Balnetar®; Estar®; Targel®

Index Terms Crude Coal Tar; LCD; Pix Carbonis

Therapeutic Category Antipsoriatic Agent, Topical; Antiseborrheic Agent, Topical

Generic Available No

Use Topically for controlling dandruff, seborrheic dermatitis, or psoriasis

Contraindications Hypersensitivity to coal tar or any ingredient in the formulation

Warnings Due to a potential carcinogenic risk, do not use around the rectum or in the genital area or groin

Precautions Do not apply to acutely inflamed skin; avoid exposure to sunlight for at least 24 hours

Adverse Reactions Dermatologic: Dermatitis, folliculitis, irritation, acneiform eruption, photosensitivity

Drug Interactions Tetracyclines, phenothiazines, tretinoin, and sulfonamides also have phototoxic potential

Mechanism of Action Reduces the number and size of epidermal cells produced

Usual Dosage Children and Adults: Topical:

Bath: 60-90 mL of a 5% to 20% solution or 15-25 mL of 30% lotion is added to bath water; soak 5-20 minutes, then pat dry; use once daily to once every 3 days

Shampoo: Apply twice weekly for the first 2 weeks then once weekly or more often if needed

Skin: Apply to the affected area 1-4 times/day; decrease frequency to 2-3 times/week once condition has been controlled

Atopic dermatitis: 2% to 5% coal tar cream may be applied once daily or every other day to reduce inflammation

Scalp psoriasis: Tar oil bath or coal tar solution may be painted sparingly to the lesions 3-12 hours before each shampoo

Psoriasis of the body, arms, legs: Apply at bedtime; if thick scales are present, use product with salicylic acid and apply several times during the day

Administration Topical:

Bath: Add appropriate amount of coal tar to lukewarm bath water and mix thoroughly

Shampoo: Rub shampoo onto wet hair and scalp, rinse thoroughly; repeat; leave on 5 minutes; rinse thoroughly

Patient Information Avoid contact with eyes, genital, or rectal area; coal tar preparations frequently stain the skin and hair; shake suspension well before use. May cause photosensitivity reactions (eg, exposure to sunlight may cause severe sunburn, skin rash, redness, or itching); avoid exposure to sunlight and artificial light sources (sunlamps, tanning booth/bed); wear protective clothing, wide-brimmed hats, sunglasses, and lip sunscreen (SPF ≥15); use a sunscreen [broad-spectrum sunscreen or physical sunscreen (preferred) or sunblock with SPF ≥15]; contact physician if reaction occurs.

Dosage Forms Excipient information presented when available (limited, particularly for generics); consult specific product labeling. [DSC] = Discontinued product

Cream:
- Fototar®: Coal tar 2% (85 g, 454 g)

Emulsion, topical:
- Cutar®: Coal tar solution 7.5% (180 mL, 3840 mL)
- Exorex®: Coal tar 1% (240 mL)

Gel, shampoo:
- DHS™ Targel: Coal tar solution 2.9% (240 mL) [equivalent to coal tar 0.5%]

Gel, topical:
- PsoriGel®: Coal tar solution 7.5% (120 g) [DSC]

Liquid:
- Doak® Tar Distillate: Coal tar 40% (60 mL) [for compounding use only]

Lotion, topical:
- MG 217®: Coal tar solution 5% (120 mL) [equivalent to coal tar 1%; contains jojoba]
- Oxipor® VHC: Coal tar solution 25% (60 mL, 120 mL) [equivalent to coal tar 5%; contains alcohol 79%]

Oil, topical:
- Balnetar®: Coal tar 2.5% (225 mL) [for use in bath]
- Doak® Tar: Coal tar distillate 2% (240 mL) [equivalent to coal tar 0.8%; for use in bath]

Ointment, topical:
- MG 217®: Coal tar solution 10% (107 g, 430 g) [equivalent to coal tar 2%]

Shampoo:
- Betatar Gel®: Coal tar solution 5% (240 mL) [equivalent to coal tar 2.5%; green apple scent]
- Denorex® Original Therapeutic Strength: Coal tar solution 12.5% (120 mL, 240 mL, 360 mL) [equivalent to coal tar 2.5%; available with or without conditioner]
- DHS™ Tar: Coal tar solution 2.9% (120 mL, 240 mL, 480 mL) [equivalent to coal tar 0.5%]
- Doak® Tar: Coal tar distillate 3% (240 mL) [equivalent to coal tar 1.2%]
- Ionil T®: Coal tar 1% (240 mL, 480 mL, 960 mL) [DSC]
- Ionil T® Plus: Coal tar 2% (240 mL)
- MG 217® Medicated Tar: Coal tar solution 15% (120 mL, 240 mL) [equivalent to coal tar 3%]
- Neutrogena® T/Gel: Coal tar 0.5% (132 mL, 255 mL, 480 mL)
- Neutrogena® T/Gel Extra Strength: Coal tar extract 4% (132 mL) [coal tar 1%]
- Neutrogena® T/Gel Stubborn Itch Control: Coal tar extract 2% (132 mL) [coal tar 0.5%]
- Pentrax®: Coal tar 5% (240 mL) [DSC]
- Polytar®: Coal tar 0.5% (177 mL)
- Reme-T™: Coal tar 5% (236 mL)
- Tera-Gel™: Solubilized coal tar 0.5% (120 mL, 240 mL)
- Zetar®: Coal tar 1% (180 mL)

Soap (Polytar®): Coal tar 0.5% (113 g)

References

Greaves MW, Weinstein GD, "Treatment of Psoriasis," *N Engl J Med*, 1995, 332(9):581-8.
Hanifin JM, "Atopic Dermatitis in Infants and Children," *Pediatr Clin North Am*, 1991, 38(4):763-89.

♦ **CO Azithromycin (Can)** *see* Azithromycin *on page 191*

Cocaine (koe KANE)

Related Information

Laboratory Detection of Drugs in Urine *on page 1928*

Index Terms Cocaine Hydrochloride

Therapeutic Category Analgesic, Topical; Local Anesthetic, Topical

Generic Available Yes

Use Topical anesthesia for mucous membranes

Restrictions C-II

Pregnancy Risk Factor C (X if nonmedical use)

Lactation Enters breast milk/contraindicated

Contraindications Hypersensitivity to cocaine or any component; systemic use

(Continued)

Cocaine *(Continued)*

Precautions Use with caution in patients with hypertension, severe cardiovascular disease, thyrotoxicosis, and in infants; use with caution in patients with severely traumatized mucosa in the region of intended application

Adverse Reactions

Cardiovascular: Hypertension, tachycardia, cardiac arrhythmias

Central nervous system: Restlessness, nervousness, euphoria, excitement, hallucinations, seizures

Gastrointestinal: Vomiting

Neuromuscular & skeletal: Tremor

Ocular: Topical: Sloughing of the corneal epithelium, ulceration of the cornea

Respiratory: Tachypnea

Drug Interactions Cytochrome P450 isoenzyme CYP3A3/4 substrate

MAO inhibitors, inhalational anesthetics, levodopa, methyldopa, sympathomimetics and ethanol may increase risk of cardiac arrhythmias; CNS stimulants; beta-adrenergic blocking agents; cholinesterase inhibitors

Stability Store in well closed, light-resistant containers

Mechanism of Action Blocks both the initiation and conduction of nerve impulses by decreasing the neuronal membrane's permeability to sodium ions. This results in inhibition of depolarization with resultant blockade of conduction; interferes with the uptake of norepinephrine by adrenergic nerve terminals producing vasoconstriction.

Pharmacodynamics Following topical administration to mucosa:

Onset of action: Within 1 minute

Maximum effect: Within 5 minutes

Duration: ≥30 minutes, depending upon route and dosage administered

Pharmacokinetics

Absorption: Well absorbed through mucous membranes; absorption is limited by drug-induced vasoconstriction and enhanced by inflammation

Distribution: V_d: ~2 L/kg; appears in breast milk (see Additional Information)

Metabolism: In the liver; major metabolites are ecgonine methyl ester and benzoyl ecgonine

Half-life: 75 minutes

Elimination: Primarily in urine as metabolites and unchanged drug (<10%); cocaine metabolites may appear in the urine of neonates for up to 5 days after birth due to maternal cocaine use shortly before birth

Usual Dosage Topical application (ear, nose, throat, bronchoscopy): Concentrations of 1% to 4% are used; use lowest effective dose; do not exceed 1 mg/kg; patient tolerance, anesthetic technique, vascularity of tissue, and area to be anesthetized will determine dose needed. Solutions >4% are not recommended due to increased risk and severity of systemic toxicities.

Administration Topical: Use only on mucous membranes of the oral, laryngeal, and nasal cavities; do not use on extensive areas of broken skin; do not apply commercially available products to the eye (an extemporaneously prepared ophthalmic product must be made)

Monitoring Parameters Heart rate, blood pressure, respiratory rate, temperature

Additional Information Repeated ophthalmic applications to the eye may cause cornea to become clouded or pitted, therefore, NS should be used to irrigate and protect cornea during surgery; not for injection; cocaine intoxication of infants who are receiving breast milk from their mothers abusing cocaine has been reported

Dosage Forms Excipient information presented when available (limited, particularly for generics); consult specific product labeling.

Powder, as hydrochloride: 1 g, 5 g, 25 g

Solution, topical, as hydrochloride: 4% [40 mg/mL] (4 mL, 10 mL); 10% [100 mg/mL] (4 mL, 10 mL)

References

Chasnoff IJ, Lewis DE, and Squires L, "Cocaine Intoxication in Breast-Fed Infants," *Pediatrics*, 1987, 80(6):836-8.

Greenglass EJ, "The Adverse Effects of Cocaine on the Developing Human," Yaffe SJ and Arana JV, eds, *Pediatric Pharmacology: Therapeutic Principles in Practice*, 2nd ed, Philadelphia, PA: WB Saunders Co, 1992, 598-604.

♦ **Cocaine Hydrochloride** *see* Cocaine *on page 395*

♦ **CO Ciprofloxacin (Can)** *see* Ciprofloxacin *on page 357*

♦ **CO Citalopram (Can)** *see* Citalopram *on page 368*

♦ **CO Clonazepam (Can)** *see* Clonazepam *on page 387*

Codeine (KOE deen)

Medication Safety Issues

Sound-alike/look-alike issues:

Codeine may be confused with Cardene®, Cophene®, Cordran®, iodine, Lodine®

Related Information

Compatibility of Medications Mixed in A Syringe *on page 1941*
Laboratory Detection of Drugs in Urine *on page 1928*
Narcotic Analgesics Comparison *on page 1705*
Overdose and Toxicology *on page 1916*

Canadian Brand Names Codeine Contin®

Index Terms Codeine Phosphate; Codeine Sulfate; Methylmorphine

Therapeutic Category Analgesic, Narcotic; Antitussive; Cough Preparation

Generic Available Yes

Use Treatment of mild to moderate pain; antitussive in lower doses (for nonproductive cough)

Restrictions C-II

Pregnancy Risk Factor C (D if used for prolonged periods or in high doses at term)

Lactation Enters breast milk/use caution (AAP rates "compatible")

Contraindications Hypersensitivity to codeine or any component (see Warnings)

Warnings Some preparations contain sulfites which may cause allergic reactions in susceptible individuals; do not discontinue abruptly after prolonged use

Precautions Use with caution in patients with hypersensitivity reactions to other phenanthrene derivative opioid agonists (morphine, hydrocodone, hydromorphone, levorphanol, oxycodone, oxymorphone); respiratory diseases including: asthma, emphysema, COPD or severe liver or renal insufficiency

Adverse Reactions

Cardiovascular: Palpitations, bradycardia, peripheral vasodilation, hypotension due to vasodilation from histamine release

Central nervous system: CNS depression, elevated intracranial pressure, dizziness, drowsiness, sedation

Dermatologic: Pruritus from histamine release

Endocrine & metabolic: Antidiuretic hormone release

Gastrointestinal: Nausea, vomiting, constipation, biliary tract spasm

Genitourinary: Urinary tract spasm

Ocular: Miosis

Respiratory: Respiratory depression

Miscellaneous: Physical and psychological dependence, histamine release

Drug Interactions Cytochrome P450 isoenzyme CYP2D6 and CYP3A3/4 substrate; isoenzyme CYP2D6 inhibitor

CNS depressants, phenothiazines, tricyclic antidepressants may potentiate the adverse effects of codeine

Mechanism of Action Binds to opiate receptors in the CNS, causing inhibition of ascending pain pathways, altering the perception of and response to pain; causes cough suppression by direct central action in the medulla; produces generalized CNS depression

Pharmacodynamics

Onset of action:

Oral: 30-60 minutes

I.M.: 10-30 minutes

Maximum effect:

Oral: 60-90 minutes

I.M.: 30-60 minutes

Duration: 4-6 hours

Pharmacokinetics

Absorption: Oral: Adequate

Distribution: Crosses the placenta; appears in breast milk

Protein binding: 7%

Metabolism: Hepatic to morphine (active); undergoes hydroxylation and O-demethylation via cytochrome P450 isoenzyme CYP2D6 and demethylation via CYP3A3/4

Bioavailability: 60% to 70%

Half-life: 2.5-3.5 hours

Elimination: 3% to 16% in urine as unchanged drug, norcodeine, and free and conjugated morphine

Usual Dosage Doses should be titrated to appropriate analgesic effect; when changing routes of administration, note that oral dose is ⅔ as effective as parenteral dose

(Continued)

Codeine *(Continued)*

Analgesic: Oral, I.M., SubQ:

Children: 0.5-1 mg/kg/dose every 4-6 hours as needed; maximum dose: 60 mg/dose

Adults: Usual: 30 mg/dose; range: 15-60 mg every 4-6 hours as needed

Antitussive: Oral (for nonproductive cough):

Infants and Children <2 years: Not recommended

Children ≥2 years: 1-1.5 mg/kg/day in divided doses every 4-6 hours as needed

Alternatively dose according to age:

2-5 years: 2.5-5 mg every 4-6 hours as needed; maximum dose: 30 mg/day

6-12 years: 5-10 mg every 4-6 hours as needed; maximum dose: 60 mg/day

Children >12 years and Adults: 10-20 mg/dose every 4-6 hours as needed; maximum dose: 120 mg/day

Dosing adjustment in renal impairment:

Cl_{cr} 10-50 mL/minute: Administer 75% of dose

Cl_{cr} <10 mL/minute: Administer 50% of dose

Administration

Oral: Administer with food or water to decrease nausea and GI upset

Parenteral: I.M., SubQ: Not intended for I.V. use due to large histamine release and cardiovascular effects

Monitoring Parameters Respiratory rate, heart rate, blood pressure, pain relief

Patient Information Increase fluid and fiber intake to avoid constipation; avoid alcohol; may cause drowsiness and impair ability to perform activities requiring mental alertness or physical coordination; may be habit-forming; avoid abrupt discontinuation after prolonged use

Nursing Implications Observe patient for excessive sedation and respiratory depression; implement safety measures; may need to assist with ambulation

Additional Information Not recommended for use for cough control in patients with a productive cough; equianalgesic doses: 120 mg codeine phosphate I.M. approximately equals morphine 10 mg I.M.

Dosage Forms Excipient information presented when available (limited, particularly for generics); consult specific product labeling. [CAN] = Canadian brand name

Injection, as phosphate: 15 mg/mL (2 mL); 30 mg/mL (2 mL) [contains sodium metabisulfite]

Tablet, as phosphate: 30 mg, 60 mg

Tablet, as sulfate: 15 mg, 30 mg, 60 mg

Tablet, controlled release (Codeine Contin®) [CAN]: 50 mg, 100 mg, 150 mg, 200 mg [not available in U.S.]

- ♦ **Codeine and Acetaminophen** *see* Acetaminophen and Codeine *on page 46*
- ♦ **Codeine and Guaifenesin** *see* Guaifenesin and Codeine *on page 746*
- ♦ **Codeine and Promethazine** *see* Promethazine and Codeine *on page 1326*
- ♦ **Codeine Contin® (Can)** *see* Codeine *on page 397*
- ♦ **Codeine Phosphate** *see* Codeine *on page 397*
- ♦ **Codeine, Promethazine, and Phenylephrine** *see* Promethazine, Phenylephrine, and Codeine *on page 1329*
- ♦ **Codeine Sulfate** *see* Codeine *on page 397*
- ♦ **Coenzyme R** *see* Biotin *on page 217*
- ♦ **CO Fluoxetine (Can)** *see* Fluoxetine *on page 681*
- ♦ **Cogentin®** *see* Benztropine *on page 208*
- ♦ **Co-Gesic®** *see* Hydrocodone and Acetaminophen *on page 779*
- ♦ **Colace® [OTC]** *see* Docusate *on page 526*
- ♦ **Colace® (Can)** *see* Docusate *on page 526*
- ♦ **Colace® Adult/Children Suppositories [OTC]** *see* Glycerin *on page 736*
- ♦ **Colace® Infant/Children Suppositories [OTC]** *see* Glycerin *on page 736*
- ♦ **Colax-C® (Can)** *see* Docusate *on page 526*

Colchicine (KOL chi seen)

Medication Safety Issues

High alert medication: The Institute for Safe Medication Practices (ISMP) includes this medication among its list of drugs which have a heightened risk of causing significant patient harm when used in error.

Therapeutic Category Anti-inflammatory Agent; Antigout Agent

Generic Available Yes

Use Treatment of acute gouty arthritis attacks and prevention of recurrences of such attacks; management of familial Mediterranean fever

Pregnancy Risk Factor D

Lactation Enters breast milk/use caution (AAP rates "compatible")

Contraindications Hypersensitivity to colchicine or any component; severe renal, GI disease, or cardiac disorders

Warnings Patients who become pregnant while receiving colchicine therapy may be at greater risk of producing trisomic offspring

Precautions Use with caution and modify dosage in patients with renal impairment

Adverse Reactions

Dermatologic: Rash, alopecia

Endocrine & metabolic: Azoospermia, hypothyroidism, metabolic acidosis

Gastrointestinal: Nausea, vomiting, diarrhea, abdominal pain, steatorrhea, paralytic ileus

Hematologic: Agranulocytosis, aplastic anemia, leukopenia

Hepatic: Elevated liver enzymes

Local: Irritation if extravasation occurs

Neuromuscular & skeletal: Myopathy, peripheral neuropathy

Renal: Hematuria, renal failure

Drug Interactions Colchicine may decrease absorption of Vitamin B_{12}

Food Interactions May need low purine diet during acute gouty attack

Stability I.V. colchicine is incompatible with dextrose or I.V. solutions with preservatives; protect from light

Mechanism of Action Decreases leukocyte motility, phagocytosis in joints and lactic acid production, thereby reducing the deposition of urate crystals that perpetuates the inflammatory response; inhibits secretion of serum amyloid A protein

Pharmacodynamics Onset of action:

Oral: Relief of pain and inflammation occurs after 24-48 hours

I.V.: 6-12 hours

Pharmacokinetics

Distribution: Concentrates in leukocytes, kidney, spleen, and liver; does not distribute in heart, skeletal muscle, and brain

Metabolism: Partially deacetylated in the liver

Half-life, terminal: 9.3-10.6 hours

Time to peak serum concentration: Oral: Within 30-120 minutes then declines for 2 hours before increasing again due to enterohepatic recycling

Elimination: Primarily in the feces via bile; 10% to 20% excreted in urine

Dialysis: Not dialyzable (0% to 5%)

Usual Dosage

Prophylaxis of familial Mediterranean fever: Oral:

- Children:
  - ≤5 years: 0.5 mg/day
  - >5 years: 1-1.5 mg/day in 2-3 divided doses
- Adults: 1-2 mg/day in 2-3 divided doses

Gouty arthritis: Acute attacks: Adults:

- Oral: Initial: 0.5-1.2 mg, then 0.5-0.6 mg every 1-2 hours or 1-1.2 mg every 2 hours until relief or GI side effects occur to a maximum total dose of 8 mg
- I.V.: Initial: 1-3 mg, then 0.5 mg every 6 hours until response, **not to exceed 4 mg/week**; if pain recurs, it may be necessary to administer a daily dose of 1-2 mg for several days, however, do not give more colchicine by any route for at least 7 days after a full course of I.V. therapy (4 mg); transfer to oral colchicine in a dose similar to that being given I.V.
- Prophylaxis of recurrent attacks: Oral: 0.5-0.6 mg every day or every other day

Dosing adjustment in renal impairment: Cl_{cr} <10 mL/minute: Decrease dose by 50%

Administration

Oral: Administer with water and maintain adequate fluid intake

Parenteral: Administer I.V. over 2-5 minutes into tubing of free-flowing I.V. with compatible fluid

Monitoring Parameters CBC with differential, urinalysis, and renal function test

Test Interactions May cause false-positive results in urine tests for erythrocytes or hemoglobin

Patient Information If taking for acute gouty attacks, discontinue if pain is relieved or if nausea, vomiting or diarrhea occur; avoid alcohol

Nursing Implications Severe local irritation can occur if inadvertently administered SubQ or I.M.; extravasation can cause tissue irritation

Dosage Forms Excipient information presented when available (limited, particularly for generics); consult specific product labeling.

Injection, solution: 0.5 mg/mL (2 mL)

Tablet: 0.6 mg

References

Levy M, Spino M, and Read SE, "Colchicine: A State-of-the-Art Review," *Pharmacotherapy*, 1991, 11(3):196-211.

(Continued)

Colchicine *(Continued)*

Majeed HA, Carroll JE, Khuffash FA, et al, "Long-term Colchicine Prophylaxis in Children With Familial Mediterranean Fever (Recurrent Hereditary Polyserositis)," *J Pediatr*, 1990, 116(6):997-9.

- **Cold-Eeze® [OTC** *see* Zinc Supplements *on page 1641*
- **CO Levetiracetam (Can)** *see* Levetiracetam *on page 922*

Colistimethate (koe lis ti METH ate)

U.S. Brand Names Coly-Mycin® M

Canadian Brand Names Coly-Mycin® M

Index Terms Colistimethate Sodium

Therapeutic Category Antibiotic, Miscellaneous

Generic Available Yes

Use Treatment of gram-negative infections due to susceptible *Pseudomonas aeruginosa, Enterobacter aerogenes, Escherichia coli,* and *Klebsiella pneumoniae*; not indicated for infections due to *Proteus* or *Neisseria* species. Parenteral use of colistimethate has mainly been replaced by less toxic antibiotics. Reserved for life-threatening infections caused by organisms resistant to the preferred drugs. Used as inhalation therapy in cystic fibrosis patients for treatment of initial colonization and management of chronic colonization with *P. aeruginosa*

Pregnancy Risk Factor C

Contraindications Hypersensitivity to colistimethate or any component

Warnings Colistimethate can cause serious nephrotoxicity and or neurotoxicity; neurotoxic reactions may be manifested by circumoral paresthesia, numbness, tingling of the extremities, pruritus, vertigo, dizziness, and slurring of speech. Dosage reduction may alleviate symptoms. Nephrotoxicity is dose-dependent and reversible if the antibiotic is discontinued. Avoid concurrent or sequential use of other nephrotoxic and neurotoxic drugs, particularly bacitracin, kanamycin, streptomycin, paromomycin, polymyxin B, tobramycin, neomycin, gentamicin, and amikacin. Neuromuscular blockade resulting in respiratory arrest has been reported in patients with neuromuscular disease (ie, myasthenia gravis) and patients receiving neuromuscular blocking agents [see Drug Interactions]; impaired renal function increases the possibility of apnea and neuromuscular blockade. Pseudomembranous colitis has been reported with colistimethate.

Precautions Use with caution and modify dosage in patients with impaired renal function

Adverse Reactions

Central nervous system: Slurred speech, dizziness, vertigo, fever, ataxia, mental confusion, seizures

Dermatologic: Pruritus, urticaria, rash

Gastrointestinal: GI upset

Local: Pain at injection site

Neuromuscular & skeletal: Paresthesia, muscle weakness, peripheral neuropathy

Renal: Elevated BUN, creatinine; decreased urine output; hematuria; albuminuria; nephrotoxicity

Respiratory: Apnea; respiratory distress; bronchospasm, cough (with inhaled colistimethate)

Drug Interactions Neuromuscular blocking agents, aminoglycosides, general anesthetics, polymyxin B, and sodium citrate potentiate the neuromuscular blocking effect; cephalothin, aminoglycosides, amphotericin B, vancomycin, and polymyxin B may potentiate nephrotoxicity (avoid concomitant use with colistimethate) (see Warnings)

Stability Store vial at room temperature; reconstituted solution is stable for 7 days when stored in the refrigerator or at room temperature.

Mechanism of Action Hydrolyzed to colistin which acts as a cationic detergent damaging the bacterial cytoplasmic membrane of gram-negative organisms causing leakage of intracellular substances and cell death

Pharmacokinetics

Absorption: Not absorbed from the GI tract, mucous membranes, or intact skin

Distribution: Widely distributed to body tissues; does not penetrate into CSF, synovial, pleural, or pericardial fluids; crosses the placenta

V_d: Adults: 0.09 ± 0.03 L/kg

Protein binding: 50%

Half-life:

Children: 2-3 hours

Adolescents and adults with cystic fibrosis: 3.5 ± 1 hour

Time to peak serum concentration: I.M.: ~2 hours

Elimination: Primarily in urine as unchanged drug

Usual Dosage Children, Adolescents, and Adults: Dosage should be based on an estimate of ideal body weight: **dosage expressed in terms of colistin:**

I.M., I.V.: 2.5-5 mg/kg/day divided every 6-12 hours
I.V.: Cystic fibrosis: 5-8 mg/kg/day divided every 8 hours; maximum dose: 160 mg/dose
Inhalation: 75 mg in NS (4 mL total volume) via nebulizer twice daily
Dosing adjustment in renal impairment: Parenteral: Adults:
S_{cr} 1.3-1.5 mg/dL: 2.5-3.8 mg/kg/day divided every 12 hours
S_{cr} 1.6-2.5 mg/dL: 2.5 mg/kg/day divided every 12-24 hours
S_{cr} 2.6-4 mg/dL: 1.5 mg/kg/dose every 36 hours

Administration
Parenteral: Reconstitute vial with 2 mL SWI resulting in a concentration of 75 mg colistin/mL; swirl gently to avoid frothing. Administer by I.M., direct I.V. injection over 3-10 minutes, intermittent infusion over 30 minutes, or by continuous I.V. infusion. For continuous I.V. infusion, one-half of the total daily dose is administered by direct I.V. injection over 3-10 minutes followed 1-2 hours later by the remaining one-half of the total daily dose diluted in a compatible I.V. solution infused over 22-23 hours. The final concentration for administration should be based on the patient's fluid needs.
Inhalation: Further dilute dose to a total volume of 4 mL in NS and administer via nebulizer.

Monitoring Parameters Renal function tests, urine output; for inhalation therapy: Pre- and post-treatment spirometry

Patient Information May impair ability to perform activities requiring mental alertness or physical coordination

Nursing Implications May premedicate with a bronchodilator to reduce the potential of bronchospasm when administering inhaled colistimethate

Dosage Forms Excipient information presented when available (limited, particularly for generics); consult specific product labeling.
Injection, powder for reconstitution: 150 mg

References
Beringer P, "The Clinical Use of Colistin in Patients With Cystic Fibrosis," *Curr Opin Pulm Med*, 2001, 7(6):434-40.
Cunningham S, Prasad A, Collyer L, et al, "Bronchoconstriction Following Nebulised Colistin in Cystic Fibrosis," *Arch Dis Child*, 2001, 84(5):432-3.
Reed MD, Stern RC, O'Riordan MA, et al, "The Pharmacokinetics of Colistin in Patients With Cystic Fibrosis," *J Clin Pharmacol*, 2001, 41(6):645-54.

- **Colistimethate Sodium** *see* Colistimethate *on page 400*
- **Colocort®** *see* Hydrocortisone *on page 781*
- **CO Lovastatin (Can)** *see* Lovastatin *on page 964*
- **Coly-Mycin® M** *see* Colistimethate *on page 400*
- **Colyte®** *see* Polyethylene Glycol-Electrolyte Solution *on page 1277*
- **Colyte™ (Can)** *see* Polyethylene Glycol-Electrolyte Solution *on page 1277*
- **Combantrin™ (Can)** *see* Pyrantel Pamoate *on page 1349*
- **Combivir®** *see* Lamivudine and Zidovudine *on page 904*
- **Compazine** *see* Prochlorperazine *on page 1321*
- **Compazine® (Can)** *see* Prochlorperazine *on page 1321*
- **Compound E** *see* Cortisone *on page 403*
- **Compound F** *see* Hydrocortisone *on page 781*
- **Compound S** *see* Zidovudine *on page 1637*
- **Compound S, Abacavir, and 3TC** *see* Abacavir, Lamivudine, and Zidovudine *on page 38*
- **Compound S, Abacavir, and Lamivudine** *see* Abacavir, Lamivudine, and Zidovudine *on page 38*
- **Compound S, ABC, and 3TC** *see* Abacavir, Lamivudine, and Zidovudine *on page 38*
- **Compound W® [OTC]** *see* Salicylic Acid *on page 1413*
- **Compound W® One Step Wart Remover [OTC]** *see* Salicylic Acid *on page 1413*
- **Compoz® Nighttime Sleep Aid [OTC]** *see* DiphenhydrAMINE *on page 509*
- **Compro™** *see* Prochlorperazine *on page 1321*
- **Comtrex® Sore Throat Maximum Strength [OTC]** *see* Acetaminophen *on page 42*
- **Comvax®** *see Haemophilus* b Conjugate and Hepatitis B Vaccine *on page 750*
- **Concerta®** *see* Methylphenidate *on page 1034*
- **Constulose** *see* Lactulose *on page 900*
- **Contac® Cold [OTC] [DSC]** *see* Pseudoephedrine *on page 1344*
- **Contac® Cold 12 Hour Relief Non Drowsy (Can)** *see* Pseudoephedrine *on page 1344*
- **ControlRx®** *see* Fluoride *on page 675*
- **CO Paroxetine (Can)** *see* Paroxetine *on page 1218*

- **Copegus®** *see* Ribavirin *on page 1378*
- **Copper Sulfate** *see* Trace Metals *on page 1558*
- **CO Pravastatin (Can)** *see* Pravastatin *on page 1300*
- **CO Ranitidine (Can)** *see* Ranitidine *on page 1366*
- **Cordarone®** *see* Amiodarone *on page 100*
- **Cordron-D NR [DSC]** *see* Carbinoxamine and Pseudoephedrine *on page 286*
- **Coreg®** *see* Carvedilol *on page 293*
- **Coreg CR™** *see* Carvedilol *on page 293*
- **Corgard®** *see* Nadolol *on page 1098*
- **Coricidin HBP® Chest Congestion and Cough [OTC]** *see* Guaifenesin and Dextromethorphan *on page 748*
- **Cormax®** *see* Clobetasol *on page 383*
- **Correctol® Tablets [OTC]** *see* Bisacodyl *on page 217*
- **Cortaid® Intensive Therapy [OTC]** *see* Hydrocortisone *on page 781*
- **Cortaid® Maximum Strength [OTC]** *see* Hydrocortisone *on page 781*
- **Cortaid® Sensitive Skin [OTC]** *see* Hydrocortisone *on page 781*
- **Cortamed® (Can)** *see* Hydrocortisone *on page 781*
- **Cortef®** *see* Hydrocortisone *on page 781*
- **Cortenema® (Can)** *see* Hydrocortisone *on page 781*
- **Corticool® [OTC]** *see* Hydrocortisone *on page 781*

Corticotropin (kor ti koe TROE pin)

Medication Safety Issues

Sound-alike/look-alike issues:

Corticotropin may be confused with corticorelin

U.S. Brand Names H.P. Acthar® Gel

Index Terms ACTH; Adrenocorticotropic Hormone; Corticotropin, Repository

Therapeutic Category Adrenal Corticosteroid; Diagnostic Agent, Adrenocortical Insufficiency; Infantile Spasms, Treatment

Generic Available No

Use Infantile spasms; diagnostic aid in adrenocortical insufficiency; acute exacerbations of multiple sclerosis; severe muscle weakness in myasthenia gravis

Pregnancy Risk Factor C

Contraindications Hypersensitivity to corticotropin, porcine proteins, or any component; scleroderma, osteoporosis, systemic fungal infections, ocular herpes simplex, peptic ulcer, hypertension, CHF

Warnings May mask signs of infection; do not administer live vaccines; long-term therapy in children may retard bone growth; acute adrenal insufficiency may occur with abrupt withdrawal after chronic use or with stress

Precautions Use with caution in patients with hypothyroidism, cirrhosis, thromboembolic disorders, seizure disorders or renal insufficiency

Adverse Reactions

Cardiovascular: Hypertension

Central nervous system: Seizures, mood swings, headache, pseudotumor cerebri

Dermatologic: Skin atrophy, bruising, hyperpigmentation, acne, hirsutism

Endocrine & metabolic: Amenorrhea, sodium and water retention, Cushing's syndrome, hyperglycemia, bone growth suppression, hypokalemia

Gastrointestinal: Abdominal distention, ulcerative esophagitis, pancreatitis

Neuromuscular & skeletal: Muscle wasting

Miscellaneous: Hypersensitivity reactions, including anaphylaxis

Drug Interactions NSAIDs (increase risk of ulcers, increase clearance of NSAIDs), loop diuretics, thiazide diuretics, amphotericin B (increases potassium wasting), antidiabetic agents (may require increased doses due to hyperglycemic activity of adrenal glucocorticoids), live virus vaccines (increase risk of viral infection), vaccines may have decreased effect

Food Interactions May increase renal loss of potassium, calcium, zinc, and vitamin C; may need to increase dietary intake or give supplements

Stability Store repository injection (gel) in the refrigerator; warm gel before administration

Mechanism of Action Stimulates the adrenal cortex to secrete adrenal steroids (including hydrocortisone, cortisone), androgenic substances, and a small amount of aldosterone. Exact mechanism of action for treatment of infantile spasms is unknown, but may be an independent antiepileptic effect (unrelated to stimulation of release of adrenocorticosteroids). One theory is that ACTH suppresses corticotropin-releasing hormone (CRH). CRH is an excitatory neuropeptide that has a greater potency in infants. Infants with infantile spasms may have increased CRH activity. ACTH may decrease CRH release and, therefore, decrease infantile spasms.

Pharmacodynamics

Maximum effect on cortisol levels: I.M., SubQ (gel): 3-12 hours

Duration: Repository (gel): 10-25 hours, up to 3 days

Pharmacokinetics

Absorption: I.M. (repository): Over 8-16 hours

Half-life: 15 minutes

Elimination: In urine

Usual Dosage

Children: I.M.: Gel (repository) formulation:

Anti-inflammatory/immunosuppressant: 0.8 units/kg/day or 25 units/m^2/day divided every 12-24 hours

Infantile spasms: Various regimens have been used. Some neurologists recommend low-dose ACTH (5-40 units/day) for short periods (1-6 weeks), while others recommend larger doses of ACTH (40-160 units/day) for long periods of treatment (3-12 months)

A prospective, single-blind study (Hrachovy, 1994) found no major difference in effectiveness between high-dose long-duration versus low-dose short-duration ACTH therapy. Hypertension, however, occurred more frequently in the high-dose group. Further studies comparing long-term outcomes are needed. Low-dose regimen used in this study:

Initial: 20 units/day for 2 weeks, if patient responds, taper and discontinue over a 1-week period; if patient does not respond, increase dose to 30 units/day for 4 weeks then taper and discontinue over a 1-week period

Usual dose: 20-40 units/day or 5-8 units/kg/day in 1-2 divided doses; range: 5-160 units/day

Adults: I.M.: Gel (repository) formulation:

Acute exacerbation of multiple sclerosis: 80-120 units/day in divided doses for 2-3 weeks

Diagnostic purposes: 25 units

Anti-inflammatory/immunosuppressant: 40-80 units every 24-72 hours

Administration Parenteral: Gel should be administered I.M. only

Monitoring Parameters Electrolytes, glucose, blood pressure, height, and weight; for infantile spasms, monitor seizure frequency, type, and duration

Test Interactions Skin tests

Patient Information Do not abruptly discontinue the medication; tell your physician you are using this drug if you are going to have skin tests, immunizations, surgery, emergency treatment, or if you have a serious infection or injury

Additional Information Cosyntropin is preferred over corticotropin for diagnostic test of adrenocortical insufficiency (cosyntropin is less allergenic and test is shorter in duration); oral prednisone (2 mg/kg/day) was as effective as I.M. ACTH gel (20 units/day) in controlling infantile spasms; corticotropin zinc hydroxide (Cortrophin® Zinc) and corticotropin aqueous (Acthar®) have been discontinued by the manufacturer

Dosage Forms Excipient information presented when available (limited, particularly for generics); consult specific product labeling.

Injection, gelatin: 80 units/mL (5 mL)

References

Haines ST and Casto DT, "Treatment of Infantile Spasms," *Ann Pharmacother*, 1994, 28(6):779-91.

Hrachovy RA and Frost JD Jr, "Infantile Spasms," *Pediatr Clin North Am*, 1989, 36(2):311-29.

Hrachovy RA, Frost JD Jr, and Glaze DG, "High-Dose, Long-Duration Versus Low-Dose, Short-Duration Corticotropin Therapy for Infantile Spasms," *J Pediatr*, 1994, 124(5 Pt 1):803-6.

Hrachovy RA, Frost JD Jr, Kellaway P, et al, "Double-Blind Study of ACTH vs Prednisone Therapy in Infantile Spasms," *J Pediatr*, 1983, 103(4):641-5.

♦ **Corticotropin, Repository** *see* Corticotropin *on page 402*

♦ **Cortifoam®** *see* Hydrocortisone *on page 781*

♦ **Cortifoam™ (Can)** *see* Hydrocortisone *on page 781*

♦ **Cortimyxin® (Can)** *see* Neomycin, (Bacitracin) Polymyxin B, and Hydrocortisone *on page 1119*

♦ **Cortisol** *see* Hydrocortisone *on page 781*

Cortisone (KOR ti sone)

Medication Safety Issues

Sound-alike/look-alike issues:

Cortisone may be confused with Cortizone®

Related Information

Corticosteroids, Systemic *on page 1685*

(Continued)

Cortisone *(Continued)*

Index Terms Compound E; Cortisone Acetate

Therapeutic Category Adrenal Corticosteroid; Anti-inflammatory Agent; Corticosteroid, Systemic; Glucocorticoid

Generic Available Yes

Use Management of adrenocortical insufficiency

Pregnancy Risk Factor D

Lactation Enters breast milk/use caution

Contraindications Hypersensitivity to cortisone, any component, or corticosteroids; serious infections, except septic shock or tuberculous meningitis; systemic fungal or viral infections

Warnings Hypothalamic-pituitary-adrenal (HPA) suppression may occur; acute adrenal insufficiency (adrenal crisis) may occur with abrupt withdrawal after long term therapy or with stress; withdrawal or discontinuation of corticosteroids should be done carefully; patients with HPA axis suppression may require increased doses of systemic glucocorticosteroids prior to, during, and after unusual stress (eg, surgery). Immunosuppression may occur; patients may be more susceptible to infections; avoid exposure to chickenpox and measles. Corticosteroids may mask signs of infection. Corticosteroids may activate latent opportunistic infections or exacerbate systemic fungal infections. May cause osteoporosis (at any age) or inhibition of bone growth in pediatric patients. Acute myopathy may occur with high doses, elevated IOP may occur (especially with prolonged use), CNS effects (ranging from euphoria to psychosis) may occur. Rare cases of anaphylactoid reactions have been reported with corticosteroids.

Precautions Avoid using higher than recommended doses; suppression of HPA axis, suppression of linear growth (ie, reduction of growth velocity), reduced bone mineral density, hypercorticism (Cushing's syndrome), hyperglycemia, or glucosuria may occur; titrate to lowest effective dose. Reduction in growth velocity may occur when corticosteroids are administered to pediatric patients by any route (monitor growth). Use with extreme caution in patients with respiratory tuberculosis, untreated systemic infections, or ocular herpes simplex; use with caution in patients with thyroid dysfunction, cirrhosis, nonspecific ulcerative colitis, hypertension, renal impairment, osteoporosis, thromboembolic tendencies, CHF, recent MI, convulsive disorders, myasthenia gravis, thrombophlebitis, peptic ulcer, diabetes, glaucoma, cataracts, or hepatic impairment. Prolonged use may result in cataracts or glaucoma.

Adverse Reactions

Cardiovascular: Edema, hypertension, CHF

Central nervous system: Vertigo, seizures, headache, psychoses, pseudotumor cerebri, euphoria, insomnia, intracranial hypertension, nervousness

Dermatologic: Acne, skin atrophy, impaired wound healing, petechiae, bruising

Endocrine & metabolic: HPA suppression, Cushing's syndrome, growth suppression, glucose intolerance, hypokalemia, alkalosis, weight gain

Gastrointestinal: Peptic ulcer, nausea, vomiting

Genitourinary: Menstrual irregularities

Neuromuscular & skeletal: Muscle weakness, osteoporosis, fractures, decreased bone mineral density

Ocular: Cataracts, elevated IOP, glaucoma

Miscellaneous: Immunosuppression, anaphylactoid reactions (rare)

Drug Interactions Cytochrome P450 isoenzyme CYP3A3/4 substrate

Barbiturates, phenytoin, rifampin, salicylates, estrogens, NSAID, diuretics (potassium depleting), anticholinesterase agents, warfarin; caffeine and alcohol may increase risk for GI ulcer; live virus vaccines (increase risk of viral infection); vaccines may have decreased effects

Food Interactions Systemic use of corticosteroids may require a diet with increased potassium, vitamins A, B_6, C, D, folate, calcium, zinc, phosphorus, and decreased sodium

Mechanism of Action Controls the rate of protein synthesis, depresses the migration of polymorphonuclear leukocytes and fibroblasts, reverses capillary permeability, and stabilizes lysosomal membranes at the cellular level to prevent or control inflammation

Pharmacodynamics

Maximum effect: Oral: Within 2 hours

Duration: 30-36 hours

Pharmacokinetics

Distribution: Crosses the placenta; appears in breast milk; distributes to muscles, liver, skin, intestines, and kidneys

Metabolism: In the liver to inactive metabolites

Half-life: 30 minutes

Elimination: In bile and urine

Usual Dosage Depends upon the condition being treated and the response of the patient. Supplemental doses may be warranted during times of stress in the course of withdrawing therapy. Oral:

Children:

Anti-inflammatory or immunosuppressive: 2.5-10 mg/kg/day or 20-300 mg/m^2/day in divided doses every 6-8 hours

Physiologic replacement: 0.5-0.75 mg/kg/day or 20-25 mg/m^2/day in divided doses every 8 hours

Adults: 20-300 mg/day divided every 12-24 hours

Administration Oral: Administer with meals, food, or milk to decrease GI effects

Monitoring Parameters Long-term use: Electrolytes, glucose, blood pressure, height, weight

Test Interactions Skin tests

Patient Information Do not discontinue or reduce dose without physician's approval; limit caffeine; avoid alcohol

Nursing Implications Taper dose gradually with long-term use

Additional Information Insoluble in water

Dosage Forms Excipient information presented when available (limited, particularly for generics); consult specific product labeling.

Tablet, as acetate: 25 mg

♦ **Cortisone Acetate** *see* Cortisone *on page 403*

♦ **Cortisporin® Cream** *see* Neomycin, (Bacitracin) Polymyxin B, and Hydrocortisone *on page 1119*

♦ **Cortisporin® Ophthalmic** *see* Neomycin, (Bacitracin) Polymyxin B, and Hydrocortisone *on page 1119*

♦ **Cortisporin® Otic** *see* Neomycin, (Bacitracin) Polymyxin B, and Hydrocortisone *on page 1119*

♦ **Cortizone®-10 Maximum Strength [OTC]** *see* Hydrocortisone *on page 781*

♦ **Cortizone®-10 Plus Maximum Strength [OTC]** *see* Hydrocortisone *on page 781*

♦ **Cortizone®-10 Quick Shot [OTC]** *see* Hydrocortisone *on page 781*

♦ **Cortrosyn®** *see* Cosyntropin *on page 405*

♦ **CO Simvastatin (Can)** *see* Simvastatin *on page 1441*

♦ **Cosmegen®** *see* Dactinomycin *on page 435*

♦ **CO Sotalol (Can)** *see* Sotalol *on page 1463*

♦ **CO Sumatriptan (Can)** *see* Sumatriptan *on page 1495*

Cosyntropin (koe sin TROE pin)

Medication Safety Issues

Sound-alike/look-alike issues:

Cortrosyn® may be confused with Cotazym®

U.S. Brand Names Cortrosyn®

Canadian Brand Names Cortrosyn®

Index Terms Synacthen; Tetracosactide

Therapeutic Category Adrenal Corticosteroid; Diagnostic Agent, Adrenocortical Insufficiency

Generic Available No

Use Diagnostic test to differentiate primary adrenal from secondary (pituitary) adrenocortical insufficiency; used in the diagnosis of congenital adrenal hyperplasia

Pregnancy Risk Factor C

Lactation Excretion in breast milk unknown/use caution

Contraindications Hypersensitivity to cosyntropin or any component

Precautions Use with caution in patients with pre-existing allergic disease or a history of allergic reactions to corticotropin

Adverse Reactions

Cardiovascular: Bradycardia, tachycardia, hypertension, peripheral edema

Dermatologic: Pruritus, flushing, rash

Miscellaneous: Hypersensitivity reactions, including anaphylaxis

Drug Interactions Cortisone, hydrocortisone, estrogens, spironolactone; use with diuretics may increase electrolyte loss

Stability Store unreconstituted vials at 15°C to 30°C (59°F to 86°F); reconstituted solution is stable for 24 hours at room temperature and 21 days when refrigerated; when diluted in NS or D_5W, I.V. infusion is stable for 12 hours at room temperature; do not add to plasma or blood infusions (inactivation by enzymes may occur)

Mechanism of Action Stimulates the adrenal cortex to secrete adrenal steroids (including hydrocortisone, cortisone), androgenic substances, and a small amount of aldosterone

(Continued)

Cosyntropin *(Continued)*

Pharmacodynamics I.M., I.V.:

Onset of action: Plasma cortisol levels rise in healthy individuals in 5 minutes

Maximum effect: Plasma cortisol levels usually peak at 45-60 minutes after the cosyntropin dose

Pharmacokinetics Metabolism: Unknown

Usual Dosage Diagnostic test doses:

Adrenocortical insufficiency: I.M., I.V.:

Preterm neonates: Dose not well defined; Korte 1996 used physiologic doses of cosyntropin (0.1 mcg/kg) to test adrenal function in VLBW infants [mean weight 900 g; mean gestational age 27 weeks (range: 23-32 weeks)]; only 36% of infants responded; increasing the dose to 0.2 mcg/kg resulted in 67% of the infants responding, but sensitivity of the test was decreased. Cole 1999 used cosyntropin doses of 3.5 mcg/kg to test adrenal function in 44 preterm infants [mean birthweight 823 g; mean gestational age 26.2 weeks; mean postmenstrual age 30.1 weeks] during inhaled beclomethasone therapy.

Neonates: 0.015 mg/kg/dose

Children ≤2 years: 0.125 mg

Children >2 years and Adults: 0.25 mg

When greater cortisol stimulation is needed, an I.V. infusion may be used: Children >2 years and Adults: 0.25 mg administered over 4-8 hours (usually 6 hours)

Congenital adrenal hyperplasia evaluation: 1 mg/m^2/dose up to a maximum of 1 mg

Administration Parenteral: Reconstitute vial with 1 mL NS; visually inspect solution for discoloration and particulate matter prior to injection

I.M.: Administer as 0.25 mg/mL concentration

I.V. push: Administer in 2-5 mL of NS over 2 minutes

I.V. infusion (Children >2 years and Adults): Dose may be added to dextrose or NS solution and administered over 4-8 hours (at a rate of approximately 0.04 mg/hour for 6 hours)

Reference Range Plasma cortisol concentrations should be measured immediately before and exactly 30 minutes after the dose; dose should be given in the early morning; normal morning baseline cortisol >5 mcg/dL (SI: >138 nmol/L); normal response 30 minutes after cosyntropin injection: an increase in serum cortisol concentration of ≥7 mcg/dL (SI: ≥193 nmol/L) or peak response >18 mcg/dL (SI: >497 nmol/L).

Nursing Implications Patient should not receive corticosteroids or spironolactone the day prior to and the day of the test

Additional Information Each 0.25 mg of cosyntropin is equivalent to 25 units of corticotropin.

Dosage Forms Excipient information presented when available (limited, particularly for generics); consult specific product labeling.

Injection, powder for reconstitution: 0.25 mg

References

Cole CH, Shah B, Abbasi S, et al, "Adrenal Function in Premature Infants During Inhaled Beclomethasone Therapy," *J Pediatr*, 1999, 135(1):65-70.

Korte C, Styne D, Merritt TA, et al, "Adrenocortical Function in the Very Low Birth Weight Infant: Improved Testing Sensitivity and Association With Neonatal Outcome," *J Pediatr*, 1996, 128(2):257-63.

♦ **Cotazym® (Can)** *see* Pancrelipase *on page 1203*
♦ **Co-Trimoxazole** *see* Sulfamethoxazole and Trimethoprim *on page 1487*
♦ **Coumadin®** *see* Warfarin *on page 1626*
♦ **Covera® (Can)** *see* Verapamil *on page 1611*
♦ **Covera-HS®** *see* Verapamil *on page 1611*
♦ **Coviracil** *see* Emtricitabine *on page 562*
♦ **CPM** *see* Cyclophosphamide *on page 419*
♦ **CPT-11** *see* Irinotecan *on page 865*
♦ **CPZ** *see* ChlorproMAZINE *on page 345*
♦ **Creomulsion® Cough [OTC]** *see* Dextromethorphan *on page 477*
♦ **Creomulsion® for Children [OTC]** *see* Dextromethorphan *on page 477*
♦ **Creon®** *see* Pancrelipase *on page 1203*
♦ **Creo-Terpin® [OTC]** *see* Dextromethorphan *on page 477*
♦ **Critic-Aid Skin Care® [OTC]** *see* Zinc Oxide *on page 1640*
♦ **Crixivan®** *see* Indinavir *on page 824*
♦ **CroFab™** *see Crotalidae* Polyvalent Immune Fab (Ovine) *on page 410*
♦ **Crolom®** *see* Cromolyn *on page 407*
♦ **Cromoglycic Acid** *see* Cromolyn *on page 407*

Cromolyn (KROE moe lin)

Medication Safety Issues

Sound-alike/look-alike issues:

Intal® may be confused with Endal®

NasalCrom® may be confused with Nasacort®, Nasalide®

Related Information

Asthma *on page 1904*

U.S. Brand Names Crolom®; Gastrocrom®; Intal®; NasalCrom® [OTC]; Opticrom®

Canadian Brand Names Apo-Cromolyn®; Intal®; Nalcrom®; Nu-Cromolyn; Opticrom®

Index Terms Cromoglycic Acid; Cromolyn Sodium; Disodium Cromoglycate; DSCG

Therapeutic Category Antiasthmatic; Inhalation, Miscellaneous

Generic Available Yes: Excludes aerosol, oral solution

Use

Oral inhalation and nebulization: Prophylactic agent used for long-term (chronic) control of persistent asthma (see Additional Information); **NOT** indicated for the relief of acute bronchospasm; also used for the prevention of allergen- or exercise-induced bronchospasm

Intranasal: Management of seasonal or perennial allergic rhinitis

Ophthalmologic: Vernal conjunctivitis, vernal keratoconjunctivitis, and vernal keratitis

Systemic: Mastocytosis, food allergy, and treatment of inflammatory bowel disease

Pregnancy Risk Factor B

Lactation Excretion in breast milk unknown/use caution

Contraindications Hypersensitivity to cromolyn or any component; primary treatment of status asthmaticus

Warnings Cromolyn is a prophylactic drug with no benefit for acute situations; rare but severe anaphylactic reactions can occur; discontinue if eosinophilic pneumonia occurs

Precautions Use with caution and decrease dose in patients with renal and hepatic impairment; use inhalation aerosol with caution in patients with coronary artery disease or history of cardiac arrhythmias (due to propellants); use with caution when tapering the dose or withdrawing the drug since symptoms may reoccur; patients should not wear contact lenses during treatment with ophthalmic solution.

Oral cromolyn increased mortality in neonatal rats when administered at ~9 times the maximum recommended daily dose for infants, but not at ~3 times the maximum recommended daily dose; use of oral cromolyn in infants and children <2 years is not recommended and should be reserved for patients with severe mastocytosis in whom potential benefits clearly outweigh the risks.

Adverse Reactions

Central nervous system: Dizziness, headache

Dermatologic: Rash, urticaria, angioedema

Gastrointestinal: Nausea, vomiting, diarrhea, xerostomia, unpleasant taste (inhalation aerosol)

Local: Nasal burning

Neuromuscular & skeletal: Arthralgia

Ocular (topical): Ocular stinging, lacrimation

Respiratory: Coughing, wheezing, sneezing, nasal congestion, throat irritation, eosinophilic pneumonia, pulmonary infiltrates, hoarseness, laryngeal edema (rare)

Miscellaneous: Anaphylaxis (rare)

Stability Protect from direct light and heat; nebulization solution is compatible with beta agonists, anticholinergic solutions, acetylcysteine and NS; incompatible with alkaline solutions, calcium and magnesium salts; store oral concentrate ampuls in foil pouch until ready for use

Mechanism of Action Prevents the mast cell release of histamine, leukotrienes and slow-reacting substance of anaphylaxis by inhibiting degranulation after contact with antigens

Pharmacodynamics Not effective for immediate relief of symptoms in acute asthmatic attacks; must be used at regular intervals for 2-4 weeks to be effective

Pharmacokinetics

Absorption:

Oral: 0.5% to 2%

Inhalation: ~8% of dose reaches the lungs upon inhalation of the powder and is well absorbed

Half-life: 80-90 minutes

Time to peak serum concentration: Within 15 minutes after inhalation

Elimination: Equally excreted unchanged in urine and feces (via bile); small amounts after inhalation are exhaled

(Continued)

Cromolyn *(Continued)*

Usual Dosage

Inhalation:

For chronic control of asthma, taper frequency to the lowest effective dose (ie, 4 times/day to 3 times/day to twice daily):

Nebulization solution: Children >2 years and Adults: Initial: 20 mg 4 times/day; usual dose: 20 mg 3-4 times/day

Metered spray:

Children 5-12 years: Initial: 2 inhalations 4 times/day; usual dose: 1-2 inhalations 3-4 times/day

Children ≥12 years and Adults: Initial: 2 inhalations 4 times/day; usual dose: 2-4 inhalations 3-4 times/day

Prevention of allergen- or exercise-induced bronchospasm: Administer 10-15 minutes prior to exercise or allergen exposure but no longer than 1 hour before:

Nebulization solution: Children >2 years and Adults: Single dose of 20 mg

Metered spray: Children >5 years and Adults: Single dose of 2 inhalations

NIH Asthma Guidelines (NAEPP, 2002):

Nebulization solution: Children and Adults: 20 mg 3-4 times/day

Metered spray:

Children ≤12 years: 1-2 inhalations 3-4 times/day

Children >12 years and Adults: 2-4 inhalations 3-4 times/day

Intranasal: Children ≥2 years and Adults: 1 spray in each nostril 3-4 times/day; maximum dose: 1 spray in each nostril 6 times/day

Ophthalmic: Children >4 years and Adults: Instill 1-2 drops 4-6 times/day

Oral:

Systemic mastocytosis:

Neonates and Preterm Infants: Not recommended

Infants and Children <2 years: Not recommended; reserve use for patients with severe disease in whom potential benefits outweigh risks (see Precautions); 20 mg/kg/day in 4 divided doses; may increase in patients 6 months to 2 years of age if benefits not seen after 2-3 weeks; do not exceed 30 mg/kg/day

Children 2-12 years: 100 mg 4 times/day; not to exceed 40 mg/kg/day

Children >12 years and Adults: 200 mg 4 times/day

Food allergy and inflammatory bowel disease:

Infants and Children <2 years: Not recommended

Children 2-12 years: Initial dose: 100 mg 4 times/day; may double the dose if effect is not satisfactory within 2-3 weeks; not to exceed 40 mg/kg/day

Children >12 years and Adults: Initial dose: 200 mg 4 times/day; may double the dose if effect is not satisfactory within 2-3 weeks; up to 400 mg 4 times/day

Once desired effect is achieved, dose may be tapered to lowest effective dose

Administration

Oral concentrate: Open ampul and squeeze contents into glass of water; stir well; administer at least 30 minutes before meals and at bedtime; do not mix with juice, milk, or food

Oral inhalation: Shake canister gently before use; do not immerse canister in water

Nasal inhalation: Clear nasal passages by blowing nose prior to use

Monitoring Parameters Asthma: Periodic pulmonary function tests; signs and symptoms of disease state when tapering dose

Patient Information May cause dry mouth. Cromolyn is not effective for the immediate relief of symptoms in acute asthmatic attacks; must be used at regular intervals for 2-4 weeks to be effective for asthma control. Cromolyn nasal spray is not effective for the immediate relief of nasal allergies; must be used at regular intervals for 1-2 weeks for optimal control of nasal allergies; to prevent nasal allergy symptoms, start using product 1-2 weeks before contact with the cause of allergies.

Additional Information The 2002 Expert Panel Report of the National Asthma Education and Prevention Program (NAEPP, 2002) no longer recommends cromolyn for initial treatment of persistent asthma in children; inhaled corticosteroids are the preferred agents; cromolyn is considered an alternative medication for the treatment of mild persistent asthma in children. Inhalation aerosol contains fluorocarbon propellants. Reserve systemic use in children <2 years of age for severe disease; avoid systemic use in premature infants.

Dosage Forms Excipient information presented when available (limited, particularly for generics); consult specific product labeling.

Aerosol, for oral inhalation, as sodium (Intal®): 800 mcg/inhalation (8.1 g) [112 metered inhalations; 56 doses], (14.2 g) [200 metered inhalations; 100 doses]

Solution for nebulization, as sodium (Intal®): 20 mg/2 mL (60s, 120s)

Solution, intranasal, as sodium [spray] (NasalCrom®): 40 mg/mL (13 mL, 26 mL) [5.2 mg/inhalation; contains benzalkonium chloride]

Solution, ophthalmic, as sodium (Crolom®, Opticrom®): 4% (10 mL) [contains benzalkonium chloride]

Solution, oral, as sodium (Gastrocrom®): 100 mg/5 mL (96s)

References

Expert Panel Report 2, "Guidelines for the Diagnosis and Management of Asthma," *Clinical Practice Guidelines*, National Institutes of Health, National Heart, Lung, and Blood Institute, NIH Publication No. 94-4051, April, 1997.

"National Asthma Education and Prevention Program. Expert Panel Report: Guidelines for the Diagnosis and Management of Asthma Update on Selected Topics--2002," *J Allergy Clin Immunol*, 2002, 110(5 Suppl):S141-219.

♦ **Cromolyn Sodium** *see* Cromolyn *on page 407*

Crotalidae Polyvalent Antivenin (Equine)

(kroe TAL ih die pol i VAY lent an tee VEN in E kwine)

Related Information

Commonly Used Antidotes for Acute Overdoses *on page 1920*

U.S. Brand Names Antivenin Polyvalent [Equine]

Index Terms Crotaline Antivenin, Polyvalent (Equine Origin); North and South American Antisnake-bite Serum; Pit Viper Antivenin; Snake (Pit Vipers) Antivenin

Therapeutic Category Antivenin

Generic Available No

Use Neutralization of venoms of North and South American crotalids: rattlesnake, copperhead, cottonmouth, tropical moccasins, fer-de-lance, bushmaster

Pregnancy Risk Factor C

Lactation Excretion in breast milk unknown/use caution

Contraindications Not effective against the venoms of coral snakes

Warnings Desensitization may need to be performed on patients with positive skin test reaction or history of sensitivity to equine serum

Precautions Patients with a negative skin test may still react when antivenin is administered; skin test should not be performed unless antivenin is to be used. If patient has a positive history for allergy and a positive skin test, antivenin administration may be dangerous. Risk of administering antivenin must be weighed against the risk of withholding it

Adverse Reactions

Cardiovascular: Flushing, cyanosis, shock, edema of the face

Central nervous system: Apprehension

Dermatologic: Urticaria

Gastrointestinal: Vomiting

Neuromuscular & skeletal: Muscle weakness, peripheral neuritis

Respiratory: Dyspnea, cough

Miscellaneous: Anaphylaxis, serum sickness (dose-related; occurs in 83% of patients receiving more than 8 vials)

Stability Avoid storage temperatures >37°C; reconstituted solutions should be used within 48 hours

Usual Dosage The initial dose of antivenin should be administered as soon as possible to be most effective (within 4 hours after the bite). Intradermal sensitivity test should be performed prior to administering antivenin; see Additional Information.

Children and Adults: I.V.:

- Minimal envenomation: 20-40 mL
- Moderate envenomation: 50-90 mL
- Severe envenomation: 100-150 mL
- See table.

Dosage Based on Severity of Clinical Picture

	Clinical Severity	# of Vials
Minimal	Symptoms confined to bite area; absent of insignificant systemic symptoms	0
Mild	Edema progressing slowly; bite site reveals small amount of ecchymosis; only systemic sign is metallic taste	5
Moderate	Tissue damage beyond immediate bite area; moderate laboratory changes; perioral fasciculation; paresthesias	10
Severe	Tissue damage to entire extremity; major systemic symptoms; significant laboratory abnormalities	>15

Gold BS and Barish RA, "Venomous Snakebites: Current Concepts in Diagnosis, Treatment, and Management," *Emerg Med Clin North Am*, 1992, 10(2):249-67.

(Continued)

Crotalidae Polyvalent Antivenin (Equine) *(Continued)*

Additional doses of antivenin are based on clinical response to the initial dose. If swelling continues to progress, symptoms increase in severity, hypotension occurs, or decrease in hematocrit appears, an additional 10-50 mL should be administered.

Administration Parenteral: Antivenin may be administered I.M. into a large muscle mass for minimal envenomation. I.V. administration of antivenin is preferred for moderate to severe envenomation or in the presence of shock; for I.V. infusion, prepare a 1:1 to 1:10 dilution of reconstituted antivenin in NS or D_5W; infuse the initial 5-10 mL dilution over 3-5 minutes while carefully observing the patient for signs and symptoms of sensitivity reactions. If no reaction occurs, continue infusion at a safe I.V. fluid delivery rate.

Monitoring Parameters Vital signs, hematocrit, hemoglobin; platelet count, prothrombin time; signs and symptoms of allergy, anaphylaxis, and serum sickness

Nursing Implications **Do not inject into a finger or toe**; immediate sensitivity reactions usually occur within 30 minutes after administration; if an immediate reaction occurs, temporarily discontinue antivenin, administer epinephrine, corticosteroid, and/or an antihistamine; then reinstate infusion at a slower rate after control of the reaction; serum-sickness reaction may occur 5-24 days after a dose

Additional Information Intradermal skin test: 0.02-0.03 mL of a 1:10 dilution of antivenin in NS. If the patient has a history of equine serum sensitivity, administer a 1:100 or greater dilution skin test. Test site is read after 5-30 minutes.

Dosage Forms Excipient information presented when available (limited, particularly for generics); consult specific product labeling.

Injection, powder for reconstitution, lyophilized serum: Equine origin: [With 10 mL SWI diluent]

Crotalidae Polyvalent Immune Fab (Ovine)

(kroe TAL ih die pol i VAY lent i MYUN fab (OE vine))

U.S. Brand Names CroFab™

Index Terms Crotalid Antivenom Ovine Fab, Polyvalent

Therapeutic Category Antivenin

Generic Available No

Use Neutralization of venoms of North American crotalids: Western diamondback rattlesnake, Eastern diamondback rattlesnake, Mojave rattlesnake, and cottonmouth or water moccasin

Pregnancy Risk Factor C

Contraindications Hypersensitivity to *Crotalidae* polyvalent immune Fab (ovine), papaya, papain, chymopapain, or any component

Warnings Recurrent coagulopathy characterized by decreased fibrinogen and platelets and elevated PT has occurred in 50% of patients studied but was only observed in patients who had experienced coagulation abnormalities during their initial treatment. Recurrent coagulopathy may persist >1-2 weeks. Evaluate patients for the need for repeat dosing.

Precautions Use with caution in patients with hypersensitivity to the pineapple enzyme bromelain, dust mite allergens, or latex allergens. *Crotalidae* polyvalent immune Fab (ovine) contains mercury in the form of ethyl mercury from thimerosal; although there is limited toxicologic data available on ethyl mercury, developing fetuses and very young children are the most susceptible to neurologic and renal toxicities associated with methyl mercury exposure. Carefully monitor all patients receiving antivenin for signs and symptoms of an anaphylactic reaction, acute allergic reaction, delayed allergic reactions (ie, serum sickness, rash, fever, myalgia, arthralgia) and infusion-related reactions. Supportive therapy and medications for the management of anaphylactic reactions should be available for immediate use. Use with caution if administering a repeat course for a subsequent envenomation episode since patients may become sensitized to the foreign protein. Skin testing is not indicated.

Adverse Reactions

Cardiovascular: Chest pain, hypotension

Central nervous system: Chills, nervousness

Dermatologic: Rash, urticaria, pruritus, erythema

Gastrointestinal: Nausea, anorexia

Hematologic: Coagulation disorder (thrombocytopenia, hypofibrinogenemia, elevated PT)

Neuromuscular & skeletal: Myalgia, paresthesia

Respiratory: Dyspnea, wheezing, cough

Miscellaneous: Serum sickness, allergic reaction, anaphylaxis

Stability Store vials at 2°C to 8°C; do not freeze; use reconstituted and diluted product within 4 hours

Mechanism of Action Antivenom composed of purified Fab fragment of IgG specific to indigenous snake species; binds and neutralizes venom toxins; facilitates their distribution away from target tissues and their elimination from the body

Pharmacodynamics

Onset of action: Within 4 hours

Duration: 6-18 hours

Pharmacokinetics

Distribution: V_d: Adults: 110 mL/kg

Half-life: 18 hours

Usual Dosage The initial dose of antivenin should be administered as soon as possible (within 6 hours after the crotalid snakebite). Skin testing prior to administering antivenin is not required.

Children and Adults: I.V.:

Initial: 4-6 vials

Observe patient for 1 hour following the completion of the first dose. If initial control is not achieved after the first dose, an additional 4-6 vials may be repeated until initial control of the envenomation syndrome has been achieved.

After initial control has been established: 2 vials every 6 hours for up to 18 hours (3 doses); an additional 2 vial dose may be administered if deemed necessary based on clinical response

Administration Parenteral: I.V. administration only; reconstitute vial with 10 mL SWI and mix by continuous gentle swirling; further dilute the number of vials needed for dose in 250 mL NS and continue to mix by gently swirling. Initial: Infuse slowly over the first 10 minutes at 25-50 mL/hour along with careful observation for any allergic reaction; if no reaction occurs, may increase to 250 mL/hour until total dose is infused

Monitoring Parameters Vital signs, PT, hematocrit, hemoglobin, platelet count, fibrin split products, fibrinogen level; signs and symptoms of allergy, anaphylaxis, and serum sickness; signs of initial control of the envenomation (arrest of local injury, systemic signs and symptoms and normalization of coagulation tests)

Patient Information Notify physician if rash, pruritus, urticaria, bruising, or bleeding occurs; bruising and bleeding may occur for up to one week or longer following initial treatment

Nursing Implications Observe patient for up to 1 hour following the completion of the first dose to determine if initial control of the envenomation has been achieved. Immediate sensitivity reactions usually occur within 30 minutes after administration; if an immediate reaction occurs, temporarily discontinue CroFab™, administer epinephrine, I.V. antihistamine, and/or albuterol

Additional Information

Definition of Minimal, Moderate, and Severe Envenomation

Envenomation Category	Definition
Minimal	Swelling, pain, and ecchymosis limited to the immediate bite site; Systemic signs and symptoms absent; Coagulation parameters normal with no clinical evidence of bleeding.
Moderate	Swelling, pain, and ecchymosis involving less than a full extremity or, if bite was sustained on the trunk, head, or neck extending less than 50 cm; Systemic signs and symptoms may be present but not life threatening, including but not limited to nausea, vomiting, oral paresthesia or unusual tastes, mild hypotension (systolic blood pressure >90 mm Hg), mild tachycardia (heart rate <150), and tachypnea; Coagulation parameters may be abnormal, but no clinical evidence of bleeding present. Minor hematuria, gum bleeding, and nosebleeds are allowed if they are not considered severe in the investigator's judgement.
Severe	Swelling, pain, and ecchymosis involving more than an entire extremity or threatening the airway; Systemic signs and symptoms are markedly abnormal, including severe alteration of mental status, severe hypotension, severe tachycardia, tachypnea, or respiratory insufficiency; Coagulation parameters are abnormal, with serious bleeding or severe threat of bleeding.

Dosage Forms Excipient information presented when available (limited, particularly for generics); consult specific product labeling.

Injection: Each vial contains up to 1 g of total protein, a maximum of 0.11 mg of mercury, and not less than the indicated number of mouse LD_{50} neutralizing units:

C. atrox (Western diamondback rattlesnake): 1350 units

C. adamanteus (Eastern diamondback rattlesnake): 800 units

(Continued)

Crotalidae Polyvalent Immune Fab (Ovine) *(Continued)*

C. scutulatus (Mojave rattlesnake): 5210 units
A. piscivorus (cottonmouth and water moccasin): 460 units

References

Clark RF, Williams SR, Nordt SP, et al, "Successful Treatment of Crotalid-Induced Neurotoxicity With a New Polyspecific Crotalid Fab Antivenom," *Ann Emerg Med*, 1997, 30(1):54-7.
Dart RC and McNally J, "Efficacy, Safety, and Use of Snake Antivenoms in the United States," *Ann Emerg Med*, 2001, 37(2):181-8.

♦ **Crotalid Antivenom Ovine Fab, Polyvalent** *see Crotalidae* Polyvalent Immune Fab (Ovine) *on page 410*
♦ **Crotaline Antivenin, Polyvalent (Equine Origin)** *see Crotalidae* Polyvalent Antivenin (Equine) *on page 409*

Crotamiton (kroe TAM i tonn)

Medication Safety Issues
Sound-alike/look-alike issues:
Eurax® may be confused with Efudex®, Eulexin®, Evoxac™, Serax®, Urex®
International issues:
Eurax® may be confused with Urex® which is a brand name for furosemide in Australia

U.S. Brand Names Eurax®

Therapeutic Category Scabicidal Agent

Generic Available No

Use Treatment of scabies (*Sarcoptes scabiei*) in infants and children; symptomatic treatment of pruritic skin

Pregnancy Risk Factor C

Lactation Excretion in breast milk unknown

Contraindications Hypersensitivity to crotamiton or any component; patients who manifest a primary irritation response to topical medications

Precautions Avoid contact with face, eyes, mucous membranes, and urethral meatus; do not apply to acutely inflamed or raw skin

Adverse Reactions
Dermatologic: Pruritus, contact dermatitis, rash
Local: Irritation
Miscellaneous: Allergic sensitivity reaction

Stability Store at room temperature.

Mechanism of Action Mechanism for scabicidal activity is unknown

Pharmacokinetics Absorption: Amount of systemic absorption following topical use has not been determined

Usual Dosage Topical: Infants, Children, and Adults:
Scabicide: Apply over entire body below the head; apply once daily for 2 days followed by a cleansing bath 48 hours after the last application; treatment may be repeated after 7-10 days if mites appear
Pruritus: Massage into affected areas until medication is completely absorbed; may repeat as necessary

Administration Topical: Wash thoroughly and scrub away loose scales, then towel dry; apply a thin layer and gently massage drug onto skin of the entire body from the neck to the toes (with special attention to skin folds, creases, and interdigital spaces); also apply cream or lotion under fingernails after trimming nails short; since scabies can affect the head, scalp, and neck in infants and young children, apply to scalp, neck, and body of this age group; do not apply to the face, eyes, mouth, mucous membranes, or urethral meatus; shake lotion well before use

Patient Information For topical use only. Not for ophthalmic, oral, or intravaginal use. All contaminated clothing and bed linen should be washed to avoid reinfestation.

Additional Information Treatment may be repeated after 7-10 days if live mites are still present

Dosage Forms Excipient information presented when available (limited, particularly for generics); consult specific product labeling.
Cream: 10% (60 g)
Lotion: 10% (60 mL, 480 mL)

References

Eichenfield LF, Honig PJ, "Blistering Disorders in Childhood," *Pediatr Clin North Am*, 1991, 38(4):959-76.
Hogan DJ, Schachner L, Tanglertsampan C, "Diagnosis and Treatment of Childhood Scabies and Pediculosis," *Pediatr Clin North Am*, 1991, 38(4):941-57.

♦ **Crude Coal Tar** *see* Coal Tar *on page 394*
♦ **Cruex® Cream [OTC]** *see* Clotrimazole *on page 393*
♦ **Crystalline Penicillin** *see* Penicillin G (Parenteral/Aqueous) *on page 1231*
♦ **Crystal Violet** *see* Gentian Violet *on page 729*

- ♦ **CsA** *see* CycloSPORINE *on page 422*
- ♦ **C-Time [OTC]** *see* Ascorbic Acid *on page 159*
- ♦ **CTM** *see* Chlorpheniramine *on page 344*
- ♦ **CTX** *see* Cyclophosphamide *on page 419*
- ♦ **Culturelle® [OTC]** *see Lactobacillus acidophilus* and *Lactobacillus bulgaricus on page 898*
- ♦ **Cupric Chloride** *see* Trace Metals *on page 1558*
- ♦ **Cuprimine®** *see* Penicillamine *on page 1227*
- ♦ **Curosurf®** *see* Poractant Alfa *on page 1280*
- ♦ **Cutar® [OTC]** *see* Coal Tar *on page 394*
- ♦ **Cutivate®** *see* Fluticasone *on page 689*
- ♦ **Cutivate™ (Can)** *see* Fluticasone *on page 689*
- ♦ **CyA** *see* CycloSPORINE *on page 422*
- ♦ **Cyanide Antidote Kit** *see* Sodium Nitrite, Sodium Thiosulfate, and Amyl Nitrite *on page 1452*
- ♦ **Cyanide Antidote Package** *see* Sodium Nitrite, Sodium Thiosulfate, and Amyl Nitrite *on page 1452*

Cyanocobalamin (sye an oh koe BAL a min)

U.S. Brand Names Nascobal®; Twelve Resin-K

Index Terms Vitamin B_{12}

Therapeutic Category Nutritional Supplement; Vitamin, Water Soluble

Generic Available Yes: Excludes nasal spray

Use Treatment of pernicious anemia; vitamin B_{12} deficiency due to dietary deficiencies or malabsorption diseases; inadequate secretion of intrinsic factor, inadequate utilization of B_{12} (eg, during neoplastic treatment); increased B_{12} requirements due to pregnancy, thyrotoxicosis, hemorrhage, malignancy, liver or kidney disease; nutritional supplement

Pregnancy Risk Factor A/C (C if dose exceeds RDA recommendation); C (intranasal)

Lactation Enters breast milk/compatible

Contraindications Hypersensitivity to cyanocobalamin, any component (see Warnings), or cobalt; patients with hereditary optic nerve atrophy (Leber's disease)

Warnings I.M./SubQ routes are used to treat pernicious anemia; oral and intranasal administration are not indicated until hematologic remission and no signs of nervous system involvement. Avoid I.V. route as has been associated with anaphylaxis. Vitamin B_{12} deficiency for >3 months results in irreversible degenerative CNS lesions; neurologic manifestations will not be prevented with folic acid unless vitamin B_{12} is also given; spinal cord degeneration might also occur when folic acid is used as a substitute for vitamin B_{12} in anemia prevention. Vegetarian diets may result in vitamin B_{12} deficiency. Injection may contain benzyl alcohol which may cause allergic reactions in susceptible individuals; large amounts of benzyl alcohol (≥99 mg/kg/day) have been associated with a potentially fatal toxicity ("gasping syndrome") in neonates; the "gasping syndrome" consists of metabolic acidosis, respiratory distress, gasping respirations, CNS dysfunction (including convulsions, intracranial hemorrhage), hypotension and cardiovascular collapse; avoid use of benzyl alcohol containing injections in neonates; *in vitro* and animal studies have shown that benzoate, a metabolite of benzyl alcohol, displaces bilirubin from protein-binding sites. Intranasal therapy is only for use in patients who are in remission following injectable treatment. Patients with early Leber's disease (hereditary optic nerve atrophy) who were treated with vitamin B_{12} suffered severe and swift optic atrophy.

Precautions Serum potassium concentrations and platelet counts should be monitored early as severe hypokalemia (sometimes fatal) and thrombocytosis have occurred after the conversion of megaloblastic anemia to normal erythropoiesis; an intradermal test dose of parenteral cyanocobalamin is recommended before initiating the nasal spray in patients suspected to be sensitive to cyanocobalamin. Vitamin B_{12} deficiency masks signs of polycythemia vera; use caution in other conditions where folic acid or vitamin B_{12} administration alone might mask true diagnosis despite hematologic response. Some parenteral products contain aluminum; use caution in neonates and patients with impaired renal function.

Adverse Reactions

Cardiovascular: Peripheral vascular thrombosis (parenteral route)
Central nervous system: Headache, dizziness
Dermatologic: Itching, urticaria, exanthema
Endocrine & metabolic: Hypokalemia
Gastrointestinal: Diarrhea (mild)
Respiratory: Rhinitis (nasal gel), pulmonary edema (parenteral route)
Miscellaneous: Anaphylactic reactions, infection

(Continued)

Cyanocobalamin *(Continued)*

Drug Interactions
Decreased absorption of cyanocobalamin from GI tract: aminoglycoside antibiotics, colchicine, extended release potassium products, aminosalicylic acid, omeprazole (and potentially other PPIs), ethanol (heavy consumption >2 weeks), phenytoin, and phenobarbital; antagonism of hematopoietic response to cyanocobalamin: chloramphenicol; chemical degradation of cyanocobalamin: large doses of ascorbic acid

Stability Store at room temperature; protect from light; injection is **incompatible** with chlorpromazine, phytonadione, prochlorperazine, warfarin, ascorbic acid, dextrose, heavy metals, oxidizing or reducing agents

Mechanism of Action Coenzyme for various metabolic functions, including fat and carbohydrate metabolism and protein synthesis, used in cell replication and hematopoiesis

Pharmacodynamics Onset of action:
Megaloblastic anemia: I.M.:
Conversion of megaloblastic to normoblastic erythroid hyperplasia within bone marrow: 8 hours
Increased reticulocytes: 2-5 days
Complicated vitamin B_{12} deficiency: I.M., SubQ: Resolution of:
Psychiatric sequelae: 24 hours
Thrombocytopenia: 10 days
Granulocytopenia: 2 weeks

Pharmacokinetics
Absorption: Oral: Drug is absorbed from the terminal ileum in the presence of calcium; for absorption to occur, gastric "intrinsic factor" must be present to transfer the compound across the intestinal mucosa
Distribution: Principally stored in the liver, also stored in the kidneys and adrenals
Protein binding: Bound to transcobalamin II
Metabolism: Converted in the tissues to active coenzymes methylcobalamin and deoxyadenosylcobalamin
Bioavailability:
Oral: Pernicious anemia: 1.2%
Intranasal gel: 8.9% (relative to I.M. formulation)
Intranasal spray: 6.1% (relative to I.M. formulation)
Time to peak serum concentration:
I.M., SubQ: 30 minutes to 2 hours
Intranasal: 1.6 hours
Elimination: 50% to 98% unchanged in the urine

Usual Dosage
Adequate intake (AI): Oral, sublingual: **Note:** Infants born to vegan mothers should be supplemented with the AI for vitamin B_{12} from birth as their vitamin B_{12} stores at birth are low and their mother's milk may supply very small amounts of the vitamin.
Infants 0-6 months: 0.4 mcg/day (0.06 mcg/kg/day)
Children 7-12 months: 0.5 mcg/day (0.06 mcg/kg/day)
Recommended daily allowance (RDA): Oral, Sublingual:
Children:
1-3 years: 0.9 mcg/day
4-8 years: 1.2 mcg/day
9-13 years: 1.8 mcg/day
Children >14 years and Adults: 2.4 mcg/day
Adults, pregnancy: 2.6 mcg/day
Adults, lactation: 2. mcg/day
Pernicious anemia: **Note:** Initial low dosage recommended due to potential hypokalemia observed during initial treatment of adults with severe anemia (Rasmussen, 2001)
Neonates and infants (congenital; if evidence of neurologic involvement): I.M., SubQ: 0.2 mcg/kg for 2 days, followed by 1000 mcg/day for 2-7 days; maintenance: 100 mcg/month
Children: I.M., SubQ: 30-50 mcg/day for 2 or more weeks (to a total dose of 1000 mcg); maintenance: 100 mcg/month
Adults: I.M., SubQ: Initial treatment: 100 mcg/day for 6-7 days; if improvement, give same dose on alternate days for 7 doses; then every 3-4 days for 2-3 weeks or as an alternative, 1000 mcg/day for 7 days followed by 1000 mcg/week for 4 weeks; follow initial therapy with maintenance treatment (see below) for life.
Maintenance:
I.M., SubQ: 100-1000 mcg/month
Intranasal: 500 mcg (1 spray) in one nostril once weekly
Oral, Sublingual: 1000-2000 mcg/day; recommended only as a option for use in patients who are very compliant; avoid use of timed release formulations

Vitamin B_{12} deficiency:

Children (dosage in children not well established): I.M., SubQ: Initial: 0.2 mcg/kg for 2 days followed by 1000 mcg/day for 2-7 days followed by 100 mcg/week for a month; for malabsorptive causes of B_{12} deficiency, monthly maintenance doses of 100 mcg have been recommended or as an alternative 100 mcg/day for 10-15 days (total dose of 1-1.5 mg), then once or twice weekly for several months; may taper to 60 mcg every month

Adults:

Uncomplicated: Initial:

Oral, Sublingual: 1000-2500 mcg/day

I.M. or deep SubQ: 100 mcg/day for 5-10 days, followed by 100-200 mcg monthly until remission is complete **or** as an alternative: 100 mcg/day for 7 days, followed by 100 mcg every other day for 2 weeks, followed by 100 mcg every 3-4 days until remission is complete

Complicated (severe anemia, CHF, thrombocytopenia with bleeding, severe neurologic damage or granulocytopenia with infection): Initial: I.M. or deep SubQ: 1000 mcg with I.M. or I.V. folic acid 15 mg as single doses, followed by 1000 mcg/day plus oral folic acid 5 mg/day for 1 week; **Note:** Oral cyanocobalamin therapy is **not** indicated for treatment of complicated deficiency due to potential poor compliance

Maintenance:

I.M., deep SubQ: 100-200 mcg monthly

Oral, Sublingual: 1000-2500 mcg/day

Intranasal: 500 mcg (1 spray) once weekly

Note: Low initial B_{12} doses combined with potassium supplementation (as needed) may prevent a hypokalemia seen in patients with severe deficiency

Dosage adjustment in renal impairment: Increased dosage may be required in vitamin B_{12}-deficient patients

Administration

Oral: Not generally recommended for treatment of severe vitamin B_{12} deficiency due to poor oral absorption (lack of intrinsic factor); oral administration may be used in less severe deficiencies and maintenance therapy; may be administered without regard to food

Sublingual: Place under the tongue and allow to dissolve; do not swallow whole, chew, or crush

Parenteral: I.M. or deep SubQ: Avoid I.V. administration due to a more rapid system elimination with resulting decreased utilization

Intranasal: Prior to initial dose, activate (prime) spray nozzle by pumping unit quickly and firmly until first appearance of spray, then prime twice more. The unit must be reprimed once immediately before each use. Administer at least one hour before or after ingestion of hot foods or liquids; hot foods can cause nasal secretions and a resulting loss of medication

Monitoring Parameters Serum potassium (particularly during initial treatment of deficiency), erythrocyte and reticulocyte count, hemoglobin, hematocrit, platelets, serum cyanocobalamin and folate concentrations; methylmalonate (MMA) and total homocysteine (elevated in Vitamin B_{12} deficiency)

Reference Range Serum vitamin B_{12} levels: Normal: >300 pg/mL; vitamin B_{12} deficiency: <200 pg/mL (200-300 pg/mL borderline result, possible deficiency); megaloblastic anemia: <100 pg/mL

Dosage Forms Excipient information presented when available (limited, particularly for generics); consult specific product labeling.

Injection, solution: 1000 mcg/mL (1 mL, 10 mL, 30 mL) [may contain benzyl alcohol and/or aluminum]

Lozenge [OTC]: 100 mcg, 250 mcg, 500 mcg

Solution, intranasal [spray]:

Nascobal®: 500 mcg/0.1 mL actuation (2.3 mL) [contains benzalkonium chloride; delivers 8 doses]

Tablet [OTC]: 50 mcg, 100 mcg, 250 mcg, 500 mcg, 1000 mcg, 5000 mcg

Twelve Resin-K: 1000 mcg [may be used as oral, sublingual, or buccal]

Tablet, extended release [OTC]: 1000 mcg, 1500 mcg

Tablet, sublingual [OTC]: 2500 mcg

References

"Dietary Reference Intakes for Thiamin, Riboflavin, Niacin, Vitamin B_6, Folate, Vitamin B_{12}, Pantothenic Acid, Biotin, and Choline," (Chapter 9) available at http://books.nap.edu/openbook/0309065542/html/306.html. Last accessed February 22, 2005.

Lane LA and Rojas-Fernandez C, "Treatment of Vitamin B(12)-Deficiency Anemia: Oral Versus Parenteral Therapy," *Ann Pharmacother*, 2002, 36(7):1268-72.

Rasmussen SA, Fernhoff PM, and Scanlon KS, "Vitamin B_{12} Deficiency in Children and Adolescents," *J Pediatr*, 2001, 138(1):10-7.

♦ **Cyanokit®** *see* Hydroxocobalamin *on page 790*

Cyclobenzaprine (sye kloe BEN za preen)

Medication Safety Issues

Sound-alike/look-alike issues:

Cyclobenzaprine may be confused with cycloSERINE, cyproheptadine

Flexeril® may be confused with Floxin®

U.S. Brand Names Fexmid™; Flexeril®

Canadian Brand Names Apo-Cyclobenzaprine®; Flexeril®; Flexitec; Gen-Cyclobenzaprine; Novo-Cycloprine; Nu-Cyclobenzaprine

Index Terms Cyclobenzaprine Hydrochloride

Therapeutic Category Skeletal Muscle Relaxant, Nonparalytic

Generic Available Yes

Use Treatment of muscle spasm associated with acute painful musculoskeletal conditions; supportive therapy in tetanus

Pregnancy Risk Factor B

Lactation Excretion in breast milk unknown/use caution

Contraindications Hypersensitivity to cyclobenzaprine or any component; hyperthyroidism, acute recovery phase of MI, CHF, arrhythmias, heart block; do not use concomitantly or within 14 days of MAO inhibitors

Warnings Abrupt withdrawal after prolonged administration may result in nausea, headache, and malaise; not effective in the treatment of spasticity due to cerebral or spinal cord disease; avoid use in patients with moderate to severe hepatic dysfunction

Precautions Use with caution in patients with urinary retention, angle-closure glaucoma and patients receiving anticholinergic medications; use with caution and reduce dosage in patients with mildly impaired liver function

Adverse Reactions

Cardiovascular: Tachycardia, hypotension, arrhythmias, edema of face/lips, syncope, palpitations

Central nervous system: Drowsiness, headache, dizziness, fatigue, nervousness, confusion, anorexia, seizures, ataxia, vertigo, insomnia, psychosis, anxiety, agitation, hallucinations

Dermatologic: Rash, pruritus, urticaria

Gastrointestinal: Dyspepsia, nausea, constipation, xerostomia, vomiting, diarrhea, paralytic ileus, dysgeusia, stomach cramps, flatulence, tongue edema

Genitourinary: Urinary frequency or retention

Hepatic: Hepatitis, cholestasis, jaundice

Neuromuscular & skeletal: Weakness, muscle twitching, tremors, paresthesia

Ocular: Diplopia

Otic: Tinnitus

Miscellaneous: Hypersensitivity reactions, angioedema

Drug Interactions Cytochrome P450 isoenzyme CYP1A2, CYP2D6, CYP3A3/4 substrate

MAO inhibitors; additive effects with sedatives, alcohol, anticholinergic agents, and other CNS depressants; due to close chemical and physiologic relationship to tricyclic antidepressants, cyclobenzaprine may share some of the same drug interactions; may increase risk of seizures with tramadol; may decrease antihypertensive effects of guanethidine

Stability Store at room temperature

Mechanism of Action Centrally-acting skeletal muscle relaxant pharmacologically related to tricyclic antidepressants; reduces tonic somatic motor activity influencing both alpha and gamma motor neurons

Pharmacodynamics

Onset of action: Within 1 hour

Duration: 12-24 hours

Pharmacokinetics

Absorption: Oral: Complete

Metabolism: Hepatic

Bioavailability: 33% to 55%

Half-life: Adults: 18 hours (range 8-37 hours)

Time to peak serum concentration: Within 3-8 hours

Elimination: Primarily renal as inactive metabolites and in the feces (via bile) as unchanged drug; may undergo enterohepatic recycling

Clearance: Adults: 0.7 L/minute

Usual Dosage Oral:

Children: Dosage has not been established

Adolescents and Adults: 5 mg 3 times/day; may increase to 10 mg 3 times/day; usage for more than 2-3 weeks is not recommended

Dosage adjustment in hepatic impairment:
Mild: 5 mg 3 times/day
Moderate to severe: Use not recommended

Administration Oral: May be administered without regard to meals

Monitoring Parameters Relief of muscle spasms and pain; improvement in physical activities

Patient Information Avoid alcohol; may cause drowsiness and impair ability to perform activities requiring mental alertness or physical coordination; may cause dry mouth

Dosage Forms Excipient information presented when available (limited, particularly for generics); consult specific product labeling.
Tablet, as hydrochloride: 5 mg, 10 mg
Fexmid™: 7.5 mg
Flexeril®: 5 mg, 10 mg

- **Cyclobenzaprine Hydrochloride** *see* Cyclobenzaprine *on page 416*
- **Cyclogyl®** *see* Cyclopentolate *on page 417*
- **Cyclomen® (Can)** *see* Danazol *on page 437*
- **Cyclomydril®** *see* Cyclopentolate and Phenylephrine *on page 418*

Cyclopentolate (sye kloe PEN toe late)

U.S. Brand Names AK-Pentolate® [DSC]; Cyclogyl®; Cylate®

Canadian Brand Names Cyclogyl®; Diopentolate®

Index Terms Cyclopentolate Hydrochloride

Therapeutic Category Anticholinergic Agent, Ophthalmic; Ophthalmic Agent, Mydriatic

Generic Available Yes

Use Diagnostic procedures requiring mydriasis and cycloplegia

Pregnancy Risk Factor C

Contraindications Hypersensitivity to cyclopentolate or any component; narrow-angle glaucoma

Warnings Use of cyclopentolate has been associated with psychotic reactions and behavioral disturbances in pediatric patients; increased susceptibility to these effects has been reported in young infants, young children, and in children with spastic paralysis or brain damage, particularly with concentrations >1%; observe neonates and infants closely for at least 30 minutes after administration; may cause transient elevation of intraocular pressure

Adverse Reactions Central nervous system and cardiovascular reactions most commonly seen in children after receiving 2% solution:
Cardiovascular: Tachycardia, hypertension
Central nervous system: Psychotic and behavioral disturbances manifested by ataxia, restlessness, hallucinations, psychosis, hyperactivity, seizures, incoherent speech
Local: Burning sensation
Ocular: Elevated intraocular pressure, loss of visual accommodation
Miscellaneous: Allergic reactions

Mechanism of Action Prevents the muscle of the ciliary body and the sphincter muscle of the iris from responding to cholinergic stimulation, causing mydriasis and cycloplegia

Pharmacodynamics
Maximum effect:
Cycloplegia: 15-60 minutes
Mydriasis: Within 15-60 minutes, with recovery taking up to 24 hours

Usual Dosage Ophthalmic:
Neonates and Infants: See Cyclopentolate and Phenylephrine *on page 418* (preferred agent for use in neonates and infants due to lower cyclopentolate concentration and reduced risk for systemic reactions)
Children: 1 drop of 0.5% or 1% in eye followed by 1 drop of 0.5% or 1% in 5 minutes, if necessary, approximately 40-50 minutes before procedure
Adults: 1 drop of 1% followed by another drop in 5 minutes; approximately 40-50 minutes prior to the procedure, may use 2% solution in heavily pigmented iris

Administration Ophthalmic: Instill drops into conjunctival sac of affected eye(s); avoid contact of bottle tip with skin or eye; to avoid excessive systemic absorption, finger pressure should be applied on the lacrimal sac during and for 1-2 minutes following application

Patient Information May cause blurred vision and increased sensitivity to light

Additional Information Pilocarpine ophthalmic drops applied after the examination may reduce recovery time to 3-6 hours

Dosage Forms Excipient information presented when available (limited, particularly for generics); consult specific product labeling. [DSC] = Discontinued product
(Continued)

Cyclopentolate *(Continued)*

Solution, ophthalmic, as hydrochloride: 1% (2 mL, 15 mL)
AK-Pentolate® [DSC], Cylate®: 1% (2 mL, 15 mL) [contains benzalkonium chloride]
Cyclogyl®: 0.5% (15 mL); 1% (2 mL, 5 mL, 15 mL); 2% (2 mL, 5 mL, 15 mL) [contains benzalkonium chloride]

Cyclopentolate and Phenylephrine

(sye kloe PEN toe late & fen il EF rin)

U.S. Brand Names Cyclomydril®

Index Terms Phenylephrine and Cyclopentolate

Therapeutic Category Adrenergic Agonist Agent, Ophthalmic; Anticholinergic Agent, Ophthalmic; Ophthalmic Agent, Mydriatic

Generic Available No

Use Diagnostic procedures requiring mydriasis and cycloplegia; preferred agent for use in neonates and infants

Pregnancy Risk Factor C

Contraindications Hypersensitivity to cyclopentolate, phenylephrine, or any component; narrow-angle glaucoma or untreated anatomically narrow angles

Warnings Use of cyclopentolate has been associated with psychotic reactions and behavioral disturbances in pediatric patients; increased susceptibility to these effects has been reported in young infants, young children, and in children with spastic paralysis or brain damage, particularly with concentrations >1%; observe neonates and infants closely for at least 30 minutes after administration; may cause transient elevation of intraocular pressure. The preservative, benzalkonium chloride, may be absorbed by soft contact lenses. Wait at least 10 minutes after instillation before reinserting lenses.

Precautions Use with caution in patient's with Down's syndrome, cardiovascular disease, hypertension, and hyperthyroidism; feeding intolerance may follow ophthalmic use of this product in neonates and infants; withhold feedings for 4 hours after examination

Adverse Reactions

Cardiovascular: Tachycardia, hypertension
Central nervous system: Psychotic and behavioral disturbances manifested by ataxia, restlessness, hallucinations, psychosis, hyperactivity, seizures, incoherent speech, hyperpyrexia
Gastrointestinal: Feeding intolerance, decreased gastric motility
Genitourinary: Urinary retention
Local: Burning sensation
Ocular: Elevated intraocular pressure, loss of visual accommodation, transient stinging, browache, photophobia, lacrimation, superficial punctate keratitis
Miscellaneous: Allergic reactions

Drug Interactions May interfere with the ocular antihypertensive action of carbachol, pilocarpine, or ophthalmic cholinesterase inhibitors

Stability Store at room temperature

Mechanism of Action See individual monographs for Cyclopentolate *on page 417* and Phenylephrine *on page 1250*

Pharmacodynamics Onset of action and duration of effect are partially dependent upon eye pigment; dark eyes have a prolonged onset of action and shorter duration than blue eyes

Onset of action: 15-60 minutes
Duration: 4-12 hours

Usual Dosage Ophthalmic:

Neonates, Infants, Children, and Adults: Instill 1 drop into the eye every 5-10 minutes, for up to 3 doses, approximately 40-50 minutes before the examination

Administration Ophthalmic: Instill drops into conjunctival sac of affected eye(s); avoid contact of bottle tip with skin or eye; to avoid excessive systemic absorption, finger pressure should be applied on the lacrimal sac during and for 1-2 minutes following application; preservative absorbed by soft contact lenses; wait at least 10 minutes before reinserting

Patient Information May cause blurred vision and increased sensitivity to light; preservative is absorbed by soft contact lenses (see Warnings)

Nursing Implications Do not repeat dosage within at least 4 hours, but preferably 24 hours, after initial treatment to prevent drug accumulation and potential systemic toxicity; see Warnings

Additional Information Cyclomydril® is the preferred agent for use in neonates and infants because lower concentrations of both cyclopentolate and phenylephrine provide optimal dilation while minimizing the systemic side effects noted with a higher concentration of each agent used alone

Dosage Forms Excipient information presented when available (limited, particularly for generics); consult specific product labeling.

Solution, ophthalmic: Cyclopentolate hydrochloride 0.2% and phenylephrine hydrochloride 1% (2 mL, 5 mL) [contains benzalkonium chloride]

♦ **Cyclopentolate Hydrochloride** *see* Cyclopentolate *on page 417*

Cyclophosphamide (sye kloe FOS fa mide)

Medication Safety Issues

Sound-alike/look-alike issues:

Cyclophosphamide may be confused with cycloSPORINE, ifosfamide

Cytoxan® may be confused with cefoxitin, Centoxin®, Ciloxan®, cytarabine, CytoGam®, Cytosar®, Cytosar-U®, Cytotec®

High alert medication: The Institute for Safe Medication Practices (ISMP) includes this medication among its list of drugs which have a heightened risk of causing significant patient harm when used in error.

Related Information

Compatibility of Chemotherapy and Related Supportive Care Medications *on page 1777*

Emetogenic Potential of Single Chemotherapeutic Agents *on page 1776*

U.S. Brand Names Cytoxan®

Canadian Brand Names Cytoxan®; Procytox®

Index Terms CPM; CTX; CYT; Neosar; NSC-26271

Therapeutic Category Antineoplastic Agent, Alkylating Agent (Nitrogen Mustard)

Generic Available Yes: Tablet

Use Treatment of Hodgkin's disease, malignant lymphomas, multiple myeloma, leukemias, sarcomas, mycosis fungoides, neuroblastoma, ovarian carcinoma, breast carcinoma, a variety of other tumors; conditioning regimen for bone marrow transplantation; nephrotic syndrome, lupus erythematosus, severe rheumatoid arthritis, and rheumatoid vasculitis

Pregnancy Risk Factor D

Lactation Enters breast milk/contraindicated

Contraindications Hypersensitivity to cyclophosphamide or any component

Warnings The FDA currently recommends that procedures for proper handling and disposal of antineoplastic agents be considered; cyclophosphamide is potentially carcinogenic and mutagenic; it may impair fertility or cause sterility and birth defects

Precautions Use with caution in patients with bone marrow suppression and impaired renal or hepatic function; modify dosage in patients with renal impairment or compromised bone marrow function. Patients with compromised bone marrow function may require a 33% to 50% reduction in initial dose.

Adverse Reactions

Cardiovascular: Cardiotoxicity with high-dose therapy, pericardial effusion, CHF

Dermatologic: Alopecia, rash, pigmentation of skin, nail changes, Stevens-Johnson syndrome (rare), toxic epidermal necrolysis (rare)

Endocrine & metabolic: Hypokalemia, amenorrhea, SIADH, hyperuricemia, hyperkalemia, hyponatremia, oligospermia, sterility (interferes with oogenesis and spermatogenesis) which may be irreversible

Gastrointestinal: Nausea, vomiting, dysgeusia, anorexia, diarrhea, mucositis

Genitourinary: Hemorrhagic cystitis (5% to 10%)

Hematologic: Leukopenia nadir at 8-15 days, hemolytic anemia, thrombocytopenia, hypothrombinemia

Hepatic: Dose-related hepatotoxicity, jaundice

Renal: Nephrotoxicity

Respiratory: Interstitial pulmonary fibrosis, nasal stuffiness

Drug Interactions Cytochrome P450 isoenzyme CYP2B6, CYP2D6, and CYP3A3/4 substrate

Allopurinol (increases myelotoxicity of cyclophosphamide); phenobarbital, phenytoin, and chloral hydrate may increase conversion of cyclophosphamide to active metabolites; chloramphenicol, phenothiazines, imipramine may inhibit the metabolism of cyclophosphamide (increased bone marrow suppression); cyclophosphamide may prolong the neuromuscular blocking activity of succinylcholine

Stability Reconstituted I.V. solution is stable for 24 hours at room temperature or 6 days if refrigerated

Mechanism of Action Interferes with the normal function of DNA by alkylation and cross-linking the strands of DNA, and by possible protein modification

Pharmacokinetics

Absorption: 75% to 95% with low doses

(Continued)

Cyclophosphamide *(Continued)*

Distribution: Crosses the placenta; appears in breast milk; distributes throughout the body including the brain and CSF, but not in concentrations high enough to treat meningeal leukemia

Protein binding: 20%; metabolite: 60%

Metabolism: Inactive prodrug must undergo hydroxylation to form active alkylating mustards; further oxidation leads to formation of inactive metabolites

Half-life: Range 3-12 hours
- Children: 4 hours
- Adults: 6-8 hours

Time to peak serum concentration: Oral: Within 1 hour

Elimination: In urine as unchanged drug (<20%) and as metabolites (85% to 90%)

Dialysis: Moderately dialyzable (20% to 50%)

Usual Dosage Refer to individual protocols

Children and Adults with no hematologic problems:

Induction:
- Oral, I.V.: Children: 2-8 mg/kg or 60-250 mg/m^2/day
- I.V.: 40-50 mg/kg (1.5-1.8 g/m^2) in divided doses over 2-5 days

Maintenance:
- Oral: Children: 2-5 mg/kg or 50-150 mg/m^2 twice weekly
- Oral: Adults: 1-5 mg/kg/day
- I.V.: 10-15 mg/kg (350-550 mg/m^2) every 7-10 days or 3-5 mg/kg (110-185 mg/m^2) twice weekly

Children:
- SLE: I.V.: 500-750 mg/m^2 every month; maximum dose: 1 g/m^2
- JRA/vasculitis: I.V.: 10 mg/kg every 2 weeks
- BMT conditioning regimen: I.V.: 50 mg/kg/day once daily for 3-4 days
- Nephrotic syndrome: Oral: 2-3 mg/kg/day every day for up to 12 weeks when corticosteroids are unsuccessful

Dosing adjustment in renal impairment:
- Cl_{cr} >10 mL/minute: Administer 100% of normal dose
- Cl_{cr} ≤10 mL/minute: Administer 75% of normal dose

Administration

Oral: Administer with food only if GI distress occurs

Parenteral: May administer IVP, I.V. intermittent, or continuous infusion at a final maximum concentration for administration of 20-25 mg/mL; usually administered as a single bolus dose or in fractionated doses over 2-3 days. Most protocols use a 30-60 minute infusion time; doses >1800 mg/m^2 need to be infused over a longer period (ie, 4- or 6-hour infusions)

Monitoring Parameters CBC with differential and platelet count, ESR, BUN, urinalysis, serum electrolytes, serum creatinine, urine specific gravity, urine output

Test Interactions Positive Coombs' [direct]

Patient Information Maintain high fluid intake and urine output. Report any difficulty or pain with urination, unusual bleeding or bruising, persistent fever or sore throat, blood in urine or stool, skin rash, or yellowing of skin or eyes. You may be more susceptible to infection; avoid crowds and unnecessary exposure to infection.

Nursing Implications Encourage adequate hydration and frequent voiding to help prevent hemorrhagic cystitis; before initiating cyclophosphamide therapy, verify that urine specific gravity is <1.010 and that urine output is >100 mL/m^2/hour (or 3 mL/kg/hour)

Additional Information Aggressive hydration using fluid containing at least 0.45% sodium chloride at 125 mL/m^2/hour, frequent emptying of the bladder, and concurrent administration of mesna are used to reduce the potential of hemorrhagic cystitis (use mesna with cyclophosphamide doses >1 g/m^2/day; doses ≤1 g/m^2/day may not require use of mesna)

Myelosuppressive effects:
- WBC: Moderate
- Platelets: Moderate
- Onset (days): 7
- Nadir (days): 8-14
- Recovery (days): 21

Dosage Forms Excipient information presented when available (limited, particularly for generics); consult specific product labeling.

Injection, powder for reconstitution:
- Cytoxan®: 500 mg, 1 g, 2 g [contains mannitol 75 mg per cyclophosphamide 100 mg

Tablet: 25 mg, 50 mg
- Cytoxan®: 25 mg, 50 mg

Extemporaneous Preparations To make a 2 mg/mL oral elixir, reconstitute a 200 mg vial with aromatic elixir, withdraw the solution, and add sufficient aromatic elixir to make a final volume of 100 mL in a graduate; store in amber glass; stable for 14 days in the refrigerator

Brook D, Davis RE, and Bequette RJ, "Chemical Stability of Cyclophosphamide in Aromatic Elixir USP," *Am J Hosp Pharm*, 1973, 30:618-20.

References

Bostrom BC, Weisdorf DJ, Kim TH, et al, "Bone Marrow Transplantation for Advanced Acute Leukemia: A Pilot Study of High-Energy Total Body Irradiation, Cyclophosphamide and Continuous Infusion Etoposide," *Bone Marrow Transplant*, 1990, 5(2):83-9.

McCune WJ, Golbus J, Zeldes W, et al, "Clinical and Immunologic Effects of Monthly Administration of Intravenous Cyclophosphamide in Severe Systemic Lupus Erythematosus," *N Engl J Med*, 1988, 318(22):1423-31.

CycloSERINE (sye kloe SER een)

Medication Safety Issues

Sound-alike/look-alike issues:

CycloSERINE may be confused with cyclobenzaprine, cycloSPORINE

U.S. Brand Names Seromycin®

Therapeutic Category Antibiotic, Miscellaneous; Antitubercular Agent

Generic Available No

Use Adjunctive treatment in pulmonary or extrapulmonary tuberculosis; treatment of acute urinary tract infections caused by *E. coli* or *Enterobacter* species when less toxic conventional therapy has failed or is contraindicated

Pregnancy Risk Factor C

Lactation Enters breast milk/compatible

Contraindications Hypersensitivity to cycloserine or any component; epilepsy, depression, severe anxiety or psychosis, severe renal insufficiency, chronic alcoholism

Precautions Dosage must be adjusted in patients with renal impairment

Adverse Reactions

Cardiovascular: Cardiac arrhythmias, CHF

Central nervous system: Drowsiness, headache, dizziness, vertigo, seizures, confusion, psychosis, paresis, coma, anxiety, nervousness, depression, personality changes

Dermatologic: Rash, photosensitivity

Endocrine & metabolic: Vitamin B_{12} deficiency, folate deficiency

Hepatic: Elevated liver enzymes

Neuromuscular & skeletal: Tremor, dysarthria

Drug Interactions Cycloserine inhibits metabolism of phenytoin; alcohol may increase risk of seizures; ethionamide, isoniazid (additive neurotoxicity with cycloserine)

Food Interactions May increase vitamin B_{12} and folic acid dietary requirements

Mechanism of Action Inhibits bacterial cell wall synthesis by competing with amino acid (D-alanine) for incorporation into the bacterial cell wall

Pharmacokinetics

Absorption: ~70% to 90% from the GI tract

Distribution: Crosses the placenta; appears in breast milk, bile, sputum, synovial fluid and CSF

Protein binding: Not plasma protein bound

Half-life: Patients with normal renal function: 10 hours

Time to peak serum concentration: Within 3-4 hours

Elimination: 60% to 70% of an oral dose excreted unchanged in urine by glomerular filtration within 72 hours, small amounts excreted in feces, remainder is metabolized

Usual Dosage Oral:

Tuberculosis:

Children: 10-20 mg/kg/day divided every 12 hours up to 1000 mg/day

Adults: Initial: 250 mg every 12 hours for 14 days, then give 500 mg to 1 g/day in 2 divided doses

Urinary tract infection: Adults: 250 mg every 12 hours for 14 days

Dosing adjustment in renal impairment:

Cl_{cr} 10-50 mL/minute: Administer every 24 hours

Cl_{cr} <10 mL/minute: Administer every 36-48 hours

Administration Oral: May administer without regard to meals

Monitoring Parameters Periodic renal, hepatic, hematological tests, and plasma cycloserine concentrations

Reference Range Adjust dosage to maintain blood cycloserine concentrations <30 mcg/mL

(Continued)

CycloSERINE *(Continued)*

Patient Information May cause drowsiness and impair ability to perform activities requiring mental alertness or physical coordination; avoid alcohol. May cause photosensitivity reactions (eg, exposure to sunlight may cause severe sunburn, skin rash, redness, or itching); avoid exposure to sunlight and artificial light sources (sunlamps, tanning booth/bed); wear protective clothing, wide-brimmed hats, sunglasses, and lip sunscreen (SPF ≥15); use a sunscreen [broad-spectrum sunscreen or physical sunscreen (preferred) or sunblock with SPF ≥15]; contact physician if reaction occurs.

Nursing Implications Some of the neurotoxic effects may be relieved or prevented by the concomitant administration of pyridoxine; sedatives may be effective in reducing anxiety or tremor

Dosage Forms Excipient information presented when available (limited, particularly for generics); consult specific product labeling.

Capsule: 250 mg

♦ **Cyclosporin A** *see* CycloSPORINE *on page 422*

CycloSPORINE (SYE kloe spor een)

Medication Safety Issues

Sound-alike/look-alike issues:

CycloSPORINE may be confused with cyclophosphamide, Cyklokapron®, cycloSERINE

CycloSPORINE modified (Neoral®, Gengraf®) may be confused with cycloSPORINE non-modified (Sandimmne®)

Gengraf® may be confused with Prograf®

Neoral® may be confused with Neurontin®, Nizoral®

Sandimmune® may be confused with Sandostatin®

Related Information

Blood Level Sampling Time Guidelines *on page 1914*

U.S. Brand Names Gengraf®; Neoral®; Restasis®; Sandimmune®

Canadian Brand Names Neoral®; Rhoxal-cyclosporine; Sandimmune® I.V.; Sandoz-Cyclosporine

Index Terms CsA; CyA; Cyclosporin A

Therapeutic Category Immunosuppressant Agent

Generic Available Yes

Use Immunosuppressant used with corticosteroids to prevent organ rejection in patients with kidney, liver, lung, heart, and bone marrow transplants; treatment of nephrotic syndrome in patients with documented focal glomerulosclerosis when corticosteroids and cyclophosphamide are unsuccessful; severe psoriasis; severe rheumatoid arthritis not responsive to methotrexate alone; severe autoimmune disease that is resistant to corticosteroids and other therapy; prevention and treatment of graft-versus-host disease in bone marrow transplant patients

Ophthalmic emulsion: Increase tear production in patients with moderate to severe keratoconjunctivitis sicca-associated ocular inflammation

Pregnancy Risk Factor C

Lactation Enters breast milk/not recommended

Contraindications Hypersensitivity to cyclosporine or any component (ie, polyoxyl 35 castor oil is an ingredient of the parenteral formulation and polyoxyl 40 hydrogenated castor oil is an ingredient of the cyclosporine capsules and solution for microemulsion). AAP considers cyclosporine to be contraindicated during breast-feeding. Concurrent therapy with PUVA or UVB, methotrexate, coal tar, or radiation therapy for use in patients with psoriasis; presence of uncontrolled hypertension, abnormal renal function, or malignancies in treatment of psoriasis or rheumatoid arthritis. Ophthalmic emulsion is contraindicated in patients with active ocular infections.

Warnings Immunosuppression with cyclosporine may result in an increased susceptibility to infection and an increased risk of malignancy (lymphomas, lymphoproliferative disorders and squamous cell carcinoma); closely monitor and be prepared to treat anaphylaxis in patients receiving I.V. cyclosporine; serious nephrotoxicity, hepatotoxicity, hypertension, and/or seizures may occur in children receiving cyclosporine; **monitor renal function and adjust dosage to avoid toxicity or possible organ rejection via cyclosporine blood or plasma concentration monitoring.**

Transplant patients: Cyclosporine may cause significant hyperkalemia and hyperuricemia. May cause seizures, particularly if used with high-dose corticosteroids. Predisposing factors associated with neurological disorders include hypertension, hypomagnesemia, hypocholesterolemia, high-dose corticosteroids, high cyclosporine serum concentration, and graft-versus-host disease.

Precautions Close monitoring and dosage adjustment is required in patients with renal and hepatic impairment. Use caution when changing dosage forms since products cannot be used interchangeably.

Adverse Reactions

Cardiovascular: Hypertension, flushing, edema, arrhythmia

Central nervous system: Seizures, headache, confusion, fever, anxiety, lethargy, dizziness, depression

Dermatologic: Hirsutism, gingival hyperplasia, acne, hypertrichosis, pruritus

Endocrine & metabolic: Hyperkalemia, hypomagnesemia, hyperuricemia, hyperchloremic metabolic acidosis, gynecomastia, hyperlipidemia (in patients receiving I.V. cyclosporine), weight loss

Gastrointestinal: Abdominal discomfort, diarrhea, nausea, vomiting, anorexia, pancreatitis, hiccups, peptic ulcer, stomatitis

Hematologic: Leukopenia, anemia, thrombocytopenia

Hepatic: Hepatotoxicity (elevated liver enzymes, hyperbilirubinemia)

Neuromuscular & skeletal: Myositis, tremor, paresthesia, leg cramps, weakness

Ocular: Ophthalmic preparation: Ocular burning, hyperemia, eye pain, pruritus, stinging

Otic: Tinnitus, hearing loss

Renal: Nephrotoxicity (elevated BUN and serum creatinine)

Respiratory: Sinusitis, cough, dyspnea

Miscellaneous: Lymphoproliferative disorder, increased susceptibility to infection, sensitivity to temperature extremes, anaphylaxis in patients receiving I.V. cyclosporine (reaction includes flushing of the face, respiratory distress with dyspnea and wheezing, hypotension, tachycardia), flu-like symptoms

Drug Interactions Cytochrome P450 isoenzyme CYP3A3/4 substrate

Ketoconazole, itraconazole, amiodarone, fluconazole, azithromycin, clarithromycin, allopurinol, erythromycin, tacrolimus, diltiazem, verapamil, and methylprednisolone increase cyclosporine concentration by inhibiting hepatic metabolism; acyclovir, amphotericin B, aminoglycosides, NSAIDs, sulfamethoxazole and trimethoprim, melphalan, ciprofloxacin, tacrolimus, and vancomycin may increase nephrotoxicity of cyclosporine; erythromycin and metoclopramide increase cyclosporine absorption; phenytoin and octreotide decrease cyclosporine bioavailability; phenytoin, phenobarbital, carbamazepine, primidone, ticlopidine, rifabutin, rifampin, trimethoprim, and nafcillin decrease cyclosporine concentration by increasing hepatic metabolism of cyclosporine; decreases clearance of digoxin, prednisolone; potassium-sparing diuretics increase risk of hyperkalemia; lovastatin, simvastatin, and cimetidine may increase cyclosporine concentration; the herbal medicine St John's wort (*Hypericum perforatum*) may significantly decrease concentrations of cyclosporine; live vaccines may be less effective (avoid vaccination during therapy); cyclosporine increases plasma levels of methotrexate; cyclosporine increases AUC of doxorubicin

Food Interactions Grapefruit and grapefruit juice may affect cyclosporine metabolism resulting in increased cyclosporine concentrations

Stability **Do not** store oral solution or oral solution for emulsion in the refrigerator; store oral solutions in original container only and use contents within 2 months after opening; store ampuls and ophthalmic emulsion-containing vials at room temperature; protect from light; I.V. cyclosporine prepared in NS is stable 6 hours in a polyvinyl chloride container or 12 hours in a glass container; I.V. cyclosporine diluted in D_5W to a final concentration of 2 mg/mL is stable for 24 hours in glass or polyvinyl chloride containers; I.V. cyclosporine may bind to the plastic tubing in I.V. administration sets and to polyvinyl chloride bags. Polyoxyethylated castor oil (Cremophor El®) surfactant in cyclosporine injection may leach phthalate from polyvinyl chloride containers such as bags and tubing.

Mechanism of Action Inhibition of production and release of interleukin II and inhibits interleukin II-induced activation of resting T lymphocytes

Pharmacokinetics

Absorption: Oral:

Cyclosporine (non-modified) solution or soft gelatin capsule: Erratically and incompletely absorbed; dependent on the presence of food, bile acids, and GI motility; larger oral doses of cyclosporine are needed in pediatric patients vs adults due to a shorter bowel length resulting in limited intestinal absorption

Cyclosporine (modified) solution in a microemulsion or soft gelatin capsule in a microemulsion: Erratically and incompletely absorbed; increased absorption, up to 30% when compared to cyclosporine (non-modified); absorption is less dependent on food intake, bile, or GI motility when compared to cyclosporine (non-modified)

Distribution: Widely distributed in tissues and body fluids including the liver, pancreas, and lungs; crosses the placenta; excreted into breast milk

V_{dss}: 4-6 L/kg in renal, liver, and marrow transplant recipients (slightly lower values in cardiac transplant patients; children <10 years of age have higher values)

(Continued)

CycloSPORINE *(Continued)*

Protein binding: 90% to 98% of dose binds to blood lipoproteins

Metabolism: Undergoes extensive first-pass metabolism following oral administration; extensively metabolized by the cytochrome P450 system in the liver; forms at least 25 metabolites

Bioavailability:

Cyclosporine (non-modified): Dependent on patient population and transplant type (<10% in adult liver transplant patients and as high as 89% in renal patients). The bioavailability of Sandimmune® capsules and oral solution are equivalent; bioavailability of oral solution is ~30% of the I.V. solution.

Children: 28% (range: 17% to 42%); with gut dysfunction commonly seen in BMT recipients, oral bioavailability is further reduced

Cyclosporine (modified): Bioavailability of Neoral® capsules and oral solution are equivalent:

Children: 43% (range: 30% to 68%)

Adults: 23% greater than with Sandimmune® in renal transplant patients, 50% greater in liver transplant patients

Half-life: May be prolonged in patients with hepatic impairment and lower in pediatric patients due to a higher metabolic rate

Cyclosporine (non-modified): Biphasic

Alpha phase: 1.4 hours

Terminal phase: 6-24 hours

Cyclosporine (modified): 8.4 hours (range: 5-18 hours)

Time to peak serum concentration:

Cyclosporine (non-modified): 2-6 hours; some patients have a second peak at 5-6 hours

Cyclosporine (modified): 1.5-2 hours (in renal transplant patients)

Elimination: Primarily biliary with 6% of the dose excreted in urine as unchanged drug (0.1%) and metabolites; clearance is more rapid in pediatric patients than in adults

Usual Dosage Children and Adults (oral dosage is ~3 times the I.V. dosage):

Transplantations:

I.V.: Cyclosporine (non-modified):

Initial: 5-6 mg/kg/dose (1/3 the oral dose) administered 4-12 hours prior to organ transplantation

Maintenance: 2-10 mg/kg/day in divided doses every 8-24 hours; patients should be switched to oral cyclosporine as soon as possible; cyclosporine doses should be adjusted to maintain whole blood HPLC trough concentrations in the reference range

Oral: Cyclosporine (non-modified):

Initial: 14-18 mg/kg/dose administered 4-12 hours prior to organ transplantation; lower initial doses of 10-14 mg/kg/day have been used for renal transplants

Maintenance, postoperative: 5-15 mg/kg/day divided every 12-24 hours; maintenance dose is usually tapered to 3-10 mg/kg/day

When using non-modified formulation, cyclosporine levels may increase in liver transplant patients when the T-tube is closed; may need to decrease dose

Oral: Cyclosporine (modified): Based on the organ transplant population:

Initial: Same as the initial dose for solution or soft gelatin capsule

or

Renal: 9 mg/kg/day (range: 6-12 mg/kg/day) divided every 12 hours

Liver: 8 mg/kg/day (range: 4-12 mg/kg/day) divided every 12 hours

Heart: 7 mg/kg/day (range: 4-10 mg/kg/day) divided every 12 hours

Note: A 1:1 ratio conversion from Sandimmune® to Neoral® has been recommended initially; however, lower doses of Neoral® may be required after conversion to prevent overdose. Total daily doses should be adjusted based on the cyclosporine trough blood concentration and clinical assessment of organ rejection. Cyclosporine blood trough levels should be determined prior to conversion. After conversion to Neoral®, cyclosporine trough levels should be monitored every 4-7 days. **Neoral® and Sandimmune® are not bioequivalent and cannot be used interchangeably.**

Focal segmental glomerulosclerosis: Oral: Initial: 3 mg/kg/day divided every 12 hours

Rheumatoid arthritis: Oral: Cyclosporine (modified): Initial: 2.5 mg/kg/day divided every 12 hours; may increase dose by 0.5-0.75 mg/kg/day if insufficient response is seen after 8 weeks of treatment; maximum dose: 4 mg/kg/day

Psoriasis: Oral: Cyclosporine (modified): Initial: 2.5 mg/kg/day divided every 12 hours; may increase dose by 0.5 mg/kg/day if insufficient response is seen after 4 weeks of treatment; maximum dose: 4 mg/kg/day

Autoimmune diseases: Oral: 1-3 mg/kg/day

Ophthalmic: Children ≥16 years and Adults: Instill one drop in affected eye(s) every 12 hours

Administration

Oral: Administer consistently at the same time twice daily; use oral syringe, glass dropper, or glass container (not plastic or styrofoam cup); to improve palatability, oral solution may be mixed with milk, chocolate milk, orange juice, or apple juice that is at room temperature; dilution of Neoral® with milk can be unpalatable; stir well and drink at once; do not allow to stand before drinking; rinse with more diluent to ensure that the total dose is taken; after use, dry outside of glass dropper, do not rinse with water or other cleaning agents

Parenteral: May administer by I.V. intermittent infusion or continuous infusion; for intermittent infusion, administer over 2-6 hours at a final concentration not to exceed 2.5 mg/mL. Anaphylaxis has been reported with I.V. use. Patients should be continuously monitored for at least the first 30 minutes of the infusion, and should be monitored frequently thereafter

Ophthalmic: Invert vial prior to use to obtain a uniform emulsion. Avoid contact of vial tip with skin or eye; remove contact lenses prior to administration; lenses may be inserted 15 minutes after instillation. May be used with artificial tears; separate administration by at least 15 minutes.

Monitoring Parameters Blood/serum drug concentration (trough), renal and hepatic function tests, serum electrolytes, lipid profile, blood pressure, heart rate

Reference Range Reference ranges are method dependent and specimen dependent; use the same analytical method consistently; trough levels should be obtained immediately prior to next dose

Therapeutic: Not well defined, dependent on organ transplanted, time after transplant, organ function, and cyclosporine toxicity. Empiric therapeutic concentration ranges for trough cyclosporine concentrations:
- Kidney: 100-200 ng/mL (serum, RIA)
- BMT: 100-250 ng/mL (serum, RIA)
- Heart: 100-200 ng/mL (serum, RIA)
- Liver: 100-400 ng/mL (blood, HPLC)

Method dependent (optimum cyclosporine trough concentrations):
- Serum, RIA: 150-300 ng/mL; 50-150 ng/mL (late post-transplant period)
- Whole blood, RIA: 250-800 ng/mL; 150-450 ng/mL (late post-transplant period)
- Whole blood, HPLC: 100-500 ng/mL

Test Interactions Cyclosporine adsorbs to silicone; specific whole blood assay for cyclosporine may be falsely elevated if sample is drawn from the same central venous line through which dose was administered (even if flush has been administered and/or dose was given hours before); cyclosporine metabolites cross-react with radioimmunoassay and fluorescence polarization immunoassay

Patient Information Avoid the herbal medicine St John's wort; take dose at the same time each day; do not allow diluted oral solution to stand before drinking; do not change brands of cyclosporine unless directed by your physician. Patients with psoriasis should avoid excessive sun exposure. Notify physician of severe headache; persistent nausea, vomiting; muscle pain or cramping; unusual swelling of extremities; chest pain or rapid heartbeat.

Nursing Implications Adequate airway, supportive measures, epinephrine and I.V. steroids for treating anaphylaxis should be present when I.V. cyclosporine is administered

Additional Information Diltiazem has been used to prevent cyclosporine nephrotoxicity, reduce the frequency of delayed graft function when administered before and after surgery, and used to treat the mild hypertension that occurs in most patients after transplantation; diltiazem increases cyclosporine blood concentration by delaying its clearance resulting in decreased dosage requirements for cyclosporine

Dosage Forms Excipient information presented when available (limited, particularly for generics); consult specific product labeling.

Capsule, soft gel, modified: 25 mg, 100 mg [contains castor oil, ethanol]
- Gengraf®: 25 mg, 100 mg [contains ethanol, castor oil, propylene glycol]
- Neoral®: 25 mg, 100 mg [contains dehydrated ethanol, corn oil, castor oil, propylene glycol]

Capsule, soft gel, non-modified (Sandimmune®): 25 mg, 100 mg [contains dehydrated ethanol, corn oil]

Emulsion, ophthalmic [preservative free, single-use vial] (Restasis®): 0.05% (0.4 mL) [contains glycerin, castor oil, polysorbate 80, carbomer 1342; 32 vials/box]

Injection, solution, non-modified (Sandimmune®): 50 mg/mL (5 mL) [contains Cremophor® EL (polyoxyethylated castor oil), ethanol]

Solution, oral, modified:
- Gengraf®: 100 mg/mL (50 mL) [contains castor oil, propylene glycol]
- Neoral®: 100 mg/mL (50 mL) [contains dehydrated ethanol, corn oil, castor oil, propylene glycol]

Solution, oral, non-modified (Sandimmune®): 100 mg/mL (50 mL) [contains olive oil, ethanol]

(Continued)

CycloSPORINE *(Continued)*

References

Burckart GJ, Canafax DM, and Yee GC, "Cyclosporine Monitoring," *Drug Intell Clin Pharm*, 1986, 20(9):649-52.

Holt DW, Mueller EA, Kovarik JM, et al, "Sandimmune® Neoral® Pharmacokinetics: Impact of the New Oral Formulation," *Transplant Proc*, 1995, 27(1):1434-7.

Lin CY and Lee SF, "Comparison of Pharmacokinetics Between CsA Capsules and Sandimmune® Neoral® in Pediatric Patients," *Transplant Proc*, 1994, 26(5):2973-4.

Niese D, "A Double-Blind Randomized Study of Sandimmune® Neoral® vs Sandimmune® in New Renal Transplant Recipients: Results After 12 Months," *Transplant Proc*, 1995, 27(2):1849-56.

Taesch S, Niese D, and Mueller EA, "Sandimmune® Neoral®, A New Oral Formulation of Cyclosporine With Improved Pharmacokinetic Characteristics: Safety and Tolerability in Renal Transplant Patients," *Transplant Proc*, 1994, 26(6):3147-9.

Wandstrat TL, Schroeder TJ, and Myre SA, "Cyclosporine Pharmacokinetics in Pediatric Transplant Recipients," *Ther Drug Monit*, 1989, 11(5):493-6.

Yee GC, "Recent Advances in Cyclosporine Pharmacokinetics," *Pharmacotherapy*, 1991, 11(5):130S-134S.

- ♦ **Cyklokapron®** *see* Tranexamic Acid *on page 1563*
- ♦ **Cylate®** *see* Cyclopentolate *on page 417*
- ♦ **Cylex® [OTC]** *see* Benzocaine *on page 204*

Cyproheptadine (si proe HEP ta deen)

Medication Safety Issues

Sound-alike/look-alike issues:

Cyproheptadine may be confused with cyclobenzaprine

Periactin may be confused with Perative®, Percodan®, Persantine®

Related Information

Overdose and Toxicology *on page 1916*

Index Terms Cyproheptadine Hydrochloride; Periactin

Therapeutic Category Antihistamine

Generic Available Yes

Use Perennial and seasonal allergic rhinitis and other allergic symptoms including urticaria; appetite stimulant (useful in the management of anorexia nervosa); prophylactic treatment of cluster and migraine headaches; spinal cord damage associated with spasticity

Pregnancy Risk Factor B

Lactation Excretion in breast milk unknown/contraindicated

Contraindications Hypersensitivity to cyproheptadine or any component; narrow-angle glaucoma, bladder neck obstruction, acute asthmatic attack, stenosing peptic ulcer, GI tract obstruction, those on MAO inhibitors

Adverse Reactions

Cardiovascular: Tachycardia, palpitations, edema

Central nervous system: Sedation, CNS stimulation, seizures, fatigue, headache, nervousness, depression

Dermatologic: Photosensitivity, rash, angioedema

Gastrointestinal: Appetite stimulation, xerostomia, nausea, diarrhea, abdominal pain

Hematologic: Hemolytic anemia, leukopenia, thrombocytopenia

Hepatic: Hepatitis

Neuromuscular & skeletal: Myalgia, paresthesia, arthralgia

Respiratory: Bronchospasm, epistaxis, pharyngitis

Miscellaneous: Allergic reactions

Drug Interactions MAO inhibitors; enhances sedative effects of other CNS depressants; enhances anticholinergic effects of other anticholinergic agents

Mechanism of Action A potent antihistamine and serotonin antagonist, competes with histamine for H_1-receptor sites on effector cells in the GI tract, blood vessels, and respiratory tract

Pharmacokinetics

Absorption: Well absorbed

Metabolism: Extensively by conjugation

Elimination: >50% excreted in urine (primarily as metabolites); approximately 25% excreted in feces

Usual Dosage Oral:

Allergic conditions:

Children: 0.25 mg/kg/day or 8 mg/m^2/day in 2-3 divided doses **or**

2-6 years: 2 mg every 8-12 hours (not to exceed 12 mg/day)

7-14 years: 4 mg every 8-12 hours (not to exceed 16 mg/day)

Adults: 4-20 mg/day divided every 8 hours (not to exceed 0.5 mg/kg/day)

Appetite stimulation (anorexia nervosa): Children >13 years and Adults: 2 mg 4 times/day; may be increased gradually over a 3-week period to 8 mg 4 times/day

Cluster headaches: Adults: 4 mg 4 times/day

Migraine headaches:
Children: 4 mg 2-3 times/day
Adults: 4-8 mg 3 times/day
Spasticity associated with spinal cord damage: Children ≥12 years and Adults: 4 mg at bedtime; increase by a 4 mg dose every 3-4 days; average daily dose: 16 mg in divided doses; not to exceed 36 mg/day

Dosage adjustment in hepatic impairment: Reduce dosage in patients with significant hepatic dysfunction

Administration Oral: Administer with food or milk

Test Interactions Diagnostic antigen skin tests; ↑ amylase (S); ↓ fasting glucose (S)

Patient Information May cause drowsiness and impair ability to perform activities requiring mental alertness or physical coordination; may cause dry mouth. May rarely cause photosensitivity reactions (eg, exposure to sunlight may cause severe sunburn, skin rash, redness, or itching); avoid direct exposure to sunlight

Dosage Forms Excipient information presented when available (limited, particularly for generics); consult specific product labeling.
Syrup, as hydrochloride: 2 mg/5 mL (473 mL) [contains alcohol 5%; mint flavor]
Tablet, as hydrochloride: 4 mg

References

Gracies JM, Nance P, Elovic E, et al, "Traditional Pharmacological Treatments for Spasticity. Part II: General and Regional Treatments," *Muscle Nerve Suppl*, 1997, 6:S92-120.

♦ **Cyproheptadine Hydrochloride** *see* Cyproheptadine *on page 426*
♦ **Cystadane®** *see* Betaine *on page 211*
♦ **Cystagon®** *see* Cysteamine *on page 427*

Cysteamine (sis TEE a meen)

U.S. Brand Names Cystagon®

Index Terms Cysteamine Bitartrate

Therapeutic Category Cystinosis, Treatment Agent

Generic Available No

Use Management of nephropathic cystinosis

Pregnancy Risk Factor C

Lactation Excretion in breast milk unknown/not recommended

Contraindications Hypersensitivity to cysteamine, penicillamine, or any component

Warnings Leukocyte cystine levels should be monitored during oral cysteamine therapy (at least every 3 months); cysteamine should be given in the lowest dose possible to achieve adequate leukocyte cystine depletion; toxicity may be reduced by initiating therapy with a slowly increasing dose schedule (see Usual Dosage); if skin rash develops, discontinue treatment until rash clears; may then resume treatment at a lower dose with a slow titration to the therapeutic dose

Precautions Use with caution in patients with a history of blood dyscrasias, gastric or duodenal ulcer, or neurologic disorder

Adverse Reactions
Cardiovascular: Hypertension
Central nervous system: Somnolence, encephalopathy, headache, seizures, ataxia, confusion, dizziness, jitteriness, nervousness, impaired cognition, emotional changes, hallucinations, nightmares, fever (22%), lethargy (11%), depression, hyperthermia
Dermatologic: Urticaria, rash (7%)
Endocrine & metabolic: Dehydration
Gastrointestinal: Bad breath, abdominal pain, dyspepsia, constipation, gastroenteritis, duodenitis, duodenal ulceration, vomiting (35%), anorexia (31%), diarrhea (16%), nausea
Hematologic: Anemia, leukopenia
Hepatic: Abnormal liver enzymes
Neuromuscular & skeletal: Tremor, hyperkinesia
Otic: Decreased hearing
Renal: Interstitial nephritis, renal failure

Stability Store at room temperature; protect from light

Mechanism of Action Reacts with cystine in the lysosome to convert it to cysteine and to a cysteine-cysteamine mixed disulfide, both of which can then exit the lysosome in patients with cystinosis, an inherited defect of lysosomal transport

Pharmacokinetics
Absorption: Rapid
Distribution: V_d: Children: 156 L
Protein binding: Mean: 52%
Half-life: 1 hour
Time to peak serum concentration: 1.4 hours
(Continued)

Cysteamine *(Continued)*

Elimination: Clearance: Children: 1.2 L/minute

Usual Dosage Oral: Initiate therapy with $^1/_4$ to $^1/_6$ of maintenance dose and titrate slowly over 4-6 weeks

Children <12 years: Initial: 1.3 g/m^2/day in 4 divided doses; may increase gradually to a maximum of 1.95 g/m^2/day

Children ≥12 years and Adults (>110 lb): 2 g/day in 4 divided doses; dosage may be increased gradually to 1.95 g/m^2/day

Approximate Cysteamine Initial Dose

Weight (lbs)	Dose (mg every 6 hrs)
≤10	100
11-20	150
21-30	200
31-40	250
41-50	300
51-70	350
71-90	400
91-110	450
>110	500

Administration Oral: Contents of capsule may be sprinkled over food

Monitoring Parameters Blood counts and liver enzymes during therapy; blood pressure; monitor leukocyte cystine measurements to determine adequate dosage and compliance (measure 5-6 hours after administration)

Reference Range Leukocyte cystine goal: <1 nmol of half-cystine/mg protein (some measurable benefits have been seen with levels <2); routine measurements are recommended every 3 months

Patient Information May cause drowsiness or impair ability to perform activities requiring mental alertness or physical coordination

Dosage Forms Excipient information presented when available (limited, particularly for generics); consult specific product labeling.

Capsule: 50 mg, 150 mg

♦ **Cysteamine Bitartrate** *see* Cysteamine *on page 427*

Cysteine (SIS teen)

Index Terms Cysteine Hydrochloride

Therapeutic Category Nutritional Supplement

Generic Available Yes

Use Supplement to crystalline amino acid solutions, in particular the specialized pediatric formulas (eg, Aminosyn® PF, TrophAmine®) to meet the intravenous amino acid nutritional requirements of infants receiving parenteral nutrition (PN)

Contraindications Hypersensitivity to cysteine or any component; patients with hepatic coma or metabolic disorders involving impaired nitrogen utilization

Warnings Metabolic acidosis has occurred in infants related to the "hydrochloride" component of cysteine; each 1 mmol cysteine (175 mg) delivers 1 mEq chloride and 1 mEq hydrogen ion; to balance the extra hydrochloride ions and prevent acidosis, addition to the PN solution of a 1 mEq acetate electrolyte salt for each mmol (175 mg) of cysteine may be needed; each 40 mg cysteine (equal to every 1 g amino acid when used in the recommended ratio) adds 0.228 mEq chloride and hydrogen

Precautions Use with caution in patients with renal dysfunction and hepatic insufficiency

Adverse Reactions

Central nervous system: Fever

Endocrine & metabolic: Metabolic acidosis (see Warnings)

Gastrointestinal: Nausea

Renal: Elevated BUN, azotemia

Stability Avoid excessive heat, do not freeze; when combined with parenteral amino acid solutions, cysteine is relatively unstable; it is intended to be added immediately prior to administration to the patient; infusion of the admixture should begin within 1 hour of mixing or refrigerated until use; stable 24 hours in PN solution; opened vials must be used within 4 hours of entry

Mechanism of Action Cysteine is a sulfur-containing amino acid synthesized from methionine via the transulfuration pathway. It is a precursor of the tripeptide glutathione and also of taurine. Newborn infants have a relative deficiency of the enzyme necessary to affect this conversion. Cysteine may be considered an essential amino acid in infants.

Usual Dosage I.V.: Neonates and Infants: Added as a fixed ratio to crystalline amino acid solution: 40 mg cysteine per g of amino acids; dosage will vary with the daily amino acid dosage (eg, 0.5-2.5 g/kg/day amino acids would result in 20-100 mg/kg/day cysteine); individual doses of cysteine of 0.8-1 mmol/kg/day have also been added directly to the daily PN solution; the duration of treatment relates to the need for PN; patients on chronic PN therapy have received cysteine until 6 months of age and in some cases until 2 years of age

Administration Parenteral: Use only after dilution into PN solution; dilute with amino acid solution in a ratio of 40 mg cysteine to 1 g amino acid: eg, 500 mg cysteine is added to 12.5 g (250 mL) of 5% amino acid solution

Monitoring Parameters BUN, ammonia, electrolytes, pH, acid-base balance, serum creatinine, liver function tests, growth curve

Additional Information Addition of cysteine to PN solutions enhances the solubility of calcium and phosphate by lowering the overall pH of the solution

Dosage Forms Excipient information presented when available (limited, particularly for generics); consult specific product labeling.

Injection, solution, as hydrochloride: 50 mg/mL (10 mL, 50 mL)

- **Cysteine Hydrochloride** *see* Cysteine *on page 428*
- **Cystospaz®** *see* Hyoscyamine *on page 798*
- **Cystospaz-M® [DSC]** *see* Hyoscyamine *on page 798*
- **CYT** *see* Cyclophosphamide *on page 419*

Cytarabine (sye TARE a been)

Medication Safety Issues

Sound-alike/look-alike issues:

Cytarabine may be confused with Cytadren®, Cytosar®, Cytoxan®, vidarabine

Cytosar-U® may be confused with cytarabine, Cytovene®, Cytoxan®, Neosar®

High alert medication: The Institute for Safe Medication Practices (ISMP) includes this medication among its list of drugs which have a heightened risk of causing significant patient harm when used in error.

Related Information

Compatibility of Chemotherapy and Related Supportive Care Medications *on page 1777*

Emetogenic Potential of Single Chemotherapeutic Agents *on page 1776*

U.S. Brand Names Cytosar-U®

Canadian Brand Names Cytosar®

Index Terms Arabinosylcytosine; Ara-C; Cytarabine Hydrochloride; Cytosine Arabinosine Hydrochloride; NSC-63878

Therapeutic Category Antineoplastic Agent, Antimetabolite

Generic Available Yes

Use Used in combination regimens for the treatment of leukemias, meningeal leukemia, Hodgkin's lymphoma, and non-Hodgkin's lymphoma

Pregnancy Risk Factor D

Lactation Excretion in breast milk unknown/not recommended

Contraindications Hypersensitivity to cytarabine or any component

Warnings The FDA currently recommends that procedures for proper handling and disposal of antineoplastic agents be considered. Must monitor for drug toxicity; drug toxicity includes bone marrow suppression with leukopenia, thrombocytopenia, and anemia along with nausea, vomiting, diarrhea, abdominal pain, oral ulceration, and hepatic dysfunction; irreversible cerebellar toxicity may occur with a cumulative dose ≥30 g/m²; cytarabine is potentially mutagenic and carcinogenic.

Precautions Marked bone marrow suppression necessitates dosage reduction or a reduction in the number of days of administration; with severe hepatic dysfunction, dosage may need to be reduced

Adverse Reactions

Cardiovascular: Cardiomegaly, chest pain, pericarditis

Central nervous system: Headache, malaise, confusion, seizures, fever, irritability, cerebral and cerebellar dysfunction (somnolence, personality changes, coma, ataxia)

Dermatologic: Alopecia, rash

Endocrine & metabolic: Hyperuricemia

Gastrointestinal: Nausea, vomiting, oral and anal inflammation with ulceration, anorexia, diarrhea, GI hemorrhage, mucositis

Hematologic: Myelosuppression (leukopenia, thrombocytopenia, anemia)

Hepatic: Hepatic dysfunction, jaundice, elevated serum bilirubin and liver enzymes

(Continued)

Cytarabine *(Continued)*

Local: Thrombophlebitis

Neuromuscular & skeletal: Myalgia, bone pain, peripheral neuropathy, weakness, gait disturbances

Ocular: Conjunctivitis, hemorrhagic conjunctivitis, corneal toxicity, photophobia, blurred vision

Respiratory: Syndrome of sudden respiratory distress progressing to pulmonary edema and diffuse interstitial pneumonitis have been reported with high-dose regimens

Miscellaneous: Ara-C syndrome (fever, myalgia, bone pain, rash, conjunctivitis, malaise occurring 6-12 hours after administration); headache and vomiting with I.T. administration; anaphylactoid reaction

Drug Interactions Decreases digoxin oral tablet absorption

Stability Reconstituted solutions containing 20-100 mg/mL cytarabine are stable for 48 hours at room temperature; I.T. Ara-C is compatible with methotrexate and hydrocortisone mixed in the same syringe; physically incompatible with fluorouracil, heparin

Mechanism of Action Converted intracellularly to the active metabolite cytarabine triphosphate; inhibits DNA polymerase by competing with deoxycytidine triphosphate resulting in inhibition of DNA synthesis; incorporated into DNA chain resulting in termination of chain elongation; cell cycle-specific for the S-phase of cell division

Pharmacokinetics

Distribution: Penetrates the CSF in limited amounts, crosses the placenta

Protein binding: 13%

Metabolism: Deactivated by cytidine deaminase primarily in the liver, but also in kidneys, GI mucosa, and granulocytes

Half-life, terminal: 1-3 hours

Elimination: ~80% of dose excreted in urine as metabolites within 24 hours; 10% excreted in urine as unchanged drug

Usual Dosage Children and Adults (refer to individual protocols):

Induction remission:

- I.V.: 200 mg/m^2/day for 5 days at 2-week intervals as a single agent; in combination chemotherapy, 100-200 mg/m^2/day for 5- to 10-day therapy course every 2-4 weeks, or every day until remission, given as an I.V. continuous drip or in 2 divided doses/day
- I.T.: 5-75 mg/m^2 every 2-7 days until CNS findings normalize

Maintenance remission:

- I.V.: 70-200 mg/m^2/day for 2-5 days at monthly intervals
- I.M., SubQ: 1-1.5 mg/kg single dose for maintenance at 1- to 4-week intervals
- I.T.: 5-75 mg/m^2 every 2-7 days until CNS findings normalize **or**
  - <1 year: 20 mg
  - 1-2 years: 30 mg
  - 2-3 years: 50 mg
  - >3 years: 70 mg

High-dose regimen: Refractory leukemias or refractory non-Hodgkin's lymphoma: I.V. infusion: 3 g/m^2/dose every 12 hours for up to 12 doses

Administration Parenteral: May administer SubQ, I.M., IVP, I.V. infusion, or I.T. at a concentration not to exceed 100 mg/mL

High-dose regimens or for use in neonates: Diluents containing benzyl alcohol should not be used to reconstitute the drug; high-dose regimens (dose >1 g/m^2) are usually administered by I.V. infusion over 2 hours or longer, or as an I.V. continuous infusion

IVP: May administer over 15 minutes; rapid administration is associated with greater neurotoxicity

I.T. administration: Reconstitute with preservative free NS, Elliotts B solution, or preservative free LR solution; use preservative free injection formulation for I.T. use; filter through a 0.22 micron filter; the volume to be given I.T. is in the range of 3-10 mL and should correspond to an equivalent volume of CSF removed; antiemetic therapy should be administered prior to intrathecal doses of cytarabine

SubQ administration: Rotate injection sites to thigh, abdomen, and flank regions; avoid repeated administration to a single site

Monitoring Parameters Liver function tests, CBC with differential and platelet count, serum creatinine, BUN, serum uric acid; signs of neurotoxicity

Patient Information Notify physician of any fever, sore throat, bleeding, or bruising

Nursing Implications Administer corticosteroid eye drops for prophylaxis of conjunctivitis around-the-clock prior to, during, and for 2-7 days after high-dose Ara-C; pyridoxine has been administered on days of high-dose Ara-C therapy for prophylaxis of CNS toxicity.

Additional Information Myelosuppressive effects:

WBC: Severe

Platelets: Severe
Onset (days): 4-7
Nadir (days): 14-18
Recovery (days): 21-28

Dosage Forms Excipient information presented when available (limited, particularly for generics); consult specific product labeling.
Injection, powder for reconstitution: 100 mg, 500 mg, 1 g, 2 g
Injection, solution: 20 mg/mL (5 mL, 25 mL, 50 mL); 100 mg/mL (20 mL)

References

Baker WJ, Royer GL, and Weiss RB, "Cytarabine and Neurologic Toxicity," *J Clinical Oncology*, 1991, 9(4):679-93.
Grossman L, Baker MA, Sutton DM, et al, "Central Nervous System Toxicity of High-Dose Cytosine Arabinoside," *Med Pediatr Oncol*, 1983, 11(4):246-50.

♦ **Cytarabine Hydrochloride** *see* Cytarabine *on page 429*
♦ **CytoGam®** *see* Cytomegalovirus Immune Globulin (Intravenous-Human) *on page 431*

Cytomegalovirus Immune Globulin (Intravenous-Human)

(sye toe meg a low VYE rus i MYUN GLOB yoo lin in tra VEE nus HYU man)

Medication Safety Issues
Sound-alike/look-alike issues:
CytoGam® may be confused with Cytoxan®, Gamimune® N

U.S. Brand Names CytoGam®

Canadian Brand Names CytoGam®

Index Terms CMV-IGIV

Therapeutic Category Immune Globulin

Generic Available No

Use Prophylaxis of cytomegalovirus disease associated with kidney, lung, liver, pancreas, heart, or bone marrow transplantation; concomitant use with ganciclovir should be considered in organ transplants other than kidney from CMV seropositive donors to CMV seronegative recipients; adjunctive treatment of CMV disease in immunocompromised patients

Pregnancy Risk Factor C

Lactation Excretion in breast milk unknown

Contraindications Hypersensitivity to CMV immune globulin, other immune globulin preparations, blood products, or any component; IgA deficiency

Warnings Renal dysfunction and/or acute renal failure has been reported with the administration of IVIG; 88% of the cases were associated with the administration of sucrose-containing IVIG products. CytoGam® contains sucrose as a stabilizing agent. May theoretically transmit blood-borne viruses and the Creutzfeldt-Jakob disease agent.

Precautions Use with caution in patients with a history of cardiovascular disease or thrombotic episodes. Rapid infusion may be a possible risk factor for vascular occlusive events. Do not exceed manufacturer's recommended initial infusion rate and advance slowly in patients at risk. Use with caution in patients at increased risk for developing acute renal failure (patients with pre-existing renal insufficiency, diabetes mellitus, volume depletion, sepsis, paraproteinemia, and concomitant nephrotoxic drugs). Assure that patients are not volume depleted prior to the initiation of a CMV-IGIV infusion.

Adverse Reactions
Cardiovascular: Flushing, hypotension, thrombosis
Central nervous system: Fever, chills, dizziness, headache, aseptic meningitis syndrome
Dermatologic: Angioneurotic edema
Gastrointestinal: Nausea, vomiting
Hematologic: Hemolysis
Neuromuscular & skeletal: Arthralgia, back pain, muscle cramps
Renal: Acute renal failure, acute tubular necrosis, elevated BUN and serum creatinine, oliguria
Respiratory: Wheezing, tightness in chest, transfusion-related acute lung injury (respiratory distress, pulmonary edema, hypoxemia)
Miscellaneous: Anaphylaxis, diaphoresis

Drug Interactions Decreased effect of live vaccines (ie, MMR, varicella) if given within 3 months of CMV-IGIV administration (defer vaccination for 6 months after CMV-IGIV infusion)

Stability Refrigerate; do not freeze; do not shake vials; do not admix or dilute with other medications prior to I.V. infusion; may piggyback into existing infusions of NS, $D_{2.5}W$, D_5W, $D_{10}W$, or $D_{20}W$ at no greater than a 1:2 dilution

Mechanism of Action CMV-IGIV contains a high titer of CMV-specific antibodies which can neutralize the CMV virus; may exert immunomodulating effects

(Continued)

Cytomegalovirus Immune Globulin (Intravenous-Human) *(Continued)*

Pharmacokinetics Half-life: 8-24 days

Usual Dosage I.V.: Children and Adults:

Prophylaxis:

Kidney transplant: 150 mg/kg within 72 hours prior to transplant; 100 mg/kg at weeks 2, 4, 6, and 8 after transplant and 50 mg/kg at weeks 12 and 16 after transplant

Liver, lung, pancreas, or heart transplant (CMV (+) donor and CMV (-) recipient): 150 mg/kg within 72 hours prior to transplant, 150 mg/kg at weeks 2, 4, 6, and 8 after transplant; 100 mg/kg at weeks 12 and 16 after transplant

Bone marrow transplant: 200 mg/kg given 6 and 8 days prior to transplant and on days 1, 7, 14, 21, 28, 42, 56, and 70 after transplant

Treatment: 100 mg/kg every other day for 3 doses, then once every week based upon CMV antigenemia assay (pp65) or EBV PCR

Severe CMV pneumonia: 400 mg/kg in combination with ganciclovir on days 1, 2, 7, or 8, followed by 200 mg/kg on days 14 and 21

Dosage adjustment in renal impairment: Use with caution and infuse at the minimum rate possible. Specific dosage adjustment recommendations are not available.

Administration Parenteral: I.V. infusion: Initial infusion is started at 15 mg/kg/hour; if there are no infusion-related reactions after 30 minutes, increase to 30 mg/kg/hour; if no infusion-related reactions after 30 minutes, increase to 60 mg/kg/hour and maintain this rate until completion of dose. Subsequent doses can be initiated at an infusion rate of 15 mg/kg/hour for the first 15 minutes, if no infusion-related reactions, increase to 30 mg/kg/hour for the next 15 minutes; if rate is tolerated, increase to 60 mg/kg/hour and maintain this rate until completion of dose; maximum infusion rate: 60 mg/kg/hour or not to exceed 75 mL/hour at a maximum concentration of 50 mg/mL. Infuse through a 0.2-15 micron in-line filter.

Monitoring Parameters Vital signs during infusion, urine output, renal function

Additional Information

IgA content: Trace

Plasma Source: 2000-5000 donors (5% with top CMV titers)

IgG subclass (%):

IgG_1: 65

IgG_2: 28

IgG_3: 5.2

IgG_4: 1.7

Monomers + dimer (%): ≥95 monomers + dimers

Gamma globulin (%): 99

Albumin: 10 mg/mL

Sodium content: 20-30 mEq/L

Sugar content: 5% sucrose

Osmolality: >200 mOsm/L

Dosage Forms Excipient information presented when available (limited, particularly for generics); consult specific product labeling.

Injection, solution [preservative free]:

CytoGam®: 50 mg ± 10 mg/mL (50 mL) [contains sodium 20-30 mEq/L, human albumin, and sucrose]

References

Bowden RA, Fisher LD, Rogers K, et al, "Cytomegalovirus (CMV)-Specific Intravenous Immunoglobulin for the Prevention of Primary CMV Infection and Disease After Marrow Transplant," *J Infect Dis*, 1991, 164(3):483-7.

Snydman DR, Werner BG, Dougherty NN, et al, "Cytomegalovirus Immune Globulin Prophylaxis in Liver Transplantation. A Randomized, Double-Blind, Placebo-Controlled Trial," *Ann Intern Med*, 1993, 119(10):984-91.

Valantine HA, Luikart H, Doyle R, et al, "Impact of Cytomegalovirus Hyperimmune Globulin on Outcome After Cardiothoracic Transplantation: A Comparative Study of Combined Prophylaxis With CMV Hyperimmune Globulin Plus Ganciclovir Versus Ganciclovir Alone," *Transplantation*, 2001, 72(10):1647-52.

♦ **Cytomel®** *see* Liothyronine *on page 943*

♦ **Cytosar® (Can)** *see* Cytarabine *on page 429*

♦ **Cytosar-U®** *see* Cytarabine *on page 429*

♦ **Cytosine Arabinosine Hydrochloride** *see* Cytarabine *on page 429*

♦ **Cytotec®** *see* Misoprostol *on page 1069*

♦ **Cytovene®** *see* Ganciclovir *on page 719*

♦ **Cytoxan®** *see* Cyclophosphamide *on page 419*

♦ **Cēpacol® Dual Action Maximum Strength [OTC]** *see* Dyclonine *on page 551*

♦ **D-3-Mercaptovaline** *see* Penicillamine *on page 1227*

♦ **d4T** *see* Stavudine *on page 1472*

- ♦ D_5W *see* Dextrose *on page 479*
- ♦ $D_{10}W$ *see* Dextrose *on page 479*
- ♦ $D_{25}W$ *see* Dextrose *on page 479*
- ♦ $D_{30}W$ *see* Dextrose *on page 479*
- ♦ $D_{40}W$ *see* Dextrose *on page 479*
- ♦ $D_{50}W$ *see* Dextrose *on page 479*
- ♦ $D_{60}W$ *see* Dextrose *on page 479*
- ♦ $D_{70}W$ *see* Dextrose *on page 479*

Dacarbazine (da KAR ba zeen)

Medication Safety Issues

Sound-alike/look-alike issues:

Dacarbazine may be confused with Dicarbosil®, procarbazine

High alert medication: The Institute for Safe Medication Practices (ISMP) includes this medication among its list of drugs which have a heightened risk of causing significant patient harm when used in error.

Related Information

Compatibility of Chemotherapy and Related Supportive Care Medications *on page 1777*

Emetogenic Potential of Single Chemotherapeutic Agents *on page 1776*

U.S. Brand Names DTIC-Dome®

Canadian Brand Names DTIC®

Index Terms DIC; Dimethyl Triazeno Imidazole Carboxamide; DTIC; Imidazole Carboxamide; Imidazole Carboxamide Dimethyltriazene; WR-139007

Therapeutic Category Antineoplastic Agent, Miscellaneous

Generic Available Yes

Use Treatment of malignant melanoma, Hodgkin's disease, soft-tissue sarcomas (fibrosarcomas, rhabdomyosarcoma), islet cell carcinoma, medullary carcinoma of the thyroid, and neuroblastoma

Pregnancy Risk Factor C

Lactation Excretion in breast milk unknown/not recommended

Contraindications Hypersensitivity to dacarbazine or any component

Warnings The FDA currently recommends that procedures for proper handling and disposal of antineoplastic agents be considered. Hematopoietic depression is common; hepatic necrosis is also possible; dacarbazine has been reported to cause sterility and is mutagenic and teratogenic in rats

Precautions Use with caution in patients with bone marrow suppression, renal and/or hepatic impairment; dosage reduction may be necessary in patients with renal or hepatic insufficiency; avoid extravasation of the drug

Adverse Reactions

Cardiovascular: Facial flushing, hypotension

Central nervous system: Malaise, headache, fever, seizure

Dermatologic: Alopecia, rash, photosensitivity

Gastrointestinal: Anorexia, nausea, vomiting, metallic taste

Hematologic: Myelosuppression (nadir: 2-4 weeks): Leukopenia, thrombocytopenia

Hepatic: Hepatotoxicity, hepatic vein thrombosis, hepatocellular necrosis

Local: Pain and burning at infusion site, thrombophlebitis

Neuromuscular & skeletal: Myalgia, paresthesia

Ocular: Blurred vision

Respiratory: Sinus congestion

Miscellaneous: Flu-like syndrome, anaphylactic reactions

Drug Interactions Phenytoin, phenobarbital may induce dacarbazine metabolism

Stability Store in refrigerator; intact vials are stable for 4 weeks at room temperature; protect dacarbazine solutions from light; reconstituted dacarbazine solution 10 mg/mL is stable for 72 hours when refrigerated or 8 hours at room temperature; drug decomposition has occurred if the solution turns pink; dacarbazine is incompatible with hydrocortisone sodium succinate

Mechanism of Action Alkylating agent which forms methyldiazonium ions that attack nucleophilic groups in DNA; inhibits DNA, RNA, and protein synthesis by cross-linking DNA strands

Pharmacokinetics

Distribution: Distributes to the liver; very little distribution into CSF with CSF concentrations ~14% of plasma concentrations

V_{dss}: Adults: 17 L/m^2

Protein binding: Minimal, 5%

Metabolism: N-demethylated in the liver by microsomal enzymes; metabolites may also have an antineoplastic effect

(Continued)

Dacarbazine *(Continued)*

Half-life, biphasic: Initial: 20-40 minutes; terminal: 5 hours (in patients with normal renal/hepatic function)

Elimination: ~30% to 50% of dose excreted in urine by tubular secretion, 15% to 25% is excreted in urine as unchanged drug

Usual Dosage I.V. (refer to individual protocols):

Children:

Pediatric solid tumors: 200-470 mg/m^2/day over 5 days every 21-28 days

Pediatric neuroblastoma: 800-900 mg/m^2 as a single dose on day 1 of therapy every 3-4 weeks in combination therapy

Hodgkin's disease: 375 mg/m^2 on days 1 and 15 of treatment course, repeat every 28 days

Adults:

Malignant melanoma: 2-4.5 mg/kg/day for 10 days, repeat in 4 weeks or may use 250 mg/m^2/day for 5 days, repeat in 3 weeks

Hodgkin's disease: 150 mg/m^2/day for 5 days, repeat every 4 weeks **or** 375 mg/m^2 on day 1, repeat in 15 days of each 28-day cycle in combination with other agents

Administration Parenteral: Reconstitute vial for IVP doses with at least 2 mL of D_5W or NS; administer dose diluted in 5-10 mL D_5W or NS by slow IVP over 2-3 minutes or by I.V. infusion over 15-120 minutes at a concentration not to exceed 10 mg/mL

Monitoring Parameters CBC with differential, erythrocytes and platelet count; liver function tests

Patient Information Restrict intake of food for 4-6 hours prior to dacarbazine dose to decrease vomiting; flu-like symptoms (ie, malaise, fever, myalgia) may occur 1 week after infusion. May cause photosensitivity reactions (eg, exposure to sunlight may cause severe sunburn, skin rash, redness, or itching); avoid exposure to sunlight and artificial light sources (sunlamps, tanning booth/bed); wear protective clothing, wide-brimmed hats, sunglasses, and lip sunscreen (SPF ≥15); use a sunscreen [broad-spectrum sunscreen or physical sunscreen (preferred) or sunblock with SPF ≥15]; contact physician if reaction occurs.

Nursing Implications Avoid extravasation; use a D_5W or NS flush before and after a dacarbazine infusion; local pain, burning sensation, and irritation at the injection site may be relieved by local application of hot packs, slowing the I.V. rate and further dilution in I.V. fluid

Dosage Forms Excipient information presented when available (limited, particularly for generics); consult specific product labeling.

Injection, powder for reconstitution: 100 mg, 200 mg, 500 mg

DTIC-Dome®: 200 mg

References

Berg SL, Grisell DL, DeLaney TF, et al, "Principles of Treatment of Pediatric Solid Tumors," *Pediatr Clin North Am*, 1991, 38(2):249-67.

Finklestein JZ, Albo V, Ertel I, et al, "5-(3,3-Dimethyl-l-triazeno) imidazole-4-carboxamide (NSC-45388) in the Treatment of Solid Tumors in Children," *Cancer Chemother Rep*, 1975, 59(2 Pt 1):351-7.

Mutz ID and Urban CE, "Dimethyl-triazeno-imidazole-carboxamide (DTIC) in Combination Chemotherapy for Childhood Neuroblastoma," *Wien Klin Wochenschr*, 1978, 90(24):867-70.

Daclizumab (da CLI zoo mab)

U.S. Brand Names Zenapax®

Canadian Brand Names Zenapax®

Therapeutic Category Immunosuppressant Agent

Generic Available No

Use In combination with an immunosuppressive regimen, including cyclosporine and corticosteroids, for prophylaxis of acute organ rejection in patients receiving renal transplants; daclizumab has also been studied in pediatric bone marrow patients; steroid-refractory graft-versus-host disease

Pregnancy Risk Factor C

Lactation Excretion in breast milk unknown/use caution

Contraindications Hypersensitivity to daclizumab or any component

Warnings Should only be used by physicians experienced in immunosuppressive therapy or management of transplant patients; adequate laboratory and supportive medical resources must be readily available in the facility for patient management; may result in an increased susceptibility to infection or an increased risk for developing lymphoproliferative disorders. Severe, acute hypersensitivity reactions, including anaphylaxis have been reported following initial exposure or following re-exposure to daclizumab. If a severe hypersensitivity reaction occurs, daclizumab should be permanently discontinued. Medications for the management of severe allergic reactions should be available for immediate use.

Adverse Reactions

Cardiovascular: Edema, hypertension (48% in pediatric patients), hypotension, tachycardia, thrombosis, chest pain, cardiac arrest

Central nervous system: Headache, dizziness, insomnia, depression, anxiety, fever, chills

Dermatologic: Impaired wound healing, acne, pruritus, rash, hirsutism

Endocrine & metabolic: Dehydration (frequency may be higher for pediatric patients than for adults), diabetes mellitus

Gastrointestinal: Constipation, nausea, diarrhea (36%), vomiting (32%), abdominal pain, abdominal distention

Genitourinary: Oliguria, dysuria

Hematologic: Bleeding

Neuromuscular & skeletal: Tremors, back pain, arthralgia, myalgia

Ocular: Blurred vision

Renal: Renal tubular necrosis, hematuria

Respiratory: Atelectasis, congestion, hypoxia, pharyngitis, pleural effusion, respiratory arrest

Miscellaneous: Anaphylaxis, diaphoresis; incidence of anti-daclizumab antibodies (children: 34%)

Stability Refrigerate; do not shake or freeze; protect from direct light; diluted daclizumab solution is stable for 24 hours if refrigerated or for 4 hours at room temperature; discard solution if colored or if particulate matter is present

Mechanism of Action A humanized IgG1 monoclonal antibody produced by recombinant DNA technology that binds specifically to the alpha subunit (p55 alpha, CD25, or Tac subunit) of the human high affinity interleukin-2 receptor (IL-2R) on the surface of activated lymphocytes inhibiting IL-2 binding; inhibits IL-2 mediated activation of lymphocytes which is involved in allograft rejection

Pharmacokinetics Daclizumab serum levels appeared to be somewhat lower in pediatric renal transplant patients than in adult transplant patients administered the same 1 mg/kg dosing regimen

Distribution: V_d: Adults: ~6 L

Half-life:

Children: 13 days

Adults: 20 days

Usual Dosage I.V. (refer to individual protocols): Children and Adults:

Initial dose: 1 mg/kg given no more than 24 hours before transplantation, followed by 1 mg/kg/dose administered every 14 days for a total of 5 doses; maximum dose: 100 mg

Steroid-refractory graft-versus-host disease: 0.5-1.5 mg/kg as a single dose administered for transient response (repeat doses have been given 11-48 days following the initial dose)

Dosing interval in renal impairment: No dosage adjustment necessary

Administration Parenteral: Daclizumab dose should be diluted in 50 mL NS solution. In fluid-restricted patients, a final concentration of 1 mg/mL can be administered over 15 minutes. When mixing the solution, gently invert the bag to avoid foaming; do not shake. Daclizumab solution should be administered within 4 hours of preparation if stored at room temperature; infuse over a 15-minute period via a peripheral or central vein. Do not mix or infuse other medications through the same I.V. line.

Monitoring Parameters CBC with differential, vital signs, immunologic monitoring of T cells, renal function tests, serum glucose

Reference Range Serum trough levels: 5-10 mcg/mL

Patient Information Women of childbearing potential should avoid becoming pregnant while on daclizumab. Use an effective form of contraception before beginning therapy, during therapy, and for 4 months following daclizumab treatment.

Dosage Forms Excipient information presented when available (limited, particularly for generics); consult specific product labeling.

Injection, solution [preservative free]: 5 mg/mL (5 mL)

References

Vincenti F, Kirkman R, Light S, et al, "Interleukin-2-Receptor Blockade With Daclizumab to Prevent Acute Rejection in Renal Transplantation. Daclizumab Triple Therapy Study Group," *N Engl J Med*, 1998, 338(3):161-5.

♦ **Dacodyl™ [OTC]** *see* Bisacodyl *on page 217*

♦ **DACT** *see* Dactinomycin *on page 435*

Dactinomycin (dak ti noe MYE sin)

Medication Safety Issues

Sound-alike/look-alike issues:

Dactinomycin may be confused with daptomycin, DAUNOrubicin

Actinomycin may be confused with Achromycin

(Continued)

Dactinomycin *(Continued)*

High alert medication: The Institute for Safe Medication Practices (ISMP) includes this medication among its list of drugs which have a heightened risk of causing significant patient harm when used in error.

Related Information

Compatibility of Chemotherapy and Related Supportive Care Medications *on page 1777*

Emetogenic Potential of Single Chemotherapeutic Agents *on page 1776*

U.S. Brand Names Cosmegen®

Canadian Brand Names Cosmegen®

Index Terms ACT; Act-D; Actinomycin; Actinomycin Cl; Actinomycin D; DACT; NSC-3053

Therapeutic Category Antineoplastic Agent, Antibiotic

Generic Available No

Use Management (either alone or in combination with other treatment modalities) of Wilms' tumor, rhabdomyosarcoma, neuroblastoma, retinoblastoma, Ewing's sarcoma, trophoblastic neoplasms, testicular tumors and uterine sarcomas

Pregnancy Risk Factor D

Lactation Excretion in breast milk unknown/contraindicated

Contraindications Hypersensitivity to dactinomycin or any component; patients with chickenpox or herpes zoster; avoid in infants <6 months of age since the incidence of adverse effects is increased in infants

Warnings The FDA currently recommends that procedures for proper handling and disposal of antineoplastic agents be considered. Dactinomycin may cause fetal harm when administered to pregnant women. Women of childbearing potential must be warned to avoid becoming pregnant. Dactinomycin is extremely irritating to tissues. If extravasation occurs during I.V. use, severe damage to soft tissue may occur leading to pain, swelling, ulceration, and necrosis. Extravasation leading to contracture of the arms has also been reported.

Reports of second primary tumors (including leukemia) following treatment with radiation and dactinomycin have occurred; long-term observation of cancer survivors is recommended. May cause potentially fatal hepatic veno-occlusive disease; reported incidence of veno-occlusive disease across different clinical studies is 2% to 13.5% with increased risk in children <4 years of age.

Precautions Use with caution in patients with hepatobiliary dysfunction or in patients who have received radiation therapy; reduce dosage in patients receiving concurrent radiation therapy and in patients with hepatobiliary dysfunction; avoid administering live virus vaccinations during therapy with dactinomycin

Adverse Reactions

Central nervous system: Fatigue, fever, chills, lethargy, malaise

Dermatologic: Alopecia, erythema, hyperpigmentation of skin, desquamation, acne, maculopapular rash

Endocrine & metabolic: Hypocalcemia, hyperuricemia, growth retardation

Gastrointestinal: Anorexia, vomiting, diarrhea, stomatitis, proctitis, nausea, dysphagia, esophagitis, GI ulceration

Hematologic: Myelosuppression (nadir: 2-3 weeks), leukopenia, agranulocytosis, thrombocytopenia, anemia

Hepatic: Hepatitis, hepatic veno-occlusive disease, elevated liver enzymes, ascites, hepatomegaly

Local: Soft tissue damage with extravasation

Neuromuscular & skeletal: Myalgia

Respiratory: Pneumonitis

Miscellaneous: Anaphylactoid reaction, immunosuppression, second primary tumors

Drug Interactions Dactinomycin potentiates the effects of radiation therapy; enflurane, halothane (increased hepatotoxicity); decreased effectiveness of vaccines given following dactinomycin

Stability Store at room temperature; protect from light and humidity. Binds to cellulose filters, therefore, avoid in-line filtration; adsorbs to glass and plastic so dactinomycin should not be given by continuous or intermittent infusion; use of a diluent containing preservatives for reconstitution may result in a precipitate; any unused portion of the reconstituted 0.5 mg/mL solution should be discarded after 24 hours

Mechanism of Action Binds to the guanine portion of DNA intercalating between guanine and cytosine base pairs blocking replication and transcription of the DNA template inhibiting RNA synthesis; causes topoisomerase-mediated single-strand breaks in DNA

Pharmacokinetics

Distribution: Concentrates in nucleated cells and bone marrow; crosses the placenta; poor penetration into CSF (CSF:plasma ratio is <10%); distributes into submaxillary gland, liver, and kidney

Metabolism: Hepatic

Half-life, terminal: 14-43 hours

Time to peak serum concentration: I.V.: Within 2-5 minutes

Elimination: ~10% of dose excreted as unchanged drug in urine; 15% recovered in feces; 50% appears in bile

Usual Dosage Dosage should be based on body surface area in obese or edematous patients

Children >6 months and Adults: I.V. (refer to individual protocols): 15 mcg/kg/day or 400-600 mcg/m^2/day (maximum dose: 500 mcg/day) for 5 days, may repeat every 3-6 weeks; or 2.5 mg/m^2 given in divided doses over 1 week; or 0.75-2 mg/m^2 as a single dose given at intervals of 3-6 weeks has been used

Administration Parenteral: I.V.: For I.V. administration only; since drug is extremely irritating to tissues, **do not give I.M. or SubQ**; avoid extravasation; use a D_5W or NS flush before and after a dactinomycin dose to ensure venous patency; administer by slow IVP over a few minutes at a concentration not to exceed 500 mcg/mL into the side-port of a freely flowing I.V. infusion

Monitoring Parameters CBC with differential and platelet count, liver function tests and renal function tests

Test Interactions May interfere with bioassays of antibacterial drug levels

Patient Information Notify physician if fever, sore throat, bleeding, or bruising occurs; report immediately any pain, burning, or swelling at the infusion site. Advise women of childbearing potential to avoid becoming pregnant while receiving dactinomycin.

Nursing Implications Dactinomycin is corrosive to soft tissue. Avoid inhalation of drug particles or vapors and contact with skin or mucous membranes, especially those of the eyes. Avoid extravasation; if extravasation occurs, apply ice to the site for 15 minutes 4 times/day for 3 days; close observation with plastic surgery consultation is recommended

Dosage Forms Excipient information presented when available (limited, particularly for generics); consult specific product labeling.

Injection, powder for reconstitution:

Cosmegen®: 0.5 mg [contains mannitol 20 mg]

References

Berg SL, Grisell DL, DeLaney TF, et al, "Principles of Treatment of Pediatric Solid Tumors," *Pediatr Clin North Am*, 1991, 38(2):249-67.

Berkowitz RS and Goldstein DP, "Gestational Trophoblastic Disease," *Cancer*, 1995, 76(10 Suppl):2079-85.

Carli M, Pastore G, Perilongo G, et al, "Tumor Response and Toxicity After Single High-Dose Versus Standard Five-Day Divided Dose Dactinomycin in Childhood Rhabdomyosarcoma," *J Clin Oncol*, 1988, 6(4):654-8.

Veal GJ, Cole M, Errington J, et al, "Pharmacokinetics of Dactinomycin in a Pediatric Patient Population: A United Kingdom Children's Cancer Study Group Study," *Clin Cancer Res*, 2005, 11(16):5893-9.

- **DAD** *see* Mitoxantrone *on page 1072*
- **Dalacin® C (Can)** *see* Clindamycin *on page 379*
- **Dalacin® T (Can)** *see* Clindamycin *on page 379*
- **Dalacin® Vaginal (Can)** *see* Clindamycin *on page 379*
- **Dalmane®** *see* Flurazepam *on page 686*
- **d-Alpha-Gems™ [OTC]** *see* Vitamin E *on page 1620*
- ***d*-Alpha Tocopherol** *see* Vitamin E *on page 1620*

Danazol (DA na zole)

Medication Safety Issues

Sound-alike/look-alike issues:

Danazol may be confused with Dantrium®

Danocrine® may be confused with Dacriose®

U.S. Brand Names Danocrine® [DSC]

Canadian Brand Names Cyclomen®; Danocrine®

Therapeutic Category Androgen

Generic Available Yes

Use Treatment of endometriosis amenable to hormonal management; fibrocystic breast disease; hereditary angioedema (see also Additional Information)

Pregnancy Risk Factor X

Lactation Enters breast milk/contraindicated

Contraindications Hypersensitivity to danazol or any component; pregnancy; undiagnosed abnormal genital bleeding; breast-feeding; porphyria; markedly impaired renal, hepatic, or cardiac function

Warnings Exposure to danazol in utero may result in androgenic effects on the female fetus; clitoral hypertrophy, labial fusion, urogenital sinus defect, vaginal atresia, and ambiguous genitalia have been reported; a sensitive test capable of determining early pregnancy is recommended immediately prior to initiation of therapy; nonhormonal

(Continued)

Danazol *(Continued)*

method of contraception should be used during treatment if indicated. Thromboembolism, thrombotic, and thrombophlebitic events have been reported (including life-threatening or fatal stroke). Long-term use has been associated with peliosis hepatis and hepatic adenoma; these conditions may be complicated by acute, potentially life-threatening intra-abdominal hemorrhage; monitor liver function. Danazol has been associated with benign intracranial hypertension (pseudotumor cerebri); monitor for early signs and symptoms including papilledema, headache, nausea, vomiting, and visual disturbances. May increase risk of atherosclerosis and CAD due to decreased HDL and possible increase LDL. May cause nonreversible androgenic effects; patients should be watched closely for signs of androgenic effects.

Precautions Use with caution in patients with seizure disorders, migraine headaches, or conditions influenced by edema

Adverse Reactions

Cardiovascular: Edema, benign intracranial hypertension (rare), flushing, hypertension, diaphoresis, thromboembolism

Central nervous system: Nervousness, emotional lability, depression, dizziness, fainting, fever (rare), headache, sleep disorders, anxiety (rare), chills (rare), seizures (rare), stroke, Guillain-Barré syndrome

Dermatologic: Acne, seborrhea, mild hirsutism, hair loss, rashes (maculopapular, vestibular, papular, purpuric, and petechial), erythema multiforme, pruritus, urticaria, photosensitivity (rare)

Endocrine & metabolic: Weight gain, menstrual irregularities (spotting, altered timing of cycle), amenorrhea, clitoral hypertrophy (rare), breast size reduction, nipple discharge, semen abnormalities (changes in volume, viscosity, sperm count, and motility), libido changes, glucose intolerance, decreased HDL, increased LDL

Gastrointestinal: Nausea, vomiting, gastroenteritis, pancreatitis (rare), appetite changes (rare), bleeding gums (rare), constipation

Genitourinary: Vaginal dryness, vaginal irritation, pelvic pain

Hematologic: Eosinophilia, erythrocytosis (reversible), leukocytosis, leukopenia, thrombocytosis, polycythemia, thrombocytopenia

Hepatic: Peliosis hepatis, hepatic adenoma, cholestatic jaundice, elevated liver enzymes

Neuromuscular & skeletal: Back pain, carpal tunnel syndrome (rare), extremity pain, joint pain, joint swelling, muscle cramps, neck pain, paresthesias, spasms, weakness, tremor

Ocular: Cataracts (rare), visual disturbances

Renal: Hematuria

Respiratory: Nasal congestion (rare)

Miscellaneous: Voice alterations (hoarseness, sore throat, instability, deepening of pitch)

Drug Interactions Cytochrome P450 isoenzyme CYP3A3/4 enzyme inhibitor

Increases effects of warfarin; increases serum concentrations of carbamazepine, cyclosporine, and tacrolimus; may increase risk of myopathy or rhabdomyolysis with HMG-CoA reductase inhibitors

Food Interactions Food delays time to peak serum level; high-fat meal increases plasma concentration

Stability Store at room temperature.

Mechanism of Action Danazol, a synthetic steroid analog, has strong antigonadotropic properties. It inhibits the mid-cycle surge of LH and FSH from the pituitary resulting in suppression of ovarian steroidogenesis. Danazol does not have any progestational or estrogenic properties but does exhibit weak anabolic and androgenic effects. Through its inactivation of the pituitary-ovarian axis, regression and atrophy of normal and ectopic endometrial tissue occurs. Danazol decreases the rate of growth of abnormal breast tissue and reduces attacks associated with hereditary angioedema by increasing levels of C4 component of complement.

Pharmacodynamics

Endometriosis:
- Onset of action: 3 weeks

Fibrocystic breast disease:
- Onset of action: 1 month
- Maximum effect: 4-6 months
- Duration: Symptoms recur in 50% of patients within one year after discontinuation of treatment

Pharmacokinetics

Absorption: Well absorbed

Metabolism: Extensive hepatic metabolism to inactive metabolites

Half-life: Adults: 4.5 hours

Time to peak serum concentration: 2 hours

Usual Dosage Adolescents and Adults: Oral: **Note:** Begin treatment during menstruation or obtain appropriate tests to ensure patient is not pregnant:

Endometriosis:

Mild case: 100-200 mg twice daily for 3-6 months; may be continued up to 9 months if necessary

Moderate to severe case: 400 mg twice daily for 3-6 months; may be continued up to 9 months if necessary

Note: A gradual downward titration to a dose sufficient to maintain amenorrhea may be considered depending upon the patient's response

Fibrocystic breast disease: 50-200 mg twice daily

Hereditary angioedema: Initial: 200 mg 2-3 times/day depending upon the patient's response; after a favorable response is obtained, decrease the dosage by 50% or less at intervals of 1-3 months or longer. If an attack occurs, the daily dosage may be increased by up to 200 mg.

Administration Oral: Avoid administration with fatty meals.

Monitoring Parameters Liver function tests, symptomatology and site of disease; serum glucose (if diabetic); HDL and LDL cholesterol; signs and symptoms of pseudotumor cerebri; androgenic effects

Test Interactions Danazol may interfere with laboratory determinations for testosterone, androstenedione, and dehydroepiandrosterone.

Patient Information Do not discontinue without consulting prescriber; therapy may take up to several months for full benefit depending upon the purpose of treatment. Report any prodromal symptoms of hepatitis (fatigue, weakness, nausea, vomiting, dark urine, or yellowing of eyes); avoid becoming pregnant while taking this medicine and for several months after stopping; use an effective form of birth control. This medication may alter hypoglycemic requirements; diabetics should monitor serum glucose closely. May cause photosensitivity reactions (eg, exposure to sunlight may cause severe sunburn, skin rash, redness, or itching); avoid direct exposure to sunlight.

Additional Information Danazol has seen limited use for treatment of ITP in children refractory to steroids. Ten children, 2.5-17 years of age were treated with 20-30 mg/kg/day in divided doses (maximum: 800 mg/day). Treatment was tapered off after patients responded to therapy (Weinblatt, 1988). Danazol has also been evaluated in hemophilia A in a randomized, double-blind placebo-controlled crossover trial in 19 children. Children <15 years received 150 mg/day and >15 years received 300 mg/day for 3 months. Factor VIII:C levels were increased (Mehta, 1992).

Dosage Forms Excipient information presented when available (limited, particularly for generics); consult specific product labeling. [DSC] = Discontinued product

Capsule: 50 mg, 100 mg, 200 mg

Danocrine®: 50 mg, 100 mg, 200 mg [DSC]

References

Mehta J, Singhal S, Kamath MV, et al, "A Randomized Placebo-Controlled Double-Blind Study of Danazol in Hemophilia A," *Acta Haematol*, 1992, 88(1):14-6.

Weinblatt ME, Kochen J, and Ortega J, "Danazol for Children With Immune Thrombocytopenic Purpura," *Am J Dis Child*, 1988, 142(12):1317-9.

♦ **Danocrine® [DSC]** *see* Danazol *on page 437*

♦ **Danocrine® (Can)** *see* Danazol *on page 437*

♦ **Dantrium®** *see* Dantrolene *on page 439*

Dantrolene (DAN troe leen)

Medication Safety Issues

Sound-alike/look-alike issues:

Dantrium® may be confused with danazol, Daraprim®

U.S. Brand Names Dantrium®

Canadian Brand Names Dantrium®

Index Terms Dantrolene Sodium

Therapeutic Category Antidote, Malignant Hyperthermia; Hyperthermia, Treatment; Skeletal Muscle Relaxant, Nonparalytic

Generic Available Yes: Capsule

Use Treatment of spasticity associated with upper motor neuron disorders such as spinal cord injury, stroke, cerebral palsy, or multiple sclerosis; treatment of malignant hyperthermia

Pregnancy Risk Factor C

Lactation Excretion in breast milk unknown/not recommended

Contraindications Hypersensitivity to dantrolene or any component; active hepatic disease such as hepatitis and cirrhosis; should not be administered where spasticity is used to maintain posture or balance

Warnings May cause hepatotoxicity; overt hepatitis has been most frequently observed between the third and twelfth month of therapy and with doses ≥800 mg/day;

(Continued)

Dantrolene *(Continued)*

hepatic injury appears to be greater in females and in patients >35 years of age; monitor LFTs. Injection is extremely irritating to peripheral veins and may cause severe tissue necrosis if extravasation occurs; administer in a fast moving I.V. solution into a large vein or into a central line.

Precautions Use with caution in patients with impaired cardiac or pulmonary function or history of previous liver disease; crosses placenta with fetal whole blood levels up to 65% of maternal at delivery

Adverse Reactions

Cardiovascular: Pericarditis (with pleural effusion), tachycardia

Central nervous system: Seizures, drowsiness, dizziness, lightheadedness, confusion, headache, fatigue, speech disturbances, mental depression, chills, fever

Dermatologic: Rash, acne-like rash, pruritus, urticaria, abnormal hair growth

Gastrointestinal: Diarrhea, nausea, vomiting, severe constipation, gastric irritation, GI bleeding, abdominal cramps, dysphagia, anorexia, swallowing difficulty, drooling

Genitourinary: Urinary retention or frequency, urinary incontinence

Hematologic: Aplastic anemia, anemia, leucopenia, lymphocytic lymphoma, thrombocytopenia

Hepatic: Hepatitis (see Warnings)

Local: Phlebitis, tissue necrosis

Neuromuscular & skeletal: Muscle weakness, myalgia, backache

Ocular: Visual disturbances, excessive tearing

Renal: Hematuria

Respiratory: Respiratory depression, pleural effusion (with pericarditis)

Drug Interactions Use with verapamil may result in hyperkalemia and myocardial depression; avoid use of calcium channel blockers with dantrolene especially as a treatment for the cardiovascular effects of malignant hyperthermia; estrogen increases incidence of hepatotoxicity when used concomitantly; additive CNS depressive effects with other CNS depressants; increased toxicity with MAO inhibitors, phenothiazines, clindamycin, warfarin, clofibrate, and tolbutamide; may prolong the paralytic effects of vecuronium

Stability Protect from light; use reconstituted injection within 6 hours; incompatible with dextrose, NS, or bacteriostatic water for injection; precipitates when placed in glass containers for infusion

Mechanism of Action Acts directly on skeletal muscle by interfering with release of calcium ion from the sarcoplasmic reticulum; prevents or reduces the increase in myoplasmic calcium ion concentration that activates the acute catabolic processes associated with malignant hyperthermia

Pharmacokinetics

Absorption: Oral: 70%

Metabolism: Extensive; metabolized to active metabolite: 5-hydroxydantrolene

Half-life:

- Neonates (at birth): ~20 hours
- Children: 10 ± 2.6 hours
- Adults: 12 hours (range: 4-21 hours)

Elimination: 25% excreted in urine as metabolites and unchanged drug; 45% to 50% excreted in feces via bile

Usual Dosage

Spasticity: Oral: **Note:** Titrate to desired effect; if no further benefit is observed at a higher dosage, decrease dose to previous lower dose.

Children: Initial: 0.5 mg/kg/dose once daily for 7 days, increase to 0.5 mg/kg/dose 3 times/day for 7 days, increase to 1 mg/kg/dose 3 times/day for 7 days, and then increase to 2 mg/kg/dose 3 times/day; not to exceed 400 mg/day

Adults: 25 mg once daily for 7 days, increase to 25 mg 3 times/day for 7 days, increase to 50 mg 3 times/day for 7 days, and then increase to 100 mg 3 times/day; not to exceed 400 mg/day

Malignant hyperthermia: Children and Adults:

Preoperative prophylaxis: No longer recommended providing that there is immediate availability of dantrolene and adequate perioperative patient management (eg, avoiding known trigger agents in susceptible patients; see Additional Information)

Oral: 4-8 mg/kg/day in 3-4 divided doses for 1-2 days prior to surgery with the last dose administered approximately 3-4 hours before scheduled surgery

I.V.: 2.5 mg/kg administered approximately 1.25 hours prior to surgery (infuse over 1 hour)

Crisis: I.V.: Malignant Hyperthermia Association of the U.S. (MHAUS) and European recommendation: 2.5 mg/kg; may repeat as often as necessary until normalization of the hypermetabolic state and the disappearance of all symptoms (typically 1-4 doses; if >20 mg/kg is used without benefit, consider other potential diagnoses)

Postcrisis: MHAUS and European recommendations differ slightly in the postcrisis treatment regimen. Both are described below.

MHAUS recommendation: I.V.: Continue therapy with 1 mg/kg/dose every 6 hours for at least 24 hours after control of symptoms

European recommendation: I.V.: Continue therapy with a continuous infusion of 10 mg/kg/day for at least 36 hours

Manufacturer's recommendation: Oral: 4-8 mg/kg/day in 4 divided doses for 1-3 days following crisis

Administration

Oral: Contents of capsule may be mixed with juice or liquid

Parenteral: Reconstitute by adding 60 mL SWI (**not bacteriostatic water for injection**), resultant concentration 0.333 mg/mL; administer by rapid I.V. injection; for infusion, do **not** further dilute with NS or dextrose; place solution in plastic container for continuous infusion

Monitoring Parameters Baseline and periodic liver function tests; temperature (hyperthermia use)

Patient Information Avoid alcohol; may cause drowsiness and impair ability to perform activities requiring mental alertness or physical coordination

Nursing Implications Avoid extravasation since dantrolene is a tissue irritant

Additional Information MHAUS provides educational and technical information to patients and healthcare providers; contact at 607-674-7901 or email to info@mhaus.org; on-call anesthesiologists available to consult in MH emergencies may be obtained 24 hours/day at 1-(800)-MH-HYPER or 1-(800)-644-9737. Triggers for the development of malignant hyperthermia in susceptible individuals include: All volatile inhalation anesthetics (desflurane, sevoflurane, isoflurane, halothane, enflurane, ether, methoxyflurane, and cyclopropane) and succinylcholine.

Dantrolene has been used successfully to treat neuroleptic malignant syndrome associated with antipsychotic agents such as prochlorperazine, promethazine, clozapine, and risperidone and also non-neuroleptic agents such as metoclopramide, amoxapine, and lithium. The recommended dose for this indication has not been established. Published case reports have used doses ranging from 1-10 mg/kg/day in divided doses both I.V. and orally.

Dosage Forms Excipient information presented when available (limited, particularly for generics); consult specific product labeling.

Capsule, as sodium: 25 mg, 50 mg, 100 mg

Dantrium®: 25 mg, 50 mg, 100 mg

Injection, powder for reconstitution, as sodium:

Dantrium®: 20 mg [contains mannitol 3 g]

Extemporaneous Preparations A 5 mg/mL suspension may be made by adding five 100 mg capsules to a citric acid solution (150 mg citric acid powder in 10 mL water) and then adding syrup to a total volume of 100 mL; shake well; stable 2 days in refrigerator. Stability is improved when syrup BP (containing 0.5% w/v methylhydroxybenzoate) is used. This solution is stable 30 days refrigerated.

Nahata, MC, Pai VB, and Hipple TF, *Pediatric Drug Formulations*, 5th ed, Cincinnati, OH: Harvey Whitney Books Co, 2004.

References

Ali SZ, Taguchi A, and Rosenberg H, "Malignant Hyperthermia," *Best Pract Res Clin Anaesthesiol*, 2003, 17(4):519-33.

Allen GC, Cattran CB, Peterson RG, et al, "Plasma Levels of Dantrolene Following Oral Administration in Malignant Hyperthermia-Susceptible Patients," *Anesthesiology*, 1988, 69(6):900-4.

Guze BH and Baxter LR Jr, "Current Concepts. Neuroleptic Malignant Syndrome," *N Engl J Med*, 1985, 313(3):163-6.

Krause T, Gerbershagen MU, Fiege M, et al, "Dantrolene - A Review of Its Pharmacology, Therapeutic Use and New Developments," *Anaesthesia*, 2004, 59(4):364-73.

Lerman J, McLeod ME, and Strong HA, "Pharmacokinetics of Intravenous Dantrolene in Children," *Anesthesiology*, 1989, 70(4):625-9.

Podranski T, Bouillon T, Schumacher PM, et al, "Compartmental Pharmacokinetics of Dantrolene in Adults: Do Malignant Hyperthermia Association Dosing Guidelines Work?" *Anesth Analg*, 2005, 101(6):1695-9.

Shime J, Gare D, Andrews J, et al, "Dantrolene in Pregnancy: Lack of Adverse Effects on the Fetus and Newborn Infant," *Am J Obstet Gynecol*, 1988, 159(4):831-4.

Susman VL, " Clinical Management of Neuroleptic Malignant Syndrome," *Psychiatr Q*, 2001, 72(4):325-36.

♦ **Dantrolene Sodium** *see* Dantrolene *on page 439*

Dapsone (DAP sone)

Medication Safety Issues

Sound-alike/look-alike issues:

Dapsone may be confused with Diprosone®

U.S. Brand Names Aczone™

Index Terms Diaminodiphenylsulfone

Therapeutic Category Antibiotic, Sulfone; Leprostatic Agent

Generic Available Yes: Tablet

(Continued)

Dapsone *(Continued)*

Use Treatment of leprosy due to susceptible strains of *M. leprae*; treatment of dermatitis herpetiformis; prophylaxis against *Pneumocystis carinii* pneumonia (PCP) in patients who cannot tolerate sulfamethoxazole and trimethoprim or aerosolized pentamidine; prophylaxis against toxoplasmic encephalitis in patients who cannot tolerate sulfamethoxazole and trimethoprim; topical treatment of acne vulgaris

Pregnancy Risk Factor C

Lactation Enters breast milk/not recommended (AAP rates "compatible")

Contraindications Hypersensitivity to dapsone or any component; patients with severe anemia

Precautions Use with caution in patients with G-6-PD deficiency, methemoglobin reductase deficiency or hemoglobin M; in patients receiving drugs capable of inducing hemolysis and in patients with severe cardiopulmonary disease; hypersensitivity to other sulfonamides; obtain G6PD levels prior to initiating dapsone therapy

Adverse Reactions

Cardiovascular: Tachycardia

Central nervous system: Psychotic episodes, hallucinations, insomnia, vertigo, irritability, depression, headache, fever, uncoordinated speech, suicidal behavior

Dermatologic: Rash, exfoliative dermatitis, erythema multiforme, toxic epidermal necrolysis, urticaria, morbilliform reactions, erythema nodosum, photosensitivity (oral)

Topical: erythema, skin peeling

Endocrine & metabolic: Hyperkalemia, hypoalbuminemia

Gastrointestinal: Nausea, vomiting, abdominal pain, anorexia, pancreatitis

Hematologic: Hemolytic anemia, methemoglobinemia, leukopenia, agranulocytosis, aplastic anemia, neutropenia

Hepatic: Hepatitis, cholestatic jaundice; elevated alkaline phosphatase, AST, bilirubin, and LDH

Neuromuscular & skeletal: Muscle weakness, peripheral neuropathy, tonic clonic movements

Ocular: Blurred vision

Otic: Tinnitus

Renal: Acute tubular necrosis, nephrotic syndrome, albuminuria

Respiratory: Pharyngitis

Miscellaneous: Lupus erythematosus, mononucleosis-like syndrome

Drug Interactions Cytochrome P450 isoenzyme CYP2C9, CYP2E1, and CYP3A3/4 substrate

Didanosine buffered formulations decrease dapsone absorption (separate buffered didanosine administration from dapsone by at least 2 hours); rifampin (decreases dapsone concentrations); trimethoprim (increases dapsone concentration); pyrimethamine, nitrofurantoin, primaquine (increase risk of hematologic side effects); rifampin, carbamazepine, fosphenytoin, oxcarbamazepine, phenobarbital, phenytoin, primidone, and St. John's wort may increase formation of dapsone metabolite, dapsone hydroxylamine, which is associated with hemolysis

Food Interactions Do not administer with antacids, alkaline foods, or alkaline drugs (may decrease dapsone absorption)

Stability Protect from freezing and light. Store at room temperature. Store gel in original box after use.

Mechanism of Action Dapsone is a sulfone antimicrobial. The mechanism of action of the sulfones is similar to that of the sulfonamides. Sulfonamides are competitive antagonists of para-aminobenzoic acid (PABA) and inhibit folic acid synthesis in susceptible organisms.

Pharmacokinetics

Absorption: Oral: 86% to 100%

Distribution: Distributes into skin, muscle, kidneys, liver, sweat, sputum, saliva, tears, and bile; distributes into breast milk; crosses the placenta

V_d: Adults: 1.5-2.5 L/kg

Protein binding: 50% to 90%

Metabolism: Acetylated and hydroxylated in the liver

Half-life:

Children: 15.1 hours

Adults: 13-83 hours (mean: 20-30 hours)

Time to peak serum concentration: Within 2-8 hours

Elimination: 5% to 20% of dose excreted in urine as unchanged drug; 70% to 85% excreted in urine as metabolites; small amount excreted in feces

Usual Dosage

Oral:

Children ≥1 month of age:

Prophylaxis for first episode of opportunistic disease due to *Toxoplasma gondii*: 2 mg/kg or 15 mg/m^2 (maximum dose: 25 mg) once daily in combination with pyrimethamine 1 mg/kg once daily and leucovorin 5 mg every 3 days

Primary and secondary PCP prophylaxis (see **Note** in Additional Information): 2 mg/kg/day once daily (maximum dose: 100 mg/day), or 4 mg/kg/dose once weekly (maximum dose: 200 mg)

Children:

Leprosy: 1-2 mg/kg/day given once daily in combination therapy; maximum dose: 100 mg/day

Adults:

Leprosy: 50-100 mg once daily; combination therapy with one or more antileprosy drugs is recommended to avoid dapsone resistance

Dermatitis herpetiformis: Initial: 50 mg once daily; maintenance dosage range: 25-400 mg/day

PCP treatment: 100 mg once daily in combination with trimethoprim

Primary and secondary PCP prophylaxis: 50 mg twice daily; or dapsone 50 mg once daily plus pyrimethamine 50 mg orally every week plus leucovorin 25 mg orally every week; or dapsone 200 mg orally plus pyrimethamine 75 mg orally plus leucovorin 25 mg orally every week

Toxoplasma gondii prophylaxis: 50 mg once daily plus pyrimethamine 50 mg orally every week, plus leucovorin 25 mg orally every week

Topical: Children ≥12 years, Adolescents, and Adults: Apply a pea-sized amount of gel to the acne-affected areas twice daily

Administration

Oral: Administer with water

Topical: Wash skin and pat dry then rub in thin layer of gel gently and completely. Wash hands after application.

Monitoring Parameters CBC with differential, platelet count, hemoglobin, reticulocyte count, hematocrit, liver function tests, and urinalysis; check G6PD levels prior to initiation of dapsone

Patient Information Notify physician if fever, sore throat, pallor, fatigue, muscle weakness, rash, purpura, or jaundice occurs. May cause photosensitivity reactions (eg, exposure to sunlight may cause severe sunburn, skin rash, redness, or itching); avoid exposure to sunlight and artificial light sources (sunlamps, tanning booth/bed); wear protective clothing, wide-brimmed hats, sunglasses, and lip sunscreen (SPF ≥15); use a sunscreen [broad-spectrum sunscreen or physical sunscreen (preferred) or sunblock with SPF ≥15]; contact physician if reaction occurs. Dapsone distributes into breast milk and may harm your baby. A decision should be made to discontinue breast-feeding or the drug.

Additional Information Note: Guidelines for prophylaxis of *Pneumocystis carinii* pneumonia: Initiate PCP prophylaxis in the following patients: In all HIV-exposed children at 4-6 weeks of age and continue through the first year of life or until HIV infection has been reasonably excluded; children 1-5 years of age with CD4+ count <500 or CD4+ percentage <15%; children 6-12 years of age with CD4+ count <200 or CD4+ percentage <15%; adolescents and adults with CD4+ count <200 or oropharyngeal candidiasis. Folinic acid (leucovorin) should be given if bone marrow suppression occurs.

Dosage Forms Excipient information presented when available (limited, particularly for generics); consult specific product labeling.

Gel, topical (Aczone™): 5% (30 g)

Tablet: 25 mg, 100 mg

Extemporaneous Preparations A 2 mg/mL oral suspension can be made using a 1:1 mixture of Ora-Sweet® and Ora-Plus®; crush eight 25 mg tablets into a fine powder in a mortar; add a small amount of vehicle and mix to make a uniform paste; mix while adding the vehicle in geometric portions to almost 100 mL; transfer to a calibrated bottle and qsad with vehicle to 100 mL; preparation is stable for 90 days when stored at room temperature or under refrigeration; label "shake well"

Jacobus Pharmaceutical Company (609) 921-7447 makes a 2 mg/mL proprietary liquid formulation available under an IND for the prophylaxis of *Pneumocystis carinii* pneumonia

Nahata MC, Morosco RS, and Trowbridge JM, "Stability of Dapsone in Two Oral Liquid Dosage Forms," *Ann Pharmacother*, 2000, 34(7-8):848-50.

References

Barnett ED, Pelton SI, Mirochnick M, et al, "Dapsone for Prevention of *Pneumocystis* Pneumonia in Children With Acquired Immunodeficiency Syndrome," *Pediatr Infect Dis J*, 1994, 13(1):72-4.

Kaplan JE, Masur H, and Holmes KK, "Guidelines for Preventing Opportunistic Infections Among HIV-Infected Persons - 2002 Recommendations of the USPHS and IDSA," *MMWR*, 2002, 51(RR-8):1-46.

Mirochnick M, Michaels M, Clarke D, et al, "Pharmacokinetics of Dapsone in Children," *J Pediatr*, 1993, 122(5 Pt 1):806-9.

(Continued)

Dapsone *(Continued)*

Stavola JJ and Noel GJ, "Efficacy and Safety of Dapsone Prophylaxis Against *Pneumocystis carinii* Pneumonia in Human Immunodeficiency Virus-Infected Children," *Pediatr Infect Dis J*, 1993, 12(8):644-7.

- **Daptacel®** *see* Diphtheria, Tetanus Toxoids, and Acellular Pertussis Vaccine *on page 517*
- **Daraprim®** *see* Pyrimethamine *on page 1354*

Darbepoetin Alfa (dar be POE e tin AL fa)

Medication Safety Issues
Sound-alike/look-alike issues:
Darbepoetin alfa may be confused with epoetin alfa

U.S. Brand Names Aranesp®

Canadian Brand Names Aranesp®

Index Terms Erythropoiesis-Stimulating Agent (ESA); Erythropoiesis-Stimulating Protein; NSC-729969

Therapeutic Category Colony-Stimulating Factor; Erythropoiesis Stimulating Protein

Generic Available No

Use Treatment of anemia associated with chronic renal failure (requiring dialysis or not) or anemia associated with concurrent chemotherapy for nonmyeloid malignancies

Pregnancy Risk Factor C

Lactation Excretion in breast milk unknown/use caution

Contraindications Hypersensitivity to darbepoetin alfa or any component; uncontrolled hypertension

Warnings Due to an increased risk of cardiac arrest, neurologic events (including seizures and stroke), exacerbations of hypertension, CHF, vascular thrombosis/ischemia/infarction, acute MI, and fluid overdose/edema in patients whose Hgb increased >12 g/dL, hemoglobin should be monitored twice weekly for 2-6 weeks following initiation and dosage adjustments. The darbepoetin alfa dosage should be decreased if the the Hgb exceeds 12 g/dL or the rate of rise of hemoglobin exceeds 1 g/dL in any 2-week period. In clinical trials, ~40% of CRF patients required initiation or intensification of antihypertensive therapy; blood pressure should be controlled adequately before initiation of darbepoetin alfa therapy; close blood pressure monitoring is recommended. Seizures have occurred during therapy; monitor closely for premonitory neurologic symptoms during the first several months of therapy. The risk of thrombotic events (eg, pulmonary emboli, thrombophlebitis, thrombosis) is increase with erythropoietic therapy. Cases of pure red cell aplasia and severe anemia with or without other cytopenias associated with neutralizing antibodies to erythropoietin have been reported in CRF patients and patients receiving other erythropoiesis-stimulating proteins. Patients who develop a sudden loss of responsiveness to darbepoetin therapy along with a severe anemia and low reticulocyte count should be evaluated for the presence of these antibodies. Withhold darbepoetin until the etiology is confirmed. Amgen can perform assays for binding and neutralizing antibodies. Darbepoetin alfa is not approved for use in patients with myeloid malignancies or in patients with cancer-related anemia who are not receiving concurrent chemotherapy.

Precautions Use with caution in patients with porphyria or a history of seizures. Darbepoetin alfa is not intended for patients who require acute corrections of anemia

Factors Limiting Response to Darbepoetin Alfa

Factor	Mechanism
Iron deficiency	Limits hemoglobin synthesis
Blood loss/hemolysis	Counteracts darbepoetin alfa-stimulated erythropoiesis
Infection/inflammation	Inhibits iron transfer from storage to bone marrow Suppresses erythropoiesis through activated macrophages
Aluminum overload	Inhibits iron incorporation into heme protein
Bone marrow replacement Hyperparathyroidism Metastatic, neoplastic disease	Limits bone marrow volume
Folic acid/vitamin B_{12} deficiency	Limits hemoglobin synthesis
Patient compliance	Self administered darbepoetin alfa or iron therapy

and is not a substitute for emergency blood transfusion. Allow sufficient time (an interval of 4-6 weeks) to determine the patient's response to a particular dosage (see Warnings regarding rapid responsiveness); patients with CRF not yet requiring dialysis may require lower maintenance doses. Assessment of iron stores and therapeutic iron supplementation is essential for optimal therapy. Iron supplementation is necessary to provide for increased requirements during expansion of the red cell mass secondary to marrow stimulation unless iron stores are already in excess.

Assessment of iron stores and therapeutic iron supplementation is essential to optimal darbepoetin alfa therapy. Iron supplementation is necessary to provide for increased requirements during expansion of the red cell mass secondary to marrow stimulation, unless iron stores are already in excess. Optimal iron stores are demonstrated by a transferrin saturation of 20% or more and a serum ferritin of 100-150 mcg/L.

Adverse Reactions

Cardiovascular: Hypertension, hypotension, edema, tachycardia, chest pain, cardiac arrhythmia, cardiac arrest, CHF, MI, TIA/CVA, venous thrombosis

Central nervous system: Fatigue, dizziness, headache, seizure, fever

Dermatologic: Pruritus, rash

Gastrointestinal: Nausea, diarrhea, vomiting, abdominal pain, constipation

Hematologic: Neutropenia, pure red cell aplasia, severe anemia (see Warnings)

Local: Pain, irritation at injection site (SubQ injection)

Neuromuscular & skeletal: Myalgia, arthralgia, back pain, limb pain

Respiratory: Cough, dyspnea, bronchitis, upper respiratory infection, pulmonary embolism

Miscellaneous: Hypersensitivity reactions, flu-like symptoms, sepsis

Stability Refrigerate; stable 7 days at room temperature; protect from light; contains no preservatives; discard after entry; may dilute with NS or bacteriostatic NS in a 1:10 ratio at the time of administration; dilution stable for 24 hours refrigerated; do not dilute with other solutions or medications

Mechanism of Action Darbepoetin alfa, manufactured by recombinant DNA technology, has the same effects as endogenous erythropoietin (EPO). It differs slightly from recombinant human erythropoietin in containing 5 N-linked oligosaccharide chains instead of 3. EPO induces erythropoiesis by stimulating the division and differentiation of committed erythroid progenitor cells. It induces the release of reticulocytes from the bone marrow into the bloodstream, where they mature to erythrocytes (dose response relationship) resulting in an increase in reticulocyte counts followed by a rise in hematocrit and hemoglobin levels. There is normally an inverse correlation between the plasma EPO level and the hemoglobin concentration (only when the hemoglobin concentration is <10.5 g/dL).

Pharmacodynamics

Onset of action: Several days

Maximum effect: 4-6 weeks

Pharmacokinetics

Absorption: SubQ: Slow and rate-limiting

Distribution: V_d:
- Children: 51.6 mL/kg (range: 21-73 mL/kg)
- Adults: 52.4 ± 6.6 mL/kg

Bioavailability: SubQ: CRF:

Children: 54% (range:32% to 70%)

Adults: ~37% (range: 30% to 50%)

Half-life:
- Children:
  - I.V.: Terminal: 22.1 hours (range: 12-30 hours)
  - SubQ: Terminal: 42.8 hours (range: 16-86 hours)
- Adults: CRF:
  - I.V.: Terminal: 21 hours
  - SubQ: Terminal: 49 ± 12.7 hours

Time to peak serum concentration: SubQ:
- CRF patients: 34 hours (range: 24-72 hours)
- Cancer patients: 90 hours (range: 71-123 hours)

Elimination:
- Clearance: I.V.:
  - Children: 2.29 mL/hour/kg (range: 1.6-3.5 mL/hour/kg)
  - Adults: 1.6 ± 1.0 mL/hour/kg

Usual Dosage Dosing schedules need to be individualized by treatment indication and patient response. Careful monitoring of hemoglobin in patients receiving the drug is recommended. The Hgb should not exceed 12 g/dL or increase by >1 g/dL in any 2-week period. See "Darbepoetin Alfa Dosage Adjustments" table on next page. Darbepoetin alfa may be ineffective if other factors such as iron or B_{12}/folate deficiency limit marrow response.

(Continued)

Darbepoetin Alfa *(Continued)*

Anemia in chronic renal failure: Children and Adults: I.V., SubQ: 0.45 mcg/kg/dose once weekly

Note: Allow at least 4 weeks to determine full effects of the new regimen. For many patients, the appropriate maintenance dose may be less than the initial dose. Patients not receiving hemodialysis may be particularly sensitive and require lower doses. SubQ dosing every two weeks has been effective in some patients.

Anemia associated with chemotherapy in patients with nonmyeloid malignancies: **Note:** Use in patients with pretreatment serum EPO levels >200 is not recommended; Children and Adults: SubQ: 2.25 mcg/kg/dose once weekly or as an alternative in adults: 500 mcg once every 3 weeks

Note: Adjust dosage depending upon response; if indicated dosage may be increased to a maximum of 4.5 mcg/kg/dose; allow at least 6 weeks of therapy before increasing the dosage

Darbepoetin Alfa Dosage Adjustments

Target hemoglobin range	9-12 g/dL; not to exceed 12 g/dL
Increase dose (not more frequently than once monthly)	By 25% when hemoglobin does not increase by 1 g/dL after 4 weeks of therapy **and** hemoglobin is below target range
Reduce dose	By 25% when hemoglobin increases >1 g/dL in any 2-week period or when hemoglobin >12 g/dL
Stop therapy	When hemoglobin continues to increase after dosage reduction; reinstate therapy at a 25% lower dose after the hemoglobin begins to decrease

Conversion From Epoetin Alfa to Darbepoetin Alfa (I.V. or SubQ)[1] (maintain the same route of administration for the conversion)

Previous Weekly Epoetin Alfa Dose (units/week)	Weekly Darbepoetin Alfa Dosage (mcg/week)[2]	
	Pediatric	Adults
<1500	—[3]	6.25
1500-2499	6.25	6.25
2500-4999	10	12.5
5000-10,999	20	25
11,000-17,999	40	40
18,000-33,999	60	60
34,000-89,999	100	100
≥90,000	200	200

[1]1 mcg darbepoetin alfa is equivalent to 200 units epoetin alfa.

[2]Due to the longer serum half-life of darbepoetin alfa, when converting from epoetin alfa, administer darbepoetin alfa once weekly if the patient was receiving epoetin alfa 2-3 times weekly and administer darbepoetin alfa once every two weeks if the patient was receiving epoetin alfa once weekly.

[3]Insufficient information to determine conversion dose.

Administration Parenteral: Do not shake as this may denature the glycoprotein rendering the drug biologically inactive. I.V.: Infuse over 1-3 minutes

Test	Initial Phase Frequency	Maintenance Phase Frequency
Hemoglobin	Once weekly until stabilized	2-4 times/month
Blood pressure	3 times/week	3 times/week
Serum ferritin	Monthly	Quarterly
Transferrin saturation	Monthly	Quarterly
Serum chemistries[1]	Regularly per routine	Regularly per routine
Reticulocyte count	Baseline prior to starting therapy	After 10 days of therapy

[1]Including CBC with differential, creatinine, BUN, potassium, phosphorus

Monitoring Parameters
Careful monitoring of blood pressure is indicated; problems with hypertension have been noted especially in renal failure patients treated with darbepoetin alfa. See table on previous page.

Patient Information Frequent blood tests are needed to determine the correct dose; notify physician if any severe headache develops; due to increased risk of seizure activity in CRF patients during the first 90 days of therapy, avoid potentially hazardous activities (eg, driving) during this period

Additional Information Optimal response is achieved when iron stores are maintained with supplemental iron if necessary; evaluate iron stores prior to and during therapy

Dosage Forms Excipient information presented when available (limited, particularly for generics); consult specific product labeling. [DSC] = Discontinued product

Injection, solution [preservative free; contains human albumin 2.5 mg/mL; single-dose vial]:
Aranesp®: 25 mcg/mL (1 mL); 40 mcg/mL (1 mL); 60 mcg/mL (1 mL); 100 mcg/mL (1 mL); 150 mcg/0.75 mL (0.75 mL); 200 mcg/mL (1 mL); 300 mcg/mL (1 mL); 500 mcg/mL (1 mL) [DSC]

Injection, solution [preservative free; contains human albumin 2.5 mg/mL; prefilled syringe; needle cover contains latex]:
Aranesp®: 25 mcg/0.42 mL (0.42 mL); 40 mcg/0.4 mL (0.4 mL); 60 mcg/0.3 mL (0.3 mL); 100 mcg/0.5 mL (0.5 mL); 150 mcg/0.3 mL (0.3 mL); 200 mcg/0.4 mL (0.4 mL); 300 mcg/0.6 mL (0.6 mL); 500 mcg/mL (1 mL) [DSC]

Injection, solution [preservative free; contains polysorbate 80; prefilled syringe; needle cover contains latex]:
Aranesp®: 25 mcg/0.42 mL (0.42 mL); 40 mcg/ 0.4 mL (0.4 mL); 60 mcg/0.3 mL (0.3 mL); 100 mcg/0.5 mL (0.5 mL); 150 mcg/0.3 mL (0.3 mL); 200 mcg/0.4 mL (0.4 mL); 300 mcg/0.6 mL (0.6 mL); 500 mcg/mL (1 mL)

Injection, solution [preservative free; contains polysorbate 80; single-dose vial]:
Aranesp®: 200 mcg/mL (1 mL); 300 mcg/mL (1 mL)

References

Joy MS, "Darbepoetin Alfa: A Novel Erythropoiesis-Stimulating Protein," *Ann Pharmacother*, 2002, 36(7):1183-92.

Lerner G, Kale AS, Warady BA, et al, "Pharmacokinetics of Darbepoetin Alfa in Pediatric Patients With Chronic Kidney Disease," *Pediatr Nephrol*, 2002, 17(11):933-7.

- **Darvocet A500™** *see* Propoxyphene and Acetaminophen *on page 1336*
- **Darvocet-N® 50** *see* Propoxyphene and Acetaminophen *on page 1336*
- **Darvocet-N® 100** *see* Propoxyphene and Acetaminophen *on page 1336*
- **Darvon®** *see* Propoxyphene *on page 1334*
- **Darvon-N®** *see* Propoxyphene *on page 1334*
- **Daunomycin** *see* DAUNOrubicin *on page 447*

DAUNOrubicin (daw noe ROO bi sin)

Medication Safety Issues
Sound-alike/look-alike issues:
DAUNOrubicin may be confused with dactinomycin, DOXOrubicin, epirubicin, idarubicin
Conventional formulations (Cerubidine®) may be confused with liposomal formulations (DaunoXome®, Doxil®)

High alert medication: The Institute for Safe Medication Practices (ISMP) includes this medication among its list of drugs which have a heightened risk of causing significant patient harm when used in error.

Related Information
Extravasation Treatment *on page 1726*

U.S. Brand Names Cerubidine®

Canadian Brand Names Cerubidine®

Index Terms Daunomycin; DNR; NSC-82151; Rubidomycin Hydrochloride

Therapeutic Category Antineoplastic Agent, Anthracycline; Antineoplastic Agent, Antibiotic

Generic Available Yes

Use In combination with other agents in the treatment of leukemias (ALL, AML)

Pregnancy Risk Factor D

Lactation Excretion in breast milk unknown/not recommended

Contraindications Hypersensitivity to daunorubicin or any component; CHF, left ventricular ejection fraction <30% to 40%, or arrhythmias; pre-existing bone marrow suppression

Warnings The FDA currently recommends that procedures for proper handling and disposal of antineoplastic agents be considered; I.V. use only; severe local tissue
(Continued)

DAUNOrubicin *(Continued)*

necrosis will result if extravasation occurs; irreversible myocardial toxicity may occur as total dosage approaches 550 mg/m^2 in adults, 400 mg/m^2 in patients receiving chest radiation, 300 mg/m^2 in children ≥2 years of age, or 10 mg/kg in children <2 years; this may occur during therapy or several months after therapy; total cumulative dose should take into account previous or concomitant treatment with cardiotoxic agents or irradiation of chest; infants and children may be more susceptible to anthracycline-induced cardiotoxicity than adults; severe myelosuppression is possible when used in therapeutic doses

Precautions Reduce dosage in patients with hepatic, biliary, or renal impairment

Adverse Reactions

Cardiovascular: Cardiotoxicity, CHF (dose-related, may occur 7-8 years after treatment), arrhythmias, EKG abnormalities

Central nervous system: Fever, chills

Dermatologic: Alopecia, hyperpigmentation of skin and nail beds, urticaria, pruritus

Endocrine & metabolic: Hyperuricemia, infertility, sterility

Gastrointestinal: Stomatitis, esophagitis, nausea, vomiting, diarrhea

Genitourinary: Discoloration of urine (red-orange)

Hematologic: Myelosuppression (thrombocytopenia, leukopenia)

Hepatic: Elevated serum bilirubin, AST, and alkaline phosphatase

Local: Severe tissue necrosis with extravasation

Stability Protect from light; reconstituted solution is stable for 48 hours when refrigerated and 24 hours at room temperature; a color change from red to blue/purple indicates decomposition of the drug; unstable in solutions with a pH >8; incompatible with heparin, sodium bicarbonate, fluorouracil, and dexamethasone

Mechanism of Action Inhibition of DNA and RNA synthesis by intercalating between DNA base pairs, uncoiling of the helix, and by steric obstruction; not cell cycle-specific for the S-phase of cell division; may cause free radical damage to DNA

Pharmacokinetics

Distribution: Widely distributed in tissues such as spleen, heart, kidneys, liver, and lungs; does not cross the blood-brain barrier; crosses the placenta

Metabolism: To daunorubicinol (active)

Half-life, terminal: 14-18.5 hours

Daunorubicinol, active metabolite: 26.7 hours

Elimination: 40% of dose excreted in bile; ~14% to 23% excreted in urine as metabolite and unchanged drug

Usual Dosage I.V. (refer to individual protocols):

Children <2 years or <0.5 m^2: Dosage should be calculated on the basis of body weight rather than body surface area: 1 mg/kg or per protocol with frequency dependent on regimen employed

Children:

ALL combination therapy: Remission induction: 25-45 mg/m^2 on days 1 and 8 of cycle, or 30-45 mg/m^2/day for 3 days every 3-4 weeks, or 25 mg/m^2 every week for 4 weeks

AML combination therapy: Induction: I.V. continuous infusion: 30-60 mg/m^2/day on days 1-3 of cycle, or 20 mg/m^2/day for 4 days every 14 days

Adults: 30-60 mg/m^2/day for 3-5 days, repeat dose in 3-4 weeks; total cumulative dose should not exceed 400-600 mg/m^2

AML: Single agent induction: 60 mg/m^2/day for 3 days; repeat every 3-4 weeks

AML: Combination therapy induction: 45 mg/m^2/day for 3 days of the first course of induction therapy; subsequent courses: Every day for 2 days

ALL: Combination therapy: Remission induction: 45 mg/m^2 on days 1, 2, and 3 of induction course

Dosing adjustment in hepatic or renal impairment: Reduce dose by 25% in patients with serum bilirubin of 1.2-3 mg/dL; reduce dose by 50% in patients with serum bilirubin and/or creatinine >3 mg/dL

Administration Parenteral: Drug is very irritating, do not inject I.M. or SubQ; administer IVP diluting the reconstituted dose in 10-15 mL NS and administering over 2-3 minutes into the tubing of a rapidly infusing I.V. solution of D_5W or NS; daunorubicin has also been diluted in 100 mL of D_5W or NS and infused over 30-45 minutes or as a continuous 24-hour infusion

Monitoring Parameters CBC with differential and platelet count, serum bilirubin, serum uric acid, liver function test, EKG, ventricular ejection fraction, renal function test; patency of I.V. line

Patient Information Transient red-orange discoloration of urine can occur for up to 48 hours after a dose; notify physician if fever, sore throat, bleeding, bruising, chills, signs of infection, abdominal pain, blood in stools, excessive fatigue, yellowing of eyes or skin, or difficulty breathing occurs

Nursing Implications Leukemic patients should receive prophylactic allopurinol to prevent acute urate nephropathy; avoid extravasation; if extravasation occurs, apply a cold compress immediately for 30-60 minutes, then alternate off/on every 15 minutes for 1 day; apply 1.5 mL of dimethylsulfoxide 99% (w/v) solution to the site every 6 hours for 14 days; allow to air-dry; do not cover

Additional Information Myelosuppressive effects:

WBC: Severe
Platelets: Severe
Onset (days): 7
Nadir (days): 10-14
Recovery (days): 21-28

Dosage Forms Excipient information presented when available (limited, particularly for generics); consult specific product labeling.

Injection, powder for reconstitution: 20 mg, 50 mg
Cerubidine®: 20 mg
Injection, solution: 5 mg/mL (4 mL, 10 mL)

References

Crom WR, Glynn-Barnhart AM, Rodman JH, et al, "Pharmacokinetics of Anticancer Drugs in Children," *Clin Pharmacokinet*, 1987, 12(3):168-213.

- **Dayhist® Allergy [OTC]** *see* Clemastine *on page 378*
- **Daypro®** *see* Oxaprozin *on page 1181*
- **Daytrana™** *see* Methylphenidate *on page 1034*
- **DDAVP®** *see* Desmopressin *on page 459*
- **ddC** *see* Zalcitabine [DSC] *on page 1634*
- **ddI** *see* Didanosine *on page 491*
- **1-Deamino-8-D-Arginine Vasopressin** *see* Desmopressin *on page 459*
- **Debrox® [OTC]** *see* Carbamide Peroxide *on page 283*
- **Deca-Durabolin® (Can)** *see* Nandrolone *on page 1105*
- **Decavac™** *see* Diphtheria and Tetanus Toxoid *on page 514*
- **Declomycin®** *see* Demeclocycline *on page 453*
- **Deep Sea [OTC]** *see* Sodium Chloride *on page 1450*

Deferasirox (de FER a sir ox)

Medication Safety Issues

Sound-alike/look-alike issues:
Deferasirox may be confused with deferoxamine

U.S. Brand Names Exjade®

Canadian Brand Names Exjade®

Index Terms ICL670

Therapeutic Category Chelating Agent, Oral

Generic Available No

Use Treatment of chronic iron overload due to blood transfusions

Pregnancy Risk Factor B

Lactation Excretion in breast milk unknown/use caution

Contraindications Hypersensitivity to deferasirox or any component

Warnings Dose-related elevations in serum creatinine have been reported; monitor and consider dose reduction, interruption, or discontinuation. Rare cases of acute renal failure (some fatalities occurring in critically ill patients) have been reported in postmarketing surveillance. Hepatitis and elevated transaminases have been reported; monitor LFTs and consider dose modifications. Auditory or ocular disturbances have been reported; monitor and consider dose reduction or treatment interruption. Do not combine with other iron chelation therapies; safety of combinations has not been established. Safety and efficacy in children <2 years of age have not been established. Rare cases of peripheral cytopenias have been reported; monitor CBC.

Precautions Use caution with hepatic impairment; limited experience. May cause skin rash (dose-related); mild-to-moderate rashes may resolve without treatment interruption; for severe rash, interrupt and consider restarting at a lower dose with dose escalation and oral steroids. May cause intermittent proteinuria; closely monitor.

Adverse Reactions

Cardiovascular: Edema
Central nervous system: Fever, headache, fatigue, dizziness, anxiety, hyperactivity, insomnia, sleep disorder
Dermatologic: Rash (dose-related), urticaria, pigment disorder, purpura
Gastrointestinal: Abdominal pain, diarrhea, nausea, vomiting, cholelithiasis, gastritis, increased hepatic transaminases
Genitourinary: Glucosuria
Hematologic: Peripheral cytopenia (rare)
Hepatic: Elevated serum transaminases
(Continued)

Deferasirox *(Continued)*

Neuromuscular & skeletal: Arthralgia, back pain

Ocular: Cataract, IOP increase, lens opacities, maculopathy, retinal disorder, visual disturbance

Otic: Ear infection, hearing loss (including high frequency)

Renal: Elevated serum creatinine, proteinuria, acute renal failure (rare)

Respiratory: Cough, nasopharyngitis, pharyngolaryngeal pain, respiratory tract infection, bronchitis, pharyngitis, acute tonsillitis, rhinitis

Miscellaneous: Influenza

Drug Interactions Aluminum-containing antacids may decrease absorption of deferasirox.

Food Interactions Bioavailability increased variably when taken with food; administer on empty stomach

Stability Store at room temperature between 15°C and 30°C (59°F and 86°F). Protect from moisture.

Mechanism of Action Selectively binds iron with a high affinity in a 2:1 ratio, forming a complex which is excreted primarily through the feces.

Pharmacokinetics

Distribution: Adults: 14 L

Protein binding: 99% to serum albumin

Metabolism: Hepatic via glucuronidation by UGT1A1 and UGT1A3; minor oxidation by CYP450; undergoes enterohepatic recirculation

Bioavailability: 70%

Half-life: 8-16 hours

Time to peak serum concentration: 1.5-4 hours (median times)

Elimination: Feces (84%), urine (6% to 8%)

Clearance: Females have moderately lower clearance than males (17.5% lower)

Usual Dosage Oral: Children ≥2 years and Adults: Initiate therapy when patient has evidence of chronic iron overload (eg, transfusion of approximately 100 mL/kg of packed RBCs and serum ferritin consistently >1000mcg/L)

Initial: 20 mg/kg daily (calculate dose to nearest whole tablet)

Maintenance: Adjust dose every 3-6 months based on serum ferritin levels; increase by 5-10 mg/kg/day (calculate dose to nearest whole tablet); titrate. Maximum dose: 30 mg/kg/day; hold dose for serum ferritin <500 mcg/L.

Note: Consider dose reduction or interruption for hearing loss or visual disturbances.

Dosage adjustment in renal impairment: Consider dose reduction, interruption, or discontinuation with serum creatinine elevation.

Dosage adjustment in hepatic impairment: Consider dose adjustment or discontinuation for severe elevations in liver function tests.

Administration Oral: **Do not chew or swallow whole tablets.** Disperse tablets in water, orange juice, or apple juice (use 3.5 ounces for total doses <1 g; 7 ounces for doses >1 g); stir to form suspension and drink entire contents. Rinse remaining residue with more fluid; drink. Administer at same time each day on an empty stomach, 30 minutes before food. Do not administer simultaneously with aluminum-containing antacids.

Monitoring Parameters

Serum creatinine (manufacturer recommends two assessments prior to initiation of therapy, weekly in the first month after initiation or with adjustment of therapy and monthly thereafter), urine protein, CBC, liver function tests, and serum ferritin monthly; baseline and annual auditory and ophthalmic function (including slit lamp examinations and dilated fundoscopy)

Patient Information May cause dizziness and impair ability to perform activities requiring physical coordination; use caution with driving or operating machinery.

Additional Information Deferasirox has a low affinity for binding with zinc and copper; may cause variable decreases in the serum concentration of these trace minerals. Deferasirox available via EPASS™ (Exjade® Patient Assistance & Support Services) network; contact at 888-903-7277.

Dosage Forms Excipient information presented when available (limited, particularly for generics); consult specific product labeling.

Tablet, for oral suspension:

Exjade®: 125 mg, 250 mg, 500 mg

References

Galanello R, Piga A, Alberti D, et al, "Safety, Tolerability, and Pharmacokinetics of ICL670, a New Orally Active Iron-Chelating Agent in Patients With Transfusion-Dependent Iron Overload Due to Beta-Thalassemia," *J Clin Pharmacol*, 2003, 43(6):565-72.

Nisbet-Brown E, Oliveri NF, Giardina PJ, et al, "Effectiveness and Safety of ICL670 in Iron-Loaded Patients With Thalassaemia: A Randomised, Double-Blind, Placebo-Controlled, Dose-Escalation Trial," *Lancet*, 2003, 361(9369):1597-602.

Rund D and Rachmilewitz E, "Beta-Thalassemia," *N Engl J Med*, 2005, 353(11):1135-46.

Deferoxamine (de fer OKS a meen)

Medication Safety Issues

Sound-alike/look-alike issues:

Deferoxamine may be confused with cefuroxime, deferasirox

Desferal® may be confused with desflurane, Dexferrum®, Disophrol®

International issues:

Desferal® may be confused with Deseril® which is a brand name for methysergide in multiple international markets

Related Information

Commonly Used Antidotes for Acute Overdoses *on page 1920*

U.S. Brand Names Desferal®

Canadian Brand Names Desferal®; PMS-Deferoxamine

Index Terms Deferoxamine Mesylate; Desferrioxamine; NSC-644468

Therapeutic Category Antidote, Aluminum Toxicity; Antidote, Iron Toxicity; Chelating Agent, Parenteral

Generic Available Yes

Use Acute iron intoxication; chronic iron overload secondary to multiple transfusions; diagnostic test for iron overload; the diagnosis and treatment of aluminum accumulation in renal failure (unlabeled use)

Pregnancy Risk Factor C

Lactation Excretion in breast milk unknown/use caution

Contraindications Hypersensitivity to deferoxamine or any component; patients with severe renal disease, anuria, or primary hemochromatosis

Warnings Cataracts, decreased visual acuity, impaired peripheral and color vision, impaired night vision, and retinal pigmentary abnormalities have been reported after usage for prolonged periods at high dosages or in patients with low ferritin levels; periodic eye exams are recommended while on chronic therapy; neurotoxicity-related auditory abnormalities have been reported including high frequency sensorineural hearing loss; periodic auditory exams are recommended. ARDS has been reported following treatment of acute iron intoxication or thalassemia with high doses of deferoxamine; flushing of the skin, urticaria, hypotension, and shock have been reported after rapid I.V. administration. High doses (>60 mg/kg), especially in patients ≤3 years of age, with resulting low ferritin levels have been associated with growth retardation; a reduction in deferoxamine dosage may partially improve growth velocity; monitor growth in children receiving chronic therapy closely.

In patients with aluminum-related encephalopathy, deferoxamine may exacerbate neurologic dysfunction (seizures) possibly due to an acute increase in circulating aluminum and also may decrease serum calcium aggravating hyperparathyroidism. Deferoxamine may precipitate the onset of dialysis dementia. Avoid deferoxamine use in patients with serum aluminium levels >200 mcg/L. Fatal mucormycosis has been reported in chronic renal failure patients receiving deferoxamine for aluminium toxicity. Ferrioxamine (chelated form of iron with deferoxamine) enhances the growth and pathogenicity of certain species of *Mucor*.

Patients with severe chronic iron overload treated with deferoxamine and high dose vitamin C have been reported to develop impaired cardiac function which is reversed after discontinuation of vitamin C; vitamin C increases the availability of iron for chelation with deferoxamine. To decrease the risk of impaired cardiac function, the manufacturer recommends: Avoiding vitamin C in patients with pre-existing cardiac failure; start vitamin C supplementation only after the first month of deferoxamine therapy; use vitamin C only if the patient is regularly receiving deferoxamine; do not exceed vitamin C doses of 50 mg/day in children <10 years, 100 mg/day in older children, and 200 mg/day in adults; monitor cardiac function.

Precautions Use with caution in patients with pyelonephritis; may increase susceptibility to *Yersinia enterocolitica* infections

Adverse Reactions

Cardiovascular: Flushing, hypotension with rapid I.V. injection, tachycardia, shock, edema, impaired cardiac function (see Warnings)

Central nervous system: Fever, seizures, dialysis dementia, headache, dizziness

Dermatologic: Erythema, urticaria, pruritus, rash, cutaneous wheal formation

Endocrine & Metabolic: Growth impairment (dose related; see Warnings)

Gastrointestinal: Abdominal discomfort, diarrhea, nausea, vomiting

Genitourinary: Discoloration of urine (reddish color), dysuria

Hematologic: Thrombocytopenia (rare), leukopenia (rare)

Local: Pain, induration at injection site

Neuromuscular & skeletal: Leg cramps, metaphyseal dysplasia, arthralgia, myalgia, paresthesia

(Continued)

Deferoxamine *(Continued)*

Ocular: Blurred vision; decreased visual acuity, dichromatopsia, maculopathy; cataracts; impaired peripheral and night vision, scotoma, visual field defects, color and night blindness; retinal pigmentary abnormalities

Otic: High frequency sensorineural hearing loss, tinnitus

Respiratory: ARDS (see Warnings), asthma

Miscellaneous: Anaphylaxis, possible increased risk of infections particularly with *Y. enterocolitica*; rare cases of mucormycosis

Drug Interactions Vitamin C (see Warnings); prochlorperazine

Stability Protect from light; do not refrigerate reconstituted solutions as they will precipitate; reconstituted solutions are stable for 7 days at room temperature; due to a lack of preservatives, the manufacturer recommends immediate use after reconstitution

Mechanism of Action Complexes with trivalent ions (ferric ions) to form ferrioxamine, which is removed by the kidneys

Pharmacokinetics

Absorption: Oral: <15%

Metabolism: By plasma enzymes to ferrioxamine

Half-life:

Deferoxamine: 6.1 hours

Ferrioxamine: 5.8 hours

Elimination: Renal excretion of the metabolite iron chelate and unchanged drug

Dialysis: Dialyzable

Usual Dosage

Acute iron intoxication: **Note:** I.V. route is used when severe toxicity is evidenced by systemic symptoms (coma, shock, metabolic acidosis, or severe GI bleeding) or potentially severe intoxications (serum iron level >500 mcg/dL). When severe symptoms are not present, the I.M. route may be preferred (per manufacturer); however, the use of I.V. deferoxamine in situations where the serum iron concentration is <500 mcg/dL or when severe toxicity is not evident is a subject of some clinical debate.

Children:

I.M.: 50 mg/kg/dose every 6 hours; maximum dose: 6 g/day or as an alternative, 90 mg/kg/dose every 8 hours; not to exceed 1 g/dose or 6 g/day

I.V.: 15 mg/kg/hour; maximum dose: 6 g/day

Alternative dosing I.M. or I.V.: 20 mg/kg or 600 mg/m^2 (not to exceed 1000 mg) initially followed by 10 mg/kg or 300 mg/m^2 (not to exceed 500 mg) at 4-hour intervals for 2 doses; subsequent doses of 10 mg/kg or 300 mg/m^2 (not to exceed 500 mg) every 4-12 hours may be repeated depending upon the clinical response; maximum dose: 6 g/day

Chronic iron overload:

I.V.: 15 mg/kg/hour; maximum dose: 12 g/day

SubQ infusion via a portable, controlled infusion device: 20-50 mg/kg/day over 8-12 hours; maximum dose: 2 g/day

Adults:

Acute iron intoxication:

I.M.: 1 g stat, then 0.5 g every 4 hours for two doses, additional doses of 0.5 g every 4-12 hours up to 6 g/day may be needed depending upon the clinical response

I.V.: 15 mg/kg/hour; maximum dose: 6 g/day

Chronic iron overload:

I.M.: 0.5-1 g/day

I.V.: 15 mg/kg/hour; maximum dose: 12 g/day

Manufacturer's recommendations: 2 g per each unit of blood transfused; maximum dose: 6 g/day if transfused or 1 g/day without transfusion

SubQ infusion via a portable, controlled infusion device: 1-2 g/day over 8-24 hours

Aluminum-induced bone disease in chronic renal failure (serum aluminium 60-200 mcg/L; do not use if baseline serum aluminium >200 mcg/L; see Warnings): Children and Adults:

Test (diagnostic) dose: 5 mg/kg as a single dose infused over the last hour of dialysis. Measure serum aluminum 2 days later. Depending upon the change in serum aluminum, treatment with deferoxamine may be indicated (see National Kidney Foundation, 2003)

Treatment of aluminum toxicity in chronic renal failure: 5-10 mg/kg as a single dose. Repeat every 7-10 days with 3-4 dialysis procedures between doses. Monitor serum aluminum levels closely. See National Kidney Foundation reference for more detailed treatment algorithms.

Administration Parenteral: Add 2 mL SWI to 500 mg vial, resulting in a 210 mg/mL solution, or 8 mL SWI to each 2 g vial, resulting in a 213 mg/mL solution; for I.M. or

SubQ administration, no further dilution is required; for I.V. infusion, may reconstitute 500 mg vial with 5 mL SWI or 2 g vial with 20 mL, resulting in 95 mg/mL concentration, then further dilute in dextrose, NS, 0.45% sodium chloride, LR 10 mg/mL (maximum concentration: 250 mg/mL); maximum rate of infusion: 15 mg/kg/hour; the manufacturer recommends using a reduced rate of infusion (not to exceed 125 mg/hour) after the first 1000 mg has been infused; local reactions at the site of subcutaneous infusion may be minimized by diluting the deferoxamine in 5-10 mL SWI and adding 1 mg hydrocortisone to each mL of deferoxamine solution (Kirking, 1991)

Monitoring Parameters Serum ferritin, iron, total iron binding capacity; body weight, growth, ophthalmologic exam, and audiometry (with chronic use); blood pressure (with I.V. infusions); aluminum level (if applicable)

Reference Range Effective plasma concentration: 3-15 mcg/mL

Test Interactions Gallium-67 imaging results may be distorted due to rapid urinary excretion of deferoxamine-bound gallium-67; discontinue deferoxamine at least 48 hours prior to imaging

Patient Information May cause dizziness or impairment of vision or hearing; report any hearing loss, night blindness, decreased visual acuity, impaired peripheral vision, or loss of color vision; may cause the urine to turn a reddish color

Nursing Implications Local injection site reactions may be minimized by daily rotation of subcutaneous injection sites and by applying topical corticosteroids; painful lumps formed under the skin may indicate that the rate of SubQ administration exceeds the rate of absorption from the injection site or the needle is inserted too close to the dermis

Dosage Forms Excipient information presented when available (limited, particularly for generics); consult specific product labeling.

Injection, powder for reconstitution, as mesylate: 500 mg, 2 g

Desferal®: 500 mg, 2 g

References

Bentur Y, McGuigan M, and Koren G, "Deferoxamine (Desferrioxamine): New Toxicities for an Old Drug," *Drug Saf*, 1991, 6(1):37-46.

Cohen AR, Mizanin J, and Schwartz E, "Rapid Removal of Excessive Iron With Daily, High-Dose Intravenous Chelation Therapy," *J Pediatr*, 1989, 115(1):151-5.

Freedman MH, Olivieri N, Benson L, et al, "Clinical Studies on Iron Chelation in Patients With Thalassemia Major," *Haematologica*, 1990, 75(Suppl 5):74-83.

Giardina PJ, Grady RW, Ehlers KH, et al, "Current Therapy of Cooley's Anemia: A Decade of Experience With Subcutaneous Desferrioxamine," *Ann N Y Acad Sci*, 1990, 612:275-85.

Kirking MH, "Treatment of Chronic Iron Overload," *Clin Pharm*, 1991, 10(10):775-83.

National Kidney Foundation, "K/DOQI Clinical Practice Guidelines for Bone Metabolism and Disease in Chronic Kidney Failure," *Am J Kidney Dis*, 2003, 42(4 Supple3):1-201.

Pippard MJ, "Iron Metabolism and Iron Chelation in the Thalassemia Disorders," *Haematologica*, 1990, 75(Suppl 5):66-71.

- **Deferoxamine Mesylate** *see* Deferoxamine *on page 451*
- **Dehydral® (Can)** *see* Methenamine *on page 1021*
- **Dehydrobenzperidol** *see* Droperidol *on page 547*
- **Del Aqua®** *see* Benzoyl Peroxide *on page 207*
- **Delatestryl®** *see* Testosterone *on page 1511*
- **Delestrogen®** *see* Estradiol *on page 605*
- **Delsym® [OTC]** *see* Dextromethorphan *on page 477*
- **Delta-9-tetrahydro-cannabinol** *see* Dronabinol *on page 546*
- **Delta-9 THC** *see* Dronabinol *on page 546*
- **Deltacortisone** *see* PredniSONE *on page 1308*
- **Deltadehydrocortisone** *see* PredniSONE *on page 1308*
- **Deltahydrocortisone** *see* PrednisoLONE *on page 1304*
- **Demadex®** *see* Torsemide *on page 1556*

Demeclocycline (dem e kloe SYE kleen)

U.S. Brand Names Declomycin®

Canadian Brand Names Declomycin®

Index Terms Demeclocycline Hydrochloride; Demethylchlortetracycline

Therapeutic Category Antibiotic, Tetracycline Derivative

Generic Available Yes

Use Treatment of susceptible bacterial infections (acne, gonorrhea, pertussis, chronic bronchitis, and urinary tract infections) caused by both gram-negative and gram-positive organisms; treatment of chronic syndrome of inappropriate antidiuretic hormone (SIADH) secretion

Pregnancy Risk Factor D

Lactation Enters breast milk/not recommended (AAP rates tetracycline "compatible")

Contraindications Hypersensitivity to demeclocycline, tetracyclines, or any component; pregnancy

(Continued)

Demeclocycline *(Continued)*

Warnings Photosensitivity reactions, characterized as severe burns of exposed surfaces, occur frequently with this drug; avoid prolonged exposure to sunlight; do not use tanning equipment. Do not administer to children ≤8 years of age; use of tetracyclines during tooth development (last half of pregnancy, infancy, and children ≤8 years of age) may cause permanent discoloration of the teeth and enamel hypoplasia; do not administer to pregnant women; use of tetracyclines in pregnant women may result in retardation of bone growth and skeletal development of the fetus; prolonged use may result in superinfection. Avoid use when possible in patients with hepatic disease. Demeclocycline may cause a reversible, dose-related diabetes insipidus syndrome. Use of outdated tetracyclines has caused a Fanconi-like syndrome.

Precautions Use with caution in patients with impaired renal or hepatic function; modify dose in patients with renal impairment

Adverse Reactions

Central nervous system: Elevated intracranial pressure, bulging fontanels in infants, headache, dizziness, vertigo

Dermatologic: Rash, pruritus, photosensitivity, exfoliative dermatitis, erythema multiforme, urticaria, discoloration of nails, Stevens-Johnson syndrome

Endocrine & metabolic: Diabetes insipidus syndrome, hyperphosphatemia

Gastrointestinal: Nausea, vomiting, diarrhea, anorexia, pancreatitis, enterocolitis

Hematologic: Leukopenia, neutropenia, thrombocytopenia, hemolytic anemia, eosinophilia

Hepatic: Hepatotoxicity, elevated liver enzymes

Neuromuscular & skeletal: Paresthesia, weakness, polyarthralgia

Ocular: Blurred vision

Renal: Azotemia, acute renal failure, nephrogenic diabetes insipidus

Miscellaneous: Anaphylaxis, lupus-like syndrome, superinfections

Drug Interactions Antacids, aluminum, calcium, magnesium, zinc, bismuth salts, and iron preparations may decrease absorption of demeclocycline; decreased effect of oral contraceptives, penicillins; increased effect of warfarin; methoxyflurane (may cause fatal nephrotoxicity)

Food Interactions Food, milk, milk formulas, dairy products, and iron decrease absorption of demeclocycline

Mechanism of Action Inhibits protein synthesis by binding with the 30S ribosomal subunits and preventing the binding of transfer RNA to those ribosomes of susceptible bacteria; may also cause alterations in the cytoplasmic membrane

Pharmacodynamics Onset of action for diuresis in SIADH: Within 5 days

Pharmacokinetics

Absorption: ~60% to 80% of dose absorbed from the GI tract; food and dairy products reduce absorption by 50% or more

Distribution: Distributes into pleural fluid, bronchial secretions, sputum, prostatic and seminal fluids, and to body tissues; crosses into breast milk

Protein binding: 36% to 91%

Metabolism: Small amounts metabolized in the liver to inactive metabolites; enterohepatically recycled

Half-life: Adults: 10-17 hours (prolonged with reduced renal function)

Time to peak serum concentration: Oral: Within 3-4 hours

Elimination: Excreted as unchanged drug (42% to 50%) in urine and 31% in feces

Usual Dosage Oral:

Children >8 years: 8-12 mg/kg/day divided every 6-12 hours

Adults: 150 mg 4 times/day or 300 mg twice daily

Uncomplicated gonorrhea: 600 mg stat, 300 mg every 12 hours for 4 days (3 g total)

SIADH: Initial: 600-1200 mg/day or 13-15 mg/kg/day divided every 6-8 hours; then decrease to 600-900 mg/day

Dosing adjustment in renal impairment: Dose and/or frequency should be modified in response to the degree of renal impairment

Dosing adjustment in hepatic impairment: Not recommended for use

Administration Oral: Administer 1 hour before or 2 hours after food or milk with plenty of fluids; do not administer with food, milk, dairy products, antacids, zinc, or iron supplements

Monitoring Parameters CBC, renal and hepatic function tests, I & O, urine output, serum sodium

Test Interactions May interfere with tests for urinary glucose (false-negative urine glucose using Clinistix®, Tes-Tape®)

Patient Information May cause photosensitivity reactions (eg, exposure to sunlight may cause severe sunburn, skin rash, redness, or itching); avoid exposure to sunlight and artificial light sources (sunlamps, tanning booth/bed); wear protective clothing, wide-brimmed hats, sunglasses, and lip sunscreen (SPF ≥15); use a sunscreen [broad-spectrum sunscreen or physical sunscreen (preferred) or sunblock with SPF ≥15]; contact physician if reaction occurs. May cause dizziness, vertigo, lightheadedness, blurred vision and impair ability to perform activities requiring mental alertness or physical coordination; may discolor fingernails. Avoid taking dosages at bedtime to reduce risk of esophageal ulceration

Dosage Forms Excipient information presented when available (limited, particularly for generics); consult specific product labeling.

Tablet, as hydrochloride: 150 mg, 300 mg

References

Abdi EA and Bishop S, "The Syndrome of Inappropriate Antidiuretic Hormone Secretion With Carcinoma of the Tongue," *Med Pediatr Oncol*, 1988, 16(3):210-5.

Troyer AD, "Demeclocycline. Treatment for Syndrome of Inappropriate Antidiuretic Hormone Secretion," *JAMA*, 1977, 237(25):2723-6.

- ♦ **Demeclocycline Hydrochloride** *see* Demeclocycline *on page 453*
- ♦ **Demerol®** *see* Meperidine *on page 1002*
- ♦ **4-Demethoxydaunorubicin** *see* Idarubicin *on page 808*
- ♦ **Demethylchlortetracycline** *see* Demeclocycline *on page 453*
- ♦ **Denavir®** *see* Penciclovir *on page 1226*
- ♦ **Denorex® Original Therapeutic Strength [OTC]** *see* Coal Tar *on page 394*
- ♦ **Denta 5000 Plus** *see* Fluoride *on page 675*
- ♦ **DentaGel** *see* Fluoride *on page 675*
- ♦ **Dentapaine [OTC]** *see* Benzocaine *on page 204*
- ♦ **Dent's Ear Wax [OTC]** *see* Carbamide Peroxide *on page 283*
- ♦ **Dent's Extra Strength Toothache [OTC]** *see* Benzocaine *on page 204*
- ♦ **Dent's Maxi-Strength Toothache [OTC]** *see* Benzocaine *on page 204*
- ♦ **2'-Deoxy-3'-Thiacytidine** *see* Lamivudine *on page 901*
- ♦ **Depacon®** *see* Valproic Acid and Derivatives *on page 1592*
- ♦ **Depakene®** *see* Valproic Acid and Derivatives *on page 1592*
- ♦ **Depakote®** *see* Valproic Acid and Derivatives *on page 1592*
- ♦ **Depakote® ER** *see* Valproic Acid and Derivatives *on page 1592*
- ♦ **Depakote® Sprinkle** *see* Valproic Acid and Derivatives *on page 1592*
- ♦ **Depen®** *see* Penicillamine *on page 1227*
- ♦ **DepoDur™** *see* Morphine Sulfate *on page 1082*
- ♦ **Depo®-Estradiol** *see* Estradiol *on page 605*
- ♦ **Depo-Medrol®** *see* MethylPREDNISolone *on page 1039*
- ♦ **Depo-Prevera® (Can)** *see* MedroxyPROGESTERone *on page 991*
- ♦ **Depo-Provera®** *see* MedroxyPROGESTERone *on page 991*
- ♦ **Depo-Provera® Contraceptive** *see* MedroxyPROGESTERone *on page 991*
- ♦ **depo-subQ provera 104™** *see* MedroxyPROGESTERone *on page 991*
- ♦ **Depotest® 100 (Can)** *see* Testosterone *on page 1511*
- ♦ **Depo®-Testosterone** *see* Testosterone *on page 1511*
- ♦ **DermaFungal [OTC]** *see* Miconazole *on page 1056*
- ♦ **Dermagran® [OTC]** *see* Antacid Preparations *on page 132*
- ♦ **Dermagran® AF [OTC]** *see* Miconazole *on page 1056*
- ♦ **Dermamycin® [OTC]** *see* DiphenhydrAMINE *on page 509*
- ♦ **Dermarest Dricort® [OTC]** *see* Hydrocortisone *on page 781*
- ♦ **Derma-Smoothe/FS®** *see* Fluocinolone *on page 672*
- ♦ **Dermazole (Can)** *see* Miconazole *on page 1056*
- ♦ **Dermoplast® Antibacterial [OTC]** *see* Benzocaine *on page 204*
- ♦ **Dermoplast® Pain Relieving [OTC]** *see* Benzocaine *on page 204*
- ♦ **Dermovate® (Can)** *see* Clobetasol *on page 383*
- ♦ **Dermtex® HC [OTC]** *see* Hydrocortisone *on page 781*
- ♦ **Desferal®** *see* Deferoxamine *on page 451*
- ♦ **Desferrioxamine** *see* Deferoxamine *on page 451*

Desipramine (des IP ra meen)

Medication Safety Issues

Sound-alike/look-alike issues:

Desipramine may be confused with clomiPRAMINE, deserpidine, diphenhydrAMINE, disopyramide, imipramine, nortriptyline

Norpramin® may be confused with clomiPRAMINE, imipramine, Norpace®, nortriptyline, Tenormin®

International issues:

Norpramin®: Brand name for omeprazole in Spain

(Continued)

Desipramine *(Continued)*

Related Information

Antidepressant Agents *on page 1681*

Medications for Which A Single Dose May Be Fatal When Ingested By A Toddler *on page 1932*

Overdose and Toxicology *on page 1916*

U.S. Brand Names Norpramin®

Canadian Brand Names Alti-Desipramine; Apo-Desipramine®; Norpramin®; Nu-Desipramine; PMS-Desipramine

Index Terms Desipramine Hydrochloride; Desmethylimipramine Hydrochloride

Therapeutic Category Antidepressant, Tricyclic

Generic Available Yes

Use Treatment of various forms of depression, often in conjunction with psychotherapy; analgesic in chronic pain, peripheral neuropathies

Medication Guide An FDA-approved patient medication guide, which is available with the product information and at http://www.fda.gov/cder/Offices/ODS/medication_guides.htm, must be dispensed with this medication for each new outpatient prescription and refill.

Pregnancy Risk Factor C

Lactation Enters breast milk/not recommended (AAP rates "of concern")

Contraindications Hypersensitivity to desipramine (cross-sensitivity with other tricyclic antidepressants may occur) or any component; use of MAO inhibitors within 14 days (potentially fatal reactions may occur, see Drug Interactions); use in patients during the acute recovery phase following MI; narrow-angle glaucoma

Warnings Desipramine is not approved for use in pediatric patients. Clinical worsening of depression or suicidal ideation and behavior may occur in children and adults with major depressive disorder. In clinical trials, antidepressants increased the risk of suicidal thinking and behavior (suicidality) in children, adolescents, and young adults (18-24 years of age) with major depressive disorder and other psychiatric disorders. This risk must be considered before prescribing antidepressants for any clinical use. Short-term studies did **not** show an increased risk of suicidality with antidepressant use in patients >24 years of age and showed a decreased risk in patients ≥65 years.

Patients of all ages who are treated with antidepressants for any indication require appropriate monitoring and close observation for clinical worsening of depression, suicidality, and unusual changes in behavior, especially during the first few months after antidepressant initiation or when the dose is adjusted. Family members and caregivers should be instructed to closely observe the patient (ie, daily) and communicate condition with healthcare provider. Patients should also be monitored for associated behaviors (eg, anxiety, agitation, panic attacks, insomnia, irritability, hostility, aggressiveness, impulsivity, akathisia, hypomania, mania) which may increase the risk for worsening depression or suicidality. Worsening depression or emergence of suicidality (or associated behaviors listed above) that is abrupt in onset, severe, or not part of the presenting symptoms, may require discontinuation or modification of drug therapy.

Do not discontinue abruptly in patients receiving high doses chronically (withdrawal symptoms may occur). To reduce risk of intentional overdose, write prescriptions for the smallest quantity consistent with good patient care. Screen individuals for bipolar disorder prior to treatment (using antidepressants alone may induce manic episodes in patients with this condition). Hypertensive episodes have been reported during surgery in patients receiving desipramine (discontinue desipramine use as soon as possible prior to elective surgery).

Precautions Use with caution in patients with cardiovascular disease, conduction disturbances, urinary retention, glaucoma, seizure disorders, hyperthyroidism or those receiving thyroid replacement

Adverse Reactions Less sedation and anticholinergic adverse effects than amitriptyline or imipramine

Cardiovascular: Arrhythmias, hypotension, edema, flushing, heart block, palpitations, MI, stroke, hypertension, tachycardia; asymptomatic EKG changes and minor increases in diastolic blood pressure and heart rate have been noted in children receiving >3.5 mg/kg/day; **Note:** 4 cases of sudden death have been reported in children 5-14 years of age; an association between desipramine and sudden death was not shown to be significant in one retrospective study; further studies are needed

Central nervous system: Sedation, confusion, dizziness, drowsiness, fatigue, headache, ataxia, incoordination, anxiety, restlessness, nervousness, agitation, insomnia, nightmares, hallucinations, hypomania, exacerbation of psychosis, extrapyramidal symptoms, seizure, drug fever; suicidal thinking and behavior (see Warnings)

Dermatologic: Photosensitivity, skin rash, urticaria, itching, petechiae

Endocrine & metabolic: SIADH, weight gain or loss, breast enlargement, galactorrhea, hyperglycemia, hypoglycemia, sexual dysfunction
Gastrointestinal: Constipation, nausea, vomiting, xerostomia, anorexia, abdominal cramps, black tongue, decreased lower esophageal sphincter tone (may cause GE reflux), diarrhea, heartburn, paralytic ileus, stomatitis, unpleasant taste
Genitourinary: Urinary retention, discoloration of urine (blue-green)
Hematologic: Agranulocytosis, eosinophilia, purpura, thrombocytopenia
Hepatic: Cholestatic jaundice, hepatitis, elevated liver enzymes
Neuromuscular & skeletal: Tremor, numbness, tingling, paresthesias of extremities, peripheral neuropathy, weakness
Ocular: Blurred vision, elevated intraocular pressure, disturbances of accommodation, mydriasis
Otic: Tinnitus
Miscellaneous: Hypersensitivity reactions, diaphoresis; withdrawal symptoms following abrupt discontinuation (see Warnings)

Drug Interactions Cytochrome P450 isoenzyme CYP1A2 and CYP2D6 substrate; isoenzyme CYP2D6 inhibitor

May decrease effects of guanethidine and clonidine. May increase effects of CNS depressants, alcohol, adrenergic agents, anticholinergic agents. With MAO inhibitors, fever, tachycardia, hypertension, seizures, and death may occur. Barbiturates may decrease TCA serum concentrations. Cimetidine may decrease desipramine clearance and increase plasma concentration. The herbal medicine St John's wort (*Hypericum perforatum*) may increase serious side effects, its use is **not** recommended. Ritonavir increases desipramine concentration by 145% (dosage reduction of desipramine is recommended); concurrent use of high dose TCAs and ritonavir may cause the serotonin syndrome. Use with other CYP2D6 inhibitors (eg, fluoxetine, quinidine) may significantly increase serum concentrations of desipramine. SSRIs may increase serotonergic effects. Interactions similar to other TCAs may occur.

Food Interactions May increase riboflavin dietary requirements

Mechanism of Action Increases the synaptic concentration of serotonin and/or norepinephrine in the CNS by inhibition of their reuptake by the presynaptic neuronal membrane

Pharmacodynamics Antidepressant effects:
Onset of action: Occasionally seen in 2-5 days
Maximum effect: After more than 2 weeks

Pharmacokinetics
Absorption: Rapidly and well absorbed from the GI tract
Distribution: V_d: Adults: 21 L/kg; distributes into breast milk (concentrations approximately equal to maternal plasma)
Protein binding: 90%
Metabolism: In the liver
Half-life, adults: 12-57 hours
Elimination: 70% in urine

Usual Dosage Oral: Depression: **Note:** Not FDA approved for use in pediatric patients; controlled clinical trials have not shown tricyclic antidepressants to be superior to placebo for the treatment of depression in children and adolescents (see Dopheide, 2006 and Wagner, 2005).
Children 6-12 years: 1-3 mg/kg/day in divided doses; monitor carefully with doses >3 mg/kg/day; maximum dose: 5 mg/kg/day
Adolescents: Initial: 25-50 mg/day; gradually increase to 100 mg/day in single or divided doses; maximum dose: 150 mg/day
Adults: Initial: 75 mg/day in divided doses; increase gradually to 150-200 mg/day in divided or single dose; maximum dose: 300 mg/day

Administration Oral: Administer with food to decrease GI upset

Monitoring Parameters Blood pressure, heart rate, EKG, mental status, weight. Monitor patient periodically for symptom resolution; monitor for worsening of depression, suicidality, and associated behaviors (especially at the beginning of therapy or when doses are increased or decreased; see Warnings)
Long-term use: Also monitor CBC with differential, liver enzymes, serum concentrations

Reference Range Plasma levels do not always correlate with clinical effectiveness.
Timing of serum samples: Draw trough just before next dose
Therapeutic: 50-300 ng/mL (SI: 188-1125 nmol/L)
Possible toxicity: >300 ng/mL (SI: >1070 nmol/L)
Toxic: >1000 ng/mL (SI: >3750 nmol/L)

Patient Information Read the patient Medication Guide that you receive with each prescription and refill of desipramine. An increased risk of suicidal thinking and behavior has been reported with the use of antidepressants in children, adolescents,
(Continued)

Desipramine *(Continued)*

and young adults (18-24 years of age). Notify physician if you feel more depressed, have thoughts of suicide, or become more agitated or irritable (see Warnings). May cause drowsiness and impair ability to perform activities requiring mental alertness or physical coordination; may cause dry mouth; avoid alcohol and the herbal medicine St John's wort; limit caffeine; may discolor urine to blue-green color; do not discontinue medication abruptly; may increase appetite. May cause photosensitivity reactions (eg, exposure to sunlight may cause severe sunburn, skin rash, redness, or itching); avoid exposure to sunlight and artificial light sources (sunlamps, tanning booth/bed); wear protective clothing, wide-brimmed hats, sunglasses, and lip sunscreen (SPF ≥15); use a sunscreen [broad-spectrum sunscreen or physical sunscreen (preferred) or sunblock with SPF ≥15]; contact physician if reaction occurs.

Dosage Forms Excipient information presented when available (limited, particularly for generics); consult specific product labeling.

Tablet, as hydrochloride: 10 mg, 25 mg, 50 mg, 75 mg, 100 mg, 150 mg

References

Biederman J, Thisted RA, Greenhill LL, et al, "Estimation of the Association Between Desipramine and the Risk for Sudden Death in 5-14 Year-Old Children," *J Clin Psychiatry*, 1995, 56(3):87-93.

Dopheide JA, "Recognizing and Treating Depression in Children and Adolescents," *Am J Health Syst Pharm*, 2006, 63(3):233-43.

Levy HB, Harper CR, and Weinberg WA, "A Practical Approach to Children Failing in School," *Pediatr Clin North Am*, 1992, 39(4):895-928.

Wagner KD, "Pharmacotherapy for Major Depression in Children and Adolescents," *Prog Neuropsychopharmacol Biol Psychiatry*, 2005, 29(5):819-26.

♦ **Desipramine Hydrochloride** *see* Desipramine *on page 455*

♦ **Desitin® [OTC]** *see* Zinc Oxide *on page 1640*

♦ **Desitin® Creamy [OTC]** *see* Zinc Oxide *on page 1640*

Desloratadine (des lor AT a deen)

U.S. Brand Names Clarinex®

Canadian Brand Names Aerius®

Therapeutic Category Antihistamine

Generic Available No

Use Symptomatic relief of nasal and non-nasal symptoms of allergic rhinitis; chronic idiopathic urticaria

Pregnancy Risk Factor C

Lactation Enters breast milk/not recommended

Contraindications Hypersensitivity to desloratadine, loratadine, or any component

Warnings Use with caution and adjust dosage in patients with liver or renal impairment. Syrup contains sodium benzoate; benzoic acid (benzoate) is a metabolite of benzyl alcohol; large amounts of benzyl alcohol (≥99 mg/kg/day) have been associated with a potentially fatal toxicity ("gasping syndrome") in neonates; the "gasping syndrome" consists of metabolic acidosis, respiratory distress, gasping respirations, CNS dysfunction (including convulsions, intracranial hemorrhage), hypotension and cardiovascular collapse; avoid use in neonates; *in vitro* and animal studies have shown that benzoate displaces bilirubin from protein binding sites

Precautions A subset of the general population (7% in clinical trials) are slow metabolizers of desloratadine; the frequency of slow metabolism appears to be higher in African Americans; patients who are slow metabolizers may be more susceptible to dose-related side effects; use with caution in "slow metabolizers." Use cautiously in patients who are also taking ketoconazole, itraconazole, fluconazole, erythromycin, clarithromycin, or other drugs which may impair desloratadine's hepatic metabolism; although increased plasma levels of desloratadine have been observed, no adverse effects with concomitant administration have been reported, including QT interval prolongation which has occurred when similar antihistamines, terfenadine and astemizole, were combined with these agents. While less sedating than other antihistamines, desloratadine may cause drowsiness and impair ability to perform hazardous activities requiring mental alertness. Use cautiously in breast-feeding women as desloratadine passes into breast milk. RediTabs® contain aspartame which is metabolized to phenylalanine and must be used with caution in patients with phenylketonuria.

Adverse Reactions

Cardiovascular: Tachycardia, edema

Central nervous system: Somnolence, fatigue, dizziness

Dermatologic: Pruritus, urticaria

Gastrointestinal: Xerostomia, nausea, dry throat

Hepatic: Elevated liver enzymes, elevated bilirubin

Neuromuscular & skeletal: Myalgia

Respiratory: Pharyngitis, dyspnea

Miscellaneous: Hypersensitivity reactions, flu-like symptoms

Drug Interactions Increased plasma concentrations and AUC of desloratadine and its active metabolite with ketoconazole and erythromycin; no change in QT_c interval or cardiac arrhythmias have been seen (see Warnings); additive CNS depression with other CNS depressants and alcohol

Food Interactions Administration with food has no effect on desloratadine's bioavailability

Stability Store at room temperature; avoid excessive heat and moisture; RediTabs® must be used immediately after removal from blister pack

Mechanism of Action Long-acting tricyclic antihistamine with selective peripheral histamine H_1-receptor antagonistic properties; active metabolite of loratadine

Pharmacodynamics

Onset of action: 1 hour

Duration: 24 hours

Pharmacokinetics

Distribution: Distributes into breast milk

Protein binding: 82% to 87% (desloratadine), 85% to 89% (metabolite)

Metabolism: Metabolized to an active metabolite (3-hydroxydesloratadine); subset of population are slow metabolizers of desloratadine (7% of patients in clinical trials were slow-metabolizers; see Precautions)

Half-life: 27 hours (both desloratadine and active metabolite)

Time to peak serum concentration: 3 hours

Elimination: 87% eliminated via urine and feces as metabolic products

Usual Dosage Oral:

Children 6-11 months: 1 mg once daily

Children 1-5 years: 1.25 mg once daily

Children 6-11 years: 2.5 mg once daily

Children ≥12 years and Adults: 5 mg once daily

Dosage adjustment in renal/hepatic impairment: Administer dosage every other day

Administration Oral: May administer without regard to food. Place RediTabs® directly on the tongue; tablet will disintegrate immediately; may be taken with or without water

Monitoring Parameters Improvement in signs and symptoms of allergic rhinitis

Reference Range Therapeutic serum levels (not used clinically): Desloratadine: 2.5-4 ng/mL

Test Interactions Antigen skin testing

Patient Information Drink plenty of water; may cause dry mouth; may cause drowsiness and impair ability to perform activities requiring mental alertness or physical coordination; avoid alcohol

Dosage Forms Excipient information presented when available (limited, particularly for generics); consult specific product labeling.

Syrup (Clarinex®): 0.5 mg/mL (120 mL, 480 mL) [bubble gum flavor]

Tablet (Clarinex®): 5 mg

Tablet, orally disintegrating (Clarinex® RediTabs®): 2.5 mg [contains phenylalanine 1.28 mg/tablet; tutti-frutti flavor]; 5 mg [contains phenylalanine 2.55 mg/tablet; tutti-frutti flavor]

References

Murdoch D, Goa KL, and Keam SJ, "Desloratadine: An Update of Its Efficacy in the Management of Allergic Disorders," *Drugs*, 2003, 63(19):2051-77.

◆ **Desmethylimipramine Hydrochloride** *see* Desipramine *on page 455*

Desmopressin (des moe PRES in)

U.S. Brand Names DDAVP®; Stimate™

Canadian Brand Names Apo-Desmopressin®; DDAVP®; Minirin®; Nove-Desmopressin®; Octostim®

Index Terms 1-Deamino-8-D-Arginine Vasopressin; Desmopressin Acetate

Therapeutic Category Antihemophilic Agent; Hemostatic Agent; Vasopressin Analog, Synthetic

Generic Available Yes

Use Treatment of diabetes insipidus, control of bleeding in hemophilia A (with factor VIII levels >5%), mild to moderate type I von Willebrand disease, and thrombocytopenia; primary nocturnal enuresis

Pregnancy Risk Factor B

Lactation Excretion in breast milk unknown/use caution

Contraindications Hypersensitivity to desmopressin or any component; avoid using in patients with severe type I, type IIB or platelet-type (pseudo) von Willebrand disease, hemophilia A with factor VIII levels ≤5% or hemophilia B; moderate-to-severe renal impairment (Cl_{cr} <50 mL/minute)

(Continued)

Desmopressin *(Continued)*

Warnings Avoid intranasal use in patients with nasal mucosa changes (scarring, edema, discharge, obstruction, or severe atopic rhinitis)

Precautions Use with caution in patients with predisposition to thrombus formation, conditions associated with fluid and electrolyte imbalance (eg, cystic fibrosis), and in patients with coronary artery disease and/or hypertensive cardiovascular disease; fluid intake may need to be reduced to decrease potential for development of water intoxication

Adverse Reactions

Cardiovascular: Facial flushing, elevated blood pressure, chest pain, palpitations, tachycardia

Central nervous system: Headache, somnolence, dizziness, insomnia, agitation

Endocrine & metabolic: Hyponatremia, water intoxication

Gastrointestinal: Nausea, abdominal cramps, dyspepsia, vomiting

Genitourinary: Vulval pain, balanitis

Local: Pain at the injection site

Ocular: Itchy or light-sensitive eyes

Respiratory: Rhinitis, upper respiratory infections, epistaxis, nasal congestion

Drug Interactions Decreased antidiuretic response with lithium, large doses of epinephrine, demeclocycline, and heparin; increased antidiuretic response with carbamazepine, chlorpropamide, fludrocortisone, and clofibrate

Stability Refrigerate injection, nasal solution and Stimate® nasal spray; nasal solution and Stimate® nasal spray are stable for 3 weeks when stored at room temperature if unopened; injection is stable for 2 weeks at room temperature; DDAVP® nasal spray is stable at room temperature

Mechanism of Action Enhances reabsorption of water in the kidneys by increasing cellular permeability of the collecting ducts; possibly causes smooth muscle constriction with resultant vasoconstriction; dose-dependent increase in plasma factor VIII and plasminogen activator

Pharmacodynamics

Oral administration:
- Onset of ADH action: 1 hour
- Maximum effect: 2-7 hours
- Duration: 6-8 hours

Intranasal administration:
- Onset of ADH action: Within 1 hour
- Maximum effect: Within 1.5 hours
- Duration: 5-21 hours

I.V. infusion:
- Onset of increased factor VIII activity: Within 15-30 minutes
- Maximum effect: 90 minutes to 3 hours

Pharmacokinetics

Absorption:
- Oral tablets: 5% to 15%
- Nasal solution: 10% to 20%
- Nasal spray (1.5 mg/mL concentration): 3.3% to 4.1%

Metabolism: Unknown

Half-life:
- Oral: 1.5-2.5 hours
- I.V.:
  - Initial: 7.8 minutes
  - Terminal: 75.5 minutes (range: 0.4-4 hours); severe renal impairment: 9 hours
- Intranasal: 3.3-3.5 hours

Time to peak serum concentration:
- Oral: 0.9 hours
- Intranasal: 1.5 hours

Excretion: Primarily in urine

Usual Dosage

Diabetes insipidus:

Oral:
- Children ≤12 years: Initial: 0.05 mg 2 times daily; titrate to desired response (range: 0.1-0.8 mg daily)
- Children >12 years and Adults: 0.05 mg 2 times daily; titrate to desired response (range: 0.1-1.2 mg divided 2-3 times/day)

Intranasal: **Note:** Use nasal solution in patients whose dosage needs are <10 mcg or are not met with 10 mcg per spray increments in spray formulation
- Children 3 months to ≤12 years: Initial: 5 mcg/day (0.05 mL/day nasal solution) divided 1-2 times/day; range: 5-30 mcg/day (0.05-0.3 mL/day nasal solution); adjust morning and evening doses separately for an adequate diurnal rhythm of water turnover

Children >12 years and Adults: Initial: 5-40 mcg (0.05-0.4 mL nasal solution) divided 1-3 times/day; adjust morning and evening doses separately for an adequate diurnal rhythm of water turnover.

I.V., SubQ: Children >12 years and Adults: 2-4 mcg/day in 2 divided doses or $^1/_{10}$ of the maintenance intranasal dose

Hemophilia:

I.V.: Children ≥3 months and Adults: 0.3 mcg/kg beginning 30 minutes before procedure; may repeat dose if needed

Intranasal: Children >12 years and Adults: Using high concentration Stimate® nasal spray:

≤50 kg: 150 mcg (1 spray)

>50 kg: 300 mcg (1 spray each nostril)

Repeat use is determined by the patient's clinical condition and laboratory work; if using preoperatively, administer 2 hours before surgery

Nocturnal enuresis (short-term treatment, 4-8 weeks):

Intranasal: Children ≥6 years: (Using 100 mcg/mL nasal solution or nasal spray): Initial: 20 mcg (0.2 mL) at bedtime; range: 10-40 mcg; for doses >10 mcg, it is recommended that $^1/_2$ of the dose be given in each nostril; use nasal solution in patients whose dosage needs are <10 mcg or are not met with 10 mcg increments in spray formulation

Oral: Children ≥6 years: 0.2-0.6 mg once before bedtime

Administration

Intranasal: Using rhinal tube delivery system, draw solution into flexible, calibrated rhinal tube; insert one end into nostril; blow on the other end to deposit the solution deep into the nasal cavity. The Stimate® spray pump must be primed prior to first use; to prime pump, press down 4 times. Avoid spray use in children <6 years of age due to difficulty in titrating dosage; discard any solution remaining after 25 or 50 doses (2.5 or 5 mL vials, respectively) because the amount delivered may be substantially less than prescribed

Parenteral: I.V.: Dilute to a maximum concentration of 0.5 mcg/mL in NS and infuse over 15-30 minutes; if desmopressin I.V. is given preoperatively, administer 30 minutes prior to surgery

Monitoring Parameters I.V. infusion: Blood pressure and pulse should be monitored

Diabetes insipidus: Fluid intake, urine volume, specific gravity, plasma and urine osmolality, serum electrolytes

Hemophilia: Factor VIII antigen levels, APTT, Factor VIII activity level

Patient Information Avoid overhydration; blow nose before using nasal solution or spray; notify physician if headache, shortness of breath, heartburn, nausea, abdominal cramps, or vulval pain occur

Dosage Forms Excipient information presented when available (limited, particularly for generics); consult specific product labeling.

Injection, solution, as acetate (DDAVP®): 4 mcg/mL (1 mL, 10 mL)

Solution, intranasal, as acetate (DDAVP®): 100 mcg/mL (2.5 mL) [with rhinal tube]

Solution, intranasal, as acetate [spray]: 100 mcg/mL (5 mL) [delivers 10 mcg/spray]

DDAVP®: 100 mcg/mL (5 mL) [delivers 10 mcg/spray]

Stimate™: 1.5 mg/mL (2.5 mL) [delivers 150 mcg/spray]

Tablet, as acetate (DDAVP®): 0.1 mg, 0.2 mg

References

Stenberg A and Läckgren G, "Desmopressin Tablets in the Treatment of Severe Nocturnal Enuresis in Adolescents," *Pediatrics*, 1994, 94(6 Pt 1):841-46.

♦ **Desmopressin Acetate** *see* Desmopressin *on page 459*
♦ **Desoxyphenobarbital** *see* Primidone *on page 1312*
♦ **Desquam-X®** *see* Benzoyl Peroxide *on page 207*
♦ **Desquam-E™** *see* Benzoyl Peroxide *on page 207*
♦ **Desyrel® [DSC]** *see* Trazodone *on page 1564*
♦ **Desyrel® (Can)** *see* Trazodone *on page 1564*
♦ **Detane® [OTC]** *see* Benzocaine *on page 204*
♦ **Detemir Insulin** *see* Insulin Detemir *on page 839*

Dexamethasone (deks a METH a sone)

Medication Safety Issues

Sound-alike/look-alike issues:

Dexamethasone may be confused with desoximetasone

Decadron® may be confused with Percodan®

Maxidex® may be confused with Maxzide®

Related Information

Corticosteroids, Systemic *on page 1685*

(Continued)

Dexamethasone *(Continued)*

U.S. Brand Names Dexamethasone Intensol™; DexPak® TaperPak®; Maxidex®

Canadian Brand Names Apo-Dexamethasone®; Dexasone®; Diodex®; Maxidex®; PMS-Dexamethasone

Index Terms Dexamethasone Sodium Phosphate

Therapeutic Category Adrenal Corticosteroid; Anti-inflammatory Agent; Anti-inflammatory Agent, Ophthalmic; Antiemetic; Corticosteroid, Ophthalmic; Corticosteroid, Systemic; Glucocorticoid

Generic Available Yes: Excludes ophthalmic suspension

Use Treatment of chronic inflammation, allergic, hematologic, dermatologic, neoplastic, rheumatic, and autoimmune diseases; may be used in management of cerebral edema, septic shock, and as a diagnostic agent; adjunctive antiemetic agent in the treatment of chemotherapy-induced emesis; treatment of airway edema prior to extubation; used in neonates with bronchopulmonary dysplasia to facilitate ventilator weaning

Pregnancy Risk Factor C

Lactation Enters breast milk/use caution

Contraindications Hypersensitivity to dexamethasone or any component (see Warnings); active untreated infections; systemic fungal infections; cerebral malaria; viral, fungal, or tuberculous diseases of the eye

Warnings Hypothalamic-pituitary-adrenal (HPA) suppression may occur; acute adrenal insufficiency (adrenal crisis) may occur with abrupt withdrawal after long term therapy or with stress; withdrawal and discontinuation of corticosteroids should be done carefully; patients with HPA axis suppression may require doses of systemic glucocorticosteroids prior to, during, and after unusual stress (eg, surgery). Immunosuppression may occur; patients may be more susceptible to infections; avoid exposure to chickenpox and measles. Corticosteroids may activate latent opportunistic infections or exacerbate systemic fungal infections. May cause osteoporosis (at any age) or inhibition of bone growth in pediatric patients. Acute myopathy may occur with high doses, elevated IOP may occur (especially with prolonged use), CNS effects (ranging from euphoria to psychosis) may occur. Rare cases of anaphylactoid reactions have been reported with corticosteroids.

Injection may contain sulfites and 0.5 mg tablet may contain tartrazine, either may cause allergic reactions in susceptible individuals. Elixir contains benzoic acid; benzoic acid (benzoate) is a metabolite of benzyl alcohol; large amounts of benzyl alcohol (≥99 mg/kg/day) have been associated with a potentially fatal toxicity ("gasping syndrome") in neonates; the "gasping syndrome" consists of metabolic acidosis, respiratory distress, gasping respirations, CNS dysfunction (including convulsions, intracranial hemorrhage), hypotension and cardiovascular collapse; use dexamethasone products containing benzoic acid with caution in neonates; *in vitro* and animal studies have shown that benzoate displaces bilirubin from protein binding sites

Precautions Avoid using higher than recommended doses; suppression of HPA function, suppression of linear growth (ie, reduction of growth velocity), reduced bone mineral density, hypercorticism (Cushing's syndrome), hyperglycemia, or glucosuria may occur; titrate to lowest effective dose. Reduction in growth velocity may occur when corticosteroids are administered to pediatric patients by any route (monitor growth). Use with extreme caution in patients with respiratory tuberculosis, untreated systemic infections, or ocular herpes simplex; use with caution in patients with thyroid dysfunction, cirrhosis, ulcerative colitis, hypertension, renal impairment, osteoporosis, thromboembolic tendencies, CHF, recent MI, convulsive disorders, myasthenia gravis, thrombophlebitis, peptic ulcer, diabetes; prolonged use may result in cataracts or glaucoma

Adverse Reactions

Cardiovascular: Edema, hypertension

Central nervous system: Headache, vertigo, seizures, euphoria, psychosis, pseudotumor cerebri, insomnia, nervousness

Dermatologic: Acne, skin atrophy

Endocrine & metabolic: HPA suppression, growth suppression, glucose intolerance, hypokalemia, alkalosis, Cushing's syndrome

Gastrointestinal: Peptic ulcer, nausea, vomiting

Neuromuscular & skeletal: Muscle weakness, osteoporosis, decreased bone mineral density, fractures

Ocular: Cataracts, increased IOP, glaucoma

Miscellaneous: Immunosuppression, anaphylactoid reactions (rare)

Drug Interactions Cytochrome P450 isoenzyme CYP3A3/4 substrate; isoenzyme CYP3A3/4 inducer; isoenzyme CYP3A3/4 inhibitor

Barbiturates, phenytoin, rifampin, ritonavir, macrolide antibiotics, ketoconazole, saquinavir, salicylates, NSAIDs, toxoids; alcohol and caffeine may increase adverse GI effects; live virus vaccines (increase risk of viral infection); vaccines may have decreased effects

Food Interactions Systemic use of corticosteroids may require a diet with increased potassium, vitamins A, B_6, C, D, folate, calcium, zinc, and phosphorus and decreased sodium

Stability Dilution of dexamethasone sodium phosphate injection with D_5W or NS is stable for at least 24 hours

Mechanism of Action Decreases inflammation by suppression of migration of polymorphonuclear leukocytes and reversal of increased capillary permeability; suppresses normal immune response

Pharmacodynamics Duration: Metabolic effects can last for 72 hours

Pharmacokinetics

Metabolism: In the liver

Half-life: Terminal:

- Extremely low birth weight infants with BPD: 9.3 hours
- Children 3 months to 16 years: 4.3 hours
- Healthy adults: 3 hours

Time to peak serum concentration:

- Oral: Within 1-2 hours
- I.M.: Within 8 hours

Elimination: In urine and bile

Usual Dosage

Neonates:

- Airway edema or extubation: I.V.: Usual: 0.25 mg/kg/dose given ~4 hours prior to scheduled extubation and then every 8 hours for 3 doses total; range: 0.25-1 mg/kg/dose for 1-3 doses; maximum dose: 1 mg/kg/day. **Note:** A longer duration of therapy may be needed with more severe cases.
- Bronchopulmonary dysplasia (to facilitate ventilator weaning): Oral, I.V.: Numerous dosing schedules have been proposed; range: 0.5-0.6 mg/kg/day given in divided doses every 12 hours for 3-7 days, then taper over 1-6 weeks

Children:

- Airway edema or extubation: Oral, I.M., I.V.: 0.5-2 mg/kg/day in divided doses every 6 hours; begin 24 hours prior to extubation and continue for 4-6 doses after extubation
- Antiemetic (chemotherapy induced): I.V.: Initial: 10 mg/m²/dose (maximum dose: 20 mg) then 5 mg/m²/dose every 6 hours
- Anti-inflammatory: Oral, I.M., I.V.: 0.08-0.3 mg/kg/day or 2.5-10 mg/m²/day in divided doses every 6-12 hours
- Bacterial meningitis: Infants and Children >2 months: I.V.: 0.6 mg/kg/day divided every 6 hours for the first 4 days of antibiotic treatment; start dexamethasone at the time of the first dose of antibiotic
- Cerebral edema: Oral, I.M., I.V.: Loading dose: 1-2 mg/kg/dose as a single dose; maintenance: 1-1.5 mg/kg/day (maximum dose: 16 mg/day) in divided doses every 4-6 hours
- Physiologic replacement: Oral, I.M., I.V.: 0.03-0.15 mg/kg/day or 0.6-0.75 mg/m²/day in divided doses every 6-12 hours

Children and Adults: Ophthalmic:

- Suspension: Instill 2 drops every hour during the day and every other hour during the night; gradually reduce dose to every 3-4 hours, then to 3-4 times/day

Adults:

- Acute nonlymphoblastic leukemia (ANLL) protocol: I.V.: 2 mg/m²/dose every 8 hours for 12 doses
- Anti-inflammatory: Oral, I.M., I.V.: 0.75-9 mg/day in divided doses every 6-12 hours
- Cerebral edema: I.V.: Initial: 10 mg then 4 mg I.M./I.V. every 6 hours
- Diagnosis for Cushing's syndrome: Oral: 1 mg at 11 PM, draw blood at 8 AM

Administration

Ophthalmic: Avoid contact of container tip with skin or eye; remove soft contact lenses prior to using solutions containing benzalkonium chloride

- Solution and suspension: Apply finger pressure to lacrimal sac during and for 1-2 minutes after instillation to decrease risk of absorption and systemic effects

Oral: May administer with food or milk to decrease GI adverse effects

Parenteral: I.V.: Administer undiluted solution (4 mg/mL) I.V. push over 1-4 minutes if dose is <10 mg; high-dose therapy must be diluted in D_5W or NS and administered by I.V. intermittent infusion over 15-30 minutes

Monitoring Parameters Hemoglobin, occult blood loss, blood pressure, serum potassium and glucose; IOP with systemic use >6 weeks; weight and height in children

Reference Range Dexamethasone suppression test: 8 AM cortisol <6 mcg/100 mL in adults given dexamethasone 1 mg at 11 PM the previous night

Test Interactions Skin tests

(Continued)

Dexamethasone *(Continued)*

Patient Information Avoid alcohol; limit caffeine; do not decrease dose or discontinue drug without physician's approval; avoid exposure to measles or chicken pox; advise physician immediately if exposed; notify physician if acute illness including fever or other signs of infection occurs. Inform physician you are taking corticosteroid prior to any surgery or with any injury

Additional Information Due to long duration of effect, not suitable for every other day dosing

Dosage Forms Excipient information presented when available (limited, particularly for generics); consult specific product labeling. [DSC] = Discontinued product

Elixir, as base: 0.5 mg/5 mL (240 mL)

Injection, solution, as sodium phosphate: 4 mg/mL (1 mL, 5 mL, 30 mL); 10 mg/mL (10 mL)

Injection, solution, as sodium phosphate [preservative free]: 10 mg/mL (1 mL)

Solution, ophthalmic, as sodium phosphate: 0.1% (5 mL)

Solution, oral: 0.5 mg/5 mL (500 mL)

Solution, oral concentrate:

Dexamethasone Intensol™: 1 mg/mL (30 mL) [contains alcohol 30%]

Suspension, ophthalmic:

Maxidex®: 0.1% (5 mL; 15 mL [DSC]) [contains benzalkonium chloride]

Tablet [scored]: 0.5 mg, 0.75 mg, 1 mg, 1.5 mg, 2 mg, 4 mg, 6 mg

DexPak® TaperPak®: 1.5 mg [51 tablets on taper dose card]

References

American Academy of Pediatrics Committee on Infectious Diseases, "Dexamethasone Therapy for Bacterial Meningitis in Infants and Children," *Pediatrics*, 1990, 86(1):130-3.

Bahal N and Nahata MC, "The Role of Corticosteroids in Infants and Children With Bacterial Meningitis," *DICP*, 1991, 25(5):542-5.

Couser RJ, Ferrara TB, Falde B, et al, "Effectiveness of Dexamethasone in Preventing Extubation Failure in Preterm Infants at Increased Risk for Airway Edema," *J Pediatr*, 1992, 121(4):591-6.

Durand M, Sardesai S, and McEvoy C, "Effects of Early Dexamethasone Therapy on Pulmonary Mechanics and Chronic Lung Disease in Very Low Birth Weight Infants: A Randomized, Controlled Trial," *Pediatrics*, 1995, 95(4):584-90.

Ng PC, "The Effectiveness and Side Effects of Dexamethasone in Preterm Infants With Bronchopulmonary Dysplasia," *Arch Dis Child*, 1993, 68(3 Spec No):330-6.

♦ **Dexamethasone and Ciprofloxacin** *see* Ciprofloxacin and Dexamethasone *on page 361*

♦ **Dexamethasone Intensol™** *see* Dexamethasone *on page 461*

Dexamethasone, Neomycin, and Polymyxin B

(deks a METH a sone, nee oh MYE sin, & pol i MIKS in bee)

Medication Safety Issues

Sound-alike/look-alike issues:

AK-Trol® may be confused with AKTob®

U.S. Brand Names AK-Trol® [DSC]; Maxitrol®; Poly-Dex™

Canadian Brand Names Dioptrol®; Maxitrol®

Index Terms Dexamethasone, Neomycin, and Polymyxin B; Polymyxin B, Neomycin, and Dexamethasone

Therapeutic Category Antibiotic, Ophthalmic; Corticosteroid, Ophthalmic

Generic Available Yes

Use Steroid-responsive inflammatory ocular conditions in which a corticosteroid is indicated and where bacterial infection or a risk of bacterial infection exists

Pregnancy Risk Factor C

Lactation Excretion in breast milk unknown/use caution

Contraindications Hypersensitivity to dexamethasone, polymyxin, neomycin, or any component; viral diseases of the cornea and conjunctiva; mycobacterial infection of the eye; fungal disease of ocular structures; dendritic keratitis; use after uncomplicated removal of a corneal foreign body

Warnings Prolonged use may result in glaucoma, defects in visual acuity, posterior subcapsular cataract formation, and secondary ocular infections

Adverse Reactions

Dermatologic: Contact dermatitis, cutaneous sensitization (sensitivity to topical neomycin has been reported to occur in 5% to 15% of patients)

Local: Pain, stinging

Ocular: Development of glaucoma, cataract, elevated intraocular pressure, optic nerve damage, visual defects, blurred vision

Miscellaneous: Delayed wound healing, secondary infections

Usual Dosage Children and Adults: Ophthalmic:

Ointment: Apply a small amount (~½") in the affected eye 3-4 times/day or apply at bedtime as an adjunct with drops

Suspension: Instill 1-2 drops into affected eye(s) every 4-6 hours; in severe disease, drops may be used hourly and tapered to discontinuation

Administration Ophthalmic: Shake suspension well before using; instill drop into affected eye; avoid contacting bottle tip with skin or eye; apply finger pressure to lacrimal sac during and for 1-2 minutes after instillation to decrease risk of absorption and systemic effects

Monitoring Parameters Intraocular pressure with use >10 days

Patient Information May cause temporary blurring of vision or stinging following administration

Dosage Forms Excipient information presented when available (limited, particularly for generics); consult specific product labeling. [DSC] = Discontinued product

Ointment, ophthalmic (Maxitrol®, Poly-Dex™): Neomycin 3.5 mg, polymyxin B sulfate 10,000 units, and dexamethasone 0.1% per g (3.5 g)

Suspension, ophthalmic (AK-Trol® [DSC], Maxitrol®, Poly-Dex™): Neomycin 3.5 mg, polymyxin B sulfate 10,000 units, and dexamethasone 0.1% per mL (5 mL) [contains benzalkonium chloride]

- ♦ **Dexamethasone, Neomycin, and Polymyxin B** *see* Dexamethasone, Neomycin, and Polymyxin B *on page 464*
- ♦ **Dexamethasone Sodium Phosphate** *see* Dexamethasone *on page 461*
- ♦ **Dexasone® (Can)** *see* Dexamethasone *on page 461*
- ♦ **Dexedrine®** *see* Dextroamphetamine *on page 469*
- ♦ **Dexferrum®** *see* Iron Supplements (Parenteral) *on page 870*

Dexmedetomidine (deks MED e toe mi deen)

Medication Safety Issues

Sound-alike/look-alike issues:

Precedex™ may be confused with Peridex®

U.S. Brand Names Precedex™

Canadian Brand Names Precedex™

Index Terms Dexmedetomidine Hydrochloride

Therapeutic Category Adrenergic Agonist Agent; Alpha-Adrenergic Agonist; Sedative

Generic Available No

Use Sedation of initially intubated and mechanically ventilated patients during treatment in an intensive care setting; duration of infusion should not exceed 24 hours

Unlabeled uses include premedication prior to anesthesia induction with thiopental; relief of pain and reduction of opioid dose following laparoscopic tubal ligation; as an adjunct anesthetic in ophthalmic surgery; treatment of shivering; premedication to attenuate the cardiostimulatory and postanesthetic delirium of ketamine

Pregnancy Risk Factor C

Lactation Excretion in breast milk unknown/use caution

Contraindications Hypersensitivity to dexmedetomidine or any component; use outside of an intensive care setting

Warnings Should be administered only by persons skilled in management of patients in intensive care setting. Patients should be continuously monitored. Episodes of bradycardia and sinus arrest have been associated with dexmedetomidine when administered rapidly I.V. (eg, bolus administration) or to patients with high vagal tone. Hypotension and bradycardia have been associated with dexmedetomidine infusion; treatment may include the use of atropine or glycopyrrolate, stopping or decreasing the infusion, increasing the rate of I.V. fluid administration, use of pressor agents, and elevation of the lower extremities. Transient hypertension has been primarily observed during the loading dose in association with the initial peripheral vasoconstrictive effects of dexmedetomidine. Treatment is usually not necessary; however, reduction of infusion rate may be desirable.

Usage for >24 hours is not recommended; abrupt discontinuation, if used for prolonged periods may result in withdrawal symptoms similar to those reported for another $alpha_2$ adrenergic agent, clonidine.

Precautions Use with caution in patients with advanced heart block, severe ventricular dysfunction, hypovolemia, diabetes mellitus, and chronic hypertension. Use with caution in patients receiving vasodilators or drugs which decrease heart rate.

Adverse Reactions

Cardiovascular: Hypotension (28%), hypertension (16%), bradycardia, atrial fibrillation, tachycardia

Central nervous system: Pain, fever, agitation, dizziness, headache, speech disorder

Endocrine & metabolic: Hyperglycemia, acidosis, hyperkalemia

Gastrointestinal: Nausea (11%), xerostomia, abdominal pain, diarrhea, vomiting

Hematologic: Anemia, hemorrhage, leukocytosis

(Continued)

Dexmedetomidine *(Continued)*

Hepatic: Elevated liver enzymes
Neuromuscular & skeletal: Pain, rigors
Ocular: Abnormal vision, photopsia
Renal: Oliguria
Respiratory: Hypoxia, pulmonary edema, pleural effusion, respiratory acidosis, apnea, bronchospasm, dyspnea, hypercapnia, hypoventilation, pulmonary congestion
Miscellaneous: Infection, thirst, diaphoresis

Drug Interactions Cytochrome P450 isoenzyme CYP2A6 substrate (major); isoenzyme CYP1A2 (weak), 2C8/9 (weak), 2D6 (strong), and 3A4 (weak) inhibitor

CYP2A6 inhibitors: May increase the levels/effects of dexmedetomidine. Example inhibitors include isoniazid, methoxsalen, and miconazole.

CYP2D6 substrates: Dexmedetomidine may increase the levels/effects of CYP2D6 substrates. Example substrates include amphetamines, selected beta-blockers, dextromethorphan, fluoxetine, lidocaine, mirtazapine, nefazodone, paroxetine, risperidone, ritonavir, thioridazine, tricyclic antidepressants, and venlafaxine.

CYP2D6 prodrug substrates: Dexmedetomidine may decrease the levels/effects of CYP2D6 prodrug substrates. Example prodrug substrates include codeine, hydrocodone, oxycodone, and tramadol.

Hypotension and/or bradycardia may be increased by vasodilators and heart rate-lowering agents.

Stability Store at room temperature; compatible when administered with LR, D_5W, NS, 20% mannitol, thiopental, etomidate, vecuronium, pancuronium, succinylcholine, atracurium, mivacurium, glycopyrrolate, phenylephrine, atropine, midazolam, morphine, and fentanyl (see manufacturer's information for more extensive compatibility listings). Incompatible when administered with amphotericin B and diazepam.

May adsorb to certain types of natural rubber; use components made with synthetic or coated natural rubber gaskets whenever possible.

Mechanism of Action Selective alpha$_2$-adrenoceptor agonist similar to clonidine, but with a much higher affinity for alpha$_2$-receptors over alpha$_1$-receptors; alpha$_1$ activity was observed at high doses or after rapid infusions; produces "arousable sedation" in which patients experience clinically effective sedation yet are easily arousable. The sedative response exhibits properties similar to natural sleep specifically simulating NREM sleep. The sedative properties result primarily from its activity in the locus ceruleus of the brain stem. Analgesic effects are produced by stimulation of the alpha$_2$-receptors in the dorsal horn of the spinal cord.

Pharmacokinetics

Distribution: V_{dss}: Approximately 118 L
Bioavailability: I.M.: 73%
Protein binding: 94%
Metabolism: Hepatic via glucuronidation and CYP2A6
Half-life: Distribution: 6 minutes; Terminal: 2 hours
Elimination: Urine (95%); feces (4%)

Clearance: Adults: 39 L/hour; hepatic impairment (Child-Pugh Class A, B, or C): mean clearance values were 74%, 64%, and 53% respectively, of those observed in healthy adults

Usual Dosage Individualize and titrate to desired clinical effect; I.V.:

Children (limited data): Loading dose: 0.5-1 mcg/kg; followed by a maintenance infusion of 0.2-0.7 mcg/kg/hour; children <1 year may require higher infusion rates; average infusion range: 0.4 mcg/kg/hour vs 0.29 mcg/kg/hour in children >1 year; doses as high as 0.75 mcg/kg/hour were used (Chrysostomou 2006)

Adults: Initial: Loading dose: 1 mcg/kg, followed by a maintenance infusion of 0.2-0.7 mcg/kg/hour

Note: The manufacturer does not recommend that the duration of infusion exceed 24 hours; however, there have been a few studies in adults demonstrating that dexmedetomidine was well tolerated in treatment periods >24 hours; titrate infusion rate so patient awakens slowly; abrupt discontinuation, particularly after prolonged infusions may result in withdrawal symptoms.

Dosage adjustment in hepatic impairment: Dosage reduction may need to be considered. No specific guidelines available.

Administration I.V.: Administer using a controlled infusion device. Dilute 200 mcg (2 mL) in 48 mL NS to achieve a final concentration of 4 mcg/mL. Infuse loading dose over 10 minutes; rapid infusions are associated with severe side effects (see Warnings). Dexmedetomidine may adhere to natural rubber; use administration components made with synthetic or coated natural rubber gaskets.

Monitoring Parameters Level of sedation, heart rate, respiration, ECG, blood pressure

Nursing Implications Continuous monitoring of vital signs, cardiac and respiratory status, and level of sedation during infusion and until full consciousness is regained. Do not discontinue abruptly (may result in rapid awakening associated with anxiety, agitation, and resistance to mechanical ventilation.

Additional Information As an adjunct to anesthesia, dexmedetomidine has been administered I.M. 0.5-1.5 mcg/kg/dose, 60 minutes prior to anesthesia.

Dosage Forms Excipient information presented when available (limited, particularly for generics); consult specific product labeling.

Injection, solution [preservative free]: 100 mcg/mL (2 mL)

References

Berkenbosch JW, Wankum PC, and Tobias JD, "Prospective Evaluation of Dexmedetomidine for Noninvasive Procedural Sedation in Children," *Pediatr Crit Care Med*, 2005, 6(4):435-9.

Buck ML, "Dexmedetomidine for Sedation in the Pediatric Intensive Care Setting," *Pedatr Pharm*, 2006, 12(1).

Chrysostomou C, Di Filippo S, Manrique AM, et al, "Use of Dexmedetomidine in Children After Cardiac and Thoracic Surgery," *Pediatr Crit Care Med*, 2006, 7(2):126-31.

Walker J, Maccalum M, Fischer C, et al, "Sedation Using Dexmedetomidine in Pediatric Burn Patients," *J Burn Care Res*, 2006, 27(2):206-10.

♦ **Dexmedetomidine Hydrochloride** *see* Dexmedetomidine *on page 465*

♦ **DexPak® TaperPak®** *see* Dexamethasone *on page 461*

Dexrazoxane (deks ray ZOKS ane)

Medication Safety Issues

Sound-alike/look-alike issues:

Zinecard® may be confused with Gemzar®

Related Information

Compatibility of Chemotherapy and Related Supportive Care Medications *on page 1777*

U.S. Brand Names Zinecard®

Canadian Brand Names Zinecard®

Index Terms ICRF-187

Therapeutic Category Antineoplastic Agent; Chelating Agent; Chemoprotectant Agent

Generic Available No

Use Reduction of anthracycline-induced (doxorubicin, daunorubicin) cardiotoxicity. Not generally recommended for use with the initiation of anthracycline therapy. Most dexrazoxane studies have been done in women with metastatic breast cancer who had received a cumulative doxorubicin dose of 300 mg/m^2.

Pregnancy Risk Factor C

Lactation Excretion in breast milk unknown/not recommended

Contraindications Hypersensitivity to dexrazoxane or any component; should only be used with chemotherapy regimens containing an anthracycline

Warnings Due to limited experience, the possibility of dexrazoxane interference with antineoplastic efficacy may exist; dose-limiting toxicity is myelosuppression; dexrazoxane may add to the myelosuppression caused by chemotherapeutic agents; dexrazoxane should be handled, prepared, and disposed as an antineoplastic agent

Precautions Do not give doxorubicin prior to dexrazoxane administration. Doxorubicin should be given within 30 minutes after the beginning of a dexrazoxane infusion.

Adverse Reactions

Central nervous system: Low grade fever

Dermatologic: Alopecia (possibly dose-related)

Endocrine/metabolic: Elevated serum iron and serum triglyceride levels, decreased serum zinc and calcium levels

Gastrointestinal: Mild nausea and vomiting, diarrhea, elevated serum amylase levels

Hepatic: Transient elevation of serum transaminase level

Hematologic: **Dose-limiting, additive myelosuppression** (leukopenia and thrombocytopenia at high doses >1000 mg/m^2)

Local: Pain at injection site (13%)

Drug Interactions Dexrazoxane can have either a synergistic or inhibitory activity with different anthracyclines

Stability Reconstituted solution is stable for 6 hours at room temperature or under refrigeration. Dexrazoxane degrades rapidly at pH >7.

Mechanism of Action Dexrazoxane is a piperazine EDTA derivative that rapidly penetrates the myocardial cell membrane. It binds intracellular iron and prevents generation of oxygen free radicals by anthracyclines. Dexrazoxane is hydrolyzed intracellularly to an open-ring chelating agent which is responsible for chelating heavy metals and preventing formation of superhydroxide free radicals believed to be

(Continued)

Dexrazoxane *(Continued)*

responsible for anthracycline-induced cardiomyopathy. Dexrazoxane may also have antitumor activity and have synergistic activity with certain cytotoxic agents.

Pharmacokinetics Minimal data in the pediatric population

Distribution: V_d:

Children: 0.67 L/kg

Adults: 1.3 L/kg

Protein binding: Insignificant

Half-life: Biphasic

Distribution half-life: 8-21 minutes

Terminal half-life: 2-3 hours

Elimination: 40% to 60% of dose excreted renally within 24 hours; removed by peritoneal or hemodialysis

Usual Dosage I.V. (refer to individual protocols):

Children: 10:1 dose ratio with doxorubicin (example: 250 mg/m^2 dexrazoxane: 25 mg/m^2 doxorubicin) is currently recommended; 20:1 ratio with doxorubicin has been studied, but due to higher incidence of adverse reactions is no longer recommended

Adults: 10:1 ratio with doxorubicin (example: 500 mg/m^2 dexrazoxane: 50 mg/m^2 doxorubicin); administer 30 minutes before doxorubicin

Administration Parenteral: Reconstitute with 0.167 Molar sodium lactate injection to a concentration of 10 mg/mL. Administer slow I.V. push or further dilute in NS or D_5W to a final concentration of 1.3-5 mg/mL and give as a rapid I.V. infusion over 15-30 minutes

Monitoring Parameters CBC with differential and platelet count; cardiac function tests; serum triglycerides, iron, calcium, and zinc levels; liver function tests

Nursing Implications To ensure optimal chemoprotectant effect, do not allow chemotherapy to be delayed following completion of dexrazoxane

Dosage Forms Excipient information presented when available (limited, particularly for generics); consult specific product labeling.

Injection, powder for reconstitution: 250 mg, 500 mg [10 mg/mL when reconstituted]

References

Sehested M, et al, "Dexrazoxane for Protection Against Cardiotoxic Effects of Anthracyclines," *J Clin Oncol*, 1996, 14:2884.

Swain SM, et al, "Cardioprotection With Dexrazoxane for Doxorubicin-Containing Therapy in Advanced Breast Cancer," *J Clin Oncol*, 1997, 15:1318-32.

Swain SM, et al, "Delayed Administration of Dexrazoxane Provides Cardioprotection for Patients With Advanced Breast Cancer Treated With Doxorubicin-Containing Therapy," *J Clin Oncol*, 1997, 15:1333-40.

Wexler LH, et al, "Randomized Trial of the Cardioprotective Agent ICRF-187 in Pediatric Sarcoma Patients Treated With Doxorubicin," *J Clin Oncol*, 1996, 14:362-72.

Dextran (DEKS tran)

Medication Safety Issues

Sound-alike/look-alike issues:

Dextran may be confused with Dexatrim®, Dexedrine®

U.S. Brand Names Gentran®; LMD®

Canadian Brand Names Gentran®

Index Terms Dextran 40; Dextran 70; Dextran, High Molecular Weight; Dextran, Low Molecular Weight

Therapeutic Category Plasma Volume Expander

Generic Available Yes

Use Fluid replacement and blood volume expander used in the treatment of hypovolemia, shock, or near shock states; dextran 40 is also indicated for use as a priming fluid in pump oxygenators during extracorporeal circulation and for venous thrombosis and pulmonary embolism prophylaxis in patients undergoing surgery associated with a high incidence of thromboembolic complications (eg, hip surgery)

Pregnancy Risk Factor C

Lactation Excretion in breast milk unknown

Contraindications Hypersensitivity to dextrans or any component; severe CHF, renal failure, severe thrombocytopenia; hypervolemia; hypofibrinogenemia; severe bleeding disorders

Warnings Use with caution in patients with CHF, pulmonary edema, renal insufficiency, thrombocytopenia, or active hemorrhage; watch for anaphylactoid reactions, have epinephrine and diphenhydramine at bedside

Precautions Use with caution in patients with extreme dehydration (renal failure may occur) and in patients with chronic liver disease

Adverse Reactions

Cardiovascular: Hypotension

Central nervous system: Fever
Dermatologic: Urticaria
Gastrointestinal: Nausea, vomiting
Hematologic: Prolongation of bleeding time with higher doses (may interfere with platelet function)
Neuromuscular & skeletal: Arthralgia
Respiratory: Wheezing, pulmonary edema with high doses, tightness of chest, dyspnea, nasal congestion
Miscellaneous: Anaphylaxis

Stability Store at room temperature; do not freeze; do not use if crystallization has occurred; discard partially used containers

Mechanism of Action Produces plasma volume expansion due to high colloidal osmotic effect (similar to albumin); draws interstitial fluid into the intravascular space; dextran 40 may also increase blood flow in microcirculation

Pharmacodynamics
Maximum effect on plasma volume:
Dextran 40: Within several minutes
Dextran 70 and dextran 75: ~1 hour

Pharmacokinetics
Metabolism: Molecules with molecular weight ≥50,000 are metabolized to glucose
Elimination:
Molecules with molecular weight ≤15,000: Rapidly eliminated in the kidney
Dextran 40: ~70% excreted in urine (unchanged) within 24 hours
Dextran 70 & 75: ~50% excreted in urine within 24 hours

Usual Dosage I.V. (dose and infusion rate are dependent upon the patient's fluid status and must be individualized):
Volume expansion/shock:
Children: Total dose should not be >20 mL/kg during first 24 hours and not >10 mL/kg/day thereafter; do not treat for >5 days
Adults: 500-1000 mL at rate of 20-40 mL/minute
Maximum daily dose: First 24 hours: 20 mL/kg and 10 mL/kg/day thereafter; therapy should not continue beyond 5 days

Administration Parenteral: I.V. infusion only; usual maximum infusion rate (adults): 4 mL/minute; maximum infusion rate in emergency situations (adults): 20-40 mL/minute

Monitoring Parameters Vital signs, signs of allergic/anaphylactoid reaction especially for 30 minutes after starting infusions; signs of circulatory overload (ie, heart rate, blood pressure, central venous pressure, hematocrit), urine output; urine specific gravity; platelets

Test Interactions Falsely elevated serum glucose when determined by methods that use high concentrations of acid (eg, sulfuric acid, acetic acid); may interfere with bilirubin assays that use alcohol and total protein assays using biuret reagents; dextran 70 may produce erythrocyte aggregation and interfere with blood typing and cross matching of blood

Nursing Implications Be prepared to treat anaphylaxis with epinephrine, antihistamines, supportive therapy, and alternative agents to dextran to maintain circulation; do not administer if cloudy or if solution contains dextran flakes; discontinue dextran if urine specific gravity is low, if oliguria or anuria occur, or if there is a rapid acute rise in central venous pressure or other signs of circulatory overload

Additional Information Dextran in sodium chloride 0.9% contains sodium chloride 154 mEq/L

Dosage Forms Excipient information presented when available (limited, particularly for generics); consult specific product labeling.
Infusion [premixed in D_5W; high molecular weight]: 6% Dextran 70 (500 mL)
Infusion [premixed in D_5W; low molecular weight] (Gentran®, LMD®): 10% Dextran 40 (500 mL)
Infusion [premixed in $D_{10}W$; high molecular weight]: 32% Dextran 70 (500 mL)
Infusion [premixed in NS; high molecular weight] (Gentran®): 6% Dextran 70 (500 mL)
Infusion [premixed in NS; low molecular weight] (Gentran®, LMD®): 10% Dextran (500 mL)

- **Dextran 40** *see* Dextran *on page 468*
- **Dextran 70** *see* Dextran *on page 468*
- **Dextran, High Molecular Weight** *see* Dextran *on page 468*
- **Dextran, Low Molecular Weight** *see* Dextran *on page 468*

Dextroamphetamine (deks troe am FET a meen)

Medication Safety Issues
Sound-alike/look-alike issues:
Dexedrine® may be confused with dextran, Excedrin®
(Continued)

Dextroamphetamine *(Continued)*

Related Information
Laboratory Detection of Drugs in Urine *on page 1928*

U.S. Brand Names Dexedrine®; Dextrostat®

Canadian Brand Names Dexedrine®

Index Terms Dextroamphetamine Sulfate

Therapeutic Category Amphetamine; Anorexiant; Central Nervous System Stimulant, Amphetamine

Generic Available Yes

Use Adjunct in treatment of attention-deficit/hyperactivity disorder (ADHD) in children, narcolepsy, exogenous obesity

Restrictions C-II

Medication Guide An FDA-approved patient medication guide, which is available with the product information and at http://www.fda.gov/cder/drug/infopage/ADHD/default.htm, must be dispensed with this medication for each new outpatient prescription and refill.

Pregnancy Risk Factor C

Lactation Enters breast milk/contraindicated

Contraindications Hypersensitivity or idiosyncrasy to dextroamphetamine, other sympathomimetic amines, or any component (see Warnings); advanced arteriosclerosis, symptomatic cardiovascular disease, moderate to severe hypertension, hyperthyroidism, glaucoma, agitated states, patients with a history of drug abuse; concurrent use or use within 14 days of MAO inhibitors (hypertensive crisis may occur)

Warnings Serious cardiovascular events including sudden death may occur in patients with pre-existing structural cardiac abnormalities or other serious heart problems. Sudden death has been reported in children and adolescents; sudden death, stroke, and MI have been reported in adults. Avoid the use of amphetamines in patients with known serious structural cardiac abnormalities, cardiomyopathy, serious heart rhythm abnormalities, coronary artery disease, or other serious cardiac problems that could place patients at an increased risk to the sympathomimetic effects of amphetamines. Patients should be carefully evaluated for cardiac disease prior to initiation of therapy.

Stimulant medications may increase blood pressure (average increase 2-4 mm Hg) and heart rate (average increase 3-6 bpm); some patients may experience greater increases; use stimulant medications with caution in patients with hypertension and other cardiovascular conditions that may be exacerbated by increases in blood pressure or heart rate; use is contraindicated in patients with moderate to severe hypertension. Psychiatric adverse events may occur. Stimulants may exacerbate symptoms of behavior disturbance and thought disorder in patients with pre-existing psychosis. New-onset psychosis or mania may occur with stimulant use. May induce mixed/manic episode in patients with bipolar disorder. May be associated with aggressive behavior or hostility (monitor for development or worsening of these behaviors).

Safety and efficacy have not been established in children <3 years of age; long-term effects in pediatric patients have not been determined. Use of stimulants in children has been associated with growth suppression (monitor growth; treatment interruption may be needed). Appetite suppression may occur; monitor weight during therapy, particularly in children. Stimulants may lower seizure threshold leading to new onset or breakthrough seizure activity (use with caution in patients with a history of seizure disorder). Visual disturbances (difficulty in accommodation and blurred vision) have been reported.

Amphetamines possess a high potential for abuse; misuse may cause sudden death and serious cardiovascular adverse events; use in weight reduction programs only when alternative therapy has been ineffective; prolonged administration may lead to drug dependence; abrupt discontinuation following high doses or for prolonged periods may result in symptoms of withdrawal; use is contraindicated in patients with history of ethanol or drug abuse. Amphetamines may impair the ability to engage in potentially hazardous activities. May exacerbate motor and phonic tics and Tourette's syndrome. Dexedrine® and Dextrostat® tablets contain and generic tablets may contain tartrazine which may cause allergic reactions in susceptible individuals.

Precautions Prescriptions should be written for the smallest quantity consistent with good patient care to minimize possibility of overdose.

Adverse Reactions
Cardiovascular: Hypertension, tachycardia, palpitations, cardiac arrhythmias; cardiomyopathy with chronic use (case reports); serious cardiovascular events including sudden death in patients with pre-existing structural cardiac abnormalities or other serious heart problems (see Warnings)

Central nervous system: Insomnia, headache, nervousness, dizziness, irritability, aggression, overstimulation, restlessness, euphoria, dyskinesia, dysphoria, depression, exacerbation of phonic and motor tics, Tourette's syndrome, seizures, psychotic episodes (rare with recommended doses); psychiatric adverse effects (see Warnings)

Dermatologic: Rash, urticaria

Endocrine & metabolic: Growth suppression, weight loss, libido changes

Gastrointestinal: Anorexia, nausea, vomiting, diarrhea, abdominal cramps, metallic taste, xerostomia, constipation

Genitourinary: Impotence

Neuromuscular & skeletal: Movement disorders, tremor

Ocular: Mydriasis, difficulty in accommodation, blurred vision

Miscellaneous: Physical and psychologic dependence with long-term use

Drug Interactions Amphetamines may decrease hypotensive effects of antihypertensives and sedative effect of antihistamines. Amphetamines may inhibit the effects of adrenergic blocking agents. May increase effects of tricyclic antidepressants or sympathomimetics; tricyclic antidepressants may enhance the CNS and cardiovascular effects of amphetamines (avoid use or monitor for CNS and cardiovascular effects). Amphetamines may potentiate the analgesic effect of meperidine and adrenergic effect of norepinephrine. Amphetamines may delay oral absorption of ethosuximide, phenobarbital, and phenytoin; may precipitate hypertensive crisis in patients receiving MAO inhibitors (avoid use within 14 days); the herbal medicine St John's wort (*Hypericum perforatum*) may increase serious side effects, its use is **not** recommended; amphetamines may precipitate arrhythmias in patients receiving general anesthetics. With propoxyphene overdose, CNS stimulation from amphetamines is potentiated (fatal convulsions may occur); chlorpromazine, haloperidol, and lithium may inhibit the CNS stimulant effects of amphetamines. Antacids may increase the oral absorption of amphetamines; urinary alkalinizers or large doses of antacids may decrease urinary excretion of amphetamines and increase their half-life and duration of action (dosage decrease may be needed). Acids or acidifiers may decrease the oral absorption of amphetamines; urinary acidifiers may increase urinary excretion of amphetamines and decrease their half-life and duration of action (dosage adjustment may be needed).

Food Interactions Acidic foods, juices, or vitamin C may decrease GI absorption. Food does not affect the rate or extent of absorption of the sustained release capsules.

Stability Store at controlled room temperature; protect from light; dispense in tightly closed container

Mechanism of Action Amphetamines are noncatecholamine, sympathomimetic amines. Blocks reuptake of dopamine and norepinephrine from the synapse, thus increases the amounts of circulating dopamine and norepinephrine in cerebral cortex to reticular activating system; inhibits the action of monoamine oxidase and causes catecholamines to be released; peripherally increases blood pressure and acts as a respiratory stimulant and weak bronchodilator

Pharmacodynamics Onset of action: Oral: 60-90 minutes

Pharmacokinetics

Distribution: V_d: Adults: 3.5-4.6 L/kg; distributes into CNS; mean CSF concentrations are 80% of plasma; enters breast milk

Metabolism: Hepatic via CYP monooxygenase and glucuronidation

Half-life: Adults: 12 hours (pH dependent)

Time to peak serum concentration: Oral: Immediate release: 3 hours; sustained release: 8 hours

Elimination: In urine as unchanged drug and inactive metabolites; urinary excretion is pH dependent and is increased with acid urine (low pH)

Usual Dosage Oral: **Note:** Use lowest effective individualized dose; administer first dose as soon as awake

ADHD: Children:

<3 years: Not recommended

3-5 years: Initial: 2.5 mg/day given every morning; increase by 2.5 mg/day at weekly intervals until optimal response is obtained, usual range is 0.1-0.5 mg/kg/dose every morning with maximum of 40 mg/day given in 1-3 divided doses per day

≥6 years: 5 mg once or twice daily; increase in increments of 5 mg/day at weekly intervals until optimal response is reached, usual range is 0.1-0.5 mg/kg/dose every morning (5-20 mg/day) with maximum of 40 mg/day given in 1-3 divided doses per day

Note: Tablets are usually dosed 2-3 times/day with first dose on awakening and additional doses (1 or 2) at intervals of 4-6 hours. Sustained release capsules are usually given 1-2 times/day.

(Continued)

Dextroamphetamine *(Continued)*

Narcolepsy:

Children 6-12 years: Initial: 5 mg/day, may increase at 5 mg increments at weekly intervals until optimal response is obtained; maximum dose: 60 mg/day

Children >12 and Adults: Initial: 10 mg/day, may increase at 10 mg increments at weekly intervals until optimal response is obtained; maximum dose: 60 mg/day

Exogenous obesity: Children >12 years and Adults: 5-30 mg/day in divided doses of 5-10 mg given 30-60 minutes before meals

Administration Oral: Sustained release preparations should be used for once daily dosing; do not crush or chew sustained release preparations; to avoid insomnia, last daily dose should be administered no less than 6 hours before retiring

Monitoring Parameters Evaluate patients for cardiac disease (see Warnings) prior to starting therapy; obtain careful history, family history and physical exam; perform EKG and echocardiogram if findings suggest cardiac disease; promptly conduct cardiac evaluation in patients who develop chest pain, unexplained syncope, or any other symptom of cardiac disease during treatment. Monitor CNS activity, blood pressure, heart rate, height, weight.

Test Interactions Amphetamines may interfere with urinary steroid measurements; may cause significant increase in plasma corticosteroid levels

Patient Information Read the patient Medication Guide that you receive with each prescription and refill of dextroamphetamine. Serious cardiac effects or psychiatric adverse effects may occur; notify your physician of any heart problems, high blood pressure, or psychiatric conditions before starting therapy. May reduce the growth rate in children and has been associated with worsening of aggressive behavior; notify your physician if your child displays aggression or hostility; make sure your physician monitors your child's weight and height. May impair ability to perform activities requiring mental alertness or physical coordination. May be habit-forming; avoid abrupt discontinuation after prolonged use. Limit caffeine; avoid alcohol and the herbal medicine St. John's wort. May cause dry mouth.

Additional Information Treatment for ADHD should include "drug holiday" or periodic discontinuation in order to assess the patient's requirements, decrease tolerance, and limit suppression of linear growth and weight. Sustained release capsule (Dexedrine® Spansule®) is formulated to release an initial dose promptly with the remaining medication gradually released over a prolonged time.

Dosage Forms Excipient information presented when available (limited, particularly for generics); consult specific product labeling. [DSC] = Discontinued product

Capsule, sustained release, as sulfate: 5 mg, 10 mg, 15 mg

Dexedrine® Spansule®: 5 mg, 10 mg, 15 mg

Tablet, as sulfate: 5 mg, 10 mg

Dexedrine®: 5 mg [contains tartrazine] [DSC]

Dextrostat®: 5 mg, 10 mg [contains tartrazine]

References

American Academy of Pediatrics, "Clinical Practice Guideline: Treatment of the School-Aged Child With Attention-Deficit/Hyperactivity Disorder," *Pediatrics*, 2001, 108(4):1033-44.

Greenhill LL, Pliszka S, Dulcan MK, et al, "Practice Parameter for the Use of Stimulant Medications in the Treatment of Children, Adolescents, and Adults," *J Am Acad Child Adolesc Psychiatry*, 2002, 41(2 Suppl):26S-49S.

Dextroamphetamine and Amphetamine

(deks troe am FET a meen & am FET a meen)

Medication Safety Issues

Sound-alike/look-alike issues:

Adderall® may be confused with Inderal®

Related Information

Dextroamphetamine *on page 469*

Laboratory Detection of Drugs in Urine *on page 1928*

U.S. Brand Names Adderall®; Adderall XR®

Canadian Brand Names Adderall XR®

Index Terms Amphetamine and Dextroamphetamine

Therapeutic Category Amphetamine; Anorexiant; Central Nervous System Stimulant, Amphetamine

Generic Available Yes: Tablet

Use Attention-deficit/hyperactivity disorder (ADHD); narcolepsy

Restrictions C-II

Medication Guide An FDA-approved patient medication guide, which is available with the product information and at http://www.fda.gov/cder/drug/infopage/ADHD/default.htm, must be dispensed with this medication for each new outpatient prescription and refill.

Pregnancy Risk Factor C

Lactation Enters breast milk/contraindicated

Contraindications Hypersensitivity or idiosyncrasy to dextroamphetamine, amphetamine, sympathomimetic amines, or any component; advanced arteriosclerosis, moderate to severe hypertension, symptomatic cardiovascular disease, hyperthyroidism, glaucoma, agitated states, history of drug abuse; concurrent use or use within 14 days of MAO inhibitors (hypertensive crisis may occur)

Warnings Serious cardiovascular events including sudden death may occur in patients with pre-existing structural cardiac abnormalities or other serious heart problems. Sudden death has been reported in children and adolescents; sudden death, stroke, and MI have been reported in adults. Avoid the use of amphetamines in patients with known serious structural cardiac abnormalities, cardiomyopathy, serious heart rhythm abnormalities, coronary artery disease, or other serious cardiac problems that could place patients at an increased risk to the sympathomimetic effects of amphetamines. Patients should be carefully evaluated for cardiac disease prior to initiation of therapy.

Stimulant medications may increase blood pressure (average increase 2-4 mm Hg) and heart rate (average increase 3-6 bpm); some patients may experience greater increases; use stimulant medications with caution in patients with hypertension and other cardiovascular conditions that may be exacerbated by increases in blood pressure or heart rate; use is contraindicated in patients with moderate to severe hypertension. Psychiatric adverse events may occur. Stimulants may exacerbate symptoms of behavior disturbance and thought disorder in patients with pre-existing psychosis. New-onset psychosis or mania may occur with stimulant use. May induce mixed/manic episode in patients with bipolar disorder. May be associated with aggressive behavior or hostility (monitor for development or worsening of these behaviors).

Safety and efficacy have not been established in children <3 years of age (use in children <3 years is **not** recommended); effects of extended-release capsule have not been studied in children 3-5 years old; long-term effects in pediatric patients have not been determined. Use of stimulants in children has been associated with growth suppression (monitor growth; treatment interruption may be needed). Appetite suppression may occur; monitor weight during therapy, particularly in children. Stimulants may lower seizure threshold leading to new onset or breakthrough seizure activity (use with caution in patients with a history of seizure disorder). Visual disturbances (difficulty in accommodation and blurred vision) have been reported.

Amphetamines possess a high potential for abuse; misuse may cause sudden death and serious cardiovascular adverse events; prolonged administration may lead to drug dependence; abrupt discontinuation following high doses or for prolonged periods may result in symptoms of withdrawal; use is contraindicated in patients with history of ethanol or drug abuse. Amphetamines may impair the ability to engage in potentially hazardous activities. May exacerbate motor and phonic tics and Tourette's syndrome.

Precautions Use with caution in patients with mild hypertension (use is contraindicated in patients with moderate to severe hypertension) and in those receiving other sympathomimetic agents. Prescribe or dispense least amount feasible to minimize chance of overdose.

Adverse Reactions

Cardiovascular system: Hypertension, tachycardia, palpitations, chest pain; cardiomyopathy with chronic use (case reports); serious cardiovascular events including sudden death in patients with pre-existing structural cardiac abnormalities or other serious heart problems (see Warnings)

Central nervous system: Insomnia, headache, nervousness, overstimulation, dizziness, lightheadedness, euphoria, dysphoria, dyskinesia, exacerbation of phonic and motor tics, Tourette's syndrome, seizures, psychotic episodes (rare at recommended doses), emotional lability, depression, anxiety, irritability, somnolence, agitation, fever

Dermatologic: Rash, urticaria, Stevens-Johnson syndrome, toxic epidermal necrolysis

Endocrine and metabolic: Growth suppression, weight loss, libido changes

Gastrointestinal: Anorexia, diarrhea, constipation, xerostomia, unpleasant taste, abdominal pain, dyspepsia, nausea, vomiting

Genitourinary: Impotence

Hepatic: Elevated transaminases

Neuromuscular and skeletal: Tremor, asthenia

Ocular: Mydriasis, difficulty in accommodation, blurred vision

Miscellaneous: Hypersensitivity reactions, angioedema, anaphylaxis, physical and psychological dependence with long-term use

Drug Interactions Dextroamphetamine: Cytochrome P450 isoenzyme CYP2D6 (major) substrate; amphetamine: Isoenzyme CYP2D6 (major) substrate and inhibitor (weak)

(Continued)

Dextroamphetamine and Amphetamine *(Continued)*

Amphetamines may decrease hypotensive effects of antihypertensives and sedative effect of antihistamines. Amphetamines may inhibit the effects of adrenergic-blocking agents. May increase effects of tricyclic antidepressants or sympathomimetics; tricyclic antidepressants may enhance the CNS and cardiovascular effects of amphetamines (avoid use or monitor for CNS and cardiovascular effects). Amphetamines may potentiate the analgesic effect of meperidine and adrenergic effect of norepinephrine. Amphetamines may delay oral absorption of ethosuximide, phenobarbital, and phenytoin; may precipitate hypertensive crisis in patients receiving MAO inhibitors (avoid use within 14 days); the herbal medicine St John's wort (*Hypericum perforatum*) may increase serious side effects, its use is **not** recommended; amphetamines may precipitate arrhythmias in patients receiving general anesthetics. With propoxyphene overdose, CNS stimulation from amphetamines is potentiated (fatal convulsions may occur); chlorpromazine, haloperidol, and lithium may inhibit the CNS stimulant effects of amphetamines. Antacids may increase the oral absorption of amphetamines; urinary alkalinizers or large doses of antacids may decrease urinary excretion of amphetamines and increase their half-life and duration of action (dosage decrease may be needed). Acids or acidifiers may decrease the oral absorption of amphetamines; urinary acidifiers may increase urinary excretion of amphetamines and decrease their half-life and duration of action (dosage adjustment may be needed).

Food Interactions Acidic foods, juices, or vitamin C may decrease oral absorption; extended release capsules: Food does not affect the extent of absorption; a high-fat meal delays the time to peak concentration of d-amphetamine by 2.5 hours and l-amphetamine by 2.1 hours; similar absorption occurs if capsule is opened and contents sprinkled on applesauce versus swallowing intact capsule on an empty stomach

Stability Store at controlled room temperature; dispense in tight, light-resistant container

Mechanism of Action Amphetamines are noncatecholamine, sympathomimetic amines. Amphetamines block the reuptake of dopamine and norepinephrine from the synapse, thus increasing the amounts of circulating dopamine and norepinephrine in cerebral cortex to reticular activating system; inhibits the action of monoamine oxidase and causes catecholamines to be released; peripherally increases blood pressure and acts as a respiratory stimulant and weak bronchodilator

Pharmacodynamics Oral:
- Onset of action: Tablet: 30-60 minutes
- Duration: Tablet: 4-6 hours

Pharmacokinetics
- Absorption: Oral: Well-absorbed
- Distribution: V_d: Adults: 3.5-4.6 L/kg; concentrates in breast milk (avoid breast-feeding); distributes into CNS, mean CSF concentrations are 80% of plasma
- Metabolism: In the liver by cytochrome P450 mono-oxygenase and glucuronidation; two active metabolites (norephedrine and 4-hydroxyamphetamine) are formed via oxidation
- Half-life:
  - d-amphetamine:
    - Children 6-12 years: 9 hours
    - Adolescents 13-17 years: 11 hours
    - Adults: 10 hours
  - l-amphetamine:
    - Children 6-12 years: 11 hours
    - Adolescents 13-17 years: 13-14 hours
    - Adults: 13 hours
- Time to peak serum concentration:
  - Tablet (immediate release): 3 hours
  - Capsule (extended release): 7 hours
- Elimination: 70% of a single dose is eliminated within 24 hours; excreted as unchanged amphetamine (30%), benzoic acid, hydroxyamphetamine, hippuric acid, norephedrine and p-hydroxynorephedrine; **Note:** Urinary recovery of amphetamine is highly dependent on urine flow rates and urinary pH; urinary recovery of amphetamine may range from 1% in alkaline urine to 75% in acidic urine
  - Clearance: Children have a higher clearance (on a mg/kg basis) than adolescents and adults

Usual Dosage Oral: **Note:** Use lowest effective individualized dose; administer first dose as soon as awake

Tablet: **Note:** Use intervals of 4-6 hours between additional doses; tablets are usually doses 1-2 times/day

ADHD:

Children <3 years: Not recommended

Children 3-5 years: Initial 2.5 mg/day given every morning; increase daily dose by 2.5 mg at weekly intervals until optimal response is obtained; maximum dose: 40 mg/day given in 1-3 divided doses per day

Children ≥6 years: Initial: 5 mg once or twice daily; increase daily dose by 5 mg at weekly intervals until optimal response is obtained; usual maximum dose: 40 mg/day given in 1-3 divided doses per day

Narcolepsy:

Children 6-12 years: Initial: 5 mg/day; increase daily dose by 5 mg at weekly intervals until optimal response is obtained; maximum dose: 60 mg/day given in 1-3 divided doses per day

Children >12 years and Adults: Initial: 10 mg/day; increase daily dose by 10 mg at weekly intervals until optimal response is obtained; maximum dose: 60 mg/day given in 1-3 divided doses per day

Extended release capsule (Adderall XR®):

ADHD:

Children <3 years: Not recommended

Children 3-5 years: Has not been studied

Children ≥6 years: Initial: 10 mg/day given every morning (may initiate with 5 mg/day given every morning if lower dose is clinically needed); increase daily dose by 5 mg or 10 mg at weekly intervals until optimal response is obtained; maximum dose: 30 mg once daily; doses >30 mg/day have not been studied; **Note:** Patients taking divided doses of immediate release tablets may be switched to extended release capsule using the same total daily dose (taken once daily); titrate dose at weekly intervals to achieve optimal response

Adolescents 13-17 years: Initial: 10 mg/day given every morning; may increase to 20 mg/day after one week if symptoms are not controlled; **Note:** Although higher doses (up to 60 mg once daily) have been studied, there is not adequate evidence that doses >20 mg/day provide additional benefit

Adults: Initial: 20 mg/day given every morning; **Note:** Although higher doses (up to 60 mg once daily) have been studied, there is not adequate evidence that doses >20 mg/day provide additional benefit

Administration Oral:

Tablet: To avoid insomnia, last daily dose should be administered no less than 6 hours before retiring

Extended release capsule: Avoid afternoon doses to prevent insomnia. Swallow capsule whole; do not chew or divide. May be administered with or without food. May open capsule and sprinkle contents on applesauce; consume applesauce/medication mixture immediately; do not store; do not chew sprinkled beads from capsule

Monitoring Parameters Evaluate patients for cardiac disease (see Warnings) prior to starting therapy; obtain careful history, family history, and physical exam; perform EKG and echocardiogram if findings suggest cardiac disease; promptly conduct cardiac evaluation in patients who develop chest pain, unexplained syncope, or any other symptom of cardiac disease during treatment. Monitor CNS activity, blood pressure, heart rate, height, weight, appetite.

Test Interactions Amphetamines may interfere with urinary steroid measurements; may cause significant increase in plasma corticosteroid levels

Patient Information Read the patient Medication Guide that you receive with each prescription and refill of dextroamphetamine and amphetamine. Serious cardiac effects or psychiatric adverse effects may occur; notify your physician of any heart problems, high blood pressure, or psychiatric conditions before starting therapy. May reduce the growth rate in children and has been associated with worsening of aggressive behavior; notify your physician if your child displays aggression or hostility; make sure your physician monitors your child's weight and height. May impair ability to perform activities requiring mental alertness or physical coordination. May be habit-forming; avoid abrupt discontinuation after prolonged use. Limit caffeine; avoid alcohol and the herbal medicine St John's wort. May cause dry mouth.

Additional Information Treatment of ADHD should include "drug holidays" or periodic discontinuation of medication in order to assess the patient's requirments, decrease tolerance, and limit suppression of linear growth and weight; the combination of equal parts of *d, l*-amphetamine aspartate, *d, l*-amphetamine sulfate, dextroamphetamine saccharate and dextroamphetamine sulfate results in a 3:1 ratio of the dextro- and levo-isomers of amphetamine.

The duration of action of Adderall® is longer than methylphenidate; behavioral effects of a single morning dose of Adderall® may last throughout the school day; a single morning dose of Adderall® has been shown in several studies to be as effective as twice daily dosing of methylphenidate for the treatment of ADHD (see Pelham, 1999a; Manos, 1999; Pliszka, 2000).

(Continued)

Dextroamphetamine and Amphetamine *(Continued)*

A recent randomized, double-blind, placebo-controlled crossover trial of Adderall® in children with ADHD demonstrated efficacy rates of 82% based on parent response, 77% based on teacher response, and 59% based on concurrence between parent and teacher response; reported side effects included decreased appetite, stomach aches, insomnia, and headaches; decreased appetite and insomnia were more problematic on the high dose (0.3 mg/kg/dose twice daily) versus the low dose (0.15 mg/kg/dose twice daily); headaches occurred more frequently on the high dose, suggesting a dose-dependency (Ahmann, 2001).

Long term use of Adderall XR® (ie, >3 weeks) has not been studied; long term usefulness should be periodically re-evaluated for the individual patient

Dosage Forms Excipient information presented when available (limited, particularly for generics); consult specific product labeling.

Capsule, extended release (Adderall XR®):

- 5 mg [dextroamphetamine sulfate 1.25 mg, dextroamphetamine saccharate 1.25 mg, amphetamine aspartate monohydrate 1.25 mg, amphetamine sulfate 1.25 mg (equivalent to amphetamine base 3.1 mg)]
- 10 mg [dextroamphetamine sulfate 2.5 mg, dextroamphetamine saccharate 2.5 mg, amphetamine aspartate monohydrate 2.5 mg, amphetamine sulfate 2.5 mg (equivalent to amphetamine base 6.3 mg)]
- 15 mg [dextroamphetamine sulfate 3.75 mg, dextroamphetamine saccharate 3.75 mg, amphetamine aspartate monohydrate 3.75 mg, amphetamine sulfate 3.75 mg (equivalent to amphetamine base 9.4 mg)]
- 20 mg [dextroamphetamine sulfate 5 mg, dextroamphetamine saccharate 5 mg, amphetamine aspartate monohydrate 5 mg, amphetamine sulfate 5 mg (equivalent to amphetamine base 12.5 mg)]
- 25 mg [dextroamphetamine sulfate 6.25 mg, dextroamphetamine saccharate 6.25 mg, amphetamine aspartate monohydrate 6.25 mg, amphetamine sulfate 6.25 mg (equivalent to amphetamine base 15.6 mg)]
- 30 mg [dextroamphetamine sulfate 7.5 mg, dextroamphetamine saccharate 7.5 mg, amphetamine aspartate monohydrate 7.5 mg, amphetamine sulfate 7.5 mg (equivalent to amphetamine base 18.8 mg)]

Tablet (Adderall®):

- 5 mg [dextroamphetamine sulfate 1.25 mg, dextroamphetamine saccharate 1.25 mg, amphetamine aspartate 1.25 mg, amphetamine sulfate 1.25 mg (equivalent to amphetamine base 3.13 mg)]
- 7.5 mg [dextroamphetamine 1.875 mg, dextroamphetamine saccharate 1.875 mg, amphetamine aspartate 1.875 mg, amphetamine sulfate 1.875 mg (equivalent to amphetamine base 4.7 mg)]
- 10 mg [dextroamphetamine sulfate 2.5 mg, dextroamphetamine saccharate 2.5 mg, amphetamine aspartate 2.5 mg, amphetamine sulfate 2.5 mg (equivalent to amphetamine base 6.3 mg)]
- 12.5 mg [dextroamphetamine sulfate 3.125 mg, dextroamphetamine saccharate 3.125 mg, amphetamine aspartate 3.125 mg, amphetamine sulfate 3.125 mg (equivalent to amphetamine base 7.8 mg)]
- 15 mg [dextroamphetamine sulfate 3.75 mg, dextroamphetamine saccharate 3.75 mg, amphetamine aspartate 3.75 mg, amphetamine sulfate 3.75 mg (equivalent to amphetamine base 9.4 mg)]
- 20 mg [dextroamphetamine sulfate 5 mg, dextroamphetamine saccharate 5 mg, amphetamine aspartate 5 mg, amphetamine sulfate 5 mg (equivalent to amphetamine base 12.6 mg)]
- 30 mg [dextroamphetamine sulfate 7.5 mg, dextroamphetamine saccharate 7.5 mg, amphetamine aspartate 7.5 mg, amphetamine sulfate 7.5 mg (equivalent to amphetamine base 18.8 mg)]

Extemporaneous Preparations A 1 mg/mL oral formulation of Adderall® in 3 different vehicles (Ora-Sweet®, Ora-Plus®, and a 1:1 mixture of Ora-Sweet® and Ora-Plus®) was found to be stable for 30 days when stored in glass bottles in the dark at 25°C and 60% relative humidity; ten 10 mg Adderall® tablets were crushed in a mortar into a fine powder; approximately 20 mL of vehicle was added to the mortar and triturated well; the contents were transferred to a 4 ounce glass prescription bottle; the mortar was rinsed with approximately 20 mL of vehicle and transferred to the bottle (this was repeated until the final volume was qsad to 100 mL); label "shake well" and "protect from light"

Justice J, Kupiec TC, Matthews P, et al, "Stability of Adderall® in Extemporaneously Compounded Oral Liquids," *Am J Health Syst Pharm*, 2001, 58(15):1418-21.

References

Ahmann PA, Theye FW, Berg R, et al, "Placebo-Controlled Evaluation of Amphetamine Mixture - Dextroamphetamine Salts and Amphetamine Salts (Adderall): Efficacy Rate and Side Effects," *Pediatrics*, 2001, 107(1), http://www.pediatrics.org/cgi/content/full/107/1/e10.

American Academy of Pediatrics, "Clinical Practice Guideline: Treatment of the School-Aged Child With Attention-Deficit/Hyperactivity Disorder," *Pediatrics*, 2001, 108(4):1033-44.

Greenhill LL, Pliszka S, Dulcan MK, et al, "Practice Parameter for the Use of Stimulant Medications in the Treatment of Children, Adolescents, and Adults," *J Am Acad Child Adolesc Psychiatry*, 2002, 41(2 Suppl):26S-49S.

Manos MJ, Short EJ, and Findling RL, "Differential Effectiveness of Methylphenidate and Adderall® in School-Age Youths With Attention-Deficit/Hyperactivity Disorder," *J Am Acad Child Adolesc Psychiatry*, 1999, 38(7):813-9.

Pelham WE, Aronoff HR, Midlam JK, et al, "A Comparison of Ritalin® and Adderall®: Efficacy and Time-Course in Children With Attention-Deficit/Hyperactivity Disorder," *Pediatrics*, 1999, 103(4):e43. URL: http://www.pediatrics.org/cgi/content/full/103/4/e43

Pelham WE, Gnagy EM, Chronis AM, et al, "A Comparison of Morning-Only and Morning/Late Afternoon Adderall® to Morning-Only, Twice-Daily, and Three Times-Daily Methylphenidate in Children With Attention-Deficit/Hyperactivity Disorder," *Pediatrics*, 1999a, 104(6):1300-11.

Pliszka SR, Browne RG, Olvera RL, et al, "A Double-Blind, Placebo-Controlled Study of Adderall® and Methylphenidate in the Treatment of Attention-Deficit/Hyperactivity Disorder," *J Am Acad Child Adolesc Psychiatry*, 2000, 39(5):619-26.

Swanson JM, Wigal S, Greenhill LL, et al, "Analog Classroom Assessment of Adderall® in Children With ADHD," *J Am Acad Child Adolesc Psychiatry*, 1998, 37(5):519-26.

♦ **Dextroamphetamine Sulfate** *see* Dextroamphetamine *on page 469*

Dextromethorphan (deks troe meth OR fan)

Medication Safety Issues

Sound-alike/look-alike issues:

Benylin® may be confused with Benadryl®, Ventolin®

Delsym® may be confused with Delfen®, Desyrel®

Related Information

OTC Cough and Cold Preparations, Pediatric *on page 1706*

U.S. Brand Names Babee® Cof Syrup [OTC]; Creomulsion® Cough [OTC]; Creomulsion® for Children [OTC]; Creo-Terpin® [OTC]; Delsym® [OTC]; ElixSure® Cough [OTC]; Hold® DM [OTC]; PediaCare® Children's Medicated Freezer Pops Long Acting Cough [OTC] [DSC]; PediaCare® Infants' Long-Acting Cough [OTC]; Robitussin® CoughGels™ [OTC]; Robitussin® Maximum Strength Cough [OTC]; Robitussin® Pediatric Cough [OTC]; Scot-Tussin DM® Cough Chasers [OTC]; Silphen DM® [OTC]; Simply Cough® [OTC] [DSC]; Triaminic® Thin Strips™ Long Acting Cough [OTC]; Vicks® 44® Cough Relief [OTC]

Index Terms DM

Therapeutic Category Antitussive; Cough Preparation

Generic Available Yes: Excludes strip, liquid freezer pop

Use Symptomatic relief of coughs caused by minor viral upper respiratory tract infections or inhaled irritants

Pregnancy Risk Factor C

Contraindications Hypersensitivity to dextromethorphan or any component (see Warnings); concomitant use or use within 14 days of MAO inhibitors

Warnings Do not use for persistent or chronic cough, or for cough accompanied by excessive secretions; Creo-Terpin® contains tartrazine which may cause allergic reactions in susceptible individuals; some products may contain sodium benzoate which may cause allergic reactions in susceptible individuals; sodium benzoate has been associated with a potentially fatal toxicity ("gasping syndrome") in neonates; *in vitro* and animal studies have shown that benzoate, a metabolite of benzyl alcohol, displaces bilirubin from protein binding sites; avoid use of products containing sodium benzoate in neonates

Precautions Anecdotal reports of abuse of dextromethorphan-containing cough/cold products have increased, especially among teenagers

Adverse Reactions

Central nervous system: Drowsiness, dizziness

Gastrointestinal: Nausea

Drug Interactions Cytochrome P450 isoenzyme CYP2D6, CYP2E1, and CYP3A3/4 substrate

MAO inhibitors (increased risk of serotonin syndrome); haloperidol and fluoxetine decrease dextromethorphan metabolism; dextromethorphan decreases fluoxetine metabolism

Mechanism of Action Non-narcotic chemical relative of morphine; controls cough by depressing the medullary cough center

Pharmacodynamics

Onset of antitussive action: Within 15-30 minutes

Duration: Up to 6 hours

Pharmacokinetics

Metabolism: In the liver

Half-Life: 1.4-3.9 hours

Time to peak serum concentration: 2-2.5 hours

Elimination: Principally in urine

(Continued)

Dextromethorphan *(Continued)*

Usual Dosage Dosage in children <2 years of age is not well established; the following dosage recommendations in children <2 years are consistent with the dosages received when using combination products containing dextromethorphan.

Oral:

Children:

1-3 months: 0.5-1 mg every 6-8 hours

3-6 months: 1-2 mg every 6-8 hours

7 months to 1 year: 2-4 mg every 6-8 hours

≥2-6 years : 2.5-7.5 mg every 4-8 hours; extended release formulation: 15 mg twice daily (maximum: 30 mg/24 hours)

7-12 years: 5-10 mg every 4 hours or 15 mg every 6-8 hours; extended release formulation: 30 mg twice daily (maximum: 60 mg/24 hours)

Children >12 years and Adults: 10-30 mg every 4-8 hours or extended release formulation: 60 mg twice daily (maximum: 120 mg/24 hours)

Administration Oral: May administer without regard to meals

Monitoring Parameters Cough, mental status

Test Interactions Can give a false-positive on phencyclidine qualitative immunoassay screen

Patient Information If cough lasts more than 1 week or is accompanied by fever or headache, notify physician

Additional Information Dextromethorphan 15-30 mg equals 8-15 mg codeine as an antitussive

Dosage Forms Excipient information presented when available (limited, particularly for generics); consult specific product labeling. [DSC] = Discontinued product

Gelcap, as hydrobromide:

Robitussin® CoughGels™: 15 mg [contains coconut oil]

Liquid, as hydrobromide:

Creo-Terpin®: 10 mg/15 mL (120 mL) [contains alcohol 25% and tartrazine]

Simply Cough®: 5 mg/5 mL (120 mL) [contains sodium benzoate; cherry berry flavor] [DSC]

Vicks® 44® Cough Relief: 10 mg/5 mL (120 mL) [contains alcohol, sodium 10 mg/5 mL, sodium benzoate]

Liquid, oral, as hydrobromide [freezer pops]:

PediaCare® Children's Medicated Freezer Pops Long Acting Cough: 7.5 mg/25 mL (8s) [alcohol free; contains sodium benzoate, berry flavor also contains benzyl alcohol; glacier grape™ and polar berry blue™ flavors] [DSC]

Liquid, oral, as hydrobromide [drops]:

PediaCare® Infants' Long-Acting Cough: 7.5 mg/0.8 mL (15 mL) [alcohol free, dye free; contains sodium benzoate; grape flavor]

Lozenge, as hydrobromide:

Hold® DM: 5 mg (10s) [cherry or original flavor]

Scot-Tussin DM® Cough Chasers: 5 mg (20s)

Strips, oral, as hydrobromide:

Triaminic® Thin Strips™ Long Acting Cough: 7.5 mg [equivalent to dextromethorphan 5 mg; cherry flavor]

Suspension, extended release:

Delsym®: Dextromethorphan polistirex [equivalent to dextromethorphan hydrobromide 30 mg/5 mL] (78 mL, 148 mL) [contains sodium 6 mg/5 mL; orange flavor]

Syrup, as hydrobromide:

Babee® Cof Syrup: 7.5 mg/5 mL (120 mL) [alcohol free, dye free; cherry flavor]

Creomulsion® Cough: 20 mg/15 mL (120 mL) [alcohol free; contains sodium benzoate]

Creomulsion® for Children: 5 mg/5 mL (120 mL) [alcohol free; contains sodium benzoate; cherry flavor]

ElixSure® Cough: 7.5 mg/5 mL (120 mL) [cherry bubble gum flavor]

Robitussin® Maximum Strength Cough: 15 mg/5 mL (120 mL, 240 mL) [contains alcohol, sodium benzoate]

Robitussin® Pediatric Cough: 7.5 mg/5 mL (120 mL) [alcohol free; contains sodium benzoate; fruit punch flavor]

Silphen DM®: 10 mg/5 mL (120 mL) [strawberry flavor]

♦ **Dextromethorphan and Guaifenesin** *see* Guaifenesin and Dextromethorphan *on page 748*

♦ **Dextropropoxyphene** *see* Propoxyphene *on page 1334*

Dextrose (DEKS trose)

Medication Safety Issues

Sound-alike/look-alike issues:

Glutose™ may be confused with Glutofac®

Related Information

Commonly Used Antidotes for Acute Overdoses *on page 1920*
Fluid and Electrolyte Requirements in Children *on page 1751*
Parenteral Nutrition (PN) *on page 1755*

Index Terms Anhydrous Glucose; Dextrose Monohydrate; D_5W; $D_{10}W$; $D_{25}W$; $D_{30}W$; $D_{40}W$; $D_{50}W$; $D_{60}W$; $D_{70}W$; Glucose; Glucose Monohydrate; Glycosum

Therapeutic Category Antidote, Insulin; Antidote, Oral Hypoglycemic; Fluid Replacement, Enteral; Fluid Replacement, Parenteral; Hyperglycemic Agent; Hyperkalemia, Adjunctive Treatment Agent; Intravenous Nutritional Therapy

Generic Available Yes

Use

5% and 10% solutions: Peripheral infusion to provide calories and fluid replacement

10% solution: Treatment of hypoglycemia in premature neonates

25% (hypertonic) solution: Treatment of acute symptomatic episodes of hypoglycemia in infants and children to restore depressed blood glucose levels; adjunctive treatment of hyperkalemia when combined with insulin

50% (hypertonic) solution: Treatment of insulin-induced hypoglycemia (hyperinsulinemia or insulin shock) and adjunctive treatment of hyperkalemia in adolescents and adults

≥10% solutions: Infusion after admixture with amino acids for nutritional support

Pregnancy Risk Factor C

Contraindications Hypersensitivity to corn or corn products; diabetic coma with hyperglycemia; hypertonic solutions in patients with intracranial or intraspinal hemorrhage; patients with delirium tremens and dehydration; patients with anuria, hepatic coma, or glucose-galactose malabsorption syndrome

Warnings Hypertonic solutions (>10%) may cause thrombosis if infused via peripheral veins; administer hypertonic solutions via a central venous catheter; rapid administration of hypertonic solutions may produce significant hyperglycemia, glycosuria, and shifts in electrolytes; this may result in dehydration, hyperosmolar syndrome, coma, and death especially in patients with chronic uremia or carbohydrate intolerance; excessive or rapid dextrose administration in very low birth weight infants has been associated with increased serum osmolality and possible intracerebral hemorrhage; hyperglycemia and glycosuria may be functions of the rate of administration of dextrose; to minimize these effects, reduce the rate of infusion; addition of insulin may be necessary; administration of potassium free I.V. dextrose solutions may result in significant hypokalemia, particularly if highly concentrated dextrose solutions are used; add potassium to dextrose solutions for patients with adequate renal function; abrupt withdrawal of dextrose solution may be associated with rebound hypoglycemia; an unexpected rise in blood glucose level in an otherwise stable patient may be an early symptom of infection; glucose is not absorbed from the buccal cavity; it must be swallowed to be effective; do not use oral forms in unconscious patients

Parenteral dextrose solutions contain aluminum which may accumulate to toxic levels with prolonged administration particularly in patients with impaired renal function. Patients with impaired renal function including premature neonates who receive aluminum at >4-5 mcg/kg/day accumulate aluminum at levels associated with CNS and bone toxicity.

Precautions Use with caution in premature infants, especially very low birth weight infants, as rapid changes is osmolality may produce profound effects on the brain, including intraventricular hemorrhage; small incremental changes in infusion rates are necessary in these patients; use with caution also in patients with diabetes mellitus

Adverse Reactions Note: Most adverse effects are associated with excessive dosage or rate of infusion

Cardiovascular: Venous thrombosis, phlebitis, hypovolemia, hypervolemia, dehydration, edema

Central nervous system: Fever, mental confusion, unconsciousness, hyperosmolar syndrome

Endocrine & metabolic: Hyperglycemia, hypokalemia, acidosis, hypophosphatemia, hypomagnesemia

Local: Pain, vein irritation, tissue necrosis

Genitourinary: Polyuria, glycosuria, ketonuria

Gastrointestinal: Polydipsia, nausea

Respiratory: Tachypnea, pulmonary edema

Drug Interactions Corticosteroids

(Continued)

Dextrose *(Continued)*

Stability Stable at room temperature; protect from freezing and extreme heat; store oral dextrose in airtight containers

Mechanism of Action Dextrose, a monosaccharide, is a source of calories and fluid for patients unable to obtain an adequate oral intake; may decrease body protein and nitrogen losses; promotes glycogen deposition in the liver; for the treatment of hyperkalemia, when combined with insulin, dextrose stimulates the uptake of potassium by cells, especially in muscle tissue

Pharmacodynamics

Onset of action: Treatment of hypoglycemia: Oral: 10 minutes

Maximum effect: Treatment of hyperkalemia: I.V.: 30 minutes

Pharmacokinetics

Absorption: Rapidly from the small intestine by an active mechanism

Metabolism: Metabolized to carbon dioxide and water

Time to peak serum concentration: Oral: 40 minutes

Usual Dosage

Hypoglycemia: Doses may be repeated in severe cases

I.V.:

Premature neonates: 0.1-0.2 g/kg/dose (1-2 mL/kg/dose of 10% solution); followed by continuous infusion at a rate of 4-6 mg/kg/minute

Infants ≤6 months: 0.25-0.5 g/kg/dose (1-2 mL/kg/dose of 25% solution; 5-10 mL/kg of 10% solution; 1-2 mL/kg of 50% solution); maximum: 25 g/dose

Infants >6 months and Children: 0.5-1 g/kg/dose (2-4 mL/kg/dose of 25% solution; 5-10 mL/kg of 10% solution; 1-2 mL/kg of 50% solution); maximum: 25 g/dose

Adolescents and Adults: 10-25 g (40-100 mL of 25% solution or 20-50 mL of 50% solution)

Oral:

Children >2 years and Adults: 10-20 g as single dose; repeat in 10 minutes if necessary

Treatment of Hyperkalemia: I.V. (in combination with insulin):

Infants and Children: 0.5-1 g/kg (using 25% or 50% solution) combined with regular insulin 1 unit for every 4-5 g dextrose given; infuse over 2 hours (infusions as short as 30 minutes have been recommended); repeat as needed

Adolescents and Adults: 25-50 g dextrose (250-500 mL $D_{10}W$) combined with 10 units regular insulin administered over 30-60 minutes; repeat as needed or as an alternative 25 g dextrose (50 mL $D_{50}W$) combined with 5-10 units regular insulin infused over 5 minutes; repeat as needed

Note: More rapid infusions (<30 minutes) may be associated with hyperglycemia and hyperosmolality and will exacerbate hyperkalemia; avoid use in patients who are already hyperglycemic

Fluid therapy: See Fluid and Electrolyte Requirements in Children *on page 1751*

Nutrition: See Parenteral Nutrition (PN) *on page 1755*

Administration

Oral: Must be swallowed to be absorbed (see Warnings)

Parenteral: Not for SubQ or I.M. administration; dilute concentrated dextrose solutions for peripheral venous administration to a maximum concentration of 12.5%; in emergency situations, 25% dextrose has been used peripherally; for direct I.V. infusion, infuse at a maximum rate of 200 mg/kg over 1 minute; continuous infusion rates very with tolerance (see Parenteral Nutrition (PN) *on page 1755*) and range from 4.5-15 mg/kg/minute; hyperinsulinemic neonates may require up to 15-25 mg/kg/minute infusion rates

Monitoring Parameters Blood and urine sugar, serum electrolytes, I & O, caloric intake

Reference Range Normal blood sugar:

Neonates: 110-270 mg/dL

0-2 years: 60-105 mg/dL

Children >2 years and Adults: 70-110 mg/dL

Additional Information Each g of I.V. dextrose contains 3.4 kcal; glucose monohydrate 1 g is equal to 1 g anhydrous dextrose; osmolarity of 10% dextrose is 505 mOsm/L and 25% dextrose is 1330 mOsm/L. Normal body fluid osmolarity is 310 mOsm/L.

Dosage Forms Excipient information presented when available (limited, particularly for generics); consult specific product labeling. [DSC] = Discontinued product

Gel, oral:

Glutose™: 40% (15 g, 45 g)

Insta-Glucose®: 40% (30 g)

Solution, oral (Glutol™): 55% [100 g dextrose/180 mL] (180 mL)

Tablet, chewable:
B-D™ Glucose: 5 g
Dex4 Glucose: 4 g

- ◆ **Dextrose Monohydrate** *see* Dextrose *on page 479*
- ◆ **Dextrostat®** *see* Dextroamphetamine *on page 469*
- ◆ **DHAD** *see* Mitoxantrone *on page 1072*
- ◆ **DHAQ** *see* Mitoxantrone *on page 1072*
- ◆ **DHE** *see* Dihydroergotamine *on page 500*
- ◆ **D.H.E. 45®** *see* Dihydroergotamine *on page 500*
- ◆ **DHPG Sodium** *see* Ganciclovir *on page 719*
- ◆ **DHS™ Sal [OTC]** *see* Salicylic Acid *on page 1413*
- ◆ **DHS™ Tar [OTC]** *see* Coal Tar *on page 394*
- ◆ **DHS™ Targel [OTC]** *see* Coal Tar *on page 394*
- ◆ **DHT™ [DSC]** *see* Dihydrotachysterol [DSC] *on page 502*
- ◆ **DHT™ Intensol™ [DSC]** *see* Dihydrotachysterol [DSC] *on page 502*
- ◆ **Diabeta** *see* GlyBURIDE *on page 734*
- ◆ **DiabetAid™ Antifungal Foot Bath [OTC]** *see* Miconazole *on page 1056*
- ◆ **Diabetic Tussin C®** *see* Guaifenesin and Codeine *on page 746*
- ◆ **Diabetic Tussin® Allergy Relief [OTC]** *see* Chlorpheniramine *on page 344*
- ◆ **Diabetic Tussin® DM [OTC]** *see* Guaifenesin and Dextromethorphan *on page 748*
- ◆ **Diabetic Tussin® DM Maximum Strength [OTC]** *see* Guaifenesin and Dextromethorphan *on page 748*
- ◆ **Diabetic Tussin® EX [OTC]** *see* Guaifenesin *on page 745*
- ◆ **Diaβeta®** *see* GlyBURIDE *on page 734*
- ◆ **Diaminocyclohexane Oxalatoplatinum** *see* Oxaliplatin *on page 1179*
- ◆ **Diaminodiphenylsulfone** *see* Dapsone *on page 441*
- ◆ **Diamode [OTC]** *see* Loperamide *on page 952*
- ◆ **Diamox® (Can)** *see* AcetaZOLAMIDE *on page 47*
- ◆ **Diamox® Sequels®** *see* AcetaZOLAMIDE *on page 47*
- ◆ **Diarr-Eze (Can)** *see* Loperamide *on page 952*
- ◆ **Diasorb® [OTC]** *see* Attapulgite *on page 184*
- ◆ **Diastat®** *see* Diazepam *on page 481*
- ◆ **Diastat® AcuDial™** *see* Diazepam *on page 481*
- ◆ **Diastat® Rectal Delivery System (Can)** *see* Diazepam *on page 481*
- ◆ **Diazemuls® (Can)** *see* Diazepam *on page 481*

Diazepam (dye AZ e pam)

Medication Safety Issues
Sound-alike/look-alike issues:
Diazepam may be confused with diazoxide, Ditropan®, lorazepam
Valium® may be confused with Valcyte™

Related Information
Febrile Seizures *on page 1898*
Laboratory Detection of Drugs in Urine *on page 1928*
Overdose and Toxicology *on page 1916*
Preprocedure Sedatives in Children *on page 1895*

U.S. Brand Names Diastat®; Diastat® AcuDial™; Diazepam Intensol®; Valium®

Canadian Brand Names Apo-Diazepam®; Diastat®; Diastat® Rectal Delivery System; Diazemuls®; Novo-Dipam; Valium®

Therapeutic Category Antianxiety Agent; Anticonvulsant, Benzodiazepine; Benzodiazepine; Hypnotic; Sedative

Generic Available Yes: Injection, tablet, solution only

Use Management of general anxiety disorders, panic disorders; to provide preoperative sedation, light anesthesia, and amnesia; treatment of status epilepticus, alcohol withdrawal symptoms; used as a skeletal muscle relaxant; rectal gel is indicated for intermittent episodes of markedly increased seizure activity in epilepsy patients on stable anticonvulsant regimens

Restrictions C-IV

Pregnancy Risk Factor D

Lactation Enters breast milk/contraindicated (AAP rates "of concern")

Contraindications Hypersensitivity to diazepam or any component (see Warnings); possible cross-sensitivity with other benzodiazepines; do not use in a comatose patient, in those with pre-existing CNS depression, respiratory depression, narrow-angle glaucoma, or severe uncontrolled pain
(Continued)

Diazepam *(Continued)*

Warnings Abrupt discontinuation may cause withdrawal symptoms or seizures. Rapid I.V. push may cause sudden respiratory depression, apnea, or hypotension. Administration of rectal gel should only be performed by individuals trained to recognize characteristic seizure activity for which the product is indicated, and who are capable of monitoring patient's response to determine need for additional medical intervention. Injection and rectal gel contain benzoic acid, benzyl alcohol, and sodium benzoate; benzyl alcohol may cause allergic reactions in susceptible individuals; benzoic acid (benzoate) is a metabolite of benzyl alcohol; large amounts of benzyl alcohol (≥99 mg/kg/day) have been associated with a potentially fatal toxicity ("gasping syndrome") in neonates; the "gasping syndrome" consists of metabolic acidosis, respiratory distress, gasping respirations, CNS dysfunction (including convulsions, intracranial hemorrhage), hypotension and cardiovascular collapse; use diazepam products containing benzoic acid, benzyl alcohol, or sodium benzoate with caution in neonates; *in vitro* and animal studies have shown that benzoate displaces bilirubin from protein binding sites. Parenteral formulation contains propylene glycol which has been associated with toxicities when administered in high dosages.

Precautions Use with caution in patients receiving other CNS depressants, patients with low albumin, renal or hepatic dysfunction, and in neonates and young infants; neonates have decreased metabolism of diazepam and desmethyldiazepam (active metabolite), both can accumulate with repeated use and cause increased toxicity; modify dosage in patients with hepatic impairment

Adverse Reactions

Cardiovascular: Cardiac arrest, hypotension, bradycardia, cardiovascular collapse

Central nervous system: Drowsiness, somnolence, confusion, dizziness, fatigue, amnesia, slurred speech, ataxia, impaired coordination, paradoxical excitement or rage (rare)

Dermatologic: Rash, dermatitis

Local: Thrombophlebitis; pain with injection; tissue necrosis may occur following extravasation

Ocular: Blurred vision, diplopia

Respiratory: Decrease in respiratory rate, apnea, laryngospasm

Miscellaneous: Physical and psychological dependence with prolonged use

Drug Interactions Cytochrome P450 isoenzyme CYP2B6, CYP2C8, CYP2C9, CYP2C19 (minor), CYP3A3/4 (minor) and CYP3A5-7 substrate; isoenzyme CYP2C19 and CYP3A3/4 inhibitor; nordiazepam is a CYP1A2 isoenzyme substrate; desmethyldiazepam is a CYP2C19 isoenzyme substrate

CNS depressants (alcohol, barbiturates, opioids) may enhance sedation and respiratory depression of diazepam; enzyme inducers may increase the hepatic metabolism of diazepam; cimetidine and erythromycin may decrease the metabolism of diazepam; valproic acid may displace diazepam from binding sites which may result in an increase in sedative effects; concurrent use of diazepam with ritonavir is not recommended

Food Interactions Grapefruit juice significantly increases oral bioavailability of diazepam

Stability

Injection: Do not mix with other medications; protect from light

Rectal gel: Store at 25°C (77°F); excursions permitted to 15°C to 30°C (59°F to 86°F)

Mechanism of Action Depresses all levels of the CNS, including the limbic and reticular formation by binding to the benzodiazepine site on the gamma-aminobutyric acid (GABA) receptor complex and modulating GABA, which is a major inhibitory neurotransmitter in the brain

Pharmacodynamics Status epilepticus:

Onset of action:
- I.V.: 1-3 minutes
- Rectal: 2-10 minutes

Duration: 15-30 minutes

Pharmacokinetics

Absorption:
- Oral: 85% to 100%
- I.M.: Poor
- Rectal (gel): Well absorbed

Distribution: Widely distributed; crosses blood-brain barrier and placenta; distributes into breast milk

Protein binding:
- Neonates: 84% to 86%
- Adults: 98%

Metabolism: In the liver to desmethyldiazepam (active metabolite) and N-methyloxazepam (active metabolite); these are metabolized to oxazepam (active) which undergoes glucuronide conjugation before being excreted

Bioavailability: Rectal (gel): 90%
Half-life:
Diazepam:
Neonates: 50-95 hours
Infants 1 month to 2 years: 40-50 hours
Children 2-12 years: 15-21 hours
Children 12-16 years: 18-20 hours
Adults: 20-50 hours
Increased half-life in those with severe hepatic disorders
Desmethyldiazepam (active metabolite): 50-100 hours; may be further prolonged in neonates
Time to peak serum concentration: Rectal (gel): 1.5 hours
Elimination: In urine, primarily as conjugated oxazepam (75%), desmethyldiazepam, and N-methyloxazepam

Usual Dosage

Children:
Conscious sedation for procedures: Oral: 0.2-0.3 mg/kg (maximum dose: 10 mg) 45-60 minutes prior to procedure
Febrile seizure prophylaxis: Oral: 1 mg/kg/day divided every 8 hours; initiate therapy at first sign of fever and continue for 24 hours after fever is gone
Sedation or muscle relaxation or anxiety:
Oral: 0.12-0.8 mg/kg/day in divided doses every 6-8 hours
I.M., I.V.: 0.04-0.3 mg/kg/dose every 2-4 hours to a maximum of 0.6 mg/kg within an 8-hour period if needed
Status epilepticus: I.V.:
Neonates: (Not recommended as a first-line agent; injection contains benzoic acid, benzyl alcohol, and sodium benzoate; see Warnings) 0.1-0.3 mg/kg/dose given over 3-5 minutes, every 15-30 minutes to a maximum total dose of 2 mg
Infants >30 days and Children <5 years: 0.05-0.3 mg/kg/dose given over 3-5 minutes, every 15-30 minutes to a maximum total dose of 5 mg **or** 0.2-0.5 mg/dose every 2-5 minutes to a maximum total dose of 5 mg; repeat in 2-4 hours as needed
Children ≥5 years: 0.05-0.3 mg/kg/dose given over 3-5 minutes, every 15-30 minutes to a maximum total dose of 10 mg **or** 1 mg/dose every 2-5 minutes to a maximum of 10 mg; repeat in 2-4 hours as needed
Muscle spasm associated with tetanus: I.V., I.M.:
Infants >30 days: 1-2 mg/dose every 3-4 hours as needed
Children ≥5 years: 5-10 mg/dose every 3-4 hours as needed
Anticonvulsant: Acute treatment:
Rectal gel formulation:
Infants <6 months: Not recommended
Children <2 years: Safety and efficacy have not been studied
Children 2-5 years: 0.5 mg/kg
Children 6-11 years: 0.3 mg/kg
Children ≥12 years and Adults: 0.2 mg/kg
Note: Round dose to 2.5, 5, 7.5, 10, 12.5, 15, 17.5, and 20 mg/dose; dose may be repeated in 4-12 hours if needed; do not use more than 5 times per month or more than once every 5 days
Rectal: Undiluted 5 mg/mL parenteral formulation (filter if using ampul): 0.5 mg/kg/dose then 0.25 mg/kg/dose in 10 minutes if needed
Adolescents: Conscious sedation for procedures:
Oral: 10 mg
I.V.: 5 mg; may repeat with 2.5 mg if needed
Adults:
Anxiety:
Oral: 2-10 mg 2-4 times/day
I.M., I.V.: 2-10 mg, may repeat in 3-4 hours if needed
Skeletal muscle relaxation:
Oral: 2-10 mg 2-4 times/day
I.M., I.V.: 5-10 mg, may repeat in 2-4 hours
Status epilepticus: I.V.: 5-10 mg every 10-15 minutes up to 30 mg in an 8-hour period; may repeat in 2-4 hours
Preoperative medication: I.M.: 10 mg before surgery

Administration

Oral: Administer with food or water; do not administer with grapefruit juice; oral concentrate solution (5 mg/mL) should be diluted or mixed with water, juice, soda, applesauce, or pudding before use
Parenteral: I.V.: Rapid injection may cause respiratory depression or hypotension; infants and children: Do not exceed 1-2 mg/minute I.V. push; adults: Maximum infusion rate: 5 mg/minute; maximum concentration for administration: 5 mg/mL

(Continued)

Diazepam *(Continued)*

Rectal:

Diastat® AcuDial™: Prior to administration, confirm that the syringe is properly set to the correct dose and that the green "ready" band is visible.

Diastat® AcuDial™ and Diastat®: Place patient on side; remove protective cap and seal pin from syringe; lubricate rectal tip with lubricating jelly (provided in twin pack); turn patient on side facing you; bend upper leg forward and separate buttocks to expose rectum; insert syringe tip gently into rectum until rim fits snug against rectal opening; administer dose while slowly counting to 3 while gently pushing on plunger; slowly count to 3 again before removing syringe; hold buttocks together while slowly counting to 3 to prevent leakage; keep patient on side, facing towards you and continue to observe patient; discard any unused medication from AcuDial™, the syringe, and all used materials safely away from children; do not reuse; see Administration and Disposal Instructions that come with product.

Monitoring Parameters Heart rate, respiratory rate, blood pressure

Reference Range Effective therapeutic range not well established

Proposed therapeutic:

Diazepam: 0.2-1.5 mcg/mL (SI: 0.7-5.3 micromoles/L)

N-desmethyldiazepam (nordiazepam): 0.1-0.5 mcg/mL (SI: 0.35-1.8 micromoles/L)

Test Interactions False-negative urinary glucose determinations with Clinistix® or Diastix®

Patient Information Avoid alcohol and grapefruit juice; limit caffeine; may cause drowsiness and impair ability to perform activities requiring mental alertness or physical coordination; may be habit-forming; avoid abrupt discontinuation after prolonged use

Nursing Implications Avoid extravasation (tissue necrosis may occur); infuse I.V. into secure line using larger veins

Additional Information Diazepam does not have any analgesic effects. Diarrhea in a 9 month old infant receiving high-dose oral diazepam was attributed to the diazepam oral solution that contained polyethylene glycol and propylene glycol (both are osmotically active); diarrhea resolved when crushed tablets were substituted for the oral solution (see Marshall, 1995).

Diastat® AcuDial™: Prescribed dose must be "dialed in" and locked before dispensing; consult package insert for directions on setting prescribed dose; confirm green "ready" band is visible prior to dispensing product.

Dosage Forms Excipient information presented when available (limited, particularly for generics); consult specific product labeling.

Gel, rectal:

Diastat®: Pediatric rectal tip [4.4 cm]: 5 mg/mL (2.5 mg, 5 mg) [contains ethyl alcohol 10%, sodium benzoate, benzyl alcohol 1.5%; twin pack]

Diastat® AcuDial™ delivery system:

10 mg: Pediatric/adult rectal tip [4.4 cm]: 5 mg/mL (delivers set doses of 5 mg, 7.5 mg, and 10 mg) [contains ethyl alcohol 10%, sodium benzoate, benzyl alcohol 1.5%; twin pack]

20 mg: Adult rectal tip [6 cm]: 5 mg/mL (delivers set doses of 10 mg, 12.5 mg, 15 mg, 17.5 mg, and 20 mg) [contains ethyl alcohol 10%, sodium benzoate, benzyl alcohol 1.5%; twin pack]

Injection, solution: 5 mg/mL (2 mL, 10 mL) [may contain benzyl alcohol, sodium benzoate, benzoic acid]

Solution, oral: 5 mg/5 mL (5 mL, 500 mL) [wintergreen-spice flavor]

Solution, oral concentrate:

Diazepam Intensol®: 5 mg/mL (30 mL)

Tablet: 2 mg, 5 mg, 10 mg

Valium®: 2 mg, 5 mg, 10 mg

References

Dreifuss FE, Rosman NP, Cloyd JC, et al, "A Comparison of Rectal Diazepam Gel and Placebo for Acute Repetitive Seizures," *N Engl J Med*, 1998, 338(26):1869-75.

Marshall JD, Farrar HC, and Kearns GL, "Diarrhea Associated With Enteral Benzodiazepine Solutions," *J Pediatr*, 1995, 126(4):657-9.

Rosman NP, Colton T, Labazzo J, et al, "A Controlled Trial of Diazepam Administered During Febrile Illnesses to Prevent Recurrence of Febrile Seizures," *N Engl J Med*, 1993, 329(2):79-84.

Zeltzer LK, Altman A, Cohen D, et al, "Report of the Subcommittee on the Management of Pain Associated With Procedures in Children With Cancer," *Pediatrics*, 1990, 86(5 Pt 2):826-31.

♦ **Diazepam Intensol®** *see* Diazepam *on page 481*

Diazoxide (dye az OKS ide)

Medication Safety Issues

Sound-alike/look-alike issues:

Diazoxide may be confused with diazepam, Dyazide®

Hyperstat® may be confused with Nitrostat®

Related Information

Antihypertensive Agents by Class *on page 1678*

U.S. Brand Names Hyperstat® [DSC]; Proglycem®

Canadian Brand Names Proglycem®

Therapeutic Category Antihypertensive Agent; Antihypoglycemic Agent; Vasodilator

Generic Available No

Use

I.V.: Emergency lowering of blood pressure

Oral: Management of hypoglycemia related to hyperinsulinism secondary to: Islet cell adenoma, carcinoma, or hyperplasia; adenomatosis; nesidioblastosis (persistent hyperinsulinemic hypoglycemia of infancy); leucine sensitivity, or extrapancreatic malignancy

Pregnancy Risk Factor C

Lactation Excretion in breast milk unknown

Contraindications Hypersensitivity to diazoxide, any component, thiazides, or other sulfonamide derivatives; I.V. diazoxide is contraindicated in patients with aortic coarctation, arteriovenous shunts, dissecting aortic aneurysm

Precautions Use with caution in patients with diabetes mellitus, renal or liver disease, coronary artery disease, or cerebral vascular insufficiency

Adverse Reactions

Cardiovascular: Hypotension, tachycardia, flushing, edema (more common in young infants and adults), arrhythmias, angina, MI; CHF (due to sodium retention)

Central nervous system: Dizziness, seizure, headache; cerebral ischemia

Dermatologic: Rash, hirsutism

Endocrine & metabolic: Hyperglycemia, ketoacidosis, hyperuricemia, sodium and water retention

Gastrointestinal: Nausea, vomiting, anorexia, constipation

Hematologic: Leukopenia, thrombocytopenia

Local: Pain, burning, cellulitis/phlebitis upon extravasation

Neuromuscular & skeletal: Weakness

Miscellaneous: Extrapyramidal symptoms and development of abnormal facies with chronic oral use

Drug Interactions Diuretics and hypotensive agents may potentiate diazoxide adverse effects; use of I.V. diazoxide within 6 hours of the administration of beta-blockers, hydralazine, methyldopa, minoxidil, nitrates, papaverine-like drugs, prazosin, or reserpine is not recommended; diazoxide may increase phenytoin metabolism or free fraction; diazoxide may decrease warfarin protein binding

Stability Protect from light, heat, and freezing; avoid using darkened solutions

Mechanism of Action Inhibits insulin release from the pancreas; produces direct smooth muscle relaxation of the peripheral arterioles which results in decrease in blood pressure and reflex increase in heart rate and cardiac output

Pharmacodynamics

Hyperglycemic effects (oral):

Onset of action: Within 1 hour

Duration (normal renal function): 8 hours

Hypotensive effects (I.V.):

Maximum effect: Within 5 minutes

Duration: Usually 3-12 hours

Pharmacokinetics

Protein binding: >90%

Half-life:

Children: 9-24 hours

Adults: 20-36 hours

Elimination: 50% excreted unchanged in urine

Usual Dosage

Hyperinsulinemic hypoglycemia: Oral (**Note**: Use lower dose listed as initial dose):

Newborns and Infants: 8-15 mg/kg/day in divided doses every 8-12 hours

Children and Adults: 3-8 mg/kg/day in divided doses every 8-12 hours

Hypertension: I.V.: Children and Adults: 1-3 mg/kg (maximum dose: 150 mg in a single injection); repeat dose in 5-15 minutes until blood pressure adequately reduced; repeat administration every 4-24 hours; monitor blood pressure closely

(Continued)

Diazoxide *(Continued)*

Administration

Oral: Administer on an empty stomach 1 hour before or 1 hour after meals; shake suspension well before use

Parenteral: Do not administer I.M. or SubQ; administer I.V. (undiluted) by rapid I.V. injection over a period of 30 seconds or less

Monitoring Parameters Blood pressure, heart rate, blood glucose, serum uric acid; CBC, platelets

Nursing Implications Avoid extravasation (injection is alkaline and irritating to tissues); patient should remain supine during and for at least 1 hour after I.V. injection

Additional Information Patients may require a diuretic with repeated I.V. doses (due to sodium retention); usual duration of I.V. therapy is <4-5 days; use of injection >10 days is not recommended

Dosage Forms Excipient information presented when available (limited, particularly for generics); consult specific product labeling. [DSC] = Discontinued product

Capsule:

Proglycem®: 50 mg [not available in the U.S.]

Injection, solution:

Hyperstat®: 15 mg/mL (20 mL) [DSC]

Suspension, oral:

Proglycem®: 50 mg/mL (30 mL) [contains alcohol 7.25%; chocolate-mint flavor]

♦ **Dibenzyline®** *see* Phenoxybenzamine *on page 1247*

Dibucaine (DYE byoo kane)

U.S. Brand Names Nupercainal® [OTC]

Therapeutic Category Analgesic, Topical; Local Anesthetic, Topical

Generic Available Yes

Use Fast, temporary relief of pain and itching due to hemorrhoids, minor burns, other minor skin conditions

Pregnancy Risk Factor C

Contraindications Hypersensitivity to dibucaine, other amide-type anesthetics, or any component (see Warnings)

Warnings Some products may contain sulfites which may cause allergic reactions in susceptible individuals

Adverse Reactions

Cardiovascular: Edema

Dermatologic: Urticaria, cutaneous lesions, contact dermatitis

Local: Burning, tenderness, irritation, inflammation

Mechanism of Action Blocks both the initiation and conduction of nerve impulses by decreasing the neuronal membrane's permeability to sodium ions, which results in inhibition of depolarization with resultant blockade of conduction

Pharmacodynamics

Onset of action: Within 15 minutes

Duration: 2-4 hours

Pharmacokinetics Absorption: Poor through intact skin, but well absorbed through mucous membranes and excoriated skin

Usual Dosage Children and Adults:

Rectal: Hemorrhoids: Administer each morning, evening, and after each bowel movement

Topical: Apply gently to the affected areas; no more than 30 g for adults or 7.5 g for children should be used in any 24-hour period

Administration

Rectal: Insert ointment into rectum using a rectal applicator

Topical: Apply gently to affected areas; do not use near the eyes or over denuded surfaces or blistered areas

Dosage Forms Excipient information presented when available (limited, particularly for generics); consult specific product labeling.

Ointment: 1% (30 g, 454 g)

Nupercainal®: 1% (30 g, 60g) [contains sodium bisulfite]

♦ **DIC** *see* Dacarbazine *on page 433*

♦ **Dichysterol** *see* Dihydrotachysterol [DSC] *on page 502*

Diclofenac (dye KLOE fen ak)

Medication Safety Issues

Sound-alike/look-alike issues:

Diclofenac may be confused with Diflucan®, Duphalac®

Cataflam® may be confused with Catapres®
Voltaren® may be confused with tramadol, Ultram®, Verelan®

U.S. Brand Names Cataflam®; Solaraze®; Voltaren®; Voltaren Ophthalmic®; Voltaren®-XR

Canadian Brand Names Apo-Diclo®; Apo-Diclo Rapide®; Apo-Diclo SR®; Cataflam®; Novo-Difenac; Novo-Difenac K; Novo-Difenac-SR; Nu-Diclo; Nu-Diclo-SR; Pennsaid®; PMS-Diclofenac; PMS-Diclofenac SR; Riva-Diclofenac; Riva-Diclofenac-K; Voltaren®; Voltaren Ophtha®; Voltaren Rapide®

Index Terms Diclofenac Potassium; Diclofenac Sodium

Therapeutic Category Analgesic, Non-narcotic; Anti-inflammatory Agent; Nonsteroidal Anti-inflammatory Drug (NSAID), Ophthalmic; Nonsteroidal Anti-inflammatory Drug (NSAID), Oral

Generic Available Yes: Excludes gel, ophthalmic solution

Use

Oral: Acute treatment of mild to moderate pain; acute and chronic treatment of rheumatoid arthritis, ankylosing spondylitis, and osteoarthritis; used for juvenile rheumatoid arthritis, gout, dysmenorrhea

Ophthalmic solution: Treatment of postoperative inflammation after cataract extraction; temporary relief of pain and photophobia in patients undergoing corneal refractive surgery

Topical: Treatment of actinic keratosis in adults

Medication Guide An FDA-approved patient medication guide, which is available with the product information and at http://www.fda.gov/cder/Offices/ODS/medication_guides.htm, must be dispensed with this medication for each new outpatient prescription and refill.

Pregnancy Risk Factor Oral: C (D in 3rd trimester); Ophthalmic: C; Topical: B

Lactation Excretion in breast milk unknown/not recommended

Contraindications Hypersensitivity to diclofenac, any component (see Warnings), aspirin, or NSAIDs; active GI bleeding; ulcer disease; patients with the "aspirin triad" [asthma, rhinitis (with or without nasal polyps) and aspirin intolerance] (fatal asthmatic and anaphylactoid reactions may occur in these patients); porphyria

Warnings In April 2005, the FDA announced product labeling changes for all NSAIDs, including COX-2 selective and OTC medications; although revised product labeling is currently not available for all products, sample labeling and a template of the required medication guide are now available. Labels for prescription nonselective NSAIDs will contain a contraindication for use in patients who have recently undergone coronary artery bypass graft (CABG) surgery and a boxed warning concerning the potential for increased risk of cardiovascular (CV) events and GI bleeding associated with NSAID use. Patients at increased risk of adverse events include patients immediately post-operative from CABG surgery, and those with existing CAD, CVD, or history of TIA or stomach ulcers. Prescribers are encouraged to use the lowest effective NSAID dose for the shortest time based on individual patient treatment goals. Medication guides will be required for all prescription products. Complete details for the labeling update can be found on the following FDA website: http://www.fda.gov/medwatch/SAFETY/2005/safety05.htm#NSAID.

Oral use: Serious GI toxicities may occur including inflammation, ulceration, bleeding, or perforation; patients with a history of PUD or GI bleeding who use NSAIDs have a >10-fold higher risk for GI bleed; other factors which may increase risk for GI bleed include: Longer duration of NSAID treatment, use of oral corticosteroids or anticoagulants, alcoholism, smoking, overall poor health, and older age. Diclofenac is not recommended for use in patients with severe renal dysfunction (if therapy is needed, close monitoring of renal function is highly recommended).

Topical gel contains benzyl alcohol which may cause allergic reactions in susceptible individuals; large amounts of benzyl alcohol (≥99 mg/kg/day) have been associated with a potentially fatal toxicity ("gasping syndrome") in neonates; avoid use of diclofenac products containing benzyl alcohol in neonates; *in vitro* and animal studies have shown that benzoate, a metabolite of benzyl alcohol, displaces bilirubin from protein binding sites

Precautions Use with caution in patients with CHF, asthma, hypertension, fluid retention, dehydration (rehydrate patient before starting therapy), mild to moderate renal dysfunction, decreased hepatic function (dosage reduction may be required), history of GI disease, or those receiving anticoagulants, ACE inhibitors, or diuretics; patients should not wear soft contact lenses while using ophthalmic solution; do not apply topical gel to open skin wounds, infections, or exfoliative dermatitis; do not allow gel to come in contact with eyes; do not use topical gel in neonates, infants, or children

Adverse Reactions

Central nervous system: Dizziness, headache

Dermatologic: Rash, pruritus; topical use: Contact dermatitis, dry skin, rash, skin exfoliation (scaling), skin irritation

(Continued)

Diclofenac *(Continued)*

Endocrine & metabolic: Fluid retention

Gastrointestinal: Abdominal pain, indigestion, peptic ulcer, GI bleeding, GI perforation, constipation, diarrhea

Hematologic: Agranulocytosis, aplastic anemia (rare), inhibition of platelet aggregation

Hepatic: Elevated ALT or AST, hepatitis, jaundice

Ocular: With ophthalmic use, itching, tearing (allergic reaction); irritation, redness, burning; ocular irritation with use of hydrogel soft contact lenses

Otic: Tinnitus

Renal: Renal impairment, nephrotic-like syndrome

Drug Interactions Cytochrome P450 isoenzyme CYP2C8 and CYP2C9 substrate; CYP2C9 isoenzyme inhibitor

Diclofenac may increase serum concentrations of digoxin, methotrexate and lithium; may increase nephrotoxicity of cyclosporine; may decrease diuretic and antihypertensive effects of thiazides and furosemide; may decrease antihypertensive effects of ACE inhibitors and angiotensin II antagonists; diclofenac plus potassium-sparing diuretics may increase serum potassium; concomitant insulin or oral hypoglycemic agents may increase or decrease serum glucose; aspirin may decrease serum concentration of diclofenac (combination not recommended); gastric irritants (eg, aspirin, other NSAIDs, potassium supplements) may increase risk of GI irritation; **Note:** Concurrent use of oral NSAIDs or aspirin with diclofenac topical gel should be minimized

Food Interactions Delayed oral absorption has been reported with food for single doses but not with chronic multiple-dose administration

Stability

Ophthalmic solution: Store at room temperature; protect from light

Tablets: Store at ≤30°C (86°F); protect from moisture; dispense in tight container

Topical gel: Store at room temperature; protect from heat; do not freeze

Mechanism of Action Inhibits prostaglandin synthesis by decreasing the activity of the enzyme, cyclooxygenase, which results in decreased formation of prostaglandin precursors

Pharmacokinetics

Absorption: Topical gel: 10%

Distribution: V_d: Adults: 1.4 L/kg

Protein binding: >99%

Metabolism: In the liver; undergoes hydroxylation then glucuronide and sulfate conjugation

Bioavailability: Oral: 50%

Half-life: Adults: 2.3 hours

Time to peak serum concentration: Adults:

- Cataflam®: 1 hour
- Voltaren®: 2.22 hours
- Voltaren®-XR: 5.25 hours

Elimination: About 65% of the dose is eliminated in the urine and ~35% in the bile (primarily as conjugated forms); little or no unchanged drug is excreted in urine or bile

Usual Dosage Note: Cataflam® tablets are immediate release and is the formulation which should be used when prompt onset of pain relief is desired; Voltaren®-XR should not be used for acute pain relief due to its extended release

Oral:

- Children: 2-3 mg/kg/day divided 2-4 times/day
- Adults:
  - Rheumatoid arthritis:
    - Cataflam® or Voltaren®: 100-200 mg/day in 2-4 divided doses; maximum dose: 225 mg/day
    - Voltaren®-XR: 100 mg/day; dose may be increased to 100 mg twice daily; maximum dose: 200 mg/day
  - Osteoarthritis:
    - Cataflam® or Voltaren®: 100-150 mg/day in 2-3 divided doses
    - Voltaren®-XR: 100 mg/day
  - Ankylosing spondylitis: Voltaren®: 100-125 mg/day in 4-5 divided doses
  - Analgesia and primary dysmenorrhea: Cataflam®: 50 mg given 3 times/day; some patients may have better relief with an initial dose of 100 mg

Ophthalmic:

- Cataract surgery: Instill 1 drop into affected eye 4 times/day beginning 24 hours after cataract surgery and continuing for 2 weeks
- Corneal refractive surgery: Instill 1-2 drops into operative eye within the hour prior to surgery, within 15 minutes after surgery, and continuing 4 times/day for up to 3 days

Topical: Adults: Apply to affected area twice daily; recommended duration of therapy: 60-90 days

Administration

Ophthalmic: Avoid contact of bottle tip with skin or eye; apply finger pressure to lacrimal sac during and for 1-2 minutes after instillation to decrease risk of absorption and systemic effects

Oral: Administer with milk or food to decrease GI upset; do not chew or crush delayed release or extended release tablets, swallow whole

Topical: Apply a small amount of gel to affected area; smooth gently over lesion; usually 0.5 g of gel is used per 5 x 5 cm lesion site

Monitoring Parameters CBC, liver enzymes; monitor urine output, BUN, serum creatinine in patients receiving diuretics

Patient Information

Oral use: Avoid alcohol; report any signs of blood in stool, GI bleeding, weight gain, edema, skin rash, yellow skin

Ophthalmic use: Do not use hydrogel soft contact lenses during ophthalmic diclofenac therapy

Topical use: Avoid exposure to sunlight or sunlamps; notify physician if rash occurs

Additional Information Vomiting, drowsiness, and acute renal failure have been reported with overdoses; the safety of concurrent use of cosmetics, sunscreens, or other topical agents with diclofenac gel is not known

Dosage Forms Excipient information presented when available (limited, particularly for generics); consult specific product labeling. [DSC] = Discontinued product

Gel, as sodium:

Solaraze®: 30 mg/g (50 g)

Solution, ophthalmic, as sodium:

Voltaren Ophthalmic®: 0.1% (2.5 mL, 5 mL)

Tablet, as potassium: 50 mg

Cataflam®: 50 mg

Tablet, delayed release, enteric coated, as sodium: 50 mg, 75 mg

Voltaren®: 25 mg [DSC], 50 mg [DSC], 75 mg

Tablet, extended release, as sodium: 100 mg

Voltaren®-XR: 100 mg

References

Brogden RN, Heel RC, Pakes GE, et al, "Diclofenac Sodium: A Review of Its Pharmacological Properties and Therapeutic Use in Rheumatic Diseases and Pain of Varying Origin," *Drugs*, 1980, 20(1):24-48.

Haapasaari J, Wuolijoki E, and Ylijoki H, "Treatment of Juvenile Rheumatoid Arthritis With Diclofenac Sodium" *Scand J Rheumatol*, 1983, 12(4):325-30.

♦ **Diclofenac Potassium** *see* Diclofenac *on page 486*

♦ **Diclofenac Sodium** *see* Diclofenac *on page 486*

Dicloxacillin (dye kloks a SIL in)

Canadian Brand Names Dycill®; Pathocil®

Index Terms Dicloxacillin Sodium

Therapeutic Category Antibiotic, Penicillin (Antistaphylococcal)

Generic Available Yes

Use Treatment of skin and soft tissue infections, pneumonia and follow-up therapy of osteomyelitis caused by susceptible penicillinase-producing staphylococci

Pregnancy Risk Factor B

Lactation Excretion in breast milk unknown (probably similar to penicillin G)

Contraindications Hypersensitivity to dicloxacillin, penicillin, or any component

Warnings Elimination is prolonged in neonates

Adverse Reactions

Central nervous system: Fever

Dermatologic: Rash

Gastrointestinal: Nausea, vomiting, diarrhea, *C. difficile* colitis

Hematologic: Eosinophilia, neutropenia, leukopenia, thrombocytopenia

Hepatic: Elevated liver enzymes

Miscellaneous: Serum sickness-like reaction

Drug Interactions Oral contraceptives (decreased effectiveness), probenecid (increase serum concentration of dicloxacillin)

Food Interactions Food decreases the rate and extent of absorption

Mechanism of Action Inhibits bacterial cell wall synthesis by binding to one or more of the penicillin-binding proteins and interfering with the final transpeptidation step of peptidoglycan synthesis

Pharmacokinetics

Absorption: 35% to 76% absorbed from the GI tract

Distribution: Into bone, bile, pleural fluid, synovial fluid, and amniotic fluid; appears in breast milk

(Continued)

Dicloxacillin *(Continued)*

Protein binding: 96% to 98%
Half-life: Adults: 0.6-0.8 hours; slightly prolonged in patients with renal impairment
Time to peak serum concentration: Within 0.5-2 hours
Elimination: Partially eliminated by the liver and excreted in bile; 31% to 65% eliminated in urine as unchanged drug and active metabolite
Neonates: Prolonged
CF patients: More rapid elimination than healthy patients
Dialysis: Not dialyzable (0% to 5%)

Usual Dosage Oral:
Children <40 kg: 25-50 mg/kg/day divided every 6 hours; doses of 50-100 mg/kg/day in divided doses every 6 hours have been used for follow-up therapy of osteomyelitis; maximum dose: 2 g/day
Children >40 kg and Adults: 125-500 mg every 6 hours; maximum dose: 2 g/day

Administration Oral: Administer with water 1 hour before or 2 hours after meals on an empty stomach

Monitoring Parameters Periodic monitoring of CBC, platelet count, BUN, serum creatinine, urinalysis, and liver enzymes during prolonged therapy

Additional Information Sodium content of 250 mg capsule: 0.6 mEq

Dosage Forms Excipient information presented when available (limited, particularly for generics); consult specific product labeling.
Capsule: 250 mg, 500 mg

♦ **Dicloxacillin Sodium** *see* Dicloxacillin *on page 489*

Dicyclomine (dye SYE kloe meen)

Medication Safety Issues
Sound-alike/look-alike issues:
Dicyclomine may be confused with diphenhydrAMINE, doxycycline, dyclonine
Bentyl® may be confused with Aventyl®, Benadryl®, Bontril®, Cantil®, Proventil®, Trental®

Related Information
Overdose and Toxicology *on page 1916*

U.S. Brand Names Bentyl®

Canadian Brand Names Bentylol®; Formulex®; Lomine; Riva-Dicyclomine

Index Terms Dicyclomine Hydrochloride; Dicycloverine Hydrochloride

Therapeutic Category Anticholinergic Agent; Antispasmodic Agent, Gastrointestinal

Generic Available Yes: Excludes syrup

Use Treatment of functional bowel/irritable bowel syndrome

Pregnancy Risk Factor B

Lactation Enters breast milk/contraindicated

Contraindications Hypersensitivity to dicyclomine or any component; narrow-angle glaucoma, tachycardia, GI obstruction, obstruction of the urinary tract, severe ulcerative colitis, myasthenia gravis; should not be used in infants <6 months of age (due to reports of respiratory distress, seizures, syncope, asphyxia, pulse rate fluctuations, muscular hypotonia, and coma), nursing mothers

Warnings Heat prostration may occur in the presence of increased environmental temperature; use caution in hot weather and/or exercise. Psychosis has been reported in patients with an extreme sensitivity to anticholinergic effects.

Precautions Use with caution in patients with hepatic or renal disease, mild-moderate ulcerative colitis, hyperthyroidism, coronary heart disease, CHF, cardiac tachyarrhythmias, hypertension, hiatal hernia, autonomic neuropathy

Adverse Reactions Children with Down's syndrome, spastic paralysis, or brain damage are more sensitive to toxic effects than adults

Cardiovascular: Tachycardia, palpitations, orthostatic hypotension
Central nervous system: Seizures, coma, nervousness, excitement, confusion, insomnia, headache, dizziness, lightheadedness, drowsiness, lethargy, speech disturbance, syncope
Dermatologic: Urticaria, pruritus, dry skin, rash
Gastrointestinal: Nausea, vomiting, constipation, xerostomia, dry throat, dysphagia, taste loss, anorexia
Genitourinary: Urinary retention
Local: Injection site reactions (I.M. injection)
Neuromuscular & skeletal: Muscular hypotonia, weakness, tingling, numbness
Ocular: Blurred vision, diplopia, mydriasis, cycloplegia, increased ocular tension, photophobia
Respiratory: Respiratory distress, asphyxia, dry nose, nasal stuffiness, apnea, sneezing

Miscellaneous: Decreased diaphoresis

Drug Interactions Additive adverse effects when given with medications with anticholinergic activity; may alter GI absorption of various drugs due to prolonged GI transit time; antacids; antagonizes effects of antiglaucoma agents

Stability Protect from light

Mechanism of Action Blocks the action of acetylcholine at parasympathetic sites in smooth muscle, secretory glands and the CNS

Pharmacodynamics

Onset of action: 1-2 hours

Duration: Up to 4 hours

Pharmacokinetics

Absorption: Oral: Well absorbed

Distribution: V_d: 3.65 L/kg

Bioavailability: 67%

Half-life:

- Initial phase: 1.8 hours
- Terminal phase: 9-10 hours

Time to peak serum concentration: Oral: 1-1.5 hours

Elimination: 80% in urine; 10% in feces

Usual Dosage

Infants >6 months: Oral: 5 mg/dose 3-4 times/day

Children: Oral: 10 mg/dose 3-4 times/day

Adults:

- Oral: Initial: 20 mg 4 times/day, then increase up to 40 mg 4 times/day
- I.M.: 20 mg/dose 4 times/day; oral therapy should replace I.M. therapy as soon as possible

Administration

Oral: Administer 30 minutes before eating

Parenteral: I.M. only; not for I.V. use

Patient Information Limit alcohol; may cause dry mouth; may cause drowsiness and impair ability to perform activities requiring mental alertness or physical coordination

Dosage Forms Excipient information presented when available (limited, particularly for generics); consult specific product labeling.

Capsule, as hydrochloride: 10 mg

- Bentyl®: 10 mg

Injection, solution, as hydrochloride: 10 mg/mL (2 mL)

- Bentyl®: 10 mg/mL (2 mL)

Syrup, as hydrochloride:

- Bentyl®: 10 mg/5 mL (480 mL)

Tablet, as hydrochloride: 20 mg

- Bentyl®: 20 mg

♦ **Dicyclomine Hydrochloride** *see* Dicyclomine *on page 490*

♦ **Dicycloverine Hydrochloride** *see* Dicyclomine *on page 490*

Didanosine (dye DAN oh seen)

Medication Safety Issues

Sound-alike/look-alike issues:

- Videx® may be confused with Lidex®

Related Information

Adult and Adolescent HIV *on page 1821*

Pediatric HIV *on page 1816*

Perinatal HIV *on page 1831*

U.S. Brand Names Videx®; Videx® EC

Canadian Brand Names Videx®; Videx® EC

Index Terms ddI; Dideoxyinosine

Therapeutic Category Antiretroviral Agent; HIV Agents (Anti-HIV Agents); Nucleoside Reverse Transcriptase Inhibitor (NRTI)

Generic Available Yes: Delayed release capsule

Use Treatment of HIV infection in combination with other antiretroviral agents; (**Note:** HIV regimens consisting of **three** antiretroviral agents are strongly recommended)

Pregnancy Risk Factor B (**Note:** Fatal lactic acidosis has been reported in pregnant women who received the combination of didanosine and stavudine with other antiretroviral agents; see Warnings)

Lactation Excretion in breast milk unknown/contraindicated

Contraindications Hypersensitivity to didanosine or any component

Warnings Fatal and nonfatal pancreatitis have been reported during therapy; risk factors for developing pancreatitis include a previous history of the condition, higher doses (eg, >10 mg/kg/day), renal impairment without dose adjustment, concurrent

(Continued)

Didanosine *(Continued)*

CMV or MAC infection, advanced HIV infection, and concomitant use of stavudine with or without hydroxyurea; use didanosine with extreme caution and only if clearly indicated in patients with risk factors for pancreatitis; discontinue didanosine if clinical signs of pancreatitis occur; only after pancreatitis has been ruled out should dosing be resumed. Dose-related (treatment-limiting) peripheral neuropathy occurs most often after 2-6 months of continuous didanosine administration; may occur more frequently in patients with a history of neuropathy, advanced HIV disease, or concurrent treatment with neurotoxic drugs, including stavudine or hydroxyurea. Retinal depigmentation in children receiving doses >300 mg/m^2/day may occur; retinal changes and optic neuritis have been reported in pediatric and adult patients.

Cases of lactic acidosis, severe hepatomegaly with steatosis, and death have been reported in patients receiving nucleoside analogs; most of these cases have been in women; prolonged nucleoside use, obesity, and prior liver disease may be risk factors; use with extreme caution in patients with other risk factors for liver disease; discontinue therapy in patients who develop laboratory or clinical evidence of lactic acidosis or pronounced hepatotoxicity. Fatal lactic acidosis has occurred in pregnant women who received didanosine plus stavudine with other antiretroviral agents; use didanosine plus stavudine with caution during pregnancy and only if benefit outweighs risks.

Precautions Use with caution in patients on sodium-restricted diets, patients with history of pancreatitis, patients with hyperuricemia, and patients with renal or hepatic impairment. Adjust dosage in patients with renal impairment or peripheral neuropathy. Monitor patients with hepatic impairment closely; these patients may be at risk for didanosine-associated liver function abnormalities, including severe and potentially fatal hepatic adverse events. Avoid using the combination of didanosine, stavudine, and hydroxyurea; fatal hepatic events were reported most often in HIV patients receiving this combination.

Fat redistribution and accumulation [ie, central obesity, peripheral wasting, facial wasting, breast enlargement, dorsocervical fat enlargement (buffalo hump), and cushingoid appearance] have been observed in patients receiving antiretroviral agents (causal relationship not established). Immune reconstitution syndrome (an acute inflammatory response to residual or indolent opportunistic infections) may occur in HIV patients during initial treatment with combination antiretroviral agents, including didanosine; this syndrome may require further patient assessment and therapy.

Safety and efficacy of didanosine delayed-release capsules have not been established in pediatric patients. **Note:** Oral chewable buffered tablets are no longer available.

Adverse Reactions

Central nervous system: Headache, insomnia, malaise, CNS depression, fever

Dermatologic: Rash, pruritus, alopecia

Endocrine & metabolic: Hypokalemia, hyperuricemia, elevated triglycerides, hyperglycemia, lactic acidosis; fat redistribution and accumulation (see Precautions)

Gastrointestinal: Diarrhea, nausea, vomiting, anorexia, stomatitis, pancreatitis [Adults: 1% to 7%; dose-related, less common in children (up to 3% with normal doses) than adults], abdominal pain

Hepatic: Elevated liver enzymes, hepatic failure, elevated amylase

Neuromuscular & skeletal: Peripheral neuropathy (dose-related), myalgia, arthritis, weakness

Ocular: Retinal depigmentation, optic neuritis

Respiratory: Cough, dyspnea

Miscellaneous: Immune reconstitution syndrome

Drug Interactions Allopurinol may significantly increase didanosine serum concentrations (coadministration is **not** recommended). Ribavirin may increase intracellular triphosphate concentrations of didanosine and increase adverse effects (concomitant use is **not** recommended). Tenofovir significantly increases didanosine peak concentrations and AUC, potentially increasing didanosine-related adverse effects, such as pancreatitis, hyperglycemia, lactic acidosis, and peripheral neuropathy; some patients have experienced decreased CD4 cell counts and/or decreased virologic response; use didanosine with great caution and reduce the dose in patients receiving tenofovir; monitor patients closely; discontinue didanosine if adverse effects/toxicity develops. Use with stavudine significantly increases risks of potentially fatal lactic acidosis and pancreatitis (concurrent use **not** recommended unless benefit clearly outweighs risks). Use with hydroxyurea significantly increases risk of pancreatitis, hepatotoxicity, and neuropathy (concurrent use **not** recommended). Avoid the combination of hydroxyurea, didanosine, and stavudine (fatal hepatic events were reported most often in patients receiving this combination).

Antacids, omeprazole, ganciclovir, cimetidine, and ranitidine may increase serum concentrations of didanosine. Methadone decreases didanosine concentration. Didanosine buffered preparations decrease absorption of ketoconazole, itraconazole, indinavir, ganciclovir, dapsone, ciprofloxacin, tetracyclines (administer at least 2 hours before or 2 hours after didanosine). Drugs associated with peripheral neuropathy (cisplatin, isoniazid, metronidazole, phenytoin, vincristine, stavudine, zalcitabine, dapsone, ethambutol, ethionamide, hydralazine, and nitrofurantoin) may increase the risk for didanosine peripheral neuropathy. Drugs associated with pancreatitis (alcohol, I.V. pentamidine, stavudine) may increase the risk of pancreatitis. Concomitant administration of didanosine and delavirdine may decrease absorption of both drugs (separate dosing by at least 2 hours). Concomitant administration of didanosine and ritonavir may decrease AUC of didanosine.

Food Interactions Food significantly decreases bioavailability. Food decreases the bioavailability of the delayed release capsules by 19%. Do not mix with fruit juice or other acid-containing liquid since didanosine is unstable in acidic solutions

Stability Undergoes rapid degradation when exposed to an acidic environment; 10% of the drug decomposes to hypoxanthine in <2 minutes at pH <3 at 37°C.

Delayed release capsules: Store in tightly closed bottles at 25°C (77°F); excursions permitted to 15°C to 30°C (59°F to 86°F).

Powder for oral solution: Unreconstituted powder should be stored at 15°C to 30°C (59°F to 86°F). Powder for oral solution is unbuffered and must be reconstituted with water and mixed with an equal volume of double-strength antacid at time of preparation. Reconstituted solution (10 mg/mL) is stable for 30 days if refrigerated; discard unused portion after 30 days. When unbuffered powder for oral solution is reconstituted and admixed with a double-strength antacid to make a 20 mg/mL solution for adult once-daily dosing, the admixture is stable for 24 hours at room temperature and for 30 days if refrigerated

Mechanism of Action A purine dideoxynucleoside analog converted within the cell to an active metabolite, dideoxyadenosine triphosphate which serves as a substrate and inhibitor of viral RNA-directed DNA polymerase resulting in premature termination of viral DNA synthesis

Pharmacokinetics

Absorption: Subject to degradation by acidic pH of stomach; some formulations are buffered to resist acidic pH. Delayed release capsules contain enteric-coated beadlets which dissolve in the small intestine.

Distribution: Extensive intracellular distribution; crosses the placenta

- CSF/plasma ratio:
  - Infants 8 months to Adolescents 19 years: 46% (range: 12% to 85%)
  - Adults: 21%
- V_d:
  - Infants 8 months to Adolescents 19 years: 28 ± 15 L/m²
  - Adults: 43.7 ± 8.9 L/m²

Protein binding: <5%

Metabolism: Converted intracellularly to active triphosphate form; presumed to be metabolized via the same metabolic pathway as endogenous purines

Bioavailability: Variable and affected by the presence of food in the GI tract, gastric pH, and the dosage form administered

- Infants 8 months to Adolescents 19 years: 25% ± 20%
- Adults: 42% ± 12%

Half-life:

- Plasma:
  - Newborns (1 day old): 2 ± 0.7 hours
  - Infants 2 weeks to 4 months: 1.2 ± 0.3 hours
  - Infants 8 months to Adolescents 19 years: 0.8 ± 0.3 hours
  - Adults with normal renal function: 1.5 ± 0.4 hours
- Intracellular: Adults: 25-40 hours

Time to peak serum concentration: Delayed release capsules: 2 hours; Oral solution: 0.25-1.5 hours

Elimination: Unchanged drug excreted in urine

- Infants 8 months to Adolescents 19 years: 18% ± 10%
- Adults: 18% ± 8%

Usual Dosage Oral: (Use in combination with other antiretroviral agents):

Neonates and Infants 2 weeks to 8 months: Oral solution: 100 mg/m²/dose every 12 hours; **Note:** Due to age-related pharmacokinetic differences, a dose of 50 mg/m²/dose every 12 hours may be more appropriate in younger infants (2 weeks to 4 months of age) (Working Group, 2006).

Infants >8 months and Children:

Oral solution: 120 mg/m²/dose every 12 hours; **Note:** Pediatric clinical studies used doses of 90-150 mg/m²/dose every 12 hours; **Note:** Once-daily dosing is **not** recommended (very limited data is available; see Additional Information)

(Continued)

Didanosine *(Continued)*

Delayed-release capsule: Not approved for use; safety and efficacy have not been established; limited published literature exists. In a single-dose pharmacokinetic study in children 4-11.5 years of age (n=10; median age 7.6 years), a dose of 240 mg/m^2 was shown to have a similar plasma AUC as compared to the buffered formulation. However, 2 patients were excluded from data analysis, one due to extremely low didanosine serum concentrations throughout the dosing interval (see King, 2002). Doses of 240 mg/m^2 once daily, with a maximum of 400 mg once daily, are being studied in pediatric clinical trials.

Adolescents and Adults:

Oral solution: **Note:** Although once-daily dosing is available, it should only be considered for adolescent/adult patients whose management requires once-daily administration (eg, to enhance compliance); the preferred dosing frequency of didanosine oral solution is twice daily because there is more evidence to support the effectiveness of this dosing frequency

<60 kg: 125 mg every 12 hours **or** 250 mg once daily

≥60 kg: 200 mg every 12 hours or 400 mg once daily using a special Videx® solution in double-strength antacid which provides 400 mg/20 mL for once-daily dosing

Delayed-release capsule:

<60 kg: 250 mg once daily

≥60 kg: 400 mg once daily

Adults: **Coadministration with tenofovir:** Reduce the dose of didanosine when used in combination with tenofovir

Adults <60 kg: Didanosine 200 mg once daily with tenofovir 300 mg once daily

Adults ≥60 kg: Didanosine 250 mg once daily with tenofovir 300 mg once daily

Dosing adjustment in renal impairment: Adults: Dosing based on patient weight, creatinine clearance, and dosage form:

Dosing for patients <60 kg:

Cl_{cr} 30-59 mL/minute:

Oral solution: 75 mg twice daily or 150 mg once daily

Delayed-release capsule: 125 once daily

Cl_{cr} 10-29 mL/minute:

Oral solution: 100 mg once daily

Delayed-release capsule: 125 mg once daily

Cl_{cr} <10 mL/minute:

Oral solution: 75 mg once daily

Delayed-release capsule: Use alternate formulation

Dosing for patients ≥60 kg:

Cl_{cr} 30-59 mL/minute:

Oral solution: 100 mg twice daily or 200 mg once daily

Delayed-release capsule: 200 mg once daily

Cl_{cr} 10-29 mL/minute:

Oral solution: 150 mg once daily

Delayed-release capsule: 125 mg once daily

Cl_{cr} <10 mL/minute:

Oral solution: 100 mg once daily

Delayed-release capsule: 125 mg once daily

Dosage adjustment in patients requiring continuous ambulatory peritoneal dialysis (CAPD) or hemodialysis: Adults: Use dosing recommendations for patients with Cl_{cr} <10 mL/minute; supplemental doses following hemodialysis are not needed

Dosing adjustment in hepatic impairment: Monitor patients with hepatic impairment closely for didanosine toxicity. Effects of hepatic impairment on didanosine pharmacokinetics are unknown. Patients with hepatic impairment may be at increased risk for didanosine toxicities (see Warnings and Precautions).

Administration Oral: Administer oral solution and delayed release capsule on an empty stomach 30 minutes before or at least 2 hours after a meal. If administered with tenofovir, the delayed release capsule may be administered with a light meal or in the fasted state. Unbuffered pediatric powder should be reconstituted with water and admixed in equal parts with a double-strength antacid to provide a final concentration of 10 mg/mL; unbuffered pediatric powder has also been reconstituted and admixed with a double-strength antacid to provide a final concentration of 20 mg/mL to be used for once-daily dosing in adults; shake oral solution well before use. Administer at least 1 hour apart from indinavir or 2 hours apart from ritonavir; didanosine should be given at least 1 hour before or 2 hours after lopinavir/ritonavir.

Monitoring Parameters Serum potassium, glucose, uric acid, lactic acid, creatinine; hemoglobin, CBC with neutrophil and platelet count, CD4 cells; HIV RNA plasma level; liver function tests, serum amylase and triglyceride levels; weight gain; perform dilated retinal exam every 6 months; signs and symptoms of peripheral neuropathy

Patient Information Didanosine is not a cure for HIV. Avoid alcohol. The buffered powder vehicle may contribute to the development of diarrhea. Inform physician if numbness, tingling or pain in hands or feet, persistent severe abdominal pain, nausea, or vomiting occurs. Shake oral solution well before use and keep refrigerated; discard solution after 30 days and obtain new supply. Take didanosine every day as prescribed; do not change dose or discontinue without physician's advice. If a dose is missed, take it as soon as possible, then return to normal dosing schedule; if a dose is skipped, do **not** double the next dose.

HIV medications may cause changes in body fat, including an increase in fat in the upper back and neck, breasts, and trunk; a loss of fat from the face, arms, and legs may also occur.

Additional Information The relative bioavailability of didanosine suspension administered once daily versus twice daily was studied in 24 children, 4.8 ± 2.9 years of age. Didanosine was administered in doses of 90 mg/m^2/dose every 12 hours and 180 mg/m^2/dose once daily. The relative bioavailability of once-daily dosing compared to twice daily dosing was 0.95 ± 0.49 (range: 0.22-1.97). The authors suggest these results support the potential clinical use of once-daily dosing in pediatric patients. However, due to the large inter- and intrasubject variability, these 2 regimens would **not** be considered to be bioequivalent based on FDA criteria (see Abreu, 2000). Further studies are needed.

A high rate of early virologic failure in therapy-naive adult HIV patients has been observed with the once-daily three-drug combination therapy of didanosine enteric-coated beadlets (Videx® EC), lamivudine, and tenofovir and the once-daily three-drug combination therapy of abacavir, lamivudine, and tenofovir. These combinations should not be used or offered at any time. Any patient currently receiving either of these regimens should be closely monitored for virologic failure and considered for treatment modification. Early virologic failure was also observed in therapy-naive adult HIV patients treated with tenofovir, didanosine enteric-coated beadlets (Videx® EC), and either efavirenz or nevirapine; rapid emergence of resistant mutations has also been reported with this combination; the combination of tenofovir, didanosine, and any non-nucleoside reverse transcriptase inhibitor is **not** recommended as initial antiretroviral therapy. **Note:** Didanosine plus tenofovir is **not** recommended as a component to any initial antiretroviral therapy regimen.

Dosage Forms Excipient information presented when available (limited, particularly for generics); consult specific product labeling.

Capsule, delayed release, enteric coated pellets: 200 mg, 250 mg, 400 mg

Capsule, delayed release, enteric coated beadlets:

Videx® EC: 125 mg, 200 mg, 250 mg, 400 mg

Powder for oral solution, pediatric:

Videx®: 2 g, 4 g [makes 10 mg/mL solution after final mixing]

References

Abreu T, Plaisance K, Rexroad V, et al, "Bioavailability of Once- and Twice-Daily Regimens of Didanosine in Human Immunodeficiency Virus-Infected Children," *Antimicrob Agents Chemother*, 2000, 44(5):1375-6.

Balis FM, Pizzo PA, Butler KM, et al, "Clinical Pharmacology of 2′, 3′-Dideoxyinosine in Human Immunodeficiency Virus-Infected Children," *J Infect Dis*, 1992, 165(1):99-104.

Briars LA, Hilao JJ, and Kraus DM, "A Review of Pediatric Human Immunodeficiency Virus Infection," *Journal of Pharmacy Practice*, 2004, 17(6):407-31.

Butler KM, Husson RN, Balis FM, et al, "Dideoxyinosine in Children With Symptomatic Human Immunodeficiency Virus Infection," *N Engl J Med*, 1991, 324(3):137-44.

King JR, Nachman S, Yogev R, et al, "Single-Dose Pharmacokinetics of Enteric-Coated Didanosine in HIV-Infected Children," *Antivir Ther*, 2002, 7(4):267-70.

Panel on Clinical Practices for Treatment of HIV Infection, "Guidelines for the Use of Antiretroviral Agents in HIV-Infected Adults and Adolescents," October 10, 2006, http://www.aidsinfo.nih.gov.

Working Group on Antiretroviral Therapy and Medical Management of HIV-Infected Children, "Guidelines for the Use of Antiretroviral Agents in Pediatric HIV Infection," October 26, 2006, http://www.aidsinfo.nih.gov.

♦ **2′,3′-didehydro-3′-deoxythymidine** *see* Stavudine *on page 1472*

♦ **Dideoxycytidine** *see* Zalcitabine [DSC] *on page 1634*

♦ **Dideoxyinosine** *see* Didanosine *on page 491*

♦ **Didronel®** *see* Etidronate Disodium *on page 622*

♦ **Differin®** *see* Adapalene *on page 57*

♦ **Differin® XP (Can)** *see* Adapalene *on page 57*

♦ **Diflucan®** *see* Fluconazole *on page 660*

♦ **Digibind®** *see* Digoxin Immune Fab *on page 498*

♦ **DigiFab™** *see* Digoxin Immune Fab *on page 498*

♦ **Digitek®** *see* Digoxin *on page 496*

Digoxin (di JOKS in)

Medication Safety Issues

Sound-alike/look-alike issues:

Digoxin may be confused with Desoxyn®, doxepin

Lanoxin® may be confused with Lasix®, Levoxyl®, Levsinex®, Lomotil®, Lonox®, Mefoxin®, Xanax®

International issues:

Dilacor®: Brand name for diltiazem in the U.S.; brand name for verapamil in Brazil; brand name for barnidipine in Argentina

Lanoxin® may be confused with Lemoxin® which is a brand bane for cefuroxime in Mexico

Lanoxin® may be confused with Limoxin® which is a brand name for amoxicillin in Mexico

Related Information

Adult ACLS Algorithms *on page 1660*

Blood Level Sampling Time Guidelines *on page 1914*

Overdose and Toxicology *on page 1916*

U.S. Brand Names Digitek®; Lanoxicaps®; Lanoxin®

Canadian Brand Names Apo-Digoxin®; Digoxin CSD; Lanoxicaps®; Lanoxin®; Novo-Digoxin; Pediatric Digoxin CSD

Therapeutic Category Antiarrhythmic Agent, Miscellaneous; Cardiac Glycoside

Generic Available Yes: Excludes capsule

Use Treatment of CHF; slows the ventricular rate in tachyarrhythmias such as atrial fibrillation, atrial flutter, supraventricular tachycardia

Pregnancy Risk Factor C

Lactation Enters breast milk (small amounts)/compatible

Contraindications Hypersensitivity to digoxin, other digitalis preparations, or any component; ventricular fibrillation, A-V block, idiopathic hypertrophic subaortic stenosis, or constrictive pericarditis

Warnings Use with extreme caution in patients with hypoxia, hypothyroidism, acute myocarditis, electrolyte disorders, acute MI

Precautions Use with caution and reduce dosage in patients with renal impairment

Adverse Reactions

Cardiovascular: Sinus bradycardia, A-V block, S-A block, atrial or nodal ectopic beats, ventricular arrhythmias, bigeminy, trigeminy, atrial tachycardia with A-V block

Central nervous system: Drowsiness, fatigue, headache, lethargy, vertigo, disorientation

Endocrine & metabolic: Hyperkalemia with acute toxicity

Gastrointestinal: Vomiting, nausea, feeding intolerance, abdominal pain, diarrhea

Neuromuscular & skeletal: Neuralgia

Ocular: Blurred vision, halos, yellow or green vision, diplopia, photophobia, flashing lights

Drug Interactions Antacids, kaolin-pectin, cholestyramine, cisapride, colestipol, sucralfate, and metoclopramide may decrease absorption of digoxin; quinidine, nifedipine, itraconazole, indomethacin, verapamil, diltiazem, flecainide, amiodarone, erythromycin, propafenone, tetracycline, and spironolactone may increase digoxin serum concentration; the herbal medicine St John's wort (*Hypericum perforatum*) may significantly decrease digoxin serum concentrations; penicillamine may decrease digoxin's pharmacologic effects; calcium (especially rapid I.V. use) may cause severe arrhythmias; paroxetine may decrease the AUC of digoxin by 15%; ritonavir may increase or decrease digoxin levels (close monitoring of digoxin levels is recommended); suspected interaction with nevirapine (careful monitoring is recommended)

Food Interactions Meals containing increased fiber (bran) or foods high in pectin, may decrease oral absorption of digoxin; avoid natural licorice (causes sodium and water retention and increases potassium loss); maintain adequate amounts of potassium in diet to decrease risk of hypokalemia (hypokalemia may increase risk of digoxin toxicity)

Stability I.V. solution compatibility: D_5W, $D_{10}W$, NS, SWI (when diluted fourfold or greater); do not mix with other drugs; store at room temperature; protect from light

Mechanism of Action Increases the influx of calcium ions, from extracellular to intracellular cytoplasm by inhibition of sodium and potassium ion movement across the myocardial membranes; this increase in calcium ions results in a potentiation of the activity of the contractile heart muscle fibers and an increase in the force of myocardial contraction (positive inotropic effect); inhibits adenosine triphosphatase (ATPase); decreases conduction through the S-A and A-V nodes

Pharmacodynamics

Onset of action:

Oral: 0.5-2 hours

I.V.: 5-30 minutes

Maximum effect:

Oral: 2-8 hours

I.V.: 1-4 hours

Duration (adults): 3-4 days

Pharmacokinetics

Distribution: Distribution phase: 6-8 hours

V_d:

Neonates, full-term: 7.5-10 L/kg

Children: 16 L/kg

Adults: 7 L/kg

Renal disease: Decreased V_d

Protein binding: 20% to 25%

Bioavailability (dependent upon formulation):

Capsules: 90% to 100%

Elixir: 70% to 85%

Tablets: 60% to 80%

Half-life, elimination (dependent upon age, renal and cardiac function):

Premature: 61-170 hours

Neonates, full-term: 35-45 hours

Infants: 18-25 hours

Children: 35 hours

Adults: 38-48 hours

Anephric adults: >4.5 days

Anuric adults: 3.5-5 days

Elimination: 50% to 70% excreted unchanged in urine

Dialysis: Nondialyzable (0% to 5%)

Usual Dosage Dosage must be individualized due to substantial individual variation; table lists dosage recommendations based on average patient response.

Dosage Recommendations for Digoxin[1]

Age	Total Digitalizing Dose[2] (mcg/kg)		Daily Maintenance Dose[3] (mcg/kg)	
	P.O.	I.V. or I.M.	P.O.	I.V. or I.M.
Neonates				
Preterm	20-30	15-25	5-7.5	4-6
Full-term	25-35	20-30	6-10	5-8
Infants and Children				
1 mo - 2 y	35-60	30-50	10-15	7.5-12
2-5 y	30-40	25-35	7.5-10	6-9
5-10 y	20-35	15-30	5-10	4-8
>10 y	10-15	8-12	2.5-5	2-3
Adults	0.75-1.5 mg	0.5-1 mg	0.125-0.5 mg	0.1-0.4 mg

[1]Based on lean body weight and normal renal function for age. Decrease maintenance dose in patients with decreased renal function and decrease total digitalizing dose by 50% in end-stage renal disease.

[2]Give one-half of the total digitalizing dose (TDD) in the initial dose, then give one-quarter of the TDD in each of two subsequent doses at 6- to 12-hour intervals. Obtain EKG 6 hours after each dose to assess potential toxicity.

[3]Divided every 12 hours in infants and children <10 years of age. Given once daily to children >10 years of age and adults.

Dosing adjustment in renal impairment: (Monitor patient closely):

Total digitalizing dose: Reduce by 50% in end-stage renal disease

Maintenance dose:

Cl_{cr} 10-50 mL/minute: Administer 25% to 75% of normal daily dose (divided and given at normal intervals) or administer normal dose every 36 hours

Cl_{cr} <10 mL/minute: Administer 10% to 25% of normal daily dose (divided and given at normal intervals) or give normal dose every 48 hours

Administration

Oral: Administer consistently with relationship to meals; avoid concurrent administration (ie, administer digoxin 1 hour before or 2 hours after) with meals high in fiber or pectin and with drugs that decrease oral absorption of digoxin

(Continued)

Digoxin *(Continued)*

Parenteral: Administer I.V. doses (undiluted or diluted at least fourfold) slowly over 5-10 minutes; avoid rapid I.V. infusion since this may result in systemic and coronary arteriolar vasoconstriction; I.M. route not usually recommended due to local irritation, pain, and tissue damage

Monitoring Parameters Heart rate and rhythm, periodic EKG; follow serum potassium, magnesium, and calcium closely (especially in patients receiving diuretics or amphotericin); decreased serum potassium and magnesium, or increased serum magnesium and calcium may increase digoxin toxicity; assess renal function (serum BUN, S_{cr}) in order to adjust dose; obtain serum drug concentrations at least 8-12 hours after a dose, preferably prior to next scheduled dose

Reference Range Therapeutic: 0.8-2 ng/mL (SI: 1.0-2.6 nmol/L); Adults: <0.5 ng/mL (SI: <0.6 nmol/L) probably indicates underdigitalization unless there are special circumstances. Toxicity usually associated with levels >2 ng/mL (SI: >2.6 nmol/L). **Note**: Serum concentration must be used in conjunction with clinical symptoms and EKG to confirm diagnosis of digoxin intoxication.

Test Interactions Spironolactone may interfere with digoxin radioimmunoassay

Patient Information Notify physician if decreased appetite, nausea, vomiting, diarrhea, or visual changes occur; avoid the herbal medicine St John's wort

Additional Information Digoxin-like immunoreactive substance (DLIS) may cross-react with digoxin immunoassay and falsely increase serum concentrations; DLIS has been found in patients with renal dysfunction, liver disease, CHF, neonates, and pregnant women (third trimester)

Dosage Forms Excipient information presented when available (limited, particularly for generics); consult specific product labeling. [CAN] = Canadian brand name

Capsule:
  Lanoxicaps®: 100 mcg, 200 mcg [contains ethyl alcohol]
Injection, solution: 250 mcg/mL (1 mL, 2 mL)
  Lanoxin®: 250 mcg/mL (2 mL) [contains alcohol 10% and propylene glycol 40%]
Injection, solution [pediatric]: 100 mcg/mL (1 mL)
Solution, oral: 50 mcg/mL (2.5 mL, 5 mL, 60 mL)
Tablet: 125 mcg, 250 mcg
  Digitek®, Lanoxin®: 125 mcg, 250 mcg
  Apo-Digoxin® [CAN]: 62.5 mcg, 125 mcg, 250 mcg

References

Bakir M and Bilgic A, "Single Daily Dose of Digoxin for Maintenance Therapy of Infants and Children With Cardiac Disease: Is It Reliable?" *Pediatr Cardiol*, 1994, 15(5):229-32.

Bendayan R and McKenzie MW, "Digoxin Pharmacokinetics and Dosage Requirements in Pediatric Patients," *Clin Pharm*, 1983, 2(3):224-35.

Johne A, Brockmoller J, Bauer S, et al, "Pharmacokinetic Interaction of Digoxin With an Herbal Extract From St John's Wort (*Hypericum perforatum*)," *Clin Pharmacol Ther*, 1999, 66(4):338-45.

Park MK, "Use of Digoxin in Infants and Children With Specific Emphasis on Dosage," *J Pediatr*, 1986, 108(6):871-7.

♦ **Digoxin CSD (Can)** *see* Digoxin *on page 496*

Digoxin Immune Fab (di JOKS in i MYUN fab)

Related Information

Commonly Used Antidotes for Acute Overdoses *on page 1920*

U.S. Brand Names Digibind®; DigiFab™

Canadian Brand Names Digibind®

Index Terms Antidigoxin Fab Fragments, Ovine

Therapeutic Category Antidote, Digoxin

Generic Available No

Use Treatment of potentially life-threatening digoxin or digitoxin intoxication in carefully selected patients; use in life-threatening ventricular arrhythmias secondary to digoxin, acute digoxin ingestion (ie, >10 mg in adults or >4 mg in children), hyperkalemia (serum potassium >5 mEq/L) in the setting of digoxin toxicity

Pregnancy Risk Factor C

Lactation Excretion in breast milk unknown/use caution

Contraindications Hypersensitivity to digoxin immune fab, ovine (sheep) proteins, or (DigiFab™ only) papain, chymopapain, other papaya extracts, or the pineapple enzyme bromelain

Warnings Hypokalemia has been reported to occur following reversal of digitalis intoxication; monitor serum potassium levels closely; Fab fragments may be eliminated more slowly in patients with renal failure; heart failure may be exacerbated as digoxin level is reduced; total serum digoxin concentration may rise precipitously following administration of digoxin immune Fab, but this will be almost entirely bound to the Fab fragment and not able to react with receptors in the body; digoxin immune

Fab will interfere with digitalis immunoassay measurements - this will result in clinically misleading serum digoxin concentrations until the Fab fragment is eliminated from the body (several days to >1 week after digoxin immune Fab administration); serum digoxin levels drawn prior to therapy may be difficult to evaluate if 6-8 hours have not elapsed after the last dose of digoxin (time to equilibration between serum and tissue); redigitalization should not be initiated until Fab fragments have been eliminated from the body, which may occur over several days or greater than a week in patients with impaired renal function

Precautions Use with caution in renal or cardiac failure; allergic reactions possible; epinephrine should be immediately available; patients may deteriorate due to withdrawal of digoxin and may require I.V. inotropic support (eg, dobutamine) or vasodilators

Adverse Reactions

Cardiovascular: Worsening of low cardiac output or CHF, rapid ventricular response in patients with atrial fibrillation as digoxin is withdrawn

Dermatologic: Urticarial rash

Endocrine & metabolic: Hypokalemia

Miscellaneous: Facial edema and redness, allergic reactions

Stability Store in refrigerator; reconstituted solutions are stable 4 hours at 2°C to 8°C

Mechanism of Action Binds with molecules of free (unbound) digoxin or digitoxin and then is removed from the body by renal excretion

Pharmacodynamics Onset of action: Improvement in signs and symptoms occurs within 2-30 minutes following I.V. infusion

Pharmacokinetics

Distribution: V_d:

Digibind®: 0.3 L/kg

DigiFab™: 0.4 L/kg

Half-life: Renal impairment prolongs the half-life of both agents:

Digibind®: 15-20 hours

DigiFab™: 15 hours

Elimination: Renal with levels declining to undetectable amounts within 5-7 days

Usual Dosage To determine the dose of digoxin immune Fab, first determine the total body load of digoxin (TBL) or digitoxin (depending upon which product was ingested) as follows (using either an approximation of the amount ingested or a postdistribution serum digoxin/digitoxin concentration (C)):

TBL of **digoxin** (in mg) = C (in ng/mL) x 5.6 x body weight (in kg)/1000

or

TBL = mg of **digoxin** ingested (as tablets or elixir) x 0.8

TBL of **digitoxin** (mg) = C (in ng/mL) x 0.56 x body weight (in kg)/1000

or

TBL of **digitoxin** (in mg) = mg digitoxin ingested

Dose of Digibind® **(in mg)** I.V. = TBL x 76

Dose of DigiFab™ **(in mg)** I.V. = TBL x 80

Dose of digoxin immune Fab (Digibind® or DigiFab™) **(# vials)** I.V. = TBL/0.5

See tables below and on next page.

Infants and Children Dose Estimates of Digoxin Immune Fab (in mg)[1] From Serum Digoxin Concentration

Patient Weight (kg)	Serum Digoxin Concentration (ng/mL) 1	2	4	8	12	16	20
1	0.4 mg[2]	1 mg[2]	1.5 mg[2]	3 mg	5 mg	6-6.5 mg	8 mg
3	1 mg[2]	2-2.5 mg[2]	5 mg	9-10 mg	14 mg	18-19 mg	23-24 mg
5	2 mg[2]	4 mg	8 mg	15-16 mg	23-24 mg	30-32 mg	38-40 mg
10	4 mg	8 mg	15-16 mg	30-32 mg	46-48 mg	61-64 mg	76-80 mg
20	8 mg	15-16 mg	30-32 mg	61-64 mg	91-96 mg	122-128 mg	152-160 mg

[1]When a range in dose is listed, the lower number represents the Digibind® dose and the higher number represents the Digifab™ dose. A single dose is the same for both products.

[2]Dilution of reconstituted vial to 1 mg/mL may be desirable.

Administration Parenteral: I.V.: Digibind® is reconstituted by adding 4 mL SWI, resulting in a 9.5 mg/mL concentration for I.V. infusion; DigiFab™ is reconstituted with 4 mL SWI, resulting in an 10 mg/mL concentration for I.V. infusion; both formulations may be further diluted with NS to a convenient volume (eg, 1 mg/mL); infuse over

(Continued)

Digoxin Immune Fab *(Continued)*

15-30 minutes; to remove protein aggregates, 0.22 micron in-line filter is needed (Digibind® only)

Adult Dose Estimate of Digoxin Immune Fab (in # of Vials) From Serum Digoxin Concentration

Patient Weight (kg)	Serum Digoxin Concentration (ng/mL)						
	1	2	4	8	12	16	20
40	0.5 v	1 v	2 v	3 v	5 v	7 v	8 v
60	0.5 v	1 v	3 v	5 v	7 v	10 v	12 v
70	1 v	2 v	3 v	6 v	9 v	11 v	14 v
80	1 v	2 v	3 v	7 v	10 v	13 v	16 v
100	1 v	2 v	4 v	8 v	12 v	16 v	20 v

v = vials

Monitoring Parameters Serum potassium; serum digoxin/digitoxin level prior to first dose of digoxin immune Fab; (digoxin levels will greatly increase with digoxin immune Fab use and are not an accurate determination of body stores); continuous EKG monitoring

Additional Information Each 38 mg vial (Digibind®) or 40 mg vial (DigiFab™) will bind approximately 0.5 mg digoxin or digitoxin; for individuals at increased risk of sensitivity (see Contraindications) an intradermal or scratch technique skin test using a 1:100 dilution of reconstituted digoxin immune Fab diluted in NS has been used. Skin test volume is 0.1 mL of 1:100 dilution; evaluate after 20 minutes.

Dosage Forms Excipient information presented when available (limited, particularly for generics); consult specific product labeling.

Injection, powder for reconstitution:
Digibind®: 38 mg
DigiFab™: 40 mg

References

Hickey AR, Wenger TL, Carpenter VP, et al, "Digoxin Immune Fab Therapy in the Management of Digitalis Intoxication: Safety and Efficacy Results of an Observational Surveillance Study," *J Am Coll Cardiol*, 1991, 17(3):590-8.

Dihydroergotamine (dye hye droe er GOT a meen)

U.S. Brand Names D.H.E. 45®; Migranal®

Canadian Brand Names Migranal®

Index Terms DHE; Dihydroergotamine Mesylate

Therapeutic Category Alpha-Adrenergic Blocking Agent, Intranasal; Alpha-Adrenergic Blocking Agent, Parenteral; Antimigraine Agent; Ergot Alkaloid and Derivative

Generic Available Yes: Injection

Use Treatment of migraine headache with or without aura; injection also indicated for treatment of cluster headaches

Pregnancy Risk Factor X

Lactation May be excreted in breast milk/contraindicated

Contraindications Hypersensitivity to dihydroergotamine, other ergot alkaloids, caffeine (nasal spray only), or any component; pregnancy; patients with uncontrolled hypertension, ischemic heart disease, angina pectoris, history of MI, silent ischemia, or coronary artery vasospasm including Prinzmetal's angina; patients with hemiplegic or basilar migraine; patients with peripheral vascular disease, sepsis, severe hepatic or renal dysfunction, and following vascular surgery; do not use within 24 hours of sumatriptan, zolmitriptan, other serotonin agonists, or ergot-like agents; do not use during or within 2 weeks of discontinuing MAO inhibitors; do not coadminister with potent cytochrome P450 isoenzyme CYP3A4 inhibitors (clarithromycin, erythromycin, itraconazole, and ketoconazole), protease inhibitors (indinavir, ritonavir, saquinavir, nelfinavir, amprenavir, lopinavir, or ritonavir), efavirenz, or delavirdine (see Drug Interactions)

Warnings May cause vasospastic reactions; persistent vasospasm may lead to gangrene or death in patients with compromised circulation; discontinue if signs of vasoconstriction develop; rare reports of increased blood pressure in patients without history of hypertension; rare reports of adverse cardiac events (acute MI, life-threatening arrhythmias, death) have been reported following use of the injection; cerebral hemorrhage, subarachnoid hemorrhage, and stroke have also occurred following use of the injection; serious and/or life-threatening cerebral and peripheral ischemia have been associated with concomitant use of dihydroergotamine with potent cytochrome P450 isoenzyme CYP3A4 inhibitors, including macrolide antibiotics (erythromycin, clarithromycin) and protease inhibitors due to increased serum levels of dihydroergotamine (see Contraindications and Drug Interactions)

Precautions Prolonged use has been associated with fibrotic changes to heart and pulmonary valves (see Adverse Reactions); use with caution and only after a satisfactory cardiovascular evaluation has been performed in patients with risk factors for CAD; it is also recommended in these patients that the healthcare provider should administer the first dose; cardiovascular status should be periodically evaluated

Adverse Reactions

Cardiovascular: Cerebral hemorrhage, coronary artery vasospasm, edema, flushing, hypertension, MI, myocardial ischemia, palpitations, subarachnoid hemorrhage, transient ventricular tachycardia, ventricular fibrillation, tachycardia, bradycardia; fibrotic thickening of the aortic, mitral, tricuspid, and/or pulmonary valves (rare)

Central nervous system: Dizziness, somnolence, anxiety, headache, stroke

Dermatologic: Rash, pruritus

Endocrine & metabolic: Hot flashes

Gastrointestinal: Nausea, taste disturbance, vomiting, diarrhea, abdominal pain, cramps, diarrhea, xerostomia

Local: Application site reaction

Neuromuscular & skeletal: Asthenia, stiffness, hyperkinesis, muscular weakness, myalgia, paresthesia, tremor

Respiratory:

Nasal spray: Pharyngitis, rhinitis, nasal congestion, rhinorrhea, sneezing, nasal edema

Injection: Pleuropulmonary fibrosis

Miscellaneous: Retroperitoneal fibrosis (injection), increased sweating

Drug Interactions Cytochrome P450 isoenzyme CYP3A inhibitor

May increase serum levels of cyclosporine and tacrolimus; increased serum levels of dihydroergotamine with macrolide antibiotics (eg, erythromycin, clarithromycin, and troleandomycin) and protease inhibitors may result in serious and/or life-threatening cerebral or peripheral ischemia (see Contraindications); MAO inhibitors; propranolol may potentiate the vasoconstrictive action of ergotamine; nicotine may increase ischemic response by provoking vasoconstriction; nitroglycerin may increase bioavailability of dihydroergotamine; dihydroergotamine decreases antianginal effects of nitrates; sumatriptan and other serotonin 5-HT_1 receptor agonists may prolong vasospastic reactions (see Contraindications); concomitant use with peripheral vasoconstrictors may cause synergistic elevation of blood pressure; use with a selective serotonin reuptake inhibitor (SSRI) (eg, dexfenfluramine, fluoxetine, paroxetine), may result in a condition known as serotonin syndrome (confusion, mental status change, diaphoresis, tremor, myoclonus, shivering, hyper-reflexia, weakness, incoordination, hypertension); delavirdine and efavirenz also increase ergotamine plasma concentrations which may result in life-threatening toxicities

Stability Store below 25°C (77°F); do not refrigerate or freeze; protect from heat and light; once the nasal spray applicator has been prepared, use within 8 hours; discard any unused nasal solution

Mechanism of Action Ergot alkaloid alpha-adrenergic blocker which aborts vascular headaches by direct vasoconstriction of vascular smooth muscle, particularly of the carotid artery bed but also peripheral and cerebral vessels, which reduces the amplitude of pulsation in the cranial arteries; it also has partial agonist or antagonist activity against tryptaminergic and dopaminergic receptors; it is less active than ergotamine

Pharmacodynamics

Onset of action:

I.M.: 15-30 minutes

Intranasal: 30 minutes

I.V.: Immediate

Duration: I.M.: 3-4 hours

Pharmacokinetics

Distribution: V_d: 14.5 L/kg (~800 L)

Bioavailability: Intranasal: 32%

Protein binding: 93%

Metabolism: Extensively in the liver; one active metabolite

Half-life: Distribution phase: 0.9-2.1 hours; terminal elimination phase: 7-32 hours

Time to peak serum concentration: I.M.: Within 15-30 minutes; intranasal: 0.5-1 hour; I.V.: 15 minutes; SubQ: 15-45 minutes

Elimination: Predominately into bile and feces and 10% excreted in urine, mostly as metabolites

Clearance: 1.5 L/minute

Usual Dosage Adolescents and Adults: Treatment should be initiated at the first symptom or sign of an attack; nasal spray may be used at any stage of a migraine attack:

(Continued)

Dihydroergotamine *(Continued)*

I.M., SubQ: 1 mg at first sign of headache; repeat hourly to a maximum total dose of 3 mg/day; do not exceed 6 mg/week

I.V.: 1 mg at first sign of headache; repeat hourly up to a maximum total dose of 2 mg/day; do not exceed 6 mg/week

Intranasal: 1 spray (0.5 mg) of nasal spray into each nostril (total: 1 mg); repeat if needed within 15 minutes; maximum: 4 sprays (2 mg/day); do not exceed 8 sprays (4 mg)/week

Dosing adjustment in renal impairment: Contraindicated in severe renal impairment

Dosing adjustment in hepatic impairment: Dosage reductions are probably necessary but specific guidelines are not available; contraindicated in severe hepatic dysfunction

Administration

Intranasal (For complete directions, see patient instruction booklet): Prior to administration, the nasal spray applicator must be primed (pumped 4 times); spray once into each nostril; avoid deep inhalation through the nose while spraying or immediately after spraying; do not tilt head back

I.M., SubQ: Administer without dilution

I.V.: Administer without dilution slowly over 2-3 minutes

Patient Information Take this drug as rapidly as possible when first symptoms occur; may cause dry mouth; may cause drowsiness and impair ability to perform activities requiring mental alertness or physical coordination; report heart palpitations, severe nausea or vomiting, or severe numbness of fingers or toes; do not assemble nasal spray until needed for use

Dosage Forms Excipient information presented when available (limited, particularly for generics); consult specific product labeling.

Injection, solution, as mesylate (D.H.E. 45®): 1 mg/mL (1 mL) [contains ethanol 94%]

Solution, intranasal spray, as mesylate (Migranal®): 4 mg/mL [0.5 mg/spray] (1 mL) [contains caffeine 10 mg/mL]

- **Dihydroergotamine Mesylate** *see* Dihydroergotamine *on page 500*
- **Dihydrohydroxycodeinone** *see* Oxycodone *on page 1189*
- **Dihydromorphinone** *see* Hydromorphone *on page 787*

Dihydrotachysterol [DSC] (dye hye droe tak IS ter ole)

U.S. Brand Names DHT™ [DSC]; DHT™ Intensol™ [DSC]; Hytakerol® [DSC]

Canadian Brand Names Hytakerol®

Index Terms Dichysterol

Therapeutic Category Nutritional Supplement; Vitamin D Analog; Vitamin, Fat Soluble

Generic Available No

Use Treatment of hypocalcemia associated with hypoparathyroidism; prophylaxis of hypocalcemic tetany following thyroid surgery; suppression of hyperparathyroidism and treatment of renal osteodystrophy in patients with chronic renal failure

Pregnancy Risk Factor C

Lactation Enters breast milk/compatible

Contraindications Hypersensitivity to dihydrotachysterol or any component; hypercalcemia

Warnings Use cautiously in patients with renal stones, renal failure, and heart disease; calcium phosphate may precipitate if the product of serum calcium multiplied by phosphate (Ca x P) >70; adequate dietary calcium is necessary for a clinical response to therapy

Adverse Reactions Related to accompanying hypercalcemia

Central nervous system: Convulsions

Endocrine & metabolic: Hypercalcemia, metastatic calcification, polydipsia, weight loss

Gastrointestinal: Nausea, vomiting, anorexia

Hematologic: Anemia

Neuromuscular & skeletal: Weakness

Renal: Renal damage, polyuria

Drug Interactions Cholestyramine may reduce absorption; clofibrate, thiazides, phenobarbital, and phenytoin decrease the half-life of dihydrotachysterol; potential dihydrotachysterol-induced hypercalcemia may precipitate arrhythmias with cardiac glycosides

Mechanism of Action A synthetic reduction product of tachysterol, a close isomer of vitamin D; stimulates calcium and phosphate absorption from the small intestine, promotes secretion of calcium from bone to blood

Pharmacodynamics
Maximum hypercalcemic effect: Within 2 weeks
Duration: As long as 9 weeks

Pharmacokinetics
Absorption: Well absorbed from the GI tract
Metabolism: Hydroxylated in liver to 25-hydroxy-dihydrotachysterol

Usual Dosage Oral:
Hypoparathyroidism:
Neonates: 0.05-0.1 mg/day
Infants and young Children: Initial: 1-5 mg/day for 4 days, then 0.5-1.5 mg/day
Older Children and Adults: Initial: 0.75-2.5 mg/day for 4 days, then 0.2-1 mg/day; maximum dose: 1.5 mg/day
Nutritional rickets: 0.5 mg as a single dose or 13-50 mcg/day until healing occurs
Renal osteodystrophy:
Children and Adolescents: 0.1-0.5 mg/day
Adults: 0.1-0.6 mg/day

Administration Oral: May administer without regard to meals

Monitoring Parameters Serum calcium and phosphate, renal function, alkaline phosphatase, 24-hour urinary calcium

Additional Information 1 mg is approximately equivalent to 120,000 international units vitamin D_2

Dosage Forms Excipient information presented when available (limited, particularly for generics); consult specific product labeling. [DSC] = Discontinued product
Capsule (Hytakerol®): 0.125 mg [contains sesame oil] [DSC]
Solution, oral concentrate (DHT™ Intensol™): 0.2 mg/mL (30 mL) [contains alcohol 20%] [DSC]
Tablet (DHT™): 0.125 mg, 0.2 mg, 0.4 mg [DSC]

- **Dihydroxyanthracenedione Dihydrochloride** *see* Mitoxantrone *on page 1072*
- **1,25 Dihydroxycholecalciferol** *see* Calcitriol *on page 259*
- **Diiodohydroxyquin** *see* Iodoquinol *on page 862*
- **Dilacor® XR** *see* Diltiazem *on page 503*
- **Dilantin®** *see* Phenytoin *on page 1253*
- **Dilaudid®** *see* Hydromorphone *on page 787*
- **Dilaudid-HP®** *see* Hydromorphone *on page 787*
- **Dilaudid-HP-Plus® (Can)** *see* Hydromorphone *on page 787*
- **Dilaudid® Sterile Powder (Can)** *see* Hydromorphone *on page 787*
- **Dilaudid-XP® (Can)** *see* Hydromorphone *on page 787*
- **Diltia XT®** *see* Diltiazem *on page 503*

Diltiazem (dil TYE a zem)

Medication Safety Issues
Sound-alike/look-alike issues:
Diltiazem may be confused with Dilantin®
Cardizem® may be confused with Cardene®, Cardene SR®, Cardizem CD®, Cardizem SR®, cardiem
Cartia XT™ may be confused with Procardia XL®
Tiazac® may be confused with Tigan®, Ziac®
Significant differences exist between oral and I.V. dosing. Use caution when converting from one route of administration to another.
International issues:
Cardizem® may be confused with Cardem® which is a brand name for celiprolol in Spain
Cartia XT™ may be confused with Cartia® which is a brand name for aspirin in multiple international markets
Dilacor®: Brand name for digoxin in Serbia, a brand name for verapamil in Brazil, and a brand name for barnidipine in Argentina
Tiazac® may be confused with Tazac® which is a brand name for nizatidine in Australia

Related Information
Adult ACLS Algorithms *on page 1660*
Antihypertensive Agents by Class *on page 1678*
Medications for Which A Single Dose May Be Fatal When Ingested By A Toddler *on page 1932*

U.S. Brand Names Cardizem®; Cardizem® CD; Cardizem® LA; Cartia XT™; Dilacor® XR; Diltia XT®; Dilt-XR; Taztia XT™; Tiazac®

Canadian Brand Names Alti-Diltiazem CD; Apo-Diltiaz®; Apo-Diltiaz CD®; Apo-Diltiaz® Injectable; Apo-Diltiaz SR®; Apo-Diltiaz TZ®; Cardizem®; Cardizem® CD;
(Continued)

Diltiazem *(Continued)*

Cardizem® SR; Diltiazem HCl ER®; Diltiazem Hydrochloride Injection; Gen-Diltiazem; Gen-Diltiazem CD; Med-Diltiazem; Novo-Diltazem; Novo-Diltazem-CD; Novo-Diltiazem HCl ER; Nu-Diltiaz; Nu-Diltiaz-CD; ratio-Diltiazem CD; Rhoxal-diltiazem CD; Rhoxal-diltiazem SR; Rhoxal-diltiazem T; Sandoz-Diltiazem CD; Sandoz-Diltiazem T; Syn-Diltiazem®; Tiazac®; Tiazac® XC

Index Terms Diltiazem Hydrochloride

Therapeutic Category Antianginal Agent; Antihypertensive Agent; Calcium Channel Blocker

Generic Available Yes: Excludes extended release tablet

Use

Oral: Treatment of chronic stable angina or angina from coronary artery spasm; hypertension (**Note:** Only extended and sustained release products are FDA approved for the treatment of hypertension)

Injection: Management of atrial fibrillation or atrial flutter; paroxysmal supraventricular tachycardias (PSVT)

Pregnancy Risk Factor C

Lactation Enters breast milk/not recommended (AAP considers "compatible")

Contraindications Hypersensitivity to diltiazem or any component; severe hypotension; second or third degree heart block; sick-sinus syndrome; acute MI with pulmonary congestion

Warnings May cause bradycardia, second or third degree heart block, hypotension, hepatic injury; may worsen CHF; use with certain medications may result in additive effects on cardiac condition (see Drug Interactions)

Precautions Use with caution in patients with CHF or impaired renal or hepatic function. Dermatologic reactions may occur; these may be transient or disappear with continued therapy; however, erythema multiforme or exfoliative dermatitis have been reported; discontinue diltiazem if skin rash persists or is severe.

Adverse Reactions **Note:** Patients with impaired ventricular function or cardiac conduction abnormalities may have higher incidence of serious adverse reactions

Cardiovascular: Arrhythmia, bradycardia, hypotension, A-V block, tachycardia (rare), flushing, peripheral edema, CHF

Central nervous system: Headache, dizziness, insomnia, nervousness

Dermatologic: Urticaria, rash; erythema multiforme, exfoliative dermatitis (rare); photosensitivity (<1%)

Gastrointestinal: Nausea, vomiting, constipation, dyspepsia, dysgeusia

Hematologic: Leukopenia (rare), thrombocytopenia (rare)

Hepatic: Mild to marked elevations in liver enzyme tests (rare)

Neuromuscular & skeletal: Gait abnormality, tremor, paresthesia, weakness, asthenia

Drug Interactions Cytochrome P450 isoenzyme CYP3A3/4 substrate; isoenzyme CYP1A2, CYP2D6, and CYP3A3/4 inhibitor

Cimetidine may increase diltiazem serum concentration; digoxin, beta-adrenergic blocking agents may increase risk of bradycardia or heart block; diltiazem may decrease metabolism and increase serum concentrations of buspirone, cyclosporine, carbamazepine, digoxin, lovastatin, midazolam, triazolam, quinidine; diltiazem may increase the effect/toxicity of digitalis glycosides, encainide, fentanyl; rifampin may decrease diltiazem serum concentrations (avoid concurrent use); cardiac effects of anesthetics may be potentiated by diltiazem (titrate doses of both carefully)

Food Interactions Food may increase absorption of diltiazem from sustained-release preparation. A high fat meal does not effect extent of absorption of Cardizem® CD, Cardizem® LA, Cartia XT™, Taztia XT™, or Tiazac®, but peak serum concentrations for Taztia XT™ and Tiazac® may occur slightly earlier. Administration of Diltia® XT with a high fat meal may increase extent of absorption and peak concentration. Avoid natural licorice (causes sodium and water retention and increases potassium loss)

Stability

Capsule, tablet: Store at controlled room temperature; avoid excessive humidity; dispense in a tight, light resistant container

Injection: Refrigerate vials; do not freeze; may store at room temperature for up to 1 month; compatible in D_5W, NS, and $D_5\frac{1}{2}NS$ at a maximum concentration of 1 mg/mL for 24 hours when stored at room temperature or under refrigeration; not compatible with furosemide

Mechanism of Action Inhibits calcium ions from entering the "slow channels" or select voltage-sensitive areas of vascular smooth muscle and myocardium during depolarization; produces a relaxation of coronary vascular smooth muscle and coronary vasodilation; increases myocardial oxygen delivery in patients with vasospastic angina

Pharmacodynamics

Onset of action:

Oral: Tablet: Immediate release: 30-60 minutes

Parenteral: I.V. (bolus): Within 3 minutes

Maximum effect:

Antiarrhythmic (I.V. bolus): 2-7 minutes

Antihypertensive (Oral): Within 2 weeks

Pharmacokinetics

Absorption: 80%

Distribution: V_d: 1.7 L/kg; appears in breast milk

Protein binding: 70% to 80%

Metabolism: Extensive first-pass effect; metabolized in the liver; desacetyldiltiazem is an active metabolite (25% to 50% as potent as diltiazem based on coronary vasodilation effects); desacetyldiltiazem may accumulate with plasma concentrations 10% to 20% of diltiazem levels

Bioavailability: Oral: ~40%

Half-life: 3-4.5 hours, up to 8 hours with chronic high dosing

Time to peak serum concentration:

Tablet: Immediate release: 2-4 hours

Cardizem® CD: 10-14 hours

Cardizem® LA: 11-18 hours

Cardizem® SR: 6-11 hours

Elimination: In urine and bile mostly as metabolites; 2% to 4% excreted as unchanged drug in urine

Dialysis: Not dialyzable

Usual Dosage

Children: Minimal information available; some centers use the following:

Hypertension: Oral: Initial: 1.5-2 mg/kg/day in 3-4 divided doses (extended release formulations may be dosed once or twice daily); maximum dose: 3.5 mg/kg/day; some centers use a maximum dose of 6 mg/kg/day up to 360 mg/day (see Flynn, 2000)

Note: Doses up to 8 mg/kg/day given in 4 divided doses have been used for investigational therapy of Duchenne muscular dystrophy

Adolescents and Adults:

Oral: Hypertension:

Capsule, extended release: **Note:** Usual dosage range: Adolescents ≥ 18 years and Adults (JNC 7): 180-420 mg once daily

Cardizem® CD, Cartia XT™: Initial: 180-240 mg once daily; may increase dose after 14 days; usual: 240-360 mg once daily; maximum: 480 mg once daily

Dilacor® XR: 180-240 mg once daily

Diltia XT®: Initial: 180-240 mg once daily; usual: 180-480 mg once daily; maximum: 540 mg once daily

Taztia XT™, Tiazac®: Initial: 120-240 mg once daily; may increase dose after 14 days; maximum: 540 mg once daily

Capsule, sustained release: Cardizem® SR: Initial: 60-120 mg twice daily; may increase dose after 14 days; usual: 240-360 mg/day

Tablet, extended release: Cardizem® LA: Initial: 180-240 mg once daily; may increase dose after 14 days; limited clinical experience with doses >360 mg/day; maximum dose: 540 mg once daily; usual dosage range for Adolescents ≥18 years and Adults (JNC 7): 120-540 mg once daily

Tablet, immediate release: 30-120 mg 3-4 times/day; dosage should be increased gradually, at 1- to 2-day intervals until optimum response is obtained; usual maintenance dose: 180-360 mg/day (see Use)

I.V. (antiarrhythmic): Initial: 0.25 mg/kg as a bolus over 2 minutes, if response is inadequate a second bolus dose (0.35 mg/kg) may be administered after 15 minutes; further bolus doses should be individualized

I.V. continuous infusion (start after I.V. bolus doses): 5-15 mg/hour for up to 24 hours

Conversion from I.V. diltiazem to oral diltiazem: Start first oral dose approximately 3 hours after bolus dose

Oral dose (mg/day) is approximately equal to [(rate in mg/hour x 3) + 3] x 10; **Note:** Dose per day may need to be divided depending on formulation used (see Usual Dosage above)

3 mg/hour = 120 mg/day

5 mg/hour = 180 mg/day

7 mg/hour = 240 mg/day

11 mg/hour = 360 mg/day (maximum recommended dose)

Administration

Oral: May be administered with or without food, but should be administered consistently with relation to meals; administer with a full glass of water; swallow extended

(Continued)

Diltiazem *(Continued)*

and sustained release preparations (CD, LA, SR, XR, XT, Tiazac®) whole, do not chew, break, or crush

Taztia XT™ and Tiazac® capsules (extended release) may be opened and sprinkled on applesauce; swallow applesauce immediately, do not chew; follow with some cool water (adults: 1 glass) to ensure complete swallowing; do not use hot applesauce; do not divide capsule contents (ie, do not administer partial doses); do not store mixture of applesauce and capsule contents, use immediately

Parenteral:

I.V. bolus: Adults: Infuse over 2 minutes

I.V. continuous infusion: May dilute with NS, D_5W, or $D_5{}^1/_2NS$; maximum final concentration: 1 mg/mL

Monitoring Parameters Blood pressure, renal function, liver enzymes; EKG with I.V. therapy

Patient Information Do not discontinue abruptly; report any dizziness, shortness of breath, palpitations, or edema; avoid alcohol. May cause photosensitivity reactions (eg, exposure to sunlight may cause severe sunburn, skin rash, redness, or itching); avoid exposure to sunlight and artificial light sources (sunlamps, tanning booth/bed); wear protective clothing, wide-brimmed hats, sunglasses, and lip sunscreen (SPF ≥15); use a sunscreen [broad-spectrum sunscreen or physical sunscreen (preferred) or sunblock with SPF ≥15]; contact physician if reaction occurs.

Nursing Implications Do not crush extended or sustained release preparations (CD, LA, SR, XR, XT, Tiazac®)

Additional Information Cartia XT™ is the generic version of Cardizem® CD; Diltia XT® and Dilt-XR are the generic versions of Dilacor XR®; Taztia XT™ is the generic version of Tiazac®

Dosage Forms Excipient information presented when available (limited, particularly for generics); consult specific product labeling.

Capsule, extended release, as hydrochloride [once-daily dosing]: 120 mg, 180 mg, 240 mg, 300 mg, 360 mg, 420 mg

Cardizem® CD: 120 mg, 180 mg, 240 mg, 300 mg, 360 mg

Cartia XT™: 120 mg, 180 mg, 240 mg, 300 mg

Dilacor® XR, Dilt-XR, Diltia XT®: 120 mg, 180 mg, 240 mg

Taztia XT™: 120 mg, 180 mg, 240 mg, 300 mg, 360 mg

Tiazac®: 120 mg, 180 mg, 240 mg, 300 mg, 360 mg, 420 mg

Capsule, sustained release, as hydrochloride [twice-daily dosing]: 60 mg, 90 mg, 120 mg

Injection, solution, as hydrochloride: 5 mg/mL (5 mL, 10 mL, 25 mL)

Injection, powder for reconstitution, as hydrochloride:

Cardizem®: 25 mg

Tablet, as hydrochloride: 30 mg, 60 mg, 90 mg, 120 mg

Cardizem®: 30 mg, 60 mg, 90 mg, 120 mg

Tablet, extended release, as hydrochloride:

Cardizem® LA: 120 mg, 180 mg, 240 mg, 300 mg, 360 mg, 420 mg

Extemporaneous Preparations A 12 mg/mL oral liquid preparation made from tablets (regular, not sustained release) and 3 different vehicles (cherry syrup, a 1:1 mixture of Ora-Sweet® and Ora-Plus®, or a 1:1 mixture of Ora-Sweet® SF and Ora-Plus®) was stable for 60 days when stored in amber plastic prescription bottles in the dark at room temperature (25°C) or under refrigeration (5°C); grind sixteen 90 mg tablets in a mortar into a fine powder; add 10 mL of the vehicle and mix well to form a uniform paste; mix while adding the vehicle in geometric proportions to **almost** 120 mL; transfer to a calibrated bottle and qsad with vehicle to 120 mL; label "shake well" and "protect from light"

Allen LV and Erickson MA, "Stability of Baclofen, Captopril, Diltiazem Hydrochloride, Dipyridamole, and Flecainide Acetate in Extemporaneously Compounded Oral Liquids," *Am J Health Sys Pharm*, 1996, 53(18):2179-84.

References

Bertorini TE, Palmieri GMA, Griffin JW, et al, "Effect of Chronic Treatment With the Calcium Antagonist Diltiazem in Duchenne Muscular Dystrophy," *Neurology*, 1988, 38(4):609-13.

Chobanian AV, Bakris GL, Black HR, et al, "The Seventh Report of the Joint National Committee on Prevention, Detection, Evaluation, and Treatment of High Blood Pressure: The JNC 7 report," *JAMA*, 2003, 289(19):2560-72.

Flynn JT and Pasko DA, "Calcium Channel Blockers: Pharmacology and Place in Therapy of Pediatric Hypertension," *Pediatr Nephrol*, 2000, 15(3-4):302-16.

♦ **Diltiazem HCl ER® (Can)** *see* Diltiazem *on page 503*

♦ **Diltiazem Hydrochloride** *see* Diltiazem *on page 503*

♦ **Diltiazem Hydrochloride Injection (Can)** *see* Diltiazem *on page 503*

♦ **Dilt-XR** *see* Diltiazem *on page 503*

♦ **Dimaphen [OTC]** *see* Brompheniramine and Pseudoephedrine *on page 235*

DimenhyDRINATE (dye men HYE dri nate)

Medication Safety Issues

Sound-alike/look-alike issues:

DimenhyDRINATE may be confused with diphenhydrAMINE

Related Information

Overdose and Toxicology *on page 1916*

U.S. Brand Names Dramamine® [OTC]; TripTone® [OTC] [DSC]

Canadian Brand Names Apo-Dimenhydrinate®; Children's Motion Sickness Liquid; Dinate®; Gravol®; Jamp® Travel Tablet; Nauseatol; Novo-Dimenate; SAB-Dimenhydrinate

Therapeutic Category Antiemetic; Antihistamine

Generic Available Yes

Use Treatment and prevention of nausea, vertigo, and vomiting associated with motion sickness

Pregnancy Risk Factor B

Contraindications Hypersensitivity to dimenhydrinate or any component (see Warnings)

Warnings Chewable tablets contain tartrazine which may cause allergic reactions in susceptible individuals

Precautions Use with caution in patients with a history of seizure disorder; may produce excitation in the young child; use with caution in any condition which may be aggravated by anticholinergic symptoms such as prostatic hypertrophy, asthma, bladder neck obstruction, narrow-angle glaucoma, etc; chewable tablets contain aspartame which is metabolized to phenylalanine and must be used with caution in patients with phenylketonuria

Adverse Reactions

Cardiovascular: Hypotension, palpitations, tachycardia

Central nervous system: Drowsiness, headache, paradoxical CNS stimulation, dizziness

Dermatologic: Photosensitivity, urticaria, rash

Gastrointestinal: Anorexia, xerostomia, dry mucous membranes, constipation

Genitourinary: Urinary frequency, dysuria

Hematologic: Hemolytic anemia

Ocular: Blurred vision, diplopia

Otic: Tinnitus

Respiratory: Chest tightness, wheezing, thickened secretions

Drug Interactions Enhances sedative effects of other CNS depressants, may potentiate anticholinergic effects; may mask early signs and symptoms of ototoxicity in patients on aminoglycosides, furosemide, etc

Mechanism of Action Competes with histamine for H_1-receptor sites on effector cells in the GI tract, blood vessels, and respiratory tract; diminishes vestibular stimulation and depresses labyrinthine function through its central anticholinergic activity; consists of equimolar proportions of diphenhydramine and chlorotheophylline

Pharmacodynamics

Onset of action: Oral: Within 15-30 minutes

Duration: ~3-6 hours

Pharmacokinetics

Absorption: Well absorbed from the GI tract

Metabolism: Extensive in the liver

Usual Dosage Oral:

Children:

2-5 years: 12.5-25 mg every 6-8 hours, maximum dose: 75 mg/day

6-12 years: 25-50 mg every 6-8 hours, maximum dose: 150 mg/day

or

Alternately: 5 mg/kg/day or 150 mg/m²/day in 4 divided doses, not to exceed 300 mg/day

Children ≥12 years and Adults: 50-100 mg every 4-6 hours, not to exceed 400 mg/day

Administration Oral: Administer with food or water

Patient Information May cause drowsiness and impair ability to perform activities requiring mental alertness or physical coordination; may cause dry mouth. May rarely cause photosensitivity reactions (eg, exposure to sunlight may cause severe sunburn, skin rash, redness, or itching); avoid direct exposure to sunlight.

Dosage Forms Excipient information presented when available (limited, particularly for generics); consult specific product labeling. [CAN] = Canadian brand name

Caplet (TripTone®): 50 mg [DSC]

Capsule, softgel (Gravol®) [CAN]: 50 mg [not available in the U.S.]

Capsule, long-acting (Gravol® L/A) [CAN]: 75 mg, 100 mg [not available in the U.S.]

(Continued)

DimenhyDRINATE *(Continued)*

Injection, solution:
Gravol® I.M. [CAN]: 50 mg/mL (1 mL, 5 mL) [not available in the U.S.]
Gravol® I.V. [CAN]: 10 mg/mL (5 mL) [not available in the U.S.]
Solution, oral (Gravol® [CAN], Children's Motion Sickness [CAN]): 3 mg/mL (75 mL) [not available in the U.S.]
Suppository, rectal (Gravol® [CAN], Sab-Dimenhydrinate [CAN]): 75 mg, 100 mg [not available in the U.S.]
Tablet:
Dinate® [CAN], Jamp® Travel Tablet [CAN], Nauseatol® [CAN]: 50 mg
Dramamine®: 50 mg
Gravol® Filmkote Jr [CAN]: 25 mg [not available in the U.S.]
Gravol® Filmkote [CAN]: 50 mg [not available in the U.S.]
Tablet, chewable:
Dramamine®: 50 mg [contains phenylalanine 1.5 mg/tablet and tartrazine; orange flavor]
Gravol® Chewable for Children [CAN]: 25 mg [not available in the U.S.]
Gravol® Chewable for Adults [CAN]: 50 mg [not available in the U.S.]

Dimercaprol (dye mer KAP role)

Related Information
Commonly Used Antidotes for Acute Overdoses *on page 1920*

U.S. Brand Names BAL in Oil®

Index Terms BAL; British Anti-Lewisite; Dithioglycerol

Therapeutic Category Antidote, Arsenic Toxicity; Antidote, Gold Toxicity; Antidote, Lead Toxicity; Antidote, Mercury Toxicity; Chelating Agent, Parenteral

Generic Available No

Use Antidote to gold, arsenic, and mercury poisoning; adjunct to edetate calcium disodium in lead poisoning

Pregnancy Risk Factor C

Contraindications Hypersensitivity to dimercaprol, peanuts (injection in peanut oil), or any component; hepatic insufficiency; do not use in iron, cadmium, or selenium poisoning; do not use iron supplements during therapy

Precautions Use with caution in patients with renal impairment or hypertension; produces hemolysis in persons with G-6-PD deficiency, especially in the presence of infection or other stressful situations; due to increased frequency of histamine-release related side effects, pretreatment with antihistamines is recommended; urine should be kept alkaline to prevent dissociation of chelate

Adverse Reactions
Cardiovascular: Hypertension, tachycardia
Central nervous system: Nervousness, seizures, fever (30% of children), headache, anxiety
Gastrointestinal: Vomiting, nausea, salivation
Hematologic: Transient neutropenia
Local: Pain at the injection site, sterile abscesses
Neuromuscular & skeletal: Paresthesia of hands
Ocular: Blepharospasm, conjunctivitis, lacrimation, burning eyes
Renal: Nephrotoxicity
Respiratory: Rhinorrhea
Miscellaneous: Burning sensation of the lips, mouth, throat, and penis

Drug Interactions Iron (chelation product toxic to kidneys)

Stability Do not mix in the same syringe with edetate calcium disodium

Mechanism of Action Sulfhydryl group combines with ions of various heavy metals (arsenic, gold, mercury, lead) to form relatively stable, nontoxic, soluble chelates which are excreted in the urine

Pharmacokinetics
Distribution: To all tissues including the brain
Metabolism: Rapid to inactive products
Time to peak serum concentration: 30-60 minutes
Elimination: In urine and feces via bile

Usual Dosage Children and Adults: I.M.:
Mild arsenic and gold poisoning: 2.5 mg/kg/dose every 6 hours for 2 days, then every 12 hours on the third day, and once daily thereafter for 10 days
Severe arsenic and gold poisoning: 3 mg/kg/dose every 4 hours for 2 days then every 6 hours on the third day, then every 12 hours thereafter for 10 days
Mercury poisoning: 5 mg/kg initially followed by 2.5 mg/kg/dose 1-2 times/day for 10 days

Lead poisoning: (use with edetate calcium disodium):
Mild: 4 mg/kg/dose for one dose then 3 mg/kg/dose every 4 hours for 2-7 days
Severe and acute encephalopathy: (**blood lead levels >70 mcg/dL**): 4 mg/kg/dose every 4 hours in combination with edetate calcium disodium for at least 72 hours; may use for up to 5 days; if additional days of therapy (>5 days) are indicated, a minimum of 2 days without treatment should elapse before considering another treatment course

Administration Parenteral: Administer undiluted, deep I.M.

Monitoring Parameters Specific heavy metal levels, urine pH

Dosage Forms Excipient information presented when available (limited, particularly for generics); consult specific product labeling.

Injection, oil: 100 mg/mL (3 mL) [contains benzyl benzoate and peanut oil]

References

"Treatment Guidelines for Lead Exposure in Children. American Academy of Pediatrics Committee on Drugs," *Pediatrics*, 1995, 96(1 Pt 1):155-60.

DiphenhydrAMINE (dye fen HYE dra meen)

Medication Safety Issues

Sound-alike/look-alike issues:

DiphenhydrAMINE may be confused with desipramine, dicyclomine, dimenhyDRINATE

Benadryl® may be confused with benazepril, Bentyl®, Benylin®, Caladryl®

Related Information

Commonly Used Antidotes for Acute Overdoses *on page 1920*
Compatibility of Chemotherapy and Related Supportive Care Medications *on page 1777*
Compatibility of Medications Mixed in A Syringe *on page 1941*
OTC Cough and Cold Preparations, Pediatric *on page 1706*
Overdose and Toxicology *on page 1916*

U.S. Brand Names Aler-Cap [OTC]; Aler-Dryl [OTC]; Aler-Tab [OTC]; AllerMax® [OTC]; Altaryl [OTC]; Banophen® [OTC]; Banophen® Anti-Itch [OTC]; Benadryl® Allergy [OTC]; Benadryl® Children's Allergy [OTC]; Benadryl® Children's Allergy Fastmelt® [OTC]; Benadryl® Children's Dye-Free Allergy [OTC]; Benadryl® Injection; Benadryl® Itch Stopping [OTC]; Benadryl® Itch Stopping Extra Strength [OTC]; Ben-Tann; Compoz® Nighttime Sleep Aid [OTC]; Dermamycin® [OTC]; Diphen® [OTC]; Diphen® AF [OTC]; Diphenhist [OTC]; Dytan™; Genahist® [OTC]; Hydramine® [OTC]; Nytol® Quick Caps [OTC]; Nytol® Quick Gels [OTC]; Siladryl® Allergy [OTC]; (Continued)

DiphenhydrAMINE *(Continued)*

Silphen® [OTC]; Simply Sleep® [OTC]; Sleep-ettes D [OTC]; Sleepinal® [OTC]; Sominex® [OTC]; Sominex® Maximum Strength [OTC]; Triaminic® Thin Strips™ Cough and Runny Nose [OTC]; Twilite® [OTC]; Unisom® Maximum Strength SleepGels® [OTC]

Canadian Brand Names Allerdryl®; Allernix; Benadryl®; Nytol®; Nytol® Extra Strength; PMS-Diphenhydramine; Simply Sleep®

Index Terms Diphenhydramine Citrate; Diphenhydramine Hydrochloride; Diphenhydramine Tannate

Therapeutic Category Antidote, Drug-induced Dystonic Reactions; Antidote, Hypersensitivity Reactions; Antihistamine; Sedative

Generic Available Yes: Excludes chewable tablet, gel, orally-disintegrating tablet, stick, strip

Use Symptomatic relief of allergic symptoms caused by histamine release which include nasal allergies and allergic dermatosis; mild nighttime sedation, prevention of motion sickness, as an antitussive; treatment of phenothiazine-induced dystonic reactions; adjunct to epinephrine in the treatment of anaphylaxis; topically for relief of pain and itching associated with insect bites, minor cuts and burns, or rashes

Pregnancy Risk Factor B

Lactation Enters breast milk/contraindicated

Contraindications Hypersensitivity to diphenhydramine or any component; should not be used in acute attacks of asthma; breast-feeding (infants may be more sensitive to the effects of antihistamines)

Warnings Topical diphenhydramine should not be used to treat chickenpox, poison ivy, or sunburn, on large areas of the body, or on blistered or oozing skin, due to potential for causing toxic psychosis, particularly in children

Precautions Use with caution in patients with angle-closure glaucoma, peptic ulcer, urinary tract obstruction, hyperthyroidism; may cause paradoxical excitation in young children; toxicity can result in hallucinations, coma, and death; chewable tablets contain phenylalanine and must be used with caution in patients with phenylketonuria

Adverse Reactions

Cardiovascular: Hypotension, palpitations, tachycardia

Central nervous system: Sedation, dizziness, paradoxical excitement, fatigue, insomnia

Dermatologic: Photosensitivity, rash, urticaria

Gastrointestinal: Nausea, vomiting, xerostomia, dry mucous membranes, anorexia, constipation, epigastric distress

Genitourinary: Urinary retention, dysuria

Hematologic: Rare: Hemolytic anemia, aplastic anemia, thrombocytopenia

Neuromuscular & skeletal: Paresthesia of hands, tremor

Ocular: Blurred vision

Respiratory: Chest tightness, thickened bronchial secretions, wheezing

Drug Interactions Cytochrome P450 isoenzyme CYP2D6 substrate

Additive sedation when given with drugs which depress the CNS; may impair absorption of aminosalicylic acid; may enhance the adverse/toxic effects of other anticholinergics; may enhance the arrhythmogenic effects of antipsychotic agents (phenothiazines); may increase the levels/effects of CYP2D6 substrates (eg, amphetamines, selected beta-blockers, dextromethorphan, fluoxetine, lidocaine, mirtazapine, nefazodone, paroxetine, risperidone, ritonavir, thioridazine, tricyclic antidepressants, venlafaxine); may decrease the levels/effects of CYP2D6 prodrug substrates (eg, codeine, hydrocodone, oxycodone, tramadol)

Stability Compatible when mixed in the same syringe: atropine, chlorpromazine, cimetidine, droperidol, fentanyl, glycopyrrolate, hydromorphone, meperidine, metoclopramide, midazolam, morphine, promethazine, and ranitidine

Mechanism of Action Competes with histamine for H_1-receptor sites on effector cells in the GI tract, blood vessels, and respiratory tract

Pharmacodynamics

Maximum sedative effect: 1-3 hours after administration

Duration: 4-7 hours

Pharmacokinetics

Absorption: Oral: Well absorbed but 40% to 60% of an oral dose reaches the systemic circulation due to first-pass metabolism

Distribution: Adults: V_d: 3-22 L/kg

Protein-binding: 78%

Metabolism: Extensive hepatic n-demethylation via CYP2D6; minor demethylation via CYP1A2, 2C9, and 2C19; significant first-pass effect

Bioavailability: ~40% to 70%

Half-life: 2-8 hours

Time to peak serum concentration: 2-4 hours

Elimination: Urine (as unchanged drug)

Usual Dosage

Oral, I.M., I.V.:

Treatment of phenothiazine dystonic reactions and moderate to severe allergic reactions:

Children: 5 mg/kg/day or 150 mg/m²/day in divided doses every 6-8 hours, not to exceed 300 mg/day

Adults: 25-50 mg every 4 hours, not to exceed 400 mg/day

Minor allergic rhinitis or motion sickness:

Children 2 to <6 years: 6.25 mg every 4-6 hours; maximum: 37.5 mg/day

Children 6 to <12 years: 12.5-25 mg [equivalent to 19-38 mg diphenhydramine citrate (Children's Benadryl® Allergy Fastmelt® 1-2 tablets)] every 4-6 hours; maximum: 150 mg/day (228 mg diphenhydramine citrate)

Children ≥12 years and Adults: 25-50 mg [equivalent to 38-76 mg diphenhydramine citrate (Children's Benadryl® Allergy Fastmelt® 2-4 tablets)] every 4-6 hours; maximum: 300 mg/day (456 mg diphenhydramine citrate)

Antitussive: Oral:

Children 2 to <6 years: 6.25 mg every 4 hours; maximum 37.5 mg/day

Children 6 to <12 years: 12.5 mg every 4 hours; maximum 75 mg/day

Children ≥12 years and Adults: 25 mg every 4 hours; maximum 150 mg/day

Night-time sleep aid: 30 minutes before bedtime:

Children 2 to <12 years: 1 mg/kg/dose; maximum: 50 mg/dose

Children ≥12 years and Adults: 50 mg

Topical cream, gel, spray, or stick:

Children ≥2 to 12 years: Apply 1% concentration not more than 3-4 times/day

Children >12 years and Adults: Apply 1% or 2% concentration not more than 3-4 times/day

Administration

Oral: Administer with food to avoid GI distress

Parenteral:

I.V.: Dilute with compatible I.V. fluid to a maximum concentration of 25 mg/mL and infuse over 10-15 minutes (maximum rate of infusion: 25 mg/minute)

I.M.: 50 mg/mL concentration by deep I.M. injection

Topical: Shake well (gel); apply thin coat to affected area (see Warnings)

Test Interactions May suppress the wheal and flare reactions to skin test antigens; discontinue 4 days prior to skin testing procedures

Patient Information May cause drowsiness and impair ability to perform activities requiring mental alertness or physical coordination; may cause dry mouth. May rarely cause photosensitivity reactions (eg, exposure to sunlight may cause severe sunburn, skin rash, redness, or itching); avoid direct exposure to sunlight.

Additional Information Diphenhydramine citrate 19 mg is equivalent to diphenhydramine hydrochloride 12.5 mg

Dosage Forms Excipient information presented when available (limited, particularly for generics); consult specific product labeling.

Caplet, as hydrochloride: 25 mg, 50 mg

Aler-Dryl, AllerMax®, Compoz® Nighttime Sleep Aid, Sleep-ettes D, Sominex® Maximum Strength, Twilite®: 50 mg

Nytol® Quick Caps, Simply Sleep®: 25 mg

Capsule, as hydrochloride: 25 mg, 50 mg

Aler-Cap, Banophen®, Benadryl® Allergy, Diphen®, Diphenhist, Genahist®: 25 mg

Sleepinal®: 50 mg

Capsule, softgel, as hydrochloride: 50 mg

Benadryl® Dye-Free Allergy: 25 mg [dye-free]

Compoz® Nighttime Sleep Aid, Nytol® Quick Gels, Sleepinal®, Unisom® Maximum Strength SleepGels®: 50 mg

Captab, as hydrochloride:

Diphenhist®: 25 mg

Cream, as hydrochloride: 2% (30 g)

Banophen® Anti-Itch: 2% (30 g) [contains zinc acetate 0.1%]

Benadryl® Itch Stopping: 1% (30 g) [contains zinc acetate 0.1%]

Benadryl® Itch Stopping Extra Strength: 2% (30 g) [contains zinc acetate 0.1%]

Diphenhist®: 2% (30 g) [contains zinc acetate 0.1%]

Elixir, as hydrochloride:

Altaryl: 12.5 mg/5 mL (120 mL, 480 mL, 3840 mL) [cherry flavor]

Banophen®: 12.5 mg/5 mL (120 mL)

Diphen AF: 12.5 mg/5 mL (120 mL, 240 mL, 480 mL) [alcohol free; cherry flavor]

Gel, topical, as hydrochloride:

Benadryl® Itch Stopping Extra Strength: 2% (120 mL)

Injection, solution, as hydrochloride: 50 mg/mL (1 mL)

Benadryl®: 50 mg/mL (1 mL; 10 mL [DSC])

(Continued)

DiphenhydrAMINE *(Continued)*

Liquid, as hydrochloride:
AllerMax®: 12.5 mg/5 mL (120 mL)
Benadryl® Allergy: 12.5 mg/5 mL (120 mL, 240 mL) [alcohol free; contains sodium benzoate; cherry flavor]
Benadryl® Children's Dye-Free Allergy: 12.5 mg/5 mL (120 mL) [alcohol free, dye free, sugar free; contains sodium benzoate; bubble gum flavor]
Genahist®: 12.5 mg/5 mL (120 mL) [alcohol free, sugar free; contains sodium benzoate; cherry flavor]
Hydramine®: 12.5 mg/5 mL (120 mL, 480 mL) [alcohol free]
Siladryl® Allergy: 12.5 mg/5 mL (120 mL, 240 mL, 480 mL) [alcohol free, sugar free; black cherry flavor]
Liquid, topical, as hydrochloride [stick]:
Benadryl® Itch Stopping Extra Strength: 2% (14 mL) [contains zinc acetate 0.1% and alcohol]
Solution, oral, as hydrochloride:
Diphenhist: 12.5 mg/5 mL (120 mL, 480 mL) [alcohol free; contains sodium benzoate]
Solution, topical, as hydrochloride [spray]:
Benadryl® Itch Stopping Extra Strength: 2% (60 mL) [contains zinc acetate 0.1% and alcohol]
Dermamycin®: 2% (60 mL) [contains menthol 1%]
Strips, oral, as hydrochloride:
Benadryl® Allergy: 25 mg (10s) [contains sodium 4 mg/strip; vanilla mint flavor]
Benadryl® Children's Allergy: 12.5 mg (10s) [vanilla mint flavor]
Triaminic® Thin Strips™ Cough and Runny Nose: 12. 5 mg (16s) [grape flavor]
Suspension, as tannate:
Ben-Tann: 25 mg/5 mL (120 ml) [contains sodium benzoate; strawberry flavor]
Dytan™: 25 mg/5 mL (120 mL) [strawberry flavor]
Syrup, as hydrochloride:
Silphen® Cough: 12.5 mg/5 mL (120 mL, 240 mL, 480 mL) [contains alcohol; 5%; strawberry flavor]
Tablet, as hydrochloride: 25 mg, 50 mg
Aler-Tab, Benadryl® Allergy, Genahist®, Sominex®: 25 mg
Tablet, chewable, as hydrochloride:
Benadryl® Children's Allergy: 12.5 mg [contains phenylalanine 4.2 mg, magnesium 15 mg, and sodium 2 mg per tablet; grape flavor]
Tablet, chewable, as tannate:
Dytan™: 25 mg [contains phenylalanine; strawberry flavor]
Tablet, orally disintegrating, as citrate:
Benadryl® Children's Allergy Fastmelt®: 19 mg [equivalent to diphenhydramine hydrochloride 12.5 mg; contains phenylalanine 4.5 mg/tablet and soy protein isolate; cherry flavor]

- **Diphenhydramine Citrate** *see* DiphenhydrAMINE *on page 509*
- **Diphenhydramine Hydrochloride** *see* DiphenhydrAMINE *on page 509*
- **Diphenhydramine Tannate** *see* DiphenhydrAMINE *on page 509*

Diphenoxylate and Atropine (dye fen OKS i late & A troe peen)

Medication Safety Issues
Sound-alike/look-alike issues:
Lomotil® may be confused with Lamictal®, Lamisil®, lamotrigine, Lanoxin®, Lasix®, ludiomil
Lonox® may be confused with Lanoxin®, Loprox®
International issues:
Lomotil® may be confused with Lemesil® which is a brand name for nimesulide in Greece
Lonox® may be confused with Flomox® which is a brand of cefcapene in Japan

U.S. Brand Names Lomotil®; Lonox®
Canadian Brand Names Lomotil®
Index Terms Atropine and Diphenoxylate
Therapeutic Category Antidiarrheal
Generic Available Yes
Use Treatment of diarrhea
Restrictions C-V
Pregnancy Risk Factor C
Lactation Enters breast milk/use caution

Contraindications Hypersensitivity to diphenoxylate, atropine, or any component; severe liver disease, obstructive jaundice, dehydration, narrow-angle glaucoma, diarrhea associated with pseudomembranous enterocolitis or enterotoxin-producing bacteria. Do not use in children <2 years of age.

Warnings Use in conjunction with fluid and electrolyte therapy in children and in adults when appropriate. In case of severe dehydration or electrolyte imbalance, withhold diphenoxylate/atropine treatment until corrective therapy has been initiated. Inhibiting peristalsis may lead to fluid retention in the intestine aggravating dehydration and electrolyte imbalance. Reduction of intestinal motility may be deleterious in diarrhea resulting from *Shigella*, *Salmonella*, toxigenic strains of *E. coli* and from pseudomembranous enterocolitis associated with broad spectrum antibiotics; use is not recommended.

Use with caution in children. Younger children (especially those with Down syndrome) may develop signs of atropinism (dry skin and mucous membranes, thirst, hyperthermia, tachycardia, urinary retention, flushing) even at the recommended dosages. Overdose in children may result in severe respiratory depression, coma, and possibly permanent brain damage.

If acute diarrhea does not clinically improve within 48 hours, this medication is unlikely to be effective and should be discontinued; if chronic diarrhea is not improved symptomatically within 10 days at maximum dosage, control is unlikely with further use. Prolonged use may result in tolerance to antidiarrheal effects and physical or psychological dependence; abrupt discontinuation may cause withdrawal symptoms.

Precautions Use with extreme caution in patients with dehydration, cirrhosis, hepatorenal disease, renal dysfunction, and acute ulcerative colitis

Adverse Reactions

Cardiovascular: Tachycardia

Central nervous system: Sedation, dizziness, euphoria, headache, depression, lethargy, confusion, restlessness, hyperthermia, flushing

Dermatologic: Pruritus, urticaria, angioneurotic edema, dry skin and mucous membranes

Gastrointestinal: Nausea, vomiting, abdominal discomfort, anorexia, paralytic ileus, pancreatitis, toxic megacolon, xerostomia, gum swelling

Genitourinary: Urinary retention

Neuromuscular & skeletal: Weakness, numbness of extremities

Ocular: Blurred vision

Respiratory: Respiratory depression (young children may be at greater risk)

Miscellaneous: Anaphylaxis; physical and psychological dependence with prolonged use

Drug Interactions MAO inhibitors (may precipitate hypertensive crisis), CNS depressants, alcohol, anticholinergic agents, naltrexone; the herbal medicine St John's wort (*Hypericum perforatum*) may increase serious side effects, its use is **not** recommended

Stability Protect from light; dispense liquid only in original container

Mechanism of Action Diphenoxylate inhibits excessive GI motility and GI propulsion; commercial preparations contain a subtherapeutic amount of atropine to discourage abuse

Pharmacodynamics Antidiarrheal effects:

Onset of action: Within 45-60 minutes

Maximum effect: Within 2 hours

Duration: 3-4 hours

Tolerance to antidiarrheal effects may occur with prolonged use

Pharmacokinetics

Atropine: See Atropine *on page 181*

Diphenoxylate:

- Absorption: Oral: Well absorbed
- Distribution: Major metabolite (diphenoxylic acid) may be excreted in breast milk
- Metabolism: Extensive in the liver via ester hydrolysis to diphenoxylic acid (active)
- Half-life:
  - Diphenoxylate: 2.5 hours
  - Diphenoxylic acid: 12-24 hours
- Time to peak serum concentration: ~2 hours
- Elimination: Primarily (49%) in feces (via bile); ~14% is excreted in urine; <1% excreted unchanged in urine

Usual Dosage Oral (as diphenoxylate):

Children 2-12 years: **Liquid: Note:** Only the liquid product is recommended for children under 13 years of age; do not exceed recommended doses; reduce dose as soon as symptoms are initially controlled; maintenance doses may be as low as 25% of initial dose; if no improvement within 48 hours of therapy, diphenoxylate is not likely to be effective

Initial: 0.3-0.4 mg/kg/day in 4 divided doses (maximum: 10 mg/day) **or**

(Continued)

Diphenoxylate and Atropine *(Continued)*

Manufacturer's recommendations: Initial:

<2 years: Not recommended
2 years (11-14 kg): 1.5-3 mL 4 times/day
3 years (12-16 kg): 2-3 mL 4 times/day
4 years (14-20 kg): 2-4 mL 4 times/day
5 years (16-23 kg): 2.5-4.5 mL 4 times/day
6-8 years (17-32 kg): 2.5-5 mL 4 times/day
9-12 years (23-55 kg): 3.5-5 mL 4 times/day

Alternative pediatric dosing: Initial:

<2 years: Not recommended
2-5 years: 2 mg 3 times/day
5-8 years: 2 mg 4 times/day
8-12 years: 2 mg 5 times/day

Adults: Initial: 5 mg (2 tablets or 10 mL) 4 times/day until control achieved (maximum: 20 mg/day); then reduced dose as needed; maintenance: 5-15 mg/day in 2-3 divided doses; some patients may be controlled on doses as low as 5 mg/day

Note: Do not exceed recommended doses; reduce dose once symptoms are initially controlled; acute diarrhea usually improves within 48 hours; if chronic diarrhea dose not improve within 10 days at maximum daily doses of 20 mg, diphenoxylate is not likely to be effective.

Administration Oral: May be administered with food to decrease GI upset; use plastic dropper provided when measuring liquid; **Note:** Dropper has a 2 mL (1 mg) capacity and is calibrated in increments of ½ mL (0.25 mg)

Monitoring Parameters Bowel frequency, signs and symptoms of atropinism, fluid and electrolytes

Patient Information Take as directed; do not exceed recommended dosage. If diarrhea does not improve within 48 hours, notify prescriber. Avoid alcohol and the herbal medicine St John's wort; may cause dizziness or drowsiness and impair ability to perform activities requiring mental alertness or physical coordination; may cause dry mouth; may be habit-forming; avoid abrupt discontinuation after prolonged use

Additional Information Naloxone reverses toxicity due to diphenoxylate; Lomotil® solution also contains sorbitol

Dosage Forms Excipient information presented when available (limited, particularly for generics); consult specific product labeling.

Solution, oral: Diphenoxylate hydrochloride 2.5 mg and atropine sulfate 0.025 mg per 5 mL (5 mL, 10 mL, 60 mL)

Lomotil®: Diphenoxylate hydrochloride 2.5 mg and atropine sulfate 0.025 mg per 5 mL (60 mL) [contains alcohol 15%; cherry flavor]

Tablet: Diphenoxylate hydrochloride 2.5 mg and atropine sulfate 0.025 mg

Lomotil®, Lonox®: Diphenoxylate hydrochloride 2.5 mg and atropine sulfate 0.025 mg

♦ **Diphenylhydantoin** *see* Phenytoin *on page 1253*

Diphtheria and Tetanus Toxoid

(dif THEER ee a & TET a nus TOKS oyd)

Related Information

Immunization Guidelines *on page 1837*

U.S. Brand Names Decavac™

Canadian Brand Names Td Adsorbed

Index Terms DT; Td; Tetanus and Diphtheria Toxoid

Therapeutic Category Vaccine

Generic Available No

Use Diphtheria and tetanus toxoids adsorbed for pediatric use (DT): Infants and Children through 6 years of age: Active immunity against diphtheria and tetanus and tetanus prophylaxis in wound management when pertussis vaccine is contraindicated

Tetanus and diphtheria toxoids adsorbed for adult use (Td) (Decavac™): Children ≥7 years of age and Adults: Active immunity against diphtheria and tetanus; tetanus prophylaxis in wound management

Pregnancy Risk Factor C [Adult formulation (Td)]

Lactation Excretion in breast milk unknown/use caution

Contraindications Hypersensitivity to diphtheria, tetanus toxoid, or any component of the formulation

Warnings Diphtheria and tetanus toxoid is available in two formulations which contain different amounts of the diphtheria toxoid; DT or "pediatric" formulation has twice the diphtheria toxoid as Td or "adult" toxoid; use of DT in children >7 years and adults is associated with more severe adverse reactions to the diphtheria toxoid than in infants and younger children. Immediate treatment for anaphylactic/anaphylactoid reaction should be available during administration of these vaccines. Patients with a history of severe local reaction (Arthus-type) or temperature of >39.4°C (103°F) following a previous dose should not be given further routine or emergency doses of Td more frequently than every 10 years. Defer administration during moderate or severe illness (with or without fever). Immune response may be decreased in immunocompromised patients. Guillain-Barré syndrome, occurring within 6 weeks of tetanus toxoid vaccination, has been reported.

Precautions Administer with caution to patients with thrombocytopenia or any coagulation disorder that would be compromised by I.M. injection; if the patient receives antihemophilia or other similar therapy, I.M. injection can be scheduled shortly after such therapy is administered.

Adverse Reactions All serious adverse reactions must be reported to the U.S. Department of Health and Human Services (DHHS) Vaccine Adverse Event Reporting System (VAERS) 1-800-822-7967.

Central nervous system: Brachial neuritis, Guillain-Barré syndrome (rare), dizziness, paresthesia, seizures, fever, malaise, EEG disturbances, encephalopathy (rare)

Dermatologic: Rash, urticaria

Gastrointestinal: Nausea, vomiting

Local: Tenderness, erythema, swelling, or pain at injection site; sterile abscess; palpable nodule at injection site

Neuromuscular & skeletal: Arthralgia, myalgia

Miscellaneous: Allergic/anaphylactic reactions, Arthus-type hypersensitivity reaction

Drug Interactions Immunosuppressant medications or therapies (antimetabolites, alkylating agents, cytotoxic drugs, corticosteroids, irradiation): The effect of the vaccine may be decreased; consider deferring vaccination for 3 months after immunosuppressant therapy is discontinued.

Stability Refrigerate; do not freeze

Usual Dosage I.M.: 0.5 mL/dose; preterm infants should be vaccinated according to their chronological age from birth

Infants and Children up to 6 years (prior to 7th birthday) with contraindication to immunization containing pertussis: Pediatric formulation (DT):

Recommended schedule: A series of 5 doses administered at 2 months, 4 months, 6 months, 15-18 months, and 4-6 years of age; the 4th dose may be administered as early as 12 months if there has been at least 6 months between the 3rd and 4th doses and the child is unlikely to return at age 15-18 months.

Catch-up schedule: Age at onset of immunization series: Children 4 months through 6 years (prior to 7th birthday): 3 doses at least 4 weeks apart followed 6 months later with dose 4; a 5th dose may be given 6 months later (the 5th dose is not necessary if the child received the 4th dose after 4 years of age)

Children ≥7 years and Adults: Adult formulation (Td):

Primary immunization: 3 total doses; 2 given at intervals of 4-6 weeks; the third 6-12 months later

Booster immunization:

Children 11-12 years: A single dose when at least 5 years have elapsed since last dose of toxoid containing vaccine

Adults: A single dose every 10 years

Tetanus prophylaxis in wound management: Use of tetanus toxoid (DT or Td) and/or tetanus immune globulin (TIG) depends upon the number of prior tetanus toxoid doses and type of wound: A single 0.5 mL dose; see table.

Tetanus Immune Globulin (TIG) and/or Tetanus Toxoid (Td) Wound Management

Number of Prior Tetanus Toxoid Doses	Clean, Minor Wounds		All Other Wounds	
	DT or Td[1]	TIG[2]	DT or Td[1]	TIG[2]
Unknown or <3	Yes	No	Yes	Yes
≥3[3]	No[4]	No	No[5]	No

[1]Use of combined antigen immunization (DT, Td, or DTaP) is preferred). Use tetanus and diphtheria toxoids formulation based upon age; use pediatric preparations (DT or DTaP) if the patient is <7 years old and Td if ≥7 years

[2]Tetanus immune globulin.

[3]If only three doses of fluid tetanus toxoid have been received, a fourth dose of toxoid, preferably an adsorbed toxoid, should be given.

[4]Yes, if >10 years since last dose.

[5]Yes, if >5 years since last dose.

Adapted from Report of the Committee on Infectious Diseases, American Academy of Pediatrics, Elk Grove Village, IL: American Academy of Pediatrics, 1986.

(Continued)

Diphtheria and Tetanus Toxoid *(Continued)*

Administration I.M. Prior to use, shake suspension well; **not for I.V. or SubQ administration**

Td: Administer in the deltoid muscle; do not inject in the gluteal area

DT: Administer in either the anterolateral aspect of the thigh or arm; do not inject in the gluteal area

Patient Information May experience mild fever or soreness, swelling, and redness/knot at the injection site usually lasting 1-2 days

Nursing Implications Federal law requires that the date of administration, the vaccine manufacturer, lot number of vaccine, and the administering person's name, title, and address be entered into the patient's permanent medical record.

Dosage Forms Excipient information presented when available (limited, particularly for generics); consult specific product labeling.

Injection, suspension, adult:

Decavac™: Diphtheria 2 Lf units and tetanus 5 Lf units per 0.5 mL (0.5 mL) [latex free prefilled syringe; contains thimerosal]

Injection, suspension, pediatric [preservative free]: Diphtheria 6.7 Lf units and tetanus 5 Lf units per 0.5 mL (0.5 mL)

References

American Academy of Pediatrics Committee on Infectious Diseases, "Recommended Immunization Schedules for Children and Adolescents - United States, 2007," *Pediatrics*, 2007, 119(1):207-8.

Atkinson WL, Pickering LK, Schwartz B, et al, "General Recommendations on Immunization. Recommendations of the Advisory Committee on Immunization Practices (ACIP) and the American Academy of Family Physicians (AAFP)," *MMWR Recomm Rep*, 2002, 51(RR-2):18.

Centers for Disease Control, "Recommended Adult Immunization Schedule, October 2004-September 2005," available at www.cdc.gov.

♦ **Diphtheria and Tetanus Toxoids and Acellular Pertussis Adsorbed, Hepatitis B (Recombinant) and Inactivated Poliovirus Vaccine Combined** *see* Diphtheria, Tetanus Toxoids, Acellular Pertussis, Hepatitis B (Recombinant), and Poliovirus (Inactivated) Vaccine *on page 516*

♦ **Diphtheria CRM_{197} Protein** *see* Pneumococcal Conjugate Vaccine (7-Valent) *on page 1271*

♦ **Diphtheria CRM_{197} Protein Conjugate** *see Haemophilus* b Conjugate Vaccine *on page 751*

Diphtheria, Tetanus Toxoids, Acellular Pertussis, Hepatitis B (Recombinant), and Poliovirus (Inactivated) Vaccine

(dif THEER ee a, TET a nus TOKS oyds, ay CEL yoo lar per TUS sis, hep a TYE tis bee ree KOM be nant, & POE lee oh VYE rus in ak ti VAY ted vak SEEN)

Related Information

Immunization Guidelines *on page 1837*

U.S. Brand Names Pediarix®

Canadian Brand Names Pediarix®

Index Terms Diphtheria and Tetanus Toxoids and Acellular Pertussis Adsorbed, Hepatitis B (Recombinant) and Inactivated Poliovirus Vaccine Combined

Therapeutic Category Vaccine

Generic Available No

Use Combination vaccine for the active immunization of infants and children 6 weeks through 6 years of age against diphtheria, tetanus, pertussis, hepatitis B virus (all known subtypes), and poliomyelitis (caused by poliovirus types 1, 2, and 3)

Pregnancy Risk Factor C

Contraindications Hypersensitivity to any component including yeast, neomycin, and polymyxin B; encephalopathy occurring within 7 days of administration of a previous dose of a pertussis-containing vaccine that is not attributable to another cause; progressive neurological disorder, including infantile spasms, uncontrolled epilepsy, or progressive encephalopathy (pertussis vaccine should be withheld until the clinical condition has stabilized); defer vaccination for persons with acute febrile illness until recovery; children ≥7 years and adults (formulation without pertussis is indicated for use in these patients)

Warnings Immediate treatment for anaphylactic/anaphylactoid reaction should be available during vaccine use. Subsequent vaccination with a pertussis containing vaccine should be carefully considered if the following reactions occur with a temporal relationship to a previous dose: Temperature ≥40.5°C (105°F) within 48 hours, not attributable to another identifiable cause, collapse, or shock-like state (hypotonic-hyporesponsive episode) within 48 hours, persistent crying lasting ≥3 hours within 48 hours, or convulsions with or without fever, occurring within 3 days. Guillain-Barré syndrome occurring within 6 weeks of vaccines containing tetanus toxoid has been reported; due to a higher rate of fever with this combination formulation than with individual vaccines, antipyretic prophylaxis at the time of and following vaccination should be considered, particularly for patients at high risk for seizures

Precautions Use with caution in patients with coagulation disorders including thrombocytopenia, due to an increased risk for bleeding following I.M. administration; if the patient receives antihemophilia or other similar therapy, I.M. injection can be scheduled shortly after such therapy is administered.

Adverse Reactions All serious adverse reactions must be reported to the U.S. Department of Health and Human Services (DHHS) Vaccine Adverse Event Reporting System (VAERS) 1-800-822-7967. See individual agents.

Drug Interactions See individual agents.

Stability Refrigerate; do not freeze

Mechanism of Action Promotes active immunity to diphtheria, tetanus, pertussis, hepatitis B and poliovirus (types 1, 2, and 3) by inducing production of specific antibodies and antitoxins.

Usual Dosage I.M.: Infants ≥6 weeks and Children <7 years: 0.5 mL per dose; preterm infants should be vaccinated according to their chronological age from birth

Recommended schedule: 3 doses repeated in 6- to 8-week intervals (preferably 8-week intervals); vaccination usually begins at 2 months, but may be started as early as 6 weeks of age.

Note: Infants ≥6 weeks and children previously vaccinated with one or more components of this combination vaccine, and who are also scheduled to receive all vaccine components, may use Pediarix™ to complete the series.

Administration Shake well; administer I.M. in either the anterolateral aspect of the thigh or arm; **not for I.V. or SubQ administration**

Patient Information May cause increased sleeping, restlessness, fussiness, decreased appetite, or fever (use antipyretic if directed by healthcare provider). May cause some redness, pain, or swelling at injection site; consult healthcare provider if excessive or persistent. Notify healthcare provider immediately of any excessive or persistent reactions (eg, fever >105°F within 48 hours, inconsolable crying that occurs within 48 hours and lasts 3 hours, seizures that occur within 3 days).

Nursing Implications Federal law requires that the date of administration, name of the vaccine manufacturer, lot number of vaccine, and the administering person's name, title, and address be entered into the patient's permanent medical record.

Additional Information Contains the following three pertussis antigens: Inactivated pertussis toxin (PT), filamentous hemagglutinin (FHA), and pertactin. Contains the same diphtheria and tetanus toxoids and pertussis antigens found in Infanrix®. Contains the same hepatitis B surface antigen (HB_sAg) found in Engerix-B® (recombinant vaccine). Thimerosal is used during manufacturing, but removed to less than detectable levels in the final suspension.

Dosage Forms Excipient information presented when available (limited, particularly for generics); consult specific product labeling.

Injection, suspension [preservative free]:

Pediarix®: Diphtheria toxoid 25 Lf, tetanus toxoid 10 Lf, inactivated PT 25 mcg, FHA 25 mcg, pertactin 8 mcg, HB_sAg 10 mcg, poliovirus type 1 40 DU, poliovirus type 2 8 DU, and poliovirus type 3 32 DU per 0.5 mL (0.5 mL) [contains aluminum, neomycin sulfate ≤0.05 ng/0.5 mL, polymyxin B ≤0.01 ng/0.5 mL, polysorbate 80, and yeast protein ≤5%; packaged in vials or prefilled syringes; the needleless prefilled syringes contain dry natural latex rubber in the tip cap and plunger]

References

American Academy of Pediatrics Committee on Infectious Diseases, "Recommended Immunization Schedules for Children and Adolescents - United States, 2007," *Pediatrics*, 2007, 119(1):207-8.

Atkinson WL, Pickering LK, Schwartz B, et al, "General Recommendations on Immunization. Recommendations of the Advisory Committee on Immunization Practices (ACIP) and the American Academy of Family Physicians (AAFP)," *MMWR Recomm Rep*, 2002, 51(RR-2):1-35.

Diphtheria, Tetanus Toxoids, and Acellular Pertussis Vaccine

(dif THEER ee a, TET a nus TOKS oyds & ay CEL yoo lar per TUS sis vak SEEN)

Medication Safety Issues

Carefully review product labeling to prevent inadvertent administration of Tdap when DTaP is indicated. Tdap contains lower amounts of diphtheria toxoid and some pertussis antigens than DTaP.

Tdap is not indicated for use in children <10 years of age

DTaP is not indicated for use in persons ≥7 years of age

Guidelines are available in case of inadvertent administration of these products; refer to ACIP recommendations, February 2006 available at http://www.cdc.gov/mmwr/preview/mmwrhtml/rr55e223a1.htm

(Continued)

Diphtheria, Tetanus Toxoids, and Acellular Pertussis Vaccine *(Continued)*

Note:

DTaP: Diphtheria and tetanus toxoids and acellular pertussis vaccine

DTP: Diphtheria and tetanus toxoids and pertussis vaccine (unspecified pertussis antigens)

DTwP: Diphtheria and tetanus toxoids and whole-cell pertussis vaccine (no longer available on U.S. market)

Tdap: Tetanus toxoid, reduced diphtheria toxoid, and acellular pertussis vaccine

Related Information

Immunization Guidelines *on page 1837*

U.S. Brand Names Adacel™; Boostrix®; Daptacel®; Infanrix®; Tripedia®

Canadian Brand Names Adacel™

Index Terms DTaP; dTpa; Tdap; Tetanus Toxoid, Reduced Diphtheria Toxoid, and Acellular Pertussis, Adsorbed

Therapeutic Category Vaccine

Generic Available No

Use

Daptacel®, Infanrix®, Tripedia®: Active immunization of children 6 weeks through 6 years of age (prior to the 7th birthday) for prevention of diphtheria, tetanus, and pertussis

Adacel™: Active booster immunization of children >11 years through adults to 64 years of age; the CDC recommends for adults 19-64 years, this vaccine replace tetanus and diphtheria toxoids (Td) vaccine if the individual has received the last dose of Td >10 years earlier and has not previously received Tdap; adults who have or who anticipate having close contact with an infant <12 months and health-care personnel who have direct patient contact should receive this vaccine

Boostrix®: Active booster immunization of children 10-18 years of age

Pregnancy Risk Factor C

Contraindications Hypersensitivity to any component; encephalopathy occurring within 7 days of administration of a previous dose of a pertussis-containing vaccine that is not attributable to another cause; progressive neurological disorder, including infantile spasms, uncontrolled epilepsy, or progressive encephalopathy; (pertussis vaccine should be withheld until the clinical condition has stabilized); defer vaccination for persons with acute febrile illness until recovery; adults (formulation without pertussis is indicated for use)

Warnings Subsequent vaccination with a pertussis containing vaccine should be carefully considered if the following reactions occur with a temporal relationship to a previous dose of DTaP: temperature ≥40.5°C (105°F) within 48 hours, not attributable to another identifiable cause, collapse or shock-like state (hypotonic-hyporesponsive episode) within 48 hours, persistent crying lasting ≥3 hours within 48 hours, or convulsions with or without fever, occurring within 3 days. Guillain Barré syndrome occurring within 6 weeks of vaccines containing tetanus toxoid has been reported. Boostrix® is a reduced antigen vaccine which is not indicated for use in the primary vaccine series (ages 6 weeks to 6 years).

Precautions A family history of seizures is not a contraindication to use of DTaP; treatment with acetaminophen or other appropriate antipyretic is recommended at the time of vaccination and for the next 24 hours afterwards to reduce the possibility of postvaccination fever; immediate treatment for anaphylactoid or acute hypersensitivity reactions should be available during vaccine use; administer with caution to patients with thrombocytopenia or any coagulation disorder that would be compromised by I.M. injection; if the patient receives antihemophilia or other similar therapy, I.M. injection can be scheduled shortly after such therapy is administered.

Adverse Reactions All serious adverse reactions must be reported to the U.S. Department of Health and Human Services (DHHS) Vaccine Adverse Event Reporting System (VAERS) 1-800-822-7967.

Central nervous system: Fever, persistent crying, high-pitched cry, fatigue, fussiness, sleepiness, Guillain-Barré, febrile seizures, autism, encephalopathy

Dermatologic: Rash, cellulitis

Gastrointestinal: Vomiting, anorexia

Hematologic: ITP

Local: Tenderness, erythema, swelling, or pain at injection site; sterile abscess; palpable nodule at injection site

Neuromuscular & skeletal: Hypotonia

Respiratory: Apnea

Miscellaneous: Hypersensitivity reactions including anaphylaxis, SIDS (causal relationship has not been demonstrated)

Drug Interactions Decreased immunologic effects with immunosuppressive agents; decreased immunologic effect in infants <15 months when Tripedia® is used to reconstitute ActHIB® vaccine (TriHIBit®) vs administered in separate injections

Stability Refrigerate; Tripedia® may be used to reconstitute ActHIB®

Usual Dosage I.M.: 0.5 mL per dose; preterm infants should be vaccinated according to their chronological age from birth

Recommended schedule: Children 6 weeks through 6 years (prior to 7th birthday): A series of five doses administered at 2 months, 4 months, 6 months, 15-18 months, and 4-6 years of age; the 4th dose may be administered as early as 12 months if there has been at least 6 months between the 3rd and 4th doses and the child is unlikely to return at age 15-18 months.

Catch-up schedule: Children 4 months through 6 years (prior to 7th birthday): 3 doses at least 4 weeks apart followed 6 months later with dose 4; a 5th dose may be given 6 months later (the 5th dose is not necessary if the child received the 4th dose after 4 years of age)

Children 10-18 years: Boostrix® or Adacel™ formulation only: A single dose; do not administer within 5 years of completion of DTaP series

Children >18 years to Adults 64 years: Adacel™ formulation only: A single dose; do not administer within 5 years of the previous dose of DTaP; may be administered within 2 years of last Td; when possible, women should receive prior to becoming pregnant or in the immediate postpartum period (CDC Recommendation)

Administration Shake vial well before withdrawing the dose; administer I.M. in either the anterolateral aspect of the thigh or arm; **not for I.V., intradermal, or SubQ administration**

Nursing Implications Federal law requires that the date of administration, the vaccine manufacturer, lot number of vaccine, and the administering person's name, title, and address be entered into the patient's permanent medical record.

Additional Information Adacel™ is formulated with the same antigens found in Daptacel® but with reduced quantities of tetanus and pertussis; Boostrix® is formulated with the same antigens found in Infanrix® but in reduced quantities. Use of Adacel™ or Boostrix® in the primary immunization series or to complete the primary series has not been evaluated.

Dosage Forms Excipient information presented when available (limited, particularly for generics); consult specific product labeling.

Injection, suspension:

Adacel™: Diphtheria 2 Lf units, tetanus 5 Lf units, and acellular pertussis 2.5 mcg per 0.5 mL (0.5 mL) [vial stopper is latex free]

Boostrix®: Diphtheria 2.5 Lf units, tetanus 5 Lf units, and acellular pertussis 8 mcg per 0.5 mL (0.5 mL) [available in vial and prefilled syringe; preservative free; contains polysorbate 80; syringe cap and rubber plunger contain natural latex rubber]

Daptacel®: Diphtheria 15 Lf units, tetanus 5 Lf units, and acellular pertussis 10 mcg per 0.5 mL (0.5 mL) [vial stopper contains natural latex rubber]

Infanrix®: Diphtheria 25 Lf units, tetanus 10 Lf units, and acellular pertussis 25 mcg per 0.5 mL (0.5 mL) [available in vial and prefilled syringe; contains polysorbate 80; syringe cap and rubber plunger contain natural latex rubber]

Tripedia®: Diphtheria 6.7 Lf units, tetanus 5 Lf units, and acellular pertussis 46.8 mcg per 0.5 mL (7.5 mL) [contains polysorbate 80 and trace amounts of thimerosal; vial stopper contains natural latex rubber]

Note: Tripedia® vaccine is also used to reconstitute ActHIB® to prepare TriHIBit® vaccine (diphtheria, tetanus toxoids, and acellular pertussis and *Haemophilus influenzae* b conjugate vaccine combination)

References

American Academy of Pediatrics Committee on Infectious Diseases, "Recommended Immunization Schedules for Children and Adolescents - United States, 2007," *Pediatrics*, 2007, 119(1):207-8.

Centers for Disease Control and Prevention, "Recommended Childhood and Adolescent Immunization Schedule - United States, July-December 2004," *MMWR Morb Mortal Wkly Rep*, 2004, 53(16):Q1-4.

Kretsinger K, Broder KR, Cortese MM, et al, "Preventing Tetanus, Diphtheria, and Pertussis Among Adults: Use of Tetanus Toxoid, Reduced Diphtheria Toxoid and Acellular Pertussis Vaccine," *MMWR Recomm Rep*, 2006, 55(RR-17):1-37.

Diphtheria, Tetanus Toxoids, and Acellular Pertussis Vaccine and *Haemophilus influenzae* b Conjugate Vaccine

(dif THEER ee a, TET a nus TOKS oyds & ay CEL yoo lar per TUS sis vak SEEN & hem OF fi lus in floo EN za bee KON joo gate vak SEEN)

Related Information

Immunization Guidelines *on page 1837*

(Continued)

Diphtheria, Tetanus Toxoids, and Acellular Pertussis Vaccine and *Haemophilus influenzae* b Conjugate Vaccine *(Continued)*

U.S. Brand Names TriHIBit®

Index Terms *Haemophilus influenzae* b Conjugate Vaccine and Diphtheria, Tetanus Toxoids, and Acellular Pertussis Vaccine

Therapeutic Category Vaccine

Generic Available No

Use Active immunization of children 15-18 months of age for prevention of diphtheria, tetanus, pertussis, and invasive disease caused by *H. influenzae* type b.

Contraindications Hypersensitivity to any component

Warnings See individual agents.

Adverse Reactions See individual agents.

Usual Dosage The combination can be used for the DTaP dose given at 15-18 months when a primary series of HIB vaccine has been given.

Children >15 months of age: I.M.: 0.5 mL

Administration Reconstitute by adding Tripedia® vaccine to ActHIB® vaccine; shake well; administer I.M. in either the anterolateral aspect of the thigh or deltoid muscle of the arm; **not for I.V. or SubQ administration**

Nursing Implications Federal law requires that the date of administration, the vaccine manufacturer, lot number of vaccine, and the administering person's name, title, and address be entered into the patient's permanent medical record.

Dosage Forms Excipient information presented when available (limited, particularly for generics); consult specific product labeling.

Injection, suspension: 5 Lf units tetanus toxoid, 6.7 Lf units diphtheria toxoid, 46.8 mcg pertussis antigens, and 10 mcg *H. influenzae* type b purified capsular polysaccharide per 0.5 mL (0.5 mL) [The combination of Tripedia® vaccine used to reconstitute ActHIB® forms TriHIBit®]

References

American Academy of Pediatrics Committee on Infectious Diseases, "Recommended Immunization Schedules for Children and Adolescents - United States, 2007," *Pediatrics*, 2007, 119(1):207-8.

Centers for Disease Control and Prevention, "Recommended Childhood and Adolescent Immunization Schedule - United States, July-December 2004," *MMWR Morb Mortal Wkly Rep*, 2004, 53(16):Q1-4.

♦ **Diphtheria Toxoid Conjugate** *see Haemophilus* b Conjugate Vaccine *on page 751*

♦ **Dipivalyl Epinephrine** *see* Dipivefrin *on page 520*

Dipivefrin (dye PI ve frin)

U.S. Brand Names Propine®

Canadian Brand Names Ophtho-Dipivefrin™; PMS-Dipivefrin; Propine®

Index Terms Dipivalyl Epinephrine; Dipivefrin Hydrochloride; DPE

Therapeutic Category Adrenergic Agonist Agent, Ophthalmic; Ophthalmic Agent, Vasoconstrictor

Generic Available Yes

Use Reduces elevated IOP in chronic open-angle glaucoma; treatment of ocular hypertension

Pregnancy Risk Factor B

Contraindications Hypersensitivity to dipivefrin, any component (see Warnings), or epinephrine; contraindicated in patients with angle-closure glaucoma

Warnings Commercial preparation contains sodium metabisulfate which may cause allergic reactions in susceptible individuals

Precautions Use with caution in patients with vascular hypertension or cardiac disorders and in aphakic patients (dipivefrin may cause cystoid macular edema in aphakic patients)

Adverse Reactions

Central nervous system: Headache

Local: Burning, stinging

Ocular: Ocular congestion, photophobia, mydriasis, blurred vision, ocular pain, bulbar conjunctival follicles, blepharoconjunctivitis, cystoid macular edema

Drug Interactions Effects of lowering IOP may be additive when used with topical miotics, timolol, betaxolol, or carbonic anhydrase inhibitors

Stability Protect from light and avoid exposure to air; discolored or darkened solutions indicate loss of potency

Mechanism of Action Dipivefrin is a prodrug of epinephrine which is the active agent that stimulates alpha- and/or beta-adrenergic receptors increasing aqueous humor outflow

Pharmacodynamics
Onset of action:
Ocular pressure effects: Within 30 minutes
Mydriasis: Within 30 minutes
Maximum effect: Ocular pressure effects: Within 1 hour
Duration:
Ocular pressure effects: 12 hours or longer
Mydriasis: Several hours

Pharmacokinetics Absorption: Rapid into the aqueous humor; converted to epinephrine

Usual Dosage Children and Adults: Ophthalmic: Initial: Instill 1 drop every 12 hours

Administration Ophthalmic: Instill drop into eye; apply finger pressure to lacrimal sac during and for 1-2 minutes after instillation to decrease risk of absorption and systemic effects; avoid contacting bottle tip with skin or eye

Monitoring Parameters IOP

Patient Information Discolored solutions should be discarded; may cause burning or stinging, blurred vision, and sensitivity to light

Dosage Forms Excipient information presented when available (limited, particularly for generics); consult specific product labeling.
Solution, ophthalmic, as hydrochloride: 0.1% (5 mL, 10 mL, 15 mL) [contains benzalkonium chloride]
Propine®: 0.1% (5 mL [DSC], 10 mL, 15 mL) [contains benzalkonium chloride]

- **Dipivefrin Hydrochloride** *see* Dipivefrin *on page 520*
- **Diprivan®** *see* Propofol *on page 1331*
- **Diprolene®** *see* Betamethasone *on page 212*
- **Diprolene® AF** *see* Betamethasone *on page 212*
- **Diprolene® Glycol (Can)** *see* Betamethasone *on page 212*
- **Dipropylacetic Acid** *see* Valproic Acid and Derivatives *on page 1592*
- **Diprosone® (Can)** *see* Betamethasone *on page 212*

Dipyridamole (dye peer ID a mole)

Medication Safety Issues
Sound-alike/look-alike issues:
Dipyridamole may be confused with disopyramide
Persantine® may be confused with Periactin®, Permitil®

Related Information
Antithrombotic Therapy in Children *on page 1804*

U.S. Brand Names Persantine®

Canadian Brand Names Apo-Dipyridamole FC®; Persantine®

Therapeutic Category Antiplatelet Agent; Vasodilator, Coronary

Generic Available Yes

Use Maintain patency after surgical grafting procedures including coronary artery bypass; with warfarin to decrease thrombosis in patients after artificial heart valve replacement; for chronic management of angina pectoris; with aspirin to prevent coronary artery thrombosis; in combination with aspirin or warfarin to prevent other thromboembolic disorders; dipyridamole may also be given 2 days prior to open heart surgery to prevent platelet activation by extracorporeal bypass pump; diagnostic agent I.V. (dipyridamole stress test) for coronary artery disease

Pregnancy Risk Factor B

Lactation Enters breast milk/use caution

Contraindications Hypersensitivity to dipyridamole or any component

Precautions Use with caution in patients with hypotension (may further decrease blood pressure due to peripheral vasodilation); use with caution in patients with CAD (may aggravate chest pain)

Adverse Reactions
Cardiovascular: Vasodilatation, flushing, syncope
Central nervous system: Dizziness, headache (dose-related)
Dermatologic: Rash, pruritus
Gastrointestinal: Abdominal distress, nausea, vomiting, diarrhea
Hepatic: Elevated liver enzymes, hepatic failure (rare)
Neuromuscular & skeletal: Weakness

Drug Interactions Heparin, warfarin, streptokinase, urokinase, alteplase, aspirin, NSAIDs, cefamandole, cefoperazone, cefotetan, and valproic acid may increase risk of bleeding; decreased coronary artery vasodilation from I.V. dipyridamole may occur in patients receiving theophylline or caffeine; dipyridamole may increase plasma concentration and effects of adenosine (reduced dose of adenosine may be needed);
(Continued)

Dipyridamole *(Continued)*

dipyridamole may counteract effect of cholinesterase inhibitors and aggravate myasthenia gravis.

Stability Do not freeze; protect I.V. preparation from light

Mechanism of Action Inhibits the activity of adenosine deaminase and phosphodiesterase, which causes an accumulation of adenosine, adenine nucleotides, and cyclic AMP; these mediators then inhibit platelet aggregation and may cause vasodilation; may also stimulate release of prostacyclin or PGD_2; causes coronary vasodilation

Pharmacokinetics Oral:

Absorption: Slow and variable

Distribution: Distributes to breast milk

V_d: Adults: 2-3 L/kg

Protein binding: 91% to 99%

Metabolism: In the liver to glucuronide conjugate

Bioavailability: 27% to 66%

Half-life, terminal: 10-12 hours

Time to peak serum concentration: Oral: 75 minutes

Elimination: In feces via bile as glucuronide conjugates and unchanged drug

Usual Dosage

Children:

Oral: 3-6 mg/kg/day in 3 divided doses

Doses of 4-10 mg/kg/day have been used investigationally to treat proteinuria in pediatric renal disease

Mechanical prosthetic heart valves: 2-5 mg/kg/day [used in combination with an oral anticoagulant in children who have systemic embolism despite adequate oral anticoagulant therapy (INR 2.5-3.5), and used in combination with low-dose oral anticoagulation (INR 2-3) plus aspirin in children in whom full-dose oral anticoagulation is contraindicated] (see Monagle, 2001). **Note:** The current *Chest* guidelines (Monagle, 2004) do not mention the use of dipyridamole for prophylaxis for mechanical prosthetic heart valves in children; an oral anticoagulant plus aspirin is recommended for the patient groups mentioned above.

Adults:

Prophylaxis of thromboembolism after cardiac valve replacement (adjunctive use): Oral: 75-100 mg 4 times/day

Dipyridamole stress test (for evaluation of myocardial perfusion): I.V.: 0.142 mg/kg/minute for a total of 4 minutes (0.57 mg/kg total); maximum dose: 60 mg; inject thallium 201 within 5 minutes after end of injection of dipyridamole

Platelet aggregation inhibitor: I.V. infusion: 250 mg/day at a rate of 10 mg/hour; maximum dose: 400 mg/day (use lower doses with aspirin)

Administration

Oral: Administer with water on an empty stomach 1 hour before or 2 hours after meals; may take with milk or food to decrease GI upset

Parenteral: I.V.: Dilute in at least a 1:2 ratio with NS, ½NS, or D_5W; infusion of undiluted dipyridamole may cause local irritation; see Usual Dosage for infusion rates

Monitoring Parameters Blood pressure, heart rate

Test Interactions Patients on theophylline may show false-negative thallium scan result on dipyridamole stress test

Patient Information Notify physician or pharmacist if taking other medications that affect bleeding, such as warfarin or NSAIDs; avoid alcohol

Dosage Forms Excipient information presented when available (limited, particularly for generics); consult specific product labeling.

Injection, solution: 5 mg/mL (2 mL, 10 mL)

Tablet: 25 mg, 50 mg, 75 mg

Persantine®: 25 mg, 50 mg, 75 mg

Extemporaneous Preparations A 10 mg/mL oral liquid preparation made from tablets and 3 different vehicles (cherry syrup, a 1:1 mixture of Ora-Sweet® and Ora-Plus®, or a 1:1 mixture of Ora-Sweet® SF and Ora-Plus®) was stable for 60 days when stored in amber plastic prescription bottles in the dark, at room temperature (25°C) or under refrigeration (5°C); grind twenty-four 50 mg tablets in a mortar into a fine powder; add 20 mL of the vehicle and mix well to form a uniform paste; mix while adding the vehicle in geometric proportions to **almost** 120 mL; transfer to a calibrated bottle and qsad with vehicle to 120 mL; label "shake well" and "protect from light"

Allen LV and Erickson MA, "Stability of Baclofen, Captopril, Diltiazem Hydrochloride, Dipyridamole, and Flecainide Acetate in Extemporaneously Compounded Oral Liquids," *Am J Health Sys Pharm*, 1996, 53(18):2179-84.

References

Monagle P, Chan A, Massicotte P, et al, "Antithrombotic Therapy in Children: The Seventh ACCP Conference on Antithrombotic and Thrombolytic Therapy," *Chest*, 2004, 126(3 Suppl):645S-687S.

Monagle P, Michelson AD, Bovill E, et al, "Antithrombotic Therapy in Children," *Chest*, 2001, 119(1 Suppl):344S-370S.

Rao PS, Solymar L, Mardini MK, et al, "Anticoagulant Therapy in Children With Prosthetic Valves," *Ann Thorac Surg*, 1989, 47(4):589-92.

Ueda N, Kawaguchi S, Niinomi Y, et al, "Effect of Dipyridamole Treatment on Proteinuria in Pediatric Renal Disease," *Nephron*, 1986, 44(3):174-9.

♦ **Disodium Cromoglycate** *see* Cromolyn *on page 407*

♦ **Disodium Thiosulfate Pentahydrate** *see* Sodium Thiosulfate *on page 1461*

♦ ***d*-Isoephedrine Hydrochloride** *see* Pseudoephedrine *on page 1344*

Disopyramide (dye soe PEER a mide)

Medication Safety Issues

Sound-alike/look-alike issues:

Disopyramide may be confused with desipramine, dipyridamole

Norpace® may be confused with Norpramin®

Related Information

Medications for Which A Single Dose May Be Fatal When Ingested By A Toddler *on page 1932*

U.S. Brand Names Norpace®; Norpace® CR

Canadian Brand Names Norpace®; Rythmodan®; Rythmodan®-LA

Index Terms Disopyramide Phosphate

Therapeutic Category Antiarrhythmic Agent, Class I-A

Generic Available Yes

Use Treatment of life-threatening ventricular arrhythmias; suppression and prevention of unifocal and multifocal ventricular premature complexes, coupled ventricular premature complexes, and/or paroxysmal ventricular tachycardia; also effective in the conversion and prevention of recurrence of atrial fibrillation, atrial flutter, and paroxysmal atrial tachycardia

Pregnancy Risk Factor C

Lactation Enters breast milk/compatible

Contraindications Hypersensitivity to disopyramide or any component; pre-existing second or third degree A-V block; congenital QT prolongation; cardiogenic shock; do not administer with clarithromycin or erythromycin (see Drug Interactions)

Precautions Use with caution in patients with pre-existing urinary retention, existing or family history of angle-closure glaucoma, myasthenia gravis, hypotension during initiation of therapy, CHF unless caused by an arrhythmia, widening of QRS complex during therapy or lengthening of QT interval (>25% to 50% of baseline QRS complex or QT interval), sick sinus syndrome, Wolf Parkinson White syndrome (WPW) or bundle-branch block; may increase ventricular rate in patients with atrial flutter who have not received digoxin; use with caution and decrease dose in patients with renal or hepatic impairment; not recommended for use 48 hours before or 24 hours after verapamil

Adverse Reactions

Cardiovascular: CHF, edema, chest pain, syncope and hypotension, conduction disturbances including A-V block, widening QRS complex and lengthening of QT interval

Central nervous system: Fatigue, headache, malaise, nervousness, acute psychosis, depression, dizziness

Dermatologic: Generalized rashes

Endocrine & metabolic: Hypoglycemia, weight gain, elevated cholesterol and triglycerides; may initiate contractions of pregnant uterus; hyperkalemia may enhance toxicities

Gastrointestinal: Xerostomia, dry throat, constipation, nausea, vomiting, diarrhea, pain, gas, anorexia

Genitourinary: Urinary retention/hesitancy

Hepatic: Elevated liver enzymes, hepatic cholestasis

Neuromuscular & skeletal: Weakness

Ocular: Blurred vision, dry eyes

Respiratory: Dyspnea (<1%), dry nasal membranes

Drug Interactions Cytochrome P450 isoenzyme CYP3A4 substrate

Hepatic microsomal enzyme inducing agents (ie, phenytoin, phenobarbital, rifampin) may increase metabolism of disopyramide and lower serum concentrations; clarithromycin and erythromycin may increase disopyramide serum concentrations which can be life-threatening (do not use with disopyramide); other antiarrhythmic agents (quinidine, procainamide, lidocaine, propranolol) may increase adverse conduction effects (widening QRS complex, lengthening QT interval); adverse effects of disopyramide may be additive with amitriptyline, imipramine, haloperidol, thioridazine, cisapride, and other drugs that prolong the QT interval; verapamil

(Continued)

Disopyramide *(Continued)*

(disopyramide is not recommended for use 48 hours before or 24 hours after verapamil)

Mechanism of Action Class IA antiarrhythmic: Decreases myocardial excitability and conduction velocity; reduces disparity in refractory period between normal and infarcted myocardium; possesses anticholinergic, peripheral vasoconstrictive and negative inotropic effects

Pharmacodynamics

Capsules, regular:

Onset of action: 30-210 minutes

Duration: 1.5-8.5 hours

Pharmacokinetics

Protein binding: Concentration dependent, stereoselective, and ranges from 20% to 60%

Distribution: V_d: Children: 1 L/kg

Metabolism: In the liver; major metabolite has anticholinergic and antiarrhythmic effects

Bioavailability: 60% to 83%

Half-life:

Children: 3.15 hours

Adults: 4-10 hours (mean: 6.7 hours), increased half-life with hepatic or renal disease

Elimination: 40% to 60% excreted unchanged in urine and 10% to 15% in feces

Clearance is greater and half-life shorter in children vs adults; clearance (children): 3.76 mL/minute/kg

Usual Dosage Oral:

Children (start with lower dose listed):

<1 year: 10-30 mg/kg/day in 4 divided doses

1-4 years: 10-20 mg/kg/day in 4 divided doses

4-12 years: 10-15 mg/kg/day in 4 divided doses

12-18 years: 6-15 mg/kg/day in 4 divided doses

Adults: **Note:** Some patients may require initial loading dose; see product information for details

<50 kg: 100 mg every 6 hours **or** 200 mg every 12 hours (controlled release)

>50 kg: 150 mg every 6 hours **or** 300 mg every 12 hours (controlled release); if no response, may increase to 200 mg every 6 hours; maximum dose required for patients with severe refractory ventricular tachycardia is 400 mg every 6 hours. **Note:** Use lower doses (100 mg of nonsustained release every 6-8 hours) in adults with cardiomyopathy or cardiac decompensation.

Adult dosing adjustment in renal impairment: 100 mg (nonsustained release) given at the following intervals: See table

Creatinine Clearance (mL/min)	Dosage Interval
30-40	Every 8 hours
15-30	Every 12 hours
<15	Every 24 hours

Administration Oral: Administer on an empty stomach; do not crush, break, or chew controlled release capsules, swallow whole

Monitoring Parameters Blood pressure, EKG, drug level; serum potassium, glucose, cholesterol, triglycerides, and liver enzymes; especially important to monitor EKG in patients with hepatic or renal disease, heart disease, or others with increased risk of adverse effects

Reference Range Therapeutic:

Atrial arrhythmias: 2.8-3.2 mcg/mL (SI: 8.3-9.4 micromoles/L)

Ventricular arrhythmias: 3.3-7.5 mcg/mL (SI: 9.7-22 micromoles/L)

Toxic: >7 mcg/mL (SI: >20.7 micromoles/L)

Patient Information Avoid alcohol; notify physician if urinary retention or worsening of CHF occurs; may cause dry mouth

Dosage Forms Excipient information presented when available (limited, particularly for generics); consult specific product labeling.

Capsule (Norpace®): 100 mg, 150 mg

Capsule, controlled release (Norpace® CR): 100 mg, 150 mg

Extemporaneous Preparations Extemporaneous suspensions in cherry syrup (1 mg/mL and 10 mg/mL) are stable for 4 weeks in amber glass bottles stored at 5°C, 30°C, or at room temperature; shake well before use; do not use extended release capsules for this suspension

Mathur LK, Lai PK, and Shively CD, "Stability of Disopyramide Phosphate in Cherry Syrup," *J Hosp Pharm*, 1982, 39(2):309-10.

References

Chiba K, Koike K, Nakamoto M, et al, "Steady-State Pharmacokinetics and Bioavailability of Total and Unbound Disopyramide in Children With Cardiac Arrhythmias," *Ther Drug Monit*, 1992, 14(2):112-8.
Echizen H, Takahashi H, Nakamura H, et al, "Stereoselective Disposition and Metabolism of Disopyramide in Pediatric Patients," *J Pharmacol Exp Ther*, 1991, 259(3):953-60.

♦ **Disopyramide Phosphate** *see* Disopyramide *on page 523*
♦ **Dithioglycerol** *see* Dimercaprol *on page 508*
♦ **Ditropan®** *see* Oxybutynin *on page 1187*
♦ **Ditropan® XL** *see* Oxybutynin *on page 1187*
♦ **Diuril®** *see* Chlorothiazide *on page 342*
♦ **Divalproex Sodium** *see* Valproic Acid and Derivatives *on page 1592*
♦ **Dixarit® (Can)** *see* Clonidine *on page 389*
♦ **5071-1DL(6)** *see* Megestrol *on page 995*
♦ ***dl*-Alpha Tocopherol** *see* Vitamin E *on page 1620*
♦ **DM** *see* Dextromethorphan *on page 477*
♦ **4-DMDR** *see* Idarubicin *on page 808*
♦ **DMSA** *see* Succimer *on page 1477*
♦ **DNase** *see* Dornase Alfa *on page 531*
♦ **DNR** *see* DAUNOrubicin *on page 447*
♦ **Doak® Tar [OTC]** *see* Coal Tar *on page 394*

DOBUTamine (doe BYOO ta meen)

Medication Safety Issues

Sound-alike/look-alike issues:

DOBUTamine may be confused with DOPamine

Related Information

Emergency Pediatric Drip Calculations *on page 1652*

Extravasation Treatment *on page 1726*

Canadian Brand Names Dobutamine Injection, USP; Dobutrex®

Index Terms Dobutamine Hydrochloride

Therapeutic Category Adrenergic Agonist Agent; Sympathomimetic

Generic Available Yes

Use Short-term management of patients with cardiac decompensation

Pregnancy Risk Factor B

Lactation Excretion in breast milk unknown

Contraindications Hypersensitivity to dobutamine or any component (see Warnings); patients with idiopathic hypertrophic subaortic stenosis (IHSS)

Warnings Potent drug; must be diluted prior to use; patient's hemodynamic status should be monitored; contains sulfites which may cause allergic reactions in susceptible individuals

Precautions Hypovolemia should be corrected prior to use; infiltration causes local inflammatory changes, extravasation may cause dermal necrosis

Adverse Reactions

Cardiovascular: Ectopic heartbeats, elevated heart rate, chest pain, palpitations, elevation in blood pressure; in higher doses ventricular tachycardia or arrhythmias may be seen; patients with atrial fibrillation or flutter are at risk of developing a rapid ventricular response

Central nervous system: Headache

Gastrointestinal: Nausea, vomiting

Local: Phlebitis

Neuromuscular & skeletal: Mild leg cramps, paresthesia

Respiratory: Dyspnea

Drug Interactions Beta-adrenergic blocking agents, general anesthetics

Stability Stable in various parenteral solutions for 24 hours; incompatible with alkaline solutions, do not give through same I.V. line as heparin, sodium bicarbonate, ethacrynic acid, cefazolin, or penicillin; compatible when coadministered with dopamine, nitroprusside, potassium chloride, protamine sulfate, tobramycin, epinephrine, atracurium, vecuronium, isoproterenol, and lidocaine; pink discoloration of dobutamine hydrochloride indicates slight oxidation, but no significant loss of potency if administered within the recommended time period

Mechanism of Action Stimulates $beta_1$-adrenergic receptors, causing increased contractility and heart rate, with little effect on $beta_2$- or alpha-receptors

Pharmacodynamics

Onset of action: I.V.: 1-10 minutes

Maximum effect: Within 10-20 minutes

(Continued)

DOBUTamine *(Continued)*

Pharmacokinetics

Metabolism: In tissues and the liver to inactive metabolites

Half-life: 2 minutes

Usual Dosage I.V. continuous infusion:

Neonates: 2-15 mcg/kg/minute, titrate to desired response

Children and Adults: 2.5-15 mcg/kg/minute, titrate to desired response; maximum dose: 40 mcg/kg/minute

Administration Parenteral: Dilute in dextrose or NS; maximum recommended concentration: 5000 mcg/mL (5 mg/mL); rate of infusion (mL/hour) = dose (mcg/kg/minute) x weight (kg) x 60 minutes/hour divided by the concentration (mcg/mL); administer into large vein; use infusion device to control rate of flow

Monitoring Parameters EKG, heart rate, CVP, MAP, urine output; if pulmonary artery catheter is in place, monitor CI, PCWP, RAP, and SVR. Dobutamine lowers central venous pressure and wedge pressure but has little effect on pulmonary vascular resistance.

Dosage Forms Excipient information presented when available (limited, particularly for generics); consult specific product labeling.

Infusion, as hydrochloride [premixed in dextrose]: 1 mg/mL (250 mL, 500 mL); 2 mg/mL (250 mL); 4 mg/mL (250 mL)

Injection, solution, as hydrochloride: 12.5 mg/mL (20 mL, 40 mL, 100 mL) [contains sodium bisulfite]

♦ **Dobutamine Hydrochloride** *see* DOBUTamine *on page 525*

♦ **Dobutamine Injection, USP (Can)** *see* DOBUTamine *on page 525*

♦ **Dobutrex® (Can)** *see* DOBUTamine *on page 525*

Docusate (DOK yoo sate)

Medication Safety Issues

Sound-alike/look-alike issues:

Docusate may be confused with Doxinate®

Colace® may be confused with Calan®

Surfak® may be confused with Surbex®

U.S. Brand Names Colace® [OTC]; Diocto® [OTC]; Docusoft-S™ [OTC]; DOK™ [OTC]; DOS® [OTC]; D-S-S® [OTC]; Dulcolax® Stool Softener [OTC]; Enemeez® [OTC]; Fleet® Sof-Lax® [OTC]; Genasoft® [OTC]; Phillips'® Stool Softener Laxative [OTC]; Silace [OTC]; Surfak® [OTC]

Canadian Brand Names Apo-Docusate-Sodium®; Colace®; Colax-C®; Novo-Docusate Calcium; Novo-Docusate Sodium; PMS-Docusate Calcium; PMS-Docusate Sodium; Regulex®; Selax®; Soflax™

Index Terms Dioctyl Calcium Sulfosuccinate; Dioctyl Sodium Sulfosuccinate; Docusate Calcium; Docusate Potassium; Docusate Sodium; DOSS; DSS

Therapeutic Category Laxative, Surfactant; Stool Softener

Generic Available Yes: Excludes gelcap

Use Stool softener in patients who should avoid straining during defecation; constipation associated with hard, dry stools; ceruminolytic

Pregnancy Risk Factor C

Lactation Excretion in breast milk unknown/compatible

Contraindications Hypersensitivity to docusate or any component; concomitant use of mineral oil; intestinal obstruction, acute abdominal pain, nausea, vomiting

Adverse Reactions

Dermatologic: Rash

Gastrointestinal: Intestinal obstruction, diarrhea, abdominal cramping

Local: Throat irritation

Drug Interactions Docusate may increase absorption of mineral oil; docusate may increase the GI toxicity of aspirin

Mechanism of Action Reduces surface tension of the oil-water interface of the stool resulting in enhanced incorporation of water and fat allowing for stool softening

Pharmacodynamics Onset of action: 12-72 hours

Usual Dosage

Infants and Children: Oral: 5 mg/kg/day in 1-4 divided doses **or** dose by age:

<3 years: 10-40 mg/day in 1-4 divided doses

3-6 years: 20-60 mg/day in 1-4 divided doses

6-12 years: 40-150 mg/day in 1-4 divided doses

Adolescents and Adults: Oral: 50-400 mg/day in 1-4 divided doses

Older Children and Adults: Rectal: Add 50-100 mg of docusate liquid (not syrup) to enema fluid (NS or water)

Administration

Oral: Administer docusate liquid (not syrup) with milk, fruit juice, or infant formula to mask the bitter taste; ensure adequate fluid intake

Rectal: Administer as a retention or flushing enema

Additional Information Docusate sodium 5-10 mg/mL **liquid** instilled in the ear as a ceruminolytic produces substantial ear wax disintegration within 15 minutes and complete disintegration after 24 hours

Dosage Forms Excipient information presented when available (limited, particularly for generics); consult specific product labeling.

Capsule, as calcium (Surfak®): 240 mg

Capsule, as sodium: 100 mg, 250 mg

Colace®: 50 mg [contains sodium 3 mg], 100 mg [contains sodium 5 mg]

Docusoft-S™: 100 mg [contains sodium 5 mg]

DOK™, Genasoft®: 100 mg

DOS®, D-S-S®: 100 mg, 250 mg

Dulcolax® Stool Softener: 100 mg [contains sodium 5 mg]

Phillips'® Stool Softener Laxative: 100 mg [contains sodium 5.2 mg]

Enema, rectal, as sodium (Enemeez®): 283 mg/5 mL 5 mL

Gelcap, as sodium (Fleet® Sof-Lax®): 100 mg

Liquid, as sodium: 150 mg/15 mL (480 mL)

Colace®: 150 mg/15 mL (30 mL) [contains sodium 1 mg/mL]

Diocto®: 150 mg/15 mL (480 mL) [vanilla flavor]

Silace: 150 mg/15 mL (480 mL) [lemon-vanilla flavor]

Syrup, as sodium: 60 mg/15 mL (480 mL)

Colace®, Diocto®: 60 mg/15 mL (480 mL) [alcohol free, sugar free; contains sodium 36 mg/5 mL]

Silace: 20 mg/5 mL (480 mL) [peppermint flavor]

References

Chen DA and Caparosa RJ, "A Nonprescription Cerumenolytic," *Am J Otol*, 1991, 12(6):475-6.

Docusate and Senna (DOK yoo sate & SEN na)

Medication Safety Issues

Sound-alike/look-alike issues:

Senokot® may be confused with Depakote®

U.S. Brand Names Peri-Colace® [OTC]; Senokot-S® [OTC]; SenoSol™-SS [OTC]

Index Terms Senna and Docusate; Senna-S

Therapeutic Category Laxative, Stimulant; Laxative, Surfactant; Stool Softener

Generic Available Yes

Use Treatment of constipation generally associated with dry, hard stools and decreased intestinal motility; prevention of opiate-induced constipation

Pregnancy Risk Factor C

Contraindications Hypersensitivity to docusate, senna, or any component; concomitant use of mineral oil; undiagnosed abdominal pain; appendicitis, intestinal obstruction or perforation; acute abdominal pain; nausea, vomiting

Warnings Do not use when abdominal pain, rectal bleeding, nausea, or vomiting are present

Precautions Avoid prolonged use (>1 week); chronic use may lead to dependency, fluid and electrolyte imbalance, vitamin and mineral deficiencies

Adverse Reactions

Dermatologic: Rash

Endocrine & metabolic: Electrolyte and fluid imbalance

Gastrointestinal: Nausea, vomiting, diarrhea, abdominal cramps, perianal irritation, discoloration of feces, melanosis coli

Genitourinary: Discoloration of urine

Hepatic: Idiosyncratic hepatitis

Drug Interactions See individual agents.

Mechanism of Action Senna's active metabolite (aglycone) acts as a local irritant on the colon and stimulates the myenteric plexus to produce peristalsis; docusate reduces surface tension of the oil-water interface of the stool resulting in enhanced incorporation of water and fat allowing for stool softening

Pharmacodynamics Onset of action: Within 6-12 hours

Pharmacokinetics Senna:

Metabolism: Senna is metabolized in the liver

Elimination: In the feces (via bile) and in urine

Usual Dosage Oral:

Children 2 to <6 years: ½ tablet once daily at bedtime; maximum: 1 tablet twice daily

Children 6 to <12 years: 1 tablet once daily at bedtime; maximum: 2 tablets twice daily

(Continued)

Docusate and Senna *(Continued)*

Children ≥12 years, Adolescents, and Adults: 2 tablets once daily at bedtime; maximum: 4 tablets twice daily

Administration Administer with water, preferably in the evening

Monitoring Parameters I & O, frequency of bowel movements, serum electrolytes if severe diarrhea develops

Patient Information May discolor urine or feces; drink plenty of fluids

Dosage Forms Excipient information presented when available (limited, particularly for generics); consult specific product labeling.

Tablet: Docusate sodium 50 mg and sennosides 8.6 mg

Peri-Colace®: Docusate sodium 50 mg and sennosides 8.6 mg

Senokot-S®: Docusate sodium 50 mg and sennosides 8.6 mg [sugar free; contains sodium 4 mg/tablet]

SenoSol™-SS: Docusate sodium 50 mg and sennosides 8.6 mg [contains sodium 3 mg/tablet]

References

Baker SS, Liptak GS, Colletti RB, et al, "Constipation in Infants and Children: Evaluation and Treatment. A Medical Position Statement of the North American Society for Pediatric Gastroenterology and Nutrition," *J Pediatr Gastroenterol Nutr*, 1999, 29(5):612-26.

Herndon CM, Jackson KC II, and Hallin PA, "Management of Opioid-Induced Gastrointestinal Effects in Patients Receiving Palliative Care," *Pharmacotherapy*, 2002, 22(2):240-50.

♦ **Docusate Calcium** *see* Docusate *on page 526*

♦ **Docusate Potassium** *see* Docusate *on page 526*

♦ **Docusate Sodium** *see* Docusate *on page 526*

♦ **Docusoft-S™ [OTC]** *see* Docusate *on page 526*

♦ **Dofus [OTC]** *see Lactobacillus acidophilus* and *Lactobacillus bulgaricus on page 898*

♦ **DOK™ [OTC]** *see* Docusate *on page 526*

Dolasetron (dol A se tron)

Medication Safety Issues

Sound-alike/look-alike issues:

Anzemet® may be confused with Aldomet® and Avandamet™

Dolasetron may be confused with granisetron, ondansetron, palonosetron

U.S. Brand Names Anzemet®

Canadian Brand Names Anzemet®

Index Terms Dolasetron Mesylate; MDL 73,147EF

Therapeutic Category 5-HT_3 Receptor Antagonist; Antiemetic

Generic Available No

Use Prevention of chemotherapy-induced nausea and vomiting; prevention and treatment of postoperative nausea and vomiting

Pregnancy Risk Factor B

Lactation Excretion in breast milk unknown/use caution

Contraindications Hypersensitivity to dolasetron or any component

Warnings Dolasetron may cause EKG interval changes (PR, QT_c, JT prolongation and QRS widening) related in magnitude and frequency to blood levels of the active metabolite, hydrodolasetron; interval prolongation could lead to cardiovascular consequences such as heart block or cardiac arrhythmias. Due to reports of arrhythmias, MI, and cardiac arrest in pediatric and adolescent patients, Canadian healthcare officials have deemed dolasetron contraindicated for the treatment of children <18 years of age, and in addition, its use in adults for the treatment of postoperative nausea and vomiting (it has never been indicated for use in children in Canada).

Precautions Use with caution in patients with, or who may develop, prolongation of cardiac conduction intervals, particularly QT_c; conditions include hypokalemia, hypomagnesemia, or congenital QT syndrome; use with caution in patients receiving antiarrhythmic or other medications known to prolong the QT interval (eg, class I or III antiarrhythmic agents) or medications known to reduce potassium or magnesium levels (eg, diuretics). Safety and efficacy in children <2 years of age has not been established.

Adverse Reactions

Cardiovascular: Prolonged QT interval and other EKG changes, MI, arrhythmias, cardiac arrest (see Warnings), hypertension, hypotension, edema, diaphoresis

Central nervous system: Headache, fatigue, dizziness, fever, chills, shivering, agitation, sleep disorder, confusion, anxiety, abnormal dreams

Dermatologic: Rash, urticaria

Gastrointestinal: Diarrhea, abdominal pain, constipation, dyspepsia, anorexia, pancreatitis (rarely), taste perversion

Genitourinary: Urinary retention, acute renal failure (rarely), polyuria (rarely), dysuria (rarely)

Hepatic: Transient elevations in liver enzymes
Local: Venous irritation
Neuromuscular & skeletal: Myalgia, arthralgia
Ocular: Photophobia (rarely), abnormal vision
Otic: Tinnitus (rarely)
Miscellaneous: Hypersensitivity reactions

Drug Interactions Cytochrome P450 isoenzyme CYP2D6 and CYP3A3/4 substrate
Increased hydrodolasetron (active metabolite) serum levels with cimetidine; decreased hydrodolasetron serum levels with rifampin; decreased clearance of hydrodolasetron with atenolol; (see Warnings and Precautions)

Stability Store at room temperature; injection is stable after dilution in NS, D_5W, $D_5{}^1/_2NS$, D_5LR, LR, and 10% mannitol injection for 24 hours at room temperature and 48 hours under refrigeration

Mechanism of Action Dolasetron and its major metabolite, hydrodolasetron, are selective 5-HT_3 receptor antagonists, blocking serotonin, both peripherally on vagal nerve terminals and centrally in the chemoreceptor trigger zone

Pharmacokinetics Due to the rapid metabolism of dolasetron to hydrodolasetron (primary active metabolite), the majority of the following pharmacokinetic parameters relate to hydrodolasetron:

Distribution:
- Children: 5.9-7.4 L/kg
- Adults: 4.15-5.5 L/kg

Metabolism: Rapidly converted by carbonyl reductase to active major metabolite, hydrodolasetron; hydrodolasetron is metabolized by the cytochrome P450 CYP2D6 and CYP3A enzyme systems and flavin mono-oxygenase
Bioavailability: Oral: Children: 59% (formulation not specified), adults: 70% to 80%
Protein binding: 69% to 77% (active metabolite)
Half-life, elimination:
- Dolasetron: <10 minutes
- Hydrodolasetron:
  - Oral: Children: 5.7 hours, adults: 8.1 hours (range: 5-10 hours)
  - I.V.: Children: 4.8 hours, adults: 7.3 hours (range: 4-8 hours)

Time to peak serum concentration:
- Oral: 1-1.5 hours
- I.V.: 0.6 hours

Elimination: Dolasetron: <1% excreted unchanged in urine; hydrodolasetron: 53% to 61% excreted unchanged in urine within 36 hours

Usual Dosage
Prevention of chemotherapy-induced nausea and vomiting: **Oral:** Administered within 1 hour before chemotherapy; or **I.V.:** Administered 30 minutes before chemotherapy:
- Children 2-16 years:
  - Oral, I.V.: 1.8 mg/kg as a single dose (maximum: 100 mg)
- Adults:
  - Oral: 100 mg as a single dose
  - I.V.: 1.8 mg/kg or alternatively 100 mg as a single dose

Prevention or treatment of postoperative nausea and vomiting: **Oral:** Administered 2 hours before surgery and; **I.V.:** Administered 15 minutes prior to cessation of anesthesia or as soon as symptoms present
- Children ≥2 to 16 years:
  - Oral: 1.2 mg/kg as a single dose (maximum: 100 mg)
  - I.V.: 0.35 mg/kg as a single dose (maximum: 12.5 mg)
- Adults:
  - Oral: 100 mg as a single dose
  - I.V.: 12.5 mg as a single dose

Dosage adjustment in hepatic or renal impairment: No dosage adjustment is indicated

Administration
Oral: May be administered with or without food; injection may be used orally, dilute injection in apple or apple-grape juice; stable for 2 hours at room temperature
Parenteral: I.V.: Infuse undiluted over 30 seconds or dilute in 50 mL compatible I.V. fluid and infuse over ≤15 minutes; do not mix with other medications

Monitoring Parameters Baseline EKG and electrolytes in high-risk patients (see Warnings and Precautions), emesis episodes

Dosage Forms Excipient information presented when available (limited, particularly for generics); consult specific product labeling.
Injection, solution, as mesylate:
- Anzemet®: 20 mg/mL (0.625 mL) [single-use Carpuject® or vial]; 20 mg/mL (5 mL) [single-use vial]; 20 mg/mL (25 mL) [multidose vial]

Tablet, as mesylate:
- Anzemet®: 50 mg, 100 mg

(Continued)

Dolasetron *(Continued)*

Extemporaneous Preparations A 10 mg/mL suspension may be made by crushing twelve 50 mg tablets; slowly add a 1:1 mixture of Ora-Plus® and Ora-Sweet® SF (or 1:1 mixture of strawberry syrup and Ora-Plus®) to a final volume of 60 mL; stable for 90 days refrigerated

Johnson CE, Wagner DS, and Bussard WE, "Stability of Dolasetron in Two Oral Liquid Vehicles," *Am J Health Syst Pharm*, 2003, 60(21):2242-4.

References

"ASHP Therapeutic Guidelines on the Pharmacologic Management of Nausea and Vomiting in Adult and Pediatric Patients Receiving Chemotherapy or Radiation Therapy or Undergoing Surgery," *Am J Health Syst Pharm*, 1999, 56(8):729-64.

Coppes MJ, Lau R, Ingram LC, et al, "Open-Label Comparison of the Antiemetic Efficacy of Single Intravenous Doses of Dolasetron Mesylate in Pediatric Cancer Patients Receiving Moderately to Highly Emetogenic Chemotherapy," *Med Pediatr Oncol*, 1999, 33(2):99-105.

Olutoye O, Jantzen EC, Alexis R, et al, "A Comparison of the Costs and Efficacy of Ondansetron and Dolasetron in the Prophylaxis of Postoperative Vomiting in Pediatric Patients Undergoing Ambulatory Surgery," *Anesth Analg*, 2003, 97(2):390-6.

◆ **Dolasetron Mesylate** *see* Dolasetron *on page 528*
◆ **Dolophine®** *see* Methadone *on page 1018*
◆ **Dom-Azithromycin (Can)** *see* Azithromycin *on page 191*
◆ **Dom-Citalopram (Can)** *see* Citalopram *on page 368*
◆ **Domeboro®** *see* Aluminum Acetate *on page 89*
◆ **Dom-Methimazole (Can)** *see* Methimazole *on page 1022*
◆ **Dom-Sumatriptan (Can)** *see* Sumatriptan *on page 1495*
◆ **Dom-Topiramate (Can)** *see* Topiramate *on page 1551*
◆ **Donnatal®** *see* Hyoscyamine, Atropine, Scopolamine, and Phenobarbital *on page 800*
◆ **Donnatal Extentabs®** *see* Hyoscyamine, Atropine, Scopolamine, and Phenobarbital *on page 800*
◆ ***L*-Dopa** *see* Levodopa *on page 926*

DOPamine (DOE pa meen)

Medication Safety Issues

Sound-alike/look-alike issues:

DOPamine may be confused with DOBUTamine, Dopram®

Related Information

Adult ACLS Algorithms *on page 1660*
Emergency Pediatric Drip Calculations *on page 1652*
Extravasation Treatment *on page 1726*

Index Terms Dopamine Hydrochloride; Intropin

Therapeutic Category Adrenergic Agonist Agent; Sympathomimetic

Generic Available Yes

Use Increase cardiac output, blood pressure, and urine flow as an adjunct in the treatment of shock or hypotension which persists after adequate fluid volume replacement; in low dosage to increase renal perfusion

Pregnancy Risk Factor C

Lactation Excretion in breast milk unknown

Contraindications Hypersensitivity to dopamine or any component (see Warnings); pheochromocytoma, or ventricular fibrillation

Warnings Potent drug; must be diluted prior to use; patient's hemodynamic status should be monitored; injection solution contains sulfites which may cause allergic reactions in susceptible individuals

Precautions Blood volume depletion should be corrected, if possible, before starting dopamine therapy. Dopamine must not be used as sole therapy in hypovolemic patients. Extravasation may cause tissue necrosis (treat extravasation with phentolamine; see Extravasation Treatment *on page 1726*); due to potential gangrene of extremities, use with caution in patients with occlusive vascular disease.

Adverse Reactions

Cardiovascular: Ectopic heartbeats, tachycardia, vasoconstriction, cardiac conduction abnormalities, widened QRS complex, hypertension, ventricular arrhythmias, gangrene of the extremities (with high doses for prolonged periods or even with low doses in patients with occlusive vascular disease), anginal pain, palpitations

Central nervous system: Anxiety, headache

Gastrointestinal: Nausea, vomiting

Genitourinary: Decreased urine output (high dose)

Neuromuscular & skeletal: Piloerection

Ocular: Dilated pupils

Renal: Azotemia

Respiratory: Dyspnea

Drug Interactions Dopamine's cardiac and pressor response are prolonged and intensified by MAO inhibitors, alpha- and beta-adrenergic agonists, and oxytocic drugs; tricyclic antidepressants may decrease effects; use with phenytoin has resulted in seizures, severe hypotension, and bradycardia; use with halogenated hydrocarbon anesthetics may lead to serious arrhythmias; dopamine's cardiac effects are antagonized by beta-adrenergic blocking agents; vasoconstrictive effects are antagonized by alpha-adrenergic blocking agents

Stability Protect from light; solutions that are darker than slightly yellow should not be used; incompatible with alkaline solutions or iron salts; compatible when coadministered with dobutamine, epinephrine, isoproterenol, lidocaine, atracurium, vecuronium

Mechanism of Action Stimulates both adrenergic and dopaminergic receptors; low doses are mainly dopaminergic which stimulate and produce renal and mesenteric vasodilation; intermediate doses stimulate both dopaminergic and $beta_1$-adrenergic receptors and produce cardiac stimulation (increased heart rate and cardiac index) and increased renal blood flow; high doses stimulate alpha-adrenergic receptors primarily (vasoconstriction and increased blood pressure)

Pharmacodynamics

Onset of action: Adults: 5 minutes

Duration: Due to its short duration of action (<10 minutes) a continuous infusion must be used

Pharmacokinetics

Metabolism: In plasma, kidneys, and liver; 75% to inactive metabolites by monoamine oxidase and catechol-o-methyltransferase and 25% to norepinephrine (active)

Half-life: 2 minutes

Clearance: Neonatal clearance varies and appears to be age related. Clearance is more prolonged with combined hepatic and renal dysfunction. Dopamine has exhibited nonlinear kinetics in children; dose changes in children may not achieve steady-state for approximately 1 hour rather than 20 minutes seen in adults.

Usual Dosage I.V. infusion:

The hemodynamic effects of dopamine are dose-dependent:

- Low dosage: 1-5 mcg/kg/minute, increased renal blood flow and urine output
- Intermediate dosage: 5-15 mcg/kg/minute, increased renal blood flow, heart rate, cardiac contractility, cardiac output, and blood pressure
- High dosage: >15 mcg/kg/minute, alpha-adrenergic effects begin to predominate, vasoconstriction, increased blood pressure

Neonates: 1-20 mcg/kg/minute continuous infusion, titrate to desired response

Infants and Children: 1-20 mcg/kg/minute, maximum dose: 50 mcg/kg/minute continuous infusion, titrate to desired response

Adults: 1 mcg/kg/minute up to 50 mcg/kg/minute, titrate to desired response

If dosages >20-30 mcg/kg/minute are needed, a more direct-acting pressor may be beneficial (ie, epinephrine, norepinephrine)

Administration Parenteral: Must be diluted prior to administration; maximum concentration: 3200 mcg/mL (3.2 mg/mL); (concentrations as high as 6000 mcg/mL have been infused into large veins, safely and with efficacy, in cases of extreme fluid restriction); rate of infusion (mL/hour) = dose (mcg/kg/minute) x weight (kg) x 60 minutes/hour divided by concentration (mcg/mL); administer into large vein to prevent the possibility of extravasation; use infusion device to control rate of flow; administration into an umbilical arterial catheter is **not** recommended

Monitoring Parameters EKG, heart rate, CVP, MAP, urine output; if pulmonary artery catheter is in place, monitor CI, PWCP, SVR, RAP, and PVR

Dosage Forms Excipient information presented when available (limited, particularly for generics); consult specific product labeling.

Infusion, as hydrochloride [premixed in D_5W]: 0.8 mg/mL (250 mL, 500 mL); 1.6 mg/mL (250 mL, 500 mL); 3.2 mg/mL (250 mL)

Injection, solution, as hydrochloride: 40 mg/mL (5 mL, 10 mL); 80 mg/mL (5 mL); 160 mg/mL (5 mL) [contains sodium metabisulfite]

References

Banner W, Jr, Vernon DD, Dean JM, et al, "Nonlinear Dopamine Pharmacokinetics in Pediatric Patients," *J Pharmacol Exp Ther*, 1989, 249(1):131-3.

♦ **Dopamine Hydrochloride** *see* DOPamine *on page 530*

♦ **Dopar® (Can)** *see* Levodopa *on page 926*

♦ **Dopram®** *see* Doxapram *on page 535*

Dornase Alfa (DOOR nase AL fa)

U.S. Brand Names Pulmozyme®

Canadian Brand Names Pulmozyme™

Index Terms DNase; Recombinant Human Deoxyribonuclease

Therapeutic Category Enzyme, Inhalant; Mucolytic Agent

Generic Available No

(Continued)

Dornase Alfa *(Continued)*

Use Management of cystic fibrosis patients to reduce the frequency of respiratory infections and to improve pulmonary function

Pregnancy Risk Factor B

Lactation Excretion in breast milk unknown

Contraindications Hypersensitivity to dornase alfa, Chinese hamster ovary cell products (eg, epoetin alfa), or any component

Warnings Safety and efficacy has not been established in children <5 years of age or in patients with forced vital capacity <40% of normal; no data exists regarding safety during lactation

Adverse Reactions

Cardiovascular: Chest pain

Dermatologic: Skin rash

Gastrointestinal: Sore throat

Hepatic: Liver disease

Ocular: Conjunctivitis

Respiratory: Increased cough, dyspnea, hemoptysis, wheezing, laryngitis, rhinitis, pharyngitis

Miscellaneous: Voice alteration, hoarseness

Drug Interactions None known at this time

Stability Must be stored in the refrigerator at 2°C to 8°C (36°F to 46°F) and protected from strong light; unopened vials left at room temperature for a total time of 24 hours should be discarded; discard solution if cloudy or discolored

Mechanism of Action Dornase alfa is a deoxyribonuclease (DNA) enzyme produced by recombinant gene technology. Dornase selectively cleaves DNA, thus reducing mucous viscosity seen in the pulmonary secretions of cystic fibrosis patients. As a result, airflow in the lung is improved and the risk of bacterial infection may be decreased.

Pharmacodynamics Onset of improved pulmonary function tests (PFTs): 3-8 days; PFTs will return to baseline 2-3 weeks after discontinuation of therapy

Pharmacokinetics Following nebulization, enzyme levels are measurable in the sputum within 15 minutes and decline rapidly thereafter

Usual Dosage

Infants and Children ≤5 years: Not approved for use, however studies using this therapy in small numbers of children as young as 3 months of age have reported efficacy and similar side effects. See References.

Children >5 years and Adults: Inhalation: 2.5 mg/day through selected nebulizers in conjunction with a Pulmo-Aide® or a Pari-Proneb® compressor; some patients, especially older than 21 years of age or with forced vital capacity (FVC) >85%, may benefit from twice daily administration

Administration Nebulization: Should not be diluted or mixed with any other drugs in the nebulizer, this may inactivate the drug

Dosage Forms Excipient information presented when available (limited, particularly for generics); consult specific product labeling.

Solution for nebulization: 1 mg/mL (2.5 mL)

References

Fuchs HJ, Borowitz DS, Christiansen DH, et al, "Effect of Aerosolized Recombinant Human DNase on Exacerbations of Respiratory Symptoms and on Pulmonary Function in Patients With Cystic Fibrosis," *N Engl J Med*, 1994, 331(10):637-42.

Mueller GA, Rubins G, Wessel D, et al, "Effects of Dornase Alfa on Pulmonary Function Tests in Infants with Cystic Fibrosis," *Am J Respir Crit Care Med*, 1996, 153:A70.

Rock M, Kirchner K, McCubbin M, et al, "Aerosol Delivery and Safety of rhDNASE in Young Children With Cystic Fibrosis: A Bronchoscopic Study," *Pediatr Pulmonol*, 1996, 13(Suppl):A268.

♦ **Doryx®** *see* Doxycycline *on page 543*

Dorzolamide (dor ZOLE a mide)

U.S. Brand Names Trusopt®

Canadian Brand Names Trusopt®

Index Terms Dorzolamide Hydrochloride

Therapeutic Category Carbonic Anhydrase Inhibitor, Ophthalmic

Generic Available No

Use Treatment of elevated intraocular pressure in patients with ocular hypertension or open-angle glaucoma

Pregnancy Risk Factor C

Lactation Excretion in breast milk unknown/not recommended

Contraindications Hypersensitivity to dorzolamide, sulfonamides, or any component

Warnings Dorzolamide, a sulfonamide, is absorbed systemically and may produce the same adverse effects seen with other sulfonamides; avoid use in patients with severe renal dysfunction (Cl_{cr} <30 mL/minute); contains the preservative benzalkonium chloride which may be absorbed by soft contact lenses; contact lenses should be removed prior to administration of the solution and may be reinserted 15 minutes following administration; concomitant use with other carbonic anhydrase inhibitors is not recommended; avoid use in patients receiving high-dose salicylate therapy (see Drug Interactions)

Precautions Use with caution in patients with hepatic impairment

Adverse Reactions

Central nervous system: Headache, fatigue, dizziness, vertigo
Dermatologic: Rash, pruritus, urticaria
Gastrointestinal: Bitter taste, nausea, throat irritation
Genitourinary: Urolithiasis
Neuromuscular & skeletal: Paresthesia
Ocular: Burning, stinging, discomfort, and pain, punctate keratitis, conjunctivitis, blurred vision, eye redness, tearing, dryness, photophobia, transient myopia, eyelid crusting, increased corneal thickness, iridocyclitis
Respiratory: Dyspnea

Drug Interactions Cytochrome P450 isoenzyme CYP2C8/9, 3A4 substrate (minor)

Increased risk of nephrolithiasis when used with topiramate; additive intraocular pressure lowering with topical β-adrenergic blocking agents; high dose salicylate therapy may result in carbonic anhydrase inhibitor accumulation and toxicity including CNS depression and metabolic acidosis

Stability Store at room temperature.

Mechanism of Action Competitive, reversible inhibition of the enzyme carbonic anhydrase in the ciliary processes of the eye resulting in decreased secretion of aqueous humor

Pharmacodynamics

Peak effect: 2 hours
Duration: 8-12 hours
Average lowering of intraoptic pressure: 3-5 mm Hg or at least 15% decrease from unmedicated baseline value

Pharmacokinetics

Absorption: Topical: Reaches systemic circulation
Distribution: Accumulates in RBCs during chronic administration
Protein binding: 33%
Metabolism: In liver to active but less potent metabolite, N-desethyl dorzolamide
Half-life: Terminal RBC half-life: 147 days
Elimination: Primarily unchanged in the urine

Usual Dosage Glaucoma: Children and Adults: 1 drop into the affected eye(s) 3 times/day

Administration Ophthalmic: Apply gentle pressure to lacrimal sac during and immediately following instillation (1 minute) or instruct patient to gently close eyelid after administration to decrease systemic absorption of ophthalmic drops; avoid contact of bottle tip with skin or eye; remove contact lenses prior to administration (see Warnings); lenses may be inserted 15 minutes after instillation; if more than one topical ophthalmic drug is being used, separate administration by at least 10 minutes

Monitoring Parameters Intraoptic pressure

Patient Information Avoid contact of bottle tip with skin or eye to prevent contamination by bacteria which may cause ocular infections; report any ocular reactions, particularly conjunctivitis and lid reactions to your physician promptly

Dosage Forms Excipient information presented when available (limited, particularly for generics); consult specific product labeling. [DSC] = Discontinued product

Solution, ophthalmic, as hydrochloride:
Trusopt®: 2% (5 mL [DSC]; 10 mL) [contains benzalkonium chloride]

References

Portellos M, Buckley EG, and Freedman SF, "Topical Versus Oral Carbonic Anhydrase Inhibitor Therapy for Pediatric Glaucoma," *J AAPOS*, 1998, 2(1):43-7.

♦ **Dorzolamide Hydrochloride** *see* Dorzolamide *on page 532*
♦ **DOS® [OTC]** *see* Docusate *on page 526*
♦ **DOSS** *see* Docusate *on page 526*

Doxacurium (doks a KYOO ri um)

Medication Safety Issues

Sound-alike/look-alike issues:
Doxacurium may be confused with doxapram, DOXOrubicin

High alert medication: The Institute for Safe Medication Practices (ISMP) includes this medication among its list of drugs which have a heightened risk of causing significant patient harm when used in error.

(Continued)

Doxacurium *(Continued)*

U.S. Brand Names Nuromax®

Index Terms Doxacurium Chloride

Therapeutic Category Neuromuscular Blocker Agent, Nondepolarizing; Skeletal Muscle Relaxant, Paralytic

Generic Available No

Use Doxacurium is indicated for use as an adjunct to general anesthesia. It provides skeletal muscle relaxation during surgery or endotracheal intubation; increases pulmonary compliance during mechanical ventilation

Pregnancy Risk Factor C

Contraindications Hypersensitivity to doxacurium or any component (see Warnings)

Warnings Use with caution in patients with neuromuscular disease such as myasthenia gravis, cardiovascular disease; use with caution and reduce dosage in patients with renal or hepatic impairment; certain clinical conditions may result in potentiation or antagonism of neuromuscular blockade, see table on next page.

Injection contains benzyl alcohol which may cause allergic reactions in susceptible individuals; large amounts of benzyl alcohol (≥99 mg/kg/day) have been associated with a potentially fatal toxicity ("gasping syndrome") in neonates; the "gasping syndrome" consists of metabolic acidosis, respiratory distress, gasping respirations, CNS dysfunction (including convulsions, intracranial hemorrhage), hypotension and cardiovascular collapse; use injection containing benzyl alcohol with caution in neonates; *in vitro* and animal studies have shown that benzoate, a metabolite of benzyl alcohol, displaces bilirubin from protein binding sites

Adverse Reactions The most frequent adverse reactions appear as an extension of the agent's neuromuscular blocking actions

Cardiovascular: Hypotension (rare), bradycardia (rare)
Central nervous system: Fever
Dermatologic: Cutaneous flushing, urticaria
Neuromuscular & skeletal: Muscle weakness
Ocular: Diplopia
Respiratory: Respiratory insufficiency and apnea, bronchospasm, wheezing

Drug Interactions See table.

Potential Drug Interactions

Potentiation	Antagonism
Inhalation anesthetics	Calcium
Desflurane, sevoflurane, enflurane and	Carbamazepine
isoflurane > halothane > nitrous	Phenytoin
oxide	Steroids (chronic administration)
Antibiotics	Theophylline
Aminoglycosides, polymyxins,	Anticholinesterases[1]
clindamycin, vancomycin, tetracycline	Neostigmine, pyridostigmine,
Magnesium	edrophonium, echothiophate
Antiarrhythmics	ophthalmic solution
Quinidine, procainamide, bretylium, and	Caffeine
possibly lidocaine	Azathioprine
Diuretics	
Furosemide, mannitol, thiazides	
Amphotericin B (secondary to hypokalemia)	
Local anesthetics	
Dantrolene (directly depresses skeletal muscle)	
Beta blockers	
Calcium channel blockers	
Ketamine	
Lithium	
Succinylcholine (when administered prior to nondepolarizing neuromuscular-blocking agent)	
Cyclosporine	

[1]Can prolong the effects of acetylcholine

Stability Stable for 24 hours at room temperature when diluted in concentrations up to 0.1 mg/mL in D_5W or NS; compatible with sufentanil, alfentanil, and fentanyl; incompatible with alkaline solutions

Clinical Conditions Affecting Neuromuscular Blockade

Potentiation	Antagonism
Electrolyte abnormalities	Alkalosis
Severe hyponatremia	Hypercalcemia
Severe hypocalcemia	Demyelinating lesions
Severe hypokalemia	Peripheral neuropathies
Hypermagnesemia	Diabetes mellitus
Neuromuscular diseases	
Acidosis	
Acute intermittent porphyria	
Renal failure	
Hepatic failure	

Mechanism of Action Doxacurium is a long-acting nondepolarizing skeletal muscle relaxant. The drug is a bis-quaternary benzylisoquinolinium diester, with a chemical structure similar to that of atracurium. Similar to other nondepolarizing neuromuscular blocking agents, doxacurium produces muscle relaxation by competing with acetylcholine for cholinergic receptor sites on the postjunctional membrane; significant presynaptic depressant activity is also observed.

Pharmacodynamics

Onset of action: 5-11 minutes

Duration: 30 minutes (range: 12-54 minutes)

Pharmacokinetics

Distribution: V_d: Adults: 0.22 L/kg

Protein binding: 30%

Half-life:

- Normal: 1.5 hours
- Renal dysfunction: 3.7 hours
- Liver dysfunction: 1.9 hours

Elimination: Primarily as unchanged drug via the kidneys (80%) and biliary tract (20%)

Usual Dosage I.V. (in obese patients, use ideal body weight):

Children 2-12 years: Initial: 0.03-0.05 mg/kg/dose (30-50 mcg/kg/dose); maintenance: 0.005-0.01 mg/kg (5-10 mcg/kg/dose) every 30-45 minutes, or as needed depending upon individual patient response

Continuous infusion: 0.1-0.2 mcg/kg/minute or 6-12 mcg/kg/hour

Children >12 years and Adults: Initial: 0.025-0.05 mg/kg/dose (25-50 mcg/kg/dose); maintenance: 0.005-0.01 mg/kg/dose (5-10 mcg/kg/dose) every 60-100 minutes

Continuous infusion: 0.1-0.2 mcg/kg/minute or 6-12 mcg/kg/hour

Dosing adjustment in renal or hepatic impairment: Reduce initial dose and titrate carefully as duration may be prolonged

Administration Parenteral: I.V.: May be administered by rapid I.V. injection undiluted

Monitoring Parameters Peripheral nerve stimulation testing (measures twitch response), heart rate, blood pressure, assisted ventilation status

Additional Information Doxacurium is a long-acting nondepolarizing neuromuscular blocker with virtually no cardiovascular side effects. The characteristics of this agent make it especially useful in procedures requiring careful maintenance of hemodynamic stability for prolonged periods

Dosage Forms Excipient information presented when available (limited, particularly for generics); consult specific product labeling.

Injection, solution, as chloride: 1 mg/mL (5 mL) [contains benzyl alcohol]

References

Martin LD, Bratton SL, and O'Rourke PP, "Clinical Uses and Controversies of Neuromuscular Blocking Agents in Infants and Children," *Crit Care Med*, 1999, 27(7):1358-68.

♦ **Doxacurium Chloride** *see* Doxacurium *on page 533*

Doxapram (DOKS a pram)

Medication Safety Issues

Sound-alike/look-alike issues:

Doxapram may be confused with doxacurium, doxazosin, doxepin, Doxinate®, DOXOrubicin

Dopram® may be confused with DOPamine

(Continued)

Doxapram *(Continued)*

U.S. Brand Names Dopram®

Index Terms Doxapram Hydrochloride

Therapeutic Category Central Nervous System Stimulant, Nonamphetamine; Respiratory Stimulant

Generic Available Yes

Use Respiratory and CNS stimulant for treatment of respiratory depression secondary to anesthesia, drug-induced CNS depression, idiopathic apnea of prematurity refractory to xanthines, and acute hypercapnia secondary to COPD (see Contraindications)

Pregnancy Risk Factor B

Lactation Excretion in breast milk unknown/use caution

Contraindications Hypersensitivity to doxapram or any component (see Warnings); epilepsy, cerebral edema, head injury, suspected or proven pulmonary embolism, pheochromocytoma, cardiovascular or coronary artery disease, severe hypertension, hyperthyroidism, cardiac arrhythmias; concomitant use with mechanical ventilation in COPD patients; patients with mechanical disorders of ventilation such as bronchial obstruction, muscle paresis (including NM blockade), flail chest, pneumothorax, pulmonary fibrosis, asthma, or other conditions resulting in restriction of chest wall muscles of respiration or alveolar expansion

Warnings Doxapram contains benzyl alcohol which may cause allergic reactions in susceptible individuals; large amounts of benzyl alcohol (≥99 mg/kg/day) have been associated with a potentially fatal toxicity ("gasping syndrome") in neonates; the "gasping syndrome" consists of metabolic acidosis, respiratory distress, gasping respirations, CNS dysfunction (including convulsions, intracranial hemorrhage), hypotension and cardiovascular collapse. Recommended doses of doxapram for treatment of neonatal apnea will deliver 5.4-27 mg/kg/day of benzyl alcohol; the use of doxapram should be reserved for neonates who are unresponsive to the treatment of apnea with therapeutic serum concentrations of theophylline or caffeine. *In vitro* and animal studies have shown that benzoate, a metabolite of benzyl alcohol, displaces bilirubin from protein-binding sites.

Doxapram is not an antagonist to muscle relaxant drugs nor a specific narcotic antagonist; doxapram alone may not stimulate adequate spontaneous breathing or provide sufficient arousal in patients who are severely depressed; use as an adjunct to establish supportive measures; since respiratory depression may recur after stimulation with doxapram, monitor closely until the patient has been fully alert for 30-60 minutes; to reduce the potential for arrhythmias, including VT and VF, in patients who have received general anesthesia with a volatile agent known to sensitize the myocardium to catecholamines, administration of doxapram should be delayed until the complete excretion of anesthetic has occurred.

Precautions Oxygen, resuscitative equipment, and anticonvulsants should be readily available to manage excessive CNS stimulation. Frequent arterial blood gas measurements are recommended to identify and prevent the development of CO_2 retention and acidosis in COPD patients with acute hypercapnia; infusion of doxapram in premature infants has been associated with a statistically significant but moderate lengthening of QT_c interval; cardiac monitoring during treatment is suggested (Maillard, 2001); use caution in patients with impaired hepatic or renal function or receiving MAOIs or sympathomimetic drugs (see Drug Interactions)

Adverse Reactions

Cardiovascular: Hypertension* (dose-related), tachycardia, arrhythmias, hypotension, flushing, chest pain, QT prolongation with heartblock*

Central nervous system: CNS stimulation, restlessness, apprehension, disorientation, lightheadedness, jitters*, hallucinations, irritability*, seizures*, headache, fever, hypothermia, excessive crying*, sleep disturbances*

Gastrointestinal: Abdominal distension*, nausea, vomiting*, retching, increased gastric residuals*, bloody stools*, necrotising enterocolitis*

Genitourinary: Urinary retention, burning sensation in genital area or perineum, spontaneous voiding

Hematologic: Hemolysis (associated with rapid infusion)

Local: Phlebitis

Metabolic: Hyperglycemia*

Neuromuscular & skeletal: Tremor, hyper-reflexia, paresthesia, involuntary movements, muscle spasticity and fasciculations, clonus, bilateral Babinski

Ocular: Lacrimation, mydriasis

Renal: Glucosuria*, albuminuria, elevated BUN

Respiratory: Coughing, laryngospasm, dyspnea, hiccups, bronchospasm, rebound hypoventilation

Miscellaneous: Diaphoresis

*Reported with infusions in premature infants

Drug Interactions Sympathomimetic drugs and MAO inhibitors may cause significant increase in blood pressure; general anesthetics (see Warnings); increased skeletal muscle activity, agitation, and hyperactivity when used with theophylline

Stability Stable at room temperature; incompatible with aminophylline, sodium bicarbonate, thiopental sodium, and other alkaline solutions

Mechanism of Action Stimulates respiration through action on respiratory center in medulla or through reflex stimulation of carotid, aortic, or other peripheral chemoreceptors; antagonizes opiate-induced respiratory depression, but does not affect analgesia

Pharmacodynamics Following a single I.V. injection:

Onset of respiratory stimulation: Within 20-40 seconds

Maximum effect: Within 1-2 minutes

Duration: 5-12 minutes

Pharmacokinetics

Metabolism: Extensive in the liver to active metabolite (keto-doxapram)

Distribution: V_d: Neonates: 4-7.3 L/kg

Half-life:

Neonates, premature: 6.6-12 hours

Adults: Mean: 3.4 hours (range: 2.4-4.1 hours)

Clearance: Neonates, premature: 0.44-0.7 L/hour/kg

Usual Dosage I.V.:

Neonatal apnea (apnea of prematurity): Initial loading dose: 2.5-3 mg/kg followed by a continuous infusion of 1 mg/kg/hour; titrate to the lowest rate at which apnea is controlled (maximum dose: 2.5 mg/kg/hour)

Respiratory depression following anesthesia: Adults: Titrate to sustain the desired level of respiratory stimulation with a minimum of side effects:

Initial: 0.5-1 mg/kg; may repeat at 5-minute intervals; maximum total dose: 2 mg/kg

I.V. infusion: Initial: 5 mg/minute until adequate response or adverse effects seen; decrease to 1-3 mg/minute; usual total infusion dose: 0.5-4 mg/kg or 300 mg

Drug-induced CNS depression: Adults: Mild to moderate depression: Initial: 1-2 mg/kg; may repeat in 5 minutes; may repeat at 1-2 hour intervals (until sustained consciousness); maximum dose: 3 g/day; if depression recurs, may repeat in 24 hours. As an alternative, after the initial doses, a continuous infusion of 1-3 mg/minute may be used. Discontinue if patient begins to waken; do not infuse for more than 2 hours.

Hypercapnia associated with COPD: Adults: Continuous infusion of 1-2 mg/minute for 2 hours; may increase to 3 mg/minute if needed. Do not infuse for more than 2 hours. Monitor arterial blood gases closely (in a minimum of 30-minute intervals)

Administration Parenteral: I.V. use only: Dilute loading dose to a maximum concentration of 2 mg/mL and infuse over 15-30 minutes; for infusion, dilute in NS or dextrose (D_5W or $D_{10}W$) to 1 mg/mL (maximum concentration: 2 mg/mL); irritating to tissues; avoid extravasation

Monitoring Parameters Pulse oximetry, blood pressure, heart rate, arterial blood gases, deep tendon reflexes; for apnea: number, duration, and severity of apneic episodes

Reference Range Initial studies suggest a therapeutic serum level of at least 1.5 mg/L; toxicity becomes frequent at serum levels >5 mg/L

Nursing Implications Doxapram is an extravasant; monitor injection site closely; rapid infusion may result in hemolysis

Dosage Forms Excipient information presented when available (limited, particularly for generics); consult specific product labeling.

Injection, solution, as hydrochloride: 20 mg/mL (20 mL) [contains benzyl alcohol]

References

Barrington KJ, Finer NN, Torok-Both G, et al, "Dose-Response Relationship of Doxapram in the Therapy for Refractory Idiopathic Apnea of Prematurity," *Pediatrics*, 1987, 80(1):22-7.

Bhatt-Mehta V and Schumacher RE, "Treatment of Apnea of Prematurity," *Paediatr Drugs*, 2003, 5(3):195-210.

Maillard C, Boutroy MJ, Fresson J, et al, "QT Interval Lengthening in Premature Infants Treated With Doxapram," *Clin Pharmacol Ther*, 2001, 70(6):540-5.

♦ **Doxapram Hydrochloride** *see* Doxapram *on page 535*

Doxepin (DOKS e pin)

Medication Safety Issues

Sound-alike/look-alike issues:

Doxepin may be confused with digoxin, doxapram, doxazosin, Doxidan®, doxycycline

Sinequan® may be confused with saquinavir, Serentil®, Seroquel®, Singulair®

Zonalon® may be confused with Zone-A Forte®

(Continued)

Doxepin *(Continued)*

International issues:

Doxal® [Finland] may be confused with Doxil® which is a brand name for doxorubicin in the U.S.

Doxal® [Finland]: Brand name for doxycycline in Austria; brand name for pyridoxine/thiamine in Brazil

Related Information

Antidepressant Agents *on page 1681*

Overdose and Toxicology *on page 1916*

U.S. Brand Names Prudoxin™; Sinequan® [DSC]; Zonalon®

Canadian Brand Names Apo-Doxepin®; Novo-Doxepin; Sinequan®; Zonalon®

Index Terms Doxepin Hydrochloride

Therapeutic Category Antianxiety Agent; Antidepressant, Tricyclic

Generic Available Yes: Capsule, solution

Use

Oral: Treatment of various forms of depression, usually in conjunction with psychotherapy; treatment of anxiety disorders; analgesic for certain chronic and neuropathic pain

Topical: Adults: Short-term (<8 days) therapy of moderate pruritus due to atopic dermatitis or lichen simplex chronicus

Medication Guide An FDA-approved patient medication guide, which is available with the product information and at http://www.fda.gov/cder/Offices/ODS/medication_guides.htm, must be dispensed with this medication for each new outpatient prescription and refill.

Pregnancy Risk Factor C (Topical: B)

Lactation Enters breast milk/not recommended (AAP rates "of concern")

Contraindications Hypersensitivity to doxepin or any component (see Warnings); cross-sensitivity with other tricyclic antidepressants may occur; narrow-angle glaucoma; patients with urinary retention

Warnings Doxepin is not approved for use in pediatric patients. Clinical worsening of depression or suicidal ideation and behavior may occur in children and adults with major depressive disorder. In clinical trials, antidepressants increased the risk of suicidal thinking and behavior (suicidality) in children, adolescents, and young adults (18-24 years of age) with major depressive disorder and other psychiatric disorders. This risk must be considered before prescribing antidepressants for any clinical use. Short-term studies did **not** show an increased risk of suicidality with antidepressant use in patients >24 years of age and showed a decreased risk in patients ≥65 years.

Patients of all ages who are treated with antidepressants for any indication require appropriate monitoring and close observation for clinical worsening of depression, suicidality, and unusual changes in behavior, especially during the first few months after antidepressant initiation or when the dose is adjusted. Family members and caregivers should be instructed to closely observe the patient (ie, daily) and communicate condition with healthcare provider. Patients should also be monitored for associated behaviors (eg, anxiety, agitation, panic attacks, insomnia, irritability, hostility, aggressiveness, impulsivity, akathisia, hypomania, mania) which may increase the risk for worsening depression or suicidality. Worsening depression or emergence of suicidality (or associated behaviors listed above) that is abrupt in onset, severe, or not part of the presenting symptoms, may require discontinuation or modification of drug therapy.

Avoid abrupt discontinuation; discontinuation symptoms (including headache, nausea, malaise) may occur if therapy is abruptly discontinued or dose reduced; taper the dose to minimize risks of discontinuation symptoms. To reduce risk of intentional overdose, write prescriptions for the smallest quantity consistent with good patient care. Screen individuals for bipolar disorder prior to treatment (using antidepressants alone may induce manic episodes in patients with this condition).

Doxepin causes a high degree of sedation (relative to other antidepressants); may cause orthostatic hypotension and anticholinergic side effects; may worsen psychosis or precipitate mania or hypomania in patients with bipolar disease; may increase the risks associated with electroconvulsive therapy. Discontinue therapy, when possible, prior to elective surgery (do not discontinue abruptly); cream contains benzyl alcohol which may cause allergic reactions in susceptible individuals; large amounts of benzyl alcohol (≥99 mg/kg/day) have been associated with a potentially fatal toxicity ("gasping syndrome") in neonates; avoid use of doxepin products containing benzyl alcohol in neonates; *in vitro* and animal studies have shown that benzoate, a metabolite of benzyl alcohol, displaces bilirubin from protein binding sites

Precautions Use with caution in patients with cardiovascular disease, conduction disturbances, seizure disorders, urinary retention, hyperthyroidism or those receiving thyroid replacement; avoid use during lactation; use with caution in pregnancy

Drowsiness and other systemic effects may occur with topical use; occlusive dressings may increase absorption of doxepin; allergic contact dermatitis may occur with topical use, risk may be increased with use >8 days. **Note:** Cream is not recommended for use in pediatric patients; overdoses from topical administration in children have been reported.

Adverse Reactions Pronounced sedation and anticholinergic adverse effects may occur

Cardiovascular: Hypotension, arrhythmias

Central nervous system: Sedation, confusion, dizziness, headache; suicidal thinking and behavior (see Warnings); drowsiness occurs in 22% of patients receiving topical cream especially if applied to >10% of body surface area; reduction in area treated, number of applications per day, amount of cream used, or discontinuation of cream may be needed if excessive drowsiness occurs

Dermatologic: Photosensitivity

Endocrine & metabolic: SIADH (rare), weight gain

Gastrointestinal: Constipation, nausea, vomiting, xerostomia, increased appetite

Genitourinary: Urinary retention

Hematologic: Blood dyscrasias (rare)

Hepatic: Hepatitis

Local: Stinging and burning at application site; exacerbation of pruritus or eczema; allergic contact dermatitis

Neuromuscular & skeletal: Fine tremor

Ocular: Blurred vision

Otic: Tinnitus

Miscellaneous: Hypersensitivity reactions; withdrawal symptoms following abrupt discontinuation (headache, nausea, malaise)

Drug Interactions Cytochrome P450 isoenzyme CYP1A2 (minor), CYP2D6 (major), and CYP3A4 (minor) substrate

CNS depressants, alcohol, or antihistamines may potentiate sedative effects; use with MAO inhibitors may cause serious side effects including death (use within 14 days is not recommended); carbamazepine, guanethidine, clonidine, antithyroid agents; cimetidine (serious anticholinergic symptoms may occur); tolazamide (severe hypoglycemia may occur); the herbal medicine St John's wort (*Hypericum perforatum*) may increase serious side effects, its use is **not** recommended; use with cytochrome P450 CYP2D6 inhibitors or substrates may increase doxepin serum concentrations or effects (monitor patient and serum concentrations); concurrent use of high-dose TCAs and ritonavir may cause the serotonin syndrome

Food Interactions Oral solution is physically incompatible with carbonated beverages and grape juice; diets rich in fiber may decrease drug effects

Stability Protect from light; store cream at ≤80°F (27°C)

Mechanism of Action Increases the synaptic concentration of serotonin and/or norepinephrine in the CNS by inhibition of their reuptake by the presynaptic neuronal membrane

Pharmacodynamics Maximum antidepressant effects: Usually occur after >2 weeks; anxiolytic effects may occur sooner

Pharmacokinetics

Distribution: Crosses the placenta; appears in breast milk

Protein binding: 80% to 85%

Metabolism: Hepatic to metabolites, including desmethyldoxepin (active)

Half-life, adults: 6-8 hours

Elimination: Renal

Usual Dosage

Oral: **Note:** Not FDA approved for use in pediatric patients; controlled clinical trials have not shown tricyclic antidepressants to be superior to placebo for the treatment of depression in children and adolescents (see Dopheide, 2006 and Wagner, 2005).

Children: 1-3 mg/kg/day in single or divided doses

Adolescents: Initial: 25-50 mg/day in single or divided doses; gradually increase to 100 mg/day

Adults: Initial: 30-150 mg/day at bedtime or in 2-3 divided doses; may increase up to 300 mg/day; single dose should not exceed 150 mg; select patients may respond to 25-50 mg/day

Topical: Adults: Apply to affected area 4 times/day

Administration

Oral: Administer with food to decrease GI upset; oral concentrate should be diluted in water, milk, or juice (but not grape juice) prior to administration (use 120 mL for adults); do not mix with carbonated beverages

Topical: Apply thin film of cream to affected area with at least 3-4 hours between applications; do not use occlusive dressings; do not use for >8 days; avoid contact with eyes

(Continued)

Doxepin *(Continued)*

Monitoring Parameters Blood pressure, heart rate, mental status, weight, liver enzymes, CBC with differential. Monitor patient periodically for symptom resolution; monitor for worsening depression, suicidality, and associated behaviors (especially at the beginning of therapy or when doses are increased or decreased; see Warnings).

Reference Range Utility of serum level monitoring controversial

Doxepin plus desmethyldoxepin:

Proposed therapeutic concentration: 110-250 ng/mL (394-895 nmol/L)

Toxic concentration: >500 ng/mL (>1790 nmol/L) (toxicities may be seen at lower concentrations in some patients)

Patient Information Read the patient Medication Guide that you receive with each prescription and refill of doxepin. An increased risk of suicidal thinking and behavior has been reported with the use of antidepressants in children, adolescents, and young adults (18-24 years of age). Notify physician if you feel more depressed, have thoughts of suicide, or become more agitated or irritable (see Warnings). May cause drowsiness and impair ability to perform activities requiring mental alertness or physical coordination; may cause dry mouth; avoid alcohol and the herbal medicine St John's wort; limit caffeine; may increase appetite; do not discontinue abruptly. May cause photosensitivity reactions (eg, exposure to sunlight may cause severe sunburn, skin rash, redness, or itching); avoid exposure to sunlight and artificial light sources (sunlamps, tanning booth/bed); wear protective clothing, wide-brimmed hats, sunglasses, and lip sunscreen (SPF ≥15); use a sunscreen [broad-spectrum sunscreen or physical sunscreen (preferred) or sunblock with SPF ≥15]; contact physician if reaction occurs.

Nursing Implications Do not use occlusive dressings with cream (increases dermal absorption)

Additional Information Safety and effectiveness of topical cream when used for >8 days has not been established; use >8 days may result in an increase in serum concentrations and systemic effects

Dosage Forms Excipient information presented when available (limited, particularly for generics); consult specific product labeling. [DSC] = Discontinued product

Capsule, as hydrochloride: 10 mg, 25 mg, 50 mg, 75 mg, 100 mg, 150 mg

Sinequan®: 10 mg, 25 mg, 50 mg, 75 mg, 100 mg, 150 mg [DSC]

Cream, as hydrochloride:

Prudoxin™: 5% (45 g) [contains benzyl alcohol]

Zonalon®: 5% (30 g, 45 g) [contains benzyl alcohol]

Solution, oral concentrate, as hydrochloride: 10 mg/mL (120 mL)

Sinequan®: 10 mg/mL (120 mL) [DSC]

References

Dopheide JA, "Recognizing and Treating Depression in Children and Adolescents," *Am J Health Syst Pharm*, 2006, 63(3):233-43.

Levy HB, Harper CR, and Weinberg WA, "A Practical Approach to Children Failing in School," *Pediatr Clin North Am*, 1992, 39(4):895-928.

Wagner KD, "Pharmacotherapy for Major Depression in Children and Adolescents," *Prog Neuropsychopharmacol Biol Psychiatry*, 2005, 29(5):819-26.

♦ **Doxepin Hydrochloride** *see* Doxepin *on page 537*

♦ **Doxidan®** **[OTC]** *see* Bisacodyl *on page 217*

DOXOrubicin (doks oh ROO bi sin)

Medication Safety Issues

Sound-alike/look-alike issues:

DOXOrubicin may be confused with dactinomycin, DAUNOrubicin, doxacurium, doxapram, doxazosin, epirubicin, idarubicin

Adriamycin PFS® may be confused with achromycin, Aredia®, Idamycin®

Rubex® may be confused with Revex®, Robaxin®

Conventional formulations (Adriamycin PFS®, Adriamycin RDF®, Rubex®) may be confused with liposomal formulations (DaunoXome®, Doxil®)

High alert medication: The Institute for Safe Medication Practices (ISMP) includes this medication among its list of drugs which have a heightened risk of causing significant patient harm when used in error.

ADR is an error-prone abbreviation

International issues:

Doxil® may be confused with Doxal® which is a brand name for doxepin in Finland, a brand name for doxycycline in Austria, and a brand name for pyridoxine/thiamine combination in Brazil

Rubex®: Brand name for ascorbic acid in Ireland

Related Information

Compatibility of Chemotherapy and Related Supportive Care Medications *on page 1777*

Emetogenic Potential of Single Chemotherapeutic Agents *on page 1776*

Extravasation Treatment *on page 1726*

U.S. Brand Names Adriamycin®; Rubex® [DSC]

Canadian Brand Names Adriamycin®

Index Terms ADR (error-prone abbreviation); Adria; Doxorubicin Hydrochloride; Hydroxydaunomycin Hydrochloride; Hydroxyldaunorubicin Hydrochloride; NSC-123127

Therapeutic Category Antineoplastic Agent, Anthracycline; Antineoplastic Agent, Antibiotic

Generic Available Yes

Use Treatment of various solid tumors including ovarian, breast, and bladder tumors; various lymphomas and leukemias (AML, ALL), soft tissue sarcomas, neuroblastoma, osteosarcoma

Pregnancy Risk Factor D

Lactation Enters breast milk/contraindicated

Contraindications Hypersensitivity to doxorubicin or any component; severe CHF, cardiomyopathy, pre-existing myelosuppression; patients who have received a total dose of 550 mg/m^2 of doxorubicin or 400 mg/m^2 in patients with previous or concomitant treatment with daunorubicin, idarubicin, mitoxantrone, cyclophosphamide, or irradiation of the cardiac region; patients who have received previous treatment with complete cumulative doses of daunorubicin, idarubicin, or other anthracycline derivatives; pregnancy

Warnings The FDA currently recommends that procedures for proper handling and disposal of antineoplastic agents be considered. **I.V. use only,** severe local tissue necrosis will result if extravasation occurs; irreversible myocardial toxicity, including potentially fatal CHF, may occur during therapy or months to years after therapy termination. The probability of developing myocardial toxicity is estimated to be 1% to 2% at a total cumulative dose of 300 mg/m^2 of doxorubicin, 3% to 5% at a total cumulative dose of 400 mg/m^2, 5% to 8% at a total cumulative dose of 450 mg/m^2, and 6% to 20% at 500 mg/m^2. Myocardial toxicity may occur at lower cumulative doses in patients with prior mediastinal irradiation, concurrent cyclophosphamide therapy, or pre-existing heart disease. Pediatric patients are at increased risk for developing delayed cardiac toxicity and CHF during early adulthood due to an increasing census of long-term survivors; periodic long-term monitoring of cardiac function is recommended. Doxorubicin may contribute to prepubertal growth failure in pediatric patients. Pediatric patients are at risk of developing secondary acute myeloid leukemia. Severe myelosuppression is also possible.

Precautions Use with caution and modify dosage in patients with impaired hepatic function

Adverse Reactions

Cardiovascular: CHF, cardiomyopathy, cardiotoxicity (transient type with abnormal EKG and arrhythmias, or a chronic, cumulative, dose-dependent type which progresses to CHF), cardiorespiratory decompensation, facial flushing

Central nervous system: Fever, chills

Dermatologic: Alopecia, hyperpigmentation of nail beds, urticaria, photosensitivity, radiation recall, urticaria

Endocrine & metabolic: Hyperuricemia, infertility, prepubertal growth failure

Gastrointestinal: Stomatitis, esophagitis, nausea, vomiting, mucositis, anorexia, diarrhea, ulceration and necrosis of the colon

Genitourinary: Discoloration of urine (red/orange), cystitis, hematuria, urinary frequency

Hematologic: Leukopenia (nadir: 10-14 days), thrombocytopenia, anemia

Hepatic: Transient elevation of liver enzymes

Local: Tissue necrosis upon extravasation, erythematous streaking along the vein if administered too rapidly, phlebitis

Ocular: Lacrimation

Miscellaneous: Anaphylaxis

Drug Interactions Cytochrome P450 isoenzyme CYP3A3/4 substrate; isoenzyme CYP2D6 inhibitor

May potentiate the toxicity of cyclophosphamide, mercaptopurine; ritonavir and cyclosporine decrease doxorubicin metabolism; doxorubicin decreases carbamazepine, digoxin, and phenytoin levels; paclitaxel decreases doxorubicin clearance resulting in increased toxicity if administered prior to doxorubicin; phenobarbital increases elimination of doxorubicin

Stability Protect from light; store vials containing powder at room temperature, refrigerate vials containing liquid; reconstituted vials stable for 7 days at room temperature

(Continued)

DOXOrubicin *(Continued)*

and 15 days if refrigerated and protected from light. Discard unused portion of preservative free injection vial. Incompatible with hydrocortisone, fluorouracil, furosemide, sodium bicarbonate, aminophylline, heparin, cephalothin, dexamethasone; unstable in solutions with a pH <3 or >7. Color change from red to purple indicates decomposition of drug.

Mechanism of Action Inhibits DNA and RNA synthesis by intercalating between DNA base pairs and by steric obstruction inducing DNA breaks; produces oxygen-free radicals which cause DNA denaturation

Pharmacokinetics

Distribution: Into breast milk; does not penetrate into CSF; distributes into cells rapidly with high concentrations in lung, kidney, muscle, spleen, and liver

Protein binding: 75%

Metabolism: In both the liver and in plasma to both active and inactive metabolites

Half-life, triphasic:

- Primary: 30 minutes
- Secondary: 3-3.5 hours for its metabolites
- Terminal: 17-30 hours for doxorubicin and its metabolites

Elimination: Undergoes triphasic elimination; 40% to 60% eventually excreted in bile and feces; <5% excreted in urine, primarily as unchanged drug and metabolites

Clearance:

- Infants <2 years: 813 mL/minute/m^2
- Children >2 years: 1540 mL/minute/m^2

Usual Dosage Patient's ideal weight should be used to calculate body surface area. Lower dose regimens should be given to patients with decreased bone marrow reserve, prior radiation therapy, or marrow infiltration with malignant cells.

I.V. (refer to individual protocols):

- Children: 35-75 mg/m^2 as a single dose, repeat every 21 days; or 20-30 mg/m^2 once weekly; or 60-90 mg/m^2 given as a continuous infusion over 96 hours every 3-4 weeks
- Adults: 60-75 mg/m^2 as a single dose, repeat every 21 days; or 20-30 mg/m^2/day for 2-3 days, repeat in 4 weeks or 20 mg/m^2 once weekly

Dosing adjustment in hepatic impairment:

- Bilirubin 1.2-3 mg/dL: Reduce dose by 50%
- Bilirubin >3 mg/dL: Reduce dose by 75%

Administration Parenteral: I.V. use only; reconstitute IVP doses with D_5W or NS to ensure isotonicity of the final solution; administer slow IVP at a rate no faster than over 3-5 minutes or by I.V. infusion over 1-4 hours at a concentration not to exceed 2 mg/mL, or by I.V. continuous infusion

Monitoring Parameters CBC with differential, erythrocyte and platelet count; serum uric acid, echocardiogram, radionuclide left ventricular ejection fraction, liver enzymes, and bilirubin; observe I.V. injection site for infiltration and vein irritation

Patient Information Transient red-orange discoloration of urine can occur for up to 48 hours after a dose; notify physician if fever, sore throat, bleeding, or bruising occurs; report any stinging sensation at the injection site during infusion. May cause photosensitivity reactions (eg, exposure to sunlight may cause severe sunburn, skin rash, redness, or itching); avoid exposure to sunlight and artificial light sources (sunlamps, tanning booth/bed); wear protective clothing, wide-brimmed hats, sunglasses, and lip sunscreen (SPF ≥15); use a sunscreen [broad-spectrum sunscreen or physical sunscreen (preferred) or sunblock with SPF ≥15]; contact physician if reaction occurs.

Nursing Implications Local erythematous streaking along the vein and/or facial flushing may indicate too rapid a rate of administration; drug is very irritating; avoid extravasation; if extravasation occurs, apply cold packs immediately for 30-60 minutes, then alternate off/on every 15 minutes for 1 day; apply 1.5 mL of dimethylsulfoxide 99% (w/v) solution to the site every 6 hours for 14 days; allow to air-dry; do not cover. Take precautions to prevent contact with the patient's urine and other body fluids for at least 5 days after each treatment.

Additional Information Myelosuppressive effects:

- WBC: Moderate
- Platelets: Moderate
- Onset (days): 7
- Nadir (days): 10-14
- Recovery (days): 21-28

Dosage Forms Excipient information presented when available (limited, particularly for generics); consult specific product labeling.

Injection, powder for reconstitution, as hydrochloride: 10 mg, 50 mg

- Adriamycin®: 10 mg, 20 mg, 50 mg, [contains lactose]
- Rubex®: 50 mg, 100 mg [contains lactose] [DSC]

Injection, solution, as hydrochloride: 2 mg/mL (5 mL, 10 mL, 25 mL, 100 mL)
Adriamycin®: 2 mg/mL (5 mL, 10 mL, 25 mL, 100 mL)

References

Berg SL, Grisell DL, DeLaney TF, et al, "Principles of Treatment of Pediatric Solid Tumors," *Pediatr Clin North Am*, 1991, 38(2):249-67.

Ishii E, Hara T, Ohkubo K, et al, "Treatment of Childhood Acute Lymphoblastic Leukemia With Intermediate Dose Cytosine Arabinoside and Adriamycin," *Med Pediatr Oncol*, 1986, 14(2):73-7.

Legha SS, Benjamin RS, Mackay B, et al, "Reduction of Doxorubicin Cardiotoxicity by Prolonged Continuous Intravenous Infusion," *Ann Intern Med*, 1982, 96(2):133-9.

♦ **Doxorubicin Hydrochloride** *see* DOXOrubicin *on page 540*

♦ **Doxy-100®** *see* Doxycycline *on page 543*

♦ **Doxycin (Can)** *see* Doxycycline *on page 543*

Doxycycline (doks i SYE kleen)

Medication Safety Issues

Sound-alike/look-alike issues:
Doxycycline may be confused with dicyclomine, doxepin, doxylamine
Doxy-100® may be confused with Doxil®
Monodox® may be confused with Maalox®

Related Information

Malaria *on page 1855*

U.S. Brand Names Adoxa®; Doryx®; Doxy-100®; Monodox®; Oracea™; Periostat®; Vibramycin®; Vibra-Tabs®

Canadian Brand Names Apo-Doxy®; Apo-Doxy Tabs®; Doxycin; Doxytec; Novo-Doxylin; Nu-Doxycycline; Periostat®; Vibra-Tabs®

Index Terms Doxycycline Calcium; Doxycycline Hyclate; Doxycycline Monohydrate

Therapeutic Category Antibiotic, Tetracycline Derivative

Generic Available Yes: Excludes capsule (variable release), powder for oral solution, syrup

Use

Children, Adolescents, Adults: Treatment of Rocky Mountain spotted fever caused by susceptible *Rickettsia*; treatment of ehrlichiosis

Older Children, Adolescents, Adults: Treatment of Lyme disease, *Mycoplasma* infection, anthrax, brucellosis, psittacosis, or *Legionella*; management of malignant pleural effusions when intrapleural therapy is indicated

Adolescents and Adults: Treatment of nongonococcal pelvic inflammatory disease and urethritis due to *Chlamydia*; nongonococcal urethritis due to *Ureaplasma urealyticum*; treatment for victims of sexual assault; relapsing fever due to *Borrelia recurrentis*; adult periodontitis

Prophylaxis: Prophylaxis of malaria due to *Plasmodium falciparum* in short-term travelers (<4 months) to areas with chloroquine and/or pyrimethamine-sulfadoxine-resistant strains

Pregnancy Risk Factor D

Lactation Enters breast milk/not recommended

Contraindications Hypersensitivity to doxycycline, tetracycline, or any component (see Warnings); children <8 years (except in treatment of anthrax exposure); severe hepatic dysfunction

Warnings Syrup contains sodium metabisulfite which may cause allergic reactions in susceptible individuals. Photosensitivity reaction may occur with this drug; avoid prolonged exposure to sunlight or tanning equipment. Do not administer to children <8 years of age (except in treatment of anthrax exposure) due to associated retardation in skeletal development and decrease in fibula growth rate; use of tetracyclines during tooth development may cause permanent discoloration of the teeth and enamel hypoplasia; staining of teeth is dose-related so that duration of therapy should be minimized; doxycycline may be less likely to stain developing teeth than tetracycline since it binds less strongly to calcium; pseudomembranous colitis has been reported with doxycycline; prolonged use may result in superinfection.

Adverse Reactions

Central nervous system: Elevated intracranial pressure, bulging fontanels in infants

Dermatologic: Rash, photosensitivity, discoloration of nails, exfoliative dermatitis urticaria, angioneurotic edema

Gastrointestinal: Nausea, vomiting, diarrhea, esophagitis and esophageal ulceration with the hyclate salt formulation; anorexia, pseudomembranous colitis, oral candidiasis

Hematologic: Neutropenia, eosinophilia, thrombocytopenia, hemolytic anemia

Hepatic: Hepatotoxicity

Local: Phlebitis, pain at the injection site

Neuromuscular & skeletal: Retardation of skeletal development in infants

Renal: Elevated BUN

(Continued)

Doxycycline *(Continued)*

Miscellaneous: May cause discoloration of teeth in children <8 years of age, anaphylaxis, serum sickness

Drug Interactions Cytochrome P450 isoenzyme CYP3A3/4 substrate; isoenzyme CYP3A4 inhibitor

Antacids containing aluminum, calcium, or magnesium, zinc, kaolin, pectin, iron, and bismuth subsalicylate may decrease doxycycline bioavailability; rifampin, barbiturates, phenytoin, and carbamazepine decrease doxycycline's half-life; doxycycline enhances the hypoprothrombinemic effect of warfarin; decreased effect of oral contraceptives. Doxycycline may decrease the therapeutic effect of penicillins.

Food Interactions Administration with iron, calcium, milk or dairy products may decrease doxycycline absorption; may decrease absorption of calcium, iron, magnesium, zinc and amino acids

Stability Reconstituted oral doxycycline suspension is stable for 2 weeks at room temperature; I.V. doxycycline solutions must be protected from direct sunlight

Mechanism of Action Inhibits protein synthesis by binding to the 30S and possibly the 50S ribosomal subunit(s) of susceptible bacteria preventing additions of amino acids to the growing peptide chain; may also cause alterations in the cytoplasmic membrane

Pharmacokinetics

Absorption: Almost completely from the GI tract; absorption can be reduced by food or milk by 20%

Distribution: Widely distributed into body tissues and fluids including synovial and pleural fluid, bile, bronchial secretions; poor penetration into the CSF; appears in breast milk

Protein binding: 80% to 85%

Metabolism: Not metabolized in the liver; partially inactivated in the GI tract by chelate formation

Bioavailability: 90% to 100%

Half-life: 12-15 hours (usually increases to 22-24 hours with multiple dosing)

Time to peak serum concentration: Oral: Within 1.5-4 hours

Elimination: In the urine (23%) and feces (30%)

Dialysis: Not dialyzable (0% to 5%)

Usual Dosage

Children ≥8 years: Oral, I.V.: 2-4 mg/kg/day divided every 12-24 hours, not to exceed 200 mg/day

Lyme disease, Q fever, or Tularemia: >45 kg: Oral: 100 mg/dose twice daily for 14-21 days

Chlamydial infections, uncomplicated: >45 kg: Oral: 100 mg/dose twice daily for 7 days

Brucellosis: Oral: 2-4 mg/kg/day divided twice daily for 6 weeks; maximum: 200 mg/day; use in combination with rifampin

Rickettsial disease or Ehrlichiosis: >45 kg: Oral, I.V.: 100 mg every 12 hours for 7-14 days

Anthrax (if strain is proven susceptible): **Note:** In the presence of systemic involvement, extensive edema, and/or lesions on head/neck, doxycycline should initially be administered I.V. Initial treatment should include two or more agents per CDC recommendations. Agents suggested for use in conjunction with doxycycline include rifampin, vancomycin, penicillin, ampicillin, chloramphenicol, imipenem, clindamycin, or clarithromycin. Continue combined therapy for 60 days.

Treatment: I.V.: 5 mg/kg/day divided every 12 hours for 60 days (switch to oral therapy when clinically appropriate); maximum dose: 200 mg/day

Inhalation (postexposure prophylaxis): Oral: 5 mg/kg/day divided every 12 hours for 60 days; maximum dose: 200 mg/day

Prophylaxis of malaria: Oral: 2 mg/kg/day once daily; maximum dose: 100 mg/day starting 1-2 days before travel to the area with endemic infection, continuing daily during travel and for 4 weeks after leaving endemic area; maximum duration of prophylaxis: 4 months

Adolescents and Adults: Oral, I.V.: 100-200 mg/day in 1-2 divided doses

Anthrax (if strain is proven susceptible): Refer to Children's dosing for "Note" on route, combined therapy, and duration

Treatment: I.V.: 100 mg every 12 hours for 60 days (substitute oral antibiotics for I.V. antibiotics as soon as clinical condition improves)

Inhalation (postexposure prophylaxis): Oral: 100 mg every 12 hours for 60 days

Lyme disease, Q fever, or Tularemia: Oral: 100 mg/dose twice daily for 14-21 days

Pelvic inflammatory disease:

Hospitalized regimen: Oral, I.V.: 100 mg every 12 hours for 14 days administered with cefoxitin or cefotetan

Outpatient regimen: Oral: 100 mg every 12 hours for 14 days plus single dose ceftriaxone

Periodontitis: Oral (Periostat®): 20 mg twice daily as an adjunct following scaling and root planing; may be administered for up to 9 months

Prophylaxis of malaria: Oral: 100 mg/dose once daily starting 1-2 days before travel to the area with endemic infection, continuing daily during travel, and for 4 weeks after leaving endemic area; maximum duration of prophylaxis: 4 months

Rickettsial disease or Ehrlichiosis: Oral, I.V.: 100 mg every 12 hours for 7-14 days

Rosacea: Oral (Oracea™): 40 mg once daily in the morning

Chlamydial infections, uncomplicated: Oral: 100 mg/dose twice daily for 7 days

Nongonococcal urethritis caused by *C. trachomatis* or *U. urealyticum*: Oral: 100 mg/dose twice daily for 7 days

Sclerosing agent for pleural effusion: 500 mg in 25-30 mL of NS instilled into the pleural space to control pleural effusions associated with metastatic tumors; or for recurrent malignant pleural effusions: 500 mg in 250 mL NS

Dosing adjustment in renal impairment: No adjustment necessary

Administration

Oral: Administer capsules or tablets with adequate amounts of fluid; avoid antacids, infant formula, milk, dairy products, and iron for 1 hour before or 2 hours after administration of doxycycline; may be administered with food to decrease GI upset; shake suspension well before use

Doryx®: May break up the tablet and sprinkle the delayed release pellets on a spoonful of applesauce. Do **not** crush or damage the delayed release pellets; loss or damage of pellets prevents using the dose. Swallow the Doryx®/applesauce mixture immediately without chewing. Discard mixture if it cannot be used immediately.

Parenteral: For I.V. use only; administer by slow I.V. intermittent infusion over a minimum of 1-2 hours at a concentration not to exceed 1 mg/mL (may be infused over 1-4 hours); concentrations <0.1 mg/mL are not recommended

Sclerosing agent:

To control pleural effusions associated with metastatic tumors: Instill into the pleural space through a thoracostomy tube following drainage of the accumulated pleural fluid; clamp the tube then remove the fluid

For recurrent malignant pleural effusions: Administer via chest tube lavage, clamp tube for 24 hours then drain

Monitoring Parameters Periodic monitoring of renal, hematologic, and hepatic function tests; observe for changes in bowel frequency

Test Interactions False-negative urine glucose using Clinistix®, Tes-Tape®; false-positive urine glucose using Clinitest®; false elevations of urinary catecholamines with fluorescence test

Patient Information May discolor teeth if <8 years of age; may discolor fingernails. May cause photosensitivity reactions (eg, exposure to sunlight may cause severe sunburn, skin rash, redness, or itching); avoid exposure to sunlight and artificial light sources (sunlamps, tanning booth/bed); wear protective clothing, wide-brimmed hats, sunglasses, and lip sunscreen (SPF ≥15); use a sunscreen [broad-spectrum sunscreen or physical sunscreen (preferred) or sunblock with SPF ≥15]; contact physician if reaction occurs.

Nursing Implications Check for signs of phlebitis; I.V. doxycycline should not be given I.M. or SubQ; avoid extravasation. Encourage patient to drink plenty of fluids with doxycycline capsules or tablets to reduce the risk of esophageal ulceration.

Additional Information Injection contains ascorbic acid

Dosage Forms Excipient information presented when available (limited, particularly for generics); consult specific product labeling. [DSC] = Discontinued product

Note: Strength expressed as base.

Capsule, as hyclate: 50 mg, 100 mg

Vibramycin®: 100 mg

Capsule, as monohydrate: 50 mg, 100 mg

Monodox®: 50 mg, 100 mg

Capsule, variable release:

Oracea™: 40 mg [30 mg (immediate-release) and 10 mg (delayed-release)]

Injection, powder for reconstitution, as hyclate: 100 mg

Doxy-100®: 100 mg

Powder for oral suspension, as monohydrate:

Vibramycin®: 25 mg/5 mL (60 mL) [raspberry flavor]

Syrup, as calcium:

Vibramycin®: 50 mg/5 mL (480 mL) [contains sodium metabisulfite; raspberry-apple flavor]

Tablet, as hyclate: 20 mg, 100 mg

Periostat®: 20 mg

Vibra-Tabs®: 100 mg

Tablet, as monohydrate: 50 mg, 75 mg, 100 mg

Adoxa®: 50 mg, 75 mg, 100 mg

Adoxa® Pak™ 1/75 [unit-dose pack]: 75 mg (31s)

(Continued)

Doxycycline *(Continued)*

Adoxa® Pak™ 1/100 [unit-dose pack]: 100 mg (31s)
Adoxa® Pak™ 1/150 [unit-dose pack]: 150 mg (30s)
Adoxa® Pak™ 2/100 [unit-dose pack]: 100 mg (60s)

Tablet, delayed-release coated pellets, as hyclate:

Doryx®: 75 mg [contains sodium 4.5 mg (0.196 mEq)], 100 mg [contains sodium 6 mg (0.261 mEq)]

References

Centers for Disease Control and Prevention, "2002 Guidelines for Treatment of Sexually Transmitted Diseases," *MMWR Morb Mortal Wkly Rep*, 2002, 51(RR-6):1-80.

Centers for Disease Control and Prevention, "Update: Investigation of Anthrax Associated with Intentional Exposure and Interim Public Health Guidelines, October 2001," *MMWR Morb Mortal Wkly Rep*, 2001, 50(41):889-93.

Inglesby TV, Henderson DA, Bartlett JG, et al, "Anthrax as a Biological Weapon: Medical and Public Health Management. Working Group on Civilian Biodefense," *JAMA*, 1999, 281(18):1735-45.

♦ **Doxycycline Calcium** *see* Doxycycline *on page 543*
♦ **Doxycycline Hyclate** *see* Doxycycline *on page 543*
♦ **Doxycycline Monohydrate** *see* Doxycycline *on page 543*
♦ **Doxytec (Can)** *see* Doxycycline *on page 543*
♦ **DPA** *see* Valproic Acid and Derivatives *on page 1592*
♦ **DPE** *see* Dipivefrin *on page 520*
♦ **D-Penicillamine** *see* Penicillamine *on page 1227*
♦ **DPH** *see* Phenytoin *on page 1253*
♦ **Dramamine® [OTC]** *see* DimenhyDRINATE *on page 507*
♦ **Dramamine® Less Drowsy Formula [OTC]** *see* Meclizine *on page 988*
♦ **Drisdol®** *see* Ergocalciferol *on page 588*
♦ **Dristan™ 12-Hour [OTC]** *see* Oxymetazoline *on page 1194*
♦ **Dristan® Long Lasting Nasal (Can)** *see* Oxymetazoline *on page 1194*
♦ **Drixoral® Nasal (Can)** *see* Oxymetazoline *on page 1194*
♦ **Drixoral® ND (Can)** *see* Pseudoephedrine *on page 1344*

Dronabinol (droe NAB i nol)

Medication Safety Issues

Sound-alike/look-alike issues:

Dronabinol may be confused with droperidol

U.S. Brand Names Marinol®

Canadian Brand Names Marinol®

Index Terms Delta-9-tetrahydro-cannabinol; Delta-9 THC; Tetrahydrocannabinol; THC

Therapeutic Category Antiemetic

Generic Available No

Use Treatment of nausea and vomiting secondary to cancer chemotherapy in patients who have not responded to conventional antiemetics; treatment of anorexia associated with weight loss in AIDS patients

Restrictions C-III

Pregnancy Risk Factor C

Lactation Enters breast milk/contraindicated

Contraindications Hypersensitivity to dronabinol, sesame oil, or any component, marijuana, or cannabinoids; should not be used in patients with a history of schizophrenia

Warnings Dronabinol has a high potential for abuse; limit antiemetic therapy availability to current cycle of chemotherapy

Precautions Use with caution in patients with heart disease, history of substance abuse, hepatic disease, or seizure disorders (may lower seizure threshold); reduce dosage in patients with severe hepatic impairment; tolerance to CNS side effects usually occurs in 1-3 days of continued use; tachyphylaxis and tolerance does not appear to develop when used as an appetite stimulant as efficacy has been documented in clinical trials for up to 5 months of treatment. Use with caution in patients with mania or depression as dronabinol may exacerbate these conditions

Adverse Reactions

Cardiovascular: Orthostatic hypotension, tachycardia, palpitations, vasodilation, hypotension, flushing

Central nervous system: Drowsiness, dizziness, vertigo, difficulty in concentrating, mood change, euphoria, detachment, depression, anxiety, paranoia, hallucinations, nervousness, ataxia, headache, memory lapse, seizures, fatigue, nightmares

Gastrointestinal: Xerostomia, diarrhea, abdominal pain

Hepatic: Elevated liver enzymes

Neuromuscular & skeletal: Myalgia, tremor, paresthesia, weakness
Ocular: Vision difficulties, conjunctivitis
Otic: Tinnitus
Respiratory: Sinusitis, cough, rhinitis
Miscellaneous: Diaphoresis

Drug Interactions Cytochrome P450 isoenzyme CYP2C18 and CYP3A3/4 substrate
Additive tachycardia, hypertension with amphetamines, cocaine, sympathomimetics, anticholinergics, tricyclic antidepressants; additive CNS effects with sedatives, antihistamines, hypnotics, psychomimetics, tricyclic antidepressants, alcohol; hypomanic state with disulfiram, fluoxetine; increases theophylline metabolism; decreases barbiturate clearance

Stability Store in a cool environment (46°F to 59°F); may be refrigerated; do not freeze

Mechanism of Action Dronabinol is the principal psychoactive substance found in *Cannabis sativa* (marijuana); its mechanism of action as an antiemetic is not well defined, it probably inhibits the vomiting center in the medulla oblongata; has complex effects on CNS including central sympathomimetic activity

Pharmacodynamics
Onset of action: 30 minutes to 1 hour
Maximum effect: 2-4 hours
Duration:
Psychoactive effects: 4-6 hours
Appetite stimulation: 24 hours

Pharmacokinetics
Absorption: Oral: 90% to 95%; first-pass metabolism results in low systemic bioavailability
Distribution: V_d: ~10L/kg
Protein binding: ~97%
Metabolism: Extensive first-pass; metabolized in the liver to several metabolites some of which are active
Bioavailability: 10% to 20%
Half-life:
Biphasic: Alpha: 4 hours
Terminal: 25-36 hours
Dronabinol metabolites: 44-59 hours
Time to peak serum concentration: Within 0.5-4 hours
Elimination: Biliary excretion is the major route of elimination; 50% excreted in feces within 72 hours; 10% to 15% excreted in urine within 72 hours
Clearance: Adults: Mean 0.2 L/kg/hour (highly variable)

Usual Dosage Oral:
Antiemetic: Children and Adults: 5 mg/m^2 1-3 hours before chemotherapy, then give 5 mg/m^2/dose every 2-4 hours after chemotherapy for a total of 4-6 doses/day; dose may be increased in 2.5 mg/m^2 increments to a maximum of 15 mg/m^2 per dose if needed
Alternative dosing: Adults: 5 mg 3-4 times/day; dosage may be escalated during a chemotherapy cycle or at subsequent cycles depending upon response
Appetite stimulant: Adults: 2.5 mg twice daily before lunch and dinner; if intolerant, a dosage of 2.5 mg once daily at night may be tried; maximum dosage (escalating): 10 mg twice daily

Administration May be administered without regard to meals; take before meals if used to stimulate appetite

Monitoring Parameters Heart rate, blood pressure

Patient Information May cause drowsiness and impair ability to perform activities requiring mental alertness or physical coordination; may cause dry mouth; avoid alcohol

Dosage Forms Excipient information presented when available (limited, particularly for generics); consult specific product labeling.
Capsule, gelatin:
Marinol®: 2.5 mg, 5 mg, 10 mg [contains sesame oil]

References
Lane M, Smith FE, Sullivan RA, et al, "Dronabinol and Prochlorperazine Alone and in Combination as Antiemetic Agents for Cancer Chemotherapy," *Am J Clin Oncol*, 1990, 13(6):480-4.

Droperidol (droe PER i dole)

Medication Safety Issues
Sound-alike/look-alike issues:
Droperidol may be confused with dronabinol
Inapsine® may be confused with Nebcin®
(Continued)

Droperidol *(Continued)*

Related Information

Compatibility of Chemotherapy and Related Supportive Care Medications *on page 1777*

Compatibility of Medications Mixed in A Syringe *on page 1941*

U.S. Brand Names Inapsine®

Canadian Brand Names Droperidol Injection, USP

Index Terms Dehydrobenzperidol

Therapeutic Category Antiemetic; Antipsychotic Agent

Generic Available Yes

Use Treatment of nausea and vomiting associated with surgical and diagnostic procedures in patients for whom other treatments are ineffective or inappropriate

Pregnancy Risk Factor C

Lactation Excretion in breast milk unknown

Contraindications Hypersensitivity to droperidol or any component; known or suspected QT prolongation; congenital long QT syndrome

Warnings Cases of QT prolongation and torsade de pointes in patients treated with droperidol in doses within or even below the approved dosage range have been reported. Some cases occurred in patients with no underlying risk factors for QT prolongation; fatalities have occurred.

Droperidol should be reserved for patients who fail other treatments. Prior to its use, all patients should undergo a 12-lead EKG. If the QT interval is prolonged, droperidol should not be used. Droperidol should be used with extreme caution in patients with risk factors for prolonged QT syndrome (ie, CHF; bradycardia; cardiac hypertrophy; any clinically significant cardiac disease; diuretic use; hypokalemia; hypomagnesemia; concomitant use of Class I or Class III antiarrhythmics, MAO inhibitors, or medications known to prolong the QT interval; age >65 years; alcohol abuse; and use of medications such as benzodiazepines, volatile anesthetics and I.V. opiates).

The dosage of droperidol should be individualized; dosages should be started low and titrated upward. Continuous EKG monitoring should be done prior to treatment and for 2-3 hours after treatment to monitor for arrhythmias. I.V. fluids and other therapy to treat hypotension should be readily available; monitor patients carefully. Use reduced initial doses of opioids, if needed. Neuromalignant syndrome may rarely occur.

Precautions Use with caution in patients with impaired hepatic or renal function; severe hypertension and tachycardia may occur in patients with pheochromocytoma

Adverse Reactions

Cardiovascular: Hypotension (especially in hypovolemic patients), tachycardia; QT prolongation, torsade de pointes, cardiac arrest, ventricular tachycardia (see Warnings)

Central nervous system: Extrapyramidal reactions such as dystonic reactions, akathisia, and oculogyric crisis; anxiety, hyperactivity, drowsiness, dizziness, hallucinations, chills, dysphoria, restlessness

Respiratory: Laryngospasm, bronchospasm

Miscellaneous: Anaphylaxis; neuromalignant syndrome (rare)

Drug Interactions Concomitant use with any drug that prolongs the QT interval is **not** recommended (see Warnings); diuretics, laxatives, and mineralocorticoids may cause hypokalemia or hypomagnesemia and increase the risk of droperidol-induced QT prolongation. Use with other CNS depressants may have additive effects (CNS, respiratory depression, etc); droperidol plus fentanyl or other analgesics may increase blood pressure; conduction anesthesia may increase hypotension; droperidol plus epinephrine may decrease blood pressure due to alpha-adrenergic blockade effects of droperidol; droperidol plus atropine may cause tachycardia

Stability Store at room temperature; protect from light. Physically compatible and chemically stable with D_5W, LR, NS at a concentration of 20 mg/L

Mechanism of Action Alters the action of dopamine in the CNS, at subcortical levels, to produce sedation and a dissociative state; also possesses alpha-adrenergic blockade effects

Pharmacodynamics

Onset of action: 3-10 minutes

Maximum effect: Within 30 minutes

Duration: 2-4 hours (up to 12 hours)

Pharmacokinetics

Metabolism: In the liver

Half-life, adults: 2.3 hours

Elimination: In urine (75%) and feces (22%)

Usual Dosage Dosage must be individualized, based on age, body weight, underlying medical conditions, physical status, concomitant medications, type of anesthesia, and surgical procedure

Children 2-12 years:

Postoperative nausea and vomiting prophylaxis for high risk surgery: I.M., I.V.: Doses as low as 0.015 mg/kg/dose may be effective; usual: 0.05-0.06 mg/kg/dose administered once; maximum initial dose: 0.1 mg/kg; administer additional doses with caution and only if potential benefit outweighs risks (see Warnings); **Note:** A recent meta-analysis of 74 randomised controlled trials (29 pediatric trials) assessed droperidol use for the prevention of postoperative nausea and vomiting; the analysis suggested that 0.075 mg/kg/dose was likely to be the most effective prophylactic dose; it was also the most frequently used dose in the trials that were assessed; however, due to side effects associated with this dose, the study considered 0.05 mg/kg/dose to be the best prophylactic dose for children in cases where sedation and drowsiness should be prevented (eg, day surgery) (see Henzi, 2000)

Postoperative nausea and vomiting (treatment): I.V.: Doses as low as 0.01-0.03 mg/kg/dose may be effective for breakthrough nausea and vomiting; maximum initial dose: 0.1 mg/kg; administer additional doses with caution and only if potential benefit outweighs risks (see Warnings)

Adults: Nausea and vomiting: I.M., I.V.: Maximum initial dose: 2.5 mg; additional doses of 1.25 mg may be administered to achieve desired effect; administer additional doses with caution and only if potential benefit outweighs risks (see Warnings)

Administration Parenteral: Administer by slow I.V. injection over 2-5 minutes; maximum concentration: 2.5 mg/mL (I.M. or I.V.)

Monitoring Parameters Prior to use: 12-lead EKG to identify patients with QT prolongation (use is contraindicated); continuous EKG during and for 2-3 hours after dosage administration is recommended. Blood pressure, heart rate, respiratory rate; serum potassium and magnesium; observe for dystonias, extrapyramidal side effects; temperature

Additional Information Does not possess analgesic effects; has little or no amnesic properties. A dose-dependent prolongation of the QT interval has been observed in adults; significant QT prolongation was noted at doses of 0.1 mg/kg, 0.175 mg/kg, and 0.25 mg/kg with prolongation of median QT_c interval by 37, 44, and 59 msec, respectively (see package insert)

Dosage Forms Excipient information presented when available (limited, particularly for generics); consult specific product labeling.

Injection, solution: 2.5 mg/mL (1 mL, 2 mL)

References

Henzi I, Sonderegger J, and Tramer MR, "Efficacy, Dose-Response, and Adverse Effects of Droperidol for Prevention of Postoperative Nausea and Vomiting," *Can J Anaesth*, 2000, 47(6):537-51.

Yaster M, Sola JE, Pegoli W Jr, et al, "The Night After Surgery: Postoperative Management of the Pediatric Outpatient - Surgical and Anesthetic Aspects," *Pediatr Clin North Am*, 1994, 41(1):199-220.

♦ **Droperidol Injection, USP (Can)** *see* Droperidol *on page 547*

Drotrecogin Alfa (Activated) (dro TRE coe jin AL fa ak ti VAY ted)

U.S. Brand Names Xigris®

Canadian Brand Names Xigris®

Index Terms Activated Protein C, Human, Recombinant; Drotrecogin Alfa, Activated; Protein C (Activated), Human, Recombinant

Therapeutic Category Biological Response Modulator

Generic Available No

Use Reduction of mortality in adult patients with severe sepsis (sepsis associated with acute organ dysfunction) who have a high risk of death (ie, as determined by APACHE II score ≥25); purpura fulminans (compassionate use protocol)

Pregnancy Risk Factor C

Lactation Excretion in breast milk unknown/not recommended

Contraindications Hypersensitivity to drotrecogin alfa or any component; patients with active internal bleeding; recent (within 3 months) hemorrhagic stroke, recent (within 2 months) intracranial or intraspinal surgery, or severe head trauma; trauma with an increased risk of life-threatening bleeding; presence of an epidural catheter; intracranial neoplasm or mass lesion or evidence of cerebral herniation

Warnings Serious bleeding was observed in 3.5% of drotrecogin alfa-treated patients and is the most common adverse effect associated with this agent. Conditions which may increase the risk of bleeding with drotrecogin alfa include concurrent heparin administration (≥15 units/kg/hour), platelet count <30,000 x 10^6/L, INR >3, recent (within 6 weeks) gastrointestinal bleeding, recent administration (within 3 days) of thrombolytic therapy, recent administration (within 7 days) of oral anticoagulants or

(Continued)

Drotrecogin Alfa (Activated) *(Continued)*

glycoprotein IIb/IIIa inhibitors, recent administration (within 7 days) of aspirin >650 mg/day, NSAIDs, clopidogrel, dipyridamole, or other platelet inhibitors, intracranial arteriovenous malformation or aneurysm, and chronic severe hepatic disease. If bleeding occurs, immediately stop the infusion. Once hemostasis has been achieved, restarting drotrecogin alfa may be considered. Stop drotrecogin alfa 2 hours prior to undergoing an invasive surgical procedure or procedure with an inherent risk of bleeding. Once hemostasis has been achieved, drotrecogin alfa may be restarted 12 hours after major invasive procedures or surgery or immediately after less invasive procedures.

Precautions Use with caution in patients at risk of bleeding, patients with chronic renal failure requiring dialysis, patients with hypercoagulable conditions (ie, hereditary deficiencies of protein C, protein S, or antithrombin III, suspected thromboembolism), or resistance to activated protein C

Adverse Reactions

Central nervous system: Intracranial hemorrhage

Gastrointestinal: GI hemorrhage

Genitourinary: GU hemorrhage

Hematologic: Bleeding, bruising

Drug Interactions Drugs affecting the coagulation system or platelet function may increase risk of bleeding (aspirin, glycoprotein IIb/IIIa antagonists, cilostazol, clopidogrel, dipyridamole, heparin, danaparoid, LMWHs, NSAIDs, thrombolytic agents, antithrombin III, warfarin)

Stability Refrigerate and protect unreconstituted vials from light. Do not freeze. Drotrecogin alfa for injection contains no preservatives. Reconstituted vial is stable for 3 hours at room temperature. Once reconstituted and further diluted with NS, infusion must be completed within 12 hours. Additional studies (data on file, Lilly Research Laboratories) show that the final solution is stable for 14 hours at room temperature. If not used immediately, a prepared solution may be stored in the refrigerator for up to 12 hours. The expiration time (refrigeration and administration) should be ≤24 hours from preparation. The only compatible solutions which can be administered through the same line as drotrecogin alfa are NS, LR, dextrose, or dextrose and saline mixtures. Avoid exposing drotrecogin alfa infusion solution to heat and/or direct sunlight.

Mechanism of Action Drotrecogin alfa, a serine protease with the same amino acid sequence as human plasma-derived activated protein C, possesses profibrinolytic, antithrombotic, and anti-inflammatory activities. Activated protein C inactivates factors Va and VIIIa decreasing generation of thrombin and ultimately decreasing fibrin/clot formation; binds to plasminogen activator type 1 enhancing the action of tissue plasminogen activator and stimulates fibrinolysis; inhibits cytokine production

Pharmacodynamics

Maximum effect on decreasing D-dimer levels: At the end of a 96-hour 24 mcg/kg/hour infusion

Duration: Nondetectable in plasma within 2 hours of discontinuation

Pharmacokinetics A phase 2 pharmacokinetic study has been performed in pediatric patients, but results from this trial are not yet available (communication with Lilly Research Laboratories, Jan 2002)

Metabolism: Plasma protease inhibitors inactivate drotrecogin alfa and endogenous activated protein C

Half-life: 1.2 hours

Usual Dosage I.V.: Continuous infusion:

Infants, Children, and Adults: Purpura fulminans: In a compassionate use program, 42 patients (range: >3 kg to 135 kg; >1 year of age) received a dose of 24 mcg/kg/hour for 96 hours. If the patient had improved after 96 hours, but had laboratory evidence of an ongoing coagulopathy, or had tissue still deemed to be at risk for necrosis, the drotrecogin alfa infusion could be continued. The maximum allowed infusion time was 168 hours.

Adults: Severe sepsis: 24 mcg/kg/hour for 4 days. Infusion should be started within 24 hours of the onset of at least three signs of systemic inflammation and evidence of at least one organ/system dysfunction

Administration Parenteral: I.V.: May administer via a dedicated I.V. line or a dedicated lumen of a central venous catheter at a final concentration between 100-1000 mcg/mL in NS. When using low concentrations <200 mcg/mL at low flow rates <5 mL/hour, the infusion set must be primed for approximately 15 minutes at a flow rate of approximately 5 mL/hour.

Monitoring Parameters Hemoglobin, hematocrit, coagulation panel, CBC with differential, platelet count, signs and symptoms of bleeding; for select patients: Plasma D-dimer levels, plasma interleukin-6 level, protein C and protein S activity; for purpura fulminans: Evaluate tissue for necrosis risk

Test Interactions Drotrecogin alfa may prolong the one-stage coagulation assay based on the APTT (such as factor VIII, IX, and XI assays) so that an apparent factor concentration appears lower than the true concentration.

Additional Information Human plasma derived protein C concentrate (an alternative, investigational product) has been used in infants and children with severe meningococcemia associated with purpura fulminans (see Ettingshausen, 1999).

Dosage Forms Excipient information presented when available (limited, particularly for generics); consult specific product labeling.

Injection, powder for reconstitution [preservative free]: 5 mg [contains sucrose 31.8 mg], 20 mg [contains sucrose 124.9 mg]

References

Alberio L, Lammle B, and Esmon CT, "Protein C Replacement in Severe Meningococcemia: Rationale and Clinical Experience," *Clin Infect Dis*, 2001, 32(9):1338-46.

Bachli EB, Vavricka SR, Walter RB, et al, "Drotrecogin Alfa (Activated) for the Treatment of Meningococcal Purpura Fulminans," *Intensive Care Med*, 2003, 29(2):337.

Bernard GR, Vincent JL, Laterre PF, et al, "Efficacy and Safety of Recombinant Human Activated Protein C for Severe Sepsis," *N Engl J Med*, 2001, 344(10):699-709.

Ettingshausen CE, Veldmann A, Beeg T, et al, "Replacement Therapy With Protein C Concentrate in Infants and Adolescents With Meningococcal Sepsis and Purpura Fulminans," *Semin Thromb Hemost*, 1999, 25(6):537-41.

Faust SN, Levin M, Harrison OB, et al, "Dysfunction of Endothelial Protein C Activation in Severe Meningococcal Sepsis," *N Engl J Med*, 2001, 345(6):408-16.

Smith KJ, Neal J, Winton EF, et al, "Purpura Fulminans and *S. pneumoniae* Sepsis With Severe Acquired Protein C Deficiency Successfully Treated With Recombinant Human Activated Protein C," *Thromb Haemost*, 1999, 82(Suppl 1):738.

- ♦ **Drotrecogin Alfa, Activated** *see* Drotrecogin Alfa (Activated) *on page 549*
- ♦ **Droxia®** *see* Hydroxyurea *on page 794*
- ♦ **Dr. Scholl's® Callus Remover [OTC]** *see* Salicylic Acid *on page 1413*
- ♦ **Dr. Scholl's® Clear Away [OTC]** *see* Salicylic Acid *on page 1413*
- ♦ **DSCG** *see* Cromolyn *on page 407*
- ♦ **DSS** *see* Docusate *on page 526*
- ♦ **D-S-S® [OTC]** *see* Docusate *on page 526*
- ♦ **DT** *see* Diphtheria and Tetanus Toxoid *on page 514*
- ♦ **DTaP** *see* Diphtheria, Tetanus Toxoids, and Acellular Pertussis Vaccine *on page 517*
- ♦ **DTIC** *see* Dacarbazine *on page 433*
- ♦ **DTIC® (Can)** *see* Dacarbazine *on page 433*
- ♦ **DTIC-Dome®** *see* Dacarbazine *on page 433*
- ♦ **DTO (error-prone abbreviation)** *see* Opium Tincture *on page 1172*
- ♦ **dTpa** *see* Diphtheria, Tetanus Toxoids, and Acellular Pertussis Vaccine *on page 517*
- ♦ **Duac™** *see* Clindamycin and Benzoyl Peroxide *on page 382*
- ♦ **Dulcolax® [OTC]** *see* Bisacodyl *on page 217*
- ♦ **Dulcolax® (Can)** *see* Bisacodyl *on page 217*
- ♦ **Dulcolax® Milk of Magnesia [OTC]** *see* Magnesium Hydroxide *on page 971*
- ♦ **Dulcolax® Milk of Magnesia [OTC]** *see* Magnesium Supplements *on page 976*
- ♦ **Dulcolax® Stool Softener [OTC]** *see* Docusate *on page 526*
- ♦ **Dull-C® [OTC]** *see* Ascorbic Acid *on page 159*
- ♦ **DuoFilm® [OTC]** *see* Salicylic Acid *on page 1413*
- ♦ **Duofilm® (Can)** *see* Salicylic Acid *on page 1413*
- ♦ **Duoforte® 27 (Can)** *see* Salicylic Acid *on page 1413*
- ♦ **DuoPlant® [DSC] [OTC]** *see* Salicylic Acid *on page 1413*
- ♦ **Durabolin® (Can)** *see* Nandrolone *on page 1105*
- ♦ **Duraclon™** *see* Clonidine *on page 389*
- ♦ **Duragesic®** *see* Fentanyl *on page 644*
- ♦ **Duralith® (Can)** *see* Lithium *on page 948*
- ♦ **Duramist® Plus [OTC]** *see* Oxymetazoline *on page 1194*
- ♦ **Duramorph®** *see* Morphine Sulfate *on page 1082*
- ♦ **Duration® [OTC]** *see* Oxymetazoline *on page 1194*
- ♦ **Duratuss® DM** *see* Guaifenesin and Dextromethorphan *on page 748*
- ♦ **Duricef®** *see* Cefadroxil *on page 302*
- ♦ **Duvoid® (Can)** *see* Bethanechol *on page 215*
- ♦ **Dycill® (Can)** *see* Dicloxacillin *on page 489*

Dyclonine (DYE kloe neen)

Medication Safety Issues

Sound-alike/look-alike issues:

Dyclonine may be confused with dicyclomine

(Continued)

Dyclonine *(Continued)*

U.S. Brand Names Cēpacol® Dual Action Maximum Strength [OTC]; Sucrets® [OTC]

Index Terms Dyclonine Hydrochloride

Therapeutic Category Local Anesthetic, Oral

Generic Available No

Use As a local anesthetic prior to laryngoscopy, bronchoscopy, or endotracheal intubation; used topically for temporary relief of pain associated with oral mucosa, skin, episiotomy, or anogenital lesions; the 0.5% topical solution may be used to block the gag reflex, and to relieve the pain of oral ulcers or stomatitis; the lozenge is used for temporary relief of sore throat pain and gum irritation

Pregnancy Risk Factor C

Contraindications Hypersensitivity to chlorobutanol (preservative used in dyclonine), dyclonine, or any component

Warnings Resuscitative equipment, oxygen and resuscitative drugs should be immediately available when dyclonine topical solution is administered to mucous membranes; may impair swallowing and enhance the danger of aspiration

Precautions Use with caution in patients with infection present in the area of application or traumatized mucosa in the area of application to avoid rapid systemic absorption; use with caution in patients with shock or heart block

Adverse Reactions Excessive dosage and rapid absorption may result in adverse CNS and cardiovascular effects

Cardiovascular: Hypotension, bradycardia, cardiac arrest, edema
Central nervous system: Excitation, drowsiness, nervousness, dizziness, seizures
Dermatologic: Rash, urticaria
Local: Slight irritation and stinging may occur when applied
Ocular: Blurred vision
Respiratory: Respiratory arrest
Miscellaneous: Allergic reactions

Stability Store in tight, light-resistant container; avoid freezing

Mechanism of Action Blocks impulses at peripheral nerve endings in skin and mucous membranes by altering cell membrane permeability to ionic transfer

Pharmacodynamics
Onset of action: Local anesthesia: 2-10 minutes
Duration: 30-60 minutes

Usual Dosage
Children and Adults:
Topical solution: Mouth sores: 5-10 mL of 0.5% or 1% to oral mucosa (swab or swish and then spit) 3-4 times/day as needed; maximum single dose: 200 mg (40 mL of 0.5% solution or 20 mL of 1% solution); solution may be diluted 1:1 with water
Bronchoscopy: Use 2 mL of the 1% solution or 4 mL of the 0.5% solution sprayed onto the larynx and trachea every 5 minutes for 2-3 applications until the reflex has been abolished
Children >3 years: Topical: Slowly dissolve 1 lozenge (1.2 mg) in mouth every 2 hours, if necessary
Children >12 years and Adults: Topical: Slowly dissolve 1 lozenge (3 mg) in mouth every 2 hours, if necessary

Administration Topical: Apply to mucous membranes of the mouth or throat area: food should not be ingested for 60 minutes following application in the mouth or throat area

Patient Information Do not chew lozenge; numbness of the tongue and buccal mucosa may result in increased risk of biting trauma; may impair swallowing

Nursing Implications Use the lowest dose needed to provide effective anesthesia; not for injection; do not apply nasally or to the eye

Dosage Forms Excipient information presented when available (limited, particularly for generics); consult specific product labeling.
Lozenge, as hydrochloride (Sucrets®): 1.2 mg [children's cherry flavor]; 2 mg [wild cherry and assorted flavors]; 3 mg [vapor black cherry and wintergreen flavors]
Spray, oral, as hydrochloride (Cēpacol® Dual Action Maximum Strength): 0.1% (120 mL) [contains glycerin 33%; cherry, honey lemon and cool menthol flavors]

References
Carnel SB, Blakeslee DB, Oswald SG, et al, "Treatment of Radiation- and Chemotherapy-Induced Stomatitis," *Otolaryngol Head Neck Surg*, 1990, 102(4):326-30.

- **Dyclonine Hydrochloride** *see* Dyclonine *on page 551*
- **Dygase** *see* Pancreatin *on page 1202*
- **Dynacin®** *see* Minocycline *on page 1066*
- **DynaCirc® [DSC]** *see* Isradipine *on page 879*
- **DynaCirc® (Can)** *see* Isradipine *on page 879*

- **DynaCirc® CR** *see* Isradipine *on page 879*
- **Dyna-Hex® [OTC]** *see* Chlorhexidine Gluconate *on page 337*
- **Dyrenium®** *see* Triamterene *on page 1571*
- **Dytan™** *see* DiphenhydrAMINE *on page 509*
- **EarSol® HC** *see* Hydrocortisone *on page 781*
- **Easprin®** *see* Aspirin *on page 163*
- **EC-Naprosyn®** *see* Naproxen *on page 1108*
- ***E. coli* Asparaginase** *see* Asparaginase *on page 161*

Econazole (e KONE a zole)

U.S. Brand Names Spectazole®
Canadian Brand Names Ecostatin®; Spectazole™
Index Terms Econazole Nitrate
Therapeutic Category Antifungal Agent, Topical
Generic Available Yes
Use Topical treatment of tinea pedis, tinea cruris, tinea corporis, tinea versicolor, and cutaneous candidiasis
Pregnancy Risk Factor C
Lactation Excretion in breast milk unknown
Contraindications Hypersensitivity to econazole or any component
Warnings Not for ophthalmic or intravaginal use
Precautions Discontinue the drug if sensitivity or chemical irritation occurs; cross-sensitization may occur with other imidazole derivatives (ie, clotrimazole, miconazole)
Adverse Reactions
Dermatologic: Pruritus, erythema, contact dermatitis
Local: Burning, stinging
Mechanism of Action Alters fungal cell wall membrane permeability; may interfere with RNA and protein synthesis, and lipid metabolism
Pharmacokinetics
Absorption: Following topical administration, <10% is percutaneously absorbed
Metabolism: In the liver to >20 metabolites
Elimination: <1% of an applied dose recovered in urine or feces
Usual Dosage Children and Adults: Topical:
Tinea cruris, corporis, pedis, and tinea versicolor: Apply once daily
Cutaneous candidiasis: Apply twice daily
Administration Topical: Apply a sufficient amount of cream to cover affected areas; do not apply to the eye or intravaginally
Patient Information For external use only. Notify physician if condition worsens or persists, or if irritation occurs.
Additional Information Candidal infections and tinea cruris, versicolor, and corporis should be treated for 2 weeks and tinea pedis for 1 month; occasionally, longer treatment periods may be required
Dosage Forms Excipient information presented when available (limited, particularly for generics); consult specific product labeling.
Cream, topical, as nitrate: 1% (15 g, 30 g, 85 g)

- **Econazole Nitrate** *see* Econazole *on page 553*
- **Econopred® Plus** *see* PrednisoLONE *on page 1304*
- **Ecostatin® (Can)** *see* Econazole *on page 553*
- **Ecotrin® [OTC]** *see* Aspirin *on page 163*
- **Ecotrin® Low Strength [OTC]** *see* Aspirin *on page 163*
- **Ecotrin® Maximum Strength [OTC]** *see* Aspirin *on page 163*
- **Ectosone (Can)** *see* Betamethasone *on page 212*
- **Edathamil Disodium** *see* Edetate Disodium *on page 555*
- **Edecrin®** *see* Ethacrynic Acid *on page 614*

Edetate Calcium Disodium (ED e tate KAL see um dye SOW dee um)

Medication Safety Issues
Sound-alike look-alike issues:
Edetate calcium disodium (CaEDTA) may be confused with edetate disodium (Na_2EDTA). CDC recommends that edetate disodium should **never** be used for chelation therapy in children. Fatal hypocalcemia may result if edetate disodium is used for chelation therapy instead of edetate calcium disodium.
Related Information
Commonly Used Antidotes for Acute Overdoses *on page 1920*
(Continued)

Edetate Calcium Disodium *(Continued)*

U.S. Brand Names Calcium Disodium Versenate®

Index Terms CaEDTA; Calcium Disodium Edetate; Calcium EDTA; EDTA (Calcium Disodium)

Therapeutic Category Antidote, Lead Toxicity; Chelating Agent, Parenteral

Generic Available No

Use Treatment of acute and chronic lead poisoning; also used as an aid in the diagnosis of lead poisoning

Pregnancy Risk Factor B

Contraindications Hypersensitivity to edetate calcium disodium or any component; severe renal disease, anuria

Warnings Do not exceed recommended daily dose; avoid rapid I.V. infusion in the management of lead encephalopathy, intracranial pressure may be increased to lethal levels; I.M. administration is the preferred route in these patients; if anuria, increasing proteinuria, or hematuria occurs during therapy, discontinue calcium EDTA

Precautions Renal tubular necrosis and fatal nephrosis may occur, especially with high doses; establish urine flow prior to administration

Adverse Reactions

Cardiovascular: Hypotension, arrhythmias, EKG changes
Central nervous system: Fever, headache, chills
Dermatologic: Skin lesions, cheilosis
Endocrine & metabolic: Hypercalcemia, zinc deficiency
Gastrointestinal: GI upset, anorexia, nausea, vomiting
Hematologic: Transient marrow suppression, anemia
Hepatic: Mild elevation in liver function tests
Local: Pain at injection site following I.M. injection, thrombophlebitis following I.V. infusion (when concentration >5 mg/mL)
Neuromuscular & skeletal: Arthralgia, tremor, numbness, paresthesia
Ocular: Lacrimation
Renal: Renal tubular necrosis, proteinuria, microscopic hematuria
Respiratory: Sneezing, nasal congestion

Drug Interactions Do not use simultaneously with zinc insulin preparations

Stability Dilute with NS or D_5W; physically incompatible with $D_{10}W$, LR; do not mix in the same syringe with dimercaprol

Mechanism of Action Calcium is displaced by divalent and trivalent heavy metals, forming a nonionizing soluble complex that is excreted in the urine

Pharmacodynamics

Onset of chelation with I.V. administration: 1 hour
Maximum excretion of chelated lead with I.V. administration: 24-48 hours

Pharmacokinetics

Absorption: I.M., SubQ: Well absorbed
Distribution: Into extracellular fluid; minimal CSF penetration
Half-life, plasma:
- I.M.: 1.5 hours
- I.V.: 20 minutes

Elimination: Rapid in urine as metal chelates or unchanged drug

Usual Dosage Several regimens have been recommended:

Diagnosis of lead poisoning: Mobilization test (not recommended by AAP guidelines):

I.M., I.V.:

Children: 500 mg/m^2/dose, (maximum dose: 1 g) as a single dose or divided into 2 doses

Adults: 500 mg/m^2/dose

Note: Urine is collected for 24 hours after first EDTA dose and analyzed for lead content; if the ratio of mcg of lead in urine to mg calcium EDTA given is >1, then test is considered positive; for convenience, an 8-hour urine collection may be done after a single 50 mg/kg I.M. (maximum dose: 1 g) or 500 mg/m^2 I.V. dose; a positive test occurs if the ratio of lead excretion to mg calcium EDTA >0.5-0.6.

Treatment of lead poisoning: Children and Adults (each regimen is specific for route):

Symptoms of lead encephalopathy and/or blood lead level >70 mcg/dL: Treat 5 days; give in conjunction with dimercaprol; wait a minimum of 2 days with no treatment before considering a repeat course:

I.M.: 250 mg/m^2/dose every 4 hours

I.V.: 50 mg/kg/day as 24-hour continuous I.V. infusion **or** 1-1.5 g/m^2 I.V. as either an 8- to 24-hour infusion or divided into 2 doses every 12 hours

Symptomatic lead poisoning **without** encephalopathy **or** asymptomatic with blood lead level >70 mcg/dL: Treat 3-5 days; treatment with dimercaprol is recommended until the blood lead level concentration <50 mcg/dL:

I.M.: 167 mg/m^2 every 4 hours

I.V.: 1 g/m^2 as an 8- to 24-hour infusion or divided every 12 hours

Asymptomatic **children** with blood lead level 45-69 mcg/dL: I.V.: 25 mg/kg/day for 5 days as an 8- to 24-hour infusion or divided into 2 doses every 12 hours

Depending upon the blood lead level, additional courses may be necessary; repeat at least 2-4 days and preferably 2-4 weeks apart

Adults with lead nephropathy: An alternative dosing regimen reflecting the reduction in renal clearance is based upon the serum creatinine (see table):

Alternative Dosing Regimen for Adults With Lead Nephropathy

Serum Creatinine (mg/dL)	Ca EDTA dosage
≤2	1 g/m^2/day for 5 days
>2-3	500 mg/m^2/day for 5 days
>3-4	500 mg/m^2/dose every 48 hours for 3 doses
>4	500 mg/m^2/week

Repeat these regimens monthly until lead excretion is reduced toward normal.

Administration Parenteral:

Intermittent I.V. infusion: Administer the dose I.V. over at least 1 hour in asymptomatic patients, 2 hours in symptomatic patients

Single daily I.V. continuous infusion: Dilute to 2-4 mg/mL in D_5W or NS and infuse over at least 8 hours, usually over 12-24 hours

I.M. injection: To minimize pain at the injection site, 1.67 mL of 2% procaine may be added to 5 mL calcium EDTA, resulting in 150 mg/mL concentration with 0.5% procaine (stable 3 months; see Nahata, 1997)

Monitoring Parameters BUN, serum creatinine, urinalysis, fluid balance, EKG, blood and urine lead concentrations

Test Interactions If calcium EDTA is given as a continuous I.V. infusion, stop the infusion for at least 1 hour before blood is drawn for lead concentration to avoid a falsely elevated value

Dosage Forms Excipient information presented when available (limited, particularly for generics); consult specific product labeling.

Injection, solution: 200 mg/mL (5 mL)

References

American Academy of Pediatrics Committee on Drugs, "Treatment Guidelines for Lead Exposure in Children," *Pediatrics*, 1995, 96(1 Pt 1):155-60.

Nahata MC and Hipple TF, *Pediatric Drug Formulations*, 3rd ed, Cincinnati, OH: Harvey Whitney Books Co, 1997.

Edetate Disodium (ED e tate dye SOW dee um)

Medication Safety Issues

Sound-alike look-alike issues:

Edetate disodium (Na_2EDTA) may be confused with edetate calcium disodium (CaEDTA). CDC recommends that edetate disodium should **never** be used for chelation therapy in children. Fatal hypocalcemia may result if edetate disodium is used for chelation therapy instead of edetate calcium disodium.

U.S. Brand Names Endrate®

Index Terms Edathamil Disodium; EDTA (Disodium); Na2EDTA; Sodium Edetate

Therapeutic Category Antidote, Hypercalcemia; Chelating Agent, Parenteral

Generic Available Yes

Use Emergency treatment of hypercalcemia; control digitalis-induced cardiac dysrhythmias (ventricular arrhythmias)

Pregnancy Risk Factor C

Contraindications Hypersensitivity to edetate disodium or any component; severe renal failure or anuria, hypocalcemia, patients with active tuberculosis or healed calcified tubercular lesions

Warnings **Not for use for chelation treatment;** severe cases of hypocalcemia have been reported. Use of this drug is recommended only when the severity of the clinical condition justifies the aggressive measures associated with this type of therapy. Use with caution in patients with intracranial lesions, seizure disorders, coronary or peripheral vascular disease; cardiac function should be evaluated prior to therapy

Precautions Sudden, precipitous decreases of serum calcium may occur, a source of I.V. calcium replacement should be readily available; blood sugar and insulin requirements may be lower when used in insulin-dependent diabetics

Adverse Reactions

Cardiovascular: Arrhythmias, hypotension

Central nervous system: Seizures, headache, chills, fever

Dermatologic: Skin eruptions

(Continued)

Edetate Disodium *(Continued)*

Endocrine & metabolic: Hypomagnesemia, hypokalemia, hypocalcemia, hyperuricemia
Gastrointestinal: Vomiting, diarrhea, abdominal cramps
Genitourinary: Urinary urgency, dysuria
Hematologic: Anemia
Local: Thrombophlebitis, pain at injection site
Neuromuscular & skeletal: Back pain, muscle cramps, paresthesia, tetany
Renal: Nephrotoxicity, acute tubular necrosis, polyuria, oliguria, glucosuria
Respiratory: Respiratory arrest

Drug Interactions May reduce insulin requirements in diabetic patients treated with insulin

Stability Physically compatible with dextrose and saline I.V. solutions

Mechanism of Action Chelates with divalent or trivalent metals to form a soluble complex that is then eliminated in urine

Pharmacokinetics
Metabolism: Not metabolized
Half-life: 20-60 minutes
Elimination: Following chelation, 95% excreted in urine as chelates within 24-48 hours

Usual Dosage I.V.:
Hypercalcemia:
Children: 40-70 mg/kg/day slow infusion over 3-4 hours or more to a maximum of 3 g/24 hours; administer for 5 days and allow 5 days between courses of therapy **or** 50 mg/kg **or** 1.5 g/m^2 as a single dose
Adults: 50 mg/kg/day over 3 or more hours to a maximum of 3 g/24 hours; administer for 5 days followed by 2 days without drug and repeat course up to 15 total doses
Digitalis-induced arrhythmias: Children and Adults: 15 mg/kg/hour (maximum dose: 60 mg/kg/day) as continuous infusion

Administration Parenteral: I.V.: Must be diluted before I.V. use in D_5W or NS to a maximum concentration of 30 mg/mL (3%) and infused over at least 3 hours; avoid extravasation; **not for I.M. use**

Monitoring Parameters Serum and urine electrolytes (including calcium and magnesium), blood pressure (during infusion), renal function (before and during therapy), liver function, EKG

Test Interactions Colorimetric, oxalate, or other precipitation methods for measuring serum calcium

Nursing Implications Patient should remain supine for a short period after infusion

Additional Information Sodium content of 1 g: 5.4 mEq

Dosage Forms Excipient information presented when available (limited, particularly for generics); consult specific product labeling.
Injection, solution: 150 mg/mL (20 mL)

♦ **Edex**® *see* Alprostadil *on page 81*

Edrophonium (ed roe FOE nee um)

Related Information
Commonly Used Antidotes for Acute Overdoses *on page 1920*
Overdose and Toxicology *on page 1916*

U.S. Brand Names Enlon®; Reversol®

Canadian Brand Names Enlon®; Tensilon®

Index Terms Edrophonium Chloride

Therapeutic Category Antidote, Neuromuscular Blocking Agent; Cholinergic Agent; Diagnostic Agent, Myasthenia Gravis

Generic Available No

Use Diagnosis of myasthenia gravis; differentiation of cholinergic crises from myasthenia crises; reversal of nondepolarizing neuromuscular blockers; treatment of paroxysmal atrial tachycardia

Pregnancy Risk Factor C

Lactation Excretion in breast milk unknown

Contraindications Hypersensitivity to edrophonium or any component; GI or GU mechanical obstruction

Warnings Overdosage can cause cholinergic crisis which may be fatal; I.V. atropine should be readily available for treatment of cholinergic reactions; injection contains sulfites which may cause allergic reactions in susceptible individuals

Precautions Use with caution in asthmatic patients, patients with cardiac dysrhythmias, and those receiving a cardiac glycoside

Adverse Reactions

Cardiovascular: Arrhythmias (especially bradycardia), hypotension, A-V block
Central nervous system: Seizures, drowsiness, headache, dysphoria
Gastrointestinal: Nausea, vomiting, diarrhea, excessive salivation, stomach cramps
Genitourinary: Urinary frequency
Local: Thrombophlebitis
Neuromuscular & skeletal: Weakness, muscle cramps, muscle spasms
Ocular: Diplopia, miosis, lacrimation, conjunctival hyperemia
Respiratory: Laryngospasm, bronchospasm, respiratory paralysis, increased bronchial secretions
Miscellaneous: Diaphoresis, hypersensitivity reactions

Drug Interactions Digoxin may enhance bradycardia potential of edrophonium; succinylcholine and decamethonium effects are prolonged by edrophonium; quinidine may antagonize effects of edrophonium; antagonizes effects of nondepolarizing muscle relaxants (eg, pancuronium, vecuronium)

Mechanism of Action Inhibits destruction of acetylcholine by acetylcholinesterase. This facilitates transmission of impulses across myoneural junction and results in increased cholinergic responses such as miosis, increased tonus of intestinal and skeletal muscles, bronchial and ureteral constriction, bradycardia, and increased salivary and sweat gland secretions

Pharmacodynamics

Onset of action:
- I.M.: 2-10 minutes
- I.V.: 30-60 seconds

Duration:
- I.M.: 5-30 minutes
- I.V.: 5-10 minutes

Pharmacokinetics

Distribution: V_d:
- Infants: 1.18 ± 0.2 L/kg
- Children: 1.22 ± 0.74 L/kg
- Adults: 0.9 ± 0.13 L/kg

Half-life:
- Infants: 73 ± 30 minutes
- Children: 99 ± 31 minutes
- Adults: 126 ± 59 minutes

Elimination: Clearance:
- Infants: 17.8 mL/kg/minute
- Children: 14.2 mL/kg/minute
- Adults: 8.3 ± 2.9 mL/kg/minute

Usual Dosage Usually administered I.V., however, if not possible, I.M. or SubQ may be used

Infants: Diagnosis of myasthenia gravis: Initial:
- I.M., SubQ: 0.5-1 mg
- I.V.: Initial: 0.1 mg, followed by 0.4 mg (if no response); total dose = 0.5 mg

Children:
- Diagnosis of myasthenia gravis: Initial:
  - I.M., SubQ: ≤34 kg: 2 mg; >34 kg: 5 mg
  - I.V.: 0.04 mg/kg given over 1 minute followed by 0.16 mg/kg given within 45 seconds (if no response) (maximum dose: 10 mg total)

    or

    Alternative (manufacturer's recommendations):
    - ≤34 kg: 1 mg; if no response after 45 seconds, it may be repeated in 1 mg increments every 30-45 seconds to a total of 5 mg
    - >34 kg: 2 mg; if no response after 45 seconds, it may be repeated in 1 mg increments every 30-45 seconds to a total of 10 mg
- Titration of oral anticholinesterase therapy: I.V.: 0.04 mg/kg once given 1 hour after oral intake of the drug being used in treatment; if strength improves, an increase in neostigmine or pyridostigmine dose is indicated

Adults:
- Diagnosis of myasthenia gravis: Initial:
  - I.M., SubQ: Initial: 10 mg; if no cholinergic reaction occurs, administer 2 mg 30 minutes later to rule out false-negative reaction
  - I.V.: 2 mg test dose administered over 15-30 seconds; 8 mg given 45 seconds later (if no response is seen); test dose may be repeated after 30 minutes.
- Titration of oral anticholinesterase therapy: I.V.: 1-2 mg given 1 hour after oral dose of anticholinesterase; if strength improves, an increase in neostigmine or pyridostigmine dose is indicated

(Continued)

Edrophonium *(Continued)*

Differentiation of cholinergic from myasthenic crisis: I.V.: 1 mg, may repeat after 1 minute (**Note:** Intubation and controlled ventilation may be required if patient has cholinergic crises.)

Reversal of nondepolarizing neuromuscular blocking agents (neostigmine with atropine usually preferred): I.V.: 10 mg over 30-45 seconds, may repeat every 5-10 minutes up to 40 mg total dose

Termination of paroxysmal atrial tachycardia: I.V.: 5-10 mg

Dosing adjustment in renal impairment: Dose may need to be reduced in patients with chronic renal failure

Administration Parenteral: Edrophonium is administered by direct I.V. or I.M. injection; see Usual Dosage

Monitoring Parameters Pre- and postinjection strength (cranial musculature is most useful); heart rate, respiratory rate, blood pressure, changes in fasciculations

Dosage Forms Excipient information presented when available (limited, particularly for generics); consult specific product labeling.

Injection, solution, as chloride:

Enlon®: 10 mg/mL (15 mL) [contains sodium sulfite]

Reversol®: 10 mg/mL (10 mL) [contains sodium sulfite]

- ♦ **Edrophonium Chloride** *see* Edrophonium *on page 556*
- ♦ **EDTA (Calcium Disodium)** *see* Edetate Calcium Disodium *on page 553*
- ♦ **EDTA (Disodium)** *see* Edetate Disodium *on page 555*
- ♦ **E.E.S.®** *see* Erythromycin *on page 595*
- ♦ **EES® (Can)** *see* Erythromycin *on page 595*

Efavirenz (eh FAH vih rehnz)

Related Information

Adult and Adolescent HIV *on page 1821*

Pediatric HIV *on page 1816*

Perinatal HIV *on page 1831*

U.S. Brand Names Sustiva®

Canadian Brand Names Sustiva®

Therapeutic Category Antiretroviral Agent; HIV Agents (Anti-HIV Agents); Non-nucleoside Reverse Transcriptase Inhibitor (NNRTI)

Generic Available No

Use Treatment of HIV-1 infection in combination with other antiretroviral agents. (**Note:** HIV regimens consisting of **three** antiretroviral agents are strongly recommended)

Pregnancy Risk Factor D

Lactation Excretion is breast milk unknown/contraindicated

Contraindications Hypersensitivity to efavirenz or any component; concurrent therapy with astemizole, bepridil, cisapride, midazolam, pimozide, triazolam, ergot derivatives, or standard doses of voriconazole (**Note:** Adjusted doses of efavirenz and voriconazole may be administered concurrently; see Usual Dosage)

Warnings Efavirenz is a mixed inducer/inhibitor of CYP450 enzymes and numerous drug interactions occur. Due to potential serious and/or life-threatening drug interactions, certain drugs are contraindicated (see Contraindications and Drug Interactions). Resistance emerges rapidly if administered as monotherapy; always use efavirenz in combination with at least two other antiretroviral agents; do not add efavirenz as a single agent to antiretroviral regimens that are failing; initiate in combination with at least one other antiretroviral agent to which the patient is naive. Immune reconstitution syndrome (an acute inflammatory response to residual or indolent opportunistic infections) may occur in HIV patients during initial treatment with combination antiretroviral agents, including efavirenz; this syndrome may require further patient assessment and therapy.

Teratogenic effects have been observed in primates receiving efavirenz; human birth defects following efavirenz exposure in the first trimester have been reported, including cases of neural tube defects (including meningomyelocele and Dandy-Walker malformation); women receiving efavirenz should avoid pregnancy; women of childbearing potential should be tested for pregnancy before starting efavirenz; barrier contraception in combination with other (hormonal) methods of contraception should be used; women who use this drug during the first trimester or who become pregnant while taking this drug should be apprised of the potential harm to the fetus

Precautions Use with caution in patients with a history of mental illness or substance abuse (delusions, inappropriate behavior, and severe acute depression may occur). Serious CNS and psychiatric symptoms may occur (see Adverse Effects). Use with caution in patients with a history of seizures (convulsions may occur). Efavirenz may decrease the serum concentrations of antiepileptic agents that are metabolized by the liver (monitor anticonvulsant levels periodically; see Drug Interactions). Discontinue efavirenz if severe rash (involving blistering, desquamation, mucosal involvement, or fever) occurs; rash is more common and more severe in children versus adults, **consider prophylaxis with antihistamines in children**. Use with caution in patients with known or suspected hepatitis B or C, those receiving other hepatotoxic medications, and those with hepatic impairment; weigh risk versus benefit in patients with persistent elevations of serum transaminases (ie, >5 times normal). Cross resistance with other non-nucleoside reverse transcriptase inhibitors may occur. Elevations of serum cholesterol and triglycerides may occur (monitor during therapy). Fat redistribution and accumulation [ie, central obesity, peripheral wasting, facial wasting, breast enlargement, dorsocervical fat enlargement (buffalo hump), and cushingoid appearance] have been observed in patients receiving antiretroviral agents (causal relationship not established).

Adverse Reactions

Central nervous system: (**Note:** Overall incidence of CNS adverse effects was 53% versus 25% in controls; nervous system symptoms in children have been reported to be 18%) somnolence, dizziness, drowsiness, abnormal dreams, insomnia, confusion, headache (children 11%), hypoesthesia, impaired concentration, abnormal thinking, agitation, amnesia, depersonalization, euphoria, hallucinations, delusions, inappropriate behavior; fever (children 21%); anxiety, nervousness; serious psychiatric adverse effects (patients with history of psychiatric disorders may be at greater risk): Suicidal ideation/attempts, severe acute depression, aggressive behavior, paranoid reactions, manic reactions; convulsions (rare)

Dermatologic: Rash, usually pruritic maculopapular skin eruptions (incidence: children 46%, adults 26%, median onset, adults: 11 days, children: 8 days [range 6-205 days], **Note:** Most rashes in children appeared within 14 days after starting therapy; median duration, adults: 16 days, children: 6 days [range 2-37 days], **Note:** Median duration of rash in children who continued therapy was 9 days; rash may be treated with antihistamines and corticosteroids and usually resolves within one month while continuing therapy; **Note:** Blistering, desquamation, fever, mucosal involvement, or ulceration may occur and requires discontinuation of drug, see Precautions); pruritus, increased sweating

Endocrine & metabolic: Hypercholesterolemia, hypertriglyceridemia, fat redistribution and accumulation (see Precautions)

Gastrointestinal: Nausea or vomiting (children 12%), diarrhea/loose stools (children 39%), abdominal pain, asymptomatic elevations in serum amylase, pancreatitis

Hepatic: Elevated liver enzymes (patients with hepatitis B or C may be at greater risk)

Respiratory: Cough (children 16%)

Miscellaneous: Alcohol intolerance, immune reconstitution syndrome (see Warnings)

Drug Interactions Cytochrome P450 isoenzyme CYP3A4 and CYP2B6 substrate; mixed inducer/inhibitor of CYP450 enzymes: Induces CYP3A4 and inhibits isoenzymes CYP2C9, 2C19, and 3A4

Concurrent use of efavirenz with astemizole, bepridil, cisapride, midazolam, pimozide, triazolam, or ergot derivatives is contraindicated (efavirenz may inhibit the metabolism of these drugs and result in serious or life-threatening effects). Efavirenz significantly decreases serum concentrations of voriconazole and voriconazole increases efavirenz concentrations (concurrent use of standard doses of voriconazole is contraindicated; adjusted doses of both drugs may be administered concurrently; see Usual Dosage).

Efavirenz may significantly decrease serum concentrations of atazanavir (atazanavir dosage adjustment with a ritonavir booster dose is recommended), indinavir (optimal concurrent indinavir dosage is not known), saquinavir (use of saquinavir as sole protease inhibitor with efavirenz is not recommended), lopinavir (an increased dose of lopinavir/ritonavir is recommended), amprenavir (including patients receiving fosamprenavir), clarithromycin, sertraline (monitor clinical response; increased sertraline doses may be needed), rifabutin (a 50% increase in the daily dose of rifabutin is recommended; a doubling of rifabutin dosage in rifabutin twice weekly or 3 times weekly regimens should be considered), and methadone (monitor patients for withdrawal, increase methadone dose as required). Efavirenz may potentially decrease serum concentrations of phenobarbital, phenytoin, or carbamazepine (optimal concurrent carbamazepine dosage is unknown; avoid concurrent carbamazepine; monitor anticonvulsant levels), antifungals such as itraconazole or ketoconazole (optimal concurrent dosage of these agents is unknown; consider alternative antifungal agents), diltiazem and other calcium channel blockers (monitor patients; dosage adjustment of calcium channel blocker may be needed), and HMG-CoA reductase inhibitors, such as atorvastatin, pravastatin, and simvastatin (monitor patients; dosage adjustment of HMG-CoA reductase inhibitor may be needed). Efavirenz increases serum concentrations of nelfinavir, ritonavir, lorazepam, ethinyl

(Continued)

Efavirenz *(Continued)*

estradiol, and 14-hydroxy metabolite of clarithromycin. Efavirenz may increase or decrease the effects of warfarin.

Saquinavir, rifampin, phenobarbital, phenytoin, carbamazepine, and other enzyme inducing agents may decrease efavirenz serum concentrations (avoid carbamazepine; monitor anticonvulsant and efavirenz serum concentrations); optimal dosage of efavirenz with rifampin has not been established; consider efavirenz dosage increase to 800 mg once daily in adults receiving rifampin and efavirenz. The herbal medicine St John's wort (*Hypericum perforatum*) may significantly decrease concentrations of efavirenz and is **not** recommended for concurrent use. Ritonavir may increase efavirenz AUC by 20%. Fluconazole may increase efavirenz AUC by 16% (but no dosage adjustment is recommended). Alcohol or other CNS depressants may increase adverse effects. Rash may be more common when efavirenz is used with clarithromycin (consider azithromycin use). Interaction with oral contraceptives is not fully characterized (use reliable barrier method).

Food Interactions

Capsules: Compared to fasting conditions, high fat/high caloric meals increase efavirenz AUC by 22% and peak concentrations by 39%; reduced fat/normal caloric meals increase efavirenz AUC by 17% and peak concentrations by 51%

Tablets: Compared to fasting conditions, high fat/high caloric meals increase efavirenz AUC by 28% and peak concentrations by 79%

Stability Store at room temperature

Mechanism of Action A non-nucleoside reverse transcriptase inhibitor which specifically binds to HIV-1 reverse transcriptase and blocks RNA-dependent and DNA-dependent DNA polymerase activity including HIV-1 replication; does not require intracellular phosphorylation for antiviral activity

Pharmacokinetics Note: Pharmacokinetics in children ≥3 years of age are thought to be similar to adults

Distribution: CSF concentrations are 0.69% of plasma (range 0.26% to 1.2%); however, CSF:plasma concentration ratio is 3 times higher than free fraction in plasma

Protein binding: 99.5% to 99.8%, primarily to albumin

Metabolism: In the liver, primarily by cytochrome P450 enzymes (mainly isoenzymes CYP3A4 and CYP2B6) to hydroxylated metabolites which then undergo glucuronidation; induces P450 enzymes and it's own metabolism

Bioavailability: 42% (increased with fatty meal)

Half-life: Adults:
- Single dose: 52-76 hours
- Multiple dose: 40-55 hours

Time to peak serum concentration: 3-5 hours

Elimination: <1% excreted unchanged in the urine; 14% to 34% excreted as metabolites in the urine and 16% to 61% in feces (primarily as unchanged drug)

Usual Dosage Oral: (use in combination with other antiretroviral agents)

Neonates, Infants, and Children <3 years: Not approved for use (no information available)

Children ≥3 years: Dose according to body weight:
- 10 kg to <15 kg: 200 mg once daily
- 15 kg to <20 kg: 250 mg once daily
- 20 kg to <25 kg: 300 mg once daily
- 25 kg to <32.5 kg: 350 mg once daily
- 32.5 kg to <40 kg: 400 mg once daily
- ≥40 kg: 600 mg once daily

Adults: 600 mg once daily

Dosage adjustment for concomitant voriconazole: Adults: Reduce efavirenz dose to 300 mg once daily (use capsule formulation) and increase voriconazole dose to 400 mg every 12 hours

Administration Administer dose at bedtime to decrease CNS adverse effects; administer with water on an empty stomach (administration with food may increase efavirenz concentrations and adverse effects; see Food Interactions). Capsules may be opened and added to small amount of food or liquid, but efavirenz tastes peppery (grape jelly may be used to improve taste). Tablets should not be broken.

Monitoring Parameters Signs and symptoms of rash; viral load; CD4 counts; serum amylase; liver enzymes in patients with known or suspected hepatitis B or C, those receiving concomitant ritonavir, and those receiving other hepatotoxic medications; serum cholesterol, triglycerides

Test Interactions False positive test for cannabinoids using the CEDIA DAU Multi-level THC assay

Patient Information May cause drowsiness and impair ability to perform activities requiring mental alertness or physical coordination; avoid alcohol; efavirenz is not a cure for HIV; notify physician immediately if rash develops; some medicines should not be taken with efavirenz; report the use of other medications, nonprescription medications and herbal or natural products to your physician and pharmacist; avoid the herbal medicine St John's wort; inform your physician if you have ever had seizures or if you now take seizure medications (blood samples to check the level of seizure medications may be needed more frequently when taking efavirenz); take efavirenz everyday as prescribed; do not change dose or discontinue without physician's advice; if a dose is missed, take it as soon as possible, then return to normal dosing schedule; if a dose is skipped, do **not** double the next dose

HIV medications may cause changes in body fat, including an increase in fat in the upper back and neck, breasts, and trunk; a loss of fat from the face, arms, and legs may also occur. Due to possible teratogenic effects, female patients of childbearing potential should be tested for pregnancy prior to starting efavirenz and should avoid pregnancy while receiving this drug; barrier contraception with other (hormonal) methods of contraception should be used (see Precautions).

Additional Information An oral liquid formulation of efavirenz (strawberry/mint-flavored solution) is available on an investigational basis from Bristol-Myers Squibb Company as part of an expanded access program for HIV-infected children and adolescents 3-16 years of age; for further details call 877-372-7097. **Note:** The bioavailability of the investigational liquid was found to be 20% lower than that of the capsules in adult volunteers; a recent pediatric study used initial doses of the liquid formulation that were 20% higher than pediatric capsule doses; these higher doses resulted in AUC values that were similar to AUCs achieved with the capsules (See Starr, 2002).

Early virologic failure and rapid emergence of resistant mutations have been observed in therapy-naive adult HIV patients treated with tenofovir, didanosine enteric-coated beadlets (Videx® EC), and either efavirenz or nevirapine; the combination of tenofovir, didanosine, and any non-nucleoside reverse transcriptase inhibitor is **not** recommended as initial antiretroviral therapy.

Dosage Forms Excipient information presented when available (limited, particularly for generics); consult specific product labeling.

Capsule:
  Sustiva®: 50 mg, 100 mg, 200 mg

Tablet:
  Sustiva®: 600 mg

References

Adkins JC and Noble S, "Efavirenz," *Drugs*, 1998, 56(6):1055-64.

Briars LA, Hilao JJ, and Kraus DM, "A Review of Pediatric Human Immunodeficiency Virus Infection," *Journal of Pharmacy Practice*, 2004, 17(6):407-31.

Collura JM and Kraus DM, "New Pediatric Antiretroviral Agents," *J Pediatr Health Care*, 2000, 14(4):183-90.

Maddocks S and Dwyer D, "The Role of Non-Nucleoside Reverse Transcriptase Inhibitors in Children With HIV-1 Infection," *Paediatr Drugs*, 2001, 3(9):681-702.

Panel on Clinical Practices for Treatment of HIV Infection, "Guidelines for the Use of Antiretroviral Agents in HIV-Infected Adults and Adolescents," October 10, 2006, http://www.aidsinfo.nih.gov.

Piscitelli SC, Burstein AH, Chaitt D, et al, "Indinavir Concentrations and St John's Wort," *Lancet*, 2000, 355(9203):547-8.

Starr SE, Fletcher CV, Spector SA, et al, "Combination Therapy With Efavirenz, Nelfinavir, and Nucleoside Reverse-transcriptase Inhibitors in Children Infected with Human Immunodeficiency Virus Type 1. Pediatric AIDS Clinical Trials Group 382 Team," *N Engl J Med* 1999, 341(25):1874-81.

Starr SE, Fletcher CV, Spector SA, et al, "Efavirenz Liquid Formulation in Human Immunodeficiency Virus-Infected Children," *Pediatr Infect Dis J*, 2002, 21(7):659-63.

Working Group on Antiretroviral Therapy and Medical Management of HIV-Infected Children, "Guidelines for the Use of Antiretroviral Agents in Pediatric HIV Infection," October 26, 2006, http://www.aidsinfo.nih.gov.

Working Group on Antiretroviral Therapy and Medical Management of HIV-Infected Children, "Guidelines for the Use of Antiretroviral Agents in Pediatric HIV Infection. Supplement I: Pediatric Antiretroviral Drug Information," October 26, 2006, http://www.aidsinfo.nih.gov.

- ♦ **Effer-K™** *see* Potassium Bicarbonate and Potassium Citrate *on page 1286*
- ♦ **Effexor®** *see* Venlafaxine *on page 1606*
- ♦ **Effexor® XR** *see* Venlafaxine *on page 1606*
- ♦ **Efudex®** *see* Fluorouracil *on page 678*
- ♦ **E-Gems® [OTC]** *see* Vitamin E *on page 1620*
- ♦ **E-Gems Elite® [OTC]** *see* Vitamin E *on page 1620*
- ♦ **E-Gems Plus® [OTC]** *see* Vitamin E *on page 1620*
- ♦ **EHDP** *see* Etidronate Disodium *on page 622*
- ♦ **Elavil** *see* Amitriptyline *on page 107*
- ♦ **Electrolyte Lavage Solution** *see* Polyethylene Glycol-Electrolyte Solution *on page 1277*
- ♦ **Elestat™** *see* Epinastine *on page 577*
- ♦ **Elestrin™** *see* Estradiol *on page 605*
- ♦ **Elidel®** *see* Pimecrolimus *on page 1262*
- ♦ **Eligard®** *see* Leuprolide *on page 918*

- **Elimite®** *see* Permethrin *on page 1243*
- **Elitek™** *see* Rasburicase *on page 1369*
- **Elixophyllin®** *see* Theophylline *on page 1520*
- **ElixSure® Cough [OTC]** *see* Dextromethorphan *on page 477*
- **ElixSure™ IB [OTC]** *see* Ibuprofen *on page 802*
- **Elocom® (Can)** *see* Mometasone Furoate *on page 1076*
- **Elocon®** *see* Mometasone Furoate *on page 1076*
- **Eloxatin®** *see* Oxaliplatin *on page 1179*
- **Elspar®** *see* Asparaginase *on page 161*
- **Eltor® (Can)** *see* Pseudoephedrine *on page 1344*
- **Eltroxin® (Can)** *see* Levothyroxine *on page 930*
- **Emend®** *see* Aprepitant *on page 153*
- **EMLA®** *see* Lidocaine and Prilocaine *on page 937*
- **Emo-Cort® (Can)** *see* Hydrocortisone *on page 781*

Emtricitabine (em trye SYE ta been)

Related Information

Adult and Adolescent HIV *on page 1821*
Pediatric HIV *on page 1816*
Perinatal HIV *on page 1831*

U.S. Brand Names Emtriva®

Canadian Brand Names Emtriva®

Index Terms BW524W91; Coviracil; FTC

Therapeutic Category Antiretroviral Agent; HIV Agents (Anti-HIV Agents); Nucleoside Reverse Transcriptase Inhibitor (NRTI)

Generic Available No

Use Treatment of HIV infection in combination with other antiretroviral agents. (**Note:** HIV regimens consisting of **three** antiretroviral agents are strongly recommended); has been used investigationally for the treatment of chronic hepatitis B infection in adults

Pregnancy Risk Factor B

Lactation Excretion in breast milk unknown/contraindicated

Contraindications Hypersensitivity to emtricitabine or any component

Warnings Cases of lactic acidosis, severe hepatomegaly with steatosis, and death have been reported in patients receiving nucleoside analogues; most of these cases have been in women; prolonged nucleoside use, obesity, and prior liver disease may be risk factors; use with extreme caution in patients with other risk factors for liver disease; discontinue therapy in patients who develop laboratory or clinical evidence of lactic acidosis or pronounced hepatotoxicity. Testing for hepatitis B is recommended prior to the initiation of emtricitabine therapy; HIV-infected patients who are coinfected with hepatitis B may experience severe acute exacerbations of hepatitis (ie, clinical symptoms or laboratory evidence of hepatitis) when emtricitabine is discontinued; monitor patients closely for at least several months after discontinuation of emtricitabine; initiate anti-hepatitis B therapy if needed

Precautions Use with caution and reduce dosage in patients with impaired renal function. Fat redistribution and accumulation [ie, central obesity, peripheral wasting, facial wasting, breast enlargement, dorsocervical fat enlargement (buffalo hump), and cushingoid appearance] have been observed in patients receiving antiretroviral agents (causal relationship not established). Immune reconstitution syndrome (an acute inflammatory response to residual or indolent opportunistic infection) may occur in HIV patients during initial treatment with combination antiretroviral agents, including emtricitabine; this syndrome may require further patient assessment and therapy. Hyperpigmentation may occur at a higher frequency in pediatric patients compared to adults (see Adverse Reactions). Do not administer with other emtricitabine or lamivudine-containing products (see Drug Interactions). Safety and efficacy have not been established in infants ≤3 months of age; recommended dosing is based on pharmacokinetic studies.

Adverse Reactions

Central nervous system: Headache, dizziness, insomnia, abnormal dreams, depression, fever

Dermatologic: Rash, pruritus, maculopapular rash, vesiculobullous rash, pustular rash; hyperpigmentation [incidence: Children: 32%; adults: 2% to 6% (may be higher in African Americans); hyperpigmentation occurs primarily of palms and/or soles but may include tongue, arms, lips, and nails; generally mild, asymptomatic, nonprogressive, and without associated local reactions such as pruritus or rash]

Endocrine & metabolic: Elevated serum triglycerides, lactic acidosis, hyperglycemia; fat redistribution and accumulation (see Precautions)

Gastrointestinal: Diarrhea, nausea, abdominal pain, dyspepsia, vomiting, gastroenteritis
Hematologic: Neutropenia, anemia
Hepatic: Elevated ALT, AST, CPK, bilirubin, lipase, and amylase; hepatic steatosis, severe hepatomegaly
Neuromuscular & skeletal: Paresthesias, peripheral neuropathy, asthenia, myalgia, arthralgia, elevated CPK
Respiratory: Cough, rhinitis
Miscellaneous: Hypersensitivity reaction, immune reconstitution syndrome

Drug Interactions Not a substrate or inhibitor of cytochrome P450 enzymes

Note: Limited drug interaction data available. No evidence of a clinically significant interaction when administered with tenofovir, indinavir, famciclovir, stavudine, or zidovudine.

Emtricitabine should **not** be used in combination with lamivudine (no potential additive benefit; similar resistance profiles). Concomitant use of ribavirin and nucleoside analogues may increase the risk of developing lactic acidosis. Drugs that decrease renal function or compete for renal elimination may decrease renal clearance of emtricitabine. Drugs with hematologic adverse effects (eg, ganciclovir, valganciclovir) may enhance hematologic toxicities of emtricitabine (avoid concurrent use).

Food Interactions

Capsules: A high fat meal decreases peak plasma concentrations, but not the extent of absorption (AUC not affected)
Oral solution: Neither a high-fat nor a low-fat meal affected peak plasma concentrations or AUC

Stability

Capsules: Store at 25°C (77°F); excursions permitted to 15°C to 30°C (59°F to 86°F).
Oral solution: Store refrigerated at 2°C to 8°C (36°F to 46°F); use within 3 months if stored at room temperature [25°C (77°F)]

Mechanism of Action A synthetic nucleoside analogue that is phosphorylated by intracellular kinases to the active triphosphate metabolite (emtricitabine 5'-triphosphate) which inhibits HIV-1 reverse transcription via viral DNA chain termination after incorporation of the nucleoside analogue. Emtricitabine triphosphate is a weak inhibitor of mammalian DNA polymerase alpha-, beta-, epsilon- and mitochondrial DNA polymerase gamma.

Pharmacokinetics

Absorption: Rapid, extensive
Distribution: Unknown if distributes into breast milk
Protein binding: <4%
Metabolism: Converted intracellularly to the active triphosphate form; undergoes minimal biotransformation via oxidation and glucuronide conjugation
Bioavailability:
- Capsules: 93%
- Oral solution: 75%
- **Note:** Relative bioavailability of solution to capsule: 80%

Half-life: Normal renal function:
- Children and Adolescents: Elimination half-life (emtricitabine):
  - Single dose: 11 hours
  - Multiple dose: 7.9"9.5 hours
  - Infants 0-3 months (n=20; median age: 26 days): 12.1 ± 3.1 hours
  - Infants 3-24 months (n=14): 8.9 ± 3.2 hours
  - Children 25 months to 6 years (n=19): 11.3 ± 6.4 hours
  - Children 7-12 years (n=17): 8.2 ± 3.2 hours
  - Adolescents 13-17 years (n=27): 8.9 ± 3.3 hours
- Adults:
  - Elimination half-life (emtricitabine): 10 hours
  - Intracellular half-life (emtricitabine 5'-triphosphate): 39 hours

Time to peak serum concentration: 1-2 hours
Elimination: Urine (86% of dose, primarily as unchanged drug; 13% as metabolites; 9% of dose as oxidative metabolite; 4% as glucuronide metabolite); feces (14% of dose)
- Clearance: Renal clearance is > creatinine clearance; thus, emtricitabine may be eliminated by both glomerular filtration and active tubular secretion

Dialysis: 30% of the dose is removed by hemodialysis (over 3 hours)

Usual Dosage Oral (use in combination with other antiretroviral agents):

Neonates and Infants 0-3 months: Oral solution: 3 mg/kg once daily
Infants ≥3 months, Children, and Adolescents <18 years: Oral solution: 6 mg/kg once daily (maximum dose: 240 mg once daily)
- Children >33 kg who can swallow capsule intact: Capsule: 200 mg once daily

Adolescents ≥18 years and Adults:
Capsules: 200 mg once daily
(Continued)

Emtricitabine *(Continued)*

Oral solution: 240 mg once daily

Dosage adjustment in renal impairment: Monitor clinical response and renal function closely:

Neonates, Infants, Children, and Adolescents <18 years: Specific dose adjustment not yet established; consider a reduction in the dose and/or an increase in the dosing interval similar to dosage adjustments for adults

Adolescents ≥18 years and Adults:

Cl_{cr} 30-49 mL/minute: Capsule: 200 mg every 48 hours; oral solution: 120 mg every 24 hours

Cl_{cr} 15-29 mL/minute: Capsule: 200 mg every 72 hours; oral solution: 80 mg every 24 hours

Cl_{cr} <15 mL/minute (including hemodialysis patients): **Note:** If dose is given on day of dialysis, administer dose after dialysis: Capsule: 200 mg every 96 hours; oral solution: 60 mg every 24 hours

Dosage adjustment in hepatic impairment: No adjustment required.

Administration May be administered without regard to food

Monitoring Parameters CBC with differential, ALT, AST, serum amylase, bilirubin; signs and symptoms of lactic acidosis, and pronounced hepatotoxicity; CD4 cell count, HIV RNA plasma levels; patients should be screened for hepatitis B infection before starting emtricitabine (see Warnings)

Patient Information Emtricitabine is not a cure for HIV. Notify physician if persistent severe abdominal pain, nausea, vomiting, rash, numbness, or tingling occur. May cause dizziness and impair ability to perform activities requiring mental alertness or physical coordination. Take emtricitabine every day as prescribed; do not change dose or discontinue without physician's advice; if a dose is missed, take it as soon as possible, then return to normal dosing schedule; if a dose is skipped, do **not** double the next dose.

HIV medications may cause changes in body fat, including an increase in fat in the upper back and neck, breasts, and trunk; a loss of fat from the face, arms, and legs may also occur. Some HIV medications (including emtricitabine) may cause a serious, but rare, condition called lactic acidosis with an increase in liver size (hepatomegaly). Before starting emtricitabine, inform your physician about your medical conditions, including any liver or kidney problems. Do not take Emtriva® with other emtricitabine-containing medications (eg, Atripla™ or Truvada®) or with medications that contain lamivudine (eg, Epivir®, Epivir-HBV®, Combivir®, Epzicom®, or Trizivir®.

Additional Information Emtricitabine is the (-) enantiomer of 2', 3'-dideoxy-5-fluoro-3'-thiacytidine (FTC), a fluorinated derivative of lamivudine.

Mutation in the HIV reverse transcriptase gene at codon 184, M184V/I (ie, substitution of methionine by valine or isoleucine) is associated with resistance to emtricitabine. Emtricitabine-resistant isolates (M184V/I) are cross-resistant to lamivudine and zalcitabine. HIV-1 isolates containing the K65R mutation show reduced susceptibility to emtricitabine.

Dosage Forms Excipient information presented when available (limited, particularly for generics); consult specific product labeling.

Excipient information presented when available (limited, particularly for generics); consult specific product labeling.

Capsule:

Emtriva®: 200 mg

Solution:

Emtriva®: 10 mg/mL (170 mL) [cotton candy flavor]

References

Bang LM and Scott LJ, "Emtricitabine: An Antiretroviral Agent for HIV Infection," *Drugs*, 2003, 63(22):2413-24.

Briars LA, Hilao JJ, and Kraus DM, "A Review of Pediatric Human Immunodeficiency Virus Infection," *Journal of Pharmacy Practice*, 2004, 17(6):407-31.

Frampton JE and Perry CM, "Emtricitabine: A Review of Its Use in the Management of HIV Infection," *Drugs*, 2005, 65(10):1427-48.

Morris JL and Kraus DM, "New Antiretroviral Therapies for Pediatric HIV Infection," *J Pediatr Pharmacol Ther*, 2005, 10:215-47.

Panel on Clinical Practices for Treatment of HIV Infection, "Guidelines for the Use of Antiretroviral Agents in HIV-Infected Adults and Adolescents," October 10, 2006, http://www.aidsinfo.nih.gov.

Wang LH, Wiznia AA, Rathore MH, et al, "Pharmacokinetics and Safety of Single Oral Doses of Emtricitabine in Human Immunodeficiency Virus-Infected Children," *Antimicrob Agents Chemother*, 2004, 48(1):183-91.

Working Group on Antiretroviral Therapy and Medical Management of HIV-Infected Children, "Guidelines for the Use of Antiretroviral Agents in Pediatric HIV Infection," October 26, 2006, http://www.aidsinfo.nih.gov.

♦ **Emtriva®** *see* Emtricitabine *on page 562*

♦ **Enalaprilat** *see* Enalapril/Enalaprilat *on page 565*

Enalapril/Enalaprilat (e NAL a pril/e NAL a pril at)

Medication Safety Issues

Sound-alike/look-alike issues:

Enalapril may be confused with Anafranil®, Elavil®, Eldepryl®, nafarelin, ramipril

Significant differences exist between oral and I.V. dosing. Use caution when converting from one route of administration to another.

International issues:

Acepril® [Hungary, Switzerland] may be confused with Accupril® which is a brand name for quinapril in the U.S.

Acepril®: Brand name for lisinopril in Denmark; brand name for captopril in Great Britain

Nacor® [Spain] may be confused with Niacor® which is a brand name for niacin in the U.S.

Related Information

Antihypertensive Agents by Class *on page 1678*

U.S. Brand Names Vasotec®

Canadian Brand Names Vasotec®

Index Terms Enalaprilat; Enalapril Maleate

Therapeutic Category Angiotensin-Converting Enzyme (ACE) Inhibitor; Antihypertensive Agent

Generic Available Yes

Use Management of mild to severe hypertension, CHF, and asymptomatic left ventricular dysfunction; has also been used to treat proteinuria in steroid-resistant nephrotic syndrome patients (see Additional Information)

Pregnancy Risk Factor C (1st trimester); D (may cause injury and death to the developing fetus when used during the 2nd and 3rd trimesters of pregnancy)

Lactation Enters breast milk/not recommended (AAP rates "compatible")

Contraindications Hypersensitivity to enalapril, enalaprilat, any component (see Warnings), or other ACE inhibitors; patients with idiopathic or hereditary angioedema or a history of angioedema with ACE inhibitors

Warnings Serious adverse effects including angioedema, anaphylactoid reactions, neutropenia, agranulocytosis, hypotension, and hepatic failure may occur (see Adverse Reactions); risk of neutropenia may be increased in patients with renal dysfunction and especially in patients with both collagen vascular disease and renal dysfunction

Injectable product contains benzyl alcohol (9 mg/mL) which may cause allergic reactions in susceptible individuals; large amounts of benzyl alcohol (≥99 mg/kg/day) have been associated with a potentially fatal toxicity ("gasping syndrome") in neonates; the "gasping syndrome" consists of metabolic acidosis, respiratory distress, gasping respirations, CNS dysfunction (including convulsions, intracranial hemorrhage), hypotension and cardiovascular collapse; use enalaprilat products containing benzyl alcohol with caution in neonates; *in vitro* and animal studies have shown that benzoate, a metabolite of benzyl alcohol, displaces bilirubin from protein binding sites

Precautions Use with caution and modify dosage in patients with renal impairment, especially renal artery stenosis; elevated BUN and S_{cr} may occur in these patients; dosage reduction or discontinuation of enalapril or discontinuation of concomitant diuretic may be needed; use with caution and modify dosage in patients with hyponatremia, hypovolemia, severe CHF, left ventricular outflow tract obstruction, or with coadministered diuretic therapy; experience in children is limited; severe hypotension may occur in patients who are sodium and/or volume depleted, initiate lower doses and monitor closely when starting therapy in these patients

Adverse Reactions

Cardiovascular: Hypotension, syncope

Central nervous system: Fatigue, vertigo, insomnia, dizziness, headache

Dermatologic: Rash, angioedema. **Note:** The relative risk of angioedema with ACE inhibitors is higher within the first 30 days of use (compared to >1 year of use), for Black Americans (compared to Whites), for lisinopril or enalapril (compared to captopril), and for patients previously hospitalized within 30 days (Brown, 1996).

Endocrine & metabolic: Hypoglycemia, hyperkalemia

Gastrointestinal: Nausea, diarrhea, ageusia

Genitourinary: Impotence

Hematologic: Agranulocytosis, neutropenia, anemia

Hepatic: Cholestatic jaundice, fulminant hepatic necrosis (rare, but potentially fatal)

Neuromuscular & skeletal: Muscle cramps

Renal: Deterioration in renal function

(Continued)

Enalapril/Enalaprilat *(Continued)*

Respiratory: Cough, dyspnea, eosinophilic pneumonitis; **Note:** An isolated dry cough lasting >3 weeks was reported in 7 of 42 pediatric patients (17%) receiving ACE inhibitors (see von Vigier, 2000)

Drug Interactions Cytochrome P450 isoenzyme CYP3A3/4 substrate

Use with potassium-sparing diuretics may result in an additive hyperkalemic effect; diuretics or other antihypertensive agents may increase hypotensive effect; indomethacin or NSAIDs may decrease hypotensive effect; enalapril may increase lithium levels; use with NSAIDs in patients with compromised renal function may increase renal dysfunction (usually reversible)

Food Interactions Food does not affect absorption; limit salt substitutes or potassium-rich diet; avoid natural licorice (causes sodium and water retention and increases potassium loss)

Stability Store vials below 86°F (30°C); solutions for I.V. infusion mixed in NS, D_5W, D_5NS, or D_5LR are stable for 24 hours at room temperature

Mechanism of Action Competitive inhibitor of angiotensin-converting enzyme (ACE); prevents conversion of angiotensin I to angiotensin II, a potent vasoconstrictor; results in lower levels of angiotensin II which causes an increase in plasma renin activity and a reduction in aldosterone secretion

Pharmacodynamics (Antihypertensive effect)

Onset of action:
- Oral: Within 1 hour
- I.V.: Within 15 minutes

Maximum effect:
- Oral: Within 4-8 hours
- I.V.: Within 1-4 hour

Duration:
- Oral: 12-24 hours
- I.V.: Dose dependent, usually 4-6 hours

Pharmacokinetics

Absorption: Oral: 55% to 75% (enalapril)

Protein binding: 50% to 60%

Metabolism: Enalapril is a prodrug (inactive) and undergoes biotransformation to enalaprilat (active) in the liver

Half-life:
- Enalapril:
  - CHF neonates 10-19 days of age (n=3): 10.3 hours (range: 4.2-13.4 hours)
  - CHF: Infants >27 days and Children ≤6.5 years of age (n=11): 2.7 hours (range: 1.3-6.3 hours)
  - Healthy adults: 2 hours
  - CHF adults: 3.4-5.8 hours
- Enalaprilat:
  - CHF neonates 10-19 days of age (n=3): 11.9 hours (range 5.9-15.6 hours)
  - CHF: Infants >27 days and Children ≤6.5 years of age (n=11): 11.1 hours (range: 5.1-20.8 hours)
  - Infants 6 weeks to 8 months: 6-10 hours
  - Adults: 35-38 hours

Time to peak serum concentration: Oral:
- Enalapril: Within 0.5-1.5 hours
- Enalaprilat (active): Within 3-4.5 hours

Elimination: Principally in urine (60% to 80%) with some fecal excretion

Usual Dosage Use lower listed initial dose in patients with hyponatremia, hypovolemia, severe CHF, decreased renal function, or in those receiving diuretics

Manufacturer's recommendations: Pediatric hypertensive patients: Oral: **Enalapril:** Initial: 0.08 mg/kg once daily (maximum dose: 5 mg); adjust dose according to blood pressure readings; doses >0.58 mg/kg (or >40 mg) have not been studied

Alternative pediatric dosing:
- Neonates:
  - Oral: **Enalapril**: Initial: 0.1 mg/kg/day given every 24 hours; increase dose and interval as required every few days (see Additional Information)
  - I.V.: **Enalaprilat**: 5-10 mcg/kg/dose administered every 8-24 hours (as determined by blood pressure readings) has been used for the treatment of neonatal hypertension; monitor patients carefully; select patients may require higher doses
- Infants and Children:
  - Oral: **Enalapril**: Initial: 0.1 mg/kg/day in 1-2 divided doses; increase as required over 2 weeks to maximum of 0.5 mg/kg/day; mean dose required for CHF improvement in 39 children (9 days to 17 years of age) was 0.36 mg/kg/day;

investigationally, select individuals have been treated with doses up to 0.94 mg/kg/day (Leversha, 1994)

I.V.: **Enalaprilat**: 5-10 mcg/kg/dose administered every 8-24 hours (as determined by blood pressure readings); monitor patients carefully; select patients may require higher doses

Adolescents and Adults:

Oral: **Enalapril**: Initial: 2.5-5 mg/day then increase as required; usual dose for hypertension: 10-40 mg/day in 1-2 divided doses; usual dosage range for hypertension in Adolescents ≥18 years and Adults (JNC 7): 2.5-40 mg/day in 1-2 divided doses; usual dose for CHF: 5-20 mg/day in 2 divided doses; maximum dose: 40 mg/day

Asymptomatic left ventricular dysfunction: Initial: 2.5 mg twice daily; increase as tolerated; usual dose: 20 mg/day in 2 divided doses

I.V.: **Enalaprilat**: 0.625-1.25 mg/dose every 6 hours; doses as high as 5 mg/dose every 6 hours have been tolerated for up to 36 hours; little experience with doses >20 mg/day

Dosing adjustment in renal impairment: Note: Use in neonates and children ≤16 years of age with GFR <30 mL/min/1.73 m^2 is not recommended (no dosing data exists)

Cl_{cr} 10-50 mL/minute: Administer 75% to 100% of dose

Cl_{cr} <10 mL/minute: Administer 50% of dose

Administration

Oral: May administer without regard to food

Parenteral: I.V.: Administer as I.V. infusion (undiluted solution or further diluted) over 5 minutes; to deliver small I.V. doses, a dilution with NS to a final concentration of 25 mcg/mL can be made

Monitoring Parameters Blood pressure, renal function, WBC, serum potassium, serum glucose

Patient Information Limit alcohol; notify physician if vomiting, diarrhea, excessive perspiration, or dehydration occurs, or if swelling of face, lips, tongue, or difficulty in breathing occurs; do not use a salt substitute (potassium-containing) without physician advice

Nursing Implications Discontinue if angioedema occurs; observe closely for hypotension within 1-3 hours of first dose or with new higher dose

Additional Information Severe hypotension was reported in a **preterm** neonate (birth weight 835 g, gestational age 26 weeks, postnatal age 9 days) who was treated with enalapril 0.1 mg/kg orally; hypotension responded to I.V. plasma and dopamine; the authors suggest starting enalapril in preterm infants at 0.01 mg/kg and increasing upwards in a stepwise fashion with very close monitoring of blood pressure and urine output. However, in this case report, oral enalapril at doses of 0.01 mg/kg to 0.04 mg/kg did not adequately control blood pressure. Further studies are needed. (Schilder, 1995)

Over the years, several pediatric studies have examined the effects of ACE inhibitors on proteinuria. In a more recent retrospective study, enalapril (in doses of 2.5-5 mg/day) administered either as monotherapy (n=17; mean age: 13.7 years; range 8-17 years) or with prednisone (n=11; mean age: 12.6 years; range: 7-16 years), significantly decreased proteinuria in normotensive proteinuric children (with or without nephrotic syndrome); no significant change in blood pressure was observed (Sasinka, 1999). In a smaller study of children with persistent proteinuria (n=7; 6 with steroid resistant nephrotic syndrome; mean age: 13.5 years; range: 7-18 years), enalapril (at mean oral doses of 0.3 mg/kg/day) significantly reduced proteinuria in 5 of the 7 patients (Lama, 2000). Another recent study assessed the effects of enalapril on urinary protein electrophoretic patterns in 13 children (mean age: 8 years; range: 1.8-12 years) with steroid resistant nephrotic syndrome; oral enalapril was initially dosed at 0.2 mg/kg/day (with a maximum dose of 30 mg/day); doses were increased each month by 0.1 mg/kg/day until the patients' urinary protein decreased by 50% from baseline; prednisone was added after 2 months in 11 of the 13 children at doses of 30 mg/m^2 given every other day; four patients had a complete remission of proteinuria after 4-12 months; an 80% decrease in urinary total protein and a 70% decrease in urinary albumin was observed in the other patients; the pattern of urinary protein shifted from a nonselective to an albumin-selective urinary protein loss in all patients; significant increases in plasma total protein and albumin occurred; it is important to note that 3 of the 13 patients (23%) required interruption of enalapril during transient acute renal failure due to an infectious disease (Delucchi, 2000). Further pediatric studies are needed to identify optimal enalapril oral doses and to establish safety and efficacy for this use.

Dosage Forms Excipient information presented when available (limited, particularly for generics); consult specific product labeling.

Injection, solution, as enalaprilat: 1.25 mg/mL (1 mL, 2 mL) [contains benzyl alcohol]

Tablet, as maleate (Vasotec®): 2.5 mg, 5 mg, 10 mg, 20 mg

(Continued)

Enalapril/Enalaprilat *(Continued)*

Extemporaneous Preparations

A 1 mg/mL oral suspension made from tablets, Bicitra®, and Ora-Sweet® SF is stable for 30 days when stored in a polyethylene terephthalate bottle under refrigeration (2°C to 8°C); place ten 20 mg tablets in a 200 mL polyethylene terephthalate bottle; add 50 mL of Bicitra®; shake well for at least 2 minutes; let stand for 1 hour then shake for one additional minute; add 150 mL of Ora-Sweet® SF and shake well; label "shake well" [Vasotec® tablets (package insert), 2001].

A 1 mg/mL oral liquid preparation made from tablets and 3 different vehicles (cherry syrup, a 1:1 mixture of Ora-Sweet® and Ora-Plus®, or a 1:1 mixture of Ora-Sweet® SF and Ora-Plus®) was stable for 60 days when stored in amber plastic prescription bottles in the dark at room temperature (25°C) or under refrigeration (5°C); grind six 20 mg tablets in a mortar into a fine powder; add 15 mL of the vehicle and mix well to form a uniform paste; mix while adding the vehicle in geometric proportions to **almost** 120 mL; transfer to a calibrated bottle and qsad with vehicle to 120 mL; label "shake well" and "protect from light" (Allen, 1998).

A 1 mg/mL oral liquid preparation made from tablets and 3 different vehicles (deionized water, citrate buffer solution at pH 5.0, or a 1:1 mixture of Ora-Sweet® and Ora-Plus®) was stable for 91 days when stored in plastic prescription bottles in the dark under refrigeration (4°C). When stored at room temperature (25°C), the preparations made in citrate buffer solution at pH 5.0 and the 1:1 mixture of Ora-Sweet® and Ora-Plus® were also stable for 91 days, but the preparation made in deionized water was stable for only 56 days. Grind twenty 10 mg tablets in a mortar; add a small amount of vehicle and mix well to form a smooth paste; mix while adding increasing amounts of the vehicle to make the mixture pourable; transfer to a graduated cylinder and qsad to 200 mL; **Note:** To prepare the isotonic citrate buffer solution (pH 5.0), see reference; label "shake well" and "protect from light" (Nahata, 1998).

A more dilute oral liquid preparation of 0.1 mg/mL made from tablets and an isotonic buffer solution at pH 5.0 was stable for 90 days when stored in amber, high density polyethylene bottles under refrigeration (5°C); grind one 20 mg tablet in a glass mortar into a fine powder; triturate with isotonic citrate buffer (pH 5.0) and filter; qsad to 200 mL with buffer solution; label "shake well" and "protect from light" (Boulton, 1994).

Allen LV and Erickson MA, "Stability of Alprazolam, Chloroquine Phosphate, Cisapride, Enalapril Maleate, and Hydralazine Hydrochloride in Extemporaneously Compounded Oral Liquids," *Am J Health Syst Pharm*, 1998, 55(18):1915-20.

Boulton DW, Woods DJ, Fawcett JP, et al, "The Stability of an Enalapril Maleate Oral Solution Prepared From Tablets," *Aust J Hosp Pharm*, 1994, 24(2):151-6.

Nahata MC, Morosco RS, and Hipple TF, "Stability of Enalapril Maleate in Three Extemporaneously Prepared Oral Liquids," *Am J Health Syst Pharm*, 1998, 55(11):1155-7.

Vasotec® (package insert), West Point, PA: Merck & Co., Inc; 2001.

References

Brown NJ, Ray WA, Snowden M, et al, "Black Americans Have an Increased Rate of Angiotensin-Converting Enzyme Inhibitor-Associated Angioedema," *Clin Pharmacol Ther*, 1996, 60(1):8-13.

Bult Y and van den Anker J, "Hypertension in a Preterm Infant Treated With Enalapril," *J Pediatr Pharm Pract*, 1997, 2(4):229-31.

Chobanian AV, Bakris GL, Black HR, et al, "The Seventh Report of the Joint National Committee on Prevention, Detection, Evaluation, and Treatment of High Blood Pressure: The JNC 7 report," *JAMA*, 2003, 289(19):2560-72.

Delucchi A, Cano F, Rodriguez E, et al, "Enalapril and Prednisone in Children With Nephrotic-Range Proteinuria," *Pediatr Nephrol*, 2000, 14(12):1088-91.

Frenneaux M, Stewart RA, Newman CM, et al, "Enalapril for Severe Heart Failure in Infancy," *Arch Dis Child*, 1989, 64(2):219-23.

Lama G, Luongo I, Piscitelli A, et al, "Enalapril: Antiproteinuric Effect in Children With Nephrotic Syndrome," *Clin Nephrol*, 2000, 53(6):432-6.

Leversha AM, Wilson NJ, Clarkson PM, et al, "Efficacy and Dosage of Enalapril in Congenital and Acquired Heart Disease," *Arch Dis Child*, 1994, 70(1):35-9.

Lloyd TR, Mahoney LT, Knoedel D, et al, "Orally Administered Enalapril for Infants With Congestive Heart Failure: A Dose Finding Study," *J Pediatr*, 1989, 114(4 Pt 1):650-4.

Marcadis ML, Kraus DM, Hatzopoulos FK, et al, "Use of Enalaprilat for Neonatal Hypertension," *J Pediatr*, 1991, 119(3):505-6.

Nakamura H, Ishii M, Sugimura T, et al, "The Kinetic Profiles of Enalapril and Enalaprilat and Their Possible Developmental Changes in Pediatric Patients With Congestive Heart Failure," *Clin Pharmacol Ther*, 1994, 56(2):160-8.

Sasinka MA, Podracka L, Boor A, et al, "Enalapril Treatment of Proteinuria in Normotensive Children," *Bratisl Lek Listy*, 1999, 100(9):476-80.

Schilder JL and Van den Anker JN, "Use of Enalapril in Neonatal Hypertension," *Acta Paediatr*, 1995, 84(12):1426-8.

von Vigier RO, Mozzettini S, Truttmann AC, et al, "Cough is Common in Children Prescribed Converting Enzyme Inhibitors," *Nephron*, 2000, 84(1):98.

Wells TG, Bunchman TE, Kearns GL, "Treatment of Neonatal Hypertension With Enalaprilat," *J Pediatr*, 1990, 117(4):664-7.

- ♦ **Enalapril Maleate** *see* Enalapril/Enalaprilat *on page 565*
- ♦ **Enbrel®** *see* Etanercept *on page 613*
- ♦ **Encort™** *see* Hydrocortisone *on page 781*
- ♦ **Endantadine® (Can)** *see* Amantadine *on page 89*
- ♦ **Endocet®** *see* Oxycodone and Acetaminophen *on page 1191*
- ♦ **Endodan®** *see* Oxycodone and Aspirin *on page 1193*
- ♦ **Endrate®** *see* Edetate Disodium *on page 555*
- ♦ **Enemeez® [OTC]** *see* Docusate *on page 526*
- ♦ **Enerjets [OTC]** *see* Caffeine *on page 255*

Enfuvirtide (en FYOO vir tide)

Related Information

Adult and Adolescent HIV *on page 1821*
Pediatric HIV *on page 1816*
Perinatal HIV *on page 1831*

U.S. Brand Names Fuzeon®

Canadian Brand Names Fuzeon®

Index Terms T-20

Therapeutic Category Antiretroviral Agent; Fusion Inhibitor; HIV Agents (Anti-HIV Agents)

Generic Available No

Use Treatment of HIV-1 infection in combination with other antiretroviral agents in treatment-experienced patients who are failing current antiretroviral therapy (**Note:** HIV regimens consisting of **three** antiretroviral agents are strongly recommended. However, in published studies, enfuvirtide was added onto a new optimized background regimen of 3-5 antiretroviral agents, in patients failing their current antiretroviral regimen. Selection of the new optimized regimen was based on medication history, genotyping, and phenotyping. Due to the lack of studies, enfuvirtide cannot be recommended as initial therapy in patients who are antiretroviral naïve.)

Pregnancy Risk Factor B

Lactation Excretion in breast milk unknown/contraindicated

Contraindications Hypersensitivity to enfuvirtide or any component

Warnings Local injection site reactions occur in the majority of patients (see Adverse Reactions); instruct patient or caregiver on proper injection method; monitor patients for local infection or cellulitis. Bacterial pneumonia was observed at a higher rate in patients receiving enfuvirtide during clinical trials; certain patients may be at greater risk (eg, those with a history of lung disease, low CD4 cell count, high initial viral load, I.V. drug use, or smoking); monitor patients closely for signs and symptoms of pneumonia. Systemic hypersensitivity reactions may occur (see Adverse Reactions); discontinue enfuvirtide and do not restart in patients with systemic hypersensitivity reactions.

Precautions Efficacy data is limited in pediatric patients ≥6 years of age; safety and pharmacokinetics in children <6 years is not established. Use of enfuvirtide may theoretically result in the production of anti-enfuvirtide antibodies, which may cross react with HIV-1 gp41; this could potentially result in a false positive ELISA test in noninfected HIV individuals; the western blot test would be expected to be negative; use of enfuvirtide in non-HIV infected individuals has not been studied.

Adverse Reactions Note: Adverse effects in pediatric patients 6-16 years of age were reported to be similar to those in adults

Central nervous system: Insomnia, depression, anxiety, dizziness

Dermatologic: Pruritus

Endocrine & metabolic: Elevated triglycerides, weight loss

Gastrointestinal: Constipation, abdominal pain, pancreatitis, taste disturbance, elevated serum amylase, elevated serum lipase, anorexia

Hematologic: Eosinophilia, anemia

Hepatic: Elevated serum transaminases

Local: Injection site reactions [98% incidence; most patients have first injection site reaction during initial week of therapy; reactions are usually mild to moderate in severity, but may be more severe; symptoms may include pain, discomfort, erythema, induration, pruritus, ecchymosis, and nodule or cyst formation; infection, including cellulitis and abscess, occur in 1.7% of patients; 11% of patients require analgesics or limitation of usual activities; reactions often occur at >1 injection site; 26% of patients have 6-14 injection site reactions and 1.3% have >14 injection site reactions at any given time; average duration of single injection site reaction is 3-7 days in 41% of patients and >7 days in 24%; 7% of patients discontinue therapy due to injection site reactions (4%) or problems with administering injections (3%)].

Neuromuscular & skeletal: Peripheral neuropathy, weakness, myalgia, elevated CPK

Ocular: Conjunctivitis

(Continued)

Enfuvirtide *(Continued)*

Respiratory: Cough, sinusitis; bacterial pneumonia (6.7 events per 100 patient years vs 0.6 events per 100 patient years in control group; about 50% of patients with pneumonia required hospitalization; see Warnings for risk factors)

Miscellaneous: Infections, flu-like symptoms, lymphadenopathy; hypersensitivity reactions (<1% incidence; symptoms may include rash, fever, chills, rigors, nausea, vomiting, hypotension, and elevated serum transaminases; other immune-mediated adverse reactions that have been reported include: primary immune complex reaction, Guillain-Barré syndrome, respiratory distress, glomerulonephritis)

Drug Interactions Not an inhibitor of cytochrome P450 enzymes; no clinically significant drug interactions have been identified

Stability Store unreconstituted vials at controlled room temperature, 25°C (77°F); excursions permitted to 15°C to 30°C (59°F to 86°F). Store reconstituted solution under refrigeration at 2°C to 8°C (36°F to 46°F); use within 24 hours.

Mechanism of Action Enfuvirtide is a synthetic protein consisting of a linear sequence of 36 amino acids. It mimics the amino acid sequence HR2 (heptad repeat 2) found in the C-terminal portion of gp41 (an HIV-1 transmembrane glycoprotein) and competitively binds with HR1 (sequence heptad repeat 1). Normally, the HR1 sequence interacts with HR2 to form a hairpin structure needed for gp41 to initiate the fusion between the HIV-1 viral membrane and host CD4 cell membrane. By mimicking HR2 and binding with HR1, enfuvirtide inhibits the fusion of viral and cellular membranes and interferes with the entry of HIV-1 into cells.

Pharmacokinetics

Absorption: SubQ: Absorption is comparable when injected into abdomen, arm, or thigh

Distribution: Adults: V_d (mean ± SD): 5.5 ± 1.1 L

Protein Binding: 92%; primarily to albumin, but also to alpha-1 acid glycoprotein (to a lesser extent); CNS penetration: Unknown (but expected to be minimal due to large molecule and high protein binding)

Metabolism: Expected to undergo catabolism via peptidases and proteinases in the liver and kidneys to amino acids; amino acids would then be recycled in the body pool. A deaminated metabolite (with 20% activity compared to parent drug) was formed via hydrolysis during *in vitro* human microsomal and hepatocyte studies.

Bioavailability:

Oral: Not bioavailable by this route

SubQ: Absolute: 84.3% ± 15.5%

Half-life: 3.8 ± 0.6 hours

Time to peak serum concentration: SubQ:

Single dose: Median: 8 hours (range: 3-12 hours)

Multiple dosing: Median: 4 hours (range: 4-8 hours)

Clearance: Plasma clearance is decreased in adults with lower body weight and in females after adjusting for body weight (clearance in adults females is 20% lower compared to adults males). However, no adjustment in dose is recommended for gender or weight.

Apparent clearance: Multiple dosing:

Children: 40 ± 17 mL/hour/kg

Adults: 30.6 ± 10.6 mL/hour/kg

Usual Dosage SubQ (use in combination with other antiretroviral agents):

Neonates, Infants, and Children <6 years: Not approved for use

Children 6-16 years: 2 mg/kg twice daily (maximum dose: 90 mg twice daily)

Adolescent >16 years and Adults: 90 mg twice daily

Dosage adjustment in renal impairment: Adults: Cl_{cr} >35 mL/minute: Clearance of enfuvirtide is not affected; no dosage adjustment required

Administration Reconstitute vial with 1.1 mL SWI to result in 90 mg/mL solution; to avoid foaming, gently tap vial for 10 seconds and roll gently between hands to ensure contact of drug with liquid; allow vial to stand until lyophilized powder goes completely into solution; this may require up to 45 minutes; to reduce reconstitution time, may gently roll vial between hands until drug is completely dissolved; visually inspect vial to ensure complete dissolution of drug; solution should be clear, colorless, and without particulate matter or bubbles; do not use vials that contain particulate matter.

Vial does not contain preservatives; reconstituted solutions should be injected immediately or refrigerated and used within 24 hours; bring refrigerated reconstituted vials to room temperature before injection and visually inspect vial again as outlined above.

Inject SubQ into upper arm, abdomen, or anterior thigh; do not inject I.M. (severity of reactions is increased); do not inject into moles, bruises, scar tissue, or the navel; rotate injection site (ie, give injections at a site different from the preceding injection site); do not inject into any site where an injection site reaction is present; after injection, apply heat or ice to injection site or gently massage area to better disperse the dose, to minimize local injection reactions; discard unused portion of the vial (vial is for single use only)

Monitoring Parameters Serum triglycerides, CBC, liver enzymes, CD4 cell count, viral load; local injection site reactions, local infection, cellulitis; signs and symptoms of pneumonia, especially in patients at risk (see Warnings)

Patient Information Enfuvirtide can only be administered by injection; follow exact injection instructions that come with your medication. Do not mix any other medications in the same syringe with enfuvirtide. Inject subcutaneously into the upper arm, abdomen, or anterior thigh; do not inject in the same area you did the time before and do not inject into the naval, scar tissue, a bruise, a mole, or where there is an injection site reaction.

Enfuvirtide may cause injection site reactions such as itching, swelling, redness, pain, hardened skin, or bumps (each local reaction usually lasts for <7 days); notify physician immediately if reaction is severe or if injection site becomes infected. Patients receiving enfuvirtide may experience bacterial pneumonia or hypersensitivity reactions; notify physician if you experience cough, fever, rapid breathing, trouble breathing, vomiting, chills, rash, blood in the urine, or swelling of the feet. Enfuvirtide may cause dizziness and impair ability to perform activities requiring mental alertness or physical coordination.

Enfuvirtide is not a cure for HIV; take enfuvirtide everyday as prescribed; do not change dose or discontinue without physician's advice; if a dose is missed, take it as soon as possible, then return to normal dosing schedule; if a dose is skipped, do not double the next dose; make sure you have adequate supply of medication; do not allow supply to run out.

Nursing Implications Teach patient or caregiver proper reconstitution, aseptic injection technique, and proper needle and syringe disposal (see Stability and Administration specifics).

Additional Information Reconstituted injection has a pH ~9.0.

Dosage Forms Excipient information presented when available (limited, particularly for generics); consult specific product labeling.

Injection, powder for reconstitution [preservative free]:

Fuzeon®: 108 mg [90 mg/mL following reconstitution; available in convenience kit of 60 vials, SWFI, syringes, alcohol wipes, patient instructions]

References

Briars LA, Hilao JJ, and Kraus DM, "A Review of Pediatric Human Immunodeficiency Virus Infection," *Journal of Pharmacy Practice*, 2004, 17(6):407-31.

Church JA, Cunningham C, Hughes M, et al, "Safety and Antiretroviral Activity of Chronic Subcutaneous Administration of T-20 in Human Immunodeficiency Virus 1-Infected Children," *Pediatr Infect Dis J*, 2002, 21(7):653-9.

Hardy H and Skolnik PR, "Enfuvirtide, a New Fusion Inhibitor for Therapy of Human Immunodeficiency Virus Infection," *Pharmacotherapy*, 2004, 24(2):198-211.

Morris JL and Kraus DM, "New Antiretroviral Therapies for Pediatric HIV Infection," *J Pediatr Pharmacol Ther*, 2005, 10:215-47.

Panel on Clinical Practices for Treatment of HIV Infections, "Guidelines for the Use of Antiretroviral Agents in HIV-Infected Adults and Adolescents," October 10, 2006, http:www.aidsinfo.nih.gov.

Soy D, Aweeka FT, Church JA, et al, "Population Pharmacokinetics of Enfuvirtide in Pediatric Patients With Human Immunodeficiency Virus: Searching for Exposure-Response Relationships," *Clin Pharmacol Ther*, 2003, 74(6):569-80.

Working Group on Antiretroviral Therapy and Medical Management of HIV-infected Children, "Guidelines for the Use of Antiretroviral Agents in Pediatric HIV Infection," October 26, 2006, http://www.aidsinfo.nih.gov.

- **Engerix-B**® *see* Hepatitis B Vaccine *on page 763*
- **Enhanced-Potency Inactivated Poliovirus Vaccine** *see* Poliovirus Vaccine (Inactivated) *on page 1275*
- **Enlon**® *see* Edrophonium *on page 556*

Enoxaparin (e noks ah PAIR in)

Medication Safety Issues

Sound-alike/look-alike issues:

Lovenox® may be confused with Lotronex®, Protonix®

High alert medication: The Institute for Safe Medication Practices (ISMP) includes this medication among its list of drugs which have a heightened risk of causing significant patient harm when used in error.

International issues:

Lovenox® may be confused with Lotanax® which is a brand name for terfenadine in the Czech Republic

Related Information

Antithrombotic Therapy in Children *on page 1804*

Commonly Used Antidotes for Acute Overdoses *on page 1920*

(Continued)

Enoxaparin *(Continued)*

U.S. Brand Names Lovenox®

Canadian Brand Names Enoxaparin Injection; Lovenox®; Lovenox® HP

Index Terms Enoxaparin Sodium

Therapeutic Category Anticoagulant; Low Molecular Weight Heparin (LMWH)

Generic Available No

Use Prophylaxis and treatment of thromboembolic disorders, specifically: (in adults) prevention of DVT following hip or knee replacement surgery, abdominal surgery in patients at thromboembolic risk (ie, >40 years of age, obese, general anesthesia >30 minutes, malignancy, history of DVT or pulmonary embolism) and in medical patients at thromboembolic risk due to severely restricted mobility during acute illness; administered with warfarin: For inpatient treatment of acute DVT (with or without pulmonary embolism) and outpatient treatment of acute DVT (without pulmonary embolism); administered with aspirin: For prevention of ischemic complications of non-Q-wave MI and unstable angina

Pregnancy Risk Factor B

Lactation Excretion in breast milk unknown/use caution

Contraindications Hypersensitivity to enoxaparin, heparin, any component (see Warnings), or pork products (enoxaparin is derived from porcine intestinal mucosa); active major bleeding; acute heparin-induced or low molecular weight heparin-induced thrombocytopenia

Warnings Bleeding or thrombocytopenia may occur; major hemorrhages (eg, intracranial and retroperitoneal bleeding) may be fatal; thrombocytopenia with thrombosis may occur and may be complicated by limb ischemia, organ infarction, or death. Use with extreme caution in patients with an increased risk of hemorrhage (eg, active GI ulceration or bleeding, angiodysplastic GI disease, bacterial endocarditis, bleeding disorders, hemorrhagic stroke); recent brain, spinal, or ophthalmological surgery; concomitant platelet inhibitor therapy (see Drug Interactions); or a history of heparin-induced thrombocytopenia. Do not use unit-for-unit in place of heparin or other low molecular weight heparins (units are not equivalent). Enoxaparin is **not** recommended for prophylaxis of thromboembolic disorders in patients with prosthetic heart valves, especially pregnant women (prosthetic heart valve thrombosis may occur; several cases occurred in pregnant women and resulted in maternal and fetal deaths; pregnant women with prosthetic heart valves may be at a higher risk for thromboembolism; use with extreme caution and monitor peak and trough anti-Factor Xa levels frequently in these patients; adjust dosage accordingly)

Epidural or spinal hematoma resulting in long-term or permanent paralysis may occur in patients receiving low molecular weight heparins or heparinoids during epidural/spinal anesthesia or spinal puncture; these patients must be monitored frequently for neurological impairment and treated immediately if compromised; the use of indwelling spinal catheters for analgesia, concomitant use of platelet inhibitors, NSAIDs, or other anticoagulants, and repeated or traumatic epidural/spinal puncture increase the risk for epidural/spinal hematoma; potential benefits must be weighed against the risks. Enoxaparin should be withheld (at least 2 doses) and antifactor Xa activity should be determined (if possible), prior to lumbar or epidural procedures.

Enoxaparin multidose vial contains benzyl alcohol which may cause allergic reactions in susceptible individuals; large amounts of benzyl alcohol (≥99 mg/kg/day) have been associated with a potentially fatal toxicity ("gasping syndrome") in neonates; the "gasping syndrome" consists of metabolic acidosis, respiratory distress, gasping respirations, CNS dysfunction (including convulsions, intracranial hemorrhage), hypotension and cardiovascular collapse; avoid use of enoxaparin products containing benzyl alcohol in neonates; use the preservative free injection; *in vitro* and animal studies have shown that benzoate, a metabolite of benzyl alcohol, displaces bilirubin from protein binding sites. Use multidose vial with caution in pregnant women and only if clearly needed (benzyl alcohol may cross the placenta).

Precautions Use with caution in patients with uncontrolled arterial hypertension, bleeding diathesis, pregnancy, history of recent GI ulceration, diabetic retinopathy, and hemorrhage; use with caution and decrease dose in patients with severe renal dysfunction (Cl_{cr} <30 mL/minute); use with caution and monitor carefully in low-weight patients (ie, women <45 kg and men <57 kg) receiving nonweight adjusted doses (an increase in enoxaparin AUC has been reported); institute appropriate therapy if thromboembolism occurs despite enoxaparin prophylaxis

Adverse Reactions

Cardiovascular: Edema

Central nervous system: Fever

Endocrine & metabolic: Hyperlipidemia (very rare)

Gastrointestinal: Nausea

Hematologic: Hemorrhage, thrombocytopenia (incidence of heparin-induced thrombocytopenia is less than with heparin therapy)

Hepatic: Elevated SGOT and SGPT (asymptomatic, fully reversible, rarely associated with elevated bilirubin levels)

Local: Irritation, pain, hematoma, ecchymosis, erythema at SubQ injection site; epidural or spinal hematoma (see Warnings)

Drug Interactions Anticoagulants, thrombolytic agents (alteplase, streptokinase, urokinase), platelet inhibitors (aspirin, salicylates, NSAIDs including ketorolac, dipyridamole, and sulfinpyrazone) may increase the risk of bleeding

Stability Store at room temperature; does not contain preservatives, discard unused portions; do not mix with other injections or infusions

Mechanism of Action Potentiates the action of antithrombin III and inactivates coagulation factor Xa; also inactivates factor IIa (thrombin), but to a much lesser degree; ratio of antifactor Xa to antifactor IIa activity is ~4:1 (ratio for unfractionated heparin is 1:1)

Pharmacodynamics Antifactor Xa and antithrombin (antifactor IIa) activities:

Maximum effect: SubQ: 3-5 hours

Duration: ~12 hours following a 40 mg daily dose given SubQ

Pharmacokinetics Based on antifactor Xa activity

Distribution: Does not cross the placental barrier

Mean V_d: Adults: 4.3 L

Protein binding: Does not bind to most heparin binding proteins

Metabolism: Primarily in the liver via desulfation and depolymerization to lower molecular weight molecules with very low biological activity

Bioavailability: Adults: SubQ: ~100%

Half-life: SubQ: Adults: Single dose: 4.5 hours; repeat dosing: 7 hours

Elimination: 40% of I.V. dose is excreted in urine as active and inactive fragments; 10% of dose is excreted by kidneys as active enoxaparin fragments; 8% to 20% of antifactor Xa activity is recovered within 24 hours in the urine

Clearance: Decreased by 30% in patients with Cl_{cr} <30 mL/minute

Usual Dosage SubQ:

Neonates, Infants, and Children: *Chest*, 2001 Recommendations:

Initial:

Infants <2 months:

Prophylaxis: 0.75 mg/kg every 12 hours

Treatment: 1.5 mg/kg every 12 hours

Infants >2 months and Children ≤18 years:

Prophylaxis: 0.5 mg/kg every 12 hours

Treatment: 1 mg/kg every 12 hours

Maintenance: See **Dosage Titration** table: **Note:** In a recent prospective study of 177 courses of enoxaparin in pediatric patients (146 treatment courses; 31 prophylactic courses) considerable variation in maintenance dosage requirements was observed (see Dix, 2000)

Enoxaparin Dosage Titration

Antifactor Xa	Dose Titration	Time to Repeat Antifactor Xa Level
<0.35 units/mL	Increase dose by 25%	4 h after next dose
0.35-0.49 units/mL	Increase dose by 10%	4 h after next dose
0.5-1 unit/mL	Keep same dosage	Next day, then 1 wk later, then monthly (4 h after dose)
1.1-1.5 units/mL	Decrease dose by 20%	Before next dose
1.6-2 units/mL	Hold dose for 3 h and decrease dose by 30%	Before next dose, then 4 h after next dose
>2 units/mL	Hold all doses until antifactor Xa is 0.5 units/mL, then decrease dose by 40%	Before next dose and every 12 h until antifactor Xa <0.5 units/mL

Modified from Monagle P, Michelson AD, Bovill E, et al, "Antithrombotic Therapy in Children," *Chest*, 2001, 119:344S-70S.

Adults: **Note:** Consider lower doses for patients <45 kg

Prevention of DVT:

Knee replacement surgery: 30 mg every 12 hours; give first dose 12-24 hours after surgery (provided hemostasis has been established); average duration 7-10 days, up to 14 days

Hip replacement surgery: Initial phase: 30 mg every 12 hours with first dose 12-24 hours after surgery (provided hemostasis has been established) or consider 40 mg once daily with first dose given 12 ± 3 hours prior to surgery; average duration of initial phase: 7-10 days, up to 14 days; after initial phase, give 40 mg once daily for 3 weeks

(Continued)

Enoxaparin *(Continued)*

Abdominal surgery in patients at risk: 40 mg once daily; give first dose 2 hours prior to surgery; average duration: 7-10 days, up to 12 days

Medical patients at risk due to severely restricted mobility during acute illness: 40 mg once daily; average duration: 6-11 days, up to 14 days

Treatment of acute DVT and pulmonary embolism: Note: Initiate warfarin therapy when appropriate (usually within 72 hours of starting enoxaparin), continue enoxaparin for a minimum of 5 days (average 7 days) until INR is therapeutic

Inpatient treatment of acute DVT with or without pulmonary embolism: 1 mg/kg every 12 hours or 1.5 mg/kg once daily

Outpatient treatment of acute DVT without pulmonary embolism: 1 mg/kg every 12 hours

Prevention of ischemic complications of non-Q-wave MI or unstable angina: 1 mg/kg every 12 hours in conjunction with oral aspirin (100-325 mg once daily); continue treatment for a minimum of 2 days until patient is clinically stabilized (usually 2-8 days; up to 12.5 days)

Dosage adjustment in renal impairment: SubQ:

Cl_{cr} ≥30 mL/minute: No specific adjustment recommended; monitor patients closely for bleeding

Cl_{cr} <30 mL/minute: **Note:** Monitor antifactor Xa activity closely

DVT prophylaxis in abdominal surgery, hip replacement, knee replacement, or in medical patients during acute illness: 30 mg once daily

DVT treatment in conjunction with warfarin (in inpatients with or without pulmonary embolism and in outpatients without pulmonary embolism): 1 mg/kg once daily

Prevention of ischemic complications of non-Q-wave MI or unstable angina (with aspirin): 1 mg/kg once daily

Administration Parenteral: For SubQ use only; do not administer I.M. or I.V.; administer by deep SubQ injection; do not rub injection site after SubQ administration as bruising may occur

Monitoring Parameters CBC with platelets, stool occult blood tests; antifactor Xa activity in select patients (eg, neonates, infants, and children, and patients with significant renal impairment, active bleeding, or abnormal coagulation parameters); **Note**: Routine monitoring of PT and APTT is not warranted since PT and APTT are relatively insensitive measures of low molecular weight heparin activity; consider monitoring bone density in infants and children with long-term use

Reference Range Antifactor Xa level of 0.5-1 unit/mL measured 4-6 hours after SubQ administration

Nursing Implications Instruct patients on proper SubQ injection technique if patient will self-inject.

Additional Information Discontinue therapy if platelets fall <100,000/mm^3; each 10 mg of enoxaparin sodium equals ~1000 international units of antifactor Xa activity.

Enoxaparin contains fragments of unfractionated heparin produced by alkaline degradation (depolymerization) of heparin benzyl ester; enoxaparin has mean molecular weights of 3500-5600 daltons, which are much lower than mean molecular weights of unfractionated heparin (12,000-15,000 daltons). Low molecular weight heparins (LMWH) have several advantages over unfractionated heparin: better SubQ bioavailability, more convenient administration (SubQ versus I.V.), longer half-life (longer dosing interval), more predictable pharmacokinetics and pharmacodynamic (anticoagulant) effect, less intensive laboratory monitoring, reduced risk of heparin-induced thrombocytopenia, potential for outpatient use, and probable reduced risk of osteoporosis (further studies are needed).

Accidental overdosage of enoxaparin may be treated with protamine sulfate; 1 mg protamine sulfate neutralizes 1 mg enoxaparin; first dose of protamine sulfate should equal the dose of enoxaparin injected, if enoxaparin was given in the previous 8 hours; use 0.5 mg protamine sulfate per 1 mg enoxaparin if enoxaparin was given >8 hours prior to protamine or if a second dose of protamine is needed; a second dose of protamine sulfate (0.5 mg per 1 mg enoxaparin) may be given if APTT remains prolonged 2-4 hours after first dose; protamine may not be required ≥12 hours after enoxaparin administration; avoid overdosage with protamine (see Protamine *on page 1342*)

Dosage Forms Excipient information presented when available (limited, particularly for generics); consult specific product labeling.

Injection, solution, as sodium [graduated prefilled syringe; preservative free]: 60 mg/0.6 mL (0.6 mL); 80 mg/0.8 mL (0.8 mL); 100 mg/mL (1 mL); 120 mg/0.8 mL (0.8 mL); 150 mg/mL (1 mL)

Injection, solution, as sodium [multidose vial]: 100 mg/mL (3 mL) [contains benzyl alcohol]

Injection, solution, as sodium [prefilled syringe; preservative free]: 30 mg/0.3 mL (0.3 mL); 40 mg/0.4 mL (0.4 mL)

References

deVeber G, Chan A, Monagle P, et al, "Anticoagulation Therapy in Pediatric Patients With Sinovenous Thrombosis: A Cohort Study," *Arch Neurol*, 1998, 55(12):1533-7.

Dix D, Andrew M, Marzinotto V, et al, "The Use of Low Molecular Weight Heparin in Pediatric Patients: A Prospective Cohort Study," *J Pediatr*, 2000, 136(4):439-45.

Hirsh J, Warkentin TE, Shaughnessy SG, et al, "Heparin and Low-Molecular-Weight Heparin: Mechanisms of Action, Pharmacokinetics, Dosing, Monitoring, Efficacy, and Safety," *Chest*, 2001, 119:64S-94S.

Martineau P and Tawil N, "Low-Molecular-Weight Heparins in the Treatment of Deep-Vein Thrombosis," *Ann Pharmacother*, 1998, 32(5):588-98, 601.

Massicotte P, Adams M, Marzinotto V, et al, "Low-Molecular-Weight Heparin in Pediatric Patients With Thrombotic Disease: A Dose Finding Study," *J Pediatr*, 1996, 128(3):313-8.

Monagle P, Michelson AD, Bovill E, et al, "Antithrombotic Therapy in Children," *Chest*, 2001, 119:344S-70S.

♦ **Enoxaparin Injection (Can)** *see* Enoxaparin *on page 571*
♦ **Enoxaparin Sodium** *see* Enoxaparin *on page 571*
♦ **Entocort® (Can)** *see* Budesonide *on page 238*
♦ **Entocort® EC** *see* Budesonide *on page 238*
♦ **Entrophen® (Can)** *see* Aspirin *on page 163*
♦ **Entsol® [OTC]** *see* Sodium Chloride *on page 1450*
♦ **Enulose** *see* Lactulose *on page 900*

Ephedrine (e FED rin)

Medication Safety Issues

Sound-alike/look-alike issues:

Ephedrine may be confused with Epifrin®, epinephrine

U.S. Brand Names Pretz-D® [OTC]

Index Terms Ephedrine Sulfate

Therapeutic Category Adrenergic Agonist Agent; Antiasthmatic; Bronchodilator; Sympathomimetic

Generic Available Yes

Use Treatment of mild asthma, nasal congestion, acute bronchospasm, idiopathic orthostatic hypotension; adjunctive agent for treatment of shock

Pregnancy Risk Factor C

Lactation Enters breast milk/not recommended

Contraindications Hypersensitivity to ephedrine or any component; patients with hypertension, cardiac arrhythmias, angle-closure glaucoma, and psychoneurosis; use during halothane or cyclopropane anesthesia (see Drug Interactions)

Warnings Use of ephedrine as a pressor is not a substitute for replacement of blood, plasma, fluids, and electrolytes; blood volume should be corrected as fully as possible before ephedrine therapy; must not be used as sole therapy in hypovolemic patients; hypoxia, hypercapnia, and acidosis may reduce the effectiveness and increase the incidence of side effects of ephedrine; may cause hypertension which may result in intracranial hemorrhage; long-term use may cause anxiety and symptoms of paranoid schizophrenia; the FDA has issued warnings concerning ephedrine-containing nonprescription products with claims of producing such effects as euphoria, increased sexual sensation, increased energy, and weight loss; healthcare professionals are urged to be aware of these products and counsel patients, when appropriate, about the potential adverse effects of ephedrine such as headache, dizziness, heart irregularities, seizures, and possibly death

Precautions Use with caution in patients with hyperthyroidism, diabetes mellitus, prostatic hypertrophy, coronary insufficiency, and angina

Adverse Reactions

Cardiovascular: Hypertension, precordial pain, edema, palpitations, tachycardia, arrhythmias

Central nervous system: Nervousness, anxiety, apprehension, fear, tension, agitation, excitation, restlessness, irritability, insomnia, dizziness, vertigo, confusion, delirium, hallucinations, euphoria, paranoid psychosis, headache

Dermatologic: Rash

Gastrointestinal: Nausea, vomiting, xerostomia, mild epigastric distress, anorexia

Genitourinary: Urinary retention

Neuromuscular & skeletal: Tremors, hyperactive reflexes, weakness

Drug Interactions Increased effects with other sympathomimetic agents; reduced pressor response to ephedrine with alpha-adrenergic blocking agents and methyldopa; increased cardiac irritability and arrhythmias with halothane and cyclopropane anesthesia; increased pressor effects with MAO inhibitors; cardiac glycosides may increase cardiac stimulation; medications which alkalinize or acidify the urine may result in increased or decreased ephedrine effects (see Pharmacokinetics); increased CNS and GI effects when used with theophylline

Stability Protect from light

(Continued)

Ephedrine *(Continued)*

Mechanism of Action Stimulates both alpha- and beta-adrenergic receptors and also stimulates the release of norepinephrine from storage sites resulting in bronchodilation, cardiac stimulation, and increased systolic and diastolic blood pressure; tachyphylaxis may occur

Pharmacodynamics

Bronchodilation:
- Onset of action: Oral: 15-60 minutes
- Duration: Oral: 2-4 hours

Pressor/cardiac effects: Duration:
- Oral: 4 hours
- I.M., SubQ: 1 hour

Pharmacokinetics

Absorption: Oral: Complete

Metabolism: Liver by oxidative deamination, demethylation, aromatic hydroxylation, and conjugation

Bioavailability: Oral: 85%

Half-life: 4.9-6.5 hours

Elimination: Dependent upon urinary pH with greatest excretion in acid pH; urine pH 5: 74% to 99% excreted unchanged; urine pH 8: 22% to 25% excreted unchanged

Usual Dosage

Bronchodilation and nasal decongestion:

Oral:
- Children >2-6 years: 2-3 mg/kg/day or 100 mg/m^2/day in 4-6 divided doses
- Children 7-11 years: 6.25-12.5 mg every 4 hours; not to exceed 75 mg/day
- Children ≥12 years and Adults: 12.5-50 mg every 3-4 hours; not to exceed 150 mg/day

Spray:
- Children 6-12 years: 1-2 sprays in each nostril not more than every 4 hours; do not exceed 3 days of therapy
- Children >12 years and Adults: 2-3 sprays in each nostril not more than every 4 hours; do not exceed 3 days of therapy

Orthostatic hypotension: Oral: Adults: 25 mg 1-4 times/day

Adjunctive agent in the treatment of shock: Use the smallest effective dose for the shortest time:
- Children <12 years: I.M., I.V., SubQ: 3 mg/kg/day in 4-6 divided doses
- Children ≥12 years and Adults:
  - I.M., SubQ: 25-50 mg (range: 10-50 mg); may repeat with a second dose of 50 mg; not to exceed 150 mg/24 hours
  - I.V.: 10-25 mg; may repeat with a second dose in 5-10 minutes of 25 mg; not to exceed 150 mg/24 hours

Administration

Oral: May be administered without regard to food

Parenteral:
- I.M., SubQ: May be administered undiluted
- I.V.: May be administered by slow I.V. push

Spray: Spray into each nostril while gently occluding the other

Monitoring Parameters Vital signs, pulmonary function tests, respiratory rate (when applicable)

Test Interactions May cause a false-positive test for amphetamine (by EMIT assay)

Patient Information Use for self-medication for asthma only under physician's direction; see Warnings; contact your physician if nervousness, tremor, insomnia, nausea, or loss of appetite occur; may cause dry mouth

Additional Information Because ephedrine has been used to synthesize methamphetamine, restrictions are in place to reduce the potential for misuse (diversion) and abuse; 24 g of ephedrine (in terms of base) is the limit for a single transaction for drug products containing ephedrine regardless of the form in which these drugs are packaged

Dosage Forms Excipient information presented when available (limited, particularly for generics); consult specific product labeling.

Capsule, as sulfate: 25 mg

Injection, solution, as sulfate: 50 mg/mL (1 mL, 10 mL)

Solution, intranasal spray, as sulfate (Pretz-D®): 0.25% (50 mL)

♦ **Ephedrine Sulfate** *see* Ephedrine *on page 575*

♦ **EpiClenz™ [OTC]** *see* Ethyl Alcohol *on page 619*

♦ **Epidermal Thymocyte Activating Factor** *see* Aldesleukin *on page 70*

Epinastine (ep i NAS teen)

U.S. Brand Names Elestat™
Index Terms Epinastine Hydrochloride
Therapeutic Category Antiallergic, Ophthalmic
Generic Available No
Use Treatment of allergic conjunctivitis
Pregnancy Risk Factor C
Lactation Excretion in breast milk unknown/use caution
Contraindications Hypersensitivity to epinastine or any component of the formulation
Warnings Not for the treatment of contact lens irritation; contains the preservative, benzalkonium chloride, which may be absorbed by soft contact lenses; wait at least 10 minutes after instillation before inserting soft contact lenses. Safety and efficacy in children <3 years of age have not been established.
Adverse Reactions
Central nervous system: Headache
Ocular: Burning sensation, folliculosis, hyperemia, pruritus
Respiratory: Cough, pharyngitis, rhinitis, sinusitis
Miscellaneous: Infection (defined as cold symptoms and upper respiratory infection)
Stability Store at controlled room temperature of 15°C to 25°C (59°F to 77°F). Keep tightly closed.
Mechanism of Action Selective H_1-receptor antagonist; inhibits release of histamine from the mast cell
Pharmacodynamics
Onset of action: 3-5 minutes
Duration: 8 hours
Pharmacokinetics
Absorption: Low systemic absorption following topical application
Distribution: Does not cross blood-brain barrier
Protein binding: 64%
Metabolism: <10% metabolized
Half-life: 12 hours
Elimination: I.V.: Urine (55%); feces (30%)
Usual Dosage Ophthalmic: Children ≥3 years and Adults: Instill 1 drop into each eye twice daily; continue throughout period of exposure, even in the absence of symptoms
Administration For ophthalmic use only; avoid touching tip of applicator to eye or other surfaces. Contact lenses should be removed prior to application; may be reinserted after 10 minutes. Do not wear contact lenses if eyes are red.
Patient Information For ophthalmic use only. Wash hands before using. Remove contact lenses before application (may be reinserted after ten minutes). May cause blurred vision, temporary stinging or burning sensation. Do not wear contact lenses if eyes are red.
Dosage Forms Excipient information presented when available (limited, particularly for generics); consult specific product labeling.
Solution, ophthalmic, as hydrochloride: 0.05% (5 mL) [contains benzalkonium chloride]

♦ **Epinastine Hydrochloride** *see* Epinastine *on page 577*

Epinephrine (ep i NEF rin)

Medication Safety Issues
Sound-alike/look-alike issues:
Epinephrine may be confused with ephedrine
Epifrin® may be confused with ephedrine, EpiPen®
EpiPen® may be confused with Epifrin®

Medication errors have occurred due to confusion with epinephrine products expressed as ratio strengths (eg, 1:1000 vs 1:10,000).
Epinephrine 1:1000 = 1 mg/mL and is most commonly used SubQ.
Epinephrine 1:10,000 = 0.1 mg/mL and is used I.V.
International issues:
EpiPen® may be confused with Epigen® which is a brand name for glycyrrhizinic acid in Mexico
EpiPen® may be confused with Epopen® which is a brand name for epoetin alfa in Spain
Related Information
Adult ACLS Algorithms *on page 1660*
Asthma *on page 1904*
(Continued)

Epinephrine *(Continued)*

CPR Pediatric Drug Dosages *on page 1650*
Emergency Pediatric Drip Calculations *on page 1652*
Extravasation Treatment *on page 1726*
Neonatal Resuscitation Algorithm *on page 1656*
Pediatric ALS Algorithms *on page 1657*

U.S. Brand Names Adrenalin®; EpiPen®; EpiPen® Jr; Primatene® Mist [OTC]; Raphon [OTC]; S2® [OTC]; Twinject™

Canadian Brand Names Adrenalin®; EpiPen®; EpiPen® Jr; Twinject™

Index Terms Adrenaline; Epinephrine Bitartrate; Epinephrine Hydrochloride; Racepinephrine

Therapeutic Category Adrenergic Agonist Agent; Antiasthmatic; Antidote, Hypersensitivity Reactions; Bronchodilator; Decongestant, Nasal; Sympathomimetic

Generic Available Yes: Solution for injection

Use Treatment of bronchospasm, anaphylactic reactions, and cardiac arrest; nasal decongestant (topical nasal formulation); upper airway obstruction and croup (racemic epinephrine)

Pregnancy Risk Factor C

Lactation Excretion in breast milk unknown

Contraindications Hypersensitivity to epinephrine or any component (see Warnings); cardiac arrhythmias, angle-closure glaucoma

Warnings Some products contain sulfites which may cause allergic reactions in susceptible individuals

Precautions Use with caution in patients with diabetes mellitus, cardiovascular disease (angina, tachycardia, MI), thyroid disease, or cerebral arteriosclerosis; rebound nasal congestion may occur after frequent nasal use

Adverse Reactions

Cardiovascular: Pallor, tachycardia, hypertension, increased myocardial oxygen consumption, cardiac arrhythmias, sudden death

Central nervous system: Anxiety, headache

Gastrointestinal: Nausea

Genitourinary: Acute urinary retention in patients with bladder outflow obstruction

Neuromuscular & skeletal: Weakness, tremor

Ocular: Precipitation of or exacerbation of narrow-angle glaucoma

Renal: Decreased renal and splanchnic blood flow

Drug Interactions Increased cardiac irritability if administered concurrently with halogenated inhalational anesthetics; beta-blocking agents (ie, propranolol); alpha-blocking agents (eg, phentolamine); alpha- and beta-blocking agents (labetalol); phenothiazines with alpha-blocking activity; tricyclic antidepressants enhance pressor response to epinephrine

Stability Protect from light; incompatible with alkaline solutions (sodium bicarbonate); compatible when coadministered with dopamine, dobutamine, inamrinone (amrinone), atracurium, pancuronium, and vecuronium

Mechanism of Action Stimulates alpha-, $beta_1$- and $beta_2$-adrenergic receptors resulting in relaxation of smooth muscle of the bronchial tree, cardiac stimulation, and dilation of skeletal muscle vasculature; small doses can cause vasodilation via $beta_2$-vascular receptors; large doses may produce constriction of skeletal and vascular smooth muscle; decreases production of aqueous humor and increases aqueous outflow; dilates the pupil by contracting the dilator muscle

Pharmacodynamics

Local vasoconstriction (topical):
- Onset of action: 5 minutes
- Duration: <1 hour

Onset of bronchodilation:
- Inhalation: Within 1 minute
- SubQ.: Within 5-10 minutes

Pharmacokinetics

Absorption: Orally ingested doses are rapidly metabolized in GI tract and liver; pharmacologically active concentrations are **not** achieved

Distribution: Crosses placenta but not blood-brain barrier

Metabolism: Extensive in the liver and other tissues by the enzymes catechol-o-methyltransferase and monoamine oxidase

Usual Dosage

Neonates: I.V., Intratracheal: 0.01-0.03 mg/kg (0.1-0.3 mL/kg of **1:10,000** solution) every 3-5 minutes as needed

Infants and Children:

Hypersensitivity reactions: **Note:** For self-administration following severe allergic reactions (eg, insect stings, food), the World Health Organization (WHO) and

Anaphylaxis Canada recommend the availability of 1 dose for every 10-20 minutes of travel time to a medical emergency facility.

I.M.: EpiPen® and EpiPen® Jr: 0.01 mg/kg

or as alternative

<30 kg: 0.15 mg

≥30 kg: 0.3 mg

I.M., SubQ: Twinject™:

Children 15-30 kg: 0.15 mg

Children >30 kg: 0.3 mg

I.V.: 0.01 mg/kg (0.1 mL/kg of **1:10,000** solution) not to exceed 0.5 mg every 20 minutes; may use continuous infusion (0.1 mcg/kg/minute) to prevent frequent doses in more severe reactions

SubQ, I.M.: 0.01 mg/kg (0.01 mL/kg/dose of **1:1000** solution) not to exceed 0.5 mg every 20 minutes

Bradycardia:

I.V.: 0.01 mg/kg (0.1 mL/kg) of **1:10,000** solution (maximum dose: 1 mg or 10 mL); may repeat every 3-5 minutes as needed

Intratracheal: 0.1 mg/kg (0.1 mL/kg) of **1:1000** solution; doses as high as 0.2 mg/kg may be effective; may repeat every 3-5 minutes as needed

Asystole or pulseless arrest:

I.V. or I.O.: 0.01 mg/kg (0.1 mL/kg) of **1:10,000** solution; may repeat every 3-5 minutes as needed; if ineffective, may increase dosage to 0.1 mg/kg (0.1 mL/kg of **1:1000** solution; doses as high as 0.2 mg/kg may be effective); repeat every 3-5 minutes as needed [increased dosage no longer routinely recommended by the American Heart Association (see References)]

Intratracheal: 0.1 mg/kg (0.1 mL/kg) of **1:1000** solution (doses as high as 0.2 mg/kg may be effective); **Note:** Recent clinical studies suggest that lower epinephrine concentrations delivered by intrathecal administration may produce transient β-adrenergic effects which may be detrimental (eg, hypotension, lower coronary artery perfusion pressure). I.V. or I.O. are the preferred methods of administration (AHA, 2005).

Inotropic support: Continuous I.V. infusion rate: 0.1-1 mcg/kg/minute; titrate dosage to desired effect

Nebulization: 0.25-0.5 mL of 2.25% **racemic epinephrine** solution diluted in 3 mL NS, or L-epinephrine at an equivalent dose; racemic epinephrine 10 mg = 5 mg L-epinephrine; use lower end of dosing range for younger infants

Nasal: Children ≥6 years and Adults: Apply drops locally as needed; do not exceed 1 mL every 15 minutes

Adults:

Asystole/pulseless arrest bradycardia, VT/VF: I.V., I.O.: 1 mg every 3-5 minutes; if this approach fails, alternative regimens include:

Intermediate: 2-5 mg every 3-5 minutes

Escalating: 1 mg, 3 mg, 5 mg at 3-minute intervals

High: 0.1 mg/kg every 3-5 minutes

Intratracheal: 1 mg (although the optimal dose is unknown, doses of 2-2.5 times the I.V. dose may be needed)

Bradycardia (symptomatic) or hypotension (not responsive to atropine or pacing): I.V. infusion: 2-10 mcg/minute; titrate to desired effect

Bronchodilator:

SubQ: 0.3-0.5 mg every 20 minutes for 3 doses

Nebulization: S2® (racemic epinephrine, OTC labeling): 0.5 mL: Repeat no more frequently than every 3-4 hours as needed.

Inhalation: Primatene® Mist (OTC labeling): One inhalation, wait at least 1 minute; if relieved, may use once more. Do not use again for at least 3 hours.

Hypersensitivity reactions: **Note:** For self-administration following severe allergic reactions (eg, insect stings, food), the World Health Organization (WHO) and Anaphylaxis Canada recommend the availability of 1 dose for every 10-20 minutes of travel time to a medical emergency facility. More than 2 doses should only be administered under direct medical supervision.

I.M.: EpiPen®: 0.3 mg

I.M., SubQ: Twinject™: 0.3 mg

I.M., SubQ: 0.3-0.5 mg (**1:1000** formulation) may repeat every 15-20 minutes, if condition requires; I.M. route is preferred

I.V.: 0.1 mg (**1:10,000** formulation); may use continuous infusion (1-4 mcg/minute) to prevent the need to repeat injections

Administration

Inhalation: Nebulization: Dilute in 3 mL NS

Intratracheal: Administer and flush with a minimum of 5 mL NS, followed by 5 manual ventilations

Nasal: Apply as drops or with sterile swab

Oral inhalation: Shake well before use; use spacer in children <8 years of age

(Continued)

Epinephrine *(Continued)*

Parenteral:

Direct I.V. or I.O. administration: Dilute to a maximum concentration of 100 mcg/mL (if using 1:10,000 concentration, no dilution is necessary)

Continuous I.V. infusion: Rate of infusion (mL/hour) = dose (mcg/kg/minute) x weight (kg) x 60 minutes/hour divided by the concentration (mcg/mL); maximum concentration: 64 mcg/mL

I.M. (EpiPen®, EpiPen® Jr, and Twinject™): Intramuscularly into anterolateral aspect of thigh

SubQ: Use only 1:1000 solution or 1:200 suspension

Monitoring Parameters EKG, heart rate, blood pressure, site of infusion for excessive blanching/extravasation

Nursing Implications Tissue irritant; extravasation may be treated by local small injections of a diluted phentolamine solution (mix 5 mg with 9 mL NS)

Dosage Forms Excipient information presented when available (limited, particularly for generics); consult specific product labeling.

Aerosol for oral inhalation:

Primatene® Mist: 0.22 mg/inhalation (15 mL, 22.5 mL) [contains CFCs]

Injection, solution [prefilled auto injector]:

EpiPen®: 0.3 mg/0.3 mL [1:1000] (2 mL) [contains sodium metabisulfite; available as single unit or in double-unit pack with training unit]

EpiPen® Jr: 0.15 mg/0.3 mL [1:2000] (2 mL) [contains sodium metabisulfite; available as single unit or in double-unit pack with training unit]

Twinject™: 0.15 mg/0.15 mL [1:1000] (1.1 mL) [contains sodium bisulfite; two 0.15 mg doses per injector]; 0.3 mg/0.3 mL [1:1000] (1.1 mL) [contains sodium bisulfite; two 0.3 mg doses per injector]

Injection, solution, as hydrochloride: 0.1 mg/mL [1:10,000] (10 mL); 1 mg/mL [1:1000] (1 mL) [products may contain sodium metabisulfite]

Adrenalin®: 1 mg/mL [1:1000] (1 mL, 30 mL) [contains sodium bisulfite]

Solution for oral inhalation, as hydrochloride:

Adrenalin®: 1% [10 mg/mL, 1:100] (7.5 mL) [contains sodium bisulfite]

Solution for oral inhalation [racepinephrine]:

S2®: 2.25% (0.5 mL, 15 mL) [as d-epinephrine 1.125% and l-epinephrine 1.125%; contains metabisulfites]

Solution, topical [racepinephrine]:

Raphon: 2.25% (15 mL) [as d-epinephrine 1.125% and l-epinephrine 1.125%; contains metabisulfites]

References

American College of Cardiology, American Heart Association Task Force, "Adult Advanced Cardiac Life Support" and "Pediatric Advanced Life Support Guidelines," *JAMA*, 1992, 268(16):2199-241 and 2262-75.

"2005 American Heart Association (AHA) Guidelines for Cardiopulmonary Resuscitation (CPR) and Emergency Cardiovascular Care (ECC) of Pediatric and Neonatal Patients: Pediatric Advanced Life Support," *Pediatrics*, 2006, 117(5):1005-28.

Waisman Y, Klein BL, Boenning DA, et al, "Prospective Randomized Double-Blind Study Comparing L-Epinephrine and Racemic Epinephrine Aerosols in the Treatment of Laryngotracheitis (Croup)," *Pediatrics*, 1992, 89(2):302-6.

♦ **Epinephrine and Lidocaine** *see* Lidocaine and Epinephrine *on page 936*
♦ **Epinephrine Bitartrate** *see* Epinephrine *on page 577*
♦ **Epinephrine Hydrochloride** *see* Epinephrine *on page 577*
♦ **EpiPen®** *see* Epinephrine *on page 577*
♦ **EpiPen® Jr** *see* Epinephrine *on page 577*
♦ **Epipodophyllotoxin** *see* Etoposide *on page 625*
♦ **Epitol®** *see* Carbamazepine *on page 279*
♦ **Epival® I.V. (Can)** *see* Valproic Acid and Derivatives *on page 1592*
♦ **Epivir®** *see* Lamivudine *on page 901*
♦ **Epivir-HBV®** *see* Lamivudine *on page 901*
♦ **EPO** *see* Epoetin Alfa *on page 580*

Epoetin Alfa (e POE e tin AL fa)

Medication Safety Issues

Sound-alike/look-alike issues:

Epoetin alfa may be confused with darbepoetin alfa

International issues:

Epopen® [Spain] may be confused with EpiPen® which is a brand name for epinephrine in the U.S.

U.S. Brand Names Epogen®; Procrit®

Canadian Brand Names Eprex®

Index Terms EPO; Erythropoiesis-Stimulating Agent (ESA); Erythropoietin; NSC-724223; *r*HuEPO-α

Therapeutic Category Colony-Stimulating Factor; Recombinant Human Erythropoietin

Generic Available No

Use Treatment of anemia associated with end-stage renal disease; anemia in cancer patients with nonmyeloid malignancies on chemotherapy; anemia related to AIDS and therapy with zidovudine-treated, HIV-infected patients; endogenous serum erythropoietin (EPO) levels which are inappropriately low for hemoglobin level (eg, anemia of neoplasia); anemia of prematurity; patients undergoing autologous blood donation prior to surgery (EPO may accelerate recovery of hemoglobin level and, in some cases, permit more units of blood to be donated)

Pregnancy Risk Factor C

Lactation Excretion in breast milk unknown/use caution

Contraindications Hypersensitivity to epoetin alfa, albumin (human) or mammalian cell-derived products, or any component of epoetin alfa (see Warnings); uncontrolled hypertension; neutropenia in newborns

Warnings Due to an increased risk of cardiac arrest, neurologic events (including seizures and stroke), exacerbations of hypertension, CHF, vascular thrombosis/ ischemia,infarction, acute MI, and fluid overdose/edema in patients whose Hgb increased >12 g/dL, hemoglobin should be monitored twice weekly for 2-6 weeks following initiation and the EPO dosage should be decreased if the Hgb exceeds 12 g/dL or the rate of rise of hemoglobin exceeds 1 g/dL in any 2 week period. Cancer patients are generally at a higher risk for thrombotic events. Blood pressure should be controlled adequately before initiation of EPO therapy particularly in CRF patients; approximately 25% of CRF patients on dialysis may require increased antihypertensive medications while receiving epoetin; hypertensive encephalopathy and seizures have been observed in CRF patients treated with epoetin; close blood pressure monitoring is recommended. Seizures have occurred during therapy; monitor closely for premonitory neurologic symptoms during the first several months of therapy. Pure red cell aplasia (PRCA) and severe anemia have been reported, predominantly in patients with CRF and patients receiving other erythropoiesis stimulating proteins. Should a sudden loss of responsiveness to epoetin alfa combined with a severe anemia and low reticulocyte count occur, temporarily discontinue epoetin and determine if anti-erythropoietin antibodies are present. Discontinue epoetin if these antibodies are detected. Prior to and during epoetin therapy, assess the patient's iron stores utilizing serum ferritin, TIBC; supplemental iron therapy is recommended to support erythropoiesis and avoid depletion of iron stores. EPO is not approved for use in patients with myeloid malignancies or in patients with cancer-related anemia who are not receiving concurrent chemotherapy.

The multidose formulation contains benzyl alcohol which may cause allergic reactions in susceptible individuals; large amounts of benzyl alcohol (≥99 mg/kg/day) have been associated with a potentially fatal toxicity ("gasping syndrome") in neonates; the "gasping syndrome" consists of metabolic acidosis, respiratory distress, gasping respirations, CNS dysfunction (including convulsions, intracranial hemorrhage), hypotension and cardiovascular collapse; avoid use of multidose formulation in neonates; *in vitro* and animal studies have shown that benzoate, a metabolite of benzyl alcohol, displaces bilirubin from protein-binding sites. Pooled use of unused portions of preservative-free EPO has resulted in microbial contamination, bacteremia, and pyrogenic reactions. Preservative-free formulations are intended for single use only.

Factors Limiting Response to Epoetin Alfa

Factor	Mechanism
Iron deficiency	Limits hemoglobin synthesis
Blood loss/hemolysis	Counteracts epoetin alfa-stimulated erythropoiesis
Infection/inflammation	Inhibits iron transfer from storage to bone marrow Suppresses erythropoiesis through activated macrophages
Aluminum overload	Inhibits iron incorporation into heme protein
Bone marrow replacement Hyperparathyroidism Metastatic, neoplastic disease	Limits bone marrow volume
Folic acid/vitamin B_{12} deficiency	Limits hemoglobin synthesis
Patient compliance	Self-administered epoetin alfa or iron therapy

(Continued)

Epoetin Alfa *(Continued)*

Precautions Use with caution in patients with porphyria or a history of seizures. EPO is not intended for patients who require acute corrections of anemia and is not a substitute for emergency blood transfusion.

Assessment of iron stores and therapeutic iron supplementation is essential to optimal EPO therapy. Iron supplementation is necessary to provide for increased requirements during expansion of the red cell mass secondary to marrow stimulation by EPO, unless iron stores are already in excess.

Adverse Reactions

Cardiovascular: Hypertension, edema, chest pain, thrombotic vascular events (eg, MI, CVA/TIA)
Central nervous system: Fatigue, dizziness, headache, seizure, fever
Dermatologic: Rash, urticaria
Gastrointestinal: Nausea, diarrhea, vomiting
Hematologic: Neutropenia, pure red cell aplasia (PRCA), anemia
Local: Pain, irritation at injection site (SubQ injection)
Neuromuscular & skeletal: Arthralgias, weakness
Respiratory: Cough
Miscellaneous: Hypersensitivity reactions

Stability Refrigerate; single-dose vials contain no preservatives; discard after entry (see Warnings). Multiple-dose vials contain benzyl alcohol preservative and are stable 2 weeks at room temperature and when refrigerated, may be used up to 21 days after initial entry. Prefilled syringes containing the preservative formulation are stable for 6 weeks refrigerated (2°C to 8°C) (Naughton, 2003). EPO is stable for 24 hours when diluted in dextrose I.V. fluid which contains at least 0.05% human albumin or parenteral nutrition solutions containing at least 0.5% amino acids. EPO may be diluted with NS or bacteriostatic NS in a 1:1 ratio at the time of SubQ administration.

Mechanism of Action Epoetin alfa, a glycoprotein manufactured by recombinant DNA technology, has the same effects as endogenous erythropoietin. EPO induces erythropoiesis by stimulating the division and differentiation of committed erythroid progenitor cells. It induces the release of reticulocytes from the bone marrow into the bloodstream, where they mature to erythrocytes (dose response relationship) resulting in an increase in reticulocyte counts followed by a rise in hematocrit and hemoglobin levels. There is normally an inverse correlation between the plasma EPO level and the hemoglobin concentration (only when the hemoglobin concentration is <10.5 g/dL).

Pharmacodynamics

Onset of action: Several days
Maximum effect: 2-6 weeks

Pharmacokinetics

Absorption: SubQ: 31.9%
Distribution: Adults: V_d: 9 L; rapid in the plasma compartment; majority of drug is taken up by the liver, kidneys, and bone marrow
Bioavailability: SubQ: ~21% to 31%
Half-life:
- Neonates: SubQ: 17.6 hours on day 3 of therapy, 11.2 hours on day 10 of therapy
- Adults: 4-13 hours in patients with chronic renal failure (CRF); half-life is 20% shorter in patients with normal renal function

Time to peak serum concentration: SubQ: 5-24 hours
Elimination: Some metabolic degradation does occur with small amounts recovered in the urine
- Clearance: Neonates: SubQ or continuous I.V. infusion: 26-35 mL/hour/kg on day 3 of therapy and 65-87 mL/hour/kg on day 10 of therapy

Note: While a much higher peak plasma concentration is achieved after I.V. bolus administration, it declines at a more rapid rate (over 2-3 days) than after subcutaneous administration (plasma concentrations greater than endogenous are maintained for at least 4 days). Subcutaneous administration is associated with a 30% to 50% lower EPO dose requirement.

Usual Dosage Dosing schedules need to be individualized and careful monitoring of patients receiving the drug is recommended. EPO may be ineffective if other factors such as iron or B_{12}/folate deficiency limit marrow response. Dosage based upon SubQ administration; use of I.V. administration may result in the need to increase doses by as much as 30% to 50% to achieve the same outcome: I.V., SubQ:

Anemia of prematurity: Neonates: Variable regimens: 25-100 units/kg/dose 3 times/week **or** 100 units/kg/dose 5 times/week **or** 200 units/kg/dose every other day for 10 doses

Anemia in cancer patients: **Note:** Use in patients with pretreatment serum EPO levels >200 is **not** recommended

Children 6 months to 18 years: Doses ranging from 25-300 units/kg 3-7 times/week have been reported

Manufacturer's recommendation: Based upon a randomized, double-blind, placebo controlled study of 222 children, 5-18 years, using I.V. administration only: 600 units/kg weekly (not to exceed 40,000 units/week); may increase to 900 units/kg weekly (not to exceed 60,000 units/week); use caution in considering this dosage for administration by the SubQ route as SubQ administration has been shown to produce effect at doses 30% to 50% lower than I.V. administration

Adults: 150 units/kg/dose 3 times/week; maximum 1200 units/kg/week; or as an alternative: 40,000 units once weekly; may increase to 60,000 units once weekly if hemoglobin is not increased by at least 1 g/dL after 4 weeks of treatment

Anemia in chronic renal failure:

Initial dose:

Children: 50 units/kg/dose 3 times/week

Adults: 50-100 units/kg/dose 3 times/week

Maintenance dose: Children and Adults: Titrate dose to response (see Epoetin Alfa Dosage Adjustments); median dose: 75 units/kg 3 times/week (range: 12.5-525 units/kg 3 times/week)

Note: Once weekly dosage has been studied in chronic renal failure patients. When transitioning from multiple doses/week to once weekly, begin with a weekly dosage equal to the current total dose per week. Allow at least 4 weeks to determine full effects of the new regimen.

Epoetin Alfa Dosage Adjustments

Target hemoglobin range	CRF, zidovudine-treated HIV: 12 g/dL Cancer: 10-12 g/dL
Reduce dose when	Target range is reached **or** hemoglobin increases >1 g/dL in any 2-week period
Increase dose when	Hemoglobin does not increase by 2 g/dL after 8 weeks of therapy **and** hemoglobin is below target range
Stop therapy when	Hemoglobin >13 g/dL; reinstate therapy at a 25% lower dose after the hemoglobin decreases to target or 12 g/dL

Zidovudine-treated, HIV-infected patients:

Children 8 months to 17 years: Limited data available; doses ranging from 50-400 units/kg 2-3 times/week have been reported

Adults (pretreatment serum EPO levels ≤500 mUnits/mL and receiving zidovudine ≤4200 mg/week): Initial: 100 units/kg/dose 3 times/week for 8 weeks; after 8 weeks of therapy the dose may be adjusted by 50-100 units/kg increments 3 times/week to a maximum dose of 300 units/kg 3 times/week

Presurgery, autologous blood donation: Adults: 300 units/kg/day for 10 days before surgery, the day of surgery, and 4 days after **or as an alternative**, 600 units/kg/week at 21-, 14-, and 7 days before surgery and on the day of surgery

Administration Parenteral: Do not shake as this may denature the glycoprotein rendering the drug biologically inactive

SubQ is the preferred route of administration; 1:1 dilution with bacteriostatic NS (containing benzyl alcohol) acts as a local anesthetic to reduce pain at the injection site. Multiple-dose vials already contain benzyl alcohol.

I.V.: Dilute with an equal volume of NS and infuse over 1-3 minutes; it may be administered into the venous line at the end of the dialysis procedure

Test	Initial Phase Frequency	Maintenance Phase Frequency
Hemoglobin	CRF: 2 times/week; Cancer, HIV: Once weekly	2-4 times/month
Blood pressure	3 times/week	3 times/week
Serum ferritin	Monthly	Quarterly
Transferrin saturation	Monthly	Quarterly
Serum chemistries including CBC with differential, creatinine, BUN, potassium, phosphorous	Regularly per routine	Regularly per routine
Reticulocyte count	Baseline prior to starting therapy	After 10 days of therapy

(Continued)

Epoetin Alfa *(Continued)*

Monitoring Parameters

Careful monitoring of blood pressure is indicated; problems with hypertension have been noted especially in renal failure patients treated with EPO. Other patients are less likely to develop this complication. See table on previous page.

Reference Range The decision to initiate EPO therapy may be made by utilizing an endogenous erythropoietin serum level measurement. Endogenous erythropoietin levels are inversely related to the hemoglobin (and hematocrit) level in anemias that are not attributed to impaired erythropoietin production (eg, iron deficiency anemia). A normal erythropoietin level, for subjects with normal hemoglobin and hematocrit, is 4.1-22.2 mIU/mL. Baseline erythropoietin levels in anemic patients may increase up to 100-1000 fold in untreated patients with a normal release of erythropoietin. The following table illustrates the "normal" response to anemia. EPO is indicated in patients who do not exhibit a normal response to anemia (eg, the measurement of endogenous erythropoietin is low relative to a normal response). If the patient has exhibited a normal response, addition of exogenous EPO may not be beneficial. Clinical studies involving the following disease states have established criteria for assessment of endogenous erythropoietin levels prior to initiating EPO therapy:

Zidovudine-treated HIV patients: Available evidence indicates patients with endogenous serum erythropoietin levels >500 mIU/mL are unlikely to respond

Cancer chemotherapy patients: Treatment of patients with endogenous serum erythropoietin levels >200 mIU/mL is not recommended.

Inverse Relationship of Endogenous Erythropoietin to Hemoglobin

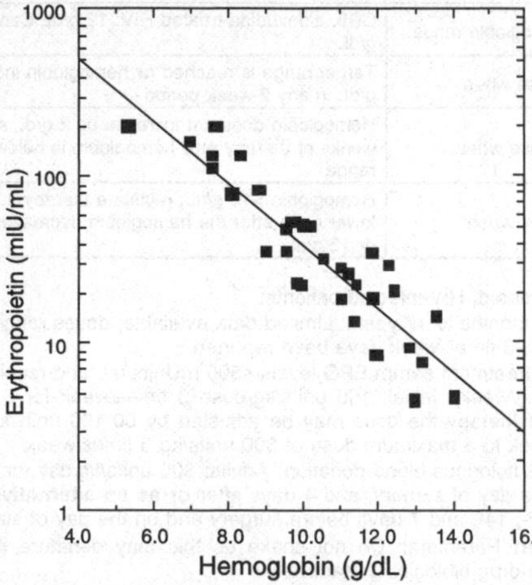

Patient Information Frequent blood tests are needed to determine the correct dose; notify physician if any severe headache develops; due to increased risk of seizure activity in CRF patients during the first 90 days of therapy, avoid potentially hazardous activities (eg, driving during this period)

Additional Information Optimal response is achieved when iron stores are maintained with supplemental iron if necessary; evaluate iron stores prior to and during therapy

Reimbursement Hotline (Epogen®): 1-800-272-9376
Professional Services [Amgen]: 1-800-77-AMGEN
Reimbursement Hotline (Procrit®): 1-800-553-3851
Professional Services [Ortho Biotech]: 1-800-325-7504

Dosage Forms Excipient information presented when available (limited, particularly for generics); consult specific product labeling.

Injection, solution [preservative free]:

Epogen®, Procrit®: 2000 units/mL (1 mL); 3000 units/mL (1 mL); 4000 units/mL (1 mL); 10,000 units/mL (1 mL); 40,000 units/mL (1 mL) [contains human albumin]

Injection, solution [with preservative]:

Epogen®, Procrit®: 10,000 units/mL (2 mL); 20,000 units/mL (1 mL) [contains human albumin and benzyl alcohol]

References

Blanche S, Caniglia M, Fischer A, et al, "Zidovudine Therapy in Children With Acquired Immunodeficiency Syndrome," *Am J Med*, 1988, 85(2A):203-7.

Halperin DS, Wacker P, Lacourt G, et al, "Effects of Recombinant Human Erythropoietin in Infants With the Anemia of Prematurity: A Pilot Study," *J Pediatr*, 1990, 116(5):779-86.

Naughton CA, Duppong LM, Forbes KD, et al, "Stability of Multidose, Preserved Formulation Epoetin Alfa in Syringes for Three and Six Weeks," *Am J Health Syst Pharm*, 2003, 60(5):464-8.

Ohls RK and Christensen, RD, "Stability of Human Recombinant Epoetin Alfa in Commonly Used Neonatal Intravenous Solutions," *Ann Pharmacother*, 1996, 30(5):466-468.

Ohls RK, Veerman MW, and Christensen RD, "Pharmacokinetics and Effectiveness of Recombinant Erythropoietin Administered to Preterm Infants by Continuous Infusion in Total Parenteral Nutrition Solution," *J Pediatr*, 1996, 128(4):518-23.

Rhondeau SM, Christensen RD, Ross MP, et al, "Responsiveness to Recombinant Human Erythropoietin of Marrow Erythroid Progenitors From Infants With the Anemia of Prematurity," *J Pediatr*, 1988, 112(6):935-40.

Shannon KM, Keith JF 3rd, Mentzer WC, et al, "Recombinant Human Erythropoietin Stimulates Erythropoiesis and Reduces Erythrocyte Transfusions in Very Low Birth Weight Preterm Infants," *Pediatrics*, 1995, 95(1):1-8.

Sinai-Trieman L, Salusky IB, and Fine RN, "Use of Subcutaneous Recombinant Human Erythropoietin in Children Undergoing Continuous Cycling Peritoneal Dialysis," *J Pediatr*, 1989, 114(4 Pt 1):550-4.

♦ **Epogen®** *see* Epoetin Alfa *on page 580*

Epoprostenol (e poe PROST en ole)

Related Information

New York Heart Association (NYHA) Classification of Functional Capacity of Patients With Diseases of the Heart, 1994 Revisions *on page 1679*

U.S. Brand Names Flolan®

Canadian Brand Names Flolan®

Index Terms Epoprostenol Sodium; PGI_2; PGX; Prostacyclin

Therapeutic Category Prostaglandin

Generic Available No

Use

Long-term I.V. treatment of primary pulmonary hypertension (PPH) and pulmonary hypertension secondary to the scleroderma spectrum of disease, in NYHA Class III and Class IV patients who are not fully responsive to other therapy.

Short-term I.V. infusion of epoprostenol in patients with pulmonary hypertension may be used diagnostically in the cardiac catheterization laboratory to screen for responsiveness to other oral vasodilating agents (eg, calcium channel blockers). **Note:** Responsiveness to short-term (acute) I.V. infusions of epoprostenol predicts responsiveness to long-term treatment with oral calcium channel blockers; however, it does not predict responsiveness to long-term I.V. epoprostenol therapy. Patients who do not respond acutely to epoprostenol, may respond to the drug when used chronically.

Other potential uses include treatment of secondary pulmonary hypertension associated with ARDS, SLE, congenital heart disease, congenital diaphragmatic hernia, neonatal pulmonary hypertension, cardiopulmonary bypass surgery, hemodialysis, peripheral vascular disorders, portal hypertension, and neonatal purpura fulminans.

Restrictions Orders for epoprostenol are distributed by two sources in the United States. Information on orders or reimbursement assistance may be obtained from either Accredo Health, Inc (1-800-935-6526) or TheraCom, Inc (1-877-356-5264).

Pregnancy Risk Factor B

Lactation Excretion in breast milk unknown/use caution

Contraindications Hypersensitivity to epoprostenol, any component, or structurally-related compounds; chronic use in patients with CHF due to severe left ventricular systolic dysfunction. **Note:** Do not use epoprostenol chronically in patients who develop pulmonary edema during dose initiation (see Warnings).

Warnings Epoprostenol **must** be reconstituted with the manufacturer-supplied sterile diluent only; do **not** reconstitute or mix with other I.V. fluids or I.V. medications prior to or during administration. Abrupt withdrawal, interruptions in drug delivery, or sudden reductions in epoprostenol dosage may result in symptoms associated with rebound pulmonary hypertension (eg, asthenia, dizziness, dyspnea) and can be potentially fatal; avoid abrupt withdrawal, interruptions in drug delivery, and sudden large reductions in dosage. Pulmonary edema, which may be associated with pulmonary veno-occlusive disease may develop in patients with pulmonary hypertension during epoprostenol dose initiation (do not use epoprostenol chronically in these patients).

Symptoms of overdose include headache, hypotension, tachycardia, nausea, vomiting, diarrhea, and flushing. Reduce the infusion rate to decrease symptoms. If symptoms do not subside or worsen, consider drug discontinuation. Fatalities due to hypoxemia, hypotension, and respiratory arrest have been reported following overdose with epoprostenol.

Precautions Use with caution and appropriately monitor patients; epoprostenol is a potent pulmonary and systemic vasodilator; it should be used only by clinicians who (Continued)

Epoprostenol *(Continued)*

are experienced in the diagnosis and treatment of pulmonary hypertension; dose initiation must occur in a setting with adequately trained personnel and proper equipment for physiologic monitoring and emergency care. Asymptomatic increases in pulmonary artery pressure, associated with increases in cardiac output, may rarely occur during dose initiation; consider dosage reduction in these patients. During chronic use, unless contraindicated, anticoagulants should be coadministered in adult patients to reduce the risk of thromboembolism [**Note:** The use of anticoagulants in **adult** patients with primary pulmonary hypertension has been shown to improve survival. Although such efficacy has **not** been demonstrated in pediatric patients, some studies have reported the routine use of warfarin in pediatric patients receiving long-term (chronic) infusions of epoprosentol for pulmonary hypertension (see Barst, 1999 and Rosenzweig, 1999), while other studies have routinely discontinued anticoagulants prior to the initiation of epoprostenol therapy (see Higenbottam, 1993); further studies are needed to assess the risks and benefits of routine anticoagulation in pediatric patients treated with epoprostenol.]

Adverse Reactions Note: Some reported adverse reactions may be related to the underlying disease (eg, chest pain, dyspnea, edema, fatigue, hypoxia, pallor, and right heart failure).

Cardiovascular: Flushing (acute: 58%; chronic 42%), hypotension, chest pain, bradycardia (vagal effect), reflex tachycardia, palpitations, arrhythmia, supraventricular tachycardia, MI

Central nervous system: Headache (acute: 49%; chronic: 83%), anxiety, nervousness, agitation, dizziness, restlessness, depression, convulsions, CVA

Dermatologic: Rash, urticaria, eczema, pruritus, skin ulcer

Endocrine & metabolic: Hypokalemia, hyperkalemia, weight reduction, weight gain

Gastrointestinal: Nausea, vomiting, diarrhea, abdominal pain, dyspepsia, anorexia, constipation, abdominal enlargement

Hematologic: Hemorrhage, thrombocytopenia

Local: Injection-site reactions: Infection (21%), pain (13%), irritation, erythema, thrombophlebitis

Neuromuscular & skeletal: Jaw pain, myalgia, musculoskeletal pain, tremor, back pain, neck pain, asthenia, hypesthesia, hyperesthesia, paresthesia, arthralgia

Ocular: Amblyopia, abnormal vision

Respiratory: Dyspnea, epistaxis, pleural effusion; pulmonary edema, which may be associated with pulmonary veno-occlusive disease (see Warnings)

Miscellaneous: Flu-like symptoms, diaphoresis, catheter-related sepsis

Drug Interactions Concurrent use of diuretics, antihypertensive agents, or other vasodilators may cause additional reduction in blood pressure. Concomitant use of antiplatelet agents or anticoagulants may increase the risk of bleeding.

Epoprostenol decreased the apparent oral clearance of digoxin by 15% and furosemide by 13% on day 2 of epoprostenol therapy; however, clearance values returned to baseline by day 87; epoprostenol may increase serum digoxin concentrations after initiation of epoprostenol therapy (monitor patients); the interaction with furosemide is not thought to be clinically significant.

Stability Store unopened vials of drug and sterile diluent at room temperature 15°C to 25°C (59°F to 77°F); protect drug vials from light; do not freeze diluent. Following reconstitution, solution must be stored under refrigeration at 2°C to 8°C (36°F to 46°F) if not used immediately; reconstituted solution is stable for up to 48 hours when refrigerated; protect from light; do not freeze (discard if solution has been frozen). Reconstituted solution (pH 10.2-10.8) is increasingly unstable at a lower pH and drug is rapidly hydrolyzed at the pH of I.V. fluids.

During use, a single reservoir of solution may be used at room temperature for a total duration of 8 hours, or used with a cold pouch for administration up to 24 hours. **Note:** Reconstituted solutions may be refrigerated for ≤40 hours prior to administration at room temperature for up to 8 hours. Reconstituted solutions may be refrigerated for ≤24 hours prior to administration with a cold pouch for up to 24 hours. Cold pouch should be changed every 12 hours and must be capable of maintaining the reconstituted solution at a temperature between 2°C to 8°C for 12 hours.

Mechanism of Action Epoprostenol (also known as prostacyclin, PGI_2 and PGX), is a metabolite of arachidonic acid and a naturally-occurring prostaglandin. It is a potent, direct-acting, vasodilator of pulmonary and systemic arterial vascular beds. In addition, it inhibits platelet aggregation and vascular smooth muscle proliferation. The reduction in platelet aggregation results from epoprostenol's activation of intracellular adenylate cyclase and the resultant increase in cyclic adenosine monophosphate concentrations within the platelets (**Note:** Patients with PPH have an imbalance in the ratio of thromboxane to prostacyclin metabolites and have a decreased amount of prostacyclin synthase in the pulmonary arteries).

Clinically, the vasodilator effects decrease right ventricular and left ventricular afterload and increase cardiac output and stroke volume. Epoprostenol decreases pulmonary vascular resistance, mean pulmonary artery pressure, and mean systemic arterial pressure. Additionally, it is capable of decreasing thrombogenesis and platelet clumping in the lungs by inhibiting platelet aggregation. Studies have demonstrated an increase in exercise capacity and improvements in dyspnea and fatigue.

Pharmacokinetics

Metabolism: Rapidly hydrolyzed at a neutral pH in blood; also metabolized by enzymatic degradation; two primary metabolites with pharmacologic activity less than epoprostenol are formed: 6-keto-PGF_{1alpha} (via spontaneous degradation) and 6,15-diketo-13,14-dihydro-PGF_{1alpha} (via enzymatic degradation); 14 minor metabolites have also been isolated in the urine

Half-life: ≤6 minutes

Elimination: Urine (84% of dose); feces (4%)

Usual Dosage I.V.: Continuous infusion: **Note:** The need for increased doses should be expected with chronic use; incremental increases occur more frequently during the first few months after the drug is initiated. The optimal dose in children is not well defined. The mean chronic dose at 1 year of therapy is 20-40 ng/kg/minute in adults, but is 50-80 ng/kg/minute in children (particularly younger children); significant variability in optimal dose occurs in pediatric patients (see Barst, 1999; Rosenweig, 1999; and Widlitz, 2003).

Children and Adults:

Chronic infusion: Initial: 1-2 ng/kg/minute, increase dose in increments of 1-2 ng/kg/minute every 15 minutes or longer until dose-limiting side effects are noted or tolerance limit to epoprostenol is observed

Dose adjustment:

Increase dose in 1-2 ng/kg/minute increments at intervals of at least 15 minutes if symptoms of pulmonary hypertension persist or recur following improvement. In clinical trials, dosing increases occurred at intervals of 24-48 hours or longer.

Decrease dose in 2 ng/kg/minute decrements at intervals of at least 15 minutes in case of dose-limiting pharmacologic (adverse) events. Avoid abrupt withdrawal or sudden large dose reductions.

Lung transplant: In patients receiving lung transplants, epoprostenol was tapered after the initiation of cardiopulmonary bypass.

Administration Reconstitute with the manufacturer-supplied sterile diluent only; do **not** reconstitute or mix with other I.V. fluids or I.V. medications prior to or during administration (epoprostenol is very unstable in neutral or acidic pH solutions). To make a 100 mL solution (daily supply) with a final concentration of 3000 ng/mL, dilute one 0.5 mg vial of epoprostenol with 5 mL of supplied diluent; withdraw 3 mL and add to sufficient diluent to make a total of 100 mL. This 100 mL 24-hour supply may be divided into 3 equal parts; one portion can be used for up to 8 hours at room temperature, and the two other portions should be stored in the refrigerator and protected from light (see Stability). During use, a single reservoir of solution may be used at room temperature for a total duration of 8 hours, or used with a cold pouch for administration up to 24 hours (see Stability). The final concentration of epoprostenol solution is determined by the minimum and maximum flow rates of the infusion pump and desired duration of infusion from the specific reservoir volume. Concentrations >15,000 ng/mL may be required for patients receiving higher infusion rates. Maximum concentration for administration: 70,000 ng/mL.

I.V.: Continuous infusion: Chronic continuous I.V. infusions of epoprostenol must be administered through a permanent indwelling central venous catheter; use an ambulatory infusion pump for patients discharged home. Peripheral infusion may be used temporarily until central line is established. Epoprostenol should be infused in a dedicated lumen exclusive of any other drugs; consider a multilumen catheter if other I.V. medications are routinely administered. Avoid abrupt withdrawal, interruptions in delivery, or sudden large reductions in dosing (see Warnings). Patients should have access to a backup infusion pump and infusion sets.

Note: The ambulatory infusion pump should be small and lightweight; be able to adjust infusion rates in 2 ng/kg/minute increments; have occlusion, end of infusion, and low battery alarms; have ±6% accuracy of the programmed rate; and be positive continuous or pulsatile pressure-driven with intervals ≤3 minutes between pulses. The reservoir should be made of polypropylene, polyvinyl chloride, or glass. The infusion pump used in the most recent clinical trial was CADD-1 HFX 5100 (Pharmacia Deltec).

Monitoring Parameters Hemodynamic effects (pulmonary vascular resistance, pulmonary arterial pressure, systemic blood pressure, heart rate). Monitor blood pressure (standing and supine) and heart rate closely for several hours following dosage adjustments. Monitor for improvements in exercise capacity, exertional dyspnea, fatigue, syncope, chest pain, and quality of life. Monitor the infusion pump device and catheters to avoid drug delivery system related failures. Monitor weight; serum potassium.

(Continued)

Epoprostenol *(Continued)*

Patient Information For most adult patients and some pediatric patients, therapy with this medication will probably be prolonged, possibly for years. This medication is infused through a permanent indwelling central venous catheter, on a continuous basis, by a small, portable infusion pump. Interruptions of the infusion (even for a brief time) may result in a rapid symptomatic deterioration of the patient. The patient or caregiver must become familiar with and perform a sterile technique to prepare and administer the medication and to care for the central venous catheter.

This medication may cause jaw pain, headache, diarrhea, nervousness, and muscular pains (use of a mild analgesia may be recommended by your prescriber); may cause dizziness and impair ability to perform activities requiring mental alertness or physical coordination. Report immediately any signs or symptoms of acute or severe headache; back pain; increased difficult breathing; flushing; fever or chills; any unusual bleeding or bruising; chest pain; palpitations; irregular, slow or fast pulse; flushing; loss of sensation; or any onset of unresolved diarrhea.

Nursing Implications Epoprostenol must be reconstituted with manufacturer-supplied sterile diluent only. When administered chronically, it must be infused through a permanent indwelling central venous catheter via a portable infusion pump. Avoid abrupt withdrawal, interruptions in drug delivery, and sudden large reductions in dosage (see Warnings); be alert for any infusion pump malfunction. Assess for signs of overdose (eg, hypotension, hypoxia, flushing, tachycardia, fever, chills, anxiety, acute headache, tremor, vomiting, diarrhea). Instruct the patient or caregiver about proper aseptic technique, appropriate catheter care, and proper drug reconstitution and administration. Instruct patient to report adverse reactions since dosage adjustments may be necessary.

Additional Information The primary role of epoprostenol is in the treatment of primary pulmonary hypertension in patients unresponsive to other therapy. Response to initial therapy is evaluated in a controlled setting before chronic therapy is administered. The role of epoprostenol in the treatment of heart failure confers a negative impact on cardiovascular morbidity and mortality. Clinical trials in adults showed improvement of heart failure symptoms and exercise tolerance, but an increase in mortality.

Dosage Forms Excipient information presented when available (limited, particularly for generics); consult specific product labeling. Available as epoprostenol sodium; mg strength refers to epoprostenol

Injection, powder for reconstitution, as sodium: 0.5 mg, 1.5 mg [provided with 50 mL sterile diluent]

References

Barst RJ, "Pharmacologically Induced Pulmonary Vasodilatation in Children and Young Adults With Primary Pulmonary Hypertension," *Chest*, 1986, 89(4):497-503.

Barst RJ, Maislin G, and Fishman AP, "Vasodilator Therapy for Primary Pulmonary Hypertension in Children," *Circulation*, 1999, 99(9):1197-208.

Barst RJ, Rubin LJ, Long WA, et al, "A Comparison of Continuous Intravenous Epoprostenol (Prostacyclin) With Conventional Therapy for Primary Pulmonary Hypertension. The Primary Pulmonary Hypertension Study Group," *N Engl J Med*, 1996, 334(5):296-302.

Higenbottam TW, Spiegelhalter D, Scott JP, et al, "Prostacyclin (Epoprostenol) and Heart-Lung Transplantation as Treatments for Severe Pulmonary Hypertension," Br Heart J, 1994, 70:366-70.

Kermode J, Butt W, and Shann F, "Comparison Between Prostaglandin E1 and Epoprostenol (Prostacyclin) in Infants After Heart Surgery," *Br Heart J*, 1991, 66(2):175-8.

Rosenzweig EB, Kerstein D, and Barst RJ, "Long-Term Prostacyclin for Pulmonary Hypertension With Associated Congenital Heart Defects," *Circulation*, 1999, 99(14):1858-65.

Widlitz A and Barst RJ, "Pulmonary Arterial Hypertension in Children," *Eur Respir J*, 2003, 21(1):155-76.

- **Epoprostenol Sodium** *see* Epoprostenol *on page 585*
- **Eprex® (Can)** *see* Epoetin Alfa *on page 580*
- **Epsilon Aminocaproic Acid** *see* Aminocaproic Acid *on page 96*
- **Epsom Salts** *see* Magnesium Sulfate *on page 974*
- **Epsom Salts (Magnesium Sulfate)** *see* Magnesium Supplements *on page 976*
- **EPT** *see* Teniposide *on page 1504*
- **Eptacog Alfa (Activated)** *see* Factor VIIa (Recombinant) *on page 631*
- **Epzicom™** *see* Abacavir and Lamivudine *on page 35*
- **Equalizer Gas Relief [OTC]** *see* Simethicone *on page 1440*
- **Equetro™** *see* Carbamazepine *on page 279*

Ergocalciferol (er goe kal SIF e role)

Medication Safety Issues

Sound-alike/look-alike issues:

Calciferol™ may be confused with calcitriol

Drisdol® may be confused with Drysol™

U.S. Brand Names Calciferol™; Drisdol®

Canadian Brand Names Drisdol®; Ostoforte®

Index Terms Activated Ergosterol; Viosterol; Vitamin D_2

Therapeutic Category Nutritional Supplement; Vitamin D Analog; Vitamin, Fat Soluble

Generic Available Yes: Capsule

Use Prevention and treatment of vitamin D deficiency; treatment of rickets or osteomalacia; treatment of familial hypophosphatemia; treatment of hypoparathyroidism; prevention and treatment of vitamin D deficiency and insufficiency in patients with chronic kidney disease (CKD); dietary supplement

Pregnancy Risk Factor A (C if dose exceeds RDA recommendation)

Lactation Enters breast milk/compatible

Contraindications Hypersensitivity to ergocalciferol or any component (see Warnings); hypercalcemia; malabsorption syndrome; evidence of vitamin D toxicity

Warnings Some products contain tartrazine which may cause allergic reactions in susceptible individuals. Serum calcium times phosphorus (Ca x P) should not exceed 65 mg^2/dL^2 for infants and children ≤12 years and 55 mg^2/dL^2 for children >12 years and adults.

Precautions Use with caution in patients with coronary artery disease, renal stones, and impaired renal function; adequate calcium intake is necessary for clinical response to ergocalciferol therapy; maintain adequate fluid intake; avoid hypercalcemia

Adverse Reactions

Cardiovascular: Hypertension, arrhythmias, hypotension

Central nervous system: Drowsiness, irritability, headache, psychosis

Dermatologic: Pruritus

Endocrine & metabolic: Mild acidosis, hypercholesterolemia, polydipsia, weight loss

Gastrointestinal: Nausea, vomiting, anorexia, constipation, metallic taste, xerostomia, pancreatitis

Genitourinary: Albuminuria, nocturia, polyuria

Neuromuscular & skeletal: Weakness, myalgia, bone pain

Ocular: Photophobia

Renal: Polyuria, nephrocalcinosis

Drug Interactions May antagonize the effects of calcium channel blockers by increasing serum calcium level; may be associated with digoxin toxicity by increasing calcium levels; may result in an additive increase in calcium levels due to decreased calcium excretion by thiazide diuretics; magnesium-containing antacids (potential development of hypermagnesemia); cholestyramine, colestipol, orlistat, and excessive use of mineral oil decrease absorption

Stability Store at room temperature; protect from light

Mechanism of Action Vitamin D stimulates calcium and phosphate absorption from the small intestine; promotes secretion of calcium from bone to blood; promotes renal tubule phosphate resorption; acts directly on bone cells (osteoblasts) to stimulate skeletal growth and on the parathyroid glands to suppress parathyroid hormone synthesis and secretion

Pharmacodynamics Maximum effect occurs in ~1 month following daily doses

Pharmacokinetics

Absorption: Readily absorbed from GI tract; absorption requires intestinal presence of bile

Metabolism: Inactive until hydroxylated in the liver and the kidney to calcifediol and then to calcitriol (most active form)

Usual Dosage Oral dosing is preferred; use I.M. only in patients with GI, liver, or biliary disease associated with malabsorption of vitamin D:

Adequate Intake (AI) (1997 National Academy of Science Recommendations):
- Neonates, Children and Adults: 200 international units/day

Dietary supplementation (each mcg = 40 USP international units):
- Premature infants: 10-20 mcg/day (400-800 international units), up to 750 mcg/day (30,000 international units)
- Infants and healthy Children: 10 mcg/day (400 international units)
- Adults: 10 mcg/day (400 international units)

Vitamin D insufficiency or deficiency associated with CKD (Stages 3-4) (K/DOQI Guidelines, 2005); serum 25 hydroxyvitamin D (25(OH)D) level <30 ng/mL: Oral:
- Serum 25(OH)D level 16-30 ng/mL:
  - Children: 2,000 international units daily for 3 months or 50,000 international units every month for 3 months
  - Adults: 50,000 international units every month for 6 months
- Serum 25(OH)D level 5-15 ng/mL:
  - Children: 4,000 international units daily for 12 weeks or 50,000 international units every other week for 12 weeks

(Continued)

Ergocalciferol *(Continued)*

Adults: 50,000 international units/week for 4 weeks followed by monthly doses for a total therapy of 6 months

Serum 25(OH)D level <5 ng/mL:

Children: 8,000 international units daily for 4 weeks or 50,000 international units/week for 4 weeks followed by 4,000 international units daily or 50,000 international units 2 times/month for a total therapy of 3 months

Adults: 50,000 international units/week for 12 weeks then monthly for a total therapy of 6 months or 500,000 international units I.M. once

Dosage adjustment: Monitor 25(OH)D, serum calcium and phosphorus levels; if serum calcium level exceeds 10.2 mg/dL or 25(OH)D level is normal, discontinue therapy; if serum phosphorus exceeds upper limit for age or 4.6 mg/dL (adults), initiate oral phosphate binder therapy.

Hypoparathyroidism:

Children: 1.25-5 mg/day (50,000-200,000 international units) with calcium supplements

Adults: 625 mcg to 5 mg/day (25,000-200,000 international units) with calcium supplements

Vitamin D-dependent rickets:

Children: 75-125 mcg/day (3000-5000 international units); maximum dose: 1500 mcg/day (60,000 international units) may be necessary

Adults: 250 mcg to 1.5 mg/day (10,000-60,000 international units); doses as high as 12.5 mg/day may be necessary

Nutritional rickets and osteomalacia:

Children and Adults (with normal absorption): 25-125 mcg/day (1000-5000 international units) for 6-12 weeks

Children with malabsorption: 250-625 mcg/day (10,000-25,000 international units)

Adults with malabsorption: 250-7500 mcg/day (10,000-300,000 international units)

Familial hypophosphatemia:

Children: Initial: 1000-2000 mcg/day (40,000-80,000 international units) with phosphate supplements; daily dosage is increased at 3- to 4-month intervals in 250-500 mcg (10,000-20,000 international units) increments

Adults: 250-1500 mcg/day (10,000-60,000 international units) with phosphate supplements

Administration

Oral: May be administered without regard to meals; for oral liquid, use accompanying dropper for dosage measurements

Parenteral: Injection for I.M. use only

Monitoring Parameters Serum calcium and phosphorus levels (in CKD: After 1 month and then at least every 3 months); alkaline phosphatase, BUN; bone x-ray (hypophosphatemia or hypoparathyroidism); 25(OH)D (in CKD: After 3 months of treatment and as needed thereafter)

Reference Range

Chronic kidney disease (CKD) is defined either as kidney damage or GFR <60 mL/minute/1.73 m^2 for ≥3 months); stages of CKD are described below:

CKD Stage 1: Kidney damage with normal or increased GFR; GFR >90 mL/minute/1.73m^2

CKD Stage 2: Kidney damage with mild decrease in GFR; GFR 60-89 mL/minute/1.73 m^2

CKD Stage 3: Moderate decrease in GFR; GFR 30-59 mL/minute/1.73 m^2

CKD Stage 4: Severe decrease in GFR; GFR 15-29 mL/minute/1.73 m^2

CKD Stage 5: Kidney failure; GFR <15 mL/minute/1.73 m^2 or dialysis

Serum 25(OH)D (goal) >30 ng/mL

Patient Information Take as directed; do not increase dosage without consulting healthcare provider. Adhere to diet as recommended (do not take any other phosphate or vitamin D-related compounds while taking ergocalciferol). You may experience nausea, vomiting, dry mouth (small frequent meals, frequent mouth care, chewing gums, or sucking lozenges may help).

Additional Information 1.25 mg ergocalciferol provides 50,000 international units of vitamin D activity; 1 drop of 8000 international units/mL = 200 international units (40 drops = 1 mL)

Dosage Forms Excipient information presented when available (limited, particularly for generics); consult specific product labeling. [DSC] = Discontinued product

Capsule (Drisdol®): 50,000 int. units [1.25 mg; contains tartrazine and soybean oil]

Injection, solution (Calciferol™): 500,000 int. units/mL [12.5 mg/mL] (1 mL) [contains sesame oil] [DSC]

Liquid, drops (Calciferol™, Drisdol®): 8000 int. units/mL [200 mcg/mL] (60 mL) [OTC]

References

"Dietary Reference Intakes for Calcium, Phosphorus, Magnesium, Vitamin D, and Fluoride. Standing Committee on the Scientific Evaluation of Dietary Reference Intakes, Food and Nutrition Board, Institute of Medicine," National Academy of Sciences, Washington, DC: National Academy Press, 1997.

"K/DOQI Clinical Practice Guidelines for Bone Metabolism and Disease in Children With Chronic Kidney Disease," *Am J Kidney Dis*, 2005, 46(4 Suppl 1):S1-121.

"K/DOQI Clinical Practice Guidelines for Bone Metabolism and Disease in Chronic Kidney Disease. Guideline 1. Evaluation of Calcium and Phosphorus Metabolism," *Am J Kidney Dis*, 2003, 42(4 Suppl 3):52-7.

"K/DOQI Clinical Practice Guidelines for Bone Metabolism and Disease in Chronic Kidney Disease. Guideline 3. Evaluation of Serum Phosphorus Levels," *Am J Kidney Dis*, 2003, 42(4 Suppl 3):62-3.

"K/DOQI Clinical Practice Guidelines for Chronic Kidney Disease: Evaluation, Classification, and Stratification, Part 4. Definition and Classification of Stages of Chronic Kidney Disease," *Am J Kidney Dis*, 2002, 39(2 Suppl 1):46-75.

Sanchez CP, "Secondary Hyperparathyroidism in Children With Chronic Renal Failure: Pathogenesis and Treatment," *Paediatr Drugs*, 2003, 5(11): 763-76.

Ziolkowska H, "Minimizing Bone Abnormalities in Children With Renal Failure," *Paediatr Drugs*, 2006, 8(4):205-22.

♦ **Ergomar®** *see* Ergotamine *on page 591*

Ergotamine (er GOT a meen)

Related Information
Overdose and Toxicology *on page 1916*

U.S. Brand Names Ergomar®

Index Terms Ergotamine Tartrate

Therapeutic Category Alpha-Adrenergic Blocking Agent, Oral; Antimigraine Agent; Ergot Alkaloid

Generic Available No

Use Prevent or abort vascular headaches, such as migraine and migraine variants also known as "histaminic cephalalgia"

Pregnancy Risk Factor X

Lactation Enters breast milk/not recommended

Contraindications Hypersensitivity to ergotamine or any component; pregnancy; peripheral vascular disease, hepatic or renal disease, hypertension, peptic ulcer disease, sepsis, coronary heart disease; concurrent therapy with protease inhibitors (indinavir, ritonavir, saquinavir, nelfinavir, amprenavir, lopinavir/ritonavir), efavirenz, or delavirdine (see Drug Interactions)

Warnings Long-term use is associated with fibrotic changes to heart, pulmonary valves, and rare cases of retroperitoneal fibrosis; chronic usage may also be harmful due to a reduction in cerebral blood flow, ECG changes, and hypertension; sustained vasoconstriction may precipitate angina or MI, aggravate intermittent claudication, or lead to ischemic colitis. Concomitant use with protease inhibitors and macrolide antibiotics has been associated with serious and/or life-threatening cerebral and peripheral ischemia; some cases have resulted in amputation (see Contraindications). Patients who take ergotamine for extended periods of time may become dependent on it and discontinuation may result in withdrawal symptoms (eg, rebound headache). Safety and efficacy have not been established in children.

Adverse Reactions

Cardiovascular: Angina-like precordial pain, transient tachycardia or bradycardia, vasospasm, vasoconstriction, claudication; fibrotic thickening of the aortic, pulmonary, mitral, and/or tricuspid valves (rare after long-term use)

Central nervous system: Rebound headaches (with abrupt withdrawal), drowsiness, dizziness

Dermatologic: Pruritus

Gastrointestinal: Nausea, vomiting, diarrhea, xerostomia, retroperitoneal fibrosis (rare)

Local: Edema

Neuromuscular & skeletal: Leg cramps, myalgia, weakness, paresthesia of the extremities

Respiratory: Pleuropulmonary fibrosis (rare)

Drug Interactions Cytochrome P450 isoenzyme CYP3A4 (major) substrate; CYP3A4 inhibitor (weak)

Serious and/or life-threatening peripheral ischemia with potent CYP3A4 inhibitors, including protease inhibitors and macrolide antibiotics (see Contraindications) due to increased blood levels of ergotamine; less potent CYP3A4 inhibitors, saquinavir, nefazodone, fluconazole, fluoxetine, fluvoxamine, zileuton, metronidazole, and clotrimazole, may also increase the risk of serious peripheral ischemia; delavirdine and efavirenz also increase ergotamine plasma concentrations potentially resulting in life-threatening toxicities; enhanced vasoconstriction with beta-blocking agents; increased vasoconstrictor effects with methysergide; serotonin antagonists (buspirone, SSRIs, TCAs, nefazodone, sumatriptan, and trazodone), MAO inhibitors, and sibutramine may increase risk of serotonin syndrome; metoclopramide and antipsychotics may diminish the effects of ergotamine; sumatriptan and other $5\text{-}HT_1$

(Continued)

Ergotamine *(Continued)*

receptor agonists may prolong vasospastic reactions (do not use within 24 hours of each other)

Food Interactions Avoid tea, cola, and coffee (caffeine may increase GI absorption of ergotamine). Avoid grapefruit juice; may cause increased blood levels of ergotamine, leading to increased toxicity

Mechanism of Action Has partial agonist and/or antagonist activity against tryptaminergic, dopaminergic and alpha-adrenergic receptors depending upon their site; is a highly active uterine stimulant; it causes constriction of peripheral and cranial blood vessels and produces depression of central vasomotor centers

Pharmacokinetics

Absorption: Oral, rectal: Erratic
Distribution: V_d: Adults: 1.85 L/kg
Metabolism: Extensive in the liver
Bioavailability: Poor overall (<5%)
Half-life: Adults: 2-2.5 hours
Time to peak serum concentration: Oral: Within 0.5-3 hours
Elimination: In bile as metabolites (90%)

Usual Dosage Adolescents and Adults: **Note:** Not for chronic daily administration: Sublingual: 1 tablet under tongue at first sign, then 1 tablet every 30 minutes; maximum: 3 tablets/24 hours, 5 tablets/week

Administration Sublingual: Place tablet under the tongue; do not crush; may administer without regard to meals

Patient Information Any symptoms such as nausea, vomiting, numbness or tingling, and chest, muscle, or abdominal pain should be reported to the physician at the first sign of an attack; do **not** exceed recommended dosage; avoid coffee, tea, cola, and grapefruit juice; may cause dry mouth

Dosage Forms Excipient information presented when available (limited, particularly for generics); consult specific product labeling.

Tablet, sublingual: Ergotamine tartrate 2 mg

Ergotamine and Caffeine (er GOT a meen & KAF een)

Medication Safety Issues

Sound-alike/look-alike issues:
Cafergot® may be confused with Carafate®

Related Information

Overdose and Toxicology *on page 1916*

U.S. Brand Names Cafergot®; Migergot

Canadian Brand Names Cafergor®

Index Terms Caffeine and Ergotamine; Ergotamine Tartrate and Caffeine

Therapeutic Category Alpha-Adrenergic Blocking Agent, Oral; Antimigraine Agent; Ergot Alkaloid

Generic Available Yes

Use Prevent or abort vascular headaches, such as migraine and migraine variants also known as "histaminic cephalalgia"

Pregnancy Risk Factor X

Lactation Enters breast milk/not recommended

Contraindications Hypersensitivity to ergotamine, caffeine, or any component; pregnancy; peripheral vascular disease, hepatic or renal disease, hypertension, peptic ulcer disease, sepsis, coronary heart disease; concurrent therapy with protease inhibitors (indinavir, ritonavir, saquinavir, nelfinavir, amprenavir, lopinavir/ritonavir), efavirenz, or delavirdine (see Drug Interactions)

Warnings Long-term use is associated with fibrotic changes to heart, pulmonary valves, and rare cases of retroperitoneal fibrosis; chronic usage may also be harmful due to a reduction in cerebral blood flow, ECG changes, and hypertension; sustained vasoconstriction may precipitate angina or MI, aggravate intermittent claudication, or lead to ischemic colitis. Concomitant use with protease inhibitors and macrolide antibiotics has been associated with serious and/or life-threatening cerebral and peripheral ischemia; some cases have resulted in amputation (see Contraindications). Patients who take ergotamine for extended periods of time may become dependent on it and discontinuation may result in withdrawal symptoms (eg, rebound headache). Safety and efficacy have not been established in children.

Adverse Reactions

Cardiovascular: Angina-like precordial pain, transient tachycardia or bradycardia, MI, vasospasm, vasoconstriction, claudication; fibrotic thickening of the aortic, pulmonary, mitral, and/or tricuspid valves (rare after long-term use)

Central nervous system: Rebound headaches (with abrupt withdrawal), drowsiness, dizziness

Dermatologic: Pruritus

Gastrointestinal: Nausea, vomiting, diarrhea, xerostomia, retroperitoneal fibrosis (rare), rectal or anal ulcers (suppository use)

Local: Edema

Neuromuscular & skeletal: Leg cramps, myalgia, weakness, paresthesia of the extremities

Respiratory: Pleuropulmonary fibrosis (rare)

Drug Interactions Ergotamine: Cytochrome P450 isoenzyme CYP3A4 (major) substrate; CYP3A4 inhibitor (weak); Caffeine: Cytochrome P450 isoenzyme 1A2 (major), 2C8/9 (minor), 2D6 (minor), 2E1 (minor), 3A4 (minor) substrate; Cytochrome P450 isoenzyme 1A2 (weak), 3A4 (moderate) inhibitor

Ergotamine: Serious and/or life-threatening peripheral ischemia with potent CYP3A4 inhibitors, including protease inhibitors and macrolide antibiotics (see Contraindications) due to increased blood levels of ergotamine; less potent CYP3A4 inhibitors, saquinavir, nefazodone, fluconazole, fluoxetine, fluvoxamine, zileuton, metronidazole, and clotrimazole, may also increase the risk of serious peripheral ischemia; delavirdine and efavirenz also increase ergotamine plasma concentrations potentially resulting in life-threatening toxicities; enhanced vasoconstriction with beta-blocking agents; increased vasoconstrictor effects with methysergide; serotonin antagonists (buspirone, SSRIs, TCAs, nefazodone, sumatriptan, and trazodone), MAO inhibitors, and sibutramine may increase risk of serotonin syndrome; metoclopramide and antipsychotics may diminish the effects of ergotamine; sumatriptan and other 5-HT_1 receptor agonists may prolong vasospastic reactions (do not use within 24 hours of each other)

Caffeine: See individual monograph for specific interactions.

Food Interactions Avoid tea, cola, and coffee (caffeine may increase GI absorption of ergotamine). Avoid grapefruit juice; may cause increased blood levels of ergotamine, leading to increased toxicity

Mechanism of Action Has partial agonist and/or antagonist activity against tryptaminergic, dopaminergic and alpha-adrenergic receptors depending upon their site; is a highly active uterine stimulant; it causes constriction of peripheral and cranial blood vessels and produces depression of central vasomotor centers; caffeine is also a vasoconstrictor which was added to potentially enhance ergotamine's effects

Pharmacokinetics

Absorption: Oral, rectal: Erratic; absorption is enhanced by caffeine coadministration

Metabolism: Extensive in the liver

Bioavailability: Poor overall (<5%)

Half-life: 2-2.5 hours

Time to peak serum concentration: Oral: Within 0.5-3 hours

Elimination: In bile as metabolites (90%)

Usual Dosage Adolescents and Adults: **Note:** Not for chronic daily administration:

Oral: 2 mg at onset of attack; then 1-2 mg every 30 minutes as needed; maximum dose: 6 mg per attack; do not exceed 10 mg/week

Rectal, suppositories: 1 suppository at first sign of an attack; follow with second dose after 1 hour, if needed; maximum dose: 2 per attack; do not exceed 5/week

Administration Oral: Tablets may be taken without regard to meals

Patient Information Any symptoms such as nausea, vomiting, numbness or tingling, and chest, muscle, or abdominal pain should be reported to the physician at the first sign of an attack; do **not** exceed recommended dosage; not for chronic daily use; avoid coffee, tea, cola, and grapefruit juice; may cause dry mouth

Dosage Forms Excipient information presented when available (limited, particularly for generics); consult specific product labeling.

Suppository, rectal:

Migergot: Ergotamine tartrate 2 mg and caffeine 100 mg (12s)

Tablet: Ergotamine tartrate 1 mg and caffeine 100 mg

Cafergot®: Ergotamine tartrate 1 mg and caffeine 100 mg

◆ **Ergotamine Tartrate** *see* Ergotamine *on page 591*

◆ **Ergotamine Tartrate and Caffeine** *see* Ergotamine and Caffeine *on page 592*

◆ **Errin™** *see* Norethindrone *on page 1148*

Ertapenem (er ta PEN em)

Medication Safety Issues

Sound-alike/look-alike issues:

Invanz® may be confused with Avinza™

(Continued)

Ertapenem *(Continued)*

U.S. Brand Names Invanz®

Canadian Brand Names Invanz®

Index Terms Ertapenem Sodium; L-749,345; MK0826

Therapeutic Category Antibiotic, Carbapenem

Generic Available No

Use Treatment of moderate to severe, complicated intra-abdominal infections, acute pelvic infections, complicated skin and skin structure infections (including diabetic foot infections without osteomyelitis), community-acquired pneumonia, and complicated urinary tract infections caused by susceptible *S. aureus* (methicillin susceptible strains only), *S. pneumoniae* (penicillin-sensitive strains), *S. agalactiae*, *S. pyogenes*, *E. coli*, *B. fragilis*, *C. clostridioforme*, *Peptostreptococcus* species, *H. influenzae* (beta-lactamase negative strains), *K. pneumoniae*, and *M. catarrhalis*; prophylaxis of surgical site infection following colorectal surgery; documented or suspected infection due to susceptible organisms for outpatient parenteral therapy

Pregnancy Risk Factor B

Lactation Enters breast milk/use caution

Contraindications Hypersensitivity to ertapenem, carbapenems, or any component; patients who have had an anaphylactoid reaction to beta-lactams; hypersensitivity to local anesthetics of the amide type for patients receiving I.M. injections

Warnings Serious and occasionally fatal hypersensitivity reactions have been reported in patients receiving beta-lactam therapy; careful inquiry should be made concerning previous hypersensitivity reactions to penicillins, cephalosporins, or other beta-lactams before initiating ertapenem. Seizures have been reported with ertapenem therapy. Pseudomembranous colitis has been reported in patients receiving ertapenem; prolonged use may result in superinfection.

Precautions Use with caution in patients with CNS disorders, history of seizures and/or compromised renal function; dosage adjustment required in patients with renal impairment

Adverse Reactions

Cardiovascular: Tachycardia, chest pain, hypotension, edema, hypertension

Central nervous system: Headache, dizziness, insomnia, seizure, anxiety, fatigue, fever, hallucinations, altered mental status, somnolence

Dermatologic: Rash, pruritus, urticaria

Genitourinary: Vaginitis

Gastrointestinal: Diarrhea, nausea, vomiting, constipation, abdominal pain, oral candidiasis, taste perversion, cholelithiasis, pancreatitis, pseudomembranous colitis

Hematologic: Elevated platelet count, elevated eosinophil count, decreased neutrophil count

Hepatic: Elevated AST, ALT, and alkaline phosphatase

Local: Pain, erythema and tenderness at injection site, phlebitis

Neuromuscular & skeletal: Arthralgia, tremor, paresthesia

Renal: Renal insufficiency, hematuria

Respiratory: Respiratory distress, dyspnea, cough, rhinitis, wheezing

Miscellaneous: Anaphylaxis

Drug Interactions Probenecid decreases clearance of ertapenem

Stability Store lyophilized powder at room temperature. Reconstituted I.V. ertapenem solution further diluted in NS is stable for 6 hours at room temperature or 24 hours if refrigerated and used within 4 hours after removal from refrigeration; do not freeze. Incompatible with dextrose-containing solutions. Reconstituted I.M. ertapenem solution should be used within 1 hour after preparation.

Mechanism of Action Inhibits cell wall synthesis by binding to penicillin-binding proteins

Pharmacokinetics

Distribution: Excreted in breast milk

V_d:

Children 3 months to 12 years: ~0.2 L/kg

Children 13-17 years: 0.16 L/kg

Adults: 0.12 L/kg

Protein binding: 85% to 95% (concentration-dependent plasma protein binding)

Metabolism: Renal metabolism to an open-ring metabolite

Bioavailability: I.M.: 90%

Half-life:

Children 3 months to 12 years: 2.5 hours

Children 13-17 years: 4 hours

Adults: 4 hours

Time to peak serum concentration: I.M.: 2.3 hours

Elimination: 80% of a dose is excreted in the urine (38% as unchanged drug) and 10% in feces; undergoes glomerular filtration and tubular secretion

Dialysis: 30% removed by hemodialysis

Usual Dosage I.M., I.V.:

Children 3 months to 12 years: 15 mg/kg/dose every 12 hours; maximum dose: 1 g/day

Adolescents and Adults:

Treatment guidelines: 1 g once daily

Total antimicrobial treatment duration for pediatric and adult patients:

Complicated intra-abdominal infections: 5-14 days

Complicated skin and skin structure infections (including diabetic foot infections): 7-14 days

Community-acquired pneumonia: 10-14 days

Complicated UTI/pyelonephritis: 10-14 days

Acute pelvic infections: 3-10 days

Prophylaxis of surgical site infection following colorectal surgery: I.V.: Single 1 g dose administered 1 hour prior to surgical procedure

Dosage adjustment in renal impairment: Adults: Cl_{cr} ≤30 mL/minute/1.73 m^2: Decrease dose 50%

Hemodialysis: Adults: If daily dose is given within 6 hours prior to hemodialysis, a supplementary dose of 150 mg should be given following hemodialysis.

Administration Parenteral:

I.M. injection: Reconstitute 1 g vial with 3.2 mL of 1% lidocaine immediately prior to administration with a resultant concentration of 312.5 mg/mL. Shake vial well. Administer I.M. injection deep into a large muscle mass such as the gluteus maximus or lateral part of the thigh.

I.V. intermittent infusion: Reconstitute 1 g vial with 10 mL SWI or NS with a resultant concentration of 100 mg/mL. Further dilute dose with NS to a final maximum concentration of 20 mg/mL and administer over 30 minutes. Do not coinfuse with other medications. **Do not infuse with dextrose-containing solutions.**

Monitoring Parameters Periodic renal, hepatic, and hematologic function tests; neurological assessment

Patient Information Inform physician of prolonged diarrhea, abdominal pain, or vomiting. Report any chest pain, respiratory difficulty, dizziness, or confusion.

Additional Information Sodium content 1 g: 6 mEq

Dosage Forms Excipient information presented when available (limited, particularly for generics); consult specific product labeling.

Injection, powder for reconstitution: 1 g [contains sodium 137 mg/g (~6 mEq/g)]

References

Curran M, Simpson D, and Perry C, "Ertapenem: A Review of Its Use in the Management of Bacterial Infections," *Drugs*, 2003, 63(17):1855-78.

Keating GM and Perry CM, "Ertapenem: A Review of Its Use in the Treatment of Bacterial Infections," Drugs, 2005, 65(15):2151-78.

Nix DE, Majumdar AK, and DiNubile MJ, "Pharmacokinetics and Pharmacodynamics of Ertapenem: An Overview for Clinicians," *J Antimicrob Chemother*, 2004, 53(Suppl 2):ii23-8.

♦ **Ertapenem Sodium** *see* Ertapenem *on page 593*

♦ **Erybid™ (Can)** *see* Erythromycin *on page 595*

♦ **Eryc® [DSC]** *see* Erythromycin *on page 595*

♦ **Eryc® (Can)** *see* Erythromycin *on page 595*

♦ **Eryderm®** *see* Erythromycin *on page 595*

♦ **Erygel®** *see* Erythromycin *on page 595*

♦ **EryPed®** *see* Erythromycin *on page 595*

♦ **Ery-Tab®** *see* Erythromycin *on page 595*

♦ **Erythrocin®** *see* Erythromycin *on page 595*

Erythromycin (er ith roe MYE sin)

Medication Safety Issues

Sound-alike/look-alike issues:

Erythromycin may be confused with azithromycin, clarithromycin, Ethmozine®

Akne-Mycin® may be confused with AK-Mycin®

E.E.S.® may be confused with DES®

Eryc® may be confused with Emcyt®, Ery-Tab®

Ery-Tab® may be confused with Eryc®

Erythrocin® may be confused with Ethmozine®

U.S. Brand Names Akne-Mycin®; E.E.S.®; Eryc® [DSC]; Eryderm®; Erygel®; EryPed®; Ery-Tab®; Erythrocin®; PCE®; Romycin®

Canadian Brand Names Apo-Erythro Base®; Apo-Erythro E-C®; Apo-Erythro-ES®; Apo-Erythro-S®; Diomycin®; EES®; Erybid™; Eryc®; Novo-Rythro Estolate;

(Continued)

Erythromycin *(Continued)*

Novo-Rythro Ethylsuccinate; Nu-Erythromycin-S; PCE®; PMS-Erythromycin; Sans Acne®

Index Terms Erythromycin Base; Erythromycin Ethylsuccinate; Erythromycin Lactobionate; Erythromycin Stearate

Therapeutic Category Antibiotic, Macrolide; Antibiotic, Ophthalmic

Generic Available Yes: Capsule, gel, ophthalmic ointment, topical solution, suspension (as ethylsuccinate), swab, tablet (as base, ethylsuccinate, and stearate)

Use Treatment of mild to moderately severe infections of the upper and lower respiratory tract and skin infections due to susceptible streptococci and staphylococci; other susceptible bacterial infections including *Mycoplasma pneumoniae*, *Legionella* pneumonia, Lyme disease, diphtheria, pertussis, chancroid, *Chlamydia*, and *Campylobacter* gastroenteritis; used in conjunction with neomycin for decontaminating the bowel for surgery.

Ophthalmic: Treatment of superficial eye infections involving the conjunctiva or cornea; prevention of gonococcal ophthalmia neonatorum

Topical: Treatment of acne vulgaris

Pregnancy Risk Factor B

Lactation Enters breast milk/use caution (AAP considers "compatible")

Contraindications Hypersensitivity to erythromycin or any component (see Warnings); hepatic impairment; concomitant administration with pimozide, astemizole, terfenadine, or cisapride

Warnings Hepatic impairment with or without jaundice has occurred primarily in older children and adults; it may be accompanied by malaise, nausea, vomiting, abdominal colic, and fever; discontinue use if these occur; risk of serious cardiac arrhythmias exist in patients receiving erythromycin and pimozide, astemizole, terfenadine, or cisapride (do not use concurrently with erythromycin). Rhabdomyolysis has been reported in seriously ill patients receiving erythromycin and lovastatin concomitantly (monitor creatine kinase and serum transaminase levels). Infantile hypertrophic pyloric stenosis with symptoms of nonbilious vomiting or irritability with feeding has been reported in 5% of infants who received erythromycin for pertussis prophylaxis.

Erythromycin lactobionate injection contains benzyl alcohol which may cause allergic reactions in susceptible individuals; large amounts of benzyl alcohol (≥99 mg/kg/day) have been associated with a potentially fatal toxicity ("gasping syndrome") in neonates; the "gasping syndrome" consists of metabolic acidosis, respiratory distress, gasping respirations, CNS dysfunction (including convulsions, intracranial hemorrhage), hypotension and cardiovascular collapse; use erythromycin lactobionate injection products containing benzyl alcohol with caution in neonates; *in vitro* and animal studies have shown that benzoate, a metabolite of benzyl alcohol, displaces bilirubin from protein binding sites

Precautions Use with caution in patients with hepatic impairment

Adverse Reactions

Cardiovascular: Ventricular arrhythmias, prolongation of the QT interval, cardiac arrest; bradycardia, hypotension with I.V. administration

Central nervous system: Fever, dizziness

Dermatologic: Skin rash, pruritus

Gastrointestinal: Abdominal pain, cramping, nausea, vomiting, diarrhea, stomatitis, pseudomembraneous colitis, infantile hypertrophic pyloric stenosis

Hematologic: Eosinophilia

Hepatic: Cholestatic hepatitis, jaundice; (incidence of erythromycin-associated hepatotoxicity is ~0.1% in children and 0.25% in adults)

Local: Thrombophlebitis (I.V. form)

Otic: Ototoxicity (after I.V. use)

Miscellaneous: Allergic reactions, anaphylaxis

Drug Interactions Cytochrome P450 isoenzyme CYP3A3/4 substrate; isoenzyme CYP1A2 and CYP3A3/4 inhibitor

Erythromycin decreases clearance of astemizole, terfenadine, carbamazepine, cisapride, cyclosporine, protease inhibitors, lovastatin, simvastatin, midazolam, phenytoin, alfentanil, and triazolam; erythromycin may decrease theophylline clearance, increase theophylline's half-life by up to 60%, and result in theophylline toxicity (patients on high dose theophylline and erythromycin or who have received erythromycin for >5 days may be at higher risk); may potentiate anticoagulant effect of warfarin; may increase toxicity of ergotamine; may increase serum levels of digoxin, disopyramide, sildenafil, and quinidine

Stability Erythromycin lactobionate should be reconstituted with SWI without preservatives to avoid gel formation; the reconstituted solution is stable for 2 weeks when refrigerated or 24 hours at room temperature. Erythromycin I.V. infusion solution is stable at pH 6-8.

Mechanism of Action Inhibits bacterial RNA-dependent protein synthesis at the chain elongation step; binds to the 50S ribosomal subunit resulting in blockage of transpeptidation

Pharmacokinetics

Absorption: Variable but better with salt forms like the estolate than with base form; 18% to 45% absorbed orally; ethylsuccinate may be better absorbed with food

Distribution: Crosses the placenta; distributes into body tissues, fluids, and breast milk with poor penetration into the CSF

V_d: 0.64 L/kg

Protein binding: 75% to 90%

Metabolism: In the liver by demethylation

Half-life:

- Neonates (≤15 days of age): 2.1 hours
- Adults: 1.5-2 hours

Time to peak serum concentration: Oral:

- Base: 4 hours
- Stearate: 3 hours
- Ethylsuccinate: 0.5-2.5 hours
- Estolate: 2-4 hours (time to peak is delayed in the presence of food except when using estolate)

Elimination: 2% to 5% unchanged drug excreted in urine, major excretion in feces (via bile)

Dialysis: Not removed by peritoneal dialysis or hemodialysis

Usual Dosage

Neonates:

- Oral: Ethylsuccinate: Postnatal age:
  - ≤7 days: 20 mg/kg/day in divided doses every 12 hours
  - >7 days, <1200 g: 20 mg/kg/day in divided doses every 12 hours
  - >7 days, 1200-2000 g: 30 mg/kg/day in divided doses every 8 hours
  - >7 days, >2000 g: 30-40 mg/kg/day in divided doses every 6-8 hours
- Ophthalmic: Prophylaxis of neonatal gonococcal ophthalmia: 0.5-1 cm ribbon of ointment should be instilled into each conjunctival sac once
- I.V.: One study (n=14, ≤15 days of age, birth weight ≤1500 g) used erythromycin lactobionate in doses of 25 or 40 mg/kg/day divided every 6 hours for treatment of *Ureaplasma urealyticum* infection
- Chlamydial conjunctivitis and pneumonia: Oral: Ethylsuccinate: 50 mg/kg/day divided every 6 hours for 14 days

Infants and Children:

- Oral:
  - Base and ethylsuccinate: 30-50 mg/kg/day divided every 6-8 hours; do not exceed 2 g/day (as base) or 3.2 g/day (as ethylsuccinate); (**Note:** Due to differences in absorption, 200 mg erythromycin ethylsuccinate produces the same serum levels as 125 mg erythromycin base or estolate)
  - Estolate: 30-50 mg/kg/day divided every 6-12 hours; do not exceed 2 g/day
  - Stearate: 30-50 mg/kg/day divided every 6 hours; do not exceed 2 g/day
- *Chlamydia trachomatis:* Oral: 50 mg/kg/day divided every 6 hours for 10-14 days
- Pertussis: Oral: 40-50 mg/kg/day divided every 6 hours for 14 days; maximum dose: 2 g/day (not preferred agent for infants <1 month)
- Preop bowel preparation: Oral: 20 mg/kg erythromycin base at 1, 2, and 11 PM on the day before surgery combined with mechanical cleansing of the large intestine and oral neomycin
- I.V.: Lactobionate: 15-50 mg/kg/day divided every 6 hours, not to exceed 4 g/day

Children and Adults:

- Ophthalmic: Instill ointment one or more times daily depending on the severity of the infection
- Topical: Apply 2% solution over the affected area twice daily after the skin has been thoroughly washed and patted dry

Adults:

- Oral:
  - Base, delayed release: 333 mg every 8 hours
  - Estolate, stearate or base: 250-500 mg every 6-12 hours
  - Ethylsuccinate: 400-800 mg every 6-12 hours
- Chancroid: Oral: Base: 500 mg 4 times/day for 7 days
- *Chlamydia trachomatis:* Oral:
  - Base: 500 mg 4 times/day for 7 days **or**
  - Ethylsuccinate: 800 mg 4 times/day for 7 days
- Pertussis: Oral: 500 mg every 6 hours for 14 days
- Preop bowel preparation: Oral: 1 g erythromycin base at 1, 2, and 11 PM on the day before surgery combined with mechanical cleansing of the large intestine and oral neomycin

(Continued)

Erythromycin *(Continued)*

I.V.: Lactobionate: 15-20 mg/kg/day divided every 6 hours or given as a continuous infusion over 24 hours, not to exceed 4 g/day

Prokinetic agent (to improve gastric emptying time and intestinal motility): **Note:** Oral route is preferred since all erythromycin-related, life-threatening, and fatal cardiac complications have been associated with I.V. erythromycin.

Infants: Oral: 10 mg/kg/dose every 8 hours (high antibacterial dose) was effective in improving gastric emptying time (*JPEN*, 2002, 34(1):23-5); a second study using low dose oral erythromycin (0.75-3 mg/kg) for two doses was not useful in very preterm infants, partially useful in older preterm infants, and useful in full-term infants in increasing duodenal contraction amplitude and amplitude/frequency of antral contractions (*JPEN*, 2002, 34(1):16-22). **Note:** Exposure to high antimicrobial doses (30-50 mg/kg/day) for ≥14 days in neonates up to 2 weeks old has been associated with a 10-fold increase in the risk of hypertrophic pyloric stenosis.

Children: Lactobionate: Initial: 1-3 mg/kg I.V. infused over 60 minutes followed by 10-20 mg/kg/day orally in 2-4 divided doses before meals, or before meals and at bedtime

Adults: Lactobionate: Initial: 200 mg I.V. followed by 250 mg orally 3 times/day 30 minutes before meals

Administration

Ophthalmic ointment for prevention of neonatal ophthalmia: Wipe each eyelid gently with sterile cotton; instill 0.5-1 cm ribbon of ointment in each lower conjunctival sac; massage eyelids gently to spread the ointment; after 1 minute, excess ointment can be wiped away with sterile cotton

Oral: Avoid milk and acidic beverages 1 hour before or after a dose; administer after food to decrease GI discomfort; ethylsuccinate chewable tablets should not be swallowed whole; do not chew or break delayed release capsule or enteric coated tablets, swallow whole

Parenteral: Administer by I.V. intermittent or continuous infusion diluted in either dextrose or saline solutions to a concentration of 1-2.5 mg/mL; maximum concentration: 5 mg/mL; I.V. intermittent infusions may be administered over 20-60 minutes; to decrease vein irritation, administer as a continuous infusion at a concentration ≤1 mg/mL; prolonging the infusion duration over 60 minutes or longer has been recommended to decrease the cardiotoxic effects of erythromycin

Topical: Apply thin film to the cleansed, affected area.

Monitoring Parameters Liver function tests; with I.V. use: Blood pressure, heart rate

Test Interactions False-positive urinary catecholamines, 17-hydroxycorticosteroids and 17-ketosteroids

Patient Information Notify physician if vomiting or irritability with feeding occurs when administered to infants.

Nursing Implications Do not crush enteric coated or delayed release drug products

Additional Information Treatment of erythromycin-associated cardiac toxicity with prolongation of the QT interval and ventricular tachydysrhythmias includes discontinuing erythromycin and administering magnesium.

Dosage Forms Excipient information presented when available (limited, particularly for generics); consult specific product labeling. [DSC] = Discontinued product; [CAN] = Canadian brand name

Note: Strength expressed as base

Capsule, delayed release, enteric-coated pellets, as base: 250 mg

Eryc®: 250 mg [DSC]

Gel, topical: 2% (30 g, 60 g)

Erygel®: 2% (30 g, 60 g) [contains alcohol 92%]

Granules for oral suspension, as ethylsuccinate:

E.E.S.®: 200 mg/5 mL (100 mL, 200 mL) [contains sodium 25.9 mg (1.1 mEq)/5 mL; cherry flavor]

Injection, powder for reconstitution, as lactobionate:

Erythrocin®: 500 mg, 1 g

Ointment, ophthalmic: 0.5% [5 mg/g] (1 g, 3.5 g)

Romycin®: 0.5% [5 mg/g] (3.5 g)

Ointment, topical:

Akne-Mycin®: 2% (25 g)

Powder for oral suspension, as ethylsuccinate:

EryPed®: 200 mg/5 mL (100 mL, 200 mL) [contains sodium 117.5 mg (5.1 mEq)/5 mL; fruit flavor]; 400 mg/5 mL (100 mL, 200 mL) [contains sodium 117.5 mg (5.1 mEq)/5 mL; banana flavor]

Powder for oral suspension, as ethylsuccinate [drops]:

EryPed®: 100 mg/2.5 mL (50 mL) [contains sodium 58.8 mg (2.6 mEq)/dropperful; fruit flavor]

Solution, topical: 2% (60 mL)

Eryderm®: 2% (60 mL) [contain alcohol]
Sans acne [CAN]: 2% (60 mL) [contains ethyl alcohol 44%; not available in U.S.]
Suspension, oral, as ethylsuccinate: 200 mg/5 mL (480 mL); 400 mg/5 mL (480 mL)
E.E.S.®: 200 mg/5 mL (100 mL, 480 mL) [fruit flavor]; 400 mg/5 mL (100 mL, 480 mL) [orange flavor]
Tablet, as base: 250 mg, 500 mg
Tablet, as base [polymer-coated particles]:
PCE®: 333 mg, 500 mg
Tablet, as ethylsuccinate: 400 mg
E.E.S.®: 400 mg
Tablet, as stearate: 250 mg, 500 mg
Erythrocin®: 250 mg, 500 mg
Tablet, delayed release, enteric coated, as base:
Ery-Tab®: 250 mg, 333 mg, 500 mg

References

Curry JI, Lander TD, and Stringer MD, "Review Article: Erythromycin as a Prokinetic Agent in Infants and Children," *Aliment Pharmacol Ther*, 2001, 15(5):595-603.
Di Lorenzo C, Lachman R, and Hyman PE, "Intravenous Erythromycin for Postpyloric Intubation," *J Pediatr Gastroenterol Nutr*, 1990, 11(1):45-7.
Patole S, Rao S, and Doherty D, "Erythromycin as a Prokinetic Agent in Preterm Neonates: A Systematic Review," *Arch Dis Child Fetal Neonatal Ed*, 2005, 90(4):F301-6.
Reid B, DiLorenzo C, Travis L, et al, "Diabetic Gastroparesis Due to Postprandial Antral Hypomotility in Childhood," *Pediatrics*, 1992, 90(1 Pt 1):43-6.
Tiwari T, Murphy TV, and Moran J, "Recommended Antimicrobial Agents for the Treatment and Postexposure Prophylaxis of Pertussis: 2005 CDC Guidelines," *MMWR Recomm Rep*, 2005, 54(RR-14):1-16.
Vanderhoof JA, Young R, Kaufman SS, et al, "Treatment of Cyclic Vomiting in Childhood With Erythromycin," *J Pediatr Gastroenterol Nutr*, 1995, 21 Suppl 1:S60-2.
Waites KB, Sims PJ, Crouse DT, et al, "Serum Concentrations of Erythromycin After Intravenous Infusion in Preterm Neonates Treated for *Ureaplasma urealyticum* Infection," *Pediatr Infect Dis J*, 1994, 13(4):287-93.

Erythromycin and Sulfisoxazole

(er ith roe MYE sin & sul fi SOKS a zole)

Medication Safety Issues
Sound-alike/look-alike issues:
Pediazole® may be confused with Pediapred®

U.S. Brand Names Pediazole® [DSC]

Canadian Brand Names Pediazole®

Index Terms Sulfisoxazole and Erythromycin

Therapeutic Category Antibiotic, Macrolide; Antibiotic, Sulfonamide Derivative

Generic Available Yes

Use Treatment of susceptible bacterial infections of the upper and lower respiratory tract; otitis media in children caused by susceptible strains of *Haemophilus influenzae*; other infections in patients allergic to penicillin

Pregnancy Risk Factor C

Lactation Enters breast milk/compatible

Contraindications Hypersensitivity to erythromycin, any component, or sulfonamides; hepatic dysfunction; infants <2 months of age (sulfas compete with bilirubin for binding sites which may result in kernicterus in newborns); patients with porphyria; pregnant women at term; mothers nursing infants <2 months of age; concomitant administration of astemizole, terfenadine, or cisapride

Warnings Risk of serious cardiac arrhythmias exist in patients receiving erythromycin, astemizole, terfenadine, or cisapride (do not use concurrently); fatalities due to Stevens-Johnson syndrome, toxic epidermal necrolysis, fulminant hepatic necrosis, agranulocytosis, and aplastic anemia have occurred with the administration of sulfonamides; prolonged use may result in superinfection or pseudomembranous colitis

Precautions Use with caution in patients with impaired renal or hepatic function, G-6-PD deficiency (hemolysis may occur)

Adverse Reactions
Cardiovascular: Tachycardia, palpitations, syncope
Central nervous system: Headache, disorientation, fever, dizziness
Dermatologic: Rash, photosensitivity, Stevens-Johnson syndrome, toxic epidermal necrolysis, pruritus, urticaria
Gastrointestinal: Abdominal cramping, nausea, vomiting, diarrhea, pseudomembranous colitis, anorexia, stomatitis, pancreatitis
Genitourinary: Crystalluria, hematuria
Hematologic: Agranulocytosis, aplastic anemia, leukopenia, eosinophilia, thrombocytopenia
Hepatic: Hepatic necrosis, jaundice
Renal: Toxic nephrosis, elevated BUN and serum creatinine, acute renal failure
Respiratory: Cough, shortness of breath, pulmonary infiltrates
(Continued)

Erythromycin and Sulfisoxazole *(Continued)*

Miscellaneous: Anaphylaxis

Drug Interactions Erythromycin is a cytochrome P450 isoenzyme CYP3A3/4 substrate; isoenzyme CYP1A2 and CYP3A3/4 inhibitor

Erythromycin decreases clearance of astemizole, terfenadine, carbamazepine, cisapride, cyclosporine, protease inhibitors, lovastatin, simvastatin, midazolam, phenytoin, alfentanil, and triazolam; erythromycin may decrease theophylline clearance, increase theophylline's half-life by up to 60%, and result in theophylline toxicity (patients on high dose theophylline and erythromycin or who have received erythromycin for >5 days may be at higher risk); may potentiate anticoagulant effect of warfarin; may increase toxicity of ergotamine; may increase serum levels of digoxin, disopyramide, and quinidine

Sulfisoxazole may decrease the amount of thiopental needed for anesthesia; sulfisoxazole may displace methotrexate from plasma protein-binding sites increasing free methotrexate concentrations; displaces tolbutamide, chlorpropamide, oral anticoagulants from protein binding sites; PABA (antagonizes the antibacterial activity of sulfas)

Stability Reconstituted suspension is stable for 14 days when refrigerated

Mechanism of Action Erythromycin inhibits bacterial protein synthesis by binding to the 50S ribosomal subunit; sulfisoxazole competitively inhibits bacterial synthesis of folic acid from para-aminobenzoic acid

Pharmacokinetics

Erythromycin ethylsuccinate:

- Absorption: Well absorbed from the GI tract
- Distribution: Widely distributed into most body tissues and fluids; poor penetration into CSF; crosses the placenta; excreted in breast milk
- Protein binding: 75% to 90%
- Metabolism: In the liver by demethylation
- Half-life: 1-1.5 hours
- Elimination: Unchanged drug is excreted and concentrated in bile; <5% of dose eliminated in urine
- Dialysis: Not removed by peritoneal dialysis or hemodialysis

Sulfisoxazole acetyl:

- Absorption: Hydrolyzed in the GI tract to sulfisoxazole which is rapidly and completely absorbed; the small intestine is the major site of absorption
- Distribution: Into extracellular space; CSF concentration ranges from 8% to 57% of blood concentration in patients with normal meninges; crosses the placenta, excreted in breast milk
- Protein binding: 85%
- Metabolism: Undergoes N-acetylation and N-glucuronide conjugation in the liver
- Half-life: 4.6-7.8 hours, prolonged in renal impairment
- Elimination: 50% in urine as unchanged drug
- Dialysis: >50% removed by hemodialysis

Usual Dosage Oral (dosage recommendation is based on the product's erythromycin content):

Children ≥2 months: 40-50 mg/kg/day in divided doses every 6-8 hours; not to exceed 2 g erythromycin or 6 g sulfisoxazole/day

Adults: 400 mg erythromycin and 1200 mg sulfisoxazole every 6 hours

Administration Oral: Administer with or without food; shake suspension well before use; maintain adequate fluid intake to prevent crystalluria and kidney stone formation

Monitoring Parameters CBC with differential and platelet count, urinalysis; periodic liver function and renal function tests; observe patient for diarrhea

Test Interactions False-positive urinary protein; false-positive urinary catecholamines, 17-hydroxycorticosteroids and 17-ketosteroids

Patient Information May cause photosensitivity reactions (eg, exposure to sunlight may cause severe sunburn, skin rash, redness, or itching); avoid exposure to sunlight and artificial light sources (sunlamps, tanning booth/bed); wear protective clothing, wide-brimmed hats, sunglasses, and lip sunscreen (SPF ≥15); use a sunscreen [broad-spectrum sunscreen or physical sunscreen (preferred) or sunblock with SPF ≥15]; contact physician if reaction occurs.

Dosage Forms Excipient information presented when available (limited, particularly for generics); consult specific product labeling. [DSC] = Discontinued product

Powder for oral suspension: Erythromycin ethylsuccinate 200 mg and sulfisoxazole acetyl 600 mg per 5 mL (100 mL, 200 mL)

Pediazole®: Erythromycin ethylsuccinate 200 mg and sulfisoxazole acetyl 600 mg per 5 mL (100 mL, 150 mL, 200 mL) [strawberry-banana flavor] [DSC]

References

Rodriguez WJ, Schwartz RH, Sait T, et al, "Erythromycin-Sulfisoxazole vs Amoxicillin in the Treatment of Acute Otitis Media in Children," *Am J Dis Child*, 1985, 139(8):766-70.

- ♦ **Erythromycin Base** *see* Erythromycin *on page 595*
- ♦ **Erythromycin Ethylsuccinate** *see* Erythromycin *on page 595*
- ♦ **Erythromycin Lactobionate** *see* Erythromycin *on page 595*
- ♦ **Erythromycin Stearate** *see* Erythromycin *on page 595*
- ♦ **Erythropoiesis-Stimulating Agent (ESA)** *see* Darbepoetin Alfa *on page 444*
- ♦ **Erythropoiesis-Stimulating Agent (ESA)** *see* Epoetin Alfa *on page 580*
- ♦ **Erythropoiesis-Stimulating Protein** *see* Darbepoetin Alfa *on page 444*
- ♦ **Erythropoietin** *see* Epoetin Alfa *on page 580*
- ♦ **Esclim®** *see* Estradiol *on page 605*
- ♦ **Eserine® (Can)** *see* Physostigmine *on page 1257*
- ♦ **Eserine Salicylate** *see* Physostigmine *on page 1257*
- ♦ **Eskalith® [DSC]** *see* Lithium *on page 948*
- ♦ **Eskalith CR® [DSC]** *see* Lithium *on page 948*

Esmolol (ES moe lol)

Medication Safety Issues

Sound-alike/look-alike issues:

Esmolol may be confused with Osmitrol®

Brevibloc® may be confused with bretylium, Brevital®, Bumex®, Buprenex®

Related Information

Antihypertensive Agents by Class *on page 1678*

Overdose and Toxicology *on page 1916*

U.S. Brand Names Brevibloc®

Canadian Brand Names Brevibloc®

Index Terms Esmolol Hydrochloride

Therapeutic Category Antiarrhythmic Agent, Class II; Antihypertensive Agent; Beta-Adrenergic Blocker

Generic Available Yes: Excludes infusion

Use Treatment of supraventricular tachycardia (primarily to control ventricular rate in patients with atrial fibrillation or flutter); noncompensatory sinus tachycardia; perioperative tachycardia and hypertension

Pregnancy Risk Factor C

Lactation Excretion in breast milk unknown/use with caution

Contraindications Hypersensitivity to esmolol, any component, or other beta-blockers; sinus bradycardia or heart block, uncompensated CHF, cardiogenic shock

Warnings Caution should be exercised when discontinuing esmolol infusions to avoid withdrawal effects

Precautions Use with extreme caution in patients with hyper-reactive airway disease; use lowest dose possible and discontinue infusion if bronchospasm occurs; use with caution in diabetes mellitus, hypoglycemia, renal failure; avoid extravasation; patients receiving beta blockers who have a history of anaphylactic reactions, may be more reactive to a repeated allergen challenge and may not be responsive to the usual epinephrine doses used to treat an allergic reaction

Adverse Reactions

Cardiovascular: Hypotension (especially with doses >200 mcg/kg/minute), bradycardia, Raynaud's phenomena, peripheral ischemia

Central nervous system: Dizziness, somnolence, confusion, lethargy, depression, headache, agitation

Gastrointestinal: Nausea, vomiting

Local: Phlebitis, inflammation, induration; skin necrosis after extravasation

Respiratory: Bronchoconstriction (less than propranolol, but more likely with higher doses)

Miscellaneous: Diaphoresis, adverse reactions similar to other beta-blockers may occur

Drug Interactions Esmolol may increase digoxin or theophylline serum concentrations; morphine may increase esmolol blood concentrations; xanthines (eg, theophylline, caffeine) may decrease effects of esmolol

Food Interactions Avoid xanthine-containing foods or beverages

Stability

Store at controlled room temperature; protect from freezing and excessive heat. Stable for at least 24 hours (under refrigeration or at controlled room temperature) at a final concentration of 10 mg/mL in the following solutions: D_5W, D_5LR, $D_5\frac{1}{2}NS$, D_5NS, LR, NS, ½NS, D_5W with KCl 40 mEq/L; **not** compatible with sodium bicarbonate 5%

Mechanism of Action Class II antiarrhythmic: Competitively blocks response to $beta_1$-adrenergic stimulation with little or no effect on $beta_2$-receptors except at high

(Continued)

Esmolol *(Continued)*

doses (ie, cardioselective at lower doses); no intrinsic sympathomimetic activity; no membrane-stabilizing activity; ultrashort-acting

Pharmacodynamics

Onset of action: I.V.: Beta blockade occurs within 2-10 minutes (onset of effects is quickest when loading doses are administered)

Duration: Short (10-30 minutes)

Pharmacokinetics

Protein binding: 55%

Distribution: V_d:

Children: 2 L/kg

Adults: 3.5 L/kg (range: 2-5 L/kg)

Metabolism: In blood by esterases

Half-life, elimination:

Children:

18 months to 14 years (n=12): 2.88 ± 2.67 minutes

2.5-16 years (n=20): 4.5 ± 2.1 minutes

Adults: 9 minutes

Elimination: ~69% of dose excreted in urine as metabolites and 2% as unchanged drug

Usual Dosage Must be adjusted to individual response and tolerance

Children: I.V.: Limited information available

Supraventricular tachycardia (SVT): Some centers have utilized initial doses of 100-500 mcg/kg given over 1 minute followed by a continuous infusion for control of SVT. One electrophysiologic study assessing esmolol-induced beta-blockade (n=20, 2-16 years of age) used an initial dose of 600 mcg/kg over 2 minutes followed by an infusion of 200 mcg/kg/minute; the infusion was titrated upward by 50-100 mcg/kg/minute every 5-10 minutes until a reduction >10% in heart rate or mean blood pressure occurred. Mean dose required: 550 mcg/kg/minute with a range of 300-1000 mcg/kg/minute (Trippel, 1991).

Postoperative hypertension: Loading doses of 500 mcg/kg/minute over 1 minute followed by a continuous infusion with doses of 50-250 mcg/kg/minute (mean 173) have been used in addition to nitroprusside in a small number of patients (7 patients, 7-19 years of age, median age 13 years) after coarctation of aorta repair (Vincent, 1990).

An open-label trial of 20 infants and children (1 month to 12 years of age; median age: 25.6 months) used the following dosing guidelines to treat postoperative hypertension following cardiac surgery: Age 0-7 days: Initial: 50 mcg/kg/minute; titrate dose by 25-50 mcg/kg/minute every 20 minutes; age 8 days to 1 month: Initial: 75 mcg/kg/minute; titrate dose by 50 mcg/kg/minute every 20 minutes; age >1 month to 1 year: Initial: 100 mcg/kg/minute; titrate dose by 50 mcg/kg/minute every 10 minutes; age >1 year to 12 years: Initial: 150 mcg/kg/minute; titrate dose by 50-100 mcg/kg/minute every 10 minutes; dose was titrated until blood pressure was ≤90th percentile for age or until maximum dose of 1000 mcg/kg/minute was reached; mean required dose: 700 mcg/kg/minute (range: 300-1000 mcg/kg/minute); final dose required was significantly higher in patients with aortic coarctation repair (mean ± SD: 830 ± 153 mcg/kg/minute) than in patients with repair of other congenital heart defects (mean ± SD: 570 ± 230 mcg/kg/minute) (Wiest, 1998)

Adults: I.V.:

Intraoperative tachycardia and/or hypertension (immediate control): Loading dose: 80 mg (~1 mg/kg) over 30 seconds; follow with a 150 mcg/kg/minute infusion, if necessary; adjust infusion rate as needed to maintain desired heart rate and/or blood pressure; maximum dose: 300 mcg/kg/minute.

Supraventricular tachycardia or gradual control of postoperative tachycardia and hypertension: Loading dose: 500 mcg/kg over 1 minute; follow with a 50 mcg/kg/minute infusion for 4 minutes; if response is inadequate, rebolus with another 500 mcg/kg loading dose over 1 minute, and increase the maintenance infusion to 100 mcg/kg/minute. Repeat this process until a therapeutic effect has been achieved or to a maximum recommended maintenance dose of 200 mcg/kg/minute. Usual dosage range: 50-200 mcg/kg/minute with average dose = 100 mcg/kg/minute.

Administration Parenteral: I.V.: The 250 mg/mL ampul is **not** for direct I.V. injection, but must first be diluted to a final concentration not to exceed 10 mg/mL (ie, 2.5 g in 250 mL or 5 g in 500 mL); infuse I.V. loading dose over 1-2 minutes

Monitoring Parameters Blood pressure, EKG, heart rate, respiratory rate, I.V. site

Nursing Implications Decrease infusion rate or discontinue if hypotension, CHF, etc occur

Dosage Forms Excipient information presented when available (limited, particularly for generics); consult specific product labeling.

Infusion [premixed in sodium chloride; preservative free]:

Brevibloc®: 2000 mg (100 mL) [20 mg/mL; double strength]; 2500 mg (250 mL) [10 mg/mL]

Injection, solution, as hydrochloride: 10 mg/mL (10 mL) [premixed in sodium chloride]

Brevibloc®: 10 mg/mL (10 mL) [alcohol free; premixed in sodium chloride]; 20 mg/mL (5 mL, 100 mL) [alcohol free; double strength; premixed in sodium chloride]; 250 mg/mL (10 mL) [contains alcohol 25%, propylene glycol 25%; concentrate]

References

Cuneo BF, Zales VR, Blahunka PC, et al, "Pharmacodynamics and Pharmacokinetics of Esmolol, A Short-Acting Beta-Blocking Agent in Children," *Pediatr Cardiol*, 1994, 15(6):296-301.

Trippel DL, Wiest DB, and Gillette PC, "Cardiovascular and Antiarrhythmic Effects of Esmolol in Children," *J Pediatr*, 1991, 119(1):142-7.

Vincent RN, Click LA, Williams HM, et al, "Esmolol As an Adjunct in the Treatment of Systemic Hypertension After Operative Repair of Coarctation of the Aorta," *Am J Cardiol*, 1990, 65(13):941-3.

Wiest DB, Garner SS, Uber WE, et al, "Esmolol for the Management of Pediatric Hypertension After Cardiac Operations," *J Thorac Cardiovasc Surg*, 1998, 115(4):890-7.

Wiest DB, Trippel DL, Gillette PC, et al, "Pharmacokinetics of Esmolol in Children," *Clin Pharmacol Ther*, 1991, 49(6):618-23.

♦ **Esmolol Hydrochloride** *see* Esmolol *on page 601*

Esomeprazole (es oh ME pray zol)

Related Information

Assessment of Liver Function *on page 1810*

U.S. Brand Names Nexium®

Canadian Brand Names Nexium®

Index Terms Esomeprazole Magnesium; Esomeprazole Sodium

Therapeutic Category Gastric Acid Secretion Inhibitor; Gastrointestinal Agent, Gastric or Duodenal Ulcer Treatment; Proton Pump Inhibitor

Generic Available No

Use

Oral formulation: Treatment and maintenance of healing of severe erosive esophagitis; treatment of symptomatic gastroesophageal reflux disease (GERD); adjunctive treatment of duodenal ulcers associated with *Helicobacter pylori*; prevention of gastric ulcers associated with continuous NSAID therapy; long term treatment of pathological hypersecretory conditions (eg, Zollinger-Ellison syndrome)

I.V. formulation: Short-term alternative treatment when oral therapy is not possible or appropriate

Pregnancy Risk Factor B

Lactation Excretion in breast milk unknown/not recommended

Contraindications Hypersensitivity to esomeprazole, substituted benzimidazole proton pump inhibitors (eg, omeprazole, lansoprazole, pantoprazole), or any component

Warnings Esomeprazole is an enantiomer of omeprazole and may share the same potential long-term side effects as omeprazole; atrophic gastritis has been noted occasionally in gastric corpus biopsies from patients treated long-term with omeprazole; in long-term (2-year) studies in rats, omeprazole produced a dose-related increase in gastric carcinoid tumors. While available endoscopic evaluations and histologic examinations of biopsy specimens from human stomachs have not detected a risk from short-term exposure to omeprazole, further human data on the effect of sustained hypochlorhydria and hypergastrinemia are needed to rule out the possibility of an increased risk for the development of tumors in humans receiving long-term therapy. Symptomatic relief does not preclude the presence of a gastric malignancy. Use of gastric acid inhibitors including proton pump inhibitors and H_2 blockers has been associated with an increased risk for development of acute gastroenteritis and community-acquired pneumonia (Canani, 2006).

Precautions Modify dosage in patients with liver impairment.

Adverse Reactions

Cardiovascular: Chest pain, tachycardia, bradycardia, flushing, hypertension

Central nervous system: Headache (8.1%), dizziness, vertigo, insomnia, anxiety, nervousness, fever, anorexia, confusion, somnolence, depression, aggression, agitation, hallucination

Dermatologic: Rash, acne, angioedema, dermatitis, pruritus, urticaria, erythema multiforme, Stevens-Johnson syndrome, toxic epidermal necrolysis, alopecia, hyperhidrosis, photosensitivity

Endocrine & metabolic: Goiter, glycosuria, hyperuricemia, hyponatremia

Gastrointestinal: Diarrhea (2%), nausea (2%), abdominal pain (2.7%), vomiting, constipation, flatulence, dyspepsia, dysphagia, epigastric pain, eructation, gastroenteritis, GI hemorrhage, hiccup, melena, irritable colon, xerostomia, anorexia, dysgeusia, abdominal pain, taste loss, taste perversion, pancreatitis, stomatitis

(Continued)

Esomeprazole *(Continued)*

Genitourinary: Dysmenorrhea, vaginitis, urinary frequency, dysuria, hematuria, gynecomastia

Hematologic: Leukopenia, pancytopenia, thrombocytopenia, anemia, leukocytosis, agranulocytosis (rare)

Hepatic: Elevated liver function tests, hepatitis (with or without jaundice)

Local: Mild erythema, pruritus (at injection site)

Neuromuscular & skeletal: Myalgia, arthralgia, back pain, arthropathy, cramps, fibromyalgia syndrome, polymyalgia rheumatica, paresthesia, weakness

Ocular: Conjunctivitis, abnormal vision

Otic: Tinnitus, earache

Renal: Hematuria, pyuria, proteinuria, interstitial nephritis (rare)

Respiratory: Cough, dyspnea, larynx edema, pharyngitis, rhinitis, sinusitis

Miscellaneous: Hypersensitivity reactions including anaphylaxis (rare), GI candidiasis

Drug Interactions Cytochrome P450 isoenzyme CYP2C19 (major) and CYP3A4 (minor) substrate (as an enantiomer of omeprazole, esomeprazole may have the same drug interaction profile); CYP2C19 inhibitor (moderate)

May decrease absorption of atazanavir, indinavir, ketoconazole, itraconazole, dapsone, and iron salts; increases half-life (decreased clearance) of diazepam; may increase absorption of digoxin; may increase warfarin effects; may increase carbamazepine, diazepam, midazolam, and triazolam levels; isoenzyme CYP2C19 inducers (eg, aminoglutethimide, carbamazepine, phenytoin, and rifampin) may decrease effects; may increase levels/effects of CYP2C19 substrates such as citalopram, diazepam, methsuximide, phenytoin, propranolol, and sertraline; may increase levels/effects of HMG-CoA reductase inhibitors; may decrease excretion of methotrexate

Food Interactions Absorption is decreased by 43% to 53% when taken with food.

Stability Store at room temperature; protect from light. Esomeprazole stability is a function of pH; it is rapidly degraded in acidic media, but has acceptable stability under alkaline conditions. Each capsule of esomeprazole contains enteric coated granules to prevent esomeprazole degradation by gastric acidity. I.V. formulation is stable at room temperature after reconstitution with NS and LR 12 hours and with D_5W 6 hours.

Mechanism of Action Esomeprazole is the S-isomer of omeprazole. Esomeprazole suppresses gastric acid secretion by inhibiting the parietal cell membrane enzyme (H^+/K^+)-ATPase or proton pump; demonstrates antimicrobial activity against *Helicobacter pylori.*

Pharmacokinetics

Distribution: Adults: V_d: 16 L

Protein binding: 97%

Metabolism: Hepatic via CYP2C19 and 3A3/4 isoenzymes to hydroxy, desmethyl, and sulfone metabolites (all inactive)

Bioavailability: 64% after a single dose; 90% with repeated administration

Half-life: Adults: 1-1.5 hours

Time to peak serum concentration: Oral: 1.5 hours

Elimination: <1% excreted unchanged in urine

Usual Dosage Oral, I.V.: **Note:** I.V. treatment should be discontinued as soon as the patient tolerates oral therapy.

GERD:

Children ≤12 years: Very limited data: Twelve children with cystinosis (mean age: 5.8 years) were successfully treated with 0.7-2.75 mg/kg/day (mean final dose: 1.7 mg/kg/day) to treat cysteamine-induced acid-hypersection (Dohil, 2005)

Children >12 to 17 years: 20-40 mg once daily for up to 8 weeks

Adults: 20 mg once daily for 4-8 weeks

Erosive esophagitis: Adults: 20-40 mg once daily for 4-8 weeks; maintenance: 20 mg once daily

Pathological hypersecretory conditions including Zollinger-Ellison syndrome: Adults: 40 mg twice daily; dosage may be increased depending upon the response to therapy; doses up to 240 mg/day have been used

Adjunctive therapy of duodenal ulcers associated with *Helicobacter pylori* (in combination with antibiotic therapy): Adults: 40 mg once daily for 10 days

Prevention of NSAID-induced gastric ulcers: Adults: 20-40 mg once daily for up to 6 months

Dosage adjustment in hepatic impairment:

Mild to moderate liver impairment (Child-Pugh Class A or B): No dosage adjustment needed

Severe liver impairment (Child-Pugh Class C): Not to exceed 20 mg daily

Administration

Oral: Administer at least 1 hour before food or meals

Capsule: Swallow whole, do not chew or crush; capsule may be opened and the enteric coated pellets may be mixed with applesauce (applesauce should not be hot) and swallowed immediately; do not store mixture for future use; esomeprazole pellets also remain intact when mixed with tap water, orange juice, apple juice, and yogurt; due to small pellet size, the entire contents of an opened capsule may be completely delivered via small caliber and standard NG tubes when mixed with 50 mL water (White, 2002); administer immediately; do not administer if the pellets have dissolved or disintegrated

Granules: Mix contents of packet with 15 mL water and leave for 2-3 minutes to thicken; stir and drink within 30 minutes. Granules may be administered by nasogastric or gastric tube: Add 15 mL of water to a syringe, add granules from packet. Shake the syringe, leave 2-3 minutes to thicken. Shake the syringe and administer through nasogastric or gastric tube (French size 6 or greater) within 30 minutes. Refill the syringe with 15 mL of water, shake and flush tube.

I.V.: Reconstitute vial (20 mg or 40 mg) with 5 mL D_5W, NS, or LR. May administer dosage without further dilution over at least 3 minutes. May also be diluted in 50 mL D_5W, NS, or LR (0.4-0.8 mg/mL) and infuse over 10-30 minutes.

Patient Information May cause dry mouth; do not chew or crush granules. May cause photosensitivity reactions (eg, exposure to sunlight may cause severe sunburn, skin rash, redness, or itching); avoid direct exposure to sunlight.

Dosage Forms Excipient information presented when available (limited, particularly for generics); consult specific product labeling.

Note: Strength expressed as base

Capsule, delayed release, as magnesium:

Nexium®: 20 mg, 40 mg

Granules, for oral suspension, delayed release, as magnesium:

Nexium®: 20 mg, 40 mg

Injection, powder for reconstitution, as sodium:

Nexium®: 20 mg, 40 mg [contains edetate sodium]

References

Canani RB, Cirillo P, Roggero P, et al, "Therapy With Gastric Acidity Inhibitors Increases the Risk of Acute Gastroenteritis and Community-Acquired Pneumonia in Children," *Pediatrics*, 2006, 117(5):e817-20.

Dohil R, Fidler M, Barshop B, et al, "Esomeprazole Therapy for Gastric Acid Hypersecretion in Children With Cystinosis," *Pediatr Nephrol*, 2005, 20(12):1786-93.

Gibbons TE and Gold BD, "The Use of Proton Pump Inhibitors in Children: A Comprehensive Review," *Paediatr Drugs*, 2003, 5(1):25-40.

Li J, Zhao J, Hamer-Maansson JE, et al, "Pharmacokinetic Properties of Esomeprazole in Adolescent Patients Aged 12 to 17 Years With Symptoms of Gastroesophageal Reflux Disease: A Randomized, Open-Label Study," *Clin Ther*, 2006, 28(3):419-27.

White CM, Kalus JS, Quercia R, et al, "Delivery of Esomeprazole Magnesium Enteric-Coated Pellets Through Small Caliber and Standard Nasogastric Tubes and Gastrostomy Tubes *In Vitro*," *Am J Health Syst Pharm*, 2002, 59(21):2085-8.

- **Esomeprazole Magnesium** *see* Esomeprazole *on page 603*
- **Esomeprazole Sodium** *see* Esomeprazole *on page 603*
- **Estar® (Can)** *see* Coal Tar *on page 394*
- **Ester-E™ [OTC]** *see* Vitamin E *on page 1620*
- **Estrace®** *see* Estradiol *on page 605*
- **Estraderm®** *see* Estradiol *on page 605*

Estradiol (es tra DYE ole)

Medication Safety Issues

Sound-alike/look-alike issues:

Alora® may be confused with Aldara™

Elestrin™ may be confused with alosetron

Estraderm® may be confused with Testoderm®

International issues:

Vivelle®: Brand name for ethinyl estradiol and norgestimate in Austria

Estring® may be confused with Estrena® [Finland]

Estrena® [Finland] may be confused with estrone in the U.S.

Transdermal patch may contain conducting metal (eg, aluminum); remove patch prior to MRI.

U.S. Brand Names Alora®; Climara®; Delestrogen®; Depo®-Estradiol; Elestrin™; Esclim®; Estrace®; Estraderm®; Estrasorb™; Estring®; EstroGel®; Femring®; Femtrace®; Gynodiol®; Menostar™; Vagifem®; Vivelle®; Vivelle-Dot®

Canadian Brand Names Climara®; Depo®-Estradiol; Estrace®; Estraderm®; Estradot®; Estring®; EstroGel®; Menostar™; Oesclim®; Sandoz-Estradiol Derm 50; Sandoz-Estradiol Derm 75; Sandoz-Estradiol Derm 100; Vagifem®

Index Terms Estradiol Acetate; Estradiol Cypionate; Estradiol Hemihydrate; Estradiol Transdermal; Estradiol Valerate

(Continued)

Estradiol *(Continued)*

Therapeutic Category Estrogen Derivative; Estrogen Derivative, Vaginal

Generic Available Yes: Oral tablet, patch

Use Treatment of hypoestrogenism (due to hypogonadism, castration, or primary ovarian failure), moderate to severe vasomotor symptoms of menopause, moderate to severe symptoms of vulvar and vaginal atrophy due to menopause; palliative treatment of breast cancer in select patients; palliative treatment of androgen-dependent prostate cancer; prevention of osteoporosis in postmenopausal women; see Warnings and Additional Information

Pregnancy Risk Factor X

Lactation Enters breast milk/use caution

Contraindications Hypersensitivity to estradiol or any component (see Warnings); history of or current DVT or PE; recent (eg, within past year) or current arterial thromboembolic disease (eg, MI, stroke); undiagnosed vaginal bleeding; pregnancy; known, suspected, or history of breast cancer (except in select patients being treated for metastatic disease); estrogen-dependent neoplasia; liver disease or dysfunction

Warnings Estrogens have been reported to increase the risk of endometrial carcinoma (the addition of a progestin has been shown to decrease the risk of estrogen-induced endometrial hyperplasia, a condition thought to be a precursor to endometrial cancer). Do not use estrogens (with or without progestins) for the prevention of cardiovascular disease; a significantly increased risk of MI, stroke, PE, DVT, and invasive breast cancer was reported in postmenopausal women receiving conjugated equine estrogens combined with medroxyprogesterone acetate (see Rossouw, 2002); use of conjugated estrogens alone significantly increased the risk of stroke in postmenopausal women, but did not affect the risk of coronary heart disease (see Women's Health Initiative Steering Committee, 2004); due to these risks, use estrogens (with or without progestins) at the lowest effective doses and for the shortest duration possible that is consistent with an individual's treatment goals and risks; periodic risk:benefit assessments should be conducted; discontinue estrogens immediately if MI, stroke, PE, or DVT occur; in order to minimize the risk of thromboembolism in patients receiving estrogens, other risk factors for venous thromboembolism (eg, obesity, SLE, personal or family history of venous thromboembolism) and arterial vascular disease (eg, diabetes mellitus, hypertension, tobacco use, obesity, and hypercholesterolemia) should be appropriately managed.

Consider topical vaginal products when estrogen is used solely for the treatment of vulvar and vaginal atrophy; if used solely for the prevention of osteoporosis in postmenopausal women, estrogens should only be considered for those at significant risk of osteoporosis and for whom nonestrogen treatment options are not considered to be appropriate. Do not use estrogens during pregnancy.

Since estrogens may increase the risk of venous thromboembolism, discontinue therapy, if possible, at least 4-6 weeks before surgery that is associated with an increased risk of thromboembolism, or during times of prolonged immobilization. Estrogens may increase the risk of breast cancer, gallbladder disease, hypercalcemia, and retinal vascular thrombosis (discontinue estrogen therapy in patients with sudden partial or complete loss of vision, sudden onset of diplopia, proptosis, or migraine, or if eye exam reveals retinal vascular lesions or papilledema). The combined use of conjugated equine estrogens and medroxyprogesterone acetate was reported to significantly increase the risk of probable dementia in postmenopausal women; it is currently not known if these findings apply to younger women or to patients receiving estrogen alone.

Absorption of topical emulsion is significantly increased by application of sunscreen (do not apply both products within close proximity of each other); estradiol may be absorbed by others upon physical contact with topical emulsion application site. Topical gel is alcohol based and is flammable; patients should avoid fire, flame, or smoking until the gel has dried (gel dries in 2-5 minutes after application); photosensitivity after gel application and effects of concurrent application of sunscreen with gel have not been evaluated; estradiol was **not** absorbed by others after physical contact with topical gel application site 1 hour after application.

Injection may contain benzyl alcohol and oral tablet may contain tartrazine, both of which may cause allergic reactions in susceptible individuals; large amounts of benzyl alcohol (≥99 mg/kg/day) have been associated with a potentially fatal toxicity ("gasping syndrome") in neonates; avoid use of estradiol products containing benzyl alcohol in neonates; *in vitro* and animal studies have shown that benzoate, a metabolite of benzyl alcohol, displaces bilirubin from protein binding sites

Precautions Use with caution in patients with asthma, epilepsy, migraines, diabetes, hypothyroidism, hypocalcemia, hypercalcemia, endometriosis, porphyria, SLE, hepatic hemangioma, history of cholestatic jaundice due to past estrogen use or pregnancy, cardiac, liver, or renal dysfunction. Estrogens may cause premature closure of the epiphyses in young individuals; may cause premature breast development in prepubertal girls or gynecomastia in boys; may include vaginal bleeding or vaginal cornification in girls; may increase risk of ovarian cancer; may increase blood pressure; may cause fluid retention; may greatly increase triglycerides and lead to pancreatitis and other problems in patients with familial defects of lipoprotein metabolism; Femring™ may not be suitable for women that have conditions which make the vagina more susceptible to vaginal ulceration or irritation, or make expulsion of the ring more likely (eg, vaginal stenosis, cervical prolapse, etc)

Adverse Reactions

Cardiovascular: Hypertension, edema, thromboembolic disorders

Central nervous system: Depression, headache, dizziness, nervousness, migraine, irritability, mood disturbances, exacerbation of epilepsy, dementia

Dermatologic: Chloasma, melasma, urticaria

Endocrine & metabolic: Breast enlargement, breast tenderness, breast pain, changes in libido, impaired glucose tolerance, hypercalcemia, hypertriglyceridemia, folate deficiency, weight gain or weight loss; increased risk of endometrial hyperplasia

Gastrointestinal: Nausea, vomiting, bloating, abdominal cramps, pancreatitis, gall bladder disease, abdominal pain

Genitourinary: Changes in menstrual flow, vaginal hemorrhage, dysmenorrhea

Hepatic: Cholestatic jaundice, enlargement of hepatic hemangiomas

Local: Pain at injection site; topical may cause burning, irritation, pruritus, redness, rash

Neuromuscular & skeletal: Premature closure of epiphyses in young patients (large and repeated doses over an extended period of time); chorea, leg cramps, arthralgia

Miscellaneous: Angioedema, anaphylactoid reaction

Drug Interactions Cytochrome P450 isoenzyme CYP1A2 and CYP3A3/4 substrate; isoenzyme CYP1A2 inhibitor

Rifampin, phenobarbital, carbamazepine, and the herbal medicine St John's wort (*Hypericum perforatum*) may decrease plasma concentrations and effects of estrogens; cytochrome P450 CYP3A4 inhibitors (eg, erythromycin, clarithromycin, ketoconazole, itraconazole, ritonavir) may increase estrogen plasma concentrations and effects; anticoagulants, bromocriptine, dantrolene (increased risk of hepatotoxicity); estrogens may decrease the clearance and increase the serum concentrations and toxic effects of corticosteroids and cyclosporine

Food Interactions Larger doses of vitamin C (eg, 1 g/day in adults) may increase the serum concentrations and adverse effects of estradiol; vitamin C supplements are not recommended, but this effect may be decreased if vitamin C supplement is given 2-3 hours after estrogen; dietary intake of folate and pyridoxine may need to be increased; grapefruit juice may possibly increase estrogen plasma concentrations and effects

Mechanism of Action Increases the synthesis of DNA, RNA, and various proteins in target tissues; reduces the release of gonadotropin-releasing hormone from the hypothalamus; reduces FSH and LH release from the pituitary

Pharmacokinetics

Absorption: Oral, topical well absorbed

Topical emulsion: Absorption is significantly increased by application of sunscreen (see Warnings)

Distribution: Widely distributes throughout the body; sex hormone target organs contain higher concentrations; distributes into breast milk

Protein binding: Primarily bound to sex hormone-binding globulin and albumin

Metabolism: Hepatic, via cytochrome P450 isoenzyme CYP3A4; estradiol is converted to estrone and estriol; estrone is also converted to estriol and is converted to estradiol (**Note:** A dynamic equilibrium of metabolic interconversions between estrogens exists in the circulation); estrogens also undergo hepatic sulfate and glucuronide conjugation and enterohepatic recirculation

Elimination: Excreted in the urine as estradiol, estrone, and estriol and glucuronide and sulfate conjugates

Usual Dosage Adolescents and Adults: **Note:** Use lowest effective dose for shortest duration possible that is consistent with an individual's treatment goals and risks; all dosage needs to be adjusted based upon the patient's response

Female hypogonadism:

I.M.:

Cypionate: 1.5-2 mg given once each month

Valerate: 10-20 mg given once each month

Oral: 0.5-2 mg/day in a cyclic regimen (3 weeks on drug, 1 week off)

Transdermal:

Once-weekly patch (Climara®): Initial: 0.025 mg/day patch applied once weekly (titrate dosage to response)

(Continued)

Estradiol *(Continued)*

Twice-weekly patch: Alora®, Esclim®, Estraderm®: Initial: 0.05 mg patch; Vivelle®, Vivelle Dot®: Initial: 0.0375 mg patch; titrate dosage to response; apply patch twice weekly in a cyclic regimen (3 weeks on drug, 1 week off) in patients with intact uterus and continuously in patients without a uterus

Vaginal and vulval atrophy: Intravaginal: Initial: 200-400 mcg of estradiol once daily for 1-2 weeks; taper dose gradually to 100-200 mcg of estradiol once daily for 1-2 weeks; maintenance, cyclic regimen (after vaginal mucosa restored): 100 mcg of estradiol 1-3 times/week for 3 weeks, then no drug for the 4th week per cycle

Vaginal ring:

Postmenopausal vaginal atrophy, urogenital symptoms: Estring®: 2 mg intravaginally; following insertion, ring should remain in place for 90 days

Moderate to severe vasomotor symptoms associated with menopause; vulvar/vaginal atrophy: Femring™: 0.05 mg intravaginally; following insertion, ring should remain in place for 3 months; dose may be increased to 0.1 mg if needed

Topical emulsion: Moderate to severe vasomotor symptoms associated with menopause: 3.84 g (contents of 2 pouches) applied once daily in the morning

Topical gel: Moderate to severe vasomotor symptoms associated with menopause or vulvar and vaginal atrophy: 1.25 g applied once daily at the same time each day

Administration

Oral: Administer with food or after a meal to reduce GI upset

Parenteral: Injection for I.M. use only

Transdermal: Apply to clean dry area; do not apply to breasts; do not apply to waistline (may loosen patch); rotate application sites

Vaginal ring: Exact positioning is not critical for efficacy, however, patient should not feel ring or discomfort once inserted. In case of discomfort, ring should be gently pushed further into vagina. If ring is expelled prior to 90 days, it may be rinsed off and reinserted.

Topical emulsion: Apply to clean dry skin on both legs while sitting. Apply contents of first pouch to top of left thigh, massage into skin of left thigh and calf until thoroughly absorbed (~3 minutes). Apply excess from hands to buttocks. Apply contents of second pouch to right thigh and calf in the same manner. Wash hands with soap and water. Allow skin to dry before covering legs with clothes. Do not apply to other areas of the body. Do not apply to red or irritated skin. Do not apply sunscreen at the same time.

Topical gel: Apply to clean, dry, unbroken skin at the same time each day. Apply gel to the arm, from the wrist to shoulder. Spread gel as thinly as possible over one arm. Allow to dry for 5 minutes prior to dressing. Wash hands with soap and water. Avoid fire, flame, or smoking until gel is dry (gel is flammable). Do not apply gel to breasts or red or irritated skin. Prior to the first use, pump must be primed by fully depressing pump twice (and discarding the gel); **Note:** Discard unused gel by rinsing down sink; avoid exposure to others and pets.

Monitoring Parameters Blood pressure, weight, serum calcium, glucose, liver enzymes; bone maturation and epiphyseal effects in young patients in whom bone growth is not complete; breast exam, mammogram, Papanicolaou smear, signs for endometrial cancer in female patients with a uterus; bone density measurement if used for prevention of osteoporosis

Test Interactions Thyroid function tests: Estrogens may increase thyroid binding globulin and circulating total thyroid hormone (when measured by T_4 RIA, T_4 by column, or by PBI); decreases free T_3 resin uptake; concentration of free T_4 is not altered; metyrapone test: Response may be reduced

Patient Information Limit alcohol, caffeine, and grapefruit juice; notify physician if sudden severe headache or vomiting, disturbance of vision or speech, numbness or weakness of extremity, sharp or crushing chest pain, calf pain, shortness of breath, severe abdominal pain or mass, mental depression, or unusual bleeding occurs

Additional Information See package insert for doses related to postmenopausal symptoms, prevention of osteoporosis in postmenopausal women, and palliative treatment of breast cancer or androgen-dependent prostate cancer in adults. Femring™ can remain in place during local treatment of vaginal infections.

Dosage Forms Excipient information presented when available (limited, particularly for generics); consult specific product labeling.

Cream, vaginal:

Estrace®: 0.1 mg/g (12 g) [refill]; 0.1 mg/g (42.5 g) [packaged with applicator]

Emulsion, topical, as hemihydrate:

Estrasorb™: 2.5 mg/g (56s) [each pouch contains 4.35 mg estradiol hemihydrate; contents of two pouches delivers estradiol 0.05 mg/day]

Gel, topical:

Elestrin™: 0.06% (144 g) [pump; delivers estradiol 0.52 mg/0.87 g; 100 actuations]

EstroGel®: 0.06% (93 g) [pump; delivers estradiol 0.75 mg/1.25 g; 64 actuations]

Injection, oil, as cypionate:
Depo®-Estradiol: 5 mg/mL (5 mL) [contains chlorobutanol; in cottonseed oil]
Injection, oil, as valerate:
Delestrogen®:
10 mg/mL (5 mL) [contains chlorobutanol; in sesame oil]
20 mg/mL (5 mL) [contains benzyl alcohol; in castor oil]
40 mg/mL (5 mL) [contains benzyl alcohol; in castor oil]
Ring, vaginal, as base:
Estring®: 2 mg [total estradiol 2 mg; releases 7.5 mcg/day over 90 days] (1s)
Ring, vaginal, as acetate:
Femring®: 0.05 mg [total estradiol 12.4 mg; releases 0.05 mg/day over 3 months] (1s); 0.1 mg [total estradiol 24.8 mg; releases 0.1 mg/day over 3 months] (1s)
Tablet, oral, as acetate:
Femtrace®: 0.45 mg, 0.9 mg, 1.8 mg
Tablet, oral, micronized: 0.5 mg, 1 mg, 2 mg
Estrace®: 0.5 mg, 1 mg, 2 mg [2 mg tablets contain tartrazine]
Gynodiol®: 0.5 mg, 1 mg, 1.5 mg, 2 mg
Tablet, vaginal, as base:
Vagifem®: 25 mcg [contains lactose]
Transdermal system: 0.025 mg/24 hours [once-weekly patch] (4s); 0.0375 mg/24 hours (4s) [once-weekly patch]; 0.05 mg/24 hours (4s) [once-weekly patch]; 0.06 mg/24 hours (4s) [once-weekly patch]; 0.075 mg/24 hours [once-weekly patch]; 0.1 mg/24 hours (4s) [once-weekly patch]
Alora® [twice-weekly patch]:
0.025 mg/24 hours [9 cm^2, total estradiol 0.77 mg] (8s)
0.05 mg/24 hours [18 cm^2, total estradiol 1.5 mg] (8s, 24s)
0.075 mg/24 hours [27 cm^2, total estradiol 2.3 mg] (8s)
0.1 mg/24 hours [36 cm^2, total estradiol 3.1 mg] (8s)
Climara® [once-weekly patch]:
0.025 mg/24 hours [6.5 cm^2, total estradiol 2.04 mg] (4s)
0.0375 mg/24 hours [9.375 cm^2, total estradiol 2.85 mg] (4s)
0.05 mg/24 hours [12.5 cm^2, total estradiol 3.8 mg] (4s)
0.06 mg/24 hours [15 cm^2, total estradiol 4.55 mg] (4s)
0.075 mg/24 hours [18.75 cm^2, total estradiol 5.7 mg] (4s)
0.1 mg/24 hours [25 cm^2, total estradiol 7.6 mg] (4s)
Esclim® [twice-weekly patch]:
0.025 mg/day [11 cm^2, total estradiol 5 mg] (8s)
0.0375 mg/day [16.5 cm^2, total estradiol 7.5 mg] (8s)
0.05 mg/day [22 cm^2, total estradiol 10 mg] (8s)
0.075 mg/day [33 cm^2, total estradiol 15 mg] (8s)
0.1 mg/day [44 cm^2, total estradiol 20 mg] (8s)
Estraderm® [twice-weekly patch]:
0.05 mg/24 hours [10 cm^2, total estradiol 4 mg] (8s)
0.1 mg/24 hours [20 cm^2, total estradiol 8 mg] (8s)
Menostar™ [once-weekly patch]: 0.014 mg/24 hours [3.25 cm^2, total estradiol 1 mg] (4s)
Vivelle® [twice-weekly patch]:
0.05 mg/24 hours [14.5 cm^2, total estradiol 4.33 mg] (8s)
0.1 mg/24 hours [29 cm^2, total estradiol 8.66 mg] (8s)
Vivelle-Dot® [twice-weekly patch]:
0.025 mg/day [2.5 cm^2, total estradiol 0.39 mg] (8s)
0.0375 mg/day [3.75 cm^2, total estradiol 0.585 mg] (8s)
0.05 mg/day [5 cm^2, total estradiol 0.78 mg] (8s)
0.075 mg/day [7.5 cm^2, total estradiol 1.17 mg] (8s)
0.1 mg/day [10 cm^2, total estradiol 1.56 mg] (8s)

References

Rossouw JE, Anderson GL, Prentice RL, et al, "Risks and Benefits of Estrogen Plus Progestin in Healthy Postmenopausal Women: Principal Results From the Women's Health Initiative Randomized Controlled Trial," *JAMA*, 2002, 288(3):321-33.

Women's Health Initiative Steering Committee, "Effects of Conjugated Equine Estrogen in Postmenopausal Women With Hysterectomy: The Women's Health Initiative Randomized Controlled Trial," *JAMA*, 2004, 291(14):1701-12.

♦ **Estradiol Acetate** *see* Estradiol *on page 605*
♦ **Estradiol Cypionate** *see* Estradiol *on page 605*
♦ **Estradiol Hemihydrate** *see* Estradiol *on page 605*
♦ **Estradiol Transdermal** *see* Estradiol *on page 605*
♦ **Estradiol Valerate** *see* Estradiol *on page 605*
♦ **Estradot® (Can)** *see* Estradiol *on page 605*
♦ **Estrasorb™** *see* Estradiol *on page 605*
♦ **Estring®** *see* Estradiol *on page 605*
♦ **EstroGel®** *see* Estradiol *on page 605*

♦ **Estrogenic Substances, Conjugated** *see* Estrogens (Conjugated/Equine) *on page 610*

Estrogens (Conjugated/Equine)

(ES troe jenz KON joo gate ed/E kwine)

Medication Safety Issues

Sound-alike/look-alike issues:

Premarin® may be confused with Primaxin®, Provera®, Remeron®

U.S. Brand Names Premarin®

Canadian Brand Names C.E.S.®; Premarin®

Index Terms CEE; C.E.S.; Estrogenic Substances, Conjugated

Therapeutic Category Estrogen Derivative; Estrogen Derivative, Vaginal

Generic Available No

Use Treatment of dysfunctional uterine bleeding, hypoestrogenism (due to hypogonadism, castration, or primary ovarian failure), moderate to severe vasomotor symptoms of menopause; moderate to severe symptoms of vulvar and vaginal atrophy due to menopause; palliative treatment of breast cancer in select patients; palliative treatment of androgen-dependent prostate cancer; prevention of osteoporosis in postmenopausal women; see Warnings and Additional Information; **Note:** Intravenous product is indicated for short-term use only

Pregnancy Risk Factor X

Lactation Enters breast milk/use caution

Contraindications Hypersensitivity to estrogens or any component (see Warnings); history of or current DVT or PE; recent (eg, within past year) or current arterial thromboembolic disease (eg, MI, stroke); undiagnosed vaginal bleeding; pregnancy; known, suspected, or history of breast cancer (except in select patients being treated for metastatic disease); estrogen-dependent neoplasia; liver disease or dysfunction

Warnings Estrogens have been reported to increase the risk of endometrial carcinoma (the addition of a progestin has been shown to decrease the risk of estrogen-induced endometrial hyperplasia, a condition thought to be a precursor to endometrial cancer). Do not use estrogens (with or without progestins) for the prevention of cardiovascular disease; a significantly increased risk of MI, stroke, PE, DVT, and invasive breast cancer was reported in postmenopausal women receiving conjugated equine estrogens combined with medroxyprogesterone acetate (see Rossouw, 2002); use of conjugated estrogens alone significantly increased the risk of stroke in postmenopausal women, but did not affect the risk of coronary heart disease (see Women's Health Initiative Steering Committee, 2004); due to these risks, use estrogens (with or without progestins) at the lowest effective doses and for the shortest duration possible that is consistent with an individual's treatment goals and risks; periodic risk:benefit assessments should be conducted; discontinue estrogens immediately if MI, stroke, PE, or DVT occur; in order to minimize the risk of thromboembolism in patients receiving estrogens, other risk factors for venous thromboembolism (eg, obesity, SLE, personal or family history of venous thromboembolism) and arterial vascular disease (eg, diabetes mellitus, hypertension, tobacco use, obesity, and hypercholesterolemia) should be appropriately managed.

Consider topical vaginal products when estrogen is used solely for the treatment of vulvar and vaginal atrophy; if used solely for the prevention of osteoporosis in postmenopausal women, estrogens should only be considered for those at significant risk of osteoporosis and for whom nonestrogen treatment options are not considered to be appropriate. Do not use estrogens during pregnancy.

Since estrogens may increase the risk of venous thromboembolism, discontinue therapy, if possible, at least 4-6 weeks before surgery that is associated with an increased risk of thromboembolism, or during times of prolonged immobilization. Estrogens may increase the risk of breast cancer, gallbladder disease, hypercalcemia, and retinal vascular thrombosis (discontinue estrogen therapy in patients with sudden partial or complete loss of vision, sudden onset of diplopia, proptosis, or migraine, or if eye exam reveals retinal vascular lesions or papilledema). The combined use of conjugated equine estrogens and medroxyprogesterone acetate was reported to significantly increase the risk of probable dementia in postmenopausal women; it is currently not known if these findings apply to younger women or to patients receiving estrogen alone.

Systemic absorption may occur with intravaginal or topical use. Diluent for injection contains benzyl alcohol which may cause allergic reactions in susceptible individuals; large amounts of benzyl alcohol (≥99 mg/kg/day) have been associated with a potentially fatal toxicity ("gasping syndrome") in neonates; avoid use of estrogen products containing benzyl alcohol in neonates; *in vitro* and animal studies have shown that benzoate, a metabolite of benzyl alcohol, displaces bilirubin from protein binding sites

Precautions Use with caution in patients with asthma, epilepsy, migraines, diabetes, hypothyroidism, hypocalcemia, hypercalcemia, endometriosis, porphyria, SLE, hepatic hemangioma, history of cholestatic jaundice due to past estrogen use or pregnancy, cardiac, liver, or renal dysfunction. Estrogens may cause premature closure of the epiphyses in young individuals; may cause premature breast development in prepubertal girls or gynecomastia in boys; may induce vaginal bleeding or vaginal cornification in girls; may increase risk of ovarian cancer. May increase blood pressure; may cause fluid retention; may greatly increase triglycerides and lead to pancreatitis and other problems in patients with familial defects of lipoprotein metabolism. Estrogen vaginal creams may contribute to the failure of barrier contraceptives by weakening condoms, diaphragms, or cervical caps made of latex or rubber.

Adverse Reactions

Cardiovascular: Hypertension, edema, thromboembolic disorder

Central nervous system: Depression, headache, dizziness, nervousness, migraine, irritability, mood disturbances, exacerbation of epilepsy, dementia

Dermatologic: Chloasma, melasma, urticaria

Endocrine & metabolic: Breast enlargement, breast tenderness, breast pain, changes in libido, impaired glucose tolerance, hypercalcemia, hypertriglyceridemia, folate deficiency, weight gain or weight loss; increased risk of endometrial hyperplasia

Gastrointestinal: Nausea, vomiting, bloating, abdominal cramps, abdominal pain, pancreatitis, gall bladder disease

Genitourinary: Changes in menstrual flow, vaginal hemorrhage, dysmenorrhea

Hepatic: Cholestatic jaundice, enlargement of hepatic hemangiomas

Local: Pain at injection site

Neuromuscular & skeletal: Premature closure of epiphyses in young patients; chorea, leg cramps, arthralgia

Miscellaneous: Angioedema, anaphylactoid reaction

Drug Interactions Cytochrome P450 isoenzyme CYP3A4 substrate

Rifampin, phenobarbital, carbamazepine, and the herbal medicine St John's wort (*Hypericum perforatum*) may decrease plasma concentrations and effects of estrogens; cytochrome P450 CYP3A4 inhibitors (eg, erythromycin, clarithromycin, ketoconazole, itraconazole, ritonavir) may increase estrogen plasma concentrations and effects; anticoagulants, bromocriptine, dantrolene (increased risk of hepatotoxicity); estrogens may decrease the clearance and increase the serum concentrations and toxic effects of corticosteroids and cyclosporine

Food Interactions Larger doses of vitamin C (eg, 1 g/day in adults) may increase the serum concentrations and adverse effects of estrogens; vitamin C supplements are not recommended, but this effect may be decreased if vitamin C supplement is given 2-3 hours after estrogen; dietary intake of folate and pyridoxine may need to be increased; grapefruit juice may possibly increase estrogen plasma concentrations and effects

Stability Injection: Store unreconstituted vials in the refrigerator at 2°C to 8°C (36°F to 46°F); if reconstituted solution is not used within a few hours, store under refrigeration; reconstituted solution is stable for 60 days when stored under refrigeration; compatible with NS, dextrose, and invert sugar solutions; **not** compatible with ascorbic acid, protein hydrolysate, or acidic pH

Mechanism of Action Increases the synthesis of DNA, RNA, and various proteins in target tissues; reduces the release of gonadotropin-releasing hormone from the hypothalamus; reduces FSH and LH release from the pituitary

Pharmacokinetics

Absorption: Oral, transmucosal, transdermal: Well absorbed

Distribution: Widely distributes throughout the body; sex hormone target organs contain higher concentrations; distributes into breast milk

Protein binding: Primarily bound to sex hormone-binding globulin and albumin

Metabolism: Hepatic, via cytochrome P450 isoenzyme CYP3A4; estradiol is converted to estrone and estriol; estrone is also converted to estriol and is converted to estradiol (**Note:** A dynamic equilibrium of metabolic interconversions between estrogens exists in the circulation); estrogens also undergo hepatic sulfate and glucuronide conjugation and enterohepatic recirculation

Elimination: Excreted in the urine as estradiol, estrone, estriol (major urinary metabolite), and glucuronide and sulfate conjugates

Usual Dosage Adolescents and Adults: **Note:** Use lowest effective dose for the shortest duration possible that is consistent with an individual's treatment goals and risks:

Female castration or primary ovarian failure: Oral: Cyclic regimen: 1.25 mg/day for 3 weeks, then no drug for the 4th week per cycle; repeat; titrate dose to response; use lowest effective dose

Female hypogonadism: Oral:

Manufacturer's recommendation: Cyclic regimen: 0.3-0.625 mg/day for 3 weeks, then no drug for the 4th week per cycle; titrate dose to response; use lowest effective dose

(Continued)

Estrogens (Conjugated/Equine) *(Continued)*

Alternative dosing: 2.5-7.5 mg/day in divided doses for 20 days, off 10 days and repeat until menses occur

Dysfunctional uterine bleeding:

Stable hematocrit: Oral: 1.25 mg twice daily for 21 days; if bleeding persists after 48 hours, increase to 2.5 mg twice daily; if bleeding persists after 48 more hours, increase to 2.5 mg 4 times/day; some recommend starting at 2.5 mg 4 times/day (**Note:** Medroxyprogesterone acetate 10 mg/day is also given on days 17-21; see Neistein, 1991)

Alternatively: Oral: 2.5-5 mg/day for 7-10 days; then decrease to 1.25 mg/day for 2 weeks

Unstable hematocrit: Oral, I.V.: 5 mg 2-4 times/day; if bleeding is profuse, 20-40 mg every 4 hours up to 24 hours may be used; **Note:** A progestational-weighted contraception pill should also be given (eg, Ovral® 2 tablets stat and 1 tablet 4 times/day or medroxyprogesterone acetate 5-10 mg 4 times/day; see Neistein, 1991)

Alternatively: I.M., I.V.: 25 mg every 6-12 hours until bleeding stops

Vaginal and vulval atrophy: Intravaginal or topical (vaginal cream): Cyclic regimen: ½ to 2 g daily (0.3125-1.25 mg/day of conjugated estrogens) for 3 weeks, then no drug for the 4th week per cycle; repeat as clinically needed

Administration

Oral: Administer with food or after eating to reduce GI upset; administration of dose at bedtime may decrease adverse effects

Intravaginal: Use marked stopping points on applicator to measure prescribed dose; to administer, lay down on back and draw knees up; gently insert applicator into vagina and press plunger downward to deliver medication; wash plunger and barrel with mild soap and water after use; do not boil or use hot water

Parenteral: Add sterile diluent provided by manufacturer and shake gently; I.V.: Administer slow I.V. to avoid vascular flushing; I.M.: may be administered I.M. for dysfunctional uterine bleeding, but I.V. use is preferred (more rapid response)

Monitoring Parameters Blood pressure, weight, serum calcium, glucose, liver enzymes; dysfunctional uterine bleeding: Hematocrit, hemoglobin, PT; bone maturation and epiphyseal effects in young patients in whom bone growth is not complete; breast exam, mammogram, Papanicolaou smear, signs for endometrial cancer in female patients with a uterus; bone density measurement if used for prevention of osteoporosis

Test Interactions Thyroid function tests: Estrogens may increase thyroid binding globulin and circulating total thyroid hormone (when measured by T_4 RIA, T_4 by column, or by PBI); decreases free T_3 resin uptake; concentration of free T_4 is not altered; metyrapone test: Response may be reduced

Patient Information Limit caffeine and grapefruit juice; notify physician if sudden severe headache, vomiting, disturbance of vision or speech, numbness or weakness of extremity, sharp or crushing chest pain, calf pain, shortness of breath, severe abdominal pain or mass, mental depression, or unusual bleeding occurs

Additional Information See package insert for doses related to postmenopausal symptoms, prevention of osteoporosis in postmenopausal women, and palliative treatment of breast cancer or androgen-dependent prostate cancer in adults.

Dosage Forms Excipient information presented when available (limited, particularly for generics); consult specific product labeling.

Cream, vaginal: 0.625 mg/g (42.5 g)

Injection, powder for reconstitution: 25 mg [contains lactose 200 mg; diluent contains benzyl alcohol]

Tablet: 0.3 mg, 0.45 mg, 0.625 mg, 0.9 mg, 1.25 mg

References

Minjarez DA and Bradshaw KD, "Abnormal Uterine Bleeding in Adolescents," *Obstet Gynecol Clin North Am*, 2000, 27(1):63-78.

Mitan LA and Slap GB, "Adolescent Menstrual Disorders. Update," *Med Clin North Am*, 2000, 84(4):851-68.

Neistein LS, *Adolescent Health Care - A Practical Guide*, 2nd ed, Baltimore: Urban & Schwarzenberg, 1991, 661-6.

Rossouw JE, Anderson GL, Prentice RL, et al, "Risks and Benefits of Estrogen Plus Progestin in Healthy Postmenopausal Women: Principal Results From the Women's Health Initiative Randomized Controlled Trial," *JAMA*, 2002, 288(3):321-33.

Women's Health Initiative Steering Committee, "Effects of Conjugated Equine Estrogen in Postmenopausal Women With Hysterectomy: The Women's Health Initiative Randomized Controlled Trial," *JAMA*, 2004, 291(14):1701-12.

♦ **ETAF** *see* Aldesleukin *on page 70*

Etanercept (et a NER cept)

U.S. Brand Names Enbrel®

Canadian Brand Names Enbrel®

Therapeutic Category Antirheumatic, Disease Modifying

Generic Available No

Use Treatment of polyarticular-course juvenile rheumatoid arthritis in patients who have had an inadequate response to one or more disease-modifying antirheumatic drugs; treatment of signs and symptoms of moderately to severely active rheumatoid arthritis in patients who have had an inadequate response to one or more disease-modifying antirheumatic drugs or in combination with methotrexate in patients who do not respond adequately to methotrexate alone; psoriatic arthritis; active ankylosing spondylitis; treatment of chronic (moderate to severe) plaque psoriasis in patients who are candidates for systemic therapy or phototherapy

Pregnancy Risk Factor B

Lactation Excretion in breast milk unknown/not recommended

Contraindications Hypersensitivity to etanercept or any component (ie, mannitol, sucrose, tromethamine, and benzyl alcohol) (see Warnings); patients with any serious active infection or sepsis

Warnings Some patients have developed serious infections and several have died from their infections while taking etanercept; patients who develop a new infection while being treated with etanercept should be monitored closely. Rate of serious infections is higher in patients on concomitant immunosuppressive therapy than with etanercept alone. Etanercept should be discontinued if a patient develops a serious infection or sepsis. Rare cases of CNS demyelinating disorders, such as multiple sclerosis, myelitis, optic neuritis, and seizure disorders have been reported in patients undergoing etanercept therapy.

A two-fold higher incidence of lymphoma has been observed in patients receiving etanercept compared to that expected in the general population. Malignancies other than lymphoma have also been observed. Long-term carcinogenic potential or effect on fertility are unknown.

Diluent for etanercept injection contains benzyl alcohol which may cause allergic reactions in susceptible individuals; large amounts of benzyl alcohol (≥99 mg/kg/day) have been associated with a potentially fatal toxicity ("gasping syndrome") in neonates; avoid use of etanercept products containing benzyl alcohol in neonates; *in vitro* and animal studies have shown that benzoate, a metabolite of benzyl alcohol, displaces bilirubin from protein binding sites; patients with latex allergy should not handle the needle cover of the diluent syringe since it contains latex

Precautions Use with caution in patients with a history of hematologic abnormalities, heart failure, or in patients with a history of recurrent infections or illnesses such as poorly controlled diabetes which predisposes the patient to infection; discontinue etanercept in a child who develops varicella infection or who has a significant exposure to varicella virus and consider prophylactic treatment with varicella-zoster immune globulin; anti-TNF therapies such as etanercept may affect host defenses against infections and malignancies

Adverse Reactions

Cardiovascular: CHF, flushing, MI

Central nervous system: Headache (19%), depression, personality disorder, dizziness, seizures, multiple sclerosis, myelitis, cerebral ischemia

Dermatologic: Rash, angioedema, cutaneous vasculitis, urticaria, pruritus

Gastrointestinal: Nausea (9%), abdominal pain (17%), vomiting (13%), pancreatitis, anorexia, diarrhea, esophagitis/gastritis, GI bleeding

Hematologic: Pancytopenia, aplastic anemia, neutropenia, thrombocytopenia

Local: Injection site reactions (erythema, discomfort, itching, swelling)

Neuromuscular & skeletal: Joint pain, paresthesia

Ocular: Optic neuritis

Respiratory: Respiratory tract infection, rhinitis, dyspnea

Miscellaneous: Allergic reaction (hives, difficulty breathing), positive antinuclear antibodies, lupus-like syndrome, positive antidouble-stranded DNA antibodies

Drug Interactions Live vaccines (do not administer live vaccines while patient is receiving etanercept; unknown whether secondary transmission of infection with live vaccines can occur); anakinra (increased rate of serious infections when used concurrently with etanercept)

Stability Store vial in the refrigerator; do not freeze; reconstituted solution prepared with bacteriostatic water for injection is stable for 14 days if refrigerated; do not shake or agitate vigorously; do not use if discolored or cloudy or if particulate matter is present; do not filter reconstituted solution; do not add or mix with other medications

(Continued)

Etanercept *(Continued)*

Mechanism of Action Binds to tumor necrosis factor (TNF) and blocks its interaction with cell surface TNF receptors rendering TNF biologically inactive; modulates biological responses that are induced or regulated by TNF

Pharmacodynamics

Onset of action: One week of treatment

Maximum effect: Full effect is usually seen within 3 months

Pharmacokinetics

Absorption: Absorbed slowly after SubQ injection

Distribution: V_d: 1.78-3.39 L/m^2

Bioavailability: SubQ: 60%

Half-life: Adults: 115 hours (range: 98-300 hours)

Time to peak serum concentration: SubQ: 72 hours (range: 48-96 hours)

Elimination: Clearance:

Children 4-17 years: 46 mL/hour/m^2

Adults: 52 mL/hour/m^2

Usual Dosage SubQ:

Children 4-17 years: Juvenile rheumatoid arthritis:

Twice-weekly dosing: 0.4 mg/kg/dose twice weekly given 72-96 hours apart; maximum dose: 25 mg

Alternative once-weekly dosing: 0.8 mg/kg/dose once weekly; maximum dose: 50 mg/week (maximum amount administered at a single injection site is 25 mg)

Adults:

Rheumatoid arthritis, psoriatic arthritis, ankylosing spondylitis:

Twice-weekly dosing: 25 mg twice weekly given 72-96 hours apart

Alternative once-weekly dosing: 50 mg once weekly; maximum amount administered at a single injection site is 25 mg

Plaque psoriasis: Initial: 50 mg twice weekly (administered 3-4 days apart) for 3 months; **Note:** Initial doses of 25 mg or 50 mg per week were also shown to be efficacious; maintenance dose: 50 mg once weekly; maximum amount administered at a single injection site: 25 mg

Administration Parenteral: Add 1 mL of bacteriostatic water for injection to 25 mg vial, resulting in 25 mg/mL solution. Administer by SubQ injection into thigh, abdomen, or upper arm; injection sites should be rotated with subsequent doses given at least 1 inch from an old site; do not inject into areas where the skin is tender, bruised, red, or hard. Do not administer >25 mg at a single injection site.

Monitoring Parameters Assess for joint swelling, pain, and tenderness; ESR or C-reactive protein level; CBC with differential and platelet count

Patient Information Notify physician if persistent fever, bruising, bleeding, or pallor occurs.

Dosage Forms Excipient information presented when available (limited, particularly for generics); consult specific product labeling.

Injection, powder for reconstitution:

Enbrel®: 25 mg [contains sucrose; diluent contains benzyl alcohol]

Injection, solution:

Enbrel®: 50 mg/mL (0.98 mL) [contains sucrose; packaging may contain dry natural rubber (latex)]

References

Ilowite NT, "Current Treatment of Juvenile Rheumatoid Arthritis," *Pediatrics*, 2002, 109(1):109-15.

Lovell DJ, Giannini EH, Reiff A, et al, "Long-Term Efficacy and Safety of Etanercept in Children With Polyarticular-Course Juvenile Rheumatoid Arthritis: Interim Results From an Ongoing Multicenter, Open-Label, Extended-Treatment Trial," *Arthritis Rheum*, 2003, 48(1):218-26.

Moreland LW, Baumgartner SW, Schiff MH, et al, "Treatment of Rheumatoid Arthritis With a Recombinant Human Tumor Necrosis Factor Receptor (p75)-Fc Fusion Protein," *N Engl J Med*, 1997, 337(3):141-7.

♦ **Ethacrynate Sodium** *see* Ethacrynic Acid *on page 614*

Ethacrynic Acid (eth a KRIN ik AS id)

Medication Safety Issues

Sound-alike/look-alike issues:

Edecrin® may be confused with Eulexin®, Ecotrin®

Related Information

Antihypertensive Agents by Class *on page 1678*

U.S. Brand Names Edecrin®

Canadian Brand Names Edecrin®

Index Terms Ethacrynate Sodium

Therapeutic Category Antihypertensive Agent; Diuretic, Loop

Generic Available No

Use Management of edema secondary to CHF, hepatic or renal disease; hypertension

Pregnancy Risk Factor B

Lactation Contraindicated

Contraindications Hypersensitivity to ethacrynic acid or any component; hypotension, hyponatremic dehydration, metabolic alkalosis with hypokalemia, or anuria

Warnings Loop diuretics are potent diuretics; excess amounts can lead to profound diuresis with fluid and electrolyte loss; close medical supervision and dose evaluation is required; may increase risk of gastric hemorrhage associated with corticosteroid treatment

Precautions Avoid use in patients with severe renal dysfunction (Cl_{cr} <10 mL/minute)

Adverse Reactions

Cardiovascular: Hypotension
Central nervous system: Headache, fatigue, mental confusion, vertigo
Dermatologic: Rash, photosensitivity
Endocrine & metabolic: Hyperglycemia, fluid and electrolyte imbalances (fluid depletion, hypokalemia, hyponatremia, hypomagnesemia, hypocalcemia), hyperuricemia
Gastrointestinal: GI irritation, diarrhea, anorexia, abdominal pain, dysphagia, GI bleed
Hematologic: Thrombocytopenia, neutropenia, agranulocytosis
Hepatic: Abnormal liver function tests, jaundice, hepatocellular damage
Local: Local irritation, pain at injection site
Otic: Ototoxicity, tinnitus
Renal: Renal injury, hematuria

Drug Interactions Additive potassium depletion with drugs which cause potassium depletion: amphotericin, steroids, corticotropin; decreased renal clearance of lithium; decreased hypoglycemic effect of insulin or oral antidiabetic agents; decreased excretion of ethacrynic acid by probenecid; increased risk of ototoxicity with aminoglycosides; increased warfarin activity due to displacement from protein-binding sites

Food Interactions Need diet rich in potassium and magnesium

Stability When reconstituted with 50 mL D_5W or NS, resultant solution (1 mg/mL) is stable for 24 hours at room temperature

Mechanism of Action Inhibits reabsorption of sodium and chloride in the ascending loop of Henle and distal renal tubule, interfering with the chloride-binding cotransport system, thus causing increased excretion of water, sodium, chloride, magnesium, and calcium

Pharmacodynamics

Onset of action:
- Oral: Within 30 minutes
- I.V.: 5 minutes

Peak effect:
- Oral: 2 hours
- I.V.: 15-30 minutes

Duration:
- Oral: 6-8 hours
- I.V.: 2 hours

Pharmacokinetics

Absorption: Oral: Rapid
Protein binding: >90%
Metabolism: In the liver to active cysteine conjugate (35% to 40%)
Elimination: In bile, 30% to 60% excreted unchanged in urine

Usual Dosage

Children:
- Oral: 1 mg/kg/dose once daily, increase at intervals of 2-3 days to a maximum of 3 mg/kg/day
- I.V.: 1 mg/kg/dose; repeat doses are not routinely recommended, however if indicated, repeat doses every 8-12 hours

Adults:
- Oral: 25-400 mg/day in 1-2 divided doses
- I.V.: 0.5-1 mg/kg/dose (maximum dose: 100 mg/dose); repeat doses not routinely recommended, however if indicated, repeat every 8-12 hours

Administration

Oral: Administer with food or milk
Parenteral: Dilute injection with 50 mL D_5W or NS (1 mg/mL concentration resulting); maximum concentration 2 mg/mL; may be injected without further dilution over a period of several minutes or infused over 20-30 minutes; tissue irritant; not to be administered I.M. or SubQ

Monitoring Parameters Serum electrolytes, blood pressure, renal function, hearing

Additional Information Injection contains thimerosal

Dosage Forms Excipient information presented when available (limited, particularly for generics); consult specific product labeling.

Injection, powder for reconstitution, as ethacrynate sodium: 50 mg
Tablet: 25 mg
(Continued)

Ethacrynic Acid *(Continued)*

Extemporaneous Preparations To make a 1 mg/mL suspension: Dissolve 120 mg ethacrynic acid powder in 13 mL alcohol, USP; add a small amount of methylparaben 0.005% and propylparaben 0.002% (final concentrations); adjust pH to 7 with 0.1N sodium hydroxide solution; add sufficient 50% sorbitol solution to make a final volume of 120 mL. Stable 220 days at room temperature. Shake well before use.

Das Gupta V, Gibbs CW Jr, and Ghanekar AG, "Stability of Pediatric Liquid Dosage Forms of Ethacrynic Acid, Indomethacin, Methyldopate Hydrochloride, Prednisone and Spironolactone," *Am J Hosp Pharm*, 1978, 35(11):1382-5.

Ethambutol (e THAM byoo tole)

Medication Safety Issues

Sound-alike/look-alike issues:

Myambutol® may be confused with Nembutal®

U.S. Brand Names Myambutol®

Canadian Brand Names Etibi®

Index Terms Ethambutol Hydrochloride

Therapeutic Category Antitubercular Agent

Generic Available Yes

Use Treatment of tuberculosis and other mycobacterial diseases in conjunction with other antimycobacterial agents

Pregnancy Risk Factor C

Lactation Enters breast milk/use caution (AAP considers "compatible")

Contraindications Hypersensitivity to ethambutol or any component; optic neuritis

Warnings Optic neuropathy including optic neuritis or retrobulbar neuritis characterized by decreased visual acuity, scotoma, color blindness, and/or visual defect has been reported with ethambutol therapy and may be related to dose and treatment duration; irreversible blindness has also been reported. Loss of visual acuity is generally reversible when ethambutol is discontinued promptly. Some patients have received ethambutol again after such recovery without recurrence of visual acuity loss. Use only in children whose visual acuity can accurately be determined and monitored; fatal hepatotoxicity has been reported; not recommended for use in children <13 years of age unless benefit outweighs risk of therapy

Precautions Use with caution in patients with ocular defects or impaired renal function; modify dose in patients with renal impairment

Adverse Reactions

Central nervous system: Malaise, mental confusion, fever, headache, dizziness

Dermatologic: Rash, pruritus

Endocrine & metabolic: Elevated uric acid levels

Gastrointestinal: Nausea, vomiting, anorexia, abdominal pain

Hematologic: Thrombocytopenia, leukopenia, eosinophilia

Hepatic: Abnormal liver function tests, hepatotoxicity

Neuromuscular & skeletal: Peripheral neuropathy, arthralgia, joint pain

Ocular: Optic neuritis, decreased visual acuity, decreased red-green color discrimination, irreversible blindness

Miscellaneous: Anaphylaxis

Stability Store tablets at controlled room temperature 20°C to 25°C (68°F to 77°F)

Mechanism of Action Suppresses mycobacterial multiplication by interfering with RNA synthesis

Pharmacokinetics

Absorption: Oral: ~80%

Distribution: Well distributed throughout the body with high concentrations in kidneys, lungs, saliva, CSF, and red blood cells; crosses the placenta; excreted into breast milk

Protein binding: 20% to 30%

Metabolism: 20% by the liver to inactive metabolite

Half-life: 2.5-3.6 hours (up to 7 hours or longer with renal impairment)

Time to peak serum concentration: Within 2-4 hours

Elimination: ~50% in urine and 20% excreted in feces as unchanged drug

Dialysis: Slightly dialyzable (5% to 20%)

Usual Dosage Oral:

Tuberculosis: Infants, Children, Adolescents, and Adults: 15-25 mg/kg/day once daily **or** 50 mg/kg/dose twice weekly, not to exceed 2.5 g/dose

Nontuberculous mycobacterial infection: Children, Adolescents, and Adults: 15 mg/kg/day, not to exceed 1 g/day

Dosing interval in renal impairment:

Cl_{cr} 10-50 mL/minute: Administer every 24-36 hours

Cl_{cr} <10 mL/minute: Administer every 48 hours and/or reduce usual dose

Administration Oral: Administer with or without food; if GI upset occurs, administer with food

Monitoring Parameters Monthly examination of visual acuity and color discrimination in patients receiving >15 mg/kg/day; periodic renal, hepatic, and hematologic function tests

Patient Information Report to physician any visual changes, numbness or tingling in hands or feet, rash, fever, and chills

Dosage Forms Excipient information presented when available (limited, particularly for generics); consult specific product labeling.

Tablet, as hydrochloride: 100 mg, 400 mg

References

American Academy of Pediatrics, Committee on Infectious Diseases, "Chemotherapy for Tuberculosis in Infants and Children," *Pediatrics*, 1992, 89(1):161-5.

Starke JR and Correa AG, "Management of Mycobacterial Infection and Disease in Children," *Pediatr Infect Dis J*, 1995, 14:455-70.

♦ **Ethambutol Hydrochloride** *see* Ethambutol *on page 616*

♦ **Ethanol** *see* Ethyl Alcohol *on page 619*

♦ **EtheDent™** *see* Fluoride *on page 675*

♦ **Ethiofos** *see* Amifostine *on page 91*

Ethionamide (e thye on AM ide)

U.S. Brand Names Trecator®

Canadian Brand Names Trecator®

Therapeutic Category Antitubercular Agent

Generic Available No

Use In conjunction with other antituberculosis agents in the treatment of tuberculosis and other mycobacterial diseases

Pregnancy Risk Factor C

Lactation Excretion in breast milk unknown/use caution

Contraindications Hypersensitivity to ethionamide or any component; severe hepatic impairment

Precautions Use with caution in patients receiving cycloserine or isoniazid or in diabetic patients

Adverse Reactions

Cardiovascular: Postural hypotension

Central nervous system: Drowsiness, dizziness, seizures, headache, encephalopathy, depression, psychotic disturbances

Dermatologic: Rash

Endocrine & metabolic: Hypoglycemia, goiter, gynecomastia, weight loss

Gastrointestinal: Nausea, vomiting, abdominal pain, diarrhea, anorexia, stomatitis, metallic taste

Hematologic: Thrombocytopenia

Hepatic: Hepatitis; jaundice; elevated AST, ALT, and serum bilirubin

Neuromuscular & skeletal: Peripheral neuropathy, tremor

Ocular: Optic neuritis

Miscellaneous: Excessive salivation

Drug Interactions Cycloserine and isoniazid may increase nervous system adverse effects; alcohol (associated with psychotic reaction)

Food Interactions Increase dietary intake of pyridoxine to prevent neurotoxic effects of ethionamide

Mechanism of Action Inhibits peptide synthesis in susceptible organisms

Pharmacokinetics

Absorption: ~80% is rapidly absorbed from the GI tract

Distribution: Crosses the placenta; widely distributed into body tissues and fluids including liver, kidneys, and CSF

Protein binding: 10%

Metabolism: In the liver to active and inactive metabolites

Bioavailability: 80%

Half-life: 2-3 hours

Time to peak serum concentration: Oral: Within 3 hours

Elimination: As metabolites (active and inactive) and parent drug in the urine

Usual Dosage Oral:

Children: 15-20 mg/kg/day in 2-3 divided doses, not to exceed 1 g/day

Adults: 500-1000 mg/day in 1-3 divided doses

Administration Oral: Administer with meals to decrease GI distress

Monitoring Parameters Initial and periodic serum AST and ALT, blood glucose, thyroid function tests, periodic ophthalmologic exams

(Continued)

Ethionamide *(Continued)*

Nursing Implications Neurotoxic effects may be relieved by the administration of pyridoxine

Dosage Forms Excipient information presented when available (limited, particularly for generics); consult specific product labeling.

Tablet: 250 mg

References

Donald PR and Seifart HI,"Cerebrospinal Fluid Concentrations of Ethionamide in Children With Tuberculous Meningitis," *J Pediatr*, 1989, 115(3):483-6.

Starke JR and Correa AG, "Management of Mycobacterial Infection and Disease in Children," *Pediatr Infect Dis J*, 1995, 14(6):455-69.

Ethosuximide (eth oh SUKS i mide)

Medication Safety Issues

Sound-alike/look-alike issues:

Ethosuximide may be confused with methsuximide

Zarontin® may be confused with Xalatan®, Zantac®, Zaroxolyn®

Related Information

Antiepileptic Drugs *on page 1902*

Blood Level Sampling Time Guidelines *on page 1914*

U.S. Brand Names Zarontin®

Canadian Brand Names Zarontin®

Therapeutic Category Anticonvulsant, Succinimide

Generic Available Yes

Use Management of absence (petit mal) seizures, myoclonic seizures, and akinetic epilepsy

Pregnancy Risk Factor D

Lactation Enters breast milk/use caution (AAP rates "compatible")

Contraindications Hypersensitivity to ethosuximide, other succinimides, or any component

Warnings Ethosuximide may increase tonic-clonic seizures in patients with mixed seizure disorders; ethosuximide must be used in combination with other anticonvulsants in patients with both absence and tonic-clonic seizures; may cause blood dyscrasias (periodic hematology tests should be performed)

Syrup may contain sodium benzoate; benzoic acid (benzoate) is a metabolite of benzyl alcohol; large amounts of benzyl alcohol (≥99 mg/kg/day) have been associated with a potentially fatal toxicity ("gasping syndrome") in neonates; the "gasping syndrome" consists of metabolic acidosis, respiratory distress, gasping respirations, CNS dysfunction (including convulsions, intracranial hemorrhage), hypotension and cardiovascular collapse; use ethosuximide products containing sodium benzoate with caution in neonates; *in vitro* and animal studies have shown that benzoate displaces bilirubin from protein binding sites

Precautions Use with caution in patients with hepatic or renal disease; abrupt withdrawal of the drug may precipitate absence status; safety and efficacy in patients <3 years of age have not been established

Adverse Reactions

Central nervous system: Sedation, dizziness, lethargy, euphoria, hallucinations, insomnia, agitation, behavioral changes, headache; increase in tonic-clonic seizures (see Warnings)

Dermatologic: Rashes, urticaria, Stevens-Johnson syndrome, hirsutism

Gastrointestinal: Nausea, vomiting, anorexia, abdominal pain, diarrhea, gum hypertrophy, tongue swelling, weight loss

Genitourinary: Vaginal bleeding

Hematologic: Rare: Leukopenia, agranulocytosis, aplastic anemia, thrombocytopenia, eosinophilia

Ocular: Myopia

Renal: Microscopic hematuria

Miscellaneous: Hiccups, allergic reactions, rarely systemic lupus erythematosus

Drug Interactions Cytochrome P450 isoenzyme CYP3A3/4 substrate

Phenytoin, carbamazepine, primidone, phenobarbital may increase the hepatic metabolism of ethosuximide; ethosuximide may increase phenytoin serum concentrations; isoniazid may inhibit hepatic metabolism with a resultant increase in ethosuximide serum concentrations; CNS depressants, alcohol may increase adverse effects; haloperidol may change the frequency or pattern of seizure activity; valproic acid (increases or decreases ethosuximide serum concentrations)

Food Interactions Folate requirements may be increased

Mechanism of Action Increases the seizure threshold and suppresses paroxysmal spike-and-wave pattern in absence seizures; depresses nerve transmission in the motor cortex

Pharmacokinetics

Distribution: V_d: Adults: 0.62-0.72 L/kg; crosses the placenta; excreted in human breast milk

Protein binding: <10%

Metabolism: ~80% metabolized in the liver to three inactive metabolites

Half-life:

Children: 30 hours

Adults: 50-60 hours

Time to peak serum concentration:

Capsule: Within 2-4 hours

Syrup: <2-4 hours

Elimination: Slow in urine as metabolites (50%) and as unchanged drug (10% to 20%); small amounts excreted in feces

Dialysis: Removed by hemodialysis and peritoneal dialysis

Usual Dosage Oral:

Children <6 years: Initial: 15 mg/kg/day in 2 divided doses (maximum dose: 250 mg/dose); increase every 4-7 days; usual maintenance dose: 15-40 mg/kg/day in 2 divided doses; maximum dose: 1.5 g/day

Children >6 years and Adults: Initial: 250 mg twice daily; increase by 250 mg/day as needed every 4-7 days up to 1.5 g/day in 2 divided doses; usual maintenance dose: 20-40 mg/kg/day in 2 divided doses

Administration Oral: Administer with food or milk to decrease GI upset

Monitoring Parameters Seizure frequency, trough serum concentrations; CBC with differential, platelets, liver enzymes, urinalysis, renal function

Reference Range

Therapeutic: 40-100 mcg/mL (SI: 280-710 micromoles/L)

Toxic: >150 mcg/mL (SI: >1062 micromoles/L)

Patient Information Avoid alcohol; may cause drowsiness and impair ability to perform activities requiring mental alertness or physical coordination; do not discontinue abruptly; notify physician if sore throat or fever occurs

Additional Information Considered to be drug of choice for simple absence seizures

Dosage Forms Excipient information presented when available (limited, particularly for generics); consult specific product labeling.

Capsule: 250 mg

Zarontin®: 250 mg

Syrup: 250 mg/5 mL (473 mL)

Zarontin®: 250 mg/5 mL [contains sodium benzoate; raspberry flavor]

References

Marquardt ED, Ishisaka DY, Batra KK, et al, "Removal of Ethosuximide and Phenobarbital by Peritoneal Dialysis in a Child," *Clin Pharm*, 1992, 11(12):1030-1.

♦ **ETH-Oxydose™** *see* Oxycodone *on page 1189*

♦ **Ethoxynaphthamido Penicillin Sodium** *see* Nafcillin *on page 1099*

Ethyl Alcohol (ETH il AL koe hol)

Medication Safety Issues

Sound-alike/look-alike issues:

Ethanol may be confused with Ethyol®, Ethamolin®

U.S. Brand Names EpiClenz™ [OTC]; GelRite [OTC]; Gel-Stat™ [OTC]; Isagel® [OTC]; Lavacol® [OTC]; Prevacare® [OTC]; Protection Plus® [OTC]; Purell® [OTC]; Purell® 2 in 1 [OTC]; Purell® with Aloe [OTC]

Canadian Brand Names Biobase™; Biobase-G™

Index Terms Alcohol, Absolute; Alcohol, Dehydrated; Ethanol; Ethyl Alcohol; EtOH

Therapeutic Category Anti-infective Agent, Topical; Antidote, Ethylene Glycol Toxicity; Antidote, Methanol Toxicity; Fat Occlusion (Central Venous Catheter), Treatment Agent; Neurolytic

Generic Available Yes

Use Antidote for the treatment of methanol and ethylene glycol intoxication; neurolysis of nerves or ganglia for the relief of intractable, chronic pain in such conditions as inoperable cancer and trigeminal neuralgia (dehydrated alcohol injection); topical anti-infective; treatment of occluded central venous catheters due to lipid deposition from fat emulsion infusion (particularly 3-in-1 admixture)

Pregnancy Risk Factor D (X if used for prolonged periods or in high doses at term)

Lactation Enters breast milk/use caution (AAP rates "compatible")

(Continued)

Ethyl Alcohol *(Continued)*

Contraindications Hypersensitivity to ethyl alcohol; seizure disorder and diabetic coma; subarachnoid injection of dehydrated alcohol in patients receiving anticoagulants

Warnings Ethyl alcohol is a flammable liquid and should be kept cool and away from any heat source; proper positioning of the patient for neurolytic administration is essential to control localization of the injection of dehydrated alcohol (which is hypobaric) into the subarachnoid space; avoid extravasation; not for SubQ administration; do not administer simultaneously with blood due to the possibility of pseudoagglutination or hemolysis; may potentiate severe hypoprothrombic bleeding; clinical evaluation and periodic lab determinations, including serum ethyl alcohol levels, are necessary to monitor effectiveness, changes in electrolyte concentrations, and acid-base balance (when used as an antidote)

Precautions Use with caution in diabetics (ethyl alcohol decreases blood sugar), hepatic impairment, patients with gout, shock, following cranial surgery, and in anticipated postpartum hemorrhage; monitor blood glucose closely, particularly in children as treatment of ingestions is associated with hypoglycemia; avoid extravasation during I.V. administration; ethyl alcohol passes freely into breast milk at a level approximately equivalent to maternal serum level; effects on the infant are insignificant until maternal blood level reaches 300 mg/dL; minimize dermal exposure of ethyl alcohol in infants as significant systemic absorption and toxicity can occur

Adverse Reactions

Cardiovascular: Tachycardia, hypertension, hypotension, arrhythmias, cardiomegaly, angina, CHF, vasodilation, flushing, hypothermia

Central nervous system: Ataxia, dementia, Wernicke-Korsakoff syndrome, amnesia, paranoia, hyperthermia, vertigo, lethargy, sedation, coma, seizures, hallucinations

Endocrine & metabolic: Hypoglycemia, acidosis, hypokalemia, hypomagnesemia, increased serum osmolality

Dermatologic: Dry skin, irritation

Gastrointestinal: Nausea, diarrhea, abdominal pain, dyspepsia, vomiting, GI hemorrhage, anorexia, pancreatitis, hiccups

Hematologic: Porphyria, megaloblastic anemia

Hepatic: Hepatic cirrhosis, fatty degeneration of liver, hepatic steatosis

Local: Phlebitis, nerve and tissue destruction (injection)

Neuromuscular & skeletal: Hypotonia, dysarthria, myopathy, neuropathy (peripheral); postinjection neuritis with persistent pain, hyperesthesia, and paresthesia (after neurolytic use)

Ocular: Eye stinging (from vapors)

Respiratory: Respiratory depression, tachypnea, bronchial irritation

Drug Interactions Increased CNS depressant effects with sedative hypnotic agents, antihistamines, antidepressants, narcotic analgesics, dronabinol, phenothiazines, benzodiazepines, and metoclopramide; disulfiram-like reaction with cephalosporins, chlorpropamide, disulfiram, furazolidone, metronidazole, and procarbazine; increased GI blood loss and bleeding time with aspirin and salicylates; altered glucose metabolism resulting in either hypoglycemic or hyperglycemic effects with insulin, phenformin, and sulfonylureas; increases phenytoin serum levels; increased oral bioavailability of ethyl alcohol with aspirin, ranitidine, cimetidine, and nizatidine; increases theophylline levels

Stability Store at room temperature (see Warnings); do not use unless solution is clear and container is intact

Mechanism of Action Competitively inhibits the oxidation of methanol and ethylene oxide by alcohol dehydrogenase to their more toxic metabolites; as a neurolytic, ethyl alcohol produces injury to tissue cells by producing dehydration and precipitation of protoplasm; when injected in close proximity to nerve cells, it produces neuritis and nerve degeneration

Pharmacokinetics

Distribution: V_d: 0.6-0.7 L/kg

Metabolism: Hepatic to acetaldehyde or acetate by alcohol dehydrogenase

Clearance: Adults: 15-20 mg/dL/hour (range: 10-34 mg/dL/hour)

Dialysis: Hemodialysis clearance: 300-400 mL/minute with an ethanol removal rate of 280 mg/minute

Usual Dosage

Absolute ethanol/ethyl alcohol (EtOH):

Treatment of methanol or ethylene glycol ingestion: Children, Adolescents, and Adults:

Loading dose (LD):

Oral: 0.8-1 mL/kg of 95% EtOH or 2 mL/kg of 40% EtOH (equivalent to 80 proof undiluted liquor) or 1.8 mL/kg of 43% EtOH (equivalent to 86 proof undiluted liquor)

I.V.: 8-10 mL/kg of 10% EtOH solution (see Administration), not to exceed 200 mL

Modified loading dose (if ingestion consists of both EtOH **and** methanol or ethylene glycol): The loading dose is reduced in a proportional manner related to the measured EtOH blood level by multiplying the calculated loading dose described above by the following factor:

$$LD \times \left[\frac{100 - (\text{patient's serum ethanol level in mg/dL})}{100}\right]$$

Maintenance dose: See table

	Non-Drinker	Average Drinker	Chronic Drinker
EtOH dosage by weight	66 mg/kg/h	110 mg/kg/h	154 mg/kg/h
Oral: 43% EtOH (34 g EtOH/dL; 86 proof undiluted liquor)	0.2 mL/kg/h	0.3 mL/kg/h	0.46 mL/kg/h
Oral: 95% EtOH (75 g EtOH/dL)	0.1 mL/kg/h	0.15 mL/kg/h	0.2 mL/kg/h
I.V.: 10% EtOH (7.9 g EtOH/dL)	0.83 mL/kg/h	1.4 mL/kg/h	2 mL/kg/h

Note: Continue therapy until methanol or ethylene glycol blood level <10 mg/dL

Dosage adjustment for hemodialysis: See table

Maintenance Dose Adjustment of Dialysis[1]:

	Non-Drinker	Chronic Drinker
EtOH dosage by weight	169 mg/kg/h	257 mg/kg/h
Oral: 43% EtOH (34 g EtOH/dL)	0.5 mL/kg/h	0.77 mL/kg/h
I.V.: 10% EtOH (7.9 g EtOH/dL)	2.13 mL/kg/h	3.26 mL/kg/h

[1]Due to considerable variability of EtOH clearance between patients, adjust dosage as needed based upon serum EtOH levels.

Treatment of fat occlusion of central venous catheters: Children and Adults: I.V. (see institutional-based protocol for catheter clearance assessment, the following assessment is a general methodology): Up to 3 mL of 70% ethanol (maximum 0.55 mL/kg); instill a volume equal to the internal volume of the catheter; may repeat if patency not restored after 30- minute dwell time; if dose repeated, reassess after 4-hour dwell time

Dehydrated alcohol injection: Therapeutic neurolysis (nerve or ganglion block): Adults: Intraneural: Dosage variable depending upon the site of injection, eg, trigeminal neuralgia: 0.05-0.5 mL as a single injection per interspace vs subarachnoid injection: 0.5-1 mL as a single injection per interspace; single doses >1.5 mL are seldom required

Liquid denatured alcohol: Topical: Children and Adults: Apply as needed

Administration

Oral: Dilute ethanol in 6 ounces orange juice and give over 30 minutes

Parenteral: Not for SubQ administration; I.V.: Dilute absolute alcohol for I.V. administration to a final concentration of 5% to 10% v/v in D_5W or $D_{10}W$ (I.V. ethanol is also available commercially in both 5% and 10% solutions; see Dosage Forms); infuse loading dose plus 1 hour of maintenance dosage over 60 minutes; for treatment of occluded central venous catheter, a 70% dilution of ethanol may be made by adding 0.8 mL SWI to 2 mL 98% ethanol; instill with a volume equal to the internal volume of the catheter; assess patency at 30 minutes (or per institutional protocol); may repeat (see Usual Dosage)

Intraneural: Separate needles should be used for each of multiple injections or sites to prevent residual alcohol deposition at sites not intended for tissue destruction; inject slowly after determining proper placement of needle; since dehydrated alcohol is hypobaric when compared with spinal fluid, proper positioning of the patient is essential to control localization of injections into the subarachnoid space

(Continued)

Ethyl Alcohol *(Continued)*

Monitoring Parameters Antidotal therapy: Blood ethanol levels (at the end of the loading dose, every hour until stabilized, and then every 8-12 hours thereafter); blood glucose, electrolytes (including serum magnesium), arterial pH, blood gases, methanol or ethylene glycol blood levels, heart rate, blood pressure

Reference Range

Symptoms associated with serum ethanol levels:

Nausea and vomiting: Serum level >100 mg/dL

Coma: Serum level >300 mg/dL

Antidote for methanol/ethylene glycol: Goal range: Blood ethanol level: 100-150 mg/dL (22-32 mmol/liter)

Patient Information May cause drowsiness and impair ability to perform activities requiring mental alertness or physical coordination

Additional Information Eighty-proof spirits contain 40% ethanol; 86 proof spirits contain 43% ethanol

Dosage Forms Excipient information presented when available (limited, particularly for generics); consult specific product labeling. [DSC] = Discontinued product

Foam, topical:

Epi-Clenz™: 62% (240 mL, 480 mL) [instant hand sanitizer; contains aloe vera and vitamin E]

Gel, topical:

Epi-Clenz™: 70% (45 mL, 120 mL, 480 mL) [instant hand sanitizer; contains aloe vera and vitamin E]

GelRite: 67% (120 mL, 480 mL, 800 mL) [instant hand sanitizer; contains vitamin E)

Gel-Stat™: 62% (120 mL, 480 mL) [instant hand sanitizer]

Isagel®: 60% (59 mL, 118 mL, 621 mL, 800 mL) [instant hand sanitizer]

Prevacare®: 60% (120 mL, 240 mL, 960 mL, 1200 mL, 1500 mL) [instant hand sanitizer]

Protection Plus®: 62% (800 mL) [instant hand sanitizer]

Purell®: 62% (15 mL, 30 mL, 59 mL, 120 mL, 236 mL, 250 mL, 360 mL, 500 mL, 800 mL, 1000 mL, 2000 mL) [instant hand sanitizer; contains moisturizers and vitamin E]

Purell® Moisture Therapy: 62% (75 mL) [instant hand sanitizer]

Purell® with Aloe: 62% (15 mL, 59 mL, 236 mL, 360 mL, 800 mL, 1000 mL, 2000 mL) [instant hand sanitizer; contains aloe and tartrazine]

Infusion [in D_5W, dehydrated]: Alcohol 5% (1000 mL)

Injection, solution [dehydrated]: 98% (1 mL, 5 mL)

Liquid, topical [denatured]: 70% (3840 mL)

Lavacol®: 70% (473 mL)

Lotion, topical:

Purell® 2 in 1: 62% (60 mL, 360 mL, 1000 mL) [instant hand sanitizer]

Towelettes, topical:

Isagel®: 60% (50s, 300s) [instant hand sanitizer]

Purell®: 62% (35s, 175s) [instant hand sanitizer]

References

Barceloux DG, Bond GR, Krenzelok EP, et al, "American Academy of Clinical Toxicology Practice Guidelines on the Treatment of Methanol Poisoning," *J Toxicol Clin Toxicol*, 2002, 40(4):415-46.

Chernow B, ed, "Poisoning", *Essentials of Critical Care Pharmacology*, 2nd ed, Baltimore: Williams & Wilkins, 1994, 501-29.

Pennington CR and Pithie AD, "Ethanol Lock in the Management of Catheter Occlusion", *JPEN J Parenter Enteral Nutr*, 1987, 11(5):507-8.

Poisoning and Drug Overdose, 2nd ed, Olson KR, ed, Norwalk, Connecticut: Appleton and Lange, 1994, 339-40.

Werlin SL, Lausten T, Jessens, et al, "Treatment of Central Venous Catheter Occlusions With Ethanol and Hydrochloric Acid", *JPEN J Parenter Enteral Nutr*, 1995, 19(5):416-8.

♦ **Ethyl Alcohol** *see* Ethyl Alcohol *on page 619*

♦ **Ethyl Aminobenzoate** *see* Benzocaine *on page 204*

♦ **Ethyol®** *see* Amifostine *on page 91*

♦ **Etibi® (Can)** *see* Ethambutol *on page 616*

Etidronate Disodium (e ti DROE nate dye SOW dee um)

Medication Safety Issues

Sound-alike/look-alike issues:

Etidronate may be confused with etidocaine, etomidate, etretinate

U.S. Brand Names Didronel®

Canadian Brand Names Didronel®; Gen-Etidronate

Index Terms EHDP; Sodium Etidronate

Therapeutic Category Antidote, Hypercalcemia; Bisphosphonate Derivative

Generic Available No

Use Symptomatic treatment of Paget's disease of bone and prevention and treatment of heterotopic ossification following spinal cord injury or total hip replacement

Pregnancy Risk Factor C

Lactation Excretion in breast milk unknown/use caution

Contraindications Hypersensitivity to etidronate, biphosphonates or any component; clinically overt osteomalacia

Warnings Response to therapy in Paget's disease may be slow in onset and continue for months after therapy is discontinued; do not increase dosage rapidly; treatment >6 months or at doses >20 mg/kg/day have been associated with osteomalacia and increased risk of fracture; hyperphosphatemia may occur at doses of 10-20 mg/kg/day due to drug-related increases in the tubular reabsorption of phosphate; serum phosphate levels usually return to normal 2-4 weeks after discontinuation of therapy; monitor serum phosphate closely

Precautions Use with caution in patients with restricted calcium and vitamin D intake; use with caution in patients with enterocolitis due to etidronate's potential to cause diarrhea particularly when using high dosages; dosage modification required in renal impairment

Adverse Reactions Generally dose-related and most significant when taking oral doses >5 mg/kg/day

Central nervous system: Fever, convulsions, pain, amnesia, confusion, depression, hallucinations

Dermatologic: Angioedema, rash, alopecia, follicular eruption

Endocrine & metabolic: Hyperphosphatemia, hypocalcemia, hypomagnesemia, fluid overload

Gastrointestinal: Diarrhea, nausea, vomiting, occult blood in stools, dysgeusia, esophagitis, glossitis

Hematologic: Agranulocytosis (rare), leukopenia (rare)

Neuromuscular & skeletal: Bone pain, increased risk of fractures, rachitic syndrome (found in children taking dosage >10 mg/kg/day over 1 year or longer); joint pain, muscle pain, paresthesia

Renal: Nephrotoxicity

Miscellaneous: Hypersensitivity reactions

Drug Interactions May increase warfarin effects; calcium, iron, magnesium, or aluminum-containing antacids may decrease absorption; separate administration by at least 2 hours

Food Interactions Avoid concurrent administration with food high in calcium (eg, milk or milk products) which may decrease absorption; separate administration by at least 2 hours

Stability Store at room temperature.

Mechanism of Action Decreases bone resorption by inhibiting osteocystic osteolysis; decreases mineral release and matrix or collagen breakdown in bone

Pharmacodynamics

Onset of therapeutic effects: Within 1-3 months of therapy

Duration: Persists for 12 months without continuous therapy

Pharmacokinetics

Absorption: ~3%

Half-life: 1-6 hours

Elimination: Primarily as unchanged drug in urine (50%) with unabsorbed drug eliminated in feces

Usual Dosage

Oral:

Heterotopic ossification: Children and Adults:

Spinal cord injury: 20 mg/kg once daily (or in divided doses if GI discomfort occurs) for 2 weeks, then 10 mg/kg/day for 10 weeks

Total hip replacement: 20 mg/kg/day 1 month before and 3 months after surgery

Note: This dosage when used in children for >1 year has been associated with a rachitic syndrome.

Paget's disease: Adults: 5-10 mg/kg once daily for no more than 6 months; may give 11-20 mg/kg/day for up to 3 months. Daily dose may be divided if adverse GI effects occur; courses of therapy should be separated by drug-free periods of at least 3 months.

Dosing adjustment in renal impairment:

S_{cr} 2.5-4.9 mg/dL: Use with caution

S_{cr} ≥5 mg/dL: **Not recommended**

Administration

Oral: Administer on an empty stomach, 2 hours before meals

Monitoring Parameters Serum calcium, phosphate, creatinine, BUN

Patient Information Maintain adequate intake of calcium and vitamin D

(Continued)

Etidronate Disodium *(Continued)*

Dosage Forms Excipient information presented when available (limited, particularly for generics); consult specific product labeling.

Tablet: 200 mg, 400 mg

- **EtOH** *see* Ethyl Alcohol *on page 619*

Etomidate (e TOM i date)

Medication Safety Issues

Sound-alike/look-alike issues:

Etomidate may be confused with etidronate

U.S. Brand Names Amidate®

Canadian Brand Names Amidate®

Therapeutic Category General Anesthetic

Generic Available Yes

Use Induction and maintenance of general anesthesia particularly in patients with diminished cardiovascular function; sedation for short procedures

Pregnancy Risk Factor C

Contraindications Hypersensitivity to etomidate or any component of the formulation

Warnings Etomidate inhibits 11-B-hydroxylase, an enzyme necessary for the production of cortisol, aldosterone, and corticosterone. A single induction dose blocks the normal stress-induced increase in adrenal cortisol production for 4-8 hours and up to 24 hours in elderly and debilitated patients. This suppression does not appear to be dose related and is unresponsive to ACTH stimulation. Since prolonged infusion of etomidate for sedation particularly in critically ill patients may prevent the response to stress, use of prolonged continuous infusions is not recommended. Consider exogenous corticosteroid replacement in patients undergoing severe stress. Etomidate does not possess analgesic activity; use in combination with narcotic analgesics to blunt the hemodynamic response to endotracheal intubation or for painful procedures.

Precautions Use with caution in patients with renal failure and hepatic cirrhosis as the duration of effect may be prolonged; use with caution in patients with seizure disorder due to its ability to increase EEG activation with epileptiform spikes; high doses of etomidate have been associated with EEG slowing and isoelectricity; involuntary muscles movements or myoclonus occur in up to 30% of patients; this may be minimized by pretreatment with benzodiazepines or fentanyl

Adverse Reactions

Cardiovascular: Bradycardia, tachycardia and other arrhythmias, hypertension, hypotension,

Central nervous system: Apnea

Endocrine & metabolic: Adrenal suppression (decreased cortisol and aldosterone levels)

Gastrointestinal: Nausea, vomiting, hiccups (10%)

Local: Pain at injection site (30% to 80%), thrombophlebitis

Neuromuscular & skeletal: Myoclonus (33%), transient skeletal movements, uncontrolled eye movements

Respiratory: Laryngospasm, hyperventilation, hypoventilation

Stability Store at room temperature. Compatible when administered by Y-site injection with: Alfentanil, atracurium, atropine, doxacurium, ephedrine, fentanyl, lidocaine, lorazepam, midazolam, mivacurium, morphine, pancuronium, phenylephrine, succinylcholine, sufentanil. Incompatible with ascorbic acid, vecuronium

Mechanism of Action A carboxylated imidazole, etomidate is an ultrashort-acting nonbarbiturate hypnotic which produces a rapid induction of anesthesia with minimal cardiovascular effects; produces EEG burst suppression at high doses; decreases intracranial pressure with no effect on cerebral perfusion or heart rate; decreases intraocular pressure; does not produce histamine release

Pharmacodynamics

Onset of action: 30-60 seconds

Maximum effect: 1 minute

Duration: Dose dependent: 2-3 minutes (0.15 mg/kg dose); 4-10 minutes (0.3 mg/kg dose); rapid recovery is due to rapid redistribution

Pharmacokinetics

Distribution: V_d: 3.6-4.5 L/kg

Protein binding: 76%; decreased protein binding resulting in an increased percentage of "free" etomidate in patients with renal failure or hepatic cirrhosis

Metabolism: Hepatic and plasma esterases

Half-life, elimination: Terminal: 2.6-3.5 hours

Time to peak serum concentration: 7 minutes

Excretion: 75% excreted in urine over 24 hours; 2% excreted unchanged

Usual Dosage I.V.:

Induction & maintenance of anesthesia: Children >10 years and Adults: Initial: 0.2-0.6 mg/kg over 30-60 seconds; maintenance: 10-20 mcg/kg/minute; smaller doses may be used to supplement subpotent anesthetic agents

Procedural sedation: Limited data in children; initial doses 0.1-0.3 mg/kg have been used (See References); repeat doses may be needed depending upon the duration of the procedure and the response of the patient

Administration I.V.: Administer I.V. push over 30-60 seconds; very irritating; avoid administration into small vessels on the dorsum of the head or hand; preadministration of lidocaine may be beneficial

Monitoring Parameters Cardiac monitoring, blood pressure, respiratory rate, sedation score (procedural sedation)

Dosage Forms Excipient information presented when available (limited, particularly for generics); consult specific product labeling.

Injection, solution: 2 mg/mL (10 mL, 20 mL) [contains propylene glycol 35% v/v]

References

Falk J and Zed PJ, "Etomidate for Procedural Sedation in the Emergency Department," *Ann Pharmacother*, 2004, 38(7-8):1272-7.

Kienstra AJ, Ward MA, Sasan F, et al, "Etomidate Versus Pentobarbital for Sedation of Children for Head and Neck CT Imaging," *Pediatr Emerg Care*, 2004, 20(8):499-506.

Tobias JD, "Etomidate: Applications in Pediatric Critical Care and Pediatric Aanesthesiology," *Pediatr Crit Care Med*, 2000, 1(2):100-6.

Etoposide (e toe POE side)

Medication Safety Issues

Sound-alike/look-alike issues:

Etoposide may be confused with teniposide

VePesid® may be confused with Versed

High alert medication: The Institute for Safe Medication Practices (ISMP) includes this medication among its list of drugs which have a heightened risk of causing significant patient harm when used in error.

Related Information

Compatibility of Chemotherapy and Related Supportive Care Medications *on page 1777*

Emetogenic Potential of Single Chemotherapeutic Agents *on page 1776*

U.S. Brand Names Toposar®; VePesid®

Canadian Brand Names VePesid®

Index Terms Epipodophyllotoxin; VP-16; VP-16-213

Therapeutic Category Antineoplastic Agent, Mitotic Inhibitor

Generic Available Yes

Use Treatment of testicular and lung carcinomas, malignant lymphoma, Hodgkin's disease, leukemias (ALL, ANLL, AML), neuroblastoma; treatment of Ewing's sarcoma, rhabdomyosarcoma, osteosarcoma, Wilms' tumor, brain tumors; conditioning regimen with hematopoietic stem cell support

Pregnancy Risk Factor D

Lactation Enters breast milk/contraindicated

Contraindications Hypersensitivity to etoposide or any component (see Warnings); pregnancy

Warnings The FDA currently recommends that procedures for proper handling and disposal of antineoplastic agents be considered. Etoposide is mutagenic, potentially carcinogenic, teratogenic, and embryotoxic. Severe myelosuppression with resulting infection or bleeding may occur; injectable etoposide contains polysorbate 80 (polysorbate 80 has caused thrombocytopenia, ascites, and renal, pulmonary, and hepatic failure in premature infants who received an injectable vitamin E product containing polysorbate 80). Higher rates of anaphylactoid reactions have been reported in children who received I.V. infusions of etoposide at higher than recommended concentrations

Etoposide injection contains benzyl alcohol which may cause allergic reactions in susceptible individuals; large amounts of benzyl alcohol (≥99 mg/kg/day) have been associated with a potentially fatal toxicity ("gasping syndrome") in neonates; the "gasping syndrome" consists of metabolic acidosis, respiratory distress, gasping respirations, CNS dysfunction (including convulsions, intracranial hemorrhage), hypotension and cardiovascular collapse; use etoposide injection containing benzyl alcohol with caution in neonates; *in vitro* and animal studies have shown that benzoate, a metabolite of benzyl alcohol, displaces bilirubin from protein binding sites

Precautions Use with caution and consider dosage reduction in patients with hepatic impairment, bone marrow suppression, and renal impairment

Adverse Reactions

Cardiovascular: Hypotension, tachycardia, facial flushing

(Continued)

Etoposide *(Continued)*

Central nervous system: Somnolence, fatigue, fever, headache, chills
Dermatologic: Alopecia, rash, urticaria, angioedema
Gastrointestinal: Nausea, vomiting, diarrhea, mucositis, anorexia, constipation
Hematologic: Myelosuppression, anemia (granulocyte nadir: ~7-14 days, platelet nadir: ~9-16 days)
Hepatic: Hepatotoxicity
Local: Thrombophlebitis
Neuromuscular & skeletal: Peripheral neuropathy, weakness
Respiratory: Bronchospasm
Miscellaneous: Anaphylactoid reactions

Drug Interactions Cytochrome P450 isoenzyme CYP3A3/4 substrate
Cyclosporine may increase the plasma levels of etoposide

Food Interactions Administration of food does not affect GI absorption with doses ≤200 mg

Stability Stability of diluted injection is concentration dependent (ie, 0.2 mg/mL: 96 hours; 0.4 mg/mL: 48 hours; 1 mg/mL: 2 hours; 2 mg/mL: 1 hour); at a concentration of 1 mg/mL in NS or D_5W, crystallization has occurred within 30 minutes; **incidence of precipitation increases when final infusion concentration is >0.4 mg/mL;** intact vials remain stable for 2 years at room temperature; refrigerate capsules

Mechanism of Action Inhibits mitotic activity; inhibits DNA type II topoisomerase producing single- and double-strand DNA breaks

Pharmacokinetics
Absorption: Oral: Large variability
Distribution: CSF concentration is <5% of plasma concentration
Children V_{dss}: 10 L/m^2
Adults: V_{dss}: 7-17 L/m^2
Protein binding: 94% to 97%
Metabolism: In the liver (with a biphasic decay)
Bioavailability: Averages 50% (range: 10% to 80%, dose-dependent)
Half-life, terminal:
Children: 6-8 hours
Adults: 4-15 hours with normal renal and hepatic function
Time to peak serum concentration: Oral: Within 1-1.5 hours
Elimination: Both unchanged drug and metabolites are excreted in urine and a small amount (2% to 16%) in feces; up to 55% of an I.V. dose is excreted unchanged in urine in children

Usual Dosage Refer to individual protocols
Children: I.V.: 60-150 mg/m^2/day for 2-5 days every 3-6 weeks
AML:
Remission induction: 150 mg/m^2/day for 2-3 days for 2-3 cycles
Intensification or consolidation: 250 mg/m^2/day for 3 days, on courses 2-5
Brain tumor: 150 mg/m^2/day on days 2 and 3 of treatment course
Neuroblastoma: 100 mg/m^2/day over 1 hour on days 1-5 of cycle; repeat cycle every 4 weeks
High-dose conditioning regimen for allogeneic BMT: 60 mg/kg/dose as a single dose
BMT conditioning regimen used in patients with rhabdomyosarcoma or neuroblastoma: I.V. continuous infusion: 160 mg/m^2/day for 4 days
Adults:
Testicular cancer: I.V.: 50-100 mg/m^2/day on days 1-5 or 100 mg/m^2/day on days 1, 3 and 5 every 3-4 weeks for 3-4 courses
Small cell lung cancer:
Oral: Twice the I.V. dose rounded to the nearest 50 mg given once daily if total dose ≤400 mg/day or in divided doses if >400 mg/day
I.V.: 35 mg/m^2/day for 4 days or 50 mg/m^2/day for 5 days every 3-4 weeks

Dosing adjustment in renal impairment:
Cl_{cr} 10-50 mL/minute: Administer 75% of normal dose
Cl_{cr} <10 mL/minute: Administer 50% of normal dose

Dosing adjustment in patients with elevated serum bilirubin: Reduce dose by 50% for bilirubin 1.5-3 mg/dL; reduce dose by 75% for bilirubin >3 mg/dL

Administration
Oral: If necessary, the injection may be used for oral administration. Mix with orange juice, apple juice, or lemonade at a final concentration not to exceed 0.4 mg/mL to prevent precipitation. Etoposide has been found to be stable with no loss of potency over 3 hours when administered in apple juice or lemonade at concentrations of 1 mg/mL.
Parenteral: I.V.: Do not administer by rapid I.V. injection or by intrathecal, intraperitoneal, or intrapleural routes due to possible severe toxicity. Administer by continuous I.V. infusion or I.V. intermittent infusion via an in-line 0.22 micron filter over at least

60 minutes at a rate not to exceed 100 mg/m²/hour (or 3.3 mg/kg/hour) to minimize the risk of hypotensive reactions at a final concentration for administration of 0.2-0.4 mg/mL in NS or D_5W. More concentrated I.V. solutions (0.6-1 mg/mL) can be infused but have shorter stability times (see Stability). For high-dose etoposide infusions, undiluted etoposide (20 mg/mL) has been infused as a single dose from a glass syringe via syringe pump through a central venous catheter over 1-4 hours. Problems associated with higher than recommended concentrations of etoposide infusions include cracking of hard plastic in chemo venting pins and infusion lines; inspect infusion solution for particulate matter and plastic devices for cracks and leaks.

Monitoring Parameters CBC with differential and platelet count, hemoglobin, vital signs (blood pressure), bilirubin, liver and renal function tests; inspect solution and tubing for precipitation before and during infusion

Patient Information Notify physician if fever, sore throat, painful/burning urination, extreme fatigue, pain or numbness in extremities, yellowing of eyes or skin, bruising, bleeding or shortness of breath occurs

Nursing Implications Adequate airway and other supportive measures and agents for treating hypotension or anaphylactoid reactions should be present when I.V. etoposide is given

Dosage Forms Excipient information presented when available (limited, particularly for generics); consult specific product labeling.

Capsule, softgel:

VePesid®: 50 mg

Injection, solution: 20 mg/mL (5 mL, 25 mL, 50 mL)

Toposar®: 20 mg/mL (5 mL, 25 mL, 50 mL) [contains alcohol 33% and polysorbate 80]

References

Berg SL, Grisell DL, DeLaney TF, et al, "Principles of Treatment of Pediatric Solid Tumors," *Pediatr Clin North Am*, 1991, 38(2):249-67.

Boos J, Krümpelmann S, Schulze-Westhoff P, et al, "Steady-State Levels and Bone Marrow Toxicity of Etoposide in Children and Infants: Does Etoposide Require Age-Dependent Dose Calculation?" *J Clin Oncol*, 1995, 13(12):2954-60.

Clark PL and Slevin ML, "The Clinical Pharmacology of Etoposide and Teniposide," *Clin Pharmacokinet*, 1987, 12(4):223-52.

Lazarus HM, Creger RJ, and Diaz D, "Simple Method for the Administration of High-Dose Etoposide During Autologous Bone Marrow Transplantation," *Cancer Treat Rep*, 1985, 70(6):819-20.

Nishikawa A, Nakamura Y, Nobori U, et al, "Acute Monocytic Leukemia in Children. Response to VP-16-213 as a Single Agent," *Cancer*, 1987, 60(9):2146-9.

O'Dwyer PJ, Leyland-Jones B, Alonso MT, et al, "Etoposide (VP-16-213): Current Status of an Active Anticancer Drug," *N Engl J Med*, 1985, 312(11):692-700.

- **Euglucon® (Can)** *see* GlyBURIDE *on page 734*
- **Eurax®** *see* Crotamiton *on page 412*
- **Evac-U-Gen [OTC]** *see* Senna *on page 1427*
- **Everone® 200 (Can)** *see* Testosterone *on page 1511*
- **Evoclin™** *see* Clindamycin *on page 379*
- **Exact® Acne Medication [OTC]** *see* Benzoyl Peroxide *on page 207*
- **Exjade®** *see* Deferasirox *on page 449*
- **ex-lax® [OTC]** *see* Senna *on page 1427*
- **ex-lax® Maximum Strength [OTC]** *see* Senna *on page 1427*
- **ex-lax® Ultra [OTC]** *see* Bisacodyl *on page 217*
- **Exorex®** *see* Coal Tar *on page 394*
- **Exsel® [DSC]** *see* Selenium Sulfide *on page 1427*
- **Exubera®** *see* Insulin Inhalation *on page 842*
- **EZ-Char™ [OTC]** *see* Charcoal, Activated *on page 328*

Ezetimibe (ez ET i mibe)

Medication Safety Issues

Sound-alike/look-alike issues:

Zetia™ may be confused with Zestril®

U.S. Brand Names Zetia™

Canadian Brand Names Ezetrol®

Therapeutic Category Antilipemic Agent; Cholesterol Absorption Inhibitor

Generic Available No

Use Adjunct to dietary therapy or in combination with HMG-CoA reductase inhibitor (atorvastatin, simvastatin) to decrease elevated serum total and low density lipoprotein cholesterol (LDL-C), apolipoprotein B (apo-B), and triglyceride levels in patients with primary hypercholesterolemia (heterozygous, familial and nonfamilial); in combination with HMG-CoA reductase inhibitor (atorvastatin, simvastatin) in the treatment of homozygous familial hypercholesterolemia; in combination with fenofibrate in the (Continued)

Ezetimibe *(Continued)*

treatment of mixed hyperlipidemia; adjunct to dietary therapy for the reduction of elevated sitosterol and campesterol levels in patients with homozygous familial sitosterolemia

Pregnancy Risk Factor C

Lactation Excretion in breast milk unknown/not recommended

Contraindications Hypersensitivity to ezetimibe or any component; active liver disease; unexplained persistent elevations of serum transaminases

Warnings The incidence of rhabdomyolysis or myopathy in clinical trials with ezetimibe was no different than that of placebo; however, rhabdomyolysis and myopathy are known adverse effects of HMG-CoA reductase inhibitors which are often used in combination with ezetimibe; follow rhabdomyolysis and myopathy monitoring recommendations for HMG-CoA reductase inhibitors when used in combination; also when ezetimibe is used in combination with HMG-CoA reductase inhibitors, the incidence of elevated serum transaminases was higher than when the HMG-CoA reductase inhibitors were used alone; monitor serum transaminases when used in combination with HMG-CoA reductase inhibitors. When studied in combination with fenofibrate, an increase in cholecystectomy rate (0.6% vs 1.7%) when compared with monotherapy was observed; monitor for signs and symptoms of cholelithiasis when used with fenofibrate.

Precautions Use with caution in patients with renal or mild hepatic impairment

Adverse Reactions

Cardiovascular: Angioedema, chest pain
Central nervous system: Fatigue, dizziness, headache
Dermatologic: Rash, urticaria
Gastrointestinal: Abdominal pain, diarrhea, cholelithiasis (when used in combination with fenofibrate; see Warnings)
Hepatic: Elevated serum transaminases (0.5%; 1.3% when used in combination with HMG-CoA reductase inhibitors)
Neuromuscular & skeletal: Arthralgia, myalgia, back pain
Respiratory: Pharyngitis, sinusitis, cough, URI
Miscellaneous: Hypersensitivity reactions, viral infections

Drug Interactions Plasma concentrations may be decreased when given with cholestyramine and colestipol (separate administration by ≥2 hours before or ≥4 hours after bile acid sequestrants); fibric acid derivatives (eg, gemfibrozil, clofibrate) and cyclosporine may increase ezetimibe serum levels

Stability Store at controlled room temperature.

Mechanism of Action Ezetimibe reduces blood cholesterol by inhibiting the absorption of cholesterol by the small intestine

Pharmacodynamics

Onset of action: Within 1 week
Maximum effect: 2-4 weeks

Pharmacokinetics

Protein binding: >90%
Metabolism: Extensively conjugated in the liver and small intestine to a pharmacologically active metabolite; may undergo enterohepatic recycling
Bioavailability: Variable
- Hepatic impairment: Child-Pugh score 7-9: AUC increased 3-4 times; Child-Pugh 10-15: AUC increased 5-6 times
- Renal impairment: Severe renal dysfunction (Cl_{cr} <30 mL/minute/1.73 m^2): AUC increased 1.5 times

Half-life: Adults: 22 hours
Time to peak serum concentration: 4-12 hours (ezetimibe); 1-2 hours (active metabolite)
Elimination: Feces (78%, 69% as ezetimibe): urine (11%, 9% as metabolite)

Usual Dosage Oral: Adolescents ≥10 years and Adults: 10 mg once daily

Dosing adjustment in renal impairment: Bioavailability increased with severe impairment; no dosage adjustment is necessary

Dosing adjustment in hepatic impairment: Bioavailability increased with moderate to severe impairment

Mild hepatic impairment (Child-Pugh score 5-6): No dosing adjustment necessary
Moderate to severe impairment (Child-Pugh score 7-15): Use of ezetimibe not recommended due to increased bioavailability (see Pharmacokinetics)

Administration Oral: May be taken without regard to meals or time of day; may be administered with an HMG-CoA inhibitor (eg, atorvastatin, simvastatin)

Monitoring Parameters Serum cholesterol (total and fractionated), CPK; liver function tests (see Precautions)

Reference Range Hypercholesterolemia: See table on next page; desired: HDL-C <40 mg/dL

Classification of Blood Cholesterol, LDL-C, and Triglyceride Concentrations[1]

Classification	Cholesterol (mg/dL)		LDL-C (mg/dL)		Triglycerides (mg/dL)
	Children	Adults	Children	Adults	Adults
Acceptable/optimal	<170	<200	<110	<100	<150
Above optimal	†	†	†	100-129	†
Borderline high	170-199	200-239	110-129	130-159	150-199
High	≥200	≥240	≥130	160-189	200-499
Very high	†	†	†	≥190	≥500

[1]Adapted from American Academy of Pediatrics Committee on Nutrition, "Cholesterol in Childhood," *Pediatrics*, 1998, 101(1 Pt 1):141-7 and "Third Report of the National Cholesterol Education Program Expert Panel on Detection, Evaluation, and Treatment of High Blood Cholesterol in Adults (Adult Treatment Panel III)," May 2001, www.nhlbi.nih.gov/guidelines/cholesterol.

†Lack of specific type of classification in either pediatric or adult recommendations.

Patient Information May cause dizziness or fatigue; may impair ability to perform activities requiring mental alertness or physical coordination

Additional Information The current recommendation for treatment of hypercholesterolemia in children is limited to children ≥10 years of age who, after a 6-month to 1-year trial of diet therapy, continue to have LDL-C concentrations greater than or equal to 190 mg/dL alone, or LDL-C concentrations ≥160 mg/dL and a family history of premature coronary artery disease or two or more other coronary artery disease risk factors (AAP Committee on Nutrition, 1998). For more specific risk assessment and treatment recommendations for adults, see the NIH Guidelines, 2001.

Dosage Forms Excipient information presented when available (limited, particularly for generics); consult specific product labeling.

Tablet: 10 mg [capsule shaped]

References

American Academy of Pediatrics Committee on Nutrition, "Cholesterol in Childhood," *Pediatrics*, 1998, 101(1 Pt 1):141-7.

American Academy of Pediatrics, "National Cholesterol Education Program: Report of the Expert Panel on Blood Cholesterol Levels in Children and Adolescents," *Pediatrics*, 1992, 89(3 Pt 2):525-84.

Gagne C, Gaudet D, Bruckert E, et al, "Efficacy and Safety of Ezetimibe Coadministered With Atorvastatin or Simvastatin in Patients With Homozygous Familial Hypercholesterolemia," *Circulation*, 2002, 105(21):2469-75.

"Third Report of the National Cholesterol Education Program Expert Panel on Detection, Evaluation, and Treatment of High Blood Cholesterol in Adults (Adult Treatment Panel III)," May 2001, www.nhlbi.nih.gov/guidelines/cholesterol.

Ezetimibe and Simvastatin (ez ET i mibe & SIM va stat in)

Medication Safety Issues

Sound-alike/look-alike issues:

Vytorin® may be confused with Vyvanse™

U.S. Brand Names Vytorin®

Therapeutic Category Antilipemic Agent; Cholesterol Absorption Inhibitor; HMG-CoA Reductase Inhibitor

Generic Available No

Use

Hyperlipidemia: Adjunct to dietary therapy to decrease elevated serum total and low density lipoprotein cholesterol (LDL-C), apolipoprotein B (apo-B), and triglyceride levels, and to increase high density lipoprotein cholesterol (HDL-C) in patients with primary hypercholesterolemia (heterozygous, familial and nonfamilial) and mixed dyslipidemia (Fredrickson types IIa and IIb); treatment of homozygous familial hypercholesterolemia; treatment of isolated hypertriglyceridemia (Fredrickson type IV) and type III hyperlipoproteinemia

Primary prevention of cardiovascular disease in high risk patients; risk factors include: Age >55 years, smoking, hypertension, low HDL-C, or family history of early coronary heart disease

Pregnancy Risk Factor X

Lactation Excretion in breast milk unknown/contraindicated

Contraindications Hypersensitivity to simvastatin, ezetimibe, or any component; active liver disease; unexplained persistent elevations of serum transaminases; pregnancy

Warnings Rhabdomyolysis with or without acute renal failure secondary to myoglobinuria has occurred rarely. Risk is increased with increasing simvastatin doses (0.02% at 20 mg, 0.07% at 40 mg, and 0.3% at 80 mg) and with concurrent use of amiodarone, clarithromycin, danazol, diltiazem, fluvoxamine, indinavir, nefazodone, nelfinavir, ritonavir, verapamil, troleandomycin, cyclosporine, fibric acid derivatives, erythromycin, niacin, or azole antifungals. Avoid concomitant use with itraconazole, ketoconazole, erythromycin, clarithromycin, telithromycin, HIV protease inhibitors,

(Continued)

Ezetimibe and Simvastatin *(Continued)*

and nefazodone. Assess the risk versus benefit before combining amiodarone, danazol, diltiazem, fluvoxamine, verapamil, cyclosporine, fibric acid derivatives, and niacin with simvastatin. A lowered dosage of simvastatin is recommended when used with some of these medications (see Usual Dosage). Discontinue Vytorin™ in any patient experiencing unexplained muscle pain, tenderness or weakness, and/or CPK level >10 times the normal range. Monitor CPK periodically in patients with complicated medical histories including renal insufficiency.

Precautions Persistent increases in serum transaminases have occurred; liver function must be monitored by laboratory assessment at the initiation of therapy and periodically thereafter for the first year of treatment or until one year after the last elevation in dose. Patients titrated to the 80 mg dose should receive an additional test at 3 months of therapy. Use with caution in patients with liver dysfunction, diabetes mellitus, and renal impairment (may be at increased risk for developing rhabdomyolysis)

Drug Interactions Cytochrome P450 isoenzyme CYP3A3/4 enzyme substrate

Plasma concentrations may be decreased when given with magnesium-aluminum hydroxide containing antacids; cholestyramine reduces absorption (separate administration either ≥2 hours before or ≥4 hours after cholestyramine); clofibrate, fenofibrate, gemfibrozil, niacin (≥1 g/day), amiodarone, and cyclosporine may increase the risk of myopathy and rhabdomyolysis (see Warnings); CYP3A3/4 inhibitors (clarithromycin, cyclosporine, danazol, diltiazem, fluconazole, fluvoxamine, erythromycin, indinavir, itraconazole, ketoconazole, miconazole, nefazodone, nelfinavir, ritonavir, saquinavir, indinavir, amprenavir, troleandomycin, and verapamil) increase simvastatin blood levels and may increase the risk of simvastatin-induced myopathy and rhabdomyolysis (see Warnings); simvastatin increases the hypoprothrombinemic response to warfarin; may increase digoxin serum level; clofibrate, gemfibrozil (fibric acid derivatives), and cyclosporine may increase ezetimibe serum levels; the herbal medicine St John's wort (*Hypericum perforatum*) may decrease simvastatin levels

Food Interactions Simvastatin serum concentration may be increased when taken with large quantities (>1 quart/day) of grapefruit juice; avoid concurrent use

Stability Tablets should be stored in well closed containers at temperatures between 5°C to 30°C (41°F to 86°F)

Mechanism of Action Ezetimibe reduces blood cholesterol by inhibiting the absorption of cholesterol by the small intestine. Simvastatin is a methylated derivative of lovastatin that acts by competitively inhibiting 3-hydroxy-3-methylglutaryl-coenzyme A (HMG-CoA) reductase, the enzyme that catalyzes the rate-limiting step in cholesterol biosynthesis.

Pharmacodynamics

Onset of action: >3 days

Maximum effect: After 2-4 weeks

Pharmacokinetics See individual agents

Usual Dosage Oral:

Hyperlipidemia: Adults: Initial: 10 mg ezetimibe/20 mg simvastatin once daily in the evening; patients requiring less aggressive LDL-C reductions may be started on 10 mg ezetimibe/10 mg simvastatin; patients who require a reduction of >55% in LDL-C may be started at 10 mg ezetimibe/40 mg simvastatin once daily

Homozygous familial hypercholesterolemia: Children ≥10 years and Adults: Ezetimibe 10 mg/simvastatin 40 mg once daily in the evening; may increase to ezetimibe 10 mg/simvastatin 80 mg once daily as needed

Dosage adjustment in patients who are concomitantly receiving cyclosporine or danazol: Adults: Not for use unless the patient has tolerated simvastatin at a does of ≥5 mg; the daily dose should not to exceed 10 mg ezetimibe/10 mg simvastatin

Dosage adjustment in patients receiving concomitant amiodarone or verapamil: Adults: The daily dose should not exceed 10 mg ezetimibe/20 mg simvastatin

Dosage adjustment with gemfibrozil: Although concurrent use is not recommended by manufacturer, the daily dose should not exceed 10 mg ezetimibe/10 mg simvastatin

Dosing adjustment in renal impairment: Adults: Because simvastatin does not undergo significant renal excretion, modification of dose should only be necessary in patients with severe renal impairment: Cl_{cr}<10 mL/minute: Not for use unless the patient has tolerated simvastatin at a dose of ≥5 mg, the daily dose should not to exceed 10 mg ezetimibe/10 mg simvastatin

Administration Oral: May be taken without regard to meals. Administration with the evening meal or at bedtime has been associated with somewhat greater LDL-C reduction.

Monitoring Parameters Serum cholesterol (total and fractionated), CPK; liver function tests (see Precautions)

Reference Range Hypercholesterolemia: as defined by serum cholesterol, LDL-C, and TG concentrations: See table; Desired: HDL-C <40 mg/dL

Classification of Blood Cholesterol, LDL-C, and Triglyceride Concentrations[1]

Classification	Cholesterol (mg/dL)		LDL-C (mg/dL)		Triglycerides (mg/dL)
	Children	Adults	Children	Adults	Adults
Acceptable/optimal	<170	<200	<110	<100	<150
Above optimal	†	†	†	100-129	†
Borderline high	170-199	200-239	110-129	130-159	150-199
High	≥200	≥240	≥130	160-189	200-499
Very high	†	†	†	≥190	≥500

[1]Adapted from American Academy of Pediatrics Committee on Nutrition, "Cholesterol in Childhood," *Pediatrics*, 1998, 101(1 Pt 1):141-7 and "Third Report of the National Cholesterol Education Program Expert Panel on Detection, Evaluation, and Treatment of High Blood Cholesterol in Adults (Adult Treatment Panel III)," May 2001, www.nhlbi.nih.gov/guidelines/cholesterol.

†Lack of specific type of classification in either pediatric or adult recommendations.

Patient Information May rarely cause photosensitivity reactions (eg, exposure to sunlight may cause severe sunburn, skin rash, redness, or itching); avoid direct exposure to sunlight. Report severe and unresolved gastric upset, any vision changes, muscle pain and weakness, changes in color of urine or stool, yellowing of skin or eyes, and any unusual bruising. Female patients of childbearing age must be counseled to use 2 effective forms of contraception simultaneously, unless absolute abstinence is the chosen method; this drug may cause severe fetal defects.

Additional Information The current recommendation for treatment of hypercholesterolemia in children is limited to children ≥10 years of age who, after a 6-month to 1-year trial of diet therapy, continue to have LDL-C concentrations ≥190 mg/dL alone, or LDL-C concentrations ≥160 mg/dL and a family history of premature coronary artery disease or two or more other coronary artery disease risk factors (AAP Committee on Nutrition, 1998). For each 1% lowering in LDL-C, the relative risk for major cardiovascular events is reduced by approximately 1%. For more specific risk assessment and treatment recommendations for adults, see NCEP ATPIII, 2004.

Dosage Forms Excipient information presented when available (limited, particularly for generics); consult specific product labeling.

Tablet:

10/10: Ezetimibe 10 mg and simvastatin 10 mg
10/20: Ezetimibe 10 mg and simvastatin 20 mg
10/40: Ezetimibe 10 mg and simvastatin 40 mg
10/80: Ezetimibe 10 mg and simvastatin 80 mg

References

American Academy of Pediatrics, Committee on Nutrition, "Cholesterol in Childhood," *Pediatrics*, 1998, 101(1 Pt 1):141-7.

"American Academy of Pediatrics, National Cholesterol Education Program: Report of the Expert Panel on Blood Cholesterol Levels in Children and Adolescents," *Pediatrics*, 1992, 89(3 Pt 2):525-84.

Dejongh S, Stalenhoef AF, Tuohy MB, et al, "Efficacy, Safety, and Tolerability of Simvastatin in Children With Familial Hypercholesterolemia: Rational, Design and Baseline Characterisitics ," *Clin Drug Invest*, 2002, 22(8):533-40.

Ducobu J, Brasseur D, Chaudron JM, et al, "Simvastatin Use in Children," *Lancet*, 1992, 339(8807):1488.

Duplaga BA, "Treatment of Childhood Hypercholesterolemia With HMG-CoA Reductase Inhibitors," *Ann Pharmacother*, 1999, 33(11):1224-7.

Gagne C, Gaudet D, Bruckert E, et al, "Efficacy and Safety of Ezetimibe Coadministered With Atorvastatin or Simvastatin in Patients With Homozygous Familial Hypercholesterolemia," *Circulation*, 2002, 105(21):2469-75.

Grundy SM, Cleeman JI, Merz CN, et al, "Implications of Recent Clinical Trials for the National Cholesterol Education Program Adult Treatment Panel III Guidelines," *Circulation*, 2004, 110(2):227-39.

"Third Report of the National Cholesterol Education Program Expert Panel on Detection, Evaluation, and Treatment of High Blood Cholesterol in Adults (Adult Treatment Panel III)," May 2001, www.nhlbi.nih.gov/guidelines/cholesterol.

♦ **Ezetrol® (Can)** *see* Ezetimibe *on page 627*

♦ **E•R•O [OTC]** *see* Carbamide Peroxide *on page 283*

♦ **F_3T** *see* Trifluridine *on page 1575*

♦ **Fabrazyme®** *see* Agalsidase Beta *on page 61*

Factor VIIa (Recombinant) (FAK ter SEV en ree KOM be nant)

Medication Safety Issues

Sound-alike/look-alike issues:

NovoSeven® may be confused with Novacet®

(Continued)

Factor VIIa (Recombinant) *(Continued)*

U.S. Brand Names NovoSeven®

Canadian Brand Names Niastase®

Index Terms Coagulation Factor VIIa; Eptacog Alfa (Activated); rFVIIa

Therapeutic Category Antihemophilic Agent; Blood Product Derivative

Generic Available No

Use Treatment of bleeding episodes in patients with hemophilia A or B when inhibitors to factor VIII or factor IX are present

Pregnancy Risk Factor C

Lactation Excretion in breast milk unknown/compatible

Contraindications Hypersensitivity to factor VII or any component of the formulation; hypersensitivity to mouse, hamster, or bovine proteins

Warnings Efficacy with prolonged infusions and data evaluating long-term adverse effects are limited.

Precautions Use with extreme caution in patients with disseminated intravascular coagulation (DIC), advanced atherosclerotic disease, sepsis, or crush injury due to the potential for an increase in thrombotic events; monitor for signs and symptoms of activation of the coagulation system or thrombosis; decrease dosage or discontinue therapy if DIC is confirmed

Adverse Reactions

Cardiovascular: Hypertension, bradycardia, hypotension, edema, MI, angina

Central nervous system: Headache, ataxia, fever, cerebrovascular events

Dermatologic: Pruritus, purpura, rash

Gastrointestinal: Vomiting

Hematologic: Hemorrhage, decreased plasma fibrinogen, coagulation disorder, disseminated intravascular coagulation (DIC), prothrombin decreased, fibrinolysis increased

Local: Injection site reactions

Neuromuscular & skeletal: Hemarthrosis, arthrosis

Renal: Abnormal renal function

Respiratory: Pneumonia, pulmonary embolism

Miscellaneous: Allergic reactions

Drug Interactions Activated prothrombin complex concentrates

Stability Store under refrigeration (2°C to 8°C/36°F to 46°F). Reconstituted solutions may be stored at room temperature or under refrigeration; do not freeze; must be infused within 3 hours of reconstitution.

Mechanism of Action Recombinant factor VIIa, a vitamin K-dependent glycoprotein, promotes hemostasis by activating the extrinsic pathway of the coagulation cascade. It replaces deficient activated coagulation factor VII, which complexes with tissue factor and may activate coagulation factor X to Xa and factor IX to IXa. When complexed with other factors, coagulation factor Xa converts prothrombin to thrombin, a key step in the formation of a fibrin-platelet hemostatic plug.

Pharmacodynamics

Onset of action: 10-20 minutes

Maximum effect: 6 hours

Pharmacokinetics

Distribution: V_d: Children: 130 mL/kg; Adults: 103-105 mL/kg (range: 78-139 mL/kg)

Half-life: Elimination: Children: 1.32 hours; Adults: 2.3 hours (range: 1.7-2.7 hours)

Time to peak serum concentration: 15 minutes

Elimination: Clearance: Children: 67 mL/kg/hour; Adults: 30-36 mL/kg/hour (range: 27-49 mL/kg/hour)

Usual Dosage I.V.: Children and Adults: 90 mcg/kg every 2 hours until hemostasis is achieved or until the treatment is judged ineffective. The dose and interval may be adjusted based upon the severity of bleeding and the degree of hemostasis achieved. The duration of therapy following hemostasis has not been fully established; in clinical trials, dosages have ranged from 35-120 mcg/kg and a decision on the outcome of treatment was reached within 8 doses in the majority of patients; adverse effects were reported most commonly in patients treated with 12 or more doses. For patients experiencing severe bleeds to maintain the hemostatic plug, dosing should be continued at 3- to 6-hour intervals; the duration of posthemostatic dosing should be minimized.

Administration Parenteral: I.V. Reconstitute 1.2 mg, 2.4 mg, and 4.8 mg vials with 2.2 mL, 4.3 mL, and 8.5 mL SWI respectively resulting in 0.6 mg/mL (600 mcg/mL) concentration; administer over 2-5 minutes within 3 hours after reconstitution

Monitoring Parameters Monitor for evidence of hemostasis; although the prothrombin time, aPTT, and factor VII clotting activity have no correlation with achieving clinical hemostasis, these parameters may be useful as adjunct tests to evaluate efficacy and guide dose or interval adjustments

Patient Information This medication can only be administered I.V. Report swelling, pain, burning, or itching at infusion site. Report acute headache, visual changes, pain in joints or muscles, respiratory difficulty, chills, back pain, dizziness, nausea, or other unusual effects; inform healthcare provider if you are or intend to become pregnant.

Additional Information Each mg factor VII contains 0.44 mEq sodium and 0.06 mEq calcium; "off-label" uses in limited patient populations have been reported (primarily adult patients) including reversal of anticoagulant over dose and reduction in bleeding associated with thrombocytopenia, trauma, hepatic dysfunction, and cardiac bypass surgery; further randomized, blinded clinical trials are needed to determine efficacy, dosage, and safety for these indications (Tobias, 2004; Ghorashian, 2004)

Dosage Forms Excipient information presented when available (limited, particularly for generics); consult specific product labeling.

Injection, powder for reconstitution [preservative free]: 1.2 mg, 2.4 mg, 4.8 mg [latex free; contains sodium 0.44 mEq/mg rFVIIa, polysorbate 80]

References

Ghorashian S and Hunt BJ, "'Off-License' Use of Recombinant Activated Factor VII," *Blood Rev*, 2004, 18(4):245-59.

Goodnough LT, Lublin DM, Zhang L, et al, "Transfusion Medicine Service Policies for Recombinant Factor VIIa Administration," *Transfusion*, 2004, 44(9):1325-31.

Tobias JD, Simsic JM, Weinstein S, et al, "Recombinant Factor VIIa to Control Excessive Bleeding Following Surgery for Congenital Heart Disease in Pediatric Patients," *J Intensive Care Med*, 2004, 19(5):270-3.

Factor IX (FAK ter nyne)

U.S. Brand Names AlphaNine® SD; BeneFix®; Mononine®

Canadian Brand Names BeneFix®; Immunine® VH; Mononine®

Therapeutic Category Antihemophilic Agent; Blood Product Derivative

Generic Available No

Use Control bleeding in patients with factor IX deficiency (hemophilia B or Christmas disease)

Pregnancy Risk Factor C

Contraindications Hypersensitivity to mouse protein (Mononine®), hamster protein (BeneFix®), or any component; DIC; fibrinolysis

Warnings Some products are prepared from pooled human plasma; such plasma may contain the causative agents of viral disease; risk of transmission is extremely rare; hypersensitivity reactions, including anaphylaxis, have been reported; these events have occurred in a close temporal relationship with the development of factor IX inhibitors; patients experiencing allergic reactions should be evaluated for the presence of inhibitors; there may be a direct relationship between the development of factor IX inhibitors and deletion mutations of the factor IX gene; patients with these deletion mutations should be observed closely for signs and symptoms of acute hypersensitivity reactions

To achieve the desired factor IX activity level, monitor factor IX activity assay; in the presence of an inhibitor, higher factor IX doses may be required

AlphaNine® SD, Mononine® contain **nondetectable levels of factors II, VII, and X** (<0.0025 units per factor IX unit using standard coagulation assays) and are **NOT INDICATED** for replacement therapy of any of these clotting factors.

BeneFix®, Mononine®, and AlphaNine® are **NOT INDICATED** in the treatment or reversal of coumarin-induced anticoagulation or in a hemorrhagic state caused by hepatitis-induced lack of production of liver dependent coagulation factors.

Precautions Due to the potential risk of thromboembolic complications, use with caution in patients with liver dysfunction, patients in the postoperative period, in neonates, or in patients at risk of thromboembolic phenomena or DIC

Adverse Reactions

Cardiovascular: Angioedema, cyanosis, flushing, hypotension, tightness in chest, thrombosis

Central nervous system: Fever, headache, chills, somnolence, dizziness, drowsiness, lightheadedness

Dermatologic: Urticaria, rash

Gastrointestinal: Nausea, vomiting, abnormal taste, diarrhea

Hematologic: DIC

Local: Injection site discomfort, phlebitis

Neuromuscular & skeletal: Tingling

Ocular: Visual disturbances

Respiratory: Dyspnea, laryngeal edema, allergic rhinitis, cough

Miscellaneous: Transient fever (following rapid administration), anaphylaxis, burning sensation in jaw/skull

Drug Interactions Aminocaproic acid may increase the risk for thrombosis.

Stability Refrigerate 2°C to 8°C (36°F to 46°F); do not freeze

(Continued)

Factor IX *(Continued)*

AlphaNine® SD: May also be stored at ≤30°C (≤86°F) for up to 3 months.
BeneFix®: May also be stored at ≤25°C (≤77°F) for up to 6 months.
Mononine®: May also be stored at ≤30°C (≤86°F) for up to 1 month.

Mechanism of Action Hemophilia B, or Christmas disease, is an X-linked inherited disorder of blood coagulation characterized by insufficient or abnormal synthesis of the clotting protein factor IX. Factor IX is a vitamin K-dependent coagulation factor which is synthesized in the liver. Factor IX is activated by factor XIa in the intrinsic coagulation pathway. Activated factor IX (IXa), in combination with factor VII, activates factor X to Xa, resulting ultimately in the conversion of prothrombin to thrombin and the formation of a fibrin clot. The infusion of exogenous factor IX to replace the deficiency present in hemophilia B temporarily restores hemostasis.

Pharmacokinetics Elimination: Half-life: 17-22 hours (range: 10-37 hours)

Usual Dosage Dosage is expressed in units of factor IX activity and must be individualized related to formulation, severity, and clinical situation. I.V. only:

Formula for units required to raise blood level %:

AlphaNine® SD, Mononine®: Children and Adults:

Number of Factor IX International Units Required = body weight (in kg) x desired Factor IX level increase (% normal) x 1 international unit/kg

For example, for a 100% level a patient who has an actual level of 20%: Number of Factor IX International Units needed = 70 kg x 80% x 1 international unit/kg = 5600 international units

BeneFix®:

Children <15 years:

Number of Factor IX International Units Required = body weight (in kg) x desired Factor IX level increase (% normal) x 1.4 international units/kg

Adults:

Number of Factor IX International Units Required = body weight (in kg) x desired Factor IX level increase (% normal) x 1.2 international units/kg

Guidelines: As a general rule, the level of factor IX required for treatment of different conditions is listed below:

Minor spontaneous hemorrhage, prophylaxis:
- Desired levels of factor IX for hemostasis: 15% to 25%
- Initial loading dose to achieve desired level: Up to 20-30 international units/kg
- Frequency of dosing: Every 12-24 hours
- Duration of treatment: 1-2 days

Moderate hemorrhage:
- Desired levels of factor IX for hemostasis: 25% to 50%
- Initial loading dose to achieve desired level: 25-50 international units/kg
- Frequency of dosing: Every 12-24 hours
- Duration of treatment: 2-7 days

Major hemorrhage:
- Desired levels of factor IX for hemostasis: >50%
- Initial loading dose to achieve desired level: 30-50 international units/kg
- Frequency of dosing: Every 12-24 hours, depending on half-life and measured factor IX levels (after 3-5 days, maintain at least 20% activity)
- Duration of treatment: 7-10 days, depending upon nature of insult

Surgery:
- Desired levels of factor IX for hemostasis: 50% to 100%
- Initial loading dose to achieve desired level: 50-100 international units/kg
- Frequency of dosing: Every 12-24 hours, depending on half-life and measured factor IX levels
- Duration of treatment: 7-10 days, depending upon nature of insult

Administration I.V.: Solution should be infused at room temperature; reconstitute with SWI; use within 3 hours of reconstitution; infuse without further dilution **slowly**. The rate of administration should be determined by the response and comfort of the patient.

Mononine®: Infuse at 2 mL/minute
Alphanine® SD: Infuse at a rate not to exceed 10 mL/minute

Monitoring Parameters Factors IX level, PTT

Reference Range Average normal factor IX levels are 50% to 150%; patients with severe hemophilia will have levels <1%, often undetectable. Moderate forms of the disease have levels of 1% to 10% while some mild cases may have 11% to 49% of normal factor IX.

Maintain factor IX plasma level at least 20% until hemostasis achieved after acute joint or muscle bleeding

In preparation for and following surgery:
- Level to prevent spontaneous hemorrhage: 5%
- Minimum level for hemostasis following trauma and surgery: 30% to 50%

Severe hemorrhage: >60%

Major surgery: ≥50% prior to procedure, 30% to 50% for several days after surgery, and >20% for 10-14 days thereafter

Additional Information

1 international unit is equal to the amount of Factor IX activity present in 1 mL of pooled, normal human plasma

Dosage Forms Excipient information presented when available (limited, particularly for generics); consult specific product labeling.

Injection, powder for reconstitution (**Note:** Exact potency labeled on each vial):

AlphaNine® SD [human derived; solvent detergent treated; virus filtered; contains nondetectable levels of factors II, VII, X; supplied with diluent]

BeneFix® [recombinant formulation; supplied with diluent]

Mononine® [human derived; monoclonal antibody purified; contains nondetectable levels of factors II, VII, X; supplied with diluent]

Factor IX Complex (Human) (FAK ter nyne KOM pleks HYU man)

U.S. Brand Names Bebulin® VH; Profilnine® SD; Proplex® T [DSC]

Index Terms Prothrombin Complex Concentrate

Therapeutic Category Antihemophilic Agent; Blood Product Derivative

Generic Available No

Use To control bleeding in patients with factor IX deficiency (hemophilia B or Christmas disease); prevention/control of bleeding in hemophilia A patients with inhibitors to factor VIII; Proplex® T is indicated to prevent or control bleeding due to factor VII deficiency

Pregnancy Risk Factor C

Contraindications Liver disease, intravascular coagulation or fibrinolysis

Precautions Use with caution in patients with liver dysfunction; risk of viral transmission is not totally eradicated, prepared from pooled human plasma

Adverse Reactions

Cardiovascular: Flushing

Central nervous system: Somnolence, fever, headache, chills

Dermatologic: Urticaria

Gastrointestinal: Nausea, vomiting

Hematologic: Disseminated intravascular coagulation, thrombosis following high dosages in hemophilia B patients

Neuromuscular & skeletal: Paresthesia

Miscellaneous: Tightness in chest and neck

Drug Interactions Increased risk of thrombosis with aminocaproic acid (some recommend to delay the administration of aminocaproic acid 8 hours after factor IX complex administration)

Stability Store unopened vials in refrigerator; do not freeze; administer within 3 hours after reconstitution; **do not refrigerate after reconstitution**; Profilnine® SD: May store unopened vials at room temperature (<30°C) for up to 3 months

Mechanism of Action Replaces deficient clotting factors including factors II, VII, IX, and X

Pharmacokinetics Cleared rapidly from the serum in two phases

Half-life:

First phase: 4-6 hours

Terminal: 22.5 hours

Usual Dosage Dose is expressed in terms of factor IX units; dose must be individualized; **Note:** 1 unit/kg raises factor IX levels 1%

Children and Adults: I.V.:

Factor IX deficiency: Hospitalized patients: 20-50 international units/kg/dose; may be higher in special cases; may be given every 24 hours or more often in special cases

Factor VIII inhibitor patients: 75-100 international units/kg/dose; may be given every 6-12 hours

Administration Parenteral: I.V. administration only; rate of administration should be individualized for patient's comfort; maximum rates of administration: Bebulin® VH: 2 mL/minute; Profilnine® SD: 10 mL/minute; Proplex® T: 3 mL/minute; use filter needle to draw product into syringe; visually inspect for particulate matter and discoloration prior to administration whenever permitted by solution or container

Monitoring Parameters Levels of factors II, IX, and X; signs/symptoms of bleeding; hemoglobin, hematocrit

Reference Range Patients with severe hemophilia will have factor IX levels <1%, often undetectable. Moderate forms of the disease have levels of 1% to 10% while some mild cases may have 11% to 49% of normal factor IX. Plasma concentration is about 4 mg/L.

(Continued)

Factor IX Complex (Human) *(Continued)*

Additional Information AlphaNine® SD and Mononine® contain only factor IX and should not be confused with factor IX **complex**

Dosage Forms Excipient information presented when available (limited, particularly for generics); consult specific product labeling. [DSC] = Discontinued product

Injection, powder for reconstitution (**Note:** Exact potency labeled on each vial):

Bebulin® VH [single-dose vial; vapor heated; supplied with sterile water for injection]

Profilnine® SD [single-dose vial; solvent detergent treated]

Proplex® T [single-dose vial; heat treated; supplied with sterile water for injection] [DSC]

References

Lusher JM, "Thrombogenicity Associated With Factor IX Complex Concentrates," *Semin Hematol*, 1991, 28(3 Suppl 6):3-5.

Shord SS and Lindley CM, "Coagulation Products and Their Uses," *Am J Health Syst Pharm*, 2000, 57(15):1403-20.

- **Factor VIII** *see* Antihemophilic Factor (Human) *on page 134*
- **Factor VIII (Human)** *see* Antihemophilic Factor/von Willebrand Factor Complex (Human) *on page 141*
- **Factor VIII (Recombinant)** *see* Antihemophilic Factor (Recombinant) *on page 138*
- **Factrel®** *see* Gonadorelin *on page 741*

Famciclovir (fam SYE kloe veer)

U.S. Brand Names Famvir®

Canadian Brand Names Apo-Famciclovir; Famvir®; PMS-Famciclovir

Therapeutic Category Antiviral Agent, Oral

Generic Available No

Use Treatment of acute herpes zoster (shingles); treatment or suppression of recurrent episodes of genital herpes in immunocompetent patients; treatment of recurrent episodes of herpes labialis (cold sores) in immunocompetent patients; treatment of recurrent episodes of mucocutaneous herpes simplex infections in HIV patients

Pregnancy Risk Factor B

Lactation Excretion in breast milk unknown/use caution

Contraindications Hypersensitivity to famciclovir, penciclovir, or any component

Precautions Use with caution and decrease dose in patients with renal dysfunction; acute renal failure has been reported in patients with renal dysfunction who received inappropriately high doses of famciclovir for their level of renal function. Dosage adjustment may be needed in patients with poorly compensated hepatic impairment. Tablets contain lactose; do not use in patients with galactose intolerance, severe lactase deficiency, or glucose-galactose malabsorption syndromes. Safety and efficacy have not been established in children <18 years of age. Efficacy has not been established in adults for treatment of initial episodes of genital herpes infection, ophthalmic zoster, disseminated zoster, or in immunocompromised patients with herpes zoster.

Adverse Reactions Note: Frequency of adverse effects vary with dose and duration; single-dose treatment of herpes labialis (cold sores) was associated with headache (10%), nausea (2%), diarrhea (2%), fatigue (1.3%), and dysmenorrhea (1%).

Central nervous system: Headache (10% to 39%), fatigue (1% to 5%), dizziness, fever, somnolence

Dermatologic: Pruritus (0 to 4%), rash (0 to 3%)

Endocrine & metabolic: Dysmenorrhea (0 to 8%)

Gastrointestinal: Nausea (2% to 13%), diarrhea (2% to 9%), vomiting (0 to 5%), constipation, anorexia, abdominal pain, flatulence

Hematologic: Neutropenia (3%), leukopenia (1%)

Hepatic: Elevated liver enzymes (2% to 3%), elevated bilirubin (2%)

Neuromuscular & skeletal: Rigors, paresthesia (0 to 3%)

Drug Interactions Probenecid may increase penciclovir serum concentrations

Food Interactions Rate of absorption and/or conversion to penciclovir and peak concentration are reduced with food, but bioavailability is not affected

Mechanism of Action Synthetic guanine derivative, prodrug for penciclovir; penciclovir has inhibitory activity against varicella zoster virus (VZV) and herpes simplex virus type 1 and 2 (HSV 1 and HSV 2); penciclovir is converted to penciclovir monophosphate (by viral thymidine kinase in VZV-, HSV 1-, and HSV 2-infected cells), then to penciclovir triphosphate which competes with deoxyguanosine triphosphate for viral DNA polymerase and incorporation into viral DNA; therefore, inhibits DNA synthesis and viral replication

Pharmacokinetics Penciclovir:

Absorption: Rapid

Distribution: V_{dss}: Healthy adults: 1.08 ± 0.17 L/kg

Protein binding: <20%

Metabolism: Famciclovir is a prodrug which is metabolized via deacetylation and oxidation in the intestinal wall and liver to penciclovir (active) during extensive first-pass metabolism

Bioavailability: 77% ± 8%

Half-life:

Serum: 2-3 hours; increased with renal dysfunction

Mean half-life, terminal:

Cl_{cr} >80 mL/minute: 2.15 hours

Cl_{cr} 60-80 mL/minute: 2.47 hours

Cl_{cr} 30-59 mL/minute: 3.87 hours

Cl_{cr} <29 mL/minute: 9.85 hours

Intracellular penciclovir triphosphate: HSV 1: 10 hours; HSV 2: 20 hours; VZV: 7 hours

Time to peak serum concentration: ~1 hour

Elimination: Primarily excreted via the kidneys; after oral administration, 73% is excreted in the urine (predominantly as penciclovir) and 27% in feces; penciclovir undergoes tubular secretion; requires dosage adjustment with renal impairment

Dialysis: Hemodialysis: May enhance elimination of penciclovir

Usual Dosage Oral:

Children and Adolescents: Insufficient clinical data exists to identify an appropriate pediatric dose (AAP, 2006):

Adults:

Herpes zoster: 500 mg every 8 hours for 7 days; initiate as soon as diagnosed; initiation of therapy within 48 hours of rash onset may be more beneficial; no efficacy data available for treatment initiated >72 hours after onset of rash

Genital herpes: Treatment of initial clinical episode: 250 mg 3 times/day for 7"10 days; **Note:** Treatment may be continued if healing is not complete after 10 days of therapy (CDC, 2006)

Recurrent genital herpes in immunocompetent patients:

Treatment: 1000 mg twice daily for 1 day or 125 mg twice daily for 5 days (CDC, 2006); initiate at first sign or symptom; efficacy is not established if treatment is started >6 hours after onset of lesions or symptoms

Suppression: 250 mg twice daily for up to 1 year

Recurrent herpes labialis (cold sores): 1500 mg as a single dose; initiate at first sign or symptom such as tingling, burning, or itching; efficacy established for initiation of treatment within 1 hour of symptom onset

Recurrent orolabial or genital herpes in HIV patients: Treatment: 500 mg twice daily for 7 days

Recurrent genital herpes in HIV patients: Suppression: 500 mg twice daily (CDC, 2006)

Dosing interval in renal impairment: Adults:

Herpes zoster:

Cl_{cr} ≥60 mL/minute: Administer 500 mg every 8 hours

Cl_{cr} 40-59 mL/minute: Administer 500 mg every 12 hours

Cl_{cr} 20-39 mL/minute: Administer 500 mg every 24 hours

Cl_{cr} <20 mL/minute: Administer 250 mg every 24 hours

Patients on hemodialysis: Administer 250 mg after each dialysis session

Recurrent genital herpes: Treatment (single day regimen):

Cl_{cr} ≥60 mL/minute: Administer 1000 mg every 12 hours for 1 day

Cl_{cr} 40-59 mL/minute: Administer 500 mg every 12 hours for 1 day

Cl_{cr} 20-39 mL/minute: Administer 500 mg as a single dose

Cl_{cr} <20 mL/minute: Administer 250 mg as a single dose

Patients on hemodialysis: Administer 250 mg as a single dose after dialysis session

Recurrent genital herpes: Suppression:

Cl_{cr} ≥40 mL/minute: Administer 250 mg every 12 hours

Cl_{cr} 20-39 mL/minute: Administer 125 mg every 12 hours

Cl_{cr} <20 mL/minute: Administer 125 mg every 24 hours

Patients on hemodialysis: Administer 125 mg after each dialysis session

Recurrent herpes labialis: Treatment (single dose regimen):

Cl_{cr} ≥60 mL/minute: Administer 1500 mg as a single dose

Cl_{cr} 40-59 mL/minute: Administer 750 mg as a single dose

Cl_{cr} 20-39 mL/minute: Administer 500 mg as a single dose

Cl_{cr} <20 mL/minute: Administer 250 mg as a single dose

Patients on hemodialysis: Administer 250 mg as a single dose after dialysis session

Recurrent orolabial or genital herpes in HIV infected patients:

Cl_{cr} ≥40 mL/minute: Administer 500 mg every 12 hours

Cl_{cr} 20-39 mL/minute: Administer 500 mg every 12 hours

Cl_{cr} <20 mL/minute: Administer 250 mg every 24 hours

Patients on hemodialysis: Administer 250 mg after each dialysis session

(Continued)

Famciclovir *(Continued)*

Administration Oral: May be administered without regard to meals; may be administered with food to decrease GI upset

Monitoring Parameters Resolution of rash, renal function, WBC, liver enzymes

Patient Information Famciclovir is not a cure for genital herpes; may cause dizziness and impair ability to perform activities requiring mental alertness or physical coordination

Dosage Forms Excipient information presented when available (limited, particularly for generics); consult specific product labeling.

Tablet: 125 mg, 250 mg, 500 mg [contains lactose]

References

Boike SC, Pue MA, and Freed MI, "Pharmacokinetics of Famciclovir in Subjects With Varying Degrees of Renal Impairment," *Clin Pharmacol Ther*, 1994, 55(4):418-26.

Centers for Disease Control and Prevention (CDC), "Sexually Transmitted Diseases Treatment Guidelines, 2006," *MMWR Recomm Rep*, 2006, 55(RR-11):1-94.

Pickering LK, ed, *2006 Red Book, Report of the Committee on Infectious Diseases*, 27th ed, Elk Grove Village IL: American Academy of Pediatrics, 2006, 787.

Spruance SL, Bodsworth N, Resnick H, et al, "Single-Dose, Patient-Initiated Famciclovir: A Randomized, Double-Blind, Placebo-Controlled Trial for Episodic Treatment of Herpes Labialis," *J Am Acad Dermatol*, 2006, 55(1):47-53.

Famotidine (fa MOE ti deen)

U.S. Brand Names Pepcid®; Pepcid® AC [OTC]

Canadian Brand Names Apo-Famotidine®; Apo-Famotidine® Injectable; Famotidine Omega; Gen-Famotidine; Novo-Famotidine; Nu-Famotidine; Pepcid®; Pepcid® AC; Pepcid® I.V.; ratio-Famotidine; Riva-Famotidine; Ulcidine

Therapeutic Category Gastrointestinal Agent, Gastric or Duodenal Ulcer Treatment; Histamine H_2 Antagonist

Generic Available Yes: Injection, tablet

Use Short-term therapy and treatment of duodenal ulcer, gastric ulcer, control gastric pH in critically ill patients, symptomatic relief in gastritis, gastroesophageal reflux disease (GERD), active benign ulcer, and pathological hypersecretory conditions; over-the-counter (OTC) formulation for use in the relief of heartburn, acid indigestion, and sour stomach

Pregnancy Risk Factor B

Lactation Enters breast milk/not recommended

Contraindications Hypersensitivity to famotidine, any component (see Warnings), or other H_2 antagonists

Warnings Use with caution and modify dose in patients with renal impairment. Use of gastric acid inhibitors including proton pump inhibitors and H_2 blockers has been associated with an increased risk for development of acute gastroenteritis and community-acquired pneumonia (Canani, 2006).

Multidose injection contains benzyl alcohol which may cause allergic reactions in susceptible individuals; large amounts of benzyl alcohol (≥99 mg/kg/day) have been associated with a potentially fatal toxicity ("gasping syndrome") in neonates; the "gasping syndrome" consists of metabolic acidosis, respiratory distress, gasping respirations, CNS dysfunction (including convulsions, intracranial hemorrhage), hypotension and cardiovascular collapse; avoid use of the multidose injection in neonates. The oral suspension contains sodium benzoate; *in vitro* and animal studies have shown that benzoate, a metabolite of benzyl alcohol, displaces bilirubin from protein binding sites; avoid use in neonates.

Precautions Pepcid® chewable tablets contain phenylalanine which should be used with caution in patients with phenylketonuria.

Adverse Reactions

Cardiovascular: Bradycardia, tachycardia, palpitations, hypertension

Central nervous system: Headache, vertigo, anxiety, dizziness, seizures, depression, insomnia, drowsiness, confusion, fever

Dermatologic: Acne, pruritus, urticaria, dry skin, alopecia

Gastrointestinal: Constipation, nausea, vomiting, diarrhea, abdominal discomfort, flatulence, belching, dysgeusia, dry mouth, anorexia

Genitourinary: Impotence

Hematologic: Thrombocytopenia, pancytopenia, leukopenia (rare)

Hepatic: Elevated liver enzymes, hepatomegaly, cholestatic jaundice

Neuromuscular & skeletal: Weakness, arthralgias, paresthesia, muscle cramps

Ocular: Orbital edema

Otic: Ototoxicity, tinnitus

Renal: Elevated BUN and serum creatinine, proteinuria

Respiratory: Bronchospasm

Drug Interactions Decreased absorption of ketoconazole, triamterene, delavirdine, itraconazole, cefpodoxime, cyanocobalamin, indomethacin, melphalan; decreased effect of tolazoline

Food Interactions Limit xanthine-containing foods and beverages

Stability Concentrate for injection must be refrigerated but is stable for 48 hours at room temperature; if concentrated injection is diluted in D_5W or NS it is stable 48 hours at room temperature; commercially available diluted solution in NS is stable at room temperature for 15 months; injection is also compatible with $D_{10}W$, LR injection, 5% bicarbonate injection, and standard parenteral nutrition solutions with electrolytes, multivitamins, and trace minerals; reconstituted oral solution is stable for 30 days at room temperature

Mechanism of Action Competitive inhibition of histamine at H_2-receptors of the gastric parietal cells, which results in inhibition of gastric acid secretion

Pharmacodynamics

Onset of GI effect: Oral, I.V.: Within 1 hour
Maximum effect:
- Oral: 1-4 hours
- I.V.: 30 minutes to 3 hours

Duration: 10-12 hours

Pharmacokinetics

Distribution: V_d:
- Infants:
  - 0-3 months: 1.4-1.8 ± 0.3-0.4 L/kg
  - >3 to 12 months: 2.3 ± 0.7 L/kg
- Children: 2 ± 1.5 L/kg
- Adults: 0.94-1.33 L/kg

Protein binding: 15% to 20%
Metabolism: 30% to 35% liver metabolism
Bioavailability: Oral: 40% to 45%
Half-life:
- Infants:
  - 0-3 months: 8.1-10.5 ± 3.5-5.4 hours
  - >3 to 12 months: 4.5 ± 1.1 hours
- Children: 3.3 ± 2.5 hours
- Adults: Injection, oral suspension, tablet: 2.5-3.5 hours; orally-disintegrating tablet: 5 hours; increases with renal impairment; if Cl_{cr} <10 mL/minute, half-life ≥20 hours
- Anuria: 24 hours

Time to peak serum concentration: Orally-disintegrating tablet: 2.5 hours
Elimination: 65% to 70% unchanged drug in urine
- Clearance:
  - Infants:
    - 0-3 months: 0.13-0.21 ± 0.06 L/hour/kg
    - >3-12 months: 0.49 ± 0.17 L/hour/kg
  - Children 1 to 11 years: 0.54 ± 0.34 L/hour/kg
  - Adults: 0.39 ± 0.14 L/hour/kg

Usual Dosage

Neonates and Infants <3 months: Oral: GERD: 0.5 mg/kg/dose once daily
Infants ≥3 months to 1 year: Oral: GERD: 0.5 mg/kg/dose twice daily
Children 1-12 years: Oral, I.V.:
- Peptic ulcer: 0.5 mg/kg/day at bedtime or divided twice daily (maximum: 40 mg/day)
- GERD: 1 mg/kg/day divided twice daily (maximum: 80 mg/day)

Children >12 years and Adults:
- Oral:
  - Duodenal ulcer, gastric ulcer: 20 mg/day at bedtime for 4-8 weeks (a regimen of 10 mg twice daily is also effective); maximum: 40 mg/day
  - Hypersecretory conditions: Initial: 20 mg every 6 hours, may increase up to 160 mg every 6 hours
  - Esophagitis: 20-40 mg twice daily for up to 12 weeks
  - GERD: 20 mg twice daily for 6 weeks
  - Acid indigestion, heartburn, or sour stomach (OTC use): 10-20 mg 15-60 minutes before eating; not more than 2 tablets per day
- I.V.: 20 mg every 12 hours

Dosing adjustment in renal impairment:
- Cl_{cr} 10-50 mL/minute: Administer normal dose every 24 hours or 50% of dose at normal dosing interval
- Cl_{cr} <10 mL/minute: Administer normal dose every 36-48 hours

Administration

Oral: May administer with food and antacids; shake suspension vigorously for 10-15 seconds prior to each use; place orally-disintegrating tablet (Fluxid™) on the top of

(Continued)

Famotidine *(Continued)*

the tongue, wait until it dissolves than swallow with saliva; tablet disintegrates in <2 minutes; do not break or chew tablet

Parenteral: I.V.: Dilute to a maximum concentration of 4 mg/mL; may be administered I.V. push at 10 mg/minute over 2 minutes or as an infusion over 15-30 minutes

Patient Information Avoid excessive amounts of coffee and aspirin; when self medicating, if the symptoms of heartburn, acid indigestion, or sour stomach persist after 2 weeks of continuous use of the drug, consult a clinician.

Dosage Forms Excipient information presented when available (limited, particularly for generics); consult specific product labeling. [DSC] = Discontinued product

Gelcap:
  Pepcid® AC: 10 mg [DSC]
Infusion [premixed in NS]: 20 mg (50 mL)
  Pepcid®: 20 mg (50 mL)
Injection, solution: 10 mg/mL (4 mL, 20 mL)
  Pepcid®: 10 mg/mL (20 mL) [contains benzyl alcohol]
Injection, solution [preservative free]: 10 mg/mL (2 mL)
  Pepcid®: 10 mg/mL (2 mL)
Powder for oral suspension:
  Pepcid®: 40 mg/5 mL (50 mL) [contains sodium benzoate; cherry-banana-mint flavor]
Tablet: 10 mg [OTC], 20 mg, 40 mg
  Pepcid®: 20 mg, 40 mg
  Pepcid® AC: 10 mg, 20 mg
Tablet, chewable:
  Pepcid® AC: 10 mg [contains phenylalanine 1.4 mg/tablet; mint flavor]

Extemporaneous Preparations An 8 mg/mL suspension may be made by crushing seventy 40 mg tablets; work into a paste with a small amount of sterile water; add a 1:1 mixture of Ora-Plus® and Ora-Sweet® to a total volume of 350 mL; stable 95 days at 23°C to 35°C

Dentinger PJ, Swenson CF, and Anaizi NH, "Stability of Famotidine in an Extemporaneously Compounded Oral Liquid," *Am J Health Syst Pharm*, 2000, 57(14):1340-2.

References

Canani RB, Cirillo P, Roggero P, et al, "Therapy With Gastric Acidity Inhibitors Increases the Risk of Acute Gastroenteritis and Community-Acquired Pneumonia in Children," *Pediatrics*, 2006, 117(5):e817-20.

James LP and Kearns GL, "Pharmacokinetics and Pharmacodynamics of Famotidine in Paediatric Patients," *Clin Pharmacokinet*, 1996, 31(2):103-10.

Treem WR, Davis PM, and Hyams JS, "Suppression of Gastric Acid Secretion by Intravenous Administration of Famotidine in Children," *J Pediatr*, 1991, 118(5):812-6.

♦ **Famotidine Omega (Can)** *see* Famotidine *on page 638*
♦ **Famvir®** *see* Famciclovir *on page 636*
♦ **Fansidar®** *see* Sulfadoxine and Pyrimethamine *on page 1486*
♦ **Fasturtec® (Can)** *see* Rasburicase *on page 1369*

Fat Emulsion (fat e MUL shun)

Related Information
Parenteral Nutrition (PN) *on page 1755*

U.S. Brand Names Intralipid®; Liposyn® III

Canadian Brand Names Intralipid®; Liposyn® II

Index Terms Intravenous Fat Emulsion

Therapeutic Category Caloric Agent; Intravenous Nutritional Therapy

Generic Available No

Use Source of calories and essential fatty acids for patients requiring parenteral nutrition of extended duration

Pregnancy Risk Factor C

Lactation Excretion in breast milk unknown/compatible

Contraindications Hypersensitivity to fat emulsion and severe egg or legume (soybean) allergies; pathologic hyperlipidemia; lipoid nephrosis; pancreatitis with hyperlipemia; 30% fat emulsions are not intended for direct I.V. infusion and dilution with another I.V. fluid (eg, NS does not produce a dilution equivalent to 10% or 20% I.V. fat emulsion); such dilutions should not be administered by direct I.V. infusion (see Additional Information)

Warnings Deaths in preterm neonates after infusion of I.V. fat emulsions have been reported. Autopsy findings included intravascular fat accumulation in the lungs. Use of I.V. fat emulsion in preterm neonates should be done carefully adhering to maximum daily dosages and infusing as slowly as possible (see Usual Dosage).

Preterm infants have a decreased ability to eliminate infused fat and must be monitored closely using triglyceride or plasma free fatty acid levels.

Precautions Use with caution in patients with severe liver damage, pulmonary disease, anemia, or blood coagulation disorder, and in jaundiced patients

Adverse Reactions

Cardiovascular: Cyanosis, flushing, chest pain

Central nervous system: Headache, fever, sleepiness, dizziness

Gastrointestinal: Nausea, vomiting

Hematologic: Hypercoagulability, thrombocytopenia, leukopenia

Hepatic: Hyperlipemia, hepatomegaly, jaundice, cholestasis, transient increases in liver enzymes

Local: Thrombophlebitis

Respiratory: Dyspnea

Miscellaneous: Sepsis, hypersensitivity reactions, diaphoresis, splenomegaly, deposition of brown pigment in the reticuloendothelial system (clinical significance unknown)

Stability May be stored at room temperature; do not use if emulsion appears to be layering out; exposure to light, particularly phototherapy light, used in treatment or prevention of hyperbilirubinemia has been associated with increased lipid oxidation; the clinical significance remains to be established; do not mix other drugs with fat emulsion; only heparin at a concentration of 1-2 units/mL may be added to fat emulsion

Mechanism of Action Fatty acids are essential for normal structure and function of cell membranes; I.V. fat emulsion provides a source of calories and essential fatty acids normally obtained in the enteral diet

Usual Dosage I.V. infusion: Fat emulsion should not exceed 60% of the total daily calories

Note: At the onset of therapy, the patient should be observed for any immediate allergic reactions such as dyspnea, cyanosis, and fever. Slower initial rates of infusion may be used for the first 10-15 minutes of the infusion (eg, 0.1 mL/minute of 10% or 0.05 mL/minute of 20% solution).

Premature infants: Initial dose: 0.25-0.5 g/kg/day, increase by 0.25-0.5 g/kg/day to a maximum of 3-4 g/kg/day; maximum rate of infusion: 0.15 g/kg/hour (0.75 mL/kg/hour of 20% solution) (see Warnings)

Infants and Children: Initial dose: 0.5-1 g/kg/day, increase by 0.5 g/kg/day to a maximum of 3-4 g/kg/day; maximum rate of infusion: 0.25 g/kg/hour (1.25 mL/kg/hour of 20% solution)

Adolescents and Adults: Initial dose: 1 g/kg/day, increase by 0.5-1 g/kg/day to a maximum of 2.5 g/kg/day; maximum rate of infusion: 0.25 g/kg/hour (1.25 mL/kg/hour of 20% solution); do not exceed 50 mL/hour (20%) or 100 mL/hour (10%)

Children and Adults: Fatty acid deficiency: 8% to 10% of total caloric intake; infuse once or twice weekly

Administration Parenteral: 10% and 20% emulsions may be simultaneously infused with amino acid, dextrose mixtures by means of Y-connector located near infusion site into either central or peripheral line; 30% emulsions must not be infused directly (see Contraindications and Additional Information)

Monitoring Parameters Serum triglycerides, free fatty acids, platelets, liver enzymes

Additional Information 10% = 1.1 Kcal/mL, 20% = 2 Kcal/mL, 30% = 3 Kcal/mL; 10% and 20% solutions are isotonic and may be administered peripherally; 30% solution is not intended for direct infusion; it must be diluted to a final concentration not to exceed 20% when added to 3-in-1 or total nutrient admixture; avoid use of 10% fat emulsion in preterm infants; a greater accumulation of plasma lipids occurs due to the greater phospholipid load of the 10% fat emulsion

Dosage Forms Excipient information presented when available (limited, particularly for generics); consult specific product labeling.

Injection, emulsion [soybean oil]:

Intralipid®: 10% [100 mg/mL] (100 mL, 250 mL, 500 mL); 20% [200 mg/mL] (50 mL, 100 mL, 250 mL, 500 mL, 1000 mL); 30% [300 mg/mL] (500 mL)

Liposyn® III: 10% [100 mg/mL] (200 mL, 500 mL); 20% [200 mg/mL] (200 mL, 500 mL); 30% [300 mg/mL] (500 mL)

References

Haumont D, Richelle M, Deckelbaum RJ, et al, "Effect of Liposomal Content of Lipid Emulsions of Plasma Lipid Concentrations in Low Birth Weight Infants Receiving Parenteral Nutrition," *J Pediatr*, 1992, 121(5 Pt 1):759-63.

Neuzil J, Darlow BA, Inder TE, et al, "Oxidation of Parenteral Lipid Emulsion by Ambient and Phototherapy Lights: Potential Toxicity of Routine Parenteral Feeding," *J Pediatr*, 1995, 126(5 Pt 1):785-90.

♦ **5-FC** *see* Flucytosine *on page 662*

♦ **Feiba VH** *see* Anti-inhibitor Coagulant Complex *on page 144*

♦ **Feiba VH Immuno (Can)** *see* Anti-inhibitor Coagulant Complex *on page 144*

Felbamate (FEL ba mate)

Related Information

Antiepileptic Drugs *on page 1902*

U.S. Brand Names Felbatol®

Therapeutic Category Anticonvulsant, Miscellaneous

Generic Available No

Use Not a first-line agent, see Warnings; reserved for patients who do not adequately respond to alternative agents and whose epilepsy is so severe that the benefit outweighs the risk of liver failure or aplastic anemia; used as monotherapy and adjunctive therapy in patients ≥14 years of age with partial seizures with and without secondary generalization; adjunctive therapy in children ≥2 years of age who have partial and generalized seizures associated with Lennox-Gastaut syndrome

Pregnancy Risk Factor C

Lactation Enters breast milk/not recommended

Contraindications Hypersensitivity to felbamate, any component, or other carbamates (eg, meprobamate); history of or current blood dyscrasia or hepatic dysfunction

Warnings Thirty-three cases of aplastic anemia (with 8 deaths) and 14 cases of hepatic failure (with 8 deaths) have been reported in patients who received felbamate. The manufacturer (Carter Wallace) and the FDA recommend the use of this agent be suspended unless withdrawal of the product would place a patient at greater risk.

Aplastic anemia: Of the 27 cases analyzed by the manufacturer, 26 occurred in adult patients (mean age: 42 years) exposed to felbamate for a mean of 170 days at a mean dose of 3168 mg/day. One case occurred in a 13-year old exposed to felbamate for 276 days at a dose of ~69 mg/kg/day. Twenty-three of 27 patients received other antiepileptic drugs (AEDs) and 9 received drugs associated with blood dyscrasias. The 8 deaths occurred in adults (mean age: 47 years). Six of the 8 patients had a history of blood dyscrasias and 6 had allergies to medications (3 to AEDs). The onset of aplastic anemia ranged from 5-30 weeks.

Hepatic failure: Of the 14 cases, 6 cases occurred in children 3-12 years of age (mean: 6 years) exposed to felbamate for 30-218 days (mean: 115 days) at a mean dose of 1520 mg/day. The overall postmarketing reported rate of hepatic failure leading to transplant or death is 6 cases per 75,000 patient years of use; this rate is underestimated due to under reporting (eg, the true rate could be as high as 1 case per 1250 patient years of use if the reporting rate is only 10%). Approximately 67% of the reported cases of hepatic failure led to liver transplantation or death, usually within 5 weeks of the onset of signs and symptoms of hepatic failure; the earliest onset of severe liver dysfunction was 3 weeks after starting felbamate; in some cases, dark urine and nonspecific prodromal symptoms (eg, malaise, anorexia, GI symptoms) preceded the onset of jaundice.

All patients receiving felbamate **must** be monitored closely; in addition, a CBC with differential and platelet count should be taken before, during, and for a significant time after discontinuing felbamate therapy; liver enzyme tests and bilirubin should be obtained before initiation and periodically during therapy. Felbamate should be immediately withdrawn if abnormal liver function tests or bone marrow suppression occur.

The FDA and the manufacturer strongly recommend that physicians discuss the risks of felbamate with each patient and a written informed consent be obtained from the patient prior to starting therapy or before continuing therapy. A patient information consent form is included as part of the package insert and is available from the local Wallace representative or by calling 609-655-6147.

Precautions Use with caution in patients concurrently receiving other antiepileptic drugs due to the potential for drug interactions; decrease dosage of phenytoin, carbamazepine, or valproic acid by 20% to 30% when felbamate is added to the regimen and when felbamate doses are titrated upwards; monitor serum levels of concomitant antiepileptic drug therapy. Use with caution and reduce dose in patients with renal dysfunction.

Adverse Reactions

Central nervous system: Headache, insomnia, somnolence, fatigue, dizziness, anxiety, drowsiness, depression, behavior changes, ataxia

Dermatologic: Acne, rash, pruritus

Endocrine & metabolic: Weight loss

Gastrointestinal: Anorexia, vomiting, nausea, diarrhea, constipation, dyspepsia, gum bleeding or hyperplasia

Hematologic: Thrombocytopenia, granulocytopenia, agranulocytosis, purpura, leukopenia, aplastic anemia (100-fold increase in risk; see Warnings)

Hepatic: Elevated liver enzymes, hepatitis, acute liver failure (may be associated with death; see Warnings)

Drug Interactions Cytochrome P450 isoenzyme CYP2C19 inhibitor

Phenytoin, carbamazepine may increase and valproic acid may decrease the clearance of felbamate; felbamate increases the concentrations of phenytoin and valproic acid; felbamate decreases carbamazepine concentrations but increases the concentration of carbamazepine epoxide (active metabolite)

Food Interactions Food does **not** affect absorption

Stability Store in tightly closed container at room temperature away from excessive heat, moisture, or direct sunlight

Mechanism of Action Mechanism of action is unknown but may be similar to other anticonvulsants; has weak inhibitory effects on GABA and benzodiazepine receptor binding; does not have activity at the MK-801 receptor binding site of the NMDA receptor-ionophore complex.

Pharmacokinetics

Absorption: Oral: Rapid and almost complete

Distribution: V_d: Adults: Mean: 0.75 L/kg; range: 0.7-1.1 L/kg

Protein binding: 20% to 25%, primarily to albumin

Metabolism: In the liver via hydroxylation and conjugation

Bioavailability: >90%

Half-life: Adults: Mean: 20-30 hours; shorter (ie, 14 hours) with concomitant enzyme-inducing drugs; half-life is prolonged (by 9-15 hours) in patients with renal dysfunction

Time to peak serum concentration: 1-4 hours

Elimination: 40% to 50% excreted as unchanged drug and 40% as inactive metabolites in urine

Clearance, apparent:

Children 2-9 years: 61.3 ± 8.2 mL/kg/hour

Children 10-12 years: 34.3 ± 4.3 mL/kg/hour

Usual Dosage See Precautions regarding concomitant antiepileptic drugs

Children 2-14 years with Lennox-Gastaut: Adjunctive therapy: Initial: 15 mg/kg/day in 3-4 divided doses; increase dose by 15 mg/kg/day increments at weekly intervals; maximum dose: 45 mg/kg/day or 3600 mg/day (whichever is less)

Children ≥14 years and Adults:

Adjunctive therapy: Initial: 1200 mg/day in 3-4 divided doses; increase daily dose by 1200 mg increments every week to a maximum dose of 3600 mg/day

Conversion to monotherapy: Initial: 1200 mg/day in 3 or 4 divided doses; at week 2, increase daily dose by 1200 mg increments every week up to a maximum dose of 3600 mg/day. Decrease dose of other anticonvulsants by $^1/_3$ their original dose at initiation of felbamate, and when felbamate dose is increased at week 2; continue to reduce other anticonvulsants as clinically needed.

Monotherapy: Initial: 1200 mg/day in 3 or 4 divided doses; titrate dosage upward according to clinical response and monitor patients closely; increase daily dose in 600 mg increments every 2 weeks to 2400 mg/day; maximum dose: 3600 mg/day

Dosage adjustment in renal impairment: Reduce initial and maintenance doses by 50%

Administration Oral: May be administered without regard to meals; shake suspension well before use

Monitoring Parameters Serum concentrations of concomitant anticonvulsant therapy; liver enzymes, bilirubin, CBC with differential, platelet count prior to therapy and periodically during therapy

Reference Range Not necessary to routinely monitor serum drug levels; dose should be titrated to clinical response; therapeutic range not fully determined; proposed 30-100 mcg/mL

Patient Information Do not abruptly discontinue, an increase in seizure activity may result; report any unusual symptoms, such as a rash, bruises, bleeding, sore throat, fever, yellow skin, GI complaints, loss of appetite, tiredness, and/or dark urine to physician immediately

Additional Information Monotherapy has not been associated with gingival hyperplasia, impaired concentration, weight gain, or abnormal thinking; felbamate has also been used in a small number of patients with infantile spasms (see Pellock, 1999); an open-label study in children with refractory partial seizures (n=30; mean age: 9 years; range: 2-17 years) found that children >10 years of age had a more favorable response; this was thought to be related to the higher felbamate serum concentrations (and lower apparent clearance) in children >10 years of age compared to those <10 years; the faster apparent clearance in children <10 years of age should be considered when using this agent (Carmant, 1994)

Dosage Forms Excipient information presented when available (limited, particularly for generics); consult specific product labeling. [DSC] = Discontinued product

(Continued)

Felbamate *(Continued)*

Suspension, oral:

Felbatol®: 600 mg/5 mL (240 mL, 960 mL)

Tablet:

Felbatol®: 400 mg; 600 mg [DSC]

References

Carmant L, Holmes GL, Sawyer S, et al, "Efficacy of Felbamate in Therapy for Partial Epilepsy in Children," *J Pediatr*, 1994, 125(3):481-6.

Dodson WE, "Felbamate in the Treatment of Lennox-Gastaut Syndrome: Results of a 12-Month Open-Label Study Following a Randomized Clinical Trial," *Epilepsia*, 1993, 34(Suppl 7):518-24.

Leppik IE, "Felbamate," *Epilepsia*, 1995, 36(Suppl 2):S66-72.

Pellock JM, "Managing Pediatric Epilepsy Syndromes With New Antiepileptic Drugs," *Pediatrics*, 1999, 104(5 Pt 1):1106-16.

The Felbamate Study Group in Lennox-Gastaut Syndrome, "Efficacy of Felbamate in Childhood Epileptic Encephalopathy (Lennox-Gastaut Syndrome)," *N Engl J Med*, 1993, 328(1):29-33.

Written Communication, Elisabeth Neumann, Director Medical Services, Wallace Laboratories, June 13, 1995.

♦ **Felbatol®** *see* Felbamate *on page 642*

♦ **Feldene®** *see* Piroxicam *on page 1268*

♦ **Fematrol [OTC]** *see* Bisacodyl *on page 217*

♦ **Femilax™ [OTC]** *see* Bisacodyl *on page 217*

♦ **Femiron® [OTC]** *see* Iron Supplements (Oral/Enteral) *on page 868*

♦ **Femring®** *see* Estradiol *on page 605*

♦ **Femtrace®** *see* Estradiol *on page 605*

Fentanyl (FEN ta nil)

Medication Safety Issues

Sound-alike/look-alike issues:

Fentanyl may be confused with alfentanil, sufentanil

Dosing of transdermal fentanyl patches may be confusing. Transdermal fentanyl patches should always be prescribed in mcg/hour, not size.

New patch dosage form of Duragesic®-12 actually delivers 12.5 mcg/hour of fentanyl. Use caution, as orders may be written as "Duragesic 12.5" which can be erroneously interpreted as a 125 mcg dose.

Iontophoretic transdermal system (Ionsys™) may contain conducting metal (eg, aluminum); remove patch prior to MRI. Transdermal patch (eg, Duragesic®) does not contain any metal-based compounds; however, the printed ink used to indicate strength on the outer surface of the patch does contain titanium dioxide, but the amount is minimal.

Related Information

Adult ACLS Algorithms *on page 1660*

Compatibility of Medications Mixed in A Syringe *on page 1941*

Narcotic Analgesics Comparison *on page 1705*

Overdose and Toxicology *on page 1916*

Preprocedure Sedatives in Children *on page 1895*

Serotonin Syndrome *on page 1955*

U.S. Brand Names Actiq®; Duragesic®; Fentora™; Ionsys™; Sublimaze®

Canadian Brand Names Actiq®; Duragesic®; Fentanyl Citrate Injection, USP

Index Terms Fentanyl Citrate; Fentanyl Hydrochloride; OTFC (Oral Transmucosal Fentanyl Citrate)

Therapeutic Category Analgesic, Narcotic; General Anesthetic

Generic Available Yes: Excludes buccal tablet and iontophoretic transdermal system

Use

Injection: Sedation; relief of pain; preoperative medication; adjunct to general or regional anesthesia

Transdermal patch (Duragesic®): Treatment of persistent, moderate-to-severe chronic pain in children ≥2 years of age and adults who are tolerant to opioid therapy and who are currently receiving opiates; see **Note**

Oral transmucosal lozenge (Actiq®): Breakthrough cancer pain in adolescents ≥16 years of age and adult patients tolerant to opioid therapy and who are currently receiving opiates for persistent cancer pain; see **Note**

Buccal tablet (Fentora™): Breakthrough cancer pain in adolescents ≥18 years of age and adult patients tolerant to opioid therapy and who are currently receiving opiates for persistent cancer pain; see **Note**

Iontophoretic transdermal system (Ionsys™): Short-term in-hospital management of acute postoperative pain in adolescents ≥18 years of age and adults

Note: Patients are considered opioid tolerant if they are receiving at least 60 mg/day of morphine, 25 mcg/hour of transdermal fentanyl, 30 mg/day of oral oxycodone, 8

mg/day of oral hydromorphone, or an equivalent dose of another opioid for 1 week or longer.

Restrictions C-II

Medication Guide An FDA-approved patient medication guide, which is available with the product information and at http://www.fda.gov/cder/Offices/ODS/medication_guides.htm, must be dispensed with the buccal tablet (Fentora™) and transmucosal lozenge (Actiq® and generic) for each new outpatient prescription and refill.

Pregnancy Risk Factor C (D if used for prolonged periods or in high doses at term)

Lactation Enters breast milk/not recommended (AAP rates "compatible")

Contraindications Hypersensitivity or intolerance to fentanyl or any component; hypersensitivity to contact adhesives (transdermal patch) or cetylpyridinium chloride (eg, Cepacol®) (iontophoretic transdermal system); increased intracranial pressure; severe respiratory depression or disease including acute or severe bronchial asthma (unless patient is mechanically ventilated); severe liver or renal insufficiency; paralytic ileus; pregnancy (prolonged use or high doses near term)

Transdermal patches, oral transmucosal lozenges (Actiq®), and buccal tablets (Fentora™) are also contraindicated in patients who are not opioid tolerant (see **Note** in Use field) and in the treatment of acute or postoperative pain; transdermal patches are also contraindicated for short-term pain management, treatment of pain following outpatient or day surgery, mild pain, or intermittent pain.

Warnings High potential for abuse; physical and psychological dependence may occur with prolonged use; abrupt discontinuation may result in withdrawal or seizures; potent opioids have a high risk of fatal overdose due to respiratory depression. Symptoms of opioid withdrawal may occur in patients after conversion of one dosage form to another or after dosage adjustment.

I.V. use: Rapid I.V. infusion may result in skeletal muscle and chest wall rigidity, impaired ventilation, respiratory distress, apnea, bronchoconstriction, laryngospasm; inject slowly over 3-5 minutes; nondepolarizing skeletal muscle relaxant may be required

Transdermal patch: Overdoses and deaths have occurred in patients using both the generic and brand name (Duragesic®) products; the directions for use must be followed exactly for safe and effective therapy. Keep used and unused patches out of the reach of children; accidental or deliberate application or ingestion by an infant, child, or adolescent may cause respiratory depression which may result in death. Should be prescribed only by specialists who are knowledgeable in treating pain with potent opioids. Use only in opioid-tolerant patients (use in nonopioid-tolerant patients may result in fatal respiratory depression). Use in pediatric patients **only** if they are opioid tolerant, receiving at least 60 mg oral morphine equivalents per day, and ≥2 years of age; safety has not been established in children <2 years. Serious or potential fatal respiratory depression may occur (even in opioid-tolerant individuals) during the initial application of the patch; patients should be monitored carefully, especially 24-72 hours after initial patch application (when peak fentanyl serum levels occur) and following increases in dosage. Monitor patients who experience adverse reactions for at least 24 hours after removal of the patch (apparent transdermal half-life is 17 hours). Serum fentanyl concentrations may increase by ~1/3 in patients with a body temperature of 104°F (40°C) secondary to temperature-dependent increases in drug released from the transdermal system and an increase in skin permeability; thus, patients with fever should be monitored for opioid adverse effects. Do not expose transdermal patch application site to direct heat sources (eg, electric blankets, heating pads, heated water beds, heat lamps, hot tubs, saunas); temperature-dependent increases in drug released from patch may result in possible overdose or death. Possible overdose or death may also occur in people accidentally exposed to the transdermal system (eg, transfer of the patch from an adult to a child while hugging). Do not place the patch in the mouth; do not chew, swallow, or use in ways that are not indicated; choking or overdose may occur and result in serious medical problems or death.

Oral transmucosal lozenge (Actiq®): Use only for the care of cancer patients who are opioid tolerant; should be prescribed only by healthcare professionals who are knowledgeable in treating cancer pain with potent opioids. Keep out of the reach of children and discard any open units properly; contains an amount of medication that can be fatal to children. Safety and efficacy have not been established for patients <16 years of age.

Buccal tablet (Fentora™): Use only for the care of cancer patients who are opioid tolerant; should be prescribed only by healthcare professionals who are knowledgeable in treating cancer pain with potent opioids. Keep out of the reach of children and discard any open units properly; contains an amount of medication that can be fatal to children. Buccal tablets have a higher bioavailability than other oral fentanyl products (including oral transmucosal lozenge); do not substitute products on a mcg per mcg basis; appropriate dosage adjustments must be made; use caution and monitor

(Continued)

Fentanyl *(Continued)*

closely when changing patients from one product to another. Safety and efficacy have not been established for patients <18 years of age.

Iontophoretic transdermal system (Ionsys™): Patients must be titrated to an acceptable level of analgesia prior to starting treatment with Ionsys™. Potentially life-threatening respiratory depression and death may occur; to avoid overdose, the patient should be the only one to activate the system; do not apply more than one system to a patient at the same time. Inappropriate use (eg, ingestion or contact with mucous membranes) or unintended exposure to fentanyl hydrogel could lead to absorption of fatal dose; hydrogel should not come in contact with fingers or mouth. Should be prescribed only by healthcare providers who are knowledgeable in treating pain with potent opioids. Should be used only in patients who are able to understand and follow instructions to operate the system. The error detection circuit uses a series of audible signals to alert the patient when a dose is not being delivered; use with caution in patients who have high frequency hearing impairment. Ionsys™ contains metal parts; remove prior to MRI procedure, cardioversion, or defibrillation. May interfere with radiographic image or CAT scan as system contains radiopaque components. Patients on chronic opioids or with a history of opioid abuse may require higher analgesic doses than Ionsys™ is able to provide. Ionsys™ is not recommended for the treatment of breakthrough pain in patients receiving chronic opioids (has not been studied). Use only in hospitalized patients under medical supervision; prior to patient's hospital discharge, the system must be removed and disposed of in accordance with State and Federal regulations for a C-II substance. Even after all 80 doses per system are used, a significant amount of fentanyl remains in the iontophoretic transdermal system and requires proper removal and disposal to avoid misuse, abuse, or diversion. Keep out of the reach of children and discard any open units properly; contains an amount of medication that can be fatal to children. Ionsys™ is not recommended for use in patients <18 years of age. **Note:** Preliminary investigations using lower doses of iontophoretically-administered fentanyl suggest that pediatric patients may be more vulnerable to application site reactions than adults (these reactions were more severe in pediatric patients than in adults).

Precautions Use with caution in patients with bradycardia; hepatic, biliary tract, renal, or respiratory disease; acute pancreatitis; cor pulmonale; significant COPD; other chronic respiratory conditions; or those with increased ICP, head injuries, or impaired consciousness. Patients must be monitored until fully recovered; decrease dose in patients with hepatic and/or renal disease; not recommended if patient received MAO inhibitors within 14 days. Frequent use of Actiq® or generic lozenge may increase risk of dental caries; Actiq® and generic lozenge contain 2 g of sugar/unit, as hydrated dextrates; patients should maintain good oral hygiene; inform diabetic patients of sugar content. Use buccal tablets with caution in patients with mucositis (no dose adjustment is needed in patients with Grade I mucositis; safety and efficacy in patients with more severe mucositis have not been studied).

Fentanyl is not recommended for analgesia during labor and delivery; transient muscular rigidity has been observed in neonates born to women who were treated with I.V. fentanyl

Adverse Reactions

Cardiovascular: Hypotension, bradycardia, flushing, cardiac arrhythmia, edema, orthostatic hypotension, hypertension, syncope, tachycardia

Central nervous system: CNS depression, drowsiness, dizziness, somnolence, confusion, sedation, euphoria, nervousness, insomnia, headache, fever, fatigue, abnormal dreams, abnormal thinking, agitation, amnesia, anxiety, hallucinations, paranoid reaction

Dermatologic: Erythema, pruritus, rash; facial pruritus with oral transmucosal product

Endocrine & metabolic: ADH release, weight loss; hypokalemia (6% with buccal tablets)

Gastrointestinal: Nausea, vomiting, constipation, biliary tract spasm, abdominal pain, xerostomia, anorexia, diarrhea, dyspepsia, flatulence, ileus; dental caries, tooth loss and gum line erosion have been reported with transmucosal lozenge containing sugar

Genitourinary: Urinary tract spasm, urinary retention

Hematologic: Anemia, neutropenia

Local:

Buccal tablet: Application-site reactions, local paresthesia, ulceration, bleeding, pain, irritation

Transdermal patch: Edema, erythema, pruritus

Iontophoretic transdermal system: Application-site reactions, erythema (14%), local edema, local sweating, vesicles, papules, pustules, hyperpigmentation (2 cases which lasted 2-3 weeks), rectangular mark at application site (3 cases which lasted up to 3 months)

Neuromuscular & skeletal: Skeletal muscle and chest wall rigidity especially following rapid I.V. administration; asthenia; back pain, abnormal coordination, abnormal gait, back pain, paresthesia, rigors, tremor

Ocular: Miosis

Respiratory: Respiratory depression, apnea, dyspnea, hemoptysis, hypoxia

Miscellaneous: Sweating, rigors, flu-like symptoms; physical and psychological dependence with prolonged use. **Note:** Neonates who receive a total fentanyl dose >1.6 mg/kg or continuous infusion duration >5 days are more likely to develop narcotic withdrawal symptoms; children 1 week to 22 months: those who receive a total dose of 1.5 mg/kg or duration >5 days have a 50% chance of developing narcotic withdrawal and those receiving a total dose >2.5 mg/kg or duration of infusion >9 days have a 100% chance of developing withdrawal. Doses should be tapered to prevent withdrawal symptoms.

Drug Interactions Cytochrome P450 isoenzyme CYP3A3/4 substrate

CNS depressants, alcohol, phenothiazines, MAO inhibitors, tricyclic antidepressants may potentiate fentanyl's adverse effects; when using fentanyl with other CNS depressants, reduce the dose of one or both agents; use of MAO inhibitors within 14 days of fentanyl is **not** recommended. Cytochrome P450 inhibitors (eg, clarithromycin, diltiazem, erythromycin, fluconazole, itraconazole, ketoconazole, nefazodone, protease inhibitors, troleandomycin, verapamil) may significantly increase or prolong the clinical or adverse effects of fentanyl; cytochrome P450 inducers (eg, carbamazepine, phenytoin, rifampin) may decrease the effect of fentanyl; close monitoring and dosage adjustment may be needed. The herbal medicine St John's wort (*Hypericum perforatum*) may increase the clearance and decrease the effects of fentanyl, its use is **not** recommended

Food Interactions Grapefruit juice may increase fentanyl serum concentrations and adverse effects.

Stability

Injection formulation: Store at controlled room temperature of 15°C to 25°C (59°F to 86°F). Protect from light.

Transdermal patch: Do not store above 25°C (77°F). Store in protective pouch until ready to use.

Transmucosal lozenge and buccal tablets: Store at controlled room temperature of 20°C to 25°C (68°F to 77°F); excursions permitted to 15°C to 30°C (56°F to 86°F); protect from freezing and moisture. Store in original child-resistant blister packaging until ready to use.

Iontophoretic transdermal system: Store at 25°C (77°F); excursions permitted to 15°C to 30°C (59°F to 86°F). Do not store unpouched.

Mechanism of Action Binds with stereospecific opioid mu receptors at many sites within the CNS, increases pain threshold, alters pain reception, inhibits ascending pain pathways

Pharmacodynamics Respiratory depressant effect may last longer than analgesic effect

Onset of action: Analgesia:
- I.M.: 7-15 minutes
- I.V.: Almost immediate
- Transdermal patch: 6-8 hours
- Transmucosal lozenge: 5-15 minutes

Maximum effect:
- Transdermal patch: 24 hours
- Transmucosal lozenge: 20-30 minutes

Duration:
- I.M.: 1-2 hours
- I.V.: 30-60 minutes
- Transdermal patch: 72 hours
- Transmucosal lozenge: 1-2 hours

Pharmacokinetics Note: Fentanyl serum concentrations were ~2 fold higher in nonopioid tolerant children 1.5-5 years old receiving the transdermal patch; pharmacokinetic parameters in older pediatric patients are similar to adults.

Absorption:
- Transmucosal lozenge: Rapid; ~25% absorbed from buccal mucosa; 75% swallowed with saliva and slowly absorbed from GI tract
- Buccal tablet: Rapid; ~50% from the buccal mucosa; 50% swallowed with saliva and slowly absorbed from GI tract
- Iontophoretic transdermal system (Ionsys™): Fentanyl levels continue to rise for 5 minutes after the completion of each 10-minute dose

Distribution: Highly lipophilic, redistributes into muscle and fat; crosses placenta; excreted in breast milk; **Note:** I.V. fentanyl exhibits a 3-compartment distribution model. Changes in blood pH may alter ionization of fentanyl and affect its distribution between plasma and CNS

(Continued)

Fentanyl *(Continued)*

V_{dss}: Children: 0.05-14 years of age (after long-term continuous infusion): ~15 L/kg (range: 5-30 L/kg)

V_{dss}: Adults: 4 L/kg

Protein binding: 80% to 85%, primarily to alpha-1-acid glycoprotein; also binds to albumin and erythrocytes; **Note:** Free fraction increases with acidosis

Metabolism: >90% metabolized in the liver via cytochrome P450 isoenzyme CYP3A4 by N-dealkylation (to norfentanyl) and hydroxylation to other inactive metabolites

Bioavailability: **Note:** Comparative studies have found the buccal tablet to have a 30% to 50% greater exposure (eg, AUC) than the transmucosal lozenge

Transmucosal lozenge: ~50% (range: 36% to 71%)

Buccal tablet: 65% ± 20%

Half-life:

Children 5 months to 4.5 years: Mean: 2.4 hours

Children 0.5-14 years (after long-term continuous infusion): ~21 hours (range: 11-36 hours)

Adults: I.V.: 2-4 hours; **Note:** Using a 3-compartment model, fentanyl displayed an initial distribution half-life of 6 minutes; second distribution half-life of 1 hour and terminal half-life of 16 hours

Transdermal patch: 17 hours (range: 13-22); apparent half-life increased with transdermal patch due to continued absorption

Transmucosal lozenge: 6.6 hours (range: 5-15 hours)

Buccal tablet: 100-200 mcg: 3-4 hours; 400-800 mcg: 11-12 hours

Iontophoretic transdermal system: 11 hours

Time to peak serum concentration:

Transdermal patch: 24-72 hours

Transmucosal lozenge: Median: 20-40 minutes (range: 20-480 minutes), measured after the start of dose administration

Buccal tablet: Median: 47 minutes (range: 20-240 minutes)

Elimination: In urine primarily as metabolites and <7% to 10% as unchanged drug

Clearance: Newborn infants: Clearance may be significantly correlated to gestational age and birth weight (see Saarenmaa, 2000)

Usual Dosage Doses should be titrated to appropriate effects; wide range of doses exist, dependent upon desired degree of analgesia/anesthesia, clinical environment, and patient's status

Neonates: Analgesia: International Evidence-Based Group for Neonatal Pain recommendations (Anand, 2001):

Intermittent doses: Slow I.V. push: 0.5-3 mcg/kg/dose

Continuous infusion: 0.5-2 mcg/kg/hour

Neonates and younger Infants:

Sedation/analgesia: Slow I.V. push: 1-4 mcg/kg/dose; may repeat every 2-4 hours

Continuous sedation/analgesia: Initial I.V. bolus: 1-2 mcg/kg, then 0.5-1 mcg/kg/hour; titrate upward

Mean required dose: Neonates with gestational age <34 weeks: 0.64 mcg/kg/hour; neonates with gestational age ≥34 weeks: 0.75 mcg/kg/hour

Continuous sedation/analgesia during ECMO: Initial I.V. bolus: 5-10 mcg/kg slow I.V. push over 10 minutes, then 1-5 mcg/kg/hour; titrate upward; tolerance may develop; higher doses (up to 20 mcg/kg/hour) may be needed by day 6 of ECMO

Older Infants and Children 1-12 years:

Sedation for minor procedures/analgesia: I.M., I.V.: 1-2 mcg/kg/dose; may repeat at 30- to 60-minute intervals. **Note:** Children 18-36 months of age may require 2-3 mcg/kg/dose.

Continuous sedation/analgesia: Initial I.V. bolus: 1-2 mcg/kg then 1 mcg/kg/hour; titrate upward; usual: 1-3 mcg/kg/hour; some require 5 mcg/kg/hour

Moderate to severe chronic pain: Transdermal patch: Children ≥2 years who are opioid tolerant and receiving at least 60 mg oral morphine equivalents per day: Initial: 25 mcg/hour system or higher, based on conversion to fentanyl equivalents and administration of equianalgesic dosage (see package insert for further information); use short-acting analgesics for first 24 hours with supplemental PRN doses thereafter (for breakthrough pain); dose may be increased after 3 days, based on the daily dose of supplementary PRN opioids required; use the ratio of 45 mg of oral morphine equivalents per day to a 12.5 mcg/hour increase in transdermal patch dosage; change patch every 72 hours; **Note:** Dosing intervals less than every 72 hours are **not** recommended for children and adolescents. Initiation of the transdermal patch in children taking <60 mg of oral morphine equivalents per day has not been studied in controlled clinical trials; in open-label trials, children 2-18 years of age who were receiving at least 45 mg of oral morphine equivalents per day were started with an initial transdermal dose of 25 mcg/hour (or higher, depending upon equianalgesic dose of opioid received).

Children >12 years and Adults:

Sedation for minor procedures/analgesia: I.V.: 0.5-1 mcg/kg/dose; may repeat after 30-60 minutes; **or** 25-50 mcg, repeat full dose in 5 minutes if needed, may repeat 4-5 times with 25 mcg at 5-minute intervals if needed. **Note:** Higher doses are used for major procedures.

Preoperative sedation, adjunct to regional anesthesia, postoperative pain: I.M., I.V.: 50-100 mcg/dose

Adjunct to general anesthesia: I.M., I.V.: 2-50 mcg/kg

General anesthesia without additional anesthetic agents: I.V. 50-100 mcg/kg with O_2 and skeletal muscle relaxant

Moderate to severe chronic pain: Transdermal patch: Patients who are opioid tolerant and receiving at least 60 mg oral morphine equivalents per day: Initial: 25 mcg/hour system or higher, based on conversion to fentanyl equivalents and administration of equianalgesic dosage (see package insert for further information); use short-acting analgesics for first 24 hours with supplemental PRN doses thereafter (for breakthrough pain); dose may be increased after 3 days based on the daily dose of supplementary PRN opioids required; use the ratio of 45 mg of oral morphine equivalents per day to a 12.5 mcg/hour increase in transdermal patch dosage; transdermal patch is usually administered every 72 hours but select **adult** patients may require every 48-hour administration; dosage increase administered every 72 hours should be tried before 48-hour schedule is used

Adolescents ≥16 years and Adults: Breakthrough cancer pain: Transmucosal lozenge (Actiq®): Titrate dose to provide adequate analgesia: Initial: 200 mcg; may repeat dose 15 minutes after completion of first dose if needed; no more than 2 units are recommended for each breakthrough cancer pain episode; titrate dose up to next higher strength if treatment of several consecutive breakthrough episodes requires >1 Actiq® per episode; evaluate each new dose over several breakthrough cancer pain episodes (generally 1-2 days) to determine proper dose of analgesia with acceptable side effects. Once dose has been determined, consumption should be limited to ≤4 units per day. Re-evaluate long-acting opioid dose if patient requires >4 units/day. If signs of excessive opioid effects occur before a dose is complete, the unit should be removed from the mouth immediately, and subsequent doses decreased.

Adolescents ≥18 years and Adults:

Breakthrough cancer pain: Buccal tablets (Fentora™): Initial dose: 100 mcg; if needed, a second 100 mcg dose may be administered 30 minutes after the start of the first dose

If needed, dose titration should be done using multiples of the 100 mcg tablets. May increase dose, if needed, to two 100 mcg tablets (one on each side of mouth). If that dose is not successful, increase dose to four 100 mcg tablets (two on each side of mouth). If titration requires >400 mcg/dose, then use 200 mcg tablets.

Conversion from transmucosal lozenge to buccal tablet (Fentora™):

If lozenge dose 200-400 mcg, then use buccal tablet 100 mcg

If lozenge dose 600-800 mcg, then use buccal tablet 200 mcg

If lozenge dose 1200 mcg, then use buccal tablet 400 mcg

Note: Four 100 mcg buccal tablets deliver approximately 12% and 13% higher values of C_{max} and AUC, respectively, compared to one 400 mcg buccal tablet. To prevent confusion, patient should only have one strength of tablets available at a time. Using more than four buccal tablets at a time has not been studied. Re-evaluate maintenance (around-the-clock) opioid dose if patient requires >4 doses of buccal tablets/day

Acute, short-term, postoperative pain: Iontophoretic transdermal system (Ionsys™): 40 mcg per activation on-demand; maximum dosing frequency: 6 doses/hour; maximum length of therapy 72 hours

Note: Patient's pain should be controlled prior to initiating system; patient should also have access to supplemental analgesia during treatment with this system. Instruct patient how to operate; only the patient should activate the dosing button. Each system operates for 24 hours or until 80 doses have been administered, whichever comes first. Patients on chronic opioids or with a history of opioid abuse may require higher analgesic doses than Ionsys™ is able to provide.

Dosing adjustment in renal impairment:

Cl_{cr} 10-50 mL/minute: Administer 75% of dose

Cl_{cr} <10 mL/minute: Administer 50% of dose

Dosing adjustment in hepatic impairment: Use with caution; specific guidelines are not available; lower dose is recommended

Administration

Parenteral: I.V.: Administer by slow I.V. push over 3-5 minutes or by continuous infusion; larger bolus doses (>5 mcg/kg) should be given slow I.V. push over 5-10 minutes (see Warnings)

(Continued)

Fentanyl *(Continued)*

Transdermal patch: Apply to nonhairy, clean, dry, nonirritated, intact skin of the flat area of front or back of upper torso, flank area, or upper arm; apply to upper back in young children or in people with cognitive impairment to decrease the potential of the patient removing the patch; monitor the adhesion of the system closely in children; clip hair prior to application, do **not** shave area; prior to application, skin may be cleaned with clear water (do not use soaps, lotions, alcohol, oils, or other substances which may irritate the skin); allow skin to dry thoroughly prior to application; apply patch immediately after removing from package; firmly press in place and hold for at least 30 seconds; change patch every 72 hours; remove old patch before applying new patch; do not apply new patch to same place as old patch; wash hands after applying patch; **Note**: Transdermal patch is a membrane-controlled system; do **not** cut the patch to deliver partial doses; do **not** use patches that are cut or damaged; do **not** use if seal of package is broken; rate of drug delivery may be significantly increased if patch is cut or damaged and result in absorption of a potentially fatal dose; reservoir contents and adhesion may be affected if cut; if partial dose is needed, surface area of patch can be blocked proportionally using adhesive bandage (see Lee, 1997). Do **not** use soap, alcohol, or other solvents to remove transdermal gel if it accidentally touches skin as they may increase transdermal absorption, use copious amounts of water. Avoid exposing application site to external heat sources (eg, electric blanket, heating pad, heat lamp, sauna, heated water bed, hot tub). Dispose of properly (see Patient Information).

Transmucosal lozenge (Actiq®): Oral: Do not use if blister package has been opened. Blister package should be opened with scissors just prior to administration; once removed, patient should place the lozenge in mouth and suck it; do not bite or chew lozenge. Place lozenge in mouth between cheek and lower gum; occasionally move lozenge from one side of the mouth to the other; consume lozenge over 15 minutes; remove lozenge from mouth if signs of excessive opioid effects appear before lozenge is totally consumed. Remove handle after lozenge is consumed or patient achieves adequate response.

Buccal tablet: Do not use if blister package has been opened or tampered with. Blister package should be opened just prior to administration. Peel back the blister backing to expose the tablet; do not push tablet through the blister (damage to the tablet may occur). Administer tablet immediately after removal from blister. Place entire tablet in the buccal cavity (above a rear molar, between the upper cheek and gum). Do not break, suck, chew, or swallow tablet (this will result in decreased effect). Tablet should dissolve in about 14-25 minutes when left between the cheek and the gum. If remnants remain after 30 minutes, they may be swallowed with a glass of water. If excessive opioid effects appear before tablet is completely dissolved (eg, dizziness, sedation, nausea), instruct patient to rinse mouth with water and spit remaining pieces of tablet into sink or toilet immediately; rinse the sink or flush toilet to dispose of tablet particles.

Iontophoretic transdermal system (Ionsys™): For transdermal use only. System should be tested prior to dispensing (see Additional Information) and must be applied by healthcare professional. The sticker on the back of the pouch is intended for use by the registered nurse; remove sticker and apply to the Ionsys™ system with date and time of application; system expires 24 hours after application. Apply to intact, nonirritated, nonirradiated skin on chest or upper outer arm. Do not apply to scarred, burned, or tattooed areas. Any excessive hair at application site should be clipped; do not shave. Wipe application site with alcohol swab; allow skin to dry completely before applying system; do not use soap, lotion, oil, or other substances that may irritate skin or change absorption characteristics. Apply to skin immediately after removing from sealed pouch; do not use if foil pouch has been broken. Open pouch by cutting on dotted line, remove and discard plastic liner covering adhesive. Do not pull on red tab while removing. Press system firmly in place with sticky side down, on skin for at least 15 seconds. Make sure all sides of outer edge stick to skin. May tape sides down if they loosen; don't tape over button or red light. To administer a dose, the patient must press the button twice firmly within 3 seconds. An audible tone (beep) indicates the start of the delivery of the dose; red light remains on throughout the 10-minute dosing period. Each system operates for 24 hours or until 80 doses have been used (whichever comes first). Rotate skin site if another system is required after the first one is finished. Do not touch sticky side of system or the gels. If the hydrogel (where fentanyl is housed) becomes separated from the delivery system during removal, use gloves or tweezers to remove the hydrogel from skin; contact with hydrogel can be harmful. Flush skin that came into contact with hydrogel thoroughly with water. Do not use soap, alcohol, or other solvents to remove the hydrogel as they can increase absorption of fentanyl. Once a system has been removed, the same system can not be reapplied. Contains metal; remove prior to MRI procedure, cardioversion, or defibrillation. Avoid exposure of system to water (may cause system to stop working or fall off).

Monitoring Parameters Respiratory rate, blood pressure, heart rate, oxygen saturation, bowel sounds, abdominal distention; signs of misuse, abuse, or addiction

Transdermal patch: Monitor patient for at least 24 hours after application of first dose

Iontophoretic transdermal system: Directly observe patient after first dose is administered to make sure system works properly and that patient understands how to use it

Patient Information All products: Report the use of other medications, nonprescription medications, and herbal or natural products to your physician and pharmacist; avoid alcohol, other CNS depressants (eg, sleep medications, tranquilizers), grapefruit juice, and the herbal medicine St John's wort. Fentanyl may cause drowsiness and impair ability to perform activities requiring mental alertness or physical coordination; may be habit-forming; avoid abrupt discontinuation after prolonged use; may cause dry mouth and constipation. Notify physician immediately or seek emergency help if acute dizziness, chest pain, slow or rapid heartbeat, shortness of breath, respiratory difficulty, confusion, or unusual symptoms occur. Notify physician if acute headache, changes in mentation, changes in voiding frequency or amount, swelling of extremities, unusual weight gain, or vision changes occur.

Transdermal patch: Keep all transdermal patches (even if used) out of the reach of children; even used patches may be dangerous or even lethal to babies, children, pets, and other adults; discard used transdermal patches immediately after removal by folding in half (so the sticky side sticks to itself) and flushing down the toilet; discard unused patches that are no longer needed in the same manner; protective pouch and liner should be thrown in garbage. Notify physician if you develop a high fever while wearing the patch. Wash skin with clear water (not soap, alcohol, or other chemicals) if gel from patch accidentally comes into contact with skin. If patch accidentally sticks to the skin of another person, take patch off immediately, wash exposed skin with water, and seek medical attention for that person. Accidental exposure or misuse may lead to serious medical problems, even death.

Transmucosal lozenge: Do not allow other people to use this product (serious adverse effects and potentially fatal overdose may occur). An Actiq® Welcome Kit and OTFC (Oral Transmucosal Fentanyl Citrate) Welcome Kit, containing a child-resistant lock, portable locking pouch, and a child-resistant temporary storage bottle (to keep medication away from children), are available from the manufacturer; these kits can be obtained by calling 1-800-896-5855. Read the patient Medication Guide that you receive with each prescription and refill of this medication. Read this guide for details on proper storage, administration, and disposal of oral transmucosal lozenges, as well as instructions about overdose management. This product contains an amount of medication that can be fatal to children; dispose of transmucosal products properly; keep all products (even if used) out of the reach of children and pets. After consumption of a complete unit, the handle may be disposed of in a trash container that is out of the reach of children and pets. For a partially-consumed unit, or a unit that still has any drug matrix remaining on the handle, the handle should be placed under hot running tap water until the drug matrix has dissolved. Use the special child-resistant container available in the Welcome Kit to temporarily store partially consumed units that cannot be disposed of immediately. Frequent use of oral transmucosal fentanyl lozenges may increase risk of dental caries; consult dentist for appropriate oral hygiene. Diabetic patients should note that oral transmucosal lozenge contains 2 grams of sugar/unit (about ½ teaspoon of sugar).

Buccal tablets: This product contains an amount of medication that can be fatal to children; keep tablets out of the reach of children. Read the patient Medication Guide that you receive with each prescription and refill of fentanyl buccal tablets. Read this guide for details on proper storage, administration, and disposal of buccal tablets, as well as instructions about overdose management. Do not allow other people to use this product (serious adverse effects and potentially fatal overdose may occur). Discard unused tablets appropriately; remove unusable tablets from blister package and flush tablets down the toilet; to dispose of excess unusable tablets call manufacturer at 1-800-896-5855.

Transdermal iontophoretic system (Ionsys™): Read the Patient Bedside Information sheet that you will receive; life-threatening breathing problems or death can occur if this medication is used in the wrong way. Do not remove or replace this system yourself. Do not allow other people to activate dosing button; do not touch sticky side of system, hydrogel compartments, or gel; do not use other than directed; do not allow other people to use this system (serious adverse effects and potentially fatal overdose may occur). If accidental exposure occurs, notify your healthcare provider right away; immediately rinse skin with large amounts of water; do not use soap, alcohol, or other chemicals. Do not leave the hospital with this system on your skin;

(Continued)

Fentanyl *(Continued)*

make sure your nurse or doctor removes this product before you leave from the hospital.

Nursing Implications An opioid antagonist, resuscitative and intubation equipment, and oxygen should be available; rapid I.V. injection may result in apnea. Patients with elevated temperature may have increased fentanyl absorption transdermally from patch; observe for adverse effects, dosage adjustment may be needed. Pharmacologic and adverse effects can be seen after discontinuation of transdermal patch and iontophoretic transdermal system; observe patients for at least 24 hours after transdermal product is removed. Do **not** cut transdermal patch or use if cut or damaged. Dispose of transdermal products properly (see Patient Information and Additional Information). Destroy unused portion of Actiq® according to hospital policy on controlled substances; partial unused doses of Actiq® can be dissolved under hot running tap water; dispose of handle properly. Keep all fentanyl products out of the reach of children; products contain an amount of medication that can be fatal to children. Assess other medications patient may be taking for additive or adverse interactions. Order safety precautions for inpatient use. Assess knowledge and teach patient appropriate use (if self-administered), adverse reactions to report, and appropriate interventions to reduce side effects.

Additional Information Fentanyl is 50-100 times as potent as morphine; morphine 10 mg I.M. = fentanyl 0.1-0.2 mg I.M. Fentanyl has less hypotensive effects than morphine or meperidine due to minimal or no histamine release. I.V. product has a pH of 4.0-7.5.

Buccal tablets (Fentora™): Product uses an effervescent reaction which may enhance the rate and extent of absorption of fentanyl through the buccal mucosa.

Iontophoretic transdermal system (Ionsys™): Each activation of the dose button delivers fentanyl 40 mcg/dose over a 10-minute period; the next dose cannot begin until the previous 10-minute delivery cycle is finished. A 3-volt lithium battery provides power for the system; the level of current is 62 microA/cm^2, which is generally imperceptible to the patient. The pharmacist should test each system before dispensing for patient. Without opening pouch, pharmacist should locate button side, find button, and firmly press and release button twice within 3 seconds. Listen for a single audible tone (beep) confirming that the system is functional. The pharmacist should sign the front of the pouch after performing the functionality test. **Note:** No drug is delivered from the system unless it is applied to the skin. Four minutes after the functionality test, the system will beep for 15 seconds indicating that it is not in contact with skin. If the system is applied to the skin within 4 minutes after the functionality test, the system will deliver the remainder of the 10-minute dose. To determine the number of doses delivered, the red light will flash between doses in one second pulses to indicate the approximate number of doses that have been administered up to the present time. Each flash indicates up to 5 doses have been administered: One flash 1-5 doses; two flashes 6-10 doses; three flashes 11-15 doses; four flashes 16-20 doses, continuing up to 16 flashes (76-80 doses). To dispose of system, wear gloves and pull the red tab to separate the bottom from the top. Fold the bottom in half with the sticky side facing in and flush down the toilet (needs to be witnessed by second healthcare provider). Dispose of top section according to hospital procedures for batteries (see also Administration).

The generic oral transmucosal lozenge is formulated as a solid drug matrix and is mounted on a plastic fracture-resistant handle; it contains sugar 2 g/unit.

Dosage Forms Excipient information presented when available (limited, particularly for generics); consult specific product labeling.

Note: Strengths expressed as base.

Infusion, as citrate [premixed in NS]: 0.05 mg (10 mL); 1 mg (100 mL); 1.25 mg (250 mL); 2 mg (100 mL); 2.5 mg (250 mL)

Injection, solution, as citrate [preservative free]: 0.05 mg/mL (2 mL, 5 mL, 10 mL, 20 mL, 30 mL, 50 mL)

Sublimaze®: 0.05 mg/mL (2 mL, 5 mL, 10 mL, 20 mL)

Lozenge, oral, as citrate [transmucosal]: 200 mcg, 400 mcg, 600 mcg, 800 mcg, 1200 mcg, 1600 mcg

Actiq®: 200 mcg, 400 mcg, 600 mcg, 800 mcg, 1200 mcg, 1600 mcg [mounted on a plastic radiopaque handle; contains sugar 2 g/unit; raspberry flavor]

Tablet, for buccal application, as citrate:

Fentora™: 100 mcg, 200 mcg, 300 mcg, 400 mcg, 600 mcg, 800 mcg

Transdermal system, topical, as base: 25 mcg/hour [6.25 cm^2] (5s); 50 mcg/hour [12.5 cm^2] (5s); 75 mcg/hour [18.75 cm^2]; 100 mcg/hour [25 cm^2] (5s)

Duragesic®: 12 [delivers 12.5 mcg/hour; 5 cm^2; contains alcohol 0.1 mL/10 cm^2] (5s); 25 [delivers 25 mcg/hour; 10 cm^2; contains alcohol 0.1 mL/10 cm^2] (5s); 50 [delivers 50 mcg/hour; 20 cm^2; contains alcohol 0.1 mL/10 cm^2] (5s); 75 [delivers

75 mcg/hour; 30 cm²; contains alcohol 0.1 mL/10 cm²]; 100 [delivers 100 mcg/hour; 40 cm²; contains alcohol 0.1 mL/10 cm²] (5s)

Transdermal iontophoretic system, topical, as hydrochloride:

Ionsys™: Fentanyl 40 mcg/dose [80 doses/patch; contains 3-volt lithium battery]

References

Anand KJ and International Evidence-Based Group for Neonatal Pain, "Consensus Statement for the Prevention and Management of Pain in the Newborn," *Arch Pediatr Adolesc Med*, 2001, 155(2):173-80.

Billmire DA, Neale HW, and Gregory RO, "Use of I.V. Fentanyl in the Outpatient Treatment of Pediatric Facial Trauma," *J Trauma*, 1985, 25(11):1079-80.

Katz R, Kelly HW, and Hsi A, "Prospective Study on the Occurrence of Withdrawal in Critically Ill Children Who Receive Fentanyl by Continuous Infusion," *Crit Care Med*, 1994, 22(5):763-7.

Lee NA and Anderson PO, "Giving Partial Doses of Transdermal Patches," *Am J Health Syst Pharm*, 1997, 54(15):1759-60.

Leuschen MP, Willett LD, Hoie EB, et al, "Plasma Fentanyl Levels in Infants Undergoing Extracorporeal Membrane Oxygenation," *J Thorac Cardiovasc Surg*, 1993, 105(5):885-91.

Roth B, Schlunder C, Houben F, et al, "Analgesia and Sedation in Neonatal Intensive Care Using Fentanyl by Continuous Infusion," *Dev Pharmacol Ther*, 1991, 17(3-4):121-7.

Saarenmaa E, Neuvonen PJ, and Fellman V, "Gestational Age and Birth Weight Effects on Plasma Clearance of Fentanyl in Newborn Infants," *J Pediatr*, 2000, 136(6):767-70.

Schechter NL, Weisman SJ, Rosenblum M, et al, "The Use of Oral Transmucosal Fentanyl Citrate for Painful Procedures in Children," *Pediatrics*, 1995, 95(3):335-9.

Zeltzer LK, Altman A, Cohen D, et al, "Report of the Subcommittee on the Management of Pain Associated With Procedures in Children With Cancer," *Pediatrics*, 1990, 86(5 Pt 2):826-31.

- **Fentanyl Citrate** *see* Fentanyl *on page 644*
- **Fentanyl Citrate Injection, USP (Can)** *see* Fentanyl *on page 644*
- **Fentanyl Hydrochloride** *see* Fentanyl *on page 644*
- **Fentora™** *see* Fentanyl *on page 644*
- **Feosol® [OTC]** *see* Iron Supplements (Oral/Enteral) *on page 868*
- **Feostat® [OTC] [DSC]** *see* Iron Supplements (Oral/Enteral) *on page 868*
- **Feratab® [OTC]** *see* Iron Supplements (Oral/Enteral) *on page 868*
- **Fer-Gen-Sol [OTC]** *see* Iron Supplements (Oral/Enteral) *on page 868*
- **Fergon® [OTC]** *see* Iron Supplements (Oral/Enteral) *on page 868*
- **Fer-In-Sol® [OTC]** *see* Iron Supplements (Oral/Enteral) *on page 868*
- **Fer-Iron® [OTC]** *see* Iron Supplements (Oral/Enteral) *on page 868*
- **Fermalac (Can)** *see* ***Lactobacillus acidophilus*** and ***Lactobacillus bulgaricus*** *on page 898*
- **Ferretts [OTC]** *see* Iron Supplements (Oral/Enteral) *on page 868*
- **Ferrex 150 [OTC]** *see* Iron Supplements (Oral/Enteral) *on page 868*
- **Ferrlecit®** *see* Iron Supplements (Parenteral) *on page 870*
- **Ferro-Sequels® [OTC]** *see* Iron Supplements (Oral/Enteral) *on page 868*
- **Ferrous Fumarate** *see* Iron Supplements (Oral/Enteral) *on page 868*
- **Ferrous Gluconate** *see* Iron Supplements (Oral/Enteral) *on page 868*
- **Ferrous Sulfate** *see* Iron Supplements (Oral/Enteral) *on page 868*
- **$FeSO_4$ (Ferrous Sulfate)** *see* Iron Supplements (Oral/Enteral) *on page 868*
- **Fe-Tinic™ 150 [OTC] [DSC]** *see* Iron Supplements (Oral/Enteral) *on page 868*
- **FeverALL® [OTC]** *see* Acetaminophen *on page 42*
- **Fexmid™** *see* Cyclobenzaprine *on page 416*

Fexofenadine (feks oh FEN a deen)

Medication Safety Issues

Sound-alike/look-alike issues:

Allegra® may be confused with Viagra®

International issues:

Allegra® may be confused with Allegro® which is a brand name for frovatriptan in Germany; a brand name for fluticasone in Israel

U.S. Brand Names Allegra®

Canadian Brand Names Allegra®

Index Terms Fexofenadine Hydrochloride

Therapeutic Category Antihistamine

Generic Available Yes: Excludes suspension

Use Symptomatic relief of seasonal allergic rhinitis and chronic idiopathic urticaria

Pregnancy Risk Factor C

Lactation Excretion in breast milk unknown/use caution (AAP rates "compatible")

Contraindications Hypersensitivity to fexofenadine, terfenadine, or any component

Warnings Adjust dosage in patients with decreased renal function

Precautions Use cautiously in patients who are also taking ketoconazole and erythromycin (see Drug Interactions); although increased plasma levels of fexofenadine have been observed, no adverse effects with concomitant administration have been reported including QT prolongation which occurred when terfenadine was combined

(Continued)

Fexofenadine *(Continued)*

with these agents; while less sedating than other antihistamines, fexofenadine may cause drowsiness and impair ability to perform hazardous activities requiring mental alertness

Adverse Reactions

Central nervous system: Headache, fever, drowsiness, fatigue, dizziness
Endocrine & metabolic: Dysmenorrhea
Gastrointestinal: Nausea, dyspepsia
Neuromuscular & skeletal: Back pain
Otic: Otitis media
Respiratory: Upper respiratory tract infection, cough, sinusitis
Miscellaneous: Hypersensitivity reactions, viral infections

Drug Interactions Cytochrome P450 isoenzyme CYP2D6 inhibitor (weak) and CYP3A3/4 substrate

Ketoconazole and erythromycin increase fexofenadine plasma levels; aluminum- and magnesium-containing antacids decrease fexofenadine absorption; the herbal medicine St John's wort (*Hypericum perforatum*) may decrease absorption; avoid alcohol (may increase sedative effects)

Food Interactions Fruit juices may reduce the bioavailability of fexofenadine by 36%

Stability Store at controlled room temperature; protect from excessive moisture

Mechanism of Action Fexofenadine is an active metabolite of terfenadine; it competes with histamine for H_1 receptor sites on effector cells in the GI tract, blood vessels, and respiratory tract; it appears that fexofenadine does not cross the blood brain barrier to any appreciable degree, resulting in a reduced potential for sedation

Pharmacodynamics

Onset of action: 1 hour
Maximum effect: 2-3 hours
Duration: ≥12 hours

Pharmacokinetics

Absorption: Rapid
Distribution: V_d: Children: 5.4-5.8 L/kg
Protein binding: 60% to 70%
Metabolism: 5% in liver; 3.5% transformed into methylester metabolite found only in feces (possibly transformed by gut microflora)
Half-life: 14-18 hours
Time to peak serum concentration: Tablets: 2.6 hours; Suspension: 1 hour
Elimination: 11% excreted unchanged in urine; 80% excreted unchanged in feces
Clearance: Children: 14-18 mL/minute/kg
Dialysis: Not effectively removed by hemodialysis

Usual Dosage Oral:

Children 6 months to <2 years: 15 mg twice daily
Children 2-11 years: 30 mg twice daily
Children ≥12 years and Adults: 60 mg twice daily or 180 mg once daily

Dosing adjustment in renal impairment:

Children 6 months to <2 years: 15 mg once daily
Children 2-11 years: 30 mg once daily
Children ≥12 years and Adults: 60 mg once daily

Administration May administer without respect to food; avoid administration with fruit juices; shake suspension well before use

Monitoring Parameters Improvement in signs and symptoms of allergic rhinitis and chronic idiopathic urticaria

Test Interactions Antigen skin testing

Patient Information May cause drowsiness and impair ability to perform activities requiring mental alertness or physical coordination; avoid alcohol

Dosage Forms Excipient information presented when available (limited, particularly for generics); consult specific product labeling.

Suspension:
Allegra®: 6 mg/mL (30 mL, 300 mL) [raspberry cream]
Tablet, as hydrochloride: 30 mg, 60 mg, 180 mg
Allegra®: 30 mg, 60 mg, 180 mg

♦ **Fexofenadine Hydrochloride** *see* Fexofenadine *on page 653*
♦ **Fiberall®** *see* Psyllium *on page 1347*
♦ **Fibro-XL [OTC]** *see* Psyllium *on page 1347*
♦ **Fibro-Lax [OTC]** *see* Psyllium *on page 1347*

Filgrastim (fil GRA stim)

Medication Safety Issues

Sound-alike/look-alike issues:

Neupogen® may be confused with Epogen®, Neumega®, Neupro®, Nutramigen®

Related Information

Compatibility of Chemotherapy and Related Supportive Care Medications *on page 1777*

U.S. Brand Names Neupogen®

Canadian Brand Names Neupogen®

Index Terms G-CSF; Granulocyte Colony Stimulating Factor; NSC-614629

Therapeutic Category Colony-Stimulating Factor

Generic Available No

Use Reduction of the duration of neutropenia and the associated risk of infection in patients with malignancies receiving myelosuppressive chemotherapeutic regimens associated with a significant incidence of severe neutropenia with fever; cancer patients receiving bone marrow transplant; severe chronic neutropenia which includes patients with congenital neutropenia, cyclic neutropenia, or idiopathic neutropenia; mobilization of peripheral blood progenitor cells into the peripheral blood for collection by leukapheresis; AIDS patients receiving zidovudine; neonatal neutropenia

Pregnancy Risk Factor C

Lactation Excretion in breast milk unknown/use caution

Contraindications Hypersensitivity to *E. coli*-derived proteins, G-CSF, or any component; use in patients receiving concomitant chemotherapy and radiation therapy

Warnings Leukocytosis (white blood cell counts ≥100,000/mm^3) has been observed in approximately 2% of patients receiving G-CSF at doses >5 mcg/kg/day

Precautions Do not administer 24 hours prior to or within 24 hours following the administration of chemotherapy; use with caution in any malignancy with myeloid characteristics due to G-CSF's potential to act as a growth factor; use with caution in patients with gout, psoriasis; monitor patients with pre-existing cardiac conditions as cardiac events (MIs, arrhythmias) have been reported in premarketing clinical studies. Be alert to the possibility of ARDS in septic patients.

Premature discontinuation of G-CSF therapy prior to the time of recovery from the expected neutrophil nadir is generally not recommended. A transient increase in neutrophil counts is typically seen 1-2 days after initiation of therapy. For a sustained therapeutic response, G-CSF should be continued until the post nadir absolute neutrophil count (ANC) reaches:

10,000/mm^3 in chemotherapy treated patients, or

>1000/mm^3 for 3 consecutive days in bone marrow transplant patients

Most patients experience a 30% to 50% decrease in circulating leukocytes within 1-2 days following discontinuation of G-CSF

Adverse Reactions

Cardiovascular: Transient decrease in blood pressure, vasculitis, chest pain

Central nervous system: Fever, headache

Dermatologic: Exacerbation of pre-existing skin disorders, alopecia, rash, pruritus

Endocrine & metabolic: Reversible elevation in uric acid

Gastrointestinal: Splenomegaly, nausea, vomiting, diarrhea, mucositis

Hematologic: Thrombocytopenia, leukocytosis

Hepatic: Elevated alkaline phosphatase, lactate dehydrogenase

Neuromuscular & skeletal: Medullary bone pain (24% incidence) is generally dose-related, localized to the lower back, posterior iliac crests, and sternum; osteoporosis

Renal: Hematuria, proteinuria

Miscellaneous: Anaphylactoid reaction (rare)

Stability Store in refrigerator; do not freeze; protect from direct sunlight; stable for 24 hours at room temperature; solutions with concentration ≥15 mcg/mL in D_5W are stable for 24 hours; incompatible with salt solutions

Mechanism of Action Stimulates the production, maturation, and activation of neutrophils; G-CSF activates neutrophils to increase both their migration and cytotoxicity

Pharmacodynamics

Onset of action: Immediate transient leukopenia with the nadir occurring 5-15 minutes after an I.V. dose or 30-60 minutes after a SubQ dose followed by a sustained elevation in neutrophil levels within the first 24 hours reaching a plateau in 3-5 days

Duration: Upon discontinuation of G-CSF, ANC decreases by 50% within 2 days and returns to pretreatment levels within 1 week; WBC counts return to normal range in 4-7 days

(Continued)

Filgrastim *(Continued)*

Pharmacokinetics

Distribution: V_d: 150 mL/kg

Bioavailability: Not bioavailable after oral administration

Half-life: Neonates: 4.4 hours; Adults: 1.8-3.5 hours

Time to peak serum concentration: SubQ: Within 2-6 hours

Elimination: No evidence of drug accumulation over a 11- to 20-day period

Usual Dosage I.V., SubQ (refer to individual protocols):

Neonates: 5-10 mcg/kg/day once daily for 3-5 days has been administered to neutropenic neonates with sepsis. There was a rapid and significant increase in peripheral neutrophil counts and the neutrophil storage pool.

Children and Adults: 5-10 mcg/kg/day (~150-300 mcg/m²/day) once daily for up to 14 days until ANC = 10,000/mm³; dose escalations at 5 mcg/kg/day may be required in some individuals when response at 5 mcg/kg/day is not adequate; in phase 3 trials, efficacy was observed at dosages of 4-8 mcg/kg/day with myelosuppressive chemotherapy

Peripheral blood progenitor cell (PBPC) mobilization: SubQ: 10 mcg/kg/day given for 4 days before the first leukapheresis procedure and continued until the last leukapheresis

Patients with congenital neutropenia: SubQ: Initial: 6 mcg/kg/dose twice daily; dosages of 2-60 mcg/kg/day individualized according to neutrophil count have been administered to children and adults

Patients with idiopathic or cyclic neutropenia: SubQ: 5 mcg/kg/day once daily

Cancer patients receiving bone marrow transplant: I.V. infusion, SubQ: 5-10 mcg/kg/day administered ≥24 hours after cytotoxic chemotherapy and ≥24 hours after bone marrow infusion

Dosage adjustment during neutrophil recovery period: see table

Filgrastim Dose Based on Neutrophil Response

Absolute Neutrophil Count (ANC)	Filgrastim Dose Adjustment
When ANC >1000/mm³ for 3 consecutive days	Reduce to 5 mcg/kg/day
If ANC remains >1000/mm³ for 3 more consecutive days	Discontinue filgrastim
If ANC decreases to <1000/mm³	Resume at 5 mcg/kg/day

If ANC decreases <1000/mm³ during the 5 mcg/kg/day dose, increase dose to 10 mcg/kg/day and follow the above steps in the table.

Administration Parenteral:

SubQ: Administer undiluted solution

SubQ continuous infusion: Dilute dose in 10 mL D_5W and infuse at a rate of 10 mL/24 hours

I.V. continuous infusion; Administer over 15-60 minutes or as a continuous I.V. infusion at a final concentration of at least 15 mcg/mL in D_5W. If the final concentration of G-CSF in D_5W is <15 mcg/mL, then add 2 mg albumin/mL to I.V. fluid; the solution is stable for 24 hours; albumin acts as a carrier molecule to prevent drug adsorption to the I.V. tubing. Albumin should be added to the D_5W prior to addition of G-CSF; final concentration of G-CSF for administration <5 mcg/mL is not recommended; do not shake solution to avoid foaming.

Monitoring Parameters Temperature, CBC with differential and platelet count, hematocrit, uric acid, urinalysis, liver function tests

Reference Range Blood samples for monitoring the hematologic effects of G-CSF should be drawn just before the next dose at least twice weekly

Patient Information Possible bone pain; notify physician of unusual fever or chills, severe bone pain, or chest pain and palpitations

Nursing Implications Bone pain management is usually successful with non-narcotic analgesic therapy

Additional Information Reimbursement hotline: 1-800-272-9376. Injection solution contains sodium 0.035 mg/mL.

Dosage Forms Excipient information presented when available (limited, particularly for generics); consult specific product labeling.

Injection, solution [preservative free]:

Neupogen®: 300 mcg/mL (1 mL, 1.6 mL) [vial; contains sodium 0.035 mg/mL and sorbitol]

Injection, solution [preservative free]:

Neupogen®: 600 mcg/mL (0.5 mL, 0.8 mL) [prefilled Singleject® syringe; contains sodium 0.035 mg/mL and sorbitol; needle cover contains latex]

References

"Update of Recommendations for the Use of Hematopoietic Colony-Stimulating Factors: Evidence-based Clinical Practice Guidelines. American Society of Clinical Oncology," *J Clin Oncol*, 1996, 14(6):1957-60.

Bonilla MA, Gillio AP, Ruggeiro M, et al, "Effects of Recombinant Human Granulocyte Colony-Stimulating Factor on Neutropenia in Patients With Congenital Agranulocytosis," *N Engl J Med*, 1989, 320(24):1574-80.

Gilmore MM, Stroncek DF, and Korones DN, "Treatment of Alloimmune Neonatal Neutropenia With Granulocyte Colony-Stimulating Factor," *J Pediatr*, 1994, 125(6 Pt 1):948-51

Hollingshead LM, Goa KL, "Recombinant Granulocyte Colony-Stimulating Factor (rG-CSF). A Review of Its Pharmacological Properties and Prospective Role in Neutropenic Conditions," *Drugs*, 1991, 42(2):300-30.

Morstyn G, Campbell L, Lieschke G, et al, "Treatment of Chemotherapy-Induced Neutropenia by Subcutaneously Administered Granulocyte Colony-Stimulating Factor With Optimization of Dose and Duration of Therapy," *J Clin Oncol*, 1989, 7(10):1554-62.

Wolach B, "Neonatal Sepsis: Pathogenesis and Supportive Therapy," *Semin Perinatol*, 1997, 21(1):28-38.

♦ **Finacea®** *see* Azelaic Acid *on page 188*
♦ **First® Testosterone** *see* Testosterone *on page 1511*
♦ **First® Testosterone MC** *see* Testosterone *on page 1511*
♦ **Fisalamine** *see* Mesalamine *on page 1011*
♦ **FK506** *see* Tacrolimus *on page 1498*
♦ **Flagyl®** *see* Metronidazole *on page 1049*
♦ **Flagyl ER®** *see* Metronidazole *on page 1049*
♦ **Flamazine® (Can)** *see* Silver Sulfadiazine *on page 1439*
♦ **Flarex®** *see* Fluorometholone *on page 677*
♦ **Flebogamma®** *see* Immune Globulin (Intravenous) *on page 818*

Flecainide (fle KAY nide)

Medication Safety Issues
Sound-alike/look-alike issues:
Flecainide may be confused with fluconazole
Tambocor™ may be confused with tamoxifen

Related Information
Medications for Which A Single Dose May Be Fatal When Ingested By A Toddler *on page 1932*

U.S. Brand Names Tambocor™

Canadian Brand Names Apo-Flecainide®; Tambocor™

Index Terms Flecainide Acetate

Therapeutic Category Antiarrhythmic Agent, Class I-C

Generic Available Yes

Use Prevention and suppression of documented life-threatening ventricular arrhythmias (ie, sustained ventricular tachycardia); prevention of symptomatic, disabling supraventricular tachycardias in patients without structural heart disease

Pregnancy Risk Factor C

Lactation Enters breast milk/compatible

Contraindications Hypersensitivity to flecainide or any component; pre-existing second or third degree A-V block; right bundle-branch block associated with left hemiblock (bifascicular block) or trifascicular block; cardiogenic shock, myocardial depression

Warnings The manufacturer and FDA recommend that this drug be reserved for life-threatening ventricular arrhythmias unresponsive to conventional therapy. Its use for symptomatic nonsustained ventricular tachycardia, frequent premature ventricular complexes (PVCs), uniform and multiform PVCs and/or coupled PVCs is no longer recommended. Flecainide can worsen or cause arrhythmias with an associated risk of death. Proarrhythmic effects range from an increased number of PVCs to more severe ventricular tachycardias (ie, tachycardias that are more sustained or more resistant to conversion to sinus rhythm).

Precautions Use with caution in patients with pacemakers, sick sinus syndrome, CHF, myocardial dysfunction, and renal and/or hepatic impairment; use decreased doses and cautiously titrate dose according to serum concentrations and clinical effects in patients with CHF, or myocardial, liver or renal dysfunction. Flecainide may cause increases in PR, QRS, and QT intervals and new first degree or bundle branch block; use with caution and consider dosing reduction when increases in such intervals occur.

Adverse Reactions
Cardiovascular: Bradycardia, heart block, worsening ventricular arrhythmias, CHF, palpitations, chest pain, edema; increased P-R interval and QRS duration
Central nervous system: Dizziness, fatigue, nervousness, hypoesthesia, headache
Dermatologic: Rash
Gastrointestinal: Nausea
Hematologic: Blood dyscrasias
Hepatic: Hepatic dysfunction
Neuromuscular & skeletal: Paresthesia, tremor
Ocular: Blurred vision
(Continued)

Flecainide *(Continued)*

Respiratory: Dyspnea

Drug Interactions Cytochrome P450 isoenzyme CYP2D6 substrate

Other antiarrhythmic agents may increase adverse cardiac effects; flecainide may increase plasma digoxin concentrations; use with beta-blockers, disopyramide, or verapamil may result in possible additive negative inotropic effects; alkalinizing agents (high-dose antacids, carbonic anhydrase inhibitors or sodium bicarbonate) may decrease flecainide's clearance; urinary acidifiers may increase flecainide's clearance; amiodarone and cimetidine increase flecainide serum concentrations; concurrent use of flecainide with ritonavir or lopinavir is not recommended

Food Interactions Dairy products (milk, infant formula, yogurt) may interfere with the absorption of flecainide in infants; there is one case report of a neonate (GA 34 weeks PNA >6 days) who required extremely large doses of oral flecainide when administered every 8 hours with feedings ("milk feeds"); changing the feedings from "milk feeds" to 5% glucose feeds alone resulted in a doubling of the flecainide serum concentration and toxicity (see Russell, 1989); clearance of flecainide may be decreased in patients with strict vegetarian diets due to urinary pH ≥8

Mechanism of Action Class IC antiarrhythmic; slows conduction in cardiac tissue by altering transport of ions across cell membranes; causes slight prolongation of refractory periods; decreases the rate of rise of the action potential without affecting its duration; increases electrical stimulation threshold of ventricle, His-Purkinje system; possesses local anesthetic and moderate negative inotropic effects

Pharmacokinetics

Absorption: Oral: Rapid and nearly complete

Distribution: V_d: Adults: 5-13.4 L/kg

Protein binding: 40% to 50% (alpha$_1$ glycoprotein)

Metabolism: In the liver

Bioavailability: 85% to 90%

Half-life, elimination: Increased half-life with CHF or renal dysfunction

- Newborns: ~29 hours
- Infants: 11-12 hours
- Children: 8 hours
- Adults: ~20 hours (range: 12-27 hours)

Time to peak serum concentration: ~3 hours (range 1-6 hours)

Elimination: In urine as unchanged drug (10% to 50%) and metabolites

Dialysis: Not dialyzable

Usual Dosage Oral:

Children: Initial: 1-3 mg/kg/day or 50-100 mg/m^2/day in 3 divided doses; usual: 3-6 mg/kg/day or 100-150 mg/m^2/day in 3 divided doses; up to 8 mg/kg/day or 200 mg/m^2/day for uncontrolled patients with subtherapeutic levels; higher doses have been reported, however they may be associated with an increased risk of proarrhythmias; a review of world literature reports the average effective dose to be 4 mg/kg/day or 140 mg/m^2/day

Adults: Life-threatening ventricular arrhythmias: Initial: 100 mg every 12 hours, increase by 100 mg/day (given in 2 doses/day) every 4 days; usual: ≤300 mg/day; maximum: 400 mg/day; for patients receiving 400 mg/day who are not controlled and have trough concentrations <0.6 mcg/mL, dosage may be increased to 600 mg/day

Prevention of paroxysmal supraventricular arrhythmias in patients with disabling symptoms but no structural heart disease: Initial: 50 mg every 12 hours; maximum dose: 300 mg/day

Dosing adjustment in renal failure:

Manufacturer recommendations: Adults: Cl_{cr} ≤35 mL/minute/1.73 m^2: Initial: 50 mg every 12 hours or 100 mg once daily; increase dose slowly at intervals >4 days; monitor plasma levels closely

Alternative adjustment: Children and Adults Cl_{cr} ≤20 mL/minute: Decrease the usual dose by 25% to 50%

Administration Oral: May be administered in children and adults without regard to food; in infants receiving milk or milk based formulas, avoid concurrent administration with feedings; monitor serum concentrations and decrease the dose when the diet changes to a decreased consumption of milk

Monitoring Parameters EKG, serum concentrations [**Note**: Obtain serum trough concentrations at steady state (after at least 3 days when doses are started or changed) or when dietary changes due to maturation or concurrent illness occur], liver enzymes, CBC with differential

Reference Range Therapeutic: 0.2-1 mcg/mL (SI: 0.4-2 micromoles/L). **Note**: Pediatric patients may respond at the lower end of the recommended therapeutic range (0.2-0.5 mcg/mL) but up to 0.8 mcg/mL may be required.

Patient Information May cause dizziness; notify physician if chest pain, faintness, palpitations, dizziness or visual disturbances occur

Additional Information Single oral dose flecainide for termination of PSVT in children and young adults (n=25) and combination therapy of flecainide with amiodarone for refractory tachyarrhythmias in infancy (n=9) have been reported (See References)

Dosage Forms Excipient information presented when available (limited, particularly for generics); consult specific product labeling.

Tablet, as acetate: 50 mg, 100 mg, 150 mg

Extemporaneous Preparations

A 5 mg/mL suspension compounded from tablets and an oral flavored commercially available diluent (Roxane®) was stable for up to 45 days when stored at 5°C or 25°C in amber glass bottles (Wiest, 1992)

A 20 mg/mL oral liquid preparation made from tablets and 3 different vehicles (cherry syrup, a 1:1 mixture of Ora-Sweet® and Ora-Plus®, or a 1:1 mixture of Ora-Sweet® SF and Ora-Plus®) was stable for 60 days when stored in amber plastic prescription bottles in the dark at room temperature (25°C) or under refrigeration (5°C); grind twenty-four 100 mg tablets in a mortar into a fine powder; add 20 mL of the vehicle and mix well to form a uniform paste; mix while adding the vehicle in geometric proportions to **almost** 120 mL; transfer to a calibrated bottle and qsad with vehicle to 120 mL; label "shake well" and "protect from light" (Allen, 1996).

Allen LV and Erickson MA, "Stability of Baclofen, Captopril, Diltiazem Hydrochloride, Dipyridamole, and Flecainide Acetate in Extemporaneously Compounded Oral Liquids," *Am J Health Syst Pharm*, 1996, 53(18):2179-84.

Wiest DB, Garner SS, and Pagacz LR, "Stability of Flecainide Acetate in an Extemporaneously Compounded Oral Suspension," *Am J Hosp Pharm*, 1992, 49(6):1467-70.

References

Fenrich AL Jr, Perry JC, and Friedman RA, "Flecainide and Amiodarone: Combined Therapy for Refractory Tachyarrhythmias in Infants," *J Am Coll Cardiol*, 1995, 25(5):1195-8.

Musto B, Cavallaro C, Musto A, et al, "Flecainide Single Oral Dose for Management of Paroxysmal Supraventricular Tachycardia in Children and Young Adults," *Am Heart J*, 1992, 124(1):110-5.

Perry JC and Garson A Jr, "Flecainide Acetate for Treatment of Tachyarrhythmias in Children: Review of World Literature on Efficacy, Safety, and Dosing," *Am Heart J*, 1992, 124(6):1614-21.

Perry JC, McQuinn RL, Smith RT Jr, et al, "Flecainide Acetate for Resistant Arrhythmias in the Young: Efficacy and Pharmacokinetics," *J Am Coll Cardiol*, 1989, 14(1):185-91.

Priestley KA, Ladusans EJ, Rosenthal E, et al, "Experience With Flecainide for the Treatment of Cardiac Arrhythmias in Children," *Eur Heart J*, 1988, 9(12):1284-90.

Russell GA and Martin RP, "Flecainide Toxicity," *Arch Dis Child*, 1989, 64(6):860-2.

Zeigler V, Gillette PC, Ross BA, et al, "Flecainide for Supraventricular and Ventricular Arrhythmias in Children and Young Adults," *Am J Cardiol*, 1988, 62(10 Pt 1):818-20.

- **Flecainide Acetate** *see* Flecainide *on page 657*
- **Fleet® Accu-Prep® [OTC]** *see* Sodium Phosphate *on page 1456*
- **Fleet® Babylax® [OTC]** *see* Glycerin *on page 736*
- **Fleet® Bisacodyl [OTC]** *see* Bisacodyl *on page 217*
- **Fleet® Enema [OTC]** *see* Sodium Phosphate *on page 1456*
- **Fleet Enema® (Can)** *see* Sodium Phosphate *on page 1456*
- **Fleet® Glycerin Suppositories [OTC]** *see* Glycerin *on page 736*
- **Fleet® Glycerin Suppositories Maximum Strength [OTC]** *see* Glycerin *on page 736*
- **Fleet® Liquid Glycerin Suppositories [OTC]** *see* Glycerin *on page 736*
- **Fleet® Mineral Oil Enema [OTC]** *see* Mineral Oil *on page 1065*
- **Fleet® Phospho-Soda® [OTC]** *see* Sodium Phosphate *on page 1456*
- **Fleet® Phospho-Soda® Oral Laxative (Can)** *see* Sodium Phosphate *on page 1456*
- **Fleet® Sof-Lax® [OTC]** *see* Docusate *on page 526*
- **Fleet® Stimulant Laxative [OTC]** *see* Bisacodyl *on page 217*
- **Fletcher's® [OTC]** *see* Senna *on page 1427*
- **Flexbumin** *see* Albumin *on page 64*
- **Flexeril®** *see* Cyclobenzaprine *on page 416*
- **Flexitec (Can)** *see* Cyclobenzaprine *on page 416*
- **Flolan®** *see* Epoprostenol *on page 585*
- **Flonase®** *see* Fluticasone *on page 689*
- **Flora-Q™ [OTC]** *see Lactobacillus acidophilus* and *Lactobacillus bulgaricus on page 898*
- **Florazole® ER (Can)** *see* Metronidazole *on page 1049*
- **Florical® [OTC]** *see* Calcium Carbonate *on page 264*
- **Florical® [OTC]** *see* Calcium Supplements *on page 272*
- **Florinef®** *see* Fludrocortisone *on page 666*
- **Flovent® Diskus® (Can)** *see* Fluticasone *on page 689*
- **Flovent® HFA** *see* Fluticasone *on page 689*
- **Floxin®** *see* Ofloxacin *on page 1161*
- **Floxin Otic Singles** *see* Ofloxacin *on page 1161*

- **Fluarix™** *see* Influenza Virus Vaccine (Inactivated) *on page 833*
- **Flubenisolone** *see* Betamethasone *on page 212*

Fluconazole (floo KOE na zole)

Medication Safety Issues

Sound-alike/look-alike issues:

Fluconazole may be confused with flecainide

Diflucan® may be confused with diclofenac, Diprivan®, disulfiram

International issues:

Canesten® [Great Britain]: Brand name for clotrimazole in multiple international markets

U.S. Brand Names Diflucan®

Canadian Brand Names Apo-Fluconazole®; Diflucan®; Fluconazole Injection; Fluconazole Omega; Gen-Fluconazole; GMD-Fluconazole; Novo-Fluconazole; Riva-Fluconazole

Therapeutic Category Antifungal Agent, Systemic

Generic Available Yes

Use Treatment of susceptible fungal infections including oropharyngeal, esophageal, and vaginal candidiasis; treatment of systemic candidal infections including urinary tract infection, peritonitis, cystitis, and pneumonia; strains of *Candida* with decreased *in vitro* susceptibility to fluconazole are being isolated with increasing frequency; fluconazole is more active against *C. albicans* than other candidal strains like *C. parapsilosis*, *C. glabrata*, and *C. tropicalis*; treatment and suppression of cryptococcal meningitis; prophylaxis of candidiasis in patients undergoing bone marrow transplantation; alternative to amphotericin B in patients with pre-existing renal impairment or when requiring concomitant therapy with other potentially nephrotoxic drugs

Pregnancy Risk Factor C

Lactation Enters breast/not recommended (AAP rates "compatible")

Contraindications Hypersensitivity to fluconazole, other azoles, or any component; concurrent use with astemizole, cisapride, and terfenadine

Warnings Rare cases, including fatalities, due to fluconazole-associated hepatotoxicity have been reported. Patients who develop abnormal liver function tests during fluconazole therapy should be monitored closely for the development of more severe hepatic injury; if clinical signs and symptoms consistent with liver disease develop that may be attributable to fluconazole, fluconazole should be discontinued. Rare cases of exfoliative skin disorders have been reported. Closely monitor patients who develop rashes during fluconazole therapy.

Fluconazole oral suspension contains sodium benzoate; benzoic acid (benzoate) is a metabolite of benzyl alcohol; large amounts of benzyl alcohol (≥99 mg/kg/day) have been associated with a potentially fatal toxicity ("gasping syndrome") in neonates; the "gasping syndrome" consists of metabolic acidosis, respiratory distress, gasping respirations, CNS dysfunction (including convulsions, intracranial hemorrhage), hypotension and cardiovascular collapse; use fluconazole oral suspension containing sodium benzoate with caution in neonates; *in vitro* and animal studies have shown that benzoate displaces bilirubin from protein binding sites

Precautions Use with caution and modify dosage in patients with impaired renal function. Use with caution in patients with hepatic dysfunction or in patients with proarrhythmic conditions.

Adverse Reactions

Cardiovascular: Pallor, angioedema, QT prolongation, torsade de pointes

Central nervous system: Dizziness, headache (1.9%), seizures

Dermatologic: Skin rash (1.8%), exfoliative skin disorders, Stevens-Johnson syndrome, pruritus

Endocrine & metabolic: Hypokalemia, hypercholesterolemia, hypertriglyceridemia

Gastrointestinal: Nausea (2%), abdominal pain (3%), vomiting (5%), diarrhea (2%), dysgeusia, dyspepsia

Hematologic: Eosinophilia, leukopenia, thrombocytopenia, neutropenia, agranulocytosis

Hepatic: Elevated AST, ALT, or alkaline phosphatase; hepatitis; cholestasis, jaundice

Miscellaneous: Anaphylaxis

Drug Interactions Cytochrome P450 isoenzyme CYP2C9 inducer; CYP2C9, CYP2C18, CYP2C19 and CYP3A3/4 (weak) isoenzyme inhibitor

Oral antidiabetic agents (fluconazole reduces the metabolism and increases the concentration of tolbutamide, glyburide, and glipizide; monitor blood glucose); hydrochlorothiazide (increases fluconazole AUC); warfarin (increased prothrombin time); fluconazole increases plasma cyclosporine, tacrolimus, midazolam, theophylline, zidovudine, cisapride, (fatal arrhythmias including ventricular tachycardia, ventricular fibrillation, torsade de pointes, and QT prolongation have been reported in patients taking cisapride concurrently with fluconazole), astemizole, terfenadine, rifabutin (uveitis has been reported when rifabutin and fluconazole are given concomitantly), and phenytoin concentrations; rifampin increases fluconazole metabolism (consider increasing fluconazole dose); antagonism may occur if amphotericin B and fluconazole are used concomitantly

Food Interactions Food decreases the rate but not the extent of absorption

Stability Store tablets, powder for oral suspension, and premixed infusion at room temperature; do not freeze. Reconstituted oral suspension is stable for 14 days at room temperature or if refrigerated.

Fluconazole injection is incompatible with ampicillin, calcium gluconate, ceftazidime, cefotaxime, cefuroxime, ceftriaxone, clindamycin, furosemide, imipenem, ticarcillin, and piperacillin

Mechanism of Action Interferes with fungal cytochrome P450 sterol C-14 alpha-demethylation activity, decreasing ergosterol synthesis (principal sterol in fungal cell membrane) and inhibiting cell membrane formation

Pharmacokinetics

Absorption: Oral: Well absorbed; food does not affect extent of absorption

Distribution: Distributes widely into body tissues and fluids including the CSF, saliva, sputum, vaginal fluid, skin, eye; excreted in breast milk

Protein binding: 11% to 12%

Bioavailability: Oral: >90%

Half-life:

- Premature newborns: 73.6 hours; 6 days PNA: 53.2 hours; 12 days PNA: 46.6 hours
- Children:
  - 9 months to 13 years: 19.5-25 hours (with oral dose)
  - 5-15 years: 15.2-17.6 hours (with multiple I.V. dosing)
- Adults: 25-30 hours with normal renal function

Time to peak serum concentration: Oral: Within 2-4 hours (1-2 hours in fasted patients)

Elimination: 80% of dose excreted unchanged in urine; 11% of dose excreted in urine as metabolites

Dialysis: Hemodialysis: 3-hour session decreases plasma concentration 50%

Usual Dosage Daily dose of fluconazole is the same for oral and I.V. administration:

Oral, I.V.:

- Premature neonates:
  - ≤29 weeks gestation:
    - Postnatal age 0-14 days: 5-6 mg/kg/dose every 72 hours
    - Postnatal age >14 days: 5-6 mg/kg/dose every 48 hours
  - 30-36 weeks gestation: Postnatal age 0-14 days: 3-6 mg/kg/dose every 48 hours
- Neonates >14 days, Infants, Children: Once daily: See table
- Safety profile of fluconazole has been studied in 577 children ages 1 day to 17 years. Doses as high as 12 mg/kg/day once daily (equivalent to adult doses of 400 mg/day) have been used to treat candidiasis in immunocompromised children; 10-12 mg/kg/day doses once daily have been used prophylactically against fungal infections in pediatric bone marrow transplantation patients. Do not exceed 600 mg/day.

Indication	Day 1	Daily Therapy	Minimum Duration of Therapy
Neonates 0-14 days: Same dosage as older children but administered every 24-72 h			
Neonates >14 days, infants, and children			
Oropharyngeal candidiasis	6 mg/kg	3 mg/kg	14 d
Esophageal candidiasis	6 mg/kg	3 mg/kg up to 12 mg/kg/d	21 d
Systemic candidiasis	6-12 mg/kg/d		28 d
Cryptococcal meningitis			
acute	12 mg/kg	6 mg/kg up to 12 mg/kg/d	10-12 wk after CSF culture becomes negative
relapse	6 mg/kg		
Adults			
Oropharyngeal candidiasis	200 mg	100 mg	14 d
Esophageal candidiasis	200 mg	100-400 mg	21 d
Systemic candidiasis	400 mg	200-800 mg	28 d
Cryptococcal meningitis			
acute	400 mg	200-800 mg	10-12 wk after CSF culture becomes negative
relapse	200 mg	200 mg	

(Continued)

Fluconazole *(Continued)*

Dose equivalency:
Pediatric patients 3 mg/kg = Adults 100 mg
Pediatric patients 6 mg/kg = Adults 200 mg
Pediatric patients 12 mg/kg = Adults 400 mg

Adults: Oral, I.V.: Once daily: See table on previous page.
Vaginal candidiasis: Oral: 150 mg single dose
Prophylaxis against fungal infections in bone marrow transplantation patients: Oral, I.V.: 400 mg/day once daily

Dosing adjustment in renal impairment: Adults:
Cl_{cr} ≤50 mL/minute (not on dialysis): Administer 50% of recommended dose
Patients receiving hemodialysis: Administer 100% of recommended dose after each dialysis treatment

Administration
Oral: Administer with or without food; shake suspension well before use
Parenteral: Fluconazole must be administered by I.V. infusion over approximately 1-2 hours at a rate not to exceed 200 mg/hour and a final concentration for administration of 2 mg/mL; for pediatric patients receiving doses ≥6 mg/kg/day, administer I.V. infusion over 2 hours

Monitoring Parameters Periodic liver function and renal function tests, serum potassium, CBC with differential, and platelet count

Patient Information Notify physician of unusual bleeding or bruising, yellowing of skin and eyes, or severe skin rash

Dosage Forms Excipient information presented when available (limited, particularly for generics); consult specific product labeling.
Infusion [premixed in sodium chloride or dextrose]: 200 mg (100 mL); 400 mg (200 mL)
Diflucan® [premixed in sodium chloride or dextrose]: 200 mg (100 mL); 400 mg (200 mL)
Powder for oral suspension: 10 mg/mL (35 mL); 40 mg/mL (35 mL)
Diflucan®: 10 mg/mL (35 mL); 40 mg/mL (35 mL) [contains sodium benzoate; orange flavor]
Tablet: 50 mg, 100 mg, 150 mg, 200 mg
Diflucan®: 50 mg, 100 mg, 150 mg, 200 mg

References

Como JA and Dismukes WE, "Oral Azole Drugs as Systemic Antifungal Therapy," *N Engl J Med*, 1993, 330(4):263-72.
Goodman JL, Winston DJ, Greenfield RA, et al, "A Controlled Trial of Fluconazole to Prevent Fungal Infections in Patients Undergoing Bone Marrow Transplantation," *N Engl J Med*, 1992, 326(13):845-51.
Lee JW, Seibel NL, Amantea M, et al, "Safety and Pharmacokinetics of Fluconazole in Children With Neoplastic Diseases," *J Pediatr*, 1992, 120(6):987-93.
Moncino MD and Gutman LT, "Severe Systemic Cryptococcal Disease in a Child: Review of Prognostic Indicators Predicting Treatment Failure and an Approach to Maintenance Therapy With Oral Fluconazole," *Pediatr Infect Dis J*, 1990, 9(5):363-8.
Viscoli C, Castagnola E, Fioredda F, et al, "Fluconazole in the Treatment of Candidiasis in Immunocompromised Children," *Antimicrob Agents Chemother*, 1991, 35(2):365-7.

♦ **Fluconazole Injection (Can)** *see* Fluconazole *on page 660*
♦ **Fluconazole Omega (Can)** *see* Fluconazole *on page 660*

Flucytosine (floo SYE toe seen)

Medication Safety Issues
Sound-alike/look-alike issues:
Flucytosine may be confused with fluorouracil
Ancobon® may be confused with Oncovin®

High alert medication: The Institute for Safe Medication Practices (ISMP) includes this medication among its list of drugs which have a heightened risk of causing significant patient harm when used in error.

Related Information
Blood Level Sampling Time Guidelines *on page 1914*

U.S. Brand Names Ancobon®
Canadian Brand Names Ancobon®
Index Terms 5-FC; 5-Fluorocytosine; 5-Flurocytosine
Therapeutic Category Antifungal Agent, Systemic
Generic Available No
Use In combination with amphotericin B in the treatment of serious Candidal or Cryptococcal pulmonary or urinary tract infections, sepsis, meningitis, or endocarditis (resistance emerges if flucytosine is used as a single agent); used in combination with another antifungal agent for treatment of chromomycosis and aspergillosis
Pregnancy Risk Factor C

Lactation Excretion in breast milk unknown/not recommended

Contraindications Hypersensitivity to flucytosine or any component

Precautions Use with extreme caution in patients with renal impairment, bone marrow suppression, patients with AIDS; monitor hematologic, renal, and hepatic function of all patients receiving flucytosine; dosage modification required in patients with impaired renal function based on serum flucytosine concentrations

Adverse Reactions

Cardiovascular: Chest pain, myocardial toxicity, ventricular dysfunction, cardiac arrest

Central nervous system: Confusion, headache, sedation, hallucinations, psychosis, seizures, vertigo, ataxia, fever

Dermatologic: Rash, pruritus, urticaria, photosensitivity

Endocrine & metabolic: Temporary growth failure, hypokalemia, hypoglycemia

Gastrointestinal: Nausea, vomiting, diarrhea, enterocolitis, anorexia, GI hemorrhage, dry mouth, duodenal ulcer

Hematologic: Bone marrow suppression (often observed after 10-26 days of therapy and occurs more frequently with sustained concentrations >100 mcg/mL), anemia, leukopenia, thrombocytopenia, agranulocytosis, eosinophilia

Hepatic: Elevated bilirubin and liver enzymes; hepatitis, jaundice

Neuromuscular & skeletal: Neuropathy, paresthesia

Otic: Hearing loss

Renal: Elevated BUN and serum creatinine, renal failure

Respiratory: Dyspnea

Miscellaneous: Anaphylaxis

Drug Interactions Increased efficacy as well as toxicity (enterocolitis, myelosuppression) with concurrent amphotericin administration; antacids and aluminum or magnesium salts delay the rate of absorption; cytosine arabinoside may inactivate flucytosine activity

Food Interactions Food decreases the rate, but not the extent of absorption

Stability Store at room temperature; protect from light

Mechanism of Action Penetrates fungal cells and is converted to fluorouracil which competes with uracil interfering with fungal RNA and protein synthesis

Pharmacokinetics

Absorption: Oral: 78% to 89%; rate of absorption is delayed in patients with renal impairment

Distribution: Widely distributed into body tissues and fluids including CSF, aqueous humor, peritoneal fluid, bronchial secretions, liver, spleen, kidney, heart, and joints

V_d: Adults: 0.68 L/kg

Protein binding: 2.9% to 4%

Metabolism: Minimal hepatic metabolism; deaminated to 5-fluorouracil (probably by gut bacteria)

Bioavailability: Decreased in neonates

Half-life:

Neonates: 4-34 hours

Infants: 7.4 hours

Adults: 2.5-6 hours (prolonged as high as 200 hours in anuria)

Time to peak serum concentration: Oral:

Children: 2.5 ± 1.3 hours

Adults: Within 2 hours

Elimination: 75% to 90% excreted unchanged in urine by glomerular filtration; small portion is excreted in the feces

Dialysis: Dialyzable (50% to 100%)

Usual Dosage Oral:

Neonates: Initial: 50-100 mg/kg/day in divided doses every 12-24 hours

Infants, Children, Adults: 100-150 mg/kg/day in divided doses every 6 hours

Dosing adjustment in renal impairment: Use lower initial dose:

Cl_{cr} 20-40 mL/minute: Administer usual individual dose every 12 hours

Cl_{cr} 10-20 mL/minute: Administer usual individual dose every 24 hours

Cl_{cr} <10 mL/minute: Administer usual individual dose every 24-48 hours

Patients receiving hemodialysis: Administer 20-50 mg/kg dose postdialysis

Administration Oral: Administer with food over a 15-minute period to decrease incidence and severity of nausea and vomiting

Monitoring Parameters Serum electrolytes, creatinine, BUN, alkaline phosphatase, AST, ALT, CBC, platelet count; serum flucytosine concentrations; *in vitro* susceptibility tests to flucytosine

Reference Range Therapeutic levels: 25-100 mcg/mL; with invasive candidiasis, maintain peak plasma concentration between 40-60 mcg/mL; increased bone marrow suppression with sustained serum flucytosine concentration >100 mcg/mL; obtain flucytosine concentration 60-120 minutes after an oral dose; obtain trough level immediately before the next dose; maintain trough ≥25 mcg/mL to prevent emergence of resistant strains

(Continued)

Flucytosine *(Continued)*

Test Interactions Flucytosine causes markedly false elevations in serum creatinine values when the Ektachem® analyzer is used

Patient Information May cause photosensitivity reactions (eg, exposure to sunlight may cause severe sunburn, skin rash, redness, or itching); avoid exposure to sunlight and artificial light sources (sunlamps, tanning booth/bed); wear protective clothing, wide-brimmed hats, sunglasses, and lip sunscreen (SPF ≥15); use a sunscreen [broad-spectrum sunscreen or physical sunscreen (preferred) or sunblock with SPF ≥15]; contact physician if reaction occurs.

Additional Information Resistance develops rapidly if used alone; more rapid emergence of fungal resistance may occur when lower doses are used

Dosage Forms Excipient information presented when available (limited, particularly for generics); consult specific product labeling.

Capsule: 250 mg, 500 mg

Extemporaneous Preparations Flucytosine oral liquid has been prepared by using the contents of ten 500 mg capsules triturated in a mortar and pestle with a small amount of distilled water; the mixture was transferred to a 500 mL volumetric flask; the mortar was rinsed several times with a small amount of distilled water and the fluid added to the flask; sufficient distilled water was added to make a total volume of 500 mL of a 10 mg/mL liquid; oral liquid was stable for 70 days when stored in glass or plastic prescription bottles at 4°C or for up to 14 days at room temperature.

Wintermeyer SM and Nahata MC, "Stability of Flucytosine in an Extemporaneously Compounded Oral Liquid," *Am J Health-Syst Pharm*, 1996, 53:407-9.

References

Baley JE, Meyers C, Kliegman RM, et al, "Pharmacokinetics, Outcome of Treatment, and Toxic Effects of Amphotericin B and 5-Fluorocytosine in Neonates," *J Pediatr*, 1990, 116(5):791-7.

Soltani M, Tobin CM, Bowker KE, et al, "Evidence of Excessive Concentrations of 5-Flucytosine in Children Aged Below 12 Years: A 12-Year Review of Serum Concentrations From a UK Clinical Assay Reference Laboratory," *Int J Antimicrob Agents*, 2006, 28(6):574-7.

♦ **Fludara®** *see* Fludarabine *on page 664*

Fludarabine (floo DARE a been)

Medication Safety Issues

Sound-alike/look-alike issues:

Fludarabine may be confused with floxuridine, Flumadine®

Fludara® may be confused with FUDR®

High alert medication: The Institute for Safe Medication Practices (ISMP) includes this medication among its list of drugs which have a heightened risk of causing significant patient harm when used in error.

Related Information

Compatibility of Chemotherapy and Related Supportive Care Medications *on page 1777*

Emetogenic Potential of Single Chemotherapeutic Agents *on page 1776*

U.S. Brand Names Fludara®

Canadian Brand Names Beneflur®; Fludara®

Index Terms Fludarabine Phosphate; NSC-312887

Therapeutic Category Antineoplastic Agent, Antimetabolite

Generic Available Yes

Use Treatment of B-cell chronic lymphocytic leukemia unresponsive to previous therapy with an alkylating agent containing regimen; non-Hodgkin's lymphoma. Fludarabine has been tested in patients with refractory acute lymphocytic leukemia and acute nonlymphocytic leukemia, but required a highly toxic dose to achieve response; used in reduced-intensity conditioning regimens prior to allogenic hematopoietic stem cell transplantation

Pregnancy Risk Factor D

Lactation Excretion in breast milk unknown/contraindicated

Contraindications Hypersensitivity to fludarabine or any component; concomitant administration with pentostatin; pregnancy

Warnings The FDA currently recommends that procedures for proper handling and disposal of antineoplastic agents be considered; doses ≥77 mg/m²/day for 5-7 days were associated with severe neurotoxicity, including blindness, coma, and death. Neurotoxicity can occur 21-60 days after completing a course of fludarabine and appears to be dose related. Severe bone marrow suppression (anemia, thrombocytopenia, and neutropenia) has been observed at therapeutic doses; bone marrow hypoplasia or aplasia resulting in death has been reported; life-threatening and sometimes fatal autoimmune hemolytic anemia has been reported after one or more cycles of treatment. Hematologic function must be frequently monitored. Concomitant therapy with pentostatin may be associated with severe pulmonary toxicity.

Precautions Use with caution in patients with pre-existing neurologic problems, patients with a fever, infection, or pre-existing hematological disorder, and in patients with renal insufficiency; dosage adjustment may be needed in patients with impaired renal function or bone marrow suppression

Adverse Reactions

Cardiovascular: Edema, CHF, angina

Central nervous system: Neurotoxicity (primarily progressive demyelinating encephalopathy with mental status deterioration), somnolence, seizures, fever, agitation, confusion, depression, chills, fatigue, headache, coma

Dermatologic: Pruritus, rash, alopecia

Endocrine & metabolic: Metabolic acidosis, tumor lysis syndrome, (hyperuricemia, hyperphosphatemia, hypocalcemia, hyperkalemia), hyperglycemia

Gastrointestinal: Nausea, vomiting, diarrhea, stomatitis, metallic taste, GI bleeding, anorexia

Genitourinary: Hemorrhagic cystitis (rare)

Hematologic: Leukopenia, neutropenia, thrombocytopenia, lymphocytopenia, autoimmune hemolytic anemia, anemia

Hepatic: Elevated transaminase levels

Neuromuscular & skeletal: Myalgia, peripheral neuropathy, weakness

Ocular: Blindness, blurred vision, photophobia

Renal: Hematuria, renal failure

Respiratory: Interstitial pneumonitis, dyspnea, cough, ARDS, pulmonary hemorrhage, pulmonary fibrosis

Drug Interactions Cytarabine when administered with or prior to a fludarabine dose competes for deoxycytidine kinase decreasing the phosphorylation of fludarabine to the active F-ara-ATP (inhibits the antineoplastic effect of fludarabine); however, administering fludarabine prior to cytarabine may stimulate activation of cytarabine, pentostatin (increased pulmonary toxicity)

Stability Store vial in refrigerator; reconstituted 25 mg/mL fludarabine solution should be used within 8 hours after preparation since it contains no preservatives. When fludarabine is diluted in D_5W or NS to a final concentration of 1 mg/mL, the solution is stable for 24 hours at room temperature. Discard solution if a slight haze develops.

Mechanism of Action F-ara-AMP is dephosphorylated to 2-fluoro-ara-A which enters the cell by a carrier mediated transport process; it is phosphorylated intracellularly to the active metabolite F-ara-ATP. F-ara-ATP competes with deoxyadenosine triphosphate for incorporation into the A-sites of the DNA strand inhibiting DNA synthesis in the S-phase via inhibition of DNA polymerases and RNA reductase.

Pharmacokinetics

Distribution: Widely distributed with extensive tissue binding

Protein binding: 19% to 29%

Half-life: Terminal (2-fluoro-ara-A):

Children: 12.4-19 hours

Adults: 7-20 hours

Elimination: Fludarabine clearance appears to be inversely correlated with serum creatinine; at a dose of 25 mg/m^2/day for 5 days, 24% of dose excreted in urine; at higher doses, 41% to 60% of dose renally excreted

Usual Dosage Not currently FDA approved for use in children (refer to individual protocols): I.V.:

Children:

Acute leukemia: 10 mg/m^2 bolus over 15 minutes followed by a continuous infusion of 30.5 mg/m^2/day for 5 days; or 10.5 mg/m^2 bolus over 15 minutes followed by a continuous infusion of 30.5 mg/m^2/day over 48 hours followed by cytarabine has been used in clinical trials

Reduced-intensity conditioning regimens prior to allogenic hematopoietic stem cell transplantation: 30 mg/m^2/day for 5 days

Solid tumors: 7-9 mg/m^2 bolus followed by 20-27 mg/m^2/day continuous infusion for 5 days

Adults:

Chronic lymphocytic leukemia: 20-25 mg/m^2/day over 30 minutes for 5 days; doses up to 30 mg/m^2/day as single daily doses for 5 days have also been used; courses are usually repeated every 28 days

Non-Hodgkin's lymphoma: Loading dose: 20 mg/m^2 followed by 30 mg/m^2/day for 48 hours

Dosing adjustment in renal impairment:

Cl_{cr} 30-70 mL/minute/1.73 m^2: Reduce dose by 20% and monitor closely for toxicity

Cl_{cr} <30 mL/minute/1.73 m^2: Not recommended

Administration Parenteral: Fludarabine phosphate has been administered by intermittent I.V. infusion over 15-30 minutes and by continuous infusion; in clinical trials the loading dose has been diluted in 20 mL D_5W and administered over 15 minutes and the continuous infusion diluted to 240 mL in D_5W and administered at a constant

(Continued)

Fludarabine *(Continued)*

rate of 10 mL/hour; in other clinical studies fludarabine has been diluted to a concentration of 0.25-1 mg/mL in D_5W or NS

Monitoring Parameters CBC with differential, platelet count, AST, ALT, creatinine, serum electrolytes, albumin, uric acid, and examination for visual changes

Patient Information Notify physician if fever, sore throat, bleeding, bruising, tachypnea, respiratory distress, or neurologic changes occur. Women of childbearing potential should be advised to avoid becoming pregnant.

Nursing Implications Prophylactic allopurinol, adequate hydration, and urinary alkalinization should be considered for patients with large initial tumor burdens

Additional Information Myelosuppressive effects:

Granulocyte nadir: 13 days (3-25)
Platelet nadir: 16 days (2-32)
Recovery: 5-7 weeks

Dosage Forms Excipient information presented when available (limited, particularly for generics); consult specific product labeling. [CAN] = Canadian brand name

Injection, powder for reconstitution, as phosphate: 50 mg
Tablet, as phosphate [CAN]: 10 mg [not available in U.S.]

References

Avramis VI, Champagne J, Sato J, et al, "Pharmacology of Fludarabine Phosphate After a Phase I/II Trial by a Loading Bolus and Continuous Infusion in Pediatric Patients," *Cancer Res*, 1990, 50(22):7226-31.
Jacobsohn DA, Emerick KM, Scholl P, et al, "Nonmyeloablative Hematopoietic Stem Cell Transplant for X-Linked Hyper-Immunoglobulin M Syndrome With Cholangiopathy," *Pediatrics*, 2004, 113(2):e122-7.
Von Hoff DD, "Phase I Clinical Trials With Fludarabine Phosphate," *Semin Oncol*, 1990, 17(5 Suppl 8):33-8.

♦ **Fludarabine Phosphate** *see* Fludarabine *on page 664*

Fludrocortisone (floo droe KOR ti sone)

Medication Safety Issues

Sound-alike/look-alike issues:
Florinef® may be confused with Fiorinal®

Related Information

Corticosteroids, Systemic *on page 1685*

U.S. Brand Names Florinef®

Canadian Brand Names Florinef®

Index Terms 9α-Fluorohydrocortisone Acetate; Fludrocortisone Acetate; Fluohydrisone Acetate; Fluohydrocortisone Acetate

Therapeutic Category Adrenal Corticosteroid; Corticosteroid, Systemic; Glucocorticoid; Mineralocorticoid

Generic Available Yes

Use Treatment of Addison's disease; partial replacement therapy for adrenal insufficiency; treatment of salt-losing forms of congenital adrenogenital syndrome; has been used in conjunction with an increased sodium intake for the treatment of idiopathic orthostatic hypotension

Pregnancy Risk Factor C

Lactation Excretion in breast milk unknown

Contraindications Hypersensitivity to fludrocortisone or any component; CHF, systemic fungal infections

Precautions Dosage should be tapered gradually if therapy is discontinued; use with caution in patients with hypertension, edema, or renal dysfunction

Adverse Reactions

Cardiovascular: Hypertension, edema, CHF
Central nervous system: Convulsions, headache
Dermatologic: Acne, rash, bruising
Endocrine & metabolic: Hypokalemic alkalosis, suppression of growth, hyperglycemia, hypothalamic-pituitary-adrenal suppression
Gastrointestinal: Peptic ulcer
Neuromuscular & skeletal: Muscle weakness
Ocular: Cataracts

Drug Interactions Digoxin (fludrocortisone-induced hypokalemia may increase digoxin toxicity); phenytoin and rifampin may increase metabolism of fludrocortisone; hypokalemia-causing medications may increase risk of hypokalemia

Food Interactions Systemic use of mineralocorticoids/corticosteroids may require a diet with increased potassium, vitamins A, B_6, C, D, folate, calcium, zinc, and phosphorus, and decreased sodium; with fludrocortisone a decrease in dietary sodium is often not required as the increased retention of sodium is usually the desired therapeutic effect

Mechanism of Action Potent mineralocorticoid with glucocorticoid activity; promotes increased reabsorption of sodium and loss of potassium from distal tubules

Pharmacodynamics Duration: 1-2 days

Pharmacokinetics

Absorption: Rapid and complete from GI tract

Protein binding: 42%

Metabolism: In the liver

Half-life:

Plasma: ~3.5 hours

Biological: 18-36 hours

Usual Dosage Oral:

Infants and Children: 0.05-0.1 mg/day

Congenital adrenal hyperplasia (salt losers): Maintenance: Range: 0.05-0.3 mg/day (AAP, 2000)

Adults: 0.05-0.2 mg/day

Administration Oral: May administer with food to decrease GI upset

Monitoring Parameters Serum electrolytes and glucose, blood pressure, serum renin

Patient Information Notify physician if dizziness, severe or continuing headache, swelling of feet or lower legs, or unusual weight gain occurs

Additional Information In patients with salt-losing forms of congenital adrenogenital syndrome, use along with cortisone or hydrocortisone; fludrocortisone 0.1 mg has sodium retention activity equal to DOCA® 1 mg

Dosage Forms Excipient information presented when available (limited, particularly for generics); consult specific product labeling.

Tablet, as acetate: 0.1 mg

References

American Academy of Pediatrics, Section on Endocrinology and Committee on Genetics, "Technical Report: Congenital Adrenal Hyperplasia," *Pediatrics*, 2000, 106(6):1511-8.

♦ **Fludrocortisone Acetate** *see* Fludrocortisone *on page 666*

♦ **FluLaval™** *see* Influenza Virus Vaccine (Inactivated) *on page 833*

♦ **Flumadine®** *see* Rimantadine *on page 1386*

Flumazenil (FLO may ze nil)

Related Information

Commonly Used Antidotes for Acute Overdoses *on page 1920*

U.S. Brand Names Romazicon®

Canadian Brand Names Anexate®; Flumazenil Injection; Flumazenil Injection, USP; Romazicon®

Therapeutic Category Antidote, Benzodiazepine

Generic Available Yes

Use Benzodiazepine antagonist; reverses sedative effects of benzodiazepines used in general anesthesia or conscious sedation; management of benzodiazepine overdose; **not indicated** for ethanol, barbiturate, general anesthetic or narcotic overdose

Pregnancy Risk Factor C

Lactation Excretion in breast milk unknown/use caution

Contraindications Hypersensitivity to flumazenil, any component, or benzodiazepines; patients given benzodiazepines for control of potentially life-threatening conditions (eg, control of intracranial pressure or status epilepticus); patients with signs of serious cyclic-antidepressant overdosage

Warnings Flumazenil may precipitate seizures in patients physically dependent on benzodiazepines, in patients treated with benzodiazepines for seizure disorders or other reasons, in overdose patients with seizure activity prior to flumazenil, in patients with serious cyclic antidepressant or mixed drug overdoses, and in patients with severe hepatic impairment; higher than normal doses of benzodiazepines may be required to treat these seizures; mixed drug overdose patients who have ingested drugs that increase the likelihood of seizures (eg, cocaine, lithium, cyclosporine, cyclic antidepressants, bupropion, methylxanthines, MAO inhibitors, isoniazid, or propoxyphene) are at extremely high risk for seizures (flumazenil may be contraindicated in these patients); flumazenil is not recommended in epileptic patients receiving chronic benzodiazepine therapy

Precautions Resedation may occur with flumazenil use (due to its short half-life in comparison to some benzodiazepines); pediatric patients (especially 1-5 years of age) may experience resedation; these patients may require repeat bolus doses or continuous infusion; monitor patients for return of sedation and respiratory depression. Flumazenil should be used with caution in the intensive care unit because of increased risk of unrecognized benzodiazepine dependence in such settings. Flumazenil may provoke panic attacks in patients with panic disorder. Do not use flumazenil until effects of neuromuscular blockers have been fully reversed. Use with

(Continued)

Flumazenil *(Continued)*

caution in patients with liver disease and decrease the amount or frequency of repeat doses.

Adverse Reactions

Cardiovascular: Arrhythmias, bradycardia, tachycardia, chest pain, hypertension, hypotension

Central nervous system: Seizures (more common in patients physically dependent on benzodiazepines or with cyclic antidepressant overdoses, see Warnings), fatigue, dizziness, headache, agitation, emotional lability, anxiety, euphoria, depression, abnormal crying

Endocrine & metabolic: Hot flashes

Gastrointestinal: Nausea, vomiting, xerostomia

Local: Pain at injection site

Ocular: Blurred vision

Miscellaneous: Increased diaphoresis, shivering, hiccups, sensation of coldness; can precipitate acute withdrawal symptoms in patients physically dependent on benzodiazepines

Drug Interactions Use with caution in mixed drug overdose; toxic effects of other drugs (especially with cyclic antidepressants) may occur with reversal of benzodiazepine effects

Stability Store at 25°C (77°F); compatible with D_5W, LR, or NS for 24 hours; discard any unused solution after 24 hours

Mechanism of Action Antagonizes the effect of benzodiazepines on the GABA/benzodiazepine receptor complex. Flumazenil is benzodiazepine specific and does not antagonize other nonbenzodiazepine GABA agonists (including ethanol, barbiturates, general anesthetics); does not reverse the effects of opiates.

Pharmacodynamics

Onset of action: Benzodiazepine reversal: Within 1-3 minutes

Maximum effect: 6-10 minutes

Duration: Usually <1 hour; duration is related to dose given and benzodiazepine plasma concentrations; reversal effects of flumazenil may wear off before effects of benzodiazepine and resedation may occur

Pharmacokinetics Follows a two compartment open model; **Note:** Clearance and V_d per kg are similar for children and adults, but children display more variability

Distribution: Distributes extensively in the extravascular space; Adults:

- Initial V_d: 0.5 L/kg
- V_{dss}: 0.9-1.1 L/kg

Protein binding: ~50%; primarily to albumin

Metabolism: In the liver to the de-ethylated free acid and its glucuronide conjugate

Half-life

- Children: Terminal: 20-75 minutes (mean: 40 minutes)
- Adults:
  - Alpha: 4-11 minutes
  - Terminal: 40-80 minutes

Elimination: 99% hepatically eliminated; <1% excreted unchanged in urine

- Clearance: Dependent upon hepatic blood flow; Adults: 0.8-1 L/hour/kg

Usual Dosage I.V.:

Children:

Reversal of benzodiazepine when used in conscious sedation or general anesthesia: Initial dose: 0.01 mg/kg (maximum dose: 0.2 mg) given over 15 seconds; may repeat 0.01 mg/kg (maximum dose: 0.2 mg) after 45 seconds, and then every minute to a maximum total cumulative dose of 0.05 mg/kg or 1 mg, whichever is lower; usual total dose: 0.08-1 mg (mean: 0.65 mg)

Management of benzodiazepine overdose: Minimal information available; initial dose: 0.01 mg/kg (maximum dose: 0.2 mg) with repeat doses of 0.01 mg/kg (maximum dose: 0.2 mg) given every minute to a maximum total cumulative dose of 1 mg; as an alternative to repeat bolus doses, follow up continuous infusions of 0.005-0.01 mg/kg/hour have been used; further studies are needed

Adults:

Reversal of benzodiazepine when used in conscious sedation or general anesthesia: 0.2 mg given over 15 seconds; may repeat 0.2 mg after 45 seconds and then every 60 seconds up to a total of 1 mg, usual total dose: 0.6-1 mg. In event of resedation, may repeat doses at 20-minute intervals with maximum of 1 mg/dose (given at 0.2 mg/minute); maximum dose: 3 mg in 1 hour.

Management of benzodiazepine overdose: 0.2 mg over 30 seconds; may give 0.3 mg dose after 30 seconds if desired level of consciousness is not obtained; additional doses of 0.5 mg can be given over 30 seconds at 1-minute intervals up to a cumulative dose of 3 mg; usual cumulative dose: 1-3 mg; rarely, patients with partial response at 3 mg may require additional titration up to total dose of 5 mg; if patient has not responded 5 minutes after cumulative dose of 5 mg, the major cause of sedation is not likely due to benzodiazepines. In the event of resedation, may repeat doses at 20-minute intervals with maximum of 1 mg/dose (given at 0.5 mg/minute); maximum dose: 3 mg in 1 hour.

Dosing adjustment in hepatic impairment: Initial dose: Use normal dose; repeat doses should be decreased in size or frequency

Administration Parenteral: For I.V. use only; administer by rapid I.V. injection over 15-30 seconds via a freely running I.V. infusion into larger vein (to decrease chance of pain, phlebitis). Children: Do not exceed 0.2 mg/minute. Adults: Repeat doses: Do not exceed 0.2 mg/minute for reversal of general anesthesia and do not exceed 0.5 mg/minute for reversal of benzodiazepine overdose.

Monitoring Parameters Level of consciousness and resedation, blood pressure, heart rate, respiratory rate, continuous pulse oximetry; monitor for resedation for 1-2 hours after reversal of sedation in patients who receive benzodiazepine sedation

Patient Information Flumazenil does not consistently reverse amnesia; do not engage in activities requiring alertness for 24 hours after discharge; resedation may occur in patients on long-acting benzodiazepines (such as diazepam); avoid alcohol or OTC medications for 24 hours after flumazenil is used or if benzodiazepine effects persist; may cause dry mouth

Nursing Implications Flumazenil does not effectively reverse hypoventilation, even in alert patients

Additional Information Flumazenil is a weak lipophilic base. In one study of conscious sedation reversal in 107 pediatric patients (1-17 years of age), resedation occurred between 19-50 minutes after the start of flumazenil. Flumazenil has been used to successfully treat paradoxical reactions in children associated with midazolam use (eg, agitation, restlessness, combativeness) (see Massanari, 1997).

Dosage Forms Excipient information presented when available (limited, particularly for generics); consult specific product labeling.

Injection, solution: 0.1 mg/mL (5 mL, 10 mL) [contains edetate sodium]

References

Baktai G, Szekely E, Marialigeti T, et al, "Use of Midazolam (Dormicum) and Flumazenil (Anexate) in Paediatric Bronchology," *Curr Med Res Opin*, 1992, 12(9):552-9.

Clark RF, Sage TA, Tunget C, et al, "Delayed Onset Lorazepam Poisoning Successfully Reversed By Flumazenil in a Child: Case Report and Review of the Literature," *Pediatr Emerg Care*, 1995, 11(1):32-4.

Jones RD, Lawson AD, Andrew LJ, et al, "Antagonism of the Hypnotic Effect of Midazolam in Children: A Randomized, Double Blind Study of Placebo and Flumazenil Administered After Midazolam-Induced Anaesthesia," *Br J Anaesth*, 1991, 66(6):660-6.

Massanari M, Novitsky J, and Reinstein LJ, "Paradoxical Reactions in Children Associated With Midazolam Use During Endoscopy," *Clin Pediatr*, 1997, 36(12):681-4.

Richard P, Autret E, Bardol J, et al, "The Use of Flumazenil in a Neonate," *J Toxicol Clin Toxicol*, 1991, 29(1):137-40.

Roald OK and Dahl V, "Flunitrazepam Intoxication in a Child Successfully Treated With the Benzodiazepine Antagonist Flumazenil," *Crit Care Med*, 1989, 17(12):1355-6.

Shannon M, Albers G, Burkhart K, et al, "Safety and Efficacy of Flumazenil in the Reversal of Benzodiazepine-Induced Conscious Sedation. The Flumazenil Pediatric Study Group," *J Pediatr*, 1997, 131(4):582-6.

Sugarman JM and Paul RI, "Flumazenil: A Review," *Pediatr Emerg Care*, 1994, 10(1):37-43.

♦ **Flumazenil Injection (Can)** *see* Flumazenil *on page 667*

♦ **Flumazenil Injection, USP (Can)** *see* Flumazenil *on page 667*

♦ **fluMist®** *see* Influenza Virus Vaccine (Live/Attenuated) *on page 835*

Flunisolide (floo NIS oh lide)

Medication Safety Issues

Sound-alike/look-alike issues:

Flunisolide may be confused with Flumadine®, fluocinonide

Nasarel® may be confused with Nizoral®

Related Information

Asthma *on page 1904*

U.S. Brand Names AeroBid®; AeroBid®-M; Aerospan™; Nasarel®

Canadian Brand Names Alti-Flunisolide; Apo-Flunisolide®; Nasalide®; PMS-Flunisolide; Rhinalar®

Therapeutic Category Adrenal Corticosteroid; Anti-inflammatory Agent; Antiasthmatic; Corticosteroid, Inhalant (Oral); Corticosteroid, Intranasal; Glucocorticoid

Generic Available Yes: Nasal spray

Use

Oral inhalation: Long-term (chronic) control of persistent bronchial asthma; **NOT** indicated for the relief of acute bronchospasm. Also used to help reduce or discontinue oral corticosteroid therapy for asthma (see Additional Information).

Intranasal: Management of seasonal or perennial rhinitis

Pregnancy Risk Factor C

Lactation Excretion in breast milk unknown/use caution

(Continued)

Flunisolide *(Continued)*

Contraindications Hypersensitivity to flunisolide or any component; primary treatment of status asthmaticus; untreated nasal mucosa infection

Warnings Fatalities have occurred due to adrenal insufficiency in asthmatic patients during and after switching from systemic corticosteroids to aerosol steroids (see Additional Information); several months may be required for full recovery of hypothalamic-pituitary-adrenal (HPA) function; patients receiving higher doses of systemic corticosteroids (eg, adults receiving ≥20 mg of prednisone per day) may be at greater risk; during this period of HPA suppression, aerosol steroids do **not** provide the systemic glucocorticoid or mineralocorticoid activity needed to treat patients requiring stress doses (ie, patients with major stress such as trauma, surgery, infections, or other conditions associated with severe electrolyte loss). When used at high doses, HPA suppression may occur; use with inhaled or systemic corticosteroids (even alternate-day dosing) may increase risk of HPA suppression. Acute adrenal insufficiency may occur with abrupt withdrawal after long-term use or with stress; withdrawal or discontinuation of corticosteroids should be done carefully; patients with HPA axis suppression may require doses of systemic glucocorticosteroids prior to, during, and after unusual stress (eg, surgery). Immunosuppression may occur; patients may be more susceptible to infections; avoid exposure to chickenpox and measles. Switching patients from systemic corticosteroids to aerosol steroids may unmask allergic conditions previously treated by the systemic steroid. Bronchospasm may occur after use of inhaled asthma medications (see Additional Information).

Precautions Avoid using higher than recommended doses; suppression of HPA function, suppression of linear growth (ie, reduction of growth velocity), reduced bone mineral density, hypercorticism (Cushing's syndrome), hyperglycemia, or glucosuria may occur; use with extreme caution in patients with respiratory tuberculosis, untreated systemic infections, or ocular herpes simplex

Adverse Reactions

Cardiovascular: Oral inhalation: Palpitations, hypertension, chest pain, edema

Central nervous system: Dizziness, headache, fever, nervousness, insomnia, migraine

Dermatologic: Rash, itching, eczema

Endocrine & metabolic: HPA suppression, Cushing's syndrome, growth suppression

Gastrointestinal: Oral candidiasis (oral inhalation), nausea, vomiting, diarrhea, upset stomach, abdominal pain, sore throat, bitter taste, aftertaste

Genitourinary: Menstrual disturbances (oral inhalation)

Local: Nasal burning

Neuromuscular & skeletal: Muscular soreness, decreased bone mineral density

Ocular: Rarely: Increased IOP, glaucoma, cataracts (oral inhalation)

Respiratory: Sneezing, nasal congestion, nasal dryness, pharyngitis, rhinitis, epistaxis, *Candida* infections of the nose or pharynx, atrophic rhinitis, upper respiratory infections

Drug Interactions Cytochrome P450 isoenzyme CYP3A4 substrate

Expected interactions similar to other corticosteroids

Stability

Aerospan™: Store at controlled room temperature; protect from freezing and direct sunlight; do not store near open heat or flame; exposure to temperatures >120°F (49°C) may cause bursting of canister; do not puncture or incinerate

Intranasal solutions: Store at 59°F to 86°F

Mechanism of Action Controls the rate of protein synthesis, depresses the migration of polymorphonuclear leukocytes and fibroblasts, reverses capillary permeability, and stabilizes lysosomal membranes at the cellular level to prevent or control inflammation

Pharmacodynamics Clinical effects are due to a direct local effect rather than systemic absorption

Onset of action: Intranasal: Within a few days

Maximum effect: Intranasal: 1-2 weeks; oral inhalation: 2-4 weeks

Pharmacokinetics

Absorption: Rapid

Distribution: Extensive; mean apparent V_d: Aerospan™: Adults: 170-350 L

Metabolism: Rapid in the liver via cytochrome P450 isoenzyme CYP3A4 to a less active metabolite (6 beta-OH flunisolide), followed by glucuronide and sulfate conjugation

Bioavailability:

- Nasal inhalation: 50%
- Oral: 20%
- Oral inhalation: AeroBid®-M: 40%; Aerospan™: <7%

Half-life: 1.8 hours

Elimination: Excreted in urine and feces; Aerospan™: <1% of dose is recovered in urine

Usual Dosage

Intranasal: Manufacturer's recommendation:

Children 6-14 years: Initial: 1 spray to each nostril 3 times/day or 2 sprays to each nostril 2 times/day; maximum dose: 4 sprays to each nostril per day; after symptoms are controlled, dose should be reduced to lowest effective amount; maintenance: 1 spray each nostril once daily

Adults: Initial: 2 sprays to each nostril twice daily; may increase in 4-7 days if needed to 2 sprays to each nostril 3 times/day; maximum dose: 8 sprays to each nostril per day; after symptoms are controlled, dose should be reduced to lowest effective amount; maintenance: 1 spray to each nostril once daily

Oral inhalation: **Note:** AeroBid® and Aerospan™ are not interchangeable on a mcg per mcg basis; dosing changes when switching from one to another. Doses should be titrated to the lowest dose once asthma is controlled:

AeroBid® and AeroBid®-M:

Manufacturer's recommendation:

Children: 6-15 years: 2 inhalations twice daily; maximum dose: 4 inhalations/day

Children ≥16 years and Adults: 2 inhalations twice daily; maximum dose: 8 inhalations/day

NIH Asthma Guidelines (NAEPP, 2002; NIH, 1997) [give in divided doses twice daily]:

Children ≤12 years:

"Low" dose: 500-750 mcg/day (2-3 puffs/day)

"Medium" dose: 1000-1250 mcg/day (4-5 puffs/day)

"High" dose: >1250 mcg/day (>5 puffs/day)

Children >12 years and Adults:

"Low" dose: 500-1000 mcg/day (2-4 puffs/day)

"Medium" dose: 1000-2000 mcg/day (4-8 puffs/day)

"High" dose: >2000 mcg/day (>8 puffs/day)

Aerospan™: Manufacturer's recommendation:

Children 6-11 years: Initial: 1 inhalation twice daily; maximum dose: 4 inhalations/day

Children ≥12 and Adults: 2 inhalations twice daily; maximum: 8 inhalations/day

Administration Shake well before use; do not spray in eyes

Oral inhalant: Rinse mouth after inhalation to decrease chance of oral candidiasis

Aerobid® and Aerobid®-M: Use a spacer for children <8 years of age

Aerospan™: Do not use with another spacer; product has a self-contained spacer; do not remove gray spacer from purple actuator; do not bite or chew gray spacer. Use at room temperature; do not use near heat or open flame. Inhaler must be primed by releasing 2 test sprays into the air (away from face) before first use and if the inhaler has not been used for >2 weeks. Begin inhalation immediately prior to actuation; a delay may reduce dose by ≥75%. Discard entire unit (metal canister, purple actuator, and gray spacer) when labeled number of metered doses has been used, even though canister is not completely empty. Do not immerse canister into water. Use by children should be supervised.

Intranasal: Clear nasal passages by blowing nose prior to use

Monitoring Parameters Check mucus membranes for signs of fungal infection; monitor growth in pediatric patients; monitor blood pressure with oral inhalation

Patient Information Notify physician if condition being treated persists or worsens; do not decrease dose or discontinue without physician approval. Avoid exposure to chicken pox or measles; if exposed, seek medical advice without delay.

Oral inhalation: Report sore mouth or mouth lesions to physician; carefully read and follow the patient instructions for use leaflet that accompanies the product

Additional Information Nasalide® and Nasarel® do not contain fluorocarbons. AeroBid® and AeroBid®-M contain fluorocarbon propellants. Aerospan™ does not contain fluorocarbons; it contains ethanol and tetrafluoroethane (HFA) as the propellent. The efficacy of Nasalide® and Nasarel® are similar; however, more nasal burning and stinging were reported with Nasalide®, and more taste problems (eg, aftertaste) were reported with Nasarel®. These differences are due to the different vehicles of the two products.

When using flunisolide oral inhalation to help reduce or discontinue oral corticosteroid therapy, begin corticosteroid taper after at least 1 week of flunisolide inhalation therapy; reduce dose of oral corticosteroid gradually, with next decrease after 1-2 weeks depending on patient's response; do not decrease prednisone faster than 2.5 mg/day on a weekly basis; monitor patients for signs of asthma instability and adrenal insufficiency (see Warnings); decrease flunisolide to lowest effective dose **after** prednisone reduction is complete. If bronchospasm with wheezing occurs after use of oral inhalation, a fast-acting bronchodilator may be used; discontinue orally inhaled corticosteroid and initiate alternative chronic therapy.

(Continued)

Flunisolide *(Continued)*

Dosage Forms Excipient information presented when available (limited, particularly for generics); consult specific product labeling.

Aerosol for oral inhalation:

AeroBid®: 250 mcg/actuation (7 g) [100 metered inhalations; contains CFCs]

AeroBid®-M: 250 mcg/actuation (7 g) [100 metered inhalations; contains CFCs; menthol flavor]

Aerospan™: 80 mcg/actuation (5.1 g) [60 metered inhalations; CFC free]; 80 mcg/actuation (8.9 g) [120 metered inhalations; CFC free]

Solution, intranasal [spray]: 29 mcg/actuation (25 mL) [200 sprays]

Nasarel®: 29 mcg/actuation (25 mL) [200 sprays; contains benzalkonium chloride]

References

Expert Panel Report 2, "Guidelines for the Diagnosis and Management of Asthma," *Clinical Practice Guidelines*, National Institutes of Health, National Heart, Lung, and Blood Institute, NIH Publication No. 94-4051, April, 1997.

"National Asthma Education and Prevention Program. Expert Panel Report: Guidelines for the Diagnosis and Management of Asthma Update on Selected Topics--2002," *J Allergy Clin Immunol*, 2002, 110(5 Suppl):S141-219.

Fluocinolone (floo oh SIN oh lone)

Medication Safety Issues

Sound-alike/look-alike issues:

Fluocinolone may be confused with fluocinonide

Related Information

Corticosteroids, Topical: Guidelines for Selection and Use *on page 1686*

U.S. Brand Names Capex™; Derma-Smoothe/FS®; Retisert™; Synalar®

Canadian Brand Names Capex™; Derma-Smoothe/FS®; Synalar®

Index Terms Fluocinolone Acetonide

Therapeutic Category Adrenal Corticosteroid; Anti-inflammatory Agent; Corticosteroid, Ophthalmic; Corticosteroid, Topical; Glucocorticoid

Generic Available Yes: Excludes ocular implant, oil, shampoo

Use Relief of susceptible inflammatory dermatosis

Capex™ shampoo: Adults: Treatment of seborrheic dermatitis of the scalp

Derma-Smoothe/FS®: Children ≥2 years: Moderate to severe atopic dermatitis (for use ≤4 weeks); Adults: Atopic dermatitis or psoriasis of the scalp

Retisert™ (ocular implant): Adults: treatment of chronic, noninfectious uveitis affecting the posterior segment of the eye

Pregnancy Risk Factor C

Lactation Excretion in breast milk unknown/use caution

Contraindications Hypersensitivity to fluocinolone or any component (see Warnings); fungal infection; TB of skin; herpes (including varicella)

Ocular implant: Additional contraindications include viral, fungal, and mycobacterial occular infections; hypersensitivity to other corticosteroids

Warnings

Topical: Infants and small children may be more susceptible to adrenal axis suppression from topical corticosteroid therapy; systemic effects may occur when used on large areas of the body, denuded areas, for prolonged periods of time, or with an occlusive dressing; Derma-Smoothe/FS® contains refined peanut oil, use with caution in patients with peanut hypersensitivity (see Additional Information). Hypothalamic pituitary adrenal (HPA) axis suppression may occur; acute adrenal insufficiency may occur with abrupt withdrawal after long term use or with stress; withdrawal or discontinuation should be done carefully; patients with HPA axis suppression may require doses of systemic glucocorticosteroids prior to, during, and after unusual stress (eg, surgery).

Ocular implant: Transient decrease in visual acuity of 1-4 weeks duration following implantation may occur. Increased IOP or glaucoma may occur; use with caution in glaucoma patients; routine monitoring of IOP is recommended; patients may require use of medications or other treatments to lower IOP. Prolonged use of ocular corticosteroids may also increase the risk of secondary occular infections, cataract formation, delayed wound healing, perforation of globe (if thinning of sclera occurs), or optic nerve damage. Unilateral implantation is recommended to minimize risk of postoperative infections in both eyes. Procedural complications with implantation may occur (eg, cataract formation, choroidal detachment, endophthalmitis, hypotony, retinal detachment, vitreous loss, or hemorrhage).

Precautions

Ocular implant: Safety and efficacy have not been established in children <12 years of age

Adverse Reactions

Topical products:

Dermatologic: Acne, hypopigmentation, allergic dermatitis, maceration of the skin, skin atrophy, folliculitis, hypertrichosis, striae, miliaria

Endocrine & metabolic: Hypothalamic-pituitary-adrenal (HPA) axis suppression, Cushing's syndrome, growth retardation

Local: Burning, itching, irritation, dryness

Miscellaneous: Secondary infection

Ocular implant:

Central nervous system: Dizziness, headache, pain, pyrexia

Dermatologic: Rash

Gastrointestinal: Nausea, vomiting

Neuromuscular and skeletal: Arthralgia, back pain, limb pain

Ocular: Cataracts, elevated IOP, glaucoma, eye pain or irritation, postprocedural complications (cataract fragments, implant migration, wound complications), decreased visual acuity, blurred vision, conjunctival hemorrhage or hyperemia, pruritus, hypotony, vitreous floaters or hemorrhage, ptosis, eye inflammation, eyelid edema, tearing, dry eye

Stability Store at controlled room temperature in tightly closed container

Ocular implant (Retisert™): Store in original container at 15°C to 25°C (59°F to 77°F); protect from freezing

Mechanism of Action Not well defined topically; possesses anti-inflammatory, antiproliferative, and immunosuppressive properties

Pharmacokinetics

Absorption:

Topical: Dependent on strength of preparation, amount applied, nature of skin at application site, vehicle, and use of occlusive dressing; increased in areas of skin damage, inflammation, or occlusion

Ocular implant: Systemic absorption is negligible

Duration: Ocular implant: Releases fluocinolone acetonide at a rate of 0.6 mcg/day, decreasing over 30 days to a steady-state release rate of 0.3-0.4 mcg/day for 30 months

Distribution:

Topical: Throughout local skin; absorbed drug is distributed rapidly into muscle, liver, skin, intestines, and kidneys

Ocular implant: Aqueous and vitreous humor

Metabolism: Primarily in skin; small amount absorbed into systemic circulation is primarily hepatic to inactive compounds

Excretion: Urine (primarily as glucuronide and sulfate, also as unconjugated products); feces (small amounts)

Usual Dosage

Children and Adults: Topical: Apply thin layer 2-4 times/day

Capex™ shampoo: Adults: Thoroughly wet hair and scalp; apply ≤1 ounce to scalp area; massage well; work into lather; allow to remain on scalp for 5 minutes; then rinse hair and scalp thoroughly; repeat daily until symptoms subside; **Note:** Once patient is symptom free, once weekly use usually keeps itching and flaking of dandruff from returning

Derma-Smoothe/FS®:

Children ≥2 years: Atopic dermatitis: Apply in a thin layer to moistened skin of affected area twice daily for ≤4 weeks

Adults:

Atopic dermatitis: Apply a thin layer to affected area 3 times/day

Scalp psoriasis: Thoroughly wet or dampen hair and scalp; apply to scalp in a thin layer, massage well, cover scalp with shower cap (supplied); leave for a minimum of 4 hours or overnight, then wash hair and rinse thoroughly

Retisert™ (ocular implant): Chronic uveitis: One silicone-encased tablet (0.59 mg) surgically implanted into the posterior segment of the eye is designed to release 0.6 mcg/day, decreasing over 30 days to a steady-state release rate of 0.3-0.4 mcg/day for 30 months. Recurrence of uveitis denotes depletion of tablet, requiring reimplantation.

Administration

Topical: Apply sparingly in a thin film; rub in lightly

Capex™ shampoo: Shake well before use; do not bandage, wrap, or cover treated scalp area unless directed by physician; discard shampoo after 3 months (**Note:** Pharmacist must empty the contents of the 12 mg fluocinolone acetonide capsule into the shampoo base before dispensing to patient)

Derma-Smoothe/FS®: Do not apply to face or diaper area; avoid application to intertriginous areas (may increase local adverse effects)

Ocular implant: Retisert™: Handle only by suture tab to avoid damaging the tablet integrity and adversely affecting release characteristics. Maintain strict adherence to aseptic handling of product; do not resterilize.

(Continued)

Fluocinolone *(Continued)*

Patient Information Topical products: Avoid contact with eyes; do not use for longer than directed; do not overuse; notify physician if condition being treated persists or worsens

Nursing Implications Do not use tight fitting diapers or plastic pants on a child being treated in diaper area; Derma-Smoothe/FS® is not recommended for diaper dermatitis

Additional Information Considered a moderate-potency steroid (Derma-Smoothe/FS® and Capex™ shampoo are considered to be low to medium potency); Derma-Smoothe/FS® is made with 48% refined peanut oil, NF (peanut protein is not detectable at 2.5 ppm)

Dosage Forms Excipient information presented when available (limited, particularly for generics); consult specific product labeling.

Cream, as acetonide: 0.01% (15 g, 60 g); 0.025% (15 g, 60 g)
  Synalar®: 0.025% (15 g, 60 g)
Oil, as acetonide:
  Derma-Smoothe/FS® [eczema oil]: 0.01% (120 mL) [contains peanut oil]
  Derma-Smoothe/FS® [scalp oil]: 0.01% (120 mL) [contains peanut oil; packaged with shower caps]
Ointment, as acetonide (Synalar®): 0.025% (15 g, 60 g)
Shampoo, as acetonide (Capex™): 0.01% (120 mL)
Solution, as acetonide: 0.01% (60 mL)
  Synalar®: 0.01% (20 mL, 60 mL)
Tablet, ocular implant, as acetonide (Retisert™): 0.59 mg [enclosed in silicone elastomer]

♦ **Fluocinolone Acetonide** *see* Fluocinolone *on page 672*

Fluocinonide (floo oh SIN oh nide)

Medication Safety Issues

Sound-alike/look-alike issues:
  Fluocinonide may be confused with flunisolide, fluocinolone
  Lidex® may be confused with Lasix®, Videx®, Wydase®

Related Information

Corticosteroids, Topical: Guidelines for Selection and Use *on page 1686*

U.S. Brand Names Lidex®; Lidex-E®; Vanos™

Canadian Brand Names Lidemol®; Lidex®; Lyderm®; Tiamol®; Topsyn®

Therapeutic Category Adrenal Corticosteroid; Anti-inflammatory Agent; Corticosteroid, Topical; Glucocorticoid

Generic Available Yes

Use Inflammation of corticosteroid-responsive dermatoses

Pregnancy Risk Factor C

Contraindications Hypersensitivity to fluocinonide or any component; viral, fungal, or tubercular skin lesions; herpes (including varicella)

Warnings Infants and small children may be more susceptible to adrenal axis suppression from topical corticosteroid therapy; systemic effects may occur when used on large areas of the body, denuded areas, for prolonged periods of time, or with occlusive dressings

Adverse Reactions

Dermatologic: Acne, hypopigmentation, allergic dermatitis, maceration of the skin, skin atrophy, folliculitis, hypertrichosis
Endocrine & metabolic: Hypothalamic-pituitary-adrenal suppression, Cushing's syndrome, growth retardation
Local: Burning, itching, irritation, dryness
Miscellaneous: Secondary infection

Mechanism of Action Not well defined topically; possesses anti-inflammatory, antiproliferative, and immunosuppressive properties

Usual Dosage Children and Adults: Topical: Apply thin layer to affected area 2-4 times/day depending on the severity of the condition

Administration Topical: Apply sparingly in a thin film; rub in lightly

Patient Information Do not overuse; avoid contact with eyes; do not use for longer than directed; avoid use on face; notify physician if condition being treated persists or worsens

Nursing Implications Do not use tight fitting diapers or plastic pants on a child being treated in the diaper area

Additional Information Considered to be a high potency steroid

Dosage Forms Excipient information presented when available (limited, particularly for generics); consult specific product labeling.

Cream, anhydrous, emollient (Lidex®): 0.05% (15 g, 30 g, 60 g)
Cream, aqueous, emollient (Lidex-E®): 0.05% (15 g, 30 g, 60 g)
Cream (Vanos™): 0.1% (30 g, 60 g)
Gel (Lidex®): 0.05% (15 g, 30 g, 60 g)
Ointment (Lidex®): 0.05% (15 g, 30 g, 60 g)
Solution (Lidex®): 0.05% (60 mL) [contains alcohol 35%]

- **Fluohydrisone Acetate** *see* Fludrocortisone *on page 666*
- **Fluohydrocortisone Acetate** *see* Fludrocortisone *on page 666*
- **Fluor-A-Day** *see* Fluoride *on page 675*

Fluoride (FLOR ide)

Medication Safety Issues
Sound-alike/look-alike issues:
Luride® may be confused with Lortab®
Phos-Flur® may be confused with PhosLo®
Thera-Flur-N® may be confused with Thera-Flu®
International issues:
Fluorex® [France] may be confused with Flarex® which is a brand name for fluorometholone in the U.S.

U.S. Brand Names ACT® [OTC]; ACT® Plus [OTC]; ACT® x2™ [OTC]; CaviRinse™; ControlRx®; Denta 5000 Plus; DentaGel; EtheDent™; Fluor-A-Day; Fluorigard® [OTC]; Fluorinse®; Flura-Drops®; Gel-Kam® [OTC]; Gel-Kam® Rinse; Just for Kids™ [OTC]; Lozi-Flur™; Luride®; Luride® Lozi-Tab®; NeutraCare®; NeutraGard® [OTC]; NeutraGard® Advanced; NeutraGard® Plus; Omnii Gel™ [OTC]; Pediaflor® [DSC]; PerioMed™; Pharmaflur®; Pharmaflur® 1.1; Phos-Flur®; Phos-Flur® Rinse [OTC]; PreviDent®; PreviDent® 5000 Plus™; StanGard®; StanGard® Perio; Stop®; Thera-Flur-N®

Canadian Brand Names Fluor-A-Day; Fluotic®

Index Terms Acidulated Phosphate Fluoride; Sodium Fluoride; Stannous Fluoride

Therapeutic Category Mineral, Oral; Mineral, Oral Topical

Generic Available Yes: Excludes lozenge, gel drops

Use Prevention of dental caries

Pregnancy Risk Factor C

Contraindications Hypersensitivity to fluoride or any component (see Warnings); when fluoride content of drinking water exceeds 0.7 ppm; low sodium or sodium-free diets; do not use 1 mg tablets in children <3 years of age or when drinking water fluoride content is ≥0.3 ppm; do not use 1 mg/5 mL rinse (as supplement) in children <6 years of age

Warnings Some products may contain tartrazine which may cause allergic reactions in susceptible individuals

Precautions Prolonged ingestion with excessive doses may result in dental fluorosis and osseous changes; dosage should be adjusted in proportion to the amount of fluoride in the drinking water; do **not** exceed recommended dosage

Adverse Reactions
Central nervous system: Headache
Dermatologic: Rash, eczema, atopic dermatitis, urticaria
Gastrointestinal: GI upset, nausea, vomiting
Miscellaneous: Products containing stannous fluoride may stain the teeth

Drug Interactions Magnesium-, aluminum-, and calcium-containing products may decrease absorption of fluoride

Food Interactions Do not administer with milk

Stability Sodium fluoride solutions decompose in glass containers; store only in tightly closed plastic containers; aqueous solutions of stannous fluoride decompose within hours of preparation; prepare solutions immediately before use

Mechanism of Action Promotes remineralization of decalcified enamel; inhibits the cariogenic microbial process in dental plaque; increases tooth resistance to acid dissolution

Pharmacokinetics
Absorption: Via GI tract, lungs, and skin
Distribution: 50% of fluoride is deposited in teeth and bone after ingestion; crosses placenta; appears in breast milk; topical application works superficially on enamel and plaque
Elimination: In urine and feces

Usual Dosage Oral:
Adequate Intake (AI) (1997 National Academy of Science Recommendations):
Children:
0-6 months: 0.01 mg/day
7-12 months: 0.5 mg/day
(Continued)

Fluoride *(Continued)*

1-3 years: 0.7 mg/day
4-8 years: 1 mg/day
9-13 years: 2 mg/day
14-18 years: 3 mg/day

Children >19 and Adults:

Males: 4 mg/day
Females: 3 mg/day

The recommended daily fluoride intake is adjusted in proportion to the fluoride content of available drinking water; see **Recommended Daily Fluoride Dose** table

Recommended Daily Fluoride Dose

Fluoride Content of Drinking Water	Daily Dose, Oral Fluoride (mg)
<0.3 ppm	
Birth - 6 mo	0
6 mo to 3 y	0.25
3-6 y	0.5
6-16 y	1
0.3-0.6 ppm	
Birth - 3 y	0
3-6 y	0.25
6-16 y	0.5
>0.6 ppm	
All ages	0

Adapted from *AAP News*, 1995, 11(2):18.

Dental rinse: See **Sodium Fluoride Dental Rinse Dosing** table

Sodium fluoride (dosage based upon concentration of solution):

Note: 2% concentrations are administered by dental personnel only

Sodium Fluoride Dental Rinse Dosing

Age	% Solution	Dosage
6 y	0.05%	10 mL daily
6-12 y	0.02%	10 mL twice daily
	0.2%	5 mL once weekly
>12 y	0.02%	10 mL twice daily
	0.2%	10 mL once weekly

Acidulated phosphate fluoride rinse: Children 6 years and Adults: 5-10 mL of 0.02% daily at bedtime

Gel:

Acidulated phosphate fluoride: Adults: 4-8 drops of 0.5% gel daily or for desensitizing exposed root surfaces, use a few drops of 0.5% to 1.2% gel applied and brushed onto affected area each night

Stannous fluoride: Children >6 years and Adults: Apply 0.4% gel to teeth once daily

Administration Oral:

Dental gel: Do **not** swallow; gel drops are placed in trough of applicator; applicator is applied over upper and lower teeth at same time; bite down for 6 minutes

Dental rinse: Swish or rinse in mouth then expectorate; do not swallow

Tablet: Dissolve in mouth, chew, swallow whole, or add to drinking water or fruit juice; administer with food (but not milk) to eliminate GI upset

Reference Range Total plasma fluoride: 0.14-0.19 mcg/mL

Dosage Forms Excipient information presented when available (limited, particularly for generics); consult specific product labeling. [DSC] = Discontinued product

Cream, oral, as sodium [toothpaste]: 1.1% (51 g) [fluoride 2.5 mg/dose]

Denta 5000 Plus: 1.1% (51g) [fluoride 2.5 mg/dose; spearmint flavor]

EtheDent™: 1.1% (51g) [fluoride 2.5 mg/dose]

Gel-drops, as sodium fluoride (Thera-Flur-N®): 1.1% (24 mL) [fluoride 0.5%; neutral pH; no artificial color or flavor]

Gel, topical, as acidulated phosphate fluoride (Phos-Flur®): 1.1% (60 g) [fluoride 0.5%; cherry and mint flavors]

Gel, topical, as sodium fluoride: 1.1% (56 g) [fluoride 2 mg/dose]

DentaGel, EtheDent™: 1.1% (56 g) [fluoride 2 mg/dose; fresh mint flavor]

NeutraCare®: 1.1% (60 g) [neutral pH; grape and mint flavors]

NeutraGard® Advanced: 1.1% (60 g) [cinnamon and mint flavors]
PreviDent®: 1.1% (60 g) [fluoride 2 mg/dose; berry, cherry, and mint flavors]
Gel, topical, as stannous fluoride:
Gel-Kam®: 0.4% (129 g) [bubble gum, cinnamon, fruit/berry, and mint flavors]
Just for Kids™: 0.4% (122 g) [bubble gum, fruit punch, and grapey grape flavors]
Omnii Gel™: 0.4% (122 g) [cinnamon, grape, natural, mint, and raspberry flavors]
StanGard®: 0.4% (122 g) [bubble gum, cherry, mint, and raspberry flavors]
Stop®: 0.4% (120 g) [bubble gum, cinnamon, grape, and mint flavors]
Lozenge, as sodium (Lozi-Flur™): 2.21 mg [fluoride 1 mg; cherry flavor]
Paste, oral, as sodium [toothpaste] (ControlRx®): 1.1% (56 g) [vanilla mint flavor]
Solution, oral drops, as sodium: 1.1 mg/mL (50 mL) [fluoride 0.5 mg/mL]
Flura-Drops®: 0.55 mg/drop (24 mL) [fluoride 0.25 mg/drop; dye free, sugar free]
Luride®: 1.1 mg/mL (50 mL) [fluoride 0.5 mg/mL; sugar free]
Pediaflor®: 1.1 mg/mL (50 mL) [fluoride 0.5 mg/mL; contains alcohol <0.5%; sugar free; cherry flavor] [DSC]
Solution, oral rinse, as sodium:
ACT®: 0.05% (530 mL) [fluoride 0.02%; bubble gum, cinnamon (contains tartrazine), and mint flavors]
ACT® Plus: 0.05% (530 mL) [fluoride 0.02%; alcohol free; icy cool mint flavor]
ACT® x2™: 0.5% (530 mL) [fluoride 0.02%; contains alcohol 11%; icy cool mint and spearmint flavors]
CaviRinse™: 0.2% (240 mL) [mint flavor]
Fluorigard®: 0.05% (480 mL) [alcohol free, sugar free; contains sodium benzoate and tartrazine; mint flavor]
Fluorinse®: 0.2% (480 mL) [alcohol free; cinnamon and mint flavors]
NeutraGard®: 0.05% (480 mL) [neutral pH; mint and tropical blast flavors]
NeutraGard® Plus: 0.2% (480 mL) [neutral pH; mint and tropical blast flavors]
Phos-Flur®: 0.44% (500 mL) [bubble gum, cherry, grape, and mint flavors]
PreviDent®: 0.2% (250 mL) [contains alcohol; mint flavor]
Solution, oral rinse concentrate, as stannous fluoride:
Gel-Kam®: 0.63% (300 mL) [fluoride 0.1%/dose; cinnamon and mint flavors]
PerioMed™: 0.63% (284 mL) [fluoride 7 mg/30 mL; alcohol free; cinnamon, mint and tropical fruit flavors]
StanGard® Perio: 0.63% (284 mL) [mint flavor]
Tablet, chewable, as sodium: 0.5 mg [fluoride 0.25 mg]; 1.1 mg [fluoride 0.5 mg]; 2.2 mg [fluoride 1 mg]
EtheDent™:
0.55 mg [fluoride 0.25 mg; sugar free; contains aspartame; vanilla flavor]
1.1 mg [fluoride 0.5 mg; sugar free; contains aspartame; grape flavor]
2.2 mg [fluoride 1 mg; sugar free; contains aspartame; cherry flavor]
Fluor-A-Day:
0.56 mg [fluoride 0.25 mg; raspberry flavor]
1.1 mg [fluoride 0.5 mg; raspberry flavor]
2.21 mg [fluoride 1 mg; raspberry flavor]
Luride® Lozi-Tab®:
0.55 mg [fluoride 0.25 mg; sugar free; vanilla flavor]
1.1 mg [fluoride 0.5 mg; sugar free; grape flavor]
2.2 mg [fluoride 1 mg; sugar free; cherry flavor]
Pharmaflur®: 2.2 mg [fluoride 1 mg; dye free, sugar free; cherry flavor]
Pharmaflur® 1.1: 1.1 mg [fluoride 0.5 mg; dye free, sugar free; grape flavor]

References

"Dietary Reference Intakes for Calcium, Phosphorus, Magnesium, Vitamin D, and Fluoride. Standing Committee on the Scientific Evaluation of Dietary Reference Intakes, Food and Nutrition Board, Institute of Medicine," National Academy of Sciences, Washington, DC: National Academy Press, 1997.

◆ **Fluorigard® [OTC]** *see* Fluoride *on page 675*
◆ **Fluorinse®** *see* Fluoride *on page 675*
◆ **5-Fluorocytosine** *see* Flucytosine *on page 662*
◆ **9α-Fluorohydrocortisone Acetate** *see* Fludrocortisone *on page 666*

Fluorometholone (flure oh METH oh lone)

Medication Safety Issues
International issues:
Flarex® may be confused with Flurets® which is a brand name for sodium fluoride in Australia
Flarex® may be confused with Fluarix® which is a brand name for influenza virus vaccine in the U.S. and in numerous international markets
Flarex® may be confused with Fluorex® which is a brand name for sodium fluoride in France
(Continued)

Fluorometholone *(Continued)*

Fluor-Op® may be confused with Fluoron® which is a brand name for fluorine in Canada

U.S. Brand Names Flarex®; FML®; FML® Forte

Canadian Brand Names Flarex®; FML®; FML Forte®; PMS-Fluorometholone

Therapeutic Category Adrenal Corticosteroid; Anti-inflammatory Agent, Ophthalmic; Corticosteroid, Ophthalmic; Glucocorticoid

Generic Available Yes: Suspension (as base)

Use Inflammatory conditions of the eye, including keratitis, iritis, cyclitis, and conjunctivitis

Pregnancy Risk Factor C

Lactation Excretion in breast milk unknown/use caution

Contraindications Hypersensitivity to fluorometholone, other corticosteroids, or any component; herpes simplex keratitis, fungal diseases of ocular structures, mycobacterial infections of the eye, and most viral diseases of cornea and conjunctiva

Warnings Not recommended for children <2 years of age

Precautions Prolonged use may result in glaucoma, increased intraocular pressure, or other ocular damage

Adverse Reactions

Local: Stinging, burning

Ocular: Elevated intraocular pressure, open-angle glaucoma, defect in visual acuity and field of vision, cataracts, photosensitivity

Mechanism of Action Decreases inflammation by suppression of migration of polymorphonuclear leukocytes and reversal of increased capillary permeability

Pharmacokinetics Absorption: Into aqueous humor with slight systemic absorption

Usual Dosage Children >2 years and Adults: Ophthalmic:

Ointment: May be applied every 4 hours in severe cases or 1-3 times/day in mild to moderate cases.

Drops: Instill 1-2 drops into conjunctival sac every hour during day, every 2 hours at night until favorable response is obtained, then use 1 drop every 4 hours; in mild or moderate inflammation: 1-2 drops into conjunctival sac 2-4 times/day.

Administration Ophthalmic: Avoid contact of medication tube or bottle tip with skin or eye; suspension: Shake well before use; apply finger pressure to lacrimal sac during and for 1-2 minutes after instillation to decrease risk of absorption and systemic effects; the preservative (benzalkonium chloride) may be absorbed by soft contact lenses; wait at least 15 minutes after administration of suspension before inserting soft contact lenses

Monitoring Parameters Intraocular pressure (if used ≥10 days)

Patient Information May cause blurring of vision; do not discontinue without consulting physician; notify physician if improvement does not occur after 2 days

Dosage Forms Excipient information presented when available (limited, particularly for generics); consult specific product labeling. [DSC] = Discontinued product

Ointment, ophthalmic, as base:

FML®: 0.1% (3.5 g)

Suspension, ophthalmic, as base: 0.1% (5 mL, 10 mL, 15 mL)

FML®: 0.1% (5 mL, 10 mL, 15 mL) [contains benzalkonium chloride]

FML® Forte: 0.25% (2 mL, 5 mL, 10 mL, 15 mL) [contains benzalkonium chloride]

Suspension, ophthalmic, as acetate:

Flarex®: 0.1% (5 mL) [contains benzalkonium chloride]

♦ **Fluoroplex®** *see* Fluorouracil *on page 678*

Fluorouracil (flure oh YOOR a sil)

Medication Safety Issues

Sound-alike/look-alike issues:

Fluorouracil may be confused with flucytosine

Efudex® may be confused with Efidac (Efidac 24®), Eurax®

High alert medication: The Institute for Safe Medication Practices (ISMP) includes this medication among its list of drugs which have a heightened risk of causing significant patient harm when used in error.

International issues:

Carac™ may be confused with Carace® which is a brand name for lisinopril in Ireland and Great Britain

Related Information

Compatibility of Chemotherapy and Related Supportive Care Medications *on page 1777*

Emetogenic Potential of Single Chemotherapeutic Agents *on page 1776*

U.S. Brand Names Adrucil®; Carac™; Efudex®; Fluoroplex®

Canadian Brand Names Efudex®

Index Terms 5-Fluorouracil; FU; 5-FU

Therapeutic Category Antineoplastic Agent, Antimetabolite

Generic Available Yes: Injection, topical solution

Use Treatment of carcinoma of stomach, colon, rectum, head and neck, breast, and pancreas; topically for management of multiple actinic or solar keratoses and superficial basal cell carcinomas

Pregnancy Risk Factor D (injection); X (topical)

Lactation Excretion in breast milk unknown/not recommended

Contraindications Hypersensitivity to fluorouracil or any component; patients with poor nutritional status, bone marrow suppression, thrombocytopenia; pregnancy; patients with dihydropyrimidine dehydrogenase (DPD) enzyme deficiency

Warnings The FDA currently recommends that procedures for proper handling and disposal of antineoplastic agents be considered; if intractable vomiting, diarrhea, stomatitis, hemorrhage, or precipitous falls in leukocyte or platelet counts occur, discontinue fluorouracil immediately

Systemic toxicity normally associated with parenteral administration (ie, neutropenia, neurotoxicity, stomatitis, diarrhea) has been reported with topical use particularly in patients with DPD enzyme deficiency. Avoid topical application to mucous membranes due to the possibility of local inflammation and ulceration.

Precautions Use with caution and modify dosage in patients with renal or hepatic impairment

Adverse Reactions

Cardiovascular: Cardiac arrhythmias, heart failure, hypotension, myocardial ischemia

Central nervous system: Headache, cerebellar ataxia (gait and speech abnormalities), somnolence, dizziness

Dermatologic: Alopecia, skin pigmentation, pruritic maculopapular rash, skin irritation, partial loss of nails or hyperpigmentation of nail bed, photosensitivity

Gastrointestinal: Nausea, vomiting, diarrhea, anorexia, GI hemorrhage, stomatitis, esophagitis

Hematologic: Myelosuppression, granulocytopenia, thrombocytopenia

Hepatic: Hepatotoxicity

Ocular: Visual disturbances, nystagmus, conjunctivitis, lacrimation

Miscellaneous: Palmar-plantar erythrodysesthesias (erythematous, desquamative rash involving hands and feet accompanied by pain, tingling, and swollen palms; this adverse effect may be treated with oral pyridoxine)

Drug Interactions Cimetidine (increases fluorouracil concentration); leucovorin may potentiate the antitumor activity of fluorouracil

Food Interactions Use of acidic solutions such as orange juice or other fruit juices to dilute fluorouracil for oral administration may result in precipitation of the drug and decreased absorption; increase dietary intake of thiamine

Stability Store at room temperature; protect from light; slight discoloration of injection during storage does not affect potency; if precipitate forms, redissolve drug by heating to 140°F, shake well; allow to cool to body temperature before administration; incompatible with cytarabine, diazepam, doxorubicin, methotrexate

Mechanism of Action A pyrimidine antimetabolite that inhibits thymidylate synthase leading to depletion of the DNA precursor thymidine; incorporated into RNA, DNA

Pharmacokinetics

Absorption: Oral: Erratic

Distribution: Into tumors, intestinal mucosa, liver, bone marrow, and CSF

Protein binding: <10%

Metabolism: Inactive metabolites are formed following metabolism in the liver

Bioavailability: 50% to 80%; variable due to saturable first-pass elimination process

Half-life, biphasic:

- Alpha: 10-20 minutes
- Terminal: 15-19 hours

Elimination: Biphasic elimination with <10% of dose excreted unchanged in the urine

Usual Dosage Children and Adults (refer to individual protocols with dose based on lean body weight):

I.V.:

- Initial: 400-500 mg/m^2/day (12 mg/kg/day; maximum dose: 800 mg/day) for 4-5 days
- Maintenance: 200-250 mg/m^2/dose (6 mg/kg) every other day for 4 doses; repeat in 4 weeks
- Single weekly bolus dose of 15 mg/kg or 500 mg/m^2 can be administered depending on the patient's reaction to the previous course of treatment; maintenance dose of 5-15 mg/kg/week as a single dose not to exceed 1 g/week

(Continued)

Fluorouracil *(Continued)*

I.V. infusion: 15 mg/kg/day or 500 mg/m^2/day (maximum daily dose: 1 g) has been given by I.V. infusion over 4 hours for 5 days; **or** 800-1200 mg/m^2 for continuous infusion over 24-120 hours

Oral: 15-20 mg/kg/day for 5-8 days has been used for colorectal carcinoma; 15 mg/kg/week for hepatoma

Topical:

Actinic keratoses:

Efudex®️ or Fluoroplex®️: Apply twice daily

Carac™: Apply once daily

Basal cell carcinoma: Efudex®️: Apply twice daily

Dosing adjustment in hepatic impairment: Bilirubin >5 mg/dL: Not recommended for use

Administration

Oral: Administer in early morning on an empty stomach; do not eat for 2 hours before and after dosage administration; dilute injectable fluorouracil solution dose in 4 oz of water or a diluted bicarbonate buffer solution to increase absorption; do not mix with orange juice or other fruit juices

Parenteral: Administer by direct I.V. injection (50 mg/mL solution needs no further dilution) over several minutes or by I.V. intermittent or continuous infusion diluted in saline or dextrose solutions; toxicity (eg, myelosuppression) may be reduced by giving the drug as a continuous infusion. Doses >750-800 mg/m^2 should be administered as a continuous infusion, **not** by bolus injection; dose-limiting toxicity with continuous infusion is mucous membrane toxicity (ie, stomatitis, diarrhea)

Topical: For external use only. Not for ophthalmic or intravaginal use. Cleanse affected area thoroughly and wait 10 minutes before applying. Apply with a nonmetallic applicator or gloved fingers in a sufficient amount to cover affected area. Avoid contact with eyes, eyelids, nostrils, and mouth. Do not cover area with an occlusive dressing

1% or 2%: Apply to lesions on the head and neck for the treatment of multiple actinic keratoses

5%: Use on lesions in areas other than the head and neck for multiple actinic keratoses; only 5% preparations are used for the treatment of superficial basal cell carcinoma

Monitoring Parameters CBC with differential and platelet count, renal function tests, liver function tests; observe for changes in bowel frequency

Patient Information Avoid alcohol; maintain adequate hydration; report signs and symptoms of infection, bleeding, bruising, vision changes, unremitting nausea, vomiting, or diarrhea, chest pain or palpitations, or CNS changes. May cause photosensitivity reactions (eg, exposure to sunlight may cause severe sunburn, skin rash, redness, or itching); avoid exposure to sunlight and artificial light sources (sunlamps, tanning booth/bed); wear protective clothing, wide-brimmed hats, sunglasses, and lip sunscreen (SPF ≥15); use a sunscreen [broad-spectrum sunscreen or physical sunscreen (preferred) or sunblock with SPF ≥15]; contact physician if reaction occurs. Women of childbearing age should be advised to avoid becoming pregnant.

Nursing Implications Wash hands immediately after topical application of the cream or solution

Additional Information Myelosuppressive effects:

WBC: Mild

Platelets: Mild

Onset (days): 7-10

Nadir (days): 9-14

Recovery (days): 21

Dosage Forms Excipient information presented when available (limited, particularly for generics); consult specific product labeling.

Cream, topical:

Carac™: 0.5% (30 g)

Efudex®️: 5% (25 g, 40 g)

Fluoroplex®️: 1% (30 g) [contains benzyl alcohol]

Injection, solution: 50 mg/mL (10 mL, 20 mL, 50 mL, 100 mL)

Adrucil®️: 50 mg/mL (10 mL, 50 mL, 100 mL)

Solution, topical (Efudex®️): 2% (10 mL); 5% (10 mL)

References

Balis FM, Holcenberg JS and Bleyer WA, "Clinical Pharmacokinetics of Commonly Used Anticancer Drugs," *Clin Pharmacokinet*, 1983, 8(3):202-32.

♦ **5-Fluorouracil** *see* Fluorouracil *on page 678*

♦ **Fluotic®️ (Can)** *see* Fluoride *on page 675*

Fluoxetine (floo OKS e teen)

Medication Safety Issues

Sound-alike/look-alike issues:

Fluoxetine may be confused with duloxetine, fluvastatin, fluvoxamine

Prozac® may be confused with Prilosec®, Proscar®, ProSom®, ProStep®

Sarafem® may be confused with Serophene®

International issues:

Fluoxin® [Czech Republic and Romania] may be confused with Floxin® which is a brand name for ofloxacin in the U.S.

Prozac® may be confused with Prazac® a brand of prazosin in Denmark

Reneuron® [Spain] may be confused with Remeron® a brand of mirtazapine in the U.S.

Related Information

Antidepressant Agents *on page 1681*

Serotonin Syndrome *on page 1955*

U.S. Brand Names Prozac®; Prozac® Weekly™; Sarafem®

Canadian Brand Names Alti-Fluoxetine; Apo-Fluoxetine®; BCI-Fluoxetine; CO Fluoxetine; FXT; Gen-Fluoxetine; Novo-Fluoxetine; Nu-Fluoxetine; PMS-Fluoxetine; Prozac®; Rhoxal-fluoxetine; Sandoz-Fluoxetine

Index Terms Fluoxetine Hydrochloride

Therapeutic Category Antidepressant, Selective Serotonin Reuptake Inhibitor (SSRI)

Generic Available Yes: Excludes delayed release capsule

Use Treatment of major depressive disorder, obsessive-compulsive disorder, bulimia nervosa, premenstrual dysphoric disorder (PMDD), panic disorder with or without agoraphobia

Medication Guide An FDA-approved patient medication guide, which is available with the product information and at http://www.fda.gov/cder/Offices/ODS/medication_guides.htm, must be dispensed with this medication for each new outpatient prescription and refill.

Pregnancy Risk Factor C

Lactation Enters breast milk/not recommended (AAP rates "of concern")

Contraindications Hypersensitivity to fluoxetine or any component; use of MAO inhibitors within 14 days (potentially fatal reactions may occur, see Drug Interactions; do not use MAO inhibitors for at least 5 weeks after fluoxetine is discontinued); concurrent use of thioridazine or use within 5 weeks after fluoxetine is discontinued (see Drug Interactions); concurrent use of pimozide

Warnings Fluoxetine is approved for use in pediatric patients only for the treatment of major depressive disorder and obsessive compulsive disorder. Clinical worsening of depression or suicidal ideation and behavior may occur in children and adults with major depressive disorder. In clinical trials, antidepressants increased the risk of suicidal thinking and behavior (suicidality) in children, adolescents, and young adults (18-24 years of age) with major depressive disorder and other psychiatric disorders. This risk must be considered before prescribing antidepressants for any clinical use. Short-term studies did **not** show an increased risk of suicidality with antidepressant use in patients >24 years of age and showed a decreased risk in patients ≥65 years.

Patients of all ages who are treated with antidepressants for any indication require appropriate monitoring and close observation for clinical worsening of depression, suicidality, and unusual changes in behavior, especially during the first few months after antidepressant initiation or when the dose is adjusted. Family members and caregivers should be instructed to closely observe the patient (ie, daily) and communicate condition with healthcare provider. Patients should also be monitored for associated behaviors (eg, anxiety, agitation, panic attacks, insomnia, irritability, hostility, aggressiveness, impulsivity, akathisia, hypomania, mania) which may increase the risk for worsening depression or suicidality. Worsening depression or emergence of suicidality (or associated behaviors listed above) that is abrupt in onset, severe, or not part of the presenting symptoms, may require discontinuation or modification of drug therapy.

Avoid abrupt discontinuation; discontinuation symptoms (including agitation, dysphoria, anxiety, confusion, dizziness, hypomania, nightmares, and other symptoms) may occur if therapy is abruptly discontinued or dose reduced; taper the dose to minimize risks of discontinuation symptoms; if intolerable symptoms occur following a decrease in dosage or upon discontinuation of therapy, consider resuming the previous dose with a more gradual taper. To reduce risk of intentional overdose, write prescriptions for the smallest quantity consistent with good patient care. Screen individuals for bipolar disorder prior to treatment (using antidepressants alone may induce manic episodes in patients with this condition). Potentially fatal serotonin syndrome may occur when SSRIs are used in combination with serotonergic drugs

(Continued)

Fluoxetine *(Continued)*

(eg, triptans) or drugs that impair the metabolism of serotonin (eg, MAO inhibitors); see Drug Interactions.

Rash or urticaria may occur along with leukocytosis, fever, edema, arthralgia, lymphadenopathy, respiratory distress, and other symptoms; rare cases of vasculitis and lupus-like syndrome have been reported; anaphylactoid reactions including laryngospasm, bronchospasm, angioedema, and urticaria may occur; discontinue use if rash or other allergic reaction occurs

Oral solution contains benzoic acid; benzoic acid (benzoate) is a metabolite of benzyl alcohol; large amounts of benzyl alcohol (≥99 mg/kg/day) have been associated with a potentially fatal toxicity ("gasping syndrome") in neonates; avoid use of fluoxetine products containing benzoic acid in neonates; *in vitro* and animal studies have shown that benzoate displaces bilirubin from protein binding sites

Precautions May cause abnormal bleeding (eg, ecchymosis, purpura, upper GI bleeding); use with caution in patients with impaired platelet aggregation and with concurrent use of aspirin, NSAIDs, or other drugs that affect coagulation. May cause insomnia, anxiety, nervousness, anorexia, or weight loss. Use with caution in patients where weight loss is undesirable. May impair cognitive or motor performance. Use with caution in patients with renal or hepatic impairment, seizure disorders, cardiac dysfunction, diabetes mellitus; use with caution during third trimester of pregnancy [newborns may experience adverse effects or withdrawal symptoms (consider risk and benefits); see Additional Information; exposure to SSRIs late in pregnancy may also be associated with an increased risk for persistent pulmonary hypertension of the newborn (see Chambers, 2006)]. Use with caution in patients receiving diuretics or those who are volume-depleted (may cause hyponatremia or SIADH). Decrease dose in liver dysfunction; use with caution in patients at high risk for suicide; add or initiate other antidepressants with caution after 5 weeks or longer after stopping fluoxetine.

Fluoxetine may cause decreased growth (smaller increases in weight and height) in children and adolescent patients; currently, no studies directly evaluate fluoxetine's long term effects on growth, development, and maturation of pediatric patients; periodic monitoring of height and weight in pediatric patients is recommended **Note:** Case reports of decreased growth in children receiving fluoxetine or fluvoxamine (n=4; age: 11.6-13.7 years) for 6 months to 5 years suggest a suppression of growth hormone secretion during SSRI therapy (see Weintrob, 2002). Further studies are needed.

Significant toxicities have been observed after exposure to fluoxetine in juvenile animals (some occurring at clinically relevant doses). Toxicities included myotoxicity (eg, skeletal muscle damage and necrosis, elevated serum CPK), impaired bone development, and long-term neurobehavioral and reproductive toxicity. The clinical significance of these findings is uncertain.

Adverse Reactions Predominant adverse effects are CNS and GI:

Cardiovascular: Vasodilation

Central nervous system: Headache, nervousness, insomnia, drowsiness, anxiety, dizziness, fatigue, sedation, somnolence, mania, hypomania, irritability, extrapyramidal reactions (rare); difficulty concentrating, abnormal dreams; suicidal thinking and behavior (see Warnings)

Note: SSRI-associated behavioral activation (ie, restlessness, hyperkinesis, hyperactivity, agitation) is 2- to 3-fold more prevalent in children compared to adolescents; it is more prevalent in adolescents compared to adults. Somnolence (including sedation and drowsiness) is more common in adults compared to children and adolescents (see Safer, 2006).

Dermatologic: Rash, urticaria, pruritus

Endocrine & metabolic: Hypoglycemia; hyponatremia, SIADH (usually in volume-depleted patients); sexual dysfunction, decreased libido, weight loss

Gastrointestinal: Nausea, diarrhea, xerostomia, anorexia, dyspepsia, constipation; decreased growth in pediatric patients

Note: SSRI-associated vomiting is 2- to 3-fold more prevalent in children compared to adolescents; it is more prevalent in adolescents compared to adults.

Hematologic: Altered platelet function (rare)

Neuromuscular & skeletal: Tremor, asthenia, weakness

Ocular: Visual disturbances

Respiratory: Rhinitis, pharyngitis, yawn

Miscellaneous: Anaphylactoid reactions, allergies, diaphoresis, flu-like syndrome; withdrawal symptoms following abrupt discontinuation (see Warnings)

Drug Interactions Cytochrome P450 isoenzyme CYP2D6 substrate (minor pathway), CYP3A3/4 substrate; CYP2C9 isoenzyme inducer; CYP1A2 (at higher doses), CYP2C9, CYP2C19, CYP2D6, CYP3A3/4 isoenzyme inhibitor (extent of CYP3A4

inhibition may not be clinically significant; however, the metabolite norfluoxetine is a more potent CYP3A inhibitor)

With MAO inhibitors, fever, tremors, seizures, delirium, coma may occur [use of MAO inhibitors within 14 days of fluoxetine use is contraindicated; do not use MAO inhibitors for at least 5 weeks after fluoxetine is discontinued (due to long elimination half-life of fluoxetine and its active metabolite)]. Tryptophan (which can be metabolized to serotonin) may increase CNS and GI toxic effects and the herbal medicine St John's wort (*Hypericum perforatum*) may increase serious side effects (the use of these agents is **not** recommended). Fluoxetine may inhibit metabolism and increase effects of tricyclic antidepressants (dosage reduction of TCA and monitoring of TCA plasma concentrations may be needed when fluoxetine is coadministered or has been recently discontinued), trazodone, phenytoin, carbamazepine, haloperidol, clozapine, alprazolam, and diazepam. Fluoxetine may inhibit the metabolism of thioridazine and increase the risk of serious adverse effects, such as QT_c prolongation, serious ventricular arrhythmias (eg, torsade de pointes) and sudden death (concurrent use of thioridazine or use within 5 weeks of discontinuation of fluoxetine is contraindicated). Concurrent use of fluoxetine with pimozide is contraindicated due to potential drug interactions or QT_c prolongation. Fluoxetine may antagonize buspirone effects; may displace highly protein bound drugs and cause adverse effects; may increase prothrombin time in patients receiving warfarin; use with NSAIDs, aspirin, or other drugs that affect coagulation may increase risk for bleeding; use with sumatriptan may cause weakness, incoordination, and hyper-reflexia; may increase or decrease serum lithium levels (monitor levels closely); concurrent use of fluoxetine with ritonavir may cause the serotonin syndrome (monitor closely)

Food Interactions Tryptophan supplements may increase CNS and GI adverse effects (eg, restlessness, agitation, GI problems); its use is **not recommended**. Food does not affect bioavailability, but may delay absorption by 1-2 hours

Stability Store at room temperature; protect tablets, immediate release capsules, and solution from light

Mechanism of Action Inhibits CNS neuron serotonin uptake; minimal or no effect on reuptake of norepinephrine or dopamine; does not significantly bind to alpha-adrenergic, histamine or cholinergic receptors; may therefore be useful in patients at risk from sedation, hypotension and anticholinergic effects of tricyclic antidepressants

Pharmacodynamics Maximum effect: Maximum antidepressant effects usually occur after >4 weeks; due to long half-life, resolution of adverse reactions after discontinuation may be slow

Pharmacokinetics Note: Average steady-state fluoxetine serum concentrations in children (n=10; 6 to <13 years of age) were 2-fold higher than in adolescents (n=11; 13 to <18 years of age); all patients received 20 mg/day; average steady-state norfluoxetine serum concentrations were 1.5-fold higher in the children compared with adolescents; differences in weight almost entirely explained the differences in serum concentrations

Absorption: Oral: Well absorbed; enteric-coated pellets contained in Prozac® Weekly™ resist dissolution until GI pH >5.5 and therefore delay onset of absorption 1-2 hours compared to immediate release formulations

Distribution: Adults: V_d: 20-45 L/kg; widely distributed

Protein binding: ~95% (albumin and alpha$_1$-glycoprotein)

Metabolism: In the liver to norfluoxetine (active) and other metabolites

Bioavailability: Capsules, tablets, solution, and weekly capsules are bioequivalent

Half-life: Adults:

- Fluoxetine: Acute dosing: 1-3 days; chronic dosing: 4-6 days; cirrhosis: 7.6 days
- Norfluoxetine: Acute and chronic dosing: 4-16 days; cirrhosis: 12 days

Time to peak serum concentration: Immediate release formulation: After 6-8 hours

Elimination: In urine as fluoxetine (2.5% to 5%) and norfluoxetine (10%)

Usual Dosage Oral:

Children and Adolescents:

Depression: 8-18 years of age: Manufacturer's recommendation: Initial: 10-20 mg/day; in patients started at 10 mg/day, may increase dose to 20 mg/day after 1 week. Lower weight children: Initial: 10 mg/day; usual: 10 mg/day; if needed, may increase dose to 20 mg/day after several weeks.

Note: Some experts recommend the following lower initial doses: Children ≤11 years: Initial: 5 mg/day; children ≥12 years: Initial: 10 mg/day; clinically, doses have been titrated up to 40 mg/day in pediatric patients (see Dopheide, 2006).

Obsessive-compulsive disorder: 7-18 years of age:

Lower weight children: Initial: 10 mg/day; if needed, may increase dose after several weeks; usual range: 20-30 mg/day; minimal experience with doses >20 mg/day; no experience with doses >60 mg/day

(Continued)

Fluoxetine *(Continued)*

Higher weight children and Adolescents: Initial: 10 mg/day; may increase dose to 20 mg/day after 2 weeks; may increase dose after several more weeks, if needed; usual range: 20-60 mg/day

Elective mutism: 6 children 6-12 years of age with elective mutism were treated with initial doses of 0.2 mg/kg/day for 1 week, then 0.4 mg/kg/day for 1 week, then 0.6 mg/kg/day for 10 weeks (Black,1994); further studies are needed

Adults:

Depression or obsessive-compulsive disorder: Initial dose: 20 mg/day administered in the morning; may increase after several weeks by 20 mg/day increments; maximum dose: 80 mg/day; doses >20 mg/day can be given either once daily (in the morning) or divided into morning or noon doses

Depression: Weekly dosing: Patients maintained on 20 mg/day may be changed to Prozac® Weekly™ 90 mg/week, starting 7 days after the last 20 mg/day dose

Bulimia nervosa: 60 mg/day administered in the morning; may need to titrate up to this dose over several days in some patients; higher doses have not been well studied

Premenstrual dysphoric disorder: 20 mg/day; given continuously (every day), **or** 20 mg/day given intermittently (starting the daily dose 14 days prior to the expected onset of menstruation with administration of daily dose through the first full day of menses); repeat with each menstrual cycle; doses >60 mg/day have not been studied; maximum dose: 80 mg/day

Panic disorder: Initial: 10 mg/day; increase dose to 20 mg/day after 1 week; if needed, may increase dose further after several weeks; doses >60 mg/day have not been evaluated

Dosage adjustment in renal impairment: Adjustment not routinely needed

Dosage adjustment in hepatic impairment: Lower doses or less frequent administration are recommended

Administration Oral: May be administered without regard to food

Monitoring Parameters Liver function, weight, serum glucose; serum sodium (in volume depleted patients); monitor for rash and signs or symptoms of anaphylactoid reactions; monitor height and weight in pediatric patients periodically. Monitor patient periodically for symptom resolution; monitor for worsening depression, suicidality, and associated behaviors (especially at the beginning of therapy or when doses are increased or decreased; see Warnings)

Reference Range

Therapeutic: Fluoxetine 100-800 ng/mL (SI: 289-2314 nmol/L); norfluoxetine 100-600 ng/mL (SI: 289-1735 nmol/L)

Toxic: (Fluoxetine plus norfluoxetine): >2000 ng/mL (SI: >5784 nmol/L)

Patient Information Read the patient Medication Guide that you receive with each prescription and refill of fluoxetine. An increased risk of suicidal thinking and behavior has been reported with the use of antidepressants in children, adolescents, and young adults (18-24 years of age). Notify physician if you feel more depressed, have thoughts of suicide, or become more agitated or irritable (see Warnings). Avoid alcohol, tryptophan supplements, and the herbal medicine St John's wort; avoid aspirin, NSAIDs, or other drugs that affect coagulation (may increase risks of bleeding); may cause dizziness or drowsiness and impair ability to perform activities requiring mental alertness or physical coordination; may cause dry mouth; inform physician immediately if hives or rash develops. Some medicines should not be taken with fluoxetine or should not be taken for a while after fluoxetine has been discontinued; report the use of other medications, nonprescription medications, and herbal or natural products to your physician and pharmacist. Take as directed; do not alter dose or frequency without consulting prescriber, avoid abrupt discontinuation.

Nursing Implications Last dose of the day should be given before 4 PM (to avoid insomnia). Assess other medications patient may be taking for possible interaction (especially MAO inhibitors, P450 inhibitors, and other CNS active agents). Assess mental status for depression, suicidal ideation, anxiety, social functioning, mania, or panic attack.

Additional Information If used for an extended period of time, long-term usefulness of fluoxetine should be periodically re-evaluated for the individual patient. A recent report describes 5 children (age: 8-15 years) who developed epistaxis (n=4) or bruising (n=1) while receiving SSRI therapy (sertraline) (Lake, 2000).

Neonates born to women receiving SSRIs later during the third trimester may experience respiratory distress, apnea, cyanosis, temperature instability, vomiting, feeding difficulty, hypoglycemia, constant crying, irritability, hypotonia, hypertonia, hyper-reflexia, tremor, jitteriness, and seizures; these symptoms may be due to a direct toxic effect, withdrawal syndrome, or (in some cases) serotonin syndrome. Withdrawal symptoms occur in 30% of neonates exposed to SSRIs *in utero*; monitor newborns for at least 48 hours after birth; long-term effects of *in utero* exposure to SSRIs are unknown (see Levinson-Castiel, 2006).

Dosage Forms Available as fluoxetine hydrochloride; mg strength refers to fluoxetine; [DSC] = Discontinued product

Capsule, as hydrochloride: 10 mg, 20 mg, 40 mg

Prozac®: 10 mg, 20 mg, 40 mg

Sarafem®: 10 mg, 20 mg

Capsule, delayed release, as hydrochloride (Prozac® Weekly™): 90 mg

Solution, oral, as hydrochloride (Prozac®): 20 mg/5 mL (120 mL) [contains alcohol 0.23% and benzoic acid; mint flavor]

Tablet, as hydrochloride: 10 mg, 20 mg

Prozac® [scored]: 10 mg [DSC]

Extemporaneous Preparations Dilutions of the commercially available oral solution may be made; 1 mg/mL and 2 mg/mL dilutions in Simple Syrup USP, Simple Syrup - British Pharmacopoeia, Aromatic Elixir USP, grape-cranberry drink (Ocean Spray® Cran-Grape), and deionized water were stable for 8 weeks when stored in amber glass bottles at 5°C and 30°C (Peterson, 1994).

Peterson JA, Risley DS, Anderson PN, et al, "Stability of Fluoxetine Hydrochloride in Fluoxetine Solution Diluted With Common Pharmaceutical Diluents," *Am J Hosp Pharm*, 1994, 51(10):1342-5.

References

Black B and Uhde TW, "Treatment of Elective Mutism With Fluoxetine: A Double Blind, Placebo-Controlled Study," *J Am Acad Child Adolesc Psychiatry*, 1994, 33(7):1000-6.

Chambers CD, Hernandez-Diaz S, Van Marter LJ, et al, "Selective Serotonin-Reuptake Inhibitors and Risk of Persistent Pulmonary Hypertension of the Newborn," *N Engl J Med*, 2006, 354(6):579-87.

Como PG and Kurlan R, "An Open-Label Trial of Fluoxetine for Obsessive-Compulsive Disorder in Gilles de la Tourette's Syndrome," *Neurology*, 1991, 41(6):872-4.

DeSilva KE, Le Flore DB, Marston BJ, et al, "Serotonin Syndrome in HIV-Infected Individuals Receiving Antiretroviral Therapy and Fluoxetine," *AIDS*, 2001, 15(10):1201-5.

Dopheide JA, "Recognizing and Treating Depression in Children and Adolescents," *Am J Health Syst Pharm*, 2006, 63(3):233-43.

Emslie GJ, Rush AJ, Weinberg WA, et al, "A Double-Blind, Randomized, Placebo-Controlled Trial of Fluoxetine in Children and Adolescents With Depression," *Arch Gen Psychiatry*, 1997, 54(11):1031-7.

Findling RL, Reed MD, and Blumer JL, "Pharmacological Treatment of Depression in Children and Adolescents," *Paediatr Drugs*, 1999, 1(3):161-82.

Kurlan R, Como PG, Deeley C, et al, "A Pilot Controlled Study of Fluoxetine for Obsessive-Compulsive Symptoms in Children With Tourette's Syndrome," *Clin Neuropharmacol*, 1993, 16(2):167-72.

Lake MB, Birmaher B, Wassick S, et al, "Bleeding and Selective Serotonin Reuptake Inhibitors in Childhood and Adolescence," *J Child Adolesc Psychopharmacol*, 2000, 10(1):35-8.

Levinson-Castiel R, Merlob P, Linder N, et al, "Neonatal Abstinence Syndrome After *in utero* Exposure to Selective Serotonin Reuptake Inhibitors in Term Infants," *Arch Pediatr Adolesc Med*, 2006, 160(2):173-6.

Riddle MA, Hardin MT, King R, et al, "Fluoxetine Treatment of Children and Adolescents With Tourette's and Obsessive-Compulsive Disorders: Preliminary Clinical Experience," *J Am Acad Child Adolesc Psychiatry*, 1990, 29(1):45-8.

Riddle MA, Scahill L, King RA, et al, "Double-Blind, Crossover Trial of Fluoxetine and Placebo in Children and Adolescents With Obsessive-Compulsive Disorder," *J Am Acad Child Adolesc Psychiatry*, 1992, 31(6):1062-9.

Safer DJ and Zito JM, "Treatment Emergent Adverse Effects of Selective Serotonin Reuptake Inhibitors by Age Group: Children vs. Adolescents," *J Child Adolesc Psychopharmacol*, 2006, 16(1/2):159-69.

Sharp SC and Hellings JA, "Efficacy and Safety of Selective Serotonin Reuptake Inhibitors in the Treatment of Depression in Children and Adolescents: Practitioner Review," *Clin Drug Investig*, 2006, 26(5):247-55.

Thomsen PH, "Obsessive-Complusive Disorder: Pharmacological Treatment," *Eur Child Adolesc Psychiatry*, 2000, 9 Suppl 1:I76-84.

Wagner KD, "Pharmacotherapy for Major Depression in Children and Adolescents," *Prog Neuropsychopharmacol Biol Psychiatry*, 2005, 29(5):819-26.

Weintrob N, Cohen D, Klipper-Aurbach Y, et al, "Decreased Growth During Therapy With Selective Serotonin Reuptake Inhibitors," *Arch Pediatr Adolesc Med*, 2002, 156(7):696-701.

♦ **Fluoxetine Hydrochloride** *see* Fluoxetine *on page 681*

Fluoxymesterone (floo oks i MES te rone)

Medication Safety Issues

Sound-alike/look-alike issues:

Halotestin® may be confused with Haldol®, haloperidol, halothane

U.S. Brand Names Halotestin®

Therapeutic Category Androgen

Generic Available Yes

Use Replacement of endogenous testicular hormone; in females used as palliative treatment of breast cancer, postpartum breast engorgement

Restrictions C-III

Pregnancy Risk Factor X

Lactation Excretion in breast milk unknown/contraindicated

Contraindications Hypersensitivity to fluoxymesterone or any component (see Warnings); serious cardiac disease, liver or kidney disease

Warnings Some tablets (brand name) contain tartrazine which may cause allergic reactions in susceptible individuals

Precautions May accelerate bone maturation without producing compensatory gain in linear growth; in prepubertal children perform radiographic examination of the hand

(Continued)

Fluoxymesterone *(Continued)*

and wrist every 6 months to determine the rate of bone maturation and to assess the effect of treatment on the epiphyseal centers

Adverse Reactions

Cardiovascular: Edema

Central nervous system: Anxiety, mental depression, headache

Dermatologic: Acne, hirsutism

Endocrine & metabolic: Gynecomastia, amenorrhea, hypercalcemia, female virilization

Gastrointestinal: Nausea

Genitourinary: Priapism

Hematologic: Polycythemia, suppression of clotting factors II, VII, IX, X

Hepatic: Cholestatic hepatitis

Neuromuscular & skeletal: Paresthesia

Miscellaneous: Hypersensitivity reactions

Drug Interactions May potentiate the action of oral anticoagulants; may decrease blood glucose concentrations and insulin requirements in patients with diabetes; may elevate cyclosporin levels; may increase extrapyramidal side effects and other CNS effects when coadministered with lithium; may potentiate respiratory depressant effects of narcotics

Mechanism of Action Synthetic androgenic anabolic steroid hormone responsible for the normal growth and development of male sex organs and maintenance of secondary sex characteristics; synthetic testosterone derivative with significant androgen activity; stimulates RNA polymerase activity resulting in an increase in protein production; increases bone development

Pharmacokinetics

Absorption: Oral: Rapid

Protein binding: 98%

Metabolism: In the liver

Half-life: 10-100 minutes

Elimination: Enterohepatic circulation and urinary excretion (90%)

Halogenated derivative of testosterone with up to 5 times the activity of methyltestosterone

Usual Dosage Adults: Oral:

Male:

Hypogonadism: 5-20 mg/day

Delayed puberty: 2.5-20 mg/day for 4-6 months

Female:

Inoperable breast carcinoma: 10-40 mg/day in divided doses for 1-3 months

Breast engorgement: 2.5 mg after delivery, 5-10 mg/day in divided doses for 4-5 days

Monitoring Parameters Periodic radiographic exams of hand and wrist (when used in children); hemoglobin, hematocrit (if receiving high dosages or long-term therapy)

Dosage Forms Excipient information presented when available (limited, particularly for generics); consult specific product labeling. [DSC] = Discontinued product

Tablet: 10 mg

Halotestin®: 2 mg, 5 mg, 10 mg [contains tartrazine; 10 mg tablet DSC]

♦ **Flura-Drops®** *see* Fluoride *on page 675*

Flurazepam (flure AZ e pam)

Medication Safety Issues

Sound-alike/look-alike issues:

Flurazepam may be confused with temazepam

Dalmane® may be confused with Demulen®, Dialume®

Related Information

Overdose and Toxicology *on page 1916*

U.S. Brand Names Dalmane®

Canadian Brand Names Apo-Flurazepam®; Dalmane®; Som Pam

Index Terms Flurazepam Hydrochloride

Therapeutic Category Benzodiazepine; Hypnotic; Sedative

Generic Available Yes

Use Short-term treatment of insomnia

Restrictions C-IV

Pregnancy Risk Factor X

Lactation Excretion in breast milk unknown/not recommended

Contraindications Hypersensitivity to flurazepam or any component (there may be cross-sensitivity with other benzodiazepines), pregnancy, pre-existing CNS depression, respiratory depression, narrow-angle glaucoma

Warnings Hypersensitivity reactions including anaphylaxis and angioedema may occur. Hazardous sleep-related activities, such as sleep-driving (driving while not fully awake without any recollection of driving), preparing and eating food, and making phone calls while asleep have also been reported. Effects with other sedative drugs or ethanol may be potentiated.

Precautions Use with caution in patients receiving other CNS depressants and in patients with low albumin or hepatic dysfunction

Adverse Reactions

Central nervous system: Drowsiness, dizziness, confusion; residual daytime sedation; paradoxical reactions, hyperactivity, and excitement (rare), ataxia

Miscellaneous: Physical and psychological dependence with prolonged use; hypersensitivity reactions, anaphylaxis, angioedema; hazardous sleep-related activities (see Warnings)

Drug Interactions Cytochrome P450 isoenzyme CYP3A3/4 substrate

Additive CNS depression with other CNS depressants, alcohol; cimetidine may decrease and enzyme inducers may increase metabolism of flurazepam; concurrent use of flurazepam with ritonavir is not recommended

Mechanism of Action Depresses all levels of the CNS, including the limbic and reticular formation, by binding to the benzodiazepine site on the gamma-aminobutyric acid (GABA) receptor complex and modulating GABA, which is a major inhibitory neurotransmitter in the brain

Pharmacodynamics Hypnotic effects:

Onset of action: 15-20 minutes

Maximum effect: 3-6 hours

Duration: 7-8 hours

Pharmacokinetics

Metabolism: In the liver to N-desalkylflurazepam (active)

Half-life, metabolite (adults): 40-114 hours

Usual Dosage Oral:

Children:

<15 years: Dose not established

≥15 years: 15 mg at bedtime

Adults: 15-30 mg at bedtime

Administration May be administered without regard to meals; administer dose at bedtime

Patient Information Avoid alcohol and other CNS depressants. May be habit-forming; avoid abrupt discontinuation after prolonged use. May cause dizziness or drowsiness and impair ability to perform activities requiring mental alertness or physical coordination. May cause hypersensitivity reactions. May cause hazardous sleep-related activities (ie, driving, preparing and eating foods, and making phone calls while not fully awake).

Additional Information In March 2007, the FDA requested that all manufacturers of sedative-hypnotic drug products, including Dalmane® (flurazepam), revise the labeling to include a greater emphasis on the risks of adverse events. The events include severe hypersensitivity reactions including anaphylaxis and/or angioedema, as well as hazardous sleep-related activities (eg, sleep-driving - driving while not fully awake after consumption of sedative-hypnotic drug, with no recollection of the event). Other activities may include preparing and ingesting food, and the use of the telephone, while asleep. These events may occur at any time during therapy including with the first dose administered.

Manufacturers must provide written notification to healthcare providers regarding the new warnings. In addition, manufacturers are to develop "Patient Medication Guides" designed to educate consumers about the potential risks and to advise them of precautionary measures that can be taken. This advice will contain recommendations on correct utilization of the medication as well as the avoidance of the consumption of ethanol and/or other CNS-depressant agents. The FDA is also recommending manufacturers conduct studies evaluating the frequencies of sleep-driving (and other sleep-related behaviors) with the individual products.

Patients should be instructed not to discontinue these medications without first speaking with their healthcare provider. Patients should also be informed of the potential for an allergic reaction, the signs and symptoms of anaphylaxis, and the appropriate emergency self-treatment of an anaphylactic reaction.

Additional information on the sedative-hypnotic products and sleep disorders is available at http://www.fda.gov/cder/drug/infopage/sedative_hypnotics/default.htm

Dosage Forms Excipient information presented when available (limited, particularly for generics); consult specific product labeling.

(Continued)

Flurazepam *(Continued)*

Capsule, as hydrochloride: 15 mg, 30 mg

Dalmane®: 15 mg, 30 mg

♦ **Flurazepam Hydrochloride** *see* Flurazepam *on page 686*

Flurbiprofen (flure BI proe fen)

Medication Safety Issues

Sound-alike/look-alike issues:

Flurbiprofen may be confused with fenoprofen

Ansaid® may be confused with Asacol®, Axid®

Ocufen® may be confused with Ocuflox®, Ocupress®

U.S. Brand Names Ansaid® [DSC]; Ocufen®

Canadian Brand Names Alti-Flurbiprofen; Ansaid®; Apo-Flurbiprofen®; Froben®; Froben-SR®; Novo-Flurprofen; Nu-Flurprofen; Ocufen®

Index Terms Flurbiprofen Sodium

Therapeutic Category Analgesic, Non-narcotic; Anti-inflammatory Agent; Anti-inflammatory Agent, Ophthalmic; Nonsteroidal Anti-inflammatory Drug (NSAID), Ophthalmic; Nonsteroidal Anti-inflammatory Drug (NSAID), Oral

Generic Available Yes

Use

Ophthalmic: For inhibition of intraoperative trauma-induced miosis; the value of flurbiprofen for the prevention and management of postoperative ocular inflammation and postoperative cystoid macular edema remains to be determined

Systemic: Management of inflammatory disease and rheumatoid disorders; dysmenorrhea; pain

Medication Guide An FDA-approved patient medication guide, which is available with the product information and at http://www.fda.gov/cder/Offices/ODS/medication_guides.htm, must be dispensed with this medication for each new outpatient prescription and refill.

Pregnancy Risk Factor B (D in 3rd trimester)

Lactation Enters breast milk/not recommended

Contraindications Hypersensitivity to flurbiprofen, any component, aspirin, or other NSAIDs; active GI bleeding, ulcer disease; patients with the "aspirin triad" [asthma, rhinitis (with or without nasal polyps), and aspirin intolerance] (fatal asthmatic and anaphylactoid reactions may occur in these patients); dendritic keratitis

Warnings In April 2005, the FDA announced product labeling changes for all NSAIDs, including COX-2 selective and OTC medications; although revised product labeling is currently not available for all products, sample labeling and a template of the required medication guide are now available. Labels for prescription nonselective NSAIDs will contain a contraindication for use in patients who have recently undergone coronary artery bypass graft (CABG) surgery and a boxed warning concerning the potential for increased risk of cardiovascular (CV) events and GI bleeding associated with NSAID use. Patients at increased risk of adverse events include patients immediately postoperative from CABG surgery, and those with existing CAD, CVD, or history of TIA or stomach ulcers. Prescribers are encouraged to use the lowest effective NSAID dose for the shortest time based on individual patient treatment goals. Medication guides will be required for all prescription products. Complete details for the labeling update can be found on the following FDA website: http://www.fda.gov/medwatch/SAFETY/2005/safety05.htm#NSAID.

Use with caution in patients with history of herpes simplex, keratitis, and patients who might be affected by inhibition of platelet aggregation; with ophthalmic use, an increased bleeding of ocular tissues may occur in conjunction with ocular surgery

Precautions Use oral form with caution in renal or hepatic impairment, GI disease, cardiac disease, and patients receiving anticoagulants

Adverse Reactions

Cardiovascular: Edema

Central nervous system: Headache, fatigue, drowsiness, vertigo

Dermatologic: Pruritus, rash

Gastrointestinal: Abdominal discomfort, nausea, heartburn, constipation, vomiting, GI bleeding, ulcers, perforation

Hematologic: Thrombocytopenia, inhibits platelet aggregation; prolongs bleeding time; agranulocytosis; increased bleeding of ocular tissues with ocular surgery (ophthalmic use)

Hepatic: Hepatitis

Ocular: Slowing of corneal wound healing, mild ocular stinging, itching, burning, ocular irritation

Otic: Tinnitus

Renal: Renal dysfunction

Drug Interactions Cytochrome P450 isoenzyme CYP2C9 substrate and inhibitor

Oral: May decrease antihypertensive effects of ACE inhibitors or angiotensin II antagonists; drug interactions similar to other NSAIDs may occur

Ophthalmic: Carbachol and acetylcholine chloride may not be effective when used concurrently with flurbiprofen

Food Interactions Food may decrease the rate but not the extent of absorption

Mechanism of Action Inhibits prostaglandin synthesis by decreasing the activity of the enzyme, cyclooxygenase, which results in decreased formation of prostaglandin precursors

Pharmacokinetics Oral:

Time to peak serum concentration: Within 1.5-2 hours

Elimination: 95% in urine

Usual Dosage

Children and Adults: Ophthalmic: Instill 1 drop every 30 minutes starting 2 hours prior to surgery (total of 4 drops to each affected eye)

Adults: Oral:

Arthritis: 200-300 mg/day in 2-4 divided doses; maximum dose: 100 mg/dose; maximum: 300 mg/day

Dysmenorrhea: 50 mg 4 times/day

Administration

Oral: Administer with food, milk, or antacid to decrease GI effects

Ophthalmic: Instill drops into affected eye(s); avoid contact of container tip with skin or eye; apply finger pressure to lacrimal sac during and for 1-2 minutes after instillation to decrease risk of absorption and systemic effects

Monitoring Parameters Systemic use: CBC, platelets, BUN, serum creatinine, liver enzymes, occult blood loss; ocular use: Periodic eye exams

Patient Information Ophthalmic solution may cause mild burning or stinging, notify physician if this becomes severe or is persistent

Dosage Forms Excipient information presented when available (limited, particularly for generics); consult specific product labeling. [DSC] = Discontinued product

Solution, ophthalmic, as sodium (Ocufen®): 0.03% (2.5 mL) [contains thimerosal]

Tablet: 50 mg, 100 mg

Ansaid®: 50 mg, 100 mg [DSC]

♦ **Flurbiprofen Sodium** *see* Flurbiprofen *on page 688*

♦ **5-Flurocytosine** *see* Flucytosine *on page 662*

Fluticasone (floo TIK a sone)

Medication Safety Issues

Sound-alike/look-alike issues:

Cutivate® may be confused with Ultravate®

International issues:

Allegro® [Israel] may be confused with Allegra® which is a brand name for fexofenadine in the U.S.

Allegro®: Brand name for frovatriptan in Germany

Flovent® may be confused with Flogen® which is a brand name for naproxen in Mexico

Related Information

Asthma *on page 1904*

Corticosteroids, Topical: Guidelines for Selection and Use *on page 1686*

U.S. Brand Names Cutivate®; Flonase®; Flovent® HFA

Canadian Brand Names Cutivate™; Flonase®; Flovent® Diskus®; Flovent® HFA

Index Terms Fluticasone Propionate

Therapeutic Category Adrenal Corticosteroid; Anti-inflammatory Agent; Antiasthmatic; Corticosteroid, Inhalant (Oral); Corticosteroid, Intranasal; Corticosteroid, Topical; Glucocorticoid

Generic Available Yes: Cream, nasal spray, ointment

Use

Oral inhalation: Long-term (chronic) control of persistent bronchial asthma; **NOT** indicated for the relief of acute bronchospasm. Also used to help reduce or discontinue oral corticosteroid therapy for asthma (see Additional Information)

Intranasal: Management of seasonal and perennial allergic and nonallergic rhinitis

Topical: Relief of inflammation and pruritus associated with corticosteroid-responsive dermatoses; atopic dermatitis [medium potency topical corticosteroid]

Pregnancy Risk Factor C

Lactation Excretion in breast milk unknown/use caution

Contraindications Hypersensitivity to fluticasone or any component (see Warnings); primary treatment of status asthmaticus

(Continued)

Fluticasone *(Continued)*

Warnings Fatalities have occurred due to adrenal insufficiency in asthmatic patients during and after switching from systemic corticosteroids to aerosol steroids (see Additional Information); several months may be required for full recovery of hypothalamic-pituitary-adrenal (HPA) function; patients receiving higher doses of systemic corticosteroids (eg, adults receiving ≥20 mg of prednisone per day) may be at greater risk; during this period of HPA suppression, aerosol steroids do **not** provide the systemic glucocorticoid or mineralocorticoid activity needed to treat patients requiring stress doses (ie, patients with major stress such as trauma, surgery, or infections, or other conditions associated with severe electrolyte loss). When used at high doses or for a prolonged time, hypercorticism and HPA suppression (including adrenal crisis) may occur; use with inhaled or systemic corticosteroids (even alternate-day dosing) may increase risk of HPA suppression. Acute adrenal insufficiency may occur with abrupt withdrawal after long-term use or with stress; withdrawal and discontinuation of corticosteroids should be done carefully; patients with HPA axis suppression may require doses of systemic glucocorticosteroids prior to, during, and after unusual stress (eg, surgery). Immunosuppression may occur; patients may be more susceptible to infections; avoid exposure to chickenpox and measles. Switching patients from systemic corticosteroids to aerosol steroids may unmask allergic conditions previously treated by the systemic steroid. Bronchospasm may occur after use of inhaled asthma medications (see Additional Information).

Powder for oral inhalation (Flovent® Diskus®) contains lactose (milk proteins) which may cause allergic reactions in patients with severe milk protein allergy. Potent inhibitors of cytochrome P450 isoenzyme CYP3A4 (eg, ritonavir) may significantly increase fluticasone serum concentrations and result in systemic corticosteroid effects (see Drug Interactions).

Topical use: Adverse systemic effects may occur when topical steroids are used on large areas of the body, denuded areas, for prolonged periods of time, with an occlusive dressing, and/or in infants or small children; infants and small children may be more susceptible to HPA axis suppression or other systemic toxicities due to a larger skin surface area to body mass ratio; use with caution in pediatric patients; do not use for the treatment of rosacea, perioral dermatitis, or in the presence of skin atrophy or infection at treatment site

Precautions Avoid using higher than recommended doses; suppression of HPA function, suppression of linear growth (ie, reduction of growth velocity), reduced bone mineral density, hypercorticism (Cushing's syndrome), hyperglycemia, or glucosuria may occur; these adverse effects (as well as intracranial hypertension) may occur with topical use and have been reported in pediatric patients (see also Additional Information); use with extreme caution in patients with respiratory tuberculosis, untreated systemic infections, or ocular herpes simplex; use with caution and monitor patients closely with hepatic dysfunction. Eosinophilic conditions (eosinophilia, vasculitic rash, cardiac complications, worsening pulmonary symptoms, and/or neuropathy) may occur and are usually associated with withdrawal or decrease of oral corticosteroids after the initiation of fluticasone (oral inhalation); a causal relationship by fluticasone has not been established

Adverse Reactions

Central nervous system: Headache, dizziness, malaise, fatigue, insomnia, agitation, aggression, anxiety, depression, restlessness; rarely: behavioral changes, irritability, hyperactivity (primarily in children)

Dermatologic:

Intranasal use: Facial edema

Inhalational use: Dermatitis, rash, facial edema

Topical use: Pruritus, dry skin, stinging at application site, excoriation, numbness of fingers, acne, hypopigmentation, allergic dermatitis, maceration of the skin, skin atrophy, striae, folliculitis, hypertrichosis, itching, telanglectasia

Endocrine & metabolic: HPA suppression, Cushing's syndrome, growth suppression, hyperglycemia

Gastrointestinal: Oral candidiasis, nausea, vomiting, diarrhea, dyspepsia

Local: Burning, irritation

Neuromuscular & skeletal: Muscular soreness, osteoporosis, decreased bone mineral density

Ocular: Eye pain, cataracts, increased IOP, glaucoma

Respiratory: Respiratory infection, pharyngitis, oropharyngeal edema, throat irritation, upper respiratory inflammation, nasal congestion, sinusitis, sinus infection, nasal discharge, rhinitis, epistaxis (intranasal), aphonia, dysphonia, or hoarseness (oral inhalation), bronchospasm, cough, bronchitis

Miscellaneous: Secondary infection, eosinophilic conditions (see Precautions); anaphylactic reaction (very rare)

Drug Interactions Cytochrome P450 isoenzyme CYP3A3/4 substrate

Ritonavir significantly increases fluticasone serum concentrations and may result in systemic corticosteroid effects (eg, Cushing's syndrome and adrenal suppression); concurrent use of ritonavir with fluticasone is **not** recommended unless benefits outweigh risks. Ketoconazole increases fluticasone serum concentrations and decreases plasma cortisol levels (but not urinary excretion of cortisol). Use fluticasone with caution in patients receiving ketoconazole or other potent cytochrome P450 3A4 isoenzyme inhibitors.

Stability

Oral inhalation: Flovent® HFA: Store at controlled room temperature of 25°C (77°F) with mouthpiece down; do not expose to temperatures >120°F; do not puncture or incinerate. Diskus®: Store at controlled room temperature; keep dry; protect from direct heat or sunlight; discard Diskus® 6 weeks (for 50 mcg strength) or 2 months (for 100 mcg and 250 mcg strengths) after opening moisture-proof foil overwrap or when dose indicator reads "0" (whichever comes first); **Note:** Diskus® device is not reusable

Intranasal: Store nasal spray between 39°F to 86°F

Topical:

Cream: Store at 2°C to 30°C (36°F to 86°F)

Lotion: Store at 15°C to 30°C (59°F to 86°F); do not refrigerate; keep tightly closed

Mechanism of Action Controls the rate of protein synthesis, depresses the migration of polymorphonuclear leukocytes and fibroblasts, reverses capillary permeability, and stabilizes lysosomal membranes at the cellular level to prevent or control inflammation

Pharmacodynamics

Oral inhalation: Clinical effects are due to direct local effect rather than systemic absorption

Onset of action: Variable; may occur within 24 hours

Maximum effect: 1-2 weeks or more

Duration after discontinuation: Several days or more

Pharmacokinetics

Distribution: V_d: Adults: 4.2 L/kg

Protein binding: 91%

Metabolism: Via cytochrome P450 3A4 pathway

Bioavailability: Oral inhalation: Flovent®: 30% of dose delivered from actuator; Flovent® HFA: 30% lower than Flovent®; Diskus®: 18%

Half-life: 7.8 hours

Usual Dosage

Intranasal: Note: For optimal effects, nasal spray should be used at regular intervals (eg, once or twice daily); however, some adolescent patients ≥12 years of age and adults with seasonal allergic rhinitis may have effective control of symptoms with prn (as needed) use of 200 mcg (2 sprays to each nostril) once daily.

Children <4 years: Not recommended

Children ≥4 years and Adolescents: Initial: 1 spray (50 mcg/spray) to each nostril daily (100 mcg/day); if response is inadequate, give 2 sprays to each nostril daily (200 mcg/day); once symptoms are controlled, reduce dose to 100 mcg/day (1 spray to each nostril daily); maximum dose: 200 mcg/day (4 sprays/day)

Adults: Initial: 200 mcg/day given as 2 sprays (50 mcg/spray) to each nostril daily or 1 spray to each nostril twice daily; dosage may be reduced to 100 mcg/day (1 spray to each nostril daily) after the first few days if symptoms are controlled; maximum dose: 200 mcg/day (4 sprays/day)

Oral inhalation: If adequate response is not seen after 2 weeks of initial dosage, increase dosage; doses should be titrated to the lowest effective dose once asthma is controlled:

Inhalation aerosol (Flovent® HFA): Manufacturer's recommendations:

Children 4-11 years: Initial: 88 mcg twice daily; maximum dose: 88 mcg twice daily

Children ≥12 years and Adults:

Patients previously treated with bronchodilators only: Initial: 88 mcg twice daily; maximum dose: 440 mcg twice daily

Patients treated with an inhaled corticosteroid: Initial: 88-220 mcg twice daily; maximum dose: 440 mcg twice daily; may start doses above 88 mcg twice daily in poorly controlled patients or in those who previously required higher doses of inhaled corticosteroids

Patients previously treated with oral corticosteroids: 440 mcg twice daily; maximum dose: 880 mcg twice daily

NIH Asthma Guidelines (NAEPP, 2002; NIH, 1997) [give in divided doses twice daily]:

Children ≤12 years:

"Low" dose: 88-176 mcg/day (44 mcg/puff: 2-4 puffs/day)

"Medium" dose: 176-440 mcg/day (44 mcg/puff: 4-10 puffs/day or 110 mcg/puff: 2-4 puffs/day)

(Continued)

Fluticasone *(Continued)*

"High" dose: >440 mcg/day (110 mcg/puff: >4 puffs/day or 220 mcg/puff: >2 puffs/day)

Children >12 years and Adults:

"Low" dose: 88-264 mcg/day (44 mcg/puff: 2-6 puffs/day or 110 mcg/puff: 2 puffs/day)

"Medium" dose: 264-660 mcg/day (110 mcg/puff: 2-6 puffs/day)

"High" dose: >660 mcg/day (110 mcg/puff: >6 puffs/day or 220 mcg/puff: >3 puffs/day)

Inhalation powder (Flovent® Diskus®): Manufacturer's recommendations:

Children 4-11 years: Patients previously treated with bronchodilators alone or inhaled corticosteroids: Initial: 50 mcg twice daily; maximum dose: 100 mcg twice daily; may start higher initial dose in poorly controlled patients or in those who previously required higher doses of inhaled corticosteroids

Adolescents and Adults:

Patients previously treated with bronchodilators alone: Initial: 100 mcg twice daily; maximum dose: 500 mcg twice daily

Patients previously treated with inhaled corticosteroids: Initial: 100-250 mcg twice daily; maximum dose: 500 mcg twice daily; may start doses above 100 mcg twice daily in poorly controlled patients or in those who previously required higher doses of inhaled corticosteroids

Patients previously treated with oral corticosteroids: Initial: 500-1000 mcg twice daily (select dose based on assessment of individual patient); maximum dose: 1000 mcg twice daily; **Note:** Inability to reduce oral corticosteroid therapy (see Additional Information) may indicate need for maximum fluticasone dose

NIH Asthma Guidelines (NAEPP, 2002) [give in divided doses twice daily]:

Children ≤12 years:

"Low" dose: 100-200 mcg/day (50 mcg/puff: 2-4 puffs/day or 100 mcg/puff: 1-2 puffs/day)

"Medium" dose: 200-400 mcg/day (50 mcg/puff: 4-8 puffs/day or 100 mcg/puff: 2-4 puffs/day)

"High" dose: >400 mcg/day (50 mcg/puff: >8 puffs/day or 100 mcg/puff: >4 puffs/day)

Children >12 years and Adults:

"Low" dose: 100-300 mcg/day (50 mcg/puff: 2-6 puffs/day or 100 mcg/puff: 1-3 puffs/day)

"Medium" dose: 300-600 mcg/day (50 mcg/puff: 6-12 puffs/day or 100 mcg/puff: 3-6 puffs/day)

"High" dose: >600 mcg/day (50 mcg/puff: >12 puffs/day or 100 mcg/puff: >6 puffs/day)

Topical:

Cream:

Infants <3 months: Not approved for use

Infants ≥3 months, Children, and Adults: **Note:** Safety and efficacy of use >4 weeks in pediatric patients have not been established:

Atopic dermatitis: Apply a thin film to affected area once or twice daily

Other dermatoses: Apply a thin film to affected area twice daily

Lotion:

Infants <1 year: Not approved for use

Children ≥1 year and Adults: **Note:** Safety of use >4 weeks has not been established:

Atopic dermatitis: Apply a thin film to affected area once daily

Ointment:

Pediatric patients: Not approved for use (due to potential for adrenal suppression)

Adults: Apply sparingly in a thin film twice daily

Dosage adjustment in hepatic impairment: Use with caution; monitor patients closely; **Note:** Fluticasone is primarily eliminated via hepatic metabolism and serum concentrations may be elevated in patients with hepatic disease

Administration

Intranasal spray: Shake bottle gently before use; clear nasal passages by blowing nose prior to use; nasal spray pump must be primed (6 actuations) before first use or after ≥1 week of nonuse; discard unit after 120 metered sprays are used

Oral inhalation: Rinse mouth with water (without swallowing) after inhalation to decrease chance of oral candidiasis

Aerosol inhalation: Shake canister well before use; use at room temperature; inhaler must be primed before first use with 4 test sprays (spray into air away from face, shake well between sprays); Flovent® HFA inhaler must be primed again with 1 test spray if not used for >7 days or if dropped. Use a spacer device for children <8 years of age; discard canister when labeled number of metered doses has been used, even though canister is not completely empty (correct amount of fluticasone per inhalation cannot be assured); do not immerse canister into water (ie, do not use "float test" to determine contents)

Powder for oral inhalation: Diskus®: Do not use with spacer device; do not exhale into Diskus®; do not wash or take apart; activate and use Diskus® in horizontal position

Topical: Apply sparingly to affected area, gently rub in until disappears; do not use on open skin; avoid application on face, underarms, or groin area unless directed by physician; avoid contact with eyes; do not occlude area unless directed; do not apply to diaper area

Monitoring Parameters Oral inhalation: Check mucus membranes for signs of fungal infection; monitor growth in pediatric patients; monitor IOP with therapy >6 weeks. Assess HPA suppression in patients using potent topical steroids applied to a large surface area or to areas under occlusion.

Patient Information Notify physician if condition being treated persists or worsens; do not decrease dose or discontinue without physician approval; avoid exposure to chicken pox or measles; if exposed, seek medical advice without delay

Oral inhalation: Report sore mouth or mouth lesions to physician; carefully read and follow the Patient's Instructions for Use leaflet that accompanies the product

Additional Information Flovent® HFA does **not** contain CFCs as the propellant; Flovent® HFA is packaged in a plastic-coated, moisture-protective foil pouch that also contains a desiccant; the desiccant should be discarded when the pouch is opened,

When using fluticasone oral inhalation to help reduce or discontinue oral corticosteroid therapy, begin prednisone taper after at least 1 week of fluticasone inhalation therapy; do not decrease prednisone faster than 2.5 mg/day on a weekly basis; monitor patients for signs of asthma instability and adrenal insufficiency (see Warnings); decrease fluticasone to lowest effective dose **after** prednisone reduction is complete. If bronchospasm with wheezing occurs after oral inhalation use, a fast-acting bronchodilator may be used; discontinue orally inhaled corticosteroid and initiate alternative chronic therapy.

Topical: HPA axis suppression occurred in 2 children (2 and 5 years old) of 43 pediatric patients treated topically with fluticasone cream for 4 weeks; application covered at least 35% of body surface area

Nasal spray: In a small pediatric study conducted over 1 year, no statistically significant effect on growth velocity or clinically relevant changes in bone mineral density or HPA axis function were observed in children 3-9 years of age receiving fluticasone nasal spray (200 mcg/day; n=56) versus placebo (n=52); effects at higher doses or in susceptible pediatric patients cannot be ruled out

Dosage Forms Excipient information presented when available (limited, particularly for generics); consult specific product labeling. [CAN] = Canadian brand name

Aerosol for oral inhalation, as propionate [CFC free]:
- Flovent® HFA: 44 mcg/inhalation (10.6 g) [120 metered doses]
- Flovent® HFA: 110 mcg/inhalation (12 g) [120 metered doses]
- Flovent® HFA: 220 mcg/inhalation (12 g) [120 metered doses]

Cream, as propionate: 0.05% (15 g, 30 g, 60 g)
- Cutivate®: 0.05% (15 g, 30 g, 60 g)

Lotion, as propionate:
- Cutivate®: 0.05% (60 mL)

Ointment, as propionate: 0.005% (15 g, 30 g, 60 g)
- Cutivate®: 0.005% (15 g, 30 g, 60 g)

Powder for oral inhalation, as propionate [prefilled blister pack]:
- Flovent® Diskus® [CAN]: 50 mcg (28s, 60s) [contains lactose] [not available in the U.S.]
- Flovent® Diskus® [CAN]: 100 mcg (28s, 60s) [contains lactose] [not available in the U.S.]
- Flovent® Diskus® [CAN]: 250 mcg (28s, 60s) [contains lactose] [not available in the U.S.]
- Flovent® Diskus® [CAN]: 500 mcg (28s, 60s) [contains lactose] [not available in the U.S.]

Suspension, intranasal spray, as propionate: 50 mcg/inhalation (16 g) [120 metered doses]
- Flonase®: 50 mcg/inhalation (16 g) [120 metered doses]

References

Expert Panel Report 2, "Guidelines for the Diagnosis and Management of Asthma," *Clinical Practice Guidelines*, National Institutes of Health, National Heart, Lung, and Blood Institute, NIH Publication No. 94-4051, April, 1997.

"National Asthma Education and Prevention Program. Expert Panel Report: Guidelines for the Diagnosis and Management of Asthma Update on Selected Topics--2002," *J Allergy Clin Immunol*, 2002, 110(5 Suppl):S141-219.

Fluticasone and Salmeterol (floo TIK a sone & sal ME te role)

Medication Safety Issues

Sound-alike/look-alike issues:

Advair may be confused with Advicor®

Related Information

Asthma *on page 1904*

U.S. Brand Names Advair Diskus®; Advair® HFA

Canadian Brand Names Advair Diskus®

Index Terms Fluticasone Propionate and Salmeterol Xinafoate; Salmeterol and Fluticasone

Therapeutic Category Adrenal Corticosteroid; Adrenergic Agonist Agent; Anti-inflammatory Agent; Antiasthmatic; Beta$_2$-Adrenergic Agonist Agent; Bronchodilator; Corticosteroid, Inhalant; Glucocorticoid

Generic Available No

Use

Advair Diskus®, Advair® HFA: Maintenance treatment of asthma

Advair Diskus®: Maintenance treatment of airflow obstruction in patients with COPD associated with chronic bronchitis

Medication Guide An FDA-approved patient medication guide, which is available with the product information and at http://www.fda.gov/cder/Offices/ODS/medication_guides.htm, must be dispensed with this medication for each new outpatient prescription and refill.

Pregnancy Risk Factor C

Lactation

Fluticasone: Excretion in breast milk unknown/use caution

Salmeterol: Enters breast milk/use caution

Contraindications Hypersensitivity to salmeterol, adrenergic amines, fluticasone, or any component; primary treatment of status asthmaticus; use with other long-acting beta$_2$-adrenergic agonists; transferring patients from systemic corticosteroid therapy (see Warnings)

Warnings Fatalities have occurred due to adrenal insufficiency in asthmatic patients during and after switching from systemic corticosteroids to aerosol steroids; several months may be required for full recovery of the adrenal glands; patients receiving higher doses of systemic corticosteroids (eg, adults receiving ≥20 mg of prednisone per day) may be at greater risk; during this period of adrenal suppression, aerosol steroids do not provide the systemic corticosteroid needed to treat patients requiring stress doses (ie, patients with major stress such as trauma, surgery, or infections); when used at high doses or for a prolonged time, hypercorticism and hypothalamic-pituitary-adrenal (HPA) suppression (including adrenal crisis) may occur; withdrawal and discontinuation of corticosteroid therapy should be done carefully. Immunosuppression may occur.

Long-acting beta$_2$ adrenergic agents (eg, salmeterol) have been associated with an increased risk of asthma-related death. Salmeterol should only be prescribed in patients not adequately controlled on other asthma-controller medications or whose disease severity clearly warrants treatment with two maintenance therapies. A medication guide is available to provide information to patients covering the risk of use.

Salmeterol/fluticasone is not meant to relieve acute asthmatic symptoms. Acute episodes should be treated with short-acting beta$_2$ agonist. Do not increase the frequency of salmeterol/fluticasone use. Paroxysmal bronchospasm (which can be fatal) has been reported with this and other inhaled beta$_2$-agonist agents. If this occurs, discontinue treatment; symptoms of laryngeal spasm, irritation, or swelling, such as stridor and choking have been reported in patients receiving fluticasone/salmeterol; if this occurs, discontinue treatment.

Precautions Use with caution in patients with cardiovascular disorders, convulsive disorders, liver dysfunction, thyrotoxicosis, or others who are sensitive to the effects of sympathomimetic amines; avoid using higher than recommended doses; suppression of HPA function, suppression of linear growth, or hypercorticism (Cushing's syndrome) may occur; use with extreme caution in patients with respiratory tuberculosis, untreated systemic infections, or ocular herpes simplex; use with caution and monitor patients closely with hepatic dysfunction; eosinophilic conditions (eosinophilia, vasculitic rash, cardiac complications, worsening pulmonary symptoms, and/or neuropathy) may occur and are usually associated with withdrawal or decrease of oral corticosteroids after the initiation of fluticasone oral inhalation; a causal relationship by fluticasone has not been established.

Adverse Reactions See Fluticasone *on page 689* and Salmeterol *on page 1415*

Drug Interactions Beta adrenergic blockers decrease effects of salmeterol component; MAO inhibitors and tricyclic antidepressants may increase cardiovascular toxicity of salmeterol (wait at least 2 weeks after discontinuation of these agents before beginning treatment with Advair Diskus® or Advair® HFA); additive potential to develop hypokalemia with diuretic use; ritonavir, azole antifungals, ciprofloxacin, clarithromycin, diclofenac, doxycycline, erythromycin, imatinib, isoniazid, nefazodone, nicardipine, propofol, protease inhibitors, quinidine, and verapamil may increase fluticasone serum levels by inhibition of cytochrome P450 isoenzyme 3A4.

Stability Store at controlled room temperature; avoid direct heat or sunlight. Advair Diskus®: Discard device 1 month after removal from the moisture-protective foil overwrap pouch or after every blister has been used (when the dose indicator reads "0") whichever comes first. Advair® HFA: Store with mouthpiece down

Mechanism of Action

Fluticasone: Controls the rate of protein synthesis, depresses the migration of polymorphonuclear leukocytes and fibroblasts, reverses capillary permeability, and stabilizes lysosomal membranes at the cellular level to prevent or control inflammation.

Salmeterol: Relaxes bronchial smooth muscle by selective action on beta$_2$-receptors with little effect on heart rate

Pharmacodynamics See Fluticasone *on page 689* and Salmeterol *on page 1415*

Pharmacokinetics See Fluticasone *on page 689* and Salmeterol *on page 1415*

Usual Dosage

Oral powder for inhalation: Advair Diskus®:

Maintenance treatment of asthma: **Note:** Titrate dosage to the lowest effective strength which maintains control of asthma

Children 4-11 years without prior inhaled corticosteroid: Fluticasone 100 mcg/salmeterol 50 mcg (Advair™ Diskus® 100/50) 1 inhalation twice daily

Children ≥12 years and Adults without prior inhaled corticosteroid: Fluticasone 100 mcg/salmeterol 50 mcg (Advair™ Diskus® 100/50) 1 inhalation twice daily

Children ≥12 years and Adults currently receiving an inhaled corticosteroid: The starting dose is dependent upon the current steroid therapy, see table.

Maintenance treatment of COPD with chronic bronchitis: Adults: Fluticasone 250 mcg/salmeterol 50 mcg (Advair Diskus® 250/50) 1 inhalation twice daily

Oral inhalation: Metered dose inhaler: Advair® HFA: Maintenance treatment of asthma:

Children ≥12 years and Adults without prior inhaled corticosteroid: 2 inhalations twice daily of either fluticasone 45 mcg/salmeterol 21 mcg (Advair® HFA 45/21) or fluticasone 115 mcg/salmeterol 21 mcg (Advair® HFA 115/21); not to exceed 2 inhalations twice daily of fluticasone 230 mcg/salmeterol 21 mcg (Advair® HFA 230/21)

Recommended Starting Dose of Fluticasone/Salmeterol (Advair Diskus®) for Patients Currently Taking Inhaled Corticosteroids

Current Daily Dose of Inhaled Corticosteroid[1]		Advair Diskus® 1 inhalation twice daily
Beclomethasone dipropionate HFA inhalation aerosal	160 mcg	100/50
	320 mcg	250/50
	640 mcg	500/50
Budesonide inhalation aerosal	≤400 mcg	100/50
	800-1200 mcg	250/50
	1600 mcg	500/50
Flunisolide inhalation aerosal	≤1000 mcg	100/50
	1250-2000 mcg	250/50
Flunisolide HFA inhalation aerosal	≤320 mcg	100/50
	640 mcg	250/50
Fluticasone propionate HFA inhalation aerosol	≤176 mcg	100/50
	440 mcg	250/50
	660-880 mcg	500/50
Fluticasone propionate inhalation powder	≤200 mcg	100/50
	500 mcg	250/50
	1000 mcg	500/50
Mometasone furoate inhalation powder	220 mcg	100/50
	440 mcg	250/50
	880 mcg	500/50
Triamcinolone acetate inhalation aerosal	≤1000 mcg	100/50
	1100-1600 mcg	250/50

[1]Not for use in patients transferring from systemic corticosteroid therapy

(Continued)

Fluticasone and Salmeterol *(Continued)*

Children ≥12 years and Adults currently receiving an inhaled corticosteroid: The starting dose is dependent upon the current steroid therapy; see table. Not to exceed 2 inhalations twice daily of fluticasone 230 mcg/salmeterol 21 mcg (Advair® HFA 230/21)

Recommended Starting Dose of Fluticasone/Salmeterol (Advair® HFA) for Patients Currently Taking Inhaled Corticosteroids

Current Daily Dose of Inhaled Corticosteroid[1]		Advair® HFA 2 inhalations twice daily
Beclomethasone dipropionate HFA inhalation aerosal	≤160 mcg	45/21
	320 mcg	115/21
	640 mcg	230/21
Budesonide inhalation powder	≤400 mcg	45/21
	800-1200 mcg	115/21
	1600 mcg	230/21
Flunisolide CFC inhalation aerosal	≤1000 mcg	45/21
	1250-2000 mcg	115/21
Flunisolide HFA inhalation aerosal	≤320 mcg	45/21
	640 mcg	115/21
Fluticasone propionate HFA inhalation aerosol	≤176 mcg	45/21
	440 mcg	115/21
	660-880 mcg	230/21
Fluticasone propionate inhalation powder	≤200 mcg	45/21
	500 mcg	115/21
	1000 mcg	230/21
Mometasone furoate inhalation powder	220 mcg	45/21
	440 mcg	115/21
	880 mcg	230/21
Triamcinolone acetonide inhalation aerosal	≤1000 mcg	45/21
	1100-1600 mcg	115/21

[1]Not for use in patients transferring from systemic corticosteroid therapy

Administration Oral inhalation:

Powder for oral inhalation: The Diskus® is a device containing a double-foil blister of a powder formulation for oral inhalation; each blister contains 1 complete dose of both medications; after the medication is opened by activating the device, the medication is dispersed into the airstream created by the patient inhaling through the mouthpiece; it may not be used with a spacer. Follow the patient directions for use which are provided with each device; do not exhale into the Diskus® or attempt to take it apart. Always activate and use the Diskus® in a level, horizontal position. Do not wash the mouthpiece or any part of the Diskus®; it must be kept dry.

Metered dose inhalation: Prime before using the first time by releasing 4 test sprays into the air away from the face, shaking well for 5 seconds before each spray. Reprime with 2 test sprays if the inhaler has been dropped or not used for more than 4 weeks; discard after 120 actuations. Never immerse canister into water. Shake well for 5 seconds before using.

Monitoring Parameters Pulmonary function tests, check mucous membranes for signs of fungal infection; monitor growth in pediatric patients

Patient Information Do not use to treat acute symptoms; do not exceed the prescribed dose of fluticasone/salmeterol; report sore mouth or mouth lesions to physician; avoid exposure to chickenpox or measles; if exposed, seek medical advice without delay; do not use with spacer (see Administration)

Additional Information When fluticasone/salmeterol is initiated in patients previously receiving a short-acting beta agonist, instruct the patient to discontinue regular use of the short-acting beta agonist and to utilize the shorter-acting agent for symptomatic acute episodes only.

Dosage Forms Excipient information presented when available (limited, particularly for generics); consult specific product labeling.

Aerosol, for oral inhalation:

Advair® HFA:

45/21: Fluticasone propionate 45 mcg and salmeterol xinafoate 30.45 mcg (12 g) [120 metered inhalations]

115/21: Fluticasone propionate 115 mcg and salmeterol xinafoate 30.45 mcg (12 g) [120 metered inhalations]

230/21: Fluticasone propionate 230 mcg and salmeterol xinafoate 30.45 mcg (12 g) [120 metered inhalations]

Powder, for oral inhalation:

Advair Diskus®:

100/50: Fluticasone propionate 100 mcg and salmeterol xinafoate 50 mcg (28s, 60s) [contains lactose; chlorofluorocarbon free]

250/50: Fluticasone propionate 250 mcg and salmeterol xinafoate 50 mcg (28s, 60s) [contains lactose; chlorofluorocarbon free]

500/50: Fluticasone propionate 500 mcg and salmeterol xinafoate 50 mcg (28s, 60s) [contains lactose; chlorofluorocarbon free]

References

"National Asthma Education and Prevention Program. Expert Panel Report: Guidelines for the Diagnosis and Management of Asthma Update on Selected Topics--2002," *J Allergy Clin Immunol*, 2002, 110(5 Suppl):S141-219.

♦ **Fluticasone Propionate** *see* Fluticasone *on page 689*

♦ **Fluticasone Propionate and Salmeterol Xinafoate** *see* Fluticasone and Salmeterol *on page 694*

♦ **Fluvirin®** *see* Influenza Virus Vaccine (Inactivated) *on page 833*

Fluvoxamine (floo VOKS a meen)

Medication Safety Issues

Sound-alike/look-alike issues:

Fluvoxamine may be confused with flavoxate, fluoxetine

Luvox may be confused with Lasix®, Levoxyl®

Related Information

Antidepressant Agents *on page 1681*

Canadian Brand Names Alti-Fluvoxamine; Apo-Fluvoxamine®; Luvox®; Novo-Fluvoxamine; Nu-Fluvoxamine; PMS-Fluvoxamine; Rhoxal-fluvoxamine; Sandoz-Fluvoxamine

Index Terms Luvox

Therapeutic Category Antidepressant, Selective Serotonin Reuptake Inhibitor (SSRI)

Generic Available Yes

Use Treatment of obsessive-compulsive disorder (OCD) in children ≥8 years of age and adults

Medication Guide An FDA-approved patient medication guide, which is available with the product information and at http://www.fda.gov/cder/Offices/ODS/medication_guides.htm, must be dispensed with this medication for each new outpatient prescription and refill.

Pregnancy Risk Factor C

Lactation Enters breast milk/not recommended (AAP rates "of concern")

Contraindications Hypersensitivity to fluvoxamine or any component; concurrent use with thioridazine, pimozide, astemizole, terfenadine, alosetron, tizanidine, mesoridazine, or cisapride; use of MAO inhibitors within 14 days (potentially fatal reactions may occur; see Drug Interactions)

Warnings Safety and efficacy in pediatric patients ≥8 years of age have been established only for the treatment of obsessive compulsive disorder; **fluvoxamine is not FDA approved for the treatment of depression in pediatric or adult patients.** Clinical worsening of depression or suicidal ideation and behavior may occur in children and adults with major depressive disorder. In clinical trials, antidepressants increased the risk of suicidal thinking and behavior (suicidality) in children, adolescents, and young adults (18-24 years of age) with major depressive disorder and other psychiatric disorders. This risk must be considered before prescribing antidepressants for any clinical use. Short-term studies did **not** show an increased risk of suicidality with antidepressant use in patients >24 years of age and showed a decreased risk in patients ≥65 years.

Patients of all ages who are treated with antidepressants for any indication require appropriate monitoring and close observation for clinical worsening of depression, suicidality, and unusual changes in behavior, especially during the first few months after antidepressant initiation or when the dose is adjusted. Family members and caregivers should be instructed to closely observe the patient (ie, daily) and communicate condition with healthcare provider. Patients should also be monitored for associated behaviors (eg, anxiety, agitation, panic attacks, insomnia, irritability, hostility, aggressiveness, impulsivity, akathisia, hypomania, mania) which may increase the risk for worsening depression or suicidality. Worsening depression or emergence of suicidality (or associated behaviors listed above) that is abrupt in onset, severe, or not part of the presenting symptoms, may require discontinuation or modification of drug therapy.

(Continued)

Fluvoxamine *(Continued)*

Avoid abrupt discontinuation; withdrawal syndrome with discontinuation symptoms (including agitation, dysphoria, anxiety, confusion, dizziness, hypomania, nightmares, irritability, sensory disturbances, headache, lethargy, emotional lability, insomnia, tinnitus, and seizures) may occur if therapy is abruptly discontinued or dose reduced; taper the dose to minimize risks of discontinuation symptoms. If intolerable symptoms occur following a decrease in dosage or upon discontinuation of therapy, consider resuming the previous dose with a more gradual taper. To reduce risk of intentional overdose, write prescriptions for the smallest quantity consistent with good patient care.

May worsen psychosis in some patients or precipitate a shift to mania or hypomania in patients with bipolar disorder. Monotherapy in patients with bipolar disorder should be avoided. Patients presenting with depressive symptoms should be screened for bipolar disorder. **Fluvoxamine is not FDA approved for the treatment of bipolar depression.**

Potentially fatal serotonin syndrome may occur when SSRIs are used in combination with serotonergic drugs (eg, triptans) or drugs that impair the metabolism of serotonin (eg, MAO inhibitors); see Drug Interactions

Precautions Fluvoxamine may cause abnormal bleeding (eg, ecchymosis, purpura, upper GI bleeding); use with caution in patients with impaired platelet aggregation and with concurrent use of aspirin, NSAIDs, or other drugs that affect coagulation. May impair cognitive or motor performance. Use with caution in patients with seizure disorders, concomitant illnesses that may effect hepatic metabolism or hemodynamic responses (eg, unstable cardiac disease, recent MI), and in suicidal patients; use with caution and decrease dose in patients with hepatic dysfunction; use with caution in patients with severe renal impairment. Use with caution in patients receiving diuretics or those who are volume depleted (may cause hyponatremia or SIADH). No clinical studies have assessed the combined use of fluvoxamine and electroconvulsive therapy; however, use with caution in patients receiving electroconvulsive therapy; may increase the risks associated with electroconvulsive therapy, consider discontinuing, when possible, prior to electroconvulsive therapy treatment.

Use with caution during third trimester of pregnancy [newborns may experience adverse effects or withdrawal symptoms (consider risk and benefits), see Additional Information; exposure to SSRIs late in pregnancy may also be associated with an increased risk for persistent pulmonary hypertension of the newborn (see Chambers, 2006)].

Adverse Reactions

Cardiovascular: Palpitations

Central nervous system: Headache, somnolence, insomnia, nervousness, dizziness, mania, hypomania, vertigo, abnormal thinking, agitation, anxiety, malaise, amnesia, yawning, hypertonia, CNS stimulation, depression, apathy, emotional lability, hyperkinesia; suicidal thinking and behavior (see Warnings)

Note: SSRI-associated behavioral activation (ie, restlessness, hyperkinesis, hyperactivity, agitation) is 2- to 3- fold more prevalent in children compared to adolescents; it is more prevalent in adolescents compared to adults. Somnolence (including sedation and drowsiness) is more common in adults compared to children and adolescents (see Safer, 2006).

Dermatologic: Rash

Endocrine & metabolic: Decreased libido, sexual dysfunction, dysmenorrhea

Gastrointestinal: Nausea, diarrhea, xerostomia, abdominal pain, vomiting, dyspepsia, constipation, abnormal taste, anorexia, flatulence, weight loss

Note: SSRI-associated vomiting is 2- to 3-fold more prevalent in children compared to adolescents; it is more prevalent in adolescents compared to adults

Genitourinary: Urinary frequency, urinary retention

Hematologic: Altered platelet function (rare), increased bleeding, bruising

Neuromuscular & skeletal: Tremors, weakness (14%)

Ocular: Blurred vision

Respiratory: Dyspnea, cough

Miscellaneous: Diaphoresis, allergic reactions (infrequent); withdrawal symptoms following abrupt discontinuation (see Warnings)

Drug Interactions Cytochrome P450 isoenzyme CYP1A2, 2D6 substrate (major); CYP1A2 (strong), 2B6 (weak), 2C9 (weak), 2C19 (strong), 2D6 (weak), 3A4 (weak) inhibitor

With MAO inhibitors, fever, tremors, seizures, delirium, coma may occur (use of MAO inhibitors within 14 days of citalopram use is contraindicated). Fluvoxamine may inhibit the metabolism of thioridazine, mesoridazine, terfenadine, astemizole, pimozide, cisapride, and increase the risk of serious adverse effects, such as QT_c prolongation, serious ventricular arrhythmias (eg, torsade de pointes) and sudden death (concurrent use of these agents with fluvoxamine is contraindicated). Fluvoxamine may significantly increase serum concentrations and serious adverse effects of alosetron, tizanidine, and ramelteon (concurrent use of fluvoxamine and alosetron or tizanidine is contraindicated; use of ramelteon is **not** recommended). Tryptophan (which can be metabolized to serotonin) and the herbal medicine St John's wort (*Hypericum perforatum*) may increase serious side effects (the use of these agents is **not** recommended).

Fluvoxamine may increase the serum concentrations or adverse effects of alprazolam (decrease initial alprazolam dose by at least 50% and titrate to lowest effective dose), diazepam (concurrent use of diazepam and fluvoxamine is not recommended), midazolam, triazolam, theophylline (reduce theophylline dose to $^1/_3$ usual and monitor serum concentrations), warfarin (monitor INR, reduce warfarin dosage), amphetamines, metoprolol, propranolol, carbamazepine, carvedilol, clozapine, mexiletine, phenytoin, dextromethorphan, haloperidol, lovastatin, simvastatin, lithium, methadone, bumetanide, furosemide, torsemide, phenothiazines, quinidine, diltiazem, ritonavir, tacrine, tacrolimus, trazodone, amitriptyline, desipramine, imipramine, nortriptyline.

Combined use of SSRIs and amphetamine, selegiline, buspirone, meperidine, methadone, sibutramine, nefazodone, serotonin agonists, sibutramine, other SSRIs, sympathomimetics, ritonavir, linezolid, lithium, tramadol, and venlafaxine may increase the risk of serotonin syndrome. Use of SSRIs with sumatriptan may cause weakness, incoordination, hyper-reflexia, and an increased risk of serotonin syndrome; use triptans with caution in patients receiving SSRIs; monitor carefully, especially during initiation of treatment and dosage increases.

Concomitant use of fluvoxamine and NSAIDs, aspirin, or other drugs affecting coagulation has been associated with an increased risk of bleeding. Combined use with warfarin may alter the hypoprothrombinemic response to warfarin. Cytochrome P450 isoenzyme CYP1A2 and CYP2D6 inhibitors may increase the levels/effects of fluvoxamine.

Food Interactions Food does not significantly affect bioavailability.

Stability Protect from high humidity and store at controlled room temperature 15°C to 30°C (59°F to 86°F). Dispense in tight containers.

Mechanism of Action Inhibits CNS neuron serotonin uptake; minimal or no effect on reuptake of norepinephrine or dopamine; does not significantly bind to alpha-adrenergic, histamine or cholinergic receptors

Pharmacodynamics

Onset of action: 1-2 weeks

Maximum effect: 8-12 weeks

Duration: 1-2 days

Pharmacokinetics Note: Steady-state plasma concentrations have been noted to be 2-3 times higher in children than those in adolescents; female children demonstrated a significantly higher AUC and peak concentration than males.

Distribution: V_d, apparent: Adults: ~25 L/kg

Protein binding: ~80%, primarily to albumin

Metabolism: Extensive via the liver; major metabolic routes are oxidative demethylation and deamination

Bioavailability: 53%; not significantly affected by food

Half-life: Adults: 15.6 hours

Time to peak serum concentration: 3-8 hours

Elimination: 94% of the dose is excreted in the urine, primarily as metabolites; 2% as unchanged drug

Clearance: Hepatic dysfunction: Decreased by 30%

Usual Dosage Oral:

Children 8-17 years: Initial: 25 mg at bedtime; adjust in 25 mg increments at 7- to 14-day intervals, as tolerated, to maximum therapeutic benefit; usual dosage range: 50-200 mg/day; daily doses >50 mg should be divided into 2 doses; administer larger portion at bedtime

Maximum: Children: 8-11 years: 200 mg/day; Adolescents: 300 mg/day; lower doses may be effective in female versus male patients

Note: Slower titration of dose every 2"4 weeks may minimize the risk of behavioral activation; behavioral activation associated with SSRI use increases the risk of suicidal behavior. Higher mg/kg doses are needed in children compared to adolescents.

Adults: Initial: 50 mg at bedtime; adjust in 50 mg increments at 4- to 7-day intervals; usual dosage range: 100-300 mg/day; daily doses >100 mg should be divided into 2 doses; administer larger portion at bedtime

Dosage adjustment in hepatic impairment: Decrease initial dose and dose titration

Monitoring Parameters Monitor patient periodically for symptom resolution; monitor for worsening depression, suicidality, and associated behaviors (especially at the beginning of therapy or when doses are increased or decreased; see Warnings).

(Continued)

Fluvoxamine *(Continued)*

Monitor for anxiety, social functioning, mania, panic attacks; akathisia, weight gain or loss, nutritional intake, sleep

Patient Information Read the patient Medication Guide that you receive with each prescription and refill of fluvoxamine. An increased risk of suicidal thinking and behavior has been reported with the use of antidepressants in children, adolescents, and young adults (18-24 years of age). Notify physician if you feel more depressed, have thoughts of suicide, or become more agitated or irritable (see Warnings). Notify physician if you experience rash, hives, or other allergic reactions. Avoid alcohol, caffeine, CNS stimulants, tryptophan supplements, and the herbal medicine St John's wort; avoid aspirin, NSAIDs, or other drugs that affect coagulation (may increase risks of bleeding); may cause dizziness or drowsiness and impair ability to perform activities requiring mental alertness or physical coordination; may cause dry mouth. Some medicines should not be taken with fluvoxamine or should not be taken for a while after fluvoxamine has been discontinued; report the use of other medications, nonprescription medications, and herbal or natural products to your physician and pharmacist. It may take 2"3 weeks to see therapeutic effects from this medication. Take as directed; do not alter dose or frequency without consulting prescriber; avoid abrupt discontinuation.

Nursing Implications Taper dosage slowly when discontinuing. Assess mental status for depression, suicidal ideation, anxiety, social functioning, mania, or panic attack.

Additional Information A recent report (Lake, 2000) describes 5 children (age 8-15 years) who developed epistaxis (n=4) or bruising (n=1) while receiving sertraline therapy. Another recent report describes the SSRI discontinuation syndrome in 6 children; the syndrome was similar to that reported in adults (see Diler, 2002). Due to limited long-term studies, the clinical usefulness of fluvoxamine should be periodically re-evaluated in patients receiving the drug for extended intervals; effects of long term use of fluvoxamine on pediatric growth, development, and maturation have not been directly assessed. **Note:** Case reports of decreased growth in children receiving fluoxetine or fluvoxamine (n=4; age: 11.6-13.7 years) for 6 months to 5 years suggest a suppression of growth hormone secretion during SSRI therapy (see Weintrob, 2002). Further studies are needed.

Neonates born to women receiving SSRIs late during the third trimester may experience respiratory distress, apnea, cyanosis, temperature instability, vomiting, feeding difficulty, hypoglycemia, constant crying, irritability, hypotonia, hypertonia, hyper-reflexia, tremor, jitteriness, and seizures; these symptoms may be due to a direct toxic effect, withdrawal syndrome, or (in some cases) serotonin syndrome. Withdrawal symptoms occur in 30% of neonates exposed to SSRIs *in utero*; monitor newborns for at least 48 hours after birth; long-term effects of *in utero* exposure to SSRIs are unknown (see Levinson-Castiel, 2006).

Dosage Forms Excipient information presented when available (limited, particularly for generics); consult specific product labeling.

Tablet, as maleate: 25 mg, 50 mg, 100 mg

References

Chambers CD, Hernandez-Diaz S, Van Marter LJ, et al, "Selective Serotonin-Reuptake Inhibitors and Risk of Persistent Pulmonary Hypertension of the Newborn," *N Engl J Med*, 2006, 354(6):579-87.

Cheer SM and Figgitt DP, "Fluvoxamine: A Review of Its Therapeutic Potential in the Management of Anxiety Disorders in Children and Adolescents," *Paediatr Drugs*, 2001, 3(10):763-81.

Cheer SM and Figgitt DP, "Spotlight on Fluvoxamine in Anxiety Disorders in Children and Adolescents," *CNS Drugs*, 2002, 16(2):139-44.

de Vries MH, Raghoebar M, Mathlener IS, et al, "Single and Multiple Oral Dose Fluvoxamine Kinetics in Young and Elderly Subjects," *Ther Drug Monit*, 1992, 14(6):493-8.

Diler R and Avci A, "Selective Serotonin Reuptake Inhibitor Discontinuation Syndrome in Children: Six Case Reports," *Current Therapeutic Research*, 2002, 63(3):188-97.

Dopheide JA, "Recognizing and Treating Depression in Children and Adolescents," *Am J of Health Syst Pharm*, 2006, 63(3):233-43.

"Fluvoxamine for the Treatment of Anxiety Disorders in Children and Adolescents. The Research Unit on Pediatric Psychopharmacology Anxiety Study Group," *N Engl J Med*, 2001, 344(17):1279-85.

Grimsley SR and Jann MW, "Paroxetine, Sertraline, and Fluvoxamine: New Selective Serotonin Reuptake Inhibitors," *Clin Pharm*, 1992, 11(11):930-57.

Lake MB, Birmaher B, Wassick S, et al, "Bleeding and Selective Serotonin Reuptake Inhibitors in Childhood and Adolescence," *J Child Adolesc Psychopharmacol*, 2000, 10(1):35-8.

Levinson-Castiel R, Merlob P, Linder N, et al, "Neonatal Abstinence Syndrome After *in utero* Exposure to Selective Serotonin Reuptake Inhibitors in Term Infants," *Arch Pediatr Adolesc Med*, 2006, 160(2):173-6.

Pass SE and Simpson RW, "Discontinuation and Reinstitution of Medications During the Perioperative Period," *Am J Health Syst Pharm*, 2004, 61(9):899-912.

Reinblatt SP and Riddle MA, "Selective Serotonin Reuptake Inhibitor-Induced Apathy: A Pediatric Case Series," *J Child Adolesc Psychopharmacol*, 2006, 16(1/2):227-33.

Riddle MA, Reeve EA, Yaryura-Tobias JA, et al, "Fluvoxamine for Children and Adolescents With Obsessive-Compulsive Disorder: A Randomized, Controlled, Multicenter Trial," *J Am Acad Child Adolesc Psychiatry*, 2001, 40(2):222-9.

Roose SP, Glassman AH, Attia E, et al, "Comparative Efficacy of Selective Serotonin Reuptake Inhibitors and Tricyclics in the Treatment of Melancholia," *Am J Psychiatry*, 1994, 151(12):1735-9.

Safer DJ and Zito JM, "Treatment Emergent Adverse Effects of Selective Serotonin Reuptake Inhibitors by Age Group: Children vs. Adolescents," *J Child Adolesc Psychopharmacol*, 2006, 16(1/2):159-69.
Weintrob N, Cohen D, Klipper-Aurbach Y, et al, "Decreased Growth During Therapy With Selective Serotonin Reuptake Inhibitors," *Arch Pediatr Adolesc Med*, 2002, 156(7):696-701.

- **Fluzone®** *see* Influenza Virus Vaccine (Inactivated) *on page 833*
- **FML®** *see* Fluorometholone *on page 677*
- **FML® Forte** *see* Fluorometholone *on page 677*
- **FML Forte® (Can)** *see* Fluorometholone *on page 677*
- **Foille® [OTC]** *see* Benzocaine *on page 204*
- **Folacin** *see* Folic Acid *on page 701*
- **Folate** *see* Folic Acid *on page 701*

Folic Acid (FOE lik AS id)

Medication Safety Issues
Sound-alike/look-alike issues:
Folic acid may be confused with folinic acid

Canadian Brand Names Apo-Folic®

Index Terms Folacin; Folate; Pteroylglutamic Acid

Therapeutic Category Nutritional Supplement; Vitamin, Water Soluble

Generic Available Yes

Use Treatment of megaloblastic and macrocytic anemias due to folate deficiency; dietary supplement to prevent neural tube defects

Pregnancy Risk Factor A (C if dose exceeds RDA recommendation)

Lactation Enters breast milk/compatible

Contraindications Hypersensitivity to folic acid or any component (see Warnings); pernicious, aplastic, or normocytic anemias

Warnings Large doses may mask the hematologic effects of B_{12} deficiency, thus obscuring the diagnosis of pernicious anemia while allowing the neurologic complications due to B_{12} deficiency to progress. Folic acid injection contains benzyl alcohol (1.5%) as preservative, which may cause allergic reactions in susceptible individuals; large amounts of benzyl alcohol (≥99 mg/kg/day) have been associated with a potentially fatal toxicity ("gasping syndrome") in neonates; the "gasping syndrome" consists of metabolic acidosis, respiratory distress, gasping respirations, CNS dysfunction (including convulsions, intracranial hemorrhage), hypotension and cardiovascular collapse; avoid use of injection in neonates; *in vitro* and animal studies have shown that benzoate, a metabolite of benzyl alcohol, displaces bilirubin from protein-binding sites

Adverse Reactions
Cardiovascular: Slight flushing
Central nervous system: Irritability, difficulty sleeping, confusion, malaise
Dermatologic: Pruritus, rash
Gastrointestinal: GI upset
Miscellaneous: Hypersensitivity reactions

Drug Interactions May decrease phenytoin serum concentration; hematologic response antagonized by chloramphenicol; folic acid antagonists (ie, methotrexate, pyrimethamine, trimethoprim) prevent the formation of tetrahydrofolic acid (active metabolite), therefore, folic acid is not effective for the treatment of overdosage of these drugs (leucovorin must be used); decreased folic acid absorption with sulfasalazine and aminosalicylic acid; decreased folic acid concentration with phenytoin, primidone, para-aminosalicylic acid

Mechanism of Action Folic acid is necessary for formation of a number of coenzymes in many metabolic systems, particularly for purine and pyrimidine synthesis; required for nucleoprotein synthesis and maintenance in erythropoiesis; stimulates WBC and platelet production in folate deficiency anemia

Pharmacodynamics Maximum effect: Oral: Within 30-60 minutes

Pharmacokinetics
Absorption: In the proximal part of the small intestine
Time to peak serum concentration: Oral: 1 hour
Elimination: Primarily via liver metabolism

Usual Dosage
Recommended daily allowance (RDA): Oral:
Premature neonates: 50 mcg (~15 mcg/kg/day)
Neonates to 6 months: 25-35 mcg
Children:
6 months to 3 years: 50 mcg
4-6 years: 75 mcg
7-10 years: 100 mcg
11-14 years: 150 mcg
(Continued)

Folic Acid *(Continued)*

Children >15 years and Adults: 200 mcg
Pregnant women: 400 mcg
Folic acid deficiency: Oral, I.M., I.V., SubQ:
Infants: 15 mcg/kg/dose daily or 50 mcg/day
Children: 1 mg/day initial dosage; maintenance dose: 1-10 years: 0.1-0.4 mg/day
Children >11 years and Adults: 1 mg/day initial dosage; maintenance dose: 0.5 mg/day

Administration
Oral: May be administered without regard to meals
Parenteral: I.V.: Dilute with SWI, dextrose or saline solution to 0.1 mg/mL; if I.M. route used, administer deep I.M.; may also administer SubQ

Monitoring Parameters CBC with differential

Reference Range Total folate: Normal: 5-15 ng/mL; folate deficiency: <5 ng/mL; megaloblastic anemia: <2 ng/mL

Additional Information Oral liquid vitamin drops (eg, Vi-Daylin®) do not contain folic acid due to the instability of folic acid in the pH of these formulations.

Dosage Forms Excipient information presented when available (limited, particularly for generics); consult specific product labeling.
Injection, solution, as sodium folate: 5 mg/mL (10 mL) [contains benzyl alcohol]
Tablet: 0.4 mg, 0.8 mg, 1 mg

Extemporaneous Preparations A 50 mcg/mL oral solution may be made by mixing 1 mL (5 mg) folic acid injection in 90 mL purified water; adjust pH to 9 with sodium hydroxide 0.1 N (approximately 2.8 mL), then add purified water to make a total volume of 100 mL; stable 30 days at room temperature
Smith SG, "A Folic Acid Solution for Oral Use," *Pharm J*, 1976, 216:108.

♦ **Folinic Acid** *see* Leucovorin *on page 916*

Fomepizole (foe ME pi zole)

Related Information
Commonly Used Antidotes for Acute Overdoses *on page 1920*

U.S. Brand Names Antizol®

Index Terms 4-Methylpyrazole; 4-MP

Therapeutic Category Antidote, Ethylene Glycol Toxicity; Antidote, Methanol Toxicity

Generic Available No

Use Antidote for ethylene glycol (antifreeze) or methanol toxicity; may be useful in propylene glycol toxicity

Pregnancy Risk Factor C

Lactation Excretion in breast milk unknown/not recommended

Contraindications Hypersensitivity to fomepizole, other pyrazoles, or any component

Warnings By inhibiting the action of alcohol dehydrogenase, fomepizole reduces the elimination of alcohol; this must be considered when using fomepizole, as alcohol is often ingested concomitantly by patients with ethylene glycol intoxication; likewise, alcohol may reduce the elimination of fomepizole by the same mechanism; safety and efficacy in pediatric patients has not been established

Precautions Management of ethylene glycol ingestion may require treatment of metabolic acidosis, acute renal failure, adult respiratory distress syndrome, and hypocalcemia; dialysis should be considered, in addition to fomepizole therapy, in patients with acute renal failure, severe metabolic acidosis, or a serum ethylene glycol concentration >50 mg/dL; adjust dosage for renal dysfunction (see Usual Dosage)

Adverse Reactions
Cardiovascular: Bradycardia, tachycardia, hypotension
Central nervous system: Headache, dizziness, seizure, slurred speech, fever, somnolence
Dermatologic: Rash
Gastrointestinal: Nausea, vomiting, diarrhea, anorexia, heartburn, metallic taste, abdominal pain
Hematologic: Eosinophilia, anemia
Hepatic: Transient elevations in transaminase levels
Local: Phlebosclerosis, vein irritation
Ocular: Nystagmus, blurred vision
Respiratory: Pharyngitis, hiccups
Miscellaneous: Hypersensitivity reactions

Drug Interactions Alcohol (see Warnings)

Stability Store at room temperature; fomepizole solidifies at temperatures <25°C (77°F); if solidification occurs, liquefy by running the vial under warm water or by holding in the hand; solidification does not affect the efficacy, safety, or stability of fomepizole; stabile diluted in NS or D_5W for 48 hours; does not contain a preservative; use within 24 hours of dilution

Mechanism of Action A competitive alcohol dehydrogenase inhibitor, fomepizole complexes and inactivates alcohol dehydrogenase thus preventing formation of the toxic metabolites of the alcohols

Pharmacokinetics

Distribution: V_d: 0.6-1.02 L/kg; rapidly distributes into total body water

Protein binding: Negligible

Metabolism: Liver; primarily to 4-carboxypyrazole; after single doses, exhibits saturable, Michaelis-Menton kinetics; with multiple dosing, fomepizole induces its own metabolism via the cytochrome P450 system; after enzyme induction elimination follows first order kinetics

Elimination: 1% to 3.5% excreted unchanged in the urine

Dialysis: Dialyzable

Usual Dosage I.V.:

Children: Has not been studied

Adults **not requiring** hemodialysis: Initial: 15 mg/kg loading dose; followed by 10 mg/kg every 12 hours for 4 doses; then 15 mg/kg every 12 hours until ethylene glycol or methanol levels have been reduced to <20 mg/dL

Adults **requiring** hemodialysis: Since fomepizole is dialyzable, follow the above dose recommendations at intervals related to institution of hemodialysis and its duration:

Dose at the beginning of hemodialysis:

If <6 hours since last fomepizole dose: Do **not** administer dose

If ≥6 hours since last fomepizole dose: Administer next scheduled dose

Dose during hemodialysis: Administer every 4 hours or as continuous infusion 1-1.5 mg/kg/hour

Dose at the time hemodialysis is completed (dependent upon the time between the last dose and the end of hemodialysis):

<1 hour: Do **not** administer at the end of hemodialysis

1-3 hours: Administer ½ of the next scheduled dose

>3 hours: Administer the next scheduled dose

Maintenance dose off hemodialysis: Give next scheduled dose 12 hours from last dose administered

Dosage adjustment in renal impairment: Fomepizole is substantially excreted by the kidney and the risk of toxic reactions to this drug may be increased in patients with impaired renal function; no dosage recommendations for patients with impaired renal function have been established

Administration Parenteral: I.V. Dilute in at least 100 mL NS or D_5W (<25 mg/mL); infuse over 30 minutes; rapid infusion of concentrations ≥25 mg/mL has been associated with vein irritation and phlebosclerosis

Monitoring Parameters Vital signs, arterial blood gases, acid-base status, urinary oxalate, anion and osmolar gaps, clinical signs and symptoms of toxicity (arrhythmias, seizures, coma); serum and urinary ethylene glycol or serum methanol level depending upon the agent ingested; formic acid level (methanol ingestion)

Reference Range Ethylene glycol or methanol serum concentration: Goal: <20 mg/dL; therapeutic plasma fomepizole level: 0.8 mcg/mL

Additional Information If ethylene glycol poisoning is left untreated, the natural progression of the poisoning leads to accumulation of toxic metabolites, including glycolic and oxalic acids; these metabolites can induce metabolic acidosis, seizures, stupor, coma, calcium oxaluria, acute tubular necrosis and death; as ethylene glycol levels diminish in the blood when metabolized to glycolate, the diagnosis of this poisoning may be difficult

Dosage Forms Excipient information presented when available (limited, particularly for generics); consult specific product labeling.

Injection, solution [preservative free]: 1 g/mL (1.5 mL)

References

Druteika DP, Zed PJ, and Ensom MH, "Role of Fomepizole in the Management of Ethylene Glycol Toxicity," *Pharmacotherapy*, 2002, 22(3):365-72.

◆ **Foradil® (Can)** *see* Formoterol *on page 703*

◆ **Foradil® Aerolizer™** *see* Formoterol *on page 703*

Formoterol (for MOH te rol)

Medication Safety Issues

Sound-alike/look-alike issues:

Foradil® may be confused with Toradol®

Foradil® capsules for inhalation are for administration via Aerolizer™ inhaler and are not for oral use.

(Continued)

Formoterol *(Continued)*

International issues:

Foradil® may be confused with Theradol® which is a brand name for tramadol in the Netherlands.

Related Information

Asthma *on page 1904*

U.S. Brand Names Foradil® Aerolizer™

Canadian Brand Names Foradil®; Oxeze® Turbuhaler®

Index Terms Formoterol Fumarate

Therapeutic Category Adrenergic Agonist Agent; Antiasthmatic; Beta$_2$-Adrenergic Agonist Agent; Bronchodilator; Sympathomimetic

Generic Available No

Use Maintenance treatment of asthma and prevention of bronchospasm in patients >5 years of age with reversible obstructive airway disease; prevention of exercise-induced bronchospasm in children >5 years of age and adults; maintenance treatment of bronchoconstriction in COPD

Medication Guide An FDA-approved patient medication guide, which is available with the product information and at http://www.fda.gov/cder/Offices/ODS/medication_guides.htm, must be dispensed with this medication for each new outpatient prescription and refill.

Pregnancy Risk Factor C

Lactation Excretion in breast milk unknown/use caution

Contraindications Hypersensitivity to formoterol, adrenergic amines, or any component; severe milk allergy (contains lactose)

Warnings Formoterol is not indicated to relieve acute asthma symptoms or for those patients who are successfully maintained with occasional use of beta$_2$ agonists. Acute asthma episodes should be treated with short-acting beta$_2$ agonists. Do not increase the frequency of formoterol use. Paroxysmal bronchospasm (which can be fatal) has been reported with this and other inhaled beta$_2$ agonists. If this occurs, discontinue treatment. Formoterol capsules should **only** be used with the Aerolizer™ inhaler and should **not** be taken orally.

Long-acting beta$_2$ agonists have been associated with an increased risk of serious asthma exacerbations and asthma-related deaths. Formoterol should only be prescribed in patients not adequately controlled on other asthma-controller medications or whose disease severity clearly warrants treatment with two maintenance therapies. A medication guide is available to provide information to patients covering the risk of use.

Precautions Use with caution in patients with cardiovascular disorders (coronary insufficiency, cardiac arrhythmias, and hypertension), convulsive disorders, thyrotoxicosis, or others who are sensitive to the effects of sympathomimetic amines

Adverse Reactions

Cardiovascular: Tachycardia, palpitations, arrhythmias, angina, hypertension, hypotension

Central nervous system: Dizziness, headache, nervousness, hyperactivity, insomnia, malaise, fatigue

Dermatologic: Rash, pruritus

Endocrine & metabolic: Hypokalemia, hyperglycemia, metabolic acidosis

Gastrointestinal: GI upset, nausea, xerostomia, tonsillitis, dysphonia

Neuromuscular & skeletal: Tremors, muscle cramps

Respiratory: Respiratory arrest, cough, pharyngitis, bronchitis, paradoxical bronchospasm (see Warnings), sinusitis, upper respiratory tract infections, rhinitis

Miscellaneous: Hypersensitivity reactions, tachyphylaxis, viral infection

Drug Interactions Cytochrome P450 isoenzyme CYP2A6, CYP2C9, CYP2C19, and CYP2D6 substrate

Additive effects with beta-adrenergic agents; MAO inhibitors and tricyclic antidepressants potentiate cardiovascular effects; beta-blocking agents antagonize effects; increased potassium losses with diuretics

Stability Store in refrigerator or at controlled room temperature; capsules should always be stored in the blister pack and only removed immediately before use

Mechanism of Action Formoterol is a long-acting selective beta$_2$-adrenergic receptor agonist. It relaxes bronchial smooth muscle by selective action on beta$_2$-receptors with little effect on heart rate

Pharmacodynamics

Onset of action: 1-3 minutes

Peak effect: 30 minutes to 1 hour

Duration: Up to 12 hours

Pharmacokinetics

Protein binding: 61% to 64%

Metabolism: Extensive via glucuronidation and o-demethylation

Half-life: Adults: 10 hours

Time to peak serum concentration: Inhalation: 5 minutes

Elimination: 10% to 18% eliminated unchanged in urine

Usual Dosage

Bronchodilation (asthma or COPD): Children ≥5 years and Adults: Inhalation, oral: 12 mcg (contents of 1 capsule aerosolized) twice daily, 12 hours apart

Prevention of exercise-induced asthma: Children ≥5 years and Adults: Inhalation: 12 mcg (contents of 1 capsule aerosolized) 15 minutes prior to exercise; additional doses should not be used for 12 hours; patients who are using formoterol twice daily should **not** use an additional formoterol dose prior to exercise; if twice daily use is not effective during exercise, consider other appropriate therapy

Administration Inhalation: The contents of a capsule are aerosolized via a device called an Aerolizer™. Place the capsule into the Aerolizer™. The capsule is pierced by pressing and releasing the buttons on the side of the Aerolizer™. The formoterol formulation is dispersed into the air stream when the patient inhales rapidly and deeply through the mouthpiece. May not be used with spacer device.

Monitoring Parameters Pulmonary function tests

Patient Information Do not use to treat acute symptoms; do not exceed the prescribed dose of formoterol; do not stop using inhaled or oral corticosteroids without medical advice even if feeling better; may cause dry mouth; the capsule is not to be taken by mouth

Additional Information When formoterol is initiated in patients previously receiving a short-acting beta agonist, instruct the patient to discontinue the regular use of the short-acting beta agonist and to utilize the shorter-acting agent for symptomatic or acute episodes only.

Dosage Forms Excipient information presented when available (limited, particularly for generics); consult specific product labeling. [CAN] = Canadian brand name

Powder for oral inhalation, as fumarate:

Foradil® Aerolizer™ [capsule]: 12 mcg (12s, 60s) [contains lactose 25 mg]

Oxeze® Turbuhaler® [CAN]: 6 mcg/inhalation [delivers 60 metered doses; contains lactose 600 mcg/dose]; 12 mcg/inhalation [delivers 60 metered doses; contains lactose 600 mcg/dose] [not available in the U.S.]

References

Bisgaard H, "Long-acting Beta$_2$-Agonists in Management of Childhood Asthma: A Critical Review of the Literature," *Pediatr Pulmonol*, 2000, 29(3):221-34

"National Asthma Education and Prevention Program. Expert Panel Report: Guidelines for the Diagnosis and Management of Asthma Update on Selected Topics--2002," *J Allergy Clin Immunol*, 2002, 110(5 Suppl):S141-219.

♦ **Formoterol Fumarate** *see* Formoterol *on page 703*
♦ **Formulation R™ [OTC]** *see* Phenylephrine *on page 1250*
♦ **Formulex® (Can)** *see* Dicyclomine *on page 490*
♦ **5-Formyl Tetrahydrofolate** *see* Leucovorin *on page 916*
♦ **Fortamet®** *see* Metformin *on page 1016*
♦ **Fortaz®** *see* Ceftazidime *on page 317*
♦ **Fortical®** *see* Calcitonin *on page 258*
♦ **Fortovase® [DSC]** *see* Saquinavir *on page 1417*
♦ **Fortovase® (Can)** *see* Saquinavir *on page 1417*

Fosamprenavir (FOS am pren a veer)

Medication Safety Issues

Sound-alike/look-alike issues:

Lexiva® may be confused with Levitra®

Related Information

Adult and Adolescent HIV *on page 1821*

Pediatric HIV *on page 1816*

Perinatal HIV *on page 1831*

U.S. Brand Names Lexiva®

Canadian Brand Names Telzir®

Index Terms Fosamprenavir Calcium; GW433908G

Therapeutic Category Antiretroviral Agent; HIV Agents (Anti-HIV Agents); Protease Inhibitor

Generic Available No

Use Treatment of HIV infection in combination with other antiretroviral agents (**Note:** HIV regimens consisting of **three** antiretroviral agents are strongly recommended)

Pregnancy Risk Factor C

Lactation Excretion in breast milk unknown/contraindicated

(Continued)

Fosamprenavir *(Continued)*

Contraindications Hypersensitivity to fosamprenavir, amprenavir or any component; concurrent therapy with cisapride, dihydroergotamine, ergonovine, ergotamine, methylergonovine, pimozide, midazolam, or triazolam; if fosamprenavir is administered with ritonavir, flecainide and propafenone are also contraindicated.

Warnings Fosamprenavir (a prodrug of amprenavir) is a potent CYP3A4 isoenzyme inhibitor that interacts with numerous drugs. Due to potential serious and/or life-threatening drug interactions, some drugs are contraindicated (see Contraindications and Drug interactions) and the following drugs require serum concentration monitoring if coadministered with fosamprenavir: Amiodarone, systemic lidocaine, tricyclic antidepressants, and quinidine. Concurrent use with rifampin, St John's wort, or certain cholesterol-lowering agents (lovastatin, simvastatin) is **not** recommended.

Severe and life-threatening skin reactions (including Stevens-Johnson syndrome) may occur; discontinue fosamprenavir in patients who develop severe or life-threatening rashes or in patients with moderate rashes and systemic symptoms. Spontaneous bleeding episodes have been reported in patients with hemophilia type A and B receiving protease inhibitors. New-onset diabetes mellitus, exacerbations of diabetes, and hyperglycemia have been reported in HIV-infected patients receiving protease inhibitors. Significant elevations of serum triglycerides and cholesterol may occur when fosamprenavir is used in combination with ritonavir (monitor and manage appropriately).

Precautions Use with caution in patients with diabetes mellitus, sulfonamide allergy (fosamprenavir is a sulfonamide), or hemophilia. Use with caution and decrease the dose in patients with hepatic impairment; patients coinfected with hepatitis B or C and those with baseline liver enzyme elevation may be at risk for elevated liver enzymes with fosamprenavir therapy. Fat redistribution and accumulation [ie, central obesity, peripheral wasting, facial wasting, breast enlargement, dorsocervical fat enlargement (buffalo hump), and cushingoid appearance] have been observed in patients receiving antiretroviral agents (causal relationship not established). Immune reconstitution syndrome (an acute inflammatory response to residual or indolent opportunistic infections) may occur in HIV patients during initial treatment with combination antiretroviral agents; this syndrome may require further patient assessment and therapy.

Adverse Reactions

Central nervous system: Depression or mood disorders (8%), headache (19%), fatigue (10%)

Dermatologic: Rash (19% to 35% incidence; usually mild to moderate, maculopapular, some pruritic; median onset: 11 days, median duration: 13 days); severe or life-threatening rash, including Stevens-Johnson syndrome (<1% of patients; see Warnings); pruritus (7%)

Endocrine & metabolic: Hyperglycemia, hypertriglyceridemia (0% to 6%), elevated serum lipase (8%); new onset diabetes, exacerbation of diabetes mellitus, ketoacidosis, elevated serum creatine phosphokinase, fat redistribution and accumulation (see Precautions)

Gastrointestinal: Nausea (39%), vomiting (16%), diarrhea (34%), abdominal pain (5%)

Hematologic: Spontaneous bleeding in hemophiliacs, neutropenia (3%), hemolytic anemia

Hepatic: Elevated liver enzymes (6%)

Neuromuscular & skeletal: Perioral paresthesia (2%)

Miscellaneous: Immune reconstitution syndrome

Drug Interactions Cytochrome P450 isoenzyme CYP2C9 (minor), CYP3A4 (major), and CYP3A5 (minor) substrate; isoenzyme CYP2C19 (weak) and CYP3A4 (strong) inhibitor

Fosamprenavir may inhibit the metabolism of the following drugs and cause serious or life-threatening adverse effects: Cisapride, dihydroergotamine, ergonovine, ergotamine, methylergonovine, pimozide, midazolam, and triazolam (concurrent therapy with these drugs and fosamprenavir is contraindicated); **Note:** If fosamprenavir and ritonavir are used concurrently, flecainide and propafenone are also contraindicated; fosamprenavir may increase the toxic effects of amiodarone, lidocaine, quinidine, warfarin, cyclosporine, tacrolimus, rapamycin, and tricyclic antidepressants (serum concentration monitoring of these drugs is necessary); fosamprenavir may increase the serum concentration of bepridil and result in life-threatening cardiac arrhythmias (use with caution; monitor closely); fosamprenavir may significantly increase concentrations of rifabutin and its metabolite (rifabutin dose should be decreased by at least $\frac{1}{2}$ the recommended dose when used in combination with fosamprenavir and by at least 75% when used in combination with fosamprenavir plus ritonavir); fosamprenavir may increase the serum concentrations or toxicity of ketoconazole, itraconazole, calcium channel blockers, benzodiazepines, trazodone (use with caution; consider trazodone dosage reduction), cholesterol-lowering agents (increased risk of myopathy and rhabdomyolysis; concurrent use of lovastatin or simvastatin is **not** recommended; use lowest possible dose of atorvastatin and carefully monitor patient; consider use of pravastatin, fluvastatin, or rosuvastatin for concurrent use with fosamprenavir), sildenafil or other phosphodiesterase-5 (PDE-5) enzyme inhibitors (use decreased dose of sildenafil or other PDE-5 enzyme inhibitor). Ritonavir significantly increases fluticasone serum concentrations and may result in systemic corticosteroid effects (eg, Cushing's syndrome and adrenal suppression); fosamprenavir plus ritonavir use with fluticasone is expected to have the same effect; concurrent use of fosamprenavir plus ritonavir with fluticasone is **not** recommended unless benefits outweigh risks; use of fosamprenavir without ritonavir may increase fluticasone serum concentrations (use with caution; consider alternative agent, especially with long-term use).

Rifampin significantly reduces amprenavir plasma concentrations and should **not** be used concurrently. Hormonal contraceptives (eg, ethinyl estradiol/norethindrone) decrease amprenavir serum concentrations; hormonal levels may also be altered; thus, hormonal contraceptive agents should **not** be used concurrently (nonhormonal contraception is recommended). Methadone may decrease the serum concentrations of amprenavir (consider alternative antiretroviral agent); fosamprenavir may decrease plasma concentrations of methadone (increase in methadone dosage may be required). Fosamprenavir may decrease serum concentrations of delavirdine and result in a loss of virological response and possible delavirdine resistance (concomitant use of amprenavir and delavirdine is **not** recommended). Fosamprenavir may decrease serum concentrations of atazanavir (appropriate dosage adjustment has not been established).

The herbal medicine St John's wort (*Hypericum perforatum*) may significantly decrease concentrations of amprenavir and is **not** recommended for concurrent use. Efavirenz and nevirapine significantly decrease the serum concentrations of amprenavir; coadministration of fosamprenavir with either efavirenz or nevirapine **without** booster doses of ritonavir is **not** recommended. **Note:** Fosamprenavir increases nevirapine serum concentrations. Saquinavir, lopinavir/ritonavir, dexamethasone, phenobarbital, phenytoin, carbamazepine, antacids, histamine H_2-receptor antagonists may decrease amprenavir concentrations. **Note:** Proton pump inhibitors may be administered at the same time as fosamprenavir without affecting amprenavir serum concentrations. Indinavir, nelfinavir, ritonavir may increase the concentration of amprenavir.

Food Interactions Food does not significantly affect absorption.

Stability Store at room temperature in tightly closed container.

Mechanism of Action Fosamprenavir is rapidly converted to amprenavir *in vivo.* Amprenavir is a protease inhibitor which acts on an enzyme (protease) late in the HIV replication process after the virus has entered into the cell's nucleus; amprenavir binds to the protease activity site and inhibits the activity of the enzyme, thus preventing cleavage of viral polyprotein precursors (gag-pol protein precursors) into individual functional proteins found in infectious HIV; this results in the formation of immature, noninfectious viral particles

Pharmacokinetics

Protein binding: 90%; primarily to $alpha_1$ acid glycoprotein; concentration dependent binding

Metabolism: Fosamprenavir is the prodrug of amprenavir; fosamprenavir is rapidly hydrolyzed to amprenavir and inorganic phosphate by cellular phosphatases in the gut epithelium as it is absorbed; amprenavir is metabolized in the liver via cytochrome P450 CYP3A4 isoenzyme system; glucuronide conjugation of oxidized metabolites also occurs

Bioavailability: Not established

Half-life: Amprenavir: Adults: 7.7 hours

Time to peak serum concentration: Amprenavir (single dose of fosamprenavir): Median: 2.5 hours; range: 1.5-4 hours

Elimination: Minimal excretion of unchanged drug in urine (1%) and feces; 75% of dose excreted as metabolites via biliary tract into feces and 14% excreted as metabolites in urine

Usual Dosage Oral (use in combination with other antiretroviral agents):

Neonates and Infants: Not approved for use; appropriate dose is unknown

Children: Not approved for use; appropriate dose is unknown; clinical studies are ongoing

Adolescents and Adults:

Antiretroviral therapy-naive patients:

Unboosted regimen (ie, regimen without ritonavir): Fosamprenavir 1400 mg twice daily

Ritonavir boosted regimens:

Once-daily regimen: Fosamprenavir 1400 mg once daily plus ritonavir 200 mg once daily

(Continued)

Fosamprenavir *(Continued)*

Twice-daily regimen: Fosamprenavir 700 mg twice daily plus ritonavir 100 mg twice daily

Protease inhibitor-experienced patients: Fosamprenavir 700 mg twice daily plus ritonavir 100 mg twice daily. **Note:** Once-daily dosing of fosamprenavir is not recommended in protease inhibitor-experienced patients.

Adults:

Concomitant therapy with efavirenz: Note: Only ritonavir boosted regimens should be used when efavirenz is used in combination with fosamprenavir.

Once-daily regimen: Fosamprenavir 1400 mg once daily plus ritonavir 300 mg once daily

Twice-daily regimen: Fosamprenavir 700 mg twice daily plus ritonavir 100 mg twice daily. **Note:** No change in ritonavir dosage is required when patients receive efavirenz with twice daily dosing of fosamprenavir with ritonavir

Concomitant therapy with nevirapine: Note: Only ritonavir boosted regimens should be used when nevirapine is used in combination with fosamprenavir.

Once-daily regimen: Not studied

Twice-daily regimen: Fosamprenavir 700 mg twice daily plus ritonavir 100 mg twice daily.

Dosage adjustment in renal impairment: No dosage adjustment required

Dosage adjustment in hepatic impairment: Use with caution: Adults: Unboosted regimens:

Mild to moderate impairment (Child-Pugh score 5-8): Reduce dosage of fosamprenavir to 700 mg twice daily (without concurrent ritonavir)

Severe impairment (Child-Pugh score 9-12): Use is not recommended

Note: No recommendations are available for dosage adjustments in patients receiving ritonavir and fosamprenavir

Administration May be administered without regard to meals; do not administer concurrently with antacids or buffered formulations of other medications (separate administration by 1 hour)

Monitoring Parameters Signs and symptoms of rash or adverse effects; serum glucose, triglycerides, cholesterol, liver enzymes, CBC with differential, CD4 cell count, viral load

Patient Information Inform your physician if you have a sulfa allergy; fosamprenavir is not a cure for HIV; notify physician immediately if rash develops; some medicines should not be taken with fosamprenavir; report the use of other medications, nonprescription medications, and herbal or natural products to your physician and pharmacist; avoid the herbal medicine St John's wort; take fosamprenavir every day as prescribed; do not change dose or discontinue without physician's advice; if a dose is missed, take it as soon as possible, then return to normal dosing schedule; if a dose is skipped, do not double the next dose.

HIV medications may cause changes in body fat, including an increase in fat in the upper back and neck, breasts, and trunk; a loss of fat from the face, arms, and legs may also occur.

Additional Information A 50 mg/mL suspension is currently under investigation. Fosamprenavir calcium 700 mg (1 tablet) is approximately equal to amprenavir 600 mg.

Dosage Forms Excipient information presented when available (limited, particularly for generics); consult specific product labeling. [CAN] = Canadian brand name

Tablet, as calcium:

Lexiva®: 700 mg

Suspension, oral, as calcium:

Telzir® [CAN]: 50 mg/mL (225 mL) [not available in the U.S.]

References

Briars LA, Hilao JJ, and Kraus DM, "A Review of Pediatric Human Immunodeficiency Virus Infection," *Journal of Pharmacy Practice*, 2004, 17(6):407-31.

Chapman TM, Plosker GL, and Perry CM, "Fosamprenavir: A Review of Its Use in the Management of Antiretroviral Therapy-Naive Patients With HIV Infection," *Drugs*, 2004, 64(18):2101-24.

Morris JL and Kraus DM, "New Antiretroviral Therapies for Pediatric HIV Infection," *J Pediatr Pharmacol Ther*, 2005, 10:215-47.

Panel on Clinical Practices for Treatment of HIV Infection, "Guidelines for the Use of Antiretroviral Agents in HIV-Infected Adults and Adolescents," October 10, 2006, http://www.aidsinfo.nih.gov.

Wire MB, Shelton MJ, and Studenberg S, "Fosamprenavir: Clinical Pharmacokinetics and Drug Interactions of the Amprenavir Prodrug," *Clin Pharmacokinet*, 2006, 45(2):137-68.

Working Group on Antiretroviral Therapy and Medical Management of HIV-Infected Children, "Guidelines for the Use of Antiretroviral Agents in Pediatric HIV Infection," October 26, 2006, http://www.aidsinfo.nih.gov.

Working Group on Antiretroviral Therapy and Medical Management of HIV-Infected Children, "Guidelines for the Use of Antiretroviral Agents in Pediatric HIV Infection. Supplement I: Pediatric Antiretroviral Drug Information," October 26, 2006, http://www.aidsinfo.nih.gov.

♦ **Fosamprenavir Calcium** *see* Fosamprenavir *on page 705*

Foscarnet (fos KAR net)

U.S. Brand Names Foscavir®

Canadian Brand Names Foscavir®

Index Terms PFA; Phosphonoformate; Phosphonoformic Acid

Therapeutic Category Antiviral Agent, Parenteral

Generic Available Yes

Use Alternative to ganciclovir for treatment of CMV infections; treatment of CMV retinitis in patients with acquired immunodeficiency syndrome; treatment of acyclovir-resistant mucocutaneous herpes simplex virus infections in immunocompromised patients and acyclovir-resistant herpes zoster infections

Pregnancy Risk Factor C

Lactation Excretion in breast milk unknown/contraindicated

Contraindications Hypersensitivity to foscarnet or any component; Cl_{cr} <0.4 mL/minute/kg

Warnings Renal impairment occurs to some degree in the majority of patients treated with foscarnet; renal impairment may occur at any time and is usually reversible within 1 week following dose adjustment or discontinuation of therapy; however, several patients have died with renal failure within 4 weeks of stopping foscarnet; foscarnet is deposited in teeth and bone of young, growing animals; it has adversely affected tooth enamel development in rats; safety and effectiveness in children has not been studied

Serum electrolyte imbalance occurs in 6% to 30% of patients (hypocalcemia, low ionized calcium, hypo- or hyperphosphatemia, hypokalemia, or hypomagnesemia). Patients with a low ionized calcium may experience perioral tingling, numbness, parasthesia, tetany, and seizures. Risk factor for seizures include a low baseline ANC, impaired renal function, and low total serum calcium.

Precautions Use with caution in patients with renal impairment, patients with altered electrolyte levels, and patients with neurologic or cardiac abnormalities; adjust dose for patients with impaired renal function; discontinue treatment in adults if serum creatinine ≥2.9 mg/dL; therapy can be restarted if serum creatinine ≤2 mg/dL

Adverse Reactions

Cardiovascular: Hypertension, palpitations, chest pain, EKG abnormalities, hypotension, flushing, arrhythmias

Central nervous system: Fatigue, fever, headache, seizures, hallucinations, dizziness, agitation, amnesia, depression

Dermatologic: Rash, pruritus

Endocrine & metabolic: Hypocalcemia, hypomagnesemia, hypokalemia, hypo- or hyperphosphatemia, weight loss

Gastrointestinal: Nausea, diarrhea, vomiting, pancreatitis, anorexia, constipation, dyspepsia, stomatitis

Genitourinary: Vulvovaginal ulceration, penile epithelium ulceration, dysuria, urethral disorder

Hematologic: Decreases in hemoglobin and hematocrit, leukopenia

Hepatic: Elevated liver enzymes, cholecystitis, hepatitis

Local: Thrombophlebitis

Neuromuscular & skeletal: Peripheral neuropathy, paresthesia, tremor

Ocular: Ocular pain, conjunctivitis

Renal: Elevated BUN and serum creatinine, polyuria, oliguria, renal failure, proteinuria

Respiratory: Coughing, dyspnea, bronchospasm

Drug Interactions Pentamidine (additive hypocalcemia); cyclosporine, aminoglycosides, amphotericin B (additive nephrotoxicity); ciprofloxacin (increases seizure potential)

Stability Store at room temperature; refrigeration may result in crystallization of the drug; incompatible with dextrose ≥30%, I.V. solutions containing calcium, magnesium, vancomycin, TPN

Mechanism of Action Pyrophosphate analog which inhibits DNA synthesis by interfering with viral DNA polymerase and reverse transcriptase

Pharmacokinetics

Distribution: V_d: Adults: 0.6 L/kg; up to 20% of cumulative I.V. dose may be deposited in bone

Protein binding: 14% to 17%

Half-life, plasma: Adults: 2-4.5 hours

Elimination: 80% to 90% excreted unchanged in urine

Usual Dosage Children and Adults: I.V.:

CMV retinitis: Induction treatment: 180 mg/kg/day divided every 8 hours for 14-21 days

Maintenance therapy: 90-120 mg/kg/day as a single infusion once daily

(Continued)

Foscarnet *(Continued)*

Acyclovir-resistant herpes simplex virus infection: 40 mg/kg/dose every 8 hours or 40-60 mg/kg/dose every 12 hours for up to 3 weeks or until lesions heal; repeat treatment may lead to the development of resistance

Dosing interval in renal impairment: See tables.

Induction Treatment

Cl_{cr} (mL/min/kg)	mg/kg/8h
≥1.6	60
1.5	56.5
1.4	53
1.3	49.4
1.2	45.9
1.1	42.4
1	38.9
0.9	35.3
0.8	31.8
0.7	28.3
0.6	24.8
0.5	21.2
0.4	17.7

Maintenance Therapy

Cl_{cr} (mL/min/kg)	mg/kg
≥1.4	90-120 q24h
1-1.4	70-90 q24h
0.8-1	50-65 q24h
0.6-0.8	80-105 q48h
0.5-0.6	60-80 q48h
0.4-0.5	50-65 q48h
<0.4	not recommended

Administration Parenteral: 24 mg/mL solution may be administered without further dilution when using a central venous catheter for infusion; for peripheral vein administration, the solution **must** be diluted to a final concentration **not to exceed** 12 mg/mL with either NS or D_5W; administer by I.V. infusion at a rate **not to exceed** 60 mg/kg/dose over 1 hour or 120 mg/kg/dose over 2 hours

Monitoring Parameters Serum creatinine, calcium, phosphorus, potassium, magnesium; hemoglobin, hematocrit, ophthalmologic exams

Reference Range Therapeutic for CMV: 150 mcg/mL

Patient Information Report any numbness in the extremities, paresthesias, perioral tingling, or seizures

Nursing Implications Provide adequate hydration with I.V. NS or D_5W prior to and during treatment to minimize nephrotoxicity

Dosage Forms Excipient information presented when available (limited, particularly for generics); consult specific product labeling.

Injection, solution: 24 mg/mL (250 mL, 500 mL)

Foscavir®: 24 mg/mL (500 mL)

References

Aweeka FT, Jacobson MA, Martin-Munley S, et al, "Effect of Renal Disease and Hemodialysis on Foscarnet Pharmacokinetics and Dosing Recommendations," *J Acquir Immune Defic Syndr Hum Retrovirol*, 1999, 20(4):350-7.

Butler KM, DeSmet MD, Husson RN, et al, "Treatment of Aggressive Cytomegalovirus Retinitis With Ganciclovir in Combination With Foscarnet in a Child Infected With Human Immunodeficiency Virus," *J Pediatr*, 1992, 120(3):483-6.

Kaplan JE, Masur H, and Holmes KK, "Guidelines for Preventing Opportunistic Infections Among HIV-Infected Persons - 2002. Recommendations of the USPHS and IDSA," *MMWR*, 2002, 51(RR-8):1-27, 29-46.

♦ **Foscavir®** *see* Foscarnet *on page 709*

Fosphenytoin (FOS fen i toyn)

Medication Safety Issues

Sound-alike/look-alike issues:

Cerebyx® may be confused with Celebrex®, Celexa™, Cerezyme®

Related Information

Blood Level Sampling Time Guidelines *on page 1914*

Phenytoin *on page 1253*

U.S. Brand Names Cerebyx®

Canadian Brand Names Cerebyx®

Index Terms Fosphenytoin Sodium

Therapeutic Category Anticonvulsant, Hydantoin

Generic Available No

Use Management of generalized convulsive status epilepticus; used for short-term parenteral administration of phenytoin; prevention and management of seizures responsive to phenytoin

Pregnancy Risk Factor D

Lactation Excretion in breast milk unknown/not recommended

Contraindications Hypersensitivity to fosphenytoin, phenytoin, other hydantoins, or any other component; second and third degree heart block, sinoatrial block, sinus bradycardia, Adams-Stokes syndrome

Warnings Abrupt withdrawal may precipitate status epilepticus; monitor blood pressure and EKG with I.V. loading doses; use with caution in patients with severe myocardial insufficiency and hypotension; discontinue if skin rash develops, do not resume drug if rash is exfoliative, purpuric, bullous, or if SLE, Stevens-Johnson syndrome, or toxic epidermal necrolysis is suspected; discontinue if acute hepatotoxicity occurs; hematologic toxicities and lymphadenopathy have been reported with phenytoin use

Precautions Use with caution in patients with porphyria; consider the amount of phosphate delivered by fosphenytoin in patients who require phosphate restriction; sensory disturbances (burning, pruritus, tingling, paresthesia) may occur especially at higher doses (≥15 mg **PE**/kg) and at maximum I.V. infusion rates (see Adverse Reactions); use with caution and modify dosage in patients with hepatic or renal dysfunction. Safety of fosphenytoin in pediatric patients has not been established.

Adverse Reactions

Cardiovascular: Hypotension (with rapid I.V. administration), vasodilation, tachycardia, bradycardia

Central nervous system: Slurred speech, dizziness, drowsiness, headache, somnolence, ataxia, fever

Dermatologic: Rash, exfoliative dermatitis, facial edema

Endocrine & metabolic: Folic acid depletion, hyperglycemia

Gastrointestinal: Nausea, vomiting, taste perversion

Genitourinary: Pelvic pain

Hematologic: Neutropenia, thrombocytopenia, anemia (megaloblastic)

Local: Pain on injection; since fosphenytoin is water soluble and has a lower pH (8.8) than phenytoin (12), irritation at injection site or phlebitis is reduced; I.M.: Local itching

Neuromuscular & skeletal: Osteomalacia

Ocular: Nystagmus, blurred vision, diplopia

Otic: Tinnitus

Miscellaneous: Lymphadenopathy; sensory disturbances (burning, pruritus, tingling, paresthesia) occur predominately in the groin area, but may occur in the lower back, abdomen, head or neck (these effects may be related to the phosphate load); paresthesia and pruritus are more common with I.V. vs I.M. administration and are dose and infusion rate related

Drug Interactions No drugs are known to interfere with the conversion of fosphenytoin to phenytoin; see Phenytoin *on page 1253* for phenytoin interactions

Stability Store unopened vials in the refrigerator; do not store unopened vials at room temperature for >48 hours; do not use vials containing particulate matter. Fosphenytoin at concentrations of 1, 8, and 20 mg phenytoin sodium equivalents **(PE)**/mL in D_5W or NS is stable for 30 days when stored at 25°C or 4°C in glass bottles or polyvinyl chloride infusion bags, and when frozen at -20°C in polyvinyl chloride infusion bags. After removal from the freezer, these solutions are stable for 7 days at 25°C or 4°C.

Undiluted fosphenytoin injection (50 mg **PE**/mL) is stable in polypropylene syringes for 30 days at 25°C, 4°C, or frozen at -20°C.

Fosphenytoin at concentrations of 1, 8, and 20 mg **PE**/mL prepared in $D_5/{}^1/_2$NS, $D_5/{}^1/_2$NS with KCl 20 mEq/L, $D_5/{}^1/_2$NS with 40 mEq/L, LR, D_5/LR, $D_{10}W$, amino acid 10%, (Continued)

Fosphenytoin *(Continued)*

mannitol 20%, hetastarch 6% in NS or Plasma-Lyte® A injection is stable in polyvinyl chloride bags for 7 days when stored at 25°C (room temperature).

Mechanism of Action Diphosphate ester salt of phenytoin which acts as a water soluble prodrug of phenytoin; after administration, plasma and tissue esterases convert fosphenytoin to phosphate, formaldehyde and phenytoin (as the active moiety); phenytoin works by stabilizing neuronal membranes and decreasing seizure activity by increasing efflux or decreasing influx of sodium ions across cell membranes in the motor cortex during generation of nerve impulses

Pharmacokinetics The pharmacokinetics of fosphenytoin-derived phenytoin are the same as those for phenytoin (see Phenytoin *on page 1253*). Parameters listed below are for fosphenytoin (the prodrug) unless otherwise noted. **Note:** The pharmacokinetics of fosphenytoin have been studied in a limited number of children 5-18 years of age and have been found to be similar to the pharmacokinetics observed in young adults (see Pellock, 1996).

Bioavailability: I.M., I.V.: 100%

Distribution: Adults: V_d: 4.3-10.8 L; V_d of fosphenytoin increases with dose and rate of administration

Protein binding: 95% to 99% primarily to albumin; binding of fosphenytoin to protein is saturable (the percent bound decreases as total concentration increases); fosphenytoin displaces phenytoin from protein binding sites; during the time fosphenytoin is being converted to phenytoin, fosphenytoin may temporarily increase the free fraction of phenytoin up to 30% unbound

Metabolism: Each millimole of fosphenytoin is metabolized to 1 millimole of phenytoin, phosphate, and formaldehyde; formaldehyde is converted to formate, which is then metabolized by a folate-dependent mechanism; conversion of fosphenytoin to phenytoin increases with increasing dose and infusion rate, most likely due to a decrease in fosphenytoin protein binding

Conversion of fosphenytoin to phenytoin: Half-life: 15 minutes

Time for complete conversion to phenytoin:

I.M.: 4 hours after injection

I.V.: 2 hours after the end of infusion

Time to peak serum concentration (phenytoin): I.M.: 3 hours

Elimination: 0% fosphenytoin excreted in urine

Usual Dosage

The dose, concentration in solutions, and infusion rates for fosphenytoin are expressed as PHENYTOIN SODIUM EQUIVALENTS (PE)

Fosphenytoin should ALWAYS be prescribed and dispensed in mg of PE; otherwise significant medication errors may occur

Neonates, Infants, and Children: I.V.: **Note:** Not FDA approved for use. A limited number of clinical studies have been conducted in pediatric patients; based on pharmacokinetic studies, experts recommend the following (see Fischer, 2003): Use the pediatric I.V. phenytoin dosing guidelines to dose fosphenytoin using doses in **PE** equal to the phenytoin doses (ie, phenytoin 1 mg = fosphenytoin 1 mg **PE**). Further pediatric studies are needed.

Adults:

Loading dose:

Status epilepticus: I.V.: 15-20 mg **PE**/kg

Nonemergent loading: I.M., I.V.: 10-20 mg **PE**/kg

Initial daily maintenance dose: I.M., I.V.: 4-6 mg **PE**/kg; I.M. dose may be administered as a single daily dose using 1 or 2 injection sites; some patients may require more frequent dosing

I.M. or I.V. substitution for oral phenytoin: Initial: Use the same total daily dose in **PE** of fosphenytoin (ie, phenytoin 1 mg = fosphenytoin 1 mg **PE**); plasma concentrations may increase slightly with this method because oral phenytoin sodium is 90% bioavailable and phenytoin derived from I.M. or I.V. fosphenytoin is 100% bioavailable. Monitor clinical response and phenytoin concentrations to further guide dosage adjustments after 3-4 days

Dosing adjustments in renal/hepatic impairment:

Cirrhosis: Phenytoin clearance may be substantially reduced and monitoring of plasma concentrations with dosage adjustments is advisable

Renal or hepatic disease and patients with hypoalbuminemia: Fosphenytoin conversion to phenytoin may be increased (due to lower protein binding) without a similar increase in phenytoin clearance, leading to a potential increase in the frequency and severity of adverse effects

Administration Dilute with D_5W or NS to 1.5-25 mg **PE**/mL

Children 5-18 years: An administration rate of 3 mg **PE**/kg/minute with a maximum of 150 mg **PE**/minute was used in 7 patients (see Pellock, 1996)

Adults: Administer at a rate of 100-150 mg **PE**/minute with a maximum infusion rate of 150 mg **PE**/minute

Monitoring Parameters Serum phenytoin concentrations, CBC with differential, platelets, serum glucose, liver enzymes; blood pressure, continuous EKG, respiratory function with I.V. loading doses; free (unbound) and total serum phenytoin concentrations in patients with hyperbilirubinemia, hypoalbuminemia, renal dysfunction, uremia, or hepatic disease

Reference Range Monitor **phenytoin** serum concentrations; obtain phenytoin concentrations 2 hours after the end of an I.V. infusion or 4 hours after an I.M. injection of fosphenytoin; see Phenytoin *on page 1253* for phenytoin reference range

Test Interactions Falsely high plasma phenytoin concentrations (due to cross-reactivity with fosphenytoin) when measured by immunoanalytical techniques (eg, TD_X®, TD_XFL_X™, Emit® 2000) prior to complete conversion of fosphenytoin to phenytoin; see Reference Range for proper times to measure phenytoin concentrations. Phenytoin may produce falsely low results for dexamethasone or metyrapone tests.

Additional Information Dosing equivalency: Fosphenytoin sodium 1.5 mg is equivalent to phenytoin sodium 1 mg which is equivalent to fosphenytoin 1 mg **PE**

Phosphate load: Each mg **PE** of fosphenytoin delivers 0.0037 mmol of phosphate

Formaldehyde production from fosphenytoin is not expected to be clinically significant in adults with short-term use (eg, 1 week); potentially harmful amounts of phosphate and formaldehyde could occur with an overdose of fosphenytoin; fosphenytoin is more water soluble than phenytoin and, therefore, the injection does not contain propylene glycol; antiarrhythmic effects should be similar to phenytoin

Overdose may result in: Lethargy, nausea, vomiting, hypotension, syncope, tachycardia, bradycardia, asystole, cardiac arrest, hypocalcemia, and metabolic acidosis; fatalities have also been reported

Dosage Forms Excipient information presented when available (limited, particularly for generics); consult specific product labeling.

Injection, solution, as sodium: 75 mg/mL [equivalent to phenytoin sodium 50 mg/mL] (2 mL, 10 mL)

References

Adams BD, Buckley NH, Kim JY, et al, "Fosphenytoin May Cause Hemodynamically Unstable Bradydysrhythmias," *J Emerg Med*, 2006, 30(1):75-9.

Fischer JH, Cwik MS, Luer MS, et al, "Stability of Fosphenytoin Sodium With Intravenous Solutions in Glass Bottles, Polyvinyl Chloride Bags, and Polypropylene Syringes," *Ann Pharmacother*, 1997, 31(5):553-9.

Koul R and Deleu D, "Subtherapeutic Free Phenytoin Levels Following Fosphenytoin Therapy in Status Epilepticus," *Neurology*, 2002, 58(1):147-8.

Kriel RL and Cifuentes RF, "Fosphenytoin in Infants of Extremely Low Birth Weight," *Pediatr Neurol*, 2001, 24(3):219-21.

McBryde KD, Wilcox J, and Kher KK, "Hyperphosphatemia Due to Fosphenytoin in a Pediatric ESRD Patient," *Pediatr Nephrol*, 2005, 20(8):1182-5.

Morton LD, "Clinical Experience With Fosphenytoin in Children," *J Child Neurol*, 1998, 13(Suppl 1):S19-22.

Ogutu BR, Newton CR, Muchohi SN, et al, "Pharmacokinetics and Clinical Effects of Phenytoin and Fosphenytoin in Children With Severe Malaria and Status Epilepticus," *Br J Clin Pharmacol*, 2003, 56(1):112-9.

Ogutu BR, Newton CR, Muchohi SN, et al, "Phenytoin Pharmacokinetics and Clinical Effects in African Children Following Fosphenytoin and Chloramphenicol Coadministration," *Br J Clin Pharmacol*, 2002, 54(6):635-42.

Pellock JM, "Fosphenytoin Use in Children," *Neurology*, 1996, 46(6 Suppl 1):S14-6.

Takeoka M, Krishnamoorthy KS, Soman TB, et al, "Fosphenytoin in Infants," *J Child Neurol*, 1998, 13(11):537-40.

- ♦ **Fosphenytoin Sodium** *see* Fosphenytoin *on page 711*
- ♦ **Fostex® 10% BPO [OTC]** *see* Benzoyl Peroxide *on page 207*
- ♦ **Fototar® [OTC]** *see* Coal Tar *on page 394*
- ♦ **Freezone® [OTC]** *see* Salicylic Acid *on page 1413*
- ♦ **Froben® (Can)** *see* Flurbiprofen *on page 688*
- ♦ **Froben-SR® (Can)** *see* Flurbiprofen *on page 688*
- ♦ **Frusemide** *see* Furosemide *on page 714*
- ♦ **FTC** *see* Emtricitabine *on page 562*
- ♦ **FU** *see* Fluorouracil *on page 678*
- ♦ **5-FU** *see* Fluorouracil *on page 678*
- ♦ **Fungi-Guard [OTC]** *see* Tolnaftate *on page 1550*
- ♦ **Fungi-Nail® [OTC]** *see* Undecylenic Acid and Derivatives *on page 1585*
- ♦ **Fungizone® (Can)** *see* Amphotericin B (Conventional) *on page 118*
- ♦ **Fung-O® [OTC]** *see* Salicylic Acid *on page 1413*
- ♦ **Fungoid® Tincture [OTC]** *see* Miconazole *on page 1056*
- ♦ **Furadantin®** *see* Nitrofurantoin *on page 1139*
- ♦ **Furazosin** *see* Prazosin *on page 1303*

Furosemide (fyoor OH se mide)

Medication Safety Issues

Sound-alike/look-alike issues:

Furosemide may be confused with torsemide

Lasix® may be confused with Esidrix®, Lanoxin®, Lidex®, Lomotil®, Luvox®, Luxiq®

International issues:

Urex® [Australia] may be confused with Eurax® which is a brand name for crotamiton in the U.S.

Urex® [Australia]: Brand name for methenamine in the U.S.

Related Information

Antihypertensive Agents by Class *on page 1678*
Tumor Lysis Syndrome, Management *on page 1803*

U.S. Brand Names Lasix®

Canadian Brand Names Apo-Furosemide®; Furosemide Injection, USP; Furosemide Special; Lasix®; Lasix® Special; Novo-Semide

Index Terms Frusemide

Therapeutic Category Antihypertensive Agent; Diuretic, Loop

Generic Available Yes

Use Management of edema associated with CHF and hepatic or renal disease; used alone or in combination with antihypertensives in treatment of hypertension

Pregnancy Risk Factor C

Lactation Enters breast milk/use caution

Contraindications Hypersensitivity to furosemide or any component; anuria

Warnings Loop diuretics are potent diuretics; excess amounts can lead to profound diuresis with fluid and electrolyte loss

Precautions Hepatic cirrhosis (rapid alterations in fluid/electrolytes may precipitate coma)

Adverse Reactions

Cardiovascular: Orthostatic hypotension

Central nervous system: Dizziness, vertigo, headache

Dermatologic: Urticaria, photosensitivity

Endocrine & metabolic: Hypokalemia, hyponatremia, hypomagnesemia, hypocalcemia, hyperglycemia, hypochloremia, alkalosis, dehydration, hyperuricemia

Gastrointestinal: Pancreatitis, nausea; oral solutions may cause diarrhea due to sorbitol content; anorexia, vomiting, constipation, abdominal cramping

Hematologic: Agranulocytosis, anemia, thrombocytopenia

Hepatic: Ischemic hepatitis, jaundice

Otic: Potential ototoxicity

Renal: Nephrocalcinosis, prerenal azotemia, interstitial nephritis, hypercalciuria

Drug Interactions Indomethacin decreases the effect of furosemide; decreased lithium excretion; decreased glucose tolerance with antidiabetic agents; increased ototoxicity with aminoglycosides and ethacrynic acid; drugs affected by potassium depletion (ie, digoxin); increased anticoagulant activity of warfarin; increased salicylate toxicity due to decreased excretion; decreased furosemide effects when administered at the same time as sucralfate

Food Interactions Do not mix with acidic solutions; limit intake of natural licorice (causes sodium and water retention and increases potassium loss)

Stability Furosemide injection should be stored at controlled room temperature and protected from light; exposure to light may cause discoloration; do not use furosemide solutions if they have a yellow color; refrigeration may result in precipitation or crystallization, however, resolubilization at room temperature or warming may be performed without affecting the stability; furosemide solutions are unstable in acidic media but very stable in basic media; I.V. infusion solution mixed in NS or D_5W solution is stable for 24 hours at room temperature

Mechanism of Action Inhibits reabsorption of sodium and chloride in the ascending loop of Henle and distal renal tubule, interfering with the chloride-binding cotransport system, thus causing increased excretion of water, potassium, sodium, chloride, magnesium, and calcium

Pharmacodynamics

Onset of action:

Oral: Within 30-60 minutes

I.M.: 30 minutes

I.V.: 5 minutes

Maximum effect: Oral: Within 1-2 hours

Duration:

Oral: 6-8 hours

I.V.: 2 hours

Pharmacokinetics

Absorption: 65% in patients with normal renal function, decreases to 45% in patients with renal failure

Protein binding: 98%

Half-life: Adults:

Normal renal function: 30 minutes

Renal failure: 9 hours

Elimination: 50% of oral dose and 80% of I.V. dose excreted unchanged in the urine within 24 hours; the remainder is eliminated by other nonrenal pathways including liver metabolism and excretion of unchanged drug in feces

Usual Dosage

Neonates, premature: (see Additional Information)

Oral: Bioavailability is poor by this route; doses of 1-4 mg/kg/dose 1-2 times/day have been used

I.M., I.V.: 1-2 mg/kg/dose given every 12-24 hours

Infants and Children:

Oral: 2 mg/kg once daily; if effective, may increase in increments of 1-2 mg/kg/dose every 6-8 hours; not to exceed 6 mg/kg/dose. In most cases, it is not necessary to exceed individual doses of 4 mg/kg or a dosing frequency of once or twice daily

I.M., I.V.: 1-2 mg/kg/dose every 6-12 hours

Continuous infusion: 0.05 mg/kg/hour; titrate dosage to clinical effect

Adults:

Oral: Initial: 20-80 mg/dose; increase in increments of 20-40 mg/dose at intervals of 6-8 hours; usual maintenance dose interval is twice daily or every day; may be titrated up to 600 mg/day with severe edematous states

Hypertension (JNC 7): 20-80 mg/day in 2 divided doses

I.M., I.V.: 20-40 mg/dose; repeat in 1-2 hours as needed and increase by 20 mg/dose until the desired effect has been obtained; usual dosing interval: 6-12 hours; for acute pulmonary edema, the usual dose is 40 mg I.V.; if not adequate, may increase dose to 80 mg; **Note:** ACC/AHA 2005 guidelines for chronic CHF recommend 40 mg I.V. dose followed by a continuous infusion (see continuous infusion)

Continuous I.V. infusion: Initial I.V. bolus dose of 20-40 mg/kg followed by continuous I.V. infusion doses of 10-40 mg/hour. If urine output is <1 mL/kg/hour, increase as necessary to a maximum of 80-160 mg/hour. The risk associated with higher infusion rates (80-160 mg/hour) must be weighed against alternative strategies. **Note:** ACC/AHA 2005 guidelines for chronic CHF recommend 40 mg I.V. dose followed by 10-40 mg/hour infusion

Refractory CHF: Oral, I.V.: Doses up to 8 g/day have been used

Dosing adjustment in renal impairment: Adults: Acute renal failure: High doses (up to 1-3 g/day - oral/I.V.) have been used to initiate desired response; avoid use in oliguric states

Dialysis: Not removed by hemo- or peritoneal dialysis; supplemental dose is not necessary

Dosing adjustment in hepatic disease: Diminished natriuretic effect with increased sensitivity to hypokalemia and volume depletion in cirrhosis; monitor effects, particularly with high doses

Administration

Oral: May administer with food or milk to decrease GI distress

Parenteral: I.V.: May be administered undiluted direct I.V. at a maximum rate of 0.5 mg/kg/minute for doses <120 mg and 4 mg/minute for doses >120 mg; may also be diluted for infusion 1-2 mg/mL (maximum concentration: 10 mg/mL) over 10-15 minutes (following maximum rate as above)

Monitoring Parameters Serum electrolytes, renal function, blood pressure, hearing (if high dosages used)

Patient Information May cause photosensitivity reactions (eg, exposure to sunlight may cause severe sunburn, skin rash, redness, or itching); avoid exposure to sunlight and artificial light sources (sunlamps, tanning booth/bed); wear protective clothing, wide-brimmed hats, sunglasses, and lip sunscreen (SPF ≥15); use a sunscreen [broad-spectrum sunscreen or physical sunscreen (preferred) or sunblock with SPF ≥15]; contact physician if reaction occurs.

Additional Information Single dose studies utilizing nebulized furosemide at 1-2 mg/kg/dose (diluted to a final volume of 2 mL with NS) have been shown to be effective in improving pulmonary function in preterm infants with bronchopulmonary dysplasia undergoing mechanical ventilation; no diuresis or systemic side effects were noted

Dosage Forms Excipient information presented when available (limited, particularly for generics); consult specific product labeling.

Injection, solution: 10 mg/mL (2 mL, 4 mL, 8 mL, 10 mL)

Solution, oral: 10 mg/mL (60 mL, 120 mL) [orange flavor]; 40 mg/5 mL (5 mL, 500 mL) [pineapple-peach flavor]

(Continued)

Furosemide *(Continued)*

Tablet (Lasix®): 20 mg, 40 mg, 80 mg

References

Chobanian AV, Bakris GL, Black HR, et al, "The Seventh Report of the Joint National Committee on Prevention, Detection, Evaluation, and Treatment of High Blood Pressure: The JNC 7 Report," *JAMA*, 2003, 289(19):2560-72.

Copeland JG, Campbell DW, Plachetka JR, et al, "Diuresis With Continuous Infusion of Furosemide After Cardiac Surgery," *Am J Surg*, 1983, 146(6):796-9.

Hunt SA, Abraham WT, Chin MH, et al, "ACC/AHA 2005 Guideline Update for the Diagnosis and Management of Chronic Heart Failure in the Adult-Summary Article: A Report of the American College of Cardiology/American Heart Association Task Force on Practice Guidelines (Writing Committee to Update the 2001 Guidelines for the Evaluation and Management of Heart Failure)," *J Am Coll Cardiol*, 2005, 46(6):1116-43.

Pai VB and Nahata MC, "Aerosolized Furosemide in the Treatment of Acute Respiratory Distress and Possible Bronchopulmonary Dysplasia in Preterm Neonates," *Ann Pharmacother*, 2000, 34(3):386-92.

Rastogi A, Luayon M, Ajayi OA, et al, "Nebulized Furosemide in Infants With Bronchopulmonary Dysplasia," *J Pediatr*, 1994, 125(6 Pt 1):976-9.

Rudy DW, Voelker JR, Greene PK, et al, "Loop Diuretics for Chronic Renal Insufficiency: A Continuous Infusion Is More Efficacious Than Bolus Therapy," *Ann Intern Med*, 1991, 115(5):360-6.

- **Furosemide Injection, USP (Can)** *see* Furosemide *on page 714*
- **Furosemide Special (Can)** *see* Furosemide *on page 714*
- **Fuzeon®** *see* Enfuvirtide *on page 569*
- **FVIII/vWF** *see* Antihemophilic Factor/von Willebrand Factor Complex (Human) *on page 141*
- **FXT (Can)** *see* Fluoxetine *on page 681*

Gabapentin (GA ba pen tin)

Medication Safety Issues

Sound-alike/look-alike issues:

Neurontin® may be confused with Neoral®, Noroxin®

Related Information

Antiepileptic Drugs *on page 1902*

U.S. Brand Names Neurontin®

Canadian Brand Names Apo-Gabapentin®; BCI-Gabapentin; Gen-Gabapentin; Neurontin®; Novo-Gabapentin; Nu-Gabapentin; PMS-Gabapentin

Therapeutic Category Anticonvulsant, Miscellaneous

Generic Available Yes: Capsule, tablet

Use Adjunct for treatment of partial seizures in children >12 years and adults (with or without secondary generalized seizures); adjunct for treatment of partial seizures in children 3-12 years of age; adjunct in the treatment of neuropathic pain; management of post-herpetic neuralgia in adults

Pregnancy Risk Factor C

Lactation Enters breast milk/use caution

Contraindications Hypersensitivity to gabapentin or any component

Warnings Neuropsychiatric adverse events, such as emotional lability (eg, behavioral problems), hostility, aggressive behaviors, thought disorder (eg, problems with concentration and school performance) and hyperkinesia (eg, hyperactivity and restlessness), have been reported in pediatric patients (see Adverse Reactions); abrupt withdrawal may precipitate status epilepticus or increase in seizures; decrease dose gradually over at least 1 week

Precautions Use with caution and decrease the dose in patients with renal dysfunction; in male (but not female) rats receiving gabapentin, a high incidence of pancreatic acinar adenocarcinoma was noted, the clinical significance in humans is unknown; effectiveness in children <3 years is not established

Adverse Reactions

Cardiovascular: Peripheral edema

Central nervous system: Somnolence, dizziness, ataxia, fatigue, depression, nervousness, fever; neuropsychiatric adverse events in children 3-12 years of age: Emotional lability (behavioral problems): 6% incidence; hostility (including aggressive behaviors): 5.2%; hyperkinesia (hyperactivity, restlessness): 4.7%; thought disorder (problems with concentration and school performance): 1.7%; **Note:** Most of these pediatric neuropsychiatric adverse events are mild to moderate in terms of intensity but discontinuation of gabapentin may be required; children with mental retardation and attention deficit disorders may be at increased risk for behavioral side effects

Dermatologic: Pruritus

Endocrine & metabolic: Weight gain

Gastrointestinal: Dyspepsia, constipation, nausea, vomiting

Genitourinary: Impotence

Hematologic: Leukopenia

Neuromuscular & skeletal: Back pain, dysarthria, tremor, myalgia
Ocular: Nystagmus, diplopia

Drug Interactions Antacids reduce the bioavailability of gabapentin by 20% (separate administration times by at least 2 hours); morphine may increase gabapentin serum concentrations (monitor patients for CNS depression; reduce morphine or gabapentin dose as appropriate); hydrocodone may increase gabapentin serum concentrations; gabapentin may decrease hydrocodone serum concentrations in a dose-dependent manner; naproxen may increase the absorption of gabapentin by 12% to 15%; cimetidine may decrease the clearance of gabapentin (minor effect); gabapentin may increase levels of norethindrone (minor effect); gabapentin does not alter the pharmacokinetics of other antiepileptic drugs

Food Interactions Food slightly increases rate and extent of absorption (AUC and peak increase by 14%)

Stability Refrigerate oral solution; store capsules and tablets at room temperature

Mechanism of Action Not fully elucidated, most likely binds to an undefined neuroreceptor in the brain that is possibly linked with, or identical to a site resembling the L-system amino acid carrier protein; although structurally similar to the inhibitory neurotransmitter, gamma-aminobutyric acid (GABA), gabapentin does not significantly affect the GABA system; it does **not** bind to GABA receptors, affect GABA neuronal uptake nor mimic GABA effects

Pharmacokinetics

Absorption: Very rapid; via an active (ie, facilitated transport) saturable process; dose-dependent

Distribution: V_d: Adults: 50-60 L or 0.65-1.04 L/kg; CSF concentrations are ~20% of plasma concentrations; distributes to breast milk

Protein binding: <3% (not clinically significant)

Metabolism: Not metabolized

Bioavailability: ~60% (300 mg dose given 3 times/day); bioavailability decreases with increasing doses; bioavailability is 27% with 1600 mg dose given 3 times/day

Time to peak serum concentration: Infants 1 month to Children 12 years and Adults: 2-3 hours

Half-life, elimination:

Infants 1 month to Children 12 years: 4.7 hours

Adults, normal: 5.3 hours (range: 5-9); increased half-life with decreased renal function; anuric adult patients: 132 hours; adults during hemodialysis: 3.8 hours

Elimination: Excreted unchanged in the urine (75% to 80%) and feces (10% to 20%)

Clearance: (**Note:** Apparent oral clearance is directly proportional to Cl_{cr}): Clearance in infants is highly variable; oral clearance (per kg) in children <5 years of age is higher than in children ≥5 years of age

Usual Dosage Oral: **Note:** Do not exceed 12 hours between doses with 3 times/day dosing:

Anticonvulsant:

Children 3-12 years: Initial: 10-15 mg/kg/day divided into 3 doses/day; titrate dose upward over ~3 days; usual dose: Children 3-4 years: 40 mg/kg/day divided into 3 doses/day; children ≥5 to 12 years: 25-35 mg/kg/day divided into 3 doses/day; doses up to 50 mg/kg/day were well tolerated in one long-term study

Children >12 years and Adults: Initial: 300 mg 3 times/day; titrate dose upward if needed; usual dose: 900-1800 mg/day divided into 3 doses/day; doses up to 2400 mg/day divided into 3 doses/day are well tolerated long-term; maximum dose: 3600 mg/day

Neuropathic pain:

Children: Limited information is available; some centers use the following doses: Initial: 5 mg/kg/dose at bedtime; day 2: Increase to 5 mg/kg/dose twice daily; day 3: Increase to 5 mg/kg/dose 3 times/day; titrate to effect; usual dosage range: 8-35 mg/kg/day divided into 3 doses/day (Galloway, 2000)

Adults: Initial: 100 mg 3 times/day; titrate to effect; doses can be increased by 300 mg/day at weekly intervals; doses of at least 900 mg/day appear to be more effective; usual dosage range: 1800-2400 mg/day divided into 3 doses/day; maximum dose: 3600 mg/day (see Laird, 2000)

Post-herpetic neuralgia: Adults: Initial: Day 1: 300 mg/day; day 2: 300 mg twice daily; day 3: 300 mg 3 times/day; titrate dose as needed for relief of pain to 600 mg 3 times/day; doses of 1800-3600 mg/day have been studied; doses >1800 mg/day did not show additional benefit

Dosing adjustment in renal impairment:

Children <12 years: Dosing in renal impairment has not been studied

Children ≥12 years and Adults: See table on next page.

Administration Oral: May be administered without regard to meals; administration with meals may decrease adverse GI effects; dose may be administered as combination of dosage forms; do not administer within 2 hours of magnesium- or aluminum-containing antacids

(Continued)

Gabapentin *(Continued)*

One pediatric study (Khurana, 1996) mixed the contents of the capsule in drinks (eg, orange juice) or food (eg, applesauce) for patients who could not swallow the capsule; oral solution is now available

Monitoring Parameters Seizure frequency and duration; renal function; weight; behavior in children

Gabapentin Dosing Adjustments in Renal Impairment

Creatinine Clearance (mL/min)	Total Daily Dose Range (mg/day)	Dosage Regimens (Maintenance Doses) (mg)				
≥60	900-3600	300 3 times/day	400 3 times/day	600 3 times/day	800 3 times/day	1200 tid
>30-59	400-1400	200 twice daily	300 twice daily	400 twice daily	500 twice daily	700 twice daily
>15-29	200-700	200 daily	300 daily	400 daily	500 daily	700 daily
15[1]	100-300	100 daily	125 daily	150 daily	200 daily	300 daily
Hemodialysis[2]		Post-Hemodialysis Supplemental Dose				
		125 mg	150 mg	200 mg	250 mg	350 mg

[1]Cl_{cr} <15 mL/minute: Reduce daily dose in proportion to creatinine clearance.

[2]Supplemental dose should be administered after each 4 hours of hemodialysis (patients on hemodialysis should also receive maintenance doses based on renal function as listed in the upper portion of the table)

Reference Range Minimum effective serum concentration may be 2 mcg/mL; **routine monitoring of drug levels is not required**

Test Interactions False positive urinary protein with N-Multistix SG® test

Patient Information Take only as prescribed; may cause dizziness or drowsiness and impair ability to perform activities requiring mental alertness or physical coordination; may cause somnolence, and other symptoms and signs of CNS depression; do not operate machinery or drive a car until you have experience with the drug

Nursing Implications Doses should be titrated based on clinical response; content of capsule is bitter tasting

Additional Information Gabapentin is not effective for absence seizures; gabapentin does not induce liver enzymes

Dosage Forms Excipient information presented when available (limited, particularly for generics); consult specific product labeling.

Capsule: 100 mg, 300 mg, 400 mg
  Neurontin®: 100 mg, 300 mg, 400 mg
Solution, oral:
  Neurontin®: 250 mg/5 mL (480 mL) [cool strawberry anise flavor]
Tablet: 100 mg, 300 mg, 400 mg, 600 mg, 800 mg
  Neurontin®: 600 mg, 800 mg

References

Andrews CO and Fischer JH, "Gabapentin: A New Agent for the Management of Epilepsy," *Ann Pharmacother*, 1994, 28(10):1188-96.

Bourgeois BF, "Antiepileptic Drugs in Pediatric Practice," *Epilepsia*, 1995, 36(Suppl 2):S34-45.

Galloway KS and Yaster M, "Pain and Symptom Control in Terminally Ill Children," *Pediatr Clin North Am*, 2000, 47(3):711-46.

Khurana DS, Riviello J, Helmers S, et al, "Efficacy of Gabapentin Therapy in Children With Refractory Partial Seizures," *J Pediatr*, 1996, 128(6):829-33.

Laird MA and Gidal BE, "Use of Gabapentin in the Treatment of Neuropathic Pain," *Ann Pharmacother*, 2000, 34(6):802-7.

Lee DO, Steingard RJ, Cesena M, et al, "Behavioral Side Effects of Gabapentin in Children," *Epilepsia*, 1996, 37(1):87-90.

Leiderman D, Garofalo E, and LaMoreaux L, "Gabapentin Patients With Absence Seizures: Two Double-Blind, Placebo Controlled Studies," *Epilepsia*, 1993, 34(Suppl 6):45 (abstract).

Pellock JM, "Managing Pediatric Epilepsy Syndromes With New Antiepileptic Drugs," *Pediatrics*, 1999, 104(5 Pt 1):1106-16.

Pressler KL, Jabbour JT, Rose DF, et al, "Gabapentin and Aggression in Pediatric Patients: A Review of the Literature," *Journal of Pediatric Pharmacy Practice*, 1998, 3(2):100-5.

♦ **Gabitril®** *see* Tiagabine *on page 1536*
♦ **Galzin™** *see* Zinc Supplements *on page 1641*
♦ **Gamimune® N (Can)** *see* Immune Globulin (Intravenous) *on page 818*
♦ **Gamma Benzene Hexachloride** *see* Lindane *on page 939*
♦ **Gamma E-Gems® [OTC]** *see* Vitamin E *on page 1620*
♦ **Gamma-E Plus [OTC]** *see* Vitamin E *on page 1620*
♦ **Gammagard® Liquid** *see* Immune Globulin (Intravenous) *on page 818*
♦ **Gammagard® S/D** *see* Immune Globulin (Intravenous) *on page 818*
♦ **Gamma Globulin** *see* Immune Globulin (Intramuscular) *on page 817*
♦ **Gammaphos** *see* Amifostine *on page 91*
♦ **Gammar®-P I.V.** *see* Immune Globulin (Intravenous) *on page 818*

- **GammaSTAN™ S/D** *see* Immune Globulin (Intramuscular) *on page 817*
- **Gamunex®** *see* Immune Globulin (Intravenous) *on page 818*

Ganciclovir (gan SYE kloe veer)

Medication Safety Issues

Sound-alike/look-alike issues:

Cytovene® may be confused with Cytosar®, Cytosar-U®

U.S. Brand Names Cytovene®; Vitrasert®

Canadian Brand Names Cytovene®; Vitrasert®

Index Terms DHPG Sodium; GCV Sodium; Nordeoxyguanosine

Therapeutic Category Antiviral Agent, Oral; Antiviral Agent, Parenteral

Generic Available Yes: Capsule

Use Treatment of cytomegalovirus (CMV) retinitis in immunocompromised patients, as well as CMV GI infections and pneumonitis; prevention of CMV disease in transplant patients who have been diagnosed with latent or active CMV; ganciclovir also has antiviral activity against herpes simplex virus types 1 and 2

Pregnancy Risk Factor C

Lactation Excretion in breast milk unknown/contraindicated

Contraindications Hypersensitivity to ganciclovir, acyclovir, or any component; absolute neutrophil count <500/mm^3; platelet count <25,000/mm^3

Warnings Ganciclovir may adversely affect spermatogenesis and fertility; due to its mutagenic potential, contraceptive precautions for female and male patients need to be followed during and for at least 90 days after therapy with the drug; ganciclovir is potentially carcinogenic

Precautions Dosage adjustment or interruption of ganciclovir therapy may be necessary in patients with neutropenia and/or thrombocytopenia and patients with impaired renal function; use with extreme caution in children since long-term safety has not been determined and due to ganciclovir's potential for long-term carcinogenic and adverse reproductive effects

Adverse Reactions

Cardiovascular: Edema, arrhythmias, hypertension

Central nervous system: Headaches, seizure, confusion, nervousness, dizziness, hallucinations, coma, fever, encephalopathy, malaise

Dermatologic: Rash, pruritus, urticaria, acne

Gastrointestinal: Nausea, vomiting, diarrhea, pancreatitis

Hematologic: Neutropenia (oral ganciclovir is associated with less neutropenia and fewer bacterial infections than I.V. ganciclovir), thrombocytopenia, leukopenia, anemia, eosinophilia

Hepatic: Elevated liver enzymes

Local: Phlebitis

Ocular: Retinal detachment, photophobia, abnormal vision, loss of vision

Renal: Hematuria, elevated BUN and serum creatinine

Respiratory: Dyspnea

Drug Interactions Zidovudine (pancytopenia), imipenem/cilastatin (seizures), immunosuppressive agents increase suppression of bone marrow; amphotericin B, tacrolimus, cyclosporine increase nephrotoxicity; probenecid decreases renal clearance of ganciclovir; increases didanosine AUC (increases risk of peripheral neuropathy, pancreatitis)

Food Interactions High fat meal may increase AUC by 22%

Stability Reconstituted solution is stable for 12 hours at room temperature; **do not refrigerate**; reconstitute with SWI **not** bacteriostatic water because parabens may cause precipitation; diluted I.V. ganciclovir solutions in D_5W or NS with a concentration <10 mg/mL are stable for 24 hours

Mechanism of Action Ganciclovir is phosphorylated to a substrate which competitively inhibits the binding of deoxyguanosine triphosphate to DNA polymerase; ganciclovir triphosphate competes with deoxyguanosine triphosphate for incorporation into viral DNA and interferes with viral DNA chain elongation resulting in inhibition of viral replication

Pharmacokinetics

Absorption: Oral: Poor

Distribution: Distributes to most body fluids, tissues, and organs including the eyes and brain

Protein binding: 1% to 2%

Bioavailability: Fasting: 5%; following food: 6% to 9%

Half-life (prolonged with impaired renal function):

Neonates 2-49 days of age: 2.4 hours

Adults: Mean: 2.5-3.6 hours (range: 1.7-5.8 hours)

Time to peak serum concentration: Oral: 2-2.5 hours

(Continued)

Ganciclovir *(Continued)*

Elimination: Majority (80% to 99%) excreted as unchanged drug in the urine
Dialysis: 40% to 50% removed by a 4-hour hemodialysis

Usual Dosage

Slow I.V. infusion:

Congenital CMV infection: Neonates and Infants: Preliminary data indicates that a higher initial dose of 15 mg/kg/day divided every 12 hours and more prolonged treatment may be more effective

Retinitis: Children >3 months and Adults:

Induction therapy: 10 mg/kg/day divided every 12 hours as a 1- to 2-hour infusion for 14-21 days

Maintenance therapy: 5 mg/kg/day as a single daily dose for 7 days/week or 6 mg/kg/day for 5 days/week

Prevention of CMV disease in transplant recipients: Children and Adults:

Initial: 10 mg/kg/day divided every 12 hours for 7-14 days, followed by 5 mg/kg/day once daily 7 days/week or 6 mg/kg/day once daily 5 days/week for 100 days

Lung/heart-lung transplant patients (CMV-positive donor with CMV-positive recipient): 6 mg/kg/day once daily for 28 days

Other CMV infections: Children and Adults: Initial: 10 mg/kg/day divided every 12 hours for 14-21 days or 7.5 mg/kg/day divided every 8 hours; maintenance therapy: 5 mg/kg/day as a single daily dose for 7 days/week or 6 mg/kg/day for 5 days/week

Oral (following induction treatment with I.V. ganciclovir):

Children: Maintenance dose, prophylaxis of CMV disease: In a study of 36 children 6 months to 16 years of age, 30 mg/kg/dose every 8 hours with food produced serum levels similar to the 1000 mg 3 times/day regimen that is effective for maintenance treatment of CMV retinitis in adults (see Frenkel, 2000).

Adults: Maintenance: 1000 mg 3 times/day **or** 500 mg 6 times/day every 3 hours during waking hours

Sustained release intravitreal implant: CMV retinitis:

Children ≥9 years: One implant every 6-9 months plus ganciclovir 30 mg/kg/dose orally 3 times/day

Adults: One implant every 6-9 months plus ganciclovir 1-1.5 g orally 3 times/day

Dosing interval in renal impairment:

Oral: Adults:

Cl_{cr} 50-69 mL/minute: Administer 1500 mg/day or 500 mg 3 times/day
Cl_{cr} 25-49 mL/minute: Administer 1000 mg/day or 500 mg twice daily
Cl_{cr} 10-24 mL/minute: Administer 500 mg/day
Cl_{cr} <10 mL/minute: Administer 500 mg 3 times/week following hemodialysis

I.V. induction:

Cl_{cr} 50-69 mL/minute: Administer 2.5 mg/kg every 12 hours
Cl_{cr} 25-49 mL/minute: Administer 2.5 mg/kg every 24 hours
Cl_{cr} 10-24 mL/minute: Administer 1.25 mg/kg every 24 hours
Cl_{cr} <10 mL/minute: Administer 1.25 mg/kg/dose 3 times/week following hemodialysis

I.V. maintenance:

Cl_{cr} 50-69 mL/minute: Administer 2.5 mg/kg/dose every 24 hours
Cl_{cr} 25-49 mL/minute: Administer 1.25 mg/kg/dose every 24 hours
Cl_{cr} 10-24 mL/minute: Administer 0.625 mg/kg/dose every 24 hours
Cl_{cr} <10 mL/minute: Administer 0.625 mg/kg/dose 3 times/week following hemodialysis

Administration Follow same precautions utilized with antineoplastic agents when preparing and administering ganciclovir

Oral: Do not open or crush ganciclovir capsules; administer with food

Parenteral: Do not administer I.M. or SubQ since the reconstituted ganciclovir injection may cause severe tissue irritation due to its high pH; administer by slow I.V. infusion over at least 1 hour at a final concentration for administration not to exceed 10 mg/mL

Monitoring Parameters CBC with differential and platelet count, urine output, serum creatinine, ophthalmologic exams, liver enzyme tests, blood pressure, urinalysis

Nursing Implications Handle and dispose according to guidelines issued for cytotoxic drugs; avoid direct contact of skin or mucous membranes with the powder contained in capsules or the I.V. solution; to minimize the risk of phlebitis, infuse through a large vein with adequate blood flow; maintain adequate patient hydration

Additional Information Sodium content of 1 g: 4 mEq

Dosage Forms Excipient information presented when available (limited, particularly for generics); consult specific product labeling. [DSC] = Discontinued product

Capsule: 250 mg, 500 mg

Cytovene®: 250 mg, 500 mg [DSC]

Implant, intravitreal (Vitrasert®): 4.5 mg [released gradually over 5-8 months]
Injection, powder for reconstitution, as sodium (Cytovene®): 500 mg

Extemporaneous Preparations A 100 mg/mL oral suspension can be prepared in a vertical flow hood by emptying eighty 250 mg capsules of ganciclovir into a glass mortar wetted and triturated with Ora-Sweet® to a smooth paste. Add 50 mL of Ora-Sweet® to the paste, mix, and transfer contents to an amber polyethylene terephthate bottle. Rinse the mortar with 50 mL of Ora-Sweet® and transfer contents to the bottle. Rinse the mortar with the last third of the vehicle and transfer contents to the bottle. Add enough vehicle to make a final volume of 200 mL. The suspension is stable for 123 days when stored at 23°C to 25°C.

Anaizi NH, Swenson CF, and Dentinger PJ, "Stability of Ganciclovir in Extemporaneously Compounded Oral Liquids," *Am J Health Syst Pharm*, 1999, 56(17):1738-41.

References

Fletcher C, Sawchuk R, Chinnock B, et al, "Human Pharmacokinetics of the Antiviral Drug DHPG," *Clin Pharmacol Ther*, 1986, 40(3):281-6.

Frenkel LM, Capparelli EV, Dankner WM, et al, "Oral Ganciclovir in Children: Pharmacokinetics, Safety, Tolerance, and Antiviral Effects," *J Infect Dis*, 2000, 182(6):1616-24.

Goodrich JM, Bowden RA, Fisher L, et al, "Ganciclovir Prophylaxis to Prevent Cytomegalovirus Disease After Allogeneic Marrow Transplant," *Ann Intern Med*, 1993, 118(3):173-8.

Gudnason T, Belani KK, and Balfour HH Jr, "Ganciclovir Treatment of Cytomegalovirus Disease in Immunocompromised Children," *Pediatr Infect Dis J*, 1989, 8(7):436-40.

Kaplan JE, Masur H, and Holmes KK, "Guidelines for Preventing Opportunistic Infections Among HIV-Infected Persons - 2002 Recommendations of the USPHS and IDSA," *MMWR*, 2002, 51(RR-8):1-46.

Merigan TC, Renlund DG, Keay S, et al, "A Controlled Trial of Ganciclovir to Prevent Cytomegalovirus Disease After Heart Transplantation," *N Engl J Med*, 1992, 326(18):1182-6.

- **Ganidin NR** *see* Guaifenesin *on page 745*
- **Gani-Tuss DM NR** *see* Guaifenesin and Dextromethorphan *on page 748*
- **Gani-Tuss® NR** *see* Guaifenesin and Codeine *on page 746*
- **Gantrisin®** *see* SulfiSOXAZOLE *on page 1491*
- **Garamycin® (Can)** *see* Gentamicin *on page 726*
- **Gardasil®** *see* Papillomavirus (Types 6, 11, 16, 18) Recombinant Vaccine *on page 1212*
- **Gas-X® [OTC]** *see* Simethicone *on page 1440*
- **Gas-X® Extra Strength [OTC]** *see* Simethicone *on page 1440*
- **Gas-X® Maximum Strength [OTC]** *see* Simethicone *on page 1440*
- **GasAid [OTC]** *see* Simethicone *on page 1440*
- **Gastrocrom®** *see* Cromolyn *on page 407*
- **Gaviscon® Tablet [OTC]** *see* Antacid Preparations *on page 132*
- **G-CSF** *see* Filgrastim *on page 655*
- **GCV Sodium** *see* Ganciclovir *on page 719*
- **GD-Sildenafil** *see* Sildenafil *on page 1435*
- **Gel-Kam® [OTC]** *see* Fluoride *on page 675*
- **Gel-Kam® Rinse** *see* Fluoride *on page 675*
- **GelRite [OTC]** *see* Ethyl Alcohol *on page 619*
- **Gel-Stat™ [OTC]** *see* Ethyl Alcohol *on page 619*
- **Gelusil® [OTC]** *see* Antacid Preparations *on page 132*

Gemcitabine (jem SITE a been)

Medication Safety Issues

Sound-alike/look-alike issues:

Gemzar® may be confused with Zinecard®

High alert medication: The Institute for Safe Medication Practices (ISMP) includes this medication among its list of drugs which have a heightened risk of causing significant patient harm when used in error.

U.S. Brand Names Gemzar®

Canadian Brand Names Gemzar®

Index Terms Gemcitabine Hydrochloride; NSC-613327

Therapeutic Category Antineoplastic Agent, Antimetabolite (Pyrimidine Antagonist)

Generic Available No

Use Treatment of locally-advanced, inoperable (stage IIIA or IIIB) or metastatic (stage IV) nonsmall cell lung cancer (NSCLC); locally advanced or metastatic pancreatic cancer; metastatic breast cancer; advanced or metastatic bladder cancer. Used in children for the treatment of refractory solid tumors (including brain tumors), refractory Hodgkin's disease, recurrent germ cell tumors, and hepatocellular carcinomas.

Pregnancy Risk Factor D

Lactation Excretion in breast milk unknown/contraindicated

Contraindications Hypersensitivity to gemcitabine or any component; pregnancy

(Continued)

Gemcitabine *(Continued)*

Warnings The FDA currently recommends that procedures for proper handling and disposal of antineoplastic agents be considered. Prolongation of the infusion time >60 minutes and more frequent than once weekly dosing have been shown to increase toxicity, including myelosuppression. Myelosuppression is usually the dose-limiting toxicity (CBC with differential and platelet count should be monitored prior to each dose of gemcitabine; reduce or withhold dose depending on the degree of hematologic toxicity). Gemcitabine has been reported to cause pulmonary toxicity, hemolytic uremic syndrome, and/or renal failure requiring dialysis or leading to death, and hepatotoxicity (including liver failure and death); discontinue gemcitabine if severe lung, renal or hepatotoxicity occurs. Gemcitabine may cause fever in the absence of clinical infection.

Precautions Use with caution in patients with renal or hepatic impairment

Adverse Reactions

Cardiovascular: CHF, arrhythmias, peripheral edema

Central nervous system: Fever, asthenia, somnolence, fatigue, lethargy

Dermatologic: Alopecia, rash, pruritus

Gastrointestinal: Constipation, diarrhea, nausea, vomiting, stomatitis

Genitourinary: Hematuria, proteinuria

Hematologic: Anemia, leukopenia, neutropenia, thrombocytopenia, hemorrhage

Hepatic: Elevated AST, ALT, bilirubin, and alkaline phosphatase; hepatotoxicity, liver failure (rare)

Neuromuscular & skeletal: Peripheral neuropathy, paresthesias

Renal: Hemolytic uremic syndrome, elevated BUN and serum creatinine, renal failure

Respiratory: Dyspnea, bronchospasm, pulmonary edema, interstitial pneumonitis, pulmonary fibrosis

Miscellaneous: Flu-like symptoms, anaphylactoid reaction, infection

Drug Interactions Warfarin (increased anticoagulant effect due to either decreased metabolism of warfarin or decreased hepatic synthesis of clotting factors)

Stability Store vial at room temperature; reconstituted vials and infusion solutions diluted in NS are stable up to 24 hours; do not refrigerate reconstituted and/or diluted solutions as crystallization may occur. Incompatible with acyclovir, cefotaxime, furosemide, ganciclovir, imipenem/cilastatin, irinotecan, methotrexate, methylprednisolone sodium succinate, piperacillin/tazobactam, and prochlorperazine

Mechanism of Action Gemcitabine undergoes intracellular phosphorylation to its corresponding diphosphate and triphosphate nucleosides which inhibit DNA polymerase and ribonucleotide reductase; results in inhibition of DNA synthesis; specific for the S-phase of the cell cycle.

Pharmacokinetics

Distribution: Widely distributed into tissues; present in ascitic fluid

V_d: Adults:

I.V. infusion <70 minutes: 50 L/m^2

I.V. infusion 70-285 minutes: 370 L/m^2

Protein binding: <10%

Metabolism: Intracellularly by nucleoside kinases to active di- and triphosphate metabolites; metabolized by cytidine deaminase to an inactive metabolite

Half-life: Adults:

I.V. infusion <70 minutes: 0.7-1.6 hours

I.V. infusion 70-285 minutes: 4.1-10.6 hours

Elimination: 92% to 98% excreted in the urine

Usual Dosage Refer to individual protocols: I.V.:

Children:

Refractory solid tumor, including Hodgkin's disease: 1000-1250 mg/m^2/dose on days 1 and 8 of a 4-week cycle; maximum single dose: 2500 mg

Refractory solid tumor in combination with docetaxel: 900 mg/m^2/dose over 60 minutes on days 1 and 8

Patients with pelvic radiation (decrease dose by 25%): 675 mg/m^2/dose over 60 minutes on days 1 and 8

Recurrent germ cell tumor: 800 mg/m^2/dose over 90 minutes on day 1

Hepatocellular carcinoma: 1000 mg/m^2/dose over 90 minutes on day 1

Dose modification for hematologic toxicity: 800 mg/m^2/dose on day 1

Adults:

Pancreatic cancer: 1000 mg/m^2 once weekly for up to 7 weeks

Nonsmall cell carcinoma: 1000 mg/m^2 on days 1,8, and 15 every 28 days in combination with cisplatin; or 1250 mg/m^2 on day 1 and 8 every 21 days in combination with cisplatin

Breast cancer: 1250 mg/m^2 on days 1 and 8 every 21 days in combination with paclitaxel

Dosing adjustment for hematologic toxicity: Adults:

Absolute granulocyte count (AGC) 500-999/mm³ or platelet count 50,000-99,000/mm³: Administer 75% of the full dose

AGC <500/mm³ or platelet count <50,000/mm³: Hold dose

Dosing adjustment in renal and/or hepatic impairment: No dosing information available

Administration I.V.: Reconstitute 200 mg vial of gemcitabine by adding 5 mL NS without preservatives or add 25 mL NS without preservatives to 1 g vial; resulting concentration is 38 mg/mL. Maximum concentration for administration: 38 mg/mL; gemcitabine can be further diluted with 50-500 mL NS to concentrations as low as 0.1 mg/mL. Infuse over 30-90 minutes based on the protocol. **Note:** Prolongation of the infusion time >60 minutes has been shown to prolong gemcitabine's half-life and increase toxicity in adults.

Monitoring Parameters CBC with differential and platelet count prior to each dose; monitor renal and hepatic function, bilirubin, LDH, and reticulocyte count

Patient Information Notify physician if extreme fatigue, severe GI upset or diarrhea, bleeding or bruising, fever, chills, sore throat, vaginal discharge, signs of fluid retention, yellowing of the skin or eyes, change in color of urine or stool, muscle or skeletal pain/weakness occur. Advise women of childbearing potential to avoid becoming pregnant while receiving gemcitabine.

Nursing Implications Maintain adequate hydration unless instructed to restrict fluid intake. If gemcitabine solution comes in contact with skin or mucosa, immediately wash the skin thoroughly with soap and water or rinse the mucosa with large amounts of water.

Dosage Forms Excipient information presented when available (limited, particularly for generics); consult specific product labeling.

Injection, powder for reconstitution:

Gemzar®: 200 mg, 1 g

References

Reid JM, Qu W, Safgren SL, et al, "Phase I Trial and Pharmacokinetics of Gemcitabine in Children With Advanced Solid Tumors," *J Clin Oncol*, 2004, 22(12):2445-51.

♦ **Gemcitabine Hydrochloride** *see* Gemcitabine *on page 721*

Gemtuzumab Ozogamicin (gem TOO zoo mab oh zog a MY sin)

Medication Safety Issues

High alert medication: The Institute for Safe Medication Practices (ISMP) includes this medication among its list of drugs which have a heightened risk of causing significant patient harm when used in error.

U.S. Brand Names Mylotarg®

Canadian Brand Names Mylotarg®

Index Terms CMA-676; NSC-720568

Therapeutic Category Antineoplastic Agent, Monoclonal Antibody

Generic Available No

Use Treatment of relapsed or *de novo* CD33-positive acute myeloid leukemia (AML)

Pregnancy Risk Factor D

Lactation Excretion in breast milk unknown/not recommended

Contraindications Hypersensitivity to gemtuzumab ozogamicin, calicheamicin derivatives, or any component; patients with anti-CD33 antibody; pregnancy

Warnings The FDA currently recommends that procedures for proper handling and disposal of antineoplastic agents be considered. Severe myelosuppression may occur at recommended doses. Severe veno-occlusive disease or hepatotoxicity has been associated with gemtuzumab.

Infusion-related events are common and generally occur with the first dose at the end of a 2-hour infusion. Infusion-related symptoms usually resolve after 2-4 hours with supportive therapy (acetaminophen, diphenhydramine, I.V. fluids). Postinfusion reactions, which include fever, chills, hypotension, and dyspnea, may occur during the first 24 hours after gemtuzumab administration. Infusion-related reactions may be severe (including anaphylaxis, pulmonary edema, or acute respiratory distress syndrome); symptomatic intrinsic lung disease or high peripheral blast counts may increase the risk of severe reactions; consider discontinuing therapy in patients who develop severe infusion-related reactions.

Precautions Use with caution in patients with pulmonary disease and renal or hepatic impairment. Tumor lysis syndrome may occur as a consequence of leukemia treatment; adequate hydration and prophylactic allopurinol must be initiated prior to starting gemtuzumab therapy. Other methods to reduce WBC <30,000 cells/mm³ (hydroxyurea or leukapheresis) may be considered to minimize tumor lysis syndrome and/or severe infusion reactions.

(Continued)

Gemtuzumab Ozogamicin *(Continued)*

Adverse Reactions

Cardiovascular: Peripheral edema, hypertension, hypotension, tachycardia

Central nervous system: Chills, fever, headache, pain, dizziness, insomnia, depression, cerebral hemorrhage, intracranial hemorrhage

Dermatologic: Rash, petechiae, ecchymosis, pruritus

Endocrine & metabolic: Hypokalemia, hypomagnesemia, hyperglycemia, hyperuricemia

Gastrointestinal: Nausea, vomiting, diarrhea, anorexia, abdominal pain, constipation, stomatitis, mucositis, abdominal distention, dyspepsia

Genitourinary: Hematuria, vaginal hemorrhage

Hematologic: Neutropenia, thrombocytopenia, anemia, bleeding, lymphopenia, hemorrhage, disseminated intravascular coagulation, elevated PT

Hepatic: Hyperbilirubinemia, elevated LDH, ALT, and AST; veno-occlusive disease (higher incidence in patients with prior history of hematopoietic stem cell transplant), hepatic failure, jaundice, hepatosplenomegaly

Neuromuscular & skeletal: Weakness, back pain, arthralgia

Renal: Renal failure secondary to tumor lysis syndrome

Respiratory: Dyspnea, epistaxis, cough, pharyngitis, rhinitis, hypoxia, acute respiratory distress syndrome, pulmonary edema

Miscellaneous: Infection, sepsis, anaphylaxis

Drug Interactions No formal drug interaction studies have been conducted.

Food Interactions Alcohol (avoid alcohol due to GI irritation)

Stability Protect from light during storage, dispensing, and administration. Refrigerate vials. Reconstituted vial is stable for 8 hours if refrigerated and protected from light.

Mechanism of Action Antibody to CD33 antigen which is expressed on leukemic blasts in >80% of AML patients, as well as normal myeloid cells. Binding results in internalization of the antibody-antigen complex, leading to the release of the calicheamicin derivative inside the myeloid cell. The calicheamicin derivative binds to DNA resulting in double strand breaks and cell death. Pluripotent stem cells and nonhematopoietic cells are not affected.

Pharmacokinetics

Half-life: Adults:

- Calicheamicin derivative: 45 hours (with repeat dose: 60 hours)
- Unconjugated derivative: 100 hours

Usual Dosage Refer to individual protocols: I.V.:

Children: Combination therapy:

- Relapsed/refractory AML:
  - Children <3 years: 0.07-0.1 mg/kg/dose
  - Children ≥3 years: 2-3 mg/m^2/dose
- Newly diagnosed childhood AML: 3 mg/m^2/dose (no dose adjustment for age or body surface area <0.6 m^2)

Children: Monotherapy: Phase I (MTD):

- Children <3 years: 0.2 mg/kg/dose for a total of 2 doses separated by 14 days
- Children >3 years: 6 mg/m^2/dose for a total of 2 doses separated by 14 days

Adults: AML in first relapse: 9 mg/m^2; full treatment course consists of a total of 2 doses separated by 14 days; maximum dose: 15 mg

Dosage adjustment in renal impairment: No recommendation (not studied)

Dosage adjustment in hepatic impairment: No recommendation (not studied)

Administration Prepare dose in a biologic safety hood with the fluorescent light turned off. Allow vial to warm to room temperature prior to reconstitution. Reconstitute vial with 5 mL SWI; reconstituted vial is stable for 8 hours if refrigerated and protected from light. Further dilute dose in 100 mL NS.

DO NOT ADMINISTER I.V. PUSH or by RAPID I.V. INJECTION; Administer via I.V. infusion over 2 hours through a dedicated line with a filter (low protein binding 1.2 micron in-line filter is recommended). May administer through a peripheral or central line. Cover dose with UV protective bag during infusion.

Monitoring Parameters Vital signs during infusion and for 4 hours following the infusion; signs and symptoms of postinfusion reaction; electrolytes, CBC with differential, platelet count, LFTs. Monitor for signs and symptoms of hepatorenal syndrome (weight gain, abdominal girth, right upper quadrant abdominal pain, hepatomegaly, ascites).

Patient Information Notify physician if fever, chills, unusual bruising or bleeding, signs of infection, dizziness, lightheadedness, difficulty breathing, or yellowing of the eyes or skin occurs. Advise women of childbearing potential to avoid becoming pregnant while receiving gemtuzumab.

Nursing Implications Handle and dispose according to guidelines issued for cytotoxic drugs. Administer diphenhydramine and acetaminophen prior to each infusion. Acetaminophen should be repeated every 4 hours for 2 additional doses as needed. Pretreatment with methylprednisolone may ameliorate infusion-related symptoms.

Dosage Forms Excipient information presented when available (limited, particularly for generics); consult specific product labeling.

Injection, powder for reconstitution:

Mylotarg®: 5 mg

References

Arceci RJ, Sande J, Lange B, et al, "Safety and Efficacy of Gemtuzumab Ozogamicin in Pediatric Patients With Advanced CD33+ Acute Myeloid Leukemia," *Blood*, 2005, 106(4):1183-8.

Buckwalter M, Dowell JA, Korth-Bradley J, et al, "Pharmacokinetics of Gemtuzumab Ozogamicin as a Single-Agent Treatment of Pediatric Patients With Refractory or Relapsed Acute Myeloid Leukemia," *J Clin Pharmacol*, 2004, 44(8):873-80.

Zwaan CM, Reinhardt D, Corbacioglu S, et al, "Gemtuzumab Ozogamicin: First Clinical Experiences in Children With Relapsed/Refractory Acute Myeloid Leukemia Treated on Compassionate-Use Basis," *Blood*, 2003, 101(10):3868-71.

♦ **Gemzar®** *see* Gemcitabine *on page 721*
♦ **Genac® [OTC]** *see* Triprolidine and Pseudoephedrine *on page 1580*
♦ **Genacote™ [OTC]** *see* Aspirin *on page 163*
♦ **Gen-Acyclovir (Can)** *see* Acyclovir *on page 54*
♦ **Genahist® [OTC]** *see* DiphenhydrAMINE *on page 509*
♦ **Gen-Alprazolam (Can)** *see* Alprazolam *on page 79*
♦ **Gen-Amiodarone (Can)** *see* Amiodarone *on page 100*
♦ **Gen-Amoxicillin (Can)** *see* Amoxicillin *on page 113*
♦ **Genapap™ [OTC]** *see* Acetaminophen *on page 42*
♦ **Genapap™ Children [OTC]** *see* Acetaminophen *on page 42*
♦ **Genapap™ Extra Strength [OTC]** *see* Acetaminophen *on page 42*
♦ **Genapap™ Infant [OTC]** *see* Acetaminophen *on page 42*
♦ **Genaphed® [OTC]** *see* Pseudoephedrine *on page 1344*
♦ **Genasal [OTC]** *see* Oxymetazoline *on page 1194*
♦ **Genasoft® [OTC]** *see* Docusate *on page 526*
♦ **Genasyme® [OTC]** *see* Simethicone *on page 1440*
♦ **Gen-Atenolol (Can)** *see* Atenolol *on page 170*
♦ **Genaton Tablet [OTC]** *see* Antacid Preparations *on page 132*
♦ **Genatuss DM® [OTC]** *see* Guaifenesin and Dextromethorphan *on page 748*
♦ **Gen-Azathioprine (Can)** *see* Azathioprine *on page 187*
♦ **Gen-Baclofen (Can)** *see* Baclofen *on page 197*
♦ **Gen-Beclo (Can)** *see* Beclomethasone *on page 200*
♦ **Gen-Budesonide AQ (Can)** *see* Budesonide *on page 238*
♦ **Gen-Buspirone (Can)** *see* BusPIRone *on page 250*
♦ **Gen-Captopril (Can)** *see* Captopril *on page 277*
♦ **Gen-Carbamazepine CR (Can)** *see* Carbamazepine *on page 279*
♦ **Gen-Cimetidine (Can)** *see* Cimetidine *on page 355*
♦ **Gen-Ciprofloxacin (Can)** *see* Ciprofloxacin *on page 357*
♦ **Gen-Citalopram (Can)** *see* Citalopram *on page 368*
♦ **Gen-Clobetasol (Can)** *see* Clobetasol *on page 383*
♦ **Gen-Clonazepam (Can)** *see* Clonazepam *on page 387*
♦ **Gen-Cyclobenzaprine (Can)** *see* Cyclobenzaprine *on page 416*
♦ **Gen-Diltiazem (Can)** *see* Diltiazem *on page 503*
♦ **Gen-Diltiazem CD (Can)** *see* Diltiazem *on page 503*
♦ **Gen-Divalproex (Can)** *see* Valproic Acid and Derivatives *on page 1592*
♦ **Genebs [OTC]** *see* Acetaminophen *on page 42*
♦ **Genebs Extra Strength [OTC]** *see* Acetaminophen *on page 42*
♦ **Generlac** *see* Lactulose *on page 900*
♦ **Gen-Etidronate (Can)** *see* Etidronate Disodium *on page 622*
♦ **Gen-Famotidine (Can)** *see* Famotidine *on page 638*
♦ **Genfiber® [OTC]** *see* Psyllium *on page 1347*
♦ **Gen-Fluconazole (Can)** *see* Fluconazole *on page 660*
♦ **Gen-Fluoxetine (Can)** *see* Fluoxetine *on page 681*
♦ **Gen-Gabapentin (Can)** *see* Gabapentin *on page 716*
♦ **Gen-Glybe (Can)** *see* GlyBURIDE *on page 734*
♦ **Gengraf®** *see* CycloSPORINE *on page 422*
♦ **Gen-Hydroxychloroquine (Can)** *see* Hydroxychloroquine *on page 792*
♦ **Gen-Hydroxyurea (Can)** *see* Hydroxyurea *on page 794*
♦ **Gen-Ipratropium (Can)** *see* Ipratropium *on page 863*
♦ **Gen-Lamotrigine (Can)** *see* Lamotrigine *on page 906*
♦ **Gen-Levothyroxine (Can)** *see* Levothyroxine *on page 930*
♦ **Gen-Lovastatin (Can)** *see* Lovastatin *on page 964*

Gentamicin (jen ta MYE sin)

Medication Safety Issues
Sound-alike/look-alike issues:
Gentamicin may be confused with kanamycin
Garamycin® may be confused with kanamycin, Terramycin®

Related Information
Blood Level Sampling Time Guidelines *on page 1914*
Overdose and Toxicology *on page 1916*

U.S. Brand Names Genoptic® [DSC]; Gentak®

Canadian Brand Names Alcomicin®; Diogent®; Garamycin®; Gentamicin Injection, USP; SAB-Gentamicin

Index Terms Gentamicin Sulfate

Therapeutic Category Antibiotic, Aminoglycoside; Antibiotic, Ophthalmic; Antibiotic, Topical

Generic Available Yes

Use Treatment of susceptible bacterial infections, normally gram-negative organisms including *Pseudomonas*, *E. coli*, *Proteus*, *Serratia*, and gram-positive *Staphylococcus*; treatment of bone infections, CNS infections, respiratory tract infections, skin and soft tissue infections, as well as abdominal and urinary tract infections, endocarditis, and septicemia; used in combination with ampicillin as empiric therapy for sepsis in newborns; prevention of bacterial endocarditis prior to surgical procedures in high risk patients; used topically to treat superficial infections of the skin or ophthalmic infections caused by susceptible bacteria

Pregnancy Risk Factor D

Lactation Enters breast milk (small amounts)/use caution (AAP rates "compatible")

Contraindications Hypersensitivity to gentamicin, any component (see Warnings), or other aminoglycosides

Warnings Parenteral aminoglycosides are associated with significant nephrotoxicity or ototoxicity; the ototoxicity is directly proportional to the amount of drug given and the duration of treatment; tinnitus or vertigo are indications of vestibular injury and impending irreversible bilateral deafness; renal damage is usually reversible and is associated with decreased creatinine clearance and urine specific gravity, elevated BUN and serum creatinine, casts in the urine, oliguria, and proteinuria; once-daily gentamicin administration has been associated with a pyrogenic endotoxin-like reaction (fever, chills, hypotension, tachycardia); some products contain sulfites which may cause allergic reactions in susceptible individuals. Aminoglycosides can cause fetal harm when administered to a pregnant woman; aminoglycosides have been associated with several reports of total irreversible bilateral congenital deafness in pediatric patients exposed *in utero.*

Precautions Use with caution in neonates due to renal immaturity that results in a prolonged gentamicin half-life and in patients with pre-existing renal impairment, auditory or vestibular impairment, hypocalcemia, myasthenia gravis, and in conditions which depress neuromuscular transmission; modify dosage in patients with renal impairment and in neonates on extracorporeal membrane oxygenation (ECMO)

Adverse Reactions

Central nervous system: Vertigo, ataxia, gait instability, dizziness, headache, fever
Dermatologic: Rash, pruritus, erythema
Endocrine & metabolic: Hypomagnesemia
Gastrointestinal: Nausea, vomiting, anorexia
Genitourinary: Decrease in urine specific gravity, casts in urine, possible electrolyte wasting
Hematologic: Granulocytopenia, thrombocytopenia, eosinophilia
Hepatic: Elevated AST and ALT
Local: Thrombophlebitis
Neuromuscular & skeletal: Neuromuscular blockade, muscle cramps, tremor, weakness
Ocular: Optic neuritis; ophthalmic use: burning, stinging, redness, lacrimation
Otic: Ototoxicity (may be associated with high serum aminoglycoside concentrations persisting for prolonged periods) with tinnitus, hearing loss; early toxicity usually affects high-pitched sound
Renal: Nephrotoxicity (high trough levels) with proteinuria, reduction in glomerular filtration rate, elevated serum creatinine

Drug Interactions Increased toxicity: Concurrent use of amphotericin B, magnesium, cephalosporins, penicillins, loop diuretics, vancomycin, cisplatin, indomethacin; potentiates effect of neuromuscular blocking agents and botulinum toxin

Stability Incompatible with penicillins, cephalosporins, heparin

Mechanism of Action Inhibits cellular initiation of bacterial protein synthesis by binding to 30S and 50S ribosomal subunits resulting in a defective bacterial cell membrane

Pharmacokinetics

Absorption: Oral: Poorly absorbed (<2%)
Distribution: Crosses the placenta; distributes primarily in the extracellular fluid volume and in most tissues; poor penetration into CSF; drug accumulates in the renal cortex; small amounts distribute into bile, sputum, saliva, tears, and breast milk
- V_d: Increased in neonates and with fever, edema, ascites, fluid overload; V_d is decreased in patients with dehydration
  - Neonates: 0.45 ± 0.1 L/kg
  - Infants: 0.4 ± 0.1 L/kg
  - Children: 0.35 ± 0.15 L/kg
  - Adolescents: 0.3 ± 0.1 L/kg
  - Adults: 0.2-0.3 L/kg

Protein binding: <30%
Half-life:
- Neonates:
  - <1 week: 3-11.5 hours
  - 1 week to 1 month: 3-6 hours
- Infants: 4 ± 1 hour
- Children: 2 ± 1 hour
- Adolescents: 1.5 ± 1 hour
- Adults with normal renal function: 1.5-3 hours
- Anuria: 36-70 hours

Time to peak serum concentration:
- I.M.: Within 30-90 minutes
- I.V.: 30 minutes after 30-minute infusion

Elimination: Clearance is directly related to renal function; eliminated almost completely by glomerular filtration of unchanged drug with excretion into urine
- Clearance:
  - Neonates: 0.045 ± 0.01 L/hour/kg
  - Infants: 0.1 ± 0.05 L/hour/kg
  - Children: 0.1 ± 0.03 L/hour/kg
  - Adolescents: 0.09 ± 0.03 L/hour/kg

Dialysis: Dialyzable (50% to 100%)

Usual Dosage Dosage should be based on an estimate of ideal body weight, except in neonates (neonatal dosage should be based on actual weight unless the patient has hydrocephalus or hydrops fetalis):

Neonates: I.M., I.V.:
- Premature neonate, <1000 g: 3.5 mg/kg/dose every 24 hours
- 0-4 weeks, <1200 g: 2.5 mg/kg/dose every 18-24 hours
- Postnatal age ≤7 days: 2.5 mg/kg/dose every 12 hours
- Postnatal age >7 days:
  - 1200-2000 g: 2.5 mg/kg/dose every 8-12 hours
  - >2000 g: 2.5 mg/kg/dose every 8 hours

(Continued)

Gentamicin *(Continued)*

Initial dose for term neonates receiving ECMO: I.V.: 2.5 mg/kg/dose every 18 hours; subsequent doses should be individualized by monitoring serum drug concentrations; when ECMO is discontinued, dosage may require readjustment due to large shifts in body water

Once daily dosing:

Premature neonates with normal renal function: 3.5-4 mg/kg/dose every 24 hours

Term neonates with normal renal function: 3.5-5 mg/kg/dose every 24 hours

Infants and Children <5 years: I.M., I.V.: 2.5 mg/kg/dose every 8 hours*

Once daily dosing in patients with normal renal function: 5-7.5 mg/kg/dose every 24 hours

Endocarditis prophylaxis (high-risk patients): 1.5 mg/kg (maximum: 120 mg) within 30 minutes of starting the procedure plus ampicillin or vancomycin (in patients allergic to ampicillin)

Pulmonary infection in cystic fibrosis: 2.5-3.3 mg/kg/dose every 6-8 hours

Patients on hemodialysis: 1.25-1.75 mg/kg/dose postdialysis

Children ≥5 years: I.M., I.V.: 2-2.5 mg/kg/dose every 8 hours*

Once daily dosing in children with normal renal function: 5-7.5 mg/kg/dose every 24 hours

Endocarditis prophylaxis (high-risk patients): 1.5 mg/kg (maximum: 120 mg) within 30 minutes of starting the procedure plus ampicillin or vancomycin (in patients allergic to ampicillin)

Pulmonary infection in cystic fibrosis: 2.5-3.3 mg/kg/dose every 6-8 hours

Patients on hemodialysis: 1.25-1.75 mg/kg/dose postdialysis

*Some patients may require larger or more frequent doses (eg, every 6 hours) if serum levels document the need (ie, cystic fibrosis, patients with major burns, or febrile granulocytopenic patients); modify dose based on individual patient requirements as determined by renal function, serum drug concentrations, and patient-specific clinical parameters

Intraventricular/intrathecal **(use a preservative free preparation)**:

Newborns: 1 mg/day

Infants >3 months and Children: 1-2 mg/day

Adults: 4-8 mg/day

Infants, Children, and Adults:

Topical: Apply 3-4 times/day

Ophthalmic:

Ointment: Apply 2-3 times/day

Solution: Instill 1-2 drops every 2-4 hours, up to 2 drops every hour for severe infections

Adults: I.M., I.V.: 3-6 mg/kg/day in divided doses every 8 hours; studies of once daily dosing have used I.V. doses of 4-6.6 mg/kg once daily

Endocarditis prophylaxis (high-risk patients): 1.5 mg/kg (maximum: 120 mg) within 30 minutes of starting the procedure plus ampicillin or vancomycin (in patients allergic to ampicillin)

Patients on hemodialysis: 0.5-0.7 mg/kg/dose postdialysis

Dosing adjustment in renal impairment: I.M., I.V.: 2.5 mg/kg** (Cl_{cr} <60 mL/minute/1.73 m^2) **or**

Cl_{cr} 40-60 mL/minute: Administer every 12 hours

Cl_{cr} 20-40 mL/minute: Administer every 24 hours

Cl_{cr} <20 mL/minute: Administer normal dose, then monitor levels

**2-3 serum level measurements should be obtained after the initial dose to measure the patient's pharmacokinetic parameters (eg, half-life, V_d) in order to determine the frequency and amount of subsequent doses

Administration

Ophthalmic: Gentamicin solution is not for subconjunctival injection. Solution may be instilled into the affected eye or a small amount of ointment may be placed into the conjunctival sac. Avoid contaminating tip of the solution bottle or ointment tube. Solution: Apply finger pressure to lacrimal sac during and for 1-2 minutes after instillation to decrease risk of absorption and systemic effects.

Parenteral: Administer by I.M., I.V. slow intermittent infusion over 30-60 minutes or by direct injection over 15 minutes; final concentration for I.V. administration should not exceed 10 mg/mL; administer other antibiotics, such as penicillins and cephalosporins, at least 1 hour before or after gentamicin

Topical: Apply a small amount gently to the cleansed affected area

Monitoring Parameters Urinalysis, urine output, BUN, serum creatinine, peak and trough serum gentamicin concentrations, hearing test, CBC with differential

Not all infants and children who receive aminoglycosides require monitoring of serum aminoglycoside concentrations. Indications for use of aminoglycoside serum concentration monitoring include:

Treatment course >5 days

Patients with decreased or changing renal function
Patients with poor therapeutic response
Infants <3 months of age
Atypical body constituency (obesity, expanded extracellular fluid volume)
Clinical need for higher doses or shorter intervals (eg, cystic fibrosis, burns, endocarditis, meningitis, critically ill patients, relatively resistant organism)
Patients on hemodialysis or chronic ambulatory peritoneal dialysis
Signs of nephrotoxicity or ototoxicity
Concomitant use of other nephrotoxic agents

Reference Range

Peak: 4-12 mcg/mL; peak values are 2-3 times greater with once daily dosing regimens
Trough: 0.5-2 mcg/mL

Test Interactions Aminoglycoside levels measured in blood taken from Silastic® central line catheters can sometimes give falsely high readings

Patient Information Report any dizziness or sensations of ringing or fullness in ears to the physician

Nursing Implications Obtain drug levels after the third or fourth dose except in neonates and patients with rapidly changing renal function in whom levels need to be measured sooner; peak gentamicin serum concentrations are drawn 30 minutes after the end of a 30-minute I.V. infusion, immediately on completion of a 1-hour I.V. infusion, or 1 hour after an intramuscular injection; trough levels are drawn within 30 minutes before the next dose; provide adequate patient hydration and perfusion

Dosage Forms Excipient information presented when available (limited, particularly for generics); consult specific product labeling. [DSC] = Discontinued product

Cream, topical, as sulfate: 0.1% (15 g, 30 g)
Infusion, as sulfate [premixed in NS]: 40 mg (50 mL); 60 mg (50 mL, 100 mL); 70 mg (50 mL); 80 mg (50 mL, 100 mL); 90 mg (100 mL); 100 mg (50 mL, 100 mL); 120 mg (100 mL)
Injection, solution, as sulfate [ADD-Vantage® vial]: 10 mg/mL (6 mL, 8 mL, 10 mL)
Injection, solution, as sulfate: 40 mg/mL (2 mL, 20 mL) [may contain sodium metabisulfite]
Injection, solution, pediatric, as sulfate: 10 mg/mL (2 mL) [may contain sodium metabisulfite]
Injection, solution, pediatric, as sulfate [preservative free]: 10 mg/mL (2 mL)
Ointment, ophthalmic, as sulfate (Gentak®): 0.3% [3 mg/g] (3.5 g)
Ointment, topical, as sulfate: 0.1% (15 g, 30 g)
Solution, ophthalmic, as sulfate: 0.3% (5 mL, 15 mL) [contains benzalkonium chloride]
Genoptic®: 0.3% (1 mL) [contains benzalkonium chloride] [DSC]
Gentak®: 0.3% (5 mL; 15 mL [DSC]) [contains benzalkonium chloride]

References

Bhatt-Mehta V, Johnson CE and Schumacher RE, "Gentamicin Pharmacokinetics in Term Neonates Receiving Extracorporeal Membrane Oxygenation," *Pharmacotherapy*, 1992, 12(1):28-32.
Gilbert DN, "Once-Daily Aminoglycoside Therapy," *Antimicrob Agents Chemother*, 1991, 35(3):399-405.
Kraus DM, Pai MP, and Rodvold KA, "Efficacy and Tolerability of Extended-Interval Aminoglycoside Administration in Pediatric Patients," *Paediatr Drugs*, 2002, 4(7):469-84.
Reimche LD, Rooney, ME, Hindmarsh KW, et al, "An Evaluation of Gentamicin Dosing According to Renal Function in Neonates With Suspected Sepsis," *Am J Perinatol*, 1987, 4(3):262-5.
Shevchuk YM and Taylor DM, "Aminoglycoside Volume of Distribution in Pediatric Patients," *DICP*, 1990, 24(3):273-6.

♦ **Gentamicin and Prednisolone** *see* Prednisolone and Gentamicin *on page 1307*
♦ **Gentamicin Injection, USP (Can)** *see* Gentamicin *on page 726*
♦ **Gentamicin Sulfate** *see* Gentamicin *on page 726*

Gentian Violet (JEN shun VYE oh let)

Index Terms Crystal Violet; Methylrosaniline Chloride

Therapeutic Category Antibacterial, Topical; Antifungal Agent, Topical

Generic Available Yes

Use Treatment of cutaneous or mucocutaneous infections caused by *Candida albicans* and other superficial skin infections refractory to topical nystatin, clotrimazole, miconazole, or econazole

Pregnancy Risk Factor C

Contraindications Hypersensitivity to gentian violet; ulcerated areas; patients with porphyria

Warnings May result in tattooing of the skin when applied to granulation tissue

Adverse Reactions

Dermatological: Staining of skin (purple), vesicle formation
Gastrointestinal: Esophagitis
(Continued)

Gentian Violet *(Continued)*

Local: Burning, irritation, vesicle formation, sensitivity reactions, ulceration of mucous membranes

Respiratory: Laryngitis, tracheitis may result from swallowing gentian violet solution, laryngeal obstruction following frequent or prolonged use

Mechanism of Action Topical antiseptic/germicide effective against some vegetative gram-positive bacteria, particularly *Staphylococcus* species, and some yeast; it is much less effective against gram-negative bacteria and is ineffective against acid-fast bacteria

Usual Dosage Topical:

Infants: Apply 3-4 drops of a 0.5% solution under the tongue or on lesion after feedings

Children and Adults: Apply 1% to 2% solution to lesion 2-3 times/day for 3 days, do not swallow

Administration Topical: Apply to lesions with cotton; do not apply to ulcerative lesions on the face

Patient Information Drug stains skin and clothing purple; proper hygiene and skin care need to be used to prevent spread of infection and reinfection

Nursing Implications Keep affected area dry and exposed to air

Additional Information 0.25% or 0.5% solution is less irritating than a 1% to 2% solution and is reported to be as effective

Dosage Forms Excipient information presented when available (limited, particularly for generics); consult specific product labeling.

Solution, topical: 1% (30 mL); 2% (30 mL)

- **Gen-Timolol (Can)** *see* Timolol *on page 1542*
- **Gentlax® (Can)** *see* Bisacodyl *on page 217*
- **Gen-Topiramate (Can)** *see* Topiramate *on page 1551*
- **Gentran®** *see* Dextran *on page 468*
- **Gen-Trazodone (Can)** *see* Trazodone *on page 1564*
- **Gen-Triazolam (Can)** *see* Triazolam *on page 1572*
- **Gen-Verapamil (Can)** *see* Verapamil *on page 1611*
- **Gen-Verapamil SR (Can)** *see* Verapamil *on page 1611*
- **Gen-Warfarin (Can)** *see* Warfarin *on page 1626*
- **Geocillin®** *see* Carbenicillin *on page 284*
- **Geri-Hydrolac™ [OTC]** *see* Lactic Acid and Ammonium Hydroxide *on page 898*
- **Geri-Hydrolac™-12 [OTC]** *see* Lactic Acid and Ammonium Hydroxide *on page 898*
- **German Measles Vaccine** *see* Rubella Virus Vaccine (Live) *on page 1410*
- **GG** *see* Guaifenesin *on page 745*
- **GI87084B** *see* Remifentanil *on page 1371*
- **Glargine Insulin** *see* Insulin Glargine *on page 840*
- **Gliadel®** *see* Carmustine *on page 290*
- **Gliadel Wafer® (Can)** *see* Carmustine *on page 290*
- **Glibenclamide** *see* GlyBURIDE *on page 734*

GlipiZIDE (GLIP i zide)

Medication Safety Issues

Sound-alike/look-alike issues:

GlipiZIDE may be confused with glimepiride, glyBURIDE
Glucotrol® may be confused with Glucophage®, Glucotrol® XL, glyBURIDE
Glucotrol® XL may be confused with Glucotrol®

High alert medication: The Institute for Safe Medication Practices (ISMP) includes this medication among its list of drugs which have a heightened risk of causing significant patient harm when used in error.

Related Information

Medications for Which A Single Dose May Be Fatal When Ingested By A Toddler *on page 1932*

U.S. Brand Names Glucotrol®; Glucotrol® XL

Index Terms Glydiazinamide

Therapeutic Category Antidiabetic Agent, Oral; Antidiabetic Agent, Sulfonylurea; Hypoglycemic Agent, Oral

Generic Available Yes

Use Management of type II diabetes mellitus (noninsulin-dependent, NIDDM) when hyperglycemia cannot be managed by diet alone; may be used concomitantly with metformin or insulin to improve glycemic control

Pregnancy Risk Factor C

Lactation Excretion in breast milk unknown/not recommended

Contraindications Hypersensitivity to glipizide, any component, or other sulfonamides; type 1 diabetes mellitus (insulin-dependent, IDDM), diabetic ketoacidosis with or without coma

Warnings Chemical similarities are present among sulfonamides, sulfonylureas, carbonic anhydrase inhibitors, thiazides, and loop diuretics (except ethacrynic acid), and although only glipizide use in patients with sulfonamide allergy is specifically contraindicated in product labeling, there is a risk of cross-reaction in patients with allergies to any of these compounds; avoid use when the previous reaction has been severe; product labeling states oral hypoglycemic drugs may be associated with an increased cardiovascular mortality as compared to treatment with diet alone or diet plus insulin; data to support this association are limited, and several studies, including a large prospective trial (UKPDS) have not supported an association

Precautions Use with caution in patients with adrenal or pituitary insufficiency; hypoglycemic reactions are more prevalent in debilitated, malnourished patients, patients with mild disease or impaired hepatic or renal function; hypoglycemia may also occur with inadequate caloric intake, strenuous exercise, or concurrent use with other hypoglycemic drugs; use of extended release formulation in patients with markedly reduced GI retention time eg, short-bowel syndrome, may potentially result in lower plasma levels and decreased effect

Adverse Reactions

Cardiovascular: Edema, flushing, hypertension, arrhythmias, syncope

Central nervous system: Headache, dizziness, drowsiness, insomnia, anxiety, depression, migraine, nervousness, confusion, somnolence, vertigo

Dermatologic: Rash, urticaria, photosensitivity, pruritus

Endocrine & metabolic: Hypoglycemia, hyponatremia, weight gain

Gastrointestinal: Anorexia, nausea, vomiting, diarrhea, epigastric fullness, flatulence, constipation, heartburn, abdominal pain

Genitourinary: Dysuria, polyuria

Hematologic: Blood dyscrasias, aplastic anemia, hemolytic anemia, bone marrow suppression, thrombocytopenia, agranulocytosis

Hepatic: Cholestatic jaundice, elevated liver enzymes

Neuromuscular & skeletal: Arthralgia, leg cramps, myalgia, tremor, hypertonia

Ocular: Blurred vision, ocular pain, conjunctivitis, retinal hemorrhage

Renal: Diuretic effect (mild), SIADH, urolithiasis

Respiratory: Rhinitis, dyspnea, pharyngitis

Miscellaneous: Diaphoresis

Drug Interactions Drugs which tend to produce hyperglycemia (eg, diuretics, corticosteroids, phenothiazines, thyroid products, estrogens, oral contraceptives, phenytoin, nicotinic acid, sympathomimetics, calcium channel-blocking drugs, rifampin, and isoniazid) may lead to a loss of glycemic control; disulfiram-like reactions with alcohol; drugs which produce an increase in glipizide's hypoglycemic effects: ACE inhibitors, cimetidine, chloramphenicol, anabolic steroids, monoamine oxidase inhibitors, fluoroquinolone antibiotics, and probenecid; since this agent is highly protein bound, use of other protein-bound drugs may result in adverse effects when glipizide therapy is initiated or discontinued; beta-adrenergic blocking agents may impair glucose tolerance, increase the frequency or severity of hypoglycemia, block hypoglycemia-induced tachycardia, delay the rate of recovery of blood glucose concentration following drug-induced hypoglycemia, and may alter the hemodynamic response to hypoglycemia; glipizide may increase cyclosporine and tacrolimus serum concentrations; cholestyramine decreases glipizide absorption; fluconazole may increase glipizide levels (mean increase in AUC: 56.9%)

Food Interactions Food delays absorption but does not affect the extent of absorption or peak levels achieved

Stability Store at room temperature; protect from light

Mechanism of Action Stimulates insulin release from the pancreatic beta cells, reduces glucose output from the liver, and increases insulin sensitivity at peripheral target sites

Pharmacodynamics

Onset of action: Immediate release formulation: 15-30 minutes; extended release formulation: 2-3 hours

Maximum effect: Immediate release formulation: Within 2-3 hours; extended release formulation: 6-12 hours

Duration: Immediate release formulation: 12-24 hours; extended release formulation: 24 hours

Average decrease in fasting blood glucose (when used as monotherapy): 60-70 mg/dL

Pharmacokinetics

Absorption: Rapid and complete

Distribution: V_d: Adults: 10 L

(Continued)

GlipiZIDE *(Continued)*

Protein binding: 98% to 99%
Metabolism: Extensive liver metabolism to inactive metabolites
Bioavailability: 80% to 100%
Half-life: Adults: 2-5 hours
Time to peak serum concentration:
Immediate release formulation: 1-3 hours
Extended release formulation: 6-12 hours
Elimination: <10% of drug excreted into urine as unchanged drug; 90% of drug excreted as metabolites in urine and 10% excreted in feces

Usual Dosage Adults: Oral:

Management of noninsulin-dependent diabetes mellitus in patients **previously untreated:** Initial: 5 mg/day immediate release or extended release tablets; adjust dosage in 2.5-5 mg daily increments in intervals of 3-7 days for immediate release tablets or 5 mg daily increments in intervals of at least 7 days for extended release tablets; if total daily dose for immediate release tablets is >15 mg, divide into twice daily dosage; maximum daily dose for immediate release tablets: 40 mg; maximum daily dose for extended release tablets: 20 mg

Note: patients may be converted from immediate release tablets to extended release tablets by giving the nearest equivalent total daily dose once daily

Management of noninsulin-dependent diabetes mellitus in patients **previously maintained on insulin:**

Insulin dosage ≤20 units/day: Use recommended initial dose and abruptly discontinue insulin

Insulin dosage >20 units/day: Use recommended initial dose and reduce daily insulin dosage by 50%; continue to withdraw daily insulin dosage gradually over several days as tolerated with incremental increases of glipizide

Dosing adjustment/comments in renal impairment: Cl_{cr} <10 mL/minute: Some investigators recommend not using

Dosing adjustment in hepatic impairment: Reduce initial dosage to 2.5 mg/day

Administration Oral: Administer immediate release tablets 30 minutes before a meal; extended release tablets should be swallowed whole and administered with breakfast; do not cut, crush, or chew

Monitoring Parameters Signs and symptoms of hypoglycemia, fasting blood glucose, glycosylated hemoglobin (hemoglobin A_{1c})

Reference Range Target range:
Blood glucose: Fasting and preprandial: 80-120 mg/dL; bedtime: 100-140 mg/dL
Glycosylated hemoglobin (hemoglobin A_{1c}): <7%

Patient Information Do not change dose or discontinue without consulting prescriber; avoid alcohol while taking this medication, may cause severe reaction; maintain regular dietary intake and exercise routine; always carry quick source of sugar; if experiencing a hypoglycemic reaction, contact prescriber immediately; report severe or persistent side effects, extended vomiting or flu-like symptoms, skin rash, easy bruising or bleeding, or change in color of urine or stool; when taking extended release tablets, it is not unusual to observe a tablet in the stool; this is the nonabsorbable shell containing the active drug which has been released. May rarely cause photosensitivity reactions (eg, exposure to sunlight may cause severe sunburn, skin rash, redness, or itching); avoid direct exposure to sunlight

Additional Information When transferring from other sulfonylurea antidiabetic agents to glyburide, with the exception of chlorpropamide, the administration of the other agent may be abruptly discontinued; due to the prolonged elimination half-life of chlorpropamide, a 2- to 3-day drug-free interval may be advisable before glipizide therapy is begun

Dosage Forms Excipient information presented when available (limited, particularly for generics); consult specific product labeling.
Tablet: 5 mg, 10 mg
Glucotrol®: 5 mg, 10 mg
Tablet, extended release: 2.5 mg, 5 mg, 10 mg
Glucotrol® XL: 2.5 mg, 5 mg, 10 mg

References

DeFronzo RA, "Pharmacologic Therapy for Type 2 Diabetes Mellitus," *Ann Intern Med*, 1999, 131(4):281-303.
"Intensive Blood-Glucose Control With Sulphonylureas or Insulin Compared With Conventional Treatment and Risk of Complications in Patients With Type 2 Diabetes (UKPDS 33) UK Prospective Diabetes Study (UKPDS) Group," *Lancet*, 1998, 352(9131):837-53.

◆ **GlucaGen®** *see* Glucagon (rDNA Origin) *on page 733*
◆ **GlucaGen® Diagnostic Kit** *see* Glucagon (rDNA Origin) *on page 733*
◆ **GlucaGen® HypoKit™** *see* Glucagon (rDNA Origin) *on page 733*
◆ **Glucagon Diagnostic Kit [DSC]** *see* Glucagon (rDNA Origin) *on page 733*

◆ **Glucagon Emergency Kit** *see* Glucagon (rDNA Origin) *on page 733*
◆ **Glucagon Hydrochloride** *see* Glucagon (rDNA Origin) *on page 733*

Glucagon (rDNA Origin) (GLOO ka gon)

Medication Safety Issues
Sound-alike/look-alike issues:
Glucagon may be confused with Glaucon®

Related Information
Commonly Used Antidotes for Acute Overdoses *on page 1920*

U.S. Brand Names GlucaGen®; GlucaGen® Diagnostic Kit; GlucaGen® HypoKit™; Glucagon Diagnostic Kit [DSC]; Glucagon Emergency Kit

Index Terms Glucagon Hydrochloride

Therapeutic Category Antihypoglycemic Agent

Generic Available No

Use Management of hypoglycemia; diagnostic aid in the radiologic examination of GI tract when a hypotonic state is needed; used with some success as a cardiac stimulant in management of severe cases of beta-adrenergic blocking agent overdosage

Pregnancy Risk Factor B

Lactation Excretion in breast milk unknown/compatible

Contraindications Hypersensitivity to glucagon or any component

Warnings Use with caution in patients with a history of insulinoma and/or pheochromocytoma; because glucagon depletes glycogen stores, the patient should be given supplemental carbohydrates as soon as physically possible

Adverse Reactions
Cardiovascular: Hypotension
Dermatologic: Urticaria
Gastrointestinal: Nausea, vomiting
Respiratory: Respiratory distress
Miscellaneous: Hypersensitivity reactions

Drug Interactions Enhances anticoagulant effect of warfarin; phenytoin inhibits the stimulant effect of glucagon on insulin release by the islet cells; propranolol partially inhibits the hyperglycemic effect of glucagon

Stability Glucagon (rDNA origin) for injection (Lilly) should be stored at controlled room temperature; glucagon (rDNA origin) for injection (GlucaGen®) should be refrigerated; both injections should be used immediately after reconstitution

Mechanism of Action Glucagon (rDNA origin) is genetically engineered and identical to human glucagon. It stimulates adenylate cyclase to produce increased cyclic AMP. It promotes hepatic glycogenolysis and gluconeogenesis, causing an increase in blood glucose levels; produces both positive inotropic and chronotropic effects.

Pharmacodynamics
Blood glucose effect (after 1 mg dosage):
Onset of action: I.M.: 8-10 minutes; I.V.: 1 minute
Duration: I.M.: 12-27 minutes; I.V.: 9-17 minutes

GI tract effect:
Onset of action: Within 1-10 minutes
Duration: 12-30 minutes

Pharmacokinetics
Distribution: V_d: 0.25 L/kg
Metabolism: Extensively degraded in liver and kidneys
Half-life, plasma: 8-18 minutes
Clearance: 13.5 mL/minute/kg

Usual Dosage
Hypoglycemia or insulin shock therapy: I.M., I.V., SubQ (may repeat in 20 minutes as needed):
Neonates, Infants and Children ≤20 kg: 0.02-0.03 mg/kg or 0.5 mg
Children >20 kg and Adults: 1 mg
Diagnostic aid: Adults: I.M., I.V.: 0.25-2 mg 10 minutes prior to procedure

Administration Parenteral: Dilute with manufacturer provided diluent resulting in 1 mg/mL; if doses exceeding 2 mg are used, dilute with SWI instead of diluent; administer by direct I.V. injection, I.M., or SubQ

Monitoring Parameters Blood glucose, blood pressure

Additional Information 1 unit = 1 mg

Dosage Forms Excipient information presented when available (limited, particularly for generics); consult specific product labeling.
Injection, powder for reconstitution, as hydrochloride:
GlucaGen®: 1 mg [equivalent to 1 unit; contains lactose 107 mg]
(Continued)

Glucagon (rDNA Origin) *(Continued)*

GlucaGen® Diagnostic Kit: 1 mg [equivalent to 1 unit; contains lactose 107 mg; packaged with sterile water]
GlucaGen® HypoKit™: 1 mg [equivalent to 1 unit; contains lactose 107 mg; packaged with prefilled syringe containing sterile water]
Glucagon®: 1 mg [equivalent to 1 unit; contains lactose 49 mg]
Glucagon Diagnostic Kit, Glucagon Emergency Kit: 1 mg [equivalent to 1 unit; contains lactose 49 mg; packaged with diluent syringe containing glycerin 12 mg/mL and water for injection]

♦ **Glucocerebrosidase** *see* Alglucerase *on page 75*
♦ **Glucophage®** *see* Metformin *on page 1016*
♦ **Glucophage® XR** *see* Metformin *on page 1016*
♦ **Glucose** *see* Dextrose *on page 479*
♦ **Glucose Monohydrate** *see* Dextrose *on page 479*
♦ **Glucotrol®** *see* GlipiZIDE *on page 730*
♦ **Glucotrol® XL** *see* GlipiZIDE *on page 730*
♦ **Glu-K® [OTC]** *see* Potassium Gluconate *on page 1289*
♦ **Glulisine Insulin** *see* Insulin Glulisine *on page 841*
♦ **Glumetza™** *see* Metformin *on page 1016*
♦ **Glumetza® (Can)** *see* Metformin *on page 1016*
♦ **Glybenclamide** *see* GlyBURIDE *on page 734*
♦ **Glybenzcyclamide** *see* GlyBURIDE *on page 734*

GlyBURIDE (GLYE byoor ide)

Medication Safety Issues
Sound-alike/look-alike issues:
GlyBURIDE may be confused with glipiZIDE, Glucotrol®
Diaβeta® may be confused with Diabinese®, Zebeta®
Micronase® may be confused with microK®, miconazole, Micronor®, Microzide™

High alert medication: The Institute for Safe Medication Practices (ISMP) includes this medication among its list of drugs which have a heightened risk of causing significant patient harm when used in error.

U.S. Brand Names Diaβeta®; Glynase® PresTab®; Micronase®

Canadian Brand Names Albert® Glyburide; Apo-Glyburide®; Diaβeta®; Euglucon®; Gen-Glybe; Novo-Glyburide; Nu-Glyburide; PMS-Glyburide; ratio-Glyburide; Sandoz-Glyburide

Index Terms Diabeta; Glibenclamide; Glybenclamide; Glybenzcyclamide

Therapeutic Category Antidiabetic Agent, Oral; Antidiabetic Agent, Sulfonylurea; Hypoglycemic Agent, Oral

Generic Available Yes

Use Management of type II diabetes mellitus (noninsulin-dependent, NIDDM) when hyperglycemia cannot be managed by diet alone; may be used concomitantly with metformin or insulin to improve glycemic control

Pregnancy Risk Factor C

Lactation Does not enter breast milk/ use caution

Contraindications Hypersensitivity to glyburide, any component, or other sulfonamides; type 1 diabetes mellitus (insulin-dependent, IDDM), diabetic ketoacidosis with or without coma

Warnings Chemical similarities are present among sulfonamides, sulfonylureas, carbonic anhydrase inhibitors, thiazides, and loop diuretics (except ethacrynic acid), and although only glyburide use in patients with sulfonamide allergy is specifically contraindicated in product labeling, there is a risk of cross-reaction in patients with allergies to any of these compounds; avoid use when the previous reaction has been severe; product labeling states oral hypoglycemic drugs may be associated with an increased cardiovascular mortality as compared to treatment with diet alone or diet plus insulin; data to support this association are limited, and several studies, including a large prospective trial (UKPDS) have not supported an association.

Precautions Use with caution in patients with adrenal or pituitary insufficiency; hypoglycemic reactions are more prevalent in debilitated, malnourished patients, patients with mild disease or impaired hepatic or renal function; hypoglycemia may also occur with inadequate caloric intake, strenuous exercise, or concurrent use with other hypoglycemic drugs

Adverse Reactions
Central nervous system: Headache, dizziness
Dermatologic: Pruritus, rash, urticaria, photosensitivity
Endocrine & metabolic: Hypoglycemia, weight gain

Gastrointestinal: Nausea, epigastric fullness, heartburn, constipation, diarrhea, anorexia
Genitourinary: Nocturia
Hematologic: Leukopenia, thrombocytopenia, hemolytic anemia, aplastic anemia, bone marrow suppression, agranulocytosis
Hepatic: Cholestatic jaundice, elevated liver enzymes
Neuromuscular & skeletal: Arthralgia, paresthesia
Ocular: Blurred vision
Renal: Diuretic effect (minor), urolithiasis

Drug Interactions Cytochrome P450 isoenzyme CYP3A3/4 enzyme substrate

Drugs which tend to produce hyperglycemia (eg, diuretics, corticosteroids, phenothiazines, thyroid products, estrogens, oral contraceptives, phenytoin, nicotinic acid, sympathomimetics, calcium channel-blocking drugs, rifampin, and isoniazid) may lead to a loss of glycemic control; disulfiram-like reactions with alcohol; drugs which produce an increase in glyburide's hypoglycemic effects: chloramphenicol, monoamine oxidase inhibitors, fluoroquinolone antibiotics, and probenecid; since this agent is highly protein bound, use of other protein-bound drugs may result in adverse effects when glyburide therapy is initiated or discontinued; beta-adrenergic blocking agents may impair glucose tolerance, increase the frequency or severity of hypoglycemia, block hypoglycemia-induced tachycardia, delay the rate of recovery of blood glucose concentration following drug-induced hypoglycemia, and may alter the hemodynamic response to hypoglycemia

Food Interactions Food does not affect absorption.

Mechanism of Action Stimulates insulin release from the pancreatic beta cells, reduces glucose output from the liver, and increases insulin sensitivity at peripheral target sites

Pharmacodynamics

Onset of action: 45-60 minutes
Maximum effect: 1.5-3 hours
Duration: Conventional formulations: 16-24 hours; micronized formulations: 12-24 hours
Average decrease in fasting blood glucose (when used as monotherapy): 60-70 mg/dL

Pharmacokinetics

Absorption: Reliably and almost completely absorbed
Distribution: V_d: 0.125 L/kg
Metabolism: Completely metabolized to one moderately active and several inactive metabolites
Protein binding: High (>99%)
Half-life: Biphasic: Terminal elimination half-life: Average: 1.4-1.8 hours (range: 0.7-3 hours); may be prolonged with renal or hepatic insufficiency
Time to peak serum concentration: Conventional formulation: 4 hours; micronized formulation: 2-3 hours
Elimination: 30% to 50% of dose excreted in the urine as metabolites in first 24 hours; the remainder of the metabolite via biliary excretion
Dialysis: Not dialyzable

Usual Dosage Adults: Oral: Formulations of micronized glyburide (Glynase® Prestab®) are **not** bioequivalent with conventional formulations (Diaβeta®, Micronase®) and dosage should be retitrated when transferring patients from one formulation to the other

Management of noninsulin-dependent diabetes mellitus in patients **previously untreated:**

Tablet (Diaβeta®, Micronase®):

Initial: 2.5-5 mg/day; in patients who are more sensitive to hypoglycemic drugs (see Precautions), start at 1.25 mg/day; increase in increments of no more than 2.5 mg/day at weekly intervals

Maintenance: 1.25-20 mg/day given as single or divided doses; maximum: 20 mg/day; doses >10 mg should be divided into twice daily doses

Micronized tablets (Glynase® Prestab®):

Initial: 1.5-3 mg/day; in patients who are more sensitive to hypoglycemic drugs (see Precautions), start at 0.75 mg/day; increase in increments of no more than 1.5 mg/day at weekly intervals

Maintenance: 0.75-12 mg/day given as a single dose or in divided doses; doses >6 mg/day should be divided into twice daily doses

Management of noninsulin-dependent diabetes mellitus in patients **previously maintained on insulin:** Initial dosage dependent upon previous insulin dosage, see table on next page.

Dosing adjustment in renal impairment: Cl_{cr} <50 mL/minute: Not recommended

Dosing adjustment in hepatic impairment: Use conservative initial and maintenance doses and avoid use in severe disease

(Continued)

GlyBURIDE *(Continued)*

Previous Daily Insulin Dosage (units)	Initial Glyburide Dosage (mg conventional formulation)	Initial Glyburide Dosage (mg micronized formulation)	Insulin Dosage Change (after glyburide started)
<20	2.5-5	1.5-3	Discontinue
20-40	5	3	Discontinue
>40	5 (increase in increments of 1.25-2.5 mg every 2-10 days)	3 (increase in increments of 0.75-1.5 mg every 2-10 days)	Reduce insulin dosage by 50% (gradually taper off insulin as glyburide dosage increased)

Administration Oral: May administer with food every morning 30 minutes before breakfast or the first main meal

Monitoring Parameters Signs and symptoms of hypoglycemia, fasting blood glucose, hemoglobin A_{1c}

Reference Range Target range:

Blood glucose: Fasting and preprandial: 80-120 mg/dL; bedtime: 100-140 mg/dL

Glycosylated hemoglobin (hemoglobin A_{1c}): <7%

Patient Information Do not change dose or discontinue without consulting prescriber; avoid alcohol while taking this medication, may cause severe reaction; maintain regular dietary intake and exercise routine; always carry quick source of sugar; if experiencing a hypoglycemic reaction, contact prescriber immediately; report severe or persistent side effects, extended vomiting or flu-like symptoms, skin rash, easy bruising or bleeding, or change in color of urine or stool. May rarely cause photosensitivity reactions (eg, exposure to sunlight may cause severe sunburn, skin rash, redness, or itching); avoid direct exposure to sunlight

Additional Information When transferring from other sulfonylurea antidiabetic agents to glyburide, with the exception of chlorpropamide, the administration of the other agent may be abruptly discontinued; due to the prolonged elimination half-life of chlorpropamide, a 2- to 3-day drug-free interval may be advisable before glyburide therapy is begun

Dosage Forms Excipient information presented when available (limited, particularly for generics); consult specific product labeling.

Tablet: 1.25 mg, 2.5 mg, 5 mg

Diaβeta®, Micronase®: 1.25 mg, 2.5 mg, 5 mg

Tablet, micronized: 1.5 mg, 3 mg, 6 mg

Glynase® PresTab®: 3 mg, 6 mg

References

DeFronzo RA, "Pharmacologic Therapy for Type 2 Diabetes Mellitus," *Ann Intern Med*, 1999, 131(4):281-303.

"Intensive Blood-Glucose Control With Sulphonylureas or Insulin Compared With Conventional Treatment and Risk of Complications in Patients With Type 2 Diabetes (UKPDS 33) UK Prospective Diabetes Study (UKPDS) Group," *Lancet*, 1998, 352(9131):837-53.

Glycerin (GLIS er in)

U.S. Brand Names Bausch & Lomb® Computer Eye Drops [OTC]; Colace® Adult/Children Suppositories [OTC]; Colace® Infant/Children Suppositories [OTC]; Fleet® Babylax® [OTC]; Fleet® Glycerin Suppositories [OTC]; Fleet® Glycerin Suppositories Maximum Strength [OTC]; Fleet® Liquid Glycerin Suppositories [OTC]; Osmoglyn® [DSC]; Sani-Supp® [OTC]

Index Terms Glycerol

Therapeutic Category Laxative, Osmotic

Generic Available Yes: Suppositories

Use Treatment of constipation; reduction of intraocular pressure; reduction of corneal edema; glycerin has been administered orally to reduce intracranial pressure; laxative used in newborns to promote bilirubin excretion by reducing enterohepatic circulation, decreasing GI transit time, and stimulating passage of meconium

Pregnancy Risk Factor C

Contraindications Hypersensitivity to glycerin or any component; severe dehydration, anuria

Precautions Use oral glycerin with caution in patients with cardiac, renal or hepatic disease and in diabetics

Adverse Reactions

Central nervous system: Dizziness, headache, confusion, disorientation

Endocrine & metabolic: Hyperglycemia, dehydration

Gastrointestinal: Diarrhea, nausea, tenesmus, thirst, cramping pain, vomiting, rectal irritation

Local: Pain/irritation with ophthalmic solution (may need to apply a topical ophthalmic anesthetic before glycerin administration)

Stability Protect from heat; freezing should be avoided

Mechanism of Action

Rectal: Osmotic dehydrating agent which increases osmotic pressure; draws fluid into colon and thus stimulates evacuation

Ophthalmic: Osmotic action reduces edema and causes clearing of corneal haze

Oral: Glycerin increases osmotic pressure of the plasma drawing water from the extravascular spaces into the blood producing a decrease in intraocular and intracranial pressure

Pharmacodynamics

Onset of action for glycerin suppository or enema: 15-30 minutes

Onset of action in decreasing intraocular pressure: Within 10-30 minutes

Duration: 4-8 hours

Increased intracranial pressure decreases within 10-60 minutes following an oral dose

Duration: ~2-3 hours

Pharmacokinetics

Absorption:

Oral: Well absorbed

Rectal: Poorly absorbed

Metabolism: Primarily in the liver with 20% metabolized in the kidney

Half-life: 30-45 minutes

Time to peak serum concentration: Oral: Within 60-90 minutes

Elimination: Only a small percentage of drug is excreted unchanged in urine

Usual Dosage

Constipation: Rectal: Administered in single doses only at infrequent intervals

Neonates: 0.5 mL/kg/dose of rectal solution as an enema

Children <6 years: 1 infant suppository as needed or 2-5 mL of rectal solution as an enema

Children ≥6 years and Adults: 1 adult suppository as needed or 5-15 mL of rectal solution as an enema

Children and Adults:

Reduction of intraocular pressure: Oral: 1-1.8 g/kg administered 1-1½ hours preoperatively; additional doses may be administered at 5-hour intervals

Reduction of intracranial pressure: Oral: 1.5 g/kg/day divided every 4 hours; 1 g/kg/dose every 6 hours has also been used

Reduction of corneal edema: Ophthalmic: Instill 1-2 drops in eye(s) every 3-4 hours

Administration

Oral: Orange or lemon juice may be added to unflavored 50% oral solution; pour solution over crushed ice and drink through a straw to improve palatability

Ophthalmic: Instill drops onto the eye; avoid contaminating tip of the solution bottle

Rectal: Insert suppository in the rectum and retain 15 minutes

Monitoring Parameters Blood glucose, intraocular pressure, evacuation of stool

Patient Information Do not use if experiencing abdominal pain, nausea, or vomiting

Nursing Implications Use caution during insertion of suppository to avoid intestinal perforation, especially in neonates; instruct patient to lie down after oral glycerin administration to prevent or relieve headaches

Dosage Forms Excipient information presented when available (limited, particularly for generics); consult specific product labeling. [DSC] = Discontinued product

Solution, ophthalmic, sterile (Bausch & Lomb® Computer Eye Drops): 1% (15 mL) [contains benzalkonium chloride]

Solution, oral (Osmoglyn®): 50% (220 mL) [lime flavor] [DSC]

Solution, rectal:

Fleet® Babylax®: 2.3 g/2.3 mL (4 mL) [6 units per box]

Fleet® Liquid Glycerin Suppositories: 5.6 g/5.5 mL (7.5 mL) [4 units per box]

Suppository, rectal: 82.5% (12s, 25s) [pediatric size]; 82.5% (12s, 24s, 25s, 50s, 100s) [adult size]

Colace® Adult/Children: 2.1 g (12s, 24s, 48s, 100s)

Colace® Infant/Children: 1.2 g (12s, 24s)

Fleet® Glycerin Suppositories: 1 g (12s) [pediatric size]; 2g (12s, 24s, 50s) [adult size]

Fleet® Glycerin Suppositories Maximum Strength: 3g (18s) [adult size]

Sani-Supp®: 82.5% (10s, 25s) [pediatric size]; 82.5% (10s, 25s, 50s) [adult size]

References

Heinemeyer G, "Clinical Pharmacokinetic Considerations in the Treatment of Increased Intracranial Pressure," *Clin Pharmacokinet*, 1987, 13(1):1-25.

Rottenberg DA, Hurwitz BJ, and Posner JB, "The Effect of Oral Glycerol on Intraventricular Pressure in Man," *Neurology*, 1977, 27(7):600-8.

(Continued)

Glycerin *(Continued)*

Zenk KE, Koeppel RM, and Liem LA, "Comparative Efficacy of Glycerin Enemas and Suppository Chips in Neonates," *Clin Pharm*, 1993, 12(11):846-8.

◆ **Glycerol** *see* Glycerin *on page 736*
◆ **Glycerol Guaiacolate** *see* Guaifenesin *on page 745*
◆ **Glyceryl Trinitrate** *see* Nitroglycerin *on page 1141*
◆ **Glycon (Can)** *see* Metformin *on page 1016*

Glycopyrrolate (glye koe PYE roe late)

Related Information
Compatibility of Medications Mixed in A Syringe *on page 1941*
Overdose and Toxicology *on page 1916*

U.S. Brand Names Robinul®; Robinul® Forte

Canadian Brand Names Glycopyrrolate Injection, USP

Index Terms Glycopyrronium Bromide

Therapeutic Category Anticholinergic Agent; Antispasmodic Agent, Gastrointestinal

Generic Available Yes

Use Adjunct in treatment of peptic ulcer disease; inhibition of salivation and excessive secretions of the respiratory tract; reversal of the muscarinic effects of cholinergic agents such as neostigmine and pyridostigmine during reversal of neuromuscular blockade

Pregnancy Risk Factor B

Lactation Excretion in breast milk unknown/use caution

Contraindications Hypersensitivity to glycopyrrolate or any component (see Warnings); narrow-angle glaucoma; acute hemorrhage; tachycardia; severe ulcerative colitis; obstructive uropathy; paralytic ileus; myasthenia gravis; intestinal atony; obstructive disease of GI tract; toxic megacolon complicating ulcerative colitis

Warnings Infants, patients with Down syndrome, and children with spastic paralysis or brain damage may be hypersensitive to antimuscarinic effects. Monitor closely in patients with renal impairment as clearance is prolonged. Paradoxical excitation may occur in infants and young children.

Precautions Use with caution in patients with fever, hyperthyroidism, hepatic or renal disease, hypertension, CHF, GI infections, diarrhea, reflux esophagitis

Adverse Reactions
Cardiovascular: Tachycardia, orthostatic hypotension, ventricular fibrillation, palpitations
Central nervous system: Drowsiness, nervousness, headache, insomnia, confusion, loss of memory, fatigue, ataxia, paradoxical excitation (infants and young children)
Dermatologic: Rash, dry skin
Gastrointestinal: Xerostomia, constipation, nausea, vomiting, dry throat, dysphagia
Genitourinary: Urinary retention, dysuria
Local: Irritation at injection site
Neuromuscular & skeletal: Weakness
Ocular: Blurred vision, light sensitivity
Respiratory: Dry nose
Miscellaneous: Decreased diaphoresis

Drug Interactions Phenothiazines, meperidine, amantadine, tricyclic antidepressants, and quinidine (additive anticholinergic effect); wax-matrix potassium chloride (increased severity of potassium-induced GI mucosal lesions); antacids (decreased absorption); decreased effect of levodopa

Stability Unstable at pH >6; compatible in the same syringe with atropine, benzquinamide, chlorpromazine, codeine, diphenhydramine, droperidol, fentanyl, hydromorphone, hydroxyzine, lidocaine, meperidine, promethazine, morphine, neostigmine, oxymorphone, procaine, prochlorperazine, promazine, pyridostigmine, scopolamine, triflupromazine, and trimethobenzamide

Mechanism of Action Inhibits the muscarinic action of acetylcholine at postganglionic parasympathetic neuroeffector sites in smooth muscle, secretory glands, and CNS

Pharmacodynamics
Onset of action:
Oral: Within 1 hour
I.M., SubQ: 15-30 minutes
I.V.: 1-10 minutes
Maximum effect: I.M., SubQ: 30-45 minutes
Duration (anticholinergic effects):
Oral: 8-12 hours
Parenteral: 7 hours

Pharmacokinetics
Absorption: Oral: Poor and erratic; 10% absorption
Distribution: Does not adequately penetrate into CNS
V_d: Adults: 0.42 ± 0.22 L/kg
Half-life:
Infants: 21.6-130 minutes
Children: 19.2-99.2 minutes
Adults: 0.83 ± 0.13 hours
Elimination: Primarily unchanged via biliary elimination (70% to 90%)
Clearance: Adults: 0.54 ± 0.14 L/kg/hour

Usual Dosage
Children:
Control of secretions:
Oral: 40-100 mcg/kg/dose 3-4 times/day
I.M., I.V.: 4-10 mcg/kg/dose every 3-4 hours
Preoperative: I.M.:
≤2 years: 4-9 mcg/kg 30-60 minutes before procedure; may repeat intraoperatively 4 mcg/kg not to exceed 0.1 mg/day in intervals of 2-3 minutes
>2 years: 4 mcg/kg 30-60 minutes before procedure; may repeat intraoperatively 4 mcg/kg not to exceed 0.1 mg/day in intervals of 2-3 minutes
Children and Adults: Reversal of muscarinic effects of cholinergic agents: I.V.: 0.2 mg for each 1 mg of neostigmine or 5 mg of pyridostigmine administered
Adults:
Peptic ulcer:
Oral: 1-2 mg 2-3 times/day
I.M., I.V.: 0.1-0.2 mg 3-4 times/day; may increase to 0.4 mg 3-4 times/day
Preoperative: I.M.: 4 mcg/kg 30-60 minutes before procedure; may repeat intraoperatively in single doses of 0.1 mg as needed in intervals of 2-3 minutes

Administration
Oral: May be administered without regard to meals
Parenteral: Dilute to a concentration of 2 mcg/mL (maximum concentration: 200 mcg/mL); infuse over 15-20 minutes; may be administered direct I.V. at a maximum rate of 20 mcg/minute; may be administered I.M.

Monitoring Parameters Heart rate

Patient Information May cause dry mouth; may cause drowsiness and blurred vision and impair ability to perform activities requiring mental alertness or physical coordination; use caution during exercise or hot weather as overheating may result in heat stroke

Dosage Forms Excipient information presented when available (limited, particularly for generics); consult specific product labeling. [DSC] = Discontinued product
Injection, solution: 0.2 mg/mL (1 mL, 2 mL, 5 mL, 20 mL)
Robinul®: 0.2 mg/mL (1 mL, 2 mL, 5 mL; 20 mL [DSC]) [contains benzyl alcohol]
Tablet: 1 mg, 2 mg
Robinul®: 1 mg
Robinul® Forte: 2 mg

- **Glycopyrrolate Injection, USP (Can)** *see* Glycopyrrolate *on page 738*
- **Glycopyrronium Bromide** *see* Glycopyrrolate *on page 738*
- **Glycosum** *see* Dextrose *on page 479*
- **Glydiazinamide** *see* GlipiZIDE *on page 730*
- **Glynase® PresTab®** *see* GlyBURIDE *on page 734*
- **Gly-Oxide® [OTC]** *see* Carbamide Peroxide *on page 283*
- **GM-CSF** *see* Sargramostim *on page 1420*
- **GMD-Azithromycin (Can)** *see* Azithromycin *on page 191*
- **GMD-Fluconazole (Can)** *see* Fluconazole *on page 660*
- **GMD-Sertraline (Can)** *see* Sertraline *on page 1429*
- **GnRH** *see* Gonadorelin *on page 741*
- **Gold Bond® Antifungal [OTC] [DSC]** *see* Tolnaftate *on page 1550*

Gold Sodium Thiomalate (gold SOW dee um thye oh MAL ate)

U.S. Brand Names Aurolate®
Canadian Brand Names Myochrysine®
Therapeutic Category Gold Compound
Generic Available No
Use Treatment of progressive rheumatoid arthritis
Pregnancy Risk Factor C
Lactation Enters breast milk/compatible (monitor closely)

(Continued)

Gold Sodium Thiomalate *(Continued)*

Contraindications Hypersensitivity to gold compounds, any component (see Warnings), or other heavy metals; severe hepatic or renal dysfunction; systemic lupus erythematosus; history of blood dyscrasias; CHF, exfoliative dermatitis, or colitis; avoid concomitant use of antimalarials, immunosuppressive agents, penicillamine, or phenylbutazone

Warnings Explain the possibility of adverse reactions before initiating therapy; signs of gold toxicity include: decrease in hemoglobin, leukocytes, granulocytes and platelets, proteinuria, hematuria, pigmentation, pruritus, stomatitis or persistent diarrhea, rash, metallic taste; advise patient to report any symptoms of toxicity

Injection contains benzyl alcohol which may cause allergic reactions in susceptible individuals; large amounts of benzyl alcohol (≥99 mg/kg/day) have been associated with a potentially fatal toxicity ("gasping syndrome") in neonates; the "gasping syndrome" consists of metabolic acidosis, respiratory distress, gasping respirations, CNS dysfunction (including convulsions, intracranial hemorrhage), hypotension and cardiovascular collapse; *in vitro* and animal studies have shown that benzoate displaces bilirubin from protein binding sites; avoid use of gold sodium thiomalate in neonates

Precautions Frequent monitoring of patients for signs and symptoms of toxicity will prevent serious adverse reactions; NSAIDs and corticosteroids may be discontinued after initiating gold therapy; must not be injected I.V.

Adverse Reactions

Cardiovascular: Flushing

Central nervous system: Seizures, headache

Dermatologic: Exfoliative urticaria, dermatitis, erythema nodosum, alopecia, shedding of nails, pruritus, gray-to-blue pigmentation of skin and mucous membranes

Gastrointestinal: Stomatitis, nausea, diarrhea, abdominal cramps, metallic taste, gingivitis, glossitis, ulcerative enterocolitis, GI hemorrhage, dysphagia

Genitourinary: Vaginitis

Hematologic: Eosinophilia, leukopenia, agranulocytosis, thrombocytopenia

Hepatic: Hepatitis

Neuromuscular & skeletal: Arthralgias, peripheral neuropathy

Ocular: Blurred vision, conjunctivitis, corneal ulcers, iritis

Renal: Hematuria, proteinuria, nephrotic syndrome

Respiratory: Interstitial pneumonitis and fibrosis

Miscellaneous: Hypersensitivity reactions including anaphylaxis (rare)

Drug Interactions Decreased effect with penicillamine, acetylcysteine

Mechanism of Action Unknown, may decrease prostaglandin synthesis or may alter cellular mechanisms by inhibiting sulfhydryl systems

Pharmacokinetics

Distribution: Breast milk to plasma ratio: 0.02-0.3

Half-life: 3-27 days (may lengthen with multiple doses)

Time to peak serum concentration: I.M.: Within 3-6 hours

Elimination: Majority (50% to 90%) excreted in urine with smaller amounts (10% to 50%) excreted in feces (via bile)

Usual Dosage I.M.:

Children: Initial: Test dose of 10 mg I.M. is recommended, followed by 1 mg/kg I.M. weekly for 20 weeks (maximum dose: 50 mg); maintenance: 1 mg/kg/dose at 2- to 4-week intervals thereafter for as long as therapy is clinically beneficial and toxicity does not develop. Administration for 2-4 months is usually required before clinical improvement is observed.

Adults: 10 mg first week; 25 mg second week; then 25-50 mg/week until clinical improvement or a 1 g cumulative dose has been given. If improvement occurs without adverse reactions, give 25-50 mg every 2 weeks for 2-20 weeks; if continues stable, give 25-50 mg every 3-4 weeks indefinitely.

Dosage adjustment in renal impairment:

Cl_{cr} 50-80 mL/minute: Administer 50% of dose

Cl_{cr} <50 mL/minute: Avoid use

Administration Parenteral: Administer I.M. only, preferably intragluteally; addition of 0.1 mL of 1% lidocaine to each injection may reduce the discomfort associated with I.M. administration; patients should be recumbent during injection and for 10 minutes afterwards; observe closely for 15 minutes after injection

Monitoring Parameters CBC, platelets, hemoglobin, urinalysis, renal and liver function tests

Reference Range Gold: Normal: 0-0.1 mcg/mL (SI: 0-0.0064 micromoles/L); Therapeutic: 1-3 mcg/mL (SI: 0.06-0.18 micromoles/L); Urine <0.1 mcg/24 hours

Dosage Forms Excipient information presented when available (limited, particularly for generics); consult specific product labeling.

Injection, solution: 50 mg/mL (1 mL, 10 mL) [contains benzyl alcohol]

♦ **GoLYTELY®** *see* Polyethylene Glycol-Electrolyte Solution *on page 1277*

Gonadorelin (goe nad oh REL in)

Medication Safety Issues

Sound-alike/look-alike issues:

Gonadorelin may be confused with gonadotropin, guanadrel

Factrel® may be confused with Sectral®

Gonadotropin may be confused with gonadorelin

U.S. Brand Names Factrel®

Canadian Brand Names Lutrepulse™

Index Terms GnRH; Gonadorelin Acetate; Gonadorelin Hydrochloride; Gonadotropin Releasing Hormone; LHRH; LRH; Luteinizing Hormone Releasing Hormone

Therapeutic Category Diagnostic Agent, Gonadotrophic Hormone; Gonadotropin

Generic Available No

Use Evaluation of hypothalamic-pituitary gonadotropic function; used to evaluate abnormal gonadotropin regulation as in precocious puberty and delayed puberty; treatment of primary hypothalamic amenorrhea

Pregnancy Risk Factor B

Lactation Excretion in breast milk unknown

Contraindications Hypersensitivity to gonadorelin or any component (see Warnings)

Warnings Anaphylactic reactions have occurred following multiple-dose administration; multiple pregnancy is a possibility with Lutrepulse®

Diluent for injection contains benzyl alcohol which may cause allergic reactions in susceptible individuals; large amounts of benzyl alcohol (≥99 mg/kg/day) have been associated with a potentially fatal toxicity ("gasping syndrome") in neonates; avoid use of gonadorelin products containing benzyl alcohol in neonates; *in vitro* and animal studies have shown that benzoate, a metabolite of benzyl alcohol, displaces bilirubin from protein binding sites

Adverse Reactions

Cardiovascular: Flushing

Central nervous system: Lightheadedness, headache

Dermatologic: Skin rash

Gastrointestinal: Nausea, abdominal discomfort

Local: Pain, pruritus, edema

Miscellaneous: Hypersensitivity reactions

Drug Interactions Androgens, estrogens, progestins, glucocorticoids affect pituitary secretion of gonadotropins; spironolactone, levodopa may increase gonadotropin levels; oral contraceptives, digoxin may suppress gonadotropin levels; phenothiazines, dopamine antagonists may blunt response to gonadorelin

Stability Prepare immediately prior to use; after reconstitution, store at room temperature and use within 1 day; discard unused portion

Mechanism of Action Stimulates the release of luteinizing hormone (LH) from the anterior pituitary gland

Pharmacodynamics

Onset of action: Following administration, maximal LH release occurs within 20 minutes

Duration: 3-5 hours

Pharmacokinetics Half-life: 4 minutes

Usual Dosage

Children: I.V. **(as hydrochloride salt)**: 100 mcg to evaluate abnormal gonadotropin regulation

Children >12 years and Adults: I.V., SubQ **(as hydrochloride salt)**: 100 mcg; administer to women during early phase of menstrual cycle (day 1-7)

Adults: I.V. **(as acetate salt)**: 5 mcg (range: 1-20 mcg) every 90 minutes for 7 days via the Lutrepulse® pump; recommended treatment interval: 21 days

Administration Parenteral:

Hydrochloride salt: Dilute in 3 mL of NS; administer I.V. push over 30 seconds

Acetate salt (Lutrepulse®): Fill presterilized reservoir bag with reconstituted solution; administer I.V. using the Lutrepulse® pump

Monitoring Parameters Plasma LH and FSH

Hypothalamic/pituitary function evaluation: Draw blood samples for LH 15 minutes before and immediately before gonadorelin dose, then at 15, 30, 45, 60, and 120 minutes after dose

Dosage Forms Excipient information presented when available (limited, particularly for generics); consult specific product labeling.

Injection, powder for reconstitution, as hydrochloride: 100 mcg [diluent contains benzyl alcohol]

(Continued)

Gonadorelin *(Continued)*

References

Pescovitz OH, Comite F, Hench K, et al, "The NIH Experience With Precocious Puberty: Diagnostic Subgroups and Response to Short-Term Luteinizing Hormone-Releasing Hormone Analogue Therapy," *J Pediatr*, 1986, 108(1):47-54.

- **Gonadorelin Acetate** *see* Gonadorelin *on page 741*
- **Gonadorelin Hydrochloride** *see* Gonadorelin *on page 741*
- **Gonadotropin Releasing Hormone** *see* Gonadorelin *on page 741*
- **Gordofilm® [OTC]** *see* Salicylic Acid *on page 1413*
- **GP 47680** *see* Oxcarbazepine *on page 1184*
- **GR38032R** *see* Ondansetron *on page 1169*

Granisetron (gra NI se tron)

Medication Safety Issues
Sound-alike/look-alike issues:
Granisetron may be confused with dolasetron, ondansetron, palonosetron

U.S. Brand Names Kytril®

Canadian Brand Names Kytril®

Index Terms BRL 43694

Therapeutic Category 5-HT_3 Receptor Antagonist; Antiemetic

Generic Available No

Use Prophylaxis and treatment of chemotherapy and radiation-related nausea and emesis; prophylaxis and treatment of postoperative nausea and vomiting

Pregnancy Risk Factor B

Lactation Excretion in breast milk unknown/use caution

Contraindications Hypersensitivity to granisetron, other 5-HT_3 receptor antagonists, or any component (see Warnings)

Warnings Some injectable products contain benzyl alcohol which may cause allergic reactions in susceptible individuals; large amounts of benzyl alcohol (≥99 mg/kg/day) have been associated with a potentially fatal toxicity ("gasping syndrome") in neonates; the "gasping syndrome" consists of metabolic acidosis, respiratory distress, gasping respirations, CNS dysfunction (including convulsions, intracranial hemorrhage), hypotension and cardiovascular collapse; avoid use of products containing benzyl alcohol in neonates. *In vitro* and animal studies have shown that benzoate, a metabolite of benzyl alcohol, displaces bilirubin from protein-binding sites; granisetron oral solution contains sodium benzoate; avoid use of oral solution in neonates

Precautions Use with caution in patients with liver disease or in pregnant patients. Use with caution in patients following abdominal surgery; may mask progressive ileus or gastric distension.

Adverse Reactions
Cardiovascular: Hypertension, hypotension, arrhythmias such as bradycardia, atrial fibrillation, A-V block, angina, syncope
Central nervous system: Agitation, anxiety, CNS stimulation, headache, insomnia, somnolence, fever, dizziness
Dermatologic: Skin rashes
Gastrointestinal: Constipation, diarrhea, dysgeusia, abdominal pain
Hepatic: Elevated liver enzymes
Neuromuscular & skeletal: Weakness, asthenia
Miscellaneous: Allergic reactions

Drug Interactions Cytochrome P450 isoenzyme CYP3A3/4 substrate
Because granisetron is metabolized by hepatic cytochrome P450 drug metabolizing enzymes, inducers or inhibitors of this system may change the clearance and half-life

Stability Tablets and injections: Store at room temperature, protect from light; injection stable when mixed in NS, D_5W for at least 24 hours; multi-use vial (with preservative) stable for 30 days after opening

Mechanism of Action Selective 5-HT_3 receptor antagonist, blocking serotonin, both peripherally on vagal nerve terminals and centrally in the chemoreceptor trigger zone

Pharmacodynamics
Onset of action: I.V.: 1-3 minutes
Duration: I.V.: ≤24 hours

Pharmacokinetics
Distribution: V_d: 2-3 L/kg; widely distributed throughout the body
Protein binding: 65%
Metabolism: Hepatic via N-demethylation, oxidation, and conjugation; some metabolites may have 5-HT_3 antagonist activity

Half-life:

Cancer patients: 10-12 hours

Healthy volunteers: 3-4 hours

Elimination: Primarily nonrenal, 8% to 15% of dose excreted unchanged in urine

Usual Dosage

Treatment of chemotherapy-induced emesis: Initial dose given just prior to chemotherapy (15-60 minutes before)

Children ≥2 years and Adults: I.V.: Manufacturer's recommendation: 10 mcg/kg; or as an alternative based on clinical research: 20-40 mcg/kg/day divided once or twice daily; maximum: 3 mg/dose or 9 mg/day

As intervention therapy for breakthrough nausea and vomiting, during the first 24 hours following chemotherapy, 2 or 3 repeat infusions (same dose) have been administered

Adults: Oral: 2 mg once daily or 1 mg twice daily

Prevention and treatment of postoperative nausea and vomiting, before induction of surgery, immediately before reversal of anesthesia, or postoperatively: I.V.:

Children ≥4 years: 20-40 mcg/kg given as a single dose; not to exceed 1 mg

Adults: 0.1 mg given as a single dose; this dosage is not yet approved by the FDA; trends in randomized, double-blind, multicenter, dose-ranging studies have shown doses of 0.1 mg, 0.2 mg, and 0.3 mg to be more effective than placebo for postoperative nausea and vomiting (Gan, 2005; Taylor, 1997; Shillington, 2005); 1 mg is the FDA approved dosage

Administration

Oral: Given at least 1 hour prior to chemotherapy and then 12 hours later; shake oral suspension well before use

Parenteral: I.V.: Infuse over 30 seconds undiluted **or** dilute in small volume NS or D_5W and administer over 5 minutes **or** dilute in 20-50 mL of NS or D_5W and infuse over 30 minutes to 1 hour

Dosage Forms Excipient information presented when available (limited, particularly for generics); consult specific product labeling.

Injection, solution: 1 mg/mL (1 mL, 4 mL) [contains benzyl alcohol]

Injection, solution [preservative free]: 0.1 mg/mL (1 mL)

Solution, oral: 2 mg/10 mL (30 mL) [contains sodium benzoate; orange flavor]

Tablet: 1 mg

Extemporaneous Preparations

A 0.2 mg/mL suspension may be made by crushing twelve 1 mg tablets. Add 30 mL distilled water, mix well, and transfer to a bottle. Rinse the mortar with 10 mL cherry syrup and add to bottle. Add enough cherry syrup to make a final volume of 60 mL. Label "shake well"; stable 14 days at room temperature or refrigerated (Quercia, 1997).

A 50 mcg/mL suspension may be made by crushing one 1 mg tablet. Add 1% methylcellulose and syrup NF to a total volume of 20 mL (may also use Ora-Sweet® or Ora-Plus® instead of methylcellulose and syrup); shake well; stable 91 days refrigerated (Nahata, 1998).

Nahata MC, Morosco RS, and Hipple TF, "Stability of Granisetron Hydrochloride in Two Oral Suspensions," *Am J Health Syst Pharm*, 1998, 55(23):2511-3.

Quercia RA, Zhang J, Fan C, et al, "Stability of Granisetron Hydrochloride in an Extemporaneously Prepared Oral Liquid," *Am J Health-Syst Pharm*, 1997, 54(12):1404-6.

References

"ASHP Therapeutic Guidelines on the Pharmacologic Management of Nausea and Vomiting in Adult and Pediatric Patients Receiving Chemotherapy or Radiation Therapy or Undergoing Surgery," *Am J Health Syst Pharm*, 1999, 56(8):729-64.

Gan TJ, Coop A, and Philip BK, "A Randomized, Double-Blind Study of Granisetron Plus Dexamethasone Versus Ondansetron Plus Dexamethasone to Prevent Postoperative Nausea and Vomiting in Patients Undergoing Abdominal Hysterectomy," *Aneth Analg*, 2005, 101(5):1323-9.

Hahlen K, Quintana E, Pinkerton CR, et al, "A Randomized Comparison of Intravenously Administered Granisetron Versus Chlorpromazine Plus Dexamethasone in the Prevention of Ifosfamide-Induced Emesis in Children," *J Pediatr*, 1995, 126(2):309-13.

Lemerle J, Amaral D, Southall DP, et al, "Efficacy and Safety of Granisetron in the Prevention of Chemotherapy-Induced Emesis in Paediatric Patients," *Eur J Cancer*, 1991, 27(9):1081-3.

Shillington A, et al, "Retrospective Cohort Study of Granisetron Administration for Postoperative Nausea and Vomiting Prophylaxis and Treatment," *Hosp Pharm*, 2005, 40(7): 592-8.

Taylor AM, Rosen M, Diemunsch PA, et al, "A Double-Blind, Parallel-Group, Placebo-Controlled, Dose-Ranging, Multicenter Study of Intravenous Granisetron in the Treatment of Postoperative Nausea and Vomiting in Patients Undergoing Surgery With General Anesthesia," *J Clin Anesth*, 1997, 9(8); 658-63.

♦ **Granulocyte Colony Stimulating Factor** *see* Filgrastim *on page 655*

♦ **Granulocyte-Macrophage Colony Stimulating Factor** *see* Sargramostim *on page 1420*

♦ **Gravol® (Can)** *see* DimenhyDRINATE *on page 507*

♦ **Grifulvin® V** *see* Griseofulvin *on page 744*

Griseofulvin (gri see oh FUL vin)

Medication Safety Issues
Sound-alike/look-alike issues:
Fulvicin® may be confused with Furacin®

U.S. Brand Names Grifulvin® V; Gris-PEG®

Index Terms Griseofulvin Microsize; Griseofulvin Ultramicrosize

Therapeutic Category Antifungal Agent, Systemic

Generic Available Yes: Suspension, ultramicrosized product

Use Treatment of tinea infections of the skin, hair, and nails caused by susceptible species of *Microsporum*, *Epidermophyton*, or *Trichophyton*

Pregnancy Risk Factor C

Lactation Excretion in breast milk unknown/use caution

Contraindications Hypersensitivity to griseofulvin or any component; severe liver disease, porphyria (interferes with porphyrin metabolism); pregnant women (may cause fetal harm)

Warnings Lupus erythematosus or lupus-like syndromes have been reported in patients receiving griseofulvin.

Precautions Avoid exposure to intense sunlight to prevent photosensitivity reactions; use with caution in patients with penicillin hypersensitivity since cross-reactivity with griseofulvin is possible

Adverse Reactions
Central nervous system: Fatigue, confusion, impaired judgment, insomnia, headache, incoordination, dizziness
Dermatologic: Rash, urticaria, photosensitivity, erythema multiforme-like drug reaction, angioneurotic edema (rare)
Endocrine & metabolic: Estrogen-like effects in children
Gastrointestinal: Nausea, vomiting, diarrhea, oral thrush
Hematologic: Leukopenia, granulocytopenia
Hepatic: Hepatotoxicity
Neuromuscular & skeletal: Paresthesia of the hand and feet (with extended therapy)
Renal: Proteinuria
Miscellaneous: Lupus-like syndrome

Drug Interactions Cytochrome P450 isoenzyme CYP1A2 inducer
Phenobarbital decreases griseofulvin concentrations; griseofulvin decreases warfarin effectiveness; griseofulvin decreases oral contraceptive efficacy; griseofulvin decreases cyclosporine concentrations; griseofulvin potentiates the effects of alcohol and causes flushing and tachycardia

Food Interactions Fatty meal will increase griseofulvin absorption

Stability Store at room temperature; protect from light

Mechanism of Action Inhibits fungal cell mitosis at metaphase by disrupting the cell's mitotic spindle structure; binds to human keratin making it resistant to fungal invasion

Pharmacokinetics
Absorption: Ultramicrosize griseofulvin absorption is almost complete; absorption of microsize griseofulvin is variable (25% to 70% of an oral dose); absorbed from the duodenum
Distribution: Deposited in the keratin layer of skin, hair, and nails; concentrates in liver, fat, and skeletal muscles; crosses the placenta
Metabolism: Extensive in the liver
Half-life: 9-22 hours
Elimination: <1% excreted unchanged in urine; also excreted in feces and perspiration

Usual Dosage Oral:
Children >2 years of age:
Microsize: 10-20 mg/kg/day in single or 2 divided doses
Ultramicrosize: 5-15 mg/kg/day once daily or in 2 divided doses; maximum dose: 750 mg/day in 2 divided doses for fungal infections like tinea pedis or tinea unguium which are more difficult to eradicate
Adults:
Microsize: 500-1000 mg/day in single or divided doses
Ultramicrosize: 330-375 mg/day in single or divided doses; doses up to 750 mg/day have been used for infections more difficult to eradicate such as tinea pedis and tinea unguium
Duration of therapy depends on the site of infection:
Tinea corporis: 2-4 weeks
Tinea capitis: 4-6 weeks or longer
Tinea pedis: 4-8 weeks
Tinea unguium: 4-6 months or longer

Administration Oral: Administer with a fatty meal (peanut butter or ice cream to increase absorption), or with food or milk to avoid GI upset; shake suspension well before use. Ultramicrosize tablets may be swallowed whole or crushed and sprinkled onto 1 tablespoonful of applesauce and taken immediately without chewing.

Monitoring Parameters Periodic renal, hepatic, and hematopoietic function tests

Test Interactions False-positive urinary VMA levels

Patient Information Avoid alcohol. May cause photosensitivity reactions (eg, exposure to sunlight may cause severe sunburn, skin rash, redness, or itching); avoid exposure to sunlight and artificial light sources (sunlamps, tanning booth/bed); wear protective clothing, wide-brimmed hats, sunglasses, and lip sunscreen (SPF ≥15); use a sunscreen [broad-spectrum sunscreen or physical sunscreen (preferred) or sunblock with SPF ≥15]; notify physician if skin rash occurs

Dosage Forms Excipient information presented when available (limited, particularly for generics); consult specific product labeling.

Suspension, oral, microsize: 125 mg/5mL (120 mL)
  Grifulvin® V: 125 mg/5 mL (120 mL) [contains alcohol 0.2%]
Tablet, microsize:
  Grifulvin® V: 500 mg
Tablet, ultramicrosize:
  Gris-PEG®: 125 mg, 250 mg

References

Fleece D, Gaughan JP, and Aronoff SC, "Griseofulvin Versus Terbinafine in the Treatment of Tinea Capitis: A Meta-analysis of Randomized, Clinical Trials," *Pediatrics*, 2004, 114(5):1312-5.

Ginsburg CM, McCracken GH Jr, Petruska M, et al, "Effect of Feeding on Bioavailability of Griseofulvin in Children," *J Pediatr*, 1983, 102(2):309-11.

♦ **Griseofulvin Microsize** *see* Griseofulvin *on page 744*
♦ **Griseofulvin Ultramicrosize** *see* Griseofulvin *on page 744*
♦ **Gris-PEG®** *see* Griseofulvin *on page 744*
♦ **Guaicon DM [OTC]** *see* Guaifenesin and Dextromethorphan *on page 748*
♦ **Guaicon DMS [OTC]** *see* Guaifenesin and Dextromethorphan *on page 748*

Guaifenesin (gwye FEN e sin)

Medication Safety Issues

Sound-alike/look-alike issues:
  Guaifenesin may be confused with guanfacine
  Mucinex® may be confused with Mucomyst®
  Naldecon® may be confused with Nalfon®
International issues:
  Mucolex® [Hong Kong] may be confused with Mycelex® which is a brand name for clotrimazole in the U.S.

Related Information

OTC Cough and Cold Preparations, Pediatric *on page 1706*

U.S. Brand Names Allfen Jr; Diabetic Tussin® EX [OTC]; Ganidin NR; Guiatuss™ [OTC]; Mucinex® [OTC]; Mucinex®, Children's [OTC]; Mucinex®, Children's Mini-Melts™ [OTC]; Mucinex®, Junior Mini-Melts™ [OTC]; Organidin® NR; Phanasin® [OTC]; Phanasin® Diabetic Choice [OTC]; Robitussin® [OTC]; Scot-Tussin® Expectorant [OTC]; Siltussin DAS [OTC]; Siltussin SA [OTC]; Vicks® Casero™ Chest Congestion Relief [OTC]; XPECT™ [OTC]

Canadian Brand Names Balminil Expectorant; Benylin® E Extra Strength; Koffex Expectorant; Robitussin®

Index Terms GG; Glycerol Guaiacolate

Therapeutic Category Expectorant

Generic Available Yes: Excludes extended release and granules

Use Expectorant used for the symptomatic treatment of coughs

Pregnancy Risk Factor C

Lactation Excretion in breast milk unknown/use caution

Contraindications Hypersensitivity to guaifenesin or any component (see Warnings)

Warnings Some products contain sodium benzoate; benzoic acid (benzoate) is a metabolite of benzyl alcohol; large amounts of benzyl alcohol (≥99 mg/kg/day) have been associated with a potentially fatal toxicity ("gasping syndrome") in neonates; *in vitro* and animal studies have shown that benzoate displaces bilirubin from protein binding sites; avoid use of products containing sodium benzoate in neonates

Precautions Some products contain phenylalanine which must be used with caution in patients with phenylketonuria.

Adverse Reactions

Central nervous system: Drowsiness, headache, dizziness
Dermatologic: Rash
Gastrointestinal: Nausea, vomiting, stomach pain

(Continued)

Guaifenesin *(Continued)*

Mechanism of Action Thought to act as an expectorant by irritating the gastric mucosa and stimulating respiratory tract secretions, thereby increasing respiratory fluid volumes and decreasing phlegm viscosity

Pharmacokinetics Absorption: Well absorbed

Usual Dosage Oral:

Children:

<2 years: 12 mg/kg/day in 6 divided doses

2-5 years: 50-100 mg every 4 hours, not to exceed 600 mg/day

6-11 years: 100-200 mg every 4 hours or as extended release product 600 mg every 12 hours; not to exceed 1.2 g/day

Children >12 years and Adults: 200-400 mg every 4 hours or as extended release product 600-1200 mg every 12 hours; not to exceed 2.4 g/day

Administration Oral: Administer with a large quantity of fluid to ensure proper action; do not crush or chew extended release tablet

Test Interactions May cause a colorimetric interference with certain laboratory determinations of 5-hydroxyindoleacetic acid (5-HIAA) and vanillylmandelic acid (VMA)

Dosage Forms Excipient information presented when available (limited, particularly for generics); consult specific product labeling.

Granules, oral:

Mucinex® Children's Mini-Melts™: 50 mg/packet (12s) [contains phenylalanine 0.6 mg/packet and magnesium 6 mg/packet; grape flavor]

Mucinex® Junior Mini-Melts™: 100 mg/packet (12s) [contains phenylalanine 1 mg/packet and magnesium 10 mg/packet; bubble gum flavor]

Liquid: 100 mg/5 mL (120 mL, 480 mL)

Diabetic Tussin EX®: 100 mg/5 mL (120 mL) [alcohol free, sugar free, dye free; contains phenylalanine 8.4 mg/5 mL]

Ganidin NR: 100 mg/5 mL (480 mL) [raspberry flavor]

Mucinex® Children's: 100 mg/5 mL (120 mL) [alcohol free; grape flavor]

Organidin® NR: 100 mg/5 mL (480 mL) [contains sodium benzoate; raspberry flavor]

Siltussin DAS: 100 mg/5 mL (120 mL) [alcohol free, dye free, sugar free; strawberry flavor]

Syrup: 100 mg/5 mL (120 mL, 480 mL)

Guiatuss™: 100 mg/5 mL (120 mL, 480 mL) [alcohol free; fruit-mint flavor]

Phanasin®: 100 mg/5 mL (120 mL, 240 mL) [alcohol free, sugar free; mint flavor]

Phanasin® Diabetic Choice: 100 mg/5 mL (120 mL) [alcohol free, sugar free; mint flavor]

Robitussin®: 100 mg/5 mL (5 mL, 10 mL, 15 mL, 30 mL, 120 mL, 240 mL, 480 mL) [alcohol free; contains sodium benzoate]

Scot-Tussin® Expectorant: 100 mg/5 mL (120 mL) [alcohol free, dye free, sugar free; contains benzoic acid; grape flavor]

Siltussin SA: 100 mg/5 mL (120 mL, 240 mL, 480 mL) [alcohol free, sugar free; strawberry flavor]

Vicks® Casero™ Chest Congestion Relief: 100 mg/6.25 mL (120 mL, 240 mL) [contains phenylalanine 5.5 mg/12.5 mL, sodium 32 mg/12.5 mL, and sodium benzoate; honey menthol flavor]

Tablet: 200 mg

Allfen Jr: 400 mg [dye free]

Organidin® NR: 200 mg

XPECT™: 400 mg

Tablet, extended release:

Mucinex®: 600 mg

♦ **Guaifenesin AC** *see* Guaifenesin and Codeine *on page 746*

Guaifenesin and Codeine (gwye FEN e sin & KOE deen)

Related Information

OTC Cough and Cold Preparations, Pediatric *on page 1706*

U.S. Brand Names Brontex®; Cheracol®; Diabetic Tussin C®; Gani-Tuss® NR; Guaifenesin AC; Guaituss AC; Kolephrin® #1; Mytussin® AC; Robafen® AC; Romilar® AC; Tussi-Organidin® NR; Tussi-Organidin® S-NR

Index Terms Codeine and Guaifenesin

Therapeutic Category Antitussive; Cough Preparation; Expectorant

Generic Available Yes

Use Temporary control of cough due to minor throat and bronchial irritation

Restrictions C-V

Pregnancy Risk Factor C

Lactation Excretion in breast milk unknown/use caution

Contraindications Hypersensitivity to guaifenesin, codeine, or any component

Warnings Some products contain sodium benzoate; benzoic acid (benzoate) is a metabolite of benzyl alcohol; large amounts of benzyl alcohol (≥99 mg/kg/day) have been associated with a potentially fatal toxicity ("gasping syndrome") in neonates; *in vitro* and animal studies have shown that benzoate displaces bilirubin from protein binding sites; avoid use of sodium benzoate products in neonates

Precautions Use with caution in patients with hypersensitivity reactions to other phenanthrene derivative opioid agonists (morphine, hydrocodone, hydromorphone, levorphanol, oxycodone, oxymorphone). Some products contain phenylalanine which must be used with caution in patients with phenylketonuria.

Adverse Reactions

Codeine:

- Cardiovascular: Palpitations, bradycardia, peripheral vasodilation
- Central nervous system: CNS depression, dizziness, drowsiness, sedation, elevated intracranial pressure
- Dermatologic: Pruritus from histamine release
- Endocrine & metabolic: Antidiuretic hormone release
- Gastrointestinal: Nausea, vomiting, constipation, biliary tract spasm
- Genitourinary: Urinary tract spasm
- Ocular: Miosis
- Respiratory: Respiratory depression
- Miscellaneous: Histamine release, physical and psychological dependence with prolonged use

Guaifenesin:

- Central nervous system: Drowsiness, headache
- Dermatologic: Rash
- Gastrointestinal: Nausea, vomiting

Drug Interactions CNS depressant medications produce additive sedative properties

Mechanism of Action See individual monographs for Guaifenesin *on page 745* and Codeine *on page 397*

Usual Dosage Oral:

Children:

- 2-6 years: 1-1.5 mg/kg codeine/day divided into 4 doses administered every 4-6 hours (maximum dose: 30 mg/24 hours)
- 6-12 years: 5 mL every 4 hours, not to exceed 30 mL/24 hours
- >12 years: 10 mL every 4 hours, up to 60 mL/24 hours

Adults: 5-10 mL or 1 tablet every 4-6 hours; not to exceed 120 mg (60 mL) codeine/day or 6 tablets/day

Administration Oral: Administer with a large quantity of fluid to ensure proper action; may administer with food to decrease nausea and GI upset from codeine

Test Interactions May cause a colorimetric interference with certain laboratory determinations of 5-hydroxy indoleacetic acid (5-HIAA) and vanillylmandelic acid (VMA)

Patient Information May be habit-forming; do not discontinue abruptly

Dosage Forms Excipient information presented when available (limited, particularly for generics); consult specific product labeling.

Liquid:

- Brontex®: Guaifenesin 75 mg and codeine phosphate 2.5 mg per 5 mL (480 mL) [alcohol free; strawberry mint flavor]
- Diabetic Tussin C®: Guaifenesin 200 mg and codeine phosphate 10 mg per 5 mL (480 mL) [contains phenylalanine 0.03 mcg/5 mL; cherry vanilla flavor]
- Gani-Tuss® NR: Guaifenesin 100 mg and codeine phosphate 10 mg per 5 mL (480 mL) [raspberry flavor]
- Guaifenesin AC: Guaifenesin 100 mg and codeine phosphate 10 mg per 5 mL (120 mL, 480 mL) [alcohol free, sugar free; raspberry flavor]
- Kolephrin® #1: Guaifenesin 100 mg and codeine phosphate 10 mg per 5 mL (120 mL) [contains sodium 1.1 mg/5 mL and sodium benzoate]
- Tussi-Organidin® NR: Guaifenesin 300 mg and codeine phosphate 10 mg per 5 mL (480 mL) [alcohol free, sugar free; contains sodium benzoate; raspberry flavor]
- Tussi-Organidin® S-NR: Guaifenesin 300 mg and codeine phosphate 10 mg per 5 mL (120 mL) [alcohol free, sugar free; contains sodium benzoate; raspberry flavor]

Syrup:

- Cheracol®: Guaifenesin 100 mg and codeine phosphate 10 mg per 5 mL (120 mL) [contains alcohol 4.75% and benzoic acid]
- Guaituss AC: Guaifenesin 100 mg and codeine phosphate 10 mg per 5 mL (120 mL, 480 mL) [contains alcohol; sugar free; fruit-mint flavor]
- Mytussin® AC: Guaifenesin 100 mg and codeine phosphate 10 mg per 5 mL (120 mL, 480 mL) [contains alcohol; sugar free; fruit flavor]
- Robafen® AC: Guaifenesin 100 mg and codeine phosphate 10 mg per 5 mL (120 mL, 480 mL)

(Continued)

Guaifenesin and Codeine *(Continued)*

Romilar® AC: Guaifenesin 100 mg and codeine phosphate 10 mg per 5 mL (480 mL) [alcohol free, sugar free, dye free; contains benzoic acid and phenylalanine; grape flavor]

Tablet: Guaifenesin 300 mg and codeine phosphate 10 mg

Brontex®: Guaifenesin 300 mg and codeine phosphate 10 mg

Guaifenesin and Dextromethorphan

(gwye FEN e sin & deks troe meth OR fan)

Medication Safety Issues

Sound-alike/look-alike issues:

Benylin® may be confused with Benadryl®, Ventolin®

Related Information

OTC Cough and Cold Preparations, Pediatric *on page 1706*

U.S. Brand Names Allfen-DM; Altarussin DM [OTC]; Amibid DM [DSC]; Cheracol® D [OTC]; Cheracol® Plus [OTC]; Coricidin HBP® Chest Congestion and Cough [OTC]; Diabetic Tussin® DM [OTC]; Diabetic Tussin® DM Maximum Strength [OTC]; Duratuss® DM; Gani-Tuss DM NR; Genatuss DM® [OTC]; Guaicon DM [OTC]; Guaicon DMS [OTC]; Guaifenex® DM; Guia-D; Guiatuss-DM® [OTC]; Hydro-Tussin™ DM; Kolephrin® GG/DM [OTC]; Mintab DM; Mucinex® Children's Cough [OTC]; Mucinex® DM [OTC]; Phanatuss® DM [OTC]; Phlemex; Respa-DM®; Robafen DM [OTC]; Robafen DM Clear [OTC]; Robitussin® Cough and Congestion [OTC]; Robitussin® DM [OTC]; Robitussin® DM Infant [OTC]; Robitussin® Sugar Free Cough [OTC]; Safe Tussin® [OTC]; Scot-Tussin® Senior [OTC]; Silexin [OTC]; Siltussin DM [OTC]; Siltussin DM DAS [OTC]; Simuc-DM; Su-Tuss DM; Touro® DM; Tussi-Organidin® DM NR; Tussi-Organidin® DM-S NR; Vicks® 44E [OTC]; Vicks® Pediatric Formula 44E [OTC]; Z-Cof LA™

Canadian Brand Names Balminil DM E; Benylin® DM-E; Koffex DM-Expectorant; Robitussin® DM

Index Terms Dextromethorphan and Guaifenesin

Therapeutic Category Antitussive; Cough Preparation; Expectorant

Generic Available Yes

Use Temporary control of cough due to minor throat and bronchial irritation

Pregnancy Risk Factor C

Lactation Excretion in breast milk unknown/use caution

Contraindications Hypersensitivity to guaifenesin, dextromethorphan, or any component; use within 14 days of MAO inhibitor therapy

Warnings Some products contain sodium benzoate; benzoic acid (benzoate) is a metabolite of benzyl alcohol; large amounts of benzyl alcohol (≥99 mg/kg/day) have been associated with a potentially fatal toxicity ("gasping syndrome") in neonates; *in vitro* and animal studies have shown that benzoate displaces bilirubin from protein binding sites; avoid use of sodium benzoate products in neonates

Precautions Some products contain phenylalanine which must be used with caution in patients with phenylketonuria.

Adverse Reactions

Central nervous system: Drowsiness, dizziness, headache

Dermatologic: Rash

Gastrointestinal: Nausea

Mechanism of Action See individual monographs for Guaifenesin *on page 745* and Dextromethorphan *on page 477*

Pharmacodynamics Onset of action: Antitussive effect: Oral (rapid release formulation): 15-30 minutes

Pharmacokinetics Absorption: Dextromethorphan is rapidly absorbed from the GI tract

Usual Dosage Oral (dose expressed in mg of **dextromethorphan**):

Children: 1-2 mg/kg/day every 6-8 hours

Children >12 years and Adults: 60-120 mg/day divided every 6-8 hours or as extended release product 30-60 mg every 12 hours; not to exceed 120 mg/day

Administration Oral: Administer without regard to meals, with a large quantity of fluid to ensure proper effect; do not crush, chew, or break extended release tablets

Test Interactions May cause a colorimetric interference with certain laboratory determinations of 5-hydroxy indoleacetic acid (5-HIAA) and vanillylmandelic acid (VMA)

Patient Information Notify healthcare provider if cough persists for greater than 7 days or if cough is associated with a fever, rash, or persistent headache

Dosage Forms Excipient information presented when available (limited, particularly for generics); consult specific product labeling. [DSC] = Discontinued product

Capsule, softgel:
- Coricidin HBP® Chest Congestion and Cough: Guaifenesin 200 mg and dextromethorphan hydrobromide 10 mg

Elixir:
- Duratuss DM®: Guaifenesin 225 mg and dextromethorphan hydrobromide 25 mg per 5 mL (480 mL) [contains sodium benzoate; grape flavor]
- Simuc-DM: Guaifenesin 225 mg and dextromethorphan hydrobromide 25 mg per 5 mL (480 mL) [grape flavor]
- Su-Tuss DM: Guaifenesin 200 mg and dextromethorphan hydrobromide 20 mg per 5 mL (480 mL) [fruit flavor]

Liquid: Guaifenesin 100 mg and dextromethorphan hydrobromide 10 mg per 5 mL (480 mL)
- Diabetic Tussin® DM: Guaifenesin 100 mg and dextromethorphan hydrobromide 10 mg per 5 mL (120 mL) [alcohol free, sugar free, dye free; contains phenylalanine 8.4 mg/5 mL]
- Diabetic Tussin® DM Maximum Strength: Guaifenesin 200 mg and dextromethorphan hydrobromide 10 mg per 5 mL (120 mL) [alcohol free, sugar free, dye free; contains phenylalanine 8.4 mg/5 mL]
- Gani-Tuss® DM NR: Guaifenesin 100 mg and dextromethorphan hydrobromide 10 mg per 5 mL (480 mL) [raspberry flavor]
- Hydro-Tussin™ DM: Guaifenesin 200 mg and dextromethorphan hydrobromide 20 mg per 5 mL (480 mL) [alcohol free, sugar free; contains sodium benzoate]
- Kolephrin® GG/DM: Guaifenesin 150 mg and dextromethorphan hydrobromide 10 mg per 5 mL (120 mL) [alcohol free; cherry flavor]
- Mucinex® Children's Cough: Guaifenesin 100 mg and dextromethorphan hydrobromide 5 mg per 5 mL (120 mL) [contains sodium 3 mg/5 mL; cherry flavor]
- Safe Tussin®: Guaifenesin 100 mg and dextromethorphan hydrobromide 15 mg per 5 mL (120 mL) [alcohol free, sodium free, sugar free, dye free; mint flavor]
- Scot-Tussin® Senior: Guaifenesin 200 mg and dextromethorphan hydrobromide 15 mg per 5 mL (120 mL) [alcohol free, sodium free, sugar free]
- Tussi-Organidin® DM NR: Guaifenesin 300 mg and dextromethorphan hydrobromide 10 mg per 5 mL (480 mL) [alcohol free, sugar free; contains sodium benzoate; grape flavor]
- Tussi-Organidin® DM-S NR: Guaifenesin 300 mg and dextromethorphan hydrobromide 10 mg per 5 mL (120 mL) [alcohol free, sugar free; contains sodium benzoate; grape flavor]
- Vicks® 44E: Guaifenesin 200 mg and dextromethorphan hydrobromide 20 mg per 15 mL (120 mL, 235 mL) [contains sodium 31 mg/15 mL, alcohol, sodium benzoate]
- Vicks® Pediatric Formula 44E: Guaifenesin 100 mg and dextromethorphan hydrobromide 10 mg per 15 mL (120 mL) [alcohol free; contains sodium 30 mg/15 mL, sodium benzoate; cherry flavor]

Liquid, oral [drops]:
- Robitussin® DM Infant: Guaifenesin 100 mg and dextromethorphan hydrobromide 5 mg per 2.5 mL (30 mL) [alcohol free; contains sodium benzoate; fruit punch flavor]

Syrup: Guaifenesin 100 mg and dextromethorphan hydrobromide 10 mg per 5 mL (120 mL, 480 mL)
- Altarussin DM: Guaifenesin 100 mg and dextromethorphan hydrobromide 10 mg per 5 mL (120 mL, 240 mL, 480 mL, 3840 mL)
- Cheracol® D: Guaifenesin 100 mg and dextromethorphan hydrobromide 10 mg per 5 mL (120 mL, 180 mL) [contains alcohol 4.75%, benzoic acid]
- Cheracol® Plus: Guaifenesin 100 mg and dextromethorphan hydrobromide 10 mg per 5 mL (120 mL) [contains alcohol 4.75%, benzoic acid]
- Genatuss DM®: Guaifenesin 100 mg and dextromethorphan hydrobromide 10 mg per 5 mL (120 mL)
- Guiatuss® DM: Guaifenesin 100 mg and dextromethorphan hydrobromide 10 mg per 5 mL (120 mL, 480 mL, 3840 mL) [alcohol free; contains sodium benzoate]
- Guaicon DM®: Guaifenesin 100 mg and dextromethorphan hydrobromide 10 mg per 5 mL (10 mL) [alcohol free]
- Guaicon DMS®: Guaifenesin 100 mg and dextromethorphan hydrobromide 10 mg per 5 mL (10 mL) [alcohol free, sugar free]
- Mintab DM: Guaifenesin 200 mg and dextromethorphan hydrobromide 10 mg per 5 mL (480 mL) [alcohol free, dye free; cherry vanilla flavor]
- Phanatuss® DM: Guaifenesin 100 mg and dextromethorphan hydrobromide 10 mg per 5 mL (120 mL) [alcohol free, sugar free]
- Robafen® DM: Guaifenesin 100 mg and dextromethorphan hydrobromide 10 mg per 5 mL (120 mL, 240 mL, 480 mL) [cherry flavor]
- Robafen® DM Clear: Guaifenesin 100 mg and dextromethorphan hydrobromide 10 mg per 5 mL (120 mL)

(Continued)

Guaifenesin and Dextromethorphan *(Continued)*

Robitussin® Cough and Congestion: Guaifenesin 100 mg and dextromethorphan hydrobromide 10 mg per 5 mL (120 mL) [alcohol free; contains sodium benzoate]
Robitussin®-DM: Guaifenesin 100 mg and dextromethorphan hydrobromide 10 mg per 5 mL (5 mL, 120 mL, 340 mL, 360 mL) [alcohol free; contains sodium benzoate]
Robitussin® Sugar Free Cough: Guaifenesin 100 mg and dextromethorphan hydrobromide 10 mg per 5 mL (120 mL) [alcohol free, sugar free; contains sodium benzoate]
Silexin: Guaifenesin 100 mg and dextromethorphan hydrobromide 10 mg per 5 mL (45 mL) [alcohol free, sugar free)]
Siltussin DM: Guaifenesin 100 mg and dextromethorphan hydrobromide 10 mg per 5 mL (120 mL, 240 mL, 480 mL) [strawberry flavor]
Siltussin DM DAS: Guaifenesin 100 mg and dextromethorphan hydrobromide 10 mg per 5 mL (120 mL) [alcohol free, dye free, sugar free; strawberry flavor]

Tablet: Guaifenesin 1000 mg and dextromethorphan hydrobromide 60 mg; guaifenesin 1200 mg and dextromethorphan hydrobromide 60 mg
Silexin: Guaifenesin 100 mg and dextromethorphan hydrobromide 10 mg

Tablet, extended release:
Amibid DM [DSC], Guaifenex® DM, Mucinex® DM, Respa-DM®: Guaifenesin 600 mg and dextromethorphan hydrobromide 30 mg
Mucophen® DM: Guaifenesin 1000 mg and dextromethorphan hydrobromide 60 mg
Phlemex: Guaifenesin 1200 mg and dextromethorphan hydrobromide 20 mg
Touro® DM: Guaifenesin 575 mg and dextromethorphan hydrobromide 30 mg

Tablet, long-acting: Guaifenesin 1000 mg and dextromethorphan hydrobromide 60 mg
Z-Cof LA [scored]: Guaifenesin 650 mg and dextromethorphan hydrobromide 30 mg

Tablet, sustained release:
Allfen-DM: Guaifenesin 1000 mg and dextromethorphan hydrobromide 55 mg
Relacon LAX: Guaifenesin 835 mg and dextromethorphan hydrobromide 30 mg
Tussi-Bid®: Guaifenesin 1200 mg and dextromethorphan hydrobromide 60 mg

Tablet, timed release [scored]: Guaifenesin 1200 mg and dextromethorphan hydrobromide 60 mg
Guia-D: Guaifenesin 1000 mg and dextromethorphan hydrobromide 60 mg [dye free]

- **Guaifenex® DM** *see* Guaifenesin and Dextromethorphan *on page 748*
- **Guaituss AC** *see* Guaifenesin and Codeine *on page 746*
- **Guia-D** *see* Guaifenesin and Dextromethorphan *on page 748*
- **Guiatuss™ [OTC]** *see* Guaifenesin *on page 745*
- **Guiatuss-DM® [OTC]** *see* Guaifenesin and Dextromethorphan *on page 748*
- **GW506U78** *see* Nelarabine *on page 1113*
- **GW433908G** *see* Fosamprenavir *on page 705*
- **Gyne-Lotrimin® 3 [OTC]** *see* Clotrimazole *on page 393*
- **Gynodiol®** *see* Estradiol *on page 605*
- **H_2O_2** *see* Hydrogen Peroxide *on page 786*

Haemophilus b Conjugate and Hepatitis B Vaccine

(he MOF i lus bee KON joo gate & hep a TYE tis bee vak SEEN)

Medication Safety Issues
Sound-alike/look-alike issues:
Comvax® may be confused with Recombivax [Recombivax HB®]

Related Information
Immunization Guidelines *on page 1837*

U.S. Brand Names Comvax®

Index Terms *Haemophilus* b (meningococcal protein conjugate) Conjugate Vaccine; Hepatitis b Vaccine (Recombinant); Hib Conjugate Vaccine

Therapeutic Category Vaccine

Generic Available No

Use Immunization against invasive disease caused by *H. influenzae* type b and against infection caused by all known subtypes of hepatitis B virus in infants 6 weeks to 15 months of age born of HB_sAg-negative mothers

Infants born of HB_sAg-positive mothers or mothers of unknown HB_sAg status should receive hepatitis B immune globulin and monovalent hepatitis B vaccine (recombinant) at birth and should complete the hepatitis B vaccination series

Pregnancy Risk Factor C

Contraindications Hypersensitivity to hepatitis vaccine, *Haemophilus* b vaccine, yeast, or any component of the formulation

Warnings Immediate treatment for anaphylactic/anaphylactoid reactions should be available during vaccine use; defer vaccination during the course of a moderate or severely febrile illness; children with chronic illness associated with increased risk of *Haemophilus influenzae* type b disease may have impaired anti-PRP antibody responses to conjugate vaccination. Examples include those with HIV infection, immunoglobulin deficiency, anatomic or functional asplenia, and sickle cell disease, as well as recipients of bone marrow transplants and recipients of chemotherapy for malignancy.

Precautions Administer with caution to patients with thrombocytopenia or any coagulation disorder that would be compromised by I.M. injection; if the patient receives antihemophilia or other similar therapy, I.M. injection can be scheduled shortly after such therapy is administered; use with caution in patients with decreased cardiopulmonary function

Adverse Reactions All serious adverse reactions must be reported to the U.S. Department of Health and Human Services (DHHS) Vaccine Adverse Event Reporting System (VAERS) 1-800-822-7967. For specific adverse reactions, see individual agents.

Drug Interactions See individual agents.

Stability Refrigerate; do not freeze

Mechanism of Action See individual agents.

Usual Dosage Infants and Children 6 weeks through 15 months: I.M.: 0.5 mL per dose

Recommended schedule: 3 doses repeated at 2, 4, and 12-15 months of age

Administration Shake well and administer I.M. in either the anterolateral aspect of the thigh or deltoid muscle of the arm; **not for I.V. or SubQ administration**

Patient Information May use antipyretics for postdose fever

Nursing Implications Federal law requires that the date of administration, the vaccine manufacturer, lot number of vaccine, and the administering person's name, title, and address be entered into the patient's permanent medical record.

Dosage Forms Excipient information presented when available (limited, particularly for generics); consult specific product labeling.

Injection, suspension [preservative free]: *Haemophilus* b PRP 7.5 mcg and HB_sAg 5 mcg per 0.5 mL (0.5 mL) [vial stopper contains latex]

References

American Academy of Pediatrics Committee on Infectious Diseases, "Recommended Immunization Schedules for Children and Adolescents - United States, 2007," *Pediatrics*, 2007, 119(1):207-8.

Centers for Disease Control and Prevention, "Recommended Childhood and Adolescent Immunization Schedule - United States, July-December 2004," *MMWR Morb Mortal Wkly Rep*, 2004, 53(16):Q1-4.

Haemophilus b Conjugate Vaccine

(he MOF fi lus bee KON joo gate vak SEEN)

Related Information

Immunization Guidelines *on page 1837*

U.S. Brand Names ActHIB®; HibTITER®; PedvaxHIB®

Canadian Brand Names ActHIB®; PedvaxHIB®

Index Terms Diphtheria CRM_{197} Protein Conjugate; Diphtheria Toxoid Conjugate; *Haemophilus* b Oligosaccharide Conjugate Vaccine; *Haemophilus* b Polysaccharide Vaccine; HbCV; HbOC; Hib Conjugate Vaccine; Hib Polysaccharide Conjugate; PRP-OMP; PRP-T

Therapeutic Category Vaccine

Generic Available No

Use Routine immunization of children 2 months to 5 years of age against invasive disease caused by *H. influenzae*

Unimmunized children ≥5 years of age with a chronic illness known to be associated with increased risk of *Haemophilus influenzae* type b disease, specifically, persons with anatomic or functional asplenia or sickle cell anemia or those who have undergone splenectomy, should receive Hib vaccine.

Adolescents and adults with specific dysfunction or certain complement deficiencies who are at especially high risk of *H. influenzae* type b infection (HIV-infected adults); patients with Hodgkin's disease (vaccinated at least 2 weeks before the initiation of chemotherapy or 3 months after the end of chemotherapy)

Pregnancy Risk Factor C

Contraindications Hypersensitivity to any component including diphtheria toxoid (HibTITER®) or tetanus toxoid (ActHIB®)

Warnings Immediate treatment for anaphylactic/anaphylactoid reactions should be available during vaccine use; defer vaccination during the course of a moderate or severely febrile illness; the carrier proteins used in Haemophilus b oligosaccharide

(Continued)

Haemophilus b Conjugate Vaccine *(Continued)*

conjugate (HbOC, HibTITER®) and polyribosylribitol phosphate-outer membrane polysaccharide conjugate (PRP-T, ActHIB®) are chemically and immunologically related to toxoids contained in DTaP vaccine. Earlier or simultaneous vaccination with diphtheria or tetanus toxoids may be required to elicit an optimal anti-PRP antibody response. In contrast, the immunogenicity of PedvaxHIB® is not affected by vaccination with DTP. In infants in whom DTaP or DT vaccination is deferred, PedvaxHIB® may be advantageous for *Haemophilus influenzae* type b vaccination.

Children with chronic illness associated with increased risk of *Haemophilus influenzae* type b disease may have impaired anti-PRP antibody responses to conjugate vaccination. Examples include those with HIV infection, immunoglobulin deficiency, anatomic or functional asplenia, and sickle cell disease, as well as recipients of bone marrow transplants and recipients of chemotherapy for malignancy. Some children with immunologic impairment may benefit from more doses of conjugate vaccine than normally indicated.

Precautions Administer with caution to patients with thrombocytopenia or any coagulation disorder that would be compromised by I.M. injection; if the patient receives antihemophilia or other similar therapy, I.M. injection can be scheduled shortly after such therapy is administered.

Adverse Reactions All serious adverse reactions must be reported to the U.S. Department of Health and Human Services (DHHS) Vaccine Adverse Event Reporting System (VAERS) 1-800-822-7967.

Cardiovascular: Edema, fever (up to 102.2°F),

Central nervous system: High pitched cry (>4 hours), irritability, lethargy, febrile seizures, fatigue

Dermatologic: Urticaria, angioedema

Gastrointestinal: Anorexia, diarrhea, vomiting

Local: Irritation, swelling, and erythema at injection site, sterile injection site abscess

Neuromuscular & skeletal: Weakness

Respiratory: Dyspnea, upper respiratory infection

Miscellaneous: Warmth, increased risk of *Haemophilus* b infections in the week after vaccination, lymphadenopathy

Drug Interactions Decreased effect with immunosuppressive agents

Stability Keep in refrigerator, do not freeze; Tripedia® may be used to reconstitute ActHIB®; ActHIB® must be administered within 24 hours of reconstitution

Mechanism of Action Stimulates production of anticapsular antibodies and provides active immunity to *Haemophilus influenzae*

Usual Dosage Children: I.M.: 0.5 mL as a single dose should be administered according to one of the following "brand-specific" schedules; preterm infants should be vaccinated according to their chronological age from birth; (see table)

Vaccination Schedule for *Haemophilus* b Conjugate Vaccines

Age at 1st Dose (mo)	ActHIB®, HibTITER®		PedvaxHIB®	
	Primary Series	Booster	Primary Series	Booster
2-6	3 doses, 2 months apart	1 dose[1]	2 doses, 2 months apart	1 dose[1]
7-11	2 doses, 2 months apart	1 dose[1]	2 doses, 2 months apart	1 dose[1]
12-14	1 dose	1 dose[1]	1 dose	1 dose[1]
15-71	1 dose	—	1 dose	—

Note: DTaP/Hib combination vaccines should not be used for infants at ages 2, 4, or 6 months but may be used as booster following any Hib vaccine.

[1]At least 2 months after previous dose and ≥12 months of age.

Administration ActHIB®: Reconstitute with provided diluent or Tripedia®; all vaccines: Shake well and administer I.M. in either the anterolateral aspect of the thigh or deltoid muscle of the arm; **not for I.V. or SubQ administration**

Nursing Implications Federal law requires that the date of administration, the vaccine manufacturer, lot number of vaccine, and the administering person's name, title, and address be entered into the patient's permanent medical record

Dosage Forms Excipient information presented when available (limited, particularly for generics); consult specific product labeling.

Injection, powder for reconstitution [preservative free]:

ActHIB®: *Haemophilus* b capsular polysaccharide 10 mcg and tetanus toxoid 24 mcg per dose [may be reconstituted with provided diluent (forms solution; vial stopper contains latex) or TriHIBit® (forms suspension)]

Injection, solution [preservative free]:

HibTITER®: *Haemophilus* b saccharide 10 mcg and diphtheria CRM 197 protein 25 mcg per 0.5 mL (0.5 mL) [vial stopper contains latex]

Injection, suspension:

PedvaxHIB®: *Haemophilus* b capsular polysaccharide 7.5 mcg and *Neisseria meningitidis* OMPC 125 mcg per 0.5 mL (0.5 mL) [contains aluminum 225 mcg/0.5 mL]

References

American Academy of Pediatrics Committee on Infectious Diseases, "Recommended Immunization Schedules for Children and Adolescents - United States, 2007," *Pediatrics*, 2007, 119(1):207-8.

Centers for Disease Control and Prevention, "Recommended Childhood and Adolescent Immunization Schedule - United States, July-December 2004," *MMWR Morb Mortal Wkly Rep*, 2004, 53(16):Q1-4.

- ***Haemophilus* b (meningococcal protein conjugate) Conjugate Vaccine** *see* *Haemophilus* b Conjugate and Hepatitis B Vaccine *on page 750*
- ***Haemophilus* b Oligosaccharide Conjugate Vaccine** *see* *Haemophilus* b Conjugate Vaccine *on page 751*
- ***Haemophilus* b Polysaccharide Vaccine** *see* *Haemophilus* b Conjugate Vaccine *on page 751*
- ***Haemophilus influenzae* b Conjugate Vaccine and Diphtheria, Tetanus Toxoids, and Acellular Pertussis Vaccine** *see* Diphtheria, Tetanus Toxoids, and Acellular Pertussis Vaccine and *Haemophilus influenzae* b Conjugate Vaccine *on page 519*
- **Halcion® [DSC]** *see* Triazolam *on page 1572*
- **Halcion® (Can)** *see* Triazolam *on page 1572*
- **Haldol®** *see* Haloperidol *on page 754*
- **Haldol® Decanoate** *see* Haloperidol *on page 754*
- **Halfprin® [OTC]** *see* Aspirin *on page 163*

Halobetasol (hal oh BAY ta sol)

Medication Safety Issues

Sound-alike/look-alike issues:

Ultravate® may be confused with Cutivate®

Related Information

Corticosteroids, Topical: Guidelines for Selection and Use *on page 1686*

U.S. Brand Names Ultravate®

Canadian Brand Names Ultravate®

Index Terms Halobetasol Propionate

Therapeutic Category Adrenal Corticosteroid; Anti-inflammatory Agent; Corticosteroid, Topical; Glucocorticoid

Generic Available Yes

Use Relief of inflammation and pruritus associated with corticosteroid-response dermatoses

Pregnancy Risk Factor C

Lactation Excretion in breast milk unknown/use caution

Contraindications Hypersensitivity to halobetasol propionate, other corticosteroids, or any component

Warnings Hypothalamic-pituitary-adrenal (HPA) axis suppression may occur with topical corticosteroid use; acute adrenal insufficiency may occur with abrupt withdrawal after long-term use or with stress; withdrawal or discontinuation should be done carefully; patients with HPA axis suppression may require increased doses of systemic glucocorticosteroids prior to, during, and after unusual stress (eg, surgery). Adverse systemic effects (including HPA axis suppression) may occur when topical steroids are used on large areas of the body, denuded areas, for prolonged periods of time, with an occlusive dressing, and/or in infants or small children; infants and small children may be more susceptible to HPA axis suppression or other systemic toxicities due to a larger skin surface area to body mass ratio; use with caution in pediatric patients; safety and efficacy have not been established in children <12 years of age (use is not recommended)

Do not use topical halobetasol for the treatment of rosacea or perioral dermatitis; do not apply to the face, groin, or axillae. Do not exceed maximum recommended dose or duration of therapy due to the potential development of HPA axis suppression.

Precautions Avoid using higher than recommended doses; suppression of HPA axis, suppression of linear growth (ie, reduction of growth velocity), reduced bone mineral, or hypercorticism (Cushing's syndrome) may occur. Discontinue treatment if local

(Continued)

Halobetasol *(Continued)*

irritation develops. Use appropriate antibacterial or antifungal agents to treat concomitant skin infections; discontinue halobetasol treatment if infection does not resolve promptly.

Adverse Reactions

Central nervous system: Intracranial hypertension (systemic effect reported in children treated with topical corticosteroids)

Dermatologic: Burning, itching, stinging, acne, dry skin, erythema, skin atrophy, leukoderma, pustulation, rash, secondary infection, striae, vesicles, telangiectasia, urticaria, miliaria, paresthesia, allergic contact dermatitis, hypopigmentation, perioral dermatitis, folliculitis, hypertrichosis

Endocrine & metabolic: Hyperglycemia, HPA axis suppression, Cushing's syndrome, growth retardation

Renal: Glycosuria

Drug Interactions None identified

Stability Store between 59°F to 86°F (15°C to 30°C)

Mechanism of Action Not well defined topically; possesses anti-inflammatory, antipruritic, antiproliferative, vasoconstrictive, and immunosuppressive properties

Pharmacokinetics

Absorption: Percutaneous absorption varies and depends on many factors including vehicle used, integrity of epidermis, dose, and use of occlusive dressing; absorption is increased by occlusive dressings or with decreased integrity of skin (eg, inflammation or skin disease)

Cream: <6% of topically applied dose enters circulation within 96 hours following application

Metabolism: Hepatic

Elimination: Renal

Usual Dosage

Children <12 years: Use not recommended (high risk of systemic adverse effects, eg, HPA axis suppression, Cushing's syndrome)

Children ≥12 years and Adults: Topical: Steroid-responsive dermatoses: Apply sparingly once or twice daily; maximum dose: 50 g/week; do not treat for >2 weeks. **Note:** To decrease risk of systemic effects, only treat small areas at any one time; discontinue therapy when control is achieved; reassess diagnosis if no improvement is seen in 2 weeks.

Administration Topical: Apply sparingly to affected area, gently rub in until disappears; do not use on open skin; do not apply to face, underarms, or groin area; avoid contact with eyes; do not occlude affected area.

Monitoring Parameters Assess HPA axis suppression in patients using potent topical steroids applied to a large surface area or to areas under occlusion (eg, ACTH stimulation test, morning plasma cortisol test, urinary free cortisol test)

Patient Information Avoid contact with eyes; do not apply to face, underarms, or groin area; do not bandage, cover, or wrap affected area unless directed by physician; do not use for longer than directed; notify physician if condition being treated persists or worsens. Do not use tight-fitting diapers or plastic pants on a child being treated in diaper area. Wash hands after applying.

Additional Information Considered to be a super high potency topical corticosteroid; patients with psoriasis who were treated with halobetasol cream or ointment in divided doses of 7 g/day for one week developed HPA axis suppression

Dosage Forms Excipient information presented when available (limited, particularly for generics); consult specific product labeling.

Cream, as propionate: 0.05% (15 g, 50 g)

Ointment, as propionate: 0.05% (15 g, 50 g)

♦ **Halobetasol Propionate** *see* Halobetasol *on page 753*

Haloperidol (ha loe PER i dole)

Medication Safety Issues

Sound-alike/look-alike issues:

Haloperidol may be confused Halotestin®

Haldol® may be confused with Halcion®, Halenol®, Halog®, Halotestin®, Stadol®

Related Information

Compatibility of Chemotherapy and Related Supportive Care Medications *on page 1777*

U.S. Brand Names Haldol®; Haldol® Decanoate

Canadian Brand Names Apo-Haloperidol®; Apo-Haloperidol LA®; Haloperidol Injection, USP; Haloperidol-LA; Haloperidol-LA Omega; Haloperidol Long Acting; Novo-Peridol; Peridol; PMS-Haloperidol LA

Index Terms Haloperidol Decanoate; Haloperidol Lactate

Therapeutic Category Antipsychotic Agent; Phenothiazine Derivative

Generic Available Yes

Use Management of schizophrenia; treatment of psychoses, Tourette's disorder, and severe behavioral problems in children; emergency sedation of severely agitated or delirious patients

Pregnancy Risk Factor C

Lactation Enters breast milk/not recommended (AAP rates "of concern")

Contraindications Hypersensitivity to haloperidol or any component (see Warnings); narrow-angle glaucoma, bone marrow suppression, CNS depression, coma, severe liver or cardiac disease, parkinsonism

Warnings May cause extrapyramidal symptoms, including pseudoparkinsonism, acute dystonic reactions, akathisia, and tardive dyskinesia (risk of these reactions is high relative to other neuroleptics). Use may be associated with neuroleptic malignant syndrome. Safety and efficacy have not been established in children <3 years of age.

Injection as deconate contains benzyl alcohol which may cause allergic reactions in susceptible individuals; large amounts of benzyl alcohol (≥99 mg/kg/day) have been associated with a potentially fatal toxicity ("gasping syndrome") in neonates; avoid use of haloperidol products containing benzyl alcohol in neonates; *in vitro* and animal studies have shown that benzoate, a metabolite of benzyl alcohol, displaces bilirubin from protein binding sites

Precautions Use with caution in patients with renal or hepatic dysfunction, thyrotoxicosis, cardiovascular disease, history of seizures, or EEG abnormalities; haloperidol may cause hypotension, precipitation of anginal pain, anticholinergic effects (low incidence relative to other neuroleptics), elevation of prolactin levels

Adverse Reactions

Cardiovascular: Tachycardia, hypotension, hypertension, EKG changes (eg, prolongation of QT interval, torsade de pointes)

Central nervous system: Extrapyramidal reactions, neuroleptic malignant syndrome, tardive dyskinesia, drowsiness, restlessness, anxiety, agitation, euphoria, insomnia, confusion, headache, lethargy, vertigo, seizures, depression, hyperpyrexia, heat stroke; exacerbation of psychotic symptoms

Dermatologic: Rash, contact dermatitis; photosensitivity (rare)

Endocrine & metabolic: Galactorrhea, gynecomastia, hyperglycemia, hypoglycemia, hyponatremia, hypomagnesemia, elevated prolactin levels, menstrual irregularities, sexual dysfunction

Gastrointestinal: Xerostomia, constipation, nausea, vomiting, diarrhea, dyspepsia, hypersalivation

Genitourinary: Urinary retention, priapism

Hematologic: Leukopenia, leukocytosis, anemia, lymphomonocytosis; agranulocytosis (rare)

Hepatic: Hepatotoxicity (rare)

Ocular: Blurred vision, retinopathy, visual disturbances

Respiratory: Bronchospasm, laryngospasm, increased depth of respiration

Miscellaneous: Diaphoresis

Drug Interactions Cytochrome P450 isoenzyme CYP1A2 (minor), CYP2D6 (minor), and CYP3A3/4 substrate; CYP2D6 isoenzyme inhibitor

CNS depressants may increase adverse effects; epinephrine may cause hypotension; fluoxetine may inhibit metabolism and increase effect of haloperidol; chlorpromazine may increase haloperidol concentrations; carbamazepine, phenobarbital, and rifampin may increase metabolism and decrease effectiveness of haloperidol; use of haloperidol with anticholinergic agents may increase intraocular pressure; concurrent use with lithium has occasionally caused acute encephalopathy-like syndrome

Food Interactions Drug may precipitate if oral concentrate is mixed with coffee or tea

Stability All dosage forms: Store at controlled room temperature; protect from light

Oral concentrate and injection, as lactate: Do not freeze

Injection, as deconate: Do not refrigerate or freeze

Mechanism of Action Competitive blockade of postsynaptic dopamine receptors in the mesolimbic dopaminergic system; depresses cerebral cortex and hypothalamus; exhibits a strong alpha-adrenergic and anticholinergic blocking activity

Pharmacokinetics

Absorption: Oral: Well absorbed, undergoes first-pass metabolism in the liver

Distribution: Crosses the placenta; appears in breast milk

Protein binding: 92%

Metabolism: In the liver, hydroxy-metabolite is active

Bioavailability: Oral: 60%

Half-life: Adults: 20 hours; range: 13-35 hours

Elimination: Excreted in urine and feces as drug and metabolites

(Continued)

Haloperidol *(Continued)*

Usual Dosage

Children:

3-12 years (15-40 kg): Oral: Initial: 0.25-0.5 mg/day given in 2-3 divided doses; increase by 0.25-0.5 mg every 5-7 days; maximum dose: 0.15 mg/kg/day; usual maintenance:

Agitation or hyperkinesia: 0.01-0.03 mg/kg/day once daily

Tourette's disorder: 0.05-0.075 mg/kg/day in 2-3 divided doses

Psychotic disorders: 0.05-0.15 mg/kg/day in 2-3 divided doses

Note: Preliminary findings of a double-blind, placebo controlled study reported the mean optimal dose in 12 schizophrenic children 5-12 years to be ~2 mg/day (range: 0.5-3.5 mg/day or 0.02-0.12 mg/kg/day) given in 3 divided doses

6-12 years: I.M. **(as lactate)**: 1-3 mg/dose every 4-8 hours to a maximum of 0.15 mg/kg/day; switch to oral therapy as soon as able

Adults:

Oral: 0.5-5 mg 2-3 times/day; usual maximum dose: 30 mg/day; some patients may require 100 mg/day

I.M.:

As **lactate:** 2-5 mg every 4-8 hours as needed

As **decanoate:** Initial: 10-15 times the individual patients' stabilized oral dose, given at 3- to 4-week intervals

Administration

Oral: Administer with food or milk to decrease GI distress; prior to administration, dilute oral concentrate with ≥2 ounces of water or acidic beverage; do not mix oral concentrate with coffee or tea

Parenteral: **Decanoate** product is for I.M. use only, do not give I.V.; although not FDA-approved, haloperidol **lactate** has been administered I.V.

Monitoring Parameters Blood pressure, heart rate, CBC with differential, liver enzymes with long-term use; serum glucose, sodium, magnesium

Patient Information Avoid alcohol; may cause drowsiness and impair ability to perform activities requiring mental alertness or physical coordination; may cause dry mouth. May rarely cause photosensitivity reactions; avoid exposure to sunlight and artificial light sources (sunlamps, tanning booth/bed); use a sunscreen; contact physician if reaction occurs

Nursing Implications Observe for extrapyramidal effects

Dosage Forms Excipient information presented when available (limited, particularly for generics); consult specific product labeling. Available as various salts; mg strength refers to haloperidol; [DSC] = Discontinued product

Note: Strength expressed as base.

Injection, oil, as decanoate: 50 mg/mL (1 mL, 5 mL); 100 mg/mL (1 mL, 5 mL)

Haldol® Decanoate: 50 mg/mL (1 mL; 5 mL [DSC]); 100 mg/mL (1 mL; 5 mL [DSC]) [contains benzyl alcohol, sesame oil]

Injection, solution, as lactate: 5 mg/mL (1 mL, 10 mL)

Haldol®: 5 mg/mL (1 mL)

Solution, oral concentrate, as lactate: 2 mg/mL (15 mL, 120 mL)

Tablet: 0.5 mg, 1 mg, 2 mg, 5 mg, 10 mg, 20 mg

References

Serrano AC, "Haloperidol - Its Use in Children," *J Clin Psychiatry*, 1981, 42(4):154-6.

Spencer EK, Kafantaris V, Padron-Gayol MV, et al, "Haloperidol in Schizophrenic Children: Early Findings From a Study in Progress," *Psychopharmacol Bull*, 1992, 28(2):183-6.

- **Haloperidol Decanoate** *see* Haloperidol *on page 754*
- **Haloperidol Injection, USP (Can)** *see* Haloperidol *on page 754*
- **Haloperidol-LA (Can)** *see* Haloperidol *on page 754*
- **Haloperidol Lactate** *see* Haloperidol *on page 754*
- **Haloperidol-LA Omega (Can)** *see* Haloperidol *on page 754*
- **Haloperidol Long Acting (Can)** *see* Haloperidol *on page 754*
- **Halotestin®** *see* Fluoxymesterone *on page 685*
- **Havrix®** *see* Hepatitis A Vaccine *on page 761*
- **HbCV** *see Haemophilus* b Conjugate Vaccine *on page 751*
- **HBIG** *see* Hepatitis B Immune Globulin *on page 762*
- **HbOC** *see Haemophilus* b Conjugate Vaccine *on page 751*
- **hCG** *see* Chorionic Gonadotropin *on page 351*
- **HCTZ (error-prone abbreviation)** *see* Hydrochlorothiazide *on page 777*
- **HDA® Toothache [OTC]** *see* Benzocaine *on page 204*
- **HDCV** *see* Rabies Virus Vaccine *on page 1364*
- **Head & Shoulders® Intensive Treatment [OTC]** *see* Selenium Sulfide *on page 1427*
- **Heavy Mineral Oil** *see* Mineral Oil *on page 1065*

- **Helixate® FS** *see* Antihemophilic Factor (Recombinant) *on page 138*
- **Hemocyte® [OTC]** *see* Iron Supplements (Oral/Enteral) *on page 868*
- **Hemofil M** *see* Antihemophilic Factor (Human) *on page 134*
- **Hemorrhoidal HC** *see* Hydrocortisone *on page 781*

Hemorrhoidal Preparations (HEM or oyd al prep a RAY shuns)

Therapeutic Category Hemorrhoidal Treatment Agent; Topical Skin Product

Use Symptomatic relief of pain and discomfort in external and internal hemorrhoids, proctitis, papillitis, cryptitis, anal fissures, incomplete fistulas and relief of local pain following anorectal surgery

Contraindications Hypersensitivity to any component (see Warnings)

Warnings Some preparations contain sulfites which may cause allergic reactions in susceptible individuals

Adverse Reactions

Dermatologic: Rash

Local: Irritation, burning, itching

Mechanism of Action

Dibucaine, benzocaine, pramoxine: Temporarily relieves pain, itching, and irritation by blocking nerve impulses at the sensory nerve endings in the skin and mucous membranes

Emollient/protectant (glycerin, lanolin, mineral oil, petrolatum, zinc oxide, cocoa butter, shark liver oil): Form a physical barrier and lubricate tissues preventing irritation of the anorectal area and water loss

Pharmacodynamics Onset of action: Topical:

Pramoxine: 3-5 minutes

Dibucaine: <15 minutes

Benzocaine: 1 minute

Usual Dosage

Children and Adults: Topical: Apply ointment as a thin layer to the perianal area and the anal canal 3-6 times/day

Benzocaine-containing preparations: Apply up to 6 times/day

Dibucaine-containing preparations: Apply ointment into the rectum each morning and evening and after each bowel movement; ointment may be applied topically to anal tissues; apply up to 3-4 times/day

Children: No more than 7.5 g in a 24-hour period

Adults: No more than 30 g in a 24-hour period

Pramoxine-containing preparations: Apply up to 5 times/day (2-3 times/day and after bowel movements)

Adults: Rectal: Insert 1 suppository in the morning and at bedtime and after each bowel movement

Administration

Rectal: Foam, ointment, and cream for rectal use are instilled using a rectal applicator. The aerosol should not be inserted into the anus.

Topical: Apply cream or ointment to affected areas and rub in gently. A small amount of foam may be applied to the affected area using a cleansing tissue or pad.

Patient Information If anorectal symptoms do not improve in 7 days, or if bleeding, protrusion or seepage occurs, consult physician; avoid contact of topical preparations to the eyes

Dosage Forms Excipient information presented when available (limited, particularly for generics); consult specific product labeling.

Foam (Perifoam®, proctoFoam®): 15 g, 45 g

Ointment:

A-Caine® Rectal, Hemocaine®, Hemet® Rectal: 30 g, 60 g

Anusol®: 30 g, 60 g

Posterisan®: 25 g

Preparation H®: 30 g, 60 g

Suppository, rectal:

Anocaine®, Hemet®

Anumed®, Anusol®, CPI®

Calmol 4®

Hem-Prep®

Pazo® Hemorrhoid

Posterisan®

Preparation H®

Rectal Medicone®

- **Hemril®-30** *see* Hydrocortisone *on page 781*
- **HepaGam B™** *see* Hepatitis B Immune Globulin *on page 762*
- **Hepalean® (Can)** *see* Heparin *on page 758*

- **Hepalean® Leo (Can)** *see* Heparin *on page 758*
- **Hepalean®-LOK (Can)** *see* Heparin *on page 758*

Heparin (HEP a rin)

Medication Safety Issues

Sound-alike/look-alike issues:

Heparin may be confused with Hespan®

High alert medication: The Institute for Safe Medication Practices (ISMP) includes this medication among its list of drugs which have a heightened risk of causing significant patient harm when used in error.

Heparin sodium injection 10,000 units/mL and Hep-Lock U/P 10 units/mL have been confused with each other. Fatal medication errors have occurred between the two whose labels are both blue. **Never rely on color as a sole indicator to differentiate product identity.**

Heparin lock flush solution is intended only to maintain patency of I.V. devices and is **not** to be used for anticoagulant therapy.

Note: The 100 unit/mL concentration should not be used in neonates or infants <10 kg. The 10 unit/mL concentration may cause systemic anticoagulation in infants <1 kg who receive frequent flushes.

Related Information

Antithrombotic Therapy in Children *on page 1804*
Commonly Used Antidotes for Acute Overdoses *on page 1920*
Compatibility of Chemotherapy and Related Supportive Care Medications *on page 1777*
Overdose and Toxicology *on page 1916*

U.S. Brand Names HepFlush®-10; Hep-Lock®; Hep-Lock U/P

Canadian Brand Names Hepalean®; Hepalean® Leo; Hepalean®-LOK

Index Terms Heparin Calcium; Heparin Lock Flush; Heparin Sodium

Therapeutic Category Anticoagulant

Generic Available Yes

Use Prophylaxis and treatment of thromboembolic disorders

Pregnancy Risk Factor C

Lactation Does not enter breast milk/compatible

Contraindications Hypersensitivity to heparin or any component (see Warnings); severe thrombocytopenia, subacute bacterial endocarditis, suspected intracranial hemorrhage, shock, severe hypotension, uncontrollable bleeding (unless secondary to disseminated intravascular coagulation)

Warnings Some preparations contain sulfites or benzyl alcohol both of which may cause allergic reactions in susceptible individuals; large amounts of benzyl alcohol (≥99 mg/kg/day) have been associated with a potentially fatal toxicity ("gasping syndrome") in neonates; the "gasping syndrome" consists of metabolic acidosis, respiratory distress, gasping respirations, CNS dysfunction (including convulsions, intracranial hemorrhage), hypotension and cardiovascular collapse; avoid use of heparin products containing benzyl alcohol in neonates (use preservative free heparin); *in vitro* and animal studies have shown that benzoate, a metabolite of benzyl alcohol, displaces bilirubin from protein binding sites

Precautions Use with caution as hemorrhage may occur; risk factors for hemorrhage include: I.M. injections; peptic ulcer disease; intermittent I.V. injections (vs continuous I.V. infusion); increased capillary permeability; menstruation; recent surgery or invasive procedures; severe renal, hepatic, or biliary disease; and indwelling catheters

Heparin does not possess fibrinolytic activity and, therefore, cannot lyse established thrombi; discontinue heparin if hemorrhage occurs; severe hemorrhage or overdosage may require protamine

Adverse Reactions

Central nervous system: Fever, headache, chills
Dermatologic: Urticaria, alopecia
Gastrointestinal: Nausea, vomiting
Hematologic: Hemorrhage, thrombocytopenia (may be more common with beef lung heparin vs porcine mucosa heparin; however, if a patient receiving beef lung heparin experiences severe thrombocytopenia it is **not** recommended to switch to porcine mucosa heparin because a similar reaction may occur)
Hepatic: Elevated liver enzymes
Local: Irritation, ulceration, cutaneous necrosis has been rarely reported with deep SubQ injections
Neuromuscular & skeletal: Osteoporosis (with long-term use)

Drug Interactions Thrombolytic agents (urokinase, streptokinase, alteplase) and drugs which affect platelet function (eg, aspirin, NSAIDs, dipyridamole) may potentiate the risk of hemorrhage; digoxin, tetracycline, nicotine, antihistamines, and I.V. nitroglycerin may decrease heparin's anticoagulant effect.

Mechanism of Action Potentiates the action of antithrombin III and thereby inactivates thrombin (as well as activated coagulation factors IX, X, XI, XII, and plasmin) and prevents the conversion of fibrinogen to fibrin; heparin also stimulates release of lipoprotein lipase (lipoprotein lipase hydrolyzes triglycerides to glycerol and free fatty acids)

Pharmacodynamics Anticoagulation effect: Onset of action:

SubQ: 20-60 minutes

I.V.: Immediate

Pharmacokinetics

Absorption: SubQ, I.M.: Erratic

Distribution: Does not cross the placenta; does not appear in breast milk

Metabolism: Believed to be partially metabolized in the reticuloendothelial system

Half-life: Mean: 90 minutes (range: 1-2 hours); affected by obesity, renal function, hepatic function, malignancy, presence of pulmonary embolism, and infections

Elimination: Renal; small amount excreted unchanged in urine

Usual Dosage

Line flushing: When using daily flushes of heparin to maintain patency of single and double lumen central catheters, 10 units/mL is commonly used for younger infants (eg, <10 kg) while 100 units/mL is used for older infants, children, and adults. Capped polyvinyl chloride catheters and peripheral heparin locks require flushing more frequently (eg, every 6-8 hours). Volume of heparin flush is usually similar to volume of catheter (or slightly greater) or may be standardized according to specific hospital's policy (eg, 2-5 mL/flush). Dose of heparin flush used should not approach therapeutic unit per kg dose. Additional flushes should be given when stagnant blood is observed in catheter, after catheter is used for drug or blood administration, and after blood withdrawal from catheter.

TPN: Heparin 1 unit/mL (final concentration) may be added to TPN solutions, both central and peripheral. (Addition of heparin to peripheral TPN has been shown to increase duration of line patency.) The final concentration of heparin used for TPN solutions may need to be decreased to 0.5 units/mL in small infants receiving larger TPN volumes in order to avoid approaching therapeutic amounts.

Arterial lines: Heparinize with a usual final concentration of 1 unit/mL; range: 0.5-2 units/mL; in order to avoid large total doses and systemic effects, use 0.5 unit/mL in low birth weight/premature newborns and in other patients receiving multiple lines containing heparin

Prophylaxis for cardiac catheterization via an artery: Newborns and Children: I.V.: Bolus: 100-150 units/kg (see Monagle, 2001)

Systemic heparinization:

Neonates and Infants <1 year: I.V. infusion: Initial loading dose: 75 units/kg given over 10 minutes; then initial maintenance dose: 28 units/kg/hour; adjust dose to maintain APTT of 60-85 seconds (assuming this reflects an antifactor Xa level of 0.3-0.7); see table.

Children >1 year:

Intermittent I.V.: Initial: 50-100 units/kg, then 50-100 units/kg every 4 hours (**Note:** Continuous I.V. infusion is preferred):

I.V. infusion: Initial loading dose: 75 units/kg given over 10 minutes, then initial maintenance dose: 20 units/kg/hour; adjust dose to maintain APTT of 60-85 seconds (assuming this reflects an antifactor Xa level of 0.3-0.7); see table.

PEDIATRIC PROTOCOL FOR SYSTEMIC HEPARIN ADJUSTMENT

To be used after initial loading dose and maintenance I.V. infusion dose (see Usual

APTT (seconds)	Dosage Adjustment	Time to Repeat APTT
<50	Give 50 units/kg bolus and increase infusion rate by 10%	4 h after rate change
50-59	Increase infusion rate by 10%	4 h after rate change
60-85	Keep rate the same	Next day
86-95	Decrease infusion rate by 10%	4 h after rate change
96-120	Hold infusion for 30 minutes and decrease infusion rate by 10%	4 h after rate change
>120	Hold infusion for 60 minutes and decrease infusion rate by 15%	4 h after rate change

Modified from Monagle P, Michelson AD, Bovill E, et al, "Antithrombotic Therapy in Children," *Chest*, 2001, 119:344S-70S.

(Continued)

Heparin *(Continued)*

Dosage listed above) to maintain APTT of 60-85 seconds (assuming this reflects antifactor Xa level of 0.3-0.7)

Obtain blood for APTT 4 hours after heparin loading dose and 4 hours after every infusion rate change

Obtain daily CBC and APTT after APTT is therapeutic

Adults:

Prophylaxis (low dose heparin): SubQ: 5000 units every 8-12 hours

Intermittent I.V.: Initial: 10,000 units, then 50-70 units/kg (5000-10,000 units) every 4-6 hours

I.V. infusion: Initial loading dose: 80 units/kg; initial maintenance dose: 18 units/kg/hour with dose adjusted according to APTT; usual range: 10-30 units/kg/hour

Adults: *Chest* 2001 Recommendations (see Hirsh, 2001):

Prophylaxis of DVT and PE: SubQ: 5000 units every 8 or 12 hours or adjusted low-dose heparin

Treatment of DVT: Initial loading dose: I.V. bolus: 5000 units, then initial maintenance dose: I.V. infusion: 32,000 units/day (1333 units/hour); adjust dose to maintain therapeutic APTT; recommendations also list SubQ 35,000-40,000 units/day (**Note:** SubQ dose which was divided into 2 daily doses, is no longer used clinically)

Unstable angina or acute MI without thrombolytic therapy: Initial loading dose: I.V. bolus: 5000 units, then initial maintenance dose: I.V. infusion: 32,000 units/day (1333 units/hour); adjust dose to maintain therapeutic APTT

Acute MI after thrombolytic therapy (role of heparin unproven): Initial loading dose: I.V. bolus: 5000 units, then initial maintenance dose: I.V. infusion: 24,000 units/day (1000 units/hour); adjust dose to maintain therapeutic APTT

Administration Parenteral: Continuous I.V. infusion is preferred vs I.V. intermittent injections; heparin lock flush solutions are intended only to maintain patency of I.V. devices and are **not** for systemic anticoagulation

Monitoring Parameters Platelet counts, signs of bleeding, hemoglobin, hematocrit, APTT; for full-dose heparin (ie, nonlow dose), the dose should be titrated according to APTT (see table). For intermittent I.V. injections, APTT is measured 3.5-4 hours after I.V. injection.

Reference Range Treatment of venous thrombotic disease: Recommended APTT should reflect a heparin level by protamine titration of 0.2-0.4 units/mL or an antifactor Xa level of 0.3-0.7 units/mL; this usually reflects an APTT of 60-85 seconds or a ratio (patient/control APTT) of 1.5-2.5; a lower therapeutic range (corresponding to antifactor Xa level of 0.14-0.34 units/mL) is recommended for patients with acute MI who received thrombolytic therapy

Test Interactions ↑ thyroxine (S) (competitive protein binding methods)

Patient Information Limit alcohol

Nursing Implications Do not administer I.M. due to pain, irritation, and hematoma formation

Additional Information To reverse the effects of heparin, use protamine (see Protamine *on page 1342* for specifics); heparin is available from beef lung and from porcine intestinal mucosa sources

Duration of heparin therapy (pediatric):

DVT: At least 5 days

Extensive DVT or pulmonary embolism (PE): 7-10 days

Note: Oral anticoagulation can be started on day 1 of heparin, except for extensive DVT or PE, when it should be delayed; oral anticoagulation should be overlapped with heparin for 5 days

Dosage Forms Excipient information presented when available (limited, particularly for generics); consult specific product labeling.

Infusion, as sodium [premixed in NaCl 0.45%; porcine intestinal mucosa source]: 12,500 units (250 mL); 25,000 units (250 mL, 500 mL)

Infusion, as sodium [preservative free; premixed in D_5W; porcine intestinal mucosa source]: 10,000 units (100 mL) [contains sodium metabisulfite]; 12,500 units (250 mL) [contains sodium metabisulfite]; 20,000 units (500 mL) [contains sodium metabisulfite]; 25,000 units (250 mL, 500 mL) [contains sodium metabisulfite]

Infusion, as sodium [preservative free; premixed in NaCl 0.9%; porcine intestinal mucosa source]: 1000 units (500 mL); 2000 units (1000 mL)

Injection, solution, as sodium [lock flush preparation; porcine intestinal mucosa source; multidose vial]: 10 units/mL (1 mL, 10 mL, 30 mL) [contains parabens]; 100 units/mL (1 mL, 5 mL) [contains parabens]

Injection, solution, as sodium [lock flush preparation; porcine intestinal mucosa source; multidose vial]: 10 units/mL (10 mL, 30 mL); 100 units/mL (10 mL, 30 mL) [contains benzyl alcohol]

Hep-Lock®: 10 units/mL (1 mL, 2 mL, 10 mL, 30 mL); 100 units/mL (1 mL, 2 mL, 10 mL, 30 mL) [contains benzyl alcohol]

Injection, solution, as sodium [lock flush preparation; porcine intestinal mucosa source; prefilled syringe]: 10 units/mL (1 mL, 2 mL, 3 mL, 5 mL); 100 units/mL (1 mL, 2 mL, 3 mL, 5 mL) [contains benzyl alcohol]

Injection, solution, as sodium [preservative free; lock flush preparation; porcine intestinal mucosa source; prefilled syringe]: 100 units/mL (5 mL)

Injection, solution, as sodium [preservative free; lock flush preparation; porcine intestinal mucosa source; vial]:

HepFlush®-10: 10 units/mL (10 mL)

Hep-Lock U/P: 10 units/mL (1 mL); 100 units/mL (1 mL)

Injection, solution, as sodium [porcine intestinal mucosa source; multidose vial]: 1000 units/mL (1 mL, 10 mL, 30 mL) [contains benzyl alcohol]; 1000 units/mL (1 mL, 10 mL, 30 mL) [contains methylparabens]; 5000 units/mL (1 mL, 10 mL) [contains benzyl alcohol]; 5000 units/mL (1 mL) [contains methylparabens]; 10,000 units/mL (1 mL, 4 mL) [contains benzyl alcohol]; 10,000 units/mL (1 mL, 5 mL) [contains methylparabens]; 20,000 units/mL (1 mL) [contains methylparabens]

Injection, solution, as sodium [porcine intestinal mucosa source; prefilled syringe]: 5000 units/mL (1 mL) [contains benzyl alcohol]

Injection, solution, as sodium [preservative free; porcine intestinal mucosa source; prefilled syringe]: 10,000 units/mL (0.5 mL)

Injection, solution, as sodium [preservative free; porcine intestinal mucosa source; vial]: 1000 units/mL (2 mL); 2000 units/mL (5 mL); 2500 units/mL (10 mL)

References

Andrew M, Marzinotto V, Massicotte P, et al, "Heparin Therapy in Pediatric Patients: A Prospective Cohort Study," *Pediatr Res*, 1994, 35(1):78-83.

Hirsh J, Warkentin TE, Shaughnessy SG, et al, "Heparin and Low-Molecular Weight-Heparin: Mechanisms of Action, Pharmacokinetics, Dosing, Monitoring, Efficacy and Safety," *Chest*, 2001, 119:64S-94S.

Monagle P, Michelson AD, Bovill E, et al, "Antithrombotic Therapy in Children," *Chest*, 2001, 119:344S-70S.

♦ **Heparin Calcium** *see* Heparin *on page 758*

♦ **Heparin Lock Flush** *see* Heparin *on page 758*

♦ **Heparin Sodium** *see* Heparin *on page 758*

Hepatitis A Vaccine (hep a TYE tis aye vak SEEN)

Related Information

Immunization Guidelines *on page 1837*

U.S. Brand Names Havrix®; VAQTA®

Canadian Brand Names Avaxim®; Avaxim®-Pediatric; Havrix®; VAQTA®

Therapeutic Category Vaccine

Generic Available No

Use Active immunization for children ≥12 months to adults against disease caused by hepatitis A virus; populations desiring protection against hepatitis A or at high risk of exposure to hepatitis A virus include: Residents and travelers to areas of high endemicity, household and sexual contacts of persons infected with hepatitis A, child daycare employees, patients with chronic liver disease, illicit drug users, male homosexuals, institutional workers (eg, institutions for the mentally and physically handicapped persons, prisons), and healthcare workers who may be exposed to hepatitis A virus (eg, laboratory employees)

Pregnancy Risk Factor C

Lactation Excretion in breast milk unknown/use caution

Contraindications Hypersensitivity to hepatitis A vaccine or any component of the formulation

Warnings Treatment for anaphylactic reactions should be immediately available; primary immunization series should be completed at least 2 weeks prior to travel to an area of high endemicity; defer vaccination during the course of a moderate or severely febrile illness

Precautions Use caution in patients with serious active infection, cardiovascular disease, or pulmonary disorders; administer with caution to patients with thrombocytopenia or any coagulation disorder that would be compromised by I.M. injection; if the patient receives antihemophilia or other similar therapy, I.M. injection can be scheduled shortly after such therapy is administered.

Adverse Reactions All serious adverse reactions must be reported to the U.S. Department of Health and Human Services (DHHS) Vaccine Adverse Event Reporting System (VAERS) 1-800-822-7967.

Cardiovascular: Syncope

Central nervous system: Headache, fatigue, fever (rare), insomnia, vertigo, seizures, encephalopathy (rare), dizziness

Dermatologic: Rash, urticaria, erythema multiforme (rare)

(Continued)

Hepatitis A Vaccine *(Continued)*

Gastrointestinal: Abdominal pain, anorexia, nausea, diarrhea, dysgeusia, vomiting, pharyngitis
Hepatic: Elevated LFTs, jaundice, hepatitis
Local: Pain, tenderness, swelling, pruritus, and erythema at injection site
Neuromuscular & skeletal: Arthralgia, myalgia, neuropathy, myelitis, paresthesia, Guillain-Barré syndrome (rare)
Ophthalmic: Photophobia
Respiratory: Dyspnea
Miscellaneous: Hypersensitivity reactions, anaphylaxis

Stability Refrigerate; do not freeze

Mechanism of Action As an inactivated virus vaccine, hepatitis A vaccine offers active immunization against hepatitis A virus infection at an effective immune response rate in up to 99% of subjects

Usual Dosage I.M.:
Havrix®:
Children 2-18 years: 0.5 mL (720 ELISA units) administered as 2 injections 6-12 months apart
Adults: 1 mL (1440 ELISA units) administered as 2 injections 6-12 months apart
VAQTA®:
Children 12 months to 17 years: 25 units (0.5 mL) administered as 2 injections 6-18 months apart
Adolescents >17 years and Adults: 50 units (1 mL) administered as 2 injections 6-18 months apart

Administration Shake well and administer I.M. in either the anterolateral aspect of the thigh or deltoid muscle of the arm; **not for I.V., intradermal, or SubQ administration**

Nursing Implications Federal law requires that the date of administration, the vaccine manufacturer, lot number of vaccine, and the administering person's name, title, and address be entered into the patient's permanent medical record.

Dosage Forms Excipient information presented when available (limited, particularly for generics); consult specific product labeling.
Injection, suspension [adult formulation; preservative free]:
Havrix®: Viral antigen 1440 ELISA units/mL (1 mL) [contains trace amounts of neomycin; syringe plunger contains latex rubber; available in prefilled syringe or single-dose vial]
VAQTA®: HAV antigen 50 units/mL (1 mL) [vial stopper and syringe plunger contain latex rubber; available in prefilled syringe or single-dose vial]
Injection, suspension [pediatric formulation; preservative free]:
Havrix®: Viral antigen 720 ELISA units/0.5 mL (0.5 mL) [contains trace amounts of neomycin; syringe plunger contains latex rubber; available in prefilled syringe or single-dose vial]
Injection, suspension [pediatric/adolescent formulation; preservative free]:
VAQTA®: HAV antigen 25 units/0.5 mL (0.5 mL) [vial stopper and syringe plunger contain latex rubber; available in prefilled syringe or single-dose vial]

References
Atkinson WL, Pickering LK, Schwartz B, et al, "General Recommendations on Immunization. Recommendations of the Advisory Committee on Immunization Practices (ACIP) and the American Academy of Family Physicians (AAFP)," *MMWR Recomm Rep*, 2002, 51(RR-2):1-35.
Bancroft WH, "Hepatitis A Vaccine," *N Engl J Med*, 1992, 327(7):488-90.
Koff RS, "Hepatitis A," *Lancet*, 1998, 351(9116):1643-9.
Lemon SM, "Inactivated Hepatitis A Vaccines," *JAMA*, 1994, 271(17):1363-4.
Niu MT, Salive M, Krueger C, et al, "Two-Year Review of Hepatitis A Vaccine Safety: Data From the Vaccine Adverse Event Reporting System (VAERS)," *Clin Infect Dis*, 1998, 26(6):1475-6.

Hepatitis B Immune Globulin (hep a TYE tis bee i MYUN GLOB yoo lin)

Related Information
Immunization Guidelines *on page 1837*
Management of Healthcare Worker Exposures to HBV, HCV, and HIV *on page 1868*

U.S. Brand Names HepaGam B™; HyperHEP B™ S/D; Nabi-HB®

Canadian Brand Names HepaGam B™; HyperHep B®

Index Terms HBIG

Therapeutic Category Immune Globulin

Generic Available No

Use Provide prophylactic passive immunity to hepatitis B infection for those individuals exposed either by direct contact with hepatitis B surface antigen positive (HB_sAg-positive) materials (blood, plasma, or serum), sexual exposure to an individual who is HB_sAg-positive, or an infant <12 months of age with close "household contact" with an individual who is HB_sAg-positive; newborns of mothers known to be HB_sAg-positive.

Note: Hepatitis B immune globulin is not indicated for treatment of active hepatitis B infection and is ineffective in the treatment of chronic active hepatitis B infection.

Pregnancy Risk Factor C

Lactation Excretion in breast milk unknown/use caution

Contraindications Hypersensitivity to hepatitis B immune globulin, thimerosal, or any component

Warnings As a product of human plasma, this product may potentially transmit infectious agents such as viruses; screening of donors, as well as testing and/or inactivation of certain viruses, has reduced this risk. Not for intravenous administration. Although extremely rare, severe hypersensitivity reactions including anaphylaxis may occur; epinephrine and other anaphylactic treatment agents should be readily available.

Precautions Administer with caution to patients with thrombocytopenia or any coagulation disorder that would be compromised by I.M. injection; administer with caution in patients with IgA deficiency or a prior history of systemic allergic reactions following the administration of human immunoglobulin preparations

Adverse Reactions

Central nervous system: Dizziness, malaise, fever, lethargy, chills, headache
Dermatologic: Urticaria, angioedema, rash, erythema
Gastrointestinal: Vomiting, nausea
Genitourinary: Nephrotic syndrome
Local: Pain, tenderness, and muscular stiffness at injection site
Neuromuscular & skeletal: Arthralgia, myalgia
Miscellaneous: Anaphylaxis

Drug Interactions Antibodies in immune globulin may interfere with the response to live viral vaccines (eg, MMR, varicella); delay administration of these vaccines for approximately 3 months following immune globulin administration

Stability Refrigerate at 2°C to 8°C (36°F to 46°F); do not freeze; use within 6 hours of puncturing the vial

Mechanism of Action Passive immunity toward hepatitis B virus

Pharmacokinetics

Absorption: I.M.: Slow
Time to peak serum concentration: I.M.: 1-6 days

Usual Dosage I.M.:

Newborns of HB_sAg-positive mothers: Hepatitis B: 0.5 mL as soon after birth as possible (within 12 hours; efficacy decreases significantly if treatment is delayed >48 hours); hepatitis B vaccine series to begin at the same time; if this series is delayed for as long as 3 months, the HBIG dose may be repeated; see Hepatitis B Vaccine *on page 763*.

Postexposure prophylaxis:

Children <12 months: 0.5 mL; initiate hepatitis vaccine series

Children ≥12 months and Adults: 0.06 mL/kg as soon as possible after exposure (ie, within 24 hours of needlestick, ocular, or mucosal exposure or within 14 days of sexual exposure); usual dose: 3-5 mL; repeat at 28-30 days after exposure

Administration I.M.: Inject only in the anterolateral aspects of the upper thigh or the deltoid muscle; multiple injections may be necessary when the dosage is a large volume (postexposure prophylaxis). Do not administer hepatitis vaccine and HBIG in same syringe (vaccine will be neutralized); hepatitis vaccine may be administered at the same time at a separate site

Dosage Forms Excipient information presented when available (limited, particularly for generics); consult specific product labeling.

Note: Potency expressed in international units (as compared to the WHO standard) is noted by individual lot on the vial label.

Injection, solution [preservative free]:

HyperHEP B™ S/D: 15% to 18% (0.5 mL, 1 mL, 5 mL)
Nabi-HB®: 5% (1 mL, 5 mL) [>312 int. units/mL; contains polysorbate 80]
HepaGam B™: 5% (1 mL, 5 mL) [>312 int. units/mL; contains maltose and polysorbate 80]

♦ **Hepatitis B Inactivated Virus Vaccine (recombinant DNA)** *see* Hepatitis B Vaccine *on page 763*

Hepatitis B Vaccine (hep a TYE tis bee vak SEEN)

Medication Safety Issues

Sound-alike/look-alike issues:

Recombivax HB® may be confused with Comvax®

Related Information

Immunization Guidelines *on page 1837*
Management of Healthcare Worker Exposures to HBV, HCV, and HIV *on page 1868*

(Continued)

Hepatitis B Vaccine *(Continued)*

U.S. Brand Names Engerix-B®; Recombivax HB®

Canadian Brand Names Engerix-B®; Recombivax HB®

Index Terms Hepatitis B Inactivated Virus Vaccine (recombinant DNA)

Therapeutic Category Vaccine

Generic Available No

Use Immunization against infection caused by all known subtypes of hepatitis B virus, in individuals considered at high risk of potential exposure to hepatitis B virus or HB_sAg-positive materials: See table.

Pre-exposure Prophylaxis for Hepatitis B
Healthcare workers with blood exposure
Special patient groups (eg, adolescents, infants born to HB_sAg-positive mothers, children born after 11/21/91, military personnel, Alaskan natives, Pacific Islanders)
Hemodialysis patients
Recipients of certain blood products
Lifestyle factors
Homosexual and bisexual men
Intravenous drug abusers
Heterosexually-active persons with multiple sexual partners or recently acquired sexually-transmitted diseases
Environmental factors
Household and sexual contacts of HBV carriers
Prison inmates
Clients and staff of institutions for the mentally handicapped
Residents, immigrants, and refugees from areas with endemic HBV infection
International travelers at increased risk of acquiring HBV infection

Pregnancy Risk Factor C

Lactation Excretion in breast milk unknown/use caution

Contraindications Hypersensitivity to hepatitis vaccine, yeast, or any component of the formulation

Warnings Immediate treatment for anaphylactic reactions should be available during vaccine use; defer vaccination for persons with acute febrile illness until recovery

Precautions Use with caution in patients with coagulation disorders including thrombocytopenia, due to an increased risk for bleeding following I.M. administration; if the patient receives antihemophilia or other similar therapy, I.M. injection can be scheduled shortly after such therapy is administered; use with caution in patients with decreased cardiopulmonary function

Adverse Reactions All serious adverse reactions must be reported to the U.S. Department of Health and Human Services (DHHS) Vaccine Adverse Event Reporting System (VAERS) 1-800-822-7967.

Cardiovascular: Hypotension, syncope, tachycardia, palpitations

Central nervous system: Agitation, chills, dizziness, fatigue, fever, flushing, headache, insomnia, irritability, lightheadedness, malaise, vertigo, encephalitis, migraine, seizures, vertigo

Dermatologic: Angioedema, petechiae, pruritus, rash, urticaria, alopecia, eczema, erythema nodosum, erythema multiforme, Stevens-Johnson syndrome, purpura, keratitis

Gastrointestinal: Abdominal pain, appetite decreased, cramps, diarrhea, dyspepsia, nausea, vomiting, constipation

Genitourinary: Dysuria

Hematologic: Thrombocytopenia

Hepatic: Elevated liver enzymes

Local: Injection site reactions: Ecchymosis, erythema, induration, pain, nodule formation, soreness, swelling, tenderness, warmth

Neuromuscular & skeletal: Achiness, arthralgia, back pain, myalgia, neck pain, neck stiffness, paresthesia, shoulder pain, weakness, arthritis, Bell's palsy, Guillain-Barré syndrome, transverse myelitis, paresthesia, hypoesthesia

Ophthalmic: Conjunctivitis, optic neuritis, visual disturbances,

Otic: Earache

Respiratory: Cough, pharyngitis, rhinitis, upper respiratory tract infection, bronchospasm

Miscellaneous: Hypersensitivity reactions, lymphadenopathy, diaphoresis, serum-sickness like syndrome (may be delayed days to weeks)

Stability Refrigerate; do not freeze

Mechanism of Action Recombinant hepatitis B vaccine is a noninfectious subunit viral vaccine. The vaccine is derived from hepatitis B surface antigen (HB_sAg) produced through recombinant DNA techniques from yeast cells. The portion of the hepatitis B gene which codes for HB_sAg is cloned into yeast which is then cultured to produce hepatitis B vaccine. Promotes immunity to hepatitis B virus by inducing the production of specific antibodies to the virus.

Usual Dosage I.M.: The strengths for each brand hepatitis B vaccine are different; however, the equivalent dose by volume is the same. Combination vaccines (eg, also containing DTaP, HIB) should not be used for the "birth" dose but may be used to complete the course beginning after the infant is 6 weeks of age.

Recommended schedule: 0.5 mL/dose in 3 total doses; special circumstances for at risk infants are described below

Infants born of HB_sAg **positive** mothers: First dose should be given within the first 12 hours of life, even if premature and regardless of birth weight (hepatitis immune globulin should also be administered at the same time/different site); the second dose is administered at 1-2 months of age and the third dose at 6 months of age; anti-HB_s and HB_sAg should be checked at 9-15 months of age. If anti-HB_s and HB_sAg are negative, reimmunize with 3 doses 2 months apart and reassess. **Note:** Premature infants <2000 g should receive 4 total doses at 0, 1, 2-3, and 6-7 months of chronological age

Infants born of HB_sAg **negative** mothers: First dose should be given prior to leaving the hospital; however, the first dose may be given at 1-2 months of age; another dose is given 1-2 months later and a final dose at 6 months of age; 4 total doses of vaccine may be given if a "birth dose" is administered and a combination vaccine is used to complete the series. **Note:** Premature infants <2000 g may have the initial dose deferred up to 30 days of chronological age.

Infants born of mothers whose HB_sAg status is unknown at birth: First dose given within 12 hours of birth even if premature regardless of birth weight, second dose following 1-2 months later; the third dose at 6 months of age; if the mother's blood HB_sAg test is positive, the infant should receive hepatitis immune globulin as soon as possible (no later than age 1 week)

Children and Adolescents ≤18 years: 0.5 mL/dose in 3 total doses; first dose given on the elected date, second dose given 1 month later, third dose given 8 weeks later and at least 16 weeks after the first dose

Adults >19 years: 1 mL/dose in 3 total doses; first dose given on the elected date, second dose given 1-2 months later, third dose given 4-6 months later

Dialysis patients: <20 years: 20 mcg/dose and >20 years: 40 mcg/dose; given at 0, 1-2, and 4-6 months; repeat dose depending upon annual assessment of hepatitis B surface antigen (anti-HB) level; if anti-HB <10 milli-international units/mL administer an additional dose

Alternative schedules per manufacturer's recommendations:

Children 5-10 years: Engerix-B®: 0.5 mL for 3 doses given 12 months apart

Adolescents 11-16 years: Engerix-B®: 1 mL for 3 doses given 12 months apart

Adolescents 11-15 years: Recombivax HB®: 1 mL/dose initially and repeated 4-6 months later

Adolescents ≥11 years and Adults with recent exposure to the virus or certain travelers to high-risk areas: Engerix-B®: 1 mL for 4 doses given at 0, 1, 2, and 12 months

Administration Shake well; administer I.M. in either the anterolateral aspect of the thigh or arm; **not for I.V. or SubQ administration**

It is possible to interchange the vaccines for completion of a series or for booster doses; the antibody produced in response to each type of vaccine is comparable

Monitoring Parameters HB_sAg and antibodies to HB_sAg (anti-HB_s) should be tested in infants born to mothers positive for HB_sAg when they are 9-15 months of age; annual anti-HB in dialysis patients

Nursing Implications Federal law requires that the date of administration, the vaccine manufacturer, lot number of vaccine, and the administering person's name, title, and address be entered into the patient's permanent medical record.

Dosage Forms Excipient information presented when available (limited, particularly for generics); consult specific product labeling.

Injection, suspension [preservative free] [recombinant DNA]:

Engerix-B®:

Adult: Hepatitis B surface antigen 20 mcg/mL (1 mL) [contains trace amounts of thimerosal; some dosage forms contain dry natural latex rubber]

Pediatric/adolescent: Hepatitis B surface antigen 10 mcg/0.5 mL (0.5 mL) [contains trace amounts of thimerosal; some dosage forms contain dry natural latex rubber]

Recombivax HB®:

Adult: Hepatitis B surface antigen 10 mcg/mL (1 mL, 3 mL)

Dialysis: Hepatitis B surface antigen 40 mcg/mL (1 mL)

Pediatric/adolescent: Hepatitis B surface antigen 5 mcg/0.5 mL (0.5 mL)

(Continued)

Hepatitis B Vaccine *(Continued)*

References

American Academy of Pediatrics Committee on Infectious Diseases, "Recommended Immunization Schedules for Children and Adolescents - United States, 2007," *Pediatrics*, 2007, 119(1):207-8.

"Prevention of Hepatitis A Through Active or Passive Immunization: Recommendations of the Advisory Committee on Immunization Practices (ACIP)," *MMWR Recomm Rep*, 1999, 48(RR-12):1-37.

Centers for Disease Control, "Recommended Adult Immunization Schedule, October 2004-September 2005," availabel at www.cdc.gov.

♦ **Hepatitis b Vaccine (Recombinant)** *see Haemophilus* b Conjugate and Hepatitis B Vaccine *on page 750*

♦ **HepFlush®-10** *see* Heparin *on page 758*

♦ **Hep-Lock®** *see* Heparin *on page 758*

♦ **Hep-Lock U/P** *see* Heparin *on page 758*

♦ **Heptovir® (Can)** *see* Lamivudine *on page 901*

♦ **HES** *see* Hetastarch *on page 766*

♦ **Hespan®** *see* Hetastarch *on page 766*

Hetastarch (HET a starch)

Medication Safety Issues

Sound-alike/look-alike issues:

Hespan® may be confused with heparin

U.S. Brand Names Hespan®; Hextend®

Canadian Brand Names Hextend®; Voluven®

Index Terms HES; Hydroxyethyl Starch

Therapeutic Category Plasma Volume Expander

Generic Available Yes: Sodium chloride infusion

Use Blood volume expander used in treatment of shock or impending shock when blood or blood products are not available; does not have oxygen-carrying capacity and is not a substitute for blood or plasma

Pregnancy Risk Factor C

Lactation Excretion in breast milk unknown/use caution

Contraindications Hypersensitivity to hetastarch or any component; severe bleeding disorders, renal failure with oliguria or anuria, or severe CHF; management of cerebral vasospasm associated with subarachnoid hemorrhage or for conditions other than leukapheresis which necessitate repeated use of the drug over several days; per manufacturer, Hextend® is contraindicated in the treatment of lactic acidosis and in leukapheresis

Warnings Anaphylactoid reactions have occurred; use with caution in patients with thrombocytopenia (may interfere with platelet function); large volume may cause drops in hemoglobin concentrations; use with caution in patients at risk from overexpansion of blood volume, including the very young or aged patients, those with CHF or pulmonary edema; large volumes (>1500 mL) may interfere with platelet function and prolong PT and PTT times; use with caution in patients with a history of liver disease

Precautions Use with caution in patients allergic to corn (may have cross allergy to hetastarch). Note electrolyte content of Hextend® including calcium, lactate, and potassium (see Additional Information); use with caution in situations where electrolyte and/or acid-base disturbances may be exacerbated (renal impairment, respiratory alkalosis).

Adverse Reactions

Cardiovascular: Heart failure, circulatory overload, peripheral edema

Central nervous system: Headache, fever, chills, intracranial bleeding

Dermatologic: Urticaria, pruritus, rash

Endocrine & metabolic: Parotid gland enlargement, hyperchloremic metabolic acidosis, hypernatremia

Gastrointestinal: Vomiting, elevated amylase levels

Hematologic: Thrombocytopenia, transient prolongation of PT, PTT, clotting time, and bleeding time, anemia, DIC (rare), hemolysis (rare)

Hepatic: Elevated indirect bilirubin

Neuromuscular & skeletal: Myalgia

Ocular: Periorbital edema

Respiratory: Wheezing

Miscellaneous: Anaphylactoid reactions, flu-like symptoms

Stability Store at room temperature; do not freeze; do not use if crystalline precipitate forms or is turbid deep brown

Mechanism of Action Hetastarch. a synthetic polymer, produces plasma volume expansion by virtue of its highly colloidal starch structure

Pharmacodynamics

Onset of volume expansion: I.V.: Within 30 minutes

Duration: 24-36 hours

Pharmacokinetics

Metabolism: Molecules >50,000 daltons require enzymatic degradation by the reticuloendothelial system or amylases in the blood prior to urinary and fecal excretion

Elimination: Smaller molecular weight molecules are readily excreted in urine; approximately 40% of dose excreted in first 24 hours in patients with normal renal function

Usual Dosage I.V. infusion:

Children: 10 mL/kg/dose; the total daily dose should not exceed 20 mL/kg

Adults: 500-1000 mL (30-60 g) per dose; the total daily dose should not exceed 1.2 g/kg or 90 g (1500 mL)

Dosing adjustment in renal impairment: Cl_{cr} <10 mL/minute: Initial dose is the same but subsequent doses should be reduced by 20% to 50% of normal

Administration Parenteral: I.V.: Maximum rate of infusion: 1.2 g/kg/hour (20 mL/kg/hour)

Monitoring Parameters Volume expansion: capillary refill time, CVP, RAP, MAP, urine output, heart rate, if pulmonary artery catheter in place, monitor PWCP, SVR, and PVR; hemoglobin, hematocrit; for leukapheresis, monitor CBC, total leukocyte and platelet counts, leukocyte differential count, hemoglobin, hematocrit, prothrombin time, and partial thromboplastin time

Additional Information Hetastarch is a synthetic polymer derived from a waxy starch composed of amylopectin, average molecular weight = 450,000; each liter of Hespan® provides 154 mEq sodium chloride; each liter of Hextend® contains the following electrolytes: Sodium 143 mEq, chloride 124 mEq, lactate 28 mEq, calcium 5 mEq, magnesium 0.9 mEq, potassium 3 mEq, and dextrose 0.99 g

Dosage Forms Excipient information presented when available (limited, particularly for generics); consult specific product labeling.

Infusion [premixed in lactated electrolyte injection] (Hextend®): 6% (500 mL)

Infusion, solution [premixed in NaCl 0.9%] (Hespan®): 6% (500 mL)

References

Brutocao D, Bratton SL, Thomas JR, et al, "Comparison of Hetastarch With Albumin for Postoperative Volume Expansion in Children After Cardiopulmonary Bypass," *J Cardiothoracic Vasc Anesth*, 1996, 10(3):348-51.

♦ **Hexachlorocyclohexane** *see* Lindane *on page 939*

Hexachlorophene (heks a KLOR oh feen)

Medication Safety Issues

Sound-alike/look-alike issues:

pHisoHex® may be confused with Fostex®, pHisoDerm®

U.S. Brand Names pHisoHex®

Canadian Brand Names pHisoHex®

Therapeutic Category Antibacterial, Topical; Soap

Generic Available No

Use Surgical scrub and as a bacteriostatic skin cleanser; to control an outbreak of gram-positive staphylococcal infection when other infection control procedures have been unsuccessful

Pregnancy Risk Factor C

Contraindications Hypersensitivity to halogenated phenol derivatives or hexachlorophene; use in premature infants; use on burned or denuded skin; use with an occlusive dressing; application to mucous membranes

Warnings Do not use for bathing infants; do not apply to mucous membranes; premature and low birth weight infants are particularly susceptible to hexachlorophene topical absorption; irritability, generalized clonic muscular contractions, decerebrate rigidity, and brain lesions in the white matter have occurred in infants following topical use of 6% hexachlorophene; exposure of preterm infants or patients with extensive burns has been associated with apnea, convulsions, agitation, and coma

Adverse Reactions

Central nervous system: CNS injury, seizures, irritability

Dermatologic: Dermatitis, erythema, dry skin, photosensitivity

Drug Interactions Polysorbate 80, nonionic detergents with concentration >8% may decrease antibacterial activity of hexachlorophene

Stability Store in nonmetallic container (incompatible with many metals); protect from light

Mechanism of Action Bacteriostatic polychlorinated biphenol which inhibits membrane-bound enzymes and disrupts the cell membrane

Pharmacokinetics

Absorption: Percutaneously through inflamed, excoriated and intact skin

(Continued)

Hexachlorophene *(Continued)*

Distribution: Crosses the placenta

Half-life, infants: 6.1-44.2 hours

Usual Dosage Children and Adults: Topical: Apply 5 mL cleanser and water to area to be cleansed; lather and rinse thoroughly under running water; for use as a surgical scrub, a second application of 5 mL cleanser should be made and the hands and forearms scrubbed for an additional 3 minutes, rinsed thoroughly with running water and dried

Administration Topical: For external use only; rinse thoroughly after each use

Patient Information Avoid prolonged contact with skin. May cause photosensitivity reactions (eg, exposure to sunlight may cause severe sunburn, skin rash, redness, or itching); avoid exposure to sunlight and artificial light sources (sunlamps, tanning booth/bed); wear protective clothing, wide-brimmed hats, sunglasses, and lip sunscreen (SPF ≥15); use a sunscreen [broad-spectrum sunscreen or physical sunscreen (preferred) or sunblock with SPF ≥15]; contact physician if reaction occurs.

Dosage Forms Excipient information presented when available (limited, particularly for generics); consult specific product labeling.

Liquid, topical: 3% (150 mL, 500 mL, 3840 mL)

References

Lester RS, "Topical Formulary for the Pediatrician," *Pediatr Clin North Am*, 1983, 30(4):749-65.

- ♦ **Hexamethylenetetramine** *see* Methenamine *on page 1021*
- ♦ **Hexit™ (Can)** *see* Lindane *on page 939*
- ♦ **Hextend®** *see* Hetastarch *on page 766*
- ♦ **hGH** *see* Human Growth Hormone *on page 769*
- ♦ **Hib Conjugate Vaccine** *see Haemophilus* b Conjugate and Hepatitis B Vaccine *on page 750*
- ♦ **Hib Conjugate Vaccine** *see Haemophilus* b Conjugate Vaccine *on page 751*
- ♦ **Hibiclens® [OTC]** *see* Chlorhexidine Gluconate *on page 337*
- ♦ **Hibidil® 1:2000 (Can)** *see* Chlorhexidine Gluconate *on page 337*
- ♦ **Hibistat® [OTC]** *see* Chlorhexidine Gluconate *on page 337*
- ♦ **Hib Polysaccharide Conjugate** *see Haemophilus* b Conjugate Vaccine *on page 751*
- ♦ **HibTITER®** *see Haemophilus* b Conjugate Vaccine *on page 751*
- ♦ **High Gamma Vitamin E Complete™ [OTC]** *see* Vitamin E *on page 1620*
- ♦ **Hiprex®** *see* Methenamine *on page 1021*
- ♦ **Histex™ SR** *see* Brompheniramine and Pseudoephedrine *on page 235*
- ♦ **Hi-Vegi-Lip [OTC]** *see* Pancreatin *on page 1202*
- ♦ **Hivid® [DSC]** *see* Zalcitabine [DSC] *on page 1634*
- ♦ **Hivid® (Can)** *see* Zalcitabine [DSC] *on page 1634*
- ♦ **HMS Liquifilm® [DSC]** *see* Medrysone *on page 992*
- ♦ **HN_2** *see* Mechlorethamine *on page 987*
- ♦ **Hold® DM [OTC]** *see* Dextromethorphan *on page 477*

Homatropine (hoe MA troe peen)

U.S. Brand Names Isopto® Homatropine

Index Terms Homatropine Hydrobromide

Therapeutic Category Anticholinergic Agent, Ophthalmic; Ophthalmic Agent, Mydriatic

Generic Available No

Use Producing cycloplegia and mydriasis for refraction; treatment of acute inflammatory conditions of the uveal tract

Pregnancy Risk Factor C

Contraindications Hypersensitivity to homatropine or any component; narrow-angle glaucoma, acute hemorrhage

Precautions Use with caution in patients with hypertension, cardiac disease, increased intraocular pressure, obstructive uropathy, paralytic ileus, or ulcerative colitis

Adverse Reactions

Cardiovascular: Vascular congestion, edema

Central nervous system: Drowsiness

Dermatologic: Eczematoid dermatitis

Ocular: Follicular conjunctivitis, blurred vision, elevated intraocular pressure, stinging, exudate

Mechanism of Action Blocks response of iris sphincter muscle and the accommodative muscle of the ciliary body to cholinergic stimulation resulting in dilation and loss of accommodation

Pharmacodynamics Ophthalmic:

Onset of accommodation and pupil action:

Maximum mydriatic effect: Within 10-30 minutes

Maximum cycloplegic effect: Within 30-90 minutes

Duration:

Mydriasis: Persists for 6 hours to 4 days

Cycloplegia: 10-48 hours

Usual Dosage Ophthalmic:

Children:

Mydriasis and cycloplegia for refraction: Instill 1 drop of 2% solution immediately before the procedure; repeat at 10-minute intervals as needed

Uveitis: Instill 1 drop of 2% solution 2-3 times/day

Adults:

Mydriasis and cycloplegia for refraction: Instill 1-2 drops of 2% solution or 1 drop of 5% solution before the procedure; repeat at 5- to 10-minute intervals as needed

Uveitis: Instill 1-2 drops of either 2% or 5% solution 2-3 times/day up to every 3-4 hours as needed

Administration Ophthalmic: Finger pressure should be applied to lacrimal sac for 1-2 minutes after instillation to decrease risk of absorption and systemic effects

Dosage Forms Excipient information presented when available (limited, particularly for generics); consult specific product labeling.

Solution, ophthalmic, as hydrobromide: 2% (5 mL); 5% (5 mL, 15 mL) [contains benzalkonium chloride]

- **Homatropine Hydrobromide** *see* Homatropine *on page 768*
- **Horse Antihuman Thymocyte Gamma Globulin** *see* Antithymocyte Globulin (Equine) *on page 146*
- **H.P. Acthar® Gel** *see* Corticotropin *on page 402*
- **HPMPC** *see* Cidofovir *on page 353*
- **HPV Vaccine** *see* Papillomavirus (Types 6, 11, 16, 18) Recombinant Vaccine *on page 1212*
- **Humalog®** *see* Insulin Lispro *on page 844*
- **Humalog® Mix 25 (Can)** *see* Insulin Lispro Protamine and Insulin Lispro *on page 845*
- **Humalog® Mix 50/50™** *see* Insulin Lispro Protamine and Insulin Lispro *on page 845*
- **Humalog® Mix 75/25™** *see* Insulin Lispro Protamine and Insulin Lispro *on page 845*
- **Human Diploid Cell Cultures Rabies Vaccine** *see* Rabies Virus Vaccine *on page 1364*

Human Growth Hormone (HYU man grothe HOR mone)

Medication Safety Issues

Sound-alike/look-alike issues:

Somatrem may be confused with somatropin

Somatropin may be confused with somatrem, sumatriptan

International issues:

Genotropin® may be confused with Genatropine® which is a brand name for atropine in France

U.S. Brand Names Genotropin®; Genotropin Miniquick®; Humatrope®; Norditropin®; Norditropin® NordiFlex®; Nutropin®; Nutropin AQ®; Omnitrope™; Saizen®; Serostim®; Tev-Tropin®; Zorbtive®

Canadian Brand Names Humatrope®; Nutropin® AQ; Nutropine®; Saizen®; Serostim®

Index Terms hGH; Human Growth Hormone; Somatrem

Therapeutic Category Growth Hormone

Generic Available No

Use

Children: Long-term treatment of growth failure as a result of lack or inadequate endogenous growth hormone secretion, Prader-Willi syndrome, birth at small for gestational age (SGA) with failure to catch-up growth by 2 years of age; chronic renal insufficiency (up until the time of renal transplantation); short stature associated with Turner syndrome (in patients whose epiphyses are not closed); idiopathic short stature (also known as nongrowth hormone-deficient short stature) defined by height more than 2.25 standard deviations below the mean for age and sex

Adults: Growth hormone deficiency as a result of pituitary disease, hypothalamic disease, surgery, radiation, or trauma

(Continued)

Human Growth Hormone *(Continued)*

Genotropin®, Norditropin®, Saizen®: Adults with growth hormone deficiency during childhood who have this deficiency confirmed as an adult prior to growth hormone replacement

Serostim®: Treatment of AIDS-related wasting or cachexia

Zorbtive™: Treatment of short-bowel syndrome (in conjunction with nutritional support)

Pregnancy Risk Factor C; Saizen®, Serostim® and Zorbtive™ (only): B

Lactation Excretion in breast milk unknown/not recommended

Contraindications Hypersensitivity to human growth hormone or any component (see Warnings); patients with Prader-Willi syndrome who are severely obese or have severe respiratory impairment; do not use for growth promotion in pediatric patients with closed epiphyses; patients with acute critical illness due to complications following open heart or abdominal surgery, multiple accidental trauma, or acute respiratory failure; patients with active neoplasia, patients with proliferative or preproliferative diabetic retinopathy

Warnings Fatalities in pediatric patients with Prader-Willi syndrome following the use of growth hormone have been reported; these fatalities occurred in patients with one or more risk factors, including severe obesity, sleep apnea, respiratory impairment, or unidentified respiratory infection. In addition, male patients may be at increased risk. Treatment interruption is recommended in patients who show signs of upper airway obstruction, including the onset of or increased snoring. In addition, evaluation of and/or monitoring for sleep apnea and respiratory infections are recommended. 35% of childhood-onset adult GH-deficient subjects treated with growth hormone 0.025 mg/kg/day for 2 years had supraphysiologic levels of insulin-like growth factor-1 (IGF-1) identified during research studies, the risks of this elevation are unknown at this time; the manufacturer recommends reduction in dosage if IGF-1 levels are excessive.

Diluents for Nutropin®, Protropin®, Saizen®, and Zorbtive™ contain benzyl alcohol which may cause allergic reactions in susceptible individuals; large amounts of benzyl alcohol (≥99 mg/kg/day) have been associated with a potentially fatal toxicity ("gasping syndrome") in neonates; the "gasping syndrome" consists of metabolic acidosis, respiratory distress, gasping respirations, CNS dysfunction (including convulsions, intracranial hemorrhage), hypotension and cardiovascular collapse; *in vitro* and animal studies have shown that benzoate, a metabolite of benzyl alcohol, displaces bilirubin from protein-binding sites; avoid use of benzyl alcohol containing diluents in neonates.

Intracranial hypertension with papilledema, visual changes, headache, nausea, and/or vomiting has been reported; this has occurred during the first 8 weeks of therapy; all reported cases were reversible upon discontinuation of therapy; baseline and regular fundoscopic exams are recommended for assistance in recognizing this potential adverse effect.

Precautions Use with caution in patients with diabetes or family history of diabetes; use with caution in patients with evidence of active malignancy, progression of any underlying intracranial lesion, or actively growing intracranial tumor; monitor these patients closely for progression or recurrence of the underlying disease process; insulin dosage may require adjustment when growth hormone therapy is instituted; patients with hypopituitarism may develop hypothyroidism during growth hormone therapy; children may develop slipped capital epiphyses during therapy; progression of scoliosis may occur in patients with a history of scoliosis

Adverse Reactions

Cardiovascular: Mild transient edema, hypertension

Central nervous system: Headache, intracranial hypertension, insomnia; Zorbtive™: Fever, malaise, dizziness

Dermatologic: Rash, increased growth of pre-existing nevi; local lipoatrophy or lipodystrophy (SubQ administration); Zorbtive™: Swelling of hands and feet; Saizen®: Exacerbation of pre-existing psoriasis

Endocrine & metabolic: Reversible hypothyroidism (reported in pituitary-derived growth hormone), mild hyperglycemia; gynecomastia (rare), hyperlipidemia

Gastrointestinal: Pancreatitis (rare); Zorbtive™: Flatulence, vomiting, nausea, abdominal pain, gastritis, gastroenteritis, pharyngitis

Hematologic: Small risk for developing leukemia

Local: Pain at injection site

Neuromuscular & skeletal: Carpal tunnel syndrome (rare); pain in hip, knee, and back; scoliosis; myalgia, weakness; Saizen® and Zorbtive™: Musculoskeletal pain, swelling, stiffness, arthralgia

Otic: Otitis media

Renal: Glucosuria

Respiratory: Rhinitis

Miscellaneous: Flu-like syndrome, hypersensitivity reactions

Drug Interactions Corticosteroids may inhibit growth hormone activity

Stability For long-term storage, refrigerate all products except Zorbtive™, do not freeze; Zorbtive™ is stable at room temperature prior to reconstitution; once reconstituted with diluents containing preservatives and refrigerated, Humotrope®, Nutropin®, Protropin®, Saizen®, Tev-Tropin™, and Zorbtive™ are stable for 14 days, Genotropin® is stable for 21 days, and Humotrope® cartridges are stable for 28 days; Nutropin® AQ (aqueous form) is stable for 28 days after initial entry; Nutropin Depot® must be used immediately after reconstitution. Genotropin MiniQuick® is stable prior to reconstitution for up to 3 months at room temperature. If diluents without preservatives are used, stability is 24 hours refrigerated. Zorbtive™ should be used immediately after reconstitution. After a Norditropen® cartridge has been inserted into the NordiPen® injector, it is stable (in the pen) refrigerated for 4 weeks. Humatrope® cartridges may only be reconstituted with provided diluent; do not substitute with diluent provided with Humatrope® multiuse vials.

Mechanism of Action Somatropin and somatrem are purified polypeptide hormones of recombinant DNA origin; somatropin contains the identical sequence of amino acids found in human growth hormone while somatrem's amino acid sequence is identical plus an additional amino acid, methionine; human growth hormone stimulates growth of linear bone, skeletal muscle, and organs; stimulates erythropoietin which increases red blood cell mass; exerts both insulin-like and diabetogenic effects; in short-bowel syndrome, growth hormone may directly stimulate receptors in the intestinal mucosa or indirectly stimulate the production of insulin-like growth factor-I which is known to mediate many of the cellular actions of growth hormone

Pharmacokinetics

Absorption: I.M., SubQ: Well absorbed

Distribution: V_d:

- Somatrem: 50 mL/kg
- Somatropin: 70 mL/kg

Metabolism: ~90% of dose metabolized in the liver and kidney cells

Bioavailability:

- SubQ:
  - Somatrem: 81% ± 20%
  - Somatropin: 75%
- I.M.: Somatropin: 63%

Half-life:

- SubQ:
  - Somatrem: 2.3 ± 0.42 hours
  - Somatropin: 3.8 hours
- I.M.: Somatropin: 4.9 hours

Elimination: 0.1% of dose excreted in urine unchanged

Usual Dosage

I.M., SubQ (preferred route); not for I.V. injection: **Note:** Human growth hormone therapy should be individualized; discontinue therapy when the patient has reached satisfactory adult height, when epiphyses have fused, or when the patient ceases to respond. Growth ≥5 cm/year is expected, if growth rate does not exceed 2.5 cm in a 6-month period, double the dose for the next 6 months, if there is still no satisfactory response, discontinue therapy.

Growth hormone inadequacy:

- Children:
  - Somatrem (Protropin®): 0.3 mg/kg (0.9 international units/kg) **weekly** divided into daily doses
  - Somatropin:
    - Genotropin®: 0.16-0.24 mg/kg **weekly** divided into daily doses (6-7 doses)
    - Humatrope®: 0.18 mg/kg (0.54 international units/kg) **weekly** divided into equal doses given either on alternate days or 6 times per week; maximum **weekly** dosage: 0.3 mg/kg (0.9 international units/kg)
    - Norditropin®: 0.024-0.034 mg/kg/dose (0.07-0.1 international units/kg/dose) 6-7 times per week
    - Nutropin®: 0.3 mg/kg (0.9 international units/kg) **weekly** divided into daily doses; in pubertal patients, dosage may be increased to 0.7 mg/kg (2.1 international units/kg) **weekly** divided into daily doses
    - Saizen®: 0.06 mg/kg (0.18 international units/kg) 3 times per week
    - Tev-Tropin™: 0.1 mg/kg (0.3 international units/kg) 3 times per week
    - Nutropin® Depot™: SubQ only:
      - Once-monthly injection: 1.5 mg/kg body weight administered on the same day of each month; patients >15 kg will require more than one injection per dose
      - Twice-monthly injection: 0.75 mg/kg body weight administered twice each month on the same days of each month (eg, days 1 and 15 of each month); patients >30 kg will require more than one injection per dose; twice monthly dosing is recommended in patients >45 kg

(Continued)

Human Growth Hormone *(Continued)*

Adults: **Note:** To minimize adverse events in older or overweight patients, reduced dosages may be necessary. During therapy, dosage should be decreased if required by the occurrence of side effects or excessive IGF-1 levels.

Norditropin®: SubQ: Initial dose ≤0.004 mg/kg/day; after 6 weeks of therapy, may increase dose to 0.016 mg/kg/day

Nutropin®, Nutropin® AQ: SubQ: ≤0.006 mg/kg/day; dose may be increased according to individual requirements, up to a maximum of 0.025 mg/kg/day in patients <35 years of age, or up to a maximum of 0.0125 mg/kg/day in patients ≥35 years of age

Humatrope®: SubQ: ≤0.006 mg/kg/day; dose may be increased according to individual requirements, up to a maximum of 0.0125 mg/kg/day

Genotropin®, Omnitrope™: SubQ: Weekly dosage: ≤0.04 mg/kg divided into 6-7 doses; dose may be increased at 4- to 8-week intervals according to individual requirements, to a maximum of 0.08 mg/kg/week

Saizen®: SubQ: ≤0.005 mg/kg/day; dose may be increased to not more than 0.01 mg/kg/day after 4 weeks, based on individual requirements.

Idiopathic short stature: Children:

Humatrope®: 0.37 mg/kg **weekly** divided into daily doses (6-7 doses)

Nutropin®, Nutropin® AQ: Up to 0.3 mg/kg **weekly** divided into daily doses

Chronic renal insufficiency: Children: Nutropin®: 0.35 mg/kg (approximately 1.05 international units/kg) **weekly**; may be continued until time of transplantation

Prader-Willi syndrome: Children: Genotropin®: 0.24 mg/kg **weekly** divided daily into 6-7 doses per week

Children SGA at birth: Genotropin®: 0.48 mg/kg **weekly** divided daily into 6-7 doses per week

Turner syndrome: Children:

Genotropin®: Weekly dosage 0.33 mg/kg divided into 6-7 doses/week

Humatrope®: Weekly dosage ≤0.375 mg/kg (1.125 international units/kg) divided into equal doses daily or on 3 alternate days

Nutropin®, Nutropin® AQ: Weekly dosage of up to 0.375 mg/kg divided into equal doses 3-7 times/week

AIDS-related wasting or cachexia: Serostim®:

Children (limited information): 0.04-0.07 mg/kg/day for 4 weeks

Adults: Administered once daily at bedtime:

<35 kg: 0.1 mg/kg

35-44 kg: 4 mg

45-55 kg: 5 mg

>55 kg: 6 mg

Short-bowel syndrome: Adults: Zorbtive™: SubQ: 0.1 mg/kg daily not to exceed 8 mg/day; treatment >4 weeks has not been studied adequately. Excessive fluid retention or arthralgias may be treated symptomatically or by a 50% dosage reduction; stop therapy for up to 5 days prior to lowering dosage if symptoms are severe; if symptoms do not resolve after 5 days or recur with the lowered dosage, discontinue treatment.

Administration Parenteral: Administer SubQ (preferred route) or I.M.; not for I.V. injection; do not shake vial; rotate injection site; administer into the thigh, buttock, or abdomen; limit SubQ injection volume to 1 mL per site

Somatrem: Protropin®: Reconstitute each 5 mg vial with 1-5 mL and each 10 mg vial with 1-10 mL bacteriostatic SWI containing benzyl alcohol; when using in neonates, reconstitute with preservative free SWI

Somatropin:

Genotropin® cartridges: Reconstitute with provided diluent resulting in the following concentrations: 1.5 mg cartridge = 1.3 mg/mL (4 international units/mL), 5.8 mg cartridge = 5 mg/mL (15 international units/mL), and 13.8 mg cartridge = 12 mg/mL (36 international units/mL)

Nutropin®: Reconstitute each 5 mg vial with 1.5-5 mL diluent

Norditropin® Cartridges: Must be used with the NordiPen® injection pen (each cartridge has a color-coded injection pen which is graduated to deliver the appropriate dose); do not interchange

Nutropin® Depot™: Reconstitute vials with provided diluent only, resulting in 19 mg/mL concentration; swirl vigorously for 2 minutes until all the powder is fully dispersed; withdraw measured dose, change to a new needle, and administer immediately to avoid settling of the suspension in the syringe; inject SubQ at a continuous rate over no more than 5 seconds

Saizen®: Reconstitute 5 mg vial with 1-3 mL provided diluent and 8.8 mg vial with 2-3 mL provided diluent (diluent contains benzyl alcohol); swirl vial with gentle rotary motion; do not shake

Tev-Tropin™: Reconstitute with 1-5 mL NS (bacteriostatic NS is provided; NS without preservative may be used in neonates); swirl gently; do not shake.

Cloudiness may occur when stored in the refrigerator after reconstitution. Allow solution to warm to room temperature. If cloudiness persists, do not use.

Zorbtive™: Reconstitute each 4 mg, 5 mg, or 6 mg vial with 0.5 mL or 1 mL preservative free SWI; reconstitute 8.8 mg vial with 1 mL or 2 mL diluent (contains benzyl alcohol)

Note: When treating chronic renal insufficiency patients, growth hormone should be administered as follows: in hemodialysis patients, administer injection at night just prior to sleeping and at least 3-4 hours after dialysis; in chronic cycling peritoneal dialysis patients, administer injection in the morning after dialysis; in chronic ambulatory peritoneal dialysis patients administer injection in the evening at the time of the overnight exchange.

Monitoring Parameters Growth curve, periodic thyroid function tests, bone age (annually), periodical urine testing for glucose, somatomedin C levels; fundoscopic exams (see Warnings); progression of scoliosis and clinical evidence of slipped capital femoral epiphysis such as a limp or hip or knee pain

Patient Information Report the development of a severe headache, acute visual changes, a limp or complaints of hip or knee pain to your physician

Additional Information SubQ administration can cause local lipoatrophy or lipodystrophy and may enhance the development of neutralizing antibodies

Dosage Forms Excipient information presented when available (limited, particularly for generics); consult specific product labeling.

Injection, powder for reconstitution [rDNA origin]:

Genotropin®: 5.8 mg [~15 int. units/mL; delivers 5 mg/mL]; 13.8 mg [~36 int. units/mL; delivers 12 mg/mL]

Genotropin Miniquick® [preservative free]: 0.2 mg, 0.4 mg, 0.6 mg, 0.8 mg, 1 mg, 1.2 mg, 1.4 mg, 1.6 mg, 1.8 mg, 2 mg [each strength delivers 0.25 mL]

Humatrope®: 5 mg [~15 int. units], 6 mg [18 int. units], 12 mg [36 int. units], 24 mg [72 int. units]

Nutropin®: 5 mg [~15 int. units; packaged with diluent containing benzyl alcohol]; 10 mg [~30 int. units; packaged with diluent containing benzyl alcohol]

Omnitrope™: 1.5 mg [~4.5 int. units; packaged with preservative free diluent]; 5.8 mg [~17.4 int. units; packaged with diluent containing benzyl alcohol]

Tev-Tropin®: 5 mg [15 int. units/mL; packaged with diluent containing benzyl alcohol]

Saizen®: 5 mg [~15 int. units; contains sucrose 34.2 mg; packaged with diluent containing benzyl alcohol]; 8.8 mg [~26.4 int. units; contains sucrose 60.2 mg; packaged with diluent containing benzyl alcohol]

Serostim®: 4 mg [12 int. units; contains sucrose 27.3 mg]; 5 mg [15 int. units; contains sucrose 34.2 mg]; 6 mg [18 int. units; contains sucrose 41 mg]

Zorbtive®: 8.8 mg [~26.4 int. units; contains sucrose 60.19 mg; packaged with diluent containing benzyl alcohol]

Injection, solution [rDNA origin]:

Norditropin®: 5 mg/1.5 mL (1.5 mL); 15 mg/1.5 mL (1.5 mL) [prefilled cartridge]

Norditropin® NordiFlex®: 5 mg/1.5 mL (1.5 mL); 10 mg/1.5 mL (1.5 mL); 15 mg/1.5 mL (1.5 mL) [prefilled pen]

Nutropin AQ®: 5 mg/mL (2 mL) [~15 int. units/mL; vial or cartridge]

References

Howrie DL, "Growth Hormone for the Treatment of Growth Failure in Children," *Clin Pharm*, 1987, 6(4):283-91.

- **Human Growth Hormone** *see* Human Growth Hormone *on page 769*
- **Human Papillomavirus Vaccine** *see* Papillomavirus (Types 6, 11, 16, 18) Recombinant Vaccine *on page 1212*
- **Humate-P®** *see* Antihemophilic Factor/von Willebrand Factor Complex (Human) *on page 141*
- **Humatin®** *see* Paromomycin *on page 1217*
- **Humatrope®** *see* Human Growth Hormone *on page 769*
- **Humegon® (Can)** *see* Chorionic Gonadotropin *on page 351*
- **Humulin® 20/80 (Can)** *see* Insulin NPH and Insulin Regular *on page 847*
- **Humulin® 50/50** *see* Insulin NPH and Insulin Regular *on page 847*
- **Humulin® 70/30** *see* Insulin NPH and Insulin Regular *on page 847*
- **Humulin® N** *see* Insulin NPH *on page 846*
- **Humulin® R** *see* Insulin Regular *on page 849*
- **Humulin® R (Concentrated) U-500** *see* Insulin Regular *on page 849*
- **Hurricaine® [OTC]** *see* Benzocaine *on page 204*

Hyaluronidase (hye al yoor ON i dase)

Medication Safety Issues
Sound-alike/look-alike issues:
Wydase may be confused with Lidex®, Wyamine®

Related Information
Extravasation Treatment *on page 1726*

U.S. Brand Names Amphadase™; Hydase™; Hylenex™; Vitrase®

Therapeutic Category Antidote, Extravasation

Generic Available No

Use Increase the dispersion and absorption of other drugs; increase rate of absorption of parenteral fluids given by hypodermoclysis; adjunct in subcutaneous urography for improving resorption of radiopaque agents; management of I.V. extravasations

Pregnancy Risk Factor C

Lactation Excretion in breast milk unknown/use caution

Contraindications Hypersensitivity to hyaluronidase or any component; do not inject in or around infected, inflamed, or cancerous areas; do not use to reduce the swelling of bites or stings; do not apply directly to the cornea; do not administer intravenously (enzyme is rapidly inactivated)

Warnings Drug infiltrates in which hyaluronidase is **not** the extravasation management of choice include dopamine and alpha agonists

Precautions Hypersensitivity reactions may occur; a preliminary intradermal skin test should be performed utilizing 0.02 mL of a 150 units/mL solution. Discontinue hyaluronidase if sensitization occurs.

Adverse Reactions
Cardiovascular: Tachycardia, hypotension
Central nervous system: Dizziness, chills
Dermatologic: Urticaria, erythema, angioedema
Gastrointestinal: Nausea, vomiting
Local: Edema

Drug Interactions Salicylates, cortisone, ACTH, estrogens, antihistamines (decrease effectiveness of hyaluronidase); hyaluronidase may increase absorption and toxicity of local anesthetics if administered together.

Stability Hyaluronidase is incompatible with furosemide, benzodiazepines and phenytoin.
Amphadase™, Hydase™, Hylenex™: Store in refrigerator; do not freeze
Vitrase®: Store unopened vial in refrigerator; after reconstitution, stable for 6 hours at room temperature.

Mechanism of Action Modifies the permeability of connective tissue through hydrolysis of hyaluronic acid, one of the chief ingredients of tissue cement which offers resistance to diffusion of liquids through tissues; hyaluronidase increases both the distribution and absorption of locally injected substances

Pharmacodynamics
Onset of action by the SubQ or intradermal routes for the treatment of extravasation: Immediate
Duration: 24-48 hours

Usual Dosage
Infants and Children: Management of I.V. extravasation: SubQ, intradermal: Take 0.1 mL of the hyaluronidase 150 units/mL solution and dilute with 0.9 mL NS to yield 15 units/mL; using a 25- or 26-gauge needle, five 0.2 mL injections are made subcutaneously or intradermally into the extravasation site at the leading edge, changing the needle after each injection; **Note**: Some centers utilize a 150 units/mL hyaluronidase solution and, without further dilution, administer 0.2 mL injections subcutaneously or intradermally into the extravasation site at the leading edge
Adults: Absorption and dispersion of drugs: I.M., SubQ: 150 units is added to the vehicle containing the drug
Urography: SubQ: Children and Adults: 75 units over each scapula followed by injection of contrast medium at the same site; patient should be in the prone position during drug administration
Hypodermoclysis: SubQ: 15 units is added to each 100 mL of I.V. fluid to be administered
Premature Infants and Neonates: Volume of a single clysis should not exceed 25 mL/kg and the rate of administration should not exceed 2 mL/minute
Children <3 years: Volume of a single clysis should not exceed 200 mL
Children ≥3 years and Adults: Rate and volume of a single clysis should not exceed those used for infusion of I.V. fluids

Administration Management of intravenous extravasations: Do not administer I.V.; stop the infusion and remove needle; elevate extremity; administer hyaluronidase within the first few minutes to 1 hour after the extravasation is recognized

Monitoring Parameters Observe appearance of lesion for induration, swelling, discoloration, blanching, and blister formation every 15 minutes for ~2 hours

Patient Information

Notify physician if pain, redness, swelling, unusual skin rash at or around injection site, swelling of mouth or lips; difficulty breathing or sudden dizziness occurs.

Dosage Forms Excipient information presented when available (limited, particularly for generics); consult specific product labeling.

Injection, powder for reconstitution:

Vitrase®: 6200 units [ovine derived; contains lactose]

Injection, solution:

Amphadase™: 150 units/mL (1 mL) [bovine derived; contains edetate disodium 1 mg, thimerosal ≤0.1 mg]

Injection, solution [preservative free]:

Hydase™: 150 units/mL (2 mL) [bovine derived; contains edetate disodium 1 mg]

Hylenex™: 150 units/mL (1 mL, 2 mL) [recombinant; contains human albumin and edetate disodium]

Vitrase®: 200 units/mL (2 mL) [ovine derived; contains lactulose]

References

Raszka WV, Keuser TK, Smith FR, et al, "The Use of Hyaluronidase in the Treatment of Intravenous Extravasation Injuries," *J Perinatol*, 1990, 10(2):146-9.

Zenk KE, "Hyaluronidase: An Antidote for Intravenous Extravasations," *CSHP Voice*, 1981, 66-8.

Zenk KE, Dungy CI, and Greene GR, "Nafcillin Extravasation Injury: Use of Hyaluronidase as an Antidote," *Am J Dis Child*, 1981, 135(12):1113-4.

♦ **Hycamptamine** *see* Topotecan *on page 1554*

♦ **Hycamtin®** *see* Topotecan *on page 1554*

♦ **hycet™** *see* Hydrocodone and Acetaminophen *on page 779*

♦ **Hycort™ (Can)** *see* Hydrocortisone *on page 781*

♦ **Hydase™** *see* Hyaluronidase *on page 774*

♦ **Hydeltra T.B.A.® (Can)** *see* PrednisoLONE *on page 1304*

♦ **Hyderm (Can)** *see* Hydrocortisone *on page 781*

HydrALAZINE (hye DRAL a zeen)

Medication Safety Issues

Sound-alike/look-alike issues:

HydrALAZINE may be confused with hydrOXYzine

Related Information

Antihypertensive Agents by Class *on page 1678*

Canadian Brand Names Apo-Hydralazine®; Apresoline®; Novo-Hylazin; Nu-Hydral

Index Terms Apresoline [DSC]; Hydralazine Hydrochloride

Therapeutic Category Antihypertensive Agent; Vasodilator

Generic Available Yes

Use Management of moderate to severe hypertension, CHF, hypertension secondary to pre-eclampsia/eclampsia, primary pulmonary hypertension

Pregnancy Risk Factor C

Lactation Enters breast milk/compatible

Contraindications Hypersensitivity to hydralazine or any component; dissecting aortic aneurysm, mitral valve rheumatic heart disease, coronary artery disease

Warnings Monitor blood pressure closely with I.V. use; modify dosage in patients with severe renal impairment

Precautions Discontinue hydralazine in patients who develop SLE-like syndrome or positive ANA; use with caution in patients with severe renal disease or cerebral vascular accidents

Adverse Reactions

Cardiovascular: Palpitations, flushing, tachycardia, edema, orthostatic hypotension (rare)

Central nervous system: Malaise, fever, headache, dizziness

Dermatologic: Rash

Gastrointestinal: Anorexia, nausea, vomiting, diarrhea

Neuromuscular & skeletal: Arthralgias, weakness, pyridoxine deficiency-induced peripheral neuropathy (paresthesia, numbness)

Miscellaneous: Positive ANA, positive LE cells, SLE-like syndrome

Drug Interactions MAO inhibitors may cause a significant decrease in blood pressure; indomethacin may decrease hypotensive effects

Food Interactions Avoid natural licorice (causes sodium and water retention and increases potassium loss); long-term use of hydralazine may cause pyridoxine deficiency resulting in numbness, tingling, and paresthesias; if symptoms develop, pyridoxine supplements may be needed

(Continued)

HydrALAZINE *(Continued)*

Stability Changes color after contact with a metal filter; do not store intact ampuls in refrigerator

Mechanism of Action Direct vasodilation of arterioles (with little effect on veins) which results in decreased systemic resistance

Pharmacodynamics

Onset of action:

- Oral: 20-30 minutes
- I.V.: 5-20 minutes

Duration:

- Oral: 2-4 hours
- I.V.: 2-6 hours

Pharmacokinetics

Distribution: Crosses placenta; appears in breast milk

Protein-binding: 85% to 90%

Metabolism: Acetylated in the liver

Bioavailability: 30% to 50%; large first-pass effect orally

Half-life, adults: 2-8 hours; half-life varies with genetically determined acetylation rates

Elimination: 14% excreted unchanged in urine

Usual Dosage

Infants and Children:

- Oral: Initial: 0.75-1 mg/kg/day in 2-4 divided doses, not to exceed 25 mg/dose; increase over 3-4 weeks to maximum of 5 mg/kg/day in infants and 7.5 mg/kg/day in children, given in 2-4 divided doses; maximum daily dose: 200 mg/day
- I.M., I.V.: Initial: 0.1-0.2 mg/kg/dose (not to exceed 20 mg) every 4-6 hours as needed; up to 1.7-3.5 mg/kg/day divided in 4-6 doses

Adults:

- Oral: Initial: 10 mg 4 times/day, increase by 10-25 mg/dose every 2-5 days to maximum of 300 mg/day; usual dosage range for hypertension (JNC 7): 25-100 mg/day in 2 divided doses
- I.M., I.V.: Hypertension: Initial: 10-20 mg/dose every 4-6 hours as needed, may increase to 40 mg/dose
- I.M., I.V.: Pre-eclampsia/eclampsia: 5 mg/dose then 5-10 mg every 20-30 minutes as needed

Dosing interval in renal impairment:

- Cl_{cr} 10-50 mL/minute: Administer every 8 hours
- Cl_{cr} <10 mL/minute: Administer every 8-16 hours in fast acetylators and every 12-24 hours in slow acetylators

Administration

Oral: Administer with food

Parenteral: I.V.: Do not exceed rate of 0.2 mg/kg/minute; maximum concentration for I.V. use: 20 mg/mL

Monitoring Parameters Heart rate, blood pressure, ANA titer

Patient Information Limit alcohol; notify physician if flu-like symptoms occur

Nursing Implications I.V. use: Monitor blood pressure closely

Additional Information Slow acetylators, patients with decreased renal function and patients receiving >200 mg/day (chronically) are at higher risk for SLE. Titrate dosage to patient's response. Usually administered with diuretic and a beta-blocker to counteract hydralazine's side effects of sodium and water retention and reflex tachycardia.

Dosage Forms Excipient information presented when available (limited, particularly for generics); consult specific product labeling.

Injection, solution, as hydrochloride: 20 mg/mL (1 mL)

Tablet, as hydrochloride: 10 mg, 25 mg, 50 mg, 100 mg

Extemporaneous Preparations

A flavored syrup (1.25 mg/mL) has been made using seventy-five hydralazine hydrochloride 50 mg tablets, dissolved in 250 mL of distilled water with 2250 g of Lycasin® (75% w/w maltitol syrup vehicle); edetate disodium 3 g and sodium saccharin 3 g dissolved in 50 mL distilled water was added; solution was preserved with 30 mL of a solution containing methylparaben 10% (w/v) and propylparaben 2% (w/v) in propylene glycol; flavored with 3 mL orange flavoring; qsad to 3 L with distilled water and then pH adjusted to pH of 3.7 using glacial acetic acid; measured stability was 5 days at room temperature (25°C); less than 2% loss of hydralazine occurred at 2 weeks when syrup was stored at 5°C (Alexander, 1993)

A 4 mg/mL oral liquid preparation made from tablets was **not** stable for very long; preparation made in cherry syrup was not even stable for 1 day; preparation made in a 1:1 mixture of Ora-Sweet® and Ora-Plus® was stable for only 1 day under refrigeration (5°C) and not even 1 day at room temperature (25°C); preparation made in a 1:1 mixture of Ora-Sweet® SF and Ora-Plus® was stable for only 2 days under refrigeration (5°C), but not even 1 day at room temperature (25°C) (Allen, 1998).

Alexander KS, Pudipeddi M, and Parker GA, "Stability of Hydralazine Hydrochloride Syrup Compounded From Tablets," *Am J Hosp Pharm*, 1993, 50(4):683-6.

Allen LV and Erickson MA, "Stability of Alprazolam, Chloroquine Phosphate, Cisapride, Enalapril Maleate, and Hydralazine Hydrochloride in Extemporaneously Compounded Oral Liquids," *Am J Health Syst Pharm*, 1998, 55(18):1915-20.

References

Chobanian AV, Bakris GL, Black HR, et al, "The Seventh Report of the Joint National Committee on Prevention, Detection, Evaluation, and Treatment of High Blood Pressure: The JNC 7 report," *JAMA*, 2003, 289(19):2560-72.

♦ **Hydralazine Hydrochloride** *see* HydrALAZINE *on page 775*
♦ **Hydramine® [OTC]** *see* DiphenhydrAMINE *on page 509*
♦ **Hydrated Chloral** *see* Chloral Hydrate *on page 331*
♦ **Hydrea®** *see* Hydroxyurea *on page 794*
♦ **Hydrisalic™ [OTC]** *see* Salicylic Acid *on page 1413*

Hydrochlorothiazide (hye droe klor oh THYE a zide)

Medication Safety Issues

Sound-alike/look-alike issues:

Hydrochlorothiazide may be confused with hydrocortisone, hydroflumethiazide

Esidrix may be confused with Lasix®

HCTZ is an error-prone abbreviation (mistaken as hydrocortisone)

Microzide™ may be confused with Micronase®

International issues:

Microzide™ may be confused with Nitrobide® which is a brand name for isosorbide dinitrate in Japan

Microzide™ may be confused with Mikrozid® which is a brand name for ethanol/propanol combination in Great Britain

Related Information

Antihypertensive Agents by Class *on page 1678*

U.S. Brand Names Microzide™

Canadian Brand Names Apo-Hydro®; Novo-Hydrazide; PMS-Hydrochlorothiazide

Index Terms HCTZ (error-prone abbreviation)

Therapeutic Category Antihypertensive Agent; Diuretic, Thiazide

Generic Available Yes

Use Management of mild to moderate hypertension; treatment of edema in CHF and nephrotic syndrome

Pregnancy Risk Factor B

Lactation Enters breast milk/use caution (AAP rates "compatible")

Contraindications Hypersensitivity to hydrochlorothiazide or any component; cross-sensitivity with other thiazides or sulfonamides; anuria

Warnings Oral solution contains sodium benzoate; benzoic acid (benzoate) is a metabolite of benzyl alcohol; large amounts of benzyl alcohol (≥99 mg/kg/day) have been associated with a potentially fatal toxicity ("gasping syndrome") in neonates; *in vitro* and animal studies have shown that benzoate displaces bilirubin from protein binding sites; avoid use in neonates

Precautions Use with caution in patients with severe renal disease (Cl_{cr} <10 mL/minute), impaired hepatic function, hepatic disease, gout, lupus erythematosus, diabetes mellitus

Adverse Reactions

Cardiovascular: Hypotension

Central nervous system: Drowsiness, vertigo, headache

Dermatologic: Photosensitivity

Endocrine & metabolic: Hypokalemia, hyperglycemia, hypochloremic metabolic alkalosis, hyperlipidemia, hyperuricemia

Gastrointestinal: Nausea, vomiting, anorexia, diarrhea, cramping, pancreatitis

Hematologic: Aplastic anemia, hemolytic anemia, leukopenia, agranulocytosis, thrombocytopenia

Hepatic: Hepatitis, intrahepatic cholestasis

Neuromuscular & skeletal: Muscle weakness, paresthesia

Renal: Polyuria, prerenal azotemia

Drug Interactions NSAIDs decrease antihypertensive effect; steroids, amphotericin B increase potassium losses; hydrochlorothiazide increases hypersensitivity reactions to allopurinol; decreased clearance of lithium; increased hyperglycemia with diazoxide; hydrochlorothiazide decreases effectiveness of antidiabetic agents in blood sugar control; cholestyramine decreases hydrochlorothiazide absorption

(Continued)

Hydrochlorothiazide *(Continued)*

Food Interactions Avoid natural licorice (causes sodium and water retention and increases potassium loss); may need to decrease sodium and calcium and increase potassium, zinc, magnesium, and riboflavin in diet

Mechanism of Action Inhibits sodium reabsorption in the distal tubules causing increased excretion of sodium and water as well as potassium, hydrogen, magnesium, phosphate, calcium, and bicarbonate ions

Pharmacodynamics

Onset of diuretic action: Oral: Within 2 hours

Maximum effect: Within 3-6 hours

Duration: 6-12 hours

Pharmacokinetics

Absorption: Oral: ~60% to 80%

Distribution: Breast milk to plasma ratio: 0.25

Half-life: 5.6-14.8 hours

Elimination: Unchanged in urine

Usual Dosage Oral:

Edema:

Neonates and Infants <6 months: 2-3.3 mg/kg/day in 2 divided doses; maximum dose: 37.5 mg/day

Infants >6 months and Children: 2 mg/kg/day in 2 divided doses; maximum dose: 200 mg/day

Adults: 25-100 mg/day in 1-2 doses; maximum dose: 200 mg/day

Hypertension:

Infants and Children: Initial: 1 mg/kg/day once daily; may increase to maximum 3 mg/kg/day; not to exceed 50 mg/day

Adults: 12.5-50 mg once daily; minimal increase in response and more electrolyte disturbances are seen with doses >50 mg/day

Dosage adjustment in renal impairment:

Cl_{cr} <25-50 mL/minute: Usually not effective

Cl_{cr} <10 mL/minute: Avoid use

Administration Oral: Administer with food or milk

Monitoring Parameters Serum electrolytes, BUN, creatinine, blood pressure, fluid balance, body weight

Patient Information May cause photosensitivity reactions (eg, exposure to sunlight may cause severe sunburn, skin rash, redness, or itching); avoid exposure to sunlight and artificial light sources (sunlamps, tanning booth/bed); wear protective clothing, wide-brimmed hats, sunglasses, and lip sunscreen (SPF ≥15); use a sunscreen [broad-spectrum sunscreen or physical sunscreen (preferred) or sunblock with SPF ≥15]; contact physician if reaction occurs.

Dosage Forms Excipient information presented when available (limited, particularly for generics); consult specific product labeling.

Capsule: 12.5 mg

Microzide™: 12.5 mg

Tablet: 25 mg, 50 mg

References

Chobanian AV, Bakris GL, Black HR, et al, "The Seventh Report of the Joint National Committee on Prevention, Detection, Evaluation, and Treatment of High Blood Pressure: The JNC 7 Report," *JAMA*, 2003, 289(19):2560-72.

National High Blood Pressure Education Program Working Group on High Blood Pressure in Children and Adolescents, "The Fourth Report on the Diagnosis, Evaluation, and Treatment of High Blood Pressure in Children and Adolescents," *Pediatrics*, 2004, 114(2 Suppl):555-76.

van der Vorst MM, Kist JE, van der Heijden AJ, et al, "Diuretics in Pediatrics: Current Knowledge and Future Prospects," *Paediatr Drugs*, 2006, 8(4):245-64.

Hydrochlorothiazide and Spironolactone

(hye droe klor oh THYE a zide & speer on oh LAK tone)

Medication Safety Issues

Sound-alike/look-alike issues:

Aldactazide® may be confused with Aldactone®

U.S. Brand Names Aldactazide®

Canadian Brand Names Aldactazide 25®; Aldactazide 50®; Novo-Spirozine

Index Terms Spironolactone and Hydrochlorothiazide

Therapeutic Category Antihypertensive Agent, Combination; Diuretic, Combination

Generic Available Yes

Use Management of mild to moderate hypertension; treatment of edema in CHF and nephrotic syndrome

Pregnancy Risk Factor C

Lactation Enters breast milk/use caution

Contraindications Hypersensitivity to hydrochlorothiazide, spironolactone, or any component; anuria, hyperkalemia, renal or hepatic failure; cross-sensitivity with other thiazides or sulfonamides; patients receiving triamterene or amiloride

Warnings This fixed combination is not indicated for initial therapy of hypertension; therapy requires titration to the individual patient; if dosage so determined represents this fixed combination, its use may be more convenient

Adverse Reactions See individual components, Hydrochlorothiazide *on page 777* and Spironolactone *on page 1469*, for full adverse drug reaction information

Drug Interactions Drugs that increase serum potassium (amiloride, triamterene, indomethacin, ACE inhibitors); digoxin decreases renal clearance; see individual components, Hydrochlorothiazide *on page 777* and Spironolactone *on page 1469*, for complete drug interaction information

Food Interactions Avoid food with high potassium content, natural licorice (causes sodium and water retention and increases potassium loss), and salt substitutes

Usual Dosage Oral: As the product is in a fixed combination of equal mg doses, the following dosages represent mg of either spironolactone **or** hydrochlorothiazide

Children: 1.5-3 mg/kg/day in 2-4 divided doses; maximum daily dosage: 200 mg
Adults: 12.5-200 mg in 1-2 divided doses

Administration Oral: Administer in the morning; administer the last dose of multiple doses before 6 PM unless instructed otherwise; administer with food or milk

Monitoring Parameters Blood pressure, serum electrolytes, renal function

Test Interactions Spironolactone may interfere with plasma and urinary cortisol levels and the radioimmunoassay for digoxin

Dosage Forms Excipient information presented when available (limited, particularly for generics); consult specific product labeling.

Tablet: Hydrochlorothiazide 25 mg and spironolactone 25 mg
Aldactazide®:
25/25: Hydrochlorothiazide 25 mg and spironolactone 25 mg
50/50: Hydrochlorothiazide 50 mg and spironolactone 50 mg

Extemporaneous Preparations A 5 mg/mL oral suspension may be compounded by crushing twenty-four 25 mg (spironolactone/HCTZ) Aldactazide® tablets; add geometric amounts of a 1:1 mixture of Ora-Sweet® and Ora-Plus®, or Ora-Sweet® SF and Ora-Plus®, or cherry syrup alone to a final volume of 120 mL; shake well, refrigerate; stable 60 days

Allen LV and Erickson MA, "Stability of Labetalol Hydrochloride, Metoprolol Tartrate, Verapamil Hydrochloride, and Spironolactone With Hydrochlorothiazide in Extemporaneously Compounded Oral Liquids," *Am J Health Syst Pharm*, 1996, 53(19):2304-9.

♦ **Hydrocil® Instant [OTC]** *see* Psyllium *on page 1347*

Hydrocodone and Acetaminophen

(hye droe KOE done & a seet a MIN oh fen)

Medication Safety Issues

Sound-alike/look-alike issues:
Lorcet® may be confused with Fioricet®
Lortab® may be confused with Cortef®, Lorabid®, Luride®
Vicodin® may be confused with Hycodan®, Hycomine®, Indocin®, Uridon®
Zydone® may be confused with Vytone®

Related Information

Narcotic Analgesics Comparison *on page 1705*
Overdose and Toxicology *on page 1916*

U.S. Brand Names Anexsia®; Ceta-Plus®; Co-Gesic®; hycet™; Lorcet® 10/650; Lorcet® Plus; Lortab®; Margesic® H; Maxidone™; Norco®; Stagesic®; Vicodin®; Vicodin® ES; Vicodin® HP; Xodol®; Xodol® 5/300; Zydone®

Index Terms Acetaminophen and Hydrocodone

Therapeutic Category Analgesic, Narcotic; Antitussive; Cough Preparation

Generic Available Yes

Use Relief of moderate to severe pain; antitussive (hydrocodone)

Restrictions C-III

Pregnancy Risk Factor C

Lactation Excretion in breast milk unknown/contraindicated

Contraindications Hypersensitivity to hydrocodone, acetaminophen, or any component; CNS depression; severe respiratory depression

Warnings Abrupt discontinuation after prolonged use may result in withdrawal symptoms or seizures
(Continued)

Hydrocodone and Acetaminophen *(Continued)*

Precautions Use with caution in patients with hypersensitivity reactions to other phenanthrene derivative opioid agonists (morphine, codeine, hydromorphone, oxycodone, oxymorphone, levorphanol)

Adverse Reactions

Cardiovascular: Hypotension, bradycardia, peripheral vasodilation

Central nervous system: CNS depression, drowsiness, dizziness, sedation, elevated intracranial pressure

Endocrine & metabolic: Antidiuretic hormone release

Gastrointestinal: Nausea, vomiting, constipation, biliary tract spasm

Genitourinary: Urinary tract spasm

Ocular: Miosis

Respiratory: Respiratory depression

Miscellaneous: Histamine release, physical and psychological dependence with prolonged use

Drug Interactions Hydrocodone is a cytochrome P450 isoenzyme CYP2D6 substrate; acetaminophen is a cytochrome P450 isoenzyme CYP1A2 substrate (minor), CYP2A6, CYP2C9, CYP2D6, CYP2E1, and CYP3A3/4 isoenzyme substrate

CNS depressants, alcohol, phenothiazines, tricyclic antidepressants may potentiate the adverse effects of hydrocodone; see also Acetaminophen *on page 42*

Food Interactions Rate of absorption of acetaminophen may be decreased when given with food high in carbohydrates

Mechanism of Action Inhibits the synthesis of prostaglandins in the CNS and peripherally blocks pain impulse generation; produces antipyresis from inhibition of hypothalamic heat-regulating center

Pharmacodynamics Narcotic analgesia: Oral:

Onset of action: Within 10-20 minutes

Duration: 3-6 hours

Usual Dosage Oral:

Antitussive (doses based on hydrocodone):

Children: 0.6 mg/kg/day or 20 mg/m^2/day divided in 3-4 doses/day

<2 years: Do not exceed 1.25 mg/single dose

2-12 years: Do not exceed 5 mg/single dose

>12 years: Do not exceed 10 mg/single dose

Analgesic: **Doses should be titrated to appropriate analgesic effect**

Children: Dose has not been well established

Adults: 1-2 tablets or capsules every 4-6 hours as needed

AHCPR dosing guidelines (doses based on hydrocodone): Opioid naive patients: (See Carr, 1992 and Jacox, 1994)

Children and Adults <50 kg: Moderate to severe pain: Usual initial dose: 0.2 mg/kg every 3-4 hours

Children and Adults ≥50 kg: Moderate to severe pain: Usual initial dose: 10 mg every 3-4 hours

Administration Oral: May administer with food or milk to decrease GI distress

Monitoring Parameters Pain relief, respiratory rate, blood pressure

Patient Information Avoid alcohol; may cause drowsiness and impair ability to perform activities requiring mental alertness or physical coordination; may be habit-forming; avoid abrupt discontinuation after prolonged use

Dosage Forms Excipient information presented when available (limited, particularly for generics); consult specific product labeling. [DSC] = Discontinued product

Capsule:

Ceta-Plus®, Margesic® H, Stagesic®: Hydrocodone bitartrate 5 mg and acetaminophen 500 mg

Elixir: Hydrocodone bitartrate 7.5 mg and acetaminophen 500 mg per 15 mL (480 mL)

Lortab®: Hydrocodone bitartrate 7.5 mg and acetaminophen 500 mg per 15 mL (480 mL) [contains alcohol 7%; tropical fruit punch flavor]

Solution, oral:

hycet™: Hydrocodone bitartrate 7.5 mg and acetaminophen 325 mg per 15 mL (480 mL) [contains alcohol 7%; tropical fruit punch flavor]

Tablet:

Hydrocodone bitartrate 2.5 mg and acetaminophen 500 mg

Hydrocodone bitartrate 5 mg and acetaminophen 325 mg

Hydrocodone bitartrate 5 mg and acetaminophen 500 mg

Hydrocodone bitartrate 7.5 mg and acetaminophen 325 mg

Hydrocodone bitartrate 7.5 mg and acetaminophen 500 mg

Hydrocodone bitartrate 7.5 mg and acetaminophen 650 mg

Hydrocodone bitartrate 7.5 mg and acetaminophen 750 mg

Hydrocodone bitartrate 10 mg and acetaminophen 325 mg

Hydrocodone bitartrate 10 mg and acetaminophen 500 mg

Hydrocodone bitartrate 10 mg and acetaminophen 650 mg

Hydrocodone bitartrate 10 mg and acetaminophen 660 mg
Hydrocodone bitartrate 10 mg and acetaminophen 750 mg
Anexsia®:
5/325: Hydrocodone bitartrate 5 mg and acetaminophen 325 mg
5/500: Hydrocodone bitartrate 5 mg and acetaminophen 500 mg [DSC]
7.5/325: Hydrocodone bitartrate 7.5 mg and acetaminophen 325 mg
7.5/650: Hydrocodone bitartrate 7.5 mg and acetaminophen 650 mg [DSC]
Co-Gesic® 5/500: Hydrocodone bitartrate 5 mg and acetaminophen 500 mg
Lorcet® 10/650: Hydrocodone bitartrate 10 mg and acetaminophen 650 mg
Lorcet® Plus: Hydrocodone bitartrate 7.5 mg and acetaminophen 650 mg
Lortab®:
5/500: Hydrocodone bitartrate 5 mg and acetaminophen 500 mg
7.5/500: Hydrocodone bitartrate 7.5 mg and acetaminophen 500 mg
10/500: Hydrocodone bitartrate 10 mg and acetaminophen 500 mg
Maxidone™: Hydrocodone bitartrate 10 mg and acetaminophen 750 mg
Norco®:
Hydrocodone bitartrate 5 mg and acetaminophen 325 mg
Hydrocodone bitartrate 7.5 mg and acetaminophen 325 mg
Hydrocodone bitartrate 10 mg and acetaminophen 325 mg
Vicodin®: Hydrocodone bitartrate 5 mg and acetaminophen 500 mg
Vicodin® ES: Hydrocodone bitartrate 7.5 mg and acetaminophen 750 mg
Vicodin® HP: Hydrocodone bitartrate 10 mg and acetaminophen 660 mg
Xodol®: Hydrocodone bitartrate 10 mg and acetaminophen 300 mg
Xodol® 5/300: Hydrocodone bitartrate 5 mg and acetaminophen 300 mg
Zydone®:
Hydrocodone bitartrate 5 mg and acetaminophen 400 mg
Hydrocodone bitartrate 7.5 mg and acetaminophen 400 mg
Hydrocodone bitartrate 10 mg and acetaminophen 400 mg

References

Carr D, Jacox A, Chapman CR, et al, "Clinical Practice Guideline Number 1: Acute Pain Management: Operative or Medical Procedures and Trauma," Rockville, Maryland: U.S. Department of Health and Human Services, Public Health Service, Agency for Health Care Policy and Research, AHCPR Publication No 92-0032, 1992.

Jacox A, Carr D, Payne R, et al, "Clinical Practice Guideline Number 9: Management of Cancer Pain," Rockville, Maryland: U.S. Department of Health and Human Services, Public Health Service, Agency for Health Care Policy and Research, AHCPR Publication No. 94-0592, 1994.

Hydrocortisone (hye droe KOR ti sone)

Medication Safety Issues

Sound-alike/look-alike issues:
Hydrocortisone may be confused with hydrocodone, hydroxychloroquine, hydrochlorothiazide
Anusol® may be confused with Anusol-HC®, Aplisol®, Aquasol®
Anusol-HC® may be confused with Anusol®
Cortef® may be confused with Lortab®
Cortizone® may be confused with cortisone
HCT (occasional abbreviation for hydrocortisone) is an error-prone abbreviation (mistaken as hydrochlorothiazide)
Hytone® may be confused with Vytone®
Proctocort® may be confused with ProctoCream®
ProctoCream® may be confused with Proctocort®

International issues:
Hytone® may be confused with Hysone® [Australia]
Nutracort® may be confused with Nitrocor® which is a brand name of nitroglycerin in Chile and Italy

Related Information

Corticosteroids, Systemic *on page 1685*
Corticosteroids, Topical: Guidelines for Selection and Use *on page 1686*

U.S. Brand Names Anucort-HC®; Anusol-HC®; Anusol® HC-1 [OTC]; Aquanil™ HC [OTC]; Beta-HC®; Caldecort® [OTC]; Cetacort®; Colocort®; Cortaid® Intensive Therapy [OTC]; Cortaid® Maximum Strength [OTC]; Cortaid® Sensitive Skin [OTC]; Cortef®; Corticool® [OTC]; Cortifoam®; Cortizone®-10 Maximum Strength [OTC]; Cortizone®-10 Plus Maximum Strength [OTC]; Cortizone®-10 Quick Shot [OTC]; Dermarest Dricort® [OTC]; Dermtex® HC [OTC]; EarSol® HC; Encort™; Hemril®-30; HydroZone Plus [OTC]; Hytone®; IvySoothe® [OTC]; Locoid®; Locoid Lipocream®; Nupercainal® Hydrocortisone Cream [OTC]; Nutracort®; Pandel®; Post Peel Healing Balm [OTC]; Preparation H® Hydrocortisone [OTC]; Proctocort®; ProctoCream® HC; Procto-Kit™; Procto-Pak™; Proctosert; Proctosol-HC®; Proctozone-HC™; Sarnol®-HC [OTC]; Solu-Cortef®; Summer's Eve® SpecialCare™ Medicated Anti-Itch Cream [OTC]; Texacort®; Tucks® Anti-Itch [OTC]; Westcort®
(Continued)

Hydrocortisone *(Continued)*

Canadian Brand Names Aquacort®; Cortamed®; Cortef®; Cortenema®; Cortifoam™; Emo-Cort®; Hycort™; Hyderm; HydroVal®; Locoid®; Prevex® HC; Sarna® HC; Solu-Cortef®; Westcort®

Index Terms A-hydroCort; Compound F; Cortisol; Hemorrhoidal HC; Hydrocortisone Acetate; Hydrocortisone Butyrate; Hydrocortisone Probutate; Hydrocortisone Sodium Succinate; Hydrocortisone Valerate

Therapeutic Category Adrenal Corticosteroid; Anti-inflammatory Agent; Anti-inflammatory Agent, Rectal; Antiasthmatic; Corticosteroid, Rectal; Corticosteroid, Systemic; Corticosteroid, Topical; Glucocorticoid

Generic Available Yes: Excludes acetate foam, butyrate cream and ointment, gel as base, otic drops as base, probutate cream, sodium succinate injection

Use Management of adrenocortical insufficiency; relief of inflammation and pruritus associated with corticosteroid-responsive dermatoses; adjunctive treatment of ulcerative colitis; septic shock

Pregnancy Risk Factor C

Lactation Excretion in breast milk unknown/use caution

Contraindications Hypersensitivity to hydrocortisone or any component (see Warnings); serious infections, except septic shock or tuberculous meningitis; viral, fungal, or tubercular skin lesions

Warnings Hypothalamic-pituitary-adrenal (HPA) suppression may occur; acute adrenal insufficiency (adrenal crisis) may occur with abrupt withdrawal after long-term therapy or with stress; withdrawal and discontinuation of corticosteroids should be done carefully; patients with HPA axis suppression may require doses of systemic glucocorticosteroids prior to, during, and after unusual stress (eg, surgery). Immunosuppression may occur; patients may be more susceptible to infections; avoid exposure to chickenpox and measles. Corticosteroids may activate latent opportunistic infections or exacerbate systemic fungal infections. May cause osteoporosis (at any age) or inhibition of bone growth in pediatric patients. Acute myopathy may occur with high doses, elevated IOP may occur (especially with prolonged use), and CNS effects (ranging from euphoria to psychosis) may occur. Rare cases of anaphylactoid reactions have been reported with corticosteroids.

Topical: Adverse systemic effects may occur when topical steroids are used in large areas of the body, denuded areas, for prolonged periods of time, with an occlusive dressing, and/or in infants and small children; infants and small children may be more susceptible to HPA axis suppression or other systemic toxicities due to larger skin surface area to body mass ratio; use with caution in pediatric patients.

Manufacturer supplied diluents for injection (eg, Solu-Cortef®) contain benzyl alcohol and topical aerosol spray and topical cream may contain benzyl alcohol which may cause allergic reactions in susceptible individuals; otic solution contains benzyl benzoate and oral suspension (see Additional Information) contains benzoic acid; benzoic acid (benzoate) is a metabolite of benzyl alcohol; large amounts of benzyl alcohol (≥99 mg/kg/day) have been associated with a potentially fatal toxicity ("gasping syndrome") in neonates; the "gasping syndrome" consists of metabolic acidosis, respiratory distress, gasping respirations, CNS dysfunction (including convulsions, intracranial hemorrhage), hypotension and cardiovascular collapse; avoid use of hydrocortisone products containing benzoic acid, benzyl alcohol, or benzyl benzoate in neonates; *in vitro* and animal studies have shown that benzoate displaces bilirubin from protein binding sites

Precautions Avoid using higher than recommended doses; suppression of HPA function, suppression of linear growth (ie, reduction of growth velocity), reduced bone mineral density, hypercorticism (Cushing's syndrome), hyperglycemia, or glucosuria may occur; titrate to lowest effective dose; these adverse effects (as well as intracranial hypertension) may also occur with topical use and have been reported in pediatric patients. Reduction in growth velocity may occur when corticosteroids are administered to pediatric patients by any route (monitor growth). Use with extreme caution in patients with respiratory tuberculosis, untreated systemic infections, or ocular herpes simplex; use with caution in patients with thyroid dysfunction, cirrhosis, nonspecific ulcerative colitis, hypertension, renal impairment, osteoporosis, thromboembolic tendencies, CHF, recent MI, convulsive disorders, myasthenia gravis, thrombophlebitis, peptic ulcer, diabetes, glaucoma, cataracts, or hepatic impairment. Prolonged use may result in cataracts or glaucoma.

Adverse Reactions

Cardiovascular: Hypertension, edema, CHF

Central nervous system: Euphoria, insomnia, headache, intracranial hypertension, vertigo, seizures, psychosis, pseudotumor cerebri, nervousness

Dermatologic: Acne, dermatitis, skin atrophy; topical use: eczema, folliculitis, pruritus, stinging, burning, dry skin, irritation, redness, hypertrichosis, hypopigmentation, maceration of the skin, striae, miliaria

Endocrine & metabolic: HPA suppression, hypokalemia, hyperglycemia, Cushing's syndrome, growth suppression, sodium and water retention

Gastrointestinal: Peptic ulcer, nausea, vomiting

Neuromuscular & skeletal: Muscle weakness, osteoporosis, decreased bone mineral density, fractures

Ocular: Cataracts, increased IOP, glaucoma

Miscellaneous: Immunosuppression, anaphylactoid reactions (rare)

Drug Interactions Cytochrome P450 isoenzyme CYP2D6 and CYP3A3/4 substrate

Barbiturates, phenytoin, rifampin, salicylates, NSAIDs, diuretics (potassium depleting), warfarin; caffeine and alcohol may increase risk for GI ulcer; live virus vaccines (increase risk of viral infection); vaccines may have decreased effects

Food Interactions Systemic use of corticosteroids may require a diet with increased potassium, vitamins A, B_6, C, D, folate, calcium, zinc, phosphorus, and decreased sodium

Stability Injection: Store at controlled room temperature 20°C to 25°C (59°F to 86°F). Reconstituted solution is clear, light yellow and heat labile.

After initial reconstitution, hydrocortisone sodium succinate solutions are stable for 3 days at room temperature or under refrigeration when protected from light. Stability of parenteral admixture (Solu-Cortef®) at room temperature (25°C) and at refrigeration temperature (4°C) is concentration-dependent:

Stability of concentration 1 mg/mL: 24 hours

Stability of concentration 2 mg/mL to 60 mg/mL: At least 4 hours

Solutions for I.V. infusion: Reconstituted solutions may be added to an appropriate volume of compatible solution for infusion. Concentration should generally not exceed 1 mg/mL. However, in adult cases where administration of a small volume of fluid is desirable, 100-3000 mg may be added to 50 mL of D_5W or NS (stability limited to 4 hours).

Mechanism of Action Decreases inflammation by suppression of migration of polymorphonuclear leukocytes and reversal of increased capillary permeability

Pharmacodynamics Anti-inflammatory effects:

Maximum effect:

Oral: 12-24 hours

I.V.: 4-6 hours

Duration: 8-12 hours

Pharmacokinetics

Absorption: Rapid by all routes, except rectally

Metabolism: In the liver

Half-life, biologic: 8-12 hours

Elimination: Renally, mainly as 17-hydroxysteroids and 17-ketosteroids

Usual Dosage Dose should be based on severity of disease and patient response; **Note:** A variety of salt forms are available and can lead to confusion in prescribing, dispensing, and administration; use the appropriate salt/dosage form for the following indications:

Acetate: For intra-articular, intrasynovial, intrabursal, intralesional, or soft tissue injection only

Cypionate: Oral suspension (see Additional Information)

Sodium succinate: For general I.V. use, I.V. use in patients allergic to sodium phosphate salt, I.V. for shock and for intrathecal use (must reconstitute with a preservative free diluent or use a preservative free product)

Acute adrenal insufficiency: I.M., I.V.:

Infants and young Children: 1-2 mg/kg/dose I.V. bolus, then 25-150 mg/day in divided doses every 6-8 hours

Older Children: 1-2 mg/kg I.V. bolus, then 150-250 mg/day in divided doses every 6-8 hours

Adults: 100 mg I.V. bolus, then 300 mg/day in divided doses every 8 hours or as a continuous infusion for 48 hours; once patient is stable change to oral, 50 mg every 8 hours for 6 doses, then taper to 30-50 mg/day in divided doses

Anti-inflammatory or immunosuppressive:

Infants and Children:

Oral: 2.5-10 mg/kg/day or 75-300 mg/m^2/day divided every 6-8 hours

I.M., I.V.: 1-5 mg/kg/day or 30-150 mg/m^2/day divided every 12-24 hours

Adolescents and Adults: Oral, I.M., I.V., SubQ: 15-240 mg every 12 hours

Congenital adrenal hyperplasia: AAP Recommendations: Oral: Initial: 10-20 mg/m^2/day in 3 divided doses; usual requirement: Infants: 2.5-5 mg 3 times/day; Children: 5-10 mg 3 times/day; **Note:** Administer morning dose as early as possible; tablets may result in more reliable serum concentrations than oral liquid formulation (see Additional Information); individualize dose by monitoring growth, hormone levels, and bone age; mineralocorticoid (eg, fludrocortisone) and sodium supplement may be required in salt losers

(Continued)

Hydrocortisone *(Continued)*

Neonatal hypoglycemia (refractory to continuous glucose infusion of >12-15 mg/kg/minute): Neonates: I.V., oral: 5 mg/kg/day divided every 8-12 hours or 1-2 mg/kg/dose every 6 hours

Physiologic replacement: Children:

Oral: 0.5-0.75 mg/kg/day or 20-25 mg/m^2/day divided every 8 hours

I.M.: 0.25-0.35 mg/kg/day or 12-15 mg/m^2/day once daily

Shock: I.V.: **Sodium succinate:**

Children: Initial: 50 mg/kg as an I.V. bolus, followed by 50 mg/kg as a 24-hour infusion (see Carcillo, 2002 and Han, 2003). Some centers use: 50 mg/kg then repeated in 4 hours and/or every 24 hours if needed

Adolescents and Adults: 500 mg to 2 g every 2-6 hours

Status asthmaticus:

Children: I.V.: Optional loading dose: 4-8 mg/kg; maximum: 250 mg; then maintenance: 2 mg/kg/dose every 6 hours

Adults: 100-500 mg every 6 hours

Adolescents and Adults: Rectal: Insert 1 application 1-2 times/day for 2-3 weeks

Ulcerative colitis: One enema nightly for 21 days, or until remission occurs; clinical symptoms should subside within 3-5 days; discontinue use if no improvement within 2-3 weeks; some patients may require 2-3 months of therapy; if therapy lasts >21 days, discontinue slowly by decreasing use to every other night for 2-3 weeks

Children and Adults: Topical: Usual: Apply 2-3 times/day (depending on severity); may be applied up to 4 times/day

Administration

Oral: Administer with food or milk to decrease GI upset (see Additional Information)

Parenteral:

I.V. bolus: Dilute to 50 mg/mL and administer over 3-5 minutes

I.V. intermittent infusion: Dilute to 1 mg/mL and administer over 20-30 minutes; usual maximum concentration: 5 mg/mL

Note: In adult patients when administration of a small volume of fluid is needed, concentrations up to 60 mg/mL (100-3000 mg in 50 mL D_5W or NS) may be administered by direct I.V. or I.V. piggyback

Rectal: Patient should lie on left side during administration and for 30 minutes after; retain enema for at least 1 hour, preferably all night

Topical: Apply a thin film to clean, dry skin and rub in gently; avoid contact with eyes. Do not apply to face, underarms, or groin unless directed by physician. Do not wrap or bandage affected area unless directed by physician. Do not apply to diaper areas because diapers or plastic pants may be occlusive.

Monitoring Parameters Blood pressure, weight, serum glucose, electrolytes; growth in pediatric patients; assess HPA axis suppression in patients using topical steroids applied to a large surface area or to areas under occlusion (eg, ACTH stimulation test, morning plasma cortisol test, urinary free cortisol test). Monitor IOP with therapy >6 weeks.

Reference Range Hydrocortisone (normal endogenous morning levels) 4-30 mcg/mL

Test Interactions Skin tests

Patient Information Limit caffeine; avoid alcohol; do not decrease dose or discontinue without physician's approval; avoid exposure to measles or chicken pox, advise physician immediately if exposed; notify physician if condition being treated persists or worsens. Topical: Avoid contact with eyes; do not use for longer than directed; contact physician if no improvement is seen in 2 weeks

Additional Information Cortef® oral suspension was reformulated in July 1998; the suspending agent was changed from tragacanth to xanthan gum; this suspension was found **not** to be bioequivalent to hydrocortisone tablets in the treatment of children with congenital adrenal hyperplasia; children required higher doses of the suspension (19.6 mg/m^2/day) compared to the tablets (15.2 mg/m^2/day); based on these findings, Cortef® suspension was voluntarily recalled from the market on July 18, 2000 (see Merke, 2001).

To facilitate retention of enema, prior antidiarrheal medication or sedation may be required (especially when beginning therapy)

Dosage Forms Excipient information presented when available (limited, particularly for generics); consult specific product labeling. [DSC] = Discontinued product

Aerosol, rectal, as acetate (Cortifoam®): 10% (15 g) [90 mg/applicator]

Cream, rectal, as acetate (Nupercainal® Hydrocortisone Cream): 1% (30 g) [strength expressed as base]

Cream, rectal, as base:

Cortizone®-10: 1% (30 g) [contains aloe]

Preparation H® Hydrocortisone: 1% (27 g)

Cream, topical, as acetate: 0.5% (9 g, 30 g, 60 g) [available with aloe]; 1% (30 g, 454 g) [available with aloe]

Cream, topical, as base: 0.5% (30 g); 1% (1.5 g, 30 g, 114 g, 454 g); 2.5% (20 g, 30 g, 454 g)

- Anusol-HC®: 2.5% (30 g) [contains benzyl alcohol]
- Caldecort®: 1% (30 g) [contains aloe vera gel]
- Cortaid® Intensive Therapy: 1% (60 g)
- Cortaid® Maximum Strength: 1% (15 g, 30 g, 40 g, 60 g) [contains aloe vera gel and benzyl alcohol]
- Cortaid® Sensitive Skin: 0.5% (15 g) [contains aloe vera gel]
- Cortizone®-10 Maximum Strength: 1% (15 g, 30 g, 60 g) [contains aloe]
- Cortizone®-10 Plus Maximum Strength: 1% (30 g, 60 g) [contains vitamins A, D, E and aloe]
- Dermarest® Dricort®: 1% (15 g, 30 g)
- HydroZone Plus, Proctocort®, Procto-Pak™: 1% (30 g)
- Hytone®: 2.5% (30 g, 60 g)
- IvySoothe®: 1% (30 g) [contains aloe]
- Post Peel Healing Balm: 1% (23 g)
- ProctoCream® HC: 2.5% (30 g) [contains benzyl alcohol]
- Procto-Kit™: 1% (30 g) [packaged with applicator tips and finger cots]; 2.5% (30 g) [packaged with applicator tips and finger cots]
- Proctosol-HC®, Proctozone-HC™: 2.5% (30 g)
- Summer's Eve® SpecialCare™ Medicated Anti-Itch Cream: 1% (30 g)

Cream, topical, as butyrate (Locoid®, Locoid Lipocream®): 0.1% (15 g, 45 g)

Cream, topical, as probutate (Pandel®): 0.1% (15 g, 45 g, 80 g)

Cream, topical, as valerate (Westcort®): 0.2% (15 g, 45 g, 60 g)

Gel, topical, as base (Corticool®): 1% (45 g)

Injection, powder for reconstitution, as sodium succinate (Solu-Cortef®): 100 mg, 250 mg, 500 mg, 1 g [diluent contains benzyl alcohol; strength expressed as base]

Lotion, topical, as base: 1% (120 mL); 2.5% (60 mL)

- Aquanil™ HC: 1% (120 mL)
- Beta-HC®, Cetacort®, Sarnol®-HC: 1% (60 mL)
- HydroZone Plus: 1% (120 mL)
- Hytone®: 2.5% (60 mL)
- Nutracort®: 1% (60 mL, 120 mL); 2.5% (60 mL, 120 mL)

Ointment, topical, as acetate: 1% (30 g) [strength expressed as base; available with aloe]

- Anusol® HC-1: 1% (21 g) [strength expressed as base]
- Cortaid® Maximum Strength: 1% (15 g, 30 g) [strength expressed as base]

Ointment, topical, as base: 0.5% (30 g); 1% (30 g, 454 g); 2.5% (20 g, 30 g, 454 g)

- Cortizone®-10 Maximum Strength: 1% (30 g, 60 g)
- Hytone®: 2.5% (30 g) [DSC]

Ointment, topical, as butyrate (Locoid®): 0.1% (15 g, 45 g)

Ointment, topical, as valerate (Westcort®): 0.2% (15 g, 45 g, 60 g)

Solution, otic, as base (EarSol® HC): 1% (30 mL) [contains alcohol 44%, benzyl benzoate, yerba santa]

Solution, topical, as base (Texacort®): 2.5% (30 mL) [contains alcohol]

Solution, topical, as butyrate (Locoid®): 0.1% (20 mL, 60 mL) [contains alcohol 50%]

Solution, topical spray, as base:

- Cortaid® Intensive Therapy: 1% (60 mL) [contains alcohol]
- Cortizone®-10 Quick Shot: 1% (44 mL) [contains benzyl alcohol]
- Dermtex® HC: 1% (52 mL) [contains menthol 1%]

Suppository, rectal, as acetate: 25 mg (12s, 24s, 100s)

- Anucort-HC®, Tucks® Anti-Itch: 25 mg (12s, 24s, 100s) [strength expressed as base; Anucort-HC® *renamed* Tucks® Anti-Itch]
- Anusol-HC®, Proctosol-HC®: 25 mg (12s, 24s)
- Encort™: 30 mg (12s)
- Hemril®-30, Proctocort®, Proctosert: 30 mg (12s, 24s)

Suspension, rectal, as base: 100 mg/60 mL (7s)

- Colocort®: 100 mg/60 mL (1s, 7s)

Tablet, as base: 20 mg

- Cortef®: 5 mg, 10 mg, 20 mg

Extemporaneous Preparations A 2.5 mg/mL oral suspension prepared from tablets (with a vehicle containing sodium carboxymethylcellulose, syrup, hydroxybenzoate 0.1% preservatives, polysorbate 80, and citric acid) and stored in the dark in amber high density polyethylene bottles was stable for 90 days when stored at 5°C or 25°C and stable for 30 days when stored at 40°C; a 2.5 mg/mL oral suspension prepared from powder and the same vehicle was stable for 90 days when stored in the dark in amber polyethylene bottles at 40°C (Fawcett, 1995).

(Continued)

Hydrocortisone *(Continued)*

Fawcett JP, Boulton DW, Jiang R, et al, "Stability of Hydrocortisone Oral Suspensions Prepared From Tablets and Powder," *Ann Pharmacother*, 1995, 29(10):987-90.

References

American Academy of Pediatrics, Section on Endocrinology and Committee on Genetics, "Technical Report: Congenital Adrenal Hyperplasia," *Pediatrics*, 2000, 106(6):1511-8.
Carcillo JA and Fields AI, "Clinical Practice Parameters for Hemodynamic Support of Pediatric and Neonatal Patients in Septic Shock," *Crit Care Med*, 2002, 30(6):1365-78.
Cowett RM and Loughead JL, "Neonatal Glucose Metabolism: Differential Diagnoses, Evaluation, and Treatment of Hypoglycemia," *Neonatal Netw*, 2002, 21(4):9-19.
Halamek LP and Stevenson DK, "Neonatal Hypoglycemia, Part II: Pathophysiology and Therapy," *Clin Pediatr (Phila)*, 1998, 37(1):11-6.
Han YY, Carcillo JA, Dragotta MA, et al, "Early Reversal of Pediatric-Neonatal Septic Shock by Community Physicians is Associated With Improved Outcome," *Pediatrics*, 2003, 112(4):793-9.
Merke DP, Cho D, Calis KA, et al, "Hydrocortisone Suspension and Hydrocortisone Tablets are not Bioequivalent in the Treatment of Children With Congenital Adrenal Hyperplasia," *J Clin Endocrinol Metab*, 2001, 86(1):441-5.

♦ **Hydrocortisone Acetate** *see* Hydrocortisone *on page 781*
♦ **Hydrocortisone and Ciprofloxacin** *see* Ciprofloxacin and Hydrocortisone *on page 362*
♦ **Hydrocortisone Butyrate** *see* Hydrocortisone *on page 781*
♦ **Hydrocortisone, Neomycin, and Polymyxin B** *see* Neomycin, (Bacitracin) Polymyxin B, and Hydrocortisone *on page 1119*
♦ **Hydrocortisone Probutate** *see* Hydrocortisone *on page 781*
♦ **Hydrocortisone Sodium Succinate** *see* Hydrocortisone *on page 781*
♦ **Hydrocortisone Valerate** *see* Hydrocortisone *on page 781*
♦ **Hydrogen Dioxide** *see* Hydrogen Peroxide *on page 786*

Hydrogen Peroxide (HYE droe jen per OKS ide)

Index Terms H_2O_2; Hydrogen Dioxide; Peroxide

Therapeutic Category Antibacterial, Otic; Antibacterial, Topical; Antibiotic, Oral Rinse

Use Cleanse wounds, suppurating ulcers, and local infections; used in the treatment of inflammatory conditions of the external auditory canal and as a mouthwash or gargle; hydrogen peroxide concentrate (30%) has been used as a hair bleach and as a tooth bleaching agent

Contraindications Should not be used in abscesses

Warnings Hydrogen peroxide concentrate (30%) is a caustic liquid; it should not be tasted since it is strongly irritating to skin or mucous membranes

Precautions Repeat use as a mouthwash or gargle may produce irritation of the buccal mucous membrane or "hairy tongue"; bandages should not be applied too quickly after its use

Adverse Reactions

Dermatologic: Bleaching effect on hair, irritating burn

Gastrointestinal: Rupture of the colon, proctitis, ulcerative colitis, gas embolism, hairy tongue

Local: Irritation of the buccal mucous membrane

Stability Protect from light and heat; decomposes upon standing, upon repeated agitation, or when in contact with oxidizing or reducing substances

Mechanism of Action Antiseptic oxidant that slowly releases oxygen and water upon contact with serum or tissue catalase

Pharmacodynamics Duration: Only while bubbling action occurs

Usual Dosage Children and Adults:

Mouthwash or gargle: Dilute the 3% solution with an equal volume of water; swish around in the mouth over the affected area for at least 1 minute and then expel; use up to 4 times/day (after meals and at bedtime)

Topical:

- 1.5% to 3% solution for cleansing wounds
- 1.5% gel for cleansing wounds or mouth/gum irritations: Apply a small amount to the affected area for at least 1 minute, then expectorate; use up to 4 times/day (after meals and at bedtime)

Administration Topical: Do not inject or instill into closed body cavities from which released oxygen cannot escape; strong solutions (30.5%) of hydrogen peroxide should not be applied undiluted to tissues

Dosage Forms

Gel, oral: 1.5% (15 g)

Solution:

- Concentrate: 30.5% (480 mL)
- Topical: 3% (120 mL, 480 mL)

♦ **Hydromorph Contin® (Can)** *see* Hydromorphone *on page 787*

♦ **Hydromorph-IR® (Can)** *see* Hydromorphone *on page 787*

Hydromorphone (hye droe MOR fone)

Medication Safety Issues

Sound-alike/look-alike issues:

Dilaudid® may be confused with Demerol®, Dilantin®

Hydromorphone may be confused with morphine; significant overdoses have occurred when hydromorphone products have been inadvertently administered instead of morphine sulfate. Commercially available prefilled syringes of both products looks similar and are often stored in close proximity to each other. **Note:** Hydromorphone 1 mg oral is approximately equal to morphine 4 mg oral; hydromorphone 1 mg I.V. is approximately equal to morphine 5 mg I.V.

Dilaudid®, Dilaudid-HP®: Extreme caution should be taken to avoid confusing the highly-concentrated (Dilaudid-HP®) injection with the less-concentrated (Dilaudid®) injectable product.

Significant differences exist between oral and I.V. dosing. Use caution when converting from one route of administration to another.

Related Information

Laboratory Detection of Drugs in Urine *on page 1928*
Narcotic Analgesics Comparison *on page 1705*
Overdose and Toxicology *on page 1916*

U.S. Brand Names Dilaudid®; Dilaudid-HP®

Canadian Brand Names Dilaudid®; Dilaudid-HP®; Dilaudid-HP-Plus®; Dilaudid® Sterile Powder; Dilaudid-XP®; Hydromorph Contin®; Hydromorph-IR®; Hydromorphone HP; Hydromorphone HP® 10; Hydromorphone HP® 20; Hydromorphone HP® 50; Hydromorphone HP® Forte; Hydromorphone Hydrochloride Injection, USP; PMS-Hydromorphone

Index Terms Dihydromorphinone; Hydromorphone Hydrochloride

Therapeutic Category Analgesic, Narcotic; Antitussive

Generic Available Yes: Excludes capsule, liquid, powder for injection

Use Management of moderate to severe pain; antitussive at lower doses. Dilaudid-HP® injection is indicated for use in opioid-tolerant patients who require larger than usual doses of opioids for pain relief.

Restrictions C-II

Pregnancy Risk Factor C

Lactation Excretion in breast milk unknown/not recommended

Contraindications Hypersensitivity to hydromorphone or any component (see Warnings); significant respiratory depression (especially in settings without resuscitative equipment or without adequate respiratory monitoring); severe CNS depression; patients with severe or acute asthma, paralytic ileus (known or suspected); pregnancy (prolonged use or high doses at term); obstetrical analgesia

Warnings Respiratory depression may occur; use with extreme caution in patients with pre-existing respiratory depression, decreased respiratory reserve, hypoxia, hypercapnia, significant COPD, or cor pulmonale. Hypotension may occur, especially in hypovolemic patients or those receiving medications that compromise vasomotor tone; use with extreme caution in patients with circulatory shock. Orthostatic hypotension may occur in ambulatory patients; physical and psychological dependence may occur; abrupt discontinuation after prolonged use may result in withdrawal symptoms or seizures; warn patient of possible impairment of alertness or physical coordination (see Patient Information); interactions with other CNS drugs may occur (see Drug Interactions). Healthcare provider should be alert to problems of abuse, misuse, and diversion. Infants born to women physically dependent on opioids will also be physically dependent and may experience respiratory difficulties or opioid withdrawal symptoms.

Do not confuse the highly-concentrated (Dilaudid-HP®) injection with the less-concentrated (Dilaudid®) injectable product; significant overdose or death could result. Extended release capsules are not recommended for use in patients with severe hepatic impairment (studies have not been conducted). Oral liquid and 8 mg tablets may contain trace amounts of sodium bisulfite which may cause allergic reactions in susceptible individuals; rubber stopper of multiple dose vials contains latex which may cause allergic reactions in susceptible individuals; avoid use in patients with allergy to latex.

Precautions Use with caution in patients with hypersensitivity reactions to other phenanthrene derivative opioid agonists (morphine, hydrocodone, levorphanol, oxycodone, oxymorphone, codeine). Use with caution and reduce the initial dose in patients

(Continued)

Hydromorphone *(Continued)*

with significant liver, respiratory, or renal disease; hypothyroidism or myxedema; head injury; increased intracranial pressure; CNS depression or coma; respiratory depression; adrenocortical insufficiency; toxic psychosis; seizures; acute abdominal conditions; post-GI surgery; biliary tract disease; pancreatitis; prostatic hypertrophy or urethral stricture; acute alcoholism; delirium tremens; kyphoscoliosis and in debilitated patients. Seizures and myoclonus have been reported in severely compromised patients receiving high doses of parenteral hydromorphone. Use with caution in patients undergoing biliary tract surgery (narcotics may cause spasm of the sphincter of Oddi).

Adverse Reactions

Cardiovascular: Palpitations, hypotension, bradycardia, peripheral vasodilation

Central nervous system: CNS depression, elevated intracranial pressure, drowsiness, dizziness, sedation

Dermatologic: Pruritus

Endocrine & metabolic: Antidiuretic hormone release

Gastrointestinal: Nausea, vomiting, constipation, biliary tract spasm

Genitourinary: Urinary tract spasm

Ocular: Miosis

Respiratory: Respiratory depression

Miscellaneous: Histamine release, physical and psychological dependence with prolonged use

Drug Interactions CNS depressants, alcohol, phenothiazines, tricyclic antidepressants, general anesthetics may potentiate the adverse effects of hydromorphone. Hydromorphone may enhance the action of neuromuscular-blocking agents resulting in excessive respiratory depression.

Food Interactions Food does not significantly affect bioavailability of extended release capsules; food decreased the peak serum concentration by 25%, prolonged the time to peak by 0.8 hours, and increased the AUC of a single tablet dose by 35% (effects may not be clinically significant).

Stability Protect from light; store suppositories in refrigerator; store other dosage forms at room temperature; a slight yellow discoloration of injection has not been associated with a loss of potency; injection is stable for at least 24 hours when protected from light and stored at 25°C in most common large volume parenteral solutions

Mechanism of Action Binds to opiate receptors in the CNS, causing inhibition of ascending pain pathways, altering the perception of and response to pain; causes cough suppression by direct central action in the medulla; produces generalized CNS depression

Pharmacodynamics Analgesic effects: Oral: Immediate release formulations:

Onset of action: Within 15-30 minutes

Maximum effect: Within 30-90 minutes

Duration: 4-5 hours; suppository may provide longer duration of effect

Pharmacokinetics

Absorption:

I.M.: Variable

Oral: Rapidly absorbed; extensive first-pass effect

Distribution: V_d: Adults: 4 L/kg; crosses the placenta; distributes into breast milk

Protein binding: ~8% to 19%

Metabolism: Primarily in the liver via glucuronidation to inactive metabolites; >95% is metabolized to hydromorphone-3-glucuronide; minor amounts as 6-hydroxy reduction metabolites

Bioavailability: Oral: 62%

Half-life: 1-3 hours

Time to peak serum concentration: Oral: 30-60 minutes

Elimination: In urine, principally as glucuronide conjugates

Usual Dosage

Antitussive: Oral:

Children 6-12 years: 0.5 mg every 3-4 hours as needed

Children >12 years and Adults: 1 mg every 3-4 hours as needed

Pain: Doses should be titrated to appropriate analgesic effects, while minimizing adverse effects; when changing routes of administration, note that oral doses are less than one-half as effective as parenteral doses (may be only $^1/_5$ as effective):

Young children:

Oral: 0.03-0.08 mg/kg/dose every 3-4 hours as needed; usual maximum dose: 5 mg/dose

I.V.: 0.015 mg/kg/dose every 3-6 hours as needed

Older Children and Adults:

Oral: Initial: Opiate-naive: 1-2 mg/dose every 3-4 hours as needed; patients with prior opiate exposure may tolerate higher initial doses; usual adult dose: 2-4 mg/dose; doses up to 8 mg have been used in adults

I.M., I.V., SubQ: Initial: Opiate-naive: 0.2-0.6 mg/dose every 2-4 hours as needed; patients with prior opiate exposure may tolerate higher initial doses

Rectal: 3 mg (1 suppository) every 6-8 hours as needed

Administration

Oral: Administer with food or milk to decrease GI upset

Parenteral: I.V.: Administer via slow I.V. injection over at least 2-3 minutes

Rectal: Insert suppository rectally and retain

Monitoring Parameters Pain relief, respiratory rate, heart rate, blood pressure

Patient Information Avoid alcohol. Hydromorphone may cause drowsiness and impair ability to perform activities requiring mental alertness or physical coordination; may be habit-forming; avoid abrupt discontinuation after prolonged use; if oral liquid spills on skin, remove contaminated clothing and rinse area with cool water

Additional Information Equianalgesic doses: Morphine 10 mg I.M. = hydromorphone 1.5 mg I.M.

Note: Palladone™ (hydromorphone extended release capsules) was voluntarily withdrawn from the United States market in July 2005. A potentially fatal adverse reaction can occur when Palladone™ is taken with alcohol or alcohol-containing medications. Alcohol interferes with the extended release mechanism of this product, causing an accelerated release, or "dose dumping," of hydromorphone. This results in dangerous increases in hydromorphone peak plasma concentrations and may lead to respiratory depression, coma, or death, even in opioid tolerant patients. The manufacturer plans to reformulate the product, but the sales and marketing of Palladone™ have been suspended during this time. The company and the FDA are considering limited distribution to hospitals and hospices until the reformulated product is available. Patients currently taking Palladone™ should consult with their healthcare provider for alternative treatments. If current supplies of Palladone™ are to be used, patients should not drink alcohol (including beer, wine, distilled spirits) or take over-the-counter medications which may contain alcohol.

Dosage Forms Excipient information presented when available (limited, particularly for generics); consult specific product labeling. [CAN] = Canadian brand name

Capsule, controlled release:

Hydromorph Contin® [CAN]: 3 mg, 6 mg, 12 mg, 18 mg, 24 mg, 30 mg [not available in U.S.]

Injection, powder for reconstitution, as hydrochloride:

Dilaudid-HP®: 250 mg

Injection, solution, as hydrochloride: 1 mg/mL (1 mL); 2 mg/mL (1 mL, 20 mL); 4 mg/mL (1 mL); 10 mg/mL (1 mL, 5 mL, 10 mL)

Dilaudid®: 1 mg/mL (1 mL); 2 mg/mL (1 mL, 20 mL) [20 mL size contains edetate sodium; vial stopper contains latex]; 4 mg/mL (1 mL)

Dilaudid-HP®: 10 mg/mL (1 mL, 5 mL, 50 mL) [50 mL packaging contains latex]

Liquid, oral, as hydrochloride:

Dilaudid®: 1 mg/mL (480 mL) [may contain trace amounts of sodium bisulfite]

Suppository, rectal, as hydrochloride: 3 mg

Dilaudid®: 3 mg (6s)

Tablet, as hydrochloride: 2 mg, 4 mg, 8 mg

Dilaudid®: 2 mg, 4 mg, 8 mg (8 mg tablets may contain trace amounts of sodium bisulfite)

References

Berde CB and Sethna NF, "Analgesics for the Treatment of Pain in Children," *N Engl J Med*, 2002, 347(14):1094-103.

Carr D, Jacox A, Chapman CR, et al, "Clinical Practice Guideline Number 1: Acute Pain Management: Operative or Medical Procedures and Trauma," Rockville, Maryland: U.S. Department of Health and Human Services, Public Health Service, Agency for Health Care Policy and Research, AHCPR Publication No 92-0032, 1992.

Jacox A, Carr D, Payne R, et al, "Clinical Practice Guideline Number 9: Management of Cancer Pain," Rockville, Maryland: U.S. Department of Health and Human Services, Public Health Service, Agency for Health Care Policy and Research, AHCPR Publication No. 94-0592, 1994.

- **Hydromorphone HP (Can)** *see* Hydromorphone *on page 787*
- **Hydromorphone HP® 10 (Can)** *see* Hydromorphone *on page 787*
- **Hydromorphone HP® 20 (Can)** *see* Hydromorphone *on page 787*
- **Hydromorphone HP® 50 (Can)** *see* Hydromorphone *on page 787*
- **Hydromorphone HP® Forte (Can)** *see* Hydromorphone *on page 787*
- **Hydromorphone Hydrochloride** *see* Hydromorphone *on page 787*
- **Hydromorphone Hydrochloride Injection, USP (Can)** *see* Hydromorphone *on page 787*
- **Hydro-Tussin™-CBX** *see* Carbinoxamine and Pseudoephedrine *on page 286*

♦ **Hydro-Tussin™ DM** *see* Guaifenesin and Dextromethorphan *on page 748*
♦ **HydroVal® (Can)** *see* Hydrocortisone *on page 781*

Hydroxocobalamin (hye droks oh koe BAL a min)

U.S. Brand Names Cyanokit®

Index Terms Vitamin B_{12a}

Therapeutic Category Antidote, Cyanide; Nutritional Supplement; Vitamin, Water Soluble

Generic Available Yes: Excludes powder for injection

Use

I.M. injection: Treatment of pernicious anemia and other vitamin B_{12} deficiency states; dietary supplement particularly in conditions of increased requirements (eg, pregnancy, thyrotoxicosis, hemorrhage, malignancy, liver or kidney disease)

I.V. infusion (Cyanokit®): Treatment of cyanide poisoning

Pregnancy Risk Factor C

Lactation Excretion in breast milk unknown/use caution

Contraindications Hypersensitivity to hydroxocobalamin, cyanocobalamin, cobalt, or any component

Warnings Anaphylactic shock has occurred after parenteral vitamin B_{12} administration; intradermal skin testing may be used prior to administration in individuals sensitive to cobalt

When using Cyanokit®: Increased blood pressure (>180 mm Hg systolic or >110 mm Hg diastolic) is associated with infusion; elevations usually noted at beginning of infusion, peak toward the end of infusion, and return to baseline within 4 hours of infusion. Collection of pretreatment blood cyanide concentrations does not preclude administration and should not delay administration in the emergency management of highly suspected or confirmed cyanide toxicity. Pretreatment levels may be useful as postinfusion levels may be inaccurate. Treatment of cyanide poisoning should include decontamination and supportive therapy. Photosensitivity is a potential concern; avoid direct sunlight while skin remains discolored. Safety and efficacy for use in children has not been established. Will produce chromaturia which may last up to 5 weeks after administration.

Precautions When using solution for I.M. injection as treatment of severe vitamin B_{12} deficiency: Serum potassium concentrations should be monitored early as severe hypokalemia has occurred after the conversion of megaloblastic anemia to normal erythropoiesis; the increase in nucleic acid degradation produced by administration of hydroxocobalamin to deficient patients may result in gout in susceptible individuals; use of hydroxocobalamin in folic acid deficient individuals may improve folate-deficient megaloblastic anemia and obscure the true diagnosis

Adverse Reactions

I.M. injection:

Cardiovascular: Peripheral vascular thrombosis
Dermatologic: Itching, exanthema, urticaria
Endocrine & metabolic: Hypokalemia
Gastrointestinal: Diarrhea
Local: Pain at injection site
Miscellaneous: Hypersensitivity reactions

I.M. infusion (Cyanokit®):

Cardiovascular: Hypertension (18% to 28%; see Warnings), chest discomfort, tachycardia, bradycardia, hot flashes, peripheral edema, angioneurotic edema
Central nervous system: Headache, dizziness, memory impairment, restlessness
Dermatologic: Erythema (94% to 100%; may last up to 2 weeks), rash (predominantly acneiform; 20% to 44%; can appear 7-28 days after administration and usually resolves within a few weeks), pruritus, urticaria; photosensitivity
Gastrointestinal: Nausea, abdominal discomfort, diarrhea, dyspepsia, dysphagia, hematochezia, vomiting
Genitourinary: Chromaturia (100%; may last up to 5 weeks after administration)
Hematologic: Decreased lymphocytes
Local: Infusion site reaction (6% to 39%)
Ocular: Irritation, redness, swelling
Respiratory: Dry throat, dyspnea, throat tightness
Miscellaneous: Hypersensitivity reactions including anaphylaxis

Drug Interactions Decreased absorption of hydroxocobalamin from GI tract by aminoglycoside antibiotics, colchicine, extended release potassium products, aminosalicylic acid, excessive alcohol use, phenytoin, and phenobarbital; antagonism of hematopoietic response to hydroxocobalamin when administered with chloramphenicol

Stability Stable at room temperature; protect from light. Cyanokit® may be exposed at short intervals to temperatures outside of room temperature:

Usual transport: <15 days at 41°F to 104°F (5°C to 40°C)

Desert transport: <4 days at 41°F to 104°F (5°C to 40°C)

Freezing/defrosting cycles: <15 days at -4°F to 104°F (-20°C to 40°C)

Reconstituted vials (Cyanokit®) are stable for 6 hours at temperatures not exceeding 104°F (40°C). Hydroxocobalamin infusion (Cyanokit®) is physically incompatible if mixed with diazapam, dobutamine, dopamine, fentanyl, nitroglycerin, pentobarbital, propofol, and thiopental. It is also chemically incompatible with sodium thiosulfate, sodium nitrate, and ascorbic acid. It should not be infused either in the same solution or into the same I.V. line with these medications.

Mechanism of Action Hydroxocobalamin (vitamin B_{12a}) is a precursor to cyanocobalamin (vitamin B_{12}). Cyanocobalamin acts as a coenzyme for various metabolic functions, including fat and carbohydrate metabolism and protein synthesis, used in cell replication and hematopoiesis. In the presence of cyanide, each hydroxocobalamin molecule can bind one cyanide ion by substituting it for the hydroxo ligand linked to the trivalent cobalt ion, forming cyanocobalamin.

Pharmacodynamics

Onset of action: I.M.:

- Megaloblastic anemia:
  - Conversion of megaloblastic to normoblastic erythroid hyperplasia within bone marrow: 8 hours
  - Increased reticulocytes: 2-5 days
- Complicated vitamin B_{12} deficiency:
  - Psychiatric sequelae: 24 hours
  - Thrombocytopenia: 10 days
  - Granulocytopenia: 2 weeks

Pharmacokinetics

Distribution: Principally stored in the liver; also stored in the kidneys and adrenals

Protein binding: I.M. solution: Bound to transcobalamin II; I.V.: Cyanokit®: Significant; forms various cobalamin-(III) complexes

Half-life: I.V.: 26-31 hours

Metabolism: Converted in the tissues to active coenzymes methylcobalamin and deoxyadenosylcobalamin

Time to peak serum concentration: 2 hours

Elimination: Urine (50% to 98%)

Usual Dosage

I.M.:

- Schilling test (diagnostic for vitamin B_{12} deficiency): Children and Adults: 1000 mcg once
- Congenital transcobalamin deficiency: Neonates: 1000 mcg twice weekly
- Vitamin B_{12} deficiency or pernicious anemia: Varying regimens:
  - Uncomplicated disease:
    - Children: Initial: 100 mcg/day for 10-15 days (total dose: 1-5 mg); maintenance: 60 mcg/month
      - **or as an alternative:** 30-50 mcg/day for at least 2 weeks (total dose: 1-5 mg); maintenance: 100 mcg/month
    - Adults: Initial: 30 mcg/day for 5-10 days; maintenance: 100-200 mcg/monthly
      - **or as an alternative:** 1000 mcg/day for 5-10 days, followed by 100-200 mcg/month
      - **or as an alternative:** 100 mcg/day for 1 week, followed by 100 mcg every other day for 2 weeks; maintenance: 100 mcg/month
  - Complicated disease (eg, severe anemia with heart failure, thrombocytopenia with bleeding, granulocytopenia with infection, severe neurologic damage): Adults: 1000 mcg plus folic acid 15 mg once, followed by 100 mcg/day plus oral folic acid 5 mg/day for 1 week; maintenance dosing as above

I.V.: Cyanide toxicity (Cyanokit®):

- Children (non-U.S. marketing experience per manufacturer): 70 mg/kg as a single infusion
- Adults: Initial: 5 g as single infusion; may repeat a second 5 g dose depending on the severity of poisoning and clinical response: maximum cumulative dose: 10 g

Dosage interval in hepatic or renal impairment: A decrease in the interval between injections may be required

Administration Parenteral:

I.M.: Administer 1000 mcg/mL injection I.M. only; do not administer SubQ

I.V.: Cyanokit®: Reconstitute 2.5 g vial with 100 mL NS, LR, or 5% dextrose; after reconstitution, repeatedly invert or "rock" solution for at least 30 seconds; do not shake. Administer over 15 minutes; if repeat dose is needed, administer second dose over 15 minutes to 2 hours depending upon the patient's clinical state

(Continued)

Hydroxocobalamin *(Continued)*

Monitoring Parameters

Anemia and deficiency states: Vitamin B_{12}, serum potassium, erythrocyte and reticulocyte counts, hemoglobin, hematocrit

Cyanide toxicity: Blood pressure and heart rate during and after infusion, serum lactate levels, venous-arterial pO_2 gradient, blood cyanide concentrations (see Warnings)

Reference Range

Vitamin B_{12}: Normal: 200-900 pg/mL; vitamin B_{12} deficiency: <200 pg/mL; megaloblastic anemia: <100 pg/mL

Cyanide toxicity: Blood cyanide levels may be used for diagnosis confirmation; however, reliable levels require prompt testing and proper storage conditions

Cyanide levels related to clinical symptomatology:

- Tachycardia/flushing: 0.5-1 mg/L
- Obtundation: 1-2.5 mg/L
- Coma: 2.5-3 mg/L
- Death: >3 mg/L

Test Interactions The following values may be affected, *in vitro*, following hydroxocobalamin 5 g dose. Interference following hydroxocobalamin 10 g dose can be expected to last up to an additional 24 hours. **Note:** Extent and duration of interference dependant on analyzer used and patient variability.

Falsely elevated:

- Basophils, hemoglobin, MCH, and MCHC [duration: 12-16 hours]
- Albumin, alkaline phosphatase, cholesterol, creatinine, glucose, total protein, and triglycerides [duration: 24 hours]
- Bilirubin [duration: up to 4 days]
- Urinalysis: Glucose, protein, erythrocytes, leukocytes, ketones, bilirubin, urobilinogen, nitrite [duration: 2-8 days]

Falsely decreased: ALT and amylase [duration: 24 hours]

Unpredictable:

- AST, CK, CKMB, LDH, phosphate, and uric acid [duration: 24 hours]
- PT (quick or INR) and aPTT [duration: 24-48 hours]
- Urine pH [duration: 2-8 days]

May also interfere with colorimetric tests

Patient Information Life-long therapy is required in patients with pernicious anemia or other absorption defects; do not discontinue therapy without consulting your physician; avoid alcohol; large doses (Cyanokit®) will result in red-colored urine for up to 5 weeks and skin and mucous membrane redness for up to 2 weeks after administration; may cause photosensitivity (eg, exposure to sunlight may cause severe sunburn, skin rash, redness, or itching) while skin is discolored; avoid exposure to sunlight and artificial light sources (sunlamps, tanning booth/bed); wear protective clothing, wide-brimmed hats, sunglasses, and lip sunscreen (SPF ≥15); use a sunscreen [broad-spectrum sunscreen or physical sunscreen (preferred) or sunblock with SPF ≥15]; contact physician if reaction occurs; an acne-like rash may occur 7-28 days after administration of Cyanokit®; this rash usually goes away without any treatment

Additional Information Cyanocobalamin is preferred over hydroxocobalamin as a treatment agent for anemia due to reports of antibody formation to the hydroxocobalamin-transcobalamin complex. Cyanide is a clear colorless gas or liquid with a faint bitter almond odor. Cyanide reacts with trivalent ions in cytochrome oxidase in the mitochondria leading to histotoxic hypoxia and lactic acidosis. Signs and symptoms of cyanide toxicity include headache, altered mental status, dyspnea, mydriasis, chest tightness, nausea, vomiting, tachycardia/hypertension (initially), bradycardia/hypotension (later), seizures, cardiovascular collapse, or coma. Expert advice from a regional poison control center for appropriate use may be obtained (1-800-222-1222).

Dosage Forms Excipient information presented when available (limited, particularly for generics); consult specific product labeling.

Injection, solution: 1000 mcg/mL (30 mL)

Injection, powder for reconstitution:

- Cyanokit®: 2.5 g (2 vials) [provided in a kit which also contains one I.V. infusion set]

◆ **Hydroxy-1,4-naphthoquinone** *see* Atovaquone *on page 178*

◆ **Hydroxycarbamide** *see* Hydroxyurea *on page 794*

Hydroxychloroquine (hye droks ee KLOR oh kwin)

Medication Safety Issues

Sound-alike/look-alike issues:

- Hydroxychloroquine may be confused with hydrocortisone
- Plaquenil® may be confused with Platinol®

Related Information
Malaria *on page 1855*
Medications for Which A Single Dose May Be Fatal When Ingested By A Toddler *on page 1932*

U.S. Brand Names Plaquenil®

Canadian Brand Names Apo-Hydroxyquine®; Gen-Hydroxychloroquine; Plaquenil®

Index Terms Hydroxychloroquine Sulfate

Therapeutic Category Antimalarial Agent; Antirheumatic, Disease Modifying

Generic Available Yes

Use Suppression or chemoprophylaxis of malaria caused by susceptible *P. vivax*, *P. ovale*, *P. malariae*, and some strains of *P. falciparum* (not active against pre-erythrocytic or exoerythrocytic tissue stages of *Plasmodium*); treatment of systemic lupus erythematosus (SLE) and rheumatoid arthritis

Pregnancy Risk Factor C

Lactation Enters breast milk/compatible

Contraindications Hypersensitivity to hydroxychloroquine, 4-aminoquinoline derivatives, or any component; retinal or visual field changes; patients with porphyria or psoriasis

Warnings Long-term use in children is **not** recommended; daily dose >6-6.5 mg/kg/day in patients with abnormal hepatic or renal function may be associated with an increased risk of retinal toxicity

Precautions Use with caution in patients with hepatic disease and G-6-PD deficiency

Adverse Reactions
Cardiovascular: Cardiomyopathy (rare)
Central nervous system: Insomnia, nervousness, nightmares, dizziness, psychosis, headache, confusion, agitation, ataxia
Dermatologic: Lichenoid dermatitis, bleaching of the hair, pruritus, alopecia, hyperpigmentation, photosensitivity, Stevens-Johnson syndrome, exfoliative dermatitis
Gastrointestinal: GI irritation, abdominal cramps, anorexia, nausea, vomiting, diarrhea
Hematologic: Bone marrow suppression, thrombocytopenia, aplastic anemia, agranulocytosis
Hepatic: Hepatic failure
Neuromuscular & skeletal: Muscle weakness, skeletal muscle palsies, neuromyopathy, depression of tendon reflexes, peripheral neuropathy
Ocular: Visual field defects, blindness, retinitis, macular degeneration, decreased night vision

Drug Interactions Increases digoxin serum levels

Food Interactions Food increases bioavailability

Stability Protect from light

Mechanism of Action Interferes with digestive vacuole function within sensitive malarial parasites by increasing the pH and interfering with lysosomal degradation of hemoglobin; inhibits locomotion of neutrophils and chemotaxis of eosinophils; impairs complement-dependent antigen-antibody reactions

Pharmacodynamics Onset of action for JRA: 2-4 months, up to 6 months

Pharmacokinetics
Absorption: Highly variable (31% to 100%)
Distribution: Extensive distribution to most body fluids and tissues; excreted into breast milk; crosses the placenta
Metabolism: In the liver
Bioavailability: Increased when administered with food
Elimination: Metabolites and unchanged drug slowly excreted in the urine

Usual Dosage Oral:
Children:
Chemoprophylaxis of malaria: 5 mg/kg **(base)** once weekly; do not exceed the recommended adult dose; begin 1-2 weeks before exposure; continue for 4 weeks after leaving endemic area
Uncomplicated acute attack of malaria: 10 mg/kg **(base)** initial dose; followed by 5 mg/kg **(base)** in 6-8 hours on day 1; 5 mg/kg **(base)** as a single dose on day 2 and on day 3
JRA or SLE: 3-5 mg/kg/day **(as sulfate)** divided 1-2 times/day to a maximum of 400 mg/day **(as sulfate)**; not to exceed 7 mg/kg/day
Adults:
Chemoprophylaxis of malaria: 310 mg **(base)** once weekly on same day each week; begin 1-2 weeks before exposure; continue for 4 weeks after leaving endemic area
Uncomplicated acute attack of malaria: 620 mg **(base)** first dose day one; 310 mg **(base)** in 6-8 hours day one; 310 mg **(base)** as a single dose day 2; and 310 mg **(base)** as a single dose on day 3

(Continued)

Hydroxychloroquine *(Continued)*

Rheumatoid arthritis: 400-600 mg/day **(as sulfate)** once daily to start; increase dose until optimum response level is reached; usually after 4-12 weeks dose should be reduced by 50% and a maintenance dose given of 200-400 mg/day **(as sulfate)** divided 1-2 times/day

Lupus erythematosus: 400 mg **(as sulfate)** every day or twice daily for several weeks depending on response; 200-400 mg/day **(as sulfate)** for prolonged maintenance therapy

Administration Oral: Administer with food or milk to decrease GI distress

Monitoring Parameters Ophthalmologic examination, CBC with differential and platelet count; check for muscular weakness with prolonged therapy

Patient Information May cause photosensitivity reactions (eg, exposure to sunlight may cause severe sunburn, skin rash, redness, or itching); avoid exposure to sunlight and artificial light sources (sunlamps, tanning booth/bed); wear protective clothing, wide-brimmed hats, sunglasses, and lip sunscreen (SPF ≥15); use a sunscreen [broad-spectrum sunscreen or physical sunscreen (preferred) or sunblock with SPF ≥15]; contact physician if reaction occurs. Notify physician if blurring of vision, vision change, or emotional change occur; may cause dizziness and vision changes, so exercise caution when driving; avoid alcohol; contraindicated during breast-feeding

Dosage Forms Excipient information presented when available (limited, particularly for generics); consult specific product labeling.

Tablet, as sulfate: 200 mg [equivalent to 155 mg base]

Extemporaneous Preparations A 25 mg/mL hydroxychloroquine sulfate suspension is made by removing the coating off of fifteen 200 mg hydroxychloroquine sulfate tablets with a towel moistened with alcohol; tablets are ground to a fine powder and levigated to a paste with 15 mL of Ora-Plus® suspending agent; add an additional 45 mL of suspending agent and levigate until a uniform mixture is obtained; qs ad to 120 mL with sterile water for irrigation; a 30 day expiration date is recommended, although stability testing has not been performed

Pesko LJ, "Compounding: Hydroxychloroquine," *Am Druggist*, 1993, 207:57.

References

Emery H, "Clinical Aspects of Systemic Lupus Erythematosus in Childhood," *Pediatr Clin North Am*, 1986, 33(5):1177-90.

Giannini EH and Cawkwell GD, "Drug Treatment in Children With Juvenile Rheumatoid Arthritis. Past, Present, and Future," *Pediatr Clin North Am*, 1995, 42(5):1099-125.

"Guidelines for the Management of Rheumatoid Arthritis. American College of Rheumatology Ad Hoc Committee on Clinical Guidelines," *Arthritis Rheum*, 1996, 39(5):713-22.

♦ **Hydroxychloroquine Sulfate** *see* Hydroxychloroquine *on page 792*

♦ **Hydroxydaunomycin Hydrochloride** *see* DOXOrubicin *on page 540*

♦ **Hydroxyethyl Starch** *see* Hetastarch *on page 766*

♦ **Hydroxyldaunorubicin Hydrochloride** *see* DOXOrubicin *on page 540*

♦ ***L*-3-Hydroxytyrosine** *see* Levodopa *on page 926*

Hydroxyurea (hye droks ee yoor EE a)

Medication Safety Issues

Sound-alike/look-alike issues:

Hydroxyurea may be confused with hydrOXYzine

High alert medication: The Institute for Safe Medication Practices (ISMP) includes this medication among its list of drugs which have a heightened risk of causing significant patient harm when used in error.

International issues:

Hydrea® may be confused with Hydra® which is a brand name for isoniazid in Japan

Related Information

Adult and Adolescent HIV *on page 1821*

Emetogenic Potential of Single Chemotherapeutic Agents *on page 1776*

U.S. Brand Names Droxia®; Hydrea®; Mylocel™

Canadian Brand Names Apo-Hydroxyurea®; Gen-Hydroxyurea; Hydrea®

Index Terms Hydroxycarbamide

Therapeutic Category Antineoplastic Agent, Miscellaneous

Generic Available Yes: Capsule

Use Treatment of chronic myelocytic leukemia (CML), melanoma, and ovarian carcinoma; used with radiation in treatment of tumors of the head and neck; adjunct in the management of sickle cell patients who have had at least three painful crises in the previous 12 months; combination therapy with didanosine for treatment of HIV infection

Pregnancy Risk Factor D

Lactation Enters breast milk/contraindicated

Contraindications Hypersensitivity to hydroxyurea or any component; severe anemia, severe bone marrow suppression; when hydroxyurea is used as an antineoplastic agent: WBC <2500/mm^3 or platelet count <100,000/mm^3; when hydroxyurea is used in patients with sickle cell anemia: Neutrophil count <2000 cells/mm^3, platelet count <80,000/mm^3, hemoglobin <9 g/dL, reticulocyte count <80,000/mm^3 when hemoglobin <9 g/dL

Warnings The FDA currently recommends that procedures for proper handling and disposal of antineoplastic agents be considered; hydroxyurea is presumed to be a human carcinogen; secondary leukemia and skin cancer have been reported in patients receiving long-term hydroxyurea therapy. Hydroxyurea impairs fertility and is embryotoxic causing fetal malformations. Vasculitic ulcerations and gangrene have been reported in patients who received hydroxyurea for myeloproliferative disorders with a previous or concurrent history of interferon use; discontinue if cutaneous vasculitic ulcerations develop.

Precautions Use with caution and modify dose in patients with renal impairment

Adverse Reactions

Central nervous system: Dizziness, disorientation, hallucinations, drowsiness, seizures, headache, fever, chills

Dermatologic: Maculopapular rash, facial erythema, thinning of the skin, pruritus, hyperpigmentation, vasculitic ulcerations, gangrene, hair loss

Endocrine & metabolic: Hyperuricemia

Gastrointestinal: Nausea, vomiting, diarrhea, constipation, anorexia, stomatitis, pancreatitis

Genitourinary: Dysuria

Hematologic: Myelosuppression (leukopenia, neutropenia, thrombocytopenia), megaloblastic anemia

Hepatic: Elevated hepatic enzymes

Renal: Renal tubular function impairment, elevated BUN, elevated serum creatinine

Respiratory: Pulmonary fibrosis (rare)

Drug Interactions Cytarabine (increases cytarabine activity); didanosine (hydroxyurea may potentiate intracellular toxicity of didanosine and precipitate didanosine-induced pancreatitis, hepatotoxicity, or neuropathy); concomitant use with didanosine is not recommended

Stability Store in a tightly sealed container since the drug is degraded by moisture; store at room temperature

Mechanism of Action Interferes with synthesis of DNA during the S-phase of cell division without interfering with RNA synthesis; inhibits ribonucleoside diphosphate reductase preventing conversion of ribonucleotides to deoxyribonucleotides; hydroxyurea also inhibits the incorporation of thymidine into DNA; in sickle cell patients, hydroxyurea increases the production of fetal hemoglobin and decreases neutrophils

Pharmacodynamics Maximum effect for sickle cell disease: 6-18 months

Pharmacokinetics

Absorption: Readily from the GI tract

Distribution: Readily crosses the blood-brain barrier and the placenta; distributes into peritoneal or pleural effusions; excreted in breast milk

Metabolism: 60% via hepatic metabolism and urease found in intestinal bacteria

Half-life: 3-4 hours

Time to peak serum concentration: Within 1-4 hours

Elimination: 50% of drug excreted unchanged in urine; renal excretion of urea (metabolite) and respiratory excretion of CO_2 (metabolic end product)

Usual Dosage Oral (refer to individual protocols): Base dosage on ideal body weight:

Children:

Treatment of pediatric astrocytoma, medulloblastoma, and primitive neuroectodermal tumors: No FDA approved dosage regimens have been established. Dosages of 1500-3000 mg/m^2 as a single dose in combination with other agents, followed by a second course 2 weeks later with subsequent courses every 4-6 weeks have been used (eight-in-one regimen).

CML: Initial: 10-20 mg/kg/day once daily; adjust dose according to hematologic response

Children and Adults: Sickle cell anemia: Initial dose: 15 mg/kg/day (range: 10-20 mg/kg/day) once daily; increase dose in increments of 5 mg/kg/day every 12 weeks to a maximum dose of 35 mg/kg/day; reduced dosage of hydroxyurea alternating with erythropoietin may decrease myelotoxicity and increase levels of fetal hemoglobin in patients who have not been helped by hydroxyurea alone

Adults:

Solid tumors:

Intermittent therapy: 80 mg/kg as a single dose every third day

Continuous therapy: 20-30 mg/kg/day given as a single dose/day

Concomitant therapy with irradiation: 80 mg/kg as a single dose every third day starting at least 7 days before initiation of irradiation

(Continued)

Hydroxyurea *(Continued)*

Resistant chronic myelocytic leukemia: 20-30 mg/kg/day once daily

HIV infection: 500 mg twice daily (15 mg/kg/day divided twice daily) in combination with didanosine 200 mg twice daily (**Note:** HIV Adult and Adolescent guidelines state that there is insufficient data to make a recommendation for or against its use; see February 4, 2002, http://www.aidsinfo.nih.gov)

Dosing adjustment in renal impairment: Adults:

Sickle cell anemia: Cl_{cr} <60 mL/minute: Reduce initial dose to 7.5 mg/kg/day

Other indications:

Cl_{cr} 10-50 mL/minute: Administer 50% of normal dose

Cl_{cr} <10 mL/minute: Administer 20% of normal dose

Hemodialysis: Administer dose following hemodialysis

Administration Oral: Administer with water on an empty stomach; for patients unable to swallow capsules, contents of capsule may be emptied into a glass of water if administered immediately

Monitoring Parameters CBC with differential and platelet count, hemoglobin, renal function and liver function tests, serum uric acid

Test Interactions False-negative triglyceride measurement by a glycerol oxidase method

Patient Information Inform physician if fever, sore throat, bruising, or bleeding develops; advise women of childbearing potential to avoid becoming pregnant while taking hydroxyurea. To minimize risk of skin exposure to hydroxyurea, wear disposable gloves when handling bottle or capsules.

Additional Information Myelosuppressive effects:

WBC: Moderate

Platelets: Moderate

Onset (days): 7

Nadir (days): 10

Recovery (days): 21

Dosage Forms Excipient information presented when available (limited, particularly for generics); consult specific product labeling.

Capsule: 500 mg

Droxia®: 200 mg, 300 mg, 400 mg

Hydrea®: 500 mg

Tablet:

Mylocel™: 1000 mg

References

Geyer JR, Finlay JL, Boyett JM, et al, "Survival of Infants With Malignant Astrocytomas. A Report From the Childrens Cancer Group," *Cancer*, 1995, 75(4):1045-50.

Geyer JR, Pendergrass TW, Milstein JM, et al, "Eight Drugs in One Day Chemotherapy in Children With Brain Tumors: A Critical Toxicity Appraisal," *J Clin Oncol*, 1988, 6(6):996-1000.

Maier-Redelsperger M, de Montalembert M, Flahault A, et al, "Fetal Hemoglobin and F-Cell Responses to Long-Term Hydroxyurea Treatment in Young Sickle Cell Patients. The French Study Group on Sickle Cell Disease," *Blood*, 1998, 91(12):4472-9.

Montaner JS, Zala C, Conway B, et al, "A Pilot Study of Hydroxyurea Among Patients With Advanced Human Immunodeficiency Virus (HIV) Disease Receiving Chronic Didanosine Therapy: Canadian HIV Trials Network Protocol 080," *J Infect Dis*, 1997, 175(4):801-6.

Panel on Clinical Practices for the Treatment of HIV Infection, "Guidelines for the Use of Antiretroviral Agents in HIV-Infected Adults and Adolescents," March 23, 2004, http://www.aidsinfo.nih.gov.

Rodgers GP, Dover GJ, Noguchi CT, et al, "Hematologic Responses of Patients With Sickle Cell Disease to Treatment With Hydroxyurea," *N Engl J Med*, 1990, 322(15):1037-45.

Rodgers GP, Dover GJ, Uyesaka N, et al, "Augmentation by Erythropoietin of the Fetal-Hemoglobin Response to Hydroxyurea in Sickle Cell Disease," *N Engl J Med*, 1993, 328(2):73-80.

HydrOXYzine (hye DROKS i zeen)

Medication Safety Issues

Sound-alike/look-alike issues:

HydrOXYzine may be confused with hydrALAZINE, hydroxyurea

Atarax® may be confused with amoxicillin, Ativan®

Vistaril® may be confused with Restoril®, Versed, Zestril®

International issues:

Vistaril® may be confused with Vastarel® which is a brand name for trimetazidine in multiple international markets

Related Information

Acute Dystonic Reactions, Management *on page 1894*

Compatibility of Chemotherapy and Related Supportive Care Medications *on page 1777*

Compatibility of Medications Mixed in A Syringe *on page 1941*

U.S. Brand Names Vistaril®

Canadian Brand Names Apo-Hydroxyzine®; Atarax®; Hydroxyzine Hydrochloride Injection, USP; Novo-Hydroxyzin; PMS-Hydroxyzine; Vistaril®

Index Terms Hydroxyzine Hydrochloride; Hydroxyzine Pamoate

Therapeutic Category Antianxiety Agent; Antiemetic; Antihistamine; Sedative

Generic Available Yes

Use Treatment of anxiety; preoperative sedative; antipruritic; antiemetic

Pregnancy Risk Factor C

Lactation Excretion in breast milk unknown/not recommended

Contraindications Hypersensitivity to hydroxyzine or any component (see Warnings); early pregnancy

Warnings Subcutaneous, intra-arterial and I.V. administration are **not** recommended since intravascular hemolysis, thrombosis, and digital gangrene can occur; extravasation can result in sterile abscess and marked tissue induration. Hydroxyzine causes sedation; caution must be used when performing tasks which require alertness (eg, operating machinery or driving). Sedative effects of CNS depressants or ethanol are potentiated (see Drug Interactions).

Injection may contain benzyl alcohol which may cause allergic reactions in susceptible individuals; syrup may contain sodium benzoate; benzoic acid (benzoate) is a metabolite of benzyl alcohol; large amounts of benzyl alcohol (≥99 mg/kg/day) have been associated with a potentially fatal toxicity ("gasping syndrome") in neonates; the "gasping syndrome" consists of metabolic acidosis, respiratory distress, gasping respirations, CNS dysfunction (including convulsions, intracranial hemorrhage), hypotension and cardiovascular collapse; avoid use of hydroxyzine products containing benzyl alcohol or sodium benzoate in neonates; *in vitro* and animal studies have shown that benzoate displaces bilirubin from protein binding sites

Precautions Use with caution in patients with narrow-angle glaucoma, prostatic hypertrophy, bladder neck obstruction, asthma, or COPD. Neonatal withdrawal symptoms, including seizures, have been reported following long-term maternal use or the use of large doses near term.

Adverse Reactions

Cardiovascular: Hypotension; supraventricular tachycardia (case report; see Wong, 2004)

Central nervous system: Drowsiness, dizziness, headache, ataxia, hallucination, seizure

Dermatologic: Pruritus, rash, urticaria

Gastrointestinal: Xerostomia

Genitourinary: Urinary retention

Local: Pain at injection site

Neuromuscular & skeletal: Weakness, involuntary movements, paresthesia, tremor

Ocular: Blurred vision

Respiratory: Thickening of bronchial secretions

Miscellaneous: Allergic reaction, anticholinergic effects

Drug Interactions Hydroxyzine may potentiate the effects of other CNS depressants or alcohol (avoid alcohol; monitor patients and use a decreased dose of CNS depressant when used concomitantly with hydroxyzine). Hydroxyzine may potentiate the effects of anticholinergics and can antagonize the vasopressor effects of epinephrine.

Stability Injection: Store at 15°C to 30°C. Protect from light

Mechanism of Action Competes with histamine for H_1-receptor sites on effector cells in the GI tract, blood vessels, and respiratory tract

Pharmacodynamics

Onset of action: Within 15-30 minutes

Duration: 4-6 hours

Pharmacokinetics

Absorption: Oral: Well absorbed

Distribution: V_d, apparent:

- Children 1-14 years: 18.5 ± 8.6 L/kg
- Adults: 16 ± 3 L/kg

Metabolism: In the liver; forms metabolites

Half-life:

- Children 1-14 years (mean age: 6.1 ± 4.6 years): 7.1 ± 2.3 hours; **Note:** Half-life increased with increasing age and was 4 hours in patients 1-year old and 11 hours in a 14-year old patient (see Simons, 1984)
- Adults: 3 hours; one study reported a terminal half-life of 20 hours (see Simons, 1984a)

Time to peak serum concentration: Oral: 2 hours

Usual Dosage

Children:

Manufacturer's recommendation:

Preoperative sedation:

Oral: 0.6 mg/kg/dose

I.M.: 0.5-1 mg/kg/dose

(Continued)

HydrOXYzine *(Continued)*

Pruritus, anxiety: Oral:
<6 years: 50 mg/day in divided doses
≥6 years: 50-100 mg/day in divided doses
Alternative dosing: Pruritus, anxiety:
Oral: 2 mg/kg/day divided every 6-8 hours
I.M.: 0.5-1 mg/kg/dose every 4-6 hours as needed
Adults:
Antiemetic: I.M.: 25-100 mg/dose every 4-6 hours as needed
Anxiety: Oral: 25-100 mg 4 times/day; maximum dose: 600 mg/day
Preoperative sedation:
Oral: 50-100 mg
I.M.: 25-100 mg
Management of pruritus: Oral: 25 mg 3-4 times/day

Dosing interval in hepatic impairment: Change dosing interval to every 24 hours in patients with primary biliary cirrhosis

Administration

Oral: May be administered without regard to food; shake suspension well before use

Parenteral: **Not** recommended for subcutaneous, intra-arterial, or I.V. administration (see Warnings). Administer I.M. deep in large muscle. For I.M. administration in children, injections should be made into the midlateral muscles of the thigh. Hydroxyzine has been administered slow I.V. to oncology patients via central venous lines without problems

Monitoring Parameters Relief of symptoms, mental status, blood pressure

Patient Information May cause drowsiness and impair ability to perform activities requiring mental alertness or physical coordination. May cause dry mouth. Avoid alcohol. Do not use other prescription or OTC medications (especially sedatives, tranquilizers, antihistamines, or pain medications) without consulting prescriber. Report hallucinations, seizure activity, tremors or involuntary movements, or loss of sensation to physician.

Dosage Forms Excipient information presented when available (limited, particularly for generics); consult specific product labeling.

Capsule, as pamoate: 25 mg, 50 mg, 100 mg
Vistaril®: 25 mg, 50 mg
Injection, solution, as hydrochloride: 25 mg/mL (1 mL); 50 mg/mL (1 mL, 2 mL, 10 mL)
Suspension, oral, as pamoate:
Vistaril®: 25 mg/5 mL (120 mL, 480 mL) [lemon flavor]
Syrup, as hydrochloride: 10 mg/5 mL (120 mL, 480 mL)
Tablet, as hydrochloride: 10 mg, 25 mg, 50 mg

References

Baumgartner TG, "Administration of Hydroxyzine Injection," *Am J Hosp Pharm*, 1979, 36(12):1660.

Berde C, Ablin A, Glazer J, et al, "American Academy of Pediatrics Report of the Subcommittee on Disease-Related Pain in Childhood Cancer," *Pediatrics*, 1990, 86(5 Pt 2):818-25.

Serreau R, Komiha M, Blanc F, et al, "Neonatal Seizures Associated With Maternal Hydroxyzine Hydrochloride in Late Pregnancy," *Reprod Toxicol*, 2005, 20(4):573-4.

Simons FE, Simons KJ, Becker AB, et al, "Pharmacokinetics and Antipruritic Effects of Hydroxyzine in Children With Atopic Dermatitis," *J Pediatr*, 1984, 104(1):123-7.

Simons FE, Simons KJ, and Frith EM, "The Pharmacokinetics and Antihistaminic of the H_1 Receptor Antagonist Hydroxyzine," *J Allergy Clin Immunol*, 1984a, 73(1 Pt 1):69-75.

Wong AR and Rasool AH, "Hydroxyzine-Induced Supraventricular Tachycardia in a Nine-Year-Old Child," *Singapore Med J*, 2004, 45(2):90-2.

♦ **Hydroxyzine Hydrochloride** *see* HydrOXYzine *on page 796*

♦ **Hydroxyzine Hydrochloride Injection, USP (Can)** *see* HydrOXYzine *on page 796*

♦ **Hydroxyzine Pamoate** *see* HydrOXYzine *on page 796*

♦ **HydroZone Plus [OTC]** *see* Hydrocortisone *on page 781*

♦ **Hylenex™** *see* Hyaluronidase *on page 774*

♦ **Hyoscine Butylbromide** *see* Scopolamine *on page 1421*

♦ **Hyoscine Hydrobromide** *see* Scopolamine *on page 1421*

Hyoscyamine (hye oh SYE a meen)

Medication Safety Issues

Sound-alike/look-alike issues:
Anaspaz® may be confused with Anaprox®, Antispas®
Levbid® may be confused with Lithobid®, Lopid®, Lorabid®
Levsinex® may be confused with Lanoxin®

U.S. Brand Names Anaspaz®; Cystospaz®; Cystospaz-M® [DSC]; Hyosine; Levbid®; Levsin®; Levsinex®; Levsin/SL®; NuLev™; Spacol [DSC]; Spacol T/S [DSC]; Symax SL; Symax SR

Canadian Brand Names Cystospaz®; Levsin®

Index Terms Hyoscyamine Sulfate; *l*-Hyoscyamine Sulfate

Therapeutic Category Anticholinergic Agent; Antispasmodic Agent, Gastrointestinal

Generic Available Yes

Use Treatment of GI tract disorders caused by spasm; adjunctive therapy for peptic ulcers and hypermotility disorders of lower urinary tract; infant colic

Pregnancy Risk Factor C

Lactation Enters breast milk/not recommended

Contraindications Hypersensitivity to hyoscyamine or any component; narrow-angle glaucoma, GI and GU obstruction, paralytic ileus, severe ulcerative colitis, myasthenia gravis

Warnings Low doses may cause a paradoxical decrease in heart rate; heat prostration may occur in hot weather. Some oral liquids contain sodium benzoate; benzoic acid (benzoate) is a metabolite of benzyl alcohol; large amounts of benzyl alcohol (≥99 mg/kg/day) have been associated with a potentially fatal toxicity ("gasping syndrome") in neonates; *in vitro* and animal studies have shown that benzoate displaces bilirubin from protein binding sites; avoid using products containing sodium benzoate in neonates

Precautions Use with caution in patients with hyperthyroidism, CHF, cardiac arrhythmias, prostatic hypertrophy, autonomic neuropathy, chronic lung disease, biliary tract disease, children with spastic paralysis. Disintegrating tablet (NuLev™) contains aspartame which is metabolized to phenylalanine and must be used with caution in patients with phenylketonuria.

Adverse Reactions

Cardiovascular: Tachycardia or palpitations, bradycardia (with very low doses), orthostatic hypotension

Central nervous system: Headache, lightheadedness, short-term memory loss, fatigue, delirium, restlessness, ataxia, dizziness, insomnia, psychosis, euphoria, nervousness, confusion, insomnia, fever

Dermatologic: Dry skin, photosensitivity, rash, urticaria

Gastrointestinal: Xerostomia, nausea, vomiting, constipation, dysphagia, dysgeusia, dry throat

Genitourinary: Difficult urination, urinary retention

Local: Irritation at injection site

Neuromuscular & skeletal: Weakness, tremor

Ocular: Blurred vision, photophobia, mydriasis, anisocoria, cycloplegia, elevated intraocular pressure

Respiratory: Dry nose

Miscellaneous: Decreased diaphoresis

Drug Interactions Decreased absorption when given with antacids; increased anticholinergic activity with amantadine, antimuscarinics, haloperidol, phenothiazines, tricyclic antidepressants, antihistamines; MAO inhibitors

Mechanism of Action Blocks the action of acetylcholine at parasympathetic sites in smooth muscle, secretory glands, and the CNS; specific anticholinergic responses are dose-related; increases cardiac output, dries secretions, antagonizes histamine and serotonin

Hyoscyamine Drops Dosage

Weight (kg)	Dose (drops)	Maximum Daily Dose (drops)
2.3	3	18
3.4	4	24
5	5	30
7	6	36
10	8	48
15	11	66

Pharmacodynamics

Onset of action:

- Oral: 20-30 minutes
- Sublingual: 5-20 minutes
- I.V.: 2-3 minutes

Duration: 4-6 hours

Pharmacokinetics

Absorption: Well absorbed from the GI tract

Distribution: Crosses the placenta; small amounts appear in breast milk

Protein binding: 50%

Metabolism: In the liver

(Continued)

Hyoscyamine *(Continued)*

Half-life: 3.5 hours

Elimination: 30% to 50% eliminated unchanged in urine within 12 hours

Usual Dosage

GI tract disorders:

Infants <2 years: Oral: The table (on previous page) lists the hyoscyamine dosage using the drop formulation; hyoscyamine drops are dosed every 4 hours as needed

Oral, S.L.:

Children 2-12 years: 0.0625-0.125 mg every 4 hours as needed; maximum daily dosage 0.75 mg **or** timed release 0.375 mg every 12 hours; maximum daily dosage 0.75 mg

Children >12 years to Adults: 0.125-0.25 mg every 4 hours as needed; maximum daily dosage 1.5 mg **or** timed release 0.375-0.75 mg every 12 hours; maximum daily dosage 1.5 mg

I.V., I.M., SubQ: Children >12 years to Adults: 0.25-0.5 mg at 4-hour intervals for 1-4 doses

Adjunct to anesthesia: I.M., I.V., SubQ: Children >2 years to Adults: 5 mcg/kg given 30-60 minutes prior to induction of anesthesia

Hypermotility of lower urinary tract: Oral, S.L.: Adults: 0.15-0.3 mg four times daily; timed release: 0.375 mg every 12 hours

Reversal of neuromuscular blockage: I.V., I.M., SubQ: 0.2 mg for every 1 mg neostigmine or equivalent dose of physostigmine

Administration

Oral: Administer before meals; timed release tablets are scored and may be cut for easier dosage titration; S.L.: Place under the tongue

Parenteral: May be administered I.M., I.V., and SubQ; no information is available for I.V. administration rate or dilution

Monitoring Parameters Pulse, anticholinergic effects, urine output, GI symptoms

Patient Information May cause dry mouth; maintain good oral hygiene habits, because lack of saliva may increase chance of cavities; notify physician if skin rash, flushing or eye pain occurs, or if difficulty in urinating, constipation, or sensitivity to light becomes severe or persists; may cause dizziness or blurred vision; may cause drowsiness and impair ability to perform activities requiring mental alertness or physical coordination. May rarely cause photosensitivity reactions (eg, exposure to sunlight may cause severe sunburn, skin rash, redness, or itching); avoid direct exposure to sunlight

Dosage Forms Excipient information presented when available (limited, particularly for generics); consult specific product labeling. [DSC] = Discontinued product

Capsule, timed release, as sulfate (Cystospaz-M® [DSC], Levsinex®): 0.375 mg

Elixir, as sulfate: 0.125 mg/5 mL (480 mL)

Hyosine: 0.125 mg/5 mL (480 mL) [contains alcohol 20% and sodium benzoate; orange flavor]

Levsin®: 0.125 mg/5 mL (480 mL) [contains alcohol 20%; orange flavor]

Injection, solution, as sulfate (Levsin®): 0.5 mg/mL (1 mL)

Liquid, as sulfate (Spacol [DSC]): 0.125 mg/5 mL (120 mL) [sugar free, alcohol free, simethicone based, bubble gum flavor]

Solution, oral drops, as sulfate: 0.125 mg/mL (15 mL)

Hyosine: 0.125 mg/mL (15 mL) [contains alcohol 5% and sodium benzoate; orange flavor]

Levsin®: 0.125 mg/mL (15 mL) [contains alcohol 5%; orange flavor]

Tablet (Cystospaz®): 0.15 mg

Tablet, as sulfate (Anaspaz®, Levsin®, Spacol [DSC]): 0.125 mg

Tablet, extended release, as sulfate (Levbid®, Symax SR, Spacol T/S [DSC]): 0.375 mg

Tablet, orally disintegrating, as sulfate (NuLev™): 0.125 mg [contains phenylalanine 1.7 mg/tablet, mint flavor]

Tablet, sublingual, as sulfate: 0.125 mg

Levsin/SL®: 0.125 mg [peppermint flavor]

Symax SL: 0.125 mg

Hyoscyamine, Atropine, Scopolamine, and Phenobarbital

(hye oh SYE a meen, A troe peen, skoe POL a meen & fee noe BAR bi tal)

Medication Safety Issues

Sound-alike/look-alike issues:

Donnatal® may be confused with Donnagel®

U.S. Brand Names Donnatal®; Donnatal Extentabs®

Index Terms Atropine, Hyoscyamine, Scopolamine, and Phenobarbital; Belladonna Alkaloids With Phenobarbital; Phenobarbital, Hyoscyamine, Atropine, and Scopolamine; Scopolamine, Hyoscyamine, Atropine, and Phenobarbital

Therapeutic Category Anticholinergic Agent; Antispasmodic Agent, Gastrointestinal

Generic Available Yes: Elixir, tablet

Use Adjunct in treatment of peptic ulcer disease, irritable bowel, spastic colitis, spastic bladder, and renal colic

Pregnancy Risk Factor C

Lactation Excretion in breast milk unknown/use caution

Contraindications Hypersensitivity to hyoscyamine, atropine, scopolamine, phenobarbital, or any component of the formulation; narrow-angle glaucoma; tachycardia; GI and GU obstruction; myasthenia gravis; paralytic ileus; intestinal atony; unstable cardiovascular status in acute hemorrhage; severe ulcerative colitis; hiatal hernia associated with reflux esophagitis; acute intermittent porphyria

Warnings Heat prostration can occur in the presence of high environmental temperature

Precautions Use with caution in patients with hepatic or renal disease, hyperthyroidism, CAD, CHF, cardiac arrhythmias, tachycardia, hypertension, autonomic neuropathy

Adverse Reactions

Cardiovascular: Tachycardia, palpitations, bradycardia (with very low doses of atropine)

Central nervous system: Headache, drowsiness, nervousness, confusion, insomnia, fever, dizziness

Gastrointestinal: Xerostomia, nausea, vomiting, constipation, dysphagia, paralytic ileus, dysgeusia

Genitourinary: Impotence, urinary retention

Neuromuscular & skeletal: Weakness, musculoskeletal pain

Ocular: Blurred vision, photophobia, mydriasis, cycloplegia, elevated intraocular pressure

Respiratory: Nasal congestion

Miscellaneous: Hypersensitivity reactions, decreased diaphoresis

Drug Interactions Phenobarbital: Cytochrome P450 isoenzyme substrate CYP2C8/9, CYP2C19, CYP2E1; inducer CYP1A2, CYP2A6, CYP2B6, CYP2C8/9, CYP3A4 (see Phenobarbital monograph for complete drug interaction profile)

Additive CNS depression with CNS depressants, antihistamines, phenothiazines, tricyclic antidepressants; additive anticholinergic activity with antihistamines, phenothiazines, amantadine

Mechanism of Action Anticholinergic agents (hyoscyamine, atropine, and scopolamine) inhibit the muscarinic actions of acetylcholine at the postganglionic parasympathetic neuroeffector sites including smooth muscle, secretory glands, and CNS sites; specific anticholinergic responses are dose-related

Pharmacokinetics Absorption: Well absorbed from the GI tract

Usual Dosage Oral:

Children: Donnatal®: 0.1 mL/kg/dose every 4 hours; maximum dose: 5 mL **or** see table for alternative.

Donnatal® Dosage

Weight (kg)	Dose (mL)	
	Every 4 Hours	Every 6 Hours
4.5	0.5	0.75
10	1	1.5
14	1.5	2
23	2.5	3.8
34	3.8	5
≥45	5	7.5

Adults: Donnatal®: 1-2 tablets or capsules 3-4 times/day **or** 5-10 mL 3-4 times/day or 1 extended release tablet every 12 hours (may increase to every 8 hours if needed)

Administration Oral: Administer 30-60 minutes before meals; do not crush or chew extended release tablets

Patient Information Maintain good oral hygiene habits because lack of saliva may increase chance of cavities; may cause dry mouth; notify physician if skin rash, flushing or eye pain occurs, or if difficulty in urinating, constipation, or sensitivity to light becomes severe or persists; observe caution while driving or performing other tasks requiring alertness, as may cause drowsiness, dizziness, or blurred vision

Dosage Forms Excipient information presented when available (limited, particularly for generics); consult specific product labeling.

Elixir (Donnatal®): Hyoscyamine sulfate 0.1037 mg, atropine sulfate 0.0194 mg, scopolamine hydrobromide 0.0065 mg, and phenobarbital 16.2 mg per 5 mL (120 mL, 480 mL) [contains alcohol 95%; grape flavor]

(Continued)

Hyoscyamine, Atropine, Scopolamine, and Phenobarbital *(Continued)*

Tablet (Donnatal®): Hyoscyamine sulfate 0.1037 mg, atropine sulfate 0.0194 mg, scopolamine hydrobromide 0.0065 mg, and phenobarbital 16.2 mg

Tablet, extended release (Donnatal Extentabs®): Hyoscyamine sulfate 0.3111 mg, atropine sulfate 0.0582 mg, scopolamine hydrobromide 0.0195 mg, and phenobarbital 48.6 mg

- ♦ **Hyoscyamine Sulfate** *see* Hyoscyamine *on page 798*
- ♦ **Hyosine** *see* Hyoscyamine *on page 798*
- ♦ **HyperHep B® (Can)** *see* Hepatitis B Immune Globulin *on page 762*
- ♦ **HyperHEP B™ S/D** *see* Hepatitis B Immune Globulin *on page 762*
- ♦ **HyperRAB™ S/D** *see* Rabies Immune Globulin (Human) *on page 1363*
- ♦ **HyperRHO™ S/D Full Dose** *see* Rh_o(D) Immune Globulin *on page 1374*
- ♦ **HyperRHO™ S/D Mini Dose** *see* Rh_o(D) Immune Globulin *on page 1374*
- ♦ **Hyperstat® [DSC]** *see* Diazoxide *on page 485*
- ♦ **HyperTET™ S/D** *see* Tetanus Immune Globulin (Human) *on page 1515*
- ♦ **Hytakerol® [DSC]** *see* Dihydrotachysterol [DSC] *on page 502*
- ♦ **Hytakerol® (Can)** *see* Dihydrotachysterol [DSC] *on page 502*
- ♦ **Hytinic® [OTC]** *see* Iron Supplements (Oral/Enteral) *on page 868*
- ♦ **Hytone®** *see* Hydrocortisone *on page 781*
- ♦ **Ibidomide Hydrochloride** *see* Labetalol *on page 895*
- ♦ **Ibu-200 [OTC]** *see* Ibuprofen *on page 802*

Ibuprofen (eye byoo PROE fen)

Medication Safety Issues

Sound-alike/look-alike issues:

Haltran® may be confused with Halfprin®

Related Information

Overdose and Toxicology *on page 1916*

U.S. Brand Names Advil® [OTC]; Advil® Children's [OTC]; Advil® Infants' [OTC]; Advil® Junior [OTC]; Advil® Migraine [OTC]; ElixSure™ IB [OTC]; Genpril® [OTC]; Ibu-200 [OTC]; I-Prin [OTC]; Midol® Cramp and Body Aches [OTC]; Motrin®; Motrin® Children's [OTC]; Motrin® IB [OTC]; Motrin® Infants' [OTC]; Motrin® Junior Strength [OTC]; NeoProfen®; Proprinal [OTC]; Ultraprin [OTC]

Canadian Brand Names Advil®; Apo-Ibuprofen®; Motrin® (Children's); Motrin® IB; Novo-Profen; Nu-Ibuprofen

Index Terms Ibuprofen Lysine; *p*-Isobutylhydratropic Acid

Therapeutic Category Analgesic, Non-narcotic; Anti-inflammatory Agent; Antipyretic; Nonsteroidal Anti-inflammatory Drug (NSAID), Oral; Nonsteroidal Anti-inflammatory Drug (NSAID), Parenteral

Generic Available Yes: Caplet, suspension, tablet

Use

Oral: Treatment of inflammatory diseases and rheumatoid disorders including juvenile rheumatoid arthritis (JRA); mild to moderate pain; migraine pain; fever; dysmenorrhea; gout

Injection: Treatment (ie, closure) of a clinically significant PDA in premature infants who weigh between 500-1500 g and who are ≤32 weeks gestational age when usual treatments are ineffective. **Note:** The prophylactic use of ibuprofen is not currently indicated nor recommended (see Shah, 2006).

Medication Guide An FDA-approved patient medication guide, which is available with the product information and at http://www.fda.gov/cder/Offices/ODS/medication_guides.htm, must be dispensed with this medication for each new outpatient prescription and refill for oral administration.

Pregnancy Risk Factor C (D if used in the 3rd trimester)

Lactation Enters breast milk/use caution (AAP rates "compatible")

Contraindications Hypersensitivity to ibuprofen, any component (see Warnings), aspirin, or other NSAIDs; active GI bleeding, ulcer disease; patients with the "aspirin triad" [asthma, rhinitis (with or without nasal polyps), and aspirin intolerance] (fatal asthmatic and anaphylactoid reactions may occur in these patients); perioperative pain in the setting of coronary artery bypass graft (CABG)

Injection (ibuprofen lysine) is contraindicated in preterm infants with untreated proven or suspected infection; congenital heart disease where patency of the PDA is necessary for pulmonary or systemic blood flow (eg, pulmonary atresia, severe tetralogy of Fallot, severe coarctation of aorta); bleeding (especially with active intracranial hemorrhage or GI bleed); thrombocytopenia; coagulation defects; proven or suspected necrotizing enterocolitis (NEC); significant renal dysfunction

Warnings NSAIDs are associated with an increased risk of adverse cardiovascular thrombotic events, including potentially fatal MI and stroke; risk may be increased with duration of use or pre-existing cardiovascular risk factors or disease; carefully evaluate cardiovascular risk profile prior to prescribing; use the lowest effective dose for the shortest duration of time, taking into consideration individual patient treatment goals; alternate therapies should be considered for patients at high risk. An increased incidence of MI and stroke was found in patients receiving COX-2 selective NSAIDs for the treatment of pain within the first 10-14 days after CABG surgery (see Contraindications). NSAIDs may cause fluid retention, edema, and new onset or worsening of pre-existing hypertension; use with caution in patients with hypertension, CHF, or fluid retention. Concurrent administration of ibuprofen, and potentially other nonselective NSAIDs, may interfere with aspirin's cardioprotective effect (see Drug Interactions).

NSAIDs may increase the risk of gastrointestinal irritation, ulceration, bleeding, and perforation. These events, which can be potentially fatal, may occur at any time during therapy, and without warning. Use NSAIDs with extreme caution in patients with a history of GI bleeding or ulcers (these patients have a 10-fold increased risk for developing a GI bleed). Use NSAIDs with caution in patients with other risk factors which may increase GI bleeding (eg, concurrent therapy with aspirin, anticoagulants, and/or corticosteroids, longer duration of NSAID use, smoking, use of alcohol, and poor general health). Use the lowest effective dose for the shortest duration of time, taking into consideration individual patient treatment goals; alternate therapies should be considered for patients at high risk.

NSAIDs may compromise existing renal function. Renal toxicity may occur in patients with impaired renal function, dehydration, heart failure, liver dysfunction, those taking diuretics and ACE inhibitors; use with caution in these patients; monitor renal function closely. NSAIDs are not recommended for use in patients with advanced renal disease. Long-term use of NSAIDs may cause renal papillary necrosis and other renal injury.

Fatal asthmatic and anaphylactoid reactions may occur in patients with the "aspirin triad" who receive NSAIDs (see Contraindications). NSAIDs may cause serious dermatologic adverse reactions including exfoliative dermatitis, Stevens-Johnson syndrome, and toxic epidermal necrolysis. Avoid use of NSAIDs in late pregnancy as they may cause premature closure of the ductus arteriosus.

Motrin® IB gelcaps contain benzyl alcohol which may cause allergic reactions in susceptible individuals. Some products contain sodium benzoate (see Dosage Forms); benzoate is a metabolite of benzyl alcohol; large amounts of benzyl alcohol (≥99 mg/kg/day) have been associated with a potentially fatal toxicity ("gasping syndrome") in neonates; the "gasping syndrome" consists of metabolic acidosis, respiratory distress, gasping respirations, CNS dysfunction (including convulsions, intracranial hemorrhage), hypotension and cardiovascular collapse; avoid use of ibuprofen products containing benzyl alcohol or sodium benzoate in neonates; *in vitro* and animal studies have shown that benzoate displaces bilirubin from protein binding sites

Precautions Use with caution in patients with decreased hepatic function; closely monitor patients with abnormal LFTs; severe hepatic reactions (eg, fulminant hepatitis, liver failure) have occurred with NSAID use, rarely; discontinue if signs or symptoms of liver disease develop, or if systemic manifestations occur. Use with caution in patients with asthma. Chewable tablets contain phenylalanine which must be avoided (or used with caution) in patients with phenylketonuria. Safety and efficacy of oral dosage forms have not been established in infants <6 months of age.

Injection: Use with caution, avoid extravasation; I.V. solution may be irritating to tissues. Use with caution in infants with controlled infection or those at risk for infection (ibuprofen may alter the usual signs of infection). May inhibit platelet aggregation; monitor for signs of bleeding. Use with caution in infants when total bilirubin is elevated (ibuprofen may displace bilirubin from albumin-binding sites). Long-term evaluations of neurodevelopmental outcome, growth, or diseases associated with prematurity (eg, chronic lung disease, retinopathy of prematurity) following treatment have not been conducted (see Additional Information).

OTC labeling: Prior to self-medication, patients should contact healthcare provider if they have had recurring stomach pain or upset, ulcers, bleeding problems, high blood pressure, heart or kidney disease, other serious medical problems, or are currently taking a diuretic. Recommended dosages should not be exceeded, due to an increased risk of GI bleeding. Consuming ≥3 alcoholic beverages/day or taking this medication longer than recommended may increase the risk of GI bleeding.

(Continued)

Ibuprofen *(Continued)*

Adverse Reactions

Oral:

Cardiovascular: Edema, hypertension

Central nervous system: Dizziness, drowsiness, fatigue, headache, nervousness; aseptic meningitis (<1%)

Dermatologic: Rash, urticaria, exfoliative dermatitis, Stevens-Johnson syndrome, toxic epidermal necrolysis

Endocrine & metabolic: Fluid retention

Gastrointestinal: Dyspepsia, heartburn, nausea, vomiting, abdominal pain, peptic ulcer, GI bleed, GI perforation, diarrhea, constipation, flatulence, epigastric pain, decreased appetite

Hematologic: Neutropenia, anemia, agranulocytosis, inhibition of platelet aggregation

Hepatic: Elevated liver enzymes; rarely: Hepatitis, jaundice, hepatic necrosis, liver failure

Ocular: Vision changes (blurred or diminished vision, changes in color vision, scotomata)

Otic: Tinnitus

Renal: Acute renal failure

Miscellaneous: Hypersensitivity reactions, anaphylactoid reactions

Injection:

Cardiovascular: Edema (4%), tachycardia, cardiac failure, hypotension

Central nervous system: Intraventricular hemorrhage (29%; grade 3/4: 15%), convulsions

Dermatologic: Skin irritation (16%)

Endocrine & metabolic: Hypocalcemia (12%), hypoglycemia (12%), adrenal insufficiency (7%), hypernatremia (7%), hyperglycemia

Gastrointestinal: GI disorders, non-NEC (22%), abdominal distension, gastroesophageal reflux, gastritis, ileus, feeding problems

Genitourinary: Urinary tract infection (9%)

Hematologic: Anemia (32%), neutropenia, thrombocytopenia

Hepatic: Cholestasis, jaundice

Local: Injection site reaction

Renal: Elevated BUN (7%), renal impairment (6%), elevated serum creatinine (3%), decreased urine output (3%; small decrease reported on days 2-6 of life with compensatory increase in output on day 9); renal failure (1%); elevated BUN with hematuria (1%), oliguria

Respiratory: Apnea (28%), respiratory infection (19%), respiratory failure (10%), atelectasis (4%); pulmonary hypertension [4 cases reported; 3 following early (prophylactic) administration of tromethamine ibuprofen and 1 case following L-lysine ibuprofen for treatment of PDA (see Bellini, 2006)]

Miscellaneous: Sepsis (43%), infection, inguinal hernia

Drug Interactions Cytochrome P450 isoenzyme CYP2C8 and CYP2C9 substrate

Ibuprofen may decrease the excretion of aminoglycosides and vancomycin; may increase digoxin, methotrexate and lithium serum concentrations; may decrease antihypertensive effects of ACE inhibitors or angiotensin II antagonists (monitor blood pressure); may decrease effects of other antihypertensive agents, furosemide, and thiazides. Other GI irritants (eg, alcohol, NSAIDs, corticosteroids, oral potassium) may increase adverse GI effects. Use with anticoagulants (warfarin, heparin, LMWHs) may increase risk of bleeding.

Ibuprofen and other COX-1 inhibitors may reduce the cardioprotective (antiplatelet effect) of aspirin depending upon when it is administered. Avoid giving these agents on a regular basis in patients requiring the antiplatelet effect of aspirin. If used occasionally, a single dose of ibuprofen should be taken 30-120 minutes after aspirin (immediate release; not enteric coated) ingestion or at least 8 hours should elapse after ibuprofen dosing before giving aspirin (see Catella-Lawson, 2001).

Food Interactions Food may decrease the rate but not the extent of oral absorption

Stability

Suspension: Store at controlled room temperature of 15°C to 30°C (59°F to 86°F).

Tablet: Store at controlled room temperature of 20°C to 25°C (68°F to 77°F).

Injection: Store at controlled room temperature of 20°C to 25°C (68°F to 77°F). Protect from light; store injection vials in carton until ready to use. Stable in I.V. dextrose or saline solutions. Following dilution, administer within 30 minutes of preparation. Discard unused portion of vial (vial does not contain preservative). **Incompatible** with TPN solution.

Mechanism of Action Inhibits prostaglandin synthesis by decreasing the activity of the enzyme, cyclooxygenase, which results in decreased formation of prostaglandin precursors

Pharmacodynamics

Fever reduction:

Onset of action (single dose 8 mg/kg):

Infants ≤1 year: Mean ± SD: 69 ± 22 minutes

Children ≥6 years: 109 ± 64 minutes

Maximum effect: 2-4 hours

Duration: 6-8 hours (dose-related)

Pharmacokinetics

Absorption: Oral: Rapid (80%)

Distribution: Ibuprofen follows a 2-compartment open model

V_d, apparent: Preterm neonates, GA: 22-31 weeks and PNA: <1 day old (n=21): 62.1 ± 3.9 mL/kg (Aranda, 1997)

V_d, central compartment: Preterm neonates, GA: 28.7 ± 1.3 weeks (n=13):

PNA 3 days old: 0.244 ± 0.084 L/kg (n=13); subset of 9 patients with ductal closure: 0.247 ± 0.102 L/kg

PNA 5 days old: 0.171 ± 0.077 L/kg (n=13); subset of 9 patients with ductal closure: 0.147 ± 0.075 L/kg

Note: The V_d of the central compartment was significantly decreased on day 5 of life versus day 3; the decrease was more pronounced in patients with ductal closure (see Van Overmeire, 2001).

V_d:

Febrile children <11 years: 0.2 L/kg

Adults: 0.12 L/kg

Protein binding: 90% to 99%

Metabolism: Oxidized in the liver; **Note:** Ibuprofen is a racemic mixture of R and S isomers; the R isomer (thought to be inactive) is slowly and incompletely (~60%) converted to the S isomer (active) in adults; the amount of conversion in children is not known, but it is thought to be similar to adults; a study in preterm neonates estimated the conversion to be 61% after prophylactic ibuprofen use and 86% after curative treatment (see Gregoire, 2004).

Half-life:

Alpha (distribution): I.V.: Preterm infants: 1.04 ± 1.48 hours (Van Overmeire, 2001)

Preterm newborn, GA: 22-31 weeks and PNA: <1 day old (n=21): Beta half-life: 30.5 ± 4.2 hours (Aranda, 1997)

Preterm neonates, GA: 28.7 ± 1.3 weeks (n=13): Beta half-life: (Van Overmeire, 2001):

PNA 3 days old: 43.1 ± 26.1 hours

PNA 5 days old: 26.8 ± 23.6 hours

Preterm neonates, GA 24-27.9 weeks (n=62): R-enantiomer: 10 hours; S-enantiomer: 25.5 hours (Gregoire, 2004)

Children: 1-2 hours; children 3 months to 10 years: Mean: 1.6 hours

Adults: 2-4 hours

Time to peak serum concentration: Tablets: 1-2 hours; suspension: Mean: 1 hour

Children with cystic fibrosis:

Suspension (n=22): 0.74 ± 0.43 hours (median: 30 minutes)

Chewable tablet (n=4): 1.5 ± 0.58 hours (median: 1.5 hours)

Tablet (n=12): 1.33 ± 0.95 hours (median: 1 hour)

Elimination: ~1% excreted as unchanged drug and 14% as conjugated ibuprofen in urine; 45% to 80% eliminated in urine as metabolites; some biliary excretion

Usual Dosage

I.V.: Infants between 500-1500 g and ≤32 weeks GA: Patent ductus arteriosus (treatment): Initial dose: Ibuprofen 10 mg/kg, followed by two doses of 5 mg/kg after 24 and 48 hours.

Note: Use birth weight to calculate all doses. Hold second or third doses if urinary output is <0.6 mL/kg/hour; may give when laboratory studies indicate renal function is back to normal. A second course of treatment, alternative pharmacologic therapy, or surgery may be needed if the ductus arteriosus fails to close or reopens following the initial course of therapy.

Oral: **Note:** To reduce the risk of adverse cardiovascular and GI effects, use the lowest effective dose for the shortest period of time

Infants and Children:

Analgesic: 4-10 mg/kg/dose every 6-8 hours; maximum daily dose: 40 mg/kg/day

Antipyretic: 6 months to 12 years: Temperature <102.5°F (39°C): 5 mg/kg/dose; temperature ≥102.5°F: 10 mg/kg/dose; give every 6-8 hours; maximum daily dose: 40 mg/kg/day

Juvenile rheumatoid arthritis: 6 months to 12 years: Usual: 30-40 mg/kg/day in 3-4 divided doses; start at lower end of dosing range and titrate; patients with milder disease may be treated with 20 mg/kg/day; doses >40 mg/kg/day may increase risk of serious adverse effects; doses >50 mg/kg/day have not been studied and are not recommended; maximum dose: 2.4 g/day

(Continued)

Ibuprofen *(Continued)*

OTC pediatric labeling (analgesic, antipyretic): 6 months to 11 years: 7.5 mg/kg/dose every 6-8 hours; maximum daily dose: 30 mg/kg

Manufacturer's recommendations: See table; use of weight to select dose is preferred; if weight is not available, then use age; doses may be repeated every 6-8 hours; maximum: 4 doses/day

Ibuprofen Dosing

Weight (lbs)	Age	Dosage (mg)
12-17	6-11 mo	50
18-23	12-23 mo	75
24-35	2-3 y	100
35-47	4-5 y	150
48-59	6-8 y	200
60-71	9-10 y	250
72-95	11 y	300

Cystic fibrosis: Ibuprofen when taken chronically (for 4 years) in doses to achieve peak plasma concentrations of 50-100 mcg/mL has been shown to slow the progression of lung disease in mild cystic fibrosis patients >5 years of age, and especially in patients who started therapy when <13 years of age. Doses administered twice daily ranged from 16.2-31.6 mg/kg/dose with 90% of patients requiring 20-30 mg/kg/dose (mean dose: ~25 mg/kg/dose), but individual patient's dose requirements were not predictable. Patients did not take pancreatic enzymes nor eat for 2 hours after the dose (Konstan, 1995). In children with cystic fibrosis, an initial ibuprofen pharmacokinetic analyses is recommended using tablet doses of 20-30 mg/kg to optimize concentrations in the therapeutic range; blood sampling is recommended at 1, 2, and 3 hours postdose. A recent pharmacokinetic study in children with cystic fibrosis demonstrated that ibuprofen oral suspension also delivers therapeutic plasma concentrations; this study recommends using a 20 mg/kg dose of ibuprofen suspension for the initial pharmacokinetic analyses and obtaining blood samples at 30, 45, and 60 minutes postdose (Scott, 1999); further studies are needed

Adolescents and Adults:

Inflammatory disease: 400-800 mg/dose 3-4 times/day; maximum dose: 3.2 g/day

Pain/fever/dysmenorrhea: 200-400 mg/dose every 4-6 hours; maximum daily dose: 1.2 g

OTC labeling (analgesic, antipyretic): 200 mg every 4-6 hours as needed (maximum: 1200 mg/24 hours)

Dosing adjustment in hepatic impairment: Severe hepatic impairment: Avoid use

Dosing adjustment in renal impairment: Advanced renal disease: Use is not recommended

Administration

Oral: Administer with food or milk to decrease GI upset; shake suspension well before use

Parenteral: I.V: For I.V. administration only; administration via umbilical arterial line has not been evaluated. Dilute with dextrose or saline to an appropriate volume. Infuse over 15 minutes through I.V. port closest to insertion site. Avoid extravasation. Do not administer simultaneously via same line with TPN. If needed, interrupt TPN for 15 minutes prior to and after ibuprofen administration, keeping line open with dextrose or saline.

Monitoring Parameters CBC, occult blood loss, liver enzymes; urine output, serum BUN, and creatinine in patients receiving I.V. ibuprofen, concurrent diuretics, those with decreased renal function, or in patients on chronic therapy. Monitor preterm infants for signs of bleeding and infection; serum electrolytes, glucose, calcium and bilirubin; vital signs; monitor I.V. site for signs of extravasation. Patients receiving long-term therapy for JRA should receive periodic ophthalmological exams.

Reference Range Plasma concentrations >200 mcg/mL may be associated with severe toxicity; cystic fibrosis: therapeutic peak plasma concentration: 50-100 mcg/mL

Patient Information Ibuprofen is a nonsteroidal anti-inflammatory drug (NSAID); NSAIDs may cause serious adverse reactions, especially with overuse; use exactly as directed; do not increase dose or frequency; do not take longer than 3 days for fever (adults and children), 10 days for pain (adults), or 3 days for pain (children) without consulting healthcare professional. NSAIDs may increase the risk for heart attack, stroke, or ulcers and bleeding in stomach or intestines; GI bleeding, ulceration, or perforation can occur with or without pain. Notify physician before use if you have hypertension, heart failure, heart or kidney disease, history of stomach ulcers or bleeding in stomach or intestines, or other medical problems. Read the patient Medication Guide that you receive with each prescription and refill of ibuprofen.

While using this medication, do not use alcohol, excessive amounts of vitamin C, other prescription or OTC medications containing aspirin or salicylate, or other NSAIDs without consulting prescriber. Ibuprofen may cause dizziness or drowsiness and impair ability to perform activities requiring mental alertness or physical coordination. Notify physician if changes in vision occur, if pain worsens or lasts >10 days in adults or >3 days in children, if fever worsens or lasts >3 days, if stomach pain or upset occurs, if swelling or redness occurs in painful area, or if any new symptoms appear. Stop taking medication and report ringing in ears; persistent cramping or stomach pain; unresolved nausea or vomiting; respiratory difficulty or shortness of breath; unusual bruising or bleeding (mouth, urine, stool); skin rash; unusual swelling of extremities; chest pain; or palpitations.

OTC (pediatrics): Do not administer to children for >3 days unless recommended by physician or other healthcare professional; notify physician if child's condition does not improve or if worsens within 24 hours

Additional Information Nystagmus, dizziness, drowsiness, seizures, vomiting, hypotension, irregular heartbeat, breathing difficulties, apnea, kidney failure, and coma have been reported with overdose. Motrin® suspension contains sucrose 0.3 g/mL and 1.6 calories/mL. Due to its effects on platelet function, ibuprofen should be withheld for at least 4-6 half-lives prior to surgical or dental procedures.

Note: A study comparing the short-term use of acetaminophen and ibuprofen in 84,192 children (6 months to 12 years of age) found no significant difference in the rates of hospitalization for acute GI bleeding, acute renal failure, anaphylaxis or Reye's syndrome. (Four of 55,785 children in the ibuprofen group and zero of 28,130 children in the acetaminophen group were hospitalized with acute GI bleeding). A low WBC occurred more frequently in the ibuprofen group (8 vs 0) (see Lesko, 1995). A subanalysis of 27,065 children <2 years of age also found no significant difference in the rates of hospitalization. (Three of 17,938 children in the ibuprofen group and zero of 9,127 children in the acetaminophen group were hospitalized with GI bleeding) (see Lesko, 1999).

There is currently no scientific evidence to support alternating acetaminophen with ibuprofen in the treatment of fever (see Mayoral, 2000)

I.V. ibuprofen is as effective as I.V. indomethacin for the treatment of PDA in preterm infants, but is less likely to cause adverse effects on renal function (eg, oliguria, increased serum creatinine) (see Van Overmeire, 2000; Lago, 2002 and Aranda, 2006). However, ibuprofen may increase the risk for the development of chronic lung disease; 4 cases of pulmonary hypertension have been reported (see Adverse Reactions; Bellini, 2006 and Ohlsson, 2006). Further studies, especially long-term studies, are needed.

Dosage Forms Excipient information presented when available (limited, particularly for generics); consult specific product labeling. [DSC] = Discontinued product

Caplet: 200 mg [OTC]
- Advil®: 200 mg [contains sodium benzoate]
- Ibu-200, Motrin® IB: 200 mg
- Motrin® Junior Strength: 100 mg

Capsule, liqui-gel:
- Advil®: 200 mg
- Advil® Migraine: 200 mg [solubilized ibuprofen; contains potassium 20 mg]

Gelcap:
- Advil®: 200 mg [contains coconut oil]

Injection, solution, as lysine [preservative free]:
- NeoProfen®: 17.1 mg/mL (2 mL) [equivalent to ibuprofen 10 mg/mL]

Suspension, oral: 100 mg/5 mL (5 mL, 120 mL, 480 mL)
- Advil® Children's: 100 mg/5 mL (60 mL, 120 mL) [contains sodium benzoate; blue raspberry, fruit, and grape flavors]
- ElixSure™ IB: 100 mg/5 mL (120 mL) [berry flavor]
- Motrin® Children's: 100 mg/5 mL (60 mL, 120 mL) [contains sodium benzoate; berry, dye free berry, bubble gum, and grape flavors]

Suspension, oral drops: 40 mg/mL (15 mL)
- Advil® Infants': 40 mg/mL (15 mL) [contains sodium benzoate; fruit and grape flavors]
- Motrin® Infants': 40 mg/mL (15 mL, 30 mL) [contains sodium benzoate; berry and dye-free berry flavors]

Tablet: 200 mg [OTC], 400 mg, 600 mg, 800 mg
- Advil®: 200 mg [contains sodium benzoate]

(Continued)

Ibuprofen *(Continued)*

Advil® Junior: 100 mg [contains sodium benzoate; coated tablets]
Genpril®, I-Prin, Midol® Cramp and Body Aches, Motrin® IB, Proprinal, Ultraprin: 200 mg
Motrin®: 400 mg [DSC], 600 mg, 800 mg

Tablet, chewable:
Advil® Children's: 50 mg [contains phenylalanine 2.1 mg; grape flavors]
Advil® Junior: 100 mg [contains phenylalanine 4.2 mg; grape flavors]
Motrin® Children's: 50 mg [contains phenylalanine 1.4 mg; grape and orange flavor]
Motrin® Junior Strength: 100 mg [contains phenylalanine 2.1 mg; grape and orange flavors]

References

Aranda JV and Thomas R, "Systematic Review: Intravenous Ibuprofen in Preterm Newborns," *Semin Perinatol*, 2006, 30(3):114-20.

Aranda JV, Varvarigou A, Beharry K, et al, "Pharmacokinetics and Protein Binding of Intravenous Ibuprofen in the Premature Newborn Infant," *Acta Paediatr*, 1997, 86(3):289-93.

Bellini C, Campone F, and Serra G, "Pulmonary Hypertension Following L-lysine Ibuprofen Therapy in a Preterm Infant With Patent Ductus Arteriosus," *CMAJ*, 2006, 174(13):1843-4.

Berde C, Ablin A, Glazer J, et al, "American Academy of Pediatrics Report of the Subcommittee on Disease-Related Pain in Childhood Cancer," *Pediatrics*, 1990, 86(5 Pt 2):818-25.

Brewer EJ, "Nonsteroidal Anti-inflammatory Agents," *Arthritis Rheum*, 1977, 20(2):513-25.

Capone ML, Sciulli MG, Tacconelli S, et al. "Pharmacodynamic Interaction of Naproxen With Low-Dose Aspirin in Healthy Subjects," *J Am Coll Cardiol*, 2005, 45(8):1295-1301.

Catella-Lawson F, Reilly MP, Kapoor SC, et al. "Cyclooxygenase Inhibitors and the Antiplatelet Effects of Aspirin," *N Engl J Med*, 2001, 345(25):1809-17.

Cryer B, Verlin RG, Cooper SA, et al. "Double-Blind, Randomized, Parallel, Placebo-Controlled Study Of Ibuprofen Effects On Thromboxane B2 Concentrations In Aspirin-Treated Healthy Adult Volunteers," *Clin Ther*, 2005, 27(2):185-191.

Gregoire N, Gualano V, Geneteau A, et al, "Population Pharmacokinetics of Ibuprofen Enantiomers in Very Premature Neonates," *J Clin Pharmacol*, 2004, 44(10):1114-24.

Kauffman RE and Nelson MV, "Effect of Age on Ibuprofen Pharmacokinetics and Antipyretic Response," *J Pediatr*, 1992, 121(6):969-73.

Konstan MW, Byard PJ, Hoppel CL, et al, "Effect of High-Dose Ibuprofen in Patients With Cystic Fibrosis," *N Engl J Med*, 1995, 332(13):848-54.

Lago P, Bettiol T, Salvadori S, et al, "Safety and Efficacy of Ibuprofen Versus Indomethacin in Preterm Infants Treated for Patent Ductus Arteriosus: A Randomised Controlled Trial," *Eur J Pediatr*, 2002, 161(4):202-7.

Lesko SM and Mitchell AA, "An Assessment of the Safety of Pediatric Ibuprofen. A Practitioner-Based Randomized Clinical Trial," *JAMA*, 1995, 273(12):929-33.

Lesko SM and Mitchell A, "The Safety of Acetaminophen and Ibuprofen Among Children Younger Than Two Years Old," *Pediatrics*, 1999, 104(4), http://www.pediatrics.org/cgi/content/full/104/4/e39.

Mayoral CE, Marino RV, Rosenfeld, W, et al, "Alternating Antipyretics: Is This an Alternative?" *Pediatrics*, 2000, 105(5):1009-12.

Ohlsson A, Walia R, and Shah S, "Ibuprofen for the Treatment of Patent Ductus Arteriosus in Preterm and/or Low Birth Weight Infants," *Cochrane Database Syst Rev*, 2005, (4):CD003481.

Scott CS, Retsch-Bogart GZ, Kustra RP, et al, "The Pharmacokinetics of Ibuprofen Suspension, Chewable Tablets, and Tablets in Children With Cystic Fibrosis," *J Pediatr*, 1999, 134(1):58-63.

Shah SS and Ohlsson A, "Ibuprofen for the Prevention of Patent Ductus Arteriosus in Preterm and/or Low Birth Weight Infants," *Cochrane Database Syst Rev*, 2006, (1):CD004213.

Van Overmeire B, Smets K, Lecoutere D, et al, "A Comparison of Ibuprofen and Indomethacin for Closure of Patent Ductus Arteriosus," *N Engl J Med*, 2000, 343(10):674-81.

Van Overmeire B, Touw D, Schepens PJ, et al, "Ibuprofen Pharmacokinetics in Preterm Infants With Patent Ductus Arteriosus," Clin Pharmacol Ther, 2001, 70(4):336-43.

- **Ibuprofen and Pseudoephedrine** *see* Pseudoephedrine and Ibuprofen *on page 1346*
- **Ibuprofen Lysine** *see* Ibuprofen *on page 802*
- **ICI-204,219** *see* Zafirlukast *on page 1632*
- **ICL670** *see* Deferasirox *on page 449*
- **ICRF-187** *see* Dexrazoxane *on page 467*
- **Idamycin® (Can)** *see* Idarubicin *on page 808*
- **Idamycin PFS®** *see* Idarubicin *on page 808*

Idarubicin (eye da ROO bi sin)

Medication Safety Issues

Sound-alike/look-alike issues:
Idarubicin may be confused with DOXOrubicin, DAUNOrubicin, epirubicin
Idamycin PFS® may be confused with Adriamycin

High alert medication: The Institute for Safe Medication Practices (ISMP) includes this medication among its list of drugs which have a heightened risk of causing significant patient harm when used in error.

Related Information

Compatibility of Chemotherapy and Related Supportive Care Medications *on page 1777*
Emetogenic Potential of Single Chemotherapeutic Agents *on page 1776*

U.S. Brand Names Idamycin PFS®

Canadian Brand Names Idamycin®

Index Terms 4-Demethoxydaunorubicin; 4-DMDR; Idarubicin Hydrochloride; IDR; IMI 30; NSC-256439; SC 33428

Therapeutic Category Antineoplastic Agent, Anthracycline; Antineoplastic Agent, Antibiotic

Generic Available Yes

Use Used in combination with other antineoplastic agents for treatment of acute leukemias (AML, ANLL, ALL)

Pregnancy Risk Factor D

Lactation Excretion in breast milk unknown

Contraindications Hypersensitivity to idarubicin or any component; patients with pre-existing bone marrow suppression unless the benefit warrants the risk; severe CHF, cardiomyopathy, or arrhythmias; pregnancy

Warnings The FDA currently recommends that procedures for proper handling and disposal of antineoplastic agents be considered; I.V. use only, severe local tissue necrosis will result if extravasation occurs; pre-existing heart disease, chest radiation, and previous therapy with anthracyclines at high cumulative doses increase risk of idarubicin-induced cardiac toxicity (manifested by potentially fatal CHF, life-threatening arrhythmias, or cardiomyopathies); the maximum lifetime anthracycline dose for idarubicin is approximately 137.5 mg/m^2; severe myelosuppression occurs in all patients given a therapeutic dose and is the dose-limiting adverse effect associated with idarubicin

Precautions Use with caution and reduce dose in patients with impaired hepatic or renal function and patients receiving concurrent radiation therapy

Adverse Reactions

Cardiovascular: Arrhythmias, EKG changes, cardiomyopathy, CHF

Dermatologic: Alopecia, rash, urticaria

Endocrine & metabolic: Hyperuricemia

Gastrointestinal: Nausea, vomiting, diarrhea, stomatitis, anorexia, mucositis

Genitourinary: Discoloration of urine (pink or red)

Hematologic: Leukopenia (nadir: 8-29 days), thrombocytopenia (nadir: 10-15 days), anemia

Hepatic: Elevated liver enzymes or bilirubin

Local: Tissue necrosis upon extravasation, erythematous streaking

Miscellaneous: Anaphylaxis

Stability Store vials under refrigeration and protect from light; incompatible with acyclovir, ceftazidime, furosemide, hydrocortisone, sodium bicarbonate and heparin; inactivated by alkaline solutions

Mechanism of Action Intercalates with DNA causing strand breakage and affects topoisomerase II activity resulting in inhibition of chain elongation and inhibition of DNA and RNA synthesis

Pharmacokinetics

Distribution:

V_d: Large volume of distribution due to extensive tissue binding; distributes into CSF

V_{dss}: 1700 L/m^2

Protein binding:

Idarubicin: 97%

Idarubicinol: 94%

Metabolism: In the liver to idarubicinol (active metabolite)

Half-life:

Children: 18.7 hours (range: 2.5-22.4 hours)

Adults: 19 hours (range: 10.5-34.7 hours)

Idarubicinol: 45-56.8 hours

Elimination: Primarily by biliary excretion; 2.3% to 6.5% of a dose is eliminated renally

Usual Dosage I.V. (refer to individual protocols):

Children:

Leukemia: 10-12 mg/m^2 once daily for 3 days of treatment course

Solid tumors: 5 mg/m^2 once daily for 3 days of treatment course

Adults: 8-12 mg/m^2 once daily for 3 days of treatment course in combination with Ara-C; reduce dose by 25% if severe mucositis is present

Dosing adjustment in hepatic and/or renal impairment:

Serum creatinine ≥2 mg/dL: Reduce dose by 25%

Bilirubin >2.5 mg/dL: Reduce dose by 50%

Bilirubin >5 mg/dL: **Do not administer**

Administration Do not administer I.M. or SubQ

Parenteral: I.V.: Administer by I.V. intermittent infusion over 10-30 minutes into a free flowing I.V. solution of NS or D_5W; administer at a final concentration of 1 mg/mL

(Continued)

Idarubicin *(Continued)*

Monitoring Parameters CBC with differential, platelet count, ECHO, EKG, serum electrolytes, creatinine, uric acid, ALT, AST, bilirubin, signs of extravasation

Patient Information Notify physician if fever, sore throat, bleeding, bruising, or pain at infusion site occurs. Urine may turn pink or red. Contraceptive measures are recommended during therapy.

Nursing Implications Maintain adequate patient hydration; local erythematous streaking along the vein may indicate too rapid a rate of administration; care should be taken to avoid extravasation; if extravasation occurs, the manufacturer recommends that the affected extremity be elevated and that topical ice packs be placed over the affected area immediately for 30 minutes, then apply for 30 minutes 4 times/day for 3 days; alternative therapy includes topical application of dimethylsulfoxide

Dosage Forms Excipient information presented when available (limited, particularly for generics); consult specific product labeling.

Injection, solution, as hydrochloride [preservative free] (Idamycin PFS®): 1 mg/mL (5 mL, 10 mL, 20 mL)

References

Dinndorf PA, Avramis VI, Wiersma S, et al, "Phase I/II Study of Idarubicin Given With Continuous Infusion Fludarabine Followed by Continuous Infusion Cytarabine in Children With Acute Leukemia: A Report From the Children's Cancer Group," *J Clin Oncol*, 1997, 15(8):2780-5.

Leahey A, Kelly K, Rorke LB, et al, "A Phase I/II Study of Idarubicin (Ida) With Continuous Infusion Fludarabine (F-ara-A) and Cytarabine (ara-C) for Refractory or Recurrent Pediatric Acute Myeloid Leukemia (AML)," *J Pediatr Hematol Oncol*, 1997, 19(4):304-8.

Reid JM, Pendergrass TW, Krailo MD, et al, "Plasma Pharmacokinetics and Cerebrospinal Fluid Concentrations of Idarubicin and Idarubicinol in Pediatric Leukemia Patients: A Children's Cancer Study Group Report," *Cancer Res*, 1990, 50(20):6525-8.

♦ **Idarubicin Hydrochloride** *see* Idarubicin *on page 808*
♦ **IDEC-C2B8** *see* Rituximab *on page 1398*
♦ **IDR** *see* Idarubicin *on page 808*
♦ **Ifex®** *see* Ifosfamide *on page 810*
♦ **IFLrA** *see* Interferon Alfa-2a *on page 854*

Ifosfamide (eye FOSS fa mide)

Medication Safety Issues

Sound-alike/look-alike issues:

Ifosfamide may be confused with cyclophosphamide

High alert medication: The Institute for Safe Medication Practices (ISMP) includes this medication among its list of drugs which have a heightened risk of causing significant patient harm when used in error.

Related Information

Compatibility of Chemotherapy and Related Supportive Care Medications *on page 1777*
Emetogenic Potential of Single Chemotherapeutic Agents *on page 1776*

U.S. Brand Names Ifex®

Canadian Brand Names Ifex®

Index Terms Isophosphamide; NSC-109724; Z4942

Therapeutic Category Antineoplastic Agent, Alkylating Agent

Generic Available Yes

Use In combination with other antineoplastics in treatment of lung cancer, Hodgkin's and non-Hodgkin's lymphoma, breast cancer, acute and chronic lymphocytic leukemia, ovarian cancer, testicular cancer, and sarcomas

Pregnancy Risk Factor D

Lactation Enters breast milk/not recommended

Contraindications Hypersensitivity to ifosfamide or any component; patients with severely depressed bone marrow function; pregnancy

Warnings The FDA currently recommends that procedures for proper handling and disposal of antineoplastic agents be considered. May require therapy cessation if confusion or coma occurs; monitor for hemorrhagic cystitis and severe myelosuppression; risk factors for ifosfamide-induced nephrotoxicity include previous or concurrent cisplatin therapy, pre-existing renal impairment, prior nephrectomy, children ≤5 years, or patients who have received high cumulative ifosfamide doses of 50 g/m^2

Precautions Use with caution in patients with impaired renal function or those with compromised bone marrow reserve

Adverse Reactions

Cardiovascular: Cardiotoxicity

Central nervous system: Somnolence, lethargy, confusion, depressive psychoses, hallucinations, dizziness, seizures, fever, ataxia, coma

Dermatologic: Alopecia, hyperpigmentation

Endocrine & metabolic: Metabolic acidosis
Gastrointestinal: Nausea, vomiting, stomatitis, diarrhea
Genitourinary: Dysuria, hemorrhagic cystitis
Hematologic: Myelosuppression (leukocyte nadir: 7-14 days), thrombocytopenia
Hepatic: Elevated liver enzymes and/or bilirubin
Local: Phlebitis
Neuromuscular & skeletal: Polyneuropathy
Renal: Renal tubular acidosis, hematuria, elevated BUN and serum creatinine

Drug Interactions Cytochrome P450 isoenzyme CYP2B6 and CYP3A3/4 substrate
Phenobarbital, phenytoin, chloral hydrate may increase the conversion of ifosfamide to active metabolites and increase toxicity; cisplatin may increase ifosfamide renal damage

Stability Reconstituted solution is stable for 7 days at room temperature and 21 days when refrigerated

Mechanism of Action Causes cross-linking of DNA strands by binding with nucleic acids and other intracellular structures; inhibits protein synthesis and DNA synthesis

Pharmacokinetics Dose-dependent pharmacokinetics:
Distribution: Unchanged ifosfamide penetrates the blood-brain barrier; excreted into breast milk
Metabolism: Requires biotransformation by the cytochrome P450 enzyme system in the liver before it can act as an alkylating agent; following hydroxylation, the metabolite breaks down to acrolein (bladder irritant) and ifosfamide mustard (active drug)
Half-life: Terminal:
Low dose (1800 mg/m^2): 4-7 hours
High dose (3800-5000 mg/m^2): 11-15 hours
Elimination: 60% to 80% of a dose is excreted in urine as unchanged drug and metabolites

Usual Dosage I.V. (refer to individual protocols):
Children: 1200-1800 mg/m^2/day for 5 days every 21-28 days or 5000 mg/m^2 as a single 24-hour infusion or 3 g/m^2/day for 2 days
Adults: 700-2000 mg/m^2/day for 5 days or 2400 mg/m^2/day for 3 days every 21-28 days; 5000 mg/m^2 as a single dose over 24 hours

Administration Parenteral: Administer as a slow I.V. intermittent infusion over at least 30 minutes at a final concentration for administration not to exceed 40 mg/mL (usual concentration for administration is between 0.6-20 mg/mL), or administer as a 24-hour infusion

Monitoring Parameters CBC with differential and platelet count, urine output, urinalysis, liver function and renal function tests, serum electrolytes

Patient Information Notify physician of pain or irritation in urination, CNS changes, fever, chills, bruising, or bleeding. Contraceptive measure are recommended during therapy.

Nursing Implications Maintain adequate patient hydration

Additional Information Usually used in combination with mesna, an agent used to prevent hemorrhagic cystitis

Dosage Forms Excipient information presented when available (limited, particularly for generics); consult specific product labeling.
Injection, powder for reconstitution: 1 g
Ifex®: 1 g, 3 g
Injection, solution: 50 mg/mL (20 mL, 60 mL)

References

Ninane J, Baurain R, and de Kraker J, "Alkylating Activity in Serum, Urine, and CSF Following High-Dose Ifosfamide in Children," *Cancer Chemother Pharmacol*, 1989, 24(Suppl 1):S2-6.
Pinkerton CR, Rogers H, James C, et al, "A Phase II Study of Ifosfamide in Children With Recurrent Solid Tumors," *Cancer Chemother Pharmacol*, 1985, 15(3):258-62.

♦ **IG** *see* Immune Globulin (Intramuscular) *on page 817*
♦ **IGIM** *see* Immune Globulin (Intramuscular) *on page 817*
♦ **IL-2** *see* Aldesleukin *on page 70*
♦ **IL-11** *see* Oprelvekin *on page 1174*
♦ **IMI 30** *see* Idarubicin *on page 808*
♦ **Imidazole Carboxamide** *see* Dacarbazine *on page 433*
♦ **Imidazole Carboxamide Dimethyltriazene** *see* Dacarbazine *on page 433*

Imiglucerase (imi GLOO ser ase)

Medication Safety Issues
Sound-alike/look-alike issues:
Cerezyme® may be confused with Cerebyx®, Ceredase®
(Continued)

Imiglucerase *(Continued)*

U.S. Brand Names Cerezyme®

Canadian Brand Names Cerezyme®

Therapeutic Category Enzyme, Glucocerebrosidase; Gaucher's Disease, Treatment Agent

Generic Available No

Use Long-term enzyme replacement therapy for patients with Type 1 Gaucher's disease

Pregnancy Risk Factor C

Lactation Excretion in breast milk unknown/use caution

Contraindications Hypersensitivity to imiglucerase or any component

Warnings During clinical trials, 16% of patients developed IgG antibodies reactive with imiglucerase; <1% of patients experienced anaphylactoid reactions; most patients may continue therapy after a reduction in the infusion rate and pretreatment with an antihistamine and/or corticosteroid; close observation for hypersensitivity reactions is recommended

Precautions Patients experiencing respiratory symptoms during treatment should be evaluated for potential pulmonary hypertension

Adverse Reactions

Cardiovascular: Systemic hypertension (mild), pulmonary hypertension, tachycardia, flushing, peripheral edema (transient)

Central nervous system: Headache, dizziness, fatigue, fever

Dermatologic: Rash, pruritus

Gastrointestinal: Nausea, abdominal pain, diarrhea, vomiting

Genitourinary: Decreased urinary frequency

Local: Burning, swelling, pruritus, sterile abscess at injection site

Neuromuscular & skeletal: Back pain

Respiratory: Dyspnea, cough

Miscellaneous: Anaphylactoid reactions (see Warnings)

Drug Interactions No information available at this time

Stability Store in refrigerator 2°C to 8°C (36°F to 46°F); after reconstitution, stable for 12 hours refrigerated or at room temperature; after dilution in NS, 40 units/mL solution is stable for 24 hours refrigerated; do not use if opaque particles or solution discoloration are seen

Mechanism of Action Imiglucerase, produced by recombinant DNA technology, is an analog of glucocerebrosidase; it acts by replacing the missing enzyme associated with Gaucher's disease; Gaucher's disease is an inherited metabolic disorder caused by the defective activity of beta-glucosidase and the resultant accumulation of glucosyl ceramide laden macrophages in the liver, bone, and spleen; this results in one or more of the following conditions: anemia, thrombocytopenia, bone disease, hepatomegaly, splenomegaly

Pharmacodynamics

Onset of significant improvement in symptoms:

Hepatosplenomegaly and hematologic abnormalities: Within 6 months

Improvement in bone mineralization: Noted at 80-104 weeks of therapy

Pharmacokinetics

Distribution: V_d: 0.09-0.15 L/kg

Half-life, elimination: 3.6-10.4 minutes

Clearance: 9.8-20.3 mL/minute/kg

Usual Dosage I.V.: Children and Adults: 30-60 units/kg every 2 weeks; range in dosage: 2.5 units/kg 3 times/week to 60 units/kg once weekly to every 4 weeks. Initial dose should be based on disease severity and rate of progression. Children at high risk for complications from Gaucher's disease (one or more of the following: symptomatic disease including manifestations of abdominal or bone pain, fatigue, exertional limitations, weakness, and cachexia; growth failure; evidence of skeletal involvement; platelet count ≤60,000 mm^3 and/or documented abnormal bleeding episode(s); Hgb ≥2.0 g/dL below lower limit for age and sex; impaired quality of life) should receive an initial dose of 60 units/kg; failure to respond to treatment within 6 months indicates the need for a higher dosage.

Maintenance: After patient response is well established a reduction in dosage may be attempted; progressive reductions may be made at intervals of 3-6 months; assess dosage frequently to maintain consistent dosage per kg body weight

Administration Parenteral: Reconstitute 200 unit vial with 5.1 mL SWI or 400 unit vial with 10.2 mL SWI resulting in a 40 units/mL concentration; further dilute in 100-200 mL NS; infuse over 1-2 hours; may filter diluted solution through an in-line low protein-binding 0.2 micron filter during administration

Monitoring Parameters CBC, platelets, liver function tests, MRI or CT scan (spleen and liver volume), skeletal x-rays

Dosage Forms Excipient information presented when available (limited, particularly for generics); consult specific product labeling.

Injection, powder for reconstitution [preservative free]: 200 units, 400 units

References

Charrow J, Andersson HC, Kaplan P, et al, "Enzyme Replacement Therapy and Monitoring for Children With Type 1 Gaucher Disease: Consensus Recommendations," *J Pediatr*, 2004, 144(1):112-20.

♦ **Imipemide** *see* Imipenem and Cilastatin *on page 813*

Imipenem and Cilastatin (i mi PEN em & sye la STAT in)

Medication Safety Issues

Sound-alike/look-alike issues:

Primaxin® may be confused with Premarin®, Primacor®

U.S. Brand Names Primaxin®

Canadian Brand Names Primaxin®; Primaxin® I.V.

Index Terms Cilastatin and Imipenem; Imipemide

Therapeutic Category Antibiotic, Carbapenem

Generic Available No

Use Treatment of documented multidrug-resistant gram-negative infection of the lower respiratory tract, urinary tract, intra-abdominal, gynecologic, bone and joint, septicemias, endocarditis, and skin and skin structure due to organisms proven or suspected to be susceptible to imipenem/cilastatin; treatment of multiple organism infection in which other agents have an insufficient spectrum of activity or are contraindicated due to toxic potential; therapeutic alternative for treatment of gram-negative sepsis in immunocompromised patients

Pregnancy Risk Factor C

Lactation Enters breast milk/use caution

Contraindications Hypersensitivity to imipenem/cilastatin or any component

Warnings Serious and occasionally fatal hypersensitivity reactions have been reported in patients receiving beta-lactam therapy; careful inquiry should be made concerning previous hypersensitivity reactions to penicillins, cephalosporins, or other beta-lactams before initiating imipenem. Seizures have been reported with imipenem therapy in children with meningitis; imipenem is not recommended in pediatric patients with CNS infections. Pseudomembranous colitis has been reported in patients receiving imipenem; prolonged use may result in superinfection.

Precautions Use with caution in patients with history of seizures or who are predisposed and in patients with a history of hypersensitivity to penicillins; use with caution and adjust dose in patients with impaired renal function

Adverse Reactions

Cardiovascular: Hypotension, tachycardia

Central nervous system: Seizures, hallucinations, altered effect, confusion, fever, dizziness

Dermatologic: Rash, pruritus, urticaria

Gastrointestinal: Nausea, vomiting, diarrhea, pseudomembranous colitis, oral candidiasis

Genitourinary: Discoloration of urine, anuria, oliguria, hematuria

Hematologic: Eosinophilia, neutropenia

Hepatic: Transient elevation in liver enzymes

Local: Phlebitis, irritation and pain at injection site

Miscellaneous: Emergence of resistant strains of *P. aeruginosa*

Drug Interactions Beta-lactam antibiotics, probenecid; ganciclovir (increased risk of seizures)

Stability

I.V.: When reconstituted suspension is further diluted with NS, it is stable for 10 hours at room temperature or 48 hours under refrigeration; when reconstituted suspension is further diluted with D_5W, $D_{10}W$, D_5NS, or $D_5\,{}^1\!/_4NS$, it is stable for 4 hours at room temperature and 24 hours under refrigeration; compatible with TPN via Y-site injection; **incompatible** when mixed directly in TPN solution; inactivated at alkaline or acidic pH

I.M.: Reconstituted I.M. suspension in lidocaine HCl should be used within 1 hour after preparation

Mechanism of Action Inhibits cell wall synthesis by binding to all of the penicillin-binding proteins with greatest affinity for PBP 1 and PBP 2; cilastatin prevents renal metabolism of imipenem by competitive inhibition of dehydropeptidase along the brush border of the proximal renal tubules

Pharmacokinetics

Absorption: I.M.:

Imipenem: 75%

Cilastatin: 95%

(Continued)

Imipenem and Cilastatin *(Continued)*

Distribution: Imipenem appears in breast milk; crosses the placenta; only low concentrations penetrate into CSF

Protein binding:

Imipenem: 13% to 21%

Cilastatin: 40%

Metabolism: Imipenem is metabolized in the kidney by dehydropeptidase; cilastatin is partially metabolized in the kidneys

Half-life, both: Prolonged with renal insufficiency

Neonates: 1.5-3 hours

Infants and Children: 1-1.4 hours

Adults: 1 hour

Elimination: When imipenem is given with cilastatin, urinary excretion of unchanged imipenem increases to 70%; 70% to 80% of a cilastatin dose is excreted unchanged in the urine

Dialysis: Moderately dialyzable (20% to 50%)

Usual Dosage Dosage recommendation based on imipenem component for non-CNS infections: I.V. infusion: (I.M. is limited to mild-moderate infections):

Neonates:

0-4 weeks, <1200 g: 20 mg/kg/dose every 18-24 hours

Postnatal age ≤7 days, 1200-1500 g: 40 mg/kg/day divided every 12 hours

Postnatal age ≤7 days, >1500 g: 50 mg/kg/day divided every 12 hours

Postnatal age >7 days, 1200-1500 g: 40 mg/kg/day divided every 12 hours

Postnatal age >7 days, >1500 g: 75 mg/kg/day divided every 8 hours

Infants 4 weeks to 3 months: 100 mg/kg/day divided every 6 hours

Infants ≥3 months and Children: 60-100 mg/kg/day divided every 6 hours; maximum dose: 4 g/day

Adults:

Serious infections: 2-4 g/day divided every 6 hours

Mild to moderate infections: 1-2 g/day in 3-4 divided doses

Dosing adjustment in renal impairment: Imipenem doses should be reduced in patients with Cl_{cr} <41-70 mL/minute/1.73 m^2: See table.

Creatinine Clearance (mL/min/1.73 m^2)	Frequency	% Decrease in Daily Maximum Dose
41-70	Every 6 hours	50
21-40	Every 8 hours	63
6-20	Every 12 hours	75

Patients with creatinine clearance ≤5 mL/minute/1.73 m^2 should not receive imipenem unless undergoing hemodialysis

Administration

I.M.: Administer suspension by deep I.M. injection into a large muscle mass such as the gluteal muscle or lateral part of the thigh; the I.M. powder for suspension should be reconstituted with lidocaine hydrochloride 1% injection (without epinephrine). **Note:** The I.M. formulation is not for I.V. use.

I.V.: Administer by I.V. intermittent infusion; final concentration should not exceed 5 mg/mL; in fluid-restricted patients, a final concentration of 7 mg/mL has been administered; doses ≤500 mg may be infused over 15-30 minutes; doses >500 mg should be infused over 40-60 minutes

Monitoring Parameters Periodic renal, hepatic, and hematologic function tests

Test Interactions Interferes with urinary glucose determination using Clinitest®; Positive Coombs' [direct]

Nursing Implications If nausea and/or vomiting occur during administration, decrease the rate of I.V. infusion

Additional Information Sodium content of 1 g I.V. formulation: 3.2 mEq; sodium content of 500 mg I.M. formulation: 1.4 mEq

Dosage Forms Excipient information presented when available (limited, particularly for generics); consult specific product labeling.

Injection, powder for reconstitution [I.M.]:

Primaxin®: Imipenem 500 mg and cilastatin 500 mg [contains sodium 32 mg (1.4 mEq)]

Injection, powder for reconstitution [I.V.]:

Primaxin®: Imipenem 250 mg and cilastatin 250 mg [contains sodium 18.8 mg (0.8 mEq)]; imipenem 500 mg and cilastatin 500 mg [contains sodium 37.5 mg (1.6 mEq)]

References

Ahonkhai VI, Cyhan GM, Wilson SE, et al, "Imipenem-Cilastatin in Pediatric Patients: An Overview of Safety and Efficacy in Studies Conducted in the United States," *Pediatr Infect Dis J*, 1989, 8(11):740-4.

Overturf GD, "Use of Imipenem-Cilastatin in Pediatrics," *Pediatr Infect Dis J*, 1989, 8(11):792-4.
Wong VK, Wright HT Jr, Ross LA, et al, "Imipenem/Cilastatin Treatment of Bacterial Meningitis in Children," *Pediatr Infect Dis J*, 1991, 10(2):122-5.

Imipramine (im IP ra meen)

Medication Safety Issues

Sound-alike/look-alike issues:

Imipramine may be confused with amitriptyline, desipramine, Norpramin®

Related Information

Antidepressant Agents *on page 1681*

Medications for Which A Single Dose May Be Fatal When Ingested By A Toddler *on page 1932*

Overdose and Toxicology *on page 1916*

U.S. Brand Names Tofranil®; Tofranil-PM®

Canadian Brand Names Apo-Imipramine®; Novo-Pramine; Tofranil®

Index Terms Imipramine Hydrochloride; Imipramine Pamoate

Therapeutic Category Antidepressant, Tricyclic

Generic Available Yes

Use Treatment of various forms of depression, often in conjunction with psychotherapy; enuresis in children; analgesic for certain chronic and neuropathic pain

Medication Guide An FDA-approved patient medication guide, which is available with the product information and at http://www.fda.gov/cder/Offices/ODS/medication_guides.htm, must be dispensed with this medication for each new outpatient prescription and refill.

Pregnancy Risk Factor D

Lactation Enters breast milk/not recommended (AAP rates "of concern")

Contraindications Hypersensitivity to imipramine (cross-sensitivity with other tricyclics may occur) or any component; use of MAO inhibitors within 14 days (potentially fatal reactions may occur, see Drug Interactions); narrow-angle glaucoma; use during acute recovery phase after MI

Warnings Imipramine is FDA approved for the treatment of nocturnal enuresis in children ≥6 years of age. Imipramine is not approved for the treatment of depression in pediatric patients. Clinical worsening of depression or suicidal ideation and behavior may occur in children and adults with major depressive disorder. In clinical trials, antidepressants increased the risk of suicidal thinking and behavior (suicidality) in children, adolescents, and young adults (18-24 years of age) with major depressive disorder and other psychiatric disorders. This risk must be considered before prescribing antidepressants for any clinical use. Short-term studies did **not** show an increased risk of suicidality with antidepressant use in patients >24 years of age and showed a decreased risk in patients ≥65 years.

Patients of all ages who are treated with antidepressants for any indication require appropriate monitoring and close observation for clinical worsening of depression, suicidality, and unusual changes in behavior, especially during the first few months after antidepressant initiation or when the dose is adjusted. Family members and caregivers should be instructed to closely observe the patient (ie, daily) and communicate condition with healthcare provider. Patients should also be monitored for associated behaviors (eg, anxiety, agitation, panic attacks, insomnia, irritability, hostility, aggressiveness, impulsivity, akathisia, hypomania, mania) which may increase the risk for worsening depression or suicidality. Worsening depression or emergence of suicidality (or associated behaviors listed above) that is abrupt in onset, severe, or not part of the presenting symptoms, may require discontinuation or modification of drug therapy.

Do not discontinue abruptly in patients receiving high doses chronically (withdrawal symptoms may occur; see Adverse Reactions). To reduce risk of intentional overdose, write prescriptions for the smallest quantity consistent with good patient care. Screen individuals for bipolar disorder prior to treatment (using antidepressants alone may induce manic episodes in patients with this condition). May worsen psychosis in some patients.

Precautions Use with caution in patients with cardiovascular disease, conduction disturbances, seizure disorders, urinary retention, anorexia, significant renal or hepatic dysfunction, hyperthyroidism or those receiving thyroid replacement; use of capsules is **not** recommended in children due to high mg strength and increased potential for acute overdose

Adverse Reactions Less sedation and anticholinergic effects than amitriptyline

Cardiovascular: Arrhythmias, hypotension (especially orthostatic)

Central nervous system: Drowsiness, sedation, confusion, dizziness, fatigue, anxiety, nervousness, sleep disorders, seizures; suicidal thinking and behavior (see Warnings)

Dermatologic: Rash, photosensitivity

(Continued)

Imipramine *(Continued)*

Endocrine & metabolic: Hyperglycemia, hypoglycemia
Gastrointestinal: Nausea, vomiting, constipation, xerostomia, decreased appetite
Genitourinary: Urinary retention
Hematologic: Blood dyscrasias
Hepatic: Hepatitis
Ocular: Blurred vision, elevated intraocular pressure
Neuromuscular & skeletal: Weakness
Miscellaneous: Hypersensitivity reactions; withdrawal symptoms following abrupt discontinuation (headache, nausea, malaise)

Drug Interactions Cytochrome P450 isoenzyme CYP1A2 (demethylation), CYP2C9 (demethylation), CYP2C19 (demethylation), CYP2D6 (hydroxylation), and CYP3A3/4 substrate

May decrease or reverse effects of guanethidine, clonidine, and similar drugs; may increase effects of CNS depressants, alcohol, adrenergic agents, anticholinergic agents, antihypertensive agents; with MAO inhibitors, fever, tachycardia, hypertension, seizures, and death may occur (do not use MAO inhibitors within 14 days of imipramine); the herbal medicine St John's wort (*Hypericum perforatum*) may increase serious side effects, its use is **not** recommended; use with cytochrome P450 CYP2D6 inhibitors or substrates may increase imipramine serum concentrations or effects (monitor patient and serum concentrations); methylphenidate may increase imipramine serum concentrations (reduction of imipramine dosage may be needed); hepatic enzyme inducers (eg, phenobarbital, phenytoin) may decrease imipramine serum concentrations (monitor patients and serum concentrations); concurrent use of high-dose TCAs and ritonavir may cause the serotonin syndrome

Food Interactions Riboflavin dietary requirements may be increased; food does not alter bioavailability

Mechanism of Action Increases the synaptic concentration of serotonin and/or norepinephrine in the CNS by inhibition of their reuptake by the presynaptic neuronal membrane

Pharmacodynamics Maximum antidepressant effects usually occur after ≥2 weeks

Pharmacokinetics

Absorption: Oral: Well absorbed
Distribution: Crosses the placenta; distributes into breast milk
V_d: Children: 14.5 L/kg; Adults: ~17 L/kg
Protein binding: >90% (primarily to $alpha_1$ acid glycoprotein and lipoproteins; to a lesser extent albumin)
Metabolism: In the liver by microsomal enzymes to desipramine (active) and other metabolites; significant first-pass effect
Bioavailability: 20% to 80%
Half-life: Adults: Range: 6-18 hours
Mean: Children: 11 hours; Adults: 16-17 hours
Desipramine (active metabolite): Adults: 22-28 hours
Time to peak serum concentration: Within 1-2 hours
Elimination: In the urine

Usual Dosage Oral:

Children:

Depression: **Note:** Not FDA approved for the treatment of depression in pediatric patients; controlled clinical trials have not shown tricyclic antidepressants to be superior to placebo for the treatment of depression in children and adolescents (see Dopheide, 2006 and Wagner, 2005).

1.5 mg/kg/day with dosage increments of 1 mg/kg every 3-4 days to a maximum dose of 5 mg/kg/day in 1-4 divided doses; monitor carefully especially with doses ≥3.5 mg/kg/day

Enuresis: ≥6 years: Initial: 10-25 mg at bedtime, if inadequate response still seen after 1 week of therapy, increase by 25 mg/day; dose should not exceed 2.5 mg/kg/day or 50 mg at bedtime if 6-12 years of age or 75 mg at bedtime if ≥12 years of age

Adjunct in the treatment of cancer pain: Initial: 0.2-0.4 mg/kg at bedtime; dose may be increased by 50% every 2-3 days up to 1-3 mg/kg/dose at bedtime

Adolescents: Initial: 25-50 mg/day; increase gradually; maximum dose: 200 mg/day in single or divided doses

Adults: Initial: 25 mg 3-4 times/day, increase dose gradually, total dose may be given at bedtime; maximum dose: 300 mg/day

Administration Oral: May administer with food to decrease GI distress

Monitoring Parameters Heart rate, EKG, supine and standing blood pressure (especially in children), liver enzymes, CBC, serum drug concentrations (see Reference Range). Monitor patient periodically for symptom resolution; monitor for worsening depression, suicidality, and associated behaviors (especially at the beginning of therapy or when doses are increased or decreased; see Warnings).

Reference Range

Therapeutic: Imipramine and desipramine 150-250 ng/mL (SI: 530-890 nmol/L); desipramine 150-300 ng/mL (SI: 560-1125 nmol/L)

Potentially toxic: >300 ng/mL (SI: >1070 nmol/L)

Toxic: >1000 ng/mL (SI: >3570 nmol/L)

Patient Information Read the patient Medication Guide that you receive with each prescription and refill of imipramine. An increased risk of suicidal thinking and behavior has been reported with the use of antidepressants in children, adolescents, and young adults (18-24 years of age). Notify physician if you feel more depressed, have thoughts of suicide, or become more agitated or irritable (see Warnings). Limit caffeine; avoid alcohol and the herbal medicine St. John's wort; may cause drowsiness and impair ability to perform activities requiring mental alertness or physical coordination; may cause dry mouth. May cause photosensitivity reactions (eg, exposure to sunlight may cause severe sunburn, skin rash, redness, or itching); avoid exposure to sunlight and artificial light sources (sunlamps, tanning booth/bed); wear protective clothing, wide-brimmed hats, sunglasses, and lip sunscreen (SPF ≥15); use a sunscreen [broad-spectrum sunscreen or physical sunscreen (preferred) or sunblock with SPF ≥15]; contact physician if reaction occurs.

Dosage Forms Excipient information presented when available (limited, particularly for generics); consult specific product labeling.

Capsule, as pamoate: 75 mg, 100 mg, 125 mg, 150 mg

Tofranil-PM®: 75 mg, 100 mg, 125 mg, 150 mg

Tablet, as hydrochloride: 10 mg, 25 mg, 50 mg

Tofranil®): 10 mg, 25 mg, 50 mg

References

Berde C, Ablin A, Glazer J, et al, "American Academy of Pediatrics Report of the Subcommittee on Disease-Related Pain in Childhood Cancer," *Pediatrics*, 1990, 86(5 Pt 2):818-25.

Dopheide JA, "Recognizing and Treating Depression in Children and Adolescents," *Am J Health Syst Pharm*, 2006, 63(3):233-43.

Levy HB, Harper CR, and Weinberg WA, "A Practical Approach to Children Failing in School," *Pediatr Clin North Am*, 1992, 39(4):895-928.

Wagner KD, "Pharmacotherapy for Major Depression in Children and Adolescents," *Prog Neuropsychopharmacol Biol Psychiatry*, 2005, 29(5):819-26.

♦ **Imipramine Hydrochloride** *see* Imipramine *on page 815*

♦ **Imipramine Pamoate** *see* Imipramine *on page 815*

♦ **Imitrex®** *see* Sumatriptan *on page 1495*

♦ **Imitrex® DF (Can)** *see* Sumatriptan *on page 1495*

♦ **Imitrex® Nasal Spray (Can)** *see* Sumatriptan *on page 1495*

Immune Globulin (Intramuscular)

(i MYUN GLOB yoo lin, IN tra MUS kyoo ler)

U.S. Brand Names BayGam® [DSC]; GammaSTAN™ S/D

Canadian Brand Names BayGam®

Index Terms Gamma Globulin; IG; IGIM; Immune Serum Globulin; ISG

Therapeutic Category Immune Globulin

Generic Available No

Use Provide passive immunity in susceptible individuals (eg, household and sexual contacts; travelers to high-risk areas; staff, attendees, and parents of diapered attendees in daycare center outbreaks; illicit drug users; staff and residents of institutions for custodial care) if given within 14 days of exposure to hepatitis A and for whom immunization is contraindicated or there is insufficient time for active immunization to take effect; prophylaxis of measles in susceptible individuals if given within 6 days of exposure; replacement therapy in antibody deficiency disorders; postexposure prophylaxis of rubella if given within 72 hours of exposure in a susceptible pregnant woman who will not consider termination of pregnancy under any circumstances

Pregnancy Risk Factor C

Contraindications Hypersensitivity to immune globulin or any component; IgA deficiency

Warnings As a product of human plasma, IGIM may potentially transmit disease; screening of donors, as well as testing and/or inactivation of certain viruses reduces this risk. Epidemiologic and laboratory data indicate current IGIM products do not have a discernible risk of transmitting HIV.

Precautions Use with caution in patients with thrombocytopenia or coagulation disorders since bleeding may occur following an I.M. injection. IGIM is **NOT** for I.V. administration.

Adverse Reactions

Cardiovascular: Flushing, chest pain

Central nervous system: Fever, chills, lethargy, headache

(Continued)

Immune Globulin (Intramuscular) *(Continued)*

Dermatologic: Urticaria, erythema, angioedema
Gastrointestinal: Nausea, vomiting
Local: Pain, tenderness, discomfort, muscle stiffness at I.M. site
Neuromuscular & skeletal: Myalgia, arthralgia
Renal: Nephrotic syndrome
Respiratory: Dyspnea
Miscellaneous: Hypersensitivity reactions, anaphylaxis

Drug Interactions May interfere with immune response to live measles, mumps, rubella, or varicella virus vaccines (defer live virus vaccine administration for at least 3 months following IGIM used for pre- or postexposure prophylaxis of hepatitis A; defer live virus vaccine administration for at least 5 months following IGIM used for measles prophylaxis in immunocompetent patients; defer live virus vaccine administration for at least 6 months following IGIM used for measles prophylaxis in immunodeficient patients)

Stability Store in refrigerator; do not freeze

Mechanism of Action Provides passive immunity by increasing the antibody titer and antigen-antibody reaction potential

Pharmacodynamics Duration: Immune effect: Usually 3-4 weeks

Pharmacokinetics

Half-life: 23 days
Time to peak serum concentration: I.M.: Within 48 hours

Usual Dosage I.M.: Infants, Children, Adolescents, and Adults:

Hepatitis A:

Pre-exposure prophylaxis upon travel into endemic areas (hepatitis A vaccine preferred):

Anticipated risk of 1-3 months: 0.02 mL/kg single dose
Anticipated risk >3 months: 0.06 mL/kg once every 4-6 months if exposure continues

Postexposure prophylaxis: 0.02 mL/kg single dose given within 14 days of exposure

Measles:

Postexposure prophylaxis: 0.25 mL/kg (~40 mg/kg IgG) single dose given within 6 days of exposure; maximum dose: 15 mL

Postexposure prophylaxis, immunocompromised host: 0.5 mL/kg (~80 mg/kg IgG) single dose given within 6 days of exposure; maximum dose: 15 mL

Rubella: Postexposure prophylaxis: 0.55 mL/kg single dose within 72 hours of exposure

Replacement therapy in antibody deficiency disorders: Initial: 1.3 mL/kg (~200 mg/kg); maintenance dose: 0.66 mL/kg (~100 mg/kg IgG) every 2-4 weeks (infants and children maximum single dose: 20-30 mL; adult maximum single dose: 30-50 mL); determine frequency of administration on the basis of trough IgG concentrations and clinical response

Administration I.M.: **Do not give I.V. or SubQ.** Administer deep I.M. into a large muscle mass; infants and small children, administer I.M. into the anterolateral aspect of the thigh; larger children and adolescents, administer into the upper outer quadrant of the gluteal region.

Limit the volume at a single injection site: Infants and small children: 1-3 mL; large child and adolescent: 5 mL; use multiple injection sites if the dose volume exceeds the recommended limit at a single injection site

Dosage Forms Excipient information presented when available (limited, particularly for generics); consult specific product labeling.

Injection, solution [preservative free]:

BayGam® [DSC], GammaSTAN™ S/D: 15% to 18% (2 mL, 10 mL)

References

Advisory Committee on Immunization Practices (ACIP), "Prevention of Hepatitis A Through Active or Passive Immunization: Recommendations of the Advisory Committee on Immunization Practices (ACIP)," *MMWR Recomm Rep*, 2006, 55(RR-7):1-23.

American Academy of Pediatrics, "Report of the Committee on Infectious Diseases," *2003 Red Book*, 26th ed, 54-6,423.

Immune Globulin (Intravenous)

(i MYUN GLOB yoo lin, IN tra VEE nus)

Medication Safety Issues

Sound-alike/look-alike issues:

Gamimune® N may be confused with CytoGam®

U.S. Brand Names Carimune™ NF; Flebogamma®; Gammagard® Liquid; Gammagard® S/D; Gammar®-P I.V.; Gamunex®; Iveegam EN; Octagam®; Panglobulin® NF; Polygam® S/D

Canadian Brand Names Gamimune® N; Gammagard® Liquid; Gammagard® S/D; Gamunex®; Iveegam Immuno®

Index Terms IVIG

Therapeutic Category Immune Globulin

Generic Available No

Use Treatment of immunodeficiency syndrome, idiopathic thrombocytopenic purpura (ITP) and B-cell chronic lymphocytic leukemia (CLL); used in conjunction with appropriate anti-infective therapy to prevent or modify acute bacterial or viral infections in patients with iatrogenically-induced or disease-associated immunodepression; autoimmune neutropenia, bone marrow transplantation patients, Kawasaki disease, pediatric HIV infection, HIV-associated thrombocytopenia, Guillain-Barré syndrome, dermatomyositis, polymyositis, demyelinating polyneuropathies

FDA and NIH Recommendations for the use of IGIV:

- Primary immunodeficiencies
- Kawasaki disease
- Pediatric HIV infection
- Chronic B-cell lymphocytic leukemia
- Recent bone marrow transplantation
- Immune-mediated thrombocytopenia
- Chronic inflammatory demyelinating polyneuropathy

Pregnancy Risk Factor C

Lactation Excretion in breast milk unknown

Contraindications Hypersensitivity to immune globulin, blood products, or any component; IgA deficiency (except with the use of Gammagard® S/D or Polygam® S/D)

Warnings Renal dysfunction and/or acute renal failure, osmotic nephrosis, and death have been reported with the administration of IVIG; 88% of the cases were associated with the administration of sucrose-containing IVIG products (Carimune™ NF, Panglobulin®, Gammar®-P I.V.). Reports of noncardiogenic pulmonary edema with severe respiratory distress, hypoxemia, and fever occurring within 1-6 hours after a dose have occurred. Thrombotic events have been reported; patients at risk include those with a history of atherosclerosis, multiple cardiovascular risk factors, impaired cardiac output, hyperviscosity/hypercoagulable disorders, and prolonged periods of immobilization.

Aseptic meningitis syndrome has been reported which usually starts within several hours to 2 days following IVIG. Symptoms include severe headache, nuchal rigidity, drowsiness, fever, photophobia, painful eye movements, nausea, and vomiting. Aseptic meningitis syndrome may occur more frequently with high dose (2 g/kg) therapy.

Precautions Use with caution in patients with a history of cardiovascular disease or thrombotic episodes. Rapid IVIG infusion may be a possible risk factor for vascular occlusive events associated with IVIG. Do not exceed manufacturer's recommended initial infusion rate, use a lower IVIG concentration, and advance slowly in patients at risk. Use with caution in patients at increased risk for developing acute renal failure (patients with pre-existing renal insufficiency, diabetes mellitus, volume depletion, sepsis, paraproteinemia, and concomitant nephrotoxic drugs). Assure that patients are not volume depleted prior to the initiation of an IVIG infusion.

Adverse Reactions

Cardiovascular: Flushing of the face, hypotension, tachycardia, pallor, cardiac arrest, chest pain, pulmonary embolism, thromboembolism

Central nervous system: Dizziness, fever, headache, chills, anxiety, seizures, lightheadedness, malaise, irritability, aseptic meningitis syndrome

Dermatologic: Urticaria, pruritus

Gastrointestinal: Nausea, vomiting, abdominal pain

Hematologic: Transient neutropenia, hemolytic anemia, leukopenia

Neuromuscular & skeletal: Myalgia, arthralgia, tremor, back pain

Renal: Acute renal failure

Respiratory: Tightness in the chest, difficulty breathing, acute respiratory distress syndrome, bronchospasm, pulmonary edema

Miscellaneous: Hypersensitivity reactions, rigors, diaphoresis, aseptic meningitis

Drug Interactions Live virus vaccines (measles, mumps, rubella)

Stability Do not mix with other drugs or I.V. infusion fluids; see table for storage

Mechanism of Action Replacement therapy for primary and secondary immunodeficiencies; interference with F_c receptors on the cells of the reticuloendothelial system for autoimmune cytopenias and ITP

Pharmacokinetics Half-life: 21-29 days

Usual Dosage Children and Adults: I.V.:

Immunodeficiency syndrome: 300-400 mg/kg/dose once a month; maintain trough IgG concentration of 500 mg/dL

(Continued)

Immune Globulin (Intravenous) *(Continued)*

Chronic lymphocytic leukemia (CLL): 400 mg/kg/dose every 3 weeks

Idiopathic thrombocytopenic purpura: 400-1000 mg/kg/day for 2-5 consecutive days; maintenance dose: 400-1000 mg/kg/dose every 3-6 weeks based on clinical response and platelet count

Pediatric HIV infection: 400 mg/kg/dose every 4 weeks in those patients with hypogammaglobulinemia (IgG concentration <250 mg/dL), those with recurrent serious bacterial infections (2 or more infections in a 1-year period), those who fail to form antibodies to common antigens such as measles vaccine, and those living in areas where measles is prevalent and have not developed an antibody response after 2 doses of MMR

HIV-associated thrombocytopenia: 500-1000 mg/kg/day for 3-5 days

Kawasaki disease: 2 g/kg as a single dose, given over 10-12 hours; if signs and symptoms persist, retreatment with a second 2 g/kg infusion should be considered

Congenital and acquired immunodeficiency syndrome: 100-400 mg/kg/dose every 3-4 weeks

Adjuvant in severe cytomegalovirus infection: 500 mg/kg/dose every other day for 7 doses

Bone marrow transplant: 400-500 mg/kg/dose every week for 3 months and then once every month

Guillain-Barré syndrome: 400 mg/kg/day for 4 days **or** 1 g/kg/day for 2 days **or** 2 g/kg as a single dose

Refractory dermatomyositis: 2 g/kg/dose every month for 3-4 doses

Refractory polymyositis: 1 g/kg/day for 2 days every month for 4 doses

Intravenous Immune Globulin Product Comparison

	Gammagard® Liquid	Gammagard® S/D	Gammar-P® IV	Gamunex®
FDA indication	Primary immuno-deficiency	Primary immuno-deficiency, ITP, CLL prophylaxis, Kawasaki disease	Primary immuno-deficiency	Primary immuno-deficiency, ITP
Contraindication	Caution in severe, selective IgA deficiency	None (caution with IgA deficiency)	IgA deficiency	Caution in severe, selective IgA deficiency
IgA content	37 mcg/mL	<2.2 mcg/mL	<50 mcg/mL	46 mcg/mL
Sugar content	0	2% glucose	5% sucrose	0
Adverse reactions	Information not available	6%	16%	Information not available
Plasma source	FDA-registered donor sites	10,000 paid donors	>1000 paid donors	Pooled donors
Half-life	35 d	24 d	40 d	36 d
IgG subclass (%)				
IgG_1 (60-70)	60.9	67 (66.8)[1]	69	65
IgG_2 (19-31)	32.1	25 (25.4)	23	26
IgG_3 (5-8.4)	5	5 (7.4)	6	5.6
IgG_4 (0.7-4)	2.1	3 (0.3)	2	2.6
Monomers	≥95% (monomer + dimer)	>96.4%	>98% (monomer + dimer)	100% (monomer + dimer)
Gammaglobulin	≥98%	>90%	>98%	>98%
Storage	2°C to 25°C	Room temp	Room temp	2°C to 8°C; may be stored at room temp for 6 months within 18 months after manufacture
Recommended **initial** infusion rate	0.5 mL/kg/h	0.5 mL/kg/h	0.01-0.02 mL/kg/min	0.01 mL/kg/min
Maximum infusion rate	4-5 mL/kg/h; <2 mL/kg/h for patients at risk for renal dysfunction or thrombotic complications	4 mL/kg/h	0.06 mL/kg/min	0.08 mL/kg/min
Maximum concentration for infusion	10%	10%	10%[2,3]	10%

[1]Skvaril F and Gardi A, "Differences Among Available Immunoglobulin Preparations for Intravenous Use," *Pediatr Infect Dis J*, 1988, 7:543-48.

[2]The 10% concentration may increase risk to patients; manufacturer strongly discourages use.

[3]Siegel J, "Intravenous Immune Globulins: Therapeutic, Pharmaceutical, & Cost Considerations," *Pharmacy Practice News*, 2006, Jan:33-7.

Reference: ASHP Commission on Therapeutics, "ASHP Therapeutic Guidelines for Intravenous Immune Globulin," *Clin Pharm*, 1992, 11:117-36.

Chronic inflammatory demyelinating polyneuropathy: 400 mg/kg/day for 5 days once each month **or** 1 g/kg/day for 2 days once each month

Severe systemic viral and bacterial infections:

Neonates: 500 mg/kg/day for 2 days then once weekly

Children: 500-1000 mg/kg/week

Prevention of gastroenteritis: Infants and Children: Oral: 50 mg/kg/day divided every 6 hours

Administration Do not administer I.M. or SubQ

I.V. infusion: For initial treatment, use a lower concentration and/or administer at the slowest infusion rate (see recommended initial infusion rate in tables) for the first 30 minutes. Titrate infusion rate up gradually to the maximum infusion rate. If an adverse reaction occurs, reduce I.V. infusion rate to previously tolerated rate. See tables on previous page and below.

Monitoring Parameters Platelet count, blood pressure, vital signs, Quantitative Immunoglobulins (QUIGS), trough IgG concentration; periodic monitoring of renal function tests, including BUN, serum creatinine, and urine output in patients with an increased risk for developing acute renal failure

Test Interactions IVIG products containing maltose (eg, Octagam®) may cause falsely elevated glucose readings when glucose dehydrogenase pyrroloquinolinequinone (GDH-PQQ) based methods are used.

Patient Information Notify physician of any sudden weight gain, fluid retention/edema, decreased urine output, and/or shortness of breath

Nursing Implications Appropriate agents for treatment of a hypersensitivity reaction (eg, epinephrine, diphenhydramine) should be readily available; patients may need to be pretreated with an antipyretic, antihistamine, and/or corticosteroid to prevent chills and fever; adverse reactions may also be alleviated by decreasing the rate or the concentration of infusion or utilizing a different IGIV preparation

Additional Information Octagam® contains sodium 30 mmol/L.

Dosage Forms Excipient information presented when available (limited, particularly for generics); consult specific product labeling.

Injection, powder for reconstitution [preservative free]:

Gammar®-P I.V.: 5 g, 10 g [stabilized with human albumin and sucrose]

Iveegam EN: 5 g [stabilized with glucose]

Injection, powder for reconstitution [preservative free, nanofiltered]:

Carimune™ NF: 3 g, 6 g, 12 g [contains sucrose]

Panglobulin® NF: 6 g, 12 g [contains sucrose]

	Iveegam EN	Polygam® S/D	Immune Globulin Intravenous (Human) Carimune™ NF or Panglobulin® NF	Octagam® 5%
FDA indication	Primary immuno-deficiency, Kawasaki syndrome	Primary immuno-deficiency, ITP, CLL, Kawasaki disease	Primary immuno-deficiency, ITP	Primary immuno-deficiency
Contraindication	IgA deficiency	None (caution with IgA deficiency)	IgA deficiency	IgA deficiency
IgA content	<10 mcg/mL	2.2 mcg/mL	720 mcg/mL	≤100 mcg/mL
Sugar content	5% glucose	2% glucose	5% sucrose	10% maltose
Adverse reactions	4%	6%	2.9%-10%	0.04%-0.16%
Plasma source	10,000 paid donors	50,000 voluntary donors	>16,000 voluntary donors	Voluntary donors
Half-life	26-29 d	24 d	23 d	40 d
IgG subclass (%)				
IgG_1 (60-70)	68.9	67	60.5 (55.3)[1]	63.6
IgG_2 (19-31)	29.3	25	30.2 (35.7)	28.3
IgG_3 (5-8.4)	0	5	6.6 (6.3)	6.9
IgG_4 (0.7-4)	1.7	3	2.8 (2.6)	1.2
Monomers	≥90% (monomer + dimer)	>96.4%	92%	>99% (monomer + dimer)
Gammaglobulin	≥95%	>90%	≥96%	≥96%
Storage	Refrigerate	Room temp	Room temp	2°C to 25°C
Recommended **initial** infusion rate	0.01 mL/kg/min	0.5 mL/kg/h	0.01-0.03 mL/kg/min	30 mg/kg/h = 0.01 mL/kg/min
Maximum infusion rate	4.8 mL/kg/h	4 mL/kg/h	2.5 mL/min	200 mg/kg/h = 0.07 mL/kg/min
Maximum concentration for infusion	5%	10%	12%	5%

[1]Skvaril F and Gardi A, "Differences Among Available Immunoglobulin Preparations for Intravenous Use," *Pediatr Infect Dis J*, 1988, 7:543-48.

Reference: ASHP Commission on Therapeutics, "ASHP Therapeutic Guidelines for Intravenous Immune Globulin," *Clin Pharm*, 1992, 11:117-36.

(Continued)

Immune Globulin (Intravenous) *(Continued)*

Injection, powder for reconstitution [preservative free, solvent detergent-treated]:
- Gammagard® S/D: 2.5 g, 5 g, 10 g [stabilized with human albumin, glycine, glucose, and polyethylene glycol]
- Polygam® S/D: 5 g, 10 g [stabilized with human albumin, glycine, glucose, and polyethylene glycol]

Injection, solution [preservative free; solvent detergent-treated]:
- Gammagard® Liquid: 10% (10 mL, 25 mL, 50 mL, 100 mL, 200 mL) [latex free, sucrose free; stabilized with glycine]
- Octagam®: 5% (20 mL, 50 mL, 100 mL, 200 mL) [sucrose free; contains sodium 30 mmol/L and maltose]

Injection, solution [preservative free]
- Flebogamma®: 5% (10 mL, 50 mL, 100 mL, 200 mL) [contains polyethylene glycol and sorbitol]
- Gamunex®: 10% (10 mL, 25 mL, 50 mL, 100 mL, 200 mL) [caprylate/chromatography purified]

References

ASHP Commission on Therapeutics, "ASHP Therapeutic Guidelines for Intravenous Immune Globulin," *Am J Hosp Pharm*, 1992, 49(3):652-4.

Blanchette VS, Luke B, Andrew M, et al, "A Prospective Randomized Trial of High-Dose Intravenous Immune Globulin G Therapy, Oral Prednisone Therapy, and No Therapy in Childhood Acute Immune Thrombocytopenic Purpura," *J Pediatr*, 1993, 123(6):989-95.

Kaplan JE, Masur H, and Holmes KK, "Guidelines for Preventing Opportunistic Infections Among HIV-Infected Persons - 2002 Recommendations of the USPHS and IDSA," *MMWR*, 2002, 51(RR-8):1-46.

NIH Consensus Conference, "Intravenous Immunoglobulin, Prevention and Treatment of Disease," *JAMA*, 1990, 264(24):3189-93.

Siegel J, "Intravenous Immune Globulins: Therapeutic, Pharmaceutical, & Cost Considerations," *Pharmacy Practice News*, 2006, Jan:33-7.

"University Hospital Consortium Expert Panel for Off-Label Use of Polyvalent Intravenously Administered Immunoglobulin Preparations Consensus Statement," *JAMA*, 1995, 273(23):1865-70.

- ♦ **Immune Serum Globulin** *see* Immune Globulin (Intramuscular) *on page 817*
- ♦ **Immunine® VH (Can)** *see* Factor IX *on page 633*
- ♦ **Imodium® (Can)** *see* Loperamide *on page 952*
- ♦ **Imodium® A-D [OTC]** *see* Loperamide *on page 952*
- ♦ **Imogam® Rabies-HT** *see* Rabies Immune Globulin (Human) *on page 1363*
- ♦ **Imogam® Rabies Pasteurized (Can)** *see* Rabies Immune Globulin (Human) *on page 1363*
- ♦ **Imovax® Rabies** *see* Rabies Virus Vaccine *on page 1364*
- ♦ **Imuran®** *see* Azathioprine *on page 187*

Inamrinone (eye NAM ri none)

Medication Safety Issues

Sound-alike/look-alike issues:

Amrinone may be confused with amiloride, amiodarone

Index Terms Amrinone Lactate

Therapeutic Category Phosphodiesterase Enzyme Inhibitor

Generic Available Yes

Use Short-term treatment of low cardiac output states (sepsis, CHF); reserved for patients who have not responded adequately to therapy with digitalis, diuretics, and vasodilators; adjunctive therapy of pulmonary hypertension

Pregnancy Risk Factor C

Contraindications Hypersensitivity to inamrinone lactate or any component (see Warnings); valvular obstructive disease

Warnings Injection contains sodium metabisulfite which may cause allergic reactions in susceptible individuals

Precautions Monitor for hypotension, thrombocytopenia, hepatotoxicity, and GI effects; discontinue inamrinone if significant increase in liver enzymes with symptoms of idiosyncratic hypersensitivity reaction (ie, eosinophilia) occurs; monitor fluids and electrolytes. Diuresis may result from improvement in cardiac output and may require dosage reduction of diuretics. Inamrinone may exacerbate myocardial ischemia or worsen ventricular ectopy.

Adverse Reactions

Cardiovascular: Hypotension (1.3% incidence), ventricular and supraventricular arrhythmias (3%); may be related to infusion rate

Gastrointestinal: Nausea (1.7%), vomiting (0.9%), abdominal pain (0.4%), anorexia (0.4%); GI effects may be due to an increase in gastric acid secretion and intestinal motility, secondary to phosphodiesterase inhibition

Hematologic: Thrombocytopenia (2.4%), may be dose-related; in one study, 8 of 16 children (1.5 months to 11.2 years of age) developed thrombocytopenia (mean count 66 x 10^9 platelets/L). Inamrinone bolus doses ranged from 1.2-3 mg/kg given in 4 divided doses over 1 hour and were followed by continuous infusions of 5-10 mcg/kg/minute. Thrombocytopenia developed 19-71 hours after starting inamrinone (mean ± SD = 51 ± 25 hours). Resolution of thrombocytopenia occurred 54 ± 15 hours after therapy was discontinued; thrombocytopenia developed in patients with a higher total dose, longer duration of infusion, higher plasma concentrations of N-acetylamrinone (major metabolite of inamrinone), and higher plasma ratios of N-acetylamrinone to inamrinone.

Hepatic: Hepatotoxicity (0.2%)

Drug Interactions Disopyramide may increase hypotension (one case report; use with caution); diuretics may cause significant hypovolemia (dosage reduction of diuretic may be required)

Stability Dilute only with NS or ½NS; do not directly dilute with dextrose-containing solutions, chemical interaction occurs; may be administered I.V. (via Y-site) into running dextrose infusions. Furosemide forms a precipitate when injected in I.V. lines containing inamrinone; incompatible with sodium bicarbonate; use diluted solutions of inamrinone (1-3 mg/mL) within 24 hours.

Mechanism of Action Inhibits phosphodiesterase III (PDE III), the major PDE in cardiac and vascular tissues. Inhibition of PDE III increases cyclic adenosine monophosphate (cAMP) which potentiates the delivery of calcium to myocardial contractile systems and results in a positive inotropic effect. Inhibition of PDE III in vascular tissue results in relaxation of vascular muscle and vasodilatation.

Pharmacodynamics

Onset of action: I.V.: Within 2-5 minutes

Maximum effect: Within 10 minutes

Duration: Dose dependent with low doses lasting ~30 minutes and higher doses lasting ~2 hours

Pharmacokinetics

Distribution: V_d:

Neonates: 1.8 L/kg

Infants: 1.6 L/kg

Adults: 1.2 L/kg

Protein binding: 10% to 49%

Metabolism: In the liver to several metabolites (N-acetate, N-glycolyl, N-glucuronide, and O-glucuronide)

Half-life:

Neonates, 1-2 weeks of age: 22.2 hours

Infants 6-38 weeks of age: 6.8 hours; negative correlation of age with half-life in infants 4-38 weeks of age

Infants and Children (1 month to 15 years of age): 2.2-10.5 hours

Adults, normal volunteers: 3.6 hours

Adults with CHF: 5.8 hours

Elimination: Excreted in urine as metabolites and unchanged drug; 10% to 40% as unchanged drug in the urine within 24 hours

Usual Dosage I.V.: **Note:** Dose should not exceed 10 mg/kg/24 hours; doses of 18 mg/kg/day have been used in adults for a short duration; titrate infusion based on patient clinical response and adverse effects

Neonates: 0.75 mg/kg I.V. bolus over 2-3 minutes followed by maintenance infusion 3-5 mcg/kg/minute; I.V. bolus may need to be repeated in 30 minutes; see Additional Information

Infants and Children: 0.75 mg/kg I.V. bolus over 2-3 minutes followed by maintenance infusion 5-10 mcg/kg/minute; I.V. bolus may need to be repeated in 30 minutes; see Additional Information

Adults: 0.75 mg/kg I.V. bolus over 2-3 minutes followed by maintenance infusion of 5-10 mcg/kg/minute; I.V. bolus may need to be repeated in 30 minutes

PALS Guidelines 2000: I.V., I.O.: Loading dose: 0.75-1 mg/kg over 5 minutes; if tolerated, loading dose may be repeated up to 2 times; maximum total loading dose: 3 mg/kg; follow with maintenance infusion of 5-10 mcg/kg/minute; **Note:** If hypotension occurs during loading dose, administer 5-10 mL/kg of NS or other appropriate fluid and position patient flat or with head down (if patient can tolerate); if hypotension continues after fluid loading, administer a vasopressor agent and do not administer further inamrinone loading doses

ACLS Guidelines 2000: Adults: 0.75 mg/kg I.V. bolus over 2-3 minutes followed by maintenance infusion of 5-15 mcg/kg/minute; I.V. bolus may need to be repeated in 30 minutes

Administration Parenteral:

I.V. bolus: Infuse over 2-3 minutes; may be administered undiluted

(Continued)

Inamrinone *(Continued)*

Continuous infusion: Dilute with NS or ½NS to final concentration of 1-3 mg/mL; use controlled infusion device (eg, I.V. pump)

Monitoring Parameters Blood pressure, heart rate, platelet count, liver enzymes, fluid status, intake and output, body weight, serum electrolytes; if Swan-Ganz catheter is present, monitor cardiac index, stroke volume, systemic vascular resistance, pulmonary vascular resistance

Reference Range Proposed: Adults: 3 mcg/mL; linear correlation with cardiac index observed from 0.5-7 mcg/mL

Nursing Implications Do **not** administer furosemide I.V. push via "Y" site into inamrinone solutions as precipitate will occur; monitor patients closely (see Monitoring Parameters)

Additional Information Preliminary pharmacokinetic studies estimate that total initial bolus doses of 3-4.5 mg/kg given in divided doses to neonates and infants are required to obtain serum concentrations similar to therapeutic adult levels. The use of these higher doses has been reported in a small number of infants and children. Some centers use a total loading dose of 3 mg/kg (administered as 4 doses of 0.75 mg/kg/dose given every 15 minutes); each of the 0.75 mg/kg doses is given over 5 minutes. Further pharmacodynamic studies are needed to define pediatric inamrinone dosing guidelines.

Use of inamrinone in controlled trials did not extend beyond 48 hours; due to potential serious adverse effects and limited experience, inamrinone should only be used in patients who have not responded to other therapies (ie, digoxin, diuretics, vasodilators). Inamrinone has not been shown to be safe or effective for long-term treatment of CHF.

Effective July 1, 2000, the nonproprietary name of the drug (amrinone) was officially changed by the U.S. Pharmacopeia (USP) Nomenclature Committee and the U.S. Adopted Names (USAN) Council to inamrinone to prevent confusion with amiodarone; other countries will still use the name amrinone

Dosage Forms Excipient information presented when available (limited, particularly for generics); consult specific product labeling.

Injection, solution, as lactate: 5 mg/mL (20 mL) [contains sodium metabisulfite]

References

Allen-Webb EM, Ross MP, Pappas JB, et al, "Age-Related Amrinone Pharmacokinetics in a Pediatric Population," *Crit Care Med*, 1994, 22(6):1016-24.

"Guidelines 2000 for Cardiopulmonary Resuscitation and Emergency Cardiovascular Care, Part 6: Advanced Cardiovascular Life Support, The American Heart Association in Collaboration With the International Liaison Committee on Resuscitation," *Circulation*, 2000, 102(8 Suppl):I86-171.

"Guidelines 2000 for Cardiopulmonary Resuscitation and Emergency Cardiovascular Care, Part 10: Pediatric Advanced Life Support, The American Heart Association in Collaboration With the International Liaison Committee on Resuscitation," *Circulation*, 2000, 102(8 Suppl): I291-342.

Lawless S, Burckart G, Diven W, et al, "Amrinone in Neonates and Infants After Cardiac Surgery," *Crit Care Med*, 1989, 17(8):751-4.

Lawless ST, Zaritsky A, and Miles MV, "The Acute Pharmacokinetics and Pharmacodynamics of Amrinone in Pediatric Patients," *J Clin Pharmacol*, 1991, 31(9):800-3.

Lynn AM, Sorensen GK, and Williams GD, "Hemodynamic Effects of Amrinone and Colloid Administration in Children Following Cardiac Surgery," *J Cardiothorac Vasc Anesth*, 1993, 7(5):560-5.

Ross MP, Allen-Webb EM, Pappas JB, et al, "Amrinone-Associated Thrombocytopenia: Pharmacokinetic Analysis," *Clin Pharmacol Ther*, 1993, 53(6):661-7.

♦ **Inapsine®** *see* Droperidol *on page 547*

♦ **Inderal®** *see* Propranolol *on page 1337*

♦ **Inderal® LA** *see* Propranolol *on page 1337*

♦ **Inderal®-LA (Can)** *see* Propranolol *on page 1337*

Indinavir (in DIN a veer)

Medication Safety Issues

Sound-alike/look-alike issues:

Indinavir may be confused with Denavir™

Related Information

Adult and Adolescent HIV *on page 1821*

Pediatric HIV *on page 1816*

Perinatal HIV *on page 1831*

U.S. Brand Names Crixivan®

Canadian Brand Names Crixivan®

Index Terms Indinavir Sulfate; L-735,524; MK-639

Therapeutic Category Antiretroviral Agent; HIV Agents (Anti-HIV Agents); Protease Inhibitor

Generic Available No

Use Treatment of HIV infection in combination with other antiretroviral agents; (**Note:** HIV regimens consisting of **three** antiretroviral agents are strongly recommended); postexposure chemoprophylaxis following occupational exposure to HIV

Pregnancy Risk Factor C

Lactation Enters breast milk/contraindicated

Contraindications Hypersensitivity to indinavir or any component; concurrent therapy with amiodarone, cisapride, dihydroergotamine, ergonovine, ergotamine, methylergonovine, midazolam, pimozide, triazolam

Warnings Indinavir is a CYP3A4 isoenzyme inhibitor that interacts with numerous drugs. Due to potential serious and/or life-threatening drug interactions, some drugs are contraindicated (see Contraindications and Drug Interactions). Concurrent use with atazanavir, rifampin, St John's wort, or certain cholesterol-lowering agents (lovastatin, simvastatin) is **not** recommended. Alteration of dose or serum concentration monitoring may be required with other medications (see Drug Interactions).

Cases of nephrolithiasis and nephrolithiasis associated with renal insufficiency, acute renal failure, or pyelonephritis with or without bacteremia have been reported. Maintain adequate hydration in all patients to minimize risk. If signs and symptoms of nephrolithiasis occur (flank pain with or without hematuria or microscopic hematuria), temporarily interrupt or discontinue therapy. Tubulointerstitial nephritis with medullary calcification and cortical atrophy has been reported in patients with asymptomatic severe leukocyturia; consider discontinuation of indinavir in patients with severe leukocyturia. Immune reconstitution syndrome (an acute inflammatory response to residual or indolent opportunistic infections) may occur in HIV patients during initial treatment with combination antiretroviral agents, including indinavir; this syndrome may require further patient assessment and therapy. Hepatitis, including hepatic failure and death, has been reported (causal relationship not established). Spontaneous bleeding episodes have been reported in patients with hemophilia A and B. New onset diabetes mellitus, exacerbation of diabetes and hyperglycemia have been reported in HIV-infected patients receiving protease inhibitors. Acute hemolytic anemia has been reported. Indirect hyperbilirubinemia and elevated serum transaminases may occur.

Precautions Use with caution in patients with hepatic impairment; modify dose in patients with impaired liver function. Use of indinavir in HIV-infected pregnant patients is **not** recommended; significantly lower serum concentrations were observed in these patients receiving standard adult doses; optimal dose is not currently known. Fat redistribution and accumulation [ie, central obesity, peripheral wasting, facial wasting, breast enlargement, dorsocervical fat enlargement (buffalo hump), and cushingoid appearance] have been observed in patients receiving antiretroviral agents (causal relationship not established).

Adverse Reactions

Central nervous system: Insomnia, dizziness, headache, somnolence, asthenia, depression

Dermatologic: Rash, dry skin, urticaria, pruritus, paronychia

Endocrine & metabolic: Rare: Hyperglycemia, diabetes, ketoacidosis; elevated serum cholesterol and triglycerides; fat redistribution and accumulation (see Precautions)

Gastrointestinal: Nausea (10%), vomiting, diarrhea, abdominal pain, dyspepsia, metallic taste, pancreatitis

Genitourinary: Dysuria, pyelonephritis

Hematologic: Hemolytic anemia, spontaneous bleeding episodes in hemophiliacs (rare)

Hepatic: Hyperbilirubinemia (14%), elevated liver function tests, jaundice, liver cirrhosis

Neuromuscular & skeletal: Arthralgia

Renal: Nephrolithiasis, urolithiasis (pediatric patients: 29%; adult patients: 12.4%); hematuria, proteinuria, renal failure, interstitial nephritis

Respiratory: Dry throat, pharyngitis

Miscellaneous: Immune reconstitution syndrome (see Warnings)

Drug Interactions Cytochrome P450 isoenzyme CYP3A3/4 substrate and inhibitor; may also be a weak inhibitor of isoenzyme CYP2D6

Indinavir may inhibit the metabolism of the following drugs and cause serious or life-threatening adverse effects: Amiodarone, cisapride, dihydroergotamine, ergonovine, ergotamine, methylergonovine, midazolam, and triazolam (concurrent therapy with these drugs and indinavir is contraindicated). Indinavir may increase the toxic effects of bepridil, lidocaine, quinidine, cyclosporine, tacrolimus, sirolimus (serum concentration monitoring of these drugs is necessary). Indinavir may increase serum concentrations or toxicity of felodipine, nifedipine, and nicardipine (use with caution; monitor closely); trazodone (use with caution; consider trazodone dosage reduction); cholesterol-lowering agents (increased risk of myopathy and rhabdomyolysis; concurrent use of lovastatin or simvastatin is not recommended; use lowest possible dose of atorvastatin and carefully monitor patient; consider use of pravastatin, fluvastatin, or

(Continued)

Indinavir *(Continued)*

rosuvastatin for concurrent use with indinavir); sildenafil or other phosphodiesterase-5 (PDE-5) enzyme inhibitors (use decreased dose of sildenafil or other PDE-5 enzyme inhibitor) and saquinavir. Ritonavir significantly increases fluticasone serum concentrations and may result in systemic corticosteroid effects (eg, Cushing's syndrome and adrenal suppression); indinavir plus ritonavir use with fluticasone is expected to have the same effect; concurrent use of indinavir plus ritonavir (or other potent CYP3A4 inhibitor) with fluticasone is **not** recommended unless benefits outweigh risks; use of indinavir without ritonavir may increase fluticasone serum concentrations (use with caution; consider alternative agent, especially with long-term use). Indinavir significantly increases serum concentrations of rifabutin and rifabutin significantly decreases indinavir concentrations (rifabutin dose should be decreased by $^1/_2$ the recommended and indinavir dose should be increased when these drugs are used in combination).

Rifampin significantly reduces indinavir plasma concentrations and should **not** be used concurrently. Efavirenz and nevirapine significantly decrease indinavir concentrations (optimal indinavir dose is unknown). Enzyme-inducing drugs, such as carbamazepine, phenobarbital, phenytoin, may decrease indinavir concentrations (use with caution). Venlafaxine may decrease indinavir serum concentrations (use with caution; clinical significance is unknown). The herbal medicine St John's wort (*Hypericum perforatum*) may significantly decrease concentrations of indinavir and lead to treatment failure; concurrent use is **not** recommended.

Delavirdine, itraconazole, and ketoconazole may increase indinavir serum concentrations (indinavir dosage reduction is recommended); nelfinavir and ritonavir may increase indinavir serum concentrations (optimal indinavir dose is unknown); indinavir may increase ritonavir serum concentrations. Clarithromycin may increase indinavir serum concentrations and indinavir may increase clarithromycin concentrations.

Coadministration with didanosine (buffered formulations) will decrease indinavir absorption (separate administration by 1 hour). Indinavir and atazanavir are both associated with indirect hyperbilirubinemia (concurrent use is **not** recommended).

Food Interactions Decreased absorption when administered with food high in calories, protein, or fat; 27% decrease in AUC when administered with grapefruit juice

Stability Store capsules at room temperature in original container with desiccant (capsules are sensitive to moisture)

Mechanism of Action A protease inhibitor which acts on an enzyme late in the HIV replication process after the virus has entered into the cell's nucleus preventing cleavage of the gag-pol protein precursors resulting in the production of immature, noninfectious virions; cross-resistance with other protease inhibitors is possible

Pharmacokinetics

Absorption: Rapid (in the fasted state); presence of food high in calories, fat, and protein significantly decreases the extent of absorption

Protein binding: 60%

Metabolism: In the liver by CYP3A4 to inactive metabolites; 6 oxidative and 1 glucuronide conjugate metabolites have been identified

Bioavailability: Wide interpatient variability in children: 15% to 50%

Half-life:

- Children 4-17 years (n=18): 1.1 hours
- Adults: 1.8 ± 0.4 hours
- Adults with mild to moderate hepatic dysfunction: 2.8 ± 0.5 hours

Time to peak serum concentration: 0.8 ± 0.3 hours

Elimination: 83% in feces as unabsorbed drug and metabolites; ~10% excreted in urine as unchanged drug

Usual Dosage Oral (use in combination with other antiretroviral agents):

Neonates: Should not be administered to neonates until further studies are performed due to side effect of hyperbilirubinemia

Children: Optimal dose not established; clinical trials used doses of 500 mg/m²/dose every 8 hours; maximum dose: 800 mg/dose every 8 hours; this dose produced AUCs and peak concentrations slightly higher than those seen in adults receiving the standard dose; however, in 50% of children studied, trough indinavir levels were lower than those observed in adults.

Note: One study in children 4-17 years of age (n=18), adjusted the indinavir dose and dosing interval to maintain trough plasma concentrations. A mean daily dose of 2043 mg/m² was required with 9 of 18 children requiring doses every 6 hours (see Fletcher, 2000). Other pediatric studies have also suggested that every 6 hour dosing may be needed in some children (see Gatti, 2000) and that a wide range of doses (1250-2450 mg/m²/day) may be required (see van Rossum, 2000). Further studies are needed.

Adolescents and Adults: 800 mg/dose every 8 hours

Adults:

Protease "boosting" by ritonavir:

Indinavir 400 mg twice daily with ritonavir 400 mg twice daily

or

Indinavir 800 mg twice daily with ritonavir 200 mg twice daily

Concomitant therapy with delavirdine, itraconazole, or ketoconazole: Reduce dose of indinavir to 600 mg every 8 hours when used in combination with delavirdine 400 mg 3 times/day, itraconazole 200 mg twice daily or ketoconazole.

Concomitant therapy with efavirenz or nevirapine: Increase dose of indinavir to 1000 mg every 8 hours

Concomitant therapy with lopinavir and ritonavir (Kaletra®): Reduce dose of indinavir to 600 mg twice daily

Concomitant therapy with nelfinavir: Increase dose of indinavir to 1200 mg twice daily

Concomitant therapy with rifabutin: Increase dose of indinavir to 1000 mg every 8 hours and reduce dose of rifabutin to 1/2 the standard dose

Dosage adjustment in mild to moderate hepatic impairment: Adults: Decrease dose from 800 mg every 8 hours to 600 mg every 8 hours

Administration Administer with water on an empty stomach or with a light snack 1 hour before or 2 hours after a meal; may administer with other liquids (ie, skim milk, coffee, tea, juice) or a light snack (ie, dry toast with jelly or cornflakes with skim milk); do not administer with grapefruit juice; if coadministered with didanosine, give at least 1 hour apart on an empty stomach. Administer every 8 hours around-the-clock to avoid significant fluctuation in serum levels.

Monitoring Parameters Serum bilirubin, cholesterol, triglycerides, amylase, lipase, liver function tests, urinalysis, blood glucose levels, CD4 cell count, plasma levels of HIV RNA, CBC

Patient Information Indinavir is not a cure for HIV. Some medicines should not be taken with indinavir; report the use of other medications, nonprescription medications, and herbal or natural products to your healthcare provider. Avoid the herbal medicine St John's wort and grapefruit juice. Take indinavir every day as prescribed; do not change dose or discontinue without physician's advice; if a dose is missed, take it as soon as possible, then return to normal dosing schedule; if a dose is skipped, do not double the next dose.

HIV medications may cause changes in body fat, including an increase in fat in the upper back and neck, breasts, and trunk; a loss of fat from the face, arms, and legs may also occur.

Nursing Implications Ensure adequate patient hydration to minimize the risk of nephrolithiasis; adults should drink at least 48 ounces of liquids per day.

Dosage Forms Excipient information presented when available (limited, particularly for generics); consult specific product labeling. Available as indinavir sulfate; mg strength refers to indinavir.

Capsule:

Crixivan®: 100 mg, 200 mg, 333 mg, 400 mg

Extemporaneous Preparations An indinavir 10 mg/mL oral solution is stable for 2 weeks stored at 4°C. The solution is made by first preparing an indinavir 100 mg/mL concentrate: Add contents of fifteen 400 mg capsules and 54 mL of purified distilled water into a 100 mL amber glass bottle. Place bottle in an ultrasonic water bath filled with water at 37°C for 60 minutes, stirring the solution every 10 minutes. Filter solution; wash bottle and filter with 6 mL purified distilled water; cool to room temperature. 50 mL of 100 mg/mL indinavir concentrate is added to 360 mL of viscous sweet base, 90 mL of simple syrup, 1.8 g citric acid, 45 mg azorubine, 0.1M sodium hydroxide solution to pH 3, and 12 drops of lemon oil to make a final volume of 500 mL. Mix solution until it is homogeneous.

Hugen PW, Burger DM, ter Hofstede HJ, et al, "Development of an Indinavir Oral Liquid for Children," *Am J Health Syst Pharm*, 2000, 57(14):1332-9.

References

Briars LA, Hilao JJ, and Kraus DM, "A Review of Pediatric Human Immunodeficiency Virus Infection," *Journal of Pharmacy Practice*, 2004, 17(6):407-31.

Fletcher CV, Brundage RC, Remmel RP, et al, "Pharmacologic Characteristics of Indinavir, Didanosine, and Stavudine in Human Immunodeficiency Virus-Infected Children Receiving Combination Therapy," *Antimicrob Agents Chemother*, 2000, 44(4):1029-34.

Gatti G, Vigano' A, Sala N, et al, "Indinavir Pharmacokinetics and Pharmacodynamics in Children With Human Immunodeficiency Virus Infection," *Antimicrob Agents Chemother*, 2000, 44(3):752-5.

Mueller BU, Smith S, Sleasman J, et al, "A Phase I/II Study of the Protease Inhibitor Indinavir (MK-0639) in Children With HIV Infection," *Eleventh International Conference on AIDS*, Vancouver, Canada, 1996.

Panel on Clinical Practices for Treatment of HIV Infection, "Guidelines for the Use of Antiretroviral Agents in HIV-Infected Adults and Adolescents," October 10, 2006, http://www.aidsinfo.nih.gov.

Piscitelli SC, Burstein AH, Chaitt D, et al, "Indinavir Concentrations and St John's Wort," *Lancet*, 2000, 355(9203):547-8.

Stein DS, Fish DG, Bilello JA, et al, "A 24-Week Open-Label Phase I/II Evaluation of the HIV Protease Inhibitor MK-639 (Indinavir)," *AIDS*, 1996, 10(5):485-92.

(Continued)

Indinavir *(Continued)*

U.S. Public Health Service, "Updated U.S. Public Health Service Guidelines for the Management of Occupational Exposures to HIV and Recommendations for Postexposure Prophylaxis," *MMWR Recomm Rep*, 2005, 54(RR-9):1-17.

van Rossum AM, Niesters HG, Geelen SP, et al, "Clinical and Virologic Response to Combination Treatment With Indinavir, Zidovudine, and Lamivudine in Children With Human Immunodeficiency Virus-1 Infection: A Multicenter Study in the Netherlands. On Behalf of the Dutch Study Group for Children with HIV-1 Infections," *J Pediatr*, 2000, 136(6):780-8.

Working Group on Antiretroviral Therapy and Medical Management of HIV-Infected Children, "Guidelines for the Use of Antiretroviral Agents in Pediatric HIV Infection," October 26, 2006, http://www.aidsinfo.nih.gov.

- **Indinavir Sulfate** *see* Indinavir *on page 824*
- **Indocid® P.D.A. (Can)** *see* Indomethacin *on page 828*
- **Indocin®** *see* Indomethacin *on page 828*
- **Indocin® I.V.** *see* Indomethacin *on page 828*
- **Indo-Lemmon (Can)** *see* Indomethacin *on page 828*
- **Indometacin** *see* Indomethacin *on page 828*

Indomethacin (in doe METH a sin)

Medication Safety Issues

Sound-alike/look-alike issues:

Indocin® may be confused with Imodium®, Lincocin®, Minocin®, Vicodin®

International issues:

Flexin® [Great Britain] may be confused with Floxin® which is a brand name for ofloxacin in the U.S.

Flexin® [Great Britain]: Brand name for orphenadrine in Israel

Related Information

Overdose and Toxicology *on page 1916*

U.S. Brand Names Indocin®; Indocin® I.V.

Canadian Brand Names Apo-Indomethacin®; Indocid® P.D.A.; Indocin®; Indo-Lemmon; Indotec; Novo-Methacin; Nu-Indo; Rhodacine®

Index Terms Indometacin; Indomethacin Sodium Trihydrate

Therapeutic Category Analgesic, Non-narcotic; Anti-inflammatory Agent; Antipyretic; Nonsteroidal Anti-inflammatory Drug (NSAID), Oral; Nonsteroidal Anti-inflammatory Drug (NSAID), Parenteral

Generic Available Yes: Capsule

Use Management of inflammatory diseases and rheumatoid disorders; moderate pain; acute gouty arthritis; I.V. form used as alternative to surgery for closure of patent ductus arteriosus (PDA) in neonates

Medication Guide An FDA-approved patient medication guide, which is available with the product information and at http://www.fda.gov/cder/Offices/ODS/medication_guides.htm, must be dispensed with this medication for each new outpatient prescription and refill.

Pregnancy Risk Factor C (D if used longer than 48 hours or after 34 weeks gestation)

Lactation Enters breast milk/use caution (AAP rates "compatible")

Contraindications Hypersensitivity to indomethacin, any component, aspirin, or other NSAIDs; active GI bleeding, ulcer disease; patients with the "aspirin triad" [asthma, rhinitis (with or without nasal polyps), and aspirin intolerance] (fatal asthmatic and anaphylactoid reactions may occur in these patients); premature neonates with necrotizing enterocolitis, impaired renal function (eg, neonates with urine output <0.6 mL/kg/hour or serum creatinine ≥1.8 mg/dL), IVH, active bleeding, thrombocytopenia

Warnings In April 2005, the FDA announced product labeling changes for all NSAIDs, including COX-2 selective and OTC medications; although revised product labeling is currently not available for all products, sample labeling and a template of the required medication guide are now available. Labels for prescription nonselective NSAIDs will contain a contraindication for use in patients who have recently undergone coronary artery bypass graft (CABG) surgery and a boxed warning concerning the potential for increased risk of cardiovascular (CV) events and GI bleeding associated with NSAID use. Patients at increased risk of adverse events include patients immediately postoperative from CABG surgery, and those with existing CAD, CVD, or history of TIA or stomach ulcers. Prescribers are encouraged to use the lowest effective NSAID dose for the shortest time based on individual patient treatment goals. Medication guides will be required for all prescription products. Complete details for the labeling update can be found on the following FDA website: http://www.fda.gov/medwatch/SAFETY/2005/safety05.htm#NSAID.

Precautions Use with caution in patients with cardiac dysfunction, hypertension, renal or hepatic impairment, epilepsy, patients receiving anticoagulants and for treatment of JRA in children (fatal hepatitis has been reported; monitor children closely; assess liver function periodically)

Adverse Reactions

Cardiovascular: Hypertension, edema

Central nervous system: Somnolence, fatigue, depression, confusion, dizziness, headache

Dermatologic: Rash

Endocrine & metabolic: Hyperkalemia, dilutional hyponatremia (I.V.), hypoglycemia (I.V.)

Gastrointestinal: Nausea, vomiting, epigastric pain, abdominal pain, anorexia; GI bleeding, ulcers, perforation; necrotizing enterocolitis

Hematologic: Hemolytic anemia, bone marrow suppression, agranulocytosis, thrombocytopenia, inhibition of platelet aggregation

Hepatic: Hepatitis

Ocular: Corneal opacities

Otic: Tinnitus

Renal: Renal failure, oliguria

Miscellaneous: Hypersensitivity reactions

Drug Interactions Cytochrome P450 isoenzyme CYP2C9 substrate

Indomethacin may increase serum concentrations of digoxin, methotrexate, lithium, and aminoglycosides (reported with I.V. use in neonates); may increase nephrotoxicity of cyclosporine; may decrease antihypertensive and diuretic effects of furosemide and thiazides; may increase serum potassium with potassium-sparing diuretics; may decrease antihypertensive effects of beta-blockers, hydralazine, ACE inhibitors and angiotensin II antagonists; aspirin may decrease and probenecid may increase indomethacin serum concentrations; other GI irritants (eg, potassium supplements, NSAIDs) may increase GI adverse effects

Food Interactions Food may decrease the rate but not the extent of absorption

Stability

Oral suspension: Store below 86°F; do not freeze

I.V. product: Protect from light; not stable in alkaline solution; reconstitute just prior to administration; discard any unused portion; do not use preservative-containing diluents for reconstitution; will precipitate if reconstituted with solutions at pH <6 (product is not buffered)

Mechanism of Action Inhibits prostaglandin synthesis by decreasing the activity of the enzyme, cyclooxygenase, which results in decreased formation of prostaglandin precursors

Pharmacokinetics

Absorption: Oral:
- Neonates: Incomplete, nonuniform
- Adults: Rapid and well absorbed

Distribution:
- Neonates: PDA: 0.36 L/kg
- Post-PDA closure: 0.26 L/kg
- Adults: 0.34-1.57 L/kg

Protein binding: 99%

Metabolism: In the liver via glucuronide conjugation and other pathways

Bioavailability: Oral:
- Neonates, premature: 13% to 20%
- Adults: ~100%

Half-life:
- Neonates:
  - Postnatal age (PNA) <2 weeks: ~20 hours
  - PNA >2 weeks: ~11 hours
- Adults: 2.6-11.2 hours

Elimination: Significant enterohepatic recycling; 33% excreted in feces as demethylated metabolites with 1.5% as unchanged drug; 60% eliminated in urine as drug and metabolites

Usual Dosage

Patent ductus arteriosus:

Neonates: I.V.: Initial: 0.2 mg/kg, followed by 2 doses depending on postnatal age (PNA):
- PNA **at time of first dose** <48 hours: 0.1 mg/kg at 12- to 24-hour intervals
- PNA **at time of first dose** 2-7 days: 0.2 mg/kg at 12- to 24-hour intervals
- PNA **at time of first dose** >7 days: 0.25 mg/kg at 12- to 24-hour intervals

In general, may use 12-hour dosing interval if urine output >1 mL/kg/hour after prior dose; use 24-hour dosing interval if urine output is <1 mL/kg/hour but >0.6 mL/kg/hour; doses should be withheld if patient has oliguria (urine output <0.6 mL/kg/hour) or anuria

(Continued)

Indomethacin *(Continued)*

Inflammatory/rheumatoid disorders: **Note:** Use lowest effective dose: Oral:
Children ≥2 years: 1-2 mg/kg/day in 2-4 divided doses; maximum dose: 4 mg/kg/day; do not exceed 150-200 mg/day
Adults: 25-50 mg/dose 2-3 times/day; maximum dose: 200 mg/day; extended release capsule should be given on a 1-2 times/day schedule

Administration
Oral: Administer with food, milk, or antacids to decrease GI adverse effects; extended release capsules must be swallowed whole, do not crush or chew
Parenteral: I.V.: Administer over 20-30 minutes at a concentration of 0.5-1 mg/mL in preservative free SWI or preservative free NS
Note: Do **not** administer via I.V. bolus or I.V. infusion via an umbilical catheter into vessels near the superior mesenteric artery, as these may cause vasoconstriction and can compromise blood flow to the intestines. Do not administer intra-arterially.

Monitoring Parameters BUN, serum creatinine, potassium, liver enzymes, CBC with differential; in addition, in neonates treated for PDA: heart rate, heart murmur, blood pressure, urine output, echocardiogram, serum sodium and glucose, platelet count, and serum concentrations of concomitantly administered drugs which are renally eliminated (eg, aminoglycosides, digoxin); periodic ophthalmic exams with chronic use

Patient Information Avoid alcohol; may cause dizziness

Additional Information Indomethacin may mask signs and symptoms of infections; fatalities in children have been reported, due to unrecognized overwhelming sepsis; drowsiness, lethargy, nausea, vomiting, seizures, paresthesia, headache, dizziness, tinnitus, GI bleeding, cerebral edema, and cardiac arrest have been reported with overdoses

Dosage Forms Excipient information presented when available (limited, particularly for generics); consult specific product labeling.
Capsule: 25 mg, 50 mg
Injection, powder for reconstitution:
Indocin® I.V: 1 mg
Suspension, oral:
Indocin®: 25 mg/5 mL (237 mL) [contains alcohol 1%; pineapple-coconut-mint flavor]

References

Coombs RC, Morgan ME, Durbin GM, et al, "Gut Blood Flow Velocities in the Newborn: Effects of Patent Ductus Arteriosus and Parenteral Indomethacin," *Arch Dis Child*, 1990, 65(10 Spec No):1067-71.
Gersony WM, Peckham GJ, Ellison RC, et al, "Effects of Indomethacin in Premature Infants With Patent Ductus Arteriosus: Results of a National Collaborative Study," *J Pediatr*, 1983, 102(6):895-906.
Kraus DM and Pham JT, "Neonatal Therapy," *Applied Therapeutics: The Clinical Use of Drugs*, 7th ed, Koda-Kimble MA, Young LY, eds, Baltimore, MD: Lippincott Williams & Wilkins, 2001.

- **Indomethacin Sodium Trihydrate** *see* Indomethacin *on page 828*
- **Indotec (Can)** *see* Indomethacin *on page 828*
- **INF-alpha 2** *see* Interferon Alfa-2b *on page 856*
- **Infanrix®** *see* Diphtheria, Tetanus Toxoids, and Acellular Pertussis Vaccine *on page 517*
- **Infantaire [OTC]** *see* Acetaminophen *on page 42*
- **Infantaire Gas Drops [OTC]** *see* Simethicone *on page 1440*
- **Infasurf®** *see* Calfactant *on page 275*
- **INFeD®** *see* Iron Supplements (Parenteral) *on page 870*
- **Inflamase® Mild (Can)** *see* PrednisoLONE *on page 1304*

Infliximab (in FLIKS e mab)

Medication Safety Issues
Sound-alike/look-alike issues:
Remicade® may be confused with Renacidin®, Rituxan®
Infliximab may be confused with rituximab

U.S. Brand Names Remicade®

Canadian Brand Names Remicade®

Index Terms Antitumor Necrosis Factor-Alpha

Therapeutic Category Antirheumatic, Disease Modifying; Gastrointestinal Agent, Miscellaneous

Generic Available No

Use Reduction of signs and symptoms of Crohn's disease in patients with moderate to severely active disease who have had an inadequate response to conventional therapy; reduction in the number of draining enterocutaneous fistulas in patients with fistulizing Crohn's disease; treatment of refractory ulcerative colitis; in combination with methotrexate for reducing signs and symptoms, inhibiting progression of structural damage, and improving physical function in patients with moderate to severe rheumatoid arthritis; reduction of signs and symptoms of ankylosing spondylitis; treatment of psoriatic arthritis

Medication Guide An FDA-approved patient medication guide, which is available with the product information and at http://www.fda.gov/cder/Offices/ODS/medication_guides.htm, must be dispensed with this medication for each new outpatient prescription and refill.

Pregnancy Risk Factor B

Lactation Excretion in breast milk unknown/not recommended

Contraindications Hypersensitivity to infliximab, murine proteins, or any component; patients with any serious active infection or sepsis; patients with moderate or severe (NYHA class III/IV) congestive heart failure. Infliximab doses >5 mg/kg should not be administered to patients with moderate to severe heart failure; doses at 10 mg/kg have been associated with an increased incidence of death and worsening heart failure (see Warnings).

Warnings Higher incidence of mortality and hospitalization for worsening heart failure have been reported in patients with CHF treated with infliximab, especially those patients treated at a higher dose of 10 mg/kg; do not initiate infliximab therapy in patients with moderate or severe CHF. Serious infections (some fatal) including sepsis, invasive fungal infections and opportunistic infections have been reported in patients receiving infliximab while on concomitant immunosuppressive therapy or another TNFα-blocking agent; combination of infliximab and anakinra is not recommended

84 cases of tuberculosis have been reported in association with infliximab therapy; the majority of cases occurred after $\leq$3 infusions of infliximab; patients should be evaluated for risk of tuberculosis prior to initiating infliximab therapy; infliximab has been associated with reactivation of hepatitis B in patients who are chronic carriers of this virus; patients who develop a new infection while receiving infliximab should be monitored closely; if a patient develops a serious infection while on treatment, infliximab therapy should be discontinued. Infliximab use has been associated with reports of leukopenia, neutropenia, thrombocytopenia, and pancytopenia (some fatal). Use with caution in patients with a history of significant hematologic abnormalities; discontinue therapy if significant hematologic abnormalities develop.

Infliximab administration has been associated with infusion-related hypersensitivity reactions which include urticaria, dyspnea, and/or hypotension that occurred during or within 2 hours of infusion; discontinue infliximab if severe reaction occurs; medications for treatment of hypersensitivity reactions must be readily available for use in case of a reaction. Rare cases of CNS demyelinating disorders, such as multiple sclerosis, optic neuritis, and seizure disorders have been reported in patients undergoing infliximab therapy; consider discontinuing therapy in patients who develop significant CNS adverse reactions. Severe hepatic reactions (some fatal), including acute liver failure, hepatitis, and cholestasis have occurred between 2 weeks to more than a year after infliximab initiation. Discontinue infliximab if jaundice and/or liver enzyme elevation ($\geq$5 times the upper limit of normal) develops.

Precautions Use with caution in patients with a history of recurrent infections or illnesses which predispose the patient to infection. An increased risk of lymphoma has been noted in infliximab clinical trials, as compared to the general population; anti-TNF therapies such as infliximab may affect host defenses against infections and malignancies

Adverse Reactions

Cardiovascular: Hypotension, hypertension, chest pain, syncope, pericardial effusion, edema, tachycardia, arrhythmia, heart failure, cardiac arrest, systemic vasculitis, pulmonary embolism

Central nervous system: Headache, dizziness, fatigue, fever, chills, seizures, anxiety, confusion, delirium, somnolence, depression, suicide attempt, multiple sclerosis, myelitis

Dermatologic: Urticaria, rash, pruritus, moniliasis, furunculosis

Endocrine & metabolic: Weight decrease, menstrual irregularity

Gastrointestinal: Nausea, vomiting, diarrhea, abdominal pain, pancreatitis, intestinal obstruction, GI hemorrhage, stomatitis, constipation

Genitourinary: Urinary tract infection

Hematologic: Anemia, thrombocytopenia, leukopenia, neutropenia, pancytopenia, hemolytic anemia

Hepatic: Cholestatic jaundice, cholecystitis, elevated AST and ALT, hepatitis, acute liver failure

Neuromuscular & skeletal: Myalgia, back pain, arthropathy, septic arthritis, chronic osteomyelitis, peripheral neuropathy

Ophthalmologic: Endophthalmitis, optic neuritis

Renal: Renal failure

(Continued)

Infliximab *(Continued)*

Respiratory: Dyspnea, cough, upper respiratory tract infections, pulmonary edema

Miscellaneous: Anaphylaxis, serum-sickness-like reaction (fever, rash, headache, sore throat, myalgias, polyarthralgias, hand and facial edema, dysphagia, antibodies to infliximab, loss of drug efficacy 3-12 days after reinstitution of infliximab following an extended period without treatment); lupus-like syndrome; infection; malignancies

Drug Interactions Live vaccines (decreased immune response may allow live vaccine to produce infection, do not administer concurrently with infliximab); immunosuppressant agents (may reduce frequency of infusion reactions and antibodies to infliximab); anakinra (may increase rate of serious infection if used concurrently with infliximab)

Stability Store vial in refrigerator; do not freeze; infliximab solution should be used immediately after reconstitution since the vial contains no preservative; do not shake or agitate vigorously; do not use if discolored or cloudy; the reconstituted dose must be further diluted in NS and the infusion should begin within 3 hours of preparation

Mechanism of Action Chimeric monoclonal antibody which binds specifically to human tumor necrosis factor alpha (TNFα); inhibits binding of TNFα with its receptors

Pharmacodynamics

Onset:

Crohn's disease: 1-2 weeks

Rheumatoid arthritis: 3-7 days

Duration:

Crohn's disease: 8-48 weeks

Rheumatoid arthritis: 6-12 weeks

Pharmacokinetics

Distribution: Within the vascular compartment

V_d: Adults: 3 L

Half-life, terminal: 8-9.5 days

Usual Dosage I.V. infusion:

Children:

Crohn's disease: 5 mg/kg/dose; in an open-label retrospective chart review (n=19; mean age: 14.4 years, range 9-19 years) patients received 1-3 infusions of infliximab for active intestinal Crohn's disease over a 12-week period for corticosteroid-resistant disease (n=7) or corticosteroid-dependence (n=12); infliximab provided rapid, short-term clinical improvement; however, additional infusion doses may be needed in some patients due to return of disease symptoms weeks to months after the initial infusion. Further studies are needed (Hyams, 2001). If the response is incomplete, dose has been increased up to 10 mg/kg (Stephens, 2003).

Juvenile idiopathic arthritis uncontrolled by conventional disease modifying drugs: Initial: 3 mg/kg; repeat 3 mg/kg/dose at 2 and 6 weeks after the first infusion, then every 8 weeks thereafter

Adults:

Crohn's disease or fistulizing disease: Initial: 5 mg/kg; repeat 5 mg/kg/dose at 2 and 6 weeks after the first infusion; maintenance: 5 mg/kg/dose every 8 weeks. If response is incomplete, may increase dose up to 10 mg/kg. Patients who do not respond by week 14 are unlikely to respond with continued infliximab dosing.

Rheumatoid arthritis (in combination with methotrexate): Initial: 3 mg/kg; repeat 3 mg/kg/dose at 2 and 6 weeks after the first infusion, then every 8 weeks thereafter. If the response is incomplete, may increase dose up to 10 mg/kg or treat as often as every 4 weeks.

Ankylosing spondylitis: Initial: 5 mg/kg; repeat 5 mg/kg/dose at 2 and 6 weeks after the first infusion, then every 6 weeks thereafter

Psoriatic arthritis: Initial: 5 mg/kg; repeat 5 mg/kg/dose at 2 and 6 weeks after the first infusion, then every 8 weeks thereafter

Ulcerative colitis: Initial: 5 mg/kg; repeat 5 mg/kg/dose at 2 and 6 weeks after the first infusion, then every 8 weeks thereafter

Administration Parenteral: Administer by I.V. infusion over 2-3 hours at a final concentration between 0.4-4 mg/mL in NS. A rate titration schedule may be used to prevent acute infusion reactions. For a total 250 mL volume to be infused, initiate at a rate of 10 mL/hour for first 15 minutes followed by 20 mL/hour for 15 minutes, 40 mL/hour for 15 minutes, 80 mL/hour for 15 minutes, 150 mL/hour for 30 minutes, and then 250 mL/hour until infusion is complete. Administer through an in-line, sterile, nonpyrogenic, low-protein-binding filter with pore size of ≤1.2 micrometers; do not infuse in the same I.V. line as other agents

Monitoring Parameters Urinalysis, blood chemistry, ESR, blood pressure, signs of infection, CBC; tuberculin skin test prior to initiation of therapy

Crohn's disease: C-reactive protein, frequency of stools, abdominal pain

Rheumatoid arthritis: C-reactive protein, rheumatoid factor, decrease in pain, swollen joints, stiffness

Patient Information Notify physician if persistent fever, bruising, cough, flu-like symptoms, severe fatigue, jaundice, abdominal pain, bleeding, pallor, shortness of breath, swelling of ankles or feet, vision change, weakness in arms and/or legs, numbness, or chest discomfort occurs.

Additional Information A retrospective study of 57 children receiving 361 infliximab infusions reported that the rate of infusion-related reactions in children was similar to that in adults (9.7% incidence shown). Female gender, immunosuppressive use for <4 months, and prior infusion reactions were risk factors for subsequent infusion reactions in children (see Crandall, 2003)

Dosage Forms Excipient information presented when available (limited, particularly for generics); consult specific product labeling.

Injection, powder for reconstitution [preservative free]:

Remicade®: 100 mg [contains sucrose and polysorbate 80]

References

Crandall WV and Mackner LM, "Infusion Reactions to Infliximab in Children and Adolescents: Frequency, Outcome and a Predictive Model," *Aliment Pharmacol Ther*, 2003, 17(1):75-84.

Hyams JS, "Use of Infliximab in the Treatment of Crohn's Disease in Children and Adolescents," *J Pediatr Gastroenterol Nutr*, 2001, 33 (Suppl 1):S36-9.

Hyams JS, Markowitz J, and Wyllie R, "Use of Infliximab in the Treatment of Crohn's Disease in Children and Adolescents," *J Pediatr*, 2000, 137(2):192-6.

Serrano MS, Schmidt-Sommerfeld E, Kilbaugh TJ, et al, "Use of Infliximab in Pediatric Patients With Inflammatory Bowel Disease," *Ann Pharmacother*, 2001, 35(7-8):823-8.

Stephens MC, Shepanski MA, Mamula P, et al, "Safety and Steroid-Sparing Experience Using Infliximab for Crohn's Disease at a Pediatric Inflammatory Bowel Disease Center," *Am J Gastroenterol*, 2003, 98(1):104-11.

Wilkinson N, Jackson G, and Gardner-Medwin J, "Biologic Therapies for Juvenile Arthritis," *Arch Dis Child*, 2003, 88(3):186-91.

Influenza Virus Vaccine (Inactivated)

(in floo EN za VYE rus vak SEEN in AK te VAT ed)

U.S. Brand Names Fluarix™; FluLaval™; Fluvirin®; Fluzone®

Index Terms Influenza Virus Vaccine (Purified Split-Virus; Purified Surface Antigen); Trivalent Inactivated Influenza Vaccine (TIV)

Therapeutic Category Vaccine; Vaccine, Inactivated Virus

Generic Available No

Use Provide active immunity to influenza virus strains contained in the vaccine

Recommendations for annual influenza vaccination:

Persons at high risk for influenza-related complications and severe disease:

- All children 6-59 months of age
- Persons ≥50 years of age
- Residents of nursing homes and other chronic-care facilities that house persons of any age with chronic medical conditions
- Adults and children with chronic disorders of the pulmonary or cardiovascular systems, including children with asthma, bronchopulmonary dysplasia, cystic fibrosis, and congenital heart disease
- Adults and children who have required regular medical follow-up or hospitalization during the preceding year because of chronic metabolic diseases (including diabetes mellitus), renal dysfunction, sickle cell disease and other hemoglobinopathies, human immunodeficiency virus (HIV) infection, or immunosuppression (including immunosuppression caused by medications)
- Children and adolescents (6 months to 18 years of age) who are receiving long-term aspirin therapy and therefore, may be at risk for developing Reye's syndrome after influenza
- Women who will be pregnant during influenza season
- Children and adults who have conditions that can compromise respiratory function or the handling of respiratory secretions or that can increase the risk for aspiration (eg, cognitive dysfunction, spinal cord injury, seizure disorder, or other neuromuscular disorders)
- Persons who live with or care for persons at high risk for influenza-related complications
- Healthy household contacts and caregivers of children aged 0-59 months and persons at high risk for severe complications from influenza
- Healthcare workers

Pregnancy Risk Factor C

Contraindications Hypersensitivity to influenza virus vaccine or any component; allergy to eggs or egg products, chicken, chicken feathers, or chicken dander; presence of acute respiratory disease or other active infections or illnesses (delay immunization in a patient with an active neurological disorder); influenza vaccines from previous seasons must not be used. **Note:** Starting July 1, 2006, no vaccines

(Continued)

Influenza Virus Vaccine (Inactivated) *(Continued)*

containing greater than trace amounts of thimerosal may be administered to pregnant women or children <3 years of age in select states (check individual state statutes).

Warnings Severe allergic reactions including anaphylaxis may occur; immediate treatment for anaphylactic/anaphylactoid reaction should be available. Antigenic response may not be as great as expected in patients receiving immunosuppressive drugs. Inactivated influenza virus vaccine is preferred over live virus vaccine for household members, healthcare workers, and others coming in close contact with severely immunosuppressed persons requiring care in a protected environment.

Precautions Use with caution in patients with history of febrile convulsions or Guillain-Barré syndrome (GBS) which has occurred within 6 weeks of receiving a prior influenza vaccine dose; patients with thrombocytopenia, any coagulation disorder, or receiving anticoagulants

Adverse Reactions All serious adverse reactions must be reported to the U.S. Department of Health and Human Services (DHHS) Vaccine Adverse Event Reporting System (VAERS) 1-800-822-7967.

Central nervous system: Fever, headache, fatigue, chills, seizures (rare), malaise (may start within 6-12 hours and last 1-2 days); Guillain-Barré syndrome (patients with a history of GBS have a greater likelihood of developing GBS than those without)

Dermatologic: Angioedema, urticaria

Local: Redness, tenderness, pain, induration at the site of injection (may last up to 2 days)

Neuromuscular & skeletal: Myalgia (may start within 6-12 hours and last 1-2 days), arthralgia

Respiratory: Cough, sore throat, dyspnea

Miscellaneous: Anaphylactoid reactions

Drug Interactions Decreased effect with immunosuppressive agents (optimal time to immunize children who must undergo chemotherapy is >3 weeks after chemotherapy has been discontinued); high-dose corticosteroids (ie, prednisone dose ≥2mg/kg or 20 mg/day) may decrease antibody response

Stability Refrigerate; do not freeze (potency is destroyed by freezing)

FluLaval™: Once multidose vial is entered, discard after 28 days

Mechanism of Action Promotes immunity to influenza virus by inducing specific antibody production

Pharmacodynamics

Onset of action: Protective antibody levels achieved ~2 weeks after vaccination

Duration: Protective antibody levels persist approximately ≥6 months

Usual Dosage I.M.: Optimal time to vaccinate is usually October and November

Fluzone®:

- Children 6-35 months: 0.25 mL (1 or 2 doses; see **Note**)
- Children 3-8 years: 0.5 mL (1 or 2 doses; see **Note**)
- Children ≥9 years and Adults: 0.5 mL (1 dose)

Fluvirin®:

- Children 4-8 years: 0.5 mL (1 or 2 doses; see **Note**)
- Children ≥9 years and Adults: 0.5 mL (1 dose)

Fluarix™, FluLaval™: Adults ≥18 years: 0.5 mL (1 dose)

Note: Previously unvaccinated children 6 months to <9 years of age should receive 2 doses, given >1 month apart in order to achieve a satisfactory antibody response. Second dose should preferably be administered before the onset of influenza season.

Administration I.M.: For I.M. administration only. Shake suspension well prior to use.

Infants and young Children: I.M. injection in the anterolateral aspect of the thigh

Older children and Adults: I.M. injection in the deltoid muscle

Patients at risk of bleeding (eg, patient receiving antihemophilic factor): Schedule vaccination shortly after factor is administered. Use a fine needle (23 gauge or smaller) for vaccination and apply firm pressure to the site (without rubbing) for at least 2 minutes.

Patient Information Notify physician if you experience a high fever, seizures, or allergic reaction (difficulty breathing, hives, weakness, dizziness, fast heart beat). Inactivated influenza virus vaccine is safe to administer to mothers who are breast-feeding.

Nursing Implications Federal law requires that the date of administration, the vaccine manufacturer, lot number of vaccine, and the administering person's name, title, and address be entered into the patient's permanent medical record.

Additional Information Influenza is highly contagious. Incubation period is 1-3 days. Patients are most contagious during the 24 hours before the onset of symptoms and during their most symptomatic period.

Dosage Forms Excipient information presented when available (limited, particularly for generics); consult specific product labeling.

Injection, solution, purified split-virus surface antigen [preservative free] (Fluvirin®): (0.5 mL) [prefilled syringe; contains thimerosal (trace amounts); manufactured using neomycin and polymyxin]; (5 mL) [multidose vial; contains thimerosal; manufactured using neomycin and polymyxin]

Injection, suspension, purified split-virus:

Fluarix™ [preservative free]: (0.5 mL) [prefilled syringe; syringe cap and rubber plunger contain natural latex rubber; may contain residual amounts of thimerosal, hydrocortisone, gentamicin, and ovalbumin]

FluLaval™: (5 mL) [TIV; latex-free; contains thimerosal; produced in chick embryo cell culture]

Fluzone®: (5 mL) [vial; contains thimerosal]

Fluzone® [preservative free]: (0.25 mL) [prefilled syringe]; (0.5 mL) [vial]

References

Advisory Committee on Immunization Practices, "Prevention and Control of Influenza: Recommendations of the Advisory Committee on Immunization Practices (ACIP)," *MMWR Recomm Rep*, 2006, 55(RR-10):1-42.

Influenza Virus Vaccine (Live/Attenuated)

(in floo EN za VYE rus vak SEEN)

U.S. Brand Names fluMist®

Index Terms Intranasal Trivalent, Cold-Adapted LAIV; LAIV; Live, Attenuated Influenza Vaccine

Therapeutic Category Vaccine; Vaccine, Live/Attenuated

Generic Available No

Use Active immunization for the prevention of influenza A and B virus strains in healthy children and adolescents, ages 5-17 years and adults, ages 18-49 years

Pregnancy Risk Factor C

Contraindications Hypersensitivity to influenza virus vaccine, egg or egg products, or any component; children receiving aspirin or aspirin-containing therapy due to the association of Reye syndrome with wild-type influenza infection; individuals who have a history of Guillain-Barré syndrome; individuals with known or suspected primary immune deficiency diseases or their close contacts; individuals with weakened immune systems due to HIV infection, malignancy, leukemia, or lymphoma; immunosuppressed individuals including patients receiving systemic corticosteroids, alkylating drugs, antimetabolites, radiation, or other immunosuppressive therapies. Do not administer to individuals with a history of asthma or reactive airway disease, patients with chronic disorders of the cardiovascular and pulmonary systems, pregnant women, patients requiring follow-up or hospitalization due to chronic metabolic diseases such as diabetes, renal dysfunction, or hemoglobinopathies such as sickle cell disease.

Warnings Children <5 years of age who received the live, attenuated influenza virus vaccine intranasally had an increased rate of asthma within 42 days of vaccination when compared to patients who received placebo.

Epinephrine injection must be readily available in the event of an acute anaphylactic reaction following vaccination.

Precautions Individuals receiving live, attenuated influenza virus vaccine intranasally should avoid close contact with immunocompromised individuals for at least 21 days. Avoid administering intranasal influenza virus vaccine during an acute phase of febrile and/or respiratory illness (postpone at least 72 hours until after the acute phase). If nasal congestion is present that might decrease delivery of the vaccine to the nasopharyngeal mucosa, postpone administration until illness resolves.

Adverse Reactions

Central nervous system: Headache, irritability, chills, fever

Gastrointestinal: Vomiting, abdominal pain, diarrhea

Neuromuscular & skeletal: Myalgia, weakness

Otic: Otitis media

Respiratory: Nasal congestion, runny nose, sore throat, cough

Miscellaneous: Anaphylaxis

Drug Interactions Concurrent antiviral therapy interferes with the immune response to influenza vaccine (wait 48 hours after cessation of antiviral therapy before administering intranasal influenza vaccine; antiviral therapy should not be administered until 2 weeks after intranasal influenza vaccine); concurrent live vaccines not administered on the same day should be separated apart by ≥4 weeks; inactivated vaccine can be administered concurrently or at any time before or after intranasal influenza virus vaccine

Stability Store at ≤15°C in a nonfrost-free freezer; do not refreeze after thawing. May thaw in a refrigerator at 2°C to 8°C and store for no more than 24 hours prior to use.

Mechanism of Action Promotes immunity to influenza virus by inducing influenza strain-specific serum antibodies

(Continued)

Influenza Virus Vaccine (Live/Attenuated) *(Continued)*

Pharmacodynamics

Onset of action: Protective antibody levels achieved ~2 weeks after vaccination

Duration: Protective antibody levels persist approximately ≥6 months

Usual Dosage Intranasal: Administer vaccine prior to exposure to influenza. Optimal time to vaccinate is usually in October and November. For children ages 5-8 years who have never received influenza vaccine, vaccinate in October or earlier since a second dose will need to be given 6-10 weeks after the initial dose.

Children 5-8 years:

Not previously vaccinated with influenza virus vaccine: 2 doses (0.5 mL each); second dose 60 days after the initial dose

Previously vaccinated with influenza virus vaccine: 1 dose (0.5 mL) per season

Children and Adolescents 9-17 years: 1 dose (0.5 mL) per season

Adults 18-49 years: 1 dose (0.5 mL) per season

Administration Intranasal: Thaw vaccine prior to use by holding the sprayer in the palm of the hand and supporting the plunger rod with the thumb; administer vaccine immediately after thawing. Administer 0.25 mL (half of the dose from a single sprayer) into each nostril while the recipient is in an upright position. Insert the tip of the sprayer just inside the nose and depress the plunger to spray. Remove dose-divider clip from the sprayer to administer the second half of the dose into the other nostril. Do not administer by the I.M., SubQ, intradermal, or I.V. route.

Patient Information If the patient sneezes after intranasal vaccine administration, the dose should not be repeated. Patients with an acute febrile illness should not receive the vaccine until symptoms improve.

Nursing Implications The used sprayer should be disposed of according to the standard procedures for biohazardous waste products. CDC has stated that the inactivated influenza virus vaccine injection is preferred over the live, intranasal influenza vaccine for physicians, nurses, family members, or individuals who will come in close contact with anyone with a weakened immune system.

Dosage Forms Excipient information presented when available (limited, particularly for generics); consult specific product labeling.

Solution, intranasal [preservative free; trivalent; live virus; spray] (fluMist®): (0.5 mL) [manufactured using eggs and gentamicin]

References

Belshe RB, Mendelman PM, Treanor J, et al, "The Efficacy of Live Attenuated, Cold-Adapted, Trivalent, Intranasal Influenza Virus Vaccine in Children," *N Engl J Med*, 1998, 338(20):1405-12.

Harper SA, Fukuda K, Cox NJ, et al, "Using Live, Attenuated Influenza Vaccine for Prevention and Control of Influenza: Supplemental Recommendations of the Advisory Committee on Immunization Practices (ACIP)," *MMWR Recomm Rep*, 2003, 52(RR-13):1-8.

♦ **Influenza Virus Vaccine (Purified Split-Virus; Purified Surface Antigen)** *see* Influenza Virus Vaccine (Inactivated) *on page 833*

♦ **Infumorph®** *see* Morphine Sulfate *on page 1082*

♦ **INH** *see* Isoniazid *on page 873*

♦ **Inhaled Insulin** *see* Insulin Inhalation *on page 842*

♦ **InnoPran XL™** *see* Propranolol *on page 1337*

Insulin Aspart (IN soo lin AS part)

Medication Safety Issues

Sound-alike/look-alike issues:

NovoLog® may be confused with Novolin®

NovoLog® Mix 70/30 may be confused with NovoLog®

High alert medication: The Institute for Safe Medication Practices (ISMP) includes this medication among its list of drugs which have a heightened risk of causing significant patient harm when used in error. ***Due to the number of insulin preparations, it is essential to identify/clarify the type of insulin to be used.***

Related Information

Insulin Regular *on page 849*

U.S. Brand Names NovoLog®

Canadian Brand Names NovoRapid®

Index Terms Aspart Insulin

Therapeutic Category Antidiabetic Agent, Parenteral; Insulin, Rapid-Acting

Generic Available No

Use Treatment of type 1 diabetes mellitus (insulin dependent, IDDM); type 2 diabetes mellitus (noninsulin dependent, NIDDM) to control hyperglycemia

Pregnancy Risk Factor B

Lactation Excretion in breast milk unknown/compatible

Contraindications Hypersensitivity insulin aspart or any component

Warnings Refer to Insulin Regular *on page 849.*

Precautions Refer to Insulin Regular *on page 849.*

Adverse Reactions Refer to Insulin Regular *on page 849.*

Drug Interactions Refer to Insulin Regular *on page 849.*

Food Interactions Refer to Insulin Regular *on page 849.*

Stability Store unopened container in refrigerator; do not freeze; protect from heat and light. Once opened (in use) vials may be stored in refrigerator or at room temperature for up to 28 days. Cartridges that are in use should be stored at room temperature and used within 28 days; do not refrigerate. Insulin in reservoir should be replaced every 48 hours. Discard if exposed to temperatures ≥37°C (98.6°F). May be mixed in the same syringe with NPH insulin.

Mechanism of Action Refer to Insulin Regular *on page 849.* Insulin aspart is a rapid-acting insulin analog.

Pharmacodynamics Onset and duration of hypoglycemic effects depend upon the route of administration (adsorption and onset of action are more rapid after deeper I.M. injections than after SubQ), site of injection (onset and duration are progressively slower with SubQ injection into the abdomen, arm, buttock, or thigh respectively), volume and concentration of injection, and the preparation administered; local heat and massage also increase the rate of absorption.

Onset of action: 0.17-0.33 hours

Maximum effect: 1-3 hours

Duration: 3-5 hours

Pharmacokinetics

Protein binding: 0% to 9%

Half-life: Adults: 81 minutes

Time to peak serum concentration: 40-50 minutes

Elimination: Urine

Clearance: Adults: 1.22 L/hour/kg

Usual Dosage Refer to Insulin Regular *on page 849.* Insulin aspart is a rapid-acting insulin analog which is normally administered as a premeal component of the insulin regimen or as a continuous SubQ infusion.

Dosing adjustment in renal impairment: Insulin requirements are reduced with renal impairment; see Insulin Regular *on page 849*

Administration Parenteral:

SubQ: Administration is usually made into the subcutaneous fat of the thighs, arms, buttocks, or abdomen, with sites rotated; cold injections should be avoided. May be mixed in the same syringe with NPH insulin. When mixing insulin aspart with NPH insulin, aspart should be drawn into the syringe first. Administer immediately before meals (within 5-10 minutes of the start of a meal). Can be infused SubQ by external insulin pump; however, when used in an external pump, it is not recommended to be diluted with other insulin.

I.V.: Insulin aspart may be administered I.V. in selected clinical situations to control hyperglycemia. Appropriate medical supervision is required. May be diluted to a concentration between 0.05 and 1 unit/mL with NS, D_5W, or $D_{10}W$

Monitoring Parameters Urine sugar and acetone, serum glucose, electrolytes, Hb A_{1c}, lipid profile; when used intravenously, close monitoring of serum glucose and potassium are required to avoid hypoglycemia and/or hypokalemia

Reference Range Refer to Insulin Regular *on page 849.*

Patient Information

Do not take any new medication during therapy unless approved by healthcare provider. This medication is used to control diabetes; it is not a cure. It is imperative to follow other components of prescribed treatment (eg, diet and exercise regimen). Take exactly as directed. Do not change dose or discontinue unless advised by healthcare provider. With insulin aspart (NovoLog®), you must start eating within 5-10 minutes after injection. If you experience hypoglycemic reaction, contact healthcare provider immediately. Always carry quick source of sugar with you. Monitor glucose levels as directed by healthcare provider. Report adverse side effects, including chest pain or palpitations; persistent fatigue, confusion, headache; skin rash or redness; numbness of mouth, lips, or tongue; muscle weakness or tremors; vision changes; respiratory difficulty; or nausea, vomiting, or flu-like symptoms.

Dosage Forms Excipient information presented when available (limited, particularly for generics); consult specific product labeling.

Injection, solution:

NovoLog®: 100 units/mL (3 mL) [FlexPen® prefilled syringe or PenFill® prefilled cartridge]; (10 mL) [vial]

♦ **Insulin Aspart and Insulin Aspart Protamine** *see* Insulin Aspart Protamine and Insulin Aspart *on page 838*

Insulin Aspart Protamine and Insulin Aspart

(IN soo lin AS part PROE ta meen & IN soo lin AS part)

Medication Safety Issues

Sound-alike/look-alike issues:

NovoLog® Mix 70/30 may be confused with Novolin® 70/30

High alert medication: The Institute for Safe Medication Practices (ISMP) includes this medication among its list of drugs which have a heightened risk of causing significant patient harm when used in error. ***Due to the number of insulin preparations, it is essential to identify/clarify the type of insulin to be used.***

Related Information

Insulin Regular *on page 849*

U.S. Brand Names NovoLog® Mix 70/30

Canadian Brand Names NovoMix® 30

Index Terms Insulin Aspart and Insulin Aspart Protamine

Therapeutic Category Antidiabetic Agent, Parenteral; Insulin, Combination

Generic Available No

Use Treatment of type 1 diabetes mellitus (insulin dependent, IDDM); type 2 diabetes mellitus (noninsulin dependent, NIDDM) to control hyperglycemia

Pregnancy Risk Factor C

Lactation Excretion in breast milk unknown/compatible

Contraindications Hypersensitivity insulin aspart, insulin aspart protamine, or to any component; hypoglycemia

Warnings Refer to Insulin Regular *on page 849*; not for I.V. infusion or use in insulin infusion pumps

Precautions Refer to Insulin Regular *on page 849.*

Adverse Reactions Refer to Insulin Regular *on page 849.*

Drug Interactions Refer to Insulin Regular *on page 849.*

Food Interactions Refer to Insulin Regular *on page 849.*

Stability Store unopened container in refrigerator; do not freeze; protect from light. If refrigeration is not possible, vial (in use) may be stored at room temperature for up to 28 days. The pen (in use) should not be refrigerated; store below 30°C (86°F) away from direct heat or light; discard after 14 days. Do not mix or dilute with other insulins.

Mechanism of Action Refer to Insulin Regular *on page 849.* Insulin aspart protamine and insulin aspart is a combination insulin product with intermediate-acting characteristics.

Pharmacodynamics

Onset of action: 10-20 minutes

Maximum effect: 1-4 hours

Duration: 18-24 hours

Pharmacokinetics

Half-life: 8-9 hours (mean)

Elimination: Urine

Usual Dosage Refer to Insulin Regular *on page 849.* Fixed ratio insulins (such as insulin aspart protamine and insulin aspart combination) are normally administered in 2 daily doses with each dose intended to cover two meals and a snack. Because of variability in the peak affect and individual patient variability in activities, meals, etc, it may be more difficult to achieve complete glycemic control using fixed combinations of insulins in all patients.

Dosing adjustment in renal impairment: Insulin requirements are reduced with renal impairment; see Insulin Regular *on page 849*

Administration

Parenteral: SubQ: Gently roll vial or pen in the palms of the hands to resuspend before use; administer into the subcutaneous fat of the thighs, arms, buttocks, or abdomen, with sites rotated. Cold injections should be avoided. Administer within 15 minutes before a meal (before breakfast and supper). Do not mix or dilute with other insulins. **Not for I.V. administration** or use in an insulin infusion pump.

Monitoring Parameters Refer to Insulin Regular *on page 849.*

Reference Range Refer to Insulin Regular *on page 849.*

Patient Information Refer to Insulin Regular *on page 849.*

Dosage Forms Excipient information presented when available (limited, particularly for generics); consult specific product labeling.

Injection, suspension (NovoLog® Mix 70/30): Insulin aspart protamine suspension 70% [intermediate acting] and insulin aspart solution 30% [rapid acting]: 100 units/mL (3 mL) [PenFill® prefilled cartridge or FlexPen® prefilled syringe]; (10 mL) [vial]

Insulin Detemir (IN soo lin DE te mir)

Medication Safety Issues

High alert medication: The Institute for Safe Medication Practices (ISMP) includes this medication among its list of drugs which have a heightened risk of causing significant patient harm when used in error. ***Due to the number of insulin preparations, it is essential to identify/clarify the type of insulin to be used.***

Note: Insulin detemir is a clear solution, but it is NOT intended for I.V. or I.M. administration.

Related Information

Insulin Regular *on page 849*

U.S. Brand Names Levemir®

Canadian Brand Names Levemir®

Index Terms Detemir Insulin

Therapeutic Category Antidiabetic Agent, Parenteral; Insulin, Intermediate-Acting

Generic Available No

Use Treatment of type 1 diabetes mellitus (insulin dependent, IDDM); type 2 diabetes mellitus (noninsulin dependent, NIDDM) to control hyperglycemia

Pregnancy Risk Factor C

Lactation Excretion in breast milk unknown/compatible

Contraindications Hypersensitivity to insulin detemir or any component; hypoglycemia

Warnings Refer to Insulin Regular *on page 849*. Safety and efficacy not established in children <6 years of age. **Not for I.V. administration** or use in insulin infusion pumps.

Precautions Refer to Insulin Regular *on page 849*.

Adverse Reactions Refer to Insulin Regular *on page 849*.

Drug Interactions Refer to Insulin Regular *on page 849*.

Food Interactions Refer to Insulin Regular *on page 849*.

Stability Store unopened vial or cartridges in refrigerator; do not freeze. Unopened vials or cartridges are stable at room temperature for 42 days. Once opened (in use), vials may be stored in refrigerator or at room temperature (below 30°C) for up to 42 days. Cartridges and prefilled syringes that are in use should be stored at room temperature and used within 42 days; do not refrigerate. Do not store with needle in place. Do not dilute or mix with other insulins or solutions.

Mechanism of Action Refer to Insulin Regular *on page 849*. The product labeling identifies this product as a long-acting insulin analog; however, its pharmacodynamic characteristics and dosing are typical of intermediate insulin forms. In some patients, or at higher dosages, it may have a duration of action approaching long-acting insulins.

Pharmacodynamics

Onset of action: 3-4 hours

Duration: 6-23 hours (dose dependent)

Pharmacokinetics

Distribution: V_d: 0.1 L/kg

Bioavailability: 60%

Half-life: SubQ: 5-7 hours (dose dependent)

Time to peak serum concentration: 6-8 hours

Elimination: Urine

Usual Dosage Also refer to Insulin Regular *on page 849*.

SubQ: Children and Adults: Type 1 or type 2 diabetes:

Previously receiving basal insulin alone (eg, insulin glargine) or basal insulin plus bolus insulin (eg, NPH + regular insulin): May be substituted on an equivalent unit-per-unit basis

Insulin-naive patients (adults with type 2 diabetes only): 0.1-0.2 units/kg once daily in the evening or 10 units once or twice daily. Adjust dose to achieve glycemic targets.

Dosage adjustment in renal impairment: Insulin requirements are reduced due to changes in insulin clearance or metabolism. See Insulin Regular *on page 849*.

Administration Parenteral: SubQ: Administer into the thighs, arms, buttocks, or abdomen, with sites rotated. Cold injections should be avoided. **Not for I.V. infusion** or use in insulin infusion pumps. May not be diluted or mixed with other insulins or solutions. When treated once daily, administer with evening meal or at bedtime. When treated twice daily, administer evening dose with evening meal, at bedtime, or 12 hours following the morning dose.

Monitoring Parameters Urine sugar and acetone, serum glucose, electrolytes, Hb A_{1c}, lipid profile

Reference Range Refer to Insulin Regular *on page 849*.

(Continued)

Insulin Detemir *(Continued)*

Patient Information Refer to Insulin Regular *on page 849.*

Dosage Forms Excipient information presented when available (limited, particularly for generics); consult specific product labeling.

Injection, solution (Levemir®): 100 units/mL (3 mL) [Innolet® prefilled syringe, Penfill® prefilled cartridge, or FlexPen® prefilled syringe]; (10 mL) [vial]

Insulin Glargine (IN soo lin GLAR jeen)

Medication Safety Issues

Sound-alike/look-alike issues:

Lantus® may be confused with Lente®

Lente® may be confused with Lantus®

High alert medication: The Institute for Safe Medication Practices (ISMP) includes this medication among its list of drugs which have a heightened risk of causing significant patient harm when used in error. ***Due to the number of insulin preparations, it is essential to identify/clarify the type of insulin to be used.***

Related Information

Insulin Regular *on page 849*

U.S. Brand Names Lantus®

Canadian Brand Names Lantus®; Lantus® OptiSet®

Index Terms Glargine Insulin

Therapeutic Category Antidiabetic Agent, Parenteral; Insulin, Long-Acting

Generic Available No

Use Treatment of type 1 diabetes mellitus (insulin dependent, IDDM); type 2 diabetes mellitus (noninsulin dependent, NIDDM) requiring basal (long-acting) insulin to control hyperglycemia

Pregnancy Risk Factor C

Lactation Excretion in breast milk unknown/compatible

Contraindications Hypersensitivity insulin glargine or any component

Warnings Refer to Insulin Regular *on page 849.* **Not for I.V. administration** or use in insulin infusion pumps

Precautions Refer to Insulin Regular *on page 849.*

Adverse Reactions Refer to Insulin Regular *on page 849.*

Drug Interactions Refer to Insulin Regular *on page 849.*

Food Interactions Refer to Insulin Regular *on page 849.*

Stability Store unopened containers or cartridges in refrigerator at 2°C to 8°C (36°F to 46°F); do not freeze; protect from direct heat or light. Once opened (in use), vials may be stored in refrigerator or at room temperature for up to 28 days. Cartridges (in use; inserted into OptiClik™ delivery system) should not be refrigerated; store below 30°C (86°F) away from direct heat or light; discard after 28 days. May **not** be mixed with any other insulin or solution.

Mechanism of Action Refer to Insulin Regular *on page 849.* Insulin glargine is a long-acting insulin formulation.

Pharmacodynamics

Onset of action: 3-4 hours

Duration: 24 hours

Pharmacokinetics

Absorption: Slow; after injection it forms microprecipitates in the skin which allow small amounts to release over time

Metabolism: Partially metabolized in the skin to form two active metabolites

Time to peak serum concentration: No pronounced peak

Elimination: Urine

Usual Dosage SubQ: Refer to Insulin Regular *on page 849*

Type 1 diabetes: Conversion from "conventional" insulin therapy to once daily insulin glargine:

Children <6 years: Limited data; thirty-five preschool-aged children (2.6-6.3 years) were converted to once-daily insulin glargine (with insulin lispro prior to each meal); 40% of the established total daily insulin dose was administered as insulin glargine. Insulin glargine was well tolerated and this regimen resulted in a reduction in hypoglycemic episodes in the nonobese group (Alemzadeh, 2005).

Children ≥6 years and Adults: Current therapy: If once-daily NPH or Ultralente® insulin: Use the same total dose of insulin glargine as NPH or Ultralente®; if twice-daily NPH or Ultralente®: Use 80% of the total daily dose of NPH or Ultralente® (eg, 20% reduction); administer once daily; adjust dosage according to patient response

Type 2 diabetes: Adults:

Patient not already on insulin: 10 units once daily, adjusted according to patient response (range in clinical study: 2-100 units/day)

Patients already on insulin: See adult type 1 diabetes recommendation above.

Dosage adjustment in renal impairment: Insulin requirements are reduced with renal impairment; see Insulin Regular *on page 849*.

Administration Parenteral: SubQ: Administer into the subcutaneous fat of the thighs, arms, buttocks, or abdomen, with sites rotated. Cold injections should be avoided. Administer once daily, at any time of day, but at the same time each day. Do not mix with any other insulin or solution.

Monitoring Parameters Urine sugar and acetone, serum glucose, electrolytes, Hb A_{1c}, lipid profile

Reference Range Refer to Insulin Regular *on page 849*.

Patient Information Refer to Insulin Regular *on page 849*.

Dosage Forms Excipient information presented when available (limited, particularly for generics); consult specific product labeling.

Injection, solution (Lantus®): 100 units/mL (3 mL) [cartridge]; (10 mL) [vial]

References

Alemzadeh R, Berhe T, and Wyatt DT, "Flexible Insulin Therapy With Glargine Insulin Improved Glycemic Control and Reduced Severe Hypoglycemia Among Preschool-Aged Children With Type 1 Diabetes Mellitus," *Pediatrics*, 2005, 115(5):1320-4.

Insulin Glulisine (IN soo lin gloo LIS een)

Medication Safety Issues

High alert medication: The Institute for Safe Medication Practices (ISMP) includes this medication among its list of drugs which have a heightened risk of causing significant patient harm when used in error. ***Due to the number of insulin preparations, it is essential to identify/clarify the type of insulin to be used.***

Related Information

Insulin Regular *on page 849*

U.S. Brand Names Apidra®

Canadian Brand Names Apidra®

Index Terms Glulisine Insulin

Therapeutic Category Insulin, Rapid-Acting

Generic Available No

Use Treatment of type 1 diabetes mellitus (insulin dependent, IDDM); type 2 diabetes mellitus (noninsulin dependent, NIDDM) to control hyperglycemia

Pregnancy Risk Factor C

Lactation Excretion in breast milk unknown/compatible

Contraindications Hypersensitivity to insulin glulisine or any component

Warnings Refer to Insulin Regular *on page 849*.

Precautions Refer to Insulin Regular *on page 849*. While regular insulin is the preferred formulation for I.V. use, insulin glulisine may be administered I.V. in carefully controlled clinical settings with medical supervision and close monitoring of blood glucose as well as serum potassium.

Adverse Reactions Refer to Insulin Regular *on page 849*.

Drug Interactions Refer to Insulin Regular *on page 849*.

Food Interactions Refer to Insulin Regular *on page 849*.

Stability Store unopened container in refrigerator; do not freeze; protect from heat and light. Once opened (in use) vials may be stored in refrigerator or or at room temperature for up to 28 days. Cartridges that are in use should be stored at room temperature and used within 28 days; do not refrigerate. Insulin glulisine in reservoir should be replaced every 48 hours. Discard if exposed to temperatures ≥37°C (98.6°F). May be mixed in the same syringe with NPH insulin.

Mechanism of Action Refer to Insulin Regular *on page 849*. Insulin glulisine is a rapid-acting insulin analog.

Pharmacodynamics Onset and duration of hypoglycemic effects depend upon the route of administration (adsorption and onset of action are more rapid after deeper I.M. injections than after SubQ), site of injection (onset and duration are progressively slower with SubQ injection into the abdomen, arm, buttock, or thigh respectively), volume and concentration of injection, and the preparation administered; local heat and massage also increase the rate of absorption.

Onset of action: 5-15 minutes

Maximum effect: 45-75 minutes

Duration: 2-4 hours

Pharmacokinetics

Distribution: V_d: Adults: 13 L

Bioavailability: ~70%

Half-life: SubQ: 42 minutes

Time to peak serum concentration: SubQ: 55 minutes (range: 34-91 minutes)

Elimination: Urine

(Continued)

Insulin Glulisine *(Continued)*

Usual Dosage Refer to Insulin Regular *on page 849*. Insulin glulisine is a rapid-acting insulin analog which is normally administered as a premeal component of the insulin regimen or as a continuous SubQ infusion. In carefully controlled clinical settings with medical supervision and close monitoring of blood glucose as well as serum potassium, insulin glulisine may also be administered I.V.

Dosing adjustment in renal impairment: Insulin requirements are reduced with renal impairment; see Insulin Regular *on page 849*.

Administration Parenteral:

SubQ: Administration is usually made into the subcutaneous fat of the thighs, arms, buttocks, or abdomen, with sites rotated; cold injections should be avoided. May be mixed in the same syringe with NPH insulin. When mixing insulin glulisine with NPH insulin, glulisine should be drawn into the syringe first. Administer 15 minutes before meals or within 20 minutes after starting a meal. Can be infused SubQ by external insulin pump; however, when used in an external pump, it is not recommended to be diluted with other insulins.

I.V.: Dilute with NS to a final concentration of 1 unit/mL and administer using PVC Viaflex infusion bags and PVC tubing into a dedicated infusion line (the use of other bags and tubing has not been studied).

Monitoring Parameters Urine sugar and acetone, serum glucose, electrolytes, Hb A_{1c}, lipid profile

Reference Range Refer to Insulin Regular *on page 849*.

Patient Information Do not take any new medication during therapy unless approved by healthcare provider. This medication is used to control diabetes; it is not a cure. It is imperative to follow other components of prescribed treatment (eg, diet and exercise regimen). Take exactly as directed. Do not change dose or discontinue unless advised by healthcare provider. With insulin glulisine (Apidra®), you must administer 15 minutes before or within 20 minutes after starting a meal. If you experience hypoglycemic reaction, contact healthcare provider immediately. Always carry quick source of sugar with you. Monitor glucose levels as directed by healthcare provider. Report adverse side effects, including chest pain or palpitations; persistent fatigue, confusion, headache; skin rash or redness; numbness of mouth, lips, or tongue; muscle weakness or tremors; vision changes; respiratory difficulty; or nausea, vomiting, or flu-like symptoms.

Dosage Forms Excipient information presented when available (limited, particularly for generics); consult specific product labeling.

Injection, solution:

Apidra®: 100 units/mL (3 mL [cartridge], 10 mL [vial])

Insulin Inhalation (IN soo lin in ha LAY shun)

Medication Safety Issues

High alert medication: The Institute for Safe Medication Practices (ISMP) includes this medication among its list of drugs which have a heightened risk of causing significant patient harm when used in error. **Due to the number of insulin preparations, it is essential to identify/clarify the type of insulin to be used. The inhalation form of insulin is expressed in milligrams rather than units, potentially leading to confusion. Absolute conversion between doses of inhalation and injection insulin is not possible.**

Related Information

Insulin Regular *on page 849*

U.S. Brand Names Exubera®

Canadian Brand Names Exubera®

Index Terms Inhaled Insulin

Therapeutic Category Antidiabetic Agent, Inhalant; Insulin, Rapid-Acting

Use Treatment of type 1 diabetes mellitus (insulin dependent, IDDM); type 2 diabetes mellitus (noninsulin dependent, NIDDM)

Medication Guide An FDA-approved patient medication guide, which is available with the product information and at http://www.fda.gov/cder/Offices/ODS/medication_guides.htm, must be dispensed with this medication for each new outpatient prescription and refill.

Pregnancy Risk Factor C

Lactation Excretion in breast milk unknown/compatible

Contraindications Hypersensitivity to insulin or any component; smokers or patients who have discontinued smoking for <6 months (see Pharmacokinetics); poorly-controlled or unstable lung disease

Warnings Also refer to Insulin Regular *on page 849*.

Due to increased systemic absorption, the risk of hypoglycemia is greatly increased in patients who smoke or who have stopped smoking for <6 months. The effect of passive exposure to smoke has not been fully evaluated but may result in alteration in absorption and/or hypoglycemia. Insulin inhalation should be immediately discontinued in any patient who resumes smoking. Conversely, normal healthy volunteers exposed to passive smoke for 2 hours, after receiving a single dose of inhaled insulin, had a 20% reduction in AUC and a 30% reduction in C_{max}. Chronic exposure to passive smoking has not been studied.

Decreases in pulmonary function have been associated with use. Due the potential impact on pulmonary function, testing should be performed prior to the initiation of inhaled insulin therapy. Not recommended for use in patients with lung disease (asthma, COPD); these patients may not only have further decreases in pulmonary function but also wide variations in pulmonary function could affect the absorption of inhaled insulin and increase the risk of hypoglycemia or hyperglycemia. Monitor closely during periods of intercurrent respiratory illness.

Precautions Use caution in renal and/or hepatic impairment.

Adverse Reactions Also refer to Insulin Regular *on page 849.*

Cardiovascular: Chest pain (5%; usually mild to moderate)

Dermatologic: Rash (rare)

Endocrine & metabolic: Hypoglycemia

Gastrointestinal: Xerostomia (2%)

Otic: Pediatric patients: Otitis media (7%), ear pain (4%), ear disorder (1%)

Respiratory: Respiratory infection (30% to 43%), cough increased (22% to 30%), pharyngitis (10% to 18%), rhinitis (9% to 15%), sinusitis (5% to 10%), dyspnea (4%), sputum increased (3% to 4%), bronchitis (3% to 5%), epistaxis (1%), laryngitis (1%), voice alteration (1%), bronchospasm (rare)

Note: Decreases in pulmonary function (reduced FEV1, DLco) have been associated with use, usually noted in the initial weeks of therapy; declines from baseline of 20% in, respectively, FEV1 and DLco, were reported in 5.1% and 1.5% of patients as compared to 3.6% and 1.3% in comparator-treated patients.

Miscellaneous: Allergic reactions, anaphylaxis (including tachycardia and hypotension), diaphoresis increased

Drug Interactions Refer to Insulin Regular *on page 849.* Bronchodilators and other inhaled medications may alter the absorption of inhaled insulin.

Food Interactions Refer to Insulin Regular *on page 849.*

Stability Store unopened blisters, in-use blisters, and inhaler at room temperature (25°C); excursions permitted to 15°C to 30°C (59°F to 86°F). Do not freeze or refrigerate. Once foil overwrap is opened, blisters should be used within 3 months. Avoid exposure to excess humidity.

Mechanism of Action Refer to Insulin Regular *on page 849.* Insulin inhalation is a rapid-acting form of human insulin.

Pharmacodynamics

Onset of action: 10-20 minutes

Maximum effect: 2 hours

Duration: ~6 hours

Pharmacokinetics

Absorption: Rapid

Bioavailability: Absolute bioavailability not defined (depends on inspiratory flow characteristics); systemic exposure may be up to 2-5 times higher in smokers

Time to peak serum concentration: 49 minutes (range: 30-90 minutes)

Elimination: Urine

Usual Dosage Inhalation: Children ≥6 years and Adults:

Initial: 0.05 mg/kg (rounded down to nearest whole milligram) 3 times/daily

Adjustment: Dosage may be increased or decreased based on serum glucose monitoring, meal size, nutrient composition, time of day, and exercise patterns.

Note: A 1 mg blister is approximately equivalent to 3 units of regular insulin, while a 3 mg blister is approximately equivalent to 8 units of regular insulin administered subcutaneously. Patients should combine 1 mg and 3 mg blisters so that the fewest blisters are required to achieve the prescribed dose. Consecutive inhalation of three 1 mg blisters results in significantly higher insulin levels as compared to inhalation of a single 3 mg blister (do not substitute). In a patient stabilized on a dosage which uses 3 mg blisters, if 3 mg blister is temporarily unavailable, inhalation of two 1 mg blisters may be substituted.

Dosing adjustment in renal impairment: Insulin requirements are reduced due to changes in insulin clearance or metabolism.

Administration Inhalation: Administer no more than 10 minutes before a meal using the Exubera® inhalation device. The Exubera® release unit in the inhaler should be changed every 2 weeks; the Exubera® inhaler may be used for 1 year. See Usual Dosage for dosage equivalency recommendations particularly as relate to the number and strength of blisters.

(Continued)

Insulin Inhalation *(Continued)*

Monitoring Parameters Pulmonary function testing at baseline and periodically during therapy; blood glucose, urine sugar and acetone, serum glucose, electrolytes, Hb A_{1c}, lipid profile

Reference Range Refer to Insulin Regular *on page 849.*

Patient Information

Do not smoke; avoid secondhand smoke. Do not take any new medication during therapy unless approved by healthcare provider. This medication is used to control diabetes; it is not a cure. It is imperative to follow other components of prescribed treatment (eg, diet and exercise regimen). Take exactly as directed. Do not change dose or discontinue unless advised by healthcare provider. When used as your mealtime insulin, take within 10 minutes before your meal. If you experience hypoglycemic reaction, contact healthcare provider immediately. Always carry quick source of sugar with you. Monitor glucose levels as directed by healthcare provider. You may experience respiratory infections, dry mouth, cough, sore throat, sinus problems, or nasal congestion. Report adverse side effects, including chest pain or palpitations; persistent fatigue, confusion, headache; skin rash or redness; numbness of mouth, lips, or tongue; muscle weakness or tremors; vision changes; respiratory difficulty; or nausea, vomiting, or flu-like symptoms.

Dosage Forms Excipient information presented when available (limited, particularly for generics); consult specific product labeling.

Combination package:

Exubera® Kit [packaged with inhaler, chamber and release unit]:
- Powder for oral inhalation [prefilled blister pack]: 1 mg/blister (180s)
- Powder for oral inhalation [prefilled blister pack]: 3 mg/blister (90s)

Exubera® Combination Pack 15 [packaged with 2 release units]:
- Powder for oral inhalation [prefilled blister pack]: 1 mg/blister (180s)
- Powder for oral inhalation [prefilled blister pack]: 3 mg/blister (90s)

Exubera® Combination Pack 12 [packaged with 2 release units]:
- Powder for oral inhalation [prefilled blister pack]: 1 mg/blister (90s)
- Powder for oral inhalation [prefilled blister pack]: 3 mg/blister (90s)

References

Skyler JS, Weinstock RS, and Raskin P, "Use of Inhaled Insulin in a Basal/Bolus Insulin Regimen in Type 1 Diabetic Subjects: A 6-Month, Randomized, Comparative Trial," *Diabetes Care*, 2005, 28(7):1630-5.

Insulin Lispro (IN su lin LIS pro)

Medication Safety Issues

Sound-alike/look-alike issues:

Humalog® may be confused with Humulin®, Humira®

High alert medication: The Institute for Safe Medication Practices (ISMP) includes this medication among its list of drugs which have a heightened risk of causing significant patient harm when used in error. ***Due to the number of insulin preparations, it is essential to identify/clarify the type of insulin to be used.***

Related Information

Insulin Regular *on page 849*

U.S. Brand Names Humalog®

Canadian Brand Names Humalog®

Index Terms Lispro Insulin

Therapeutic Category Antidiabetic Agent, Parenteral; Insulin, Rapid-Acting

Generic Available No

Use Treatment of type 1 diabetes mellitus (insulin dependent, IDDM); type 2 diabetes mellitus (noninsulin dependent, NIDDM) to control hyperglycemia

Pregnancy Risk Factor B

Lactation Excretion in breast milk unknown/compatible

Contraindications Hypersensitivity lispro insulin or any component; hypoglycemia

Warnings Refer to Insulin Regular *on page 849.*

Precautions Refer to Insulin Regular *on page 849.*

Adverse Reactions Refer to Insulin Regular *on page 849.*

Drug Interactions Refer to Insulin Regular *on page 849.*

Food Interactions Refer to Insulin Regular *on page 849.*

Stability Store unopened container in refrigerator; do not freeze; protect from heat and light. Once opened (in use) vials may be stored in refrigerator or at room temperature for up to 28 days. Cartridges that are in use should be stored at room temperature and used within 28 days; do not refrigerate. Insulin in reservoir should be replaced every 48 hours. Discard if exposed to temperatures ≥37°C (98.6°F). May be mixed in the same syringe with Humulin® N, Humulin® U and NPH insulins. A sterile diluent is available from the manufacturer for preparing dilutions of Humalog®.

Mechanism of Action Refer to Insulin Regular *on page 849*. Insulin lispro is a rapid-acting form of insulin.

Pharmacodynamics Onset and duration of hypoglycemic effects depend upon the route of administration (adsorption and onset of action are more rapid after deeper I.M. injections than after SubQ), site of injection (onset and duration are progressively slower with SubQ injection into the abdomen, arm, buttock, or thigh respectively), volume and concentration of injection, and the preparation administered; local heat, and massage also increase the rate of absorption.

Onset of action: 15-30 minutes
Maximum effect: 0.5-2.5 hours
Duration: 3-6.5 hours

Pharmacokinetics

Distribution: V_d: 0.26-0.36 L/kg
Bioavailability: 55% to 77%
Half-life: SubQ: 1 hour
Excretion: Urine

Usual Dosage Refer to Insulin Regular *on page 849*. Insulin lispro is a rapid-acting insulin analog which is normally administered as a premeal component of the insulin regimen or as a continuous SubQ infusion.

Dosing adjustment in renal impairment: Insulin requirements are reduced due to changes in insulin clearance or metabolism. Refer to Insulin Regular *on page 849*.

Administration Parenteral: SubQ: Administration is usually made into the subcutaneous fat of the thighs, arms, buttocks, or abdomen, with sites rotated; cold injections should be avoided. May be mixed in the same syringe with Humulin® N, Humulin® U, or NPH insulin. When mixing insulin lispro with other insulins, lispro should be drawn into the syringe first. Administer 15 minutes before meals or immediately after. Can be infused SubQ by external insulin pump; however, when used in an external pump, it is not recommended to be diluted with other insulins.

Monitoring Parameters Urine sugar and acetone, serum glucose, electrolytes, Hb A_{1c}, lipid profile

Reference Range Refer to Insulin Regular *on page 849* monograph.

Patient Information Do not take any new medication during therapy unless approved by healthcare provider. This medication is used to control diabetes; it is not a cure. It is imperative to follow other components of prescribed treatment (eg, diet and exercise regimen). Take exactly as directed. Do not change dose or discontinue unless advised by healthcare provider. With insulin lispro (Humalog®), you must administer 15 minutes before meals or immediately after. If you experience hypoglycemic reaction, contact healthcare provider immediately. Always carry quick source of sugar with you. Monitor glucose levels as directed by healthcare provider. Report adverse side effects, including chest pain or palpitations; persistent fatigue, confusion, headache; skin rash or redness; numbness of mouth, lips, or tongue; muscle weakness or tremors; vision changes; respiratory difficulty; or nausea, vomiting, or flu-like symptoms.

Dosage Forms Excipient information presented when available (limited, particularly for generics); consult specific product labeling.

Injection, solution (Humalog®): 100 units/mL (3 mL) [prefilled cartridge or prefilled disposable pen]; (10 mL) [vial]

♦ **Insulin Lispro and Insulin Lispro Protamine** *see* Insulin Lispro Protamine and Insulin Lispro *on page 845*

Insulin Lispro Protamine and Insulin Lispro

(IN soo lin LYE sproe PROE ta meen & IN soo lin LYE sproe)

Medication Safety Issues

Sound-alike/look-alike issues:

Humalog® Mix 75/25™ may be confused with Humulin® 70/30.

High alert medication: The Institute for Safe Medication Practices (ISMP) includes this medication among its list of drugs which have a heightened risk of causing significant patient harm when used in error. ***Due to the number of insulin preparations, it is essential to identify/clarify the type of insulin to be used.***

Related Information

Insulin Regular *on page 849*

U.S. Brand Names Humalog® Mix 50/50™; Humalog® Mix 75/25™

Canadian Brand Names Humalog® Mix 25

Index Terms Insulin Lispro and Insulin Lispro Protamine

Therapeutic Category Antidiabetic Agent, Parenteral; Insulin, Combination

Generic Available No

Use Treatment of type 1 diabetes mellitus (insulin dependent, IDDM); type 2 diabetes mellitus (noninsulin dependent, NIDDM) to control hyperglycemia

(Continued)

Insulin Lispro Protamine and Insulin Lispro *(Continued)*

Pregnancy Risk Factor B

Lactation Excretion in breast milk unknown/compatible

Contraindications Hypersensitivity to insulin lispro, insulin lispro protamine, or any component; hypoglycemia

Warnings Refer to Insulin Regular *on page 849.* Not for I.V. infusion or use in insulin infusion pumps

Precautions Refer to Insulin Regular *on page 849.*

Adverse Reactions Refer to Insulin Regular *on page 849.*

Drug Interactions Refer to Insulin Regular *on page 849.*

Food Interactions Refer to Insulin Regular *on page 849.*

Stability Store unopened container or pen in refrigerator; do not freeze; protect from light. If refrigeration is not possible, vial (in use) may be stored at room temperature for up to 28 days. The pen (in use) should **not** be refrigerated; store below 30°C (86°F) away from direct heat or light; discard after 10 days. Do not mix or dilute with other insulins.

Mechanism of Action Refer to Insulin Regular *on page 849.* Insulin lispro protamine and insulin lispro is a combination product with a rapid onset and a duration of action which is similar to intermediate-acting insulin products.

Pharmacodynamics

Onset of action: 0.25-0.5 hours

Maximum effect: 2 hours

Duration: 18-24 hours

Pharmacokinetics

Time to peak serum concentration: 1 hour (median; range: 0.5-4 hours)

Elimination: Urine

Usual Dosage Refer to Insulin Regular *on page 849.* Fixed ratio insulins (such as insulin lispro protamine and insulin lispro combination) are normally administered in 2 daily doses with each dose intended to cover two meals and a snack. Because of variability in the peak affect and individual patient variability in activities, meals, etc, it may be more difficult to achieve complete glycemic control with fixed combination formulations in all patients.

Dosage adjustment in renal impairment: Insulin requirements are reduced with renal impairment; see Insulin Regular *on page 849.*

Administration Parenteral: SubQ: Gently roll vial or pen in the palms of the hands to resuspend before use; administer into the subcutaneous fat of the thighs, arms, buttocks, or abdomen, with sites rotated. Cold injections should be avoided. Administer within 15 minutes before a meal (breakfast and supper). Do not mix or dilute with other insulins. **Not for I.V. administration** or use in an insulin infusion pump.

Monitoring Parameters Refer to Insulin Regular *on page 849.*

Reference Range Refer to Insulin Regular *on page 849.*

Patient Information Refer to Insulin Regular *on page 849.*

Dosage Forms Excipient information presented when available (limited, particularly for generics); consult specific product labeling.

Injection, suspension:

Humalog® Mix 50/50™: Insulin lispro protamine suspension 50% [intermediate acting] and insulin lispro solution 50% [rapid acting]: 100 units/mL (3 mL) [disposable pen]

Humalog® Mix 75/25™: Insulin lispro protamine suspension 75% [intermediate acting] and insulin lispro solution 25% [rapid acting]: 100 units/mL (3 mL) [disposable pen]; (10 mL) [vial]

Insulin NPH (IN soo lin N P H)

Medication Safety Issues

Sound-alike/look-alike issues:

Humulin® may be confused with Humalog®, Humira®

Novolin® may be confused with NovoLog®

High alert medication: The Institute for Safe Medication Practices (ISMP) includes this medication among its list of drugs which have a heightened risk of causing significant patient harm when used in error. ***Due to the number of insulin preparations, it is essential to identify/clarify the type of insulin to be used.***

Related Information

Insulin Regular *on page 849*

U.S. Brand Names Humulin® N; Novolin® N
Canadian Brand Names Humulin® N; Novolin® ge NPH
Index Terms Isophane Insulin; NPH Insulin
Therapeutic Category Antidiabetic Agent, Insulin; Insulin, Intermediate-Acting
Generic Available No
Use Treatment of type 1 diabetes mellitus (insulin dependent, IDDM); type 2 diabetes mellitus (noninsulin dependent, NIDDM) to control hyperglycemia
Pregnancy Risk Factor B
Lactation Excretion in breast milk unknown/compatible
Contraindications Hypersensitivity to NPH insulin or any component
Warnings Refer to Insulin Regular *on page 849.*
Precautions Refer to Insulin Regular *on page 849.*
Adverse Reactions Refer to Insulin Regular *on page 849.*
Drug Interactions Refer to Insulin Regular *on page 849.*
Food Interactions Refer to Insulin Regular *on page 849.*
Stability Store unopened containers in refrigerator at 2°C to 8°C (36°F to 46°F); do not freeze; protect from direct heat or light. Once opened (in use), vials may be stored in refrigerator or at room temperature for up to 28 days. Cartridges should not be refrigerated; store below 30°C (86°F) away from direct heat or light; discard after 14 days. May be mixed with regular insulin, insulin lispro, insulin aspart, and insulin glulisine (always add the NPH insulin to the mixture last). A sterile diluent is available from the manufacturer for preparing dilutions of Humulin® N.
Mechanism of Action Refer to Insulin Regular *on page 849.* Insulin NPH is an intermediate-acting form of insulin.
Pharmacodynamics
Onset of action: 1-2 hours
Maximum effect: 6-14 hours
Duration: 18 to >24 hours
Pharmacokinetics
Elimination: Urine
Usual Dosage Refer to Insulin Regular *on page 849.* Insulin NPH is an intermediate-acting insulin formulation which is usually administered 1-2 times daily.
Dosing adjustment in renal impairment: Insulin requirements are reduced due to changes in insulin clearance or metabolism.
Administration Parenteral: SubQ: Gently roll vial or pen in the palms of the hands to resuspend before use; administer into the subcutaneous fat of the thighs, arms, buttocks, or abdomen, with sites rotated. Cold injections should be avoided. Administer within 15 minutes before a meal (before breakfast and supper). May be mixed with regular insulin, insulin aspart, insulin lispro, and insulin glulisine. **Not for I.V. administration** or use in insulin infusion pumps.
Monitoring Parameters Urine sugar and acetone, serum glucose, electrolytes, Hb A_{1c}, lipid profile
Reference Range Refer to Insulin Regular *on page 849.*
Patient Information Do not take any new medication during therapy unless approved by healthcare provider. This medication is used to control diabetes; it is not a cure. It is imperative to follow other components of prescribed treatment (eg, diet and exercise regimen). Take exactly as directed. Do not change dose or discontinue unless advised by healthcare provider. If you experience hypoglycemic reaction, contact healthcare provider immediately. Always carry quick source of sugar with you. Monitor glucose levels as directed by healthcare provider. Report adverse side effects, including chest pain or palpitations; persistent fatigue, confusion, headache; skin rash or redness; numbness of mouth, lips, or tongue; muscle weakness or tremors; vision changes; respiratory difficulty; or nausea, vomiting, or flu-like symptoms.
Dosage Forms Excipient information presented when available (limited, particularly for generics); consult specific product labeling. [CAN] = Canadian brand name
Injection, suspension:
Humulin® N: 100 units/mL (3 mL) [disposable pen]; (10 mL) [vial]
Novolin® ge NPH [CAN]: 100 units/mL (3 mL) [NovolinSet® prefilled syringe or PenFill® prefilled cartridge]; 10 mL [vial]
Novolin® N: 100 units/mL (3 mL) [InnoLet® prefilled syringe or PenFill® prefilled cartridge]; (10 mL) [vial]

Insulin NPH and Insulin Regular
(IN soo lin N P H & IN soo lin REG yoo ler)

Medication Safety Issues
Sound-alike/look-alike issues:
Humulin® 70/30 may be confused with Humalog® Mix 75/25
(Continued)

Insulin NPH and Insulin Regular *(Continued)*

Novolin® 70/30 may be confused with NovoLog® Mix 70/30

High alert medication: The Institute for Safe Medication Practices (ISMP) includes this medication among its list of drugs which have a heightened risk of causing significant patient harm when used in error. ***Due to the number of insulin preparations, it is essential to identify/clarify the type of insulin to be used.***

Related Information

Insulin Regular *on page 849*

U.S. Brand Names Humulin® 50/50; Humulin® 70/30; Novolin® 70/30

Canadian Brand Names Humulin® 20/80; Humulin® 70/30; Novolin® ge 10/90; Novolin® ge 20/80; Novolin® ge 30/70; Novolin® ge 40/60; Novolin® ge 50/50

Index Terms Insulin Regular and Insulin NPH; Isophane Insulin and Regular Insulin; NPH Insulin and Regular Insulin

Therapeutic Category Antidiabetic Agent, Parenteral; Insulin, Combination

Generic Available No

Use Treatment of type 1 diabetes mellitus (insulin dependent, IDDM); type 2 diabetes mellitus (noninsulin dependent, NIDDM) to control hyperglycemia

Pregnancy Risk Factor C

Contraindications Hypersensitivity to regular insulin, NPH insulin, or any component; hypoglycemia

Warnings Refer to Insulin Regular *on page 849*. Not for I.V. infusion or use in insulin infusion pumps.

Precautions Refer to Insulin Regular *on page 849.*

Adverse Reactions Refer to Insulin Regular *on page 849.*

Drug Interactions Refer to Insulin Regular *on page 849.*

Food Interactions Refer to Insulin Regular *on page 849.*

Stability Store unopened container in refrigerator; do not freeze; protect from light. If refrigeration is not possible, vial (in use) may be stored at room temperature for up to 28 days. The pen (in use) should **not** be refrigerated; store below 30°C (86°F) away from direct heat or light; discard after 10 days. Do not mix or dilute with other insulins.

Mechanism of Action Refer to Insulin Regular *on page 849*. Insulin NPH and insulin regular is a combination insulin product with intermediate-acting characteristics.

Pharmacodynamics

Onset of action:

Novolin® 70/30, Humulin® 70/30: 0.5 hours

Humulin® 50/50: 0.5-1 hour

Maximum effect:

Novolin® 70/30, Humulin® 70/30: 1.5-12 hours

Humulin® 50/50: 1.5-4.5 hours

Duration:

Novolin® 70/30, Humulin® 70/30: Up to 24 hours

Humulin® 50/50: 7.5-24 hours

Pharmacokinetics

Elimination: Urine

Usual Dosage Refer to Insulin Regular *on page 849*. Fixed ratio insulins (such as insulin aspart protamine and insulin aspart combination) are normally administered in 2 daily doses with each dose intended to cover two meals and a snack. Because of variability in the peak affect and individual patient variability in activities, meals, etc, it may be more difficult to achieve complete glycemic control using fixed combinations of insulins in all patients.

Dosing adjustment in renal impairment: Insulin requirements are reduced with renal impairment; see Insulin Regular *on page 849*

Administration Parenteral: SubQ: Gently roll vial or pen in the palms of the hands to resuspend before use; administer into the subcutaneous fat of the thighs, arms, buttocks, or abdomen, with sites rotated. Cold injections should be avoided. Administer within 15 minutes before a meal (before breakfast and supper). Do not mix or dilute with other insulins. **Not for I.V. administration** or use in an insulin infusion pump.

Monitoring Parameters Refer to Insulin Regular *on page 849.*

Reference Range Refer to Insulin Regular *on page 849.*

Patient Information Refer to Insulin Regular *on page 849.*

Dosage Forms Excipient information presented when available (limited, particularly for generics); consult specific product labeling.

Injection, suspension:

Humulin® 50/50: Insulin NPH suspension 50% [intermediate acting] and insulin regular solution 50% [short acting]: 100 units/mL (10 mL) [vial]

Humulin® 70/30: Insulin NPH suspension 70% [intermediate acting] and insulin regular solution 30% [short acting]: 100 units/mL (3 mL) [disposable pen]; (10 mL) [vial]

Novolin® 70/30: Insulin NPH suspension 70% [intermediate acting] and insulin regular solution 30% [short acting]: 100 units/mL (3 mL) [InnoLet® prefilled syringe or PenFill® prefilled cartridge]; (10 mL) [vial]

Additional formulations available in Canada: Injection, suspension:

Humulin® 20/80: Insulin regular solution 20% [short acting] and insulin NPH suspension 80% [intermediate acting]: 100 units/mL (3 mL) [PenFill® prefilled cartridge]

Novolin® ge 10/90: Insulin regular solution 10% [short acting] and insulin NPH suspension 90% [intermediate acting]: 100 units/mL (3 mL) [PenFill® prefilled cartridge]

Novolin® ge 20/80: Insulin regular solution 20% [short acting] and insulin NPH suspension 80% [intermediate acting]: 100 units/mL (3 mL) [PenFill® prefilled cartridge]

Novolin® ge 30/70: Insulin regular solution 30% [short acting] and insulin NPH suspension 70% [intermediate acting]: 100 units/mL (3 mL) [prefilled syringe or PenFill® prefilled cartridge]; (10 mL) [vial]

Novolin® ge 40/60: Insulin regular solution 40% [short acting] and insulin NPH suspension 60% [intermediate acting]: 100 units/mL (3 mL) [PenFill® prefilled cartridge]

Novolin® ge 50/50: Insulin regular solution 50% [short acting] and insulin NPH suspension 50% [intermediate acting]: 100 units/mL (3 mL) [PenFill® prefilled cartridge]

Insulin Regular (IN soo lin REG yoo ler)

Medication Safety Issues

Sound-alike/look-alike issues:

Humulin® may be confused with Humalog®, Humira®

Novolin® may be confused with NovoLog®

High alert medication: The Institute for Safe Medication Practices (ISMP) includes this medication among its list of drugs which have a heightened risk of causing significant patient harm when used in error. ***Due to the number of insulin preparations, it is essential to identify/clarify the type of insulin to be used.***

Concentrated solutions (eg, U-500) should not be available in patient care areas.

Related Information

Insulin Aspart *on page 836*
Insulin Aspart Protamine and Insulin Aspart *on page 838*
Insulin Detemir *on page 839*
Insulin Glargine *on page 840*
Insulin Glulisine *on page 841*
Insulin Inhalation *on page 842*
Insulin Lispro *on page 844*
Insulin Lispro Protamine and Insulin Lispro *on page 845*
Insulin NPH *on page 846*
Insulin NPH and Insulin Regular *on page 847*

U.S. Brand Names Humulin® R; Humulin® R (Concentrated) U-500; Novolin® R

Canadian Brand Names Humulin® R; Novolin® ge Toronto

Index Terms Regular Insulin

Therapeutic Category Antidiabetic Agent, Parenteral; Antidote; Hyperkalemia, Adjunctive Treatment Agent; Insulin, Short-Acting

Generic Available No

Use Treatment of insulin-dependent diabetes mellitus, also noninsulin-dependent diabetes mellitus unresponsive to treatment with diet and/or oral hypoglycemics; to assure proper utilization of glucose and reduce glucosuria in nondiabetic patients receiving parenteral nutrition (glucosuria cannot be adequately controlled with infusion rate adjustments or requires assistance in achieving optimal caloric intakes); treatment of hyperkalemia (use with glucose to shift potassium into cells to lower serum potassium levels)

Pregnancy Risk Factor B

Lactation Excretion in breast milk unknown/compatible

Contraindications Hypersensitivity to regular insulin or any component; hypoglycemia

Warnings Hypoglycemia is the most common adverse effect of insulin. The timing of hypoglycemia differs among various insulin formulations. Any change of insulin should be made cautiously; changing manufacturers, type, and/or method of manufacture may result in the need for a change of dosage. Human insulin differs from

(Continued)

Insulin Regular *(Continued)*

animal-source insulin. Hypoglycemia may result from increased work or exercise without eating; use of long-acting insulin preparations (insulin glargine, Ultralente®) with regular insulin may delay recovery from hypoglycemia.

Precautions Use with caution and adjust dosage in patients with renal impairment; use with caution and monitor closely in patient with hepatic impairment. While regular insulin is the preferred formulation for I.V. administration, both insulin aspart and insulin glulisine have been approved for I.V. use in selected clinical situations with close medical supervision and monitoring of serum potassium.

Adverse Reactions Primarily symptoms of hypoglycemia

Cardiovascular: Palpitation, pallor, tachycardia

Central nervous system: Fatigue, headache, hypothermia, loss of consciousness, mental confusion

Dermatologic: Urticaria, redness

Endocrine & metabolic: Hypoglycemia, hypokalemia

Gastrointestinal: Hunger, nausea, numbness of mouth

Local: Atrophy or hypertrophy of SubQ fat tissue; edema, itching, pain or warmth at injection site; stinging

Neuromuscular & skeletal: Muscle weakness, paresthesia, tremor

Ocular: Transient presbyopia or blurred vision

Miscellaneous: Anaphylaxis, diaphoresis, local and/or systemic hypersensitivity reactions

Drug Interactions Cytochrome P450 isoenzyme CYP1A2 inducer (weak)

Drugs which **DECREASE** hypoglycemic effect of insulin: Acetazolamide, alcohol (chronic use), antiretrovirals, asparaginases, calcitonin, contraceptives (oral), corticosteroids, cyclophosphamide, danazol, diazoxide, diltiazem, dobutamine, epinephrine, ethacrynic acid, isoniazid, lithium, morphine, niacin, nicotine, phenothiazines, phenytoin, somatropin, terbutaline, thiazide diuretics, thyroid hormone

Drugs which **INCREASE** hypoglycemic effect of insulin: ACE inhibitors, alcohol (acute use), alpha-blockers, anabolic steroids, beta-blockers, calcium, chloroquine, clofibrate, fluoxetine, guanethidine, lithium, MAO inhibitors, mebendazole, octreotide, pentamidine, phenylbutazone, propoxyphene, pyridoxine, salicylates, sulfinpyrazone, sulfonamides, and tetracyclines.

Note: Nonselective beta-blockers may delay recovery from hypoglycemic episodes and mask signs/symptoms of hypoglycemia. Cardioselective agents may be alternatives. Insulin increases the risk of hypoglycemia associated with oral hypoglycemic agents (including sulfonylureas, metformin, pioglitazone, rosiglitazone, and troglitazone).

Food Interactions Use caution with chromium, garlic, gymnema (may increase hypoglycemia).

Stability Store unopened containers in refrigerator at 2°C to 8°C (36°F to 46°F); do not freeze; protect from direct heat or light. Once opened (in use) vials may be stored in refrigerator or at room temperature for up to 28 days. Regular insulin should only be used if clear. May be mixed in the same syringe with NPH, Lente®, and Ultralente® insulins. For I.V. continuous infusion, may be diluted in NS, $^1/_2$NS, D_5W, or $D_{10}W$.

Stability of parenteral admixture of regular insulin in NS or $^1/_2$NS at room temperature (25°C) and at refrigeration temperature (4°C): 24 hours; all bags should be prepared fresh; tubing should be flushed 30 minutes prior to administration to allow adsorption as time permits. See Administration.

Mechanism of Action Insulin acts via specific membrane-bound receptors on target tissues to regulate metabolism of carbohydrate, protein, and fats. Insulin facilitates entry of glucose into muscle, adipose, and other tissues via hexose transporters, including GLUT4. Insulin stimulates the cellular uptake of amino acids and increases cellular permeability to several ions, including potassium, magnesium, and phosphate. By activating sodium-potassium ATPases, insulin promotes the intracellular movement of potassium.

Target organs for insulin include the liver, skeletal muscle, and adipose tissue. Within the liver, insulin stimulates hepatic glycogen synthesis through the activation of the enzymes hexokinase, phosphofructokinase, and glycogen synthase as well as the inhibition of glucose-6 phosphatase. Insulin promotes hepatic synthesis of fatty acids, which are released into the circulation as lipoproteins. Skeletal muscle effects of insulin include increased protein synthesis and increased glycogen synthesis. Within adipose tissue, insulin stimulates the processing of circulating lipoproteins to provide free fatty acids, facilitating triglyceride synthesis and storage by adipocytes. Insulin also directly inhibits the hydrolysis of triglycerides.

Normally secreted by the pancreas, insulin products are manufactured for pharmacologic use through recombinant DNA technology using either *E. coli* or *Saccharomyces cerevisiae*. Insulins are categorized based on promptness and duration of effect, including rapid-, short-, intermediate-, and long-acting insulins. Regular insulin is considered a "short-acting" insulin.

Pharmacodynamics Onset and duration of hypoglycemic effects depend upon the route of administration (adsorption and onset of action are more rapid after deeper I.M. injections than after SubQ), site of injection (onset and duration are progressively slower with SubQ injection into the abdomen, arm, buttock, or thigh respectively), volume and concentration of injection, and the preparation administered; local heat and massage also increase the rate of absorption.

Onset of action: Approximately 30-60 minutes

Maximum effect: 1-5 hours

Duration: 6-10 hours (may increase with dose)

Pharmacokinetics

Distribution: V_d: 0.26-0.36 L/kg

Half-life: SubQ: 1.5 hours

Excretion: Urine

Usual Dosage The general objective of insulin replacement therapy is to approximate the physiologic pattern of insulin secretion. This requires a basal level of insulin throughout the day, supplemented by additional insulin at mealtimes. Since combinations using different types of insulins are frequently used, dosage adjustment must address the individual component of the insulin regimen which most directly influences the blood glucose value in question, based on the known onset and duration of the insulin component. The frequency of doses and monitoring must be individualized in consideration of the patient's ability to manage therapy. Diabetic education and nutritional counseling are essential to maximize the effectiveness of therapy.

Type 1 diabetes mellitus: Children and Adults: **Note:** Multiple daily doses guided by blood glucose monitoring are the standard of diabetes care. The following daily doses are expressed as the total units/kg/day of all insulin formulations used.

Initial dose: SubQ: 0.2-0.6 units/kg/day in divided doses. Conservative initial doses of 0.2-0.4 units/kg/day are often recommended to avoid the potential for hypoglycemia. Regular insulin may be the only insulin formulation used initially.

Division of daily insulin requirement ("conventional therapy"): Generally, 50% to 75% of the daily insulin dose is given as an intermediate- or long-acting form of insulin (in 1-2 daily injections). The remaining portion of the 24-hour insulin requirement is divided and administered as either regular insulin or a rapid acting form of insulin at the same time before breakfast and dinner.

Division of daily insulin requirement ("intensive therapy"): Basal insulin delivery with one or two doses of intermediate- or long-acting insulin formulations superimposed with doses of rapid or very rapid-acting insulin formulations three or more times daily.

Adjustment of dose: Dosage must be titrated to achieve glucose control and avoid hypoglycemia. Adjust dose to maintain premeal and bedtime glucose in target range (see Reference Range). Since combinations of agents are frequently used, dosage adjustment must address the individual component of the insulin regimen which most directly influences the blood glucose value in question, based on the known onset and duration of the insulin component.

Usual maintenance range: 0.5-1 unit/kg/day in divided doses. An estimate of anticipated needs may be based on body weight and/or activity factors as follows:

Adolescents: May require ≤1.2 units/kg/day during growth spurts

Nonobese: 0.4-0.6 units/kg/day

Obese: 0.8-1.2 units/kg/day

Continuous SubQ insulin infusion (insulin pump): Regular insulin, insulin lispro, insulin aspart, and insulin glulisine: Combination of a "basal" continuous insulin infusion rate using one of these insulin formulations with preprogrammed, premeal bolus doses which are patient controlled. When converting from multiple daily SubQ doses of maintenance insulin, it is advisable to reduce the basal rate to less than the equivalent of the total daily units of longer acting insulin, eg NPH. Divide the total number of units by 24 to get the basal rate in units/hour. Do not include the total units of regular insulin or other rapid-acting insulin formulations in this calculation. The same premeal regular insulin dosage may be used.

Type 2 diabetes mellitus: Augmentation therapy (patients for which diet, exercise, weight reduction, and oral hypoglycemics have not been adequate): Adults: Initial dosage of 0.15-0.2 units/kg/day (10-12 units) of an intermediate- or long-acting insulin administered at bedtime has been recommended. As an alternative, regular insulin or rapid-acting insulin formulations administered before meals have also been used. Dosage must be carefully adjusted.

Diabetic ketoacidosis:

Children: I.V. continuous infusion: 0.05-0.1 units/kg/hour (range: 0.05-0.2 units/kg/hour) depending upon the rate of decrease of serum glucose (decreasing the serum glucose level too rapidly may lead to cerebral edema; optimum rate of

(Continued)

Insulin Regular *(Continued)*

decrease of serum glucose 80-100 mg/dL/hour). Continue infusion until acidosis clears (pH >7.3 and HCO_3 >25 mEq/L), not when the blood glucose normalizes. SubQ therapy may begin when the HCO_3 >16 mE/L, pH >7.3, and/or anion gap <16mEq/L. Continue I.V. insulin infusion until the onset of the SubQ insulin dose (for regular insulin: 30-60 minutes).

Adults: I.V.: Regular insulin 0.15 units/kg (approximately 15-20 units) initially followed by an infusion of 0.1 units/kg/hour (approximately 7 units/hour); increase infusion rate achieve glucose serum reduction of 50-70 mg/dL/hour. Decrease dose to 0.05-0.1 units/kg/hour once serum glucose reaches 250 mg/dL and ketoacidosis/acid-base abnormalities have resolved.

Note: Newly-diagnosed patients with IDDM presenting in DKA and patients with blood sugars <800 mg/dL may be relatively "sensitive" to insulin and should receive loading and initial maintenance doses ~50% of those indicated.

Optimization of caloric intake while on parenteral nutrition: Neonates: Continuous I.V. infusion: 0.01-0.1 units/kg/hour; neonates are very sensitive to insulin; start at low end of infusion rate and monitor closely

Hyperkalemia (after treatment with calcium and sodium bicarbonate; unlabeled use):

Children: Dextrose 0.5-1 g/kg (using 25% or 50% dextrose) combined with regular insulin 1 unit for every 4-5 g dextrose; infuse over 2 hours **OR** as an alternative, dextrose 0.5-1 g/kg infused over 15-30 minutes followed by 0.1 unit/kg insulin SubQ or I.V.

Adults: I.V.: 50% dextrose at 0.1-1 mL/kg and regular insulin 1 unit for every 4-5 g dextrose administered

Dosing adjustment in renal impairment (regular): Insulin requirements are reduced due to changes in insulin clearance or metabolism

Cl_{cr} 10-50 mL/minute: Administer at 75% of recommended dose

Cl_{cr} <10 mL/minute: Administer at 25% to 50% of recommended dose and monitor glucose closely

Hemodialysis: Because of a large molecular weight (6000 daltons), insulin is not significantly removed by either peritoneal or hemodialysis; supplemental dose is not necessary

Peritoneal dialysis: Supplemental dose is not necessary

Continuous arteriovenous or venovenous hemofiltration effects: Supplemental dose is not necessary

Administration Parenteral:

SubQ, I.M.: Administration is usually made into the subcutaneous fat of the thighs, arms, buttocks, or abdomen, with sites rotated; may be administered I.M. however, SubQ is the preferred route. When mixing regular insulin with other insulin preparations, regular insulin should be drawn into the syringe first; administer 30-60 minutes before meals. May be infused SubQ by external insulin pump; however, when used in an external pump, it is not recommended to be diluted with other solutions.

I.V.: Regular insulin is the preferred insulin formulation approved for I.V. administration (insulin aspart and insulin glulisine have been approved for I.V. administration in carefully controlled clinical settings with medical supervision and close monitoring of blood glucose as well as serum potassium); to minimize absorption of insulin to I.V. solution bag or tubing:

If new tubing is **not** needed: Wait a minimum of 30 minutes between the preparation of the solution and the initiation of the infusion.

If new tubing is needed: After receiving the insulin continuous infusion solution, the administration set should be attached to the I.V. container and the line should be flushed with the insulin solution, wait 30 minutes, then flush the line again with the insulin solution prior to initiating the infusion.

Because of adsorption, the actual amount of insulin being administered could be substantially less than the apparent amount. Therefore, adjustment of the insulin drip rate should be based on the effect and not solely on the apparent insulin dose. Furthermore, the apparent I.V. infusion dose should not be used as the basis for determining the subsequent insulin dose upon discontinuing the insulin drip. Dosage adjustment requires continuous medical supervision.

Monitoring Parameters Urine sugar and acetone, serum glucose, electrolytes, Hb A_{1c}, lipid profile

DKA: Arterial blood gases (initial), venous pH, CBC with differential, urinalysis, serum glucose (baseline and every hour until reaches 250 mg/dL), BUN, creatinine, electrolytes, anion gap, I&O

Hyperkalemia: Serum potassium and glucose must be closely monitored to avoid hypoglycemia and/or hypokalemia.

Reference Range

Glucose, fasting:

Newborns: 30-90 mg/dL

Adults: 70-110 mg/dL

Recommendations for glycemic control with type 1 diabetes:

Hb A_{1c}:

<6 years: ≤8.5% and ≥7.5%

6-12 years: <8%

13-19 years: <7.5%

Adults: <7%

Plasma glucose*:

Preprandial:

<6 years: 90-130 mg/dL

6-12 years: 90-180 mg/dL

13 years to Adults: 90-130 mg/dL

Bedtime and overnight:

<6 years: 110-200 mg/dL

6-12 years: 100-180 mg/dL

13-19 years: 90-150 mg/dL

Peak postprandial** : Adults: <180 mg/dL

*Plasma glucose concentrations are generally 10% to 15% higher than those in whole blood

**Peak postprandial plasma glucose is measured 1-2 hours after a meal

Criteria for diagnosis of DKA:

Serum glucose:

Children: >200 mg/dL

Adults: >250 mg/dL

Arterial pH:

Children: <7.3

Adults: <7-7.24

Bicarbonate:

Children: <15 mEq/L

Adults: <10-15 mEq/L

Moderate ketonuria or ketonemia

Patient Information Do not take any new medication during therapy unless approved by healthcare provider. This medication is used to control diabetes; it is not a cure. It is imperative to follow other components of prescribed treatment (eg, diet and exercise regimen). Take exactly as directed. Do not change dose or discontinue unless advised by healthcare provider. If you experience hypoglycemic reaction, contact healthcare provider immediately. Always carry quick source of sugar with you. Monitor glucose levels as directed by healthcare provider. Report adverse side effects, including chest pain or palpitations; persistent fatigue, confusion, headache; skin rash or redness; numbness of mouth, lips, or tongue; muscle weakness or tremors; vision changes; respiratory difficulty; or nausea, vomiting, or flu-like symptoms.

Additional Information In mild diabetic ketoacidosis or unusual circumstances, for patients without I.V. access, SubQ or I.M. regular insulin has been used. Doses are similar to the doses recommended for bolus and the hourly infusion (total dose administered once per hour). If volume depletion and secondary sympathetic activation decrease local perfusion, insulin absorption may be inconsistent. For this reason, many clinicians do not recommend this approach.

Dosage Forms Excipient information presented when available (limited, particularly for generics); consult specific product labeling.

Injection, solution:

Humulin® R: 100 units/mL (10 mL) [vial]

Novolin® R: 100 units/mL (3 mL) [InnoLet® prefilled syringe or PenFill® prefilled cartridge]; (10 mL) [vial]

Injection, solution [concentrate]:

Humulin® R U-500: 500 units/mL (20 mL vial)

References

American Diabetes Association, "Standards of Medical Care in Diabetes," *Diabetes Care*, 2007, 30(Suppl 1):4-41.

Simeon PS, Geffner ME, Levin SR, et al, "Continuous Insulin Infusions in Neonates: Pharmacologic Availability of Insulin in Intravenous Solutions," *J Pediatr*, 1994, 124(5 Pt 1):818-20.

♦ **Insulin Regular and Insulin NPH** *see* Insulin NPH and Insulin Regular *on page 847*

♦ **Intal®** *see* Cromolyn *on page 407*

♦ **α-2-interferon** *see* Interferon Alfa-2b *on page 856*

Interferon Alfa-2a (in ter FEER on AL fa too aye)

Medication Safety Issues
Sound-alike/look-alike issues:
Interferon alfa-2a may be confused with interferon alfa-2b, interferon alfa-n3, pegylated interferon alfa-2b
Roferon-A® may be confused with Rocephin®
International issues:
Interferon alfa-2a may be confused with interferon alpha multi-subtype which is available in international markets

U.S. Brand Names Roferon®-A

Canadian Brand Names Roferon®-A

Index Terms IFLrA; Interferon Alpha-2a; NSC-367982; rIFN-A

Therapeutic Category Antineoplastic Agent, Miscellaneous; Biological Response Modulator; Interferon

Generic Available No

Use FDA approved in patients >18 years of age: Hairy cell leukemia, AIDS-related Kaposi's sarcoma, chronic hepatitis C, Philadelphia chromosome-positive chronic myelogenous leukemia (within 1 year of diagnosis); multiple unlabeled uses: hemangiomas of infancy

Medication Guide An FDA-approved patient medication guide, which is available with the product information and at http://www.fda.gov/cder/Offices/ODS/medication_guides.htm, must be dispensed with this medication for each new outpatient prescription and refill.

Pregnancy Risk Factor C

Lactation Enters breast milk/not recommended (AAP rates "compatible")

Contraindications Hypersensitivity to alpha interferon or any component (see Warnings); autoimmune hepatitis, hepatic decompensation (Child-Pugh class B and C)

Warnings The FDA currently recommends that procedures for proper handling and disposal of antineoplastic agents be considered. Interferon alfa-2a may cause life-threatening neuropsychiatric, autoimmune, and infectious disorders. Depression, suicidal ideation, suicidal attempts, and suicides in association with interferon alfa-2a therapy in patients with and without previous psychiatric symptoms have been reported. Patients should be monitored closely and those patients with persistently severe or worsening symptoms of these conditions should be withdrawn from therapy. Alpha interferons suppress bone marrow function which may result in severe cytopenias or aplastic anemia. Discontinue alpha interferon in patients who develop severe decreases in neutrophil count or platelet counts. Ophthalmologic disorders including vision loss, retinopathy, optic neuritis, and papilledema have occurred; close monitoring is advised. Development of autoimmune diseases including vasculitis, ITP, rheumatoid arthritis, SLE, and hepatitis have been reported in patients on alfa interferon. Safety and efficacy in children <18 years of age have not been established.

Interferon alfa-2a injection contains benzyl alcohol which may cause allergic reactions in susceptible individuals; large amounts of benzyl alcohol (≥99 mg/kg/day) have been associated with a potentially fatal toxicity ("gasping syndrome") in neonates; the "gasping syndrome" consists of metabolic acidosis, respiratory distress, gasping respirations, CNS dysfunction (including convulsions, intracranial hemorrhage), hypotension and cardiovascular collapse; use interferon alfa-2a products containing benzyl alcohol with caution in neonates; *in vitro* and animal studies have shown that benzoate, a metabolite of benzyl alcohol, displaces bilirubin from protein binding sites

Precautions Use with caution in patients with seizure disorders, pulmonary function impairment, psychiatric disorders, brain metastases, multiple sclerosis, compromised CNS, and patients with pre-existing cardiac disease, myelosuppression, or severe renal impairment (Cl_{cr} <50 mL/minute) and hepatic impairment. Use with caution in patients with diabetes or pre-existing thyroid disease. Discontinue if unexplained or persistent pulmonary infiltrates are noted.

Adverse Reactions Flu-like symptoms (fever, fatigue/malaise, myalgia, chills, headache, arthralgia, rigors) begin about 2-6 hours after the dose is given and may persist as long as 24 hours; severity of flu-like symptoms increase with higher dosages; usually patient can build up a tolerance to side effects

Cardiovascular: Tachycardia, arrhythmias, hypotension, edema, chest pain, syncope, cardiomyopathy, MI, vasculitis
Central nervous system: Fatigue/malaise, dizziness, depression, confusion, sensory neuropathy, psychiatric symptoms (psychosis, mania, depression, suicidal behavior), fever, headache, EEG abnormalities, chills, impaired memory, agitation
Dermatologic: Partial alopecia, rash, dry skin, pruritus, urticaria, angioedema

Endocrine & metabolic: Elevated uric acid level, thyroid dysfunction, hyperglycemia, hypertriglyceridemia, weight loss, growth retardation

Gastrointestinal: Anorexia, xerostomia, nausea, vomiting, diarrhea, abdominal cramps, dysgeusia, stomatitis, GI hemorrhage, ulcerative colitis, pancreatitis

Hematologic: Leukopenia (mainly neutropenia); anemia; thrombocytopenia; neutralizing antibodies

Hepatic: Elevated ALT and AST, hepatitis, ascites

Local: Burning, pain, erythema, pruritus, rash at the site of injection

Neuromuscular & skeletal: Myalgia, arthralgia, rigors, leg cramps, spastic diplegia

Ocular: Blurred vision, retinal hemorrhage, optic neuritis, papilledema

Renal: Proteinuria, elevated BUN and serum creatinine, interstitial nephritis

Respiratory: Coughing, nasal congestion, dyspnea, pulmonary infiltrates, interstitial pneumonitis

Miscellaneous: Diaphoresis, anaphylaxis, SLE, flu-like symptoms

Drug Interactions Cytochrome P450 isoenzyme CYP1A2 inhibitor (weak)

Interferon Alfa-2b: Possible competitive binding to same receptors

Acyclovir: Possible synergistic effects

Interleukin-2: May increase risk of renal failure.

Theophylline: Clearance of theophylline is reduced

Vinblastine: May increase interferon toxicity; increased neurotoxicity

Zidovudine: Possible additive myelosuppression

Stability Store in refrigerator; do not freeze; do not shake; after reconstitution stable at room temperature for 24 hours; do not store in syringes for prolonged periods

Mechanism of Action Inhibits cellular growth, alters the state of cellular differentiation, interferes with oncogene expression, alters cell surface antigen expression, increases phagocytic activity of macrophages and augments cytotoxicity of lymphocytes for target cells

Pharmacokinetics

Absorption: I.M., SubQ: >80%

Metabolism: In the kidney, filtered, and absorbed at the renal tubule

Half-life:

- I.M., I.V.: 2 hours
- SubQ: 3 hours

Time to peak serum concentration: Within 3-8 hours

Usual Dosage Refer to individual protocols

Infants and Children:

- Hemangiomas of infancy, pulmonary hemangiomatosis: SubQ: 1-3 million units/m^2/day once daily
- Philadelphia chromosome-positive CML: I.M., SubQ: 2.5-5 million units/m^2 daily
- Chronic hepatitis B: SubQ: 5-10 million units/m^2 3 times/week
- Chronic hepatitis C: SubQ: 3 million units/m^2 3 times/week

Children >18 years and Adults: I.M., SubQ:

- Hairy cell leukemia: Induction dose is 3 million units/day for 16-24 weeks; maintenance: 3 million units 3 times/week
- AIDS-related Kaposi's sarcoma: Induction dose: 36 million units/day for 10-12 weeks; maintenance: 36 million units 3 times/week (may begin with dose escalation from 3 to 9 to 18 million units each day over 3 consecutive days followed by 36 million units/day for the remainder of the 10-12 weeks of induction); **or** 20 million units/m^2 daily for 4 weeks, then if responding, 20 million units/m^2 3 times/week
- CML: 9 million units daily
- Hepatitis C: Initial: 6 million units 3 times/week for 3 months followed by 3 million units 3 times/week for 9 months or 3 million units 3 times/week for 12 months

Melanoma: 12 million units/m^2 3 times/week for 3 months

Administration Parenteral: SubQ (rather than I.M.) administration is suggested for those patients who are at risk for bleeding or are thrombocytopenic; rotate SubQ injection site to help minimize local reactions

Monitoring Parameters Baseline EKG, CBC with differential and platelet count, hemoglobin, hematocrit, blood glucose, electrolytes, TSH levels, triglyceride levels, liver and renal function tests, weight, neuropsychiatric monitoring (including depressive symptomatology), chest x-ray, ophthalmologic exam

Patient Information Do not change brands as changes in dosage may result; possible mental status changes may occur while on therapy. Report any signs of depression or suicidal ideation to your physician. May cause drowsiness and dizziness impairing ability to perform activities requiring mental alertness or physical coordination. May cause dry mouth

Nursing Implications Patient should be well hydrated; pretreatment with NSAIDs or acetaminophen can decrease fever and its severity and alleviate headache

Additional Information Indications and dosage regimens are specific for a particular brand of interferon; other brands of interferon (ie, Intron® A) have different indications

(Continued)

Interferon Alfa-2a *(Continued)*

and dosage guidelines; do not change brands of interferon as changes in dosage may result

Dosage Forms Excipient information presented when available (limited, particularly for generics); consult specific product labeling.

Injection, solution:

Roferon®-A: 3 million units/0.5 mL (0.5 mL) [contains benzyl alcohol and polysorbate 80]; 6 million units/0.5 mL (0.5 mL) [contains benzyl alcohol and polysorbate 80]; 9 million units/0.5 mL (0.5 mL) [contains benzyl alcohol and polysorbate 80]

References

Ezekowitz RAB, Mulliken JB, and Folkman J, "Interferon Alfa-2a Therapy for Life-Threatening Hemangiomas of Infancy," *N Engl J Med*, 1992, 326(22):1456-63.

Jonas MM, Ott MJ, Nelson SP, et al, "Interferon-Alpha Treatment of Chronic Hepatitis C Virus Infection in Children," *Pediatr Infect Dis J*, 1998, 17(3):241-6.

Ozen H, Kocak N, Yuce A, et al, "Retreatment With Higher Dose Interferon Alpha in Children With Chronic Hepatitis B Infection," *Pediatr Infect Dis J*, 1999, 18(8):694-7.

White CW, Sondheimer HM, Crouch EC, et al, "Treatment of Pulmonary Hemangiomatosis With Recombinant Interferon Alfa-2a," *N Engl J Med*, 1989, 320(18):1197-200.

Interferon Alfa-2b (in ter FEER on AL fa too bee)

Medication Safety Issues

Sound-alike/look-alike issues:

Interferon alfa-2b may be confused with interferon alfa-2a, interferon alfa-n3, pegylated interferon alfa-2b

Intron® A may be confused with PEG-Intron®

International issues:

Interferon alfa-2b may be confused with interferon alpha multi-subtype which is available in international markets

U.S. Brand Names Intron® A

Canadian Brand Names Intron® A

Index Terms α-2-interferon; INF-alpha 2; Interferon Alpha-2b; NSC-377523; rLFN-α2

Therapeutic Category Antineoplastic Agent, Miscellaneous; Biological Response Modulator; Interferon

Generic Available No

Use

Patients ≥1 year of age: Chronic hepatitis B

Patients ≥18 years of age: Induce hairy cell leukemia remission; treatment of AIDS-related Kaposi's sarcoma; condylomata acuminata; adjuvant therapy of melanoma following surgical excision; chronic hepatitis C

Multiple unlabeled uses: Hemangiomas of infancy

Medication Guide An FDA-approved patient medication guide, which is available with the product information and at http://www.fda.gov/cder/Offices/ODS/medication_guides.htm, must be dispensed with this medication for each new outpatient prescription and refill.

Pregnancy Risk Factor C

Lactation Enters breast milk/not recommended (AAP rates "compatible")

Contraindications Hypersensitivity to interferon alfa or any component (see Warnings); autoimmune hepatitis, hepatic decompensation, immunosuppressed transplant patients, patients with visceral AIDS-related Kaposi's sarcoma associated with rapidly-progressing or life-threatening disease

Warnings Safety and efficacy in children <18 years of age have not been established. The FDA currently recommends that procedures for proper handling and disposal of antineoplastic agents be considered. Alpha interferons suppress bone marrow function which may result in severe cytopenias or aplastic anemia. Alpha interferons may cause or aggravate fatal or life-threatening neuropsychiatric, autoimmune, ischemic, and infectious disorders. Depression, suicidal ideation, suicidal attempts, and suicides in association with interferon alfa therapy in patients with and without previous psychiatric symptoms has been reported. Suicidal ideation or attempts may occur more frequently in pediatric patients as compared to adults. Patients should be monitored closely and those patients with severe or worsening signs or symptoms of these conditions should be withdrawn from therapy.

Ophthalmologic disorders including vision loss, retinopathy, optic neuritis, and papilledema have occurred; close monitoring is advised. Development of autoimmune diseases including vasculitis, ITP, rheumatoid arthritis, SLE, and hepatitis have been reported in patients on alfa interferon. Avoid use in patients with autoimmune disorders.

Diluent for interferon alfa-2b injection may contain benzyl alcohol which can cause allergic reactions in susceptible individuals; large amounts of benzyl alcohol (≥99 mg/kg/day) have been associated with a potentially fatal toxicity ("gasping syndrome") in neonates; the "gasping syndrome" consists of metabolic acidosis, respiratory distress, gasping respirations, CNS dysfunction (including convulsions, intracranial hemorrhage), hypotension and cardiovascular collapse; avoid use of interferon alfa-2b products containing benzyl alcohol in neonates; *in vitro* and animal studies have shown that benzoate, a metabolite of benzyl alcohol, displaces bilirubin from protein binding sites

Precautions Use with caution in patients with pulmonary function impairment, seizure disorders, brain metastases, compromised CNS, multiple sclerosis, arrhythmias, and patients with pre-existing cardiac disease, severe renal dysfunction (Cl_{cr} <50 mL/minute), hepatic impairment, or myelosuppression. Use caution in patients with diabetes, pre-existing thyroid disease, coagulopathy, hypertension, or in patients receiving drugs that may cause lactic acidosis.

Adverse Reactions Flu-like symptoms (fever, fatigue/malaise, myalgia, chills, headache, arthralgia, rigors) begin about 2-6 hours after the dose is given and may persist as long as 24 hours; usually patient can build up a tolerance to side effects

Cardiovascular: Tachycardia, arrhythmias, hypotension, edema, chest pain, syncope, cardiomyopathy, MI, vasculitis

Central nervous system: Fatigue/malaise, dizziness, depression, confusion, sensory neuropathy, psychiatric symptoms (psychosis, mania, depression, suicidal behavior), fever, headache, EEG abnormalities, chills, impaired memory, agitation

Dermatologic: Partial alopecia, rash, pruritus, dry skin, urticaria, angioedema

Endocrine & metabolic: Elevated uric acid level, thyroid dysfunction, hyperglycemia, hypertriglyceridemia, weight loss, growth retardation

Gastrointestinal: Anorexia, xerostomia, nausea, vomiting, diarrhea, abdominal cramps, dysgeusia, stomatitis, GI hemorrhage, ulcerative colitis, pancreatitis

Hematologic: Leukopenia (mainly neutropenia); anemia; thrombocytopenia; neutralizing antibodies

Hepatic: Elevated ALT and AST, hepatitis, ascites

Local: Burning, pain, erythema, pruritus, rash at the site of injection

Neuromuscular & skeletal: Myalgia, arthralgia, rigors, leg cramps, tendonitis, spondylitis

Ocular: Blurred vision, retinal hemorrhage, optic neuritis, papilledema

Renal: Proteinuria, elevated BUN and serum creatinine, interstitial nephritis

Respiratory: Coughing, nasal congestion, dyspnea, pulmonary infiltrates, interstitial pneumonitis

Miscellaneous: Diaphoresis, anaphylaxis, flu-like symptoms, SLE

Drug Interactions Cytochrome P450 isoenzyme CYP1A2 inhibitor (weak)

Interferon Alfa-2a: May competitively bind to same receptors

Interleukin 2: May increase risk of renal failure

Acyclovir: Possible synergistic effect

Theophylline: Clearance of theophylline is reduced

Vinblastine: May increase interferon toxicity; increased neurotoxicity

Zidovudine: Possible additive myelosuppression

Stability Refrigerate; do not freeze; do not shake; reconstituted solution from powder for injection is stable for 24 hours when refrigerated; after first use of prefilled pen, discard unused portion after 1 month

Mechanism of Action Inhibits cellular growth, alters the state of cellular differentiation, interferes with oncogene expression, alters cell surface antigen expression, increases phagocytic activity of macrophages, and augments cytotoxicity of lymphocytes for target cells

Pharmacokinetics

Metabolism: Majority of dose is thought to be metabolized in the kidney, filtered and absorbed at the renal tubule

Bioavailability:
- I.M.: 83%
- SubQ: 90%

Half-life, elimination:
- I.M., I.V.: 2 hours
- SubQ: 3 hours

Time to peak serum concentration: I.M., SubQ: ~3-8 hours

Usual Dosage Refer to individual protocols:

Children: SubQ:
- Chronic hepatitis B: 3-10 million units/m^2 3 times/week
- Chronic hepatitis C: 3-5 million units/m^2 3 times/week
- Hemangiomas: 3 million units/m^2 daily

Adults:
- Hairy cell leukemia: I.M., SubQ: 2 million units/m^2 3 times/week
- AIDS-related Kaposi's sarcoma: I.M., SubQ: 30 million units/m^2 3 times/week or 50 million units/m^2 I.V. 5 days/week every other week

(Continued)

Interferon Alfa-2b *(Continued)*

Condylomata acuminata: Intralesionally: 1 million units/lesion 3 times/week for 3 weeks; not to exceed 5 million units per treatment (maximum dose: 5 lesions at one time) (use only the 10 million units vial)

Chronic hepatitis B: I.M., SubQ: 5 million units given once daily **or** 10 million units given 3 times/week for 4 months

Chronic hepatitis C: I.M., SubQ: 3 million units 3 times/week for approximately a 6-month course; relapse of hepatitis has occurred after treatment was stopped

Melanoma adjuvant therapy:

Induction: I.V.: 20 million units/m^2/day 5 days/week for 4 weeks

Maintenance: SubQ: 10 million units/m^2/day 3 days/week for 48 weeks

Administration Parenteral: SubQ (rather than I.M.) administration is suggested for those patients who are at risk for bleeding or are thrombocytopenic; rotate SubQ injection site to help minimize local reactions

Monitoring Parameters Baseline EKG, CBC with differential and platelet count, hemoglobin, hematocrit, blood glucose, liver function tests, renal function tests, TSH levels, triglyceride levels, electrolytes, weight, chest x-ray, neuropsychiatric monitoring (including depressive symptomatology), ophthalmologic examination

Patient Information Read the patient Medication Guide that you receive with each prescription and refill of interferon alfa-2a. Do not change brands of interferon as changes in dosage may result; do not operate heavy machinery while on therapy since changes in mental status may occur; may cause dry mouth. Report any signs of depression or suicidal ideation to your physician.

Nursing Implications Patient should be well hydrated; may pretreat with NSAID or acetaminophen to decrease fever and its severity and to alleviate headache

Additional Information Myelosuppressive effects:

WBC: Mild

Platelets: Mild

Onset (days): 7-10

Nadir (days): 14

Recovery (days): 21

Dosage Forms Excipient information presented when available (limited, particularly for generics); consult specific product labeling.

Injection, powder for reconstitution:

Intron® A: 10 million units; 18 million units; 50 million units [contains human albumin]

Injection, solution [multidose prefilled pen]:

Intron® A:

Delivers 3 million units/0.2 mL (1.5 mL) [delivers 6 doses; 18 million units; contains polysorbate 80; edetate disodium]

Delivers 5 million units/0.2 mL (1.5 mL) [delivers 6 doses; 30 million units; contains polysorbate 80; edetate disodium]

Delivers 10 million units/0.2 mL (1.5 mL) [delivers 6 doses; 60 million units; contains polysorbate 80; edetate disodium]

Injection, solution [multidose vial]:

Intron® A: 6 million units/mL (3 mL); 10 million units/mL (2.5 mL) [contains polysorbate 80; edetate disodium]

Injection, solution [single-dose vial]:

Intron® A: 10 million units/ mL (1 mL) [contains polysorbate 80; edetate disodium]

See also Interferon Alfa-2b and Ribavirin Combination Pack monograph.

References

Davis GL, Balart LA, Schiff ER, et al, "Treatment of Chronic Hepatitis C With Recombinant Interferon Alfa. A Multicenter Randomized, Controlled Trial. Hepatitis Interventional Therapy Group," *N Engl J Med*, 1989, 321(22):1501-6.

Garmendia G, Miranda N, Borroso S, et al, "Regression of Infancy Hemangiomas With Recombinant IFN-Alpha 2b," *J Interferon Cytokine Res*, 2001, 21(1):31-8.

Gurakan F, Kocak N, Ozen H, et al, "Comparison of Standard and High Dosage Recombinant Interferon Alpha 2b for Treatment of Children With Chronic Hepatitis B Infection," *Pediatr Infect Dis J*, 2000, 19(1):52-6.

Kirkwood JM, Ibrahim JG, Sondak VK, et al, "High- and Low-Dose Interferon Alfa-2b in High-Risk Melanoma: First Analysis of Intergroup Trial E1690/S9111/C9190," *J Clin Oncol*, 2000, 18(12):2444-58.

Zwiener RJ, Fielman BA, Cochran C, et al, "Interferon-Alpha-2b Treatment of Chronic Hepatitis C in Children With Hemophilia," *Pediatr Infect Dis J*, 1996, 15(10):906-8.

- **Interferon Alpha-2a** *see* Interferon Alfa-2a *on page 854*
- **Interferon Alpha-2b** *see* Interferon Alfa-2b *on page 856*
- **Interleukin-2** *see* Aldesleukin *on page 70*
- **Interleukin-11** *see* Oprelvekin *on page 1174*
- **Intralipid®** *see* Fat Emulsion *on page 640*
- **Intranasal Trivalent, Cold-Adapted LAIV** *see* Influenza Virus Vaccine (Live/Attenuated) *on page 835*
- **Intravenous Fat Emulsion** *see* Fat Emulsion *on page 640*

- ♦ **Intron® A** *see* Interferon Alfa-2b *on page 856*
- ♦ **Intropin** *see* DOPamine *on page 530*
- ♦ **Invanz®** *see* Ertapenem *on page 593*
- ♦ **Invirase®** *see* Saquinavir *on page 1417*
- ♦ **Iodex [OTC]** *see* Iodine *on page 859*

Iodine (EYE oh dyne)

Medication Safety Issues

Sound-alike/look-alike issues:

Iodine may be confused with codeine, Iopidine®, Lodine®

U.S. Brand Names Iodex [OTC]; Iodoflex™; Iodosorb®

Therapeutic Category Topical Skin Product

Generic Available Yes: Tincture

Use Used topically as an antiseptic in the management of minor, superficial skin wounds and has been used to disinfect the skin preoperatively

Pregnancy Risk Factor D

Lactation Enters breast milk/use caution (AAP rates "compatible")

Contraindications Hypersensitivity to iodine preparations or any component; neonates; Hashimoto thyroiditis, history of Grave's disease, or nontoxic nodular goiter

Warnings May be highly toxic if ingested; iodine may be absorbed systemically, especially when large wounds are treated or when used in neonates. Not for application to large areas of the body or for use with tight or air-excluding bandages. When used for self medication (OTC), do not use on deep wounds, puncture wounds, animal bites, or serious burns without consulting with healthcare provider. Notify healthcare provider if condition does not improve within 7 days. Iodosorb® is for use as topical application to wet wounds only.

Precautions Use with caution in patients with renal dysfunction; since iodine may be absorbed systemically, thyroid function may need to be monitored when used chronically or over a large area.

Adverse Reactions

Endocrine & metabolic: Increase TSH

Local: Skin irritation, discoloration, eczema, edema, pain, redness

Miscellaneous: Hypersensitivity, allergic reactions

Drug Interactions Not for concomitant use with mercurial antiseptics (eg, Mercurochrome®, thimerosal)

Stability Store at room temperature.

Mechanism of Action Free iodine oxidizes microbial protoplasm making it effective against bacteria, fungi, yeasts, protozoa, and viruses; complexes with amino groups in tissue compounds to form iodophors from which the iodine is slowly released causing a sustained action. Iodosorb® and Iodoflex™ contain iodine in hydrophilic beads of cadexomer which allows a slow release of iodine into the wound.

Pharmacokinetics

Absorption: Topical: Amount absorbed systemically depends upon the iodine concentration and skin characteristics

Metabolism: Degraded by amylases normally present in wound fluid

Excretion: Urine (>90%)

Usual Dosage Children and Adults:

Antiseptic for minor cuts, scrapes: Apply small amount to affected area 1-3 times/day

Cleaning wet ulcers and wounds (Iodosorb®, Iodoflex™): Apply to clean wound; maximum: 50 g/application and 150 g/week. Change dressing ~3 times/week; reduce applications as exudate decreases. Do not use for >3 months; discontinue when wound is free of exudate.

Administration Topical: Apply to affected areas; avoid tight bandages because iodine may cause burns on occluded skin.

Iodosorb®: Apply 1/8' to 1/4' thickness to dry sterile gauze, then place prepared gauze onto clean wound. Change dressing when gel changes color from brown to yellow/gray (~3 times/week). Remove with sterile water, saline, or wound cleanser; gently blot fluid from surface leaving wound slightly moist before reapplying gel.

Patient Information May stain skin and clothing; may experience transient pain within the first hour after application

Additional Information Sodium thiosulfate inactivates iodine and is an effective chemical antidote for iodine poisoning; solutions of sodium thiosulfate may be used to remove iodine stains from skin and clothing

Dosage Forms Excipient information presented when available (limited, particularly for generics); consult specific product labeling.

Dressing, topical [gel pad] (Iodoflex™): 0.9% (5 g, 10 g)

Gel, topical (Iodosorb®): 0.9% (40 g)

Ointment, topical (Iodex): 4.7% (30 g, 720 g)

Tincture, topical: 2% (30 mL, 480 mL); 7% (30 mL, 480 mL)

♦ **Iodine Sodium** *see* Trace Metals *on page 1558*

Iodixanol (EYE oh dix an ole)

Medication Safety Issues
Not for intrathecal use

U.S. Brand Names Visipaque™

Therapeutic Category Radiological/Contrast Media, Nonionic

Generic Available No

Use Nonionic contrast media for radiological use intra-arterially: Digital subtraction angiography; angiocardiography (left ventriculography and selective coronary arteriography), peripheral arteriography, visceral arteriography, and cerebralarteriography. Intravenously: Contrast enhanced computed tomography (CECT) imaging of the head and body, excretory urography, and peripheral venography

Pregnancy Risk Factor B

Lactation Excretion in breast milk unknown/not recommended

Contraindications Hypersensitivity to iodixanol or any component; intrathecal administration; administration to children who have experienced prolonged fasting or received recent laxative dose(s)

Warnings For I.V. or intra-arterial use only; **may be fatal if given intrathecally;** intrathecal injection has also resulted in serious reactions (seizures, cerebral hemorrhage, coma, paralysis, arachnoiditis, ARF, cardiac arrest, rhabdomyolysis, hyperthermia, and brain edema). May cause rare but serious thromboembolic events including MI and stroke. Iodinated contrast media has been associated with severe hypersensitivity reactions including anaphylaxis; immediate treatment for anaphylactic reactions should be available during administration of iodixanol. Use with extreme caution in patients with or suspected of having pheochromocytoma; the amount of iodixanol used should be kept to an absolute minimum and blood pressure should be closely monitored throughout the procedure in these patients. Contrast media when administered intravascularly may promote sickling in patients who are homozygous for sickle cell disease. May worsen renal insufficiency in patients with multiple myeloma. Avoid use in patients with homocystinuria due to the risk of inducing thrombosis and embolism. Avoid extravasation.

Precautions Use with caution in children with asthma, hypersensitivity to other medication and/or allergens, cyanotic and acyanotic heart disease, CHF, serum creatinine >1.5 mg/dL, and neonates (immature renal function) due to an increased risk of adverse effects with iodixanol. Dehydration, particularly in children, may also increase the risk of adverse effects. Patients should be adequately hydrated both prior to and after iodixanol administration. Use caution in thyroid disease; thyroid storm has been reported in patients with history of hyperthyroidism.

Adverse Reactions
Cardiovascular: Cardiac arrest, chest pain, angina, syncope, arrhythmias, cardiac failure, hypotension, hypertension, MI, flushing, peripheral ischemia
Central nervous system: Agitation, anxiety, insomnia, nervousness, dizziness, headache, migraine, vertigo, fatigue, malaise, seizures, cerebral vascular disorder, stupor, confusion, amnesia
Dermatologic: Rash, pruritus, urticaria
Endocrine & metabolic: Hypoglycemia
Gastrointestinal: Diarrhea, nausea, vomiting, taste perversion, dyspepsia, pharyngeal edema
Genitourinary: Hematuria
Hematologic: DIC
Local: Injection site reactions (discomfort/pain/warmth)
Neuromuscular & skeletal: Back pain, dyskinesia, polymyalgia rheumatica
Ocular: Abnormal vision, cortical blindness (rare)
Otic: Tinnitus
Renal: Acute renal failure, abnormal renal function
Respiratory: Asthma, bronchitis, dyspnea, pulmonary edema, rhinitis, respiratory depression
Miscellaneous: Hypersensitivity reactions including anaphylaxis, diaphoresis

Drug Interactions Oral cholecystographic contrast agents (may have increased risk of renal toxicity); do not administer intravascular contrast to patients who have recently received an oral cholecystographic contrast agent

Stability Store at room temperature; do not mix with or inject in I.V. lines with other medications, solutions, or TPN solutions

Mechanism of Action Iodixanol is a nonionic, isosmolar, water soluble, iodinated x-ray contrast media for intravascular administration. It opacifies vessels in the path of flow permitting radiographic visualization of internal structures.

Pharmacodynamics Following administration, the increase in tissue density is related to blood flow, the concentration of the iodixanol solution used, and the extraction of iodixanol by various interstitial tissues. The degree of enhancement is directly related to the iodine content in an administered dose.

Kidney:

Visualization: Renal parenchyma: 30-60 seconds; calyces and pelves (normal renal function): 1-3 minutes

Optimum contrast: 5-15 minutes

Pharmacokinetics

Distribution: V_d: Adults: 0.26 L/kg

Metabolism: Metabolites have not been identified.

Time to peak level: I.V.: Children: 0.75-1.25 hours

Half-life:

Newborns to Infants <2 months: 4.1 ± 1.4 hours

Infants 2-6 months: 2.8 ± 0.6 hours

Infants 6-12 months: 2.4 ± 0.4 hours

Children 1 to <3 years: 2.2 ± 0.5 hours

Children 3 to <12 years: 2.3 ± 0.5 hours

Adults: 2.1 ± 0.1 hours

Elimination: 97% excreted unchanged in the urine within 24 hours; <2% excreted in feces

Clearance: Adults: 110 mL/minute

Dialysis: Dialyzable (36% to 49% depending upon the membrane)

Usual Dosage The concentration and volume of iodixanol to be used should be individualized depending upon age, weight, size of vessel, and rate of blood flow within the vessel.

Children >1 year:

Intra-arterial: Cerebral, cardiac chambers and related major arteries, and visceral studies: **320 mg iodine/mL**: 1-2 mL/kg; not to exceed 4 mL/kg

I.V.: Contrast-enhanced computerized tomography or excretory urography: **270 mg iodine/mL**: 1-2 mL/kg; not to exceed 2 mL/kg

Children >12 years and Adults: Maximum recommended total dose of iodine: 80 g

Intra-arterial: Iodixanol **320 mg iodine/mL**: Dose individualized based on injection site and study type; refer to product labeling

I.V.: Iodixanol **270 mg and 320 mg iodine /mL**: concentration and dose vary based on study type; refer to product labeling.

Dosage adjustment in renal impairment: Not studied; use caution

Administration I.V. or intra-arterial: Administer without further dilution. **Not for intrathecal administration** (see Warnings). Avoid extravasation.

Monitoring Parameters Monitor signs and symptoms of hypersensitivity reactions

Test Interactions False positive result for urine protein when using Multistix®; may affect urine specific gravity results immediately following administration (refractometry or urine osmolality may be used as an alternative); protein-bound iodine and radioactive iodine will not accurately reflect thyroid function for at least 16 days following iodixanol administration

Patient Information Inform healthcare provider if you are allergic to any drugs or food, or if you have had any reactions to previous injections of dyes used for x-ray procedures.

Dosage Forms Excipient information presented when available (limited, particularly for generics); consult specific product labeling.

Injection, solution [preservative free]:

270: 550 mg/mL (100 mL, 125 mL, 150 mL, 200 mL) [provides organically-bound iodine 270 mg/mL; contains tromethamine 1.2 mg/mL, edetate calcium disodium]

320: 652 mg/mL (50 mL, 100 mL, 125 mL, 150 mL, 200 mL) [provides organically-bound iodine 320 mg/mL; contains tromethamine 1.2 mg/mL, edetate calcium disodium]

References

Johnson WH, Lloyd TR, Victorica BE, et al, "Iodixanol Pharmacokinetics in Children," *Pediatr Cardiol*, 2001, 22(3):223-7.

♦ **Iodoflex**™ *see* Iodine *on page 859*

♦ **Iodopen**® *see* Trace Metals *on page 1558*

Iodoquinol (eye oh doe KWIN ole)

U.S. Brand Names Yodoxin®
Canadian Brand Names Diodoquin®
Index Terms Diiodohydroxyquin
Therapeutic Category Amebicide
Generic Available No
Use Treatment of acute and chronic intestinal amebiasis due to *Entamoeba histolytica*; asymptomatic cyst passers; *Blastocystis hominis* infections; iodoquinol alone is ineffective for amebic hepatitis or hepatic abscess
Pregnancy Risk Factor C
Lactation Excretion in breast milk unknown
Contraindications Hypersensitivity to iodine, iodoquinol, or any component; hepatic or renal damage; pre-existing optic neuropathy
Precautions Use with caution in patients with thyroid disease or neurological disorders
Adverse Reactions
Central nervous system: Agitation, retrograde amnesia, fever, chills, headache, ataxia
Dermatologic: Anal pruritus, rash, acne
Endocrine & metabolic: Enlargement of the thyroid
Gastrointestinal: Nausea, vomiting, diarrhea, gastritis, anorexia, constipation
Neuromuscular & skeletal: Weakness, peripheral neuropathy, myalgia
Ocular: Optic neuritis, optic atrophy, visual impairment
Mechanism of Action Contact amebicide that works in the lumen of the intestine by an unknown mechanism
Pharmacokinetics
Absorption: Oral: Poor and irregular
Metabolism: In the liver
Elimination: In feces; metabolites appear in urine
Usual Dosage Oral:
Children: 30-40 mg/kg/day in 3 divided doses for 20 days; not to exceed 1.95 g/day
Adults: 650 mg 3 times/day after meals for 20 days; not to exceed 2 g/day
Administration Oral: Administer medication after meals; tablets may be crushed and mixed with applesauce or chocolate syrup
Monitoring Parameters Ophthalmologic exam
Test Interactions May increase protein-bound serum iodine concentrations reflecting a decrease in iodine 131 uptake; false-positive ferric chloride test for phenylketonuria
Patient Information Notify physician if rash occurs
Dosage Forms Excipient information presented when available (limited, particularly for generics); consult specific product labeling.
Tablet: 210 mg, 650 mg

- **Iodosorb®** *see* Iodine *on page 859*
- **Ionil® [OTC]** *see* Salicylic Acid *on page 1413*
- **Ionil® Plus [OTC]** *see* Salicylic Acid *on page 1413*
- **Ionil T® [OTC]** *see* Coal Tar *on page 394*
- **Ionil T® Plus [OTC]** *see* Coal Tar *on page 394*
- **Ionsys™** *see* Fentanyl *on page 644*
- **Iosat™ [OTC]** *see* Potassium Iodide *on page 1290*

Ipecac Syrup (IP e kak SIR up)

Index Terms Syrup of Ipecac
Therapeutic Category Antidote, Emetic
Generic Available Yes
Use Treatment of acute oral drug overdosage and certain poisonings; use only in alert conscious patients who have ingested potentially toxic amounts of substance
Pregnancy Risk Factor C
Lactation Excretion in breast milk unknown/use caution
Contraindications Hypersensitivity to ipecac syrup or any component; do not use in unconscious patients, patients with absent gag reflex or seizures; ingestion of strong bases or acids, other corrosive substances, volatile oils, hydrocarbons with high potential for aspiration
Warnings Avoid use in patients with coagulopathy or bleeding problems (risk of gastroesophageal hemorrhage) and in patients receiving calcium channel blockers, beta-blockers, clonidine, or digitalis glycosides (risk of exaggerated vagal stimulation

with gagging, resulting in severe bradycardia); do not confuse ipecac syrup with ipecac fluid extract; fluid extract is 14 times more potent than syrup

Precautions Use with caution in patients with cardiovascular disease and bulimics

Adverse Reactions

Cardiovascular: Cardiotoxicity

Central nervous system: Lethargy, drowsiness

Gastrointestinal: Protracted vomiting, diarrhea; Mallory-Weiss syndrome, gastric rupture

Neuromuscular & skeletal: Myopathy

Respiratory: Aspiration (can be fatal)

Drug Interactions Activated charcoal may decrease effectiveness

Food Interactions Milk, carbonated beverages may decrease effectiveness

Mechanism of Action Irritates the gastric mucosa and stimulates the medullary chemoreceptor trigger zone to induce vomiting

Pharmacodynamics

Onset of vomiting after oral dose: Within 15-30 minutes; usual: 20 minutes

Duration: 20-25 minutes; can last longer, up to 1-2 hours

Usual Dosage Oral:

Children:

- <6 months: Not recommended
- 6-12 months: 5-10 mL followed by 10-20 mL/kg or 120-240 mL of water; repeat dose one time if vomiting does not occur within 20-30 minutes
- 1-12 years: 15 mL followed by 10-20 mL/kg or 120-240 mL of water; repeat dose one time if vomiting does not occur within 20-30 minutes

Adolescents and Adults: 30 mL followed by 240 mL of water; repeat dose one time if vomiting does not occur within 20-30 minutes

Administration Oral: Administer within 60 minutes of ingestion; follow administration with water; do not administer with milk or carbonated beverages

Nursing Implications Do **not** administer to unconscious patients

Additional Information Patients should be kept active and moving following administration of ipecac; if vomiting does not occur after second dose, gastric lavage may be considered to remove ingested substance

The Position Statement of The American Academy of Clinical Toxicology and The European Association of Poisons Centres and Clinical Toxicologists does **not** recommend **routine** administration of ipecac syrup to poisoned patients; scientific literature does not support that ipecac improves patient outcome; this paper states that the **routine** administration of ipecac syrup in the emergency room should be abandoned. Also, scientific literature cannot support or exclude giving ipecac syrup soon after toxic ingestions; administration of ipecac syrup may delay the administration or decrease the effectiveness of activated charcoal, oral antidotes, or whole bowel irrigation; its use should be considered only if it can be given within 60 minutes after ingestion of poison.

A recent study suggests that the use of syrup of ipecac, selectively administered at home, does **not** improve patient outcome or reduce utilization of emergency services; thus, clear evidence of the benefit of at home use of ipecac syrup is lacking (see Bond, 2003). Furthermore, the American Academy of Pediatrics now recommends that ipecac syrup should no longer be used routinely as a home treatment strategy and that existing ipecac syrup in the home should be disposed of safely (see AAP, 2003).

Dosage Forms Excipient information presented when available (limited, particularly for generics); consult specific product labeling.

Syrup: 70 mg/mL (30 mL) [contains alcohol]

References

American Academy of Pediatrics Committee on Injury, Violence, and Poison Prevention, "Poison Treatment in the Home," *Pediatrics*, 2003, 112(5):1182-5.

Bond GR, "Home Syrup of Ipecac Use Does Not Reduce Emergency Department Use or Improve Outcome," *Pediatrics*, 2003, 112(5):1061-4.

"Position Statement: Ipecac Syrup. American Academy of Clinical Toxicology; European Association of Poisons Centres and Clinical Toxicologists," *J Toxicol Clin Toxicol*, 1997, 35(7):699-709.

Quang LS and Woolf AD, "Past, Present, and Future Role of Ipecac Syrup," *Curr Opin Pediatr*, 2000, 12(2):153-62.

Shannon M, "Ingestion of Toxic Substances by Children," *N Engl J Med*, 2000, 342(3):186-91.

♦ **IPOL®** *see* Poliovirus Vaccine (Inactivated) *on page 1275*

Ipratropium (i pra TROE pee um)

Medication Safety Issues

Sound-alike/look-alike issues:

Atrovent® may be confused with Alupent®

(Continued)

Ipratropium *(Continued)*

Related Information
Asthma *on page 1904*

U.S. Brand Names Atrovent®; Atrovent® HFA

Canadian Brand Names Alti-Ipratropium; Apo-Ipravent®; Atrovent®; Atrovent® HFA; Gen-Ipratropium; Novo-Ipramide; Nu-Ipratropium; PMS-Ipratropium

Index Terms Ipratropium Bromide

Therapeutic Category Antiasthmatic; Anticholinergic Agent; Bronchodilator

Generic Available Yes: Excludes solution for oral inhalation, aerosol for oral inhalation

Use Anticholinergic bronchodilator used in bronchospasm associated with asthma, COPD, bronchitis, and emphysema; symptomatic relief of rhinorrhea associated with allergic and nonallergic rhinitis (nasal spray)

Pregnancy Risk Factor B

Lactation Excretion in breast milk unknown/use caution

Contraindications Hypersensitivity to ipratropium, atropine, or any component; hypersensitivity to soya lecithin and related food products such as soybeans and peanuts (MDI formulation only)

Warnings Not indicated for the initial treatment of acute episodes of bronchospasm

Precautions Use with caution in patients with narrow-angle glaucoma, bladder neck obstruction, or prostatic hypertrophy

Adverse Reactions

Note: Ipratropium is poorly absorbed from the lung, so systemic effects are rare

Cardiovascular: Palpitations, tachycardia (including SVT), flushing, hypotension, hypertension, atrial fibrillation, angioedema
Central nervous system: Nervousness, dizziness, headache, fatigue, drowsiness, insomnia
Dermatologic: Rash, pruritus, alopecia, urticaria
Gastrointestinal: Nausea, xerostomia, constipation
Genitourinary: Dysuria, urinary retention
Ocular: Blurred vision, mydriasis
Respiratory: Cough, hoarseness, dry secretions, epistaxis (with nasal spray), laryngospasm, bronchospasm
Miscellaneous: Hypersensitivity reactions

Drug Interactions Additive effects with anticholinergics or drugs with anticholinergic properties

Stability Store at room temperature; compatible for 1 hour when mixed with albuterol or metaproterenol in a nebulizer

Mechanism of Action Blocks the action of acetylcholine at parasympathetic sites in bronchial smooth muscle causing bronchodilation; inhibits secretions from the serous and seromucous glands lining the nasal mucosa

Pharmacodynamics

Onset of bronchodilation: 1-3 minutes after administration
Maximum effect: Maximal effect within 1.5-2 hours
Duration: Bronchodilation persists for up to 4-6 hours

Pharmacokinetics

Absorption: Not readily absorbed into the systemic circulation from the surface of the lung or from the GI tract
Distribution: Following inhalation, 15% of dose reaches the lower airways
Half-life: 2 hours

Usual Dosage

Neonates: Nebulization: 25 mcg/kg/dose 3 times/day
Infants: Nebulization: 125-250 mcg 3 times/day
Acute exacerbation of asthma (NIH guidelines):
- Children: Nebulization: 250 mcg every 20 minutes for 3 doses then every 2-4 hours
  - Metered inhaler: 4-8 puffs as needed
- Children >12 years and Adults: Nebulization: 500 mcg every 30 minutes for 3 doses then every 2-4 hours as needed
  - Metered inhaler: 4-8 puffs as needed

Maintenance treatments (nonacute) (NIH guidelines):
- Children:
  - Nebulization: 250-500 mcg every 6 hours
  - Metered inhaler: 1-2 inhalations every 6 hours; not to exceed 12 inhalations/day
- Children ≥12 years and Adults:
  - Nebulization: 250 mcg every 6 hours
  - Metered inhaler: 2-3 inhalations every 6 hours; not to exceed 12 inhalations/day

Nasal spray:
- Children >6 years and Adults: 0.03%: 2 sprays in each nostril 2-3 times/day
- Children >5 years and Adults: 0.06%: 2 sprays in each nostril 3-4 times/day

Administration

Nasal spray: Pump must be primed before usage by 7 actuations into the air away from the face; if not used for >24 hours, pump must be reprimed with 2 actuations; if not used >7 days, reprime with 7 actuations

Nebulization: May be administered with or without dilution in NS; use of a nebulizer with a mouth piece rather than a face mask may be preferred to prevent contact with eyes

Oral Inhalation: Shake well before use (Atrovent® only; Atrovent® HFA does not require shaking); use spacer device in children <8 years

Patient Information May cause dry mouth; avoid spraying aerosol in eyes as this may cause blurred vision, eye pain or discomfort, and precipitate or worsen glaucoma in susceptible patients

Dosage Forms Excipient information presented when available (limited, particularly for generics); consult specific product labeling.

Aerosol for oral inhalation, as bromide:

Atrovent® HFA: 17 mcg/actuation (12.9 g)

Solution for nebulization, as bromide: 0.02% (2.5 mL)

Solution, intranasal, as bromide [spray]:

Atrovent®: 0.03% (30 mL); 0.06% (15 mL)

References

"Guidelines for the Diagnosis and Management of Asthma. NAEPP Expert Panel Report 2," July 1997, www.nhlbi.nih.gov/guidelines/asthma/asthgdln.pdf.

Henry RI, Hiller EG, Milner AD, et al, "Nebulised Ipratropium Bromide and Sodium Cromoglycate in the First 2 Years of Life," *Arch Dis Child*, 1984, 59(1):54-7.

Mann NP and Hiller RG, "Ipratropium Bromide in Children With Asthma," *Thorax*, 1982, 37(1):72-4.

"National Asthma Education and Prevention Program. Expert Panel Report: Guidelines for the Diagnosis and Management of Asthma Update on Selected Topics--2002," *J Allergy Clin Immunol*, 2002, 110(5 Suppl):S141-219.

Schuh S, Johnson DW, Callahan S, et al, "Efficacy of Frequent Nebulized Ipratropium Added to Frequent High-Dose Albuterol Therapy in Severe Childhood Asthma," *J Pediatr*, 1995, 126(4):639-45.

Schuh S, Johnson D, Canny G, et al, "Efficacy of Adding Nebulized Ipratropium Bromide to Nebulized Albuterol Therapy in Acute Bronchiolitis," *Pediatrics*, 1992, 90(6): 920-3.

Wang EE, Milner R, Allen U, et al, "Bronchodilators for Treatment of Mild Bronchiolitis: A Factorial Randomized Trial," *Arch Dis Child*, 1992, 67(3):289-93.

Wilkie RA and Bryan MH, "Effect of Bronchodilators on Airway Resistance in Ventilator-dependent Neonates With Chronic Lung Disease," *J Pediatr*, 1987, 111(2):278-82.

♦ **Ipratropium Bromide** *see* Ipratropium *on page 863*

♦ **I-Prin [OTC]** *see* Ibuprofen *on page 802*

♦ **Iproveratril Hydrochloride** *see* Verapamil *on page 1611*

♦ **IPV** *see* Poliovirus Vaccine (Inactivated) *on page 1275*

♦ **Iquix®** *see* Levofloxacin *on page 927*

♦ **Ircon® [OTC]** *see* Iron Supplements (Oral/Enteral) *on page 868*

Irinotecan (eye rye no TEE kan)

Medication Safety Issues

High alert medication: The Institute for Safe Medication Practices (ISMP) includes this medication among its list of drugs which have a heightened risk of causing significant patient harm when used in error.

Related Information

Compatibility of Chemotherapy and Related Supportive Care Medications *on page 1777*

U.S. Brand Names Camptosar®

Canadian Brand Names Camptosar®; Irinotecan Hydrochloride Trihydrate

Index Terms Camptothecin-11; CPT-11; NSC-616348

Therapeutic Category Antineoplastic Agent, Topoisomerase Inhibitor

Generic Available No

Use Childhood refractory solid tumors including neuroblastoma, hepatocellular tumor, Wilms' tumor, osteosarcoma, and rhabdomyosarcoma; recurrent or refractory CNS tumors such as medulloblastoma, ependymoma, brain stem glioma, or astrocytoma; adult brain tumors; colorectal, breast, and prostate cancer; leukemia, lymphoma, small and nonsmall cell lung cancer, and gastric, ovarian, and cervical cancer

Pregnancy Risk Factor D

Lactation Excretion in breast milk unknown/not recommended

Contraindications Hypersensitivity to irinotecan or any component; pregnancy; concurrent use with St John's wort or ketoconazole (see Drug Interactions)

Warnings The FDA currently recommends that procedures for proper handling and disposal of antineoplastic agents be considered. Irinotecan is potentially embryotoxic and teratogenic if administered to pregnant women.

Early and late forms of severe diarrhea have been reported with irinotecan administration. Early diarrhea has occurred during or shortly after infusion and may be (Continued)

Irinotecan *(Continued)*

accompanied by symptoms of rhinitis, increased salivation, miosis, lacrimation, diaphoresis, flushing, and abdominal cramping. Atropine 0.01 mg/kg I.V. (maximum dose: 0.4 mg) may be used to prevent or treat symptoms of early diarrhea. Late diarrhea has occurred >24 hours after irinotecan administration and can be prolonged leading to life-threatening dehydration and electrolyte imbalance. Treat late diarrhea promptly with loperamide until a normal pattern of bowel movements returns (see Additional Information for loperamide dosing recommendation); fluid and electrolyte replacement may be needed for dehydration. Provide antibiotic support if patient develops ileus, fever, or severe neutropenia. Interrupt or reduce subsequent irinotecan doses if National Cancer Institute (NCI) grade 3 (increase of 7-9 stools daily, or incontinence, or severe cramping) or grade 4 (increase ≥10 stools daily, grossly bloody stool, or need for parenteral support) late diarrhea occurs.

Deaths due to sepsis following severe myelosuppression have been reported with irinotecan administration. Patients with abnormal glucuronidation of bilirubin, such as Gilbert's syndrome, may also be at greater risk of myelosuppression when receiving irinotecan. Temporarily discontinue therapy if neutropenic fever occurs or if absolute neutrophil count is <1000/mm^3; reduce subsequent doses depending upon level of neutropenia observed.

Precautions Use with caution and reduce initial irinotecan dose in patients with elevated total serum bilirubin concentration (1-2 mg/dL) who previously received pelvic/abdominal radiation therapy or in patients with baseline total serum bilirubin concentration >2 mg/dL.

Adverse Reactions

Cardiovascular: Facial flushing, bradycardia

Central nervous system: Fever, asthenia, tremor, headache, dizziness, confusion, insomnia

Dermatologic: Alopecia, rash

Endocrine & metabolic: Hyponatremia, hypernatremia, hypokalemia, metabolic acidosis

Gastrointestinal: Diarrhea (see Warnings), nausea, vomiting, abdominal pain, anorexia, constipation, mucositis, colitis, ileus, GI bleeding

Genitourinary: Hematuria, proteinuria, glucosuria

Hematologic: Leukopenia, neutropenia, thrombocytopenia, thromboembolism, anemia, lymphocytopenia

Hepatic: Elevated transaminases, alkaline phosphatase, bilirubin

Local: Pain at infusion site

Renal: Elevated serum creatinine, acute renal failure (rare)

Respiratory: Pulmonary infiltrates, pneumonitis, dyspnea, cough

Miscellaneous: Anaphylaxis, cholinergic symptoms (rhinitis, increased salivation, diaphoresis, miosis, lacrimation)

Drug Interactions Cytochrome P450 isoenzyme CYP2B6 and CYP3A3/4 substrate

Concurrent administration of erythromycin, ciprofloxacin, clarithromycin, doxycycline, imatinib, isoniazid, propofol, protease inhibitors, verapamil, cimetidine, fluconazole, or itraconazole with irinotecan may result in increased exposure to irinotecan; nevirapine, rifampin, rifabutin, phenytoin, phenobarbital, and carbamazepine may decrease systemic exposure to SN-38, the active metabolite (consider substituting a nonCYP3A4-inducing medication at least 2 weeks prior to starting irinotecan); prochlorperazine may increase incidence of akathisia; ketoconazole may increase exposure to irinotecan and SN-38 (concomitant therapy with irinotecan is contraindicated; discontinue ketoconazole at least 1 week prior to starting irinotecan); St John's wort may reduce exposure to active metabolite SN-38 (concomitant therapy with irinotecan is contraindicated; discontinue St John's wort at least 2 weeks prior to the first cycle of irinotecan).

Stability Store unopened vials at room temperature; protect from light. Once injectable solution is mixed with D_5W, solution is stable for 24 hours if stored at room temperature or 48 hours if stored refrigerated. Injectable solution mixed with NS is stable for 24 hours if stored at room temperature. Do not refrigerate solutions mixed in NS since visible particulates may develop.

Mechanism of Action Prodrug undergoes de-esterification by cellular carboxylesterases to a potent active metabolite (SN-38) which is a topoisomerase I inhibitor. Binds to topoisomerase I-DNA complex preventing religation of single-strand DNA breaks.

Pharmacokinetics

Protein binding:

- Irinotecan: 30% to 68%
- SN-38 (active metabolite): 95%

Half-life, terminal: Adults:

- Irinotecan: 6-12 hours
- SN-38 (active metabolite): 10-20 hours

Metabolism: Irinotecan is converted to its active metabolite SN-38 by carboxylesterase-mediated cleavage of the carbamate bond. SN-38 undergoes conjugation to a glucuronide metabolite in the liver. Irinotecan also undergoes oxidation by cytochrome P450 3A4 to yield to 2 inactive metabolites.

Elimination: 11% to 20% of irinotecan and <1% SN-38 is excreted in the urine

Usual Dosage I.V. infusion (refer to individual protocols):

Children:

Refractory solid tumor (low-dose, protracted schedule): 20 mg/m^2/day for 5 days for 2 consecutive weeks followed by a week of rest; repeat cycle every 3 weeks

Refractory solid tumor or CNS tumor: 50 mg/m^2/day for 5 days; repeat cycle every 21 days; or for heavily pretreated patients: 125 mg/m^2/dose once weekly for 4 weeks, repeat cycle every 6 weeks; less heavily pretreated patients: 160 mg/m^2/dose once weekly for 4 weeks, repeat cycle every 6 weeks

Adults:

Colorectal cancer that has recurred or progressed following fluorouracil-containing chemotherapy: 300-350 mg/m^2/dose once every 3 weeks or 125 mg/m^2/dose once weekly (maximum dose: 150 mg/m^2) for 4 weeks followed by a 2-week rest period; repeat courses every 6 weeks (4 weeks of therapy followed by 2 weeks off)

Small cell lung cancer: 100-125 mg/m^2/dose once weekly (maximum dose: 150 mg/m^2) or 350 mg/m^2/dose once every 3 weeks; or 60-70 mg/m^2 once weekly for 3 weeks in combination with other agents

Note: A new cycle of irinotecan therapy should not begin until serious treatment-induced toxicity has fully resolved, granulocyte count recovers to ≥1500/mm^3, and platelet count recovers to ≥100,000/mm^3. Treatment should be delayed 1-2 weeks to allow for recovery from treatment-related toxicities. If the patient has not recovered after a 2-week delay, consider discontinuing irinotecan.

Administration Parenteral: I.V. infusion: Irinotecan can be further diluted in D_5W (preferred diluent) or NS to a final concentration of 0.12-2.8 mg/mL. Infuse over 60-90 minutes depending on protocol. Higher incidence of cholinergic symptoms have been reported with more rapid infusion rates.

Monitoring Parameters Signs of diarrhea and dehydration, serum electrolytes, serum BUN and creatinine; infusion site for signs of inflammation; CBC with differential and platelet count, hemoglobin, liver function tests, and serum bilirubin

Patient Information Advise women of childbearing potential to avoid becoming pregnant while receiving irinotecan. Avoid the use of laxatives. Notify physician if diarrhea, vomiting, fever, or symptoms of dehydration such as fainting, lightheadedness, or dizziness occur. Initiate loperamide therapy at the first episode of poorly formed or loose stools after irinotecan administration (see Additional Information).

Nursing Implications Avoid extravasation. If extravasation occurs, flush the site with sterile water and apply an ice pack. To prevent emesis, pretreat with a 5-HT_3 antagonist and dexamethasone 30 minutes prior to irinotecan therapy.

Additional Information Loperamide dosing for treatment of late diarrhea: Oral:

8-10 kg: 1 mg after the first loose bowel movement followed by 0.5 mg every 3 hours until a normal pattern of bowel movement returns. Take 0.75 mg every 4 hours during the night rather than every 3 hours.

10.1-20 kg: 1 mg after the first loose bowel movement followed by 1 mg every 3 hours until a normal pattern of bowel movement returns. Take 1 mg every 4 hours during the night rather than every 3 hours.

20.1-30 kg: 2 mg after the first loose bowel movement followed by 1 mg every 3 hours until a normal pattern of bowel movement returns. Take 2 mg every 4 hours during the night rather than every 3 hours.

30.1-43 kg: 2 mg after the first loose bowel movement followed by 1 mg every 2 hours until a normal pattern of bowel movement returns. Take 2 mg every 4 hours during the night rather than every 2 hours.

>43 kg: 4 mg after the first loose bowel movement followed by 2 mg every 2 hours until the patient is diarrhea free for 12 hours. Take 4 mg every 4 hours during the night rather than every 2 hours.

Dosage Forms Excipient information presented when available (limited, particularly for generics); consult specific product labeling.

Injection, solution, as hydrochloride:

Camptosar®: 20 mg/mL (2 mL, 5 mL) [contains sorbitol 45 mg/mL]

References

Bomgaars L, Kerr J, Berg S, et al, "A Phase I Study of Irinotecan Administered on a Weekly Schedule in Pediatric Patients," *Pediatr Blood Cancer*, 2005, Mar 14.

Cosetti M, Wexler LH, Calleja E, et al, "Irinotecan for Pediatric Solid Tumors: The Memorial Sloan-Kettering Experience," *J Pediatr Hematol Oncol*, 2002, 24(2):101-5.

Gajjar A, Chintagumpala MM, Bowers DC, et al, "Effect of Intrapatient Dosage Escalation of Irinotecan on Its Pharmacokinetics in Pediatric Patients Who Have High-Grade Gliomas and Receive Enzyme-Inducing Anticonvulsant Therapy," *Cancer*, 2003, 97(9 Suppl):2374-80.

♦ **Irinotecan Hydrochloride Trihydrate (Can)** *see* Irinotecan *on page 865*

- **Iron Dextran** *see* Iron Supplements (Parenteral) *on page 870*
- **Iron Sucrose** *see* Iron Supplements (Parenteral) *on page 870*
- **Iron Sulfate (Ferrous Sulfate)** *see* Iron Supplements (Oral/Enteral) *on page 868*

Iron Supplements (Oral/Enteral) (EYE ern SUP la ments)

Related Information

Overdose and Toxicology *on page 1916*

U.S. Brand Names Femiron® [OTC]; Feosol® [OTC]; Feostat® [OTC] [DSC]; Feratab® [OTC]; Fer-Gen-Sol [OTC]; Fergon® [OTC]; Fer-In-Sol® [OTC]; Fer-Iron® [OTC]; Ferretts [OTC]; Ferrex 150 [OTC]; Ferro-Sequels® [OTC]; Fe-Tinic™ 150 [OTC] [DSC]; Hemocyte® [OTC]; Hytinic® [OTC]; Ircon® [OTC]; Nephro-Fer® [OTC]; Niferex® [OTC]; Niferex® 150 [OTC]; Nu-Iron® 150 [OTC]; Slow FE® [OTC]

Index Terms Ferrous Fumarate; Ferrous Gluconate; Ferrous Sulfate; $FeSO_4$ (Ferrous Sulfate); Iron Sulfate (Ferrous Sulfate)

Therapeutic Category Iron Salt; Mineral, Oral

Generic Available Yes

Use Prevention and treatment of iron deficiency anemias; supplemental therapy for patients receiving epoetin alfa

Pregnancy Risk Factor A

Contraindications Hypersensitivity to iron salts or any component (see Warnings); hemochromatosis, hemolytic anemia

Warnings Avoid use in premature infants until the vitamin E stores, deficient at birth, are replenished; some products contain sulfites and/or tartrazine which may cause allergic reactions in susceptible individuals

Precautions Avoid using for longer than 6 months, except in patients with conditions that require prolonged therapy; avoid in patients with peptic ulcer, enteritis, or ulcerative colitis; avoid in patients receiving frequent blood transfusions

Adverse Reactions

Gastrointestinal: GI irritation, epigastric pain, nausea, diarrhea, dark stools, constipation

Genitourinary: Discoloration of urine (black or dark)

Miscellaneous: Liquid preparations may temporarily stain the teeth

Drug Interactions Absorption of oral preparation of iron and tetracyclines are decreased when both of these drugs are given together; concurrent administration of antacids and cimetidine may decrease iron absorption; iron may decrease absorption of penicillamine, levothyroxine, methyldopa, and levodopa when given at the same time; response to iron therapy may be delayed in patients receiving chloramphenicol; concurrent administration of ≥200 mg vitamin C per 30 mg elemental iron increases absorption of oral iron; absorption of quinolones may be decreased due to formation of a ferric ion-quinolone complex

Food Interactions Milk, cereals, dietary fiber, tea, coffee, or eggs decrease absorption of iron

Mechanism of Action Iron is released from the plasma and eventually replenishes the depleted iron stores in the bone marrow where it is incorporated into hemoglobin

Recommended Daily Allowance of Iron (dosage expressed as elemental iron)

Age	RDA (mg)
<5 mo	5
5 mo to 10 y	10
Male	
11-18 y	12
>18 y	10
Female	
11-50 y	15
>50 y	10

Pharmacodynamics

Onset of action: Hematologic response to either oral or parenteral iron salts is essentially the same; red blood cell form and color changes within 3-10 days

Maximum effect: Peak reticulocytosis occurs in 5-10 days, and hemoglobin values increase within 2-4 weeks

Pharmacokinetics

Absorption: Oral: Iron is absorbed in the duodenum and upper jejunum; in persons with normal iron stores 10% of an oral dose is absorbed, this is increased to 20% to

30% in persons with inadequate iron stores; food and achlorhydria will decrease absorption

Elimination: Iron is largely bound to serum transferrin and excreted in the urine, sweat, sloughing of intestinal mucosa, and by menses

Usual Dosage Note: Multiple salt forms of iron exist; close attention must be paid to the salt form when ordering and administering iron; incorrect selection or substitution of one salt for another without proper dosage adjustment may result in serious over- or underdosing.

Oral (dose expressed in terms of **elemental** iron):

Recommended Daily Allowance, see table on previous page.

Premature neonates: 2-4 mg elemental iron/kg/day divided every 12-24 hours (maximum dose: 15 mg/day)

Infants and Children:

Severe iron deficiency anemia: 4-6 mg elemental iron/kg/day in 3 divided doses

Mild to moderate iron deficiency anemia: 3 mg elemental iron/kg/day in 1-2 divided doses

Prophylaxis: 1-2 mg elemental iron/kg/day up to a maximum of 15 mg elemental iron/day

Adults:

Iron deficiency: 2-3 mg/kg/day or 60-100 mg elemental iron twice daily up to 60 mg elemental iron 4 times/day, or 50 mg elemental iron (extended release) 1-2 times/day

Prophylaxis: 60-100 mg elemental iron/day; see table

Elemental Iron Content of Iron Salts

Iron Salt	Elemental Iron Content (% of salt form)	Approximate Equivalent Doses (mg of iron salt)
Ferrous fumarate	33	197
Ferrous gluconate	11.6	560
Ferrous sulfate	20	324
Ferrous sulfate, exsiccated	30	217

Administration Oral: Do not chew or crush sustained release preparations; administer with water or juice between meals for maximum absorption; may administer with food if GI upset occurs; do not administer with milk or milk products

Monitoring Parameters Serum iron, total iron binding capacity, reticulocyte count, hemoglobin, ferritin

Reference Range

Serum iron:

Newborns: 110-270 mcg/dL

Infants: 30-70 mcg/dL

Children: 55-120 mcg/dL

Adults: Male: 75-175 mcg/dL; Female: 65-165 mcg/dL

Total iron binding capacity:

Newborns: 59-175 mcg/dL

Infants: 100-400 mcg/dL

Children and Adults: 230-430 mcg/dL

Transferrin: 204-360 mg/dL

Percent transferrin saturation: 20% to 50%

Iron levels >300 mcg/dL may be considered toxic; should be treated as an overdosage

Ferritin: 13-300 ng/mL

Test Interactions False-positive for blood in stool by the guaiac test

Patient Information May color the stools and urine black; do not take within 2 hours of tetracyclines or fluoroquinolones, do not take with milk or antacids; keep out of reach of children

Additional Information When treating iron deficiency anemias, treat for 3-4 months after hemoglobin/hematocrit return to normal in order to replenish total body stores; elemental iron dosages as high as 15 mg/kg/day have been used to supplement neonates receiving concomitant epoetin alpha in the treatment of anemia of prematurity

Dosage Forms Excipient information presented when available (limited, particularly for generics); consult specific product labeling. [DSC] = Discontinued product.

Ferrous fumarate:

Tablet: 324 mg [elemental iron 106 mg]

Femiron®: 63 mg [elemental iron 20 mg]

Ferretts: 325 mg [elemental iron 106 mg]

Hemocyte®: 324 mg [elemental iron 106 mg]

(Continued)

Iron Supplements (Oral/Enteral) *(Continued)*

Ircon®: 200 mg [elemental iron 66 mg]
Nephro-Fer®: 350 mg [elemental iron 115 mg; contains tartrazine]
Tablet, chewable (Feostat®): 100 mg [elemental iron 33 mg; chocolate flavor] [DSC]
Tablet, timed release (Ferro-Sequels®): 150 mg [elemental iron 50 mg; contains docusate sodium and sodium benzoate]

Ferrous gluconate:
Tablet: 246 mg [elemental iron 28 mg]; 300 mg [elemental iron 34 mg]; 325 mg [elemental iron 36 mg]
Fergon®: 240 mg [elemental iron 27 mg]

Ferrous sulfate:
Elixir: 220 mg/5 mL (480 mL) [elemental iron 44 mg/5 mL; contains alcohol]
Liquid, oral drops: 75 mg/0.6 mL (50 mL) [elemental iron 15 mg/0.6 mL]
Fer-Gen-Sol: 75 mg/0.6 mL (50 mL) [elemental iron 15 mg/0.6 mL]
Fer-In-Sol®: 75 mg/0.6 mL (50 mL) [elemental iron 15 mg/0.6 mL; contains alcohol 0.2% and sodium bisulfite]
Fer-Iron®: 75 mg/0.6 mL (50 mL) [elemental iron 15 mg/0.6 mL]
Tablet: 324 mg [elemental iron 65 mg]; 325 mg [elemental iron 65 mg]
Feratab®: 300 mg [elemental iron 60 mg]
Tablet, exsiccated (Feosol®): 200 mg [elemental iron 65 mg]
Tablet, exsiccated, timed release (Slow FE®): 160 mg [elemental iron 50 mg]

Polysaccharide - iron complex:
Capsule (Ferrex 150, Fe-Tinic™ 150 [DSC], Hytinic®, Niferex® 150, Nu-Iron® 150): Elemental iron 150 mg
Elixir (Niferex®): Elemental iron 100 mg/5 mL (240 mL) [contains alcohol 10%]
Tablet (Niferex®): Elemental iron 50 mg

Iron Supplements (Parenteral) (EYE ern SUP la ments)

U.S. Brand Names Dexferrum®; Ferrlecit®; INFeD®; Venofer®
Index Terms Iron Dextran; Iron Sucrose; Sodium Ferric Gluconate
Therapeutic Category Iron Salt, Parenteral; Mineral, Parenteral
Generic Available No
Use

Iron dextran: Treatment of microcytic, hypochromic anemia resulting from iron deficiency when oral iron administration is infeasible or ineffective

Ferric gluconate: Treatment of microcytic, hypochromic anemia resulting from iron deficiency in combination with erythropoietin in hemodialysis patients when iron administration is not feasible or ineffective

Iron sucrose: Treatment of microcytic, hypochromic anemia resulting from iron deficiency in chronic kidney disease patients, either dialysis-dependent or nondialysis-dependent, who may or may not be receiving erythropoietin

Pregnancy Risk Factor B (ferric gluconate, iron sucrose); C (iron dextran)

Contraindications Hypersensitivity to the iron formulation or any component (see Warnings); anemias that are not associated with iron deficiency; hemochromatosis; hemolytic anemia; iron overload

Warnings Deaths associated with parenteral iron administration following anaphylactic-type reactions have been reported; treatment agents for anaphylactic reactions (eg, epinephrine, steroids, diphenhydramine) should be immediately available; a test dose is recommended prior to initial therapy; rapid I.V. administration is associated with flushing, fatigue, weakness, chest, back, groin, or flank pain, and hypotension; use parenteral iron only in patients where the iron deficient state is not amenable to oral iron therapy; only iron dextran is approved for I.M. administration.

Ferric gluconate formulation contains benzyl alcohol which may cause allergic reactions in susceptible individuals; large amounts of benzyl alcohol (≥99 mg/kg/day) have been associated with a potentially fatal toxicity ("gasping syndrome") in neonates; the "gasping syndrome" consists of metabolic acidosis, respiratory distress, gasping respirations, CNS dysfunction (including convulsions, intracranial hemorrhage), hypotension and cardiovascular collapse; *in vitro* and animal studies have shown that benzoate, a metabolite of benzyl alcohol, displaces bilirubin from protein-binding sites; avoid use of ferric gluconate formulation in neonates. NEC was reported in five premature neonates who had received iron sucrose; no causal relationship has been established.

Precautions Use with caution in patients with histories of significant allergies, asthma, hepatic impairment, rheumatoid arthritis

Adverse Reactions Anaphylactoid reactions: Respiratory difficulties and cardiovascular collapse have been reported and occur most frequently within the first several minutes of administration

Cardiovascular: Cardiovascular collapse, hypotension, flushing, chest pain, syncope, tachycardia, MI, hypovolemia, hypertension, thrombosis
Central nervous system: Dizziness, fever, headache, chills, shivering, malaise, insomnia, agitation, somnolence
Dermatologic: Urticaria, pruritus, rash
Gastrointestinal: Nausea, vomiting, diarrhea, metallic taste, abdominal pain, dyspepsia, flatulence, eructation, melena, pharyngitis
Genitourinary: Discoloration of urine
Hematologic: Leukocytosis
Hepatic: Elevated liver enzymes
Local: Pain, staining of skin at the site of I.M. injection, phlebitis
Neuromuscular & skeletal: Arthralgia, arthritic reactivation in patients with quiescent arthritis, backache, paresthesia, leg cramps, weakness
Ocular: Blurred vision, conjunctivitis
Renal: Hematuria
Respiratory: Dyspnea, cough, rhinitis, upper respiratory infection, pulmonary edema, pneumonia
Miscellaneous: Lymphadenopathy, diaphoresis
Note: Sweating, urticaria, arthralgia, fever, chills, dizziness, headache, and nausea may be delayed 24-48 hours after I.V. administration or 3-4 days after I.M. administration

Stability Store at room temperature; use immediately after dilution in NS; product literature states parenteral iron formulations should not be mixed with other medications or in parenteral nutrition solutions

Mechanism of Action Replaces iron found in hemoglobin, myoglobin, and specific enzymes; allows transportation of oxygen via hemoglobin

Pharmacodynamics
Onset of action: Hematologic response to either oral or parenteral iron salts is essentially the same; red blood cell form and color changes within 3-10 days
Maximum effect: Peak reticulocytosis occurs in 5-10 days, and hemoglobin values increase within 2-4 weeks

Pharmacokinetics
Absorption: I.M.: 60% absorbed after 3 days; 90% after 1-3 weeks, the balance is slowly absorbed over months
Following I.V. doses, the uptake of iron by the reticuloendothelial system appears to be constant at about 40-60 mg/hour
Half-life:
Iron dextran: 48 hours
Iron sucrose: 6 hours
Ferric gluconate: 1.31 hours
Elimination: By the reticuloendothelial system and excreted in urine and feces (via bile)
Dialysis: Not dialyzable

Usual Dosage Multiple forms for parenteral iron exist; close attention must be paid to the specific product when ordering and administering; incorrect selection or substitution of one form for another without proper dosage adjustment may result in serious over or under dosing; test doses are recommended before starting therapy

Ferric gluconate: Dosage expressed in mg elemental iron: I.V.:
Children: 1.5 mg/kg (0.12 mL/kg Ferrlecit®) repeated at each of 8 sequential dialysis sessions not to exceed 125 mg (10 mL) per dose
Adults: 125 mg (10 mL) during hemodialysis; most patients will require a cumulative dose of 1 g over ~8 sequential dialysis treatments to achieve a favorable response
Note: A test dose (25 mg in adult patients) previously recommended in product literature is no longer listed. No pediatric test dose has been recommended by the manufacturer

Iron dextran:
Iron deficiency anemia:
I.M., I.V.: Test dose (given 1 hour prior to starting iron dextran therapy):
Infants: 12.5 mg (0.25 mL)
Children, Adolescents, and Adults: 25 mg (0.5 mL)
Total replacement dosage of iron dextran for iron deficiency anemia:
(mL) = 0.0476 x LBW (kg) x (Hb_n - Hb_o) + 1 mL/per 5 kg LBW (up to maximum of 14 mL)
LBW = lean body weight
Hb_n = desired hemoglobin (g/dL) = 12 if <15 kg or 14.8 if >15 kg
Hb_o = measured hemoglobin (g/dL)
Total iron replacement dosage for acute blood loss: Assumes 1 mL of normocytic, normochromic red cells = 1 mg elemental iron: Iron dextran (mL) = 0.02 x blood loss (mL) x hematocrit (expressed as a decimal fraction)
(Continued)

Iron Supplements (Parenteral) *(Continued)*

Note: Total dose infusions have been used safely and are the preferred method of administration

I.M.: Maximum daily dose: Injected in daily or less frequent increments:
- Infants <5 kg: 25 mg
- Children 5-10 kg: 50 mg
- Children >10 kg and Adults: 100 mg

Anemia of prematurity: I.V.: Neonates: 0.2-1 mg/kg/day or 20 mg/kg/week with epoetin alfa therapy

Anemia of chronic renal failure: I.V.: Children and Adults: 2 mg/kg three times/week with epoetin alfa therapy

Iron sucrose: I.V.:

Children: Limited data on 14 children (ages 2-14 years) with ESRD were treated with iron sucrose in 3 dosages: 3 mg/kg/dialysis (repletion treatment), 1 mg/kg/dialysis (repletion treatment), and 0.3 mg/kg/dialysis (maintenance treatment). Iron overload expressed by serum ferritin >400, occurred in all patients receiving 3 mg/kg dosage. The lower dosage (1 mg/kg) successfully increased ferritin therapeutic levels. The 0.3 mg/kg dose was successful in maintaining ferritin between 193-250 mcg/L (Leijn, 2004).

Adults **(doses expressed in mg of elemental iron)**: Test dose: 50 mg (while product labeling does not indicate need for a test dose in product-naive patients, test doses were administered in some clinical trials)

Hemodialysis-dependent chronic renal failure: 100 mg (5 mL) administered 1-3 times/week during dialysis, for a total dose of 1000 mg (10 doses); administer no more than 3 times/week; may continue to administer at lowest dose necessary to maintain target hemoglobin, hematocrit, and iron storage parameters

Nonhemodialysis-dependent chronic renal failure: 200 mg (10 mL) administered on 5 different days over a 2-week period (total dose: 1000 mg). Single doses of 500 mg administered for 2 doses (day 1 and day 14) have been done in a limited number of patients, 6% (2/30) experienced hypotension (manufacturer's information)

Administration Parenteral: Avoid dilution in dextrose due to an increased incidence of local pain and phlebitis

Iron dextran:

I.M.: Use Z-track technique for I.M. administration (deep into the upper outer quadrant of buttock)

I.V.: Infuse test dose over at least 5 minutes; dilute replacement dose in NS (50-100 mL), maximum concentration 50 mg/mL and infuse over 1-6 hours at a maximum rate of 50 mg/minute

Ferric gluconate:

I.V. infusion: Dilute test dose in 50 mL NS and infuse over 1 hour; dilute repletion dose in 25-100 mL NS and infuse over at least 1 hour; do not exceed 12.5 mg/minute; **not for I.M. administration**

Slow I.V. injection: 1 mL (12.5 mg iron) of undiluted solution per minute (5 minutes/vial)

Iron sucrose:

Slow I.V. injection: 100-200 mg (5-10 mL) over 2-5 minutes

Infusion: Dilute 1 vial (5 mL) in maximum of 100 mL NS; infuse over at least 15 minutes; large doses (500 mg) should be diluted in 250 mL NS and infused over 3.5-4 hours (limited experience in adult patients with the large-dose infusion; see Usual Dosage in non-hemodialysis-dependent chronic renal failure patients) **not for I.M. administration**

Monitoring Parameters Vital signs and other symptoms of anaphylactoid reactions (during I.V. infusion); reticulocyte count, serum ferritin, hemoglobin, serum iron concentrations, and TIBC may not be meaningful for 3 weeks after administration, especially after large I.V. doses

Reference Range

Serum iron:
- Newborns: 110-270 mcg/dL
- Infants: 30-70 mcg/dL
- Children: 55-120 mcg/dL
- Adults: Male: 75-175 mcg/dL; female: 65-165 mcg/dL

Total iron binding capacity:
- Newborns: 59-175 mcg/dL
- Infants: 100-400 mcg/dL
- Children and Adults: 230-430 mcg/dL

Transferrin: 204-360 mg/dL

Percent transferrin saturation: 20% to 50%

Iron levels >300 mcg/dL may be considered toxic; should be treated as an overdosage

Ferritin: 13-300 ng/mL

Test Interactions May cause falsely elevated values of serum bilirubin and falsely decreased values of serum calcium

Nursing Implications Only iron dextran is approved for I.M. administration

Additional Information Iron storage may lag behind the appearance of normal red blood cell morphology; use periodic hematologic determination to assess therapy; VLBW infants receiving I.V. iron sucrose 2 mg/kg/day with erythropoietin showed improved erythropoiesis when compared with oral iron supplementation and erythropoietin (Pollak, et al)

Dosage Forms Excipient information presented when available (limited, particularly for generics); consult specific product labeling. Expressed as mg of **elemental iron:**

Injection, solution, as **ferric gluconate** (Ferrlecit®): 12.5 mg/mL (5 mL) [contains benzyl alcohol and sucrose 20%]

Injection, solution, as **iron dextran**:

Dexferrum®: 50 mg/mL (1 mL, 2 mL)

INFeD®: 50 mg/mL (2 mL)

Injection, solution, as **iron sucrose** [preservative free] (Venofer®): 20 mg/mL (5 mL)

References

Auerbach M, Witt D, Toler W, et al, "Clinical Use of the Total Dose Intravenous Infusion of Iron Dextran," *J Lab Clin Med*, 1988, 111(5):566-70.

Benito RP and Guerrero TC, "Response to a Single Intravenous Dose Versus Multiple Intramuscular Administration of Iron-Dextran Complex: A Comparative Study," *Curr Ther Res Clin Exp*, 1973, 15(7):373-82.

Leijn E, Monnens LA, and Cornelissen EA, "Intravenous Iron Supplementation in Children on Hemodialysis," *J Nephrol*, 2004, 17(3):423-6.

Pollak A, Hayde M, Hayn M, et al, "Effect of Intravenous Iron Supplementation on Erythropoiesis in Erythropoietin-Treated Premature Infants," *Pediatrics*, 2001, 107(1):78-85.

Seligman PA, Dahl NV, Strobos J, et al, "Single-Dose Pharmacokinetics of Sodium Ferric Gluconate Complex in Iron-Deficient Subjects," *Pharmacotherapy*, 2004, 24(5):574-83.

♦ **Isagel® [OTC]** *see* Ethyl Alcohol *on page 619*

♦ **ISG** *see* Immune Globulin (Intramuscular) *on page 817*

♦ **Isoamyl Nitrite** *see* Amyl Nitrite *on page 130*

Isoniazid (eye soe NYE a zid)

Medication Safety Issues

International issues:

Hydra® [Japan] may be confused with Hydrea®

Related Information

Commonly Used Antidotes for Acute Overdoses *on page 1920*

Overdose and Toxicology *on page 1916*

U.S. Brand Names Nydrazid® [DSC]

Canadian Brand Names Isotamine®; PMS-Isoniazid

Index Terms INH; Isonicotinic Acid Hydrazide

Therapeutic Category Antitubercular Agent

Generic Available Yes

Use Treatment of susceptible mycobacterial infection due to *M. tuberculosis* and prophylactically to those individuals exposed to tuberculosis

Pregnancy Risk Factor C

Lactation Enters breast milk/compatible

Contraindications Hypersensitivity to isoniazid or any component; acute liver disease; previous history of hepatic damage during isoniazid therapy

Warnings Severe and sometimes fatal hepatitis may occur or develop even after many months of treatment; the administration of isoniazid in combination with rifampin is associated with an increased incidence of hepatotoxicity if isoniazid dose is >10 mg/kg/day; patients must report any prodromal symptoms of hepatitis such as fatigue, weakness, malaise, anorexia, nausea, vomiting, dark urine, or yellowing of eyes

Precautions Use with caution in patients with renal impairment and chronic liver disease

Adverse Reactions

Central nervous system: Seizure, stupor, dizziness, agitation, euphoria, psychosis, fever, ataxia

Dermatologic: Skin eruptions, rash, acne

Endocrine & metabolic: Hyperglycemia, metabolic acidosis, pellagra

Gastrointestinal: Nausea, vomiting, epigastric distress; diarrhea (associated with administration of syrup formulation)

Hematologic: Agranulocytosis, hemolytic anemia, aplastic anemia, thrombocytopenia, eosinophilia, leukopenia

Hepatic: Hepatitis, 3% to 10% of children experience transient elevated liver transaminase levels

Local: Irritation at I.M. injection site

(Continued)

Isoniazid *(Continued)*

Neuromuscular & skeletal: Peripheral neuropathy
Ocular: Optic neuritis
Otic: Tinnitus
Miscellaneous: Hypersensitivity reaction

Drug Interactions Cytochrome P450 isoenzyme CYP2E1 substrate; isoenzyme CYP2E1 inducer; isoenzyme CYP1A2, CYP2C, CYP2C9, CYP2C19, and CYP3A3/4 inhibitor

May increase serum concentrations of phenytoin, carbamazepine, diazepam; aluminum salts may decrease isoniazid absorption; prednisolone may increase isoniazid metabolism; cycloserine, ethionamide (additive CNS toxicity); disulfiram (coordination difficulty, psychotic episode); meperidine (serotonin syndrome); rifampin (increased hepatotoxicity)

Food Interactions Rate and extent of isoniazid absorption may be reduced when administered with food; avoid foods with histamine or tyramine (cheese, broad beans, dry sausage, salami, nonfresh meat, liver pate, soya bean, liquid and powdered protein supplements, wine); increase dietary intake of folate, niacin, magnesium, and pyridoxine; the American Academy of Pediatrics recommends that pyridoxine supplementation (1-2 mg/kg/day) should be administered to patients with nutritional deficiencies including all symptomatic HIV-infected children, children or adolescents on meat or milk-deficient diets, breast-feeding infants and their mothers, pregnant adolescents and women, and those predisposed to neuritis to prevent peripheral neuropathy

Stability Protect from light and excessive heat; avoid freezing

Mechanism of Action Inhibits mycolic acid synthesis resulting in disruption of the bacterial cell wall

Pharmacokinetics

Absorption: Oral, I.M.: Rapid and complete
Distribution: Crosses the placenta; appears in breast milk; distributes into most body tissues and fluids including the CSF
Protein binding: 10% to 15%
Metabolism: By the liver to acetylisoniazid with decay rate determined genetically by acetylation phenotype; undergoes further hydrolysis to isonicotinic acid and acetylhydrazine
Half-life: May be prolonged in patients with impaired hepatic function or severe renal impairment
- Fast acetylators: 30-100 minutes
- Slow acetylators: 2-5 hours

Time to peak serum concentration: Oral: Within 1-2 hours
Elimination: 75% to 95% excreted in urine as unchanged drug and metabolites; small amounts excreted in feces and saliva
Dialysis: Dialyzable (50% to 100%)

Usual Dosage Oral, I.M.:

Infants and Children:
- Treatment: 10-15 mg/kg/day in 1-2 divided doses; maximum dose: 300 mg/day
- Prophylaxis: 10 mg/kg/day given once daily, not to exceed 300 mg/day

Adults:
- Treatment: 5 mg/kg/day given daily (usual dose: 300 mg)
- Disseminated disease: 10 mg/kg/day in 1-2 divided doses
- Prophylaxis: 300 mg/day given daily

American Thoracic Society and CDC currently recommend twice weekly therapy as part of a short-course regimen which follows 1-2 months of daily treatment for uncomplicated pulmonary tuberculosis in **compliant** patients
- Children: 20-30 mg/kg/dose (up to 900 mg/dose) twice weekly
- Adults: 15 mg/kg/dose (up to 900 mg/dose) twice weekly

Duration of therapy:
- Asymptomatic infection (positive skin test):
  - Isoniazid susceptible: 9 months of isoniazid
  - Isoniazid resistant: 9 months of rifampin
- Pulmonary, hilar adenopathy, and extrapulmonary infection other than meningitis, bone/joint, or disseminated infection:
  - **6 months** which includes 2-month therapy of isoniazid, rifampin, and pyrazinamide daily followed by 4 months of isoniazid and rifampin daily **or** 2 months of isoniazid, rifampin, and pyrazinamide daily, followed by 4 months of isoniazid and rifampin twice weekly under direct observation
  - **alternatively**
  - **9 months** of isoniazid and rifampin daily **or** 1 month of isoniazid and rifampin daily followed by 8 months of isoniazid and rifampin twice weekly under direct observation; if isoniazid resistance is identified, rifampin and ethambutol should be continued for a maximum of 12 months

Note: If drug resistance is possible, ethambutol or streptomycin should be added to the initial therapy regimen until susceptibility is determined

Meningitis, bone/joint, and disseminated infection:

12 months which includes 2 months of isoniazid, rifampin, pyrazinamide, and streptomycin daily followed by 10 months of isoniazid and rifampin daily **or** 2 months of isoniazid, rifampin, pyrazinamide, and streptomycin daily followed by 10 months of isoniazid and rifampin twice weekly under direct observation

Administration

Oral: Administer 1 hour before or 2 hours after meals with water; administration of isoniazid syrup has been associated with diarrhea

Parenteral: I.M.: Administer I.M. when oral therapy is not possible

Monitoring Parameters Periodic liver function tests; monitor for prodromal signs of hepatitis; ophthalmologic exam; chest x-ray

Test Interactions False-positive urinary glucose with Clinitest®

Patient Information Report any prodromal symptoms of hepatitis (fatigue, weakness, nausea, vomiting, dark urine, or yellowing of eyes) or any burning, tingling, or numbness in the extremities; avoid alcohol

Dosage Forms Excipient information presented when available (limited, particularly for generics); consult specific product labeling. [DSC] = Discontinued product

Injection, solution (Nydrazid®): 100 mg/mL (10 mL) [DSC]

Syrup: 50 mg/5 mL (473 mL) [orange flavor]

Tablet: 100 mg, 300 mg

References

Ad Hoc Committee of the Scientific Assembly on Microbiology, Tuberculosis, and Pulmonary Infections, "Treatment of Tuberculosis and Tuberculosis Infection in Adults and Children," *Clin Infect Dis*, 1995, 21:9-27.

American Academy of Pediatrics, Committee on Infectious Diseases, "Chemotherapy for Tuberculosis in Infants and Children," *Pediatrics*, 1992, 89(1):161-5.

Starke JR, "Modern Approach to the Diagnosis and Treatment of Tuberculosis in Children," *Pediatr Clin North Am*, 1988, 35(3):441-64.

Starke JR, "Multidrug Therapy for Tuberculosis in Children," *Pediatr Infect Dis J*, 1990, 9(11):785-93.

Van Scoy RE and Wilkowske CJ, "Antituberculous Agents: Isoniazid, Rifampin, Streptomycin, Ethambutol, and Pyrazinamide," *Mayo Clin Proc*, 1983, 58(4):233-40.

- **Isonicotinic Acid Hydrazide** *see* Isoniazid *on page 873*
- **Isonipecaine Hydrochloride** *see* Meperidine *on page 1002*
- **Isophane Insulin** *see* Insulin NPH *on page 846*
- **Isophane Insulin and Regular Insulin** *see* Insulin NPH and Insulin Regular *on page 847*
- **Isophosphamide** *see* Ifosfamide *on page 810*

Isoproterenol (eye soe proe TER e nole)

Medication Safety Issues

Sound-alike/look-alike issues:

Isuprel® may be confused with Disophrol®, Ismelin®, Isordil®

Related Information

Asthma *on page 1904*

Commonly Used Antidotes for Acute Overdoses *on page 1920*

Emergency Pediatric Drip Calculations *on page 1652*

U.S. Brand Names Isuprel®

Index Terms Isoproterenol Hydrochloride

Therapeutic Category Adrenergic Agonist Agent; Antiasthmatic; $Beta_1$ & $Beta_2$-Adrenergic Agonist Agent; Bronchodilator; Sympathomimetic

Generic Available Yes

Use Treatment of asthma or COPD (reversible airway obstruction); ventricular arrhythmias due to A-V nodal block; hemodynamically compromised bradyarrhythmias or atropine-resistant bradyarrhythmias, temporary use in third degree A-V block until pacemaker insertion; low cardiac output or vasoconstrictive shock states

Pregnancy Risk Factor C

Lactation Excretion in breast milk unknown

Contraindications Hypersensitivity to isoproterenol, other sympathomimetic amines, or any component (see Warnings); angina, pre-existing cardiac arrhythmias (ventricular); tachycardia or A-V block caused by cardiac glycoside intoxication; narrow-angle glaucoma

Warnings Tolerance may occur with prolonged use; when discontinuing an isoproterenol continuous infusion used for bronchodilation, the infusion **must** be gradually tapered over a 24- to 48-hour period to prevent rebound bronchospasm; injection contains sulfites which may cause allergic reactions in susceptible individuals

Precautions Use with caution in diabetics, renal or cardiovascular disease, hyperthyroidism, prostatic hypertrophy

(Continued)

Isoproterenol *(Continued)*

Adverse Reactions

Cardiovascular: Flushing of the face or skin, ventricular arrhythmias, tachycardia, hypotension, chest pain, palpitations, hypertension

Central nervous system: Nervousness, restlessness, anxiety, dizziness, headache, vertigo, insomnia

Endocrine & metabolic: Parotid glands swelling

Gastrointestinal: Heartburn, GI distress, nausea, vomiting, dry throat, xerostomia

Neuromuscular & skeletal: Tremor, weakness, trembling

Miscellaneous: Diaphoresis

Drug Interactions Additive effects and increased cardiotoxicity when administered concomitantly with other sympathomimetic amines; beta-adrenergic blocking agents may decrease effectiveness due to beta blockade; may increase theophylline elimination

Mechanism of Action Stimulates $beta_1$- and $beta_2$-receptors resulting in relaxation of bronchial, GI, and uterine smooth muscle; increases heart rate and contractility; causes vasodilation of peripheral vasculature

Pharmacodynamics

Onset of action: I.V.: Immediately

Duration: I.V. (single dose): Few minutes

Pharmacokinetics

Metabolism: By conjugation in many tissues including the liver and lungs

Half-life: 2.5-5 minutes

Elimination: In urine principally as sulfate conjugates

Usual Dosage

Neonates, Infants, and Children: I.V. infusion: 0.05-2 mcg/kg/minute; rate (mL/hour) = dose (mcg/kg/minute) x weight (kg) x 60 minutes/hour divided by concentration (mcg/mL)

Adults: I.V. infusion: 2-20 mcg/minute

Administration Parenteral: For continuous infusions, dilute in dextrose or NS to a maximum concentration of 20 mcg/mL; concentrations as high as 64 mcg/mL have been used safely and with efficacy in situations of extreme fluid restriction

Monitoring Parameters Heart rate, blood pressure, respiratory rate, arterial blood gases, central venous pressure, EKG

Patient Information May cause dry mouth

Additional Information Hypotension is more common in hypovolemic patients

Dosage Forms Excipient information presented when available (limited, particularly for generics); consult specific product labeling.

Injection, solution, as hydrochloride: 0.02 mg/mL (10 mL); 0.2 mg/mL (1:5000) (1 mL, 5 mL) [contains sodium metabisulfite]

References

"National Asthma Education and Prevention Program. Expert Panel Report: Guidelines for the Diagnosis and Management of Asthma Update on Selected Topics--2002," *J Allergy Clin Immunol*, 2002, 110(5 Suppl):S141-219.

Rachelefsky GS and Siegel SC, "Asthma in Infants and Children - Treatment of Childhood Asthma: Part 1l," *J Allergy Clin Immunol*, 1985, 76(3):409-25.

♦ **Isoproterenol Hydrochloride** *see* Isoproterenol *on page 875*

♦ **Isoptin® SR** *see* Verapamil *on page 1611*

♦ **Isopto® Atropine** *see* Atropine *on page 181*

♦ **Isopto® Carpine** *see* Pilocarpine *on page 1260*

♦ **Isopto® Eserine (Can)** *see* Physostigmine *on page 1257*

♦ **Isopto® Homatropine** *see* Homatropine *on page 768*

♦ **Isopto® Hyoscine** *see* Scopolamine *on page 1421*

♦ **Isotamine® (Can)** *see* Isoniazid *on page 873*

Isotretinoin (eye soe TRET i noyn)

Medication Safety Issues

Sound-alike/look-alike issues:

Accutane® may be confused with Accolate®, Accupril®

U.S. Brand Names Accutane®; Amnesteem™; Claravis™; Sotret®

Canadian Brand Names Accutane®; Clarus™; Isotrex®

Index Terms 13-*cis*-Retinoic Acid

Therapeutic Category Acne Products; Retinoic Acid Derivative; Vitamin A Derivative

Generic Available Yes

Use Treatment of severe recalcitrant cystic and/or conglobate acne unresponsive to conventional therapy; used investigationally for the treatment of children with high-risk neuroblastoma that does not respond to conventional therapy

Restrictions iPLEDGE is a risk minimization program designed by the FDA to decrease fetal exposures to isotretinoin. iPLEDGE requires that all wholesalers, prescribers, patients, and dispensing pharmacies register with a central clearinghouse. Registration will be accessible through the internet at http://www.ipledgeprogram.com or by calling 866-495-0654. The Responsible Site Pharmacist must activate the iPLEDGE registration. Prescriptions for isotretinoin may not be dispensed unless authorized by the iPLEDGE system. Prescriptions may not be written for more than a 1-month supply. The iPLEDGE system will automatically calculate and provide the "Do Not Dispense To Patient After" date to the pharmacist. The pharmacist must not dispense the prescription after this date. Refills are not allowed.

Prescribers will be provided with qualification stickers after they have read the details of the program and have signed and mailed to the manufacturer their agreement to participate. Audits of pharmacies will be conducted to monitor program compliance.

Medication Guide An FDA-approved patient medication guide, which is available with the product information and at http://www.fda.gov/cder/Offices/ODS/medication_guides.htm, must be dispensed with this medication for each new outpatient prescription and refill.

Pregnancy Risk Factor X

Lactation Excretion in breast milk unknown/contraindicated

Contraindications Hypersensitivity to isotretinoin, parabens, vitamin A or other retinoids; patients who are pregnant or intend to become pregnant during treatment; nursing mothers

Warnings Major human fetal abnormalities to isotretinoin administration have been documented; during pregnancy, it can cause fetal defects in the CNS (cerebral abnormalities, hydrocephalus, microcephaly, cranial nerve deficit, cerebellar malformation), skull, ear, eye, and cardiovascular systems, cleft palate, and parathyroid hormone deficiency; not to be used in women of childbearing potential unless woman is capable of complying with effective contraceptive measures. Prescription for isotretinoin should not be issued until a female patient has had negative results from 2 urine or serum pregnancy tests, one performed in the prescriber's office when the patient is qualified for therapy, the second one performed on the second day of next normal menstrual period or 11 days after the last unprotected act of sexual intercourse, whichever is later. Effective contraception must be used for at least 1 month before beginning therapy, during therapy, and for 1 month after discontinuation of therapy. Isotretinoin may cause depression, psychosis, and suicidal ideations; concomitant use with tetracyclines has been associated with cases of pseudotumor cerebri; avoid concomitant treatment with tetracyclines

Precautions Use with caution in patients with diabetes mellitus or hypertriglyceridemia; history of childhood osteoporosis, osteomalacia, or other disorders of bone metabolism including patients with anorexia nervosa or patients receiving drugs that cause osteoporosis/osteomalacia or affect vitamin D metabolism (ie, corticosteroids, anticonvulsants)

Adverse Reactions

- Cardiovascular: Palpitations, tachycardia, vascular thrombotic stroke, edema, vasculitis
- Central nervous system: Fatigue, headache, dizziness, pseudotumor cerebri, psychosis, mental depression, suicidal ideation, seizures, insomnia
- Dermatologic: Pruritus, alopecia, cheilitis, photosensitivity, rash
- Endocrine & metabolic: Hypertriglyceridemia, hyperuricemia, hyperglycemia, hypercalcemia
- Gastrointestinal: Xerostomia, anorexia, nausea, vomiting, inflammatory bowel syndrome, acute pancreatitis
- Hematologic: Elevation in erythrocyte sedimentation rate, decrease in hemoglobin and hematocrit, neutropenia
- Hepatic: Hepatitis; elevated AST, ALT, and alkaline phosphatase
- Neuromuscular & skeletal: Bone pain, arthralgia, myalgia, skeletal hyperostosis, premature epiphyseal closure, rhabdomyolysis (rare)
- Ocular: Conjunctivitis, corneal opacities, cataracts, blurred vision, decreased night vision
- Otic: Hearing impairment
- Renal: Hematuria, proteinuria
- Respiratory: Epistaxis, bronchospasm
- Miscellaneous: Hypersensitivity reactions

Drug Interactions Increased clearance of carbamazepine; vitamin A supplements increase toxic effects; alcohol may potentiate an increase in serum triglycerides;

(Continued)

Isotretinoin *(Continued)*

concomitant use with tetracyclines has been associated with cases of pseudotumor cerebri (avoid tetracyclines)

Food Interactions Food or milk increases isotretinoin bioavailability

Stability Protect from light

Mechanism of Action Reduces sebaceous gland size and reduces sebum production; regulates cell proliferation and differentiation

Pharmacokinetics

Absorption: Oral: Demonstrates biphasic absorption

Distribution: Crosses the placenta; appears in breast milk, bile

Protein binding: 99% to 100%

Metabolism: In the liver; major metabolite: 4-oxo-isotretinoin (active); undergoes enterohepatic circulation

Half-life, terminal: 10-20 hours for isotretinoin, and 17-50 hours for its metabolite

Time to peak serum concentration: Within 3 hours

Elimination: Excreted in feces as unchanged drug and in urine as metabolites

Usual Dosage Oral:

Children: Maintenance therapy for neuroblastoma: 160 mg/m^2/day in 2 divided doses for 14 consecutive days in a 28-day cycle has been used investigationally

Children and Adults: Acne: 0.5-2 mg/kg/day in 2 divided doses (dosages as low as 0.05 mg/kg/day have been reported to be beneficial) for 15-20 weeks or until the total cyst count decreases by 70%, whichever is sooner

Administration Oral: Capsules can be swallowed or chewed and swallowed; the capsule may be opened with a large needle and the contents placed on apple sauce or ice cream for patients unable to swallow the capsule; administer with meals

Monitoring Parameters CBC with differential, platelet count, baseline ESR, serum triglyceride, liver enzymes, CPK, ophthalmologic exam, blood glucose; pregnancy test in female patients of childbearing potential (see Warnings); bone density measurement

Patient Information Read the patient Medication Guide that you receive with each prescription and refill of isotretinoin. Do not take vitamin supplements containing vitamin A; use caution when driving at night since decreased night vision can develop suddenly; patients who wear contact lenses may experience decreased tolerance to the lenses; avoid alcohol; may cause dry mouth; notify physician of any headache, blurred vision, yellowing of skin or eyes, bone or muscle pain, vision changes, suicidal thoughts, dark urine, abdominal pain, rectal bleeding, or severe diarrhea; female patients of childbearing potential must be counseled to use 2 effective forms of contraception simultaneously, unless absolute abstinence is the chosen method; patients should not self-medicate with St John's wort due to a possible interaction with hormonal contraceptives; provide female patients instruction to join the Accutane® survey and watch a videotape that provides information about contraceptive methods; inform patients not to donate blood during therapy and for 1 month following discontinuation of therapy

May cause photosensitivity reactions (eg, exposure to sunlight may cause severe sunburn, skin rash, redness, or itching); avoid exposure to sunlight and artificial light sources (sunlamps, tanning booth/bed); wear protective clothing, wide-brimmed hats, sunglasses, and lip sunscreen (SPF ≥15); use a sunscreen [broad-spectrum sunscreen or physical sunscreen (preferred) or sunblock with SPF ≥15]; contact physician if reaction occurs.

Dosage Forms Excipient information presented when available (limited, particularly for generics); consult specific product labeling.

Capsule:

Accutane®: 10 mg, 20 mg, 40 mg [contains soybean oil and parabens]

Amnesteem™: 10 mg, 20 mg, 40 mg [contains soybean oil]

Claravis™: 10 mg, 20 mg, 40 mg

Sotret®: 10 mg, 20 mg, 30 mg, 40 mg [contains soybean oil]

References

American Academy of Pediatrics Committee on Drugs, "Retinoid Therapy for Severe Dermatological Disorders," *Pediatrics*, 1992, 90(1 Pt 1):119-20.

DiGiovanna JJ and Peck GL, "Oral Synthetic Retinoid Treatment in Children," *Pediatr Dermatol*, 1983, 1(1):77-88.

Matthay KK, Villablanca JG, Seeger RC, et al, "Treatment of High-Risk Neuroblastoma With Intensive Chemotherapy, Radiotherapy, Autologous Bone Marrow Transplantation, and 13-cis-Retinoic Acid. Children's Cancer Group," *N Engl J Med*, 1999, 341:1165-73.

Reynolds CP, Kane DJ, Einhorn PA, et al, "Response of Neuroblastoma to Retinoic Acid *In Vitro*, and *In Vivo*," *Prog Clin Biol Res*, 1991, 366:203-11

♦ **Isotrex® (Can)** *see* Isotretinoin *on page 876*

Isradipine (iz RA di peen)

Medication Safety Issues

Sound-alike/look-alike issues:

DynaCirc® may be confused with Dynabac®, Dynacin®

Related Information

Antihypertensive Agents by Class *on page 1678*

U.S. Brand Names DynaCirc® [DSC]; DynaCirc® CR

Canadian Brand Names DynaCirc®

Therapeutic Category Antihypertensive Agent; Calcium Channel Blocker

Generic Available Yes: Capsule

Use Treatment of hypertension

Pregnancy Risk Factor C

Lactation Excretion in breast milk unknown/not recommended

Contraindications Hypersensitivity to isradipine or any component

Warnings Symptomatic hypotension may occur; syncope and severe dizziness have been rarely reported, especially after initiation of recommended doses. May cause negative inotropic effects in some patients (use with caution in patients with CHF, especially when used in combination with beta-blockers). Dose-related peripheral edema may occur (use caution in differentiating this adverse effect from decreasing left ventricular function in patients with CHF).

Capsules may contain benzyl alcohol which may cause allergic reactions in susceptible individuals; large amounts of benzyl alcohol (≥99 mg/kg/day) have been associated with a potentially fatal toxicity ("gasping syndrome") in neonates; the "gasping syndrome" consists of metabolic acidosis, respiratory distress, gasping respirations, CNS dysfunction (including convulsions, intracranial hemorrhage), hypotension and cardiovascular collapse; use isradipine capsules containing benzyl alcohol with caution in neonates; *in vitro* and animal studies have shown that benzoate, a metabolite of benzyl alcohol, displaces bilirubin from protein binding sites

Precautions Use with caution in patients with CHF or hepatic dysfunction. Use controlled release tablets with caution in patients with severe GI narrowing (obstructive symptoms have occurred in patients with GI strictures after ingestion of other nondeformable controlled release products). Safety and efficacy have not been established in pediatric patients.

Adverse Reactions

Cardiovascular: Edema (dose related, 1% to 9%), palpitation (dose related, 1% to 5%), flushing (dose related, 1% to 5%), tachycardia, chest pain; syncope (rare); slight prolongation of QT_c interval of 3% in one study

Central nervous system: Headache, dizziness, fatigue (dose related, 1% to 9%)

Dermatologic: Rash

Gastrointestinal: Nausea, abdominal discomfort, vomiting, diarrhea, constipation, abdominal distention

Genitourinary: Increased urinary frequency

Neuromuscular & skeletal: Weakness

Respiratory: Dyspnea

Drug Interactions Cytochrome P450 isoenzyme CYP3A4 (major) substrate; isoenzyme CYP3A4 (weak) inhibitor

Concomitant antihypertensive agents or diuretics may increase the hypotensive effects of isradipine; anesthetic doses of fentanyl with concurrent use of a beta-blocker and calcium channel blocker may cause severe hypotension (administration of IV fluids may be required). Calcium may decrease or reverse the effects of calcium channel blockers, especially hypotension. Isradipine may increase propranolol serum concentrations.

Concurrent use with cimetidine or cytochrome P450 isoenzyme CYP3A4 inhibitors (eg, azole antifungals, clarithromycin, erythromycin, isoniazid, propofol, protease inhibitors, quinidine) may increase serum concentrations or effects of isradipine (monitor closely; dosage adjustment may be needed). Cytochrome P450 isoenzyme CYP3A4 inducers [eg, carbamazepine, phenobarbital, phenytoin, rifampin, the herbal medicine St. John's wort (*Hypericum perforatum*)] may decrease serum concentrations or effects of isradipine (monitor closely; dosage increase of isradipine may be needed).

Food Interactions

Capsules: Food decreases the rate, but not the extent of absorption

Controlled release tablets: Food decreases bioavailability by up to 25%

Stability

Capsules: Store at controlled room temperature; dispense in a tight, light-resistant container

(Continued)

Isradipine *(Continued)*

Controlled release tablets: Store below 30°C (86°F), in a tight container; protect from moisture and humidity

Mechanism of Action Inhibits calcium ions from entering the "slow channels" or select voltage-sensitive areas of vascular smooth muscle and myocardium during depolarization; produces a relaxation of coronary vascular smooth muscle and coronary vasodilation; increases myocardial oxygen delivery in patients with vasospastic angina

Pharmacodynamics

Onset of action:
- Immediate release capsule: ~1 hour
- Controlled release tablet: 2 hours

Maximum effect: **Note:** Full hypotensive effect may not occur for 2-4 weeks
- Immediate release capsule (single dose): 2-3 hours
- Controlled release tablet (single dose): 8-10 hours

Duration:
- Immediate release capsule: >12 hours
- Controlled release tablet: 24 hours

Pharmacokinetics

Absorption: 90% to 95%, but large first-pass effect

Distribution: V_d (apparent): 3 L/kg; crosses the placenta

Protein binding: 95%

Metabolism: Extensive first-pass effect; hepatically metabolized via cytochrome P450 isoenzyme CYP3A4; major metabolic pathways include oxidation and ester cleavage; six inactive metabolites have been identified

Bioavailability: Oral: 15% to 24%
- Patients with renal dysfunction (Cl_{cr} 30-80 mL/minute): Increased by 45%
- Patients with severe renal failure (Cl_{cr} < 10 mL/minute) who are on hemodialysis: Decreased by 20% to 50%
- Patients with hepatic impairment: Increased by 52%

Half-life: Alpha half-life: 1.5-2 hours; terminal half-life: 8 hours

Time to peak serum concentration:
- Immediate release capsule: 1.5 hours
- Controlled release tablet: Plateaus between 7-18 hours

Elimination: 60% to 65% of the dose is eliminated in the urine (none as unchanged drug); 25% to 30% in the feces

Dialysis: Not significantly removed by hemodialysis (supplemental dose not required)

Usual Dosage

Children: Limited information exists; dose is not well established; only 3 retrospective pediatric studies have been published (see Johnson, 1997; Strauser, 2000; Flynn, 2002); further studies are needed. Some experts recommend the following:
- Immediate release capsules (or extemporaneously prepared suspension): Initial: 0.05-0.15 mg/kg/dose given 3-4 times/day; titrate dose to response; usual dose: 0.3-0.4 mg/kg/day divided every 8 hours; maximum dose 0.8 mg/kg/day up to 20 mg/day (see Flynn, 2000)
- Controlled release tablet: Children who receive a total daily dose of 5 or 10 mg of an immediate release formulation may be switched to an equivalent daily dose of the controlled release tablets administered once or twice daily (Flynn, 2002).

Adults:
- Immediate release capsules: Initial: 2.5 mg twice daily; titrate dose to response; may increase dose in increments of 5 mg/day at 2-4 week intervals; usual dosage range (JNC 7): 2.5-10 mg/day in 2 divided doses; maximum: 20 mg/day; **Note:** Most patients do not have any additional response to doses >10 mg/day, but may have increased adverse effects.
- Controlled release tablet: Initial: 5 mg once daily; titrate dose to response; may increase dose in increments of 5 mg/day at 2-4 week intervals; maximum: 20 mg/day; **Note:** Doses >10 mg/day are associated with increased adverse effects.

Administration May be administered without regard to meals; swallow controlled release tablet whole, do not crush, break, chew, or divide.

Monitoring Parameters Blood pressure, heart rate, liver and renal function

Patient Information May cause dizziness and impair ability to perform activities requiring mental alertness or physical coordination. Do not discontinue abruptly. Report unrelieved headache, dizziness, shortness of breath, rapid heart beat, chest pain, swelling of extremities, or sudden weight gain. Some medicines may interact with isradipine; report the use of other medications, nonprescription medications, and herbal or natural products to your physician and pharmacist; avoid the herbal medicine St John's wort. Empty controlled release tablets may appear in stool after medication is absorbed (this is normal).

Nursing Implications Assess therapeutic effectiveness and adverse reactions on a regular basis during therapy. Monitor blood pressure. Instruct patient on appropriate use, side effects, appropriate interventions, and adverse symptoms to report.

Additional Information DynaCirc® CR is an osmotic controlled-release formulation; the tablet is nondeformable; drug is released from the tablet at a constant rate that is dependent on the osmotic gradient between the contents of the bilayer active drug core of the tablet and the fluid in the GI tract; drug release is independent of pH or GI motility.

Dosage Forms Excipient information presented when available (limited, particularly for generics); consult specific product labeling.

Capsule: 2.5 mg, 5 mg

DynaCirc®: 2.5 mg [DSC], 5 mg [DSC]

Tablet, controlled release:

DynaCirc® CR: 5 mg, 10 mg

Extemporaneous Preparations A 1 mg/mL oral suspension made from isradipine capsules and simple syrup, NF was stable for 35 days when stored in amber glass prescription bottles in the dark at 4°C. Empty the contents of ten 5 mg isradipine capsules into a glass mortar; wet the powder with glycerin, USP and triturate to a fine paste; add 15 mL of simple syrup and triturate well; transfer contents to a 60 mL amber glass prescription bottle; use 10 mL of simple syrup to rinse the mortar and transfer to the prescription bottle; repeat and qsad to a final volume of 50 mL; label "refrigerate" and "shake well".

MacDonald JL, Johnson CE, and Jacobson P, "Stability of Isradipine in Extemporaneously Compounded Oral Liquids," *Am J Hosp Pharm*, 1994, 51(19):2409-11.

References

Ahmed K, Michael B, and Burke JF Jr, "Effects of Isradipine on Renal Hemodynamics in Renal Transplant Patients Treated With Cyclosporine," *Clin Nephrol*, 1997, 48(5):307-10.

Chobanian AV, Bakris GL, Black HR, et al, "The Seventh Report of the Joint National Committee on Prevention, Detection, Evaluation, and Treatment of High Blood Pressure: The JNC 7 Report," *JAMA*, 2003, 289(19):2560-72.

Flynn JT and Pasko DA, "Calcium Channel Blockers: Pharmacology and Place in Therapy of Pediatric Hypertension," *Pediatr Nephrol*, 2000, 15(3-4):302-16.

Flynn JT and Warnick SJ, "Isradipine Treatment of Hypertension in Children: A Single-Center Experience," *Pediatr Nephrol*, 2002, 17(9):748-53.

Johnson CE, Jacobson PA, and Song MH, "Isradipine Therapy in Hypertensive Pediatric Patients," *Ann Pharmacother*, 1997, 31(6):704-7.

McCrea JB, Francos GF, and Burke JF, "The Beneficial Effects of Isradipine on Renal Hemodynamics in Cyclosporine-Treated Renal Transplant Recipients," *Transplantation*, 1992, 55(3):273-4.

Rodicio JL, "Calcium Antagonists and Renal Protection From Cyclosporine Nephrotoxicity: Long-Term Trial in Renal Transplantation Patients," *J Cardiovasc Pharmacol*, 2000, 35(3 Suppl 1):S7-11.

Steele RM, Schuna AA, and Schreiber RT, "Calcium Antagonist-Induced Gingival Hyperplasia," *Ann Intern Med*, 1994, 120(8):663-4.

Strauser LM, Groshong T, and Tobias JD, "Initial Experience With Isradipine for the Treatment of Hypertension in Children," *South Med J*, 2000, 93(3):287-93.

♦ **Istalol™** *see* Timolol *on page 1542*

♦ **Isuprel®** *see* Isoproterenol *on page 875*

Itraconazole (i tra KOE na zole)

Medication Safety Issues

Sound-alike/look-alike issues:

Sporanox® may be confused with Suprax®

U.S. Brand Names Sporanox®

Canadian Brand Names Sporanox®

Therapeutic Category Antifungal Agent, Systemic

Generic Available No

Use Treatment of susceptible systemic fungal infections in immunocompromised and nonimmunocompromised patients including blastomycosis, coccidioidomycosis, paracoccidioidomycosis, histoplasmosis, and aspergillosis in patients who do not respond to or cannot tolerate amphotericin B; treatment of oropharyngeal or esophageal candidiasis (oral solution only)

Pregnancy Risk Factor C

Lactation Enters breast milk/not recommended

Contraindications Hypersensitivity to itraconazole or any component; concomitant administration with terfenadine, astemizole, cisapride, pimozide, quinidine, dofetilide, alprazolam, triazolam, or HMG-CoA reductase inhibitors metabolized by CYP3A4 isoenzyme (ie, lovastatin, simvastatin)

Warnings Itraconazole has induced bone defects (decreased bone plate activity, thinning of the zona compacta of large bones, increased bone fragility) and changes in tooth appearance in rats. Severe cardiovascular effects including QT interval

(Continued)

Itraconazole *(Continued)*

prolongation, ventricular tachycardia, ventricular fibrillation, cardiac arrest, palpitations, syncope, and death have occurred in patients receiving itraconazole concomitantly with terfenadine, astemizole, or cisapride; **Itraconazole solution and capsules should not be used interchangeably**

Precautions Use with caution in patients with hypersensitivity to other azole antifungal agents, patients with left ventricular dysfunction or a history of CHF, and in patients with hepatic impairment; discontinue if signs and symptoms of liver disease or CHF develop

Adverse Reactions

Cardiovascular: Hypertension, ventricular fibrillation, edema, CHF

Central nervous system: Headache, dizziness, somnolence, fever, fatigue

Dermatologic: Rash, pruritus, urticaria, angioedema, toxic epidermal necrolysis

Endocrine & metabolic: Hypokalemia, adrenal insufficiency, gynecomastia

Gastrointestinal: Nausea, vomiting, diarrhea, abdominal pain, anorexia

Hematologic: Thrombocytopenia, leukopenia

Hepatic: Elevated liver enzymes, hepatitis

Otic: Tinnitus

Renal: Albuminuria

Drug Interactions Cytochrome P450 isoenzyme CYP3A3/4 substrate; isoenzyme CYP3A3/4 inhibitor

Decreased effect of itraconazole with rifampin, rifabutin, carbamazepine, isoniazid, phenytoin, and phenobarbital (increases itraconazole's metabolism); H_2 antagonists, omeprazole, antacids, didanosine (decreases absorption)

Increased effect of cyclosporine, tacrolimus (interferes with clearance); digoxin, warfarin, amlodipine, buspirone, corticosteroids, protease inhibitors (ie, indinavir), and hypoglycemic agents (decreased metabolism)

Increased toxicity of terfenadine, astemizole, alprazolam, triazolam, oral midazolam, cisapride, lovastatin, simvastatin, vinca alkaloids; see Warnings

Food Interactions Grapefruit juice decreases itraconazole AUC by 30%; avoid drinking grapefruit juice while taking oral itraconazole; absorption of capsule and oral solution are increased when taken with a cola beverage

Capsule: Food increases bioavailability

Solution: 31% increase in AUC if taken without food

Stability Store at room temperature; protect from light. Avoid freezing. A precise mixing ratio of itraconazole injection to NS diluent resulting in a 3.33 mg/mL concentration is required for a stable admixture. Following dilution of itraconazole injection in NS, the solution is stable for up to 48 hours when refrigerated and protected from light.

Mechanism of Action Inhibits ergosterol synthesis in fungal cell membranes by inhibiting fungal cytochrome P450

Pharmacokinetics

Absorption:

Capsule: Rapid and complete when capsule is given immediately after a meal (bioavailability: 100%); decreased absorption reported when administered via nasogastric tube

Oral solution: Solution better absorbed on empty stomach

Distribution: High affinity for tissues (liver, lung, kidney, adipose tissue, brain, vagina, dermis, epidermis); poor penetration into CSF, eye fluid, saliva; distributes into breast milk, bronchial exudate, and sputum

Protein binding: 99%

Metabolism: Saturable hepatic metabolism to active and inactive metabolites

Bioavailability: Capsules:

Fasted state: 40%

Fed state: Dose administered immediately after a meal: 100%

Half-life: 17-30 hours

Elimination: Metabolites are excreted in urine (35%) and bile (55%)

Dialysis: Nondialyzable

Usual Dosage

Oral:

Children: Efficacy of itraconazole has not been established; a limited number of children have been treated with itraconazole using doses of 3-5 mg/kg/day once daily; doses as high as 5-10 mg/kg/day divided every 12-24 hours have been used in 32 patients with chronic granulomatous disease for prophylaxis against *Aspergillus* infection; doses of 6-8 mg/kg/day have been used in the treatment of disseminated histoplasmosis

Prophylaxis for first episode of *Cryptococcus neoformans* or *Histoplasma capsulatum* in HIV-infected infants and children: 2-5 mg/kg/dose every 12-24 hours

Prophylaxis for recurrence of opportunistic disease in HIV-infected infants and children:

Cryptococcus neoformans: 2-5 mg/kg/dose every 12-24 hours

Histoplasma capsulatum: 2-5 mg/kg/dose every 12-48 hours

Adults:

Blastomycosis and nonmeningeal histoplasmosis: Initial: 200 mg once daily; if poor response, increase dose in 100 mg increments to a maximum of 400 mg/day in 2 divided doses

Life-threatening infection and aspergillosis: Initial loading dose can be administered as follows: 600 mg/day in 3 divided doses for the first 3-4 days; maintenance dose: 200-400 mg/day in 2 divided doses; maximum dose: 600 mg/day in 3 divided doses

Esophageal candidiasis: Vigorously swish 10 mL in the mouth for several seconds and then swallow daily; maximum dose: 200 mg/day

Oropharyngeal candidiasis: Vigorously swish 10 mL in the mouth for several seconds at a time once daily (20 mL total daily dose), or 10 mL twice daily in patients refractory to oral fluconazole

I.V.: Adults: Blastomycosis, aspergillosis, or histoplasmosis: 200 mg twice daily for 4 doses then decrease dose to 200 mg once daily. Safety and efficacy of I.V. itraconazole administered for longer than 14 days has not been established; therapy should be completed using oral itraconazole

Dosing adjustment in renal impairment: Cl_{cr} <30 mL/minute: Itraconazole injection is not recommended.

Administration

Oral: Avoid grapefruit juice

Capsules: Administer with food

Solution: Administer on an empty stomach

Parenteral I.V. infusion: Dilute entire contents of an ampul (250 mg) in 50 mL of NS diluent provided by the manufacturer to provide a solution with a final concentration of 3.33 mg/mL. Calculate itraconazole dosage volume needed and infuse over 60 minutes using the infusion set provided by the manufacturer and a dedicated I.V. line. Do not mix with other drugs. After completion of infusion, flush infusion set with 15-20 mL NS over 5-15 minutes via the two-way stopcock, then discard the entire I.V. line. Do not flush the infusion set with bacteriostatic NS.

Monitoring Parameters Periodic liver function tests, serum potassium; monitor for prodromal signs of hepatitis

Reference Range Therapeutic blood level: >250 ng/mL

Patient Information Report any prodromal symptoms of hepatitis (fatigue, weakness, nausea, vomiting, dark urine, or yellowing of eyes); avoid grapefruit juice

Nursing Implications Do not administer with antacids or H_2 antagonists

Dosage Forms Excipient information presented when available (limited, particularly for generics); consult specific product labeling.

Capsule: 100 mg

Injection, solution: 10 mg/mL (25 mL) [packaged in a kit containing sodium chloride 0.9% (50 mL); filtered infusion set (1)]

Solution, oral: 100 mg/10 mL (150 mL) [cherry flavor]

References

Cowie F, Meller ST, Cushing P, et al, "Chemoprophylaxis for Pulmonary Aspergillosis During Intensive Chemotherapy," *Arch Dis Child*, 1994, 70(2):136-8.

Mouy R, Veber F, Blanche S, et al, "Long-Term Itraconazole Prophylaxis Against *Aspergillus* Infections in Thirty-Two Patients With Chronic Granulomatous Disease," *J Pediatr*, 1994, 125(6 Pt 1):998-1003.

Tobon AM, Franco L, Espinal D, et al, "Disseminated Histoplasmosis in Children: The Role of Itraconazole Therapy," *Pediatr Infect Dis J*, 1996; 15:1002-8.

"1999 USPHS/IDSA Guidelines for the Prevention of Opportunistic Infections in Persons Infected With Human Immunodeficiency Virus. USPHS/IDSA Prevention of Opportunistic Infections Working Group," *MMWR Morb Mortal Wkly Rep*, 1999, 48 (RR-10):1-66.

◆ **Iveegam EN** *see* Immune Globulin (Intravenous) *on page 818*
◆ **Iveegam Immuno® (Can)** *see* Immune Globulin (Intravenous) *on page 818*
◆ **IVIG** *see* Immune Globulin (Intravenous) *on page 818*
◆ **Ivy-Rid® [OTC]** *see* Benzocaine *on page 204*
◆ **IvySoothe® [OTC]** *see* Hydrocortisone *on page 781*
◆ **Jamp® Travel Tablet (Can)** *see* DimenhyDRINATE *on page 507*
◆ **Jantoven™** *see* Warfarin *on page 1626*

Japanese Encephalitis Virus Vaccine (Inactivated)

(jap a NEESE en sef a LYE tis VYE rus vak SEEN, in ak ti VAY ted)

Related Information

Immunization Guidelines *on page 1837*

(Continued)

Japanese Encephalitis Virus Vaccine (Inactivated) *(Continued)*

U.S. Brand Names JE-VAX®

Canadian Brand Names JE-VAX®

Index Terms JE Vaccine

Therapeutic Category Vaccine

Generic Available No

Use Active immunization against Japanese encephalitis for persons 1 year of age and older who plan to spend 1 month or more in endemic areas in Asia, especially persons traveling during the transmission season or visiting rural areas; depending upon the epidemic circumstances, vaccination may be indicated for shorter trips to epidemic areas or extensive outdoor activities in rural endemic areas; elderly (>55 years of age) individuals should be considered for vaccination, since they have increased risk of developing symptomatic illness after infection; those planning travel to or residence in endemic areas should consult the Travel Advisory Service (Central Campus) for specific advice

Pregnancy Risk Factor C

Contraindications Hypersensitivity to the vaccine, any component, or to proteins of rodent or neural origin

Warnings Severe adverse reactions manifesting as generalized urticaria or angioedema may occur within minutes following vaccination, or up to 17 days later; most reactions occur within 10 days, with the majority within 48 hours; observe vaccinees for 30 minutes after vaccination; warn them of the possibility of delayed generalized urticaria and to remain where medical care is readily available for 10 days following any dose of the vaccine; immediate treatment for severe hypersensitivity reactions should be available during vaccine use. Due to the potential for severe adverse reactions, Japanese encephalitis (JE) vaccine is **not** recommended for all persons traveling to or residing in Asia; safety and efficacy in infants <1 year of age have not been established; therefore, immunization of infants should be deferred whenever possible; it is not known whether the vaccine is excreted in breast milk

Precautions The CDC recommends that the following individuals should not generally receive JE vaccine unless the benefit to the individual clearly outweighs the risk: Individuals acutely ill or with active infections, heart, kidney, or liver disorders, generalized malignancies such as leukemia or lymphoma, a history of multiple allergies, urticaria after hymenoptera envenomation, and pregnant women (unless there is a very high risk of Japanese encephalitis during the woman's stay in Asia). Unusual alcohol intake immediately after vaccination has been associated with an increased incidence of hypersensitivity reactions; avoid excessive alcohol intake during the 48 hours following vaccination. Individuals receiving other vaccinations within 7 days prior to this vaccine also had an increased incidence of hypersensitivity reactions; where possible, JE vaccine should be administered concurrently with other vaccines.

Adverse Reactions Report allergic or unusual adverse reactions to the Vaccine Adverse Event Reporting System (VAERS) 1-800-822-7967.

Cardiovascular: Hypotension, angioedema (rare)

Central nervous system: Fever, headache, malaise, chills, dizziness, seizure (rare), encephalitis (rare), encephalopathy (rare)

Dermatologic: Rash, urticaria, itching with or without accompanying rash, facial swelling, erythema multiforme (rare), erythema nodosum (rare)

Gastrointestinal: Nausea, vomiting, abdominal pain

Local: Tenderness, redness, and swelling at injection site

Neuromuscular & skeletal: Myalgia, peripheral neuropathy (rare), joint swelling (rare)

Respiratory: Dyspnea

Miscellaneous: Severe hypersensitivity reactions including anaphylaxis (see Warnings)

Drug Interactions Hypersensitivity reactions may be increased when given within 7 days of other vaccines (see Precautions)

Stability Refrigerate; do not freeze; discard 8 hours after reconstitution

Mechanism of Action An inactivated vaccine prepared from the homogenate of infected mice brains which offers immunity to disease caused by the Japanese encephalitis virus.

Usual Dosage SubQ:

Children 1-3 years: Three 0.5 mL doses given on days 0, 7, and 30

Children >3 years and Adults: Three 1 mL doses given on days 0, 7, and 30

An abbreviated schedule with the third dose administered on day 14 should be used only when time does not permit waiting; 2 doses a week apart produce immunity in about 80% of recipients; the longest regimen yields highest titers after 6 months.

Booster dose: Give after 2 years, or according to current recommendation

Note: Travel should not commence for at least 10 days after the last dose of vaccine, to allow adequate antibody formation and recognition of any delayed adverse reaction

Administration Parenteral: Use entire contents of provided diluent to reconstitute vaccine; gently agitate to mix thoroughly; discard if powder does not dissolve; use within 8 hours following reconstitution; administer by SubQ injection into the anterolateral aspect of the thigh or arm; **not for I.V. administration**

Patient Information Adverse reactions may occur shortly after vaccination or up to 17 days (usually within 10 days) after vaccination; advise concurrent use of other means to reduce the risk of mosquito exposure when possible, including bed nets, insect repellents, protective clothing, avoidance of travel in endemic areas, and avoidance of outdoor activity during twilight and evening periods

Nursing Implications Federal law requires that the date of administration, name of manufacturer, lot number, and administering person's name, title and address be entered into patient's permanent medical record.

Additional Information Japanese encephalitis vaccine is currently available only from the Centers for Disease Control. Contact Centers for Disease Control at (404) 639-6370 (Mon-Fri) or (404) 639-2888 (nights, weekends, or holidays).

Dosage Forms Excipient information presented when available (limited, particularly for generics); consult specific product labeling.

Injection, powder for reconstitution:

JE-VAX®: Nakayama-NIH strain (1 mL) [contains mouse serum protein, thimerosal, gelatin, polysorbate 80]

References

Centers for Disease Control, "Recommendations of the Advisory Committee on Immunization Practices (ACIP): General Recommendations on Immunization," *MMWR Recomm Rep*, 1994, 43(RR-1):23.

Ketamine (KEET a meen)

Medication Safety Issues

Sound-alike/look-alike issues:

Ketalar® may be confused with Kenalog®

Related Information

Adult ACLS Algorithms *on page 1660*
Preprocedure Sedatives in Children *on page 1895*

U.S. Brand Names Ketalar®

Canadian Brand Names Ketalar®; Ketamine Hydrochloride Injection, USP

Index Terms Ketamine Hydrochloride

Therapeutic Category General Anesthetic

Generic Available Yes

Use Anesthesia, short surgical procedures, dressing changes

Restrictions C-III

Pregnancy Risk Factor D

Contraindications Hypersensitivity to ketamine or any component; elevated intracranial pressure; patients with hypertension, aneurysms, thyrotoxicosis, CHF, angina, psychotic disorders

Warnings Use only by or under the direct supervision of physicians experienced in administering general anesthetics. Resuscitative equipment should be available for use; respiratory depression may occur with rapid administration rates or with overdose. Postanesthetic emergence reactions which can manifest as vivid dreams, hallucinations and/or frank delirium occur in 12% of patients; these reactions are less common in pediatric patients; emergence reactions may occur up to 24 hours postoperatively and may be reduced by minimization of verbal, tactile, and visual patient stimulation during recovery, or by pretreatment with a benzodiazepine (using lower recommended doses of ketamine). Severe emergent reactions may require treatment with a small hypnotic dose of a short or ultra-short acting barbiturate. Prolonged use may cause physical dependence (withdrawal symptoms on discontinuation) and tolerance.

Precautions Use with caution in patients with gastroesophageal reflux; use with caution and decrease the dose in patients with hepatic dysfunction; use with caution in patients with a full stomach, patients should fast (ie, be NPO) for an appropriate time before being sedated for elective procedures; use with caution in patients with elevated CSF pressure, chronic alcoholics, and in acutely intoxicated patients; do not use as sole anesthetic in surgery or diagnostic procedures of the pharynx, larynx, or bronchial tree or in surgical procedures involving visceral pain pathways

Adverse Reactions

Cardiovascular: Hypertension, tachycardia, increased cardiac output, paradoxical direct myocardial depression, hypotension, bradycardia, increases cerebral blood flow, arrhythmias

Central nervous system: Tonic-clonic movements, elevated intracranial pressure, hallucinations

Dermatologic: Transient erythema, morbilliform rash

Endocrine & metabolic: Increased metabolic rate

Gastrointestinal: Hypersalivation, vomiting, postoperative nausea, anorexia

Local: Pain and exanthema at injection site

Neuromuscular & skeletal: Increased skeletal muscle tone, tremor, purposeless movement, fasciculations

Ocular: Diplopia, nystagmus, elevated intraocular pressure

Respiratory: Increased airway resistance, cough reflex may be depressed, decreased bronchospasm; respiratory depression or apnea with large doses or rapid infusions, laryngospasm; increased bronchial mucous gland secretion

Miscellaneous: Emergence reactions; anaphylaxis; physical and psychological dependence with prolonged use

Drug Interactions Cytochrome P450 isoenzyme CYP3A substrate

Barbiturates, narcotics, hydroxyzine prolong recovery from anesthesia

Stability Protect from light; do not mix with barbiturates or diazepam as precipitation may occur

Mechanism of Action Produces dissociative anesthesia by direct action on the cortex and limbic system; does not usually impair pharyngeal or laryngeal reflexes

Pharmacodynamics

Onset of action:

- Anesthesia:
  - I.M.: 3-4 minutes
  - I.V.: Within 30 seconds
- Analgesia:
  - Oral: Within 30 minutes

I.M.: Within 10-15 minutes
Duration: Following single dose:
Anesthesia:
I.M.: 12-25 minutes
I.V.: 5-10 minutes
Analgesia: I.M.: 15-30 minutes
Recovery:
I.M.: 3-4 hours
I.V.: 1-2 hours

Pharmacokinetics
Metabolism: In the liver via N-dealkylation, hydroxylation of cyclohexone ring, glucuronide conjugation, and dehydration of hydroxylated metabolites
Half-life:
Alpha: 10-15 minutes
Terminal: 2.5 hours

Usual Dosage Titrate dose to effect
Children:
Oral: 6-10 mg/kg for 1 dose (mixed in cola or other beverage) given 30 minutes before the procedure
I.M.: 3-7 mg/kg
I.V.: Range: 0.5-2 mg/kg, use smaller doses (0.5-1 mg/kg) for sedation for minor procedures; usual induction dosage: 1-2 mg/kg
Continuous I.V. infusion: Sedation: 5-20 mcg/kg/minute; start at lower dosage listed and titrate to effect
Adults:
I.M.: 3-8 mg/kg
I.V.: Range: 1-4.5 mg/kg; usual induction dosage: 1-2 mg/kg
Children and Adults: Maintenance: Supplemental doses of $^1/_3$ to $^1/_2$ of initial dose

Administration
Oral: Use 100 mg/mL I.V. solution and mix the appropriate dose in 0.2-0.3 mL/kg of cola or other beverage
Parenteral: I.V.: Administer slowly, do not exceed 0.5 mg/kg/minute; do not administer faster than 60 seconds; maximum concentration for slow I.V. push: 50 mg/mL; **Note:** Do not inject 100 mg/mL concentration I.V. without proper dilution; dilute with an equal volume of SWI, NS, or D_5W to produce 50 mg/mL concentration for slow I.V. push. Maximum concentration for intermittent or continuous infusion: 2 mg/mL

Monitoring Parameters Cardiovascular effects, heart rate, blood pressure, respiratory rate, transcutaneous O_2 saturation

Patient Information May cause drowsiness and impair ability to perform activities requiring mental alertness or physical coordination; do not engage in such activities for at least 24 hours after ketamine anesthesia.

Nursing Implications Resuscitative equipment should be available for use. Ensure that outpatients have fully recovered from ketamine anesthesia before being released and that they are accompanied by a responsible adult.

Additional Information Used in combination with anticholinergic agents to decrease hypersalivation; should not be used for sedation for procedures that require a total lack of movement (eg, MRI, radiation therapy) due to association with purposeless movements

Dosage Forms Excipient information presented when available (limited, particularly for generics); consult specific product labeling.
Injection, solution: 50 mg/mL (10 mL); 100 mg/mL (5 mL)
Ketalar®: 10 mg/mL (20 mL); 50 mg/mL (10 mL); 100 mg/mL (5 mL)

References

Cote CJ, "Sedation for the Pediatric Patient: A Review," *Pediatr Clin North Am*, 1994, 41(1):31-58.
Gutstein HB, Johnson KL, Heard MN, et al, "Oral Ketamine Premedication in Children," *Anesthesiology*, 1992, 76(1):28-33.
Tobias JD, Phipps S, Smith B, et al, "Oral Ketamine Premedication to Alleviate the Distress of Invasive Procedures in Pediatric Oncology Patients," *Pediatrics*, 1992, 90(4):537-41.
Tobias JD and Rasmussen GE, "Pain Management and Sedation in the Pediatric Intensive Care Unit," *Pediatr Clin North Am*, 1994, 41(6):1269-92.

♦ **Ketamine Hydrochloride** *see* Ketamine *on page 886*
♦ **Ketamine Hydrochloride Injection, USP (Can)** *see* Ketamine *on page 886*

Ketoconazole (kee toe KOE na zole)

Medication Safety Issues
Sound-alike/look-alike issues:
Nizoral® may be confused with Nasarel®, Neoral®, Nitrol®

U.S. Brand Names Kuric™; Nizoral®; Nizoral® A-D [OTC]; Xolegel™

Canadian Brand Names Apo-Ketoconazole®; Ketoderm®; Novo-Ketoconazole; Xolegel™

(Continued)

Ketoconazole *(Continued)*

Therapeutic Category Antifungal Agent, Systemic; Antifungal Agent, Topical

Generic Available Yes: Cream, shampoo, tablet

Use Treatment of susceptible fungal infections, including candidiasis, oral thrush, blastomycosis, histoplasmosis, paracoccidioidomycosis, chronic mucocutaneous candidiasis, as well as certain recalcitrant cutaneous dermatophytoses; used topically for treatment of tinea corporis, tinea cruris, tinea versicolor, and cutaneous candidiasis; shampoo is used for dandruff

Pregnancy Risk Factor C

Lactation Enters breast milk/not recommended

Contraindications Hypersensitivity to ketoconazole or any component; single agent in the treatment of CNS fungal infections (due to poor CNS penetration); concomitant administration of astemizole, terfenadine, cisapride, or irinotecan (see Drug Interactions)

Warnings Has been associated with hepatotoxicity, including some fatalities; perform periodic liver function tests; high doses of ketoconazole may depress adrenocortical function and decrease serum testosterone concentrations; risk of serious cardiac arrhythmias in patients receiving ketoconazole and astemizole, terfenadine, or cisapride

Precautions Gastric acidity is necessary for the dissolution and absorption of ketoconazole; avoid concomitant (within 2 hours) administration of antacids, H_2 blockers, anticholinergics; use with caution in patients with impaired hepatic function

Adverse Reactions

Central nervous system: Lethargy, nervousness, headache, dizziness, somnolence, fever, chills, bulging fontanelles

Dermatologic: Pruritus, rash, dry skin

Endocrine & metabolic: Adrenocortical insufficiency, gynecomastia, decreased libido

Gastrointestinal: Nausea, vomiting, abdominal discomfort, GI bleeding, diarrhea

Genitourinary: Oligospermia

Hematologic: Leukopenia, thrombocytopenia, hemolytic anemia

Hepatic: Hepatotoxicity; elevated AST, ALT, and alkaline phosphatase; jaundice

Local: Irritation, stinging

Miscellaneous: Anaphylaxis

Drug Interactions Cytochrome P450 isoenzyme CYP3A3/4 substrate; CYP1A2, CYP2A6, CYP2B6 (weak), CYP2C8/9, CYP2C19, CYP2D6, CYP3A3/4 isoenzyme inhibitor

Drugs that decrease ketoconazole absorption (raise gastric pH) such as antacids, didanosine, sodium bicarbonate, omeprazole, H_2-receptor blockers; sucralfate decreases absorption of ketoconazole by 20%; drugs that decrease serum concentrations of ketoconazole (rifampin, nevirapine, isoniazid, phenytoin, St John's wort); drug concentrations that are increased by ketoconazole (phenytoin, astemizole, buspirone, busulfan (avoid concurrent use), cisapride, digoxin, cyclosporine, sirolimus, tacrolimus, triazolam, temazepam, diazepam, alprazolam, midazolam, HMG-CoA reductase inhibitors, corticosteroids, terfenadine, indinavir, saquinavir, sildenafil, nifedipine, verapamil, vinca alkaloids, docetaxel, warfarin); drugs that cause hepatotoxicity; alcohol may cause disulfiram-like reactions; increased trough concentrations of delavirdine if given with ketoconazole (see Warnings). Ketoconazole may increase exposure to irinotecan and SN-38 (see Contraindications; discontinue ketoconazole at least 1 week prior to starting irinotecan).

Food Interactions Food may increase ketoconazole absorption; administration with an acidic beverage (eg, Coca-Cola, Pepsi, citrus juice) increases ketoconazole absorption

Mechanism of Action Alters the permeability of the cell wall; inhibits fungal biosynthesis of triglycerides and phospholipids; inhibits several fungal enzymes that results in a build-up of toxic concentrations of hydrogen peroxide

Pharmacokinetics

Absorption: Oral: Rapid (~75%)

Distribution: Minimal penetration into the CNS; distributes to bile, saliva, urine, sweat, synovial fluid, lungs, liver, kidney and bone marrow

Protein binding: 84% to 99%

Metabolism: Partially in the liver via CYP3A4 to inactive compounds

Bioavailability: Decreases as pH of the gastric contents increase

Half-life, biphasic:

- Alpha: 2 hours
- Terminal: 8 hours

Time to peak serum concentration: Oral: Within 1-2 hours

Elimination: Primarily in feces (57%) with smaller amounts excreted in urine (~13%)

Dialysis: Not dialyzable (0% to 5%)

Usual Dosage

Infants and Children: Oral: 3.3-6.6 mg/kg/day once daily

Prophylaxis for recurrence of mucocutaneous candidiasis with HIV infection: 5-10 mg/kg/day divided every 12-24 hours; maximum: 800 mg/day divided twice daily

Adults: Oral: 200-400 mg/day as a single daily dose; maximum: 800 mg/day divided twice daily

Children and Adults:

Shampoo: Shampoo twice weekly (at least 3 days should elapse between each shampoo) for 4 weeks

Topical: Apply once daily to twice daily

Administration

Oral: May administer with or without food or with juice; administer with food to decrease nausea and vomiting; administer 2 hours prior to antacids, didanosine, proton pump inhibitors, or H_2-receptor antagonists to prevent decreased ketoconazole absorption; shake suspension well before use

Shampoo: Apply to wet hair and massage over entire scalp for 1 minute; rinse hair thoroughly and reapply shampoo for 3 minutes; rinse

Topical: Apply a sufficient amount and rub gently into the affected and surrounding area

Monitoring Parameters Liver function tests, signs of adrenal dysfunction

Patient Information Cream is for topical application to the skin only; avoid contact with the eye; notify physician of unusual fatigue, weakness, vomiting, dark urine, or yellowing of eyes; avoid alcohol

Dosage Forms Excipient information presented when available (limited, particularly for generics); consult specific product labeling.

Cream, topical: 2% (15 g, 30 g, 60 g)

Kuric™: 2%: (25 g, 75 g)

Gel, topical:

Xolegel™: 2% (15 g) [contains dehydrated alcohol 34%]

Shampoo, topical: 1% (120 mL), 2% (120 mL)

Nizoral® : 2% (120 mL)

Nizoral® A-D: 1% (120 mL, 210 mL)

Tablet: 200 mg

Nizoral®: 200 mg

Extemporaneous Preparations A 20 mg/mL suspension may be made by pulverizing twelve 200 mg ketoconazole tablets to a fine powder; add 40 mL Ora-Plus® in small portions with thorough mixing; incorporate Ora-Sweet® to make a final volume of 120 mL and mix thoroughly; shake well before using; protect from light; stable for 60 days when stored without light at 5°C and 25°C

Allen LV and Erickson MA, "Stability of Ketoconazole, Metolazone, Metronidazole, Procainamide, Hydrochloride, and Spironolactone in Extemporaneously Compounded Oral Liquids," *AM J Health-Syst Pharm*, 1996, 53:2073-8.

References

Como JA and Dismukes WE, "Oral Azole Drugs as Systemic Antifungal Therapy," *N Engl J Med*, 1994, 330(4):263-72.

Ginsburg AM, McCracken GH Jr, and Olsen K, "Pharmacology of Ketoconazole Suspension in Infants and Children," *Antimicrob Agents Chemother*, 1983, 23(5):787-9.

Herrod HG, "Chronic Mucocutaneous Candidiasis in Childhood and Complications of non-*Candida* Infection: A Report of the Pediatric Immunodeficiency Collaborative Study Group," *J Pediatr*, 1990, 116(3):377-82.

♦ **Ketoderm® (Can)** *see* Ketoconazole *on page 887*

Ketorolac (KEE toe role ak)

Medication Safety Issues

Sound-alike/look-alike issues:

Acular® may be confused with Acthar®, Ocular®

Toradol® may be confused with Foradil®, Inderal®, Tegretol®, Torecan®, tramadol

International issues:

Toradol® may be confused with Theradol® which is a brand name for tramadol in the Netherlands

U.S. Brand Names Acular®; Acular LS™; Acular® PF; Toradol®

Canadian Brand Names Acular®; Acular LS™; Apo-Ketorolac®; Apo-Ketorolac Injectable®; Ketorolac Tromethamine Injection, USP; Novo-Ketorolac; ratio-Ketorolac; Toradol®; Toradol® IM

Index Terms Ketorolac Tromethamine

Therapeutic Category Analgesic, Non-narcotic; Anti-inflammatory Agent; Antipyretic; Nonsteroidal Anti-inflammatory Drug (NSAID), Ophthalmic; Nonsteroidal Anti-inflammatory Drug (NSAID), Oral; Nonsteroidal Anti-inflammatory Drug (NSAID), Parenteral

Generic Available Yes: Injection, tablet

(Continued)

Ketorolac *(Continued)*

Use

Oral, I.M., I.V.: Short-term (≤5 days) management of moderate to severe pain, usually postoperative pain; has also been used to treat visceral pain associated with cancer, pain associated with trauma. **Note:** In adults, oral ketorolac is indicated only as continuation therapy to I.M. or I.V. ketorolac; the combined duration of oral and parenteral ketorolac should not be >5 days due to the increased risk of serious adverse effects. Only single-dose ketorolac injection is approved for use in children 2-16 years of age.

Ophthalmic:

Acular®: Treatment of ocular itch associated with seasonal allergic conjunctivitis; postoperative inflammation following cataract extraction

Acular LS™: Reduction of ocular pain, burning, and stinging after corneal refractive surgery

Acular® P.F.: Reduction of ocular pain and photophobia after incisional refractive surgery

Medication Guide An FDA-approved patient medication guide, which is available with the product information and at http://www.fda.gov/cder/Offices/ODS/medication_guides.htm, must be dispensed with this medication for each new outpatient prescription and refill.

Pregnancy Risk Factor C (D if used in 3rd trimester)

Lactation Enters breast milk/contraindicated

Contraindications Hypersensitivity to ketorolac, any component, aspirin, or other NSAIDs; patients with the "aspirin triad" [asthma, rhinitis (with or without nasal polyps), and aspirin intolerance] (fatal asthmatic and anaphylactoid reactions may occur in these patients); patients with active peptic ulcer disease (PUD), recent GI bleeding or perforation, or history of PUD or GI bleeding; advanced renal dysfunction; patients at risk for renal failure due to hypovolemia; women in late pregnancy; women in labor and delivery or breast-feeding; preoperative or intraoperative use; patients with cerebrovascular bleeding, incomplete hemostasis, hemorrhagic diathesis, or at high risk of bleeding; contraindicated for epidural or intrathecal use due to alcohol content; do not administer with aspirin, NSAIDs, or probenecid

Warnings In April 2005, the FDA announced product labeling changes for all NSAIDs, including COX-2 selective and OTC medications; although revised product labeling is currently not available for all products, sample labeling and a template of the required medication guide are now available. Labels for prescription nonselective NSAIDs will contain a contraindication for use in patients who have recently undergone coronary artery bypass graft (CABG) surgery and a boxed warning concerning the potential for increased risk of cardiovascular (CV) events and GI bleeding associated with NSAID use. Patients at increased risk of adverse events include patients immediately postoperative from CABG surgery, and those with existing CAD, CVD, or history of TIA or stomach ulcers. Prescribers are encouraged to use the lowest effective NSAID dose for the shortest time based on individual patient treatment goals. Medication guides will be required for all prescription products. Complete details for the labeling update can be found on the following FDA website: http://www.fda.gov/medwatch/SAFETY/2005/safety05.htm#NSAID.

Serious GI adverse effects (eg, GI bleeding, ulceration, perforation) may occur; these effects may be related to dose and duration of therapy. Ketorolac may inhibit platelet aggregation; pediatric patients may be at a greater risk for bleeding when using ketorolac following tonsillectomy (see Additional Information). Anaphylactoid reactions may occur (even in patients without previous exposure or hypersensitivity to aspirin, ketorolac, or other NSAIDs). Decreased renal function or acute renal failure may occur (patients with impaired renal function, dehydration, heart failure, liver impairment, or patients taking diuretics may be at greatest risk); correct hypovolemia before starting ketorolac. Fluid retention, edema, and sodium retention may occur; use with caution in patients with CHF, hypertension, cardiac decompensation, or similar conditions.

Precautions Use with caution and reduce dose in patients with decreased renal function; use with caution in patients with hepatic impairment and in patients in whom prolongation of bleeding time would cause adverse effects; not recommended after plastic or neurosurgery due to increased risk of bleeding.

Use ocular product with caution in patients with complicated ocular surgeries, corneal denervation or epithelial defects, ocular surface diseases (eg, dry eye syndrome), repeated ocular surgeries within a short period of time, diabetes mellitus, rheumatoid arthritis; these patients may be at risk for corneal adverse events that may be sight threatening (see Adverse Reactions)

Adverse Reactions

Cardiovascular: Edema (4%), hypertension

Central nervous system: Somnolence, drowsiness (6%), dizziness (7%), headache (17%), insomnia, euphoria, hallucinations, malaise (<1%)
Dermatologic: Rash, pruritus, purpura, urticaria
Gastrointestinal: Dyspepsia (12%), nausea (12%), diarrhea (7%), GI pain, peptic ulcer, melena, rectal bleeding, constipation, vomiting
Genitourinary: Urinary frequency
Hematologic: Inhibits platelet aggregation, may prolong bleeding time
Hepatic: Elevated liver enzymes
Local: Pain at injection site (2%)
Ocular: Blurred vision; ocular use: Transient stinging, burning, corneal edema or infiltrates, conjunctival hyperemia, allergic reactions; ocular irritation, pain, edema, or inflammation; delayed ocular healing; keratitis; epithelial breakdown, corneal thinning, erosion, ulceration, or perforation in susceptible patients (may be sight threatening; discontinue use; monitor closely); **Note:** Use >24 hours before surgery and >14 days after surgery may increase risk of corneal adverse events
Renal: Oliguria, interstitial nephritis, acute renal failure (rare)
Respiratory: Dyspnea, wheezing
Miscellaneous: Anaphylaxis, hypersensitivity reactions

Drug Interactions Warfarin, heparin, lithium, methotrexate, salicylates, NSAIDs, GI irritants (eg, potassium supplements), probenecid (significantly increases ketorolac half-life and plasma levels), furosemide, phenytoin, carbamazepine; ketorolac may decrease antihypertensive effects of ACE inhibitors and angiotensin II antagonists

Food Interactions High-fat meals may delay time to peak (by ~1 hour) and decrease peak concentrations

Stability Protect from light; Injection: Color change indicates degradation; do not administer in same syringe with narcotics; ketorolac will precipitate if mixed with morphine, meperidine, promethazine, or hydroxyzine. Discard single-use Acular® P.F. vial immediately after administration (solution does not contain preservative).

Mechanism of Action Inhibits prostaglandin synthesis by decreasing the activity of the enzyme, cyclooxygenase, which results in decreased formation of prostaglandin precursors

Pharmacodynamics Analgesia:
Onset of action:
Oral: 30-60 minutes
I.M., I.V.: ~30 minutes
Maximum effect:
Oral: 1.5-4 hours
I.M., I.V.: 1-2 hours
Duration: 4-6 hours

Pharmacokinetics
Absorption:
Oral: Well absorbed; 100%
I.M.: Rapid and complete
Distribution: Crosses placenta, crosses into breast milk, poor penetration into CSF; follows two-compartment model
V_d beta:
Children 4-8 years: 0.19-0.44 L/kg (mean: 0.26 L/kg)
Adults: 0.11-0.33 L/kg (mean: 0.18 L/kg)
Protein binding: 99%
Metabolism: In the liver; undergoes hydroxylation and glucuronide conjugation; in children 4-8 years, V_{dss} and plasma clearance were twice as high as adults, but terminal half-life was similar
Bioavailability: Oral, I.M.: 100%
Half-life, terminal:
Children 4-8 years: ~6 hours; range: 3.5-10 (n=10)
Adults: Mean: ~5 hours; range: 4-9 hours
With renal impairment: S_{cr} 1.9-5 mg/dL: Mean: ~11 hours; range: 4-19 hours
Renal dialysis patients: Mean: ~14 hours; range: 8-40 hours
Time to peak serum concentration:
Oral: ~45 minutes
I.M.: 30-45 minutes
I.V.: 1-3 minutes
Elimination: Renal excretion: 60% in urine as unchanged drug with 40% as metabolites; 6% of dose excreted in feces

Usual Dosage Note: Ketorolac injection is approved for use in pediatric patients only as a single I.M. or I.V. dose in children 2-16 years of age; the use of ketorolac injection in children <2 years of age, the use of multiple doses of the injection in children <16 years of age, and the use of the tablets in children <16 years of age are outside of product labeling; ophthalmic solutions are approved for use in children ≥3 years of age
(Continued)

Ketorolac *(Continued)*

Children 2-16 years: **Do not exceed adult doses**; see Additional Information

Single-dose treatment:

Manufacturer's recommendations:

I.M.: 1 mg/kg as a single dose; maximum dose: 30 mg

I.V.: 0.5 mg/kg as a single dose; maximum dose: 15 mg

Alternative dosing:

I.M., I.V.: 0.4-1 mg/kg as a single dose; **Note:** Limited information exists. Single I.V. doses of 0.5 mg/kg, 0.75 mg/kg, 0.9 mg/kg and 1 mg/kg have been studied in children 2-16 years of age for postoperative analgesia. One study (Maunuksela, 1992) used a titrating dose starting with 0.2 mg/kg I.V. up to a total of 0.5 mg/kg (median dose required: 0.4 mg/kg).

Oral: One study used 1 mg/kg as a single dose for analgesia in 30 children (mean ± SD age: 3 ± 2.5 years) undergoing bilateral myringotomy

Multiple-dose treatment: I.M., I.V., Oral: No pediatric studies exist; one report (Buck, 1994) of the clinical experience with ketorolac in 112 children, 6 months to 19 years of age (mean: 9 years), described usual I.V. maintenance doses of 0.5 mg/kg every 6 hours (mean dose: 0.52 mg/kg; range: 0.17-1 mg/kg)

Children >16 years and >50 kg and Adults <65 years:

Single-dose treatment:

I.M.: 60 mg as a single dose

I.V.: 30 mg as a single dose

Multiple-dose treatment:

I.M., I.V.: 30 mg every 6 hours; maximum dose: 120 mg/day

Oral: Initial: 20 mg, then 10 mg every 4-6 hours; maximum dose: 40 mg/day

Adults ≥65 years, renally impaired, or <50 kg:

Single-dose treatment:

I.M.: 30 mg as a single dose

I.V.: 15 mg as a single dose

Multiple-dose treatment:

I.M., I.V.: 15 mg every 6 hours; maximum dose: 60 mg/day

Oral: 10 mg every 4-6 hours; maximum dose: 40 mg/day

Children ≥3 years and Adults: Ophthalmic:

Seasonal allergic conjunctivitis (Acular®): Instill 1 drop in eye(s) 4 times/day

Postoperative inflammation (Acular®): Instill 1 drop in affected eye(s) 4 times/day starting 24 hours after cataract surgery and through 14 days after surgery

Postoperative pain, burning, and stinging (Acular LS™): Instill 1 drop in affected eye 4 times/day as needed for up to 4 days after corneal refractive surgery

Postoperative pain and photophobia (Acular® P.F.): Instill 1 drop in affected eye(s) 4 times/day as needed for up to 3 days after incisional refractive surgery

Administration

Ophthalmic: Instill drops into affected eye(s); avoid contact of container tip with skin or eyes; apply finger pressure to lacrimal sac during and for 1-2 minutes after instillation to decrease risk of absorption and systemic effects. Acular® P.F.: Administer to one or both eyes immediately after opening single-use vial; discard vial immediately after use

Oral: May administer with food or milk to decrease GI upset

Parenteral:

I.M.: Administer slowly and deeply into muscle; 60 mg/2 mL vial is for I.M. use only

I.V. bolus: Administer over at least 15 seconds; maximum concentration: 30 mg/mL; **Note:** I.V. ketorolac has been infused over 1-5 minutes in children

Monitoring Parameters Signs of pain relief (eg, increased appetite and activity); BUN, serum creatinine, liver enzymes, occult blood loss, urinalysis, urine output

Reference Range Serum concentration:

Therapeutic: 0.3-5 mcg/mL

Toxic: >5 mcg/mL

Patient Information Avoid alcohol; may cause dizziness or drowsiness and impair ability to perform activities requiring mental alertness or physical coordination; do not exceed 5 days total use (I.M., I.V., oral). Do not use ophthalmic solution while wearing contact lenses.

Additional Information 30 mg provides analgesia comparable to 12 mg of morphine or 100 mg of meperidine; ketorolac may possess an opioid-sparing effect; diarrhea, pallor, vomiting, and labored breathing may occur with overdose

Note: A single I.V. dose of ketorolac (0.75 mg/kg) in 21 children (2.5-9 years of age) undergoing outpatient strabismus surgery was associated with less postoperative emesis than morphine plus metoclopramide (Munro, 1994). However, a single dose of I.V. ketorolac (1 mg/kg) in 25 children (2-15 years of age) undergoing tonsillectomy was associated with an increase in surgical bleeding, more patients requiring extra hemostatic measures (eg, synthetic collagen, extra Neo-Synephrine® packing), and a higher estimated blood loss compared to rectal acetaminophen (Rusy, 1995); further studies are needed.

Dosage Forms Excipient information presented when available (limited, particularly for generics); consult specific product labeling. [DSC] = Discontinued product

Injection, solution, as tromethamine: 15 mg/mL (1 mL); 30 mg/mL (1 mL, 2 mL, 10 mL) [contains alcohol]

Solution, ophthalmic, as tromethamine:

Acular®: 0.5% (3 mL, 5 mL, 10 mL) [contains benzalkonium chloride]

Acular LS™: 0.4% (5 mL) [contains benzalkonium chloride]

Acular® P.F. [preservative free]: 0.5% (0.4 mL)

Tablet, as tromethamine: 10 mg

Toradol®: 10 mg [DSC]

References

Buck ML, "Clinical Experience With Ketorolac in Children," *Ann Pharmacother*, 1994, 28(9):1009-13.

Maunuksela E, Kokki H, and Bullingham RES, "Comparison of Intravenous Ketorolac With Morphine for Postoperative Pain in Children," *Clin Pharmacol Ther*, 1992, 52(4):436-43.

Munro HM, Reigger LQ, Reynolds PI, et al, "Comparison of the Analgesic and Emetic Properties of Ketorolac and Morphine for Paediatric Outpatient Strabismus Surgery," *Br J Anaesth*, 1994, 72(6):624-8.

Rusy LM, Houck CS, Sullivan LJ, et al, "A Double-Blind Evaluation of Ketorolac Tromethamine Versus Acetaminophen in Pediatric Tonsillectomy: Analgesia and Bleeding," *Anesth Analg*, 1995, 80(2):226-9.

Watcha MF, Jones MB, Lagueruela RG, et al, "Comparison of Ketorolac and Morphine as Adjuvants During Pediatric Surgery," *Anesthesiology*, 1992, 76(3):368-72.

♦ **Ketorolac Tromethamine** *see* Ketorolac *on page 889*

♦ **Ketorolac Tromethamine Injection, USP (Can)** *see* Ketorolac *on page 889*

Ketotifen (kee toe TYE fen)

U.S. Brand Names Alaway™ [OTC]; Zaditor® [OTC]

Canadian Brand Names Apo-Ketotifen®; Novo-Ketotifen; Zaditen®; Zaditor®

Index Terms Ketotifen Fumarate

Therapeutic Category Antiallergic, Ophthalmic; Histamine H_1 Antagonist, Ophthalmic

Generic Available Yes

Use Temporary prevention of eye itching due to allergic conjunctivitis

Pregnancy Risk Factor C

Lactation Use caution

Contraindications Hypersensitivity to ketotifen or any component

Warnings Not indicated for use in eye irritation due to contact lenses; patients should be advised not to wear contact lens if their eye is red; solution contains benzalkonium chloride which may be absorbed by soft contact lenses; wait at least 10 minutes after administration before inserting contact lenses

Adverse Reactions

Central nervous system: Headache

Dermatologic: Rash

Gastrointestinal: Pharyngitis

Local: Stinging, burning sensation

Ocular: Conjunctivitis, conjunctival injection, eye discharge, dry eyes, eye pain, eyelid disorder, itching, keratitis, lacrimation disorder, mydriasis, photophobia

Respiratory: Rhinitis

Miscellaneous: Flu-like syndrome, hypersensitivity reactions

Drug Interactions None known

Stability Store at controlled room temperature (59°F to 77°F).

Mechanism of Action Ketotifen is an H_1 receptor antagonist and mast cell stabilizer which inhibits the release of mediators from cells involved in hypersensitivity reactions. Decreased chemotaxis and activation of eosinophils has also been demonstrated.

Pharmacodynamics

Onset of action: 5-15 minutes

Duration: 5-8 hours

Usual Dosage Ophthalmic: Children ≥3 years and Adults: Instill 1 drop into lower conjunctival sac of affected eye(s) twice daily, every 8-12 hours

Administration Ophthalmic: Instill into conjunctival sac avoiding contact of bottle tip with skin or eye; apply finger pressure to lacrimal sac during and for 1-2 minutes after instillation to decrease risk of absorption and systemic effects. Administer other topical ophthalmic medications at least 5 minutes apart.

Monitoring Parameters Improvement in symptomatology (eg, reduction in itching, tearing, and hyperaemia)

Patient Information Do not let tip of the applicator touch eye; do not contaminate tip of applicator (may cause eye infection, eye damage, or vision loss); wait at least 10

(Continued)

Ketotifen *(Continued)*

minutes before putting soft contact lenses in; do not wear contact lenses if eyes are red

Dosage Forms Excipient information presented when available (limited, particularly for generics); consult specific product labeling.

Solution, ophthalmic: 0.025% (5 mL)

Alaway™: 0.025% (10 mL) [contains benzalkonium chloride]

Zaditor®: 0.025% (5 mL) [contains benzalkonium chloride]

References

Horak F, et al, "Onset and Duration of Action of Ketotifen 0.025% and Emedastine 0.05% in Seasonal Allergic Conjunctivitis," *Clin Drug Invest*, 2003, 23(5): 329-37.

- ♦ **Ketotifen Fumarate** *see* Ketotifen *on page 893*
- ♦ **Key-E® [OTC]** *see* Vitamin E *on page 1620*
- ♦ **Key-E® Kaps [OTC]** *see* Vitamin E *on page 1620*
- ♦ **KI** *see* Potassium Iodide *on page 1290*
- ♦ **Kidkare Decongestant [OTC]** *see* Pseudoephedrine *on page 1344*
- ♦ **Kidrolase® (Can)** *see* Asparaginase *on page 161*
- ♦ **Kionex™** *see* Sodium Polystyrene Sulfonate *on page 1460*
- ♦ **Kivexa™ (Can)** *see* Abacavir and Lamivudine *on page 35*
- ♦ **Klaron®** *see* Sulfacetamide *on page 1483*
- ♦ **Klean-Prep® (Can)** *see* Polyethylene Glycol-Electrolyte Solution *on page 1277*
- ♦ **Klonopin®** *see* Clonazepam *on page 387*
- ♦ **K-Lor®** *see* Potassium Chloride *on page 1287*
- ♦ **Klor-Con®** *see* Potassium Chloride *on page 1287*
- ♦ **Klor-Con® 8** *see* Potassium Chloride *on page 1287*
- ♦ **Klor-Con® 10** *see* Potassium Chloride *on page 1287*
- ♦ **Klor-Con®/25** *see* Potassium Chloride *on page 1287*
- ♦ **Klor-Con® M** *see* Potassium Chloride *on page 1287*
- ♦ **Klor-Con®/EF** *see* Potassium Bicarbonate and Potassium Citrate *on page 1286*
- ♦ **K-Lyte®** *see* Potassium Bicarbonate and Potassium Citrate *on page 1286*
- ♦ **K-Lyte/Cl®** *see* Potassium Bicarbonate and Potassium Chloride *on page 1285*
- ♦ **K-Lyte®/Cl (Can)** *see* Potassium Chloride *on page 1287*
- ♦ **K-Lyte® DS** *see* Potassium Bicarbonate and Potassium Citrate *on page 1286*
- ♦ **Kodet SE [OTC]** *see* Pseudoephedrine *on page 1344*
- ♦ **Koffex DM-Expectorant (Can)** *see* Guaifenesin and Dextromethorphan *on page 748*
- ♦ **Koffex Expectorant (Can)** *see* Guaifenesin *on page 745*
- ♦ **Kogenate® (Can)** *see* Antihemophilic Factor (Recombinant) *on page 138*
- ♦ **Kogenate® FS** *see* Antihemophilic Factor (Recombinant) *on page 138*
- ♦ **Kolephrin® #1** *see* Guaifenesin and Codeine *on page 746*
- ♦ **Kolephrin® GG/DM [OTC]** *see* Guaifenesin and Dextromethorphan *on page 748*
- ♦ **Konakion (Can)** *see* Phytonadione *on page 1258*
- ♦ **Kondremul® [OTC]** *see* Mineral Oil *on page 1065*
- ♦ **Konsyl® [OTC]** *see* Psyllium *on page 1347*
- ♦ **Konsyl-D® [OTC]** *see* Psyllium *on page 1347*
- ♦ **Konsyl® Easy Mix [OTC]** *see* Psyllium *on page 1347*
- ♦ **Konsyl® Orange [OTC]** *see* Psyllium *on page 1347*
- ♦ **Koāte®-DVI** *see* Antihemophilic Factor (Human) *on page 134*
- ♦ **K-Pek II [OTC]** *see* Loperamide *on page 952*
- ♦ **K-Phos® MF** *see* Potassium Phosphate and Sodium Phosphate *on page 1296*
- ♦ **K-Phos® Neutral** *see* Potassium Phosphate and Sodium Phosphate *on page 1296*
- ♦ **K-Phos® No. 2** *see* Potassium Phosphate and Sodium Phosphate *on page 1296*
- ♦ **K+ Potassium** *see* Potassium Chloride *on page 1287*
- ♦ **Kristalose®** *see* Lactulose *on page 900*
- ♦ **K-Tab®** *see* Potassium Chloride *on page 1287*
- ♦ **Kuric™** *see* Ketoconazole *on page 887*
- ♦ **kutrase®** *see* Pancreatin *on page 1202*
- ♦ **ku-zyme®** *see* Pancreatin *on page 1202*
- ♦ **ku-zyme® HP** *see* Pancrelipase *on page 1203*
- ♦ **Kwellada-P™ (Can)** *see* Permethrin *on page 1243*
- ♦ **Kytril®** *see* Granisetron *on page 742*
- ♦ **L-735,524** *see* Indinavir *on page 824*
- ♦ **L-749,345** *see* Ertapenem *on page 593*
- ♦ **L-M-X™ 4 [OTC]** *see* Lidocaine *on page 933*

- **L-M-X™ 5 [OTC]** *see* Lidocaine *on page 933*
- **L 754030** *see* Aprepitant *on page 153*

Labetalol (la BET a lole)

Medication Safety Issues

Sound-alike/look-alike issues:

Labetalol may be confused with betaxolol, Hexadrol®, lamotrigine

Trandate® may be confused with tramadol, Trendar®, Trental®, Tridrate®

Significant differences exist between oral and I.V. dosing. Use caution when converting from one route of administration to another.

Related Information

Antihypertensive Agents by Class *on page 1678*

Overdose and Toxicology *on page 1916*

U.S. Brand Names Trandate®

Canadian Brand Names Apo-Labetalol®; Labetalol Hydrochloride Injection, USP; Normodyne®; Trandate®

Index Terms Ibidomide Hydrochloride; Labetalol Hydrochloride

Therapeutic Category Alpha-/Beta- Adrenergic Blocker; Antihypertensive Agent

Generic Available Yes

Use Treatment of mild to severe hypertension; I.V. for hypertensive emergencies

Pregnancy Risk Factor C

Lactation Enters breast milk/use caution (AAP rates "compatible")

Contraindications Hypersensitivity to labetalol or any component; asthma, obstructive airway disease, cardiogenic shock, uncompensated CHF, bradycardia, pulmonary edema, or heart block; history of asthma or obstructive airway disease

Warnings Orthostatic hypotension may occur with I.V. administration; patient should remain supine during and for up to 3 hours after I.V. administration; use with extreme caution when reducing severely elevated blood pressure; cerebral and cardiac adverse effects (infarction/ischemia) may occur if blood pressure is decreased too rapidly; blood pressure should be lowered over as long a period of time that is compatible with the status of the patient

Tablets may contain sodium benzoate; benzoic acid (benzoate) is a metabolite of benzyl alcohol; large amounts of benzyl alcohol (≥99 mg/kg/day) have been associated with a potentially fatal toxicity ("gasping syndrome") in neonates; the "gasping syndrome" consists of metabolic acidosis, respiratory distress, gasping respirations, CNS dysfunction (including convulsions, intracranial hemorrhage), hypotension and cardiovascular collapse; avoid use of labetalol products containing sodium benzoate in neonates; *in vitro* and animal studies have shown that benzoate displaces bilirubin from protein binding sites

Precautions Paradoxical increase in blood pressure has been reported with treatment of pheochromocytoma or clonidine withdrawal syndrome; use with extreme caution in patients with hyper-reactive airway disease, CHF, diabetes mellitus, hepatic dysfunction

Adverse Reactions

Cardiovascular: Orthostatic hypotension especially with I.V. administration, edema, CHF, A-V conduction disturbances (but less than with propranolol), bradycardia

Central nervous system: Drowsiness, fatigue, dizziness, behavior disorders, headache

Dermatologic: Rash, tingling in scalp or skin (transient with initiation of therapy)

Gastrointestinal: Nausea, xerostomia

Genitourinary: Sexual dysfunction, urinary problems

Neuromuscular & skeletal: Reversible myopathy has been reported in 2 children, paresthesia

Respiratory: Bronchospasm, nasal congestion

Drug Interactions Cytochrome P450 isoenzyme CYP2D6 substrate and inhibitor

Cimetidine may potentiate labetalol action; additive hypotensive effects with other hypotensive drugs; halothane may cause synergistic hypotension; tricyclic antidepressants; beta agonists; nitroglycerin; calcium antagonists

Food Interactions Avoid natural licorice (causes sodium and water retention and increases potassium loss); food may increase bioavailability

Stability

Injection: Store at room temperature; do not freeze; protect from light; stable in D_5W, NS, dextrose/saline combinations, D_5/LR, D_5/Ringer's, LR, and Ringer's injection for 24 hours; incompatible with sodium bicarbonate, furosemide; most stable in pH of 2-4

Tablets: Store at room temperature; protect unit dose boxes from excessive moisture

Mechanism of Action Blocks alpha-, beta$_1$- and beta$_2$-adrenergic receptor sites; elevated renins are reduced

(Continued)

Labetalol *(Continued)*

Pharmacodynamics

Onset of action:
- Oral: 20 minutes to 2 hours
- I.V.: 2-5 minutes

Maximum effect:
- Oral: 1-4 hours
- I.V.: 5-15 minutes

Duration:
- Oral: 8-24 hours (dose dependent)
- I.V.: 2-4 hours

Pharmacokinetics

Distribution: Crosses the placenta; small amounts in breast milk
- V_d: Adults: 3-16 L/kg; mean: 9.4 L/kg

Protein-binding: 50%

Metabolism: In the liver primarily via glucuronide conjugation; extensive first-pass effect

Bioavailability: Oral: 25%; increased bioavailability with liver disease, elderly

Half-life: 5-8 hours

Elimination: Possible decreased clearance in neonates/infants; <5% excreted in urine unchanged

Dialysis: Not removed by hemo- or peritoneal dialysis; supplemental dose is not necessary

Usual Dosage

Children: **Note**: Limited information regarding labetalol use in pediatric patients is currently available in the literature; labetalol should be initiated cautiously in pediatric patients (using the lower doses listed) with careful dosage adjustment and blood pressure monitoring

- Oral: Some centers recommend initial oral doses of 4 mg/kg/day in 2 divided doses. (Reported oral doses have started at 3 mg/kg/day and 20 mg/kg/day and have increased up to 40 mg/kg/day.)
- I.V., intermittent bolus doses: Initial doses of 0.2-0.5 mg/kg/dose with a range of 0.2-1 mg/kg/dose have been suggested; maximum dose: 20 mg/dose
- Treatment of pediatric hypertensive emergencies: Initial continuous infusions of 0.4-1 mg/kg/hour with a maximum of 3 mg/kg/hour have been used; one study used initial bolus dose of 0.2-1 mg/kg (maximum dose: 20 mg, mean: 0.5 mg/kg) followed by a continuous infusion of 0.25-1.5 mg/kg/hour (mean: 0.78 mg/kg/hour)

Adults:

- Oral:
  - **Outpatient:** Initial: 100 mg twice daily, may increase as needed every 2-3 days by 100 mg until desired response is obtained; usual dose: 200-400 mg twice daily; not to exceed 2.4 g/day; usual dosage range (JNC 7): 200-800 mg/day in 2 divided doses
  - **Inpatient (following acute loading with I.V. infusion):** Initial: 200 mg; administer next dose as 200 mg or 400 mg after 6-12 hours, depending on blood pressure response; thereafter, for **inpatient** titration of dose, dose may be increased at 1-day intervals to obtain desired blood pressure control; increase dose as needed according to the following: 400 mg/day given in 2-3 divided doses; 800 mg/day given in 2-3 divided doses; 1600 mg/day given in 2-3 divided doses; up to a maximum of 2400 mg/day given in 2-3 divided doses (see above for outpatient dosing).
- I.V.: Initial: 20 mg; may give 40-80 mg at 10-minute intervals, up to 300 mg total dose
- I.V. infusion (acute loading): Initial: 2 mg/minute; titrate to response; usual effective total dose: 50-200 mg total; maximum: 300 mg total dose; discontinue infusion and start oral tablets once satisfactory response in blood pressure is obtained.

Note: Only acute loading dose infusions are described in the I.V. product labeling. Limited documentation of prolonged continuous infusions exists. In rare clinical situations, higher dosages (2-6 mg/**minute**) have been used in the critical care setting (eg, in patients with aortic dissection). Continuous infusions at relatively low doses (2-6 mg/**hour** - note difference in units) have been used in some settings (eg, following loading infusion in patients who are unable to be converted to oral regimens or as a continuation of outpatient oral regimens). These prolonged infusions should not be confused with loading infusions. Careful clarification of orders and specific infusion rates/units is required to avoid confusion.

Dosage adjustment in hepatic impairment: Dosage reduction may be necessary.

Administration

Oral: May administer with food but should be administered in a consistent manner with regards to meals

Parenteral:

I.V. bolus: Administer over 2-3 minutes; do not administer faster than 2 mg/minute; maximum concentration: 5 mg/mL

I.V. continuous infusion: Dilute to 1 mg/mL; undiluted labetalol injection (5 mg/mL) has been administered to a very small number of adult patients who were extremely fluid restricted

Monitoring Parameters Blood pressure, heart rate, pulse, EKG; **Note:** I.V. use: Monitor closely; due to the prolonged duration of action, careful monitoring should be extended for the duration of the infusion and for several hours after the infusion; excessive administration may result in prolonged hypotension and/or bradycardia

Test Interactions False-positive urine catecholamines, VMA if measured by fluorometric or photometric methods; use HPLC or specific catecholamine radioenzymatic technique

Patient Information Limit alcohol; may cause dizziness or drowsiness and impair ability to perform activities requiring mental alertness or physical coordination; do not stop medication abruptly; may cause dry mouth

Nursing Implications Instruct patient regarding compliance; do **not** abruptly withdraw medication in patients with ischemic heart disease; labetalol may mask other signs and symptoms of diabetes mellitus, but sweating can still occur

Dosage Forms Excipient information presented when available (limited, particularly for generics); consult specific product labeling.

Injection, solution, as hydrochloride: 5 mg/mL (4 mL, 20 mL, 40 mL)

Trandate®: 5 mg/mL (20 mL, 40 mL)

Tablet, as hydrochloride: 100 mg, 200 mg, 300 mg

Trandate®: 100 mg, 200 mg [contains sodium benzoate], 300 mg

Extemporaneous Preparations

A 40 mg/mL labetalol hydrochloride oral liquid preparation made from tablets and 3 different vehicles (cherry syrup, a 1:1 mixture of Ora-Sweet® and Ora-Plus®, or a 1:1 mixture of Ora-Sweet® SF and Ora-Plus®) was stable for 60 days when stored in amber plastic prescription bottles in the dark at room temperature (25°C) or under refrigeration (5°C); grind sixteen 300 mg tablets in a mortar into a fine powder; add 20 mL of the vehicle and mix well to form a uniform paste; mix while adding the vehicle in geometric proportions to **almost** 120 mL; transfer to a calibrated bottle and qsad with vehicle to make 120 mL; label "shake well" and "protect from light" (Allen, 1996).

Extemporaneously prepared solutions of labetalol hydrochloride (approximate concentrations 7-10 mg/mL) prepared in distilled water, simple syrup, apple juice, grape juice, and orange juice were stable for 4 weeks when stored in amber glass or plastic prescription bottles at 23°C and 4°C (Nahata, 1991).

Allen LV and Erickson MA, "Stability of Labetalol Hydrochloride, Metoprolol Tartrate, Verapamil Hydrochloride, and Spironolactone With Hydrochlorothiazide in Extemporaneously Compounded Oral Liquids," *Am J Health Syst Pharm*, 1996, 53(19):2304-9.

Nahata MC, "Stability of Labetolol Hydrochloride in Distilled Water, Simple Syrup, and Three Fruit Juices," *DICP*, 1991, 25(5):465-9.

References

Bunchman TE, Lynch RE, and Wood EG, "Intravenously Administered Labetalol for Treatment of Hypertension in Children," *J Pediatr*, 1992, 120(1):140-4.

Chobanian AV, Bakris GL, Black HR, et al, "The Seventh Report of the Joint National Committee on Prevention, Detection, Evaluation, and Treatment of High Blood Pressure: The JNC 7 report," *JAMA*, 2003, 289(19):2560-72.

Farine M, and Arbus GS, "Management of Hypertensive Emergencies in Children," *Pediatr Emerg Care*, 1989, 5(1):51-5.

Ishisaka DY, Yonan CD, Housel BF, "Labetalol for Treatment of Hypertension in a Child," *Clin Pharm*, 1991, 10(7):500-1 (case report).

Jones SE, "Coarctation in Children. Controlled Hypotension Using Labetalol and Halothane," *Anaesthesia*, 1979, 34(10):1052-5.

Jureidini KF, "Oral Labetalol in a Child With Phaeochromocytoma and Five Children With Renal Hypertension," *N Z Med J*, 1980, 10:479 (abstract).

Mueller JB and Solhaug MJ, "Labetalol in Pediatric Hypertensive Emergencies," *Pediatr Res*, 1988, 23(Pt 2):543A (abstract).

Wesley AG, Hariparsad D, Pather M, et al, "Labetalol in Tetanus. The Treatment of Sympathetic Nervous System Overactivity," *Anaesthesia*, 1983, 38(3):243-9.

♦ **Labetalol Hydrochloride** *see* Labetalol *on page 895*

♦ **Labetalol Hydrochloride Injection, USP (Can)** *see* Labetalol *on page 895*

♦ **Lac-Hydrin®** *see* Lactic Acid and Ammonium Hydroxide *on page 898*

♦ **Lac-Hydrin® Five [OTC]** *see* Lactic Acid and Ammonium Hydroxide *on page 898*

♦ **LAClotion™** *see* Lactic Acid and Ammonium Hydroxide *on page 898*

Lactic Acid and Ammonium Hydroxide

(LAK tik AS id with a MOE nee um hye DROKS ide)

U.S. Brand Names AmLactin® [OTC]; Geri-Hydrolac™ [OTC]; Geri-Hydrolac™-12 [OTC]; Lac-Hydrin®; Lac-Hydrin® Five [OTC]; LAClotion™

Index Terms Ammonium Lactate

Therapeutic Category Topical Skin Product

Generic Available Yes

Use Topical humectant used in the treatment of ichthyosis vulgaris, ichthyosis xerosis, and dry skin conditions

Pregnancy Risk Factor B

Lactation Use caution

Contraindications Hypersensitivity to ammonium lactate, parabens, or any component

Warnings May cause photosensitivity reaction (see Patient Information)

Precautions Use with caution on face due to potential irritation, particularly in fair-skinned individuals

Adverse Reactions

Dermatologic: Rash, erythema, peeling, photosensitivity

Local: Burning, stinging

Drug Interactions Mixture of calcipotriene ointment with ammonium lactate lotion may result in a significant decrease in the calcipotriene concentration within 24 hours and continued decrease over the next 10 days

Stability Store at room temperature

Mechanism of Action Ammonium lactate is a formulation of lactic acid neutralized with ammonium hydroxide. Lactic acid is an alpha-hydroxy acid which increases hydration of the skin, decreases corneocyte adhesion, reduces excessive epidermal keratinization in hyperkeratotic conditions, and induces synthesis of mucopolysaccharides and collagen in photodamaged skin.

Pharmacodynamics Onset of action: Ichthyosis xerosis: 3-7 days

Pharmacokinetics Bioavailability: 6%

Usual Dosage Infants, Children, and Adults: Topical: Apply twice daily

Administration Topical: Apply a small amount to the affected area(s) and rub in thoroughly; avoid contact with eyes, lips, or mucous membranes; shake lotion well before use

Monitoring Parameters Physical examination of skin condition

Patient Information Avoid contact with eyes, lips, or mucous membranes; may cause stinging or burning when applied to skin with fissures, erosions, or abrasions. May cause photosensitivity reactions (eg, exposure to sunlight may cause severe sunburn, skin rash, redness, or itching); avoid exposure to sunlight and artificial light sources (sunlamps, tanning booth/bed); wear protective clothing, wide-brimmed hats, sunglasses, and lip sunscreen (SPF ≥15); use a sunscreen [broad-spectrum sunscreen or physical sunscreen (preferred) or sunblock with SPF ≥15]; contact physician if reaction occurs. Do not use cosmetics or other skin care products on the treated skin area.

Dosage Forms Excipient information presented when available (limited, particularly for generics); consult specific product labeling.

Cream, topical: Lactic acid 12% with ammonium hydroxide (140 g, 280 g, 385 g)

AmLactin®: Lactic acid 12% with ammonium hydroxide (140 g)

Lac-Hydrin®: Lactic acid 12% with ammonium hydroxide (280 g, 385 g)

Lotion, topical (AmLactin®, Lac-Hydrin®, LAClotion™): Lactic acid 12% with ammonium hydroxide (225 g, 400 g)

Geri-Hydrolac™, Lac-Hydrin® Five: Lactic acid 5% with ammonium hydroxide (120 mL, 240 mL)

Geri-Hydrolac™-12: Lactic acid 12% with ammonium hydroxide (120 mL, 240 mL)

♦ **Lactinex™ [OTC]** *see Lactobacillus acidophilus* and *Lactobacillus bulgaricus on page 898*

♦ ***Lactobacillus acidophilus*** *see Lactobacillus acidophilus* and *Lactobacillus bulgaricus on page 898*

Lactobacillus acidophilus and *Lactobacillus bulgaricus*

(lak toe ba SIL us as i DOF fil us & lak toe ba SIL us bul GAR i cus)

U.S. Brand Names Bacid® [OTC]; Culturelle® [OTC]; Dofus [OTC]; Flora-Q™ [OTC]; Kala® [OTC]; Lactinex™ [OTC]; Lacto-Bifidus [OTC]; Lacto-Key [OTC]; Lacto-Pectin [OTC]; Lacto-TriBlend [OTC]; Megadophilus® [OTC]; MoreDophilus® [OTC]; Superdophilus® [OTC]

Canadian Brand Names Bacid®; Fermalac

Index Terms *Lactobacillus acidophilus*; *Lactobacillus bifidus*; *Lactobacillus bulgaricus*; *Lactobacillus casei*; *Lactobacillus paracasei*; *Lactobacillus reuteri*; *Lactobacillus rhamnosus* GG

Therapeutic Category Antidiarrheal

Generic Available Yes

Use Treatment of uncomplicated diarrhea particularly that caused by antibiotic therapy; re-establish normal physiologic and bacterial flora of the intestinal tract

Contraindications Allergy to milk or lactose

Warnings Discontinue if high fever present

Adverse Reactions Gastrointestinal: Intestinal flatus

Stability Store in the refrigerator

Mechanism of Action Creates an environment unfavorable to potentially pathogenic fungi or bacteria through the production of lactic acid, and favors establishment of an aciduric flora, thereby suppressing the growth of pathogenic microorganisms; helps re-establish normal intestinal flora

Pharmacokinetics

Absorption: Not orally absorbed

Distribution: Locally, primarily in the colon

Elimination: In feces

Usual Dosage Children and Adults: Oral:

Capsule: 1-2 capsules 2-4 times/day

Granules: 1 packet added to or taken with cereal, food, milk, fruit juice, or water, 3-4 times/day

Powder: $^1/_4$-1 teaspoon 1-3 times/day with liquid

Tablet, chewable: 4 tablets 3-4 times/day; may follow each dose with a small amount of milk, fruit juice, or water

Recontamination protocol for BMT unit: 1 packet 3 times/day for 6 doses for those patients who refuse yogurt

Administration Oral: Granules, powder, or contents of capsules may be added to or administered with cereal, food, milk, fruit juice, or water

Dosage Forms Excipient information presented when available (limited, particularly for generics); consult specific product labeling.

Capsule:

Culturelle®: *L. rhamnosus* GG 10 billion colony-forming units [contains casein and whey]

Dofus: *L. acidophilus* and *L. bifidus* 10:1 ratio [beet root powder base]

Flora-Q™: *L. acidophilus* and *L. paracasei* ≥8 billion colony-forming units [also contains *Bifidobacterium* and *S. thermophilus*]

Lacto-Key:

100: *L. acidophilus* 1 billion colony-forming units [milk, soy, and yeast free; rice derived]

600: *L. acidophilus* 6 billion colony-forming units [milk, soy, and yeast free; rice derived]

Lacto-Bifidus:

100: *L. bifidus* 1 billion colony-forming units [milk, soy, and yeast free; rice derived]

600: *L. bifidus* 6 billion colony-forming units [milk, soy, and yeast free; rice derived]

Lacto-Pectin: *L. acidophilus* and *L. casei* ≥5 billion colony-forming units [also contains *Bifidobacterium lactis* and citrus pectin cellulose complex]

Lacto-TriBlend:

100: *L. acidophilus, L. bifidus,* and *L. bulgaricus* 1 billion colony-forming units [milk, soy and yeast free; rice derived]

600: *L. acidophilus, L. bifidus,* and *L. bulgaricus* 6 billion colony-forming units [milk, soy and yeast free; rice derived]

Megadophilus®, Superdophilus®: *L. acidophilus* 2 billion units [available in dairy based or dairy free formulations]

Capsule, softgel: *L. acidophilus* 100 active units

Caplet (Bacid®): *L. acidophilus 80%* and *L. bulgaricus* 10% [also contains *Bifidobacterium biffidum* 5% and *S. thermophilus* 5%]

Granules (Lactinex™): *L. acidophilus* and *L. bulgaricus* 100 million live cells per 1 g packet (12s) [contains whey, evaporated milk, soy peptone, lactose, and beef extract]

Powder:

Lacto-TriBlend: *L. acidophilus, L. bifidus,* and *L. bulgaricus* 10 billion colony-forming units per $^1/_4$ teaspoon (60 g) [milk, soy, and yeast free; rice derived]

(Continued)

Lactobacillus acidophilus and *Lactobacillus bulgaricus* *(Continued)*

Megadophilus®, Superdophilus®: *L. acidophilus* 2 billion units per half-teaspoon (49 g, 70 g, 84 g, 126 g) [available in dairy based or dairy free (garbanzo bean) formulations]

MoreDophilus®: *L. acidophilus* 12.4 billion units per teaspoon (30 g, 120 g) [dairy free, yeast free; soy and carrot derived]

Tablet:

Kala®: *L. acidophilus* 200 million units [dairy free, yeast free; soy based]

Lactinex™: *L. acidophilus* and *L. bulgaricus* 1 million live cells [contains whey, evaporated milk, soy peptone, lactose, and beef extract; contains sodium 5.6 mg/4 tablets]

Tablet, chewable: *L. reuteri* 100 million organisms

Wafer: *L. acidophilus* 90 mg and *L. bifidus* 25 mg (100s) [provides 1 billion organisms/wafer at time of manufacture; milk free]

Lactulose (LAK tyoo lose)

Medication Safety Issues

Sound-alike/look-alike issues:

Lactulose may be confused with lactose

U.S. Brand Names Constulose; Enulose; Generlac; Kristalose®

Canadian Brand Names Acilac; Apo-Lactulose®; Laxilose; PMS-Lactulose

Therapeutic Category Ammonium Detoxicant; Hyperammonemia Agent; Laxative, Miscellaneous

Generic Available Yes

Use Adjunct in the prevention and treatment of portal-systemic encephalopathy (PSE); treatment of chronic constipation

Pregnancy Risk Factor B

Lactation Excretion in breast milk unknown

Contraindications Hypersensitivity to lactulose or any component; galactosemia or patients requiring low galactose diet

Warnings Accumulation of hydrogen gas in intestine could result in an explosion if the patient were to undergo electrocautery procedure

Precautions Use with caution in patients with diabetes mellitus; do not use with other laxatives especially when initiating PSE treatment as increased loose stools may falsely suggest adequate lactulose dosage

Adverse Reactions Gastrointestinal: Flatulence, abdominal discomfort, diarrhea, nausea, vomiting

Drug Interactions Oral antibiotics may interfere with desired degradation of lactulose by eliminating key GI bacteria; nonabsorbable antacids may eliminate desired lactulose-induced decreased GI tract pH

Food Interactions Contraindicated in patients on galactose-restricted diet

Stability Store at room temperature to reduce viscosity; discard solution if cloudy or very dark

Mechanism of Action The bacterial degradation of lactulose resulting in an acidic pH inhibits the diffusion of NH_3 into the blood by causing the conversion of NH_3 to NH_4+;

also enhances the diffusion of NH_3 from the blood into the gut where conversion to NH_4+ occurs; produces an osmotic effect in the colon with resultant distention promoting peristalsis and elimination of NH_4+ from the body

Pharmacokinetics

Absorption: Oral: Not absorbed appreciably

Metabolism: By colonic flora to lactic acid and acetic acid

Elimination: Primarily in feces and urine (~3%)

Usual Dosage

Prevention and treatment of portal systemic encephalopathy (PSE): Oral:

Infants: 2.5-10 mL/day divided 3-4 times/day, adjust dosage to produce 2-3 soft stools per day

Children: 40-90 mL/day divided 3-4 times/day, adjust dosage to produce 2-3 soft stools per day

Adults:

Oral:

Acute episodes of PSE: 30-45 mL (20-30 g) at 1- to 2-hour intervals until laxative effect observed, then adjust dosage to produce 2-3 soft stools per day

Chronic therapy: 30-45 mL/dose (20-30 g/dose) 3-4 times/day; titrate dose every 1-2 days to produce 2-3 soft stools per day

Rectal: 300 mL diluted with 700 mL of water or NS, and given via a rectal balloon catheter and retained for 30-60 minutes; may give every 4-6 hours

Constipation: Oral:

Children: 7.5 mL/day (5 g/day) after breakfast

Adults: 15-30 mL/day (10-20 g/day); increase to a maximum of 60 mL/day (40 g/day) if needed

Administration

Oral: Administer with juice, milk, or water; dissolve crystals in 4 ounces of water or juice

Rectal: See Usual Dosage

Monitoring Parameters Serum ammonia, serum potassium, fluid status, stool output

Additional Information Upon discontinuation of therapy, allow 24-48 hours for resumption of normal bowel movements

Dosage Forms Excipient information presented when available (limited, particularly for generics); consult specific product labeling.

Crystals for solution, oral:

Kristalose®: 10 g/packet (30s), 20 g/packet (30s)

Syrup: 10 g/15 mL (15 mL, 30 mL, 237 mL, 473 mL, 946 mL, 1890 mL)

Constulose: 10 g/15 mL (240 mL, 960 mL)

Enulose: 10 g/15 mL (480 mL)

Generlac: 10 g/15 mL (480 mL, 1920 mL)

♦ **LAIV** *see* Influenza Virus Vaccine (Live/Attenuated) *on page 835*

♦ **L-AmB** *see* Amphotericin B Liposome *on page 122*

♦ **Lamictal®** *see* Lamotrigine *on page 906*

Lamivudine (la MI vyoo deen)

Medication Safety Issues

Sound-alike/look-alike issues:

Lamivudine may be confused with lamotrigine

Epivir® may be confused with Combivir®

Related Information

Adult and Adolescent HIV *on page 1821*

Pediatric HIV *on page 1816*

Perinatal HIV *on page 1831*

U.S. Brand Names Epivir®; Epivir-HBV®

Canadian Brand Names Heptovir®; 3TC®

Index Terms 2'-Deoxy-3'-Thiacytidine; 3TC

Therapeutic Category Antiretroviral Agent; HIV Agents (Anti-HIV Agents); Nucleoside Reverse Transcriptase Inhibitor (NRTI)

Generic Available No

Use Treatment of HIV infection in combination with other antiretroviral agents. (**Note:** HIV regimens consisting of **three** antiretroviral agents are strongly recommended); chemoprophylaxis after occupational exposure to HIV; management of chronic hepatitis B infection associated with evidence of hepatitis B viral replication and active liver inflammation

Pregnancy Risk Factor C

Lactation Enters breast milk/contraindicated

Contraindications Hypersensitivity to lamivudine or any component

(Continued)

Lamivudine *(Continued)*

Warnings The major clinical toxicity of lamivudine in pediatric patients is pancreatitis which has occurred in 14% of patients in one open-label, uncontrolled study; discontinue lamivudine therapy if clinical signs, symptoms, or laboratory abnormalities suggestive of pancreatitis occur. Cases of lactic acidosis, severe hepatomegaly with steatosis, and death have been reported in patients receiving nucleoside analogues; most of these cases have been in women; prolonged nucleoside use, obesity, and prior liver disease may be risk factors; use with extreme caution in patients with other risk factors for liver disease; discontinue therapy in patients who develop laboratory or clinical evidence of lactic acidosis or pronounced hepatotoxicity.

If treatment doses used for chronic hepatitis B are administered as monotherapy to a patient with unrecognized or untreated HIV infection, rapid emergence of HIV resistance will occur. HIV-infected patients who are coinfected with hepatitis B may experience clinical symptoms or laboratory evidence of hepatitis when lamivudine is discontinued; most cases are self-limited, but fatalities have been reported; monitor patients closely for at least several months after discontinuation of lamivudine. Concomitant use of combination antiretroviral therapy with interferon alfa (with or without ribavirin) has resulted in hepatic decompensation (with some fatalities) in patients coinfected with HIV and HCV; monitor patients closely, especially for hepatic decompensation; consider discontinuation of lamivudine if needed; consider dose reduction or discontinuation of interferon alfa, ribavirin, or both if clinical toxicities, including hepatic decompensation, worsen.

Precautions Use with extreme caution and only if there is no satisfactory alternative therapy in pediatric patients with a history of pancreatitis or other significant risk factors for the development of pancreatitis. Use with caution and reduce dosage in patients with impaired renal function. Fat redistribution and accumulation [ie, central obesity, peripheral wasting, facial wasting, breast enlargement, dorsocervical fat enlargement (buffalo hump), and cushingoid appearance] have been observed in patients receiving antiretroviral agents (causal relationship not established). Immune reconstitution syndrome (an acute inflammatory response to residual or indolent opportunistic infections) may occur in HIV patients during initial treatment with combination antiretroviral agents; this syndrome may require further patient assessment and therapy.

Adverse Reactions

Central nervous system: Headache, fatigue, insomnia, fever, psychomotor disorders, dizziness, depressive disorder

Dermatologic: Rash, pruritus, urticaria, alopecia

Endocrine & metabolic: Lactic acidosis, hyperglycemia; fat redistribution and accumulation (see Precautions)

Gastrointestinal: Nausea, feeding problem, abdominal discomfort, pancreatitis (children: 14%; primarily seen in children with advanced HIV receiving multiple medications), diarrhea, vomiting, anorexia, stomatitis

Hematologic: Neutropenia, anemia, thrombocytopenia

Hepatic: Elevated ALT, AST, bilirubin, and amylase; hepatic steatosis, severe hepatomegaly

Neuromuscular & skeletal: Paresthesias, peripheral neuropathy, musculoskeletal pain, gait disorder, myalgia, muscle weakness, rhabdomyolysis, elevated CPK

Respiratory: Cough, wheezing

Miscellaneous: Immune reconstitution syndrome

Drug Interactions Coadministration with trimethoprim/sulfamethoxazole increases the AUC of lamivudine by 44% (significance is unknown); when used with zidovudine, lamivudine may prevent emergence of zidovudine resistance; lamivudine and zalcitabine may inhibit intracellular phosphorylation of each other (concurrent use of lamivudine and zalcitabine is **not** recommended). Ribavirin may decrease the intracellular phosphorylation of lamivudine (*in vitro* data); however, one clinical study did not identify a pharmacokinetic or pharmacodynamic interaction. Concomitant use of lamivudine with interferon alfa (with or without ribavirin) in patients coinfected with HIV and HCV, may result in hepatic decompensation which may be fatal (see Warnings).

Food Interactions Food delays the rate but not the extent of absorption (bioavailability is not significantly affected).

Stability Store tablets and oral solution at room temperature in tightly closed bottles

Mechanism of Action A synthetic nucleoside analogue that is converted intracellularly to the active triphosphate metabolite which inhibits reverse transcription via viral DNA chain termination after incorporation of the nucleoside analogue. Lamivudine triphosphate is a weak inhibitor of DNA polymerase alpha- and beta-mitochondrial DNA polymerase.

Pharmacokinetics

Absorption: Oral: Rapid

Distribution: Into extravascular spaces; distributes into breast milk

Children (n=38): CSF/plasma ratio: Median: 0.12; range: 0.04-0.47
V_d: Adults: 1.3 ± 0.4 L/kg
Protein binding: <36%
Metabolism: Converted intracellularly to the active triphosphate form
Bioavailability:
Children: Oral solution: 66% ± 26%
Adolescents and Adults:
150 mg tablet: 86% ± 16%
Oral solution: 87% ± 13%
Half-life:
Intracellular: 10-15 hours
Elimination:
Children 4 months to 14 years: 2 ± 0.6 hours
Adults with normal renal function: 5-7 hours
Time to peak serum concentration:
Fasting state: 0.9 hours
Fed state: 3.2 hours
Elimination: 70% of dose eliminated unchanged in urine via active organic secretion; 5.2% of dose is eliminated as a trans-sulfoxide metabolite

Usual Dosage Oral (use in combination with other antiretroviral agents):

HIV:
Neonates <30 days: 2 mg/kg/dose twice daily
Infants >3 months and Children <16 years: 4 mg/kg/dose twice daily; maximum dose: 150 mg every 12 hours
Adolescents ≥16 years and Adults, body weight <50 kg: 4 mg/kg/dose twice daily; maximum dose: 150 mg every 12 hours
Adolescents ≥16 years and Adults, body weight ≥50 kg: 150 mg twice daily or 300 mg once daily

HIV postexposure prophylaxis: Adolescents ≥16 years and Adults: 150 mg/dose twice daily or 300 mg/dose once daily (in combination with zidovudine, tenofovir, stavudine, or didanosine, with or without a protease inhibitor depending on risk)

Chronic hepatitis B infection: Note: Patients coinfected with HIV and hepatitis B should receive HIV doses of lamivudine (see above).
Children 2-17 years: 3 mg/kg/dose once daily; maximum dose: 100 mg/day
Adolescents ≥16 years and Adults: 100 mg/dose once daily

Dosing adjustment in renal impairment for HIV: Adolescents and Adults:
Cl_{cr} 30-49 mL/minute: 150 mg once daily
Cl_{cr} 15-29 mL/minute: 150 mg first dose, then 100 mg once daily
Cl_{cr} 5-14 mL/minute: 150 mg first dose, then 50 mg once daily
Cl_{cr} <5 mL/minute: 50 mg first dose, then 25 mg once daily
Note: Additional dose of lamivudine after routine (4 hour) peritoneal or hemodialysis is not required

Dosing adjustment in renal impairment for chronic hepatitis B: Adults:
Cl_{cr} 30-49 mL/minute: 100 mg first dose, then 50 mg once daily
Cl_{cr} 15-29 mL/minute: 100 mg first dose, then 25 mg once daily
Cl_{cr} 5-14 mL/minute: 35 mg first dose, then 15 mg once daily
Cl_{cr} <5 mL/minute: 35 mg first dose, then 10 mg once daily

Dosing adjustment in hepatic impairment: Dosage adjustment not required; use with caution in patients with decompensated liver disease (safety and efficacy not established with these patients)

Administration Oral: May be administered without regard to meals

Monitoring Parameters CBC with differential, hemoglobin, ALT, AST, serum amylase, bilirubin; signs and symptoms of pancreatitis, lactic acidosis, and pronounced hepatotoxicity; CD4 cell count, HIV RNA plasma levels in patients with HIV; HIV patients should be screened for hepatitis B infection before starting lamivudine (see Warnings)

Patient Information Lamivudine is not a cure for HIV; notify physician if persistent severe abdominal pain, nausea, vomiting, numbness, or tingling occur; avoid alcohol. Take lamivudine every day as prescribed; do not change dose or discontinue without physician's advice; if a dose is missed, take it as soon as possible, then return to normal dosing schedule; if a dose is skipped, do **not** double the next dose.

HIV medications may cause changes in body fat, including an increase in fat in the upper back and neck, breasts, and trunk; a loss of fat from the face, arms, and legs may also occur.

Additional Information Epivir® oral solution contains sucrose 1 g/5 mL.

A high rate of early virologic failure in therapy-naive adult HIV patients has been observed with the once-daily three-drug combination therapy of didanosine enteric-coated beadlets (Videx® EC), lamivudine, and tenofovir and the once-daily three-drug combination therapy of abacavir, lamivudine, and tenofovir. These combinations should not be used as a new treatment regimen for naive or pretreated
(Continued)

Lamivudine *(Continued)*

patients. Any patient currently receiving either of these regimens should be closely monitored for virologic failure and considered for treatment modification.

Dosage Forms Excipient information presented when available (limited, particularly for generics); consult specific product labeling.

Solution, oral:

Epivir®: 10 mg/mL (240 mL) [strawberry-banana flavor]

Epivir-HBV®: 5 mg/mL (240 mL) [strawberry-banana flavor]

Tablet:

Epivir®: 150 mg, 300 mg

Epivir-HBV®: 100 mg

References

Briars LA, Hilao JJ, and Kraus DM, "A Review of Pediatric Human Immunodeficiency Virus Infection," *Journal of Pharmacy Practice*, 2004, 17(6):407-31.

Eron JJ, Benoit SL, Jemsek J, et al, "Treatment With Lamivudine, Zidovudine, or Both in HIV-Positive Patients With 200 to 500 CD4+ Cells Per Cubic Millimeter," *N Engl J Med*, 1995, 333(25):1662-9.

Lai CL, Chien RN, Leung NW, et al, "A One-Year Trial of Lamivudine for Chronic Hepatitis B," *N Engl J Med*, 1998, 339(2):61-8.

Lewis LL, Mueller B, Schock R, et al, "A Phase I/II Study to Evaluate the Safety, Toxicity, and Preliminary Efficacy of Combinations of Lamivudine (3TC), Zidovudine (AZT) and Didanosine (ddI) in Children With HIV Infection," Natl Conf Hum Retroviruses Relat Infect (2nd), 1995, Jan 29-Feb 2:103.

Lewis LL, Venzon D, Church J, et al, "Lamivudine in Children With Human Immunodeficiency Virus Infection: A Phase I/II Study," *J Infect Dis*, 1996, 174(1):16-25.

Panel on Clinical Practices for Treatment of HIV Infection, "Guidelines for the Use of Antiretroviral Agents in HIV-Infected Adults and Adolescents," October 10, 2006, http://www.aidsinfo.nih.gov.

"Updated U.S. Public Health Service Guidelines for the Management of Occupational Exposures to HIV and Recommendations for Postexposure Prophylaxis," *MMWR Recomm Rep*, 2005, 54(RR-9):1-17.

Working Group on Antiretroviral Therapy and Medical Management of HIV-Infected Children, "Guidelines for the Use of Antiretroviral Agents in Pediatric HIV Infection," October 26, 2006, http://www.aidsinfo.nih.gov.

♦ **Lamivudine, Abacavir, and Zidovudine** *see* Abacavir, Lamivudine, and Zidovudine *on page 38*

♦ **Lamivudine and Abacavir** *see* Abacavir and Lamivudine *on page 35*

Lamivudine and Zidovudine (la MI vyoo deen & zye DOE vyoo deen)

Medication Safety Issues

Sound-alike/look-alike issues:

Combivir® may be confused with Combivent®, Epivir®

AZT is an error-prone abbreviation (mistaken as azathioprine, aztreonam)

U.S. Brand Names Combivir®

Canadian Brand Names Combivir®

Index Terms AZT and 3TC; 3TC and AZT; 3TC and ZDV; ZDV and 3TC; Zidovudine and Lamivudine

Therapeutic Category Antiretroviral Agent; HIV Agents (Anti-HIV Agents); Nucleoside Reverse Transcriptase Inhibitor (NRTI)

Generic Available No

Use Treatment of HIV-1 infection in combination with at least one other antiretroviral agent; (**Note:** HIV regimens consisting of **three** antiretroviral agents are strongly recommended)

Pregnancy Risk Factor C

Lactation See individual agents.

Contraindications Hypersensitivity to lamivudine, zidovudine, or any component

Warnings This product contains lamivudine and zidovudine as a fixed-dose combination; ordinarily, concomitant use of Combivir® with either lamivudine or zidovudine is not recommended. The major clinical toxicity of lamivudine in pediatric patients is pancreatitis; discontinue therapy if clinical signs, symptoms, or laboratory abnormalities suggestive of pancreatitis occur. HIV-infected patients who are coinfected with hepatitis B may experience clinical symptoms or laboratory evidence of hepatitis when a lamivudine-containing medication is discontinued; most cases are self-limited, but fatalities have been reported; monitor patients closely for at least several months after discontinuation of lamivudine and zidovudine. Concomitant use of combination antiretroviral therapy with interferon alfa (with or without ribavirin) has resulted in hepatic decompensation (with some fatalities) in patients coinfected with HIV and HCV; monitor patients closely, especially for hepatic decompensation, neutropenia, and anemia; consider discontinuation of lamivudine and zidovudine if needed; consider dose reduction or discontinuation of interferon alfa, ribavirin, or both if clinical toxicities, including hepatic decompensation, worsen.

Zidovudine is associated with hematologic toxicity including granulocytopenia and severe anemia requiring transfusions; use with caution in patients with ANC <1000 cells/mm^3 or hemoglobin <9.5 g/dL; discontinue treatment in children with an ANC

<500 cells/mm^3 until marrow recovery is observed; use of erythropoietin, filgrastim, or reduced zidovudine dosage may be necessary in some patients; prolonged use of zidovudine may cause myositis and myopathy; zidovudine has been shown to be carcinogenic in rats and mice.

Cases of lactic acidosis, severe hepatomegaly with steatosis, and death have been reported with the use of lamivudine, zidovudine and other antiretroviral agents; most of these cases have been in women; prolonged nucleoside use, obesity, and prior liver disease may be risk factors; use with extreme caution in patients with other risk factors for liver disease; discontinue therapy in patients who develop laboratory or clinical evidence of lactic acidosis or pronounced hepatotoxicity.

Precautions Always use Combivir® in combination with another antiretroviral agent; use with extreme caution and only if there is no satisfactory alternative therapy in pediatric patients with a history of pancreatitis or other significant risk factors for pancreatitis; use with caution in patients with bone marrow compromise or in patients with impaired renal or hepatic function. The dose of lamivudine should be reduced in patients with renal dysfunction; the dose of zidovudine should be reduced or therapy interrupted in patients with anemia, granulocytopenia, myopathy, renal or hepatic impairment, or liver cirrhosis; use of the fixed-dose combination product (Combivir®) is **not** recommended for patients who need a dosage reduction (use individual antiretroviral agents to appropriately adjust dosages).

Fat redistribution and accumulation [ie, central obesity, peripheral wasting, facial wasting, breast enlargement, dorsocervical fat enlargement (buffalo hump), and cushingoid appearance] have been observed in patients receiving antiretroviral agents (causal relationship not established). Immune reconstitution syndrome (an acute inflammatory response to residual or indolent opportunistic infections) may occur in HIV patients during initial treatment with combination antiretroviral agents; this syndrome may require further patient assessment and therapy.

Adverse Reactions See Lamivudine *on page 901* and Zidovudine *on page 1637*

Drug Interactions See Lamivudine *on page 901* and Zidovudine *on page 1637*

Food Interactions Food does not affect the extent of of absorption

Mechanism of Action See Lamivudine *on page 901* and Zidovudine *on page 1637*

Pharmacokinetics One Combivir® tablet is bioequivalent to one lamivudine 150 mg tablet plus one zidovudine 300 mg tablet; see Lamivudine *on page 901* and Zidovudine *on page 1637*

Usual Dosage Oral (use in combination with at least one other antiretroviral agent): Adolescents ≥12 years and Adults: One tablet twice daily

Dosage adjustment in hepatic impairment: Mild to moderate hepatic dysfunction or liver cirrhosis: Not recommended (use individual antiretroviral agents to reduce dosage)

Dosage adjustment in renal impairment: Cl_{cr} ≤50 mL/minute: Not recommended (use individual antiretroviral agents to reduce dosage)

Administration Oral: May be administered without regard to meals

Monitoring Parameters CBC with differential, hemoglobin, MCV, reticulocyte count, liver enzymes, serum amylase, bilirubin, CD4 cell count, HIV RNA plasma levels, renal and hepatic function tests; signs and symptoms of pancreatitis, lactic acidosis, pronounced hepatotoxicity, anemia, and bone marrow suppression; HIV patients should be screened for hepatitis B infection before starting lamivudine (see Warnings)

Patient Information Avoid alcohol; Combivir® is not a cure; notify physician if persistent severe abdominal pain, nausea, or vomiting occurs; take Combivir® every day as prescribed; do not change dose or discontinue without physician's advice. If a dose is missed, take it as soon as possible, then return to normal dosing schedule; if a dose is skipped, do **not** double the next dose

HIV medications may cause changes in body fat, including an increase in fat in the upper back and neck, breasts, and trunk; a loss of fat from the face, arms, and legs may also occur.

Dosage Forms Excipient information presented when available (limited, particularly for generics); consult specific product labeling.

Tablet:

Combivir®: Zidovudine 300 mg and lamivudine 150 mg

References

Briars LA, Hilao JJ, and Kraus DM, "A Review of Pediatric Human Immunodeficiency Virus Infection," *Journal of Pharmacy Practice*, 2004, 17(6):407-31.

♦ **Lamivudine, Zidovudine, and Abacavir** *see* Abacavir, Lamivudine, and Zidovudine *on page 38*

Lamotrigine (la MOE tri jeen)

Medication Safety Issues

Sound-alike/look-alike issues:

Lamotrigine may be confused with labetalol, Lamisil®, lamivudine, Lomotil®, ludiomil

Lamictal® may be confused with Lamisil®, Lomotil®, ludiomil

Related Information

Antiepileptic Drugs *on page 1902*

Assessment of Liver Function *on page 1810*

U.S. Brand Names Lamictal®

Canadian Brand Names Apo-Lamotrigine®; Gen-Lamotrigine; Lamictal®; Novo-Lamotrigine; PMS-Lamotrigine; ratio-Lamotrigine

Index Terms BW-430C; LTG

Therapeutic Category Anticonvulsant, Miscellaneous

Generic Available Yes: Chewable tablet

Use Adjunctive treatment of generalized seizures of Lennox-Gastaut syndrome, primary generalized tonic-clonic seizures, and partial seizures in children ≥2 years of age and adults; monotherapy of partial seizures in adults who are converted from valproic acid or a single enzyme-inducing AED (specifically, carbamazepine, phenytoin, phenobarbital, or primidone); maintenance treatment of bipolar disorder in adults

Note: Preliminary investigations have shown potential efficacy as add-on therapy for absence, atypical absence, atonic, tonic, and myoclonic seizures; and as monotherapy in adults and adolescents for idiopathic generalized tonic-clonic seizures; additional studies are underway

Pregnancy Risk Factor C

Lactation Enters breast milk/not recommended (AAP rates "of concern")

Contraindications Hypersensitivity to lamotrigine or any component

Warnings Skin rash may occur (10% incidence in patients with epilepsy; 14% incidence in patients with bipolar disorder); skin rash can be serious enough to require hospitalization or discontinuation of drug; serious skin rashes (including Stevens-Johnson syndrome) occur in 0.8% of pediatric and 0.3% of adult epilepsy patients and in up to 0.13% of adult patients treated for bipolar and other mood disorders; rare cases of toxic epidermal necrolysis have been reported; rash-related deaths have occurred in pediatric and adult patients. In addition to pediatric age, the risk of rash may be increased in patients receiving valproic acid, high initial doses, or with rapid dosage increases; rash usually appears in the first 2-8 weeks of therapy, but may occur after prolonged treatment (eg, 6 months). Benign rashes may occur, but one cannot predict which rashes will become serious or life-threatening; the manufacturer recommends (ordinarily) discontinuation of lamotrigine at the first sign of rash (unless rash is clearly not drug related); discontinuation of lamotrigine may not prevent rash from becoming life-threatening or permanently disfiguring or disabling

Potentially fatal hypersensitivity reactions may occur; these may include multiorgan failure or dysfunction; early symptoms of hypersensitivity reaction (eg, lymphadenopathy, fever) may occur without rash; discontinue lamotrigine if another cause for symptoms cannot be established. Blood dyscrasias may occur.

Preliminary data from the North American Antiepileptic Drug Pregnancy Registry (NAAED) suggest a possible association of lamotrigine exposure in the first trimester of pregnancy with an increased chance of cleft lip and/or cleft palate. More research and data collection is needed to confirm this possible association. Pregnant women who are currently taking lamotrigine or who are thinking about taking lamotrigine should talk with their physician first, before stopping or starting this medication.

Precautions Use with caution and decrease the dose in patients with renal or moderate to severe hepatic dysfunction. Use with caution in patients with impaired cardiac function (clinical experience is limited). Use with caution and adjust the dose in patients receiving estrogen-containing oral contraceptives (see Drug Interactions). Patients treated for bipolar disorder should be monitored closely for clinical worsening of depressive symptoms or suicidality, especially with initiation of therapy or dosage changes; prescriptions should be written for the smallest quantity consistent with good patient care.

Do not abruptly discontinue; when discontinuing therapy, gradually reduce the dose by ~50% per week and taper over at least 2 weeks unless safety concerns require a more rapid withdrawal. Lamotrigine should **not** be restarted in patients who discontinued therapy due to lamotrigine-associated rash, unless benefits clearly outweigh risks; if restarting lamotrigine after withholding for >5 half-lives, use the initial dosing recommendations and titrate dosage accordingly (ie, do **not** restart at the previous maintenance dose). Lamotrigine binds to melanin and may possibly accumulate in the eye and other tissues rich in melanin; long-term ophthalmologic effects are unknown.

Lamotrigine is **not** approved for acute treatment of mood episodes or for use in epilepsy as initial monotherapy, conversion to monotherapy from AEDs other than carbamazepine, phenytoin, phenobarbital, primidone, or valproic acid, or for conversion to monotherapy from 2 or more AEDs (safety and efficacy is not established). Safety and efficacy have not been established for the treatment of seizure disorders in children <2 years of age or for the treatment of bipolar disorder in children <18 years of age.

Adverse Reactions

Cardiovascular: Edema, chest pain, facial edema

Central nervous system: Dizziness, sedation, somnolence, headache, agitation, irritability, emotional lability, abnormal gait, ataxia, fever; incoordination, insomnia, depression, nervousness, anxiety, vertigo, difficulty concentrating, speech disorder; exacerbation of seizures has been reported

Dermatologic: Rash (higher incidence in children and in patients receiving valproic acid, high initial lamotrigine doses, or rapid dosage increases), angioedema, Stevens-Johnson syndrome, pruritus, photosensitivity; toxic epidermal necrolysis (rare)

Endocrine & metabolic: Dysmenorrhea, amenorrhea, vaginitis, weight loss

Gastrointestinal: Nausea, vomiting, diarrhea, abdominal pain, dyspepsia, constipation, anorexia, xerostomia

Hematologic: Leukopenia, neutropenia, anemia, thrombocytopenia, pancytopenia, aplastic anemia (rare), pure red cell aplasia (rare)

Neuromuscular & skeletal: Tremor, asthenia, arthralgia

Ocular: Diplopia, amblyopia, nystagmus, blurred vision, abnormal vision

Miscellaneous: Hypersensitivity reactions, lymphadenopathy, tooth disorder; acute multiorgan failure (rare)

Drug Interactions Enzyme-inducing AEDs (eg, carbamazepine, phenytoin, phenobarbital, primidone) may increase the clearance of lamotrigine, decrease lamotrigine's half-life by ~50%, and decrease lamotrigine serum concentrations by ~40% (dosage adjustment of lamotrigine is required). Carbamazepine, when administered at the same time as lamotrigine, may increase adverse effects such as dizziness, diplopia, ataxia (space administration of drugs by at least 1 hour). Acetaminophen and rifampin may increase the clearance of lamotrigine and decrease lamotrigine serum concentrations.

Estrogen-containing oral contraceptives may decrease the serum concentration of lamotrigine; dosage adjustment of lamotrigine will be necessary in most women when starting or stopping estrogen-containing oral contraceptives; lamotrigine plasma concentrations may increase (as high as twofold) during the inactive (pill-free) week of oral combination hormonal contraceptives; dose dependent adverse effects (dizziness, ataxia, diplopia) may occur during that time. Efficacy of oral contraceptives may be decreased with lamotrigine use (patients should report any changes in menstrual pattern, eg, breakthrough bleeding).

Valproic acid decreases the clearance of lamotrigine (whether given with or without enzyme-inducing AEDs) and increases half-life and serum concentrations of lamotrigine (dosage adjustment of lamotrigine is required; inhibition of lamotrigine clearance by valproic acid appears to be maximal at doses of 250-500 mg/day in adults). Valproic acid may increase the incidence of lamotrigine rash (see Warnings). Lamotrigine may increase the clearance of valproic acid. Lamotrigine may increase topiramate serum concentrations by 15% (not expected to be clinically relevant). Drugs that induce or inhibit glucuronidation may affect the clearance of lamotrigine (monitor closely; dosage adjustment may be needed). Use with other sedative agents or ethanol may increase CNS sedation. Use with oxcarbazepine may increase CNS adverse effects.

Food Interactions Absorption is not affected by food

Stability Store at room temperature in a dry place away from heat and light

Mechanism of Action A triazine derivative which affects voltage-sensitive sodium channels and inhibits presynaptic release of glutamate and aspartate (excitatory amino acid CNS neurotransmitters); mechanism of action for treatment of bipolar disorder has not been established

Pharmacokinetics

Absorption: Oral: Rapid, 97.6% absorbed

Distribution: V_d: Adults: 1.1 L/kg; range: 0.9-1.3 L/kg; crosses into breast milk

Protein binding: 55% (primarily albumin)

Metabolism: >75% metabolized in the liver via glucuronidation; autoinduction may occur

Bioavailability: 98%

(Continued)

Lamotrigine *(Continued)*

Half-life:

Infants and children:

With enzyme-inducing AEDs (ie, phenytoin, phenobarbital, carbamazepine, primidone):

Infants 10 months of age to children 5.3 years: 7.7 hours (range: 6-11 hours)

Children 5-11 years: 7 hours (range: 4-10 hours)

With enzyme-inducing AED and valproic acid (VPA): Children 5-11 years: 19 hours (range: 7-31 hours)

With VPA:

Infants 10 months of age to children 5.3 years: 45 hours (range: 30-52 hours)

Children 5-11 years: 66 hours (range 50-74 hours)

Adults:

Normal: Single dose: 33 hours; multiple dose: ~25 hours (range: 12-62 hours)

With enzyme-inducing AEDs: 13 hours (range: 8-23 hours)

With enzyme-inducing AED and VPA: ~27 hours (range: 11-52 hours)

With VPA: 59 hours (range: 30-89 hours)

Hepatic dysfunction: Child-Pugh classification:

Mild liver impairment: 46 ± 20 hours

Moderate liver impairment: 72 ± 44 hours

Severe liver impairment without ascites: 67± 11 hours

Severe liver impairment with ascites: 100 ± 48 hours

Renal dysfunction (Cl_{cr} 13 mL/minute): ~43 hours

Severe renal dysfunction (Cl_{cr} <10 mL/minute): 57.4 hours

During dialysis: 13 hours

Time to peak serum concentration: Oral: ~2 hours (range: 1.4-4.8 hours); select patients may have second peak at 4-6 hours due to enterohepatic recirculation

Elimination: 75% to 90% excreted as glucuronide metabolites and 10% as unchanged drug

Dialysis: ~20% is removed during 4-hour hemodialysis period

Usual Dosage Note: Dosage depends on patient's concomitant medications, ie, valproic acid; enzyme-inducing AEDs (specifically phenytoin, phenobarbital, carbamazepine, and primidone); or AEDS other than carbamazepine, phenytoin, phenobarbital, primidone, or valproic acid.

Anticonvulsant: Adjunctive (add-on) therapy:

Children 2-12 years: **Note: Only whole tablets should be used for dosing**; children 2-6 years will likely require maintenance doses at the higher end of recommended range; patients weighing <30 kg may need as much as a 50% increase in maintenance dose, compared with patients weighing >30 kg; titrate dose to clinical effect

Patients receiving AEDs **other than carbamazepine, phenytoin, phenobarbital, primidone, or valproic acid:**

Weeks 1 and 2: 0.3 mg/kg/day in 1-2 divided doses; round dose down to the nearest whole tablet

Weeks 3 and 4: 0.6 mg/kg/day in 2 divided doses; round dose down to the nearest whole tablet

Maintenance dose: Titrate dose to effect; after week 4, increase dose every 1-2 weeks by a calculated increment; calculate increment as 0.6 mg/kg/day rounded down to the nearest whole tablet; add this amount to the previously administered daily dose; usual maintenance: 4.5-7.5 mg/kg/day in 2 divided doses; maximum: 300 mg/day

Patients receiving AED regimens **containing valproic acid**:

Weeks 1 and 2: 0.15 mg/kg/day in 1-2 divided doses; round dose down to the nearest whole tablet; use 2 mg every other day for patients weighing >6.7 kg and <14 kg

Weeks 3 and 4: 0.3 mg/kg/day in 1-2 divided doses; round dose down to the nearest whole tablet

Maintenance dose: Titrate dose to effect; after week 4, increase dose every 1-2 weeks by a calculated increment; calculate increment as 0.3 mg/kg/day rounded down to the nearest whole tablet; add this amount to the previously administered daily dose; usual maintenance: 1-5 mg/kg/day in 1-2 divided doses; maximum: 200 mg/day. **Note:** Usual maintenance dose in children adding lamotrigine to valproic acid **alone**: 1-3 mg/kg/day

Patients receiving **enzyme-inducing** AED regimens **without valproic acid**:

Weeks 1 and 2: 0.6 mg/kg/day in 2 divided doses; round dose down to the nearest whole tablet

Weeks 3 and 4: 1.2 mg/kg/day in 2 divided doses; round dose down to the nearest whole tablet

Maintenance dose: Titrate dose to effect; after week 4, increase dose every 1-2 weeks by a calculated increment; calculate increment as 1.2 mg/kg/day rounded down to the nearest whole tablet; add this amount to the previously administered daily dose; usual maintenance: 5-15 mg/kg/day in 2 divided doses; maximum: 400 mg/day

Children >12 years and Adults:

Patients receiving AEDs **other than carbamazepine, phenytoin, phenobarbital, primidone, or valproic acid:**

Weeks 1 and 2: 25 mg every day

Weeks 3 and 4: 50 mg every day

Maintenance dose: Titrate dose to effect; after week 4, increase dose every 1-2 weeks by 50 mg/day; usual maintenance: 225-375 mg/day in 2 divided doses

Patients receiving AED regimens **containing valproic acid**:

Weeks 1 and 2: 25 mg every other day

Weeks 3 and 4: 25 mg every day

Maintenance dose: Titrate dose to effect; after week 4, increase dose every 1-2 weeks by 25-50 mg/day; usual maintenance: 100-400 mg/day in 1-2 divided doses; usual maintenance in patients adding lamotrigine to valproic acid **alone**: 100-200 mg/day

Patients receiving **enzyme-inducing** AED regimens **without valproic acid**:

Weeks 1 and 2: 50 mg/day

Weeks 3 and 4: 100 mg/day in 2 divided doses

Maintenance dose: Titrate dose to effect; after week 4, increase dose every 1-2 weeks by 100 mg/day; usual maintenance: 300-500 mg/day in 2 divided doses; doses as high as 700 mg/day in 2 divided doses have been used

Anticonvulsant: Monotherapy: Children ≥16 years and Adults:

Conversion from adjunctive therapy with a **single enzyme-inducing** AED to lamotrigine monotherapy: **Note:** First add lamotrigine and titrate it (as outlined below) to the recommended maintenance monotherapy dose (500 mg/day in 2 divided doses), while maintaining the enzyme-inducing AED at a fixed level; then gradually taper the enzyme-inducing AED by 20% decrements each week to fully withdraw over a 4-week period

Weeks 1 and 2: 50 mg/day

Weeks 3 and 4: 100 mg/day in 2 divided doses

Maintenance dose: After week 4, increase dose every 1-2 weeks by 100 mg/day; recommended maintenance monotherapy dose: 500 mg/day in 2 divided doses

Conversion from adjunctive therapy with **valproate** to lamotrigine monotherapy:

Note: This is a 4 step conversion process to achieve the lamotrigine recommended monotherapy dose (500 mg/day in 2 divided doses)

First: Add lamotrigine and titrate it to a dose of 200 mg/day as follows (if not already receiving 200 mg/day), while maintaining the valproate dose at a fixed level:

Weeks 1 and 2: 25 mg every other day

Weeks 3 and 4: 25 mg every day

Then increase dose every 1-2 weeks by 25-50 mg/day

Second: Keep lamotrigine dose at 200 mg/day; slowly taper valproate dose in decrements of ≤500 mg/day per week, to a dose of 500 mg/day; maintain this dose for one week

Third: Increase lamotrigine to 300 mg/day and decrease valproate to 250 mg/day; maintain this dose for one week

Fourth: Discontinue valproate and increase lamotrigine by 100 mg/day at weekly intervals to achieve recommended maintenance monotherapy dose of 500 mg/day in 2 divided doses

Conversion from adjunctive therapy with AEDs other than enzyme-inducing AEDs or valproate to lamotrigine monotherapy: No specific guidelines available

Bipolar disorder: Adolescents ≥18 years and Adults:

Patients **not** receiving enzyme-inducing drugs (eg, carbamazepine) or valproate:

Weeks 1 and 2: 25 mg/day

Weeks 3 and 4: 50 mg/day

Week 5: 100 mg/day

Week 6 and thereafter: 200 mg/day

Patients receiving **valproate**:

Weeks 1 and 2: 25 mg every other day

Weeks 3 and 4: 25 mg/day

Week 5: 50 mg/day

Week 6 and thereafter: 100 mg/day

Note: If valproate is discontinued, increase daily lamotrigine dose in 50 mg increments at weekly intervals until dosage of 200 mg/day is attained.

Patients receiving **enzyme-inducing drugs** (eg, carbamazepine) **without valproate:**

Weeks 1 and 2: 50 mg/day

Weeks 3 and 4: 100 mg/day in divided doses

(Continued)

Lamotrigine *(Continued)*

Week 5: 200 mg/day in divided doses
Week 6: 300 mg/day in divided doses
Week 7 and thereafter: May increase to 400 mg/day in divided doses
Note: If carbamazepine (or other enzyme-inducing drug) is discontinued, maintain current lamotrigine dose for 1 week, then decrease daily lamotrigine dose in 100 mg increments at weekly intervals until dosage of 200 mg/day is attained.

Dosage adjustment with concomitant estrogen-containing oral contraceptives: Follow initial dosing guidelines, maintenance dose should be adjusted as follows:

Patients **taking** carbamazepine, phenytoin, phenobarbital, primidone, or rifampin: No dosing adjustment required

Patients **not taking** carbamazepine, phenytoin, phenobarbital, primidone, or rifampin: If already taking estrogen-containing oral contraceptives, the maintenance dose of lamotrigine may need to be increased by as much as twofold over the target maintenance dose listed above. If already taking a stable dose of lamotrigine and starting an oral contraceptive agent, the lamotrigine maintenance dose may need to be increased by as much as twofold. Dose increases should start when contraceptive agent is started and titrated to clinical response increasing no more rapidly than 50-100 mg/day every week. Gradual increases of lamotrigine plasma levels may occur during the inactive "pill-free" week and will be greater when dose increases are made the week before. If increased adverse events consistently occur during "pill-free" week, overall dose adjustments may be required. Dose adjustments during "pill-free" week are not recommended. When discontinuing combination hormonal contraceptive, dose of lamotrigine may need decreased by as much as 50%; do not decrease by more than 25% of total daily dose over a 2-week period unless clinical response or plasma levels indicate otherwise.

Dosage adjustment in renal impairment: Use with caution; decreased dosage may be effective in patients with significant renal impairment

Dosage adjustment in hepatic impairment:

Mild hepatic impairment: No dosage adjustment required

Moderate and severe hepatic impairment without ascites: Reduce initial, escalation, and maintenance doses by ~25%

Severe hepatic impairment with ascites: Reduce initial escalation, and maintenance doses by 50%

Note: Adjust escalation and maintenance doses by clinical response

Administration Oral: May be administered without regard to food

Regular tablet: Do not chew, as a bitter taste may result

Chewable, dispersible tablet: Only whole tablets should be administered; may swallow whole, chew, or disperse in water or diluted fruit juice; if chewed, administer a small amount of water or diluted fruit juice to help in swallowing. To disperse, add tablets to a small amount of liquid (~1 teaspoon or enough to cover the medication); when the tablets are completely dispersed (in about 1 minute), swirl the solution and administer the entire amount immediately. Do not attempt to administer partial quantities of dispersed tablets.

Monitoring Parameters All patients: Monitor for hypersensitivity reactions, especially rash; CBC with differential; liver and renal function

Epilepsy: Seizure frequency, duration, and severity; serum levels of concurrent anticonvulsants

Bipolar disorder: Clinical worsening of depressive symptoms or suicidality, especially with initiation of therapy or dosage changes

Reference Range The clinical value of monitoring lamotrigine plasma concentrations has not been established. Dosing should be based on therapeutic response. Proposed therapeutic range: 1-5 mcg/mL. Lamotrigine plasma concentrations of 0.25-29.1 mcg/mL have been reported in the literature.

Patient Information Take exactly as directed; do not increase dose or frequency or discontinue without consulting prescriber. Taking other medications may require a dosage change in lamotrigine; report the use of other medications, nonprescription medications, and herbal or natural products to your physician and pharmacist; do not use alcohol and other prescription or OTC medications (especially pain medications, sedatives, antihistamines, or hypnotics) without consulting prescriber. Notify physician if you will be starting or stopping oral contraceptives or other female hormonal products (a dosage adjustment of lamotrigine may be needed; efficacy of oral contraceptives may be decreased; report any changes in menstrual pattern such as breakthrough bleeding). Report any rash, fever, or swelling of glands to the physician immediately (skin rash may indicate a serious medical problem). Lamotrigine may cause dizziness, drowsiness, or blurred vision and impair ability to perform activities requiring mental alertness or physical coordination. May cause photosensitivity reactions (eg, exposure to sunlight may cause severe sunburn, skin rash, redness, or itching); avoid exposure to sunlight and artificial light sources (sunlamps, tanning booth/bed); wear protective clothing, wide-brimmed hats, sunglasses, and lip sunscreen (SPF ≥15); use a sunscreen [broad-spectrum sunscreen or physical sunscreen (preferred) or sunblock with SPF ≥15]; contact physician if reaction occurs. Report CNS changes, mentation changes, or changes in cognition; persistent GI symptoms (cramping, constipation, vomiting, anorexia); swelling of face, lips, or tongue; easy bruising or bleeding (mouth, urine, stool); vision changes; worsening of seizure activity, or loss of seizure control to prescriber.

Additional Information Low water solubility. Does **not** induce P450 microsomal enzymes. The clinical usefulness of lamotrigine should be periodically re-evaluated in patients with bipolar disorder who are receiving the drug for extended intervals (ie, >18 months).

Three different lamotrigine "Starter Kits" are available for adult patients; each starter kit contains a blisterpack with a certain number and mg strength of tablets that are specific for initiating doses in different patient populations (see Dosage Forms).

Dosage Forms Excipient information presented when available (limited, particularly for generics); consult specific product labeling.

Tablet:
- Lamictal®: 25 mg, 100 mg, 150 mg, 200 mg

Tablet, combination package [each unit-dose starter kit contains]:
- Lamictal® (blue kit; for patients taking valproic acid):
  - Tablet: Lamotrigine 25 mg (35s)
- Lamictal® (green kit; for patients taking carbamazepine, phenytoin, phenobarbital, primidone, or rifampin **and not** taking valproic acid):
  - Tablet: Lamotrigine 25 mg (84s)
  - Tablet: Lamotrigine 100 mg (14s)
- Lamictal® (orange kit; for patients **not** taking carbamazepine, phenytoin, phenobarbital, primidone, rifampin, or valproic acid):
  - Tablet: Lamotrigine 25 mg (42s)
  - Tablet: Lamotrigine 100 mg (7s)

Tablet, dispersible/chewable: 5 mg, 25 mg
- Lamictal®: 2 mg, 5 mg, 25 mg [black currant flavor]

Extemporaneous Preparations A 1 mg/mL oral suspension made from tablets and 2 different vehicles (a 1:1 mixture of Ora-Sweet® and Ora-Plus®, or a 1:1 mixture of Ora-Sweet® SF and Ora-Plus®) was stable for 91 days when stored in amber plastic prescription bottles at room temperature (25°C) or under refrigeration (4°C); grind one 100 mg tablet in a mortar into a fine powder; add a small amount of the vehicle and mix well to form a uniform paste; mix while adding the vehicle in geometric proportions to **almost** 100 mL; transfer the mixture to a graduated cylinder and qsad with vehicle to make 100 mL; label "shake well" and "protect from light" (Nahata, 1999)

Nahata MC, Morosco RS, and Hipple TF, "Stability of Lamotrigine in Two Extemporaneously Prepared Oral Suspensions at 4°C and 25°C," *Am J Health Syst Pharm*, 1999, 56(3):240-2.

References

Battino D, Estienne M, and Avanzini G, "Clinical Pharmacokinetics of Antiepileptic Drugs in Paediatric Patients: Part II. Phenytoin, Carbamazepine, Sulthiame, Lamotrigine, Vigabatrin, Oxcarbazepine, and Felbamate," *Clin Pharmacokinet*, 1995, 29(5):341-69.

Besag FM, Wallace SJ, Dulac O, et al, "Lamotrigine for the Treatment of Epilepsy in Childhood," *J Pediatr*, 1995, 127(6):991-7.

Burstein AH, "Lamotrigine," *Pharmacotherapy*, 1995, 15(2):129-43.

Dooley J, Camfield P, Gordon K, et al, "Lamotrigine-Induced Rash in Children," *Neurology*, 1996, 46(1):240-2.

Fitton A, and Goa KL, "Lamotrigine: An Update of its Pharmacology and Therapeutic Use in Epilepsy," *Drugs*, 1995, 50(4):691-713.

Messenheimer JA, "Lamotrigine," *Epilepsia*, 1995, 36(Suppl 2):S87-94.

Messenheimer JA, Giorgi L, and Risner ME, "The Tolerability of Lamotrigine in Children," *Drug Saf*, 2000, 22(4):303-12.

Nahata MC, Morosco RS, and Hipple RT, "Stability of Lamotrigine in Two Extemporaneously Prepared Oral Suspensions at 4°C and 25°C," *Am J Health Syst Pharm*, 1999, 56(93):240-2.

♦ **Lanacane® [OTC]** *see* Benzocaine *on page 204*

♦ **Lanacane® Maximum Strength [OTC]** *see* Benzocaine *on page 204*

♦ **Lanoxicaps®** *see* Digoxin *on page 496*

♦ **Lanoxin®** *see* Digoxin *on page 496*

Lansoprazole (lan SOE pra zole)

Medication Safety Issues

Sound-alike/look-alike issues:

Prevacid® may be confused with Pravachol®, Prevpac®, Prilosec®, Prinivil®

(Continued)

Lansoprazole *(Continued)*

U.S. Brand Names Prevacid®; Prevacid® SoluTab™

Canadian Brand Names Prevacid®

Therapeutic Category Gastric Acid Secretion Inhibitor; Gastrointestinal Agent, Gastric or Duodenal Ulcer Treatment; Proton Pump Inhibitor

Generic Available No

Use

Oral: Short-term treatment (up to 4 weeks) for healing and symptomatic relief of active duodenal ulcer; short-term treatment (up to 8 weeks) for healing and symptomatic relief of all grades of erosive esophagitis; maintenance of healed erosive esophagitis; treatment of pathological hypersecretory conditions, including Zollinger-Ellison syndrome; adjuvant therapy in the treatment of *Helicobacter pylori*-associated antral gastritis; short-term treatment of symptomatic gastroesophageal reflux disease (GERD); prevention and treatment of NSAID-associated gastric ulcers

I.V.: Short-term treatment of all grades of erosive esophagitis

Pregnancy Risk Factor B

Lactation Excretion in breast milk unknown/not recommended

Contraindications Hypersensitivity to lansoprazole, pantoprazole, esomeprazole, omeprazole, or any component

Warnings Long-term effects are not known; enterochromaffin (ECF)-like hyperplasia and subsequent carcinoids have developed in rats following lifetime exposure to high doses (150 mg/kg/day). Use of gastric acid inhibitors including proton pump inhibitors and H_2 blockers has been associated with an increased risk for development of acute gastroenteritis and community-acquired pneumonia (Canani, 2006).

Precautions Symptomatic response to therapy does not preclude the presence of gastric malignancy; use with caution in patients with liver disease, reduce dosage with severe impairment; Prevacid® SoluTabs™ contain aspartame which is metabolized to phenylalanine and must be used with caution in patients with phenylketonuria

Adverse Reactions

Cardiovascular: Angina, hypertension, hypotension, palpitations, tachycardia, edema, bradycardia, syncope, MI

Central nervous system: Fatigue, dizziness, headache, insomnia, chills, fever, malaise, confusion, depression, hallucinations

Dermatologic: Rash, erythema multiforme, Stevens-Johnson syndrome, toxic epidermal necrolysis

Endocrine & metabolic: Hyperglycemia, hypoglycemia

Gastrointestinal: Abdominal pain, nausea, vomiting, melena, anorexia, cholelithiasis, xerostomia, dyspepsia, eructation, discoloration of feces, flatulence, hypergastrinemia, increased appetite, diarrhea, constipation, pancreatitis, taste perversion, halitosis, cholelithasis, gastritis

Genitourinary: Urinary retention

Hematologic (rare): Agranulocytosis, aplastic anemia, hemolytic anemia, leukopenia, neutropenia, pancytopenia, thrombocytopenia, thrombotic thrombocytopenic purpura

Hepatic: Elevated serum transaminases

Local: Pain at injection site, injection site reactions

Neuromuscular & skeletal: Paresthesia, tremor, hypertonia, neck pain, leg cramps, myalgia

Ocular: Diplopia, dry eyes, eye pain, photophobia

Otic: Tinnitus, deafness

Renal: Proteinuria

Miscellaneous: Hypersensitivity reactions, flu-like syndrome

Drug Interactions Cytochrome P450 isoenzyme CYP2C19 and CYP3A3/4 substrate

Due to profound and long-lasting inhibition of gastric acid secretion, potential for interfering with the absorption of drugs where acid pH is important exists (such as ketoconazole, itraconazole, ampicillin, iron salts, and digoxin); may decrease the absorption of some protease inhibitors (atazanavir and indinavir); may decrease the execretion of methotrexate (antirheumatic doses of methotrexate probably hold minimal risk); sucralfate delays and decreases lansoprazole absorption by 30%; lansoprazole increases theophylline clearance mildly (~10%); may increase warfarin effects; may increase the serum concentration of HMG-CoA reductase inhibitors; may increase the levels/effects of CYP2C19 substrates (examples include citalopram, diazepam, methsuximide, phenytoin, propranolol, and sertraline); CYP3A4 and CYP2C19 inducers (eg, aminoglutethimide, carbamazepine, nafcillin, nevirapine, phenobarbital, phenytoin, and rifamycins) may decrease the levels/effects of lansoprazole.

Food Interactions Food decreases lansoprazole's bioavailability by 50%

Stability Store at room temperature; protect from light and moisture; oral lansoprazole is unstable in acidic media (eg, stomach contents) and is available only as enteric coated granules; I.V. formulation is stable for 1 hour after initial reconstitution; when further diluted in NS or LR, it is stable for 24 hours and in D_5W, 8-12 hours at room temperature

Mechanism of Action Suppresses gastric acid secretion by selectively inhibiting the parietal cell membrane enzyme (H+, K+)-ATPase or proton pump; demonstrates antimicrobial activity against *Helicobacter pylori*

Pharmacodynamics

Duration of antisecretory activity: ≥24 hours

Relief of symptoms:

Gastric or duodenal ulcers: 1 week

Reflux esophagitis: 1-4 weeks

Ulcer healing:

Duodenal: 2 weeks

Gastric: 4 weeks

Pharmacokinetics

Absorption: Extremely acid labile and will degrade in acid pH of stomach; enteric coated granules improve bioavailability (80%)

Distribution: V_d:

Children: 0.61-0.9 L/kg

Adults: 15.7 ± 1.9 L

Protein binding: 97%

Metabolism: Extensive by the liver to inactive metabolites; in acid media of gastric parietal cell, lansoprazole is transformed to active sulfanilamide metabolite

Bioavailability: 80% (reduced by 50% if given 30 minutes after food)

Half-life:

Children: 1.2-1.5 hours

Adults: 1.3-1.7 hours

Time to peak serum concentration: 1.7 hours

Elimination: 14% to 25% in urine as metabolites; <1% as unchanged drug; biliary excretion is major route of elimination

Clearance:

Children: 0.57-0.71 L/hour/kg

Adults: 11.1 ± 3.8 L/hour

Adults: Hepatic impairment: 3.2-7.2 hours

Usual Dosage

Children: Oral: Limited data in single dose studies in children 3 months to 14 years; dosing range used: 0.5-1.6 mg/kg; limited multiple dose studies in pediatric patients 1-11 years of age for GERD treatment:

<10 kg: 7.5 mg once daily

10-30 kg: 15 mg once or twice daily

≥30 kg: 30 mg once or twice daily

Children ≥12 years and Adults:

Duodenal ulcer: Oral: 15 mg once daily for 4 weeks; maintenance therapy: 15 mg once daily

Primary gastric ulcer (and also associated with NSAID use): Oral: 30 mg once daily for up to 8 weeks

Erosive esophagitis:

Oral: 30 mg once daily for up to 8 weeks; additional 8 weeks may be tried in those patients who failed to respond or for a recurrence of esophagitis; maintenance: 15 mg once daily

I.V.: 30 mg once daily for up to 7 days; switch to the oral route as soon as the patient can tolerate oral administration

GERD: Oral: 15 mg once daily for up to 8 weeks

Pathological hypersecretory conditions: Oral: Initial: 60 mg once daily; adjust dosage based upon patient response; doses of 90 mg twice daily have been used; administer doses >120 mg/day in divided doses

Reflux esophagitis: Oral: 30-60 mg once daily for 8 weeks

Helicobacter pylori-associated antral gastritis: Oral: 30 mg twice daily for 2 weeks (in combination with 1 g amoxicillin and 500 mg clarithromycin given twice daily for 14 days). Alternatively, in patients allergic to or intolerant of clarithromycin or in whom resistance to clarithromycin is known or suspected, lansoprazole 30 mg every 8 hours and amoxicillin 1 g every 8 hours may be given for 2 weeks

NSAID-associated gastric ulcer: Oral:

Healing: 30 mg once daily for up to 8 weeks

Prevention: 15 mg once daily for up to 12 weeks

Dosage adjustment in hepatic impairment: Reduce dosage for severe impairment

Administration

Oral: Administer before eating

Capsules: Capsules may be opened and mixed with small amount of applesauce prior to administration without affecting the bioavailability; do not chew or crush granules; for nasogastric tube administration, the capsules can be opened, the

(Continued)

Lansoprazole *(Continued)*

granules mixed with 40 mL of apple, cranberry, grape, orange, pineapple, prune, tomato, and V-8® vegetable juice, and then administered through the NG tube; granules remain intact when mixed and stored for up to 30 minutes

Granules for oral suspension: Mix in 2 tablespoons (30 mL) water. Do not mix with other liquids or foods; stir well and drink immediately; do not chew granules. If any material remains after drinking, add more water and drink immediately. This product is not intended to be administered through a feeding tube due to increased viscosity from xanthan gum used in formulation and resulting blockage of tube.

Tablet, orally-disintegrating: Place the tablet on the tongue and allow to disintegrate with or without water until the particles can be swallowed; do not chew or crush

I.V.: Reconstitute with 5 mL SWI **only**, resulting in 6 mg/mL solution; further dilute in 50 mL NS, D_5W, or LR (see Stability) and infuse over 30 minutes; in-line filter (1.2 microns) must be used. Do not infuse with other medications.

Monitoring Parameters Patients with Zollinger-Ellison syndrome should be monitored for gastric acid output, which should be maintained at 10 mEq/hour or less during the last hour before the next lansoprazole dose; lab monitoring should include CBC, liver function, renal function, and serum gastrin levels

Reference Range Plasma levels do not correlate with pharmacologic activity

Patient Information May cause dry mouth

Dosage Forms Excipient information presented when available (limited, particularly for generics); consult specific product labeling.

Capsule, delayed release:
- Prevacid®: 15 mg, 30 mg

Granules, for oral suspension, delayed release:
- Prevacid®: 15 mg/packet (30s), 30 mg/packet (30s) [strawberry flavor]

Injection, powder for reconstitution:
- Prevacid®: 30 mg [contains mannitol 60 mg]

Tablet, orally disintegrating:
- Prevacid® SoluTab™: 15 mg [contains phenylalanine 2.5 mg; strawberry flavor]; 30 mg [contains phenylalanine 5.1 mg; strawberry flavor]

Extemporaneous Preparations A 3 mg/mL suspension of lansoprazole is prepared by emptying the contents of ten 30 mg capsules and adding 100 mL 8.4% sodium bicarbonate solution; stir for 30 minutes; protect from light; stable for 8 hours at room temperature and for 14 days refrigerated (DiGiacinto, 2000). **Note:** The same formulation was studied by Phillips, et al. A 2-week stability at room temperature and 4-week stability under refrigeration were reported.

DiGiacinto JL, Olsen KM, Bergman KL, et al, "Stability of Suspension Formulations of Lansoprazole and Omeprazole Stored in Amber-Colored Plastic Oral Syringes," *Ann Pharmacother*, 2000, 34(5):600-4.

Phillips JO, Metzler MH, and Olsen K, "The Stability of SImplified Lansoprazole Suspension (SLS)," *Gastroen*, 1999, 116:A89.

References

Canani RB, Cirillo P, Roggero P, et al, "Therapy With Gastric Acidity Inhibitors Increases the Risk of Acute Gastroenteritis and Community-Acquired Pneumonia in Children," *Pediatrics*, 2006, 117(5):e817-20.

Chun AH, Eason CJ, Shi HH, et al, "Lansoprazole: An Alternative Method of Administration of a Capsule Dosage Formulation," *Clin Ther*, 1995, 17(3):441-7.

Gibbons TE and Gold BD, "The Use of Proton Pump Inhibitors in Children: A Comprehensive Review," *Paediatr Drugs*, 2003, 5(1):25-40.

Oderda G, Chiorboli E, Haitink AR, "Inhibition of Hastric ACidity in Children by Lansoprazole Granules," *Gastroent*, 1998, 114(4pt2):A295.

Scott LJ, "Lansoprazole: In the Management of Gastroesophageal Reflux Disease in Children," *Paediatr Drugs*, 2003, 5(1):57-61.

Tran A, et al, "Pharmacokinetics/Pharmacodynamics Study of Oral Lansoprazole in Children," *Fundam Clin Pharmacol*, 1996, 10:A221.

♦ **Lantus®** *see* Insulin Glargine *on page 840*

♦ **Lantus® OptiSet® (Can)** *see* Insulin Glargine *on page 840*

♦ **Lanvis® (Can)** *see* Thioguanine *on page 1527*

♦ **Lapase** *see* Pancreatin *on page 1202*

♦ **Largactil® (Can)** *see* ChlorproMAZINE *on page 345*

♦ **Lariam®** *see* Mefloquine *on page 993*

♦ **Larodopa® (Can)** *see* Levodopa *on page 926*

Laronidase (lair OH ni days)

U.S. Brand Names Aldurazyme®

Canadian Brand Names Aldurazyme®

Index Terms Recombinant α-L-Iduronidase (Glycosaminoglycan α-L-Iduronohydrolase)

Therapeutic Category Enzyme; Mucopolysaccharidosis I (MPS I) Disease, Treatment Agent

Generic Available No

Use Treatment of patients with mucopolysaccharidosis I (MPS I) lysosomal storage disease who have one of the following clinical syndromes: Hurler's syndrome (severe), Hurler-Scheie syndrome (intermediate), or patients with the Scheie form who have moderate to severe symptoms

Pregnancy Risk Factor B

Lactation Excretion in breast milk unknown/use caution

Contraindications Hypersensitivity to laronidase or any component

Warnings Hypersensitivity reactions can occur at any time during laronidase therapy. Resuscitation equipment, oxygen, diphenhydramine, and a corticosteroid should be readily available to treat hypersensitivity or anaphylactic reactions. Use epinephrine with caution in patients with MPS I due to an increased prevalence of coronary artery disease in these patients.

Precautions The risks and benefits of administering laronidase following a severe anaphylactic or hypersensitivity reaction should be considered. If laronidase is to be readministered, use caution and have appropriate resuscitation measures available.

Adverse Reactions

Cardiovascular: Flushing, chest pain, edema, hypotension
Central nervous system: Chills, fever, headache
Dermatologic: Rash, urticaria, pruritus, angioedema
Hematologic: Thrombocytopenia
Local: Injection site reaction
Neuromuscular & skeletal: Hyper-reflexia, paresthesia
Respiratory: Dyspnea, cough, bronchospasm
Miscellaneous: Anaphylaxis, antibodies to laronidase

Drug Interactions No information available at this time.

Stability Store vials in refrigerator at 2°C to 8°C (36°F to 46°F). Do not freeze or shake. Diluted infusion solution is stable for up to 32 hours when stored at 2°C to 8°C (36°F to 46°F). Do not mix laronidase with any other drugs.

Mechanism of Action MPS I is a mucopolysaccharide storage disorder caused by a deficiency of the lysosomal enzyme, α-L-iduronidase which is required for the catabolism of glycosaminoglycans (GAG). Laronidase catalyses the hydrolysis of terminal α-L-iduronic acid residues of dermatan sulfate and heparan sulfate decreasing the accumulation of GAG substrates.

Pharmacokinetics

Distribution: V_d: 0.24 to 0.6 L/kg
Half-life: 1.5-3.6 hours
Clearance: Plasma: 1.7 to 2.7 mL/minute/kg

Usual Dosage Children, Adolescents, and Adults: I.V. infusion:

Patients ≤20 kg: 0.58 mg/kg/dose once weekly. Dose is delivered in a total volume of 100 mL.

Patients >20 kg: 0.58 mg/kg/dose once weekly. Dose is delivered in a total volume of 250 mL.

Administration I.V. infusion:

Determine the number of vials to be diluted. Remove vials from the refrigerator and allow them to reach room temperature. Do not use if the solution is discolored or contains particulate matter. Determine the total infusion volume based on the patient's weight (dose delivered in a total volume of 100 mL or 250 mL); prepare an infusion bag of 0.1% albumin in NS; gently rotate infusion bag after addition of albumin.

Remove and discard volume of 0.1% albumin in NS equal to volume of laronidase injection solution to be added to the infusion bag. Add laronidase; do not agitate solution as it denatures the enzyme. Administer with an in-line, low protein binding 0.2 micron filter.

An initial 10 mcg/kg/hour infusion rate may be incrementally increased every 15 minutes during the first hour if tolerated; increase to a maximum infusion rate of 200 mcg/kg/hour which is maintained for the remainder of the infusion (approximately 3 hours). See the following:

Initial infusion rate: 10 mcg/kg/hour for 15 minutes: If stable, increase rate to:
20 mcg/kg/hour for 15 minutes: If stable, increase rate to:
50 mcg/kg/hour for 15 minutes: If stable, increase rate to:
100 mcg/kg/hour for 15 minutes: If stable, increase rate to:
200 mcg/kg/hour for ~3 hours (remainder of the infusion)

Monitoring Parameters Vital signs, FVC, height, weight, range of motion, serum antibodies to α-L-iduronidase, urine levels of glycosaminoglycans (GAG), change in liver size

Nursing Implications Premedication with acetaminophen and/or diphenhydramine should be administered 30-60 minutes prior to starting infusion. If an infusion reaction

(Continued)

Laronidase *(Continued)*

occurs, decrease the infusion rate, temporarily stop the infusion, and/or administer antipyretics, antihistamines, and/or steroids

Dosage Forms Excipient information presented when available (limited, particularly for generics); consult specific product labeling.

Injection, solution [preservative free]: 2.9 mg/5 mL (5 mL)

References

Kakkis ED, Muenzer J, Tiller GE, et al, "Enzyme-Replacement Therapy in Mucopolysaccharidosis I," *N Engl J Med*, 2001, 344(3):182-8.

- ♦ **Lasix®** *see* Furosemide *on page 714*
- ♦ **Lasix® Special (Can)** *see* Furosemide *on page 714*
- ♦ **LASP** *see* Asparaginase *on page 161*
- ♦ **L-asparaginase** *see* Asparaginase *on page 161*
- ♦ **Lassar's Zinc Paste** *see* Zinc Oxide *on page 1640*
- ♦ **Lavacol® [OTC]** *see* Ethyl Alcohol *on page 619*
- ♦ **Laxilose (Can)** *see* Lactulose *on page 900*
- ♦ ***l*-Bunolol Hydrochloride** *see* Levobunolol *on page 925*
- ♦ **L-Carnitine** *see* Carnitine *on page 292*
- ♦ **LCD** *see* Coal Tar *on page 394*
- ♦ **LCR** *see* VinCRIStine *on page 1617*
- ♦ **Lepargylic Acid** *see* Azelaic Acid *on page 188*

Leucovorin (loo koe VOR in)

Medication Safety Issues

Sound-alike/look-alike issues:

Leucovorin may be confused with Leukeran®, Leukine®

Folinic acid may be confused with folic acid

Related Information

Compatibility of Chemotherapy and Related Supportive Care Medications *on page 1777*

Index Terms Calcium Leucovorin; Citrovorum Factor; Folinic Acid; 5-Formyl Tetrahydrofolate; Leucovorin Calcium

Therapeutic Category Antidote, Methotrexate; Folic Acid Derivative

Generic Available Yes

Use Reduce toxic effects of methotrexate ("leucovorin rescue"); antidote for folic acid antagonist overdosage; treatment of folate deficient megaloblastic anemias of infancy, sprue, or pregnancy; nutritional deficiency when oral folate therapy is not possible; adjunctive treatment with sulfadiazine and pyrimethamine to prevent hematologic toxicity

Pregnancy Risk Factor C

Lactation Enters breast milk/compatible

Contraindications Hypersensitivity to leucovorin or any component; pernicious anemia and other megaloblastic anemias secondary to the lack of vitamin B_{12}; not to be administered by intrathecal or intraventricular route

Warnings Administer promptly; when the time interval between administration of folic acid antagonists and leucovorin rescue increases, its effectiveness in treatment of toxicity diminishes

Adverse Reactions

Dermatologic: Rash, pruritus, erythema, urticaria

Hematologic: Thrombocytosis

Respiratory: Wheezing

Miscellaneous: Anaphylactoid reactions

Drug Interactions Leucovorin enhances the toxicity of fluorouracil; high doses of leucovorin may reduce the efficacy of intrathecally administered methotrexate

Stability When powder for injection is reconstituted with bacteriostatic SWI, stability is 7 days at room temperature; protect from light; when doses >10 mg/m^2 are used, prepare leucovorin with preservative free SWI to decrease the amount of benzyl alcohol intake; do not mix in the same solution with 5-fluorouracil as precipitation occurs

Mechanism of Action A derivative of tetrahydrofolic acid, a reduced form of folic acid; does not require a reduction by dihydrofolate reductase for activation; allows for purine and thymidine synthesis, a necessity for normal erythropoiesis; leucovorin supplies the necessary cofactor blocked by methotrexate, enters the cells via the same active transport system as methotrexate

Pharmacodynamics Onset of action:

Oral: Within 30 minutes

I.V.: Within 5 minutes

Pharmacokinetics

Absorption: Oral, I.M.: Rapid

Metabolism: Rapidly converted to (5MTHF) 5-methyl-tetrahydrofolate (active) in the intestinal mucosa and by the liver

Bioavailability:

Oral absorption is saturable in doses >25 mg; apparent bioavailability:

Tablet, 25 mg: 97%

Tablet, 50 mg: 75%

Tablet, 100 mg: 37%

Tablet, 200 mg: 31%

Injection solution, when administered orally, provides equivalent bioavailability

Half-life:

Leucovorin: 15 minutes

5MTHF: 33-35 minutes

Elimination: Primarily in urine (80% to 90%) with small losses appearing in feces (5% to 8%)

Usual Dosage Children and Adults:

Treatment of folic acid antagonist overdosage (eg, pyrimethamine, trimethoprim): Oral: 2-15 mg/day for 3 days or until blood counts are normal or 5 mg every 3 days; doses of 6 mg/day are needed for patients with platelet counts <100,000/mm^3

Folate deficient megaloblastic anemia: I.M.: 1 mg/day

Megaloblastic anemia secondary to congenital deficiency of dihydrofolate reductase: I.M.: 3-6 mg/day

Leucovorin rescue: I.V.: 10 mg/m^2 to start, then 10 mg/m^2 every 6 hours orally for 72 hours; if serum creatinine 24 hours after methotrexate administration is elevated ≥50% **or** the serum methotrexate concentration is >5 x 10^{-6} M, increase leucovorin dose to 100 mg/m^2/dose every 3 hours until serum methotrexate level is less than 1 x 10^{-8} M (see graph for further dosing recommendations as a function of plasma methotrexate level vs. time)

LEUCOVORIN RESCUE DOSE

(Determined by Plasma Methotrexate Level and Time After Start of Methotrexate Infusion)

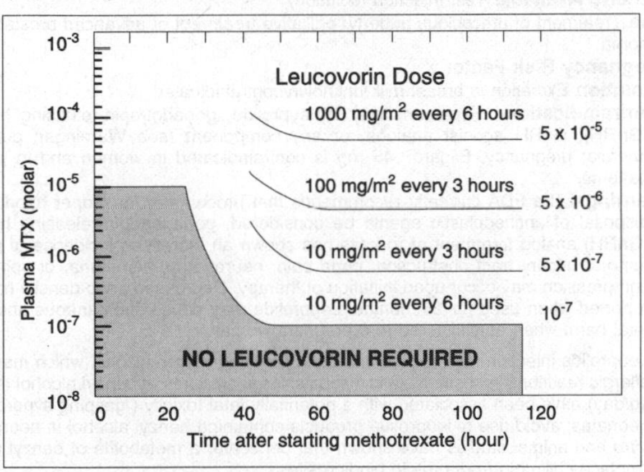

Adjunctive treatment with sulfadiazine to prevent hematologic toxicity (for toxoplasmosis): Infants, Children, and Adults: Oral, I.V.: 5-10 mg once daily; repeat every 3 days (see Sulfadiazine *on page 1485*)

Adjunctive treatment with pyrimethamine to prevent hematologic toxicity (*Pneumocystis carinii*): Adolescents and Adults: Oral, I.V.: 25 mg once weekly

Investigational: Post I.T. methotrexate: Oral, I.V.: 12 mg/m^2 as a single dose; post high-dose methotrexate: 100-1000 mg/m^2/dose until the serum methotrexate level is less than 1 x 10^{-7} molar

Administration

Oral: **This drug should be given parenterally instead of orally in patients with GI toxicity, nausea, vomiting, and when individual doses are >25 mg.**

Parenteral: I.M., I.V.: Reconstitute 50 mg or 100 mg powder for injection vials with 5-10 mL SWI (350 mg vial requires 17 mL diluent resulting in 20 mg/mL final concentration); for I.V. administration, infuse at a maximum rate of 160 mg/minute; not for intrathecal or intraventricular administration.

(Continued)

Leucovorin *(Continued)*

Monitoring Parameters CBC with differential; plasma methotrexate concentration as a therapeutic guide to high-dose methotrexate therapy with leucovorin rescue. Leucovorin is continued until the plasma methotrexate level is less than 1 x 10^{-7} molar. Each dose of leucovorin is increased if the plasma methotrexate concentration is excessively high. With 4- to 6-hour high-dose methotrexate infusions, plasma drug values in excess of 5 x 10^{-5} and 10^{-6} molar at 24 and 48 hours after starting the infusion, respectively, are often predictive of delayed methotrexate clearance; see leucovorin rescue dose graph.

Dosage Forms Excipient information presented when available (limited, particularly for generics); consult specific product labeling.

Injection, powder for reconstitution, as calcium: 50 mg, 100 mg, 200 mg, 350 mg, 500 mg

Injection, solution, as calcium: 10 mg/mL (50 mL)

Tablet, as calcium: 5 mg, 10 mg, 15 mg, 25 mg

♦ **Leucovorin Calcium** *see* Leucovorin *on page 916*

♦ **Leukeran**® *see* Chlorambucil *on page 333*

♦ **Leukine**® *see* Sargramostim *on page 1420*

Leuprolide (loo PROE lide)

Medication Safety Issues

Sound-alike/look-alike issues:

Lupron® may be confused with Nuprin®

Lupron Depot®-3 Month may be confused with Lupron Depot-Ped®

U.S. Brand Names Eligard®; Lupron®; Lupron Depot®; Lupron Depot-Ped®; Viadur®

Canadian Brand Names Eligard®; Lupron®; Lupron® Depot®; Viadur®

Index Terms Abbott-43818; Leuprolide Acetate; Leuprorelin Acetate; NSC-377526; TAP-144

Therapeutic Category Antineoplastic Agent, Hormone (Gonadotropin Hormone-Releasing Analog); Luteinizing Hormone-Releasing Hormone Analog

Generic Available Yes: Injection (solution)

Use Treatment of precocious puberty; palliative treatment of advanced prostate carcinoma

Pregnancy Risk Factor X

Lactation Excretion in breast milk unknown/contraindicated

Contraindications Hypersensitivity to leuprolide, gonadotropin-releasing hormone (GnRH), GnRH agonist analogs, or any component (see Warnings); pernicious anemia; pregnancy. Eligard® 45 mg is contraindicated in women and in pediatric patients.

Warnings The FDA currently recommends that procedures for proper handling and disposal of antineoplastic agents be considered; gonadotropin-releasing hormone (GnRH) analog treatment of rodents has shown an increased incidence of pituitary tumors; urinary tract obstruction, bone pain, neuropathy, hematuria, or spinal cord compression may occur upon initiation of therapy. Decreased bone density has been reported when used for ≥6 months. Leuprolide may cause spontaneous abortion or fetal harm when administered to a pregnant woman.

Leuprolide injection for subcutaneous use contains benzyl alcohol which may cause allergic reactions in susceptible individuals; large amounts of benzyl alcohol (≥99 mg/kg/day) have been associated with a potentially fatal toxicity ("gasping syndrome") in neonates; avoid use of leuprolide products containing benzyl alcohol in neonates; *in vitro* and animal studies have shown that benzoate, a metabolite of benzyl alcohol, displaces bilirubin from protein binding sites

Precautions Long-term safety of leuprolide in children has not been established

Adverse Reactions

Cardiovascular: Edema, cardiac arrhythmias, hypertension, hypotension

Central nervous system: Dizziness, lethargy, insomnia, headache, pain, depression, emotional lability, memory disorders

Dermatologic: Rash, pruritus, acne

Endocrine & metabolic: Estrogenic effects (gynecomastia, breast tenderness), hot flashes, hyperglycemia

Gastrointestinal: Nausea, vomiting, diarrhea, GI bleeding, constipation, anorexia

Genitourinary: Urinary frequency, vaginitis

Hematologic: Decreased hemoglobin and hematocrit

Neuromuscular & skeletal: Myalgia, paresthesia, bone pain, weakness, neuropathy, arthralgia, decreased bone density

Ocular: Blurred vision

Renal: Hematuria, elevated BUN

Miscellaneous: Diaphoresis, anaphylaxis

Stability Refrigerate leuprolide acetate injection; leuprolide (Depot®) powder for suspension and its diluent may be stored at room temperature; upon reconstitution, the suspension is stable for 24 hours; protect from light and heat; do not freeze vials; leuprolide implant may be stored at room temperature

Mechanism of Action Continuous daily administration results in suppression of ovarian and testicular steroidogenesis due to decreased levels of LH and FSH so that puberty and the pubertal growth spurt are arrested; produces a "medical castration" in prostate cancer patients; inhibits pituitary gonadotropin secretion

Pharmacodynamics Onset of action: Serum testosterone levels first increase within 3 days of therapy, then decrease after 2-4 weeks with continued therapy

Pharmacokinetics

- Absorption: Requires parenteral administration since it is rapidly destroyed within the GI tract
- Protein binding: 43% to 49%
- Bioavailability:
  - Oral: 0%
  - SubQ: 94%
- Half-life: 3 hours
- Elimination: Not well defined

Usual Dosage Refer to individual protocol

- Children: Precocious puberty:
  - I.M. (Depot®) formulation: 0.15-0.3 mg/kg/dose given every 28 days; minimum dose: 7.5 mg; younger children generally require higher dosages on a mg/kg basis than older children. Consider discontinuing leuprolide therapy in girls by age 11 and boys by age 12.
    - Initial dose for girls <8 years or boys <9 years (titrate dose in 3.75 mg increments every 4 weeks until clinical or laboratory tests indicate no disease progression):
      - <25 kg: 7.5 mg every 4 weeks
      - 25-37.5 kg: 11.25 mg every 4 weeks
      - >37.5 kg: 15 mg every 4 weeks
  - SubQ: 35-50 mcg/kg once daily; may titrate dose upward by 10 mcg/kg/day if suppression of ovarian or testicular steroidogenesis is not achieved.
- Adults: Advanced prostatic carcinoma:
  - I.M. (Depot® formulation): 7.5 mg/dose given monthly, **or** 22.5 mg once every 3 months, **or** 30 mg once every 4 months
  - Implant: Insert 65 mg implant subcutaneously every 12 months
  - SubQ: 1 mg/day
  - SubQ (Eligard™ Depot): 7.5 mg/dose given monthly, **or** 22.5 mg once every 3 months, **or** 30 mg once every 4 months, **or** 45 mg once every 6 months

Administration

- Implant: Insert subcutaneously in the inner aspect of the upper arm. Keep site clean and dry for 24 hours after insertion. Remove at 12-month intervals.
- Parenteral: Do not administer I.V.:
  - Eligard®: Packaged in 2 syringes whose contents are mixed immediately prior to administration; one contains the Atrigel polymer system, and the second contains leuprolide acetate powder. Must be administered within 30 minutes of mixing. Injection site should be rotated periodically.
  - Lupron Depot®: I.M.: Diluent is added to the vial to form a milky suspension; reconstitute only with diluent provided. Do not use needles smaller than 22 gauge.
  - Lupron®: SubQ: 5 mg/mL solution is administered undiluted into areas on the arm, thigh, or abdomen

Monitoring Parameters Precocious puberty: Height, weight, bone age, Tanner staging test, GnRH testing (blood LH and FSH levels), testosterone in males and estradiol in females; closely monitor patients with prostatic carcinoma for plasma testosterone, acid phosphatase, and signs of weakness, paresthesias, and urinary tract obstruction during the first few weeks of therapy

Test Interactions Interferes with diagnostic tests of pituitary gonadotropic and gonadal function for up to 3 months after therapy

Patient Information Female patients should be informed that menstruation or spotting may occur for the first 2 months of therapy; notify physician if vaginal bleeding continues after 2 months of drug therapy

Nursing Implications Rotate SubQ and I.M. injection sites periodically

Dosage Forms Excipient information presented when available (limited, particularly for generics); consult specific product labeling.

- Implant (Viadur®): 65 mg [released over 12 months; packaged with administration kit]
- Injection, solution, as acetate (Lupron®): 5 mg/mL (2.8 mL) [contains benzyl alcohol; packaged with syringes and alcohol swabs]

(Continued)

Leuprolide *(Continued)*

Injection, powder for reconstitution, as acetate [depot formulation; prefilled syringe]:
Eligard®:
7.5 mg [released over 1 month]
22.5 mg [released over 3 months]
30 mg [released over 4 months]
45 mg [released over 6 months]
Lupron Depot®: 3.75 mg, 7.5 mg [released over 1 month; contains polysorbate 80]
Lupron Depot®-3 Month: 11.25 mg, 22.5 mg [released over 3 months; contains polysorbate 80]
Lupron Depot®-4 Month: 30 mg [released over 4 months; contains polysorbate 80]
Lupron Depot-Ped®: 7.5 mg, 11.25 mg, 15 mg [released over 1 month; contains polysorbate 80]

References

Kappy MS, Stuart T, and Perelman A, "Efficacy of Leuprolide Therapy in Children With Central Precocious Puberty," *Am J Dis Child*, 1988, 142(10):1061-4.

Lee PA and Page JG, "Effects of Leuprolide in the Treatment of Central Precocious Puberty," *J Pediatr*, 1989, 114(2):321-4.

♦ **Leuprolide Acetate** *see* Leuprolide *on page 918*
♦ **Leuprorelin Acetate** *see* Leuprolide *on page 918*
♦ **Leurocristine Sulfate** *see* VinCRIStine *on page 1617*
♦ **Leustatin®** *see* Cladribine *on page 373*

Levalbuterol (leve al BYOO ter ole)

Medication Safety Issues
Sound-alike/look-alike issues:
Xopenex® may be confused with Xanax®

U.S. Brand Names Xopenex®; Xopenex HFA™

Canadian Brand Names Xopenex®

Index Terms Levalbuterol Hydrochloride; Levalbuterol Tartrate; R-albuterol

Therapeutic Category Adrenergic Agonist Agent; Antiasthmatic; Beta$_2$-Adrenergic Agonist Agent; Bronchodilator; Sympathomimetic

Generic Available No

Use Treatment and prevention of bronchospasm in patients with reversible obstructive airway disease

Pregnancy Risk Factor C

Lactation Excretion in breast milk unknown/use caution

Contraindications Hypersensitivity to levalbuterol, any component, albuterol, or adrenergic amine

Warnings Paradoxical bronchospasm may occur, especially with the first use. Excessive use of inhaled sympathomimetics has been associated with death possibly due to cardiac arrest.

Precautions Use with caution in patients with hyperthyroidism, hypokalemia, diabetes mellitus, cardiovascular disorders including coronary insufficiency, hypertension, or history of cardiac arrhythmias; excessive or prolonged use can lead to tolerance

Adverse Reactions
Cardiovascular: Tachycardia, hypertension, hypotension, syncope, EKG abnormalities, chest pain, angioedema, arrhythmias
Central nervous system: Nervousness, dizziness, anxiety, headache, insomnia
Dermatologic: Rash, urticaria
Endocrine & metabolic: Hyperglycemia, hypokalemia, dysmenorrhea
Gastrointestinal: Dyspepsia, diarrhea, xerostomia, dry throat, gastroenteritis, nausea, pharyngitis, constipation
Genitourinary: Hematuria, vaginal moniliasis
Neuromuscular & skeletal: Leg cramps, pain, tremor
Ocular: Eye itching, conjunctivitis
Otic: Ear pain
Respiratory: Cough, rhinitis, sinusitis, turbinate edema, paradoxical bronchospasm, dyspnea
Miscellaneous: Hypersensitivity reactions, flu-like syndrome

Drug Interactions Action of levalbuterol is antagonized by beta-adrenergic blocking agents such as propranolol; cardiovascular effects are potentiated in patients also receiving MAO inhibitors or tricyclic antidepressants; concomitant administration of sympathomimetics may result in enhanced cardiovascular effects; may decrease serum digoxin level; may enhance hypokalemic effects of diuretics

Food Interactions Caffeinated beverages may increase side effects of levalbuterol

Stability Store all formulations at room temperature; protect from light; discard nebulized solution if it is not colorless; after the foil covering is opened, use within 2 weeks;

if removed from the foil pouch, use within 1 week; vials of concentrated solution should be used immediately after removing from foil pouch; store aerosol with mouth-piece up; discard after 200 actuations

Mechanism of Action R-enantiomer of racemic albuterol; relaxes bronchial smooth muscle by action on $beta_2$-receptors with little effect on heart rate

Pharmacodynamics

Onset of action: Nebulized: 10-17 minutes; aerosol: 5.5-10 minutes

Maximum effect: Nebulized: 1.5 hours; aerosol: 77 minutes

Duration: Nebulized: 5-6 hours; aerosol: 3-6 hours

Pharmacokinetics Nebulization:

Distribution: V_d: Adults: 1900 L

Metabolism: In the liver to an inactive sulfate

Half-life: 3.3-4.0 hours

Time to peak serum concentration: 0.2-1.8 hours

Elimination: 3% to 6% excreted unchanged in urine

Usual Dosage

Inhalation by nebulization (**dosage expressed in terms of mg levalbuterol**):

Children 2-11 years: In a randomized, double-blind, single dose, crossover study (Gawchik, 1999), doses ranging from 0.16-1.25 mg were used safely with clinically significant improvements in pulmonary function tests

Children 6-11 years: 0.31 mg 3 times/day, every 6-8 hours; not to exceed 0.63 mg 3 times/day

Children ≥12 years and Adults: 0.63 mg 3 times/day, every 6-8 hours; may be increased to 1.25 mg 3 times/day

Metered dose inhalation: Children ≥4 years and Adults: 1-2 puffs every 4-6 hours

Administration

Inhalation: Nebulization: dilution required for concentrated solution

Oral inhalation: Prime the inhaler (before first use or if it has not been used for more than 2 weeks) by releasing 4 test sprays into the air away from the face; shake well before use; use spacer for children <8 years of age

Monitoring Parameters Serum potassium, heart rate, asthma symptoms, pulmonary function tests, respiratory rate; arterial or capillary blood gases (if patient's condition warrants)

Patient Information Do not exceed recommended dosage; may cause dry mouth; rinse mouth with water following each inhalation to help with dry throat and mouth; if more than one inhalation is necessary, wait at least 1 full minute between inhalations; notify physician if palpitations, tachycardia, chest pain, muscle tremors, dizziness, or headache occur, or if breathing difficulty persists; limit caffeinated beverages

Additional Information 0.63 mg levalbuterol comparable to 1.25 mg albuterol (Lotvall, 2001)

Dosage Forms Excipient information presented when available (limited, particularly for generics); consult specific product labeling.

Note: Strength expressed as base.

Aerosol, oral, as tartrate:

Xopenex HFA™: 45 mcg/actuation (15 g) [200 doses; chlorofluorocarbon free]

Solution for nebulization, as hydrochloride:

Xopenex®: 0.31 mg/3 mL (24s); 0.63 mg/3 mL (24s); 1.25 mg/3 mL (24s)

Solution for nebulization, concentrate, as hydrochloride:

Xopenex®: 1.25 mg/0.5 mL (30s)

References

Gawchik SM, Saccar CL, Noonan M, et al, "The Safety and Efficacy of Nebulized Levalbuterol Compared With Racemic Albuterol and Placebo in the Treatment of Asthma in Pediatric Patients," *J Allergy Clin Immunol*, 1999, 103(4):615-21.

Lotvall J, Palmqvist M, Arvidsson P, et al, "The Therapeutic Ratio of R-Albuterol is Comparable With That of RS-Albuterol in Asthmatic Patients," *J Allergy Clin Immunol*, 2001, 108(5):726-31.

Milgrom H, Skoner DP, Bensch G, et al, "Low-Dose Levalbuterol in Children With Asthma: Safety and Efficacy in Comparison With Placebo and Racemic Albuterol," *J Allergy Clin Immunol*, 2001, 108(6):938-45.

"National Asthma Education and Prevention Program. Expert Panel Report: Guidelines for the Diagnosis and Management of Asthma Update on Selected Topics--2002," *J Allergy Clin Immunol*, 2002, 110(5 Suppl):S141-219.

♦ **Levalbuterol Hydrochloride** *see* Levalbuterol *on page 920*

♦ **Levalbuterol Tartrate** *see* Levalbuterol *on page 920*

♦ **Levaquin®** *see* Levofloxacin *on page 927*

♦ **Levarterenol Bitartrate** *see* Norepinephrine *on page 1147*

♦ **Levate® (Can)** *see* Amitriptyline *on page 107*

♦ **Levbid®** *see* Hyoscyamine *on page 798*

♦ **Levemir®** *see* Insulin Detemir *on page 839*

Levetiracetam (lee va tye RA se tam)

Medication Safety Issues

Sound-alike/look-alike issues:

Potential for dispensing errors between Keppra® and Kaletra® (lopinavir/ritonavir)

U.S. Brand Names Keppra®

Canadian Brand Names CO Levetiracetam; Keppra®

Therapeutic Category Anticonvulsant, Miscellaneous

Generic Available No

Use

Oral: Adjunctive therapy in the treatment of partial onset seizures in children ≥4 years and adults; adjunctive therapy in the treatment of juvenile myoclonic epilepsy in adolescents ≥12 years and myoclonic seizures in adults

I.V.: Adjunctive therapy in the treatment of partial onset seizures in adolescents ≥16 years and adults; temporary use in patients in whom oral administration is not feasible

Note: Studies have reported the use of oral levetiracetam as adjunctive therapy for the treatment of generalized seizures, generalized epilepsy with photosensitivity, generalized idiopathic epilepsies, and Lennox-Gastaut syndrome; has also been used investigationally as monotherapy for the treatment of various seizures types. Studies have also reported its use for treatment of tics in patients with Tourette syndrome; prophylaxis in pediatric migraine; and bipolar disorder.

Pregnancy Risk Factor C

Lactation Enters breast milk/not recommended

Contraindications Hypersensitivity to levetiracetam or any component

Warnings Neuropsychiatric adverse events including somnolence, fatigue, coordination difficulties, behavioral abnormalities (eg, aggression, agitation, anxiety, anger, hostility, depression) and psychotic symptoms (psychosis, hallucinations) may occur; incidence of behavioral abnormalities may be increased in children; dosage reductions may be required. Do not abruptly discontinue therapy; withdraw gradually to lessen chance for increased seizure frequency.

Precautions Use with caution and decrease dose in patients with renal dysfunction. Hematologic abnormalities (small but statistically significant decreases in RBC count, Hgb, Hct, WBC count, and neutrophils) may occur. Safety and efficacy of oral formulation in children <4 years and I.V. formulation in children <16 years have not been established.

Adverse Reactions Note: Adverse reactions are listed for oral levetiracetam when used to treat partial onset seizures; spectrum and frequency of adverse reactions is expected to be similar for treatment of myoclonic epilepsy and with I.V. use. The most frequently reported adverse reactions in pediatric clinical trials were somnolence, accidental injury, hostility, nervousness, and asthenia; unless otherwise noted, percent incidence is from pediatric studies; in adults, asthenia, somnolence, dizziness, and coordination difficulties occurred most frequently during the first 4 weeks of therapy (but may occur at anytime during treatment)

Cardiovascular: Facial edema (2%)

Central nervous system: Behavioral symptoms (agitation, aggression, anger, anxiety, apathy, depersonalization, depression, emotional lability, hostility, hyperkinesias, irritability, nervousness, neurosis, and personality disorder; incidence: adults 13%; children 38%); somnolence (adults 15%; children 23%); headache (adults 14%); hostility (adults 2%; children 12%); nervousness (adults 4%; children 10%); dizziness (adults 9%; children 7%); personality disorder (8%); pain (adults 7%; children 6%); agitation (6%); emotional lability (adults 2%; children 6%); depression (adults 4%; children 3%); ataxia (adults 3%); vertigo (adults 3%); amnesia (adults 2%); anxiety (adults 2%); confusion (2%); psychotic symptoms (adults 0.7%)

Dermatologic: Bruising (4%), pruritus (2%), rash (2%), skin discoloration (2%)

Gastrointestinal: Vomiting (15%), anorexia (adults 3%; children 13%), diarrhea (8%), gastroenteritis (4%), constipation (3%), dehydration (2%)

Hematologic: Decreased leukocytes (3%)

Neuromuscular & skeletal: Asthenia (adults 15%; children 9%), neck pain (2%), paresthesia (adults 2%), reflexes increased (2%)

Ocular: Conjunctivitis (3%), diplopia (adults 2%), amblyopia (2%)

Otic: Ear pain (2%)

Renal: Albuminuria (4%), urine abnormality (2%)

Respiratory: Rhinitis (adults 4%; children 13%), cough (adults 2%; children 11%), pharyngitis (adults 6%; children 10%), asthma (2%), sinusitis (adults 2%)

Miscellaneous: Accidental injury (children 17%); infection (adults 13%; children 2%); flu-like symptoms (3%); attempted suicide, suicidal ideation (rare)

Drug Interactions Levetiracetam and its major metabolite are neither inhibitors of nor substrates for cytochrome P450 isoenzymes, epoxide hydrolase, or UDP-glucuronide enzymes.

No pharmacokinetic interactions were observed in adult clinical trials when levetiracetam was used with other anticonvulsants, including phenytoin, valproic acid, carbamazepine, phenobarbital, lamotrigine, gabapentin, and primidone. However, in pediatric patients, coadministration of enzyme-inducing antiepileptic drugs increased the total body clearance of levetiracetam by 22% (dosage adjustments are not recommended); levetiracetam did not effect plasma concentrations of carbamazepine, lamotrigine, topiramate, or valproic acid.

Ethanol may increase CNS adverse effects. Case reports suggest that levetiracetam may possibly increase the adverse effects of carbamazepine or topiramate (dosage reduction of carbamazepine or topiramate may be needed; see Patsalos, 2004).

Food Interactions Food delays the rate, but not the extent of absorption (bioavailability is not affected).

Stability

Oral solution, tablets: Store at 25°C (77°F), away from heat and light

I.V. solution: Store at 25°C (77°F); dilute dose in 100 mL of D_5W, NS, or LR; admixed solution is stable for at least 24 hours in polyvinyl chloride bags stored at controlled room temperature. Stable when mixed with lorazepam, diazepam, or valproate sodium (concentrations not specified; see package insert)

Mechanism of Action The exact mechanism of the antiepileptic effects of levetiracetam is unknown. Several studies suggest one or more of the following central pharmacologic effects may be involved: Inhibition of voltage-dependent N-type calcium channels; blockade of GABA-ergic inhibitory transmission through displacement of negative modulators; reversal of the inhibition of glycine currents; reduction of delayed rectifier potassium current; and/or binding to synaptic proteins which modulate neurotransmitter release.

Pharmacokinetics

Absorption: Oral: Rapid and complete

Distribution: V_d approximates volume of intracellular and extracellular water; V_d Adults: 0.5-0.7 L/kg

Protein binding: <10%

Metabolism: Not extensive; 24% of dose is metabolized by enzymatic hydrolysis of acetamide group (major metabolic pathway; hydrolysis occurs primarily in the blood; not cytochrome P450 dependent); two minor metabolites (one via hydroxylation of 2-oxo-pyrrolidine ring and one via opening of the 2-oxo-pyrrolidine ring in position 5) are also formed; metabolites are inactive and renally excreted

Bioavailability: Oral: 100%; tablets, oral solution, and injection are bioequivalent

Half-life: Increased in patients with renal dysfunction
- Children 4-12 years: 5 hours
- Adults: 6-8 hours

Time to peak serum concentration: Fasting adults and children: Oral: 1 hour

Excretion: 66% excreted in urine as unchanged drug and 27% as inactive metabolites; undergoes glomerular filtration and subsequent partial tubular reabsorption
- Clearance: Correlated with creatinine clearance; clearance is decreased in patients with renal dysfunction
  - Children 6-12 years: 40% higher than adults on a per kg basis

Dialysis: Hemodialysis: Standard 4-hour treatment removes ~50% of the drug from the body; supplemental doses after dialysis are recommended

Usual Dosage Anticonvulsant:

Oral:

Infants 6 months of age to Children 4 years: Not approved for use; limited information is available from prospective open-label clinical trials that involved a wider age range of children: Initial: 5-10 mg/kg/day given in 2-3 divided doses; may increase every week by 10 mg/kg/day, if tolerated, to a maximum of 60 mg/kg/day (see Grosso, 2005 and Lagae, 2005).

Myoclonic seizures: Children ≥12 years: Initial 500 mg twice daily; increase dosage every 2 weeks by 500 mg/dose given twice daily, to the recommended dose of 1500 mg twice daily. Efficacy of doses >3000 mg/day has not been established.

Partial onset seizures:

Children 4 to <16 years: Initial: 10 mg/kg/dose given twice daily; may increase every 2 weeks by 10 mg/kg/dose given twice daily, if tolerated, to a maximum of 30 mg/kg/dose twice daily (60 mg/kg/day); mean required dose: 52 mg/kg/day.

Adolescents ≥16 years and Adults: Initial: 500 mg twice daily; may increase every 2 weeks by 500 mg/dose given twice daily, if tolerated, to a maximum of 1500 mg twice daily. Doses >3000 mg/day have been used in trials; however, there is no evidence of increased benefit.

I.V.: Partial onset seizures: Adolescents ≥16 years and Adults: Initial: 500 mg twice daily; may increase every 2 weeks by 500 mg/dose given twice daily, if tolerated, to a maximum of 1500 mg twice daily. Oral doses >3000 mg/day have been used in trials; however, there is no evidence of increased benefit.

(Continued)

Levetiracetam *(Continued)*

Note: When switching from oral to I.V. formulation, the total daily dose should be the same

Dosing adjustment in renal impairment: Adults:

Cl_{cr} >80 mL/minute: 500-1500 mg every 12 hours

Cl_{cr} 50-80 mL/minute: 500-1000 mg every 12 hours

Cl_{cr} 30-50 mL/minute: 250-750 mg every 12 hours

Cl_{cr} <30 mL/minute: 250-500 mg every 12 hours

End-stage renal disease patients using dialysis: 500-1000 mg every 24 hours; a supplemental dose of 250-500 mg following dialysis is recommended

Administration

Oral: May be administered without regard to meals; swallow tablets whole, do not break, crush, or chew

Parenteral: I.V.: **Injection is for I.V. use only and must be diluted prior to use.** In patients ≥16 years, dilute dose in 100 mL of D_5W, NS, or LR; infuse over 15 minutes. Do not use if solution contains particulate matter or is discolored. Discard unused portion of vial (does not contain preservative).

Monitoring Parameters Seizure frequency, duration, and severity; behavioral abnormalities and neuropsychiatric adverse events (see Warnings); renal function; CBC

Reference Range Therapeutic range and benefit of therapeutic drug monitoring have not been established; concentrations of 6-20 mg/L (35-120 micromol/L) were attained in adult study patients receiving doses of 1000-3000 mg/day

Patient Information May cause dizziness or drowsiness and impair ability to perform activities requiring mental alertness or physical coordination. Avoid abrupt discontinuation after prolonged use. Inform healthcare provider if any of the following symptoms occur: Extreme weakness, tiredness, or sleepiness; problems walking or moving; unusual thoughts or depression; changes in behavior or mood (such as aggression, agitation, anger, anxiety, apathy, hostility, and irritability). Avoid ethanol (may increase adverse effects). Inform healthcare provider if taking other prescription and nonprescription medications, especially pain medications, sedatives, antihistamines, or hypnotics, which may increase adverse effects.

Nursing Implications Doses should be titrated based on clinical response. Be aware of neuropsychiatric adverse events (see Warnings). Taper dosage slowly when discontinuing therapy. Injection must be diluted before I.V. use.

Additional Information In a preliminary report, levetiracetam-associated behavioral abnormalities were successfully treated with pyridoxine in 5 of 6 children, 2-10 years of age; further studies are needed before this treatment can be recommended (see Miller, 2002). Levetiracetam- induced psychosis (including visual and auditory hallucinations and persecutive delusions) has been reported in pediatric patients (see Kossoff, 2001).

Injection solution for I.V. administration is buffered to a pH of ~5.5

Dosage Forms Excipient information presented when available (limited, particularly for generics); consult specific product labeling.

Injection, solution:

Keppra®: 100 mg/mL (5 mL)

Solution, oral:

Keppra®: 100 mg/mL (480 mL) [dye free; grape flavor]

Tablet:

Keppra®: 250 mg, 500 mg, 750 mg, 1000 mg

References

Awaad Y, Michon AM, and Minarik S, "Use of Levetiracetam to Treat Tics in Children and Adolescents With Tourette Syndrome," *Mov Disord*, 2005, 20(6):714-8.

Glauser TA, Pellock JM, Bebin EM, et al, "Efficacy and Safety of Levetiracetam in Children with Partial Seizures: An Open-Label Trial," *Epilepsia*, 2002, 43(5):518-24.

Grosso S, Franzoni E, Coppola G, et al, "Efficacy and Safety of Levetiracetam: An Add-On Trial in Children With Refractory Epilepsy," *Seizure*, 2005, 14(4):248-53.

Grunewald R, "Levetiracetam in the Treatment of Idiopathic Generalized Epilepsies," *Epilepsia*, 2005, 46(Suppl 9):154-60.

Kossoff EH, Bergey GK, Freeman JM, et al, "Levetiracetam Psychosis in Children With Epilepsy," *Epilepsia*, 2001, 42(12):1611-3.

Lagae L, Buyse G, and Ceulemans B, "Clinical Experience With Levetiracetam in Childhood Epilepsy: An Add-On and Monotherapy Trial," *Seizure*, 2005, 14(1):66-71.

Mandelbaum DE, Bunch M, Kugler SL, et al, "Efficacy of Levetiracetam at 12 Months in Children Classified By Seizure Type, Cognitive Status, and Previous Anticonvulsant Drug Use," *J Child Neurol*, 2005, 20(7):590-4.

Miller GS, "Pyridoxine Ameliorates Adverse Behavioral Effects of Levetiracetam in Children," *Epilepsia*, 2002, 43(Suppl 7):S62.

Miller GS, "Efficacy and Safety of Levetiracetam in Pediatric Migraine," *Headache*, 2004, 44(3):238-43.

Opp J, Tuxhorn I, May T, et al, "Levetiracetam in Children With Refractory Epilepsy: A Multicenter Open Label Study in Germany," *Seizure*, 2005, 14(7):476-84.

Patsalos PN, "Clinical Pharmacokinetics of Levetiracetam," *Clin Pharmacokinet*, 2004, 43(11):707-24.

Sankar R and Holmes GL, "Mechanisms of Action for the Commonly Used Antiepileptic Drugs: Relevance to Antiepileptic Drug-Associated Neurobehavioral Adverse Effects," *J Child Neurol*, 2004, 19(Suppl 1):6-14.

Vigevano F, "Levetiracetam in Pediatrics," *J Child Neurol*, 2005, 20(2):87-93.

Levobunolol (lee voe BYOO noe lole)

Medication Safety Issues

Sound-alike/look-alike issues:

Levobunolol may be confused with levocabastine

Betagan® may be confused with Betadine®

International issues:

Betagan® may be confused with Betagon® which is a brand name for mepindolol in Italy

U.S. Brand Names Betagan®

Canadian Brand Names Apo-Levobunolol®; Betagan®; Novo-Levobunolol; Optho-Bunolol®; PMS-Levobunolol; Sandoz-Levobunolol

Index Terms *l*-Bunolol Hydrochloride; Levobunolol Hydrochloride

Therapeutic Category Beta-Adrenergic Blocker, Ophthalmic

Generic Available Yes

Use To lower intraocular pressure in chronic open-angle glaucoma or ocular hypertension

Pregnancy Risk Factor C

Contraindications Hypersensitivity to levobunolol or any component (see Warnings); asthma, severe COPD, sinus bradycardia, second or third degree A-V block, cardiogenic shock

Warnings Contains metabisulfite which may cause allergic reactions in susceptible individuals; use only in combination with miotic for patients with angle closure glaucoma; products contain sulfites which may cause allergic reactions in susceptible individuals

Precautions Use with caution in patients with CHF, diabetes mellitus, hyperthyroidism, myasthenia gravis

Adverse Reactions

Cardiovascular: Bradycardia, arrhythmias, hypotension, palpitations, cerebral ischemia, cerebral vascular accident, syncope, heart block, CHF

Central nervous system: Dizziness, headache, depression, ataxia, cerebral ischemia

Dermatologic: Rash, alopecia, itching

Endocrine & metabolic: Masked symptoms of hypoglycemia in diabetics

Gastrointestinal: Nausea, heartburn, diarrhea

Ocular: Stinging, burning, erythema, itching, blepharoconjunctivitis, keratitis, ptosis, decreased visual acuity, conjunctivitis, tearing

Respiratory: Bronchospasm

Drug Interactions May have additive toxicity with systemic beta-adrenergic blocking drugs; ophthalmic epinephrine decreases effectiveness

Mechanism of Action A nonselective beta-adrenergic blocking agent that lowers intraocular pressure by reducing aqueous humor production

Pharmacodynamics

Onset of action: Following ophthalmic instillation, decreases in intraocular pressure can be noted within 1 hour

Maximum effect: Within 2-6 hours

Maximal effectiveness: 2-3 weeks

Duration: 1-7 days

Pharmacokinetics

Absorption: May be absorbed systemically and produce systemic side effects

Metabolism: Extensively metabolized into several metabolites; primary metabolite (active) dihydrolevobunolol

Elimination: Not well defined

Usual Dosage Adults: 1-2 drops of 0.5% solution in eye(s) once daily or 1-2 drops of 0.25% solution twice daily; may increase to 1 drop of 0.5% solution twice daily

Administration Intraocular: Apply drops into conjunctival sac of affected eye(s); avoid contacting bottle tip with skin; apply gentle pressure to lacrimal sac during and immediately following instillation (1-2 minutes) to decrease systemic absorption; see manufacturer's information regarding proper usage of C Cap (compliance cap)

Monitoring Parameters Intraocular pressure

Dosage Forms Excipient information presented when available (limited, particularly for generics); consult specific product labeling.

Solution, ophthalmic, as hydrochloride: 0.25% (5 mL, 10 mL); 0.5% (5 mL, 10 mL, 15 mL) [contains benzalkonium chloride and sodium metabisulfite]

Betagan®: 0.25% (5 mL, 10 mL); 0.5% (2 mL, 5 mL, 10 mL, 15 mL) [contains benzalkonium chloride and sodium metabisulfite]

♦ **Levobunolol Hydrochloride** *see* Levobunolol *on page 925*

Levodopa (lee voe DOE pa)

Related Information
Serotonin Syndrome *on page 1955*

Canadian Brand Names Dopar®; Larodopa®

Index Terms *L*-3-Hydroxytyrosine; *L*-Dopa

Therapeutic Category Anti-Parkinson's Agent; Diagnostic Agent, Growth Hormone Function

Generic Available No

Use Diagnostic agent for growth hormone deficiency; treatment of Parkinson's disease

Pregnancy Risk Factor C

Contraindications Hypersensitivity to levodopa or any component; narrow-angle glaucoma, use of MAO inhibitors within prior 14 days (however, may be administered concomitantly with the manufacturer's recommended dose of a MAO inhibitor with selectivity for MAO type B), melanomas, or any undiagnosed skin lesions

Warnings GI hemorrhage has occurred in patients with a history of peptic ulcer disease; sudden discontinuation of levodopa may cause a worsening of Parkinson's disease

Precautions Use cautiously in patients with severe cardiovascular disease or pulmonary disease, asthma, occlusive cerebrovascular disease, renal, hepatic, or endocrine disease, affective disorders, major psychoses, cardiac arrhythmias, and chronic wide-angle glaucoma; use with caution in patients with risk of hypotension; may cause orthostatic hypotension

Adverse Reactions

Cardiovascular: Orthostatic hypotension, palpitations, cardiac arrhythmias, hypertension

Central nervous system: Memory loss, nervousness, anxiety, insomnia, fatigue, hallucinations, dystonic movements, ataxia, headache, confusion

Endocrine & metabolic: Hyperhomocysteinemia

Gastrointestinal: Nausea, vomiting, GI bleeding, constipation, anorexia, xerostomia

Hematologic: Hemolytic anemia

Neuromuscular & skeletal: Muscle twitching

Ocular: Blurred vision, eyelid spasms

Miscellaneous: Discoloration of sweat

Drug Interactions Antacids and metoclopramide increase bioavailability of levodopa; benzodiazepines, antipsychotics, clonidine, tacrine, hydantoins, methionine, papaverine, and pyridoxine decrease levodopa's effectiveness; iron salts, TCAs, and anticholinergics decrease GI absorption of levodopa; MAO inhibitors and linezolid may increase hypertensive reaction; levodopa may decrease metoclopramide's effects; methyldopa may have additive hypotensive effects

Food Interactions High protein diets may decrease the efficacy of levodopa when used for parkinsonism via competition with amino acids in crossing the blood-brain barrier; avoid foods high in pyridoxine content such as liver, fish, whole grain cereals, peas, and beans

Mechanism of Action Increases dopamine levels in the brain; stimulates dopaminergic receptors in the basal ganglia to improve the balance between cholinergic and dopaminergic activity

Pharmacokinetics

Metabolism: Majority of drug is peripherally decarboxylated to dopamine; small amounts of levodopa reach the brain where it is also decarboxylated to active dopamine

Half-life: 1.2-2.3 hours

Time to peak serum concentration: Oral: Within 1-2 hours

Elimination: Primarily in urine (80%) as dopamine, norepinephrine, and homovanillic acid

Usual Dosage Oral:

Diagnostic agent for growth hormone deficiency: Children: 0.5 g/m^2 as a single dose, not to exceed 500 mg **or** as an alternative
<30 lb: 125 mg
30-70 lb: 250 mg
>70 lb: 500 mg

Parkinson's disease: Adults: 500-1000 mg/day in divided doses every 6-12 hours; increase by 100-750 mg/day every 3-7 days until response or total dose of 8000 mg is reached

Administration Oral: Administer with food

Monitoring Parameters Growth hormone level

Test Interactions False-positive reaction for urinary glucose with Clinitest®; false-negative reaction using Clinistix®; false-positive urine ketones with Acetest®,

Ketostix®, Labstix®; false-positive Coombs' test; false increase in uric acid with colorimetric method

Patient Information May cause dry mouth

Dosage Forms Excipient information presented when available (limited, particularly for generics); consult specific product labeling.

Capsule: 100 mg, 250 mg, 500 mg

Tablet: 100 mg, 250 mg, 500 mg

References

Cara JF and Johanson HJ, "Growth Hormone for Short Stature Not Due to Classic Growth Hormone Deficiency," *Pediatr Clin North Am*, 1990, 37(6):1229-54.

Levofloxacin (lee voe FLOKS a sin)

U.S. Brand Names Iquix®; Levaquin®; Quixin™

Canadian Brand Names Levaquin®; Novo-Levofloxacin

Therapeutic Category Antibiotic, Ophthalmic; Antibiotic, Quinolone

Generic Available No

Use Treatment of acute maxillary sinusitis, lower respiratory tract infections, skin and skin structure infections, complicated urinary tract infections and acute pyelonephritis due to multidrug-resistant organisms susceptible to levofloxacin including *Streptococcus pneumoniae* (including penicillin-resistant strains), *S. aureus, Haemophilus influenzae, H. parainfluenzae, Moraxella catarrhalis, Klebsiella pneumoniae, Legionella pneumophila, Chlamydia pneumoniae, Mycoplasma pneumoniae, E. coli, Enterococcus fecalis, S. pyogenes, Proteus mirabilis, Enterobacter cloacae,* (less active than ciprofloxacin against *Pseudomonas aeruginosa*; combination therapy with a beta-lactam antipseudomonal is recommended); treatment of community-acquired pneumonia; infectious diarrhea due to enterotoxigenic *E. coli, Shigella, Salmonella, Campylobacter* spp, *Vibrio parahaemolyticus*; postexposure prevention of inhalational anthrax.

Used ophthalmically for treatment of bacterial conjunctivitis due to *S. aureus* (methicillin-susceptible strains), *S. epidermidis, S. pneumoniae, Streptococcus* (groups C/F), *Streptococcus* (group G), Viridans group *Streptococci, Corynebacterium* spp, *H. influenzae, Acinetobacter iwoffii,* or *Serratia marcescens*; treatment of bacterial corneal ulcer due to susceptible organisms

Pregnancy Risk Factor C

Lactation Excretion in breast milk unknown/not recommended

Contraindications Hypersensitivity to levofloxacin, any component, or other quinolones; not recommended for use in pregnant women or during breast-feeding

Warnings Oral and parenteral formulations are not recommended in children <18 years of age; levofloxacin increased osteochondrosis in immature rats and dogs. Fluoroquinolones have caused arthropathy with erosions of the cartilage in weight-bearing joints of immature animals; Achilles tendonitis and tendon rupture have been reported with fluoroquinolones with risk increased in patients taking concomitant corticosteroids; prolonged use may result in superinfection; CNS stimulation and increased intracranial pressure may occur resulting in tremors, restlessness, confusion, and rarely hallucinations, depression, nightmares, suicidal ideation, or convulsive seizures; serious and occasionally fatal hypersensitivity and/or anaphylactic reactions have been reported often following the first dose. If these reactions occur, discontinue levofloxacin.

Oral solution contains benzyl alcohol and propylene glycol which may be toxic to newborns in high doses; benzyl alcohol may cause allergic reactions in susceptible individuals; large amounts of benzyl alcohol (≥99 mg/kg/day) have been associated with a potentially fatal toxicity ("gasping syndrome") in neonates; the "gasping syndrome" consists of metabolic acidosis, respiratory distress, gasping respirations, CNS dysfunction (including convulsions, intracranial hemorrhage), hypotension and cardiovascular collapse; *in vitro* and animal studies have shown that benzoate, a metabolite of benzyl alcohol, displaces bilirubin from protein binding sites

Precautions Use with caution in patients with known or suspected CNS disorders, seizure disorders, severe cerebral arteriosclerosis, or renal impairment; modify dosage in patients with renal impairment. Rare cases of torsade de pointes have been reported in patients taking levofloxacin so use with caution in patients on concurrent therapy with Class Ia or Class III antiarrhythmics or in patients with known prolongation of QT interval, bradycardia, cardiomyopathy, hypokalemia, or hypomagnesemia

Adverse Reactions

Cardiovascular: Cardiac failure, hypertension, hypotension, bradycardia, tachycardia, edema, torsade de pointes (rare), prolongation of QT interval

Central nervous system: Dizziness, fever, headache, insomnia, increased intracranial pressure, seizures, fatigue, nervousness, restlessness, confusion, hallucinations,

(Continued)

Levofloxacin *(Continued)*

anxiety, lightheadedness, suicidal thoughts, depression, encephalopathy, abnormal EEG

Dermatologic: Photosensitivity, pruritus, urticaria, rash, angioedema, Stevens-Johnson syndrome, toxic epidermal necrolysis, erythema multiforme

Endocrine & metabolic: Hypoglycemia, hyperglycemia, electrolyte abnormality

Gastrointestinal: Nausea, vomiting, diarrhea, constipation, anorexia, abdominal pain, pseudomembranous colitis, pancreatitis

Genitourinary: Vaginitis

Hematologic: Granulocytopenia, leukopenia, thrombocytopenia, hemolytic anemia

Hepatic: Elevated liver enzymes, hepatic failure, jaundice

Local: With I.V.: Phlebitis, burning, pain, erythema, swelling

Neuromuscular & skeletal: Tremor, arthralgia, tendonitis, tendon rupture, myalgia, peripheral neuropathy

Ocular: Ophthalmic solution: Foreign body sensation, transient decreased vision; ocular pain, burning, itching, dryness, discomfort, photophobia, corneal erosion, hyperemia, lid edema, lid erythema

Renal: Interstitial nephritis, acute renal insufficiency

Respiratory: Bronchospasm, respiratory distress, dyspnea

Miscellaneous: Anaphylaxis, serum sickness

Drug Interactions Cytochrome P450 isoenzyme CYP1A2 enzyme inhibitor (minor)

Decreased absorption with antacids containing aluminum, magnesium, and/or calcium, sucralfate, metal cations (ie, zinc, iron, copper, magnesium), and didanosine; may decrease serum levels of phenytoin; cimetidine and probenecid increase serum levels and half-life of levofloxacin; concomitant use with foscarnet or NSAIDs may increase risk of seizures; may enhance hypoprothrombinemic effect of warfarin; may alter blood glucose concentrations in diabetic patients receiving levofloxacin and antidiabetic medications concurrently; concurrent use with corticosteroids may increase the risk of tendon rupture

Food Interactions Iron and mineral supplements decrease levofloxacin concentrations

Stability Store ophthalmic solution, vial, premixed injection, tablet, and oral solution at room temperature; protect from light. Injection is stable for 72 hours when diluted to 5 mg/mL in a compatible I.V. fluid (ie, D_5W, NS, D_5W with NaCl and KCl, D_5LR) and stored at room temperature; stable for 14 days when stored under refrigeration; incompatible with mannitol, sodium bicarbonate, multivalent cations (eg, magnesium).

Mechanism of Action L-isomer of the racemate, ofloxacin, levofloxacin inhibits DNA gyrase (bacterial topoisomerase II) thereby inhibiting relaxation of supercoiled DNA and promoting breakage of DNA strands. DNA gyrase maintains the superhelical structure of DNA and is required for DNA replication, transcription, repair, recombination and transposition.

Pharmacokinetics

Absorption: Well absorbed; levofloxacin oral tablet and solution formulations are bioequivalent

Distribution: Widely distributed in the body including blister fluid, skin tissue, macrophages, prostate, lung tissue; excreted in breast milk

V_d: Adults: 1.25 L/kg

Protein binding: 24% to 38%

Bioavailability: Oral: 99%

Half-life: 6-8 hours

Time to peak serum concentration: Oral: Within 1-2 hours; food prolongs the time to peak by approximately 1 hour and decreases the peak concentration by 14%

Elimination: 87% excreted unchanged in urine over 48 hours by tubular secretion and glomerular filtration

Dialysis: Not removed by hemodialysis or peritoneal dialysis

Usual Dosage

Oral, I.V.:

Children: **Note:** Limited information regarding levofloxacin use in pediatric patients is currently available in the literature; some centers recommend the following dose:

Children 6 months to 5 years: 10 mg/kg/dose every 12 hours

Children ≥5 years: 10 mg/kg/dose every 24 hours; maximum dose: 500 mg

Adults:

Chronic bacterial prostatitis: 500 mg every 24 hours for 28 days

Chronic bronchitis: 500 mg every 24 hours for 7 days

Community-acquired pneumonia: 500 mg every 24 hours for 7-14 days or 750 mg every 24 hours for 5 days

Nosocomial pneumonia: 750 mg every 24 hours for 7-14 days

Acute maxillary sinusitis: 500 mg every 24 hours for 10-14 days

Complicated skin infection: 750 mg every 24 hours for 7-14 days
Uncomplicated skin infections: 500 mg every 24 hours for 7-10 days
Complicated UTI or acute pyelonephritis: 250 mg every 24 hours for 10 days
Uncomplicated UTI: 250 mg every 24 hours for 3 days
Drug-resistant tuberculosis: 500-1000 mg every 24 hours (maximum dose: 1 g)
Travelers' diarrhea: 500 mg every 24 hours for up to 3 days
Inhalational anthrax (postexposure): 500 mg every 24 hours for 60 days beginning as soon as possible after exposure

Ophthalmic:
Children ≥1 year and Adults: Bacterial conjunctivitis: 0.5% solution:
Treatment day 1 and day 2: Instill 1-2 drops into affected eye(s) every 2 hours while awake, up to 8 times/day
Treatment day 3 through 7: Instill 1-2 drops into affected eye(s) every 4 hours while awake, up to 4 times/day
Children ≥6 years and Adults: Bacterial corneal ulcer: 1.5% solution
Treatment days 1-3: Instill 1-2 drops into affected eye(s) every 30 minutes to 2 hours while awake and ~4 and 6 hours after retiring
Treatment day 4 through treatment completion: Instill 1-2 drops into affected eye(s) every 1-4 hours while awake

Dosing interval in renal impairment:
Complicated UTI/pyelonephritis, chronic bronchitis, community-acquired pneumonia, acute maxillary sinusitis, uncomplicated skin infection, chronic bacterial prostatitis, or inhalational anthrax:
Cl_{cr} 20-49 mL/minute: Administer 250 mg every 24 hours (initial dose: 500 mg)
Cl_{cr} 10-19 mL/minute: Administer 250 mg every 48 hours (initial dose: 500 mg for most infections; 250 mg for UTI or pyelonephritis)
Uncomplicated UTI: No dosing adjustment required
Complicated skin infection, nosocomial pneumonia:
Cl_{cr} 20-49 mL/minute: Administer 750 mg every 48 hours
Cl_{cr} 10-19 mL/minute: Administer 500 mg every 48 hours

Administration
Oral: May administer levofloxacin tablets with or without food; administer levofloxacin oral solution 1 hour before or 2 hours after eating; avoid antacid use within 2 hours of administration; drink plenty of fluids to maintain proper hydration and urine output
Parenteral: I.V. infusion: Not for I.M., SubQ, or intrathecal administration; final concentration for administration should not exceed 5 mg/mL; administer by slow I.V. infusion over 60-90 minutes (250-500 mg over 60 minutes; 750 mg over 90 minutes); avoid rapid or bolus I.V. infusion due to risk of hypotension
Ophthalmic: Not for subconjunctival injection or for use into anterior chamber of the eye. Contact lenses should not be worn during treatment; instill drops into conjunctival sac of affected eye(s); apply finger pressure to lacrimal sac during and for 1-2 minutes after instillation to decrease risk of absorption and systemic effects; avoid contacting bottle tip with skin

Monitoring Parameters Patient receiving concurrent levofloxacin and theophylline should have serum levels of theophylline monitored; monitor INR in patients receiving warfarin; monitor blood glucose in patients receiving antidiabetic agents; monitor renal, hepatic, and hematopoietic function periodically; number and type of stools/day for diarrhea

Patient Information Drink plenty of fluids; may cause dizziness or lightheadedness and impair ability to perform activities requiring mental alertness or physical coordination; notify physician if tendon pain or swelling occurs; or if palpitations or chest pain, signs of allergy, burning, tingling, numbness, or weakness develops; difficulty breathing, or persistent diarrhea occurs. May cause photosensitivity reactions (eg, exposure to sunlight may cause severe sunburn, skin rash, redness, or itching); avoid exposure to sunlight and artificial light sources (sunlamps, tanning booth/bed); wear protective clothing, wide-brimmed hats, sunglasses, and lip sunscreen (SPF ≥15); use a sunscreen [broad-spectrum sunscreen or physical sunscreen (preferred) or sunblock with SPF ≥15]; contact physician if reaction occurs.

Nursing Implications Do not administer antacids containing calcium, aluminum, or magnesium, iron, sucralfate, multivitamin preparations with zinc, or didanosine chewable/buffered tablets or pediatric powder for oral solution with or within 2 hours before or 2 hours after a levofloxacin dose; ensure adequate patient hydration

Dosage Forms Excipient information presented when available (limited, particularly for generics); consult specific product labeling.
Infusion [premixed in D_5W] (Levaquin®): 250 mg (50 mL); 500 mg (100 mL); 750 mg (150 mL)
Injection, solution [preservative free] (Levaquin®): 25 mg/mL (20 mL, 30 mL)
Solution, ophthalmic:
Iquix®: 1.5% (5 mL)
Quixin™: 0.5% (5 mL) [contains benzalkonium chloride]
Solution, oral (Levaquin®): 25 mg/mL (480 mL) [contains benzyl alcohol]
(Continued)

Levofloxacin *(Continued)*

Tablet (Levaquin®): 250 mg, 500 mg, 750 mg

Levaquin® Leva-Pak: 750 mg (5s)

Extemporaneous Preparations A 50 mg/mL oral suspension made from tablets and two different vehicles (a 1:1 mixture of Ora-Plus® and strawberry syrup NF) was stable for 57 days when stored in amber plastic prescription bottles at room temperature (23°C to 25°C) or under refrigeration (3°C to 5°C); crush six 500 mg tablets in a mortar into a fine powder; add a small amount of the vehicle and mix well to form a uniform paste; mix while adding the vehicle in geometric proportions to **almost** 60 mL; transfer the mixture to a graduated cylinder and qsad with vehicle to make 60 mL; label "shake well."

VandenBussche HL, Johnson CE, Fontana EM, et al, "Stability of Levofloxacin in an Extemporaneously Compounded Oral Liquid," *Am J Health Syst Pharm*, 1999, 56(22):2316-8.

References

Chien S, Wells TG, Blumer JL, et al, "Levofloxacin Pharmacokinetics in Children," *J Clin Pharmacol*, 2005, 45(2):153-60.

Ernst ME, Ernst EJ, and Klepser ME, "Levofloxacin and Trovafloxacin: The Next Generation of Fluoroquinolones?" *Am J Health Syst Pharm*, 1997, 54(22):2569-84.

Schaad UB, "Role of the New Quinolones in Pediatric Practice," *Pediatr Infect Dis J*, 1992, 11(12):1043-6.

♦ **Levophed®** *see* Norepinephrine *on page 1147*

♦ **Levothroid®** *see* Levothyroxine *on page 930*

Levothyroxine (lee voe thye ROKS een)

Medication Safety Issues

Sound-alike/look-alike issues:

Levothyroxine may be confused with liothyronine

Levoxyl® may be confused with Lanoxin®, Luvox®

Synthroid® may be confused with Symmetrel®

To avoid errors due to misinterpretation of a decimal point, always express dosage in mcg (**not** mg).

Significant differences exist between oral and I.V. dosing. Use caution when converting from one route of administration to another.

U.S. Brand Names Levothroid®; Levoxyl®; Synthroid®; Unithroid®

Canadian Brand Names Eltroxin®; Gen-Levothyroxine; Levothyroxine Sodium; Synthroid®

Index Terms Levothyroxine Sodium; *L*-Thyroxine Sodium; T_4

Therapeutic Category Thyroid Product

Generic Available Yes

Use Replacement or supplemental therapy in congenital or acquired hypothyroidism; treatment or prevention of euthyroid goiters (TSH suppression) including thyroid nodules and chronic lymphocytic thyroiditis; as adjunctive therapy with surgery and radioiodine in the management of thyrotropin-dependent well-differentiated thyroid cancer

Pregnancy Risk Factor A

Lactation Enters breast milk/compatible

Contraindications Hypersensitivity to levothyroxine sodium or any component; recent MI or thyrotoxicosis; uncorrected adrenal insufficiency; untreated subclinical thyrotoxicosis (suppressed TSH levels with normal T_3 and T_4 levels)

Warnings Not for use in the treatment of obesity or for weight loss; in euthyroid patients, doses within the range of daily hormonal requirements are ineffective for weight reduction; larger doses may produce serious or even life-threatening toxic effects particularly when used with some anorectic drugs (sympathomimetic amines). Overtreatment may result in craniosynostosis in infants and premature closure of epiphyses in children; monitor use closely.

Precautions Use with extreme caution in patients with cardiovascular disease, adrenal insufficiency, hypertension or coronary artery disease; patients with diabetes mellitus and insipidus may have their symptoms exaggerated or aggravated; in the first 2 weeks of therapy, neonates and infants should be monitored for cardiac overload, arrhythmias, and aspiration from avid suckling

Adverse Reactions

Cardiovascular: Palpitations, tachycardia, cardiac arrhythmias, angina, CHF, hypertension

Central nervous system: Nervousness, insomnia, fever, headache, pseudotumor cerebri

Dermatologic: Alopecia

Endocrine & metabolic: Weight loss

Gastrointestinal: Diarrhea, abdominal cramps, increased appetite

Neuromuscular & skeletal: Tremor, slipped capital femoral epiphysis
Miscellaneous: Diaphoresis

Drug Interactions Antacids (aluminum-, magnesium-, and calcium carbonate-containing), cholestyramine resin, iron salts, sodium polystyrene sulfonate, and sucralfate decrease absorption; estrogens, clofibrate, methadone, fluorouracil, mitotane, tamoxifen, and imatinib may increase thyroid requirements; levothyroxine increases effect of oral anticoagulants; phenytoin, carbamazepine, phenobarbital, rifampin, amiodarone, propylthiouracil, and β-adrenergic antagonists may decrease levothyroxine levels; androgens, anabolic steroids, asparaginase, glucocorticoids, and slow-release nicotinic acid decrease thyroid requirements; concurrent use with sympathomimetics, TCAs, and SSRIs may enhance the toxic effects of both drugs; use with ketamine may produce significant tachycardia and hypertension; may increase insulin and other antidiabetic agent requirements

Food Interactions Limit intake of goitrogenic foods (asparagus, cabbage, peas, turnip greens, broccoli, spinach, brussel sprouts, lettuce, soybeans); soybean-based formulas, cottonseed meal, walnuts, and dietary fiber may decrease absorption

Stability Store at room temperature; protect from light and moisture; I.V. form must be administered immediately after preparation

Mechanism of Action Primary active compound is T_3 (triiodothyronine), which may be converted from T_4 (thyroxine) by deiodination in liver and peripheral tissues; exact mechanism of action is unknown; however, it is believed the thyroid hormone exerts its many metabolic effects through control of DNA transcription and protein synthesis; involved in normal metabolism, growth, and development; promotes gluconeogenesis, increases utilization and mobilization of glycogen stores, and stimulates protein synthesis, increases basal metabolic rate

Pharmacodynamics

Onset of action:
- Oral: 3-5 days for therapeutic effects
- I.V.: Within 6-8 hours

Maximum effect: 4-6 weeks

Pharmacokinetics

Absorption: Oral: Erratic (40% to 80%); decreases with age
Protein binding: >99%
Metabolism: In the liver and other peripheral sites by deiodination to triiodothyronine (active) T_3
Half-life: 6-7 days
Time to peak serum concentration: Within 2-4 hours
Elimination: Thyroid hormones are eliminated primarily in urine with 20% of T_4 excreted in feces

Usual Dosage

Neonates, Infants, and Children: Daily dosage:
- Oral:
  - 0-3 months: 10-15 mcg/kg; if the infant is at risk for development of cardiac failure use a lower starting dose ~25 mcg/day; if the initial serum T_4 is very low (<5 mcg/dL) begin treatment at a higher dosage ~50 mcg/day
  - >3-6 months: 8-10 mcg/kg or 25-50 mcg
  - >6-12 months: 6-8 mcg/kg or 50-75 mcg
  - >1-5 years: 5-6 mcg/kg or 75-100 mcg
  - 6-12 years: 4-5 mcg/kg or 100-125 mcg
  - >12 years: 2-3 mcg/kg or ≥150 mcg
  - Growth and puberty complete: 1.7 mcg/kg
  - **Note:** Hyperactivity in older children may be minimized by starting at one-quarter of the recommended dose and increasing each week by that amount until the full dose is achieved (4 weeks)
- I.V., I.M.: 50% to 75% of the oral dose

Adults:
- Hypothyroidism:
  - Oral: 1.7 mcg/kg/day or 100-200 mcg/day; if severe hypothyroidism, use 12.5-50 mcg/day to start, then increase by 25-50 mcg/day at intervals of 2-4 weeks
  - I.V., I.M.: 50% of the oral dose
- Subclinical hypothyroidism (if treated): Oral: 1 mcg/kg
- Myxedema coma or stupor: I.V.: 200-500 mcg one time, then 75-300 mcg daily; due to potential poor absorption of oral levothyroxine, avoid oral use in acute treatment
- Thyroid suppression therapy: Oral: 2-6 mcg/kg/day for 7-10 days

Administration

Oral: Administer on an empty stomach; 1-1.5 hours prior to breakfast
Parenteral: Dilute vial with 5 mL NS; use immediately after reconstitution; administer by direct I.V. infusion over 2- to 3-minute period; may administer I.M.

(Continued)

Levothyroxine *(Continued)*

Monitoring Parameters T_4, TSH, heart rate, blood pressure, clinical signs of hypo- and hyperthyroidism; growth, bone development (children); TSH is the most reliable guide for evaluating adequacy of thyroid replacement dosage. TSH may be elevated during the first few months of thyroid replacement despite patients being clinically euthyroid. In cases where T_4 remains low and TSH is within normal limits, an evaluation of "free" (unbound) T_4 is needed to evaluate further increase in dosage.

In congenital hypothyroidism, adequacy of replacement should be determined using both TSH and total- or free-T_4. During the first 3 years of life, total- or free-T_4 should be maintained in the upper ½ of the normal range; this should result in normalization of the TSH. In some patients, TSH may not normalize due to a resetting of the pituitary-thyroid feedback as a result of *in utero* hypothyroidism.

Suggested frequency for monitoring thyroid function tests in children: Every 1-2 months during the first year of life, every 2-3 months between ages 1-3 years, and every 3-12 months thereafter until growth is completed; repeat tests two weeks after any change in dosage.

Reference Range See normal values in Normal Laboratory Values for Children *on page 1881*

Test Interactions Many drugs may have effects on thyroid function tests: para-aminosalicylic acid, aminoglutethimide, amiodarone, barbiturates, carbamazepine, chloral hydrate, clofibrate, colestipol, corticosteroids, danazol, diazepam, estrogens, ethionamide, fluorouracil, I.V. heparin, insulin, lithium, methadone, methimazole, mitotane, nitroprusside, oxyphenbutazone, phenylbutazone, PTU, perphenazine, phenytoin, propranolol, salicylates, sulfonylureas, and thiazides

Patient Information Do not change brands without physician's knowledge; report immediately to physician any chest pain, increased pulse, palpitations, heat intolerances, excessive sweating; do not discontinue without notifying physician

Additional Information 15-37.5 mcg liothyronine = 50-60 mcg levothyroxine = 60 mg thyroid USP = 45 mg Thyroid Strong® = 60 mg thyroglobulin = 50-60 mcg liotrix

Dosage Forms Excipient information presented when available (limited, particularly for generics); consult specific product labeling.

Injection, powder for reconstitution, as sodium: 0.2 mg, 0.5 mg

Tablet, as sodium: 25 mcg, 50 mcg, 75 mcg, 88 mcg, 100 mcg, 112 mcg, 125 mcg, 137 mcg, 150 mcg, 175 mcg, 200 mcg, 300 mcg

- Levothroid®: 25 mcg, 50 mcg, 75 mcg, 88 mcg, 100 mcg, 112 mcg, 125 mcg, 150 mcg, 175 mcg, 200 mcg, 300 mcg
- Levoxyl®: 25 mcg, 50 mcg, 75 mcg, 88 mcg, 100 mcg, 112 mcg, 125 mcg, 137 mcg, 150 mcg, 175 mcg, 200 mcg; 300 mcg [DSC]
- Synthroid®: 25 mcg, 50 mcg, 75 mcg, 88 mcg, 100 mcg, 112 mcg, 125 mcg, 137 mcg, 150 mcg, 175 mcg, 200 mcg, 300 mcg
- Unithroid®: 25 mcg, 50 mcg, 75 mcg, 88 mcg, 100 mcg, 112 mcg, 125 mcg, 150 mcg, 175 mcg, 200 mcg, 300 mcg

Extemporaneous Preparations A 25 mcg/mL extemporaneous suspension may be compounded by crushing twenty-five 0.1 mg tablets; measure 40 mL glycerol; triturate powder into a pourable suspension with a small amount of glycerol and transfer to a calibrated 100 mL amber bottle; rinse the mortar with about 10 mL of the glycerol and pour into the bottle; repeat until the glycerol is used up; add water to bring the oral liquid to a total volume of 100 mL; label "shake well" and "refrigerate". The suspension is stable 8 days refrigerated.

Boulton DV, Fawcett JP, and Woods DJ, "Stability of an Extemporaneously Compounded Levothyroxine Sodium Oral Liquid," *Am J Health-Syst Pharm*, 1996; 53:1157-61.

References

de Groot JW, Zonnenberg BA, Plukker JT, et al, "Imatinib Induces Hypothyroidism in Patients Receiving Levothyroxine," *Clin Pharmacol Ther*, 2005, 78(4):433-8.

♦ **Lidex-E®** *see* Fluocinonide *on page 674*

Lidocaine (LYE doe kane)

Medication Safety Issues

High alert medication: The Institute for Safe Medication Practices (ISMP) includes this medication (I.V. formulation) among its list of drugs which have a heightened risk of causing significant patient harm when used in error.

Transdermal patch may contain conducting metal (eg, aluminum); remove patch prior to MRI.

International issues:

Lidpen® may be confused with Linoten® which is a brand name for pamidronate in Spain

Related Information

Adult ACLS Algorithms *on page 1660*
CPR Pediatric Drug Dosages *on page 1650*
Emergency Pediatric Drip Calculations *on page 1652*
Pediatric ALS Algorithms *on page 1657*

U.S. Brand Names Anestacon®; Band-Aid® Hurt-Free™ Antiseptic Wash [OTC]; Burnamycin [OTC]; Burn Jel [OTC]; Burn-O-Jel [OTC]; LidaMantle®; Lidoderm®; L-M-X™ 4 [OTC]; L-M-X™ 5 [OTC]; LTA® 360; Premjact® [OTC]; Solarcaine® Aloe Extra Burn Relief [OTC]; Topicaine® [OTC]; Xylocaine®; Xylocaine® MPF; Xylocaine® Viscous; Zilactin-L® [OTC]

Canadian Brand Names Betacaine®; Lidodan™; Lidoderm®; Xylocaine®; Xylocard®; Zilactin®

Index Terms Lidocaine Hydrochloride; Lignocaine Hydrochloride

Therapeutic Category Analgesic, Topical; Antiarrhythmic Agent, Class I-B; Local Anesthetic, Injectable; Local Anesthetic, Topical

Generic Available Yes: Cream, infusion, injection, jelly, lotion, ointment, solution

Use Treatment of ventricular ectopy, ventricular tachycardia (VT), ventricular fibrillation (VF); local anesthetic; pain relief of postherpetic neuralgia

Lidocaine is recommended in the PALS guidelines for cardiac arrest with pulseless VT or VF (unresponsive to defibrillation, CPR, and vasopressor administration); to be considered in patients with cocaine overdose to prevent arrhythmias secondary to MI. It is recommended in the ACLS guidelines as an alternative to amiodarone for cardiac arrest with pulseless VT or VF (unresponsive to defibrillation, CPR, and vasopressor administration); it is not considered to be the drug of choice, but may be considered for the following: Stable monomorphic VT (in patients with preserved ventricular function), polymorphic VT (with normal baseline or prolonged QT interval)

Pregnancy Risk Factor B

Lactation Enters breast milk (small amounts)/use caution (AAP rates "compatible")

Contraindications Hypersensitivity to lidocaine, amide-type local anesthetics, or any component (see Warnings); patients with Adams-Stokes syndrome, Wolff-Parkinson-White syndrome, or with severe degree of S-A, A-V, or intraventricular heart block (without a pacemaker)

Warnings Decrease dose in patients with decreased cardiac output or hepatic disease; do not use lidocaine solutions containing epinephrine for treatment of arrhythmias; do not use preservative-containing solution for I.V. use; do not apply patch to larger areas or for longer than recommended (toxicities may result)

Topical use prior to cosmetic procedures can result in high systemic levels and lead to toxic effects (eg, arrhythmias, seizures, coma, respiratory depression, and death). Toxic effects may occur particularly when topical anesthetics are applied in large amounts or to large areas of the skin; left on for long periods of time; used with materials, wraps, or dressings to cover the skin after application; or applied to broken skin, rashes, or areas of skin irritation. These practices may increase the degree of systemic absorption and should be avoided. The FDA recommends that consumers consult their healthcare provider for instructions on safe use, prior to applying topical anesthetics for medical or cosmetic purposes. Use of products with the lowest amount of anesthetic and applying the least amount possible to relieve pain is also recommended.

Premixed infusions containing dextrose may cause hypersensitivity reactions in patients allergic to corn or corn products; topical gel may contain tartrazine or benzyl alcohol; topical and rectal creams may contain benzyl alcohol; tartrazine and benzyl alcohol may cause allergic reactions in susceptible individuals; large amounts of benzyl alcohol (≥99 mg/kg/day) have been associated with a potentially fatal toxicity ("gasping syndrome") in neonates; the "gasping syndrome" consists of metabolic acidosis, respiratory distress, gasping respirations, CNS dysfunction (including convulsions, intracranial hemorrhage), hypotension and cardiovascular collapse; (Continued)

Lidocaine *(Continued)*

avoid use of lidocaine products containing benzyl alcohol in neonates; *in vitro* and animal studies have shown that benzoate, a metabolite of benzyl alcohol, displaces bilirubin from protein binding sites

Precautions Hepatic disease, heart failure, marked hypoxia, severe respiratory depression, hypovolemia or shock; incomplete heart block or bradycardia, atrial fibrillation

Adverse Reactions

Cardiovascular: Bradycardia, hypotension, heart block, arrhythmias, cardiovascular collapse

Central nervous system: Lethargy, coma, agitation, slurred speech, seizures, anxiety, euphoria, hallucinations

Gastrointestinal: Nausea, vomiting

Local: Thrombophlebitis; with patch: Erythema, edema, abnormal sensation

Neuromuscular & skeletal: Paresthesia, muscle twitching

Ocular: Blurred vision, diplopia

Respiratory: Respiratory depression or arrest

Miscellaneous: Allergic and anaphylactoid reactions (rare)

Drug Interactions Cytochrome P450 isoenzyme CYP1A2, CYP2B6, CYP2D6, and CYP3A3/4 substrate; isoenzyme CYP1A2 inhibitor

Cimetidine or beta-blockers may increase lidocaine serum concentration and toxicity; Class I antiarrhythmic agents (mexiletine, phenytoin, procainamide, quinidine, tocainide), amiodarone, or other antiarrhythmics may increase adverse or toxic effects

Mechanism of Action Class IB antiarrhythmic; suppresses automaticity of conduction tissue by increasing electrical stimulation threshold of ventricle, His-Purkinje system, and spontaneous depolarization of the ventricles during diastole by a direct action on the tissues; blocks both the initiation and conduction of nerve impulses by decreasing the neuronal membrane's permeability to sodium ions, which results in inhibition of depolarization with resultant blockade of conduction

Pharmacodynamics

Antiarrhythmic effect:

- Onset of action (single I.V. bolus dose): 45-90 seconds
- Duration: 10-20 minutes

Local anesthetic effect: Duration: 1-2 hours

Pharmacokinetics

Distribution: V_d alterable by many patient factors; decreased V_d in CHF and liver disease

Protein binding: 60% to 80%; binds to alpha$_1$-acid glycoprotein

Metabolism: 90% in the liver; active metabolites monoethylglycinexylidide (MEGX) and glycinexylidide (GX) can accumulate and may cause CNS toxicity

Half-life, biphasic:

- Alpha: 7-30 minutes
- Beta, terminal:
  - Infants, premature: 3.2 hours
  - Adults: 1.5-2 hours
- CHF, liver disease, shock, severe renal disease: Prolonged half-life

Elimination: <10% excreted unchanged in urine

Dialysis: Dialyzable (0% to 5%)

Usual Dosage

Children and Adults:

- Topical: Apply to affected area as needed; maximum dose: 3 mg/kg/dose; do not repeat within 2 hours
- Injectable local anesthetic: Dose varies with procedure, degree of anesthesia needed, vascularity of tissue, duration of anesthesia required, and physical condition of patient; maximum dose: 4.5 mg/kg/dose; do not repeat within 2 hours

Children (PALS 2005 guidelines):

- I.V., I.O.: (**Note:** For use in pulseless VT or VF, give after defibrillation and epinephrine): Loading dose: 1 mg/kg (maximum: 100 mg/dose); follow with continuous infusion; may administer second bolus of 0.5-1 mg/kg if delay between bolus and start of infusion is >15 minutes; continuous infusion: 20-50 mcg/kg/minute. Use 20 mcg/kg/minute in patients with shock, hepatic disease, cardiac arrest, mild CHF; moderate to severe CHF may require ½ loading dose and lower infusion rates to avoid toxicity.
- E.T.: 2-3 mg; flush with 5 mL of NS and follow with 5 assisted manual ventilations

Adults (decrease the dose in patients with CHF, acute MI with hypotension, shock, poor peripheral perfusion states, or hepatic disease; usual bolus dose, but 1/2 of normal maintenance infusion should be used in these patients):

I.V.:

Antiarrhythmic: Initial bolus: 1-1.5 mg/kg; may repeat doses of 0.5-0.75 mg/kg every 5-10 minutes if needed to a total of 3 mg/kg; continuous infusion: Initial: 1-4 mg/minute

Ventricular fibrillation or pulseless VT (after defibrillation and epinephrine or vasopressin) (ACLS 2005 guidelines): Initial dose: I.V./I.O.: 1-1.5 mg/kg; may repeat 0.5-0.75 mg at 5-10 minute intervals; maximum total dose: 3 mg/kg; follow with continuous I.V. infusion after return of perfusion; continuous I.V. infusion: 1-4 mg/min; **Note:** Use only bolus doses for cardiac arrest caused by VF or pulseless VT

Patients with impaired cardiac function: Initial bolus: 0.5-0.75 mg/kg IVP; may repeat every 5-10 minutes; follow with continuous infusion: Initial: 1-4 mg/min; maximum total dose: 3 mg/kg (administered over 1 hour)

Prevention of ventricular fibrillation: I.V.: Initial bolus: 0.5 mg/kg; repeat every 5-10 minutes to a total dose of 2 mg/kg

E.T.: 2-2.5 times the I.V. bolus dose; dilute in 10 mL NS or distilled water

I.M.: Prehospital post-MI antiarrhythmic prophylaxis: 300 mg

Lidoderm® patch: Postherpetic neuralgia: Apply patch to most painful areas; up to 3 patches may be applied per application; patch may remain in place for up to 12 hours in any 24-hour period

Administration

Endotracheal:

Children: Flush with 5 mL of NS after E.T. administration; follow with 5 assisted manual ventilations

Adults: Dilute in 10 mL NS or distilled water prior to E.T. administration (**Note:** Use of distilled water results in greater absorption, but a greater adverse effect on PaO_2)

Parenteral: I.V.: Solutions of 40-200 mg/mL must be diluted for I.V. use; final concentration not to exceed 20 mg/mL for I.V. push or 8 mg/mL for I.V. infusion; I.V. push rate of administration should not exceed 0.7 mg/kg/minute or 50 mg/minute, whichever is less; I.V. continuous infusion must be administered with a calibrated infusion device

Transdermal: Apply patch to intact skin so most painful area is covered; do not apply to broken or inflamed skin; patch may be cut to appropriate size; remove immediately if burning sensation occurs; wash hands after applying patch; avoid eye contact; keep out of the reach of children; dispose of used patch properly (see Additional Information)

Monitoring Parameters Monitor EKG continuously; serum concentrations with continuous infusion; I.V. site (local thrombophlebitis may occur with prolonged infusions)

Reference Range

Therapeutic: 1.5-5 mcg/mL (SI: 6-21 micromoles/L)

Potentially toxic: >6 mcg/mL (SI: >26 micromoles/L)

Toxic: >9 mcg/mL (SI: >38 micromoles/L)

Nursing Implications Multiple products and concentrations exist; use of an I.V. fluid filter is recommended where possible

Additional Information Transdermal patches (both used and unused) may cause toxicities in children; used patches still contain large amounts of lidocaine; store and dispose patches out of the reach of children

Dosage Forms Excipient information presented when available (limited, particularly for generics); consult specific product labeling. [DSC] = Discontinued product

Cream, rectal (L-M-X™ 5): 5% (15 g) [contains benzyl alcohol; packaged with applicator]; (30 g) [contains benzyl alcohol]

Cream, topical (L-M-X™ 4): 4% (5 g) [contains benzyl alcohol; packaged with Tegaderm™ dressing]; (15 g, 30 g) [contains benzyl alcohol]

Cream, topical, as hydrochloride: 3% (30 g)

LidaMantle®: 3% (30 g, 85 g)

Gel, topical:

Burn-O-Jel: 0.5% (90 g)

Topicaine®: 4% (10 g, 30 g, 113 g) [contains alcohol 35%, benzyl alcohol, aloe vera, and jojoba]

Gel, topical, as hydrochloride:

Burn Jel: 2% (3.5 g, 120 g)

Solarcaine® Aloe Extra Burn Relief: 0.5% (113 g, 226 g) [contains aloe vera gel and tartrazine]

Infusion, as hydrochloride [premixed in D_5W]: 0.4% [4 mg/mL] (250 mL, 500 mL); 0.8% [8 mg/mL] (250 mL, 500 mL)

(Continued)

Lidocaine *(Continued)*

Injection, solution, as hydrochloride: 0.5% [5 mg/mL] (50 mL); 1% [10 mg/mL] (2 mL, 10 mL, 20 mL, 30 mL, 50 mL); 2% [20 mg/mL] (2 mL, 5 mL, 20 mL, 50 mL)
 Xylocaine®: 0.5% [5 mg/mL] (50 mL); 1% [10 mg/mL] (10 mL, 20 mL, 50 mL); 2% [20 mg/mL] (1.8 mL, 10 mL, 20 mL, 50 mL)
Injection, solution, as hydrochloride [preservative free]: 0.5% [5 mg/mL] (50 mL); 1% [10 mg/mL] (2 mL, 5 mL, 30 mL); 1.5% [15 mg/mL] (20 mL); 2% [20 mg/mL] (2 mL, 5 mL, 10 mL); 4% [40 mg/mL] (5 mL)
 Xylocaine®: 10% [100 mg/mL] (5 mL) [for ventricular arrhythmias]
 Xylocaine® MPF: 0.5% [5 mg/mL] (50 mL); 1% [10 mg/mL] (2 mL, 5 mL, 10 mL, 30 mL); 1.5% [15 mg/mL] (10 mL, 20 mL); 2% [20 mg/mL] (2 mL, 5 mL, 10 mL); 4% [40 mg/mL] (5 mL)
Injection, solution, as hydrochloride [premixed in $D_{7.5}W$, preservative free]: 5% (2 mL)
 Xylocaine® MPF: 1.5% (2 mL) [DSC]
Jelly, topical, as hydrochloride: 2% (5 mL, 30 mL)
 Anestacon®: 2% (15 mL) [contains benzalkonium chloride]
 Xylocaine®: 2% (5 mL, 30 mL)
Liquid, topical (Zilactin®-L): 2.5% (7.5 mL)
Lotion, topical, as hydrochloride (LidaMantle®): 3% (177 mL)
Ointment, topical: 5% (37 g, 50 g)
Solution, topical, as hydrochloride: 4% [40 mg/mL] (50 mL)
 Band-Aid® Hurt-Free™ Antiseptic Wash: 2% (180 mL)
 LTA® 360: 4% [40 mg/mL] (4 mL) [packaged with cannula for laryngotracheal administration]
 Xylocaine®: 4% [40 mg/mL] (50 mL)
Solution, viscous, as hydrochloride: 2% [20 mg/mL] (20 mL, 100 mL)
 Xylocaine® Viscous: 2% [20 mg/mL] (100 mL, 450 mL)
Spray, topical:
 Burnamycin: 0.5% (60 mL) [contains aloe vera gel and menthol]
 Premjact®: 9.6% (13 mL)
 Solarcaine® Aloe Extra Burn Relief: 0.5% (127 g) [contains aloe vera]
Transdermal system, topical (Lidoderm®): 5% (30s)

References

American Heart Association Emergency Cardiovascular Care Committee, " 2005 American Heart Association (AHA) Guidelines for Cardiopulmonary Resuscitation (CPR) and Emergency Cardiovascular Care (ECC), Part 7.2: Management of Cardiac Arrest, Part 7.3: Management of Symptomatic Bradycardia and Tachycardia, and Part 12: Pediatric Advanced Life Support," *Circulation*, 2005, 112(24 Suppl):IV58-77,167-87.

Lidocaine and Epinephrine (LYE doe kane & ep i NEF rin)

Medication Safety Issues
Transdermal patch may contain conducting metal (eg, aluminum); remove patch prior to MRI.

U.S. Brand Names LidoSite™; Xylocaine® MPF With Epinephrine; Xylocaine® With Epinephrine

Canadian Brand Names Xylocaine® With Epinephrine

Index Terms Epinephrine and Lidocaine

Therapeutic Category Local Anesthetic, Injectable

Generic Available Yes: Excludes transdermal system

Use Local infiltration anesthesia

Pregnancy Risk Factor B

Lactation Enters breast milk/compatible

Contraindications Hypersensitivity to epinephrine, lidocaine, amide-type local anesthetics, or any component (see Warnings)

Warnings Topical use prior to cosmetic procedures can result in high systemic levels and lead to toxic effects (eg, arrhythmias, seizures, coma, respiratory depression, and death). Toxic effects may occur particularly when topical anesthetics are applied in large amounts or to large areas of the skin; left on for long periods of time; used with materials, wraps, or dressings to cover the skin after application; or applied to broken skin, rashes, or areas of skin irritation. These practices may increase the degree of systemic absorption and should be avoided. The FDA recommends that consumers consult their healthcare provider for instructions on safe use, prior to applying topical anesthetics for medical or cosmetic purposes. Use of products with the lowest amount of anesthetic and applying the least amount possible to relieve pain is also recommended.

Some products contain sodium metabisulfite which may cause allergic reactions in susceptible individuals

Precautions Do not use solutions in distal portions of the body (digits, nose, ears, penis); do not use large doses in patients with conduction defects (ie, heart block)

Adverse Reactions
Cardiovascular: Hypotension, bradycardia
Central nervous system: Lightheadedness, nervousness, confusion, dizziness, drowsiness, convulsions
Dermatologic: Urticaria
Neuromuscular & skeletal: Tremor
Ocular: Blurred vision
Otic: Tinnitus

Mechanism of Action Lidocaine blocks both the initiation and conduction of nerve impulses via decreased permeability of sodium ions; epinephrine increases the duration of action of lidocaine by causing vasoconstriction (via alpha effects) which slows the vascular absorption of lidocaine

Pharmacodynamics
Maximum effect: Within 5 minutes
Duration: 2-6 hours, dependent on dose and anesthetic procedure

Usual Dosage Dosage varies with the anesthetic procedure
Children: Use lidocaine concentrations of 0.5% or 1% (or even more dilute) to decrease possibility of toxicity; lidocaine dose (when using combination product of lidocaine and epinephrine) should not exceed 7 mg/kg/dose; do not repeat within 2 hours

Administration Local injection: Before injecting, withdraw syringe plunger to make sure that injection is not into vein or artery; do not administer I.V. or intra-arterially

Additional Information Use preservative free solutions for epidural or caudal use

Dosage Forms Excipient information presented when available (limited, particularly for generics); consult specific product labeling.

Injection, solution:
0.5% / 1:200,000: Lidocaine hydrochloride 0.5% and epinephrine 1:200,000 (50 mL)
1% / 1:100,000: Lidocaine hydrochloride 1% and epinephrine 1:100,000 (20 mL, 30 mL, 50 mL)
1% / 1:200,000: Lidocaine hydrochloride 1% and epinephrine 1:200,000 (30 mL)
1.5% / 1:200,000: Lidocaine hydrochloride 1.5% and epinephrine 1:200,000 (30 mL)
2% / 1:50,000: Lidocaine hydrochloride 2% and epinephrine 1:50,000 (1.8 mL)
2% / 1:100,000: Lidocaine hydrochloride 2% and epinephrine 1:100,000 (1.8 mL, 30 mL, 50 mL)
2% / 1:200,000: Lidocaine hydrochloride 2% and epinephrine 1:200,000 (20 mL)

Xylocaine® with Epinephrine:
0.5% / 1:200,000: Lidocaine hydrochloride 0.5% and epinephrine 1:200,000 (50 mL) [contains methylparaben]
1% / 1:100,000: Lidocaine hydrochloride 1% and epinephrine 1:100,000 (10 mL, 20 mL, 50 mL) [contains methylparaben]
2% / 1:50,000: Lidocaine hydrochloride 2% and epinephrine 1:50,000 (1.8 mL) [contains sodium metabisulfite]
2% / 1:100,000: Lidocaine hydrochloride 2% and epinephrine 1:100,000 (1.8 mL) [contains sodium metabisulfite]; (10 mL, 20 mL, 50 mL) [contains methylparaben]

Xylocaine®-MPF with Epinephrine:
1% / 1:200,000: Lidocaine hydrochloride 1% and epinephrine 1:200,000 (5 mL, 10 mL, 30 mL) [contains sodium metabisulfite]
1.5% / 1:200,000: Lidocaine hydrochloride 1.5% and epinephrine 1:200,000 (5 mL, 10 mL, 30 mL) [contains sodium metabisulfite]
2% / 1:200,000: Lidocaine hydrochloride 2% and epinephrine 1:200,000 (5 mL, 10 mL, 20 mL) [contains sodium metabisulfite]

Transdermal system (LidoSite™): Lidocaine hydrochloride 10% and epinephrine 0.1% (25s) [contains sodium metabisulfite; for use only with LidoSite™ controller]

Lidocaine and Prilocaine (LYE doe kane & PRIL oh kane)

U.S. Brand Names EMLA®; Oraquix®
Canadian Brand Names EMLA®
Index Terms Prilocaine and Lidocaine
Therapeutic Category Analgesic, Topical; Antipruritic, Topical; Local Anesthetic, Topical
Generic Available Yes: Cream
Use Topical anesthetic for use on normal intact skin to provide local analgesia for minor procedures such as I.V. cannulation or venipuncture; topical anesthetic for superficial minor surgery of genital mucous membranes and as an adjunct for local infiltration anesthesia in genital mucous membranes; has also been used for painful procedures such as lumbar puncture and skin graft harvesting
(Continued)

Lidocaine and Prilocaine *(Continued)*

Pregnancy Risk Factor B

Lactation Enters breast milk/compatible

Contraindications Hypersensitivity to lidocaine, prilocaine, amide-type local anesthetics, or any component; patients with congenital or idiopathic methemoglobinemia, neonates <37 weeks gestation, infants <12 months of age who are receiving concurrent treatment with methemoglobin-inducing agents (ie, sulfas, acetaminophen, benzocaine, chloroquine, dapsone, nitrofurantoin, nitroglycerin, nitroprusside, phenobarbital, phenytoin, primaquine, quinine)

Warnings Topical use prior to cosmetic procedures can result in high systemic levels and lead to toxic effects (eg, arrhythmias, seizures, coma, respiratory depression, and death). Toxic effects may occur particularly when topical anesthetics are applied in large amounts or to large areas of the skin; left on for long periods of time; used with materials, wraps, or dressings to cover the skin after application; or applied to broken skin, rashes, or areas of skin irritation. These practices may increase the degree of systemic absorption and should be avoided. The FDA recommends that consumers consult their healthcare provider for instructions on safe use, prior to applying topical anesthetics for medical or cosmetic purposes. Use of products with the lowest amount of anesthetic and applying the least amount possible to relieve pain is also recommended.

Precautions Use with caution in patients with severe hepatic disease, patients with G-6-PD deficiency, and patients taking drugs associated with drug-induced methemoglobinemia; adjust dosage by using smaller areas for application in small children (especially infants <3 months of age) or patients with impaired renal or hepatic function

Adverse Reactions

Cardiovascular: Bradycardia, hypotension, shock, angioedema

Central nervous system: Nervousness, euphoria, confusion, dizziness, drowsiness, convulsions, CNS excitation, alteration in temperature sensation

Dermatologic: Rash, urticaria

Hematologic: Methemoglobinemia

Local: Blanching, itching, erythema, edema

Neuromuscular & skeletal: Tremor

Ocular: Blurred vision

Otic: Tinnitus

Respiratory: Respiratory depression, bronchospasm

Drug Interactions Class IB antiarrhythmic drugs (tocainide, mexiletine): toxic effects are additive; drugs known to induce methemoglobinemia (see Contraindications)

Stability Store at room temperature

Mechanism of Action Local anesthetic action occurs by stabilization of neuronal membranes and inhibiting the ionic fluxes required for the initiation and conduction of impulses

Pharmacodynamics

Onset of action: 1 hour for sufficient dermal analgesia

Maximum effect: 2-3 hours

Duration: 1-2 hours after removal of the cream

Pharmacokinetics

Absorption: Topical: Related to the duration of application and to the area over which it is applied

- 3-hour application: 3.6% lidocaine and 6.1% prilocaine were absorbed
- 24-hour application: 16.2% lidocaine and 33.5% prilocaine were absorbed

Distribution: Both cross the blood-brain barrier; lidocaine and probably prilocaine are excreted in breast milk; V_d:

- Lidocaine: 1.1-2.1 L/kg
- Prilocaine: 0.7-4.4 L/kg

Protein binding:

- Lidocaine: 70%
- Prilocaine: 55%

Metabolism:

- Lidocaine: Metabolized by the liver to inactive and active metabolites
- Prilocaine: Metabolized in both the liver and kidneys

Half-life:

- Lidocaine: 65-150 minutes, prolonged with cardiac or hepatic dysfunction
- Prilocaine: 10-150 minutes, prolonged in hepatic or renal dysfunction

Usual Dosage Topical:

Newborns ≥37 weeks gestation, Infants, Children, and Adults: For minor procedures, apply 2.5 g/site for at least 60 minutes; for painful procedures, apply 2 g/10 cm^2 of skin and leave on for at least 2 hours; see table on next page.

Note: Preliminary results in a study of 30 preterm neonates (n=30) using a single 0.5 g dose of EMLA® applied to the heel for 1 hour resulted in no measurable changes in methemoglobin levels

EMLA® Cream Maximum Recommended Dose and Application Area for Infants and Children Based on Application to Intact Skin

Age and Body Weight Requirements	Maximum Total Dose of EMLA®	Maximum Application Area	Maximum Application Time
Birth to 3 mo or <5 kg	1g	10 cm^2	1 h
3-12 mo and >5 kg	2 g	20 cm^2	4 h
1-6 y and >10 kg	10 g	100 cm^2	4 h
7-12 y and >20 kg	20 g	200 cm^2	4 h

Adult male genital skin as an adjunct prior to local anesthetic infiltration: Apply 1 g/ 10 cm^2 to skin surface for 15 minutes followed immediately by local anesthetic infiltration after removal of EMLA® cream

Administration Topical: Do not use on mucous membranes or the eyes; apply a thick layer of cream to intact skin and cover with an occlusive dressing

Patient Information Not for ophthalmic use; for external use only. EMLA® may block sensation in the treated skin.

Nursing Implications In small infants and children, an occlusive bandage should be placed over the EMLA® cream to prevent the child from placing the cream in his/her mouth or smearing the cream on the eyes

Dosage Forms Excipient information presented when available (limited, particularly for generics); consult specific product labeling.

Cream, topical: Lidocaine 2.5% and prilocaine 2.5% (5 g, 30 g)

EMLA®: Lidocaine 2.5% and prilocaine 2.5% (5 g, 30 g) [each packaged with Tegaderm® dressings]

Disc, topical: Lidocaine 2.5% and prilocaine 2.5% per disc (2s, 10s) [each 1 g disc is 10 cm^2]

Gel, periodontal: Lidocaine 2.5% and prilocaine 2.5% (1.7 g) [cartridge]

References

Broadman LM, Soliman IE, Hannallah RS, et al, "Analgesic Efficacy of Eutectic Mixture of Local Anesthetics (EMLA®) vs Intradermal Infiltration Prior to Venous Cannulation in Children," *Am J Anaesth*, 1987, 34:S56.

Halperin DL, Koren G, Attias D, et al, "Topical Skin Anesthesia for Venous Subcutaneous Drug Reservoir and Lumbar Puncture in Children," *Pediatrics*, 1989, 84(2):281-4.

Robieux I, Kumar R, Radhakrishnan S, et al, "Assessing Pain and Analgesia With a Lidocaine-Prilocaine Emulsion in Infants and Toddlers During Venipuncture," *J Pediatr*, 1991, 118(6):971-3.

Taddio A, Shennan AT, Stevens B, et al, "Safety of Lidocaine-Prilocaine Cream in the Treatment of Preterm Neonates," *J Pediatr*, 1995, 127(6):1002-5.

♦ **Lidocaine Hydrochloride** *see* Lidocaine *on page 933*

♦ **Lidodan™ (Can)** *see* Lidocaine *on page 933*

♦ **Lidoderm®** *see* Lidocaine *on page 933*

♦ **LidoSite™** *see* Lidocaine and Epinephrine *on page 936*

♦ **LID-Pack® (Can)** *see* Bacitracin and Polymyxin B *on page 196*

♦ **Lignocaine Hydrochloride** *see* Lidocaine *on page 933*

♦ **Lin-Amox (Can)** *see* Amoxicillin *on page 113*

♦ **Lin-Buspirone (Can)** *see* BusPIRone *on page 250*

Lindane (LIN dane)

Canadian Brand Names Hexit™; PMS-Lindane

Index Terms Benzene Hexachloride; Gamma Benzene Hexachloride; Hexachlorocyclohexane

Therapeutic Category Antiparasitic Agent, Topical; Pediculocide; Scabicidal Agent; Shampoos

Generic Available Yes

Use Alternative treatment of scabies (*Sarcoptes scabiei*), *Pediculus capitis* (head lice), and *Pediculus pubis* (crab lice); (the AAP and CDC consider permethrin 5% to be the scabicide of choice due to its safety and efficacy profile; many clinicians no longer recommend lindane as initial therapy for pediculosis due to reports of resistance and neurotoxicity)

Medication Guide An FDA-approved patient medication guide, which is available with the product information and at http://www.fda.gov/cder/Offices/ODS/medication_guides.htm, must be dispensed with this medication for each new outpatient prescription and refill.

Pregnancy Risk Factor B

(Continued)

Lindane *(Continued)*

Lactation Enters breast milk/contraindicated

Contraindications Hypersensitivity to lindane or any component; premature neonates; pregnant or lactating women; acutely inflamed skin or raw, weeping surfaces

Warnings Avoid contact with the face, eyes, mucous membranes, and urethral meatus

Precautions Use with caution in infants, small children and patients with pre-existing seizure disorders due to its potential for neurologic toxicity; if used in young children, cover hands to prevent accidental lindane ingestion from thumbsucking; **consider alternative therapy for the treatment of scabies in infants and young children <2 years of age (ie, permethrin)**

Adverse Reactions

Cardiovascular: Cardiac arrhythmia

Central nervous system: Dizziness, restlessness, seizures, headache, ataxia

Dermatologic: Eczematous eruptions, contact dermatitis, rash

Gastrointestinal: Nausea, vomiting

Hematologic: Aplastic anemia

Hepatic: Hepatitis

Local: Burning and stinging

Ocular: Conjunctivitis

Renal: Hematuria

Respiratory: Pulmonary edema

Mechanism of Action Directly absorbed by parasites and ova through the exoskeleton; stimulates the nervous system resulting in seizures and death of parasitic arthropods

Pharmacokinetics

Absorption: Topical: Up to 13% absorbed systemically (absorption is greater when applied to damaged skin, face, scalp, neck, or scrotum)

Distribution: Stored in body fat and accumulates in the brain; skin and adipose tissue may act as repositories

Metabolism: By the liver

Half-life, children: 17-22 hours

Time to peak serum concentration: Children: Topical: 6 hours

Elimination: In urine and feces

Usual Dosage Children and Adults: Topical:

Scabies: Apply a thin layer of lotion and massage it on skin from the neck to the toes (head to toe in infants).

Infants: Wash off 6 hours after application

Children: Wash off 6-8 hours after application

Adults: Bathe and remove drug 8-12 hours after application

Do not reapply sooner than 1 week later if live mites appear

Pediculosis: 15-30 mL of shampoo is applied and lathered for 4 minutes; rinse hair thoroughly and comb with a fine tooth comb to remove nits; repeat treatment in 7 days if lice or nits are still present

Pediculosis of the eyelashes: Do not treat with lindane; instead, apply an occlusive ophthalmic ointment like petrolatum to the eyelid margins twice daily for 10 days

Administration

For topical use only; do not apply to face; avoid getting in eyes; do **not** apply lotion immediately after a hot, soapy bath; lotion should be applied to dry, cool skin

Before applying lindane shampoo, wash hair with a plain shampoo, then dry

Patient Information Read the patient Medication Guide that you receive with each prescription and refill of lindane. Clothing and bedding should be washed in hot water or by dry cleaning to kill the scabies mite; combs and brushes may be washed with lindane shampoo then thoroughly rinsed with water

Nursing Implications

Children <6 years: ~30 mL lotion is sufficient volume for one application

Children ≥6 years and Adults: ~30-60 mL lotion is sufficient volume for one application

Pruritus associated with scabies or pediculosis may persist for longer than 1 week following treatment with drug. Oral antihistamine and/or topical corticosteroid may be used to help relieve pruritus.

Additional Information Excessive absorption may result in overdose with signs and symptoms which include nausea, vomiting, seizures, headaches, arrhythmias, apnea, pulmonary edema, hematuria, hepatitis, coma, and even death

Dosage Forms Excipient information presented when available (limited, particularly for generics); consult specific product labeling.

Lotion, topical: 1% (60 mL)

Shampoo, topical: 1% (60 mL) [contains alcohol 0.5%]

References

Eichenfield LF, Honig PJ, "Blistering Disorders in Childhood," *Pediatr Clin North Am*, 1991, 38(4):959-76.

Hogan DJ, Schachner L, Tanglertsampan C, "Diagnosis and Treatment of Childhood Scabies and Pediculosis," *Pediatr Clin North Am*, 1991, 38(4):941-57.

Pramanik AK and Hansen RC, "Transcutaneous Gamma Benzene Hexachloride Absorption and Toxicity in Infants and Children," *Arch Dermatol*, 1979, 115(10):1224-5.

Linezolid (li NE zoh lid)

Medication Safety Issues

Sound-alike/look-alike issues:

Zyvox® may be confused with Vioxx®, Ziox™, Zosyn®, Zovirax®

U.S. Brand Names Zyvox®

Canadian Brand Names Zyvoxam®

Index Terms PNU-100766

Therapeutic Category Antibiotic, Oxazolidinone

Generic Available No

Use Treatment of community-acquired pneumonia, hospital-acquired pneumonia, complicated and uncomplicated skin and soft tissue infections (including diabetic foot infections without concomitant osteomyelitis), bacteremia caused by susceptible vancomycin-resistant *Enterococcus faecium* (VREF), *Enterococcus faecalis*, *Streptococcus pneumoniae* including multidrug resistant strains, *Staphylococcus aureus* including MRSA, *Streptococcus pyogenes*, or *Streptococcus agalactiae*. **Note:** There have been reports of vancomycin-resistant *E. faecium* and *S. aureus* (methicillin-resistant) developing resistance to linezolid during its clinical use.

Pregnancy Risk Factor C

Lactation Excretion in breast milk unknown/use caution

Contraindications Hypersensitivity to linezolid or any component; since therapeutic linezolid concentrations were not consistently achieved or maintained in the CSF of pediatric patients with ventriculoperitoneal shunts, use of linezolid for the empiric treatment of pediatric CNS infections is not recommended

Warnings Linezolid is a reversible, nonselective MAO inhibitor with the potential to have the same interactions as other MAO inhibitors. Avoid use with serotonergic agents such as tricyclic antidepressants, venlafaxine, trazodone, sibutramine, meperidine, dextromethorphan, and SSRIs. Thrombocytopenia, anemia, leukopenia, and pancytopenia have been reported in patients receiving linezolid and may be dependent on duration of therapy (generally >2 weeks of treatment); monitor patients' CBC weekly during linezolid therapy; discontinuation of therapy may be required; *C. difficile*-associated colitis has been reported. Peripheral and optic neuropathy with vision loss have been reported primarily in patients treated for longer then 28 days with linezolid. Cases of lactic acidosis in which patients experienced repeated episodes of nausea and vomiting, acidosis, and low bicarbonate levels have been reported. Oral suspension contains sodium benzoate; benzoic acid (benzoate) is a metabolite of benzyl alcohol; large amounts of benzyl alcohol (≥99 mg/kg/day) have been associated with a potentially fatal toxicity ("gasping syndrome") in neonates; use caution when administering oral suspension containing sodium benzoate to neonates; *in vitro* and animal studies have shown that benzoate displaces bilirubin from protein binding sites

Precautions Use with caution in patients with uncontrolled hypertension, history of seizures, pheochromocytoma, carcinoid syndrome, severe renal or hepatic impairment, pre-existing myelosuppression, patients receiving other drugs which may cause bone marrow suppression, or untreated hyperthyroidism; linezolid suspension contains aspartame which is metabolized to phenylalanine and must be used with caution in patients with phenylketonuria.

Adverse Reactions

Cardiovascular: Hypertension

Central nervous system: Headache, insomnia, dizziness, fever, vertigo, seizures

Dermatologic: Rash, pruritus

Endocrine & metabolic: Lactic acidosis

Gastrointestinal: Nausea, diarrhea, vomiting, constipation, pseudomembranous colitis, dyspepsia, taste alteration, tongue discoloration, pancreatitis, abdominal pain

Genitourinary: Vaginal moniliasis

Hematologic: Neutropenia, thrombocytopenia, anemia, leukopenia, pancytopenia, eosinophilia

Hepatic: Elevated ALT

Neuromuscular & skeletal: Peripheral neuropathy

Ocular: Optic neuropathy, blurred vision, loss of vision

Renal: Elevated BUN and creatinine

Respiratory: Dyspnea

Drug Interactions Linezolid is a reversible, nonselective inhibitor of monoamine oxidase: Enhanced vasopressor effects if used with sympathomimetic agents such as dopamine, phenylpropanolamine, epinephrine, pseudoephedrine; serotonin (Continued)

Linezolid *(Continued)*

syndrome (hyperpyrexia, myoclonus, tremor, hyper-reflexia, cognitive dysfunction) if used in patients receiving concomitant serotonergic agents including tricyclic antidepressants, venlafaxine, tramadol, trazodone, sibutramine, meperidine, dextromethorphan, and SSRIs (see Warnings); myelosuppressive drugs (may increase risk of myelosuppression with linezolid)

Food Interactions Ingestion of tyramine-containing foods may cause hypertensive crisis; limit intake of tyramine-containing foods to less than 100 mg/meal

Stability Store at room temperature; protect from light. Store infusion bags in overwrap until ready for use. The yellow color of the injectable solution may intensify over time without adversely affecting potency. Store reconstituted oral suspension at room temperature and use within 21 days. Linezolid injection is physically incompatible with amphotericin B, chlorpromazine, diazepam, erythromycin lactobionate, pentamidine, phenytoin, sulfamethoxazole and trimethoprim, and ceftriaxone. Linezolid injection is compatible with D_5W, NS, and LR.

Mechanism of Action Inhibits initiation of protein synthesis by binding to a site on the bacterial 23S ribosomal RNA of the 50S subunit preventing the formation of a functional 70S initiation complex which is an essential component of the bacterial translation process

Pharmacokinetics

Absorption: Well absorbed orally

Distribution: Well-perfused tissues

- V_d: Children: 0.73 ± 0.18 L/kg

Protein binding: 31%

Metabolism: Oxidation to 2 inactive metabolites

Bioavailability: 100%

Half-life:

- Preterm neonate <1 week: 5.6 hours
- Full term neonate <1 week: 3 hours
- Full term neonate ≥1 week to ≤28 days: 1.5 hours
- Infants: 1.8 hours
- Children: 3 ± 1.1 hours
- Adolescents: 4.1 hours
- Adults: 4-5 hours

Time to peak serum concentration: Oral: 1-2 hours

Elimination: 65% nonrenal; 30% renal; 2 metabolites of linezolid may accumulate in patients with severe renal impairment

- Clearance: Children: 0.34 ± 0.15 L/hour/kg

Dialysis: 30% removed in a 3-hour hemodialysis session (linezolid dose should be given after hemodialysis)

Usual Dosage Note: No dosage adjustment needed when switching from I.V. to oral

Neonates 0-4 weeks and birthweight <1200 g: Oral, I.V.: 10 mg/kg/dose every 8-12 hours (**Note:** Use every 12 hours in patients <34 weeks gestation and <1 week of age)

Neonates <7 days and birthweight ≥1200 g: Oral, I.V.: 10 mg/kg/dose every 8-12 hours (**Note:** Use every 12 hours in patients <34 weeks gestation and <1 week of age)

Neonates ≥7 days and birthweight ≥1200 g, Infants, and Children:

- Complicated skin and skin structure infections, nosocomial or community-acquired pneumonia including concurrent bacteremia: Oral, I.V.: 10 mg/kg/dose every 8 hours for 10-14 days
- VREF: Oral, I.V.: 10 mg/kg/dose every 8 hours for 14-28 days
- Uncomplicated skin and skin structure infections: Oral:
  - Children <5 years: 10 mg/kg/dose every 8 hours for 10-14 days
  - Children 5-11 years: 10 mg/kg/dose every 12 hours for 10-14 days
- Sixty-six children 12 months to 17 years of age with community-acquired pneumonia were enrolled in a Phase II, open-label multicenter study of I.V. linezolid followed by oral linezolid with a mean total treatment duration of 12.2 ± 6.2 days (range: 6-41 days); 92.4% of patients were considered cured, one failed (methicillin-resistant *Staphylococcus aureus*) and 4 were considered indeterminate (Kaplan, 2001); pharmacokinetic data obtained in pediatric patients 0.3-16 years of age support an I.V. linezolid dose of 10 mg/kg/dose 2-3 times/day (Kearns, 2000)

Children ≥12 years and Adolescents:

- Uncomplicated skin and skin structure infections: Oral: 600 mg every 12 hours for 10-14 days
- Complicated skin and skin structure infections, nosocomial or community-acquired pneumonia including concurrent bacteremia: Oral, I.V.: 600 mg every 12 hours for 10-14 days
- VREF infections: Oral, I.V.: 600 mg every 12 hours for 14-28 days

Adults:

Uncomplicated skin and skin structure infections: Oral: 400 mg every 12 hours for 10-14 days

Complicated skin and skin structure infection, nosocomial or community-acquired pneumonia including concurrent bacteremia: Oral, I.V.: 600 mg every 12 hours for 10-14 days

VREF infections: Oral, I.V.: 600 mg every 12 hours for 14-28 days

Dosage adjustment in renal impairment: No adjustment is recommended

Dosage adjustment in hepatic impairment: Mild to moderate impairment (Child Pugh class A or B): No adjustment is recommended

Administration

Oral: Administer with or without food. Gently invert suspension bottle 3-5 times before use. Do not shake. Store at room temperature.

Parenteral: I.V.: Infuse over 30-120 minutes. 2 mg/mL infusion should be administered without further dilution. Do not mix or infuse with other medications. Flush line before and after infusion with a linezolid-compatible I.V. solution like D_5W, NS, or LR.

Monitoring Parameters CBC; platelet counts and hemoglobin, particularly in patients at increased risk for bleeding, patients with pre-existing thrombocytopenia or myelosuppression, patients with chronic infection who have received or who are on concomitant antibiotics, or concomitant medications that decrease platelet count or function or produce bone marrow suppression, and inpatients requiring >2 weeks of therapy; number and type of stools/day for diarrhea; visual function in patients requiring ≥3 months of therapy or in patients reporting new visual symptoms

Patient Information Avoid alcohol and excessive amounts of tyramine-containing foods while taking linezolid: Red wine, aged cheese, smoked or pickled fish, beef or chicken liver, sauerkraut, soy sauce, dried sausage, fava or broad bean pods; notify physician of changes in vision, persistent or worsening symptoms of infection, diarrhea, nausea, or vomiting; complete entire course of therapy even if symptoms improve

Dosage Forms Excipient information presented when available (limited, particularly for generics); consult specific product labeling. [CAN] = Canadian brand name

Infusion [premixed]:

Zyvox®: 200 mg (100 mL) [contains sodium 1.7 mEq]

Zyvox® [CAN]: 600 mg (300 mL) [contains sodium 5 mEq] [not available in the U.S.]

Powder for oral suspension:

Zyvox®: 20 mg/mL (150 mL) [contains phenylalanine 20 mg/5 mL, sodium benzoate, and sodium 0.4 mEq/5 mL; orange flavor]

Tablet:

Zyvox®: 600 mg [contains sodium 0.1 mEq/tablet]

References

Clemett D and Markham A, "Linezolid," *Drugs*, 2000, 59(4):815-27.

Kaplan SL, Patterson L, Edwards KM, et al, "Linezolid for the Treatment of Community-Acquired Pneumonia in Hospitalized Children. Linezolid Pediatric Pneumonia Study Group," *Pediatr Infect Dis J*, 2001, 20(5):488-94.

Kearns GL, Jungbluth GL, Abdel-Rahman SM, et al, "Impact of Ontogeny on Linezolid Disposition in Neonates and Infants," *Clin Pharmacol Ther*, 2003, 74(5):413-22.

Kearns GL, Abdel-Rahman SM, Blumer JL, et al, "Single Dose Pharmacokinetics of Linezolid in Infants and Children," *Pediatr Infect Dis J*, 2000, 19(12):1178-84.

Tan TQ, "Update on the Use of Linezolid: A Pediatric Perspective," *Pediatr Infect Dis J*, 2004, 23(10):955-6.

Taylor JJ, Wilson JW, and Estes LL, "Linezolid and Serotonergic Drug Interactions: A Retrospective Survey," *Clin Infect Dis*, 2006, 43(2):180-7.

♦ **Lin-Sotalol (Can)** *see* Sotalol *on page 1463*

♦ **Lioresal®** *see* Baclofen *on page 197*

♦ **Liotec (Can)** *see* Baclofen *on page 197*

Liothyronine (lye oh THYE roe neen)

Medication Safety Issues

Sound-alike/look-alike issues:

Liothyronine may be confused with levothyroxine

T3 is an error-prone abbreviation (mistaken as acetaminophen and codeine [ie, Tylenol® #3])

U.S. Brand Names Cytomel®; Triostat®

Canadian Brand Names Cytomel®

Index Terms Liothyronine Sodium; Sodium *L*-Triiodothyronine; T_3 Sodium (error-prone abbreviation)

Therapeutic Category Thyroid Product

Generic Available No

Use Replacement or supplemental therapy in congenital or acquired hypothyroidism, treatment or prevention of euthyroid goiters including thyroid nodules and chronic

(Continued)

Liothyronine *(Continued)*

lymphocytic thyroiditis; as a diagnostic aid in suppression tests to differentiate suspected mild hyperthyroidism or thyroid gland autonomy

Pregnancy Risk Factor A

Lactation Enters breast milk (small amounts)/compatible

Contraindications Hypersensitivity to liothyronine sodium or any component; recent MI or thyrotoxicosis; uncorrected adrenal insufficiency

Warnings Not for use in the treatment of obesity or for weight loss; in euthyroid patients, doses within the range of daily hormonal requirements are ineffective for weight reduction; larger doses may produce serious or even life-threatening toxic effects particularly when used with some anorectic drugs (sympathomimetic amines). Short duration of action permits more rapid assessment of dosage changes and rapid diminution of adverse effects upon discontinuation; transient partial loss of hair in pediatrics may be seen in the first few months of therapy.

Precautions Use with extreme caution in patients with cardiovascular disease, adrenal insufficiency, or coronary artery disease; use with extreme caution in patients receiving digoxin or vasopressors (see Drug Interactions); use with caution in patients with diabetes mellitus and diabetes insipidus as symptoms of their disease may be exaggerated or aggravated; myxedematous patients are very sensitive to thyroid supplements; initiate therapy at very low doses and increase gradually

Adverse Reactions

Cardiovascular: Palpitations, tachycardia, cardiac arrhythmias, angina, CHF, hypertension

Central nervous system: Nervousness, insomnia, fever, headache, irritability

Dermatologic: Alopecia, dermatitis herpetiformis, hair loss (transient)

Endocrine & metabolic: Weight loss

Gastrointestinal: Diarrhea, abdominal cramps, increased appetite

Local: Phlebitis with parenteral form

Neuromuscular & skeletal: Tremor

Miscellaneous: Diaphoresis

Drug Interactions Antacids (aluminum-, magnesium-, and calcium carbonate-containing), cholestyramine resin, iron salts, sodium polystyrene sulfonate, and sucralfate decrease absorption; estrogens, clofibrate, methadone, fluorouracil, mitotane, and tamoxifen increase thyroid requirements; liothyronine increases effect of oral anticoagulants; phenytoin, carbamazepine, phenobarbital, rifampin, amiodarone, propylthiouracil, and β-adrenergic antagonists may decrease thyroid levels; androgens, anabolic steroids, asparaginase, glucocorticoids, and slow-release nicotinic acid decrease thyroid requirements; concurrent use with sympathomimetics, TCAs, and SSRIs may enhance the toxic effects of both drugs; use with ketamine may produce significant tachycardia and hypertension; may increase insulin and other antidiabetic agent requirements; increases the adrenergic effect of catecholamines (epinephrine, norepinephrine); may potentiate the toxic effects of digoxin

Food Interactions Limit intake of goitrogenic foods (asparagus, cabbage, peas, turnip greens, broccoli, spinach, brussel sprouts, lettuce, soybeans)

Stability Store tablets at controlled room temperature; refrigerate parenteral solution at temperatures between 2°C and 8°C (36°F to 46°F)

Mechanism of Action Primary active compound is T_3 (triiodothyronine), which may be converted from T_4 (thyroxine) by deiodination in liver and peripheral tissues; exact mechanism of action is unknown; however, it is believed the thyroid hormone exerts its many metabolic effects through control of DNA transcription and protein synthesis; involved in normal metabolism, growth, and development; promotes gluconeogenesis, increases utilization and mobilization of glycogen stores, and stimulates protein synthesis, increases basal metabolic rate

Pharmacodynamics I.V., Oral:

Onset of action: Within a few hours

Maximum effect: Within 48 hours

Duration: Up to 72 hours

Pharmacokinetics

Absorption: Oral: Well absorbed (~85% to 90%)

Metabolism: In the liver to inactive compounds

Half-life: 25 hours (range: 16-49 hours); hypothyroid 1.4 days; hyperthyroid 0.6 days

Elimination: 76% to 83% In urine

Usual Dosage

Congenital hypothyroidism (Cretinism): Neonates, Infants, and Children <3 years: Oral: 5 mcg/day; increase by 5 mcg every 3 days to a maximum dosage of 20 mcg/day for neonates and infants, 50 mcg/day for children 1-3 years of age

Hypothyroidism:

Children: Oral: 5 mcg/day increase in 5 mcg/day increments every 3-4 days; Usual maintenance dose:

Infants: 20 mcg/day

Children 1-3 years: 50 mcg/day

Children >3 years: Full adult dosage may be necessary

Adults: Oral: 25 mcg/day increase in 12.5-25 mcg/day increments every 1-2 weeks to a maximum of 100 mcg/day

Goiter, nontoxic:

Children: Oral: 5 mcg/day increase in 5 mcg/day increments every 1-2 weeks; usual maintenance dose 15-20 mcg/day

Adults: Oral: 5 mcg/day; increase in 5-10 mcg/day increments every 1-2 weeks; when 25 mcg is reached, increase dosage in 12.5-25 mcg increments every 1-2 weeks; usual maintenance dosage: 75 mcg/day

T_3 suppression test: Adults: Oral: 75-100 mcg/day for 7 days

Myxedema coma: Adults:

I.V.: 25-50 mcg; reduce dosage in patients with known or suspected cardiovascular disease to 10-20 mcg

Note: Normally, at least 4 hours should be allowed between I.V. doses to adequately assess therapeutic response and no more than 12 hours should elapse between doses to avoid fluctuations in hormone levels.

Oral (**Note:** Due to potential poor oral absorption in the acute phase of myxedema, oral therapy should be avoided until the clinical situation has been stabilized): 5 mcg/day; increase in 5-10 mcg/day increments every 1-2 weeks; when 25 mcg/day is reached; increase by 5-25 mcg/day increments every 1-2 weeks; usual maintenance dose: 50-100 mcg/day

Administration

Oral: Administer on an empty stomach

Parenteral: I.V.: For I.V. use only; do not administer SubQ or I.M.; should not be admixed with other solutions

Monitoring Parameters T_3, TSH, heart rate, blood pressure, clinical signs of hypo- and hyperthyroidism; TSH is the most reliable guide for evaluating adequacy of thyroid replacement dosage. TSH may be elevated during the first few months of thyroid replacement despite patients being clinically euthyroid.

Suggested frequency for monitoring thyroid function tests in children: Every 1-2 months during the first year of life, every 2-3 months between ages 1-3 years, and every 3-12 months thereafter until growth is completed; repeat tests two weeks after any change in dosage.

Reference Range See normal values in Normal Laboratory Values for Children *on page 1881*

Test Interactions Many drugs may have effects on thyroid function tests (ie, para-aminosalicylic acid, aminoglutethimide, amiodarone, barbiturates, carbamazepine, chloral hydrate, clofibrate, colestipol, corticosteroids, danazol, diazepam, estrogens, ethionamide, fluorouracil, I.V. heparin, insulin, lithium, methadone, methimazole, mitotane, nitroprusside, oxyphenbutazone, phenylbutazone, PTU, perphenazine, phenytoin, propranolol, salicylates, sulfonylureas, and thiazides)

Patient Information Do not change brands without physician's knowledge; report immediately to physician any chest pain, increased pulse, palpitations, heat intolerance, excessive sweating; do not discontinue without notifying physician

Additional Information 15-37.5 mcg liothyronine = 50-60 mcg levothyroxine = 60 mg thyroid USP

Dosage Forms Excipient information presented when available (limited, particularly for generics); consult specific product labeling.

Injection, solution, as sodium (Triostat®): 10 mcg/mL (1 mL) [contains alcohol 6.8%]

Tablet, as sodium (Cytomel®): 5 mcg, 25 mcg, 50 mcg

- ♦ **Liothyronine Sodium** *see* Liothyronine *on page 943*
- ♦ **Lipancreatin** *see* Pancrelipase *on page 1203*
- ♦ **Lipitor®** *see* Atorvastatin *on page 175*
- ♦ **Liposyn® II (Can)** *see* Fat Emulsion *on page 640*
- ♦ **Liposyn® III** *see* Fat Emulsion *on page 640*
- ♦ **Lipram 4500** *see* Pancrelipase *on page 1203*
- ♦ **Lipram-CR** *see* Pancrelipase *on page 1203*
- ♦ **Lipram-PN** *see* Pancrelipase *on page 1203*
- ♦ **Lipram-UL** *see* Pancrelipase *on page 1203*
- ♦ **Liquid Antidote** *see* Charcoal, Activated *on page 328*
- ♦ **Liqui-Doss® [OTC]** *see* Mineral Oil *on page 1065*
- ♦ **Liquid Paraffin** *see* Mineral Oil *on page 1065*

Lisinopril (lyse IN oh pril)

Medication Safety Issues

Sound-alike/look-alike issues:

Lisinopril may be confused with fosinopril, Lioresal®, Risperdal®

Prinivil® may be confused with Plendil®, Pravachol®, Prevacid®, Prilosec®, Proventil®

Zestril® may be confused with Desyrel®, Restoril®, Vistaril®, Zetia™, Zostrix®

International issues:

Acepril® [Denmark] may be confused with Accupril® which is a brand name for quinapril in the U.S.

Acepril®: Brand name for enalapril in Hungary and Switzerland; brand name for captopril in Great Britain

Carace® [Ireland; Great Britain] may be confused with Carac™ which is a brand name for fluorouracil in the U.S.

Zetril® may be confused with Nostril® which is a brand name for chlorhexidine/cetrimonium in France

Related Information

Antihypertensive Agents by Class *on page 1678*

U.S. Brand Names Prinivil®; Zestril®

Canadian Brand Names Apo-Lisinopril®; Prinivil®; Zestril®

Therapeutic Category Angiotensin-Converting Enzyme (ACE) Inhibitor; Antihypertensive Agent

Generic Available Yes

Use Management of hypertension; adjunctive treatment of CHF; adjunctive therapy in hemodynamically stable post MI patients to improve survival

Pregnancy Risk Factor C (1st trimester); D (may cause injury and death to the developing fetus when used during the 2nd and 3rd trimesters of pregnancy)

Lactation Excretion in breast milk unknown/not recommended

Contraindications Hypersensitivity to lisinopril, any component, or other ACE inhibitors; patients with idiopathic or hereditary angioedema or a history of angioedema with previous ACE inhibitor use

Warnings Serious adverse effects including angioedema, anaphylactoid reactions, neutropenia, agranulocytosis, hypotension, and hepatic failure may occur (see Adverse Reactions). Angioedema may occur in the head, neck, extremities, or intestines; angioedema of the larynx, glottis, or tongue may cause airway obstruction, especially in patients with a history of airway surgery; prolonged monitoring may be required, even in patients with swelling of only the tongue (ie, without respiratory distress) because treatment with corticosteroids and antihistamines may not be sufficient; very rare fatalities have occurred with angioedema of the larynx or tongue; appropriate treatment (eg, establishing patent airway and/or SubQ epinephrine) should be readily available for patients with angioedema of larynx, glottis, or tongue, in whom airway obstruction is likely to occur. Risk of neutropenia may be increased in patients with renal dysfunction, especially if the patients have collagen vascular diseases.

Precautions Use with caution and modify dosage in patients with renal impairment, especially renal artery stenosis; elevated BUN and S_{cr} may occur in these patients; discontinuation of concomitant diuretic or lisinopril may be needed; use with caution and modify dosage in patients with hyponatremia, hypovolemia, severe CHF, left ventricular outflow tract obstruction, or with coadministered diuretic therapy. Severe hypotension may occur in patients who are sodium and/or volume depleted; initiate lower doses and monitor closely when starting therapy in these patients.

Adverse Reactions **Note:** No relevant differences in adverse reactions between pediatric and adult patients has been identified.

Cardiovascular: Hypotension, chest discomfort, orthostatic hypotension, syncope

Central nervous system: Dizziness, headache, fatigue

Dermatologic: Rash, angioedema (see Warnings); **Note:** The relative risk of angioedema with ACE inhibitors is higher within the first 30 days of use (compared to >1 year of use), for Black Americans (compared to Whites), for lisinopril or enalapril (compared to captopril), and for patients previously hospitalized within 30 days (Brown, 1996).

Endocrine & metabolic: Hyperkalemia

Gastrointestinal: Diarrhea, nausea, vomiting, ageusia, intestinal angioedema (rare)

Hematologic: Neutropenia, agranulocytosis

Hepatic: Cholestatic jaundice, hepatitis, fulminant hepatic necrosis (rare, but potentially fatal)

Renal: Elevated BUN, elevated serum creatinine

Respiratory: Cough, dyspnea, eosinophilic pneumonitis; **Note:** An isolated dry cough lasting >3 weeks was reported in 7 of 42 pediatric patients (17%) receiving ACE inhibitors (see von Vigier, 2000)

Neuromuscular & skeletal: Weakness
Miscellaneous: Anaphylactoid reactions

Drug Interactions Use with potassium-sparing diuretics may result in an additive hyperkalemic effect; diuretics and other antihypertensive agents may increase hypotensive effect; indomethacin or NSAIDs may decrease hypotensive effect; lisinopril may increase lithium levels; use with NSAIDs in patients with renal impairment may further decrease renal function (usually reversible)

Food Interactions Food does not effect oral absorption; limit salt substitutes or potassium-rich diet; avoid natural licorice (causes sodium and water retention and increases potassium loss)

Mechanism of Action Competitive inhibitor of angiotensin-converting enzyme (ACE); prevents conversion of angiotensin I to angiotensin II, a potent vasoconstrictor; results in lower levels of angiotensin II which causes an increase in plasma renin activity and a reduction in aldosterone secretion

Pharmacodynamics
Onset of action (decrease in blood pressure): 1 hour
Maximum effect: 6-8 hours
Duration: 24 hours

Pharmacokinetics
Absorption: Oral:
Children 6-16 years: 28%
Adults: 25% (range: 6% to 60%)
Protein binding: 25%
Half-life: 11-13 hours; half-life increases with renal dysfunction
Time to peak serum concentration:
Children 6-16 years: Within 6 hours
Adults: Within 7 hours
Elimination: Excreted in urine as unchanged drug
Dialysis: Removable by hemodialysis

Usual Dosage Oral: Dosage must be titrated according to patient's response; **use lower doses (~1/2 of those listed) for patients with hyponatremia, hypovolemia, severe CHF, decreased renal function, or in those receiving diuretics:**
Hypertension (**Note:** If possible, discontinue diuretics 2-3 days prior to initiating lisinopril; restart diuretic, if needed, after blood pressure is stable):
Children <6 years: No dosing information available; manufacturer does not recommend use
Children ≥6 years: Initial: 0.07 mg/kg once daily; maximum initial dose: 5 mg once daily; increase dose at 1- to 2-week intervals; doses >0.61 mg/kg or >40 mg have not been evaluated
Adults: Initial: 10 mg/day given once daily; increase dose by 5-10 mg/day at 1- to 2-week intervals; usual dose: 20-40 mg/day given once daily; doses up to 80 mg/day have been used, but do not appear to have a greater effect; usual dosage range (JNC 7): 10-40 mg once daily
CHF: Adults: Initial: 5 mg once daily (with diuretics and digitalis); increase dose by ≤10 mg/day at ≥2 week intervals based on clinical response; usual dose: 5-40 mg/day given once daily; maximum dose: 40 mg/day

Dosing adjustment in renal impairment:
Children: Cl_{cr} <30 mL/minute/1.73 m^2: Use is not recommended
Adults:
Hypertension: Modify initial dose and cautiously titrate dose based on clinical response; maximum dose: 40 mg once daily
Cl_{cr} >30 mL/minute: Usual: 10 mg once daily
Cl_{cr} 10-30 mL/minute: Initial: 5 mg once daily
Cl_{cr} <10 mL/minute (usually on hemodialysis): Initial: 2.5 mg once daily
CHF: Cl_{cr} <30 mL/minute or serum creatinine >3 mg/dL: Initial: 2.5 mg/day

Administration Oral: May be administered without regard to food

Monitoring Parameters Blood pressure, BUN, serum creatinine, renal function, WBC, and serum potassium

Patient Information Limit alcohol; notify physician if vomiting, diarrhea, excessive perspiration, or dehydration occurs or if swelling of face, lips, tongue or difficulty in breathing occurs; do not use a salt substitute (potassium-containing) without physician advice

Nursing Implications Discontinue if angioedema occurs; observe closely for hypotension after the first dose or initiation of a new higher dose (keep in mind that maximum effect on blood pressure occurs at 6-8 hours)

Dosage Forms Excipient information presented when available (limited, particularly for generics); consult specific product labeling. [DSC] = Discontinued product
Tablet: 2.5 mg, 5 mg, 10 mg, 20 mg, 30 mg, 40 mg
Prinivil®: 5 mg, 10 mg, 20 mg, 30 mg; 40 mg [DSC]
Zestril®: 2.5 mg, 5 mg, 10 mg, 20 mg, 30 mg, 40 mg
(Continued)

Lisinopril *(Continued)*

Extemporaneous Preparations

A 1 mg/mL lisinopril suspension made from tablets, Bicitra®, and Ora-Sweet SF™ is stable for up to 4 weeks when stored at ≤25°C (77°F) in a polyethylene terephthalate bottle; add 10 mL of purified water (USP) to a bottle containing ten 20 mg lisinopril tablets; shake for ≥1 minute; add 30 mL of Bicitra® and 160 mL of Ora-Sweet SF™ to the mixture in the bottle; shake gently to suspend the contents; label "shake well" [Prinivil® (package insert), 2003 and Zestril® (package insert), 2003].

A 2 mg/mL lisinopril syrup made from powder (Sigma Chemical Company, St. Louis, MO) and simple syrup was stable for 30 days when stored in amber plastic prescription bottles at room temperature (23°C) or under refrigeration (5°C); dissolve 1 gram of lisinopril powder in 30 mL of distilled water; incorporate resultant solution into syrup using geometric dilution and qsad to 500 mL; label "shake well" and "refrigerate"; **Note:** Although no visual evidence of microbial growth was observed, the authors recommend storage at 5°C to inhibit microbial growth (Webster, 1997).

Webster AA, English BA, and Rose DJ, "The Stability of Lisinopril as an Extemporaneous Syrup," *Intr J Pharmaceut Compound*, 1997, 1:352-3.

Prinivil® (package insert), Whitehouse Station, NJ: Merck & Co, Inc, 2003.

Zestril® (package insert), Wilmington, DE: AstraZeneca Pharmaceuticals, 2003.

References

Brown NJ, Ray WA, Snowden M, et al, "Black Americans Have an Increased Rate of Angiotensin-Converting Enzyme Inhibitor-Associated Angioedema," *Clin Pharmacol Ther*, 1996, 60(1):8-13.

Chase SL and Sutton JD, "Lisinopril: A New Angiotensin-Converting Enzyme Inhibitor," *Pharmacotherapy*, 1989, 9(3):120-30.

Chobanian AV, Bakris GL, Black HR, et al, "The Seventh Report of the Joint National Committee on Prevention, Detection, Evaluation, and Treatment of High Blood Pressure: The JNC 7 report," *JAMA*, 2003, 289(19):2560-72.

Raia JJ Jr, Barone JA, Byerly WG, et al, "Angiotensin-Converting Enzymes Inhibitors: A Comparative Review," *DICP*, 1990, 24(5):506-25.

von Vigier RO, Mozzettini S, Truttmann AC, et al, "Cough is Common in Children Prescribed Converting Enzyme Inhibitors," *Nephron*, 2000, 84(1):98.

♦ **Lispro Insulin** *see* Insulin Lispro *on page 844*

♦ **Lithane™ (Can)** *see* Lithium *on page 948*

Lithium (LITH ee um)

Medication Safety Issues

Sound-alike/look-alike issues:

Eskalith® may be confused with Estratest®

Lithobid® may be confused with Levbid®, Lithostat®

Do not confuse **mEq** (milliequivalent) with **mg** (milligram). **Note:** 8 mEq lithium carbonate equals 300 mg lithium carbonate. Dosage should be written in **mg** (milligrams) to avoid confusion. Check prescriptions for unusually high volumes of the syrup for dosing errors.

Related Information

Serotonin Syndrome *on page 1955*

U.S. Brand Names Eskalith® [DSC]; Eskalith CR® [DSC]; Lithobid®

Canadian Brand Names Apo-Lithium® Carbonate; Apo-Lithium® Carbonate SR; Carbolith™; Duralith®; Lithane™; PMS-Lithium Carbonate; PMS-Lithium Citrate

Index Terms Lithium Carbonate; Lithium Citrate

Therapeutic Category Antidepressant, Miscellaneous; Antimanic Agent

Generic Available Yes

Use Management of acute manic episodes; mania in individuals with bipolar disorder (maintenance treatment diminishes or prevents intensity of subsequent manic episodes); depression; has been used investigationally to treat severe aggression in children and adolescents with conduct disorder (see Additional Information)

Pregnancy Risk Factor D

Lactation Enters breast milk/contraindicated

Contraindications Hypersensitivity to lithium or any component (see Warnings). Generally, avoid use in patients with severe cardiovascular or renal disease, severe dehydration or debilitation, sodium depletion, and in patients receiving ACE inhibitors or diuretics (these patients are at very high risk of lithium toxicity)

Warnings Lithium toxicity is closely related to serum levels and can occur at therapeutic doses; serum lithium determinations are required to monitor therapy; chronic lithium therapy may result in diminished renal concentrating ability (eg, nephrogenic diabetes insipidus). An encephalopathic syndrome (resembling neuroleptic malignant syndrome) may occur in patients receiving lithium with haloperidol or other antipsychotic agents (see Drug Interactions).

Capsule may contain benzyl alcohol which may cause allergic reactions in susceptible individuals; large amounts of benzyl alcohol (≥99 mg/kg/day) have been associated with a potentially fatal toxicity ("gasping syndrome") in neonates; avoid use of lithium products containing benzyl alcohol in neonates; *in vitro* and animal studies have shown that benzoate, a metabolite of benzyl alcohol, displaces bilirubin from protein binding sites

Precautions Use with caution in patients with cardiovascular or thyroid disease, patients receiving medications that alter sodium excretion (eg, diuretics, ACE inhibitors, or NSAIDs), and in patients with significant fluid loss (protracted sweating, diarrhea, or prolonged fever); monitor lithium levels closely, lithium dosage reduction or temporary cessation may be required. Use with caution and modify dose in patients with renal dysfunction.

Adverse Reactions

Cardiovascular: Arrhythmias, sinus node dysfunction, hypotension, severe bradycardia, syncope

Central nervous system: Sedation, confusion, somnolence, seizures, fatigue, headache, vertigo, dizziness, slurred speech, blackout spells, restlessness, ataxia, dystonia

Dermatologic: Rash, drying and thinning of hair, alopecia, anesthesia of skin, chronic folliculitis, exacerbation of psoriasis

Endocrine & metabolic: Nephrogenic diabetes insipidus (thirst, polyuria, polydipsia), goiter, hypothyroidism; rarely hyperthyroidism

Gastrointestinal: Nausea, diarrhea, vomiting, xerostomia, anorexia, gastritis, salivary gland swelling, excessive salivation

Genitourinary: Oliguria, polyuria, albuminuria, glycosuria

Hematologic: Leukocytosis

Neuromuscular & skeletal: Muscle hyperirritability, muscle weakness, tremor, choreoathetoid movements

Ocular: Nystagmus, blurred vision

Miscellaneous: Coldness and painful discoloration of fingers and toes

Drug Interactions Diuretics, indomethacin, NSAIDs, cyclooxygenase-2 (COX-2) inhibitors, ACE inhibitors, angiotensin II receptor antagonists (eg, losartan), metronidazole may decrease lithium renal excretion and enhance lithium toxicity (monitor lithium levels closely); iodide salts (or iodine) may increase hypothyroid effects; use with haloperidol or other antipsychotic agents may result in an encephalopathic syndrome and irreversible brain damage (monitor patients closely; discontinue therapy promptly if neurological toxicity occurs); lithium may prolong the effects of neuromuscular blocking agents (use with caution; monitor closely); carbamazepine, calcium channel blocking agents, methyldopa may increase neurotoxic side effects; acetazolamide, alkalinizing agents (eg, sodium bicarbonate), urea and xanthine products may increase urinary lithium excretion and decrease lithium serum concentrations; fluoxetine may increase or decrease lithium serum concentrations (monitor closely); use of lithium with SSRIs may increase GI and CNS adverse effects; phenytoin may increase lithium toxicity

Food Interactions Avoid changes in sodium content of diet (reduction in sodium intake can increase lithium toxicity); syrup may precipitate in tube feedings

Stability Store at controlled room temperature; protect slow-release tablets from moisture

Mechanism of Action Alters cation transport across cell membrane in nerve and muscle cells and influences reuptake of serotonin and/or norepinephrine

Pharmacokinetics

Distribution: Crosses the placenta; appears in breast milk at 35% to 50% of the concentrations in serum

Adults:

V_d: Initial: 0.3-0.4 L/kg

V_{dss}: 0.7-1 L/kg

Half-life, terminal: Adults: 18-24 hours, can increase to more than 36 hours in patients with renal impairment

Time to peak serum concentration (nonsustained release product): Within 0.5-2 hours

Elimination: 90% to 98% of a dose is excreted in the urine as unchanged drug; other excretory routes include feces (1%) and sweat (4% to 5%)

Dialysis: Dialyzable (50% to 100%)

Usual Dosage Oral: Monitor serum concentrations and clinical response (efficacy and toxicity) to determine proper dose

Children: 15-60 mg/kg/day in 3-4 divided doses; dose not to exceed usual adult dosage; initiate at lower dose and adjust dose weekly based on levels

Adolescents: 600-1800 mg/day in 3-4 divided doses for regular tablets or 2 divided doses for sustained release tablets

Adults: 300 mg 3-4 times/day; usual maximum maintenance dose: 2.4 g/day or 450-900 mg of sustained release tablets twice daily

(Continued)

Lithium *(Continued)*

Dosing adjustment in renal impairment:

Cl_{cr} 10-50 mL/minute: Administer 50% to 75% of normal dose

Cl_{cr} <10 mL/minute: Administer 25% to 50% of normal dose

Administration Oral: Administer with meals to decrease GI upset; do not crush or chew slow- or controlled-release dosage form, swallow whole

Monitoring Parameters Serum lithium every 3-4 days during initial therapy; once patient is clinically stable and serum concentrations are stable, serum lithium may be obtained every 1-2 months; obtain lithium serum concentrations 8-12 hours postdose (ie, just before next dose); renal, hepatic, thyroid and cardiovascular function; CBC with differential, urinalysis, serum sodium, calcium, potassium

Reference Range

Therapeutic: Acute mania: 0.6-1.2 mEq/L (SI: 0.6-1.2 mmol/L); protection against future episodes in most patients with bipolar disorder: 0.8-1 mEq/L (SI: 0.8-1 mmol/L). A higher rate of relapse is described in subjects who are maintained <0.4 mEq/L (SI: <0.4 mmol/L)

Toxic: >2 mEq/L (SI: >2 mmol/L)

Concentration-related adverse effects:

GI complaints/tremor: 1.5-2 mEq/L

Confusion/somnolence: 2-2.5 mEq/L

Seizures/death: >2.5 mEq/L

Patient Information Limit caffeine; limit alcohol; avoid tasks requiring psychomotor coordination until CNS effects are known; may cause dry mouth; blood level monitoring is required to determine the proper dose; maintain a steady salt and fluid intake especially during the summer months; avoid dehydration; notify physician if vomiting, diarrhea, muscle weakness, tremor, drowsiness, or ataxia occur (these may be signs of lithium toxicity)

Nursing Implications Avoid dehydration

Additional Information In terms of efficacy, the results of studies using lithium to treat severe aggression in children and adolescents with conduct disorders, are mixed. A double-blind, placebo-controlled trial in patients 10-17 years of age (n=40) demonstrated efficacy for lithium in reducing aggressive behavior in psychiatrically hospitalized patients with conduct disorder and severe aggression. Lithium was initiated at 600 mg/day and titrated upwards by 300 mg/day. Final lithium carbonate doses ranged from 900-2100 mg/day divided into 3 doses/day (mean ± SD: 1425 ± 321 mg/day); serum lithium concentrations ranged from 0.78-1.55 mmol/L (mean ± SD: 1.07 ± 0.19 mmol/L) (see Malone, 2000). In an earlier double-blind, placebo-controlled study in 50 children 5-12 years of age (mean ± SD: 9.4 ± 1.8 years), lithium was also initiated at 600 mg/day in 3 divided doses. Doses were titrated upwards in 300 mg/day increments. The mean optimal lithium dose was 1248 mg/day (range: 600-1800 mg/day); serum lithium concentrations ranged from 0.53-1.79 mmol/L (mean: 1.12 mmol/L). Doses >1500 mg/day and serum concentrations >1.13 mmol/L did not provide additional benefit (see Campbell, 1995). Several other studies have not demonstrated efficacy; further studies are needed.

Dosage Forms Excipient information presented when available (limited, particularly for generics); consult specific product labeling. [DSC] = Discontinued product

Capsule, as carbonate: 150 mg, 300 mg, 600 mg

Eskalith®: 300 mg [contains benzyl alcohol] [DSC]

Solution, as citrate: 300 mg/5 mL (5 mL, 500 mL) [equivalent to amount of lithium in lithium carbonate]

Syrup, as citrate: 300 mg/5 mL (480 mL) [equivalent to amount of lithium in lithium carbonate]

Tablet, as carbonate: 300 mg

Tablet, controlled release, as carbonate: 450 mg

Eskalith CR®: 450 mg [DSC]

Tablet, slow release, as carbonate: 300 mg

Lithobid®: 300 mg

References

Campbell M, Adams PB, Small AM, et al, "Lithium in Hospitalized Aggressive Children With Conduct Disorder: A Double-Blind and Placebo-Controlled Study," *J Am Acad Child Adolesc Psychiatry*, 1995, 34(4):445-53.

Campbell M, Kafantaris V, and Cueva JE, "An Update on the Use of Lithium Carbonate in Aggressive Children and Adolescents With Conduct Disorder," *Psychopharmacol Bull*, 1995a, 31(1):93-102.

Levy HB, Harper CR, and Weinberg WA, "A Practical Approach to Children Failing in School," *Pediatr Clin North Am*, 1992, 39(4):895-928.

Malone RP, Delaney MA, Luebbert JF, et al, "A Double-Blind Placebo-Controlled Study of Lithium in Hospitalized Aggressive Children and Adolescents With Conduct Disorder," *Arch Gen Psychiatry*, 2000, 57(7):649-54.

Weller EB, Weller RA, and Fristad MA, "Lithium Dosage Guide for Prepubertal Children: A Preliminary Report," *J Am Acad Child Psychiatry*, 1986, 25(1):92-5.

♦ **Lithium Carbonate** *see* Lithium *on page 948*

- **Lithium Citrate** *see* Lithium *on page 948*
- **Lithobid®** *see* Lithium *on page 948*
- **Live, Attenuated Influenza Vaccine** *see* Influenza Virus Vaccine (Live/Attenuated) *on page 835*
- **LMD®** *see* Dextran *on page 468*
- **Locoid®** *see* Hydrocortisone *on page 781*
- **Locoid Lipocream®** *see* Hydrocortisone *on page 781*
- **Lodrane®** *see* Brompheniramine and Pseudoephedrine *on page 235*
- **Lodrane® 12D** *see* Brompheniramine and Pseudoephedrine *on page 235*
- **Lodrane® 24D** *see* Brompheniramine and Pseudoephedrine *on page 235*
- **Lodrane® D** *see* Brompheniramine and Pseudoephedrine *on page 235*
- **LoHist 12D** *see* Brompheniramine and Pseudoephedrine *on page 235*
- **LoHist LQ** *see* Brompheniramine and Pseudoephedrine *on page 235*
- **LoHist PD** *see* Brompheniramine and Pseudoephedrine *on page 235*
- **L-OHP** *see* Oxaliplatin *on page 1179*
- **Lomine (Can)** *see* Dicyclomine *on page 490*
- **Lomotil®** *see* Diphenoxylate and Atropine *on page 512*

Lomustine (loe MUS teen)

Medication Safety Issues

Sound-alike/look-alike issues:

Lomustine may be confused with carmustine

High alert medication: The Institute for Safe Medication Practices (ISMP) includes this medication among its list of drugs which have a heightened risk of causing significant patient harm when used in error.

Lomustine should only be administered as a single dose once every 6 weeks; serious errors have occurred when lomustine was inadvertently administered daily.

Related Information

Emetogenic Potential of Single Chemotherapeutic Agents *on page 1776*

U.S. Brand Names CeeNU®

Canadian Brand Names CeeNU®

Index Terms CCNU; NSC-79037

Therapeutic Category Antineoplastic Agent, Alkylating Agent (Nitrosourea)

Generic Available No

Use Treatment of brain tumors, Hodgkin's disease, non-Hodgkin's lymphomas, melanoma, renal carcinoma, lung cancer, colon cancer

Pregnancy Risk Factor D

Lactation Enters breast milk/contraindicated

Contraindications Hypersensitivity to lomustine or any component; pregnancy

Warnings The FDA currently recommends that procedures for proper handling and disposal of antineoplastic agents be considered. Lomustine should be administered under the supervision of a physician experienced in the use of cancer chemotherapy agents. Bone marrow suppression, notably thrombocytopenia and leukopenia, may lead to bleeding and overwhelming infections in an already compromised patient; nadir: ~6 weeks; do not give courses more frequently than every 6 weeks because the toxicity is cumulative; pulmonary toxicity from lomustine appears to be dose-related; lomustine has been found to be mutagenic, teratogenic, embryotoxic, and carcinogenic in animals.

Precautions Use with caution in patients with depressed platelet, leukocyte or erythrocyte counts; reduced dosages are recommended. Use with caution in patients with renal or hepatic impairment.

Adverse Reactions

Central nervous system: Disorientation, lethargy, ataxia

Dermatologic: Alopecia

Gastrointestinal: Nausea and vomiting (usually within 3-6 hours after oral administration), stomatitis, anorexia, diarrhea

Hematologic: Anemia, thrombocytopenia, leukopenia, myelosuppression (occurs 4-6 weeks after a dose and may persist 1-2 weeks)

Hepatic: Hepatotoxicity; elevation of hepatic enzymes, alkaline phosphatase, and bilirubin

Neuromuscular & skeletal: Dysarthria

Ocular: Blindness, optic atrophy

Renal: Renal failure, interstitial nephritis, azotemia

Respiratory: Pulmonary fibrosis with total cumulative dose >1 g/m^2 with onset occurring after 6 months or longer from the start of therapy; delayed-onset fibrosis may occur up to 17 years after treatment

(Continued)

Lomustine *(Continued)*

Miscellaneous: Secondary malignancies

Drug Interactions Cytochrome P450 isoenzyme CYP2D6 inhibitor

Phenobarbital may increase metabolism and reduce activity of lomustine; cimetidine may decrease metabolism and increase myelotoxicity of lomustine

Food Interactions Avoid concurrent administration of food/drugs that cause vomiting

Stability Store at 15°C to 30°C. Avoid exposure to excessive heat (>40°C) and prolonged exposure to moisture

Mechanism of Action Inhibits DNA and RNA synthesis through DNA alkylation and DNA cross-linking; carbamoylates amine groups on proteins; inhibits DNA polymerase activity, RNA and protein synthesis

Pharmacokinetics

Absorption: Rapid and complete absorption from the GI tract (30-60 minutes)

Distribution: Lomustine and/or its metabolites penetrate into the CNS; metabolites are present in breast milk

Metabolism: Rapid conversion to 4-hydroxy metabolites (active) partially by liver microsomal enzymes during first pass through the liver

Half-life, terminal (active metabolite): 1.3-2 days

Time to peak serum concentration (of active metabolite): Within 3 hours

Elimination: Excreted primarily in urine as metabolites; <5% fecal excretion

Usual Dosage Oral (refer to individual protocol):

Children: 75-150 mg/m^2 as a single dose every 6 weeks; subsequent doses are readjusted after initial treatment according to platelet and leukocyte counts

Subsequent dosing adjustment based on nadir:

Platelet nadirs 50,000-74,999/mm^3: Reduce dosage by 25%

Platelet nadirs 25,000-49,999/mm^3: Reduce dosage by 50%

Platelet nadirs <25,000/mm^3: Reduce dosage by 75%

Adults: 100-130 mg/m^2 as a single dose every 6 weeks; readjust after initial treatment according to platelet and leukocyte counts. Repeat courses should only be administered after adequate recovery: WBC >4000/mm^3 and platelet count >100,00/mm^3

With compromised marrow function: Initial dose: 100 mg/m^2 as a single dose every 6 weeks

Subsequent dosing adjustment based on nadir:

Leukocytes 2000-2999/mm^3, platelets 25,000-74,999/mm^3: Administer 70% of prior dose

Leukocytes <2000/mm^3, platelets <25,000/mm^3: Administer 50% of prior dose

Administration Oral: Administer with fluids on an empty stomach; do not administer food or drink for 2 hours after lomustine administration to decrease incidence of nausea and vomiting

Monitoring Parameters CBC with differential and platelet count, hepatic and renal function tests, pulmonary function tests (forced vital capacity, carbon monoxide diffusing capacity)

Patient Information Wear gloves when handling lomustine capsules. Notify physician if fever, chills, sore throat, bleeding, bruising, dry cough, swelling of feet or lower legs, shortness of breath, mental confusion, or yellowing of the eyes or skin occur; avoid alcohol for short periods after taking lomustine. Women of childbearing potential should be advised to avoid becoming pregnant while taking lomustine.

Dosage Forms Excipient information presented when available (limited, particularly for generics); consult specific product labeling.

Capsule:

CeeNU®: 10 mg, 40 mg, 100 mg

Capsule [dose pack]:

CeeNU®: 10 mg (2s); 40 mg (2s); 100 mg (2s)

References

Berg SL, Grisell DL, DeLaney TF, et al, "Principles of Treatment of Pediatric Solid Tumors," *Pediatr Clin North Am*, 1991, 38(2):249-67.

Pendergrass TW, Milstein JM, Geyer JR, et al, "Eight Drugs in One Day Chemotherapy for Brain Tumors: Experience in 107 Children and Rationale for Preradiation Chemotherapy," *J Clin Oncol*, 1987, 5(8):1221-31.

♦ **Lonox®** *see* Diphenoxylate and Atropine *on page 512*

♦ **Loperacap (Can)** *see* Loperamide *on page 952*

Loperamide (loe PER a mide)

Medication Safety Issues

Sound-alike/look-alike issues:

Imodium® A-D may be confused with Indocin®, Ionamin®

International issues:

Diasorb®: Brand name for attapulgite in the U.S.

U.S. Brand Names Diamode [OTC]; Imodium® A-D [OTC]; Kao-Paverin® [OTC]; K-Pek II [OTC]

Canadian Brand Names Apo-Loperamide®; Diarr-Eze; Imodium®; Loperacap; Novo-Loperamide; PMS-Loperamine; Rho®-Loperamine; Riva-Loperamine

Index Terms Loperamide Hydrochloride

Therapeutic Category Antidiarrheal

Generic Available Yes

Use Treatment of acute diarrhea and chronic diarrhea associated with inflammatory bowel disease; chronic functional diarrhea (idiopathic), chronic diarrhea caused by bowel resection or organic lesions; to decrease the volume of ileostomy discharge

Pregnancy Risk Factor C

Lactation Enters breast milk/not recommended.

Contraindications Hypersensitivity to loperamide or any component; abdominal pain in the absence of diarrhea; children <24 months of age; acute ulcerative colitis; patients who must avoid constipation; infectious diarrhea resulting from organisms that penetrate the intestinal mucosa (eg, *Shigella*, *Salmonella*); patients with pseudomembranous colitis; bloody diarrhea

Warnings Discontinue therapy if constipation, abdominal distension, or ileus develop. HIV-positive patients should have therapy discontinued with early signs of abdominal distension due to reports of toxic megacolon in these patients who, while receiving loperamide, developed infectious colitis from both viral and bacterial pathogens.

Imodium® A-D contains benzoic acid and sodium benzoate; benzoic acid (benzoate) is a metabolite of benzyl alcohol; large amounts of benzyl alcohol (≥99 mg/kg/day) have been associated with a potentially fatal toxicity ("gasping syndrome") in neonates; *in vitro* and animal studies have shown that benzoate displaces bilirubin from protein binding sites; avoid use in neonates

Precautions If clinical improvement in acute diarrhea is not observed in 48 hours, discontinue use; use with caution and monitor patients with hepatic dysfunction closely for CNS toxicity

Adverse Reactions

Central nervous system: Sedation, fatigue, dizziness

Dermatologic: Rash, pruritus, urticaria, angioedema, erythema multiforme (rare), Stevens-Johnson syndrome (rare), toxic epidermal necrolysis (rare)

Gastrointestinal: Nausea, vomiting, constipation, abdominal cramping, xerostomia, toxic megacolon, paralytic ileus

Genitourinary: Urinary retention

Miscellaneous: Hypersensitivity reactions

Drug Interactions Cytochrome P450 isoenzyme CYP2C8 and CYP3A4 substrate (major) and CYP2D6 and CYP2B6 substrate (minor)

Additive CNS toxicity with CNS depressants, phenothiazines, tricyclic antidepressants, alcohol; quinidine and ritonavir increase loperamide plasma levels; reduce loperamide dosage if used concomitantly; loperamide may reduce saquinavir exposure by 54%

Mechanism of Action Acts directly on intestinal muscles to inhibit peristalsis and prolong transit time

Pharmacodynamics Onset of action: Within 30-60 minutes

Pharmacokinetics

Absorption: Oral: 40%

Protein binding: 97%

Metabolism: Hepatic (>50%) to inactive compounds

Half-life: Adults: 10.8 hours (range 9.1-14.4 hours)

Time to peak serum concentration:

- Capsules: 5 hours
- Liquid: 2.5 hours

Elimination: Fecal and urinary (1%) excretion of metabolites and unchanged drug (30% to 40%)

Usual Dosage Oral:

Acute diarrhea:

- Children: Initial doses (in first 24 hours):
  - 2-5 years (13-20 kg): 1 mg 3 times/day
  - 6-8 years (21-30): 2 mg twice daily
  - 9-12 years (>30 kg): 2 mg 3 times/day
  - After initial dosing, 0.1 mg/kg doses after each loose stool but not exceeding initial dosage
- Children >12 years and Adults: 4 mg initially, followed by 2 mg after each loose stool, up to 16 mg/day

Chronic diarrhea:

- Children: 0.08-0.24 mg/kg/day divided 2-3 times/day, maximum: 2 mg/dose
- Adults: 4 mg initially followed by 2 mg after each unformed stool until diarrhea is controlled; reduce dosage to meet individual requirements. When optimal dosage

(Continued)

Loperamide *(Continued)*

is determined, may administer total dosage once daily or in divided doses. Average daily maintenance dosage: 4-8 mg; if improvement is not seen with 16 mg/day for at least 10 days, symptoms are unlikely to be controlled by further therapy

Administration Oral: Drink plenty of fluids to help prevent dehydration

Patient Information Do not exceed maximum daily dosage; may cause drowsiness and impair ability to perform activities requiring mental alertness or physical coordination; if acute diarrhea lasts longer than 48 hours, consult physician; may cause dry mouth; avoid alcohol

Dosage Forms Excipient information presented when available (limited, particularly for generics); consult specific product labeling.

Caplet, as hydrochloride: 2 mg

Diamode, Imodium® A-D, Kao-Paverin®: 2 mg

Capsule, as hydrochloride: 2 mg

Liquid, oral, as hydrochloride: 1 mg/5 mL (5 mL, 10 mL, 120 mL)

Imodium® A-D: 1 mg/5 mL (60 mL, 120 mL) [contains alcohol, sodium benzoate, benzoic acid; cherry mint flavor]

Imodium® A-D [new formulation]: 1 mg/7.5 mL (60 mL, 120 mL, 360 mL) [contains sodium 10 mg/30 mL, sodium benzoate; creamy mint flavor]

Tablet, as hydrochloride: 2 mg

K-Pek II: 2 mg

♦ **Loperamide Hydrochloride** *see* Loperamide *on page 952*

Lopinavir and Ritonavir (lop IN uh veer & rit ON uh veer)

Medication Safety Issues

Sound-alike/look-alike issues:

Potential for dispensing errors between Kaletra™ and Keppra® (levetiracetam)

Related Information

Adult and Adolescent HIV *on page 1821*

Pediatric HIV *on page 1816*

Perinatal HIV *on page 1831*

U.S. Brand Names Kaletra®

Canadian Brand Names Kaletra®

Index Terms ABT-378/Ritonavir; Ritonavir and Lopinavir

Therapeutic Category Antiretroviral Agent; HIV Agents (Anti-HIV Agents); Protease Inhibitor

Generic Available No

Use Treatment of HIV infection in combination with other antiretroviral agents (**Note:** HIV regimens consisting of three antiretroviral agents are strongly recommended)

Pregnancy Risk Factor C

Lactation Excretion in breast milk unknown/contraindicated

Contraindications Hypersensitivity to lopinavir, ritonavir, or any component; concurrent therapy with medications that largely rely on cytochrome P450 isoenzymes CYP3A for clearance and that have an association between increased plasma concentrations and serious or life-threatening effects (eg, astemizole, cisapride, dihydroergotamine, ergonovine, ergotamine, methylergonovine, midazolam, pimozide, terfenadine, triazolam). **Note:** Lopinavir/ritonavir was found **not** to inhibit P450 isoenzyme CYP2D6 at clinically relevant concentrations, thus, flecainide and propafenone are no longer listed as being contraindicated in the product labeling. However, these 2 drugs are still listed as drugs that should not be used with lopinavir/ritonavir in the current HIV guidelines.

Warnings Lopinavir and ritonavir are potent CYP3A isoenzyme inhibitors that interact with numerous drugs. Due to potential serious and/or life-threatening drug interactions, some drugs are contraindicated (see Contraindications and Drug Interactions) and other medications may require concentration monitoring or dosage adjustment if coadministered with lopinavir and ritonavir (see Drug Interactions). Concomitant use with certain medications may require dosage adjustment of lopinavir and ritonavir (see Drug Interactions).

Potentially fatal pancreatitis may occur; markedly elevated serum triglycerides is a risk factor for developing pancreatitis; advanced HIV disease or a history of pancreatitis may also place patients at increased risk; discontinue lopinavir and ritonavir therapy if clinical signs, symptoms, or laboratory abnormalities suggestive of pancreatitis occur. New onset diabetes mellitus, exacerbations of diabetes, and hyperglycemia have been reported in HIV-infected patients receiving protease inhibitors. Immune reconstitution syndrome (an acute inflammatory response to residual or indolent opportunistic infections) may occur in HIV patients during initial treatment with combination antiretroviral agents, including lopinavir/ritonavir; this syndrome may require further patient assessment and therapy.

Precautions Use with caution in patients with hepatic impairment (lopinavir and ritonavir are primarily metabolized by the liver); hepatitis or markedly elevated transaminases prior to therapy may increase risk for further elevations in liver enzymes or for hepatic decompensation; hepatic dysfunction (including fatalities) have been reported; in general, these occurred in patients with advanced HIV disease who were taking multiple concomitant medications and who had underlying chronic hepatitis or cirrhosis; a causal relationship with lopinavir/ritonavir has not been established; consider more frequent monitoring of liver enzymes in these patients, especially during the first few months of lopinavir/ritonavir therapy. Spontaneous bleeding episodes have been reported in patients with hemophilia type A and B receiving protease inhibitors. Large increases in total cholesterol and triglycerides have been reported; patients should be monitored prior to therapy and periodically during treatment. Fat redistribution and accumulation [ie, central obesity, peripheral wasting, facial wasting, breast enlargement, dorsocervical fat enlargement (buffalo hump), and cushingoid appearance] have been observed in patients receiving antiretroviral agents (causal relationship not established).

Adverse Reactions

Central nervous system: Headache (2% to 7%), insomnia (1% to 2%), pain

Dermatologic: Rash (1% to 4%; children 3%)

Endocrine & metabolic: Hyperglycemia (1% to 5%), hypertriglyceridemia (9% to 36%), hypercholesterolemia (9% to 39%), hyperuricemia (up to 3%); new onset diabetes, exacerbation of diabetes mellitus; decreased serum phosphorus (up to 2%); fat redistribution and accumulation (see Precautions)

Gastrointestinal: Nausea (5% to 16%), vomiting (2% to 12%), diarrhea (16% to 27%; **Note:** In one study, incidence of diarrhea was higher in patients receiving once-daily dosing compared to twice daily dosing), abdominal pain (2% to 10%), elevated amylase (3% to 8%)

Hematologic: Decreased platelets (children 4%), decreased neutrophils (1% to 5%), hemolytic anemia, spontaneous bleeding in hemophiliacs

Hepatic: Elevated liver enzymes, elevated bilirubin (children 3%); hepatitis (may be life-threatening in rare cases)

Neuromuscular & skeletal: Asthenia (up to 9%)

Miscellaneous: Immune reconstitution syndrome (see Warnings)

Drug Interactions Cytochrome P450 isoenzyme CYP3A substrate and inhibitor; may induce glucuronidation; does not inhibit CYP1A2, CYP2B6, CYP2C9, CYP2C19, CYP2D6, or CYP2E1 at clinically obtained concentrations

Lopinavir/ritonavir may inhibit the metabolism of the following drugs and cause serious or life-threatening adverse effects: Astemizole, cisapride, dihydroergotamine, ergonovine, ergotamine, methylergonovine, midazolam, pimozide, terfenadine, triazolam (concurrent therapy with these drugs and lopinavir/ritonavir is contraindicated). Lopinavir/ritonavir may increase the toxic effects of amiodarone, bepridil, systemic lidocaine, quinidine, warfarin, cyclosporine, tacrolimus, rapamycin (serum concentration monitoring of these drugs is necessary). Lopinavir/ritonavir may increase the concentrations of the following drugs: Clarithromycin (decrease clarithromycin dosage in patients with renal impairment), ketoconazole (high dose ketoconazole is not recommended), itraconazole (high dose itraconazole is not recommended), trazodone (use reduced dose of trazodone), rifabutin and rifabutin metabolite (rifabutin dose should be decreased by at least 75% of the normal dose; further reduction in dosage may be needed, monitor closely for adverse effects). Lopinavir/ritonavir may also increase serum concentrations or toxicity of lovastatin or simvastatin (concurrent use of these agents is not recommended), atorvastatin or cerivastatin (use lowest possible dose of these agents, monitor closely; consider use of pravastatin, fluvastatin), nifedipine, felodipine, nicardipine, sildenafil, or other phosphodiesterase-5 (PDE-5) enzyme inhibitors (use decreased dose of sildenafil or other PDE-5 enzyme inhibitor). Ritonavir significantly increases fluticasone serum concentrations and may result in systemic corticosteroid effects (eg, Cushing's syndrome and adrenal suppression); lopinavir/ritonavir use with fluticasone is expected to have the same effect; concurrent use of lopinavir/ritonavir with fluticasone is **not** recommended unless benefits outweigh risks.

Lopinavir/ritonavir will increase the serum concentrations of amprenavir, indinavir, nelfinavir, and saquinavir (decreased doses of these other protease inhibitors are recommended when used concomitantly with lopinavir/ritonavir). Lopinavir/ritonavir increases tenofovir serum concentrations (monitor closely). Amprenavir, fosamprenavir, nelfinavir, efavirenz, and nevirapine decrease lopinavir concentrations (an increased dose of lopinavir/ritonavir is recommended). Lopinavir/ritonavir may decrease the concentration and effect of amprenavir when administered as fosamprenavir. Delavirdine and ritonavir may increase lopinavir concentrations.

(Continued)

Lopinavir and Ritonavir *(Continued)*

Lopinavir/ritonavir may decrease the concentrations of atovaquone and methadone (increased doses of these agents may be needed). Lopinavir/ritonavir may decrease the efficacy of estrogen-based oral contraceptives or contraceptive patch (alternative nonhormonal contraceptive methods should be used). Lopinavir/ritonavir may potentially decrease abacavir and zidovudine concentrations through induction of glucuronidation (clinical significance unknown). Lopinavir/ritonavir may decrease voriconazole concentrations (use of voriconazole is not recommended).

Rifampin may significantly reduce lopinavir/ritonavir plasma concentrations and should not be used concurrently. The herbal medicine St John's wort (*Hypericum perforatum*) may significantly decrease concentrations of lopinavir/ritonavir and is not recommended for concurrent use. Phenobarbital, phenytoin, carbamazepine, dexamethasone may decrease lopinavir concentrations (these agents may decrease effectiveness of lopinavir/ritonavir, use with caution).

Oral solution contains alcohol and may produce disulfiram-like reaction when coadministered with disulfiram or metronidazole. Didanosine should be given at least 1 hour before or 2 hours after lopinavir/ritonavir capsules and oral solution; didanosine may be taken at the same time as lopinavir/ritonavir tablets without food.

Food Interactions Compared to fasting, a moderate fat meal increased lopinavir AUC by 80% (oral solution), but by only 26.9% for the tablets; a high fat meal increased lopinavir AUC by 130% (oral solution), but by only 18.9% for the tablets

Stability

Oral solution: Store at 2°C to 8°C (36°F to 46°F) until dispensed; refrigerated products are stable until labeled expiration date; stability at room temperature: 2 months; avoid exposure to excessive heat; dispense solution in original container.

Tablets: Store at controlled room temperature 20°C to 25°C (68°F to 77°F) in original container. Do not expose to high humidity outside original container for >2 weeks.

Mechanism of Action This product is a fixed-dose combination of lopinavir and ritonavir; antiretroviral effects are due to lopinavir, a protease inhibitor; lopinavir acts on an enzyme (protease) late in the HIV replication process after the virus has entered into the cell's nucleus. Lopinavir binds to the protease activity site and inhibits the activity of the enzyme, thus preventing cleavage of viral polyprotein precursors (gag-pol protein precursors) into individual functional proteins found in infectious HIV. This results in the formation of immature, noninfectious viral particles. Ritonavir inhibits the metabolism of lopinavir via the cytochrome P450 CYP3A isoenzyme pathway and significantly increases plasma concentrations of lopinavir.

Pharmacokinetics Information below refers to Lopinavir; see Ritonavir *on page 1395* for additional information.

Protein binding: 98% to 99%; binds to both alpha$_1$ - acid glycoprotein and albumin; higher affinity for alpha$_1$-acid glycoprotein; decreased protein binding in patients with mild to moderate hepatic impairment

Metabolism: Primarily oxidative, via cytochrome P450 CYP3A isoenzyme; 13 oxidative metabolites identified; may induce its own metabolism

Bioavailability: Absolute bioavailability not established; AUC for oral solution was 22% lower than capsule when given under fasting conditions; concentrations were similar under nonfasting conditions

Half-life: Adults: Mean: 5-6 hours

Elimination: 2.2% of dose eliminated unchanged in urine; 83% of dose eliminated in feces

Clearance: (Apparent oral): Adults: 6-7 L/hour

Dialysis: Unlikely to remove significant amounts of drug (due to high protein binding)

Usual Dosage Oral (use in combination with other antiretroviral agents):

Neonates and Infants <6 months: Not approved for use; investigational dose of lopinavir 300 mg per m^2/ritonavir 75 mg per m^2 given twice daily is currently being studied

Children 6 months to 12 years: Dosage based on weight and lopinavir component:

Note: Once-daily dosing has not been studied in pediatric patients and therefore, is not recommended

Patients receiving concomitant antiretroviral therapy **without amprenavir, efavirenz, or nevirapine:**

7 to <15 kg: Lopinavir 12 mg/kg twice daily

15-40 kg: Lopinavir 10 mg/kg twice daily

>40 kg: Lopinavir 400 mg (2 tablets or 5 mL) twice daily

Patients receiving concomitant antiretroviral therapy **with amprenavir, efavirenz, or nevirapine:** (or treatment-experienced patients in whom decreased susceptibility to lopinavir is suspected; Working Group, 2006):

7 to <15 kg: Lopinavir 13 mg/kg twice daily

15-45 kg: Lopinavir 11 mg/kg twice daily

>45 kg: Lopinavir 533 mg (6.5 mL) twice daily; **Note:** Children ≤12 years who are >40 kg may receive the adult dose of 2 tablets twice daily (manufacturer's recommendation); the NIH guidelines recommend that children ≤12 years who are >50 kg receive 6.5 mL or 3 tablets twice daily (Working Group, 2006)

Children >12 years and Adults:

Patients receiving concomitant antiretroviral therapy **without amprenavir, fosamprenavir, efavirenz, nelfinavir, or nevirapine:** Lopinavir 400 mg/ritonavir 100 mg (2 tablets or 5 mL) twice daily

Once-daily dosing: Adults: **Antiretroviral-naive patients only**: Lopinavir 800 mg/ritonavir 200 mg (4 tablets or 10 mL) once daily; **Note:** Once-daily dosing is not recommended for pediatric or antiretroviral-experienced patients, or for patients receiving carbamazepine, phenobarbital, or phenytoin; once-daily dosing has not been evaluated with concurrent use of indinavir or saquinavir

Patients receiving concomitant antiretroviral therapy **with amprenavir, fosamprenavir, efavirenz, nelfinavir, or nevirapine: Note:** Once-daily dosing is **not** recommended:

Oral solution: Lopinavir 533 mg/ritonavir 133 mg (6.5 mL) twice daily

Tablets:

Antiretroviral-naive patients only: Lopinavir 400 mg/ritonavir 100 mg (2 tablets) twice daily

Treatment experience patients: Lopinavir 600 mg/ritonavir 150 mg (3 tablets) twice daily

Dosing adjustment in renal impairment: Has not been studied in patients with renal impairment; however, a decrease in clearance is not expected

Dosing adjustment in hepatic impairment: Plasma levels are increased in patients with hepatic impairment; use with caution

Administration Oral:

Oral solution: Administer with food to enhance bioavailability and decrease kinetic variability

Tablets: May be administered without regard to meals; swallow tablets whole, do not crush, break, or chew

Monitoring Parameters Signs and symptoms of pancreatitis; serum electrolytes, glucose, triglycerides, cholesterol, liver enzymes, bilirubin, amylase, CBC with differential, platelets, CD4 cell count, viral load

Patient Information Lopinavir and ritonavir is not a cure for HIV; notify physician if symptoms of pancreatitis occur (nausea, vomiting, abdominal pain); report the use of other medications, nonprescription medications and herbal or natural products to your physician and pharmacist; avoid the herbal medicine St John's wort; take lopinavir and ritonavir everyday as prescribed; do not change dose or discontinue without physician's advice; if a dose is missed, take it as soon as possible, then return to normal dosing schedule; if a dose is skipped, do not double the next dose

HIV medications may cause changes in body fat, including an increase in fat in the upper back and neck, breasts, and trunk; a loss of fat from the face, arms, and legs may also occur.

Additional Information Oral solution contains 42.4% alcohol (v/v); overdose in a child may cause potentially lethal alcohol toxicity; treatment should be supportive and include general poisoning management; activated charcoal may help remove unabsorbed medication; dialysis unlikely to be of benefit

Preliminary studies have reported response rates (defined as viral loads <400 copies/mL) of 91%, 81%, and 33% for patients with 0-5, 6-7, and 8-10 protease mutations at baseline, respectively (see Hurst, 2000)

Dosage Forms Excipient information presented when available (limited, particularly for generics); consult specific product labeling.

Solution, oral:

Kaletra®: Lopinavir 80 mg and ritonavir 20 mg per mL (160 mL) [contains alcohol 42.4%]

Tablet:

Kaletra®: Lopinavir 200 mg and ritonavir 50 mg

References

Briars LA, Hilao JJ, and Kraus DM, "A Review of Pediatric Human Immunodeficiency Virus Infection," *Journal of Pharmacy Practice*, 2004, 17(6):407-31.

Hurst M and Faulds D, "Lopinavir," *Drugs*, 2000, 60(6):1371-9.

Mangum EM and Graham KK, "Lopinavir-Ritonavir: A New Protease Inhibitor," *Pharmacotherapy*, 2001, 21(11):1352-63.

Morris JL and Kraus DM, "New Antiretroviral Therapies for Pediatric HIV Infection," *J Pediatr Pharmacol Ther*, 2005, 10:215-47.

Panel on Clinical Practices for Treatment of HIV Infection, "Guidelines for the Use of Antiretroviral Agents in HIV-Infected Adults and Adolescents," October 10, 2006, http://www.aidsinfo.nih.gov.

Piscitelli SC, Burstein AH, Chaitt D, et al, "Indinavir Concentrations and St John's Wort," *Lancet*, 2000, 355(9203):547-8.

Working Group on Antiretroviral Therapy and Medical Management of HIV-Infected Children, "Guidelines for the Use of Antiretroviral Agents in Pediatric HIV Infection," October 26, 2006, http://www.aidsinfo.nih.gov.

(Continued)

Lopinavir and Ritonavir *(Continued)*

Working Group on Antiretroviral Therapy and Medical Management of HIV-Infected Children, "Guidelines for the Use of Antiretroviral Agents in Pediatric HIV Infection. Supplement I: Pediatric Antiretroviral Drug Information," October 26, 2006, http://www.aidsinfo.nih.gov.

- **Lopremone** *see* Protirelin *on page 1343*
- **Lopressor®** *see* Metoprolol *on page 1046*
- **Lorabid® [DSC]** *see* Loracarbef [DSC] *on page 958*
- **Lorabid® (Can)** *see* Loracarbef [DSC] *on page 958*

Loracarbef [DSC] (lor a KAR bef)

Medication Safety Issues

Sound-alike/look-alike issues:

Lorabid® may be confused with Levbid®, Lopid®, Lortab®, Slo-bid™

U.S. Brand Names Lorabid® [DSC]

Canadian Brand Names Lorabid®

Therapeutic Category Antibiotic, Carbacephem

Generic Available No

Use Treatment of mild to moderate community-acquired infections of the respiratory tract, skin and skin structure, and urinary tract that are caused by susceptible *S. pneumoniae, H. influenzae, M. catarrhalis, S. aureus, S. pyogenes*, and *E. coli*

Pregnancy Risk Factor B

Lactation Excretion in breast milk unknown/use caution

Contraindications Hypersensitivity to loracarbef, any component, or cephalosporins

Warnings Prolonged use may result in superinfection or pseudomembranous colitis

Precautions Use with caution in patients with a previous history of hypersensitivity to other beta-lactam antibiotics (eg, penicillins); use with caution in patients with impaired renal function and patients with a history of colitis; modify dosage in patients with renal impairment

Adverse Reactions

Cardiovascular: Vasodilation

Central nervous system: Headache, somnolence, nervousness, dizziness, insomnia

Dermatologic: Skin rashes, urticaria, pruritus, erythema multiforme, Stevens-Johnson syndrome

Gastrointestinal: Diarrhea, nausea, vomiting, abdominal pain, anorexia, pseudomembranous colitis

Genitourinary: Candidal vaginitis

Hematologic: Transient thrombocytopenia, leukopenia, eosinophilia, prolongation of prothrombin time

Hepatic: Transient elevations of ALT, AST, alkaline phosphatase; cholestasis, jaundice

Renal: Transient elevation of BUN and serum creatinine

Respiratory: Rhinitis

Miscellaneous: Anaphylaxis, superinfection

Drug Interactions Probenecid inhibits renal excretion and increases the serum concentration of loracarbef

Food Interactions Administration with food decreases and delays the peak plasma concentration

Stability After reconstitution, suspension may be stored at room temperature for 14 days

Mechanism of Action Inhibits bacterial cell wall synthesis by binding to one or more of the penicillin binding proteins; inhibits the final transpeptidation step of peptidoglycan synthesis in bacterial cell walls, thus inhibiting cell wall biosynthesis. Upon exposure to beta-lactam antibiotics, bacteria eventually lyse due to ongoing activity of cell wall autolytic enzymes (autolysins and murein hydrolases) while cell wall assembly is arrested.

Pharmacokinetics

Absorption: Oral: Rapid; 90% absorbed from the GI tract

Distribution: Loracarbef middle-ear fluid concentration approximates 48% of the plasma concentration 2 hours after a dose in pediatric patients

Protein binding: 25%

Bioavailability: 90%

Half-life, elimination:

Children (suspension): ~0.78-0.85 hours

Adults, normal renal function: ~1 hour

Time to peak serum concentration: 0.5-1 hour after administration

Elimination: Primarily by the kidneys as unchanged drug in the urine

Usual Dosage Oral:

Children 6 months to 12 years:

Acute otitis media: 30 mg/kg/day divided every 12 hours for 10 days (should be treated with the **suspension** which results in higher peak plasma concentrations than the capsule)

Acute maxillary sinusitis: 30 mg/kg/day divided every 12 hours for 10 days

Pharyngitis/tonsillitis/skin and skin structure infections: 15 mg/kg/day divided every 12 hours

Adults:

Pneumonia, chronic bacterial bronchitis, sinusitis: 400 mg every 12 hours

Acute bacterial bronchitis: 200-400 mg every 12 hours

Uncomplicated urinary tract infections: 200 mg once daily for 7 days

Skin and skin structure: 200 mg every 12 hours

Uncomplicated pyelonephritis: 400 mg every 12 hours for 14 days

Dosing adjustment in renal impairment:

Cl_{cr} 10-49 mL/minute: 50% of usual dose at usual interval or usual dose given half as often

Cl_{cr} <10 mL/minute: Give usual dose every 3-5 days

Hemodialysis: Removed by hemodialysis; postdialysis dose should be administered when appropriate

Administration Oral: Administer on an empty stomach at least 1 hour before or 2 hours after meals; shake suspension well before use

Monitoring Parameters Observe patient for diarrhea; with prolonged therapy, monitor renal function periodically

Dosage Forms Excipient information presented when available (limited, particularly for generics); consult specific product labeling. [DSC] = Discontinued product

Capsule:

Lorabid®: 200 mg, 400 mg [DSC]

Powder for oral suspension:

Lorabid®: 100 mg/5 mL (100 mL); 200 mg/5 mL (100 mL) [strawberry bubble gum flavor] [DSC]

References

Force RW and Nahata MC, "Loracarbef: A New Orally Administered Carbacephem Antibiotic," *Ann Pharmacother*, 1993, 27(3):321-9.

Foshee WS, "Loracarbef (LY163892) Versus Amoxicillin-Clavulanate in the Treatment of Acute Otitis Media With Effusion," *J Pediatr*, 1992, 120(6):980-6.

Nelson JD, Shelton S, and Kusmiesz H, "Pharmacokinetics of LY163892 in Infants and Children," *Antimicrob Agents Chemother*, 1988, 32(11):1738-9.

Loratadine (lor AT a deen)

Medication Safety Issues

Sound-alike/look-alike issues:

Dimetapp® may be confused with Dermatop®, Dimetabs®, Dimetane®

Related Information

OTC Cough and Cold Preparations, Pediatric *on page 1706*

U.S. Brand Names Alavert® [OTC]; Claritin® 24 Hour Allergy [OTC]; Claritin® Hives Relief [OTC]; Tavist® ND [OTC]; Triaminic® Allerchews™ [OTC]

Canadian Brand Names Apo-Loratadine®; Claritin®; Claritin® Kids

Therapeutic Category Antihistamine

Generic Available Yes

Use Symptomatic relief of nasal and non-nasal symptoms of allergic rhinitis; treatment of chronic idiopathic urticaria

Pregnancy Risk Factor B

Lactation Enters breast milk/not recommended (AAP rates "compatible")

Contraindications Hypersensitivity to loratadine or any component

Warnings Use with caution and adjust dosage in patients with severe liver impairment or renal impairment; Claritin® syrup contains sodium benzoate; benzoic acid (benzoate) is a metabolite of benzyl alcohol; large amounts of benzyl alcohol (≥99 mg/kg/day) have been associated with a potentially fatal toxicity ("gasping syndrome") in neonates; *in vitro* and animal studies have shown that benzoate displaces bilirubin from protein binding sites; avoid use in neonates

Precautions Use cautiously in patients who are also taking ketoconazole, itraconazole, fluconazole, erythromycin, clarithromycin, or other drugs which may impair loratadine's hepatic metabolism; although increased plasma levels of loratadine have been observed, no adverse effects with concomitant administration have been reported including QT interval prolongation which has occurred when similar antihistamines, terfenadine and astemizole, were combined with these agents; while less sedating than other antihistamines, loratadine may cause drowsiness and impair ability to perform hazardous activities requiring mental alertness. Use cautiously in breast-feeding women as breast milk levels of loratadine are equivalent

(Continued)

Loratadine *(Continued)*

to serum levels. Some tablets contain phenylalanine which must be avoided (or used with caution) in patients with phenylketonuria.

Adverse Reactions

Cardiovascular: Hypotension, hypertension, palpitations, tachycardia, chest pain, syncope

Central nervous system: Headache, somnolence, fatigue, anxiety, depression, dizziness, fever, migraine, agitation, nervousness, hyperactivity

Dermatologic: Alopecia, dermatitis, dry skin, rash, pruritus, photosensitivity

Gastrointestinal: Xerostomia, nausea, vomiting, gastritis, abdominal pain, diarrhea

Endocrine & metabolic: Breast pain and enlargement (rare), menorrhagia, dysmenorrhea

Neuromuscular & skeletal: Hyperkinesia, arthralgias, myalgias, leg cramps

Ocular: Blurred vision, altered lacrimation, eye pain, conjunctivitis

Genitourinary: Discoloration of urine

Respiratory: Nasal dryness, pharyngitis, dyspnea, nasal congestion, wheezing, nose bleed

Miscellaneous: Diaphoresis

Drug Interactions Cytochrome P450 isoenzyme CYP2D6 and CYP3A3/4 substrate

Increased plasma concentrations and AUC of loratadine and its active metabolite with ketoconazole, erythromycin, and cimetidine; no change in QT_c interval or cardiac arrhythmias have been seen (see Warnings); a prolonged QT interval was reported in one patient who was receiving quinidine and loratadine; additive CNS depression with other CNS depressants, alcohol, and procarbazine; prolonged anticholinergic effects with MAO inhibitors

Food Interactions Administration with food increases loratadine's bioavailability by 40%

Mechanism of Action Long-acting tricyclic antihistamine with selective peripheral histamine H_1 receptor antagonistic properties

Pharmacodynamics

Onset of action: Within 1-3 hours

Maximum effect: 8-12 hours

Duration: >24 hours

Pharmacokinetics

Absorption: Rapid; food increases total bioavailability (AUC) by 40%

Distribution: Binds preferentially to peripheral nervous system H_1 receptors; no appreciable entry into CNS; loratadine and metabolite pass easily into breast milk and achieve concentrations equivalent to plasma levels; breast milk to plasma ratio: 1.17

Protein binding: 97% (loratadine), 73% to 77% (metabolite)

Metabolism: Extensive first-pass metabolism by cytochrome P450 system to an active metabolite (descarboethoxyloratadine)

Half-life: 8.4 hours (loratadine), 28 hours (metabolite)

Time to peak serum concentration: 1-2 hours

Elimination: 80% eliminated via urine & feces as metabolic products

Usual Dosage Oral:

Children 2-5 years: 5 mg once daily

Children ≥6 years and Adults: 10 mg once daily

Dosing interval in renal (GFR <30 mL/minute) or hepatic impairment: Administer dosage every other day

Administration Oral: Administer on an empty stomach or before meals; place Claritin® RediTab® (rapidly disintegrating tablet) on the tongue; tablet disintegration occurs rapidly; may administer with or without water

Monitoring Parameters Improvement in signs and symptoms of allergic rhinitis or chronic idiopathic urticaria

Reference Range Therapeutic serum levels (not used clinically): Loratadine: 2.5-100 ng/mL; active metabolite: 0.5-100 ng/mL

Test Interactions Antigen skin testing

Patient Information Drink plenty of water; may cause dry mouth; may color urine; may cause drowsiness and impair ability to perform activities requiring mental alertness or physical coordination; notify physician if fainting episode occurs; avoid alcohol. May rarely cause photosensitivity reactions (eg, exposure to sunlight may cause severe sunburn, skin rash, redness, or itching); avoid direct exposure to sunlight

Dosage Forms Excipient information presented when available (limited, particularly for generics); consult specific product labeling.

Syrup: 1 mg/mL (120 mL)

Claritin®: 1 mg/mL (120 mL) [contains sodium benzoate; fruit flavor]; (60 mL, 120 mL) [alcohol free, dye free, sugar free; contains sodium 6 mg/5 mL and sodium benzoate; grape flavor]

Tablet: 10 mg
Alavert®, Claritin®, Claritin® Hives Relief, Claritin® 24 Hour Allergy, Tavist® ND: 10 mg
Tablet, rapidly disintegrating: 10 mg
Alavert®: 10 mg [contains phenylalanine 8.4 mg/tablet; mint and citrus burst flavors]
Claritin® RediTabs®: 10 mg [mint flavor]
Triaminic® Allerchews™: 10 mg

References

Lin CC, Radwanski E, Affrime M, et al, "Pharmacokinetics of Loratadine in Pediatric Subjects," *Am J Therapeut*, 1995, 2:504-8.

Luck JC and Evrard HM, "Atrial Fibrillation Associated With Loratadine Use," *J Allergy Clin Immunol*, 1995, 95(2):282.

Lutsky BN, Klose P, Melon J, et al, "A Comparative Study of the Efficacy and Safety of Loratadine Syrup and Terfenadine Suspension in the Treatment of 3 to 6 Year Old Children With Seasonal Allergic Rhinitis," *Clin Ther*, 1993, 15(5):855-65.

Salmun LM, Herron JM, Banfield C, et al, "The Pharmacokinetics, Electrocardiographic Effects, and Tolerability of Loratadine Syrup in Children Aged 2 to 5 Years," *Clin Ther*, 2000, 22(5):613-21.

Loratadine and Pseudoephedrine

(lor AT a deen & soo doe e FED rin)

Related Information

OTC Cough and Cold Preparations, Pediatric *on page 1706*

U.S. Brand Names Alavert™ Allergy and Sinus [OTC]; Claritin-D® 12-Hour [OTC]; Claritin-D® 24-Hour [OTC]

Canadian Brand Names Chlor-Tripolon ND®; Claritin® Extra; Claritin® Liberator

Index Terms Pseudoephedrine and Loratadine

Therapeutic Category Antihistamine/Decongestant Combination

Generic Available Yes

Use Symptomatic relief of symptoms of seasonal allergic rhinitis and nasal congestion

Pregnancy Risk Factor B

Lactation Enters breast milk/not recommended

Contraindications Hypersensitivity to loratadine, pseudoephedrine, or any component; MAO inhibitor therapy; severe hypertension; severe coronary artery disease; narrow-angle glaucoma

Precautions Use with caution and adjust dosage in patients with renal impairment; use with caution in patients with hyperthyroidism, diabetes mellitus, prostatic hypertrophy, mild to moderate hypertension, arrhythmias; use cautiously in patients who are also taking ketoconazole, itraconazole, fluconazole, erythromycin, clarithromycin, or other drugs which may impair loratadine's hepatic metabolism; although increased plasma levels of loratadine have been observed, no adverse effects with concomitant administration have been reported including QT interval prolongation which has occurred when similar antihistamines, terfenadine and astemizole, were combined with these agents; while less sedating than other antihistamines, loratadine may cause drowsiness and impair ability to perform hazardous activities requiring mental alertness, the CNS stimulant properties of pseudoephedrine may counteract this effect. Use cautiously in breast-feeding women as breast milk levels of loratadine are equivalent to serum levels.

Adverse Reactions See individual monographs for Loratadine *on page 959* and Pseudoephedrine *on page 1344*.

Drug Interactions See individual monographs for Loratadine *on page 959* and Pseudoephedrine *on page 1344*.

Food Interactions Administration with food increases loratadine's bioavailability by 40%

Mechanism of Action Loratadine is a long-acting tricyclic antihistamine with selective peripheral histamine H_1-receptor antagonistic properties. Pseudoephedrine directly stimulates alpha-adrenergic receptors of respiratory mucosa causing vasoconstriction and directly stimulates beta-adrenergic receptors causing bronchial relaxation, increased heart rate and contractility

Pharmacokinetics See individual monographs for Loratadine *on page 959* and Pseudoephedrine *on page 1344*.

Usual Dosage Oral: Children ≥12 years and Adults:
Claritin-D® 12-Hour: 1 tablet every 12 hours
Claritin-D® 24-Hour: 1 tablet every 24 hours
Dosage adjustment in renal impairment: Cl_{cr} <30 mL/minute:
Claritin-D® 12-Hour: 1 tablet every 24 hours
Claritin-D® 24-Hour: 1 tablet every other day

Administration Oral: Administer on an empty stomach or before meals; swallow extended release tablets whole, do not chew or crush

Monitoring Parameters Improvement in signs and symptoms of allergic rhinitis or nasal congestion

(Continued)

Loratadine and Pseudoephedrine *(Continued)*

Reference Range Therapeutic serum levels (not used clinically): Loratadine: 2.5-100 ng/mL; active metabolite: 0.5-100 ng/mL

Test Interactions Antigen skin testing; false-positive test for amphetamines by EMIT assay

Patient Information Drink plenty of water; may cause dry mouth; may color urine; notify physician if fainting episode occurs; avoid alcohol. May rarely cause photosensitivity reactions (eg, exposure to sunlight may cause severe sunburn, skin rash, redness, or itching); avoid direct exposure to sunlight

Dosage Forms Excipient information presented when available (limited, particularly for generics); consult specific product labeling.

Tablet, extended release: Loratadine 10 mg and pseudoephedrine sulfate 240 mg

Alavert™ Allergy and Sinus, Claritin-D® 12-hour: Loratadine 5 mg and pseudoephedrine sulfate 120 mg

Claritin-D® 24-hour: Loratadine 10 mg and pseudoephedrine sulfate 240 mg

Lorazepam (lor A ze pam)

Medication Safety Issues

Sound-alike/look-alike issues:

Lorazepam may be confused with alprazolam, clonazepam, diazepam, temazepam

Ativan® may be confused with Atarax®, Atgam®, Avitene®

Injection dosage form contains propylene glycol. Monitor for toxicity when administering continuous lorazepam infusions.

Related Information

Compatibility of Chemotherapy and Related Supportive Care Medications *on page 1777*

Overdose and Toxicology *on page 1916*

Preprocedure Sedatives in Children *on page 1895*

U.S. Brand Names Ativan®; Lorazepam Intensol®

Canadian Brand Names Apo-Lorazepam®; Ativan®; Lorazepam Injection, USP; Novo-Lorazepam; Nu-Loraz; PMS-Lorazepam; Riva-Lorazepam

Therapeutic Category Antianxiety Agent; Anticonvulsant, Benzodiazepine; Antiemetic; Benzodiazepine; Hypnotic; Sedative

Generic Available Yes

Use Management of anxiety; status epilepticus; preoperative sedation and amnesia

Restrictions C-IV

Pregnancy Risk Factor D

Lactation Enters breast milk/not recommended (AAP rates "of concern")

Contraindications Hypersensitivity to lorazepam or any component (see Warnings); there may be a cross-sensitivity with other benzodiazepines; do not use in a comatose patient, those with pre-existing CNS depression, narrow-angle glaucoma, severe uncontrolled pain, severe hypotension

Warnings Dilute injection prior to I.V. use with equal volume of compatible diluent (D_5W, NS, SWI); do not inject intra-arterially, arteriospasm and gangrene may occur; abrupt discontinuation after prolonged use may result in withdrawal symptoms or seizures

Injection contains 2% benzyl alcohol, polyethylene glycol, and propylene glycol, which may be toxic to newborns in high doses; benzyl alcohol may cause allergic reactions in susceptible individuals; large amounts of benzyl alcohol (≥99 mg/kg/day) have been associated with a potentially fatal toxicity ("gasping syndrome") in neonates; the "gasping syndrome" consists of metabolic acidosis, respiratory distress, gasping respirations, CNS dysfunction (including convulsions, intracranial hemorrhage), hypotension and cardiovascular collapse; use lorazepam products containing benzyl alcohol with caution in neonates; *in vitro* and animal studies have shown that benzoate, a metabolite of benzyl alcohol, displaces bilirubin from protein binding sites

Precautions Use with caution in neonates, especially in preterm infants (several cases of neurotoxicity and myoclonus have been reported); use with caution in patients with renal or hepatic impairment, compromised pulmonary function, or those receiving other CNS depressants

Adverse Reactions

Cardiovascular: Bradycardia, circulatory collapse, hypertension, or hypotension

Central nervous system: Confusion, CNS depression, sedation, drowsiness, lethargy, hangover effect, dizziness, transitory hallucinations, ataxia, rhythmic myoclonic jerking in preterm infants

Gastrointestinal: Constipation, xerostomia, nausea, vomiting

Genitourinary: Urinary incontinence or retention

Local: Pain with injection
Ocular: Diplopia, nystagmus
Respiratory: Respiratory depression, apnea
Miscellaneous: Physical and psychological dependence with prolonged use

Drug Interactions Other CNS or respiratory depressants may increase adverse effects

Stability Do not use if injection is discolored or contains precipitate; protect from light; refrigerate injectable form and oral solution; injection is stable at room temperature for 8 weeks

Mechanism of Action Depresses all levels of the CNS, including the limbic and reticular formation, by binding to the benzodiazepine site on the gamma-aminobutyric acid (GABA) receptor complex and modulating GABA, which is a major inhibitory neurotransmitter in the brain

Pharmacodynamics Sedation:
Onset of action:
Oral: Within 60 minutes
I.M.: 30-60 minutes
I.V.: 15-30 minutes
Duration: 8-12 hours

Pharmacokinetics
Absorption: Oral, I.M.: Rapid, complete
Distribution: Crosses into placenta; crosses into breast milk
V_d:
Neonates: 0.76 L/kg
Adults: 1.3 L/kg
Protein binding: ~85%
Metabolism: Primarily by glucuronide conjugation in the liver
Bioavailability: Oral: 90% to 93%
Half-life:
Full-term neonates: 40.2 hours; range: 18-73 hours
Older Children: 10.5 hours; range: 6-17 hours
Adults: 12.9 hours; range: 10-16 hours
Elimination: In urine primarily as the glucuronide conjugate

Usual Dosage
Adjunct to antiemetic therapy:
Children: I.V.: Limited information exists in the literature, especially for multiple doses:
Single dose: 0.04-0.08 mg/kg/dose prior to chemotherapy (maximum dose: 4 mg)
Multiple doses: Some centers use 0.02-0.05 mg/kg/dose (maximum dose: 2 mg) every 6 hours as needed
Adults: Oral, I.V.: 0.5-2 mg every 4-6 hours as needed
Anxiety/sedation:
Infants and Children: Oral, I.V.: Usual: 0.05 mg/kg/dose (maximum dose: 2 mg/dose) every 4-8 hours; range: 0.02-0.1 mg/kg
Adults: Oral: 1-10 mg/day in 2-3 divided doses; usual dose: 2-6 mg/day in divided doses
Insomnia: Adults: Oral: 2-4 mg at bedtime
Operative amnesia: Adults: I.V.: up to 0.05 mg/kg; maximum dose: 4 mg/dose
Preoperative: Adults: I.M.: 0.05 mg/kg administered 2 hours before surgery; maximum dose: 4 mg/dose; I.V.: 0.044 mg/kg 15-20 minutes before surgery; usual maximum dose: 2 mg/dose
Sedation (preprocedure): Infants and Children:
Oral, I.M., I.V.: Usual: 0.05 mg/kg; range: 0.02-0.09 mg/kg
I.V.: may use smaller doses (eg, 0.01-0.03 mg/kg) and repeat every 20 minutes, as needed to titrate to effect
Status epilepticus: I.V.:
Neonates: 0.05 mg/kg over 2-5 minutes; may repeat in 10-15 minutes (see warning regarding benzyl alcohol)
Infants and Children: 0.1 mg/kg slow I.V. over 2-5 minutes, do not exceed 4 mg/single dose; may repeat second dose of 0.05 mg/kg slow I.V. in 10-15 minutes if needed
Adolescents: 0.07 mg/kg slow I.V. over 2-5 minutes; maximum dose: 4 mg/dose; may repeat in 10-15 minutes
Adults: 4 mg/dose given slowly over 2-5 minutes; may repeat in 10-15 minutes; usual total maximum dose per 12-hour period: 8 mg

Administration
Oral: May administer with food to decrease GI distress; dilute oral solution in water, juice, soda, or semisolid food (eg, applesauce, pudding)
Parenteral:
I.V.: Do not exceed 2 mg/minute or 0.05 mg/kg over 2-5 minutes; dilute I.V. dose with equal volume of compatible diluent (D_5W, NS, SWI); administer I.V. using

(Continued)

Lorazepam *(Continued)*

repeated aspiration with slow I.V. injection, to make sure the injection is not intra-arterial and that perivascular extravasation has not occurred

I.M.: Administer undiluted by deep injection into muscle mass

Monitoring Parameters Respiratory rate, blood pressure, heart rate; CBC with differential and liver function with long-term use

Patient Information Avoid alcohol; limit caffeine; may be habit-forming; avoid abrupt discontinuation after prolonged use; may cause drowsiness and impair ability to perform activities requiring mental alertness or physical coordination; may cause dry mouth

Additional Information Single oral doses >0.09 mg/kg produced increased ataxia without increasing sedative benefit vs lower doses; since both strengths of injection contain 2% benzyl alcohol, Neofax® recommends using the 4 mg/mL strength for dilution with **preservative free** SWI to make a 0.4 mg/mL dilution for I.V. use in neonates (in order to decrease the amount of benzyl alcohol delivered to the neonate); however, the stability of this dilution has not been studied. Diarrhea in a 9 month old infant receiving high-dose oral lorazepam was attributed to the lorazepam oral solution that contained polyethylene glycol and propylene glycol (both are osmotically active); diarrhea resolved when crushed tablets were substituted for the oral solution (see Marshall, 1995).

Dosage Forms Excipient information presented when available (limited, particularly for generics); consult specific product labeling.

Injection, solution: 2 mg/mL (1 mL, 10 mL); 4 mg/mL (1 mL, 10 mL)

Ativan®: 2 mg/mL (1 mL, 10 mL); 4 mg/mL (1 mL, 10 mL) [contains benzyl alcohol, propylene glycol, and propylene glycol]

Solution, oral concentrate:

Lorazepam Intensol®: 2 mg/mL (30 mL) [alcohol free, dye free]

Tablet: 0.5 mg, 1 mg, 2 mg

Ativan®: 0.5 mg, 1 mg, 2 mg

References

Crawford TO, Mitchell WG, and Snodgrass SR, "Lorazepam in Childhood Status Epilepticus and Serial Seizures: Effectiveness and Tachyphylaxis," *Neurology*, 1987, 37(2):190-5.

Deshmukh A, Wittert W, Schnitzler E, et al, "Lorazepam in the Treatment of Refractory Neonatal Seizures: A Pilot Study," *Am J Dis Child*, 1986, 140(10):1042-4.

Henry DW, Burwinkle JW, and Klutman NE, "Determination of Sedative and Amnestic Doses of Lorazepam in Children," *Clin Pharm*, 1991, 10(8):625-9.

Lee DS, Wong HA, and Knoppert DC, "Myoclonus Associated With Lorazepam Therapy in Very-Low-Birth-Weight Infants," *Biol Neonate*, 1994, 66(6):311-5.

Marshall JD, Farrar HC, and Kearns GL, "Diarrhea Associated With Enteral Benzodiazepine Solutions," *J Pediatr*, 1995, 126(4):657-9.

McDermott CA, Kowalczyk AL, Schnitzler ER, et al, "Pharmacokinetics of Lorazepam in Critically Ill Neonates With Seizures," *J Pediatr*, 1992, 120(3):479-83.

- **Lorazepam Injection, USP (Can)** *see* Lorazepam *on page 962*
- **Lorazepam Intensol®** *see* Lorazepam *on page 962*
- **Lorcet® 10/650** *see* Hydrocodone and Acetaminophen *on page 779*
- **Lorcet® Plus** *see* Hydrocodone and Acetaminophen *on page 779*
- **Loroxide® [OTC]** *see* Benzoyl Peroxide *on page 207*
- **Lortab®** *see* Hydrocodone and Acetaminophen *on page 779*
- **Losec® (Can)** *see* Omeprazole *on page 1167*
- **Losec MUPS® (Can)** *see* Omeprazole *on page 1167*
- **Lotio Calaminae** *see* Calamine Lotion *on page 257*
- **Lotrimin® AF Athlete's Foot Cream [OTC]** *see* Clotrimazole *on page 393*
- **Lotrimin® AF Athlete's Foot Solution [OTC]** *see* Clotrimazole *on page 393*
- **Lotrimin® AF Jock Itch Cream [OTC]** *see* Clotrimazole *on page 393*
- **Lotrimin® AF Jock Itch Powder Spray [OTC]** *see* Miconazole *on page 1056*
- **Lotrimin® AF Powder/Spray [OTC]** *see* Miconazole *on page 1056*

Lovastatin (LOE va sta tin)

Medication Safety Issues

Sound-alike/look-alike issues:

Lovastatin may be confused with Leustatin®, Livostin®, Lotensin®

Mevacor® may be confused with Mivacron®

International issues:

Lovacol® [Chile and Finland] may be confused with Levatol® which is a brand name for penbutolol in the U.S.

Lovastin® [Poland] may be confused with Livostin® which is a brand name for levocabastine in the U.S.

U.S. Brand Names Altoprev®; Mevacor®

Canadian Brand Names Apo-Lovastatin®; CO Lovastatin; Gen-Lovastatin; Mevacor®; Novo-Lovastatin; Nu-Lovastatin; PMS-Lovastatin; RAN™-Lovastatin; ratio-Lovastatin; Riva-Lovastatin; Sandoz-Lovastatin

Index Terms Mevinolin; Monacolin K

Therapeutic Category Antilipemic Agent; HMG-CoA Reductase Inhibitor

Generic Available Yes: Immediate release tablet

Use Hyperlipidemia: Adjunct to dietary therapy to decrease elevated serum total and low density lipoprotein cholesterol (LDL-C), apolipoprotein B (apo-B), and triglyceride levels, and to increase high density lipoprotein cholesterol (HDL-C) in patients with primary hypercholesterolemia (heterozygous, familial and nonfamilial) and mixed dyslipidemia (Fredrickson types IIa and IIb); treatment of isolated hypertriglyceridemia (Fredrickson type IV) and type III hyperlipoproteinemia; treatment of primary dysbetalipoproteinemia (Fredrickson Type III)

Primary prevention of cardiovascular disease in high risk patients; risk factors include: Age ≥55 years, smoking, hypertension, low HDL-C or family history of early coronary heart disease

Pregnancy Risk Factor X

Lactation Excretion unknown/contraindicated

Contraindications Hypersensitivity to lovastatin or any component; active liver disease; unexplained persistent elevations of serum transaminases; pregnancy; breast-feeding

Warnings Rhabdomyolysis with or without acute renal failure secondary to myoglobinuria has occurred rarely and is dose-related. Risk is increased with concurrent use of clarithromycin, danazol, diltiazem, fluvoxamine, indinavir, nefazodone, nelfinavir, ritonavir, verapamil, troleandomycin, cyclosporine, fibric acid derivatives, erythromycin, niacin, azole antifungals and large quantities of grapefruit juice (>1 quart/day). Assess the risk versus benefit before combining any of these drugs with lovastatin. Temporarily discontinue lovastatin in any patient experiencing an acute or serious condition predisposing to renal failure secondary to rhabdomyolysis.

Precautions Persistent increases in serum transaminases have occurred; liver function must be monitored by laboratory assessment at the initiation of therapy in patients with a history of liver disease, prior to use of doses ≥40 mg daily or as clinically indicated. Use with caution in patients with history of heavy alcohol use or have a previous history of liver disease; use with caution and modify dose in patients with renal impairment or receiving concomitant amiodarone, cyclosporine, danazol, fibrates, lipid-lowering doses of niacin, or verapamil. Lovastatin is less effective in patients with rare **homozygous** familial hypercholesterolemia and may be more likely to elevate serum transaminases.

Adverse Reactions

Cardiovascular: Chest pain

Central nervous system: Headache, dizziness, insomnia, tremor, vertigo, memory loss, psychic disturbances, anxiety, depression

Dermatologic: Rash, alopecia, pruritus, dermatomyositis

Endocrine & metabolic: Gynecomastia, abnormal thyroid function tests

Gastrointestinal: Abdominal pain, constipation, diarrhea, dyspepsia, flatulence, nausea, acid regurgitation, xerostomia, vomiting, anorexia

Hepatic: Hepatitis, cholestatic jaundice, cirrhosis, hepatic necrosis, hepatoma, elevated hepatic enzymes

Neuromuscular & skeletal: Increased CPK, myalgia, weakness, muscle cramps, leg pain, arthralgia, paresthesia, rhabdomyolysis

Ocular: Blurred vision, eye irritation, cataracts, ophthalmoplegia

Miscellaneous: Hypersensitivity syndrome (including one or more of the following features: Anaphylaxis, angioedema, lupus erythematous-like syndrome, polymyalgia rheumatica, dermatomyositis, vasculitis, purpura, leukopenia, hemolytic anemia, erythema multiforme)

Drug Interactions Cytochrome P450 isoenzyme CYP3A3/4 substrate

Plasma concentrations may be decreased when given with magnesium-aluminum hydroxide containing antacids; cholestyramine reduces absorption; amiodarone, clofibrate, danazol, fenofibrate, gemfibrozil, niacin (1 g/day), and cyclosporine may increase the risk of myopathy and rhabdomyolysis (see Warnings); CYP3A3/4 inhibitors (clarithromycin, cyclosporine, danazol, diltiazem, fluconazole, fluvoxamine, erythromycin, indinavir, itraconazole, ketoconazole, miconazole, nefazodone, nelfinavir, ritonavir, saquinavir, indinavir, amprenavir, troleandomycin, and verapamil) increase lovastatin blood levels and may increase the risk of lovastatin-induced myopathy and rhabdomyolysis (see Warnings); lovastatin may increase the hypoprothrombinemic response to warfarin; the herbal medicine St John's wort (*Hypericum perforatum*) may decrease lovastatin levels

(Continued)

Lovastatin *(Continued)*

Food Interactions Food **increases** the absorption of lovastatin immediate release tablets (serum concentrations of active drug under fasting conditions are approximately two-thirds of that when administered with food). Food **decreases** the absorption of lovastatin extended release tablets. Lovastatin serum concentrations may be increased if taken with grapefruit juice; the risk of myopathy/rhabdomyolysis is increased with daily intake of large quantities of grapefruit juice (>1 quart/day); avoid concurrent use.

Stability Immediate release tablets should be stored at temperatures between 5°C to 30°C (41°F to 86°F); extended release tablets should be stored at temperatures between 20°C to 25°C (68°F to 77°F); avoid excessive heat and humidity

Mechanism of Action Lovastatin acts by competitively inhibiting 3-hydroxyl-3-methylglutaryl-coenzyme A (HMG-CoA) reductase, the enzyme that catalyzes the rate-limiting step in cholesterol biosynthesis

Pharmacodynamics

Onset of action: 3 days

Maximum effect: 4-6 weeks

LDL-C reduction: 40 mg/day: 31% (for each doubling of this dose, LDL-C is lowered by ~6%)

Average HDL-C increase: 5% to 15%

Average triglyceride reduction: 7% to 30%

Pharmacokinetics

Absorption: Oral: 30% absorbed but less than 5% reaches the systemic circulation due to an extensive first-pass effect; absorption increased with extended release tablets

Protein binding: 95%

Half-life: 1.1-1.7 hours

Time to peak serum concentration: 2-4 hours

Elimination: ~80% to 85% of dose excreted in feces and 10% in urine

Usual Dosage Oral:

Treatment of heterozygous familial hypercholesterolemia: Children and Adolescents 10-17 years: Begin treatment if after adequate trial of diet the following are present: LDL-C >189 mg/dL or LDL-C remains >160 mg/dL and positive family history of premature cardiovascular disease or meets NCEP classification (see Chart):

Initial (using immediate release formulation): 10 mg once daily, increase to 20 mg once daily after 8 weeks and 40 mg once daily after 16 weeks as needed. (**Note:** Girls must be at least 1 year post-menarche)

Adults: Initial:

Immediate release tablet: 20 mg once daily; adjust dosage at 4-week intervals; range: 10-80 mg/day in single or 2 divided doses; maximum dose: 80 mg/day; for patients requiring LDL-C reductions <20%, a lower initial dose of 10 mg once daily may be used.

Extended release tablet: 20 mg once daily; adjust dosage at 4-week intervals; maximum dose: 60 mg/day

Dosing adjustment in patients who are concomitantly receiving amiodarone or verapamil: Dose should not exceed 40 mg/day

Dosage adjustment in patients who are concomitantly receiving cyclosporine or danazol: Initial: 10 mg once daily, not to exceed 20 mg/day

Dosage adjustment in patients who are concomitantly receiving fibrates or lipid-lowering doses of niacin (≥1 g/day): Dose should not exceed 20 mg/day

Dosing adjustment in renal impairment: Cl_{cr} <30 mL/minute: Doses exceeding 20 mg/day should be carefully considered and implemented cautiously

Classification of Blood Cholesterol, LDL-C, and Triglyceride Concentrations[1]

Classification	Cholesterol (mg/dL)		LDL-C (mg/dL)		Triglycerides (mg/dL)
	Children	Adults	Children	Adults	Adults
Acceptable/optimal	<170	<200	<110	<100	<150
Above optimal	†	†	†	100-129	†
Borderline high	170-199	200-239	110-129	130-159	150-199
High	≥200	≥240	≥130	160-189	200-499
Very high	†	†	†	≥190	≥500

[1]Adapted from American Academy of Pediatrics Committee on Nutrition, "Cholesterol in Childhood," *Pediatrics*, 1998, 101(1 Pt 1):141-7 and "Third Report of the National Cholesterol Education Program Expert Panel on Detection, Evaluation, and Treatment of High Blood Cholesterol in Adults (Adult Treatment Panel III)," May 2001, www.nhlbi.nih.gov/guidelines/cholesterol.

†Lack of specific type of classification in either pediatric or adult recommendations.

Administration Oral: Administer immediate release tablets with the evening meal. Administer extended release tablet at bedtime; do not crush or chew; avoid administration with grapefruit juice

Monitoring Parameters Serum cholesterol (total and fractionated), creatine phosphokinase levels (CPK); liver function tests (see Precautions)

Reference Range Hypercholesterolemia as defined by serum cholesterol, LDL-C, and TG concentrations: See table on previous page; desired HDL-C <40 mg/dL

Patient Information Avoid grapefruit juice and the herbal medicine, St John's wort. Report severe and unresolved gastric upset, any vision changes, unexplained muscle pain or weakness, changes in color of urine or stool, yellowing of skin or eyes, and any unusual bruising. Female patients of childbearing age must be counseled to use 2 effective forms of contraception simultaneously, unless absolute abstinence is the chosen method; this drug may cause severe fetal defects.

Additional Information The current recommendation for treatment of hypercholesterolemia in children is limited to children ≥10 years of age who, after a 6-month to 1-year trial of diet therapy, continue to have LDL-C concentrations ≥190 mg/dL alone, or LDL-C concentrations ≥160 mg/dL and a family history of premature coronary artery disease, or two or more other coronary artery disease risk factors (AAP Committee on Nutrition, 1998). For each 1% lowering in LDL-C, the relative risk for major cardiovascular events is reduced by approximately 1%. For more specific risk assessment and treatment recommendations for adults, see NCEP ATPIII.

Dosage Forms Excipient information presented when available (limited, particularly for generics); consult specific product labeling.

Tablet: 10 mg, 20 mg, 40 mg

Mevacor®: 20 mg, 40 mg

Tablet, extended release:

Altoprev®: 20 mg, 40 mg, 60 mg

References

American Academy of Pediatrics Committee on Nutrition, "Cholesterol in Childhood," *Pediatrics*, 1998, 101(1 Pt 1):141-7.

American Academy of Pediatrics, "National Cholesterol Education Program: Report of the Expert Panel on Blood Cholesterol Levels in Children and Adolescents," *Pediatrics*, 1992, 89(3 Pt 2):525-84.

Duplaga BA, "Treatment of Childhood Hypercholesterolemia With HMG-CoA Reductase Inhibitors," *Ann Pharmacother*, 1999, 33(11):1224-7.

Grundy SM, Cleeman JI, Merz CN, et al, "Implications of Recent Clinical Trials for the National Cholesterol Education Program Adult Treatment Panel III Guidelines," *Circulation*, 2004, 110(2):227-39.

Lambert M, Lupien PJ, Gagne C, et al, "Treatment of Familial Hypercholesterolemia in Children and Adolescents: Effect of Lovastatin. Canadian Lovastatin in Children Study Group," *Pediatrics*, 1996, 97(5):619-28.

Stein EA, Illingworth DR, Kwiterovich PO Jr, et al, "Efficacy and Safety of Lovastatin in Adolescent Males With Heterozygous Familial Hypercholesterolemia: A Randomized Controlled Trial," *JAMA*, 1999, 281(2):137-44.

"Third Report of the National Cholesterol Education Program Expert Panel on Detection, Evaluation, and Treatment of High Blood Cholesterol in Adults (Adult Treatment Panel III)," May 2001, www.nhlbi.nih.gov/guidelines/cholesterol.

- **Lovenox®** *see* Enoxaparin *on page 571*
- **Lovenox® HP (Can)** *see* Enoxaparin *on page 571*
- **Lozi-Flur™** *see* Fluoride *on page 675*
- **L-PAM** *see* Melphalan *on page 997*
- **LRH** *see* Gonadorelin *on page 741*
- **L-Sarcolysin** *see* Melphalan *on page 997*
- **LTA® 360** *see* Lidocaine *on page 933*
- **LTG** *see* Lamotrigine *on page 906*
- **Lugol's Solution** *see* Potassium Iodide and Iodine *on page 1292*
- **Luminal® Sodium** *see* Phenobarbital *on page 1245*
- **LupiCare™ II Psoriasis [OTC]** *see* Salicylic Acid *on page 1413*
- **LupiCare™ Dandruff [OTC]** *see* Salicylic Acid *on page 1413*
- **LupiCare™ Psoriasis [OTC]** *see* Salicylic Acid *on page 1413*
- **Lupron®** *see* Leuprolide *on page 918*
- **Lupron Depot®** *see* Leuprolide *on page 918*
- **Lupron® Depot® (Can)** *see* Leuprolide *on page 918*
- **Lupron Depot-Ped®** *see* Leuprolide *on page 918*
- **Luride®** *see* Fluoride *on page 675*
- **Luride® Lozi-Tab®** *see* Fluoride *on page 675*
- **LuSonal™** *see* Phenylephrine *on page 1250*
- **Luteinizing Hormone Releasing Hormone** *see* Gonadorelin *on page 741*
- **Lutrepulse™ (Can)** *see* Gonadorelin *on page 741*
- **Luvox** *see* Fluvoxamine *on page 697*
- **Luvox® (Can)** *see* Fluvoxamine *on page 697*
- **Luxiq®** *see* Betamethasone *on page 212*

- ♦ **LY139603** *see* Atomoxetine *on page 172*
- ♦ **Lyderm® (Can)** *see* Fluocinonide *on page 674*
- ♦ **Lymphocyte Immune Globulin** *see* Antithymocyte Globulin (Equine) *on page 146*
- ♦ **Lymphocyte Mitogenic Factor** *see* Aldesleukin *on page 70*
- ♦ **M-M-R® II** *see* Measles, Mumps, and Rubella Vaccines (Combined) *on page 980*
- ♦ **Maalox® [OTC]** *see* Antacid Preparations *on page 132*
- ♦ **Maalox® Max [OTC]** *see* Antacid Preparations *on page 132*
- ♦ **Maalox® Quick Dissolve [OTC]** *see* Calcium Supplements *on page 272*
- ♦ **Maalox® Regular Chewable [OTC]** *see* Calcium Carbonate *on page 264*
- ♦ **Maalox® Total Stomach Relief® [OTC]** *see* Bismuth *on page 219*
- ♦ **Macrobid®** *see* Nitrofurantoin *on page 1139*
- ♦ **Macrodantin®** *see* Nitrofurantoin *on page 1139*

Mafenide (MA fe nide)

U.S. Brand Names Sulfamylon®

Index Terms Mafenide Acetate

Therapeutic Category Antibiotic, Topical

Generic Available No

Use Adjunct in the treatment of second and third degree burns to prevent septicemia caused by susceptible organisms such as *Pseudomonas aeruginosa*

Pregnancy Risk Factor C

Lactation Excretion in breast milk unknown/not recommended

Contraindications Hypersensitivity to mafenide or any component (see Warnings)

Warnings Superinfection with nonsusceptible organisms has occurred in burn wounds treated with mafenide; some products contain sulfites which may cause allergic reactions in susceptible individuals

Precautions Use with caution in patients with renal impairment and in patients with G-6-PD deficiency

Adverse Reactions

Dermatologic: Erythema, rash, pruritus, urticaria

Endocrine & metabolic: Hyperchloremia, metabolic acidosis

Hematologic: Bone marrow suppression, hemolytic anemia, bleeding, porphyria, eosinophilia

Local: Burning sensation, excoriation, pain, swelling

Respiratory: Hyperventilation, tachypnea

Miscellaneous: Hypersensitivity reactions, facial edema

Stability Prepared topical solution is stable for 48 hours at room temperature

Mechanism of Action Interferes with bacterial cellular metabolism and bacterial folic acid synthesis through competitive inhibition of para-aminobenzoic acid

Pharmacokinetics

Absorption: Diffuses through devascularized areas and is rapidly absorbed from burned surface

Metabolism: To para-carboxybenzene sulfonamide which is a carbonic anhydrase inhibitor

Time to peak serum concentration: Topical: 2-4 hours

Elimination: In urine as metabolites

Usual Dosage Children ≥3 months and Adults: Topical

Cream: Apply once or twice daily; apply to a thickness of approximately 16 mm; the burned area should be covered with cream at all times

Solution: Irrigate dressing every 4 hours or as needed to keep gauze moistened

Administration Topical:

Cream: Apply to cleansed, debrided, burned area with a sterile-gloved hand

Solution: Reconstitute 50 g powder by adding to 1 liter sterile water or 1 liter NS for irrigation; mix until completely dissolved; filter solution through a 0.22 micron filter before use; cover area with gauze and the dressing wetted with mafenide solution; wound dressing may be left undisturbed for up to 5 days

Monitoring Parameters Acid base balance, improvement of wound healing

Patient Information Inform physician if rash, blisters, or swelling appear

Nursing Implications For external use only

Dosage Forms Excipient information presented when available (limited, particularly for generics); consult specific product labeling.

Cream, topical:

Sulfamylon®: 85 mg/g (60 g, 120 g, 454 g) [contains sodium metabisulfite]

Powder, for topical solution, as acetate:

Sulfamylon®: 50 g/packet (5s)

- ♦ **Mafenide Acetate** *see* Mafenide *on page 968*

Magnesium Chloride (mag NEE zhum KLOR ide)

U.S. Brand Names Chloromag®; Mag 64™ [OTC]; Mag Delay® [OTC]; Slow-Mag® [OTC]

Therapeutic Category Electrolyte Supplement, Oral; Electrolyte Supplement, Parenteral; Magnesium Salt

Generic Available Yes

Use Treatment and prevention of hypomagnesemia; dietary supplement

Pregnancy Risk Factor C

Lactation Enters breast milk/compatible

Contraindications Hypersensitivity to magnesium salt(s) or any component (see Warnings); serious renal impairment, myocardial damage, heart block; patients with colostomy or ileostomy, intestinal obstruction, impaction, or perforation, appendicitis, abdominal pain

Warnings Multiple salt forms of magnesium exist; close attention must be paid to the salt form when ordering and administering magnesium; **incorrect selection or substitution of one salt for another without proper dosage adjustment may result in serious over- or under-dosing**

Magnesium chloride injection contains benzyl alcohol which may cause allergic reactions in susceptible individuals; large amounts of benzyl alcohol (≥99 mg/kg/day) have been associated with a potentially fatal toxicity ("gasping syndrome") in neonates; the "gasping syndrome" consists of metabolic acidosis, respiratory distress, gasping respirations, CNS dysfunction (including convulsions, intracranial hemorrhage), hypotension and cardiovascular collapse; avoid or use magnesium chloride injection with caution in neonates

Precautions See Magnesium Supplements *on page 976.*

Adverse Reactions See Magnesium Supplements *on page 976.*

Drug Interactions See Magnesium Supplements *on page 976.*

Mechanism of Action Magnesium is important as a cofactor in many enzymatic reactions in the body. There are at least 300 enzymes which are dependent upon magnesium for normal functioning. Actions on lipoprotein lipase have been found to be important in reducing serum cholesterol. Magnesium is necessary for the maintaining of serum potassium and calcium levels due to its effect on the renal tubule. In the heart, magnesium acts as a calcium channel blocker. It also activates sodium potassium ATPase in the cell membrane to promote resting polarization and produce arrhythmias.

Pharmacodynamics See Magnesium Supplements *on page 976.*

Pharmacokinetics See Magnesium Supplements *on page 976.*

Usual Dosage

Hypomagnesemia:

Neonates: I.V.: **Magnesium chloride:** 0.2-0.4 mEq/kg/dose every 8-12 hours for 2-3 doses

Children:

I.M., I.V.: **Magnesium chloride:** 0.2-0.4 mEq/kg/dose every 4-6 hours for 3-4 doses; maximum single dose: 16 mEq

Oral: **Note:** Achieving optimal magnesium levels using oral therapy may be difficult due to the propensity for magnesium to cause diarrhea; I.V. replacement may be more appropriate particularly in situations of severe deficit: **Magnesium chloride:** 10-20 mg/kg elemental magnesium per dose up to 4 times/day

Dietary supplement: Adults: Oral: (Mag 64™, Mag Delay®, Slow-Mag®): 2 tablets once daily

(Continued)

Magnesium Chloride *(Continued)*

Daily maintenance magnesium: I.V.: **Magnesium chloride:**
Neonates, Infants, and Children ≤45 kg: 0.25-0.5 mEq/kg/day
Adolescents >45 kg and Adults: 0.2-0.5 mEq/kg/day or 3-10 mEq/1000 kcal/day (maximum: 8-20 mEq/day)

Dosing adjustment in renal impairment: Patients in severe renal failure should not receive magnesium due to toxicity from accumulation. Patients with a Cl_{cr} <25 mL/minute receiving magnesium should have serum magnesium levels monitored.

Administration
Oral: Tablet: Take with full glass of water; do not chew or crush sustained release formulations
Parenteral: Intermittent infusion: Dilute to a concentration of 0.5 mEq/mL (maximum concentration: 1.6 mEq/mL, and infuse over 2-4 hours; do not exceed 1 mEq/kg/hour; in severe circumstances, half of the dosage to be administered may be infused over the first 15-20 minutes

Monitoring Parameters See Magnesium Supplements *on page 976.*
Reference Range See Magnesium Supplements *on page 976.*
Additional Information Magnesium chloride 500 mg = 59 mg **elemental** magnesium= 4.9 mEq magnesium
Dosage Forms Excipient information presented when available (limited, particularly for generics); consult specific product labeling.
Injection, solution: 200 mg/mL [1.97 mEq/mL] (50 mL)
Chloromag®: 200 mg/mL [1.97 mEq/mL] (50 mL)
Tablet [enteric coated]:
Slow-Mag®: Elemental magnesium 64 mg [contains elemental calcium 106 mg]
Tablet, delayed release:
Mag 64™, Mag Delay®: Magnesium chloride hexahydrate 535 mg [equivalent to elemental magnesium 64 mg; contains elemental calcium 110 mg]

Magnesium Citrate (mag NEE zhum SIT rate)

U.S. Brand Names Citroma® [OTC]
Canadian Brand Names Citro-Mag®
Index Terms Citrate of Magnesia
Therapeutic Category Laxative, Osmotic; Magnesium Salt
Generic Available Yes
Use Short-term treatment of constipation
Pregnancy Risk Factor B
Contraindications Hypersensitivity to magnesium salt(s) or any component (see Warnings); serious renal impairment, myocardial damage, heart block; patients with colostomy or ileostomy, intestinal obstruction, impaction, or perforation, appendicitis, abdominal pain
Warnings Multiple salt forms of magnesium exist; close attention must be paid to the salt form when ordering and administering magnesium; **incorrect selection or substitution of one salt for another without proper dosage adjustment may result in serious over- or under-dosing**
Precautions See Magnesium Supplements *on page 976.*
Adverse Reactions See Magnesium Supplements *on page 976.*
Drug Interactions See Magnesium Supplements *on page 976.*
Mechanism of Action Promotes bowel evacuation by causing osmotic retention of fluid which distends the colon and produces increased peristaltic activity when taken orally.
Pharmacodynamics See Magnesium Supplements *on page 976.*
Pharmacokinetics See Magnesium Supplements *on page 976.*
Usual Dosage Cathartic: Oral:
Children <6 years: 2-4 mL/kg/dose given once or in divided doses
Children 6-12 years: 100-150 mL/dose given once or in divided doses
Children >12 years and Adults: 150-300 mL/dose given once or in divided doses

Dosing adjustment in renal impairment: Patients in severe renal failure should not receive magnesium due to toxicity from accumulation. Patients with a Cl_{cr} <25 mL/minute receiving magnesium should have serum magnesium levels monitored.

Administration Oral:
Solution: Mix with water and administer on an empty stomach.
Tablet: Take with full glass of water.
Monitoring Parameters See Magnesium Supplements *on page 976.*
Reference Range See Magnesium Supplements *on page 976.*
Dosage Forms Excipient information presented when available (limited, particularly for generics); consult specific product labeling.

Solution, oral: 290 mg/5 mL (300 mL) [cherry and lemon flavors]
Citroma®: 290 mg/5 mL (300 mL) [contains magnesium 48 mg and potassium 13 mg per 5 mL; cherry and lemon flavors]; (300 mL) [contains magnesium 48 mg and sodium 7.5 mg per 5 mL; grape and lemony flavors]
Tablet: 100 mg [as elemental magnesium]

Magnesium Gluconate (mag NEE zhum GLOO koe nate)

U.S. Brand Names Almora® [OTC]; Mag G® [OTC]; Magonate® [OTC]; Magtrate® [OTC]

Therapeutic Category Electrolyte Supplement, Oral; Magnesium Salt

Generic Available Yes: Tablet

Use Treatment and prevention of hypomagnesemia; dietary supplement

Lactation Enters breast milk/compatible

Contraindications Hypersensitivity to magnesium salt(s) or any component (see Warnings); serious renal impairment, myocardial damage, heart block; patients with colostomy or ileostomy, intestinal obstruction, impaction, or perforation, appendicitis, abdominal pain

Warnings Multiple salt forms of magnesium exist; close attention must be paid to the salt form when ordering and administering magnesium; **incorrect selection or substitution of one salt for another without proper dosage adjustment may result in serious over- or under-dosing**

Magonate® solution contains sodium benzoate; benzoic acid (benzoate) is a metabolite of benzyl alcohol; large amounts of benzyl alcohol (≥99 mg/kg/day) have been associated with a potentially fatal toxicity ("gasping syndrome") in neonates; *in vitro* and animal studies have shown that benzoate displaces bilirubin from protein binding sites; avoid use of Magonate® solution in neonates

Precautions See Magnesium Supplements *on page 976.*

Adverse Reactions See Magnesium Supplements *on page 976.*

Drug Interactions See Magnesium Supplements *on page 976.*

Mechanism of Action Magnesium is important as a cofactor in many enzymatic reactions in the body. There are at least 300 enzymes which are dependent upon magnesium for normal functioning. Actions on lipoprotein lipase have been found to be important in reducing serum cholesterol. Magnesium is necessary for the maintaining of serum potassium and calcium levels due to its effect on the renal tubule. In the heart, magnesium acts as a calcium channel blocker. It also activates sodium potassium ATPase in the cell membrane to promote resting polarization and produce arrhythmias.

Pharmacodynamics See Magnesium Supplements *on page 976.*

Pharmacokinetics See Magnesium Supplements *on page 976.*

Usual Dosage Oral: **Note:** Achieving optimal magnesium levels using oral therapy may be difficult due to the propensity for magnesium to cause diarrhea: I.V. replacement may be more appropriate particularly in situations of severe deficit.

Prevention and treatment of hypomagnesemia:
Children: 10-20 mg/kg **elemental** magnesium per dose up to 4 times/day
Adults: 500-1000 mg 3 times/day

Dosing adjustment in renal impairment: Patients in severe renal failure should not receive magnesium due to toxicity from accumulation. Patients with a Cl_{cr} <25 mL/minute receiving magnesium should have serum magnesium levels monitored.

Administration Oral:
Solution: Mix with water and administer on an empty stomach.
Tablet: Take with full glass of water.

Monitoring Parameters See Magnesium Supplements *on page 976.*

Reference Range See Magnesium Supplements *on page 976.*

Additional Information Magnesium gluconate 500 mg = 27 mg **elemental** magnesium = 2.4 mEq magnesium

Dosage Forms Excipient information presented when available (limited, particularly for generics); consult specific product labeling.

Solution:
Magonate®: 1000 mg/5 mL (480 mL) [magnesium 4.8 mEq/5 mL; equivalent to elemental magnesium 54 mg/5 mL; contains sodium benzoate]
Tablet: 500 mg [magnesium 2.4 mEq; equivalent to elemental magnesium 27 mg]
Almora®, Mag G®, Magonate®, Magtrate®): 500 mg [magnesium 2.4 mEq; equivalent to elemental magnesium 27 mg]

Magnesium Hydroxide (mag NEE zhum hye DROKS ide)

U.S. Brand Names Dulcolax® Milk of Magnesia [OTC]; Phillips'® Milk of Magnesia [OTC]; Phillips'® M-O [OTC]

(Continued)

Magnesium Hydroxide *(Continued)*

Index Terms Magnesia Magma; Milk of Magnesia; MOM

Therapeutic Category Antacid; Laxative, Osmotic

Generic Available Yes: Liquid

Use Short-term treatment of constipation; treatment of hyperacidity symptoms

Pregnancy Risk Factor B

Contraindications Hypersensitivity to magnesium salt(s) or any component (see Warnings); serious renal impairment, myocardial damage, heart block; patients with colostomy or ileostomy, intestinal obstruction, impaction, or perforation, appendicitis, abdominal pain

Warnings Multiple salt forms of magnesium exist; close attention must be paid to the salt form when ordering and administering magnesium; **incorrect selection or substitution of one salt for another without proper dosage adjustment may result in serious over- or under-dosing**

Precautions See Magnesium Supplements *on page 976.*

Adverse Reactions See Magnesium Supplements *on page 976.*

Drug Interactions See Magnesium Supplements *on page 976.*

Mechanism of Action Promotes bowel evacuation by causing osmotic retention of fluid which distends the colon and produces increased peristaltic activity when taken orally. To reduce stomach acidity, it reacts with hydrochloric acid in stomach to form magnesium chloride.

Pharmacodynamics See Magnesium Supplements *on page 976.*

Pharmacokinetics See Magnesium Supplements *on page 976.*

Usual Dosage Oral:

Liquid: Dosage based upon regular strength liquid (400 mg/5 mL); when using concentrated magnesium hydroxide solution, reduce recommended dose by 1/2:
- Children <2 years: 0.5 mL/kg/dose
- Children 2-5 years: 5-15 mL/day once before bedtime or in divided doses
- Children 6-11 years: 15-30 mL/day once before bedtime or in divided doses
- Children ≥12 years and Adults: 30-60 mL/day once before bedtime or in divided doses

Tablet:
- Children 2-5 years: 311-622 mg (1-2 tablets) once before bedtime or in divided doses
- Children 6-11 years: 933-1244 mg (3-4 tablets) once before bedtime or in divided doses
- Children ≥12 years and Adults: 1866-2488 mg (6-8 tablets) once before bedtime or in divided doses

Magnesium hydroxide and mineral oil (Phillips'® M-O) (infant dosage to provide equivalent dosage of magnesium hydroxide listed above):
- Children <2 years: 0.6 mL/kg/dose
- Children 2-5 years: 5-15 mL/day once or in divided doses
- Children 6-11 years: 15-30 mL/day once or in divided doses
- Children ≥12 years and Adults: 30-60 mL once or in divided doses

Antacid: Oral:
- Children:
  - Liquid: 2.5-5 mL/dose, up to 4 times/day
  - Tablet: 311 mg (1 tablet) up to 4 times/day
- Adults:
  - Liquid: 5-15 mL/dose, up to 4 times/day
  - Liquid concentrate: 2.5-7.5 mL/dose, up to 4 times/day
  - Tablet: 622-1244 mg/dose (2-4 tablets) up to 4 times/day

Dosing adjustment in renal impairment: Patients in severe renal failure should not receive magnesium due to toxicity from accumulation. Patients with a Cl_{cr} <25 mL/minute receiving magnesium should have serum magnesium levels monitored.

Administration Oral:

Solution: Mix with water and administer on an empty stomach.

Tablet: Take with full glass of water.

Monitoring Parameters See Magnesium Supplements *on page 976.*

Reference Range See Magnesium Supplements *on page 976.*

Dosage Forms Excipient information presented when available (limited, particularly for generics); consult specific product labeling.

Magnesium hydroxide:
- Liquid, oral: 400 mg/5 mL (360 mL, 480 mL, 960 mL, 3780 mL)
  - Dulcolax® Milk of Magnesia: 400 mg/5 mL (360 mL, 780 mL) [regular and mint flavors]
  - Phillips'® Milk of Magnesia: 400 mg/5 mL (120 mL, 360 mL, 780 mL) [original, French vanilla, cherry, and mint flavors]
- Liquid, oral concentrate: 800 mg/5 mL (100 mL, 400 mL)

Phillips'® Milk of Magnesia [concentrate]: 800 mg/5 mL (240 mL) [strawberry créme flavor]

Tablet, chewable (Phillips'® Milk of Magnesia): 311 mg [mint flavor]

Magnesium hydroxide and mineral oil:

Suspension, oral (Phillips'® M-O): Magnesium hydroxide 300 mg and mineral oil 1.25 mL per 5 mL (360 mL, 780 mL) [original and mint flavors]

Magnesium L-aspartate Hydrochloride

(mag NEE zhum el as PAR tate hye droe KLOR ide)

U.S. Brand Names Maginex™ [OTC]; Maginex™ DS [OTC]

Index Terms MAH

Therapeutic Category Electrolyte Supplement, Oral; Magnesium Salt

Generic Available No

Use Magnesium supplement

Lactation Enters breast milk/compatible

Contraindications Hypersensitivity to magnesium salt(s) or any component (see Warnings); serious renal impairment, myocardial damage, heart block; patients with colostomy or ileostomy, intestinal obstruction, impaction, or perforation, appendicitis, abdominal pain

Warnings Multiple salt forms of magnesium exist; close attention must be paid to the salt form when ordering and administering magnesium; **incorrect selection or substitution of one salt for another without proper dosage adjustment may result in serious over- or under-dosing**

Precautions See Magnesium Supplements *on page 976.*

Adverse Reactions See Magnesium Supplements *on page 976.*

Drug Interactions See Magnesium Supplements *on page 976.*

Mechanism of Action Magnesium is important as a cofactor in many enzymatic reactions in the body. There are at least 300 enzymes which are dependent upon magnesium for normal functioning. Actions on lipoprotein lipase have been found to be important in reducing serum cholesterol. Magnesium is necessary for the maintaining of serum potassium and calcium levels due to its effect on the renal tubule. In the heart, magnesium acts as a calcium channel blocker. It also activates sodium potassium ATPase in the cell membrane to promote resting polarization and produce arrhythmias.

Pharmacodynamics See Magnesium Supplements *on page 976.*

Pharmacokinetics See Magnesium Supplements *on page 976.*

Usual Dosage Oral:

Hypomagnesemia: **Note:** Achieving optimal magnesium levels using oral therapy may be difficult due to the propensity for magnesium to cause diarrhea: I.V. replacement may be more appropriate particularly in situations of severe deficit:

Children: 10-20 mg/kg elemental magnesium per dose up to 4 times/day

Dietary supplement: Adults: 1230 mg up to 3 times/day

Dosing adjustment in renal impairment: Patients in severe renal failure should not receive magnesium due to toxicity from accumulation. Patients with a Cl_{cr} <25 mL/minute receiving magnesium should have serum magnesium levels monitored.

Administration Oral:

Granules: Mix each packet in 4 ounces water or juice prior to administration

Tablet: Take with full glass of water

Monitoring Parameters See Magnesium Supplements *on page 976.*

Reference Range See Magnesium Supplements *on page 976.*

Additional Information Magnesium L-aspartate 500 mg = 49.6 mg **elemental** magnesium = 4.1 mEq magnesium

Dosage Forms Excipient information presented when available (limited, particularly for generics); consult specific product labeling.

Granules:

Maginex™ DS: 1230 mg [magnesium 10 mEq; equivalent to magnesium 122 mg; lemon flavor]

Tablet [enteric coated]:

Maginex™: 615 mg [magnesium 5 mEq; equivalent to magnesium 61 mg]

Magnesium Oxide (mag NEE zhum OKS ide)

U.S. Brand Names Mag-Caps [OTC]; MagGel™ [OTC]; Mag-Ox® 400 [OTC]; Uro-Mag® [OTC]

Therapeutic Category Electrolyte Supplement, Oral; Laxative, Osmotic; Magnesium Salt

Generic Available Yes

(Continued)

Magnesium Oxide *(Continued)*

Use Magnesium supplement; short-term treatment of constipation; treatment of hyperacidity symptoms

Lactation Enters breast milk/compatible

Contraindications Hypersensitivity to magnesium salt(s) or any component (see Warnings); serious renal impairment, myocardial damage, heart block; patients with colostomy or ileostomy, intestinal obstruction, impaction, or perforation, appendicitis, abdominal pain

Warnings Multiple salt forms of magnesium exist; close attention must be paid to the salt form when ordering and administering magnesium; **incorrect selection or substitution of one salt for another without proper dosage adjustment may result in serious over- or under-dosing**

Precautions See Magnesium Supplements *on page 976.*

Adverse Reactions See Magnesium Supplements *on page 976.*

Drug Interactions See Magnesium Supplements *on page 976.*

Mechanism of Action Magnesium is important as a cofactor in many enzymatic reactions in the body. There are at least 300 enzymes which are dependent upon magnesium for normal functioning. Actions on lipoprotein lipase have been found to be important in reducing serum cholesterol. Magnesium is necessary for the maintaining of serum potassium and calcium levels due to its effect on the renal tubule. In the heart, magnesium acts as a calcium channel blocker. It also activates sodium potassium ATPase in the cell membrane to promote resting polarization and produce arrhythmias. Promotes bowel evacuation by causing osmotic retention of fluid which distends the colon and produces increased peristaltic activity when taken orally. To reduce stomach acidity, it reacts with hydrochloric acid in the stomach to form magnesium chloride

Pharmacodynamics See Magnesium Supplements *on page 976.*

Pharmacokinetics See Magnesium Supplements *on page 976.*

Usual Dosage Oral:

Antacid: Adults: 140 mg 3-4 times/day or 400-840 mg/day

Cathartic: Adults: 2-4 g at bedtime

Hypomagnesemia: **Note:** Achieving optimal magnesium levels using oral therapy may be difficult due to the propensity for magnesium to cause diarrhea: I.V. replacement may be more appropriate particularly in situations of severe deficit.
Children: 10-20 mg/kg elemental magnesium per dose up to 4 times/day

Dosing adjustment in renal impairment: Patients in severe renal failure should not receive magnesium due to toxicity from accumulation. Patients with a Cl_{cr} <25 mL/minute receiving magnesium should have serum magnesium levels monitored.

Administration Oral: Tablet: Take with full glass of water.

Monitoring Parameters See Magnesium Supplements *on page 976.*

Reference Range See Magnesium Supplements *on page 976.*

Additional Information Magnesium oxide 500 mg = 302 mg **elemental** magnesium = 25 mEq magnesium

Dosage Forms Excipient information presented when available (limited, particularly for generics); consult specific product labeling.

Caplet: 250 mg

Capsule:

- Mag-Caps: Elemental magnesium 85 mg
- Uro-Mag®: 140 mg [magnesium 7 mEq; equivalent to elemental magnesium 84.5 mg]

Capsule, softgel:

- MagGel™: 600 mg [magnesium 28.64 mEq; equivalent to elemental magnesium 348 mg]

Tablet: 400 mg [magnesium 20 mEq; equivalent to elemental magnesium 242 mg], 500 mg

- Mag-Ox® 400: 400 mg [magnesium 20 mEq; equivalent to elemental magnesium 242 mg]

Magnesium Sulfate (mag NEE zhum SUL fate)

Medication Safety Issues

Sound-alike/look-alike issues:

Magnesium sulfate may be confused with manganese sulfate, morphine sulfate
$MgSO_4$ is an error-prone abbreviation (mistaken as morphine sulfate)

High alert medication: The Institute for Safe Medication Practices (ISMP) includes this medication (I.V. formulation) among its list of drugs which have a heightened risk of causing significant patient harm when used in error.

Related Information

Adult ACLS Algorithms *on page 1660*

CPR Pediatric Drug Dosages *on page 1650*
Pediatric ALS Algorithms *on page 1657*

Index Terms Epsom Salts; $MgSO_4$ (error-prone abbreviation)

Therapeutic Category Anticonvulsant; Electrolyte Supplement, Oral; Electrolyte Supplement, Parenteral; Magnesium Salt

Generic Available Yes

Use Treatment and prevention of hypomagnesemia, treatment of hypertension, torsade de pointes, and encephalopathy and seizures associated with acute nephritis; prevention and treatment of seizures in severe pre-eclampsia or eclampsia; prevention of premature labor

Unlabeled use: Adjunctive treatment for bronchodilation in moderate to severe acute asthma

Pregnancy Risk Factor A

Lactation Enters breast milk/compatible

Contraindications Hypersensitivity to magnesium salt(s) or any component (see Warnings); serious renal impairment, myocardial damage, heart block; patients with colostomy or ileostomy, intestinal obstruction, impaction, or perforation, appendicitis, abdominal pain

Warnings Multiple salt forms of magnesium exist; close attention must be paid to the salt form when ordering and administering magnesium; **incorrect selection or substitution of one salt for another without proper dosage adjustment may result in serious over- or under-dosing**

Precautions See Magnesium Supplements *on page 976.*

Adverse Reactions See Magnesium Supplements *on page 976.*

Drug Interactions See Magnesium Supplements *on page 976.*

Mechanism of Action Magnesium is important as a cofactor in many enzymatic reactions in the body. There are at least 300 enzymes which are dependent upon magnesium for normal functioning. Actions on lipoprotein lipase have been found to be important in reducing serum cholesterol. Magnesium is necessary for the maintaining of serum potassium and calcium levels due to its effect on the renal tubule. In the heart, magnesium acts as a calcium channel blocker. It also activates sodium potassium ATPase in the cell membrane to promote resting polarization and produce arrhythmias. Magnesium prevents premature labor by inhibiting myometrial contractions. In the CNS, magnesium prevents or controls seizures by blocking neuromuscular transmission and decreasing the amount of acetylcholine liberated at the end-plate by the motor nerve impulse. It also has a depressant effect on the CNS.

Pharmacodynamics See Magnesium Supplements *on page 976.*

Pharmacokinetics See Magnesium Supplements *on page 976.*

Usual Dosage

Hypomagnesemia:

- Neonates: I.V.: 25-50 mg/kg/dose (0.2-0.4 mEq/kg/dose) every 8-12 hours for 2-3 doses
- Children: I.M., I.V.: 25-50 mg/kg/dose (0.2-0.4 mEq/kg/dose) every 4-6 hours for 3-4 doses; maximum single dose: 2000 mg (16 mEq)
- Adults: I.M., I.V.: 1 g every 6 hours for 4 doses, or 250 mg/kg over a 4-hour period; for severe hypomagnesemia: 8-12 g/day in divided doses has been used

Daily maintenance magnesium: I.V.:

- Neonates, Infants, and Children ≤45 kg: 0.25-0.5 mEq/kg/day
- Adolescents >45 kg and Adults: 0.2-0.5 mEq/kg/day or 3-10 mEq/1000 kcal/day (maximum: 8-24 mEq/day)

Management of seizures and hypertension: I.M., I.V.:

- Children: 20-100 mg/kg/dose every 4-6 hours as needed; in severe cases, doses as high as 200 mg/kg/dose have been used
- Adults: 1 g every 6 hours for 4 doses as needed

Prevention of premature labor: I.V.: Adolescents and Adults: Initial loading dose: 4-6 g followed by a continuous infusion of 2-3 g/hour

Treatment and prevention of seizures in severe pre-eclampsia or eclampsia: I.V.: Adolescents and Adults: Initial loading dose: 4-6 g followed by a continuous infusion of 2 g/hour; alternatively, following the loading dose, 4-5 g I.M. into alternate buttocks every 4 hours has been used

Treatment of torsade de pointes VT: I.V.:

- Infants and Children: 25-50 mg/kg/dose; not to exceed 2 g/dose
- Adults: 1-2 g/dose

Bronchodilation (adjunctive treatment in moderate to severe acute asthma): I.V.:

- Children: 25 mg/kg/dose (maximum dose: 2 g) as a single dose
- Adults: 2 g as a single dose

Note: Literature evaluating magnesium sulfate's efficacy in the relief of bronchospasm has utilized single dosages in patients with acute symptomatology who have received aerosol β-agonist therapy (see References) with inconsistent results. A recent study (Ciarallo, 2000) showed significant improvement in

(Continued)

Magnesium Sulfate *(Continued)*

pulmonary function in children who received a single dose of 40 mg/kg magnesium sulfate vs. placebo; pulmonary index scores after magnesium sulfate 75 mg/kg (maximum: 2.5 g) vs. placebo were not statistically different in 54 children between 1-18 years of age (Scarfone, 2000). See Additional Information.

Dosing adjustment in renal impairment: Patients in severe renal failure should not receive magnesium due to toxicity from accumulation. Patients with a Cl_{cr} <25 mL/minute receiving magnesium should have serum magnesium levels monitored.

Administration Parenteral:

Intermittent infusion: Dilute to a concentration of 0.5 mEq/mL (60 mg/mL of **magnesium sulfate**) (maximum concentration: 1.6 mEq/mL, 200 mg/mL of magnesium sulfate) and infuse over 2-4 hours; do not exceed 1 mEq/kg/hour (125 mg/kg/hour of magnesium sulfate); in severe circumstances, half of the dosage to be administered may be infused over the first 15-20 minutes; in medical emergencies (eg, prevention of seizures in pre-eclampsia), the loading dose (4-6 g) may be infused over 15-20 minutes (smaller doses, eg, treatment of torsade de pointes, may be infused over 5-20 minutes).

For I.M. administration, dilute magnesium sulfate to a maximum concentration of 200 mg/mL prior to injection

Monitoring Parameters See Magnesium Supplements *on page 976.*

Reference Range See Magnesium Supplements *on page 976.*

Additional Information Magnesium sulfate 500mg = 49.3 mg **elemental** magnesium = 4.1 mEq magnesium. Nebulized magnesium sulfate in varying concentrations/dosages has been used successfully with and without $beta_2$-adrenergic agonists in the treatment of acute asthma (Blitz, 2006).

Dosage Forms Excipient information presented when available (limited, particularly for generics); consult specific product labeling.

Infusion [premixed in D_5W]: 10 mg/mL (100 mL); 20 mg/mL (500 mL, 1000 mL)

Infusion [premixed in water for injection]: 40 mg/mL (100 mL, 500 mL, 1000 mL); 80 mg/mL (50 mL)

Injection, solution: 125 mg/mL (8 mL); 500 mg/mL (2 mL, 5 mL, 10 mL, 20 mL, 50 mL)

Powder, oral/topical: Magnesium sulfate USP (227 g, 454 g, 480 g, 1810 g, 1920 g, 2720 g)

References

"2005 American Heart Association (AHA) Guidelines for Cardiopulmonary Resuscitation (CPR) and Emergency Cardiovascular Care (ECC) of Pediatric and Neonatal Patients: Pediatric Advanced Life Support," *Pediatrics*, 2006, 117(5):1005-28.

Blitz M, Blitz S, Beasely R, et al, "Inhaled Magnesium Sulfate in the Treatment of Acute Asthma," *Cochrane Database Syst Rev*, 2005, 19(4):CD003898.

Briggs GG and Wan SR, "Drug Therapy During Labor and Delivery, Part 2," *Am J Health Syst Pharm*, 2006, 63(12):1131-9.

Bloch H, Silverman R, Mancherje N, et al, "Intravenous Magnesium Sulfate as an Adjunct in the Treatment of Acute Asthma," *Chest*, 1995, 107(6):1576-81.

Chernow B, Smith J, Rainey TG, et al, "Hypomagnesemia: Implications for the Critical Care Specialist," *Crit Care Med*, 1982, 10(3):193-6.

Cheuk DK, Chau TC, and Lee SL, "A Meta-analysis on Intravenous Magnesium Sulphate for Treating Acute Asthma," *Arch Dis Child*, 2005, 90(1):74-7

Ciarallo L, Brousseau D, and Reinert S, "Higher-Dose Intravenous Magnesium Therapy for Children With Moderate to Severe Acute Asthma," *Arch Pediatr Adolesc Med*, 2000, 154(10):979-83.

Ciarallo L, Sauer AH, and Shannon MW, "Intravenous Magnesium Therapy for Moderate to Severe Pediatric Asthma: Results of a Randomized, Placebo-Controlled Trial," *J Pediatr*, 1996, 129(6):809-14.

"Dietary Reference Intakes for Calcium, Phosphorus, Magnesium, Vitamin D, and Fluoride. Standing Committee on the Scientific Evaluation of Dietary Reference Intakes, Food and Nutrition Board, Institute of Medicine," National Academy of Sciences, Washington, DC: National Academy Press, 1997.

Scarfone RJ, Loiselle JM, Joffe MD, et al, "A Randomized Trial of Magnesium in the Emergency Department Treatment of Children With Asthma," *Ann Emerg Med*, 2000, 36(6):572-8.

Magnesium Supplements (mag NEE zee um SUP la ments)

Related Information

Magnesium Chloride *on page 969*
Magnesium Citrate *on page 970*
Magnesium Gluconate *on page 971*
Magnesium Hydroxide *on page 971*
Magnesium L-aspartate Hydrochloride *on page 973*
Magnesium Oxide *on page 973*
Magnesium Sulfate *on page 974*

U.S. Brand Names Almora® [OTC]; Chloromag®; Dulcolax® Milk of Magnesia [OTC]; Mag Delay® [OTC]; Mag G® [OTC]; MagGel™ [OTC]; Maginex™ [OTC]; Maginex™ DS [OTC]; Magonate® [OTC]; Magonate® Sport [OTC] [DSC]; Mag-Ox 400® [OTC]; Magtrate® [OTC]; May-SR® [OTC]; Phillips'® Milk of Magnesia [OTC]; Phillips'® M-O [OTC]; Slow-Mag® [OTC]; Uro-Mag® [OTC]

Index Terms Citrate of Magnesia (Magnesium Citrate); Epsom Salts (Magnesium Sulfate); Magnesia Magma (Magnesium Hydroxide); Milk of Magnesia (Magnesium Hydroxide); MOM (Magnesium Hydroxide)

Therapeutic Category Antacid; Anticonvulsant, Miscellaneous; Electrolyte Supplement, Oral; Electrolyte Supplement, Parenteral; Laxative, Osmotic; Magnesium Salt

Generic Available Yes

Use

Treatment and prevention of hypomagnesemia **(see individual monographs for magnesium chloride, magnesium sulfate, magnesium gluconate, magnesium l-aspartate hydrochloride, and magnesium oxide)**

Treatment of hypertension **(see individual monograph for magnesium sulfate)**

Treatment of torsade de pointes **(see individual monograph for magnesium sulfate)**

Treatment of encephalopathy and seizures associated with acute nephritis **(see individual monograph for magnesium sulfate)**

Short-term treatment of constipation **(see individual monographs for magnesium citrate, magnesium hydroxide, and magnesium oxide)**

Treatment of hyperacidity symptoms **(see individual monographs for magnesium hydroxide and magnesium oxide)**

Unlabeled use: Adjunctive treatment for bronchodilation in moderate to severe acute asthma **(see individual monograph for magnesium sulfate)**

Pregnancy Risk Factor B

Contraindications Hypersensitivity to magnesium salt(s) or any component (see Warnings); serious renal impairment, myocardial damage, heart block; patients with colostomy or ileostomy, intestinal obstruction, impaction, or perforation, appendicitis, abdominal pain

Warnings Multiple salt forms of magnesium exist; close attention must be paid to the salt form when ordering and administering magnesium; **incorrect selection or substitution of one salt for another without proper dosage adjustment may result in serious over- or under-dosing.**

Precautions Use with caution in patients with impaired renal function (accumulation of magnesium may lead to magnesium intoxication); use with caution in digitalized patients (may alter cardiac conduction leading to heart block)

Adverse Reactions Adverse effects with magnesium therapy are primarily related to the magnesium serum level

>3 mg/dL: Depressed CNS, blocked peripheral neuromuscular transmission leading to anticonvulsant effects
>5 mg/dL: Depressed deep tendon reflexes, flushing, somnolence
>12 mg/dL: Respiratory paralysis, complete heart block

Other effects:
- Cardiovascular: Hypotension
- Endocrine & metabolic: Hypermagnesemia
- Gastrointestinal: Diarrhea, abdominal cramps, gas formation
- Neuromuscular & skeletal: Muscle weakness

Drug Interactions Magnesium salts, when given orally, may decrease the absorption of the following: H_2 antagonists, phenytoin, iron salts, penicillamine, tetracycline, ciprofloxacin, benzodiazepines, chloroquine, steroids, and glyburide; systemic magnesium may enhance the effects of calcium channel blockers and neuromuscular blockers; may share additive CNS depressant effects with CNS depressants; if sufficient alkalinization of the urine by magnesium salts occurs, the excretion of salicylates is enhanced and the tubular reabsorption of quinidine is enhanced (increased effect)

Pharmacodynamics

Onset of action:
- Anticonvulsant:
  - I.M.: 60 minutes
  - I.V.: Immediately
- Laxative: Oral: 4-8 hours

Duration: Anticonvulsant:
- I.M.: 3-4 hours
- I.V.: 30 minutes

Pharmacokinetics

Absorption: Oral: Up to 30%

Elimination: Renal with unabsorbed drug excreted in feces

Usual Dosage

Recommended daily allowance of magnesium: Oral: See table on next page.

Treatment and prevention of hypomagnesemia:

I.V.: See magnesium chloride *on page 969* and magnesium sulfate *on page 974*

(Continued)

Magnesium Supplements *(Continued)*

Magnesium - Recommended Daily Allowance (RDA) and Estimated Average Requirement (EAR) (in terms of elemental magnesium)

Age	RDA (mg/day)	EAR (mg/day)
<6 mo	40	30
6-12 mo	60	75
1-3 y	80	65
4-8 y	130	110
Male		
9-13 y	240	200
14-18 y	410	340
19-30 y	400	330
Female		
9-13 y	240	200
14-18 y	360	300
19-30 y	310	255

Elemental Magnesium Content of Magnesium Salts

Magnesium Salt	Elemental Magnesium (mg per 500 mg salt)	mEq Magnesium per 500 mg salt
Magnesium chloride	59	4.9
Magnesium gluconate	27	2.4
Magnesium L-aspartate	49.6	4.1
Magnesium oxide	302	25
Magnesium sulfate	49.3	4.1

Oral: See magnesium chloride *on page 969*, magnesium gluconate *on page 971*, magnesium L-aspartate *on page 973*, and magnesium oxide *on page 973*.

Management of hypertension & seizures: I.V.: See magnesium sulfate *on page 974*

Treatment of torsade de pointes VT: I.V.: See magnesium sulfate *on page 974*

Bronchodilation: I.V: See magnesium sulfate *on page 974*

Cathartic: Oral: See magnesium citrate *on page 970*, magnesium hydroxide *on page 971*, and magnesium oxide *on page 973*

Antacid: Oral: See magnesium hydroxide *on page 971* and magnesium oxide *on page 973*

Administration See individual monographs.

Monitoring Parameters Serum magnesium, deep tendon reflexes, respiratory rate, renal function, blood pressure, stool output (laxative use)

Reference Range

Neonates and Infants: 1.5-2.3 mEq/L

Children: 1.5-2.0 mEq/L

Adults: 1.4-2.0 mEq/L

Additional Information 1 g elemental magnesium = 83.3 mEq = 41.1 mmol

Dosage Forms See individual monographs.

References

"2005 American Heart Association (AHA) Guidelines for Cardiopulmonary Resuscitation (CPR) and Emergency Cardiovascular Care (ECC) of Pediatric and Neonatal Patients: Pediatric Advanced Life Support," *Pediatrics*, 2006, 117(5):1005-28.

Bloch H, Silverman R, Mancherje N, et al, "Intravenous Magnesium Sulfate as an Adjunct in the Treatment of Acute Asthma," *Chest*, 1995, 107(6):1576-81.

Chernow B, Smith J, Rainey TG, et al, "Hypomagnesemia: Implications for the Critical Care Specialist," *Crit Care Med*, 1982, 10(3):193-6.

Ciarallo L, Brousseau D, and Reinert S, "Higher-Dose Intravenous Magnesium Therapy for Children With Moderate to Severe Acute Asthma," *Arch Pediatr Adolesc Med*, 2000, 154(10):979-83.

Ciarallo L, Sauer AH, and Shannon MW, "Intravenous Magnesium Therapy for Moderate to Severe Pediatric Asthma: Results of a Randomized, Placebo-Controlled Trial," *J Pediatr*, 1996, 129(6):809-14.

"Dietary Reference Intakes for Calcium, Phosphorus, Magnesium, Vitamin D, and Fluoride. Standing Committee on the Scientific Evaluation of Dietary Reference Intakes, Food and Nutrition Board, Institute of Medicine," National Academy of Sciences, Washington, DC: National Academy Press, 1997.

Engel J, "Normal Laboratory Values," *Pocket Guide to Pediatric Assessment*, St Louis, MO: CV Mosby, 1989, 259.

Scarfone RJ, Loiselle JM, Joffe MD, et al, "A Randomized Trial of Magnesium in the Emergency Department Treatment of Children With Asthma," *Ann Emerg Med*, 2000, 36(6):572-8.

- ♦ **Magonate® [OTC]** *see* Magnesium Gluconate *on page 971*
- ♦ **Magonate® [OTC]** *see* Magnesium Supplements *on page 976*
- ♦ **Magonate® Sport [OTC] [DSC]** *see* Magnesium Supplements *on page 976*
- ♦ **Mag-Ox® 400 [OTC]** *see* Magnesium Oxide *on page 973*
- ♦ **Mag-Ox 400® [OTC]** *see* Magnesium Supplements *on page 976*
- ♦ **Magtrate® [OTC]** *see* Magnesium Gluconate *on page 971*
- ♦ **Magtrate® [OTC]** *see* Magnesium Supplements *on page 976*
- ♦ **MAH** *see* Magnesium L-aspartate Hydrochloride *on page 973*
- ♦ **Maldemar™** *see* Scopolamine *on page 1421*
- ♦ **Mandelamine®** *see* Methenamine *on page 1021*
- ♦ **Mandrake** *see* Podophyllum Resin *on page 1275*
- ♦ **Manganese Chloride** *see* Trace Metals *on page 1558*
- ♦ **Manganese Sulfate** *see* Trace Metals *on page 1558*

Mannitol (MAN i tole)

Medication Safety Issues

Sound-alike/look-alike issues:

Osmitrol® may be confused with esmolol

Related Information

Antihypertensive Agents by Class *on page 1678*

U.S. Brand Names Osmitrol®; Resectisol®

Canadian Brand Names Osmitrol®

Index Terms *D*-Mannitol

Therapeutic Category Diuretic, Osmotic

Generic Available Yes

Use Reduction of increased intracranial pressure (ICP) associated with cerebral edema; promotion of diuresis in the prevention and/or treatment of oliguria or anuria due to acute renal failure; reduction of increased intraocular pressure; promotion of urinary excretion of toxic substances. Resectisol® is used for urologic irrigation for transurethral prostatic resection (see package insert for further information on this use).

Pregnancy Risk Factor C

Lactation Excretion in breast milk unknown/use caution

Contraindications Hypersensitivity to mannitol or any component; severe renal disease, dehydration, active intracranial bleeding, severe pulmonary edema or congestion

Adverse Reactions

Cardiovascular: Circulatory overload, CHF (due to inadequate urine output and overexpansion of extracellular fluid)

Central nervous system: Convulsions, headache

Endocrine & metabolic: Fluid and electrolyte imbalance, hyponatremia or hypernatremia, hypokalemia or hyperkalemia, water intoxication, dehydration and hypovolemia secondary to rapid diuresis

Gastrointestinal: Xerostomia

Local: Tissue necrosis

Respiratory: Pulmonary edema

Miscellaneous: Allergic reactions

Drug Interactions Lithium

Stability Store at room temperature (15°C to 30°C); protect from freezing; crystallization may occur at low temperatures; do not use solutions that contain crystals; heating in a hot water bath and vigorous shaking may be utilized for resolubilization of crystals; cool solutions to body temperature before using; incompatible with strongly acidic or alkaline solutions; potassium chloride or sodium chloride may cause precipitation of mannitol 20% or 25% solution

Mechanism of Action Increases the osmotic pressure of glomerular filtrate, which inhibits tubular reabsorption of water and electrolytes and increases urinary output

Pharmacodynamics After I.V. injection:

Diuresis: Onset of action: Within 1-3 hours

Reduction in ICP:

Onset of action: Within 15 minutes

Duration: 3-6 hours

Pharmacokinetics

Distribution: Remains confined to extracellular space; does not penetrate blood-brain barrier (except in very high concentrations or with acidosis)

Metabolism: Minimal amounts in the liver to glycogen

Half-life: 1.1-1.6 hours

Elimination: Primarily unchanged in urine by glomerular filtration

(Continued)

Mannitol *(Continued)*

Usual Dosage I.V.:

Children:

Test dose (to assess adequate renal function): 200 mg/kg (maximum dose: 12.5 g) over 3-5 minutes to produce a urine flow of at least 1 mL/kg/hour for 1-3 hours

Initial: 0.5-1 g/kg

Maintenance: 0.25-0.5 g/kg every 4-6 hours

Adults:

Test dose: 12.5 g (200 mg/kg) over 3-5 minutes to produce a urine flow of at least 30-50 mL of urine per hour over the next 2-3 hours

Initial: 0.5-1 g/kg

Maintenance: 0.25-0.5 g/kg every 4-6 hours

Administration Parenteral: In-line filter set (≤5 micron) should always be used for mannitol infusion with concentrations ≥20%; administer test dose (for oliguria) I.V. push over 3-5 minutes; for cerebral edema or elevated ICP, administer over 20-30 minutes; maximum concentration for administration: 25%

Monitoring Parameters Renal function, daily fluid intake and output, serum electrolytes, serum and urine osmolality; for treatment of elevated intracranial pressure, maintain serum osmolality 310-320 mOsm/kg

Patient Information May cause dry mouth

Nursing Implications Avoid extravasation; crenation and agglutination of red blood cells may occur if administered with whole blood

Additional Information Approximate osmolarity: Mannitol 20%: 1100 mOsm/L; mannitol 25%: 1375 mOsm/L

Dosage Forms Excipient information presented when available (limited, particularly for generics); consult specific product labeling.

Injection, solution: 5% [50 mg/mL] (1000 mL); 10% [100 mg/mL] (500 mL, 1000 mL); 15% [150 mg/mL] (500 mL); 20% [200 mg/mL] (150 mL, 250 mL, 500 mL); 25% [250 mg/mL] (50 mL)

Osmitrol®: 5% [50 mg/mL] (1000 mL); 10% [100 mg/mL] (500 mL, 1000 mL); 15% [150 mg/mL] (500 mL); 20% [200 mg/mL] (250 mL, 500 mL)

Solution, urogenital (Resectisol®): 5% [50 mg/mL] (2000 mL, 4000 mL)

♦ **Mapap [OTC]** *see* Acetaminophen *on page 42*
♦ **Mapap Children's [OTC]** *see* Acetaminophen *on page 42*
♦ **Mapap Extra Strength [OTC]** *see* Acetaminophen *on page 42*
♦ **Mapap Infants [OTC]** *see* Acetaminophen *on page 42*
♦ **Mapezine® (Can)** *see* Carbamazepine *on page 279*
♦ **Marcaine®** *see* Bupivacaine *on page 244*
♦ **Marcaine® Spinal** *see* Bupivacaine *on page 244*
♦ **Margesic® H** *see* Hydrocodone and Acetaminophen *on page 779*
♦ **Marinol®** *see* Dronabinol *on page 546*
♦ **Matulane®** *see* Procarbazine *on page 1320*
♦ **3M™ Avagard™ [OTC]** *see* Chlorhexidine Gluconate *on page 337*
♦ **Maxair™ Autohaler™** *see* Pirbuterol *on page 1267*
♦ **Maxidex®** *see* Dexamethasone *on page 461*
♦ **Maxidone™** *see* Hydrocodone and Acetaminophen *on page 779*
♦ **Maxipime®** *see* Cefepime *on page 306*
♦ **Maxitrol®** *see* Dexamethasone, Neomycin, and Polymyxin B *on page 464*
♦ **May Apple** *see* Podophyllum Resin *on page 1275*
♦ **May-SR® [OTC]** *see* Magnesium Supplements *on page 976*
♦ **MCT** *see* Medium Chain Triglycerides *on page 989*
♦ **MCT Oil® [OTC]** *see* Medium Chain Triglycerides *on page 989*
♦ **MCT Oil® (Can)** *see* Medium Chain Triglycerides *on page 989*
♦ **MCV4** *see* Meningococcal Polysaccharide (Groups A / C / Y and W-135) Diphtheria Toxoid Conjugate Vaccine *on page 999*
♦ **MDL 73,147EF** *see* Dolasetron *on page 528*

Measles, Mumps, and Rubella Vaccines (Combined)

(MEE zels, mumpz & roo BEL a vak SEENS, kom BINED)

Related Information

Immunization Guidelines *on page 1837*

U.S. Brand Names M-M-R® II

Canadian Brand Names M-M-R® II; Priorix™

Index Terms MMR; Mumps, Measles and Rubella Vaccines, Combined; Rubella, Measles and Mumps Vaccines, Combined

Therapeutic Category Vaccine

Generic Available No

Use Provide active immunity to measles, mumps, and rubella viruses in individuals ≥12 months of age

Pregnancy Risk Factor C

Lactation

Measles/mumps: Excretion in breast milk unknown/use caution

Rubella: Enters breast milk/use caution

Contraindications Hypersensitivity to measles, mumps, and rubella vaccine, gelatin or any component of the formulation; history of anaphylactic reactions to neomycin; individuals with blood dyscrasias, leukemia, lymphomas, or other malignant neoplasms affecting the bone marrow or lymphatic systems; concurrent immunosuppressive therapy; primary and acquired immunodeficiency states; family history of congenital or hereditary immunodeficiency; active/untreated tuberculosis; current febrile illness or active febrile infection; pregnancy; known anaphylactoid reaction to eggs

Warnings Avoid pregnancy for 3 months following vaccination; women who are pregnant when vaccinated or who become pregnant within 28 days of vaccination should be counseled on the theoretical risks to the fetus. Use in patients with existing thrombocytopenia may result in more severe reduction in platelets; avoid use in patients with previous history of postvaccination thrombocytopenia, as rechallenge has resulted in recurrence of thrombocytopenia; severe allergic reactions including anaphylaxis have been reported rarely. Immediate treatment for anaphylactic/anaphylactoid reaction should be available during vaccine use. Use with extreme caution in patients with immediate-type hypersensitivity reactions to eggs.

MMR vaccine should not be administered to severely immunocompromised persons with the exception of asymptomatic children with HIV. Severely immunocompromised patients and symptomatic HIV-infected patients who are exposed to measles should receive immune globulin, regardless of prior vaccination status. Patients with minor illnesses (diarrhea, mild upper respiratory tract infection with or without low grade fever or other illnesses with low-grade fever) may receive vaccine. Leukemia patients who are in remission and who have not received chemotherapy for at least 3 months may be vaccinated.

Precautions Use with caution in patients with history of cerebral injury, convulsions, or other conditions where stress due to fever should be avoided; defer vaccination for at least 3 months after receiving blood and plasma transfusions or immune globulin (See Appendix Immunization Guidelines, "Suggested Intervals Between Administration of Immune Globulin Preparations for Various Indications and Measles Immunization").

Adverse Reactions All serious adverse reactions must be reported to the U.S. Department of Health and Human Services (DHHS) Vaccine Adverse Event Reporting System (VAERS) 1-800-822-7967.

Cardiovascular: Syncope, vasculitis

Central nervous system: Ataxia, dizziness, febrile convulsions, fever, encephalitis (rare), encephalopathy (rare), Guillain-Barré syndrome (rare), headache, irritability, malaise, measles inclusion body encephalitis, polyneuritis, polyneuropathy, seizures, subacute sclerosing panencephalitis

Dermatologic: Angioneurotic edema, erythema multiforme, purpura, rash, Stevens-Johnson syndrome, urticaria

Endocrine & metabolic: Diabetes mellitus, parotitis

Gastrointestinal: Diarrhea, nausea, pancreatitis, sore throat, vomiting

Genitourinary: Orchitis

Hematologic: Leukocytosis, thrombocytopenia

Local: Injection site reactions which include burning, induration, redness, stinging, swelling, tenderness, wheal and flare, vesiculation

Neuromuscular & skeletal: Arthralgia/arthritis (variable; highest rates in women, 12% to 26% versus children, up to 3%), myalgia, paresthesia

Ocular: Ocular palsies

Otic: Otitis media

Renal: Conjunctivitis, retinitis, optic neuritis, papillitis, retrobulbar neuritis

Respiratory: Bronchospasm, cough, pneumonitis, rhinitis

Miscellaneous: Anaphylactoid reactions, anaphylaxis, atypical measles, panniculitis, regional lymphadenopathy, aseptic meningitis (associated with Urabe strain of mumps vaccine)

Drug Interactions Immunosuppressant medications may decrease the effectiveness of the vaccine; avoid high doses of systemic corticosteroids for ≥14 days, wait at least

(Continued)

Measles, Mumps, and Rubella Vaccines (Combined) *(Continued)*

1 month between discontinuing steroid therapy and administering vaccine. Immune globulin may decrease effectiveness of vaccine; do not administer together; vaccination should be deferred for at least 3 months following immune globulin administration (See Appendix Immunization Guidelines, "Suggested Intervals Between Administration of Antibody-Containing Products for Different Indications and Measles Immunization")

Stability Prior to reconstitution, store the powder at 2°C to 8°C (36°F to 46°F) or colder (freezing does not affect potency). Protect from light. Diluent may be stored with powder or at room temperature. Discard if not used within 8 hours of reconstitution.

Mechanism of Action As a live, attenuated vaccine, MMR vaccine offers active immunity to disease caused by the measles, mumps, and rubella viruses.

Usual Dosage SubQ: 0.5 mL per dose

Infants <12 months: If there is risk of exposure to measles, single-antigen measles vaccine should be administered at 6-11 months of age with a second dose (of MMR) at ≥12 months of age.

Children ≥12 months: 2 doses, the first at 12 months of age, then repeated at 4-6 years of age. If the second dose was not received, the schedule should be completed by the 11- to 12-year old visit. (The second dose may be administered at any time provided at least 4 weeks have elapsed since the first dose.)

Adults: Adults born in or after 1957 (adults born before 1957 are generally considered to be immune to measles and mumps) without documentation of live vaccine on or after first birthday, or without physician-diagnosed measles or mumps, or without laboratory evidence of immunity, should be vaccinated with at least one dose; a second dose, separated by no less than 1 month, is indicated for those previously vaccinated with one dose of measles vaccine, students entering institutions of higher learning, recently exposed in an outbreak setting, healthcare workers at time of employment, and for travelers to endemic areas.

Administration Use entire contents of the provided diluent to reconstitute vaccine. Gently agitate to mix thoroughly. Discard if powder does not dissolve. Use as soon as possible following reconstitution; administer by SubQ injection into the anterolateral aspect of the thigh or arm; **not for I.V. administration**

Test Interactions Temporary suppression of TB skin test reactivity with onset approximately 3 days after administration

Patient Information Soreness or swelling may occur at the site of injection; fever, mild rash, swelling in the glands of the cheeks or neck, and temporary pain or stiffness in the joints may occur. Some effects may not occur until 1-2 weeks after the injection. Notify your healthcare provider immediately if these effects continue or are severe, or for a high fever, seizures or allergic reaction (respiratory difficulty, hives, weakness, dizziness, fast heartbeat). Not to be used during pregnancy; do not get pregnant for 28 days after getting the vaccine. Pregnant women should wait until after giving birth to get the vaccine.

Nursing Implications Federal law requires that the date of administration, the vaccine manufacturer, lot number of vaccine, and the administering person's name, title, and address be entered into the patient's permanent medical record.

Additional Information Using separate sites and syringes, MMR may be administered concurrently with DTaP or *Haemophilus* b conjugate vaccine (PedvaxHIB®). Varicella vaccine may be administered with MMR using separate sites and syringes; however, if not administered simultaneously, doses should be separated by at least 30 days. Unless otherwise specified, MMR should be given 1 month before or 1 month after live viral vaccines.

Dosage Forms Excipient information presented when available (limited, particularly for generics); consult specific product labeling.

Injection, powder for reconstitution [preservative free]:

M-M-R® II: Measles virus 1000 $TCID_{50}$, mumps virus 20,000 $TCID_{50}$, and , rubella virus 1000 $TCID_{50}$ [contains neomycin 25 mcg, gelatin, human albumin, and bovine serum; produced in chick embryo cell culture]

References

American Academy of Pediatrics Committee on Infectious Diseases, "Recommended Immunization Schedules for Children and Adolescents - United States, 2007," *Pediatrics*, 2007, 119(1):207-8.

Centers for Disease Control, "Recommended Adult Immunization Schedule by Age Group and Medical Conditions, United States, 2003-2004," available at www.cdc.gov.

Measles, Mumps, Rubella, and Varicella Virus Vaccine

(MEE zels, mumpz, roo BEL a, & var i SEL a VYE rus vak SEEN)

Related Information

Immunization Guidelines *on page 1837*

U.S. Brand Names ProQuad®

Index Terms Mumps, Rubella, Varicella, and Measles Vaccine; Rubella, Varicella, Measles, and Mumps Vaccine; Varicella, Measles, Mumps, and Rubella Vaccine

Therapeutic Category Vaccine

Generic Available No

Use To provide active immunity to measles, mumps, rubella, and varicella viruses to children between the ages of 12 months to 12 years of age

Pregnancy Risk Factor C

Lactation

Measles, mumps, varicella: Excretion in breast milk unknown/use caution

Rubella: Enters breast milk/use caution

Contraindications Hypersensitivity to any component of the vaccine including gelatin; known anaphylactic reaction to neomycin; individuals with blood dyscrasias, leukemia, lymphomas, or other malignant neoplasms affecting the bone marrow or lymphatic systems; concurrent immunosuppressive therapy; primary and acquired immunodeficiency states including those who are immunosuppressed in association with HIV; family history of congenital or hereditary immunodeficiency; active untreated tuberculosis; current febrile illness; pregnancy; known anaphylactic reaction to eggs

Warnings Individuals of childbearing age should avoid pregnancy for 3 months following vaccination; individuals who are pregnant when vaccinated or who become pregnant within 28 days of vaccination should be counseled on the theoretical risks to the fetus. Immediate treatment for anaphylactic/anaphylactoid reaction should be available during vaccine use. Use extreme caution in patients with immediate-type hypersensitivity reactions to eggs. Varicella virus transmission may occur; vaccinated individuals should not have close association with susceptible high risk individuals (newborns, pregnant women, immunocompromised persons) for 6 weeks following vaccination. While safety and efficacy of this combination vaccine has not been established in patients with HIV infection, MMR and varicella individual vaccines have been recommended in children with HIV infection who are asymptomatic and not immunosuppressed (CDC immunologic category 1). Avoid use of salicylates for 6 weeks following vaccination; varicella may increase the risk of Reye's syndrome.

Precautions Use caution with history of cerebral injury, seizures, or other conditions where stress due to fever should be avoided. Use caution in patients with thrombocytopenia and those who develop thrombocytopenia after first dose; thrombocytopenia may worsen. Defer vaccination at least 3 months after receiving blood and plasma transfusions or immune globulin (see Appendix Immunization Guidelines "Suggested Intervals Between Administration of Immune Globulin Preparations for Various Indications and Measles Immunization")

Adverse Reactions All serious adverse reactions must be reported to the U.S. Department of Health and Human Services (DHHS) Vaccine Adverse Event Reporting System (VAERS) 1-800-822-7967.

With the exception of fever and measles-like rash, the incidence of adverse events was similar to that reported in patients receiving M-M-R® II and Varivax®. Also refer to M-M-R® II and Varivax® monographs for additional adverse reactions reported with those agents. Local injection site reactions appear to be slightly less than reported with individual vaccine formulations.

Central nervous system: Fever ≥38.9°C (≥102°F) (22%), irritability (7%), crying, insomnia, malaise, sleep disorder, somnolence

Dermatologic: Measles-like rash (3%), varicella-like rash (2%), rash (2%), viral exanthema (1%), miliaria rubra, rubella-like rash

Gastrointestinal: Diarrhea (1%), anorexia, vomiting, pharyngitis

Local: Injection site reaction including pain, tenderness, soreness (22%); erythema (14%), swelling (8%), bruising (2%)

Otic: Otitis media

Respiratory: Upper respiratory tract infection (1%), cough, nasal congestion, respiratory congestion, rhinorrhea

Miscellaneous: Hypersensitivity reactions

Drug Interactions Salicylates may increase the risk of Reye's syndrome following varicella vaccination; avoid use of salicylates for 6 weeks following vaccination. Immunosuppressant medications may decrease the effectiveness of the vaccine; avoid high doses of systemic corticosteroids for ≥ 14days, wait at least 1 month between discontinuing steroid therapy and administering vaccine. Immune globulin may decrease effectiveness of vaccine; do not administer together; vaccination should be deferred for at least 3 months following immune globulin administration (see Appendix Immunization Guidelines "Suggested Intervals Between Administration of Immune Globulin Preparations for Various Indications and Measles Immunization").

Vaccines: May be administered concomitantly with *Haemophilus* b conjugate (PedvaxHIB®) vaccine and hepatitis B recombinant vaccine (using separate sites and syringes)

(Continued)

Measles, Mumps, Rubella, and Varicella Virus Vaccine *(Continued)*

Allow at least 1 month between administering a dose of a measles-containing vaccine (ie, M-M-R® II) and ProQuad®

Allow at least 3 months between administering a varicella-containing vaccine (ie, Varivax®) and ProQuad®

Stability Vaccine: Stable in a freezer for up to 18 months at temperatures at or below -15°C (-5°F). Do not store in refrigerator; discard if refrigerated. During shipment, powder should be stored at or below -20°C (-4°F). Protect from light; use within 30 minutes following reconstitution.

Diluent: Store at under refrigeration at 2°C to 8°C (36°F to 46°F) or at room temperature of 20°C to 25°C (68°F to 77°F).

Mechanism of Action A live, attenuated virus; offers active immunity to disease caused by the measles, mumps, rubella, and varicella-zoster virus.

Usual Dosage SubQ: Children 12 months to 12 years: One dose (0.5 mL)

Allow at least 1 month between administering a dose of a measles-containing vaccine (eg, M-M-R® II) and ProQuad®.

Allow at least 3 months between administering a varicella-containing vaccine (eg, Varivax®) and ProQuad®.

Administration Parenteral: Use entire contents of provided diluent to reconstitute vaccine. Gently agitate to mix thoroughly. Discard if powder does not dissolve. Use as soon as possible following reconstitution; administer by SubQ injection into the anterolateral aspect of the thigh or arm; **not for I.V. administration**

Test Interactions Temporary suppression of TB skin test reactivity with onset approximately 3 days after administration.

Patient Information Soreness or swelling may occur at the site of injection; fever, mild rash, swelling in the glands of the cheeks or neck, and temporary pain or stiffness in the joints may occur. Some effects may not occur until 1-2 weeks after the injection. Notify your healthcare provider immediately if these effects continue or are severe, or for a high fever, seizures, or allergic reaction (respiratory difficulty, hives, weakness, dizziness, fast heartbeat) occurs. Not to be given during pregnancy; do not get pregnant for 28 days after getting the vaccine. Do not use aspirin or aspirin-containing products for 6 weeks following vaccination.

Nursing Implications

Federal law requires that the date of administration, name of manufacturer, lot number, and administering person's name, title, and address be entered into patient's permanent medical record.

Dosage Forms Excipient information presented when available (limited, particularly for generics); consult specific product labeling.

Injection, powder for reconstitution [preservative free]:

ProQuad®: Measles virus ≥3.00 $\log_{10}$ TCID50, mumps virus ≥4.3 $\log_{10}$ TCID50, rubella virus ≥3.0 $\log_{10}$ TCID50, and varicella virus ≥3.99 $\log_{10}$ plaque-forming units [contains neomycin, sucrose, gelatin, human albumin, and bovine serum; produced in chick embryo cell culture]

Measles Virus Vaccine (Live) (MEE zels VYE rus vak SEEN, live)

Medication Safety Issues

Sound-alike/look-alike issues:

Attenuvax® may be confused with Meruvax®

Related Information

Immunization Guidelines *on page 1837*

U.S. Brand Names Attenuvax®

Index Terms More Attenuated Enders Strain; Rubeola Vaccine

Therapeutic Category Vaccine

Generic Available No

Use Provide active immunity to measles virus in persons ≥12 months of age; immunization is also recommended for infants 6-12 months of age in outbreak situations; revaccination is recommended for students entering colleges and other institutions of higher education, for healthcare workers at the time of employment, and for international travelers who visit endemic areas. Adults born before 1957 are generally considered to be immune.

MMR is the vaccine of choice if recipients are likely to be susceptible to rubella and/or mumps as well as to measles. Persons vaccinated between 1963 and 1967 with a killed measles vaccine, followed by live vaccine within 3 months, or with a vaccine of unknown type, should be revaccinated with live measles virus vaccine.

Pregnancy Risk Factor C

Lactation Excretion in breast milk unknown/use caution

Contraindications Hypersensitivity to neomycin, gelatin, or any component of the formulation; acute respiratory infections, active, untreated tuberculosis, immunosuppressed patients; pregnancy; patients with blood dyscrasias, leukemia, lymphomas, or other malignant neoplasms affecting the bone marrow or lymphatic systems, primary and acquired immunodeficiency states, including HIV, cellular immune deficiencies, hypogammaglobulinemic and dysgammaglobulinemic states; known anaphylactoid reaction to eggs

Warnings Use in patients with existing thrombocytopenia may result in more severe reduction in platelets; avoid use in patients with previous history of postvaccination thrombocytopenia as rechallenge has resulted in recurrence of thrombocytopenia; avoid pregnancy for 3 months following vaccination; severe allergic reactions including anaphylaxis have been reported rarely; use with extreme caution in patients with immediate-type hypersensitivity reactions to eggs

Precautions Use with caution in patients with history of cerebral injury or seizures; defer vaccination for at least 3 months after receiving blood and plasma transfusions or immune globulin (See Appendix Immunization Guidelines, "Suggested Intervals Between Administration of Immune Globulin Preparations for Various Indications and Measles Immunization")

Adverse Reactions All serious adverse reactions must be reported to the U.S. Department of Health and Human Services (DHHS) Vaccine Adverse Event Reporting System (VAERS) 1-800-822-7967.

Cardiovascular: Edema, vasculitis, angioneurotic edema

Central nervous system: Fever between 100°F and 103°F usually between 5th and 12th days postvaccination, fatigue, convulsions, encephalitis, confusion, severe headache, ataxia, syncope, dizziness, malaise, irritability, Guillain-Barré syndrome, subacute sclerosing panencephalitis

Dermatologic: Rash (rarely generalized), pruritus, reddening of skin (especially around ears and eyes), erythema multiforme, urticaria, thrombocytopenic purpura, Stevens-Johnson syndrome

Gastrointestinal: Diarrhea

Hematologic: Thrombocytopenia

Local: Burning or stinging, induration, vesiculation at injection site

Neuromuscular & skeletal: Palsies, stiff neck

Ocular: Diplopia, coryza, ocular palsies, retinitis, optic neuritis, papillitis, retrobulbar neuritis, conjunctivitis

Respiratory: Cough, rhinitis, bronchospasm

Miscellaneous: Anaphylaxis and anaphylactoid reactions, lymphadenopathy

Drug Interactions Immunosuppressant medications may decrease the effectiveness of the vaccine; avoid high doses of systemic corticosteroids for ≥14 days, wait at least 1 month between discontinuing steroid therapy and administering vaccine. Immune globulin may decrease effectiveness of vaccine; do not administer together; vaccination should be deferred for at least 3 months following immune globulin administration (See Appendix Immunization Guidelines, "Suggested Intervals Between Administration of Antibody-Containing Products for Different Indications and Measles-Containing and Varicella Vaccine")

Stability Refrigerate at 2°C to 8°C (36°F to 46°F); discard if left at room temperature for over 8 hours; protect from light

Mechanism of Action Promotes active immunity to measles virus by inducing specific measles IgG and IgM antibodies.

Usual Dosage Children ≥15 months and Adults: SubQ: 0.5 mL

Administration Reconstitute with provided diluent only; agitate to mix thoroughly until completely dissolved; administer by SubQ injection into the anterolateral aspect of the thigh or arm; **not for I.V. administration**

Test Interactions May temporarily depress tuberculin skin test sensitivity

Patient Information Parents should monitor children closely for fever for 5-11 days after vaccination; females should not become pregnant within 3 months of vaccination

Nursing Implications Federal law requires that the date of administration, the vaccine manufacturer, lot number of vaccine, and the administering person's name, title, and address be entered into the patient's permanent medical record

Additional Information Contains 25 mcg neomycin per dose. Measles vaccine given immediately after exposure to natural measles may provide some protection if the vaccine is administered within 72 hours of exposure; vaccination even a few days prior to natural exposure may provide significant protection; DTP, IPV, Hib, and hepatitis B vaccines may be given concurrently

Dosage Forms Excipient information presented when available (limited, particularly for generics); consult specific product labeling.

(Continued)

Measles Virus Vaccine (Live) *(Continued)*

Injection, powder for reconstitution [preservative free]:

Attenuvax®: ≥1000 $TCID_{50}$/0.5 mL (0.5 mL) [contains human albumin, bovine serum, neomycin, gelatin, neomycin, sorbitol, and sucrose; produced in chick embryo cell culture]

References

American Academy of Pediatrics Committee on Infectious Diseases, "Recommended Immunization Schedules for Children and Adolescents - United States, 2007," *Pediatrics*, 2007, 119(1):207-8.

Centers for Disease Control, "Recommendations of the Advisory Committee on Immunization Practices (ACIP): General Recommendations on Immunization," *MMWR Recomm Rep*, 1994, 43(RR-1):23.

Centers for Disease Control, "Recommended Adult Immunization Schedule by Age Group and Medical Conditions, United States, 2003-2004," available at www.cdc.gov.

Gardner P and Schaffner W, "Immunization of Adults," *N Engl J Med*, 1993, 328(17):1252-8.

♦ **Mebaral®** *see* Mephobarbital *on page 1004*

Mebendazole (me BEN da zole)

U.S. Brand Names Vermox® [DSC]

Canadian Brand Names Vermox®

Therapeutic Category Anthelmintic

Generic Available Yes

Use Treatment of enterobiasis (pinworm infection), trichuriasis (whipworm infection), ascariasis (roundworm infection), and hookworm infections caused by *Necator americanus* or *Ancylostoma duodenale*; drug of choice in the treatment of capillariasis

Pregnancy Risk Factor C

Lactation Excretion in breast milk unknown/use caution

Contraindications Hypersensitivity to mebendazole or any component

Warnings Pregnancy and children <2 years of age are relative contraindications since safety has not been established

Adverse Reactions

Central nervous system: Dizziness, fever, headache

Dermatologic: Rash, pruritus, alopecia

Gastrointestinal: Diarrhea, abdominal pain, nausea, vomiting

Hematologic: Neutropenia, anemia, leukopenia

Hepatic: Transient abnormalities in liver function tests

Otic: Tinnitus

Renal: Hematuria

Drug Interactions Anticonvulsants such as carbamazepine and phenytoin may increase metabolism of mebendazole

Food Interactions Food increases mebendazole absorption

Mechanism of Action Selectively and irreversibly blocks uptake of glucose and other nutrients in susceptible intestine-dwelling helminths

Pharmacokinetics

Absorption: Oral: 2% to 10%

Distribution: To liver, fat, muscle, plasma, and hepatic cysts

Protein binding: 95%

Metabolism: Extensive in the liver

Half-life: 2.8-9 hours

Time to peak serum concentration: Variable (0.5-7 hours)

Elimination: Primarily in feces as inactive metabolites with 5% to 10% eliminated in urine

Dialysis: Not dialyzable

Usual Dosage Children and Adults: Oral:

Pinworms: Single chewable tablet (100 mg); may need to repeat after 2 weeks

Whipworms, roundworms, hookworms: 100 mg twice daily, morning and evening on 3 consecutive days; if patient is not cured within 3-4 weeks, a second course of treatment may be administered

Capillariasis: 200 mg twice daily for 20 days

Administration Oral: Administer with food; tablet can be crushed and mixed with food, swallowed whole, or chewed

Monitoring Parameters For treatment of trichuriasis, ascariasis, hookworm, or mixed infections, check for helminth ova in the feces within 3-4 weeks following the initial therapy

Dosage Forms Excipient information presented when available (limited, particularly for generics); consult specific product labeling.

Tablet, chewable: 100 mg

References

Hotez PJ, "Hookworm Disease in Children," *Pediatr Infect Dis J*, 1989, 8(8):516-20.

Mechlorethamine (me klor ETH a meen)

Medication Safety Issues

High alert medication: The Institute for Safe Medication Practices (ISMP) includes this medication among its list of drugs which have a heightened risk of causing significant patient harm when used in error.

Related Information

Compatibility of Chemotherapy and Related Supportive Care Medications *on page 1777*
Emetogenic Potential of Single Chemotherapeutic Agents *on page 1776*
Extravasation Treatment *on page 1726*

U.S. Brand Names Mustargen®

Canadian Brand Names Mustargen®

Index Terms Chlorethazine; Chlorethazine Mustard; HN_2; Mechlorethamine Hydrochloride; Mustine; Nitrogen Mustard; NSC-762

Therapeutic Category Antineoplastic Agent, Alkylating Agent (Nitrogen Mustard)

Generic Available No

Use Combination therapy of Hodgkin's disease, brain tumors, non-Hodgkin's lymphoma, and malignant lymphomas; palliative treatment of lung, breast, and ovarian carcinoma; sclerosing agent in intracavitary therapy of pleural, pericardial, and other malignant effusions

Pregnancy Risk Factor D

Lactation Excretion in breast milk unknown/not recommended

Contraindications Hypersensitivity to mechlorethamine or any component; pre-existing profound myelosuppression; pregnancy

Warnings The FDA currently recommends that procedures for proper handling, administration, and disposal of mechlorethamine powder and solution be followed. Avoid inhalation of dust or vapors and contact with skin or mucous membranes. Mechlorethamine is potentially carcinogenic, teratogenic, and mutagenic. It may cause permanent sterility and birth defects. Extravasation of the drug into subcutaneous tissues results in painful inflammation, erythema, and induration; sloughing may occur; promptly infiltrate the area with sterile isotonic sodium thiosulfate ($^1/_6$ molar) and apply a cold compress for 6-12 hours. See Extravasation Treatment *on page 1726*.

Precautions Use with caution in patients with myelosuppression; patients with lymphoma should receive adequate hydration, alkalinization of the urine and/or prophylactic allopurinol to prevent complications such as uric acid nephropathy and hyperuricemia

Adverse Reactions

Cardiovascular: Thrombosis

Central nervous system: Vertigo, fever, headache, drowsiness, lethargy, encephalopathy (high dose)

Dermatologic: Rash, alopecia

Endocrine & metabolic: Amenorrhea, impaired spermatogenesis, hyperuricemia

Gastrointestinal: Nausea, vomiting, anorexia, diarrhea, metallic taste, mucositis

Hematologic: Myelosuppression (leukopenia, thrombocytopenia), hemolytic anemia

Local: Thrombophlebitis, tissue necrosis upon extravasation

Neuromuscular & skeletal: Weakness

Ocular: Lacrimation

Otic: Tinnitus, deafness

Miscellaneous: Hypersensitivity reactions, diaphoresis, anaphylaxis

Stability Highly unstable in neutral or alkaline solutions; use immediately after reconstitution; discard any unused drug after 60 minutes (although manufacturer reports only 15 minutes of stability after reconstitution, other studies indicate it is stable longer)

Mechanism of Action Alkylating agent that inhibits DNA and RNA synthesis via formation of carbonium ions which can attach to nucleic acids at the N^7 position of guanine; cross-links strands of DNA causing miscoding, breakage, and failure of replication

Pharmacokinetics

Absorption: Incomplete after intracavitary administration secondary to rapid deactivation by body fluids

Distribution: Following I.V. administration, drug undergoes rapid hydrolysis to a highly reactive alkylating intermediate; unchanged drug is undetectable in the blood within a few minutes

Half-life: <1 minute

Elimination: <0.01% of unchanged drug is recovered in urine

Usual Dosage Refer to individual protocols

(Continued)

Mechlorethamine *(Continued)*

Children:

Lymphoma: MOPP regimen: Mustargen® (mechlorethamine), Oncovin® (vincristine), procarbazine, and prednisone: I.V.: 6 mg/m² on days 1 and 8 of a 28-day cycle

Brain tumors: MOPP regimen: I.V.: 3 mg/m² on days 1 and 8 of a 28-day cycle

Adults:

I.V.: 0.4 mg/kg or 12-16 mg/m² as a single monthly dose or divided into 0.1 mg/kg/day once daily for 4 days, repeated at 4- to 6-week intervals

Intracavitary: 10-30 mg or 0.2-0.4 mg/kg

Administration

Intracavitary: Dilute dose in up to 100 mL NS; paracentesis is performed to remove most of the fluid from the cavity prior to administration; inject drug slowly with frequent aspiration to ensure that a free flow of fluid is present; change patient's position every 5-10 minutes for 1 hour following injection to distribute drug uniformly throughout the cavity

Parenteral: **DO NOT ADMINISTER I.M. or SubQ** Administer I.V. push through a side port of an established I.V. line over 1-5 minutes at a concentration not to exceed 1 mg/mL

Monitoring Parameters CBC with differential and platelet count, hemoglobin; serum uric acid in lymphoma patients

Patient Information Report to physician any pain or irritation at the site of injection, fever, sore throat, bruising, bleeding, shortness of breath, itching, or wheezing

Nursing Implications Avoid extravasation, inhalation of vapors, or contact with skin, mucous membranes, and eyes since mechlorethamine is a potent vesicant. If accidental eye contact occurs, copious irrigation for at least 15 minutes with NS or a balanced salt ophthalmic irrigating solution should be instituted immediately followed by prompt ophthalmologic consultation. If accidental skin contact occurs, irrigate the affected area with copious amounts of water for at least 15 minutes while removing contaminated clothing, followed by application of a 2% sodium thiosulfate solution; contaminated clothing should be destroyed. Medical attention should be sought immediately. For mechlorethamine extravasations, infiltrate area with a $^1/_6$ molar sodium thiosulfate solution and apply cold compresses for 6-12 hours; $^1/_6$ molar sodium thiosulfate solution can be prepared by diluting 4 mL of 10% sodium thiosulfate injection with 6 mL of SWI; Dorr recommends to inject 2 mL of the $^1/_6$ molar solution into site for each milligram of mechlorethamine extravasated

Additional Information Myelosuppressive effects:

WBC: Severe

Platelets: Severe

Onset (days): 4-7

Nadir (days): 14

Recovery (days): 21

Dosage Forms Excipient information presented when available (limited, particularly for generics); consult specific product labeling.

Injection, powder for reconstitution, as hydrochloride: 10 mg

References

Ater JL, van Eys J, Woo SY, et al, "MOPP Chemotherapy Without Irradiation as Primary Postsurgical Therapy for Brain Tumors in Infants and Young Children," *J Neurooncol*, 1997, 32(3):243-52.

Berg SL, Grisell DL, DeLaney TF, et al, "Principles of Treatment of Pediatric Solid Tumors," *Pediatr Clin North Am*, 1991, 38(2):249-67.

Dorr RT, Soble M, and Alberts DS, "Efficacy of Sodium Thiosulfate as a Local Antidote to Mechlorethamine Skin Toxicity in the Mouse," *Cancer Chemother Pharmacol*, 1988, 22(4):299-302.

Krischer JP, Ragab AH, Kun L, et al, "Nitrogen Mustard, Vincristine, Procarbazine, and Prednisone as Adjuvant Chemotherapy in the Treatment of Medulloblastoma. A Pediatric Oncology Group Study," *J Neurosurg*, 1991, 74(6):905-9.

♦ **Mechlorethamine Hydrochloride** *see* Mechlorethamine *on page 987*

Meclizine (MEK li zeen)

Medication Safety Issues

Sound-alike/look-alike issues:

Antivert® may be confused with Axert™

Related Information

Overdose and Toxicology *on page 1916*

U.S. Brand Names Antivert®; Bonine® [OTC]; Dramamine® Less Drowsy Formula [OTC]

Canadian Brand Names Bonamine™; Bonine®

Index Terms Meclizine Hydrochloride; Meclozine Hydrochloride

Therapeutic Category Antiemetic; Antihistamine

Generic Available Yes

Use Prevention and treatment of motion sickness; management of vertigo

Pregnancy Risk Factor B

Lactation Excretion in breast milk unknown/not recommended

Contraindications Hypersensitivity to meclizine or any component

Precautions Use with caution in patients with angle-closure glaucoma or obstructive diseases of the GI or GU tract

Adverse Reactions

Cardiovascular: Hypotension, palpitations, tachycardia

Central nervous system: Drowsiness, fatigue, auditory and visual hallucinations, restlessness, excitation, insomnia, nervousness

Dermatologic: Urticaria, rash

Endocrine & metabolic: Weight gain

Gastrointestinal: Xerostomia, anorexia, nausea, vomiting, diarrhea, constipation, appetite increase

Hepatic: Cholestatic jaundice, hepatitis

Neuromuscular & skeletal: Myalgia, tremor, paresthesia

Ocular: Blurred vision, diplopia

Otic: Tinnitus

Respiratory: Bronchospasm, epistaxis

Drug Interactions Additive sedation with CNS depressants (eg, sedatives, alcohol, antihistamines)

Mechanism of Action Has central anticholinergic action and CNS depressant activity; decreases excitability of the middle ear labyrinth and blocks conduction in the middle ear vestibular-cerebellar pathways

Pharmacodynamics

Onset of action: Oral: 30-60 minutes

Duration: 12-24 hours

Pharmacokinetics

Metabolism: In the liver

Half-life: 6 hours

Elimination: As metabolites in urine and as unchanged drug in feces

Usual Dosage Children >12 years and Adults: Oral:

Motion sickness: 25-50 mg 1 hour before travel, repeat dose every 24 hours if needed

Vertigo: 25-100 mg/day in divided doses

Administration Oral: Administer with food to decrease GI distress

Patient Information May cause drowsiness and impair ability to perform activities requiring mental alertness or physical coordination; may cause dry mouth; avoid alcohol

Dosage Forms Excipient information presented when available (limited, particularly for generics); consult specific product labeling.

Tablet, as hydrochloride: 12.5 mg, 25 mg

- Antivert®: 12.5 mg, 25 mg, 50 mg
- Dramamine® Less Drowsy Formula: 25 mg

Tablet, chewable, as hydrochloride (Bonine®): 25 mg

- ♦ **Meclizine Hydrochloride** *see* Meclizine *on page 988*
- ♦ **Meclozine Hydrochloride** *see* Meclizine *on page 988*
- ♦ **Med-Diltiazem (Can)** *see* Diltiazem *on page 503*
- ♦ **Medicinal Carbon** *see* Charcoal, Activated *on page 328*
- ♦ **Medicinal Charcoal** *see* Charcoal, Activated *on page 328*
- ♦ **Medicone® Suppositories [OTC]** *see* Phenylephrine *on page 1250*
- ♦ **Medi-Phenyl [OTC]** *see* Phenylephrine *on page 1250*
- ♦ **Mediplast® [OTC]** *see* Salicylic Acid *on page 1413*

Medium Chain Triglycerides (mee DEE um chane trye GLIS er ides)

U.S. Brand Names MCT Oil® [OTC]

Canadian Brand Names MCT Oil®

Index Terms MCT; Triglycerides, Medium Chain

Therapeutic Category Caloric Agent; Nutritional Supplement

Generic Available No

Use Nutritional supplement for those who cannot digest long chain fats; malabsorption associated with disorders such as pancreatic insufficiency, bile salt deficiency, and bacterial overgrowth of the small bowel; induce ketosis as a prevention for seizures (akinetic, clonic, and petit mal)

Pregnancy Risk Factor C

(Continued)

Medium Chain Triglycerides *(Continued)*

Contraindications Hypersensitivity to medium chain triglycerides or any component; should not be used in patients with hepatic encephalopathy due to earlier observations which report that short chain fatty acids may have a narcotic effect on the CNS and inhibit oxidative phosphorylation

Warnings Patients with cirrhosis demonstrate higher concentrations of medium chain fatty acids in the serum and CSF than normal individuals; impaired hepatic clearance of medium chain fatty acids due to parenchymal dysfunction of medium chain fatty acid oxidation, portal systemic shunt, and impaired protein binding of fatty acid enhance the passive diffusion of medium chain fatty acids into the CSF

Precautions Use with caution in patients with hepatic cirrhosis and complications such as portacaval shunts or encephalopathy

Adverse Reactions

Central nervous system: Sedation, narcosis, coma (cirrhotics)

Endocrine & metabolic: Ketosis

Gastrointestinal: Nausea, vomiting, abdominal pain, diarrhea, borborygmi

Mechanism of Action A semisynthetic class of lipids; medium chain triglycerides (MCT) are composed of fatty acids with chain length varying from 6-12 carbon atoms; preparations contain approximately 75% octanoic (caprylic), 20% to 25% decanoic (capric), 1% hexanoic (caproic), and 1% dodecanoic (lauric) acids

MCT are hydrolyzed in the stomach and in the small intestine by pancreatic lipase to form medium chain fatty acids; the medium chain fatty acids are incorporated into bile salts for more rapid solubilization and entrance into the mucosal cell and into the portal venous blood; MCT can also be absorbed unchanged as a triglycerides into the mucosal cell; medium chain fatty acids presented to the liver are minimally converted to hepatic lipid and are rapidly oxidized to carbon dioxide, ketones, and acetate; the medium chain fatty acids are also esterified to long chain triglycerides

Pharmacodynamics Onset of action: Octanoic acid appeared in each subject by 30 minutes following ingestion; effect on seizures in children: Within 6 weeks

Pharmacokinetics

Absorption: Up to 30% of dose can be absorbed unchanged as a triglyceride in the mucosal cell

Metabolism: Almost entirely oxidized by the liver to acetyl CoA fragments and to carbon dioxide; little deposited in adipose tissue or elsewhere

Elimination: As much as 20% of oral dose of MCT, recovered in expired CO_2 in 50 minutes; <10% elimination of medium chain fatty acids in feces

Usual Dosage Oral:

Infants: Nutritional supplement: Initial: 0.5 mL every other feeding, then advance to every feeding, then increase in increments of 0.25-0.5 mL/feeding at intervals of 2-3 days as tolerated

Children: Seizures: About 40 mL with each meal or 50% to 70% (800-1120 kcal) of total calories (1600 kcal) as the oil will induce the ketosis necessary for seizure control

Children and Adults: Cystic fibrosis: 3 tablespoons/day in divided doses

Adults: Malabsorption syndromes: 15 mL 3-4 times/day

Administration Oral:

Dilute with at least an equal volume of water or mix with some other vehicle such as fruit juice (should not be cold; flavoring may be added); mixture should be sipped slowly; administer no more than 15-20 mL at any one time (up to 100 mL may be administered in divided doses in a 24-hour period)

Possible GI side effects from medication can be prevented if therapy is initiated with small supplements at meals and gradually increased according to patient's tolerance

Monitoring Parameters

Nutritional supplement and malabsorption: Weight gain, height, stool output

Seizure treatment: Reduction in seizures, urine ketones

Patient Information GI symptoms may occur during the first few days of administration and then disappear; it is important to continue therapy with at least the smallest dose

Additional Information Does not provide any essential fatty acids; contains only saturated fats; supplementation with safflower, corn oil, or other polyunsaturated vegetable oil must be given to provide the patient with the essential fatty acids; caloric content: 8.3 calories/g; 115 calories/15 mL

Dosage Forms Excipient information presented when available (limited, particularly for generics); consult specific product labeling.

Oil: 14 g/15 mL (960 mL) [115 calories/15 mL; derived from coconut oil]

◆ **Medrol®** *see* MethylPREDNISolone *on page 1039*

MedroxyPROGESTERone (me DROKS ee proe JES te rone)

Medication Safety Issues

Sound-alike/look-alike issues:

MedroxyPROGESTERone may be confused with hydroxyprogesterone, methylPREDNISolone, methylTESTOSTERone

Provera® may be confused with Covera®, Parlodel®, Premarin®

The injection dosage form is available in different formulations. Carefully review prescriptions to assure the correct formulation and route of administration.

U.S. Brand Names Depo-Provera®; Depo-Provera® Contraceptive; depo-subQ provera 104™; Provera®

Canadian Brand Names Alti-MPA; Apo-Medroxy®; Depo-Prevera®; Depo-Provera®; Gen-Medroxy; Novo-Medrone; Provera®; Provera-Pak

Index Terms Acetoxymethylprogesterone; Medroxyprogesterone Acetate; Methylacetoxyprogesterone; MPA

Therapeutic Category Contraceptive, Progestin Only; Progestin

Generic Available Yes

Use Secondary amenorrhea or abnormal uterine bleeding due to hormonal imbalance; prevention of pregnancy; reduction of endometrial hyperplasia in nonhysterectomized postmenopausal women receiving conjugated estrogens; endometrial or renal carcinoma; management of endometriosis-associated pain

Pregnancy Risk Factor X

Lactation Enters breast milk/compatible

Contraindications Hypersensitivity to medroxyprogesterone or any component; thrombophlebitis; cerebral vascular disease, undiagnosed vaginal bleeding, liver dysfunction, thromboembolic disorders, breast cancer, pregnancy (known or suspected)

Warnings Discontinue if there is a sudden partial or complete loss of vision, proptosis, diplopia, migraine, if papilledema or retinal vascular lesions are present, or any other symptom of a thromboembolic event. Prolonged use of medroxyprogesterone as a contraceptive reduces estrogen levels and has been associated with increased bone mineral density (BMD) losses. Use as a long-term contraceptive agent (≥2 years) should be reserved for situations when other contraceptives are not effective or contraindicated. Monitor BMD if prolonged use is necessary.

Precautions Use with caution in patients with mental depression, diabetes, epilepsy, asthma, migraines, renal or cardiac dysfunction

Adverse Reactions

Cardiovascular: Edema, thromboembolic disorders, chest pain, tachycardia

Central nervous system: Depression, dizziness, nervousness, fever, insomnia, seizures, somnolence

Dermatologic: Melasma, chloasma, urticaria, acne, alopecia, hirsutism, dry skin

Endocrine & metabolic: Menstrual irregularities, amenorrhea, breakthrough bleeding, breast tenderness, weight gain or loss, bone mineral density loss (contraceptive use), ectopic pregnancy, decreased glucose tolerance, galactorrhea, increased libido, oligomenorrhea

Gastrointestinal: Anorexia, rectal bleeding

Hepatic: Cholestatic jaundice

Local: Pain at injection site, thrombophlebitis

Neuromuscular & skeletal: Weakness, osteoporotic fractures (contraceptive use), paresthesia

Miscellaneous: Anaphylaxis

Drug Interactions Aminoglutethimide depresses serum concentrations of medroxyprogesterone acetate

Mechanism of Action Inhibits secretion of pituitary gonadotropins, which prevents follicular maturation and ovulation, transforms a proliferative endometrium into a secretory one

Pharmacodynamics Time to ovulation (after last injection): 10 months (range: 6-12 months)

Pharmacokinetics

Absorption: I.M.: Slow

Protein binding: 86% to 90%

Metabolism: In the liver

Bioavailability: 0.6% to 10%

Half-life: 30 days

Time to peak serum concentration: SubQ (depo-subQ provera 104™): 1 week

Elimination: Oral: In urine and feces

Usual Dosage

Adolescents and Adults:

Amenorrhea: Oral: 5-10 mg/day for 5-10 days or 2.5 mg/day

(Continued)

MedroxyPROGESTERone *(Continued)*

Abnormal uterine bleeding: Oral: 5-10 mg for 5-10 days starting on day 16 or day 21 of menstrual cycle

Contraception: **Note:** First dose to be given only during first 5 days of normal menstrual period; only within 5 days postpartum if not breast-feeding, or only at sixth postpartum week if exclusively breast-feeding. When switching from other contraceptive methods, depo-subQ provera 104™ should be administered within 7 days after the last day of using the last method (pill, ring, patch).

I.M. (Depo-Provera®): 150 mg every 3 months

SubQ (depo-subQ provera 104™): 104 mg every 3 months (every 12-14 weeks)

Endometriosis-associated pain: SubQ (depo-subQ provera 104™): 104 mg every 3 months; treatment longer than 2 years is not recommended due to impact of long-term use on bone mineral density

Adults: Accompanying cyclic estrogen therapy (postmenopausal): Oral: 5-10 mg for 12-14 consecutive days each month, starting on day 1 or day 16 of cycle; lower doses may be used if given with estrogen continuously throughout the cycle

Administration

Oral: Administer with food

Parenteral: I.M. injection, suspension only: In upper arm or buttock; SubQ (depo-subQ provera 104™ only): Into anterior thigh or abdomen; not for I.V. use; shake well before drawing into syringe

Monitoring Parameters BMD (see Warnings), menstrual bleeding patterns

Test Interactions Altered thyroid and liver function tests, prothrombin time, factors VII, VIII, IX, X, metyrapone test

Patient Information Notify physician if sudden loss of vision, severe headache, sharp chest pain, coughing up blood, weakness or numbness in an arm or leg, severe pain or swelling in calf, unusual heavy vaginal bleeding or severe pain or tenderness in lower abdominal area

Additional Information I.M. dosing is recommended only for contraceptive purposes or in the treatment of endometrial or renal carcinoma

Dosage Forms Excipient information presented when available (limited, particularly for generics); consult specific product labeling.

Injection, suspension, as acetate: 150 mg/mL (1 mL)

Depo-Provera®: 400 mg/mL (2.5 mL)

Depo-Provera® Contraceptive: 150 mg/mL (1 mL) [prefilled syringe or vial]

depo-subQ provera 104™: 104 mg/0.65 mL (0.65 mL) [prefilled syringe]

Tablet, as acetate (Provera®): 2.5 mg, 5 mg, 10 mg

♦ **Medroxyprogesterone Acetate** *see* MedroxyPROGESTERone *on page 991*

Medrysone (ME dri sone)

U.S. Brand Names HMS Liquifilm® [DSC]

Therapeutic Category Anti-inflammatory Agent, Ophthalmic; Corticosteroid, Ophthalmic

Generic Available No

Use Treatment of allergic conjunctivitis, vernal conjunctivitis, episcleritis, ophthalmic epinephrine sensitivity reaction

Pregnancy Risk Factor C

Lactation Excretion in breast milk unknown/use caution

Contraindications Hypersensitivity to medrysone or any component; ocular fungal, viral, or tuberculosis infections; acute superficial herpes simplex

Warnings Medrysone is not recommended for use in uveitis or iritis (effectiveness has not been established); may delay healing after cataract surgery and increase risk of bleb formation; effectiveness and safety have not been established in children <3 years of age

Precautions Prolonged use has been associated with the development of glaucoma, corneal or scleral perforation, and posterior subcapsular cataracts; use with caution in patients with glaucoma (monitor IOP frequently); may mask or enhance the establishment of acute purulent untreated infections of the eye; dose should be tapered to avoid disease exacerbation; re-evaluate patient if symptoms do not improve after 2 days; secondary ocular infections may occur (especially with prolonged use)

Adverse Reactions

Endocrine & metabolic: Systemic hypercorticoidism (rare)

Local: Stinging, burning

Ocular: Corneal thinning, elevated intraocular pressure, glaucoma, damage to the optic nerve, defects in visual activity, cataracts, foreign body sensation, acute anterior uveitis, perforation of the globe; rarely: Keratitis, corneal ulcers, conjunctivitis, mydriasis, ptosis, conjunctival hyperemia, loss of accommodation

Miscellaneous: Hypersensitivity reactions

Stability Store at temperatures up to 25°C (77°F); do not freeze

Mechanism of Action Inhibits inflammatory response by suppression of migration of polymorphonuclear leukocytes and reversal of increased capillary permeability

Pharmacokinetics

Absorption: Through aqueous humor

Metabolism: In the liver

Elimination: By the kidneys and feces

Usual Dosage Children ≥3 years and Adults: Ophthalmic: Instill 1 drop in conjunctival sac 2-4 times/day up to every 4 hours; may use every 1-2 hours during first 1-2 days

Administration Ophthalmic: Shake well before use; do not touch dropper to the eye or skin; finger pressure should be applied to lacrimal sac during and for 1-2 minutes after instillation to decrease risk of absorption and systemic reactions

Monitoring Parameters Monitor IOP if duration of therapy is >10 days; periodic examination of lens (with prolonged use)

Patient Information If eye pain or inflammation persists >48 hours or becomes worse, discontinue medrysone and contact physician.

Additional Information Medrysone is a synthetic corticosteroid; structurally related to progesterone; duration of therapy: 3-4 days to several weeks dependent on type and severity of disease

Dosage Forms Excipient information presented when available (limited, particularly for generics); consult specific product labeling. [DSC] = Discontinued product

Solution, ophthalmic: 1% (5 mL, 10 mL) [contains benzalkonium chloride] [DSC]

Mefloquine (ME floe kwin)

Related Information

Malaria *on page 1855*

U.S. Brand Names Lariam®

Canadian Brand Names Apo-Mefloquine®; Lariam®

Index Terms Mefloquine Hydrochloride

Therapeutic Category Antimalarial Agent

Generic Available Yes

Use Treatment of acute malarial infections and prevention of malaria; prevention of chloroquine-resistant *Plasmodium falciparum* malaria. Malaria prophylaxis for women who are pregnant or likely to become pregnant if exposure to chloroquine-resistant *P. falciparum* cannot be avoided.

Restrictions A medication guide and wallet card must be provided to patients when mefloquine is dispensed for prevention of malaria. An FDA-approved medication guide is available at http://www.fda.gov/cder/Offices/OdS/labeling.htm.

Pregnancy Risk Factor C

Lactation Enters breast milk/not recommended

Contraindications Hypersensitivity to mefloquine, related compounds such as quinine and quinidine, or any component; history of convulsions, cardiac conduction abnormalities, or severe psychiatric disorder (including active or recent history of depression, generalized anxiety disorder, psychosis, or schizophrenia); use with halofantrine

Warnings Mefloquine may cause a range of psychiatric symptoms (anxiety, paranoia, depression, hallucinations and psychosis). Rare cases of suicidal ideation and suicide have been reported (no causal relationship established). The appearance of psychiatric symptoms such as acute anxiety, depression, restlessness, or confusion may be considered a prodrome to more serious events. When used as prophylaxis, substitute an alternative medication. Discontinue if unexplained neuropsychiatric disturbances occur. Dizziness, loss of balance, and other CNS disorders have been reported; due to long half-life, effects may persist long after mefloquine has been discontinued.

Precautions Use with caution in patients with a previous history of depression (see Contraindications regarding severe psychiatric illness, including active/recent depression). Use caution in patients with significant cardiac disease. If mefloquine is to be used for a prolonged period, periodic evaluations including liver function tests and ophthalmic examinations should be performed. In cases of life-threatening, serious, or overwhelming malaria infections due to *Plasmodium falciparum*, patients should be treated with an intravenous malarial drug. Mefloquine may be given orally to complete the course. Use caution in activities requiring mental alertness and fine motor coordination such as driving or operating machinery.

Adverse Reactions

Cardiovascular: Bradycardia, extrasystoles, syncope, hypotension, AV block, chest pain, edema, palpitations, tachycardia, flushing

Central nervous system: Headache, fever, chills, fatigue, dizziness, emotional lability, seizure, abnormal dreams, aggressive behavior, agitation, anxiety, confusion,

(Continued)

Mefloquine *(Continued)*

depression, encephalopathy, hallucinations, psychosis, somnolence, insomnia, suicidal ideation, mood changes, panic attacks, paranoia, vertigo

Dermatologic: Rash, alopecia, pruritus, erythema multiforme, Stevens-Johnson syndrome, urticaria

Gastrointestinal: Vomiting, diarrhea, abdominal pain, nausea, decreased appetite, dyspepsia

Hematologic: Leukocytosis, thrombocytopenia, leukopenia

Hepatic: Cholestasis, elevated bilirubin, hepatitis

Neuromuscular & skeletal: Myalgia, weakness, arthralgia, ataxia, muscle cramps, paresthesia, tremor

Ophthalmic: Visual disturbances, blurred vision

Otic: Tinnitus, hearing impairment

Respiratory: Dyspnea

Miscellaneous: Anaphylaxis

Drug Interactions Cytochrome P450 CYP3A4 substrate, CYP2D6 and CYP3A4 inhibitor

Chloroquine, quinine, quinidine increase toxicity of mefloquine (hold mefloquine for at least 12 hours after these drugs have been given); increased toxicity, potentially fatal prolongation of the QT_c interval with halofantrine (concurrent use is contraindicated; see Contraindications); CYP3A4 inhibitors (azole antifungals, ciprofloxacin, clarithromycin, diclofenac, doxycycline, erythromycin, imatinib, isoniazid, nefazodone, nicardipine, propofol, protease inhibitors, quinidine, and verapamil) may increase mefloquine levels

Mefloquine may decrease the effect of valproic acid, carbamazepine, phenobarbital, phenytoin. CYP3A4 inducers (aminoglutethimide, carbamazepine, nafcillin, nevirapine, phenobarbital, phenytoin, rifampin) may decrease levels of mefloquine. May interfere with antibody response to oral typhoid vaccine (delay oral typhoid vaccine dose by at least 24 hours after a dose of mefloquine).

Food Interactions Food increases bioavailability of mefloquine by ~40%.

Stability Store at room temperature. Protect from light.

Mechanism of Action Mefloquine which is structurally similar to quinine, destroys the asexual blood forms of *Plasmodium falciparum, P. vivax, P. malariae, P. ovale*; interferes with the malaria parasite's ability to metabolize and utilize erythrocyte hemoglobin; produces swelling of the parasitic food vacuoles

Pharmacokinetics Absorption: Slowly absorbed; more complete absorption when administered as a suspension compared with tablets

Distribution: Distributes into tissues, erythrocytes, urine, CSF; excreted into breast

V_d:

Children 6-24 months of age: 11.95 L/kg

Children 5-12 years: 8.84 L/kg

Adults: 19 L/kg

Protein binding: 98%

Metabolism: Hepatic; main metabolite is inactive

Half-life:

Children: 9.8-10.7 days

Adults: 21-22 days (range: 13-33 days)

Time to peak serum concentration: 6-24 hours (median: ~17 hours)

Elimination: Primarily bile and feces; urine (9% as unchanged drug, 4% as primary metabolite)

Dialysis: Not removed by hemodialysis

Usual Dosage Oral (dose is expressed in terms of mefloquine hydrochloride):

Children: ≥6 months and >5 kg:

Treatment: 15 mg/kg/dose (maximum: 750 mg) followed 6-12 hours later by 10 mg/kg/dose (maximum: 500 mg). If clinical improvement is not seen within 48-72 hours, an alternative therapy should be used for retreatment.

Dosing for Mefloquine Prophylaxis

Weight	Dose
<5 kg	5 mg/kg/dose once weekly
5-10 kg	1/8 of a 250 mg tablet once weekly
11-20 kg	1/4 of a 250 mg tablet once weekly
21-30 kg	1/2 of a 250 mg tablet once weekly
31-45 kg	3/4 of a 250 mg tablet once weekly
>45 kg	One 250 mg tablet once weekly

Prophylaxis: 5 mg/kg/dose once weekly on the same day each week (maximum dose: 250 mg) starting 1-2 weeks before arrival in the area with endemic infection, continuing weekly during travel, and for 4 weeks after leaving endemic area. CDC suggests that mefloquine be considered for use in children <5 kg, regardless of weight or age restrictions, when travel cannot be avoided to areas where chloroquine-resistant *P. falciparum* exists.

Alternatively, the following doses may be used: See table on previous page.

Adults:

Treatment (mild to moderate infection): 5 tablets (1250 mg) as a single dose **or** 750 mg followed 6-12 hours later by 500 mg. If clinical improvement is not seen within 48-72 hours, an alternative therapy should be used for retreatment.

Prophylaxis: 250 mg once weekly on the same day each week, starting 1-2 weeks before arrival in endemic area, continuing weekly during travel, and for 4 weeks after leaving endemic area

Dosage adjustment in renal impairment: No dosage adjustment needed.

Dosage adjustment in hepatic impairment: Half-life may be prolonged and plasma levels may be higher.

Administration Oral: Administer with food and an ample amount of water, at least 8 oz of water for adults. If vomiting occurs within 30 minutes after a dose, repeat dose. If vomiting occurs within 30-60 minutes after a dose, an additional half-dose should be administered. If vomiting recurs, monitor closely and consider alternative treatment. Administering mefloquine on a full stomach may minimize nausea and vomiting. For patients unable to swallow tablets or unable to tolerate its bitter taste, crush tablets and mix with a small amount of water, milk, applesauce, chocolate syrup, jelly, or food immediately before administration. Pulverized dose of mefloquine can be enclosed in a gelatin capsule to mask bitter taste.

Monitoring Parameters Sequential blood smears for percent parasitemia; periodic hepatic function tests, ophthalmologic exam

Patient Information Do not take mefloquine on an empty stomach. May cause dizziness or drowsiness and impair ability to perform activities requiring mental alertness or physical coordination. Advise women of childbearing potential to use effective contraceptive measures during malaria prophylaxis and for 3 months after the last dose. Report any symptoms of anxiety, confusion, depression, or restlessness.

Additional Information Information on recommendations for travelers can be accessed by contacting the Centers for Disease Control and Prevention (CDC) Malaria Hotline (770-488-7788) or visit the CDC website: http://www.cdc.gov/travel/diseases.htm#malaria.

Dosage Forms Excipient information presented when available (limited, particularly for generics); consult specific product labeling.

Tablet, as hydrochloride: 250 mg [equivalent to 228 mg base]

References

Dubos F, Delattre P, Demer M, et al, "Safety of Mefloquine in Infants With Acute Falciparum Malaria," *Pediatr Infect Dis J*, 2004, 23(7):679-81.

Fryauff DJ, Owusu-agyei S, Utz G, et al, "Mefloquine Treatment for Uncomplicated Falciparum Malaria in Young Children 6-24 months of Age in Northern Ghana," *Am J Trop Med Hyg*, 2007, 76 (2):224-31.

♦ **Mefloquine Hydrochloride** *see* Mefloquine *on page 993*

♦ **Mefoxin®** *see* Cefoxitin *on page 313*

♦ **Megace®** *see* Megestrol *on page 995*

♦ **Megace® ES** *see* Megestrol *on page 995*

♦ **Megace® OS (Can)** *see* Megestrol *on page 995*

♦ **Megadophilus® [OTC]** *see Lactobacillus acidophilus* and *Lactobacillus bulgaricus on page 898*

Megestrol (me JES trole)

Medication Safety Issues

Sound-alike/look-alike issues:

Megace® may be confused with Reglan®

U.S. Brand Names Megace®; Megace® ES

Canadian Brand Names Apo-Megestrol®; Megace®; Megace® OS; Nu-Megestrol

Index Terms 5071-1DL(6); Megestrol Acetate; NSC-71423

Therapeutic Category Antineoplastic Agent, Miscellaneous; Progestin

Generic Available Yes

Use Appetite stimulation and promotion of weight gain in cachexia (particularly in HIV patients) which is unresponsive to nutritional supplementation; palliative treatment of breast and endometrial carcinomas

Pregnancy Risk Factor X

Lactation Enters breast milk/contraindicated

(Continued)

Megestrol *(Continued)*

Contraindications Hypersensitivity to megestrol or any component; pregnancy (known or suspected); concomitant use with dofetilide

Warnings The FDA currently recommends that procedures for proper handling and disposal of antineoplastic agents be considered. May cause fetal harm when administered during pregnancy; women of childbearing age should use appropriate contraceptive measures. May suppress HPA axis during chronic administration; acute adrenal insufficiency may occur with abrupt withdrawal after long-term use or with stress; withdrawal or discontinuation of megestrol should be done carefully. Consider providing exogenous glucocorticoids during periods of stress or severe infection.

Oral suspensions contain sodium benzoate; benzoic acid (benzoate) is a metabolite of benzyl alcohol; large amounts of benzyl alcohol (≥99 mg/kg/day) have been associated with a potentially fatal toxicity ("gasping syndrome") in neonates; *in vitro* and animal studies have shown that benzoate, a metabolite of benzyl alcohol, displaces bilirubin from protein-binding sites; avoid use of products containing sodium benzoate in neonates. Megestrol may inhibit the elimination of dofetilide resulting in increased dofetilide plasma concentrations and potential serious ventricular arrhythmias associated with QT interval prolongation; concomitant use with dofetilide is not recommended. Megestrol may reduce indinavir serum levels resulting in a need for increase in indinavir dose.

Precautions Use with caution in patients with history of thromboembolic disease and diabetes mellitus

Adverse Reactions

Cardiovascular: Cardiomyopathy, palpitations, edema, hypertension, chest pain

Central nervous system: Insomnia, depression, fever, headache, confusion, mood changes, lethargy, malaise, asthenia

Dermatologic: Rash, alopecia, pruritus

Endocrine & metabolic: Breakthrough bleeding and amenorrhea, spotting, changes in menstrual flow or vaginal bleeding pattern, changes in cervical erosion and secretions, increased breast tenderness, hyperglycemia, HPA axis suppression, adrenal insufficiency, Cushing's syndrome, hypercalcemia, weight gain

Gastrointestinal: Constipation, xerostomia, nausea, vomiting, diarrhea, flatulence, abdominal pain, dyspepsia

Genitourinary: Impotence, gynecomastia, urinary incontinence

Hematologic: Leukopenia, anemia

Hepatic: Hepatomegaly, cholestatic jaundice, hepatotoxicity

Local: Thrombophlebitis

Neuromuscular & skeletal: Weakness, paresthesia, carpal tunnel syndrome

Ocular: Amblyopia

Respiratory: Hyperpnea, dyspnea, pulmonary embolism, hyperventilation

Miscellaneous: Diaphoresis

Drug Interactions Megestrol may inhibit the elimination of dofetilide resulting in increased dofetilide plasma concentrations and potential serious ventricular arrhythmias associated with QT interval prolongation. May reduce plasma levels of indinavir.

Food Interactions Food significantly increases plasma levels

Stability Store tablets and oral suspension at room temperature; protect from heat

Mechanism of Action A synthetic progestin with antiestrogenic properties which disrupt the estrogen receptor cycle. Megestrol interferes with the normal estrogen cycle and results in a lower LH titer. It may also have a direct effect on the endometrium. As an antineoplastic progestin, it is thought to act through an antileutenizing effect mediated via the pituitary. The exact mechanism for appetite stimulation has not been determined but is postulated to be due in part to a direct effect on the hypothalamus.

Pharmacodynamics Onset of action:

Antineoplastic: 2 months of continuous therapy

Weight gain: 2-4 weeks

Pharmacokinetics

Absorption: Well absorbed

Metabolism: In the liver

Half-life: Adults: 10-120 hours

Time to peak serum concentration:

Tablet: 2-3 hours

Suspension: 3-5 hours

Elimination: In urine (57% to 78%) and feces (8% to 30%) within 10 days

Usual Dosage Oral: **Note:** Megace® ES is not equivalent mg per mg with other megestrol formulations (625 mg Megace® ES is equivalent to 800 mg megestrol tablets or suspension).

Appetite stimulant in cachexia: Titrate dosage to response; decrease dose if weight gain is excessive:

Children: Limited data has been reported in cachectic children with cystic fibrosis, HIV, and solid tumors: 7.5-10 mg/kg/day in 1-4 divided doses; not to exceed 800 mg/day or 15 mg/kg/day

Adolescents and Adults:

Megestrol (tablets or 40 mg/mL suspension): 800 mg/day in 1-4 divided doses; titrate dose to response; doses between 400-800 mg/day have been clinically effective

Megace® ES: 625 mg once daily

Breast carcinoma: Female Adults: 40 mg 4 times/day

Endometrial carcinoma: Female Adults: 40-320 mg/day in divided doses; not to exceed 800 mg/day

Uterine bleeding: Female Adults: 40 mg 2-4 times/day

Administration Oral: Shake oral suspension well before administering; administer without regard to food

Monitoring Parameters Monitor for signs of thromboembolic phenomena and adrenal axis suppression

Appetite stimulation: Weight, caloric intake, basal cortisol level

Antineoplastic: Tumor response

Patient Information Follow dosage schedule and do not take more than prescribed. May cause photosensitivity reactions (eg, exposure to sunlight may cause severe sunburn, skin rash, redness, or itching); avoid exposure to sunlight and artificial light sources (sunlamps, tanning booth/bed); wear protective clothing, wide-brimmed hats, sunglasses, and lip sunscreen (SPF ≥15); use a sunscreen [broad-spectrum sunscreen or physical sunscreen (preferred) or sunblock with SPF ≥15]; contact physician if reaction occurs. May cause dry mouth. Report absent or altered menses, abdominal pain, vaginal itching, irritation, or discharge; report warmth, redness, or swelling of extremities, sudden onset of difficulty breathing, severe headache, or change in vision. May cause fetal harm particularly in the first 4 months of pregnancy; use appropriate contraception.

Dosage Forms Excipient information presented when available (limited, particularly for generics); consult specific product labeling.

Suspension, oral, as acetate: 40 mg/mL (10 mL, 240 mL, 480 mL)

Megace®: 40 mg/mL (240 mL) [contains alcohol 0.06% and sodium benzoate; lemon-lime flavor]

Megace® ES: 125 mg/mL (150 mL) [contains alcohol 0.06% and sodium benzoate; lemon-lime flavor]

Tablet, as acetate: 20 mg, 40 mg

References

Eubanks V, Koppersmith N, Wooldridge N, et al, "Effects of Megestrol Acetate on Weight Gain, Body Composition, and Pulmonary Function In Patients With Cystic Fibrosis," *J Pediatr*, 2002, 140(4):439-44.

Nasr SZ, Hurwitz ME, Brown RW, et al, "Treatment of Anorexia and Weight Loss With Megestrol Acetate in Patients With Cystic Fibrosis," *Pediatr Pulmonol*, 1999, 28(5):380-2.

Stockheim JA, Daaboul JJ, Yogev R, et al, "Adrenal Suppression in Children With the Human Immunodeficiency Virus Treated With Megestrol Acetate," *J Pediatr*, 1999, 134(3):368-70.

Tchekmedyian NS, Hickman M, and Heber D, "Treatment of Anorexia and Weight Loss With Megestrol Acetate in Patients With Cancer or Acquired Immunodeficiency Syndrome," *Semin Oncol*, 1991, 18(1 Suppl 2):35-42.

♦ **Megestrol Acetate** *see* Megestrol *on page 995*

♦ **Mellaril® (Can)** *see* Thioridazine *on page 1530*

Melphalan (MEL fa lan)

Medication Safety Issues

Sound-alike/look-alike issues:

Melphalan may be confused with Mephyton®, Myleran®

Alkeran® may be confused with Alferon®, Leukeran®

High alert medication: The Institute for Safe Medication Practices (ISMP) includes this medication among its list of drugs which have a heightened risk of causing significant patient harm when used in error.

Related Information

Compatibility of Chemotherapy and Related Supportive Care Medications *on page 1777*

Emetogenic Potential of Single Chemotherapeutic Agents *on page 1776*

U.S. Brand Names Alkeran®

Canadian Brand Names Alkeran®

Index Terms L-PAM; L-Sarcolysin; NSC-8806; Phenylalanine Mustard

Therapeutic Category Antineoplastic Agent, Alkylating Agent (Nitrogen Mustard)

Generic Available No

(Continued)

Melphalan *(Continued)*

Use Palliative treatment of multiple myeloma and nonresectable epithelial ovarian carcinoma; neuroblastoma, rhabdomyosarcoma, breast cancer, sarcoma; I.V. formulation: Use in patients in whom oral therapy is not appropriate

Pregnancy Risk Factor D

Lactation Excretion in breast milk unknown/not recommended

Contraindications Hypersensitivity to melphalan or any component; severe bone marrow suppression; patients whose disease was resistant to prior therapy; pregnancy

Warnings The FDA currently recommends that procedures for proper handling and disposal of antineoplastic agents be considered; potentially mutagenic, carcinogenic, and teratogenic; long-term oral dosing can increase the chance of developing secondary leukemia; produces amenorrhea

Precautions Cross-sensitivity may exist between melphalan and chlorambucil; reduce dosage or discontinue therapy if leukocyte count is <3000/mm^3 or platelet count is <100,000/mm^3; use with caution in patients with bone marrow suppression and impaired renal function; dosage reduction may be necessary in patients with impaired renal function

Adverse Reactions

Cardiovascular: Vasculitis, chest pain; hypotension, diaphoresis, and cardiac arrest have been reported following I.V. administration

Dermatologic: Alopecia, rash, pruritus, vesiculation of skin, urticaria

Endocrine & metabolic: Amenorrhea, sterility, SIADH

Gastrointestinal: Nausea, vomiting, diarrhea, stomatitis, mucositis, anorexia

Hematologic: Leukopenia, thrombocytopenia, anemia, agranulocytosis, hemolytic anemia

Hepatic: Hepatic veno-occlusive disease, hepatitis, jaundice

Local: Burning, discomfort, skin ulceration at injection site, tissue necrosis

Respiratory: Pulmonary fibrosis, interstitial pneumonitis, dyspnea

Miscellaneous: Hypersensitivity reaction

Drug Interactions Cyclosporine (development of severe renal failure); cimetidine and other H_2 antagonists decrease bioavailability of oral melphalan; nalidixic acid may increase incidence of severe hemorrhagic necrotic enterocolitis

Food Interactions Food interferes with oral absorption

Stability Protect from light and store at room temperature; reconstituted 5 mg/mL solution for injection is stable 90 minutes at room temperature; do not refrigerate since it may precipitate; once reconstituted solution is further diluted for I.V. infusion with NS, administration must be completed within 1 hour

Mechanism of Action Alkylating agent that inhibits DNA and RNA synthesis via formation of carbonium ions; cross-links strands of DNA

Pharmacokinetics

Absorption: Oral: Variable and incomplete

Distribution: Distributes throughout total body water; V_{dss}: 0.5 L/kg

Protein binding: 60% to 90%

Metabolism: Nonenzymatic hydrolysis to mono- or dihydroxy products; some conjugation to glutathione

Bioavailability: Ranges from 49% to 95% depending on the presence of food; average: 60%

Half-life, terminal: 75-120 minutes

Time to peak serum concentration: Oral: Within 2 hours

Elimination: 10% to 15% of dose excreted unchanged in urine; after oral administration, 20% to 50% excreted in stool

Usual Dosage Refer to individual protocols

Children:

- I.V.:
  - Pediatric rhabdomyosarcoma: 10-35 mg/m^2/dose every 21-28 days
  - High-dose melphalan with bone marrow transplantation for neuroblastoma: 70-100 mg/m^2/day on day 7 and 6 before BMT; or 140-220 mg/m^2 single dose before BMT; or 50 mg/m^2/day for 4 days; or 70 mg/m^2/day for 3 days
- Oral: 4-20 mg/m^2/day for 1-21 days

Adults:

- Multiple myeloma:
  - Oral: 6 mg/day once daily initially adjusted as indicated or 0.15 mg/kg/day for 7 days; or 0.25 mg/kg/day for 4 days or 8-10 mg/m^2 for 4 days, repeat at 4- to 6-week intervals
  - I.V.: 16 mg/m^2/dose every 2 weeks for 4 doses, then repeat monthly as per protocol for multiple myeloma
- Ovarian carcinoma: Oral: 0.2 mg/kg/day for 5 days, repeat in 4-5 weeks

Dosing adjustment in renal impairment:

BUN >30 mg/dL: Reduce dose by 50%

Serum creatinine >1.5 mg/dL: Reduce dose by 50%

Administration

Oral: Administer on an empty stomach

Parenteral: I.V.: Reconstitute 50 mg vial for injection with special diluent to yield a 5 mg/mL solution; dilute the reconstituted solution with NS to a final concentration not to exceed 2 mg/mL for I.V. central line administration or 0.45 mg/mL for peripheral I.V. administration; administer by I.V. infusion over 15-30 minutes at a rate not to exceed 10 mg/minute but total infusion should be administered within 1 hour

Monitoring Parameters CBC with differential and platelet count, serum electrolytes, hemoglobin

Test Interactions Positive Coombs' [direct]

Patient Information Notify physician if fever, shortness of breath, persistent cough, sore throat, bleeding, or bruising occurs

Nursing Implications Ensure adequate patient hydration; care should be taken to avoid extravasation

Additional Information Myelosuppressive effects:

WBC: Moderate
Platelets: Moderate
Onset (days): 7
Nadir (days): 14-21
Recovery (days): 42-50

Dosage Forms Excipient information presented when available (limited, particularly for generics); consult specific product labeling.

Injection, powder for reconstitution: 50 mg [diluent contains ethanol and propylene glycol]

Tablet: 2 mg

References

Berg SL, Grisell DL, DeLaney TF, et al, "Principles of Treatment of Pediatric Solid Tumors," *Pediatr Clin North Am*, 1991, 38(2):249-67.

Pole JG, Casper J, Elfenbein G, et al, "High-Dose Chemoradiotherapy Supported by Marrow Infusions for Advanced Neuroblastoma: A Pediatric Oncology Group Study," *J Clin Oncol*, 1991, 9(1):152-8.

Schroeder H, Pinkerton CR, Powles RL, et al, "High-Dose Melphalan and Total Body Irradiation With Autologous Marrow Rescue in Childhood Acute Lymphoblastic Leukemia After Relapse," *Bone Marrow Transplant*, 1991, 7(1):11-15.

♦ **Menactra®** *see* Meningococcal Polysaccharide (Groups A / C / Y and W-135) Diphtheria Toxoid Conjugate Vaccine *on page 999*

Meningococcal Polysaccharide (Groups A / C / Y and W-135) Diphtheria Toxoid Conjugate Vaccine

(me NIN joe kok al pol i SAK a ride groops aye, see, why & dubl yoo won thur tee fyve dif THEER ee a TOKS oyds KON joo gate vak SEEN)

Medication Safety Issues

Administration issue:

Menactra® (MCV4) should be administered by intramuscular (I.M.) injection only. Inadvertent subcutaneous (SubQ) administration has been reported; possibly due to confusion of this product with Menomume® (MPSV4), also a meningococcal polysaccharide vaccine, which is administered by the SubQ route.

Related Information

Immunization Guidelines *on page 1837*

U.S. Brand Names Menactra®

Index Terms MCV4; Quadrivalent Meningococcal Conjugate Vaccine

Therapeutic Category Vaccine

Generic Available No

Use Prevention of invasive meningococcal disease in adolescents and adults (11-55 years of age) at risk; individuals with anatomic or functional asplenia, those with terminal complement component or properdin deficiencies, and residents of or travelers to epidemic or highly endemic areas. The American College Health Association recommends immunization of college students who will be living in dormitories for the first time.

Vaccinations should be considered for household or institutional contacts of persons with meningococcal disease as an adjunct to appropriate antibiotic chemoprophylaxis as well as medical and laboratory personnel at risk of exposure to meningococcal disease.

Pregnancy Risk Factor C

Lactation Excretion in breast milk unknown/use caution

Contraindications Hypersensitivity to any component of the formulation including diphtheria toxoid; individuals with history of latex allergy (stopper contains latex); defer vaccination for persons with acute febrile illness until recovery

(Continued)

Meningococcal Polysaccharide (Groups A / C / Y and W-135) Diphtheria Toxoid Conjugate Vaccine *(Continued)*

Warnings Immediate treatment for anaphylactoid or acute hypersensitivity reactions should be available during vaccine use; patients receiving immunosuppressive therapy may have diminished response; Guillain-Barré syndrome (GBS) has been reported in a temporal relationship following Menactra® administration. Individuals with a previous history of GBS should not receive this vaccine. Safety and efficacy in children <11 years of age have not been established.

Precautions Use with caution in patients with coagulation disorders including thrombocytopenia, due to an increased risk for bleeding following I.M. administration; if the patient receives antihemophilia or other similar therapy, I.M. injection can be scheduled shortly after such therapy is administered

Adverse Reactions **All serious adverse reactions must be reported to the U.S. Department of Health and Human Services (DHHS) Vaccine Adverse Event Reporting System (VAERS) 1-800-822-7967.** Incidence of erythema, swelling, or tenderness may be higher in children

Central nervous system: Headache, malaise, fever, chills, Guillain-Barré syndrome

Local: Tenderness, pain at injection site, erythema, induration

Neuromuscular & skeletal: Transverse myelitis

Drug Interactions Immunosuppressant medications may decrease the effectiveness of the vaccine

Stability Store at 2°C to 8°C (35°F to 46°F); do not freeze; protect from light

Mechanism of Action Induces the formation of bactericidal antibodies to meningococcal antigens; the presence of these antibodies is strongly correlated with immunity to meningococcal disease caused by *Neisseria meningitidis* groups A, C, Y and W-135.

Usual Dosage I.M.: Adolescents and Adults >11-55 years of age: 0.5 mL; the need for booster is unknown, but may be considered in high-risk individuals, particularly children first vaccinated at <4 years of age. May be administered to those vaccinated 3 or more years earlier with Menomune®

Administration Administer by I.M. injection; **not for intradermal, subcutaneous, or I.V. administration**

Patient Information Inform patients about common side effects; patients should report serious and unusual effects to physician

Nursing Implications Federal law requires that the date of administration, the vaccine manufacturer, lot number of vaccine, and the administering person's name, title, and address be entered into the patient's permanent medical record.

Dosage Forms Excipient information presented when available (limited, particularly for generics); consult specific product labeling.

Injection, solution:

Menactra®: 4 mcg each of polysaccharide antigen groups A, C, Y, and W-135 per 0.5 mL [conjugated to diphtheria toxoid protein 48 mcg; adjuvant and preservative free; vial stopper contains dry, natural latex rubber]

References

American Academy of Pediatrics Committee on Infectious Diseases, "Recommended Immunization Schedules for Children and Adolescents - United States, 2007," *Pediatrics*, 2007, 119(1):207-8.

Centers for Disease Control and Prevention, "Recommended Childhood and Adolescent Immunization Schedule - United States, July-December 2004," *MMWR Morb Mortal Wkly Rep*, 2004, 53(16):Q1-4.

Centers for Disease Control, "Recommended Adult Immunization Schedule, October 2004-September 2005," available at www.cdc.gov.

Meningococcal Polysaccharide Vaccine (Groups A / C / Y and W-135)

(me NIN joe kok al pol i SAK a ride vak SEEN groops aye, see, why & dubl yoo won thur tee fyve)

Medication Safety Issues

Administration issue:

Menomume® (MPSV4) should be administered by subcutaneous (SubQ) injection. Menactra® (MCV4), also a meningococcal polysaccharide vaccine, is to be administered by intramuscular (I.M.) injection only.

Related Information

Immunization Guidelines *on page 1837*

U.S. Brand Names Menomune®-A/C/Y/W-135

Index Terms MPSV4; Quadrivalent Meningococcal Conjugate Vaccine

Therapeutic Category Vaccine

Generic Available No

Use Provide active immunity to meningococcal serogroups contained in the vaccine; prevention and control of outbreaks of serogroup C meningococcal disease; recommended for use in children ≥2 years and adults at risk (anatomic or functional asplenia, those with terminal complement component or properdin deficiencies), and residents of or travelers to epidemic or highly endemic areas. The American College Health Association recommends immunization of college students who will be living in dormitories for the first time.

Vaccinations should be considered for household or institutional contacts of persons with meningococcal disease as an adjunct to appropriate antibiotic chemoprophylaxis as well as medical and laboratory personnel at risk of exposure to meningococcal disease.

Pregnancy Risk Factor C

Lactation Excretion in breast milk unknown/use caution

Contraindications Hypersensitivity to any component of the formulation; defer vaccination for persons with acute febrile illness until recovery

Warnings Avoid administration at the same time as whole-cell pertussis or whole-cell typhoid vaccines due to the combined endotoxin content; patients receiving immunosuppressive therapy may have diminished response. Safety and efficacy in pediatric patients <2 years of age have not been established. Some dosage forms contain thimerosal.

Precautions Immediate treatment for anaphylactoid or acute hypersensitivity reactions should be available during vaccine use.

Adverse Reactions All serious adverse reactions must be reported to the U.S. Department of Health and Human Services (DHHS) Vaccine Adverse Event Reporting System (VAERS) 1-800-822-7967. Incidence of erythema, swelling, or tenderness may be higher in children.

Central nervous system: Headache, malaise, fever, chills

Local: Tenderness, pain at injection site, erythema, induration

Drug Interactions Immunosuppressant medications may decrease the effectiveness of the vaccine; increased adverse effects due to combined endotoxin content when administered at the same time as whole-cell pertussis or whole-cell typhoid vaccines

Stability Prior to and following reconstitution, store at 2°C to 8°C (35°F to 46°F); single use vial stable for 30 minutes after reconstitution; multidose vial stable 10 days after reconstitution; use multidose vial within 35 days of reconstitution

Mechanism of Action Induces the formation of bactericidal antibodies to meningococcal antigens; the presence of these antibodies is strongly correlated with immunity to meningococcal disease caused by *Neisseria meningitidis* groups A, C, Y and W-135.

Pharmacodynamics

Onset of action: Antibody levels: 7-10 days

Duration: Antibodies against group A and C polysaccharides decline markedly (to prevaccination levels) over the first 3 years following a single dose of vaccine, especially in children <4 years of age

Usual Dosage SubQ: Children ≥2 years and Adults: 0.5 mL; the need for booster is unknown, but may be considered in high-risk individuals, particularly children first vaccinated at <4 years of age.

Administration Reconstitute using provided diluent; shake well; administer by SubQ injection; **not for intradermal, I.M., or I.V. administration**

Patient Information Inform patients about common side effects; patients should report serious and unusual effects to physician

Nursing Implications Federal law requires that the date of administration, the vaccine manufacturer, lot number of vaccine, and the administering person's name, title and address be entered into the patient's permanent medical record.

Dosage Forms Excipient information presented when available (limited, particularly for generics); consult specific product labeling.

Injection, powder for reconstitution: 50 mcg each of polysaccharide antigen groups A, C, Y, and W-135 [contains lactose; packaged with 0.78 mL preservative free diluent or 6 mL diluent containing thimerosal; vial stoppers contain dry, natural latex rubber]

References

American Academy of Pediatrics Committee on Infectious Diseases, "Recommended Immunization Schedules for Children and Adolescents - United States, 2007," *Pediatrics*, 2007, 119(1):207-8.

Centers for Disease Control and Prevention, "Recommended Childhood and Adolescent Immunization Schedule - United States, July-December 2004," *MMWR Morb Mortal Wkly Rep*, 2004, 53(16):Q1-4.

Centers for Disease Control, "Recommended Adult Immunization Schedule, October 2004-September 2005," available at www.cdc.gov.

♦ **Menomune®-A/C/Y/W-135** *see* Meningococcal Polysaccharide Vaccine (Groups A / C / Y and W-135) *on page 1000*

♦ **Menostar™** *see* Estradiol *on page 605*

Meperidine (me PER i deen)

Medication Safety Issues

Sound-alike/look-alike issues:

Meperidine may be confused with meprobamate

Demerol® may be confused with Demulen®, Desyrel®, dicumarol, Dilaudid®, Dymelor®, Pamelor®

Related Information

Adult ACLS Algorithms *on page 1660*

Compatibility of Medications Mixed in A Syringe *on page 1941*

Narcotic Analgesics Comparison *on page 1705*

Overdose and Toxicology *on page 1916*

Preprocedure Sedatives in Children *on page 1895*

Serotonin Syndrome *on page 1955*

U.S. Brand Names Demerol®; Meperitab®

Canadian Brand Names Demerol®

Index Terms Isonipecaine Hydrochloride; Meperidine Hydrochloride; Pethidine Hydrochloride

Therapeutic Category Analgesic, Narcotic

Generic Available Yes

Use Management of moderate to severe pain; adjunct to anesthesia and preoperative sedation

Restrictions C-II

Pregnancy Risk Factor C (D if used for prolonged periods or in high doses at term)

Lactation Enters breast milk/contraindicated (AAP rates "compatible")

Contraindications Hypersensitivity to meperidine or any component (see Warnings); use of MAO inhibitors within 14 days (potentially fatal reactions may occur, see Drug Interactions)

Warnings Abrupt discontinuation after prolonged use may cause withdrawal symptoms or seizures; multiple dose vial may contain sulfites which may cause allergic reactions in susceptible individuals; syrup contains benzoic acid and oral solution may contain sodium benzoate; benzoic acid (benzoate) is a metabolite of benzyl alcohol; large amounts of benzyl alcohol (≥99 mg/kg/day) have been associated with a potentially fatal toxicity ("gasping syndrome") in neonates; the "gasping syndrome" consists of metabolic acidosis, respiratory distress, gasping respirations, CNS dysfunction (including convulsions, intracranial hemorrhage), hypotension and cardiovascular collapse; use meperidine products containing benzoic acid or sodium benzoate with caution in neonates; *in vitro* and animal studies have shown that benzoate displaces bilirubin from protein binding sites

Precautions Use with great caution (and only if essential) in patients with head injury, increased ICP, or other intercranial lesions (potential to depress respiration and increase ICP may be greatly exaggerated in these patients); use with caution in neonates and young infants (these patients may be at higher risk for adverse effects, especially respiratory depression, due to decreased elimination); use with caution in patients with pulmonary, hepatic, or renal disorders; use with caution in patients with tachycardias, biliary colic, seizure disorders or those receiving high-dose meperidine [normeperidine (an active metabolite and CNS stimulant) may accumulate and precipitate twitches, tremors, or seizures]; decrease the dose in patients with renal or hepatic impairment (normeperidine metabolite may accumulate in these patients); use with caution and decrease initial dose in patients with sickle cell anemia, Addison's disease, hypothyroidism, urethral stricture, prostatic hypertrophy, or pheochromocytoma (meperidine may precipitate hypertension in patients with pheochromocytoma)

Adverse Reactions

Cardiovascular: Palpitations, hypotension, bradycardia, peripheral vasodilation, tachycardia

Central nervous system: CNS depression, dizziness, drowsiness, sedation, elevated intracranial pressure; active metabolite (normeperidine) may precipitate twitches, tremors, or seizures

Dermatologic: Pruritus

Endocrine & metabolic: Antidiuretic hormone release

Gastrointestinal: Nausea, vomiting, constipation, biliary tract spasm

Genitourinary: Urinary tract spasm

Local: Induration, irritation (repeated SubQ use)

Ocular: Miosis

Respiratory: Respiratory depression

Miscellaneous: Physical and psychological dependence, histamine release

Drug Interactions Cytochrome P450 isoenzyme CYP2D6 substrate

May aggravate the adverse effects of isoniazid; MAO inhibitors greatly potentiate the effects of meperidine (acute opioid overdosage symptoms can be seen, including severe toxic reactions; the use of MAO inhibitors within 14 days of meperidine use is contraindicated); the herbal medicine St John's wort (*Hypericum perforatum*) may increase serious side effects, its use is **not** recommended; CNS depressants, alcohol, tricyclic antidepressants, phenothiazines may potentiate the effects of meperidine; phenytoin may increase the hepatic metabolism of meperidine and result in decreased analgesic effects (and increased concentrations of normeperidine); ritonavir may increase plasma concentrations of meperidine or normeperidine (concurrent use is not recommended); acyclovir may increase plasma concentrations of meperidine and normeperidine (use with caution); cimetidine may decrease the clearance of meperidine and the formation of normeperidine (use with caution)

Stability Incompatible with aminophylline, heparin, phenobarbital, phenytoin, and sodium bicarbonate

Mechanism of Action Binds to opiate receptors in the CNS, causing inhibition of ascending pain pathways, altering the perception of and response to pain; produces generalized CNS depression

Pharmacodynamics Analgesia:

Onset of action:
- Oral, I.M., SubQ: Within 10-15 minutes
- I.V.: Within 5 minutes

Maximum effect:
- Oral, I.M., SubQ: Within 1 hour
- I.V.: 5-7 minutes

Duration:
- Oral, I.M., SubQ: 2-4 hours
- I.V.: 2-3 hours

Pharmacokinetics

Distribution: Crosses the placenta; appears in breast milk

V_{dss}:
- Neonates: Preterm 1-7 days: 8.8 L/kg; term 1-7 days: 5.6 L/kg
- Infants: 1 week to 2 months: 8 L/kg; 3-18 months: 5 L/kg; 5-8 years: 2.8 L/kg
- Adults: 3-4 L/kg

Protein binding: (to alpha$_1$-acid glycoprotein)
- Neonates: 52%
- Infants: 3-18 months: 85%
- Adults: ~60% to 80%

Metabolism: In the liver via hydrolysis and N-demethylation

Bioavailability: ~50% to 60%, increased bioavailability with liver disease

Half-life, terminal:
- Preterm infants 3.6-65 days of age: 11.9 hours (range: 3.3-59.4 hours)
- Term infants:
  - 0.3-4 days of age: 10.7 hours (range: 4.9-16.8 hours)
  - 26-73 days of age: 8.2 hours (range: 5.7-31.7 hours)
- Neonates: 23 hours (range: 12-39 hours)
- Infants 3-18 months: 2.3 hours
- Children 5-8 years: 3 hours
- Adults: 2.5-4 hours
- Adults with liver disease: 7-11 hours
- Normeperidine (active metabolite): Neonates: 30-85 hours; Adults: 8-16 hours; normeperidine half-life is dependent on renal function and can accumulate with high doses or in patients with decreased renal function; normeperidine may precipitate tremors or seizures

Elimination: ~5% meperidine eliminated unchanged in urine

Usual Dosage Doses should be titrated to appropriate analgesic effect; **when changing route of administration, note that oral doses are about half as effective as parenteral dose**

Children:
- Oral, I.M., I.V., SubQ: Usual: 1-1.5 mg/kg/dose every 3-4 hours as needed; 1-2 mg/kg as a single dose preoperative medication may be used; maximum dose: 100 mg/dose
- I.V. continuous infusion: Loading dose: 0.5-1 mg/kg followed by initial rate: 0.3 mg/kg/hour; titrate dose to effect; may require 0.5-0.7 mg/kg/hour

Adults: Oral, I.M., I.V.: SubQ: 50-150 mg/dose every 3-4 hours as needed

AHCPR dosing guidelines: Opioid naive patients: **Note:** Oral route not recommended (See Carr, 1992 and Jacox, 1994):
- Children and Adults <50 kg: Moderate to severe pain: I.M., I.V., SubQ: Usual initial dose: 0.75 mg/kg every 2-3 hours

(Continued)

Meperidine *(Continued)*

Children and Adults ≥50 kg: Moderate to severe pain: I.M., I.V., SubQ: Usual initial dose: 100 mg every 3 hours

Dosing adjustment in renal impairment:

Cl_{cr} 10-50 mL/minute: Administer 75% of normal dose

Cl_{cr} <10 mL/minute: Administer 50% of normal dose

Administration

Oral: Administer with water; dilute syrup in water prior to use (use 4 oz water for adults)

Parenteral:

Slow I.V. push: Do not administer rapid I.V., administer over at least 5 minutes and dilute to ≤10 mg/mL

Intermittent infusion: Dilute to 1 mg/mL and administer over 15-30 minutes

Monitoring Parameters Respiratory and cardiovascular status; relief of pain, level of sedation

Patient Information Avoid alcohol and the herbal medicine St John's wort; may be habit-forming; avoid abrupt discontinuation after prolonged use; may cause drowsiness and impair ability to perform activities requiring mental alertness or physical coordination

Additional Information Equianalgesic doses: morphine 10 mg I.M. = meperidine 75-100 mg I.M.. **Note**: Although meperidine has been used in combination with chlorpromazine and promethazine as a premedication ("Lytic Cocktail"), this combination may have a higher rate of adverse effects compared to alternative sedatives and analgesics (See American Academy of Pediatrics Committee on Drugs, 1995)

Dosage Forms Excipient information presented when available (limited, particularly for generics); consult specific product labeling.

Injection, solution, as hydrochloride [ampul]: 25 mg/0.5 mL (0.5 mL); 25 mg/mL (1 mL); 50 mg/mL (1 mL, 1.5 mL, 2 mL); 75 mg/mL (1 mL); 100 mg/mL (1 mL)

Injection, solution, as hydrochloride [prefilled syringe]: 25 mg/mL (1 mL); 50 mg/mL (1 mL); 75 mg/mL (1 mL); 100 mg/mL (1 mL)

Injection, solution, as hydrochloride [for PCA pump]: 10 mg/mL (30 mL, 50 mL, 60 mL)

Injection, solution, as hydrochloride [vial]: 25 mg/mL (1 mL); 50 mg/mL (1 mL, 30 mL); 75 mg/mL (1 mL); 100 mg/mL (1 mL, 20 mL) [may contain sodium metabisulfite]

Solution, oral, as hydrochloride: 50 mg/5 mL (500 mL)

Syrup, as hydrochloride:

Demerol®: 50 mg/5 mL (480 mL) [contains benzoic acid; banana flavor]

Tablet, as hydrochloride: 50 mg, 100 mg

Demerol®, Meperitab®: 50 mg, 100 mg

References

American Academy of Pediatrics Committee on Drugs, "Reappraisal of Lytic Cocktail/Demerol®, Phenergan®, and Thorazine® (DPT) for the Sedation of Children," *Pediatrics*, 1995, 95(4):598-602.

Carr D, Jacox A, Chapman CR, et al, "Clinical Practice Guideline Number 1: Acute Pain Management: Operative or Medical Procedures and Trauma," Rockville, Maryland: U.S. Department of Health and Human Services, Public Health Service, Agency for Health Care Policy and Research, AHCPR Publication No 92-0032, 1992.

Cole TB, Sprinkle RH, Smith SJ, et al, "Intravenous Narcotic Therapy for Children With Severe Sickle Cell Pain Crisis," *Am J Dis Child*, 1986, 140(12):1255-9.

Jacox A, Carr D, Payne R, et al, "Clinical Practice Guideline Number 9: Management of Cancer Pain," Rockville, Maryland: U.S. Department of Health and Human Services, Public Health Service, Agency for Health Care Policy and Research, AHCPR Publication No. 94-0592, 1994.

Olkkola KT, Hamunen K, and Maunuksela EL, "Clinical Pharmacokinetics and Pharmacodynamics of Opioid Analgesics in Infants and Children," *Clin Pharmacokinet*, 1995, 28(5):385-404.

Pokela ML, Olkkola KT, Koivisto ME, et al, "Pharmacokinetics and Pharmacodynamics of Intravenous Meperidine in Neonates and Infants," *Clin Pharmacol Ther*, 1992, 52(4):342-9.

♦ **Meperidine Hydrochloride** *see* Meperidine *on page 1002*

♦ **Meperitab®** *see* Meperidine *on page 1002*

Mephobarbital (me foe BAR bi tal)

Medication Safety Issues

Sound-alike/look-alike issues:

Mephobarbital may be confused with methocarbamol

Mebaral® may be confused with Medrol®, Mellaril®, Tegretol®

U.S. Brand Names Mebaral®

Canadian Brand Names Mebaral®

Index Terms Methylphenobarbital

Therapeutic Category Anticonvulsant, Barbiturate; Barbiturate; Sedative

Generic Available No

Use Treatment of generalized tonic-clonic and simple partial seizures

Restrictions C-IV

Pregnancy Risk Factor D

Contraindications Hypersensitivity to mephobarbital or any component; pre-existing CNS depression; respiratory depression; severe uncontrolled pain; history of porphyria

Precautions Use with caution in patients with hepatic or renal impairment or respiratory diseases

Adverse Reactions

Central nervous system: Drowsiness, lethargy, paradoxical excitement (especially in children)

Dermatologic: Rash, including Stevens-Johnson syndrome or erythema multiforme

Gastrointestinal: Nausea, vomiting

Hematologic: Agranulocytosis, thrombocytopenic purpura

Miscellaneous: Psychological and physical dependence

Drug Interactions Cytochrome P450 isoenzyme CYP2C, CYP2C8, and CYP2C19 substrate

Mephobarbital is expected to have similar drug interactions as phenobarbital, since mephobarbital is metabolized in the liver to phenobarbital (see Phenobarbital *on page 1245*)

Food Interactions High doses of pyridoxine may decrease drug effect; barbiturates may increase the metabolism of vitamin D & K; dietary requirements of vitamin D, K, C, B_{12}, folate and calcium may be increased with long-term use

Mechanism of Action Increases seizure threshold in the motor cortex; depresses monosynaptic and polysynaptic transmission in the CNS; depresses CNS activity by binding to barbiturate site at GABA-receptor complex enhancing GABA activity; depresses reticular activating system; higher doses may be gabamimetic

Pharmacokinetics Values listed are for mephobarbital; see also Phenobarbital *on page 1245*

Absorption: Oral: ~50%

Metabolism: In the liver via N-demethylation to phenobarbital

Usual Dosage Epilepsy: Oral:

Children: 4-10 mg/kg/day in 2-4 divided doses

Adults: 200-600 mg/day in 2-4 divided doses

Administration Oral: Administer with water, milk, or juice

Monitoring Parameters Phenobarbital serum concentrations; CBC with differential, platelet count, hepatic and renal function

Reference Range Phenobarbital level should be in the range of 15-40 mcg/mL (SI: 65-172 micromoles/L)

Patient Information May cause drowsiness and impair ability to perform activities requiring mental alertness or physical coordination; avoid alcohol; limit caffeine; may be habit-forming; avoid abrupt discontinuation after prolonged use

Additional Information Sometimes used in specific patients who have excessive sedation or hyperexcitability from phenobarbital

Dosage Forms Excipient information presented when available (limited, particularly for generics); consult specific product labeling.

Tablet: 32 mg, 50 mg, 100 mg

♦ **Mephyton®** *see* Phytonadione *on page 1258*

Mepivacaine (me PIV a kane)

Medication Safety Issues

Sound-alike/look-alike issues:

Mepivacaine may be confused with bupivacaine

Polocaine® may be confused with prilocaine

U.S. Brand Names Carbocaine®; Polocaine®; Polocaine® Dental; Polocaine® MPF

Canadian Brand Names Carbocaine®; Polocaine®

Index Terms Mepivacaine Hydrochloride

Therapeutic Category Local Anesthetic, Injectable

Generic Available No

Use Local or regional analgesia; anesthesia by local infiltration, peripheral and central neural techniques including epidural and caudal blocks; **not** for use in spinal anesthesia

Pregnancy Risk Factor C

Lactation Excretion in breast milk unknown/use caution

Contraindications Hypersensitivity to mepivacaine, other amide-type local anesthetics, or any component

Warnings Local anesthetics have been associated with rare occurrences of sudden respiratory arrest; convulsions due to systemic toxicity leading to cardiac arrest have been reported presumably due to intravascular injection. A test dose is recommended

(Continued)

Mepivacaine *(Continued)*

prior to epidural administration and all reinforcing doses with continuous catheter technique. Do not use solutions containing preservatives for caudal or epidural block.

Precautions Use with extreme caution as lumbar or caudal anesthesia in patients with existing neurologic disease, spinal deformities, or severe hypertension. Use with caution in patients with cardiac disease, hepatic or renal disease. Use caution in debilitated, elderly, or acutely-ill patients; dose reduction may be required.

Adverse Reactions Degree of adverse effects in the CNS and cardiovascular system is directly related to the blood levels of mepivacaine, route of administration, and physical status of the patient. The effects below are more likely to occur after systemic administration rather than infiltration.

Cardiovascular: Bradycardia, cardiac arrest, decreased cardiac output, heart block, hypertension, hypotension, myocardial depression, syncope, tachycardia, ventricular arrhythmias

Central nervous system: Anxiety, chills, seizures, depression, dizziness, excitation, restlessness, tremors, fever, headache

Dermatologic: Angioneurotic edema, erythema, pruritus, urticaria

Gastrointestinal: Fecal incontinence, nausea, vomiting

Genitourinary: Incontinence, urinary retention

Neuromuscular & skeletal: Paralysis, tremors, paresthesia, weakness

Ocular: Blurred vision, pupil constriction

Otic: Tinnitus

Respiratory: Apnea, hypoventilation, sneezing

Miscellaneous: Allergic reaction, anaphylactoid reaction, diaphoresis

Stability Store at controlled room temperature of 15°C to 30°C (59°F to 86°F). Brief exposure up to 40°C (104°F) does not adversely affect the product. Solutions may be sterilized.

Mechanism of Action Blocks both the initiation and conduction of nerve impulses by decreasing the neuronal membrane's permeability to sodium ions, which results in inhibition of depolarization with resultant blockade of conduction

Pharmacodynamics Route and dose dependent:

Onset of action: Range: 3-20 minutes

Duration: 2-2.5 hours

Pharmacokinetics

Protein binding: ~75%

Metabolism: Primarily hepatic via N-demethylation, hydroxylation, and glucuronidation

Half-life:

- Neonates: 8.7-9 hours
- Adults: 1.9-3 hours

Elimination: Urine (95% as metabolites)

Usual Dosage Injectable local anesthetic: Dose varies with procedure, degree of anesthesia needed, vascularity of tissue, duration of anesthesia required, and physical condition of patient. The smaller dose/concentration (0.5%) will produce more superficial blockade, a higher dose (1%) will block sensory and sympathetic conduction without loss of motor function, a higher dose (1.5%) will provide extensive and often complete motor blockade, and 2% will produce complete sensory and motor blockade. The smallest dose and concentration required to produce the desired effect should be used.

Children: Maximum dose: 5-6 mg/kg; only concentrations <2% should be used in children <3 years or <14 kg (30 lbs)

Adults: Maximum dose: 400 mg; do not exceed 1000 mg/24 hours

- Cervical, brachial, intercostal, pudendal nerve block: 5-40 mL of a 1% solution (maximum: 400 mg) **or** 5-20 mL of a 2% solution (maximum: 400 mg). For pudendal block: Inject $^1/_2$ the total dose each side.
- Transvaginal block (paracervical plus pudendal): Up to 30 mL (both sides) of a 1% solution (maximum: 300 mg). Inject $^1/_2$ the total dose into each side.
- Paracervical block: Up to 20 mL (both sides) of a 1% solution (maximum: 200 mg). Inject $^1/_2$ the total dose into each side. This is the maximum recommended dose per 90-minute procedure; inject slowly with 5 minutes between sides.
- Caudal and epidural block (**preservative free solutions only**): 15-30 mL of a 1% solution (maximum: 300 mg) **or** 10-25 mL of a 1.5% solution (maximum: 375 mg) **or** 10-20 mL of a 2% solution (maximum: 400 mg)
- Infiltration: Up to 40 mL of a 1% solution (maximum: 400 mg)
- Therapeutic block (pain management): 1-5 mL of a 1% solution (maximum: 50 mg) **or** 1-5 mL of a 2% solution (maximum: 100 mg)

Administration Parenteral: Administer in small incremental doses; when using continuous intermittent catheter techniques, use frequent aspirations before and during the injection to avoid intravascular injection

Monitoring Parameters
Blood pressure, heart rate, respiration, signs of CNS toxicity (lightheadedness, dizziness, tinnitus, restlessness, tremors, twitching, drowsiness, circumoral paresthesia)

Patient Information You will experience decreased sensation to pain, heat, or cold in the area and/or decreased muscle strength (depending on area of application) until effects wear off; use necessary caution to reduce incidence of possible injury until full sensation returns. Report irritation, pain, burning at injection site; chest pain or palpitations; or respiratory difficulty.

Oral injection: This will cause numbness of your mouth. Do not eat or drink for 1 hour after use. Take small sips of water at first to ensure that you can swallow without difficulty. Your tongue and/or mouth may be numb, use caution to avoid biting yourself. Report irritation, pain, burning at injection site; chest pain or palpitations; or respiratory difficulty.

Dosage Forms Excipient information presented when available (limited, particularly for generics); consult specific product labeling.

Injection, solution, as hydrochloride [contains methylparabens]:
- Carbocaine®: 1% (50 mL); 2% (50 mL)
- Polocaine®: 1% (50 mL); 2% (50 mL)

Injection, solution, as hydrochloride [preservative free]:
- Carbocaine®: 1% (30 mL); 1.5% (30 mL); 2% (20 mL); 3% (1.8 mL) [dental cartridge]
- Polocaine® Dental: 3% (1.8 mL) [dental cartridge]
- Polocaine® MPF: 1% (30 mL); 1.5% (30 mL); 2% (20 mL)

References
Dodson WE, Hillman RE, and Hillman LS, "Brain Tissue Levels in a Fatal Case of Neonatal Mepivacaine (Carbocaine®) Poisoning," *J Pediatr*, 1975, 86(4):624-7.

Torres MJ, Garcia JJ, del Cano Moratinos AM, et al, "Fixed Drug Eruption Induced by Mepivacaine," *J Allergy Clin Immunol*, 1995, 96(1):130-1.

♦ **Mepivacaine Hydrochloride** *see* Mepivacaine *on page 1005*
♦ **Mepron®** *see* Atovaquone *on page 178*

Mercaptopurine (mer kap toe PYOOR een)

Medication Safety Issues
Sound-alike/look-alike issues:
- Purinethol® may be confused with propylthiouracil

High alert medication: The Institute for Safe Medication Practices (ISMP) includes this medication among its list of drugs which have a heightened risk of causing significant patient harm when used in error.

To avoid potentially serious dosage errors, the terms "6-mercaptopurine" or "6-MP" should be avoided; use of these terms has been associated with sixfold overdosages.

Azathioprine is metabolized to mercaptopurine; concurrent use of these commercially-available products has resulted in profound myelosuppression.

Related Information
Emetogenic Potential of Single Chemotherapeutic Agents *on page 1776*

U.S. Brand Names Purinethol®

Canadian Brand Names Purinethol®

Index Terms 6-Mercaptopurine (error-prone abbreviation); 6-MP (error-prone abbreviation); NSC-755

Therapeutic Category Antineoplastic Agent, Antimetabolite; Antineoplastic Agent, Purine

Generic Available Yes

Use Use in conjunction with methotrexate for maintenance therapy in childhood ALL; use in combination regimens for the treatment of AML, CML; non-Hodgkin's lymphoma

Pregnancy Risk Factor D

Lactation Enters breast milk/contraindicated

Contraindications Hypersensitivity to mercaptopurine or any component; severe liver disease; severe bone marrow suppression; patients whose disease showed prior resistance to mercaptopurine or thioguanine

Warnings The FDA currently recommends that procedures for proper handling and disposal of antineoplastic agents be considered; mercaptopurine may cause birth defects; potentially carcinogenic

Avoid using the terms "6-mercaptopurine" or "6-MP" which have been associated with medication errors resulting in sixfold overdosages.
(Continued)

Mercaptopurine *(Continued)*

Precautions Use with caution and adjust dosage in patients with renal impairment or hepatic failure; patients who receive allopurinol concurrently should have the mercaptopurine dose reduced by 66% to 75%

Adverse Reactions

Central nervous system: Drug fever
Dermatologic: Rash, hyperpigmentation, alopecia
Endocrine & metabolic: Hyperuricemia
Gastrointestinal: Mild nausea or vomiting, diarrhea, stomatitis, anorexia
Genitourinary: Oligospermia
Hematologic: Myelosuppression (leukopenia, thrombocytopenia, anemia), eosinophilia
Hepatic: Hepatotoxicity, hyperbilirubinemia, jaundice, elevation of liver enzymes
Renal: Renal toxicity (oliguria, hematuria)

Drug Interactions Allopurinol may potentiate the effect of bone marrow suppression (blocks metabolism of **orally** administered mercaptopurine by inhibiting xanthine oxidase); mercaptopurine decreases anticoagulant effect of warfarin; doxorubicin, hepatotoxic drugs (may potentiate liver toxicity)

Food Interactions Food decreases bioavailability

Stability Intact vials and tablets should be stored at room temperature and protected from light; reconstitute 500 mg vial with 49.8 mL SWI; the 10 mg/mL solution is stable for 24 hours

Mechanism of Action Prodrug incorporated into DNA and RNA; blocks purine synthesis and inhibits DNA and RNA synthesis

Pharmacokinetics

Absorption: Oral: Variable and incomplete (16% to 50%)
Distribution: Distributed throughout total body water; penetrates into CSF at low concentrations
Protein binding: 19%
Metabolism: Undergoes first-pass metabolism in the GI mucosa and liver; metabolized in the liver to sulfate conjugates, 6-thiouric acid, and other inactive compounds
Bioavailability: Oral: <20% (variable)
Half-life: Age dependent
- Children: <60 minutes
- Adults: 36-90 minutes

Time to peak serum concentration: Oral: Within 2 hours
Elimination: 20% excreted unchanged in urine

Usual Dosage Refer to individual protocols

Children:
- Oral:
  - Induction: 2.5-5 mg/kg/day given once daily, or 70-100 mg/m^2/day once daily
  - Maintenance: 1.5-2.5 mg/kg/day given once daily or 50-75 mg/m^2/day once daily
- I.V. continuous infusion (investigational; distributed under the auspices of the NCI for authorized studies): 50 mg/m^2/hour for 24-48 hours, or 1000 mg/m^2/day for 24 hours

Adults: Oral:
- Induction: 2.5-5 mg/kg/day given once daily, or 80-100 mg/m^2/day given once daily
- Maintenance: 1.5-2.5 mg/kg/day given once daily

Dosing adjustment in renal impairment: Children and Adults:
- Cl_{cr} <50 mL/minute: Administer every 48 hours

Administration

Oral: Do not administer with meals. For pediatric patients with ALL, studies suggest that evening administration may lower the risk of relapse compared to morning administration.

Parenteral: Administer by slow I.V. push over several minutes or by slow I.V. continuous infusion to reduce the incidence of vein irritation; further dilute the 10 mg/mL reconstituted solution in NS or D_5W to a final concentration for administration of 1-2 mg/mL

Monitoring Parameters CBC with differential and platelet count, liver function tests, uric acid, urinalysis

Patient Information Report to physician if fever, sore throat, bleeding, bruising, shortness of breath, or painful urination occurs; avoid alcohol

Nursing Implications Avoid extravasation

Additional Information Myelosuppressive effects:

WBC: Moderate
Platelets: Moderate
Onset (days): 7-10
Nadir (days): 14
Recovery (days): 21

Dosage Forms Excipient information presented when available (limited, particularly for generics); consult specific product labeling.

Tablet [scored]: 50 mg

Extemporaneous Preparations A 50 mg/mL oral suspension can be prepared in a vertical flow hood using a 1:1 mixture of methylcellulose 1% and simple syrup; crush thirty 50 mg tablets into a fine powder in a mortar; add a small amount of methylcellulose and simple syrup mixture to make a uniform paste; mix while adding 1:1 mixture of methylcellulose 1% and simple syrup to a final volume of 30 mL. **Note:** May use ultrasonication dispersal. Preparation is stable for 14 days when stored at room temperature; label "shake well" and "caution chemotherapy"

Nahata MC and Hipple TF, *Pediatric Drug Formulations*, 4th ed, Cincinnati, OH: Harvey Whitney Books, 2000.

References

Zimm S, Ettinger LJ, Holcenberg JS, et al, "Phase I and Clinical Pharmacological Study of Mercaptopurine Administered as a Prolonged Intravenous Infusion," *Cancer Res*, 1988, 45(4):1869-73.

♦ **6-Mercaptopurine (error-prone abbreviation)** *see* Mercaptopurine *on page 1007*

♦ **Mercapturic Acid** *see* Acetylcysteine *on page 51*

Meropenem (mer oh PEN em)

U.S. Brand Names Merrem® I.V.

Canadian Brand Names Merrem®

Index Terms SM-7338

Therapeutic Category Antibiotic, Carbapenem

Generic Available No

Use Treatment of multidrug-resistant gram-negative and gram-positive aerobic and anaerobic pathogens documented or suspected to be susceptible to meropenem; used in treatment of meningitis, lower respiratory tract infections, urinary tract infections, intra-abdominal infections, complicated skin and skin structure infections and sepsis caused by susceptible *S. aureus*, *S. pyogenes*, *S. agalactiae*, *S. pneumoniae*, *H. influenzae*, *N. meningitidis*, *M. catarrhalis*, *E. coli*, *Klebsiella*, *Enterobacter*, *Serratia*, *P. aeruginosa*, *B. cepacia*, and *B. fragilis*

Pregnancy Risk Factor B

Lactation Excretion in breast milk unknown/use caution

Contraindications Hypersensitivity to meropenem, any component, other carbapenems, or in patients who have experienced anaphylactic reactions to beta-lactams

Warnings Safety and efficacy in children <3 months of age have not been established; pseudomembranous colitis has been reported with the use of meropenem; prolonged use may result in superinfection. Seizures and other CNS adverse events have been reported, most commonly in patients with renal impairment and/or underlying neurologic disorders. Thrombocytopenia has been reported in patients with renal dysfunction who are receiving meropenem.

Precautions Use with caution in patients with a history of seizures, CNS disease, CNS infection, and/or compromised renal function; dosage adjustment required in patients with renal impairment

Adverse Reactions

Cardiovascular: Hypotension, chest pain, bradycardia, syncope

Central nervous system: Seizures (<0.38%), headache, pain, insomnia, dizziness, agitation, fever, chills, hallucinations, somnolence

Dermatologic: Rash (1.4%), pruritus, urticaria, toxic epidermal necrolysis, Stevens-Johnson syndrome

Gastrointestinal: Nausea, vomiting (1%), diarrhea (4.3%), melena, constipation, oral moniliasis, GI hemorrhage

Hematologic: Leukopenia, neutropenia, anemia, thrombocytopenia

Hepatic: Elevated AST, ALT, alkaline phosphatase, LDH, and bilirubin; cholestatic jaundice

Local: Phlebitis (1.2%); pain, edema, and inflammation at the injection site

Renal: Elevated BUN and serum creatinine

Respiratory: Dyspnea, apnea

Drug Interactions Probenecid inhibits renal excretion of meropenem (increases meropenem half-life 38%); meropenem may reduce valproic acid to subtherapeutic serum levels

Stability Store intact vials at room temperature. Meropenem reconstituted with SWI is stable for up to 2 hours at room temperature or for up to 12 hours when refrigerated; when reconstituted with NS to a final concentration between 2.5-50 mg/mL, the solution is stable for up to 2 hours at room temperature or 18 hours when refrigerated; when reconstituted with D_5W to a final concentration between 2.5-50 mg/mL, the solution is stable for up to 1 hour at room temperature or 8 hours when refrigerated; solutions prepared for infusion in plastic I.V. bags with NS at concentrations ranging (Continued)

Meropenem *(Continued)*

from 2.5-20 mg/mL are stable for 4 hours at room temperature or 24 hours when refrigerated

Mechanism of Action Inhibits cell wall synthesis by binding to penicillin-binding proteins (PBPs) with its strongest affinities for PBPs 2, 3 and 4 of *E. coli* and *P. aeruginosa* and PBPs 1, 2 and 4 of *S. aureus*

Pharmacokinetics

Distribution: Penetrates into most tissues and body fluids including CSF, urinary tract, peritoneal fluid, bone, bile, lung, bronchial mucosa, muscle tissue, and heart valves

Protein binding: 2%

Metabolism: 20% is hydrolyzed in plasma to an inactive metabolite

Half-life:

- Premature newborns: 3 hours
- Full-term newborns: 2 hours
- Infants 3 months to 2 years: 1.5 hours
- Children 2-12 years and Adults: 1 hour

Time to peak tissue and fluid levels: 1 hour after the start of infusion except in bile, lung, muscle, and CSF which peak at 2-3 hours

Elimination: Cleared by the kidney with 70% excreted unchanged in urine

Usual Dosage I.V.:

Neonates:

- Postnatal age 0-7 days: 20 mg/kg/dose every 12 hours
- Postnatal age >7 days:
  - Weight 1200-2000 g: 20 mg/kg/dose every 12 hours
  - Weight >2000 g: 20 mg/kg/dose every 8 hours

Children ≥3 months:

- Complicated skin and skin structure infection: 10 mg/kg/dose every 8 hours; maximum dose: 500 mg
- Intra-abdominal infection: 20 mg/kg/dose every 8 hours; maximum dose: 1 g
- Meningitis: 40 mg/kg/dose every 8 hours; maximum dose: 2 g

Adults:

- Complicated skin and skin structure infection: 500 mg every 8 hours
- Intra-abdominal infection: 1 g every 8 hours
- Meningitis: 2 g every 8 hours

Dosage adjustment in renal impairment: Adults:

- Cl_{cr} 26-50 mL/minute: Standard dose every 12 hours
- Cl_{cr} 10-25 mL/minute: One-half dose every 12 hours
- Cl_{cr} <10 mL/minute: One-half dose every 24 hours

Continuous arteriovenous or venous hemofiltration: Dose as Cl_{cr} 10-50 mL/minute

Administration Administer by I.V. push or I.V. intermittent infusion; final concentration for administration should not exceed 50 mg/mL; infuse I.V. push injection over 3-5 minutes; intermittent infusion dose should be administered over 15-30 minutes

Monitoring Parameters Periodic renal, hepatic, and hematologic function tests. Observe for changes in bowel frequency.

Test Interactions Positive Coombs' [direct]

Additional Information Sodium content 1 g: 3.92 mEq

Dosage Forms Excipient information presented when available (limited, particularly for generics); consult specific product labeling.

Injection, powder for reconstitution: 500 mg [contains sodium 45.1 mg as sodium carbonate (1.96 mEq)]; 1 g [contains sodium 90.2 mg as sodium carbonate (3.92 mEq)]

References

Blummer JL, "Pharmacokinetic Determinants of Carbapenem Therapy in Neonates and Children," *Pediatr Infect Dis J*, 1996, 15(8):733-7.

Blummer JL, Reed MD, Kearns GL, et al, "Sequential, Single-Dose Pharmacokinetic Evaluation of Meropenem in Hospitalized Infants and Children," *Antimicrob Agents Chemother*, 1995, 39(8):1721-5.

Bradley, JS, "Meropenem: A New, Extremely Broad Spectrum Beta-lactam Antibiotic for Serious Infections in Pediatrics," *Pediatr Infect Dis J*, 1997, 16:263-8.

Odio CM, Puig JR, Feris JM, et al, "Prospective, Randomized, Investigator-Blinded Study of the Efficacy and Safety of Meropenem vs. Cefotaxime Therapy in Bacterial Meningitis in Children. Meropenem Meningitis Study Group," *Pediatr Infect Dis J*, 1999, 18(7):581-90.

Ververs TF, van Dijk A, Vinks SA, et al, "Pharmacokinetics and Dosing Regimen of Meropenem in Critically Ill Patients Receiving Continuous Venovenous Hemofiltration," *Crit Care Med*, 2000, 28(10):3412-6.

Wiseman LR, Wagstaff AJ, Brogden RN, et al, "Meropenem. A Review of its Antibacterial Activity, Pharmacokinetic Properties and Clinical Efficacy," *Drugs*, 1995, 50(1):73-101.

♦ **Merrem® (Can)** *see* Meropenem *on page 1009*

♦ **Merrem® I.V.** *see* Meropenem *on page 1009*

♦ **Meruvax® II** *see* Rubella Virus Vaccine (Live) *on page 1410*

Mesalamine (me SAL a meen)

Medication Safety Issues

Sound-alike/look-alike issues:

Mesalamine may be confused with mecamylamine

Asacol® may be confused with Ansaid®, Os-Cal®

Lialda™ may be confused with Aldara™

U.S. Brand Names Asacol®; Canasa™; Lialda™; Pentasa®; Rowasa®

Canadian Brand Names Asacol®; Asacol® 800; Mesasal®; Novo-5 ASA; Pendo-5 ASA; Pentasa®; Quintasa®; Rowasa®; Salofalk®

Index Terms 5-Aminosalicylic Acid; 5-ASA; Fisalamine; Mesalazine

Therapeutic Category 5-Aminosalicylic Acid Derivative; Anti-inflammatory Agent; Anti-inflammatory Agent, Rectal

Generic Available Yes: Rectal suspension

Use Treatment of ulcerative colitis (UC), proctosigmoiditis, and proctitis

Pregnancy Risk Factor B

Lactation Enters breast milk/use caution

Contraindications Hypersensitivity to mesalamine, salicylates, or any component (see Warnings); Canasa™ suppositories contain saturated vegetable fatty acid esters (contraindicated in patients with allergy to these components)

Warnings Myocarditis and pericarditis should be considered in patients with chest pain; this cardiac hypersensitivity reaction has occurred rarely with mesalamine-containing products; pancreatitis should be considered in any patient with new abdominal complaints; has been implicated in the production of an acute intolerance syndrome or exacerbation of colitis (<3%), prompt discontinuation is required if this develops.

Some products may contain sulfites which may cause allergic reactions in susceptible individuals. Rowasa® suspension contains sodium benzoate; benzoic acid (benzoate) is a metabolite of benzyl alcohol; large amounts of benzyl alcohol (≥99 mg/kg/day) have been associated with a potentially fatal toxicity ("gasping syndrome") in neonates; *in vitro* and animal studies have shown that benzoate displaces bilirubin from protein binding sites; avoid use of Rowasa® suspension in neonates.

Precautions Use with caution in patients with hypersensitivity to sulfasalazines or patients with renal or hepatic impairment and patients with conditions predisposing to the development of myocarditis or pericarditis; use delayed release formulations with caution in patients with pyloric stenosis due to prolonged gastric retention

Adverse Reactions

Cardiovascular: Pericarditis, chest pain, myocarditis, T-wave abnormalities, edema

Central nervous system: Chills, dizziness, fever, headache, insomnia, malaise, anxiety, depression, somnolence

Dermatologic: Psoriasis, rash, acne, prurigo, dry skin, urticaria, pyoderma gangrenosum, erythema nodosum, photosensitivity, lichen planus, alopecia

Endocrine & metabolic: Amenorrhea, menorrhagia, breast pain

Gastrointestinal: Abdominal pain, cramps, flatulence, bloody diarrhea, anal irritation, anorexia, pancreatitis, gastritis, dyspepsia, eructation, vomiting, hemorrhoids, constipation, dysgeusia, pharyngolaryngeal pain, exacerbation of colitis (see Warnings)

Genitourinary: Epididymitis, dysuria, discoloration of urine (yellow-brown)

Hematologic: Rare: Agranulocytosis, thrombocytopenia, eosinophilia, aplastic anemia

Hepatic: Elevated liver enzymes, jaundice, cholestatic jaundice, liver necrosis/failure

Neuromuscular & skeletal: Weakness, tremor

Otic: Ear pain

Renal: Interstitial nephritis, renal papillary necrosis, nephrotic syndrome

Respiratory: Interstitial pneumonitis, pulmonary infiltrates, sinusitis, asthma exacerbation, pleuritis, fibrosing alveolitis

Miscellaneous: Kawasaki-like syndrome, lupus-like syndrome

Drug Interactions Decreased digoxin bioavailability; use with NSAIDs or other potentially nephrotoxic drugs may increase the risk of renal adverse effects; mesalamine may increase the risk of myelosuppression with azathioprine, mercaptopurine, thioguanine

Stability Store tablets and capsules at room temperature; unstable in presence of water or light; once foil has been removed, unopened bottles have an expiration of 1 year following the date of manufacture; store suppositories at room temperature; do not refrigerate

Mechanism of Action Mesalamine (5-aminosalicylic acid) is the active component of sulfasalazine; the specific mechanism of action of mesalamine is unknown; however, it is thought that it modulates local chemical mediators of the inflammatory response, especially leukotrienes; action appears topical rather than systemic

(Continued)

Mesalamine *(Continued)*

Pharmacokinetics

Absorption:

Capsule: 20% to 30%

Rectal: ~15%; variable and dependent upon retention time, underlying GI disease, and colonic pH

Tablet: 28%

Distribution: Breast milk to plasma ratio:

5-ASA: 0.27

Acetyl 5-ASA: 5.1

Protein binding: 43%

Metabolism: In the liver by acetylation to acetyl-5-aminosalicylic acid (acetyl-5-ASA, an active metabolite) and to glucuronide conjugates; intestinal metabolism may also occur

Half-life:

5-ASA: 0.5-1.5 hours

Acetyl 5-ASA: 5-10 hours

Time to peak serum concentration: Capsule: Pentasa®: 3 hours; rectal: Within 4-7 hours; delayed release tablet: Asacol®: 4-12 hours; Lialda™: 9-12 hours (average)

Elimination: Most metabolites are excreted in urine with <2% appearing in feces

Usual Dosage Oral (usual course of therapy is 3-6 weeks):

(Oral products are formulated to slowly release therapeutic quantities of drug throughout the GI tract):

Capsule (ethylcellulose-coated, controlled release):

Children: 50 mg/kg/day divided every 6-12 hours

Adults: 1 g 4 times/day for up to 8 weeks

Tablet (coated with acrylic-based resin; drug released after reaches terminal ileum):

Children: 50 mg/kg/day divided every 8-12 hours

Adults: Treatment:

Asacol®: 800 mg 3 times/day for 6 weeks; maintenance for remission of UC: 1.6 g daily in divided doses up to 6 months

Lialda™: 2.4-4.8 g once daily for up to 8 weeks

Retention enema: Adults: 60 mL (4 g) at bedtime, retained overnight, approximately 8 hours for 3-6 weeks

Rectal suppository: Adults: Insert 1 suppository (500 mg) in rectum twice daily or 1 suppository (1000 mg) in rectum once daily at bedtime, for 3-6 weeks; may increase to 3 times daily (500 mg only) if ineffective response noted after 2 weeks of therapy

Administration

Oral: Administer with food; swallow tablets or capsules whole, do not chew or crush; do not break outer coating of Asacol® or Lialda™ tablets

Rectal: Retain enema for 8 hours or as long as practical; shake rectal suspension well before use; retain suppository for 1-3 hours

Patient Information May discolor urine yellow-brown. May rarely cause photosensitivity reactions (eg, exposure to sunlight may cause severe sunburn, skin rash, redness, or itching); avoid direct exposure to sunlight. Suppositories will cause staining of direct contact surfaces including fabrics.

Dosage Forms Excipient information presented when available (limited, particularly for generics); consult specific product labeling.

Capsule, controlled release:

Pentasa®: 250 mg, 500 mg

Suppository, rectal:

Canasa™: 500 mg [DSC], 1000 mg [contains saturated vegetable fatty acid esters]

Suspension, rectal: 4 g/60 mL (7s, 28s) [contains potassium metabisulfite and sodium benzoate]

Rowasa®: 4 g/60 mL (7s, 28s) [contains potassium metabisulfite and sodium benzoate]

Tablet, delayed release [enteric coated]:

Asacol®: 400 mg

Lialda™: 1.2 g

References

Grand RJ, Ramakrishna J, and Calenda KA, "Inflammatory Bowel Disease in the Pediatric Patient," *Gastroenterol Clin North Am*, 1995, 24(3):613-32.

♦ **Mesalazine** *see* Mesalamine *on page 1011*

♦ **Mesasal® (Can)** *see* Mesalamine *on page 1011*

♦ **M-Eslon® (Can)** *see* Morphine Sulfate *on page 1082*

Mesna (MES na)

Related Information

Compatibility of Chemotherapy and Related Supportive Care Medications *on page 1777*

U.S. Brand Names Mesnex®

Canadian Brand Names Mesnex®; Uromitexan

Index Terms Sodium 2-Mercaptoethane Sulfonate

Therapeutic Category Antidote, Cyclophosphamide-induced Hemorrhagic Cystitis; Antidote, Ifosfamide-induced Hemorrhagic Cystitis

Generic Available Yes

Use Detoxifying agent used as a protectant against hemorrhagic cystitis induced by ifosfamide and cyclophosphamide

Pregnancy Risk Factor B

Lactation Excretion in breast milk unknown/not recommended

Contraindications Hypersensitivity to mesna, other thiol compounds, or any component (see Warnings)

Warnings Mesna injection contains benzyl alcohol which may cause allergic reactions in susceptible individuals; large amounts of benzyl alcohol (≥99 mg/kg/day) have been associated with a potentially fatal toxicity ("gasping syndrome") in neonates; the "gasping syndrome" consists of metabolic acidosis, respiratory distress, gasping respirations, CNS dysfunction (including convulsions, intracranial hemorrhage), hypotension and cardiovascular collapse; avoid use of mesna products containing benzyl alcohol in children <2 years of age; a benzyl alcohol free (preservative free) injection is available (see Additional Information); *in vitro* and animal studies have shown that benzoate, a metabolite of benzyl alcohol, displaces bilirubin from protein binding sites

Precautions Examine morning urine specimen for hematuria prior to ifosfamide or cyclophosphamide treatment; if hematuria develops, reduce the ifosfamide/cyclophosphamide dose or discontinue the drug and consider increasing the mesna dosage

Adverse Reactions

Cardiovascular: Hypotension

Central nervous system: Malaise, headache

Dermatologic: Skin rash

Gastrointestinal: Diarrhea, nausea, vomiting, dysgeusia

Neuromuscular & skeletal: Limb pain

Stability Diluted solutions in D_5W, D_5/NS, NS, or LR are chemically and physically stable for 48 hours at room temperature; compatible with solutions containing ifosfamide or cyclophosphamide; incompatible with cisplatin

Mechanism of Action In the urinary bladder, mesna binds with and detoxifies acrolein and other urotoxic metabolites of ifosfamide and cyclophosphamide via an active sulfhydryl group on mesna

Pharmacokinetics

Distribution: No tissue penetration; following glomerular filtration, mesna disulfide is reduced in the renal tubules back to mesna and delivered to the bladder in the active form

Bioavailability: Oral: 50%

Half-life: 24 minutes (mesna); after I.V. administration, mesna is rapidly oxidized intravascularly to mesna disulfide (half-life: 72 minutes)

Elimination: Unchanged drug and metabolite are excreted primarily in the urine; time for maximum urinary mesna excretion: 1 hour after I.V. and 2-3 hours after an oral mesna dose

Usual Dosage Children and Adults (refer to individual protocols): **Mesna dose depends on dose of antineoplastic agent used:**

When used with ifosfamide: I.V.: Mesna dose is 20% w/w of ifosfamide dose 15 minutes before and 4 and 8 hours later or combined with ifosfamide administration; for high-dose ifosfamide, mesna has been administered at a dose of 20% w/w 15 minutes before and every 3 hours for 3-6 doses or combined with ifosfamide administration; (**Note:** In clinical protocols, total daily mesna dose ranged between 60% to 160% w/w of the daily ifosfamide dose)

When used with cyclophosphamide: I.V.: Mesna dose is 20% w/w of cyclophosphamide dose 15 minutes before and every 3 hours for 3-4 doses or combined with cyclophosphamide administration; (**Note:** In clinical protocols, total daily mesna dose ranged between 60% to 160% w/w of the daily cyclophosphamide dose)

I.V. continuous infusion: Mesna doses equivalent to 60% to 100% of the ifosfamide or cyclophosphamide dose have been used

Oral: Mesna dose is 40% w/w of the antineoplastic agent dose in 3 doses at 4-hour intervals or 20 mg/kg/dose every 4 hours x 3 (oral mesna is not recommended for the first dose before ifosfamide or cyclophosphamide)

(Continued)

Mesna *(Continued)*

Administration

Oral: Dilute mesna solution before oral administration to decrease sulfur odor; mesna can be diluted 1:1 to 1:10 in carbonated cola drinks, fruit juices (grape, apple, tomato, and orange juice) or in plain or chocolate milk (most palatable in chilled grape juice)

Parenteral: Administer by I.V. infusion over 15-30 minutes, or by continuous I.V. infusion, or per protocol; mesna may be diluted in D_5W or NS to a final concentration of 1-20 mg/mL; may be added to solutions containing ifosfamide or cyclophosphamide

Monitoring Parameters Urinalysis

Test Interactions False-positive urinary ketones with Chemstrip®, Multistix®, or Labstix®

Nursing Implications Used concurrently with and/or following high-dose ifosfamide or cyclophosphamide; ensure adequate patient hydration; report vomiting within 1 hour of an oral mesna dose to physician so that I.V. mesna can be administered

Additional Information pH of the commercial 100 mg/mL solution: 6.5-8.5. A preservative free formulation of Mesnex® injection may be obtained directly from the manufacturer. It is restricted for use in children <2 years and others who are sensitive to benzyl alcohol. Contact Bristol-Myers Squibb Company at 800-437-0994 for additional information.

Dosage Forms Excipient information presented when available (limited, particularly for generics); consult specific product labeling.

Injection, solution: 100 mg/mL (10 mL) [contains benzyl alcohol]

Tablet: 400 mg

References

Ben Yehuda A, Heyman A and Steiner Salz D, "False Positive Reaction for Urinary Ketones With Mesna," *Drug Intell Clin Pharm*, 1987, 21(6): 547-8.

Brock N and Pohl J, "The Development of Mesna for Regional Detoxification," *Cancer Treat Rev*, 1983, 10(Suppl A):33-43.

"Cancer Chemotherapy," *Med Lett Drugs Ther*, 1989, 31(793):49-56.

Schoenike SE and Dana WJ, "Ifosfamide and Mesna," *Clin Pharm*, 1990, 9(3):179-91.

♦ **Mesnex®** *see* Mesna *on page 1013*
♦ **Mestinon®** *see* Pyridostigmine *on page 1351*
♦ **Mestinon®-SR (Can)** *see* Pyridostigmine *on page 1351*
♦ **Mestinon® Timespan®** *see* Pyridostigmine *on page 1351*
♦ **Metacortandralone** *see* PrednisoLONE *on page 1304*
♦ **Metadate® CD** *see* Methylphenidate *on page 1034*
♦ **Metadate® ER** *see* Methylphenidate *on page 1034*
♦ **Metadol™ (Can)** *see* Methadone *on page 1018*
♦ **Metamucil® [OTC]** *see* Psyllium *on page 1347*
♦ **Metamucil® (Can)** *see* Psyllium *on page 1347*
♦ **Metamucil® Plus Calcium [OTC]** *see* Psyllium *on page 1347*
♦ **Metamucil® Smooth Texture [OTC]** *see* Psyllium *on page 1347*

Metaproterenol (met a proe TER e nol)

Medication Safety Issues

Sound-alike/look-alike issues:

Metaproterenol may be confused with metipranolol, metoprolol

Alupent® may be confused with Atrovent®

Related Information

Asthma *on page 1904*

U.S. Brand Names Alupent®

Canadian Brand Names Apo-Orciprenaline®; Ratio-Orciprenaline®; Tanta-Orciprenaline®

Index Terms Metaproterenol Sulfate; Orciprenaline Sulfate

Therapeutic Category Adrenergic Agonist Agent; Antiasthmatic; $Beta_2$-Adrenergic Agonist Agent; Bronchodilator; Sympathomimetic

Generic Available Yes: Excludes inhaler

Use Bronchodilator in reversible airway obstruction due to asthma or COPD

Pregnancy Risk Factor C

Lactation Excretion in breast milk unknown

Contraindications Hypersensitivity to metaproterenol or any component; pre-existing cardiac arrhythmias associated with tachycardia; narrow-angle glaucoma

Warnings Excessive use may result in cardiac arrest and death; do not use concurrently with other sympathomimetic bronchodilators. Some products contain sodium benzoate; benzoic acid (benzoate) is a metabolite of benzyl alcohol; large amounts of benzyl alcohol (≥99 mg/kg/day) have been associated with a potentially fatal toxicity ("gasping syndrome") in neonates; *in vitro* and animal studies have shown that benzoate displaces bilirubin from protein binding sites; avoid use of sodium benzoate containing products in neonates.

Precautions Use with caution in patients with ischemic heart disease, hypertension, hyperthyroidism, seizure disorders, CHF, cardiac arrhythmias, and diabetes mellitus

Adverse Reactions

Cardiovascular: Tachycardia, palpitations, hypertension

Central nervous system: Nervousness, dizziness, headache, fatigue, vertigo

Gastrointestinal: Nausea, vomiting, diarrhea, GI distress, xerostomia, dysgeusia, throat irritation

Neuromuscular & skeletal: Tremor, weakness, muscle cramps

Respiratory: Exacerbation of asthma, hoarseness, cough, nasal congestion

Drug Interactions Beta-adrenergic blockers (eg, propranolol) may antagonize metaproterenol's effects; sympathomimetics may increase adverse effects if administered concomitantly; MAO inhibitors may cause hypertensive crisis

Stability Protect from light

Mechanism of Action Relaxes bronchial smooth muscle and peripheral vasculature by action on $beta_2$-receptors

Pharmacodynamics

Onset of bronchodilation:

Oral: Within 30 minutes

Inhalation: Within 60 seconds

Maximum effect: Oral: Within 1 hour

Duration: (approximately 1-5 hours) regardless of route administered

Pharmacokinetics

Absorption: Oral: Well absorbed

Metabolism: Extensive first-pass in the liver (~40% of oral dose is available)

Elimination: Mainly as glucuronic acid conjugates

Usual Dosage

Oral:

Children:

<2 years: 0.4 mg/kg/dose given 3-4 times/day; in infants, the dose can be given every 8-12 hours

2-6 years: 1.3-2.6 mg/kg/day divided every 6-8 hours

6-9 years: 10 mg/dose given 3-4 times/day

Children >9 years and Adults: 20 mg/dose given 3-4 times/day

Inhalation: Children >12 years and Adults: 2-3 inhalations every 3-4 hours, up to 12 inhalations in 24 hours

Nebulizer:

Infants and Children: 0.01-0.02 mL/kg (0.5-1 mg/kg) of 5% solution; minimum dose: 0.1 mL (5 mg); maximum dose: 0.3 mL (15 mg) every 4-6 hours (may be given more frequently according to need); equivalent doses using more dilute solutions may be administered at the same frequency

Adolescents and Adults: 0.2 to 0.3 mL (10-15 mg) of 5% metaproterenol every 4-6 hours (can be given more frequently according to need); equivalent doses using more dilute solutions may be administered at the same frequency

Administration

Nebulization: Dilute 5% solution in 2-3 mL NS; more dilute solutions may be used without dilution

Oral: Administer with food to decrease GI distress

Monitoring Parameters Heart rate, respiratory rate, blood pressure, arterial or capillary blood gases if applicable, pulmonary function tests

Patient Information May cause dry mouth

Dosage Forms Excipient information presented when available (limited, particularly for generics); consult specific product labeling.

Aerosol for oral inhalation, as sulfate (Alupent®): 0.65 mg/inhalation (14 g) [200 doses]

Solution for nebulization, as sulfate [preservative free]: 0.4% [4 mg/mL] (2.5 mL); 0.6% [6 mg/mL] (2.5 mL)

Syrup, as sulfate: 10 mg/5 mL (480 mL) [may contain sodium benzoate]

Tablet, as sulfate: 10 mg, 20 mg

References

"National Asthma Education and Prevention Program. Expert Panel Report: Guidelines for the Diagnosis and Management of Asthma Update on Selected Topics--2002," *J Allergy Clin Immunol*, 2002, 110(5 Suppl):S141-219.

♦ **Metaproterenol Sulfate** *see* Metaproterenol *on page 1014*

Metformin (met FOR min)

Medication Safety Issues
Sound-alike/look-alike issues:
Metformin may be confused with metronidazole
Glucophage® may be confused with Glucotrol®, Glutofac®

U.S. Brand Names Fortamet®; Glucophage®; Glucophage® XR; Glumetza™; Riomet™

Canadian Brand Names Alti-Metformin; Apo-Metformin®; BCI-Metformin; Gen-Metformin; Glucophage®; Glumetza®; Glycon; Novo-Metformin; Nu-Metformin; PMS-Metformin; RAN™-Metformin; ratio-Metformin; Rho®-Metformin; Sandoz-Metformin FC

Index Terms Metformin Hydrochloride

Therapeutic Category Antidiabetic Agent, Biguanide; Antidiabetic Agent, Oral; Hypoglycemic Agent, Oral

Generic Available Yes: Excludes solution

Use Management of type II diabetes mellitus (noninsulin-dependent, NIDDM) as monotherapy when hyperglycemia cannot be managed with diet and exercise alone; may be used concomitantly with a sulfonylurea or insulin to improve glycemic control

Pregnancy Risk Factor B

Lactation Enters breast milk/not recommended

Contraindications Hypersensitivity to metformin or any component; renal disease or renal dysfunction (S_{cr} ≥1.5 mg/dL in males or ≥1.4 mg/dL in females) or abnormal creatinine clearance which may result from clinical conditions such as cardiovascular collapse, respiratory failure, acute MI, acute CHF, and septicemia (see Warnings); acute or chronic metabolic acidosis with or without coma (including diabetic ketoacidosis)

Warnings Lactic acidosis is a rare, but potentially severe consequence of therapy with metformin; withhold therapy in clinical conditions which may predispose to the development of lactic acidosis (eg, hypoxemia, dehydration, hypoperfusion, sepsis) or in any patient with CHF requiring pharmacologic management; the risk of accumulation and lactic acidosis increases with the degree of impairment of renal function and age; avoid use in patients with renal function below the limit of normal for their age; measure baseline renal function and monitor annually; more frequent monitoring may be necessary depending upon the patient's clinical condition; therapy should be suspended for any surgical procedures (resume only after normal intake resumed and normal renal function is verified); temporarily discontinue therapy for 48 hours in patients undergoing radiologic studies involving the intravascular administration of iodinated contrast materials (potential for acute alteration in renal function); avoid use in patients with impaired liver function; avoid excessive acute or chronic alcohol use (alcohol potentiates the effect of metformin on lactate metabolism); lactic acidosis should be suspected in any diabetic patient receiving metformin who has evidence of acidosis when evidence of ketoacidosis is lacking

Precautions Use with caution in patients receiving medications that may affect renal function, particularly tubular secretion, as they may also affect metformin disposition; hypoglycemia (rare with metformin) may occur with inadequate caloric intake, strenuous exercise, or concurrent use with other hypoglycemic drugs

Adverse Reactions
Cardiovascular: Chest discomfort, flushing, palpitation
Central nervous system: Headache, chills, dizziness, lightheadedness
Dermatologic: Rash, urticaria
Endocrine & metabolic: Hypoglycemia (rare), lactic acidosis
Gastrointestinal: Anorexia, nausea, vomiting, diarrhea, flatulence, indigestion, abdominal discomfort, abdominal distention, abnormal stools, constipation, dyspepsia, heartburn, metallic taste
Hematologic: Megaloblastic anemia (rare)
Neuromuscular & skeletal: Weakness, myalgia
Respiratory: Dyspnea, upper respiratory tract infection
Miscellaneous: Decreased vitamin B_{12} levels, increased sweating, flu-like syndrome, nail disorder

Drug Interactions Drugs which tend to produce hyperglycemia (eg, diuretics, corticosteroids, phenothiazines, thyroid products, estrogens, oral contraceptives, phenytoin, nicotinic acid, sympathomimetics, calcium channel blocking drugs, isoniazid) may lead to a loss of glycemic control; alcohol potentiates the effects of metformin on lactate metabolism; cationic drugs (eg, amiloride, digoxin, morphine, procainamide, quinidine, quinine, ranitidine, triamterene, trimethoprim, and vancomycin) which are eliminated by renal tubular secretion have the potential for interaction with metformin by competing for common renal tubular transport systems; cimetidine increases (by 60%) peak metformin blood concentrations; in a single dose study, furosemide increased the metformin blood concentration without altering metformin renal clearance; nifedipine may enhance the absorption of metformin; metformin may interfere with vitamin B_{12} absorption

Food Interactions Food decreases the extent and slightly delays the absorption (clinical significance unknown); may decrease absorption of vitamin B_{12} and folic acid

Stability Tablets and oral solution: Store at 20°C to 25°C (68°F to 77°F); protect from light

Mechanism of Action Decreases hepatic glucose production, decreases intestinal absorption of glucose, and improves insulin sensitivity (increases peripheral glucose uptake and utilization)

Pharmacodynamics

Onset of action: Within days, maximum effects up to 2 weeks

Average decrease in fasting blood glucose: Children >10 years and Adults: 60-70 mg/dL

Pharmacokinetics

Absorption: Oral: Slowly and incompletely absorbed

Distribution: Adults: V_d: 654 ± 358 L

Protein binding, plasma: Negligible

Bioavailability: Oral: 50% to 60% (under fasting conditions)

Half-life, plasma elimination: 3-6 hours

Time to peak serum concentration: Immediate release formulation: 2-4 hours; extended release formulation: 4-8 hours (median: 7 hours)

Elimination: Renal; tubular secretion is major route; excretion: 90% in urine as unchanged drug

Dialysis: Removed by hemodialysis; clearance up to 170 mL/minute

Usual Dosage Oral: **Note:** While significant responses may not be seen at doses <1500 mg daily, a lower recommended starting dose and gradual increase in dosage is recommended to minimize GI symptoms

Treatment of type 2 diabetes mellitus (noninsulin-dependent) in previously untreated patients or patients currently receiving sulfonylurea oral antidiabetic agents:

Children 10-16 years: Initial: 500 mg twice daily; dosage increases should be made weekly, in increments of 500 mg/day in divided doses, up to a maximum of 2000 mg/day.

Children ≥17 years and Adults:

Initial: 500 mg twice daily; dosage increases should be made weekly, in increments of 500 mg/day in 2 divided doses, up to a maximum of 2500 mg/day; doses >2000 mg/day may be better tolerated divided 3 times/day

Alternative dose: Initial: 850 mg once daily; dosage increases should be made in increments of 850 mg every 2 weeks, given in divided doses, up to a maximum of 2550 mg/day

Glucophage® XR (extended release tablets): Initial: 500 mg once daily; dosage may be increased by 500 mg weekly; maximum dose: 2000 mg once daily. If glycemic control is not achieved at maximum dose, may divide dose to 1000 mg twice daily; if doses >2000 mg/day are needed, switch to regular release tablets and titrate to maximum dose of 2550 mg/day

Glumetza™ (extended release tablet): Initial: 1000 mg once daily; may increase weekly as needed in 500 mg increments; not to exceed 2000 mg/day; if 2000 mg/day is ineffective, may consider using 1000 mg twice daily

Adjunctive agent to diabetic patient receiving insulin: Children ≥17 years and Adults: Initial: 500 mg metformin or metformin extended release once daily, continue current insulin dose; increase by 500 mg every week; maximum dose: 2500 mg metformin or 2000 mg metformin extended release; decrease insulin dose by 10% to 25% when fasting blood glucose <120 mg/dL

Dosing adjustment in renal impairment: Metformin is contraindicated in the presence of renal dysfunction (see Contraindications)

Dosing adjustment in hepatic impairment: Avoid metformin; liver disease is a risk factor for the development of lactic acidosis during metformin therapy.

Administration Oral:

Glucophage®, Riomet™: Administer in divided doses with meals

Glucophage® XR, Glumetza™: Administer with evening meal; extended release tablets should be swallowed whole; do not cut, crush, or chew

Monitoring Parameters Fasting blood glucose, hemoglobin A_{1c}, initial and periodic monitoring of hemoglobin, hematocrit, and red blood cell indices; renal function (baseline and annually)

Reference Range Target range:

Blood glucose: Fasting and preprandial: 80-120 mg/dL; bedtime: 100-140 mg/dL

Glycosylated hemoglobin (hemoglobin A_{1c}): <7%

Patient Information Do not change dose or discontinue without consulting prescriber; avoid alcohol while taking this medication, could cause severe reaction; maintain regular dietary intake and exercise routine; always carry quick source of sugar with (Continued)

Metformin *(Continued)*

you; during the first weeks of therapy, side effects such as headache, nausea, vomiting, or diarrhea may occur; consult prescriber if these persist; report severe or persistent side effects, extended vomiting or flu-like symptoms, skin rash, easy bruising or bleeding, or change in color of urine or stool; contact your healthcare provider immediately if you feel very weak, tired, or uncomfortable, have unusual muscle pain, trouble breathing, unusual stomach discomfort, are dizzy or lightheaded, or suddenly develop a slow or irregular heartbeat; parts of the extended release tablet (which do not contain active ingredient) may be found excreted in the stool

Additional Information When transferring therapy from chlorpropamide to metformin, monitor the patient closely during the first 2 weeks due to the prolonged retention of chlorpropamide in the body, leading to overlapping drug effects and possible hypoglycemia; if the patient has not responded to 4 weeks at the maximum metformin dosage, consider a gradual addition of a sulfonylurea antidiabetic agent, even if prior primary or secondary failure to a sulfonylurea has occurred; continue metformin at the maximum dose

Dosage Forms Excipient information presented when available (limited, particularly for generics); consult specific product labeling.

Solution, oral, as hydrochloride:

Riomet™: 100 mg/mL (118 mL, 473 mL) [contains saccharin; cherry flavor]

Tablet, as hydrochloride: 500 mg, 850 mg, 1000 mg

Glucophage®: 500 mg, 850 mg, 1000 mg

Tablet, extended release, as hydrochloride: 500 mg, 750 mg

Fortamet®: 500 mg, 1000 mg

Glucophage® XR: 500 mg, 750 mg

Glumetza™: 500 mg

References

DeFronzo RA, "Pharmacologic Therapy for Type 2 Diabetes Mellitus," *Ann Intern Med*, 1999, 131(4):281-303.

Jones K, Arlanian S, McVie R, et al, "Metformin Improves Glycemic Control in Children With Type 2 Diabetes," *Diabetes*, 2000, 49(Suppl 1):A75.

"Type 2 Diabetes in Children and Adolescents. American Diabetes Association," *Diabetes Care*, 2000, 23(3):381-9.

♦ **Metformin Hydrochloride** *see* Metformin *on page 1016*

Methadone (METH a done)

Medication Safety Issues

Sound-alike/look-alike issues:

Methadone may be confused with Mephyton®, methylphenidate, Metadate®, and Metadate® ER

Related Information

Compatibility of Chemotherapy and Related Supportive Care Medications *on page 1777*

Medications for Which A Single Dose May Be Fatal When Ingested By A Toddler *on page 1932*

Narcotic Analgesics Comparison *on page 1705*

Overdose and Toxicology *on page 1916*

U.S. Brand Names Dolophine®; Methadone Diskets®; Methadone Intensol™; Methadose®

Canadian Brand Names Metadol™

Index Terms Methadone Hydrochloride

Therapeutic Category Analgesic, Narcotic

Generic Available Yes

Use Management of moderate to severe pain unresponsive to non-narcotics; used in narcotic detoxification maintenance programs and for the treatment of iatrogenic narcotic dependency

Restrictions C-II

Treatment of narcotic addiction (detoxification or maintenance programs): Methadone may only be dispensed by pharmacies or maintenance programs certified by the Federal Substance Abuse and Mental Health Service Administration, registered by the Drug Enforcement Agency, and approved by the designated state authority. Exceptions include: During inpatient care, when patients are admitted for conditions other than concurrent opioid addiction (parenteral methadone may be used for those patients unable to take oral methadone) and during an emergency period ≤3 days while opioid addiction treatment is being sought in an appropriately licensed facility.

Pregnancy Risk Factor B (D if used for prolonged periods or in high doses at term)

Lactation Enters breast milk/not recommended (AAP rates "compatible")

Contraindications Hypersensitivity to methadone or any component; severe respiratory depression (in absence of resuscitative equipment or ventilatory support); acute or severe asthma; hypercarbia

Warnings Death and life-threatening adverse events (eg, respiratory depression, cardiac arrhythmias) in patients receiving methadone for pain control have been reported. These events may be the result of unintentional overdoses, drug interactions, and cardiac toxicities associated with methadone (QT prolongation, torsade de pointes). Particular vigilance and patient monitoring is necessary during treatment initiation (including conversion from another opioid) and dose titration. Incomplete cross-tolerance between methadone and other opioids may occur; fatalities have been reported when converting patients from chronic, high dose treatment with other opioids to methadone; knowledge of the pharmacokinetics of methadone is essential for appropriate conversion from other opioids (see package insert for conversion tables). Methadone's elimination half-life is significantly longer than its duration of analgesic action. The respiratory depressant effects of methadone occur later and persist longer than its peak analgesic effects. Carefully select initial methadone dose for pain control and slowly titrate to analgesic effect in all patients, including those who are opioid-tolerant. Instruct patients to take methadone as prescribed; do not take more methadone than prescribed without first talking with physician.

Methadone may cause prolongation of the QT interval or torsade de pointes (especially at higher doses, eg, in adults with doses >200 mg/day); use with caution in patients at risk for QT prolongation (eg, patients with cardiac hypertrophy, hypokalemia, hypomagnesemia, concomitant diuretic use), with medications known to prolong the QT interval, or with history of conduction abnormalities. May cause respiratory depression; use with extreme caution in patients with respiratory disease or pre-existing respiratory depression; methadone's effect on respiration lasts longer than analgesic effects. Use with extreme caution (and only if essential) in patients with head injury, increased ICP, or other intracranial lesions. May cause severe hypotension; use with caution in patients with severe volume depletion or circulatory shock. Tablets are to be used only for oral administration and **must not** be used for injection. Abrupt discontinuation after prolonged use may result in withdrawal symptoms or seizures.

Precautions Due to the cumulative effects of methadone, the dose and frequency of administration need to be reduced with repeated use; use with caution in patients with hepatic, renal, pulmonary, or cardiovascular disease; use with caution and decrease dose in patients who are debilitated and those with severe renal or hepatic dysfunction, hypothyroidism, Addison's disease, urethral stricture, or prostatic hypertrophy.

Adverse Reactions

Cardiovascular: Hypotension, bradycardia, peripheral vasodilation; prolongation of QT interval, torsade de pointes (see Warnings)

Central nervous system: CNS depression, elevated intracranial pressure, drowsiness, dizziness, sedation (marked sedation seen after repeated administration)

Endocrine & metabolic: Antidiuretic hormone release

Gastrointestinal: Nausea, vomiting, constipation, xerostomia, biliary tract spasm

Genitourinary: Urinary tract spasm

Ocular: Miosis

Respiratory: Respiratory depression

Miscellaneous: Histamine release, physical and psychological dependence with prolonged use

Drug Interactions Cytochrome P450 isoenzyme CYP1A2, CYP2D6, CYP3A3/4 substrate; CYP2D6 isoenzyme inhibitor

CNS depressants, alcohol, phenothiazines, tricyclic antidepressants may potentiate the adverse effects of methadone; barbiturates, carbamazepine, phenytoin, primidone, efavirenz, nevirapine, ritonavir, nelfinavir, amprenavir, lopinavir, rifampin, or other enzyme inducers may increase the metabolism of methadone and may precipitate withdrawal (monitor patients, larger doses of methadone may be required); the herbal medicine St John's wort (*Hypericum perforatum*) may decrease methadone serum concentrations and precipitate withdrawal; CYP3A4 or CYP2D6 enzyme inhibitors may decrease the metabolism of methadone and increase adverse effects; methadone may decrease stavudine (no dosage adjustment needed) and didanosine concentrations (consider increase in didanosine dose); methadone may increase zidovudine and desipramine serum concentrations; medications known to prolong the QT interval (eg, TCAs, certain neuroleptics, calcium channel blockers, astemizole, class I and III antiarrhythmics, erythromycin) and drugs which may cause hypomagnesemia or hypokalemia (eg, diuretics, laxatives, mineralocorticoids) may increase risk for QT prolongation and torsade de pointes (avoid concurrent use with methadone or use with extreme caution)

Stability Store at controlled room temperature; protect from light

Tablets: Protect from moisture

(Continued)

Methadone *(Continued)*

Mechanism of Action Binds to opiate receptors in the CNS, causing inhibition of ascending pain pathways, altering the perception of and response to pain; produces generalized CNS depression

Pharmacodynamics Analgesia:

Onset of action:

Oral: Within 30-60 minutes

Parenteral: Within 10-20 minutes

Maximum effect: Parenteral: 1-2 hours

Duration: Oral: 6-8 hours; after repeated doses, duration increases to 22-48 hours

Pharmacokinetics

Distribution: Crosses the placenta; appears in breast milk

V_d: (Mean ± SD)

Children: 7.1 ± 2.5 L/kg

Adults: 6.1 ± 2.4 L/kg

V_{dss}: Adults: 2-6 L/kg

Protein binding: 85% to 90% (primarily to alpha$_1$-acid glycoprotein)

Metabolism: N-demethylated in the liver to an inactive metabolite

Half-life: May be prolonged with alkaline pH

Children: 19 ± 14 hours (range: 4-62 hours)

Adults: 35 ± 22 hours (range: 9-87 hours)

Elimination: In urine (<10% as unchanged drug); increased renal excretion with urine pH <6; **Note:** Methadone may persist in the liver and other tissues; slow release from tissues may prolong the pharmacologic effect despite low serum concentrations

Dialysis: Hemodialysis, peritoneal dialysis: Not established as effective for increasing the elimination of methadone (or metabolite)

Usual Dosage Doses should be titrated to appropriate effects:

Neonatal abstinence syndrome: Oral, I.V.: Initial: 0.05-0.2 mg/kg/dose given every 12-24 hours or 0.5 mg/kg/day divided every 8 hours; individualize dose and tapering schedule to control symptoms of withdrawal; usually taper dose by 10% to 20% per week over 1 to 1½ months. **Note**: Due to long elimination half-life, tapering is difficult; consider alternate agent.

Children:

Analgesia: **Note:** Dosing interval may range from 4-12 hours during initial therapy; decrease in dose or frequency may be required (~2-5 days after initiation of therapy or dosage increase) due to accumulation with repeated doses

I.V.: Initial: 0.1 mg/kg/dose every 4 hours for 2-3 doses, then every 6-12 hours as needed; maximum dose: 10 mg/dose

Oral, I.M., SubQ: Initial: 0.1 mg/kg/dose every 4 hours for 2-3 doses, then every 6-12 hours as needed or 0.7 mg/kg/24 hours divided every 4-6 hours as needed; maximum dose: 10 mg/dose

Iatrogenic narcotic dependency: Oral: Controlled studies have not been conducted; several clinically used dosing regimens have been reported. Methadone dose **must be individualized** and will depend upon patient's previous narcotic dose and severity of opioid withdrawal; patients who have received higher doses of narcotics will require higher methadone doses.

General guidelines: Initial: 0.05-0.1 mg/kg/dose every 6 hours; increase by 0.05 mg/kg/dose until withdrawal symptoms are controlled; after 24-48 hours, the dosing interval can be lengthened to every 12-24 hours; to taper dose, wean by 0.05 mg/kg/day; if withdrawal symptoms recur, taper at a slower rate

Adults:

Analgesia:

Oral: Initial 5-10 mg; dosing interval may range from 4-12 hours during initial therapy; decrease in dose or frequency may be required (~2-5 days after initiation of therapy or dosage increase) due to accumulation with repeated doses

Manufacturer's recommendations: 2.5-10 mg every 3-4 hours as needed

I.V.: Manufacturer's recommendations: Opioid-naive patients: Initial: 2.5-10 mg every 8-12 hours; titrate slowly to effect; may also be administered by SubQ or I.M. injection

Detoxification: Oral: 15-40 mg/day

Maintenance of opiate dependence: Oral: 20-120 mg/day

Dosing adjustment in renal impairment: Children and Adults:

Cl_{cr} <10 mL/minute: Administer 50% to 75% of normal dose

Administration Oral: Administer with juice or water; dispersible tablet should be completely dissolved before administration; oral dose for detoxification and maintenance may be administered in Tang®, Kool-Aid®, apple juice, grape Crystal Light®

Monitoring Parameters Respiratory, cardiovascular, and mental status, pain relief (if used for analgesia), abstinence scoring system (if used for neonatal abstinence syndrome)

Patient Information Avoid alcohol; may be habit-forming; avoid abrupt discontinuation after prolonged use; may cause drowsiness and impair ability to perform activities requiring mental alertness or physical coordination; may cause dry mouth; may cause postural hypotension (use with caution when changing positions from lying or sitting to standing); seek medical attention immediately if you experience heart palpitations, dizziness, lightheadedness, or fainting (these may be symptoms of an arrhythmia)

Additional Information Methadone accumulates with repeated doses and dosage may need to be adjusted downward after 3-5 days to prevent toxic effects. Some patients may benefit from every 8- to 12-hour dosing interval (pain control).

Methadone 10 mg I.M. = morphine 10 mg I.M.

Dosage Forms Excipient information presented when available (limited, particularly for generics); consult specific product labeling.

Injection, solution, as hydrochloride: 10 mg/mL (20 mL)

Solution, oral, as hydrochloride: 5 mg/5 mL (500 mL); 10 mg/5 mL (500 mL) [contains alcohol 8%; citrus flavor]

Solution, oral, as hydrochloride [concentrate]: 10 mg/mL (946 mL)
- Methadone Intensol™: 10 mg/mL (30 mL)
- Methadose®: 10 mg/mL (1000 mL) [cherry flavor]
- Methadose®: 10 mg/mL (1000 mL) [dye free, sugar free, unflavored]

Tablet, as hydrochloride: 5 mg, 10 mg
- Dolophine®: 5 mg, 10 mg
- Methadose®: 5 mg, 10 mg [DSC]

Tablet, dispersible, as hydrochloride: 40 mg
- Methadose®: 40 mg
- Methadone Diskets®: 40 mg [orange-pineapple flavor]

References

Anand KJ and Arnold JH, "Opioid Tolerance and Dependence in Infants and Children," *Crit Care Med*, 1994, 22(2):334-42.

Berde C, Ablin A, Glazer J, et al, "American Academy of Pediatrics Report of the Subcommittee on Disease-Related Pain in Childhood Cancer," *Pediatrics*, 1990, 86(5 Pt 2):818-25.

Krantz MJ, Lewkowiez L, Hays H, et al, "Torsade de Pointes Associated With Very-High-Dose Methadone," *Ann Intern Med*, 2002, 137(6):501-4.

Lauriault G, LeBelle MJ, Lodge BA, et al, "Stability of Methadone in Four Vehicles for Oral Administration," *Am J Hosp Pharm*, 1991, 48(6):1252-6.

Olkkola KT, Hamunen K, and Maunuksela EL, "Clinical Pharmacokinetics and Pharmacodynamics of Opioid Analgesics in Infants and Children," *Clin Pharmacokinet*, 1995, 28(5):385-404.

♦ **Methadone Diskets®** *see* Methadone *on page 1018*

♦ **Methadone Hydrochloride** *see* Methadone *on page 1018*

♦ **Methadone Intensol™** *see* Methadone *on page 1018*

♦ **Methadose®** *see* Methadone *on page 1018*

Methenamine (meth EN a meen)

Medication Safety Issues

Sound-alike/look-alike issues:
- Methenamine may be confused with methazolamide, methionine
- Urex® may be confused with Eurax®, Serax®

International issues:
- Urex®: Brand name for furosemide in Australia

U.S. Brand Names Hiprex®; Mandelamine®; Urex®

Canadian Brand Names Dehydral®; Hiprex®; Mandelamine®; Urasal®; Urex®

Index Terms Hexamethylenetetramine; Methenamine Hippurate; Methenamine Mandelate

Therapeutic Category Antibiotic, Miscellaneous

Generic Available Yes

Use Prophylaxis or suppression of recurrent urinary tract infections

Pregnancy Risk Factor C

Lactation Enters breast milk/compatible

Contraindications Hypersensitivity to methenamine or any component (see Warnings); severe dehydration, renal insufficiency (methenamine is ineffective in patients with renal impairment), hepatic insufficiency in patients receiving hippurate salt; concurrent therapy with sulfonamides

Warnings Dosage of 8 g/day for 3-4 weeks has been associated with bladder irritation, albuminuria, and hematuria; Hiprex® tablets contain tartrazine which may cause allergic reactions in susceptible individuals

(Continued)

Methenamine *(Continued)*

Precautions Use with caution in patients with hepatic impairment. Use care to maintain an acidic pH of the urine when treating infections due to urea-splitting organisms such as *Proteus* and *Pseudomonas*.

Adverse Reactions

Central nervous system: Headache
Dermatologic: Rash, pruritus, urticaria
Gastrointestinal: Nausea, vomiting, diarrhea, abdominal cramping, anorexia, stomatitis
Genitourinary: Bladder irritation, painful and frequent micturition, dysuria, crystalluria
Hepatic: Elevated AST and ALT (with hippurate formulation)
Otic: Tinnitus
Renal: Hematuria
Respiratory: Lipoid pneumonitis (with mandelate suspension), dyspnea

Drug Interactions Sulfonamides (may form an insoluble precipitate with formaldehyde in urine); sodium bicarbonate, acetazolamide (decrease effect of methenamine)

Food Interactions Foods/diets which alkalinize urine pH >5.5 decrease activity of methenamine; cranberry juice can be used to acidify urine and increase activity of methenamine

Stability Protect from excessive heat

Mechanism of Action Methenamine is hydrolyzed to formaldehyde and ammonia in acidic urine; formaldehyde has nonspecific bactericidal action

Pharmacokinetics

Absorption: Readily from the GI tract; 10% to 30% of the drug will be hydrolyzed by gastric juices unless it is protected by an enteric coating
Distribution: Distributes into breast milk; crosses the placenta
Metabolism: ~10% to 25% in the liver
Half-life: 3-6 hours
Elimination: Excretion occurs via glomerular filtration and tubular secretion with ~70% to 90% of dose excreted unchanged in urine within 24 hours

Usual Dosage Oral:

Children >2 years to 12 years: Mandelate: 50-75 mg/kg/day divided every 6-8 hours; maximum dose: 4 g/day
Children 6-12 years: Hippurate: 0.5-1 g twice daily
Children >12 years and Adults:
Hippurate: 1 g twice daily
Mandelate: 1 g 4 times/day after meals and at bedtime

Administration Oral: Administer with food to minimize GI upset; shake suspension well before use; patient should drink plenty of fluids to ensure adequate urine flow; administer with cranberry juice, ascorbic acid, or ammonium chloride to acidify urine; avoid intake of alkalinizing agents (sodium bicarbonate, antacids)

Monitoring Parameters Urinary pH, urinalysis, urine cultures, periodic liver function tests in patients receiving hippurate salt

Test Interactions Formaldehyde interferes with fluorometric procedures causing falsely increased results for catecholamines and VMA (U); falsely decreased urine estriol concentration with tests using acid hydrolysis

Nursing Implications Urine should be acidic, pH <5.5 for maximum effect

Additional Information Should not be used to treat infections outside of the lower urinary tract (ie, pyelonephritis)

Dosage Forms Excipient information presented when available (limited, particularly for generics); consult specific product labeling.

Tablet, as hippurate (Hiprex®, Urex®): 1 g [Hiprex® contains tartrazine dye]
Tablet, enteric coated, as mandelate (Mandelamine®): 500 mg, 1 g

References

"Practice Parameter: The Diagnosis, Treatment, and Evaluation of the Initial Urinary Tract Infection in Febrile Infants and Young Children. American Academy of Pediatrics. Committee on Quality Improvement. Subcommittee on Urinary Tract Infection," *Pediatrics*, 1999, 103(4 Pt 1):843-52.

♦ **Methenamine Hippurate** *see* Methenamine *on page 1021*
♦ **Methenamine Mandelate** *see* Methenamine *on page 1021*

Methimazole (meth IM a zole)

Medication Safety Issues

Sound-alike/look-alike issues:
Methimazole may be confused with metolazone

U.S. Brand Names Tapazole®

Canadian Brand Names Dom-Methimazole; PHL-Methimazole; Tapazole®

Index Terms Thiamazole

Therapeutic Category Antithyroid Agent

Generic Available Yes

Use Palliative treatment of hyperthyroidism, to return the hyperthyroid patient to a normal metabolic state prior to thyroidectomy, and to control thyrotoxic crisis that may accompany thyroidectomy

Pregnancy Risk Factor D

Lactation Enters breast milk/contraindicated (AAP rates "compatible")

Contraindications Hypersensitivity to methimazole or any component, nursing mothers per manufacturer, however, expert analysis and the American Academy of Pediatrics state this drug may be used with caution in nursing mothers (see Breast-Feeding and Drugs *on page 1933*)

Precautions Use with extreme caution in patients receiving other drugs known to cause agranulocytosis

Adverse Reactions

Cardiovascular: Edema, periarteritis

Central nervous system: Drowsiness, vertigo, headache, CNS stimulation, neuropathies, CNS depression, fever, dizziness

Dermatologic: Rash, urticaria, pruritus, alopecia, skin pigmentation, exfoliative dermatitis

Endocrine & metabolic: Weight gain, goiter

Gastrointestinal: Ageusia, nausea, vomiting, epigastric distress, splenomegaly, constipation

Hematologic: Agranulocytosis, hypoprothrombinemia

Hepatic: Cholestatic jaundice, hepatitis

Neuromuscular & skeletal: Arthralgia, myalgia, paresthesia, neuritis

Renal: Nephritis

Respiratory: Interstitial pneumonitis

Miscellaneous: Lupus-like syndrome, lymphadenopathy, insulin autoimmune syndrome

Drug Interactions Lithium and potassium iodide may potentiate hypothyroid effects; potentiates warfarin's anticoagulant effects

Mechanism of Action Inhibits the synthesis of thyroid hormones by blocking the oxidation of iodine in the thyroid gland, blocking iodine's ability to combine with tyrosine to form thyroxine (T_4) and triiodothyronine (T_3)

Pharmacodynamics Antithyroid effect:

Onset of action: 12-18 hours

Duration: 36-72 hours

Pharmacokinetics

Distribution: Found in high concentrations in breast milk; breast milk to plasma ratio: 1.0

Bioavailability: 80% to 95%

Half-life: 5-13 hours

Time to peak serum concentration: 1 hour

Elimination: <12% excreted in urine

Usual Dosage Oral:

Children:

Initial: 0.4 mg/kg/day in 3 divided doses; maintenance: 0.2 mg/kg/day in 3 divided doses

or

Initial: 0.5-0.7 mg/kg/day or 15-20 mg/m²/day in 3 divided doses

Maintenance: ⅓ to ⅔ of initial dose; maximum dose: 30 mg/day

Adults: Initial: 5 mg every 8 hours; 10 mg every 8 hours for moderately severe disease and up to 20 mg every 8 hours for severe hyperthyroidism; maintenance: 5-15 mg/day

Administration Oral: Administer with meals

Monitoring Parameters CBC with differential, liver function (baseline and as needed); serum thyroxine, free thyroxine index, prothrombin time

Patient Information Notify physician of fever, sore throat, unusual bleeding or bruising, headache, rash, or yellowing of skin

Dosage Forms Excipient information presented when available (limited, particularly for generics); consult specific product labeling.

Tablet: 5 mg, 10 mg, 20 mg

Tapazole® 5 mg, 10 mg

References

Raby C, Lagorce JF, Jambut-Absil AC, et al, "The Mechanism of Action of Synthetic Antithyroid Drugs: Iodine Complexation During Oxidation of Iodide," *Endocrinology*, 1990, 126(3):1683-91.

Methocarbamol (meth oh KAR ba mole)

Medication Safety Issues

Sound-alike/look-alike issues:

Methocarbamol may be confused with mephobarbital

Robaxin® may be confused with Rubex®

U.S. Brand Names Robaxin®

Canadian Brand Names Robaxin®

Therapeutic Category Skeletal Muscle Relaxant, Nonparalytic

Generic Available Yes: Tablet

Use Treatment of muscle spasm associated with acute painful musculoskeletal conditions; supportive therapy in tetanus

Pregnancy Risk Factor C

Lactation Excretion in breast milk unknown/use caution

Contraindications Hypersensitivity to methocarbamol or any component; injectable formulation in patients with renal impairment

Warnings Solution is hypertonic, avoid extravasation; avoid using injection in patients with impaired renal function because the polyethylene glycol vehicle may be irritating to the kidneys

Precautions Use injectable form cautiously in patients with suspected or known seizure disorders; use with caution in myasthenia gravis patients receiving pyridostigmine (see Drug Interactions); use oral formulation with caution in patients with renal or hepatic impairment; monitor these patients closely

Adverse Reactions

Cardiovascular: Syncope, bradycardia, hypotension

Central nervous system: Drowsiness, dizziness, lightheadedness, headache, fever, vertigo, seizures, amnesia, confusion

Dermatologic: Urticaria, pruritus, rash

Gastrointestinal: Nausea, metallic taste, GI upset, vomiting, dyspepsia

Genitourinary: Discoloration of urine (brown, black, or green)

Hematologic: Leukopenia

Hepatic: Cholestatic jaundice

Local: Pain and phlebitis at injection site, thrombophlebitis

Ocular: Blurred vision, conjunctivitis, nystagmus, diplopia

Respiratory: Nasal congestion

Miscellaneous: Hypersensitivity reactions including anaphylaxis and angioneurotic edema

Drug Interactions Additive effects with other CNS depressants; may inhibit effects of pyridostigmine

Stability Injection when diluted to 4 mg/mL in SWI, D_5W, or NS is stable for 6 days at room temperature; do **not** refrigerate after dilution

Mechanism of Action CNS depressant with sedative and skeletal muscle relaxant effects; exact mechanism of action is unknown

Pharmacodynamics Onset of action: 30 minutes

Pharmacokinetics Oral:

Protein binding: 46% to 50%

Metabolism: Extensive in the liver via dealkylation and hydroxylation

Half-life: 1-2 hours

Time to peak serum concentration: Within ~1-2 hours

Elimination: Clearance: Adults: 0.2-0.8 L/hour/kg

Usual Dosage

Tetanus: I.V.:

Children (recommended **only** for use in tetanus): 15 mg/kg/dose or 500 mg/m²/dose, may repeat every 6 hours if needed; maximum dose: 1.8 g/m²/day for 3 days only

Adults: 1-2 g by direct I.V. injection followed by additional 1-2 g (maximum dose: 3 g total); repeat with 1-2 g every 6 hours until NG tube or oral therapy possible; total daily dose of up to 24 g may be needed

Muscle spasm: Adults:

Oral: 1.5 g 4 times/day for 2-3 days (up to 8 g/day may be used for severe conditions); decrease dose to 4-4.5 g/day as 1 g 4 times/day or 750 mg every 4 hours or 1.5 g 3 times/day

I.M., I.V.: 1 g every 8 hours if oral not possible; maximum dose: 3 g/day for 3 consecutive days (except when treating tetanus); may be reinstituted after 2 drug-free days

Dosing adjustment in renal impairment: Clearance is reduced by as much as 40% in patients with renal failure on hemodialysis; avoid use or reduce dosage and monitor closely; do not administer parenteral formulation to patients with renal dysfunction

Dosing adjustment in hepatic impairment: Clearance may be reduced by as much as 70% in cirrhotic patients; avoid use or reduce dosage and monitor patient closely

Administration

Parenteral: I.V.: May be injected directly I.V. without dilution at a maximum rate of 180 mg/m^2/minute but not >3 mL/minute; may also be diluted in NS or D_5W to a concentration of 4 mg/mL and infused more slowly; patient should be in the recumbent position during and for 10-15 minutes after I.V. administration

I.M.: Do not inject more than 3 mL per site; not recommended for SubQ administration

Test Interactions May cause color interference in certain screening tests for 5-hydroxyindoleacetic acid (5-HIAA) using nitrosonaphthol reagent and in screening tests for vanillylmandelic acid (VMA) using the Gitlow method

Patient Information May cause drowsiness and impair ability to perform activities requiring mental alertness or physical coordination; urine may darken to brown, black, or green

Nursing Implications Avoid infiltration, extremely irritating to tissues

Dosage Forms Excipient information presented when available (limited, particularly for generics); consult specific product labeling.

Injection, solution: 100 mg/mL (10 mL) [in polyethylene glycol; vial stopper contains latex]

Tablet: 500 mg, 750 mg

Methohexital (meth oh HEKS i tal)

Medication Safety Issues

Sound-alike/look-alike issues:

Brevital® may be confused with Brevibloc®

Related Information

Adult ACLS Algorithms *on page 1660*

Preprocedure Sedatives in Children *on page 1895*

U.S. Brand Names Brevital® Sodium

Canadian Brand Names Brevital®

Index Terms Methohexital Sodium

Therapeutic Category Barbiturate; General Anesthetic; Sedative

Generic Available No

Use Induction and maintenance of general anesthesia for short procedures; induction of hypnotic state

Restrictions C-IV

Pregnancy Risk Factor B

Contraindications Hypersensitivity to methohexital, barbiturates, or any component; porphyria; patients in whom general anesthesia is contraindicated

Warnings Continuously monitor respiratory function, pulse oximetry, and cardiac function. Resuscitative drugs, ventilation and intubation equipment, and trained personnel should be immediately available. For deep sedation, a designated individual (other than the person performing the procedure) should be present to continuously monitor the patient.

Precautions Use with extreme caution in patients with liver impairment, asthma, cardiovascular instability; may precipitate seizures in patients with history of convulsions, especially partial seizure disorders; prolonged administration may result in increased CNS, respiratory, and cardiovascular effects; use with caution in patients with obstructive pulmonary disease, severe hypertension or hypotension, myocardial disease, CHF, severe anemia, extreme obesity, renal impairment, or endocrine disorders

Adverse Reactions

Cardiovascular: Hypotension, peripheral vascular collapse, tachycardia (following induction)

Central nervous system: Seizures, headache, somnolence, unconsciousness

Gastrointestinal: Nausea, vomiting, abdominal pain

Hepatic: Elevated liver enzymes

Local: Pain on I.M. injection, thrombophlebitis

Neuromuscular & skeletal: Twitching, rigidity, tremor, involuntary muscle movement

Respiratory: Apnea, respiratory depression, laryngospasm, coughing

Miscellaneous: Hiccups

Drug Interactions CNS depressants may increase effects; prior chronic use of phenytoin, barbiturates, or other enzyme inducing agents may decrease effect of methohexital; methohexital may affect absorption or elimination of phenytoin, anticoagulants, corticosteroids, halothane, ethanol, propylene glycol containing solutions

(Continued)

Methohexital *(Continued)*

Stability Do not dilute with solutions containing bacteriostatic agents; acceptable diluents: D_5W, NS, SWI, or accompanying diluent (for 500 mg vial to make a 1% solution); SWI is the preferred diluent except for making the 0.2% solution for I.V. continuous infusion (use of SWI to make the 0.2% solution will result in extreme hypotonicity; D_5W or NS should be used). Do not use I.V./I.M. solutions if not clear and colorless. Solutions are alkaline (pH 9.5-11) and incompatible with acids (eg, atropine sulfate, succinylcholine chloride); incompatible with phenol-containing solutions, silicone, and LR

Mechanism of Action Ultra short-acting I.V. barbiturate anesthetic; depresses CNS activity by binding to barbiturate site at GABA-receptor complex enhancing GABA activity; depresses reticular activating system; higher doses may be gabamimetic

Pharmacodynamics

Onset of action:
- I.M. (pediatric patients): 2-10 minutes
- I.V.: 1 minute
- Rectal (pediatric patients): 5-15 minutes

Duration:
- I.M.: 1-1.5 hours
- I.V.: 7-10 minutes
- Rectal: 1-1.5 hours

Pharmacokinetics

Metabolism: In the liver via demethylation and oxidation

Bioavailability: Rectal: 17%

Elimination: Through the kidney via glomerular filtration

Usual Dosage Doses must be titrated to effect

Manufacturer's recommendations:
- Infants <1 month: Safety and efficacy not established
- Infants ≥1 month and Children:
  - I.M.: Induction: 6.6-10 mg/kg of a 5% solution
  - Rectal: Induction: Usual: 25 mg/kg of a 1% solution

Alternative pediatric dosing:
- Children 3-12 years:
  - I.M.: Preoperative: 5-10 mg/kg/dose
  - I.V.: Induction: 1-2 mg/kg/dose (additional studies are needed)
  - Rectal: Preoperative/induction: 20-35 mg/kg/dose; usual: 25 mg/kg/dose; maximum dose: 500 mg/dose; give as 10% aqueous solution

Adults: I.V.:
- Induction: Range: 50-120 mg or 1-1.5 mg/kg; usual: 70 mg (**Note:** This provides anesthesia for 5-7 minutes)
- Maintenance: Intermittent I.V. bolus injection: 20-40 mg (2-4 mL of a 1% solution) every 4-7 minutes **OR** Continuous infusion: Average dose: 6 mg/minute (eg, 3 mL/minute of a 0.2% solution); titrate to effect; reduce administration rate gradually for longer surgical procedures

Administration

Parenteral:
- I.M.: Reconstitute with NS to a maximum concentration of 50 mg/mL (5% solution)
- I.V.: Adults:
  - Bolus: Dilute with SWI (preferred), NS, or D_5W to a maximum concentration of 10 mg/mL (1% solution); for induction, infuse a 1% solution at a rate of 1 mL/5 seconds
  - Continuous Infusion: Dilute with D_5W or NS to prepare a 0.2% solution (see Usual Dosage)

Rectal: Dilute with acceptable diluent (see Stability) to a recommended concentration of 10 mg/mL (1% solution)

Monitoring Parameters Blood pressure, heart rate, respiratory rate, oxygen saturation, pulse oximetry

Patient Information May cause drowsiness and impair ability to perform activities requiring mental alertness or physical coordination; do not drive a motor vehicle or operate machinery until 8-12 hours after medication was administered, or until normal functions return (whichever is longer)

Nursing Implications Check catheter placement prior to I.V. injection; avoid extravasation; avoid intra-arterial administration (thrombosis, necrosis, and gangrene may occur)

Additional Information Does not possess analgesic properties; Brevital® has FDA-approved labeling for I.V. use in adults, and for rectal and I.M. use only in pediatric patients >1 month of age; 100 pediatric patients (3 months to 5 years of age) received rectal methohexital (25 mg/kg) for sedation prior to computed tomography (CT) scan; sedation was adequate in 95% of patients; mean time for full sedation = 8.2 ± 3.9 minutes; mean duration of action = 79.3 ± 30.9 minutes; 10% of patients had transient side effects (see Pomeranz, 2000)

Dosage Forms Excipient information presented when available (limited, particularly for generics); consult specific product labeling.

Injection, powder for reconstitution, as sodium: 500 mg, 2.5 g, 5 g

References

Cote' CJ, "Sedation for the Pediatric Patient," *Pediatr Clin North Am*, 1994, 41(1):31-58.

Pomeranz ES, Chudnofsky CR, Deegan TJ, et al, "Rectal Methohexital Sedation for Computed Tomography Imaging of Stable Pediatric Emergency Department Patients," *Pediatrics*, 2000, 105(5):1110-4.

♦ **Methohexital Sodium** *see* Methohexital *on page 1025*

Methotrexate (meth oh TREKS ate)

Medication Safety Issues

Sound-alike/look-alike issues:

Methotrexate may be confused with metolazone, mitoxantrone

MTX is an error-prone abbreviation (mistaken as mitoxantrone)

High alert medication: The Institute for Safe Medication Practices (ISMP) includes this medication among its list of drugs which have a heightened risk of causing significant patient harm when used in error.

Errors have occurred (resulting in death) when methotrexate was administered as "daily" dose instead of the recommended "weekly" dose.

International issues:

Trexall™ may be confused with Truxal® which is a brand name for chlorprothixene in Belgium

Trexall™ may be confused with Trexol® which is a brand name for tramadol in Mexico

Related Information

Compatibility of Chemotherapy and Related Supportive Care Medications *on page 1777*

Emetogenic Potential of Single Chemotherapeutic Agents *on page 1776*

U.S. Brand Names Rheumatrex®; Trexall™

Canadian Brand Names Apo-Methotrexate®; ratio-Methotrexate

Index Terms Amethopterin; Methotrexate Sodium; MTX (error-prone abbreviation); NSC-740

Therapeutic Category Antineoplastic Agent, Antimetabolite; Antirheumatic, Disease Modifying

Generic Available Yes

Use Treatment of trophoblastic neoplasms, leukemias, meningeal leukemia, histiocytoses, osteosarcoma, breast cancer, head and neck cancer, non-Hodgkin's lymphoma; psoriasis; children with severe polyarticular juvenile rheumatoid arthritis who have failed to respond to other agents

Pregnancy Risk Factor X (psoriasis, rheumatoid arthritis)

Lactation Enters breast milk/contraindicated

Contraindications Hypersensitivity to methotrexate or any component (see Warnings); severe renal or hepatic impairment; pre-existing profound bone marrow suppression; high-dose methotrexate (>1 g/m^2) should not be administered to patients with a creatinine clearance of <50% to 75% of normal; pregnancy; nursing mothers

Warnings The FDA currently recommends that procedures for proper handling and disposal of antineoplastic agents be considered. Due to the possibility of severe toxic reactions, fully inform patient of the risks involved; do not use in women of child-bearing age unless benefit outweighs risks; methotrexate has been reported to cause fetal death and/or congenital anomalies; women of childbearing potential should not be started on methotrexate until pregnancy is excluded. May cause hepatotoxicity, fibrosis and cirrhosis, along with marked bone marrow suppression; death from intestinal perforation may occur. Methotrexate-induced lung disease may occur at any time during therapy with doses as low as 7.5 mg/week. Neurotoxicity manifested as generalized or focal seizures has been reported in pediatric patients with acute lymphoblastic leukemia treated with I.V. methotrexate (1 g/m^2). Symptomatic patients were commonly noted to have leukoencephalopathy and/or microangiopathic calcifications. An acute, neurologic syndrome (confusion, hemiparesis, transient blindness, seizures, coma) has been reported in patients receiving high-dose methotrexate.

Some injections contain benzyl alcohol which may cause allergic reactions in susceptible individuals; large amounts of benzyl alcohol (≥99 mg/kg/day) have been associated with a potentially fatal toxicity ("gasping syndrome") in neonates; the "gasping syndrome" consists of metabolic acidosis, respiratory distress, gasping respirations, CNS dysfunction (including convulsions, intracranial hemorrhage), hypotension and cardiovascular collapse; avoid use of methotrexate products containing benzyl

(Continued)

Methotrexate *(Continued)*

alcohol in neonates; *in vitro* and animal studies have shown that benzoate, a metabolite of benzyl alcohol, displaces bilirubin from protein binding sites. Methotrexate formulations and diluents containing preservatives must not be used for intrathecal or high-dose methotrexate therapy.

Precautions Use with caution in patients with peptic ulcer disease, ulcerative colitis, pre-existing bone marrow suppression; use with caution and reduce dosage in patients with renal or hepatic impairment, ascites, and pleural effusion

Adverse Reactions

Cardiovascular: Vasculitis, pericarditis, hypotension

Central nervous system: Malaise, fatigue, dizziness, encephalopathy, seizures, confusion, fever, headache, chills

I.T.: Acute chemical arachnoiditis (headache, back pain, nuchal rigidity); leukoencephalopathy (confusion, irritability, somnolence, ataxia, dementia, seizures, coma)

Dermatitis: Alopecia, rash, depigmentation or hyperpigmentation of skin, photosensitivity, pruritus, urticaria, Stevens-Johnson syndrome, toxic epidermal necrolysis, exfoliative dermatitis, erythema multiforme

Endocrine & metabolic: Hyperuricemia

Gastrointestinal: Nausea, vomiting, diarrhea, anorexia, stomatitis, enteritis

Genitourinary: Cystitis

Hematologic: Myelosuppression, leukopenia, thrombocytopenia, neutropenia, aplastic anemia, anemia, hemorrhage

Hepatic: Hepatotoxicity, elevated liver enzymes, hyperbilirubinemia; hepatic fibrosis or cirrhosis (in psoriatic patients, hepatotoxicity has occurred after ≥2 years and after a total dose of at least 1.5 g)

Neuromuscular & skeletal: Arthralgia

I.T.: Subacute myelopathy (paraparesis/paraplegia)

Ocular: Blurred vision, conjunctivitis

Renal: Nephropathy (azotemia, hematuria, renal failure)

Respiratory: Interstitial pneumonitis, cough, dyspnea, hypoxemia

Miscellaneous: Anaphylaxis

Drug Interactions Salicylates may delay methotrexate's clearance; sulfonamides, salicylates, phenytoin displace methotrexate from protein binding sites; live virus vaccines (may result in vaccinia infection), pyrimethamine, fluorouracil; NSAIDs increase toxicity of methotrexate by elevating serum methotrexate concentrations (do not use NSAIDs with high-dose methotrexate therapy); penicillins may decrease renal clearance of methotrexate; probenecid decreases the renal elimination of methotrexate; methotrexate may decrease theophylline clearance (monitor theophylline levels)

Food Interactions Milk-rich foods may decrease methotrexate absorption; folate may decrease drug response; folate deficiency states may increase methotrexate toxicity

Stability Protect from light; incompatible with fluorouracil, cytarabine, prednisolone, and sodium phosphate

Mechanism of Action An antimetabolite that binds to dihydrofolate reductase blocking the reduction of dihydrofolate to tetrahydrofolic acid; depletion of tetrahydrofolic acid leads to depletion of DNA precursors and inhibition of DNA and purine synthesis

Pharmacodynamics Approximate time to benefit in treatment of rheumatoid arthritis: 3-6 weeks

Pharmacokinetics

Absorption:

Oral: Average: 30%; variable absorption at low doses (<30 mg/m^2); incomplete absorption after large doses

I.M.: Completely absorbed

Distribution: Small amounts excreted into breast milk; crosses the placenta; does not achieve therapeutic concentrations in the CSF; sustained concentrations are retained in the kidney and liver

Metabolism: In the liver to 7-hydroxymethotrexate

Protein binding: 50% to 60%

Time to peak serum concentration:

Oral: 0.5-4 hours

Parenteral: 0.5-2 hours

Half-life (terminal): Low dose <30 mg/m^2: 3-10 hours; high dose: 8-15 hours

Elimination: Small amounts in feces; primarily excreted unchanged in urine (90%) via glomerular filtration and active secretion by the renal tubule; 1% to 11% of a dose is excreted as the 7-hydroxy metabolite

Usual Dosage Refer to individual protocols:

Children:

Dermatomyositis: Oral: 15-20 mg/m^2/week as a single dose once weekly or 0.3-1 mg/kg/dose once weekly

Juvenile rheumatoid arthritis: Oral, I.M., SubQ: 5-15 mg/m^2/week as a single dose or in 3 divided doses given 12 hours apart; folic acid 1 mg daily or folinic acid ≤5 mg weekly are often used to prevent folate depletion from methotrexate

Antineoplastic dosage range:

Oral, I.M.: 7.5-30 mg/m^2/week or every 2 weeks

I.V.: 10 mg to 33,000 mg/m^2 bolus dosing or continuous infusion over 6-42 hours

Antineoplastic dosing schedules (adapted from Dorr RT and Von Hoff DD, *Cancer Chemotherapy Handbook*, 2nd ed, 1994): See table

Methotrexate Dosing Schedules

	Dose	Route	Frequency
Conventional dose	15-20 mg/m^2	Oral	Twice weekly
	30-50 mg/m^2	Oral, I.V.	Weekly
	15 mg/day for 5 days	Oral, I.M.	Every 2-3 weeks
Intermediate dose	50-150 mg/m^2	I.V. push	Every 2-3 weeks
	240 mg/m^2*	I.V. infusion	Every 4-7 days
	0.5-1 g/m^2*	I.V. infusion	Every 2-3 weeks
High dose	1-12 g/m^2*	I.V. infusion	Every 1-3 weeks

*Followed with leucovorin rescue

Pediatric solid tumors:

<12 years: 12 g/m^2 (dosage range: 12-18 g)

≥12 years: 8 g/m^2 (maximum dose: 18 g)

Meningeal leukemia: I.T.: 10-15 mg/m^2 (maximum: 15 mg) by protocol **or**

≤3 months: 3 mg dose

4-11 months: 6 mg dose

1 year: 8 mg dose

2 years: 10 mg dose

≥3 years: 12 mg dose

I.T. doses are administered at 2- to 5-day intervals until CSF counts return to normal followed by a dose once weekly for 2 weeks then monthly thereafter

ALL (high-dose): I.V.: Loading dose: 200 mg/m^2 followed by a 24-hour infusion of 1200 mg/m^2/day

ANLL: I.V.: 7.5 mg/m^2/day on days 1-5 of treatment course

Resistant ANLL: I.V.: 100 mg/m^2/dose on day 1 of treatment course

Non-Hodgkin's lymphoma: I.V.: 200-500 mg/m^2; repeat every 28 days

Induction of remission in acute lymphoblastic leukemias: Oral: 3.3 mg/m^2/day for 4-6 weeks

Remission maintenance: Oral, I.M.: 20-30 mg/m^2 2 times/week

Adults:

Trophoblastic neoplasms: Oral, I.M.: 15-30 mg/day for 5 days, repeat in 7 days for 3-5 courses

Head and neck cancer: Oral, I.M., I.V.: 25-50 mg/m^2 once weekly

Rheumatoid arthritis: Oral: 7.5 mg once weekly or 2.5 mg every 12 hours for 3 doses/week; not to exceed 20 mg/week

Psoriasis: Oral: 2.5-5 mg/dose every 12 hours for 3 doses given weekly

or

Oral, I.M.: 10-25 mg given once weekly

Dosing adjustment in renal impairment:

Cl_{cr} 61-80 mL/minute: Decrease dose by 25%

Cl_{cr} 51-60 mL/minute: Decrease dose by 33%

Cl_{cr} 10-50 mL/minute: Decrease dose by 50% to 70%

Administration Parenteral:

Methotrexate may be administered I.V. push, I.V. intermittent infusion, or I.V. continuous infusion at a concentration <25 mg/mL; doses >100-300 mg/m^2 are usually administered by I.V. continuous infusion and are followed by a course of leucovorin rescue

For intrathecal use, mix methotrexate without preservatives with NS, Elliotts B solution, or LR to a concentration not greater than 2 mg/mL

Monitoring Parameters CBC with differential and platelet count, creatinine clearance, serum creatinine, BUN, hepatic function tests, serum electrolytes, urinalysis, plasma methotrexate concentrations (see Leucovorin rescue graph> to evaluate plasma methotrexate concentration versus leucovorin rescue dose); periodic liver

(Continued)

Methotrexate *(Continued)*

biopsy for psoriatic patients receiving long-term treatment; chest x-ray; pulmonary function tests if methotrexate-induced lung disease is suspected

Reference Range Serum levels >1 x 10^{-7} mol/L for more than 40 hours are toxic

Patient Information Report to physician any fever, sore throat, black or tarry stools, yellowing of skin or eyes, bleeding or bruising, shortness of breath, painful urination; avoid alcohol. May cause photosensitivity reactions (eg, exposure to sunlight may cause severe sunburn, skin rash, redness, or itching); avoid exposure to sunlight and artificial light sources (sunlamps, tanning booth/bed); wear protective clothing, wide-brimmed hats, sunglasses, and lip sunscreen (SPF ≥15); use a sunscreen [broad-spectrum sunscreen or physical sunscreen (preferred) or sunblock with SPF ≥15]; contact physician if reaction occurs. Pregnancy should be avoided if either partner is receiving methotrexate; effective contraceptive measures must be used; avoid pregnancy for a minimum of 3 months after completion of therapy in male patients and for at least one ovulatory cycle in female patients.

Nursing Implications Intensive hydration should be administered and urine should be alkalinized prior to high doses to enhance methotrexate solubility

Additional Information Myelosuppressive effects:

WBC: Mild
Platelets: Moderate
Onset (days): 7
Nadir (days): 10
Recovery (days): 21

Dosage Forms Excipient information presented when available (limited, particularly for generics); consult specific product labeling.

Injection, powder for reconstitution [preservative free]: 20 mg, 1 g
Injection, solution: 25 mg/mL (2 mL, 10 mL) [contains benzyl alcohol]
Injection, solution [preservative free]: 25 mg/mL (2 mL, 4 mL, 8 mL, 10 mL)
Tablet: 2.5 mg
  Trexall™: 5 mg, 7.5 mg, 10 mg, 15 mg
Tablet, as sodium [dose pack] (Rheumatrex® Dose Pack): 2.5 mg (4 cards with 2, 3, 4, 5, or 6 tablets each)

References

Berg SL, Grisell DL, DeLaney TF, et al, "Principles of Treatment of Pediatric Solid Tumors," *Pediatr Clin North Am*, 1991, 38(2):249-67.
Bleyer WA, "Clinical Pharmacology of Intrathecal Methotrexate II. An Approved Dosage Regimen Derived From Age-Related Pharmacokinetics," *Cancer Treat Rep*, 1977, 61(8):1419-25.
Crom WR, Glynn-Barnhart AM, Rodman JH, et al, "Pharmacokinetics of Anticancer Drugs in Children," *Clin Pharmacokinet*, 1987, 12(3):168-213.
Giannini EH, Brewer EJ, Kuzmina N, et al, "Methotrexate in Resistant Juvenile Rheumatoid Arthritis. Results of the USA-USSR Double-Blind, Placebo-Controlled Trial," *N Engl J Med*, 1992, 326(16):1043-9.
Greaves MW and Weinstein GD, "Treatment of Psoriasis," *N Engl J Med*, 1995, 332(9):581-8.
Rose CD, Singsen BH, and Eichenfield AH, "Safety and Efficacy of Methotrexate Therapy for Juvenile Rheumatoid Arthritis," *J Pediatr*, 1990, 117(4):653-9.

♦ **Methotrexate Sodium** *see* Methotrexate *on page 1027*

Methsuximide (meth SUKS i mide)

Medication Safety Issues

Sound-alike/look-alike issues:
  Methsuximide may be confused with ethosuximide

Related Information

Antiepileptic Drugs *on page 1902*

U.S. Brand Names Celontin®

Canadian Brand Names Celontin®

Therapeutic Category Anticonvulsant, Succinimide

Generic Available No

Use Control of absence (petit mal) seizures; useful adjunct in refractory, partial complex (psychomotor) seizures

Pregnancy Risk Factor C

Contraindications Hypersensitivity to methsuximide, other succinimides, or any component

Warnings Blood dyscrasias (sometimes fatal) have been reported (monitor hematologic function periodically); SLE has been reported with the use of succinimides

Precautions Use with caution in patients with hepatic or renal disease; avoid abrupt withdrawal. Methsuximide may increase tonic clonic seizures in some patients.

Adverse Reactions

Central nervous system: Dizziness, drowsiness, lethargy, euphoria, nervousness, hallucinations, insomnia, mental confusion, headache, ataxia
Dermatologic: Rash, urticaria, Stevens-Johnson syndrome
Gastrointestinal: Nausea, vomiting, anorexia, diarrhea, abdominal pain

Genitourinary: Microscopic hematuria, proteinuria
Hematologic: Leukopenia, thrombocytopenia, eosinophilia, pancytopenia, monocytosis
Ocular: Periorbital edema
Miscellaneous: Hiccups

Drug Interactions Methsuximide may increase phenytoin and phenobarbital serum concentrations (monitor serum levels)

Stability Store at room temperature; protect from light, moisture, and heat; **Note:** Methsuximide has a relatively low melting temperature (124°F); do not store in conditions that promote high temperatures (eg, in a closed vehicle)

Mechanism of Action Increases the seizure threshold and suppresses paroxysmal spike-and-wave pattern in absence seizures; depresses nerve transmission in the motor cortex

Pharmacokinetics
Metabolism: Rapidly demethylated in the liver to N-desmethylmethsuximide (active metabolite)
Half-life: 2-4 hours
N-desmethylmethsuximide:
Children: 26 hours
Adults: 28-80 hours
Time to peak serum concentration: Within 1-3 hours
Elimination: <1% in urine as unchanged drug

Usual Dosage Oral:
Children: Initial: 10-15 mg/kg/day in 3-4 divided doses; increase weekly up to maximum of 30 mg/kg/day; mean dose required:
<30 kg: 20 mg/kg/day
>30 kg: 14 mg/kg/day
Adults: 300 mg/day for the first week; may increase by 300 mg/day at weekly intervals up to 1.2 g in 2-4 divided doses/day

Administration Oral: Administer with food

Monitoring Parameters CBC with differential, liver enzymes, urinalysis; measure trough serum levels for efficacy and 3-hour postdose concentrations for toxicity

Reference Range Measure N-desmethylmethsuximide concentrations:
Therapeutic: 10-40 mcg/mL (SI: 53-212 micromoles/L)
Toxic: >40 mcg/mL (SI: >212 micromoles/L)

Patient Information May cause drowsiness and impair ability to perform activities requiring mental alertness or physical coordination; do not discontinue abruptly; notify physician if sore throat or fever develop; do not store capsules in conditions that promote high temperatures (eg, in closed cars or other vehicles), as medication may melt

Dosage Forms Excipient information presented when available (limited, particularly for generics); consult specific product labeling.
Capsule: 150 mg, 300 mg

References

Miles MV, Tennison MB, and Greenwood RS, "Pharmacokinetics of N-desmethylmethsuximide in Pediatric Patients," *J Pediatr*, 1989, 114(4 Pt 1):647-50.

Tennison MB, Greenwood RS, Miles MV, "Methsuximide for Intractable Childhood Seizures," *Pediatrics*, 1991, 87(2):186-9.

♦ **Methylacetoxyprogesterone** *see* MedroxyPROGESTERone *on page 991*

Methyldopa (meth il DOE pa)

Medication Safety Issues
Sound-alike/look-alike issues:
Methyldopa may be confused with L-dopa, levodopa

Related Information
Antihypertensive Agents by Class *on page 1678*

Canadian Brand Names Apo-Methyldopa®; Nu-Medopa

Index Terms Aldomet; Methyldopate Hydrochloride

Therapeutic Category Alpha-Adrenergic Inhibitors, Central; Antihypertensive Agent

Generic Available Yes

Use Management of moderate to severe hypertension

Pregnancy Risk Factor B

Lactation Enters breast milk/compatible

Contraindications Hypersensitivity to methyldopa or any component (see Warnings); liver disease, pheochromocytoma

Warnings Injection contains sodium bisulfite which may cause allergic reactions in susceptible individuals

Precautions Use with caution and adjust dose in patients with renal dysfunction; active metabolite may accumulate in uremia
(Continued)

Methyldopa *(Continued)*

Adverse Reactions

Cardiovascular: Orthostatic hypotension, bradycardia, edema

Central nervous system: Drowsiness, sedation, vertigo, headache, depression, memory lapse, fever

Dermatologic: Rash

Endocrine & metabolic: Gynecomastia, sexual dysfunction, sodium retention

Gastrointestinal: Nausea, vomiting, diarrhea, xerostomia, "black" tongue

Genitourinary: Discoloration of urine (red or brown)

Hematologic: Hemolytic anemia, positive Coombs' test, leukopenia

Hepatic: Hepatitis, elevated liver enzymes, jaundice, cirrhosis

Neuromuscular & skeletal: Weakness

Respiratory: Nasal congestion

Drug Interactions May increase lithium toxicity; concomitant oral administration of iron salts may decrease oral absorption of methyldopa and result in an increase in blood pressure, spacing drugs 2 hours apart may decrease this effect

Food Interactions Avoid natural licorice (causes sodium and water retention and increases potassium loss); dietary requirements for vitamin B_{12} and folate may be increased with high doses of methyldopa

Mechanism of Action Stimulates inhibitory alpha-adrenergic receptors via alpha-methylnorepinephrine (false transmitter); this results in a decreased sympathetic outflow to the heart, kidneys, and peripheral vasculature; may decrease plasma renin activity

Pharmacodynamics Hypotensive effects:

Maximum effect: Oral, I.V.: Single-dose: Within 3-6 hours; multiple-dose: 2-3 days

Duration:

Oral: Single-dose: 12-24 hours; multiple-dose: 1-2 days

I.V.: 10-16 hours

Pharmacokinetics

Absorption: Oral: ~50%

Distribution: Crosses placenta; appears in breast milk

Protein binding: <15%

Metabolism: In the intestine and the liver

Half-life: Elimination:

Neonates: 10-20 hours

Adults: 1-3 hours

Elimination: ~70% of systemic dose eliminated in urine as drug and metabolites

Dialysis: Slightly dialyzable (5% to 20%)

Usual Dosage

Children:

Oral: Initial: 10 mg/kg/day in 2-4 divided doses; increase every 2 days as needed to maximum dose of 65 mg/kg/day; do not exceed 3 g/day

I.V.: Initial: 2-4 mg/kg/dose; if response is not seen within 4-6 hours, may increase to 5-10 mg/kg/dose; administer doses every 6-8 hours; maximum daily dose: 65 mg/kg or 3 g, whichever is less

Adults:

Oral: Initial: 250 mg 2-3 times/day; increase every 2 days as needed; usual dose 500 mg to 2 g daily in 2-4 divided doses; maximum dose: 3 g/day; usual dosage range (JNC 7): 250-1000 mg/day in 2 divided doses

I.V.: 250-1000 mg every 6-8 hours; maximum dose: 4 g/day

Dosing interval in renal impairment: Children and Adults:

Cl_{cr} >50 mL/minute: Administer normal dose every 8 hours

Cl_{cr} 10-50 mL/minute: Administer normal dose every 8-12 hours

Cl_{cr} <10 mL/minute: Administer normal dose every 12-24 hours

Administration

Oral: May be administered without regard to food; administer new dosage increases in the evening to minimize sedation

Parenteral: I.V.: Infuse I.V. dose slowly over 30-60 minutes at a concentration ≤10 mg/mL

Monitoring Parameters Blood pressure, CBC with differential, hemoglobin, hematocrit, Coombs' test [direct], liver enzymes

Test Interactions Urinary uric acid, serum creatinine (alkaline picrate method), AST (colorimetric method), and urinary catecholamines (falsely high levels)

Patient Information Avoid alcohol; may cause drowsiness and impair ability to perform activities requiring mental alertness or physical coordination; may cause dry mouth; rise slowly from prolonged sitting or lying position; may cause urine to turn red or brown; notify physician of unexplained prolonged general tiredness, fever, or jaundice

Nursing Implications Transient sedation or depression may occur for first 72 hours of therapy, or when doses are increased

Additional Information Most effective if used with diuretic; titrate dose to optimal blood pressure control with minimal side effects

Dosage Forms Excipient information presented when available (limited, particularly for generics); consult specific product labeling.

Injection, solution, as methyldopate hydrochloride: 50 mg/mL (5 mL) [contains sodium bisulfite]

Tablet: 250 mg, 500 mg

Extemporaneous Preparations A 50 mg/mL oral liquid preparation made from tablets and 2 different vehicles [unpreserved simple syrup (Syrup, USP) and a 1:1 mixture of simple syrup (containing 0.5% citric acid) and hydrochloric acid 0.2 N] was stable for 14 days when stored in glass prescription bottles in the dark, at room temperature (25°C) or under refrigeration (5°C); grind ten 250 mg tablets in a glass mortar into a fine powder. To make formulation with unpreserved simple syrup (Syrup, USP), levigate with Syrup, USP to form a uniform paste; add a small amount of Syrup, USP; mix well; transfer to a calibrated bottle; rinse the mortar and pestle several times with vehicle; transfer to calibrated bottle and qsad to 50 mL. To make formulation with second vehicle, levigate powdered tablets with 25 mL of hydrochloric acid 0.2 N (0.73% w/v); dilute this mixture to 50 mL with simple syrup containing 0.5% citric acid by the method described above. Label "shake well" and "protect from light."

Newton DW, Rogers AG, Becker CH, et al, "Extemporaneous Preparation of Methyldopa in Two Syrup Vehicles," *Am J Hosp Pharm*, 1975, 32(8):817-21.

References

Chobanian AV, Bakris GL, Black HR, et al, "The Seventh Report of the Joint National Committee on Prevention, Detection, Evaluation, and Treatment of High Blood Pressure: The JNC 7 report," *JAMA*, 2003, 289(19):2560-72.

♦ **Methyldopate Hydrochloride** *see* Methyldopa *on page 1031*

Methylene Blue (METH i leen bloo)

Medication Safety Issues Due to potential toxicity (hemolytic anemia), do not use methylene blue to color enteral feedings to detect aspiration.

U.S. Brand Names Urolene Blue®

Therapeutic Category Antidote, Cyanide; Antidote, Drug-induced Methemoglobinemia

Generic Available Yes: Injection

Use Antidote for cyanide poisoning and drug-induced methemoglobinemia, indicator dye, bacteriostatic genitourinary antiseptic

Pregnancy Risk Factor C (D if injected intra-amniotically)

Contraindications Hypersensitivity to methylene blue or any component; renal insufficiency

Warnings Do not inject subcutaneously or intrathecally as necrotic abscesses (SubQ) and neural damage (I.T.) including paraplegia have occurred

Precautions Use with caution in patients with G-6-PD deficiency; continued use can cause profound anemia

Adverse Reactions

Cardiovascular: Hypertension, cyanosis, large I.V. doses have been associated with precordial pain

Central nervous system: Dizziness, mental confusion, headache, fever

Dermatologic: Stains skin

Gastrointestinal: Nausea, vomiting, abdominal pain, diarrhea, discoloration of feces (blue-green)

Genitourinary: Bladder irritation, discoloration of urine (blue-green)

Hematologic: Formation of methemoglobin

Miscellaneous: Diaphoresis

Mechanism of Action Weak germicide; in low concentrations hastens the conversion of methemoglobin to hemoglobin; has opposite effect at high concentrations by converting ferrous iron of reduced hemoglobin to ferric iron to form methemoglobin; in cyanide toxicity, it combines with cyanide to form cyanmethemoglobin preventing the interference of cyanide with the cytochrome system

Pharmacokinetics

Absorption: Well absorbed from GI tract

Elimination: In bile, feces, and urine

Usual Dosage

Methemoglobinemia: Children and Adults: I.V.: 1-2 mg/kg or 25-50 mg/m^2; may be repeated after 1 hour if necessary

Chronic methemoglobinemia: Adults: Oral: 100-300 mg/day

NADPH-methemoglobin reductase deficiency: Children: Oral: 1-1.5 mg/kg/day (maximum dose: 300 mg/day) given with 5-8 mg/kg/day ascorbic acid

Genitourinary antiseptic: Adults: Oral: 65-130 mg 3 times/day; maximum dose: 390 mg/day

(Continued)

Methylene Blue *(Continued)*

Chronic urolithiasis: Adults: Oral: 65 mg 3 times/day

Administration

Parenteral: Administer undiluted by direct I.V. injection over several minutes

Oral: Administer after meals with a full glass of water

Patient Information May discolor urine and feces blue-green; may discolor skin on contact

Additional Information Has been used topically (0.1% solutions) in conjunction with polychromatic light to photoinactivate viruses such as herpes simplex (this is an unlabeled indication); has been used alone or in combination with vitamin C for the management of chronic urolithiasis; skin stains may be removed using a hypochlorite solution

Dosage Forms Excipient information presented when available (limited, particularly for generics); consult specific product labeling.

Injection, solution: 10 mg/mL (1 mL, 10 mL)

Tablet:

Urolene Blue®: 65 mg

♦ **Methylin®** *see* Methylphenidate *on page 1034*

♦ **Methylin® ER** *see* Methylphenidate *on page 1034*

♦ **Methylmorphine** *see* Codeine *on page 397*

Methylphenidate (meth il FEN i date)

Medication Safety Issues

Sound-alike/look-alike issues:

Methylphenidate may be confused with methadone

Ritalin® may be confused with Ismelin®, Rifadin®

U.S. Brand Names Concerta®; Daytrana™; Metadate® CD; Metadate® ER; Methylin®; Methylin® ER; Ritalin®; Ritalin® LA; Ritalin-SR®

Canadian Brand Names Apo-Methylphenidate®; Apo-Methylphenidate® SR; Biphentin®; Concerta®; PMS-Methylphenidate; Riphenidate; Ritalin®; Ritalin® SR

Index Terms Methylphenidate Hydrochloride

Therapeutic Category Central Nervous System Stimulant, Nonamphetamine

Generic Available Yes: Immediate release tablet, extended release 20 mg tablet

Use Attention-deficit/hyperactivity disorder (ADHD); narcolepsy

Restrictions C-II

Medication Guide An FDA-approved patient medication guide, which is available with the product information and at http://www.fda.gov/cder/drug/infopage/ADHD/default.htm, must be dispensed with this medication for each new outpatient prescription and refill.

Pregnancy Risk Factor C

Lactation Enters breast milk/use caution

Contraindications Hypersensitivity to methylphenidate or any component; glaucoma; motor tics; Tourette's syndrome (diagnosis or family history); patients with marked agitation, tension, and anxiety; use of MAO inhibitors within 14 days (hypertensive crisis may occur)

Metadate® CD is also contraindicated in patients with severe hypertension, heart failure, arrhythmia, hyperthyroidism, recent MI, or angina.

Warnings Serious cardiovascular events including sudden death may occur in patients with pre-existing structural cardiac abnormalities or other serious heart problems. Sudden death has been reported in children and adolescents; sudden death, stroke, and MI have been reported in adults. Avoid the use of amphetamines in patients with known serious structural cardiac abnormalities, cardiomyopathy, serious heart rhythm abnormalities, coronary artery disease, or other serious cardiac problems that could place patients at an increased risk to the sympathomimetic effects of amphetamines. Patients should be carefully evaluated for cardiac disease prior to initiation of therapy. EKG abnormalities and 4 cases of sudden cardiac death have been reported in children receiving clonidine with methylphenidate; reduce dose of methylphenidate by 40% when used concurrently with clonidine; consider EKG monitoring.

Stimulant medications may increase blood pressure (average increase 2-4 mm Hg) and heart rate (average increase 3-6 bpm); some patients may experience greater increases; use stimulant medications with caution in patients with hypertension and other cardiovascular conditions that may be exacerbated by increases in blood pressure or heart rate. Psychiatric adverse events may occur. Stimulants may exacerbate symptoms of behavior disturbance and thought disorder in patients with pre-existing psychosis. New-onset psychosis or mania may occur with stimulant use. May induce mixed/manic episode in patients with bipolar disorder. May be associated with aggressive behavior or hostility (monitor for development or worsening of these behaviors).

Safety and efficacy have not been established in children <6 years of age (use is **not** recommended in children <6 years of age). Long-term effects in pediatric patients have not been determined. Use of stimulants in children has been associated with growth suppression (monitor growth; treatment interruption may be needed). Appetite suppression may occur; monitor weight during therapy, particularly in children. Stimulants may lower seizure threshold leading to new onset or breakthrough seizure activity (use with caution in patients with a history of seizure disorder). Visual disturbances (difficulty in accommodation and blurred vision) have been reported.

Amphetamines possess a high potential for abuse; misuse may cause sudden death and serious cardiovascular adverse events; prolonged administration may lead to drug dependence; abrupt discontinuation following high doses or for prolonged periods may result in symptoms of withdrawal; use with caution in patients with history of ethanol or drug abuse. Do not use for severe depression or normal fatigue states.

A potential for GI obstruction exists with Concerta® (tablet is nondeformable); do not ordinarily use in patients with severe GI narrowing (eg, esophageal motility disorders, small bowel inflammatory disease, short gut syndrome, history of cystic fibrosis, peritonitis, chronic intestinal pseudo-obstruction, or Meckel's diverticulum). Transdermal system may cause allergic contact sensitization, characterized by intense local reactions (edema, vesicles, papules); remove patch and monitor application site if reaction occurs; seek further evaluation if erythema, edema, and/or papules do not significantly decrease or resolve within 24 hours of patch removal. Allergic sensitization may subsequently manifest systemically when methylphenidate is administered orally or via other routes; systemic sensitization reactions may include dermatitis, generalized skin eruptions, headache, fever, vomiting, diarrhea, arthralgia, or malaise; initiate oral methylphenidate under close medical supervision in patients who have experienced a contact sensitization to the transdermal system; some of these patients may **not** be able to take methylphenidate in any dosage form. Do not expose transdermal application site to direct external heat sources (eg, electric blankets, heating pads, heated water beds); a >2-fold increase in drug release may occur.

Precautions Use with caution in patients with heart failure, recent MI, hyperthyroidism, seizures, acute stress reactions, emotional instability; hematological monitoring is advised with long term use (see Monitoring Parameters)

Chewable tablets contain aspartame which is metabolized to phenylalanine and must be avoided (or used with caution) in patients with phenylketonuria. Chewable tablets must be taken with adequate amount of liquid, otherwise tablet may swell and block the throat or esophagus and cause choking; do not use chewable tablets in patients who have difficulty swallowing; instruct patients to seek immediate medical attention if chest pain, vomiting, difficulty in breathing or swallowing occur after taking chewable tablet.

Adverse Reactions

Cardiovascular: Tachycardia, hypertension, hypotension, palpitations, angina, cardiac arrhythmias; cerebral arteritis, cerebral occlusion (case reports); serious cardiovascular events including sudden death in patients with pre-existing structural cardiac abnormalities or other serious heart problems (see Warnings)

Central nervous system: Nervousness, insomnia, irritability, aggression, emotional lability, dizziness, drowsiness, movement disorders, motor tics, precipitation of Tourette's syndrome; fever, headache, toxic psychosis (rare); neuroleptic malignant syndrome (very rare and usually in patients receiving medications associated with the syndrome; one case with concurrent first dose of venlafaxine has been reported); transient depression

Dermatologic: Rash, urticaria, exfoliative dermatitis, erythema multiforme, necrotizing vasculitis, scalp hair loss

Endocrine & metabolic: Growth suppression, weight loss

Gastrointestinal: Anorexia, nausea, vomiting, abdominal pain, diarrhea, potential for GI obstruction with Concerta® (see Warnings)

Hematologic: Thrombocytopenia, anemia, leukopenia, thrombocytopenic purpura

Hepatic: Abnormal liver function, elevated transaminases, hepatic coma

Local: Transdermal system: Application site reactions, erythema, itching; papules, edema, vesicles (allergic contact dermatitis)

Neuromuscular & skeletal: Arthralgia, dyskinesia

Ocular: Visual disturbances, blurred vision, problems with accommodation

Miscellaneous: Hypersensitivity reactions; physical and psychological dependence

Drug Interactions Use with clonidine may potentially increase EKG effects (see Warnings). Methylphenidate increases serum concentrations of tricyclic antidepressants, selective serotonin reuptake inhibitors, phenylbutazone, warfarin, phenytoin, phenobarbital and primidone (a decrease in the dose of these agents may be

(Continued)

Methylphenidate *(Continued)*

required, monitor closely). Use of MAO inhibitors within 14 days may result in hypertensive crisis; use of MAOI within 14 days of methylphenidate is contraindicated. The herbal medicine St John's wort (*Hypericum perforatum*) may increase serious side effects; its use is **not** recommended. Effects of guanethidine, other antihypertensive agents, bretylium may be antagonized by methylphenidate. Use with vasopressor agents may further increase blood pressure (use with caution).

Food Interactions Food may increase oral absorption

Concerta®: A high fat meal does not alter pharmacokinetics or pharmacodynamics; no evidence of dose dumping occurs when administered with or without food

Metadate® CD: Food delays the early peak by ~1 hour; a high fat meal increases peak concentrations by 30% and AUC by 17%; one adult study showed no difference in bioavailability when Metadate® CD capsules were opened and contents sprinkled onto 1 tablespoon of applesauce (compared to fasting conditions; see Pentikin, 2002).

Methylin®:

Chewable tablets: A high fat meal delays peak concentrations by ~1 hour, but increases AUC by ~20% (**Note:** Magnitude of food effect is similar to immediate release tablets).

Oral solution: A high fat meal delays peak concentrations by ~1 hour, but increases peak by ~13% and AUC by ~25% (**Note:** Increase in peak concentration and AUC are similar to immediate release tablets).

Ritalin® LA: Compared to fasting, food does not affect the first peak concentration, extent of absorption, or time to second peak concentration; however, the second peak was 25% lower. A high fat meal delays absorption. Compared to fasting, no differences in pharmacokinetics occurred when Ritalin® LA capsules were administered with applesauce. No evidence of dose dumping occurs when administered with or without food.

Stability Store at room temperature; dispense oral formulations in tight, light-resistant container; **Note:** Metadate® CD should be dispensed in the original dose pack of 30 capsules

Methylin® chewable tablets, Methylin® ER, Ritalin-SR®: Protect from moisture

Concerta®: Protect from humidity

Transdermal system: Keep patches stored in protective pouch; use patches within 2 months after tray is opened

Mechanism of Action Produces stimulant effect by activating the brain stem arousal system and cerebral cortex; blocks the reuptake of norepinephrine and dopamine into presynaptic neurons, thus increasing the concentrations of these neurotransmitters in the extraneuronal space.

Pharmacodynamics Cerebral stimulation:

Maximum effect:

Immediate release tablet: Within 2 hours

Sustained release tablet: Within 4-7 hours

Duration (AAP, 2001):

Immediate release tablet (short-acting): Methylin®, Ritalin®: 3-5 hours

Sustained release, extended release (intermediate-acting): Metadate® ER, Methylin® ER, Ritalin-SR®: 3-8 hours

Extended release (long-acting): Concerta®, Metadate® CD, Ritalin® LA: 8-12 hours

Pharmacokinetics

Absorption: Oral:

Immediate release products: Readily absorbed

Transdermal: Absorption is increased when applied to inflamed skin or exposed to heat; transdermal absorption may increase with chronic therapy

Protein binding: 15%

Metabolism: In the liver via hydroxylation (de-esterification) to ritalinic acid (alpha-phenyl-2-piperidine acetic acid), which has little or no pharmacologic activity

Bioavailability: Chewable tablets and oral solution are bioequivalent to immediate release tablets. **Note:** A much lower first pass effect occurs with transdermal (vs oral) administration; thus, much lower doses (on a mg/kg basis) given via the transdermal route may still produce higher AUCs, compared to the oral route.

Half-life: 2-4 hours

Time to peak serum concentration:

Chewable tablets, oral solution: 1-2 hours

Extended release tablet (Concerta®): 6-10 hours

Elimination: 90% of dose is eliminated in the urine as metabolites and unchanged drug; main urinary metabolite (ritalinic acid) accounts for 80% of the dose; drug is also excreted in feces via bile

Usual Dosage Note: Discontinue medication if no improvement is seen after appropriate dosage adjustment over a one-month period of time:

Oral:

Immediate release product (Methylin®, Ritalin®):

Children ≥6 years: ADHD: Initial: 0.3 mg/kg/dose or 2.5-5 mg/dose given before breakfast and lunch; increase by 0.1 mg/kg/dose or by 5-10 mg/day at weekly intervals; usual dose: 0.3-1 mg/kg/day; maximum dose: 2 mg/kg/day or 60 mg/day; specific patients may require 3 doses/day (ie, additional dose at 4 PM)

Adults: Narcolepsy: 10 mg 2-3 times/day; maximum dose: 60 mg/day

Metadate® ER, Methylin® ER, Ritalin-SR®: Children ≥6 years and Adults: Sustained release and extended release tablets (duration of action ~8 hours) may be given in place of regular tablets, once the daily dose is titrated using the regular tablets and the titrated 8-hour dosage corresponds to sustained release tablet size

Concerta®: Children ≥6 years and Adults:

Initial: Methylphenidate naive patients: 18 mg once daily

Switching from methylphenidate immediate release 5 mg 2-3 times/day: Concerta® 18 mg once daily

Switching from methylphenidate immediate release 10 mg 2-3 times/day: Concerta® 36 mg once daily

Switching from methylphenidate immediate release 15 mg 2-3 times/day: Concerta® 54 mg once daily

Dosage adjustment: May increase by 18 mg/day increments at weekly intervals

Maximum dose:

Children 6-12 years: 54 mg/day

Adolescent and Adults: 72 mg/day; do not exceed 2 mg/kg/day

Metadate® CD: Children ≥6 years and Adults: Initial: 20 mg once daily; may increase by 20 mg/day increments at weekly intervals; maximum dose: 60 mg once daily

Ritalin® LA: Children ≥6 years and Adults:

Methylphenidate naive patients: Initial: 20 mg once daily; may increase by 10 mg/day increments at weekly intervals; maximum dose: 60 mg once daily; **Note:** If a lower initial dose is desired, patients may begin with Ritalin® LA 10 mg once daily. Alternatively, patients may begin therapy with an immediate release product, and switch to Ritalin® LA once immediate release dosage is titrated to 5 mg twice daily (see below)

Patients currently receiving methylphenidate: Initial dose: See table; may increase by 10 mg/day increments at weekly intervals; maximum dose: 60 mg once daily

Recommended Ritalin® LA Dose for Patients Receiving Methylphenidate

Previous Methylphenidate Dose	Recommended Ritalin® LA Dose
5 mg methylphenidate twice daily	10 mg once daily
10 mg methylphenidate twice daily or 20 mg methylphenidate sustained release	20 mg once daily
15 mg methylphenidate twice daily	30 mg once daily
20 mg methylphenidate twice daily or 40 mg methylphenidate sustained release	40 mg once daily
30 mg methylphenidate twice daily or 60 mg methylphenidate sustained release	60 mg once daily

Transdermal (Daytrana™): Children 6-12 years: Initial: 10 mg patch once daily; apply to hip 2 hours before effect is needed and remove 9 hours after application (see Administration); titrate dose based on response and tolerability; may increase to next transdermal patch dosage size no more frequently than every week. **Note:** Doses >20 mg/9 hours do not appear to provide additional benefit. Patch may be removed before 9 hours if a shorter duration of action is required or if late day adverse effects appear. Plasma concentrations usually start to decline when the patch is removed but drug absorption may continue for several hours after patch removal.

Administration

Oral: Immediate and sustained release tablets: Administer on an empty stomach ~30-45 minutes before meals; do not crush, chew, or break sustained or extended release dosage form, swallow whole; to avoid insomnia, last daily dose should be administered several hours before retiring.

Concerta®: May be administered without regard to food, but must be taken with water, milk, or juice; administer dose once daily in the morning; do not crush, chew, or divide tablets

Metadate® CD: Administer dose once daily in the morning, before breakfast, with water, milk, or juice; capsule may be swallowed whole or opened and contents

(Continued)

Methylphenidate *(Continued)*

sprinkled on a small amount (one tablespoonful) of applesauce; immediately consume drug/applesauce mixture; do not store for future use; drink fluids after consuming drug/applesauce mixture to ensure complete swallowing of beads; do not crush, chew, or divide capsules or its contents

Methylin® chewable tablet: Children and Adults: Administer with at least 8 ounces of water or other fluid (choking may occur if not enough fluids are taken; see Precautions)

Ritalin® LA: Administer dose once daily in the morning; may be administered with or without food (but some food may delay absorption); capsule may be swallowed whole or may be opened and contents sprinkled on a small amount (one spoonful) of applesauce (**Note:** Applesauce should not be warm); immediately consume drug/applesauce mixture; do not store for future use; do not crush, chew, or divide capsule or its contents

Topical: Transdermal (Daytrana™): Apply patch immediately after opening pouch and removing protective liner; do not use patch if pouch seal is broken; do not use patches that are cut or damaged. Apply to clean, dry, healthy skin on the hip; do not apply to oily, damaged, or irritated skin; do not apply to the waistline. Apply at the same time each day, 2 hours before effect is needed. Alternate site of application daily (ie, use alternate hip). Press patch firmly for 30 seconds to ensure proper adherence. Remove patch 9 hours after application. Patch may be removed earlier if a shorter duration of action is required or if late day adverse effects occur.

Avoid exposure of application site to external heat source (eg, electric blankets, heating pads, heated water beds), which may significantly increase the amount of drug absorbed. If patch should become dislodged, may replace with new patch (to different site) but total wear time should not exceed 9 hours. If adhesive residue remains on child's skin after patch removal, use oil or lotion and gently rub area to remove adhesive. Avoid touching the sticky side of the patch. Wash hands with soap and water after handling.

Dispose of used patch by folding adhesive side onto itself, and discard in toilet or appropriate lidded container; discard unused patches that are no longer needed in the same manner; protective pouch and liner should be discarded in an appropriate lidded container. **Note:** Used patches contain residual drug; keep all transdermal patches out of the reach of children.

Monitoring Parameters Evaluate patients for cardiac disease (see Warnings) prior to starting therapy; obtain careful history, family history and physical exam; perform EKG and echocardiogram if findings suggest cardiac disease; promptly conduct cardiac evaluation in patients who develop chest pain, unexplained syncope, or any other symptom of cardiac disease during treatment. Monitor CBC with differential, platelet count, blood pressure, heart rate, height, weight, appetite. Transdermal system: Also monitor the application site for local adverse reactions and allergic contact sensitization (see Warnings).

Patient Information Read the patient Medication Guide that you receive with each prescription and refill of methylphenidate. Serious cardiac effects or psychiatric adverse effects may occur; notify your physician of any heart problems, high blood pressure, or psychiatric conditions before starting therapy. May reduce the growth rate in children and has been associated with worsening of aggressive behavior; notify your physician if your child displays aggression or hostility; make sure your physician monitors your child's weight and height. Avoid caffeine and the herbal medicine St John's wort. May be habit-forming; avoid abrupt discontinuation after prolonged use. May cause dizziness or drowsiness and impair ability to perform activities requiring mental alertness or physical coordination. Notify physician if blurred vision occurs. Intact Concerta® tablet shell may appear in stool (this is normal). Report the use of other medications and herbal or natural products to your physician and pharmacist. Seek immediate medical attention if chest pain, vomiting, or difficulty in breathing or swallowing occur after taking chewable tablet. When using transdermal patches, avoid exposing application site to external heat sources (eg, electric blankets, heating pads, heated water bed); patches may be irritating to the skin; inform physician if skin rash or irritation occurs; do not use patch if swelling or blistering occurs; see Administration for details of patch application

Additional Information Methylphenidate is a racemic mixture of d- and l-enantiomers; the d-enantiomer is more active than the l-enantiomer. Treatment with methylphenidate should include "drug holidays" or periodic discontinuation in order to assess the patient's requirements, decrease tolerance and limit suppression of linear growth and weight. Concerta®, Metadate® CD, and Ritalin® LA are formulated to deliver methylphenidate in a biphasic release profile; Concerta® is an osmotic controlled release formulation, with an immediate release (within 1 hour) outer coating; once daily Concerta® has been shown to be as effective as immediate release methylphenidate tablets administered 3 times/day (see Pelham, 2001). Metadate® CD capsules contain both immediate release beads (30% of the dose) and extended release beads (70% of the dose). Ritalin® LA capsules contain both immediate release beads (50% of the dose) and enteric coated, delayed release beads (50% of the dose). Methylin®, Methylin® ER, and Ritalin-SR® tablets are color and additive free; Methylin® oral solution is colorless. Concerta® tablets may be seen on abdominal x-ray under certain conditions (eg, when digital enhancing techniques are used).

Daytrana™ Transdermal System consists of an adhesive-based matrix containing active drug which is dispersed in acrylic adhesive that is dispersed in a silicone adhesive. The patch consists of 3 layers: A polyester/ethylene vinyl acetate laminate (outside) film backing, the adhesive layer containing methylphenidate, and a flouropolymer-coated polyester protective liner (which must be removed before application). Long-term use of the transdermal system (ie, >7 weeks) has not been studied; long-term usefulness should be periodically re-evaluated for the individual patient.

Dosage Forms Excipient information presented when available (limited, particularly for generics); consult specific product labeling.

Capsule, extended release, as hydrochloride:
- Metadate® CD: 10 mg, 20 mg, 30 mg, 40 mg, 50 mg, 60 mg
- Ritalin® LA: 10 mg, 20 mg, 30 mg, 40 mg

Solution, oral, as hydrochloride:
- Methylin®: 5 mg/5 mL (500 mL) [grape flavor]; 10 mg/5 mL (500 mL) [grape flavor]

Tablet, as hydrochloride: 5 mg, 10 mg, 20 mg
- Methylin®, Ritalin®: 5 mg, 10 mg, 20 mg

Tablet, chewable, as hydrochloride:
- Methylin®: 2.5 mg [contains phenylalanine 0.42 mg; grape flavor]; 5 mg [contains phenylalanine 0.84 mg; grape flavor]; 10 mg [contains phenylalanine 1.68 mg; grape flavor]

Tablet, extended release, as hydrochloride: 20 mg
- Concerta®: 18 mg, 27 mg, 36 mg, 54 mg [osmotic controlled release]
- Metadate® ER, Methylin® ER: 10 mg, 20 mg

Tablet, sustained release, as hydrochloride:
- Ritalin-SR®: 20 mg [dye free]

Transdermal system [once-daily patch]:
- Daytrana™: 10 mg/9 hours (10s, 30s) [12.5 cm^2, total methylphenidate 27.5 mg]; 15 mg/9 hours (10s, 30s) [18.75 cm^2, total methylphenidate 41.3 mg]; 20 mg/9 hours (10s, 30s) [25 cm^2, total methylphenidate 55 mg]; 30 mg/9 hours (10s, 30s) [37.5 cm^2, total methylphenidate 82.5 mg]

References

American Academy of Pediatrics. Subcommittee on Attention-Deficit/Hyperactivity Disorder, "Clinical Practice Guideline: Treatment of the School-Aged Child With Attention-Deficit/Hyperactivity Disorder," *Pediatrics*, 2001, 108(4):1033-44.

Greenhill LL, "Pharmacologic Treatment of Attention Deficit Hyperactivity Disorder," *Psychiatr Clin North Am*, 1992, 15(1):1-27.

Greenhill LL, Pliszka S, Dulcan MK, et al, "Practice Parameter for the Use of Stimulant Medications in the Treatment of Children, Adolescents, and Adults," *J Am Acad Child Adolesc Psychiatry*, 2002, 41(2 Suppl):26S-49S.

Kelly DP and Aylward GP, "Attention Deficits in School-Aged Children and Adolescents," *Pediatr Clin North Am*, 1992, 39(3):487-512.

Pelham WE, Gnagy EM, Burrows-Maclean L, et al, "Once-a-Day Concerta Methylphenidate Versus Three-Times-Daily Methylphenidate in Laboratory and Natural Settings," *Pediatrics*, 2001, 107(6), http://www.pediatrics.org/cgi/content/full/107/6/e105.

Pentikis HS, Simmons RD, Benedict MF, et al, "Methylphenidate Bioavailability in Adults When an Extended-Release Multiparticulate Formulation is Administered Sprinkled on Food or as an Intact Capsule," *J Am Acad Child Adolesc Psychiatry*, 2002, 41(4):443-9.

Wilens TE and Biederman J, "The Stimulants," *Psychiatr Clin North Am*, 1992, 15(1):191-222.

♦ **Methylphenidate Hydrochloride** *see* Methylphenidate *on page 1034*
♦ **Methylphenobarbital** *see* Mephobarbital *on page 1004*
♦ **Methylphenoxy-Benzene Propanamine** *see* Atomoxetine *on page 172*
♦ **Methylphenyl Isoxazolyl Penicillin** *see* Oxacillin *on page 1178*
♦ **Methylphytyl Napthoquinone** *see* Phytonadione *on page 1258*

MethylPREDNISolone (meth il pred NIS oh lone)

Medication Safety Issues

Sound-alike/look-alike issues:
- MethylPREDNISolone may be confused with medroxyPROGESTERone, predniSONE
- Depo-Medrol® may be confused with Solu-Medrol®
- Medrol® may be confused with Mebaral®
- Solu-Medrol® may be confused with Depo-Medrol®

International issues:
- Medor® may be confused with Medral® which is a brand name for omeprazole in Mexico

(Continued)

MethylPREDNISolone *(Continued)*

Related Information

Asthma *on page 1904*

Corticosteroids, Systemic *on page 1685*

U.S. Brand Names Depo-Medrol®; Medrol®; Solu-Medrol®

Canadian Brand Names Depo-Medrol®; Medrol®; Methylprednisolone Acetate; Solu-Medrol®

Index Terms 6-α-Methylprednisolone; A-Methapred; Methylprednisolone Acetate; Methylprednisolone Sodium Succinate

Therapeutic Category Adrenal Corticosteroid; Anti-inflammatory Agent; Antiasthmatic; Corticosteroid, Systemic; Glucocorticoid

Generic Available Yes: Sodium succinate injection, tablet

Use Anti-inflammatory or immunosuppressant agent in the treatment of a variety of diseases including those of hematologic, allergic, inflammatory, neoplastic, and autoimmune origin

Pregnancy Risk Factor C

Lactation Excretion in breast milk unknown

Contraindications Hypersensitivity to methylprednisolone or any component (see Warnings); systemic fungal infections; varicella infections; live or live, attenuated virus vaccines (with immunosuppressive doses of corticosteroids)

Warnings Hypothalamic pituitary adrenal (HPA) suppression may occur; acute adrenal insufficiency (adrenal crisis) may occur with abrupt withdrawal after long-term therapy or with stress; withdrawal or discontinuation of corticosteroids should be done carefully; patients with HPA axis suppression may require increased doses of systemic glucocorticosteroids prior to, during, and after unusual stress (eg, surgery). Immunosuppression may occur; patients may be more susceptible to infections; avoid exposure to chickenpox and measles. Corticosteroids may mask signs of infection. Corticosteroids may activate latent opportunistic infections or exacerbate systemic fungal infections. May cause osteoporosis (at any age) or inhibition of bone growth in pediatric patients. Acute myopathy may occur with high doses, elevated IOP may occur (especially with prolonged use), CNS effects (ranging from euphoria to psychosis) may occur. Rare cases of anaphylactoid reactions have been reported with corticosteroids.

Methylprednisolone **acetate** I.M. injection (multiple-dose vial) and the diluent for methylprednisolone **sodium succinate** injection contain benzyl alcohol which may cause allergic reactions in susceptible individuals; large amounts of benzyl alcohol (≥99 mg/kg/day) have been associated with a potentially fatal toxicity ("gasping syndrome") in neonates; the "gasping syndrome" consists of metabolic acidosis, respiratory distress, gasping respirations, CNS dysfunction (including convulsions, intracranial hemorrhage), hypotension and cardiovascular collapse; avoid use of methylprednisolone products containing benzyl alcohol in neonates; *in vitro* and animal studies have shown that benzoate, a metabolite of benzyl alcohol, displaces bilirubin from protein binding sites

Precautions Avoid using higher than recommended doses; suppression of HPA axis, suppression of linear growth (ie, reduction of growth velocity), reduced bone mineral density, or hypercorticism (Cushing's syndrome), hyperglycemia, glucosuria, may occur; titrate to lowest effective dose. Reduction in growth velocity may occur when corticosteroids are administered to pediatric patients by any route (monitor growth). Use with extreme caution in patients with respiratory tuberculosis, untreated systemic infections, or ocular herpes simplex; use with caution in patients with thyroid dysfunction, cirrhosis, nonspecific ulcerative colitis, hypertension, renal impairment, osteoporosis, thromboembolic tendencies, CHF, recent MI, convulsive disorders, myasthenia gravis, thrombophlebitis, peptic ulcer, diabetes, glaucoma, cataracts, or hepatic impairment. Prolonged use may result in cataracts or glaucoma.

Adverse Reactions

Cardiovascular: Edema, hypertension, CHF

Central nervous system: Vertigo, seizures, psychoses, pseudotumor cerebri, headache, euphoria, insomnia, intracranial hypertension, nervousness

Dermatologic: Acne, skin atrophy, impaired wound healing, petechiae, bruising

Endocrine & metabolic: HPA axis suppression, Cushing's syndrome, growth suppression, glucose intolerance, hypokalemia, alkalosis, sodium and water retention

Gastrointestinal: Peptic ulcer, nausea, vomiting

Hematologic: Transient leukocytosis

Neuromuscular & skeletal: Muscle weakness, osteoporosis, fractures, decreased bone mineral density

Ocular: Cataracts, elevated IOP, glaucoma

Miscellaneous: Immunosuppression, anaphylactoid reactions (rare)

Drug Interactions Cytochrome P450 isoenzyme CYP3A3/4 substrate (minor); **Note:** Unclear if methylprednisolone is a CYP3A3/4 inducer (like other corticosteroids) or inhibitor (weak)

Barbiturates, phenytoin, rifampin may increase the clearance of methylprednisolone; salicylates; methylprednisolone may increase cyclosporine serum concentrations. Live or live, attenuated virus vaccines (these increase the risk of viral infection and are contraindicated with immunosuppressive doses of corticosteroids); toxoids and vaccines may have decreased effects; reactions to skin tests may be suppressed.

Food Interactions Systemic use of corticosteroids may require a diet with increased potassium, vitamins A, B_6, C, D, folate, calcium, zinc and phosphorus and decreased sodium; grapefruit juice may significantly increase the bioavailability of oral methylprednisolone

Mechanism of Action Decreases inflammation by suppression of migration of polymorphonuclear leukocytes and reversal of increased capillary permeability

Pharmacodynamics The time of maximum effects and the duration of these effects is dependent upon the route of administration. See table.

Route	Maximum Effect	Duration
Oral	1-2 h	30-36 h
I.M. (acetate)	4-8 d	1-4 wk
Intra-articular	1 wk	1-5 wk

Usual Dosage Note: Only sodium succinate salt may be given I.V.

NIH Asthma Guidelines (NAEPP, 2002):

Children ≤12 years:

Asthma exacerbations (emergency medical care or hospital doses): Oral, I.V.: 1 mg/kg every 6 hours for 48 hours; then 1-2 mg/kg/day (maximum: 60 mg/day) in divided doses given twice daily until peak expiratory flow is 70% of predicted or personal best

Short-course "burst" (acute asthma):

Oral: 1-2 mg/kg/day in divided doses 1-2 times/day for 3-10 days; longer treatment may be required; usually given for 5 days; maximum dose: 60 mg/day

I.M. **(acetate):** 7.5 mg/kg as a one-time dose; maximum dose: 240 mg (**Note:** This may be given in place of short-course "burst" of oral steroids in patients who are vomiting or if compliance is a problem)

Long-term treatment: Oral: 0.25-2 mg/kg/day given as a single dose in the morning or every other day as needed for asthma control; maximum dose: 60 mg/day

Children >12 years and Adults:

Asthma exacerbations (emergency medical care or hospital doses): Oral, I.V.: 120-180 mg/day in divided doses 3-4 times/day for 48 hours; then 60-80 mg/day in divided doses given twice daily until peak expiratory flow is 70% of predicted or personal best

Short-course "burst" (acute asthma):

Oral: 40-60 mg/day in divided doses 1-2 times/day for 3-10 days; longer treatment may be required; usually given for 5 days

I.M. **(acetate)**: 240 mg as a one time dose (**Note:** This may be given in place of short-course "burst" of oral steroids in patients who are vomiting or if compliance is a problem)

Long-term treatment: Oral: 7.5-60 mg daily given as a single dose in the morning or every other day as needed for asthma control

Children:

Anti-inflammatory or immunosuppressive: Oral, I.M., I.V.: 0.5-1.7 mg/kg/day or 5-25 mg/m²/day in divided doses every 6-12 hours

"Pulse" therapy: 15-30 mg/kg/dose over ≥30 minutes given once daily for 3 days

Status asthmaticus: I.V.: Loading dose: 2 mg/kg/dose, then 0.5-1 mg/kg/dose every 6 hours

Lupus nephritis: I.V.: 30 mg/kg over ≥30 minutes every other day for 6 doses

Acute spinal cord injury: I.V.: 30 mg/kg over 15 minutes followed in 45 minutes by a continuous infusion of 5.4 mg/kg/hour for 23 hours

Adults:

Oral: 2-60 mg/day in 1-4 divided doses

High-dose therapy: I.V.: 30 mg/kg over ≥30 minutes; repeat as needed every 4-6 hours for 48-72 hours

I.M. **(acetate):** 10-80 mg/day once daily

I.V.: 40-250 mg every 4-6 hours

Lupus nephritis: High-dose "pulse" therapy: I.V.: 1 g/day for 3 days

Intra-articular, intralesional: 4-40 mg, up to 80 mg for large joints every 1-5 weeks

(Continued)

MethylPREDNISolone *(Continued)*

Administration

Oral: Administer after meals or with food or milk; do not administer with grapefruit juice

Parenteral: I.V.: **Succinate:** Low dose (eg, ≤1.8 mg/kg or ≤125 mg/dose): I.V. push over 3-15 minutes; moderate dose (eg, ≥2 mg/kg or 250 mg/dose): administer over 15-30 minutes; high dose (eg, 15 mg/kg or ≥500 mg/dose): administer over ≥30 minutes; doses >15 mg/kg or ≥1 g: administer over 1 hour. Do **not** administer high-dose I.V. push; hypotension, cardiac arrhythmia, and sudden death have been reported in patients given high-dose methylprednisolone I.V. push over <20 minutes; administer intermittent infusion over 15-60 minutes; maximum concentration: I.V. push: 125 mg/mL; I.V. infusion: 2.5 mg/mL. **Do not give acetate form I.V.**

Monitoring Parameters Blood pressure, serum glucose, and electrolytes

Test Interactions Interferes with skin tests

Patient Information Avoid alcohol; avoid grapefruit juice if taking oral methylprednisolone; limit caffeine; do not decrease or discontinue dose without physician's approval

Additional Information Sodium content of 1 g sodium succinate injection: 2.01 mEq; methylprednisolone sodium succinate 53 mg = methylprednisolone base 40 mg

Dosage Forms Excipient information presented when available (limited, particularly for generics); consult specific product labeling.

Injection, powder for reconstitution, as sodium succinate: 125 mg [strength expressed as base]

Solu-Medrol®: 40 mg, 125 mg, 500 mg, 1 g, 2 g [packaged with diluent; diluent contains benzyl alcohol; strength expressed as base]

Solu-Medrol®: 500 mg, 1 g

Injection, suspension, as acetate (Depo-Medrol®): 20 mg/mL (5 mL); 40 mg/mL (5 mL); 80 mg/mL (5 mL) [contains benzyl alcohol; strength expressed as base]

Injection, suspension, as acetate [single-dose vial] (Depo-Medrol®): 40 mg/mL (1 mL, 10 mL); 80 mg/mL (1 mL)

Tablet: 4 mg

Medrol®: 2 mg, 4 mg, 8 mg, 16 mg, 32 mg

Tablet, dose-pack: 4 mg (21s)

Medrol® Dosepack™: 4 mg (21s)

References

"National Asthma Education and Prevention Program. Expert Panel Report: Guidelines for the Diagnosis and Management of Asthma Update on Selected Topics--2002," *J Allergy Clin Immunol*, 2002, 110(5 Suppl):S141-219.

♦ **6-α-Methylprednisolone** *see* MethylPREDNISolone *on page 1039*
♦ **Methylprednisolone Acetate** *see* MethylPREDNISolone *on page 1039*
♦ **Methylprednisolone Sodium Succinate** *see* MethylPREDNISolone *on page 1039*
♦ **4-Methylpyrazole** *see* Fomepizole *on page 702*
♦ **Methylrosaniline Chloride** *see* Gentian Violet *on page 729*

Metoclopramide (met oh kloe PRA mide)

Medication Safety Issues

Sound-alike/look-alike issues:

Metoclopramide may be confused with metolazone

Reglan® may be confused with Megace®, Regonol®, Renagel®

Related Information

Compatibility of Chemotherapy and Related Supportive Care Medications *on page 1777*

Compatibility of Medications Mixed in A Syringe *on page 1941*

U.S. Brand Names Reglan®

Canadian Brand Names Apo-Metoclop®; Metoclopramide Hydrochloride Injection; Nu-Metoclopramide

Therapeutic Category Antiemetic; Gastrointestinal Agent, Prokinetic

Generic Available Yes

Use Treatment of gastroesophageal reflux; prevention of nausea and vomiting associated with chemotherapy; prevention of postoperative nausea and vomiting; facilitates intubation of the small intestine and symptomatic treatment of diabetic gastric stasis

Pregnancy Risk Factor B

Lactation Enters breast milk/use caution

Contraindications Hypersensitivity to metoclopramide or any component; GI obstruction, pheochromocytoma, history of seizure disorder or patients receiving drugs likely to cause extrapyramidal reactions

Warnings Rare reports of neuroleptic malignant syndrome; patients with NADH-cytochrome b5 reductase deficiency are at increased risk for developing methemoglobinemia and/or sulfhemoglobinemia

Some products contain sodium benzoate; benzoic acid (benzoate) is a metabolite of benzyl alcohol; large amounts of benzyl alcohol (≥99 mg/kg/day) have been associated with a potentially fatal toxicity ("gasping syndrome") in neonates; *in vitro* and animal studies have shown that benzoate displaces bilirubin from protein binding sites; avoid use of sodium benzoate containing products in neonates.

Precautions Use with caution and reduce dosage in patients with renal impairment, hypertension, or depression; transient increases in plasma aldosterone may occur which could result in fluid retention or volume overload. Patients with CHF or cirrhosis of the liver may be at increased risk for development of fluid retention and volume overload. Use with caution in these patients and discontinue therapy if symptoms of excessive body fluids occurs.

Adverse Reactions Extrapyramidal reactions occur most frequently in children and young adults and following I.V. administration of high doses, usually within 24-48 hours after starting therapy

Cardiovascular: Hypertension, hypotension, SVT, bradycardia, A-V block, CHF

Central nervous system: Drowsiness, fatigue, restlessness, anxiety, agitation, depression, tardive dyskinesia, dystonia, seizures, hallucinations, neuroleptic malignant syndrome (rare)

Endocrine & metabolic: Gynecomastia, amenorrhea, galactorrhea, hyperprolactinemia

Gastrointestinal: Constipation, diarrhea

Genitourinary: Urinary frequency, impotence

Hematologic: Methemoglobinemia (see Warnings), sulfhemoglobinemia (see Warnings), neutropenia, leukopenia, agranulocytosis

Hepatic: Porphyria, jaundice

Ocular: Visual disturbances

Miscellaneous: Hypersensitivity reactions

Drug Interactions Cytochrome P450 isoenzyme CYP1A2 and CYP2D6 substrate

Decreased cimetidine and digoxin GI absorption; increased cyclosporine GI absorption; levodopa decreases metoclopramide effects; increases hypertensive episodes with MAO inhibitors; increased neuromuscular blocking effects of succinylcholine; anticholinergics and narcotic analgesics antagonize GI motility effects of metoclopramide; metoclopramide may increase tacrolimus serum levels

Stability Protect from light; stable for 48 hours at room temperature when admixed with ascorbic acid, cimetidine (in NS only), cytarabine, dexamethasone sodium phosphate, diphenhydramine, doxorubicin, heparin, benztropine, dexamethasone hydrochloride, hydrocortisone sodium phosphate, lidocaine, magnesium sulfate, mannitol, potassium acetate, potassium chloride, and potassium phosphate; stable for 24 hours at room temperature when admixed with clindamycin (in NS only) and cyclophosphamide; incompatible with cephalothin, chloramphenicol, and sodium bicarbonate

Mechanism of Action Potent dopamine receptor antagonist; blocks dopamine receptors in chemoreceptor trigger zone of the CNS, preventing emesis; accelerates gastric emptying and intestinal transit time without stimulating gastric, biliary, or pancreatic secretions

Pharmacodynamics

Onset of action:
- Oral: Within 30-60 minutes
- I.M.: Within 10-15 minutes
- I.V.: Within 1-3 minutes

Duration: Therapeutic effects persist for 1-2 hours, regardless of route administered

Pharmacokinetics

Distribution: V_d: 3.5 L/kg; crosses the placenta; appears in breast milk; breast milk to plasma ratio: 0.5-4.06

Protein binding: 30%

Bioavailability: Oral: 80 ± 15.5%

Half-life: 2.5-6 hours (half-life and clearance may be dose-dependent)

Elimination: Primarily as unchanged drug in the urine and feces

Usual Dosage

Intubation of small intestine to facilitate radiographic examination of upper GI tract:
- I.V.:
  - Children:
    - <6 years: 0.1 mg/kg
    - 6-14 years: 2.5-5 mg
  - Children >14 years and Adults: 10 mg

Gastroesophageal reflux: Oral, I.M., I.V.:
- Neonates, Infants and Children: 0.4-0.8 mg/kg/day in 4 divided doses
- Adults: 10-15 mg 4 times/day

(Continued)

Metoclopramide *(Continued)*

Postoperative nausea and vomiting: I.V.:
Children: 0.1-0.2 mg/kg/dose; repeat every 6-8 hours as needed
Children >14 years and Adults: 10 mg; repeat every 6-8 hours as needed
Antiemetic **(chemotherapy-induced emesis)**: Oral, I.V.:
Children and Adults: 1-2 mg/kg/dose every 2-4 hours; pretreatment with diphenhydramine will decrease risk of extrapyramidal reactions to this dosage
Diabetic gastroparesis: Adults: Oral, I.V.: 10 mg before each meal and at bedtime for 2-8 weeks

Dosing adjustment in renal impairment: Children and Adults:
Cl_{cr} 40-50 mL/minute: Administer 75% of recommended dose
Cl_{cr} 10-40 mL/minute: Administer 50% of recommended dose
Cl_{cr} <10 mL/minute: Administer 25% to 50% of recommended dose

Administration
Oral: Administer 30 minutes before meals and at bedtime
Parenteral: Dilute to 0.2 mg/mL (maximum concentration: 5 mg/mL) and infuse over 15-30 minutes (maximum rate of infusion: 5 mg/minute); rapid I.V. administration is associated with a transient but intense feeling of anxiety and restlessness, followed by drowsiness

Monitoring Parameters Renal function; blood pressure and heart rate (when rapid I.V. administration is used)

Patient Information May cause drowsiness and impair ability to perform activities requiring mental alertness or physical coordination

Dosage Forms Excipient information presented when available (limited, particularly for generics); consult specific product labeling.
Injection, solution (Reglan®): 5 mg/mL (2 mL, 10 mL, 30 mL)
Syrup: 5 mg/5 mL (10 mL, 480 mL)
Tablet (Reglan®): 5 mg, 10 mg

♦ **Metoclopramide Hydrochloride Injection (Can)** *see* Metoclopramide *on page 1042*

Metolazone (me TOLE a zone)

Medication Safety Issues
Sound-alike/look-alike issues:
Metolazone may be confused with metaxalone, methazolamide, methimazole, methotrexate, metoclopramide, metoprolol, minoxidil
Zaroxolyn® may be confused with Zarontin®

Related Information
Antihypertensive Agents by Class *on page 1678*

U.S. Brand Names Zaroxolyn®
Canadian Brand Names Zaroxolyn®
Therapeutic Category Antihypertensive Agent; Diuretic, Miscellaneous
Generic Available Yes
Use Management of mild to moderate hypertension (Zaroxolyn® only); treatment of edema in CHF, nephrotic syndrome, and impaired renal function
Pregnancy Risk Factor B
Lactation Enters breast milk/not recommended
Contraindications Hypersensitivity to metolazone, any component, other thiazide diuretics, or sulfonamide-derived drugs; anuria; patients with hepatic coma
Warnings Chemical similarities are present among sulfonamides, sulfonylureas, carbonic anhydrase inhibitors, thiazides, and loop diuretics (except ethacrynic acid). Use in patients with thiazide or sulfonamide allergy is specifically contraindicated in product labeling, however, there is potential for cross-reaction with any of these compounds; avoid use in patients allergic to these compounds particularly if the reaction was severe. Large or prolonged fluid and electrolyte losses may occur with concomitant furosemide administration.
Precautions Use with caution in patients with severe renal disease, impaired hepatic function, gout, lupus erythematosus, diabetes mellitus, moderate-high cholesterol concentrations, and/or high triglycerides

Adverse Reactions
Cardiovascular: Palpitations, chest pain, orthostatic hypotension, precordial pain, syncope, venous thrombosis, necrotizing angiitis
Central nervous system: Vertigo, headache, chills, drowsiness, fatigue, restlessness, depression, dizziness
Dermatologic: Rash, dry skin, photosensitivity, toxic epidermal necrolysis, Stevens-Johnson syndrome, cutaneous vasculitis, urticaria
Endocrine & metabolic: Hypokalemia, hyponatremia, hypochloremia, metabolic alkalosis, hyperglycemia, hyperuricemia, hypomagnesemia, gout, hypercalcemia

Gastrointestinal: Abdominal bloating, GI irritation, bitter taste, nausea, vomiting, anorexia, xerostomia, abdominal pain, epigastric distress

Hematologic: Blood dyscrasias, aplastic anemia, hemolytic anemia, leukopenia, agranulocytosis, thrombocytopenia

Hepatic: Hepatitis, cholestatic jaundice

Neuromuscular & skeletal: Arthralgia, back pain, paresthesias, joint pain, muscle cramps/spasm, weakness

Ocular: Eye itching, transient blurred vision

Otic: Tinnitus

Renal: Polyuria, prerenal azotemia, uremia

Respiratory: Cough, sinus congestion, epistaxis

Drug Interactions Increased digoxin toxicity (due to potassium and magnesium depletion); increased lithium toxicity; additive potassium losses with amphotericin B and steroids; salicylates and NSAIDs decrease antihypertensive effects; allopurinol increases hypersensitivity reactions; rare occurrence of hemolytic anemia with methyldopa; cholestyramine and colestipol decrease metolazone absorption

Food Interactions Avoid natural licorice (causes sodium and water retention and increases potassium loss); avoid garlic (may have increased antihypertensive effect); avoid ephedra, yohimbe, ginseng (may worsen hypertension)

Mechanism of Action Inhibits sodium reabsorption in the cortical diluting site and proximal convoluted tubules causing increased excretion of sodium and water as well as potassium and hydrogen ions

Pharmacodynamics

Onset of action: 1 hour

Duration: 12-24 hours

Pharmacokinetics

Absorption: Oral: Rate and extent vary with the preparation

Protein binding: 95%

Half-life: 6-20 hours

Elimination: Enterohepatic recycling; 70% to 95% excreted unchanged in urine

Usual Dosage Oral:

Children: 0.2-0.4 mg/kg/day divided every 12-24 hours

Adults:

- Edema: 5-10 mg/dose every 24 hours
- Edema associated with renal disease or cardiac failure (ACC/AHA 2005 Heart Failure Guidelines): 2.5-20 mg/dose every 24 hours
- Hypertension: 2.5-5 mg/dose every 24 hours

Administration Oral: Administer with food to decrease GI distress; administer early in day to avoid nocturia

Monitoring Parameters Serum electrolytes, renal function, blood pressure, body weight, fluid balance

Patient Information May cause dry mouth; may cause drowsiness and impair ability to perform activities requiring mental alertness or physical coordination. May cause photosensitivity reactions (eg, exposure to sunlight may cause severe sunburn, skin rash, redness, or itching); avoid exposure to sunlight and artificial light sources (sunlamps, tanning booth/bed); wear protective clothing, wide-brimmed hats, sunglasses, and lip sunscreen (SPF ≥15); use a sunscreen [broad-spectrum sunscreen or physical sunscreen (preferred) or sunblock with SPF ≥15]; contact physician if reaction occurs.

Additional Information Metolazone 5 mg is approximately equivalent to hydrochlorothiazide 50 mg

Dosage Forms Excipient information presented when available (limited, particularly for generics); consult specific product labeling.

Tablet: 2.5 mg, 5 mg, 10 mg

Zaroxolyn®: 2.5 mg, 5 mg, 10 mg

Extemporaneous Preparations

A 1 mg/mL suspension may be made by crushing twelve 10 mg Zaroxolyn® tablets; add Ora-Sweet®, Ora-Sweet® SF, Ora-Plus®, or cherry syrup diluted 1:4 with simple syrup to total volume of 120 mL. Label "shake well"; stable 60 days refrigerated.

A 0.25 mg/mL suspension may be made by crushing one 2.5 mg tablet; add 1:1 mixture 1% methylcellulose:simple syrup mixture to a total volume of 10 mL; label "shake well"; refrigerate; stable 91 days refrigerated; 28 days at room temperature in plastic and 14 days at room temperature in glass.

Nahata, MC, Pai VB, and Hipple TF, *Pediatric Drug Formulations*, 5th ed, Cincinnati, OH: Harvey Whitney Books Co, 2004.

References

Arnold WC, "Efficacy of Metolazone and Furosemide in Children With Furosemide-Resistant Edema," *Pediatrics*, 1984, 74(5):872-5.

(Continued)

Metolazone *(Continued)*

Chobanian AV, Bakris GL, Black HR, et al, "The Seventh Report of the Joint National Committee on Prevention, Detection, Evaluation, and Treatment of High Blood Pressure: The JNC 7 Report," *JAMA*, 2003, 289(19):2560-72.

Wells TG, "The Pharmacology and Therapeutics of Diuretics in the Pediatric Patient," *Pediatr Clin North Am*, 1990, 37(2):463-504.

♦ **Metopirone®** *see* Metyrapone *on page 1051*

Metoprolol (me toe PROE lole)

Medication Safety Issues

Sound-alike/look-alike issues:

Metoprolol may be confused with metaproterenol, metolazone, misoprostol

Toprol-XL® may be confused with Tegretol®, Tegretol®-XR, Topamax®

Significant differences exist between oral and I.V. dosing. Use caution when converting from one route of administration to another.

Related Information

Antihypertensive Agents by Class *on page 1678*

U.S. Brand Names Lopressor®; Toprol-XL®

Canadian Brand Names Apo-Metoprolol®; Betaloc®; Betaloc® Durules®; Lopressor®; Metoprolol Tartrate Injection, USP; Novo-Metoprolol; Nu-Metop; PMS-Metoprolol; Sandoz-Metoprolol; Toprol-XL®

Index Terms Metoprolol Succinate; Metoprolol Tartrate

Therapeutic Category Antianginal Agent; Antiarrhythmic Agent, Class II; Antihypertensive Agent; Antimigraine Agent; Beta-Adrenergic Blocker

Generic Available Yes

Use Management of hypertension, angina pectoris, and arrhythmias (such as multifocal atrial tachycardia); prevention of MI and migraine headaches; extended release tablets are also indicated to reduce mortality and hospitalization in adults with CHF (stable NYHA Class II or III) who are receiving ACE inhibitors, diuretics, and/or digoxin

Pregnancy Risk Factor C (D if used in 2nd of 3rd trimester)

Lactation Enters breast milk/use caution (AAP rates "compatible")

Contraindications Hypersensitivity to metoprolol or any component; sinus bradycardia; heart block greater then first degree; sick sinus syndrome (except in patients with a functioning artificial pacemaker); cardiogenic shock; uncompensated CHF

Warnings May depress myocardial activity and precipitate or worsen CHF; use with caution and monitor closely, especially in patients with compensated heart failure and during upwards titration of dose; if CHF worsens, may need to increase diuretics and not advance the dose of metoprolol; a reduction in dose or discontinuation of metoprolol may be needed. In patients with coronary artery disease, exacerbation of angina and, in some cases, MI may occur following abrupt discontinuation of therapy. Beta-blockers should generally be avoided in patients with bronchospastic disease; metoprolol, with relative beta$_1$ selectivity, should be used with caution and closely monitored in patients with bronchospastic disease; beta$_2$ stimulants and the lowest possible dose of metoprolol should be used in these patients. Metoprolol may block hypoglycemia-induced tachycardia and blood pressure changes; use with caution in patients with diabetes mellitus. Metoprolol decreases the ability of the heart to respond to reflex adrenergic stimuli and may increase the risk of general anesthesia and surgical procedures. May mask clinical signs of hyperthyroidism (exacerbation of symptoms of hyperthyroidism, including thyroid storm, may occur following abrupt discontinuation). Use with caution with verapamil, diltiazem, or anesthetic agents that decrease myocardial function (bradycardia or heart block may occur).

Precautions Use with caution in patients with hepatic dysfunction and in patients with peripheral vascular disease (beta-blockers may aggravate arterial insufficiency). Patients who have a history of severe anaphylactic hypersensitivity reactions to various substances may be more reactive while receiving beta-blockers; these patients may not be responsive to the normal doses of epinephrine used to treat hypersensitivity reactions. Use with caution in patients with pheochromocytoma; these patients should receive an alpha-blocking agent before receipt of any beta-blocking agent.

Adverse Reactions

Cardiovascular: Bradycardia, reduced peripheral circulation, palpitations, CHF, hypotension, peripheral edema, worsening of AV conduction disturbances, heart block (second and third degree)

Central nervous system: Dizziness, tiredness, depression, mental confusion, insomnia

Dermatologic: Rash, pruritus, worsening of psoriasis

Gastrointestinal: Diarrhea, nausea, abdominal pain, xerostomia, constipation, vomiting

Hematologic (potential): Agranulocytosis, thrombocytopenia

Hepatic: Hepatitis, hepatic dysfunction, jaundice; rare: elevated transaminase, alkaline phosphatase, LDH

Respiratory: Bronchospasm, wheezing, dyspnea

Drug Interactions Cytochrome P450 isoenzyme CYP2D6 substrate

Catecholamine-depleting drugs, such as reserpine or MAO inhibitors, may have additive effects (hypotension, bradycardia); hypotensive agents, diuretics, cardiac glycosides, amiodarone, calcium channel blockers, agents that slow AV conduction, and myocardial depressant general anesthetics may have additive effects with beta-blockers; verapamil may significantly increase the oral bioavailability of metoprolol (avoid concomitant use or reduce metoprolol dose and monitor closely); cimetidine, ciprofloxacin, fluoxetine, hydralazine, oral contraceptives, propoxyphene, and quinidine may increase metoprolol serum concentrations and effects. Abrupt withdrawal of clonidine while receiving beta-blockers may result in an exaggerated hypertensive crisis; NSAIDs may decrease the antihypertensive effects of beta-blockers; barbiturates and rifampin may increase the metabolism of metoprolol and decrease metoprolol serum concentrations; metoprolol may increase lidocaine serum concentrations

Food Interactions

Metoprolol tartrate: Food may enhance the extent of oral absorption

Metoprolol succinate (extended release tablets): Food does not significantly affect bioavailability

Stability

Tablets and extended release tablets: Store at controlled room temperature 15°C to 30°C (59°F to 86°F)

Tablets: Protect from moisture and dispense in tight, light-resistant container

Injection: Do not store above 30°C (86°F); protect from light

Mechanism of Action Selective inhibitor of beta$_1$-adrenergic receptors at lower doses; competitively blocks beta$_1$ adrenergic receptors with little or no effect on beta$_2$-receptors at doses in adults <100 mg/day; inhibits beta$_2$- receptors at higher doses; does not exhibit membrane stabilizing or intrinsic sympathomimetic activity

Pharmacodynamics

Beta blockade:

Onset of action: Oral: Metoprolol tartrate tablets: Within 1 hour

Maximum effect: I.V.: 20 minutes

Duration: Dose dependent

Antihypertensive effect:

Onset of action: Oral: Metoprolol tartrate tablets: Within 15 minutes

Maximum effect: Oral (multiple dosing): After 1 week

Duration: Oral: Metoprolol tartrate tablets (single dose): 6 hours; metoprolol succinate (extended release tablets): Up to 24 hours

Pharmacokinetics

Absorption: Rapid and complete, with large first-pass effect

Distribution: Crosses the blood brain barrier; CSF concentrations are 78% of plasma concentrations

Protein binding: 12% bound to albumin

Metabolism: Significant first-pass metabolism; extensive metabolism in the liver via isoenzyme CYP2D6

Bioavailability: Oral: 50%

Half-Life:

Neonates: 5-10 hours

Adults: 3-7 hours

Adults with chronic renal failure: Similar to normal adults

Elimination: 10% of an I.V. dose and <5% of an oral dose is excreted unchanged in the urine

Usual Dosage (See Additional Information)

Oral: Hypertension:

Children and Adolescents 1-17 years: Tablets (nonsustained release): Initial: 1-2 mg/kg/day, administered in 2 divided doses; maximum 6 mg/kg/day (≤200 mg/day) (National High Blood Pressure Education Program Working Group on High Blood Pressure in Children and Adolescents, 2004)

Note: Limited pediatric studies are available. A recent article examined the use of metoprolol extended release tablets in children 6-16 years of age (mean age: 12.5 ± 2.8 years). In part 1 (a 4-week double-blind dose ranging study), patients were randomized to receive placebo (n=23) or metoprolol 0.2 mg/kg/day (n=45), 1 mg/kg/day (n=23), or 2 mg/kg/day (n=49) given as once daily dosing. For patients in the higher dosing groups, doses were initiated at 0.5 mg/kg/day, and increased after 1 week to 1 mg/kg/day if tolerated. Doses were increased again after 1 week to 2 mg/kg/day if tolerated in the 2 mg/kg/day dosing group. At the

(Continued)

Metoprolol *(Continued)*

end of 4 weeks, metoprolol significantly decreased systolic blood pressure in the 1 mg/kg/day and 2 mg/kg/day groups compared to placebo. Diastolic blood pressure was significantly reduced only in the 2 mg/kg/day group. In part 2 (a 52-week open label trial), 100 patients received initial doses of 25 mg or 12.5 mg once daily; doses were increased every 2 weeks in 25 mg or 50 mg increments based on blood pressure and tolerability, to a maximum dose of 200 mg once daily. The mean doses were: 37 ± 33 mg at study entry, 97 ± 64 mg at week 16, and 112 ± 69 mg at study end (see Batisky, 2007). In an older study using nonsustained release tablets, sixteen hypertensive adolescents (≥13 years of age) were treated with an initial metoprolol dose of 50 mg twice daily; patients were seen every 4-6 weeks and doses were increased to 100 mg twice daily if blood pressure was not controlled (see Falkner, 1982).

Adults:

Tablets (nonsustained release): Initial: 100 mg/day in single or divided doses, increase at weekly intervals to desired effect; usual dosage range: 100-450 mg/day; doses >450 mg/day have not been studied; usual dosage range (JNC 7): 50-100 mg/day in 1-2 divided doses

Note: Lower once-daily dosing (especially 100 mg/day) may not control blood pressure for 24 hours; larger or more frequent dosing may be needed. Patients with bronchospastic diseases should receive the lowest possible daily dose; dose should initially be divided into 3 doses per day (to avoid high plasma concentrations).

Extended release tablets: Initial: 25-100 mg/day as a single dose; increase at weekly intervals to desired effect; doses >400 mg/day have not been studied; usual dosage range (JNC 7): 50-100 mg once daily

Oral: Congestive heart failure: Adults: Extended release tablets: Initial: NYHA Class II heart failure: 25 mg once daily; more severe heart failure: 12.5 mg once daily; may double the dose every 2 weeks as tolerated; maximum: 200 mg/day

Administration Oral:

Metoprolol tartrate tablets: Administer with food or immediately after meals

Metoprolol succinate extended release tablets: May be administered without regard to meals; do not chew, crush, or break extended release tablets

Monitoring Parameters Blood pressure, heart rate, respirations, circulation in extremities

Additional Information Do not abruptly discontinue therapy, taper dosage gradually over 1-2 weeks. Beta-blockers without intrinsic sympathomimetic activity (such as metoprolol) have been shown to decrease morbidity and mortality when initiated in the acute treatment of MI and continued long term; metoprolol injection is used for early treatment of definitive or suspected MI; consult adult reference for further information.

Limited pediatric dosing information is available in the literature; in one case report, oral metoprolol (2 mg/kg/day in 3 divided doses) helped control paroxysmal supraventricular tachycardia in a 6 month old infant receiving digoxin (see Hepner, 1983). Low dose oral metoprolol (initial: 0.1 mg/kg/dose given twice daily, then increased slowly as needed to a maximum of 0.9 ± 0.7 mg/kg/day) was used to treat severe CHF that failed conventional therapy in 4 children (mean age: 7.8 years) with cardiomyopathy who were under consideration for heart transplantation (see Shaddy, 1998). A follow-up report in 15 children, 2.5-15 years of age (mean: 8.6 ± 1.3 years), used low dose oral metoprolol [Initial: 0.1-0.2 mg/kg/dose given twice daily, then increased slowly as needed to a maximum of 1.1 ± 0.1 mg/kg/day (range: 0.5-2.3 mg/kg/day)] to treat dilated cardiomyopathy and CHF; all patients received ACE inhibitors, digoxin, and diuretics before starting metoprolol (see Shaddy, 1999). Two studies (Muller, 1993; O'Marcaigh, 1994) assessed metoprolol for unexplained syncope in children at I.V. doses of 0.1 to 0.2 mg/kg for tilt table testing; in both studies, oral metoprolol was given after tilt table testing to select patients; initial oral doses of 0.8-2.8 mg/kg/day were used in 15 patients (8-20 years of age), but treatment was discontinued in 3 patients receiving 1.8-2.8 mg/kg/day due to adverse effects (Muller, 1993); oral doses of 1 to 2 mg/kg/day, rounded to the nearest 25 mg/day and divided into 2 doses daily were used in 19 patients (7-18 years of age) with unexplained syncope; the mean effective dose was 1.5 mg/kg/day (O'Marcaigh, 1994). High-dose beta-blocker therapy has been recommended to treat childhood hypertrophic cardiomyopathy (see Ostman-Smith, 1999). Further pediatric studies are required before these doses can be recommended.

Dosage Forms Excipient information presented when available (limited, particularly for generics); consult specific product labeling.

Injection, solution, as tartrate: 1 mg/mL (5 mL)

Lopressor®: 1 mg/mL (5 mL)

Tablet, as tartrate: 25 mg, 50 mg, 100 mg

Lopressor®: 50 mg, 100 mg

Tablet, extended release, as succinate: 25 mg, 50 mg, 100 mg, 200 mg [expressed as mg equivalent to tartrate]

Toprol-XL®: 25 mg, 50 mg, 100 mg, 200 mg [expressed as mg equivalent to tartrate]

Extemporaneous Preparations A 10 mg/mL metoprolol tartrate oral liquid preparation made with twelve 100 mg tablets and qsad to 120 mL with 3 different vehicles (a 1:1 mixture of Ora-Sweet® and Ora-Plus®, a 1:1 mixture of Ora-Sweet® SF and Ora-Plus®, or cherry syrup) was found to be stable for 60 days when stored in amber plastic bottles in the dark at 5°C and 25°C. Microbial growth was not determined. Label "shake well" and "protect from light".

Allen LV and Erickson MA, "Stability of Labetalol Hydrochloride, Metoprolol Tartrate, Verapamil Hydrochloride, and Spironolactone With Hydrochlorothiazide in Extemporaneously Compounded Oral Liquids," *Am J Health Syst Pharm*, 1996, 53(19):2304-9.

References

Batisky DL, Sorof JM, Sugg J, et al, "Efficacy and Safety of Extended Release Metoprolol Succinate in Hypertensive Children 6 to 16 Years of Age: A Clinical Trial Experience," *J Pediatr*, 2007, 150(2):134-9.

Chobanian AV, Bakris GL, Black HR, et al, "The Seventh Report of the Joint National Committee on Prevention, Detection, Evaluation, and Treatment of High Blood Pressure: The JNC 7 report," *JAMA*, 2003, 289(19):2560-72.

Falkner B, Lowenthal DT, and Affrime MB, "The Pharmacodynamic Effectiveness of Metoprolol in Adolescent Hypertension," *Pediatr Pharmacol (New York)*, 1982, 2(1):49-55.

Hepner SI, and Davoli E, "Successful Treatment of Supraventricular Tachycardia With Metoprolol, a Cardioselective Beta Blocker," *Clin Pediatr (Phila)*, 1983, 22(7):522-3.

Morselli PL, Boutroy MJ, Bianchetti G, et al, "Pharmacokinetics of Antihypertensive Drugs in the Neonatal Period," *Dev Pharmacol Ther*, 1989, 13(2-4):190-8.

Muller G, Deal BJ, Strasburger JF, et al, "Usefulness of Metoprolol for Unexplained Syncope and Positive Response to Tilt Testing in Young Persons," *Am J Cardiol*, 1993, 71(7):592-5.

National High Blood Pressure Education Program Working Group on High Blood Pressure in Children and Adolescents, "The Fourth Report on the Diagnosis, Evaluation, and Treatment of High Blood Pressure in Children and Adolescents," *Pediatrics*, 2004, 114(2 Suppl 4th Report):555-76.

O'Marcaigh AS, MacLellan-Tobert SG, and Porter CJ, "Tilt-Table Testing and Oral Metoprolol Therapy in Young Patients With Unexplained Syncope," *Pediatrics*, 1994, 93(2):278-83.

Ostman-Smith I, Wettrell G, and Riesenfield T, "A Cohort Study of Childhood Hypertrophic Cardiomyopathy: Improved Survival Following High-Dose Beta-Adrenoceptor Antagonist Treatment," *J Am Coll Cardiol*, 1999, 34(6):1813-22.

Shaddy RE, "Beta-Blocker Therapy in Young Children With Congestive Heart Failure Under Consideration for Heart Transplantation," *Am Heart J*, 1998, 136(1):19-21.

Shaddy RE, Tani LY, Gidding SS, et al, "Beta-Blocker Treatment of Dilated Cardiomyopathy With Congestive Heart Failure in Children: A Multi-Institutional Experience," *J Heart Lung Transplant*, 1999, 18(3):269-74.

- **Metoprolol Succinate** *see* Metoprolol *on page 1046*
- **Metoprolol Tartrate** *see* Metoprolol *on page 1046*
- **Metoprolol Tartrate Injection, USP (Can)** *see* Metoprolol *on page 1046*
- **MetroCream®** *see* Metronidazole *on page 1049*
- **MetroGel®** *see* Metronidazole *on page 1049*
- **Metrogel® (Can)** *see* Metronidazole *on page 1049*
- **MetroGel-Vaginal®** *see* Metronidazole *on page 1049*
- **MetroLotion®** *see* Metronidazole *on page 1049*

Metronidazole (me troe NI da zole)

Medication Safety Issues

Sound-alike/look-alike issues:

Metronidazole may be confused with metformin.

Related Information

Compatibility of Chemotherapy and Related Supportive Care Medications *on page 1777*

U.S. Brand Names Flagyl®; Flagyl ER®; MetroCream®; MetroGel®; MetroGel-Vaginal®; MetroLotion®; Noritate®; Vandazole™

Canadian Brand Names Apo-Metronidazole®; Flagyl®; Florazole® ER; MetroCream®; Metrogel®; Nidagel™; Noritate®; Trikacide

Index Terms Metronidazole Hydrochloride

Therapeutic Category Amebicide; Antibiotic, Anaerobic; Antibiotic, Topical; Antiprotozoal

Generic Available Yes: Capsule, cream, gel, infusion, lotion, tablet

Use Treatment of susceptible anaerobic bacterial and protozoal infections in the following conditions: amebiasis (liver abscess, dysentery), giardiasis, symptomatic and asymptomatic trichomoniasis; skin and skin structure infections, CNS infections, intra-abdominal infections, and systemic anaerobic bacterial infections; topically for the treatment of acne rosacea; treatment of antibiotic-associated pseudomembranous colitis (AAPC) caused by *C. difficile*; bacterial vaginosis

Pregnancy Risk Factor B

(Continued)

Metronidazole *(Continued)*

Lactation Enters breast milk/not recommended (AAP rates "of concern")

Contraindications Hypersensitivity to metronidazole or any component; 1st trimester of pregnancy

Warnings Has been shown to be carcinogenic in rodents

Precautions Use with caution in patients with liver impairment, blood dyscrasias, CNS disease; metronidazole injection should be used with caution in patients receiving corticosteroids or patients predisposed to edema (injection contains 28 mEq of sodium/g metronidazole); reduce dosage in patients with severe liver impairment; dosage adjustment is not necessary in patients with moderate to severe renal insufficiency

Adverse Reactions

Central nervous system: Dizziness, confusion, seizures, headache, insomnia, hallucinations, paresthesias

Dermatologic: Rash

Endocrine & Metabolic: Disulfiram-type reaction with alcohol

Gastrointestinal: Metallic taste, nausea, xerostomia, diarrhea, furry tongue, vomiting

Genitourinary: Urethral burning, discoloration of urine (dark or reddish brown)

Hematologic: Leukopenia, neutropenia

Local: Thrombophlebitis

Neuromuscular & skeletal: Peripheral neuropathy

Drug Interactions Disulfiram (psychotic episodes); phenobarbital and rifampin (may increase metabolism of metronidazole); increased levels/toxicity of phenytoin, lithium, warfarin; alcohol may cause disulfiram-like reactions

Food Interactions Peak concentration is decreased and delayed when administered with food

Stability Do not refrigerate neutralized solution because precipitation may occur; reconstituted vials are chemically stable for 96 hours when stored at room temperature; protect from light

Mechanism of Action Reduced to a product which interacts with DNA to cause a loss of helical DNA structure and strand breakage resulting in inhibition of protein synthesis and cell death in susceptible organisms

Pharmacokinetics

Absorption: Oral: Well absorbed

Distribution: Excreted in breast milk; widely distributed into body tissues, fluids including bile, liver, bone, pleural fluid, vaginal secretions, CSF, erythrocytes, and hepatic abscesses

Protein binding: <20%

Metabolism: 30% to 60% in the liver to hydroxylated metabolite (60% to 80% bioactive), acetic acid metabolites, glucuronide, and sulfated conjugates

Half-life (increases with hepatic impairment):
- Neonates: 25-75 hours
- Children and Adults:
  - Metronidazole: 6-12 hours
  - Hydroxymetronidazole: 9.5-20 hours

Time to peak serum concentration: Within 1-2 hours

Elimination: Excreted via the urine (20% as unchanged drug) and feces (6% to 15%)

Dialysis: Extensively removed by hemodialysis and peritoneal dialysis

Usual Dosage

Neonates: Anaerobic infections: Oral, I.V.:
- 0-4 weeks, <1200 g: 7.5 mg/kg every 48 hours
- Postnatal age ≤7 days:
  - 1200-2000 g: 7.5 mg/kg/day given every 24 hours
  - >2000 g: 15 mg/kg/day in divided doses every 12 hours
- Postnatal age >7 days:
  - 1200-2000 g: 15 mg/kg/day in divided doses every 12 hours
  - >2000 g: 30 mg/kg/day in divided doses every 12 hours

Infants and Children:
- Amebiasis: Oral: 35-50 mg/kg/day in divided doses every 8 hours
- Other parasitic infections: Oral: 15-30 mg/kg/day in divided doses every 8 hours
- Anaerobic infections: Oral, I.V.: 30 mg/kg/day in divided doses every 6 hours; maximum dose: 4 g/day
- AAPC: Oral: 30 mg/kg/day divided every 6 hours for 7-10 days
- *Helicobacter pylori* infection (has been used in combination with amoxicillin and bismuth subsalicylate): Oral: 15-20 mg/kg/day in 2 divided doses for 4 weeks

Adults:
- Amebiasis: Oral: 500-750 mg every 8 hours
- Other parasitic infections: Oral: 250 mg every 8 hours or 2 g as a single dose
- Anaerobic infections: Oral, I.V.: 30 mg/kg/day in divided doses every 6 hours; not to exceed 4 g/day

AAPC: Oral: 250-500 mg 3-4 times/day for 10-14 days
Helicobacter pylori infection: Oral: 250-500 mg 3 times/day in combination with at least one other agent active against *H. pylori*
STD prophylaxis for acute sexual assault: Oral: 2 g in a single dose in combination with ceftriaxone and doxycycline
Topical: Apply a thin film twice daily to affected areas
Vaginal: One applicatorful (5 g) intravaginally 2 times/day for 5 days

Dosing adjustment in hepatic impairment: 50% to 67% decrease in dosage

Administration

Intravaginal: Use only **vaginal gel** intravaginally; do not apply to the eye
Oral: Administer on an empty stomach; may administer with food if GI upset occurs
Parenteral: Administer I.V. by slow intermittent infusion over 30-60 minutes at a final concentration for administration of 5-8 mg/mL
Topical: Wash affected areas with a mild cleanser; wait 15-20 minutes, then apply a thin film of drug to the affected area and rub in. Do not apply to the eye.

Monitoring Parameters WBC count

Test Interactions May cause falsely decreased AST and ALT levels

Patient Information May discolor urine dark or reddish brown; avoid alcohol; do not take alcohol for at least 48 hours after the last dose; may cause dry mouth

Nursing Implications Avoid contact between the drug and aluminum in the infusion set

Additional Information Sodium content of 500 mg ready-to-use vial: 14 mEq

Dosage Forms Excipient information presented when available (limited, particularly for generics); consult specific product labeling.

Capsule: 375 mg
Flagyl®: 375 mg
Cream, topical: 0.75% (45 g)
MetroCream®: 0.75% (45 g) [contains benzyl alcohol]
Noritate®: 1% (60 g)
Gel, topical: 0.75% (45 g)
MetroGel®: 1% (46 g, 60 g) [60 g tube also packaged in a kit with Cetaphil® skin cleanser]
Gel, vaginal: 0.75% (70 g)
MetroGel-Vaginal®, Vandazole™: 0.75% (70 g)
Infusion [premixed iso-osmotic sodium chloride solution]: 500 mg (100 mL)
Lotion, topical: 0.75% (60 mL)
MetroLotion®: 0.75% (60 mL) [contains benzyl alcohol]
Tablet: 250 mg, 500 mg
Flagyl®: 250 mg, 500 mg
Tablet, extended release:
Flagyl® ER: 750 mg

Extemporaneous Preparations A 50 mg/mL oral suspension can be made using a 1:1 mixture of Ora-Sweet® and Ora-Plus®; crush twenty-four 250 mg tablets into a fine powder in a mortar; add a small amount of vehicle and mix to make a uniform paste; mix while adding the vehicle in geometric portions to almost 120 mL; transfer to a calibrated bottle and qsad with vehicle to 120 mL; preparation is stable for 60 days when stored at room temperature or under refrigeration; label "shake well"

Allen LV Jr and Erickson MA III, "Stability of Ketoconazole, Metolazone, Metronidazole, Procainamide Hydrochloride, and Spironolactone in Extemporaneously Compounded Oral Liquids," *Am J Health Syst Pharm*, 1996, 53(17):2073-8.

References

Committee on Adolescence, American Academy of Pediatrics, "Sexual Assault and the Adolescent," *Pediatrics*, 1994, 94(5):761-5.
Israel DM and Hassall E, "Treatment and Long-Term Follow-up of *Helicobacter pylori*-Associated Duodenal Ulcer Disease in Children," *J Pediatr*, 1993, 123(1):53-8.
Kelly CP, Pothoulakis C, and LaMont JT, "*Clostridium difficile* Colitis," *N Engl J Med*, 1994, 330(4):257-62.
Oldenburg B and Speck WT, "Metronidazole," *Pediatr Clin North Am*, 1983, 30(1):71-5.

◆ **Metronidazole Hydrochloride** *see* Metronidazole *on page 1049*

Metyrapone (me TEER a pone)

Medication Safety Issues

Sound-alike/look-alike issues:
Metyrapone may be confused with metyrosine

U.S. Brand Names Metopirone®

Therapeutic Category Diagnostic Agent, Hypothalamic-Pituitary ACTH Function

Generic Available No

Use Diagnostic drug for testing hypothalamic-pituitary ACTH function

Pregnancy Risk Factor C

Lactation Excretion in breast milk unknown/use caution

(Continued)

Metyrapone *(Continued)*

Contraindications Hypersensitivity to metyrapone or any component; adrenal cortical insufficiency

Warnings All corticosteroid therapy should be discontinued prior to and during the metyrapone test; administration of metyrapone may induce acute adrenal insufficiency in patients with reduced adrenal secretory capacity; patients with suspected adrenocortical insufficiency should be observed closely over 24 hours

Precautions The test may be abnormal in the presence of thyroid dysfunction; demonstrate the ability of the adrenals to respond to exogenous ACTH before using metyrapone

Adverse Reactions

Cardiovascular: Hypotension, tachycardia

Central nervous system: Dizziness, headache, sedation

Dermatologic: Rash

Gastrointestinal: Abdominal discomfort, nausea, vomiting

Hematologic: Bone marrow suppression (rare)

Drug Interactions Phenytoin, chlorpromazine, amitriptyline, cyproheptadine, estrogens, phenobarbital may reduce test effectiveness; metyrapone inhibits glucuronidation of acetaminophen

Stability Protect from light

Mechanism of Action Reduces cortisol and corticosterone production by inhibition of 11-beta-hydroxylation of precursors in the adrenal cortex. Continued inhibition stimulates increased ACTH production by the pituitary; increased precursor levels have a weak suppressive activity on ACTH release. Elevated levels of precursor metabolites (17-hydroxycorticosteroids [17-OHCS] or 17-ketogenic steroids [17-KGS]) appear in the urine which can easily serve as an index of pituitary ACTH responsiveness. Production of aldosterone may also be suppressed by metyrapone. The adrenal cortex must have the ability to respond to ACTH before metyrapone is employed to test the capacity of the pituitary to respond to a decreased concentration of plasma cortisol.

Pharmacodynamics Maximum effect: Peak excretion of steroid during the first 24 hours after administration

Pharmacokinetics

Absorption: Oral: Well absorbed

Half-life, elimination: 1.9 ± 0.7 hours

Time to peak serum concentration: 1 hour

Elimination: 5.3% of dose excreted in urine unchanged

Usual Dosage Oral:

Children: 15 mg/kg/dose or 300 mg/m^2/dose every 4 hours for 6 doses; minimum: 250 mg/dose **or as an alternative** 30 mg/kg as a single dose (maximum: 3 g) given at midnight the night before the test

Adults: 750 mg every 4 hours for 6 doses **or as an alternative** 3 g as a single dose given at midnight the night before the test

Administration Oral: May administer with food or milk to reduce GI irritation

Reference Range

Normal response to metyrapone:

Plasma ACTH: 44 pmol/L (200 ng/L)

Plasma II desoxycortisol: 0.2 micromoles/L (70 mcg/L)

24 hour urinary excretion of 17-OHCS: 2-4 time increase

24 hour urinary excretion of 17-KGS: 2 time increase

A subnormal response may be indicative of panhypopituitarism or partial hypopituitarism. An excessive response is suggestive of Cushing's syndrome associated with adrenal hyperplasia.

Patient Information Arise slowly from prolonged sitting or lying position; may cause drowsiness and impair ability to perform activities requiring mental alertness or physical coordination

Dosage Forms Excipient information presented when available (limited, particularly for generics); consult specific product labeling.

Capsule: 250 mg

- **Mevacor®** *see* Lovastatin *on page 964*
- **Mevinolin** *see* Lovastatin *on page 964*
- **Mexar™ Wash** *see* Sulfacetamide *on page 1483*

Mexiletine (MEKS i le teen)

U.S. Brand Names Mexitil® [DSC]

Canadian Brand Names Novo-Mexiletine

Therapeutic Category Antiarrhythmic Agent, Class I-B

Generic Available Yes

Use Management of serious ventricular arrhythmias; suppression of premature ventricular contractions; diabetic neuropathy

Pregnancy Risk Factor C

Lactation Enters breast milk/compatible

Contraindications Hypersensitivity to mexiletine or any component; cardiogenic shock; second or third degree heart block (except in patients with a functioning artificial pacemaker)

Warnings Exercise extreme caution in patients with pre-existing sinus node dysfunction; mexiletine can worsen bradycardias and other arrhythmias; blood dyscrasias (including leukopenia, agranulocytosis, and thrombocytopenia) have been reported

Precautions Use with caution in patients with seizure disorders, severe CHF, hypotension, hepatic impairment; avoid dietary regimens or concomitant drug therapy that markedly change urine pH (see Drug and Food Interactions)

Adverse Reactions

Cardiovascular: Palpitations, bradycardia, chest pain, syncope, hypotension, atrial or ventricular arrhythmias

Central nervous system: Dizziness, confusion, ataxia

Dermatologic: Rash

Gastrointestinal: Nausea, vomiting, diarrhea

Hematologic: Rarely thrombocytopenia, leukopenia, agranulocytosis

Hepatic: Elevated liver enzymes, hepatitis

Neuromuscular & skeletal: Paresthesia, tremor

Ocular: Diplopia

Otic: Tinnitus

Respiratory: Dyspnea

Miscellaneous: Positive antinuclear antibody

Drug Interactions Cytochrome P450 isoenzyme CYP1A2 and CYP2D6 substrate; CYP1A2 isoenzyme inhibitor

Phenobarbital, phenytoin, rifampin, and other hepatic enzyme inducers may lower mexiletine plasma levels; cimetidine, fluvoxamine, and other enzyme inhibitors may increase mexiletine plasma levels; antacids, narcotics, or anticholinergics may decrease rate of absorption; metoclopramide may increase rate of absorption; drugs which affect urine pH can increase or decrease excretion of mexiletine; mexiletine may increase the serum concentrations of theophylline and caffeine

Food Interactions Food may decrease the rate, but not the extent of oral absorption; diets which affect urine pH can increase or decrease excretion of mexiletine; avoid dietary changes that alter urine pH

Mechanism of Action Class IB antiarrhythmic; structurally related to lidocaine; may cause increase in systemic vascular resistance and decrease in cardiac output; no significant negative inotropic effect

Pharmacodynamics Onset of action: Oral: 30-120 minutes

Pharmacokinetics

Distribution: V_d: 5-7 L/kg; found in breast milk in similar concentrations as plasma

Protein-binding: 50% to 70%

Metabolism: Extensive in the liver (some minor active metabolites)

Bioavailability: Oral: 88%

Half-life, adults: 10-14 hours; increase in half-life with hepatic or heart failure

Elimination: 10% to 15% excreted unchanged in urine; urinary acidification increases excretion

Usual Dosage Oral:

Children: Range: 1.4-5 mg/kg/dose (mean: 3.3 mg/kg/dose) given every 8 hours; start with lower initial dose and increase according to effects and serum concentrations

Adults: Initial: 200 mg every 8 hours (may load with 400 mg if necessary); adjust dose every 2-3 days; usual dose: 200-300 mg every 8 hours; some patients may respond to the same daily dose divided every 12 hours; maximum dose: 1.2 g/day

Dosing adjustment in renal impairment: Children and Adults: Cl_{cr} <10 mL/minute: Administer 50% to 75% of normal dose

Dosing adjustment in hepatic disease: Children and Adults: Administer 25% to 30% of normal dose; patients with severe liver disease may require even lower doses, monitor closely

Administration Oral: Administer with food, milk, or antacids to decrease GI upset

Monitoring Parameters Liver enzymes, CBC, EKG, heart rate, serum concentrations

(Continued)

Mexiletine *(Continued)*

Reference Range

Therapeutic range: 0.5-2 mcg/mL

Potentially toxic: >2 mcg/mL

Patient Information Limit caffeine; may cause dizziness; notify physician if persistent abdominal pain, nausea, vomiting, yellowing of the eyes or skin, pale stools, dark urine, fever, sore throat, bleeding, or bruising occurs

Additional Information I.V. form under investigation

Dosage Forms Excipient information presented when available (limited, particularly for generics); consult specific product labeling. [DSC] = Discontinued product

Capsule, as hydrochloride: 150 mg, 200 mg, 250 mg

Mexitil®: 150 mg, 200 mg, 250 mg [DSC]

Extemporaneous Preparations A 10 mg/mL oral suspension can be made using capsules and distilled water or sorbitol USP; grind the contents of eight 150 mg capsules to a powder in a mortar and pestle; then add a small amount of distilled water or sorbitol; mix to make a uniform paste; add distilled water or sorbitol in geometric amounts (while mixing) to **almost** 120 mL; transfer to a graduated cylinder and qsad 120 mL while mixing; suspension made with sorbitol is stable in plastic prescription bottles for 2 weeks at room temperature (25°C) and 4 weeks if refrigerated (4°C); suspension made with distilled water is stable in plastic prescription bottles for 7 weeks at room temperature (25°C) and 13 weeks if refrigerated (4°C); extended storage at 4°C is recommended to minimize microbial contamination; shake well before use

Nahata MC, Morosco RS, and Hipple TF, "Stability of Mexiletine in Two Extemporaneous Liquid Formulations Stored Under Refrigeration and at Room Temperature," *J Am Pharm Assoc*, 2000, 40(2):257-9.

References

Moak JP, Smith RT, and Garson A Jr, "Mexiletine: An Effective Antiarrhythmic Drug for Treatment of Ventricular Arrhythmias in Congenital Heart Disease," *J Am Coll Cardiol*, 1987, 10(4):824-9.

- **Mexitil® [DSC]** *see* Mexiletine *on page 1053*
- **MG 217® [OTC]** *see* Coal Tar *on page 394*
- **MG 217® Medicated Tar [OTC]** *see* Coal Tar *on page 394*
- **MG217 Sal-Acid® [OTC]** *see* Salicylic Acid *on page 1413*
- **$MgSO_4$ (error-prone abbreviation)** *see* Magnesium Sulfate *on page 974*
- **Miacalcin®** *see* Calcitonin *on page 258*
- **Miacalcin® NS (Can)** *see* Calcitonin *on page 258*
- **Mi-Acid [OTC]** *see* Antacid Preparations *on page 132*
- **Mi-Acid Maximum Strength [OTC]** *see* Antacid Preparations *on page 132*
- **Micaderm® [OTC]** *see* Miconazole *on page 1056*

Micafungin (mi ka FUN gin)

U.S. Brand Names Mycamine®

Index Terms Micafungin Sodium

Therapeutic Category Antifungal Agent, Echinocandin; Antifungal Agent, Systemic

Generic Available No

Use Treatment of patients with esophageal candidiasis; prophylaxis of *Candida* infections in patients undergoing hematopoietic stem cell transplant; treatment of invasive aspergillosis (unlabeled use)

Pregnancy Risk Factor C

Lactation Excretion in breast milk unknown/use caution

Contraindications Hypersensitivity to micafungin or any component

Warnings Cases of hypersensitivity reactions including anaphylactoid reactions and anaphylaxis with shock have been reported in patients who received micafungin; if reaction occurs, discontinue infusion and provide appropriate treatment. Rare cases of acute intravascular hemolysis, hemoglobinuria, and hemolytic anemia have been reported; monitor for evidence of worsening of these conditions.

Precautions Use with caution in patients with renal impairment, hepatic impairment, and in patients receiving concomitant hepatotoxic drugs; monitor for evidence of worsening function.

Adverse Reactions

Cardiovascular: Vasodilation, facial swelling, shock

Central nervous system: Fever, rigors, headache, dizziness, somnolence, delirium

Dermatologic: Rash, pruritus

Gastrointestinal: Nausea, vomiting, abdominal pain, diarrhea

Hematologic: Leukopenia, neutropenia, thrombocytopenia, anemia, lymphopenia, hemolytic anemia

Hepatic: Elevated alkaline phosphatase, AST, ALT, and blood LDH; hepatitis, hyperbilirubinemia

Local: Infusion site inflammation, phlebitis, thrombophlebitis (local reactions occur more frequently when micafungin is administered via peripheral line)

Renal: Elevated BUN and serum creatinine, acute renal failure

Respiratory: Epistaxis

Miscellaneous: Histamine-mediated reaction

Drug Interactions Cytochrome P450 isoenzyme CYP3A substrate and inhibitor (weak)

May increase serum concentration of sirolimus and nifedipine (monitor for sirolimus or nifedipine toxicity; sirolimus or nifedipine dosage reduction may be required)

Stability Store unopened vials at room temperature; reconstituted solution may be stored in the original vial for up to 24 hours at room temperature; diluted infusion may be stored for up to 24 hours at room temperature; protect from light.

Mechanism of Action Inhibits synthesis of beta (1,3)-D-glucan, an essential cell wall component of susceptible fungi, disrupting the cell wall structure and leading to osmotic stress and lysis of the fungal cell.

Pharmacokinetics

Distribution: Distributes into lung, liver, spleen, and kidney

Children 2-8 years: V_{dss}: 0.35 ± 0.18 L/kg

Children 9-17 years: V_{dss}: 0.28 ± 0.09 L/kg

Adults : V_d: 0.39 ± 0.11 L/kg

Protein binding: >99% to albumin

Metabolism: In the liver to M-1, catechol form by arylsulfatase; further metabolized to M-2, methoxy form by catechol-O-methyltransferase; hydroxylation to M-5 by CYP3A

Half-life:

Children 2-8 years: 11.6 ± 2.8 hours

Children 9-17 years: 13.3 ± 4.3 hours

Healthy Adults: 14-15 hours

Adults receiving bone marrow or peripheral stem-cell transplantation: 10.7-13.5 hours

Elimination: <15% of dose is eliminated unchanged renally; 40% is eliminated as parent drug and metabolites in the bile

Clearance:

Children 2-8 years: 0.385 ± 0.15 mL/minute/kg

Children 9-17 years: 0.285 ± 0.12 mL/minute/kg

Dialysis: Not dialyzable

Usual Dosage I.V.:

Neonates <1000 g: 8-10 mg/kg/dose once daily is currently under investigation

Neonates >1000 g: 5-7 mg/kg/dose once daily is currently under investigation

Infants and Children <2 years: 6 mg/kg/dose once daily

Children 2-8 years:

Treatment of esophageal candidiasis: 3 mg/kg/dose once daily; maximum daily dose: 150 mg

Prophylaxis of *Candida* infections in hematopoietic stem cell transplant recipients: 1-2 mg/kg/dose once daily; maximum daily dose: 50 mg

Treatment of invasive aspergillosis: 3-4 mg/kg/day once daily is currently under investigation

Children >8 years, Adolescents, and Adults:

Treatment of esophageal candidiasis: 150 mg once daily for 15 days (range:10-30 days)

Prophylaxis of *Candida* infections in hematopoietic stem cell transplant recipients: 50 mg once daily for 19 days (range: 6-51 days)

Treatment of invasive aspergillosis: 150 mg once daily dose is currently under investigation

Dosing adjustment in renal impairment: No adjustment needed

Dosing adjustment in hepatic impairment: No adjustment needed in mild-to-moderate hepatic impairment; the effect of severe hepatic impairment on micafungin pharmacokinetics has not been studied

Administration Parenteral: I.V.: Flush line with NS prior to administration. Infuse over one hour at a final concentration of 0.5-1.5 mg/mL in NS or D_5W; more rapid infusions may result in a higher incidence of histamine-mediated reactions. Do not coinfuse with other medications since precipitation may occur.

Reconstitute vial with NS or D_5W by gently dissolving powder by swirling the vial. Do **not** vigorously shake the vial. Further dilute the reconstituted solution in 100 mL of NS or D_5W or to a final concentration between 0.5-1.5 mg/mL.

Monitoring Parameters Periodic liver function tests, renal function tests, CBC with differential

(Continued)

Micafungin *(Continued)*

Nursing Implications
Infuse slowly over 1 hour; possible histamine-mediated reactions have been reported to occur with more rapid infusions.

Dosage Forms Excipient information presented when available (limited, particularly for generics); consult specific product labeling.

Injection, powder for reconstitution, as sodium [preservative-free]:
Mycamine®: 50 mg, 100 mg [contains lactose]

References

Antachopoulos C and Walsh TJ, "New Agents for Invasive Mycoses in Children," *Curr Opin Pediatr*, 2005, 17(1):78-87.

Carver PL, "Micafungin," *Ann Pharmacother*, 2004, 38(10):1707-21.

Heresi GP, Gerstmann DR, Reed MD, et al, "The Pharmacokinetics and Safety of Micafungin, a Novel Echinocandin, in Premature Infants," *Pediatr Infect Dis J*, 2006, 25(12):1110-5.

Seibel NL, Schwartz C, Arrieta A, et al, "Safety, Tolerability, and Pharmacokinetics of Micafungin (FK463) in Febrile Neutropenic Pediatric Patients," *Antimicrob Agents Chemother*, 2005, 49(8):3317-24.

van Burik JA, Ratanatharathorn V, Stepan DE, et al, "Micafungin Versus Fluconazole for Prophylaxis Against Invasive Fungal Infections During Neutropenia in Patients Undergoing Hematopoietic Stem Cell Transplantation," *Clin Infect Dis*, 2004, 39(10):1407-16.

♦ **Micafungin Sodium** *see* Micafungin *on page 1054*
♦ **Micatin® (Can)** *see* Miconazole *on page 1056*
♦ **Micatin® Athlete's Foot [OTC]** *see* Miconazole *on page 1056*
♦ **Micatin® Jock Itch [OTC]** *see* Miconazole *on page 1056*

Miconazole (mi KON a zole)

Medication Safety Issues
Sound-alike/look-alike issues:
Miconazole may be confused with Micronase®, Micronor®
Lotrimin® may be confused with Lotrisone®, Otrivin®
Micatin® may be confused with Miacalcin®

U.S. Brand Names Aloe Vesta® 2-n-1 Antifungal [OTC]; Baza® Antifungal [OTC]; Carrington Antifungal [OTC]; DermaFungal [OTC]; Dermagran® AF [OTC]; DiabetAid™ Antifungal Foot Bath [OTC]; Fungoid® Tincture [OTC]; Lotrimin® AF Jock Itch Powder Spray [OTC]; Lotrimin® AF Powder/Spray [OTC]; Micaderm® [OTC]; Micatin® Athlete's Foot [OTC]; Micatin® Jock Itch [OTC]; Micro-Guard® [OTC]; Mitrazol™ [OTC]; Monistat® 1 Combination Pack [OTC]; Monistat® 3 [OTC]; Monistat® 3 Combination Pack [OTC]; Monistat® 7 [OTC]; Monistat-Derm® [DSC]; Neosporin® AF [OTC]; Podactin Cream [OTC]; Secura® Antifungal [OTC]; Zeasorb®-AF [OTC]

Canadian Brand Names Dermazole; Micatin®; Micozole; Monistat®; Monistat® 3

Index Terms Miconazole Nitrate

Therapeutic Category Antifungal Agent, Topical; Antifungal Agent, Vaginal

Generic Available Yes

Use Treatment of vulvovaginal candidiasis; topical treatment of superficial fungal infections

Pregnancy Risk Factor C

Lactation Excretion in breast milk unknown/use caution

Contraindications Hypersensitivity to miconazole or any component; vaginal preparation should not be used in the first trimester of pregnancy unless the drug is essential to patient's welfare

Warnings The safety of miconazole in infants <1 year of age has not been established

Precautions Use with caution in patients allergic to other imidazole-derivative antifungals (eg, clotrimazole, econazole, ketoconazole)

Adverse Reactions
Central nervous system: Headache
Dermatologic: Maceration, urticaria, rash, pruritus, allergic contact dermatitis
Genitourinary: Pelvic cramps
Local: Irritation, burning, itching, phlebitis

Drug Interactions Cytochrome P450 isoenzyme CYP3A3/4 substrate; isoenzyme CYP2C, CYP3A3/4 (moderate), and CYP3A5-7 inhibitor
Enhanced hypoprothrombinemia with warfarin; oral sulfonylureas (severe hypoglycemia); may be antagonistic with amphotericin B; inhibits cisapride metabolism

Stability Store at room temperature

Mechanism of Action Inhibits biosynthesis of ergosterol, damaging the fungal cell wall membrane which increases permeability and causes leaking of nutrients

Pharmacokinetics
Absorption: Vaginal: Small amount absorbed systemically
Distribution: Into body tissues, joints, and fluids; poor penetration into sputum, saliva, urine, and CSF
Protein binding: 91% to 93%

Metabolism: In the liver
Half-life: Multiphasic degradation:
Alpha: 40 minutes
Beta: 126 minutes
Terminal: 24 hours
Elimination: ~50% excreted in feces and <1% in urine as unchanged drug

Usual Dosage

Infants, Children, Adolescents, and Adults: Topical:
Tinea pedis and tinea corporis: Apply twice daily for 4 weeks
Tinea cruris: Apply twice daily for 2 weeks

Adolescents and Adults:
Vaginal: Insert contents of 1 applicator of 2% vaginal cream or 100 mg vaginal suppository at bedtime for 7 days; or 1 applicator of 4% vaginal cream or 200 mg vaginal suppository at bedtime for 3 days; or 1200 mg vaginal suppository one-time dose at bedtime or during the day

Note: Many products are available as a combination pack (contains a suppository for vaginal instillation and external cream which is applied twice daily for up to 7 days to relieve external symptoms)

Administration For external use only.

Topical: Apply sparingly to the cleansed, dry affected area; if intertriginous areas are involved, rub cream gently into the skin

Vaginal: Wash hands before using; gently insert tablet or full applicator of cream high into vagina at bedtime. Wash applicator with soap and water following use. Remain lying down for 30 minutes following administration.

Monitoring Parameters Hematocrit, hemoglobin, serum electrolytes and lipids

Patient Information Avoid contact with the eyes; do not use vaginal cream or suppositories for self-medication if patient has abdominal pain, fever, or malodorous vaginal discharge; inform physician if abdominal pain, hives, skin rash, vaginal pruritus or discomfort occurs; avoid intercourse during therapy if using vaginal product. Condoms and diaphragms may not be effective if using vaginal product. Do not use tampons, douches, spermicides, or other vaginal products during treatment. Use deodorant-free sanitary napkins or pads instead.

Dosage Forms Excipient information presented when available (limited, particularly for generics); consult specific product labeling. [DSC] = Discontinued product

Combination products: Miconazole nitrate vaginal suppository 200 mg (3s) and miconazole nitrate external cream 2%
Monistat® 1 Combination Pack: Miconazole nitrate vaginal insert 1200 mg (1) and miconazole nitrate external cream 2% (5 g) [Note: Do not confuse with 1-Day™ (formerly Monistat® 1) which contains tioconazole]
Monistat® 3 Combination Pack:
Miconazole nitrate vaginal insert 200 mg (3s) and miconazole nitrate external cream 2%
Miconazole nitrate vaginal cream 4% and miconazole nitrate external cream 2%
Monistat® 7 Combination Pack:
Miconazole nitrate vaginal suppository 100 mg (7s) and miconazole nitrate external cream 2%
Miconazole nitrate vaginal cream 2% (7 prefilled applicators) and miconazole nitrate external cream 2%

Cream, topical, as nitrate: 2% (15 g, 30 g, 45 g)
Baza® Antifungal: 2% (4 g, 57 g, 142 g) [zinc oxide based formula]
Carrington Antifungal: 2% (150 g)
Micaderm®, Neosporin® AF, Podactin: 2% (30 g)
Micatin® Athlete's Foot, Micatin® Jock Itch: 2% (15 g)
Micro-Guard®, Mitrazol™: 2% (60 g)
Monistat-Derm®: 2% (15 g, 30 g, 85 g) [DSC]
Secura® Antifungal: 2% (60 g, 98 g)

Cream, vaginal, as nitrate [prefilled or refillable applicator]: 2% (45 g)
Monistat® 3: 4% (15 g, 25 g)
Monistat® 7: 2% (45 g)

Liquid, spray, topical, as nitrate:
Micatin® Athlete's Foot: 2% (90 mL) [contains alcohol]
Neosporin AF®: 2% (105 mL)

Lotion, powder, as nitrate (Zeasorb®-AF): 2% (56 g) [contains alcohol 36%]

Ointment, topical, as nitrate:
Aloe Vesta® 2-n-1 Antifungal: 2% (60 g, 150 g)
DermaFungal: 2% (113 g)
Dermagran® AF: (113 g) [contains vitamin A and zinc]

Powder, topical, as nitrate:
Lotrimin® AF: 2% (160 g)
Micro-Guard®: 2% (90 g)
Mitrazol™: 2% (30 g)

(Continued)

Miconazole *(Continued)*

Zeasorb®-AF: 2% (70 g)

Powder spray, topical, as nitrate:

Lotrimin® AF, Lotrimin® AF Jock Itch: 2% (140 g)

Micatin® Athlete's Foot, Micatin® Jock Itch: 2% (90 g) [contains alcohol]

Neosporin® AF: 2% (85 g)

Suppository, vaginal, as nitrate: 100 mg (7s); 200 mg (3s)

Monistat® 3: 200 mg (3s)

Monistat® 7: 100 mg (7s)

Tablet, for solution, topical, as nitrate [effervescent]:

DiabetAid™ Antifungal Foot Bath: 2% (10s)

Tincture, topical, as nitrate (Fungoid®): 2% (30 mL, 473 mL) [contains isopropyl alcohol 30%]; 30 mL size also available in a treatment kit which contains nail scrub and nail brush]

- **Miconazole Nitrate** *see* Miconazole *on page 1056*
- **Micozole (Can)** *see* Miconazole *on page 1056*
- **MICRhoGAM®** *see* Rh_0(D) Immune Globulin *on page 1374*
- **Micro-Guard® [OTC]** *see* Miconazole *on page 1056*
- **microK®** *see* Potassium Chloride *on page 1287*
- **microK® 10** *see* Potassium Chloride *on page 1287*
- **Micro-K Extencaps® (Can)** *see* Potassium Chloride *on page 1287*
- **Micronase®** *see* GlyBURIDE *on page 734*
- **Micronor®** *see* Norethindrone *on page 1148*
- **Microzide™** *see* Hydrochlorothiazide *on page 777*
- **Midamor® [DSC]** *see* Amiloride *on page 95*

Midazolam (MID aye zoe lam)

Medication Safety Issues

Sound-alike/look-alike issues:

Versed may be confused with VePesid®, Vistaril®

Related Information

Adult ACLS Algorithms *on page 1660*

Compatibility of Medications Mixed in A Syringe *on page 1941*

Overdose and Toxicology *on page 1916*

Preprocedure Sedatives in Children *on page 1895*

Canadian Brand Names Apo-Midazolam®; Midazolam Injection

Index Terms Midazolam Hydrochloride; Versed

Therapeutic Category Anticonvulsant, Benzodiazepine; Benzodiazepine; Hypnotic; Sedative

Generic Available Yes

Use Sedation, anxiolysis, amnesia prior to procedure or before induction of anesthesia; conscious sedation prior to diagnostic or radiographic procedures; continuous I.V. sedation of intubated and mechanically ventilated patients; status epilepticus

Restrictions C-IV

Pregnancy Risk Factor D

Lactation Enters breast milk/not recommended (AAP rates "of concern")

Contraindications Hypersensitivity to midazolam, any component (see Warnings), or cherries (syrup); cross-sensitivity with other benzodiazepines may occur; uncontrolled pain; existing CNS depression; shock; narrow-angle glaucoma

Warnings Midazolam may cause respiratory depression/arrest; deaths and hypoxic encephalopathy have resulted when these were not promptly recognized and treated appropriately; dose must be individualized and patients must be appropriately monitored; serious respiratory adverse events occur most often when midazolam is used in combination with other CNS depressants; personnel and equipment needed for standard respiratory resuscitation should be immediately available during midazolam use; a dedicated individual (other than the one performing the procedure) should monitor the deeply sedated pediatric patient throughout the procedure

Syrup contains sodium benzoate and injection may contain benzyl alcohol which may cause allergic reactions in susceptible individuals; large amounts of benzyl alcohol (≥99 mg/kg/day) have been associated with a potentially fatal toxicity ("gasping syndrome") in neonates; the "gasping syndrome" consists of metabolic acidosis, respiratory distress, gasping respirations, CNS dysfunction (including convulsions, intracranial hemorrhage), hypotension and cardiovascular collapse; avoid use of midazolam products containing benzyl alcohol or sodium benzoate in neonates; a benzyl alcohol free (preservative free) injection is available; *in vitro* and animal studies have shown that benzoate, a metabolite of benzyl alcohol, displaces bilirubin from protein binding sites

Precautions Use with caution in patients with CHF, renal impairment, pulmonary disease, hepatic dysfunction and in neonates (especially premature neonates); several cases of myoclonus have been reported in premature infants; benzodiazepine withdrawal may occur if abruptly discontinued in patients receiving prolonged I.V. continuous infusions; doses should be tapered slowly with prolonged use; do not administer by rapid I.V. injection (especially in neonates where severe hypotension and seizures have occurred after rapid I.V. administration)

Adverse Reactions

Cardiovascular: Cardiac arrest, hypotension, bradycardia

Central nervous system: Drowsiness, sedation, amnesia, dizziness, paradoxical excitement, hyperactivity, combativeness, headache, ataxia, rhythmic myoclonic jerking in preterm infants (~8% incidence), nystagmus

Gastrointestinal: Nausea, vomiting

Local:

I.M., I.V.: Pain and local reactions at injection site (severity less than diazepam)

Nasal: Burning, irritation, discomfort

Neuromuscular & skeletal: Tonic/clonic movements, muscle tremor

Ocular: Blurred vision, diplopia, lacrimation

Respiratory: Respiratory depression, oxygen desaturation, apnea, laryngospasm, bronchospasm, cough

Miscellaneous: Physical and psychological dependence with prolonged use, hiccups

Drug Interactions Cytochrome P450 isoenzyme CYP3A3/4 substrate

CNS depressants, alcohol may increase sedation and respiratory depression; narcotic agents may increase hypotension (especially in neonates); doses of anesthetic agents should be reduced when used in conjunction with midazolam; cimetidine, ranitidine, erythromycin, diltiazem, verapamil, fluconazole, ketoconazole, itraconazole may increase midazolam serum concentrations; theophylline may antagonize the sedative effects of midazolam; rifampin reduces the plasma concentration of oral midazolam by >90%; carbamazepine and phenytoin may increase hepatic metabolism of midazolam; protease inhibitors (indinavir, nelfinavir, ritonavir, saquinavir) and delavirdine may decrease midazolam's metabolism and increase midazolam serum concentrations; concurrent use of midazolam with protease inhibitors or delavirdine is not recommended. Long-term administration (≥2 weeks) of the herbal medicine St John's wort (*Hypericum perforatum*) may significantly decrease serum concentrations of oral midazolam (Wang, 2001).

Food Interactions Grapefruit juice delays the absorption and significantly increases bioavailability of oral midazolam

Stability Stable at a concentration of 0.5 mg/mL for 24 hours in D_5W or NS and for 4 hours in LR

Mechanism of Action Depresses all levels of the CNS, including the limbic and reticular formation, by binding to the benzodiazepine site on the gamma-aminobutyric acid (GABA) receptor complex and modulating GABA, which is a major inhibitory neurotransmitter in the brain

Pharmacodynamics Sedation:

Onset of action:

- Oral: Children: Within 10-20 minutes
- I.M.:
  - Children: Within 5 minutes
  - Adults: Within 15 minutes
- I.V.: Within 1-5 minutes
- Intranasal: Within 5 minutes

Maximum effect:

- I.M.:
  - Children: 15-30 minutes
  - Adults: 30-60 minutes
- I.V.: 5-7 minutes
- Intranasal: 10 minutes

Duration:

- I.M.: Mean: 2 hours, up to 6 hours
- I.V.: 20-30 minutes
- Intranasal: 30-60 minutes

Note: Full recovery may take more than 24 hours

Pharmacokinetics

Absorption: Oral, nasal: Rapid

Distribution: V_d:

- Preterm infants (n=24; GA: 26-34 weeks; PNA: 3-11 days): Median: 1.1 L/kg (range: 0.4-4.2 L/kg)
- Infants and Children 6 months to 16 years: 1.24-2.02 L/kg
- Adults: 1-3.1 L/kg

(Continued)

Midazolam *(Continued)*

Increased V_d with CHF and chronic renal failure; widely distributed in body including CSF and brain; crosses placenta; enters fetal circulation; crosses into breast milk

Protein binding: Children >1 year and Adults: 97%; primarily to albumin

Metabolism: Extensive in the liver via cytochrome P450 CYP3A4 enzyme; undergoes hydroxylation and then glucuronide conjugation; primary metabolite (alpha-hydroxy-midazolam) is active and equipotent to midazolam

Bioavailability: Oral: 15% to 45% (syrup: 36%); I.M.: >90%; intranasal: ~60%; rectal: ~40% to 50%

Half-life, elimination: Increased half-life with cirrhosis, CHF, obesity, elderly, and acute renal failure

Preterm infants (n=24; GA: 26-34 weeks; PNA: 3-11 days): Median: 6.3 hours (range: 2.6-17.7 hours)

Neonates: 4-12 hours; seriously ill neonates: 6.5-12 hours

Children: I.V.: 2.9-4.5 hours; syrup: 2.2-6.8 hours

Adults: 3 hours (range: 1.8-6.4 hours)

Elimination: 63% to 80% excreted as alpha-hydroxy-midazolam glucuronide in urine; ~2% to 10% in feces, <1% eliminated as unchanged drug in the urine

Clearance:

Preterm infants (n=24; GA: 26-34 weeks; PNA: 3-11 days): Median: 1.8 mL/minute/kg (range: 0.7-6.7 mL/minute/kg)

Neonates <39 weeks GA: 1.17 mL/minute/kg

Neonates >39 weeks GA: 1.84 mL/minute/kg

Seriously ill neonates: 1.2-2 mL/minute/kg

Infants >3 months: 9.1 mL/minute/kg

Children >1 year: 3.2-13.3 mL/minute/kg

Healthy adults: 4.2-9 mL/minute/kg

Adults with acute renal failure: 1.9 mL/minute/kg

Usual Dosage Dosage must be individualized and based on patient's age, underlying diseases, concurrent medications, and desired effect; decrease dose (by ~30%) if narcotics or other CNS depressants are administered concomitantly; use multiple small doses and titrate to desired sedative effect; allow 3-5 minutes between doses to decrease the chance of oversedation

Neonates:

Conscious sedation during mechanical ventilation: I.V. continuous infusion:

<32 weeks: Initial: 0.03 mg/kg/hour (0.5 mcg/kg/minute)

>32 weeks: Initial: 0.06 mg/kg/hour (1 mcg/kg/minute)

Note: Do not use I.V. loading doses in neonates; for faster achievement of sedation, infuse the continuous infusion at a faster rate for the first several hours; use the smallest dose possible

Infants >2 months and Children:

Status epilepticus refractory to standard therapy: I.V.: Loading dose: 0.15 mg/kg followed by a continuous infusion of 1 mcg/kg/minute; titrate dose upward every 5 minutes until clinical seizure activity is controlled; mean infusion rate required in 24 children was 2.3 mcg/kg/minute with a range of 1-18 mcg/kg/minute (Rivera, 1993)

Infants ≥6 months and Children:

Sedation, anxiolysis, and amnesia prior to procedure or before induction of anesthesia: Oral: Single dose; 0.25-0.5 mg/kg, depending on patient status and desired effect, usual: 0.5 mg/kg; maximum dose: 20 mg;

Patient-specific dosing:

Infants 6 months to <6 years, and less cooperative patients: Higher doses (up to 1 mg/kg) may be required

Children 6 to ≥16 years, or cooperative patients (especially if intensity and duration of sedation is less critical): 0.25 mg/kg may suffice

High risk pediatric patients (respiratory or cardiac compromised, concomitant CNS depressants, higher risk surgical patients): 0.25 mg/kg should be considered

Children:

Preoperative sedation or conscious sedation for procedures:

I.M.: Usual: 0.1-0.15 mg/kg 30-60 minutes before surgery or procedure; range: 0.05-0.15 mg/kg; doses up to 0.5 mg/kg have been used in more anxious patients; maximum total dose: 10 mg

I.V.:

Infants <6 months: Limited information is available in nonintubated infants; dosing recommendations are unclear; infants <6 months are at higher risk for airway obstruction and hypoventilation; titrate dose with small increments to desired clinical effect; monitor carefully

Infants 6 months to Children 5 years: Initial: 0.05-0.1 mg/kg; titrate dose carefully; total dose of 0.6 mg/kg may be required; usual total dose maximum dose: 6 mg

Children 6-12 years: Initial: 0.025-0.05 mg/kg; titrate dose carefully; total doses of 0.4 mg/kg may be required; usual total dose maximum: 10 mg

Children 12-16 years: Dose as adults; usual total dose maximum: 10 mg

Intranasal: Usual: 0.2 mg/kg; may repeat in 5-15 minutes; range: 0.2-0.3 mg/kg/dose

Conscious sedation during mechanical ventilation: I.V.: Continuous infusion: Loading dose: 0.05-0.2 mg/kg given slow I.V. over 2-3 minutes, then follow with initial continuous infusion: 0.06-0.12 mg/kg/hour (1-2 mcg/kg/minute); titrate to the desired effect; range: 0.4-6 mcg/kg/minute

Adults:

Preoperative sedation: I.M.: 0.07-0.08 mg/kg 30-60 minutes presurgery; usual dose: 5 mg

Conscious sedation: I.V.: Titrate dose slowly to desired effect; administer slowly over at least 2 minutes and wait another 2 or more minutes to evaluate effect. Some adults may respond to doses as low as 1 mg; do not give more than 2.5 mg over a period of 2 minutes. Titrate as needed, using small increments every 2-3 minutes. Usual total dose: 2.5-5 mg; total dose >5 mg is generally not needed; maintenance doses may be given by slow titration, if needed, in increments of 25% of the original dose used to reach sedative endpoint.

Conscious sedation during mechanical ventilation: I.V.: Optional loading dose: 0.01-0.05 mg/kg (~0.5-4 mg/dose); may repeat at 10- to 15-minute intervals until patient is adequately sedated, then begin continuous infusion

Continuous infusion: Initial: 0.02-0.1 mg/kg/hour (1-7 mg/hour); use lowest doses listed for patients receiving other sedatives, or opioids, or having residual anesthetic effects; titrate the infusion to achieve adequate level of sedation; use lowest effective dose

Administration

Intranasal: Administer using a 1 mL needleless syringe into the nares over 15 seconds; use the 5 mg/mL injection; ½ of the dose may be administered to each nare; **Note:** The 5 mg/mL injection has also been administered as a nasal spray using a graded pump device (see Ljungman, 2000)

Oral: Administer on empty stomach (feeding is usually contraindicated prior to sedation for procedures); do not administer with grapefruit juice

Parenteral:

I.V.: Administer by slow I.V. injection over at least 2-5 minutes at a concentration of 1-5 mg/mL (maximum concentration: 5 mg/mL) or by I.V. infusion; avoid extravasation; do not administer intra-arterially

I.M.: Maximum concentration: 1 mg/mL

Monitoring Parameters Level of sedation, respiratory rate, heart rate, blood pressure, oxygen saturation (ie, pulse oximetry)

Patient Information Report the use of other medications, nonprescription medications, and herbal or natural products to your physician and pharmacist; avoid alcohol; avoid grapefruit juice if taking oral midazolam

Nursing Implications Abrupt discontinuation after prolonged use may result in withdrawal symptoms

Additional Information Sodium content of injection: 0.14 mEq/mL. For Neonates: Since both concentrations of Versed® injection contain 1% benzyl alcohol, use the 5 mg/mL injection and dilute to 0.5 mg/mL with SWI without preservatives to decrease the amount of benzyl alcohol delivered to the neonate, or use preservative free injection. With continuous infusion, midazolam may accumulate in peripheral tissues; use lowest effective infusion rate to reduce accumulation effects. Midazolam is 3-4 times as potent as diazepam. Paradoxical reactions associated with midazolam use in children (eg, agitation, restlessness, combativeness) have been successfully treated with flumazenil (see Massanari, 1997)

Dosage Forms Excipient information presented when available (limited, particularly for generics); consult specific product labeling.

Injection, solution: 1 mg/mL (2 mL, 5 mL, 10 mL); 5 mg/mL (1 mL, 2 mL, 5 mL, 10 mL) [contains benzyl alcohol 1%]

Injection, solution [preservative free]: 1 mg/mL (2 mL, 5 mL); 5 mg/mL (1 mL, 2 mL)

Syrup: 2 mg/mL (118 mL) [contains sodium benzoate; cherry flavor]

References

Adrian ER, "Intranasal Versed®: The Future of Pediatric Conscious Sedation," *Pediatr Nurs*, 1994, 20(3):287-92.

Booker PD, Beechey A, and Lloyd-Thomas AR, "Sedation of Children Requiring Artificial Ventilation Using an Infusion of Midazolam," *Br J Anaesth*, 1986, 58(10):1104-8.

Burtin P, Jacqz-Aigrain E, Girard P, et al, "Population Pharmacokinetics of Midazolam in Neonates," *Clin Pharmacol Ther*, 1994, 56(6 Pt 1):615-25.

de Wildt SN, Kearns GL, Hop WC, et al, "Pharmacokinetics and Metabolism of Intravenous Midazolam in Preterm Infants," *Clin Pharmacol Ther*, 2001, 70(6):525-31.

(Continued)

Midazolam *(Continued)*

Jacqz-Algrain E, Daoud P, Burtin P, et al, "Placebo-Controlled Trial of Midazolam Sedation in Mechanically Ventilated Newborn Babies," *Lancet*, 1994, 344(8923):646-50.

Kupietzky A and Houpt MI, "Midazolam: A Review of Its Use for Conscious Sedation of Children," *Pediatr Dent*, 1993, 15(4):237-41.

Ljungman G, Kreuger A, Andreasson S, et al, "Midazolam Nasal Spray Reduces Procedural Anxiety in Children," *Pediatrics*, 2000, 105(1 Pt 1):73-8.

Lugo RA, Fishbein M, Nahata MC, et al, "Complication of Intranasal Midazolam," *Pediatrics*, 1993, 92(4):638.

Magny JF, Zupan V, Dehan M, et al, "Midazolam and Myoclonus in Neonate," *Eur J Pediatr*, 1994, 153(5):389-90.

Malinovsky JM, Populaire C, Cozian A, et al, "Premedication With Midazolam in Children, Effect of Intranasal, Rectal and Oral Routes on Plasma Midazolam Concentrations," *Anaesthesia*, 1995, 50(4):351-4.

Massanari M, Novitsky J, and Reinstein LJ, "Paradoxical Reactions in Children Associated With Midazolam Use During Endoscopy," *Clin Pediatr*, 1997, 36(12):681-4.

Riva J, Lejbusiewicz G, Papa M, et al, "Oral Premedication With Midazolam in Paediatric Anaesthesia. Effects on Sedation and Gastric Contents," *Paediatr Anaesth*, 1997, 7(3):191-6.

Rivera R, Segnini M, Baltodano A, et al, "Midazolam in the Treatment of Status Epilepticus in Children," *Crit Care Med*, 1993, 21(7):991-4.

Silvasi DL, Rosen DA, and Rosen KR, "Continuous Intravenous Midazolam Infusion for Sedation in the Pediatric Intensive Care Unit," *Anesth Analg*, 1988, 67(3):286-8.

Wang Z, Gorski JC, Hamman MA, et al, "The Effects of St John's Wort (*Hypericum perforatum*) on Human Cytochrome P450 Activity," *Clin Pharmacol Ther*, 2001, 70(4):317-26.

♦ **Midazolam Hydrochloride** *see* Midazolam *on page 1058*
♦ **Midazolam Injection (Can)** *see* Midazolam *on page 1058*
♦ **Midol® Cramp and Body Aches [OTC]** *see* Ibuprofen *on page 802*
♦ **Midol® Extended Relief** *see* Naproxen *on page 1108*
♦ **Migergot** *see* Ergotamine and Caffeine *on page 592*
♦ **Migranal®** *see* Dihydroergotamine *on page 500*
♦ **Mild-C® [OTC]** *see* Ascorbic Acid *on page 159*
♦ **Milk of Magnesia** *see* Magnesium Hydroxide *on page 971*
♦ **Milk of Magnesia (Magnesium Hydroxide)** *see* Magnesium Supplements *on page 976*

Milrinone (MIL ri none)

Medication Safety Issues
Sound-alike/look-alike issues:
Primacor® may be confused with Primaxin®

U.S. Brand Names Primacor®

Canadian Brand Names Milrinone Lactate Injection; Primacor®

Index Terms Milrinone Lactate

Therapeutic Category Phosphodiesterase Enzyme Inhibitor

Generic Available Yes

Use Short-term treatment of acute decompensated heart failure

Pregnancy Risk Factor C

Lactation Excretion in breast milk unknown

Contraindications Hypersensitivity to milrinone, any component, or inamrinone (amrinone)

Warnings Longer treatment of heart failure (>48 hours) has not been shown to be safe and effective (there are no controlled trials using milrinone infusions for >48 hours); long-term oral use for heart failure was associated with no improvement in symptoms, increased risk of hospitalization, and increased risk of sudden death; monitor EKG continuously to promptly detect and manage ventricular arrhythmias

Precautions Avoid use in patients with severe obstructive aortic or pulmonic valvular disease; use in patients with hypertrophic subaortic stenosis may increase outflow tract obstruction; use with caution in patients with a history of ventricular arrhythmias, atrial fibrillation, or atrial flutter; use with caution and modify dosage in patients with impaired renal function

Adverse Reactions
Central nervous system: Headaches (mild to moderate, 2.9%)
Cardiovascular: Ventricular arrhythmias (12.1%) including ventricular ectopic activity (8.5%), nonsustained ventricular tachycardia (2.8%), sustained ventricular tachycardia (1%), and ventricular fibrillation (0.2%); supraventricular arrhythmias (3.8%); hypotension (2.9%); angina/chest pain (1.2%); torsade de pointes (rare)
Dermatologic: Rash
Endocrine & metabolic: Hypokalemia (0.6%)
Hematologic: Thrombocytopenia (0.4%)
Hepatic: Abnormal liver function tests
Neuromuscular & skeletal: Tremor (0.4%)
Respiratory: Bronchospasm (rare)
Miscellaneous: Anaphylactic shock (rare)

Stability Incompatible with furosemide (a precipitate forms when furosemide is injected into I.V. lines containing milrinone); compatible with ½NS, NS, and D_5W

Mechanism of Action Inhibits phosphodiesterase III (PDE III), the major PDE in cardiac and vascular tissues. Inhibition of PDE III increases cyclic adenosine monophosphate (cAMP) which potentiates the delivery of calcium to myocardial contractile systems and results in a positive inotropic effect. Inhibition of PDE III in vascular tissue results in relaxation of vascular muscle and vasodilatation.

Pharmacodynamics Onset of action (improved hemodynamic function): Within 5-15 minutes

Pharmacokinetics

Distribution: V_d beta
- Infants (after cardiac surgery): 0.9 ± 0.4 L/kg
- Children (after cardiac surgery): 0.7 ± 0.2 L/kg
- Adults:
  - After cardiac surgery: 0.3 ± 0.1 L/kg
  - CHF (with single injection): 0.38 L/kg
  - CHF (with infusion): 0.45 L/kg

Protein binding: 70%

Half-life:
- Infants (after cardiac surgery): 3.15 ± 2 hours
- Children (after cardiac surgery): 1.86 ± 2 hours
- Adults:
  - After cardiac surgery: 1.69 ± 0.18 hours
  - CHF: 2.3-2.4 hours
- Renal impairment: Prolonged half-life

Elimination: Excreted in the urine as unchanged drug (83%) and glucuronide metabolite (12%)
- Clearance:
  - Infants (after cardiac surgery): 3.8 ± 1 mL/kg/minute
  - Children (after cardiac surgery): 5.9 ± 2 mL/kg/minute
  - Children (with septic shock): 10.6 ± 5.3 mL/kg/minute
  - Adults:
    - After cardiac surgery: 2 ± 0.7 mL/kg/minute
    - CHF: 2.2-2.3 mL/kg/minute
  - Renal impairment: Decreased clearance

Usual Dosage

Neonates, Infants, and Children: I.V.: A limited number of studies have used different dosing schemes (see Additional Information). Two recent pharmacokinetic studies propose per kg doses for pediatric patients with septic shock that are greater than those recommended for adults (Lindsay, 1998) and in infants and children after cardiac surgery (Ramamoorthy, 1998). Further pharmacodynamic studies are needed to define pediatric milrinone guidelines. Several centers are using the following guidelines:

Loading dose: 50 mcg/kg administered over 15 minutes followed by a continuous infusion of 0.5 mcg/kg/minute; range: 0.25-0.75 mcg/kg/minute; titrate dose to effect

PALS Guidelines 2000: I.V., I.O.: Loading dose: 50-75 mcg/kg administered over 15 minutes followed by a continuous infusion of 0.5-0.75 mcg/kg/minute

Adults: I.V.: Loading dose: 50 mcg/kg slow I.V. over 10 minutes, followed by a continuous infusion of 0.5 mcg/kg/minute; range: 0.375-0.75 mcg/kg/minute; titrate does to effect; maximum daily dose: 1.13 mg/kg/day

Dosing adjustment in renal impairment: For continuous infusion:
- Cl_{cr} 50 mL/minute/1.73 m^2: Administer 0.43 mcg/kg/minute
- Cl_{cr} 40 mL/minute/1.73 m^2: Administer 0.38 mcg/kg/minute
- Cl_{cr} 30 mL/minute/1.73 m^2: Administer 0.33 mcg/kg/minute
- Cl_{cr} 20 mL/minute/1.73 m^2: Administer 0.28 mcg/kg/minute
- Cl_{cr} 10 mL/minute/1.73 m^2: Administer 0.23 mcg/kg/minute
- Cl_{cr} 5 mL/minute/1.73 m^2: Administer 0.2 mcg/kg/minute

Administration

Loading dose: Administer slow I.V. push over 15 minutes for pediatric patients and over 10 minutes in adults; loading dose may be given as undiluted solution, but may dilute to 10-20 mL (in adults) for ease of administration.

I.V. continuous infusion: Dilute with ½NS, NS, or D_5W and administer via infusion pump or syringe pump; usual concentration: ≤200 mcg/mL; 250 mcg/mL in NS has been used (see Barton, 1996). **Note:** Some pediatric centers use a concentration of 500 mcg/mL but only if infused via a central line.

Monitoring Parameters Blood pressure, heart rate, cardiac output, CI, SVR, PVR, CVP, EKG, platelet count, serum potassium, renal function; clinical signs and symptoms of CHF

(Continued)

Milrinone *(Continued)*

Nursing Implications Do not administer furosemide I.V. push via "Y" site into milrinone solutions as precipitate will occur; decrease the infusion rate if significant hypotension occurs

Additional Information Dosing schemes and proposed dosing based on pharmacokinetic data:

Neonates: A loading dose of 50 mcg/kg administered over 15 minutes, followed by a continuous infusion of 0.5 mcg/kg/minute for 30 minutes in 10 neonates (3-27 days old, median age 5 days) improved hemodynamic parameters and was well tolerated (see Chang, 1995). Further neonatal studies of longer duration are needed.

Infants and children with septic shock: Twelve patients (9 months to 15 years of age) were administered a loading dose of 50 mcg/kg, followed by a continuous infusion of 0.5 mcg/kg/minute. At 1 hour after the loading dose, if patients did not respond (defined as a ≥20% increase in CI or an improvement in peripheral perfusion), an additional loading dose of 25 mcg/kg was given and the infusion rate was increased to 0.75 mcg/kg/minute. Nine of 12 patients required the additional loading dose and increased rate of infusion (see Barton 1996). A subsequent pharmacokinetic analysis of these patients recommended larger loading doses of 75 mcg/kg and infusion rates of 0.75-1 mcg/kg/minute. However, these doses were based on a one-compartment pharmacokinetic model and are higher then the mean infusion rate of 0.69 mcg/kg/minute used in the study (see Lindsay 1998). Further studies are needed.

Infants and Children after open heart surgery: A prospective, open-label trial compared a lower dose of milrinone (Group A) to a higher dose (Group B). Group A: Eleven patients received a loading dose of 25 mcg/kg given over 5 minutes followed by an infusion of 0.25 mcg/kg/minute; 30 minutes later, a second 25 mcg/kg loading dose was given and the infusion was increased to 0.5 mcg/kg/minute. Group B: 8 patients received a loading dose of 50 mcg/kg given over 10 minutes followed by an infusion of 0.5 mcg/kg/minute; 30 minutes later, a second loading dose of 25 mcg/kg was given and the infusion was increased to 0.75 mcg/kg/minute. Patients in both groups received a third loading dose of 25 mcg/kg if needed. A two-compartment model and NONMEM pharmacokinetic analyses were performed. Based on the NONMEM analysis, the authors propose the following doses: Infants: Loading dose: 104 mcg/kg and continuous infusion of 0.49 mcg/kg/minute; children: loading dose: 67 mcg/kg and continuous infusion of 0.61 mcg/kg/minute (see Ramamoorthy). Further studies are needed before these proposed doses can routinely be used in the pediatric population.

A double-blind placebo-controlled trial, compared low dose (loading dose: 25 mcg/kg given over 60 minutes followed by an infusion of 0.25 mcg/kg/minute for 35 hours) with high-dose (loading dose: 75 mcg/kg given over 60 minutes followed by an infusion of 0.75 mcg/kg/minute for 35 hours) milrinone for the prevention of low cardiac output syndrome in 227 pediatric patients, ranging in age from 2 days to 6.9 years (median age: 3 months). High-dose milrinone decreased the risk of low cardiac output syndrome by 48% (see Hoffman, 2003). Further studies are needed.

Dosage Forms Excipient information presented when available (limited, particularly for generics); consult specific product labeling. Available as milrinone lactate; mg strength refers to milrinone; [DSC] = Discontinued product.

Infusion [premixed in D_5W]: 200 mcg/mL (100 mL, 200 mL)
  Primacor®: 200 mcg/mL (100 mL [DSC], 200 mL)
Injection, solution: 1 mg/mL (10 mL, 20 mL, 50 mL)
  Primacor®: 1 mg/mL (10 mL, 20 mL)

References

Barton P, Garcia J, Kouatli A, et al, "Hemodynamic Effects of I.V. Milrinone Lactate in Pediatric Patients With Septic Shock. A Prospective Double-Blinded, Randomized, Placebo-Controlled, Interventional Study," *Chest*, 1996, 109(5):1302-12.

Chang AC, Atz AM, Wernovsky G, et al, "Milrinone: Systemic and Pulmonary Hemodynamic Effects in Neonates After Cardiac Surgery," *Crit Care Med*, 1995, 23(11):1907-14.

"Guidelines 2000 for Cardiopulmonary Resuscitation and Emergency Cardiovascular Care, Part 10: Pediatric Advanced Life Support, The American Heart Association in Collaboration With the International Liaison Committee on Resuscitation," *Circulation*, 2000, 102(8 Suppl): I291-342.

Hoffman TM, Wernovsky G, Atz AM, et al, "Efficacy and Safety of Milrinone in Preventing Low Cardiac Output Syndrome in Infants and Children After Corrective Surgery for Congenital Heart Disease," *Circulation*, 2003, 107(7):996-1002.

Hoffman TM, Wernovsky G, Atz AM, et al, "Prophylactic Intravenous Use of Milrinone After Cardiac Operation in Pediatrics (PRIMACORP) Study," *Am Heart J*, 2002, 143(1):15-21.

Lindsay CA, Barton P, Lawless S, et al, "Pharmacokinetics and Pharmacodynamics of Milrinone Lactate in Pediatric Patients With Septic Shock," *J Pediatr*, 1998, 132(2):329-34.

Ramamoorthy C, Anderson GD, Williams GD, et al, "Pharmacokinetics and Side Effects of Milrinone in Infants and Children After Open Heart Surgery," *Anesth Analg*, 1998, 86(2):283-9.

♦ **Milrinone Lactate** *see* Milrinone *on page 1062*

♦ **Milrinone Lactate Injection (Can)** *see* Milrinone *on page 1062*

Mineral Oil (MIN er al oyl)

U.S. Brand Names Fleet® Mineral Oil Enema [OTC]; Kondremul® [OTC]; Liqui-Doss® [OTC]

Index Terms Heavy Mineral Oil; Liquid Paraffin; White Mineral Oil

Therapeutic Category Laxative, Lubricant

Generic Available Yes: Oral oil

Use Temporary relief of constipation, to relieve fecal impaction, preparation for bowel studies or surgery

Pregnancy Risk Factor C

Contraindications Patients with a colostomy or an ileostomy, appendicitis, ulcerative colitis, diverticulitis, dysphagia or hiatal hernia

Warnings Oral form should be avoided in children <4 years of age because of the risk of aspiration

Adverse Reactions

Gastrointestinal: Nausea, vomiting, diarrhea, abdominal cramps, anal itching, anal seepage

Respiratory: Lipid pneumonitis with aspiration

Drug Interactions May impair absorption of fat-soluble vitamins, oral contraceptives, coumarin; increased absorption with docusate

Food Interactions May decrease absorption of fat-soluble vitamins, carotene, calcium, and phosphorus

Mechanism of Action Eases passage of stool by decreasing water absorption, softens stool, and lubricates the intestine

Pharmacodynamics Onset of action: ~6-8 hours

Pharmacokinetics

Absorption: Minimal following oral or rectal administration

Distribution: Into intestinal mucosa, liver, spleen, and mesenteric lymph nodes

Elimination: In feces

Usual Dosage

Children:

Oral: 5-11 years: 5-15 mL once daily or in divided doses; should not be used for longer than 1 week

Rectal: 2-11 years: 30-60 mL as a single dose

Children ≥12 years and Adults:

Oral: 15-45 mL/day once daily or in divided doses; should not be used for longer than 1 week

Rectal: Contents of one retention enema (range 60-150 mL)/day as a single dose

Administration

Oral: Nonemulsified mineral oil may be administered at bedtime on an empty stomach; emulsified mineral oil should be shaken before using; may be administered with meals (more palatable than nonemulsified mineral oil)

Rectal: Gently insert enema tip into rectum with a slight side-to-side movement with tip pointing toward the navel; have patient bear down

Monitoring Parameters Evacuation of stool; anal leakage indicates dose too high or need for disimpaction

Patient Information Do not take if experiencing abdominal pain, nausea, or vomiting. Rectal enema: Do not take if experiencing rectal bleeding

Dosage Forms Excipient information presented when available (limited, particularly for generics); consult specific product labeling.

Liquid, oral:

Liqui-Doss®: 13.5 mL/15 mL (480 mL) [self-emulsifying oily liquid; alcohol free, sugar free]

Microemulsion, oral:

Kondremul®: 2.5 mL/5 mL (480 mL) [sugar free; mint flavor]

Oil, rectal [enema]:

Fleet® Mineral Oil: 100% (118 mL)

Oil, oral: 100% (30 mL, 480 mL, 3840 mL)

References

Baker SS, Liptak GS, Colletti RB, et al, "A Medical Position Statement of the North American Society for Pediatric Gastroenterology and Nutrition; Constipation in Infants and Children: Evaluation and treatment," www.naspgn.org/constipation, 2000, 1-34.

♦ **Minipress®** *see* Prazosin *on page 1303*
♦ **Minirin® (Can)** *see* Desmopressin *on page 459*
♦ **Minitran™** *see* Nitroglycerin *on page 1141*
♦ **Minocin® (Can)** *see* Minocycline *on page 1066*
♦ **Minocin® PAC** *see* Minocycline *on page 1066*

Minocycline (mi noe SYE kleen)

Medication Safety Issues

Sound-alike/look-alike issues:

Dynacin® may be confused with Dyazide®, Dynabac®, DynaCirc®, Dynapen®

Minocin® may be confused with Indocin®, Lincocin®, Minizide®, Mithracin®, niacin

U.S. Brand Names Dynacin®; Minocin® PAC; myrac™; Solodyn™

Canadian Brand Names Alti-Minocycline; Apo-Minocycline®; Gen-Minocycline; Minocin®; Novo-Minocycline; PMS-Minocycline; Rhoxal-minocycline; Sandoz-Minocycline

Index Terms Minocycline Hydrochloride

Therapeutic Category Antibiotic, Tetracycline Derivative

Generic Available Yes: Excludes extended release tablet

Use Treatment of susceptible gram-negative and gram-positive infections, including *Burkholderia cepacia, Burkholderia mallei, Nocardia* species, *Stenotrophomonas maltophilia*; treatment of anthrax (inhalational, cutaneous, and gastrointestinal); inflammatory acne vulgaris; *Mycobacterium marinum* cutaneous infections; asymptomatic meningococcal carrier state; Rickettsial diseases (including Rocky Mountain spotted fever, typhus fever, Q fever); nongonococcal urethritis and gonorrhea

Pregnancy Risk Factor D

Lactation Enters breast milk/not recommended

Contraindications Hypersensitivity to minocycline, other tetracyclines, or any component; pregnancy; children ≤8 years unless safer, effective alternative is not available

Warnings Use of tetracyclines during tooth development may cause permanent discoloration of the teeth (yellow-gray to brown) and enamel hypoplasia; adult-onset tooth discoloration following long-term minocycline administration has also been reported. Do not administer to children <8 years of age due to permanent discoloration of teeth and retardation of skeletal development and bone growth (risk being greatest for children <4 years and in those receiving high doses). Minocycline has been associated with increases in BUN secondary to antianabolic effects. Pseudotumor cerebri has been reported rarely in infants and adolescents; use with isotretinoin has been associated with cases of pseudotumor cerebri; avoid concomitant treatment with isotretinoin. CNS effects (lightheadedness, vertigo) may occur; patients must be cautioned about performing tasks which require mental alertness. Photosensitivity reaction may occur; avoid prolonged exposure to sunlight or tanning equipment; discontinue if skin erythema occurs. Prolonged use may result in superinfection. Minocycline has been shown to be embryotoxic, fetal toxic, and impair fertility in animals.

Precautions Use with caution in patients with renal or hepatic impairment; consider dosage modification in patients with renal impairment

Adverse Reactions

Cardiovascular: Myocarditis, pericarditis, vasculitis

Central nervous system: Bulging fontanels, seizure, dizziness, fever, headache, pseudotumor cerebri, sedation, vertigo

Dermatologic: Alopecia, angioedema, epidermal necrolysis, erythema nodosum, rash, exfoliative dermatitis, hyperpigmentation of nails, photosensitivity, pruritus, Stevens-Johnson syndrome, erythema multiforme, skin hyperpigmentation (blue-black), urticaria

Endocrine & metabolic: Thyroid dysfunction, thyroid gland discoloration (brown-black)

Gastrointestinal: Nausea, vomiting, diarrhea, stomatitis, anorexia, dyspepsia, esophagitis, pancreatitis, pseudomembranous colitis, oral cavity discoloration, moniliasis

Genitourinary: Balanitis, vulvovaginitis

Hematologic: Agranulocytosis; eosinophilia, hemolytic anemia, leukopenia, neutropenia, pancytopenia, thrombocytopenia

Hepatic: Hepatic cholestasis, hepatic failure, hepatitis, hyperbilirubinemia, jaundice, elevated liver enzymes

Neuromuscular & skeletal: Paresthesia, hypoesthesia, arthralgia, arthritis, bone discoloration, joint stiffness, myalgia, injury to growing bones and teeth

Otic: Hearing loss, tinnitus

Renal: Acute renal failure, elevated BUN, interstitial nephritis

Respiratory: Asthma, bronchospasm, cough, dyspnea, pneumonitis, pulmonary infiltrates with eosinophilia

Miscellaneous: Anaphylaxis, systemic lupus erythematosus, serum sickness, enamel hypoplasia, tooth discoloration

Drug Interactions Minocycline may enhance the hypoprothrombinemic effect of warfarin; isotretinoin, retinoic acid derivatives, and vitamin A may increase risk of pseudotumor cerebri; methoxyflurane may produce nephrotoxicity; may reduce efficacy of penicillins and cephalosporins. Calcium-, magnesium-, or aluminum-containing antacids, bile acid sequestrants, bismuth, iron, zinc may decrease minocycline absorption. Minocycline may decrease efficacy of live, attenuated oral typhoid vaccine.

Food Interactions Administration with iron, calcium, milk or dairy products may decrease minocycline absorption; minocycline may decrease absorption of calcium, iron, magnesium and zinc.

Stability Store at room temperature; protect from light, moisture, and excessive heat

Mechanism of Action Inhibits bacterial protein synthesis by binding with the 30S and possibly the 50S ribosomal subunit(s) of susceptible bacteria

Pharmacokinetics

Absorption: Well absorbed

Distribution: Widely distributed to most body fluids, bile, and tissues; poor CNS penetration; deposits in fat for extended periods; crosses placenta; appears in breast milk

Protein binding: 55% to 88%

Bioavailability: 90%

Half-life: Adults: 17 hours (range:11-26 hours)

Time to peak serum concentration:

- Capsules and pellet filled capsules: 1-4 hours
- Tablet: 1-3 hours
- Extended release tablet: 3.5-4 hours

Elimination: 4% to 19% excreted in urine; 20% to 34% excreted in feces

Usual Dosage Oral:

Children >8 years: Initial: 4 mg/kg followed by 2 mg/kg/dose every 12 hours

Children ≥12 years and Adults: Inflammatory, non-nodular, moderate-to-severe acne:

- Extended release tablet:
- 45-59 kg: 45 mg once daily
- 60-90 kg: 90 mg once daily
- 91-136 kg: 135 mg once daily
- **Note:** Therapy should be continued for 12 weeks. Higher doses do not confer greater efficacy.

Adults: Infections: Initial: 200 mg, followed by 100 mg every 12 hours; maximum: 400 mg/day

- Acne: 50-100 mg once or twice daily
- Chlamydial or *Ureaplasma urealyticum* infection, uncomplicated: Urethral, endocervical, or rectal: 100 mg every 12 hours for at least 7 days
- Gonococcal infection, uncomplicated (males): Without urethritis or anorectal infection: Initial: 200 mg, followed by 100 mg every 12 hours for at least 4 days
- Gonococcal infection, uncomplicated urethritis: 100 mg every 12 hours for 5 days
- Asymptomatic meningococcal carrier state: 100 mg every 12 hours for 5 days
- *Mycobacterium marinum* cutaneous infection: 100 mg every 12 hours for 6-8 weeks (**Note:** Optimal dosing has not been established)
- Syphilis: Initial: 200 mg, followed by 100 mg every 12 hours for 10-15 days

Dosage adjustment in renal impairment: Consider decreasing dose or extending interval between doses; maximum dose: 200 mg/day (minocycline serum level may need to be monitored)

Administration Oral: Administer with adequate fluid to decrease the risk of esophageal irritation and ulceration. Administer tablets and pellet-filled capsule 1 hour before or 2 hours after meals; capsule and extended release tablet may be taken with or without food or milk

Monitoring Parameters Renal, hepatic and hematologic function tests

Test Interactions May cause interference with fluorescence test for urinary catecholamines (false elevation)

Patient Information May discolor nails, skin and teeth. May cause photosensitivity reactions (eg, exposure to sunlight may cause severe sunburn, skin rash, redness, or itching); avoid exposure to sunlight and artificial light sources (sunlamps, tanning booth/bed); wear protective clothing, wide-brimmed hats, sunglasses, and lip sunscreen (SPF ≥15); use a sunscreen [broad-spectrum sunscreen or physical sunscreen (preferred) or sunblock with SPF ≥15]; contact physician if reaction occurs. May cause lightheadedness/dizziness and impair ability to perform activities requiring mental alertness or physical coordination. Women of childbearing potential should be advised to avoid becoming pregnant.

Dosage Forms Excipient information presented when available (limited, particularly for generics); consult specific product labeling.

Capsule: 50 mg, 75 mg, 100 mg

- Dynacin®: 75 mg, 100 mg

Capsule, pellet filled: 50 mg, 100 mg

- Minocin® PAC: 50 mg, 100 mg [packaged with wipes, serum, and masque]

Tablet: 50 mg, 75 mg, 100 mg

- Dynacin®, myrac™: 50 mg, 75 mg, 100 mg

(Continued)

Minocycline *(Continued)*

Tablet, extended release:
Solodyn™: 45 mg, 90 mg, 135 mg

References

Sanchez AR, Rogers RS 3rd, and Sheridan PJ, "Tetracycline and Other Tetracycline-Derivative Staining of the Teeth and Oral Cavity," *Int J Dermatol*, 2004, 43(10):709-15.
Zouboulis CC and Piquero-Martin J, "Update and Future of Systemic Acne Treatment," *Dermatology*, 2003, 206(1):37-53.

- **Minocycline Hydrochloride** *see* Minocycline *on page 1066*
- **Minox (Can)** *see* Minoxidil *on page 1068*

Minoxidil (mi NOKS i dil)

Medication Safety Issues
Sound-alike/look-alike issues:
Minoxidil may be confused with metolazone, Monopril®, Noxafil®
International issues:
Noxidil® [Thailand] may be confused with Noxafil® which is a brand name for posaconazole in the U.S.

Related Information
Antihypertensive Agents by Class *on page 1678*

U.S. Brand Names Rogaine® Extra Strength for Men [OTC]; Rogaine® for Men [OTC]; Rogaine® for Women [OTC]

Canadian Brand Names Apo-Gain®; Minox; Rogaine®

Therapeutic Category Antihypertensive Agent; Vasodilator

Generic Available Yes

Use Management of severe hypertension; topically for management of alopecia or male pattern alopecia

Pregnancy Risk Factor C

Contraindications Hypersensitivity to minoxidil or any component; pheochromocytoma

Warnings May cause pericarditis, pericardial effusion and tamponade, angina, and sodium and water retention; use of minoxidil should be reserved for treatment of hypertension in patients who have not adequately responded to maximum doses of a diuretic and 2 other antihypertensive agents; minoxidil is usually used with a beta-blocker (to treat minoxidil-induced tachycardia) and a diuretic (for treatment of water retention/edema); avoid concomitant use of minoxidil with guanethidine (see Drug Interactions); minoxidil may rapidly control blood pressure; too rapid control of blood pressure may lead to syncope, CVA, MI, or ischemia

Precautions Use with caution in patients with coronary artery disease or with recent MI, pulmonary hypertension, significant renal dysfunction, CHF; renal failure or dialysis patients may require dosage reduction

Adverse Reactions
Cardiovascular: Edema, CHF, tachycardia, angina, pericardial effusion and tamponade, EKG changes
Central nervous system: Dizziness, fatigue, headache
Dermatologic: Hypertrichosis (commonly occurs within 1-2 months of therapy), coarsening facial features, dermatologic reactions, rash, Stevens-Johnson syndrome, photosensitivity
Endocrine & metabolic: Sodium and water retention, weight gain
Respiratory: Pulmonary hypertension, pulmonary edema

Drug Interactions Concurrent administration with guanethidine may cause profound orthostatic hypotensive effects; additive hypotensive effects with other hypotensive agents or diuretics

Food Interactions Avoid natural licorice (causes sodium and water retention and increases potassium loss)

Stability Store at controlled room temperature 20°C to 25°C (68°F to 77°F); topical 5% solution is flammable, keep away from fire or flame

Mechanism of Action Produces vasodilation by directly relaxing arteriolar smooth muscle, with little effect on veins; effects may be mediated by cyclic AMP; stimulation of hair growth is secondary to vasodilation, increased cutaneous blood flow and stimulation of resting hair follicles

Pharmacodynamics Hypotensive effects:
Onset of action: Oral: Within 30 minutes
Maximum effect: Within 2-8 hours
Duration: Up to 2-5 days

Pharmacokinetics
Metabolism: 88% primarily via glucuronidation
Protein-binding: None

Bioavailability: Oral: 90%
Half-life, adults: 3.5-4.2 hours
Elimination: 12% excreted unchanged in urine
Dialysis: Dialyzable (50% to 100%)

Usual Dosage
Hypertension: Oral:
Children <12 years: Initial: 0.1-0.2 mg/kg once daily; maximum dose: 5 mg/day; increase gradually every 3 days; usual dosage: 0.25-1 mg/kg/day in 1-2 divided doses; maximum dose: 50 mg/day
Children >12 years and Adults: Initial: 5 mg once daily, increase gradually every 3 days; usual dose: 10-40 mg/day in 1-2 divided doses; maximum dose: 100 mg/day; **Note:** Usual dosage range for Adolescents ≥18 years and Adults (JNC 7): 2.5-80 mg/day in 1-2 divided doses
Alopecia: Adults: Topical: Apply twice daily

Administration Oral: May be administered without regard to food

Monitoring Parameters Fluids and electrolytes, body weight, blood pressure

Patient Information May cause dizziness; rise slowly from prolonged lying or sitting position. May cause photosensitivity reactions (eg, exposure to sunlight may cause severe sunburn, skin rash, redness, or itching); avoid exposure to sunlight and artificial light sources (sunlamps, tanning booth/bed); wear protective clothing, wide-brimmed hats, sunglasses, and lip sunscreen (SPF ≥15); use a sunscreen [broad-spectrum sunscreen or physical sunscreen (preferred) or sunblock with SPF ≥15]; contact physician if reaction occurs.

Additional Information May take 1-6 months for hypertrichosis to totally reverse after oral minoxidil therapy is discontinued

Dosage Forms Excipient information presented when available (limited, particularly for generics); consult specific product labeling.
Aerosol, topical [foam]:
Men's Rogaine®: 5% (60 g)
Solution, topical: 2% (60 mL); 5% (60 mL)
Rogaine® for Men, Rogaine® for Women: 2% (60 mL) [supplied with dropper applicator]
Rogaine® Extra Strength for Men: 5% (60 mL) [supplied with dropper applicator]
Tablet: 2.5 mg, 10 mg

References

Chobanian AV, Bakris GL, Black HR, et al, "The Seventh Report of the Joint National Committee on Prevention, Detection, Evaluation, and Treatment of High Blood Pressure: The JNC 7 report," *JAMA*, 2003, 289(19):2560-72.

◆ **Mintab DM** *see* Guaifenesin and Dextromethorphan *on page 748*
◆ **Mintezol®** *see* Thiabendazole *on page 1525*
◆ **Mintox Extra Strength [OTC]** *see* Antacid Preparations *on page 132*
◆ **Mintox Plus [OTC]** *see* Antacid Preparations *on page 132*
◆ **Miochol®-E** *see* Acetylcholine *on page 50*
◆ **MiraLax™** *see* Polyethylene Glycol-Electrolyte Solution *on page 1277*

Misoprostol (mye soe PROST ole)

Medication Safety Issues
Sound-alike/look-alike issues:
Misoprostol may be confused with metoprolol
Cytotec® may be confused with Cytoxan®, Sytobex®

U.S. Brand Names Cytotec®

Canadian Brand Names Apo-Misoprostol®; Novo-Misoprostol

Therapeutic Category Gastrointestinal Agent, Gastric Ulcer Treatment; Prostaglandin

Generic Available Yes

Use Prevention of NSAID-induced gastric ulcers; improvement in fat absorption in cystic fibrosis patients when used in conjunction with pancreatic enzyme supplements (unlabeled use)

Pregnancy Risk Factor X

Lactation Excretion in breast milk unknown/contraindicated

Contraindications Hypersensitivity to misoprostol or any component; pregnancy

Warnings Not to be used for reducing the risk of NSAID-induced ulcers in pregnant women or women of childbearing potential unless the woman is capable of complying with effective contraceptive measures; women should have a negative serum pregnancy test within 2 weeks prior to initiating therapy with therapy begun on the second or third day of next menstrual period; may cause abortion, premature labor, or birth defects if given to pregnant women
(Continued)

Misoprostol *(Continued)*

Precautions Use with caution in patients with inflammatory bowel disease (due to potential for development of diarrhea with misoprostol) and renal impairment

Adverse Reactions

Cardiovascular: Chest pain, hypotension, hypertension, arrhythmia, MI, syncope; thromboembolism events including pulmonary embolism, arterial thrombosis, and CVA

Central nervous system: Headache, fever, anxiety, depression, drowsiness, dizziness, confusion

Dermatologic: Rash, dermatitis, alopecia

Endocrine & metabolic: Glycosuria, gout

Gastrointestinal: Nausea, vomiting, constipation, flatulence, diarrhea, abdominal pain, dyspepsia, GI bleeding, GI inflammation, abnormal taste

Genitourinary: Uterine stimulation, cramps, vaginal bleeding, menstrual irregularities, uterine rupture (when taken after the eighth week of pregnancy), polyuria, dysuria, urinary tract infection

Hematologic: Anemia, thrombocytopenia, purpura

Neuromuscular & skeletal: Arthralgia, myalgia, back pain

Ophthalmologic: Conjunctivitis

Otic: Tinnitus, earache

Miscellaneous: Hypersensitivity reactions

Drug Interactions Magnesium containing antacids enhance diarrhea associated with misoprostol

Food Interactions Misoprostol peak serum concentrations may be decreased if taken with food (not clinically significant)

Mechanism of Action Misoprostol, a gastric antisecretory agent, is a synthetic prostaglandin E_1 analog that replaces the protective prostaglandins consumed with prostaglandin-inhibiting therapies (eg, NSAIDs) resulting in reduction of acid secretion from the gastric parietal cell and stimulation of bicarbonate production from the gastric and duodenal mucosa

Pharmacodynamics Inhibition of gastric acid secretion:

Onset of action: 30 minutes

Maximum effect: 60-90 minutes

Duration: 3 hours

Pharmacokinetics

Absorption: Rapid

Protein binding (misoprostol acid): 80% to 90%

Metabolism: Extensive "first pass" de-esterification to misoprostol acid (active metabolite)

Bioavailability: 88%

Half-life (metabolite): Terminal: 20-40 minutes

Time to peak serum concentration (active metabolite): Within 15-30 minutes

Elimination: In urine (64% to 73% in 24 hours) and feces (15% in 24 hours)

Usual Dosage Oral:

Prevention of NSAID-induced ulcers: Adults: 200 mcg 4 times/day; if not tolerated, may decrease dose to 100 mcg 4 times/day or 200 mcg twice daily; take for the duration of NSAID therapy

Improvement of fat malabsorption in cystic fibrosis (limited data available in children): Children 8-16 years: 100 mcg four times daily

Administration Oral: Administer after meals and at bedtime

Patient Information May initially cause diarrhea which usually resolves after 8 days of therapy; avoid taking with magnesium-containing antacids; do not take if you are pregnant

Nursing Implications Incidence of diarrhea may be lessened by having patient take dose right after meals

Dosage Forms Excipient information presented when available (limited, particularly for generics); consult specific product labeling.

Tablet: 100 mcg, 200 mcg

References

Cleghorn GJ, Shepherd RW, and Holt TL, "The Use of a Synthetic Prostaglandin E1 Analogue (Misoprostol) as an Adjunct to Pancreatic Enzyme Replacement in Cystic Fibrosis," *Scand J Gastroenterol Suppl*, 1988, 143:142-7.

Robinson PJ, Smith AL, and Sly PD, "Duodenal pH in Cystic Fibrosis and Its Relationship to Fat Malabsorption," *Dig Dis Sci*, 1990, 35(10):1299-304.

Mitomycin (mye toe MYE sin)

Medication Safety Issues

Sound-alike/look-alike issues:

Mitomycin may be confused with mithramycin, mitotane, mitoxantrone

High alert medication: The Institute for Safe Medication Practices (ISMP) includes this medication among its list of drugs which have a heightened risk of causing significant patient harm when used in error.

Related Information

Compatibility of Chemotherapy and Related Supportive Care Medications *on page 1777*
Emetogenic Potential of Single Chemotherapeutic Agents *on page 1776*

U.S. Brand Names Mutamycin®

Canadian Brand Names Mutamycin®

Index Terms Mitomycin-C; Mitomycin-X; MTC; NSC-26980

Therapeutic Category Antineoplastic Agent, Antibiotic

Generic Available Yes

Use Therapy of disseminated adenocarcinoma of stomach, colon, or pancreas in combination with other approved chemotherapeutic agents; bladder cancer, breast cancer

Pregnancy Risk Factor D

Lactation Enters breast milk/contraindicated

Contraindications Hypersensitivity to mitomycin or any component; platelet counts <75,000/mm^3; leukocyte counts <3000/mm^3 or serum creatinine >1.7 mg/dL; coagulation disorders; pregnancy

Warnings The FDA currently recommends that procedures for proper handling and disposal of antineoplastic agents be considered. Bone marrow suppression, notably thrombocytopenia and leukopenia, may contribute to the development of a secondary infection; hemolytic uremic syndrome, a serious and often fatal syndrome consisting of microangiopathic hemolytic anemia, thrombocytopenia, and irreversible renal failure has occurred in patients receiving systemic therapy; the risk of hemolytic uremic syndrome increases with a total cumulative dose >50 mg/m^2; mitomycin is potentially mutagenic and teratogenic.

Precautions Use with caution in patients with myelosuppression, impaired renal or hepatic function; modify dosage in patients with myelosuppression or renal impairment

Adverse Reactions

Cardiovascular: CHF (rare)
Central nervous system: Fever, headache, confusion
Dermatologic: Alopecia, pruritus
Gastrointestinal: Nausea, vomiting, mouth ulcers, diarrhea, anorexia
Hematologic: Bone marrow suppression (leukopenia, thrombocytopenia), microangiopathic hemolytic anemia
Hepatic: Veno-occlusive disease
Local: Thrombophlebitis; necrosis and sloughing of tissue with extravasation
Neuromuscular & skeletal: Paresthesia, weakness
Renal: Hemolytic uremic syndrome, nephrotoxicity, elevated serum creatinine
Respiratory: Pulmonary toxicity, interstitial pneumonia, bronchospasm, dyspnea, cough

Drug Interactions Anthracyclines (may enhance cardiotoxicity)

Stability Store intact vials at room temperature; protect from light; reconstitute vial with SWI to a concentration of 0.5 mg/mL; the reconstituted solution must be protected from light if not used within 24 hours; stable for 7 days at room temperature and 14 days when refrigerated; I.V. infusion in D_5W is stable for 3 hours at room temperature; in NS solution is stable for 12 hours at room temperature; physically compatible with ondansetron for 4 hours

Mechanism of Action Inhibits DNA and RNA synthesis by alkylating and cross-linking the strands of DNA

Pharmacokinetics

Distribution: Into bile and ascites fluid; high drug concentrations found in kidney, muscle, heart, and lung tissue
Metabolism: Primarily hepatic with metabolism also occurring in other tissues
Half-life, terminal: 50 minutes
Elimination: Primarily by hepatic metabolism followed by urinary excretion (<10% as unchanged drug) and to a small extent biliary excretion

Nadir After Prior Dose/mm^3		% of Prior Dose to Be Given
Leukocytes	Platelets	
4000	>100,000	100
3000-3999	75,000-99,999	100
2000-2999	25,000-74,999	70
2000	<25,000	50

(Continued)

Mitomycin *(Continued)*

Usual Dosage Children and Adults: I.V. (refer to individual protocols): 10-20 mg/m^2/dose every 6-8 weeks, or 3 mg/m^2/day for 5 days every 4-6 weeks; subsequent doses should be adjusted to platelet and leukocyte response; see table on previous page. Very high doses (40-50 mg/m^2 as a single dose) have been administered by hepatic artery infusion followed by autologous bone marrow transplantation.

Dosing adjustment in renal impairment: Cl_{cr} <10 mL/minute: Administer 75% of normal dose

Administration Parenteral: Administer by short I.V. infusion over 30-60 minutes or by slow I.V. push over 5-10 minutes through a Y-site of a running I.V.; short I.V. infusions are usually administered at a final concentration of 20-40 mcg/mL (in 50-250 mL of D_5W or NS); I.V. slow push can be administered at a concentration not to exceed 0.5 mg/mL

Monitoring Parameters Platelet count, CBC with differential, hemoglobin, prothrombin time, renal and pulmonary function tests; observe I.V. injection site for infiltration and vein irritation

Patient Information Notify physician if fever, sore throat, bruising, bleeding, shortness of breath, or painful urination occur

Nursing Implications Care should be taken to avoid extravasation since ulceration and tissue sloughing can occur; mitomycin extravasation has been treated using a 99% (w/v) solution of dimethylsulfoxide (DMSO); apply 1.5 mL to the site every 6 hours for 14 days; allow to air-dry; do not cover

Additional Information Bladder fibrosis/contraction which in rare cases required cystectomy has been reported with intravesical administration of mitomycin (non-FDA approved route of administration).

Myelosuppressive effects:

WBC: Moderate
Platelets: Severe
Onset (days): 21
Nadir (days): 36
Recovery (days): 42-56

Dosage Forms Excipient information presented when available (limited, particularly for generics); consult specific product labeling.

Injection, powder for reconstitution: 5 mg, 20 mg, 40 mg

References

Alberts DS and Dorr RT, "Case Report: Topical DMSO for Mitomycin C-Induced Skin Ulceration," *Oncol Nurs Forum*, 1991, 18(4):693-5.

◆ **Mitomycin-X** *see* Mitomycin *on page 1070*

◆ **Mitomycin-C** *see* Mitomycin *on page 1070*

Mitoxantrone (mye toe ZAN trone)

Medication Safety Issues

Sound-alike/look-alike issues:

Mitoxantrone may be confused with methotrexate, mitomycin

High alert medication: The Institute for Safe Medication Practices (ISMP) includes this medication among its list of drugs which have a heightened risk of causing significant patient harm when used in error.

Related Information

Compatibility of Chemotherapy and Related Supportive Care Medications *on page 1777*

Emetogenic Potential of Single Chemotherapeutic Agents *on page 1776*

U.S. Brand Names Novantrone®

Canadian Brand Names Mitoxantrone Injection®; Novantrone®

Index Terms DAD; DHAD; DHAQ; Dihydroxyanthracenedione Dihydrochloride; Mitoxantrone Hydrochloride CL-232315; Mitozantrone; NSC-301739

Therapeutic Category Antineoplastic Agent, Anthracenedione; Antineoplastic Agent, Antibiotic

Generic Available Yes

Use For remission-induction therapy of acute nonlymphocytic leukemia (ANLL) and acute myelogenous leukemia (AML); mitoxantrone is also active against other leukemias, lymphoma, breast cancer, and moderately active against pediatric sarcoma; initial chemotherapy for patients with pain related to advanced hormone refractory prostate cancer; reducing neurologic disability and/or frequency of clinical relapses in patients with secondary progressive, progressive relapsing, or worsening relapsing-remitting multiple sclerosis

Pregnancy Risk Factor D (may cause fetal harm when administered to a pregnant woman)

Lactation Enters breast milk/contraindicated

Contraindications Hypersensitivity to mitoxantrone or any component; patients with multiple sclerosis who have hepatic impairment, baseline left ventricular ejection fraction (LVEF) <50%, cumulative lifetime mitoxantrone dose ≥140 mg/m^2, or neutrophil counts <1500 cells/mm^3 should not receive mitoxantrone; pregnancy; discontinue breast-feeding before starting mitoxantrone

Warnings Mitoxantrone can cause severe myelosuppression (avoid in patients with pre-existing myelosuppression); mitoxantrone has been associated with cardiotoxicity which can occur at any time during therapy or years after therapy termination. The predisposing factors for mitoxantrone-induced cardiotoxicity include prior anthracycline therapy, prior cardiovascular disease, concomitant use of other cardiotoxic drugs, and mediastinal irradiation. The risk of developing cardiotoxicity is <3% when the cumulative mitoxantrone dose is <140 mg/m^2; baseline LVEF by ECG or multigated radionuclide angiography (MUGA) should be performed and re-evaluated prior to each dose of mitoxantrone administered to patients with multiple sclerosis. Interstitial pneumonitis has been reported in patients receiving combination chemotherapy that included mitoxantrone; extravasation can result in tissue necrosis with resultant need for debridement and skin grafting

The FDA currently recommends that procedures for proper handling and disposal of antineoplastic agents be considered. Secondary acute myelogenous leukemia has been reported in patients treated with mitoxantrone (monitor CBC, platelet count; signs and symptoms of infection prior to each course and after discontinuation of mitoxantrone); occurrence of secondary leukemia is more common when anthracyclines are given in combination with DNA-damaging agents, when patients have been heavily pretreated with cytotoxic drugs, or when anthracycline doses have been escalated. Intrathecal administration is not recommended since local nerve demyelinization, seizures, coma, and paraplegia have been reported with this route.

Precautions Dosage should be reduced in patients with pre-existing bone marrow suppression, previous treatment with cardiotoxic agents, and patients with impaired hepatobiliary function

Adverse Reactions

Cardiovascular: Cardiotoxicity (arrhythmias, CHF), hypotension, tachycardia, cardiomyopathy

Central nervous system: Seizures, headache

Dermatologic: Alopecia, pruritus, skin desquamation, rash, discoloration of skin (blue-green)

Endocrine & metabolic: Menstrual disorder, amenorrhea

Gastrointestinal: Nausea, diarrhea, vomiting, stomatitis (occurs more frequently with "daily times 3 day" regimens than once every 3 week schedules), mucositis, constipation

Genitourinary: Discoloration of urine (blue-green)

Hematologic: Myelosuppression (leukopenia, neutropenia, pancytopenia), mild anemia, thrombocytopenia

Hepatic: Transient elevation of liver enzymes, jaundice

Local: Phlebitis, tissue necrosis with extravasation

Respiratory: Interstitial pneumonitis, dyspnea

Miscellaneous: Anaphylaxis

Drug Interactions Cytochrome P450 isoenzyme CYP2E1 inducer (weak)

High-dose cytarabine (therapeutic synergy)

Stability After penetration of the stopper, undiluted mitoxantrone solution is stable for 7 days at room temperature or 14 days when refrigerated; incompatible with heparin; physically compatible with ondansetron for at least 4 hours

Mechanism of Action Inhibits DNA and RNA synthesis by intercalating with DNA and causing template disordering and steric obstruction; replication is decreased by binding to DNA topoisomerase II (enzyme responsible for DNA helix supercoiling); active throughout entire cell cycle. Mitoxantrone inhibits B cell, T cell, and macrophage proliferation; impairs antigen presentation and secretion of interferon gamma, TNF_{α}, IL-2.

Pharmacokinetics

Distribution: Distributes into thyroid, liver, pancreas, spleen, heart, bone marrow, and red blood cells; prolonged retention in tissues; excreted in breast milk

V_{dss} Adults: >1000 L/m^2

Protein binding: 78%

Half-life, terminal: Adults: 23-215 hours (median: 75 hours); may be prolonged with liver impairment

Elimination: 11% of dose excreted in urine (65% as unchanged drug) and 25% in bile as unchanged drug and metabolites

Usual Dosage I.V. (refer to individual protocols):

Leukemias:

Children ≤2 years: 0.4 mg/kg/day once daily for 3-5 days

(Continued)

Mitoxantrone *(Continued)*

Children >2 years and Adults: 12 mg/m²/day once daily for 2-3 days; acute leukemia in relapse: 8-12 mg/m²/day once daily for 4-5 days; ANLL: 10 mg/m²/day once daily for 3-5 days

Solid tumors:

Children: 18-20 mg/m² once every 3-4 weeks

Adults: 12-14 mg/m² once every 3-4 weeks

Multiple sclerosis: Adults: 12 mg/m²/dose every 3 months; maximum cumulative dose: 140 mg/m²

Dosing adjustment in hepatic impairment: Although official dosage adjustment recommendations have not been established, dosage reduction of 50% in patients with serum bilirubin of 1.5-3 mg/dL and dosage reduction of 75% in patients with serum bilirubin >3 mg/dL have been recommended

Administration **Do not administer by SubQ, I.M., intrathecal, or intra-arterial injection** (intra-arterial injection has resulted in local/regional neuropathy; seizures, coma, paralysis with bowel and bladder dysfunction, and neurotoxicity have been reported following intrathecal injection of mitoxantrone).

Parenteral: I.V.: Do **not** administer I.V. push over <3 minutes; may administer by I.V. bolus over 5-15 minutes, I.V. intermittent infusion over 15-60 minutes or I.V. continuous infusion at a concentration of 0.02-0.5 mg/mL in D_5W or NS

Monitoring Parameters CBC with differential, platelet count, serum uric acid, liver function tests, echocardiogram with monitoring of left ventricular ejection fraction at baseline and prior to each dose; signs or symptoms of CHF; women with multiple sclerosis of childbearing potential must have a pregnancy test prior to each dose; injection site for signs of extravasation

Patient Information May discolor skin, sclera, tears, sweat, and urine to a blue-green color; women of child-bearing potential should be advised to avoid becoming pregnant; contraceptive measures are recommended during therapy; do not breast-feed. Notify physician if fever, chills, sore throat, cough, pain with urinating, trouble breathing, swelling of legs or ankles, uneven or fast heartbeat, unusual bleeding or bruising occurs.

Nursing Implications Mitoxantrone is a nonvesicant; if extravasation occurs, the drug should be discontinued and restarted in another vein; extravasation may result in erythema, swelling, pain, burning, and/or a blue discoloration of the skin. If extravasation occurs, place ice pack over the affected area and elevate extremity.

Additional Information Myelosuppression (leukocyte nadir: 10-14 days; recovery: 21 days); injection contains 0.14 mEq of sodium/mL

Dosage Forms Excipient information presented when available (limited, particularly for generics); consult specific product labeling.

Injection, solution: 2 mg/mL (10 mL, 12.5 mL, 15 mL)

Novantrone®: 2 mg/mL (10 mL, 12.5 mL, 15 mL)

References

Koeller J and Eble M, "Mitoxantrone: A Novel Anthracycline Derivative," *Clin Pharm*, 1988, 7(8):574-81.

Pratt CB, Vietti TJ, Etcubanas E, et al, "Novantrone® for Childhood Malignant Solid Tumors. A Pediatric Oncology Group Phase II Study," *Invest New Drugs*, 1986, 4(1):43-8.

Stevens RF, Hann IM, Wheatley K, et al, "Marked Improvements in Outcome With Chemotherapy Alone in Paediatric Acute Myeloid Leukemia: Results of the United Kingdom Medical Research Council's 10th AML Trial. MRC Childhood Leukaemia Working Party," *Br J Haematol*, 1998, 101(1):130-40.

Wells RJ, Adams MT, Alonzo TA, et al, "Mitoxantrone and Cytarabine Induction, High-Dose Cytarabine, and Etoposide Intensification for Pediatric Patients With Relapsed or Refractory Acute Myeloid Leukemia: Children's Cancer Group Study 2951," *J Clin Oncol*, 2003, 21(15):2940-7.

♦ **Mitoxantrone Hydrochloride CL-232315** *see* Mitoxantrone *on page 1072*

♦ **Mitoxantrone Injection® (Can)** *see* Mitoxantrone *on page 1072*

♦ **Mitozantrone** *see* Mitoxantrone *on page 1072*

♦ **Mitrazol™ [OTC]** *see* Miconazole *on page 1056*

♦ **Mivacron® [DSC]** *see* Mivacurium [DSC] *on page 1074*

♦ **Mivacron® (Can)** *see* Mivacurium [DSC] *on page 1074*

Mivacurium [DSC] (mye va KYOO ree um)

Medication Safety Issues

Sound-alike/look-alike issues:

Mivacron® may be confused with Mevacor®

High alert medication: The Institute for Safe Medication Practices (ISMP) includes this medication among its list of drugs which have a heightened risk of causing significant patient harm when used in error.

U.S. Brand Names Mivacron® [DSC]

Canadian Brand Names Mivacron®

Index Terms Mivacurium Chloride

Therapeutic Category Neuromuscular Blocker Agent, Nondepolarizing; Skeletal Muscle Relaxant, Paralytic

Generic Available No

Use Short-acting nondepolarizing neuromuscular blocking agent used as an adjunct to general anesthesia; facilitates endotracheal intubation; provides skeletal muscle relaxation during surgery or mechanical ventilation

Pregnancy Risk Factor C

Lactation Excretion in breast milk unknown/use caution

Contraindications Hypersensitivity to mivacurium chloride, any component (see Warnings), or other benzylisoquinolinium agents

Warnings Multidose vials contain benzyl alcohol which may cause allergic reactions in susceptible individuals; large amounts of benzyl alcohol (≥99 mg/kg/day) have been associated with a potentially fatal toxicity ("gasping syndrome") in neonates; the "gasping syndrome" consists of metabolic acidosis, respiratory distress, gasping respirations, CNS dysfunction (including convulsions, intracranial hemorrhage), hypotension and cardiovascular collapse; avoid use of multidose vials in neonates. *In vitro* and animal studies have shown that benzoate, a metabolite of benzyl alcohol, displaces bilirubin from protein-binding sites.

Precautions Use cautiously in patients with reduced plasma cholinesterase activity, asthma, severe cardiovascular disease

Adverse Reactions

Cardiovascular: Hypotension, bradycardia, tachycardia, flushing, cardiac arrhythmias

Central nervous system: Dizziness

Dermatologic: Cutaneous erythema, rash

Local: Injection site reaction

Neuromuscular & skeletal: Muscle spasms

Respiratory: Bronchospasm, wheezing

Miscellaneous: Endogenous histamine release

Drug Interactions See table.

Potential Drug Interactions

Potentiation	Antagonism
Inhalation anesthetics	Calcium
Desflurane, sevoflurane, enflurane and isoflurane > halothane > nitrous oxide	Carbamazepine
Antibiotics	Phenytoin
Aminoglycosides, polymyxins, clindamycin, vancomycin, tetracycline	Steroids (chronic administration)
Magnesium	Theophylline
Antiarrhythmics	Anticholinesterases[1]
Quinidine, procainamide, bretylium, and possibly lidocaine	Neostigmine, pyridostigmine, edrophonium, echothiophate ophthalmic solution
Diuretics	Caffeine
Furosemide, mannitol, thiazides	Azathioprine
Amphotericin B (secondary to hypokalemia)	
Local anesthetics	
Dantrolene (directly depresses skeletal muscle)	
Beta blockers	
Calcium channel blockers	
Ketamine	
Lithium	
Succinylcholine (when administered prior to nondepolarizing neuromuscular-blocking agent)	
Cyclosporine	

[1]Can prolong the effects of acetylcholine

Stability Store at room temperature; stable in D_5W, D_5/LR, NS for 24 hours; avoid exposure to direct ultraviolet light; incompatible with alkaline solutions; compatible with Y-site administration with sufentanil, fentanyl, alfentanil, midazolam, droperidol
(Continued)

Mivacurium [DSC] *(Continued)*

Mechanism of Action Mivacurium is a short-acting, nondepolarizing, neuromuscular-blocking agent. Like other nondepolarizing drugs, mivacurium antagonizes acetylcholine by competitively binding to cholinergic sites on motor endplates in skeletal muscle.

Pharmacodynamics

Onset of action: 1-3 minutes

Duration: Short due to rapid hydrolysis by plasma cholinesterases; recovery from muscular paralysis occurs within 9-20 minutes

Pharmacokinetics Mivacurium exists as a mixture of isomers; the most potent are the *trans-trans* and *cis-trans* isomers

Distribution: V_d: *Trans-trans* isomer: 0.15 L/kg; *cis-trans* isomer: 0.27 L/kg

Metabolism: Enzymatic hydrolysis by plasma cholinesterase

Half-life: *Trans-trans* isomer: 2.3 minutes (range: 1.4-3.6); *cis-trans* isomer: 2.1 minutes (range: 0.8-4.8)

Clearance: *Trans-trans* isomer: 53 mL/minute/kg; *cis-trans* isomer: 99 mL/minute/kg

Usual Dosage Children require higher doses mg/kg than adults and more frequent maintenance doses; I.V.:

Children 2-12 years: 0.2 mg/kg; continuous infusion: 10-14 mcg/kg/minute; doses as high as 31 mcg/kg/minute have been used

Adults: 0.15-0.2 mg/kg; for prolonged neuromuscular block, continuous infusion: 9-10 mcg/kg/minute

Administration Parenteral: Administer undiluted by rapid I.V. injection; infusions diluted in D_5W to a maximum concentration of 0.5 mg/mL

Monitoring Parameters Assisted ventilation status, heart rate, blood pressure, peripheral nerve stimulator measuring twitch response

Nursing Implications Does not alter the patient's state of consciousness; addition of sedation is recommended

Dosage Forms Excipient information presented when available (limited, particularly for generics); consult specific product labeling.

Injection, solution [preservative free]:

Mivacron®: 2 mg/mL (5 mL, 10 mL) [DSC]

Injection, solution:

Mivacron®: 2 mg/mL (20 mL, 50 mL) [with benzyl alcohol] [DSC]

References

Martin LD, Bratton SL, and O'Rourke PP, "Clinical Uses and Controversies of Neuromuscular Blocking Agents in Infants and Children," *Crit Care Med*, 1999, 27(7):1358-68.

♦ **Mivacurium Chloride** *see* Mivacurium [DSC] *on page 1074*
♦ **MK-639** *see* Indinavir *on page 824*
♦ **MK0826** *see* Ertapenem *on page 593*
♦ **MK 869** *see* Aprepitant *on page 153*
♦ **MMF** *see* Mycophenolate *on page 1093*
♦ **MMR** *see* Measles, Mumps, and Rubella Vaccines (Combined) *on page 980*
♦ **Modane® Bulk [OTC]** *see* Psyllium *on page 1347*
♦ **Molypen®** *see* Trace Metals *on page 1558*
♦ **MOM** *see* Magnesium Hydroxide *on page 971*

Mometasone Furoate (moe MET a sone FYOOR oh ate)

Medication Safety Issues

Sound-alike/look-alike issues:

Elocon® lotion may be confused with ophthalmic solutions. Manufacturer's labeling emphasizes the product is **NOT** for use in the eyes.

Related Information

Corticosteroids, Topical: Guidelines for Selection and Use *on page 1686*

U.S. Brand Names Asmanex® Twisthaler®; Elocon®; Nasonex®

Canadian Brand Names Elocom®; Nasonex®; PMS-Mometasone; ratio-Mometasone; Taro-Mometasone

Index Terms Mometasone Furoate

Therapeutic Category Adrenal Corticosteroid; Anti-inflammatory Agent; Antiasthmatic; Corticosteroid, Inhalant (Oral); Corticosteroid, Intranasal; Corticosteroid, Topical; Glucocorticoid

Generic Available Yes: Ointment

Use

Oral inhalation: Long-term (chronic) control of persistent bronchial asthma; **NOT** indicated for the relief of acute bronchospasm. Also used to help reduce or discontinue oral corticosteroid therapy for asthma (see Additional Information)

Intranasal: Treatment of seasonal and perennial allergic rhinitis in children ≥2 years and adults; prevention of seasonal allergic rhinitis in adolescents ≥12 years and adults; treatment of nasal polyps in adults

Topical: Relief of the inflammation and pruritus associated with corticosteroid-responsive dermatoses [medium potency topical corticosteroid]; **Note:** Due to lack of established safety and efficacy in specific age groups, the cream and ointment are not recommended for use in children <2 years of age and the lotion is not recommended for use in children <12 years of age (see also Additional Information)

Pregnancy Risk Factor C

Lactation Excretion in breast milk unknown/use caution

Contraindications Hypersensitivity to mometasone or any component (see Warnings); primary treatment of status asthmaticus

Warnings

Oral inhalation: Fatalities have occurred due to adrenal insufficiency in asthmatic patients during and after switching from systemic corticosteroids to aerosol steroids (see Additional Information); several months may be required for full recovery of hypothalamic-pituitary-adrenal (HPA) function; patients receiving higher doses of systemic corticosteroids (eg, adults receiving ≥20 mg of prednisone per day) may be at greater risk; during this period of HPA suppression, aerosol steroids do **not** provide the systemic glucocorticoid or mineralocorticoid activity needed to treat patients requiring stress doses (ie, patients with major stress such as trauma, surgery, infections, or other conditions associated with severe electrolyte loss). When used at high doses or for a prolonged time, hypercorticism and HPA suppression (including adrenal crisis) may occur; use with inhaled or systemic corticosteroids (even alternate-day dosing) may increase risk of HPA suppression. Acute adrenal insufficiency may occur with abrupt withdrawal after long-term use or with stress; withdrawal and discontinuation of corticosteroids should be done carefully; patients with HPA axis suppression may require doses of systemic glucocorticosteroids prior to, during, and after unusual stress (eg, surgery). Immunosuppression may occur; patients may be more susceptible to infections; avoid exposure to chickenpox and measles. Switching patients from systemic corticosteroids to aerosol steroids may unmask allergic conditions previously treated by the systemic steroid. Bronchospasm may occur after use of inhaled asthma medications (see Additional Information).

Powder for oral inhalation (Asmanex® Twisthaler®) contains lactose (milk proteins) which may cause allergic reactions in patients with severe milk protein allergy.

Nasal: Acute adrenal insufficiency or corticosteroid withdrawal may occur when replacing a systemic corticosteroid with a nasal corticosteroid; hypothalamic-pituitary-adrenal (HPA) axis suppression or hypercorticism may occur, especially in younger children or in patients receiving high doses for a prolonged period of time. Immunosuppression may occur; avoid exposure to chickenpox and measles.

Topical: Adverse systemic effects may occur when topical steroids are used on large areas of the body, denuded areas, for prolonged periods of time, with an occlusive dressing, and/or in infants or small children; infants and small children may be more susceptible to HPA axis suppression or other systemic toxicities due to a larger skin surface area to body mass ratio; use with caution in pediatric patients and for no longer than 3 weeks

Precautions Avoid using higher than recommended doses; suppression of HPA axis function, suppression of linear growth (ie, reduction of growth velocity), reduced bone mineral density, hypercorticism (Cushing's syndrome), hyperglycemia, or glucosuria may occur; titrate to lowest effective dose; these adverse effects (as well as intracranial hypertension) may also occur with topical use and have been reported in pediatric patients (see also Additional Information). Do not use topical mometasone furoate products for the treatment of diaper dermatitis. Use with extreme caution in patients with respiratory tuberculosis, untreated systemic infections, ocular herpes simplex. Nasal corticosteroids are not recommended for patients with recent nasal trauma, nasal surgery, or nasal septum ulcers, due to inhibition of wound healing. Rarely, local fungal infections, immediate hypersensitivity reactions, nasal septum perforation, or increased intraocular pressure may occur with intranasal corticosteroid use; glaucoma and/or cataracts have also been reported.

Adverse Reactions

Nasal/oral inhalation:

Cardiovascular: Chest pain

Central nervous system: Headache; fatigue (oral inhalation), depression (oral inhalation), insomnia (oral inhalation)

Endocrine & metabolic: Dysmenorrhea; HPA suppression, Cushing's syndrome, growth suppression (oral inhalation)

Gastrointestinal: Vomiting, nausea, diarrhea, dyspepsia, abdominal pain, oral candidiasis; taste disturbance (rare)

(Continued)

Mometasone Furoate *(Continued)*

Neuromuscular & skeletal: Musculoskeletal pain, arthralgia, myalgia; decreased bone mineral density (oral inhalation)
Ocular: Conjunctivitis, rarely: Increased IOP, glaucoma, cataracts (oral inhalation)
Otic: Earache, otitis media
Respiratory: Pharyngitis, cough, epistaxis, upper respiratory tract infection, sinusitis, asthma, bronchitis, nasal irritation, rhinitis, wheezing; nasal burning and irritation; nasal ulcers (rare), nasal candidiasis (rare), nasal septum perforation (rare), smell disturbance (rare)
Miscellaneous: Viral infection, flu-like symptoms; cases of anaphylaxis and angioedema have been reported

Topical use: Dermatologic: Bacterial skin infection, burning, tingling, stinging, furunculosis, pruritus, skin atrophy, folliculitis, moniliasis, paresthesia, skin depigmentation, acneform reaction, itching, rosacea

Drug Interactions Cytochrome P450 isoenzyme CYP3A4 substrate

Ketoconazole increases mometasone furoate serum concentrations and decreases plasma cortisol levels; use ketoconazole with caution in patients receiving mometasone

Stability

Cream: Store between 2°C to 25°C (36°F to 77°F)
Lotion: Store between 2°C to 30°C (36°F to 86°F)
Nasal spray: Store between 2°C to 25°C (36°F to 77°F); protect from light
Ointment: Store at 25°C (77°F); excursions permitted to 15°C to 30°C (59°F to 86°F)
Oral inhaler: Store at 25°C (77°F) in a dry place; excursions permitted to 15°C to 30°C (59°F to 86°F); discard inhaler 45 days after opening foil pouch (or when dose counter reads "00")

Mechanism of Action Controls the rate of protein synthesis, depresses the migration of polymorphonuclear leukocytes and fibroblasts, reverses capillary permeability, and stabilizes lysosomal membranes at the cellular level to prevent or control inflammation

Pharmacodynamics Clinical effects are due to direct local effect rather than systemic absorption

Onset of action: Intranasal: Improvement in allergic rhinitis symptoms may be seen within 11 hours
Maximum effect: Intranasal: Within 1-2 weeks after starting therapy; oral inhalation: 1-2 weeks or more
Duration after discontinuation: Oral inhalation: Several days or more

Pharmacokinetics

Absorption:
Intranasal: Undetectable in plasma
Topical: 0.4% of the applied dose of the cream and 0.7% of the applied dose of the ointment enter the circulation after 8 hours of contact with normal skin (without occlusion); absorption is increased by occlusive dressings or with decreased integrity of skin (eg, inflammation or skin disease)
Distribution: V_{dss}: Adults: 152 L
Protein binding: 98% to 99%
Metabolism: Extensive in the liver to multiple metabolites; no major metabolites are detectable in the plasma; *in vitro* incubation studies identified one minor metabolite, 6 Beta-hydroxymometasone furoate, formed via cytochrome P450 CYP3A4 pathway
Bioavailability: Oral inhalation: Single dose: <1%
Half-life: Adults: Mean: 5 hours
Elimination: Metabolites are excreted primarily via the bile with a limited amount via urine; after oral inhalation 74% of the dose was excreted in the feces and 8% in the urine (none as unchanged drug)

Usual Dosage

Nasal spray: Titrate to lowest effective dose
Allergic rhinitis:
Children 2-11 years: 1 spray (50 mcg) in each nostril once daily
Children ≥12 years and Adults: 2 sprays (100 mcg) in each nostril once daily; when used for the prevention of allergic rhinitis, treatment should begin 2-4 weeks prior to pollen season
Nasal polyps: Adults ≥18 years: 2 sprays (100 mcg) in each nostril twice daily; 2 sprays (100 mcg) in each nostril once daily may be effective in some patients
Oral inhalation: Children ≥12 years and Adults: **Note:** Maximum effects may not be seen until 1-2 weeks or longer; doses should be titrated to the lowest effective dose once asthma is controlled:
Patients previously treated with bronchodilators only or with inhaled corticosteroids: Initial: 1 inhalation (220 mcg) once daily, administered in the evening.

Maximum dose: 2 inhalations/day (440 mcg /day); may be administered as 1 inhalation twice daily or 2 inhalations once daily in the evening

Patients previously treated with oral corticosteroids: Initial: 2 inhalations (440 mcg) twice daily. Maximum dose: 4 inhalations/day (880 mcg/day)

Topical: Apply sparingly, do not use occlusive dressings. Discontinue therapy when control is achieved; reassess diagnosis if no improvement is seen in 2 weeks.

Cream, ointment: Children ≥2 years and Adults: Apply a thin film to affected area once daily; do not use in pediatric patients for >3 weeks

Lotion: Children ≥12 years and Adults: Apply a few drops to affected area once daily; massage lightly into skin

Administration

Oral inhalation: Remove inhaler from foil pouch; write date on cap label. Keep inhaler upright while removing cap, twisting in a counterclockwise direction; lifting the cap loads the device with the medication. Exhale fully prior to bringing the inhaler up to the mouth. Place inhaler in mouth, while holding it in a horizontal position. Close lips around the mouthpiece and inhale quickly and deeply. Remove the inhaler from your mouth and hold your breath for about 10 seconds, if possible. Do not exhale into inhaler. Wipe the mouthpiece dry and replace the cap immediately after each inhalation; rotate fully until click is heard. Rinse mouth with water (without swallowing) after inhalation to decrease chance of oral candidiasis. Avoid contact of the inhaler with any liquids; do not wash; wipe with dry cloth or tissue if needed. Discard the inhaler 45 days after opening foil pouch or when dose counter reads "00".

Intranasal spray: Shake well prior to each use; clear nasal passages by blowing nose prior to use; occlude one nostril while administering to the other. Nasal spray must be primed before first use (10 actuations or until a fine spray appears) or after >1 week of nonuse (2 actuations or until a fine spray appears); discard unit after 120 metered sprays are used. Spray should be administered once or twice daily, at a regular interval. Do not spray into eyes or directly onto nasal septum. After removing nasal spray from container, avoid prolonged exposure of product to direct light; brief exposure to light (with normal use) is acceptable.

Topical: Apply sparingly; avoid contact with eyes. Do not apply to face, underarms, or groin unless directed by physician. Do not wrap or bandage affected area unless directed by physician. Do not use for treatment of diaper dermatitis or in diaper area.

Lotion: Hold nozzle of bottle close to affected area and gently squeeze bottle

Monitoring Parameters Monitor growth in pediatric patients; assess HPA axis suppression in patients using topical steroids applied to a large surface area or to areas under occlusion. Intranasal and oral inhalation: Check mucous membranes for signs of fungal infection. Oral inhalation: Monitor for decreased bone density in patients at higher risk (eg, family history of osteoporosis; prolonged immobilization; chronic use of anticonvulsants, corticosteroids or other medications that can reduce bone mass).

Patient Information Notify physician if condition being treated persists or worsens. Do not decrease dose or discontinue without physician approval. Avoid exposure to chickenpox or measles; if exposed, seek medical advice without delay

Oral inhalation: Report sore mouth or mouth lesions to physician; carefully read and follow the Patient's Instructions for Use leaflet that accompanies the product

Topical: Avoid contact with eyes; do not use occlusive dressings or other corticosteroid-containing products unless directed by physician; do not use for longer than directed; contact physician if no improvement is seen in 2 weeks

Additional Information When using mometasone oral inhalation to help reduce or discontinue oral corticosteroid therapy, begin prednisone taper after at least 1 week of mometasone inhalation therapy; do not decrease prednisone faster than 2.5 mg/day on a weekly basis; monitor patients for signs of asthma instability and adrenal insufficiency (see Warnings); decrease mometasone to lowest effective dose **after** prednisone reduction is complete. If bronchospasm with wheezing occurs after oral inhalation use, a fast-acting bronchodilator may be used; discontinue orally inhaled corticosteroid and initiate alternative chronic therapy.

Several studies conducted in children 6-23 months of age with atopic dermatitis demonstrated a high incidence of adrenal suppression when topical mometasone furoate products were applied once daily for approximately 3 weeks over an average body surface area of about 40%. Of the patients with normal baseline adrenal function, adrenal suppression occurred in 16% of patients using the cream, 27% of patients using the ointment, and 29% of patients using the lotion. Follow-up testing 2-4 weeks after discontinuation of therapy demonstrated suppressed HPA axis function in 1 of 5 patients who used the cream, 3 of 8 patients who used the ointment, and 1 of 8 patients who used the lotion.

Dosage Forms Excipient information presented when available (limited, particularly for generics); consult specific product labeling.

(Continued)

Mometasone Furoate *(Continued)*

Cream, topical, as furoate:
Elocon®: 0.1% (15 g, 45 g)
Lotion, topical, as furoate:
Elocon®: 0.1% (30 mL, 60 mL) [contains isopropyl alcohol 40%]
Ointment, topical, as furoate: 0.1% (15 g, 45 g)
Elocon®: 0.1% (15 g, 45 g)
Powder for oral inhalation, as furoate:
Asmanex® Twisthaler®: 220 mcg (14 units, 30 units, 60 units, 120 units) [contains lactose]
Suspension, intranasal, as furoate [spray]:
Nasonex®: 50 mcg/spray (17 g) [delivers 120 sprays; contains benzalkonium chloride]

- **Mometasone Furoate** *see* Mometasone Furoate *on page 1076*
- **MOM (Magnesium Hydroxide)** *see* Magnesium Supplements *on page 976*
- **Monacolin K** *see* Lovastatin *on page 964*
- **Monarc-M™** *see* Antihemophilic Factor (Human) *on page 134*
- **Monistat® (Can)** *see* Miconazole *on page 1056*
- **Monistat® 1 Combination Pack [OTC]** *see* Miconazole *on page 1056*
- **Monistat® 3 [OTC]** *see* Miconazole *on page 1056*
- **Monistat® 3 (Can)** *see* Miconazole *on page 1056*
- **Monistat® 3 Combination Pack [OTC]** *see* Miconazole *on page 1056*
- **Monistat® 7 [OTC]** *see* Miconazole *on page 1056*
- **Monistat-Derm® [DSC]** *see* Miconazole *on page 1056*
- **Monoclate-P®** *see* Antihemophilic Factor (Human) *on page 134*
- **Monoclonal Antibody** *see* Muromonab-CD3 *on page 1092*
- **Monodox®** *see* Doxycycline *on page 543*
- **Mononine®** *see* Factor IX *on page 633*

Montelukast (mon te LOO kast)

Medication Safety Issues
Sound-alike/look-alike issues:
Singulair® may be confused with Sinequan®
Related Information
Asthma *on page 1904*
U.S. Brand Names Singulair®
Canadian Brand Names Singulair®
Index Terms Montelukast Sodium
Therapeutic Category Antiasthmatic; Leukotriene Receptor Antagonist
Generic Available No
Use Prophylaxis and chronic treatment of asthma; relief of symptoms of seasonal and perennial allergic rhinitis; prevention of exercise-induced bronchospasm in patients ≥15 years
Pregnancy Risk Factor B
Lactation Excretion in breast milk unknown/use caution
Contraindications Hypersensitivity to montelukast or any component
Warnings Montelukast is not indicated for use in the reversal of bronchospasm in acute asthma attacks, including status asthmaticus; therapy with montelukast can be continued during acute exacerbations of asthma; rare cases of systemic eosinophilia, sometimes presenting with clinical features of vasculitis (consistent with Churg-Strauss syndrome) have been reported; these reactions may also be associated with a reduction in oral corticosteroid dosage; a causal association with montelukast has not been established
Precautions Phenobarbital reduces the AUC of montelukast ~40% following a single 10 mg dosage; no dosage adjustment of montelukast is indicated, however, appropriate clinical monitoring is indicated when potent cytochrome P450 enzyme inducers, such as phenobarbital or rifampin, are coadministered with montelukast. Chewable tablets contain phenylalanine which must be avoided (or used with caution) in patients with phenylketonuria.
Adverse Reactions
Cardiovascular: Palpitations, edema, vasculitis (rare)
Central nervous system: Headache, fever, dizziness, drowsiness, irritability, restlessness, insomnia, dream abnormalities, hallucinations, seizure (rare), agitation
Dermatologic: Rash
Gastrointestinal: Diarrhea, nausea, abdominal pain, dyspepsia, pancreatitis (rare)
Hematologic: Eosinophilia

Hepatic: Elevated liver enzymes, hepatic eosinophilic infiltration, cholestatic hepatitis (rare)

Neuromuscular & skeletal: Myalgia, cramps, paresthesia, hypoesthesia, arthralgia

Otic: Otitis

Respiratory: Sinusitis, laryngitis, nasal congestion, cough, rhinorrhea

Miscellaneous: Viral infection, influenza, hypersensitivity reactions

Drug Interactions Cytochrome P450 isoenzyme CYP2A6, CYP2C9, and CYP3A3/4 substrate

Phenobarbital and rifampin (see Precautions)

Stability Store at room temperature; protect from moisture and light; granules must be administered within 15 minutes of opening the packet

Mechanism of Action Montelukast is a selective leukotriene receptor antagonist that inhibits the cysteinyl leukotriene $CysLT_1$ receptor. This activity produces inhibition of the effects of this leukotriene on bronchial smooth muscle resulting in the attenuation of bronchoconstriction and decreased vascular permeability, mucosal edema, and mucus production.

Pharmacokinetics

Absorption: Rapid

Distribution: V_d: Adults: 8-11 L

Protein binding: >99%

Metabolism: Extensive by cytochrome P450 3A4 and 2C9

Bioavailability: Tablet:
- 5 mg: 63% to 73%
- 10 mg: 64%

Time to peak serum concentration: Tablet:
- 4 mg: 2 hours
- 5 mg: 2-2.5 hours
- 10 mg: 3-4 hours

Elimination: Exclusively via bile; <0.2% excreted in urine

Usual Dosage Oral:

Treatment of asthma and allergic rhinitis (safety and efficacy for treatment of asthma in children <12 months or perennial allergic rhinitis in infants <6 months has not been established):

Children
- 6 months to 5 years: 4 mg/day
- 6-14 years: 5 mg/day

Adolescents >14 years and Adults: 10 mg/day

Prevention of exercise-induced bronchospasm: Adolescents ≥15 years and Adults: 10 mg at least 2 hours prior to exercise; additional doses should not be administered within 24 hours. Daily administration to prevent exercise-induced bronchospasm has not been evaluated.

Note: None of the clinical trials evaluated the safety and efficacy of therapy with morning dosing; the pharmacokinetics of montelukast are similar whether dosed in the morning or evening

Administration Oral: Administer in the evening without regard to meals. Granules may be administered directly into the mouth or mixed in cold or room temperature soft foods; based on stability studies, only applesauce, mashed carrots, rice, and ice cream should be used; granules are not intended to be dissolved in liquid and must be administered within 15 minutes of opening the packet; liquids may be taken subsequent to administration

Monitoring Parameters Pulmonary function tests (FEV-1), improvement in asthma symptoms

Patient Information Take regularly as prescribed, even during symptom-free periods. Do not use to treat acute episodes of asthma. Do not decrease the dose or stop taking any other asthma medications unless instructed by a physician.

Additional Information Recent studies of montelukast use in acute asthma and RSV bronchiolitis have shown promising results. Pulmonary function tests improved significantly in adult patients receiving a single dose (10 mg) montelukast along with I.V. prednisolone at the onset of an acute asthma exacerbation (Cylly, 2003). Pediatric patients with RSV positive bronchiolitis receiving daily montelukast demonstrated fewer symptoms when compared with placebo treated controls (Bisgaard, 2003).

Dosage Forms Excipient information presented when available (limited, particularly for generics); consult specific product labeling.

Granules:
- Singulair®: 4 mg/packet

Tablet:
- Singulair®: 10 mg

Tablet, chewable:
- Singulair®: 4 mg [contains phenylalanine 0.674 mg; cherry flavor]; 5 mg [contains phenylalanine 0.842 mg; cherry flavor]

(Continued)

Montelukast *(Continued)*

References

Bisgaard H, "A Randomized Trial of Montelukast in Respiratory Syncytial Virus Postbronchiolitis," *Am J Respir Crit Care Med*, 2003, 167(3):379-83.

Cylly A, Kara A, Ozdemir T, et al, "Effects of Oral Montelukast on Airway Function in Acute Asthma," *Respir Med*, 2003, 97(5):533-6.

"National Asthma Education and Prevention Program. Expert Panel Report: Guidelines for the Diagnosis and Management of Asthma Update on Selected Topics--2002," *J Allergy Clin Immunol*, 2002, 110(5 Suppl):S141-219.

♦ **Montelukast Sodium** *see* Montelukast *on page 1080*

♦ **More Attenuated Enders Strain** *see* Measles Virus Vaccine (Live) *on page 984*

♦ **MoreDophilus® [OTC]** *see Lactobacillus acidophilus* and *Lactobacillus bulgaricus on page 898*

♦ **Morphine HP® (Can)** *see* Morphine Sulfate *on page 1082*

♦ **Morphine LP® Epidural (Can)** *see* Morphine Sulfate *on page 1082*

Morphine Sulfate (MOR feen SUL fate)

Medication Safety Issues

Sound-alike/look-alike issues:

Morphine may be confused with hydromorphone
Morphine sulfate may be confused with magnesium sulfate
MSO_4 is an error-prone abbreviation (mistaken as magnesium sulfate)
Avinza® may be confused with Evista®, Invanz®
Roxanol™ may be confused with OxyFast®, Roxicet™

Use care when prescribing and/or administering morphine solutions. These products are available in different concentrations. Always prescribe dosage in mg; **not** by volume (mL).

Use caution when selecting a morphine formulation for use in neurologic infusion pumps (eg, Medtronic delivery systems). The product should be appropriately labeled as "preservative-free" and suitable for intraspinal use via continuous infusion. In addition, the product should be formulated in a pH range that is compatible with the device operation specifications.

Significant differences exist between oral and I.V. dosing. Use caution when converting from one route of administration to another.

Related Information

Adult ACLS Algorithms *on page 1660*
Compatibility of Medications Mixed in A Syringe *on page 1941*
Laboratory Detection of Drugs in Urine *on page 1928*
Medications for Which A Single Dose May Be Fatal When Ingested By A Toddler *on page 1932*
Narcotic Analgesics Comparison *on page 1705*
Overdose and Toxicology *on page 1916*
Preprocedure Sedatives in Children *on page 1895*

U.S. Brand Names Astramorph/PF™; Avinza®; DepoDur™; Duramorph®; Infumorph®; Kadian®; MS Contin®; Oramorph SR®; RMS®; Roxanol™

Canadian Brand Names Kadian®; M-Eslon®; Morphine HP®; Morphine LP® Epidural; M.O.S.® 10; M.O.S.® 20; M.O.S.® 30; M.O.S.-SR®; M.O.S.-Sulfate®; MS Contin®; MS-IR®; PMS-Morphine Sulfate SR; ratio-Morphine SR; Statex®; Zomorph®

Index Terms MSO_4 (error-prone abbreviation and should not be used)

Therapeutic Category Analgesic, Narcotic

Generic Available Yes: Excludes capsule, controlled release tablet, sustained release tablet, extended release liposomal suspension for injection

Use Relief of moderate to severe acute and chronic pain; pain of MI; relieves dyspnea of acute left ventricular failure and pulmonary edema; preanesthetic medication

DepoDur™: Epidural (at the lumbar level) single-dose management of surgical pain in adults; may be used in women undergoing cesarean section following clamping of the umbilical cord (not for use in vaginal labor and delivery)

Duramorph®: I.V., epidural, or intrathecal (both at the lumbar level) management of pain unresponsive to non-narcotic analgesics in adults

Infumorph®: Intrathecal (at the lumbar level) or epidural infusion via microinfusion device for the treatment of intractable chronic pain in adults

Restrictions C-II

Pregnancy Risk Factor C (D if used for prolonged periods or in high doses at term)

Lactation Enters breast milk/use caution (AAP rates "compatible")

Contraindications Hypersensitivity to morphine sulfate or any component (see Warnings); severe respiratory depression; acute or severe asthma; upper airway obstruction; severe liver or renal insufficiency; GI obstruction especially known or suspected paralytic ileus; pregnancy (prolonged use or high doses at term). DepoDur™ is also contraindicated in patients with suspected or known CNS injury, increased ICP, circulatory shock, or conditions that preclude an epidural injection. Duramorph® is also labeled as being contraindicated in patients with depleted blood volume or concurrent administration of phenothiazines or general anesthetics (severe hypotension may occur).

Warnings CNS and respiratory depression may occur; neonates and infants <3 months of age are more susceptible to respiratory depression, use with caution and in reduced doses in this age group. Use only preservative free injections for epidural or intrathecal administration and in neonates. Abrupt discontinuation after prolonged use may result in withdrawal symptoms. Use with extreme caution in patients with COPD, cor pulmonale, hypoxia, hypercapnia, pre-existing respiratory depression, significantly decreased respiratory reserve, head injury, increased ICP, other intracranial lesions. Severe hypotension may occur; use with caution in patients with circulatory shock, hypovolemia, impaired myocardial function or those receiving drugs which may exaggerate hypotensive effects (including phenothiazines or general anesthetics). Morphine may obscure diagnosis or clinical course of patients with acute abdominal conditions.

A toxic or potentially fatal dose of morphine may be rapidly released if extended, sustained, or controlled release products are chewed, crushed, broken or dissolved; consumption of alcoholic beverages or ethanol-containing products (prescription or nonprescription) while receiving Avinza® therapy may disrupt the extended-release formulation, causing a rapid release of morphine and potentially fatal overdose.

Prior to administration via epidural or intrathecal route, evaluate benefits versus risks in patients with infection at injection site, bleeding diatheses, or anticoagulation therapy. Only physicians experienced in the techniques and familiar with the clinical management of the adverse effects of epidural and intrathecal drug administration should administer drugs via the intraspinal route. When morphine is used via the epidural or intrathecal routes, severe adverse effects may occur, including significant respiratory depression; facilities must be properly equipped to resuscitate patients; monitor patients for delayed sedation. When DepoDur™ is used, patients must be closely monitored for a minimum of 48 hours (due to prolonged effects of extended release epidural preparation). Monitor patients closely for a minimum of 24 hours after the initial epidural or intrathecal dose of Duramorph®. When Infumorph® is used, patients must be closely monitored for a minimum of 24 hours after the initial (single) test dose and as appropriate for the first several days after catheter implantation. Due to fewer potential adverse effects, the epidural route is preferred over the intrathecal route (intrathecal route is associated with a higher incidence of respiratory depression). Tolerance to morphine and increased epidural or intrathecal dosage requirements may occur (patients may require hospitalization and detoxification). Seizures may occur with high doses of intraspinal morphine. Myoclonic spasm of the lower extremities has been reported in adults receiving high doses of intrathecal morphine. Safety and efficacy of spinal morphine products have not been established in pediatric patients. Freezing may adversely affect modified-release mechanism of Depo-Dur™; check freeze indicator within carton prior to administration (see Stability).

Parenteral products are designed for administration by specific routes (I.V., intrathecal, epidural). Use caution when prescribing, dispensing, or administering so as to use formulations only by intended route(s). Injection may contain sodium metabisulfite which may cause allergic reactions in susceptible individuals; oral solution may contain sodium benzoate; benzoic acid (benzoate) is a metabolite of benzyl alcohol; large amounts of benzyl alcohol (≥99 mg/kg/day) have been associated with a potentially fatal toxicity ("gasping syndrome") in neonates; the "gasping syndrome" consists of metabolic acidosis, respiratory distress, gasping respirations, CNS dysfunction (including convulsions, intracranial hemorrhage), hypotension and cardiovascular collapse; avoid use of morphine sulfate products containing sodium benzoate in neonates; *in vitro* and animal studies have shown that benzoate displaces bilirubin from protein binding sites

Precautions Use with caution in patients with hypersensitivity reactions to other phenanthrene derivative opioid agonists (codeine, hydrocodone, hydromorphone, levorphanol, oxycodone, oxymorphone). Use with caution in patients with biliary tract disease or acute pancreatitis (morphine may cause spasm of the sphincter of Oddi); use with caution and decrease the dose in patients with Addison's disease, hypothyroidism, renal impairment, hepatic dysfunction (eg, cirrhosis), urethral stricture, prostatic hypertrophy, or in debilitated patients; use with caution in patients with CNS depression, toxic psychosis, seizure disorders, acute alcoholism, and delirium tremens. MS Contin® 100 mg or 200 mg tablets are for use only in opioid-tolerant patients requiring >400 mg/day of morphine. Kadian® should be discontinued 24 hours prior to cordotomy or other interruption of pain transmission pathways (use parenteral short-acting opioids to control pain).
(Continued)

Morphine Sulfate *(Continued)*

When administered to a pregnant woman, I.V., epidural, and intrathecal morphine readily pass into the fetal circulation and may result in respiratory depression in the newborn; resuscitative equipment and naloxone should be available for the neonate

Adverse Reactions

Cardiovascular: Palpitations, hypotension, syncope, bradycardia, peripheral vasodilation, orthostatic hypotension, atrial fibrillation, chest pain, edema, tachycardia

Central nervous system: CNS depression, drowsiness, dizziness, sedation, elevated intracranial pressure, headache (especially following epidural or intrathecal use), amnesia, anxiety, apathy, ataxia, chills, depression, euphoria, fever, hypoesthesia, insomnia, lethargy, malaise, restlessness, seizure, vertigo; dysphoric reactions and toxic psychoses have been reported

Dermatologic: Pruritus (more common with epidural or intrathecal administration; may be due to histamine release; may be dose-related), urticaria

Endocrine & metabolic: Antidiuretic hormone release, hyponatremia, gynecomastia

Gastrointestinal: Nausea, vomiting, constipation, xerostomia, biliary tract spasm, intestinal obstruction, paralytic ileus, anorexia, dyspepsia, dysphagia, GERD, GI irritation

Genitourinary: Urinary tract spasm (may be more common with epidural or intrathecal administration), urinary retention (may be prolonged, up to 20 hours, following epidural or intrathecal use), decreased urination

Hematologic: Anemia, leukopenia, thrombocytopenia

Hepatic: Elevated liver enzymes

Local: Pain at injection site

Neuromuscular & skeletal: Weakness, arthralgia, back pain, bone pain, paresthesia, trembling

Ocular: Miosis, vision problems

Respiratory: Respiratory depression, asthma, atelectasis, dyspnea, hiccups, hypoxia, noncardiogenic pulmonary edema, rhinitis

Miscellaneous: Diaphoresis, physical and psychological dependence, histamine release, flu-like syndrome

Drug Interactions

Drug Interactions Cytochrome P450 isoenzyme CYP2D6 substrate

CNS depressants, alcohol, phenothiazines, tricyclic antidepressants may potentiate the adverse effects of morphine. MAO inhibitors may significantly potentiate the effects of morphine (do not use DepoDur™ within 14 days of MAO inhibitors). Morphine associated respiratory depression may delay spontaneous pulmonary ventilation recovery from neuromuscular blocking agents. Alcoholic beverages or ethanol-containing products (prescription or nonprescription) may disrupt the extended-release formulation of Avinza® and result in the rapid release of the total morphine dose (this could result in the absorption of a potentially fatal morphine dose).

DepoDur™: Administration of an epidural test dose (lidocaine 1.5% and epinephrine 1:200,000) may affect the release of morphine from the liposomal preparation and increase morphine peak serum concentrations (delaying the administration of DepoDur™ for ≥15 minutes after the test dose minimizes this interaction). Do not use other epidural local anesthetics before or after DepoDur™. Do not administer any other medication into the epidural space for at least 48 hours after DepoDur™.

Food Interactions

Avinza®: A high fat meal may delay absorption

Kadian®: Food may decrease the rate, but not the extent of absorption

MS Contin®: A fatty meal may slightly decrease peak plasma concentrations

Oral solution: Food may increase bioavailability

Oramorph SR®: Food has little to no effect on bioavailability

Stability

Suppositories: Refrigerate; do not freeze

Injection: Store at controlled room temperature. Protect from light. Degradation depends on pH and presence of oxygen; relatively stable in pH ≤4; darkening of solutions indicates degradation. Morphine solutions for injection are stable in D_5¼NS, D_5½NS, D_5NS, D_5W, D_{10}W, LR, D_5LR, ½NS, NS, dextran 6% in dextrose, dextran 6% in NS.

Avinza® and Kadian®: Store at controlled room temperature. Protect from light and moisture

Duramorph®: Store in carton at controlled room temperature of 20°C to 25°C (65°F to 77°F); excursions permitted to 15°C to 30°C (59°F to 86°F). Protect from light; do not freeze. Discard unused portion of vial (vial does not contain preservative). Do not heat sterilize.

DepoDur™: Store in carton under refrigeration, 2°C to 8°C (36°F to 46°F). Do not freeze; do not use if product has been frozen or is suspected of having been frozen. Check freeze indicator (located on carton) before administration; do not administer if indicator bulb is pink or purple (this indicates drug may have been frozen). May store unopened vials at room temperature for up to 7 days. After withdrawal from vial, drug may be held at room temperature for ≤4 hours before use. Do not heat or gas sterilize. Discard unused portion of vial (vial does not contain preservatives). Do not mix with other medications.

Mechanism of Action Binds to opiate receptors in the CNS, causing inhibition of ascending pain pathways, altering the perception of and response to pain; produces generalized CNS depression

Pharmacodynamics See table.

Dosage Form/Route	Analgesia Peak	Analgesia Duration
Tablets	1 h	3-5 h
Oral solution	1 h	3-5 h
Epidural	1 h	12-20 h
Extended release tablets	3-4 h	8-12 h
Suppository	20-60 min	3-7 h
Subcutaneous injection	50-90 min	3-5 h
I.M. injection	30-60 min	3-5 h
I.V. injection	20 min	3-5 h

Pharmacokinetics

Absorption: Oral: Variable

Distribution: Distributes to skeletal muscle, liver, kidneys, lungs, intestinal tract, spleen, brain, and into breast milk; crosses placenta

V_d, apparent: Children 1.7-18.7 years with cancer: Median: 5.2 L/kg; a significantly higher V_d was observed in children <11 years (median: 7.1 L/kg) versus >11 years (median: 4.7 L/kg) (see Hunt, 1999)

V_d, apparent: Adults: 1-4.7 L/kg

Protein binding:

Premature Infants: <20%

Adults: 20% to 35%

Metabolism: In the liver via glucuronide conjugation to morphine-6-glucuronide (active) and morphine-3-glucuronide (inactive)

Half-life:

Preterm: 10-20 hours

Neonates: 7.6 hours (range: 4.5-13.3 hours)

Infants 1-3 months: 6.2 hours (range: 5-10 hours)

Infants 6 months to Children 2.5 years: 2.9 hours (range: 1.4-7.8 hours)

Preschool Children: 1-2 hours

Children 6-19 years with sickle cell disease: Mean ~1.3 hours

Adults: 2-4 hours

Elimination: Excreted unchanged in urine:

Neonates: 3% to 15%

Adults: 2% to 12%

Clearance: **Note:** Adult values are reached by 6 months to 2.5 years of age

Preterm: 0.5-3 mL/minute/kg

Neonates 1-7 days: Median: 5.5 mL/minute/kg (range: 3.2-8.4 mL/minute/kg)

Neonates 8-30 days: Median: 7.4 mL/minute/kg (range: 3.4-13.8 mL/minute/kg)

Infants 1-3 months: Median: 10.5 mL/minute/kg (range: 9.8-20.1 mL/minute/kg)

Infants 3-6 months: Median: 13.9 mL/minute/kg (range: 8.3-24.1 mL/minute/kg)

Infants 6 months to Children 2.5 years: Median: 21.7 mL/minute/kg (range: 5.8-28.6 mL/minute/kg)

Preschool Children: 20-40 mL/minute/kg

Children 1.7-18.7 years with cancer: Median: 23.1 mL/minute/kg; a significantly higher clearance was observed in children <11 years (median: 37.4 mL/minute/kg) versus >11 years (median: 21.9 mL/minute/kg) (see Hunt, 1999)

Children 6-19 years with sickle cell disease: Mean ~36 mL/minute/kg (range: 6-59 mL/minute/kg)

Adults: 10-20 mL/minute/kg

Usual Dosage Doses should be titrated to appropriate effect; when changing routes of administration in chronically treated patients, please note that oral doses are approximately one-half as effective as parenteral dose

Neonates (see Warnings; use preservative free formulation):

I.M., I.V., SubQ: Initial: 0.05 mg/kg every 4-8 hours; titrate carefully to effect; maximum dose: 0.1 mg/kg/dose

(Continued)

Morphine Sulfate *(Continued)*

I.V. continuous infusion: Initial: 0.01 mg/kg/hour (10 mcg/kg/hour); do **not** exceed infusion rates of 0.015-0.02 mg/kg/hour due to decreased elimination, increased CNS sensitivity, and adverse effects; **Note:** Some centers may use slightly higher doses, especially in neonates who develop tolerance

International Evidence-Based Group for Neonatal Pain recommendations (Anand, 2001): I.V.:

Intermittent dose: 0.05-0.1 mg/kg/dose

Continuous infusion: Range: 0.01-0.03 mg/kg/hour

Infants and Children:

Oral: Tablet and solution (prompt release): 0.2-0.5 mg/kg/dose every 4-6 hours as needed

I.M., I.V., SubQ: 0.1-0.2 mg/kg/dose every 2-4 hours as needed; may initiate at 0.05 mg/kg/dose; usual maximum dose: 15 mg/dose

I.V., SubQ continuous infusion:

Sickle cell or cancer pain: Initial: Infants: 0.02 mg/kg/hour (20 mcg/kg/hour); Children: 0.03 mg/kg/hour (30 mcg/kg/hour); conversion from intermittent I.V. morphine: Administer the patient's total daily I.V. morphine dose over 24 hours as a continuous infusion; titrate dose to appropriate effect; in one study (Miser, 1980), children with severe pain from terminal cancer required a median dose of 0.04-0.07 mg/kg/hour (40-70 mcg/kg/hour); range: 0.025-2.6 mg/kg/hour

Postoperative pain: 0.01-0.04 mg/kg/hour

Sedation/analgesia for procedures: I.V.: 0.05-0.1 mg/kg 5 minutes before the procedure

Epidural (use preservative free): 0.03-0.05 mg/kg (30-50 mcg/kg); maximum dose: 0.1 mg/kg (100 mcg/kg) or 5 mg/24 hours

Children: Oral: Controlled release tablet: 0.3-0.6 mg/kg/dose every 12 hours

Conversion from prompt release tablets and solution: Administer $^1/_2$ of the patient's total daily oral morphine dose every 12 hours or $^1/_3$ of the patient's total daily oral morphine dose every 8 hours

Adolescents >12 years: Sedation/analgesia for procedures: I.V.: 3-4 mg; may repeat in 5 minutes if necessary

Adults:

Oral:

Prompt release: 10-30 mg every 4 hours as needed

Controlled release: 15-30 mg every 8-12 hours

Avinza® extended release capsules (chronic pain): Conversion from other oral morphine products: Administer the patient's total daily oral morphine dose as Avinza® capsules once daily; do not administer more often than every 24 hours; supplemental pain medication may be needed (up to 4 days) until response to daily Avinza® dosage has been stabilized; see package insert for more details; maximum dose: 1600 mg/day; higher doses contain quantity of fumaric acid that may result in nephrotoxicity

Kadian® sustained release capsules (chronic pain): Conversion from other oral morphine products: Administer $^1/_2$ of the patient's total daily oral morphine dose as Kadian® capsules every 12 hours or administer the total daily oral morphine dose as Kadian® capsules every 24 hours; do not administer more often than every 12 hours; see package insert for more details

I.M., I.V., SubQ: 2.5-20 mg/dose every 2-6 hours as needed; usual: 10 mg/dose every 4 hours as needed

I.V., SubQ continuous infusion: 0.8-10 mg/hour; may increase depending on pain relief/adverse effects; usual range up to 80 mg/hour

Epidural (use preservative free; use lower doses and with extreme caution in debilitated patients):

Duramorph®:

Single dose: Initial: 5 mg in lumbar region; if inadequate pain relief within 1 hour, give 1-2 mg; maximum dose: 10 mg/24 hours

Continuous infusion: Initial: 2 mg/24 hours to 4 mg/24 hours; may give further doses of 1-2 mg if pain relief is not achieved initially; maximum total dose: 10 mg/24 hours

DepoDur™ (extended release liposome injection): Surgical pain: Single-dose:

Cesarean section: 10 mg

Lower abdominal or pelvic surgery: 10-15 mg; **Note:** Some patients may benefit from a 20 mg dose; however, the incidence of adverse respiratory effects may be increased

Major orthopedic surgery of the lower extremity: 15 mg

Intrathecal (1/10 of epidural dose, use preservative free; use lower doses and with extreme caution in debilitated patients): 0.2-1 mg/dose; repeat doses **not** recommended; **Note:** Consider use of low-dose continuous naloxone infusion (0.6 mg/hour) for 24 hours to help reduce potential side effects

Dosing adjustment in renal impairment: Children and Adults:

Cl_{cr} 10-50 mL/minute: Administer 75% of normal dose

Cl_{cr} <10 mL/minute: Administer 50% of normal dose

Dosing adjustment in hepatic impairment: Use with caution; specific guidelines are not available; clearance is decreased in patients with cirrhosis; accumulation of morphine is not expected with single-dose use, but may occur with multiple doses; lower doses may be needed with multiple dose regimens

Administration

Oral: Administer with food; swallow extended, sustained, and controlled release products whole; do not chew, crush, break, or dissolve (this would result in rapid release and absorption of a potentially toxic dose of drug)

Avinza® and Kadian® capsules may be administered without regard to meals. Do not administer Avinza® with alcohol (see Patient Information). Avinza® (extended release capsules) and Kadian® (sustained release capsules) may be opened and contents sprinkled on a small amount of applesauce immediately prior to ingestion; swallow mixture; rinse mouth with water and swallow to ensure all beads have been ingested; do not chew, crush, or dissolve beads or pellets from capsule (this would result in rapid release and absorption of a potentially toxic dose of drug). Kadian® capsules may be opened and contents sprinkled into ~10 mL of water, then flushed while swirling through a pre-wetted 16-French gastrostomy tube fitted with a funnel at the port end; flush with water to transfer all pellets and flush the tube; do not attempt to administer via NG tube.

Parenteral: **Note:** Solutions for injection should be visually inspected for particulate matter and discoloration prior to administration. Do not use if contains a precipitate or is darker in color than pale yellow or discolored in any other way.

I.V. push: Administer over at least 5 minutes at a final concentration of 0.5-5 mg/mL (rapid I.V. administration may increase adverse effects)

Intermittent infusion: Administer over 15-30 minutes at a final concentration of 0.5-5 mg/mL

Continuous I.V. infusion: 0.1-1 mg/mL in D_5W, $D_{10}W$, or NS

Epidural and intrathecal: Use only preservative free injections. Adults: Infumorph® was developed for use in continuous microinfusion devices only; it may require dilution before use, as determined by the individual patient's dosage requirements and the characteristics of the continuous microinfusion device; not recommended for single dose I.V., I.M., or SubQ administration; filter through ≤5 micron microfilter before injecting into microinfusion device

Epidural, extended release liposome suspension (DepoDur™): Adults: For epidural use only (at the lumbar level); do not administer I.V., I.M., or by the intrathecal route; not recommended for administration into thoracic epidural space or higher (has not been studied). Do not use if suspect vial has been frozen (see Stability). Gently invert vial to resuspend particles immediately before use (avoid aggressive agitation). May administer undiluted or may dilute up to 5 mL total volume in preservative free NS. Product does not contain preservative; drug must be administered within 4 hours after withdrawal from vial. Do not use in-line filter during administration. Do not administer within 15 minutes of epidural lidocaine and epinephrine (see Drug Interactions); do not administer any other medication into the epidural space for at least 48 hours after DepoDur™

Monitoring Parameters Respiratory and cardiovascular status, oxygen saturation, pain relief (if used for analgesia), level of sedation. **Note:** Resedation may occur following epidural administration; when DepoDur™ is used, monitor patients closely for ≥48 hours due to prolonged effects of extended release epidural preparation. Monitor patients receiving Infumorph® closely for ≥24 hours after initiation and as appropriate for the first several days after catheter implantation.

Patient Information Avoid alcohol. Do not drink any alcohol (including beer, wine, distilled spirits) or take over-the-counter or other prescription medications which may contain alcohol, when taking Avinza® (alcohol may cause a sudden and dangerous release of medication from this product which may cause decreased breathing, coma, or death). Morphine may cause drowsiness and impair ability to perform activities requiring mental alertness or physical coordination; may be habit-forming; avoid abrupt discontinuation after prolonged use

Nursing Implications Do not administer rapidly I.V. Accidental dermal exposure to Duramorph® should be treated by removing contaminated clothing and rinsing the affected area with water. See also Monitoring Parameters.

Additional Information Less adverse effects are associated with epidural compared to intrathecal route of administration; equianalgesic doses: Codeine: 120 mg I.M. = morphine 10 mg I.M. = single dose oral morphine 60 mg **or** chronic dosing oral morphine 15-25 mg

(Continued)

Morphine Sulfate *(Continued)*

DepoDur™ is an extended release sterile suspension of multivesicular liposomes in NS; liposomes range in size from 17-23 micrometers (median diameter); the pharmacokinetics, safety, and efficacy of DepoDur™ have not been studied in patients <18 years of age and use in these patients is **not** recommended

Avinza® capsules contain both immediate release and extended release beads; also contains fumaric acid (as an osmotic agent and local pH modifier); this product is intended for once daily oral administration only; not for PRN or postoperative use. Kadian® capsules contain sustained release pellets that are polymer-coated; this product is intended for every 12 hour or every 24 hour dosing. The pharmacokinetics of Avinza® and Kadian® have not been studied in patients <18 years of age; the available capsule mg strength may not be appropriate for pediatric patients who are very young; sprinkling capsule contents on applesauce is **not** a suitable alternative for these patients; other oral products should be used.

Dosage Forms Excipient information presented when available (limited, particularly for generics); consult specific product labeling.

Capsule, extended release:
- Avinza®: 30 mg, 60 mg, 90 mg, 120 mg

Capsule, sustained release:
- Kadian®: 20 mg, 30 mg, 50 mg, 60 mg, 80 mg, 100 mg, 200 mg

Infusion [premixed in D_5W]: 1 mg/mL (100 mL, 250 mL)

Injection, extended release liposomal suspension [lumbar epidural injection, preservative free]:
- DepoDur™: 10 mg/mL (1 mL, 1.5 mL, 2 mL)

Injection, solution: 2 mg/mL (1 mL); 4 mg/mL (1 mL); 5 mg/mL (1 mL); 8 mg/mL (1 mL); 10 mg/mL (1 mL, 10 mL); 15 mg/mL (1 mL, 20 mL); 25 mg/mL (4 mL, 10 mL, 20 mL, 40 mL, 50 mL, 100 mL, 250 mL); 50 mg/mL (20 mL, 40 mL) [some preparations contain sodium metabisulfite]

Injection, solution [epidural, intrathecal, or I.V. infusion; preservative free]:
- Astramorph/PF™: 0.5 mg/mL (2 mL, 10 mL); 1 mg/mL (2 mL, 10 mL)
- Duramorph®: 0.5 mg/mL (10 mL); 1 mg/mL (10 mL)

Injection, solution [epidural or intrathecal infusion via microinfusion device; preservative free]:
- Infumorph®: 10 mg/mL (20 mL); 25 mg/mL (20 mL)

Injection, solution [I.V. infusion via PCA pump]: 0.5 mg/mL (30 mL); 1 mg/mL (30 mL, 50 mL); 2 mg/mL (30 mL); 5 mg/mL (30 mL, 50 mL)

Injection, solution [preservative free]: 0.5 mg/mL (10 mL); 1 mg/mL (10 mL); 25 mg/mL (4 mL, 10 mL, 20 mL)

Solution, oral: 10 mg/5 mL (5 mL, 10 mL, 100 mL, 500 mL); 20 mg/5 mL (100 mL, 500 mL); 20 mg/mL (30 mL, 120 mL, 240 mL)
- Roxanol™: 20 mg/mL (30 mL, 120 mL); 100 mg/5 mL (240 mL) [with calibrated spoon]

Suppository, rectal: 5 mg (12s), 10 mg (12s), 20 mg (12s), 30 mg (12s)
- RMS®: 5 mg (12s), 10 mg (12s), 20 mg (12s), 30 mg (12s)

Tablet: 10 mg, 15 mg, 30 mg

Tablet, controlled release:
- MS Contin®: 15 mg, 30 mg, 60 mg, 100 mg, 200 mg

Tablet, extended release: 15 mg, 30 mg, 60 mg, 100 mg, 200 mg

Tablet, sustained release:
- Oramorph SR®: 15 mg, 30 mg, 60 mg, 100 mg

References

Berde C, Ablin A, Glazer J, et al, "American Academy of Pediatrics Report of the Subcommittee on Disease-Related Pain in Childhood Cancer," *Pediatrics*, 1990, 86(5 Pt 2):818-25.

Dampier CD, Setty BN, Logan J, et al, "Intravenous Morphine Pharmacokinetics in Pediatric Patients With Sickle Cell Disease," *J Pediatr*, 1995, 126(3):461-7.

Henneberg SW, Hole P, Madsen de Haas I, et al, "Epidural Morphine for Postoperative Pain Relief in Children," *Acta Anaesthesiol Scand*, 1993, 37(7):664-7.

Hunt A, Joel S, Dick G, et al, "Population Pharmacokinetics of Oral Morphine and Its Glucuronides in Children Receiving Morphine as Immediate-Release Liquid or Sustained-Release Tablets for Cancer Pain," *J Pediatr*, 1999, 135(1):47-55.

McRorie TI, Lynn AM, Nespeca MK, et al, "The Maturation of Morphine Clearance and Metabolism," *Am J Dis Child*, 1992, 147(8):972-6.

Miser AW, Davis DM, Hughes CS, et al, "Continuous Subcutaneous Infusion of Morphine in Children With Cancer," *Am J Dis Child*, 1983, 137(4):383-5.

Miser AW, Miser JS, and Clark BS, "Continuous Intravenous Infusion of Morphine Sulfate for Control of Severe Pain in Children With Terminal Malignancy," *J Pediatr*, 1980, 96(5):930-2.

Olkkola KT, Hamunen K, and Maunuksela EL, "Clinical Pharmacokinetics and Pharmacodynamics of Opioid Analgesics in Infants and Children," *Clin Pharmacokinet*, 1995, 28(5):385-404.

♦ **M.O.S.® 10 (Can)** *see* Morphine Sulfate *on page 1082*

♦ **M.O.S.® 20 (Can)** *see* Morphine Sulfate *on page 1082*

♦ **M.O.S.® 30 (Can)** *see* Morphine Sulfate *on page 1082*

♦ **Mosco® Corn and Callus Remover [OTC]** *see* Salicylic Acid *on page 1413*

Mumps Virus Vaccine (Live/Attenuated)

(mumpz VYE rus vak SEEN, live, a ten YOO ate ed)

Related Information

Immunization Guidelines *on page 1837*

U.S. Brand Names Mumpsvax®

Therapeutic Category Vaccine

Generic Available No

Use Mumps prophylaxis by promoting active immunity in children ≥12 months and adults

Note: Trivalent measles-mumps-rubella (MMR) vaccine is the preferred agent for most children and many adults; persons born prior to 1957 are generally considered immune and need not be vaccinated

Pregnancy Risk Factor C

Lactation

Excretion in breast milk unknown/use caution

(Continued)

Mumps Virus Vaccine (Live/Attenuated) *(Continued)*

Contraindications Hypersensitivity to mumps vaccine, gelatin, or any component of the formulation; history of anaphylactic reactions to neomycin; individuals with blood dyscrasias, leukemia, lymphomas, or other malignant neoplasms affecting the bone marrow or lymphatic systems; concurrent immunosuppressive therapy; primary and acquired immunodeficiency states; family history of congenital or hereditary immunodeficiency; active/untreated tuberculosis; current febrile illness or active febrile infection

Warnings Avoid pregnancy for 3 months following vaccination; use in patients with existing thrombocytopenia may result in more severe reduction in platelets; avoid use in patients with previous history of post vaccination thrombocytopenia, as rechallenge has resulted in recurrence of thrombocytopenia; severe allergic reactions including anaphylaxis have been reported rarely. Immediate treatment for anaphylactic/anaphylactoid reaction should be available during vaccine use. Use extreme caution in patients with immediate-type hypersensitivity reactions to eggs.

Mumps vaccine should not be administered to severely immunocompromised persons with the exception of asymptomatic children with HIV. Patients with minor illnesses (diarrhea, mild upper respiratory tract infection with or without low grade fever or other illnesses with low-grade fever) may receive vaccine. Leukemia patients who are in remission and who have not received chemotherapy for at least 3 months may be vaccinated.

Precautions Immediate treatment for anaphylactic reactions should be available during vaccine use; defer vaccination for persons with acute febrile illness until recovery

Adverse Reactions All serious adverse reactions must be reported to the U.S. Department of Health and Human Services (DHHS) Vaccine Adverse Event Reporting System (VAERS) 1-800-822-7967.

Cardiovascular: Vasculitis

Central nervous system: Fever, seizures, syncope, irritability, confusion, headache, encephalitis, Guillain-Barré syndrome

Dermatologic: Rash, Stevens-Johnson syndrome, erythema multiforme, urticaria

Endocrine & metabolic: Parotitis

Genitourinary: Orchitis in postpubescent and adult males

Gastrointestinal: Pancreatitis, diarrhea, parotitis

Hematologic: Thrombocytopenia, purpura, leukocytosis

Local: Burning or stinging at injection site

Ocular: Ocular palsies, optic neuritis, papillitis, retrobulbar neuritis, conjunctivitis

Otic: Nerve deafness, otitis media

Respiratory: Cough, rhinitis

Miscellaneous: Hypersensitivity reactions, lymphadenopathy

Drug Interactions Immunosuppressive medications may decrease the effectiveness of the vaccine; avoid high doses of corticosteroids for ≥14 days, wait at least 1 month between discontinuing steroid therapy and administering vaccine; immune globulin may decrease effectiveness; defer vaccination for 3 months following immune globulin administration

Stability Prior to reconstitution, store the powder at 2°C to 8°C (36°F to 46°F) or colder (freezing does not affect potency). Protect from light. Diluent may be stored with powder or at room temperature. Discard if not used within 8 hours of reconstitution.

Mechanism of Action Promotes active immunity to mumps virus by inducing specific antibodies.

Usual Dosage Children ≥12 months and Adults: SubQ: 0.5 mL as a single dose

Administration Use entire contents of the provided diluent to reconstitute vaccine. Gently agitate to mix thoroughly. Discard if powder does not dissolve. Use as soon as possible following reconstitution; discard if not used within 8 hours; administer by SubQ injection into the anterolateral aspect of the thigh or arm; **not for I.M. or I.V. administration**

Test Interactions Temporary suppression of tuberculosis skin test

Patient Information Pregnancy should be avoided for 3 months following vaccination. A little swelling of the glands in the cheeks and under the jaw may occur that lasts for a few days; this could happen from 1-2 weeks after getting the mumps vaccine; this happens rarely.

Nursing Implications Federal law requires that the date of administration, the vaccine manufacturer, lot number of vaccine, and the administering person's name, title, and address be entered into the patient's permanent medical record.

Additional Information All adults without documentation of live vaccine on or after the first birthday or physician-diagnosed mumps, or laboratory evidence or immunity (particularly males and young adults who work in or congregate in hospitals, colleges, and on military bases) should be vaccinated. It is reasonable to consider persons born before 1957 immune, but there is no contraindication to vaccination of older persons. Susceptible travelers should be vaccinated.

Dosage Forms Excipient information presented when available (limited, particularly for generics); consult specific product labeling.

Injection, powder for reconstitution [preservative free]:

Mumpsvax®: $TCID_{50}$ 20,000 [contains human albumin, bovine serum, gelatin, neomycin; packaged with diluent]

References

American Academy of Pediatrics Committee on Infectious Diseases, "Recommended Childhood and Adolescent Immunization Schedule - United States, January-June 2004," *Pediatrics*, 2004, 113(1 Pt 1):142-7.

Centers for Disease Control and Prevention, "Recommended Childhood and Adolescent Immunization Schedule - United States, July-December 2004," *MMWR Morb Mortal Wkly Rep*, 2004, 53(16):Q1-4.

Centers for Disease Control, "Recommended Adult Immunization Schedule, October 2004-September 2005," available at www.cdc.gov.

Mupirocin (myoo PEER oh sin)

Medication Safety Issues

Sound-alike/look-alike issues:

Bactroban® may be confused with bacitracin, baclofen

U.S. Brand Names Bactroban®; Bactroban® Nasal; Centany™

Canadian Brand Names Bactroban®

Index Terms Mupirocin Calcium; Pseudomonic Acid A

Therapeutic Category Antibiotic, Topical

Generic Available Yes: Topical ointment

Use Ointment: Topical treatment of impetigo caused by *Staphylococcus aureus* and *Streptococcus pyogenes*; topical treatment of folliculitis, furunculosis, minor wounds, burns, and ulcers caused by susceptible organisms; Cream: Treatment of secondarily-infected traumatic skin lesions due to susceptible strains of *S. aureus* and *S. pyogenes*; prophylactic agent applied to intravenous catheter exit sites; Intranasal ointment: Eradication of *S. aureus* from nasal and perineal carriage sites

Pregnancy Risk Factor B

Lactation Excretion in breast milk unknown/use caution

Contraindications Hypersensitivity to mupirocin, polyethylene glycol, or any component

Warnings Potentially toxic amounts of polyethylene glycol (PEG) contained in the vehicle may be absorbed percutaneously in patients with extensive burns or open wounds; the PEG vehicle may irritate mucous membranes and increase nasal secretions if applied intranasally; prolonged use may result in overgrowth of nonsusceptible organisms

Precautions Use with caution in patients with impaired renal function and in burn patients

Adverse Reactions

Dermatologic: Pruritus, rash, erythema, dry skin

Local: Burning, stinging, pain, tenderness, local edema

Stability Do not mix with Aquaphor®, coal tar solution, or salicylic acid

Mechanism of Action Binds to bacterial isoleucyl transfer-RNA synthetase preventing isoleucine incorporation resulting in the inhibition of protein and RNA synthesis

Pharmacokinetics

Absorption: Following topical administration, penetrates the outer layers of the skin; systemic absorption is minimal through intact skin

Protein binding: 95%

Metabolism: Extensive in the liver and skin to monic acid

Half-life: 17-36 minutes

Elimination: Metabolite is excreted in urine

Usual Dosage

Intranasal: Children and Adults: Apply small amount 2-4 times/day for 5-14 days

Topical:

Cream: Infants ≥3 months, Children, and Adults: Apply small amount 3 times/day for 10 days

Ointment: Infants ≥2 months, Children, and Adults: Apply a small amount 3-5 times/day for 5-14 days

Administration Cream and ointment: For topical use only; do not apply into the eye; may cover with gauze dressing; Intranasal: Avoid contact with eyes; apply one-half of the ointment from the single-use tube into each nostril

Additional Information Contains polyethylene glycol vehicle

Dosage Forms Excipient information presented when available (limited, particularly for generics); consult specific product labeling.

Note: Strength expressed as base

(Continued)

Mupirocin *(Continued)*

Cream, topical, as calcium:
  Bactroban®: 2% (15 g, 30 g) [contains benzyl alcohol]
Ointment, intranasal, as calcium:
  Bactroban® Nasal: 2% (1 g) [single-use tube]
Ointment, topical: 2% (0.9 g, 22 g)
  Bactroban®: 2% (22 g) [contains polyethylene glycol]
  Centany™: 2% (15 g, 30 g)

References

Britton JW, Fajardo JE, and Krafte-Jacobs B, "Comparison of Mupirocin and Erythromycin in the Treatment of Impetigo," *J Pediatr*, 1990, 117(5):827-9.

Hayakawa T, Hayashidera T, Katsura S, et al, "Nasal Mupirocin Treatment of Pharynx-Colonized Methicillin Resistant *Staphylococcus aureus*: Preliminary Study With 10 Carrier Infants," *Pediatr Int*, 2000, 42(1):67-70.

Hitomi S, Kubota M, Mori N, et al, "Control of a Methicillin-Resistant *Staphylococcus aureus* Outbreak in a Neonatal Intensive Care Unit by Unselective Use of Nasal Mupirocin Ointment," *J Hosp Infect*, 2000, 46(2):123-9.

Oh J, von Baum H, Klaus G, et al, "Nasal Carriage of *Staphylococcus aureus* in Families of Children on Peritoneal Dialysis. European Pediatric Peritoneal Dialysis Study Group (EPPS)," *Adv Perit Dial*, 2000, 16:324-7.

♦ **Mupirocin Calcium** *see* Mupirocin *on page 1091*

♦ **Murine® Ear Wax Removal System [OTC]** *see* Carbamide Peroxide *on page 283*

♦ **Muro 128® [OTC]** *see* Sodium Chloride *on page 1450*

Muromonab-CD3 (myoo roe MOE nab see dee three)

U.S. Brand Names Orthoclone OKT® 3

Canadian Brand Names Orthoclone OKT® 3

Index Terms Monoclonal Antibody; OKT3

Therapeutic Category Immunosuppressant Agent

Generic Available No

Use Treatment of acute allograft rejection in renal transplant patients; effective in reversing acute hepatic, cardiac, and bone marrow transplant rejection episodes resistant to conventional treatment

Pregnancy Risk Factor C

Lactation Excretion in breast milk unknown/contraindicated

Contraindications Hypersensitivity to OKT3 or any Murine® product; patients in fluid overload or those with >3% weight gain within 1 week prior to start of OKT3

Warnings May result in an increased susceptibility to infection; severe pulmonary edema has occurred in patients with fluid overload; first-dose effect (flu-like symptoms, anaphylactic-type reaction) may occur within 30 minutes to 6 hours, up to 24 hours after the first dose. Cardiopulmonary resuscitation may be needed. Methylprednisolone sodium succinate given prior to first OKT3 dose and I.V. hydrocortisone sodium succinate given 30 minutes after administration are strongly recommended to decrease the incidence of reactions to the first dose.

Precautions Dosage of concomitant immunosuppressants should be reduced by 50%, and cyclosporine discontinued or decreased by 50% during OKT3 therapy (see Additional Information); maintenance immunosuppression and cyclosporine should be resumed about 3 days before stopping OKT3 to protect against rebound rejection

Adverse Reactions

Cardiovascular: Tachycardia, hypertension, hypotension, perioral and peripheral cyanosis
Central nervous system: Aseptic meningitis, seizures, headache, pyrexia, confusion
Dermatologic: Pruritus, rash
Gastrointestinal: Diarrhea, nausea, vomiting
Neuromuscular & skeletal: Arthralgia, tremor, myalgia
Ocular: Photophobia
Renal: Elevated BUN, elevated serum creatinine
Respiratory: Dyspnea, chest pain, tightness, wheezing, pulmonary edema
Miscellaneous: Flu-like symptoms (ie, fever, chills), anaphylactic-type reactions

Stability Store in refrigerator; do not freeze or shake; OKT3 left out of the refrigerator for more than 4 hours must not be used

Mechanism of Action Coats the circulating T lymphocytes subjecting these cells to opsonization by the reticuloendothelial system; modulates the T lymphocyte antigen receptor CD3 complex which results in the removal of all CD3 molecules from the cell surface so that the cell lacks the ability to function as a T lymphocyte

Pharmacokinetics

Distribution: V_d is closely related to the apparent volume of distribution for albumin
Half-life: 18 hours

Elimination: Binds to T lymphocytes with resultant opsonization and removal by the reticuloendothelial system

Usual Dosage I.V. (refer to individual protocols):

Note: Children and Adults: Methylprednisolone sodium succinate 1 mg/kg I.V. given 2-6 hours prior to first OKT3 administration and I.V. hydrocortisone sodium succinate 50-100 mg given 30 minutes after administration are strongly recommended to decrease the incidence of reactions to the first dose; patient temperature should not exceed 37.8°C (100°F) at time of administration

Children <12 years: 0.1 mg/kg/day once daily for 10-14 days **or** patients ≤30 kg: 2.5 mg once daily for 10-14 days; patients >30 kg: 5 mg once daily for 10-14 days

Children ≥12 years and Adults: 5 mg/day once daily for 10-14 days

Administration Parenteral: Filter each dose through a low protein-binding 0.22 micron filter (Millex GV) before administration; administer I.V. push over 1 minute at a final concentration of 1 mg/mL

Monitoring Parameters Chest x-ray, weight gain, CBC with differential, BUN and S_{cr}, vital signs (blood pressure, temperature, pulse, respiration) and immunologic monitoring of T cells, serum levels of OKT3, CD3+ cell count

Reference Range Mean serum trough levels rise during the first 3 days, then average 0.9 mcg/mL on days 3-14; if serum trough OKT3 concentrations are maintained at 1 mcg/mL, then CD3 counts remain low

Nursing Implications Inform patient of expected first dose effects which may include fever, chills, chest tightness, wheezing, nausea, vomiting, and diarrhea; first-dose reaction usually starts 40-60 minutes after the injection and lasts for several hours; first-dose effects are markedly reduced with subsequent doses; monitor patient closely for 48 hours after the first dose; corticosteroids are recommended; acetaminophen and antihistamines can be given concomitantly with OKT3 to reduce early reactions

Additional Information Recommend decreasing dose of prednisone to 0.5 mg/kg, azathioprine to 0.5 mg/kg (approximate 50% decrease in dose), and discontinuing cyclosporine or decreasing cyclosporine dose by 50% while patient is receiving OKT3

Dosage Forms Excipient information presented when available (limited, particularly for generics); consult specific product labeling.

Injection, solution: 1 mg/mL (5 mL) [contains sodium 43 mg/5 mL]

References

Ettenger RB, Marik JL, Rosenthal JT, et al, "OKT_3 for Rejection Reversal in Pediatric Renal Transplantation," *Clin Transpl*, 1988, 2:180-4.

Hooks MA, Wade CS, and Millikan WJ Jr, "Muromonab CD-3: A Review of Its Pharmacology, Pharmacokinetics, and Clinical Use in Transplantation," *Pharmacotherapy*, 1991, 11(1):26-37.

Niaudet P, Murcia I, Jean G, et al, "A Comparative Trial of OKT_3 and Antilymphocyte Serum in the Preventive Treatment of Rejection After Kidney Transplantation in Children," *Ann Pediatr Paris*, 1990, 37(2):83-5.

Todd PA and Brogden RN, "Muromonab CD3 A Review of Its Pharmacology and Therapeutic Potential," *Drugs*, 1989, 37(6):871-99.

- ♦ **Muse®** *see* Alprostadil *on page 81*
- ♦ **Muse® Pellet (Can)** *see* Alprostadil *on page 81*
- ♦ **Mustargen®** *see* Mechlorethamine *on page 987*
- ♦ **Mustine** *see* Mechlorethamine *on page 987*
- ♦ **Mutamycin®** *see* Mitomycin *on page 1070*
- ♦ **Myambutol®** *see* Ethambutol *on page 616*
- ♦ **Mycamine®** *see* Micafungin *on page 1054*
- ♦ **Mycelex®** *see* Clotrimazole *on page 393*
- ♦ **Mycelex®-7 [OTC]** *see* Clotrimazole *on page 393*
- ♦ **Mycelex® Twin Pack [OTC]** *see* Clotrimazole *on page 393*
- ♦ **Mycinaire™ [OTC]** *see* Sodium Chloride *on page 1450*
- ♦ **Mycinettes® [OTC]** *see* Benzocaine *on page 204*
- ♦ **Mycobutin®** *see* Rifabutin *on page 1382*
- ♦ **Mycocide® NS [OTC]** *see* Tolnaftate *on page 1550*

Mycophenolate (mye koe FEN oh late)

U.S. Brand Names CellCept®; Myfortic®

Canadian Brand Names CellCept®; Myfortic®

Index Terms MMF; MPA; Mycophenolate Mofetil; Mycophenolate Sodium; Mycophenolic Acid

Therapeutic Category Immunosuppressant Agent

Generic Available No

Use Immunosuppressant agent used in conjunction with other immunosuppressive therapies (eg, cyclosporine and corticosteroids with or without antithymocyte induction) for the prophylaxis of organ rejection in patients receiving allogeneic renal, (Continued)

Mycophenolate *(Continued)*

hepatic, or cardiac transplants; add-on immunosuppressant agent that is typically used in place of azathioprine in combination regimens for the treatment of refractory acute kidney graft rejection; use of mycophenolate is also being studied in bone marrow transplant patients

Pregnancy Risk Factor C

Lactation Excretion in breast milk unknown/not recommended

Contraindications Hypersensitivity to mycophenolate mofetil, mycophenolate sodium, mycophenolic acid, polysorbate 80 (I.V. formulation), or any component

Warnings Immunosuppression with mycophenolate may result in an increased susceptibility to infection and an increased risk of developing lymphomas and other malignancies, particularly of the skin; risk appears to be associated with the intensity and duration of immunosuppression. Mycophenolate has been shown to have teratogenic effects and causes fetal harm; in women of childbearing potential, effective contraception must be initiated before starting mycophenolate therapy and continued for 6 weeks after it has been discontinued.

Precautions Use with caution in patients with active serious digestive disease and in patients with renal impairment; modify dosage in patients with severe chronic renal impairment (GFR <25 mL/minute/1.73 m^2 outside of the immediate post-transplant period) and in patients with neutropenia. Avoid use in patients with rare hereditary deficiency of hypoxanthineguanine phosphoribosyl-transferase (HGPRT) such as Lesch-Nyhan and Kelley-Seegmiller syndrome. The oral suspension contains aspartame which is metabolized to phenylalanine and must be used with caution in patients with phenylketonuria.

Adverse Reactions

Cardiovascular: Hypertension, chest pain, peripheral edema, tachycardia

Central nervous system: Insomnia, dizziness, fever, headache, anxiety

Dermatologic: Rash, acne

Endocrine & metabolic: Hypercholesterolemia, hypophosphatemia, hypokalemia, hyperkalemia, hyperglycemia

Gastrointestinal: Diarrhea, constipation, nausea, vomiting, oral moniliasis, abdominal pain, dyspepsia, GI tract hemorrhage, colitis, pancreatitis, anorexia, intestinal perforation, gastric and duodenal ulcers

Genitourinary: Hematuria, urinary tract infection

Hematologic: Leukopenia, neutropenia, anemia, thrombocytopenia, leukocytosis

Local: Phlebitis, thrombosis

Neuromuscular & skeletal: Tremor, back pain, myalgia, weakness

Renal: Renal tubular necrosis

Respiratory: Dyspnea, cough, pharyngitis, pulmonary fibrosis

Miscellaneous: 1% incidence of lymphoproliferative disease

Drug Interactions Aluminum- and magnesium-containing antacids decrease mycophenolate absorption; cholestyramine decreases mycophenolate bioavailability by 40% (interrupts enterohepatic recirculation of mycophenolic acid); acyclovir and ganciclovir may compete with mycophenolic acid glucuronide (MPAG) for renal tubular secretion resulting in increased concentrations of both drugs and MPAG; drugs which inhibit renal tubular secretion (probenecid) increase mycophenolate and MPAG concentrations; azathioprine (potential for additive bone marrow suppression); live vaccines (vaccination may be less effective, but influenza vaccine may be of value)

Food Interactions Presence of food decreases mycophenolate peak concentration by 40% but has no effect on the extent of absorption

Stability Store at room temperature

Suspension: Store reconstituted suspension in refrigerator or at room temperature; stable for 60 days after reconstitution

Injection: Mycophenolate I.V. infusion solution is stable for 12 hours at room temperature after preparation; administration of the infusion solution should be within 4 hours from reconstitution and dilution of the drug. Do not mix mycophenolate with any other drugs.

Mechanism of Action Hydrolyzed to form mycophenolic acid (MPA), the active metabolite, which is a potent, uncompetitive reversible inhibitor of inosine monophosphate dehydrogenase (IMPDH) in the purine biosynthesis pathway; inhibition of IMPDH results in a depletion of guanosine triphosphate and deoxyguanosine triphosphate, thereby inhibiting T- and B-cell proliferation, cytotoxic T-cell generation and antibody secretion.

Pharmacokinetics

Absorption: Rapid and extensive; early post-transplant period MPA AUC values are approximately 45% to 53% lower than later post-transplant period (>3 months) MPA AUC values in pediatric patients 1-18 years.

Distribution: Mean V_d (adults): 4 L/kg

Protein binding:
Mycophenolate: 97%
Mycophenolate glucuronide: 82%

Metabolism: Mycophenolate mofetil undergoes hydrolysis to mycophenolic acid (MPA is the active metabolite); MPA is metabolized by glucuronyl transferase to mycophenolic acid glucuronide (MPAG is inactive). MPAG is converted to MPA via enterohepatic recirculation.

Bioavailability: 94% based on MPA; enterohepatic recirculation contributes to MPA concentration; two 500 mg tablets have been shown to be bioequivalent to four 250 mg capsules or 1000 mg of oral suspension

Half-life:
Oral: 17.9 hours
I.V.: 16.6 hours

Time to peak serum concentration: Mycophenolate mofetil: 0.5-1 hour; mycophenolate sodium: 1.5-2.75 hours

Elimination: 93% of dose recovered in urine, 6% in feces; 87% of mycophenolic acid dose recovered as MPAG in urine; <1% of dose excreted as MPA in urine

Dialysis: Not dialyzable

Usual Dosage

Oral: Mycophenolate mofetil tablets, capsules, and suspension should **not** be used interchangeably with the delayed-release tablet formulation due to differences in the rate of absorption.

Children:

Mycophenolate mofetil: 600 mg/m^2/dose twice daily; maximum dose: 2 g/day; **Note:** Limited information regarding mycophenolate use in pediatric patients is currently available in the literature: 32 pediatric patients (14 underwent living donor and 18 receiving cadaveric donor renal transplants) received mycophenolate 8-30 mg/kg/dose orally twice daily with cyclosporine, prednisone, and Atgam® induction. However, pharmacokinetic studies suggest that doses of mycophenolate adjusted to body surface area resulted in AUCs which better approximated those of adults versus doses adjusted for body weight which resulted in lower AUCs in pediatric patients.

or

BSA 1.25 m^2 to 1.5 m^2: 750 mg twice daily
BSA >1.5 m^2: 1 g twice daily

Mycophenolate delayed-release tablet: 400 mg/m^2/dose twice daily; maximum dose: 720 mg
BSA <1.19 m^2: Use of this formulation is not recommended.

or

BSA 1.19-1.58 m^2: 540 mg twice daily
BSA >1.58 m^2: 720 mg twice daily

Adults:

Mycophenolate mofetil:
Renal transplant: 1 g twice daily in combination with corticosteroids and cyclosporine; dosages as high as 3-3.5 g/day were used in clinical trials, but no efficacy advantage was established
Cardiac transplant: 1.5 g twice daily
Hepatic transplant: 1.5 g twice daily

Mycophenolate delayed-release tablet: 720 mg twice daily

I.V. infusion (administer within 24 hours following transplantation; can be given for up to 14 days; patients should be switched to oral formulation as soon as oral medication is tolerated):

Adults:
Renal transplant: 1 g twice daily
Cardiac transplant: 1.5 g twice daily
Hepatic transplant: 1 g twice daily

Dosing adjustment in renal impairment: Renal transplant: GFR <25 mL/minute/1.73 m^2 outside the immediate post-transplant period:
Mycophenolate mofetil: Avoid doses >1 g twice daily
Mycophenolate delayed-release tablet: Monitor carefully

Administration

Oral: Administer on an empty stomach one hour before or two hours after food; one center has mixed the contents of the capsule in chocolate syrup; mycophenolate suspension can be administered orally or via a nasogastric tube with a minimum size of 8 French; shake suspension well before use. Swallow delayed-release tablet whole; do not crush, chew, or cut.

I.V.: Reconstitute vial with D_5W and further dilute to a final concentration of 6 mg/mL using D_5W. Administer by slow I.V. infusion over a period of no less than 2 hours.

Monitoring Parameters CBC with differential, platelet count, serum electrolytes, glucose, phosphate, cholesterol, and renal function tests; blood pressure. Pregnancy

(Continued)

Mycophenolate *(Continued)*

test in female patients of childbearing potential within 1 week prior to beginning therapy.

Patient Information Do not take within 1 hour before or 2 hours after antacids or cholestyramine; maintain adequate hydration. You will be susceptible to infection (avoid crowds and people with infections). Report to physician any chest pain, acute headache or dizziness, respiratory infection symptoms, difficulty breathing, or unusual bleeding or bruising. You may be at increased risk for skin cancer (wear protective clothing and use sunscreen). Women of childbearing age should use 2 effective forms of contraception simultaneously unless abstinence is the chosen method before starting mycophenolate therapy, during therapy, and for 6 weeks after discontinuing mycophenolate.

Nursing Implications Mycophenolate capsules should not be opened or crushed; avoid inhalation or direct contact of the capsule contents with skin or mucous membranes; mycophenolate tablets should not be crushed

Dosage Forms Excipient information presented when available (limited, particularly for generics); consult specific product labeling.

Capsule, as mofetil (CellCept®): 250 mg

Injection, powder for reconstitution, as mofetil hydrochloride (CellCept®): 500 mg [contains polysorbate 80]

Powder for oral suspension, as mofetil (CellCept®): 200 mg/mL (225 mL) [provides 175 mL suspension following reconstitution; contains phenylalanine 0.56 mg/mL; mixed fruit flavor]

Tablet, as mofetil (CellCept®): 500 mg [may contain ethyl alcohol]

Tablet, delayed release, as mycophenolic acid (Myfortic®): 180 mg, 360 mg [formulated as a sodium salt]

Extemporaneous Preparations A 50 mg/mL suspension can be prepared in a vertical flow hood by emptying six 250 mg mycophenolate mofetil capsules into a mortar wetted and triturated with 7.5 mL Ora-Plus® to a smooth paste. Add 15 mL of cherry syrup and triturate to make a final volume of 30 mL. The suspension is stable for 210 days when stored at 5°C, stable for 28 days when stored at 37°C or 25°C, and stable for 11 days when stored at 45°C.

Venkataramanan R, McCombs JR, Zudarnan S, et al, "Stability of Mycophenolate Mofetil as an Extemporaneous Suspension," *Ann Pharmacother*, 1998, 32:755-7.

References

Ettenger R, Warshaw B, Menster M, et al, "Mycophenolate Mofetil in Pediatric Renal Transplantation: A Report of the Ped MMF Study Group." Abstract: 1996, Annual Meeting, ASTP.

Sollinger HW, "Mycophenolate Mofetil for the Prevention of Acute Rejection in Primary Cadaveric Renal Allograft Recipients. U.S. Renal Transplant Mycophenolate Mofetil Study Group," *Transplantation*, 1995, 60:225-32.

Nabilone (NA bi lone)

U.S. Brand Names Cesamet™
Canadian Brand Names Cesamet™
Therapeutic Category Antiemetic
Generic Available No
Use Treatment of refractory nausea and vomiting associated with cancer chemotherapy
Restrictions C-II
Pregnancy Risk Factor C
Lactation Excretion in breast milk unknown/not recommended
Contraindications Hypersensitivity to nabilone, cannabinoids, tetrahydrocannabinol, or any component
Warnings Nabilone has potential for abuse and/or dependence; use caution in patients with substance abuse history; limit antiemetic therapy availability to current cycle of chemotherapy. Safety and efficacy in children have not been established.
Precautions Use with caution in patients with cardiovascular disease (may cause tachycardia and orthostatic hypotension), history of substance abuse, and those with pre-existing CNS depression; use caution with current or previous history of mental illness; cannabinoid use may reveal symptoms of psychiatric disorders. Psychiatric adverse reactions may persist for up to 3 days after discontinuing treatment.
Adverse Reactions

Cardiovascular: Orthostatic hypotension, arrhythmia, chest pain, hypertension, syncope, tachycardia

Central nervous system: Dizziness (59%), drowsiness (52% to 66%), vertigo (52% to 59%), euphoria (11% to 38%), ataxia, depression, concentration decreased, sleep disturbance, dysphoria, headache, sedation, depersonalization, disorientation, abnormal dreams, anxiety, apathy, cerebral vascular accident, chills, fatigue, fever, emotional disorder, emotional lability, hallucinations, insomnia, mood swings, memory disturbance, nervousness, neurosis (phobic), panic disorder, paranoia, psychosis (toxic)

Dermatologic: Photosensitivity, rash, pruritus

Gastrointestinal: Xerostomia (22% to 36%), anorexia, nausea, appetite increased, abdominal pain, aphthous ulcer, constipation, diarrhea, dyspepsia, gastritis, epistaxis, mouth irritation, taste perversion, vomiting

Genitourinary: Urinary retention, polyuria

Hematologic: Anemia, leukopenia

Neuromuscular & skeletal: Weakness, akathisia, back pain, dystonia, joint pain, muscle pain, neck pain, numbness, paresthesia, tremor

Ocular: Visual disturbance (13%), amblyopia, eye irritation, xerophthalmia, photophobia, pupil dilation

Otic: Tinnitus

Respiratory: Cough, dyspnea, nasal congestion, wheezing

Miscellaneous: Hypersensitivity reactions, diaphoresis, anhydrosis

Drug Interactions Cytochrome P450 isoenzyme CYP2C8 and CYP2C9 inhibitor (moderate) and CYP2E1 and 3A4 inhibitor (weak)

Additive tachycardia and hypertension with amphetamines, cocaine, sympathomimetics, anticholinergics, tricyclic antidepressants; additive CNS effects with sedatives, antihistamines, hypnotics, psychomimetics, tricyclic antidepressants, and alcohol; may potentiate and have cross-tolerance to opioids; naltrexone may enhance cannabinoid effects via opioid receptor blockade; may increase metabolism of theophylline

Stability Store at room temperature between 15°C and 30°C (59°F and 86°F).
Mechanism of Action Not fully characterized; antiemetic activity may be due to effect on cannabinoid receptors (CB1) within the central nervous system
Pharmacokinetics

Absorption: Rapid and complete

Distribution: ~12.5 L/kg

Metabolism: To several active metabolites by oxidation and stereospecific enzyme reduction; CYP450 enzymes may also be involved

Half-life: Parent compound: 2 hours; Metabolites: 35 hours

Time to peak serum concertration: Within 2 hours

Elimination: Feces (~60%); renal (~24%)

Usual Dosage

Oral:

Children >4 years (unlabeled use):

- <18 kg: 0.5 mg twice daily
- 18-30 kg: 1 mg twice daily
- >30 kg: 1 mg 3 times/day

(Continued)

Nabilone *(Continued)*

Adults: 1-2 mg twice daily (maximum: 6 mg divided in 3 doses daily)

Dosage adjustment in renal impairment: No adjustment required.

Administration Oral: Initial dose should be given 1-3 hours before chemotherapy; may be given 2-3 times/day during the entire chemotherapy course and for up to 48 hours after the last dose of chemotherapy; a dose the night before chemotherapy may be useful

Monitoring Parameters Blood pressure, heart rate; signs and symptoms of excessive use, abuse, or misuse

Patient Information May cause drowsiness and impair ability to perform activities requiring mental alertness or physical coordination; may cause dry mouth; avoid alcohol. May cause photosensitivity reactions; avoid exposure to sunlight and artificial light sources. Report excessive or persistent CNS changes (euphoria, anxiety, depression, memory lapse, bizarre thought patterns, excitability, inability to control thoughts or behavior, fainting); respiratory difficulties; rapid heartbeat; or other adverse reactions.

Dosage Forms Excipient information presented when available (limited, particularly for generics); consult specific product labeling.

Capsule:

Cesamet™: 1 mg

References

Chan HS, Correia JA, and MacLeod SM, "Nabilone Versus Prochlorperazine for Control of Cancer Chemotherapy-Induced Emesis in Children: A Double-Blind, Crossover Trial," *Pediatrics*, 1987, 79(6):946-52.

Dupuis LL and Nathan PC, "Options for the Prevention and Management of Acute Chemotherapy-Induced Nausea and Vomiting in Children," *Pediatr Drug*, 2003, 5(9):597-613.

Tramer MR, Carroll D, Campbell FA, et al, "Cannabinoids for Control of Chemotherapy Induced Nausea and Vomiting: Quantitative Systematic Review," *BMJ*, 2001, 323(7303):16-21.

Ward A and Holmes B, "Nabilone: A Preliminary Review of Its Pharmacological Properties and Therapeutic Use," *Drugs*, 1985, 30(2):127-44.

◆ **NAC** *see* Acetylcysteine *on page 51*

◆ ***N*-Acetyl-L-cysteine** *see* Acetylcysteine *on page 51*

◆ ***N*-Acetylcysteine** *see* Acetylcysteine *on page 51*

◆ **N-Acetyl-P-Aminophenol** *see* Acetaminophen *on page 42*

◆ **NaCl** *see* Sodium Chloride *on page 1450*

Nadolol (nay DOE lole)

Medication Safety Issues

Sound-alike/look-alike issues:

Nadolol may be confused with Mandol®

Corgard® may be confused with Cognex®

Related Information

Antihypertensive Agents by Class *on page 1678*

Overdose and Toxicology *on page 1916*

U.S. Brand Names Corgard®

Canadian Brand Names Alti-Nadolol; Apo-Nadol®; Corgard®; Novo-Nadolol

Therapeutic Category Antianginal Agent; Antiarrhythmic Agent, Class II; Antihypertensive Agent; Antimigraine Agent; Beta-Adrenergic Blocker

Generic Available Yes

Use Treatment of hypertension and angina pectoris; prophylaxis of migraine headaches

Pregnancy Risk Factor C

Lactation Enters breast milk/use caution (AAP rates "compatible")

Contraindications Hypersensitivity to nadolol or any component; uncompensated CHF, cardiogenic shock, bradycardia or heart block, bronchial asthma, bronchospasms

Precautions Therapy should not be discontinued abruptly; reduce dosage gradually over a period of 1-2 weeks; increase dosing interval in patients with renal dysfunction; use with caution in patients with diabetes mellitus

Adverse Reactions

Cardiovascular: Persistent bradycardia, orthostatic hypotension, Raynaud's syndrome, CHF, edema

Central nervous system: Fatigue, dizziness

Dermatological: Rash

Gastrointestinal: GI discomfort

Respiratory: Bronchospasm

Drug Interactions Other hypotensive agents, diuretics and phenothiazines may increase hypotensive effects of nadolol; abrupt withdrawal of clonidine while receiving beta-blockers may result in an exaggerated hypertensive crisis; nadolol may enhance neuromuscular blocking agents and will antagonize beta-sympathomimetic drugs; other drug interactions similar to propranolol may occur

Food Interactions Avoid natural licorice (causes sodium and water retention and increases potassium loss)

Mechanism of Action Competitively blocks response to beta-adrenergic stimulation; nonselective beta-blocker

Pharmacodynamics Duration: 24 hours

Pharmacokinetics

Absorption: Oral: 30% to 40%

Distribution: Concentration in human breast milk is 4.6 times higher than serum

Protein-binding: 28%

Half-life, elimination:

Increased half-life with decreased renal function

Infants 3-22 months (n=3): 3.2-4.3 hours

Children 10 years (n=1): 15.7 hours

Children ~15 years (n=1): 7.3 hours

Adults: 10-24 hours

Dialysis: Moderately dialyzable (20% to 50%)

Usual Dosage Oral:

Children: Very limited information (ie, one study) regarding pediatric dosage currently available in literature: The study used oral nadolol to control supraventricular tachycardia (SVT) in 26 children 3 months to 15 years of age. SVT was well controlled in 23 out of 26 children; recommended initial dose: 0.5-1 mg/kg once daily; monitor carefully, gradually increase dose; median dose required: 1 mg/kg/day; maximum dose: 2.5 mg/kg/day.

Adults: Initial: 40 mg once daily; increase gradually; usual dosage: 40-80 mg/day; may need up to 240-320 mg/day; doses as high as 640 mg/day have been used; usual dosage range for hypertension (JNC 7): 40-120 mg once daily

Dosage adjustment in adults with renal impairment:

Cl_{cr} 10-50 mL/minute: Administer 50% of normal dose

Cl_{cr} <10 mL/minute: Administer 25% of normal dose

Administration Oral: May administer without regard to meals

Monitoring Parameters Blood pressure, heart rate, fluid intake and output, weight

Patient Information Limit alcohol; do not abruptly discontinue; may mask symptoms of hypoglycemia, but sweating may still occur

Dosage Forms Excipient information presented when available (limited, particularly for generics); consult specific product labeling. [DSC] = Discontinued product

Tablet: 20 mg, 40 mg, 80 mg, 120 mg, 160 mg

Corgard®: 20 mg, 40 mg, 80 mg, 120 mg [DSC], 160 mg [DSC]

References

Chobanian AV, Bakris GL, Black HR, et al, "The Seventh Report of the Joint National Committee on Prevention, Detection, Evaluation, and Treatment of High Blood Pressure: The JNC 7 report," *JAMA*, 2003, 289(19):2560-72.

Devlin RG and Duchin KL, "Nadolol in Human Serum and Breast Milk," *Br J Clin Pharmacol*, 1981, 12(3):393-6.

Mehta AV and Chidambaram B, "Efficacy and Safety of Intravenous and Oral Nadolol for Supraventricular Tachycardia in Children," *J Am Coll Cardiol*, 1992, 19(3):630-5.

Mehta AV and Chidambaram B, and Rice PJ, "Pharmacokinetics of Nadolol in Children With Supraventricular Tachycardia," *J Clin Pharmacol*, 1992, 32(1):1023-7.

Nafcillin (naf SIL in)

Related Information

Extravasation Treatment *on page 1726*

Canadian Brand Names Nallpen®; Unipen®

Index Terms Ethoxynaphthamido Penicillin Sodium; Nafcillin Sodium; Nallpen; Sodium Nafcillin

Therapeutic Category Antibiotic, Penicillin (Antistaphylococcal)

Generic Available Yes

Use Treatment of bacterial infections such as osteomyelitis, septicemia, endocarditis, and CNS infections due to susceptible penicillinase-producing strains of *Staphylococcus*

Pregnancy Risk Factor B

Lactation Enters breast milk/use caution

Contraindications Hypersensitivity to nafcillin, any component, or penicillins. Premixed nafcillin solutions containing dextrose may be contraindicated in patients with allergies to corn or corn products.

Warnings Elimination rate will be decreased in neonates; avoid using in neonates during the first 2 weeks of life. Serious hypersensitivity reactions including anaphylaxis have been reported; immediate treatment for anaphylactic reaction should be

(Continued)

Nafcillin *(Continued)*

available during administration. Pseudomembranous colitis has been reported in patients receiving nafcillin.

Precautions Extravasation of I.V. infusions should be avoided; modification of dosage is necessary in patients with both severe renal and hepatic impairment; use with caution in patients with cephalosporin hypersensitivity

Adverse Reactions

Central nervous system: Fever, seizures
Dermatologic: Skin rash
Endocrine & metabolic: Hypokalemia
Gastrointestinal: Nausea, diarrhea, pseudomembranous colitis
Hematologic: Neutropenia, anemia, eosinophilia
Hepatic: Elevated AST
Local: Pain, thrombophlebitis
Neuromuscular & skeletal: Arthralgia, myalgia
Renal: Acute interstitial nephritis (rare), hematuria
Miscellaneous: Hypersensitivity reactions

Drug Interactions Cytochrome P450 isoenzyme CYP3A3/4 inducer

Probenecid (decreases rate of nafcillin elimination), oral anticoagulants (may decrease half-life and effects of warfarin), may increase hepatic metabolism of cyclosporine. Tetracyclines may decrease the bactericidal effect of penicillin. Nafcillin may decrease levels/effects of CYP3A3/4 substrates including benzodiazepines, calcium channel blockers, cyclosporine, clarithromycin, erythromycin, estrogens, mirtazapine, nefazodone, nevirapine, protease inhibitors, tacrolimus, venlafaxine.

Food Interactions Food decreases GI absorption

Stability Reconstituted nafcillin 250 mg/mL solution for injection is stable for 3 days at room temperature and 7 days when refrigerated; when diluted for I.V. intermittent infusion in D_5W or NS, solution is stable for 24 hours at room temperature and 96 hours when refrigerated. Thawed premixed frozen solution is stable for 21 days under refrigeration or 72 hours at room temperature. Incompatible with aminoglycosides.

Mechanism of Action Interferes with bacterial cell wall synthesis during active multiplication by binding to one or more of the penicillin-binding proteins; inhibits the final transpeptidation step of peptidoglycan synthesis causing cell wall death and resultant bactericidal activity against susceptible bacteria

Pharmacokinetics

Distribution: Distributes into bile, synovial, pleural, ascitic, and pericardial fluids and into bone and liver; CSF penetration is poor unless meninges are inflamed; crosses the placenta; excreted into breast milk

V_d:
- Neonates: 0.24-0.53 L/kg
- Children: 0.85-0.91 L/kg
- Adults: 0.57-1.55 L/kg

Protein binding: 90%
Metabolism: 70% to 90%
Half-life:
- Neonates:
  - <3 weeks: 2.2-5.5 hours
  - 4-9 weeks: 1.2-2.3 hours
- Children 1 month to 14 years: 0.75-1.9 hours
- Adults with normal renal and hepatic function: 0.5-1.5 hours

Time to peak serum concentration: I.M.: Within 30-60 minutes
Elimination: Primarily in bile and 10% to 30% in urine as unchanged drug; undergoes enterohepatic recycling
Dialysis: Not dialyzable (0% to 5%)

Usual Dosage

Neonates: I.M., I.V.:
- 0-4 weeks, <1200 g: 50 mg/kg/day in divided doses every 12 hours
- ≤7 days:
  - 1200-2000 g: 50 mg/kg/day in divided doses every 12 hours
  - >2000 g: 75 mg/kg/day in divided doses every 8 hours
- >7 days:
  - 1200-2000 g: 75 mg/kg/day in divided doses every 8 hours
  - >2000 g: 100-140 mg/kg/day in divided doses every 6 hours

Children:
- I.M., I.V.:
  - Mild to moderate infections: 50-100 mg/kg/day in divided doses every 6 hours
  - Severe infections: 100-200 mg/kg/day in divided doses every 4-6 hours
    - Maximum dose: 12 g/day

Staphylococcal endocarditis:

Native valve: 200 mg/kg/day in divided doses every 4-6 hours for 6 weeks

Prosthetic valve: 200 mg/kg/day in divided doses every 4-6 hours for 6 weeks or longer with rifampin and with gentamicin for the first 2 weeks of therapy

Adults:

I.M.: 500 mg every 4-6 hours

I.V.: 500-2000 mg every 4-6 hours

Dosing adjustment in patients with both severe renal/hepatic impairment: Use lower range of usual dose or reduce dose 33% to 50%

Administration Parenteral:

I.M.: Administer deep I.M. into a large muscle (ie, gluteus maximus) using a solution containing 250 mg/mL

I.V.: Nafcillin may be administered by I.V. push over 5-10 minutes or by I.V. intermittent infusion over 15-60 minutes at a final concentration not to exceed 40 mg/mL; in fluid-restricted patients, a maximum concentration of 100 mg/mL may be administered

Monitoring Parameters Periodic CBC with differential, urinalysis, BUN, serum creatinine, AST, and ALT; initial culture and susceptibility test

Test Interactions False-positive urinary and serum proteins

Patient Information Report any redness, swelling, burning, or pain at injection site; report any difficulty in swallowing or respiration.

Nursing Implications Extravasation may cause tissue sloughing and necrosis; hyaluronidase infiltration may help avoid injury

Additional Information Sodium content of 1 g injection: 3.33 mEq

Dosage Forms Excipient information presented when available (limited, particularly for generics); consult specific product labeling.

Infusion [premixed iso-osmotic dextrose solution]: 1 g (50 mL); 2 g (100 mL)

Injection, powder for reconstitution, as sodium: 1 g, 2 g, 10 g

References

Banner W Jr, Gooch WM 3d, Burckart G, et al, "Pharmacokinetics of Nafcillin in Infants With Low Birth Weights," *Antimicrob Agents Chemother*, 1980, 17(4):691-4.

Zenk KE, Dungy CL, and Greene CR, "Nafcillin Extravasation Injury: Use of Hyaluronidase as an Antidote," *Am J Dis Child*, 1981, 135(12):1113-4.

♦ **Nafcillin Sodium** *see* Nafcillin *on page 1099*

♦ **$NaHCO_3$** *see* Sodium Bicarbonate *on page 1448*

Nalbuphine (NAL byoo feen)

Medication Safety Issues

Sound-alike/look-alike issues:

Nubain® may be confused with Navane®, Nebcin®

U.S. Brand Names Nubain®

Index Terms Nalbuphine Hydrochloride

Therapeutic Category Analgesic, Narcotic; Opiate Partial Agonist

Generic Available Yes

Use Relief of moderate to severe pain; supplement to balanced anesthesia [for preoperative and postoperative analgesia, and obstetrical analgesia (during labor and delivery)]; prevention or treatment of opioid-induced pruritus

Pregnancy Risk Factor B (D if used for prolonged periods or in high doses at term)

Lactation Enters breast milk/use caution

Contraindications Hypersensitivity to nalbuphine or any component

Warnings Abrupt discontinuation after prolonged use may result in narcotic withdrawal; administration to patients receiving chronic opiates may precipitate narcotic withdrawal

Neonatal and fetal adverse reactions have occurred after administration of nalbuphine to pregnant women during labor; these adverse reactions, which may be life-threatening, include: Bradycardia, respiratory depression, apnea, cyanosis, and hypotonia; use with caution in pregnancy; monitor neonates closely with maternal use in labor and delivery.

Precautions Reduce dose in patients with hepatic impairment; use with caution in patients with CNS depression, impaired respiration, recent MI, or biliary tract surgery; may produce respiratory depression or bradycardia; use with caution in patients with a history of drug dependence, head trauma or increased intracranial pressure, decreased hepatic or renal function, or patients suspected to be opioid dependent

Adverse Reactions

Cardiovascular: Hypotension, tachycardia, bradycardia, peripheral vasodilation

Central nervous system: CNS depression, drowsiness, headache, dizziness, sedation, elevated ICP

Dermatologic: Urticaria, pruritus, rash

(Continued)

Nalbuphine *(Continued)*

Gastrointestinal: Anorexia, nausea, vomiting, xerostomia, biliary tract spasm
Genitourinary: Urinary tract spasm, urinary retention
Ocular: Blurred vision, miosis
Respiratory: Respiratory depression
Miscellaneous: Histamine release, physical and psychological dependence, narcotic withdrawal in patients receiving opiate agonists chronically, sweating; anaphylaxis, anaphylactoid reactions (may be life-threatening)

Drug Interactions CNS depressants, alcohol, phenothiazine, tricyclic antidepressants may potentiate adverse effects

Stability Store at controlled room temperature at 25°C (77°F); protect from excessive light; store product in carton until used; not physically compatible with nafcillin and ketorolac

Mechanism of Action Binds to opiate receptors in the CNS, causing inhibition of ascending pain pathways, altering the perception of and response to pain; produces generalized CNS depression; opiate antagonistic effect may result from competitive inhibition at the opiate mu receptor

Pharmacodynamics

Onset of action:
- I.M., SubQ: Within 15 minutes
- I.V.: 2-3 minutes

Maximum effect:
- I.M.: 30 minutes
- I.V.: 1-3 minutes

Duration: 3-6 hours

Pharmacokinetics

Distribution: Crosses placenta; distributes into breast milk in small amounts (<1% of dose)
Metabolism: In the liver; extensive first-pass metabolism
Protein binding: ~50%
Half-life, terminal:
- Children 1-8 years: 0.9 hours
- Adults 23-32 years: ~2 hours; range: 3.5-5 hours
- Adults 65-90 years: 2.3 hours

Time to peak serum concentration:
- I.M.: 30 minutes
- I.V.: 1-3 minutes

Elimination: Metabolites primarily in feces (via bile) and in urine; 4% to 7% eliminated unchanged in the urine

Usual Dosage

Children 1-14 years: Premedication: I.M., I.V., SubQ: 0.2 mg/kg; maximum dose: 20 mg/dose
Children: Analgesia: I.M., I.V., SubQ: 0.1-0.15 mg/kg every 3-6 hours as needed; maximum single-dose: 20 mg/dose; maximum daily dose: 160 mg/day
Adults:
- Analgesia: I.M., I.V., SubQ: 10 mg/70 kg every 3-6 hours as needed; maximum single-dose: 20 mg/dose; maximum daily dose: 160 mg/day
- Surgical anesthesia supplement: I.V.: Induction: 0.3-3 mg/kg administered over 10-15 minutes; maintenance doses of 0.25-0.5 mg/kg may be given as required
- Opioid-induced pruritus: I.V.: 2.5-5 mg; may repeat dose (see Cohen, 1992)

Administration Parenteral: I.V.: Administer over 5-10 minutes; larger doses should be administered over 10-15 minutes

Monitoring Parameters Relief of pain, respiratory and mental status, blood pressure

Test Interactions May interfere with certain enzymatic methods used to detect opioids, depending on sensitivity and specificity of the test (refer to test manufacturer for details)

Patient Information Avoid alcohol; may cause drowsiness and impair ability to perform activities requiring mental alertness or physical coordination; may impair judgment; may be habit-forming; avoid abrupt discontinuation after prolonged use; will cause withdrawal in patients currently dependent on narcotics; may cause dry mouth

Nursing Implications Observe patient for excessive sedation, respiratory depression, implement safety measures, assist with ambulation; observe for narcotic withdrawal (nausea, vomiting, abdominal cramps, lacrimation, rhinorrhea, piloerection, anxiety, restlessness, increased temperature)

Additional Information Analgesic potency: 1 mg nalbuphine ~1 mg morphine

Dosage Forms Excipient information presented when available (limited, particularly for generics); consult specific product labeling. [DSC] = Discontinued product
Injection, solution, as hydrochloride: 10 mg/mL (10 mL); 20 mg/mL (10 mL)
- Nubain®: 10 mg/mL (10 mL) [DSC]; 20 mg/mL (10 mL)

Injection, solution, as hydrochloride [preservative free]: 10 mg/mL (1 mL); 20 mg/mL (1 mL)

Nubain®: 10 mg/mL (1 mL); 20 mg/mL (1 mL)

References

Cohen SE, Ratner EF, Kreitzman TR, et al, "Nalbuphine is Better Than Naloxone for Treatment of Side Effects After Epidural Morphine," *Anesth Analg*, 1992, 75(5):747-52.

Jaillon P, Gardin ME, Lecocq B, et al, "Pharmacokinetics of Nalbuphine in Infants, Young Healthy Volunteers, and Elderly Patients," *Clin Pharmacol Ther*, 1989, 46(2):226-33.

Kendrick WD, Woods AM, Daly MY, et al, "Naloxone Versus Nalbuphine Infusion for Prophylaxis of Epidural Morphine-Induced Pruritus," *Anesth Analg*, 1996, 82:641-7.

Kjellberg F and Tramer MR, "Pharmacological Control of Opioid-Induced Pruritus: A Quantitative Systematic Review of Randomized Trials," *Eur J Anaesthesiol*, 2001, 18(6):346-57.

Nakatsuka N, Minogue SC, Lim J, et al, "Intravenous Nalbuphine 50 Microg x kg(-1) is Ineffective for Opioid-Induced Pruritus in Pediatrics," *Can J Anaesth*, 2006, 53(11):1103-10.

- **Nalbuphine Hydrochloride** *see* Nalbuphine *on page 1101*
- **Nalcrom® (Can)** *see* Cromolyn *on page 407*
- **Nallpen** *see* Nafcillin *on page 1099*
- **Nallpen® (Can)** *see* Nafcillin *on page 1099*
- ***N*-allylnoroxymorphine Hydrochloride** *see* Naloxone *on page 1103*

Naloxone (nal OKS one)

Medication Safety Issues

Sound-alike/look-alike issues:

Naloxone may be confused with naltrexone

Narcan® may be confused with Marcaine®, Norcuron®

International issues:

Narcan® may be confused with Marcen® which is a brand name for ketazolam in Spain

Related Information

Commonly Used Antidotes for Acute Overdoses *on page 1920*

CPR Pediatric Drug Dosages *on page 1650*

Canadian Brand Names Naloxone Hydrochloride Injection®

Index Terms *N*-allylnoroxymorphine Hydrochloride; Naloxone Hydrochloride; Narcan

Therapeutic Category Antidote for Narcotic Agonists

Generic Available Yes

Use Reverses CNS and respiratory depression in suspected narcotic overdose; neonatal opiate depression; coma of unknown etiology; used as low dose I.V. continuous infusion for the prevention and treatment of narcotic-induced pruritus; adjunct in the treatment of septic shock (see Additional Information); used investigationally for phencyclidine and alcohol ingestion

Pregnancy Risk Factor B

Lactation Excretion in breast milk unknown/not recommended

Contraindications Hypersensitivity to naloxone or any component

Warnings May precipitate withdrawal symptoms (hypertension, sweating, agitation, irritability, shrill cry, failure to feed) in patients with physical dependence to opiates (including newborns of narcotic dependent mothers)

Precautions Use with caution in patients with chronic cardiac or pulmonary disease or coronary artery disease. Following the use of narcotics during surgery, naloxone may reverse analgesia and increase blood pressure; use with caution and administer in smaller increments to patients suspected to be opioid dependent and in postoperative patients (to avoid large cardiovascular changes)

Adverse Reactions

Cardiovascular: Hypertension, hypotension, tachycardia, ventricular arrhythmias, cardiac arrest

Gastrointestinal: Nausea, vomiting

Miscellaneous: Increased diaphoresis

Stability Protect from light; stable in NS and D_5W at 4 mcg/mL for 24 hours; do not mix with alkaline solutions

Mechanism of Action Competes and displaces narcotics at narcotic receptor sites

Pharmacodynamics

Onset of action:

E.T., I.M., SubQ: Within 2-5 minutes

I.V.: Within 2 minutes

Duration: (20-60 minutes) is shorter than that of most opioids; therefore, repeated doses are usually needed

Pharmacokinetics

Distribution: Crosses the placenta

Metabolism: Primarily by glucuronidation in the liver

(Continued)

Naloxone *(Continued)*

Half-life:

Neonates: 1.2-3 hours

Adults: 0.5-1.5 hours (mean: ~1 hour)

Elimination: In urine as metabolites

Usual Dosage

PALS 2000 Guidelines: I.V. (**Note:** May be administered I.M., SubQ, or E.T., but onset of action may be delayed, especially if patient has poor perfusion; recommended PALS E.T. doses are 2-10 times the I.V. dose; see also Administration):

For total reversal of narcotic effect: **Note:** Doses may need to be repeated:

Infants and Children ≤ 5 years or ≤20 kg: 0.1 mg/kg

Children >5 years or >20 kg: 2 mg/dose

Alternative dosing to avoid sudden hemodynamic effects from opioid reversal: Use repeated doses of 0.01-0.03 mg/kg

Neonatal opioid-induced depression: I.V., I.M., SubQ: Manufacturer's recommendations: Initial: Usual: 0.01 mg/kg; may repeat every 2-3 minutes as needed based on response; may need to repeat every 1-2 hours

I.M., I.V. (preferred), E.T. (preferred if I.V. route not available), SubQ: **Note:** The dose for pediatric postoperative narcotic reversal is **one-tenth** of the dose used for opiate intoxication:

Opiate intoxication:

Birth (including premature infants) to 5 years or <20 kg: 0.1 mg/kg; repeat every 2-3 minutes if needed; may need to repeat doses every 20-60 minutes

>5 years or ≥20 kg: 2 mg/dose; if no response, repeat every 2-3 minutes; may need to repeat doses every 20-60 minutes

Children and Adults: I.V. continuous infusion: If continuous infusion is required, calculate the initial dosage/hour based on the effective intermittent dose used and duration of adequate response seen; titrate dose; a range of: 2.5-160 mcg/kg/hour has been reported; taper continuous infusion gradually to avoid relapse

Adults: 0.4-2 mg every 2-3 minutes as needed; may need to repeat doses every 20-60 minutes; **Note:** Use 0.1-0.2 mg increments in patients who are opioid dependent and in postoperative patients to avoid large cardiovascular changes

Postanesthesia narcotic reversal: Infants and Children: **0.01 mg/kg**; may repeat every 2-3 minutes as needed based on response

Manufacturer's recommendations (postoperative opioid depression): I.V.: Initial: 0.005-0.01 mg/dose every 2-3 minutes as needed based on response; may need to repeat every 1-2 hours

Narcotic-induced pruritus:

Children and Adolescents: Limited pediatric information is available

Prevention: One double-blind, prospective, randomized, placebo-controlled study used the following dose: Children and adolescents 6"17 years (n=20): I.V.: Continuous infusion: 0.25 mcg/kg/hour; **Note:** Patients who received this dose experienced a lower incidence and severity of opioid-induced side effects (ie, pruritis, nausea) without a loss of pain control (see Maxwell, 2005).

Treatment: One retrospective study reported the following doses: Children and Adolescents 3-20 years (n=30): I.V.: Continuous infusion: Initial: 2 mcg/kg/hour; **Note:** Most initial nonresponders received antihistamines; may increase by 0.5 mcg/kg/hour every few hours if pruritus continues; mean (± SD) dose: 2.3 ± 0.68 mcg/kg/hour; monitor closely; doses ≥3 mcg/kg/hour may increase risk for loss of pain control and patients may require an increase in opioid dose (see Vrchoticky, 2000).

Adults: I.V.: Continuous infusion: Initial 0.25 mcg/kg/hour; **Note:** Doses ranging from 0.25-2.4 mcg/kg/hour have been used in randomized clinical trials; monitor closely; doses ≥2 mcg/kg/hour may increase risk for loss of pain control and patients may require an increase in opioid dose (see Kjellberg, 2001).

Administration

Endotracheal: Dilute to 1-2 mL with NS; PALS Guidelines 2000 recommendations: Dilute to 3-5 mL with NS; follow with several positive-pressure ventilations

Parenteral:

I.V. continuous infusion: Dilute to 4 mcg/mL in D_5W or NS

I.V. push: Administer over 30 seconds as undiluted preparation

Note: I.M. or SubQ administration in hypotensive patients or patients with peripheral vasoconstriction or hypoperfusion may result in erratic or delayed absorption

Monitoring Parameters Respiratory rate, heart rate, blood pressure

Nursing Implications Use of neonatal naloxone (0.02 mg/mL) is no longer recommended because unacceptably high fluid volumes will result, especially in small neonates; the 0.4 mg/mL preparation is available and can be accurately dosed with appropriately sized syringes (1 mL)

Additional Information Contains methyl and propylparabens. Naloxone has been used to increase blood pressure in patients with septic shock; increases in blood pressure may last several hours; however, an increase in patient survival has not been demonstrated and in some studies serious adverse effects (eg, agitation, pulmonary edema, hypotension, cardiac arrhythmias, seizures) have been reported; naloxone should be used with caution for septic shock, especially in patients with underlying pain or opioid tolerance; optimal dosage for this indication has not been established; one neonatal study (n=2) reported a positive blood pressure response, but one neonate developed intractable seizures and died.

Dosage Forms Excipient information presented when available (limited, particularly for generics); consult specific product labeling.

Injection, solution, as hydrochloride: 0.4 mg/mL (1 mL, 10 mL); 1 mg/mL (2 mL)

References

American Academy of Pediatrics Committee on Drugs, "Naloxone Dosage and Route of Administration for Infants and Children: Addendum to Emergency Drug Doses for Infants and Children," *Pediatrics*, 1990, 86(3):484-5.

Chamberlain JM and Klein BL, "A Comprehensive Review of Naloxone for the Emergency Physician," *Am J Emerg Med*, 1994, 12(6):650-60.

"Guidelines 2000 for Cardiopulmonary Resuscitation and Emergency Cardiovascular Care, Part 10: Pediatric Advanced Life Support, The American Heart Association in Collaboration With the International Liaison Committee on Resuscitation," *Circulation*, 2000, 102(8 Suppl): I291-342.

"Guidelines 2000 for Cardiopulmonary Resuscitation and Emergency Cardiovascular Care, Part 11: Neonatal Resuscitation, The American Heart Association in Collaboration With the International Liason Committee on Resuscitation," *Circulation*, 2000, 102(8 Suppl): I343-357.

Kjellberg F and Tramer MR, "Pharmacological Control of Opioid-Induced Pruritus: A Quantitative Systematic Review of Randomized Trials," *Eur J Anaesthesiol*, 2001, 18(6):346-57.

Maxwell LG, Kaufmann SC, and Bitzer S, "The Effects of a Small-Dose Naloxone Infusion on Opioid-Induced Side Effects and Analgesia in Children and Adolescents Treated With Intravenous Patient-controlled Analgesia: A Double-Blind, Prospective, Randomized, Controlled Study," *Anesth Analg*, 2005, 100(4):953-8.

Vrchoticky T, "Naloxone for the Treatment of Narcotic Indiced Pruritus," *Journal of Pediatric Pharmacy Practice*, 2000, 5(2):92-7.

- **Naloxone and Buprenorphine** *see* Buprenorphine and Naloxone *on page 249*
- **Naloxone Hydrochloride** *see* Naloxone *on page 1103*
- **Naloxone Hydrochloride and Pentazocine Hydrochloride** *see* Pentazocine *on page 1237*
- **Naloxone Hydrochloride Dihydrate and Buprenorphine Hydrochloride** *see* Buprenorphine and Naloxone *on page 249*
- **Naloxone Hydrochloride Injection® (Can)** *see* Naloxone *on page 1103*

Nandrolone (NAN droe lone)

Canadian Brand Names Deca-Durabolin®; Durabolin®

Index Terms Nandrolone Decanoate; Nandrolone Phenpropionate

Therapeutic Category Androgen, Anabolic Steroid

Generic Available Yes

Use Management of anemia of renal insufficiency

Restrictions C-III

Pregnancy Risk Factor X

Lactation Excretion in breast milk unknown/contraindicated

Contraindications Hypersensitivity to nandrolone or any component; pregnancy; male patients with carcinoma of breast or prostate; female patients with carcinoma of the breast and hypercalcemia; nephrosis

Warnings Use has been associated with peliosis hepatitis (a condition where liver and sometimes splenic tissue is replaced with blood-filled cysts) and liver cell tumors; these conditions may be complicated by acute, potentially life-threatening intra-abdominal hemorrhage and liver failure; monitor liver function. May increase risk of atherosclerosis and CAD due to decreased HDL and possible increase LDL. May cause virilization (deepening of the voice, hirsutism, acne, clitoromegaly and menstrual irregularities) in women; discontinue therapy when virilization is mild to prevent irreversible effects. Nandrolone has not been shown to be safe and effective for the enhancement of athletic performance.

May accelerate bone maturation without producing compensating gain in linear growth; perform radiographic examination of the hand and wrist every 6 months to determine the rate of bone maturation (when using in prepubertal children). Exposure to nandrolone in utero may result in androgenic effects on the female fetus; clitoral hypertrophy, labial fusion, urogenital sinus defect, vaginal atresia, and ambiguous genitalia; a sensitive test capable of determining early pregnancy is recommended immediately prior to initiation of therapy; nonhormonal method of contraception should be used during treatment if indicated. Some injections (200 mg/mL) contain benzyl alcohol which may cause allergic reactions in susceptible individuals. Safety and efficacy in children <2 years of age has not been established.

(Continued)

Nandrolone *(Continued)*

Precautions Use with caution in patients with cardiac, renal, or hepatic disease. May cause fluid retention; may alter insulin or oral hypoglycemic drug dosages in diabetic patients. May cause hypercalcemia in breast cancer patients. Decreases levels of thyroxine-binding globulin resulting in decreased total T4 serums levels and increased resin uptake of T3 and T4. Free thyroid hormone levels remain unchanged and there is no clinical evidence of thyroid dysfunction.

Adverse Reactions

Cardiovascular: Edema, MI

Central nervous system: Habituation, excitation, insomnia, depression

Dermatologic: Mild hirsutism, hair loss, acne, oily skin

Endocrine & metabolic: Decreased glucose tolerance, gynecomastia, menstrual irregularities, weight gain

Gastrointestinal: Nausea, vomiting, diarrhea

Genitourinary:

Prepubertal males: Penile enlargement and increased frequency of erections

Postpubertal males: Inhibition of testicular function, testicular atrophy, oligospermia, impotence, chronic priapism, epididymitis, bladder irritability

Women: Clitoral enlargement

Both Sexes: Increased or decreased libido

Hepatic: Peliosis hepatis, liver tumors, cholestatic jaundice, elevated liver enzymes, hypertriglyceridemia, increased LDL, decreased HDL, suppression of clotting factors (Factors II, VII, and X)

Local: Swelling, pain at injection site

Neuromuscular & skeletal: Premature epiphyses closure (pediatric use)

Drug Interactions Nandrolone may potentiate the effects of oral anticoagulants, insulins, and oral hypoglycemic agents.

Stability

Store at room temperature and protect from light.

Mechanism of Action Anabolic steroid (synthetic derivative of testosterone) that suppresses gonadotropic functions of the pituitary; increases production of erythropoietin, causes protein anabolism; increases hemoglobin and RBC volume

Pharmacodynamics Anemia of chronic renal failure:

Maximum effect: 3-6 months

Pharmacokinetics

Absorption: I.M.: 77%

Metabolism: In liver

Half-life: Adults: 6-8 days

Time to peak serum concentration: I.M. variable: 6-24 hours

Elimination: Clearance: Adults: 1.6 L/hour

Usual Dosage I.M.:

Children 2-13 years: 25-50 mg every 3-4 weeks

Females >14 years and Adults: 50-100 mg every 1-4 weeks

Males >14 years and Adults: 50-200 mg every 1-4 weeks

Administration Parenteral: I.M.: Administer deep I.M.; not for I.V. or SubQ administration

Monitoring Parameters CBC, liver function tests, serum glucose (if diabetic); HDL and LDL cholesterol; androgenic effects

Patient Information Therapy may take up to several months for full benefit. Report any prodromal symptoms of hepatitis (fatigue, weakness, nausea, vomiting, dark urine, or yellowing of eyes); avoid becoming pregnant while taking this medicine and for several months after stopping; use an effective form of birth control. This medication may alter hypoglycemic requirements; diabetics should monitor serum glucose closely.

Dosage Forms Excipient information presented when available (limited, particularly for generics); consult specific product labeling.

Injection, solution, as decanoate [in sesame oil]: 100 mg/mL (2 mL); 200 mg/mL (1 mL) [contains benzyl alcohol] [DSC]

- **Nandrolone Decanoate** *see* Nandrolone *on page 1105*
- **Nandrolone Phenpropionate** *see* Nandrolone *on page 1105*
- **NAPA and NABZ** *see* Sodium Phenylacetate and Sodium Benzoate *on page 1453*

Naphazoline (naf AZ oh leen)

U.S. Brand Names AK-Con™; Albalon®; Clear eyes® for Dry Eyes and ACR Relief [OTC]; Clear eyes® for Dry Eyes and Redness Relief [OTC]; Clear eyes® Redness Relief [OTC]; Clear eyes® Seasonal Relief [OTC]; Naphcon® [OTC]; Privine® [OTC]

Canadian Brand Names Naphcon Forte®; Vasocon®

Index Terms Naphazoline Hydrochloride

Therapeutic Category Adrenergic Agonist Agent, Ophthalmic; Decongestant, Nasal; Nasal Agent, Vasoconstrictor; Ophthalmic Agent, Vasoconstrictor

Generic Available No

Use Topical ocular vasoconstrictor (to soothe, refresh, moisturize, and relieve redness due to minor eye irritation); temporarily relieves nasal congestion associated with rhinitis, sinusitis, hay fever, or the common cold

Pregnancy Risk Factor C

Lactation Excretion in breast milk unknown/use caution

Contraindications Hypersensitivity to naphazoline or any component; narrow-angle glaucoma; prior to peripheral iridectomy (in patients susceptible to angle block)

Warnings Excessive dosage may cause marked sedation in children, particularly infants

Precautions Rebound congestion may occur with extended use (use no longer than 3-5 days); use with caution in the presence of hypertension, diabetes mellitus, hyperthyroidism, heart disease, coronary artery disease, cerebral arteriosclerosis, or long-standing asthma

Adverse Reactions

Cardiovascular: Systemic cardiovascular stimulation (rare), pallor

Central nervous system: Dizziness, headache, nervousness, anxiety, tenseness, drowsiness, hallucinations, convulsions, CNS depression, prolonged psychosis

Gastrointestinal: Nausea, vomiting

Local: Transient stinging, nasal mucosa irritation, dryness

Ocular: Mydriasis, elevated intraocular pressure, blurring of vision, blepharospasm (ophthalmic formulations)

Respiratory: Respiratory difficulty, sneezing, rebound nasal congestion (nasal formulations)

Miscellaneous: Diaphoresis

Drug Interactions Anesthetics (discontinue naphazoline prior to use of anesthetics that sensitize the myocardium to sympathomimetics, ie, cyclopropane, halothane); MAO inhibitors, methyldopa, tricyclic antidepressants increase hypertensive response

Mechanism of Action Stimulates alpha-adrenergic receptors in the arterioles of the conjunctiva and the nasal mucosa to produce vasoconstriction

Pharmacodynamics

Onset of action: Following topical administration, decongestion occurs within 10 minutes

Duration: 2-6 hours

Pharmacokinetics Elimination: Not well defined

Usual Dosage

Nasal: Intranasal not recommended for use in children <6 years of age (especially in infants) due to CNS depression; therapy should not exceed 3-5 days

Children 6-12 years: 0.05%, 1 drop or spray every 6 hours if needed

Children >12 years to Adults: 0.05%, 1-2 drops or sprays every 3-6 hours if needed

Ophthalmic: Therapy should generally not exceed 3-4 days; not recommended for use in children <6 years of age due to CNS depression (especially in infants)

Children >6 years and Adults (0.01% to 0.1%): Instill 1-2 drops every 3-4 hours

Administration

Ophthalmic: Instill drops into conjunctival sac of affected eye; finger pressure should be applied to lacrimal sac during and for 1-2 minutes after instillation to decrease risk of absorption and systemic reactions; avoid contact of bottle tip with skin or eye

Nasal: Spray or drop medication into one nostril while gently occluding the other; then reverse procedure

Patient Information Discontinue eye drops if visual changes or ocular pain occur

Dosage Forms Excipient information presented when available (limited, particularly for generics); consult specific product labeling.

Solution, intranasal, as hydrochloride [drops]:

Privine®: 0.05% (25 mL)

Solution, intranasal, as hydrochloride [spray]:

Privine®: 0.05% (20 mL)

Solution, ophthalmic, as hydrochloride:

AK-Con™, Albalon®: 0.1% (15 mL) [contains benzalkonium chloride]

Clear eyes® for Dry Eyes and ACR Relief: 0.025% (15 mL) [contains hypromellose, and zinc sulfate]

Clear eyes® for Dry Eyes and Redness Relief: 0.012% (15 mL) [contains hypromellose, glycerin and benzalkonium chloride]

Clear eyes® Redness Relief: 0.012% (6 mL, 15 mL, 30 mL) [contains glycerin and benzalkonium chloride]

(Continued)

Naphazoline *(Continued)*

Clear eyes® Seasonal Relief: 0.012% (15 mL, 30 mL) [contains glycerin, zinc sulfate and benzalkonium chloride]

Naphcon®: 0.012% (15 mL) [contains benzalkonium chloride]

♦ **Naphazoline Hydrochloride** *see* Naphazoline *on page 1106*
♦ **Naphcon® [OTC]** *see* Naphazoline *on page 1106*
♦ **Naphcon Forte® (Can)** *see* Naphazoline *on page 1106*
♦ **Naprelan®** *see* Naproxen *on page 1108*
♦ **Naprosyn®** *see* Naproxen *on page 1108*

Naproxen (na PROKS en)

Medication Safety Issues

Sound-alike/look-alike issues:

Naproxen may be confused with Natacyn®, Nebcin®
Aleve® may be confused with Alesse®
Anaprox® may be confused with Anaspaz®, Avapro®
Naprelan® may be confused with Naprosyn®
Naprosyn® may be confused with Naprelan®, Natacyn®, Nebcin®

International issues:

Flogen® [Mexico] may be confused with Flovent® which is a brand name for fluticasone in the U.S.

Flogen® [Mexico] may be confused with Floxin® which is a brand name for ofloxacin in the U.S.

Related Information

Overdose and Toxicology *on page 1916*

U.S. Brand Names Aleve® [OTC]; Anaprox®; Anaprox® DS; EC-Naprosyn®; Midol® Extended Relief; Naprelan®; Naprosyn®; Pamprin® Maximum Strength All Day Relief [OTC]

Canadian Brand Names Anaprox®; Anaprox® DS; Apo-Napro-Na®; Apo-Napro-Na DS®; Apo-Naproxen®; Apo-Naproxen EC®; Apo-Naproxen SR®; Gen-Naproxen EC; Naprosyn®; Naxen®; Naxen® EC; Novo-Naproc EC; Novo-Naprox; Novo-Naprox Sodium; Novo-Naprox Sodium DS; Novo-Naprox SR; Nu-Naprox; Riva-Naproxen

Index Terms Naproxen Sodium

Therapeutic Category Analgesic, Non-narcotic; Anti-inflammatory Agent; Antipyretic; Nonsteroidal Anti-inflammatory Drug (NSAID), Oral

Generic Available Yes

Use Management of inflammatory disease and rheumatoid disorders (including rheumatoid arthritis, juvenile rheumatoid arthritis, osteoarthritis, ankylosing spondylitis); acute gout; mild to moderate pain; primary dysmenorrhea; fever; tendonitis, bursitis. **Note:** Due to delayed absorption, the delayed"release tablets are **not** recommended for initial treatment of pain

Medication Guide An FDA-approved patient medication guide, which is available with the product information and at http://www.fda.gov/cder/Offices/ODS/medication_guides.htm, must be dispensed with this medication for each new outpatient prescription and refill.

Pregnancy Risk Factor C (D if used in the 3rd trimester)

Lactation Enters breast milk/not recommended (AAP rates "compatible")

Contraindications Hypersensitivity to naproxen, any component, aspirin, or other NSAIDs; active GI bleeding, ulcer disease; patients with the "aspirin triad" [asthma, rhinitis (with or without nasal polyps), and aspirin intolerance] (fatal asthmatic and anaphylactoid reactions may occur in these patients); perioperative pain in the setting of coronary artery bypass graft (CABG)

Warnings NSAIDs are associated with an increased risk of adverse cardiovascular thrombotic events, including potentially fatal MI and stroke; risk may be increased with duration of use or pre-existing cardiovascular risk factors or disease; carefully evaluate cardiovascular risk profile prior to prescribing; use the lowest effective dose for the shortest duration of time, taking into consideration individual patient treatment goals; alternate therapies should be considered for patients at high risk. An increased incidence of MI and stroke was found in patients receiving COX-2 selective NSAIDs for the treatment of pain within the first 10-14 days after CABG surgery (see Contraindications). NSAIDs may cause fluid retention, edema, and new onset or worsening of pre-existing hypertension; use with caution in patients with hypertension, CHF or fluid retention; be aware of sodium content of sodium naproxen products in patients with sodium restriction.

NSAIDs may increase the risk of gastrointestinal irritation, ulceration, bleeding, and perforation. These events, which can be potentially fatal, may occur at any time during therapy and without warning. Use NSAIDs with extreme caution in patients with a history of GI bleeding or ulcers (these patients have a 10-fold increased risk for developing a GI bleed). Use NSAIDs with caution in patients with other risk factors which may increase GI bleeding (eg, concurrent therapy with aspirin, anticoagulants and/or corticosteroids, longer duration of NSAID use, smoking, use of alcohol, and poor general health). Use the lowest effective dose for the shortest duration of time, taking into consideration individual patient treatment goals; alternate therapies should be considered for patients at high risk.

NSAIDs may compromise existing renal function. Renal toxicity may occur in patients with impaired renal function, dehydration, salt depletion, heart failure, liver dysfunction, those taking diuretics and ACE inhibitors; use with caution in these patients; monitor renal function closely. Naproxen is not recommended for use in patients with moderate to severe or severe renal impairment (Cl_{cr} <30 mL/minute). Long-term use of NSAIDs may cause renal papillary necrosis and other renal injury.

Fatal asthmatic and anaphylactoid reactions may occur in patients with the "aspirin triad" who receive NSAIDs (see Contraindications). NSAIDs may cause serious dermatologic adverse reactions including exfoliative dermatitis, Stevens-Johnson syndrome, and toxic epidermal necrolysis. Avoid use of NSAIDs in late pregnancy as they may cause premature closure of the ductus arteriosus.

Precautions Use with caution in patients with decreased hepatic function; closely monitor patients with abnormal LFTs; severe hepatic reactions (eg, fulminant hepatitis, liver failure) have occurred with NSAID use, rarely; discontinue if signs or symptoms of liver disease develop, or if systemic manifestations occur. Use with caution in patients with asthma. Safety and efficacy have not been established in children <2 years of age.

OTC labeling: Prior to self-medication, patients should contact healthcare provider if they have had recurring stomach pain or upset, ulcers, bleeding problems, high blood pressure, heart or kidney disease, other serious medical problems, or are currently taking a diuretic. Recommended dosages should not be exceeded, due to an increased risk of GI bleeding. Consuming ≥3 alcoholic beverages/day or taking this medication longer than recommended may increase the risk of GI bleeding. Not for OTC use in children <12 years of age without consulting with physician.

Adverse Reactions

Cardiovascular: Edema, hypertension, palpitations

Central nervous system: Fatigue, drowsiness, vertigo, headache; aseptic meningitis (<1%)

Dermatologic: Pruritus, rash; pseudoporphyria (ie, increased skin fragility and blistering with scarring in sun-exposed skin), incidence: 12% in naproxen-treated children with JRA (discontinue therapy if this occurs); exfoliative dermatitis, Stevens-Johnson syndrome, toxic epidermal necrolysis

Endocrine & metabolic: Fluid retention

Gastrointestinal: Abdominal pain, nausea, heartburn, constipation, vomiting, GI bleed, ulcers, perforation, diarrhea, dyspepsia, stomatitis

Hematologic: Thrombocytopenia, anemia, inhibition of platelet aggregation, prolongation of bleeding time, agranulocytosis

Hepatic: Elevated liver enzymes; rarely: hepatitis, jaundice, hepatic necrosis, liver failure

Ocular: Visual disturbances

Otic: Tinnitus

Renal: Renal dysfunction

Miscellaneous: Hypersensitivity reactions, anaphylactoid reactions

Drug Interactions Cytochrome P450 isoenzyme CYP2C8 (5-hydroxylation), CYP2C9 (5-hydroxylation), and CYP2C18 substrate

Naproxen may increase methotrexate and lithium serum concentrations. May decrease antihypertensive effects of ACE inhibitors or angiotensin II antagonists; may decrease effects of other antihypertensive agents, furosemide, and thiazides (monitor blood pressure). Concomitant use with antacids, sucralfate, or cholestyramine may delay the absorption of naproxen (separate administration by 2 hours). Concomitant use of H_2-blockers, sucralfate, or intensive antacid therapy is not recommended with naproxen delayed-release tablets (due to effects of these agents on gastric pH). Probenecid may increase naproxen serum concentrations. Other GI irritants (eg, aspirin, alcohol, NSAIDs, corticosteroids, oral potassium supplements) may increase GI adverse effects. Use with anticoagulants (warfarin, heparin, LMWHs) may increase risk of bleeding. Due to high protein binding of naproxen, interactions with other drugs that are highly protein bound may occur. **Note:** Ibuprofen and other COX-1 inhibitors may reduce the cardioprotective (antiplatelet effect) of aspirin if administered concurrently (see Ibuprofen monograph).

Food Interactions Delayed-release tablets: Food delays the time to peak concentrations.

(Continued)

Naproxen *(Continued)*

Stability Store tablets and suspension at room temperature [15°C to 30°C (59°F to 86°F)]; avoid exposure of suspension to excessive heat >40°C (104°F); dispense naproxen tablets and suspension in light-resistant, well-closed containers

Mechanism of Action Inhibits prostaglandin synthesis by decreasing the activity of the enzyme, cyclooxygenase, which results in decreased formation of prostaglandin precursors

Pharmacokinetics

Absorption: Oral: Almost 100%

Distribution: Crosses the placenta; ~1% distributed into breast milk

V_d: Adults: 0.16 L/kg

Protein binding: >99%

Metabolism: Extensively metabolized in the liver to 6-0-desmethyl naproxen; parent drug and desmethyl metabolite undergo further metabolism to their respective acylglucuronide conjugated metabolites

Bioavailability: 95%

Half-life, elimination: Children: Range: 8-17 hours

Children 8-14 years: 8-10 hours

Adults: 12-17 hours

Time to peak serum concentration:

Tablets, naproxen: 2-4 hours

Tablets, naproxen sodium: 1-2 hours

Tablets, delayed-release (empty stomach): 4-6 hours; range 2-12 hours

Tablets, delayed-release (with food): 12 hours; range: 4-24 hours

Suspension: 1-4 hours

Elimination: 95% excreted in urine (<1% as unchanged drug; <1% as 6-0-desmethyl naproxen; 66% to 92% as their conjugates); ≤3% excreted in feces

Usual Dosage Note: Dosage expressed as naproxen base; 200 mg naproxen base is equivalent to 220 mg naproxen sodium

Oral:

Children >2 years:

Analgesia: 5-7 mg/kg/dose every 8-12 hours

Inflammatory disease, including JRA: Usual: 10-15 mg/kg/day in 2 divided doses; range: 7-20 mg/kg/day; maximum dose: 1000 mg/day. Manufacturer's recommendation for JRA: 10 mg/kg/day in 2 divided doses

Children >12 and Adults ≤65 years: OTC labeling for pain and fever: 200 mg every 8-12 hours; if needed may take 400 mg for the initial dose; maximum dose: 600 mg/day

Adults:

Rheumatoid arthritis, osteoarthritis, and ankylosing spondylitis: 500-1000 mg/day in 2 divided doses

Acute gout: Initial: 750 mg, followed by 250 mg every 8 hours until attack subsides. **Note:** Delayed release tablet is not recommended due to delayed absorption.

Mild to moderate pain, dysmenorrhea, acute tendonitis, or bursitis: Initial: 500 mg, then 500 mg every 12 hours or 250 mg every 6-8 hours as needed; maximum dose: 1250 mg/day initially, then 1000 mg/day thereafter. **Note:** Delayed release tablet is not recommended for treatment of acute pain, due to delayed absorption

Dosage adjustment in renal impairment: Moderate to severe and severe renal impairment (Cl_{cr} <30 mL/minute): Not recommended for use

Administration Oral: Administer with food, milk, or antacids to decrease GI adverse effects. Shake suspension well before use. Do not chew, crush, or break delayed or controlled release tablet, swallow whole.

Monitoring Parameters CBC with differential, platelets, BUN, serum creatinine, liver enzymes, occult blood loss, periodic ophthalmologic exams, hemoglobin, hematocrit, blood pressure

Test Interactions Naproxen may interfere with urinary tests for 17-ketogenic steroids, due to an interaction with m-di-nitrobenzene; interaction with the measurement of 17-hydroxy-corticosteroids does not appear to occur; however, naproxen should be discontinued 72 hours before adrenal function testing if the Porter-Silber test is used. Naproxen may interfere with urinary assays of 5-hydroxy indoleacetic acid (5HIAA).

Patient Information Naproxen is a nonsteroidal anti-inflammatory drug (NSAID); NSAIDs may cause serious adverse reactions, especially with overuse; use exactly as directed; do not increase dose or frequency; do not take longer than 3 days for fever (adults and children), 10 days for pain (adults), or 3 days for pain (children) without consulting healthcare professional. NSAIDs may increase the risk for heart attack, stroke, or ulcers and bleeding in stomach or intestines; GI bleeding, ulceration, or perforation can occur with or without pain. Notify physician before use if you have hypertension, heart failure, heart or kidney disease, history of stomach ulcers or bleeding in stomach or intestines, or other medical problems. Read the patient Medication Guide that you receive with each prescription and refill of naproxen.

While using this medication, do not use alcohol, excessive amounts of vitamin C, other prescription or OTC medications containing aspirin or salicylate, or other NSAIDs without consulting prescriber. Naproxen may cause dizziness or drowsiness and impair ability to perform activities requiring mental alertness or physical coordination. Children with JRA: Protect skin from sun; use sunscreen, wide-brimmed hats, etc.

Notify physician if changes in vision occur, if pain worsens or lasts >10 days in adults or >3 days in children, if fever worsens or lasts >3 days, if stomach pain or upset occurs, if swelling or redness occurs in painful area, or if any new symptoms appear. Stop taking medication and report ringing in ears; persistent cramping or stomach pain; unresolved nausea or vomiting; respiratory difficulty or shortness of breath; unusual bruising or bleeding (mouth, urine, stool); skin rash; unusual swelling of extremities; chest pain; or palpitations. Report weight gain or edema to physician.

OTC (pediatrics): Do not administer to children for >3 days unless recommended by physician or other healthcare professional; notify physician if child's condition does not improve or if worsens within 24 hours

Additional Information In a multicenter, retrospective chart review, 19 children, 4-14 years of age (mean: 9.1 ± 2.9) with rheumatic fever (but without carditis, chorea, or rashes), were treated solely with naproxen (10-20 mg/kg/day divided in 2 doses) until ESR normalized (between 4-8 weeks); fever and arthritis resolved within a median of 1 day of starting therapy; no patient had side effects, or developed carditis over the following 6 months; comparative studies with aspirin that include patients with mild carditis are needed to confirm these findings (see Uziel, 2000)

Due to its effects on platelet function, naproxen should be withheld for at least 4-6 half-lives prior to surgical or dental procedures.

Dosage Forms Excipient information presented when available (limited, particularly for generics); consult specific product labeling.

Caplet, as sodium (Aleve®, Midol® Extended Relief, Pamprin® Maximum Strength All Day Relief): 220 mg [equivalent to naproxen 200 mg and sodium 20 mg]

Gelcap, as sodium (Aleve®): 220 mg [equivalent to naproxen 200 mg and sodium 20 mg]

Suspension, oral (Naprosyn®): 125 mg/5 mL (480 mL) [contains sodium 0.3 mEq/mL; orange-pineapple flavor]

Tablet (Naprosyn®): 250 mg, 375 mg, 500 mg

Tablet, as sodium: 220 mg [equivalent to naproxen 200 mg and sodium 20 mg]; 275 mg [equivalent to naproxen 250 mg and sodium 25 mg]; 550 mg [equivalent to naproxen 500 mg and sodium 50 mg]

Aleve®: 220 mg [equivalent to naproxen 200 mg and sodium 20 mg]

Anaprox®: 275 mg [equivalent to naproxen 250 mg and sodium 25 mg]

Anaprox® DS: 550 mg [equivalent to naproxen 500 mg and sodium 50 mg]

Tablet, controlled release, as sodium: 550 mg [equivalent to naproxen 500 mg and sodium 50 mg]

Naprelan®: 421.5 mg [equivalent to naproxen 375 mg and sodium 37.5 mg]; 550 mg [equivalent to naproxen 500 mg and sodium 50 mg]

Tablet, delayed release (EC-Naprosyn®): 375 mg, 500 mg

References

Berde C, Ablin A, Glazer J, et al, "American Academy of Pediatrics Report of the Subcommittee on Disease-Related Pain in Childhood Cancer," *Pediatrics*, 1990, 86(5 Pt 2):818-25.

Lang BA and Finlayson LA, "Naproxen-Induced Pseudoporphyria in Patients With Juvenile Rheumatoid Arthritis," *J Pediatr*, 1994, 124(4):639-42.

Uziel Y, Hashkes PJ, Kassem E, et al, "The Use of Naproxen in the Treatment of Children With Rheumatic Fever," *J Pediatr*, 2000, 137(2):269-71.

Wells TG, Mortensen ME, Dietrich A, et al, "Comparison of the Pharmacokinetics of Naproxen Tablets and Suspension in Children," *J Clin Pharmacol*, 1994, 34(1):30-3.

♦ **Naproxen Sodium** *see* Naproxen *on page 1108*
♦ **Narcan** *see* Naloxone *on page 1103*
♦ **Naropin®** *see* Ropivacaine *on page 1404*
♦ **Nasacort® AQ** *see* Triamcinolone *on page 1568*
♦ **NaSal™ [OTC]** *see* Sodium Chloride *on page 1450*
♦ **NasalCrom® [OTC]** *see* Cromolyn *on page 407*
♦ **Nasalide® (Can)** *see* Flunisolide *on page 669*
♦ **Nasal Moist® [OTC]** *see* Sodium Chloride *on page 1450*
♦ **Nasarel®** *see* Flunisolide *on page 669*
♦ **Nascobal®** *see* Cyanocobalamin *on page 413*
♦ **Nasonex®** *see* Mometasone Furoate *on page 1076*
♦ **Natulan® (Can)** *see* Procarbazine *on page 1320*
♦ **Natural Fiber Therapy [OTC]** *see* Psyllium *on page 1347*
♦ **Natural Lung Surfactant** *see* Beractant *on page 210*
♦ **Nauseatol (Can)** *see* DimenhyDRINATE *on page 507*

- **Navane®** *see* Thiothixene *on page 1534*
- **Naxen® (Can)** *see* Naproxen *on page 1108*
- **Naxen® EC (Can)** *see* Naproxen *on page 1108*
- **Na-Zone® [OTC]** *see* Sodium Chloride *on page 1450*
- **NebuPent®** *see* Pentamidine *on page 1236*

Nedocromil (ne doe KROE mil)

Related Information
Asthma *on page 1904*

U.S. Brand Names Alocril®; Tilade®

Canadian Brand Names Alocril®; Tilade®

Index Terms Nedocromil Sodium

Therapeutic Category Antiallergic, Ophthalmic; Antiasthmatic; Inhalation, Miscellaneous

Generic Available No

Use
Aerosol: Maintenance therapy in patients with mild to moderate asthma
Ophthalmic: Treatment of itching associated with allergic conjunctivitis

Pregnancy Risk Factor B

Lactation Excretion in breast milk unknown/use caution

Contraindications Hypersensitivity to nedocromil or any component

Warnings If systemic or inhaled steroid therapy is at all reduced, monitor patients carefully; nedocromil is **not** a bronchodilator and, therefore, should not be used for reversal of acute bronchospasm

Precautions Refrain from wearing contact lenses while exhibiting the signs and symptoms of allergic conjunctivitis

Adverse Reactions
Cardiovascular: Chest pain
Central nervous system: Dizziness, dysphonia, headache, fatigue
Dermatologic: Rash
Gastrointestinal: Nausea, vomiting, dyspepsia, diarrhea, abdominal pain, xerostomia, dysgeusia, unpleasant taste
Hepatic: Elevated ALT
Neuromuscular and skeletal: Arthritis, tremor
Ocular: Burning, irritation, stinging, conjunctivitis, eye redness, photophobia (ophthalmic formulation)
Respiratory: Cough, pharyngitis, rhinitis, bronchitis, upper respiratory infection, bronchospasm, increased sputum production, pneumonitis with eosinophilia (PIE syndrome) (inhalation formulation)

Stability Store at room temperature; do not freeze; the remaining contents of Alocril® unit dose solution should be discarded immediately after use

Mechanism of Action Inhibits the activation of and mediator release from a variety of inflammatory cell types associated with asthma including eosinophils, neutrophils, macrophages, mast cells, monocytes, and platelets; it inhibits the release of histamine, leukotrienes, and slow-reacting substance of anaphylaxis; it inhibits the development of early and late bronchoconstriction responses to inhaled antigen

Pharmacodynamics Inhalation: Duration: 2 hours; maximum therapeutic benefit is seen after at least 1 week of therapy

Pharmacokinetics
Absorption: Systemic: Inhalation: 7% to 9%; ophthalmic: <4%
Protein binding, plasma: 89%
Elimination: Excreted unchanged in urine 70%; feces 30%

Usual Dosage
Inhalation: Children ≥6 years and Adults: 2 inhalations 4 times/day; may reduce dosage to 2-3 times/day once desired clinical response to initial dose is observed
Ophthalmic: Children ≥3 years and Adults: 1-2 drops in each eye twice daily throughout the period of exposure to allergen

Administration
Oral inhalation: Shake well before use; must be primed by 3 actuations prior to first use; if canister remains unused for >7 days, reprime with 3 actuations; discard canister after 104 actuations
Ophthalmic: Instill drops into conjunctival sac; avoid contact of bottle tip with skin or eye

Patient Information May cause dry mouth

Additional Information Has no known therapeutic systemic activity when delivered by inhalation

Dosage Forms Excipient information presented when available (limited, particularly for generics); consult specific product labeling.

Aerosol for oral inhalation, as sodium (Tilade®): 1.75 mg/activation (16.2 g)
Solution, ophthalmic, as sodium (Alocril®): 2% (5 mL) [contains benzalkonium chloride]

♦ **Nedocromil Sodium** *see* Nedocromil *on page 1112*

Nelarabine (nel AY re been)

Medication Safety Issues
High alert medication: The Institute for Safe Medication Practices (ISMP) includes this medication among its list of drugs which have a heightened risk of causing significant patient harm when used in error.

U.S. Brand Names Arranon®

Index Terms 2-Amino-6-Methoxypurine Arabinoside; GW506U78; 506U78

Therapeutic Category Antineoplastic Agent, Antimetabolite

Generic Available No

Use Treatment of relapsed or refractory T-cell acute lymphoblastic leukemia (ALL) and T-cell lymphoblastic lymphoma; treatment of CML (Philadelphia Chromosome positive) T-cell blast phase

Pregnancy Risk Factor D

Lactation Excretion in breast milk unknown/not recommended

Contraindications Hypersensitivity to nelarabine or any component

Warnings The FDA currently recommends that procedures for proper handling and disposal of antineoplastic agents be considered. Neurotoxicity is the dose-limiting toxicity (monitor closely for signs and symptoms of neurotoxicity which include somnolence, confusion, convulsions, ataxia, paresthesia, hypoesthesia, coma, status epilepticus, craniospinal demyelination, or ascending neuropathy similar in appearance to Guillain-Barré syndrome). Risk of neurotoxicity may increase in patients with concurrent or previous intrathecal chemotherapy or history of craniospinal irradiation. Discontinue nelarabine for neurologic events of NCI Common Toxicity Criteria ≥2. Nelarabine should be administered under the supervision of a physician experienced in the use of cancer chemotherapy agents.

Precautions Use extreme caution in patients with elevated uric acid, gout, and history of uric acid stones (monitor for hyperuricemia, consider allopurinol, and hydrate accordingly). Use caution in patients with renal impairment and severe hepatic impairment. Avoid administration of live vaccines in immunocompromised patients on nelarabine therapy.

Adverse Reactions
Cardiovascular: Peripheral edema, edema, hypotension, tachycardia, chest pain
Central nervous system: Fatigue, fever, somnolence (7%), lethargy, dizziness, headache (17%), progressive multifocal leukoencephalopathy, seizures (6%), coma, cerebral hemorrhage, ataxia (2%), confusion, insomnia, depression, amnesia, hydrocephalus, hemiparesis, nerve palsy, aphasia
Dermatologic: Petechiae
Endocrine & metabolic: Hypokalemia (11%), hypocalcemia (8%), dehydration, hyperglycemia, hypoglycemia (6%), hypomagnesemia (6%)
Gastrointestinal: Nausea, diarrhea, vomiting (10%), constipation, abdominal pain, anorexia, stomatitis, abdominal distention, taste perversion
Hematologic: Anemia (95%), leukopenia (38%), neutropenia (94%), thrombocytopenia (88%)
Hepatic: Elevated AST and ALT (12%), hyperbilirubinemia (10%), hypoalbuminemia (10%)
Neuromuscular & skeletal: Peripheral neuropathy (12%), paresthesia (4%), hypoesthesia (6%), weakness, myalgia, motor dysfunction (4%), neuropathic pain, sciatica, arthralgia, back pain, rigors, limb pain, abnormal gait (6%), tremor (4%), dysarthria, hyporeflexia, hypertonia, incoordination
Ocular: Nystagmus, blurred vision
Renal: Elevated serum creatinine (6%)
Respiratory: Cough, dyspnea, pleural effusion, epistaxis, pneumonia, sinusitis, wheezing
Miscellaneous: Infection

Drug Interactions Pentostatin (inhibitor of adenosine deaminase which may reduce conversion of the prodrug nelarabine to its active form resulting in reduced efficacy; concurrent administration with pentostatin is not recommended)

Stability Store unopened vials at room temperature. Undiluted injection solution is stable in a PVC infusion bag or glass container for up to 8 hours at room temperature.

Mechanism of Action Nelarabine is a prodrug that is demethylated by adenosine deaminase to ara-G. Ara-G is phosphorylated by deoxyguanosine kinase and deoxycytidine kinase to ara-GTP (active). Ara-GTP is incorporated into the DNA of leukemic blasts leading to inhibition of DNA synthesis and cell death. Ara-GTP appears to

(Continued)

Nelarabine *(Continued)*

accumulate at higher levels in T-cells compared with B-cells correlating to its differential activity.

Pharmacokinetics

Distribution: V_{ss}:

Nelarabine: Adults: 197 ± 216 L/m^2; Children: 213 ± 358 L/m^2

Ara-G: Adults: 50 ± 24 L/m^2; Children: 33 ± 9.3 L/m^2

Protein binding: Nelarabine and ara-G: <25%

Metabolism: Nelarabine is O-demethylated to ara-G by adenosine deaminase; ara-G undergoes hydrolysis to guanine; guanine is N-deaminated to xanthine which is further oxidized to form uric acid and then oxidized to form allantoin

Half-life: Adults:

Nelarabine: 30 minutes

Ara-G: 3 hours

Elimination: Nelarabine 6.6% and ara-G 27% are excreted in urine within 24 hours of infusion on day 1

Clearance: Nelarabine clearance is ~30% higher in children (259 ± 409 L/hour/m^2) than in adults (197 ± 189 L/hour/m^2); ara-G clearance in children (11.3 ± 4.2 L/hour/m^2) is similar to adults (10.5 ± 4.5 L/hour/m^2)

Usual Dosage Refer to individual protocols: I.V.:

T-cell ALL, T-cell lymphoblastic lymphoma:

Children: 650 mg/m^2/day on days 1 through 5; repeat cycle every 21 days

Adults: 1500 mg/m^2/day on days 1, 3, and 5; repeat cycle every 21 days

Dosage adjustment for toxicity:

For neurologic toxicity ≥ grade 2 of NCI Common Toxicity Criteria: Discontinue treatment

For hematologic or other non-neurologic toxicity: Consider treatment delay

Dosage adjustment in renal impairment:

Cl_{cr} <50 mL/minute: Safety has not been established

Cl_{cr} <30 mL/minute: Closely monitor

Dosage adjustment in hepatic impairment: Safety has not been established

Bilirubin >3 mg/dL: Closely monitor

Administration I.V.: The appropriate nelarabine dose is transferred into an empty PVC infusion bag or glass container and administered undiluted.

Children: Infuse over 1 hour daily for 5 consecutive days

Adults: Infuse over 2 hours on days 1, 3, and 5

Monitoring Parameters Monitor for neurologic toxicity (severe somnolence, seizure, peripheral neuropathy, confusion, ataxia, paresthesia, hypoesthesia, coma, or craniospinal demyelination); signs and symptoms of tumor lysis syndrome; hydration status; CBC with platelet counts, renal and liver function tests

Patient Information May cause drowsiness and impair ability to perform activities requiring mental alertness or physical coordination. Notify physician if unusual bleeding, bruising, breathing difficulty, somnolence, confusion, seizures, coma, peripheral neuropathy (numbness and tingling in the hands, fingers, feet, or toes), problems with fine motor skills, unsteady gait, weakness, or paralysis occurs. Women of childbearing potential should be advised to avoid becoming pregnant while receiving nelarabine treatment.

Nursing Implications Appropriate measures must be taken to prevent hyperuricemia in patients at risk for tumor lysis syndrome (eg, hydration, urine alkalinization, and prophylaxis with allopurinol).

Dosage Forms Excipient information presented when available (limited, particularly for generics); consult specific product labeling.

Injection, solution: 5 mg/mL (50 mL)

References

Berg SL, Blaney SM, Devidas M, et al, "Phase II Study of Nelarabine (Compound 506U78) in Children and Young Adults With Refractory T-Cell Malignancies: A Report From the Children's Oncology Group," *J Clin Oncol*, 2005, 23(15):3376-82.

Gandhi V, Plunkett W, Weller S, et al, "Evaluation of the Combination of Nelarabine and Fludarabine in Leukemias: Clinical Response, Pharmacokinetics, and Pharmacodynamics in Leukemia Cells," *J Clin Oncol*, 2001, 19(8):2142-52.

Kurtzberg J, Ernst TJ, Keating MJ, et al, "Phase I Study of 506U78 Administered on a Consecutive 5-Day Schedule in Children and Adults With Refractory Hematologic Malignancies," *J Clin Oncol*, 2005, 23(15):3396-403.

Nelfinavir (nel FIN a veer)

Medication Safety Issues

Sound-alike/look-alike issues:

Nelfinavir may be confused with nevirapine

Viracept® may be confused with Viramune®

Related Information
Adult and Adolescent HIV *on page 1821*
Pediatric HIV *on page 1816*
Perinatal HIV *on page 1831*

U.S. Brand Names Viracept®

Canadian Brand Names Viracept®

Index Terms NFV

Therapeutic Category Antiretroviral Agent; HIV Agents (Anti-HIV Agents); Protease Inhibitor

Generic Available No

Use Treatment of HIV infection in combination with other antiretroviral agents. (**Note:** HIV regimens consisting of **three** antiretroviral agents are strongly recommended)

Pregnancy Risk Factor B

Lactation Excretion in breast milk unknown/contraindicated

Contraindications Hypersensitivity to nelfinavir or any component; concurrent therapy with amiodarone, dihydroergotamine, ergonovine, ergotamine, midazolam, methylergonovine, pimozide, quinidine, or triazolam

Warnings Nelfinavir inhibits cytochrome P450 isoenzyme CYP3A and interacts with numerous drugs. Due to potential serious and/or life-threatening drug interactions, some drugs are contraindicated (see Contraindications and Drug Interactions) and the following drugs should **not** be coadministered with nelfinavir: Astemizole, cisapride, terfenadine, rifampin, St John's wort, lovastatin, simvastatin, or proton pump inhibitors; concurrent use with some anticonvulsants may significantly limit nelfinavir's effectiveness. Spontaneous bleeding episodes have been reported in patients with hemophilia type A and B receiving protease inhibitors. New onset diabetes mellitus, exacerbations of diabetes, and hyperglycemia have been reported in HIV-infected patients receiving protease inhibitors.

Precautions Use with caution in patients with hepatic insufficiency since nelfinavir is metabolized in the liver. Fat redistribution and accumulation [ie, central obesity, peripheral wasting, facial wasting, breast enlargement, dorsocervical fat enlargement (buffalo hump), and cushingoid appearance] have been observed in patients receiving antiretroviral agents (causal relationship not established). Immune reconstitution syndrome (an acute inflammatory response to residual or indolent opportunistic infections) may occur in HIV patients during initial treatment with combination antiretroviral agents, including nelfinavir; this syndrome may require further patient assessment and therapy. Powder formulation contains aspartame which is metabolized to phenylalanine and should be avoided or used with caution in patients with phenylketonuria.

Adverse Reactions Note: Adverse effects are similar in children and adults, with diarrhea being the most common adverse effect in both age groups

Cardiovascular: Hypertension

Central nervous system: Decreased concentration, anxiety, depression, dizziness, emotional lability, hyperkinesia, insomnia, migraine, seizures, sleep disorder, somnolence, suicide ideation, fever, headache, asthenia, malaise

Dermatologic: Rash, pruritus, urticaria, diaphoresis

Endocrine & metabolic: Hyperlipemia, hyperuricemia; rare: hyperglycemia, diabetes, ketoacidosis; fat redistribution and accumulation (see Precautions)

Gastrointestinal: Diarrhea (Adults: 14% to 20%; children: 39% to 47%; **Note:** Diarrhea may be more frequent in patients receiving 625 mg tablets due to increased bioavailability), nausea, flatulence, abdominal pain, anorexia, dyspepsia, epigastric pain, mouth ulceration, GI bleeding, pancreatitis, vomiting

Genitourinary: Kidney calculus, sexual dysfunction

Hematologic: Anemia, leukopenia, thrombocytopenia; rare: spontaneous bleeding episodes in hemophiliacs

Hepatic: Hepatitis, elevated liver function tests, worsening of chronic liver disease

Neuromuscular & skeletal: Weakness, arthralgia, arthritis, cramps, myalgia, myasthenia, myopathy, paresthesia, back pain

Ocular: Acute iritis

Respiratory: Dyspnea, pharyngitis, rhinitis, sinusitis

Drug Interactions Cytochrome P450 isoenzyme CYP3A3/4 and CYP2C19 substrate; isoenzyme CYP3A3/4 inhibitor

Nelfinavir inhibits the metabolism and increases the serum concentrations of cisapride, terfenadine, astemizole, amiodarone, quinidine, lovastatin, simvastatin, ergot derivatives, pimozide, midazolam, and triazolam (concurrent use of these drugs is contraindicated or not recommended; see Contraindications and Warnings). Nelfinavir may increase serum concentrations or adverse effects of azithromycin (monitor closely for adverse effects); cyclosporine, tacrolimus, sirolimus (monitor serum concentrations and adjust dose); sildenafil; atorvastatin (monitor carefully, use lowest atorvastatin dose possible or alternative agent); fluticasone

(Continued)

Nelfinavir *(Continued)*

(use with caution; consider alternative agent, especially with long-term use); trazodone (use with caution, monitor carefully, consider lower dose of trazodone). Nelfinavir increases rifabutin plasma AUC by 207% (reduce rifabutin dose by 50% when coadministering with nelfinavir).

Rifampin decreases nelfinavir plasma AUC by ~83% (concurrent use is **not** recommended). The herbal medicine St John's wort (*Hypericum perforatum*) may significantly decrease serum concentrations of nelfinavir (concurrent use is **not** recommended). Omeprazole significantly decreases nelfinavir plasma concentrations (concurrent use of proton pump inhibitors with nelfinavir is **not** recommended). Antacids may decrease serum concentrations of nelfinavir (avoid coadministration). Phenobarbital, phenytoin, and carbamazepine may significantly decrease nelfinavir serum concentrations. Indinavir and ritonavir increase nelfinavir concentrations. Nelfinavir decreases hormone levels of oral contraceptives (ethinyl estradiol, norethindrone; alternative or additional methods of contraception should be used). Nelfinavir increases serum concentrations of saquinavir and indinavir. Coadministration with delavirdine increases nelfinavir concentrations by twofold and decreases delavirdine concentrations by 50%. If coadministered with didanosine, administer nelfinavir 2 hours before or 1 hour after didanosine. Nelfinavir may decrease serum concentrations of phenytoin (monitor levels; dosage adjustment may be needed) or methadone (increase in methadone dose may be required).

Food Interactions Food enhances bioavailability and decreases pharmacokinetic variability. A bitter taste will result if the oral powder formulation is mixed with acidic food or juice (see Administration)

Stability Store at room temperature of 15°C to 30°C (59°F to 86°F). Dispense in original container; keep container tightly closed.

Mechanism of Action A protease inhibitor which acts on an enzyme (protease) late in the HIV replication process after the virus has entered into the cell's nucleus; nelfinavir binds to the protease activity site and inhibits the activity of the enzyme, thus preventing cleavage of viral polyprotein precursors (gag-pol protein precursors) into individual functional proteins found in infectious HIV; this results in the formation of immature, noninfectious viral particles

Pharmacokinetics

Absorption: AUC is two- to threefold higher under fed conditions versus fasting; AUC is highly variable in pediatric patients due to increased clearance, problems with compliance, and inconsistent food intake with dosing

Distribution: V_d: Adults: 2-7 L/kg

Protein binding: >98%

Metabolism: Via multiple cytochrome P450 isoforms including CYP3A4 and CYP2C19; one active oxidative metabolite with comparable activity to the parent drug and several minor oxidative metabolites are formed

Bioavailability: The 250 mg and 625 mg tablets are **not** bioequivalent; the AUC for the 625 mg tablets is 34% higher than the 250 mg tablets in fasted adults and 24% higher than the 250 mg tablets under fed conditions

Half-life: Adults: 3.5-5 hours

Time to peak serum concentration: 2-4 hours

Elimination: 98% to 99% excreted in feces (78% as metabolites and 22% as unchanged nelfinavir); 1% to 2% excreted in urine (primarily as unchanged drug)

Usual Dosage Oral (use in combination with other antiretroviral agents):

Neonates and Infants: Not approved for use; a reliable, effective dose has not been established. **Note:** 40 mg/kg/dose twice daily given to neonates and infants (age: birth to 6 weeks) resulted in high interpatient variability in serum drug concentrations; nelfinavir dosing is problematic in young infants, since the drug is best absorbed when taken with a high fat meal; higher doses are currently being studied. **Note:** Three times daily dosing may be required in infants <2 months of age; further studies are needed (see Hirt, 2006).

Infants and Children <2 years: Not approved for use; a reliable, effective dose has not been established. **Note:** Current guidelines recommend nelfinavir only for initial therapy in children >2 years of age; this is due to a lower virologic response observed in children <2 years and the lack of appropriate dosing recommendations.

Children 2-13 years (oral powder or 250 mg tablets): 45-55 mg/kg/dose (maximum: 1250 mg) twice daily or 25-35 mg/kg/dose (maximum: 750 mg) 3 times/day; **Note:** Doses >2500 mg/day have not been studied in children

Adolescents ≥14 years and Adults: 1250 mg/dose twice daily or 750 mg 3 times/day

Dosing adjustment in hepatic impairment: Use with caution; **Note:** Pharmacokinetics of multiple doses of nelfinavir in patients with hepatic impairment has not been studied

Dosing adjustment in renal impairment: Has not been studied; however, since <2% of the drug is eliminated in the urine, renal impairment should have minimal effect on nelfinavir elimination

Administration Administer with food to enhance bioavailability and decrease kinetic variability. **Note:** Due to problems with administration of the oral powder to infants, use of the tablets may be preferred. Tablets can be readily dissolved in water and consumed or mixed with milk or chocolate milk; consume immediately; rinse glass with water and swallow to make sure total dose is consumed; tablets can also be crushed and administered with pudding. Oral powder can be mixed with a small amount of water, milk, formula, dietary supplements, ice cream, or pudding; mixture must be stored under refrigeration if not used immediately; do not store mixture for more than 6 hours; do not mix oral powder with any acidic food or juice (eg, grapefruit, orange, or apple juice or applesauce) because of resulting bitter taste. If coadministered with didanosine, nelfinavir should be administered 2 hours before or 1 hour after didanosine.

Monitoring Parameters Liver function tests, blood glucose levels, CBC with differential, CD4 cell count, plasma levels of HIV RNA

Patient Information Nelfinavir is not a cure for HIV. Some medications should not be taken with nelfinavir; report the use of other medications, nonprescription medications, and herbal or natural products to your physician and pharmacist; avoid the herbal medicine St John's wort. Use an alternative method of contraception to birth control pills during nelfinavir therapy. If a nelfinavir dose is missed, take the dose as soon as possible and then return to the normal schedule. However, if a dose is skipped, do not double the next dose.

HIV medications may cause changes in body fat, including an increase in fat in the upper back and neck, breasts, and trunk; a loss of fat from the face, arms, and legs may also occur.

Nursing Implications Do not add water to bottles of oral powder; a special scoop is provided with powder for measuring purposes. If diarrhea occurs, it may be treated with an antimotility agent like loperamide

Additional Information Due to the higher variability of nelfinavir plasma concentrations in infants and children, dosage adjustment utilizing measurement of plasma concentrations and pharmacokinetics may be beneficial (see Crommentuyn, 2006). Further studies are needed.

Dosage Forms Excipient information presented when available (limited, particularly for generics); consult specific product labeling.

Powder, oral:

Viracept®: 50 mg/g (144 g) [contains phenylalanine 11.2 mg/g]

Tablet:

Viracept®: 250 mg, 625 mg

References

Briars LA, Hilao JJ, and Kraus DM, "A Review of Pediatric Human Immunodeficiency Virus Infection," *Journal of Pharmacy Practice*, 2004, 17(6):407-31.

Crommentuyn KM, Scherpbier HJ, Kuijpers TW, et al, "Population Pharmacokinetics and Pharmacodynamics of Nelfinavir and Its Active Metabolite M8 in HIV-1-Infected Children," *Pediatr Infect Dis J*, 2006, 25(6):538-43.

Hirt D, Urien S, Jullien V, et al, "Age-Related Effects on Nelfinavir and M8 Pharmacokinetics: A Population Study With 182 Children," *Antimicrob Agents Chemother*, 2006, 50(3):910-6.

McDonald CK and Kuritzkes DR, "Human Immunodeficiency Virus Type I Protease Inhibitors," *Arch Intern Med*, 1997, 157(9):951-9.

Panel on Clinical Practices for Treatment of HIV Infection, "Guidelines for the Use of Antiretroviral Agents in HIV-Infected Adults and Adolescents," October 10, 2006, http://www.aidsinfo.nih.gov.

Working Group on Antiretroviral Therapy and Medical Management of HIV-Infected Children, "Guidelines for the Use of Antiretroviral Agents in Pediatric HIV Infection," October 26, 2006, http://www.aidsinfo.nih.gov.

♦ **Nembutal®** *see* Pentobarbital *on page 1239*

♦ **Nembutal® Sodium (Can)** *see* Pentobarbital *on page 1239*

♦ **NeoCeuticals™ Acne Spot Treatment [OTC]** *see* Salicylic Acid *on page 1413*

♦ **Neo-Fradin™** *see* Neomycin *on page 1117*

♦ **Neofrin™** *see* Phenylephrine *on page 1250*

Neomycin (nee oh MYE sin)

Medication Safety Issues

Sound-alike/look-alike issues:

Myciguent may be confused with Mycitracin®

Related Information

Emetogenic Potential of Single Chemotherapeutic Agents *on page 1776*

Overdose and Toxicology *on page 1916*

(Continued)

Neomycin *(Continued)*

U.S. Brand Names Neo-Fradin™; Neo-Rx

Index Terms Neomycin Sulfate

Therapeutic Category Ammonium Detoxicant; Antibiotic, Aminoglycoside; Antibiotic, Topical; Hyperammonemia Agent

Generic Available Yes

Use Administered orally to prepare GI tract for surgery; treat minor skin infections; treat diarrhea caused by *E. coli*; adjunct in the treatment of hepatic encephalopathy

Pregnancy Risk Factor C

Lactation Excretion in breast milk unknown

Contraindications Hypersensitivity to neomycin or any component; patients with intestinal obstruction

Warnings Neomycin is more toxic than other aminoglycosides when given parenterally; **do not administer parenterally**; topical neomycin is a contact sensitizer with sensitivity occurring in 5% to 15% of patients treated with the drug; systemic absorption can occur when neomycin is utilized for irrigation of wounds or surgical sites

Precautions Use with caution in patients with renal impairment, pre-existing hearing impairment, neuromuscular disorders; modify dosage in patients with renal impairment

Adverse Reactions

Dermatologic: Contact dermatitis, erythema, rash, urticaria
Gastrointestinal: Nausea, vomiting, diarrhea, colitis, malabsorption
Local: Burning
Neuromuscular & skeletal: Neuromuscular blockade
Ocular: Contact conjunctivitis
Otic: Ototoxicity
Renal: Nephrotoxicity
Miscellaneous: Candidiasis

Drug Interactions Oral neomycin may potentiate the effects of oral anticoagulants; may decrease GI absorption of digoxin and methotrexate; synergistic effects seen with penicillins; increase adverse effects with other neurotoxic, ototoxic or nephrotoxic drugs

Stability Reconstituted neomycin solution is stable for 7 days when refrigerated

Mechanism of Action Interferes with bacterial protein synthesis by binding to 30S ribosomal subunits

Pharmacokinetics

Absorption: Poor orally (3%) or percutaneously; readily absorbed through denuded or abraded skin and body cavities
Distribution: V_d: 0.36 L/kg
Half-life: 2-3 hours (age and renal function dependent)
Time to peak serum concentration:
- I.M.: Within 2 hours
- Oral: 1-4 hours

Elimination: In urine (30% to 50% as unchanged drug); 97% of an oral dose eliminated unchanged in feces
Dialysis: Dialyzable (50% to 100%)

Usual Dosage

Neonates: Oral: Diarrhea: 50 mg/kg/day divided every 6 hours
Children: Oral: 50-100 mg/kg/day in divided doses every 6-8 hours
- Preoperative bowel antisepsis: 90 mg/kg/day divided every 4 hours for 2 days; or 25 mg/kg at 1, 2, and 11 PM on the day preceding surgery as an adjunct to mechanical cleansing of the intestine and in combination with erythromycin base
- Hepatic coma: 2.5-7 g/m^2/day divided every 4-6 hours for 5-6 days not to exceed 12 g/day
- Diarrhea caused by enteropathogenic *E. coli*: 50 mg/kg/day divided every 6 hours for 2-3 days

Children and Adults: Topical: Apply ointment 1-3 times/day; topical solutions containing 0.1% to 1% neomycin have been used for irrigation
Adults: Oral: 500-2000 mg every 6-8 hours
- Preoperative bowel antisepsis: 1 g each hour for 4 doses then 1 g every 4 hours for 5 doses; or 1 g at 1 PM, 2 PM, and 11 PM with oral erythromycin on day preceding surgery as an adjunct to mechanical cleansing of the bowel; or 6 g/day divided every 4 hours for 2-3 days
- Hepatic coma: 4-12 g/day divided every 4-6 hours
- Diarrhea caused by enteropathogenic *E. coli*: 3 g/day divided every 6 hours

Monitoring Parameters Renal function tests

Patient Information Notify physician if ringing in the ears, hearing impairment, or dizziness occurs

Dosage Forms Excipient information presented when available (limited, particularly for generics); consult specific product labeling.

Powder, micronized, as sulfate [for prescription compounding] (Neo-Rx): (10 g, 100 g)

Solution, oral, as sulfate (Neo-Fradin™): 125 mg/5 mL (60 mL, 480 mL) [contains benzoic acid; cherry flavor]

Tablet, as sulfate: 500 mg

References

Feigin RD and Cherry JD, *Textbook of Pediatric Infectious Diseases*, 4th ed, Philadelphia, PA: WB Saunders Co, 1997.

Neomycin and Polymyxin B (nee oh MYE sin & pol i MIKS in bee)

U.S. Brand Names Neosporin® G.U. Irrigant

Canadian Brand Names Neosporin® Irrigating Solution

Index Terms Polymyxin B and Neomycin

Therapeutic Category Antibiotic, Topical; Antibiotic, Urinary Irrigation; Genitourinary Irrigant

Generic Available Yes: Irrigation solution 1 mL package size

Use Short-term use as a continuous irrigant or rinse in the urinary bladder to prevent bacteriuria and gram-negative rod septicemia associated with the use of indwelling catheters

Pregnancy Risk Factor D if used as GU irrigant

Lactation Excretion in breast milk unknown

Contraindications Hypersensitivity to neomycin, polymyxin B, or any component; ophthalmic use; irrigation should be avoided in patients with defects in the bladder mucosa or wall

Warnings Topical neomycin is a contact sensitizer

Precautions Use with caution in patients with impaired renal function, dehydrated patients, burn patients, and patients receiving a high dose for prolonged treatment

Adverse Reactions

Dermatologic: Contact dermatitis, erythema, rash, urticaria

Genitourinary: Bladder irritation

Local: Burning

Neuromuscular & skeletal: Neuromuscular blockade

Otic: Ototoxicity

Renal: Nephrotoxicity

Stability Store irrigant solution in the refrigerator

Mechanism of Action Neomycin inhibits bacterial protein synthesis by binding to the 30S ribosomal subunits; polymyxin B interacts with phospholipid components in the cytoplasmic membranes of susceptible bacteria disrupting the osmotic integrity of the cell membrane

Pharmacokinetics Absorption: Not absorbed following topical application to intact skin; absorbed through denuded or abraded skin, peritoneum, wounds, or ulcers

Usual Dosage Children and Adults: Bladder irrigation: 1 mL is added to 1 L of NS with administration rate adjusted to patient's urine output; usually administered via a 3-way catheter (approximately 40 mL/hour); continuous irrigation or rinse of the urinary bladder should not exceed 10 days

Administration Bladder irrigant: Do not inject irrigant solution; concentrated irrigant solution must be diluted in 1 liter NS before administration; connect irrigation container to the inflow lumen of a 3-way catheter to permit continuous irrigation of the urinary bladder

Monitoring Parameters Urinalysis, renal function

Patient Information Notify physician if condition worsens or if rash/irritation develops

Additional Information GU irrigant contains methylparaben

Dosage Forms Excipient information presented when available (limited, particularly for generics); consult specific product labeling.

Solution, irrigant: Neomycin 40 mg and polymyxin B 200,000 units per mL (1 mL)

Neosporin® G.U. Irrigant: Neomycin 40 mg and polymyxin B 200,000 units per mL (1 mL, 20 mL)

◆ **Neomycin, Bacitracin, and Polymyxin B** *see* Neomycin, Polymyxin B, and Bacitracin *on page 1121*

Neomycin, (Bacitracin) Polymyxin B, and Hydrocortisone

(nee oh MYE sin, bas i TRAY sin, pol i MIKS in bee, & hye droe KOR ti sone)

U.S. Brand Names Cortisporin® Cream; Cortisporin® Ophthalmic; Cortisporin® Otic; PediOtic®

(Continued)

Neomycin, (Bacitracin) Polymyxin B, and Hydrocortisone *(Continued)*

Canadian Brand Names Cortimyxin®; Cortisporin® Otic

Index Terms Hydrocortisone, Neomycin, and Polymyxin B; Polymyxin B, Neomycin, and Hydrocortisone

Therapeutic Category Antibacterial, Otic; Antibiotic, Ophthalmic; Antibiotic, Otic; Antibiotic, Topical; Corticosteroid, Ophthalmic; Corticosteroid, Otic; Corticosteroid, Topical

Generic Available Yes

Use Steroid-responsive inflammatory condition for which a corticosteroid is indicated and where bacterial infection or a risk of bacterial infection exists

Pregnancy Risk Factor C

Contraindications Hypersensitivity to hydrocortisone, polymyxin B sulfate, bacitracin, neomycin sulfate, or any component (see Warnings); herpes simplex, vaccinia and varicella; otic use: perforated tympanic membrane

Warnings Neomycin may cause cutaneous and conjunctival sensitization; children are more susceptible to topical corticosteroid-induced hypothalamic pituitary-adrenal axis suppression and Cushing's syndrome; otic solution contains potassium metabisulfate which may cause allergic reactions in susceptible individuals

Precautions Use with caution in patients with chronic otitis media and when the integrity of the tympanic membrane is in question

Adverse Reactions

Dermatologic: Contact dermatitis

Local: Itching, pain, stinging, burning, local edema

Ocular: Elevated intraocular pressure, glaucoma, cataracts, conjunctival erythema; blurring of vision (ophthalmic formulation)

Otic: Ototoxicity

Miscellaneous: Sensitization to neomycin, secondary infections

Usual Dosage

Children: Otic: Solution and suspension: 3 drops into affected ear 3-4 times/day

Adults: Otic: Solution and suspension: 4 drops into affected ear 3-4 times/day

Children and Adults:

Topical ointment: Apply thin layer to affected area 2-4 times/day

Ophthalmic:

Ointment: Apply $^1/_2$" ribbon to inside of lower lid every 3-4 hours until improvement occurs then 1-3 times/day

Suspension: Instill 1-2 drops in the affected eye every 3-4 hours

Administration Shake ophthalmic and otic suspension well before use

Ophthalmic: Avoid contamination of the tip of the eye dropper or ointment tube; solution and suspension: Apply finger pressure to lacrimal sac during and for 1-2 minutes after instillation to decrease risk of absorption and systemic effects

Otic: Drops can be instilled directly into the affected ear, or a cotton wick may be saturated with suspension and inserted in ear canal. Keep wick moist with suspension every 4 hours; wick should be replaced every 24 hours.

Topical: Apply a thin layer to the cleansed, dry affected area; may cover with a sterile bandage

Patient Information Ophthalmic: May cause sensitivity to bright light; may cause temporary blurring of vision or stinging following administration

Additional Information Otic **suspension** is the preferred otic preparation; otic **suspension** can be used for the treatment of infections of mastoidectomy and fenestration cavities caused by susceptible organisms; otic **solution** is used **only** for superficial infections of the external auditory canal (ie, swimmer's ear)

Dosage Forms Excipient information presented when available (limited, particularly for generics); consult specific product labeling.

Cream, topical (Cortisporin®): Neomycin 3.5 mg, polymyxin B 10,000 units, and hydrocortisone acetate 5 mg per g (7.5 g)

Solution, otic (Cortisporin®): Neomycin 3.5 mg, polymyxin B 10,000 units, and hydrocortisone 10 mg per mL (10 mL) [contains potassium metabisulfite]

Suspension, ophthalmic (Cortisporin®): Neomycin 3.5 mg, polymyxin B 10,000 units, and hydrocortisone 10 mg per mL (7.5 mL) [contains thimerosal]

Suspension, otic: Neomycin 3.5 mg, polymyxin B 10,000 units, and hydrocortisone 10 mg per mL (10 mL)

Cortisporin®: Neomycin 3.5 mg, polymyxin B 10,000 units, and hydrocortisone 10 mg per mL (10 mL) [contains thimerosal]

PediOtic®: Neomycin 3.5 mg, polymyxin B 10,000 units, and hydrocortisone 10 mg per mL (7.5 mL) [contains thimerosal]

Neomycin, Polymyxin B, and Bacitracin

(nee oh MYE sin, pol i MIKS in bee, & bas i TRAY sin)

U.S. Brand Names Neosporin® Neo To Go® [OTC]; Neosporin® Ophthalmic Ointment [DSC]; Neosporin® Topical [OTC]

Canadian Brand Names Neosporin® Ophthalmic Ointment

Index Terms Neomycin, Bacitracin, and Polymyxin B; Polymyxin B, Bacitracin, and Neomycin; Triple Antibiotic

Therapeutic Category Antibiotic, Ophthalmic; Antibiotic, Topical

Generic Available Yes

Use Help prevent infection in minor cuts, scrapes and burns; short-term treatment of superficial external ocular infections caused by susceptible organisms

Pregnancy Risk Factor C

Lactation Excretion in breast milk unknown/use caution

Contraindications Hypersensitivity to neomycin, polymyxin B, zinc bacitracin, or any component

Warnings Symptoms of neomycin sensitization include itching, reddening, edema, failure to heal; ophthalmic ointments may retard corneal healing

Precautions Prolonged use may result in overgrowth of nonsusceptible organisms

Adverse Reactions

Local: Rash and hypersensitivity reactions ranging from generalized itching, local edema, and erythema have been reported; contact dermatitis

Ocular: Conjunctival sensitization, blurring of vision (ophthalmic formulation)

Usual Dosage Children and Adults:

Ophthalmic ointment: Instill into the conjunctival sac 1 or more times daily every 3-4 hours for 7-10 days

Topical: Apply 1-3 times/day

Administration

Ophthalmic: Avoid contamination of the tip of the ointment tube

Topical: Apply a thin layer to the cleansed affected area; may cover with a sterile bandage

Patient Information Ophthalmic: May cause sensitivity to bright light; may cause temporary blurring of vision or stinging following administration

Dosage Forms Excipient information presented when available (limited, particularly for generics); consult specific product labeling. [DSC] = Discontinued product

Ointment, ophthalmic (Neosporin® [DSC]): Bacitracin 400 units, neomycin 3.5 mg, and polymyxin B 10,000 units per g (3.5 g)

Ointment, topical: Bacitracin 400 units, neomycin 3.5 mg, and polymyxin B 5000 units per g (0.9 g, 15 g, 30 g, 454 g)

Neosporin®: Bacitracin 400 units, neomycin 3.5 mg, and polymyxin B 5000 units per g (15 g, 30 g)

Neosporin® Neo To Go®: Bacitracin 400 units, neomycin 3.5 mg, and polymyxin B 5000 units per g (0.9 g)

Neomycin, Polymyxin B, and Prednisolone

(nee oh MYE sin, pol i MIKS in bee, & pred NIS oh lone)

U.S. Brand Names Poly-Pred®

Index Terms Polymyxin B, Neomycin, and Prednisolone; Prednisolone, Neomycin, and Polymyxin B

Therapeutic Category Antibiotic, Ophthalmic; Corticosteroid, Ophthalmic

Generic Available No

Use Used for steroid-responsive inflammatory ocular condition in which bacterial infection or a risk of bacterial ocular infection exists

Pregnancy Risk Factor C

Contraindications Hypersensitivity to neomycin, polymyxin B, prednisolone, or any component; dendritic keratitis, viral disease of the cornea and conjunctiva, mycobacterial infection of the eye, fungal disease of the ocular structure, or after uncomplicated removal of a corneal foreign body

Warnings Symptoms of neomycin sensitization include itching, reddening, edema, or failure to heal

Precautions Prolonged use may result in overgrowth of nonsusceptible organisms, glaucoma, damage to the optic nerve, defects in visual acuity, and cataract formation

Adverse Reactions

Dermatologic: Cutaneous sensitization, skin rash, delayed wound healing

Ocular: Elevated intraocular pressure, glaucoma, optic nerve damage, cataracts, conjunctival sensitization

(Continued)

Neomycin, Polymyxin B, and Prednisolone *(Continued)*

Usual Dosage Children and Adults:

Ophthalmic: Instill 1-2 drops every 3-4 hours; acute infections may require every 30-minute instillation initially with frequency of administration reduced as the infection is brought under control

To treat the eye lids: Instill 1-2 drops every 3-4 hours, close the eye and rub the excess on the lids and lid margins.

Administration Ophthalmic: Avoid contamination of the dropper tip; shake suspension well before using; apply finger pressure to lacrimal sac during and for 1-2 minutes after instillation to decrease risk of absorption and systemic effects

Patient Information Ophthalmic: May cause sensitivity to bright light; may cause temporary blurring of vision or stinging following administration

Dosage Forms Excipient information presented when available (limited, particularly for generics); consult specific product labeling.

Suspension, ophthalmic: Neomycin 0.35%, polymyxin B 10,000 units per mL, and prednisolone acetate 0.5% (5 mL; 10 mL [DSC]) [contains thimerosal]

- **Neomycin Sulfate** *see* Neomycin *on page 1117*
- **Neonatal Trace Metals** *see* Trace Metals *on page 1558*
- **NeoProfen®** *see* Ibuprofen *on page 802*
- **Neoral®** *see* CycloSPORINE *on page 422*
- **Neo-Rx** *see* Neomycin *on page 1117*
- **Neosar** *see* Cyclophosphamide *on page 419*
- **Neosporin® AF [OTC]** *see* Miconazole *on page 1056*
- **Neosporin® G.U. Irrigant** *see* Neomycin and Polymyxin B *on page 1119*
- **Neosporin® Irrigating Solution (Can)** *see* Neomycin and Polymyxin B *on page 1119*
- **Neosporin® Neo To Go® [OTC]** *see* Neomycin, Polymyxin B, and Bacitracin *on page 1121*
- **Neosporin® Ophthalmic Ointment [DSC]** *see* Neomycin, Polymyxin B, and Bacitracin *on page 1121*
- **Neosporin® Ophthalmic Ointment (Can)** *see* Neomycin, Polymyxin B, and Bacitracin *on page 1121*
- **Neosporin® Topical [OTC]** *see* Neomycin, Polymyxin B, and Bacitracin *on page 1121*

Neostigmine (nee oh STIG meen)

Medication Safety Issues

Sound-alike/look-alike issues:

Prostigmin® may be confused with physostigmine

Related Information

Commonly Used Antidotes for Acute Overdoses *on page 1920*

Overdose and Toxicology *on page 1916*

U.S. Brand Names Prostigmin®

Canadian Brand Names Prostigmin®

Index Terms Neostigmine Bromide; Neostigmine Methylsulfate

Therapeutic Category Antidote, Neuromuscular Blocking Agent; Cholinergic Agent; Diagnostic Agent, Myasthenia Gravis

Generic Available Yes: Injection

Use Treatment of myasthenia gravis; prevention and treatment of postoperative bladder distention and urinary retention; reversal of the effects of nondepolarizing neuromuscular blocking agents after surgery

Pregnancy Risk Factor C

Lactation Excretion in breast milk unknown/not recommended

Contraindications Hypersensitivity to neostigmine, bromides, or any component; GI or GU obstruction, peritonitis

Warnings Does **not** antagonize, and may prolong the phase I block of depolarizing muscle relaxants (eg, succinylcholine); adequate facilities should be available for cardiopulmonary resuscitation when testing and adjusting dose for myasthenia gravis; have atropine and epinephrine ready to treat hypersensitivity reactions; anticholinesterase insensitivity can develop for brief or prolonged periods

Precautions Use with caution in patients with epilepsy, asthma, bradycardia, hyperthyroidism, cardiac arrhythmias, peptic ulcer, vagotonia, or recent coronary occlusion

Adverse Reactions

Cardiovascular: Bradycardia, hypotension, asystole, A-V block, nodal rhythms, flushing, syncope

Central nervous system: Restlessness, agitation, seizures, dysphonia, dizziness, drowsiness, headache

Dermatologic: Rash, urticaria
Gastrointestinal: Hyperperistalsis, nausea, vomiting, diarrhea, dysphagia, flatulence, abdominal cramps; increased salivary, gastric, and intestinal secretions
Genitourinary: Urinary frequency and incontinence
Local: Thrombophlebitis
Neuromuscular & skeletal: Weakness, muscle cramps, arthralgia, tremor, dysarthria
Ocular: Miosis, lacrimation, diplopia, conjunctival hyperemia
Respiratory: Bronchoconstriction, increased secretions, laryngospasm, dyspnea, respiratory arrest, bronchospasm, respiratory paralysis
Miscellaneous: Allergic reactions, diaphoresis

Drug Interactions Antagonizes effects of nondepolarizing muscle relaxants (eg, pancuronium, tubocurarine); atropine and magnesium antagonize the muscarinic effects of neostigmine; corticosteroids may decrease neostigmine effects; prolongs effects of depolarizing muscle relaxants (eg, succinylcholine)

Mechanism of Action Competitively inhibits the hydrolysis of acetylcholine by acetylcholinesterase facilitating transmission of impulses across the myoneural junction and producing cholinergic activity

Pharmacodynamics

Onset of action:
- Oral: 45-75 minutes
- I.M.: Within 20-30 minutes
- I.V.: Within 1-20 minutes

Duration:
- Oral: 2-4 hours
- I.M.: 2-4 hours
- I.V.: 1-2 hours

Pharmacokinetics

Absorption: Oral: Poor (~1% to 2%)
Metabolism: In the liver
Half-life: 0.5-2.1 hours
Elimination: 50% excreted renally as unchanged drug

Usual Dosage

Myasthenia gravis:
- Diagnosis: I.M. (all cholinesterase medications should be discontinued at least 8 hours before; atropine should be administered I.V. immediately prior to or I.M. 30 minutes before neostigmine):
  - Children: 0.025-0.04 mg/kg as a single dose
  - Adults: 0.02 mg/kg as a single dose
- Treatment (dosage requirements are variable; adjust dosage so patient takes larger doses at times of greatest fatigue):
  - Children:
    - Oral: 2 mg/kg/day or 60 mg/m^2/day every 3-4 hours; not to exceed 375 mg/day
    - I.M., I.V., SubQ: 0.01-0.04 mg/kg every 2-4 hours
  - Adults:
    - Oral: Initial: 15 mg/dose every 3-4 hours, gradually increase every 1-2 days; usual daily range: 15-375 mg
    - I.M., I.V., SubQ: 0.5-2.5 mg every 1-3 hours up to 10 mg/24 hours maximum

Reversal of nondepolarizing neuromuscular blockade after surgery in conjunction with atropine or glycopyrrolate: I.V.:
- Infants: 0.025-0.1 mg/kg/dose
- Children: 0.025-0.08 mg/kg/dose
- Adults: 0.5-2.5 mg; total dose not to exceed 5 mg

Bladder atony: Adults: I.M., SubQ:
- Prevention: 0.25 mg every 4-6 hours for 2-3 days
- Treatment: 0.5-1 mg every 3 hours for 5 doses after bladder has emptied

Dosing adjustment in renal impairment:
- Cl_{cr} 10-50 mL/minute: Administer 50% of normal dose
- Cl_{cr} <10 mL/minute: Administer 25% of normal dose

Administration

Parenteral: May be administered undiluted by slow I.V. injection over several minutes; may be administered I.M. or SubQ
Oral: Divide dosages so patient receives larger doses at times of greatest fatigue; may be administered with or without food

Monitoring Parameters Muscle strength, heart rate, respiratory rate

Patient Information The side effects are generally due to exaggerated pharmacologic effects; the most common side effects are salivation and muscle fasciculations; notify physician if nausea, vomiting, muscle weakness, severe abdominal pain, or difficulty breathing occurs

Dosage Forms Excipient information presented when available (limited, particularly for generics); consult specific product labeling.
(Continued)

Neostigmine *(Continued)*

Injection, solution, as methylsulfate: 0.5 mg/mL (1 mL, 10 mL); 1 mg/mL (10 mL)
Tablet, as bromide: 15 mg

- ♦ **Neostigmine Bromide** *see* Neostigmine *on page 1122*
- ♦ **Neostigmine Methylsulfate** *see* Neostigmine *on page 1122*
- ♦ **Neo-Synephrine® (Can)** *see* Phenylephrine *on page 1250*
- ♦ **Neo-Synephrine® 12 Hour [OTC]** *see* Oxymetazoline *on page 1194*
- ♦ **Neo-Synephrine® 12 Hour Extra Moisturizing [OTC]** *see* Oxymetazoline *on page 1194*
- ♦ **Neo-Synephrine® Extra Strength [OTC]** *see* Phenylephrine *on page 1250*
- ♦ **Neo-Synephrine® Injection** *see* Phenylephrine *on page 1250*
- ♦ **Neo-Synephrine® Mild [OTC]** *see* Phenylephrine *on page 1250*
- ♦ **Neo-Synephrine® Regular Strength [OTC]** *see* Phenylephrine *on page 1250*
- ♦ **Neotrace-4®** *see* Trace Metals *on page 1558*
- ♦ **Nephro-Calci® [OTC]** *see* Calcium Carbonate *on page 264*
- ♦ **Nephro-Calci® [OTC]** *see* Calcium Supplements *on page 272*
- ♦ **Nephro-Fer® [OTC]** *see* Iron Supplements (Oral/Enteral) *on page 868*
- ♦ **Nesacaine®** *see* Chloroprocaine *on page 339*
- ♦ **Nesacaine®-CE (Can)** *see* Chloroprocaine *on page 339*
- ♦ **Nesacaine®-MPF** *see* Chloroprocaine *on page 339*
- ♦ **Neumega®** *see* Oprelvekin *on page 1174*
- ♦ **Neupogen®** *see* Filgrastim *on page 655*
- ♦ **Neurontin®** *see* Gabapentin *on page 716*
- ♦ **Neut®** *see* Sodium Bicarbonate *on page 1448*
- ♦ **NeutraCare®** *see* Fluoride *on page 675*
- ♦ **NeutraGard® [OTC]** *see* Fluoride *on page 675*
- ♦ **NeutraGard® Advanced** *see* Fluoride *on page 675*
- ♦ **NeutraGard® Plus** *see* Fluoride *on page 675*
- ♦ **Neutra-Phos® [OTC]** *see* Potassium Phosphate and Sodium Phosphate *on page 1296*
- ♦ **Neutra-Phos®-K [OTC]** *see* Potassium Phosphate *on page 1293*
- ♦ **Neutrogena® Acne Mask [OTC]** *see* Benzoyl Peroxide *on page 207*
- ♦ **Neutrogena® Acne Wash [OTC]** *see* Salicylic Acid *on page 1413*
- ♦ **Neutrogena® Body Clear™ [OTC]** *see* Salicylic Acid *on page 1413*
- ♦ **Neutrogena® Clear Pore [OTC]** *see* Salicylic Acid *on page 1413*
- ♦ **Neutrogena® Clear Pore Shine Control [OTC]** *see* Salicylic Acid *on page 1413*
- ♦ **Neutrogena® Healthy Scalp [OTC]** *see* Salicylic Acid *on page 1413*
- ♦ **Neutrogena® Maximum Strength T/Sal® [OTC]** *see* Salicylic Acid *on page 1413*
- ♦ **Neutrogena® On The Spot® Acne Patch [OTC]** *see* Salicylic Acid *on page 1413*
- ♦ **Neutrogena® On The Spot® Acne Treatment [OTC]** *see* Benzoyl Peroxide *on page 207*
- ♦ **Neutrogena® T/Gel [OTC]** *see* Coal Tar *on page 394*
- ♦ **Neutrogena® T/Gel Extra Strength [OTC]** *see* Coal Tar *on page 394*
- ♦ **Neutrogena® T/Gel Stubborn Itch Control [OTC]** *see* Coal Tar *on page 394*

Nevirapine (ne VYE ra peen)

Medication Safety Issues

Sound-alike/look-alike issues:

Nevirapine may be confused with nelfinavir

Viramune® may be confused with Viracept®

Related Information

Adult and Adolescent HIV *on page 1821*

Pediatric HIV *on page 1816*

Perinatal HIV *on page 1831*

U.S. Brand Names Viramune®

Canadian Brand Names Viramune®

Index Terms NVP

Therapeutic Category Antiretroviral Agent; HIV Agents (Anti-HIV Agents); Non-nucleoside Reverse Transcriptase Inhibitor (NNRTI)

Generic Available No

Use Treatment of HIV infection in combination with other antiretroviral agents. **(Note:** HIV regimens consisting of **three** antiretroviral agents are strongly recommended). Do not start nevirapine therapy in women with $CD4^+$ counts >250 cells/mm^3 or in men with $CD4^+$ counts >400 cells/mm^3 unless benefit of therapy outweighs the risk (see

Warnings). Nevirapine is also used as chemoprophylaxis to prevent maternal-fetal HIV transmission (see Related Information, Perinatal HIV).

Medication Guide An FDA-approved patient medication guide, which is available with the product information and at http://www.fda.gov/cder/Offices/ODS/medication_guides.htm, must be dispensed with this medication for each new outpatient prescription and refill.

Pregnancy Risk Factor C

Lactation Enters breast milk/contraindicated

Contraindications Hypersensitivity to nevirapine or any component; concurrent therapy with ketoconazole (see Drug Interactions)

Warnings Severe and life-threatening skin reactions (eg, Stevens-Johnson syndrome, toxic epidermal necrolysis) have occurred in patients receiving nevirapine. Discontinue nevirapine in patients who develop a severe rash or rash accompanied by fever, blistering, oral lesions, conjunctivitis, swelling, muscle or joint aches, or malaise. Initiating therapy at a lower dose for the first 14 days of therapy has been shown to reduce the frequency of rash. Concomitant use of prednisone during the first 6 weeks of therapy was associated with an increase in incidence and severity of rash. Use of prednisone to prevent nevirapine-associated rash is not recommended.

Severe, life-threatening, and fatal cases of hepatotoxicity have been reported with the use of nevirapine. Hepatitis or hepatic failure may be associated with hypersensitivity reactions and may include severe rash, rash with fever, malaise, fatigue, blisters, oral lesions, conjunctivitis, facial edema, muscle of joint aches, eosinophilia, granulocytopenia, lymphadenopathy, renal dysfunction. Intensive monitoring is required during the initial 18 weeks of therapy to detect potentially life-threatening hepatotoxicity or skin reactions. The greatest risk for these reactions occurs in the first 6 weeks of therapy. Patients with elevated AST or ALT levels, coinfection with hepatitis B or C, women with $CD4^+$ counts >250 cells/mm^3, and men with $CD4^+$ counts >400 cells/mm^3 may be at higher risk for rash-associated hepatic adverse events. Women with high $CD4^+$ counts are at the greatest risk of hepatotoxicity including potentially fatal hepatic events. Serious hepatotoxicity has been reported in patients receiving multiple dose regimens of nevirapine for postexposure prophylaxis. Symptomatic liver toxicity has **not** been reported after single doses of nevirapine (when used for chemoprophylaxis) and may be less common in HIV-infected children. Permanently discontinue nevirapine therapy if clinical hepatotoxicity, severe skin reactions, or hypersensitivity reactions occur and do not restart after recovery.

Nevirapine induces hepatic cytochrome P450 3A and has the potential for interacting with numerous drugs; drugs having suspected interactions and that should only be used with careful monitoring include rifampin, rifabutin, triazolam, midazolam, oral contraceptives, oral anticoagulants, digoxin, phenytoin, and theophylline.

Precautions Fat redistribution and accumulation [ie, central obesity, peripheral wasting, facial wasting, breast enlargement, dorsocervical fat enlargement (buffalo hump), and cushingoid appearance] have been observed in patients receiving antiretroviral agents (causal relationship not established). Use with caution in patients with either renal or hepatic dysfunction; not recommended for use in patients with severe hepatic impairment; elevated AST or ALT levels and/or a history of chronic hepatitis (B or C) infection are associated with a greater risk of hepatic adverse events; nevirapine may accumulate in patients with worsening hepatic function and ascites

Adverse Reactions

Central nervous system: Headache, fever, sedation, malaise

Dermatologic: Rash (usually maculopapular erythematous cutaneous eruptions with or without pruritus, located on the trunk, face, and extremities; women may be at a higher risk for development of rash; 19% of pediatric patients developed rash), toxic epidermal necrolysis, angioedema, Stevens-Johnson syndrome (see Warnings)

Endocrine & metabolic: Fat redistribution and accumulation (see Precautions)

Gastrointestinal: Nausea, diarrhea, vomiting, abdominal pain

Hematologic: Eosinophilia, granulocytopenia (more common in children receiving nevirapine with zidovudine), thrombocytopenia

Hepatic: Elevated liver enzymes, liver failure, cholestatic hepatitis, hepatic necrosis, jaundice (see Warnings)

Neuromuscular & skeletal: Myalgia, arthralgia, paresthesia

Miscellaneous: Anaphylaxis, hypersensitivity reactions

Drug Interactions Cytochrome P450 isoenzyme CYP3A3/4 substrate, inducer, and inhibitor; CYP2B6 substrate and inducer

Cimetidine, ketoconazole (not recommended for concurrent use), macrolides increase nevirapine plasma concentrations; rifabutin, rifampin decrease nevirapine plasma concentrations; nevirapine decreases metabolism of rifampin and rifabutin (dosage adjustments of these drugs may be needed when administered with nevirapine); nevirapine decreases indinavir and saquinavir concentrations; decreases hormonal contraceptive efficacy; decreases metabolism of triazolam,

(Continued)

Nevirapine *(Continued)*

midazolam, oral anticoagulants, digoxin, phenytoin, theophylline; the herbal medicine St John's wort (*Hypericum perforatum*) may decrease serum concentration of nevirapine and is not recommended for concurrent use; increased incidence and severity of rash when nevirapine is used with prednisone; nevirapine may reduce plasma concentration of methadone (avoid concurrent use since acute withdrawal symptoms have been reported); monitor closely for withdrawal if concurrent use cannot be avoided and adjust methadone dosage accordingly

Stability Store at room temperature

Mechanism of Action A non-nucleoside reverse transcriptase inhibitor which specifically binds to HIV-1 reverse transcriptase blocking the RNA-dependent and DNA-dependent DNA polymerase activity and disrupting the virus' life cycle. Nevirapine does not inhibit HIV-2 reverse transcriptase or human DNA polymerase.

Pharmacokinetics

Absorption: Rapid and readily absorbed

Distribution: V_d: 1.21 L/kg; widely distributed; crosses the placenta; excreted in breast milk; 45% of the plasma concentration in CSF

Metabolism: Metabolized by cytochrome P450 isozymes from the CYP3A family to hydroxylated metabolites; autoinduction of metabolism occurs in 2-4 weeks with a 1.5-2 times increase in clearance; nevirapine is more rapidly metabolized in pediatric patients than in adults

Protein binding, plasma: 60%

Bioavailability: 91% to 93%

Half-life: Single dose (45 hours); multiple dosing (25-30 hours)

Time to peak serum concentration: 4 hours

Elimination: 81.3% in urine as metabolites, 10.1% in feces; <3% of the total dose is eliminated in urine as parent drug

Usual Dosage Oral (use in combination with other antiretroviral agents for treatment of HIV infection; for use in prevention of perinatal HIV infection see Related Information): **Note:** If nevirapine therapy is interrupted for >7 days, restart at the initial recommended dose (ie, once daily for the first 14 days) before increasing to twice daily dosing

Neonates to 2 months (Investigational, under study in PACTG 365): 5 mg/kg/dose or 120 mg/m^2/dose once daily for 14 days, followed by 120 mg/m^2/dose every 12 hours for 14 days, followed by 200 mg/m^2/dose every 12 hours

Children 2 months to 8 years: Initial: 4 mg/kg/dose once daily for the first 14 days of therapy; increase to 7 mg/kg/dose every 12 hours if no rash or other adverse effects occur; maximum: 200 mg/dose

Children ≥8 years: Initial: 4 mg/kg/dose once daily for the first 14 days of therapy; increase to 4 mg/kg/dose every 12 hours if no rash or other adverse effects occur; maximum: 200 mg/dose

Note: Alternative pediatric dosing (Working Group, 2005): Initial: 120 mg/m^2/dose (maximum: 200 mg/dose) once daily for the first 14 days of therapy; increase to 120-200 mg/m^2/dose every 12 hours if no rash or other adverse effects occur (maximum: 200 mg/dose); children <8 years of age may require the higher dose (ie, 200 mg/m^2/dose) every 12 hours. Some clinicians prefer using the mg/m^2 dosing regimen because the majority of pediatric clinical trials used this regimen; it also avoids the abrupt decrease in dosage that would occur at 8 years of age with the mg/kg dosing regimen. However, other clinicians prefer to use the mg/kg dosing regimen, but do not decrease the patient's dose at 8 years of age; instead, they allow the child to gradually gain weight and grow into the lower mg/kg/dose.

Adolescents and Adults: Initial: 200 mg/dose once daily for the first 14 days; increase to 200 mg every 12 hours if no rash or other adverse effects occur

Dosage adjustment in renal impairment: Adults:

Cl_{cr} ≥20 mL/minute: No dosage adjustment required

Hemodialysis: An additional 200 mg dose is recommended following dialysis.

Administration Oral: May be administered with water, milk, or soda, with or without meals; may be administered with an antacid or didanosine; shake suspension gently prior to administration

Monitoring Parameters Clinical chemistry tests, CD4 cell count, plasma levels of HIV RNA; liver function tests at baseline, closely during first 18 weeks of treatment, prior to dose escalation, 2 weeks postdose escalation, and at frequent intervals thereafter; obtain liver function tests immediately if patient develops signs or symptoms consistent with hepatitis or hypersensitivity reactions

Patient Information Nevirapine is not a cure for HIV; take nevirapine as prescribed; read the patient Medication Guide that you receive with each prescription and refill of nevirapine; avoid the herbal medicine St John's wort; inform physician immediately of any rash or symptoms of fatigue, malaise, jaundice, liver tenderness, anorexia, or nausea; use an alternative method of contraception from birth control pills during nevirapine therapy; if a dose is missed, take the next dose as soon as possible, however, if a dose is skipped, do not double the next dose

HIV medications may cause changes in body fat, including an increase in fat in the upper back and neck, breasts, and trunk; a loss of fat from the face, arms, and legs may also occur.

Additional Information Early virologic failure and rapid emergence of resistant mutations have been observed in therapy-naive adult HIV patients treated with tenofovir, didanosine enteric-coated beadlets (Videx® EC) and either efavirenz or nevirapine; the combination of tenofovir, didanosine, and any non-nucleoside reverse transcriptase inhibitor is **not** recommended as initial antiretroviral therapy.

Dosage Forms Excipient information presented when available (limited, particularly for generics); consult specific product labeling. Suspension is available as nevirapine hemihydrate; mg strength refers to nevirapine.

Suspension, oral:
  Viramune®: 50 mg/5 mL (240 mL)

Tablet:
  Viramune®: 200 mg

References

Briars LA, Hilao JJ, and Kraus DM, "A Review of Pediatric Human Immunodeficiency Virus Infection," *Journal of Pharmacy Practice*, 2004, 17(6):407-31.

D'Aquila RT, Hughes MD, Johnson VA, et al, "Nevirapine, Zidovudine, and Didanosine Compared With Zidovudine and Didanosine in Patients With HIV-1 Infection. A Randomized, Double-Blind, Placebo-Controlled Trial. National Institute of Allergy and Infectious Diseases AIDS Clinical Trials Group Protocol 241 Investigators," *Ann Intern Med*, 1996, 124(12):1019-30.

Mueller BU, Sei S, Anderson B, et al, "Comparison of Virus Burden in Blood and Sequential Lymph Node Biopsy Specimens From Children Infected With Human Immunodeficiency Virus," *J Pediatr*, 1996, 129(3):410-8.

Panel on Clinical Practices for Treatment of HIV Infection, "Guidelines for the Use of Antiretroviral Agents in HIV-Infected Adults and Adolescents," October 10, 2006, http://www.aidsinfo.nih.gov.

Working Group on Antiretroviral Therapy and Medical Management of HIV-Infected Children, "Guidelines for the Use of Antiretroviral Agents in Pediatric HIV Infection," October 26, 2006, http://www.aidsinfo.nih.gov.

♦ **Nexium®** *see* Esomeprazole *on page 603*

♦ **NFV** *see* Nelfinavir *on page 1114*

♦ **NH_4Cl** *see* Ammonium Chloride *on page 112*

Niacin (NYE a sin)

Medication Safety Issues

Sound-alike/look-alike issues:
  Niacin may be confused with Minocin®, Niaspan®, Nispan®
  Niaspan® may be confused with niacin
  Nicobid® may be confused with Nitro-Bid®

International issues:
  Niacor® may be confused with Nacor® which is a brand name for enalapril in Spain

U.S. Brand Names Niacor®; Niaspan®; Slo-Niacin® [OTC]

Canadian Brand Names Niaspan®

Index Terms Nicotinic Acid; Vitamin B_3

Therapeutic Category Antilipemic Agent; Nutritional Supplement; Vitamin, Water Soluble

Generic Available Yes

Use Adjunctive treatment of hyperlipidemias; peripheral vascular disease and circulatory disorders; treatment of pellagra; dietary supplement; **Note:** Niacin may be used in combination with lovastatin or bile acid sequestrants for treatment of hyperlipidemias in patients who fail monotherapy; combination therapy is not indicated as initial therapy

Pregnancy Risk Factor A (C if used in doses greater than RDA suggested doses)

Lactation Enters breast milk/consult prescriber

Contraindications Hypersensitivity to niacin or any component; significant liver disease, active peptic ulcer, severe hypotension, arterial hemorrhaging; GERD (relative contraindication)

Warnings Hepatotoxicity may occur and may be more common if extended release product is substituted for immediate release product at same dosage; do not interchange extended or sustained release products for immediate release at same dosage. Rare cases of rhabdomyolysis have occurred during concomitant use of niacin with HMG-CoA reductase inhibitors; monitor patients receiving both medications for clinical signs of rhabdomyolysis (muscle pain, tenderness, or weakness) and serum CPK and potassium.

Precautions May elevate uric acid levels, use with caution in patients predisposed to gout; large doses should be administered with caution to patients with gallbladder disease, jaundice, liver disease, diabetes, unstable angina, MI, renal dysfunction or

(Continued)

Niacin *(Continued)*

heavy alcohol use; niacin may cause small increases in prothrombin time (use with caution in patients receiving anticoagulants; monitor closely)

Adverse Reactions

Cardiovascular: Flushing, hypotension, tachycardia, syncope, vasovagal attacks, arrhythmias, palpitations, orthostasis, edema

Central nervous system: Dizziness, headache, chills, insomnia, nervousness

Dermatologic: Pruritus, increased sebaceous gland activity, tingling skin, burning, acanthosis nigricans (reversible), dry skin, rash, urticaria, hyperpigmentation

Endocrine & metabolic: Hyperuricemia, hyperglycemia, transient hypophosphatemia

Gastrointestinal: GI upset, nausea, vomiting, heartburn, diarrhea, anorexia, peptic ulcers, eructation, flatulence

Hematologic: Slight reduction in platelet counts, small increases in prothrombin time

Hepatic: Abnormal liver function tests, jaundice, chronic liver damage, hepatitis

Neuromuscular & skeletal: Asthenia, myalgia, myasthenia, leg cramps, paresthesia

Ocular: Blurred vision

Respiratory: Dyspnea

Miscellaneous: Sweating, hypersensitivity reactions (rare)

Drug Interactions May inhibit uricosuric effects of sulfinpyrazone and probenecid; adrenergic blocking agents and other vasodilating drugs may cause additive vasodilating effect and postural hypotension; bile acid sequestrants may decrease the absorption of niacin (separate administration by at least 4-6 hours); vitamins containing large amounts of niacin, nicotinamide, and related substances may increase adverse effects; use with lipid-lowering agents will enhance antilipid effects; HMG-CoA reductase inhibitors may increase risk of rhabdomyolysis, myopathy; use with anticoagulants may have additive effect on prothrombin time (monitor closely)

Food Interactions Concurrent intake of hot drinks or alcohol may increase flushing and pruritus (avoid around the time of niacin administration)

Mechanism of Action Component of two coenzymes necessary for tissue respiration, lipid metabolism, and glycogenolysis; inhibits the synthesis of very low density lipoproteins

Pharmacodynamics Vasodilation:

Onset of action: Within 20 minutes

Extended release: Within 1 hour

Duration: 20-60 minutes

Extended release: 8-10 hours

Pharmacokinetics

Absorption: Oral: Rapid and extensive; ≥60% to 76% of dose is absorbed

Distribution: Crosses into breast milk

Metabolism: Extensive first-pass effect; niacin in smaller doses is converted to niacinamide which is metabolized in the liver; niacin undergoes conjugation with glycine to form nicotinuric acid; nicotinamide, nicotinamide adenine dinucleotide (NAD), and other niacin metabolites are formed via saturable pathways; **Note:** It is not clear whether nicotinamide is formed before or after the synthesis of NAD

Bioavailability: Single dose studies indicate that Niaspan® tablet strengths are **not** interchangeable (eg, three 500 mg tablets are **not** equivalent to two 750 mg tablets)

Half-life: 45 minutes

Time to peak serum concentration: Immediate release: ~45 minutes; extended release: 4-5 hours

Elimination: In urine, with ~33% as unchanged drug; with larger doses, a greater percentage is excreted unchanged in urine

Usual Dosage Oral:

Children:

Recommended daily allowances (RDA):

0-0.5 years: 5 mg/day

0.5-1 year: 6 mg/day

1-3 years: 9 mg/day

4-6 years: 12 mg/day

7-10 years: 13 mg/day

Male:

11-14 years: 17 mg/day

15-18 years: 20 mg/day

19-24 years: 19 mg/day

Female: 11-24 years: 15 mg/day

Hyperlipidemia: Initial: 100-250 mg/day (maximum dose: 10 mg/kg/day) in 3 divided doses with meals; increase weekly by 100 mg/day or increase every 2-3 weeks by 250 mg/day as tolerated; evaluate efficacy and adverse effects with laboratory tests at 20 mg/kg/day or 1000 mg/day (whichever is less); continue to increase if needed and as tolerated; re-evaluate at each 500 mg increment; doses up to

2250 mg/day have been used; **Note:** Routine use in children and adolescents is not recommended due to limited safety and efficacy information

Pellagra: 50-100 mg/dose 3 times/day

Adults:

Recommended daily allowances (RDA):

Male:

25-50 years: 19 mg/day

>51 years: 15 mg/day

Female:

25-50 years: 15 mg/day

>51 years: 13 mg/day

Hyperlipidemia:

Immediate release products: Initial: 50-100 mg twice daily for 1 week; increase slowly over 1 month (by doubling daily dose every week) to 1-1.5 g/day divided in 2-3 doses; assess therapy at 4 and 8 weeks of therapy; if needed, dose may be increased slowly to 3 g/day or until desired result is attained; maximum dose: 3 g/day in 3 divided doses; **Note:** Some patients may require a slower dose titration

Extended release products: Initial: 500 mg/day divided in 2 doses for 1 week; increase to 500 mg twice daily for 3 weeks; if needed, dose may be increased to 2 g/day or until desired result is attained; maximum dose: 2 g/day

Niaspan®: Initial: 500 mg daily at bedtime for 4 weeks; increase to 1 g daily at bedtime for 4 weeks; adjust dose to patient response and tolerance; may increase by 500 mg/day at 4-week intervals; maximum dose: 2 g/day; **Note:** Women may respond at lower doses than men.

Niacin deficiency: 10-20 mg/day, maximum dose: 100 mg/day

Pellagra: 50-100 mg 3-4 times/day, maximum dose: 500 mg/day

Dosage adjustment in renal impairment: Use with caution

Dosage adjustment in hepatic impairment: Contraindicated in patients with significant or unexplained hepatic dysfunction; use with caution in patients with history of liver disease or unexplained transaminase elevations

Administration Oral: Administer with food or milk to decrease GI upset; swallow timed release tablet and capsule whole; do not chew or crush; to minimize flushing, administer dose at bedtime, take aspirin (adults: 325 mg) 30 minutes before niacin, and avoid alcohol or hot drinks around the time of administration

Monitoring Parameters Blood glucose; serum uric acid, periodic liver function tests (with large doses or prolonged therapy); Treatment of hyperlipidemias: Baseline: Liver enzymes, uric acid, fasting glucose, and minimum of 2 fasting lipid profiles; repeat 4-6 weeks after dose is stabilized; once LDL-C goal is reached, repeat every 2-3 months for first year and then every 6-12 months if no sign of toxicity develops and dose remains stable

Reference Range Hypercholesterolemia: See table below; HDL-C <40 mg/dL

Classification of Blood Cholesterol, LDL-C, and Triglyceride Concentrations[1]

Classification	Cholesterol (mg/dL)		LDL-C (mg/dL)		Triglycerides (mg/dL)
	Children	Adults	Children	Adults	Adults
Acceptable/optimal	<170	<200	<110	<100	<150
Above optimal	†	†	†	100-129	†
Borderline high	170-199	200-239	110-129	130-159	150-199
High	≥200	≥240	≥130	160-189	200-499
Very high	†	†	†	≥190	≥500

[1]Adapted from American Academy of Pediatrics Committee on Nutrition, "Cholesterol in Childhood," *Pediatrics*, 1998, 101(1 Pt 1):141-7 and "Third Report of the National Cholesterol Education Program Expert Panel on Detection, Evaluation, and Treatment of High Blood Cholesterol in Adults (Adult Treatment Panel III)," May 2001, www.nhlbi.nih.gov/guidelines/cholesterol.

†Lack of specific type of classification in either pediatric or adult recommendations.

Test Interactions False elevations in some fluorometric determinations of urinary catecholamines; false-positive urine glucose (Benedict's reagent)

Patient Information Transient flushing of the skin and a sensation of warmth (especially of face and upper body), itching, tingling or headache may occur; if dizziness occurs, avoid sudden changes in posture and notify physician; notify physician if taking vitamins or other products that contain niacin or nicotinamide; do not change brands once dosage is stabilized; report signs and symptoms of hepatotoxicity (nausea, vomiting, loss of appetite, yellow skin, dark urine, general feeling of weakness) to physician

Additional Information Discontinue use if liver enzymes increase to ≥3 times the upper limit of normal

(Continued)

Niacin *(Continued)*

Dosage Forms Excipient information presented when available (limited, particularly for generics); consult specific product labeling.

Capsule, extended release: 125 mg, 250 mg, 400 mg, 500 mg
Capsule, timed release: 250 mg
Tablet: 50 mg, 100 mg, 250 mg, 500 mg
Niacor®: 500 mg
Tablet, controlled release (Slo-Niacin®): 250 mg, 500 mg, 750 mg
Tablet, extended release (Niaspan®): 500 mg, 750 mg, 1000 mg
Tablet, timed release: 250 mg, 500 mg, 750 mg, 1000 mg

References

American Academy of Pediatrics Committee on Nutrition, "Cholesterol in Childhood," *Pediatrics*, 1998, 101(1 Pt 1):141-7.
"ASHP Therapeutic Position Statement on the Safe Use of Niacin in the Management of Dyslipidemias. American Society of Health-System Pharmacists," *Am J Health Syst Pharm*, 1997, 54(24):2815-9.
Colletti RB, Neufeld EJ, Roff NK, et al, "Niacin Treatment of Hypercholesterolemia in Children." *Pediatrics*, 1993, 92(1):78-82.
Schuna AA, "Safe Use of Niacin," *Am J Health Syst Pharm*, 1997, 54(24):2803.
"Third Report of the National Cholesterol Education Program Expert Panel on Detection, Evaluation, and Treatment of High Blood Cholesterol in Adults (Adult Treatment Panel III)," May 2001, www.nhlbi.nih.gov/guidelines/cholesterol.

♦ **Niacor®** *see* Niacin *on page 1127*
♦ **Niaspan®** *see* Niacin *on page 1127*
♦ **Niastase® (Can)** *see* Factor VIIa (Recombinant) *on page 631*

NiCARdipine (nye KAR de peen)

Medication Safety Issues

Sound-alike/look-alike issues:
NiCARdipine may be confused with niacinamide, NIFEdipine, nimodipine
Cardene® may be confused with Cardizem®, Cardura®, codeine
International issues:
Cardene® may be confused with Cardem® which is a brand name for celiprolol in Spain
Cardene® may be confused with Cardin® which is a brand name for methyldopa in Brazil and a brand name for simvastatin in Poland

Significant differences exist between oral and I.V. dosing. Use caution when converting from one route of administration to another.

Related Information

Antihypertensive Agents by Class *on page 1678*

U.S. Brand Names Cardene®; Cardene® I.V.; Cardene® SR

Index Terms Nicardipine Hydrochloride

Therapeutic Category Antianginal Agent; Antihypertensive Agent; Calcium Channel Blocker

Generic Available Yes: Capsule

Use

Immediate release product: Treatment of chronic stable angina; hypertension
Sustained release product: Treatment of hypertension
Parenteral: Short-term treatment of hypertension when oral treatment is not possible

Pregnancy Risk Factor C

Lactation Enters breast milk/not recommended

Contraindications Hypersensitivity to nicardipine or any component; advanced aortic stenosis

Warnings Symptomatic hypotension may occur; monitor blood pressure carefully (see Monitoring Parameters); lowering of blood pressure should be done at a rate appropriate for the patient's condition; rapid drops in blood pressure may lead to arterial insufficiency; avoid systemic hypotension in patients following an acute cerebral infarct or hemorrhage.

Nicardipine may increase frequency, duration, or severity of angina with initiation of therapy or dosage increase (use with caution in patients with CAD). May cause negative inotropic effects in some patients (use with caution in patients with CHF or significant left ventricular dysfunction, especially when used in combination with beta-blockers).

Precautions Use with caution and carefully titrate the dose in patients with cardiac, renal, or hepatic dysfunction or reduced liver blood flow; decrease the starting dose for patients with severe hepatic dysfunction. Use I.V. formulation with caution in patients with pheochromocytoma (limited clinical experience) and portal hypertension (may cause increase hepatic venous pressure gradient). Peripheral infusion sites (for I.V. therapy) should be changed every 12 hours to minimize venous irritation. Abrupt withdrawal may cause rebound angina in patients with CAD. Use of immediate release product for treatment of hypertension may result in relatively large differences in peak and trough blood pressures (compared to sustained release product). Safety and efficacy have not been demonstrated in pediatric patients.

Adverse Reactions

Cardiovascular: Flushing, vasodilation, palpitation, tachycardia, peripheral edema (dose related), increased angina (dose related), hypotension (I.V.: 6%), orthostasis, syncope, abnormal EKG, facial edema, MI

Central nervous system: Headache, dizziness, somnolence, paresthesia, nervousness, insomnia, abnormal dreams; intracranial hemorrhage (I.V.: 0.7%)

Dermatologic: Rash

Endocrine & metabolic: Hypokalemia (I.V.: 0.7%)

Gastrointestinal: Nausea, vomiting, dyspepsia, xerostomia, constipation, diarrhea, abdominal pain; gingival hyperplasia (1 case report)

Genitourinary: Polyuria, nocturia; hematuria (I.V.: 0.7%)

Local: Injection site reaction (I.V. 1.4%); injection site pain (0.7%)

Neuromuscular & skeletal: Asthenia, myalgia, malaise, tremor, hypesthesia

Ocular: Blurred vision

Respiratory: Dyspnea

Miscellaneous: Diaphoresis

Drug Interactions Cytochrome P450 isoenzyme CYP1A2 (minor), CYP2C8/9 (minor), CYP2D6 (minor), CYP2E1 (minor), CYP3A4 (major) substrate; isoenzyme CYP2C8/9 (strong), CYP2C19 (moderate), CYP2D6 (moderate), CYP3A4 (strong) inhibitor

Concomitant antihypertensive agents or diuretics may increase the hypotensive effects of nicardipine; ethanol may increase CNS depression; anesthetic doses of fentanyl with concurrent use of a beta-blocker and calcium channel blocker may cause severe hypotension (administration of I.V. fluids may be required). Calcium may decrease or reverse the effects of calcium channel blockers, especially hypotension.

Nicardipine may increase cyclosporine serum concentrations (monitor cyclosporine levels; a decrease in cyclosporine dose may be needed); nicardipine may increase metoprolol serum concentrations by 25%; I.V. nicardipine may increase vecuronium serum concentrations or effects (dosage reduction of vecuronium is recommended); although nicardipine does not usually alter digoxin serum concentrations, digoxin levels should be monitored in patients after therapy with nicardipine is started.

Concurrent use with cimetidine or cytochrome P450 isoenzyme CYP3A4 inhibitors (eg, azole antifungals, clarithromycin, erythromycin, isoniazid, propofol, protease inhibitors, quinidine) may increase serum concentrations or effects of nicardipine (monitor closely; dosage adjustment may be needed). Cytochrome P450 isoenzyme CYP3A4 inducers [eg, carbamazepine, phenobarbital, phenytoin, rifampin, the herbal medicine St John's wort (*Hypericum perforatum*)] may decrease serum concentrations or effects of nicardipine.

Nicardipine may increase the serum concentration or effects of cytochrome P450 isoenzyme CYP2C8/9 substrates (eg, amiodarone, fluoxetine, phenytoin, sertraline, warfarin), CYP2C19 substrates (eg, citalopram, diazepam, phenytoin, propranolol, sertraline), CYP2D6 substrates (eg, amphetamines, selected beta-blockers, fluoxetine, lidocaine, paroxetine, risperidone, ritonavir, thioridazine, TCAs, venlafaxine), and CYP3A4 substrates (eg, benzodiazepines, other calcium channel blockers, tacrolimus, and venlafaxine). Selected benzodiazepines (midazolam and triazolam), cisapride, ergot alkaloids, selected HMG-CoA reductase inhibitors (lovastatin and simvastatin), and pimozide are generally contraindicated with strong CYP3A4 inhibitors.

Nicardipine may decrease serum concentrations or effects of CYP2D6 prodrug substrates (eg, codeine, hydrocodone, oxycodone, and tramadol).

Food Interactions A high-fat meal may decrease nicardipine peak concentrations and the extent of absorption; however, in the clinical trials that established safety and efficacy, the immediate and sustained release capsules were administered without regard to meals. Administration of sustained release capsule with a high-fat meal reduces fluctuations in serum concentrations.

Grapefruit juice may increase nicardipine serum concentrations (avoid concurrent use); avoid natural licorice (causes sodium and water retention and increases potassium loss)

Stability

Capsules (immediate and sustained-release): Store at 15°C to 30°C (59°F to 86°F); dispense in light-resistant container

Injection: Store at room temperature; protect from light (store ampuls in carton before use); avoid exposure to elevated temperatures; freezing does not affect stability; diluted solution (0.1 mg/mL) is stable for 24 hours at room temperature

(Continued)

NiCARdipine *(Continued)*

Compatible in D_5W, D_5W with KCl 40 mEq, D_5NS, D_5½NS, NS, ½NS for 24 hours when stored at controlled room temperature in glass or polyvinyl chloride containers; **not** compatible with sodium bicarbonate 5% or LR

Y-site administration: Compatible: Diltiazem, dobutamine, dopamine, epinephrine, fentanyl, gatifloxacin, hydromorphone, labetalol, linezolid, lorazepam, midazolam, milrinone, morphine, nitroglycerin, norepinephrine, ranitidine, vecuronium. **Incompatible:** Furosemide, heparin, thiopental

Mechanism of Action Inhibits calcium ions from entering the "slow channels" or select voltage-sensitive areas of vascular smooth muscle and myocardium during depolarization; produces a relaxation of coronary vascular smooth muscle and coronary vasodilation; increases myocardial oxygen delivery in patients with vasospastic angina

Pharmacodynamics Antihypertensive effects:

Onset of action:

I.V.: Within minutes

Oral: 0.5-2 hours

Maximum effect:

Immediate capsules: 1-2 hours

Sustained release capsules (at steady state): Sustained from 2-6 hours postdose

I.V. continuous infusion: 50% of the maximum effect is seen by 45 minutes; final effect of a continuously infused dose is seen by 50 hours

Duration:

Immediate release capsules: <8 hours

Sustained release capsules: 12 hours

I.V.: Single dose: 3 hours

I.V. continuous infusion: Upon discontinuation, a 50% decrease in effect is seen in ~30 minutes with gradual discontinuing antihypertensive effects for ~50 hours.

Pharmacokinetics Absorption: Oral: ~100%, but large first-pass effect

Distribution: V_d: Adults: 8.3 L/kg

Protein binding: >95%

Metabolism: Extensive, saturable, first-pass effect; dose-dependent (nonlinear) pharmacokinetics; extensive hepatic metabolism; major pathway is via cytochrome P450 isoenzyme CYP3A4

Bioavailability: Oral: 35%

Half-life: Follows dose-dependent (nonlinear) pharmacokinetics; "apparent" or calculated half-life is dependant upon serum concentrations. Half-life over the first 8 hours after oral dosing is 2-4 hours; terminal half-life (oral): 8.6 hours. After I.V. infusion, serum concentrations decrease tri-exponentially; alpha half-life: 2.7 minutes; beta half-life: 44.8 minutes; terminal half-life: 14.4 hours (**Note:** Terminal half-life can only be seen after long-term infusions)

Time to peak serum concentration: Oral:

Immediate release capsule: 30-120 minutes (mean: 1 hour)

Sustained release capsule: 1-4 hours

Elimination: 60% of an oral dose is excreted in the urine (<1% as unchanged drug); 35% excreted in feces.

Clearance: Decreased in patients with hepatic dysfunction; may be decreased in patients with renal impairment

Usual Dosage Note: Oral and I.V. doses are **not** equivalent on a mg per mg basis.

Neonates: **Note:** Very limited information exists

I.V. continuous infusion: One prospective open-label study of 20 hypertensive neonates (15 preterm; median PNA 15 days) used initial nicardipine doses of 0.5 mcg/kg/minute (n = 17). Doses were titrated according to blood pressure; the mean maximal required dose was 0.74 ± 0.41 mcg/kg/minute (range: 0.5-2 mcg/kg/minute) and occurred at 12 ± 19 hours of nicardipine infusion. The median duration of treatment was 11 days (range: 2-43 days) (see Milou, 2000). Similar doses were required in a smaller study of 8 preterm infants and in one case report of a neonate who received ECMO therapy (see Gouyon, 1997 and McBride, 2003). Further studies are needed.

Oral: No information is available.

Children: Note: Limited information exists; dose is not well established. Further studies are needed.

I.V. continuous infusion: Some experts recommend the following: Initial: 0.5-1 mcg/kg/minute; titrate dose according to blood pressure; rate of infusion may be increased every 15-30 minutes; maximum dose: 4-5 mcg/kg/minute (see Flynn, 2000 and Flynn, 2001; see also Additional Information).

Note: Other smaller studies support the use of an initial pediatric nicardipine dose of 1 mcg/kg/minute (see Nakagawa, 2004 and Treluyer, 1993). However, several studies used a higher initial dose of 5 mcg/kg/minute; once blood pressure was controlled, the dose was decreased to a lower maintenance dose. Mean maintenance doses have been reported to be 2.4 mcg/kg/minute (range: 1-5 mcg/kg/minute in 10 PICU patients) and 3 mcg/kg/minute (range: 2.1-5.5 mcg/kg/minute in 9 post-op cardiac surgery patients) (see Tobias, 2001).

Oral: One case report used 20 mg every 8 hours in a 14-year old boy following cardiac transplant (see Larsen, 1994). Another case used 30 mg every 8 hours in a 14-year old girl with renal disease (see Michael, 1998).

Adults:

Oral:

Immediate release: Initial: 20 mg 3 times/day; titrate to response; usual: 20-40 mg 3 times/day; allow at least 3 days between increases in dose

Sustained release: Initial: 30 mg twice daily; titrate to response; usual: 30-60 mg twice daily; **Note:** Usual dosage range (JNC 7): 30-60 mg twice daily.

Note: Use caution and re-examine blood pressure control when converting patients from the immediate release to the sustained release product; the total daily dose of immediate release product may not be equivalent to the daily sustained-release dose.

I.V. continuous infusion:

Hypertension in patients **not** receiving oral nicardipine: Initial: 5 mg/hour; titrate dose according to blood pressure; increase infusion by 2.5 mg/hour every 15 minutes to a maximum of 15 mg/hour; may increase infusion rate every 5 minutes if a more rapid blood pressure reduction is required; once desired blood pressure is achieved, decrease infusion rate to 3 mg/hour. Monitor and titrate to lowest dose necessary to maintain stable blood pressure.

Substitution for oral nicardipine therapy (approximate equivalents):

Oral dose of 20 mg every 8 hours = 0.5 mg/hour I.V. infusion

Oral dose of 30 mg every 8 hours = 1.2 mg/hour I.V. infusion

Oral dose of 40 mg every 8 hours = 2.2 mg/hour I.V. infusion

Dosing adjustment in renal impairment: Specific guidelines are not available; careful monitoring and dosage adjustment is warranted. Adult: Oral: Titrate dose carefully beginning with usual initial dose.

Dosing adjustment in hepatic impairment: Specific guidelines are not available; use with caution in patients with severe hepatic impairment; careful monitoring and dosage adjustment is warranted. Adult: Oral: Initial:

Immediate release: Titrate dose carefully beginning with 20 mg twice daily

Sustained release: Has not been studied

Administration

Oral: May be administered without regard to meals; avoid concurrent administration with high-fat meals or grapefruit juice. Swallow sustained release capsule whole; do not crush, break, or chew.

I.V.: Administer by slow I.V. continuous infusion; I.V. product must be diluted prior to administration; may dilute with D_5W, D_5W with KCl 40 mEq, D_5NS, $D_5\frac{1}{2}NS$, NS, ½NS; manufacturer recommended concentration for infusion: 0.1 mg/mL; **Note:** One pediatric study used infusions of 0.5 mg/mL in D_5W, NS, or other compatible solution (see Flynn, 2001). Avoid extravasation.

Monitoring Parameters Blood pressure, heart rate, liver and renal function; **Note:** Monitor blood pressure carefully during initiation of therapy and with dosage adjustments.

Immediate release product: Measure blood pressure at peak effects (1-2 hours after the dose) especially during initiation of therapy, and just prior to the next dose (to ensure control of blood pressure throughout dosing interval).

Sustained release product: Measure blood pressure 2-4 hours after the first dose or dosage increase and just prior to the next dose

I.V.: Monitor infusion site for extravasation; monitor blood pressure continuously during I.V. administration

Patient Information May cause dizziness or drowsiness and impair ability to perform activities requiring mental alertness or physical coordination; may cause dry mouth. May cause low blood pressure upon standing; rise slowly from prolonged sitting or lying position. Avoid alcohol and grapefruit juice.

Do not discontinue abruptly; report any dizziness, shortness of breath, palpitations, chest pain, rapid heart beat, swelling of extremities, muscle weakness or pain, or nervousness. Some medicines may interact with nicardipine; report the use of other medications, nonprescription medications, and herbal or natural products to your physician and pharmacist; avoid the herbal medicine St John's wort.

Nursing Implications Do not crush or break sustained release capsules.

I.V.: Avoid extravasation; closely monitor I.V. site for swelling, redness, burning, or pain; change peripheral infusion sites every 12 hours

Assess therapeutic effectiveness, and adverse reactions on a regular basis during therapy. Monitor blood pressure (see Monitoring Parameters). Instruct patient on

(Continued)

NiCARdipine *(Continued)*

appropriate use, side effects, appropriate interventions, and adverse symptoms to report.

Additional Information A retrospective study in 29 hypertensive children (mean age: 7.8 years; range: 2 days to 18 years) used initial nicardipine doses of 0.5-1 mcg/kg/minute; doses were titrated according to blood pressure and the rate of infusion was increased every 15"30 minutes; the mean effective dose was 1.8 ± 0.3 mcg/kg/minute (range: 0.3-4 mcg/kg/minute); blood pressure was controlled within 2.7 ± 2.1 hours (range: 0.5"9 hours) after starting nicardipine continuous infusion (see Flynn, 2001). Nicardipine has also been used in children for controlled hypotension to limit intraoperative blood loss (see Tobias, 2002).

The sustained release capsule contains a powder component (containing 25% of the dose) and a spherical granule component (containing 75% of the dose). The I.V. product is buffered to a pH of 3.5.

Dosage Forms Excipient information presented when available (limited, particularly for generics); consult specific product labeling.

Capsule (Cardene®): 20 mg, 30 mg

Capsule, sustained release (Cardene® SR): 30 mg, 45 mg, 60 mg

Injection, solution (Cardene® IV): 2.5 mg/mL (10 mL)

References

Chobanian AV, Bakris GL, Black HR, et al, "The Seventh Report of the Joint National Committee on Prevention, Detection, Evaluation, and Treatment of High Blood Pressure: The JNC 7 Report," *JAMA*, 2003, 289(19):2560-72.

Flynn JT and Pasko DA, "Calcium Channel Blockers: Pharmacology and Place in Therapy of Pediatric Hypertension," *Pediatr Nephrol*, 2000, 15(3-4):302-16.

Flynn JT, Mottes TA, Brophy PD, et al, "Intravenous Nicardipine for Treatment of Severe Hypertension in Children," *J Pediatr*, 2001, 139(1):38-43.

Gouyon JB, Geneste B, Semama DS, et al, "Intravenous Nicardipine in Hypertensive Preterm Infants," *Arch Dis Child Fetal Neonatal Ed*, 1997, 76(2):F126-7.

Larsen A and Tobias J, "Nicardipine for the Treatment of Hypertension Following Cardiac Transplantation in a 14-Year-Old Boy," *Clin Pediatr (Phila)*, 1994, 33(5):309-11.

McBride BF, White CM, Campbell M, et al, "Nicardipine to Control Neonatal Hypertension During Extracorporeal Membrane Oxygen Support," *Ann Pharmacother*, 2003, 37(5):667-70.

Michael J, Groshong T, and Tobias JD, "Nicardipine for Hypertensive Emergencies in Children With Renal Disease," *Pediatr Nephrol*, 1998, 12(1):40-2.

Milou C, Debuche-Benouachkou V, Semama DS, et al, "Intravenous Nicardipine as a First-Line Antihypertensive Drug in Neonates," *Intensive Care Med*, 2000, 26(7):956-8.

Nakagawa TA, Sartori SC, Morris A, et al, "Intravenous Nicardipine for Treatment of Postcoarctectomy Hypertension in Children," *Pediatr Cardiol*, 2004, 25(1):26-30.

Steele RM, Schuna AA, and Schreiber RT, "Calcium Antagonist-Induced Gingival Hyperplasia," *Ann Intern Med*, 1994, 120(8):663-4.

Tobias JD, "Nicardipine to Control Mean Arterial Pressure After Cardiothoracic Surgery in Infants and Children," *Am J Ther*, 2001, 8(1):3-6.

Treluyer JM, Hubert P, Jouvet P, et al, "Intravenous Nicardipine in Hypertensive Children," *Eur J Pediatr*, 1993, 152(9):712-4.

♦ **Nicardipine Hydrochloride** *see* NiCARdipine *on page 1130*
♦ **Nicotinic Acid** *see* Niacin *on page 1127*
♦ **Nidagel™ (Can)** *see* Metronidazole *on page 1049*
♦ **Nifediac™ CC** *see* NIFEdipine *on page 1134*
♦ **Nifedical™ XL** *see* NIFEdipine *on page 1134*

NIFEdipine (nye FED i peen)

Medication Safety Issues

Sound-alike/look-alike issues:

NIFEdipine may be confused with niCARdipine, nimodipine, nisoldipine

Procardia XL® may be confused with Cartia® XT

International issues:

Nipin® [Italy and Singapore] may be confused with Nipent® which is a brand name for pentostatin in the U.S.

Related Information

Antihypertensive Agents by Class *on page 1678*

Medications for Which A Single Dose May Be Fatal When Ingested By A Toddler *on page 1932*

U.S. Brand Names Adalat® CC; Afeditab™ CR; Nifediac™ CC; Nifedical™ XL; Procardia®; Procardia XL®

Canadian Brand Names Adalat® XL®; Apo-Nifed®; Apo-Nifed PA®; Novo-Nifedin; Nu-Nifed; Procardia®

Therapeutic Category Antianginal Agent; Antihypertensive Agent; Calcium Channel Blocker

Generic Available Yes

Use Treatment of angina, hypertrophic cardiomyopathy; hypertension (extended release only)

Pregnancy Risk Factor C

Lactation Enters breast milk/compatible

Contraindications Hypersensitivity to nifedipine or any component (see Warnings); recent MI

Warnings Excessive hypotension may occur, especially during initiation of therapy or dosage increase (more common with concurrent beta-blocker therapy; monitor blood pressure closely); profound hypotension, MI, and death have been reported in adults when immediate release nifedipine has been used (orally or sublingually) for acute reduction of blood pressure (manufacturer does **not** recommended use of capsules for acute reduction of blood pressure); immediate release nifedipine is not FDA approved for long-term control of essential hypertension (appropriate studies to determine optimal dose or dosing interval have not been conducted); 90 mg tablet may contain tartrazine which may cause allergic reactions in susceptible individuals (see Dosage Forms)

Precautions May increase frequency, duration, and severity of angina or precipitate acute MI during initiation of therapy; use with caution in patients with CHF or aortic stenosis (especially with concomitant beta-blocker)

Adverse Reactions

Cardiovascular: Flushing, hypotension, tachycardia, palpitations, syncope, peripheral edema

Central nervous system: Dizziness, fever, headache, chills

Dermatologic: Dermatitis, urticaria, purpura; photosensitivity (rare)

Gastrointestinal: Nausea, diarrhea, constipation, gingival hyperplasia

Hematologic: Thrombocytopenia, leukopenia, anemia

Hepatic: Elevated liver enzymes, cholestasis, jaundice; allergic hepatitis (rare)

Neuromuscular & skeletal: Joint stiffness, arthritis with elevated ANA

Ocular: Blurred vision, transient blindness

Respiratory: Shortness of breath

Miscellaneous: Diaphoresis

Drug Interactions Cytochrome P450 isoenzyme CYP3A3/4 and CYP3A5-7 substrate; isoenzyme CYP3A4 inhibitor

Beta-blockers may increase cardiovascular adverse effects; anesthetic doses of fentanyl may cause hypotension; severe hypotension may occur in patients taking immediate release nifedipine concurrently with beta blockers when undergoing CABG with high dose fentanyl (consider tapering off nifedipine >36 hours before surgery with high dose fentanyl in patients receiving nifedipine); enzyme inhibitors (cimetidine, quinidine, verapamil, diltiazem, erythromycin, azole antifungals, protease inhibitors, nefazodone, valproic acid, quinupristin/dalfopristin) and cyclosporine may significantly increase nifedipine serum concentrations; enzyme inducers [phenobarbital, phenytoin, rifampin, carbamazepine and the herbal medicine St John's wort (*Hypericum perforatum*)] may significantly decrease nifedipine serum concentrations; nifedipine may increase phenytoin, cyclosporine, tacrolimus, vincristine, and possibly digoxin serum concentrations; nifedipine may decrease quinidine serum concentrations; combined use of nifedipine with cyclosporine may significantly increase gingival hyperplasia; alpha 1-blockers, magnesium salts may enhance the effects of nifedipine; calcium may decrease the effect of nifedipine; nifedipine may enhance the effect of neuromuscular-blocking agents (nondepolarizing)

Food Interactions Capsule is rapidly absorbed orally if it is administered without food but may result in vasodilator side effects; administration with low-fat meals may decrease flushing; grapefruit juice may significantly increase the oral bioavailability of nifedipine (avoid concurrent use); food may decrease the rate but not the extent of absorption of Procardia XL®; a high fat meal does not effect the extent of absorption of Adalat® CC, but delays the time to peak and increases the peak concentration

Stability Store at room temperature; protect from light and moisture

Mechanism of Action Inhibits calcium ions from entering the "slow channels" or select voltage-sensitive areas of vascular smooth muscle and myocardium during depolarization; produces a relaxation of coronary vascular smooth muscle and coronary vasodilation; increases myocardial oxygen delivery in patients with vasospastic angina

Pharmacodynamics

Onset of action:

- S.L. or "bite and swallow": Within 1-5 minutes
- Oral:
  - Immediate release: Within 20-30 minutes
  - Extended release: 2-2.5 hours

Duration:

- Immediate release: 4-8 hours
- Extended release: 24 hours

(Continued)

NIFEdipine *(Continued)*

Pharmacokinetics

Protein-binding: 92% to 98% (concentration-dependent); **Note:** Protein-binding may be significantly decreased in patients with renal or hepatic impairment

Metabolism: In the liver to inactive metabolites

Bioavailability:

Capsules: 45% to 75%

Extended release: 65% to 89% relative to immediate release capsules

Half-life:

Normal adults: 2-5 hours

Cirrhosis: 7 hours

Elimination: In the urine with >90% of the dose excreted as inactive metabolites

Usual Dosage Oral, S.L. or "bite and swallow" (eg, patient bites capsule to release liquid contents and then swallows) (see Warnings):

Note: Doses are usually titrated upward over 7 to 14 days; may increase over 3 days if clinically necessary:

Children:

Hypertensive emergencies: 0.25-0.5 mg/kg/dose; maximum dose: 10 mg/dose; may repeat if needed every 4-6 hours; monitor carefully; maximum dose: 1-2 mg/kg/day

Hypertrophic cardiomyopathy: 0.6-0.9 mg/kg/24 hours in 3-4 divided doses

Hypertension (chronic treatment): Limited information is available; some centers use the following:

Extended release: Initial: 0.25-0.5 mg/kg/day given once daily or divided in 2 doses per day; titrate dose to effect; maximum dose: 3 mg/kg/day up to 180 mg/day (see Flynn, 2000)

Adolescents and Adults:

Capsules: Initial: 10 mg 3 times/day; maintenance: 10-30 mg 3-4 times/day; maximum dose: 180 mg/24 hours

Extended release tablet: Initial: 30 mg once daily; usual dosage range for hypertension (JNC 7): Adolescents ≥18 years and Adults: 30-60 mg once daily; maximum dose: 120 mg/day

Administration Oral: Administer with food; Adalat® CC: Administer on an empty stomach; do not administer nifedipine with grapefruit juice; swallow sustained release tablets whole, do not crush, break, or chew; liquid-filled capsule may be punctured and drug solution administered sublingually or orally; when measuring smaller doses from the liquid-filled capsules, consider the following concentrations (for Procardia®) 10 mg capsule = 10 mg/0.34 mL; 20 mg capsule = 20 mg/0.45 mL

Note: When nifedipine is administered sublingually, only a small amount is absorbed sublingually; the observed effects are actually due to swallowing of the drug with subsequent rapid oral absorption

Monitoring Parameters Blood pressure, CBC, platelets, periodic liver enzymes

Patient Information Avoid alcohol and grapefruit juice; rise slowly from prolonged sitting or lying position; insoluble shell of extended release tablet may appear in the stool (this is normal). May rarely cause photosensitivity reactions; avoid exposure to sunlight and artificial light sources (sunlamps, tanning booth/bed); use a sunscreen; contact physician if reaction occurs

Dosage Forms Excipient information presented when available (limited, particularly for generics); consult specific product labeling.

Capsule, softgel: 10 mg, 20 mg

Procardia®: 10 mg

Tablet, extended release: 30 mg, 60 mg, 90 mg

Adalat® CC, Procardia XL®: 30 mg, 60 mg, 90 mg

Afeditab™ CR, Nifedical™ XL: 30 mg, 60 mg

Nifediac™ CC: 30 mg, 60 mg, 90 mg [90 mg tablet contains tartrazine]

References

Adcock KG and Wilson JT, "Nifedipine Labeling Illustrates the Pediatric Dilemma for Off-Patent Drugs," *Pediatrics*, 2002, 109(2):319-21.

Chobanian AV, Bakris GL, Black HR, et al, "The Seventh Report of the Joint National Committee on Prevention, Detection, Evaluation, and Treatment of High Blood Pressure: The JNC 7 report," *JAMA*, 2003, 289(19):2560-72.

Dilmen U, Cagfülar MK, Senses A, et al, "Nifedipine in Hypertensive Emergencies of Children," *Am J Dis Child*, 1983, 137(12):1162-5.

Flynn JT and Pasko DA, "Calcium Channel Blockers: Pharmacology and Place in Therapy of Pediatric Hypertension," *Pediatr Nephrol*, 2000, 15(3-4):302-16.

Lopez-Herce J, Albajara L, Cagigas P, et al, "Treatment of Hypertensive Crisis in Children With Nifedipine," *Intensive Care Med*, 1988, 14(5):519-21.

Rosen WJ and Johnson CE, "Evaluation of Five Procedures for Measuring Nonstandard Doses of Nifedipine Liquid," *Am J Hosp Pharm*, 1989, 46(11):2313-7.

♦ **Niferex® [OTC]** *see* Iron Supplements (Oral/Enteral) *on page 868*

♦ **Niferex® 150 [OTC]** *see* Iron Supplements (Oral/Enteral) *on page 868*

- **Nilstat (Can)** *see* Nystatin *on page 1156*
- **Nimbex®** *see* Cisatracurium *on page 364*
- **Niravam™** *see* Alprazolam *on page 79*
- **Nitalapram** *see* Citalopram *on page 368*

Nitazoxanide (nye ta ZOX a nide)

U.S. Brand Names Alinia®

Index Terms NTZ

Therapeutic Category Antiprotozoal

Generic Available No

Use Treatment of diarrhea caused by *Cryptosporidium parvum* or *Giardia lamblia* in immunocompetent patients; manufacturer is pursuing approval for treatment of *Cryptosporidium*-induced diarrhea in HIV-infected patients and patients with immunodeficiency; treatment of intestinal amebiasis; treatment of refractory or recurrent *Clostridium difficile*-associated diarrhea

Pregnancy Risk Factor B

Lactation Excretion in breast milk unknown/use caution

Contraindications Hypersensitivity to nitazoxanide or any component

Warnings Suspension contains sodium benzoate; benzoic acid (benzoate) is a metabolite of benzyl alcohol; large amounts of benzyl alcohol (≥99 mg/kg/day) have been associated with a potentially fatal toxicity ("gasping syndrome") in neonates; avoid use of sodium benzoate containing products in neonates; *in vitro* and animal studies have shown that benzoate displaces bilirubin from protein binding sites

Precautions Use with caution in patients with renal, hepatic, or biliary disease since pharmacokinetics of nitazoxanide have not been studied in these patients. Use suspension dosage form with caution in diabetic patients due to sucrose content.

Adverse Reactions

Cardiovascular: Tachycardia, syncope, hypertension

Central nervous system: Headache (1.1%), fever, malaise, dizziness, chills, somnolence, insomnia

Dermatologic: Pruritus, rash

Endocrine and metabolic: Amenorrhea

Gastrointestinal: Abdominal pain (7.8%), diarrhea (2.1%), vomiting (1.1%), nausea, anorexia, flatulence, constipation

Genitourinary: Discoloration of urine (bright yellow), dysuria

Hepatic: Elevated ALT

Neuromuscular and skeletal: Myalgia, leg cramps

Ophthalmologic: Discoloration of eye (yellow sclerae)

Renal: Elevated serum creatinine

Miscellaneous: Diaphoresis

Drug Interactions Concurrent use with other highly plasma protein-bound drugs may affect protein binding or serum concentration of other drug

Food Interactions

Suspension: Administration with food increases AUC two-fold and peak concentrations by 50%

Tablet: Administration with food increases AUC by 45% to 50% and peak concentrations by ≤10%

Stability Store tablets and powder for oral suspension at room temperature. Reconstituted oral suspension is stable for 7 days at room temperature.

Mechanism of Action Appears to interfere with the pyruvate:ferredoxin oxidoreductase (PFOR) enzyme-dependent electron transfer reaction which is essential for anaerobic energy metabolism

Pharmacokinetics

Protein binding: Tizoxanide: >99%

Metabolism: Hydrolyzed in plasma to tizoxanide (active); conjugated to tizoxanide glucuronide in the liver

Bioavailability: Relative bioavailability of the suspension to the tablet is 70%

Half-life: Tizoxanide: 1-1.6 hours

Time to peak serum concentration: Tizoxanide: 1-4 hours

Elimination: Tizoxanide is excreted in urine (<10%), bile, and feces (60%); tizoxanide glucuronide is excreted in urine and bile

Usual Dosage Oral:

Diarrhea caused by *Cryptosporidium parvum* or *Giardia lamblia*:

Children 12-47 months: 100 mg every 12 hours for 3 days

Children 4-11 years: 200 mg every 12 hours for 3 days

Children ≥12 years, Adolescents, and Adults: 500 mg every 12 hours for 3 days

C. difficile-associated diarrhea: Adults: 500 mg every 12 hours for 7-10 days

(Continued)

Nitazoxanide *(Continued)*

Dosage adjustment in renal and/or hepatic impairment: Specific recommendations are not available; use with caution

Administration Minimize gastric irritation by administering with food; shake suspension well prior to use

Monitoring Parameters Periodic liver function tests, stool frequency

Patient Information May discolor eyes or urine to a yellow tint

Additional Information The oral suspension contains sucrose 1.48 g/5 mL.

A randomized, placebo-controlled study of 89 adults and adolescents receiving a 3-day course of nitazoxanide 500 mg twice daily for 3 days to treat enteric protozoa found a cure rate of 81% versus a cure rate of 40% for placebo (Rossignol, 2001).

Dosage Forms Excipient information presented when available (limited, particularly for generics); consult specific product labeling.

Powder for oral suspension: 100 mg/5 mL (60 mL) [contains sucrose 1.48 g/5 mL, sodium benzoate; strawberry flavor]

Tablet: 500 mg

Alinia® 3-Day Therapy Packs™ [unit-dose pack]: 500 mg (6s)

References

Bobak DA, "Use of Nitazoxanide for Gastrointestinal Tract Infections: Treatment of Protozoan Parasitic Infection and Beyond," *Curr Infect Dis Rep*, 2006, 8(2):91-5.

Rossignol JF, Ayoub A, and Ayers MS, "Treatment of Diarrhea Caused by *Giardia intestinalis* and *Entamoeba histolytica* or *E. dispar*: A Randomized, Double-Blind, Placebo-Controlled Study of Nitazoxanide," *J Infect Dis*, 2001, 184(3):381-4.

Nitisinone (ni TIS i known)

U.S. Brand Names Orfadin®

Therapeutic Category Tyrosinemia Type 1, Treatment Agent

Generic Available No

Use Adjunct to dietary restriction of tyrosine and phenylalanine in the treatment of hereditary tyrosinemia type 1 (HT-1)

Pregnancy Risk Factor C

Lactation Excretion in breast milk unknown/use caution

Contraindications Hypersensitivity to nitisinone or any component

Warnings Nitisinone therapy should be initiated by individuals experienced in the treatment of HT-1. Dietary restriction of tyrosine and phenylalanine must be used in conjunction with nitisinone; inadequate dietary restriction can result in elevations in plasma tyrosine leading to toxic ophthalmic effects (corneal ulcers, corneal opacities, keratitis, conjunctivitis, eye pain, and photophobia), skin effects (painful hyperkeratotic plaques on the soles and palms), and variable degrees of mental retardation and developmental delay. Nitisinone dosage should not be adjusted in order to lower the plasma tyrosine level. Transient thrombocytopenia has been reported; platelet and WBC counts should be monitored regularly during nitisinone therapy.

Precautions Slit-lamp examination of the eyes should be done prior to initiation of nitisinone therapy; patients who develop photophobia, eye pain or signs of inflammation such as redness, swelling, or burning of the eyes during treatment should be re-examined and a plasma tyrosine level measured; if the plasma tyrosine level is >500 micromoles/L a more restrictive diet is indicated. Patients with HT-1 are at risk for developing porphyric crises, liver failure, or hepatic neoplasm; regular liver monitoring by imaging (ultrasound, CT scan, MRI), liver function tests, and measurement of serum alpha-fetoprotein concentration is recommended; an increase in serum alpha-fetoprotein or signs of nodules in the liver during treatment may be a sign of inadequate therapy or hepatic malignancy.

Adverse Reactions Many adverse reactions noted in clinical trials are consistent with symptomatology of HT-1

Cardiovascular: Cyanosis

Central nervous system: Headache, seizures, encephalopathy, brain tumor, nervousness, somnolence

Endocrine & metabolic: Dehydration, hypoglycemia, amenorrhea

Dermatologic: Pruritus, exfoliative dermatitis, dry skin, maculopapular rash, alopecia

Gastrointestinal: Abdominal pain, diarrhea, gastritis, gastroenteritis, GI hemorrhage, melena, tooth discoloration

Hematologic: Thrombocytopenia, leukopenia, porphyria

Hepatic: Liver failure, hepatic neoplasm, hepatomegaly, elevated liver enzymes

Ocular: Conjunctivitis, corneal opacity, keratitis, photophobia, blepharitis, eye pain, cataracts

Respiratory: Bronchitis, respiratory insufficiency, epistaxis

Miscellaneous: Infection, septicemia

Drug Interactions None as yet have been identified

Stability Store in refrigerator 2°C to 8°C (36°F to 46°F)

Mechanism of Action Nitisinone is a competitive inhibitor of 4-hydroxyphenyl-pyruvate dioxygenase, an enzyme of the tyrosine metabolic pathway. Hereditary tyrosinemia type 1 occurs due to a deficiency in fumarylacetoacetase (FAH) the final enzyme in the tyrosine metabolic pathway. This deficiency results in an accumulation of maleylacetoacetate and fumarylacetoacetate. These catabolic intermediates are converted to the toxic metabolites succinylacetone and succinylacetoacetate which are responsible for progressive liver failure, increased risk of hepatocellular carcinoma, coagulopathy, painful neurologic crises, and renal tubular dysfunction with rickets. Nitisinone prevents the formation of these toxic metabolites.

Pharmacokinetics

Half-life: Adults: 54 hours

Time to peak serum concentration: 3 hours

Usual Dosage Oral: Infants, Children, and Adults: 1 mg/kg/day twice daily; may increase after 1 month of treatment to 1.5 mg/kg/day if needed; not to exceed 2 mg/kg/day

Administration Oral: Administer on an empty stomach, at least one hour before a meal. Capsules may be opened and mixed with a small amount of water, formula, or applesauce immediately before use.

Monitoring Parameters Urine succinylacetone level, alpha-fetoprotein, plasma tyrosine level, liver function, CBC, platelets, ophthalmic exams (see Warnings and Precautions)

Reference Range Plasma tyrosine level <500 micromoles/L

Patient Information Advise patients and caregivers of the need to maintain a diet low in tyrosine and phenylalanine; report eye symptoms (see Precautions), rash, jaundice, or excessive bleeding to a physician promptly

Dosage Forms Excipient information presented when available (limited, particularly for generics); consult specific product labeling.

Capsule: 2 mg, 5 mg, 10 mg

References

Holme E and Lindstedt S, "Diagnosis and Management of Tyrosinemia Type I," *Curr Opin Pediatr*, 1995, 7(6):726-32.

- ♦ **Nitrek® [DSC]** *see* Nitroglycerin *on page 1141*
- ♦ **Nitro-Bid®** *see* Nitroglycerin *on page 1141*
- ♦ **Nitro-Dur®** *see* Nitroglycerin *on page 1141*

Nitrofurantoin (nye troe fyoor AN toyn)

Medication Safety Issues

International issues:

Macrobid® may be confused with Mikrozid® which is a brand name for ethanol/propanol combination in Great Britain

U.S. Brand Names Furadantin®; Macrobid®; Macrodantin®

Canadian Brand Names Apo-Nitrofurantoin®; Macrobid®; Macrodantin®; Novo-Furantoin

Therapeutic Category Antibiotic, Miscellaneous

Generic Available Yes: Excludes suspension

Use Prevention and treatment of urinary tract infections caused by susceptible gram-negative and some gram-positive organisms including *E. coli*, *Klebsiella*, *Enterobacter*, enterococci, and *S. aureus*; *Pseudomonas*, *Serratia*, and most species of *Proteus* are generally resistant to nitrofurantoin

Pregnancy Risk Factor B; contraindicated in pregnant women at term and during labor (due to possible hemolytic anemia in the neonate)

Lactation Enters breast milk/not recommended (infants <1 month); AAP rates "compatible"

Contraindications Hypersensitivity to nitrofurantoin or any component; anuria, oliguria, or significant renal impairment (Cl_{cr} <60 mL/minute); infants <1 month of age (due to the possibility of hemolytic anemia); pregnant patients at term; during labor and delivery; should not be used to treat UTI in febrile infants and young children in whom renal involvement is likely

Warnings Therapeutic concentrations of nitrofurantoin are not attained in the urine of patients with renal insufficiency (Cl_{cr} <60 mL/minute, anuria, or oliguria). Acute, subacute, or chronic (usually after 6 months of therapy) pulmonary reactions, including fatalities have been reported; monitor for dyspnea, cough, fever, malaise, radiologic evidence of diffuse interstitial pneumonitis or fibrosis; if these reactions occur, discontinue nitrofurantoin immediately. Hepatitis, cholestatic jaundice, chronic active hepatitis (onset may be insidious) and hepatic necrosis resulting in death may occur; monitor patients for changes in liver function; if hepatitis occurs, discontinue nitrofurantoin immediately. Peripheral neuropathy may occur; risk is increased by renal

(Continued)

Nitrofurantoin *(Continued)*

impairment, anemia, diabetes mellitus, electrolyte imbalance, vitamin B deficiency, and debilitating disease. Optic neuritis has been reported.

Precautions Use with caution in patients with G-6-PD deficiency, patients with anemia, vitamin B deficiency, diabetes mellitus, or electrolyte abnormalities

Adverse Reactions

Cardiovascular: Chest pain, cyanosis, EKG changes (associated with pulmonary toxicity)

Central nervous system: Dizziness, headache, chills, fever, vertigo, drowsiness, malaise, pseudotumor cerebri, confusion, depression, psychotic reactions

Dermatologic: Rash, exfoliative dermatitis, urticaria, pruritus, alopecia, Stevens-Johnson syndrome, angioedema, erythema multiforme

Gastrointestinal: Nausea, vomiting, anorexia, pancreatitis, pseudomembranous colitis (rare), diarrhea, abdominal pain, flatulence, dyspepsia, constipation

Genitourinary: Discoloration of urine (dark yellow or brown), crystalluria

Hematologic: Hemolytic anemia, eosinophilia, leukopenia, granulocytopenia, thrombocytopenia, megaloblastic anemia, methemoglobinemia

Hepatic: Hepatotoxicity, cholestatic jaundice, hepatitis; elevated AST, ALT, and alkaline phosphatase

Neuromuscular & skeletal: Arthralgia, peripheral neuropathy, muscle weakness, asthenia, paresthesia, myalgia

Ocular: Optic neuritis (rare), amblyopia, nystagmus

Respiratory: Interstitial pneumonitis and/or fibrosis, dyspnea, cough

Miscellaneous: Hypersensitivity reactions, lupus-like syndrome, anaphylaxis

Drug Interactions Probenecid decreases renal excretion of nitrofurantoin; antacids decrease extent and rate of absorption of nitrofurantoin (avoid taking antacids containing magnesium trisilicate); drugs which delay gastric emptying increase the extent of nitrofurantoin absorption; quinolones (nitrofurantoin may antagonize antibacterial activity of quinolones)

Food Interactions Food increases the total amount absorbed; cranberry juice and other urinary acidifiers may enhance the action of nitrofurantoin; ensure diet is adequate in protein and vitamin B complex

Stability Protect from light; store at room temperature

Mechanism of Action Inhibits several bacterial enzyme systems including acetyl coenzyme A; reduced by bacterial enzymes to active intermediates that may alter ribosomal proteins resulting in inhibition of protein, DNA, RNA, and cell wall synthesis

Pharmacokinetics

Absorption: Well absorbed from the GI tract; macrocrystalline form is absorbed more slowly due to slower dissolution, but causes less GI distress than formulations containing microcrystals of the drug

Distribution: V_d: 0.8 L/kg; crosses the placenta; appears in breast milk and bile

Protein binding: ~40% to 60%

Metabolism: Partially in the liver

Bioavailability: Presence of food increases bioavailability

Half-life: 20-60 minutes and is prolonged with renal impairment

Elimination: As metabolites and unchanged drug (40%) in the urine and small amounts in the bile; renal excretion is via glomerular filtration and tubular secretion

Usual Dosage Oral:

Infants >1 month and Children: 5-7 mg/kg/day divided every 6 hours; maximum dose: 400 mg/day

Prophylaxis of UTI: 1-2 mg/kg/day as a single daily dose; maximum dose: 100 mg/day

Adults: 50-100 mg/dose every 6 hours; macrocrystal/monohydrate: 100 mg twice daily for 7 days

Prophylaxis of UTI: 50-100 mg/dose at bedtime

Dosing adjustment in renal impairment: Cl_{cr} <60 mL/minute: Avoid use

Administration Oral: Administer with food or milk; suspension may be mixed with water, milk, fruit juice, or infant formula. Shake suspension well before use.

Monitoring Parameters Signs of pulmonary reaction; signs of numbness or tingling of the extremities; periodic liver and renal function tests; CBC; urine culture and *in vitro* susceptibility tests

Test Interactions Causes false-positive urine glucose with Clinitest®

Patient Information May discolor urine to a dark yellow or brown color; avoid alcohol

Dosage Forms Excipient information presented when available (limited, particularly for generics); consult specific product labeling.

Capsule [macrocrystal]: 50 mg, 100 mg

Macrodantin®: 25 mg, 50 mg, 100 mg

Capsule [macrocrystal/monohydrate]: 100 mg [nitrofurantoin macrocrystal 25% and nitrofurantoin monohydrate 75%]

Macrobid®: 100 mg [nitrofurantoin macrocrystal 25% and nitrofurantoin monohydrate 75%]

Suspension, oral:

Furadantin®: 25 mg/5 mL (470 mL)

References

Brendstrup L, Hjelt K, Petersen KE, et al, "Nitrofurantoin Versus Trimethoprim Prophylaxis in Recurrent Urinary Tract Infections in Children," *Acta Paediatr Scand*, 1990. 79(12):1225-34.

Coraggio MJ, Gross TP, and Roscelli JD, "Nitrofurantoin Toxicity in Children," *Pediatr Infect Dis J*, 1989, 8(3):163-6.

"Practice Parameter: The Diagnosis, Treatment, and Evaluation of the Initial Urinary Tract Infection in Febrile Infants and Young Children. American Academy of Pediatrics. Committee on Quality Improvement. Subcommittee on Urinary Tract Infection," *Pediatrics*, 1999, 103(4 Pt 1):843-52.

♦ **Nitrogen Mustard** *see* Mechlorethamine *on page 987*

Nitroglycerin (nye troe GLI ser in)

Medication Safety Issues

Sound-alike/look-alike issues:

Nitroglycerin may be confused with nitroprusside
Nitro-Bid® may be confused with Nicobid®
Nitroderm may be confused with NicoDerm®
Nitrol® may be confused with Nizoral®
Nitrostat® may be confused with Hyperstat®, Nilstat®, nystatin

Nitroglycerin transdermal patches should be removed prior to defibrillation or MRI study.

International issues:

Nitrocor® [Chile and Italy] may be confused with Natrecor® which is a brand name for nesiritide in the U.S.

Nitrocor® [Chile and Italy] may be confused with Nutracort® which is a brand name for hydrocortisone in the U.S.

Nitro-Dur® may be confused with Nitrocor® [Chile and Italy]

Related Information

Antihypertensive Agents by Class *on page 1678*

U.S. Brand Names Minitran™; Nitrek® [DSC]; Nitro-Bid®; Nitro-Dur®; Nitrolingual®; NitroMist™; NitroQuick®; Nitrostat®; NitroTime®

Canadian Brand Names Gen-Nitro; Minitran™; Nitro-Dur®; Nitroglycerin Injection, USP; Nitrol®; Nitrostat™; Rho®-Nitro; Transderm-Nitro®; Trinipatch® 0.2; Trinipatch® 0.4; Trinipatch® 0.6

Index Terms Glyceryl Trinitrate; Nitroglycerol; NTG

Therapeutic Category Antianginal Agent; Antihypertensive Agent; Nitrate; Vasodilator; Vasodilator, Coronary

Generic Available Yes: Capsule, injection, patch, tablet

Use Acute treatment and prophylaxis of angina pectoris; I.V. for treatment of CHF (especially when associated with acute MI); pulmonary hypertension; hypertensive emergencies occurring perioperatively (especially during cardiovascular surgery)

Pregnancy Risk Factor C

Lactation Excretion in breast milk unknown/use caution

Contraindications Hypersensitivity to nitroglycerin, organic nitrates, or any component (including adhesives in transdermal patches); glaucoma; severe anemia; increased ICP; concurrent use with sildenafil or other phosphodiesterase-5 (PDE-5) inhibitors (see Drug Interactions); I.V. product is also contraindicated in hypotension, uncontrolled hypokalemia, pericardial tamponade, or constrictive pericarditis

Warnings May cause severe hypotension; use with caution in hypovolemia, hypotension, and right ventricular infarctions

Adverse Reactions

Cardiovascular: Flushing, hypotension, pallor, reflex tachycardia, cardiovascular collapse; severe hypotension, bradycardia, and acute coronary vascular insufficiency with abrupt withdrawal

Central nervous system: Dizziness, restlessness, headache

Dermatologic: Allergic contact dermatitis, exfoliative dermatitis

Endocrine & metabolic: Alcohol intoxication from one I.V. formulation

Gastrointestinal: Nausea, vomiting

Miscellaneous: Perspiration

Drug Interactions I.V. nitroglycerin may antagonize the anticoagulant effect of heparin, monitor closely, may need to decrease heparin dosage when nitroglycerin is discontinued. Alcohol, beta-blockers, calcium channel blockers may enhance nitroglycerin's hypotensive effect. Sildenafil and other phosphodiesterase-5 (PDE-5) inhibitors may increase vasodilatory effects of nitroglycerin and result in severe hypotension (use of these agents with nitroglycerin is contraindicated).

(Continued)

Nitroglycerin *(Continued)*

Stability Nitroglycerin adsorbs to plastics; I.V. must be prepared in glass bottles and special administration sets intended for nitroglycerin (nonpolyvinyl chloride) must be used; do not mix with other drugs; store sublingual tablets and ointment in tightly closed container; store at 15°C to 30°C

Mechanism of Action Reduces cardiac oxygen demand by decreasing left ventricular end diastolic pressure and systemic vascular resistance; dilates coronary arteries and improves collateral flow to ischemic regions; vasodilates veins more than arteries

Pharmacodynamics Onset and duration of action is dependent upon dosage form administered; see table.

Nitroglycerin[1]

Dosage Form	Onset (min)	Duration
I.V.	1-2	3-5 min
Sublingual	1-3	30-60 min
Translingual spray	2	30-60 min
Buccal, extended release	2-3	3-5 h
Oral, sustained release	40	4-8 h
Topical ointment	20-60	2-12 h
Transdermal	40-60	18-24 h

[1]Hemodynamic and antianginal tolerance often develops within 24-48 h of continuous nitrate administration.

Adapted from Corwin S and Reiffel, JA, "Nitrate Therapy for Angina Pectoris," *Arch Intern Med,* 1985, 145:538-43 and Franciosa JA, "Nitroglycerin and Nitrates in Congestive Heart Failure," *Heart and Lung,* 1980, 9(5):873-82.

Pharmacokinetics

Protein binding: 60%

Metabolism: Extensive first-pass

Half-life: 1-4 minutes

Elimination: Excretion of inactive metabolites in urine

Usual Dosage Tolerance to the hemodynamic and antianginal effects can develop within 24-48 hours of continuous use

Children: I.V. continuous infusion: Initial: 0.25-0.5 mcg/kg/minute; titrate by 0.5-1 mcg/kg/minute every 3-5 minutes as needed; usual dose: 1-3 mcg/kg/minute; usual maximum dose: 5 mcg/kg/minute; doses up to 20 mcg/kg/minute may be used

Adults:

Oral: 2.5-9 mg every 8-12 hours

I.V. continuous infusion: Initial: 5 mcg/minute, increase by 5 mcg/minute every 3-5 minutes to 20 mcg/minute, then increase as needed by 10 mcg/minute every 3-5 minutes, up to 200 mcg/minute

Sublingual: 0.2-0.6 mg every 5 minutes for maximum of 3 doses in 15 minutes

Ointment: 1" to 2" every 8 hours

Patch, transdermal: Initial: 0.2-0.4 mg/hour, titrate to 0.4-0.8 mg/hour; use a "patch-on" period of 12-14 hours per day and a "patch-off" period of 10-12 hours per day to minimize tolerance

Lingual: 1-2 sprays into mouth onto or under tongue every 3-5 minutes for maximum of 3 sprays in 15 minutes; may administer 5-10 minutes before activities that may precipitate angina

Buccal: Initial: 1 mg every 5 hours while awake (3 times/day); titrate dosage upward if angina occurs with tablet in place

Administration

Oral:

Buccal tablet: Place in buccal pouch and allow to dissolve; do not swallow, chew, or crush

Lingual spray: Do not shake container. Pump spray must be primed prior to first use with 5 sprays; direct priming sprays into the air, away from patient and others; if unused for 6 weeks, a single priming spray is needed; storage >6 weeks without use may require up to 5 repriming sprays. Monitor amount of medication in container; the end of the pump should be covered by the fluid in the bottle; replace container when fluid falls below the level of the center tub. To administer dose, spray onto or under tongue with container as close to mouth as possible; do not inhale spray; avoid swallowing immediately after spray; do not expectorate or rinse mouth for 5-10 minutes after use

Sublingual tablet: Place under tongue and allow to dissolve, do not swallow, chew, or crush; do not eat or drink while tablet dissolves

Regular or sustained release capsule/tablet: Administer with a full glass of water on an empty stomach; swallow sustained release capsules/tablets whole, do not crush or chew

Parenteral: I.V. continuous infusion: Dilute in D_5W or NS to 50-100 mcg/mL; maximum concentration not to exceed 400 mcg/mL; rate of infusion (mL/hour) = dose (mcg/kg/minute) x weight (kg) x 60 minutes/hour divided by the concentration (mcg/mL); administer via controlled infusion device

Transdermal: Place on hair-free area of skin; rotate patch sites; **Note:** Some products are a membrane-controlled system (eg, Transderm-Nitro®); do **not** cut these patches to deliver partial doses; rate of drug delivery, reservoir contents, and adhesion may be affected; if partial dose is needed, surface area of patch can be blocked proportionally using adhesive bandage (see Lee, 1997 and see specific product labeling)

Monitoring Parameters Blood pressure, heart rate (continuously with I.V. use)

Patient Information Avoid alcohol; may cause dizziness, headache; if no relief of chest pains after 3 sublingual doses, seek emergency care immediately

Nursing Implications Transdermal patches are now labeled as mg/hour (rates of release used to be described as mg/24 hours)

Additional Information I.V. preparations contain alcohol and/or propylene glycol; may need to use nitrate-free interval (10-12 hours/day) to avoid tolerance development; tolerance may possibly be reversed with acetylcysteine; gradually decrease dose in patients receiving NTG for prolonged period to avoid withdrawal reaction; lingual spray contains 20% alcohol, do not spray toward flames

Dosage Forms Excipient information presented when available (limited, particularly for generics); consult specific product labeling.

Capsule, extended release: 2.5 mg, 6.5 mg, 9 mg

Nitro-Time®: 2.5 mg, 6.5 mg, 9 mg

Infusion [premixed in D_5W]: 25 mg (250 mL) [0.1 mg/mL]; 50 mg (250 mL) [0.2 mg/mL]; 50 mg (500 mL) [0.1 mg/mL]; 100 mg (250 mL) [0.4 mg/mL]; 200 mg (500 mL) [0.4 mg/mL]

Injection, solution: 5 mg/mL (5 mL, 10 mL) [contains alcohol and propylene glycol]

Ointment, topical:

Nitro-Bid®: 2% [20 mg/g] (1 g, 30 g, 60 g)

Solution, translingual [spray]:

Nitrolingual®: 0.4 mg/metered spray (4.9 g) [contains alcohol 20%; 60 metered sprays]; (12 g) [contains alcohol 20%; 200 metered sprays]

NitroMist™:0.4 mg/metered spray (8.5 g) [230 metered sprays]

Tablet, sublingual:

NitroQuick®, Nitrostat®: 0.3 mg, 0.4 mg, 0.6 mg

Transdermal system [once-daily patch]: 0.1 mg/hour (30s); 0.2 mg/hour (30s); 0.4 mg/hour (30s); 0.6 mg/hour (30s)

Minitran™: 0.1 mg/hour (30s); 0.2 mg/hour (30s); 0.4 mg/hour (30s); 0.6 mg/hour (30s)

Nitrek®: 0.2 mg/hour (30s); 0.4 mg/hour (30s); 0.6 mg/hour (30s) [DSC]

Nitro-Dur®: 0.1 mg/hour (30s); 0.2 mg/hour (30s); 0.3 mg/hour (30s); 0.4 mg/hour (30s); 0.6 mg/hour (30s); 0.8 mg/hour (30s)

References

Elkayam U, "Tolerance to Organic Nitrates: Evidence, Mechanisms, Clinical Relevance, and Strategies for Prevention," *Ann Intern Med*, 1991, 114(8):667-77.

Lee HA and Anderson PO, "Giving Partial Doses of Transdermal Patches," *Am J Health Syst Pharm*, 1997, 54(15):1759-60.

♦ **Nitroglycerin Injection, USP (Can)** *see* Nitroglycerin *on page 1141*

♦ **Nitroglycerol** *see* Nitroglycerin *on page 1141*

♦ **Nitrol® (Can)** *see* Nitroglycerin *on page 1141*

♦ **Nitrolingual®** *see* Nitroglycerin *on page 1141*

♦ **NitroMist™** *see* Nitroglycerin *on page 1141*

♦ **Nitropress®** *see* Nitroprusside *on page 1143*

Nitroprusside (nye troe PRUS ide)

Medication Safety Issues

Sound-alike/look-alike issues:

Nitroprusside may be confused with nitroglycerin

High alert medication: The Institute for Safe Medication Practices (ISMP) includes this medication among its list of drugs which have a heightened risk of causing significant patient harm when used in error.

Related Information

Antihypertensive Agents by Class *on page 1678*

(Continued)

Nitroprusside *(Continued)*

U.S. Brand Names Nitropress®

Index Terms Nitroprusside Sodium; Sodium Nitroferricyanide; Sodium Nitroprusside

Therapeutic Category Antihypertensive Agent; Vasodilator

Generic Available Yes

Use Management of hypertensive crises; CHF; used for controlled hypotension during anesthesia

Pregnancy Risk Factor C

Lactation Excretion in breast milk unknown

Contraindications Hypersensitivity to nitroprusside or any component; decreased cerebral perfusion; arteriovenous shunt or coarctation of the aorta (ie, compensatory hypertension)

Warnings Use only as an infusion with D_5W; continuously monitor patient's blood pressure; excessive amounts of nitroprusside can cause cyanide toxicity (usually in patients with decreased liver function) or thiocyanate toxicity (usually in patients with decreased renal function, or in patients with normal renal function but prolonged nitroprusside use)

Precautions Use with caution in patients with severe renal impairment, hepatic failure, hypothyroidism, hyponatremia, increased intracranial pressure

Adverse Reactions

Cardiovascular: Excessive hypotensive response, palpitations, substernal distress
Central nervous system: Restlessness, disorientation, psychosis, headache, elevated intracranial pressure
Endocrine & metabolic: Thyroid suppression
Gastrointestinal: Nausea, vomiting
Hematologic: Thiocyanate toxicity
Neuromuscular & skeletal: Weakness
Miscellaneous: Diaphoresis, cyanide toxicity

Stability Discard solution 24 hours after reconstitution and dilution; discard highly colored solutions

Mechanism of Action Causes peripheral vasodilation by direct action on venous and arteriolar smooth muscle, thus reducing peripheral resistance; will increase cardiac output by decreasing afterload; reduces aortal and left ventricular impedance

Pharmacodynamics Hypotensive effects:

Onset of action: Within 2 minutes
Duration: 1-10 minutes

Pharmacokinetics

Metabolism: Converted to cyanide by erythrocyte and tissue sulfhydryl group interactions; cyanide is converted in the liver by the enzyme rhodanase to thiocyanate
Half-life: <10 minutes
Thiocyanate: 2.7-7 days
Elimination: Thiocyanate is excreted in the urine

Usual Dosage Children and Adults: I.V. continuous infusion: Start 0.3-0.5 mcg/kg/minute, titrate to effect; usual dose: 3 mcg/kg/minute; rarely need >4 mcg/kg/minute; maximum dose: 8-10 mcg/kg/minute

Rate (mL/hour) = dose (mcg/kg/minute) x weight (kg) x 60 minutes/hour divided by concentration (mcg/mL)

Administration Parenteral: I.V. continuous infusion only via controlled infusion device; not for direct injection; dilute in plain dextrose solutions only (eg, D_5W); solution should be protected from light, but not necessary to wrap administration set or I.V. tubing. Final concentration for administration: Usual maximum: 200 mcg/mL; in fluid restricted patients a final maximum concentration of 1000 mcg/mL in D_5W has been used. Do not add other medications to nitroprusside solutions.

Monitoring Parameters Blood pressure, heart rate; monitor for cyanide and thiocyanate toxicity; monitor acid-base status as acidosis can be the earliest sign of cyanide toxicity; monitor thiocyanate levels if requiring prolonged infusion (>3 days) or dose ≥4 mcg/kg/minute or patient has renal dysfunction; monitor cyanide blood levels in patients with decreased hepatic function

Reference Range

Thiocyanate:
Toxic: 35-100 mcg/mL
Fatal: >200 mcg/mL
Cyanide:
Normal <0.2 mcg/mL
Normal (smoker): <0.4 mcg/mL
Toxic: >2 mcg/mL
Potentially lethal: >3 mcg/mL

Additional Information Thiocyanate toxicity includes psychoses, blurred vision, confusion, weakness, tinnitus, seizures; cyanide toxicity includes metabolic acidosis, tachycardia, pink skin, decreased pulse, decreased reflexes, altered consciousness, coma, almond smell on breath, methemoglobinemia, dilated pupils

Dosage Forms Excipient information presented when available (limited, particularly for generics); consult specific product labeling.
Injection, solution, as sodium: 25 mg/mL (2 mL)

- **Nitroprusside Sodium** *see* Nitroprusside *on page 1143*
- **NitroQuick®** *see* Nitroglycerin *on page 1141*
- **Nitrostat®** *see* Nitroglycerin *on page 1141*
- **Nitrostat™ (Can)** *see* Nitroglycerin *on page 1141*
- **NitroTime®** *see* Nitroglycerin *on page 1141*
- **Nix® [OTC]** *see* Permethrin *on page 1243*
- **Nix® (Can)** *see* Permethrin *on page 1243*

Nizatidine (ni ZA ti deen)

Medication Safety Issues
Sound-alike/look-alike issues:
Axid® may be confused with Ansaid®
International issues:
Tazac® [Australia] may be confused with Tiazac® which is a brand name for diltiazem in the U.S.

U.S. Brand Names Axid®; Axid® AR [OTC]

Canadian Brand Names Apo-Nizatidine®; Axid®; Gen-Nizatidine; Novo-Nizatidine; Nu-Nizatidine; PMS-Nizatidine

Therapeutic Category Gastrointestinal Agent, Gastric or Duodenal Ulcer Treatment; Histamine H_2 Antagonist

Generic Available Yes: Capsule

Use Treatment and maintenance therapy of duodenal ulcer; treatment of active benign gastric ulcer; esophagitis; gastroesophageal reflux disease (GERD); over-the-counter (OTC) formulation for use in the relief of heartburn, acid indigestion, and sour stomach; adjunctive therapy in the treatment of *Helicobacter pylori*-associated duodenal ulcer

Pregnancy Risk Factor B

Lactation Enters breast milk/may be compatible

Contraindications Hypersensitivity to nizatidine, H_2 antagonists, or any component

Warnings Use of gastric acid inhibitors including proton pump inhibitors and H_2 blockers has been associated with an increased risk for development of acute gastroenteritis and community-acquired pneumonia (Canani, 2006). A large epidemiological study has suggested an increased risk for developing pneumonia in patients receiving H_2 receptor antagonists; however, a causal relationship with nizatidine has not been demonstrated.

Precautions Use with caution and modify dosage in patients with impaired renal function

Adverse Reactions
Cardiovascular: Chest pain, ventricular tachycardia (short, asymptomatic episodes)
Central nervous system: Headache, fever, dizziness, insomnia, somnolence, anxiety, nervousness, irritability
Dermatologic: Rash, pruritus
Endocrine & metabolic: Hyperuricemia
Gastrointestinal: Nausea, vomiting, diarrhea, flatulence, dyspepsia, constipation, dry mouth, anorexia, abdominal pain
Genitourinary: Impotence
Hematologic: Anemia, thrombocytopenia, eosinophilia, leukopenia
Hepatic: Elevated liver enzymes, jaundice, hepatitis
Neuromuscular & skeletal: Back pain, asthenia, myalgia
Ocular: Amblyopia
Respiratory: Rhinitis, pharyngitis, sinusitis, cough, nasal congestion, pneumonia (causal relationship has not been established; see Warnings)
Miscellaneous: Hypersensitivity reactions, serum sickness

Drug Interactions May increase salicylate serum concentration (high-dose salicylate therapy); decreases absorption of itraconazole, delavirdine, and ketoconazole

Food Interactions Limit xanthine-containing foods and beverages; administration with apple juice decreases absorption by 27%

Stability Nizatidine is stable for 48 hours at room temperature when the contents of a capsule are mixed in Gatorade® lemon-lime, Cran-Grape® grape-cranberry drink, V8®, or aluminum- and magnesium hydroxide suspension (approximate concentration 2.5 mg/mL)
(Continued)

Nizatidine *(Continued)*

Mechanism of Action Competitive inhibition of histamine at H_2-receptors of the gastric parietal cells, which inhibits gastric acid secretion

Pharmacodynamics Maximum effect: Duodenal ulcer: 4 weeks

Pharmacokinetics

Distribution: V_d: Adults: 0.8-1.5 L/kg; breast milk: 0.1% excreted into breast milk
Protein binding: 35%
Bioavailability: Oral: 70%
Half-life, elimination: Adults: 1-2 hours; anuric: 3.5-11 hours
Time to peak serum concentration: 0.5-3 hours
Elimination: 60% excreted unchanged in urine

Usual Dosage Oral:

Infants 6 months to Children 11 years: Limited information available: 5-10 mg/kg/day divided twice daily (see References)
GERD, esophagitis: Children ≥12 years and Adults: 150 mg twice daily
Active duodenal and gastric ulcers: Adults: 300 mg once daily at bedtime or 150 mg twice daily
Maintenance of healed duodenal ulcer: Adults: 150 mg once daily
Relief of heartburn, acid indigestion, sour stomach (OTC use): Adults: 75 mg 30-60 minutes before meals; no more than 2 tablets/day
Helicobacter pylori-associated duodenal ulcer (limited information): Adults: 150 mg twice daily for 4 weeks (combined with clarithromycin and bismuth formulation; followed by 300 mg/day)

Dosing adjustment in renal impairment: Adults:

Active treatment:
Cl_{cr} 20-50 mL/minute: 150 mg once daily
Cl_{cr} <20 mL/minute: 150 mg every other day

Maintenance treatment:
Cl_{cr} 20-50 mL/minute: 150 every other day
Cl_{cr} <20 mL/minute: 150 mg every 3 days

Administration Oral: May administer with or without food; do not administer or mix with apple juice (see Food Interactions and Stability)

Test Interactions False-positive urobilinogen with Multistix®

Patient Information Avoid excessive amounts of caffeinated beverages and aspirin; do not take with apple juice; with self medication, if the symptoms of heartburn, acid indigestion, or sour stomach persist after 2 weeks of continuous use of the drug, consult clinician

Dosage Forms Excipient information presented when available (limited, particularly for generics); consult specific product labeling.

Capsule (Axid®): 150 mg, 300 mg
Solution, oral (Axid®): 15 mg/mL (120 mL, 480 mL) [bubble gum flavor]
Tablet (Axid® AR): 75 mg

Extemporaneous Preparations A 2.5 mg/mL solution may be made by opening a 300 mg capsule into a mortar and grinding to a fine powder. Add incremental amounts of Gatorade® lemon-lime, Ocean Spray® cran-grape, apple juice, or V8® 100% vegetable juice to a total volume of 120 mL; shake well; stable for 2 days refrigerated.

Nahata, MC, Pai VB, and Hipple TF, *Pediatric Drug Formulations*, 5th ed, Cincinnati, OH: Harvey Whitney Books Co, 2004.

References

Canani RB, Cirillo P, Roggero P, et al, "Therapy With Gastric Acidity Inhibitors Increases the Risk of Acute Gastroenteritis and Community-Acquired Pneumonia in Children," *Pediatrics*, 2006, 117(5):e817-20.
Mikawa K, Nishina K, Maekawa N, et al, "Effects of Oral Nizatidine on Preoperative Gastric Fluid pH and Volume in Children," *Br J Anaesth*, 1994, 73(5):600-4.
Simeone D, Caria MC, Miele E, et al, "Treatment of Childhood Peptic Esophagitis: A Double-Blind Placebo-Controlled Trial of Nizatidine," *J Pediatr Gastroenterol Nur*, 1997, 25(1):51-5.

♦ **Nizoral®** *see* Ketoconazole *on page 887*
♦ **Nizoral® A-D [OTC]** *see* Ketoconazole *on page 887*
♦ **N-Methylhydrazine** *see* Procarbazine *on page 1320*
♦ **No Doz® Maximum Strength [OTC]** *see* Caffeine *on page 255*
♦ **Nora-BE™** *see* Norethindrone *on page 1148*
♦ **Noradrenaline** *see* Norepinephrine *on page 1147*
♦ **Noradrenaline Acid Tartrate** *see* Norepinephrine *on page 1147*
♦ **Norco®** *see* Hydrocodone and Acetaminophen *on page 779*
♦ **Norcuron® [DSC]** *see* Vecuronium *on page 1604*
♦ **Norcuron® (Can)** *see* Vecuronium *on page 1604*
♦ **Nordeoxyguanosine** *see* Ganciclovir *on page 719*
♦ **Norditropin®** *see* Human Growth Hormone *on page 769*
♦ **Norditropin® NordiFlex®** *see* Human Growth Hormone *on page 769*

Norepinephrine (nor ep i NEF rin)

Related Information

Emergency Pediatric Drip Calculations *on page 1652*

Extravasation Treatment *on page 1726*

U.S. Brand Names Levophed®

Canadian Brand Names Levophed®

Index Terms Levarterenol Bitartrate; Noradrenaline; Noradrenaline Acid Tartrate; Norepinephrine Bitartrate

Therapeutic Category Adrenergic Agonist Agent; Alpha-Adrenergic Agonist; Sympathomimetic

Generic Available Yes

Use Treatment of shock which persists after adequate fluid volume replacement; severe hypotension; cardiogenic shock

Pregnancy Risk Factor C

Lactation Excretion in breast milk unknown

Contraindications Hypersensitivity to norepinephrine or any component (see Warnings)

Warnings Potent drug; must be diluted prior to use; monitor hemodynamic status; injection contains sodium metabisulfite which may cause allergic reactions in susceptible individuals

Precautions Blood/volume depletion should be corrected, if possible, before norepinephrine therapy; extravasation may cause severe tissue necrosis; do **not** give to patients with peripheral or mesenteric vascular thrombosis because ischemia may be increased and the area of infarct extended; use with caution during cyclopropane or halothane anesthesia and in patients with occlusive vascular disease

Adverse Reactions

Cardiovascular: Cardiac arrhythmias, palpitations, bradycardia, tachycardia, hypertension, chest pain, pallor

Central nervous system: Anxiety, headache

Endocrine & metabolic: Uterine contractions

Gastrointestinal: Vomiting

Local: Organ ischemia (due to vasoconstriction of renal and mesenteric arteries), ischemic necrosis and sloughing of superficial tissue after extravasation

Ocular: Photophobia

Respiratory: Respiratory distress

Miscellaneous: Diaphoresis

Drug Interactions Atropine sulfate may block the reflex bradycardia caused by norepinephrine and enhance the pressor response; tricyclic antidepressants, MAO inhibitors, antihistamines (diphenhydramine, tripelennamine), guanethidine, ergot alkaloids, and methyldopa may potentiate the effect of norepinephrine

Stability Readily oxidized, do not use if brown coloration; dilute with D_5W or D_5W/NS; not recommended for dilution in NS; not stable with alkaline solutions

Mechanism of Action Stimulates $beta_1$-adrenergic receptors and alpha-adrenergic receptors causing increased contractility and heart rate as well as vasoconstriction, thereby increasing systemic blood pressure and coronary blood flow; clinically, alpha effects (vasoconstriction) are greater than beta effects (inotropic and chronotropic effects)

Pharmacodynamics

Onset of action: Very rapid

Duration: Limited duration following I.V. injection

Pharmacokinetics

Metabolism: By catechol-o-methyltransferase (COMT) and monoamine oxidase (MAO)

Elimination: In urine (84% to 96% as inactive metabolites)

Usual Dosage I.V. (dose stated in terms of **norepinephrine base**):

Children: Initial: 0.05-0.1 mcg/kg/minute, titrate to desired effect; maximum dose: 1-2 mcg/kg/minute

Rate (mL/hour) = dose (mcg/kg/minute) x weight (kg) x 60 minutes/hour divided by concentration (mcg/mL)

Adults: Initial: 4 mcg/minute; titrate to desired response; usual dose: 8-12 mcg/minute as an infusion

ACLS Guidelines 2000: Initial 0.5-1 mcg/minute; titrate to effect

Refractory shock: 8-30 mcg/minute may be required

Administration Parenteral: Administer into large vein to avoid potential extravasation; standard concentration: 4 mcg/mL but 16 mcg/mL has been used safely and with efficacy in situations of extreme fluid restriction

Monitoring Parameters Blood pressure, heart rate, urine output, peripheral perfusion

(Continued)

Norepinephrine *(Continued)*

Additional Information Treat extravasations with local injections of phentolamine (see Extravasation Treatment *on page 1726*)

Dosage Forms Excipient information presented when available (limited, particularly for generics); consult specific product labeling.

Injection, solution, as bitartrate: 1 mg/mL (4 mL) [contains sodium metabisulfite]

♦ **Norepinephrine Bitartrate** *see* Norepinephrine *on page 1147*

Norethindrone (nor eth IN drone)

Medication Safety Issues

Sound-alike/look-alike issues:

Micronor® may be confused with miconazole, Micronase®

U.S. Brand Names Aygestin®; Camila™; Errin™; Jolivette™; Micronor®; Nora-BE™; Nor-QD®

Canadian Brand Names Micronor®; Norlutate®

Index Terms Norethindrone Acetate; Norethisterone

Therapeutic Category Contraceptive, Oral; Contraceptive, Progestin Only; Progestin

Generic Available Yes

Use Treatment of amenorrhea, abnormal uterine bleeding, endometriosis, oral contraceptive

Pregnancy Risk Factor X

Lactation Enters breast milk/use caution

Contraindications Hypersensitivity to norethindrone or any component; thromboembolic disorders, severe hepatic disease, breast cancer, cerebral hemorrhage, undiagnosed vaginal bleeding; known or suspected pregnancy; as a diagnostic test for pregnancy

Warnings Discontinue if sudden partial or complete loss of vision, proptosis, diplopia, or migraine occur; **there is a higher rate of failure with progestin only contraceptives**; progestin-induced withdrawal bleeding occurs within 3-7 days after discontinuation of drug

Precautions Use with caution in patients with asthma, diabetes mellitus, seizure disorder, migraine, cardiac or renal dysfunction, psychic depression; may affect lipid and carbohydrate metabolism; women with diabetes mellitus or hyperlipidemias should be monitored closely

Adverse Reactions

Cardiovascular: Edema, thromboembolic disorders, hypertension

Central nervous system: Mental depression, nervousness, dizziness, fatigue, headache

Dermatologic: Hirsutism, rash, melasma or chloasma

Endocrine & metabolic: Breakthrough bleeding, spotting, changes in menstrual flow, weight gain or loss

Hepatic: Cholestatic jaundice

Drug Interactions Rifampin decreases pharmacologic effect of norethindrone

Food Interactions High-dose vitamin C (1 g/day) may increase adverse effects; increase dietary intake of folate and pyridoxine

Mechanism of Action Inhibits secretion of pituitary gonadotropin (LH) which prevents follicular maturation and ovulation; in the presence of adequate endogenous estrogen, transforms a proliferative endometrium to a secretory one

Pharmacokinetics

Protein binding: 80%

Metabolism: In the liver

Half-life: 5-14 hours

Time to peak serum concentration: 0.5-4 hours

Usual Dosage Adolescents and Adults: Oral:

Amenorrhea and abnormal uterine bleeding: Norethindrone acetate 2.5-10 mg/day for 5-10 days beginning during the latter half of the menstrual cycle

Endometriosis: Norethindrone acetate 5 mg/day for 14 days; increase at increments of 2.5 mg/day every 2 weeks up to 15 mg/day

Contraception: Progesterone only: Norethindrone 0.35 mg every day of the year starting on first day of menstruation

Administration Oral: Administer with food

Test Interactions Thyroid function test, metyrapone test, liver function tests, coagulation tests (prothrombin time, factors VII, VIII, IX, X)

Patient Information Progestin-induced withdrawal bleeding occurs within 3-7 days after discontinuation of the drug; when used for contraception, if one dose is missed take as soon as remembered, then take the next tablet at the regular time; if two

(Continued)

doses are missed, take one of the missed doses, discard the other, and take daily dose at usual time; if three doses are missed, use another form of birth control until menses appear or pregnancy is ruled out; limit caffeine

Dosage Forms Excipient information presented when available (limited, particularly for generics); consult specific product labeling.

Tablet (Camila™, Errin™, Jolivette™, Micronor®, Nora-BE™, Nor-QD®): 0.35 mg

Tablet, as acetate (Aygestin®): 5 mg

- **Norethindrone Acetate** *see* Norethindrone *on page 1148*
- **Norethisterone** *see* Norethindrone *on page 1148*
- **Noritate®** *see* Metronidazole *on page 1049*
- **Norlutate® (Can)** *see* Norethindrone *on page 1148*
- **Normal Human Serum Albumin** *see* Albumin *on page 64*
- **Normal Saline** *see* Sodium Chloride *on page 1450*
- **Normal Serum Albumin (Human)** *see* Albumin *on page 64*
- **Normodyne® (Can)** *see* Labetalol *on page 895*
- **Norpace®** *see* Disopyramide *on page 523*
- **Norpace® CR** *see* Disopyramide *on page 523*
- **Norpramin®** *see* Desipramine *on page 455*
- **Nor-QD®** *see* Norethindrone *on page 1148*
- **Nortemp Children's [OTC]** *see* Acetaminophen *on page 42*
- **North and South American Antisnake-bite Serum** *see Crotalidae* Polyvalent Antivenin (Equine) *on page 409*

Nortriptyline (nor TRIP ti leen)

Medication Safety Issues

Sound-alike/look-alike issues:

Nortriptyline may be confused with amitriptyline, desipramine, Norpramin®

Aventyl® HCl may be confused with Bentyl®

Pamelor® may be confused with Demerol®, Dymelor®

Related Information

Antidepressant Agents *on page 1681*

U.S. Brand Names Pamelor®

Canadian Brand Names Alti-Nortriptyline; Apo-Nortriptyline®; Aventyl®; Gen-Nortriptyline; Norventyl; Novo-Nortriptyline; Nu-Nortriptyline; PMS-Nortriptyline

Index Terms Nortriptyline Hydrochloride

Therapeutic Category Antidepressant, Tricyclic

Generic Available Yes: Excludes solution

Use Treatment of various forms of depression, often in conjunction with psychotherapy; nocturnal enuresis

Medication Guide An FDA-approved patient medication guide, which is available with the product information and at http://www.fda.gov/cder/Offices/ODS/medication_guides.htm, must be dispensed with this medication for each new outpatient prescription and refill.

Pregnancy Risk Factor D

Lactation Enters breast milk/contraindicated (AAP rates "of concern")

Contraindications Hypersensitivity to nortriptyline or amitriptyline (cross-sensitivity with other tricyclics may occur) or any component (see Warnings); angle-closure glaucoma, use of MAO inhibitors within 14 days (potentially fatal reactions may occur, see Drug Interactions)

Warnings Nortriptyline is not approved for use in pediatric patients. Clinical worsening of depression or suicidal ideation and behavior may occur in children and adults with major depressive disorder. In clinical trials, antidepressants increased the risk of suicidal thinking and behavior (suicidality) in children, adolescents, and young adults (18-24 years of age) with major depressive disorder and other psychiatric disorders. This risk must be considered before prescribing antidepressants for any clinical use. Short-term studies did **not** show an increased risk of suicidality with antidepressant use in patients >24 years of age and showed a decreased risk in patients ≥65 years.

Patients of all ages who are treated with antidepressants for any indication require appropriate monitoring and close observation for clinical worsening of depression, suicidality, and unusual changes in behavior, especially during the first few months after antidepressant initiation or when the dose is adjusted. Family members and caregivers should be instructed to closely observe the patient (ie, daily) and communicate condition with healthcare provider. Patients should also be monitored for associated behaviors (eg, anxiety, agitation, panic attacks, insomnia, irritability, hostility, aggressiveness, impulsivity, akathisia, hypomania, mania) which may increase the risk for worsening depression or suicidality. Worsening depression or

(Continued)

Nortriptyline *(Continued)*

emergence of suicidality (or associated behaviors listed above) that is abrupt in onset, severe, or not part of the presenting symptoms, may require discontinuation or modification of drug therapy.

Do not discontinue abruptly in patients receiving high doses chronically (withdrawal symptoms may occur). To reduce risk of intentional overdose, write prescriptions for the smallest quantity consistent with good patient care. Screen individuals for bipolar disorder prior to treatment (using antidepressants alone may induce manic episodes in patients with this condition). May worsen psychosis in some patients.

Use with extreme caution with renal or hepatic impairment. Capsule may contain sodium bisulfite and/or benzyl alcohol, both of which may cause allergic reactions in susceptible individuals; solution contains benzoic acid; benzoic acid (benzoate) is a metabolite of benzyl alcohol; large amounts of benzyl alcohol (≥99 mg/kg/day) have been associated with a potentially fatal toxicity ("gasping syndrome") in neonates; avoid use of nortriptyline products containing benzoic acid or benzyl alcohol in neonates; *in vitro* and animal studies have shown that benzoate displaces bilirubin from protein binding sites

Precautions Use with caution in patients with cardiac conduction disturbances, cardiovascular disease, seizure disorder, history of urinary retention, hyperthyroidism, or those receiving thyroid hormone replacement

Adverse Reactions Nortriptyline has lower anticholinergic and sedative effects compared to amitriptyline

Cardiovascular: Postural hypotension, arrhythmias, tachycardia, sudden death

Central nervous system: Sedation, fatigue, anxiety, impaired cognitive function, seizures; suicidal thinking and behavior (see Warnings)

Dermatologic: Photosensitivity

Endocrine & metabolic: SIADH (rare), weight gain

Gastrointestinal: Xerostomia, constipation, increased appetite

Genitourinary: Urinary retention

Hematologic: Rarely agranulocytosis, leukopenia, eosinophilia

Hepatic: Cholestatic jaundice, elevated liver enzymes

Neuromuscular & skeletal: Tremor, weakness

Ocular: Blurred vision, elevated intraocular pressure

Miscellaneous: Allergic reactions

Drug Interactions Cytochrome P450 isoenzyme CYP1A2 and CYP2D6 (hydroxylation) substrate

Nortriptyline may decrease the effects of guanethidine and clonidine (use with clonidine may result in possible hypertensive crisis); nortriptyline may increase the effects of other CNS depressants (including alcohol), adrenergic agents (epinephrine, isoproterenol), anticholinergic agents and warfarin

With MAO inhibitors, hyperpyrexia, hypertension, tachycardia, confusion, seizures, and death have been reported (see Contraindications); concurrent use of high-dose TCAs and ritonavir may cause the serotonin syndrome; the herbal medicine St John's wort (*Hypericum perforatum*) may increase serious side effects, its use is **not** recommended

Cimetidine, fluoxetine, and methylphenidate may decrease the metabolism and phenobarbital may increase the metabolism of nortriptyline

Food Interactions Riboflavin dietary requirements may be increased

Stability Protect from light

Mechanism of Action Increases the synaptic concentration of serotonin and/or norepinephrine in the CNS by inhibition of their reuptake by the presynaptic neuronal membrane

Pharmacodynamics Onset of action: Therapeutic antidepressant effects begin in 7-21 days; maximum effects may not occur for ≥2-3 weeks

Pharmacokinetics

Absorption: Oral: Rapid; well absorbed

Distribution: V_d: 14-22 L/kg; crosses placenta; enters breast milk

Protein binding: 93% to 95%

Metabolism: Undergoes significant first-pass metabolism; primarily detoxified in the liver via hydroxylation followed by glucuronide conjugation

Half-life:

Children (mean ± SD): 18 ± 4 hours

Adults (mean ± SD): 46 ± 24 hours

Time to peak serum concentration: Oral: Within 7-8.5 hours

Elimination: Metabolites and small amounts of unchanged drug excreted in urine; small amounts of biliary elimination occur

Dialysis: Not Dialyzable

Usual Dosage Oral:

Nocturnal enuresis: Children (give dose 30 minutes before bedtime):

- 6-7 years (20-25 kg): 10 mg/day
- 8-11 years (25-35 kg): 10-20 mg/day
- >11 years (35-54 kg): 25-35 mg/day

Depression: **Note:** Not FDA approved for use in pediatric patients; controlled clinical trials have not shown tricyclic antidepressants to be superior to placebo for the treatment of depression in children and adolescents (see Dopheide, 2006 and Wagner, 2005).

- Children 6-12 years: 1-3 mg/kg/day or 10-20 mg/day in 3-4 divided doses
- Adolescents: 1-3 mg/kg/day or 30-50 mg/day in 3-4 divided doses; usual maximum dose: 150 mg/day
- Adults: 25 mg 3-4 times/day up to 150 mg/day

Dosing adjustment in hepatic impairment: Use lower doses and slower titration; individualization of dosage is recommended

Administration Oral: May administer with food to decrease GI upset; dilute oral solution in water, milk, or fruit juice immediately before use; do not dilute in grape juice or carbonated beverages

Monitoring Parameters Heart rate, blood pressure, mental status, weight, plasma concentrations. Monitor patient periodically for symptom resolution; monitor for worsening depression, suicidality, and associated behaviors (especially at the beginning of therapy or when doses are increased or decreased; see Warnings).

Reference Range Therapeutic: 50-150 ng/mL (SI: 190-570 nmol/L)

Patient Information Read the patient Medication Guide that you receive with each prescription and refill of nortriptyline. An increased risk of suicidal thinking and behavior has been reported with the use of antidepressants in children, adolescents, and young adults (18-24 years of age). Notify physician if you feel more depressed, have thoughts of suicide, or become more agitated or irritable (see Warnings). Avoid alcohol and the herbal medicine St John's wort; limit caffeine; do not discontinue medication abruptly; may cause drowsiness and impair ability to perform activities requiring mental alertness or physical coordination; may cause dry mouth. May cause photosensitivity reactions (eg, exposure to sunlight may cause severe sunburn, skin rash, redness, or itching); avoid exposure to sunlight and artificial light sources (sunlamps, tanning booth/bed); wear protective clothing, wide-brimmed hats, sunglasses, and lip sunscreen (SPF ≥15); use a sunscreen [broad-spectrum sunscreen or physical sunscreen (preferred) or sunblock with SPF ≥15]; contact physician if reaction occurs.

Nursing Implications Treatment duration of nocturnal enuresis is usually ≤3 months

Dosage Forms Excipient information presented when available (limited, particularly for generics); consult specific product labeling.

Capsule, as hydrochloride: 10 mg, 25 mg, 50 mg, 75 mg

Pamelor®: 10 mg, 25 mg, 50 mg, 75 mg [may contain benzyl alcohol; 50 mg may also contain sodium bisulfite]

Solution, as hydrochloride (Pamelor®): 10 mg/5 mL (473 mL) [contains alcohol 4% and benzoic acid]

References

Dopheide JA, "Recognizing and Treating Depression in Children and Adolescents," *Am J Health Syst Pharm*, 2006, 63(3):233-43.

Levy HB, Harper CR, and Weinberg WA, "A Practical Approach to Children Failing in School," *Pediatr Clin North Am*, 1992, 39(4):895-928

Wagner KD, "Pharmacotherapy for Major Depression in Children and Adolescents," *Prog Neuropsychopharmacol Biol Psychiatry*, 2005, 29(5):819-26.

- ♦ **Nortriptyline Hydrochloride** *see* Nortriptyline *on page 1149*
- ♦ **Norvasc®** *see* Amlodipine *on page 109*
- ♦ **Norventyl (Can)** *see* Nortriptyline *on page 1149*
- ♦ **Norvir®** *see* Ritonavir *on page 1395*
- ♦ **Norvir® SEC (Can)** *see* Ritonavir *on page 1395*
- ♦ **Novamoxin® (Can)** *see* Amoxicillin *on page 113*
- ♦ **Novantrone®** *see* Mitoxantrone *on page 1072*
- ♦ **Novarel®** *see* Chorionic Gonadotropin *on page 351*
- ♦ **Novasen (Can)** *see* Aspirin *on page 163*
- ♦ **Nove-Desmopressin® (Can)** *see* Desmopressin *on page 459*
- ♦ **Novo-5 ASA (Can)** *see* Mesalamine *on page 1011*
- ♦ **Novo-Alprazol (Can)** *see* Alprazolam *on page 79*
- ♦ **Novo-Amiodarone (Can)** *see* Amiodarone *on page 100*
- ♦ **Novo-Ampicillin (Can)** *see* Ampicillin *on page 123*
- ♦ **Novo-Atenol (Can)** *see* Atenolol *on page 170*
- ♦ **Novo-Azathioprine (Can)** *see* Azathioprine *on page 187*
- ♦ **Novo-Azithromycin (Can)** *see* Azithromycin *on page 191*

- ♦ **Nu-Sucralate (Can)** *see* Sucralfate *on page 1480*
- ♦ **Nu-Sundac (Can)** *see* Sulindac *on page 1493*
- ♦ **Nu-Tetra (Can)** *see* Tetracycline *on page 1518*
- ♦ **Nu-Timolol (Can)** *see* Timolol *on page 1542*
- ♦ **Nutracort®** *see* Hydrocortisone *on page 781*
- ♦ **Nutralox® [OTC]** *see* Calcium Carbonate *on page 264*
- ♦ **Nutralox® [OTC]** *see* Calcium Supplements *on page 272*
- ♦ **Nu-Trazodone (Can)** *see* Trazodone *on page 1564*
- ♦ **Nutropin®** *see* Human Growth Hormone *on page 769*
- ♦ **Nutropin AQ®** *see* Human Growth Hormone *on page 769*
- ♦ **Nutropin® AQ (Can)** *see* Human Growth Hormone *on page 769*
- ♦ **Nutropine® (Can)** *see* Human Growth Hormone *on page 769*
- ♦ **Nu-Verap (Can)** *see* Verapamil *on page 1611*
- ♦ **NVP** *see* Nevirapine *on page 1124*
- ♦ **Nyaderm (Can)** *see* Nystatin *on page 1156*
- ♦ **Nyamyc™** *see* Nystatin *on page 1156*
- ♦ **Nydrazid® [DSC]** *see* Isoniazid *on page 873*

Nystatin (nye STAT in)

Medication Safety Issues
Sound-alike/look-alike issues:
Nystatin may be confused with Nilstat®, Nitrostat®
Nilstat may be confused with Nitrostat®, nystatin

U.S. Brand Names Bio-Statin®; Mycostatin®; Nyamyc™; Nystat-Rx®; Nystop®; Pedi-Dri®

Canadian Brand Names Candistatin®; Nilstat; Nyaderm; PMS-Nystatin

Therapeutic Category Antifungal Agent, Oral Nonabsorbed; Antifungal Agent, Topical; Antifungal Agent, Vaginal

Generic Available Yes: Cream, ointment, powder, suspension, tablet

Use Treatment of susceptible cutaneous, mucocutaneous, oral cavity and vaginal fungal infections normally caused by the *Candida* species

Pregnancy Risk Factor C

Lactation Does not enter breast milk/compatible (not absorbed orally)

Contraindications Hypersensitivity to nystatin or any component

Adverse Reactions
Dermatologic: Contact dermatitis, Stevens-Johnson syndrome, pruritus, rash
Gastrointestinal: Nausea, vomiting, diarrhea
Local: Irritation, burning, pain

Stability Store vaginal inserts in refrigerator; protect from moisture and light

Mechanism of Action Binds to sterols in fungal cell membrane, changing the cell wall permeability allowing for leakage of cellular contents

Pharmacodynamics Onset of action: Symptomatic relief from candidiasis: Within 24-72 hours

Pharmacokinetics
Absorption: Not absorbed through mucous membranes or intact skin; poorly absorbed from the GI tract
Elimination: In feces as unchanged drug

Usual Dosage
Oral candidiasis:
Neonates: 100,000 units 4 times/day or 50,000 units to each side of mouth 4 times/day
Infants: 200,000 units 4 times/day or 100,000 units to each side of mouth 4 times/day
Children and Adults: 400,000-600,000 units 4 times/day
Cutaneous candidal infections: Children and Adults: Topical: Apply 2-4 times/day
Intestinal infections: Adults: Oral: 500,000-1,000,000 units every 8 hours
Vaginal infections: Adolescents and Adults: Vaginal tablets: Insert 1 tablet/day at bedtime for 2 weeks

Administration
Oral: Shake suspension well before use; suspension should be swished about the mouth and retained in the mouth for as long as possible (several minutes) before swallowing. For neonates and infants, paint nystatin suspension into recesses of the mouth.
Topical:
Cream or ointment: Gently massage formulation into the skin
Intravaginal: Insert vaginal tablet high in the vagina

Powder: Dust in shoes, in stockings, and on feet for treatment of candidal infection of the feet; also used on very moist lesions

Monitoring Parameters KOH smears or cultures should be used to confirm diagnosis of cutaneous or mucocutaneous candidiasis

Patient Information Inform physician if irritation or sensitization occur during therapy

Dosage Forms Excipient information presented when available (limited, particularly for generics); consult specific product labeling.

Capsule:
- Bio-Statin®: 500,000 units, 1 million units

Cream: 100,000 units/g (15 g, 30 g)
- Mycostatin®: 100,000 units/g (30 g)

Ointment, topical: 100,000 units/g (15 g, 30 g)

Powder, for prescription compounding: 50 million units (10 g); 150 million units (30 g); 500 million units (100 g); 2 billion units (400 g)
- Nystat-Rx®: 50 million units (10 g); 150 million units (30 g); 500 million units (100 g); 1 billion units (190 g); 2 billion units (350 g)

Powder, topical:
- Mycostatin®: 100,000 units/g (15 g) [contains talc]
- Nyamyc™: 100,000 units/g (15 g, 30 g) [contains talc]
- Nystop®: 100,000 units/g (15 g, 30 g, 60 g) [contains talc]
- Pedi-Dri®: 100,000 units/g (56.7 g) [contains talc]

Suspension, oral: 100,000 units/mL (5 mL, 60 mL, 480 mL)

Tablet: 500,000 units

Tablet, vaginal: 100,000 units (15s) [packaged with applicator]

References

Dismukes WE, Wade JS, Lee JY, et al, "A Randomized, Double-Blind Trial of Nystatin Therapy for the Candidiasis Hypersensitivity Syndrome," *N Engl J Med*, 1990, 323(25):1717-23.

- ♦ **Nystat-Rx®** *see* Nystatin *on page 1156*
- ♦ **Nystop®** *see* Nystatin *on page 1156*
- ♦ **Nytol® (Can)** *see* DiphenhydrAMINE *on page 509*
- ♦ **Nytol® Extra Strength (Can)** *see* DiphenhydrAMINE *on page 509*
- ♦ **Nytol® Quick Caps [OTC]** *see* DiphenhydrAMINE *on page 509*
- ♦ **Nytol® Quick Gels [OTC]** *see* DiphenhydrAMINE *on page 509*
- ♦ **NāSop™** *see* Phenylephrine *on page 1250*
- ♦ **Nōstrilla® [OTC]** *see* Oxymetazoline *on page 1194*
- ♦ **OCBZ** *see* Oxcarbazepine *on page 1184*
- ♦ **Occlusal®-HP [OTC]** *see* Salicylic Acid *on page 1413*
- ♦ **Occlusal™-HP (Can)** *see* Salicylic Acid *on page 1413*
- ♦ **Ocean® [OTC]** *see* Sodium Chloride *on page 1450*
- ♦ **Oceant® for Kids [OTC]** *see* Sodium Chloride *on page 1450*
- ♦ **Octagam®** *see* Immune Globulin (Intravenous) *on page 818*
- ♦ **Octostim® (Can)** *see* Desmopressin *on page 459*

Octreotide Acetate (ok TREE oh tide AS e tate)

Medication Safety Issues

Sound-alike/look-alike issues:
- Sandostatin® may be confused with Sandimmune®

U.S. Brand Names Sandostatin®; Sandostatin LAR®

Canadian Brand Names Octreotide Acetate Injection; Octreotide Acetate Omega; Sandostatin®; Sandostatin LAR®

Index Terms NSC-671663; Octreotide Acetate

Therapeutic Category Antidiarrheal; Antisecretory Agent; Somatostatin Analog

Generic Available Yes: Solution

Use Control of symptoms in patients with metastatic carcinoid, vasoactive intestinal peptide-secreting tumors (VIPomas), and secretory diarrhea; acromegaly

Unlabeled use: AIDS-associated secretory diarrhea, control of bleeding of esophageal varices, breast cancer, cryptosporidiosis, Cushing's syndrome, insulinomas, small bowel fistulas, postgastrectomy dumping syndrome, chemotherapy-induced diarrhea, GVHD-induced diarrhea, Zollinger-Ellison syndrome, persistent hyperinsulinemic hypoglycemia of infancy (nesidioblastosis), postoperative chylothorax, treatment of sulfonylurea overdosage; hypothalamic obesity

Pregnancy Risk Factor B

Lactation Excretion in breast milk unknown/use caution

Contraindications Hypersensitivity to octreotide or any component

Warnings Dosage adjustment may be required to maintain symptomatic control; octreotide may affect glucose regulation; insulin requirements may be reduced in type I diabetic patients; symptomatic hypoglycemia which may be severe, has been

(Continued)

Octreotide Acetate *(Continued)*

reported; in nondiabetics and type II diabetics with partially intact insulin reserves, octreotide may decrease insulin levels and hyperglycemia may occur; monitor glucose tolerance and antidiabetic treatment closely

Precautions Patients must be monitored closely for biliary tract abnormalities (including biliary obstruction, cholecystitis, and cholelithiasis), hypothyroidism, and glucose tolerance; use with caution in patients with renal impairment and consider dosage modification in patients with severe renal failure requiring dialysis; use with caution in diabetic patients with gastroparesis; chronic usage is associated with depressed vitamin B_{12} levels; monitor vitamin B_{12} levels in patients receiving long-term therapy; suppression of growth hormone (animal data) is of concern when used as long-term therapy in children

Adverse Reactions

Cardiovascular: Flushing, edema, chest pain, hypertension, palpitations, CHF, orthostatic hypotension, syncope, bradycardia, arrhythmias, conduction abnormalities

Central nervous system: Dizziness, fatigue, anxiety, headache, depression, insomnia, fever, chills, seizures, vertigo, hyperesthesia, Bell's palsy

Dermatologic: Erythema, alopecia, bruising, pruritus, rash

Endocrine & metabolic: Hypoglycemia, hyperglycemia (see Warnings), galactorrhea, hypothyroidism

Gastrointestinal: Nausea, diarrhea, abdominal pain, vomiting, constipation, flatulence, fat malabsorption, GI bleeding (rare), xerostomia, dyspepsia, steatorrhea, cholelithiasis (33% in pediatric trial), biliary sludge, pancreatitis

Genitourinary: Prostatitis

Hepatic: Hepatitis, jaundice, elevated liver enzymes

Local: Injection site pain, thrombophlebitis

Neuromuscular & skeletal: Weakness, increased CPK, backache, muscle spasm, muscle cramps, arthralgia, tremor, numbness

Ocular: Visual disturbance, ocular burning

Renal: Oliguria, urinary hyperosmolarity

Respiratory: Shortness of breath, rhinorrhea

Drug Interactions Cytochrome P450 isoenzyme CYP2D6 (high dose) and CYP3A inhibitor

Increases the bioavailability of bromocriptine; may decrease quinidine clearance and also the clearance of other drugs metabolized by isoenzyme CYP3A4; may decrease cyclosporine levels (case report of a transplant rejection) possibly due to decreased cyclosporine bioavailability; may alter insulin and oral hypoglycemic agent requirements (see Warnings)

Food Interactions Schedule injections between meals to decrease GI effects; may decrease vitamin B_{12} levels and decrease absorption of dietary fats. Avoid hypoglycemic herbs, including alfalfa, aloe, bilberry, bitter melon, burdock, celery, damiana, fenugreek, garcinia, garlic, ginger, ginseng, gymnema, marshmallow, and stinging nettle (may enhance the hypoglycemic effect of octreotide).

Stability Store in refrigerator; Sandostatin® injection is stable 14 days at room temperature if protected from light; stable in NS for 4 days and D_5W for 24 hours at room temperature; not compatible in TPN solutions due to glycosyl octreotide conjugate which may have decreased activity; Sandostatin LAR® Depot must be used immediately after reconstitution

Mechanism of Action A synthetic polypeptide which mimics natural somatostatin by inhibiting serotonin release, and the secretion of gastrin, vasoactive intestinal peptide (VIP), insulin, glucagon, secretin, motilin, thyrotropin, cholecystokinin, serotonin, and pancreatic polypeptide; in animals, also a potent inhibitor of growth hormone; decreases GI motility and inhibits intestinal secretion of water and electrolytes, and decreases splanchnic blood flow

Pharmacodynamics Duration (immediate release formulation): SubQ: 6-12 hours

Pharmacokinetics

Absorption:

- SubQ: Rapid
- I.M. (Sandostatin LAR® Depot): 60% to 63% when compared with SubQ immediate release formulation

Distribution: V_d:

- Adults: 13.6 L/kg
- Adults with acromegaly: 21.6 ± 8.5 L

Metabolism: Extensive by the liver

Half-life: 1.7 hours

Time to peak serum concentration: SubQ: 0.4 hours

Elimination: 32% excreted unchanged in urine

Clearance:

- Adults: 10 L/hour
- Adults with acromegaly: 18 L/hour

Note: When using Sandostatin LAR® Depot formulation, steady state levels are achieved after 3 injections (3 months of therapy)

Usual Dosage Dosage should be individualized according to the patient's response

Sandostatin®:

Diarrhea:

Infants and Children (limited data from case reports):

I.V., SubQ: Doses of 1-10 mcg/kg every 12 hours have been used in children beginning at the low end of the range and increasing based upon the clinical response

I.V. continuous infusion: An initial 1 mcg/kg bolus dose followed by a continuous infusion of 1 mcg/kg/hour has been used successfully in several cases of severe diarrhea secondary to graft vs host disease

Adults:

SubQ: Initial: 50 mcg 1-2 times/day

I.V.: Initial: 50-100 mcg every 8 hours; increase by 100 mcg/dose at 48-hour intervals; maximum dose: 500 mcg every 8 hours

The following are effective dosing ranges for specific therapies: SubQ, I.V.:

Children (limited data in case reports):

Persistent hyperinsulinemic hypoglycemia of infancy (nesidioblastosis): 2-10 mcg/kg/day initially divided every 12 hours; increase dosage depending upon patient response by either using a more frequent interval (every 6-8 hours) or larger dose; doses of 40 mcg/kg/day have been used

GI bleed: 1 mcg/kg initial bolus followed by 1 mcg/kg/hour continuous infusion; titrate infusion rate to response; taper dose by 50% every 12 hours when no active bleeding occurs for 24 hours; may discontinue when dose is 25% of initial dose

Chylothorax: 0.5-4 mcg/kg/hour continuous infusion; titrate dose to response; case reports of effective dosage ranging between 0.3-40 mcg/kg/hour; treatment duration is usually 1-2 weeks but may vary with the clinical response

Treatment of sulfonylurea overdose: 1 mcg/kg/dose every 12 hours or a single 25 mcg dose; the duration of treatment is dependent upon the sulfonylurea ingested and its half-life.

Adults:

Carcinoid: 100-600 mcg/day in 2-4 divided doses

Chylothorax: 50-100 mcg every 8 hours; treatment duration is usually 1-2 weeks but may vary with the clinical response

VIPomas: 200-300 mcg/day in 2-4 divided doses; tachyphylaxis may occur requiring an increase in dosage up to 1000 mcg/day

Esophageal varices bleeding: I.V. bolus: 25-50 mcg followed by continuous I.V. infusion of 25-50 mcg/hour for 48 hours

Acromegaly: 50 mcg 3 times/day; increase as needed (usual requirement: 100 mcg 3 times/day); maximum dose: 500 mcg 3 times/day; hold dose for 4 weeks per year in patients who have been irradiated, to assess disease activity; resume therapy if growth hormone or somatomedin C (IGF-I) levels increase and signs and symptoms recur

AIDS-related diarrhea: 50-250 mcg every 8 hours; doses as high as 1500 mcg/day have been used; an improved response rate is reported in patients without infection-related diarrhea

Sandostatin LAR® Depot: May be used in patients who have responded to the immediate release formulation; Adults: I.M.:

Acromegaly: Initial: 20 mg at 4-week intervals for 3 months; dosage may be adjusted based upon the following:

Maintain same dosage **IF**: Growth hormone level <2.5 ng/mL, IGF-I normal, and clinical symptoms controlled

Increase dosage to 30 mg **IF**: Growth hormone level >2.5 ng/mL, IGF-I elevated, and clinical symptoms uncontrolled

Reduce dosage to 10 mg **IF**: Growth hormone level ≤1 ng/mL, IGF-I normal, and clinical symptoms controlled

[May increase dosage to maximum 40 mg every 4 weeks if 30 mg dosage ineffective; it is not recommended to administer dosage at intervals >4 weeks; hold dose for 8 weeks per year in patients who have been irradiated, to assess disease activity; resume therapy if growth hormone or somatomedin C (IGF-I) levels increase and signs and symptoms recur.]

VIPomas, carcinoid: Initial: 20 mg at 4-week intervals; due to the need for serum octreotide to reach therapeutically effective levels following initial injection for Sandostatin LAR® Depot, subcutaneous Sandostatin® injection should be continued at the current dosage **at the same time** for at least the first 2 weeks of therapy (some patients may require 3 or 4 weeks of such therapy). Adjust Sandostatin LAR® Depot dosage after 2 months of therapy depending upon patient response; doses >30 mg are not recommended

(Continued)

Octreotide Acetate *(Continued)*

Dosage adjustment in renal impairment: Clearance is decreased by 50% in patients with severe renal failure requiring dialysis; consider dosage modification in these patients

Administration Parenteral: Only Sandostatin® injection may be administered I.V., I.M., and SubQ; Sandostatin LAR® Depot may only be administered I.M.

I.V. infusion: Dilute Sandostatin® injection in 50-200 mL NS or D_5W and infuse over 15-30 minutes or over 24 hours as a continuous infusion; in emergency situations, may be administered undiluted by direct I.V. push over 3 minutes; see Stability for compatibility information; allow solution to come to room temperature before administration

I.M. administration: Reconstitute with provided diluent; see detailed instruction booklet for complete instructions; use immediately after reconstitution; administer into gluteal area only (avoid deltoid injections due to significant pain and discomfort at injection site)

Monitoring Parameters Baseline and periodic ultrasound evaluations for cholelithiasis, blood sugar, baseline and periodic thyroid function tests, fluid and electrolyte balance, fecal fat, and serum carotene determinations; for carcinoid, monitor urinary 5-hydroxyindole acetic acid (5-HIAA), plasma serotonin, plasma substance P; for VIPoma, monitor VIP; vitamin B_{12} levels (chronic therapy); for acromegaly: growth hormone levels, IGF-I (somatomedin C)

Reference Range Vasoactive intestinal peptide (VIP): <75 ng/L; levels vary considerably between laboratories; growth hormone level: <5 ng/mL; IGF-I (somatomedin C): males: <1.9 units/mL, females: <2.2 units/mL

Patient Information May cause dry mouth

Dosage Forms Excipient information presented when available (limited, particularly for generics); consult specific product labeling.

Injection, microspheres for suspension, as acetate [depot formulation]:
Sandostatin LAR®: 10 mg, 20 mg, 30 mg [with diluent and syringe]

Injection, solution, as acetate: 0.2 mg/mL (5 mL); 1 mg/mL (5 mL)
Sandostatin®: 0.2 mg/mL (5 mL); 1 mg/mL (5 mL)

Injection, solution, as acetate [preservative free]: 0.05 mg/mL (1 mL); 0.1 mg/mL (1 mL); 0.5 mg/mL (1 mL)
Sandostatin®: 0.05 mg/mL (1 mL); 0.1 mg/mL (1 mL); 0.5 mg/mL (1 mL)

References

Beckman RA, Siden R, Yanik GA, et al, "Continuous Octreotide Infusion for the Treatment of Secretory Diarrhea Caused by Acute Intestinal Graft-Versus-Host Disease in a Child," *J Pediatr Hematol Oncol*, 2000, 22(4):344-50.

Cheung Y, Leung MP, and Yip M, "Octreotide for Treatment of Postoperative Chylothorax," *J Pediatr*, 2001, 139(1):157-9.

Couper RT, Berzen A, Berall G, et al, "Clinical Response to the Long-Acting Somatostatin Analogue SMS 201-995 in a Child With Congenital Microvillus Atrophy," *Gut*, 1989, 30(7):1020-4.

Jaros W, Biller J, Greer S, et al, "Successful Treatment of Idiopathic Secretory Diarrhea of Infancy With the Somatostatin Analogue SMS 201-995," *Gastroenterology*, 1988, 94(1):189-93.

Katz MD and Erstad BL, "Octreotide, A New Somatostatin Analogue," *Clin Pharm*, 1989, 8(4):255-73.

Kalomenidis I, "Octreotide and chylothorax," Curr Opin Pulm Med, 2006, 12(4):264-7.

Pratap U, Slavik Z, Ofoe VD, et al, "Octreotide to Treat Postoperative Chylothorax After Cardiac Operations in Children," *Ann Thorac Surg*, 2001, 72(5):1740-2.

Siafakas C, Fox VL, and Nurko S, "Use of Octreotide for the Treatment of Severe Gastrointestinal Bleeding in Children," *J Pediatr Gastroenterol Nutr*, 1998, 26(3):356-9.

Stanley CA, "Hyperinsulinism in Infants and Children," *Pediatr Clin North Am*, 1997, 44(2):363-74.

♦ **Octreotide Acetate** *see* Octreotide Acetate *on page 1157*

♦ **Octreotide Acetate Injection (Can)** *see* Octreotide Acetate *on page 1157*

♦ **Octreotide Acetate Omega (Can)** *see* Octreotide Acetate *on page 1157*

♦ **Ocufen®** *see* Flurbiprofen *on page 688*

♦ **Ocuflox®** *see* Ofloxacin *on page 1161*

Ocular Lubricant (OK yoo lar LOO bri kant)

Index Terms Petrolatum White and Mineral Oil Ophthalmic Ointment

Therapeutic Category Lubricant, Ocular; Ophthalmic Agent, Miscellaneous

Use Ocular lubricant

Contraindications Hypersensitivity to any component

Warnings Discontinue if eye pain, vision change, redness or eye irritation occurs or if condition worsens or persists >72 hours

Adverse Reactions Ocular: Temporary blurring of vision, irritation

Stability Store away from heat

Mechanism of Action Forms an occlusive film on the surface of the eye to lubricate and protect the eye from drying

Usual Dosage Children and Adults: Ophthalmic: Apply 1/4" of ointment to the inside of the lower lid as needed

Administration Ophthalmic: Do not use with contact lenses; to avoid contamination, do not touch tip of container to any surface

Additional Information Contains petrolatum, mineral oil, chlorobutanol and lanolin alcohols

Dosage Forms Excipient information presented when available (limited, particularly for generics); consult specific product labeling.

Ointment, ophthalmic: 3.5 g

- **OcuNefrin™ [OTC]** *see* Phenylephrine *on page 1250*
- **Oesclim® (Can)** *see* Estradiol *on page 605*

Ofloxacin (oh FLOKS a sin)

Medication Safety Issues

Sound-alike/look-alike issues:

Floxin® may be confused with Flexeril®

Ocuflox® may be confused with Ocufen®

International issues:

Floxin® may be confused with Flogen® which is a brand name for naproxen in Mexico

Floxin® may be confused with Fluoxin® which is a brand name for fluoxetine in the Czech Republic and Romania

Floxin® may be confused with Flexin® which is a brand name for orphenadrine in Israel and indomethacin in Great Britain

U.S. Brand Names Floxin®; Ocuflox®

Canadian Brand Names Apo-Oflox®; Apo-Ofloxacin®; Floxin®; Novo-Ofloxacin; Ocuflox®; PMS-Ofloxacin

Index Terms Floxin Otic Singles

Therapeutic Category Antibiotic, Ophthalmic; Antibiotic, Otic; Antibiotic, Quinolone

Generic Available Yes: Tablet, ophthalmic solution

Use Treatment of acute bacterial exacerbations of chronic bronchitis, community-acquired pneumonia, uncomplicated skin and skin structure infections, urethral and cervical gonorrhea (acute, uncomplicated), urethritis and cervicitis (nongonococcal), pelvic inflammatory disease, uncomplicated cystitis, complicated urinary tract infections, and prostatitis caused by susceptible organisms including *S. pneumoniae, S. aureus, S. pyogenes, C. koseri, E. aerogenes, E. coli, H. influenzae, K. pneumoniae, N. gonorrhoeae, P. mirabilis, C. trachomatis,* and *P. aeruginosa*

Ophthalmic: Treatment of bacterial keratitis due to susceptible organisms including *P. aeruginosa, Propionibacterium acnes, S. marcescens, S. aureus, S. epidermidis,* and *S. pneumoniae*; treatment of severe bacterial conjunctivitis due to susceptible organisms including *Enterobacter cloacae, H. influenzae, P. mirabilis, P. aeruginosa, S. aureus, S. epidermidis,* or *S. pneumoniae*

Otic: Treatment of chronic suppurative otitis media with or without perforation of the tympanic membrane; instillation into the ear canal of patients with tympanostomy tubes for treatment of acute otitis media caused by susceptible *S. aureus, S. pneumoniae, H. influenzae, M. catarrhalis,* or *P. aeruginosa*; otitis externa caused by susceptible *S. aureus* or *P. aeruginosa*

Pregnancy Risk Factor C

Lactation Enters breast milk/not recommended (AAP rates "compatible")

Contraindications Hypersensitivity to ofloxacin, any component, or other quinolones; not recommended for use in pregnant women or during breast-feeding

Otic formulation: Patients with viral infections of the external ear canal

Warnings Oral formulation not recommended for use in children <18 years of age; ofloxacin has caused osteochondrosis in immature rats and dogs. Fluoroquinolones have caused arthropathy with erosions of the cartilage in weight-bearing joints of immature animals; Achilles tendonitis and tendon rupture have been reported with fluoroquinolones with risk increased in patients taking concomitant corticosteroids; prolonged use may result in superinfection; CNS stimulation and increased intracranial pressure may occur resulting in tremors, restlessness, confusion, and rarely hallucinations, depression, nightmares, suicidal ideation, or convulsive seizures; serious and occasionally fatal hypersensitivity and/or anaphylactic reactions have been reported often following the first dose. If these reactions occur, discontinue ofloxacin.

Precautions Use with caution in patients with known or suspected CNS disorders, seizure disorders, severe cerebral arteriosclerosis or renal impairment; modify dosage in patients with renal impairment. Rare cases of torsade de pointes have been reported in patients taking ofloxacin so use with caution in patients on concurrent therapy with Class Ia or Class III antiarrhythmics or in patients with known prolongation of QT interval, bradycardia, cardiomyopathy, hypokalemia, or hypomagnesemia

(Continued)

Ofloxacin *(Continued)*

Adverse Reactions

Cardiovascular: Cardiac failure, hypertension, hypotension, bradycardia, tachycardia, edema, torsade de pointes (rare), prolongation of QT interval, chest pain

Central nervous system: Dizziness, lightheadedness, vertigo, insomnia (more common with ofloxacin than other quinolones), fever, headache, increased intracranial pressure, seizures, fatigue, nervousness, restlessness, confusion, hallucinations, anxiety, suicidal thoughts, depression, encephalopathy, abnormal EEG

Dermatologic: Rash, pruritus, Stevens-Johnson syndrome, photosensitivity, urticaria, angioedema, toxic epidermal necrolysis, erythema multiforme

Endocrine & metabolic: Hypoglycemia, hyperglycemia, electrolyte abnormality

Gastrointestinal: Bitter taste, nausea, vomiting, diarrhea, constipation, anorexia, abdominal pain, pseudomembraneous colitis, pancreatitis

Genitourinary: Vaginitis

Hematologic: Granulocytopenia, leukopenia, thrombocytopenia, hemolytic anemia

Hepatic: Elevated liver enzymes, hepatic failure, jaundice

Neuromuscular & skeletal: Tremor, arthralgia, tendonitis, tendon rupture, myalgia, peripheral neuropathy

Ocular: Ophthalmic solution: Burning, stinging, itching, foreign body sensation, conjunctival hyperemia, ocular edema, redness, photophobia, blurred vision

Otic: Otic solution: Earache, tinnitus, otorrhagia

Renal: Interstitial nephritis, acute renal insufficiency, hematuria

Respiratory: Bronchospasm, respiratory distress, dyspnea

Miscellaneous: Anaphylaxis, serum sickness syndrome

Drug Interactions Cytochrome P450 isoenzyme CYP1A2 enzyme inhibitor

May alter blood glucose concentrations in diabetic patients receiving ofloxacin and antidiabetic medications concurrently. Concomitant use with corticosteroids may increase the risk of tendon rupture. May increase serum levels of cyclosporine, theophylline, methylxanthines, warfarin, and glyburide. Probenecid may increase ofloxacin levels. Decreased absorption with antacids containing aluminum, magnesium, and/or calcium, sucralfate, metal cations (ie, zinc, iron, copper, magnesium), and didanosine. Concomitant use with foscarnet or NSAIDs may increase risk of CNS stimulation and seizures. Concomitant use with other QT_c-prolonging agents (eg, Class Ia and Class III antiarrhythmics, erythromycin, cisapride, antipsychotics, and cyclic antidepressants) may result in arrhythmias such as torsade de pointes.

Food Interactions Calcium, dairy products, iron, mineral supplements, and enteral products may decrease ofloxacin concentrations.

Stability Store tablets, ophthalmic solution, and otic solution at room temperature.

Mechanism of Action Ofloxacin inhibits DNA gyrase (bacterial topoisomerase II) thereby inhibiting relaxation of supercoiled DNA and promoting breakage of DNA strands. DNA gyrase maintains the superhelical structure of DNA and is required for DNA replication, transcription, repair, recombination, and transposition.

Pharmacokinetics

Absorption:

- Oral: Well absorbed
- Ocular: Minimal absorption unless inflammation or epithelial defect is present
- Otic: Minimal absorption unless tympanic membrane is perforated

Distribution: Widely distributed into body tissues and fluids including blister fluid, cervix, lung, ovary, prostatic tissue, skin, and sputum; crosses the placenta; excreted into breast milk

- V_d: 2.4-3.5 L/kg

Protein binding: 20% to 32%

Bioavailability: Oral: 98%

Half-life, biphasic: 4-7.4 hours and 20-25 hours; prolonged with renal impairment

Time to peak serum concentration: Oral 1-2 hours

Elimination: 68% to 90% is excreted unchanged in urine; 4% to 8% excreted in feces; <10% is metabolized

Usual Dosage

Oral:

- Children: **Note:** Limited information regarding ofloxacin use in pediatric patients is currently available in the literature; some centers recommend doses of 15 mg/kg/day divided every 12 hours
- Adults:
  - Chronic bronchitis (acute exacerbation), community-acquired pneumonia, skin and skin structure infections (uncomplicated): 400 mg every 12 hours for 10 days
  - Urethral and cervical gonorrhea (acute, uncomplicated): 400 mg as a single dose
  - Cervicitis/urethritis (nongonococcal) due to *C. trachomatis* or mixed infections due to *C. trachomatis* and *N. gonorrhoeae*: 300 mg every 12 hours for 7 days
  - Pelvic inflammatory disease: 400 mg every 12 hours for 10-14 days

Cystitis (uncomplicated): 200 mg every 12 hours for 3-7 days
UTI (complicated): 200 mg every 12 hours for 10 days
Prostatitis: 300 mg every 12 hours for 6 weeks

Ophthalmic: Children >1 year and Adults:

Conjunctivitis: Instill 1-2 drops in affected eye(s) every 2-4 hours while awake for the first 2 days, then 4 times/day for an additional 5 days

Corneal ulcer: Instill 1-2 drops in affected eye(s) every 30 minutes while awake and every 4-6 hours at night for the first 2 days; then starting day 3, instill 1-2 drops every hour while awake for 4-6 additional days; thereafter, 1-2 drops 4 times/day until clinical cure is achieved.

Otic:

Acute otitis media with tympanostomy tubes: Children >1 year to 12 years: Instill 5 drops (0.25 mL) into the affected ear(s) twice daily for 10 days

Chronic suppurative otitis media with perforated tympanic membranes: Adolescents ≥12 years and Adults: Instill 10 drops (0.5 mL) into the affected ear(s) twice daily for 10-14 days

Otitis externa:

Children 6 months to 13 years: Instill 5 drops into the affected ear(s) once daily for 7 days

Adolescents ≥13 years and Adults: Instill 10 drops into the affected ear(s) once daily for 7 days

Dosage adjustment in renal impairment: Adults: Oral:

Cl_{cr} 20-50 mL/minute: Administer usual dose every 24 hours
Cl_{cr} <20 mL/minute: Administer half the usual dose every 24 hours

Dosage adjustment in hepatic impairment: Severe impairment: Maximum dose: 400 mg/day

Administration

Oral: May administer ofloxacin tablets with or without food; avoid antacids, vitamins with iron or minerals, sucralfate, or didanosine; use within 2 hours of administration; drink plenty of fluids to maintain proper hydration and urine output

Ophthalmic: Not for subconjunctival or direct injection into the anterior chamber of the eye. Apply gentle pressure to lacrimal sac during and immediately following instillation (1 minute) or instruct patient to gently close eyelid after administration, to decrease systemic absorption of ophthalmic drops; avoid contact of bottle tip with skin or eye. Remove contact lenses prior to administration (ophthalmic solution contains benzalkonium chloride which may adsorb to soft contact lenses); lenses may be inserted 15 minutes after administration.

Otic: Not for ophthalmic use or injection. Gently clean any discharge that can be easily removed from the outer ear. Warm otic solution by holding bottle in hand for 1-2 minutes prior to instillation. The tip of the bottle should not touch the fingers, ear, or any surface. Patient should lie on side with affected ear upward. For middle ear infections, gently press the tragus 4 times in a pumping motion to allow the drops to pass through the hole or tube in the eardrum and into the middle ear. For otitis externa infection, pull the outer ear upward and backward to allow the ear drops to flow down into the ear canal. Patient should remain on his/her side for at least 5 minutes. If necessary, repeat procedure for the other ear.

Monitoring Parameters Patients receiving concurrent ofloxacin and theophylline should have serum levels of theophylline monitored; monitor INR in patients receiving warfarin; monitor blood glucose in patients receiving antidiabetic agents; monitor renal, hepatic, hematopoietic function, and electrolytes periodically; number and type of stools/day for diarrhea

Ophthalmic: Slit-lamp biomicroscopy and fluorescein staining may be necessary
Otic: Presence of otorrhea, cultures

Patient Information Avoid contaminating otic and ophthalmic solution containers. Drink plenty of fluids; may cause dizziness or lightheadedness and impair ability to perform activities requiring mental alertness or physical coordination; notify physician if tendon pain or swelling, burning, tingling, numbness, or weakness develops, or if palpitations, chest pains, signs of allergy occurs; burning, tingling, numbness, or weakness develop; difficulty breathing, or persistent diarrhea occurs. May cause photosensitivity reactions (eg, exposure to sunlight may cause severe sunburn, skin rash, redness, or itching); avoid exposure to sunlight and artificial light sources (sunlamps, tanning booth/bed); wear protective clothing, wide-brimmed hats, sunglasses, and lip sunscreen (SPF ≥15); use a sunscreen [broad-spectrum sunscreen or physical sunscreen (preferred) or sunblock with SPF ≥15]; contact physician if reaction occurs.

Nursing Implications Do not administer antacids containing calcium, aluminum, or magnesium, iron, sucralfate, multivitamin preparations with zinc, didanosine chewable/buffered tablets or pediatric powder for oral solution with or within 2 hours before or 2 hours after a ofloxacin dose; ensure adequate patient hydration

Dosage Forms Excipient information presented when available (limited, particularly for generics); consult specific product labeling. [DSC] = Discontinued product
(Continued)

Ofloxacin *(Continued)*

Solution, ophthalmic (Ocuflox®): 0.3% (5 mL; 10 mL [DSC]) [contains benzalkonium chloride]

Solution, otic:

Floxin®: 0.3% (5 mL, 10 mL) [contains benzalkonium chloride]

Floxin® Otic Singles™: 0.3% (0.25 mL) [contains benzalkonium chloride; packaged as 2 single-dose containers per pouch, 10 pouches per carton, total net volume 5 mL]

Tablet (Floxin®): 200 mg, 300 mg, 400 mg

References

Alghasham AA and Nahata MC, "Clinical Use of Fluoroquinolones in Children," *Ann Pharmacother*, 2000, 34(3):347-59.

♦ **OKT3** *see* Muromonab-CD3 *on page 1092*

♦ **Oleovitamin A** *see* Vitamin A *on page 1619*

♦ **Oleum Ricini** *see* Castor Oil *on page 300*

Olsalazine (ole SAL a zeen)

Medication Safety Issues

Sound-alike/look-alike issues:

Olsalazine may be confused with olanzapine

Dipentum® may be confused with Dilantin®

U.S. Brand Names Dipentum®

Canadian Brand Names Dipentum®

Index Terms Olsalazine Sodium

Therapeutic Category 5-Aminosalicylic Acid Derivative; Anti-inflammatory Agent

Generic Available No

Use Maintenance of remission of ulcerative colitis in patients intolerant to sulfasalazine

Pregnancy Risk Factor C

Lactation Enters breast milk/use caution (monitor for diarrhea)

Contraindications Hypersensitivity to olsalazine, salicylates, or any component

Warnings Diarrhea is a common adverse effect of olsalazine

Precautions Use with caution in patients with hypersensitivity to sulfasalazine, salicylates, or mesalamine

Adverse Reactions

Cardiovascular: Pericarditis, heart block, hypertension, orthostatic hypotension, edema, chest pain, tachycardia

Central nervous system: Headache, fatigue, drowsiness, depression, insomnia, vertigo, fever

Dermatologic: Erythema nodosum, photosensitivity, rash, pruritus

Gastrointestinal: Diarrhea, cramps, nausea, dyspepsia, bloating, vomiting, pancreatitis, rectal bleeding, xerostomia

Genitourinary: Urinary frequency, dysuria

Hematologic: Leukopenia, neutropenia, lymphopenia, eosinophilia, thrombocytopenia

Hepatic: Mild cholestatic hepatitis, elevated AST and ALT

Neuromuscular & skeletal: Arthralgia, tremor, paresthesia

Ocular: Blurred vision, dry eyes

Renal: Hematuria, proteinuria

Respiratory: Bronchospasm, respiratory infection

Drug Interactions Increases effects of warfarin

Mechanism of Action Olsalazine is a sodium salt of a salicylate compound that is effectively bioconverted by colonic bacteria to 5-aminosalicylic acid (5-ASA). The exact mechanism of action appears to be topical rather than systemic. It may diminish colonic inflammation by blocking cyclooxygenase and inhibiting colon prostaglandin production in the bowel mucosa.

Pharmacokinetics

Absorption: <3%; very little intact olsalazine is systemically absorbed

Protein binding: >99%

Metabolism: Mostly by colonic bacteria to the active drug, 5-aminosalicylic acid

Bioavailability: 2.4%

Half-life, elimination: 56 minutes (in serum)

Elimination: Primarily in feces; <1% eliminated in urine

Usual Dosage Adults: Oral: 1 g/day in 2 divided doses

Administration Oral: Administer with food in evenly divided doses

Patient Information Contact physician if diarrhea occurs. May cause dry mouth. May rarely cause photosensitivity reactions (eg, exposure to sunlight may cause severe sunburn, skin rash, redness, or itching); avoid direct exposure to sunlight.

Dosage Forms Excipient information presented when available (limited, particularly for generics); consult specific product labeling.
Capsule, as sodium: 250 mg

- **Olsalazine Sodium** *see* Olsalazine *on page 1164*
- **Olux®** *see* Clobetasol *on page 383*
- **Olux-E™** *see* Clobetasol *on page 383*

Omalizumab (oh mah lye ZOO mab)

U.S. Brand Names Xolair®
Canadian Brand Names Xolair®
Index Terms rhuMAb-E25
Therapeutic Category Monoclonal Antibody, Anti-Asthmatic
Generic Available No
Use Treatment of moderate to severe, persistent allergic asthma not adequately controlled with inhaled corticosteroids
Pregnancy Risk Factor B
Lactation Excretion in breast milk unknown/use caution
Contraindications Hypersensitivity to omalizumab or any component
Warnings Not indicated for use in the control of acute asthma symptoms. Anaphylaxis, including delayed-onset anaphylaxis, has been reported following administration; reactions usually occur within 2 hours of administration, but may occur up to 24 hours and in some cases >24 hours after treatment. Patients should receive treatment only under direct medical supervision and be observed for a minimum of 2 hours following administration; providers and patients should have appropriate treatment for anaphylaxis available. Hypersensitivity reactions may occur following any dose, even during chronic therapy; discontinue therapy following any severe reaction. Injection site reactions typically occur within 1 hour postinjection, last <8 days, and generally decrease in frequency after subsequent doses. Safety and efficacy in children <12 years of age has not been established.

Malignant neoplasms of varying types (breast, nonmelanoma skin, prostate, and parotid) were observed in 0.5% of patients during clinical trials (compared with 0.2% in controls); the majority of these patients received omalizumab for <1 year; risk of long-term exposure to omalizumab is not known. Systemic or inhaled corticosteroid use should not be abruptly discontinued upon initiation of omalizumab therapy; gradual tapering under medical supervision is recommended. In a one year clinical trial in Brazil, patients with increased risk of geohelminthic infections (roundworm, hookworm, whipworm, threadworm) experienced an increase in geohelminthic infections when compared with the control group (42% vs 53%).

Precautions Dosage and frequency of administration are dependent upon the serum total IgE level and body weight. Total IgE level must be measured prior to beginning treatment. Total IgE levels are elevated during treatment and remain elevated for up to one year after the discontinuation of treatment. Remeasurement of IgE levels during omalizumab treatment should not be used as a guide to dosage. Remeasurement of IgE levels may be used after treatment has been discontinued for at least one year.

Adverse Reactions
Central nervous system: Headache, dizziness, fatigue
Dermatologic: Urticaria, dermatitis, pruritus
Local: Injection site reactions (bruising, redness, warmth, burning, stinging, pain, induration, and inflammation)
Neuromuscular & skeletal: Arthralgia, leg pain, arm pain
Respiratory: Upper respiratory infections, sinusitis, pharyngitis
Miscellaneous: Anaphylaxis, hypersensitivity reactions, viral infections

Drug Interactions None as yet have been identified
Stability Store in refrigerator at 2°C to 8°C (36°F to 46°F); omalizumab is provided in a single use vial with no preservatives; the reconstituted solution is stable for 4 hours at room temperature and 8 hours refrigerated
Mechanism of Action Omalizumab is an IgG monoclonal antibody which binds to free (unbound) IgE and prevents the binding of IgE to the high-affinity IgE receptor on the surface of mast cells and basophils. By decreasing bound IgE, the activation and release of mediators in the allergic response (early and late phase) is limited. Both the free (unbound) IgE serum level and the number of high-affinity IgE receptors are decreased. Long-term treatment in patients with allergic asthma showed a decrease in asthma exacerbations and corticosteroid usage.
Pharmacokinetics
Absorption: Slow after SubQ administration
Distribution: V_d: 78 ± 32 mL/kg
(Continued)

Omalizumab *(Continued)*

Metabolism: Hepatic: IgG degradation by reticuloendothelial system and endothelial cells
Bioavailability: Absolute: 68%
Half-life: Adults: 1-4 weeks
Time to peak serum concentration: 7-8 days
Excretion: Primarily via hepatic degradation; intact IgG may be secreted in bile
Clearance: 2.4 ± 1.1 mL/kg/day

Usual Dosage Dosage and frequency of administration are dependent upon the serum total IgE level and body weight. Measure total IgE level prior to beginning treatment. Total IgE levels are elevated during treatment and remain elevated for up to one year after the discontinuation of treatment. Remeasurement of IgE levels during omalizumab treatment should not be used as a guide to dosage.

SubQ: Children ≥12 years and Adults: Asthma:
IgE ≥30-100 international units/mL:
30-90 kg: 150 mg every 4 weeks
>90-150 kg: 300 mg every 4 weeks
IgE >100-200 international units/mL:
30-90 kg: 300 mg every 4 weeks
>90-150 kg: 225 mg every 2 weeks
IgE >200-300 international units/mL:
30-60 kg: 300 mg every 4 weeks
>60-90 kg: 225 mg every 2 weeks
>90-150 kg: 300 mg every 2 weeks
IgE >300-400 international units/mL:
30-70 kg: 225 mg every 2 weeks
>70-90 kg: 300 mg every 2 weeks
>90 kg: Do not use*
IgE >400-500 international units/mL:
30-70 kg: 300 mg every 2 weeks
>70-90 kg: 375 mg every 2 weeks
>90 kg: Do not use*
IgE >500-600 international units/mL:
30-60 kg: 300 mg every 2 weeks
>60-70 kg: 375 mg every 2 weeks
>70 kg: Do not use*
IgE >600-700 international units/mL:
30-60 kg: 375 mg every 2 weeks
>60 kg: Do not use*

*Dosage has not been studied and approved for this weight and IgE level

Administration SubQ: Reconstitute 150 mg vial with 1.4 mL SWI; swirl vial for approximately 1 minute to evenly wet powder; repeat swirling for 5-10 seconds every 5 minutes in order to dissolve remaining solids; dissolution time is at least 20 minutes. Reconstituted solution will be viscous with no visible gel-like particles present in solution. Do not use if contents of vial do not dissolve within 40 minutes. Resulting concentration is 150 mg/1.2 mL (125 mg/mL). Due to viscosity, injection may take 5-10 seconds to administer. Doses >150 mg should be divided into more than one injection site.

Monitoring Parameters Baseline total serum IgE, pulmonary function tests

Reference Range See Usual Dosage

Patient Information Do not alter asthma medications without consulting physician.

Additional Information Omalizumab was used successfully in a double-blind, randomized, placebo-controlled study of 334 children between the ages of 6-12 years; omalizumab dosage was based on body weight and initial serum total IgE. Patients received omalizumab at either 2- or 4-week intervals with a dosage equal to 0.016 mg/kg/IgE (international units/mL) per 4 weeks. 55% of patients were able to discontinue corticosteroid use (Milgrom, 2003).

Dosage Forms Excipient information presented when available (limited, particularly for generics); consult specific product labeling.
Injection, powder for reconstitution [preservative free]:
Xolair®: 150 mg [contains sucrose 145.5 g]

References

Berger W, Gupta N, McAlary M, et al, "Evaluation of Long-Term Safety of the Anti-IgE Antibody, Omalizumab, in Children with Allergic Asthma," *Ann Allergy Asthma Immunol*, 2003, 91(2):182-8.

Casale TB, Condemi J, LaForce C, et al, "Effect of Omalizumab on Symptoms of Seasonal Allergic Rhinitis: A Randomized Controlled Trial," *JAMA*, 2001, 286(23):2956-67.

Milgrom H, Berger W, Nayak A, et al, "Treatment of Childhood Asthma With Anti-Immunoglobulin E Antibody (Omalizumab)," *Pediatrics*, 2001, 108(2):E36.

Milgrom H, Fick RB Jr, Su JQ, et al, "Treatment of Allergic Asthma With Monoclonal Anti-IgE Antibody. rhuMAb-E25 Study Group," *Engl J Med*, 1999, 341(26):1966-73.

Omeprazole (oh ME pray zol)

Medication Safety Issues

Sound-alike/look-alike issues:

Prilosec® may be confused with Plendil®, Prevacid®, predniSONE, prilocaine, Prinivil®, Proventil®, Prozac®

International issues:

Norpramin®: Brand name for desipramine in the U.S.

U.S. Brand Names Prilosec®; Prilosec OTC™ [OTC]

Canadian Brand Names Apo-Omeprazole®; Losec®; Losec MUPS®

Therapeutic Category Gastric Acid Secretion Inhibitor; Gastrointestinal Agent, Gastric or Duodenal Ulcer Treatment; Proton Pump Inhibitor

Generic Available Yes: Delayed release capsule

Use Treatment and maintenance of healing of severe erosive esophagitis (grade 2 or above); treatment of active duodenal ulcer; treatment of active benign gastric ulcers; treatment of symptomatic gastroesophageal reflux disease (GERD); treatment of pathological hypersecretory conditions; treatment of peptic ulcer disease; adjunctive treatment of duodenal ulcers associated with *Helicobacter pylori*; relief of frequent heartburn (OTC use)

Pregnancy Risk Factor C

Lactation Enters breast milk/not recommended

Contraindications Hypersensitivity to omeprazole, substituted benzimidazole proton pump inhibitors (eg, esomeprazole, lansoprazole), or any component; Zegerid™ use in patients with metabolic alkalosis and hypocalcemia

Warnings In long-term (2-year) studies in rats, omeprazole produced a dose-related increase in gastric carcinoid tumors. While available endoscopic evaluations and histologic examinations of biopsy specimens from human stomachs have not detected a risk from short-term exposure to omeprazole, further human data on the effect of sustained hypochlorhydria and hypergastrinemia are needed to rule out the possibility of an increased risk for the development of tumors in humans receiving long-term therapy. Symptomatic response to therapy does not prelude the presence of GI malignancy. Use of gastric acid inhibitors including proton pump inhibitors and H_2 blockers has been associated with an increased risk for development of acute gastroenteritis and community-acquired pneumonia (Canani, 2006). Powder for suspension (Zegerid™) contains sodium bicarbonate; chronic use may lead to systemic alkalosis, edema, and weight gain.

Precautions Use powder for suspension (Zegerid™) with caution in patients with Bartter's syndrome, hypokalemia, and respiratory alkalosis due to high content of sodium bicarbonate; avoid use in patient's on sodium restrictive diets

Adverse Reactions

Cardiovascular: Chest pain, tachycardia, bradycardia, palpitations, hypertension, edema (see Warnings)

Central nervous system: Headache, dizziness, vertigo, insomnia, confusion, anxiety, hemifacial dysesthesia, nervousness, fever, fatigue, malaise, depression, aggression, hallucinations

Dermatologic: Rash, dry skin, urticaria, pruritus, alopecia, toxic epidermal necrolysis (rare), Stevens-Johnson syndrome (rare), erythema multiforme, hyperhydrosis

Endocrine & metabolic: Hypoglycemia, hyponatremia, weight gain, gynecomastia, metabolic alkalosis (Zegerid™; see Warnings)

Gastrointestinal: Diarrhea, nausea, abdominal pain, vomiting, constipation, flatulence, discoloration of feces, irritable colon, xerostomia, anorexia, dysgeusia, abdominal pain, atrophic gastritis, pancreatitis (some fatal), anorexia, fecal discoloration, gastric fundic polyps, mucosal atrophy of tongue, taste perversion

Genitourinary: Urinary frequency

Hematologic: Agranulocytosis, pancytopenia, thrombocytopenia, anemia, leukocytosis, hemolytic anemia

Hepatic: Hepatitis, elevated liver function tests, jaundice, liver necrosis

Neuromuscular & skeletal: Muscle cramps, myalgia, arthralgia, leg pain, paresthesia, back pain, joint pain

Ocular: Blurred vision, ocular irritation, optic atrophy, dry eyes, anterior ischemic optic neuropathy, optic neuritis, double vision

Otic: Tinnitus, otitis media

Renal: Hematuria, pyuria, proteinuria, glycosuria, interstitial nephritis, UTI, elevated serum creatinine

Respiratory: Pharyngeal pain, cough, epistaxis, URI

Miscellaneous: Hypersensitivity reactions

Drug Interactions Cytochrome P450 isoenzyme CYP1A2 inducer; isoenzyme CYP2C8, CYP2C18, CYP2C19, and CYP3A3/4 substrate; isoenzyme CYP2C9, CYP3A3/4, CYP2C8, and CYP2C19 inhibitor

(Continued)

Omeprazole *(Continued)*

Omeprazole inhibits oxidative metabolism; the full potential related to specific drugs remains to be determined; decreases absorption of ketoconazole, itraconazole, iron salts, ampicillin esters; increases half-life (decreased clearance) of diazepam, phenytoin, and warfarin; may increase absorption of digoxin and didanosine; may decrease elimination of methotrexate; clarithromycin may increase bioavailability of omeprazole

Food Interactions A 25% reduction in peak plasma concentration was measured when the 20 mg capsule was mixed with applesauce; there was no change in AUC; the clinical significance is unknown. There was no change in peak plasma level or AUC when the 40 mg capsule was mixed with applesauce. Administration of omeprazole powder for suspension (Zegerid™) 1 hour after a meal reduced the AUC by 24% and peak plasma level by 63%.

Stability Omeprazole stability is a function of pH; it is rapidly degraded in acidic media, but has acceptable stability under alkaline conditions. Each capsule of omeprazole contains enteric coated granules to prevent omeprazole degradation by gastric acidity.

Mechanism of Action Suppresses gastric acid secretion by inhibiting the parietal cell membrane enzyme (H^+/K^+)-ATPase or proton pump; demonstrates antimicrobial activity against *Helicobacter pylori*

Pharmacodynamics

Onset of action: 1 hour
Maximum effect: 2 hours
Duration: 72 hours
Maximum secretory inhibition: 4 days

Pharmacokinetics

Absorption: Rapid
Protein binding: 95%
Metabolism: Extensive first-pass metabolism in the liver
Bioavailability: 30% to 40%; improves slightly with repeated administration; excreted into breast milk (peak concentration in breast milk <7% of corresponding peak plasma concentration)
Half-life: Adults: 0.5-1 hour; chronic hepatic disease: 3 hours
Time to peak serum concentration: 0.5-3.5 hours
Elimination:
Clearance: Adults: 500-600 mL/minute; chronic hepatic disease: 70 mL/minute

Note: Half-life and AUC were significantly reduced for omeprazole suspension when compared with an equivalent dose via the commercially available capsule in 7 adults (Song, 2001).

Usual Dosage Oral:

GERD, ulcers, esophagitis:

Children: 1 mg/kg/day once or twice daily; range of effective dosages in the literature: 0.2-3.5 mg/kg/day (Hassall, 2000; Zimmermann, 2001). Higher doses may be necessary in children between 1-6 years of age due to increased metabolic clearance (Andersson, 2000). In critically ill children to maintain gastric pH >5, administration every 6-8 hours may be necessary (1.5-2 mg/kg/day) (Kaufman, 2002)

Manufacturer's recommendations (as an alternative): Children ≥2 years:
≤20 kg: 10 mg once daily
>20 kg: 20 mg once daily

Adolescents and Adults:
Active duodenal ulcer: 20 mg/day for 4-8 weeks
Gastric ulcers: 40 mg/day for 4-8 weeks
GERD or severe erosive esophagitis: 20 mg/day for 4-8 weeks
Maintenance of healing of erosive esophagitis: 20 mg/day
Pathological hypersecretory conditions: 60 mg/day to start; doses up to 120 mg 3 times/day have been administered; administer daily doses >80 mg in divided doses
Frequent heartburn (≥2 times/week): 20 mg/day for 14 days

Adjunctive therapy of duodenal ulcers associated with *Helicobacter pylori* [in combination with antibiotic therapy either clarithromycin or clarithromycin and amoxicillin]:

Children (Gottrand, 2001):
15-30 kg: 10 mg twice daily
>30 kg: 20 mg twice daily

Adults: 20 mg twice daily for 10 days (in combination with two antibiotics) or 40 mg once daily for 14 days

Note: If an ulcer is present at the time of initial therapy the recommended duration of treatment should be extended an additional 18 days (dual therapy) or 14 days (triple therapy)

Administration Oral: Administer before food or meals; capsule should be swallowed whole, do not chew or crush; because the enteric coating of granules will dissolve in alkaline pH, administration via NG tube should be in acidic juice (eg, apple juice or cranberry juice); stable 30 minutes after mixing; may add contents of capsule to applesauce and swallow immediately; do not crush or chew granules; to administer via jejunostomy tube, crush the granules and dissolve in a mixture of water to which a crushed 650 mg sodium bicarbonate tablet has been added. Dilute 20 mg or 40 mg packet of powder for suspension (Zegerid®) in 15-30 mL water; stir and drink immediately; refill cup with water and drink again; do not mix with other liquids. When administering powder for suspension through a feeding tube, dilute in 20 mL water. For patients receiving continuous feedings, hold feedings for 3 hours before and 1 hour after administration of omeprazole.

Patient Information May cause dry mouth; do not chew or crush granules

Dosage Forms Excipient information presented when available (limited, particularly for generics); consult specific product labeling.

Capsule, delayed release: 10 mg, 20 mg

Prilosec®: 10 mg, 20 mg, 40 mg

Tablet, delayed release:

Prilosec OTC™: 20 mg

Extemporaneous Preparations Omeprazole 2 mg/mL suspension may be made by adding 100 mL 8.4% sodium bicarbonate solution to the contents of ten 20 mg omeprazole capsules; stir for 30 minutes; protect from light; stable 14 days at room temperature and 45 days refrigerated

DiGiacinto JL, Olsen KM, Bergman KL, et al, "Stability of Suspension Formulations of Lansoprazole and Omeprazole Stored in Amber-colored Plastic Oral Syringes," *Ann Pharmacother*, 2000, 34(5):600-4.

References

Andersson T, Hassall E, Lundborg P, et al, "Pharmacokinetics of Orally Administered Omeprazole in Children. International Pediatric Omeprazole Pharmacokinetic Group," *Am J Gastroenterol*, 2000, 95(11):3101-6.

Canani RB, Cirillo P, Roggero P, et al, "Therapy With Gastric Acidity Inhibitors Increases the Risk of Acute Gastroenteritis and Community-Acquired Pneumonia in Children," *Pediatrics*, 2006, 117(5):e817-20.

Gibbons TE and Gold BD, "The Use of Proton Pump Inhibitors in Children: A Comprehensive Review," *Paediatr Drugs*, 2003, 5(1):25-40.

Gottrand F, Kalach N, Spyckerelle C, et al, "Omeprazole Combined With Amoxicillin and Clarithromycin in the Eradication of *Helicobacter pylori* in Children With Gastritis: A Prospective Randomized Double-Blind Trial," *J Pediatr*, 2001, 139(5):664-8.

Gunasekaran TS and Hassall EG, "Efficacy and Safety of Omeprazole for Severe Gastroesophageal Reflux in Children," *J Pediatr*, 1993, 123(1):148-54.

Hassall E, Israel D, Shepherd R, "Omeprazole for Treatment of Chronic Erosive Esophagitis in Children: A Multicenter Study of Efficacy, Safety, Tolerability and Dose Requirements. International Pediatric Omeprazole Study Group," *J Pediatr*, 2000, 137(6):800-7.

Kane DL, "Administration of Omeprazole (Prilosec™) in the Atypical Patient," *Int J Pharm Compounding*, 1997, 1(1):13.

Kato S, Ebina K, Fujii K, et al, "Effect of Omeprazole in the Treatment of Refractory Acid-Related Diseases in Childhood: Endoscopic Healing and Twenty-Four Hour Intragastric Acidity," *J Pediatr*, 1996, 128(3):415-21.

Kaufman SS, Lyden ER, Brown CR, et al, "Omeprazole Therapy in Pediatric Patients After Liver and Intestinal Transplantation," *J Pediatr Gastroenterol Nutr*, 2002, 34(2):194-8.

Song JC, Quercia RA, Fan C, et al, "Pharmacokinetic Comparison of Omeprazole Capsules and a Simplified Omeprazole Suspension," *Am J Health Syst Pharm*, 2001, 58(8):689-94.

Zimmermann AE, Walters JK, Katona BG, et al, "A Review of Omeprazole Use in the Treatment of Acid-Related Disorders in Children," *Clin Ther*, 2001, 23(5):660-79.

- **Omnicef®** *see* Cefdinir *on page 305*
- **Omnil Gel™ [OTC]** *see* Fluoride *on page 675*
- **Omnitrope™** *see* Human Growth Hormone *on page 769*
- **Oncaspar®** *see* Pegaspargase *on page 1224*

Ondansetron (on DAN se tron)

Medication Safety Issues

Sound-alike/look-alike issues:

Ondansetron may be confused with dolasetron, granisetron, palonosetron

Zofran® may be confused with Zantac®, Zosyn®

Related Information

Compatibility of Chemotherapy and Related Supportive Care Medications *on page 1777*

U.S. Brand Names Zofran®; Zofran® ODT

Canadian Brand Names Apo-Ondansetron®; Zofran®; Zofran® ODT

Index Terms GR38032R; Ondansetron Hydrochloride

Therapeutic Category 5-HT_3 Receptor Antagonist; Antiemetic

Generic Available Yes

(Continued)

Ondansetron *(Continued)*

Use Prevention of nausea and vomiting associated with highly emetogenic cancer chemotherapy or radiotherapy; prevention of postoperative nausea and vomiting; treatment of hyperemesis gravidarum (unlabeled use)

Pregnancy Risk Factor B

Lactation Excretion in breast milk unknown/use caution

Contraindications Hypersensitivity to ondansetron, other 5-HT_3 receptor antagonists, or any component

Warnings Zofran® solution contains sodium benzoate; benzoic acid (benzoate) is a metabolite of benzyl alcohol; large amounts of benzyl alcohol (≥99 mg/kg/day) have been associated with a potentially fatal toxicity ("gasping syndrome") in neonates; *in vitro* and animal studies have shown that benzoate displaces bilirubin from protein binding sites; avoid use of Zofran® solution in neonates.

Precautions Zofran® ODT tablets contain aspartame; use with caution in patients with phenylketonuria

Adverse Reactions

Cardiovascular: Tachycardia, bradycardia, angina, syncope, flushing, hypotension, palpitation

Central nervous system: Lightheadedness, seizures, headache, dizziness, drowsiness, sedation, fatigue, fever, shivers

Dermatologic: Rash, local injection site reaction, urticaria

Endocrine & metabolic: Hypokalemia (rare)

Gastrointestinal: Constipation, diarrhea, abdominal pain, xerostomia, hiccups

Hepatic: Transient elevations in liver enzymes

Neuromuscular & skeletal: Weakness, musculoskeletal pain, tremor, twitching, ataxia, acute dystonic reaction (rare)

Ocular: Blurred vision (transient, following infusion), oculogyric crisis

Respiratory: Bronchospasm, dyspnea, laryngeal edema, laryngospasm, stridor

Miscellaneous: Hypersensitivity reactions

Drug Interactions Cytochrome P450 isoenzyme CYP1A2, CYP2D6, CYP2E1, and CYP3A3/4 substrate

No documented drug interactions; however, ondansetron does contain the same imidazole nucleus as cimetidine and omeprazole; patients receiving concurrent theophylline, phenytoin, or warfarin should be followed closely

Stability

Compatible for 7 days at room temperature when diluted in saline or dextrose solutions; Y-site injection compatibility with bleomycin, carboplatin, carmustine, chlorpromazine, cisplatin, cyclophosphamide, cytarabine, dacarbazine, dactinomycin, daunorubicin, dexamethasone, diphenhydramine, doxorubicin, droperidol, etoposide, fludarabine, ifosfamide, mechlorethamine, methotrexate, mesna, metoclopramide, mitoxantrone, prochlorperazine, promethazine, teniposide, vinblastine, and vincristine

Incompatible with acyclovir, ampicillin, aminophylline, furosemide, ganciclovir, lorazepam, methylprednisolone, and piperacillin

Mechanism of Action Selective 5-HT_3 receptor antagonist, blocking serotonin, both peripherally on vagal nerve terminals and centrally in the chemoreceptor trigger zone

Pharmacokinetics

Absorption: Oral: 100%; nonlinear absorption occurs with increasing oral doses; Zofran® ODT tablets are bioequivalent to Zofran® tablets; absorption does not occur via oral mucosa

Distribution: V_d:
- Children: Surgical patients:
  - 1-4 months: 3.5 L/kg
  - 5-24 months: 2.3 L/kg
  - 3-12 years: 1.65 L/kg
- Children: Cancer patients: 4-18 years: 1.9 L/kg
- Adults: 1.9 L/kg

Protein binding, plasma: 70% to 76%

Metabolism: Extensive first-pass metabolism; primarily by hydroxylation, followed by glucuronidation and sulfate conjugation

Bioavailability: Oral: 50% to 70% due to significant first-pass metabolism; in cancer patients (adult) 85% to 87% bioavailability possibly related to changes in metabolism

Half-life:
- Children: 1-4 months: 6.7 hours; 5 months to 12 years: 2.9 hours
- Adults: 3.5-5.5 hours

Elimination: In urine and feces; <5% of the parent drug is recovered unchanged in urine

Clearance:
Children: Surgical patients:
1-4 months: 0.401 L/kg/hour
5-24 months: 0.581 L/kg/hour
3-12 years: 0.439 L/kg/hour
Children: Cancer patients: 4-18 years: 0.599 L/kg/hour
Adults (normal):
19-40 years: 0.381 L/kg/hour
61-74 years: 0.319 L/kg/hour
>75 years: 0.262 L/kg/hour

Usual Dosage

Prevention of chemotherapy- or radiotherapy-induced nausea and vomiting:
Oral (all doses given 30 minutes before chemotherapy or 1-2 hours prior to radiotherapy and repeated at 8-hour intervals):
Children <4 years: No FDA-approved oral dosage; however, the following dosages based upon body surface area have been used:
<0.3 m^2: 1 mg 3 times/day
0.3-0.6 m^2: 2 mg 3 times/day
0.6-1 m^2: 3 mg 3 times/day
>1 m^2: 4 mg 3 times/day
or
Children 4-11 years: 4 mg 3 times/day
Children >11 years and Adults: 8 mg 3 times/day or 24 mg once daily
Adults: Total body irradiation: 8 mg 1-2 hours before each fraction of radiotherapy administered each day
Single high-dose fraction radiotherapy to abdomen: 8 mg 1-2 hours before irradiation, then 8 mg every 8 hours after first dose for 1-2 days after completion of radiotherapy
Daily fractionated radiotherapy to abdomen: 8 mg 1-2 hours before irradiation, then 8 mg every 8 hours after first dose for each day of radiotherapy
I.V.:
Children 6 months to 18 years: 0.15 mg/kg/dose infused 30 minutes before the start of emetogenic chemotherapy, with subsequent doses administered 4 and 8 hours after the first dose
Adults: A single 32 mg dose/day or 0.15 mg/kg/dose or 45-80 kg: 8 mg, >80 kg: 12 mg infused 30 minutes before the start of emetogenic chemotherapy with subsequent doses administered 4 and 8 hours after the first dose; a few studies have evaluated a single 8 mg loading dose followed by a continuous 1 mg/hour infusion
Prevention of postoperative nausea and vomiting: I.V., I.M. (this route has only been recommended in adults): Give immediately before induction of anesthesia, or postoperatively if the patient is symptomatic:
Children ≥2 years <40 kg: 0.1 mg/kg
Children >40 kg and Adults: 4 mg
Note: Repeating a second ondansetron dose in patients who did not achieve adequate control of postoperative nausea and vomiting after a single dose will not provide additional control.
Treatment of hyperemesis gravidarum (unlabeled use): I.V.: 8 mg every 12 hours or 1 mg/hour infused continuously for up to 24 hours
Dosing adjustment in severe hepatic impairment (Child-Pugh score ≥10): Adults: Once daily dosage; maximum 8 mg per dose

Administration

Oral: May administer without regard to meals; Zofran® ODT tablet: Place tablet on tongue, it will disintegrate immediately; may also swallow with fluids as whole tablet
Parenteral:
I.V.: Dilute in 50 mL I.V. fluid (maximum concentration: 1 mg/mL) and infuse over 15 minutes; single doses for prevention of postoperative nausea/vomiting may be administered I.V. undiluted over 2-5 minutes
I.M.: Administer as undiluted injection

Patient Information May cause dry mouth

Dosage Forms Excipient information presented when available (limited, particularly for generics); consult specific product labeling.
Infusion [premixed in D_5W, preservative free]: 32 mg (50 mL)
Zofran®: 32 mg (50 mL)
Injection, solution: 2 mg/mL (2 mL, 20 mL)
Zofran®: 2 mg/mL (2 mL, 20 mL)
Solution, oral: 4 mg/5 mL (50 mL)
Zofran®: 4 mg/5 mL (50 mL) [contains sodium benzoate; strawberry flavor]
Tablet: 4 mg; 8 mg
Zofran®: 4 mg; 8 mg
Tablet, orally disintegrating: 4 mg; 8 mg
(Continued)

Ondansetron *(Continued)*

Zofran® ODT: 4 mg, 8 mg [each strength contains phenylalanine <0.03 mg/tablet; strawberry flavor]

References

"ASHP Therapeutic Guidelines on the Pharmacologic Management of Nausea and Vomiting in Adult and Pediatric Patients Receiving Chemotherapy or Radiation Therapy or Undergoing Surgery," *Am J Health Syst Pharm*, 1999, 56(8):729-64.

Carden PA, Mitchell SL, Waters KD, et al, "Prevention of Cyclophosphamide/Cytarabine-Induced Emesis With Ondansetron in Children With Leukemia," *J Clin Oncol*, 1990, 8(9):1531-5.

Marty M, Pouillart P, Scholl S, et al, "Comparison of the 5-hydroxytryptamine 3 (Serotonin) Antagonist Ondansetron (GR 38032F) With High-Dose Metoclopramide in the Control of Cisplatin-Induced Emesis," *N Engl J Med*, 1990, 322(12):816-21.

Pinkerton CR, Williams D, Wootton C, et al, "5-HT_3 Antagonist Ondansetron - An Effective Outpatient Antiemetic in Cancer Treatment," *Arch Dis Child*, 1990, 65(8):822-5.

Roila F and Del Favero A, "Ondansetron Clinical Pharmacokinetics," *Clin Pharmacokinet*, 1995, 29(2):95-109.

Seynaeve C, Schuller J, Buser K, et al, "Comparison of the Anti-emetic Efficacy of Different Doses of Ondansetron, Given as Either a Continuous Infusion or a Single Intravenous Dose, in Acute Cisplatin-Induced Emesis," *Br J Cancer* 1992, 66(1):192-7.

Spahr-Schopfer IA, Lerman J, Sikich N, et al, "Pharmacokinetics of Intravenous Ondansetron in Healthy Children Undergoing Ear, Nose, and Throat Surgery," *Clin Pharmacol Ther*, 1995, 58(3):316-21.

Spector JI, Lester EP, Chevlen EM, et al, "A Comparison of Oral Ondansetron and Intravenous Granisetron for the Prevention of Nausea and Emesis Associated With Cisplatin-Based Chemotherapy," *Oncologist*, 1998, 3(6):432-438.

- ♦ **Ondansetron Hydrochloride** *see* Ondansetron *on page 1169*
- ♦ **One Gram C [OTC]** *see* Ascorbic Acid *on page 159*
- ♦ **Onxol™** *see* Paclitaxel *on page 1196*
- ♦ **Operand® Chlorhexidine Gluconate [OTC]** *see* Chlorhexidine Gluconate *on page 337*
- ♦ **Ophthetic®** *see* Proparacaine *on page 1331*
- ♦ **Ophtho-Dipivefrin™ (Can)** *see* Dipivefrin *on page 520*
- ♦ **Ophtho-Tate® (Can)** *see* PrednisoLONE *on page 1304*
- ♦ **Opium and Belladonna** *see* Belladonna and Opium *on page 202*

Opium Tincture (OH pee um TING chur)

Medication Safety Issues

Sound-alike/look-alike issues:

Opium tincture may be confused with camphorated tincture of opium (paregoric)

Use care when prescribing opium tincture; each mL contains the equivalent of morphine 10 mg; paregoric contains the equivalent of morphine 0.4 mg/mL

DTO is an error-prone abbreviation (mistaken as Diluted Tincture of Opium; dose equivalency of paregoric)

Related Information

Overdose and Toxicology *on page 1916*

Index Terms DTO (error-prone abbreviation); Opium Tincture, Deodorized

Therapeutic Category Analgesic, Narcotic; Antidiarrheal

Generic Available Yes

Use Treatment of diarrhea or relief of pain; **a 25-fold dilution with water** (final concentration 0.4 mg/mL morphine) can be used to treat neonatal abstinence syndrome (opiate withdrawal)

Restrictions C-II

Pregnancy Risk Factor B (D if used for prolonged periods or in high doses at term)

Lactation Enters breast milk/use caution

Contraindications Hypersensitivity to opium, morphine, or any component; diarrhea caused by poisoning until the toxic material has been removed; increased intracranial pressure, severe respiratory depression, severe liver or renal insufficiency

Warnings Do not confuse opium tincture with paregoric; opium tincture is 25 times as potent as paregoric; opium shares the toxic potential of opiate agonists, usual precautions of opiate agonist therapy should be observed; opium may mask dehydration by producing fluid retention in the bowel; monitor patients with prolonged or severe diarrhea carefully; abrupt discontinuation after prolonged use may result in withdrawal symptoms

Precautions Use with caution in patients with respiratory, hepatic, or renal dysfunction, severe prostatic hypertrophy, or history of narcotic abuse; infants <3 months of age are more susceptible to respiratory depression, use with caution and in reduced doses in this age group

Adverse Reactions

Cardiovascular: Hypotension, bradycardia, peripheral vasodilation

Central nervous system: CNS depression, elevated intracranial pressure, drowsiness, dizziness, sedation

Dermatologic: Pruritus
Endocrine & metabolic: Antidiuretic hormone release
Gastrointestinal: Nausea, vomiting, constipation
Genitourinary: Urinary tract spasm, urinary retention
Hepatic: Biliary tract spasm
Ocular: Miosis
Respiratory: Respiratory depression
Miscellaneous: Physical and psychological dependence, histamine release

Drug Interactions CNS depressants (eg, alcohol, narcotics, benzodiazepines, tricyclic antidepressants, MAO inhibitors, phenothiazines) may increase effects/toxicity

Stability Protect from light and excessive heat; do not refrigerate, decreased solubility and precipitation may occur

Mechanism of Action Contains many narcotic alkaloids including morphine; gastric motility inhibition is primarily due to morphine content; decreases digestive secretions, increases GI muscle tone, and reduces GI propulsion

Pharmacodynamics Duration: 4-5 hours

Pharmacokinetics

Absorption: Variable from GI tract
Metabolism: In the liver
Elimination: In urine and bile

Usual Dosage Oral:

Neonates (full-term): Neonatal abstinence syndrome (opiate withdrawal): **Use a 25-fold dilution of opium tincture** (final concentration: 0.4 mg/mL morphine); Initial: Give 0.1 mL/kg or 2 drops/kg of the 25-fold dilution per dose with feedings every 3-4 hours; increase as needed by 0.1 mL/kg or 2 drops/kg of the 25-fold dilution every 3-4 hours until withdrawal symptoms are controlled; usual dose: 0.2-0.5 mL of the 25-fold dilution per dose given every 3-4 hours; it is rare to exceed 0.7 mL of the 25-fold dilution per dose; stabilize withdrawal symptoms for 3-5 days, then gradually decrease the dosage (keeping the same dosage interval) over a 2- to 4- week period

Children:

Diarrhea: 0.005-0.01 mL/kg/dose every 3-4 hours for a maximum of 6 doses/24 hours

Analgesia: 0.01-0.02 mL/kg/dose every 3-4 hours

Adults:

Diarrhea: Usual: 0.6 mL/dose; range: 0.3-1 mL/dose every 3-6 hours to maximum of 6 mL/24 hours

Analgesia: 0.6-1.5 mL/dose every 3-4 hours; usual maximum dose: 6 mL/24 hours

Administration Oral: May administer with food to decrease GI upset; for neonatal abstinence syndrome (opiate withdrawal), use a 25-fold dilution of opium tincture

Monitoring Parameters Respiratory rate, blood pressure, heart rate, resolution of diarrhea or pain, mental status; if using a 25-fold dilution to treat neonatal abstinence syndrome, monitor for resolution of withdrawal symptoms (such as irritability, high-pitched cry, stuffy nose, rhinorrhea, vomiting, poor feeding, diarrhea, sneezing, yawning etc), and signs of overtreatment (such as bradycardia, lethargy, hypotonia, irregular respirations, respiratory depression etc). An abstinence scoring system (eg, Finnegan abstinence scoring system) can be used to more objectively assess neonatal opiate withdrawal symptoms and the need for dosage adjustment. Monitor fluid and electrolyte balance in young children being treated for prolonged or severe diarrhea.

Patient Information Avoid alcohol; may cause drowsiness and impair ability to perform activities requiring mental alertness or physical coordination; may be habit-forming; avoid abrupt discontinuation after prolonged use

Nursing Implications Observe patient for excessive sedation, respiratory depression; implement safety measures; assist with ambulation; do not abruptly discontinue after prolonged use

Additional Information Opium tincture contains 10 mg/mL morphine and 17% to 21% alcohol; for treatment of neonatal abstinence syndrome, a 25-fold dilution of opium tincture (final concentration: 0.4 mg/mL morphine) is preferred over paregoric; the 25-fold dilution of opium tincture contains the same morphine concentration as paregoric, but without the high amount of alcohol or additives of paregoric

Dosage Forms Excipient information presented when available (limited, particularly for generics); consult specific product labeling.

Liquid: 10% (120 mL, 480 mL) [0.6 mL equivalent to morphine 6 mg; contains alcohol 19%]

References

Kraus DM and Pham JT, "Neonatal Therapy," *Applied Therapeutics: The Clinical Use of Drugs*, 7th ed, Koda-Kimble MA, Young LY, eds, Baltimore, MD: Lippincott Williams & Wilkins, 2001.

Levy M and Spino M, "Neonatal Withdrawal Syndrome: Associated Drugs and Pharmacologic Management," *Pharmacotherapy*, 1993, 13(3):202-11.

(Continued)

Opium Tincture *(Continued)*

"Neonatal Drug Withdrawal. American Academy of Pediatrics Committee on Drugs," *Pediatrics*, 1998, 101(6):1079-88.

♦ **Opium Tincture, Deodorized** *see* Opium Tincture *on page 1172*

Oprelvekin (oh PREL ve kin)

Medication Safety Issues
Sound-alike/look-alike issues:
Oprelvekin may be confused with aldesleukin, Proleukin®
Neumega® may be confused with Neulasta®, Neupogen®

U.S. Brand Names Neumega®

Index Terms IL-11; Interleukin-11; NSC-722848; Recombinant Human Interleukin-11; Recombinant Interleukin-11; rhIL-11; rIL-11

Therapeutic Category Biological Response Modulator; Thrombopoietic Growth Factor

Generic Available No

Use Prevention of severe thrombocytopenia and the reduction of the need for platelet transfusions following myelosuppressive chemotherapy in adult patients with nonmyeloid malignancies who are at high risk of severe thrombocytopenia

Pregnancy Risk Factor C

Lactation Excretion in breast milk unknown/not recommended

Contraindications Hypersensitivity to oprelvekin or any component

Warnings Treatment has been associated with severe hypersensitivity reactions including anaphylaxis; permanently discontinue oprelvekin in any patient developing an allergic reaction. Not indicated following myeloablative chemotherapy as effectiveness was not significant vs placebo and toxicity (edema, conjunctival bleeding, hypotension, and tachycardia) was increased vs placebo in these patients. Severe hypokalemia and/or sudden death have been reported in patients receiving chronic diuretic therapy, ifosfamide, and oprelvekin. Moderate decreases in hemoglobin, hematocrit, and RBC without a decrease in red cell mass have been observed; this is predominately related to an increase in plasma volume (dilutional anemia) from renal sodium and water retention. Onset of dilutional anemia is within 3-5 days of oprelvekin therapy and is reversible over approximately 7 days following discontinuation of oprelvekin. Stroke has been reported in patients who develop atrial fibrillation/flutter while receiving oprelvekin. Animal studies were predictive of an effect of oprelvekin on developing bone in children; thickening of femoral and tibial growth plates was noted. Papilledema has been reported in 2% of adult patients and 16% of pediatric patients receiving oprelvekin; use with caution in patients with pre-existing papilledema, as this may worsen with oprelvekin therapy. Per the manufacturer, oprelvekin should not be used in children, particularly those <12 years of age, except as part of a controlled clinical trial.

Precautions Oprelvekin may cause serious fluid retention resulting in peripheral edema, facial edema, dyspnea on exertion, pulmonary edema, capillary leak syndrome, atrial arrhythmias, and exacerbation of pre-existing pleural effusions. Use cautiously in patients with conditions where expansion of plasma volume should be avoided (eg, left ventricular dysfunction, CHF, hypertension). Use caution in patients with cardiac arrhythmias or conduction defects (ventricular arrhythmias generally occurring within 2-7 days of initiation of treatment have been reported postmarketing); use with caution in patients with respiratory disease; history of thromboembolic problems or stroke, and hepatic or renal dysfunction; modify dosage in patients with severe renal dysfunction

Adverse Reactions
Cardiovascular: Tachycardia (children: 84%), palpitation, atrial arrhythmias, peripheral edema, syncope, stroke, cardiomegaly (children: 21%), CHF, palpitations, pericardial effusion
Central nervous system: Headache, dizziness, insomnia, fatigue, fever
Dermatologic: Rash, skin discoloration, exfoliative dermatitis
Endocrine & metabolic: Fluid retention, hypokalemia, hypocalcemia
Gastrointestinal: Nausea, vomiting, anorexia, weight gain, oral moniliasis, mucositis
Hematologic: Anemia (dilutional; see Warnings)
Local: Injection site reactions
Neuromuscular & skeletal: Arthralgia, myalgia, periosteal changes (children: 11%), paresthesia
Ocular: Papilledema (frequency estimated to be up to 16% in children, 2% in adults); conjunctival injection (children: 57%), amblyopia
Renal: Renal failure
Respiratory: Dyspnea, pleural effusion, pulmonary edema, capillary leak syndrome, pneumonia, rhinitis, cough, pharyngitis

Miscellaneous: Hypersensitivity reactions including anaphylaxis, facial edema

Drug Interactions Diuretics: Oprelvekin may increase the risk of hypokalemia in patients receiving chronic diuretic therapy; monitor electrolytes closely.

Stability Store vials under refrigeration between 2°C to 8°C (36°F to 46°F); protect from light; do not freeze. Use reconstituted oprelvekin within 3 hours of reconstitution and store in the vial at either 2°C to 8°C (36°F to 46°F) or room temperature (≤25°C/70°F). Do not freeze reconstituted solution.

Mechanism of Action Oprelvekin stimulates multiple stages of megakaryocytopoiesis and thrombopoiesis, resulting in proliferation of megakaryocyte progenitors and megakaryocyte maturation

Pharmacodynamics

Onset of action: 5-9 days

Maximum effect: 14-19 days

Duration: Up to 7 days after discontinuation

Pharmacokinetics

Distribution: V_d: Adults: 112-152 mL/kg

Bioavailability: >80%

Metabolism: Uncertain

Half-life: Terminal: 6.9-8.1 hours

Time to peak serum concentration: 3.2 ± 2.4 hours

Elimination: Urine (primarily as metabolites)

Clearance: Adults: 2.2-2.7 mL/min/kg; clearance decreases with age and is about 1.2-1.6 times faster in children than in adults

Usual Dosage SubQ: **Note:** First dose should not be administered until 6-24 hours after the end of chemotherapy. Discontinue the drug at least 48 hours before beginning the next cycle of chemotherapy.

Children: 75-100 mcg/kg once daily for 10-21 days (until postnadir platelet count ≥50,000 cells/μL)

Note: The manufacturer states that, until efficacy/toxicity parameters are established, the use of oprelvekin in pediatric patients (particularly those <12 years of age) should be restricted to use in controlled clinical trials.

Adults: 50 mcg/kg once daily for 10-21 days (until postnadir platelet count ≥50,000 cells/μL)

Dosage adjustment in renal failure: Adults: Cl_{cr} <30 mL/minute: 25 mcg/kg

Administration SubQ: Reconstitute to a final concentration of 5 mg/mL with SWI; gently swirl, do not shake; administer subcutaneously in either the abdomen, thigh, hip, or upper arm (if not self-injected)

Monitoring Parameters Monitor electrolytes and fluid balance during therapy; obtain a CBC at regular intervals during therapy; monitor platelet counts until adequate recovery has occurred

Patient Information Report any swelling in the arms or legs (peripheral edema), shortness of breath (congestive failure, anemia), irregular heartbeat, headaches, or hypersensitivity reactions.

Dosage Forms Excipient information presented when available (limited, particularly for generics); consult specific product labeling.

Injection, powder for reconstitution:

Neumega®: 5 mg [packaged with diluent]

References

Du X and Williams DA, "Interleukin-11: Review of Molecular, Cell Biology, and Clinical Use," *Blood*, 1997, 89(11):3897-908.

Gordon MS, "Thrombopoietic Activity of Recombinant Human Interleukin 11 in Cancer Patients Receiving Chemotherapy," *Cancer Chemother Pharmacol*, 1996, 38 (Suppl):96-8.

Milman E, Berdon WE, Garvin JH, et al, "Periostitis Secondary to Interleukin-11 (Oprelvekin, Neumega®). Treatment for Thrombocytopenia in Pediatric Patients," *Pediatr Radiol*, 2003, 33(7):450-2.

Tepler I, Elias L, Smith JW 2d, et al, "A Randomized Placebo-Controlled Trial of Recombinant Human Interleukin-11 in Cancer Patients With Severe Thrombocytopenia Due to Chemotherapy," *Blood*, 1996, 87(9):3607-14.

Teramura M, Kobayashi S, Yoshinaga K, et al, "Effect of Interleukin 11 on Normal and Pathological Thrombopoiesis," *Cancer Chemother Pharmacol*, 1996, 38 (Suppl):99-102.

- **Optho-Bunolol® (Can)** *see* Levobunolol *on page 925*
- **Opticrom®** *see* Cromolyn *on page 407*
- **Optimyxin® (Can)** *see* Bacitracin and Polymyxin B *on page 196*
- **Optivar®** *see* Azelastine *on page 189*
- **Orabase® with Benzocaine [OTC]** *see* Benzocaine *on page 204*
- **Oracea™** *see* Doxycycline *on page 543*
- **Oracort (Can)** *see* Triamcinolone *on page 1568*
- **Orajel® Baby Daytime and Nighttime [OTC]** *see* Benzocaine *on page 204*
- **Orajel® Baby Teething [OTC]** *see* Benzocaine *on page 204*
- **Orajel® Baby Teething Nighttime [OTC]** *see* Benzocaine *on page 204*
- **Orajel® Denture Plus [OTC]** *see* Benzocaine *on page 204*

- ♦ **Orajel® Maximum Strength [OTC]** *see* Benzocaine *on page 204*
- ♦ **Orajel® Medicated Toothache [OTC]** *see* Benzocaine *on page 204*
- ♦ **Orajel® Mouth Sore [OTC]** *see* Benzocaine *on page 204*
- ♦ **Orajel® Multi-Action Cold Sore [OTC]** *see* Benzocaine *on page 204*
- ♦ **Orajel® Perioseptic® Spot Treatment [OTC]** *see* Carbamide Peroxide *on page 283*
- ♦ **Orajel PM® [OTC]** *see* Benzocaine *on page 204*
- ♦ **Orajel® Ultra Mouth Sore [OTC]** *see* Benzocaine *on page 204*
- ♦ **Oramorph SR®** *see* Morphine Sulfate *on page 1082*
- ♦ **Oranyl [OTC]** *see* Pseudoephedrine *on page 1344*
- ♦ **Orapred®** *see* PrednisoLONE *on page 1304*
- ♦ **Orapred ODT™** *see* PrednisoLONE *on page 1304*
- ♦ **Oraquix®** *see* Lidocaine and Prilocaine *on page 937*
- ♦ **Orazinc® [OTC]** *see* Zinc Supplements *on page 1641*
- ♦ **Orciprenaline Sulfate** *see* Metaproterenol *on page 1014*
- ♦ **Orfadin®** *see* Nitisinone *on page 1138*
- ♦ **ORG 946** *see* Rocuronium *on page 1402*
- ♦ **Organidin® NR** *see* Guaifenesin *on page 745*
- ♦ **ORG NC 45** *see* Vecuronium *on page 1604*
- ♦ **ORO-Clense (Can)** *see* Chlorhexidine Gluconate *on page 337*
- ♦ **Orthoclone OKT® 3** *see* Muromonab-CD3 *on page 1092*
- ♦ **Os-Cal® (Can)** *see* Calcium Carbonate *on page 264*
- ♦ **Os-Cal® 500 [OTC] [DSC]** *see* Calcium Carbonate *on page 264*
- ♦ **Os-Cal® 500 [OTC]** *see* Calcium Supplements *on page 272*

Oseltamivir (o sel TAM e veer)

Medication Safety Issues

Sound-alike/look-alike issues:

Tamiflu® may be confused with Thera-Flu®

U.S. Brand Names Tamiflu®

Canadian Brand Names Tamiflu®

Therapeutic Category Antiviral Agent, Oral; Neuraminidase Inhibitor

Generic Available No

Use Treatment of uncomplicated acute illness due to influenza A and B infection in patients who have been symptomatic for **no more than 2 days**; prophylaxis of influenza A and B exposures that occur before (or less than 2 weeks after) vaccination with inactivated vaccine, or in years when circulating strains differ from those included in the vaccine (oseltamivir is not a substitute for annual flu vaccination)

Pregnancy Risk Factor C

Lactation Excretion in breast milk unknown/not recommended

Contraindications Hypersensitivity to oseltamivir, any component, or other sialic acid-based neuraminidase inhibitors

Warnings Oral suspension contains sodium benzoate; benzoic acid (benzoate) is a metabolite of benzyl alcohol; large amounts of benzyl alcohol (≥99 mg/kg/day) have been associated with a potentially fatal toxicity ("gasping syndrome") in neonates; use oral suspension containing sodium benzoate with caution in neonates; *in vitro* and animal studies have shown that benzoate displaces bilirubin from protein binding sites

Precautions Use with caution and modify dosage in patients with renal impairment; oseltamivir does not prevent complication of serious bacterial infection which may begin with or coexist with influenza

Adverse Reactions

Cardiovascular: Unstable angina, arrhythmia

Central nervous system: Dizziness, headache, fatigue, insomnia, vertigo, seizure, confusion, delirium, self-injury

Dermatologic: Rash, toxic epidermal necrolysis

Endocrine & metabolic: Aggravation of diabetes mellitus

Gastrointestinal: Nausea, vomiting, diarrhea, abdominal pain, pseudomembranous colitis

Hematologic: Anemia

Hepatic: Hepatitis

Ocular: Conjunctivitis

Respiratory: Bronchitis, epistaxis

Miscellaneous: Swelling of face or tongue

Drug Interactions Probenecid (increases serum oseltamivir carboxylate concentration due to decreased tubular secretion in the kidney); live-attenuated vaccine

(oseltamivir decreases efficacy of fluMist®; discontinue oseltamivir 48 hours before and do not restart for at least 1-2 weeks after fluMist® administration)

Food Interactions Food has no significant effect on peak oseltamivir plasma concentration or AUC

Stability Store capsule and powder for oral suspension at room temperature. Reconstituted oral suspension is stable for 10 days if refrigerated; do not freeze.

Mechanism of Action Inhibits influenza virus neuraminidase which is responsible for detachment of virions from the infected cell's membrane and for viral penetration through respiratory secretions resulting in the inability of the virus to spread within the respiratory tract

Pharmacodynamics Reduction in the median time to improvement: 1.3 days

Pharmacokinetics

Absorption: Well absorbed from the GI tract

Distribution: Adults: V_{dss}: 23-26 L

Protein binding: 3% (oseltamivir carboxylate); 42% (oseltamivir phosphate)

Metabolism: Prodrug oseltamivir phosphate is metabolized by hepatic esterases to oseltamivir carboxylate (active); neither oseltamivir phosphate or oseltamivir carboxylate are a substrate, inducer, or inhibitor of cytochrome P450 isoenzymes

Half-life:

- Oseltamivir phosphate: 1-3 hours
- Oseltamivir carboxylate: 6-10 hours

Elimination: >99% of oseltamivir carboxylate is eliminated by renal excretion via glomerular filtration and tubular secretion

Usual Dosage Oral:

Treatment of influenza (treatment should begin within 2 days of onset of flu symptoms):

- Children ≥1-12 years:
  - ≤15 kg: 2 mg/kg/dose (maximum dose: 30 mg) twice daily for 5 days
  - >15 kg to 23 kg: 45 mg/dose twice daily for 5 days
  - >23 kg to 40 kg: 60 mg/dose twice daily for 5 days
  - >40 kg: 75 mg/dose twice daily for 5 days
- Children >12 years and Adults: 75 mg/dose twice daily for 5 days

Prophylaxis of influenza: Children ≥13 years and Adults: 75 mg/dose once daily for at least 7 days or for up to 6 weeks; therapy should begin within 2 days of exposure.

Dosing adjustment in renal impairment: Adults:

- Cl_{cr} 10-30 mL/minute:
  - Treatment of influenza: 75 mg/dose once daily
  - Prophylaxis of influenza: 75 mg/dose every other day
- Cl_{cr} <10 mL/minute: No recommended dosage regimens are available for patients with end-stage renal disease

Administration May administer with or without food; may decrease stomach upset if administered with food; shake suspension well before use

Monitoring Parameters Renal function, serum glucose in patients with diabetes mellitus

Patient Information Oseltamivir is not a substitute for the annual flu vaccination. Report any unusual behavior to physician.

Dosage Forms Excipient information presented when available (limited, particularly for generics); consult specific product labeling.

Capsule, as phosphate:
- Tamiflu®: 75 mg

Powder for oral suspension:
- Tamiflu®: 12 mg/mL (25 mL) [contains sodium benzoate; tutti-frutti flavor]

References

Hayden FG, Atmar RL, Schilling M, et al, "Use of the Selective Oral Neuraminidase Inhibitor Oseltamivir to Prevent Influenza," *N Engl J Med*, 1999, 341(18):1336-43.

Treanor JJ, Hayden FG, Vrooman PS, et al, "Efficacy and Safety of the Oral Neuraminidase Inhibitor Oseltamivir in Treating Acute Influenza: A Randomized Controlled Trial. US Oral Neuraminidase Study Group," *JAMA*, 2000, 283(8):1016-24.

♦ **Osmitrol®** *see* Mannitol *on page 979*
♦ **Osmoglyn® [DSC]** *see* Glycerin *on page 736*
♦ **OsmoPrep™** *see* Sodium Phosphate *on page 1456*
♦ **Osteocit® (Can)** *see* Calcium Citrate *on page 267*
♦ **Ostoforte® (Can)** *see* Ergocalciferol *on page 588*
♦ **OTFC (Oral Transmucosal Fentanyl Citrate)** *see* Fentanyl *on page 644*
♦ **Oticaine** *see* Benzocaine *on page 204*
♦ **Otocaine™** *see* Benzocaine *on page 204*
♦ **Outgro® [OTC]** *see* Benzocaine *on page 204*
♦ **Ovace®** *see* Sulfacetamide *on page 1483*
♦ **Ovace® Wash** *see* Sulfacetamide *on page 1483*

♦ **Ovol® (Can)** *see* Simethicone *on page 1440*

Oxacillin (oks a SIL in)

Index Terms Methylphenyl Isoxazolyl Penicillin; Oxacillin Sodium
Therapeutic Category Antibiotic, Penicillin (Antistaphylococcal)
Generic Available Yes
Use Treatment of bacterial infections such as osteomyelitis, septicemia, endocarditis, and CNS infections due to susceptible penicillinase-producing strains of *Staphylococcus*
Pregnancy Risk Factor B
Lactation Enters breast milk/compatible
Contraindications Hypersensitivity to oxacillin, other penicillins, or any component
Warnings Prolonged use may result in superinfection. Elimination rate will be decreased in neonates; monitor patients closely.
Precautions Use with caution in patients with hypersensitivity to cephalosporins, severe renal impairment; dosage modification required in patients with renal impairment
Adverse Reactions
Central nervous system: Fever
Dermatologic: Rash, urticaria, pruritus
Gastrointestinal: Diarrhea, nausea, vomiting, *C. difficile* colitis
Hematologic: Mild leukopenia, agranulocytosis, thrombocytopenia, neutropenia, eosinophilia
Hepatic: Elevated AST, hepatotoxicity
Local: Thrombophlebitis
Renal: Acute interstitial nephritis; hematuria and azotemia have occurred in neonates and infants receiving high-dose oxacillin; albuminuria
Miscellaneous: Hypersensitivity reactions, serum sickness-like reactions, anaphylaxis
Drug Interactions Probenecid (decreases oxacillin elimination rate); tetracycline may antagonize the bactericidal effect of oxacillin
Stability Reconstituted oxacillin 250 mg/1.5 mL solution for injection is stable for 3 days at room temperature or 7 days when refrigerated; injection is incompatible with aminoglycosides and tetracyclines
Mechanism of Action Interferes with bacterial cell wall synthesis during active multiplication by binding to one or more of the penicillin-binding proteins; inhibits the final transpeptidation step of peptidoglycan synthesis causing cell wall death and resultant bactericidal activity against susceptible bacteria
Pharmacokinetics
Distribution: Distributes into bile, pleural, synovial, and pericardial fluids and into lungs and bone; penetrates the blood-brain barrier only when meninges are inflamed; crosses the placenta; appears in breast milk
Protein binding: 90% to 95%
Metabolism: In the liver to active and inactive metabolites
Half-life (prolonged with reduced renal function):
- Neonates 8-15 days: 1.6 hours
- Children 1 week to 2 years: 0.9-1.8 hours
- Adults: 0.3-0.8 hours

Time to peak serum concentration: I.M.: Within 30-60 minutes
Elimination: By the kidneys and to small degree via bile as parent drug and metabolites
Dialysis: Not dialyzable (0% to 5%)
Usual Dosage
Neonates: I.M., I.V.:
- 0-4 weeks, <1200 g: 50 mg/kg/day in divided doses every 12 hours
- Postnatal age <7 days:
  - 1200-2000 g: 50-100 mg/kg/day in divided doses every 12 hours
  - >2000 g: 75-150 mg/kg/day in divided doses every 8 hours
- Postnatal age ≥7 days:
  - 1200-2000 g: 75-150 mg/kg/day in divided doses every 8 hours
  - >2000 g: 100-200 mg/kg/day in divided doses every 6 hours

Infants and Children: I.M., I.V.:
- Mild to moderate infections: 100-150 mg/kg/day in divided doses every 6 hours; maximum dose: 4 g/day
- Severe infections: 150-200 mg/kg/day in divided doses every 4-6 hours; maximum dose: 12 g/day

Adults: I.M., I.V.:
- Mild to moderate infections: 500 mg to 1 g/dose every 6 hours
- Severe infections: 1-2 g/dose every 4-6 hours

Dosing interval in renal impairment: Cl_{cr} <10 mL/minute: Use lower range of the usual dosage

Administration Parenteral:

I.M. injection: Reconstitute each gram of oxacillin with 5.7 mL of SWI to make a 167 mg/mL solution; shake well until a clear solution is obtained. Administer by deep I.M. injection into a large muscle mass (eg, gluteus maximus).

I.V. push: Administer over 10 minutes at a maximum concentration of 100 mg/mL

I.V. intermittent infusion: Administer over 15-30 minutes at a final concentration ≤40 mg/mL

I.M. injection: May dilute with SWI to a final concentration of 167 mg/mL; administer I.M. injections deep into a large muscle mass

Monitoring Parameters Periodic CBC with differential, urinalysis, BUN, serum creatinine, AST and ALT; number and type of stools/day for diarrhea

Test Interactions False-positive urinary and serum proteins

Additional Information Sodium content: 1 g injection: 2.5 mEq

Dosage Forms Excipient information presented when available (limited, particularly for generics); consult specific product labeling.

Infusion [premixed iso-osmotic dextrose solution]: 1 g (50 mL); 2 g (50 mL)

Injection, powder for reconstitution, as sodium: 1 g, 2 g, 10 g

References

Olans RN and Weiner LB, "Reversible Oxacillin Hepatotoxicity," *J Pediatr*, 1976, 89(5):835-8.

Prober CG, Stevenson DK, and Benitz WE, "The Use of Antibiotics in Neonates Weighing Less Than 1200 Grams," *Pediatr Infect Dis J*, 1990, 9(2):111-21.

♦ **Oxacillin Sodium** *see* Oxacillin *on page 1178*

Oxaliplatin (ox AL i pla tin)

Medication Safety Issues

Sound-alike/look-alike issues:

Oxaliplatin may be confused with Aloxi®, carboplatin

High alert medication: The Institute for Safe Medication Practices (ISMP) includes this medication among its list of drugs which have a heightened risk of causing significant patient harm when used in error.

U.S. Brand Names Eloxatin®

Index Terms Diaminocyclohexane Oxalatoplatinum; L-OHP; NSC-266046

Therapeutic Category Antineoplastic Agent, Alkylating Agent

Generic Available No

Use Treatment of advanced colon cancer and advanced rectal carcinoma; treatment of head and neck cancer, nonsmall cell lung cancer, non-Hodgkin's lymphoma, ovarian cancer, relapsed/refractory childhood solid tumors including CNS and non-CNS tumors

Pregnancy Risk Factor D

Lactation Excretion in breast milk unknown/not recommended

Contraindications Hypersensitivity to oxaliplatin, other platinum-containing compounds, or any component; pregnancy; grade 3 to 4 neuropathy usually due to prior exposure

Warnings The FDA currently recommends that procedures for proper handling and disposal of antineoplastic agents be considered. Oxaliplatin should be administered under the supervision of a physician experienced in the use of cancer chemotherapy agents. Anaphylactic-like reactions may occur within minutes of oxaliplatin administration; manage reactions with supportive therapy, epinephrine, corticosteroids, and antihistamines. Two different types of neuropathy may occur: 1) an acute (within first 2 days), reversible (resolves within 14 days) sensory neuropathy with peripheral symptoms that are often exacerbated by cold (may include pharyngolaryngeal dysesthesia); 2) persistent (>14 days) sensory neuropathy which presents with paresthesias, dysesthesias, hypoesthesias, and impaired proprioception that often interferes with daily activities (eg, writing, buttoning, swallowing); these symptoms may improve upon discontinuing treatment. May cause pulmonary fibrosis or hepatotoxicity. The presence of hepatic vascular disorders, including veno-occlusive disease, should be considered, especially in individuals developing portal hypertension or who present with elevated liver function tests. When administered as sequential infusions, taxane derivatives (docetaxel, paclitaxel) should be administered before platinum derivatives to limit myelosuppression and enhance efficacy. Oxaliplatin may cause fetal harm (pregnancy should be avoided during therapy).

Precautions Use caution in patients with renal impairment since increased toxicity may occur.

Adverse Reactions

Cardiovascular: Edema, chest pain, peripheral edema, flushing, thromboembolism, hypotension

(Continued)

Oxaliplatin *(Continued)*

Central nervous system: Fatigue, fever, pain, headache, insomnia, dizziness
Dermatologic: Rash, alopecia, hand-foot syndrome, angioedema, urticaria, pruritus, erythema
Endocrine & metabolic: Dehydration, hypokalemia, metabolic acidosis
Gastrointestinal: Nausea, diarrhea, vomiting, abdominal pain, constipation, anorexia, stomatitis, dyspepsia, taste perversion, gastroesophageal reflux, mucositis, dysphagia, colitis, ileus, pancreatitis, GI bleed
Genitourinary: Dysuria, hematuria
Hematologic: Anemia, thrombocytopenia, leukopenia, neutropenia, hemolytic anemia
Hepatic: Elevated AST, ALT, bilirubin, alkaline phosphatase; veno-occlusive liver disease, hepatotoxicity
Local: Injection site reaction, erythema, swelling, pain
Neuromuscular & skeletal: Rigors, arthralgia, peripheral neuropathy, back pain, paresthesia, dysesthesia, hypoesthesia, jaw spasm
Ocular: Abnormal lacrimation, optic neuritis, decreased visual acuity, visual field disturbance, ocular pain
Renal: Elevated serum creatinine
Respiratory: Dyspnea, cough, URI, rhinitis, epistaxis, pharyngitis, pharyngolaryngeal dysesthesia, shortness of breath, bronchospasm, pulmonary fibrosis, interstitial lung disease
Miscellaneous: Anaphylaxis, hiccup

Drug Interactions Nephrotoxic agents may increase oxaliplatin toxicity; live vaccines (increased risk of infection)

Stability Store at room temperature; protect from light; do not freeze. Diluted solution is stable up to 6 hours at room temperature or up to 24 hours under refrigeration. Do not dilute using chloride-containing solutions (eg, NaCl). Diluted infusion solutions do not require protection from light. Do not reconstitute or dilute oxaliplatin using needles containing aluminum. Incompatible with alkaline solutions (eg, fluorouracil), chloride-containing solutions, and diazepam.

Mechanism of Action Oxaliplatin, an alkylating agent, binds to DNA forming cross-links which inhibit DNA replication and transcription, resulting in cell death.

Pharmacokinetics

Distribution: V_d: Adults: 440 L
Protein binding: >90%
Metabolism: Nonenzymatic biotransformation (rapid and extensive), forms active and inactive derivatives
Half-life:
- Adults: Oxaliplatin ultrafilterable platinum:
  - Distribution:
    - Alpha phase: 0.4 hours
    - Beta phase: 16.8 hours
  - Terminal: 391 hours
- Children:
  - Oxaliplatin: Beta: 200.6 hours (median range: 162.5-299 hours)
  - Oxaliplatin ultrafilterable platinum: Beta: 217.6 hours (median range: 79.7-936.6 hours)

Elimination: Primarily in urine (54%); feces (2%)

Usual Dosage I.V.: Refer to individual protocols

Children: Protocol ADVL0421 for relapsed/recurrent childhood solid tumors:
- ≤12 months: 4.3 mg/kg over 2 hours every 3 weeks
- >12 months: 130 mg/m^2 over 2 hours every 3 weeks

Adults:
- Combination therapy: 85-100 mg/m^2 every 2-3 weeks (ie, GEMOX or FOLFOX4)
- Single agent therapy: 130 mg/m^2 every 2-3 weeks (ie, ADVL0421)
- Stage III colon cancer and colorectal cancer: 85 mg/m^2 every 2 weeks
- Unlabeled doses: 20-25 mg/m^2 days 1-5 every 3 weeks or 100-130 mg/m^2 every 2-3 weeks

Dosage adjustments for toxicity: Adults:
- Persistent grade 2 neurosensory event: Reduce dose to 75 mg/m^2 for Stage III colon cancer or 65 mg/m^2 for advanced colorectal cancer
- Grade 3 neurosensory event: Consider discontinuing therapy
- Recovery from grade 3/4 GI or grade 4 neutropenia or grade 3/4 thrombocytopenia: Reduce dose to 75 mg/m^2 for Stage III colon cancer
- Recovery from grade 3/4 GI or grade 4 neutropenia or grade 3/4 thrombocytopenia: Reduce dose to 65 mg/m^2 for advanced colorectal cancer; next dose should be delayed until neutrophils >1.5 x10^9/L and platelets >75 x10^9/L

Dosage adjustment in renal impairment: Adults: Consider omitting dose or changing chemotherapy regimen if Cl_{cr} ≤19 mL/minute

Administration I.V.: Administer as I.V. infusion over 2-6 hours. The final concentration should not be less than 0.2 mg/mL. For patients in which volume may be of concern, a final concentration of 0.3-0.6 mg/mL is acceptable. Flush infusion line with D_5W prior to administration of any concomitant medication. Do **not** use I.V. administration sets containing aluminum.

Monitoring Parameters CBC with differential, hemoglobin, platelet count, serum creatinine, liver function tests; signs of neuropathy, hypersensitivity reaction, and respiratory effects. Delay dosage until recovery of neutrophils >1.5 x 10^9/L and platelets >75 x10^9/L

Patient Information Maintain adequate hydration. Inform physician of sore throat, fever, chills, unusual fatigue or unusual bruising/bleeding, persistent diarrhea, rash, cough, swelling of throat, difficulty breathing, muscle cramps or twitching, tingling/numbness in arms, fingers, legs, or toes (avoid exposure to cold temperature, cold drinks, or cold objects since symptoms of acute sensory neuropathy may be exacerbated by cold temperature). Avoid becoming pregnant during or for 1 month following therapy; effective contraceptive measures must be used. Do not breast-feed.

Nursing Implications Patients should receive an antiemetic premedication regimen. Longer infusion times (up to 6 hours) may mitigate acute toxicities. Observe closely for anaphylactic-like reactions which can occur within minutes of administration. Extravasation may result in tissue necrosis; care should be taken to avoid extravasation. If skin or mucous membranes come in contact with oxaliplatin, thoroughly wash skin immediately with soap and water; flush mucous membranes with water. Do not use ice for mucositis prophylaxis.

Dosage Forms Excipient information presented when available (limited, particularly for generics); consult specific product labeling. [DSC] = Discontinued product

Injection, powder for reconstitution:
- Eloxatin®: 50 mg, 100 mg [contains lactose] [DSC]

Injection, solution [preservative free]:
- Eloxatin®: 5 mg/mL (10 mL, 20 mL)

References

Fouladi M, Blaney SM, Poussaint TY, et al, "Phase II Study of Oxaliplatin in Children with Recurrent or Refractory Medulloblastoma, Supratentorial Primitive Neuroectodermal Tumors, and Atypical Teratoid Rhabdoid Tumors " A Pediatric Brain Tumor Consortium Study," *Cancer* 2006, 107(9):2291-7.

Iacono LC, Spunt SL, Pratt CB, et al, "Pharmacokinetics of Oxaliplatin in Children With Solid Tumors," *Proc Am Soc Clin Oncol*, 2002, 21(abstr 2170).

Oxaprozin (oks a PROE zin)

Medication Safety Issues

Sound-alike/look-alike issues:
- Daypro® may be confused with Diupres®
- Oxaprozin may be confused with oxazepam

U.S. Brand Names Daypro®

Canadian Brand Names Apo-Oxaprozin®; Daypro®

Therapeutic Category Analgesic, Non-narcotic; Anti-inflammatory Agent; Nonsteroidal Anti-inflammatory Drug (NSAID), Oral

Generic Available Yes

Use Symptomatic relief of the signs and symptoms of osteoarthritis; adult and juvenile rheumatoid arthritis

Medication Guide An FDA-approved patient medication guide, which is available with the product information and at http://www.fda.gov/cder/Offices/ODS/medication_guides.htm, must be dispensed with this medication for each new outpatient prescription and refill.

Pregnancy Risk Factor C (D if used in the third trimester)

Lactation Excretion in breast milk unknown/not recommended

Contraindications Hypersensitivity to oxaprozin, any component, aspirin, or other NSAIDs; active GI bleeding, ulcer disease; patients with the "aspirin triad" [asthma, rhinitis (with or without nasal polyps), and aspirin intolerance] (fatal asthmatic and anaphylactoid reactions may occur in these patients)

Warnings In April 2005, the FDA announced product labeling changes for all NSAIDs, including COX-2 selective and OTC medications; although revised product labeling is currently not available for all products, sample labeling and a template of the required medication guide are now available. Labels for prescription nonselective NSAIDs will contain a contraindication for use in patients who have recently undergone coronary artery bypass graft (CABG) surgery and a boxed warning concerning the potential for increased risk of cardiovascular (CV) events and GI bleeding associated with NSAID use. Patients at increased risk of adverse events include patients immediately postoperative from CABG surgery, and those with existing CAD, CVD, or history of TIA or stomach ulcers. Prescribers are encouraged to use the lowest effective NSAID dose for the shortest time based on individual patient treatment goals. Medication guides will be required for all prescription products. Complete details for the labeling update

(Continued)

Oxaprozin *(Continued)*

can be found on the following FDA website: http://www.fda.gov/medwatch/SAFETY/2005/safety05.htm#NSAID.

Serious GI toxicities may occur including ulceration, bleeding, or perforation; patients with a history of PUD or GI bleeding who use NSAIDs have a >10-fold higher risk for GI bleed; other factors which may increase risk for GI bleed include: Longer duration of NSAID treatment, use of oral corticosteroids or anticoagulants, alcoholism, smoking, overall poor health, and older age. To decrease the risk of GI adverse effects, use the lowest effective dose for the shortest duration possible.

Anaphylactoid reactions may occur. Oxaprozin is not recommended for use in patients with severe renal dysfunction (if therapy is needed, close monitoring of renal function is highly recommended). Oxaprozin is not recommended for use in late pregnancy (premature closure of the ductus arteriosus may occur).

Precautions Fluid retention, edema, hypertension, mild photosensitivity reactions, rash, or severe hepatic reactions (rare) may occur. Use with caution in patients with CHF, asthma, hypertension, fluid retention, dehydration (rehydrate patient before starting therapy), mild to moderate renal dysfunction, hepatic dysfunction, history of GI disease, coagulation disorders, or those receiving anticoagulants, ACE inhibitors, or diuretics. Long-term use of NSAIDs may result in renal injury, including renal papillary necrosis. Safety and efficacy in pediatric patients <6 years of age have not been established.

Adverse Reactions Note: Adverse reactions occurred in 45% of JRA patients, compared to ~30% of adult rheumatoid arthritis patients (see also Additional Information)

Cardiovascular: Fluid retention, edema, hypertension

Central nervous system: Confusion, depression, dizziness, headache, sedation, sleep disturbance, somnolence

Dermatologic: Pruritus, rash; mild photosensitivity reactions (reported in 30% of JRA patients; see Additional Information)

Gastrointestinal: Abdominal distress, abdominal pain, anorexia, constipation, diarrhea, flatulence, dyspepsia, nausea, vomiting; GI ulcer, bleeding or perforation

Hematologic: Anemia, increased bleeding time, inhibition of platelet aggregation; agranulocytosis, aplastic anemia (rare)

Hepatic: Elevated liver enzymes; Rarely: Severe hepatic reactions (jaundice, fatal fulminant hepatitis, liver necrosis, hepatic failure)

Ocular: Blurred vision, conjunctivitis

Otic: Tinnitus

Renal: Dysuria, renal dysfunction, urinary frequency, acute renal failure; renal injury, renal papillary necrosis (long-term use)

Miscellaneous: Anaphylaxis, anaphylactoid reactions

Drug Interactions Oxaprozin may increase serum concentrations of lithium (monitor lithium concentrations) or methotrexate (consider methotrexate dosage reduction); use with anticoagulants (warfarin, heparin, LMWH) or antiplatelet drugs may increase risk of bleeding; oxaprozin displaces salicylates from protein binding sites (avoid concurrent use with aspirin or other salicylates; increased toxicities are expected); use with other gastric irritants (eg, alcohol, corticosteroids) may increase risk of GI irritation or bleed; oxaprozin may decrease the antihypertensive effects of ACE inhibitors, beta blockers, thiazide diuretics, or furosemide (monitor blood pressure); oxaprozin may decrease serum concentrations of enalapril, but increase serum concentrations of its active metabolite, enalaprilat; oxaprozin may alter pharmacokinetics of glyburide (monitor blood glucose); cimetidine or ranitidine decrease the total body clearance of oxaprozin (unlikely to be clinically significant)

Food Interactions Food may decrease the rate, but not the extent of oral absorption

Stability Store at 25°C (77°F); protect from light; keep bottle tightly closed

Mechanism of Action Inhibits prostaglandin synthesis by decreasing the activity of the enzyme, cyclooxygenase, which results in decreased formation of prostaglandin precursors

Pharmacodynamics Maximum effect: Due to its long half-life, several days of treatment are required for oxaprozin to reach its full effect

Pharmacokinetics

Absorption: Oral: 95%

Distribution: Distributes into synovial tissues at twice the concentration of plasma and 3 times the concentration of synovial fluid; expected to distribute into breast milk (exact amount not known)

V_d (apparent): Adults: 11-17 L per 70 kg

Protein binding: 99%, primarily to albumin; protein binding is saturable (nonlinear protein binding)

Metabolism: Hepatic via microsomal oxidation (65%) and conjugation with glucuronic acid (35%); major conjugated metabolites are ester and ether glucuronide (inactive); small amounts of an active phenolic metabolite is produced (<5%) but has limited contribution to overall activity

Half-life: Adults: 41-55 hours

Time to peak serum concentration: 2.4-3.1 hours

Elimination: Excreted in the urine (5% as unchanged drug, 65% as metabolites) and feces (35% as metabolites)

Clearance: After adjusting for body weight, no clinically important age-related differences in apparent clearance of unbound drug were identified between adult and pediatric patients ≥6 years of age

Dialysis: Not significantly removed by hemodialysis or CAPD due to high protein binding

Usual Dosage Note: Use lowest effective dose; dose may be divided if patient does not tolerate once daily dosing; Oral:

Children 6-16 years: JRA: Dose according to body weight. **Note:** Doses greater than 1200 mg have not been evaluated:

22-31 kg: 600 mg once daily

32-54 kg: 900 mg once daily

≥55 kg: 1200 mg once daily

Adults: Osteoarthritis or Rheumatoid arthritis: Usual: 1200 mg once daily; titrate to lowest effective dose; patients with low body weight should start with 600 mg daily; a one-time loading dose of 1200 mg to 1800 mg or 26 mg/kg (whichever is lower) may be given if needed; maximum daily dose: 1800 mg or 26 mg/kg (whichever is lower) in divided doses

Note: Chronic administration of doses >1200 mg/day should be reserved for adult patients >50 kg with severe disease, low risk for peptic ulcer disease, and normal hepatic and renal function; ensure that patient tolerates lower doses before advancing to larger dose

Dosing adjustment in renal impairment: Severe renal impairment or patients on dialysis: Initial: 600 mg once daily; may increase dose if needed to 1200 mg once daily with close monitoring

Dosing adjustment in hepatic impairment: Use with caution in patients with severe hepatic dysfunction (dosage reduction is not required in patients with well compensated cirrhosis)

Administration May be administered without regard to food; administer with food or milk to decrease GI distress

Monitoring Parameters CBC, occult blood loss, liver enzymes, renal function tests; blood pressure, signs and symptoms of GI bleeding

Test Interactions False-positive urine immunoassay screening test for benzodiazepines may occur; test may remain positive for several days after discontinuing oxaprozin

Patient Information May cause dizziness and impair ability to perform activities requiring mental alertness or physical coordination; avoid alcohol; report any signs of blood in stool, GI bleeding, weight gain, edema, skin rash, unusual fatigue, persistent abdominal pain/tenderness or yellow skin to physician. May cause photosensitivity reactions (eg, exposure to sunlight may cause severe sunburn, skin rash, redness, or itching); avoid exposure to sunlight and artificial light sources (sunlamps, tanning booth/bed); wear protective clothing, wide-brimmed hats, sunglasses, and lip sunscreen (SPF ≥15); use a sunscreen [broad-spectrum sunscreen or physical sunscreen (preferred) or sunblock with SPF ≥15]; contact physician if reaction occurs.

Additional Information An open-label study of oxaprozin (10-20 mg/kg/dose once daily) in 59 JRA patients [3-16 years of age (mean age: 9 years)], reported adverse events in 58% of patients; GI symptoms occurred at a higher incidence than historically reported in adults; 9 of 30 patients (30%) who continued therapy for a total of 19-48 weeks, developed a vesicular rash on sun-exposed areas of skin; 5 of these 9 patients with rash discontinued the drug (see Bass, 1985).

Dosage Forms Excipient information presented when available (limited, particularly for generics); consult specific product labeling.

Tablet: 600 mg

References

Bass JC, Athreya BH, Brewer EJ, et al, "A Once-Daily Anti-Inflammatory Drug, Oxaprozin, in the Treatment of Juvenile Rheumatoid Arthritis," *J Rheumatol*, 1985, 12(2):384-6.

Oxcarbazepine (ox car BAZ e peen)

U.S. Brand Names Trileptal®

Canadian Brand Names Trileptal®

Index Terms GP 47680; OCBZ

Therapeutic Category Anticonvulsant, Miscellaneous

Generic Available No

Use Treatment of partial seizures in patients with epilepsy (as monotherapy in children ≥4 years of age and adults, and as adjunctive therapy in children ≥2 years of age and adults)

Pregnancy Risk Factor C

Lactation Enters breast milk/not recommended

Contraindications Hypersensitivity to oxcarbazepine or any component

Warnings Significant hyponatremia may occur; a serum sodium <125 mEq/L has been reported in 2.5% of patients; consider monitoring serum sodium especially in patients who receive other drugs that may cause hyponatremia and in patients with symptoms of hyponatremia (eg, nausea, headache, malaise, confusion, lethargy, obtundation, or an increase in seizure frequency or severity). Do not abruptly discontinue therapy, withdraw gradually to lessen chance for increased seizure frequency (unless a more rapid withdrawal is required due to safety concerns). Serious dermatologic reactions (including potentially fatal Stevens-Johnson syndrome and toxic epidermal necrolysis) have been reported (median onset 19 days); consider discontinuation of oxcarbazepine and alternative therapy in patients who develop skin reactions. Cross-hypersensitivity reactions with carbamazepine may occur (incidence: 25% to 30%); serious and potentially fatal multiorgan hypersensitivity reactions have also been reported (see Adverse Reactions); discontinue oxcarbazepine immediately if signs or symptoms of hypersensitivity develop

Precautions CNS adverse effects may occur including somnolence, fatigue, coordination abnormalities (ataxia and gait disturbances), and cognitive symptoms (difficulty concentrating, speech or language problems, and psychomotor slowing); these effects may be more common when oxcarbazepine is used as add-on therapy versus monotherapy. Use with caution and modify dose in patients with renal impairment. Multiple drug interactions may occur (see Drug Interactions).

Adverse Reactions

Central nervous system: Headache, dizziness, somnolence (incidence in children: Up to 34.8%), fatigue, ataxia or gait disturbances (children: Up to 23.2%), tremor, insomnia, cognitive symptoms (children: Up to 5.8%; psychomotor slowing, difficulty concentrating, speech or language problems), vertigo, anxiety, nervousness, emotional lability

Dermatologic: Rash, maculopapular rash; rare: Stevens-Johnson syndrome, erythema multiforme, toxic epidermal necrolysis

Endocrine and Metabolic: Hyponatremia (incidence: 2.5%; usually occurs within the first 3 months of therapy, but has been reported in patients more than 1 year after starting medication; serum sodium returns towards normal after discontinuation, reduction of dose, or with conservative treatment such as fluid restriction); reduction in T_4 levels

Gastrointestinal: Nausea, vomiting, abdominal pain, dyspepsia

Neuromuscular & skeletal: Abnormal gait

Ocular: Diplopia, abnormal vision, nystagmus

Miscellaneous: Hypersensitivity reactions; a rare, multiorgan hypersensitivity reaction with rash, lymphadenopathy, fever, abnormal liver function tests, hepatitis, nephritis, oliguria, hepatorenal syndrome, hematological abnormalities, pruritus, asthenia, and/or arthralgia has also been reported (median time to detection: 13 days post-therapy initiation)

Drug Interactions Cytochrome P450 isoenzyme CYP2C19 inhibitor; CYP3A4 and CYP3A5 inducer

Oxcarbazepine may inhibit hepatic metabolism and increase the serum concentrations of phenobarbital (by 14%) and phenytoin (by 40% with high-dose oxcarbazepine; dosage reduction of phenytoin may be needed); may induce hepatic metabolism and decrease serum concentrations of felodipine, lamotrigine, and oral contraceptives such as ethinyl estradiol and levonorgestrel (alternative methods of contraception are recommended); use with alcohol may increase sedative effects

P450 enzyme inducers such as carbamazepine, phenobarbital, and phenytoin, may significantly decrease MHD concentrations by 25% to 40%; valproic acid decreases MHD concentrations by 18% and verapamil decreases MHD concentrations by 20%

Food Interactions

Tablets: Food does not affect rate or extent of absorption

Suspension: Effect of food has not been studied, but bioavailability is not likely to be affected

Stability Store at controlled room temperature (25°C); dispense in tight container; suspension is stable for 7 weeks after first opening the bottle

Mechanism of Action Active 10-monohydroxy metabolite (MHD) is primarily responsible for anticonvulsant activity; exact mechanism unknown; both MHD and oxcarbazepine are thought to decrease the spread of seizure activity by blockade of sodium channels; also increases conductance of potassium and modulates activity of high-voltage activated calcium channels

Pharmacokinetics

Absorption: Oral: Complete

Distribution: MHD: V_d (apparent): Adults: 49 L

Protein binding: Oxcarbazepine: 67%; MHD: 40%, primarily to albumin; parent drug and metabolite do not bind to alpha-1 acid glycoprotein

Metabolism: Oxcarbazepine is extensively metabolized in the liver to its active 10-monohydroxy metabolite (MHD); MHD undergoes further metabolism via glucuronide conjugation; 4% of dose is oxidized to the 10,11-dihydroxy metabolite (DHD) (inactive); 70% of serum concentration appears as MHD, 2% as unchanged oxcarbazepine, and the rest as minor metabolites; **Note:** Unlike carbamazepine, autoinduction of metabolism has not been observed and biotransformation of oxcarbazepine does not result in an epoxide metabolite

Bioavailability: Tablets and suspension have similar bioavailability (based on MDH serum concentrations)

Half-life:

Adults:

Oxcarbazepine: 2 hours

MHD: 9 hours

Adults with renal impairment (Cl_{cr} <30 mL/minute): MHD: 19 hours

Time to peak serum concentration: Adults:

Tablets: 3-13 hours (median: 4.5 hours)

Suspension: Median: 6 hours

Elimination: >95% of dose is excreted in the urine with <1% as unchanged parent drug, 27% as unchanged MHD, 49% as MHD glucuronides, 3% as DHD (inactive), and 13% as conjugate of oxcarbazepine and MHD; <4% excreted in feces

Clearance (per body weight):

Children 2 to <4 years: Increased by ~80% compared to adults

Children 4-12 years: Increased by ~40% compared to adults

Children ≥13 years: Values approach adult clearance

Hepatic impairment: Mild to moderate: No effect on pharmacokinetics; Severe: Not studied

Usual Dosage Oral: **Note:** Oral suspension and tablets are interchangeable on a mg per mg basis:

Neonates, Infants, and Children <2 years: Not approved for use; limited information is available

Children 2-16 years:

Adjunctive therapy:

Children 2 to <4 years: Initial dose: 8-10 mg/kg/day given in 2 divided doses (usual maximum: 600 mg/day); for children <20 kg, consider initial dose of 16"20 mg/kg/day given in 2 divided doses; increase dose slowly over 2"4 weeks; do not exceed 60 mg/kg/day in 2 divided doses

Children 4-16 years: Initial dose: 8-10 mg/kg/day given in 2 divided doses (usual maximum: 600 mg/day); increase dose slowly over 2 weeks to the following weight-dependent target maintenance dose:

20-29 kg: 900 mg/day in 2 divided doses

29.1-39 kg: 1200 mg/day in 2 divided doses

>39 kg: 1800 mg/day in 2 divided doses

Note: Use of these pediatric target maintenance doses in one clinical trial resulted in doses ranging from 6-51 mg/kg/day (median dose: 31 mg/kg/day) in children 4"16 years of age (see Glauser, 2000). In children 2"4 years of age, 50% of patients were titrated to a final dose of at least 55 mg/kg/day with target dose of 60 mg/kg/day. Due to a higher drug clearance, children 2 to <4 years of age may require up to twice the dose per body weight compared to adults; children 4 to ≤12 years of age may require a 50% higher dose per body weight compared to adults (see product information).

Children 4-16 years:

Conversion to monotherapy: Initial: 8-10 mg/kg/day given in 2 divided doses, with a simultaneous initial reduction of the dose of concomitant antiepileptic drugs (AEDs); withdraw concomitant AEDs completely over 3-6 weeks, while increasing oxcarbazepine dose as needed by no more than 10 mg/kg/day at approximately weekly intervals; increase oxcarbazepine dose to achieve the recommended monotherapy maintenance dose by weight (listed on next page).

(Continued)

Oxcarbazepine *(Continued)*

Initiation of monotherapy: Initial: 8-10 mg/kg/day given in 2 divided doses; increase dose every third day by 5 mg/kg/day to achieve the recommended monotherapy maintenance dose by weight, as follows:
20 kg: 600-900 mg/day in 2 divided doses
25-30 kg: 900-1200 mg/day in 2 divided doses
35-40 kg: 900-1500 mg/day in 2 divided doses
45 kg: 1200-1500 mg/day in 2 divided doses
50-55 kg: 1200-1800 mg/day in 2 divided doses
60-65 kg: 1200-2100 mg/day in 2 divided doses
70 kg: 1500-2100 mg/day in 2 divided doses

Adults:

Adjunctive therapy: Initial: 300 mg twice daily; increase if needed by no more than 600 mg/day at approximately weekly intervals; recommended maintenance dose: 600 mg twice daily; **Note:** Doses >1200 mg/day may have greater efficacy, but most patients are not able to tolerate 2400 mg/day (mostly due to CNS effects); monitor patient closely and measure concentrations of concomitant antiepileptic agents during dosage titration and especially with oxcarbazepine doses >1200 mg/day

Conversion to monotherapy: Initial: 300 mg twice daily with a simultaneous initial reduction of the dose of concomitant antiepileptic drugs (AEDs); withdraw concomitant AEDs completely over 3-6 weeks, while increasing oxcarbazepine dose as needed by no more than 600 mg/day at approximately weekly intervals; recommended oxcarbazepine dose (1200 mg twice daily) should be reached in about 2-4 weeks; **Note:** A lower dose (1200 mg/day) was effective in one study in patients who initiated oxcarbazepine monotherapy

Initiation of monotherapy: Initial: 300 mg twice daily; increase by 300 mg/day every third day to 1200 mg/day; a higher dose (2400 mg/day) was effective in patients who were converted from other AEDs to oxcarbazepine monotherapy.

Dosing adjustment in renal impairment: Cl_{cr} <30 mL/minute: Initial dose: Administer 50% of the normal starting dose; slowly increase the dose if needed, using a slower dosage titration than normal

Dosing adjustment in hepatic impairment:
Mild to moderate hepatic impairment: No dosage adjustment recommended
Severe hepatic impairment: Not evaluated

Administration Oral: May be taken without regard to meals

Suspension: Prior to using for the first time, firmly insert the manufacturer supplied plastic adapter into the neck of the bottle; cover the adapter with child-resistant cap when not in use; shake suspension well (for at least 10 seconds) before use; remove child-resistant cap and insert manufacturer supplied oral syringe to withdraw appropriate dose; dose may be administered directly from syringe or mixed in a small amount of water immediately prior to use; after use, rinse oral syringe with warm water and allow to dry thoroughly; discard any unused portion 7 weeks after first opening bottle

Monitoring Parameters Seizure frequency, duration and severity; symptoms of CNS depression (dizziness, headache, somnolence) and allergic reaction; consider monitoring serum sodium (particularly during first three months of therapy) especially in patients who receive other drugs that may cause hyponatremia and in patients with symptoms of hyponatremia (see Warnings)

Patient Information Inform prescriber if allergic to carbamazepine; do not abruptly discontinue, an increase in seizure activity may result; report excessive somnolence or allergic reactions to physician immediately; report unusual symptoms such as nausea, headache, malaise, confusion, lethargy, obtundation, or a worsening of seizures to physician immediately (blood test for serum sodium may be needed); report skin rash, fever, itching, joint pain, abdominal pain, lack of urination, and swollen glands to physician immediately (these may be signs of a serious or potentially fatal multiorgan hypersensitivity reaction); avoid alcohol; may cause drowsiness and impair ability to perform activities requiring mental alertness or physical coordination; oxcarbazepine may decrease the effectiveness of oral contraceptives (use an alternative, nonhormonal, form of contraception)

Additional Information Symptoms of overdose may include CNS depression (somnolence, ataxia, obtundation); treatment is symptomatic and supportive; consider general poisoning management (eg, gastric lavage, activated charcoal); largest reported overdose is 24 g; oxcarbazepine is a keto analogue of carbamazepine

Dosage Forms Excipient information presented when available (limited, particularly for generics); consult specific product labeling.

Suspension, oral: 300 mg/5 mL (250 mL) [contains ethanol; packaged with oral syringe]

Tablet: 150 mg, 300 mg, 600 mg

References

Glauser TA, Nigro M, Sachdeo R, et al, "Adjunctive Therapy With Oxcarbazepine in Children With Partial Seizures. The Oxcarbazepine Pediatric Study Group," *Neurology*, 2000, 54(12):2237-44.
Tecoma ES, "Oxcarbazepine," *Epilepsia*, 1999, 40(Suppl 5): S37-46.

♦ **Oxeze® Turbuhaler® (Can)** *see* Formoterol *on page 703*
♦ **Oxipor® VHC [OTC]** *see* Coal Tar *on page 394*
♦ **Oxpentifylline** *see* Pentoxifylline *on page 1241*
♦ **Oxy 10® Balanced Medicated Face Wash [OTC]** *see* Benzoyl Peroxide *on page 207*
♦ **Oxy 10® Balance Spot Treatment [OTC]** *see* Benzoyl Peroxide *on page 207*
♦ **Oxy Balance® [OTC]** *see* Salicylic Acid *on page 1413*
♦ **Oxy Balance® Deep Pore [OTC]** *see* Salicylic Acid *on page 1413*

Oxybutynin (oks i BYOO ti nin)

Medication Safety Issues

Sound-alike/look-alike issues:

Oxybutynin may be confused with OxyContin®
Ditropan® may be confused with Detrol®, diazepam, Diprivan®, dithranol

Transdermal patch may contain conducting metal (eg, aluminum); remove patch prior to MRI.

U.S. Brand Names Ditropan®; Ditropan® XL; Oxytrol®

Canadian Brand Names Apo-Oxybutynin®; Ditropan®; Ditropan® XL; Gen-Oxybutynin; Novo-Oxybutynin; Nu-Oxybutyn; Oxytrol®; PMS-Oxybutynin; Uromax®

Index Terms Oxybutynin Chloride

Therapeutic Category Antispasmodic Agent, Urinary

Generic Available Yes: Excludes transdermal patch

Use Relief of bladder spasms associated with voiding in patients with uninhibited and reflex neurogenic bladder; treatment of overactive bladder with symptoms of urge urinary incontinence, urgency, and frequency

Pregnancy Risk Factor B

Lactation Excretion in breast milk unknown/use caution

Contraindications Hypersensitivity to oxybutynin or any component; glaucoma (angle-closure), partial or complete GI obstruction, GU obstruction; toxic megacolon

Warnings Transdermal patch may contain conducting metal (eg, aluminum); remove patch prior to MRI. The extended release formulation consists of drug within a nondeformable matrix; following drug release/absorption, the matrix/shell is expelled in the stool.

Precautions Use with caution in patients with hepatic or renal disease, myasthenia gravis, heart disease, hyperthyroidism, reflux esophagitis, hypertension, prostatic hypertrophy, autonomic neuropathy, ulcerative colitis, intestinal atony

Adverse Reactions

Cardiovascular: Tachycardia, palpitations, vasodilation, myocarditis, arrhythmias, peripheral edema

Central nervous system: Drowsiness, dizziness, insomnia, fever, hallucinations, headache, somnolence, confusion, seizures

Dermatologic: Rash

Endocrine & metabolic: Hot flashes, suppressed lactation

Gastrointestinal: Xerostomia, nausea, vomiting, constipation, decreased GI motility, abdominal pain, dyspepsia, diarrhea, flatulence

Genitourinary: Impotence, urinary hesitancy or retention, urinary tract infections

Local: Application site reactions, such as rash, macular rash, pruritus, erythema, and burning (transdermal formulation)

Neuromuscular & skeletal: Weakness

Ocular: Blurred vision, mydriasis, decreased lacrimation, amblyopia, cycloplegia

Respiratory: Dry nasal and sinus mucous membranes

Miscellaneous: Hypersensitivity reactions, decreased diaphoresis

Drug Interactions Cytochrome P450 isoenzyme CYP3A4 substrate

Additive sedation with CNS depressants and alcohol; additive anticholinergic effects with antihistamines and anticholinergic agents; ketoconazole and other CYP3A4 inhibitors (eg, itraconazole, macrolide antibiotics) may increase serum oxybutynin levels

Food Interactions Food may slightly delay absorption and reduce bioavailability of immediate release formulation by 25%. Absorption of extended release formulation is not affected by food.

Stability Store at controlled room temperature; protect syrup from light; keep transdermal patch in sealed pouch; protect from moisture or humidity

(Continued)

Oxybutynin *(Continued)*

Mechanism of Action Direct antispasmodic effect on smooth muscle, also inhibits the action of acetylcholine on smooth muscle; does not block effects at skeletal muscle or at autonomic ganglia; increases bladder capacity, decreases uninhibited contractions, and delays desire to void resulting in decreased urgency and frequency

Pharmacodynamics

Immediate release formulation:

Onset of action: Oral: Within 30-60 minutes

Maximum effect: 3-6 hours

Duration: 6-10 hours

Extended release formulation: Maximum effects: 3 days

Transdermal formulation: Duration: 96 hours

Pharmacokinetics

Absorption: Oral: Rapid and well absorbed

Distribution: V_d: Adults: 193 L

Metabolism: Hepatic via cytochrome isozyme CYP3A4 found mostly in liver and gut wall; extensive first pass effect (not with I.V. or transdermal use); metabolized in the liver to active and inactive metabolites

Bioavailability: Oral: Immediate release: 6% (range: 1.6% to 10.9%)

Half-life: Adults: 2-3 hours

Time to peak serum concentration:

Immediate release: Within 60 minutes

Extended release: 4-6 hours

Transdermal: 24-48 hours

Elimination: <0.1% excreted unchanged in urine

Usual Dosage

Children: Oral:

Immediate release:

1-5 years: 0.2 mg/kg/dose 2-3 times/day

>5 years: 5 mg twice daily, up to 5 mg 3 times/day

Extended release: ≥6 years: 5 mg once daily; increase as tolerated in 5 mg increments to a maximum of 20 mg/day

Adults:

Oral: 5 mg 2-3 times/day up to 5 mg 4 times/day maximum **or** extended release tablet (Ditropan® XL) 5-10 mg once daily; increase in 5 mg increments to a maximum of 30 mg/day

Transdermal: 3.9 mg/day system applied twice weekly (every 3-4 days)

Note: Should be discontinued periodically to determine whether the patient can manage without the drug and to minimize tolerance to the drug

Administration

Oral: Administer immediate release formulation on an empty stomach; extended release formulation may be administered with or without food; swallow extended release tablets whole; do not chew or crush.

Transdermal: Apply to dry intact skin on the abdomen, hip, or buttock. Rotate site of application with each administration and avoid application to the same site within 7 days

Patient Information May cause drowsiness and impair ability to perform activities requiring mental alertness or physical coordination; may cause heat prostration (fever and heat stroke due to decreased sweating) when used in hot climates; avoid alcohol; may cause dry mouth; nonabsorbable tablet shell may be seen in stool, but active drug has been released

Dosage Forms Excipient information presented when available (limited, particularly for generics); consult specific product labeling.

Syrup, as chloride: 5 mg/5 mL (473 mL)

Ditropan®: 5 mg/5 mL (473 mL)

Tablet, as chloride: 5 mg

Ditropan®: 5 mg

Tablet, extended release, as chloride: 5 mg, 10 mg, 15 mg

Ditropan® XL: 5 mg, 10 mg, 15 mg

Transdermal system:

Oxytrol®: 3.9 mg/day (8s) [39 cm^2; total oxybutynin 36 mg]

References

Humphreys MR and Reinberg YE, "Contemporary and Emerging Drug Treatments for Urinary Incontinence in Children," *Paediatr Drugs*, 2005, 7(3):151-62.

◆ **Oxybutynin Chloride** *see* Oxybutynin *on page 1187*

◆ **Oxycocet® (Can)** *see* Oxycodone and Acetaminophen *on page 1191*

◆ **Oxycodan® (Can)** *see* Oxycodone and Aspirin *on page 1193*

Oxycodone (oks i KOE done)

Medication Safety Issues

Sound-alike/look-alike issues:

Oxycodone may be confused with OxyContin®

OxyContin® may be confused with oxybutynin, oxycodone

OxyFast® may be confused with Roxanol™

U.S. Brand Names ETH-Oxydose™; OxyContin®; OxyFast®; OxyIR®; Roxicodone®

Canadian Brand Names OxyContin®; Oxy.IR®; Supeudol®

Index Terms Dihydrohydroxycodeinone; Oxycodone Hydrochloride

Therapeutic Category Analgesic, Narcotic

Generic Available Yes

Use Relief of moderate to severe pain

Controlled release tablets (OxyContin®) are indicated for around-the-clock management of moderate to severe pain when an analgesic is needed for an extended period of time; **Note:** OxyContin® is not intended for use as a PRN analgesic or for treatment of mild pain, pain that is not expected to persist for an extended period of time, or for immediate postoperative pain (within 12-24 hours after surgery); OxyContin® may be used for postoperative pain only if the patient received it prior to surgery or if moderate to severe persistent pain is anticipated.

Restrictions C-II

Pregnancy Risk Factor B (D if used for prolonged periods or in high doses at term)

Lactation Enters breast milk/use caution

Contraindications Hypersensitivity to oxycodone or any component (see Warnings); significant respiratory depression (in settings without resuscitative equipment or without adequate respiratory monitoring); patients with hypercarbia, severe or acute asthma, paralytic ileus (known or suspected)

Warnings Respiratory depression may occur; use with extreme caution in patients with pre-existing respiratory depression, decreased respiratory reserve, hypoxia, hypercapnia, significant COPD, or cor pulmonale. Hypotension may occur, especially in hypovolemic patients or those receiving medications that compromise vasomotor tone; use with extreme caution in patients with circulatory shock; orthostatic hypotension may occur in ambulatory patients. Physical and psychological dependence may occur; abrupt discontinuation after prolonged use may result in withdrawal symptoms; use of agonist/antagonist analgesics may precipitate withdrawal symptoms and/or reduce the analgesic efficacy in patients who have received or who are receiving a pure opioid agonist such as oxycodone. Warn patient of possible impairment of alertness or physical coordination (see Patient Information); interactions with other CNS drugs may occur (see Drug Interactions). Controlled release 60 mg, 80 mg, and 160 mg tablets should only be used in patients who are opioid tolerant (administration of these tablet strengths to opioid naive patients may cause fatal respiratory depression). Healthcare provider should be alert to problems of abuse, misuse, and diversion.

Oral concentrate contains sodium benzoate; benzoic acid (benzoate) is a metabolite of benzyl alcohol; large amounts of benzyl alcohol (≥99 mg/kg/day) have been associated with a potentially fatal toxicity ("gasping syndrome") in neonates; the "gasping syndrome" consists of metabolic acidosis, respiratory distress, gasping respirations, CNS dysfunction (including convulsions, intracranial hemorrhage), hypotension and cardiovascular collapse; avoid use of oxycodone products containing sodium benzoate in neonates; *in vitro* and animal studies have shown that benzoate displaces bilirubin from protein binding sites. Oral dropper for OxyFast® oral concentrate contains natural rubber latex which may cause allergic reactions in susceptible individuals; avoid use in patients with allergy to latex.

Precautions Use with caution in patients with hypersensitivity to other phenanthrene derivative opioid agonists (morphine, codeine, hydrocodone, hydromorphone, oxymorphone, levorphanol). Use with caution in patients with head injury; increased intracranial pressure; CNS depression; respiratory depression; coma; toxic psychosis; seizures; acute abdominal conditions; biliary tract disease, pancreatitis; severe renal, respiratory, or hepatic insufficiency; hypothyroidism; Addison's disease; urethral stricture and in debilitated patients. Use care in prescribing, dispensing, and administering the oral concentrated solution, inappropriate use may cause overdose.

Adverse Reactions

Cardiovascular system: Hypotension, orthostatic hypotension, bradycardia, peripheral vasodilation

Central nervous system: CNS depression, elevated intracranial pressure, dizziness, drowsiness, insomnia, somnolence, nervousness, fever, chills, confusion, anxiety, sedation, lightheadedness, dysphoria, headache, fatigue, abnormal dreams, abnormal thoughts

Dermatologic: Pruritus, skin rash

(Continued)

Oxycodone *(Continued)*

Endocrine & metabolic: Antidiuretic hormone release
Gastrointestinal: Nausea, vomiting, constipation, biliary tract spasm, xerostomia, anorexia, abdominal pain, dyspepsia, gastritis
Genitourinary: Urinary tract spasm, urinary retention
Neuromuscular & skeletal: Asthenia
Ocular: Miosis
Respiratory: Respiratory depression, dyspnea, hiccups
Miscellaneous: Physical and psychological dependence, histamine release, diaphoresis; anaphylaxis, anaphylactoid reactions

Drug Interactions Cytochrome P450 isoenzyme CYP2D6 substrate
CNS depressants, phenothiazines, tricyclic antidepressants may potentiate the CNS adverse effects of oxycodone (dosage reduction of one or both agents is recommended; some recommend starting opioid analgesics at $^1/_3$ to $^1/_2$ of the normal dose in patients receiving other CNS depressants). Agonist/antagonist analgesics (eg, pentazocine, nalbuphine, butorphanol) may precipitate withdrawal symptoms and/or reduce analgesic efficacy.

Food Interactions Food does not significantly affect absorption of controlled release tablets; high fat meal may increase peak concentrations of OxyContin® 160 mg tablet by 25%

Stability Store at room temperature; protect from light and moisture
OxyFast® oral concentrate: Stable for 90 days after opening

Mechanism of Action Binds to opiate receptors in the CNS, causing inhibition of ascending pain pathways, altering the perception of and response to pain; produces generalized CNS depression

Pharmacodynamics Duration of pain relief: Oral:
Immediate release: 4-5 hours
Controlled release: 12 hours

Pharmacokinetics
Distribution: Distributes into skeletal muscle, liver, intestinal tract, lungs, spleen, brain, and breast milk; V_{dss}:
Children 2-10 years: Mean: 2.1 L/kg; range: 1.2-3.7 L/kg
Adults: 2.6 L/kg
Protein binding: 38% to 45%
Metabolism: In the liver primarily to noroxycodone (via demethylation) and oxymorphone (via CYP2D6); noroxycodone is the major circulating metabolite, but has much weaker activity than oxycodone; oxymorphone is active, but present in low concentrations; <15% of the dose is metabolized to oxymorphone via CYP2D6; drug and metabolites undergo glucuronide conjugation
Bioavailability: Adults: 60% to 87%
Half-life, apparent: Adults:
Immediate release: 3.2 hours
Controlled release (OxyContin®): 4.5 hours
Half-life, elimination:
Children 2-10 years: 1.8 hours; range: 1.2-3 hours
Adults: 3.7 hours
Adults with renal dysfunction (Cl_{cr} <60 mL/minute): Half-life increases by 1 hour, but peak oxycodone concentrations increase by 50% and AUC increases by 60%
Adults with mild to moderate hepatic dysfunction: Half-life increases by 2.3 hours, peak oxycodone concentrations increase by 50%, and AUC increases by 95%
Elimination: In the urine as unchanged drug (≤19%) and metabolites: Conjugated oxycodone (≤50%), conjugated oxymorphone (≤14%), noroxycodone, and conjugated noroxycodone

Usual Dosage Oral: **Doses should be titrated to appropriate effect:**
Immediate release products:
Children: 0.05-0.15 mg/kg/dose every 4-6 hours as needed
Adults: Initial: 5 mg every 6 hours as needed; usual: 10-30 mg every 4 hours as needed; more severe pain: ≥30 mg every 4 hours
AHCPR dosing guidelines: Opioid naive patients: (See Carr, 1992 and Jacox, 1994)
Children and Adults <50 kg: Moderate to severe pain: Usual initial dose: 0.2 mg/kg every 3-4 hours
Children and Adults ≥50 kg: Moderate to severe pain: Usual initial dose: 10 mg every 3-4 hours
Controlled release product: Adolescents ≥18 years and Adults: Initial: 10 mg every 12 hours; use immediate-release analgesics as needed for rescue from breakthrough pain or prior to predictable pain from procedures or activities; rescue analgesic should be $^1/_4$ to $^1/_3$ of the 12-hour controlled release oxycodone dose; increase the dose of controlled release oxycodone if >2 doses of rescue analgesic are required within 24 hours; dose of controlled release oxycodone may be adjusted every 1-2

days by 25% to 50% (initial increase may be from 10 mg to 20 mg every 12 hours). Mean doses used in open-label trials: Opioid naive patients: 40 mg/day; cancer patients: 105 mg/day (range: 20-720 mg/day)

Note: To convert patients from other opioid or nonopioid analgesics to oxycodone controlled release tablets: See OxyContin® package insert

Dosing adjustment in renal impairment: Cl_{cr} <60 mL/minute: Initiate doses conservatively and carefully titrate dose to appropriate effect

Dosing adjustment in hepatic impairment: Initial: 1/3 to 1/2 of the usual dose; carefully titrate dose to appropriate effect

Administration May administer with food to decrease GI upset; swallow controlled (sustained) release tablets whole; do not crush, chew, or break (this would result in rapid release and absorption of a potentially fatal dose of drug); avoid high fat meals when initiating controlled release 160 mg tablets

Monitoring Parameters Pain relief, respiratory rate, mental status, blood pressure

Patient Information May cause dry mouth; may cause drowsiness and impair ability to perform activities requiring mental alertness or physical coordination; may cause postural hypotension (use caution when changing positions from lying or sitting to standing); avoid alcohol; report the use of other prescription and nonprescription medications to your physician and pharmacist. May be habit-forming; do not discontinue abruptly if therapy lasts more than a few weeks; dose should be tapered to prevent withdrawal. Do not crush, chew, or break controlled release tablets (OxyContin®), as risk of overdose (and possibly death) may occur. Empty controlled release tablets may appear in stool after medication is absorbed (this is normal). Do not share OxyContin® with others (sharing is illegal and may cause severe medical adverse effects, including death).

Additional Information OxyContin® tablets deliver medication over 12 hours; release is pH independent. Equianalgesic doses: oral oxycodone 30 mg = morphine 10 mg I.M. = single oral dose morphine 60 mg **or** chronic dosing oral morphine 30 mg

Dosage Forms Excipient information presented when available (limited, particularly for generics); consult specific product labeling.

Capsule, as hydrochloride: 5 mg
- OxyIR®: 5 mg

Solution, oral, as hydrochloride: 5 mg/5 mL (500 mL)
- Roxicodone®: 5 mg/5 mL (5 mL, 500 mL) [contains alcohol]

Solution, oral, as hydrochloride [concentrate]: 20 mg/mL (30 mL)
- ETH-Oxydose™: 20 mg/mL (1 mL, 30 mL) [contains sodium benzoate; berry flavor]
- OxyFast®: 20 mg/mL (30 mL) [contains sodium benzoate and dry natural rubber]
- Roxicodone®: 20 mg/mL (30 mL) [contains sodium benzoate]

Tablet, as hydrochloride: 5 mg, 15 mg, 30 mg
- Roxicodone®: 5 mg, 15 mg, 30 mg

Tablet, controlled release, as hydrochloride:
- OxyContin®: 10 mg, 20 mg, 40 mg, 60 mg, 80 mg, 160 mg

Tablet, extended release, as hydrochloride: 10 mg, 20 mg, 40 mg, 80 mg

References

Carr D, Jacox A, Chapman CR, et al, "Clinical Practice Guideline Number 1: Acute Pain Management: Operative or Medical Procedures and Trauma," Rockville, Maryland: U.S. Department of Health and Human Services, Public Health Service, Agency for Health Care Policy and Research, AHCPR Publication No 92-0032, 1992.

Jacox A, Carr D, Payne R, et al, "Clinical Practice Guideline Number 9: Management of Cancer Pain," Rockville, Maryland: U.S. Department of Health and Human Services, Public Health Service, Agency for Health Care Policy and Research, AHCPR Publication No. 94-0592, 1994.

Olkkola KT, Hamunen K, and Maunuksela EL, "Clinical Pharmacokinetics and Pharmacodynamics of Opioid Analgesics in Infants and Children," *Clin Pharmacokinet*, 1995, 28(5):385-404.

Olkkola KT, Hamunen K, Seppala T, et al, "Pharmacokinetics and Ventilatory Effects of Intravenous Oxycodone in Postoperative Children," *Br J Clin Pharmacol*, 1994, 38(1):71-6.

Oxycodone and Acetaminophen

(oks i KOE done & a seet a MIN oh fen)

Medication Safety Issues

Sound-alike/look-alike issues:
- Percocet® may be confused with Percodan®
- Roxicet™ may be confused with Roxanol™
- Tylox® may be confused with Trimox®, Tylenol®, Wymox®, Xanax®

Related Information

Narcotic Analgesics Comparison *on page 1705*

Overdose and Toxicology *on page 1916*

U.S. Brand Names Endocet®; Percocet®; Roxicet™; Roxicet™ 5/500; Tylox®

Canadian Brand Names Endocet®; Oxycocet®; Percocet®; Percocet®-Demi; PMS-Oxycodone-Acetaminophen

(Continued)

Oxycodone and Acetaminophen *(Continued)*

Index Terms Acetaminophen and Oxycodone

Therapeutic Category Analgesic, Narcotic

Generic Available Yes: Excludes caplet and solution

Use Relief of moderate to severe pain

Restrictions C-II

Pregnancy Risk Factor C

Lactation Enters breast milk/use caution

Contraindications Hypersensitivity to oxycodone, acetaminophen, or any component (see Warnings); severe respiratory depression, severe liver or renal insufficiency

Warnings Abrupt discontinuation after prolonged use may result in withdrawal symptoms; some preparations contain sodium metabisulfite which may cause allergic reactions in susceptible individuals; capsule may contain sodium benzoate; benzoic acid (benzoate) is a metabolite of benzyl alcohol; large amounts of benzyl alcohol (≥99 mg/kg/day) have been associated with a potentially fatal toxicity ("gasping syndrome") in neonates; the "gasping syndrome" consists of metabolic acidosis, respiratory distress, gasping respirations, CNS dysfunction (including convulsions, intracranial hemorrhage), hypotension and cardiovascular collapse; avoid use of oxycodone and acetaminophen products containing sodium benzoate in neonates; *in vitro* and animal studies have shown that benzoate displaces bilirubin from protein binding sites

Precautions Use with caution in patients with hypersensitivity to other phenanthrene derivative opioid agonists (morphine, codeine, hydrocodone, hydromorphone, oxymorphone, levorphanol)

Adverse Reactions

Cardiovascular: Hypotension, bradycardia, peripheral vasodilation

Central nervous system: CNS depression, elevated intracranial pressure, drowsiness, sedation

Dermatologic: Pruritus

Endocrine & metabolic: Antidiuretic hormone release

Gastrointestinal: Nausea, vomiting, constipation, biliary tract spasm

Genitourinary: Urinary tract spasm

Ocular: Miosis

Respiratory: Respiratory depression

Miscellaneous: Physical and psychological dependence, histamine release

Drug Interactions See Acetaminophen *on page 42* and Oxycodone *on page 1189*

Food Interactions Rate of absorption of acetaminophen may be decreased when given with food high in carbohydrates

Mechanism of Action See Acetaminophen *on page 42* and Oxycodone *on page 1189*

Pharmacodynamics

Onset of action: Within 10-15 minutes

Maximum effect: Within 1 hour

Duration: 3-6 hours

Pharmacokinetics See Acetaminophen *on page 42* and Oxycodone *on page 1189*

Usual Dosage Oral (titrate dose to appropriate analgesic effects):

Children: Based on **oxycodone component**: 0.05-0.15 mg/kg/dose up to 5 mg/dose every 4-6 hours as needed

Adults: 1-2 tablets every 4-6 hours as needed for pain; maximum daily dose of acetaminophen: 4 g/day

Administration Oral: May administer with food or milk to decrease GI upset

Monitoring Parameters Pain relief, respiratory rate, mental status, blood pressure

Patient Information Avoid alcohol; may cause drowsiness and impair ability to perform activities requiring mental alertness or physical coordination. May be habit-forming; do not discontinue abruptly if therapy lasts more than a few weeks; dose should be tapered to prevent narcotic withdrawal.

Dosage Forms Excipient information presented when available (limited, particularly for generics); consult specific product labeling.

Caplet:

Roxicet™ 5/500: Oxycodone hydrochloride 5 mg and acetaminophen 500 mg

Capsule: 5/500: Oxycodone hydrochloride 5 mg and acetaminophen 500 mg

Tylox®: 5/500: Oxycodone hydrochloride 5 mg and acetaminophen 500 mg [contains sodium benzoate and sodium metabisulfite]

Solution, oral:

Roxicet™: Oxycodone hydrochloride 5 mg and acetaminophen 325 mg per 5 mL (5 mL, 500 mL) [contains alcohol <0.5%]

Tablet: 5/325: Oxycodone hydrochloride 5 mg and acetaminophen 325 mg; 7.5/325: Oxycodone hydrochloride 7.5 mg and acetaminophen 325 mg; 7.5/500: Oxycodone hydrochloride 7.5 mg and acetaminophen 500 mg; 10/325: Oxycodone hydrochloride 10 mg and acetaminophen 325 mg; 10/650: Oxycodone hydrochloride 10 mg and acetaminophen 650 mg

Endocet® 5/325 [scored]: Oxycodone hydrochloride 5 mg and acetaminophen 325 mg

Endocet® 7.5/325: Oxycodone hydrochloride 7.5 mg and acetaminophen 325 mg

Endocet® 7.5/500: Oxycodone hydrochloride 7.5 mg and acetaminophen 500 mg

Endocet® 10/325: Oxycodone hydrochloride 10 mg and acetaminophen 325 mg

Endocet® 10/650: Oxycodone hydrochloride 10 mg and acetaminophen 650 mg

Percocet® 2.5/325: Oxycodone hydrochloride 2.5 mg and acetaminophen 325 mg

Percocet® 5/325 [scored]: Oxycodone hydrochloride 5 mg and acetaminophen 325 mg

Percocet® 7.5/325: Oxycodone hydrochloride 7.5 mg and acetaminophen 325 mg

Percocet® 7.5/500: Oxycodone hydrochloride 7.5 mg and acetaminophen 500 mg

Percocet® 10/325: Oxycodone hydrochloride 10 mg and acetaminophen 325 mg

Percocet® 10/650: Oxycodone hydrochloride 10 mg and acetaminophen 650 mg

Roxicet™ [scored]: Oxycodone hydrochloride 5 mg and acetaminophen 325 mg

References

Olkkola KT, Hamunen K, and Maunuksela EL, "Clinical Pharmacokinetics and Pharmacodynamics of Opioid Analgesics in Infants and Children," *Clin Pharmacokinet*, 1995, 28(5):385-404.

Oxycodone and Aspirin (oks i KOE done & AS pir in)

Medication Safety Issues

Sound-alike/look-alike issues:

Percodan® may be confused with Decadron®, Percocet®, Percogesic®, Periactin®

Related Information

Overdose and Toxicology *on page 1916*

U.S. Brand Names Endodan®; Percodan®

Canadian Brand Names Endodan®; Oxycodan®; Percodan®

Index Terms Aspirin and Oxycodone

Therapeutic Category Analgesic, Narcotic

Generic Available Yes

Use Relief of moderate to moderately severe pain

Restrictions C-II

Pregnancy Risk Factor D

Lactation Enters breast milk/use caution

Contraindications Hypersensitivity to oxycodone, salicylates, other NSAIDs, or any component; patients with the aspirin "triad" [asthma, rhinitis (with or without nasal polyps), and aspirin intolerance] (fatal asthmatic and anaphylactoid reactions may occur in these patients); severe respiratory depression; hypercarbia; severe or acute asthma; paralytic ileus (known or suspected); severe liver or renal insufficiency; bleeding disorders

Warnings Contains aspirin, do not use aspirin-containing products in children <16 years of age for chickenpox or flu symptoms due to the association with Reye's syndrome. Contains oxycodone; respiratory depression may occur; use with extreme caution in patients with pre-existing respiratory depression, decreased resiratory reserve, hypoxia, hypercapnia, significant COPD, or cor pulmonale. Hypotension may occur, especially in hypovolemic patients or those receiving medications that compromise vasomotor tone; use with extreme caution in patients with circulatory shock. Orthostatic hypotension may occur in ambulatory patients; physical and psychological dependence may occur; abrupt discontinuation after prolonged use may result in withdrawal symptoms; warn patients of possible impairment of alertness or physical coordination (see Patient Information); interactions with other CNS drugs may occur (see Drug Interactions). Healthcare provider should be alert to problems of abuse, misuse, and diversion.

Precautions Contains aspirin, use with caution in patients with impaired hepatic or renal function, erosive gastritis, peptic ulcer, gout. Contains oxycodone. Use with caution in patients with hypersensitivity to other phenanthrene derivative opioid agonists (morphine, codeine, hydrocodone, hydromorphone, oxymorphone, levorphanol). Use with caution in patients with head injury; increased intracranial pressure; CNS depression; respiratory depression; coma; toxic psychosis; seizures; acute abdominal conditions; biliary tract disease, pancreatitis; severe renal, respiratory, or hepatic insufficiency; hypothyroidism; Addison's disease; urethral stricture and in debilitated patients.

Adverse Reactions

Cardiovascular: Hypotension, bradycardia, peripheral vasodilation

Central nervous system: CNS depression, elevated intracranial pressure, drowsiness, sedation

Dermatologic: Pruritus, rash

(Continued)

Oxycodone and Aspirin *(Continued)*

Endocrine & metabolic: Antidiuretic hormone release
Gastrointestinal: Nausea, vomiting, constipation, biliary tract spasm, GI distress, GI bleeding, ulcers
Genitourinary: Urinary tract spasm
Hematologic: Inhibition of platelet aggregation (due to aspirin)
Hepatic: Hepatotoxicity (due to aspirin)
Ocular: Miosis
Respiratory: Respiratory depression, bronchospasm
Miscellaneous: Histamine release, physical and psychological dependence

Drug Interactions See Aspirin *on page 163* and Oxycodone *on page 1189*

Food Interactions Aspirin may increase renal excretion of vitamin C and may decrease serum folate levels

Mechanism of Action See Aspirin *on page 163* and Oxycodone *on page 1189*

Pharmacokinetics See Aspirin *on page 163* and Oxycodone *on page 1189*

Usual Dosage Oral: Based on **oxycodone-combined salt component**:

Children: 0.05-0.15 mg/kg/dose every 4-6 hours as needed; maximum dose: 5 mg/dose (1 tablet Percodan®)

Adults: Percodan®: 1 tablet every 6 hours as needed for pain; **Note:** Maximum aspirin dose should not exceed 4 g/day

Dosing adjustment in renal impairment: Cl_{cr} <60 mL/minute: Initiate doses conservatively and carefully titrate dose to appropriate effect

Dosing adjustment in hepatic impairment: Initial: 1/3 to 1/2 of the usual dose; carefully titrate dose to appropriate effect

Administration Oral: May administer with food or milk to decrease GI upset

Monitoring Parameters Pain relief, respiratory rate, mental status, blood pressure

Patient Information Avoid alcohol; may cause drowsiness and impair ability to perform activities requiring mental alertness or physical coordination. May be habit-forming; do not discontinue abruptly if therapy lasts more than a few weeks; dose should be tapered to prevent narcotic withdrawal.

Additional Information One generic tablet contains ~5 mg oxycodone as combined salt

Dosage Forms Excipient information presented when available (limited, particularly for generics); consult specific product labeling.

Tablet: Oxycodone hydrochloride 4.5 mg, oxycodone terephthalate 0.38 mg, and aspirin 325 mg

Endodan®, Percodan®: Oxycodone hydrochloride 4.8355 mg and aspirin 325 mg

- **Oxycodone Hydrochloride** *see* Oxycodone *on page 1189*
- **OxyContin®** *see* Oxycodone *on page 1189*
- **Oxyderm™ (Can)** *see* Benzoyl Peroxide *on page 207*
- **OxyFast®** *see* Oxycodone *on page 1189*
- **OxyIR®** *see* Oxycodone *on page 1189*
- **Oxy.IR® (Can)** *see* Oxycodone *on page 1189*

Oxymetazoline (oks i met AZ oh leen)

Medication Safety Issues

Sound-alike/look-alike issues:

Oxymetazoline may be confused with oxymetholone
Afrin® may be confused with aspirin
Visine® may be confused with Visken®

Related Information

OTC Cough and Cold Preparations, Pediatric *on page 1706*

U.S. Brand Names Afrin® Extra Moisturizing [OTC]; Afrin® Original [OTC]; Afrin® Severe Congestion [OTC]; Afrin® Sinus [OTC]; Dristan™ 12-Hour [OTC]; Duramist® Plus [OTC]; Duration® [OTC]; Genasal [OTC]; Neo-Synephrine® 12 Hour [OTC]; Neo-Synephrine® 12 Hour Extra Moisturizing [OTC]; Nōstrilla® [OTC]; NRS® [OTC]; Vicks Sinex® 12 Hour [OTC]; Vicks Sinex® 12 Hour Ultrafine Mist [OTC]; Visine® L.R. [OTC]; 4-Way® 12 Hour [OTC]

Canadian Brand Names Claritin® Allergic Decongestant; Dristan® Long Lasting Nasal; Drixoral® Nasal

Index Terms Oxymetazoline Hydrochloride

Therapeutic Category Adrenergic Agonist Agent; Decongestant, Nasal; Nasal Agent, Vasoconstrictor; Vasoconstrictor, Nasal; Vasoconstrictor, Ophthalmic

Generic Available Yes: Nasal spray

Use Symptomatic relief of nasal mucosal congestion associated with acute or chronic rhinitis, the common cold, sinusitis, hay fever, or other allergies

Pregnancy Risk Factor C

Contraindications Hypersensitivity to oxymetazoline or any component (see Warnings); patients on MAO inhibitor therapy

Warnings Use for periods exceeding 3 days may result in severe rebound nasal congestion; excessive dosage in children may cause profound CNS depression. Some products contain benzyl alcohol which may cause allergic reactions in susceptible individuals; large amounts of benzyl alcohol (≥99 mg/kg/day) have been associated with a potentially fatal toxicity ("gasping syndrome") in neonates; the "gasping syndrome" consists of metabolic acidosis, respiratory distress, gasping respirations, CNS dysfunction (including convulsions, intracranial hemorrhage), hypotension and cardiovascular collapse; *in vitro* and animal studies have shown that benzoate, a metabolite of benzyl alcohol, displaces bilirubin from protein binding sites; avoid use of these products in neonates

Precautions Use with caution in patients with hyperthyroidism, heart disease, hypertension, diabetes mellitus, increased intraocular pressure, or prostatic hypertrophy

Adverse Reactions

Cardiovascular: Hypertension, palpitations, reflex bradycardia, pallor

Central nervous system: Nervousness, dizziness, insomnia, headache, anxiety, tenseness, drowsiness, CNS depression, convulsions, hallucinations

Gastrointestinal: Nausea, vomiting

Ocular: Stinging to eye, mydriasis, elevated intraocular pressure, blurred vision

Respiratory: Sneezing, respiratory difficulty, rebound congestion with prolonged use, dryness of nasal mucosa

Miscellaneous: Diaphoresis

Drug Interactions Anesthetics (discontinue oxymetazoline prior to use of anesthetics that sensitize the myocardium to sympathomimetics, ie, cyclopropane, halothane); MAO inhibitors, methyldopa, tricyclic antidepressants increase hypertensive response

Mechanism of Action Stimulates alpha-adrenergic receptors in the arterioles of the nasal mucosa and arterioles of the conjunctiva to produce vasoconstriction

Pharmacodynamics

Onset of action: Intranasal: Within 5-10 minutes

Duration: 5-6 hours

Pharmacokinetics Metabolic fate is unknown

Usual Dosage

Nasal: Therapy should not exceed 3-5 days; avoid use in children <6 years of age

Children ≥6 years and Adults: 2-3 drops or 2-3 sprays or 1-2 metered sprays (Nōstrilla®) into each nostril twice daily

Ophthalmic: Children ≥6 years and Adults: Instill 1-2 drops into the affected eye(s) 2-4 times/day (≥6 hours apart)

Administration

Nasal: Spray or apply drops into each nostril while gently occluding the other

Ophthalmic: Instill drops into conjunctival sac of affected eye(s); avoid contact of bottle tip with skin or eye; finger pressure should be applied to lacrimal sac during and for 1-2 minutes after instillation to decrease the risk of absorption and systemic reactions

Dosage Forms Excipient information presented when available (limited, particularly for generics); consult specific product labeling.

Solution, intranasal, as hydrochloride [spray]: 0.05% (15 mL, 30 mL)

Afrin® Extra Moisturizing: 0.05% (15 mL) [contains benzyl alcohol and glycerin; regular or no drip formula]

Afrin® Original: 0.05% (15 mL, 30 mL) [contains benzalkonium chloride]

Afrin® Original: 0.05% (15 mL) [contains benzyl alcohol and benzalkonium chloride; no drip formula]

Afrin® Severe Congestion: 0.05% (15 mL) [contains benzyl alcohol and menthol; regular or no drip formula]

Afrin® Sinus: 0.05% (15 mL) [contains benzyl alcohol, benzalkonium chloride, camphor, phenol; regular or no drip formula]

Dristan™ 12-Hour: 0.05% (15 mL) [contains benzyl alcohol and benzalkonium chloride]

Duramist® Plus, Neo-Synephrine® 12 Hour, Nōstrilla®, Vicks Sinex® 12 Hour Ultrafine Mist, Vicks Sinex® 12 Hour, 4-Way® 12 Hour: 0.05% (15 mL) [contains benzalkonium chloride]

Duration®: 0.05% (30 mL) [contains benzalkonium chloride]

Genasal, NRS®: 0.05% (15 mL, 30 mL) [contains benzalkonium chloride]

Neo-Synephrine® 12 Hour Extra Moisturizing: 0.05% (15 mL) [contains glycerin]

Solution, ophthalmic, as hydrochloride (Visine® L.R.): 0.025% (15 mL, 30 mL) [contains benzalkonium chloride]

♦ **Oxymetazoline Hydrochloride** *see* Oxymetazoline *on page 1194*

♦ **Oxytrol®** *see* Oxybutynin *on page 1187*

♦ **Oysco 500 [OTC]** *see* Calcium Carbonate *on page 264*

- ♦ **Oysco® 500 [OTC]** *see* Calcium Supplements *on page 272*
- ♦ **Oyst-Cal 500 [OTC]** *see* Calcium Carbonate *on page 264*
- ♦ **Oyst-Cal 500 [OTC]** *see* Calcium Supplements *on page 272*
- ♦ **P-071** *see* Cetirizine *on page 327*
- ♦ **Pacerone®** *see* Amiodarone *on page 100*

Paclitaxel (PAK li taks el)

Medication Safety Issues

Sound-alike/look-alike issues:

Paclitaxel may be confused with paroxetine, Paxil®

Paclitaxel (conventional) may be confused with paclitaxel (protein-bound)

Taxol® may be confused with Abraxane®, Paxil®, Taxotere®

High alert medication: The Institute for Safe Medication Practices (ISMP) includes this medication among its list of drugs which have a heightened risk of causing significant patient harm when used in error.

Related Information

Compatibility of Chemotherapy and Related Supportive Care Medications *on page 1777*

U.S. Brand Names Onxol™; Taxol®

Canadian Brand Names Apo-Paclitaxel®; Taxol®

Index Terms NSC-125973; NSC-673089

Therapeutic Category Antineoplastic Agent, Antimicrotubular

Generic Available Yes

Use Treatment of advanced metastatic breast cancer, metastatic ovarian cancer, and AIDS-related Kaposi's sarcoma that is refractory to conventional therapy; active in lung cancer, head and neck cancer, bladder cancer, malignant melanoma, and other refractory solid tumors, and leukemias

Pregnancy Risk Factor D

Lactation Excretion in breast milk unknown/contraindicated

Contraindications Hypersensitivity to paclitaxel, Cremophor® EL (polyoxyethylated castor oil) or any component

Warnings The FDA currently recommends that procedures for proper handling and disposal of antineoplastic agents be considered. Anaphylaxis and severe hypersensitivity reactions have occurred in 2% of patients receiving paclitaxel in clinical trials during first or subsequent infusions. **All patients should be premedicated with a corticosteroid, diphenhydramine, and an H_2-receptor antagonist to prevent hypersensitivity reactions.** Patients who experience severe hypersensitivity reactions to paclitaxel should not be rechallenged with the drug. Be prepared to treat a severe hypersensitivity reaction with epinephrine, I.V. fluids, diphenhydramine and a corticosteroid.

CNS toxicity has been reported in pediatric patients receiving high doses of paclitaxel (350-420 mg/m^2 as a 3-hour infusion) which may have resulted from the ethanol contained in the formulation. Severe bone marrow suppression (primarily neutropenia) with resulting infection may occur. In general, do not administer paclitaxel to patients with baseline neutrophil counts <1500/mm^3.

Precautions Use with caution in patients with moderate or severe hepatic impairment; dosage adjustment may be necessary in patients with hepatic impairment, severe neutropenia, or peripheral neuropathy

Adverse Reactions

Cardiovascular: Hypotension or hypertension, bradycardia, arrhythmias, flushing, syncope, edema

Central nervous system: Seizures, ataxia, fatigue, headache, fever, confusion

Dermatologic: Alopecia, rash, changes in nail pigmentation

Endocrine & metabolic: Elevations in serum triglyceride levels

Gastrointestinal: Mild to moderate nausea/vomiting, diarrhea, mucositis

Hematologic: Severe neutropenia (dose-limiting toxicity), leukopenia, thrombocytopenia, anemia

Hepatic: Elevated AST, alkaline phosphatase, bilirubin

Local: Erythema, tenderness, swelling at the injection site

Neuromuscular & skeletal: Peripheral neuropathy (dose-dependent, characterized by paresthesia with numbness and tingling in a stocking-and-glove distribution), myalgia, muscle weakness, motor dysfunction, arthralgia

Ocular: Loss of visual acuity, diplopia

Renal: Elevated serum creatinine

Respiratory: Dyspnea

Miscellaneous: Anaphylactoid reactions (dyspnea, bronchospasm, hypotension, generalized urticaria), ethanol intoxication

Drug Interactions Cytochrome P450 isoenzyme CYP2C8 and CYP3A3/4 substrate

Paclitaxel clearance decreases approximately 33% when administered following cisplatin. Since paclitaxel is metabolized by cytochrome P450 3A4 and 2C8 isozymes, potential drug interactions can occur with agents that are isoenzyme inducers which reduce plasma paclitaxel concentration (ie, phenytoin) or inhibitors (ie, ketoconazole, verapamil, diazepam, cyclosporine, vincristine, etoposide, dexamethasone) which may increase plasma paclitaxel concentration; opiates, antihistamines, or other CNS depressants may potentiate CNS depression caused by ethanol in the paclitaxel formulation

Stability Refrigerate intact vials or store at room temperature; undiluted vials of paclitaxel may precipitate upon refrigeration, but will redissolve at room temperature with no loss in potency; dilution of paclitaxel from 0.3 mg/mL to 1.2 mg/mL in NS or D_5W is stable for up to 48 hours at room temperature; incompatible with amphotericin B, chlorpromazine, hydroxyzine, methylprednisolone, and mitoxantrone

Mechanism of Action An antimicrotubule agent that promotes the assembly of microtubules from tubulin dimers and stabilizes microtubules by preventing depolymerization; results in the inhibition of mitotic cellular functions and cell replication by blocking cells in the late G2 phase and M phase of the cell cycle

Pharmacokinetics

Distribution: Biphasic with initial rapid distribution to the peripheral compartment; later phase is a slow efflux of paclitaxel from the peripheral compartment

V_d: 227-688 L/m^2

Protein binding: 89% to 98%

Metabolism: Cytochrome P450 hepatic isoenzymes metabolize paclitaxel to 6 alpha-hydroxypaclitaxel

Half-life (varies with dose and infusion duration):

Children: 4.6-17 hours

Adults: 1.5-8.4 hours

Elimination: Urinary recovery of unchanged drug: 1.3% to 12.6%

Dialysis: No significant drug removal by hemodialysis

Usual Dosage I.V. infusion (refer to individual protocols):

Children:

Treatment for refractory leukemia is still undergoing investigation: 250-360 mg/m^2/dose infused over 24 hours every 14 days

Recurrent Wilms' tumor: 250-350 mg/m^2/dose infused over 24 hours every 3 weeks

Adults:

Ovarian carcinoma: 135-175 mg/m^2/dose infused over 1-24 hours every 3 weeks

Metastatic breast cancer: 175 mg/m^2/dose infused over 3 hours every 3 weeks (protocols have used dosages ranging between 135-250 mg/m^2/dose over 1-24 hours every 3 weeks)

Kaposi's sarcoma: 135 mg/m^2/dose infused over 3 hours every 3 weeks, or 100 mg/m^2/dose infused over 3 hours every 2 weeks

Dosage adjustment in renal impairment: None

Dosage adjustment in hepatic impairment:

Total bilirubin ≤1.5 mg/dL and AST >2x normal limits: Total dose <135 mg/m^2

Total bilirubin 1.6-3.0 mg/dL: Total dose ≤75 mg/m^2

Total bilirubin ≥3.1 mg/dL: Total dose ≤50 mg/m^2

Administration Parenteral: I.V.: Patients should be premedicated with a corticosteroid, diphenhydramine and an H_2-receptor antagonist 30-60 minutes prior to paclitaxel administration. To minimize patient exposure to the plasticizer diethylhexylphthalate (DEHP) from polyoxyl 35 castor oil-induced leaching of polyvinyl chloride-containing I.V. infusion bags and administration sets, prepare paclitaxel infusions in glass or in polypropylene or polyolefin bags and administer through polyethylene lined administration sets with a 0.22 micron in-line filter. Paclitaxel can be further diluted in D_5W, NS, D_5/NS or D_5 in Ringer's injection to a final concentration of 0.3-1.2 mg/mL. Paclitaxel has been infused over short (1-3 hours) and long periods (24, 72, and 96 hours to 14 days continuous infusion)

Monitoring Parameters CBC with differential, platelet count, vital signs, ECG, liver function test; observe I.V. injection site for extravasation

Patient Information Avoid alcohol; may cause drowsiness and impair ability to perform activities requiring mental alertness or physical coordination

Dosage Forms Excipient information presented when available (limited, particularly for generics); consult specific product labeling.

Injection, solution: 6 mg/mL (5 mL, 16.7 mL, 25 mL, 50 mL) [contains alcohol and purified Cremophor® EL (polyoxyethylated castor oil)]

Onxol™: 6 mg/mL (5 mL, 25 mL, 50 mL) [contains alcohol and purified Cremophor® EL (polyoxyethylated castor oil)]

Taxol®: 6 mg/mL (5 mL, 16.7 mL, 50 mL) [contains alcohol and purified Cremophor® EL (polyoxyethylated castor oil)]

References

Woo MH, Gregornik D, Shearer PD, et al, "Pharmacokinetics of Paclitaxel in an Anephric Patient," *Cancer Chemother Pharmacol*, 1999, 43(1):92-6.

- **Pain Eze [OTC]** *see* Acetaminophen *on page 42*
- **Palcaps** *see* Pancrelipase *on page 1203*
- **Palgic®** *see* Carbinoxamine *on page 285*
- **Palgic®-D [DSC]** *see* Carbinoxamine and Pseudoephedrine *on page 286*
- **Palgic®-DS [DSC]** *see* Carbinoxamine and Pseudoephedrine *on page 286*

Palivizumab (pah li VIZ u mab)

Medication Safety Issues
Sound-alike/look-alike issues:
Synagis® may be confused with Synalgos®-DC, Synvisc®

U.S. Brand Names Synagis®

Canadian Brand Names Synagis®

Therapeutic Category Monoclonal Antibody

Generic Available No

Use Prevention of serious lower respiratory tract disease caused by respiratory syncytial virus (RSV) in infants and children <2 years of age with chronic lung disease who have required medical therapy for their chronic lung disease within 6 months before the anticipated RSV season; prevention of serious RSV disease in patients with a history of prematurity (≤28 weeks gestation) up to 12 months of age or infants born at 29-32 weeks of gestation up to 6 months of age; prophylaxis may be considered in infants (<6 months of age) born between 32 and 35 weeks of gestation who are at greatest risk of severe infection (risk factors include childcare attendance, school-age siblings, exposure to environmental air pollutants, congenital abnormalities of the airways, or severe neuromuscular disease; see *AAP Red Book*, 2006); prevention of serious RSV disease in children with hemodynamically significant congenital heart disease; prophylaxis of infants with severe immune deficiency exposed to RSV

Pregnancy Risk Factor C

Contraindications Hypersensitivity to palivizumab or any component

Warnings Rare cases of anaphylaxis have been reported following re-exposure to palivizumab. Severe acute hypersensitivity reactions have also been reported following administration of palivizumab. Palivizumab should be permanently discontinued if a severe hypersensitivity reaction occurs. If anaphylaxis or severe allergic reaction occurs, administer epinephrine (1:1000) and provide supportive care as required.

Precautions Use with caution in patients with thrombocytopenia or any coagulation disorder. Safety and efficacy have not been demonstrated for treatment of established RSV disease.

Adverse Reactions
Dermatologic: Rash
Gastrointestinal: Diarrhea, vomiting
Hepatic: Elevated SGOT
Local: Injection site reaction, erythema, induration
Respiratory: Upper respiratory infection, otitis media, rhinitis, pharyngitis, cough
Miscellaneous: Anaphylaxis

Drug Interactions No formal drug interaction studies have been conducted. Note: No interference with measles, mumps, and rubella vaccines (combined) and varicella vaccine occurs

Stability Store in refrigerator at a temperature between 2°C to 8°C (35.6°F to 46.4°F) in original container; do not freeze; the single-use vial does not contain a preservative; solution should be administered within 6 hours of reconstitution

Mechanism of Action Humanized monoclonal antibody directed to an epitope in the A antigenic site of the respiratory syncytial virus F protein resulting in neutralizing and fusion-inhibitory activity against RSV

Pharmacokinetics
Half-life:
Children <24 months: 20 days
Adults: 18 days
Time to achieve adequate serum antibody titers: 48 hours

Usual Dosage Children:
I.M.: 15 mg/kg once monthly during RSV season
I.V. (I.V. route is investigational): 15 mg/kg has been administered to patients who could not receive I.M. injections; use has been investigated in hematopoietic stem cell transplant patients with active RSV upper respiratory tract infection.

Administration Parenteral:
Lyophilized product: Reconstitute by adding 0.6 mL of SWI to each 50 mg vial or by adding 1 mL of SWI to each 100 mg vial; swirl vial gently for 30 seconds to avoid foaming. Do not shake vial. Allow solution to stand at room temperature for 20 minutes until it clears

Solution: Administer undiluted solution

I.M.: Administer I.M., preferably in the anterolateral aspect of the thigh; gluteal muscle should not be used routinely as an injection site because of the risk of damage to the sciatic nerve; injection volume over 1 mL should be given as a divided dose

I.V. (I.V. route is investigational): Administer IVP or I.V. intermittent infusion at a rate not to exceed 1-2 mL/minute at a final concentration of 20 mg/mL in SWI. Filter through a 0.22 micron low protein binding filter (Millex-GV) prior to administration.

Monitoring Parameters Observe for anaphylactic or severe allergic reactions

Additional Information RSV prophylaxis should be initiated at the onset of the RSV season. In most areas of the United States, onset of RSV outbreaks is October to December, and termination is March to May, but regional differences occur.

Dosage Forms Excipient information presented when available (limited, particularly for generics); consult specific product labeling. [DSC] = Discontinued product

Injection, powder for reconstitution:

Synagis®: 50 mg, 100 mg [DSC]

Injection, solution [preservative free]:

Synagis®: 50 mg/0.5 mL (0.5 mL); 100 mg/mL (1 mL)

References

American Academy of Pediatrics, "Report of the Committee on Infectious Diseases," *2006 Red Book*, 27th ed, 2006.

Boeckh M, Berrey MM, Bowden RA, et al, "Phase 1 Evaluation of the Respiratory Syncytial Virus-Specific Monoclonal Antibody Palivizumab in Recipients of Hematopoietic Stem Cell Transplants," *J Infect Dis*, 2001, 184(3):350-4.

Feltes TF, Cabalka AK, Meissner HC, et al, "Palivizumab Prophylaxis Reduces Hospitalization Due to Respiratory Syncytial Virus in Young Children With Hemodynamically Significant Congenital Heart Disease," *J Pediatr*, 2003, 143(4):532-40.

"Palivizumab, a Humanized Respiratory Syncytial Virus Monoclonal Antibody, Reduces Hospitalization From Respiratory Syncytial Virus Infection in High-Risk Infants. The Impact-RSV Study Group," *Pediatrics*, 1998, 102(3 Pt 1):531-7.

"Prevention of Respiratory Syncytial Virus Infections: Indications for the Use of Palivizumab and Update on the Use of RSV-IGIV. American Academy of Pediatrics Committee on Infectious Diseases and Committee on Fetus and Newborn," *Pediatrics*, 1998, 102(5):1211-6.

♦ **Palmer's® Skin Success Acne [OTC]** *see* Benzoyl Peroxide *on page 207*

♦ **Palmer's® Skin Success Acne Cleanser [OTC]** *see* Salicylic Acid *on page 1413*

♦ **Palmitate-A® [OTC]** *see* Vitamin A *on page 1619*

Palonosetron (pal oh NOE se tron)

Medication Safety Issues

Sound-alike/look-alike issues:

Aloxi® may be confused with oxaliplatin

Palonosetron may be confused with dolasetron, granisetron, ondansetron

U.S. Brand Names Aloxi®

Index Terms Palonosetron Hydrochloride; RS-25259; RS-25259-197

Therapeutic Category 5-HT$_3$ Receptor Antagonist; Antiemetic

Generic Available No

Use Prevention of acute and delayed chemotherapy-induced nausea and vomiting

Pregnancy Risk Factor B

Lactation Excretion in breast milk unknown/not recommended

Contraindications Hypersensitivity to palonosetron or any component

Warnings Palonosetron may cause EKG interval changes (PR, QT$_c$, JT prolongation and QRS widening); interval prolongation could lead to cardiovascular consequences such as heart block or cardiac arrhythmias; hypersensitivity reactions may occur in patients who have exhibited hypersensitivity to other 5-HT$_3$ antagonists (eg, ondansetron, dolasetron)

Precautions Use with caution in patients with, or who may develop, prolongation of cardiac conduction intervals, particularly QT$_c$; conditions include hypokalemia, hypomagnesemia, or congenital QT syndrome; use with caution in patients receiving antiarrhythmic or other medications known to prolong the QT interval (eg, class I or III antiarrhythmic agents) or medications known to reduce potassium or magnesium levels (eg, diuretics)

Adverse Reactions

Cardiovascular: Prolonged QT interval and other EKG changes (see Warnings), tachycardia, hypotension, hypertension, myocardial ischemia, extrasystoles

Central nervous system: Headache, fatigue, dizziness, insomnia, fever, anxiety, euphoria

Dermatologic: Rash

Endocrine & metabolic: Hyperkalemia, hyperglycemia, metabolic acidosis

Gastrointestinal: Diarrhea, abdominal pain, constipation, dyspepsia, xerostomia, hiccups, flatulence

Genitourinary: Urinary retention

Hepatic: Transient elevations in liver enzymes

(Continued)

Palonosetron *(Continued)*

Local: Vein discoloration
Neuromuscular & skeletal: Weakness, myalgia
Ocular: Eye irritation, amblyopia
Otic: Tinnitus
Miscellaneous: Hypersensitivity reactions, flu-like syndrome

Drug Interactions Cytochrome P450 isoenzyme CYP1A2 (minor), CYP2D6 (primary), and CYP3A3/4 (minor) substrate
No drug interactions have been identified.

Stability Store at room temperature; protect from light; do not mix with other drugs

Mechanism of Action Palonosetron is a selective 5-HT_3 receptor antagonist, blocking serotonin, both peripherally on vagal nerve terminals and centrally in the chemoreceptor trigger zone

Pharmacokinetics
Distribution: Adults: 8.3 ± 2.5 L/kg
Protein binding: 62%
Metabolism: Metabolized to 2 minimally active metabolites (<1% activity of palonosetron)
Half-life, elimination: Terminal: 40 hours
Elimination: Urine 80% (40% as unchanged drug)
Clearance: Adults: Total body: 160 mL/h/kg

Usual Dosage I.V.: Prevention of acute and delayed chemotherapy-induced nausea and vomiting: Adults: 0.25 mg as a single dose administered 30 minutes before chemotherapy; (repeated doses of palonosetron within a seven day interval are not recommended because the safety and efficacy of repeated doses have not been evaluated)
Dosage adjustment in hepatic or renal impairment: No dosage adjustment is indicated

Administration Parenteral: I.V.: Infuse undiluted over 30 seconds; do not mix with other medications

Monitoring Parameters Baseline EKG in high-risk patients (see Warnings and Precautions), emesis episodes

Patient Information May cause dry mouth

Dosage Forms Excipient information presented when available (limited, particularly for generics); consult specific product labeling.
Injection, solution:
Aloxi®: 0.05 mg/mL (5 mL) [contains disodium edetate]

References

Eisenberg P, Figueroa-Vadillo J, Zamora R, et al, "Improved Prevention of Moderately Emetogenic Chemotherapy-Induced Nausea and Vomiting With Palonosetron, a Pharmacologically Novel 5-HT_3 Receptor Antagonist: Results of a Phase III, Single-Dose Trial Versus Dolasetron," *Cancer*, 2003, 98(11):2473-82.
Gralla R, Lichinitser M, Van Der Vegt S, et al, "Palonosetron Improves Prevention of Chemotherapy-Induced Nausea and Vomiting Following Moderately Emetogenic Chemotherapy: Results of a Double-Blind Randomized Phase III Trial Comparing Single Doses of Palonosetron With Ondansetron," *Ann Oncol*, 2003, 14(10):1570-7.
Siddiqui MA and Scott LJ, "Palonosetron," *Drugs*, 2004, 64(10):1125-32.

♦ **Palonosetron Hydrochloride** *see* Palonosetron *on page 1199*
♦ **2-PAM** *see* Pralidoxime *on page 1299*
♦ **Pamelor®** *see* Nortriptyline *on page 1149*

Pamidronate (pa mi DROE nate)

Medication Safety Issues
Sound-alike/look-alike issues:
Aredia® may be confused with Adriamycin, Meridia®
International issues:
Linoten® [Spain] may be confused with Lidopen® which is a brand name for lidocaine in the U.S.

U.S. Brand Names Aredia®

Canadian Brand Names Aredia®; Pamidronate Disodium®; Rhoxal-pamidronate

Index Terms Pamidronate Disodium

Therapeutic Category Antidote, Hypercalcemia; Bisphosphonate Derivative

Generic Available Yes

Use Symptomatic treatment of moderate to severe Paget's disease; hypercalcemia associated with malignancy; treatment of osteolytic bone lesions associated with multiple myeloma or metastatic breast cancer
Investigation use: Inhibit bone resorption in severe osteogenesis imperfecta

Pregnancy Risk Factor D

Lactation Excretion in breast milk unknown/use caution

Contraindications Hypersensitivity to pamidronate or any component; pregnancy; severe renal impairment

Warnings Leukopenia has been observed with oral pamidronate; monitoring of white blood cell counts is suggested; vein irritation and thrombophlebitis may occur with I.V. infusions; due to increased potential for renal toxicity, single doses should not exceed 90 mg; monitor serum creatinine prior to each dose; avoid use in patients with severe renal impairment; in patients receiving pamidronate for bone metastases who experience deterioration in renal function, hold treatment until renal function returns to baseline

Osteonecrosis of the jaw has been reported in cancer patients receiving biphosphonates; many of these patients were also receiving corticosteroids and chemotherapy, the majority of cases were associated with dental procedures; a dental exam should be considered prior to treatment in cancer patients, especially those with risk factors (chemotherapy, corticosteroids, poor oral hygiene); while on treatment, avoid invasive dental procedures

Precautions Use with caution in patients with renal impairment; maintain adequate hydration and urinary output during treatment; use with caution with other potentially nephrotoxic drugs

Adverse Reactions

Cardiovascular: Tachycardia, hypertension, syncope
Central nervous system: Malaise, fever, fatigue, somnolence, insomnia, seizures
Dermatologic: Rash
Endocrine & metabolic: Hypocalcemia, hypophosphatemia, hypothyroidism, hypokalemia, hypomagnesemia, fluid overload
Gastrointestinal: Nausea, anorexia, constipation, GI hemorrhage, abdominal pain, occult blood in stools, abnormal taste
Hematologic: Leukopenia, anemia
Local: Vein irritation, thrombophlebitis
Neuromuscular & skeletal: Bone pain, myalgia, osteonecrosis of the jaw
Ocular: Scleritis, uveitis, conjunctivitis
Renal: Uremia
Respiratory: Rales, rhinitis
Miscellaneous: Moniliasis (associated with 90 mg dosage)

Stability Reconstituted solution stable for 24 hours at room temperature or refrigerated; incompatible with calcium-containing I.V. fluids (ie, Ringer's solution)

Mechanism of Action Pamidronate, a biphosphonate, lowers serum calcium concentrations by binding to bone and inhibiting osteoclast-mediated calcium resorption; this agent does not appear to produce any significant effect on renal tubular calcium handling

Pharmacodynamics

Onset of hypocalcemic action: 24-48 hours
Maximum effect: 5-7 days

Pharmacokinetics

Absorption: Poorly from the GI tract; pharmacokinetic studies are lacking
Bone half-life: 300 days
Half-life, elimination: Adults with cancer: 28 ± 7 hours
Elimination:
- Biphasic: ~50% excreted unchanged in urine within 72 hours
- Clearance: Adults with cancer: Total: 107 ± 50 mL/minute; renal: 49 ± 28 mL/minute

Usual Dosage

Hypercalcemia: I.V.: **Note:** Due to increased risk of nephrotoxicity, doses should not exceed 90 mg
- Children (limited experience): 0.5-1 mg/kg
- Adults: Dosage based upon serum calcium measurement:
  - Serum calcium 12-13.5 mg/dL: 60-90 mg
  - Serum calcium >13.5 mg/dL: 90 mg
  - Consider retreatment if the serum calcium becomes elevated again; allow a minimum of 7 days between each treatment to allow for a full response to the initial treatment

Osteogenesis imperfecta:
- Children (limited experience): 0.5-3 mg/kg/day for 3 days; may repeat in 4- to 6-month intervals; or as an alternative 10-30 mg/m² monthly

Osteopenia in nonambulatory children with cerebral palsy: Limited experience (Henderson, 2002); 1 mg/kg/day for 3 days; each dose not <15 mg/day or >30 mg/day; repeat at 3-month intervals

Osteolytic bone lesions of breast cancer or multiple myeloma: Adults: 90 mg/month

Paget's disease: Adults: 30 mg for 3 consecutive days

Dosing adjustment in renal impairment: Not recommended for use in patients with severe renal impairment; safety and efficacy have not been established in patients

(Continued)

Pamidronate *(Continued)*

with serum creatinine >5 mg/dL; limited studies have reported successful use in multiple myeloma patients with serum creatinine ≥3 mg/dL

Administration Reconstitute each vial with 10 mL SWI; dilute further in 250-1000 mL D_5W, ½NS, or NS; do not mix with calcium-containing solutions (eg, LR); infuse over 2-24 hours; longer infusions (>2 hours) may reduce the risk for renal toxicity, particularly in patients with pre-existing renal insufficiency

Monitoring Parameters Monitor serum creatinine prior to each dose; serum calcium, phosphate, potassium, magnesium, hemoglobin, hematocrit, CBC with differential; in addition (Paget's disease) serum alkaline phosphatase, urinary hydroxyproline excretion

Dosage Forms Excipient information presented when available (limited, particularly for generics); consult specific product labeling.

Injection, powder for reconstitution, as disodium: 30 mg, 90 mg

Aredia®: 30 mg, 90 mg

Injection, solution: 3 mg/mL (10 mL); 6 mg/mL (10 mL); 9 mg/mL (10 mL)

References

Falk MJ, Heeger S, Lynch KA, et al, "Intravenous Bisphosphonate Therapy in Children With Osteogenesis Imperfecta," *Pediatrics*, 2003, 111(3):573-8.

Glorieux FH, Bishop NH, Plotkin H, et al, "Cyclic Administration of Pamidronate in Children With Severe Osteogenesis Imperfecta," *N Engl J Med*, 1998, 339(14):947-52.

Henderson RC, Lark RK, Kecskemethy HH, et al, "Bisphosphonates to Treat Osteopenia in Children With Quadriplegic Cerebral Palsy: A Randomized, Placebo-Controlled Clinical Trial," *J Pediatr*, 2002, 141(5):644-51.

Lteif AN and Zimmerman D, "Bisphosphonates for Treatment of Childhood Hypercalcemia," *Pediatrics*, 1998, 102(4 Pt 1):990-3.

♦ **Pamidronate Disodium** *see* Pamidronate *on page 1200*
♦ **Pamidronate Disodium® (Can)** *see* Pamidronate *on page 1200*
♦ **Pamprin® Maximum Strength All Day Relief [OTC]** *see* Naproxen *on page 1108*
♦ **Pan-2400™ [OTC]** *see* Pancreatin *on page 1202*
♦ **Pan-B Antibody** *see* Rituximab *on page 1398*
♦ **Pancrease® (Can)** *see* Pancrelipase *on page 1203*
♦ **Pancrease® MT** *see* Pancrelipase *on page 1203*

Pancreatin (PAN kree a tin)

Medication Safety Issues

Sound-alike/look-alike issues:

Pancreatin may be confused with Panretin®

U.S. Brand Names Dygase; Hi-Vegi-Lip [OTC]; kutrase®; ku-zyme®; Lapase; Pan-2400™ [OTC]; Pancreatin 4X [OTC]; Pancreatin 8X [OTC]; Veg-Pancreatin 4X [OTC]

Therapeutic Category Enzyme, Pancreatic; Pancreatic Enzyme

Generic Available Yes

Use Replacement therapy in symptomatic treatment of malabsorption syndrome caused by pancreatic enzyme insufficiency

Pregnancy Risk Factor C

Lactation Excretion in breast milk unknown/use caution

Contraindications Hypersensitivity to pancreatin, any component, or to bovine or pork protein; acute pancreatitis; acute exacerbations of chronic pancreatic diseases

Warnings Pancreatin is inactivated by acids; use microencapsulated products whenever possible, since these products permit better dissolution of enzymes in the duodenum and protect the enzyme preparations from acid degradation in the stomach; these products are not bioequivalent, do not substitute without consulting a physician or pharmacist; do not substitute generic pancreatic enzymes for brand name products

Colonic strictures have been reported in several pediatric patients. There is a possible association between the development of strictures and a high lipase intake (mean >16,000 units/kg/meal). Patients receiving doses >2500 lipase units/kg/meal or 4000 lipase units/g fat/day should be re-evaluated or titrated downward to lowest effective dose.

Precautions Do not spill powder on hands as is a skin irritant; inhalation of powder may produce an asthmatic attack

Adverse Reactions

Dermatologic: Rash

Endocrine & metabolic: Hyperuricemia

Gastrointestinal: Nausea, abdominal cramps, constipation, diarrhea, colonic strictures, mouth irritation, greasy stools, perianal irritation/inflammation, flatulence

Ocular: Lacrimation

Renal: Hyperuricosuria
Respiratory: Sneezing, bronchospasm
Miscellaneous: Hypersensitivity reactions

Drug Interactions Calcium carbonate, magnesium hydroxide may decrease effectiveness of enzymes; pancreatin may decrease the response to oral iron therapy; H_2 antagonists (eg, ranitidine, cimetidine) increase effectiveness of pancreatic enzymes

Food Interactions Avoid placing contents of opened capsules on alkaline foods (pH >5.5), such as dairy products (milk, custard, or ice cream); see Administration

Mechanism of Action Replaces endogenous pancreatic enzymes to assist in digestion of protein, starch and fats

Pharmacokinetics

Absorption: Not absorbed, acts locally in the GI tract
Elimination: In feces

Usual Dosage Oral: The following dosage recommendations are only an approximation for initial dosages. The actual dosage will depend on the digestive requirements of the individual patient. Adjust dose based upon body weight and stool fat content. Oral: Total daily dose in children and adults is divided into 3 meals/day plus 2-3 snacks/day with half the meal-time dose given with the snack:

Infants: 2000-4000 lipase units/120 mL (4 ounce) formula
Children ≤4 years: 1000 lipase units/kg/meal (maximum: 2500 lipase units/kg), with 1/2 dose with each snack
Children >4 years and Adults: 400-500 lipase units/kg/meal (maximum: 2500 lipase units/kg), with 1/2 dose with each snack

Administration Oral: Swallow capsules/tablets whole; retention in the mouth before swallowing may cause mucosal irritation and stomatitis; administer before or with meals; when administering to infants, may open capsule and spread over acidic foods (applesauce, mashed fruits, rice cereal) in a rubber-tipped teaspoon (use mixture immediately, do not make ahead of time). Place mixture onto the middle of the infant's tongue and then give bottle or breast. As an alternative, the parent may dip a clean finger into the food/enzyme mixture and then place finger into the infant's mouth and allow infant to suck on. Check infant's mouth after eating for lodged enzyme beads and remove.

Monitoring Parameters Stool fat content

Additional Information Concomitant administration of conventional pancreatin enzymes with an H_2-receptor antagonist has been used to decrease acid inactivation of enzyme activity.

Dosage Forms Excipient information presented when available (limited, particularly for generics); consult specific product labeling.

Capsule: Lipase 8500 units, protease 50,000 units, amylase 50,000 units [pancreatin 500 mg]
- Dygase, kutrase®: Lipase 2400 units, protease 30,000 units, amylase 30,000 units
- ku-zyme®: Lipase 1200 units, protease 15,000 units, amylase 15,000 units
- Lapase: Lipase 1200 units, protease 15,000 units, and amylase 15,000 units [contains tartrazine]
- Pan-2400™: Lipase 9816 units, protease 60,214 units, amylase 75,900 units [pancreatin 2400 mg]

Tablet: Lipase 565 units, protease 8200 units, amylase 8200 units [pancreatin 325 mg]; lipase 2400 units, protease 30,000 units, amylase 30,000 units [pancreatin 1200 mg]
- Hi-Vegi-Lip: Lipase 4800 units, protease 60,000 units, amylase 60,000 units [pancreatin 2400 mg; vegetable source]
- Pancreatin 4X: Lipase 4800 units, protease 60,000 units, amylase 60,000 units [pancreatin 600 mg]
- Pancreatin 8X: Lipase 14,400 units, protease 180,000 units, amylase 180,000 units [pancreatin 900 mg]
- Veg-Pancreatin 4X: Lipase 5500 units, protease 690,000 units, amylase 690,000 units [pancreatin 690 mg; vegetable source]

References

Pettei MJ, Leonidas JC, Levinne JJ, et al, "Pancolonic Disease in Cystic Fibrosis and High-Dose Pancreatic Enzyme Therapy," *J Pediatr*, 1994, 125(4):587-9.
Taylor CJ, "Colonic Strictures in Cystic Fibrosis," *Lancet*, 1994, 343(8898):615-6.

♦ **Pancreatin 4X [OTC]** *see* Pancreatin *on page 1202*
♦ **Pancreatin 8X [OTC]** *see* Pancreatin *on page 1202*
♦ **Pancrecarb MS®** *see* Pancrelipase *on page 1203*

Pancrelipase (pan kre LI pase)

Related Information

Pancreatin *on page 1202*
(Continued)

Pancrelipase *(Continued)*

U.S. Brand Names Creon®; ku-zyme® HP; Lipram 4500; Lipram-CR; Lipram-PN; Lipram-UL; Palcaps; Pancrease® MT; Pancrecarb MS®; Pangestyme™ CN; Pangestyme™ EC; Pangestyme™ MT; Pangestyme™ UL; Panocaps; Panocaps MT; Panokase®; Panokase® 16; Plaretase® 8000; Ultracaps MT; Ultrase®; Ultrase® MT; Viokase®

Canadian Brand Names Cotazym®; Creon®; Pancrease®; Pancrease® MT; Ultrase®; Ultrase® MT; Viokase®

Index Terms Lipancreatin

Therapeutic Category Enzyme, Pancreatic; Pancreatic Enzyme

Generic Available Yes: Excludes powder

Use Replacement therapy in symptomatic treatment of malabsorption syndrome caused by pancreatic enzyme insufficiency; open occluded feeding tubes

Pregnancy Risk Factor C

Lactation Excretion in breast milk unknown/use caution

Contraindications Hypersensitivity to pancrelipase, any component, or to pork protein; acute pancreatitis; acute exacerbations of chronic pancreatic diseases

Warnings Pancrelipase is inactivated by acids; use microencapsulated products whenever possible, since these products permit better dissolution of enzymes in the duodenum and protect the enzyme preparations from acid degradation in the stomach; products are not bioequivalent, do not substitute without consulting a physician or pharmacist; do not substitute generic enzymes for brand name products

Colonic strictures have been reported in several pediatric patients. There is a possible association between the development of strictures and a high lipase intake (mean >16,000 units/kg/meal). Patients receiving doses >2500 lipase units/kg/meal or 4000 lipase units/g fat/day should be re-evaluated or titrated downward to lowest effective dose.

Precautions Do not spill powder on hands as is skin irritant; inhalation of powder may produce an asthmatic attack

Adverse Reactions

Dermatologic: Rash

Endocrine & metabolic: Hyperuricemia

Gastrointestinal: Nausea, abdominal cramps, constipation, diarrhea, colonic strictures, mouth irritation, greasy stools, perianal irritation/inflammation, flatulence

Ocular: Lacrimation

Renal: Hyperuricosuria

Respiratory: Sneezing, bronchospasm

Miscellaneous: Hypersensitivity reactions

Drug Interactions Calcium carbonate, magnesium hydroxide may decrease effectiveness of enzymes; may decrease the response to oral iron therapy; H_2 antagonists (eg, ranitidine, cimetidine) may increase effectiveness of pancreatic enzymes

Food Interactions Avoid placing contents of opened capsules on alkaline foods (pH >5.5), such as dairy products (milk, custard, or ice cream); see Administration

Mechanism of Action Replaces endogenous pancreatic enzymes to assist in digestion of protein, starch and fats

Pharmacokinetics

Absorption: Not absorbed, acts locally in the GI tract

Elimination: In feces

Usual Dosage The following dosage recommendations are only an approximation for initial dosages. The actual dosage will depend on the digestive requirements of the individual patient. Adjust dose based upon body weight and stool fat content. Oral: Total daily dose in children and adults is divided into 3 meals/day plus 2-3 snacks/day with half the meal-time dose given with the snack:

Infants: 2000-4000 lipase units/120 mL (4 ounce) formula

Children ≤4 years: 1000 lipase units/kg/meal (maximum: 2500 lipase units/kg), with ½ dose with each snack

Children >4 years and Adults: 400-500 lipase units/kg/meal (maximum: 2500 lipase units/kg), with ½ dose with each snack

Occluded feeding tubes: Children and Adults: One tablet of Viokase® crushed with one 325 mg tablet of sodium bicarbonate (to activate the Viokase®) in 5 mL of water can be instilled into the nasogastric tube and clamped for 5 minutes; then flushed with 50 mL of water

Administration Oral: Swallow tablets and capsules whole; do not chew the microspheres or microtablets; retention in the mouth before swallowing may cause mucosal irritation and stomatitis; administer before or with meals; when administering to infants, may open capsule and spread over acidic foods (applesauce, mashed fruits, rice cereal) in a rubber-tipped teaspoon (use mixture immediately, do not make ahead of time). Place mixture onto the middle of the infant's tongue and then give bottle or breast. As an alternative, the parent may dip a clean finger into the food/

enzyme mixture and then place finger into the infant's mouth and allow infant to suck on. Check infant's mouth after eating for lodged enzyme beads and remove.

Monitoring Parameters Stool fat content

Additional Information Concomitant administration of conventional pancreatin enzymes with an H_2-receptor antagonist has been used to decrease acid inactivation of enzyme activity. Colonic strictures have been reported in several pediatric patients. There is a possible association between the development of strictures and a high lipase intake (mean >16,000 units/kg/meal). Patients receiving doses >2500 lipase units/kg/meal or 4000 lipase units/g fat/day should be re-evaluated or titrated downward to lowest effective dose

Dosage Forms Excipient information presented when available (limited, particularly for generics); consult specific product labeling. [DSC] = Discontinued product

Capsule:

- ku-zyme® HP: Lipase 8000 units, protease 30,000 units, and amylase 30,000 units

Capsule, delayed release, enteric coated granules:

- Pangestyme™ CN-10: Lipase 10,000 units, protease 37,500 units, amylase 33,200 units
- Pangestyme™ CN-20: Lipase 20,000 units, protease 75,000 units, amylase 66,400 units
- Pangestyme™ EC: Lipase 4500 units, protease 25,000 units, and amylase 20,000 units
- Pangestyme™ MT16: Lipase 16,000 units, protease 48,000 units, and amylase 48,000 units
- Pangestyme™ UL 12: Lipase 12,000 units, protease 39,000 units, and amylase 39,000 units
- Pangestyme™ UL 18: Lipase 18,000 units, protease 58,500 units, and amylase 58,500 units
- Pangestyme™ UL 20: Lipase 20,000 units, protease 65,000 units, and amylase 65,000 units

Capsule, delayed release, enteric coated microspheres: Lipase 4500 units, protease 25,000 units, and amylase 20,000 units

- Creon® 5: Lipase 5000 units, protease 18,750 units, and amylase 16,600 units
- Creon® 10, Palcaps 10: Lipase 10,000 units, protease 37,500 units, and amylase 33,200 units
- Creon® 20, Palcaps 20: Lipase 20,000 units, protease 75,000 units, and amylase 66,400 units
- Lipram 4500, Panocaps: Lipase 4500 units, protease 25,000 units, and amylase 20,000 units
- Lipram-CR10: Lipase 10,000 units, protease 37,500 units, and amylase 33,200 units
- Lipram-CR20: Lipase 20,000 units, protease 75,000 units, and amylase 66,400 units
- Lipram-PN10: Lipase 10,000 units, protease 30,000 units, and amylase 30,000 units
- Lipram-PN16, Panocap MT 16: Lipase 16,000 units, protease 48,000 units, and amylase 48,000 units
- Lipram-PN20, Panocap MT 20: Lipase 20,000 units, protease 44,000 units, and amylase 56,000 units
- Lipram-UL20, Ultracaps MT 20: Lipase 20,000 units, protease 65,000 units, and amylase 65,000 units
- Pancrecarb MS-4®: Lipase 4000 units, protease 25,000 units, and amylase 25,000 units [buffered]
- Pancrecarb MS-8®: Lipase 8000 units, protease 45,000 units, and amylase 40,000 units [buffered]
- Pancrecarb MS-16® Lipase 16,000 units, protease 52,000 units, and amylase 52,000 units [buffered]

Capsule, enteric coated microspheres:

- Ultrase®: Lipase 4500 units, protease 25,000 units, and amylase 20,000 units

Capsule, enteric coated microtablets:

- Pancrease® MT 4: Lipase 4000 units, protease 12,000 units, and amylase 12,000 units
- Pancrease® MT 10: Lipase 10,000 units, protease 30,000 units, and amylase 30,000 units
- Pancrease® MT 16: Lipase 16,000 units, protease 48,000 units, and amylase 48,000 units
- Pancrease® MT 20: Lipase 20,000 units, protease 44,000 units, and amylase 56,000 units

Capsule, enteric coated minitablets:

- Ultrase® MT12: Lipase 12,000 units, protease 39,000 units, and amylase 39,000 units

(Continued)

Pancrelipase *(Continued)*

Ultrase® MT18: Lipase 18,000 units, protease 58,500 units, and amylase 58,500 units

Ultrase® MT20: Lipase 20,000 units, protease 65,000 units, and amylase 65,000 units

Powder (Viokase®): Lipase 16,800 units, protease 70,000 units, and amylase 70,000 units per 0.7 g (227 g)

Tablet: Lipase 8000 units, protease 30,000 units, and amylase 30,000 units

Panokase®: Lipase 8000 units, protease 30,000 units, and amylase 30,000 units

Panokase® 16: Lipase 16,000 units, protease 60,000 units, and amylase 60,000 units

Plaretase™ 8000: Lipase 8000 units, protease 30,000 units, and amylase 30,000 units

Viokase® 8: Lipase 8000 units, protease 30,000 units, and amylase 30,000 units

Viokase® 16: Lipase 16,000 units, protease 60,000 units, and amylase 60,000 units

References

Pettei MJ, Leonidas JC, Levinne JJ, et al, "Pancolonic Disease in Cystic Fibrosis and High-Dose Pancreatic Enzyme Therapy," *J Pediatr*, 1994, 125(4):587-9.

Taylor CG, "Colonic Strictures in Cystic Fibrosis," *Lancet*, 1994, 343(8898):615-6.

Pancuronium (pan kyoo ROE nee um)

Medication Safety Issues

Sound-alike/look-alike issues:

Pancuronium may be confused with pipecuronium

High alert medication: The Institute for Safe Medication Practices (ISMP) includes this medication among its list of drugs which have a heightened risk of causing significant patient harm when used in error.

Canadian Brand Names Pancuronium Bromide®

Index Terms Pancuronium Bromide; Pavulon [DSC]

Therapeutic Category Neuromuscular Blocker Agent, Nondepolarizing; Skeletal Muscle Relaxant, Paralytic

Generic Available Yes

Use Produces skeletal muscle relaxation during surgery after induction of general anesthesia, increases pulmonary compliance during assisted mechanical respiration, facilitates endotracheal intubation

Pregnancy Risk Factor C

Lactation Excretion in breast milk unknown/not recommended

Contraindications Hypersensitivity to pancuronium, bromide, or any component (see Warnings)

Warnings Ventilation must be supported during neuromuscular blockade; electrolyte imbalance alters blockade; contains benzyl alcohol which may cause allergic reactions in susceptible individuals; large amounts of benzyl alcohol (≥99 mg/kg/day) have been associated with a potentially fatal toxicity ("gasping syndrome") in neonates; the "gasping syndrome" consists of metabolic acidosis, respiratory distress, gasping respirations, CNS dysfunction (including convulsions, intracranial hemorrhage), hypotension and cardiovascular collapse; *in vitro* and animal studies have shown that benzoate, a metabolite of benzyl alcohol, displaces bilirubin from protein binding sites; avoid use of benzyl alcohol containing products in neonates

Precautions Use with caution and decrease dose in patients with decreased renal function; many clinical conditions may affect the response to neuromuscular blockade, see table.

Clinical Conditions Affecting Neuromuscular Blockade

Potentiation	Antagonism
Electrolyte abnormalities	Alkalosis
Severe hyponatremia	Hypercalcemia
Severe hypocalcemia	Demyelinating lesions
Severe hypokalemia	Peripheral neuropathies
Hypermagnesemia	Diabetes mellitus
Neuromuscular diseases	
Acidosis	
Acute intermittent porphyria	
Renal failure	
Hepatic failure	

Adverse Reactions Most frequent adverse reactions are related to prolongation of pharmacologic actions

Cardiovascular: Tachycardia, hypertension
Dermatologic: Rash, erythema
Gastrointestinal: Excessive salivation
Local: Burning sensation along the vein
Neuromuscular & skeletal: Muscle weakness
Respiratory: Wheezes, bronchospasm
Miscellaneous: Hypersensitivity reactions

Drug Interactions See table.

Potential Drug Interactions

Potentiation	Antagonism
Inhalation anesthetics	Calcium
Desflurane, sevoflurane, enflurane and isoflurane > halothane > nitrous oxide	Carbamazepine
	Phenytoin
	Steroids (chronic administration)
Antibiotics	Theophylline
Aminoglycosides, polymyxins, clindamycin, vancomycin, tetracycline	Anticholinesterases[1]
	Neostigmine, pyridostigmine, edrophonium, echothiophate ophthalmic solution
Magnesium	
Antiarrhythmics	
Quinidine, procainamide, bretylium, and possibly lidocaine	Caffeine
	Azathioprine
Diuretics	
Furosemide, mannitol, thiazides	
Amphotericin B (secondary to hypokalemia)	
Local anesthetics	
Dantrolene (directly depresses skeletal muscle)	
Beta blockers	
Calcium channel blockers	
Ketamine	
Lithium	
Succinylcholine (when administered prior to nondepolarizing neuromuscular-blocking agent)	
Cyclosporine	

[1]Can prolong the effects of acetylcholine

Stability Refrigerate; however, stable for up to 6 months at room temperature; compatible with D_5W, NS, D_5NS, and LR injections

Mechanism of Action Nondepolarizing neuromuscular blocker which blocks acetylcholine from binding to receptors on motor endplate thus inhibiting depolarization

Pharmacodynamics

Maximum effect: I.V. injection: Within 2-3 minutes
Duration: 40-60 minutes (dose dependent)

Pharmacokinetics

Distribution: V_d: Adult: 0.23 L/kg
Protein binding: 87%
Metabolism: 30% to 40% metabolized in liver
Half-life: 110 minutes
Elimination: Primarily in urine (60%) as unchanged drug and bile (40%)
Clearance: Adult: 1.9 mL/kg/minute

Usual Dosage I.V.:

Neonates and Infants: 0.1 mg/kg every 30-60 minutes as needed or as continuous infusion of 0.02-0.04 mg/kg/hour or 0.4-0.6 mcg/kg/minute

Children: 0.15 mg/kg every 30-60 minutes as needed or as continuous infusion 0.03-0.1 mg/kg/hour or 0.5-1.7 mcg/kg/minute

Adolescents and Adults: 0.15 mg/kg every 30-60 minutes as needed or as a continuous infusion 0.02-0.04 mg/kg/hour or 0.4-0.6 mcg/kg/minute

Dosing adjustment in renal impairment:

Cl_{cr} 10-50 mL/minute: Administer 50% of normal dose
Cl_{cr} <10 mL/minute: Do not use

Administration Parenteral: May be administered undiluted by rapid I.V. injection; for continuous infusion, dilute to 0.01-0.8 mg/mL in D_5NS, D_5W, LR, or NS.

(Continued)

Pancuronium *(Continued)*

Monitoring Parameters Heart rate, blood pressure, assisted ventilation status, peripheral nerve stimulator measuring twitch response

Nursing Implications Does not alter the patient's state of consciousness; addition of sedation and analgesia are recommended

Additional Information Patients with hepatic and biliary disease have a larger V_d which may result in a higher total initial dose and possibly a slower onset of effect; the duration of neuromuscular blocking effects may be prolonged in patients with hepatic, biliary, or renal dysfunction

Dosage Forms Excipient information presented when available (limited, particularly for generics); consult specific product labeling.

Injection, solution, as bromide: 1 mg/mL (10 mL); 2 mg/mL (2 mL, 5 mL) [may contain benzyl alcohol]

References

Martin LD, Bratton SL, and O'Rourke PP, "Clinical Uses and Controversies of Neuromuscular Blocking Agents in Infants and Children," *Crit Care Med*, 1999, 27(7):1358-68.

- ♦ **Pancuronium Bromide** *see* Pancuronium *on page 1206*
- ♦ **Pancuronium Bromide® (Can)** *see* Pancuronium *on page 1206*
- ♦ **Pandel®** *see* Hydrocortisone *on page 781*
- ♦ **Pangestyme™ CN** *see* Pancrelipase *on page 1203*
- ♦ **Pangestyme™ EC** *see* Pancrelipase *on page 1203*
- ♦ **Pangestyme™ MT** *see* Pancrelipase *on page 1203*
- ♦ **Pangestyme™ UL** *see* Pancrelipase *on page 1203*
- ♦ **Panglobulin® NF** *see* Immune Globulin (Intravenous) *on page 818*
- ♦ **Panixine DisperDose™ [DSC]** *see* Cephalexin *on page 324*
- ♦ **Panocaps** *see* Pancrelipase *on page 1203*
- ♦ **Panocaps MT** *see* Pancrelipase *on page 1203*
- ♦ **Panokase®** *see* Pancrelipase *on page 1203*
- ♦ **Panokase® 16** *see* Pancrelipase *on page 1203*
- ♦ **PanOxyl®** *see* Benzoyl Peroxide *on page 207*
- ♦ **PanOxyl®-AQ** *see* Benzoyl Peroxide *on page 207*
- ♦ **PanOxyl® Aqua Gel** *see* Benzoyl Peroxide *on page 207*
- ♦ **PanOxyl® Bar [OTC]** *see* Benzoyl Peroxide *on page 207*
- ♦ **Panto™ IV (Can)** *see* Pantoprazole *on page 1208*
- ♦ **Pantoloc® (Can)** *see* Pantoprazole *on page 1208*
- ♦ **Pantoloc® M (Can)** *see* Pantoprazole *on page 1208*

Pantoprazole (pan TOE pra zole)

Medication Safety Issues

Sound-alike/look-alike issues:

Protonix® may be confused with Lotronex®, Lovenox®, protamine

Vials containing Protonix® I.V. for injection are not recommended for use with spiked I.V. system adaptors. Nurses and pharmacists have reported breakage of the glass vials during attempts to connect spiked I.V. system adaptors, which may potentially result in injury to healthcare professionals.

International issues:

Protonix® may be confused with Pretanix® which is a brand name for indapamide in Hungary

U.S. Brand Names Protonix®

Canadian Brand Names Panto™ IV; Pantoloc®; Pantoloc® M; PMS-Pantoprazole; Protonix®

Therapeutic Category Gastric Acid Secretion Inhibitor; Gastrointestinal Agent, Gastric or Duodenal Ulcer Treatment; Proton Pump Inhibitor

Generic Available No

Use

Oral: Treatment and maintenance of healing of erosive esophagitis associated with gastroesophageal reflux disease (GERD); treatment of pathological hypersecretory conditions including Zollinger-Ellison syndrome; adjunctive therapy of duodenal ulcers associated with *Helicobacter pylori* (unlabeled use)

I.V.: Short-term treatment (7-10 days) of patients with GERD with a history of erosive esophagitis; an alternative to oral therapy in patients who are unable to continue taking oral pantoprazole; treatment of pathological hypersecretory conditions associated with Zollinger-Ellison syndrome or other neoplastic conditions

Pregnancy Risk Factor B

Lactation Enters breast milk/not recommended

Contraindications Hypersensitivity to pantoprazole, substituted benzimidazole proton pump inhibitors (eg, esomeprazole, omeprazole, lansoprazole), or any component

Warnings In long-term (2-year) studies in rodents, pantoprazole was carcinogenic and caused rare types of gastrointestinal tumors. While available endoscopic evaluations and histologic examinations of biopsy specimens from human stomachs have not detected a risk from short-term exposure to pantoprazole, further human data on the effect of sustained hypochlorhydria and hypergastrinemia are needed to rule out the possibility of an increased risk for the development of tumors in humans receiving long-term therapy. Symptomatic response to therapy does not preclude the presence of gastric malignancy. Use of gastric acid inhibitors including proton pump inhibitors and H_2 blockers has been associated with an increased risk for development of acute gastroenteritis and community-acquired pneumonia (Canani, 2006).

Precautions Long-term treatment (>3 years) may lead to malabsorption of cyanocobalamin (vitamin B_{12}) caused by hypo or achlorhydria. Injection contains edetate sodium (EDTA); EDTA is a potent chelator of metal ions, particularly zinc; use with caution in patients prone to zinc deficiency or receiving other EDTA-containing products. Zinc supplementation may be necessary.

Adverse Reactions

Cardiovascular: Chest pain, tachycardia, angina, palpitations, hypertension, hypotension, syncope

Central nervous system: Headache, dizziness, vertigo, insomnia, anxiety, fever, nervousness, confusion, depression, emotional lability, hallucinations, migraine, speech disorder

Dermatologic: Urticaria, pruritus, acne, alopecia, dry skin, maculopapular rash; rare severe dermatologic conditions such as Stevens-Johnson syndrome, erythema multiforme, toxic epidural necrolysis

Endocrine & metabolic: Hyperglycemia, hyperlipemia, goiter, gout

Gastrointestinal: Diarrhea, nausea, abdominal pain, vomiting, constipation, flatulence, dyspepsia, eructation, xerostomia, anorexia, dysgeusia, duodenitis, dysphagia, glossitis, halitosis, abnormal stools, tongue discoloration, ulcerative colitis, taste perversion, pancreatitis (rare), increased salivation

Genitourinary: Urinary frequency, UTI, interstitial nephritis (rare)

Hematologic: Thrombocytopenia, leukopenia, leukocytosis, anemia, pancytopenia (rare), pernicious anemia (see Precautions)

Hepatic: Hepatitis, elevated liver function tests, cholestatic jaundice, biliary pain, hyperbilirubinemia, hepatic failure (rare)

Local: I.V.: Thrombophlebitis, abscess

Neuromuscular & skeletal: Muscle cramps, myalgia, arthralgia, neck pain, hypertonia, back pain, paresthesias, decreased reflexes, leg cramps, bone pain, bursitis, elevated CPK, rhabdomyolysis (rare)

Ocular: Amblyopia, diplopia, extraocular palsy, glaucoma, anterior ischemic optic neuropathy (rare), blurred vision

Otic: Ear pain, tinnitus

Renal: Hematuria, pyuria, proteinuria, glycosuria, interstitial nephritis (rare)

Respiratory: Rhinitis, bronchitis, cough, dyspnea, pharyngitis, sinusitis, URI

Miscellaneous: Anaphylaxis (I.V. formulation), flu-like syndrome, infection

Drug Interactions Cytochrome P450 isoenzyme CYP1A2 (weak) and CYP3A4 (weak) inducer; isoenzyme 2C8/9 inhibitor (moderate); isoenzyme CYP2C19 (major), and CYP3A4, CYP2D6, and CYP2C9 (minor) substrate

The full potential for drug interactions remains to be determined; due to profound and long-lasting inhibition of gastric acid secretion, pantoprazole may decrease the absorption of atazanavir, indinavir, ketoconazole, itraconazole, iron salts, and ampicillin esters; isoenzyme 2C19 inducers such as aminoglutethemide, carbamazepine, phenytoin, and rifampin may decrease its effects; may increase the anticoagulant effects of warfarin (monitor INR closely)

Stability Protect from light; store tablets at room temperature; refrigerate powder for injection (36°F to 46°F). Reconstituted injection is stable at room temperature for 24 hours; do not freeze; after further dilution with I.V. fluid, the solution is stable at room temperature for 24 hours. Neither the reconstituted solution or diluted solution need be protected from light. Pantoprazole stability is a function of pH; it is rapidly degraded in acidic media, but has acceptable stability under alkaline conditions. Each tablet of pantoprazole is enteric coated to prevent degradation by gastric acidity.

Mechanism of Action Suppresses gastric acid secretion by inhibiting the parietal cell membrane enzyme (H^+/K^+)-ATPase or proton pump; demonstrates antimicrobial activity against *Helicobacter pylori*

Pharmacodynamics Acid secretion:

Onset of action:

Oral: 2.5 hours

I.V.: 15-30 minutes

Maximum effect: I.V.: 2 hours

(Continued)

Pantoprazole *(Continued)*

Duration: Oral, I.V.: 24 hours

Pharmacokinetics

Distribution: V_d: Adults: 11-23.6 L

Protein binding: 98%

Metabolism: Extensive liver metabolism; no evidence of active metabolites

Bioavailability: ~77%

Half-life: Adults: 1 hour; prolonged half-life (3.5-10 hours) in slow metabolizers

Time to peak serum concentration: Oral: 2.5 hours

Elimination: Renal: 71% (as metabolites); biliary/fecal: 18%

Clearance: Adults: 7.6-14 L/hour

Dialysis: Not appreciably removed by hemodialysis

Usual Dosage I.V. therapy should be discontinued as soon as the patient tolerates oral therapy

Erosive esophagitis associated with GERD:

Children: Oral: Limited data; 20 mg once daily (0.5-1 mg/kg/day) was used in 15 children, 6-13 years of age (20-40 kg) for 28 days (Madrazo-De La Garza, 2003)

Adults: Treatment and maintenance:

Oral: 40 mg/day for up to 8 weeks; in mild GERD, 20 mg/day has been effective

I.V.: 40 mg/day for 7-10 days

Hypersecretory conditions (including Zollinger-Ellison syndrome): Adults:

Oral: Initial: 40 mg twice daily; adjust dose based on patient response; doses up to 240 mg/day have been used

I.V.: Initial: 80 mg twice daily; adjust dosage to maintain acid output below 10 mEq/hour; doses up to 80 mg every 8 hours have been used; doses >240 mg/day or treatment duration >6 days have not been studied

Adjunctive therapy of duodenal ulcers associated with *Helicobacter pylori* (in combination with antibiotic therapy) (unlabeled use): Adults: Oral: 40 mg once or twice daily

Administration

I.V.: Reconstitute powder for injection with 10 mL NS; further dilute in NS, D_5W, or LR to a final concentration 0.4-0.8 mg/mL; infuse over 15 minutes at a rate not to exceed 7 mL/minute; for more rapid infusion, dilute reconstituted solution to a final concentration of 4 mg/mL and infuse over 2 minutes; not for I.M. or SubQ use

Oral: Administer without regard to food; tablet should be swallowed whole, do not chew or crush; may be administered with antacids

Test Interactions Reports of false-positive urine screening tests for tetrahydrocannabinol in patients receiving pantoprazole

Patient Information May cause dry mouth; do not chew or crush tablets

Dosage Forms Excipient information presented when available (limited, particularly for generics); consult specific product labeling. [CAN] = Canadian brand name

Note: Strength expressed as base

Injection, powder for reconstitution, as sodium:

Protonix®: 40 mg [contains edetate sodium 1 mg]

Tablet, delayed release, as sodium:

Protonix®: 20 mg, 40 mg

Tablet, enteric coated, as magnesium (Pantoloc® M) [CAN]: 40 mg [not available in the U.S.]

Extemporaneous Preparations A 2 mg/mL oral liquid may be prepared by first removing the Protonix® imprint from twenty 40 mg tablets by gently rubbing the tablets on a paper towel dampened with alcohol; allow to air dry; (this eliminates dark flecks in final product). Crush the tablets; place coarse powder in 600 mL beaker and add 340 mL SWI. Place beaker on a magnetic stirrer. While stirring, add 16.8 g sodium bicarbonate powder and stir for about 20 minutes until the tablet remnants have disintegrated and the coating has dissolved. While continuing to stir, add another 16.8 g sodium bicarbonate powder and stir for an additional 5 minutes until the powder dissolves. Add enough SWI to bring the final volume to 400 mL. Mix well. Stable 62 days refrigerated and protected from light. Label "shake well."

Dentinger PJ, Swenson CF, and Anaizi NH, "Stability of Pantoprazole in an Extemporaneously Compounded Oral Liquid," *Am J Health Syst Pharm*, 2002, 59(10):953-6.

References

Canani RB, Cirillo P, Roggero P, et al, "Therapy With Gastric Acidity Inhibitors Increases the Risk of Acute Gastroenteritis and Community-Acquired Pneumonia in Children," *Pediatrics*, 2006, 117(5):e817-20.

Madrazo-De La Garza A, Dibildox M, Vargas A, et al, "Efficacy and Safety of Oral Pantoprazole 20 mg Given Once Daily for Reflux Esophagitis in Children," *J Pediatr Gastroenterol Nutr*, 2003, 36(2):261-5.

Papaverine (pa PAV er een)

U.S. Brand Names Para-Time SR®
Index Terms Papaverine Hydrochloride; Pavabid [DSC]
Therapeutic Category Antimigraine Agent; Vasodilator
Generic Available Yes
Use Relief of peripheral and cerebral ischemia associated with arterial spasm; investigationally for prophylaxis of migraine headache; intracavernosal injection for impotence
Pregnancy Risk Factor C
Lactation Excretion in breast milk unknown/not recommended
Contraindications Hypersensitivity to papaverine or any component; complete atrioventricular block; Parkinson's disease
Precautions Use with caution in patients with glaucoma; administer I.V. slowly and with caution since arrhythmias and apnea may occur with rapid I.V. use; should **not** be used in neonates due to the increased risk of drug-induced cerebral vasodilation and possibility of an intracranial bleed
Adverse Reactions
Cardiovascular: Flushing of the face, tachycardia, hypotension, arrhythmias with rapid I.V. use
Central nervous system: Depression, dizziness, vertigo, drowsiness, sedation, lethargy, headache
Dermatologic: Pruritus
Gastrointestinal: Xerostomia, nausea, constipation
Hepatic: Hepatic hypersensitivity
Local: Thrombosis at the I.V. administration site
Respiratory: Apnea with rapid I.V. use
Miscellaneous: Diaphoresis
Drug Interactions Cytochrome P450 isoenzyme CYP2D6 substrate
Additive effects with CNS depressants or morphine; papaverine decreases the effects of levodopa
Stability Protect from heat or freezing; do not refrigerate injection; solutions should be clear to pale yellow; precipitates with LR
Mechanism of Action Smooth muscle spasmolytic producing a generalized smooth muscle relaxation including vasodilatation, GI sphincter relaxation, bronchiolar muscle relaxation, and potentially a depressed myocardium
Pharmacodynamics Onset of action: Oral: Rapid
Pharmacokinetics
Protein binding: 90%
Metabolism: Rapid in the liver
Bioavailability: Oral: ~54%
Half-life: 30-120 minutes
Elimination: Primarily as metabolites in urine
Usual Dosage
Children: I.M., I.V.: 1.5 mg/kg 4 times/day
Migraine prophylaxis: 6-15 years: Oral: Initial: 5 mg/kg/day given once daily; range: 5-10 mg/kg/day divided into 2-3 doses/day
Adults:
Oral: 75-300 mg 3-5 times/day
Oral, sustained release: 150-300 mg every 12 hours
I.M., I.V.: 30-120 mg every 3 hours as needed
Administration
Oral: Administer after or with meals, milk or antacids to decrease nausea; swallow sustained release capsule whole, do not crush or chew
Parenteral: Rapid I.V. administration may result in arrhythmias and fatal apnea; administer slow I.V. over 1-2 minutes
Monitoring Parameters Liver enzymes; intraocular pressure in glaucoma patients
Patient Information May cause dizziness, flushing, headache; may cause drowsiness and impair ability to perform activities requiring mental alertness or physical coordination; may cause dry mouth
Additional Information Evidence of therapeutic value of systemic use for relief of peripheral and cerebral ischemia related to arterial spasm is lacking

Further studies are needed to determine the benefit of adding papaverine (60 mg/500 mL) to arterial catheter infusions containing NS or ½NS and heparin 1 unit/mL. One investigation showed a lower risk of arterial catheter failure and longer duration of arterial catheter function in patients 7 months to 5.5 years of age who received papaverine in their arterial catheter solutions; these results should be verified by additional studies before the addition of papaverine to arterial catheter solutions can be recommended.
(Continued)

Papaverine *(Continued)*

Dosage Forms Excipient information presented when available (limited, particularly for generics); consult specific product labeling.

Capsule, sustained release, as hydrochloride: 150 mg

Para-Time SR®: 150 mg

Injection, solution, as hydrochloride: 30 mg/mL (2 mL, 10 mL)

References

Heulitt MJ, Farrington EA, O'Shea TM, et al, "Double-Blind, Randomized, Controlled Trial of Papaverine-Containing Infusions to Prevent Failure of Arterial Catheters in Pediatric Patients," *Crit Care Med*, 1993, 21(6):825-9.

Sillanpää M and Koponen M, "Papaverine in the Prophylaxis of Migraine and Other Vascular Headache in Children," *Acta Paediatr Scand*, 1978, 67(2):209-12.

♦ **Papaverine Hydrochloride** *see* Papaverine *on page 1211*

Papillomavirus (Types 6, 11, 16, 18) Recombinant Vaccine

(pap ih LO ma VYE rus typs six e LEV en SIX teen aye teen ree KOM be nant vak SEEN)

Related Information

Immunization Guidelines *on page 1837*

U.S. Brand Names Gardasil®

Index Terms HPV Vaccine; Human Papillomavirus Vaccine; Papillomavirus Vaccine, Recombinant; Quadrivalent Human Papillomavirus Vaccine

Therapeutic Category Vaccine

Generic Available No

Use Prevention of cervical cancer, vulvar and vaginal precancers, genital warts, and low-grade cervical lesions caused by human papillomavirus (HPV) types 6, 11, 16, and 18 in girls and women 9-26 years of age.

Pregnancy Risk Factor B

Lactation Excretion in breast milk unknown/use caution. Infants had a higher incidence of acute respiratory illness when breast-fed by mothers within 30 days postvaccination.

Contraindications Hypersensitivity to human papillomavirus vaccine or any component

Warnings Administration of HPV vaccine during pregnancy is not recommended. Pregnancies detected within 30 days of vaccination had a higher rate of congenital anomalies (pyloric stenosis, congenital megacolon, congenital hydronephrosis, hip dysplasia, club foot) than the placebo group. Pregnancies with onset beyond 30 days of vaccination had a rate of congenital anomalies consistent with the general population. A registry has been established for women exposed to the HPV vaccine during pregnancy (1-800-986-8999).

Immediate treatment for anaphylactic reactions should be available during vaccine use. There is no evidence that individuals already infected with HPV will be protected. Consider deferring vaccination for patients with serious illness. May vaccinate patients with mild concurrent febrile illness.

Precautions Use with caution in patients with bleeding disorders such as hemophilia or thrombocytopenia or patients on anticoagulant therapy, due to an increased risk for bleeding following I.M. administration.

Adverse Reactions All serious adverse reactions must be reported to the U.S. Department of Health and Human Services (DHHS) Vaccine Adverse Event Reporting System (VAERS) 1-800-822-7967.

Central nervous system: Fever, dizziness, malaise, insomnia, headache

Gastrointestinal: Nausea, diarrhea, vomiting, toothache, appendicitis, gastroenteritis

Genitourinary: Pelvic inflammatory disease

Local: Injection site pain, swelling, erythema, pruritus

Neuromuscular & skeletal: Arthralgia

Respiratory: Cough, nasal congestion, asthma, bronchospasm

Drug Interactions Immunosuppressive therapies (eg, antimetabolites, alkylating agents, cytotoxic drugs, irradiation, corticosteroids) may decrease the effectiveness of the vaccine. HPV vaccine may be administered with hepatitis B vaccine using separate injection sites and syringes if both vaccines are indicated.

Stability Store in the refrigerator; do not freeze. Protect from light.

Mechanism of Action Promotes immunity to human HPV types 6, 11, 16, and 18 by inducing the production of neutralizing antibodies to the virus types

Usual Dosage I.M.: 0.5 mL

Preadolescent girls ≥9 years, Adolescent girls, and Women ≤26 years: Initial dose: 0.5 mL followed by a second dose 2 months after first dose; third dose 6 months after first dose (immunization with HPV vaccine is usually initiated at 11-12 years; optimally, vaccination should be completed prior to onset of sexual activity)

Administration I.M.: Shake suspension well prior to use; do not use suspension if it is discolored or contains particulate matter; administer I.M. into the deltoid region of the upper arm or in the higher anterolateral area of the thigh; **not for I.V. or SubQ administration**

Patient Information This vaccine does not substitute for regular, routine cervical cancer screening; the vaccine is not intended for the treatment of active genital warts or cervical cancer. This vaccine may be given during a minor illness, such as a cold or low-grade fever. Three doses will be required for effective immunity. Inform prescriber immediately if difficulty breathing, chest pain, acute headache, rash, difficulty swallowing, or excessive pain/swelling at injection site occurs.

Nursing Implications Federal law requires that the date of administration, the vaccine manufacturer, lot number of vaccine, and the administering person's name, title and address be entered into the patient's permanent medical record.

Dosage Forms Excipient information presented when available (limited, particularly for generics); consult specific product labeling.

Injection, suspension [preservative free]:

Gardasil®: HPV 6 L1 protein 20 mcg, HPV 11 L1 protein 40 mcg, HPV 16 L1 protein 40 mcg, and HPV 18 L1 protein 20 mcg per 0.5 mL (0.5 mL) [contains aluminum, polysorbate 80; manufactured using *S. cerevisiea* (bakers yeast)]

References

Block SL, Nolan T, Sattler C, et al, "Comparison of the Immunogenicity and Reactogenicity of a Prophylactic Quadrivalent Human Papillomavirus (Types 6, 11, 16, and 18) L1 Virus-Like Particle Vaccine in Male and Female Adolescents and Young Adult Women," *Pediatrics*, 2006, 118(5):2135-45.

Centers for Disease Control and Prevention (CDC), "CDC's Advisory Committee Recommends Human Papillomavirus Virus Vaccination," available at http://www.cdc.gov/od/oc/media/pressrel/r060629.htm, accessed Jul 3, 2006.

♦ **Papillomavirus Vaccine, Recombinant** *see* Papillomavirus (Types 6, 11, 16, 18) Recombinant Vaccine *on page 1212*

♦ **Paracetamol** *see* Acetaminophen *on page 42*

♦ **Parafon Forte® (Can)** *see* Chlorzoxazone *on page 348*

♦ **Parafon Forte® DSC** *see* Chlorzoxazone *on page 348*

♦ **Paraplatin® [DSC]** *see* Carboplatin *on page 288*

♦ **Paraplatin-AQ (Can)** *see* Carboplatin *on page 288*

♦ **Para-Time SR®** *see* Papaverine *on page 1211*

Paregoric (par e GOR ik)

Medication Safety Issues

Sound-alike/look-alike issues:

Camphorated tincture of opium is an error-prone synonym (mistaken as opium tincture)

Paregoric may be confused with Percogesic®

Use care when prescribing opium tincture; each mL contains the equivalent of morphine 10 mg; paregoric contains the equivalent of morphine 0.4 mg/mL

Related Information

Overdose and Toxicology *on page 1916*

Index Terms Camphorated Tincture of Opium (error-prone synonym)

Therapeutic Category Analgesic, Narcotic; Antidiarrheal

Generic Available Yes

Use Treatment of diarrhea or relief of pain; neonatal abstinence syndrome (neonatal opiate withdrawal)

Restrictions C-III

Pregnancy Risk Factor B (D when used for long-term or in high-doses)

Lactation Enters breast milk/use caution

Contraindications Hypersensitivity to opium or any component (see Warnings and Additional Information); diarrhea caused by poisoning until the toxic material has been removed

Warnings Abrupt discontinuation after prolonged use may result in symptoms of withdrawal; paregoric contains benzoic acid; benzoic acid (benzoate) is a metabolite of benzyl alcohol; large amounts of benzyl alcohol (≥99 mg/kg/day) have been associated with a potentially fatal toxicity ("gasping syndrome") in neonates; the "gasping syndrome" consists of metabolic acidosis, respiratory distress, gasping respirations, CNS dysfunction (including convulsions, intracranial hemorrhage), hypotension and cardiovascular collapse; use paregoric products containing benzoic acid with caution in neonates; *in vitro* and animal studies have shown that benzoate displaces bilirubin from protein binding sites

Precautions Use with caution in patients with respiratory, hepatic or renal dysfunction, severe prostatic hypertrophy, or history of narcotic abuse; opium shares the toxic potential of opiate agonists, usual precautions of opiate agonist therapy should be (Continued)

Paregoric *(Continued)*

observed; infants <3 months of age are more susceptible to respiratory depression, use with caution and in reduced doses in this age group

Adverse Reactions

Cardiovascular: Hypotension, bradycardia, vasodilation

Central nervous system: CNS depression, elevated intracranial pressure, drowsiness, dizziness, sedation

Endocrine & metabolic: Antidiuretic hormone release

Gastrointestinal: Nausea, vomiting, constipation, biliary tract spasm

Genitourinary: Urinary tract spasm, urinary retention

Ocular: Miosis

Respiratory: Respiratory depression

Miscellaneous: Physical and psychological dependence, histamine release

Drug Interactions CNS depressants (eg, alcohol, narcotics, benzodiazepines, tricyclic antidepressants, MAO inhibitors, phenothiazines) may increase effects/toxicity

Stability Store in light-resistant, tightly closed container; protect from freezing

Mechanism of Action Increases smooth muscle tone in GI tract, decreases motility and peristalsis, diminishes digestive secretions

Pharmacokinetics

Metabolism: Opium is metabolized in the liver

Elimination: In urine, primarily as morphine glucuronide conjugates and as parent compound (morphine, codeine, papaverine, etc)

Usual Dosage Oral:

Neonates (full term): (See Additional Information): Neonatal abstinence syndrome (opiate withdrawal): Initial: 0.1 mL/kg or 2 drops/kg with feedings every 3-4 hours; increase dosage by 0.1 mL/kg or 2 drops/kg every 3-4 hours until withdrawal symptoms are controlled; it is rare to exceed 0.7 mL/dose. Stabilize withdrawal symptoms for 3-5 days, then gradually decrease the dosage (keeping the same dosing interval) over a 2- to 4-week period.

Children: 0.25-0.5 mL/kg 1-4 times/day

Adults: 5-10 mL 1-4 times/day

Administration Oral: May administer with food to decrease GI upset; shake well before use

Monitoring Parameters Respiratory rate, blood pressure, heart rate, level of sedation; neonatal abstinence syndrome (opiate withdrawal): Monitor for resolution of withdrawal symptoms (such as irritability, high-pitched cry, stuffy nose, rhinorrhea, vomiting, poor feeding, diarrhea, sneezing, yawning, etc) and signs of over treatment (such as bradycardia, lethargy, hypotonia, irregular respirations, respiratory depression, etc); an abstinence scoring system (eg, Finnegan abstinence scoring system) can be used to more objectively assess neonatal opiate withdrawal symptoms and the need for dosage adjustment

Patient Information Avoid alcohol; may cause drowsiness and impair ability to perform activities requiring mental alertness or physical coordination; may be habit-forming; avoid abrupt discontinuation after prolonged use

Additional Information Do **not** confuse this product with opium tincture which is 25 times **more** potent; each 5 mL of paregoric contains 2 mg morphine equivalent, 0.02 mL anise oil, 20 mg benzoic acid, 20 mg camphor, 0.2 mL glycerin and alcohol; final alcohol content 45%; paregoric also contains papaverine and noscapine; because all of these additives may be harmful to neonates, **a 25-fold dilution of opium tincture** is often preferred for treatment of neonatal abstinence syndrome (opiate withdrawal); see Opium Tincture *on page 1172*

Dosage Forms Excipient information presented when available (limited, particularly for generics); consult specific product labeling.

Liquid, oral: Morphine equivalent 2 mg/5 mL (473 mL) [equivalent to opium 20 mg powder; contains alcohol 45% and benzoic acid]

References

Kraus DM and Pham JT, "Neonatal Therapy," *Applied Therapeutics: The Clinical Use of Drugs*, 7th ed, Koda-Kimble MA, Young LY, eds, Baltimore, MD: Lippincott Williams & Wilkins, 2001.

Levy M and Spino M, "Neonatal Withdrawal Syndrome: Associated Drugs and Pharmacologic Management," *Pharmacotherapy*, 1993, 13(3):202-11.

"Neonatal Drug Withdrawal. American Academy of Pediatrics Committee on Drugs," *Pediatrics*, 1998, 101(6):1079-88.

Paricalcitol (pah ri KAL si tole)

U.S. Brand Names Zemplar®

Canadian Brand Names Zemplar®

Therapeutic Category Vitamin D Analog; Vitamin, Fat Soluble

Generic Available No

Use

I.V.: Prevention and treatment of secondary hyperparathyroidism associated with stage 5 chronic kidney disease (CKD)

Oral: Prevention and treatment of secondary hyperparathyroidism associated with stages 3 and 4 chronic kidney disease (CKD)

Pregnancy Risk Factor C

Lactation Excretion in breast milk unknown/not recommended

Contraindications Hypersensitivity to paricalcitol or any component; vitamin D toxicity; hypercalcemia

Warnings Excessive administration may lead to over suppression of PTH, hypercalcemia, hypercalciuria, hyperphosphatemia, and adynamic bone disease. Acute hypercalcemia may increase risk of cardiac arrhythmias and seizures. Chronic hypercalcemia may lead to generalized vascular and other soft-tissue calcification. Phosphate and vitamin D (and its derivatives) should be withheld during therapy to avoid hypercalcemia. Safety and efficacy in pediatric patients (oral formulation) and in children <5 years of age (I.V. formulation) have not been established. Not indicated for use in patients with rapidly worsening kidney function or those who are noncompliant with medications or follow-up (K/DOQI Guidelines, 2003).

Precautions Hypercalcemia potentiates digoxin toxicity; use concomitantly with caution

Adverse Reactions

Cardiovascular: Edema, hypertension, hypotension, palpitation, chest pain, syncope, cardiomyopathy, MI, postural hypotension, CHF, arrhythmias

Central nervous system: Chills, dizziness, headache, lightheadedness, vertigo, fever, depression, insomnia, hyperthermia, psychosis (rare)

Dermatologic: Rash, skin ulcer, pruritus, skin hypertrophy, urticaria, facial edema

Endocrine & metabolic: Dehydration, acidosis, hypokalemia

Gastrointestinal: Nausea (6% to 13%), vomiting, diarrhea, GI bleeding, abdominal pain, xerostomia, constipation, gastroenteritis, dyspepsia, gastritis, taste perversion (metallic), anorexia, weight loss, pancreatitis

Genitourinary: Urinary tract infection

Neuromuscular & skeletal: Arthritis, back pain, leg cramps, weakness, neuropathy

Ocular: Amblyopia, retinal disorder, conjunctivitis (calcific), photophobia

Respiratory: Pneumonia, rhinitis, sinusitis, bronchitis, cough, epistaxis, rhinorrhea

Miscellaneous: Infection (bacterial, fungal, viral); allergic reaction, flu-like syndrome, sepsis

Drug Interactions Cytochrome P450 isoenzyme CYP3A4 substrate(major)

CYP3A4 inhibitors (azole antifungals, ciprofloxacin, clarithromycin, diclofenac, doxycycline, erythromycin, imatinib, isoniazid, nefazodone, nicardipine, propofol, protease inhibitors, quinidine, and verapamil) may increase the levels/effects of paricalcitol. Ketoconazole may increase paricalcitol levels/effects.

Stability Store at room temperature.

Mechanism of Action Paricalcitol is a synthetic analog of cacitriol (1,25-hydroxy vitamin D_3) which binds to and activates the vitamin D receptor in kidney, parathyroid gland, intestine, and bone, thus reducing PTH levels and improving calcium and phosphate homeostasis. Decreased renal conversion of vitamin D to its primary active metabolite (1,25-hydroxyvitamin D) in chronic renal failure leads to reduced activation of vitamin D receptor, which subsequently removes inhibitory suppression of parathyroid hormone (PTH) release; increased serum PTH (secondary hyperparathyroidism) reduces calcium excretion and enhances bone resorption. Paricalcitol appears to have less effects on serum calcium and/or phosphorus levels than calcitriol.

Pharmacokinetics

Distribution: V_d:

- Healthy subjects: Oral: 34 L; I.V.: 24 L
- Stage 3 and 4 CKD: Oral: 44-46 L
- Stage 5 CKD: I.V.: 31-35 L

Protein binding: >99%

Metabolism: Hydroxylation and glucuronidation via hepatic and nonhepatic enzymes, including CYP24, CYP3A4, UGT1A4; forms metabolites (at least one active)

Bioavailability: Oral: ~72% in healthy subjects

Time to peak serum concentration: Oral: 3 hours

Half-life: Adults:

- Healthy subjects: Oral: 4-6 hours; I.V.: 5-7 hours
- Stage 3 and 4 CKD: Oral: 17-20 hours
- Stage 5 CKD: I.V.: 14-15 hours

Elimination: Healthy subjects: Feces (Oral: 70% to 74%; I.V.: 63%); urine (Oral: 16% to 18%, I.V.: 19%); 51% to 59% as metabolites

Usual Dosage If hypercalcemia or Ca x P >75 is observed, reduce or interrupt dosing until parameters are normalized.

(Continued)

Paricalcitol *(Continued)*

Secondary hyperparathyroidism associated with chronic renal failure (stage 5 CKD): Children ≥5 years (limited small studies) and Adults: I.V.: 0.04-0.1 mcg/kg no more frequently than every other day; dose may be increased by 2-4 mcg every 2-4 weeks; doses as high as 0.24 mcg/kg (16.8 mcg) have been administered safely; children may require higher weight-based doses; 0.2 ± 0.7 mcg/kg/dose (Seeherunvong, 2006); the dose of paricalcitol should be adjusted based on serum intact parathyroid hormone (iPTH) levels, as follows:

Same or increasing iPTH level: Increase paricalcitol dose

iPTH level decreased by <30%: Increase paricalcitol dose

iPTH level decreased by >30% and <60%: Maintain paricalcitol dose

iPTH level decrease by >60%: Decrease paricalcitol dose

iPTH level 1.5-3 times upper limit of normal: Maintain paricalcitol dose

Secondary hyperparathyroidism associated with stage 3 and 4 CKD: Adults:

Oral: Initial dose based on baseline serum iPTH:

iPTH ≤500 pg/mL: 1 mcg/day or 2 mcg 3 times/week*

iPTH >500 pg/mL: 2 mcg/day or 4 mcg 3 times/week*

*Do not administer 3 times/week regimen more frequently than every other day

Dosage adjustment based on iPTH level relative to baseline, adjust dose at 2-4 week intervals:

iPTH same or increased: Increase paricalcitol dose by 1 mcg/day or 2 mcg 3 times/week

iPTH decreased by <30%: Increase paricalcitol dose by 1 mcg/day or 2 mcg 3 times/week

iPTH decreased by ≥30% or ≤60%: Maintain paricalcitol dose

iPTH decreased by >60%: Decrease paricalcitol dose by 1 mcg/day* or 2 mcg 3 times/week

iPTH <60 pg/mL: Decrease paricalcitol dose by 1 mcg/day* or 2 mcg 3 times/ week

*If patient is taking the lowest dose on an every other day regimen, but further dose reduction is needed, decrease dose to 1 mcg 3 times/week. If further dose reduction is required, withhold drug as needed and restart at a lower dose. If applicable, calcium-phosphate binder dosing may also be adjusted or withheld, or switch to noncalcium-based binder.

Dosage adjustment in hepatic impairment: Adjustment not needed for mild-to-moderate impairment. Paricalcitol has not been evaluated in severe hepatic impairment.

Administration Oral: May be administered with or without food. With the 3 times/week dosing schedule, doses should not be given more frequently than every other day.

Parenteral: Administer undiluted as an I.V. bolus dose at anytime during dialysis. Doses should not be administered more often than every other day.

Monitoring Parameters Signs and symptoms of vitamin D intoxication

Serum calcium and phosphorus:

I.V. therapy: Twice weekly during initial phase, then at least monthly once dose established

Oral therapy: At least every 2 weeks for 3 months or following dose adjustment, then monthly for 3 months, then every 3 months

Serum or plasma intact parathyroid hormone (iPTH): At least every 2 weeks for 3 months or following dose adjustment, then monthly for 3 months, then as per K/DOQI Guidelines below

Per Kidney Disease Outcome Quality Initiative Practice Guidelines - Children (K/DOQI, 2005):

Stage 3 CKD: iPTH every 6 months

Stage 4 CKD: iPTH every 3 months

Stage 5 CKD: iPTH every 3 months

Per Kidney Disease Outcome Quality Initiative Practice Guidelines - Adults (K/DOQI, 2003):

Stage 3 CKD: iPTH every 12 months

Stage 4 CKD: iPTH every 3 months

Stage 5 CKD: iPTH every 3 months

Reference Range Chronic kidney disease (CKD) is defined either as kidney damage or GFR <60 mL/minute/1.73 m^2 for ≥3 months); stages of CKD are described below:

CKD Stage 1: Kidney damage with normal or increased GFR; GFR ≥90 mL/minute/1.73 m^2

CKD Stage 2: Kidney damage with mild decrease in GFR; GFR 60-89 mL/minute/1.73 m^2

CKD Stage 3: Moderate decrease in GFR; GFR 30-59 mL/minute/1.73 m^2

CKD Stage 4: Severe decrease in GFR; GFR 15-29 mL/minute/1.73 m^2

CKD Stage 5: Kidney failure; GFR <15 mL/minute/1.73 m^2 or dialysis

Target range for iPTH:
Stage 2 CKD: Children: 35-70 pg/mL (3.85-7.7 pmol/L)
Children and Adults:
Stage 3 CKD: Children and Adults: 35-70 pg/mL (3.85-7.7 pmol/L)
Stage 4 CKD: Children and Adults: 70-110 pg/mL (7.7-12.1 pmol/L)
Stage 5 CKD:
Children: 200-300 pg/mL (22-33 pmol/L)
Adults: 150-300 pg/mL (16.5-33 pmol/L)
Serum phosphorous:
Stages 1-4 CKD: Children: At or above the age-appropriate lower limits and no higher than age-appropriate upper limits
Stage 3 and 4 CKD: Adults: ≥2.7 to <4.6 mg/dL (≥0.87 to <1.49 mmol/L)
Stage 5 CKD:
Children 1-12 years: 4-6 mg/dL (1.29-1.94 mmol/L)
Children >12 years and Adults: 3.5-5.5 mg/dL (1.13-1.78 mmol/L)

Patient Information Take as directed; do not increase dosage without consulting prescriber. Adhere to diet as recommended (do not take any other phosphate or vitamin D related compounds while taking paricalcitol). You may experience nausea, vomiting, dry mouth (small frequent meals, frequent mouth care, chewing gums, or sucking lozenges may help); swelling of extremities (elevate feet when sitting); or lightheadedness or dizziness (use caution when driving or engaging in tasks requiring alertness until response to drug is known). Report persistent fever, gastric disturbances, abdominal pain or blood in stool, chest pain or palpitations, bone pain, irritability, muscular twitching, weakness, or signs of respiratory infection or flu.

Dosage Forms Excipient information presented when available (limited, particularly for generics); consult specific product labeling.
Capsule, gelatin: 1 mcg, 2 mcg, 4 mcg [contains alcohol and coconut or palm kernel oil]
Injection, solution: 2 mcg/mL (1 mL); 5 mcg/mL (1 mL, 2 mL) [contains alcohol 20% v/v and propylene glycol 30% v/v]

References

"K/DOQI Clinical Practice Guidelines for Bone Metabolism and Disease in Children With Chronic Kidney Disease," *Am J Kidney Dis*, 2005, 46(4 Suppl 1):S1-121.
"K/DOQI Clinical Practice Guidelines for Bone Metabolism and Disease in Chronic Kidney Disease. Guideline 1. Evaluation of Calcium and Phosphorus Metabolism," *Am J Kidney Dis* , 2003, 42(4 Suppl 3):52-7.
"K/DOQI Clinical Practice Guidelines for Bone Metabolism and Disease in Chronic Kidney Disease. Guideline 3. Evaluation of Serum Phosphorus Levels," *Am J Kidney Dis* , 2003, 42(4 Suppl 3):62-3.
"K/DOQI Clinical Practice Guidelines for Chronic Kidney Disease: Evaluation, Classification, and Stratification, Part 4. Definition and Classification of Stages of Chronic Kidney Disease," *Am J Kidney Dis*, 2002, 39(2 Suppl 1):46-75.
Sanchez CP, "Secondary Hyperparathyroidism in Children With Chronic Renal Failure: Pathogenesis and Treatment," *Paediatr Drugs*, 2003, 5(11): 763-76.
Seeherunvong W, Nwobi, O, Abitbol CL, et al, "Paricalcitol Versus Calcitriol Treatment for Hyperparathyroidism in Pediatric Hemodialysis Patients," *Pediatr Nephrol*, 2006, 21(10):1434-9.
Ziolkowska H, "Minimizing Bone Abnormalities in Children With Renal Failure," *Paediatr Drugs*, 2006, 8(4):205-22.

♦ **Pariet® (Can)** *see* Rabeprazole *on page 1362*
♦ **Pariprazole** *see* Rabeprazole *on page 1362*
♦ **Parlodel®** *see* Bromocriptine *on page 232*
♦ **Parlodel® SnapTabs®** *see* Bromocriptine *on page 232*

Paromomycin (par oh moe MYE sin)

U.S. Brand Names Humatin®
Canadian Brand Names Humatin®
Index Terms Paromomycin Sulfate
Therapeutic Category Amebicide
Generic Available Yes
Use Treatment of acute and chronic intestinal amebiasis due to susceptible *Entamoeba histolytica* (not effective in the treatment of extraintestinal amebiasis); tapeworm infestations; adjunctive management of hepatic coma; treatment of cryptosporidial diarrhea
Pregnancy Risk Factor C
Lactation Does not enter breast milk/compatible
Contraindications Hypersensitivity to paromomycin or any component; intestinal obstruction
Warnings May result in overgrowth of nonsusceptible organisms
Precautions Use with caution in patients with impaired GI motility or possible or proven ulcerative bowel lesions; use with caution in patients with impaired renal function
Adverse Reactions
Central nervous system: Headache, vertigo
(Continued)

Paromomycin *(Continued)*

Dermatologic: Exanthema, rash, pruritus
Endocrine & metabolic: Hypocholesterolemia
Gastrointestinal: Diarrhea, abdominal cramps, nausea, vomiting, anorexia, steatorrhea, secondary enterocolitis, pancreatitis
Hematologic: Eosinophilia
Otic: Ototoxicity
Renal: Hematuria

Drug Interactions May decrease digoxin level; increased effect of oral anticoagulants

Food Interactions Paromomycin may cause malabsorption of xylose, sucrose, and fats

Mechanism of Action Acts directly on ameba in the intestinal lumen; interferes with bacterial protein synthesis by binding to 30S ribosomal subunit of susceptible bacteria

Pharmacokinetics
Absorption: Poor from the GI tract
Elimination: Excreted unchanged in feces; portion of oral dose that may be absorbed is excreted in urine

Usual Dosage Oral:
Children:
Intestinal amebiasis (*Entamoeba histolytica*): 25-35 mg/kg/day divided every 8 hours for 7 days
Dientamoeba fragilis infection: 25-30 mg/kg/day divided every 8 hours for 7 days
Tapeworm:
T. saginata, *T. solium*, *D. latum*: 11 mg/kg/dose every 15 minutes for 4 doses
H. nana: 45 mg/kg/day once daily for 5-7 days
Adults:
Intestinal amebiasis (*Entamoeba histolytica*): 25-35 mg/kg/day divided every 8 hours for 7 days
Dientamoeba fragilis infection: 25-30 mg/kg/day divided every 8 hours for 7 days
Tapeworm:
T. saginata, *T. solium*, *D. latum*: 1 g every 15 minutes for 4 doses
H. nana: 45 mg/kg/day once daily for 5-7 days
Hepatic coma: 4 g/day in 2-4 divided doses for 5-6 days
Cryptosporidial diarrhea: 1.5-2 g/day in 3-4 divided doses for 10-14 days

Administration Oral: Administer with or after meals

Monitoring Parameters Periodic urinalysis and renal function tests; be alert to ototoxicity

Patient Information Notify physician if ringing in ears, hearing loss, or dizziness occurs

Additional Information With the treatment of cestodiasis caused by *T. solium*, paromomycin may cause disintegration of worm segments and release of viable eggs resulting in an increased risk for the development of cysticercosis

Dosage Forms Excipient information presented when available (limited, particularly for generics); consult specific product labeling.
Capsule: 250 mg

References

Danziger LH, Kanyok TP, and Novak RM, "Treatment of Cryptosporidial Diarrhea in an AIDS Patient With Paromomycin," *Ann Pharmacother*, 1993, 27(12):1460-2.
Liu LX and Weller PF, "Antiparasitic Drugs," *N Engl J Med*, 1996, 334(18):1178-84.

♦ **Paromomycin Sulfate** *see* Paromomycin *on page 1217*

Paroxetine (pa ROKS e teen)

Medication Safety Issues
Sound-alike/look-alike issues:
Paroxetine may be confused with paclitaxel, pyridoxine
Paxil® may be confused with Doxil®, paclitaxel, Plavix®, Taxol®

Related Information
Antidepressant Agents *on page 1681*
Serotonin Syndrome *on page 1955*

U.S. Brand Names Paxil®; Paxil CR®; Pexeva®

Canadian Brand Names Apo-Paroxetine®; CO Paroxetine; Gen-Paroxetine; Novo-Paroxetine; Paxil®; Paxil CR®; PMS-Paroxetine; ratio-Paroxetine; Rhoxal-paroxetine; Sandoz-Paroxetine

Index Terms Paroxetine Hydrochloride; Paroxetine Mesylate

Therapeutic Category Antidepressant, Selective Serotonin Reuptake Inhibitor (SSRI)

Generic Available Yes: Tablet, as hydrochloride

Use Treatment of depression, obsessive compulsive disorder, panic disorder, social anxiety disorder, generalized anxiety disorder, and post-traumatic stress disorder

Paxil CR®: Treatment of depression, panic disorder, social anxiety disorder, premenstrual dysphoric disorder

Pexeva®: Treatment of depression, obsessive compulsive disorder, panic disorder, generalized anxiety disorder

Medication Guide An FDA-approved patient medication guide, which is available with the product information and at http://www.fda.gov/cder/Offices/ODS/medication_guides.htm, must be dispensed with this medication for each new outpatient prescription and refill.

Pregnancy Risk Factor D

Lactation Enters breast milk/use caution (AAP rates "of concern")

Contraindications Hypersensitivity to paroxetine or any component; use of MAO inhibitors within 14 days (potentially fatal reactions may occur, see Drug Interactions); concurrent use of thioridazine or pimozide (see Drug Interactions)

Warnings Paroxetine is not approved for use in pediatric patients. Clinical worsening of depression or suicidal ideation and behavior may occur in children and adults with major depressive disorder. In clinical trials, antidepressants increased the risk of suicidal thinking and behavior (suicidality) in children, adolescents, and young adults (18-24 years of age) with major depressive disorder and other psychiatric disorders. This risk must be considered before prescribing antidepressants for any clinical use. Short-term studies did **not** show an increased risk of suicidality with antidepressant use in patients >24 years of age and showed a decreased risk in patients ≥65 years.

Patients of all ages who are treated with antidepressants for any indication require appropriate monitoring and close observation for clinical worsening of depression, suicidality, and unusual changes in behavior, especially during the first few months after antidepressant initiation or when the dose is adjusted. Family members and caregivers should be instructed to closely observe the patient (ie, daily) and communicate condition with healthcare provider. All patients should also be monitored for associated behaviors (eg, anxiety, agitation, panic attacks, insomnia, irritability, hostility, aggressiveness, impulsivity, akathisia, hypomania, mania) which may increase the risk for worsening depression or suicidality. Worsening depression or emergence of suicidality (or associated behaviors listed above) that is abrupt in onset, severe, or not part of the presenting symptoms, may require discontinuation or modification of drug therapy.

Avoid abrupt discontinuation; discontinuation symptoms (including agitation, dysphoria, anxiety, confusion, dizziness, hypomania, nightmares, and other symptoms) may occur if therapy is abruptly discontinued or dose reduced; taper dosage gradually in patients receiving >20 mg/day to minimize risks of discontinuation symptoms; if intolerable symptoms occur following a decrease in dosage or upon discontinuation of therapy, consider resuming the previous dose with a more gradual taper. To reduce risk of intentional overdose, write prescriptions for the smallest quantity consistent with good patient care.

Screen individuals for bipolar disorder prior to treatment (using antidepressants alone may induce manic episodes in patients with this condition). Potentially fatal serotonin syndrome may occur when SSRIs are used in combination with serotonergic drugs (eg, triptans) or drugs that impair the metabolism of serotonin (eg, MAO inhibitors); see Drug Interactions.

An increased risk of birth defects (specifically cardiovascular malformations) has been reported when paroxetine was taken during the first trimester of pregnancy. The majority of heart defects were ventricular and atrial septal defects (VSD and ASD), some of which required surgical correction. Use paroxetine during pregnancy only if the potential benefits to the mother outweigh the possible risks to the fetus. Administration of paroxetine during late third trimester may result in adverse effects or paroxetine withdrawal syndrome in the newborn (consider risks and benefits; use with caution during late third trimester; see Additional Information). Exposure to SSRIs late in pregnancy may also be associated with an increased risk for persistent pulmonary hypertension of the newborn (see Chambers, 2006). Postmarketing reports of premature births in pregnant women receiving paroxetine or other SSRIs have been noted.

Precautions Use with caution in patients with a history of seizures, mania, renal disease, cardiac disease, or hepatic disease and in suicidal patients, children, or during breast-feeding in lactating women. Modify dosage in patients with renal or hepatic impairment. May cause hyponatremia, use with caution in patients with volume depletion or diuretic use. May cause abnormal bleeding (eg, ecchymosis, purpura, upper GI bleeding); use with caution in patients with impaired platelet aggregation and with concurrent use of aspirin, NSAIDs, or other drugs that affect coagulation. May cause akathisia (psychomotor restlessness), usually within the first few weeks of initiation of therapy. No clinical studies have assessed the combined use of paroxetine and electroconvulsive therapy

(Continued)

Paroxetine *(Continued)*

Adverse Reactions

Cardiovascular: Palpitations, tachycardia, vasodilation, postural hypotension, bradycardia, hypotension

Central nervous system: Headache, somnolence, dizziness, insomnia, nervousness, agitation, anxiety, migraine, impaired concentration, yawning, emotional lability, hostility, hyperkinesias, akathisia (psychomotor restlessness), hallucinations; suicidal thinking and behavior (see Warnings)

Note: SSRI-associated behavioral activation (ie, restlessness, hyperkinesis, hyperactivity, agitation) is 2- to 3-fold more prevalent in children compared to adolescents; it is more prevalent in adolescents compared to adults. Somnolence (including sedation and drowsiness) is more common in adults compared to children and adolescents (see Safer, 2006).

Dermatologic: Alopecia, purpura, ecchymosis, photosensitivity

Endocrine & metabolic: Hyponatremia (volume-depleted patients), SIADH, sexual dysfunction

Gastrointestinal: Nausea, xerostomia, constipation, vomiting, diarrhea, anorexia, flatulence, gastritis, abdominal pain

Note: SSRI-associated vomiting is 2- to 3-fold more prevalent in children compared to adolescents; it is more prevalent in adolescents compared to adults.

Hematologic: Anemia, leukopenia

Neuromuscular & skeletal: Weakness, tremor, arthritis, paresthesia, asthenia

Ocular: Eye pain, blurred vision

Otic: Ear pain

Respiratory: Asthma, rhinitis

Miscellaneous: Diaphoresis, thirst, bruxism, akinesia; withdrawal symptoms following abrupt discontinuation (see Warnings)

Drug Interactions Cytochrome P450 isoenzyme CYP2D6 substrate (minor); CYP2D6, CYP1A2 (high dose) (weak), and CYP3A3/4 (weak) isoenzyme inhibitor

With MAO inhibitors, fever, tremors, seizures, hypertension, delirium, coma may occur (use of MAO inhibitors within 14 days of paroxetine use is contraindicated). Tryptophan (which can be metabolized to serotonin) and the herbal medicine St John's wort (*Hypericum perforatum*) may increase serious serotonin side effects (serotonin syndrome); the use of these agents is **not** recommended.

Combined use of SSRIs and amphetamine, buspirone, dextromethorphan, meperidine, nefazodone, serotonin agonists, sibutramine, other SSRIs, sympathomimetics, ritonavir, linezolid, lithium, tramadol, and venlafaxine may increase the risk of serotonin syndrome. Use of SSRIs with sumatriptan may cause weakness, incoordination, hyper-reflexia, and an increased risk of serotonin syndrome; use triptans with caution in patients receiving SSRIs; monitor carefully, especially during initiation of treatment and dosage increases.

Increased effect/toxicity of paroxetine occurs with alcohol, cimetidine, phenothiazines, type 1C antiarrhythmics. Increased effect/toxicity of tricyclic antidepressants, risperidone, atomoxetine (a lower initial dose of atomoxetine is recommended; further dosage adjustment may be needed), fluoxetine, sertraline, theophylline, warfarin, NSAIDs, aspirin, other drugs that affect coagulation (increased risk for bleeding), thioridazine (paroxetine may inhibit the metabolism of thioridazine and increase the risk of serious cardiac effects such as prolongation of the QT_c interval, ventricular arrhythmias, torsade de pointes, and sudden death; concurrent use of thioridazine and paroxetine is contraindicated), pimozide (paroxetine may increase serum concentrations of pimozide and increase serious adverse effects; concurrent use of pimozide and paroxetine is contraindicated); the combination of paroxetine and pimozide resulted in an oculogyric crisis in a 9-year old boy (Horrigan, 1994)

Decreased effect with phenobarbital, phenytoin (may also decrease phenytoin levels). Fosamprenavir, coadministered with ritonavir, significantly decreases serum concentrations of paroxetine. Cyproheptadine may decrease or antagonize effects of paroxetine; paroxetine may decrease the AUC of digoxin by 15%; paroxetine may increase or worsen lysergic acid diethylamide (LSD) flashbacks

Food Interactions Tryptophan supplements may increase serious side effects; its use is **not recommended.**

Immediate release: Food or milk does not significantly affect extent of absorption; food may slightly increase AUC (by 6%), increase peak concentration by 29%, and decrease time to peak from 6.4 hours to 4.9 hours postdose

Controlled release: Bioavailability is not affected by food

Stability

Immediate release tablet: Hydrochloride: Store between 15°C to 30°C (59°F to 86°F); mesylate: Store at 25°C (77°F); excursions permitted to 15°C to 30°C (59°F to 86°F); protect from humidity

Oral suspension and controlled release tablet: Store ≤25°C (77°F)

Mechanism of Action Paroxetine is a selective serotonin reuptake inhibitor (SSRI), chemically unrelated to tricyclic, tetracyclic, or other antidepressants; the inhibition of serotonin reuptake from CNS neuronal synapses potentiates serotonin activity in the brain

Pharmacodynamics

Onset of action: Antidepressant effects: Within 1-4 weeks

Antiobsessional and antipanic effects: Up to several weeks

Pharmacokinetics

Absorption: Oral: Well absorbed

Distribution: V_d (adults): Mean: 8.7 L/kg; range: 3-28 L/kg

Protein binding: 95%

Metabolism: Extensive by cytochrome P450 enzymes via oxidation and methylation followed by glucuronide and sulfate conjugation; nonlinear kinetics may be seen with higher doses and longer duration of therapy due to saturation of P450 2D6 (CYP2D6), an enzyme partially responsible for metabolism. **Note:** Paroxetine pharmacokinetics have not been studied in patients deficient in CYP2D6 (ie, poor metabolizers)

Bioavailability: Immediate release tablet and oral suspension have equal bioavailability

Half-life: Adults: Mean: 21 hours; range: 3-65 hours

Time to peak serum concentration:

Immediate release tablet:

As hydrochloride: Mean: 5.2 hours

As mesylate: Mean: 8.1 hours

Controlled release tablet: 6-10 hours

Elimination: Metabolites are excreted in urine and bile; 2% of drug excreted unchanged in urine

Usual Dosage Oral: **Note:** For maintenance therapy, use lowest effective dose and periodically reassess need for continued treatment

Children and Adolescents: **Note:** Not FDA approved; see Warnings. Limited information is available.

Depression: The FDA recommends that paroxetine not be used in pediatric patients for the treatment of depression. Three well-controlled trials in pediatric patients with depression have failed to show therapeutic superiority over placebo; in addition, an increased risk for suicidal behavior was observed in patients receiving paroxetine when compared to other SSRIs (see Dopheide, 2006).

Obsessive-compulsive disorder (OCD): A 12-week open-label trial of paroxetine in 20 outpatients 8-17 years of age demonstrated the potential clinical usefulness in pediatric OCD; doses were initiated at 10 mg/day and could be increased every 2 weeks by no more than 10 mg/day increments, to a maximum of 60 mg/day (see Rosenberg, 1999). Efficacy of paroxetine was demonstrated in a 10-week, randomized, double-blind, placebo-controlled trial conducted in 207 pediatric patients (aged 7-17 years) with OCD; paroxetine doses were initiated at 10 mg/day and could be increased no more often than every 7 days by 10 mg/day increments, to a maximum dose of 50 mg/day; the overall mean dose was 20.3 mg/day for children and 26.8 mg/day for adolescents (see Geller, 2004). Further studies are needed.

Self-injurious behavior: A 15-year old autistic male with self-injurious behavior was successfully treated with paroxetine 20 mg/day (Snead, 1994). Further studies are needed.

Social phobia: A small case series reported the effective use of paroxetine in 5 pediatric patients with social phobia [2 children (7 and 11 years of age) and 3 adolescents (16, 17, and 18 years of age)]; comorbid diagnoses (obsessive compulsive disorder and/or dysthymia) existed in 3 patients; doses were adjusted on an individual basis; the 7-year old was started on 2.5 mg/day and increased to 5 mg/day after 4 weeks; the 11-year old was started on 5 mg/day and the dose was titrated upwards by 5 mg/day increments every 3-4 weeks to 15 mg/day; adolescents were started on ≤20 mg/day (see Mancini, 1999). A 16-week multicenter, randomized, double-blind, placebo-controlled trial reported the efficacy of paroxetine in pediatric patients (aged 8-17 years) with social anxiety disorder; 163 patients were randomized to receive paroxetine; doses were initiated at 10 mg/day and could be increased every 7 days by 10 mg/day increments, to a maximum dose of 50 mg/day; the overall mean dose was 21.7 mg/day for children and 26.1 mg/day for adolescents (see Wagner, 2004). Further studies are needed.

Adults:

Depression:

Paxil®, Pexeva®: Initial: 20 mg/day given once daily preferably in the morning; increase if needed by 10 mg/day increments at intervals of at least 1 week; maximum dose: 50 mg/day

(Continued)

Paroxetine *(Continued)*

Paxil CR®: Initial: 25 mg/day given once daily preferably in the morning; increase if needed by 12.5 mg/day increments at intervals of at least 1 week; maximum dose: 62.5 mg/day

Generalized anxiety disorder: Paxil®, Pexeva®: Initial: 20 mg/day given once daily preferably in the morning; recommended dose: 20 mg/day; range: 20-50 mg/day; doses >20 mg may not have additional benefit; if dose is increased, adjust in increments of 10 mg/day at intervals of at least 1 week

Obsessive compulsive disorder: Paxil®, Pexeva®: Initial: 20 mg/day given once daily preferably in the morning; increase by 10 mg/day increments at intervals of at least 1 week; recommended dose: 40 mg/day; range: 20-60 mg/day; maximum dose: 60 mg/day

Panic disorder:

Paxil®, Pexeva®: Initial: 10 mg/day given once daily preferably in the morning; increase by 10 mg/day increments at intervals of at least 1 week; recommended dose: 40 mg/day; range: 10-60 mg/day; maximum dose: 60 mg/day

Paxil CR®: Initial: 12.5 mg/day given once daily preferably in the morning; increase if needed by 12.5 mg/day increments at intervals of at least 1 week; maximum dose: 75 mg/day

Post-traumatic stress disorder: Paxil®: Initial: 20 mg/day given once daily preferably in the morning; recommended dose: 20 mg/day; range: 20-50 mg/day; doses of 40 mg/day have not been shown to be of greater benefit than 20 mg/day; if indicated, increase dose by 10 mg/day increments at intervals of at least 1 week

Premenstrual dysphoric disorder: Paxil CR®: Initial: 12.5 mg/day given once daily preferably in the morning; increase if needed to 25 mg/day after at least 1 week; may be given daily throughout the menstrual cycle **or** limited to the luteal phase

Social anxiety disorder:

Paxil®: Initial: 20 mg/day given once daily preferably in the morning; recommended dose: 20 mg/day; range: 20-60 mg/day; doses >20 mg may not have additional benefit

Paxil CR®: Initial: 12.5 mg/day given once daily preferably in the morning; increase if needed by 12.5 mg/day increments at intervals of at least 1 week; maximum dose: 37.5 mg/day

Dosing adjustment in severe hepatic or renal impairment: Adults:

Paxil®, Pexeva®: Initial: 10 mg/day; increase if needed by 10 mg/day increments at intervals of at least 1 week; maximum dose: 40 mg/day

Paxil CR®: Initial: 12.5 mg/day; increase if needed by 12.5 mg/day increments at intervals of at least 1 week; maximum dose: 50 mg/day

Administration May be administered without regard to meals; administration with food may decrease GI side effects; shake suspension well before use. Do not chew or crush immediate or controlled release tablet, swallow whole

Monitoring Parameters Blood pressure, heart rate, liver and renal function. Monitor patient periodically for symptom resolution; monitor for worsening depression, suicidality, and associated behaviors (especially at the beginning of therapy or when doses are increased or decreased; see Warnings)

Patient Information Read the patient Medication Guide that you receive with each prescription and refill of paroxetine. An increased risk of suicidal thinking and behavior has been reported with the use of antidepressants in children, adolescents, and young adults (18-24 years of age). Notify physician if you feel more depressed, have thoughts of suicide, or become more agitated or irritable (see Warnings). Avoid alcohol, tryptophan supplements, and the herbal medicine St John's wort; avoid aspirin, NSAIDs, or other drugs that affect coagulation (may increase risks of bleeding); may cause dizziness or drowsiness and impair ability to perform activities requiring mental alertness or physical coordination; may cause photosensitivity reactions; avoid exposure to sunlight and artificial light sources (sunlamps, tanning booth/bed); use a sunscreen; contact physician if reaction occurs; may cause dry mouth. Some medicines should not be taken with paroxetine or should not be taken for a while after paroxetine has been discontinued; report the use of other medications, nonprescription medications, and herbal or natural products to your physician and pharmacist. Take as directed; do not alter dose or frequency without consulting prescriber; avoid abrupt discontinuation.

Nursing Implications Assess other medications patient may be taking for possible interaction (especially MAO inhibitors, P450 inhibitors, and other CNS active agents). Assess mental status for depression, suicidal ideation, anxiety, social functioning, mania, or panic attack.

Additional Information Paroxetine is more potent and more selective than other SSRIs (eg, fluoxetine, fluvoxamine, sertraline, and clomipramine) in the inhibition of serotonin reuptake. If used for an extended period of time, long-term usefulness of paroxetine should be periodically re-evaluated for an individual patient. Paxil CR® tablets contain a degradable polymeric matrix (that controls the dissolution rate over ~4-5 hours) and an entering coating (that delays drug release until tablets leave the stomach). A recent report describes 5 children (age: 8-15 years) who developed epistaxis (n=4) or bruising (n=1) while receiving SSRI therapy (sertraline) (Lake, 2000). Another recent report describes the SSRI discontinuation syndrome in 6 children; the syndrome was similar to that reported in adults (see Diler, 2002).

Neonates born to women receiving SSRIs late during the third trimester may experience respiratory distress, apnea, cyanosis, temperature instability, vomiting, feeding difficulty, hypoglycemia, constant crying, irritability, hypotonia, hypertonia, hyper-reflexia, tremor, jitteriness, and seizures; these symptoms may be due to a direct toxic effect, withdrawal syndrome, or (in some cases) serotonin syndrome. Withdrawal symptoms occur in 30% of neonates exposed to SSRIs *in utero*; monitor newborns for at least 48 hours after birth; long-term effects of *in utero* exposure to SSRIs are unknown (see Levinson-Castiel, 2006).

Dosage Forms Excipient information presented when available (limited, particularly for generics); consult specific product labeling.

Note: Strength expressed as base:

Suspension, oral, as hydrochloride:

Paxil®: 10 mg/5 mL (250 mL) [orange flavor]

Tablet, as hydrochloride: 10 mg, 20 mg, 30 mg, 40 mg

Paxil®: 10 mg, 20 mg, 30 mg, 40 mg

Tablet, as mesylate:

Pexeva®: 10 mg, 20 mg, 30 mg, 40 mg

Tablet, controlled release, as hydrochloride:

Paxil CR®: 12.5 mg, 25 mg, 37.5 mg

References

Chambers CD, Hernandez-Diaz S, Van Marter LJ, et al, "Selective Serotonin-Reuptake Inhibitors and Risk of Persistent Pulmonary Hypertension of the Newborn," *N Engl J Med*, 2006, 354(6):579-87.

Diler RS and Avci A, "Selective Serotonin Reuptake Inhibitor Discontinuation Syndrome in Children: Six Case Reports," *Current Therapeutic Reseach*, 2002, 63(3):188-97.

Dopheide JA, "Recognizing and Treating Depression in Children and Adolescents," *Am J Health Syst Pharm*, 2006, 63(3):233-43.

Findling RL, Reed MD, and Blumer JL, "Pharmacological Treatment of Depression in Children and Adolescents," *Paediatr Drugs*, 1999, 1(3):161-82.

Geller DA, Wagner KD, Emslie G, et al, "Paroxetine Treatment in Children and Adolescents With Obsessive-Compulsive Disorder: A Randomized, Multicenter, Double-Blind, Placebo-Controlled Trial," *J Am Acad Child Adolesc Psychiatry*, 2004, 43(11):1387-96.

Horrigan JP and Barnhill LJ, "Paroxetine-Pimozide Drug Interactions," *J Am Acad Child Adolesc Psychiatry*, 1994, 33(7):1060-1.

Keller MB, Ryan ND, Strober M, et al, "Efficacy of Paroxetine in the Treatment of Adolescent Major Depression: A Randomized, Controlled Trial," *J Am Acad Child Adolesc Psychiatry*, 2001, 40(7):762-72.

Lake MB, Birmaher B, Wassick S, et al, "Bleeding and Selective Serotonin Reuptake Inhibitors in Childhood and Adolescence," *J Child Adolesc Psychopharmacol*, 2000, 10(1):35-8.

Levinson-Castiel R, Merlob P, Linder N, et al, "Neonatal Abstinence Syndrome After *in utero* Exposure to Selective Serotonin Reuptake Inhibitors in Term Infants," *Arch Pediatr Adolesc Med*, 2006, 160(2):173-6.

Mancini C, Van Ameringen M, Oakman JM, et al, "Serotonergic Agents in the Treatment of Social Phobia in Children and Adolescents: A Case Series," *Depress Anxiety*, 1999, 10(1):33-9.

Markel H, Lee A, Holmes RD, et al, "LSD Flashback Syndrome Exacerbated by Selective Serotonin Reuptake Inhibitor Antidepressants in Adolescents," *J Pediatr*, 1994, 125(5 Pt 1):817-9.

Rey-Sanchez F and Guitierrez-Cassares JR, "Paroxetine in Children With Major Depressive Disorder: An Open Trial," *J Am Acad Child Adolesc Psychiatry*, 1997, 36(10):1443-7.

Rosenberg DR, Stewart CM, Fitzgerald KD, et al, "Paroxetine Open-Label Treatment of Pediatric Outpatients With Obsessive-Compulsive Disorder," *J Am Acad Child Adolesc Psychiatry*, 1999, 38(9):1180-5.

Safer DJ and Zito JM, "Treatment Emergent Adverse Effects of Selective Serotonin Reuptake Inhibitors by Age Group: Children vs. Adolescents," *J Child Adolesc Psychopharmacol*, 2006, 16(1/2):159-69.

Sharp SC and Hellings JA, "Efficacy and Safety of Selective Serotonin Reuptake Inhibitors in the Treatment of Depression in Children and Adolescents: Practitioner Review," *Clin Drug Investig*, 2006, 26(5):247-55.

Snead RW, Boon F, and Presberg J, "Paroxetine for Self-Injurious Behavior," *J Am Acad Child Adolesc Psychiatry*, 1994, 33(6):909-10.

Stiskal JA, Kulin N, Koren G, et al, "Neonatal Paroxetine Withdrawal Syndrome," *Arch Dis Child Fetal Neonatal Ed*, 2001, 84(2):F134-5.

Wagner KD, Berard R, Stein MB, et al, "A Multicenter, Randomized, Double-Blind, Placebo-Controlled Trial of Paroxetine in Children and Adolescents With Social Anxiety Disorder," *Arch Gen Psychiatry*, 2004, 61(11):1153-62.

Wagner KD, "Pharmacotherapy for Major Depression in Children and Adolescents," *Prog Neuropsychopharmacol Biol Psychiatry*, 2005, 29(5):819-26.

♦ **Paroxetine Hydrochloride** *see* Paroxetine *on page 1218*
♦ **Paroxetine Mesylate** *see* Paroxetine *on page 1218*
♦ **Parvolex® (Can)** *see* Acetylcysteine *on page 51*
♦ **Pathocil® (Can)** *see* Dicloxacillin *on page 489*
♦ **Pavabid [DSC]** *see* Papaverine *on page 1211*
♦ **Pavulon [DSC]** *see* Pancuronium *on page 1206*
♦ **Paxil®** *see* Paroxetine *on page 1218*
♦ **Paxil CR®** *see* Paroxetine *on page 1218*
♦ **PCA (error-prone abbreviation)** *see* Procainamide *on page 1315*

- **PCE®** *see* Erythromycin *on page 595*
- **PCEC** *see* Rabies Virus Vaccine *on page 1364*
- **PCV** *see* Penciclovir *on page 1226*
- **PCV7** *see* Pneumococcal Conjugate Vaccine (7-Valent) *on page 1271*
- **PediaCare® Children's Medicated Freezer Pops Long Acting Cough [OTC] [DSC]** *see* Dextromethorphan *on page 477*
- **PediaCare® Decongestant Infants [OTC]** *see* Pseudoephedrine *on page 1344*
- **PediaCare® Infants' Long-Acting Cough [OTC]** *see* Dextromethorphan *on page 477*
- **Pediaflor® [DSC]** *see* Fluoride *on page 675*
- **Pediapred®** *see* PrednisoLONE *on page 1304*
- **Pediarix®** *see* Diphtheria, Tetanus Toxoids, Acellular Pertussis, Hepatitis B (Recombinant), and Poliovirus (Inactivated) Vaccine *on page 516*
- **PediaTan™** *see* Chlorpheniramine *on page 344*
- **Pediatex™-D [DSC]** *see* Carbinoxamine and Pseudoephedrine *on page 286*
- **Pediatric Digoxin CSD (Can)** *see* Digoxin *on page 496*
- **Pediatrix (Can)** *see* Acetaminophen *on page 42*
- **Pediazole® [DSC]** *see* Erythromycin and Sulfisoxazole *on page 599*
- **Pediazole® (Can)** *see* Erythromycin and Sulfisoxazole *on page 599*
- **Pedi-Dri®** *see* Nystatin *on page 1156*
- **PediOtic®** *see* Neomycin, (Bacitracin) Polymyxin B, and Hydrocortisone *on page 1119*
- **Pedisilk® [OTC]** *see* Salicylic Acid *on page 1413*
- **Pedtrace-4®** *see* Trace Metals *on page 1558*
- **PedvaxHIB®** *see Haemophilus* b Conjugate Vaccine *on page 751*
- **PEG-L-asparaginase** *see* Pegaspargase *on page 1224*

Pegaspargase (peg AS par jase)

Medication Safety Issues

Sound-alike/look-alike issues:

Pegaspargase may be confused with asparaginase

High alert medication: The Institute for Safe Medication Practices (ISMP) includes this medication among its list of drugs which have a heightened risk of causing significant patient harm when used in error.

Related Information

Emetogenic Potential of Single Chemotherapeutic Agents *on page 1776*

U.S. Brand Names Oncaspar®

Index Terms NSC-644954; PEG-L-asparaginase

Therapeutic Category Antineoplastic Agent, Miscellaneous

Generic Available No

Use First-line treatment of newly diagnosed acute lymphoblastic leukemia (ALL) as part of a multiple chemotherapeutic drug regimen; induction treatment of acute lymphoblastic leukemia in combination with other chemotherapeutic agents in patients who have developed hypersensitivity to native forms of L-asparaginase derived from *E. coli* and/or *Erwinia chrysanthemia*; treatment of lymphoma

Pregnancy Risk Factor C

Lactation Excretion in breast milk unknown; since potential for serious adverse reaction in nursing infant exists, breast-feeding is not recommended

Contraindications Hypersensitivity to pegaspargase or any component; pancreatitis or history of pancreatitis; patients who have had significant thrombosis or hemorrhagic events associated with prior L-asparaginase therapy

Warnings The FDA currently recommends that procedures for proper handling and disposal of antineoplastic agents be considered; inhalation of vapors and contact with skin, eyes, or mucous membranes must be avoided; be prepared to treat anaphylaxis at each administration. Risk of serious allergic reactions is higher in patients with hypersensitivity to other forms of L-asparaginase. Serious thrombotic events can occur in patients receiving pegaspargase. Pancreatitis can occur in patients receiving pegaspargase. Discontinue pegaspargase if anaphylaxis or serious allergic reaction, thrombosis, or pancreatitis occur.

Glucose intolerance can occur in patients receiving pegaspargase. Coagulopathy with elevated prothrombin time, partial thromboplastin time, and hypofibrinogenemia can occur in patients receiving pegaspargase (monitor coagulation parameters at baseline and periodically during and after treatment). In patients with severe or symptomatic coagulopathy, treat with fresh-frozen plasma.

Precautions Use with caution in patients with an underlying coagulopathy or previous hematologic complication from asparaginase; patients receiving anticoagulation therapy, aspirin, or NSAIDs; use with caution in patients with hyperglycemia, diabetes, hepatic dysfunction, or in patients receiving hepatotoxic agents

Adverse Reactions Incidence of coagulopathy, hepatotoxicity, nephrotoxicity, and adverse GI effects is less for I.M. pegaspargase administration than for I.V. use.

Cardiovascular: Hypotension, chest pain, tachycardia, edema, stroke

Central nervous system: Somnolence, confusion, seizures, fever, chills, headache, dizziness, malaise, coma, mental status changes, CNS thrombosis

Dermatologic: Rash, pruritus, urticaria, erythema

Endocrine & metabolic: Hyperglycemia, transient diabetes mellitus, hyperammonemia, hyperuricemia

Gastrointestinal: Protracted nausea and vomiting, abdominal pain, constipation, diarrhea, anorexia, pancreatitis

Genitourinary: Hemorrhagic cystitis

Hematologic: Leukopenia, anemia, thrombocytopenia; prolonged prothrombin, thrombin and partial thromboplastin times; decreased fibrinogen; thrombosis; hemorrhage

Hepatic: Hepatotoxicity, jaundice, elevated ALT and AST, hyperbilirubinemia

Neuromuscular & skeletal: Paresthesia, weakness, arthralgia, myalgia

Renal: Elevated BUN, elevated serum creatinine, renal failure

Respiratory: Cough, bronchospasm, epistaxis, laryngeal edema, dyspnea

Miscellaneous: Anaphylaxis

Drug Interactions Methotrexate (decreases antineoplastic effect if given immediately prior to methotrexate); vincristine (increases toxicity if given concomitantly); prednisone (increases hyperglycemic effect); may increase toxicity of highly protein bound drugs; may increase bleeding in patients receiving warfarin, heparin, aspirin, NSAID, or dipyridamole

Stability Store vials in refrigerator; do not freeze; do not administer if there is any indication that the drug has been frozen or if stored at room temperature for >48 hours; avoid excessive agitation, do not shake; do not use if cloudy or if precipitate is present; use of a 0.2 micron filter may result in some loss of potency

Mechanism of Action Hydrolyzes asparagine to aspartic acid and ammonia depleting the exogenous asparagine supply needed by leukemic cells for protein synthesis

Pharmacokinetics

Absorption: Not absorbed from the GI tract; therefore, requires parenteral administration

Distribution: Apparent V_d: Plasma volume

Half-life: 5.8 days; 3.24 ± 1.83 days in patients who previously had a hypersensitivity reaction to asparaginase

Elimination: Clearance is unaffected by age, renal function, or hepatic function; not detected in urine

Usual Dosage Refer to individual protocols; I.M., I.V. (I.M. administration is preferred over I.V. due to lower incidence of adverse effects):

Children:

- BSA <0.6 m^2: 82.5 units/kg/dose every 14 days
- BSA ≥0.6 m^2: 2500 units/m^2/dose every 14 days

Adults: 2500 units/m^2/dose every 14 days

Administration

I.M.: Preferred route of administration due to the lower incidence of hepatotoxicity, coagulopathy, and GI and renal disorders compared to the I.V. route; for I.M. administration, limit the volume at a single injection site to 2 mL; if the volume to be administered is >2 mL, use multiple injection sites

I.V.: Administer dose as an I.V. infusion in 100 mL of D_5W or NS over a period of 1-2 hours

Monitoring Parameters Vital signs during administration, CBC with differential, platelet count, urinalysis, serum amylase, liver enzymes, bilirubin, prothrombin time, renal function tests, urine glucose, blood glucose, uric acid, fibrinogen levels

Patient Information Notify physician if fever, sore throat, severe abdominal pain, excessive thirst, painful/burning urination, increase in frequency of urination, severe headache, bruising, bleeding, chest tightness, rash, swelling, or shortness of breath occurs

Nursing Implications Patients should be observed for 1 hour following injection; appropriate agents for maintenance of an adequate airway and treatment of a hypersensitivity reaction (antihistamine, epinephrine, oxygen, I.V. corticosteroids) should be readily available

Dosage Forms Excipient information presented when available (limited, particularly for generics); consult specific product labeling.

Injection, solution [preservative free]:

Oncaspar®: 750 units/mL (5 mL)

(Continued)

Pegaspargase *(Continued)*

References

Asselin BL, Whitin JC, Cappola DJ, et al, "Comparative Pharmacokinetic Studies of Three Asparaginase Preparations," *J Clin Oncol*, 1993, 11(9):1780-6.

Avramis VI and Panosyan EH, "Pharmacokinetic/Pharmacodynamic Relationships of Asparaginase Formulations: The Past, the Present and Recommendations for the Future," *Clin Pharmacokinet*, 2005, 44(4):367-93.

Capizzi RL, "Asparaginase Revisited," *Leuk Lymphoma*, 1993, 10(Suppl):147-50.

Jarrar M, Gaynon PS, Periclou AP, et al, "Asparagine Depletion After Pegylated *E. coli* Asparaginase Treatment and Induction Outcome in Children With Acute Lymphoblastic Leukemia in First Bone Marrow Relapse: A Children's Oncology Group Study (CCG-1941)," *Pediatr Blood Cancer*, 2006, 47(2):141-6.

♦ **PegLyte® (Can)** *see* Polyethylene Glycol-Electrolyte Solution *on page 1277*

Pemirolast (pe MIR oh last)

U.S. Brand Names Alamast®

Canadian Brand Names Alamast®

Therapeutic Category Antiallergic, Ophthalmic; Ophthalmic Agent, Miscellaneous

Generic Available No

Use Prevention of itching of the eye due to allergic conjunctivitis

Pregnancy Risk Factor C

Lactation Excretion in breast milk unknown/use caution

Contraindications Hypersensitivity to pemirolast or any component

Warnings Not for treatment of contact lens related irritation; the preservative in pemirolast, lauralkonium chloride, may be absorbed by soft contact lenses; wait at least 10 minutes after administration before inserting soft contact lenses.

Adverse Reactions

Central nervous system: Headache, fever

Ocular: Burning, dry eyes, ocular discomfort, foreign body sensation

Respiratory: Rhinitis, bronchitis, cough, sinusitis, nasal congestion

Miscellaneous: Hypersensitivity reactions; cold/flu-like symptoms

Drug Interactions None identified

Stability Store at controlled room temperature

Mechanism of Action Pemirolast is a mast cell stabilizer that inhibits immediate hypersensitivity reactions by preventing the release of antigen-induced inflammatory mediators (eg, histamine, leukotriene C_4, D_4, E_4). It also inhibits the chemotaxis of eosinophils into ocular tissue and blocks the release of mediators from eosinophils.

Pharmacodynamics

Onset of action: A few days

Maximum effect: Up to 4 weeks

Pharmacokinetics

Half-life: Adults: 4.5 ± 0.2 hours

Excretion: 10% to 15% excreted unchanged in the urine

Usual Dosage Ophthalmic: Children >3 years and Adults: 1-2 drops into affected eye(s) four times daily

Administration Ophthalmic: Apply finger pressure to lacrimal duct during and for 1-2 minutes after instillation to decrease risk of systemic effects; avoid contact of bottle tip with skin or eye; the preservative in pemirolast, lauralkonium chloride, may be absorbed by soft contact lenses; wait at least 10 minutes after administration before inserting soft contact lenses.

Monitoring Parameters Local symptomatology

Patient Information May cause dry eyes

Dosage Forms Excipient information presented when available (limited, particularly for generics); consult specific product labeling.

Solution, ophthalmic, as potassium: 0.1% (10 mL) [contains lauralkonium chloride]

Penciclovir (pen SYE kloe veer)

Medication Safety Issues

Sound-alike/look-alike issues:

Denavir® may be confused with indinavir

U.S. Brand Names Denavir®

Index Terms PCV

Therapeutic Category Antiviral Agent, Topical

Generic Available No

Use Topical treatment of recurrent herpes labialis (cold sores, fever blisters)

Pregnancy Risk Factor B

Lactation Excretion in breast milk unknown

Contraindications Hypersensitivity to penciclovir or any component; previous or significant adverse reactions to famciclovir

Precautions No data available on safety and efficacy of penciclovir application to mucous membranes. Efficacy has not been established in immunocompromised patients or children <18 years of age.

Adverse Reactions

Central nervous system: Headache

Dermatologic: Erythematous rash

Local: Local anesthesia, application site reaction

Stability Store at room temperature; do not freeze

Mechanism of Action In cells infected with HSV-1 or HSV-2, viral thymidine kinase phosphorylates penciclovir to a monophosphate form which is converted to penciclovir triphosphate by cellular kinases. Penciclovir triphosphate inhibits HSV polymerase by competing with deoxyguanosine triphosphate inhibiting viral DNA synthesis and replication.

Pharmacodynamics Resolution of pain and cutaneous healing: 3.5-4.8 days

Pharmacokinetics Absorption: Topical: Negligible

Usual Dosage Topical: Adolescents and Adults: Apply every 2 hours during waking hours for 4 days

Administration Topical: Apply only to herpes labialis on the lips and face. Apply sufficient amount to cover lesions and gently rub into the affected area. Avoid application in or near eyes since it may cause irritation.

Monitoring Parameters Resolution of pain and healing of cold sore lesion

Patient Information Start treatment at the first sign or symptom of cold sore; report if you experience significant burning, itching, stinging, or redness when applying this medication

Additional Information Penciclovir is the active metabolite of the prodrug famciclovir.

Dosage Forms Excipient information presented when available (limited, particularly for generics); consult specific product labeling.

Cream: 1% (1.5 g)

References

Dekker CL and Prober CG, "Pediatric Uses of Valacyclovir, Penciclovir and Famciclovir," *Pediatr Infect Dis J*, 2001, 20(11):1079-81.

♦ **Pendo-5 ASA (Can)** *see* Mesalamine *on page 1011*

Penicillamine (pen i SIL a meen)

Medication Safety Issues

Sound-alike/look-alike issues:

Penicillamine may be confused with penicillin

Depen® may be confused with Endal®

International issues:

Depen® may be confused with Depon® which is a brand name for acetaminophen in Greece

Depen® may be confused with Dipen® which is a brand name for diltiazem in Greece

Pemine® [Italy] may be confused with Pamine® which is a brand name for methscopolamine in the U.S.

Related Information

Commonly Used Antidotes for Acute Overdoses *on page 1920*

Overdose and Toxicology *on page 1916*

U.S. Brand Names Cuprimine®; Depen®

Canadian Brand Names Cuprimine®; Depen®

Index Terms β,β-Dimethylcysteine; D-3-Mercaptovaline; D-Penicillamine

Therapeutic Category Antidote, Copper Toxicity; Antidote, Lead Toxicity; Chelating Agent, Oral

Generic Available No

Use Treatment of Wilson's disease, cystinuria, adjunct in the treatment of severe rheumatoid arthritis; lead poisoning, primary biliary cirrhosis (as adjunctive therapy following initial treatment with calcium EDTA or BAL)

Pregnancy Risk Factor D

Lactation Excretion in breast milk unknown/contraindicated

Contraindications Hypersensitivity to penicillamine, any component, and possibly penicillin (although this is rare due to synthetic production of penicillamine); rheumatoid arthritic patients with renal insufficiency; patients with previous penicillamine-related aplastic anemia or agranulocytosis; concomitant administration with other hematopoietic-depressant drugs (eg, gold, immunosuppressants, antimalarials,

(Continued)

Penicillamine *(Continued)*

phenylbutazone), pregnancy (except for the treatment of Wilson's disease or certain cases of cystinuria), breast-feeding

Warnings Penicillamine has been associated with fatalities due to agranulocytosis, aplastic anemia, thrombocytopenia, Goodpasture's syndrome, and myasthenia gravis; discontinue therapy if WBC <3500/mm^3; temporarily discontinue treatment if the platelet count <100,000/mm^3; patients should be warned to promptly report any symptoms suggesting toxicity; due to the potential severity of these effects, patients should be monitored closely (see Monitoring Parameters). Proteinuria and/or hematuria may develop and are early warning signs of membraneous glomerulopathy which can progress to nephrotic syndrome; these symptoms may disappear with continued therapy; close observation is warranted; follow 24 hour urine protein excretion rates; excretion of >1 g protein in urine per 24 hours or proteinuria which is progressively increasing requires decreasing the dosage or discontinuation in patients treated for rheumatoid arthritis; in Wilson's disease and cystinuria, the risks versus benefits of continuing must be considered.

Drug fever, sometimes accompanied with a skin eruption, necessitates temporary discontinuation of penicillamine in Wilson's disease and cystinuria patients and discontinuation in rheumatoid arthritic patients. Treatment may be resumed with a small dose and gradually increased to the desired dose once the symptoms have subsided. Early rashes (first few months) associated with penicillamine usually disappear within days after discontinuation of therapy and seldom return when treatment is restarted at a lower dose; late rashes (>6 months of treatment) require discontinuation of therapy.

Interruption of continuous therapy for Wilson's disease or cystinuria even for a few days has been associated with sensitivity reactions upon reinstitution of therapy; approximately 33% of patients will experience an allergic reaction. When used for cystinuria, renal stones may develop; an annual x-ray for renal stones is recommended

Precautions Patients on penicillamine for Wilson's disease or cystinuria should receive pyridoxine supplementation 25-50 mg/day; when treating rheumatoid arthritis, daily pyridoxine supplementation is also recommended. A positive ANA for lupus erythematosus may occur possibly progressing to a lupus-like syndrome.

Adverse Reactions

Cardiovascular: Edema of the face, feet, or lower legs

Central nervous system: Fever, chills, myasthenic syndrome, fatigue

Dermatologic: Rash, pruritus, pemphigus, increased friability of the skin, (dose-related) exfoliative dermatitis, alopecia, angioedema

Endocrine & metabolic: Iron deficiency, hypoglycemia, thyroiditis, weight gain

Gastrointestinal: Oral ulcerations, (dose-related) nausea, vomiting (in children with doses >60 mg/kg/day), epigastric pain, colitis, dysgeusia, ageusia, pancreatitis, sore throat, cheilosis (rare), glossitis, gingivostomatitis

Genitourinary: Urinary incontinence, bloody or cloudy urine

Hematologic: Leukopenia (5%), thrombocytopenia (5%), eosinophilia, aplastic anemia, agranulocytosis, hemolytic anemia

Hepatic: Hepatic cholestasis, hepatitis

Neuromuscular & skeletal: Arthralgia, dermatomyositis, polymyositis, peripheral neuropathy, myasthenia syndrome

Ocular: Optic neuritis

Otic: Tinnitus

Renal: Nephrotic syndrome, renal vasculitis, Goodpasture's syndrome, proteinuria, hematuria

Respiratory: Obliterative bronchiolitis, pulmonary fibrosis, interstitial pneumonitis, coughing, wheezing

Miscellaneous: Lymphadenopathy, allergic reactions, SLE-like syndrome, white spots on lips or mouth

Drug Interactions Gold, antimalarials, immunosuppressants, phenylbutazone are associated with similar serious hematologic reactions; iron salts, zinc salts, and antacids decrease penicillamine absorption (separate administration times by at least 2 hours); decreases serum digoxin levels; increases pyridoxine requirements

Food Interactions Do not administer with milk or food; iron and zinc may decrease drug action; increase dietary intake of pyridoxine; for Wilson's disease, decrease copper in diet and omit chocolate, nuts, shellfish, mushrooms, liver, raisins, broccoli, and molasses; for lead poisoning, decrease calcium in diet

Mechanism of Action Chelates with lead, copper, mercury, iron, and other heavy metals to form stable, soluble complexes that are excreted in the urine; depresses circulating IgM rheumatoid factor levels and *in vitro*, depresses T-cell but not B-cell activity; combines with cystine to form a more soluble compound which prevents the formation of cystine calculi

Pharmacodynamics Onset of action:

Rheumatoid arthritis: 2-3 months

Wilson's disease: 1-3 months

Pharmacokinetics

Absorption: 40% to 70%

Protein binding: 80%

Metabolism: In the liver

Half-life: 1.7-3.2 hours

Time to peak serum concentration: Within 1-3 hours

Elimination: Primarily (30% to 60%) in urine as unchanged drug

Usual Dosage Oral:

Rheumatoid arthritis: **Note:** The optimal duration of therapy has not been determined; in patients experiencing a remission for ≥6 months, the daily dosage may be decreased in a stepwise fashion in 3-month intervals:

Children: Initial: 3 mg/kg/day (≤250 mg/day) for 3 months, then 6 mg/kg/day (≤500 mg/day) in 2 divided doses for 3 months to a maximum of 10 mg/kg/day (≤1-1.5 g/day) in 3-4 divided doses

Adults: 125-250 mg/day, may increase dose by 125-250 mg/day; if therapy still ineffective after 2-3 months of treatment and no signs of adverse effects, increases of 250 mg/day at 2-3 month intervals up to a maximum daily dose of 1.5 g may be done; doses >500 mg/day should be given in divided doses

Wilson's disease (doses titrated to maintain urinary copper excretion >2 mg/day):

Infants and Children: 20 mg/kg/day in 2-4 doses; maximum dose: 1 g/day

Adults: 1 g/day in 4 divided doses; maximum dose: 2 g/day; in pregnant patients, limit daily dose to 1 g; if a cesarean section is planned, limit daily dose to 250 mg during the last 6 weeks before delivery and postoperatively until the wound has healed

Cystinuria (doses titrated to maintain urinary cystine excretion at <100-200 mg/day in patients without a history of stones and <100 mg/day in patients who have had stone formation and/or pain):

Children: 30 mg/kg/day in 4 divided doses; maximum dose: 4 g/day

Adults: Initial: 2 g/day divided every 6 hours (range: 1-4 g/day)

Lead poisoning (treatment duration varies from 4-12 weeks depending upon the pretreatment blood lead level; goal of therapy is to reduce the total body content so that the blood lead level does not rebound to unacceptable levels post-treatment):

Children: 20-30 mg/kg/day in 3-4 divided doses; initiating treatment at 25% of this dose and gradually increasing to the full dose over 2-3 weeks may minimize adverse reactions; maximum dose: 1.5 g/day; a reduced dosage of 15 mg/kg/day in 2 divided doses has been shown to be effective in the treatment of mild to moderate lead poisoning (blood lead concentration 20-40 mcg/dL) with a reduction in adverse effects (Shannon, 2000)

Adults: 1-1.5 g/day in 3-4 divided doses; initiating treatment at 25% of this dose and gradually increasing to the full dose over 2-3 weeks may minimize adverse reactions

Primary biliary cirrhosis: Adults: 250 mg/day to start, increase by 250 mg every 2 weeks up to a maintenance dose of 1 g/day, as 250 mg 4 times/day

Arsenic poisoning: Children: 100 mg/kg/day divided every 6 hours for 5 days; not to exceed 1 g/day

Dosing adjustment in renal impairment: Cl_{cr} <50 mL/minute: Avoid use

Administration Oral: Administer on an empty stomach 1 hour before or 2 hours after meals, milk, or other medications; patients unable to swallow capsules may mix contents of capsule with fruit juice or chilled pureed fruit; patients with cystinuria should drink copious amounts of water

Monitoring Parameters Urinalysis, CBC with differential, hemoglobin, and platelet count are recommended twice weekly for the first month then every 2 weeks for 6 months and monthly thereafter; in addition, monitor the patient's skin, lymph nodes, and body temperature; liver function tests are recommended every 6 months; weekly measurements of urinary and blood concentrations of the intoxicating metal are indicated; quantitative 24-hour urine protein at 1- to 2-week intervals initially (first 2-3 months); annual x-ray for renal stones (when used for cystinuria); Wilson's disease: 24-hour urinary copper excretion

Reference Range Wilson's disease: Adequate treatment: "Free" (unbound) serum copper <10 mcg/dL (Free serum copper = Total copper - ceruloplasmin copper)

Patient Information Possible severe allergic reaction if patient allergic to penicillin; notify physician if unusual bleeding or bruising, or persistent fever, sore throat, or fatigue occur. Report any unexplained cough, shortness of breath, or rash; loss of taste may occur; do not skip or miss doses or discontinue without notifying physician; cystinuric patients should drink copious amounts of fluid particularly before bed and once during the night

Dosage Forms Excipient information presented when available (limited, particularly for generics); consult specific product labeling. [DSC] = Discontinued product

(Continued)

Penicillamine *(Continued)*

Capsule (Cuprimine®): 125 mg [DSC], 250 mg
Tablet (Depen®): 250 mg

Extemporaneous Preparations A 50 mg/mL suspension may be made by mixing sixty 250 mg capsules with 3 g carboxymethylcellulose, 150 g sucrose, 300 mg citric acid, parabens (methylparaben 120 mg, propylparaben 12 mg, propylene glycol qsad to 100 mL), and purified water to a total volume of 300 mL; cherry flavor may be added. Stability is 30 days refrigerated.

DeCastro FJ, Jaeger RQ, and Rolfe UT, "An Extemporaneously Prepared Penicillamine Suspension Used to Treat Lead Intoxication," *Hosp Pharm*, 1977, 2:446-8.

References

Piomelli S, "Childhood Lead Poisoning," *Pediatr Clin North Am*, 2002, 49(6):1285-304.
Shannon MW and Townsend MK, "Adverse Effects of Reduced-Dose d-Penicillamine in Children With Mild-to-Moderate Lead Poisoning," *Ann Pharmacother*, 2000, 34(1):15-8.
"Treatment Guidelines for Lead Exposure in Children. American Academy of Pediatrics Committee on Drugs," *Pediatrics*, 1995, 96(1 Pt 1):155-60.

Penicillin G Benzathine (pen i SIL in jee BENZ a theen)

Medication Safety Issues

Sound-alike/look-alike issues:

Penicillin may be confused with penicillamine
Bicillin® may be confused with Wycillin®
Bicillin® C-R (penicillin G benzathine and penicillin G procaine) may be confused with Bicillin® L-A (penicillin G benzathine). Penicillin G benzathine is the only product currently approved for the treatment of syphilis. Administration of penicillin G benzathine and penicillin G procaine combination instead of Bicillin® L-A may result in inadequate treatment response.

Penicillin G benzathine may only be administered by deep intramuscular injection; intravenous administration of penicillin G benzathine has been associated with cardiopulmonary arrest and death.

U.S. Brand Names Bicillin® L-A

Canadian Brand Names Bicillin® L-A

Index Terms Benzathine Benzylpenicillin; Benzathine Penicillin G; Benzylpenicillin Benzathine

Therapeutic Category Antibiotic, Penicillin

Generic Available No

Use Active against most gram-positive organisms and some spirochetes; treatment of syphilis; used only for the treatment of mild to moderately severe infections (ie, *Streptococcus* pharyngitis) caused by organisms susceptible to low concentrations of penicillin G, or for prophylaxis of infections caused by these organisms such as rheumatic fever prophylaxis

Pregnancy Risk Factor B

Lactation Enters breast milk/compatible

Contraindications Hypersensitivity to penicillin or any component

Precautions Use with caution in patients with impaired renal function, impaired cardiac function, pre-existing seizure disorder, or hypersensitivity to cephalosporins

Adverse Reactions

Central nervous system: Convulsions, confusion, lethargy, fever, dizziness
Dermatologic: Rash
Hematologic: Hemolytic anemia
Local: Pain at injection site
Neuromuscular & skeletal: Myoclonus
Renal: Interstitial nephritis
Miscellaneous: Jarisch-Herxheimer reaction, hypersensitivity reactions, anaphylaxis

Drug Interactions Probenecid increases serum concentration of penicillin; antibacterial activity with aminoglycosides is synergistic; tetracyclines, chloramphenicol, and erythromycin may antagonize the activity of penicillin

Stability Store in the refrigerator; avoid freezing

Mechanism of Action Inhibits bacterial cell wall synthesis by binding to one or more of the penicillin-binding proteins; inhibits the final transpeptidation step of peptidoglycan synthesis in bacterial cell wall

Pharmacokinetics

Absorption: I.M.: Slow
Distribution: Minimal concentrations attained in CSF with inflamed or uninflamed meninges
Time to peak serum concentration: Within 12-24 hours; serum levels are usually detectable for 1-4 weeks depending on the dose; larger doses result in more sustained levels rather than higher levels

Elimination: Penicillin G is detected in urine for up to 12 weeks after a single I.M. injection; renal clearance is delayed in neonates, young infants, and patients with impaired renal function

Usual Dosage I.M. (dosage frequency depends on infection being treated):

Neonates >1200 g: Asymptomatic congenital syphilis: 50,000 units/kg for 1 dose

Infants and Children:

- Group A streptococcal upper respiratory infection: 25,000-50,000 units/kg as a single dose; maximum dose: 1.2 million units/dose **or**
  - Children <27 kg: 300,000-600,000 units as a single dose
  - Children ≥27 kg: 900,000 units as a single dose
- Prophylaxis of recurrent rheumatic fever: 25,000-50,000 units/kg every 3-4 weeks; maximum dose: 1.2 million units/dose
- Congenital syphilis: 50,000 units/kg every week for 3 weeks; maximum dose: 2.4 million units/dose
- Syphilis of more than 1-year duration: 50,000 units/kg every week for 3 successive weeks; maximum dose: 2.4 million units/dose

Adults:

- Group A streptococcal upper respiratory infection: 1.2 million units as a single dose
- Prophylaxis of recurrent rheumatic fever: 1.2 million units every 3-4 weeks or 600,000 units twice monthly
- Early syphilis: 2.4 million units as a single dose in 2 injection sites
- Syphilis of more than 1-year duration: 2.4 million units (in 2 injection sites) once weekly for 3 doses

Administration Parenteral: I.M.: Give undiluted injection; administer by deep I.M. injection in the upper outer quadrant of the buttock (adolescents and adults) or into the midlateral muscle of the thigh (infants and children); do **not** give I.V., intra-arterially or SubQ; **inadvertent I.V. administration has resulted in thrombosis, severe neurovascular damage, cardiac arrest, and death**

Monitoring Parameters CBC, urinalysis, renal function tests

Test Interactions Positive Coombs' [direct], false-positive urinary and/or serum proteins

Nursing Implications SubQ administration may cause pain and induration; avoid repeated I.M. injections into the anterolateral thigh in neonates and infants since quadriceps femoris fibrosis and atrophy may occur

Additional Information Use a penicillin G benzathine/penicillin G procaine combination (ie, Bicillin® C-R) to achieve early peak levels in acute infections. Do not administer Bicillin® C-R to treat patients infected with syphilis since this may result in inadequate treatment.

Dosage Forms Excipient information presented when available (limited, particularly for generics); consult specific product labeling.

Injection, suspension [prefilled syringe]: 600,000 units/mL (1 mL, 2 mL, 4 mL)

References

Kaplan EL, Berrios X, Speth J, et al, "Pharmacokinetics of Benzathine Penicillin G: Serum Levels During the 28 Days After Intramuscular Injection of 1,200,000 Units," *J Pediatr*, 1989, 115(1):146-50.

Paryani SG, Vaughn AJ, Crosby M, et al, "Treatment of Asymptomatic Congenital Syphilis: Benzathine Versus Procaine Penicillin G Therapy," *J Pediatr*, 1994, 125(3):471-5.

WHO Study Group, "Rheumatic Fever and Rheumatic Heart Disease," *World Health Organ Tech Rep Ser*, 1988, 764:1-58.

Penicillin G (Parenteral/Aqueous)

(pen i SIL in jee, pa REN ter al, AYE kwee us)

Medication Safety Issues

Sound-alike/look-alike issues:

Penicillin may be confused with penicillamine

U.S. Brand Names Pfizerpen®

Canadian Brand Names Pfizerpen®

Index Terms Benzylpenicillin Potassium; Benzylpenicillin Sodium; Crystalline Penicillin; Penicillin G Potassium; Penicillin G Sodium

Therapeutic Category Antibiotic, Penicillin

Generic Available Yes

Use Treatment of sepsis, meningitis, pericarditis, endocarditis, pneumonia, and other infections due to susceptible gram-positive organisms (except *Staphylococcus aureus*), some gram-negative organisms such as *Neisseria gonorrhoeae*, or *N. meningitidis* and some anaerobes and spirochetes

Pregnancy Risk Factor B

Lactation Enters breast milk/compatible

Contraindications Hypersensitivity to penicillin or any component

Precautions Use with caution in patients with renal impairment, hypersensitivity to cephalosporins, or pre-existing seizure disorder; dosage modification required in

(Continued)

Penicillin G (Parenteral/Aqueous) *(Continued)*

patients with renal impairment; further dosage reduction recommended in patients with impaired hepatic and renal function

Adverse Reactions

Central nervous system: Convulsions, confusion, lethargy, fever, dizziness
Dermatologic: Rash, urticaria
Endocrine & metabolic: Electrolyte imbalance
Gastrointestinal: Diarrhea
Hematologic: Hemolytic anemia, neutropenia
Local: Thrombophlebitis
Neuromuscular & skeletal: Myoclonus
Renal: Acute interstitial nephritis
Miscellaneous: Jarisch-Herxheimer reaction, hypersensitivity reactions, anaphylaxis

Drug Interactions Probenecid increases serum concentration of penicillin; antibacterial activity with aminoglycosides is synergistic; tetracyclines, chloramphenicol, and erythromycin may antagonize the activity of penicillin

Food Interactions Food or milk decreases absorption

Stability Reconstituted parenteral solution is stable for 7 days when refrigerated; incompatible with aminoglycosides; inactivated in acidic or alkaline solutions

Mechanism of Action Inhibits bacterial cell wall synthesis by binding to one or more of the penicillin-binding proteins; inhibits the final transpeptidation step of peptidoglycan synthesis in bacterial cell wall

Pharmacokinetics

Absorption: Oral: <30%
Distribution: Penetration across the blood-brain barrier is poor with uninflamed meninges; crosses the placenta; appears in breast milk
Protein binding: 65%
Metabolism: In the liver (10% to 30%) to penicilloic acid
Half-life:
- Neonates:
  - <6 days: 3.2-3.4 hours
  - 7-13 days: 1.2-2.2 hours
  - >14 days: 0.9-1.9 hours
- Infants and Children: 0.5-1.2 hours
- Adults: 0.5-0.75 hours with normal renal function

Time to peak serum concentration:
- Oral: Within 30-60 minutes
- I.M.: Within 30 minutes

Elimination: Penicillin G and its metabolites are excreted in urine mainly by tubular secretion
Dialysis: Moderately dialyzable (20% to 50%)

Usual Dosage

Neonates: I.M., I.V.:
- Postnatal age ≤7 days:
  - ≤2000 g: 50,000 units/kg/day in divided doses every 12 hours
    - Meningitis: 100,000 units/kg/day in divided doses every 12 hours
  - >2000 g: 75,000 units/kg/day in divided doses every 8 hours
    - Meningitis: 150,000 units/kg/day in divided doses every 8 hours
  - Congenital syphilis: 100,000 units/kg/day in divided doses every 12 hours
  - Group B streptococcal meningitis: 250,000-450,000 units/kg/day in divided doses every 8 hours
- Postnatal age >7 days:
  - <1200 g: 50,000 units/kg/day in divided doses every 12 hours
    - Meningitis: 100,000 units/kg/day in divided doses every 12 hours
  - 1200-2000 g: 75,000 units/kg/day in divided doses every 8 hours
    - Meningitis: 150,000 units/kg/day in divided doses every 8 hours
  - >2000 g: 100,000 units/kg/day in divided doses every 6 hours
    - Meningitis: 200,000 units/kg/day in divided doses every 6 hours
  - Congenital syphilis: 150,000 units/kg/day in divided doses every 8 hours
  - Group B streptococcal meningitis: I.V.: 450,000 units/kg/day in divided doses every 6 hours

Infants and Children:
- I.M., I.V.: 100,000 to 250,000 units/kg/day in divided doses every 4-6 hours
- Severe infections: 250,000-400,000 units/kg/day in divided doses every 4-6 hours; maximum dose: 24 million units/day

Adults: I.M., I.V.: 2-24 million units/day in divided doses every 4-6 hours

Dosing interval in renal impairment:
- Cl_{cr} 10-30 mL/minute: Administer normal dose every 8-12 hours
- Cl_{cr} <10 mL/minute: Administer normal dose every 12-18 hours

Administration Parenteral: Administer by I.V. intermittent infusion over 15-60 minutes at a final concentration for administration of 100,000-500,000 units/mL. A final concentration of 50,000 units/mL infused over 15-30 minutes is recommended for neonates and infants. The potassium or sodium content of the dose should be considered when determining the infusion rate.

Monitoring Parameters Periodic serum electrolytes, renal and hematologic function tests

Test Interactions False-positive or negative urinary glucose determination using Clinitest®; positive Coombs' [direct]; false-positive urinary and/or serum proteins

Additional Information

Penicillin G potassium: 1.7 mEq of potassium and 0.3 mEq of sodium per 1 million units of penicillin G

Penicillin G sodium: 2 mEq of sodium per 1 million units of penicillin G

Dosage Forms Excipient information presented when available (limited, particularly for generics); consult specific product labeling.

Infusion, as potassium [premixed iso-osmotic dextrose solution, frozen]: 1 million units (50 mL), 2 million units (50 mL), 3 million units (50 mL) [contains sodium 1.02 mEq and potassium 1.7 mEq per 1 million units]

Injection, powder for reconstitution, as potassium (Pfizerpen®): 5 million units, 20 million units [contains sodium 6.8 mg (0.3 mEq) and potassium 65.6 mg (1.68 mEq) per 1 million units]

Injection, powder for reconstitution, as sodium: 5 million units [contains sodium 1.68 mEq per 1 million units]

References

American Academy of Pediatrics Committee on Infectious Diseases, "Treatment of Bacterial Meningitis," *Pediatrics*, 1988, 81(6):904-7.

Prober CG, Stevenson DK, and Benitz WE, "The Use of Antibiotics in Neonates Weighing Less Than 1200 Grams," *Pediatr Infect Dis J*, 1990, 9(2):111-21.

♦ **Penicillin G Potassium** *see* Penicillin G (Parenteral/Aqueous) *on page 1231*

Penicillin G Procaine (pen i SIL in jee PROE kane)

Medication Safety Issues

Sound-alike/look-alike issues:

Penicillin G procaine may be confused with penicillin V potassium

Wycillin® may be confused with Bicillin®

Canadian Brand Names Pfizerpen-AS®; Wycillin®

Index Terms APPG; Aqueous Procaine Penicillin G; Procaine Benzylpenicillin; Procaine Penicillin G; Wycillin [DSC]

Therapeutic Category Antibiotic, Penicillin

Generic Available Yes

Use Moderately severe infections due to *Treponema pallidum* and other penicillin G-sensitive microorganisms that are susceptible to low but prolonged serum penicillin concentrations

Pregnancy Risk Factor B

Lactation Enters breast milk/compatible

Contraindications Hypersensitivity to penicillin, procaine, or any component (see Warnings)

Warnings Some formulations contain sulfites which may cause allergic reactions in susceptible individuals

Precautions Use with caution in patients with renal impairment, hypersensitivity to cephalosporins, or history of seizures; modify dosage in patients with severe renal impairment

Adverse Reactions

Cardiovascular: Myocardial depression, vasodilation, conduction disturbances

Central nervous system: Seizures, confusion, lethargy, dizziness, disorientation, agitation, hallucinations

Hematologic: Hemolytic anemia

Local: Sterile abscess and pain at injection site

Neuromuscular & skeletal: Myoclonus

Renal: Interstitial nephritis

Miscellaneous: Pseudoanaphylactic reactions, Jarisch-Herxheimer reaction, hypersensitivity reactions

Drug Interactions Probenecid increases serum concentration of penicillin; antibacterial activity with aminoglycosides is synergistic; tetracyclines, chloramphenicol, and erythromycin may antagonize the activity of penicillin

Stability Store in refrigerator

Mechanism of Action Inhibits bacterial cell wall synthesis by binding to one or more of the penicillin-binding proteins; inhibits the final transpeptidation step of peptidoglycan synthesis in bacterial cell wall

(Continued)

Penicillin G Procaine *(Continued)*

Pharmacokinetics

Absorption: I.M.: Slow

Distribution: Penetration across the blood-brain barrier is poor, despite inflamed meninges; appears in breast milk

Time to peak serum concentration: Within 1-4 hours and can persist within the therapeutic range for 15-24 hours

Elimination: Renal clearance is delayed in neonates, young infants, and patients with impaired renal function

Dialysis: Moderately dialyzable (20% to 50%)

Usual Dosage I.M.:

Neonates ≥1200 g: Avoid using in this age group since sterile abscesses and procaine toxicity occur more frequently with neonates than older patients

Congenital syphilis: 50,000 units/kg/day once daily for 10 days; if more than 1 day of therapy is missed, the entire course should be restarted

Infants and Children: 25,000-50,000 units/kg/day in divided doses every 12-24 hours; not to exceed 4.8 million units/24 hours

Congenital syphilis: 50,000 units/kg/day once daily for 10 days; if more than 1 day of therapy is missed, the entire course should be restarted

Adults: 0.6-4.8 million units/day in divided doses every 12-24 hours

When used in conjunction with an aminoglycoside for the treatment of endocarditis caused by susceptible *S. viridans*: 1.2 million units every 6 hours for 2-4 weeks

Neurosyphilis: 2.4 million units once daily for 10 days with probenecid 500 mg every 6 hours

Administration Parenteral: **Do not give I.V., intra-arterially, or SubQ**; procaine suspension for deep I.M. injection only; inadvertent I.V. administration has resulted in neurovascular damage; in infants and children it is preferable to administer I.M. into the midlateral muscles of the thigh; in adults, administer into the gluteus maximus or into the midlateral muscles of the thigh

Monitoring Parameters Periodic renal and hematologic function tests with prolonged therapy

Test Interactions Positive Coombs' [direct], false-positive urinary and/or serum proteins

Nursing Implications Avoid repeated I.M. injections into the anterolateral thigh in neonates and infants since quadriceps femoris fibrosis and atrophy may occur

Dosage Forms Excipient information presented when available (limited, particularly for generics); consult specific product labeling.

Injection, suspension: 600,000 units/mL (1 mL, 2 mL)

References

Paryani SG, Vaughn AJ, Crosby M, et al, "Treatment of Asymptomatic Congenital Syphilis: Benzathine Versus Procaine Penicillin G Therapy," *J Pediatr*, 1994, 125(3):471-5.

♦ **Penicillin G Sodium** *see* Penicillin G (Parenteral/Aqueous) *on page 1231*

Penicillin V Potassium (pen i SIL in vee poe TASS ee um)

Medication Safety Issues

Sound-alike/look-alike issues:

Penicillin V procaine may be confused with penicillin G potassium

Canadian Brand Names Apo-Pen VK®; Novo-Pen-VK; Nu-Pen-VK

Index Terms Pen VK; Phenoxymethyl Penicillin

Therapeutic Category Antibiotic, Penicillin

Generic Available Yes

Use Treatment of mild to moderately severe susceptible bacterial infections involving the upper respiratory tract, skin, and urinary tract; prophylaxis of pneumococcal infections and rheumatic fever

Pregnancy Risk Factor B

Lactation Enters breast milk (other penicillins are compatible with breast-feeding)

Contraindications Hypersensitivity to penicillin or any component

Warnings Oral solution contains sodium benzoate; benzoic acid (benzoate) is a metabolite of benzyl alcohol; large amounts of benzyl alcohol (≥99 mg/kg/day) have been associated with a potentially fatal toxicity ("gasping syndrome") in neonates; the "gasping syndrome" consists of metabolic acidosis, respiratory distress, gasping respirations, CNS dysfunction (including convulsions, intracranial hemorrhage), hypotension and cardiovascular collapse; use oral solution containing sodium benzoate with caution in neonates; *in vitro* and animal studies have shown that benzoate displaces bilirubin from protein binding sites

Precautions Use with caution in patients with renal impairment, hypersensitivity to cephalosporins, or history of seizures; dosage adjustment may be necessary in patients with renal impairment; oral solution may contain aspartame which is metabolized to phenylalanine and must be avoided (or used with caution) in patients with phenylketonuria

Adverse Reactions

Central nervous system: Convulsions, fever

Dermatologic: Rash

Gastrointestinal: Nausea, diarrhea, vomiting, black hairy tongue, pseudomembranous colitis

Hematologic: Hemolytic anemia

Renal: Acute interstitial nephritis

Miscellaneous: Hypersensitivity reactions, anaphylaxis

Drug Interactions Probenecid (higher, prolonged penicillin serum concentration)

Food Interactions Food or milk may decrease absorption

Stability Refrigerate suspension after reconstitution; discard after 14 days

Mechanism of Action Interferes with bacterial cell wall synthesis during active multiplication by binding to one or more of the penicillin-binding proteins; inhibits the final transpeptidation step of peptidoglycan synthesis causing cell wall death and resultant bactericidal activity against susceptible bacteria

Pharmacokinetics

Absorption: Oral: 60% to 73% from the GI tract

Distribution: Widely distributed to kidneys, liver, skin, tonsils, and into synovial, pleural, and pericardial fluids; appears in breast milk

Protein binding: 80%

Metabolism: 10% to 30%

Half-life: 30 minutes and is prolonged in patients with renal impairment

Time to peak serum concentration: Within 30-60 minutes

Elimination: Penicillin V and its metabolites are excreted in urine mainly by tubular secretion

Usual Dosage Oral:

Systemic infections:

Children <12 years: 25-50 mg/kg/day in divided doses every 6-8 hours; maximum dose: 3 g/day

Children ≥12 years and Adults: 125-500 mg every 6-8 hours

Primary prevention of rheumatic fever (treatment of streptococcal tonsillopharyngitis):

Children: 250 mg 2-3 times/day for 10 days

Adolescents and Adults: 500 mg 2-3 times/day for 10 days

Prophylaxis of pneumococcal infections in children with sickle cell disease and functional or anatomic asplenia: Children:

Before 2 months of age or as soon as sickle cell disease or asplenia occurs to 3 years: 125 mg twice daily

>3-5 years: 250 mg twice daily; may discontinue penicillin prophylaxis after 5 years of age in children who have not experienced invasive pneumococcal infection and have received recommended pneumococcal immunizations

Recurrent rheumatic fever, prophylaxis: Children and Adults: 250 mg twice daily

Administration Oral: Administer with water on an empty stomach 1 hour before or 2 hours after meals; may be administered with food to decrease GI upset

Monitoring Parameters Periodic renal and hematologic function tests during prolonged therapy

Test Interactions False-positive or negative urinary glucose determination using Clinitest®; positive Coombs' [direct]; false-positive urinary and/or serum proteins

Additional Information 0.7 mEq of potassium/250 mg penicillin V; 250 mg = 400,000 units of penicillin

Dosage Forms Excipient information presented when available (limited, particularly for generics); consult specific product labeling.

Note: 250 mg = 400,000 units

Powder for oral solution: 125 mg/5 mL (100 mL, 200 mL); 250 mg/5 mL (100 mL, 200 mL)

Tablet: 250 mg, 500 mg

References

"American Academy of Pediatrics. Committee on Infectious Diseases. Policy Statement: Recommendations for the Prevention of Pneumococcal Infections, Including the Use of Pneumococcal Conjugate Vaccine (Prevnar™), Pneumococcal Polysaccharide Vaccine, and Antibiotic Prophylaxis," *Pediatrics*, 2000, 106(2 Pt 1):362-6.

Dajani A, Taubert K, Ferrieri P, et al, "Treatment of Acute Streptococcal Pharyngitis and Prevention of Rheumatic Fever: A Statement for Health Professionals. Committee on Rheumatic Fever, Endocarditis, and Kawasaki Disease of the Council on Cardiovascular Disease in the Young, the American Heart Association," *Pediatrics*, 1995, 96(4 Pt 1):758-64.

♦ **Penicilloyl-polylysine** *see* Benzylpenicilloyl-polylysine [DSC] *on page 210*

♦ **Pennsaid® (Can)** *see* Diclofenac *on page 486*

♦ **Pentahydrate** *see* Sodium Thiosulfate *on page 1461*

◆ **Pentam-300®** *see* Pentamidine *on page 1236*

Pentamidine (pen TAM i deen)

U.S. Brand Names NebuPent®; Pentam-300®
Index Terms Pentamidine Isethionate
Therapeutic Category Antibiotic, Miscellaneous; Antiprotozoal
Generic Available No
Use Treatment and prevention of pneumonia caused by *Pneumocystis carinii* in patients who cannot tolerate or who fail to respond to sulfamethoxazole and trimethoprim; treatment of African trypanosomiasis; treatment of visceral leishmaniasis caused by *L. donovani*
Pregnancy Risk Factor C
Lactation Excretion in breast milk unknown/contraindicated
Contraindications Hypersensitivity to pentamidine isethionate or any component (inhalation and injection); do not use concomitantly with didanosine since both drugs can cause pancreatitis
Warnings Healthcare personnel who administer aerosolized pentamidine inhalation therapy, a cough-producing procedure, should be aware of the possibility of secondary exposure to tuberculosis or other infections from patients with undiagnosed pulmonary disease
Precautions Use with caution in patients with diabetes mellitus, renal or hepatic dysfunction, hypertension or hypotension; adjust dose in renal impairment
Adverse Reactions
Cardiovascular: Hypotension, tachycardia, cardiac arrhythmias
Central nervous system: Dizziness, fever, fatigue, delirium
Dermatologic: Rash, itching
Endocrine & metabolic: Hypoglycemia, hyperglycemia, hypocalcemia, hyperkalemia
Gastrointestinal: Nausea, vomiting, metallic taste, pancreatitis
Hematologic: Megaloblastic anemia, neutropenia, leukopenia, thrombocytopenia
Hepatic: Mild hepatic injury
Local: Pain at injection site, thrombophlebitis, sterile abscess, erythema
Renal: Nephrotoxicity, elevated BUN, elevated serum creatinine
With aerosolized pentamidine: Irritation of the airway, cough, transient arterial desaturation, bronchospasm, fatigue, conjunctivitis
Miscellaneous: Jarisch-Herxheimer-like reaction
Drug Interactions Cytochrome P450 isoenzyme CYP2C19 substrate
Aminoglycosides, amphotericin B, cisplatin and vancomycin (additive nephrotoxicity); didanosine (additive toxicity)
Stability Reconstituted solution is stable for 48 hours at room temperature when protected from light; do not refrigerate due to the possibility of crystallization
Mechanism of Action Interferes with RNA/DNA, phospholipids and protein synthesis through inhibition of oxidative phosphorylation and/or interference with incorporation of nucleotides and nucleic acids into RNA and DNA, in protozoa
Pharmacokinetics
Absorption: I.M.: Well absorbed; limited systemic absorption following pentamidine inhalation therapy
Distribution: Binds to tissues and plasma protein; high concentrations are found in the liver, kidney, adrenals, spleen, lungs and pancreas; poor penetration into CNS; following oral inhalation, high concentrations are found in bronchoalveolar fluid
Half-life, terminal: 6.4-9.4 hours; half-life may be prolonged in patients with severe renal impairment
Elimination: 33% to 66% in urine as unchanged drug
Dialysis: Not appreciably removed by hemodialysis or peritoneal dialysis
Usual Dosage
Children:
Treatment of *Pneumocystis carinii* pneumonia: I.M., I.V. (I.V. preferred): 4 mg/kg/day once daily for 14-21 days
Prophylaxis for *Pneumocystis carinii* pneumonia (See **Note** in Additional Information):
I.M., I.V.: 4 mg/kg/dose every 2-4 weeks **or**
Inhalation: Every month via Respirgard® II nebulizer
Infants <1 year: Aerosolized pentamidine is administered at doses adjusted for minute ventilation and weight
Infant dose = 2.27 mg/kg x nebulizer output (L/minute) x wt (kg) divided by alveolar ventilation (L/minute)
Children <5 years: Some institutions have used a dose of 8 mg/kg
Children ≥5 years: 300 mg/dose
Treatment of trypanosomiasis: I.M.: 4 mg/kg/day once daily for 10 days

Treatment of visceral leishmaniasis: I.M.: 2-4 mg/kg/day once daily or every 2 days for up to 15 doses

Adults:

Treatment: I.M., I.V. (I.V. preferred): 4 mg/kg/day once daily for 14 days

Prevention: Inhalation: 300 mg every 4 weeks via Respirgard® II nebulizer

Dosing adjustment in renal impairment:

Cl_{cr} 10-30 mL/min: Administer normal dose once every 36 hours

Cl_{cr} <10 mL/min: Administer normal dose once every 48 hours

Administration

Oral inhalation: Safe and effective administration via nebulization in children is dependent on patients wearing an appropriately sized pediatric face mask

Parenteral: May administer deep I.M. or by slow I.V. infusion; rapid I.V. administration can cause severe hypotension; infuse I.V. slowly over a period of at least 60 minutes at a final concentration for administration not to exceed 6 mg/mL

Monitoring Parameters Liver function tests, renal function tests, blood glucose, serum potassium and calcium, CBC with differential and platelet count, EKG, blood pressure

Patient Information Maintain adequate fluid intake; notify physician if fever, cough, or shortness of breath occurs; avoid alcohol

Nursing Implications Patients should receive parenteral pentamidine while lying down and blood pressure should be monitored closely during administration and after completion of the infusion until blood pressure is stabilized; if hypotension occurs due to rapid I.V. administration, slow infusion rate to administer dose over 1-2 hours

Additional Information

Note: Guidelines for prophylaxis of *Pneumocystis carinii* pneumonia: Initiate PCP prophylaxis for the following patients: All HIV-exposed children at 4-6 weeks of age and continue through the first year of life or until HIV infection has been reasonably excluded; children 1-5 years of age with CD4+ count <500 or CD4+ percentage <15%; children 6-12 years of age with CD4+ count <200 or CD4+ percentage <15%; for children who had a CD4+ count <750 or a CD4+ percentage <15% in the first year of life, prophylaxis should be continued until 2 years of age

1 mg pentamidine: 1.74 mg pentamidine isethionate

Dosage Forms Excipient information presented when available (limited, particularly for generics); consult specific product labeling.

Injection, powder for reconstitution, as isethionate [preservative free]:

Pentam-300®: 300 mg

Powder for nebulization, as isethionate [preservative free]:

NebuPent®: 300 mg

References

Hand IL, Wiznia AA, Porricolo M, et al, "Aerosolized Pentamidine for Prophylaxis of *Pneumocystis carinii* Pneumonia in Infants With Human Immunodeficiency Virus Infection," *Pediatr Infect Dis J*, 1994, 13(2):100-4.

Hughes WT, "*Pneumocystis carinii* Pneumonia: New Approaches to Diagnosis, Treatment, and Prevention," *Pediatr Infect Dis J*, 1991, 10(5):391-9.

"1999 USPHS/IDSA Guidelines for the Prevention of Opportunistic Infections in Persons Infected With Human Immunodeficiency Virus," *MMWR Morb Mortal Wkly Rep*, 1999, 48(RR-10):1-66.

♦ **Pentamidine Isethionate** *see* Pentamidine *on page 1236*

♦ **Pentamycetin® (Can)** *see* Chloramphenicol *on page 335*

♦ **Pentasa®** *see* Mesalamine *on page 1011*

♦ **Pentavalent Human-Bovine Reassortant Rotavirus Vaccine** *see* Rotavirus Vaccine (Live/Pentavalent) *on page 1408*

Pentazocine (pen TAZ oh seen)

Related Information

Compatibility of Medications Mixed in A Syringe *on page 1941*

Narcotic Analgesics Comparison *on page 1705*

U.S. Brand Names Talwin®; Talwin® NX

Canadian Brand Names Talwin®

Index Terms Naloxone Hydrochloride and Pentazocine Hydrochloride; Pentazocine Hydrochloride; Pentazocine Hydrochloride and Naloxone Hydrochloride; Pentazocine Lactate

Therapeutic Category Analgesic, Narcotic; Opiate Partial Agonist; Sedative

Generic Available Yes: Tablet

Use Relief of moderate to severe pain; a sedative prior to surgery; supplement to surgical anesthesia

Restrictions C-IV

Pregnancy Risk Factor B (D if used for prolonged periods or in high doses at term)

Lactation Excretion in breast milk unknown/use caution

Contraindications Hypersensitivity to pentazocine or any component (see Warnings)

(Continued)

Pentazocine *(Continued)*

Warnings Pentazocine may precipitate opiate withdrawal symptoms in patients who have been receiving opiates regularly; injection may contain sodium bisulfite which may cause allergic reactions in susceptible individuals

Precautions Use with caution in seizure-prone patients, acute MI, patients undergoing biliary tract surgery, patients with renal and hepatic dysfunction, and patients with a history of prior opioid dependence or abuse; decrease dosage in patients with decreased hepatic or renal function

Adverse Reactions

Cardiovascular: Palpitations, hypotension, tachycardia, peripheral vasodilation

Central nervous system: CNS depression, drowsiness, sedation, dizziness, euphoria, headache, insomnia, chills, lightheadedness (more frequently than morphine), hallucinations, confusion, disorientation, elevated intracranial pressure; seizures may occur in seizure-prone patients especially with large I.V. doses

Dermatologic: Pruritus, rash; serious skin reactions (eg, toxic epidermal necrolysis, Stevens-Johnson syndrome, erythema multiforme)

Endocrine & metabolic: Antidiuretic hormone release

Gastrointestinal: Nausea (more frequently than morphine), vomiting, constipation, biliary tract spasm

Genitourinary: Urinary tract spasm, urinary retention

Local: Tissue damage and irritation with I.M./SubQ use

Neuromuscular & skeletal: Paresthesia, weakness

Ocular: Miosis

Respiratory: Respiratory depression, laryngospasm

Miscellaneous: Physical and psychological dependence, histamine release

Drug Interactions Cytochrome P450 isoenzyme CYP2D6 substrate

May potentiate or reduce analgesic effect of opiate agonist (ie, morphine), depending on patient's tolerance to opiates; additive effects seen with other CNS depressants; tripelennamine potentiates pentazocine effects and lethality and the two have been abused in combination (Ts and blues) I.V. to provide effects similar to heroin

Stability Store injection at room temperature; do not mix injection with barbiturates, precipitation will occur

Mechanism of Action Binds to opiate receptors in the CNS, causing inhibition of ascending pain pathways, altering the perception of and response to pain; produces generalized CNS depression

Pharmacodynamics

Onset of action:

- Oral, I.M., SubQ: Within 15-30 minutes
- I.V.: Within 2-3 minutes

Duration:

- Oral: 4-5 hours
- Parenteral: 2-3 hours

Pharmacokinetics

Protein binding: 60%

Metabolism: In the liver via oxidative and glucuronide conjugation pathways

Bioavailability: Oral: ~20% due to large first-pass effect; increased oral bioavailability to 60% to 70% in patients with cirrhosis

Half-life: Increased half-life with decreased hepatic function

- Children 4-8 years (mean ± SD): 3 ± 1.5 hours
- Adults: 2-3 hours

Elimination: Small amounts excreted unchanged in urine

Usual Dosage

Children: Limited information available

Preoperative sedation: Manufacturer recommendations:

- Infants <1 year: Safety and efficacy not established
- Children 1-16 years: I.M.: 0.5 mg/kg as a single dose
- **Note:** In 300 children (1-14 years) I.M. doses ranging from approximately 0.45-1.5 mg/kg in children <27 kg to 0.65-1.9 mg/kg in children >27 kg were used preoperatively (Rita, 1970)

Postoperative pain: I.M.: Doses of 15 mg for children 5-8 years of age and 30 mg for children 9-14 years of age have been used (n=30) (Waterworth, 1974)

Intraoperative analgesia: I.V.: Titrating doses of 0.5 mg/kg every 30-45 minutes as needed have been given in 50 children 5-9 years of age; total dose required: 1-1.5 mg/kg (Ray, 1994)

Children >14 years and Adults: Oral: 50 mg every 3-4 hours; may increase to 100 mg/dose if needed; maximum dose: 600 mg/day

Adults:

- I.M., SubQ: 30-60 mg every 3-4 hours; maximum: 360 mg/day
- I.V.: 30 mg every 3-4 hours; maximum: 360 mg/day

Dosing adjustment in renal impairment: Children and Adults:
Cl_{cr} 10-50 mL/minute: Administer 75% of normal dose
Cl_{cr} <10 mL/minute: Administer 50% of normal dose

Administration
Oral: May be administered with food or milk to decrease GI upset
Parenteral: SubQ route not advised due to tissue damage; rotate injection site for I.M., SubQ use; avoid intra-arterial injection

Monitoring Parameters Respiratory and cardiovascular status; level of pain relief and sedation; blood pressure

Patient Information Avoid alcohol; may cause drowsiness and impair ability to perform activities requiring mental alertness or physical coordination; may be habit-forming; avoid abrupt discontinuation after prolonged use; will cause narcotic withdrawal symptoms in patients currently dependent on narcotics

Additional Information Use only in patients who are not tolerant to or physically dependent upon narcotics

Talwin® NX tablet (pentazocine hydrochloride with naloxone) was formulated to decrease abuse potential of dissolving tablets in water and using as injection

Dosage Forms Excipient information presented when available (limited, particularly for generics); consult specific product labeling.
Injection, solution:
Talwin®: 30 mg/mL (1 mL, 10 mL) [10 mL size contains sodium bisulfite]
Tablet: Pentazocine 50 mg and naloxone 0.5 mg
Talwin® NX: Pentazocine 50 mg and naloxone 0.5 mg

References
Hamunen K, Olkkola KT, Seppala T, et al, "Pharmacokinetics and Pharmacodynamics of Pentazocine in Children," *Pharmacol Toxicol*, 1993, 73(2):120-3.
Ray AD and Gupta M, "Clinical Trial of Pentazocine as Analgesic in Pediatric Cases," *J Indian Med Assoc*, 1994, 92(3):77-9.
Rita L, Seleny FL, and Levin RM, "A Comparison of Pentazocine and Morphine for Pediatric Premedication," *Anesth Analg*, 1970, 49(3):377-82.
Waterworth TA, "Pentazocine (Fortal) as Postoperative Analgesic in Children," *Arch Dis Child*, 1974, 49(6):488-90.

♦ **Pentazocine Hydrochloride** *see* Pentazocine *on page 1237*
♦ **Pentazocine Hydrochloride and Naloxone Hydrochloride** *see* Pentazocine *on page 1237*
♦ **Pentazocine Lactate** *see* Pentazocine *on page 1237*

Pentobarbital (pen toe BAR bi tal)

Medication Safety Issues
Sound-alike/look-alike issues:
Pentobarbital may be confused with phenobarbital
Nembutal® may be confused with Myambutol®

Related Information
Compatibility of Medications Mixed in A Syringe *on page 1941*
Laboratory Detection of Drugs in Urine *on page 1928*
Overdose and Toxicology *on page 1916*
Preprocedure Sedatives in Children *on page 1895*

U.S. Brand Names Nembutal®

Canadian Brand Names Nembutal® Sodium

Index Terms Pentobarbital Sodium

Therapeutic Category Anticonvulsant, Barbiturate; Barbiturate; General Anesthetic; Hypnotic; Sedative

Generic Available No

Use Preoperative sedation; high-dose barbiturate coma for treatment of increased intracranial pressure or status epilepticus unresponsive to other therapy

Restrictions C-II

Pregnancy Risk Factor D

Lactation Enters breast milk/contraindicated

Contraindications Hypersensitivity to barbiturates or any component; marked liver function impairment or latent porphyria; chronic or acute pain

Warnings Abrupt discontinuation after prolonged use may result in withdrawal symptoms or seizures; commercially available injection contains 40% propylene glycol

Precautions Use with caution in patients with hypovolemic shock, CHF, or hepatic impairment

Adverse Reactions
Cardiovascular: Arrhythmias, bradycardia, hypotension
Central nervous system: Drowsiness, lethargy, CNS excitation or depression, impaired judgment, hypothermia
Dermatologic: Rash
(Continued)

Pentobarbital *(Continued)*

Gastrointestinal: Nausea, vomiting

Local: Arterial spasm, gangrene with inadvertent intra-arterial injection, thrombophlebitis

Renal: Oliguria

Respiratory: Laryngospasm, respiratory depression, apnea (especially with rapid I.V. use)

Miscellaneous: Physical and psychological dependency with chronic use

Drug Interactions Barbiturates are enzyme inducers (monitor patient closely for decreased effect of concomitantly administered medications or increased effect when barbiturates are discontinued); carbamazepine, chloramphenicol, cimetidine, corticosteroids, CNS depressants, alcohol, doxycycline, warfarin, valproic acid

Food Interactions High doses of pyridoxine may decrease drug effect; barbiturates may increase the metabolism of vitamins D and K; dietary requirements of vitamins D, K, C, B_{12}, folate, and calcium may be increased with long-term use

Stability Protect from light; aqueous solutions are not stable; low pH may cause precipitate; use only clear solution

Mechanism of Action Short-acting barbiturate with sedative, hypnotic, and anticonvulsant properties; depresses CNS activity by binding to barbiturate site at GABA-receptor complex enhancing GABA activity; depresses reticular activating system; higher doses may be gabamimetic

Pharmacodynamics

Onset of action:

- I.M.: Within 10-15 minutes
- I.V.: Within 1 minute

Duration: I.V.: 15 minutes

Pharmacokinetics

Distribution: V_d:

- Children: 0.8 L/kg
- Adults: 1 L/kg

Protein binding: 35% to 55%

Metabolism: Extensive in the liver via hydroxylation and oxidation pathways

Half-life, terminal:

- Children: 25 hours
- Normal adults: 22 hours; range: 35-50 hours

Elimination: <1% excreted unchanged renally

Usual Dosage

Infants ≥6 months and Children: (**Note:** Limited information is available for infants <6 months of age):

- Preoperative/preprocedure sedation:
  - I.M.: 2-6 mg/kg; maximum dose: 100 mg/dose
  - I.V.: 1-3 mg/kg to a maximum of 100 mg until asleep

Children:

- Hypnotic: I.M.: 2-6 mg/kg; maximum dose: 100 mg/dose
- Conscious sedation prior to a procedure: Children >18 months: I.V.: Initial: 2 mg/kg, additional doses of 1-2 mg/kg may be given every 5-10 minutes until adequate sedation is achieved; maximum total dose: 6 mg/kg or 150-200 mg; mean total dose required (for CT scan sedation): 3.3-4.5 mg/kg

Adolescents: Conscious sedation: I.V.: 100 mg prior to a procedure

Children and Adults: Pentobarbital coma: I.V. (see Additional Information):

- Loading dose: 10-15 mg/kg given slowly over 1-2 hours; monitor blood pressure and respiratory rate
- Maintenance infusion: Initial: 1 mg/kg/hour; may increase to 2-3 mg/kg/hour; maintain burst suppression on EEG

Adults:

- Hypnotic:
  - I.M.: 150-200 mg
  - I.V.: Initial: 100 mg, may repeat every 1-3 minutes up to 200-500 mg total
- Preoperative sedation: I.M.: 150-200 mg

Administration

Parenteral: I.V.: Do not inject >50 mg/minute; rapid I.V. injection may cause respiratory depression, apnea, laryngospasm, bronchospasm, and hypotension; administer over 10-30 minutes; maximum concentration: 50 mg/mL for slow I.V. push; may dilute in D_5W, $D_{10}W$, NS, ½NS, LR, Ringer's injection, D_5LR, and dextrose/saline combinations for continuous infusion

Monitoring Parameters Vital signs, respiratory status (includes pulse oximetry for conscious sedation), cardiovascular status, CNS status; monitor ICP and cerebral perfusion pressure (CPP) (CPP = MAP - ICP) when using pentobarbital coma to reduce ICP

Reference Range Therapeutic:

Sedation: 1-5 mcg/mL (SI: 4-22 micromoles/L)

Sleep: 5-15 mcg/mL (SI: 22-66 micromoles/L)

Coma: 20-40 mcg/mL (SI: 88-177 micromoles/L)

Patient Information Avoid alcohol; limit caffeine; may be habit-forming; avoid abrupt discontinuation after prolonged use; may cause drowsiness and impair ability to perform activities requiring mental alertness or physical coordination

Nursing Implications Parenteral solutions are very alkaline; avoid extravasation; avoid intra-arterial injection

Additional Information Tolerance to hypnotic effect can occur; taper dose to prevent withdrawal; **Note**: Loading doses of 15-35 mg/kg (given over 1-2 hours) have been utilized in pediatric patients for pentobarbital coma but these higher loading doses often cause hypotension requiring vasopressor therapy

I.V. continuous infusions of pentobarbital using initial bolus doses of 1-2 mg/kg followed by initial continuous infusions of 1-2 mg/kg/hour have been used for PICU sedation in six intubated, mechanically ventilated infants (age: 2-17 months) who "failed" sedation with fentanyl and midazolam infusions; doses were titrated to effect and supplemental boluses were administered as needed; further studies are needed (see Tobias, 1995)

Dosage Forms Excipient information presented when available (limited, particularly for generics); consult specific product labeling.

Injection, solution, as sodium: 50 mg/mL (20 mL, 50 mL) [contains alcohol 10% and propylene glycol 40%]

References

Fischer JH and Raineri DL, "Pentobarbital Anesthesia for Status Epilepticus," *Clin Pharm*, 1987, 6(8):601-2.

Hubbard AM, Markowitz RI, Kimmel B, et al, "Sedation for Pediatric Patients Undergoing CT and MRI," *J Comput Assist Tomogr*, 1992, 16(1):3-6.

Pereira JK, Burrows PE, Richards HM, et al, "Comparison of Sedation Regimens for Pediatric Outpatient CT," *Pediatr Radiol*, 1993, 23(5):341-4.

Schaible DH, Cupit GC, Swedlow DB, et al, "High-Dose Pentobarbital Pharmacokinetics in Hypothermic Brain-Injured Children," *J Pediatr*, 1982, 100(4):655-60.

Tobias JD, Deshpande JK, Pietsch JB, et al, "Pentobarbital Sedation for Patients in the Pediatric Intensive Care Unit," *South Med J*, 1995, 88(3):290-4.

♦ **Pentobarbital Sodium** *see* Pentobarbital *on page 1239*

♦ **Pentothal®** *see* Thiopental *on page 1529*

Pentoxifylline (pen toks I fi leen)

Medication Safety Issues

Sound-alike/look-alike issues:

Pentoxifylline may be confused with tamoxifen

Trental® may be confused with Bentyl®, Tegretol®, Trandate®

U.S. Brand Names Pentoxil®; Trental®

Canadian Brand Names Albert® Pentoxifylline; Apo-Pentoxifylline SR®; Nu-Pentoxifylline SR; ratio-Pentoxifylline; Trental®

Index Terms Oxpentifylline

Therapeutic Category Blood Viscosity Reducer Agent

Generic Available Yes

Use Symptomatic management of peripheral vascular disease, mainly intermittent claudication

Investigational use: AIDS patients with increased tumor necrosis factor, cerebrovascular accidents, cerebrovascular diseases, new onset type I diabetes mellitus, diabetic atherosclerosis, diabetic neuropathy, gangrene, cutaneous polyarteritis nodosa, hemodialysis shunt thrombosis, cerebral malaria, septic shock, sepsis in premature neonates, sickle cell syndromes, vasculitis, Kawasaki disease, Raynaud's syndrome, cystic fibrosis, bone marrow transplant-related toxicities (ie, graft-versus-host disease, veno-occlusive disease, and interstitial pneumonitis), and persistent pulmonary hypertension of the newborn

Pregnancy Risk Factor C

Lactation Enters breast milk/not recommended

Contraindications Hypersensitivity to pentoxifylline, any component, or other xanthine derivatives (eg, caffeine, theophylline, theobromine); recent cerebral or retinal hemorrhage

Warnings Use with caution in patients with renal or hepatic impairment, insulin-treated diabetics, chronic occlusive arterial disease of the limbs, recent surgery, or peptic ulcerations

Adverse Reactions

Cardiovascular: Mild hypotension, angina

Central nervous system: Headache, dizziness, agitation

Gastrointestinal: Dyspepsia, nausea, vomiting

(Continued)

Pentoxifylline *(Continued)*

Ocular: Blurred vision

Drug Interactions Cimetidine may increase plasma concentrations of pentoxifylline; pentoxifylline may increase the effect of antihypertensive agents, warfarin, heparin; pentoxifylline may increase serum theophylline levels and toxicity (monitor closely, dosage adjustment of theophylline may be needed)

Food Interactions Food may decrease rate but not extent of absorption

Mechanism of Action Mechanism of action remains unclear; is thought to reduce blood viscosity and improve blood flow by altering the rheology of red blood cells; inhibits production of tumor necrosis factor-alpha; inhibits neutrophil activation and adhesion; increases tissue oxygen levels in patients with peripheral arterial disease; inhibits platelet aggregation

Pharmacodynamics Onset of action: 2-4 weeks with multiple doses

Pharmacokinetics

Absorption: Oral: Well absorbed

Distribution: Pentoxifylline and metabolites distribute into breast milk

Metabolism: Undergoes first-pass in the liver, dose-related (nonlinear) pharmacokinetics

Half-life, apparent:

Parent drug: 24-48 minutes

Metabolites: 60-96 minutes

Time to peak serum concentration: Within 2-4 hours

Elimination: Metabolites excreted in urine; 0% eliminated unchanged in the urine

Usual Dosage Oral:

Children: Minimal information available; one investigation (Furukawa, 1994) found a lower incidence of coronary artery lesions in 22 children (mean age 2 years) treated for acute Kawasaki disease with versus without pentoxifylline 20 mg/kg/day (given in 3 divided doses); all patients received aspirin and I.V. gamma globulin therapy; a lower dose (10 mg/kg/day) was not effective; higher doses have been used investigationally for the treatment of cystic fibrosis (Aronoff 1994)

Adults: 400 mg 3 times/day with meals; decrease to 400 mg twice daily if CNS or GI side effects occur. **Note:** Although clinical benefit may be seen within 2-4 weeks, treatment should be continued for at least 8 weeks

Administration Oral: Administer with food or antacids to decrease GI upset. Do not crush, break, or chew extended or controlled release tablet, swallow whole.

Test Interactions False positive theophylline level

Patient Information Limit caffeine; if GI or CNS side effects continue, contact physician; while beneficial effects may be seen in 2-4 weeks, continue treatment for at least 8 weeks

Dosage Forms Excipient information presented when available (limited, particularly for generics); consult specific product labeling.

Tablet, controlled release:

Trental®: 400 mg

Tablet, extended release: 400 mg

Pentoxil®: 400 mg

References

Aronoff SC, Quinn FJ, Carpenter LS, et al, "Effects of Pentoxifylline on Sputum Neutrophil Elastase and Pulmonary Function in Patients With Cystic Fibrosis: Preliminary Observations," *J Pediatr*, 1994, 125(6 Pt 1):992-7.

Berman W Jr, Berman N, Pathak D, et al, "Effects of Pentoxifylline (Trental®) on Blood Flow, Viscosity, and Oxygen Transport in Young Adults With Inoperable Cyanotic Congenital Heart Disease," *Pediatr Cardiol*, 1994, 15(2):66-70.

Furukawa S, Matsubara T, Umezawa Y, et al, "Pentoxifylline and Intravenous Gamma Globulin Combination Therapy for Acute Kawasaki Disease," *Eur J Pediatr*, 1994, 153(9):663-7.

Lauterbach R, "Pentoxifylline Treatment of Persistent Pulmonary Hypertension of Newborn," *Eur J Pediatr*, 1993, 152(5):460. (I.V. use)

Lauterbach R, Pawlik D, Tomaszczyk B, et al, "Pentoxifylline Treatment of Sepsis of Premature Infants; Preliminary Clinical Observations," *Eur J Pediatr*, 1994, 153(9):672-4. (I.V. use)

MacDonald MJ, Shahidi NT, Allen DB, et al, "Pentoxifylline in the Treatment of Children With New-Onset Type I Diabetes Mellitus," *JAMA*, 1994, 271(1):27-8.

- **Pentoxil®** *see* Pentoxifylline *on page 1241*
- **Pen VK** *see* Penicillin V Potassium *on page 1234*
- **Pepcid®** *see* Famotidine *on page 638*
- **Pepcid® AC [OTC]** *see* Famotidine *on page 638*
- **Pepcid® AC (Can)** *see* Famotidine *on page 638*
- **Pepcid® I.V. (Can)** *see* Famotidine *on page 638*
- **Pepto-Bismol® [OTC]** *see* Bismuth *on page 219*
- **Pepto-Bismol® Maximum Strength [OTC]** *see* Bismuth *on page 219*
- **Percocet®** *see* Oxycodone and Acetaminophen *on page 1191*
- **Percocet®-Demi (Can)** *see* Oxycodone and Acetaminophen *on page 1191*

- ♦ **Percodan®** *see* Oxycodone and Aspirin *on page 1193*
- ♦ **Perdiem® Overnight Relief [OTC]** *see* Senna *on page 1427*
- ♦ **Periactin** *see* Cyproheptadine *on page 426*
- ♦ **Peri-Colace® [OTC]** *see* Docusate and Senna *on page 527*
- ♦ **Peridex®** *see* Chlorhexidine Gluconate *on page 337*
- ♦ **Peridol (Can)** *see* Haloperidol *on page 754*
- ♦ **PerioChip®** *see* Chlorhexidine Gluconate *on page 337*
- ♦ **PerioGard®** *see* Chlorhexidine Gluconate *on page 337*
- ♦ **PerioMed™** *see* Fluoride *on page 675*
- ♦ **Periostat®** *see* Doxycycline *on page 543*

Permethrin (per METH rin)

U.S. Brand Names A200® Lice [OTC]; Acticin®; Elimite®; Nix® [OTC]; Rid® Spray [OTC]

Canadian Brand Names Kwellada-P™; Nix®

Therapeutic Category Antiparasitic Agent, Topical; Pediculocide; Scabicidal Agent

Generic Available Yes: Excludes spray

Use Single application treatment of infestation with *Pediculus humanus capitis* (head louse) and its nits; treatment of *Sarcoptes scabiei* (scabies)

Pregnancy Risk Factor B

Lactation Effect on infant unknown

Contraindications Hypersensitivity to pyrethroid, pyrethrin, any component, or to chrysanthemums

Precautions For external use only; do not use near the eyes or on mucous membranes such as inside the nose, mouth, or vagina

Adverse Reactions

Dermatologic: Pruritus, erythema, rash of the scalp

Local: Burning, stinging, pain, edema, tingling, numbness, scalp discomfort

Mechanism of Action Inhibits sodium ion influx through nerve cell membrane channels in parasites resulting in delayed repolarization, paralysis, and death of organism

Pharmacokinetics

Absorption: Topical: Minimal (<2%)

Metabolism: By ester hydrolysis to inactive metabolites

Usual Dosage Topical: Children >2 months and Adults:

Head lice: After hair has been washed with shampoo, rinsed with water and towel dried, apply a sufficient volume of creme rinse to saturate the hair and scalp; also apply behind the ears and at the base of the neck; leave on hair for 10 minutes before rinsing off with water; remove remaining nits. May repeat in 1 week if lice or nits still present; in areas of head lice resistance to 1% permethrin, 5% permethrin has been applied to clean, dry hair and left on overnight (8-14 hours) under a shower cap.

Scabies: Apply cream from head to toe; leave on for 8-14 hours before washing off with water; for infants, also apply on the hairline, neck, scalp, temple, and forehead; may reapply in 1 week if live mites appear. Permethrin 5% cream was shown to be safe and effective when applied to an infant <1 month of age with neonatal scabies; time of application was limited to 6 hours before rinsing with soap and water.

Administration Topical: Avoid contact with eyes during application; shake creme rinse well before using

Patient Information Clothing and bedding should be washed in hot water or by dry cleaning to kill the scabies mite

Nursing Implications

To remove nits: Comb hair with a fine-toothed nit comb and apply a damp towel to the scalp for 30-60 minutes

For infestation of eyelashes: Apply petroleum ointment to eyelashes 3-4 times/day for 8-10 days; remove nits mechanically from the eyelashes

For scabies: Itching may continue for several weeks despite successful treatment; oral antihistamines and/or topical corticosteroids may be helpful in relieving symptoms

Additional Information Topical cream formulation contains formaldehyde which is a contact allergen

Dosage Forms Excipient information presented when available (limited, particularly for generics); consult specific product labeling.

Cream, topical (Acticin®, Elimite®): 5% (60 g) [contains coconut oil]

Lotion, topical: 1% (59 mL)

Liquid, topical [creme rinse formulation] (Nix®): 1% (60 mL) [contains isopropyl alcohol 20%]

(Continued)

Permethrin *(Continued)*

Solution, spray [for bedding and furniture]:
- A200® Lice: 0.5% (180 mL)
- Nix®: 0.25% (148 mL)
- Rid®: 0.5% (150 mL)

References

"Drugs for Head Lice," *Med Lett Drugs Ther,* 1997, 39(992):6-7.

Hogan DJ, Schachner L, Tanglertsampan C, "Diagnosis and Treatment of Childhood Scabies and Pediculosis," *Pediatr Clin North Am,* 1991, 38(4):941-57.

Krowchuk DP, Tunnessen WW Jr, and Hurwitz S, "Pediatric Dermatology Update," *Pediatrics,* 1992, 90(2 Pt 1):259-64.

Quarterman MJ and Lesher JL, "Neonatal Scabies Treated With Permethrin 5% Cream," *Pediatr Dermatol,* 1994, 11(3):264-6.

- ♦ **Peroxide** *see* Hydrogen Peroxide *on page 786*
- ♦ **Persantine®** *see* Dipyridamole *on page 521*
- ♦ **Pethidine Hydrochloride** *see* Meperidine *on page 1002*
- ♦ **Petrolatum White and Mineral Oil Ophthalmic Ointment** *see* Ocular Lubricant *on page 1160*
- ♦ **Pexeva®** *see* Paroxetine *on page 1218*
- ♦ **Pexicam® (Can)** *see* Piroxicam *on page 1268*
- ♦ **PFA** *see* Foscarnet *on page 709*
- ♦ **Pfizerpen®** *see* Penicillin G (Parenteral/Aqueous) *on page 1231*
- ♦ **Pfizerpen-AS® (Can)** *see* Penicillin G Procaine *on page 1233*
- ♦ **PGE_1** *see* Alprostadil *on page 81*
- ♦ **PGI_2** *see* Epoprostenol *on page 585*
- ♦ **PGX** *see* Epoprostenol *on page 585*
- ♦ **Phanasin® [OTC]** *see* Guaifenesin *on page 745*
- ♦ **Phanasin® Diabetic Choice [OTC]** *see* Guaifenesin *on page 745*
- ♦ **Phanatuss® DM [OTC]** *see* Guaifenesin and Dextromethorphan *on page 748*
- ♦ **Pharmaflur®** *see* Fluoride *on page 675*
- ♦ **Pharmaflur® 1.1** *see* Fluoride *on page 675*
- ♦ **Phazyme™ (Can)** *see* Simethicone *on page 1440*
- ♦ **Phazyme® Quick Dissolve [OTC]** *see* Simethicone *on page 1440*
- ♦ **Phazyme® Ultra Strength [OTC]** *see* Simethicone *on page 1440*
- ♦ **Phenadoz™** *see* Promethazine *on page 1324*
- ♦ **Phenazo™ (Can)** *see* Phenazopyridine *on page 1244*

Phenazopyridine (fen az oh PEER i deen)

Medication Safety Issues

Sound-alike/look-alike issues:

Pyridium® may be confused with Dyrenium®, Perdiem®, pyridoxine, pyrithione

U.S. Brand Names AZO-Gesic® [OTC]; AZO-Standard® [OTC]; Baridium® [OTC]; Prodium® [OTC]; Pyridium®; ReAzo [OTC]; Uristat® [OTC]; UTI Relief® [OTC]

Canadian Brand Names Phenazo™

Index Terms Phenazopyridine Hydrochloride; Phenylazo Diamino Pyridine Hydrochloride

Therapeutic Category Analgesic, Urinary; Local Anesthetic, Urinary

Generic Available Yes

Use Symptomatic relief of urinary burning, itching, frequency and urgency in association with urinary tract infection, or following urologic procedures

Pregnancy Risk Factor B

Lactation Excretion in breast milk unknown

Contraindications Hypersensitivity to phenazopyridine or any component; liver or kidney disease (do not use in patients with Cl_{cr} <50 mL/minute)

Warnings Does not treat infection, acts only as an analgesic; drug should be discontinued if skin or sclera develop a yellow color.

Precautions Use with caution in patients with renal impairment (Cl_{cr} 50-80 mL/minute)

Adverse Reactions

Central nervous system: Vertigo, headache

Dermatologic: Skin pigmentation, rash, pruritus

Gastrointestinal: Stomach cramps

Genitourinary: Discoloration of urine (orange or red)

Hematologic: Methemoglobinemia, hemolytic anemia

Hepatic: Hepatitis

Renal: Transient acute renal failure

Mechanism of Action Exerts local topical anesthetic or analgesic action on urinary tract mucosa through an unknown mechanism

Pharmacokinetics

Metabolism: In the liver and other tissues

Elimination: In urine (where it exerts its action); renal excretion (as unchanged drug) is rapid and accounts for 65% of the drug's elimination

Usual Dosage Oral:

Children: 12 mg/kg/day in 3 divided doses for 2 days if used concomitantly with an antibacterial agent for UTI

Adults: 95-200 mg 3-4 times/day for 2 days if used concomitantly with an antibacterial agent for UTI

Dosing interval in renal impairment:

Cl_{cr} 50-80 mL/minute: Administer every 8-16 hours

Cl_{cr} <50 mL/minute: Avoid use

Administration Oral: Administer with food to decrease GI distress

Test Interactions False-negative Clinistix®, Tes-Tape®, Ictotest®, Acetest®, Ketostix®, urinalysis based upon spectrometry or color reactions

Patient Information May discolor urine orange or red; may stain contact lenses and fabric; not an antibiotic and does not treat infection; contact physician for antibiotic therapy

Dosage Forms Excipient information presented when available (limited, particularly for generics); consult specific product labeling.

Tablet, as hydrochloride: 100 mg, 200 mg

AZO-Gesic®, AZO-Standard®, Prodium®, ReAzo, Uristat®: 95 mg

Baridium®, UTI Relief®: 97.2 mg

Pyridium®: 100 mg, 200 mg

Extemporaneous Preparations A 10 mg/mL suspension may be made by crushing three 200 mg tablets. Mix with a small amount of distilled water or glycerin. Add 20 mL Cologel® [DSC] and levigate until a uniform mixture is obtained. Add sufficient 2:1 simple syrup/cherry syrup mixture to make a final volume of 60 mL. Store in an amber container. Label "shake well". Stability is 60 days refrigerated.

Handbook on Extemporaneous Formulations, Bethesda MD: American Society of Hospital Pharmacists, 1987.

♦ **Phenazopyridine Hydrochloride** *see* Phenazopyridine *on page 1244*

♦ **Phenergan®** *see* Promethazine *on page 1324*

Phenobarbital (fee noe BAR bi tal)

Medication Safety Issues

Sound-alike/look-alike issues:

Phenobarbital may be confused with pentobarbital

Luminal® may be confused with Tuinal®

Related Information

Antiepileptic Drugs *on page 1902*

Blood Level Sampling Time Guidelines *on page 1914*

Febrile Seizures *on page 1898*

Laboratory Detection of Drugs in Urine *on page 1928*

Overdose and Toxicology *on page 1916*

U.S. Brand Names Luminal® Sodium

Canadian Brand Names PMS-Phenobarbital

Index Terms Phenobarbital Sodium; Phenobarbitone; Phenylethylmalonylurea

Therapeutic Category Anticonvulsant, Barbiturate; Barbiturate; Hypnotic; Sedative

Generic Available Yes

Use Management of generalized tonic-clonic (grand mal) and partial seizures; neonatal seizures; febrile seizures in children; sedation; may also be used for prevention and treatment of neonatal hyperbilirubinemia and lowering of bilirubin in chronic cholestasis

Restrictions C-IV

Pregnancy Risk Factor D

Lactation Enters breast milk/not recommended (AAP recommends use "with caution")

Contraindications Hypersensitivity to phenobarbital or any component; pre-existing CNS depression, severe uncontrolled pain, porphyria, severe respiratory disease with dyspnea or obstruction

Warnings Abrupt withdrawal may precipitate status epilepticus

Precautions Use with caution in patients with renal or hepatic impairment

Adverse Reactions

Cardiovascular: Hypotension, circulatory collapse

(Continued)

Phenobarbital *(Continued)*

Central nervous system: Drowsiness, paradoxical excitement, hyperkinetic activity, cognitive impairment, defects in general comprehension, short-term memory deficits, decreased attention span, ataxia
Dermatologic: Skin eruptions, skin rash, exfoliative dermatitis
Hematologic: Megaloblastic anemia
Hepatic: Hepatitis
Respiratory: Respiratory depression, apnea (especially with rapid I.V. use)
Miscellaneous: Psychological and physical dependence

Drug Interactions Cytochrome P450 isoenzyme CYP1A2, CYP2B6, CYP2C8, CYP2C9, CYP2C18, CYP2C19, CYP3A3/4, and CYP3A5-7 inducer

Phenobarbital may decrease the serum concentration or effect of lamotrigine, ritonavir, saquinavir, delavirdine, ethosuximide, warfarin, oral contraceptives, chloramphenicol, griseofulvin, doxycycline, beta-blockers, theophylline, corticosteroids, teniposide, etoposide, doxorubicin, vincristine, methotrexate, tricyclic antidepressants, cyclosporin, quinidine, haloperidol, and phenothiazines

Valproic acid, methylphenidate, chloramphenicol, felbamate, and propoxyphene may inhibit the metabolism of phenobarbital with resultant increase in phenobarbital serum concentration; ritonavir may affect the metabolism of phenobarbital; phenobarbital and benzodiazepines or other CNS depressants may increase CNS and respiratory depression (especially with I.V. loading doses of phenobarbital)

Food Interactions High doses of pyridoxine may decrease drug effect; barbiturates may increase the metabolism of vitamins D and K; dietary requirements of vitamins D, K, C, B_{12}, folate, and calcium may be increased with long-term use

Stability Protect elixir from light; not stable in aqueous solutions; use only clear solutions; do not add to acidic solutions, precipitation may occur

Mechanism of Action Depresses CNS activity by binding to barbiturate site at GABA-receptor complex enhancing GABA activity; depresses reticular activating system; higher doses may be gabamimetic

Pharmacodynamics Hypnosis:

Onset of action:
- Oral: Within 20-60 minutes
- I.V.: Within 5 minutes

Maximum effect: I.V.: Within 30 minutes

Duration:
- Oral: 6-10 hours
- I.V.: 4-10 hours

Pharmacokinetics

Absorption: Oral: 70% to 90%

Distribution: V_d:
- Neonates: 0.8-1 L/kg
- Infants: 0.7-0.8 L/kg
- Children: 0.6-0.7 L/kg

Protein binding: 35% to 50%, decreased protein binding in neonates

Metabolism: In the liver via hydroxylation and glucuronide conjugation

Half-life:
- Neonates: 45-200 hours
- Infants: 20-133 hours
- Children: 37-73 hours
- Adults: 53-140 hours

Time to peak serum concentration: Oral: Within 1-6 hours

Elimination: 20% to 50% excreted unchanged in urine; clearance can be increased with alkalinization of urine or with oral multiple-dose activated charcoal

Dialysis: Moderately dialyzable (20% to 50%)

Usual Dosage

Anticonvulsant: Status epilepticus: **Loading dose:** I.V.:
- Neonates: 15-20 mg/kg in a single or divided dose
- Infants, Children, and Adults: 15-18 mg/kg in a single or divided dose; usual maximum loading dose: 20 mg/kg
  - **Note:** In select patients, may give additional 5 mg/kg/dose every 15-30 minutes until seizure is controlled or a total dose of 30 mg/kg is reached; be prepared to support respirations

Anticonvulsant **maintenance dose**: Oral, I.V. (**Note:** Maintenance dose usually starts 12 hours after loading dose):
- Neonates: 3-4 mg/kg/day given once daily; assess serum concentrations; increase to 5 mg/kg/day if needed (usually by second week of therapy)
- Infants: 5-6 mg/kg/day in 1-2 divided doses
- Children:
  - 1-5 years: 6-8 mg/kg/day in 1-2 divided doses
  - 5-12 years: 4-6 mg/kg/day in 1-2 divided doses

>12 years and adults: 1-3 mg/kg/day in 1-2 divided doses

Children:

Sedation: Oral: 2 mg/kg 3 times/day

Hypnotic: I.M., I.V., SubQ: 3-5 mg/kg at bedtime

Hyperbilirubinemia: <12 years: Oral: 3-8 mg/kg/day in 2-3 divided doses; doses up to 12 mg/kg/day have been used

Preoperative sedation: Oral, I.M., I.V.: 1-3 mg/kg 1-1.5 hours before procedure

Adults:

Sedation: Oral, I.M.: 30-120 mg/day in 2-3 divided doses

Hypnotic: Oral, I.M., I.V., SubQ: 100-320 mg at bedtime

Hyperbilirubinemia: Oral: 90-180 mg/day in 2-3 divided doses

Preoperative sedation: I.M.: 100-200 mg 1-1.5 hours before procedure

Administration

Oral: Administer elixir with water, milk, or juice

Parenteral: Do not inject I.V. faster than 1 mg/kg/minute with a maximum of 30 mg/minute for infants and children and 60 mg/minute for adults >60 kg; do not administer intra-arterially; avoid extravasation; use only powder for injection for SubQ use, not solutions for injection

Monitoring Parameters CNS status, seizure activity, liver enzymes, CBC with differential, renal function, serum concentrations; I.V. use: Respiratory rate, heart rate, blood pressure; hyperbilirubinemia: bilirubin (total and direct)

Reference Range

Therapeutic: 15-40 mcg/mL (SI: 65-172 micromoles/L)

Potentially toxic: >40 mcg/mL (SI: >172 micromoles/L)

Coma: >50 mcg/mL (SI: >215 micromoles/L)

Potentially lethal: >80 mcg/mL (SI: >344 micromoles/L)

Patient Information Avoid alcohol; limit caffeine; may be habit-forming; avoid abrupt discontinuation after prolonged use; may cause dizziness or drowsiness and impair ability to perform activities requiring mental alertness or physical coordination

Nursing Implications Parenteral solutions are very alkaline

Additional Information A recent study (Relling, 2000) demonstrated that enzyme-inducing antiepileptic drugs (AEDs) (carbamazepine, phenobarbital, and phenytoin) increased systemic clearance of antileukemic drugs (teniposide and methotrexate) and were associated with a worse event-free survival, CNS relapse, and hematologic relapse (ie, lower efficacy), in B-lineage ALL children receiving chemotherapy; the authors recommend using nonenzyme-inducing AEDs in patients receiving chemotherapy for ALL.

Dosage Forms Excipient information presented when available (limited, particularly for generics); consult specific product labeling.

Elixir: 20 mg/5 mL (5 mL, 7.5 mL, 15 mL) [contains alcohol]

Injection, solution, as sodium: 65 mg/mL (1 mL); 130 mg/mL (1 mL) [contains alcohol and propylene glycol]

Luminal® Sodium: 60 mg/mL (1 mL); 130 mg/mL (1 mL) [contains alcohol 10% and propylene glycol]

Tablet: 15 mg, 30 mg, 60 mg, 100 mg

References

Relling MV, Pui CH, Sandlund JT, et al, "Adverse Effect of Anticonvulsants on Efficacy of Chemotherapy for Acute Lymphoblastic Leukaemia," *Lancet*, 2000, 356(9226):285-90.

♦ **Phenobarbital, Hyoscyamine, Atropine, and Scopolamine** *see* Hyoscyamine, Atropine, Scopolamine, and Phenobarbital *on page 800*

♦ **Phenobarbital Sodium** *see* Phenobarbital *on page 1245*

♦ **Phenobarbitone** *see* Phenobarbital *on page 1245*

Phenoxybenzamine (fen oks ee BEN za meen)

Related Information

Antihypertensive Agents by Class *on page 1678*

Overdose and Toxicology *on page 1916*

U.S. Brand Names Dibenzyline®

Canadian Brand Names Dibenzyline®

Index Terms Phenoxybenzamine Hydrochloride

Therapeutic Category Alpha-Adrenergic Blocking Agent, Oral; Antihypertensive Agent; Vasodilator

Generic Available No

Use Symptomatic management of hypertension and sweating in patients with pheochromocytoma

Pregnancy Risk Factor C

Contraindications Hypersensitivity to phenoxybenzamine or any component (see Warnings); shock

(Continued)

Phenoxybenzamine *(Continued)*

Warnings Capsule contains benzyl alcohol which may cause allergic reactions in susceptible individuals; large amounts of benzyl alcohol (≥99 mg/kg/day) have been associated with a potentially fatal toxicity ("gasping syndrome") in neonates; avoid use of phenoxybenzamine products containing benzyl alcohol in neonates; *in vitro* and animal studies have shown that benzoate, a metabolite of benzyl alcohol, displaces bilirubin from protein binding sites

Precautions Use with caution in patients with renal dysfunction, cerebral or coronary arteriosclerosis

Adverse Reactions

Cardiovascular: Postural hypotension, tachycardia, syncope, shock
Central nervous system: Lethargy, headache, dizziness
Gastrointestinal: Vomiting, nausea, diarrhea
Neuromuscular & skeletal: Weakness
Ocular: Miosis
Respiratory: Nasal congestion

Drug Interactions Antagonizes effects of alpha-adrenergic stimulating sympathomimetic agents

Mechanism of Action Produces long-lasting noncompetitive alpha-adrenergic blockade of postganglionic synapses in exocrine glands and smooth muscle

Pharmacodynamics Oral:

Onset of action: Within 2 hours
Maximum effect: Within 4-6 hours
Duration: Effects can continue for up to 4 days

Pharmacokinetics

Absorption: Oral: ~20% to 30%
Distribution: Distributes to and may accumulate in adipose tissues
Half-life: Adults: 24 hours
Elimination: Primarily in urine and bile

Usual Dosage Oral:

Children: Initial: 0.2 mg/kg once daily; maximum dose: 10 mg/dose; increase every 4 days by 0.2 mg/kg/day increments; usual maintenance dose: 0.4-1.2 mg/kg/day every 6-8 hours; maximum doses of up to 2-4 mg/kg/day have been recommended

Adults: Initial: 10 mg twice daily; increase dose every other day to usual dose of 10-40 mg every 8-12 hours; higher doses may be needed

Administration Oral: May administer with milk to decrease GI upset

Monitoring Parameters Blood pressure, orthostasis, heart rate

Patient Information Avoid alcohol; may cause dizziness; avoid sudden changes in posture; may cause nasal congestion and constricted pupils; avoid cough, cold, or allergy medications containing sympathomimetics

Dosage Forms Excipient information presented when available (limited, particularly for generics); consult specific product labeling.

Capsule, as hydrochloride: 10 mg [contains benzyl alcohol]

Extemporaneous Preparations

A 2 mg/mL oral liquid preparation made from capsules and with 1% propylene glycol and 0.15% citric acid in distilled water was stable for 7 days when stored in amber glass prescription bottles under refrigeration (4°C). The vehicle is made by dissolving 150 mg of citric acid in a minimal amount of distilled water; then 1 mL of propylene glycol is added and the solution is mixed well; qsad to 100 mL with distilled water. Grind the contents of two 10 mg capsules in a mortar into a fine powder; add a small amount of the vehicle and mix well; transfer to a graduated cylinder and qsad with vehicle to 10 mL; transfer to an amber glass prescription bottle with tight-fitting cap; label "shake well" and "refrigerate" (Lim, 1997).

A stock solution of 10 mg/mL in propylene glycol was stable for 30 days when stored under refrigeration (4°C); when this stock solution was diluted 1:4 (v/v) with syrup (66.7% sucrose) to 2 mg/mL, the preparation was stable for 1 hour at 4°C (see Lim, 1997). **Note**: Although the stock solution is stable for 30 days, it **must be diluted** before administration to decrease the amount of propylene glycol delivered to the patient.

Lim LY, Tan LL, Chan EW, et al "Stability of Phenoxybenzamine Hydrochloride in Various Vehicles," *Am J Health Syst Pharm*, 1997, 54(18):2073-8.

♦ **Phenoxybenzamine Hydrochloride** *see* Phenoxybenzamine *on page 1247*
♦ **Phenoxymethyl Penicillin** *see* Penicillin V Potassium *on page 1234*

Phentolamine (fen TOLE a meen)

Medication Safety Issues

Sound-alike/look-alike issues:

Phentolamine may be confused with phentermine, Ventolin®

Related Information

Antihypertensive Agents by Class *on page 1678*
Extravasation Treatment *on page 1726*
Overdose and Toxicology *on page 1916*

Canadian Brand Names Regitine®; Rogitine®

Index Terms Phentolamine Mesylate; Regitine [DSC]

Therapeutic Category Alpha-Adrenergic Blocking Agent, Parenteral; Antidote, Extravasation; Antihypertensive Agent; Diagnostic Agent, Pheochromocytoma; Vasodilator

Generic Available Yes

Use Diagnosis of pheochromocytoma; treatment of hypertension associated with pheochromocytoma or other causes of excess sympathomimetic amines; local treatment and prevention of dermal necrosis after extravasation of drugs with alpha-adrenergic effects (dobutamine, dopamine, epinephrine, metaraminol, norepinephrine, phenylephrine) (see Additional Information)

Pregnancy Risk Factor C

Lactation Excretion in breast milk unknown

Contraindications Hypersensitivity to phentolamine or any component; renal impairment; coronary or cerebral arteriosclerosis; MI

Precautions Use with caution in patients with gastritis, peptic ulcer; history of cardiac arrhythmias; MI, cerebrovascular spasm, and cerebrovascular occlusion may occur

Adverse Reactions

Cardiovascular: Hypotension, tachycardia, angina, arrhythmias
Central nervous system: Dizziness, headache
Gastrointestinal: Nausea, vomiting, diarrhea, exacerbation of peptic ulcer
Neuromuscular & skeletal: Weakness
Respiratory: Nasal congestion

Stability Reconstituted solution is stable for 48 hours at room temperature and 1 week when refrigerated

Mechanism of Action

Systemic: Competitively blocks alpha-adrenergic receptors to produce brief antagonism of circulating epinephrine and norepinephrine; reduces hypertension caused by alpha effects of catecholamines; also has positive inotropic and chronotropic effects on the heart

SubQ: Blocks alpha-adrenergic receptors and reverses vasoconstriction caused by extravasation of medications with alpha-adrenergic effects

Pharmacodynamics

Onset of action:
- I.M.: Within 15-20 minutes
- I.V.: Immediate

Maximum effect:
- I.M.: Within 20 minutes
- I.V.: Within 2 minutes

Duration:
- I.M.: 30-45 minutes
- I.V.: Within 15-30 minutes

Pharmacokinetics

Metabolism: In the liver
Half-life: Adults: 19 minutes
Elimination: 10% to 13% excreted in urine as unchanged drug

Usual Dosage

Treatment of alpha-adrenergic drug extravasation: SubQ:

Neonates: Infiltrate area with a small amount (eg, 1 mL) of solution (made by diluting 2.5-5 mg in 10 mL of preservative free NS) within 12 hours of extravasation; do not exceed 0.1 mg/kg or 2.5 mg total

Infants, Children, and Adults: Infiltrate area with a small amount (eg, 1 mL) of solution (made by diluting 5-10 mg in 10 mL of NS) within 12 hours of extravasation; do not exceed 0.1-0.2 mg/kg or 5 mg total

Diagnosis of pheochromocytoma: I.M., I.V.:

Children: 0.05-0.1 mg/kg/dose, maximum single dose: 5 mg
Adults: 5 mg

Hypertension (prior to surgery for pheochromocytoma): I.M., I.V.:

Children: 0.05-0.1 mg/kg/dose given 1-2 hours before pheochromocytomectomy; repeat as needed to control blood pressure; maximum single dose: 5 mg

Adults: 5 mg given 1-2 hours before pheochromocytomectomy; repeat as needed to control blood pressure

Hypertensive crisis due to MAO inhibitor/sympathomimetic amine interaction: I.M., I.V.: Adults: 5-20 mg

Administration Parenteral: Treatment of extravasation: Infiltrate area of extravasation with multiple small injections of a diluted solution (see Usual Dosage); use 27- or

(Continued)

Phentolamine *(Continued)*

30-gauge needles and change needle between each skin entry; do not inject a volume such that swelling of the extremity or digit with resultant compartment syndrome occurs

Monitoring Parameters Blood pressure, heart rate, orthostasis; treatment of extravasation: site of extravasation, skin color, local perfusion

Nursing Implications Monitor the site of extravasation closely, as repeat doses of SubQ phentolamine may be needed

Additional Information When drugs with alpha-adrenergic effects extravasate, they cause local vasoconstriction which causes blanching of the skin and a pale, cold, hard appearance; SubQ phentolamine blocks the alpha-adrenergic receptors and reverses the vasoconstriction; the extravasation area should "pink up" and return to normal skin color following SubQ administration of phentolamine. Dobutamine primarily stimulates $beta_1$-adrenergic receptors, but does possess alpha (and $beta_2$) adrenergic effects; the alpha-adrenergic effects (vasoconstriction) may be seen when dobutamine extravasates (since high concentrations of dobutamine would be present locally); although infrequent, cases of dermal necrosis from dobutamine extravasation have been reported; thus, phentolamine may help prevent dermal necrosis following dobutamine extravasations (see MacCara, 1983; Hoff, 1979). Injection contains mannitol 25 mg/vial

Dosage Forms Excipient information presented when available (limited, particularly for generics); consult specific product labeling.

Injection, powder for reconstitution, as mesylate: 5 mg

References

Hoff JV, Peatty PA, and Wade JL, "Dermal Necrosis From Dobutamine," *N Engl J Med*, 1979, 300(22):1280.

MacCara ME, "Extravasation: A Hazard of Intravenous Therapy," *Drug Intell Clin Pharm*, 1983, 17(10):713-7.

- **Phentolamine Mesylate** *see* Phentolamine *on page 1248*
- **Phenylalanine Mustard** *see* Melphalan *on page 997*
- **Phenylazo Diamino Pyridine Hydrochloride** *see* Phenazopyridine *on page 1244*

Phenylephrine (fen il EF rin)

Medication Safety Issues

Sound-alike/look-alike issues:

Mydfrin® may be confused with Midrin®

Related Information

Extravasation Treatment *on page 1726*

OTC Cough and Cold Preparations, Pediatric *on page 1706*

U.S. Brand Names Ah-Chew D®; AK-Dilate®; Altafrin; Anu-Med [OTC]; Dimetapp® Toddler's [OTC]; Formulation R™ [OTC]; LuSonal™; Medicone® Suppositories [OTC]; Medi-Phenyl [OTC]; Mydfrin®; NāSop™; Neofrin™; Neo-Synephrine® Extra Strength [OTC]; Neo-Synephrine® Injection; Neo-Synephrine® Mild [OTC]; Neo-Synephrine® Regular Strength [OTC]; OcuNefrin™ [OTC]; Preparation H® [OTC]; Rectacaine [OTC]; Relief® [OTC]; Rhinall [OTC]; Sudafed PE™ [OTC]; Tronolane® Suppository [OTC]; Tur-bi-kal® [OTC]; Vicks® Sinex® Nasal Spray [OTC]; Vicks® Sinex® UltraFine Mist [OTC]; 4 Way® Fast Acting [OTC]; 4 Way® Menthol [OTC]; 4 Way® No Drip [OTC]

Canadian Brand Names Dionephrine®; Mydfrin®; Neo-Synephrine®

Index Terms Phenylephrine Hydrochloride; Phenylephrine Tannate

Therapeutic Category Adrenergic Agonist Agent; Adrenergic Agonist Agent, Ophthalmic; Alpha-Adrenergic Agonist; Hemorrhoidal Treatment Agent; Nasal Agent, Vasoconstrictor; Ophthalmic Agent, Mydriatic; Sympathomimetic

Generic Available Yes: Excludes cream, filmstrip, liquid, suspension

Use Treatment of hypotension and vascular failure in shock; supraventricular tachycardia; as a vasoconstrictor in regional analgesia; symptomatic relief of nasal and nasopharyngeal mucosal congestion; as a mydriatic in ophthalmic procedures and treatment of wide-angle glaucoma; symptomatic relief of hemorrhoidal symptoms (rectal cream and ointment)

Pregnancy Risk Factor C

Lactation Excretion in breast milk unknown/not recommended

Contraindications Hypersensitivity to phenylephrine or any component (see Warnings); pheochromocytoma, severe hypertension, ventricular tachycardia; acute pancreatitis, hepatitis; peripheral or mesenteric vascular thrombosis, myocardial disease, severe coronary disease, asthma, narrow-angle glaucoma (ophthalmic preparation); MAO inhibitor therapy or within 2 weeks of discontinuation of MAO inhibitor

Warnings Do not use if solution turns brown or contains a precipitate. Injection and ophthalmic agents may contain sulfites which may cause allergic reactions in susceptible individuals. Some formulations contain sodium benzoate; benzoic acid (benzoate) is a metabolite of benzyl alcohol; large amounts of benzyl alcohol (≥99 mg/kg/day) have been associated with a potentially fatal toxicity ("gasping syndrome") in neonates; *in vitro* and animal studies have shown that benzoate displaces bilirubin from protein binding sites; avoid use of benzyl alcohol containing products in neonates. Rebound nasal congestion may occur if abruptly discontinued after prolonged use.

Precautions Use as pressor therapy for treatment of hypotension and vascular failure is **not** a substitute for replacement of blood, plasma, and body fluids; use with caution in patients with hyperthyroidism, bradycardia, partial heart block, myocardial disease, or severe arteriosclerosis; infuse into large veins to prevent extravasation which may cause severe necrosis

Adverse Reactions

Cardiovascular: Hypertension, angina, reflex severe bradycardia, arrhythmias, peripheral vasoconstriction, precordial pain

Central nervous system: Restlessness, excitability, headache, anxiety, nervousness, dizziness

Dermatologic: Pilomotor response, skin blanching

Local: Necrosis if extravasation occurs

Neuromuscular & skeletal: Tremor

Ocular: (Ophthalmic preparation): Transient stinging, browache, blurred vision, photophobia, lacrimation

Respiratory: Respiratory distress, rebound nasal congestion, sneezing, burning, stinging, dryness

Drug Interactions With alpha- and beta-adrenergic blocking agents, may see decreased actions; with oxytocic drugs, may see increased actions; with sympathomimetics and halogenated hydrocarbon anesthetics, tachycardia or arrhythmias may occur; with MAO inhibitors, guanethidine, and bretylium, actions may be potentiated

Stability Store at room temperature; protect from light; compatible when admixed with dextrose, dextrose-saline, Ringer's, LR, NS, and 1/6 M sodium lactate injection; do not use if solution turns brown or contains a precipitate

Mechanism of Action Potent, direct-acting alpha-adrenergic stimulator with weak beta-adrenergic activity; causes vasoconstriction of the arterioles of the nasal mucosa and conjunctiva; activates the dilator muscle of the pupil to cause contraction; produces systemic arterial vasoconstriction

Pharmacodynamics

Onset of action:

- I.M.: Within 10-15 minutes
- I.V.: Following parenteral injection, effects occur immediately
- Oral: 15-20 minutes
- SubQ: 10-15 minutes

Duration:

- I.M.: 30 minutes to 2 hours
- I.V.: 15-20 minutes
- Oral: 2-4 hours
- SubQ: 1 hour

Pharmacokinetics

Metabolism: In the liver and intestine by the enzyme monoamine oxidase

Half-life: 2.5 hours

Elimination: Metabolites, routes, and rates of excretion have not been identified

Usual Dosage

Ophthalmic procedures:

- Infants <1 year: Instill 1 drop of 2.5% 15-30 minutes before procedures
- Children and Adults: Instill 1 drop of 2.5% or 10% solution, may repeat in 10-60 minutes as needed

Ophthalmic irritation (OTC formulation for relief of eye redness): Adults: Instill 1-2 drops 0.12% solution into affected eye, up to 4 times/day; do not use for >72 hours

Nasal decongestant: Intranasal (therapy should not exceed 3-5 days): **Note:** 0.16% and 0.125% nasal solutions/sprays are no longer commercially available; may dilute 0.25% or 0.5% with NS to achieve desired concentration:

- Infants >6 months: 1-2 drops of 0.16% every 3 hours
- Children:
  - 1-6 years: 2-3 drops every 4 hours of 0.125% solution as needed
  - 6-12 years: 2-3 drops every 4 hours of 0.25% solution as needed
- Children >12 years and Adults: 2-3 drops or 1-2 sprays every 4 hours of 0.25% to 0.5% solution as needed; 1% solution may be used in adults in cases of extreme nasal congestion

Nasal decongestant: Oral: Manufacturer's recommendations:

- Phenylephrine hydrochloride salt:
  - Dimetapp® Toddler's: Children 2-6 years: 2.5 mg (1.6 mL) every 4 hours; not to exceed 6 doses/24 hours

(Continued)

Phenylephrine *(Continued)*

NāSop™ tablets:
Children 2-6 years: 5 mg every 4 hours
Children 6-12 years: 10 mg every 4 hours
Children >12 years and Adults: 10-20 mg every 4 hours

Phenylephrine tannate salt:
NāSop™ suspension:
Children 2-6 years: 1.88-3.75 mg every 12 hours
Children 6-12 years: 3.75-7.5 mg every 12 hours
Children >12 years and Adults: 7.5-15 mg every 12 hours

Ah-Chew D®:
Children 6-12 years: 5-10 mg (2.5-5 mL) every 12 hours
Children >12 years and Adults: 10-20 mg (5-10 mL) every 12 hours

Hypotension/shock:
Children:
I.M., SubQ: 0.1 mg/kg/dose or 3 mg/m^2/dose every 1-2 hours as needed; (maximum dose: 5 mg)
I.V. bolus: 5-20 mcg/kg/dose every 10-15 minutes as needed
I.V. infusion: 0.1-0.5 mcg/kg/minute, titrate to desired effect
Adults:
I.M., SubQ: 2-5 mg/dose every 1-2 hours as needed; reported effective dosage range: 1-10 mg; (initial dose should not exceed 5 mg)
I.V. bolus: 0.2 mg/dose (range: 0.1-0.5 mg/dose) every 10-15 minutes as needed (initial dose should not exceed 0.5 mg)
I.V. infusion: 100-180 mcg/minute, titrate to desired effect; once stabilized, a maintenance rate of 40-60 mcg/minute is usually effective

Paroxysmal supraventricular tachycardia: I.V.:
Children: 5-10 mcg/kg over 20-30 seconds
Adults: Initial: 0.25-0.5 mg over 20-30 seconds; subsequent doses may be increased in 0.1-0.2 mg increments; not to exceed 1 mg/dose (maximum dose of 2 mg is recommended by some clinicians)

Treatment of hemorrhoidal symptoms: Children ≥12 years and Adults: Apply to rectal area or by applicator into rectum up to 4 times/day

Administration

Intranasal: Spray or apply drops into each nostril while gently occluding the other

Ophthalmic: Instill drops into conjunctival sac of affected eye(s); avoid contact of bottle tip with skin or eye; finger pressure should be applied to the lacrimal sac during and for 1-2 minutes after instillation to decrease risk of absorption and systemic reactions

Oral: Administer without regard to food; place orally dissolving tablet (NāSop™) on tongue and allow to dissolve

Parenteral: For direct I.V. administration, dilute to 1 mg/mL by adding 1 mL to 9 mL of SWI, then administer dose over 20-30 seconds; continuous infusion concentrations are usually 20-60 mcg/mL by adding 5 mg to 250 mL I.V. solution (20 mcg/mL) or 15 mg to 250 mL (60 mcg/mL); rate of infusion (mL/hour) = dose (mcg/kg/minute) x weight (kg) x 60 minutes/hour divided by concentration (mcg/mL); administer into a large vein to prevent the possibility of extravasation; use infusion device to control rate of flow; administration into an umbilical arterial catheter is **not** recommended

Rectal: Apply to clean and dry rectal area at night, in the morning, or after each bowel movement; when using applicator, remove protective cover from applicator and attach to tube. Lubricate applicator well, then gently insert into rectum. Thoroughly cleanse applicator after each use and replace protective cover.

Monitoring Parameters Heart rate, blood pressure, central venous pressure, arterial blood gases (hypotension/shock treatment)

Nursing Implications Extravasant; avoid I.V. infiltration; extravasation may be treated with local infiltration of phentolamine 5-10 mg diluted in 10-15 mL NS solution

Dosage Forms Excipient information presented when available (limited, particularly for generics); consult specific product labeling. [DSC] = Discontinued product

Cream, rectal, as hydrochloride:
Formulation R™: 0.25% (54 g) [contains sodium benzoate]

Filmstrip, orally disintegrating:
Sudafed PE™: 10 mg (5s, 10s) [contains phenylalanine 1 mg/strip; cherry menthol flavor]

Injection, solution, as hydrochloride: 1% [10 mg/mL] (1 mL, 5 mL, 10 mL) [may contain sodium metabisulfite]
Neo-Synephrine®: 1% (1 mL) [contains sodium metabisulfite]

Liquid, oral:
LuSonal™: 7.5 mg/5 mL (480 mL) [contains phenylalanine; strawberry flavor]

Liquid, oral [drops]:
Dimetapp® Toddler's: 1.25 mg/0.8 mL (15 mL) [alcohol free; contains sodium benzoate; grape flavor]
Ointment, rectal, as hydrochloride:
Formulation R™, Preparation H®: 0.25% (30 g, 60 g) [contains benzoic acid]
Rectacaine: 0.25% (30 g)
Solution, intranasal, as hydrochloride [drops]:
Neo-Synephrine® Extra Strength: 1% (15 mL) [contains benzalkonium chloride]
Neo-Synephrine® Regular Strength: 0.5% (15 mL) [contains benzalkonium chloride]
Rhinall: 0.25% (30 mL) [contains benzalkonium chloride and sodium bisulfite]
Tur-bi-kal®: 0.17% (30 mL) [contains benzalkonium choride]
Solution, intranasal, as hydrochloride [spray]:
4 Way® Fast Acting: 1% (15 mL, 30 mL) [contains benzalkonium chloride]
4 Way® Menthol: 1% (15 mL) [contains benzalkonium chloride and menthol]
4 Way® No Drip: 1% (15 mL) [contains benzalkonium chloride]
Neo-Synephrine® Extra Strength: 1% (15 mL) [contains benzalkonium chloride]
Neo-Synephrine® Mild: 0.25% (15 mL) [contains benzalkonium chloride]
Neo-Synephrine® Regular Strength: 0.5% (15 mL) [contains benzalkonium chloride]
Rhinall: 0.25% (40 mL) [contains benzalkonium chloride and sodium bisulfite]
Vicks® Sinex®, Vicks® Sinex® UltraFine Mist: 0.5% (15 mL) [contains benzalkonium chloride]
Solution, ophthalmic, as hydrochloride: 2.5% (2 mL, 3 mL, 5 mL, 15 mL) [may contain sodium bisulfite]
AK-Dilate®: 2.5% (2 mL, 15 mL); 10% (5 mL) [contains benzyl alcohol]
Altrafrin: 0.12% (15 mL) [OTC]; 2.5% (15 mL) [RX; contains benzalkonium chloride]; 10% (5 mL) [RX; contains benzalkonium chloride]
Mydfrin®: 2.5% (3 mL, 5 mL) [contains sodium bisulfite]
Neofrin™: 2.5% (15 mL); 10% (15 mL)
OcuNefrin™: 0.12% (15 mL)
Relief®: 0.12% (15 mL) [contains benzalkonium chloride]
Suppository, rectal, as hydrochloride: 0.25% (12s)
Anu-Med: 0.25% (12s)
Formulation R™, Preparation H®: 0.25% (12s, 24s, 48s)
Medicone®, Tronolane®: 0.25% (12s, 24s)
Rectacaine: 0.25% (12s)
Suspension, oral, as tannate:
Ah-Chew D®: Phenylephrine tannate (120 mL) [equivalent to phenylephrine hydrochloride 10 mg/5 mL]
NāSop™: 7.5 mg/5 mL (120 mL) [orange flavor]
Tablet, as hydrochloride: 10 mg
Medi-Phenyl: 5 mg
Sudafed PE™: 10 mg
Tablet, orally dissolving, as hydrochloride:
NāSop™: 10 mg [contains phenylalanine 4 mg/tablet; bubble gum flavor]

- **Phenylephrine and Cyclopentolate** *see* Cyclopentolate and Phenylephrine *on page 418*
- **Phenylephrine and Promethazine** *see* Promethazine and Phenylephrine *on page 1328*
- **Phenylephrine Hydrochloride** *see* Phenylephrine *on page 1250*
- **Phenylephrine, Promethazine, and Codeine** *see* Promethazine, Phenylephrine, and Codeine *on page 1329*
- **Phenylephrine Tannate** *see* Phenylephrine *on page 1250*
- **Phenylethylmalonylurea** *see* Phenobarbital *on page 1245*
- **Phenytek**® *see* Phenytoin *on page 1253*

Phenytoin (FEN i toyn)

Medication Safety Issues
Sound-alike/look-alike issues:
Phenytoin may be confused with phenelzine, phentermine
Dilantin® may be confused with Dilaudid®, diltiazem, Dipentum®
International issues:
Dilantin® may be confused with Dolantine® which is a brand name for pethidine in Belgium and Switzerland

Related Information
Adult ACLS Algorithms *on page 1660*
Antiepileptic Drugs *on page 1902*
Blood Level Sampling Time Guidelines *on page 1914*
(Continued)

Phenytoin *(Continued)*

Overdose and Toxicology *on page 1916*

U.S. Brand Names Dilantin®; Phenytek®

Canadian Brand Names Dilantin®

Index Terms Diphenylhydantoin; DPH; Phenytoin Sodium; Phenytoin Sodium, Extended; Phenytoin Sodium, Prompt

Therapeutic Category Antiarrhythmic Agent, Class I-B; Anticonvulsant, Hydantoin

Generic Available Yes: Excludes chewable tablet

Use Management of generalized tonic-clonic (grand mal), simple partial and complex partial seizures; prevention of seizures following head trauma/neurosurgery; ventricular arrhythmias, including those associated with digitalis intoxication, prolonged QT interval and surgical repair of congenital heart diseases in children; epidermolysis bullosa

Pregnancy Risk Factor D

Lactation Enters breast milk/not recommended (AAP rates "compatible")

Contraindications Hypersensitivity to phenytoin or any component; heart block, sinus bradycardia

Warnings Dilantin® 30 mg capsule and oral suspension contain sodium benzoate; benzoic acid (benzoate) is a metabolite of benzyl alcohol; large amounts of benzyl alcohol (≥99 mg/kg/day) have been associated with a potentially fatal toxicity ("gasping syndrome") in neonates; the "gasping syndrome" consists of metabolic acidosis, respiratory distress, gasping respirations, CNS dysfunction (including convulsions, intracranial hemorrhage), hypotension and cardiovascular collapse; use phenytoin products containing sodium benzoate with caution in neonates; *in vitro* and animal studies have shown that benzoate displaces bilirubin from protein binding sites. Injection contains 40% propylene glycol and 10% alcohol.

Precautions Use with caution in patients with porphyria; discontinue if rash or lymphadenopathy occurs; modify dosage in patients with hepatic or renal dysfunction

Adverse Reactions

Dose-related:

- Central nervous system: Slurred speech, dizziness, drowsiness, lethargy, coma, ataxia, dyskinesias
- Ocular: Nystagmus, blurred vision, diplopia

Cardiovascular: I.V.: Hypotension, bradycardia, arrhythmias, cardiovascular collapse (especially with rapid I.V. use)

Central nervous system: Fever, mood changes

Dermatologic: Hirsutism, coarsening of facial features, Stevens-Johnson syndrome, rash, exfoliative dermatitis

Endocrine & metabolic: Folic acid depletion, hyperglycemia

Gastrointestinal: Nausea, vomiting, gingival hyperplasia, gum tenderness

Hematologic: Blood dyscrasias, pseudolymphoma, lymphoma

Hepatic: Hepatitis

Local: Venous irritation and pain, thrombophlebitis

Neuromuscular & skeletal: Peripheral neuropathy, osteomalacia

Miscellaneous: Lymphadenopathy, SLE-like syndrome

Drug Interactions Cytochrome P450 isoenzyme CYP2C9 and CYP2C19 substrate; CYP1A2, CYP2B6, CYP2C8, CYP2C9, CYP2C18, CYP2C19, CYP3A3/4, and CYP3A5-7 isoenzyme inducer

Phenytoin may decrease the serum concentration or effectiveness of lamotrigine, ritonavir, saquinavir, delavirdine, felbamate, valproic acid, ethosuximide, primidone, warfarin, oral contraceptives, corticosteroids, teniposide, etoposide, doxorubicin, vincristine, methotrexate, cyclosporine, theophylline, chloramphenicol, rifampin, doxycycline, quinidine, mexiletine, disopyramide, dopamine, or nondepolarizing skeletal muscle relaxants; protein binding of phenytoin can be affected by valproic acid or salicylates; serum phenytoin concentrations may be increased by cimetidine, chloramphenicol, felbamate, zidovudine, isoniazid, trimethoprim, or sulfonamides and decreased by rifampin, zidovudine, cisplatin, vinblastine, bleomycin, antacids (concurrent administration), folic acid, or continuous NG feeds; suspected interaction with nevirapine (monitor closely); ritonavir may affect the metabolism of phenytoin

Food Interactions Food may effect absorption of phenytoin, depending on product formulation; a high fat meal decreases the rate, but not the extent of absorption of 100 mg Dilantin® Kapseals (Cook, 2001); a high fat meal decreased the bioavailability of a generic extended phenytoin sodium capsule (Mylan) by 13% compared to Dilantin® Kapseals; when taken with a high fat meal, substituting the generic product for Dilantin® could result in a 37% decrease in serum phenytoin concentrations; substituting Dilantin® for the generic could result in a 102% increase in plasma phenytoin concentrations; thus, when taking phenytoin sodium with food, switching products may result in decreased efficacy or increased toxicity (see Wilder, 2001)

Tube feedings decrease phenytoin bioavailability; to avoid decreased serum levels with continuous NG feeds, hold feedings for 2 hours prior to and 2 hours after phenytoin administration, if possible; phenytoin may increase the metabolism of vitamins D and K; dietary requirements of vitamins D, K, B_{12}, folate, and calcium may be increased with long-term use; high doses of folate may decrease bioavailability of phenytoin; avoid giving calcium or magnesium supplements at the same time as phenytoin, space administration by ≥2 hours

Stability Parenteral solution may be used as long as there is no precipitate and it is not hazy; slightly yellowed solution may be used; refrigeration may cause precipitate, sometimes the precipitate is resolved by allowing the solution to reach room temperature again; drug may precipitate with pH ≤11.5; do not mix with other medications. I.V. intermittent infusion: No consensus exists in the literature regarding phenytoin stability in I.V. solutions; due to a low solubility, phenytoin may precipitate in aqueous solutions; some centers have successfully used dilutions of 1-10 mg/mL in NS or LR; infusions should begin as soon as possible after preparation (eg, within 1 hour); diluted solutions should **not** be refrigerated; inspect for particulate matter; discard 4 hours after preparation (see Gannaway, 1983).

Mechanism of Action Stabilizes neuronal membranes and decreases seizure activity by increasing efflux or decreasing influx of sodium ions across cell membranes in the motor cortex during generation of nerve impulses; prolongs effective refractory period and suppresses ventricular pacemaker automaticity, shortens action potential in the heart

Pharmacokinetics

Absorption: Oral: Slow, variable; dependent on product formulation (see Food Interactions); decreased in neonates

Distribution: V_d:
- Neonates:
  - Premature: 1-1.2 L/kg
  - Full-term: 0.8-0.9 L/kg
- Infants: 0.7-0.8 L/kg
- Children: 0.7 L/kg
- Adults: 0.6-0.7 L/kg

Protein binding: Adults: 90% to 95%; increased free fraction (decreased protein binding) in neonates (up to 20% free), infants (up to 15% free), and patients with hyperbilirubinemia, hypoalbuminemia, renal dysfunction, or uremia

Metabolism: Follows dose-dependent (Michaelis-Menten) pharmacokinetics; "apparent" or calculated half-life is dependent upon serum concentration, therefore, metabolism is best described in terms of K_m and V_{max}; V_{max} is increased in infants >6 months and children compared to adults; major metabolite (via oxidation) HPPA undergoes enterohepatic recycling and elimination in urine as glucuronides

Bioavailability: Formulation dependent

Time to peak serum concentration: Oral: Dependent upon formulation
- Extended release capsule: Within 4-12 hours
- Immediate release preparation: Within 2-3 hours

Elimination: <5% excreted unchanged in urine; increased clearance and decreased serum concentrations with febrile illness; highly variable clearance, dependent upon intrinsic hepatic function and dose administered

Usual Dosage

Status epilepticus: I.V.:
- **Loading dose:**
  - Neonates: 15-20 mg/kg in a single or divided dose;
  - Infants, Children, and Adults: 15-18 mg/kg in a single or divided dose
- **Maintenance dose**, anticonvulsant (**Note:** Maintenance dose usually starts 12 hours after the loading dose):
  - Neonates: Initial: 5 mg/kg/day in 2 divided doses; usual: 5-8 mg/kg/day in 2 divided doses; some patients may require dosing every 8 hours
  - Infants and Children: Initial: 5 mg/kg/day in 2-3 divided doses; usual doses:
  - 0.5-3 years: 8-10 mg/kg/day
  - 4-6 years: 7.5-9 mg/kg/day
  - 7-9 years: 7-8 mg/kg/day
  - 10-16 years: 6-7 mg/kg/day
  - Some patients require every 8 hours dosing due to fast apparent half-life
  - Adults: Usual: 300 mg/day or 4-6 mg/kg/day in 2-3 divided doses

Anticonvulsant: Infants, Children and Adults: Oral:
- **Loading dose:** 15-20 mg/kg; based on phenytoin serum concentrations and recent dosing history; administer oral loading dose in 3 divided doses given every 2-4 hours to decrease GI adverse effects and to ensure complete oral absorption
- **Maintenance dose:** Same as I.V. maintenance dose/day listed above. Divide daily dose into 3 doses/day when using suspension, chewable tablets or nonextended release preparations. Extended release preparations may be dosed in adults

(Continued)

Phenytoin *(Continued)*

every 12 or 24 hours if patient is not receiving concomitant enzyme-inducing drugs and apparent half-life is sufficiently long.

Arrhythmias:

Children and Adults: Loading dose: I.V.: 1.25 mg/kg every 5 minutes, may repeat up to total loading dose: 15 mg/kg

Children: Maintenance dose: Oral, I.V.: 5-10 mg/kg/day in 2-3 divided doses

Adults: Loading dose: Oral: 250 mg 4 times/day for 1 day, 250 mg twice daily for 2 days, then maintenance at 300-400 mg/day in divided doses 1-4 times/day

Administration

Oral: To ensure consistent absorption, phenytoin should be administered at the same time with regards to meals; may administer with food or milk to decrease GI upset; 100 mg Dilantin® Kapseals may be administered without regard to meals; shake oral suspension well prior to each dose; separate administration of antacids or tube feedings and oral phenytoin by 2 hours

Parenteral: I.V.: Neonates: Do not exceed I.V. infusion rate of 0.5 mg/kg/minute; Infants, Children, Adults: Do not exceed I.V. infusion rate of 1-3 mg/kg/minute, maximum rate: 50 mg/minute; I.V. injections should be followed by NS flushes through the same needle or I.V. catheter to avoid local irritation of the vein; I.V. intermittent infusion: Dilute with NS to a concentration of 1-10 mg/mL (see Stability), use an in-line 0.22 micron filter; avoid extravasation; avoid I.M. use due to erratic absorption, pain on injection, and precipitation of drug at injection site

Monitoring Parameters Serum concentrations, CBC with differential, liver enzymes; blood pressure with I.V. use; free and total serum concentrations in patients with hyperbilirubinemia, hypoalbuminemia, renal dysfunction, or uremia

Reference Range

Neonates: Therapeutic: 8-15 mcg/mL

Children and Adults:

Therapeutic: 10-20 mcg/mL (SI: 40-79 micromoles/L); toxicity is measured clinically, some patients require levels outside the suggested therapeutic range

Toxic: >20 mcg/mL (SI: >79 micromoles/L)

Lethal: >100 mcg/mL (SI: >400 micromoles/L)

Commonly accepted therapeutic free (unbound) concentration: 1-2 mcg/mL

Patient Information Avoid alcohol; do not change brand or dosage without consulting physician; maintain good oral hygiene

Additional Information The 30 mg/5 mL oral suspension is no longer made; possible permanent cerebellum damage may occur with chronic toxic serum concentrations

A recent study (Relling, 2000) demonstrated that enzyme-inducing antiepileptic drugs (AEDs) (carbamazepine, phenobarbital, and phenytoin) increased systemic clearance of antileukemic drugs (teniposide and methotrexate) and were associated with a worse event-free survival, CNS relapse, and hematologic relapse, (ie, lower efficacy), in B-lineage ALL children receiving chemotherapy; the authors recommend using nonenzyme-inducing AEDs in patients receiving chemotherapy for ALL.

Dosage Forms Excipient information presented when available (limited, particularly for generics); consult specific product labeling.

Capsule, extended release, as sodium: 100 mg

Dilantin®: 30 mg [contains sodium benzoate], 100 mg

Phenytek®: 200 mg, 300 mg

Capsule, prompt release, as sodium: 100 mg

Injection, solution, as sodium: 50 mg/mL (2 mL, 5 mL) [contains alcohol and propylene glycol]

Suspension, oral: 100 mg/4 mL (4 mL); 125 mg/5 mL (240 mL)

Dilantin®: 125 mg/5 mL (240 mL) [contains alcohol <0.6%, sodium benzoate; orange vanilla flavor]

Tablet, chewable:

Dilantin®: 50 mg

References

Bauer LA and Blouin RA, "Phenytoin Michaelis-Menten Pharmacokinetics in Caucasian Pediatric Patients," *Clin Pharmacokinet*, 1983, 8(6):545-9.

Chiba K, Ishizaki T, Miura H, et al, "Michaelis-Menten Pharmacokinetics of Diphenylhydantoin and Application in the Pediatric Age Patient," *J Pediatr*, 1980, 96(3 Pt 1):479-84.

Cook J, Randinitis E, and Wilder BJ, "Effect of Food on the Bioavailability of 100-mg Dilantin® Kapseals," *Neurology*, 2001, 57(4):698-700.

Gannaway WL, Wilding DC, Siepler JK, et al, "Clinical Use of Intravenous Phenytoin Sodium Infusions," *Clin Pharm*, 1983, 2(2):135-8.

Relling MV, Pui CH, Sandlund JT, et al, "Adverse Effect of Anticonvulsants on Efficacy of Chemotherapy for Acute Lymphoblastic Leukaemia," *Lancet*, 2000, 356(9226):285-90.

Suzuki Y, Mimaki T, Cox S, et al, "Phenytoin Age-Dose-Concentration Relationship in Children," *Ther Drug Monit*, 1994, 16(2):145-50.

Wilder BJ, Leppik I, Hietpas TJ, et al, "Effect of Food on Absorption of Dilantin® Kapseals and Mylan Extended Phenytoin Sodium Capsules," *Neurology*, 2001, 57(4):582-9.

♦ **Phenytoin Sodium** *see* Phenytoin *on page 1253*

- **Phenytoin Sodium, Extended** *see* Phenytoin *on page 1253*
- **Phenytoin Sodium, Prompt** *see* Phenytoin *on page 1253*
- **Phillips'® M-O [OTC]** *see* Magnesium Hydroxide *on page 971*
- **Phillips'® M-O [OTC]** *see* Magnesium Supplements *on page 976*
- **Phillips'® Milk of Magnesia [OTC]** *see* Magnesium Hydroxide *on page 971*
- **Phillips'® Milk of Magnesia [OTC]** *see* Magnesium Supplements *on page 976*
- **Phillips'® Stool Softener Laxative [OTC]** *see* Docusate *on page 526*
- **pHisoHex®** *see* Hexachlorophene *on page 767*
- **PHL-Amoxicillin (Can)** *see* Amoxicillin *on page 113*
- **PHL-Azithromycin (Can)** *see* Azithromycin *on page 191*
- **PHL-Citalopram (Can)** *see* Citalopram *on page 368*
- **Phlemex** *see* Guaifenesin and Dextromethorphan *on page 748*
- **PHL-Methimazole (Can)** *see* Methimazole *on page 1022*
- **PHL-Sumatriptan (Can)** *see* Sumatriptan *on page 1495*
- **PHL-Topiramate (Can)** *see* Topiramate *on page 1551*
- **Phos-Flur®** *see* Fluoride *on page 675*
- **Phos-Flur® Rinse [OTC]** *see* Fluoride *on page 675*
- **PhosLo®** *see* Calcium Acetate *on page 263*
- **PhosLo®** *see* Calcium Supplements *on page 272*
- **Phos-NaK** *see* Potassium Phosphate and Sodium Phosphate *on page 1296*
- **Phospha 250™ Neutral** *see* Potassium Phosphate and Sodium Phosphate *on page 1296*
- **Phosphate, Potassium** *see* Potassium Phosphate *on page 1293*
- **Phosphonoformate** *see* Foscarnet *on page 709*
- **Phosphonoformic Acid** *see* Foscarnet *on page 709*
- **Phoxal-timolol (Can)** *see* Timolol *on page 1542*
- ***p*-Hydroxyampicillin** *see* Amoxicillin *on page 113*
- **Phyllocontin® (Can)** *see* Aminophylline *on page 98*
- **Phyllocontin®-350 (Can)** *see* Aminophylline *on page 98*
- **Phylloquinone** *see* Phytonadione *on page 1258*

Physostigmine (fye zoe STIG meen)

Medication Safety Issues

Sound-alike/look-alike issues:

Physostigmine may be confused with Prostigmin®, pyridostigmine

Related Information

Commonly Used Antidotes for Acute Overdoses *on page 1920*

Overdose and Toxicology *on page 1916*

Canadian Brand Names Eserine®; Isopto® Eserine

Index Terms Eserine Salicylate; Physostigmine Salicylate; Physostigmine Sulfate

Therapeutic Category Antidote, Anticholinergic Agent; Cholinergic Agent; Cholinergic Agent, Ophthalmic

Generic Available Yes

Use Reverse toxic CNS and cardiac effects caused by anticholinergics and tricyclic antidepressants

Pregnancy Risk Factor C

Lactation Excretion in breast milk unknown

Contraindications Hypersensitivity to physostigmine or any component (see Warnings); GI or GU obstruction, asthma, diabetes mellitus, gangrene, severe cardiovascular disease; patients receiving depolarizing neuromuscular blockers (eg, succinylcholine)

Warnings Because physostigmine has the potential for producing severe adverse effects, (ie, seizures, bradycardia), routine use as an antidote is controversial; atropine should be readily available to treat severe adverse effects. Injection contains benzyl alcohol and bisulfite which may cause allergic reactions in susceptible individuals; large amounts of benzyl alcohol (≥99 mg/kg/day) have been associated with a potentially fatal toxicity ("gasping syndrome") in neonates; the "gasping syndrome" consists of metabolic acidosis, respiratory distress, gasping respirations, CNS dysfunction (including convulsions, intracranial hemorrhage), hypotension and cardiovascular collapse; *in vitro* and animal studies have shown that benzoate, a metabolite of benzyl alcohol, displaces bilirubin from protein-binding sites; use injection with caution in neonates.

Precautions Use with caution in patients with epilepsy, narrow-angle glaucoma, marked vagotonia, parkinsonism, bradycardia

(Continued)

Physostigmine *(Continued)*

Adverse Reactions
Cardiovascular: Palpitations, bradycardia
Central nervous system: Restlessness, hallucinations, seizures, nervousness
Dermatologic: Burning, redness
Gastrointestinal: Nausea, vomiting, epigastric pain, salivation, diarrhea
Neuromuscular & skeletal: Weakness, muscle twitching
Ocular: Miosis, lacrimation
Respiratory: Dyspnea, bronchospasm, respiratory paralysis, pulmonary edema
Miscellaneous: Diaphoresis

Drug Interactions Additive cholinergic activity with bethanechol and methacholine; succinylcholine

Mechanism of Action Inhibits destruction of acetylcholine by acetylcholinesterase which prolongs the central and peripheral effects of acetylcholine

Pharmacodynamics Parenteral:
Onset of action: Within 3-8 minutes
Duration: 30 minutes to 1 hour

Pharmacokinetics
Distribution: Widely distributed throughout the body; crosses into the CNS
Half-life: 1-2 hours
Elimination: Via hydrolysis by cholinesterases

Usual Dosage
Reversal of toxic anticholinergic effects:
Children: Reserve for life-threatening situations only: I.V.: 0.01-0.03 mg/kg/dose; may repeat after 15-20 minutes to a maximum total dose of 2 mg
Adults: I.M., I.V., SubQ: 0.5-2 mg initially, repeat every 20 minutes until response or adverse effect occurs; repeat 1-4 mg every 30-60 minutes as life-threatening signs (arrhythmias, seizures, deep coma) recur
Preanesthetic reversal: Children and Adults:
I.M., I.V.: Give twice the dose, on a weight basis, of the anticholinergic drug (atropine, scopolamine)

Administration Parenteral: Infuse slowly I.V. without additional dilution at a maximum rate of 0.5 mg/minute in children or 1 mg/minute in adults

Monitoring Parameters Heart rate, respiratory rate

Dosage Forms Excipient information presented when available (limited, particularly for generics); consult specific product labeling.
Injection, solution, as salicylate: 1 mg/mL (2 mL) [contains benzyl alcohol and sodium metabisulfite]

♦ **Physostigmine Salicylate** *see* Physostigmine *on page 1257*
♦ **Physostigmine Sulfate** *see* Physostigmine *on page 1257*
♦ **Phytomenadione** *see* Phytonadione *on page 1258*

Phytonadione (fye toe na DYE one)

Medication Safety Issues
Sound-alike/look-alike issues:
Mephyton® may be confused with melphalan, methadone

Related Information
Compatibility of Chemotherapy and Related Supportive Care Medications *on page 1777*

U.S. Brand Names Mephyton®

Canadian Brand Names AquaMEPHYTON®; Konakion; Mephyton®

Index Terms Methylphytyl Napthoquinone; Phylloquinone; Phytomenadione; Vitamin K_1

Therapeutic Category Nutritional Supplement; Vitamin, Fat Soluble

Generic Available Yes

Use Prevention and treatment of hypoprothrombinemia caused by vitamin K deficiency or anticoagulant-induced hypoprothrombinemia; hemorrhagic disease of the newborn

Pregnancy Risk Factor C

Lactation Enters breast milk/use caution (APP rates "compatible")

Contraindications Hypersensitivity to phytonadione or any component (see Warnings)

Warnings Ineffective in hereditary hypoprothrombinemia and hypoprothrombinemia caused by severe liver disease; severe hemolytic anemia and hyperbilirubinemia has been reported rarely in neonates following large doses (10-20 mg) of phytonadione. Injection contains 0.9% benzyl alcohol which may cause allergic reactions in susceptible individuals; large amounts of benzyl alcohol (≥99 mg/kg/day) have been associated with a potentially fatal toxicity ("gasping syndrome") in neonates; the "gasping syndrome" consists of metabolic acidosis, respiratory distress, gasping respirations, CNS dysfunction (including convulsions, intracranial hemorrhage), hypotension and cardiovascular collapse; *in vitro* and animal studies have shown that benzoate, a metabolite of benzyl alcohol, displaces bilirubin from protein-binding sites; injection is safe in neonates when used in appropriate doses.

Precautions Severe reactions resembling anaphylaxis or hypersensitivity have occurred rarely during or immediately after I.V. administration (even with proper dilution and rate of administration) and with I.M. administration; restrict I.V. and I.M. administration for situations where the subcutaneous route is not feasible

Adverse Reactions See Warnings and Precautions

Cardiovascular: Flushing, hypotension, cyanosis
Central nervous system: Dizziness
Endocrine & metabolic: Hyperbilirubinemia (neonates; greater than recommended dose)
Gastrointestinal: GI upset, dysgeusia, hyperbilirubinemia (neonates)
Hematologic: Hemolysis, hemolytic anemia (neonates; greater than recommended dose)
Local: Pain, edema, tenderness at injection site
Respiratory: Dyspnea
Miscellaneous: Anaphylactoid reactions, diaphoresis

Drug Interactions Antagonizes action of warfarin; mineral oil decreases phytonadione absorption; orlistat may reduce absorption; separate administration by at least 2 hours

Stability Stable at room temperature; protect from light

Mechanism of Action Cofactor in the liver synthesis of clotting factors (II, VII, IX, X)

Pharmacodynamics Onset of action: Blood coagulation factors increase within 6-12 hours after oral doses and within 1-2 hours following parenteral administration; after parenteral administration prothrombin time may become normal after 12-14 hours

Pharmacokinetics

Absorption: Oral: From the intestines in the presence of bile
Metabolism: Rapidly in the liver
Elimination: In bile and urine

Usual Dosage SubQ route is preferred; I.V. and I.M. routes should be restricted for situations when the SubQ route is not feasible

Hemorrhagic disease of the newborn: Neonates: SubQ, I.M.:
- Prophylaxis: 0.5-1 mg within 1 hour of birth; may repeat if necessary 6-8 hours later
- Treatment: 1-2 mg/day

Oral anticoagulant overdose:
- Infants and Children:
  - No bleeding, rapid reversal needed, patient will require further oral anticoagulant therapy: SubQ, I.V.: 0.5-2 mg
  - No bleeding, rapid reversal needed, patient will **not** require further oral anticoagulant therapy: SubQ, I.V.: 2-5 mg
  - Significant bleeding, not life-threatening: SubQ, I.V.: 0.5-2 mg
  - Significant bleeding, life-threatening: I.V.: 5 mg
- Adults: SubQ, I.V.: 2.5-10 mg/dose (rarely up to 25-50 mg has been used); may repeat in 6-8 hours if given by SubQ, I.V. route; may repeat 12-48 hours after oral route

Vitamin K deficiency due to drugs, malabsorption, or decreased synthesis of vitamin K:
- Infants and Children:
  - Oral: 2.5-5 mg/24 hours
  - SubQ, I.M., I.V.: 1-2 mg/dose as a single dose
- Adults:
  - Oral: 2.5-25 mg/24 hours
  - SubQ, I.M., I.V.: 10 mg

Minimum daily requirement: Oral: Not well established
- Infants: 1-5 mcg/kg/day
- Adults: 0.03 mcg/kg/day

Adequate intake:
- 0-6 months: 2 mcg/day
- 7-12 months: 2.5 mcg/day
- 1-3 years: 30 mcg/day
- 4-8 years: 55 mcg/day
- 9-13 years: 60 mcg/day
- 14-18 years: 75 mcg/day
- Adults, male: 120 mcg/day
- Adults, female: 90 mcg/day
- Pregnant, <18 years of age: 75 mcg/day
- Pregnant, >19 years of age: 90 mcg/day
- Breast-feeding, <18 years of age: 75 mcg/day

(Continued)

Phytonadione *(Continued)*

Breast-feeding, >19 years of age: 90 mcg/day

Administration

Oral: May be administered with or without food

Parenteral: SubQ administration is the preferred method (see Precautions); for I.V. administration, dilute in 5-10 mL I.V. fluid (D_5W or NS) (maximum concentration: 10 mg/mL); infuse over 15-30 minutes; maximum rate of infusion: 1 mg/minute

Monitoring Parameters PT, INR (if applicable)

Additional Information Phytonadione is more effective and is preferred to other vitamin K preparations in the presence of impending hemorrhage; oral absorption depends on the presence of bile salts

Dosage Forms Excipient information presented when available (limited, particularly for generics); consult specific product labeling.

Injection, aqueous colloidal: 2 mg/mL (0.5 mL); 10 mg/mL (1 mL)

Tablet: 100 mcg [OTC]

Mephyton®: 5 mg

Extemporaneous Preparations A 1 mg/mL suspension may be made by crushing six 5 mg tablets, add 5 mL purified water and 5 mL 1% methylcellulose, mix well, add 70% sorbitol to a total volume of 30 mL; shake well, refrigerate, expected stability: 3 days.

Nahata, MC, Pai VB, and Hipple TF, *Pediatric Drug Formulations*, 5th ed, Cincinnati, OH: Harvey Whitney Books Co, 2004.

References

Michelson AD, Bovill E, Monagle P, et al, "Antithrombic Therapy in Children," *Chest*, 1998, 114(5 Suppl):748S-69S.

Pilocarpine (pye loe KAR peen)

Medication Safety Issues

Sound-alike/look-alike issues:

Isopto® Carpine may be confused with Isopto® Carbachol

Salagen® may be confused with Salacid®, selegiline

International issues:

Salagen® may be confused with Poagen® which is a brand name for grass pollen extract in Portugal

U.S. Brand Names Isopto® Carpine; Pilopine HS®; Salagen®

Canadian Brand Names Diocarpine; Isopto® Carpine; Pilopine HS®; Salagen®

Index Terms Pilocarpine Hydrochloride

Therapeutic Category Cholinergic Agent; Cholinergic Agent, Ophthalmic; Ophthalmic Agent, Miotic

Generic Available Yes: Hydrochloride solution, tablet

Use

Ophthalmic: Management of chronic simple glaucoma, chronic and acute angle-closure glaucoma; counter effects of cycloplegics

Oral: Symptomatic treatment of xerostomia caused by salivary gland hypofunction resulting from radiotherapy for cancer of the head and neck; and in Sjögren's syndrome

Pregnancy Risk Factor C

Lactation Excretion in breast milk unknown/not recommended

Contraindications Hypersensitivity to pilocarpine or any component; when cholinergic effects such as constriction are undesirable, eg, acute inflammatory disease of anterior chamber, acute iritis; severe hepatic impairment (oral use)

Warnings Reduce dosage in hepatic impairment

Precautions Use with caution in patients with pre-existing retinal disease, CHF, asthma, peptic ulcer, urinary tract obstruction, Parkinson's disease, corneal abrasion, or those predisposed to retinal tears; may occasionally precipitate angle closure by increased resistance to aqueous flow from the posterior to anterior eye chamber

Adverse Reactions

Cardiovascular: Rare hypertension, tachycardia, flushing

Central nervous system: Headache, chills, dizziness

Gastrointestinal (rare): Nausea, vomiting, diarrhea, salivation

Genitourinary: Polyuria

Local: Stinging, burning

Neuromuscular & skeletal: Weakness

Ocular: Ophthalmic formulation: Miosis, ciliary spasm, blurred vision, retinal detachment, photophobia, acute iritis, keratitis, corneal opacities, lacrimation, browache, conjunctival and ciliary congestion early in therapy

Otic: Tinnitus

Respiratory: Rhinitis

Miscellaneous: Hypersensitivity reactions, diaphoresis

Drug Interactions Topical NSAIDs may decrease pilocarpine effect; increased toxicities when combined with other parasympathomimetics; decreased effectiveness with anticholinergics; use with β-blockers may increase risk of conduction disturbances

Food Interactions High fat meals decrease the rate of oral absorption and maximum serum concentration; the time to reach maximum concentrations is also increased

Mechanism of Action Directly stimulates cholinergic receptors in the eye causing miosis (by contraction of the iris sphincter), loss of accommodation (by constriction of ciliary muscle), and lowering of intraocular pressure (with decreased resistance to aqueous humor outflow)

Pharmacodynamics

Ophthalmic solution instillation: Miosis:
- Onset of action: Within 10-30 minutes
- Duration: 4-8 hours

Intraocular pressure reduction:
- Onset of action: 1 hour
- Duration: 4-12 hours

Oral: Increased salivary flow
- Onset of action: 20 minutes
- Maximum effect: 1 hour
- Duration: 3-5 hours

Pharmacokinetics Adults:

Half-life, elimination: Oral: 0.76-1.35 hours
- Mild to moderate hepatic impairment: 2.1 hours

Elimination: Urine

Usual Dosage

Ophthalmic: Children and Adults:
- Gel: 0.5" (1.3 cm) ribbon applied to lower conjunctival sac once daily at bedtime; adjust dosage as required to control elevated intraocular pressure
- Solution: Instill 1-2 drops up to 6 times/day; adjust the concentration and frequency as required to control elevated intraocular pressure
- To counteract the mydriatic effects of sympathomimetic agents: Instill 1 drop of a 1% solution in the affected eye

Xerostomia: Adults: Oral:
- Following head and neck cancer: 5 mg 3 times/day, titration up to 10 mg 3 times/day may be considered for patients who have not responded adequately; not to exceed 10 mg/dose
- Sjögren's syndrome: 5 mg 4 times/day

Dosage adjustment in hepatic impairment: Adults: Oral: Patients with moderate impairment 5 mg 2 times/day regardless of indication; avoid use in severe hepatic impairment

Administration

Ophthalmic gel: Instill gel into affected eye(s); close the eye for 1-2 minutes and instruct patient to roll the eyeball in all directions; avoid contact of bottle tip with eye or skin

Ophthalmic solution: Shake well before use; instill into affected eye(s); apply finger pressure to lacrimal sac during and for 1-2 minutes after instillation to decrease drainage into the nose and throat and minimize possible systemic absorption

Oral: May be administered with or without food; avoid administration with high fat meal

Monitoring Parameters Intraocular pressure, funduscopic exam, visual field testing; salivation (xerostomia treatment)

Patient Information May sting on instillation; notify physician of sweating, urinary retention; usually causes difficulty in dark adaptation; use caution when driving at night or doing hazardous activities in poor light

Dosage Forms Excipient information presented when available (limited, particularly for generics); consult specific product labeling.

Gel, ophthalmic, as hydrochloride (Pilopine HS®): 4% (4 g) [contains benzalkonium chloride]

Solution, ophthalmic, as hydrochloride: 0.5% (15 mL); 1% (2 mL, 15 mL); 2% (2 mL, 15 mL); 3% (15 mL); 4% (2 mL, 15 mL); 6% (15 mL) [may contain benzalkonium chloride]
- Isopto® Carpine: 1% (15 mL); 2% (15 mL); 4% (15 mL) [contains benzalkonium chloride]

Tablet, as hydrochloride: 5 mg, 7.5 mg
- Salagen®: 5 mg, 7.5 mg

♦ **Pilocarpine Hydrochloride** *see* Pilocarpine *on page 1260*

♦ **Pilopine HS®** *see* Pilocarpine *on page 1260*

♦ **Pima®** *see* Potassium Iodide *on page 1290*

Pimecrolimus (pim e KROE li mus)

U.S. Brand Names Elidel®
Canadian Brand Names Elidel®
Index Terms SDZ ASM 981
Therapeutic Category Immunomodulating Agent, Topical
Generic Available No

Use Second-line agent for short-term and intermittent treatment of mild to moderate atopic dermatitis in nonimmunocompromised patients unresponsive to, or intolerant of other treatments

Medication Guide An FDA-approved patient medication guide, which is available with the product information and at http://www.fda.gov/cder/Offices/ODS/medication_guides.htm, must be dispensed with this medication for each new outpatient prescription and refill.

Pregnancy Risk Factor C

Lactation Excretion in breast milk unknown/not recommended

Contraindications Hypersensitivity to pimecrolimus or any component; Netherton's syndrome due to potential for increased systemic absorption; application to site with active cutaneous viral infection (treat and clear infection prior to the start of therapy)

Warnings Pimecrolimus therapy may be associated with an increased risk for eczema herpeticum, varicella zoster, or herpes simplex virus infection; consider discontinuing therapy in patients who develop lymphadenopathy or in patients who have skin papillomas which worsen. Cream contains benzyl alcohol which may cause allergic reactions in susceptible individuals; large amounts of benzyl alcohol (≥99 mg/kg/day) have been associated with a potentially fatal toxicity ("gasping syndrome") in neonates; the "gasping syndrome" consists of metabolic acidosis, respiratory distress, gasping respirations, CNS dysfunction (including convulsions, intracranial hemorrhage), hypotension and cardiovascular collapse.

Precautions Use with caution in immunocompromised patients and in patients who have experienced adverse effects to topical cyclosporine or tacrolimus.

Adverse Reactions

Central nervous system: Headache
Dermatologic: Pruritus, acne, infected hair follicles, skin cancer
Gastrointestinal: Nausea
Local: Burning sensation, stinging
Miscellaneous: Lymphoma

Drug Interactions Cytochrome P450 isoenzyme CYP3A3/4 substrate

No drug interactions have been reported with topical pimecrolimus. However, patients with erythrodermic disease who may experience increased absorption of pimecrolimus should be monitored for evidence of pimecrolimus toxicity when coadministered with a CYP3A4 inhibitor such as erythromycin, itraconazole, ketoconazole, fluconazole, cimetidine, or calcium channel blockers.

Stability Store at room temperature; do not freeze

Mechanism of Action Binds with high affinity to macrophilin-12 (FKBP-12) inhibiting the calcium-dependent phosphatase activity of calcineurin. Inhibits T-cell activation by blocking the transcription and synthesis in human T-cells of early cytokines interleukin-2, interferon gamma (T_h1-type), interleukin-4, and interleukin-10 (T_h2-type). Prevents the release of inflammatory cytokines and mediators from mast cells after stimulation by antigen/IgE.

Pharmacodynamics Onset of action: Time to significant improvement: 8 days

Pharmacokinetics

Absorption: Topical: Low systemic absorption; blood concentration of pimecrolimus was routinely <2 ng/mL with treatment of atopic dermatitis in adult patients (13% to 62% BSA involvement); blood concentration of pimecrolimus was <3 ng/mL in 26 pediatric patients 2-14 years of age with atopic dermatitis (20% to 69% BSA involvement)
Protein binding: 74% to 87%
Metabolism: In the liver by the cytochrome P450 3A4 system
Half-life: Terminal: 30-40 hours
Time to peak serum concentration: Topical: 2-6 hours
Elimination: Primarily in the feces as metabolites

Usual Dosage Children ≥2 years of age and Adults: Topical: Apply twice daily; continue therapy for as long as symptoms persist; re-evaluate patient at 6 weeks. **Note:** Pimecrolimus is not approved for use in children <2 years of age since the drug's long-term effect on the developing immune system is unknown. Children <2 years of age treated with pimecrolimus had a higher rate of upper respiratory infections than those treated with placebo.

Administration Topical: Avoid contact with eyes, nose, mouth, and cut, scraped, or infected skin areas. Wash hands with soap and water prior to and after cream application. Apply thin layer of cream by gently rubbing it in over affected skin surfaces which may include head and neck areas. The use of occlusive dressings is not recommended.

Monitoring Parameters Check skin for signs of worsening condition (increase in pruritus, erythema, excoriation, and lichenification)

Patient Information Avoid exposure to sunlight and artificial light sources (sunlamps, tanning booth/bed); wear protective clothing, wide-brimmed hats, and lip sunscreen (SPF ≥15); use a sunscreen [broad-spectrum sunscreen or physical sunscreen (preferred) or sunblock with SPF ≥15]; contact physician if any signs of serious infection occurs

Dosage Forms Excipient information presented when available (limited, particularly for generics); consult specific product labeling.

Cream, topical: 1% (30 g, 60 g, 100 g)

References

Eichenfield LF, Lucky AW, Boguniewicz M, et al, "Safety and Efficacy of Pimecrolimus (ASM 981) Cream 1% in the Treatment of Mild and Moderate Atopic Dermatitis in Children and Adolescents," *J Am Acad Dermatol*, 2002, 46(4):495-504.

Wahn U, Bos JD, Goodfield M, et al, "Efficacy and Safety of Pimecrolimus Cream in the Long-Term Management of Atopic Dermatitis in Children," *Pediatrics*, 2002, 110(1 Pt 1):e2.

Wellington K and Jarvis B, "Topical Pimecrolimus: A Review of Its Clinical Potential in the Management of Atopic Dermatitis," *Drugs*, 2002, 62(5):817-40.

♦ **Pin-X® [OTC]** *see* Pyrantel Pamoate *on page 1349*

♦ **Pink Bismuth** *see* Bismuth *on page 219*

Piperacillin (pi PER a sil in)

Canadian Brand Names Piperacillin for Injection, USP

Index Terms Piperacillin Sodium

Therapeutic Category Antibiotic, Penicillin (Antipseudomonal)

Generic Available Yes

Use Treatment of serious infections caused by susceptible strains of gram-positive, gram-negative, and anaerobic bacilli; mixed aerobic-anaerobic bacterial infections or empiric antibiotic therapy in granulocytopenic patients. Primary use is in the treatment of serious carbenicillin-resistant or ticarcillin-resistant *Pseudomonas aeruginosa* infections susceptible to piperacillin.

Pregnancy Risk Factor B

Lactation Enters breast milk (small amounts - other penicillins are compatible with breast-feeding)

Contraindications Hypersensitivity to piperacillin, penicillins, or any component

Warnings Superinfection has been reported in up to 6% to 8% of patients receiving an extended spectrum penicillin; piperacillin therapy has been associated with an increased incidence of fever and rash in cystic fibrosis patients

Precautions Use with caution in patients with hypersensitivity to cephalosporins; dosage modification required in patients with impaired renal function

Adverse Reactions

Central nervous system: Seizures, fever, headache, dizziness, confusion, drowsiness

Dermatologic: Rash, exfoliative dermatitis

Endocrine & metabolic: Hypokalemia

Gastrointestinal: Diarrhea, vomiting

Hematologic: Hemolytic anemia, eosinophilia, neutropenia, prolonged bleeding time, thrombocytopenia

Hepatic: Elevated liver enzymes, cholestatic hepatitis

Local: Thrombophlebitis

Neuromuscular & skeletal: Myoclonus

Renal: Acute interstitial nephritis

Miscellaneous: Hypersensitivity reactions, anaphylaxis, serum sickness-like reaction

Drug Interactions Aminoglycosides (antibacterial activity is synergistic), probenecid (increases serum concentration of piperacillin), vecuronium (prolongs neuromuscular blockade)

Stability Reconstituted piperacillin solution is stable for 24 hours at room temperature and 7 days when refrigerated; incompatible with aminoglycosides

Mechanism of Action Inhibits bacterial cell wall synthesis by binding to one or more of the penicillin-binding proteins; inhibits the final transpeptidation step of peptidoglycan synthesis in bacterial cell walls

Pharmacokinetics

Absorption: I.M.: 70% to 80%

Distribution: Crosses the placenta; distributes into breast milk at low concentrations; penetration across the blood-brain barrier is poor when meninges are uninflamed; good biliary concentration (30-60 times higher than serum concentration)

Protein binding: 22%

(Continued)

Piperacillin *(Continued)*

Metabolism: 5% to 10%

Half-life: Prolonged with moderately severe renal or hepatic impairment

Neonates:

1-5 days: 3.6 hours

>6 days: 2.1-2.7 hours

Children:

1-6 months: 0.5-1 hours

6 months to 12 years: 0.39-0.5 hours

Adults: 36-80 minutes (dose-dependent)

Time to peak serum concentration: I.M.: Within 30-50 minutes

Elimination: Principally in urine and partially in feces (via bile)

Dialysis: Dialyzable (20% to 50%)

Usual Dosage Safety and efficacy in children <12 years of age has not been established

I.M., I.V.:

Neonates:

≤7 days: 150 mg/kg/day divided every 8 hours

>7 days: 200 mg/kg/day divided every 6 hours

Infants and Children: 200-300 mg/kg/day in divided doses every 4-6 hours; maximum dose: 24 g/day

Higher doses have been used in cystic fibrosis: 350-500 mg/kg/day in divided doses every 4 hours

Adults: 2-4 g/dose every 4-8 hours; maximum dose: 24 g/day

Dosing interval in renal impairment:

Cl_{cr} 20-40 mL/minute: Administer every 8 hours

Cl_{cr} <20 mL/minute: Administer every 12 hours

Administration Parenteral:

I.M.: Reconstitute each gram of piperacillin with at least 2 mL of SWI, NS, or 0.5% or 1% lidocaine hydrochloride (without epinephrine) to make a 400 mg/mL solution; administer by deep I.M. injection into the gluteus maximus

I.V. push: Administer over 3-5 minutes at a maximum concentration of 200 mg/mL

I.V. intermittent infusion: Administer over 30-60 minutes at a final concentration ≤20 mg/mL

Monitoring Parameters Serum electrolytes, bleeding time especially in patients with renal impairment; periodic tests of renal, hepatic and hematologic function

Test Interactions False-positive urinary and serum proteins, positive Coombs' [direct]

Nursing Implications If the patient is on concurrent aminoglycoside therapy, separate piperacillin administration from the aminoglycoside by at least 30-60 minutes

Additional Information Sodium content of 1 g: 1.85 mEq

Dosage Forms Excipient information presented when available (limited, particularly for generics); consult specific product labeling.

Injection, powder for reconstitution: 2 g, 3 g, 4 g, 40 g

References

Placzek M, Whitelaw A, Want S, et al, "Piperacillin in Early Neonatal Infection," *Arch Dis Child*, 1983, 58(12):1006-9.

Prince AS and Neu HC, "Use of Piperacillin, A Semisynthetic Penicillin, in the Therapy of Acute Exacerbations of Pulmonary Disease in Patients With Cystic Fibrosis," *J Pediatr*, 1980, 97(1):148-51.

Thirumoorthi MC, Asmar BI, Buckley JA, et al, "Pharmacokinetics of Intravenously Administered Piperacillin in Preadolescent Children," *J Pediatr*, 1983, 102(6):941-6.

Piperacillin and Tazobactam (pi PER a sil in & ta zoe BAK tam)

Medication Safety Issues

Sound-alike/look-alike issues:

Zosyn® may be confused with Zofran®, Zyvox®

U.S. Brand Names Zosyn®

Canadian Brand Names Tazocin®

Index Terms Piperacillin Sodium and Tazobactam Sodium; Tazobactam and Piperacillin

Therapeutic Category Antibiotic, Beta-lactam and Beta-lactamase Inhibitor Combination; Antibiotic, Penicillin (Antipseudomonal)

Generic Available No

Use Treatment of sepsis, postpartum endometritis or pelvic inflammatory disease, intra-abdominal infections, including appendicitis (complicated by rupture or abscess) and peritonitis; uncomplicated or complicated infections involving skin and skin structures, the lower respiratory tract, and urinary tract caused by piperacillin-resistant, beta-lactamase-producing strains that are piperacillin/tazobactam susceptible. Tazobactam expands activity of piperacillin to include beta-lactamase producing strains of *S. aureus*, *H. influenzae*, *B. fragilis*, *Klebsiella*, *E. coli*, and *Acinetobacter*.

When piperacillin and tazobactam is used to treat nosocomial pneumonia caused by *P. aeruginosa*, combination therapy with an aminoglycoside is recommended.

Pregnancy Risk Factor B

Lactation Enters breast milk/use caution

Contraindications Hypersensitivity to piperacillin, tazobactam, penicillins, cephalosporins, beta-lactamase inhibitors, or any component

Warnings Prolonged use may result in superinfection, including pseudomembranous colitis; abnormal platelet aggregation and prolonged bleeding have been reported in patients with renal failure; piperacillin therapy has been associated with an increased incidence of fever and rash in cystic fibrosis patients. Severe anaphylactic reactions, including shock, have been reported in patients receiving piperacillin and tazobactam; be prepared to treat anaphylaxis when administering Zosyn®

Precautions Use with caution in patients requiring restricted salt intake, and in patients with renal impairment or pre-existing seizure disorder; dosage modification required in patients with impaired renal function

Adverse Reactions

Cardiovascular: Hypertension, hypotension, edema, chest pain, arrhythmia, tachycardia, cardiac arrest

Central nervous system: Insomnia, headache, dizziness, agitation, confusion, fever, anxiety, convulsions, confusion

Dermatologic: Rash, pruritus, erythema multiforme, Stevens-Johnson syndrome, urticaria

Endocrine & metabolism: Hypokalemia

Gastrointestinal: Diarrhea, constipation, nausea, vomiting, dyspepsia, melena, abdominal pain, pseudomembranous colitis

Hematologic: Leukopenia, thrombocytopenia, neutropenia, decrease in hemoglobin/hematocrit, eosinophilia, prolonged prothrombin time, hemolytic anemia, agranulocytosis

Hepatic: Elevated AST, ALT, bilirubin; hepatitis, cholestatic jaundice

Local: Phlebitis, pain, injection site reaction

Otic: Tinnitus

Renal: Elevated BUN and serum creatinine, interstitial nephritis, renal failure

Respiratory: Dyspnea, rhinitis, pharyngitis

Miscellaneous: Hypersensitivity reactions, anaphylaxis

Drug Interactions Probenecid prolongs half-life of piperacillin/tazobactam; vecuronium (prolongs neuromuscular blockade); aminoglycosides (antibacterial activity is synergistic); may decrease renal clearance of methotrexate; heparin, oral anticoagulants (may increase risk of bleeding)

Stability Reconstituted piperacillin/tazobactam solution is stable for 24 hours at room temperature and 2 days when refrigerated; incompatible with LR solution and aminoglycosides (especially tobramycin)

Note: Reformulated Zosyn® containing EDTA has been shown to be compatible *in vitro* for Y-site infusion with amikacin and gentamicin, but not compatible with tobramycin.

Premixed solution: Store frozen; thawed solution is stable for 24 hours at room temperature or 14 days refrigerated; do not refreeze

Mechanism of Action Inhibits bacterial cell wall synthesis by binding to one or more of the penicillin-binding proteins; inhibits the final transpeptidation step of peptidoglycan synthesis in bacterial cell walls; tazobactam prevents degradation of piperacillin by binding to beta-lactamases

Pharmacokinetics Both AUC and peak concentrations are dose proportional

Distribution: Widely distributed into tissues and body fluids including lungs, intestinal mucosa, female reproductive tissues, interstitial fluid, gallbladder, and bile; penetration into CSF is poor when meninges are uninflamed; piperacillin and tazobactam cross the placenta; piperacillin is excreted into breast milk

V_d: Children and Adults: 0.243 L/kg

Protein binding:

Piperacillin: ~26% to 33%

Tazobactam: 31% to 32%

Metabolism:

Piperacillin: 6% to 9% to desethyl metabolite (weak activity)

Tazobactam: ~22% to inactive metabolite

Bioavailability: I.M.:

Piperacillin: 71%

Tazobactam: 84%

Half-life:

Piperacillin:

Infants 2-5 months: 1.4 hours

Children 6-23 months: 0.9 hour

Children 2-12 years: 0.7 hour

(Continued)

Piperacillin and Tazobactam *(Continued)*

Adults: 0.7-1.2 hours
Metabolite: 1-1.5 hours
Tazobactam:
Infants 2-5 months: 1.6 hours
Children 6-23 months: 1 hour
Children 2-12 years: 0.8-0.9 hour
Adults: 0.7-0.9 hour

Elimination: Piperacillin and tazobactam are both eliminated by renal tubular secretion and glomerular filtration. Piperacillin, tazobactam, and desethylpiperacillin are also secreted into bile.
Piperacillin: 50% to 70% eliminated unchanged in urine
Tazobactam: Found in urine at 24 hours, with 20% as the inactive metabolite and 80% as unchanged drug
Clearance: Children 9 months to 12 years: 5.64 mL/minute/kg

Dialysis: Hemodialysis removes 30% to 40% of a piperacillin/tazobactam dose; peritoneal dialysis removes 21% of tazobactam and 6% of piperacillin

Usual Dosage Zosyn® (piperacillin and tazobactam) is a combination product; each 3.375 g vial contains 3 g piperacillin sodium and 0.375 g tazobactam sodium in a 8:1 ratio. Dosage recommendations are based on the **piperacillin** component.

Infants <6 months of age: I.V.: 150-300 mg of piperacillin component/kg/day in divided doses every 6-8 hours

Infants and Children ≥6 months: I.V.: 240 mg of piperacillin component/kg/day in divided doses every 8 hours; higher doses have been used for serious pseudomonal infections: 300-400 mg of piperacillin component/kg/day in divided doses every 6 hours; maximum dose: 18 g of piperacillin component/day

Appendicitis and/or peritonitis:
Infants 2-9 months: 240 mg of piperacillin component/kg/day in divided doses every 8 hours
Children ≥9 months and ≤40 kg: 300 mg piperacillin component/kg/day in divided doses every 8 hours
Children >40 kg and Adults: I.V.: 3.375 g (3 g piperacillin/0.375 g tazobactam) every 6 hours; maximum dose: 18 g of piperacillin component/day

Adults: Nosocomial pneumonia: I.V.: 4.5 g (4 g piperacillin/0.5 g tazobactam) every 6 hours for 7-14 days

Dosing adjustment in renal impairment: Adults:
Cl_{cr} 20-40 mL/minute: Decrease dose by 30% and administer every 6 hours
Cl_{cr} <20 mL/minute: Decrease dose by 30% and administer every 8 hours

Hemodialysis: Adults: Administer 2.25 g every 8-12 hours with an additional dose of 0.75 g after each dialysis

CAPD: Adults: Administer 2.25 g every 8-12 hours

Dosage adjustment in patients with hepatic cirrhosis: No dosing adjustment required

Administration Parenteral: I.V. intermittent infusion: May administer over 30 minutes at a maximum concentration of 200 mg/mL (piperacillin component); however, concentrations ≤20 mg/mL are preferred. Piperacillin has been shown to inactivate aminoglycosides *in vitro*. Concurrent aminoglycoside administration with piperacillin may pose a risk of reduced antibacterial efficacy *in vivo*, particularly in patients with end-stage renal disease requiring hemodialysis. If the patient is on concurrent aminoglycoside therapy, separate piperacillin and tazobactam administration from the aminoglycoside by at least 30-60 minutes.

Monitoring Parameters Serum electrolytes, bleeding time especially in patients with renal impairment; periodic tests of renal, hepatic, and hematologic function; observe for changes in bowel frequency

Test Interactions Positive Coombs' [direct], false-positive urinary and serum proteins; false-positive urine glucose using Clinitest®; false positive test results using the Platelia® *Aspergillus* enzyme immunoassay (EIA)

Additional Information Sodium content of 1 g piperacillin component in the combination product: 2.79 mEq

Dosage Forms Excipient information presented when available (limited, particularly for generics); consult specific product labeling.

Note: 8:1 ratio of piperacillin sodium/tazobactam sodium

Infusion [premixed iso-osmotic solution, frozen]:
2.25 g: Piperacillin 2 g and tazobactam 0.25 g (50 mL) [contains sodium 5.58 mEq (128 mg) and EDTA]
3.375 g: Piperacillin 3 g and tazobactam 0.375 g (50 mL) [contains sodium 8.38 mEq (192 mg) and EDTA]
4.5 g: Piperacillin 4 g and tazobactam 0.5 g (50 mL) [contains sodium 11.17 mEq (256 mg) and EDTA]

Injection, powder for reconstitution:
2.25 g: Piperacillin 2 g and tazobactam 0.25 g [contains sodium 5.58 mEq (128 mg) and EDTA]
3.375 g: Piperacillin 3 g and tazobactam 0.375 g [contains sodium 8.38 mEq (192 mg) and EDTA]
4.5 g: Piperacillin 4 g and tazobactam 0.5 g [contains sodium 11.17 mEq (256 mg) and EDTA]
40.5 g: Piperacillin 36 g and tazobactam 4.5 g [contains sodium 100.4 mEq (2304 mg) and EDTA; bulk pharmacy vial]

References

Bryson HM and Brogden RN, "Piperacillin/Tazobactam. A Review of its Antibacterial Activity, Pharmacokinetic Properties, and Therapeutic Potential," *Drugs*, 1994, 47(3):506-35.
Reed MD, Goldfarb J, Yamashita T, et al, "Single-Dose Pharmacokinetics of Piperacillin and Tazobactam in Infants and Children," *Antimicrob Agents Chemother*, 1994, 38(12):2817-26.

♦ **Piperacillin for Injection, USP (Can)** *see* Piperacillin *on page 1263*
♦ **Piperacillin Sodium** *see* Piperacillin *on page 1263*
♦ **Piperacillin Sodium and Tazobactam Sodium** *see* Piperacillin and Tazobactam *on page 1264*

Pirbuterol (peer BYOO ter ole)

U.S. Brand Names Maxair™ Autohaler™
Index Terms Pirbuterol Acetate
Therapeutic Category Adrenergic Agonist Agent; Antiasthmatic; $Beta_2$-Adrenergic Agonist Agent; Bronchodilator; Sympathomimetic
Generic Available No
Use Prevention and treatment of bronchospasm in patients with reversible airway obstruction due to asthma or COPD
Pregnancy Risk Factor C
Lactation Excretion in breast milk unknown
Contraindications Hypersensitivity to pirbuterol or or any component
Warnings Paradoxical bronchospasm may occur, especially with the first use of a new cannister
Precautions Use with caution in patients with hyperthyroidism, diabetes mellitus, cardiovascular disorders (including coronary insufficiency or hypertension); excessive or prolonged use can lead to tolerance
Adverse Reactions
Cardiovascular: Tachycardia, palpitations, hypertension, chest pain
Central nervous system: Nervousness, CNS stimulation, anxiety, syncope, hyperactivity, insomnia, dizziness, depression, lightheadedness, drowsiness, headache
Dermatologic: Rash, pruritus, alopecia
Endocrine & metabolic: Hypokalemia
Gastrointestinal: GI upset, xerostomia, glossitis, abdominal pain, vomiting, nausea, unusual taste, hoarseness
Neuromuscular & skeletal: Tremor, weakness, muscle cramping
Respiratory: Irritation of oropharynx, cough, paradoxical bronchospasm
Miscellaneous: Diaphoresis
Drug Interactions Action of pirbuterol is antagonized by beta-adrenergic blocking agents such as propranolol; cardiovascular effects are potentiated in patients also receiving MAO inhibitors or tricyclic antidepressants; concomitant administration of sympathomimetics may result in enhanced cardiovascular effects
Stability Store at room temperature
Mechanism of Action Relaxes bronchial smooth muscle by action on $beta_2$-adrenergic receptors with little effect on heart rate
Pharmacodynamics
Onset of action: 5 minutes
Maximum effect: 30-60 minutes
Duration: 5 hours
Pharmacokinetics
Metabolism: Liver (by sulfate conjugation)
Half-life: 2 hours
Elimination: 51% excreted in the urine as pirbuterol plus its sulfate conjugate
Usual Dosage Oral inhalation:
Acute asthma exacerbation (NIH guidelines):
Children: 4-8 inhalations every 20 minutes for 3 doses then every 1-4 hours
Children >12 years and Adults: 4-8 inhalations every 20 minutes for up to 4 hours then every 1-4 hours
Maintenance therapy (nonacute) (NIH guidelines): Children and Adults: 2 inhalations 3-4 times/day
(Continued)

Pirbuterol *(Continued)*

Administration Oral inhalation: Shake well before administration; "prime" (test spray) inhaler prior to first use and if it has not been used for 48 hours; use spacer for children <8 years of age (Maxair™ Inhaler only); Maxair™ Autohaler™ is breath activated; after sealing lips around mouthpiece, inhale deeply with steady, moderate force; inhalation triggers the release "puff" of medication; do not stop inhalation when puff occurs, but continue to take a deep, full breath; hold breath for 10 seconds, then exhale slowly

Monitoring Parameters Serum potassium, heart rate, pulmonary function tests, respiratory rate; arterial or capillary blood gases (if patient's condition warrants)

Patient Information Do not exceed recommended dosage; may cause dry mouth; rinse mouth with water following each inhalation to help with dry throat and mouth; if more than one inhalation is necessary, wait at least 1 full minute between inhalations; notify physician if palpitations, tachycardia, chest pain, muscle tremors, dizziness, headache, flushing occur, or if breathing difficulty persists

Dosage Forms Excipient information presented when available (limited, particularly for generics); consult specific product labeling.

Aerosol for oral inhalation, as acetate:

Maxair™ Autohaler™: 200 mcg/actuation (14 g) [400 actuations; contains chlorofluorocarbons]

References

"National Asthma Education and Prevention Program. Expert Panel Report: Guidelines for the Diagnosis and Management of Asthma Update on Selected Topics--2002," *J Allergy Clin Immunol*, 2002, 110(5 Suppl):S141-219.

♦ **Pirbuterol Acetate** *see* Pirbuterol *on page 1267*

Piroxicam (peer OKS i kam)

Medication Safety Issues

International issues:

Flogene® [Brazil] may be confused with Florone® which is a brand name for diflorasone in the U.S.

Related Information

Overdose and Toxicology *on page 1916*

U.S. Brand Names Feldene®

Canadian Brand Names Apo-Piroxicam®; Gen-Piroxicam; Novo-Pirocam; Nu-Pirox; Pexicam®

Therapeutic Category Analgesic, Non-narcotic; Anti-inflammatory Agent; Nonsteroidal Anti-inflammatory Drug (NSAID), Oral

Generic Available Yes

Use Management of inflammatory diseases and rheumatoid disorders; dysmenorrhea

Medication Guide An FDA-approved patient medication guide, which is available with the product information and at http://www.fda.gov/cder/Offices/ODS/medication_guides.htm, must be dispensed with this medication for each new outpatient prescription and refill.

Pregnancy Risk Factor C (D if used in the 3rd trimester)

Lactation Enters breast milk (small amounts)/not recommended (AAP rates "compatible")

Contraindications Hypersensitivity to piroxicam, any component, aspirin, or other NSAIDs; active GI bleeding, ulcer disease; patients with the "aspirin triad" [asthma, rhinitis (with or without nasal polys), and aspirin intolerance] (fatal asthmatic and anaphylactoid reactions may occur in these patients)

Warnings In April 2005, the FDA announced product labeling changes for all NSAIDs, including COX-2 selective and OTC medications; although revised product labeling is currently not available for all products, sample labeling and a template of the required medication guide are now available. Labels for prescription nonselective NSAIDs will contain a contraindication for use in patients who have recently undergone coronary artery bypass graft (CABG) surgery and a boxed warning concerning the potential for increased risk of cardiovascular (CV) events and GI bleeding associated with NSAID use. Patients at increased risk of adverse events include patients immediately postoperative from CABG surgery, and those with existing CAD, CVD, or history of TIA or stomach ulcers. Prescribers are encouraged to use the lowest effective NSAID dose for the shortest time based on individual patient treatment goals. Medication guides will be required for all prescription products. Complete details for the labeling update can be found on the following FDA website: http://www.fda.gov/medwatch/SAFETY/2005/safety05.htm#NSAID.

Precautions Use with caution in patients with impaired cardiac function, hypertension, impaired renal function, GI disease and patients receiving anticoagulants

Adverse Reactions

Cardiovascular: Edema

Central nervous system: Dizziness, headache

Dermatologic: Rash, phototoxic skin eruptions, photosensitivity

Gastrointestinal: Nausea, epigastric distress, anorexia, abdominal discomfort, vomiting, GI bleeding, ulcers, perforation

Hematologic: Reduction in hemoglobin and hematocrit, inhibition of platelet aggregation

Hepatic: Elevated liver enzymes, hepatitis

Renal: Acute renal failure, elevated BUN, elevated serum creatinine

Miscellaneous: Anaphylactoid reactions

Drug Interactions Cytochrome P450 isoenzyme CYP2C9 and CYP2C18 substrate

May increase serum concentrations of lithium; aspirin may decrease piroxicam serum concentrations; GI irritants (eg, potassium supplements) may increase GI adverse effects; piroxicam may decrease antihypertensive effects of ACE inhibitors or angiotensin II antagonists; drug interactions similar to other NSAIDs may also occur; concurrent use of piroxicam with ritonavir is not recommended

Food Interactions Food may decrease the rate but not the extent of absorption

Mechanism of Action Inhibits prostaglandin synthesis by decreasing the activity of the enzyme, cyclooxygenase, which results in decreased formation of prostaglandin precursors

Pharmacodynamics Analgesia:

Onset of action: Oral: Within 1 hour

Maximum effect: 3-5 hours

Pharmacokinetics

Distribution: Distributes into breast milk at a concentration of about 1% to 3% of maternal plasma

V_d: Adults: 0.14 L/kg

Protein binding: 99%

Metabolism: In the liver

Half-life: Adults: 50 hours

Elimination: Excreted as metabolites and unchanged drug (~5% to 10%) in the urine; small amount excreted in feces

Usual Dosage Oral:

Children: 0.2-0.3 mg/kg/day once daily; maximum dose: 15 mg/day

Adults: 10-20 mg/day once daily; although associated with increase in GI adverse effects, doses >20 mg/day have been used (ie, 30-40 mg/day)

Administration Oral: May administer with food or milk to decrease GI upset

Monitoring Parameters CBC, BUN, serum creatinine, liver enzymes; periodic ophthalmologic exams with chronic use

Patient Information Avoid alcohol. May cause photosensitivity reactions (eg, exposure to sunlight may cause severe sunburn, skin rash, redness, or itching); avoid exposure to sunlight and artificial light sources (sunlamps, tanning booth/bed); wear protective clothing, wide-brimmed hats, sunglasses, and lip sunscreen (SPF ≥15); use a sunscreen [broad-spectrum sunscreen or physical sunscreen (preferred) or sunblock with SPF ≥15]; contact physician if reaction occurs.

Dosage Forms Excipient information presented when available (limited, particularly for generics); consult specific product labeling.

Capsule: 10 mg, 20 mg

- ♦ ***p*-Isobutylhydratropic Acid** *see* Ibuprofen *on page 802*
- ♦ **Pitressin®** *see* Vasopressin *on page 1602*
- ♦ **Pitrex (Can)** *see* Tolnaftate *on page 1550*
- ♦ **Pit Viper Antivenin** *see* *Crotalidae* Polyvalent Antivenin (Equine) *on page 409*
- ♦ **Pix Carbonis** *see* Coal Tar *on page 394*
- ♦ **Plantago Seed** *see* Psyllium *on page 1347*
- ♦ **Plantain Seed** *see* Psyllium *on page 1347*
- ♦ **Plaquenil®** *see* Hydroxychloroquine *on page 792*
- ♦ **Plaretase® 8000** *see* Pancrelipase *on page 1203*
- ♦ **Plasbumin®** *see* Albumin *on page 64*
- ♦ **Plasbumin®-5 (Can)** *see* Albumin *on page 64*
- ♦ **Plasbumin®-25 (Can)** *see* Albumin *on page 64*
- ♦ **Platinol®-AQ [DSC]** *see* Cisplatin *on page 366*
- ♦ **PMPA** *see* Tenofovir *on page 1506*
- ♦ **PMS-Amantadine (Can)** *see* Amantadine *on page 89*
- ♦ **PMS-Amiodarone (Can)** *see* Amiodarone *on page 100*
- ♦ **PMS-Amitriptyline (Can)** *see* Amitriptyline *on page 107*
- ♦ **PMS-Amoxicillin (Can)** *see* Amoxicillin *on page 113*

- ♦ **PMS-Atenolol (Can)** *see* Atenolol *on page 170*
- ♦ **PMS-Azithromycin (Can)** *see* Azithromycin *on page 191*
- ♦ **PMS-Baclofen (Can)** *see* Baclofen *on page 197*
- ♦ **PMS-Bethanechol (Can)** *see* Bethanechol *on page 215*
- ♦ **PMS-Brimonidine Tartrate (Can)** *see* Brimonidine *on page 231*
- ♦ **PMS-Bromocriptine (Can)** *see* Bromocriptine *on page 232*
- ♦ **PMS-Buspirone (Can)** *see* BusPIRone *on page 250*
- ♦ **PMS-Captopril (Can)** *see* Captopril *on page 277*
- ♦ **PMS-Carbamazepine (Can)** *see* Carbamazepine *on page 279*
- ♦ **PMS-Carvedilol (Can)** *see* Carvedilol *on page 293*
- ♦ **PMS-Cefaclor (Can)** *see* Cefaclor *on page 301*
- ♦ **PMS-Chloral Hydrate (Can)** *see* Chloral Hydrate *on page 331*
- ♦ **PMS-Cholestyramine (Can)** *see* Cholestyramine Resin *on page 349*
- ♦ **PMS-Cimetidine (Can)** *see* Cimetidine *on page 355*
- ♦ **PMS-Ciprofloxacin (Can)** *see* Ciprofloxacin *on page 357*
- ♦ **PMS-Citalopram (Can)** *see* Citalopram *on page 368*
- ♦ **PMS-Clonazepam (Can)** *see* Clonazepam *on page 387*
- ♦ **PMS-Deferoxamine (Can)** *see* Deferoxamine *on page 451*
- ♦ **PMS-Desipramine (Can)** *see* Desipramine *on page 455*
- ♦ **PMS-Dexamethasone (Can)** *see* Dexamethasone *on page 461*
- ♦ **PMS-Diclofenac (Can)** *see* Diclofenac *on page 486*
- ♦ **PMS-Diclofenac SR (Can)** *see* Diclofenac *on page 486*
- ♦ **PMS-Diphenhydramine (Can)** *see* DiphenhydrAMINE *on page 509*
- ♦ **PMS-Dipivefrin (Can)** *see* Dipivefrin *on page 520*
- ♦ **PMS-Docusate Calcium (Can)** *see* Docusate *on page 526*
- ♦ **PMS-Docusate Sodium (Can)** *see* Docusate *on page 526*
- ♦ **PMS-Erythromycin (Can)** *see* Erythromycin *on page 595*
- ♦ **PMS-Famciclovir (Can)** *see* Famciclovir *on page 636*
- ♦ **PMS-Flunisolide (Can)** *see* Flunisolide *on page 669*
- ♦ **PMS-Fluorometholone (Can)** *see* Fluorometholone *on page 677*
- ♦ **PMS-Fluoxetine (Can)** *see* Fluoxetine *on page 681*
- ♦ **PMS-Fluvoxamine (Can)** *see* Fluvoxamine *on page 697*
- ♦ **PMS-Gabapentin (Can)** *see* Gabapentin *on page 716*
- ♦ **PMS-Glyburide (Can)** *see* GlyBURIDE *on page 734*
- ♦ **PMS-Haloperidol LA (Can)** *see* Haloperidol *on page 754*
- ♦ **PMS-Hydrochlorothiazide (Can)** *see* Hydrochlorothiazide *on page 777*
- ♦ **PMS-Hydromorphone (Can)** *see* Hydromorphone *on page 787*
- ♦ **PMS-Hydroxyzine (Can)** *see* HydrOXYzine *on page 796*
- ♦ **PMS-Ipratropium (Can)** *see* Ipratropium *on page 863*
- ♦ **PMS-Isoniazid (Can)** *see* Isoniazid *on page 873*
- ♦ **PMS-Lactulose (Can)** *see* Lactulose *on page 900*
- ♦ **PMS-Lamotrigine (Can)** *see* Lamotrigine *on page 906*
- ♦ **PMS-Levobunolol (Can)** *see* Levobunolol *on page 925*
- ♦ **PMS-Lindane (Can)** *see* Lindane *on page 939*
- ♦ **PMS-Lithium Carbonate (Can)** *see* Lithium *on page 948*
- ♦ **PMS-Lithium Citrate (Can)** *see* Lithium *on page 948*
- ♦ **PMS-Loperamine (Can)** *see* Loperamide *on page 952*
- ♦ **PMS-Lorazepam (Can)** *see* Lorazepam *on page 962*
- ♦ **PMS-Lovastatin (Can)** *see* Lovastatin *on page 964*
- ♦ **PMS-Metformin (Can)** *see* Metformin *on page 1016*
- ♦ **PMS-Methylphenidate (Can)** *see* Methylphenidate *on page 1034*
- ♦ **PMS-Metoprolol (Can)** *see* Metoprolol *on page 1046*
- ♦ **PMS-Minocycline (Can)** *see* Minocycline *on page 1066*
- ♦ **PMS-Mometasone (Can)** *see* Mometasone Furoate *on page 1076*
- ♦ **PMS-Morphine Sulfate SR (Can)** *see* Morphine Sulfate *on page 1082*
- ♦ **PMS-Nizatidine (Can)** *see* Nizatidine *on page 1145*
- ♦ **PMS-Nortriptyline (Can)** *see* Nortriptyline *on page 1149*
- ♦ **PMS-Nystatin (Can)** *see* Nystatin *on page 1156*
- ♦ **PMS-Ofloxacin (Can)** *see* Ofloxacin *on page 1161*
- ♦ **PMS-Oxybutynin (Can)** *see* Oxybutynin *on page 1187*
- ♦ **PMS-Oxycodone-Acetaminophen (Can)** *see* Oxycodone and Acetaminophen *on page 1191*
- ♦ **PMS-Pantoprazole (Can)** *see* Pantoprazole *on page 1208*

- ♦ **PMS-Paroxetine (Can)** *see* Paroxetine *on page 1218*
- ♦ **PMS-Phenobarbital (Can)** *see* Phenobarbital *on page 1245*
- ♦ **PMS-Pravastatin (Can)** *see* Pravastatin *on page 1300*
- ♦ **PMS-Pseudoephedrine (Can)** *see* Pseudoephedrine *on page 1344*
- ♦ **PMS-Ranitidine (Can)** *see* Ranitidine *on page 1366*
- ♦ **PMS-Risperidone ODT (Can)** *see* Risperidone *on page 1388*
- ♦ **PMS-Salbutamol (Can)** *see* Albuterol *on page 66*
- ♦ **PMS-Sertraline (Can)** *see* Sertraline *on page 1429*
- ♦ **PMS-Simvastatin (Can)** *see* Simvastatin *on page 1441*
- ♦ **PMS-Sodium Polystyrene Sulfonate (Can)** *see* Sodium Polystyrene Sulfonate *on page 1460*
- ♦ **PMS-Sotalol (Can)** *see* Sotalol *on page 1463*
- ♦ **PMS-Sucralate (Can)** *see* Sucralfate *on page 1480*
- ♦ **PMS-Sumatriptan (Can)** *see* Sumatriptan *on page 1495*
- ♦ **PMS-Theophylline (Can)** *see* Theophylline *on page 1520*
- ♦ **PMS-Timolol (Can)** *see* Timolol *on page 1542*
- ♦ **PMS-Tobramycin (Can)** *see* Tobramycin *on page 1545*
- ♦ **PMS-Topiramate (Can)** *see* Topiramate *on page 1551*
- ♦ **PMS-Trazodone (Can)** *see* Trazodone *on page 1564*
- ♦ **PMS-Valproic Acid (Can)** *see* Valproic Acid and Derivatives *on page 1592*
- ♦ **PMS-Valproic Acid E.C. (Can)** *see* Valproic Acid and Derivatives *on page 1592*
- ♦ **Pneumo 23™ (Can)** *see* Pneumococcal Polysaccharide Vaccine (Polyvalent) *on page 1273*
- ♦ **Pneumococcal 7-Valent Conjugate Vaccine** *see* Pneumococcal Conjugate Vaccine (7-Valent) *on page 1271*

Pneumococcal Conjugate Vaccine (7-Valent)

(noo moe KOK al KON ju gate vak SEEN, seven vay lent)

Medication Safety Issues

Sound-alike/look-alike issues:

Prevnar® may be confused with PREVEN®

Related Information

Immunization Guidelines *on page 1837*

U.S. Brand Names Prevnar®

Canadian Brand Names Prevnar®

Index Terms Diphtheria CRM_{197} Protein; PCV7; Pneumococcal 7-Valent Conjugate Vaccine

Therapeutic Category Vaccine

Generic Available No

Use

Immunization of infants and toddlers against *Streptococcus pneumoniae* infection caused by serotypes included in the vaccine

Advisory Committee on Immunization Practices (ACIP) guidelines recommend PCV7 for use in:

All infants and children 2-23 months

Children ≥2-59 months with cochlear implants

Children ages 24-59 months with: Sickle cell disease (including other sickle cell hemoglobinopathies, asplenia, splenic dysfunction), HIV infection, immunocompromising conditions (congenital immunodeficiencies, renal failure, nephrotic syndrome, diseases associated with immunosuppressive or radiation therapy, solid organ transplant), chronic illnesses (cardiac disease, cerebrospinal fluid leaks, diabetes mellitus, pulmonary disease excluding asthma unless on high dose corticosteroids)

Consider use in all children 24-59 months with priority given to:

Children 24-35 months

Children 24-59 months who are of Alaska native, American Indian, or African-American descent

Children 24-59 months who attend group day care centers

Pregnancy Risk Factor C

Lactation

Excretion in breast milk unknown/not recommended

Contraindications Hypersensitivity to pneumococcal vaccine or any component of the formulation, including diphtheria toxoid; defer vaccination for persons with acute febrile illness until recovery

(Continued)

Pneumococcal Conjugate Vaccine (7-Valent) *(Continued)*

Warnings Immediate treatment for anaphylactoid or acute hypersensitivity reactions should be available during vaccine use; children with impaired immune responsiveness may have a reduced response to active immunization; use of this vaccine does not replace the use of 23-valent pneumococcal polysaccharide vaccine in children >24 months of age with sickle cell disease, asplenia, HIV infection, chronic illness, or who are immunocompromised

Precautions Administer with caution to patients with thrombocytopenia or any coagulation disorder that would be compromised by I.M. injection; if the patient receives antihemophilia or other similar therapy, I.M. injection can be scheduled shortly after such therapy is administered.

Adverse Reactions All serious adverse reactions must be reported to the U.S. Department of Health and Human Services (DHHS) Vaccine Adverse Event Reporting System (VAERS) 1-800-822-7967.

Central nervous system: Fever, irritability, drowsiness, restlessness

Dermatologic: Erythema, rash

Gastrointestinal: Decreased appetite, vomiting, diarrhea

Local: Induration, tenderness, nodules

Drug Interactions Immunosuppressants: May decrease response to active immunizations

Stability Store refrigerated at 2°C to 8°C (36°F to 46°F).

Mechanism of Action Contains saccharides of capsular antigens of serotypes 4, 6B, 9V, 18C, 19F, and 23F, individually conjugated to CRM197 protein

Usual Dosage I.M.: 0.5 mL; **Note:** Preterm infants should be vaccinated according to their chronological age from birth

Recommended schedule: Age at initiation of immunization: (**Note:** For "catch up" schedule recommendations See Appendix, Immunization Guidelines)

Infants 2-6 months: 4 total doses with the first three doses at least 6-8 weeks apart and the last dose at 12-15 months of age (eg, at ages 2, 4, 6, and 12-15 months); the first dose may be given as young as 6 weeks of age, but is typically given at 2 months of age. In case of a moderate shortage of vaccine, defer the fourth dose until shortage is resolved; in case of a severe shortage of vaccine, defer third and fourth doses until shortage is resolved.

7-11 months: 3 total doses; 2 doses at least 6-8 weeks apart, followed by a third dose at 12-15 months; in case of a severe shortage of vaccine, defer the third dose until shortage is resolved.

12-23 months: 2 total doses, at least 6-8 weeks apart. In case of a severe shortage of vaccine, defer the second dose until shortage is resolved.

24-59 months:

Healthy Children: 1 dose. In case of a severe shortage of vaccine, defer dosing until shortage is resolved.

Children with sickle cell disease, asplenia, HIV infection, chronic illness, or immunocompromising conditions: 2 total doses at least 6-8 weeks apart

Children 24-59 months of age at high risk for pneumococcal disease but have already received the 23-valent pneumococcal polysaccharide vaccine (PS23) may benefit from the immunologic response induced by PCV7. Suggested dosing: Starting ≥2 months after last PPV23 dose: One dose of PCV7, followed by a second dose ≥2 months later.

Children ≥5 years: Children at high risk for pneumococcal disease due to chronic underlying disease may benefit from PCV7 and the 23-valent pneumococcal polysaccharide vaccine (PS23): One dose PCV7; followed with one dose PS23 6-8 weeks later

Administration I.M.: Shake vial well before withdrawing the dose; administer I.M. in either the anterolateral aspect of the thigh or arm; **not for I.V. or SubQ administration**

Patient Information This vaccine is used to prevent bacterial meningitis and ear infections in infants and toddlers. This vaccine will help prevent the disease and stop its spread from person to person. It may be given with other childhood vaccines. Children who are moderately to severely ill should not get this vaccine until they have recovered. This vaccine may be given during a minor illness, such as a cold. Side effects from this vaccine include redness, tenderness, or swelling at the injection site and mild fever. Contact your healthcare provider immediately for high fever, unusual behavior, or signs of allergic reaction (respiratory difficulty, hoarseness or wheezing, hives, paleness, weakness, fast heartbeat, dizziness, or swelling of the throat).

Nursing Implications Federal law requires that the date of administration, the vaccine manufacturer, lot number of vaccine, and the administering person's name, title and address be entered into the patient's permanent medical record

Dosage Forms Excipient information presented when available (limited, particularly for generics); consult specific product labeling.

Injection, suspension:

Prevnar®: 2 mcg of each saccharide for serotypes 4, 9V, 14, 18C, 19F, and 23F, and 4 mcg of serotype 6B per 0.5 mL (0.5 mL) [contains 16 mcg total saccharide; also contains diphtheria CRM197 carrier protein ~20 mcg/0.5 mL and aluminum 0.125 mg/0.5 mL (as aluminum phosphate adjuvant); serotypes grown in soy peptone broth; packaging contains latex]

References

Advisory Committee on Immunization Practices, "Preventing Pneumococcal Disease Among Infants and Young Children. Recommendations of the Advisory Committee on Immunization Practices (ACIP)," *MMWR Recomm Rep*, 2000, 49(RR-9):1-35.

American Academy of Pediatrics Committee on Infectious Diseases, "Recommended Immunization Schedules for Children and Adolescents - United States, 2007," *Pediatrics*, 2007, 119(1):207-8.

Centers for Disease Control and Prevention (CDC), Advisory Committee on Immunization Practices, "Pneumococcal Vaccination for Cochlear Implant Candidates and Recipients: Updated Recommendations of the Advisory Committee on Immunization Practices," *MMWR Morb Mortal Wkly Rep*, 2003, 52(31):739-40.

Centers for Disease Control and Prevention (CDC), "Notice to Readers: Limited Supply of Pneumococcal Conjugate Vaccine: Suspension of Recommendation for Fourth Dose," *MMWR Morb Mortal Wkly Rep*, 53(05);108-9, available at: http://www.cdc.gov/mmwr/preview/mmwrhtml/mm5305a6.htm, last accessed February 13, 2004.

Centers for Disease Control and Prevention (CDC), "Notice to Readers: Pneumococcal Conjugate Vaccine Shortage Resolved," *MMWR Morb Mortal Wkly Rep*, 53(36):851-2, available at: http://www.cdc.gov/mmwr/preview/mmwrhtml/mm5336a8.htm, last accessed September 16, 2004.

Center for Disease Control and Prevention (CDC), "Notice to Readers: Updated Recommendations for Use of Pneumococcal Conjugate Vaccine: Reinstatement of the Third Dose," *MMWR Morb Mortal Wkly Rep*, 53(26):589-90; available at: http://www.cdc.gov/mmwr/preview/mmwrhtml/mm5326a7.htm, last accessed July 12, 2004.

Centers for Disease Control and Prevention (CDC), "Updated Recommendations on the Use of Pneumococcal Conjugate Vaccine: Suspension of Recommendation for Third and Fourth Dose," *MMWR Dispatch*, 53(Dispatch):1-2, available at: http://www.cdc.gov/mmwr/preview/mmwrhtml/mm53d302a1.htm, last accessed March 3, 2004.

Centers for Disease Control and Prevention, "Recommended Childhood and Adolescent Immunization Schedule - United States, July-December 2004," *MMWR Morb Mortal Wkly Rep*, 2004, 53(16):Q1-4.

"Pneumococcal Vaccination for Cochlear Implant Recipients," *MMWR Morb Mortal Wkly Rep*, 2002, 51(41):931.

Reefhuis J, Honein MA, Whitney CG, et al, "Risk of Bacterial Meningitis in Children With Cochlear Implants," *N Engl J Med*, 2003, 349(5):435-45.

Pneumococcal Polysaccharide Vaccine (Polyvalent)

(noo moe KOK al pol i SAK a ride vak SEEN, pol i VAY lent)

Related Information

Immunization Guidelines *on page 1837*

U.S. Brand Names Pneumovax® 23

Canadian Brand Names Pneumo 23™; Pneumovax® 23

Index Terms PPV23; 23PS; 23-Valent Pneumococcal Polysaccharide Vaccine

Therapeutic Category Vaccine

Generic Available No

Use

Children >2 years of age and adults who are at increased risk of pneumococcal disease and its complications due to underlying health conditions (including patients with sickle cell disease, splenectomy, HIV infection, leukemia, lymphoma, Hodgkin's disease, multiple myeloma, generalized immunosuppression, and those receiving immunosuppressive chemotherapy, and patients with cochlear implants)

Current Advisory Committee on Immunization Practices (ACIP) guidelines recommend **pneumococcal 7-valent conjugate vaccine (PCV7)** be used for children 2-23 months of age and, in certain situations, children up to 59 months of age

Pregnancy Risk Factor C

Lactation Excretion in breast milk unknown/use caution

Contraindications Hypersensitivity to pneumococcal vaccine or any component of the formulation; defer vaccination for persons with acute febrile illness until recovery

Warnings Immediate treatment for anaphylactoid or acute hypersensitivity reactions should be available during vaccine use; intradermal administration may cause severe local reactions

Precautions Use caution in patients with severe cardiovascular or pulmonary disease where a systemic reaction may pose a significant risk. Patients who will be receiving immunosuppressive therapy (including Hodgkin's disease, cancer chemotherapy, or transplantation) should be vaccinated at least 2 weeks prior to the initiation of immunosuppressive therapy. Immune responses may be impaired for several months following intensive immunosuppressive therapy (up to 2 years in Hodgkin's disease patients). Patients who will undergo splenectomy should also be vaccinated at least 2 weeks prior to surgery, if possible. Patients with HIV should be vaccinated as soon as possible (following confirmation of the diagnosis). Not recommended in children ≤2 years of age.

(Continued)

Pneumococcal Polysaccharide Vaccine (Polyvalent) *(Continued)*

Administer with caution to patients with thrombocytopenia or any coagulation disorder that would be compromised by I.M. injection; if the patient receives antihemophilia or other similar therapy, I.M. injection can be scheduled shortly after such therapy is administered.

Adverse Reactions All serious adverse reactions must be reported to the U.S. Department of Health and Human Services (DHHS) Vaccine Adverse Event Reporting System (VAERS) 1-800-822-7967.

Central nervous system: Fever, malaise, headache, Guillain-Barré syndrome
Dermatologic: Rash, cellulitis, urticaria
Gastrointestinal: Nausea, vomiting
Hematologic: Thrombocytopenia (stabilized ITP patients); hemolytic anemia (patients with previous history of hematologic disorders)
Local: Erythema, induration and soreness at the injection site (~72%) (2-3 days)
Neuromuscular & skeletal: Arthralgia, myalgia, arthritis, paresthesia, radiculoneuropathy
Miscellaneous: Anaphylaxis, serum sickness, angioneurotic edema

Drug Interactions Decreased effect with immunosuppressive agents

Stability Refrigerate

Mechanism of Action Although there are more than 80 known pneumococcal capsular types, pneumococcal disease is mainly caused by only a few types of pneumococci. Pneumococcal vaccine contains capsular polysaccharides of 23 pneumococcal types which represent at least 98% of pneumococcal disease isolates in the United States and Europe. The pneumococcal vaccine with 23 pneumococcal capsular polysaccharide types became available in 1983. The 23 capsular pneumococcal vaccine contains purified capsular polysaccharides of pneumococcal types 1, 2, 3, 4, 5, 8, 9, 12, 14, 17, 19, 20, 22, 23, 26, 34, 43, 51, 56, 57, 67, 70 (American Classification). These are the main pneumococcal types associated with serious infections in the United States.

Usual Dosage I.M., SubQ: 0.5 mL

Children ≥2 years at high risk for pneumococcal disease:
- One dose PS23 6-8 weeks after last of 1-4 doses of PCV7; revaccinate with PPV23 3-5 years later
- One dose PS23 followed by 2 doses PCV7 6-8 weeks apart; revaccinate with PS23 3-5 years later
- Following bone marrow transplant: Administer one dose PPV23 at 12- and 24-months following BMT

Adults <65 years at high risk for pneumococcal disease: One dose; revaccinate 5 years later

Administration Administer SubQ or I.M. either the anterolateral aspect of the thigh or arm; **not for I.V. or intradermal administration**

Patient Information This vaccine is used to prevent pneumococcal disease which causes bacterial meningitis and pneumonia. Side effects from this vaccine include redness, tenderness, or swelling at the injection site and mild fever. Contact your healthcare provider immediately for high fever or signs of allergic reaction (respiratory difficulty, hoarseness or wheezing, hives, paleness, weakness, fast heartbeat, dizziness, swelling of the throat).

Nursing Implications Federal law requires that the date of administration, the vaccine manufacturer, lot number of vaccine, and the administering person's name, title, and address be entered into the patient's permanent medical record.

Dosage Forms Excipient information presented when available (limited, particularly for generics); consult specific product labeling.

Injection, solution: 25 mcg each of 23 polysaccharide isolates/0.5 mL (0.5 mL, 2.5 mL)

References

Advisory Committee on Immunization Practices, "Preventing Pneumococcal Disease Among Infants and Young Children. Recommendations of the Advisory Committee on Immunization Practices (ACIP)," *MMWR Recomm Rep*, 2000, 49(RR-9):1-35.

American Academy of Pediatrics Committee on Infectious Diseases, "Recommended Immunization Schedules for Children and Adolescents - United States, 2007," *Pediatrics*, 2007, 119(1):207-8.

Centers for Disease Control, "Recommended Adult Immunization Schedule, October 2004-September 2005," available at www.cdc.gov.

Davidson M, Bulkow LR, Grabman J, et al, "Immunogenicity of Pneumococcal Revaccination in Patients With Chronic Disease," *Arch Intern Med*, 1994, 154(19):2209-14.

Gardner P and Schaffner W, "Immunization of Adults," *N Engl J Med*, 1993, 328(17):1252-8.

"Pneumococcal Vaccination for Cochlear Implant Recipients," *MMWR Morb Mortal Wkly Rep*, 2002, 51(41):931.

"Prevention of Pneumococcal Disease: Recommendations of the Advisory Committee on Immunization Practices (ACIP)," *MMWR Recomm Rep*, 1997, 46(RR-8):1-24.

♦ **Pneumovax® 23** *see* Pneumococcal Polysaccharide Vaccine (Polyvalent) *on page 1273*

- **PNU-100766** *see* Linezolid *on page 941*
- **Podactin Cream [OTC]** *see* Miconazole *on page 1056*
- **Podactin Powder [OTC]** *see* Tolnaftate *on page 1550*
- **Podocon-25®** *see* Podophyllum Resin *on page 1275*
- **Podofilm® (Can)** *see* Podophyllum Resin *on page 1275*
- **Podophyllin** *see* Podophyllum Resin *on page 1275*

Podophyllum Resin (po DOF fil um REZ in)

U.S. Brand Names Podocon-25®

Canadian Brand Names Podofilm®

Index Terms Mandrake; May Apple; Podophyllin

Therapeutic Category Keratolytic Agent

Generic Available No

Use Topical treatment of benign growths including external genital and perianal warts (condylomata acuminata), papillomas, fibroids

Pregnancy Risk Factor X

Lactation Enters breast milk/contraindicated

Contraindications Not to be used on birthmarks, moles, or warts with hair growth; cervical, urethral, oral warts; not to be used by diabetic patients or patients with poor circulation; pregnant women; do not apply to normal tissue

Warnings Avoid contact with the eyes as it can cause severe corneal damage; 25% solution should not be applied to or near mucous membranes; podophyllum resin has caused teratogenic effects (skin tags, polyneuritis, limb malformations, septal heart defects) and fetal death when used during pregnancy

Precautions Topical application to large areas or in excessive amounts for prolonged periods should be avoided

Adverse Reactions

Central nervous system: Confusion, lethargy, hallucinations, ataxia, apnea, agitation, seizures

Dermatologic: Pruritus, erythema, scarring

Gastrointestinal: Nausea, vomiting, abdominal pain, diarrhea

Hematologic: Leukopenia, thrombocytopenia

Hepatic: Hepatotoxicity

Local: Pain, local edema

Neuromuscular & skeletal: Peripheral neuropathy, weakness

Renal: Renal failure

Stability Protect from light; avoid exposure to excessive heat

Mechanism of Action Directly affects epithelial cell metabolism by arresting mitosis through binding to a protein subunit of spindle microtubules (tubulin)

Usual Dosage Children and Adults: Topical: 10% to 25% solution in compound benzoin tincture; use 1 drop at a time allowing drying between drops until area is covered; total volume should be limited to <0.5 mL to an area <10 cm^2 for genital or perianal warts or <2 cm^2 for vaginal warts per treatment session; therapy may be repeated once weekly for up to 4 applications for the treatment of genital or perianal warts; use 10% solution when applied to or near mucous membranes

Verrucae: 25% solution is applied directly to the wart; remove drug from area of application within 6 hours

Administration Topical: Shake well before using; use protective occlusive dressing around warts to prevent contact with unaffected skin; apply drug to dry surface of affected area

Patient Information Notify physician if undue skin irritation develops

Nursing Implications Solution should be washed off within 1-4 hours for genital and perianal warts and within 1-2 hours for accessible meatal warts

Dosage Forms Excipient information presented when available (limited, particularly for generics); consult specific product labeling.

Liquid, topical: 25% (15 mL) [in benzoin tincture]

References

Goldfarb MT, Gupta AK, Gupta MA, et al, "Office Therapy for Human Papillomavirus Infection in Nongenital Sites," *Dermatol Clin*, 1991, 9(2):287-96.

"1993 Sexually Transmitted Diseases Treatment Guidelines," *MMWR Morb Mortal Wkly Rep*, 1993, 42(RR-14):1-102.

Poliovirus Vaccine (Inactivated)

(POE lee oh VYE rus vak SEEN, in ak ti VAY ted)

Related Information

Immunization Guidelines *on page 1837*

(Continued)

Poliovirus Vaccine (Inactivated) *(Continued)*

U.S. Brand Names IPOL®

Canadian Brand Names IPOL®

Index Terms Enhanced-Potency Inactivated Poliovirus Vaccine; IPV; Salk Vaccine

Therapeutic Category Vaccine

Generic Available No

Use Provide active immunity to poliovirus

Pregnancy Risk Factor C

Lactation Excretion into breast milk unknown/use caution

Contraindications Hypersensitivity to any component including neomycin, streptomycin, or polymyxin B; defer vaccination for persons with acute febrile illness until recovery

Warnings Although there is no convincing evidence documenting adverse effects of polio vaccine to the pregnant woman or developing fetus, it is prudent on theoretical grounds to avoid vaccinating pregnant women unless the woman is at increased risk of infection and requires immediate protection.

Adverse Reactions All serious adverse reactions must be reported to the U.S. Department of Health and Human Services (DHHS) Vaccine Adverse Event Reporting System (VAERS) 1-800-822-7967.

Central nervous system: Fever (>101.3°F), crying, fatigue, fussiness, sleepiness, Guillain-Barré

Dermatologic: Rash, erythema

Gastrointestinal: Decreased appetite

Local: Tenderness or pain at injection site, reddening of skin

Respiratory: Dyspnea

Drug Interactions Decreased effect with immunosuppressive agents, immune globulin, cholera vaccine; separate by 1 month if possible

Stability Refrigerate

Usual Dosage SubQ: 0.5 mL per dose

Infants and Children: Recommended schedule: A total of 4 doses administered at 2 months, 4 months, between 6-18 months, and between 4-6 years of age

Catch-up schedule: **Note:** Age at initiation of vaccination series:

4 months-17 years: A total of 3 injections 4 weeks apart

Adolescents ≥18 years and Adults: Not routinely recommended unless at increased risk of exposure; a total of 3 doses with second and third doses administered 1-2 months and 6-12 months later; if sufficient time is not available, alternative schedules with three doses given 1 month apart, or two doses given 1 month apart or a single dose have been used depending upon the expediency desired

Administration Administer subcutaneously in either the anterolateral aspect of the thigh or arm; **not for I.V. administration**

Test Interactions May temporarily suppress tuberculin skin test sensitivity (4-6 weeks)

Nursing Implications Federal law requires that the date of administration, the vaccine manufacturer, lot number of vaccine, and the administering person's name, title, and address be entered into the patient's permanent medical record.

Additional Information DTP, MMR, HIB, and hepatitis B vaccines may be given concurrently if at different sites; oral polio vaccine (OPV) is no longer distributed in the United States; OPV is the vaccine of choice for global eradication in areas with continued or recent circulation of wild-type poliovirus, most developing countries where the higher cost of IPV prohibits its use or where inadequate sanitation necessitates an optimal barrier to wild-type virus circulation. (American Academy of Pediatrics, *Red Book*, 26th ed)

Dosage Forms Excipient information presented when available (limited, particularly for generics); consult specific product labeling.

Injection, suspension:

IPOL®: Type 1 poliovirus 40 D antigen units, type 2 poliovirus 8 D antigen units, and type 3 poliovirus 32 D antigen units per 0.5 mL (0.5 mL, 5 mL) [contains 2-phenoxyethanol, formaldehyde, calf serum protein, neomycin, streptomycin, and polymyxin B; packaging contains natural latex rubber]

References

American Academy of Pediatrics Committee on Infectious Diseases, "Recommended Immunization Schedules for Children and Adolescents - United States, 2007," *Pediatrics*, 2007, 119(1):207-8.

Committee on Infectious Diseases, American Academy of Pediatrics, *Red Book: 2003 Report of the Committee on Infectious Diseases*, 26th ed, Pickering L, ed, Elk Grove Village, IL: American Academy of Pediatrics, 2003, 508.

Centers for Disease Control, "Recommended Adult Immunization Schedule by Age Group and Medical Conditions, United States, 2003-2004," available at www.cdc.gov.

Centers for Disease Control and Prevention, "Recommended Childhood and Adolescent Immunization Schedule - United States, July-December 2004," *MMWR Morb Mortal Wkly Rep*, 2004, 53(16):Q1-4.

Gardner P and Schaffner W, "Immunization of Adults," *N Engl J Med*, 1993, 328(17):1252-8.

- **Polocaine®** *see* Mepivacaine *on page 1005*
- **Polocaine® Dental** *see* Mepivacaine *on page 1005*
- **Polocaine® MPF** *see* Mepivacaine *on page 1005*
- **Poly-Dex™** *see* Dexamethasone, Neomycin, and Polymyxin B *on page 464*

Polyethylene Glycol-Electrolyte Solution

(pol i ETH i leen GLY kol ee LEK troe lite soe LOO shun)

Medication Safety Issues

Sound-alike/look-alike issues:

GoLYTELY® may be confused with NuLYTELY®

NuLYTELY® may be confused with GoLYTELY®

U.S. Brand Names Colyte®; GoLYTELY®; MiraLax™; MoviPrep®; NuLYTELY®; TriLyte™

Canadian Brand Names Colyte™; Klean-Prep®; PegLyte®

Index Terms Electrolyte Lavage Solution

Therapeutic Category Laxative, Bowel Evacuant; Laxative, Osmotic

Generic Available Yes

Use Bowel cleansing prior to GI examination (products containing electrolyte supplements only); treatment of occasional constipation (MiraLax™)

Pregnancy Risk Factor C

Lactation Excretion in breast milk unknown/use caution

Contraindications Hypersensitivity to polyethylene glycol or any component; GI obstruction, ileus, gastric retention, bowel perforation, toxic colitis, megacolon

Warnings Seizures associated with electrolyte abnormalities (eg, hyponatremia, hypokalemia) have been reported. Do not add flavorings as additional ingredients before use

Precautions May interfere with barium coating of intestinal wall using the double contrast technique; use with caution in patients with ulcerative colitis; use with caution and observe in patients with impaired gag reflex or those who are otherwise prone to regurgitation or aspiration during administration; treatment duration for occasional constipation should not exceed 2 weeks. Use MoviPrep® with caution in patients with G6PD deficiency; contains ascorbic acid. MoviPrep® contains phenylalanine which must be avoided (or used with caution) in patients with phenylketonuria.

Adverse Reactions

Central nervous system: Malaise, dizziness, headache

Dermatologic: Irritative perineal rashes

Endocrine & metabolic: Mild metabolic acidosis with prolonged irrigation periods, electrolyte disturbances

Gastrointestinal: Nausea, cramps, vomiting, abdominal distention, bloating, dyspepsia

Neuromuscular & skeletal: Rigors

Drug Interactions Increased peristalsis may decrease absorption of oral medications given within 1 hour of beginning lavage solution

Stability

Store at room temperature before reconstitution; use Colyte®, GoLYTELY®, NuLYTELY®, and TriLyte™ within 48 hours of reconstitution; use MoviPrep® within 24 hours of preparation; refrigerate reconstituted solution

Mechanism of Action Induces catharsis by strong electrolyte and osmotic effects

Pharmacodynamics Onset of action: Bowel cleansing: Within 1-2 hours; constipation: 2-4 days

Usual Dosage

Bowel cleansing (to prevent excessive fluid and electrolyte changes, use only products containing supplemental electrolytes for bowel cleansing): Patient should fast at least 2 hours (preferably 3-4 hours) prior to ingestion:

Children: Oral, nasogastric: Colyte®, GoLYTELY®, NuLYTELY®, and TriLyte™: 25-40 mL/kg/hour until rectal effluent is clear (usually in 4-10 hours)

Adults:

Oral: Drink 240 mL (8 oz) every 10 minutes until 4 liters are consumed or the rectal effluent is clear

Nasogastric: 20-30 mL/minute (1.2-1.8 L/hour) until 4 liters are administered

MoviPrep®: Split-dose regimen: The evening prior to colonoscopy: 1 L over 1 hour (one 8 oz glass every 15 minutes) followed by 0.5 L (16 oz) clear fluid; repeat the morning of the study and complete at least 1 hour prior to the start of the study

MoviPrep® Full-dose regimen: Beginning at 6 pm the night before the study and completed before bed: 1 L over 1 hour (one 8 oz glass every 15 minutes) followed 1.5 hours later with a second 1 L over 1 hour; administer an additional 1 L (approximately 32 oz) clear fluid

(Continued)

Polyethylene Glycol-Electrolyte Solution *(Continued)*

Occasional constipation: MiraLax™:
Children >4 years: 0.7-1.5 g/kg daily; not to exceed 17 g/day
Adults: Oral: 17 g (~1 heaping tablespoon) daily

Administration Oral: Colyte®, GoLYTELY®, NuLYTELY®, and TriLyte™: Add tap water to "fill-line" for reconstitution of powder for solution; MoviPrep®: Add 1 L lukewarm water to the contents of 1 pouch A and 1 pouch B and mix together. No solid foods for 2 hours prior to initiation of therapy; rapid drinking is preferred to drinking small amounts continuously; chilled solution often more palatable; do not add flavorings as additional ingredients before use; MiraLax™ 17 g (dose may be measured using bottle cap) added to 8 oz of water

Monitoring Parameters Electrolytes, BUN, serum glucose, urine osmolality

Patient Information Chilled solution is often more palatable

Nursing Implications First bowel movement should occur in 1 hour

Dosage Forms Excipient information presented when available (limited, particularly for generics); consult specific product labeling.

Powder, for oral solution: PEG 3350 240 g, sodium sulfate 22.72 g, sodium bicarbonate 6.72 g, sodium chloride 5.84 g, and potassium chloride 2.98 g (4000 mL)

Colyte®:

PEG 3350 240 g, sodium sulfate 22.72 g, sodium bicarbonate 6.72 g, sodium chloride 5.84 g, and potassium chloride 2.98 g (4000 mL) [available with citrus berry, lemon lime, cherry, and pineapple flavor packets]

PEG 3350 227.1 g, sodium sulfate 21.5 g, sodium bicarbonate 6.36 g, sodium chloride 5.53 g, and potassium chloride 2.82 g (4000 mL) [regular and pineapple flavor]

GoLYTELY®:

Disposable jug: PEG 3350 236 g, sodium sulfate 22.74 g, sodium bicarbonate 6.74 g, sodium chloride 5.86 g, and potassium chloride 2.97 g (4000 mL) [regular and pineapple flavor]

Packets: PEG 3350 227.1 g, sodium sulfate 21.5 g, sodium bicarbonate 6.36 g, sodium chloride 5.53 g, and potassium chloride 2.82 g (4000 mL) [regular flavor]

MiraLax™: PEG 3350 17 g/packet (12s) [DSC]; PEG 3350 255 g (14 oz); PEG 3350 527 g (26 oz) [DSC]

MoviPrep®: Disposable jug: Pouch A: PEG 3350 100 g, sodium sulfate 7.5 g, sodium chloride 2.69 g, potassium chloride 1.015 g; Pouch B: Ascorbic acid 4.7 g, sodium ascorbate 5.9 g (1000 mL) [contains phenylalanine 2.33 mg/treatment; lemon flavor; packaged with 2 of Pouch A and 2 of Pouch B in carton]

NuLYTELY®: PEG 3350 420 g, sodium bicarbonate 5.72 g, sodium chloride 11.2 g, and potassium chloride 1.48 (4000 mL) [cherry, lemon-lime, and orange flavors]

TriLyte™: PEG 3350 420 g, sodium bicarbonate 5.72 g, sodium chloride 11.2 g, and potassium chloride 1.48 (4000 mL) [supplied with flavor packets]

References

Loening-Baucke V and Pashankar DS, "A Randomized, Prospective, Comparison Study of Polyethylene Glycol 3350 Without Electrolytes and Milk of Magnesia for Children With Constipation and Fecal Incontinence," *Pediatrics*, 2006, 118(2):528-35.

North American Society for Pediatric Gastroenterology, Hepatology and Nutrition, "Evaluation and Treatment of Constipation in Children: Summary of Updated Recommendations of the North American Society for Pediatric Gastroenterology, Hepatology and Nutrition," *J Pediatr Gastroenterol Nutr*, 2006, 43(3):405-7.

Sondheimer JM, Sokol RJ, Taylor SF, et al, "Safety, Efficacy and Tolerance of Intestinal Lavage in Pediatric Patients Undergoing Diagnostic Colonoscopy," *J Pediatr*, 1991, 119(1):148-52.

Tuggle DW, Hoelzer DJ, Tunell WP, et al, "The Safety and Cost-Effectiveness of Polyethylene Glycol Electrolyte Solution Bowel: Preparation in Infants and Children," *J Pediatr Surg*, 1987, 22(6):513-5.

♦ **Polygam® S/D** *see* Immune Globulin (Intravenous) *on page 818*

Polymyxin B (pol i MIKS in bee)

U.S. Brand Names Poly-Rx

Index Terms Polymyxin B Sulfate

Therapeutic Category Antibiotic, Miscellaneous; Antibiotic, Ophthalmic; Antibiotic, Urinary Irrigation

Generic Available Yes

Use Topically for wound irrigation and bladder irrigation against *Pseudomonas aeruginosa*; used occasionally for gut decontamination. Parenteral use of polymyxin B has mainly been replaced by less toxic antibiotics. Reserved for life-threatening infections caused by organisms resistant to the preferred drugs; used as inhalation therapy for gram-negative respiratory infections resistant to preferred drugs; used intrathecally for meningeal infections due to susceptible organisms which are resistant to less toxic antibiotics

Pregnancy Risk Factor B

Lactation Excretion in breast milk unknown/use caution

Contraindications Hypersensitivity to polymyxin or any component

Warnings Polymyxin B can cause serious nephrotoxicity and or neurotoxicity; neurotoxic reactions may be manifested by irritability, weakness, drowsiness, ataxia, perioral paresthesia, numbness of the extremities and blurring of vision. These reactions are usually associated with high serum levels found in patients with impaired renal function or nephrotoxicity. Avoid concurrent or sequential use of other nephrotoxic and neurotoxic drugs, particularly bacitracin, kanamycin, streptomycin, paromomycin, colistin, tobramycin, neomycin, gentamicin, and amikacin. The drug's neurotoxicity can result in respiratory paralysis from neuromuscular blockade, especially when the drug is given soon after anesthesia or muscle relaxants. Polymyxin B sulfate is toxic when given parenterally; **avoid parenteral use whenever possible.**

Precautions Use with caution in patients with myasthenia gravis, patients receiving neuromuscular blocking agents or anesthetics, and in patients with impaired renal function; modify dosage in patients with renal impairment; **I.M. use is not recommended in infants and children due to severe pain at injection site**

Adverse Reactions

Cardiovascular: Facial flushing

Central nervous system: Drowsiness, ataxia, fever, dizziness

Dermatologic: Rash, urticaria

Endocrine & metabolic: Hypocalcemia, hyponatremia, hypokalemia, hypochloremia

Local: Pain at injection site, thrombophlebitis

Neuromuscular & skeletal: Neuromuscular blockade, paresthesia

Ocular: Diplopia

Renal: Nephrotoxicity (hematuria, proteinuria, azotemia)

Respiratory: Respiratory arrest

Miscellaneous: Hypersensitivity reactions

Drug Interactions Neuromuscular blocking agents, anesthetics (increase skeletal muscle relaxation); aminoglycosides, colistin, sodium citrate, parenteral quinidine

Stability Protect from light; incompatible with calcium, magnesium, cephalothin, chloramphenicol, heparin, penicillins; inactivated by acidic or alkaline solutions

Mechanism of Action Binds to phospholipids, alters permeability and damages the bacterial cytoplasmic membrane permitting leakage of intracellular constituents

Pharmacokinetics

Absorption: Well absorbed from the peritoneum; minimal absorption (<10%) from the GI tract (except in neonates), from mucous membranes or intact skin

Distribution: Widely distributed to body tissues in the liver, kidneys, heart, muscle; does not penetrate into CSF or synovial fluid; does not cross the placenta

Half-life: 4.5-6 hours, increased with reduced renal function

Time to peak serum concentration: I.M.: Within 2 hours

Elimination: Primarily as unchanged drug (>60%) in urine via glomerular filtration

Dialysis: Not removed by hemodialysis

Usual Dosage Note: Avoid parenteral use when possible

Infants <2 years:

I.M.: 25,000-40,000 units/kg/day divided every 6 hours

I.V.: 15,000-45,000 units/kg/day by continuous I.V. infusion or divided every 12 hours

Intrathecal: 20,000 units once daily for 3-4 days or 25,000 units once every other day; continue 25,000 units once every other day for at least 2 weeks after cultures of the CSF are negative

Children ≥2 years and Adults:

I.M.: 25,000-30,000 units/kg/day divided every 6 hours

I.V.: 15,000-25,000 units/kg/day divided every 12 hours or by continuous infusion; total daily dose should not exceed 2,000,000 units/day

Bladder irrigation: Continuous irrigation of the urinary bladder for up to 10 days using 20 mg (equal to 200,000 units) added to 1 L of NS; usually no more than 1 L of irrigant is used per day unless urine flow rate is high; administration rate is adjusted to patient's urine output

Topical irrigation or topical solution: 0.1% to 0.3% solution used to irrigate infected wounds; should not exceed 2 million units/day in adults

Gut sterilization: Oral: 100,000-200,000 units/kg/day divided every 6-8 hours

Inhalation: 2-2.5 mg/kg/day divided every 6 hours; final concentration for administration should not exceed 10 mg/mL

Intrathecal: 50,000 units once daily for 3-4 days, then reduce to once every other day for at least 2 weeks after cultures of the CSF are negative

Dosing adjustment in renal impairment:

Cl_{cr} 5-20 mL/minute: Administer 50% of usual daily dose divided every 12 hours

Cl_{cr} <5 mL/minute: Administer 15% of the usual daily dose divided every 12 hours

(Continued)

Polymyxin B *(Continued)*

Administration Parenteral (avoid parenteral use whenever possible):

I.M.: Not recommended for routine use in infants and children because of the severe pain which occurs with I.M. injection; administer I.M. injections deep into the upper outer quadrant of the gluteal muscles at a final concentration of 250,000 units/mL

I.V.: Infuse drug slowly over 60-90 minutes or by continuous infusion at a concentration of 1000-1667 units/mL in D_5W

Intrathecal: Reconstitute vial with 10 mL NS without preservatives to provide a final concentration of 50,000 units/mL

Monitoring Parameters WBC, serum electrolytes, renal function tests, serum drug concentration, urine output

Reference Range Serum concentration >5 mcg/mL are toxic in adults

Additional Information 1 mg = 10,000 units; neuromuscular blockade may be reversed with calcium chloride

Dosage Forms Excipient information presented when available (limited, particularly for generics); consult specific product labeling.

Injection, powder for reconstitution: 500,000 units

Powder [for prescription compounding]:

Poly-Rx: 100 million units (13 g)

- **Polymyxin B and Bacitracin** *see* Bacitracin and Polymyxin B *on page 196*
- **Polymyxin B and Neomycin** *see* Neomycin and Polymyxin B *on page 1119*
- **Polymyxin B, Bacitracin, and Neomycin** *see* Neomycin, Polymyxin B, and Bacitracin *on page 1121*
- **Polymyxin B, Neomycin, and Dexamethasone** *see* Dexamethasone, Neomycin, and Polymyxin B *on page 464*
- **Polymyxin B, Neomycin, and Hydrocortisone** *see* Neomycin, (Bacitracin) Polymyxin B, and Hydrocortisone *on page 1119*
- **Polymyxin B, Neomycin, and Prednisolone** *see* Neomycin, Polymyxin B, and Prednisolone *on page 1121*
- **Polymyxin B Sulfate** *see* Polymyxin B *on page 1278*
- **Poly-Pred®** *see* Neomycin, Polymyxin B, and Prednisolone *on page 1121*
- **Poly-Rx** *see* Polymyxin B *on page 1278*
- **Polysporin® [OTC]** *see* Bacitracin and Polymyxin B *on page 196*
- **Polytar® [OTC]** *see* Coal Tar *on page 394*
- **Pontocaine®** *see* Tetracaine *on page 1517*
- **Pontocaine® Niphanoid®** *see* Tetracaine *on page 1517*

Poractant Alfa (por AKT ant AL fa)

U.S. Brand Names Curosurf®

Canadian Brand Names Curosurf®

Index Terms Porcine Lung Surfactant

Therapeutic Category Lung Surfactant

Generic Available No

Use Treatment of respiratory distress syndrome (RDS) in premature infants

Warnings Rapidly affects oxygenation and lung compliance and should be restricted to a highly supervised use in a clinical setting with immediate availability of clinicians experienced with intubation and ventilatory management of premature infants; if transient episodes of bradycardia and decreased oxygen saturation occur, discontinue the dosing procedure and initiate measures to alleviate the condition; produces rapid improvements in lung oxygenation and compliance that may require immediate reductions in ventilator settings and FiO_2.

Precautions Correction of acidosis, hypotension, anemia, hypoglycemia, and hypothermia is recommended prior to administration

Adverse Reactions

Cardiovascular: Transient bradycardia, hypotension

Local: Endotracheal tube blockage

Respiratory: Oxygen desaturation

Stability Store in refrigerator; protect from light; prior to administration, allow to slowly warm to room temperature; artificial warming methods should **not** be used; unused, unopened vials warmed to room temperature may be returned to the refrigerator within 24 hours of warming only once

Mechanism of Action Poractant alfa, an extract of natural porcine lung surfactant, replaces deficient or ineffective endogenous lung surfactant in neonates with respiratory distress syndrome (RDS); surfactant prevents the alveoli from collapsing during expiration by lowering surface tension between air and alveolar surfaces

Usual Dosage Neonates: Intratracheal: Initial: 2.5 mL/kg/dose (200 mg/kg/dose); may repeat 1.25 mL/kg/dose (100 mg/kg/dose) at 12-hour intervals for up to 2 additional doses; maximum total dose: 5 mL/kg

Administration Intratracheal: For intratracheal administration only; suction infant prior to administration; inspect solution to verify complete mixing of the suspension; do not shake; gently turn vial upside-down to obtain uniform suspension; administer intratracheally by instillation through a 5-French end-hole catheter inserted into the infant's endotracheal tube; each dose should be administered as two aliquots, with each aliquot administered into one of the two main bronchi by positioning the infant with either the right or left side dependent; alternatively, it may be administered through a secondary lumen of a dual lumen endotracheal tube as a single dose administered over 1 minute without interrupting mechanical ventilation

Monitoring Parameters Continuous heart rate and transcutaneous O_2 saturation should be monitored during administration; frequent ABG sampling is necessary to prevent postdosing hyperoxia and hypocarbia

Dosage Forms Excipient information presented when available (limited, particularly for generics); consult specific product labeling.

Suspension, intratracheal [preservative free; porcine derived]:

Curosurf®: 80 mg/mL (1.5 mL, 3 mL)

♦ **Porcine Lung Surfactant** *see* Poractant Alfa *on page 1280*

Posaconazole (poe sa KON a zole)

Medication Safety Issues

Sound-alike/look-alike issues:

Noxafil® may be confused with minoxidil

International issues:

Noxafil® may be confused with Noxidil® which is a brand name for minoxidil in Thailand

U.S. Brand Names Noxafil®

Index Terms SCH 56592

Therapeutic Category Antifungal Agent, Systemic; Antifungal Agent, Triazole

Generic Available No

Use Prophylaxis of invasive *Aspergillus* and *Candida* infections in high-risk, severely immunocompromised patients such as hematopoietic stem cell transplant recipients with graft-versus-host disease or those with hematologic malignancies with prolonged neutropenia secondary to chemotherapy; treatment of oropharyngeal candidiasis (including patients refractory to itraconazole and/or fluconazole); treatment of serious invasive fungal infections, including zygomycosis and coccidioidomycosis in patients intolerant of, or refractory to, conventional antifungal therapy

Pregnancy Risk Factor C

Lactation Excretion in breast milk unknown/use caution

Contraindications Hypersensitivity to posaconazole or any component; concurrent therapy with ergot alkaloids (see Drug Interactions); coadministration with terfenadine, astemizole, cisapride, pimozide, halofantrine, or quinidine (posaconazole may increase plasma concentrations of these agents resulting in QT_c prolongation and rarely, torsade de pointes)

Warnings Hepatotoxicity including hepatitis, cholestasis, hepatic failure and elevations in ALT, AST, alkaline phosphatase, and total bilirubin have been reported. Liver function tests and bilirubin should be monitored at the start and during posaconazole therapy.

Elevated cyclosporine levels resulting in nephrotoxicity, leukoencephalopathy, and death have been reported in patients on concurrent therapy with posaconazole. Dose adjustment and more frequent clinical monitoring of cyclosporine, tacrolimus, and sirolimus should be performed when posaconazole therapy is initiated in patients on these medications.

Oral suspension contains sodium benzoate; benzoic acid (benzoate) is a metabolite of benzyl alcohol; large amounts of benzyl alcohol (≥99 mg/kg/day) have been associated with a potentially fatal toxicity ("gasping syndrome") in neonates; use oral suspension containing sodium benzoate with caution in neonates; *in vitro* and animal studies have shown that benzoate displaces bilirubin from protein-binding sites

Precautions Use caution in patients with hypersensitivity to other azole antifungal agents since cross-reaction may occur but has not yet been established. Use with caution in patients with proarrhythmic conditions since posaconazole has been associated with QT interval prolongation and torsade de pointes; do not administer with medications known to prolong the QT_c interval and are metabolized through the CYP3A4 system. Use with caution in patients with hepatic impairment or severe renal impairment (CL_{cr} <20 mL/minute/1.73m^2); monitor for breakthrough fungal infection in patients with severe renal impairment.

(Continued)

Posaconazole *(Continued)*

Adverse Reactions

Cardiovascular: Edema, hypertension, tachycardia, QT/QT_c prolongation

Central nervous system: Headache, fever, dizziness, fatigue, insomnia, anxiety

Dermatologic: Rash, pruritus

Endocrine & metabolic: Hypokalemia, hypomagnesemia, hyperglycemia, hypocalcemia

Gastrointestinal: Nausea, vomiting, abdominal pain, diarrhea, dry mouth, anorexia, mucositis, dyspepsia, taste perversion, constipation

Hematologic: Anemia, neutropenia, thrombocytopenia

Hepatic: Elevated bilirubin, ALT, AST, and alkaline phosphatase; hepatitis

Neuromuscular & skeletal: Weakness, myalgia, tremor, arthralgia

Ocular: Blurred vision

Renal: Elevated serum creatinine

Respiratory: Coughing, dyspnea

Drug Interactions Coadministration with cimetidine, rifabutin, or phenytoin may decrease posaconazole levels (avoid concomitant use with posaconazole unless benefit outweighs the risks); posaconazole may increase cyclosporine, tacrolimus levels (adjust cyclosporine or tacrolimus dose; monitor blood trough concentrations of cyclosporine and tacrolimus frequently). Posaconazole may increase rifabutin concentration (avoid concomitant use if possible; if coadministration is required, frequent monitoring of CBC and signs of uveitis is recommended); posaconazole may increase midazolam or phenytoin concentrations (adjust dose; frequent monitoring for adverse effects related to these agents and monitoring phenytoin concentrations).

Posaconazole may increase levels of terfenadine, astemizole, pimozide, cisapride, and quinidine which can lead to QT prolongation (coadministration with posaconazole is contraindicated); posaconazole increases levels of ergot alkaloids which may lead to ergotism (coadministration of ergot alkaloids with posaconazole is contraindicated). Posaconazole may increase levels of vincristine, vinblastine, sirolimus, HMG-CoA reductase inhibitors (statins), and calcium channel blockers metabolized through CYP3A4 which includes felodipine, nifedipine, and verapamil (consider dose reduction of these drugs, frequent monitoring of adverse events related to these agents, and monitoring sirolimus concentrations).

Food Interactions Posaconazole AUC and C_{max} are 3 times higher when administered with a nonfat meal and 4 times higher if administered with a high fat meal relative to a fasted state

Stability Store at room temperature; do not freeze.

Mechanism of Action Inhibits the enzyme 14 α-sterol demethylase, an essential enzyme in ergosterol biosynthesis resulting in the inhibition of fungal cell membrane formation.

Pharmacokinetics

Absorption: Food and/or liquid nutritional supplements increase absorption

Distribution: V_d: Adults: 1774 L; extensive extravascular distribution and penetration into body tissues

Protein binding: >98%

Metabolism: Undergoes hepatic glucuronidation to form glucuronide conjugates; substrate for p-glycoprotein efflux

Half-life: 35 hours (range: 20-66 hours)

Time to peak serum concentration: 3-5 hours

Elimination: 71% (66% as unchanged drug) eliminated in feces; <0.2% as unchanged drug excreted in urine

Dialysis: Not removed by hemodialysis

Usual Dosage Oral: Children ≥13 years and Adults:

Prophylaxis of invasive *Aspergillus* and *Candida* infections: 200 mg 3 times/day

Treatment of refractory invasive fungal infections: 800 mg/day in divided doses (ie, 400 mg 2 times/day or 200 mg 4 times/day)

Treatment of oropharyngeal candidiasis: Initial: 100 mg 2 times/day on day 1; maintenance: 100 mg once daily for 13 days

Treatment of refractory oropharyngeal candidiasis: 400 mg 2 times/day

Dosage adjustment in renal impairment: No adjustment is necessary; monitor for breakthrough fungal infection in patients with CL_{cr} <20 mL/minute/1.73 m^2

Dosage adjustment in hepatic impairment: No adjustment necessary

Administration Oral: Shake suspension before use. Administer with a full meal or with a liquid nutritional supplement. For patients who cannot tolerate a full meal or an oral liquid nutritional supplement, alternative antifungal therapy should be considered.

Monitoring Parameters Hepatic function tests and bilirubin, serum electrolytes, serum creatinine, ECG

Patient Information Inform physician if severe diarrhea or vomiting, chest pain or palpitations, yellowing of eyes or skin, changes in color of urine or stool, weakness or tremor, or changes in vision occur.

Additional Information Dextrose content (oral suspension): 350 mg/mL

Dosage Forms Excipient information presented when available (limited, particularly for generics); consult specific product labeling.

Suspension, oral:

Noxafil®: 40 mg/mL (123 mL) [contains sodium benzoate; delivers 105 mL of suspension; cherry flavor; packaged with calibrated dosing spoon]

References

Greenberg RN, Mullane K, vanBurik JA, et al, "Posaconazole As Salvage Therapy for Zygomycosis," *Antimicrob Agents Chemother*, 2006, 50(1):126-33.

Gubbins PO, Krishna G, Sansone-Parsons A, et al, "Pharmacokinetics and Safety of Oral Posaconazole in Neutropenic Stem Cell Transplant Recipients," *Antimicrob Agents Chemother*, 2006, 50(6):1993-9.

Walsh TJ, Raad I, Patterson TF, et al, "Treatment of Invasive Aspergillosis With Posaconazole in Patients Who Are Refractory to or Intolerant of Conventional Therapy: An Externally Controlled Trial," *Clin Infect Dis*, 2007, 44(1):2-12.

♦ **Post Peel Healing Balm [OTC]** *see* Hydrocortisone *on page 781*

♦ **Posture® [OTC]** *see* Calcium Phosphate, Tribasic *on page 271*

♦ **Posture®** *see* Calcium Supplements *on page 272*

Potassium Acetate (poe TASS ee um AS e tate)

Medication Safety Issues

Consider special storage requirements for intravenous potassium salts; I.V. potassium salts have been administered IVP in error, leading to fatal outcomes.

Therapeutic Category Electrolyte Supplement, Parenteral

Generic Available Yes

Use Treatment and prevention of hypokalemia when it is necessary to avoid chloride or acid/base status requires an additional source of bicarbonate

Pregnancy Risk Factor C

Contraindications Hypersensitivity to any component of the potassium supplement; severe renal impairment, untreated Addison's disease, heat cramps, hyperkalemia, severe tissue trauma

Warnings Potassium acetate should be administered only in patients with adequate urine flow; must be diluted before I.V. use and infused slowly (see Administration)

Precautions Use with caution in patients with cardiac disease, patients receiving potassium-sparing drugs; patients should be on a cardiac monitor during intermittent infusions for doses >0.5 mEq/kg/hour or 5mEq/hour (adults); solution for injection contains aluminum; use caution with impaired renal function and in premature infants

Adverse Reactions

Cardiovascular (with rapid I.V. administration): Arrhythmias and cardiac arrest, heart block, hypotension

Central nervous system: Mental confusion

Endocrine & metabolic: Hyperkalemia, metabolic alkalosis

Local: Pain at the site of injection, phlebitis

Neuromuscular & skeletal: Muscle weakness, paresthesia, flaccid paralysis

Respiratory: Dyspnea

Drug Interactions Potassium-sparing diuretics, salt substitutes, and ACE inhibitors may result in increased serum potassium.

Stability Store at room temperature; do not freeze

Mechanism of Action Potassium is the major cation of intracellular fluid and is essential for the conduction of nerve impulses in heart, brain, and skeletal muscle; contraction of cardiac, skeletal, and smooth muscles; maintenance of normal renal function, acid-base balance, carbohydrate metabolism, and gastric secretion

Pharmacokinetics

Distribution: Enters cells via active transport from extracellular fluid

Elimination: Primarily urine; skin and feces (small amounts); most intestinal potassium reabsorbed

Usual Dosage I.V. doses should be incorporated into the patient's maintenance I.V. fluids; intermittent I.V. potassium administration should be reserved for severe depletion situations; continuous EKG monitoring should be used for intermittent doses >0.5 mEq/kg/hour. **Note:** Doses listed as mEq of **potassium**.

Normal daily requirement: I.V.:

Neonates >24 hours of age and Infants: 2-6 mEq/kg/day

Children: 2-3 mEq/kg/day

Adults: 40-80 mEq/day

(Continued)

Potassium Acetate *(Continued)*

Treatment of hypokalemia:

Neonates, Infants, and Children:

I.V. intermittent infusion (must be diluted prior to administration): 0.5-1 mEq/kg/dose (maximum dose: 40 mEq) to infuse at 0.3-0.5 mEq/kg/hour (maximum dose/rate: 1 mEq/kg/hour); then repeated as needed based on frequently obtained lab values; severe depletion or ongoing losses may require >200% of normal daily limit needs

Adults:

I.V. intermittent infusion: 5-10 mEq/hour (continuous cardiac monitor recommended for rates >5 mEq/hour), not to exceed 40 mEq/hour; usual adult maximum per 24 hours: 400 mEq

Potassium dosage/rate of infusion guidelines:

Serum potassium ≥2.5 mEq/L (and <desired): 10 mEq with additional doses if needed; maximum infusion rate: 10 mEq/hour; maximum 24-hour dose: 200 mEq

Serum potassium <2.5 mEq/L: Up to 40 mEq with additional doses based upon frequent lab monitoring; maximum infusion rate: 40 mEq/hour; maximum 24-hour dose: 400 mEq; deficits at a plasma level of 2 mEq/L may be as high as 400-800 mEq of potassium

Administration Parenteral: Potassium must be diluted prior to parenteral administration; maximum recommended concentration (peripheral line): 80 mEq/L; maximum recommended concentration (central line): 150 mEq/L or 15 mEq/100 mL; in severely fluid-restricted patients (with central lines): 200 mEq/L or 20 mEq/100 mL has been used; maximum rate of infusion, see Usual Dosage, I.V. intermittent infusion

Monitoring Parameters Serum potassium, glucose, chloride, pH, urine output (if indicated), cardiac monitor [if intermittent I.V. infusion or potassium I.V. infusion rates >0.5 mEq/kg/hour or 5 mEq/hour (adults)]

Additional Information 1 mEq of acetate is equivalent to the alkalinizing effect of 1 mEq of bicarbonate. Hypokalemia is highly arrhythmogenic, particularly in the setting of ischemia or digitalis toxicity. ECG evidence of hypokalemia includes flattening of the T wave. As the T wave shrinks, U waves may appear. There is no prolongation of the QT interval. Hyperkalemia may present as tall peaked symmetrical T waves. S-T elevation may present in severe hyperkalemia. QRS complex progressively widens with eventual apparent sine waves on the ECG. Hyperkalemia will also induce cardiac slowing and AV conduction abnormalities.

Dosage Forms Excipient information presented when available (limited, particularly for generics); consult specific product labeling.

Injection, solution: 2 mEq/mL (20 mL, 50 mL, 100 mL) [contains aluminum]

Injection, solution [concentrate]: 4 mEq/mL (50 mL) [contains aluminum]

References

Hamill RJ, Robinson LM, Wexler HR, et al, "Efficacy and Safety of Potassium Infusion Therapy in Hypokalemic Critically Ill Patients," *Crit Care Med*, 1991, 19(5):694-9.

Khilnani P, "Electrolyte Abnormalities in Critically Ill Children," *Crit Care Med*, 1992, 20(2):241-50.

Potassium Bicarbonate (poe TASS ee um bye KAR bun ate)

Therapeutic Category Electrolyte Supplement, Oral

Generic Available Yes

Use Treatment and prevention of hypokalemia when it is necessary to avoid chloride or acid/base status requires bicarbonate

Pregnancy Risk Factor C

Contraindications Hypersensitivity to any component of the potassium supplement; severe renal impairment, untreated Addison's disease, heat cramps, hyperkalemia, severe tissue trauma; solid oral dosage forms are contraindicated in patients in whom there is a structural, pathological, and/or pharmacologic cause for delay or arrest in passage through the GI tract

Precautions Use with caution in patients with cardiac and/or renal disease, patients receiving potassium-sparing drugs

Adverse Reactions

Central nervous system: Mental confusion

Endocrine & metabolic: Hyperkalemia, metabolic alkalosis

Gastrointestinal: Nausea, vomiting, diarrhea, abdominal pain, GI lesions, flatulence

Neuromuscular & skeletal: Muscle weakness, paresthesia, flaccid paralysis

Drug Interactions Potassium-sparing diuretics, salt substitutes, and ACE inhibitors may result in increased serum potassium.

Stability Store at room temperature.

Mechanism of Action Potassium is the major cation of intracellular fluid and is essential for the conduction of nerve impulses in heart, brain, and skeletal muscle; contraction of cardiac, skeletal, and smooth muscles; maintenance of normal renal function, acid-base balance, carbohydrate metabolism, and gastric secretion. Bicarbonate neutralizes hydrogen ion concentration and raises blood and urinary pH .

Pharmacokinetics

Absorption: Well absorbed from upper GI tract

Distribution: Enters cells via active transport from extracellular fluid

Elimination: Primarily urine; skin and feces (small amounts); most intestinal potassium reabsorbed

Usual Dosage Oral (doses listed as mEq of **potassium**):

Normal daily requirement:

Children: 2-3 mEq/kg/day

Adults: 40-80 mEq/day

Prevention of hypokalemia during diuretic therapy:

Children: 1-2 mEq/kg/day in 1-2 divided doses

Adults: 25-100 mEq/day in 2-4 divided doses

Administration Oral: Dissolve completely in 3-8 oz cold water, juice, or other suitable beverage and drink slowly

Monitoring Parameters Serum potassium, chloride, glucose, pH, urine output (if indicated)

Additional Information Hypokalemia is highly arrhythmogenic, particularly in the setting of ischemia or digitalis toxicity. ECG evidence of hypokalemia includes flattening of the T wave. As the T wave shrinks, U waves may appear. There is no prolongation of the QT interval. Hyperkalemia may present as tall peaked symmetrical T waves. S-T elevation may present in severe hyperkalemia. QRS complex progressively widens with eventual apparent sine waves on the ECG. Hyperkalemia will also induce cardiac slowing and AV conduction abnormalities.

Dosage Forms Excipient information presented when available (limited, particularly for generics); consult specific product labeling.

Tablet for oral solution, effervescent: Potassium 25 mEq

Potassium Bicarbonate and Potassium Chloride

(poe TASS ee um bye KAR bun ate & poe TASS ee um KLOR ide)

Related Information

Potassium Bicarbonate *on page 1284*

Potassium Chloride *on page 1287*

U.S. Brand Names K-Lyte/Cl®

Index Terms Potassium Bicarbonate and Potassium Chloride (Effervescent)

Therapeutic Category Electrolyte Supplement, Oral

Generic Available Yes

Use Treatment or prevention of hypokalemia

Pregnancy Risk Factor C

Lactation Enters breast milk/compatible

Contraindications Hypersensitivity to any component of the potassium supplement; severe renal impairment, untreated Addison's disease, heat cramps, hyperkalemia, severe tissue trauma

Precautions Use with caution in patients with cardiac and/or renal disease, patients receiving potassium-sparing drugs

Adverse Reactions

Central nervous system: Mental confusion

Endocrine & metabolic: Hyperkalemia, metabolic alkalosis

Gastrointestinal: Nausea, vomiting, diarrhea, abdominal pain, GI lesions, flatulence

Neuromuscular & skeletal: Muscle weakness, paresthesia, flaccid paralysis

Drug Interactions Potassium-sparing diuretics, salt substitutes, and ACE inhibitors may result in increased serum potassium.

Stability Store at room temperature.

Usual Dosage Oral (doses listed as mEq of **potassium**):

Normal daily requirement:

Children: 2-3 mEq/kg/day

Adults: 40-80 mEq/day

Prevention of hypokalemia during diuretic therapy:

Children: 1-2 mEq/kg/day in 1-2 divided doses

Adults: 25-100 mEq/day in 2-4 divided doses

Administration Dissolve tablets in 3-4 ounces cold water or juice; solution should be sipped slowly, over 5-10 minutes; administer with meals

Monitoring Parameters Serum potassium, glucose, chloride, pH, urine output (if indicated)

Additional Information Hypokalemia is highly arrhythmogenic, particularly in the setting of ischemia or digitalis toxicity. ECG evidence of hypokalemia includes flattening of the T wave. As the T wave shrinks, U waves may appear. There is no

(Continued)

Potassium Bicarbonate and Potassium Chloride *(Continued)*

prolongation of the QT interval. Hyperkalemia may present as tall peaked symmetrical T waves. S-T elevation may present in severe hyperkalemia. QRS complex progressively widens with eventual apparent sine waves on the ECG. Hyperkalemia will also induce cardiac slowing and AV conduction abnormalities.

Dosage Forms Excipient information presented when available (limited, particularly for generics); consult specific product labeling.

Tablet for solution, oral [effervescent]: Potassium chloride 25 mEq [potassium bicarbonate 0.5 g and potassium chloride 1.5 g]

K-Lyte/Cl®: Potassium chloride 25 mEq [potassium bicarbonate 0.5 g and potassium chloride 1.5 g; citrus or fruit punch flavor]

♦ **Potassium Bicarbonate and Potassium Chloride (Effervescent)** *see* Potassium Bicarbonate and Potassium Chloride *on page 1285*

Potassium Bicarbonate and Potassium Citrate

(poe TASS ee um bye KAR bun ate & poe TASS ee um SIT rate)

Medication Safety Issues

Sound-alike/look-alike issues:

Klor-Con® may be confused with Klaron®, K-Lor®

Related Information

Potassium Bicarbonate *on page 1284*

U.S. Brand Names Effer-K™; Klor-Con®/EF; K-Lyte®; K-Lyte® DS

Index Terms Potassium Bicarbonate and Potassium Citrate (Effervescent)

Therapeutic Category Electrolyte Supplement, Oral

Generic Available Yes

Use Treatment or prevention of hypokalemia, particularly when it is necessary to avoid chloride or the acid/base status requires bicarbonate

Pregnancy Risk Factor C

Contraindications Hypersensitivity to any component of the potassium supplement; severe renal impairment, untreated Addison's disease, heat cramps, hyperkalemia, severe tissue trauma

Precautions Use with caution in patients with cardiac and/or renal disease, patients receiving potassium-sparing drugs

Adverse Reactions

Central nervous system: Mental confusion

Endocrine & metabolic: Hyperkalemia, metabolic alkalosis

Gastrointestinal: Nausea, vomiting, diarrhea, abdominal pain, GI lesions, flatulence

Neuromuscular & skeletal: Muscle weakness, paresthesia, flaccid paralysis

Drug Interactions Potassium-sparing diuretics, salt substitutes, and ACE inhibitors may result in increased serum potassium.

Stability Store at room temperature.

Mechanism of Action Potassium is the major cation of intracellular fluid and is essential for the conduction of nerve impulses in heart, brain, and skeletal muscle; contraction of cardiac, skeletal, and smooth muscles; maintenance of normal renal function, acid-base balance, carbohydrate metabolism, and gastric secretion. Bicarbonate neutralizes hydrogen ion concentration and raises blood and urinary pH

Pharmacokinetics

Absorption: Well absorbed from upper GI tract

Distribution: Enters cells via active transport from extracellular fluid

Elimination: Primarily urine; skin and feces (small amounts); most intestinal potassium reabsorbed

Usual Dosage Oral (doses listed as mEq of **potassium**):

Normal daily requirement:

Children: 2-3 mEq/kg/day

Adults: 40-80 mEq/day

Prevention of hypokalemia during diuretic therapy:

Children: 1-2 mEq/kg/day in 1-2 divided doses

Adults: 25-100 mEq/day in 2-4 divided doses

Administration Oral: Dissolve completely in 3-8 oz cold water, juice, or other suitable beverage and drink slowly.

Monitoring Parameters Serum potassium, chloride, glucose, pH, urine output (if indicated)

Additional Information Hypokalemia is highly arrhythmogenic, particularly in the setting of ischemia or digitalis toxicity. ECG evidence of hypokalemia includes flattening of the T wave. As the T wave shrinks, U waves may appear. There is no prolongation of the QT interval. Hyperkalemia may present as tall peaked symmetrical T waves. S-T elevation may present in severe hyperkalemia. QRS complex progressively widens with eventual apparent sine waves on the ECG. Hyperkalemia will also induce cardiac slowing and AV conduction abnormalities.

Dosage Forms Excipient information presented when available (limited, particularly for generics); consult specific product labeling.

Tablet, effervescent:

Effer-K™: Potassium 25 mEq [cherry berry, lemon citrus, orange, or unflavored]

Klor-Con®/EF: Potassium 25 mEq [sugar free; orange flavor]

K-Lyte®: Potassium 25 mEq [orange flavor]

K-Lyte® DS: Potassium 50 mEq [orange flavor]

♦ **Potassium Bicarbonate and Potassium Citrate (Effervescent)** *see* Potassium Bicarbonate and Potassium Citrate *on page 1286*

Potassium Chloride (poe TASS ee um KLOR ide)

Medication Safety Issues

Sound-alike/look-alike issues:

Kaon-Cl-10® may be confused with kaolin

KCl may be confused with HCl

K-Dur® may be confused with Cardura®, Imdur®

K-Lor® may be confused with Kaochlor®, Klor-Con®

Klor-Con® may be confused with Klaron®, K-Lor®

Klotrix® may be confused with liotrix

microK® may be confused with Micronase®

High alert medication: The Institute for Safe Medication Practices (ISMP) includes this medication (I.V. formulation) among its list of drugs which have a heightened risk of causing significant patient harm when used in error.

Per JCAHO recommendations, concentrated electrolyte solutions should not be available in patient care areas.

Consider special storage requirements for intravenous potassium salts; I.V. potassium salts have been administered IVP in error, leading to fatal outcomes.

U.S. Brand Names Kaon-Cl-10®; Kaon-Cl® 20; Kay Ciel®; K-Dur® 10; K-Dur® 20; K-Lor®; Klor-Con®; Klor-Con® 8; Klor-Con® 10; Klor-Con®/25; Klor-Con® M; K+ Potassium; K-Tab®; microK®; microK® 10; Rum-K®

Canadian Brand Names Apo-K®; K-10®; K-Dur®; K-Lor®; K-Lyte®/Cl; Micro-K Extencaps®; Roychlor®; Slo-Pot; Slow-K®

Index Terms KCl

Therapeutic Category Electrolyte Supplement, Oral; Electrolyte Supplement, Parenteral

Generic Available Yes

Use Treatment or prevention of hypokalemia

Pregnancy Risk Factor C

Contraindications Hypersensitivity to any component of the potassium supplement; severe renal impairment, untreated Addison's disease, heat cramps, hyperkalemia, severe tissue trauma; solid oral dosage forms are contraindicated in patients in whom there is a structural, pathological, and/or pharmacologic cause for delay or arrest in passage through the GI tract; an oral liquid potassium preparation should be used in patients with esophageal compression or delayed gastric emptying time

Warnings Potassium chloride injection should be administered only in patients with adequate urine flow; injection must be diluted before I.V. use and infused slowly (see Administration)

Precautions Use with caution in patients with cardiac disease and/or renal disease, patients receiving potassium-sparing drugs; patients should be on a cardiac monitor during intermittent infusions for doses >0.5 mEq/kg/hour

Adverse Reactions

Cardiovascular (with rapid I.V. administration): Arrhythmias and cardiac arrest, heart block, hypotension

Central nervous system: Mental confusion

Endocrine & metabolic: Hyperkalemia

Gastrointestinal (with oral administration): Nausea, vomiting, diarrhea, abdominal pain, GI lesions, flatulence

Local: Pain at the site of injection, phlebitis

Neuromuscular & skeletal: Muscle weakness, paresthesia, flaccid paralysis

Drug Interactions Potassium-sparing diuretics, salt substitutes, and ACE inhibitors may result in increased serum potassium.

Stability Store at room temperature; do not freeze

Mechanism of Action Potassium is the major cation of intracellular fluid and is essential for the conduction of nerve impulses in heart, brain, and skeletal muscle; (Continued)

Potassium Chloride *(Continued)*

contraction of cardiac, skeletal, and smooth muscles; maintenance of normal renal function, acid-base balance, carbohydrate metabolism, and gastric secretion

Pharmacokinetics

Absorption: Well absorbed from upper GI tract; enters cells via active transport from extracellular fluid

Distribution: Enters cells via active transport from extracellular fluid

Elimination: Primarily urine; skin and feces (small amounts); most intestinal potassium reabsorbed

Usual Dosage I.V. doses should be incorporated into the patient's maintenance I.V. fluids; intermittent I.V. potassium administration should be reserved for severe depletion situations; continuous EKG monitoring should be used for intermittent doses >0.5 mEq/kg/hour. Doses listed as mEq of **potassium**. When using microencapsulated or wax matrix formulations, use no more than 20 mEq as a single dose.

Normal daily requirements: Oral, I.V.:

Neonates >24 hours of age and Infants: 2-6 mEq/kg/day

Children: 2-3 mEq/kg/day

Adults: 40-80 mEq/day

Prevention of hypokalemia during diuretic therapy: Oral:

Neonates, Infants, and Children: 1-2 mEq/kg/day in 1-2 divided doses

Adults: 20-40 mEq/day in 1-2 divided doses

Treatment of hypokalemia:

Neonates, Infants, and Children:

Oral: 2-5 mEq/kg/day in divided doses; not to exceed 1-2 mEq/kg as a single dose; if deficits are severe or ongoing losses are great, I.V. route should be considered preferred route of administration

I.V. intermittent infusion (must be diluted prior to administration): 0.5-1 mEq/kg/dose (maximum dose: 40 mEq) to infuse at 0.3-0.5 mEq/kg/hour (maximum dose/rate: 1 mEq/kg/hour); then repeated as needed based on frequently obtained lab values; severe depletion or ongoing losses may require >200% of normal daily limit needs

Adults:

I.V. intermittent infusion: 5-10 mEq/hour (continuous cardiac monitor recommended for rates >5 mEq/hour), not to exceed 40 mEq/hour; usual adult maximum per 24 hours: 400 mEq

Potassium dosage/rate of infusion guidelines:

Serum potassium ≥2.5 mEq/L (and <desired): 10 mEq with additional doses if needed; maximum infusion rate: 10 mEq/hour; maximum 24-hour dose: 200 mEq

Serum potassium <2.5 mEq/L: Up to 40 mEq, with additional doses based upon frequent lab monitoring; maximum infusion rate: 40 mEq/hour; maximum 24-hour dose: 400 mEq; deficits at a plasma level of 2 mEq/L may be as high as 400-800 mEq of potassium

Oral:

Serum potassium ≥2.5 mEq/L (and <desired):

60-80 mEq/day plus additional amounts if needed

Serum potassium <2.5 mEq/L:

Up to 40-60 mEq initial dose, followed by further doses based on lab values

Administration

Oral: Sustained release and wax matrix tablets should be swallowed whole, do not crush or chew; administer with food; powder should be dissolved in water or juice; do not administer liquid full strength, must be diluted in 2-6 parts of water or juice

Parenteral: Potassium must be diluted prior to parenteral administration; maximum recommended concentration (peripheral line): 80 mEq/L; maximum recommended concentration (central line): 150 mEq/L or 15 mEq/100 mL; in severely fluid-restricted patients (with central lines): 200 mEq/L or 20 mEq/100 mL has been used; maximum rate of infusion, see Usual Dosage, I.V. intermittent infusion

Monitoring Parameters Serum potassium, glucose, chloride, pH, urine output (if indicated), cardiac monitor [if intermittent I.V. infusion or potassium I.V. infusion rates >0.5 mEq/kg/hour or 5 mEq/hour (adults)]

Additional Information Hypokalemia is highly arrhythmogenic, particularly in the setting of ischemia or digitalis toxicity. ECG evidence of hypokalemia includes flattening of the T wave. As the T wave shrinks, U waves may appear. There is no prolongation of the QT interval. Hyperkalemia may present as tall peaked symmetrical T waves. S-T elevation may present in severe hyperkalemia. QRS complex progressively widens with eventual apparent sine waves on the ECG. Hyperkalemia will also induce cardiac slowing and AV conduction abnormalities.

Dosage Forms Excipient information presented when available (limited, particularly for generics); consult specific product labeling. [DSC] = Discontinued product

Capsule, extended release: 10 mEq [750 mg]

microK® [microencapsulated]: 8 mEq [600 mg]
microK® 10 [microencapsulated]: 10 mEq [750 mg]

Infusion [premixed in D_5W]: 20 mEq (1000 mL); 30 mEq (1000 mL); 40 mEq (1000 mL)

Infusion [premixed in D_5W and LR]: 20 mEq (1000 mL); 30 mEq (1000 mL); 40 mEq (1000 mL)

Infusion [premixed in D_5W and ¼NS]: 10 mEq (500 mL, 1000 mL); 20 mEq (250 mL, 500 mL, 1000 mL); 30 mEq (1000 mL); 40 mEq (1000 mL)

Infusion [premixed in D_5W and ½NS]: 10 mEq (500 mL, 1000 mL); 20 mEq (500 mL, 1000 mL); 30 mEq (1000 mL); 40 mEq (1000 mL)

Infusion [premixed in D_5 and NS]: 20 mEq (1000 mL); 40 mEq (1000 mL)

Infusion [premixed in D_5W and sodium chloride 0.3%]: 10 mEq (500 mL); 20 mEq (1000 mL); 30 mEq (1000 mL); 40 mEq (1000 mL)

Infusion [premixed in $D_{10}W$ and sodium chloride 0.2%]: 20 mEq (250 mL)

Infusion [premixed in NS]: 20 mEq (1000 mL); 40 mEq (1000 mL)

Infusion [premixed in SWFI; concentrate]: 10 mEq (50 mL, 100 mL); 20 mEq (50 mL, 100 mL); 30 mEq (100 mL); 40 mEq (100 mL)

Injection, solution [concentrate]: 2 mEq/mL (5 mL, 10 mL, 15 mL, 20 mL, 30 mL, 250 mL, 500 mL)

Powder, for oral solution: 20 mEq/packet (30s, 100s, 1000s)
K-Lor™: 20 mEq/packet (30s, 100s) [fruit flavor]
K+ Potassium: 20 mEq/packet (30s) [orange flavor]
Kay Ciel® 10%: 20 mEq/packet (30s, 100s) [sugar free]
Klor-Con®: 20 mEq/packet (30s, 100s) [sugar free; fruit flavor]
Klor-Con®/25: 25 mEq/packet (30s, 100s) [sugar free; fruit flavor]

Solution, oral: 20 mEq/15 mL (480 mL, 3840 mL); 40 mEq/15 mL (480 mL)
Kaon-Cl® 20: 40 mEq/15 mL (480 mL) [sugar free; contains alcohol; cherry flavor]
Kay Ciel®: 10%: 20 mEq/15 mL (480 mL) [sugar free; contains alcohol] [DSC]
Rum-K®: 20 mEq/10 mL (480 mL) [alcohol free, sugar free; butter/rum flavor]

Tablet, extended release: 8 mEq [600 mg]; 10 mEq [750 mg]; 20 mEq [1500 mg]
K-Dur® 10 [microencapsulated]: 10 mEq [750 mg]
K-Dur® 20 [microencapsulated]: 20 mEq [1500 mg; scored]
K-Tab®: 10 mEq [750 mg]
Kaon-Cl® 10: 10 mEq [750 mg]
Klor-Con® 8: 8 mEq [600 mg; wax matrix]
Klor-Con® 10: 10 mEq [750 mg; wax matrix]
Klor-Con® M10 [microencapsulated]: 10 mEq [750 mg]
Klor-Con® M15 [microencapsulated]: 15 mEq [1125 mg; scored]
Klor-Con® M20 [microencapsulated]: 20 mEq [1500 mg; scored]

References

Hamill RJ, Robinson LM, Wexler HR, et al, "Efficacy and Safety of Potassium Infusion Therapy in Hypokalemic Critically Ill Patients," *Crit Care Med*, 1991, 19(5):694-9.

Khilnani P, "Electrolyte Abnormalities in Critically Ill Children," *Crit Care Med*, 1992, 20(2):241-50.

Potassium Gluconate (poe TASS ee um GLOO coe nate)

U.S. Brand Names Glu-K® [OTC]

Therapeutic Category Electrolyte Supplement, Oral

Generic Available Yes

Use Treatment or prevention of hypokalemia

Pregnancy Risk Factor A

Contraindications Hypersensitivity to any component of the potassium supplement; severe renal impairment, untreated Addison's disease, heat cramps, hyperkalemia, severe tissue trauma; solid oral dosage forms are contraindicated in patients in whom there is a structural, pathological, and/or pharmacologic cause for delay or arrest in passage through the GI tract

Precautions Use with caution in patients with cardiac and/or renal disease, patients receiving potassium-sparing drugs

Adverse Reactions

Central nervous system: Mental confusion
Endocrine & metabolic: Hyperkalemia
Gastrointestinal: Nausea, vomiting, diarrhea, abdominal pain, GI lesions, flatulence
Neuromuscular & skeletal: Muscle weakness, paresthesia, flaccid paralysis

Drug Interactions Potassium-sparing diuretics, salt substitutes, and ACE inhibitors may result in increased serum potassium.

Stability Store at room temperature.

Mechanism of Action Potassium is the major cation of intracellular fluid and is essential for the conduction of nerve impulses in heart, brain, and skeletal muscle; contraction of cardiac, skeletal, and smooth muscles; maintenance of normal renal function, acid-base balance, carbohydrate metabolism, and gastric secretion

(Continued)

Potassium Gluconate *(Continued)*

Pharmacokinetics

Absorption: Well absorbed from upper GI tract

Distribution: Enters cells via active transport from extracellular fluid

Elimination: Primarily urine; skin and feces (small amounts); most intestinal potassium reabsorbed

Usual Dosage Oral (doses listed as mEq of **potassium**):

Normal daily requirement:

Children: 2-3 mEq/kg/day

Adults: 40-80 mEq/day

Prevention of hypokalemia during diuretic therapy:

Children: 1-2 mEq/kg/day in 1-2 divided doses

Adults: 20-40 mEq/day in 1-2 divided doses

Treatment of hypokalemia:

Children: 2-5 mEq/kg/day in divided doses; not to exceed 1-2 mEq/kg as a single dose; if deficits are severe or ongoing losses are great, I.V. route should be considered preferred route of administration

Adults: 40-100 mEq/day in 2-4 divided doses

Administration Oral: Sustained release and wax matrix tablets should be swallowed whole, do not crush or chew; administer with food

Monitoring Parameters Serum potassium, chloride, glucose, pH, urine output (if indicated)

Additional Information 9.4 g potassium gluconate is approximately equal to 40 mEq potassium (4.3 mEq potassium/g potassium gluconate). Hypokalemia is highly arrhythmogenic, particularly in the setting of ischemia or digitalis toxicity. ECG evidence of hypokalemia includes flattening of the T wave. As the T wave shrinks, U waves may appear. There is no prolongation of the QT interval. Hyperkalemia may present as tall peaked symmetrical T waves. S-T elevation may present in severe hyperkalemia. QRS complex progressively widens with eventual apparent sine waves on the ECG. Hyperkalemia will also induce cardiac slowing and AV conduction abnormalities.

Dosage Forms Excipient information presented when available (limited, particularly for generics); consult specific product labeling.

Tablet: 500 mg, 610 mg

Glu-K®: 486 mg

Tablet, timed release: 595 mg

Potassium Iodide (poe TASS ee um EYE oh dide)

Medication Safety Issues

Sound-alike/look-alike issues:

Potassium iodide products, including saturated solution of potassium iodide (SSKI®) may be confused with potassium iodide and iodine (Strong Iodide Solution or Lugol's solution)

U.S. Brand Names Iosat™ [OTC]; Pima®; SSKI®; ThyroSafe™ [OTC]; ThyroShield™ [OTC]

Index Terms KI

Therapeutic Category Antithyroid Agent; Expectorant

Use Expectorant for the symptomatic treatment of chronic pulmonary diseases complicated by mucous; reduce thyroid vascularity prior to thyroidectomy and management of thyrotoxic crisis; block thyroidal uptake of radioactive isotopes of iodine in a radiation emergency or other exposure to radioactive iodine; treat cutaneous sporotrichosis (unlabeled use)

Pregnancy Risk Factor D

Lactation Enters breast milk/use caution (AAP rates "compatible")

Contraindications Hypersensitivity to iodides or any component; hyperkalemia, pulmonary edema, hyperthyroidism, impaired renal function, iodine-induced goiter, dermatitis herpetiformis, hypocomplementemic vasculitis

Warnings Prolonged use can lead to hypothyroidism.

Precautions Use with caution in patients with cystic fibrosis (may have exaggerated susceptibility to goitrogenic effects); use caution in patients with myotonia congenital, patients with a history of thyroid disease, and in patients with cardiac disease, Addison's disease, tuberculosis, or acute bronchitits; treatment may cause flare-up of acne

Adverse Reactions

Cardiovascular: Arrhythmia

Central nervous system: Fever, headache, confusion

Dermatologic: Urticaria, acne, angioedema, cutaneous hemorrhage

Endocrine & metabolic: Goiter with hypothyroidism, thyroid adenoma, acute parotitis

Gastrointestinal: Metallic taste, GI upset, GI bleeding, soreness of teeth and gums, cutaneous and mucosal hemorrhage, nausea, vomiting, diarrhea
Hematologic: Eosinophilia
Neuromuscular & skeletal: Arthralgia, numbness, paresthesia
Respiratory: Rhinitis, wheezing
Miscellaneous: Lymph node enlargement, swelling of face, lips, tongue, throat, hands, and feet

Drug Interactions Potassium-containing medications, ACE inhibitors, and potassium-sparing diuretics may increase serum potassium; lithium and antithyroid drugs may potentiate hypothyroid and goitrogenic effects

Stability Store at room temperature; SSKI® if exposed to cold temperatures may develop crystallization; warming with shaking will redissolve crystals; if solution becomes brown/yellow in color, it should be discarded

Mechanism of Action Reduces viscosity of mucus by increasing respiratory tract secretions; inhibits the release of thyroid hormone; following radioactive iodine exposure, potassium iodide blocks the uptake of radioiodine by the thyroid, reducing the risk of thyroid cancer

Pharmacodynamics Antithyroid effects:
Onset of action: 24-48 hours
Maximum effect: 10-15 days after continuous therapy
Duration: May persist up to 6 weeks

Usual Dosage Oral:
Expectorant:
Children:
SSKI®: 60-250 mg 4 times/day; maximum single dose: 500 mg
Pima®:
<3 years: 162 mg 3 times/day
>3 years: 325 mg 3 times/day
Adults:
SSKI®: 300-600 mg 3-4 times/day
Pima®: 325-650 mg 3 times/day
Preoperative thyroidectomy: Children and Adults: Given 10-14 days before surgery: 50-250 mg (1-5 drops, 1 g/mL SSKI®) 3 times/day
Thyrotoxic crisis:
Infants <1 year: 150-250 mg (3-5 drops, 1 g/mL SSKI®) 3 times/day
Children and Adults: 300-500 mg (6-10 drops 1 g/mL SSKI®) 3 times/day
Cutaneous Sporotrichosis:
Children: 250-500 mg (5-10 drops, 1 g/mL SSKI®) 3 times/day; increase gradually to a maximum of 1.25-2 g (25-40 drops SSKI®)
Adults: 250-500 mg (5-10 drops, 1 g/mL SSKI®) 3 times/day; increase gradually to a maximum of 2-2.5 g (40-50 drops SSKI®)
Note: Therapy is continued at the maximum tolerated dosage until the cutaneous lesions have resolved, usually 6-12 weeks
Radiation protectant to radioactive isotopes of iodine (Pima®):
Infants and children <1 year: 65 mg once daily for 10 days; start 24 hours prior to exposure
Children >1 year: 130 mg once daily for 10 days; start 24 hours prior to exposure
Adults: 195 mg once daily for 10 days; start 24 hours prior to exposure
Prevention of thyroidal uptake of radioactive isotopes of iodine to reduce risk of thyroid cancer following nuclear accident (Iosat™, ThyroSafe™, ThyroShield™):
Infants <1 month: 16.25 mg once daily
Infants ≥1 month and Children <3 years: 32.5 mg once daily
Children 3-18 years (≤150 lbs): 65 mg once daily
Children >18 years (>150 lbs) and Adults (including pregnant and lactating women): 130 mg once daily
Note: Treatment should continue until the risk of exposure has passed and/or until other measures (evacuation, sheltering, control of the food and milk supply) have been successfully implemented.

Administration Oral: Administer after meals with food or milk or dilute with a large quantity of water, fruit juice, milk, or broth

Monitoring Parameters Thyroid function tests; sign/symptoms of hyperthyroidism; thyroid function should be monitored in pregnant women, neonates, and young infants if repeat doses are required following radioactive iodine exposure

Additional Information 10 drops SSKI® = potassium iodide 500 mg

Dosage Forms Excipient information presented when available (limited, particularly for generics); consult specific product labeling.
Solution, oral:
SSKI®: 1 g/mL (30 mL, 240 mL) [contains sodium thiosulfate]
ThyroShield™: 65 mg/mL (30 mL) [black raspberry flavor]
(Continued)

Potassium Iodide *(Continued)*

Syrup (Pima®): 325 mg/5 mL (473 mL) [equivalent to iodide 249 mg/5 mL; black raspberry flavor]

Tablet:

Iosat™: 130 mg

ThyroSafe™: 65 mg [equivalent to iodine 50 mg]

Extemporaneous Preparations Preparation of oral solution:

Concentration of 16.25 mg/5 mL oral solution: Crush one 130 mg tablet into a fine powder. Add 20 mL of water and mix until powder is dissolved. Add an additional 20 mL of low-fat milk (white or chocolate), orange juice, flat soda, raspberry syrup, or infant formula. Final concentration will be 16.25 mg/5 mL.

Concentration of 8.125 mg/5 mL oral solution: Crush one 65 mg tablet into a fine powder. Add 20 mL of water and mix until powder is dissolved. Add an additional 20 mL of low-fat milk (white or chocolate), orange juice, flat soda, raspberry syrup, or infant formula. Final concentration will be 8.125 mg/5 mL.

References

"American Academy of Pediatrics Committee on Environmental Health. Radiation Disasters and Children," *Pediatrics*, 2003, 111(6 Pt 1):1455-66.

Kauffman CA, Hajjeh R, and Chapman SW, "Practice Guidelines for the Management of Patients With Sporotrichosis. For the Mycoses Study Group. Infectious Diseases Society of America," *Clin Infect Dis*, 2000, 30(4):684-7.

"Potassium Iodide as a Thyroid Blocking Agent in a Radiation Emergency: Final Recommendations on Use," Washington DC, Bureau of Radiological Health and Bureau of Drugs, Food and Drug Administration, 1982.

U.S. Food and Drug Administration, "FDA's Guidance on Protection of Children and Adults Against Thyroid Cancer in Case of Nuclear Accident," FDA Talk Paper. Available at: http://www.fda.gov/bbs/topics/answers/2001/ans01126.html. Accessed January 11, 2002.

Potassium Iodide and Iodine

(poe TASS ee um EYE oh dide & EYE oh dine)

Medication Safety Issues

Sound-alike/look-alike issues:

Potassium iodide and iodine (Strong Iodide Solution or Lugol's solution) may be confused with potassium iodide products, including saturated solution of potassium iodide (SSKI®)

Index Terms Lugol's Solution; Strong Iodine Solution

Therapeutic Category Antithyroid Agent

Generic Available Yes

Use Reduce thyroid vascularity prior to thyroidectomy and management of thyrotoxic crisis

Pregnancy Risk Factor D (potassium iodide)

Lactation Enters breast milk/use caution (AAP rates "compatible")

Contraindications Hypersensitivity to iodine or any component; hyperkalemia, pulmonary edema, hyperthyroidism, impaired renal function, iodine-induced goiter, dermatitis herpetiformis, hypocomplementemic vasculitis

Warnings Prolonged use can lead to hypothyroidism.

Precautions Use with caution in patients with cystic fibrosis (may have exaggerated susceptibility to goitrogenic effects); use caution in patients with myotonia congenital, patients with a history of thyroid disease, and in patients with cardiac disease, Addison's diseases, tuberculosis, or acute bronchitis; treatment may cause flare-up of acne

Adverse Reactions

Cardiovascular: Arrhythmia

Central nervous system: Fever, headache, confusion

Dermatologic: Urticaria, acne, angioedema, cutaneous hemorrhage, skin rash

Endocrine & metabolic: Goiter with hypothyroidism, thyroid adenoma, acute parotitis

Gastrointestinal: Metallic taste, GI upset, GI bleeding, soreness of teeth and gums, cutaneous and mucosal hemorrhage, nausea, vomiting, diarrhea

Hematologic: Eosinophilia

Neuromuscular & skeletal: Arthralgia, numbness, paresthesia

Respiratory: Rhinitis, wheezing

Miscellaneous: Lymph node enlargement, swelling of face, lips, tongue, throat, hands, and feet

Drug Interactions Potassium-containing medications, ACE inhibitors, and potassium-sparing diuretics may increase serum potassium; lithium and antithyroid drugs may potentiate hypothyroid and goitrogenic effects

Stability Store at room temperature; excursions permitted to 15°C to 30°C (59°F to 86°F); protect from light and keep container tightly closed

Mechanism of Action Inhibits the release of thyroid hormone; following radioactive iodine exposure, potassium iodide blocks the uptake of radioiodine by the thyroid, reducing the risk of thyroid cancer

Pharmacodynamics Antithyroid effects:

Onset of action: 24-48 hours

Maximum effect: 10-15 days after continuous therapy

Duration: May persist up to 6 weeks

Usual Dosage Oral:

Preoperative thyroidectomy: Children and Adults: Given 10-14 days before surgery: 0.1-0.3 mL (3-5 drops) strong iodine (Lugol's solution) 3 times/day

Graves' disease in neonates: 1 drop strong iodine (Lugol's solution) 3 times/day

Thyrotoxic crisis: Children and Adults: 1 mL strong iodine (Lugol's solution) 3 times/day

Administration Oral: Administer after meals with food or milk or dilute with a large quantity of water, fruit juice, milk, or broth

Monitoring Parameters

Thyroid function tests, signs/symptoms of hyperthyroidism; thyroid function should be monitored in pregnant women, neonates, and young infants if repeat doses are required following radioactive iodine exposure

Dosage Forms Excipient information presented when available (limited, particularly for generics); consult specific product labeling.

Solution, oral (Lugol's solution, strong iodine): Potassium iodide 100 mg/mL and iodine 50 mg/mL (15 mL, 480 mL)

References

"American Academy of Pediatrics Committee on Environmental Health. Radiation Disasters and Children," *Pediatrics*, 2003, 111(6 Pt 1):1455-66.

Kauffman CA, Hajjeh R, and Chapman SW, "Practice Guidelines for the Management of Patients With Sporotrichosis. For the Mycoses Study Group. Infectious Diseases Society of America," *Clin Infect Dis*, 2000, 30(4):684-7.

"Potassium Iodide as a Thyroid Blocking Agent in a Radiation Emergency: Final Recommendations on Use," Washington DC, Bureau of Radiological Health and Bureau of Drugs, Food and Drug Administration, 1982.

U.S. Food and Drug Administration, "FDA's Guidance on Protection of Children and Adults Against Thyroid Cancer in Case of Nuclear Accident," FDA Talk Paper. Available at: http://www.fda.gov/bbs/topics/answers/2001/ans01126.html. Accessed January 11, 2002.

Potassium Phosphate (poe TASS ee um FOS fate)

Medication Safety Issues

Sound-alike/look-alike issues:

Neutra-Phos®-K may be confused with K-Phos Neutral®

High alert medication: The Institute for Safe Medication Practices (ISMP) includes this medication (I.V. formulation) among its list of drugs which have a heightened risk of causing significant patient harm when used in error.

Per JCAHO recommendations, concentrated electrolyte solutions should not be available in patient care areas.

Consider special storage requirements for intravenous potassium salts; I.V. potassium salts have been administered IVP in error, leading to fatal outcomes.

U.S. Brand Names Neutra-Phos®-K [OTC]

Index Terms Phosphate, Potassium

Therapeutic Category Electrolyte Supplement, Oral; Electrolyte Supplement, Parenteral; Phosphate Salt; Potassium Salt

Generic Available Yes: Injection

Use Treatment and prevention of hypophosphatemia; source of phosphate in large volume I.V. fluids

Pregnancy Risk Factor C

Contraindications Hypersensitivity to phosphate (salts) or any component; hyperphosphatemia, hyperkalemia, hypocalcemia, hypomagnesemia, severe renal impairment, severe tissue trauma, heat cramps, CHF, patients with phosphate kidney stones

Warnings Parenteral **potassium** salt forms should be administered only in patients with adequate urine flow; must be diluted before I.V. use and infused slowly (see Administration), and patients must be on a cardiac monitor during intermittent infusions

Precautions Use with caution in patients with renal impairment, patients receiving potassium-sparing drugs (potassium salt forms), patients with adrenal insufficiency, cirrhosis

(Continued)

Potassium Phosphate *(Continued)*

Adverse Reactions

Cardiovascular: Hypotension, edema, arrhythmias, heart block, cardiac arrest

Central nervous system: Tetany, mental confusion, seizures, dizziness, headache

Endocrine & metabolic: Hyperphosphatemia, hyperkalemia, hypocalcemia

Gastrointestinal: Nausea, vomiting, diarrhea, flatulence (oral use)

Local: Phlebitis (parenteral forms)

Neuromuscular & skeletal: Paresthesia, bone and joint pain, arthralgia, weakness, muscle cramps

Renal: Acute renal failure

Clinical manifestations of hypophosphatemia by systems:

Neuromuscular: Muscle weakness, anorexia, tremor, paresthesia, convulsions, coma, hyporeflexia, irritability, numbness, abnormal EEG, cardiomyopathy, respiratory failure, inability to wean from ventilator

Hematologic: Rhabdomyolysis, hemolytic anemia, decreased oxygen release, decreased chemotaxis, decreased phagocytosis, decreased platelet survival, myoglobinuria, thrombocytopenia

Skeletal: Osteomalacia, joint arthralgias, pathologic fractures

Drug Interactions Do not give orally at the same time as aluminum- and magnesium-containing antacids or sucralfate which can act as phosphate binders; use of potassium phosphate with potassium-sparing diuretics, ACE inhibitors, or salt substitutes may result in hyperkalemia.

Food Interactions Avoid giving with oxalate (ie, berries, nuts, chocolate, beans, celery, tomatoes) or phytate-containing foods (ie, bran, whole wheat)

Stability Phosphate salts may precipitate when mixed with calcium salts; solubility is improved in parenteral nutrition solutions which contain amino acids; check with a pharmacist to determine compatibility

Mechanism of Action Phosphorus is an essential mineral that is usually found in nature combined with oxygen as phosphate. It participates in bone deposition, calcium metabolism, as part of molecules that regulate many coenzymes, steps in the clotting cascade, and functions of the immune system. It is a component of the lipid bilayer of cell membranes in the form of phospholipids and of other intracellular compounds like nucleic acids and nucleoproteins. It acts as a buffer for the maintenance of plasma and urinary pH.

Pharmacokinetics

Absorption: Oral: 1% to 20%

Elimination: Oral forms excreted in feces; I.V. forms are excreted in the urine with over 80% to 90% of dose reabsorbed by the kidney

Usual Dosage Note: Consider the contribution of potassium when determining the appropriate phosphate replacement.

Phosphorus - Recommended Daily Allowance (RDA) and Estimated Average Requirement (EAR):

0-6 months:
- EAR: 3.2 mmol/day (adequate intake)

7-12 months:
- EAR: 8.9 mmol/day (adequate intake)

1-3 years:
- RDA: 14.8 mmol/day
- EAR: 12.3 mmol/day

4-8 years:
- RDA: 16.1 mmol/day
- EAR: 13.1 mmol/day

9-18 years:
- RDA: 40.3 mmol/day
- EAR: 34 mmol/day

19-30 years:
- RDA: 22.6 mmol/day
- EAR: 18.7 mmol/day

Hypophosphatemia: Hypophosphatemia does not necessarily equate with phosphate depletion. Hypophosphatemia may occur in the presence of low, normal, or high total body phosphate and conversely, phosphate depletion may exist with normal, low, or elevated levels of serum phosphate (Gaasbeek, 2005). It is difficult to provide concrete guidelines for the treatment of severe hypophosphatemia because the extent of total body deficits and response to therapy are difficult to predict. Aggressive doses of phosphate may result in a transient serum elevation followed by redistribution into intracellular compartments or bone tissue. Various regimens for replacement of phosphate in adults have been studied. The regimens below have only been studied in adult patients, however, many institutions have used them in children safely and successfully.

I.V. doses may be incorporated into the patient's maintenance I.V. fluids; intermittent I.V. infusion should be reserved for severe depletion situations. **Note:** Doses listed as mmol of **phosphate** (see also Additional Information).

Intermittent I.V. infusion: It is recommended that repletion of severe hypophosphatemia be done I.V. because large doses of oral phosphate may cause diarrhea and intestinal absorption may be unreliable.

Children and Adults: **Note:** There are no prospective studies of parenteral phosphate replacement in children. The following weight-based guidelines for adult dosing may be cautiously employed in pediatric patients. Guidelines differ based on degree of illness, use of TPN, and severity of hypophosphatemia.

General replacement guidelines (Lentz, 1978): **Note:** The initial dose may be increased by 25% to 50% if the patient is symptomatic secondary to hypophosphatemia and lowered by 25% to 50% if the patient is hypercalcemic.

Low dose: 0.08 mmol/kg over 6 hours; use if losses are recent and uncomplicated

Intermediate dose: 0.16-0.24 mmol/kg over 4-6 hours; use if serum phosphorus level 0.5-1 mg/dL (0.16-0.32 mmol/L)

High dose: 0.36 mmol/kg over 6 hours; use if serum phosphorus <0.5 mg/dL (<0.16 mmol/L)

Patients receiving TPN (Clark, 1995):

Low dose: 0.16 mmol/kg over 4-6 hours; use if serum phosphorus level 2.3-3 mg/dL (0.73- 0.96 mmol/L)

Intermediate dose: 0.32 mmol/kg over 4-6 hours; use if serum phosphorus level 1.6-2.2 mg/dL (0.51-0.72 mmol/L)

High dose: 0.64 mmol/kg over 8-12 hours; use if serum phosphorus <1.5 mg/dL (< 0.5 mmol/L)

Critically ill adult trauma patients receiving TPN (Brown, 2006):

Low dose: 0.32 mmol/kg over 4-6 hours; use if serum phosphorus level 2.3-3 mg/dL (0.73-0.96 mmol/L)

Intermediate dose: 0.64 mmol/kg over 4-6 hours; use if serum phosphorus level 1.6-2.2 mg/dL (0.51-0.72 mmol/L)

High dose: 1 mmol/kg over 8-12 hours; use if serum phosphorus <1.5 mg/dL (< 0.5 mmol/L)

Alternative method in critically ill patients (Kingston, 1985):

Low dose: 0.25 mmol/kg over 4 hours; use if serum phosphorus level 0.5-1 mg/dL (0.16-0.32 mmol/L)

Moderate dose: 0.5 mmol/kg over 4 hours; use if serum phosphorus level <0.5 mg/dL (<0.16 mmol/L)

Adults: 15 mmol/dose over 2 hours; use if serum phosphorus <2 mg/dL (0.65 mmol/L); may repeat in 6- to 8-hour intervals if repeat serum phosphorus (at least 6 hours postdose) <2 mg/dL (0.65 mmol/L); not to exceed 45 mmol/24 hours (Rosen, 1995)

Maintenance:

Children:

I.V.:

Neonates: 0.8-1.5 mmol/kg/day

Infants and Children < 25 kg: 0.5-1.5 mmol/kg/day

Children 25-45 kg: 0.5-1 mmol/kg/day

Oral: 2-3 mmol/kg/day in divided doses (including dietary intake; see Additional Information)

Adults:

I.V.: 50-70 mmol/day

Oral: 50-150 mmol/day in divided doses (including dietary intake; see Additional Information)

(Continued)

Potassium Phosphate *(Continued)*

Administration

Oral: Administer with food to reduce the risk of diarrhea; contents of 1 packet should be diluted in 75 mL water before administration; administer tablets with a full glass of water; maintain adequate fluid intake

Parenteral: For intermittent I.V. infusion: Peripheral line: Dilute to a maximum concentration of 0.05 mmol/mL; Central line: Dilute to a maximum concentration of 0.12 mmol/mL (maximum concentrations were determined with consideration for maximum potassium concentrations); maximum rate of infusion: 0.06 mmol/kg/hour; do **not** infuse with calcium-containing I.V. fluids

Monitoring Parameters Serum potassium, calcium, phosphorus, renal function, reflexes; cardiac monitor (when intermittent infusion or high-dose I.V. replacement of potassium salts needed)

Reference Range Note: There is a diurnal variation with the nadir at 1100, plateau at 1600, and peak in the early evening (Gaasbeek, 2005); 1 mmol/L phosphate = 3.1 mg/dL phosphorus

Newborns: 4.2-9 mg/dL phosphorus (1.36-2.91 mmol/L phosphate)
6 weeks to 18 months: 3.8-6.7 mg/dL phosphorus (1.23-2.16 mmol/L phosphate)
18 months to 3 years: 2.9-5.9 mg/dL phosphorus (0.94-1.91 mmol/L phosphate)
3-15 years: 3.6-5.6 mg/dL phosphorus (1.16-1.81 mmol/L phosphate)
>15 years: 2.5-5 mg/dL phosphorus (0.81-1.62 mmol/L phosphate)

Hypophosphatemia:
Moderate: 1-2 mg/dL phosphorus (0.32-0.65 mmol/L phosphate)
Severe: <1 mg/dL phosphorus (<0.32 mmol/L phosphate)

Additional Information Each mmol of phosphate contains 31 mg elemental phosphorus; 1 mmol/L phosphate = 3.1 mg/dL phosphorus; cow's milk is a good source of phosphate with 1 mg elemental (0.032 mmol) elemental phosphate per mL

With orders for I.V. phosphate, there is considerable confusion associated with the use of millimoles (mmol) versus milliequivalents (mEq) to express the phosphate requirement. Because inorganic phosphate exists as monobasic and dibasic anions, with the mixture of valences dependent on pH, ordering by mEq amounts is unreliable and may lead to large dosing errors. In addition, I.V. phosphate is available in the sodium and potassium salt; therefore, the content of these cations must be considered when ordering phosphate. The most reliable method of ordering I.V. phosphate is by millimoles, then specifying the potassium or sodium salt.

Dosage Forms Excipient information presented when available (limited, particularly for generics); consult specific product labeling.

Injection, solution: Potassium 4.4 mEq and phosphorus 3 mmol per mL (5 mL, 15 mL, 50 mL) [equivalent to potassium 170 mg and phosphate 285 mg per mL]

Powder for oral solution [packet] (Neutra-Phos®-K): Monobasic potassium phosphate and dibasic potassium phosphate/packet (100s) [equivalent to elemental potassium 556 mg (14.2 mEq) and phosphorus 250 mg per packet; sodium and sugar free; fruit flavor]

References

Brown KA, Dickerson, RN, Morgan, RN, et al, "A New Graduated Dosing Regimen for Phosphorus Replacement in Patients Receiving Nutrition Support," *JPEN*, 2006, 30(3):209-14.

Clark CL, Sacks GS, Dickerson RN, et al, "Treatment of Hypophosphatemia in Patients Receiving Specialized Nutrition Support Using a Graduated Dosing Scheme: Results From a Prospective Clinical Trial," *Crit Care Med*, 1995, 23(9):1504-11.

"Dietary Reference Intakes for Calcium, Phosphorus, Magnesium, Vitamin D, and Fluoride. Standing Committee on the Scientific Evaluation of Dietary Reference Intakes, Food and Nutrition Board, Institute of Medicine," National Academy of Sciences, Washington, DC: National Academy Press, 1997.

Gaasbeek A and Meinders AE, "Hypophosphatemia: An Update on Its Etiology and Treatment," Am J Med, 2005, 118(10):1094-101.

Kingston M and Al-Siba'i MB, "Treatment of Severe Hypophosphatemia," *Crit Care Med*, 1985, 13(1):16-8

Lentz RD, Brown DM, and Kjellstrand CM, "Treatment of Severe Hypophosphatemia," *Ann Intern Med*, 1978, 89(6):941-4.

Lloyd CW and Johnson CE, "Management of Hypophosphatemia," *Clin Pharm*, 1988, 7(2):123-8.

Rosen GH, Boullata JI, O'Rangers EA, et al, "Intravenous Phosphate Repletion Regimen for Critically Ill Patients With Moderate Hypophosphatemia," *Crit Care Med*, 1995, 23(7):1204-10.

Potassium Phosphate and Sodium Phosphate

(poe TASS ee um FOS fate & SOW dee um FOS fate)

Medication Safety Issues

Sound-alike/look-alike issues:
K-Phos® Neutral may be confused with Neutra-Phos-K®

U.S. Brand Names K-Phos® MF; K-Phos® Neutral; K-Phos® No. 2; Neutra-Phos® [OTC]; Phos-NaK; Phospha 250™ Neutral; Uro-KP-Neutral®

Index Terms Sodium Phosphate and Potassium Phosphate

Therapeutic Category Electrolyte Supplement, Oral; Phosphate Salt; Potassium Salt; Sodium Salt

Generic Available Yes

Use Treatment and prevention of hypophosphatemia; short-term treatment of constipation

Pregnancy Risk Factor C

Contraindications

Hypersensitivity to phosphate (salts) or any component; hyperphosphatemia, hyperkalemia, hypocalcemia, hypomagnesemia, hypernatremia, severe renal impairment, severe tissue trauma, heat cramps, CHF, patients with phosphate kidney stones

Precautions Use with caution in patients with renal impairment, patients receiving potassium-sparing drugs (potassium salt forms), patients with adrenal insufficiency, cirrhosis

Adverse Reactions

Cardiovascular: Hypotension, edema, arrhythmias, heart block, cardiac arrest

Central nervous system: Tetany, mental confusion, seizures, dizziness, headache

Endocrine & metabolic: Hyperphosphatemia, hyperkalemia, hypocalcemia, hypernatremia

Gastrointestinal: Nausea, vomiting, diarrhea, flatulence (oral use)

Neuromuscular & skeletal: Paresthesia, bone and joint pain, arthralgia, weakness, muscle cramps

Renal: Acute renal failure

Drug Interactions Do not give orally at the same time as aluminum- and magnesium-containing antacids or sucralfate which can act as phosphate binders; use of potassium phosphate with potassium-sparing diuretics, ACE inhibitors, or salt substitutes may result in hyperkalemia

Food Interactions Avoid giving with oxalate (ie, berries, nuts, chocolate, beans, celery, tomatoes) or phytate-containing foods (ie, bran, whole wheat)

Stability Store at room temperature.

Mechanism of Action Phosphorus is an essential mineral that is usually found in nature combined with oxygen as phosphate. It participates in bone deposition, calcium metabolism, as part of molecules that regulate many coenzymes, steps in the clotting cascade, and functions of the immune system. It is a component of the lipid bilayer of cell membranes in the form of phospholipids and of other intracellular compounds like nucleic acids and nucleoproteins. It acts as a buffer for the maintenance of plasma and urinary pH. When administered orally or rectally as a laxative, it exerts osmotic effect in the small intestine by drawing water into the lumen of the gut, producing distension, promoting peristalsis, and evacuation of the bowel.

Pharmacodynamics Onset of action (catharsis):

Oral: 3-6 hours

Pharmacokinetics

Absorption: Oral: 1% to 20%

Elimination: Oral forms excreted in feces

Usual Dosage Note: Consider the contribution of sodium and potassium cations when determining appropriate phosphate replacement.

Phosphorus-Recommended Daily Allowance (RDA) and Estimated Average Requirement (EAR)

0-6 months:

EAR: 3.2 mmol/day (adequate intake)

7-12 months:

EAR: 8.9 mmol/day (adequate intake)

1-3 years:

RDA: 14.8 mmol/day

EAR: 12.3 mmol/day

(Continued)

Potassium Phosphate and Sodium Phosphate *(Continued)*

4-8 years:
RDA: 16.1 mmol/day
EAR: 13.1 mmol/day
9-18 years:
RDA: 40.3 mmol/day
EAR: 34 mmol/day
19-30 years:
RDA: 22.6 mmol/day
EAR: 18.7 mmol/day

Maintenance: Oral:
Children: 2-3 mmol/kg/day in divided doses
Adults: 50-150 mmol/day in divided doses

Laxative: Oral: Uro-KP-Neutral®:
Children ≤ 4 years: 1 capsule or packet (250 mg phosphorus/8 mmol) 4 times/day; dilute as instructed
Children >4 years and Adults: 1-2 capsules or packets (250-500 mg phosphorus/8-16 mmol) 4 times/day; dilute as instructed

Administration Oral: Administer with food to reduce the risk of diarrhea; contents of 1 packet should be diluted in 75 mL water before administration; administer tablets/caplets with a full glass of water; maintain adequate fluid intake; dilute oral solution with an equal volume of cool water

Monitoring Parameters Serum potassium, sodium, calcium, phosphorus, renal function, reflexes; stool output (laxative use)

Reference Range Note: There is a diurnal variation with the nadir at 1100, plateau at 1600, and peak in the early evening (Gaasbeek, 2005); 1 mmol/L phosphate = 3.1 mg/dL phosphorus
Newborns: 4.2-9 mg/dL phosphorus (1.36-2.91 mmol/L phosphate)
6 weeks to 18 months: 3.8-6.7 mg/dL phosphorus (1.23-2.16 mmol/L phosphate)
18 months to 3 years: 2.9-5.9 mg/dL phosphorus (0.94-1.91 mmol/L phosphate)
3-15 years: 3.6-5.6 mg/dL phosphorus (1.16-1.81 mmol/L phosphate)
>15 years: 2.5-5 mg/dL phosphorus (0.81-1.62 mmol/L phosphate)

Hypophosphatemia:
Moderate: 1-2 mg/dL phosphorus (0.32-0.65 mmol/L phosphate)
Severe: <1 mg/dL phosphorus (<0.32 mmol/L phosphate)

Additional Information Each mmol of phosphate contains 31 mg elemental phosphorus; 1 mmol/L phosphate = 3.1 mg/dL phosphorus; cow's milk is a good source of phosphate with 1 mg elemental (0.032 mmol) elemental phosphate per mL

Dosage Forms Excipient information presented when available (limited, particularly for generics); consult specific product labeling.
Caplet:
Uro-KP-Neutral®: Sodium phosphate monobasic, dipotassium phosphate, and disodium phosphate [equivalent to elemental phosphorus 258 mg, sodium 262.4 mg (10.8 mEq), and potassium 49.4 mg (1.3 mEq)]
Powder, for oral solution:
Neutra-Phos®, Phos-NaK): Monobasic sodium, dibasic sodium, and potassium phosphate/packet (100s) [equivalent to elemental phosphorus 250 mg, sodium 164 mg (7.1 mEq), and potassium 278 mg (7.1 mEq) per packet]
Tablet:
K-Phos® MF: Potassium acid phosphate 155 mg and sodium acid phosphate 350 mg [equivalent to elemental phosphorus 125.6 mg, sodium 67 mg (2.9 mEq), and potassium 44.5 mg (1.1 mEq)]
K-Phos® Neutral: Dibasic sodium phosphate 852 mg, monobasic potassium phosphate 155 mg, and monobasic sodium phosphate 130 mg [equivalent to elemental phosphorus 250 mg, sodium 298 mg (13 mEq), and potassium 45 mg (1.1 mEq)]
K-Phos® No. 2: Potassium acid phosphate 305 mg and sodium acid phosphate 700 mg [equivalent to elemental phosphorus 250 mg, sodium 134 mg (5.8 mEq), and potassium 88 mg (2.3 mEq)]
Phospha 250™ Neutral: Dibasic sodium phosphate 852 mg, monobasic potassium phosphate 155 mg, and monobasic sodium phosphate 130 mg [equivalent to elemental phosphorus 250 mg, sodium 298 mg (13 mEq), and potassium 45 mg (1.1 mEq)]

References

Gaasbeek A and Meinders AE, "Hypophosphatemia: An Update on Its Etiology and Treatment," *Am J Med*, 2005, 118(10):1094-101.

♦ **PPL** *see* Benzylpenicilloyl-polylysine [DSC] *on page 210*
♦ **PPV23** *see* Pneumococcal Polysaccharide Vaccine (Polyvalent) *on page 1273*

Pralidoxime (pra li DOKS eem)

Medication Safety Issues
Sound-alike/look-alike issues:
Pralidoxime may be confused with pramoxine, pyridoxine
Protopam® may be confused with Proloprim®, protamine, Protropin®

Related Information
Commonly Used Antidotes for Acute Overdoses *on page 1920*

U.S. Brand Names Protopam®

Canadian Brand Names Protopam®

Index Terms 2-PAM; Pralidoxime Chloride; 2-Pyridine Aldoxime Methochloride

Therapeutic Category Antidote, Anticholinesterase; Antidote, Organophosphate Poisoning

Generic Available No

Use Reverse muscle paralysis associated with toxic exposure to organophosphate anticholinesterase pesticides and chemicals; control of overdosage by anticholinesterase drugs used to treat myasthenia gravis (neostigmine, pyridostigmine)

Pregnancy Risk Factor C

Lactation Excretion in breast milk unknown/not recommended

Contraindications Hypersensitivity to pralidoxime or any component; poisonings due to phosphorus, inorganic phosphates, or organic phosphates without anticholinesterase activity

Warnings Not indicated as an antidote for carbamate classes of pesticides and may increase toxicity of carbaryl

Precautions Use with caution in patients with myasthenia gravis; dosage modification required in patients with impaired renal function; use with caution in patients receiving theophylline, succinylcholine, phenothiazines, respiratory depressants (eg, narcotic, barbiturates); rapid I.V. infusion has been associated with tachycardia, laryngospasm, and muscle rigidity

Adverse Reactions
Cardiovascular: Tachycardia (after rapid I.V. infusion), hypertension
Central nervous system: Dizziness, headache, drowsiness
Dermatologic: Rash
Gastrointestinal: Nausea
Local: Pain at injection site after I.M. use
Neuromuscular & skeletal: Muscular weakness, muscle rigidity (after rapid I.V. infusion), transient elevated CPK
Ocular: Blurred vision, diplopia
Respiratory: Hyperventilation, laryngospasm (after rapid I.V. administration)

Drug Interactions Barbiturates potentiated by anticholinesterases

Mechanism of Action Reactivates cholinesterase that had been inactivated by phosphorylation as a result of exposure to organophosphate pesticides; removes the phosphoryl group from the active site of the inactivated enzyme

Pharmacokinetics
Half-life: 74-77 minutes
Time to peak serum concentration: I.V.: Within 5-15 minutes
Elimination: 80% to 90% excreted unchanged in urine 12 hours after administration

Usual Dosage
Organophosphate poisoning:
Children: I.M., I.V. (use in conjunction with atropine): 20-50 mg/kg/dose; repeat in 1-2 hours if muscle weakness has not been relieved, then at 10- to 12-hour intervals if cholinergic signs recur
Adults: I.M., I.V. (use in conjunction with atropine): 1-2 g; repeat in 1-2 hours if muscle weakness has not been relieved, then at 10- to 12-hour intervals if cholinergic signs recur
Treatment of toxicity from medications used to treat myasthenia gravis: Adults: I.V.: 1-2 g followed by increments of 250 mg every 5 minutes

Administration Parenteral: Reconstitute with 20 mL SWI (preservative free) resulting in 50 mg/mL solution; dilute in NS to 20 mg/mL and infuse over 15-30 minutes; if a more rapid onset of effect is desired or in a fluid-restricted situation, the maximum concentration is 50 mg/mL; the maximum rate of infusion is over 5 minutes and not exceeding 200 mg/minute

Monitoring Parameters Heart rate, respiratory rate, blood pressure, continuous EKG, muscle strength

Dosage Forms Excipient information presented when available (limited, particularly for generics); consult specific product labeling.
Injection, powder for reconstitution, as chloride: 1 g

♦ **Pralidoxime Chloride** *see* Pralidoxime *on page 1299*

- ♦ **Prandase® (Can)** *see* Acarbose *on page 41*
- ♦ **Pravachol®** *see* Pravastatin *on page 1300*

Pravastatin (PRA va stat in)

Medication Safety Issues
Sound-alike/look-alike issues:
Pravachol® may be confused with Prevacid®, Prinivil®, propranolol

U.S. Brand Names Pravachol®

Canadian Brand Names Apo-Pravastatin®; CO Pravastatin; Novo-Pravastatin; PMS-Pravastatin; Pravachol®; ratio-Pravastatin; Riva-Pravastatin; Sandoz-Pravastatin

Index Terms Pravastatin Sodium

Therapeutic Category Antilipemic Agent; HMG-CoA Reductase Inhibitor

Generic Available Yes

Use Hyperlipidemia: Adjunct to dietary therapy to decrease elevated serum total and low density lipoprotein cholesterol (LDL-C), apolipoprotein B (apo-B), and triglyceride levels, and to increase high density lipoprotein cholesterol (HDL-C) in patients with primary hypercholesterolemia (heterozygous, familial and nonfamilial) and mixed dyslipidemia (Fredrickson types IIa and IIb); treatment of homozygous familial hypercholesterolemia; treatment of isolated hypertriglyceridemia (Fredrickson type IV) and type III hyperlipoproteinemia; treatment of primary dysbetalipoproteinemia (Fredrickson Type III)

Primary prevention of cardiovascular disease in high risk patients; risk factors include: Age ≥55 years, smoking, hypertension, low HDL-C or family history of early coronary heart disease

Pregnancy Risk Factor X

Lactation Enters breast milk/contraindicated

Contraindications Hypersensitivity to pravastatin or any component; active liver disease; unexplained persistent elevations of serum transaminases; pregnancy; breast-feeding

Warnings Rhabdomyolysis with or without acute renal failure secondary to myoglobinuria has occurred rarely. Risk is increased with concurrent use of HMG-CoA reductase inhibitors and amiodarone, clarithromycin, danazol, diltiazem, fluvoxamine, amprenavir, delavirdine, indinavir, nefazodone, nelfinavir, ritonavir, verapamil, troleandomycin, cyclosporine, fibric acid derivatives, erythromycin, niacin, or azole antifungals. Assess the risk versus benefit before combining any of these medications with pravastatin. Temporarily discontinue pravastatin in any patient experiencing an acute or serious condition predisposing to renal failure secondary to rhabdomyolysis (eg, sepsis, hypotension, major surgery, trauma, severe metabolic, endocrine or electrolyte disorders, or uncontrolled seizures).

Precautions Persistent increases in serum transaminases have occurred (incidence in clinical trials ≤1.2%); liver function tests must be monitored at the initiation of therapy, prior to an increase in dosage, and then periodically (eg, semiannually), thereafter. Use with caution in patients with a recent history of liver disease, clinical signs of liver disease, or heavy users of alcohol.

Adverse Reactions
Cardiovascular: Angina, chest pain
Central nervous system: Dizziness, headache, somnolence, fatigue, sleep disturbances, depression, anxiety, nervousness, libido change, fever, vertigo
Dermatologic: Rash, pruritus, urticaria, dry skin, alopecia, dermatitis; rare: Photosensitivity, toxic epidermal necrolysis, erythema multiforme including Stevens-Johnson syndrome
Endocrine & metabolic: Gynecomastia
Gastrointestinal: Constipation, heartburn, flatulence, abdominal pain, diarrhea, nausea, pancreatitis, gastroenteritis, vomiting, decreased appetite, taste perversion
Genitourinary: Urinary frequency, dysuria, nocturia
Hematologic: Hemolytic anemia (rare)
Hepatic: Elevated serum transaminases, hepatitis, cholestatic jaundice; rare: Cirrhosis, fulminant hepatic necrosis, hepatoma
Neuromuscular & skeletal: Elevated CPK, myalgia, muscle cramps, myopathy, peripheral nerve palsy, rhabdomyolysis, arthralgias, muscle weakness, dermatomyositis
Ocular: Blurred vision, diplopia
Respiratory: Rhinitis, cough, dyspnea, URI
Miscellaneous: Hypersensitivity reactions, influenza, lupus erythematosus-like syndrome

Drug Interactions Cytochrome P450 isoenzyme CYP3A3/4 enzyme substrate; isoenzyme CYP3A4, CYP2C8/9, and CYP2D6 inhibitor

Cholestyramine and colestipol reduce pravastatin absorption (administer pravastatin at least 1 hour before or 4 hours after); pravastatin may share the same potential drug interactions as other HMG-CoA reductase inhibitors with clofibrate, fenofibrate, gemfibrozil, niacin (≥1 g/day), and amiodarone resulting in an increase in pravastatin serum concentrations and consequent increased risk of myopathy and rhabdomyolysis (see Warnings); cyclosporine, imidazole antifungals (itraconazole, ketoconazole), rifampin, and phenytoin may increase pravastatin serum concentrations; the herbal medicine St John's wort may decrease pravastatin serum concentration

Stability Tablets should be stored in well closed containers at controlled room temperature between 20°C to 25°C (68°F to 77°F); protect from light

Mechanism of Action Pravastatin is a selective, competitive inhibitor of 3-hydroxy-3-methylglutaryl-coenzyme A (HMG-CoA) reductase, the enzyme that catalyzes the rate-limiting step in cholesterol biosynthesis

Pharmacodynamics

Onset of action: 2 weeks
Maximum effect: After 4 weeks
LDL-reduction: 40 mg/day: 34% (for each doubling of this dose, LDL-C is lowered by ~6%)

Pharmacokinetics

Absorption: Oral: Rapidly absorbed
Distribution: V_d: Adults: 0.46 L/kg
Protein binding: 43% to 55%
Metabolism: Extensive first-pass metabolism to metabolites with minimal activity
Bioavailability: Absolute: 17%
Half-life:
Children: 1.6 hours (range: 0.85-4.2 hours)
Adults: 2.6-3.2 hours
Time to peak serum concentration: 1-1.5 hours
Elimination: ~20% excreted in urine unchanged and 70% in feces

Usual Dosage Oral: Dosage should be individualized according to the baseline LDL-C level, the recommended goal of therapy, and patient response; adjustments should be made at intervals of 4 weeks

Hyperlipidemia:
Children 8-13 years: 20 mg once daily; doses >20 mg have not been studied
Adolescents 14-18 years: 40 mg once daily; doses >40 mg have not been studied
Adolescents >18 years and Adults: 40 mg once daily; may increase dosage up to 80 mg once daily as indicated

Dosing adjustment in renal impairment: Adults: Initiate dosage at 10 mg once daily

Dosing adjustment in hepatic impairment: Adults: Initiate dosage at 10 mg once daily; avoid use in active liver disease

Dosing adjustment in patient's receiving concomitant cyclosporine: 20 mg once daily

Administration Oral: May be taken without regard to meals or time of day

Monitoring Parameters Serum cholesterol (total and fractionated), CPK; liver function tests (see Precautions)

Reference Range Hypercholesterolemia as defined by serum cholesterol, LDL-C, and TG concentrations: See table; desired: HDL-C <40 mg/dL

Classification of Blood Cholesterol, LDL-C, and Triglyceride Concentrations[1]

Classification	Cholesterol (mg/dL)		LDL-C (mg/dL)		Triglycerides (mg/dL)
	Children	Adults	Children	Adults	Adults
Acceptable/optimal	<170	<200	<110	<100	<150
Above optimal	†	†	†	100-129	†
Borderline high	170-199	200-239	110-129	130-159	150-199
High	≥200	≥240	≥130	160-189	200-499
Very high	†	†	†	≥190	≥500

[1]Adapted from American Academy of Pediatrics Committee on Nutrition, "Cholesterol in Childhood," *Pediatrics*, 1998, 101(1 Pt 1):141-7 and "Third Report of the National Cholesterol Education Program Expert Panel on Detection, Evaluation, and Treatment of High Blood Cholesterol in Adults (Adult Treatment Panel III)," May 2001, www.nhlbi.nih.gov/guidelines/cholesterol.

†Lack of specific type of classification in either pediatric or adult recommendations.

Patient Information May rarely cause photosensitivity reactions (eg, exposure to sunlight may cause severe sunburn, skin rash, redness, or itching); avoid direct exposure to sunlight. Report severe and unresolved gastric upset, any vision changes, muscle pain and weakness, changes in color of urine or stool, yellowing of skin or eyes, and any unusual bruising. Female patients of childbearing age must be counseled to use 2 effective forms of contraception simultaneously, unless absolute

(Continued)

Pravastatin *(Continued)*

abstinence is the chosen method; this drug may cause severe fetal defects. Avoid the herbal medicine St John's wort.

Additional Information The current recommendation for treatment of hypercholesterolemia in children is limited to children ≥10 years of age who, after a 6-month to 1-year trial of diet therapy, continue to have LDL-C concentrations ≥190 mg/dL alone, or LDL-C concentrations ≥160 mg/dL and a family history of premature coronary artery disease or two or more other coronary artery disease risk factors (AAP Committee on Nutrition, 1998). For each 1% lowering of LDL-C, the relative risk for major cardiovascular events is reduced by approximately 1%. For more specific risk assessment and treatment recommendations for adults, see NCEP ATPIII.

Dosage Forms Excipient information presented when available (limited, particularly for generics); consult specific product labeling.

Tablet, as sodium: 10 mg, 20 mg, 40 mg

Pravachol®: 10 mg, 20 mg, 40 mg, 80 mg

References

American Academy of Pediatrics. Committee on Nutrition, "Cholesterol in Childhood," *Pediatrics*, 1998, 101(1 Pt 1):141-7.

American Academy of Pediatrics, "National Cholesterol Education Program: Report of the Expert Panel on Blood Cholesterol Levels in Children and Adolescents," *Pediatrics*, 1992, 89(3 Pt 2):525-84.

Duplaga BA, "Treatment of Childhood Hypercholesterolemia With HMG-CoA Reductase Inhibitors," *Ann Pharmacother*, 1999, 33(11):1224-7.

Grundy SM, Cleeman JI, Merz CN, et al, "Implications of Recent Clinical Trials for the National Cholesterol Education Program Adult Treatment Panel III Guidelines," *Circulation*, 2004, 110(2):227-39.

Hedman M, Neuvonen PJ, Neuvonen M, et al, "Pharmacokinetics and Pharmacodynamics of Pravastatin in Children With Familial Hypercholesterolemia," *Clin Pharmacol Ther*, 2003, 74(2):178-85.

"Third Report of the National Cholesterol Education Program Expert Panel on Detection, Evaluation, and Treatment of High Blood Cholesterol in Adults (Adult Treatment Panel III)," May 2001, www.nhlbi.nih.gov/guidelines/cholesterol.

Wiegman A, Hutten BA, de Groot E, et al, "Efficacy and Safety of Statin Therapy in Children With Familial Hypercholesterolemia: A Randomized Controlled Trial," *JAMA*, 2004, 292(3):331-7.

♦ **Pravastatin Sodium** *see* Pravastatin *on page 1300*

Praziquantel (pray zi KWON tel)

U.S. Brand Names Biltricide®

Canadian Brand Names Biltricide®

Therapeutic Category Anthelmintic

Generic Available No

Use Treatment of all stages of schistosomiasis caused by *Schistosoma* species pathogenic to humans; also active in the treatment of clonorchiasis, opisthorchiasis, cysticercosis, and many intestinal tapeworm and trematode infections

Pregnancy Risk Factor B

Lactation Enters breast milk

Contraindications Hypersensitivity to praziquantel or any component; ocular cysticercosis, spinal cysticercosis

Precautions Use with caution in patients with severe hepatic disease and in patients with a history of seizures

Adverse Reactions

Central nervous system: Dizziness, drowsiness, fever, headache, vertigo, malaise, CSF reaction syndrome in patients being treated for neurocysticercosis (syndrome includes headache, seizures, intracranial hypertension, elevated CSF protein concentrations, hyperthermia)

Dermatologic: Urticarial rash, itching

Gastrointestinal: Abdominal pain, nausea, vomiting, anorexia, diarrhea

Hematologic: Eosinophilia

Miscellaneous: Diaphoresis

Drug Interactions Alcohol may increase CNS depression; phenytoin and carbamazepine may induce metabolism of praziquantel and decrease its activity; cimetidine increases praziquantel serum concentrations

Mechanism of Action Increases the cell permeability to calcium in schistosomes; causes strong contractions and paralysis of worm musculature leading to detachment of suckers from the blood vessel walls and to dislodgment

Pharmacokinetics

Absorption: Oral: ~80%

Distribution: CSF concentration is 14% to 20% of plasma concentration; excreted in breast milk

Protein binding: ~80%

Metabolism: Extensive first-pass effect; metabolized by the liver to hydroxylated and conjugated metabolites

Half-life: 0.8-1.5 hours

Metabolites: 4.5 hours

Time to peak serum concentration: Within 1-3 hours

Elimination: Praziquantel and metabolites excreted mainly in urine (99% as metabolites)

Usual Dosage Children and Adults: Oral:

Schistosomiasis:

S. mansoni, *S. haematobium*: 20 mg/kg/dose twice daily for 1 day

S. japonicum, *S. mekongi*: 20 mg/kg/dose 3 times/day for 1 day at 4- to 6-hour intervals

Flukes:

Liver, intestine: 75 mg/kg/day divided every 8 hours for 1 day

Lung: 75 mg/kg/day divided every 8 hours for 2 days

Nanophyetus salmincola: 60 mg/kg/day divided every 8 hours for 1 day

Cysticercosis: 50 mg/kg/day divided every 8 hours for 15 days (adjunctive therapy with dexamethasone is recommended for patients with numerous cysts and for those in whom neurologic symptoms or intracranial hypertension develops); for neurocysticercosis, steroids should be administered **prior** to starting praziquantel

Tapeworms: 5-10 mg/kg as a single dose (25 mg/kg for *H. nana*)

Administration Oral: Administer with food; tablets can be halved or quartered; do not chew tablets due to bitter taste

Patient Information Avoid alcohol (increased CNS depression); may cause drowsiness and impair ability to perform activities requiring mental alertness or physical coordination

Dosage Forms Excipient information presented when available (limited, particularly for generics); consult specific product labeling.

Tablet [tri-scored]: 600 mg

References

King CH and Mahmoud AA, "Drug Five Years Later: Praziquantel," *Ann Intern Med*, 1989, 110(4):290-6.

Liu LX and Weller PF, "Antiparasitic Drug," *N Engl J Med*, 1996, 334(18):1178-84.

Prazosin (PRA zoe sin)

Medication Safety Issues

Sound-alike/look-alike issues:

Prazosin may be confused with predniSONE

International issues:

Prazac® [Denmark] may be confused with Prozac® which is a brand name for fluoxetine in the U.S.

Prazepam [multiple international markets] may be confused with prazosin.

Related Information

Antihypertensive Agents by Class *on page 1678*

Overdose and Toxicology *on page 1916*

U.S. Brand Names Minipress®

Canadian Brand Names Apo-Prazo®; Minipress®; Novo-Prazin; Nu-Prazo

Index Terms Furazosin; Prazosin Hydrochloride

Therapeutic Category Alpha-Adrenergic Blocking Agent, Oral; Antihypertensive Agent; Vasodilator

Generic Available Yes

Use Management of hypertension; severe CHF (in conjunction with diuretics and cardiac glycosides)

Pregnancy Risk Factor C

Lactation Excretion in breast milk unknown/use caution

Contraindications Hypersensitivity to prazosin, quinazolines, or any component

Precautions Marked orthostatic hypotension, syncope, and loss of consciousness may occur with first dose ("first dose phenomenon"). This reaction is more likely to occur in patients receiving beta-blockers, diuretics, low sodium diets or larger first doses (ie, >1 mg/dose in adults); avoid rapid increase in dose; use with caution in patients with renal impairment.

Adverse Reactions

Cardiovascular: Orthostatic hypotension, syncope, palpitations, tachycardia, edema

Central nervous system: Dizziness, lightheadedness, nightmares, drowsiness, headache, hypothermia

Dermatologic: Rash

Endocrine & metabolic: Fluid retention, sexual dysfunction

Gastrointestinal: Nausea, xerostomia

Genitourinary: Urinary frequency

Neuromuscular & skeletal: Weakness

Respiratory: Nasal congestion

Drug Interactions Diuretics and antihypertensive medications (especially beta-blockers) may increase prazosin's hypotensive effect

(Continued)

Prazosin *(Continued)*

Food Interactions Avoid natural licorice (causes sodium and water retention and increases potassium loss); food has variable effects on absorption

Mechanism of Action Competitively inhibits postsynaptic alpha-adrenergic receptors which results in vasodilation of veins and arterioles and a decrease in total peripheral resistance and blood pressure

Pharmacodynamics Hypotensive effect:
Onset of action: Within 2 hours
Maximum decrease: 2-4 hours
Duration: 10-24 hours

Pharmacokinetics
Distribution: V_d: 0.5 L/kg (hypertensive adults)
Protein-binding: 92% to 97%
Metabolism: Extensive in the liver, metabolites may be active
Bioavailability, oral: 43% to 82%
Half-life, adults: 2-4 hours, increased half-life with CHF
Elimination: 6% to 10% excreted renally as unchanged drug

Usual Dosage Oral:
Children: Initial: 5 mcg/kg/dose (to assess hypotensive effects); usual dosing interval every 6 hours; increase dosage gradually up to 25 mcg/kg/dose every 6 hours; maximum daily dose: 15 mg or 0.4 mg/kg/day (400 mcg/kg/day); may be divided in 2 or 3 doses/day for treatment of hypertension
Adults: Initial: 1 mg/dose 2-3 times/day; usual maintenance dose: 3-15 mg/day in divided doses 2-4 times/day; maximum daily dose: 20 mg; usual dosage range for hypertension (JNC 7): 2-20 mg/day in 2-3 divided doses

Administration Oral: Administer in a consistent manner with respect to meals

Monitoring Parameters Blood pressure (standing and sitting or supine)

Test Interactions False positive screening tests for pheochromocytoma (increases urinary VMA by 17%; increases norepinephrine metabolite by 42%)

Patient Information Avoid alcohol; rise slowly from sitting or lying position; may cause dizziness or drowsiness and impair ability to perform activities requiring mental alertness or physical coordination; may cause dry mouth

Nursing Implications Be aware of "first-dose phenomenon" (see Precautions); syncope may occur usually within 90 minutes of initial dose

Dosage Forms Excipient information presented when available (limited, particularly for generics); consult specific product labeling.
Capsule, as hydrochloride: 1 mg, 2 mg, 5 mg

References

Chobanian AV, Bakris GL, Black HR, et al, "The Seventh Report of the Joint National Committee on Prevention, Detection, Evaluation, and Treatment of High Blood Pressure: The JNC 7 report," *JAMA*, 2003, 289(19):2560-72.

Friedman WF and George BL, "New Concepts and Drugs in the Treatment of Congestive Heart Failure," *Pediatr Clin North Am*, 1984, 31(6):1197-227.

Sinaiko AR, "Pharmacologic Management of Childhood Hypertension," *Pediatr Clin North Am*, 1993, 40(1):195-212.

♦ **Prazosin Hydrochloride** *see* Prazosin *on page 1303*
♦ **Precedex™** *see* Dexmedetomidine *on page 465*
♦ **Precose®** *see* Acarbose *on page 41*
♦ **Pred Forte®** *see* PrednisoLONE *on page 1304*
♦ **Pred-G®** *see* Prednisolone and Gentamicin *on page 1307*
♦ **Pred Mild®** *see* PrednisoLONE *on page 1304*

PrednisoLONE (pred NIS oh lone)

Medication Safety Issues
Sound-alike/look-alike issues:
PrednisoLONE may be confused with predniSONE
Pediapred® may be confused with Pediazole®

Related Information
Asthma *on page 1904*
Corticosteroids, Systemic *on page 1685*

U.S. Brand Names Econopred® Plus; Orapred®; Orapred ODT™; Pediapred®; Pred Forte®; Pred Mild®; Prelone®

Canadian Brand Names Diopred®; Hydeltra T.B.A.®; Inflamase® Mild; Novo-Prednisolone; Ophtho-Tate®; Pediapred®; Pred Forte®; Pred Mild®; Sab-Prenase

Index Terms Deltahydrocortisone; Metacortandralone; Prednisolone Acetate; Prednisolone Acetate, Ophthalmic; Prednisolone Sodium Phosphate; Prednisolone Sodium Phosphate, Ophthalmic

Therapeutic Category Adrenal Corticosteroid; Anti-inflammatory Agent; Anti-inflammatory Agent, Ophthalmic; Antiasthmatic; Corticosteroid, Ophthalmic; Corticosteroid, Systemic; Glucocorticoid

Generic Available Yes

Use Treatment of endocrine disorders, rheumatic disorders, collagen diseases, dermatologic diseases, allergic states, ophthalmic diseases, respiratory diseases, hematologic disorders, neoplastic diseases, edematous states, and GI diseases

Ophthalmic: Treatment of palpebral and bulbar conjunctivitis; corneal injury from chemical, radiation, thermal burns, or foreign body penetration

Pregnancy Risk Factor C

Lactation Enters breast milk/use caution (AAP rates "compatible")

Contraindications Hypersensitivity to prednisolone or any component (see Warnings); acute superficial herpes simplex keratitis; systemic fungal infections; varicella infections; live or live, attenuated virus vaccines (with immunosuppressive doses of corticosteroids)

Warnings Hypothalamic-pituitary-adrenal (HPA) suppression may occur; acute adrenal insufficiency (adrenal crisis) may occur with abrupt withdrawal after long term therapy or with stress; withdrawal or discontinuation of corticosteroids should be done carefully; patients with HPA axis suppression may require increased doses of systemic glucocorticosteroids prior to, during, and after unusual stress (eg, surgery). Immunosuppression may occur; patients may be more susceptible to infections; avoid exposure to chickenpox and measles. Corticosteroids may mask signs of infection. Corticosteroids may activate latent opportunistic infections or exacerbate systemic fungal infections. May cause osteoporosis (at any age) or inhibition of bone growth in pediatric patients. Acute myopathy may occur with high doses, elevated IOP may occur (especially with prolonged use), and CNS effects (ranging from euphoria to psychosis) may occur. Rare cases of anaphylactoid reactions have been reported with corticosteroids.

Ophthalmic suspension may contain sodium bisulfite which may cause allergic reactions in susceptible individuals; Orapred® oral solution contains sodium benzoate and Prelone® syrup contains benzoic acid; benzoic acid (benzoate) is a metabolite of benzyl alcohol; large amounts of benzyl alcohol (≥99 mg/kg/day) have been associated with a potentially fatal toxicity ("gasping syndrome") in neonates; the "gasping syndrome" consists of metabolic acidosis, respiratory distress, gasping respirations, CNS dysfunction (including convulsions, intracranial hemorrhage), hypotension and cardiovascular collapse; use prednisolone products containing sodium benzoate or benzoic acid with caution in neonates; *in vitro* and animal studies have shown that benzoate displaces bilirubin from protein binding sites

Precautions Avoid using higher than recommended doses; suppression of HPA axis, suppression of linear growth (ie, reduction of growth velocity), reduced bone mineral density, hypercorticism (Cushing's syndrome), hyperglycemia, or glucosuria may occur; titrate to lowest effective dose. Reduction in growth velocity may occur when corticosteroids are administered to pediatric patients by any route (monitor growth). Use with extreme caution in patients with respiratory tuberculosis, untreated systemic infections, or ocular herpes simplex; use with caution in patients with thyroid dysfunction, cirrhosis, nonspecific ulcerative colitis, hypertension, renal impairment, osteoporosis, thromboembolic tendencies, CHF, recent MI, convulsive disorders, myasthenia gravis, thrombophlebitis, peptic ulcer, diabetes, glaucoma, cataracts, or hepatic impairment. Prolonged use may result in cataracts or glaucoma.

Adverse Reactions

Cardiovascular: Edema, hypertension, CHF

Central nervous system: Vertigo, seizures, psychoses, pseudotumor cerebri, headache, euphoria, insomnia, intracranial hypertension, nervousness

Dermatologic: Acne, skin atrophy, impaired wound healing, petechiae, bruising

Endocrine & metabolic: HPA suppression, Cushing's syndrome, growth suppression, glucose intolerance, hypokalemia, alkalosis, sodium and water retention

Gastrointestinal: Peptic ulcer, nausea, vomiting

Genitourinary: Menstrual irregularities

Neuromuscular & skeletal: Muscle weakness, osteoporosis, fractures, decreased bone mineral density

Ocular: Cataracts, elevated IOP, glaucoma

Miscellaneous: Immunosuppression, anaphylactoid reactions (rare)

Drug Interactions Cytochrome P450 isoenzyme CYP3A3/4 substrate and inducer

Enzyme-inducing agents (eg, barbiturates, phenytoin, rifampin) may decrease prednisolone serum concentrations. Estrogens and ketoconazole may decrease the hepatic metabolism of corticosteroids and increase corticosteroid serum concentrations and adverse effects (monitor). Cyclosporine may increase corticosteroid serum concentrations and corticosteroids may increase cyclosporine concentrations (monitor closely; convulsions have been reported with concurrent use). Use with aspirin, salicylates, or NSAIDs may increase risk of GI side effects. Caffeine

(Continued)

PrednisoLONE *(Continued)*

and alcohol may increase risk for GI ulcer. Use of corticosteroids with potassium-depleting drugs (eg, diuretics, amphotericin B) may increase risk for hypokalemia. Use with anticholinesterase agents may produce severe weakness in patients with myasthenia gravis. Corticosteroids may decrease effect of warfarin (monitor INR). Live or live, attenuated virus vaccines (these increase the risk of viral infection and are contraindicated with immunosuppressive doses of corticosteroids); toxoids and vaccines may have decreased effects; reactions to skin tests may be suppressed.

Food Interactions Systemic use of corticosteroids may require a diet with increased potassium, vitamins A, B_6, C, D, folate, calcium, zinc, and phosphorus and decreased sodium

Stability Dispense oral liquid formulations in tight, light-resistant containers. Storage: Prelone® syrup: Store at room temperature, do not refrigerate; Pediapred® oral solution: Store at 4°C to 24°C (39°F to 77°F), may be refrigerated; Orapred® oral solution: Store in refrigerator [2°C to 8°C (36°F to 46°F)]; Orapred ODT™: Store at controlled room temperature at 20°C to 25°C (68°F to 77°F) in blister pack; protect from moisture

Mechanism of Action Decreases inflammation by suppression of migration of polymorphonuclear leukocytes and reversal of increased capillary permeability; suppresses the immune system by reducing activity and volume of the lymphatic system

Pharmacokinetics

Absorption: Oral: Well absorbed

Protein binding: 70% to 90% (concentration dependent)

Metabolism: Primarily in the liver, but also metabolized in most tissues, to inactive compounds

Half-life: Adults (serum): 2-4 hours

Elimination: In urine, principally as glucuronide and sulfate-conjugated metabolites

Usual Dosage Dose depends upon condition being treated and response of patient; dosage for infants and children should be based on disease severity and patient response rather than by rigid adherence to dosage guidelines by age, weight, or body surface area. Consider alternate day therapy for long-term therapy. Discontinuation of long-term therapy requires gradual withdrawal by tapering the dose.

NIH Asthma Guidelines (NAEPP, 2002): Oral:

Children ≤12 years:

Asthma exacerbations (emergency care or hospital doses): 1 mg/kg every 6 hours for 48 hours; then 1-2 mg/kg/day (maximum: 60 mg/day) in divided doses given twice daily until peak expiratory flow is 70% of predicted or personal best

Short-course "burst" (acute asthma): 1-2 mg/kg/day in divided doses 1-2 times/day for 3-10 days; longer treatment may be required; usually given for 5 days; maximum dose: 60 mg/day

Long-term treatment: 0.25-2 mg/kg/day given as a single dose in the morning or every other day as needed for asthma control; maximum dose: 60 mg/day

Children >12 years and Adults:

Asthma exacerbations (emergency care or hospital doses): 120-180 mg/day in divided doses 3-4 times/day for 48 hours; then 60-80 mg in divided doses given twice daily until peak expiratory flow is 70% of predicted or personal best

Short-course "burst" (acute asthma): 40-60 mg/day in divided doses 1-2 times/day for 3-10 days; longer treatment may be required; usually given for 5 days

Long-term treatment: 7.5-60 mg daily given as a single dose in the morning or every other day as needed for asthma control

Children: Oral:

Anti-inflammatory or immunosuppressive dose: 0.1-2 mg/kg/day in divided doses 1-4 times/day

Nephrotic syndrome:

Pediatric Nephrology Panel recommendations (Hogg, 2000):

Initial: 2 mg/kg/day or 60 mg/m²/day given every day in 1-3 divided doses (maximum dose: 80 mg/day) until urine is protein free or for 4-6 weeks; followed by maintenance dose: 2 mg/kg/dose or 40 mg/m²/dose given every other day in the morning; gradually taper and discontinue after 4-6 weeks; **Note:** 6-week daily therapy followed by 6-week alternate day therapy may induce a higher rate of long remission compared to the standard of 4 weeks of daily therapy followed by 4 weeks of alternate day therapy; however, a higher incidence of adverse effects may be seen with the longer regimen and the clinical benefit may be variable

Relapse: Use high-dose daily steroid regimen (listed above) until urine is protein free for 3 days; follow with maintenance-tapering course of alternate day therapy (maintenance dose listed above) for 4-6 weeks; subsequent therapy is determined by individual's response and number of relapses (see Hogg, 2000)

British Pediatric Nephrology Consensus Statement (Report of a Workshop by the British Association for Paediatric Nephrology and Research Unit, 1994):

First 3 episodes: Initial: 2 mg/kg/day or 60 mg/m²/day given every day (maximum dose: 80 mg/day) until urine is protein free for 3 consecutive days (maximum dose: 28 days); followed by 1-1.5 mg/kg/dose or 40 mg/m²/dose (maximum: 60 mg/dose) given every other day for 4 weeks

Frequent relapses (long-term maintenance dose): 0.5-1 mg/kg/dose given every other day for 3-6 months

Adults: Oral: 5-60 mg/day

Children and Adults: Ophthalmic suspension: Instill 1-2 drops into conjunctival sac every hour during day, every 2 hours at night until favorable response is obtained, then use 1 drop every 4 hours

Administration

Oral: Administer after meals or with food or milk to decrease GI upset

Orapred ODT™: Do not cut, split, or break tablets; do not use partial tablets. Remove tablet from blister pack immediately prior to use. May swallow tablet whole or allow to dissolve on tongue

Ophthalmic: Shake suspension well before use; instill drops into affected eye(s); avoid contact of container tip with skin or eye; apply finger pressure to lacrimal sac during and for 1-2 minutes after instillation to decrease risk of absorption and systemic effects

Monitoring Parameters Blood pressure, weight, electrolytes, serum glucose; IOP (use >6 weeks); bone mineral density (long-term use); children's height and growth

Test Interactions Skin tests

Patient Information Avoid alcohol; limit caffeine; do not decrease dose or discontinue without physician's approval; avoid exposure to chicken pox or measles, if exposed, seek medical advice without delay

Dosage Forms Excipient information presented when available (limited, particularly for generics); consult specific product labeling.

Solution, ophthalmic, as sodium phosphate: 1% (5 mL, 10 mL, 15 mL) [contains benzalkonium chloride]

Solution, oral, as sodium phosphate: Prednisolone base 5 mg/5 mL (120 mL)

Orapred®: 20 mg/5 mL (20 mL, 240 mL) [equivalent to prednisolone base 15 mg/5 mL; dye free; contains alcohol 2%, sodium benzoate; grape flavor]

Pediapred®: 6.7 mg/5 mL (120 mL) [equivalent to prednisolone base 5 mg/5 mL; dye free; raspberry flavor]

Suspension, ophthalmic, as acetate: 1% (5 mL, 10 mL, 15 mL)

Econopred® Plus: 1% (5 mL, 10 mL) [contains benzalkonium chloride]

Pred Forte®: 1% (1 mL, 5 mL, 10 mL, 15 mL) [contains benzalkonium chloride and sodium bisulfite]

Pred Mild®: 0.12% (5 mL, 10 mL) [contains benzalkonium chloride and sodium bisulfite]

Syrup, as base: 5 mg/5 mL (120 mL); 15 mg/5 mL (240 mL, 480 mL)

Prelone®: 15 mg/5 mL (240 mL, 480 mL) [contains alcohol 5%, benzoic acid; cherry flavor]

Tablet, as base: 5 mg

Tablet, orally disintegrating, as base:

Orapred ODT™: 10 mg, 15 mg, 30 mg [grape flavor]

References

Hogg RJ, Portman RJ, Milliner D, et al, "Evaluation and Management of Proteinuria and Nephrotic Syndrome in Children: Recommendations From a Pediatric Nephrology Panel Established at the National Kidney Foundation Conference on Proteinuria, Albuminuria, Risk, Assessment, Detection, and Elimination (PARADE)," *Pediatrics*, 2000, 105(6):1242-9.

"National Asthma Education and Prevention Program. Expert Panel Report: Guidelines for the Diagnosis and Management of Asthma Update on Selected Topics--2002," *J Allergy Clin Immunol*, 2002, 110(5 Suppl):S141-219.

Report of a Workshop by the British Association for Paediatric Nephrology and Research Unit, Royal College of Physicians, "Consensus Statement on Management and Audit Potential for Steroid Responsive Nephrotic Syndrome," *Arch Dis Child*, 1994, 70(2):151-7.

♦ **Prednisolone Acetate** *see* PrednisoLONE *on page 1304*

♦ **Prednisolone Acetate, Ophthalmic** *see* PrednisoLONE *on page 1304*

Prednisolone and Gentamicin (pred NIS oh lone & jen ta MYE sin)

U.S. Brand Names Pred-G®

Index Terms Gentamicin and Prednisolone

Therapeutic Category Antibiotic, Ophthalmic; Corticosteroid, Ophthalmic

Generic Available No

(Continued)

Prednisolone and Gentamicin *(Continued)*

Use Treatment of steroid responsive inflammatory conditions and superficial ocular infections due to strains of microorganisms susceptible to gentamicin such as *Staphylococcus*, *E. coli*, *H. influenzae*, *Klebsiella*, *Neisseria*, *Pseudomonas*, *Proteus*, and *Serratia* species

Pregnancy Risk Factor C

Lactation Excretion in breast milk unknown/not recommended

Contraindications Hypersensitivity to prednisolone, gentamicin, or any component; dendritic keratitis, fungal diseases, vaccinia, varicella, most other viral infections, and mycobacterial infection of the eye. Contraindicated after uncomplicated removal of a corneal foreign body.

Warnings Prolonged use may result in glaucoma, damage to the optic nerve, defects in visual acuity, posterior subcapsular cataract formation, and secondary ocular infections

Adverse Reactions

Local: Burning, stinging, redness

Ocular: Elevation of intraocular pressure, glaucoma, infrequent optic nerve damage, posterior subcapsular cataract formation, superficial punctate keratitis, increased lacrimation

Miscellaneous: Development of secondary infection, allergic sensitization, delayed wound healing

Mechanism of Action See individual monographs for Prednisolone *on page 1304* and Gentamicin *on page 726*

Usual Dosage Children and Adults: Ophthalmic: Instill 1 drop 2-4 times/day; during the initial 24-48 hours, the dosing frequency may be increased if necessary, up to 1 drop every hour; or small amount (½" ribbon) of ointment can be applied into the conjunctival sac 1-3 times/day

Administration Suspension: Shake well before using; instill drop into affected eye; avoid contacting bottle tip with skin or eye; apply finger pressure to lacrimal sac during and for 1-2 minutes after instillation to decrease risk of absorption and systemic effects

Monitoring Parameters With use >10 days, monitor intraocular pressure

Dosage Forms Excipient information presented when available (limited, particularly for generics); consult specific product labeling.

Ointment, ophthalmic: Prednisolone acetate 0.6% and gentamicin sulfate 0.3% (3.5 g)

Suspension, ophthalmic: Prednisolone acetate 1% and gentamicin sulfate 0.3% (2 mL, 5 mL, 10 mL) [contains benzalkonium chloride]

- **Prednisolone, Neomycin, and Polymyxin B** *see* Neomycin, Polymyxin B, and Prednisolone *on page 1121*
- **Prednisolone Sodium Phosphate** *see* PrednisoLONE *on page 1304*
- **Prednisolone Sodium Phosphate, Ophthalmic** *see* PrednisoLONE *on page 1304*

PredniSONE (PRED ni sone)

Medication Safety Issues

Sound-alike/look-alike issues:

PredniSONE may be confused with methylPREDNISolone, Pramosone®, prazosin, prednisoLONE, Prilosec®, primidone, promethazine

Related Information

Asthma *on page 1904*

Corticosteroids, Systemic *on page 1685*

U.S. Brand Names Prednisone Intensol™; Sterapred®; Sterapred® DS

Canadian Brand Names Apo-Prednisone®; Novo-Prednisone; Winpred™

Index Terms Deltacortisone; Deltadehydrocortisone

Therapeutic Category Adrenal Corticosteroid; Anti-inflammatory Agent; Antiasthmatic; Corticosteroid, Systemic; Glucocorticoid

Generic Available Yes

Use Management of adrenocortical insufficiency; used for its anti-inflammatory or immunosuppressant effects

Pregnancy Risk Factor C

Lactation Enters breast milk/compatible

Contraindications Hypersensitivity to prednisone or any component; serious infections, except septic shock or tuberculous meningitis; systemic fungal infections; varicella infections; live or live, attenuated virus vaccines (with immunosuppressive doses of corticosteroids)

Warnings Hypothalamic pituitary adrenal (HPA) suppression may occur; acute adrenal insufficiency (adrenal crisis) may occur with abrupt withdrawal after long term therapy or with stress; withdrawal or discontinuation of corticosteroids should be done carefully; patients with HPA axis suppression may require increased doses of systemic glucocorticosteroids prior to, during, and after unusual stress (eg, surgery). Immunosuppression may occur; patients may be more susceptible to infections; avoid exposure to chickenpox and measles. Corticosteroids may mask signs of infection. Corticosteroids may activate latent opportunistic infections or exacerbate systemic fungal infections. May cause osteoporosis (at any age) or inhibition of bone growth in pediatric patients. Acute myopathy may occur with high doses, elevated IOP may occur (especially with prolonged use), CNS effects (ranging from euphoria to psychosis) may occur. Rare cases of anaphylactoid reactions have been reported with corticosteroids.

Oral solution contains sodium benzoate; benzoic acid (benzoate) is a metabolite of benzyl alcohol; large amounts of benzyl alcohol (≥99 mg/kg/day) have been associated with a potentially fatal toxicity ("gasping syndrome") in neonates; the "gasping syndrome" consists of metabolic acidosis, respiratory distress, gasping respirations, CNS dysfunction (including convulsions, intracranial hemorrhage), hypotension and cardiovascular collapse; use prednisone products containing sodium benzoate with caution in neonates; *in vitro* and animal studies have shown that benzoate displaces bilirubin from protein binding sites

Precautions Avoid using higher than recommended doses; suppression of HPA axis, suppression of linear growth (ie, reduction of growth velocity), reduced bone mineral density, hypercorticism (Cushing's syndrome), hyperglycemia, or glucosuria may occur; titrate to lowest effective dose. Reduction in growth velocity may occur when corticosteroids are administered to pediatric patients by any route (monitor growth). Use with extreme caution in patients with respiratory tuberculosis, untreated systemic infections, or ocular herpes simplex; use with caution in patients with thyroid dysfunction, cirrhosis, nonspecific ulcerative colitis, hypertension, renal impairment, osteoporosis, thromboembolic tendencies, CHF, recent MI, convulsive disorders, myasthenia gravis, thrombophlebitis, peptic ulcer, diabetes, glaucoma, cataracts, or hepatic impairment. Prolonged use may result in cataracts or glaucoma.

Adverse Reactions

Cardiovascular: Edema, hypertension, CHF

Central nervous system: Vertigo, seizures, psychoses, pseudotumor cerebri, headache, euphoria, insomnia, intracranial hypertension, nervousness

Dermatologic: Acne, skin atrophy, impaired wound healing, petechiae, bruising

Endocrine & metabolic: HPA suppression, Cushing's syndrome, growth suppression, glucose intolerance, hypokalemia, alkalosis, sodium and water retention

Gastrointestinal: Peptic ulcer, nausea, vomiting

Genitourinary: Menstrual irregularities

Neuromuscular & skeletal: Muscle weakness, osteoporosis, fractures, decreased bone mineral density

Ocular: Cataracts, elevated IOP, glaucoma

Miscellaneous: Immunosuppression, anaphylactoid reactions (rare)

Drug Interactions Cytochrome P450 isoenzyme CYP3A3/4 substrate and inducer

Barbiturates, phenytoin, rifampin, salicylates, toxoids, NSAIDs, diuretics (potassium depleting); caffeine and alcohol may increase risk for GI ulcer; live or live, attenuated virus vaccines (these increase the risk of viral infection and are contraindicated with immunosuppressive doses of corticosteroids); toxoids and vaccines may have decreased effects; reactions to skin tests may be suppressed.

Food Interactions Systemic use of corticosteroids may require a diet with increased potassium, vitamins A, B_6, C, D, folate, calcium, zinc, and phosphorus and decreased sodium

Mechanism of Action Decreases inflammation by suppression of migration of polymorphonuclear leukocytes and reversal of increased capillary permeability; suppresses the immune system by reducing activity and volume of the lymphatic system

Pharmacokinetics Converted rapidly in the liver to prednisolone (active)

Usual Dosage Dose depends upon condition being treated and response of patient; dosage for infants and children should be based on disease severity and patient response rather than by rigid adherence to dosage guidelines by age, weight, or body surface area. Consider alternate day therapy for long-term therapy. Discontinuation of long-term therapy requires gradual withdrawal by tapering the dose. Oral:

NIH Asthma Guidelines (NAEPP, 2002):

Children ≤12 years:

Asthma exacerbations (emergency care or hospital doses): 1 mg/kg every 6 hours for 48 hours; then 1-2 mg/kg/day (maximum: 60 mg/day) in divided doses given twice daily until peak expiratory flow is 70% of predicted or personal best

(Continued)

PredniSONE *(Continued)*

Short-course "burst" (acute asthma): 1-2 mg/kg/day in divided doses 1-2 times/day for 3-10 days; longer treatment may be required; usually given for 5 days; maximum dose: 60 mg/day

Long-term treatment: 0.25-2 mg/kg/day given as a single dose in the morning or every other day as needed for asthma control; maximum dose: 60 mg/day

Children >12 years and Adults:

Asthma exacerbations (emergency care or hospital doses): 120-180 mg/day in divided doses 3-4 times/day for 48 hours; then 60-80 mg in divided doses given twice daily until peak expiratory flow is 70% of predicted or personal best

Short-course "burst" (acute asthma): 40-60 mg/day in divided doses 1-2 times/day for 3-10 days; longer treatment may be required; usually given for 5 days

Long-term treatment: 7.5-60 mg daily given as a single dose in the morning or every other day as needed for asthma control

Children:

Alternative asthma dosing by age:

Short-course "burst" (acute asthma):

<1 year: 10 mg every 12 hours
1-4 years: 20 mg every 12 hours
5-13 years: 30 mg every 12 hours
>13 years: 40 mg every 12 hours

Long-term treatment:

<1 year: 10 mg every other day
1-4 years: 20 mg every other day
5-13 years: 30 mg every other day
>13 years: 40 mg every other day

Anti-inflammatory or immunosuppressive: 0.05-2 mg/kg/day divided 1-4 times/day

Nephrotic syndrome:

Pediatric Nephrology Panel recommendations (Hogg, 2000):

Initial: 2 mg/kg/day or 60 mg/m²/day given every day in 1-3 divided doses (maximum dose: 80 mg/day) until urine is protein free or for 4-6 weeks; followed by maintenance dose: 2 mg/kg/dose or 40 mg/m²/dose given every other day in the morning; gradually taper and discontinue after 4-6 weeks; **Note:** 6-week daily therapy followed by 6-week alternate day therapy may induce a higher rate of long remission compared to the standard of 4 weeks of daily therapy followed by 4 weeks of alternate day therapy; however, a higher incidence of adverse effects may be seen with the longer regimen and the clinical benefit may be variable

Relapse: Use high-dose daily steroid regimen (listed above) until urine is protein free for 3 days; follow with maintenance-tapering course of alternate day therapy (maintenance dose listed above) for 4-6 weeks; subsequent therapy is determined by individual's response and number of relapses (see Hogg, 2000)

British Pediatric Nephrology Consensus Statement (Report of a Workshop by the British Association for Paediatric Nephrology and Research Unit, 1994):

First 3 episodes: Initial: 2 mg/kg/day or 60 mg/m²/day given every day (maximum dose: 80 mg/day) until urine is protein free for 3 consecutive days (maximum dose: 28 days); followed by 1-1.5 mg/kg/dose or 40 mg/m²/dose (maximum: 60 mg/dose) given every other day for 4 weeks

Frequent relapses (long-term maintenance dose): 0.5-1 mg/kg/dose given every other day for 3-6 months

Children and Adults: Physiologic replacement: 4-5 mg/m²/day

Adults: 5-60 mg/day in divided doses 1-4 times/day

Administration Oral: Administer after meals or with food or milk to decrease GI upset

Monitoring Parameters Blood pressure, weight, serum electrolytes, glucose; children's height and growth

Test Interactions Skin tests

Patient Information Avoid alcohol; limit caffeine; do not decrease dose or discontinue without physician's approval

Dosage Forms Excipient information presented when available (limited, particularly for generics); consult specific product labeling.

Solution, oral: 1 mg/mL (5 mL, 120 mL, 500 mL) [contains alcohol 5%, sodium benzoate; vanilla flavor]

Solution, oral concentrate (Prednisone Intensol™): 5 mg/mL (30 mL) [contains alcohol 30%]

Tablet: 1 mg, 2.5 mg, 5 mg, 10 mg, 20 mg, 50 mg

Sterapred®: 5 mg [supplied as 21 tablet 6-day unit-dose package or 48 tablet 12-day unit-dose package]

Sterapred® DS: 10 mg [supplied as 21 tablet 6-day unit-dose package or 48 tablet 12-day unit-dose package]

References

Hogg RJ, Portman RJ, Milliner D, et al, "Evaluation and Management of Proteinuria and Nephrotic Syndrome in Children: Recommendations From a Pediatric Nephrology Panel Established at the National Kidney Foundation Conference on Proteinuria, Albuminuria, Risk, Assessment, Detection, and Elimination (PARADE)," *Pediatrics*, 2000, 105(6):1242-9.

Murphy CM, Coonce SL, and Simon PA, "Treatment of Asthma in Children," *Clin Pharm*, 1991, 10(9):685-703.

"National Asthma Education and Prevention Program. Expert Panel Report: Guidelines for the Diagnosis and Management of Asthma Update on Selected Topics--2002," *J Allergy Clin Immunol*, 2002, 110(5 Suppl):S141-219.

Report of a Workshop by the British Association for Paediatric Nephrology and Research Unit, Royal College of Physicians, "Consensus Statement on Management and Audit Potential for Steroid Responsive Nephrotic Syndrome," *Arch Dis Child*, 1994, 70(2):151-7.

- **Prednisone Intensol™** *see* PredniSONE *on page 1308*
- **Pregnyl®** *see* Chorionic Gonadotropin *on page 351*
- **Prelone®** *see* PrednisoLONE *on page 1304*
- **Premarin®** *see* Estrogens (Conjugated/Equine) *on page 610*
- **Premjact® [OTC]** *see* Lidocaine *on page 933*
- **Preparation H® [OTC]** *see* Phenylephrine *on page 1250*
- **Preparation H® Hydrocortisone [OTC]** *see* Hydrocortisone *on page 781*
- **Pre-Pen® [DSC]** *see* Benzylpenicilloyl-polylysine [DSC] *on page 210*
- **Pressyn® (Can)** *see* Vasopressin *on page 1602*
- **Pressyn® AR (Can)** *see* Vasopressin *on page 1602*
- **Pretz® [OTC]** *see* Sodium Chloride *on page 1450*
- **Pretz-D® [OTC]** *see* Ephedrine *on page 575*
- **Prevacare® [OTC]** *see* Ethyl Alcohol *on page 610*
- **Prevacid®** *see* Lansoprazole *on page 911*
- **Prevacid® SoluTab™** *see* Lansoprazole *on page 911*
- **Prevalite®** *see* Cholestyramine Resin *on page 349*
- **Prevex® B (Can)** *see* Betamethasone *on page 212*
- **Prevex® HC (Can)** *see* Hydrocortisone *on page 781*
- **PreviDent®** *see* Fluoride *on page 675*
- **PreviDent® 5000 Plus™** *see* Fluoride *on page 675*
- **Prevnar®** *see* Pneumococcal Conjugate Vaccine (7-Valent) *on page 1271*
- **Prilocaine and Lidocaine** *see* Lidocaine and Prilocaine *on page 937*
- **Prilosec®** *see* Omeprazole *on page 1167*
- **Prilosec OTC™ [OTC]** *see* Omeprazole *on page 1167*
- **Primaclone** *see* Primidone *on page 1312*
- **Primacor®** *see* Milrinone *on page 1062*

Primaquine (PRIM a kween)

Related Information
Malaria *on page 1855*

Index Terms Primaquine Phosphate; Prymaccone

Therapeutic Category Antimalarial Agent

Generic Available Yes

Use In conjunction with a blood schizonticidal agent to provide radical cure of *P. vivax* or *P. ovale* malaria after a clinical attack has been confirmed by blood smear or serologic titer; prevention of relapse of *P. ovale* or *P. vivax* malaria; malaria postexposure prophylaxis

Pregnancy Risk Factor C

Lactation Excretion in breast milk unknown

Contraindications Acutely ill patients who have a tendency to develop granulocytopenia (rheumatoid arthritis, SLE); patients receiving other drugs capable of depressing the bone marrow; patients receiving quinacrine

Precautions Use with caution in patients with G6PD deficiency or NADH methemoglobin reductase deficiency

Adverse Reactions
Cardiovascular: Arrhythmias, hypertension
Central nervous system: Headache
Dermatologic: Pruritus
Gastrointestinal: Nausea, vomiting, abdominal cramps
Hematologic: Hemolytic anemia, methemoglobinemia, leukocytosis, leukopenia, agranulocytosis
Ocular: Interference with visual accommodation

Drug Interactions Quinacrine (increased toxicity of primaquine)

Stability Protect from light

(Continued)

Primaquine *(Continued)*

Mechanism of Action Eliminates the primary tissue exoerythrocytic forms of *P. falciparum*, *P. malariae*, *P. ovale*, and *P. vivax*; interferes with plasmodial DNA

Pharmacokinetics

Absorption: Oral: Well absorbed

Metabolism: Liver metabolism to carboxyprimaquine, an active metabolite

Half-life: 3.7-9.6 hours

Time to peak serum concentration: Within 6 hours

Elimination: Small amount of unchanged drug excreted in urine

Usual Dosage Oral:

Children: 0.3 mg base/kg/day once daily for 14 days not to exceed 15 mg base/day, or 0.9 mg base/kg once weekly for 8 weeks not to exceed 45 mg base/week

Adults: 15 mg/day (base) once daily for 14 days or 45 mg base once weekly for 8 weeks

Administration Oral: Administer with meals to decrease adverse GI effects; drug has a bitter taste

Monitoring Parameters Periodic CBC, visual color check of urine, hemoglobin

Patient Information Notify physician if a darkening of the urine occurs

Dosage Forms Excipient information presented when available (limited, particularly for generics); consult specific product labeling.

Tablet, as phosphate: 26.3 mg [15 mg base]

References

Lynk A and Gold R, "Review of 40 Children With Imported Malaria," *Pediatr Infect Dis J*, 1989, 8(11):745-50.

Wyler DJ, "Malaria Chemoprophylaxis for the Traveler," *N Engl J Med*, 1993, 329(1):31-7.

♦ **Primaquine Phosphate** *see* Primaquine *on page 1311*

♦ **Primatene® Mist [OTC]** *see* Epinephrine *on page 577*

♦ **Primaxin®** *see* Imipenem and Cilastatin *on page 813*

♦ **Primaxin® I.V. (Can)** *see* Imipenem and Cilastatin *on page 813*

Primidone (PRI mi done)

Medication Safety Issues

Sound-alike/look-alike issues:

Primidone may be confused with predniSONE

Related Information

Antiepileptic Drugs *on page 1902*

U.S. Brand Names Mysoline®

Canadian Brand Names Apo-Primidone®

Index Terms Desoxyphenobarbital; Primaclone

Therapeutic Category Anticonvulsant, Barbiturate; Barbiturate

Generic Available Yes

Use Management of generalized tonic-clonic (grand mal), complex partial and simple partial (focal) seizures

Pregnancy Risk Factor D

Lactation Enters breast milk/not recommended (AAP recommends use "with caution")

Contraindications Hypersensitivity to primidone or any component; porphyria

Warnings Generic tablet may contain sodium benzoate; benzoic acid (benzoate) is a metabolite of benzyl alcohol; large amounts of benzyl alcohol (≥99 mg/kg/day) have been associated with a potentially fatal toxicity ("gasping syndrome") in neonates; the "gasping syndrome" consists of metabolic acidosis, respiratory distress, gasping respirations, CNS dysfunction (including convulsions, intracranial hemorrhage), hypotension and cardiovascular collapse; avoid use of primidone products containing sodium benzoate in neonates; *in vitro* and animal studies have shown that benzoate displaces bilirubin from protein binding sites

Precautions Use with caution in patients with renal or hepatic impairment; abrupt discontinuation may precipitate status epilepticus

Adverse Reactions

Central nervous system: Drowsiness, vertigo, lethargy, behavior change, ataxia

Dermatologic: Rash

Gastrointestinal: Nausea, vomiting

Hematologic: Leukopenia, malignant lymphoma-like syndrome, megaloblastic anemia

Ocular: Diplopia, nystagmus

Miscellaneous: Systemic lupus-like syndrome

Drug Interactions Cytochrome P450 isoenzyme CYP1A2, CYP2B6, CYP2C, CYP2C8, CYP3A3/4, and CYP3A5-7 inducer

Primidone may decrease serum concentrations of ethosuximide, valproic acid, griseofulvin; methylphenidate may increase primidone serum concentrations; phenytoin may decrease primidone serum concentrations; valproic acid may increase phenobarbital concentrations derived from primidone

Food Interactions May increase the metabolism of vitamins D and K; dietary requirements of vitamins D, K, B_{12}, folate, and calcium may be increased with long-term use

Mechanism of Action Decreases neuron excitability, raises seizure threshold similar to phenobarbital

Pharmacokinetics

Distribution: V_d: Adults: 2-3 L/kg

Protein-binding: 99%

Metabolism: In the liver to phenobarbital (active) and phenylethylmalonamide (PEMA)

Bioavailability: 60% to 80%

Half-life:

- Primidone: 10-12 hours
- PEMA: 16 hours
- Phenobarbital: 52-118 hours (age-dependent)

Time to peak serum concentration: Oral: Within 4 hours

Elimination: Urinary excretion of both active metabolites and unchanged primidone (15% to 25%)

Usual Dosage Oral:

Neonates: 12-20 mg/kg/day in divided doses 2-4 times/day; start with lower dosage and titrate upward

Children <8 years: Initial: 50-125 mg/day given at bedtime; increase by 50-125 mg/day increments every 3-7 days; usual dose: 10-25 mg/kg/day in divided doses 3-4 times/day

Children ≥8 years and Adults: Initial: 125-250 mg/day at bedtime; increase by 125-250 mg/day every 3-7 days; usual dose: 750-1500 mg/day in divided doses 3-4 times/day with maximum dosage of 2 g/day

Administration Oral: Administer with food to decrease GI upset

Monitoring Parameters Serum primidone and phenobarbital concentrations; CBC with differential; neurological status, seizure frequency, duration, severity

Reference Range Monitor both primidone and phenobarbital concentrations (see Phenobarbital *on page 1245*); Primidone:

Therapeutic: 5-12 mcg/mL (SI: 23-55 micromoles/L)

Toxic effects rarely present with levels <10 mcg/mL (SI: 46 micromoles/L) if phenobarbital concentrations are low

Toxic: >15 mcg/mL (SI: >69 micromoles/L)

Patient Information Avoid alcohol; limit caffeine; may cause drowsiness and impair ability to perform activities requiring mental alertness or physical coordination; do not abruptly discontinue or change dose without physician approval

Additional Information Mysoline® suspension was discontinued in February 2001

Dosage Forms Excipient information presented when available (limited, particularly for generics); consult specific product labeling.

Tablet: 50 mg, 250 mg [generic tablet may contain sodium benzoate]

Dosage forms available in Canada: Tablet: 125 mg, 250 mg. **Note:** 50 mg tablet is **not** available in Canada.

- ♦ **Primsol®** *see* Trimethoprim *on page 1578*
- ♦ **Prinivil®** *see* Lisinopril *on page 946*
- ♦ **Priorix™ (Can)** *see* Measles, Mumps, and Rubella Vaccines (Combined) *on page 980*
- ♦ **Pristinamycin** *see* Quinupristin/Dalfopristin *on page 1360*
- ♦ **Privine® [OTC]** *see* Naphazoline *on page 1106*
- ♦ **ProAir™ HFA** *see* Albuterol *on page 66*

Probenecid (proe BEN e sid)

Medication Safety Issues

Sound-alike/look-alike issues:

Probenecid may be confused with Procanbid®

Canadian Brand Names Benuryl™

Index Terms Benemid [DSC]

Therapeutic Category Adjuvant Therapy, Penicillin Level Prolongation; Antigout Agent; Uric Acid Lowering Agent; Uricosuric Agent

Generic Available Yes

Use Treatment of hyperuricemia associated with gout and gouty arthritis; adjuvant to therapy with penicillins or cephalosporins to prolong serum levels

Pregnancy Risk Factor B

Lactation Excretion in breast milk unknown

Contraindications Hypersensitivity to probenecid or any component; children <2 years of age; individuals with blood dyscrasias or uric acid kidney stones

(Continued)

Probenecid *(Continued)*

Warnings Salicylates may diminish the therapeutic effect of probenecid; this effect may be more pronounced with high, chronic doses; however, the manufacturer recommends the use of an alternative analgesic even in place of small doses of aspirin; therapy with probenecid should not be initiated until an acute gouty attack has subsided; if an acute attack occurs during probenecid therapy, usage may continue but other appropriate agents (eg, colchicine) should be used to control the acute attack

Precautions Use with caution in patients with peptic ulcer; hematuria, renal colic; formation of uric acid stones associated with the use of probenecid may be prevented by liberal fluid intake and alkalinization of urine; may not be effective when Cl_{cr} <30 mL/minute

Adverse Reactions

Cardiovascular: Flushing
Central nervous system: Dizziness, headache, fever
Dermatologic: Rash, alopecia, dermatitis, pruritus
Gastrointestinal: Anorexia, nausea, vomiting, sore gums
Genitourinary: Urinary frequency, hematuria
Hematologic: Anemia, leukopenia, aplastic anemia, hemolytic anemia (possibly related to G-6-PD deficiency)
Hepatic: Hepatic necrosis
Neuromuscular & skeletal: Costovertebral pain, gouty arthritis (acute)
Renal: Nephrotic syndrome, renal colic, uric acid stones
Miscellaneous: Hypersensitivity reactions

Drug Interactions Salicylates and probenecid inhibit the uricosuric actions of each other (see Warnings); probenecid may increase the plasma levels (decrease the excretion) of acyclovir, penicillins, ciprofloxacin, ganciclovir, cephalosporins, methotrexate, dapsone, NSAIDs, carbapenem antibiotics (eg, ertapenem, imipenem, meropenem), and dapsone; may decrease the metabolism of zidovudine, benzodiazepines, and thiopental; sulfonylureas may have an increase in half-life; clofibrate may have an increased accumulation of its active metabolite; avoid concomitant use with ketorolac since its half-life is increased twofold and levels and toxicity are significantly increased; niacin may inhibit uricosuric effects of probenecid

Mechanism of Action Competitively inhibits the reabsorption of uric acid at the proximal convoluted tubule, thereby promoting its excretion and reducing serum uric acid levels; increases plasma levels of weak organic acids (penicillins, cephalosporins, or other beta-lactam antibiotics) by competitively inhibiting their renal tubular secretion

Pharmacodynamics Exerts maximal effects on penicillin levels after 2 hours; produces maximal renal clearance of uric acid in 30 minutes

Pharmacokinetics

Absorption: Rapid and complete from GI tract
Protein binding: 85% to 95%
Metabolism: In the liver
Half-life: 6-12 hours
Time to peak serum concentration: Within 2-4 hours

Usual Dosage Oral:

Prolongation of penicillin serum levels:

Children 2-14 years: Initial: 25 mg/kg/dose or 0.7 g/m^2/dose as a single dose; maintenance: 40 mg/kg/day or 1.2 g/m^2/day in 4 divided doses (maximum single dose: 500 mg)

Adults: 500 mg 4 times/day

Hyperuricemia: Adults: Initial: 250 mg twice daily for 1 week; increase to 500 mg twice daily; may increase in 500 mg increments every 4 weeks if needed to a maximum of 2-3 g/day; begin therapy 2-3 weeks after an acute gouty attack

Gonorrhea: Children >45 kg and Adults: CDC guidelines (alternative regimen): 1 g before appropriate antibiotic (eg, cefoxitin)

Pelvic inflammatory disease: CDC guidelines (alternative regimen): 1 g before appropriate antibiotic (eg, cefoxitin)

Neurosyphilis: CDC guidelines (alternative regimen): 500 mg 4 times/day plus procaine penicillin 2.4 million units/day I.M. for 10-14 days

Dosing adjustment in renal impairment: Cl_{cr} <30 mL/minute: Avoid use

Administration Oral: Administer with food or antacids to minimize GI effects

Monitoring Parameters Uric acid, renal function, CBC

Test Interactions False-positive glucosuria with Clinitest®; falsely elevated serum theophylline level (Schack & Waxler technique); inhibits renal excretion of phenosulfonphythalein (PSP), 17-ketosteroids, and sulfobromophthalein (BSP)

Patient Information Drink plenty of fluids to reduce the risk of uric acid stones; the frequency of acute gouty attacks may increase during the first 6-12 months of therapy; avoid taking large doses of aspirin or other salicylates; avoid alcohol

Dosage Forms Excipient information presented when available (limited, particularly for generics); consult specific product labeling.

Tablet: 500 mg

References

Centers for Disease Control and Prevention, "Sexually Transmitted Diseases Treatment Guidelines, 2006," *MMWR Recomm Rep*, 2006, 55(RR-11):1-94.

Procainamide (proe kane A mide)

Medication Safety Issues

Sound-alike/look-alike issues:

Procanbid® may be confused with probenecid

Pronestyl® may be confused with Ponstel®

PCA is an error-prone abbreviation (mistaken as patient controlled analgesia)

Related Information

Adult ACLS Algorithms *on page 1660*

CPR Pediatric Drug Dosages *on page 1650*

Medications for Which A Single Dose May Be Fatal When Ingested By A Toddler *on page 1932*

Pediatric ALS Algorithms *on page 1657*

U.S. Brand Names Procanbid®

Canadian Brand Names Apo-Procainamide®; Procainamide Hydrochloride Injection, USP; Procan® SR; Pronestyl®-SR

Index Terms PCA (error-prone abbreviation); Procainamide Hydrochloride; Procaine Amide Hydrochloride

Therapeutic Category Antiarrhythmic Agent, Class I-A

Generic Available Yes

Use Treatment of ventricular tachycardia, premature ventricular contractions, paroxysmal atrial tachycardia, and atrial fibrillation; to prevent recurrence of ventricular tachycardia, paroxysmal supraventricular tachycardia, atrial fibrillation or flutter; **Note:** Due to proarrhythmic effects, use should be reserved for life-threatening arrhythmias

Procainamide is recommended in the PALS guidelines for tachycardia with pulses and poor perfusion [SVT (unresponsive to vagal maneuvers and adenosine) and VT (unresponsive to synchronized cardioversion or adenosine)]. It is recommended in the ACLS guidelines as one of several drugs that can be considered for treatment of the following arrhythmias in patients with preserved ventricular function: Stable monomorphic VT; atrial fibrillation or atrial flutter, including pre-excitation syndrome; AV re-entrant narrow complex tachycardias (eg, re-entrant SVT), uncontrolled by adenosine and vagal maneuvers; and stable wide complex regular tachycardia (likely VT).

Pregnancy Risk Factor C

Lactation Enters breast milk/use caution (AAP rates "compatible")

Contraindications Hypersensitivity to procainamide, procaine, related drugs, or any component (see Warnings); complete heart block; second or third degree heart block without pacemaker; "torsade de pointes" (twisting of the points), an unusual ventricular tachycardia; pre-existing QT prolongation; myasthenia gravis; SLE

Warnings Serious blood dyscrasias may occur (see Adverse Reactions); long-term administration leads to the development of a positive antinuclear antibody (ANA) test in 50% of patients which may lead to a lupus erythematosus-like syndrome (in 20% to 30% of patients); assess relative benefits and risks if ANA titer becomes positive and consider alternative agent; discontinue procainamide if SLE symptoms develop and change to alternative agent; do not use sustained release preparation for initial therapy; injection contains sulfites which may cause allergic reactions in susceptible individuals

Precautions Use with caution in patients with marked A-V conduction disturbances, bundle-branch block or severe cardiac glycoside intoxication, ventricular arrhythmias in patients with organic heart disease or coronary occlusion, CHF, supraventricular tachyarrhythmias unless digitalis glycoside levels are adequate to prevent marked increases in ventricular rates; drug may accumulate in patients with renal or hepatic dysfunction, dosage adjustment required

Adverse Reactions

Cardiovascular: Hypotension, tachycardia, arrhythmias, A-V block, QT prolongation, widening QRS complex

Central nervous system: Confusion, disorientation, drug fever

Gastrointestinal: Nausea, vomiting, GI complaints

Hematologic: Agranulocytosis, neutropenia, thrombocytopenia, hypoplastic anemia

Hepatic: Hepatomegaly, elevated liver enzymes

Miscellaneous: Lupus-like syndrome (arthralgia, positive Coombs' test, thrombocytopenia, rash, myalgia, fever, pericarditis, pleural effusion)

(Continued)

Procainamide *(Continued)*

Drug Interactions Cimetidine, ranitidine, amiodarone, beta-blocking agents, trimethoprim may increase plasma procainamide and NAPA concentrations, procainamide dosage adjustment may be required; procainamide may potentiate skeletal muscle relaxants; anticholinergic drugs may have enhanced effects

Food Interactions Procanbid® extended release tablets: A high fat meal may increase extent of absorption by ~20%

Stability Use only clear or slightly yellow solutions; stability of parenteral admixture with D_5W at room temperature (25°C) is 24 hours but 7 days at refrigerated temperature (2°C to 8°C)

Mechanism of Action Class IA antiarrhythmic with anticholinergic and local anesthetic effects; decreases myocardial excitability and conduction velocity and depresses myocardial contractility, by increasing the electrical stimulation threshold of ventricle, His-Purkinje system and through direct cardiac effects

Pharmacodynamics Onset of action: I.M. 10-30 minutes

Pharmacokinetics

Absorption: Oral: Well absorbed; Procanbid®: Absorption is sustained over 12 hours

Distribution: V_d (decreased with CHF or shock):
- Children: 2.2 L/kg
- Adults: 2 L/kg

Protein binding: 15% to 20%

Metabolism: By acetylation in the liver to produce N-acetyl procainamide (NAPA) (active metabolite)

Bioavailability, oral: 75% to 95%

Half-life:
- Procainamide (dependent upon hepatic acetylator phenotype, cardiac function, and renal function):
  - Children: 1.7 hours
  - Adults with normal renal function: 2.5-4.7 hours
- NAPA (dependent upon renal function):
  - Children: 6 hours
  - Adults with normal renal function: 6-8 hours

Time to peak serum concentration:
- Oral (capsule): Within 45 minutes to 2.5 hours
- I.M.: 15-60 minutes

Elimination: Urinary excretion (25% as NAPA)

Dialysis: Moderately dialyzable by hemodialysis (20% to 50%), but not dialyzable by peritoneal dialysis

Usual Dosage Must be titrated to patient's response

Children:
- Oral: 15-50 mg/kg/day divided every 3-6 hours; maximum 4 g/day
- I.M.: 20-30 mg/kg/day divided every 4-6 hours; maximum 4 g/day
- I.V.:
  - Loading dose: 3-6 mg/kg/dose over 5 minutes, not to exceed 100 mg/dose; may repeat every 5-10 minutes to maximum total loading dose of 15 mg/kg; do not exceed 500 mg in 30 minutes
  - Maintenance: Continuous I.V. infusion: 20-80 mcg/kg/minute; maximum dose: 2 g/day
- PALS Guidelines 2005 (for perfusing tachycardias): **Note:** Use extreme caution when administering procainamide with other drugs that prolong QT interval (eg, amiodarone); consider consulting with expert
  - I.V., I.O.: Loading dose: 15 mg/kg infused over 30-60 minutes; monitor EKG and blood pressure; stop the infusion if hypotension occurs or QRS complex widens by >50% of baseline

Adults:
- Oral: Immediate release products: 250-500 mg/dose every 3-6 hours; sustained release: 500 mg to 1 g every 6 hours; extended release (Procanbid®): 1-2 g every 12 hours; usual dose: 50 mg/kg/day or 2-4 g/day
- I.V.: **Note:** Reduce loading dose to 12 mg/kg in patients with severe renal or cardiac impairment; reduce maintenance infusion by one-third in patients with moderate renal or cardiac impairment and by two-thirds in patients with severe renal or cardiac impairment
  - Loading dose: 50-100 mg/dose, repeated every 5-10 minutes until patient controlled; or load with 15-18 mg/kg; maximum loading dose: 1-1.5 g
  - Maintenance: Continuous I.V. infusion: 3-4 mg/minute; range: 1-6 mg/minute; monitor levels and do not exceed 3 mg/minute for >24 hours in adults with renal failure
- Refractory ventricular fibrillation:
  - Loading dose: 30 mg/minute up to a total of 17 mg/kg

I.V. maintenance infusion: 1-4 mg/minute; monitor levels and do not exceed 3 mg/minute for >24 hours in adults with renal failure

ACLS guidelines 2005:

I.V.: Loading dose: Infuse 20 mg/minute until arrhythmia is controlled, hypotension occurs, QRS complex widens by 50% of its original width, or total of 17 mg/kg is given

I.V. maintenance infusion: 1-4 mg/minute; decrease dose in patients with renal failure

Dosing interval in renal impairment:

Oral:

Cl_{cr} 10-50 mL/minute: Administer normal dose every 6-12 hours

Cl_{cr} <10 mL/minute: Administer normal dose every 8-24 hours

I.V.: Adults:

Loading dose: Reduce dose to 12 mg/kg in severe renal impairment.

Maintenance infusion: Reduce dose by one-third in patients with mild renal impairment. Reduce dose by two-thirds in patients with severe renal impairment.

Dialysis:

Procainamide: Moderately hemodialyzable (20% to 50%): Adults: 200 mg supplemental dose posthemodialysis is recommended.

N-acetylprocainamide: Not dialyzable (0% to 5%)

Procainamide/N-acetylprocainamide: Not peritoneal dialyzable (0% to 5%)

Procainamide/N-acetylprocainamide: Replace by blood level during continuous arteriovenous or venovenous hemofiltration

Dosing adjustment in hepatic impairment: Reduce dose by 50%.

Administration

Oral: Administer with water on an empty stomach; if GI distress occurs may administer with food or milk to decrease GI upset; swallow extended and sustained release tablets whole, do not chew, break, or crush

Parenteral: I.V.: Do not administer faster than 20-30 mg/minute; severe hypotension can occur with rapid I.V. administration; administer I.V. push over at least 5 minutes; administer I.V. loading doses and intermittent infusions over 25-30 minutes; use concentration of 20-30 mg/mL for loading dose and 2-4 mg/mL for maintenance infusions; rate of infusion (mL/hour) = dose (mcg/kg/minute) x weight (kg) x 60 minutes/hour divided by the concentration

Monitoring Parameters EKG, blood pressure, CBC with differential, platelet count, antinuclear antibody test (ANA); serum drug concentrations, procainamide and NAPA, especially in patients with renal failure or those receiving higher maintenance doses (eg, adults: >3 mg/minute) for >24 hours

Reference Range

Therapeutic:

Procainamide: 4-10 mcg/mL (SI: 15-37 micromoles/L)

Sum of procainamide and N-acetyl procainamide: 10-30 mcg/mL (SI: <110 micromoles/L)

Optimal ranges must be ascertained for individual patients, with EKG monitoring

Toxic (procainamide): >10-12 mcg/mL (SI: >37-44 micromoles/L)

Patient Information Limit alcohol; some sustained release tablets have a wax core that slowly releases the drug, this wax core is not absorbed and will be eliminated in the stool; inform physician if symptoms such as fever, sore throat, chills, bruising, or bleeding occur

Dosage Forms Excipient information presented when available (limited, particularly for generics); consult specific product labeling.

Capsule, as hydrochloride: 250 mg, 500 mg

Injection, solution, as hydrochloride: 100 mg/mL (10 mL); 500 mg/mL (2 mL) [contains sodium metabisulfite]

Tablet, extended release, as hydrochloride: 500 mg, 750 mg, 1000 mg

Procanbid®: 500 mg, 1000 mg

Extemporaneous Preparations Note: Several formulations have been described, some being more complex; for all formulations, the pH must be 4-6 to prevent degradation; some preparations require adjustment of pH; **label all preparations "shake well before use"**

A 50 mg/mL oral liquid preparation made from the contents of capsules and 3 different vehicles (cherry syrup, a 1:1 mixture of Ora-Sweet® and Ora-Plus®, or a 1:1 mixture of Ora-Sweet® SF and Ora-Plus®) was stable for 60 days when stored in amber plastic prescription bottles in the dark at room temperature (25°C) or under refrigeration (5°C); empty the contents of twenty-four 250 mg capsules into a mortar; break up the powder and pulverize it; add 20 mL of the vehicle and mix well to form a uniform paste; mix while adding the vehicle in geometric proportions to **almost** 120 mL; transfer to a calibrated bottle and qsad with vehicle to 120 mL; label "protect from light" (Allen, 1996)

(Continued)

Procainamide *(Continued)*

A suspension of 50 mg/mL can be made with the capsules, distilled water, and a 2:1 simple syrup/cherry syrup mixture; stability 2 weeks under refrigeration (ASHP, 1987)

Concentrations of 5, 50, and 100 mg/mL oral liquid preparations, (made with the capsules, sterile water for irrigation and cherry syrup) stored at 4°C to 6°C (pH 6) were stable for at least 6 months (Metras, 1992)

A sucrose-based syrup (procainamide 50 mg/mL) made with capsules, distilled water, simple syrup, parabens, and cherry flavoring had a calculated stability of 456 days at 25°C and measured stability of 42 days at 40°C (pH ~5) while a maltitol-based syrup (procainamide 50 mg/mL) made with capsules, distilled water, Lycasin® (a syrup vehicle with 75% w/w maltitol), parabens, sodium bisulfate, saccharin, sodium acetate, pineapple and apricot flavoring, FD & C yellow number 6, (pH adjusted to 5 with glacial acetic acid) had a calculated stability of 97 days at 25°C and a measured stability of 94 days at 40°C. The maltitol-based syrup was more stable than the sucrose-based syrup when temperature was >37°C, but the sucrose-based syrup was more stable at temperatures <37°C (Alexander, 1993)

Alexander KS, Pudipeddi M, and Parker GA, "Stability of Procainamide Hydrochloride Syrups Compounded From Capsules," *Am J Hosp Pharm*, 1993, 50(4):693-8.

Allen LV and Erickson MA, "Stability of Ketoconazole, Metolazone, Metronidazole, Procainamide Hydrochloride, and Spironolactone in Extemporaneously Compounded Oral Liquids," *Am J Health Syst Pharm*, 1996, 53(17):2073-8.

Handbook in Extemporaneous Formulations, Bethesda, MD: American Society of Hospital Pharmacists, 1987.

Metras JI, Swenson CF, and MacDermott MP, "Stability of Procainamide Hydrochloride in an Extemporaneously Compounded Oral Liquid," *Am J Hosp Pharm*, 1992, 49(7):1720-4.

Swenson CF, "Importance of Following Instructions When Compounding," *Am J Hosp Pharm*, 1993, 50(2):261.

References

American Heart Association Emergency Cardiovascular Care Committee, " 2005 American Heart Association (AHA) Guidelines for Cardiopulmonary Resuscitation (CPR) and Emergency Cardiovascular Care (ECC), Part 7.2: Management of Cardiac Arrest, Part 7.3: Management of Symptomatic Bradycardia and Tachycardia, and Part 12: Pediatric Advanced Life Support," *Circulation*, 2005, 112(24 Suppl):IV58-77,167-87.

Singh S, Gelband H, Mehta AV, et al, "Procainamide Elimination Kinetics in Pediatric Patients," *Clin Pharmacol Ther*, 1982, 32(5):607-11.

♦ **Procainamide Hydrochloride** *see* Procainamide *on page 1315*

♦ **Procainamide Hydrochloride Injection, USP (Can)** *see* Procainamide *on page 1315*

Procaine (PROE kane)

U.S. Brand Names Novocain®

Index Terms Procaine Hydrochloride

Therapeutic Category Local Anesthetic, Injectable

Generic Available No

Use Production of local or regional analgesia and anesthesia by local infiltration and peripheral nerve block techniques

Pregnancy Risk Factor C

Lactation Excretion in breast milk unknown

Contraindications Hypersensitivity to procaine, PABA, parabens, any anesthetic of the ester type, or any component; cerebrospinal diseases such as meningitis or syphilis and septicemia (spinal anesthetic use)

Warnings Convulsions and cardiac arrhythmias, due to systemic toxicity leading to cardiac arrest have been reported, presumably following unintentional I.V. injection; should be administered in small incremental doses

Precautions Use with extreme caution as lumbar or caudal anesthesia in patients with existing neurologic disease, spinal deformities, or severe hypertension. Use with caution in patients with cardiac disease, hepatic or renal disease. Use caution in debilitated, elderly, or acutely-ill patients; dose reduction may be required. Some preparations contain metabisulfite which may cause allergic reactions in susceptible individuals.

Adverse Reactions Degree of adverse effects in the CNS and cardiovascular system is directly related to the blood level of procaine, route of administration, and physical status of the patient. The effects below are more likely to occur after systemic administration rather than infiltration.

Cardiovascular: Bradycardia, cardiac arrest, decreased cardiac output, heart block, hypertension, hypotension, myocardial depression, syncope, tachycardia, ventricular arrhythmias

Central nervous system: Anxiety, chills, seizures, depression, dizziness, excitation, restlessness, tremors, fever, headache

Dermatologic: Angioneurotic edema, erythema, pruritus, urticaria

Gastrointestinal: Fecal incontinence, nausea, vomiting

Genitourinary: Incontinence, urinary retention

Neuromuscular & skeletal: Paralysis, tremors, paresthesia, weakness

Ocular: Blurred vision, pupil constriction

Otic: Tinnitus

Respiratory: Apnea, hypoventilation, sneezing

Miscellaneous: Allergic reaction, anaphylactoid reaction, diaphoresis

Drug Interactions Decreased effect of sulfonamides with the PABA metabolite of procaine

Stability Store at controlled room temperature of 15°C to 30°C (59°F to 86°F); protect from light. Solutions may be sterilized by autoclaving for 15 minutes; reautoclaving increases the likelihood of crystal formation. Stable in dextrose, dextran 6% in NS, D_5LR, $D_5{}^1/_4NS$, $D_5{}^1/_2NS$, D_5NS, D_5W, $D_{10}W$, LR, $^1/_2NS$, NS.

Mechanism of Action Blocks both the initiation and conduction of nerve impulses by decreasing the neuronal membrane's permeability to sodium ions, which results in inhibition of depolarization with resultant blockade of conduction

Pharmacodynamics

Onset of action: 2-5 minutes

Duration (patient, type of block, concentration, and method of anesthesia dependent): 1 hour

Pharmacokinetics

Metabolism: Rapidly hydrolyzed by plasma enzymes to para-aminobenzoic acid and diethylaminoethanol (80% conjugated before elimination)

Half-life (*in vitro*):

Neonates: 84 ± 30 seconds

Adults: 40 ± 9 seconds

Elimination: Urine (as metabolites and some unchanged drug)

Usual Dosage Dose varies with procedure, desired depth, and duration of anesthesia, desired muscle relaxation, vascularity of tissues, physical condition, and age of patient. The smallest dose and concentration required to produce the desired effect should be used.

Children: Maximum dose: 15 mg/kg of 0.5% solution

Adults: Maximum dose: 1000 mg per treatment

Infiltration anesthesia: 0.25% to 0.5% solution: 350-600 mg

Peripheral nerve block: 0.5% (up to 200 mL), 1% (up to 100 mL), 2% (up to 50 mL)

Spinal anesthesia: Using 10% (diluted prior to use with NS, SWI, spinal fluid; and for hyperbaric technique, sterile dextrose solution):

Extent of anesthesia: Perineum: 0.5 mL (50 mg) diluent volume 0.5 mL

Perineum and local extremities: 1 mL (100 mg) diluent volume 1 mL

Up to costal margin: 2 mL (200 mg) diluent volume 1 mL

Administration Parenteral: Administer in small incremental doses; when using continuous intermittent catheter techniques, use frequent aspirations before and during the injection to avoid intravascular injection; for spinal anesthesia, inject 1 mL per 5 seconds

Monitoring Parameters Blood pressure, heart rate, respiration, signs of CNS toxicity (lightheadedness, dizziness, tinnitus, restlessness, tremors, twitching, drowsiness, circumoral paresthesia)

Patient Information You will experience decreased sensation to pain, heat, or cold in the area and/or decreased muscle strength (depending on area of application) until effects wear off; use necessary caution to reduce incidence of possible injury until full sensation returns. Report irritation, pain, burning at injection site; chest pain or palpitations; or respiratory difficulty.

Dosage Forms Excipient information presented when available (limited, particularly for generics); consult specific product labeling.

Injection, solution, as hydrochloride: 1% [10 mg/mL] (2 mL) [contains sodium bisulfite]; 10% (2 mL) [contains sodium bisulfite]

- **Procaine Amide Hydrochloride** *see* Procainamide *on page 1315*
- **Procaine Benzylpenicillin** *see* Penicillin G Procaine *on page 1233*
- **Procaine Hydrochloride** *see* Procaine *on page 1318*
- **Procaine Penicillin G** *see* Penicillin G Procaine *on page 1233*
- **Procanbid®** *see* Procainamide *on page 1315*
- **Procan® SR (Can)** *see* Procainamide *on page 1315*

Procarbazine (proe KAR ba zeen)

Medication Safety Issues

Sound-alike/look-alike issues:

Procarbazine may be confused with dacarbazine

Matulane® may be confused with Modane®

High alert medication: The Institute for Safe Medication Practices (ISMP) includes this medication among its list of drugs which have a heightened risk of causing significant patient harm when used in error.

Related Information

Emetogenic Potential of Single Chemotherapeutic Agents *on page 1776*

U.S. Brand Names Matulane®

Canadian Brand Names Matulane®; Natulan®

Index Terms Benzmethyzin; N-Methylhydrazine; NSC-77213; Procarbazine Hydrochloride

Therapeutic Category Antineoplastic Agent, Miscellaneous

Generic Available No

Use Treatment of Hodgkin's disease, non-Hodgkin's lymphoma, brain tumor, bronchogenic carcinoma

Pregnancy Risk Factor D

Lactation Excretion in breast milk unknown/not recommended

Contraindications Hypersensitivity to procarbazine or any component; pre-existing bone marrow aplasia

Warnings The FDA currently recommends that procedures for proper handling and disposal of antineoplastic agents be considered; procarbazine is a carcinogen which may cause a secondary acute nonlymphocytic leukemia; procarbazine may cause infertility and is potentially teratogenic

Precautions May potentiate CNS depression when used with phenothiazine derivatives, barbiturates, narcotics, alcohol, tricyclic antidepressants, methyldopa; use with caution in patients with pre-existing renal or hepatic impairment; reduce dosage in patients with marrow disorders, renal impairment (serum creatinine >2 mg/dL and/or a blood urea nitrogen >40 mg/dL), or decreased hepatic function (total bilirubin >3 mg/dL)

Adverse Reactions

Central nervous system: CNS depression, somnolence, confusion, nervousness, irritability, cerebellar ataxia, hallucinations, seizures, nightmares, headache, chills, fever, dizziness

Dermatologic: Dermatitis, alopecia, hypersensitivity rash, pruritus

Endocrine & metabolic: Disulfiram-like reaction, amenorrhea

Gastrointestinal: Nausea, vomiting, diarrhea, stomatitis, anorexia

Genitourinary: Azoospermia, ovarian failure

Hematologic: Myelosuppression, thrombocytopenia, pancytopenia, hemolysis

Neuromuscular & skeletal: Arthralgia, myalgia, tremor, neuropathy, weakness

Ocular: Nystagmus, diplopia, photophobia

Miscellaneous: Flu-like syndrome

Drug Interactions Alcohol (disulfiram-like reaction with nausea, vomiting, headache, sedation, and visual disturbances); MAO inhibitors, tricyclic antidepressants, ephedrine, epinephrine, isoproterenol (hypertensive crisis, tremor, excitation, cardiac palpitations, angina); narcotics, phenothiazines, barbiturates, methyldopa (additive CNS depression); phenytoin, phenobarbital (increases cytotoxic activity of procarbazine)

Food Interactions Avoid food with high tyramine content (cheese, tea, dark beer, coffee, cola drinks, wine, bananas) as hypertensive crisis, tremor, excitation, cardiac palpitations, and angina may occur

Stability Unstable in water or aqueous solution; avoid contact of the drug with moisture

Mechanism of Action Inhibits DNA, RNA, and protein synthesis; may damage DNA directly via free-radical formation and suppress mitosis

Pharmacokinetics

Absorption: Oral: Well absorbed

Distribution: Crosses the blood-brain barrier and distributes into CSF, liver, kidney, intestine, and skin

Metabolism: In the liver; first-pass conversion to cytotoxic metabolites

Half-life: 10 minutes

Time to peak serum concentration: Within 1 hour

Elimination: In urine (<5% as unchanged drug) and 70% as metabolites

Usual Dosage Oral (refer to individual protocols; base dosage on ideal body weight):

Children:

Hodgkin's disease: 50-100 mg/m²/day once daily for 10-14 days of a 28-day cycle

BMT aplastic anemia conditioning regimen: 12.5 mg/kg/dose every other day for 4 doses

Brain tumor: 75 mg/m² at hour 1 on day 1; repeat cycle every 2-4 weeks if tolerated; **or** 100 mg/m² on days 1-14 of a treatment course

Neuroblastoma and medulloblastoma: Doses as high as 100-200 mg/m²/day once daily have been used

Adults: Initial: 2-4 mg/kg/day in single or divided doses for 7 days then increase dose to 4-6 mg/kg/day until response is obtained or leukocyte count decreases to <4000/mm³ or the platelet count decreases to <100,000/mm³; maintenance: 1-2 mg/kg/day

Administration Oral: Administer with food or after meals; total daily dose may be administered at a single time or in divided doses throughout the day to minimize GI toxicity

Monitoring Parameters CBC with differential, platelet count, and reticulocyte count; urinalysis, liver function test, renal function test

Patient Information Notify physician of fever, sore throat, bleeding, or bruising; avoid alcohol (disulfiram-like reaction with nausea, vomiting, headache, sedation, and visual disturbances)

Additional Information Myelosuppressive effects:

WBC: Moderate
Platelets: Moderate
Onset (days): 14
Nadir (days): 21
Recovery (days): 28

Dosage Forms Excipient information presented when available (limited, particularly for generics); consult specific product labeling.

Capsule, as hydrochloride:
Matulane®: 50 mg

References

Longo DL, Young RC, Wesley M, et al, "Twenty Years of MOPP Therapy for Hodgkin's Disease," *J Clin Oncol*, 1986, 4(9):1295-306.

Rodriguez LA, Prados M, Silver P, et al, "Re-evaluation of Procarbazine for the Treatment of Recurrent Malignant Central Nervous System Tumors," *Cancer*, 1989, 64(12):2420-3.

◆ **Procarbazine Hydrochloride** *see* Procarbazine *on page 1320*
◆ **Procardia**® *see* NIFEdipine *on page 1134*
◆ **Procardia XL**® *see* NIFEdipine *on page 1134*

Prochlorperazine (proe klor PER a zeen)

Medication Safety Issues

Sound-alike/look-alike issues:

Prochlorperazine may be confused with chlorproMAZINE
Compazine® may be confused with Copaxone®, Coumadin®

CPZ (occasional abbreviation for Compazine®) is an error-prone abbreviation (mistaken as chlorpromazine)

Related Information

Compatibility of Chemotherapy and Related Supportive Care Medications *on page 1777*
Compatibility of Medications Mixed in A Syringe *on page 1941*
Overdose and Toxicology *on page 1916*

U.S. Brand Names Compro™

Canadian Brand Names Apo-Prochlorperazine®; Compazine®; Nu-Prochlor; Stemetil®

Index Terms Chlormeprazine; Compazine; Prochlorperazine Edisylate; Prochlorperazine Maleate

Therapeutic Category Antiemetic; Antipsychotic Agent; Phenothiazine Derivative

Generic Available Yes: Injection, tablet, suppository

Use Management of nausea and vomiting; acute and chronic psychosis; treatment of intractable migraine headaches

Pregnancy Risk Factor C

Lactation Excretion in breast milk unknown/use caution

Contraindications Hypersensitivity to prochlorperazine or any component (see Warnings); cross-sensitivity with other phenothiazines may exist; avoid use in patients with narrow-angle glaucoma; severe liver or cardiac disease, severe toxic CNS depression or coma; pediatric surgery

Warnings High incidence of extrapyramidal reactions especially in children, reserve use in children <5 years of age to those who are unresponsive to other antiemetics; incidence of extrapyramidal reactions is increased with acute illnesses such as chicken pox, measles, CNS infections, gastroenteritis, and dehydration; extrapyramidal reactions may also be confused with CNS signs of Reye's syndrome or other encephalopathies; avoid use in these clinical conditions
(Continued)

Prochlorperazine *(Continued)*

Injection contains benzyl alcohol which may cause allergic reactions in susceptible individuals; large amounts of benzyl alcohol (≥99 mg/kg/day) have been associated with a potentially fatal toxicity ("gasping syndrome") in neonates; the "gasping syndrome" consists of metabolic acidosis, respiratory distress, gasping respirations, CNS dysfunction (including convulsions, intracranial hemorrhage), hypotension and cardiovascular collapse; avoid use of injection in neonates; syrup contains sodium benzoate; *in vitro* and animal studies have shown that benzoate, a metabolite of benzyl alcohol, displaces bilirubin from protein binding sites; avoid use of syrup in neonates.

Lowers seizure threshold, use cautiously in patients with seizure history; discontinue use at least 48 hours before myelography and do not resume therapy until 24 hours post myelography. Use of antipsychotics in combination with lithium has been associated with an encephalopathy syndrome similar to NMS; monitor patients closely and discontinue treatment if encephalopathic symptomatology develops.

Precautions Safety and efficacy have not been established in children <9 kg or <2 years of age

Adverse Reactions Incidence of extrapyramidal reactions are higher with prochlorperazine than chlorpromazine

Cardiovascular: Hypotension (especially with I.V. use); orthostatic hypotension; tachycardia, arrhythmias, sudden death

Central nervous system: Sedation, drowsiness, restlessness, anxiety; extrapyramidal reactions which include dystonic reactions such as spasm of neck muscles, torticollis, extensor rigidity of back muscles, opisthotonos, trismus, and mandibular tics; pseudoparkinsonian signs and symptoms, tardive dyskinesia, neuroleptic malignant syndrome, seizures, altered central temperature regulation

Dermatologic: Hyperpigmentation, pruritus, rash, photosensitivity

Endocrine & metabolic: Amenorrhea, galactorrhea, gynecomastia, abnormal glucose tolerance, weight gain

Gastrointestinal: GI upset, xerostomia, constipation

Genitourinary: Impotence, urinary retention

Hematologic: Agranulocytosis, leukopenia (usually in patients with large doses for prolonged periods), thrombocytopenia, hemolytic anemia, eosinophilia

Hepatic: Cholestatic jaundice

Ocular: Retinal pigmentation, blurred vision

Miscellaneous: Anaphylactoid reactions

Drug Interactions Phenothiazines inhibit the ability of bromocriptine to lower serum prolactin concentrations; benztropine (and other anticholinergics) may inhibit the therapeutic response to prochlorperazine; sulfadoxine-pyrimethamine, propranolol, and chloroquine may increase prochlorperazine concentrations; cigarette smoking may enhance the hepatic metabolism of prochlorperazine; concurrent use of prochlorperazine and antihypertensives may produce additive hypotensive effects; antihypertensive effects of guanethidine and guanadrel may be inhibited by prochlorperazine; concurrent use with TCAs may produce increased toxicity or altered therapeutic response; prochlorperazine may inhibit the antiparkinsonian effect of levodopa; prochlorperazine plus lithium may rarely produce encephalopathy similar to NMS; barbiturates may reduce prochlorperazine concentrations; prochlorperazine and CNS depressants (ethanol, narcotics) may produce additive CNS depressant effects; prochlorperazine and trazodone may produce additive hypotensive effects; use with cisapride may increase the risk of malignant arrhythmias

Food Interactions Increase dietary intake of riboflavin

Stability Protect from light; clear or slightly yellow solutions may be used; incompatible with aminophylline, amphotericin B, ampicillin, calcium salts, cephalothin, foscarnet (Y-site), furosemide, hydrocortisone, hydromorphone, methohexital, midazolam, penicillin G, pentobarbital, phenobarbital, thiopental

Mechanism of Action Blocks postsynaptic mesolimbic dopaminergic receptors in the brain, including the medullary chemoreceptor trigger zone; exhibits a strong alpha-adrenergic blocking effect and depresses the release of hypothalamic and hypophyseal hormones

Pharmacodynamics

Onset of action:

- Oral: 30-40 minutes
- I.M.: Within 10-20 minutes
- Rectal: Within 60 minutes

Duration:

- I.M., oral extended release: 12 hours
- Rectal, oral immediate release: 3-4 hours

Usual Dosage

Antiemetic:

Children >10 kg:

Oral, rectal: 0.4 mg/kg/day in 3-4 divided doses; **or** as an alternative:

10-14 kg: 2.5 mg every 12-24 hours as needed; maximum dose: 7.5 mg/day

15-18 kg: 2.5 mg every 8-12 hours as needed; maximum dose: 10 mg/day

19-39 kg: 2.5 mg every 8 hours or 5 mg every 12 hours as needed; maximum dose: 15 mg/day

I.M., I.V.: 0.1-0.15 mg/kg/dose every 8-12 hours; not to exceed 40 mg/day

Adults:

Oral: 5-10 mg 3-4 times/day; usual maximum dose: 40 mg/day

Oral, extended release: 10 mg twice daily or 15 mg once daily

I.M.: 5-10 mg every 3-4 hours; usual maximum dose: 40 mg/day

I.V.: 2.5-10 mg; maximum 10 mg/dose or 40 mg/day; may repeat dose every 3-4 hours as needed

Rectal: 25 mg twice daily

Treatment of intractable migraine headaches (limited information available): I.V.: Children: 0.15 mg/kg as a single dose in 20 children between the ages of 8-17 years combined with I.V. hydration has been used (Kabbouche, 2001)

Treatment of psychoses:

Children 2-12 years:

Oral, rectal: 2.5 mg 2-3 times/day, increase dosage as needed to a maximum daily dose of 20 mg for 2-5 years and 25 mg for 6-12 years

I.M.: 0.13 mg/kg/dose, change to oral as soon as possible

Adults:

Oral: 5-10 mg 3-4 times/day, increase as needed to a daily maximum dose of 150 mg

I.M.: 10-20 mg every 4 hours as needed, change to oral as soon as possible

Administration

Oral: Administer with food or water

Parenteral: I.M. is preferred; avoid I.V. administration; if necessary, may be administered by direct I.V. injection at a maximum rate of 5 mg/minute; do not administer by SubQ route (tissue damage may occur)

Monitoring Parameters CBC with differential and periodic ophthalmic exams (if chronically used)

Test Interactions False-positives for phenylketonuria, urinary amylase, uroporphyrins, urobilinogen

Patient Information Limit caffeine; may cause drowsiness and impair ability to perform activities requiring mental alertness or physical coordination; may cause dry mouth. May cause photosensitivity reactions (eg, exposure to sunlight may cause severe sunburn, skin rash, redness, or itching); avoid exposure to sunlight and artificial light sources (sunlamps, tanning booth/bed); wear protective clothing, wide-brimmed hats, sunglasses, and lip sunscreen (SPF ≥15); use a sunscreen [broad-spectrum sunscreen or physical sunscreen (preferred) or sunblock with SPF ≥15]; contact physician if reaction occurs.

Nursing Implications Avoid skin contact with oral solution or injection, contact dermatitis has occurred

Additional Information Use lowest possible dose in pediatric patients to try to decrease incidence of extrapyramidal reactions

Dosage Forms Excipient information presented when available (limited, particularly for generics); consult specific product labeling.

Injection, solution, as edisylate: 5 mg/mL (2 mL, 10 mL) [contains benzyl alcohol]

Suppository, rectal: 2.5 mg (12s), 5 mg (12s), 25 mg (12s) [may contain coconut and palm oil]

Compro™: 25 mg (12s) [contains coconut and palm oils]

Tablet, as maleate: 5 mg, 10 mg

References

Kabbouche MA, Vockell AL, LeCates SL, et al, "Tolerability and Effectiveness of Prochlorperazine for Intractable Migraine in Children," *Pediatrics*, 2001, 107(4):E62, www.pediatrics.org/cgi/content/full/107/4/e62.

- **Prochlorperazine Edisylate** *see* Prochlorperazine *on page 1321*
- **Prochlorperazine Maleate** *see* Prochlorperazine *on page 1321*
- **Procrit®** *see* Epoetin Alfa *on page 580*
- **Proctocort®** *see* Hydrocortisone *on page 781*
- **ProctoCream® HC** *see* Hydrocortisone *on page 781*
- **Procto-Kit™** *see* Hydrocortisone *on page 781*
- **Procto-Pak™** *see* Hydrocortisone *on page 781*
- **Proctosert** *see* Hydrocortisone *on page 781*
- **Proctosol-HC®** *see* Hydrocortisone *on page 781*

- **Proctozone-HC™** *see* Hydrocortisone *on page 781*
- **Procytox® (Can)** *see* Cyclophosphamide *on page 419*
- **Prodium® [OTC]** *see* Phenazopyridine *on page 1244*
- **Profasi® HP (Can)** *see* Chorionic Gonadotropin *on page 351*
- **Profilnine® SD** *see* Factor IX Complex (Human) *on page 635*
- **Proflavanol C™ (Can)** *see* Ascorbic Acid *on page 159*
- **Proglycem®** *see* Diazoxide *on page 485*
- **Prograf®** *see* Tacrolimus *on page 1498*
- **Proleukin®** *see* Aldesleukin *on page 70*
- **Proloprim®** *see* Trimethoprim *on page 1578*

Promethazine (proe METH a zeen)

Medication Safety Issues

Sound-alike/look-alike issues:

Promethazine may be confused with chlorproMAZINE, predniSONE, promazine

Phenergan® may be confused with Phenaphen®, Phrenilin®, Theragran®

Administration issues:

To prevent or minimize tissue damage during I.V. administration, the Institute for Safe Medication Practices (ISMP) has the following recommendations:

Limit concentration available to the 25 mg/mL product

Consider limiting initial doses to 6.25-12.5 mg

Further dilute the 25 mg/mL strength into 10-20 mL NS

Administer through a large bore vein (not hand or wrist)

Administer via running I.V. line at port furthest from patient's vein

Consider administering over 10-15 minutes

Instruct patients to report immediately signs of pain or burning

Related Information

Compatibility of Chemotherapy and Related Supportive Care Medications *on page 1777*

Compatibility of Medications Mixed in A Syringe *on page 1941*

Overdose and Toxicology *on page 1916*

U.S. Brand Names Phenadoz™; Phenergan®; Promethegan™

Canadian Brand Names Phenergan®

Index Terms Promethazine Hydrochloride

Therapeutic Category Antiemetic; Phenothiazine Derivative; Sedative

Generic Available Yes

Use Symptomatic treatment of various allergic conditions and motion sickness; sedative; antiemetic

Pregnancy Risk Factor C

Lactation Excretion in breast milk unknown/use caution

Contraindications Hypersensitivity to promethazine or any component (cross reactivity with other phenothiazines may occur); severe toxic CNS depression or coma; children <2 years (see Warnings)

Warnings Use with extreme caution in children and avoid use in children <2 years of age, due to the potential for severe and potentially fatal respiratory depression; a wide range of weight based doses have resulted in respiratory depression; excessively high doses have been associated with sudden death in children; use the lowest effective dose in children >2 years of age and avoid concomitant use with other medications having respiratory depressant effects. Injection may contain sodium metabisulfite which may cause allergic reactions in susceptible individuals. Do not give SubQ or intra-arterially due to severe local reactions including necrosis; rapid I.V. administration may produce a transient fall in blood pressure; slow I.V. administration may produce a slightly elevated blood pressure. Neuroleptic malignant syndrome (NMS) has been reported with promethazine when used alone or in combination with antipsychotic drugs. Children with dehydration are at increased risk for development of dystonic reactions.

Precautions Use with caution in patients with cardiovascular disease, narrow-angle glaucoma, prostatic hypertrophy, GI or GU obstruction, bone marrow depression, impaired liver function, asthma, peptic ulcer, sleep apnea, and hypertensive crisis; avoid in patients with suspected Reye's syndrome; promethazine may lower the seizure threshold; use with caution in patients with seizure disorders or receiving other medications which may also lower the seizure threshold

Adverse Reactions

Cardiovascular: Tachycardia, bradycardia, hypotension (rapid I.V. administration), hypertension (slow I.V. administration), palpitations, angioneurotic edema

Central nervous system: Sedation (pronounced), drowsiness, confusion, fatigue, excitation (paradoxical), extrapyramidal reactions, dystonia, tardive dyskinesia, NMS, hallucinations, insomnia, seizures, catatonic-like states, hysteria
Dermatologic: Photosensitivity, rash, angioedema, urticaria
Endocrine & metabolic: Weight gain
Gastrointestinal: Xerostomia, GI upset, increased appetite, abdominal pain, diarrhea, nausea
Genitourinary: Urinary retention
Hematologic: Thrombocytopenia, leukopenia, agranulocytosis (rare)
Hepatic: Cholestatic jaundice, hepatitis
Local: Thrombophlebitis (injection)
Neuromuscular & skeletal: Arthralgia, tremor, paresthesia, myalgia
Ocular: Blurred vision, diplopia
Otic: Tinnitus
Respiratory: Thickening of bronchial secretions, pharyngitis, respiratory depression, and apnea (particularly severe in children, see Warnings)
Miscellaneous: Allergic reactions

Drug Interactions Cytochrome P450 isoenzyme CYP2D6 enzyme substrate

Phenothiazines inhibit the ability of bromocriptine to lower serum prolactin concentrations; benztropine (and other anticholinergics) may inhibit the therapeutic response to promethazine; sulfadoxine-pyrimethamine, propranolol, and chloroquine may increase promethazine concentrations; cigarette smoking may enhance the hepatic metabolism of promethazine; concurrent use of promethazine with an antihypertensive may produce additive hypotensive effects; antihypertensive effects of guanethidine and guanadrel may be inhibited by promethazine; concurrent use with TCA may produce increased toxicity or altered therapeutic response; promethazine may inhibit the antiparkinsonian effect of levodopa; promethazine plus lithium may rarely produce neurotoxicity; barbiturates may reduce promethazine concentrations; promethazine may reverse the pressor effects of epinephrine; promethazine and CNS depressants (ethanol, narcotics) may produce additive CNS depressant effects; promethazine and trazodone may produce additive hypotensive effects; use with cisapride may increase the risk of malignant arrhythmias; additive effects when used with anticholinergic medications; increased extrapyramidal effects when used with MAO inhibitors

Food Interactions Increase dietary intake of riboflavin

Stability Protect from light; store injection and tablets at controlled room temperature; refrigerate suppositories; **compatible** (when comixed in the same syringe) with atropine, chlorpromazine, diphenhydramine, droperidol, fentanyl, glycopyrrolate, hydromorphone, hydroxyzine hydrochloride, meperidine, midazolam, nalbuphine, pentazocine, prochlorperazine, scopolamine; **incompatible** when mixed with aminophylline, cefoperazone (Y-site), chloramphenicol, dimenhydrinate (same syringe), foscarnet (Y-site), furosemide, heparin, hydrocortisone, methohexital, penicillin G, pentobarbital, phenobarbital, thiopental

Mechanism of Action Blocks postsynaptic mesolimbic dopaminergic receptors in the brain; exhibits a strong alpha-adrenergic blocking effect and depresses the release of hypothalamic and hypophyseal hormones; competes with histamine for the H_1-receptor

Pharmacodynamics

Onset of action:
- Oral, I.M.: Within 20 minutes
- I.V.: 3-5 minutes

Duration: Oral: 4-6 hours

Pharmacokinetics

Absorption: 88%
Bioavailability: 25% (due to first pass metabolism)
Half-life: 9-16 hours
Metabolism: In the liver
Elimination: Principally as inactive metabolites in the urine and in the feces

Usual Dosage

Children ≥2 years (use with extreme caution utilizing the lowest most effective dose; see Warnings):
- Antihistamine: Oral: 0.1 mg/kg/dose (not to exceed 12.5 mg) every 6 hours during the day and 0.5 mg/kg/dose (not to exceed 25 mg) at bedtime as needed
- Antiemetic: Oral, I.M., I.V., rectal: 0.25-1 mg/kg (not to exceed 25 mg) 4-6 times/day as needed
- Motion sickness: Oral, rectal: 0.5 mg/kg (not to exceed 25 mg) 30 minutes to 1 hour before departure, then every 12 hours as needed
- Sedation: Oral, I.M., I.V., rectal: 0.5-1 mg/kg/dose (not to exceed 50 mg) every 6 hours as needed

(Continued)

Promethazine *(Continued)*

Adults:
Antihistamine:
Oral, rectal: 6.25-12.5 mg 3 times/day and 25 mg at bedtime
I.M., I.V.: 25 mg, may repeat in 2 hours when necessary; switch to oral route as soon as feasible
Antiemetic: Oral, I.M., I.V., rectal: 12.5-25 mg every 4 hours as needed
Motion sickness: Oral: 25 mg twice daily with the first dose 30 minutes to 1 hour before departure, then repeat 8-12 hours later as needed
Sedation: Oral, I.M., I.V., rectal: 25-50 mg/dose; repeat every 4-6 hours if needed

Administration
Oral: Administer with food, water, or milk to decrease GI distress
Parenteral: I.M. administration is preferred; avoid I.V. use (see Warnings); in selected patients, promethazine has been administered I.V. diluted to a maximum concentration of 25 mg/mL and infused at a maximum rate of 25 mg/minute; not for SubQ administration, promethazine is a chemical irritant which may produce necrosis

Test Interactions Alters the flare response in intradermal allergen tests; false negative and positive reactions with pregnancy tests relying on immunological reactions between hCG and anti-hCG

Patient Information May cause drowsiness and impair ability to perform activities requiring mental alertness or physical coordination; notify physician of involuntary movements or feelings of restlessness; may cause dry mouth. May cause photosensitivity reactions (eg, exposure to sunlight may cause severe sunburn, skin rash, redness, or itching); avoid exposure to sunlight and artificial light sources (sunlamps, tanning booth/bed); wear protective clothing, wide-brimmed hats, sunglasses, and lip sunscreen (SPF ≥15); use a sunscreen [broad-spectrum sunscreen or physical sunscreen (preferred) or sunblock with SPF ≥15]; contact physician if reaction occurs.

Additional Information Although promethazine has been used in combination with meperidine and chlorpromazine as a premedication (lytic cocktail), this combination may have a higher rate of adverse effects compared to alternative sedative/analgesics

Dosage Forms Excipient information presented when available (limited, particularly for generics); consult specific product labeling. [DSC] = Discontinued product
Injection, solution, as hydrochloride: 25 mg/mL (1 mL); 50 mg/mL (1 mL)
Phenergan®: 25 mg/mL (1 mL); 50 mg/mL (1 mL) [contains sodium metabisulfite]
Suppository, rectal, as hydrochloride: 12.5 mg, 25 mg, 50 mg
Phenadoz™: 12.5 mg, 25 mg
Phenergan®: 25 mg, 50 mg [DSC]
Promethegan™: 12.5 mg, 25 mg, 50 mg
Syrup, as hydrochloride: 6.25 mg/5 mL (120 mL, 480 mL) [contains alcohol]
Tablet, as hydrochloride: 12.5 mg, 25 mg, 50 mg
Phenergan®: 25 mg [DSC]

References
Strenkoski-Nix LC, Ermer J, DeCleene S, et al, "Pharmacokinetics of Promethazine Hydrochloride After Administration of Rectal Suppositories and Oral Syrup to Healthy Subjects," *Am J Health Syst Pharm*, 2000, 57(16):1499-505.

Promethazine and Codeine (proe METH a zeen & KOE deen)

Medication Safety Issues
Sound-alike/look-alike issues:
Phenergan® may be confused with Phenaphen®, Phrenilin®, Theragran®

Index Terms Codeine and Promethazine

Therapeutic Category Antitussive; Cough Preparation; Phenothiazine Derivative

Generic Available Yes

Use Temporary relief of coughs and upper respiratory symptoms associated with allergy or the common cold

Restrictions C-V

Pregnancy Risk Factor C

Lactation Enters breast milk (codeine)/not recommended

Contraindications Hypersensitivity to promethazine, codeine, or any component; children <16 years of age (see Warnings); cross reactivity with other phenothiazines may occur; lower respiratory tract symptoms, including asthma; concurrent use of MAO inhibitors

Warnings Avoid use in children <16 years of age, due to the potential for severe and potentially fatal respiratory depression associated with the combination of promethazine and other respiratory depressants (eg, codeine); fatalities associated with promethazine use alone in children <2 years of age have also been reported. Dose should not be increased if cough does not respond; re-evaluate within 5 days for possible underlying pathology. Codeine is not recommended for cough control in patients with a productive cough. Neuroleptic malignant syndrome (NMS) has been reported with promethazine when used alone or in combination with antipsychotic drugs. May alter temperature regulation or mask toxicity of other drugs due to antiemetic effects. May alter cardiac conduction (life-threatening arrhythmias have occurred with therapeutic doses of phenothiazines).

Precautions Use with caution in patients with cardiovascular disease, narrow-angle glaucoma, prostatic hypertrophy, GI or GU obstruction, bone marrow depression, impaired liver function, asthma, peptic ulcer, sleep apnea, and hypertensive crisis; avoid in patients with suspected Reye's syndrome; promethazine may lower the seizure threshold; use with caution in patients with seizure disorders or receiving other medications which may also lower the seizure threshold; use with caution in patients with hypersensitivity reactions to morphine, hydrocodone, hydromorphone, levorphanol, oxycodone, oxymorphone. May cause orthostatic hypotension, use with caution in patients at risk of hypotension or where transient hypotensive episodes would be poorly tolerated (cardiovascular disease or cerebrovascular disease). May cause drowsiness and impair ability to perform hazardous activities requiring mental alertness.

Adverse Reactions

Promethazine:

- Cardiovascular: Tachycardia, bradycardia, palpitations, arrhythmias, orthostatic hypotension
- Central nervous system: Sedation (pronounced), confusion, drowsiness, restlessness, anxiety, extrapyramidal reactions, tardive dyskinesia, seizures, hallucinations, NMS
- Dermatologic: Rash, photosensitivity
- Endocrine & metabolic: Antidiuretic hormone release
- Gastrointestinal: GI upset, xerostomia, constipation
- Genitourinary: Urinary retention
- Hematologic: Agranulocytosis, leukopenia (rare), thrombocytopenia
- Hepatic: Cholestatic jaundice, hepatitis
- Neuromuscular & skeletal: Arthralgia, tremor, paresthesia, myalgia
- Ocular: Blurred vision
- Respiratory: Thickening of bronchial secretions, pharyngitis
- Miscellaneous: Allergic reactions

Codeine:

- Cardiovascular: Palpitations, orthostatic hypotension, tachycardia or bradycardia, peripheral vasodilation
- Central nervous system: CNS depression, dizziness, sedation, euphoria, hallucination, seizures
- Dermatologic: Pruritus
- Gastrointestinal: Nausea, vomiting, constipation, biliary tract spasm
- Genitourinary: Urinary tract spasm
- Ocular: Miosis
- Respiratory: Respiratory depression
- Miscellaneous: Physical and psychological dependence, histamine release, allergic reactions

Drug Interactions See Promethazine *on page 1324* and Codeine *on page 397*

Food Interactions Increase fluids, fiber intake, and riboflavin in diet

Mechanism of Action See individual monographs for Codeine *on page 397* and Promethazine *on page 1324*

Usual Dosage Oral (**in terms of codeine**):

Children >16 years and Adults: 10-20 mg/dose every 4-6 hours as needed; maximum dose: 120 mg codeine/day; or 5-10 mL every 4-6 hours as needed

Administration Oral: Administer with food or water to decrease GI upset

Test Interactions Alters the flare response in intradermal allergen tests; false negative and positive reactions with pregnancy tests relying on immunological reactions between hCG and anti-hCG

Patient Information May cause drowsiness and impair ability to perform activities requiring mental alertness or physical coordination; may cause dry mouth; may be habit-forming; do not discontinue abruptly. May cause photosensitivity reactions (eg, exposure to sunlight may cause severe sunburn, skin rash, redness, or itching); avoid exposure to sunlight and artificial light sources (sunlamps, tanning booth/bed); wear protective clothing, wide-brimmed hats, sunglasses, and lip sunscreen (SPF ≥15); use a sunscreen [broad-spectrum sunscreen or physical sunscreen (preferred) or sunblock with SPF ≥15]; contact physician if reaction occurs.

Dosage Forms Excipient information presented when available (limited, particularly for generics); consult specific product labeling.

Syrup: Promethazine hydrochloride 6.25 mg and codeine phosphate 10 mg per 5 mL (120 mL, 473 mL) [contains alcohol]

Promethazine and Phenylephrine (proe METH a zeen & fen il EF rin)

Related Information
Phenylephrine *on page 1250*
Promethazine *on page 1324*

Index Terms Phenylephrine and Promethazine

Therapeutic Category Antihistamine/Decongestant Combination

Generic Available Yes

Use Temporary relief of upper respiratory symptoms associated with allergy or the common cold

Pregnancy Risk Factor C

Lactation Excretion in breast milk unknown/not recommended

Contraindications Hypersensitivity to promethazine, phenylephrine, or any component; cross reactivity with other phenothiazines may occur; asthma, peripheral vascular disease, severe hypertension, cardiovascular disease, liver disease, patients receiving MAO inhibitors; children <2 years (see Warnings)

Warnings Use with extreme caution in children and avoid use in children <2 years of age, due to the potential for severe and potentially fatal respiratory depression; a wide range of weight based doses have resulted in respiratory depression; excessively high doses have been associated with sudden death in children; use the lowest effective dose in children >2 years of age and avoid concomitant use with other medications having respiratory depressant effects. Neuroleptic malignant syndrome (NMS) has been reported with promethazine when used alone or in combination with antipsychotic drugs. Children with dehydration are at increased risk for development of dystonic reactions.

Precautions Use with caution in patients with cardiovascular disease, narrow-angle glaucoma, prostatic hypertrophy, GI or GU obstruction, bone marrow depression, impaired liver function, asthma, peptic ulcer, sleep apnea, and hypertensive crisis; avoid in patients with suspected Reye's syndrome; promethazine may lower the seizure threshold; use with caution in patients with seizure disorders or receiving other medications which may also lower the seizure threshold

Adverse Reactions

Promethazine:
- Cardiovascular: Hypertension, hypotension, tachycardia
- Central nervous system: Sedation (pronounced), drowsiness, confusion, fatigue, excitation, extrapyramidal reactions, dystonia, tardive dyskinesia, hallucinations, NMS
- Dermatologic: Photosensitivity, rash, angioedema
- Endocrine & metabolic: Weight gain
- Gastrointestinal: Xerostomia, GI upset, increased appetite, abdominal pain, diarrhea, nausea
- Genitourinary: Urinary retention
- Hematologic: Thrombocytopenia, leukopenia, agranulocytosis (rare)
- Hepatic: Cholestatic jaundice, hepatitis
- Ocular: Blurred vision
- Neuromuscular & skeletal: Arthralgia, tremor, paresthesia, myalgia
- Respiratory: Thickening of bronchial secretions, pharyngitis
- Miscellaneous: Allergic reactions

Phenylephrine:
- Cardiovascular: Hypertension, angina, reflex severe bradycardia, arrhythmias, peripheral vasoconstriction
- Central nervous system: Restlessness, excitability, headache, anxiety, nervousness, dizziness
- Dermatologic: Pilomotor response, skin blanching
- Neuromuscular & skeletal: Tremor
- Respiratory: Respiratory distress, rebound nasal congestion, sneezing, burning, stinging, dryness

Drug Interactions See Promethazine *on page 1324* and Phenylephrine *on page 1250*

Food Interactions Increase dietary intake of riboflavin

Usual Dosage Oral:

Children:
- 2-6 years: 1.25 mL every 4-6 hours, not to exceed 7.5 mL in 24 hours
- 6-12 years: 2.5 mL every 4-6 hours, not to exceed 15 mL in 24 hours

Children >12 years and Adults: 5 mL every 4-6 hours, not to exceed 30 mL in 24 hours

Administration Oral: Administer with food, water, or milk to decrease GI distress

Test Interactions Alters the flare response in intradermal allergen tests; false negative and positive reactions with pregnancy tests relying on immunological reactions between hCG and anti-hCG

Patient Information May cause drowsiness and impair ability to perform activities requiring mental alertness or physical coordination; may cause dry mouth. May cause photosensitivity reactions (eg, exposure to sunlight may cause severe sunburn, skin rash, redness, or itching); avoid exposure to sunlight and artificial light sources (sunlamps, tanning booth/bed); wear protective clothing, wide-brimmed hats, sunglasses, and lip sunscreen (SPF ≥15); use a sunscreen [broad-spectrum sunscreen or physical sunscreen (preferred) or sunblock with SPF ≥15]; contact physician if reaction occurs.

Dosage Forms Excipient information presented when available (limited, particularly for generics); consult specific product labeling.

Syrup: Promethazine hydrochloride 6.25 mg and phenylephrine hydrochloride 5 mg per 5 mL (473 mL) [contains alcohol]

♦ **Promethazine Hydrochloride** *see* Promethazine *on page 1324*

Promethazine, Phenylephrine, and Codeine

(proe METH a zeen, fen il EF rin, & KOE deen)

Index Terms Codeine, Promethazine, and Phenylephrine; Phenylephrine, Promethazine, and Codeine

Therapeutic Category Antihistamine/Decongestant Combination; Antitussive; Cough Preparation

Generic Available Yes

Use Temporary relief of coughs and upper respiratory symptoms including nasal congestion in children >16 years and adults

Restrictions C-V

Pregnancy Risk Factor C

Lactation Enters breast milk/not recommended

Contraindications Hypersensitivity to promethazine, codeine, phenylephrine, or any component; cross reactivity with other phenothiazines may occur; children <16 years of age; asthma, peripheral vascular disease; patients receiving MAO inhibitors

Warnings Avoid use in children <16 years of age, due to the potential for severe and potentially fatal respiratory depression associated with the combination of promethazine and other respiratory depressants (eg, codeine); fatalities associated with promethazine use alone in children <2 years of age have also been reported. Dose should not be increased if cough does not respond; re-evaluate within 5 days for possible underlying pathology. Codeine is not recommended for cough control in patients with a productive cough. Neuroleptic malignant syndrome (NMS) has been reported with promethazine when used alone or in combination with antipsychotic drugs. May alter temperature regulation or mask toxicity of other drugs due to antiemetic effects. May alter cardiac conduction (life-threatening arrhythmias have occurred with therapeutic doses of phenothiazines).

Precautions Use with caution in patients with cardiovascular disease, narrow-angle glaucoma, prostatic hypertrophy, GI or GU obstruction, bone marrow depression, impaired liver function, asthma, hyperthyroidism, diabetes mellitus, peptic ulcer, sleep apnea, and hypertensive crisis; avoid in patients with suspected Reye's syndrome; promethazine may lower the seizure threshold; use with caution in patients with seizure disorders or receiving other medications which may also lower the seizure threshold; use with caution in patients with hypersensitivity reactions to morphine, hydrocodone, hydromorphone, levorphanol, oxycodone, oxymorphone. May cause orthostatic hypotension, use with caution in patients at risk of hypotension or where transient hypotensive episodes would be poorly tolerated (cardiovascular disease or cerebrovascular disease). May cause drowsiness and impair ability to perform hazardous activities requiring mental alertness.

Adverse Reactions See individual monographs for Promethazine *on page 1324*, Phenylephrine *on page 1250*, and Codeine *on page 397*

Drug Interactions See individual monographs for Promethazine *on page 1324*, Phenylephrine *on page 1250*, and Codeine *on page 397*

Food Interactions Increase fluids, fiber intake, and riboflavin in diet

Usual Dosage Oral: Children ≥16 years and Adults: 5 mL every 4-6 hours, not to exceed 30 mL/24 hours

Administration Oral: Administer with food or water to decrease GI upset

Patient Information May cause drowsiness and impair ability to perform activities requiring mental alertness or physical coordination; may cause dry mouth; may be habit-forming; do not discontinue abruptly. May cause photosensitivity reactions (eg, exposure to sunlight may cause severe sunburn, skin rash, redness, or itching); avoid exposure to sunlight and artificial light sources (sunlamps, tanning booth/bed); wear

(Continued)

Promethazine, Phenylephrine, and Codeine *(Continued)*

protective clothing, wide-brimmed hats, sunglasses, and lip sunscreen (SPF ≥15); use a sunscreen [broad-spectrum sunscreen or physical sunscreen (preferred) or sunblock with SPF ≥15]; contact physician if reaction occurs.

Dosage Forms Excipient information presented when available (limited, particularly for generics); consult specific product labeling.

Syrup: Promethazine hydrochloride 6.25 mg, phenylephrine hydrochloride 5 mg, and codeine phosphate 10 mg per 5 mL (480 mL) [contains alcohol and sodium benzoate]

♦ **Promethegan™** *see* Promethazine *on page 1324*
♦ **Pronap-100®** *see* Propoxyphene and Acetaminophen *on page 1336*
♦ **Pronestyl®-SR (Can)** *see* Procainamide *on page 1315*
♦ **Propaderm® (Can)** *see* Beclomethasone *on page 200*

Propantheline (proe PAN the leen)

Index Terms Propantheline Bromide

Therapeutic Category Anticholinergic Agent; Antispasmodic Agent, Gastrointestinal; Antispasmodic Agent, Urinary

Generic Available Yes

Use Adjunctive treatment of peptic ulcer, irritable bowel syndrome, pancreatitis, ureteral and urinary bladder spasm; to reduce duodenal motility during diagnostic radiologic procedures

Pregnancy Risk Factor C

Lactation Excretion in breast milk unknown

Contraindications Hypersensitivity to propantheline or any component; narrow-angle glaucoma; ulcerative colitis; toxic megacolon; obstructive disease of the GI or urinary tract

Warnings Infants, patients with Down's syndrome, and children with spastic paralysis or brain damage may be hypersensitive to antimuscarinic effects

Precautions Use with caution in febrile patients, patients with hyperthyroidism, hepatic, cardiac, or renal disease, hypertension, GI infections, diarrhea, reflux esophagitis

Adverse Reactions

Cardiovascular: Tachycardia, palpitations, flushing
Central nervous system: Insomnia, drowsiness, dizziness, nervousness, headache
Dermatologic: Rash, dry skin
Endocrine & metabolic: Suppression of lactation
Gastrointestinal: Xerostomia, nausea, vomiting, constipation, dry throat, dysphagia
Genitourinary: Impotence, urinary retention
Ocular: Mydriasis, blurred vision
Neuromuscular & skeletal: Weakness
Respiratory: Dry nose
Miscellaneous: Allergic reactions, diaphoresis (decreased)

Drug Interactions May increase potential of potassium chloride wax-matrix preparations to cause intestinal lesions due to decreased peristalsis; increased effect/toxicity with anticholinergics, disopyramide, narcotic analgesics, bretylium, type I antiarrhythmics, antihistamines, phenothiazines, tricyclic antidepressants, corticosteroids (increased IOP), CNS depressants (sedation), adenosine, amiodarone, beta-blockers, amoxapine

Mechanism of Action Competitively blocks the action of acetylcholine at postganglionic parasympathetic receptor sites

Pharmacodynamics

Onset of action: Within 30-45 minutes
Duration: 4-6 hours

Pharmacokinetics

Metabolism: In the liver and GI tract
Elimination: In urine, bile, and other body fluids

Usual Dosage Oral:

Antisecretory:
- Children: 1-2 mg/kg/day in 3-4 divided doses
- Adults: 15 mg 3 times/day before meals or food and 30 mg at bedtime; for mild manifestations: 7.5 mg 3 times/day

Antispasmodic:
- Children: 2-3 mg/kg/day in divided doses every 4-6 hours and at bedtime
- Adults: 15 mg 3 times/day before meals or food and 30 mg at bedtime

Administration Oral: Administer 30 minutes before meals and at bedtime

Patient Information May cause drowsiness and impair ability to perform activities requiring mental alertness or physical coordination; notify physician if skin rash, flushing, or eye pain occurs; or if difficulty in urinating, constipation, or sensitivity to light becomes severe or persists; may cause dry mouth; maintain good oral hygiene habits, because lack of saliva may increase chance of cavities

Dosage Forms Excipient information presented when available (limited, particularly for generics); consult specific product labeling.

Tablet, as bromide: 15 mg [contains lactose 23.2 mg]

- **Propantheline Bromide** *see* Propantheline *on page 1330*
- **Propa pH [OTC]** *see* Salicylic Acid *on page 1413*

Proparacaine (proe PAR a kane)

Medication Safety Issues

Sound-alike/look-alike issues:

Proparacaine may be confused with propoxyphene

U.S. Brand Names Alcaine®; Ophthetic®

Canadian Brand Names Alcaine®; Diocaine®

Index Terms Proparacaine Hydrochloride; Proxymetacaine

Therapeutic Category Local Anesthetic, Ophthalmic

Generic Available Yes

Use Local anesthesia for tonometry, gonioscopy; suture removal from cornea; removal of corneal foreign body; cataract extraction, glaucoma surgery; short operative procedure involving the cornea and conjunctiva

Pregnancy Risk Factor C

Contraindications Hypersensitivity to proparacaine or any component

Precautions Use with caution in patients with cardiac disease, hyperthyroidism

Adverse Reactions

Dermatologic: Allergic contact dermatitis

Local: Irritation, stinging, sensitization

Ocular: Keratitis, iritis, erosion of the corneal epithelium, conjunctival congestion and hemorrhage, corneal opacification

Stability Refrigerate and protect from light

Mechanism of Action Local anesthetic; prevents initiation and transmission of impulse at the nerve cell membrane by decreasing ion permeability

Pharmacodynamics

Onset of action: Within 20 seconds of instillation

Duration: 15-20 minutes

Usual Dosage Children and Adults:

Ophthalmic surgery: Instill 1 drop of 0.5% solution in eye every 5-10 minutes for 5-7 doses

Tonometry, gonioscopy, suture removal: Instill 1-2 drops of 0.5% solution in eye just prior to procedure

Administration Ophthalmic: Instill drops into affected eye(s); avoid contact of bottle tip with skin or eye

Patient Information Do not rub eye until anesthesia has worn off

Dosage Forms Excipient information presented when available (limited, particularly for generics); consult specific product labeling.

Solution, ophthalmic, as hydrochloride: 0.5% (15 mL) [contains benzalkonium chloride]

- **Proparacaine Hydrochloride** *see* Proparacaine *on page 1331*
- **Propine®** *see* Dipivefrin *on page 520*
- **Proplex® T [DSC]** *see* Factor IX Complex (Human) *on page 635*

Propofol (PROE po fole)

Medication Safety Issues

Sound-alike/look-alike issues:

Diprivan® may be confused with Diflucan®, Ditropan®

U.S. Brand Names Diprivan®

Canadian Brand Names Diprivan®

Therapeutic Category General Anesthetic

Generic Available Yes

Use Induction of anesthesia in children ≥3 years and adults; maintenance of anesthesia in children ≥2 months and adults; initiation and maintenance of monitored anesthesia care sedation in adults; continuous sedation of adult intensive care unit patients

Pregnancy Risk Factor B

(Continued)

Propofol *(Continued)*

Lactation Enters breast milk/not recommended

Contraindications Hypersensitivity to propofol or any component (see Warnings); patients who are not intubated or mechanically ventilated; other contraindications to general anesthesia or sedation apply

Warnings Diprivan® contains egg lecithin, soybean oil, and disodium edetate; generic products may contain egg lecithin, soybean oil, or sodium metabisulfite; any of which may cause allergic reactions in susceptible individuals. Generic products may also contain benzyl alcohol or sodium benzoate; benzoic acid (benzoate) is a metabolite of benzyl alcohol; large amounts of benzyl alcohol (≥99 mg/kg/day) have been associated with a potentially fatal toxicity ("gasping syndrome") in neonates; the "gasping syndrome" consists of metabolic acidosis, respiratory distress, gasping respirations, CNS dysfunction (including convulsions, intracranial hemorrhage), hypotension, and cardiovascular collapse; use propofol products containing benzyl alcohol or sodium benzoate with caution in neonates; *in vitro* and animal studies have shown that benzoate displaces bilirubin from protein binding sites

Not recommended for induction of anesthesia in children <3 years or for maintenance of anesthesia in infants <2 months of age; not recommended for monitored anesthesia care sedation in children; **not recommended for sedation of PICU patients. Note: The FDA is very concerned about the safety of propofol in PICU patients.** The results of a manufacturer's randomized controlled clinical trial (n=327) revealed an increase in the number of deaths in PICU patients treated with Diprivan® versus other standard sedative agents. Diprivan® was administered at initial infusion rates of 5.5 mg/kg/hour and titrated to maintain a standardized level of sedation. Twenty-one of the 25 deaths occurred in patients who received propofol. The FDA's review of the data did not find a correlation of the deaths with an underlying disease state, nor did the review identify a definite pattern to the causes of death. A new clinical trial will be conducted to address this issue (see http://www.FDA.gov/medwatch/safety/2001/dipvivan_deardoc.pdf). The use of propofol in PICU patients, especially at high doses for prolonged periods of time may be associated with certain toxicities; metabolic acidosis with fatal cardiac failure has occurred in several children (4 weeks to 11 years of age) who received propofol infusions at average rates of infusion of 4.5-10 mg/kg/hour for 66-115 hours (maximum rates of infusion 6.2-11.5 mg/kg/hour); see Parke, 1992; Strickland, 1995; and Bray, 1995.

Patients require continuous monitoring and airway management; cardiovascular and respiratory resuscitation equipment should be available; decrease the dose in ASA III or IV, elderly, debilitated, or hypovolemic patients; not recommended for use in obstetrics, cesarean deliveries, lactating women, patients with increased ICP or impaired cerebral circulation. Abrupt discontinuation may result in rapid awakening, anxiety, agitation, and resistance to mechanical ventilation. Although products contain preservatives, rapid growth of micro-organisms can occur; failure to use aseptic technique can result in microbial contamination and fever, sepsis, infection, life-threatening illnesses, or death; discard I.V. tubing and unused portions after 12 hours; **do not use if microbial contamination is suspected**.

Propofol should be administered by qualified healthcare professionals trained in advanced cardiac life support and anesthetic drug use (when used for general anesthesia and monitored anesthesia care sedation) or management of critically ill patients (when used for sedation in intensive care patient).

Precautions Use with caution in patients with seizures or history of epilepsy, or severe cardiac or respiratory disease; I.V. injection may produce transient local pain; perioperative myoclonia may occur; decrease dose and rate of infusion for elderly, debilitated, or ASA III/IV patients. Abrupt discontinuation in pediatric patients may cause agitation, hyperirritability, tremulousness, and flushing of hands and feet. Increased frequency of bradycardia, jitteriness, and agitation have also been observed.

Diprivan® contains disodium edetate which can chelate trace metals, including zinc; as much as 10 mg of elemented zinc may be lost per day when calcium disodium edetate is used in gram doses to treat heavy metal poisonings; no reports of zinc deficiency or low zinc levels have been reported with Diprivan®, however, the manufacturer recommends that Diprivan® not be infused for >5 days without giving a "drug holiday"; during this time off of Diprivan®, replacement of estimated or measured urine zinc losses is recommended.

Adverse Reactions

Cardiovascular: Hypotension (dose related), bradycardia, myocardial depression, flushing

Central nervous system: Fever, headache, dizziness

Dermatologic: Rash, pruritus

Endocrine & metabolic: Hyperlipidemia; fatal metabolic acidosis has been reported

Gastrointestinal: Nausea, vomiting, abdominal cramping

Genitourinary: Discoloration of urine (green)

Local: Pain at injection site (especially when administered via small vein); **Note:** Dilution with D_5W or administration of lidocaine pretreatment may decrease local pain

Neuromuscular & skeletal: Myalgia, twitching, clonic/myoclonic movement

Respiratory: Respiratory acidosis, respiratory depression, apnea

Miscellaneous: Anaphylaxis, anaphylactoid reactions

Drug Interactions Theophylline may antagonize the CNS effects of propofol; propofol may increase serum concentrations of alfentanil; increased toxicity may occur with acetazolamide (cardiorespiratory instability), CNS depressants, atracurium (anaphylaxis), phenothiazines, fentanyl (increased concentration of propofol), guanabenz, MAO inhibitors, narcotic analgesics, vecuronium (increased neuromuscular blockade); in pediatric patients, concurrent use of propofol with fentanyl may cause serious bradycardia

Stability Does not require refrigeration; protect from light; do not use if there is evidence of separation of phases of emulsion, particulate matter, or discoloration; discard unused portions at end of surgical procedure; ICU use: Discard tubing and unused portions after 12 hours; dilute with D_5W only; do not dilute to <2 mg/mL; diluted emulsion is more stable in glass; stability in plastic: 95% potency after 2 hours; may administer with D_5W, LR, D_5LR, $D_5/{}^1/_2NS$, $D_5/{}^1/_4NS$; do not administer with blood or blood products through the same I.V. catheter; do not mix with other drugs

Mechanism of Action Propofol is a hindered phenolic compound with intravenous general anesthetic properties. The drug is unrelated to any of the currently used barbiturate, opioid, benzodiazepine, arylcyclohexylamine, or imidazole intravenous anesthotic agents

Pharmacodynamics

Onset of anesthesia: Within 30 seconds after bolus infusion

Duration: ~3-10 minutes depending on the dose, rate and duration of administration; with prolonged use (eg, 10 days ICU sedation), propofol accumulates in tissues and redistributes into plasma when the drug is discontinued, so that the time to awakening (duration of action) is increased; however, if dose is titrated on a daily basis, so that the minimum effective dose is utilized, time to awakening may be within 10-15 minutes even after prolonged use

Pharmacokinetics

Distribution: Large volume of distribution; highly lipophilic

- V_d (apparent): Children 4-12 years: 5-10 L/kg
- V_{dss}:
  - Adults: 170-350 L
  - Adults (10-day infusion): 60 L/kg

Protein binding: 97% to 99%

Metabolism: In the liver via glucuronide and sulfate conjugation

Half-life (three-compartment model):

- Alpha: 2-8 minutes
- Beta (second distribution): ~40 minutes
- Terminal: ~200 minutes; range: 300-700 minutes
- Terminal (after 10-day infusion): 1-3 days

Elimination: ~90% excreted in urine as metabolites and <1% as unchanged drug

Usual Dosage Dosage must be individualized based on total body weight and titrated to the desired clinical effect; wait at least 3-5 minutes between dosage adjustments to clinically assess drug effects; smaller doses are required when used with narcotics; the following are general dosing guidelines:

General anesthesia:

I.V. induction: (See "Symbols and Abbreviations Used in This Handbook" in front section of this book for explanation of ASA classes):

- Children ≥3 years, ASA I or II: 2.5-3.5 mg/kg; use a lower dose for children ASA III or IV
- Adults, ASA I or II, <55 years: 2-2.5 mg/kg (~40 mg every 10 seconds until onset of induction)
- Elderly, debilitated, hypovolemic, or ASA III or IV: 1-1.5 mg/kg (~20 mg every 10 seconds until onset of induction)
- Cardiac anesthesia: 0.5-1.5 mg/kg (~20 mg every 10 seconds until onset of induction)
- Neurosurgical patients: 1-2 mg/kg (~20 mg every 10 seconds until onset of induction)

Maintenance: I.V. infusion:

- Infants ≥2 months to Children 16 years, ASA I or II: Initial: 200-300 mcg/kg/minute; decrease dose after 30 minutes if clinical signs of light anesthesia are absent; usual infusion rate: 125-150 mcg/kg/minute; younger pediatric patients may require larger infusion rates compared to older children

(Continued)

Propofol *(Continued)*

Adults, ASA I or II, <55 years: Initial: 150-200 mcg/kg/minute for 10-15 minutes; decrease by 30% to 50% during first 30 minutes of maintenance; usual infusion rate: 100-200 mcg/kg/minute

Elderly, debilitated, hypovolemic, ASA III or IV: 50-100 mcg/kg/minute

Cardiac anesthesia:

Low dose propofol with primary opioid: 50-100 mcg/kg/minute (see manufacturer's labeling)

Primary propofol with secondary opioid: 100-150 mcg/kg/minute

Neurosurgical patients: 100-200 mcg/kg/minute

Maintenance: I.V. intermittent bolus: Adults, ASA I or II, <55 years: 20-50 mg increments as needed

Monitored Anesthesia Care sedation:

Initiation:

Adults, ASA I or II, <55 years: Slow I.V. infusion: 100-150 mcg/kg/minute for 3-5 minutes; slow injection: 0.5 mg/kg over 3-5 minutes

Elderly, debilitated, neurosurgical, or ASA III or IV patients: Use similar doses to healthy adults; avoid rapid I.V. boluses

Maintenance:

Adults, ASA I or II, <55 years: I.V. infusion using variable rates (preferred over intermittent boluses): 25-75 mcg/kg/minute; incremental bolus doses: 10 mg or 20 mg

Elderly, debilitated, neurosurgical, or ASA III or IV patients: Use 80% of healthy adult dose; **do not** use rapid bolus doses (single or repeated)

ICU sedation in intubated mechanically ventilated patients: Avoid rapid bolus injection; individualize dose and titrate to response

Adults: Continuous infusion: Initial: 0.3 mg/kg/hour; increase by 0.3-0.6 mg/kg/hour every 5-10 minutes until desired sedation level is achieved; usual maintenance: 0.3-3 mg/kg/hour or higher; reduce dose by 80% in elderly, debilitated, and ASA III or IV patients; reduce dose after adequate sedation established and adjust to response (ie, evaluate frequently to use minimum dose for sedation)

Administration Parenteral: I.V.: Shake injection well before use; administer pediatric induction doses over 20-30 seconds; do not administer via filter with <5-micron pore size

Monitoring Parameters Respiratory rate, blood pressure, heart rate, oxygen saturation, ABGs, depth of sedation; serum lipids or triglycerides with use >24 hours

Nursing Implications May change urine color to green

Additional Information Due to poor water solubility, the I.V. formulation is an isotonic oil-in-water emulsion and contains soybean oil, glycerol, egg lecithin, and sodium hydroxide (for pH adjustment); the brand name and generic product differ in the preservative used; Diprivan® contains 0.005% disodium edetate, while the generic product contains sodium metabisulfite (0.25 mg/mL); propofol injection contains ~0.1 g of fat/mL (1.1 kcal/mL)

Dosage Forms Excipient information presented when available (limited, particularly for generics); consult specific product labeling.

Injection, emulsion: 10 mg/mL (20 mL, 50 mL, 100 mL) [products may contain egg lecithin, and soybean oil; may contain benzyl alcohol, sodium benzoate, or sodium metabisulfite]

Diprivan®: 10 mg/mL (20 mL, 50 mL, 100 mL) [contains egg lecithin, soybean oil, and disodium edetate]

References

Bray RJ, "Fatal Myocardial Failure Associated With a Propofol Infusion in a Child," *Anaesthesia*, 1995, 50(1):94.

Parke TJ, Stevens JE, Rice ASC, et al, "Metabolic Acidosis and Fatal Myocardial Failure After Propofol Infusion in Children: Five Case Reports," *BMJ*, 1992, 305(6854):613-6.

Strickland RA and Murray MJ, "Fatal Metabolic Acidosis in a Pediatric Patient Receiving an Infusion of Propofol in the Intensive Care Unit: Is There a Relationship?" *Crit Care Med*, 1995, 23(2):405-9.

Propoxyphene (proe POKS i feen)

Medication Safety Issues

Sound-alike/look-alike issues:

Propoxyphene may be confused with proparacaine

Darvon® may be confused with Devrom®, Diovan®

Darvon-N® may be confused with Darvocet-N®

Related Information

Overdose and Toxicology *on page 1916*

U.S. Brand Names Darvon®; Darvon-N®
Canadian Brand Names Darvon-N®; 642® Tablet
Index Terms Dextropropoxyphene; Propoxyphene Hydrochloride; Propoxyphene Napsylate
Therapeutic Category Analgesic, Narcotic
Generic Available Yes: Capsule
Use Management of mild to moderate pain
Restrictions C-IV
Pregnancy Risk Factor C (D if used for prolonged periods)
Lactation Enters breast milk/use caution (AAP rates "compatible")
Contraindications Hypersensitivity to propoxyphene or any component
Warnings Do not exceed recommended dosage; abrupt discontinuation after prolonged use may result in withdrawal symptoms
Precautions Use with caution in patients with renal or hepatic dysfunction, or when substituting propoxyphene for opiates in narcotic dependent patients; reduce dose in patients with hepatic dysfunction; avoid use in patients with Cl_{cr} <10 mL/minute
Adverse Reactions

Central nervous system: Dizziness, lightheadedness, sedation, paradoxical excitement and insomnia, headache
Dermatologic: Rashes
Gastrointestinal: GI upset, nausea, vomiting, constipation
Hepatic: Elevated liver enzymes
Neuromuscular & skeletal: Weakness
Miscellaneous: Psychologic and physical dependence

Drug Interactions Cytochrome P450 Isoenzyme CYP2C9, CYP2D6, CYP3A3/4, and CYP3A5-7 inhibitor

CNS depressants, alcohol, MAO inhibitors, may potentiate adverse effects; propoxyphene may inhibit the metabolism and increase the serum concentrations of carbamazepine, phenobarbital, tricyclic antidepressants, and warfarin; concurrent use of propoxyphene with ritonavir is not recommended

Food Interactions Food may decrease rate of absorption, but may slightly increase bioavailability
Mechanism of Action Binds to opiate receptors in the CNS, causing inhibition of ascending pain pathways, altering the perception of and response to pain; produces generalized CNS depression
Pharmacodynamics

Onset of action: Oral: Within 30-60 minutes
Duration: 4-6 hours

Pharmacokinetics

Metabolism: In the liver to an active metabolite (norpropoxyphene) and inactive metabolites
Bioavailability: Oral: 30% to 70% due to first-pass effect
Half-life, adults: 8-24 hours (mean: ~15 hours)
Norpropoxyphene, adults: 34 hours
Dialysis: Not dialyzable (0% to 5%)

Usual Dosage Oral:

Children: Dose not well established; doses of propoxyphene hydrochloride of 2-3 mg/kg/day divided every 6 hours have been used
Adults:
Hydrochloride: 65 mg every 3-4 hours as needed for pain; maximum dose: 390 mg/day
Napsylate: 100 mg every 4 hours as needed for pain; maximum dose: 600 mg/day
Dosing adjustment in renal impairment: Cl_{cr} <10 mL/minute: Avoid use
Dosing adjustment in hepatic impairment: Reduced doses should be used

Administration Oral: May administer with food to decrease GI upset
Monitoring Parameters Pain relief, respiratory rate, blood pressure, mental status; liver enzymes with long-term use
Test Interactions False-positive methadone test
Patient Information Avoid alcohol; may be habit-forming; avoid abrupt discontinuation after prolonged use; may cause dizziness or drowsiness and impair ability to perform activities requiring mental alertness or physical coordination
Additional Information Propoxyphene does not possess any anti-inflammatory or antipyretic actions; it possesses little, if any, antitussive effects; propoxyphene napsylate 100 mg is equivalent to 65 mg of propoxyphene hydrochloride; several cases utilizing propoxyphene in children for opioid detoxification have been reported (see References)
Dosage Forms Excipient information presented when available (limited, particularly for generics); consult specific product labeling.

Capsule, as hydrochloride (Darvon®): 65 mg
(Continued)

Propoxyphene *(Continued)*

Tablet, as napsylate (Darvon-N®): 100 mg

References

Hasday JD and Weintraub M, "Propoxyphene in Children With Iatrogenic Morphine Dependence," *Am J Dis Child*, 1983, 137(8):745-8.

Propoxyphene and Acetaminophen

(proe POKS i feen & a seet a MIN oh fen)

Medication Safety Issues

Sound-alike/look-alike issues:

Darvocet-N® may be confused with Darvon-N®

Related Information

Narcotic Analgesics Comparison *on page 1705*

Overdose and Toxicology *on page 1916*

U.S. Brand Names Balacet 325™; Darvocet A500™; Darvocet-N® 50; Darvocet-N® 100; Pronap-100®

Canadian Brand Names Darvocet-N® 50; Darvocet-N® 100

Index Terms Acetaminophen and Propoxyphene; Propoxyphene Hydrochloride and Acetaminophen; Propoxyphene Napsylate and Acetaminophen

Therapeutic Category Analgesic, Narcotic

Generic Available Yes

Use Management of mild to moderate pain

Restrictions C-IV

Pregnancy Risk Factor C

Lactation Enters breast milk/compatible

Contraindications Hypersensitivity to propoxyphene, acetaminophen, or any component

Warnings Do not exceed recommended dosage; abrupt discontinuation after prolonged use may result in withdrawal symptoms

Precautions Use with caution in patients with renal or hepatic dysfunction, or when substituting propoxyphene for opiates in narcotic dependent patients; consider dosage reduction in patients with renal or hepatic dysfunction; propoxyphene should be avoided in patients with Cl_{cr} <10 mL/minute

Adverse Reactions

Propoxyphene:

- Central nervous system: Dizziness, lightheadedness, sedation, paradoxical excitement, insomnia, headache
- Dermatologic: Rashes
- Gastrointestinal: GI upset, nausea, vomiting, constipation
- Hepatic: Elevated liver enzymes
- Neuromuscular & skeletal: Weakness
- Miscellaneous: Psychologic and physical dependence

Acetaminophen:

- Dermatologic: Rash
- Hematologic: Blood dyscrasias (neutropenia, pancytopenia, leukopenia)
- Hepatic: Hepatic necrosis with overdose
- Renal: Renal injury with chronic use
- Miscellaneous: Hypersensitivity reactions (rare)

Drug Interactions See Propoxyphene *on page 1334* and Acetaminophen *on page 42*

Food Interactions Food may decrease rate of absorption of propoxyphene, but may slightly increase bioavailability; the rate of absorption of acetaminophen may be decreased when given with food high in carbohydrates

Pharmacodynamics See individual monographs for Propoxyphene *on page 1334* and Acetaminophen *on page 42*

Pharmacokinetics See individual monographs for Propoxyphene *on page 1334* and Acetaminophen *on page 42*

Usual Dosage Adults: Oral:

Darvocet-N® 50: 1-2 tablets every 4 hours as needed; maximum: 600 mg propoxyphene napsylate/day

Darvocet A500™, Darvocet-N® 100: 1 tablet every 4 hours as needed; maximum: 600 mg propoxyphene napsylate/day

Dosing adjustment in renal impairment: Serum concentrations of propoxyphene may be increased or elimination may be delayed; consider dosage reduction; specific dosing recommendations not available

Cl_{cr} <10 mL/minute: Avoid use

Dosing adjustment in hepatic impairment: Serum concentrations of propoxyphene and acetaminophen may be increased or elimination may be delayed; consider dosage reduction; specific dosing recommendations not available

Administration Oral: Administer with water on an empty stomach; may administer with food to decrease GI upset

Monitoring Parameters Pain relief, respiratory rate, blood pressure, mental status; liver enzymes with long-term use

Test Interactions False-positive methadone test

Patient Information Avoid alcohol; may be habit-forming; avoid abrupt discontinuation after prolonged use; may cause dizziness or drowsiness and impair ability to perform activities requiring mental alertness or physical coordination

Additional Information Propoxyphene napsylate 100 mg is equivalent to 65 mg of propoxyphene hydrochloride; Wygesic® tablets were discontinued in May 2001

Dosage Forms Excipient information presented when available (limited, particularly for generics); consult specific product labeling.

Tablet: Propoxyphene hydrochloride 65 mg and acetaminophen 650 mg, propoxyphene napsylate 100 mg, and acetaminophen 650 mg

Balacet 325™: Propoxyphene napsylate 100 mg and acetaminophen 325 mg

Darvocet A500™: Propoxyphene napsylate 100 mg and acetaminophen 500 mg [contains lactose]

Darvocet-N® 50: Propoxyphene napsylate 50 mg and acetaminophen 325 mg

Darvocet-N® 100, Pronap-100®: Propoxyphene napsylate 100 mg and acetaminophen 650 mg

♦ **Propoxyphene Hydrochloride** *see* Propoxyphene *on page 1334*

♦ **Propoxyphene Hydrochloride and Acetaminophen** *see* Propoxyphene and Acetaminophen *on page 1336*

♦ **Propoxyphene Napsylate** *see* Propoxyphene *on page 1334*

♦ **Propoxyphene Napsylate and Acetaminophen** *see* Propoxyphene and Acetaminophen *on page 1336*

Propranolol (proe PRAN oh lole)

Medication Safety Issues

Sound-alike/look-alike issues:

Propranolol may be confused with Pravachol®, Propulsid®

Inderal® may be confused with Adderall®, Enduron®, Enduronyl®, Imdur®, Imuran®, Inderide®, Isordil®, Toradol®

Inderal® 40 may be confused with Enduronyl® Forte

Significant differences exist between oral and I.V. dosing. Use caution when converting from one route of administration to another.

International issues:

Inderal® may be confused with Indiaral® which is a brand name for loperamide in France

Related Information

Antihypertensive Agents by Class *on page 1678*

Overdose and Toxicology *on page 1916*

U.S. Brand Names Inderal®; Inderal® LA; InnoPran XL™

Canadian Brand Names Apo-Propranolol®; Inderal®; Inderal®-LA; Novo-Pranol; Nu-Propranolol; Propranolol Hydrochloride Injection, USP

Index Terms Propranolol Hydrochloride

Therapeutic Category Antianginal Agent; Antiarrhythmic Agent, Class II; Antihypertensive Agent; Antimigraine Agent; Beta-Adrenergic Blocker

Generic Available Yes

Use Management of hypertension, angina pectoris, pheochromocytoma, essential tremor, tetralogy of Fallot cyanotic spells, and arrhythmias (such as atrial fibrillation and flutter, A-V nodal re-entrant tachycardias, and catecholamine-induced arrhythmias); prevention of MI, migraine headache; symptomatic treatment of hypertrophic subaortic stenosis; short-term adjunctive therapy of thyrotoxicosis

Pregnancy Risk Factor C

Lactation Enters breast milk/use caution (AAP rates "compatible")

Contraindications Hypersensitivity to propranolol or any component; uncompensated CHF, cardiogenic shock, bradycardia or heart block, asthma, hyperactive airway disease, chronic obstructive lung disease, Raynaud's syndrome

Warnings May depress myocardial activity and precipitate or worsen CHF; use with caution and monitor closely, especially in patients with compensated heart failure. In patients with angina pectoris, exacerbation of angina and, in some cases, MI occurred following abrupt discontinuance of therapy. Beta-blockers should generally be avoided in patients with bronchospastic disease (nonallergic bronchospasm, (Continued)

Propranolol *(Continued)*

chronic bronchitis, emphysema), as bronchospasm may occur. Hypoglycemia may occur, particularly in infants and children (whether the patient has diabetes mellitus or not), especially during fasting before surgery; hypoglycemia may also occur after prolonged physical exertion and in patients with renal dysfunction. Propranolol decreases the ability of the heart to respond to reflex adrenergic stimuli and may increase the risks of general anesthesia and surgical procedures. Propranolol may mask clinical signs of hyperthyroidism (exacerbation of symptoms of hyperthyroidism, including thyroid storm, may occur following abrupt discontinuation). Severe bradycardia (requiring pacemaker) may occur in patients with Wolff-Parkinson-White syndrome.

Precautions Propranolol may block hypoglycemia-induced tachycardia and blood pressure changes, use with caution in patients with diabetes mellitus; acute elevations in blood pressure have been reported after insulin-induced hypoglycemia in patients receiving propranolol. Use with caution in patients with peripheral vascular disease (beta-blockers may aggravate arterial insufficiency). Use with caution in patients with renal or hepatic dysfunction; consider dosage reduction in patients with hepatic insufficiency. Avoid I.V. use in patients receiving calcium channel blockers (eg, verapamil) (effects may be potentiated). Patients receiving beta-blockers who have a history of anaphylactic reactions, may be more reactive to a repeated allergen challenge and may not be responsive to the usual epinephrine doses used to treat an allergic reaction

Adverse Reactions

Cardiovascular: Hypotension, impaired myocardial contractility, CHF, bradycardia, worsening of A-V conduction disturbances

Central nervous system: Lightheadedness, insomnia, vivid dreams, lethargy, depression, fatigue, dizziness

Endocrine & metabolic: Hypoglycemia [also blunts warning signs of hypoglycemia (eg, tachycardia)], hyperglycemia, hyperkalemia

Gastrointestinal: Nausea, vomiting, diarrhea, GI distress, constipation

Hematologic: Agranulocytosis

Hepatic: Elevated liver enzymes

Neuromuscular & skeletal: Weakness

Respiratory: Bronchospasm

Miscellaneous: Cold extremities

Drug Interactions Cytochrome P450 isoenzyme CYP1A2, CYP2C18, CYP2C19, and CYP2D6 substrate

Phenobarbital, rifampin, or other enzyme inducers may increase propranolol clearance and decrease its activity; amiodarone, cimetidine, ciprofloxacin, fluconazole, fluoxetine, fluvoxamine, imipramine, isoniazid, paroxetine, quinidine, ritonavir, teniposide, theophylline, tolbutamide, and zileuton may increase serum concentrations or toxicity of propranolol; propranolol significantly increases the serum concentrations or toxicities of propafenone, theophylline, lidocaine, nifedipine, diazepam, thioridazine, warfarin; use with chlorpromazine may increase serum concentrations of both drugs; coadministration with cholestyramine or colestipol may decrease propranolol concentrations; aluminum-containing antacid may reduce GI absorption of propranolol; ACE inhibitors, disopyramide, digoxin, diltiazem, flecainide, hydralazine, prazosin, quinidine, MAO inhibitors, TCAs, haloperidol, verapamil may increase cardiovascular adverse effects; concurrent use with ACE inhibitors may increase bronchial hyperreactivity; abrupt withdrawal of clonidine while receiving beta-blockers may result in an exaggerated hypertensive crisis; NSAIDs, indomethacin may decrease the antihypertensive effect of propranolol

Food Interactions Avoid natural licorice (causes sodium and water retention and increases potassium loss); protein-rich foods may increase bioavailability; a change in diet from high carbohydrate/low protein to low carbohydrate/high protein may result in increased oral clearance; a high fat meal decreases the rate but not the extent of oral absorption of the extended release capsules

Stability Injection: Store at controlled room temperature; protect from freezing or excessive heat; protect from light; injection is compatible in D_5W, NS, D_5/NS, D_5/ $^1/_2$NS, $^1/_2$NS, LR; incompatible with bicarbonate

Mechanism of Action Nonselective beta-adrenergic blocker (class II antiarrhythmic); competitively blocks response to $beta_1$ and $beta_2$-adrenergic stimulation which results in a decrease in heart rate, myocardial contractility, blood pressure, and myocardial oxygen demand. Beta-adrenergic blocking effects are due to the S (-) enantiomer. Propranolol also exerts a quinidine-like or anesthetic-like membrane action at doses higher than those required for beta blockade; this affects the cardiac action potential (clinical significance is uncertain).

Pharmacodynamics Beta blockade: Oral (immediate release):

Onset of action: Within 1-2 hours

Duration: ~6 hours

Pharmacokinetics

Distribution: V_d: Adults: 3.9 L/kg; crosses the placenta; small amounts appear in breast milk

Protein-binding (Alpha$_1$-acid glycoprotein and albumin): **Note:** The S-isomer of propranolol preferentially binds to alpha$_1$-acid glycoprotein and the R-isomer preferentially binds to albumin

Newborns: 60% to 68%

Adults: 93%

Metabolism: Extensive first-pass effect, metabolized in the liver to active and inactive compounds; the 3 main metabolic pathways include: Aromatic hydroxylation (primarily 4-hydroxylation), N-dealkylation followed by further side-chain oxidation and direct glucuronidation; the 4 primary metabolites include: Propranolol glucuronide, naphthyloxylactic acid, and sulfate and glucuronic acid conjugates of 4-hydroxy propranolol; **Note:** Aromatic hydroxylation is catalyzed primarily by isoenzyme CYP2D6; side chain oxidation is mainly via CYP1A2, but also CYP2D6; 4-hydroxypropranolol possesses beta-adrenergic receptor blocking activity and is a weak inhibitor of CYP2D6.

Bioavailability: 30% to 40%; oral bioavailability may be increased in Down syndrome children

Half-life, distribution: I.V.: 5"10 minutes

Half-life, elimination (prolonged with hepatic dysfunction):

Neonates and Infants: Possible increased half-life

Children: 3.9-6.4 hours

Adults: 4-6 hours

Elimination: Metabolites are excreted primarily in urine (96% to 99%); <1% excreted in urine as unchanged drug

Clearance: Decreased in hepatic dysfunction and in chronic renal failure

Dialysis: Not dialyzable: (0% to 5%)

Usual Dosage

Neonates:

Oral: Initial: 0.25 mg/kg/dose every 6-8 hours; increase slowly as needed to maximum of 5 mg/kg/day

I.V.: Initial: 0.01 mg/kg slow I.V. push over 10 minutes; may repeat every 6-8 hours as needed; increase slowly to maximum of 0.15 mg/kg/dose every 6-8 hours

Arrhythmias:

Oral:

Children: Initial: 0.5-1 mg/kg/day in divided doses every 6-8 hours; titrate dosage upward every 3-5 days; usual dose: 2-4 mg/kg/day; higher doses may be needed; do not exceed 16 mg/kg/day or 60 mg/day

Adults: Initial: 10-20 mg/dose every 6-8 hours, increase gradually; usual range: 40-320 mg/day

I.V.:

Children: 0.01-0.1 mg/kg slow I.V. over 10 minutes; maximum dose: 1 mg (infants); 3 mg (children)

Adults: 1 mg/dose slow I.V.; repeat every 5 minutes up to a total of 5 mg

Hypertension: Oral:

Children: Initial: 0.5-1 mg/kg/day in divided doses every 6-12 hours; increase gradually every 5-7 days; usual dose: 1-5 mg/kg/day; maximum dose: 8 mg/kg/day

Adults: Initial: 40 mg twice daily or 60-80 mg once daily as sustained or extended release capsules; increase dosage every 3-7 days; usual dose: Immediate release products: ≤320 mg divided in 2-3 doses/day; sustained or extended release products: 120-160 mg once daily; maximum daily dose: 640 mg; usual dosage range (JNC 7): Immediate release products: 20-80 mg twice daily; sustained or extended release products: 60-180 mg once daily

Migraine headache prophylaxis: Oral:

Children: 0.6-1.5 mg/kg/day divided every 8 hours; maximum dose: 4 mg/kg/day **or**

≤35 kg: 10-20 mg 3 times/day

>35 kg: 20-40 mg 3 times/day

Adults: Initial: 80 mg/day divided every 6-8 hours (or once daily as sustained release capsule); increase by 20-40 mg/dose every 3-4 weeks to a maximum of 160-240 mg/day given in divided doses every 6-8 hours (or once daily as sustained release capsules)

Tetralogy spells: Infants and Children:

Oral: Palliation: Initial: 0.25 mg/kg/dose every 6 hours (1 mg/kg/day); if ineffective within first week of therapy, may increase by 1 mg/kg/day every 24 hours to maximum of 5 mg/kg/day; if patient becomes refractory may increase slowly to a maximum of 10-15 mg/kg/day but must carefully monitor heart rate, heart size, and cardiac contractility; average dose: 2.3 mg/kg/day; range: 0.8-5 mg/kg/day (see Garson, 1981). Some centers use: Initial: 0.5-1 mg/kg/dose every 6 hours; usual: 1-2 mg/kg/dose every 6 hours.

(Continued)

Propranolol *(Continued)*

I.V.: 0.01-0.02 mg/kg/dose infused over 10 minutes; maximum initial dose: 1 mg (Committee on Drugs, 1998). Some centers use: 0.15-0.25 mg/kg/dose slow I.V.; may repeat in 15 minutes

Thyrotoxicosis:

Neonates: Oral: 2 mg/kg/day in divided doses every 6-12 hours; occasionally higher doses may be required

Adolescents and Adults: Oral: 10-40 mg/dose every 6 hours

Adults: I.V.: 1-3 mg/dose slow I.V. as a single dose

Administration

Oral: Administer with food; administer extended release capsules consistently either with food or on an empty stomach; do not chew or crush sustained or extended release capsules, swallow whole; mix concentrated oral solution with water, fruit juice, liquid, or semisolid food before administration

Parenteral: I.V. administration should not exceed 1 mg/minute; administer slow I.V. over 10 minutes in children; maximum concentration for injection: 1 mg/mL

Monitoring Parameters EKG, blood pressure

Reference Range Therapeutic: 50-100 ng/mL (SI: 190-390 nmol/L) at end of dosing interval

Patient Information Avoid alcohol; do not discontinue abruptly; may mask fast heart rate of hypoglycemia, but sweating will still occur

Nursing Implications The I.V. dose is much smaller than oral dose

Additional Information Not indicated for hypertensive emergencies. Do not abruptly discontinue therapy, taper dosage gradually over 2 weeks. The pH of solution for injection is adjusted with citric acid.

Dosage Forms Excipient information presented when available (limited, particularly for generics); consult specific product labeling. [DSC] = Discontinued product

Capsule, extended release, as hydrochloride: 60 mg, 80 mg, 120 mg, 160 mg

InnoPran XL™: 80 mg, 120 mg

Capsule, sustained release, as hydrochloride:

Inderal® LA: 60 mg, 80 mg, 120 mg, 160 mg

Injection, solution, as hydrochloride: 1 mg/mL (1 mL)

Inderal®: 1 mg/mL (1 mL)

Solution, oral, as hydrochloride: 4 mg/mL (500 mL); 8 mg/mL (500 mL) [strawberry-mint flavor; contains alcohol 0.6%]

Tablet, as hydrochloride: 10 mg, 20 mg, 40 mg, 80 mg

Inderal®: 10 mg [DSC], 20 mg [DSC], 40 mg, 60 mg, 80 mg

References

Chobanian AV, Bakris GL, Black HR, et al, "The Seventh Report of the Joint National Committee on Prevention, Detection, Evaluation, and Treatment of High Blood Pressure: The JNC 7 report," *JAMA*, 2003, 289(19):2560-72.

Committee on Drugs, "Drugs for Pediatric Emergencies," *Pediatrics*, 1998, 101(1):E13

Garson A Jr, Gillette PC, and McNamara DG, "Propranolol: The Preferred Palliation for Tetralogy of Fallot," *Am J Cardiol*, 1981, 47(5):1098-104.

Lai CW, Ziegler DK, Lansky LL, et al, "Hemiplegic Migraine in Childhood: Diagnostic and Therapeutic Aspects," *J Pediatr*, 1982, 101(5):696-9.

Pickoff AS, Zies L, Ferrer PL, et al, "High-Dose Propranolol Therapy in the Management of Supraventricular Tachycardia," *J Pediatr*, 1979, 94(1):144-6.

Rasoulpour M and Marinelli KA, "Systemic Hypertension," *Clin Perinatol*, 1992, 19(1):121-37.

Sinaiko AR, "Pharmacologic Management of Childhood Hypertension," *Pediatr Clin North Am*, 1993, 40(1):195-212.

♦ **Propranolol Hydrochloride** *see* Propranolol *on page 1337*

♦ **Propranolol Hydrochloride Injection, USP (Can)** *see* Propranolol *on page 1337*

♦ **Proprinal [OTC]** *see* Ibuprofen *on page 802*

♦ **Proprinal® Cold and Sinus [OTC]** *see* Pseudoephedrine and Ibuprofen *on page 1346*

♦ **Propulsid®** *see* Cisapride ***U.S. - Available Via Limited-Access Protocol Only*** *on page 363*

♦ **2-Propylpentanoic Acid** *see* Valproic Acid and Derivatives *on page 1592*

Propylthiouracil (proe pil thye oh YOOR a sil)

Medication Safety Issues

Sound-alike/look-alike issues:

Propylthiouracil may be confused with Purinethol®

PTU is an error-prone abbreviation (mistaken as mercaptopurine [Purinethol®; 6-MP])

Canadian Brand Names Propyl-Thyracil®

Index Terms PTU (error-prone abbreviation)

Therapeutic Category Antithyroid Agent

Generic Available Yes

Use Palliative treatment of hyperthyroidism; adjunct to ameliorate hyperthyroidism in preparation for surgical treatment or radioactive iodine therapy; management of thyrotoxic crisis

Pregnancy Risk Factor D

Lactation Enters breast milk/use caution (AAP rates "compatible")

Contraindications Hypersensitivity to propylthiouracil or any component

Warnings May cause agranulocytosis, thyroid hyperplasia, thyroid carcinoma (usage >1 year); discontinue in the presence of agranulocytosis, aplastic anemia, ANCA-positive vasculitis, hepatitis, unexplained fever, or exfoliative dermatitis

Precautions Use with caution in patients receiving other drugs known to cause agranulocytosis

Adverse Reactions

Cardiovascular: Edema, cutaneous vasculitis

Central nervous system: Drowsiness, vertigo, dizziness, headache, drug fever

Dermatologic: Rash, urticaria, pruritus, exfoliative dermatitis, alopecia, skin pigmentation

Gastrointestinal: Nausea, vomiting, ageusia, sialoadenopathy, constipation

Hematologic: Agranulocytosis, leukopenia, thrombocytopenia, bleeding, hypoprothrombinemia

Hepatic: Jaundice, hepatitis

Neuromuscular & skeletal: Arthralgia, paresthesia, neuritis

Renal: Nephritis

Respiratory: Interstitial pneumonitis

Miscellaneous: Lymphadenopathy

Drug Interactions Anticoagulants (enhanced anticoagulant activity); correction of hyperthyroidism may alter the disposition of beta-blockers, digoxin, and theophylline, necessitating a dose reduction in these agents

Mechanism of Action Inhibits the synthesis of thyroid hormones by blocking the oxidation of iodine in the thyroid gland; blocks synthesis of thyroxine and triiodothyronine

Pharmacodynamics For significant therapeutic effects 24-36 hours are required; remission of hyperthyroidism usually does not occur before 4 months of continued therapy

Pharmacokinetics

Distribution: Breast milk to plasma ratio: 0.1

Protein binding: 75% to 80%

Metabolism: Hepatic

Bioavailability: 80% to 95%

Half-life: 1.5-5 hours

End-stage renal disease: 8.5 hours

Time to peak serum concentration: Oral: Within 1 hour; persists for 2-3 hours

Elimination: 35% excreted in urine

Usual Dosage Oral:

Neonates: 5-10 mg/kg/day in divided doses every 8 hours

Children: 5-7 mg/kg/day in divided doses every 8 hours **or**

6-10 years: 50-150 mg/day divided every 8 hours

≥10 years: 150-300 mg/day divided every 8 hours

Maintenance: $^1/_3$-$^2/_3$ of the initial dose in divided doses every 8-12 hours; this begins usually after 2 months on an effective initial dosage

Adults: Initial: 300-450 mg/day in divided doses every 8 hours (doses of 600-1200 mg/day are sometimes needed); maintenance: 100-150 mg/day in divided doses every 8-12 hours

Dosing adjustment in renal impairment: Adjustment is not necessary

Administration Oral: Administer with food

Monitoring Parameters CBC with differential, liver function tests, platelets, thyroid function tests (TSH, T_3, T_4), prothrombin time

Reference Range See normal values for thyroid function in Normal Laboratory Values for Children *on page 1881*

Patient Information Do not exceed prescribed dosage; take at regular intervals around-the-clock; notify physician or pharmacist if fever, sore throat, unusual bleeding or bruising, headache, or general malaise occurs

Dosage Forms Excipient information presented when available (limited, particularly for generics); consult specific product labeling.

Tablet: 50 mg

Extemporaneous Preparations A 5 mg/mL oral suspension may be made by crushing twenty 50 mg propylthiouracil tablets; add by geometric proportions 1:1 mixture of Ora-Plus® and Ora-Sweet® to a final volume of 200 mL; stable 91 days at 4°C and 70 days at 25°C

(Continued)

Propylthiouracil *(Continued)*

Nahata MC, Morosco RS, and Trowbridge JM, "Stability of Propylthiouracil in Extemporaneously Prepared Oral Suspensions at 4 and 25 Degrees C," *Am J Health Syst Pharm*, 2000, 57(12):1141-3.

References

Raby C, Lagorce JF, Jambut-Absil AC, et al, "The Mechanism of Action of Synthetic Antithyroid Drugs: Iodine Complexation During Oxidation of Iodide," *Endocrinology*, 1990, 126(3):1683-91.

- **Propyl-Thyracil® (Can)** *see* Propylthiouracil *on page 1340*
- **2-Propylvaleric Acid** *see* Valproic Acid and Derivatives *on page 1592*
- **ProQuad®** *see* Measles, Mumps, Rubella, and Varicella Virus Vaccine *on page 982*
- **Proquin® XR** *see* Ciprofloxacin *on page 357*
- **Prostacyclin** *see* Epoprostenol *on page 585*
- **Prostaglandin E_1** *see* Alprostadil *on page 81*
- **Prostigmin®** *see* Neostigmine *on page 1122*
- **Prostin® VR (Can)** *see* Alprostadil *on page 81*
- **Prostin VR Pediatric®** *see* Alprostadil *on page 81*

Protamine (PROE ta meen)

Medication Safety Issues

Sound-alike/look-alike issues:

Protamine may be confused with ProAmatine®, protamine, Protopam®, Protropin®

Therapeutic Category Antidote, Heparin

Generic Available Yes

Use Treatment of heparin overdosage; neutralize heparin during surgery or dialysis procedures

Pregnancy Risk Factor C

Lactation Excretion in breast milk unknown

Contraindications Hypersensitivity to protamine or any component

Warnings Heparin rebound associated with anticoagulation and bleeding has been reported to occur occasionally; symptoms typically occur 8-9 hours after protamine administration, but may occur as long as 18 hours later

Precautions Use with caution in patients allergic to fish, with prior history of vasectomy, patients receiving protamine-containing insulin or previous protamine therapy

Adverse Reactions

Cardiovascular: Hypotension, bradycardia, flushing, pulmonary hypertension

Central nervous system: Lassitude

Gastrointestinal: Nausea, vomiting

Neuromuscular & skeletal: Back pain

Respiratory: Dyspnea

Miscellaneous: Hypersensitivity reactions

Stability Refrigerate; stable for at least 2 weeks at room temperature

Mechanism of Action Combines with strongly acidic heparin to form a stable complex (salt) neutralizing the anticoagulant activity of both drugs

Pharmacodynamics Onset of action: Heparin neutralization occurs within 5 minutes following I.V. injection

Pharmacokinetics Elimination: Unknown

Usual Dosage I.V.: Protamine dosage is determined by the most recent dosage of heparin or low molecular weight heparin (LMWH); 1 mg of protamine neutralizes 90 USP units of heparin (lung), 115 USP units of heparin (intestinal), and 1 mg (100 units) LMWH; maximum dose: 50 mg

Heparin overdosage: Since blood heparin concentrations decrease rapidly **after** heparin administration, adjust the protamine dosage depending upon the duration of time since heparin administration as follows (see table):

Time Since Last Heparin Dose (min)	Dose of Protamine (mg) to Neutralize 100 units of Heparin
<30	1
30-60	0.5-0.75
60-120	0.375-0.5
>120	0.25-0.375

If heparin is administered by deep SubQ injection, use 1-1.5 mg protamine per 100 units heparin; this may be done by administering a portion of the dose (eg, 25-50 mg) slowly I.V. followed by the remaining portion as a continuous infusion over 8-16 hours (the expected absorption time of the SubQ heparin dose)

LMWH overdosage: If most recent LMWH dose has been administered within the last 4 hours, use 1 mg protamine per 1 mg (100 units) LMWH; a second dose of 0.5 mg protamine per 1 mg (100 units) LMWH may be given if APTT remains prolonged 2-4 hours after the first dose

Administration Parenteral: Reconstitute vial with 5 mL SWI; if using protamine in neonates, reconstitute with preservative free SWI; resulting solution equals 10 mg/mL; inject without further dilution over 10 minutes not to exceed 5 mg/minute; maximum of 50 mg in any 10-minute period

Monitoring Parameters Coagulation tests, APTT or ACT, cardiac monitor, and blood pressure monitor required during administration

Dosage Forms Excipient information presented when available (limited, particularly for generics); consult specific product labeling.

Injection, solution, as sulfate [preservative free]: 10 mg/mL (5 mL, 25 mL)

References

Monagle P, Michelson AD, Bovill E, et al, "Antithrombic Therapy in Children," *Chest*, 2001, 119:344S-70S.

♦ **Protection Plus® [OTC]** *see* Ethyl Alcohol *on page 619*

♦ **Protein C (Activated), Human, Recombinant** *see* Drotrecogin Alfa (Activated) *on page 549*

♦ **Prothrombin Complex Concentrate** *see* Factor IX Complex (Human) *on page 635*

Protirelin (proe TYE re lin)

U.S. Brand Names Thyrel® TRH [DSC]

Canadian Brand Names Relefact® TRH

Index Terms Lopremone; Thyrotropin Releasing Hormone; TRH

Therapeutic Category Diagnostic Agent, Thyroid Function

Generic Available No

Use Adjunct in the diagnostic assessment of thyroid function, and an adjunct to other diagnostic procedures in assessment of patients with pituitary or hypothalamic dysfunction; also causes release of prolactin from the pituitary and is used to detect defective control of prolactin secretion.

Pregnancy Risk Factor C

Contraindications Hypersensitivity to protirelin or any component

Warnings Due to transient changes in blood pressure (both increases and decreases), monitor blood pressure frequently during and at frequent intervals during first 15 minutes after administration; patient should be supine before, during, and immediately after administration; do not administer to patients in whom marked changes in blood pressure may cause serious risk

Precautions Thyroid hormones reduce TSH response to protirelin; when using diagnostically, discontinue thyroid hormones (liothyronine 7 days prior to testing and levothyroxine 14 days prior to testing); do not discontinue thyroid hormones when using protirelin to evaluate the effectiveness of thyroid suppression by thyroid hormone in patients with nodular or diffuse goiter or for an adjustment of thyroid hormone dosage in primary hypothyroidism

Adverse Reactions

Cardiovascular: Marked changes in blood pressure (hypotension or hypertension), flushing, chest tightness

Central nervous system: Lightheadedness, anxiety, seizures (rare), drowsiness, headache

Endocrine & metabolic: Breast enlargement

Gastrointestinal: Nausea, dysgeusia, abdominal discomfort, xerostomia

Genitourinary: Urinary frequency

Miscellaneous: Diaphoresis

Drug Interactions Aspirin in therapeutic doses, pharmacologic doses of steroids, levodopa, and thyroid hormones reduce TSH response to protirelin

Mechanism of Action Increases release of thyroid stimulating hormone (TSH) and prolactin from the anterior pituitary

Pharmacodynamics Maximum TSH levels occur in 20-30 minutes; TSH returns to baseline after about 3 hours

Pharmacokinetics Mean plasma half-life: 5 minutes

Usual Dosage I.V.:

Infants and Children: 7 mcg/kg to a maximum dose of 500 mcg

Adults: 500 mcg (range 200-500 mcg)

Administration Parenteral: Administer undiluted direct I.V. over 15-30 seconds with the patient remaining supine for an additional 15 minutes (see Warnings)

Monitoring Parameters Blood pressure, prolactin, TSH (drawn immediately prior to injection and 30 minutes after), T_4, and T_3

Reference Range See table on next page.

Patient Information May cause dry mouth; fast or eat low fat meal before test

(Continued)

Protirelin *(Continued)*

Characterization Based on Serum TSH Levels at Baseline and 30 Minutes After Protirelin

	Baseline Serum TSH (μU/mL)	Change of Serum TSH (μU/mL) at 30 minutes
Euthyroidism (normal thyroid function)	≤10 (usually ≤6); 20% have <1.5 μU/mL)	≥2 (usually 6-30)
Hyperthyroidism	≤10 (usually ≤4)	<2
Primary Hypothyroidism (Thyroidal)	>10 (usually 15-100)	≥2 (usually ≥20)
Secondary Hypothyroidism (Pituitary)	≤10 (usually ≤6)	<2 (59%) 2-50 (41%)
Tertiary Hypothyroidism (Hypoalamic)	≤10 (often <2)	≥2

Nursing Implications Keep patient supine during drug administration; have patient urinate prior to administration

Additional Information TSH response is reduced by repetitive protirelin administration; do not repeat test for at least 7 days

Dosage Forms Excipient information presented when available (limited, particularly for generics); consult specific product labeling.
Injection, solution: 500 mcg/mL (1 mL)

- ♦ **Protonix®** *see* Pantoprazole *on page 1208*
- ♦ **Protopam®** *see* Pralidoxime *on page 1299*
- ♦ **Protopic®** *see* Tacrolimus *on page 1498*
- ♦ **Proventil®** *see* Albuterol *on page 66*
- ♦ **Proventil® HFA** *see* Albuterol *on page 66*
- ♦ **Provera®** *see* MedroxyPROGESTERone *on page 991*
- ♦ **Provera-Pak (Can)** *see* MedroxyPROGESTERone *on page 991*
- ♦ **Proxymetacaine** *see* Proparacaine *on page 1331*
- ♦ **Prozac®** *see* Fluoxetine *on page 681*
- ♦ **Prozac® Weekly™** *see* Fluoxetine *on page 681*
- ♦ **PRP-OMP** *see* *Haemophilus* b Conjugate Vaccine *on page 751*
- ♦ **PRP-T** *see* *Haemophilus* b Conjugate Vaccine *on page 751*
- ♦ **Prudoxin™** *see* Doxepin *on page 537*
- ♦ **Prymaccone** *see* Primaquine *on page 1311*
- ♦ **23PS** *see* Pneumococcal Polysaccharide Vaccine (Polyvalent) *on page 1273*

Pseudoephedrine (soo doe e FED rin)

Medication Safety Issues
Sound-alike/look-alike issues:
Dimetapp® may be confused with Dermatop®, Dimetabs®, Dimetane®
Sudafed® may be confused with Sufenta®

Related Information
OTC Cough and Cold Preparations, Pediatric *on page 1706*

U.S. Brand Names Contac® Cold [OTC] [DSC]; Dimetapp® 12-Hour Non-Drowsy Extentabs® [OTC] [DSC]; Dimetapp® Decongestant Infant [OTC] [DSC]; Genaphed® [OTC]; Kidkare Decongestant [OTC]; Kodet SE [OTC]; Oranyl [OTC]; PediaCare® Decongestant Infants [OTC]; Silfedrine Children's [OTC]; Simply Stuffy™ [OTC] [DSC]; Sudafed® 12 Hour [OTC]; Sudafed® 24 Hour [OTC]; Sudafed® Children's [OTC]; Sudafed® Maximum Strength Nasal Decongestant [OTC]; Sudodrin [OTC]; SudoGest [OTC]; Sudo-Tab® [OTC]

Canadian Brand Names Balminil Decongestant; Benylin® D for Infants; Contac® Cold 12 Hour Relief Non Drowsy; Drixoral® ND; Eltor®; PMS-Pseudoephedrine; Pseudofrin; Robidrine®; Sudafed® Decongestant

Index Terms *d*-Isoephedrine Hydrochloride; Pseudoephedrine Hydrochloride; Pseudoephedrine Sulfate

Therapeutic Category Adrenergic Agonist Agent; Decongestant; Sympathomimetic

Generic Available Yes: Liquid, tablet

Use Temporary symptomatic relief of nasal congestion due to common cold, upper respiratory allergies, and sinusitis; also promotes nasal or sinus drainage

Pregnancy Risk Factor C

Lactation Enters breast milk/use caution (AAP rates "compatible")

Contraindications Hypersensitivity to pseudoephedrine or any component; MAO inhibitor therapy, severe hypertension, severe coronary artery disease

Warnings Some products contain sodium benzoate; benzoic acid (benzoate) is a metabolite of benzyl alcohol; large amounts of benzyl alcohol (≥99 mg/kg/day) have been associated with a potentially fatal toxicity ("gasping syndrome") in neonates; *in vitro* and animal studies have shown that benzoate displaces bilirubin from protein binding sites; avoid use of sodium benzoate containing products in neonates

Precautions Use with caution in patients with hyperthyroidism, diabetes mellitus, prostatic hypertrophy, mild-moderate hypertension, arrhythmias. Chewable tablets contain phenylalanine; avoid or use with caution in patients with phenylketonuria.

Adverse Reactions

Cardiovascular: Tachycardia, palpitations, arrhythmias

Central nervous system: Nervousness, excitability, dizziness, insomnia, drowsiness, headache, seizures, hallucinations

Gastrointestinal: Nausea, vomiting

Neuromuscular & skeletal: Tremor, weakness

Miscellaneous: Diaphoresis

Drug Interactions Additive effects with other sympathomimetics; hypertensive crisis with MAO inhibitors; phenothiazines and tricyclic antidepressants potentiate pressor effects; propranolol (beta-blockers)

Mechanism of Action Directly stimulates alpha-adrenergic receptors of respiratory mucosa causing vasoconstriction; directly stimulates beta-adrenergic receptors causing bronchial relaxation, increased heart rate and contractility

Pharmacodynamics

Onset of action: Oral: Decongestant effects occur within 15-30 minutes

Duration: 4-6 hours (up to 12 hours with extended release formulation administration)

Pharmacokinetics

Distribution: Children: V_d: 2.4-2.6 L/kg; breast milk to plasma ratio: 2.6-3.3

Metabolism: Incomplete in the liver to inactive metabolite

Half-life:
- Children 3.1 hours
- Adults: 9-16 hours

Elimination: 55% to 75% of dose excreted unchanged in urine
- Clearance:
  - Children: 9.2-10.3 mL/minute/kg
  - Adults: 7.3-7.6 mL/minute/kg

Usual Dosage Oral:

Children:
- <2 years: 4 mg/kg/day in divided doses every 6 hours
- 2-5 years: 15 mg every 6 hours; maximum dose: 60 mg/24 hours
- 6-12 years: 30 mg every 6 hours; maximum dose: 120 mg/24 hours

Children >12 years and Adults: 60 mg every 6 hours; maximum dose: 240 mg/day; using extended release products: 120 mg every 12 hours or 240 mg once daily

Administration Oral: Administer with water or milk to decrease GI distress; swallow timed release tablets or capsules whole, do not chew or crush

Test Interactions False-positive test for amphetamines by EMIT assay

Dosage Forms Excipient information presented when available (limited, particularly for generics); consult specific product labeling. [DSC] = Discontinued product

Caplet, extended release, as hydrochloride:
- Contac® Cold [DSC], Sudafed® 12 Hour: 120 mg

Liquid, as hydrochloride: 30 mg/5 mL (120 mL, 480 mL)
- Silfedrine Children's: 15 mg/5 mL (120 mL, 480 mL) [alcohol and sugar free; grape flavor]
- Simply Stuffy™: 15 mg/5 mL (120 mL) [alcohol free; contains sodium benzoate; cherry berry flavor] [DSC]
- Sudafed® Children's: 15 mg/5 mL (120 mL) [alcohol and sugar free; contains sodium benzoate; grape flavor]

Liquid, oral, as hydrochloride [drops]:
- Dimetapp® Decongestant Infant Drops: 7.5 mg/0.8 mL (15 mL) [alcohol free; contains sodium benzoate; grape flavor] [DSC]
- Kidkare Decongestant: 7.5 mg/0.8 mL (30 mL) [alcohol free; contains benzoic acid and sodium benzoate; cherry flavor]
- PediaCare® Decongestant: 7.5 mg/0.8 mL (15 mL) [alcohol free, dye free; contains benzoic acid, sodium benzoate; fruit flavor]

Tablet, as hydrochloride: 30 mg, 60 mg
- Genaphed®, Kodet SE, Oranyl, Sudafed®, Sudodrin, Sudo-Tab®: 30 mg
- SudoGest: 30 mg, 60 mg

Tablet, chewable, as hydrochloride:
- Sudafed® Children's: 15 mg [sugar free; contains phenylalanine 0.78 mg/tablet; orange flavor]

(Continued)

Pseudoephedrine *(Continued)*

Tablet, extended release, as hydrochloride:
Dimetapp® 12-Hour Non-Drowsy Extentabs®: 120 mg [DSC]
Sudafed® 24 Hour: 240 mg

References

Simons FE, Gu X, Watson WT, et al, "Pharmacokinetics of the Orally Administered Decongestants Pseudoephedrine and Phenylpropanolamine in Children," *J Pediatr*, 1996, 129(5):729-34.

♦ **Pseudoephedrine and Brompheniramine** *see* Brompheniramine and Pseudoephedrine *on page 235*

♦ **Pseudoephedrine and Carbinoxamine** *see* Carbinoxamine and Pseudoephedrine *on page 286*

Pseudoephedrine and Ibuprofen

(soo doe e FED rin & eye byoo PROE fen)

U.S. Brand Names Advil® Cold & Sinus [OTC]; Advil® Cold, Children's [OTC]; Motrin® Cold and Sinus [OTC]; Motrin® Cold, Children's [OTC]; Proprinal® Cold and Sinus [OTC]

Canadian Brand Names Advil® Cold & Sinus; Children's Advil® Cold; Sudafed® Sinus Advance

Index Terms Ibuprofen and Pseudoephedrine

Therapeutic Category Decongestant/Analgesic

Generic Available Yes: Caplet

Use Temporary relief of cold, sinus, and flu symptoms (including nasal congestion, headache, sore throat, minor body aches and pains, and fever)

Pregnancy Risk Factor Ibuprofen: B/D (3rd trimester)

Contraindications Hypersensitivity to pseudoephedrine, ibuprofen, or any component, aspirin, or other NSAIDs; active GI bleeding, ulcer disease; patients with the "aspirin triad" [asthma, rhinitis (with or without nasal polyps), and aspirin intolerance] (fatal asthmatic and anaphylactoid reactions may occur in these patients); MAO inhibitor therapy, severe hypertension, severe coronary artery disease

Warnings Some products contain sodium benzoate (see Dosage Forms); benzoic acid (benzoate) is a metabolite of benzyl alcohol; large amounts of benzyl alcohol (≥99 mg/kg/day) have been associated with a potentially fatal toxicity ("gasping syndrome") in neonates; the "gasping syndrome" consists of metabolic acidosis, respiratory distress, gasping respirations, CNS dysfunction (including convulsions, intracranial hemorrhage), hypotension and cardiovascular collapse; avoid use of formulations containing sodium benzoate in neonates; *in vitro* and animal studies have shown that benzoate displaces bilirubin from protein binding sites

Precautions Use with caution in patients with mild-moderate hypertension, heart disease, arrhythmias, diabetes mellitus, thyroid disease, asthma, glaucoma, prostatic hypertrophy, CHF, decreased renal or hepatic function, dehydration, history of GI disease (bleeding or ulcers), or those receiving anticoagulants.

Adverse Reactions See individual monographs for Pseudoephedrine *on page 1344* and Ibuprofen *on page 802.*

Drug Interactions See individual monographs for Pseudoephedrine *on page 1344* and Ibuprofen *on page 802.*

Pharmacodynamics See individual monographs for Pseudoephedrine *on page 1344* and Ibuprofen *on page 802.*

Pharmacokinetics See individual monographs for Pseudoephedrine *on page 1344* and Ibuprofen *on page 802.*

Usual Dosage Oral:

Manufacturer's recommendations:
- Children's Advil® Cold (suspension) and Advil® Cold & Sinus (capsules):
  - Children 2-5 years (10-20 kg): 5 mL (pseudoephedrine 15 mg/ibuprofen 100 mg) every 6 hours; not to exceed 4 doses/day
  - Children 6-11 years: 10 mL (pseudoephedrine 30 mg/ibuprofen 200 mg) every 6 hours; not to exceed 4 doses/day
  - Children >12 years and Adults: 1 capsule (pseudoephedrine 30 mg/ibuprofen 200 mg) every 4-6 hours; if symptoms do not respond; may use 2 capsules/dose; not to exceed 6 capsules/day

Alternative pediatric dosing: May dose according to the pseudoephedrine component:
- Infants and Children <2 years: 4 mg/kg/day in divided doses every 6 hours
- Children 2-5 years: 15 mg every 6 hours; maximum dose: 60 mg/24 hours
- Children 6-12 years: 30 mg every 6 hours or extended release product 60 mg every 12 hours; maximum dose: 120 mg/24 hours
- Children >12 years and Adults: 30-60 mg every 6 hours; maximum dose: 240 mg/24 hours

Administration Oral: Administer with food

Test Interactions False-positive test for amphetamines by EMIT assay

Dosage Forms Excipient information presented when available (limited, particularly for generics); consult specific product labeling. [DSC] = Discontinued product

Caplet:

Advil® Cold and Sinus [DSC], Motrin® Cold and Sinus, Proprinal® Cold and Sinus: Pseudoephedrine hydrochloride 30 mg and ibuprofen 200 mg

Capsule, liquid filled:

Advil® Cold and Sinus: Pseudoephedrine hydrochloride 30 mg and ibuprofen 200 mg [solubilized ibuprofen as free acid and potassium salt; contains coconut oil]

Suspension:

Advil® Cold, Children's: Pseudoephedrine hydrochloride 15 mg and ibuprofen 100 mg per 5 mL (120 mL) [alcohol free; contains sodium benzoate; grape flavor]

Motrin® Cold, Children's: Pseudoephedrine hydrochloride 15 mg and ibuprofen 100 mg per 5 mL (120 mL) [contains sodium benzoate; berry, dye free berry, and grape flavors]

Tablet:

Advil® Cold and Sinus: Pseudoephedrine hydrochloride 30 mg and ibuprofen 200 mg [DSC]

♦ **Pseudoephedrine and Loratadine** *see* Loratadine and Pseudoephedrine *on page 961*

♦ **Pseudoephedrine and Triprolidine** *see* Triprolidine and Pseudoephedrine *on page 1580*

♦ **Pseudoephedrine Hydrochloride** *see* Pseudoephedrine *on page 1344*

♦ **Pseudoephedrine Sulfate** *see* Pseudoephedrine *on page 1344*

♦ **Pseudofrin (Can)** *see* Pseudoephedrine *on page 1344*

♦ **Pseudomonic Acid A** *see* Mupirocin *on page 1091*

♦ **PsoriGel® [OTC] [DSC]** *see* Coal Tar *on page 394*

Psyllium (SIL i yum)

Medication Safety Issues

Sound-alike/look-alike issues:

Fiberall® may be confused with Feverall®

Hydrocil® may be confused with Hydrocet®

Modane® may be confused with Matulane®, Moban®

Perdiem® may be confused with Pyridium®

U.S. Brand Names Fiberall®; Fibro-Lax [OTC]; Fibro-XL [OTC]; Genfiber® [OTC]; Hydrocil® Instant [OTC]; Konsyl® [OTC]; Konsyl-D® [OTC]; Konsyl® Easy Mix [OTC]; Konsyl® Orange [OTC]; Metamucil® [OTC]; Metamucil® Plus Calcium [OTC]; Metamucil® Smooth Texture [OTC]; Modane® Bulk [OTC]; Natural Fiber Therapy [OTC]; Reguloid® [OTC]; Serutan® [OTC]

Canadian Brand Names Metamucil®

Index Terms Plantago Seed; Plantain Seed; Psyllium Hydrophilic Mucilloid

Therapeutic Category Laxative, Bulk-Producing

Generic Available Yes: Capsule, powder

Use Treatment of chronic atonic or spastic constipation and in constipation associated with rectal disorders; management of irritable bowel syndrome; adjunctive treatment with low cholesterol and saturated fat diet to reduce risk of coronary artery disease

Pregnancy Risk Factor B

Lactation Excretion in breast milk unknown/compatible

Contraindications Hypersensitivity to psyllium or any component; fecal impaction, GI obstruction

Warnings Inhalation of psyllium powder may produce allergic reactions in susceptible individuals

Precautions Use with caution in patients with esophageal strictures, ulcers, stenosis, or intestinal adhesions. Products may contain aspartame which is metabolized to phenylalanine and must be avoided (or used with caution) in patients with phenylketonuria.

Adverse Reactions

Gastrointestinal: Esophageal or bowel obstruction, diarrhea, constipation, abdominal cramps

Respiratory: Bronchospasm

Miscellaneous: Rhinoconjunctivitis, anaphylaxis upon inhalation in susceptible individuals

Drug Interactions Decreased effect of warfarin, digitalis, potassium-sparing diuretics, salicylates, tetracyclines, nitrofurantoin

Mechanism of Action Adsorbs water in the intestine to form a viscous liquid which promotes peristalsis and reduces transit time

(Continued)

Psyllium *(Continued)*

Pharmacodynamics

Onset of action: 12-24 hours

Maximum effect: May take 2-3 days

Pharmacokinetics Absorption: Oral: Generally not absorbed; small amounts of grain extract present in the preparation have been reportedly absorbed following colonic hydrolysis

Usual Dosage Oral (3.4 g psyllium hydrophilic mucilloid/7 g powder is equivalent to a rounded teaspoonful or 1 packet or 1 wafer):

Constipation:

Children 6-11 years: ½-1 rounded teaspoonful in 4 oz glass of liquid 1-3 times/day

Adults: 1-2 rounded teaspoonfuls or 1-2 packets or 1-2 wafers 1-4 times/day; 5 capsules up to 3 times/day

Fiber supplementation: Children ≥12 years and Adults: 2-6 capsules up to 3 times/day

Administration Oral: Granules and powder must be mixed in an 8 ounce glass of water or juice; drink a 8 ounce glass of liquid with each dose of wafers or capsules

Monitoring Parameters Stool output and frequency

Patient Information Each dose must be taken with an 8 ounce glass of water; inadequate fluid intake may result in throat swelling and choking

Nursing Implications Inhalation of psyllium dust may cause sensitivity to psyllium (runny nose, watery eyes, wheezing)

Dosage Forms Excipient information presented when available (limited, particularly for generics); consult specific product labeling.

Capsule:

Fibro XL: 675 mg

Metamucil®: 0.52 g [contains potassium 5 mg/capsule; provides 3 g dietary fiber 2.4 g per 6 capsules]

Metamucil® Plus Calcium: 0.42 g [contains potassium 6 mg/capsule; provides dietary fiber 2.1 g and calcium 300 mg per 5 capsules]

Granules (Serutan®): 2.5 g/teaspoon (510 g) [contains sodium benzoate]

Powder: 3.4 g/dose (390 g, 570 g)

Bulk-K: 4.725 g/dose (392 g)

Fiberall®: 3.5 g/dose (454 g) [sugar free; contains phenylalanine; orange flavor]

Fibro-Lax: 4.725 g /dose (140 g, 392g)

Genfiber®: 3.4 g/dose (397 g, 595 g) [regular flavor]

Genfiber®: 3.5 g/dose (283 g) [sugar free; orange flavor]

Hydrocil® Instant: 3.5 g/dose (3.7 g unit-dose packets, 300 g) [sugar free]

Konsyl®: 6 g/dose (6 g unit-dose packets, 300 g, 450 g) [sugar free; contains sodium 4.1 mg/dose; regular flavor]

Konsyl-D®: 3.4 g/dose (6.5 g unit-dose packets, 325 g, 397 g, 500 g) [contains sodium 2.3 mg/dose and dextrose]

Konsyl® Easy Mix: 6 g/dose (6 g unit-dose packets, 250 g) [sugar free; contains sodium 4.4 mg/dose]

Konsyl® Orange: 3.4 g/dose (12 g unit-dose packets, 538 g) [contains sodium 2.3 mg/dose and sucrose; orange flavor]

Konsyl® Orange: 3.4 g/dose (425 g) [sugar free; contains sodium 2.3 mg/dose; orange flavor]

Metamucil®: 3.4 g/dose:

(390 g, 570 g, 870 g) [contains sodium 3 mg and potassium 30 mg per dose; regular flavor]

(570 g, 870 g, 1254 g) [contains sodium 5 mg and potassium 30 mg per dose; orange flavor]

Metamucil® Smooth Texture: 3.4 g/dose:

(unit-dose packets, 609 g, 912 g, 1446 g) [contains sodium 5 mg and potassium 30 mg per dose; orange flavor]

(300 g, 450 g, 690 g) [contains sodium 4 mg and potassium 30 mg per dose; regular flavor]

(unit-dose packets, 183 g, 300 g, 450 g, 699 g, 1104 g) [sugar free; contains phenylalanine 25 mg, sodium 5 mg, and potassium 30 mg per dose; orange flavor]

Modane® Bulk: 3.4 g/dose (390 g) [contains dextrose; flavor free]

Natural Fiber Therapy: 3.4 g/dose (369 g, 539 g) [natural and orange flavors]

Reguloid®: 3.4 g/dose (300 g, 450 g) [sugar free; regular or orange flavors]; (390 g, 570g) [regular or orange flavors]

Wafers (Metamucil®): 3.4 g/dose (24s) [one dose = 2 wafers; contains sodium 20 mg and potassium 60 mg per dose; apple crisp and cinnamon spice flavors]

♦ **Psyllium Hydrophilic Mucilloid** *see* Psyllium *on page 1347*

♦ **P.T.E.-4®** *see* Trace Metals *on page 1558*

♦ **P.T.E.-5®** *see* Trace Metals *on page 1558*

Pyrantel Pamoate (pi RAN tel PAM oh ate)

U.S. Brand Names Pin-X® [OTC]; Reese's® Pinworm Medicine [OTC]

Canadian Brand Names Combantrin™

Therapeutic Category Anthelmintic

Generic Available No

Use Roundworm (*Ascaris lumbricoides*), pinworm (*Enterobius vermicularis*), and hookworm (*Ancylostoma duodenale* and *Necator americanus*) infestations; trichostrongyliasis and moniliformis infections

Pregnancy Risk Factor C

Contraindications Hypersensitivity to pyrantel pamoate or any component

Warnings Pin-X® contains sodium benzoate; benzoic acid (benzoate) is a metabolite of benzyl alcohol; large amounts of benzyl alcohol (≥99 mg/kg/day) have been associated with a potentially fatal toxicity ("gasping syndrome") in neonates; the "gasping syndrome" consists of metabolic acidosis, respiratory distress, gasping respirations, CNS dysfunction (including convulsions, intracranial hemorrhage), hypotension and cardiovascular collapse; avoid use of pyrantel pamoate products containing sodium benzoate in neonates; *in vitro* and animal studies have shown that benzoate displaces bilirubin from protein binding sites

Precautions Use with caution in patients with liver impairment, anemia, malnutrition. The chewable tablet contains aspartame which is metabolized to phenylalanine and must be avoided or used with caution in patients with phenylketonuria.

Adverse Reactions

Central nervous system: Dizziness, drowsiness, insomnia, headache, fever
Dermatologic: Rash
Gastrointestinal: Nausea, vomiting, anorexia, diarrhea, abdominal cramps, tenesmus
Hepatic: Elevated liver enzymes
Neuromuscular & skeletal: Weakness

Drug Interactions Piperazine (antagonist)

Stability Store at room temperature. Protect from light.

Mechanism of Action Promotes release of acetylcholine and inhibits cholinesterase causing neuromuscular paralysis of susceptible helminths

Pharmacokinetics

Absorption: Oral: Poor
Metabolism: Undergoes partial hepatic metabolism
Time to peak serum concentration: Within 1-3 hours
Elimination: In feces (50% as unchanged drug) and urine (7% as unchanged drug and metabolites)

Usual Dosage Children and Adults: Oral:

Roundworm, pinworm, or trichostrongyliasis: 11 mg pyrantel base/kg administered as a single dose; maximum dose: 1 g; dosage should be repeated after 2 weeks for pinworm infection

Hookworm: 11 mg pyrantel base/kg/day once daily for 3 days
Maximum daily dose: 1 g

Moniliformis infection: 11 mg pyrantel base/kg as a single dose; repeat this dose twice at 2-week intervals

Administration Oral: May mix drug with milk or fruit juice; may administer with or without food; shake suspension well before use. Chewable tablet must be chewed thoroughly before swallowing.

Monitoring Parameters Stool for presence of eggs, worms, and occult blood; serum AST and ALT

Patient Information Hygienic precaution is essential to prevent reinfection. Disinfect toilets; change and wash underclothes, bed linens, towels, and clothes daily. Wash

(Continued)

Pyrantel Pamoate *(Continued)*

your hands with soap often, especially before eating and after using the toilet. Do not scratch the infected area or place your fingers in your mouth. May cause dizziness or drowsiness and impair ability to perform activities requiring mental alertness or physical coordination.

Nursing Implications Fasting or purgation is not required prior to administration

Dosage Forms Excipient information presented when available (limited, particularly for generics); consult specific product labeling.

Caplet, as pamoate:

Reese's® Pinworm Medicine: 180 mg [equivalent to pyrantel base 62.5 mg/tablet]

Suspension, oral as pamoate:

Pin-X®: 144 mg/mL (30 mL, 60 mL) [equivalent to pyrantel base 50 mg/mL; sugar free; contains sodium benzoate; caramel flavor]

Reese's® Pinworm Medicine: 144 mg/mL (30 mL) [equivalent to pyrantel base 50 mg/mL]

Tablet, chewable, as pamoate:

Pin-X®: 720.5 mg [equivalent to pyrantel base 250 mg/tablet; contains aspartame; orange flavor]

Pyrazinamide (peer a ZIN a mide)

Canadian Brand Names Tebrazid™

Index Terms Pyrazinoic Acid Amide

Therapeutic Category Antitubercular Agent

Generic Available Yes

Use In combination with other antituberculosis agents in the treatment of *Mycobacterium* tuberculosis infection (especially useful in disseminated and meningeal tuberculosis); CDC currently recommends a 3 or 4 multidrug regimen which includes pyrazinamide, rifampin, INH, and at times ethambutol or streptomycin for the treatment of tuberculosis

Pregnancy Risk Factor C

Lactation Enters breast milk/use caution

Contraindications Hypersensitivity to pyrazinamide or any component; severe hepatic damage

Warnings Two-month rifampin-pyrazinamide regimen for the treatment of latent tuberculosis infection (LTBI) has been associated with severe and fatal liver injuries. The IDSA and CDC now recommend that this regimen should not generally be used in patients with LTBI.

Precautions Use with caution in patients with renal failure, gout, diabetes mellitus, patients receiving concurrent medications associated with liver injury (particularly with rifampin), or in patients with a history of alcoholism

Adverse Reactions

Central nervous system: Malaise, fever

Dermatologic: Urticaria, rash, photosensitivity

Endocrine & metabolic: Gout, hyperuricemia

Gastrointestinal: Nausea, vomiting, anorexia, abdominal pain

Hepatic: Hepatotoxicity (increased incidence with doses >30 mg/kg/day), jaundice

Neuromuscular & skeletal: Arthralgia

Drug Interactions Isoniazid (decreased INH serum levels); combination therapy with rifampin has been associated with severe and fatal hepatotoxic reactions

Mechanism of Action Converted to pyrazinoic acid in susceptible strains of *Mycobacterium* which lowers the pH of the environment

Pharmacokinetics

Absorption: Oral: Well absorbed

Distribution: Widely distributed into body tissues and fluids including the liver, lung, and CSF

Protein binding: 50%

Metabolism: In the liver

Half-life: 9-10 hours, prolonged with reduced renal or hepatic function

Time to peak serum concentration: Within 2 hours

Elimination: In urine (4% as unchanged drug)

Usual Dosage Oral:

Infants, Children, and Adolescents: 20-40 mg/kg/day in divided doses every 12-24 hours for the first 2 months of active treatment; daily dose not to exceed 2 g; **or** daily pyrazinamide for 2 weeks followed by directly observed therapy of 50 mg/kg/dose twice weekly to a maximum of 2 g/dose for 6 weeks

Adults: 15-30 mg/kg/day in 1-4 divided doses for the first 2 months of active treatment; maximum daily dose: 3 g/day; or daily pyrazinamide for 2 weeks followed by directly observed therapy of 50-70 mg/kg/dose twice weekly to a maximum of 4 g/dose for 6 weeks

Monitoring Parameters Periodic liver function tests, serum uric acid

Patient Information Notify physician if fatigue, weakness, nausea, abdominal pain, jaundice, vomiting, or joint pain and swelling occur. May cause photosensitivity reactions (eg, exposure to sunlight may cause severe sunburn, skin rash, redness, or itching); avoid exposure to sunlight and artificial light sources (sunlamps, tanning booth/bed); wear protective clothing, wide-brimmed hats, sunglasses, and lip sunscreen (SPF ≥15); use a sunscreen [broad-spectrum sunscreen or physical sunscreen (preferred) or sunblock with SPF ≥15]; contact physician if reaction occurs.

Dosage Forms Excipient information presented when available (limited, particularly for generics); consult specific product labeling.

Tablet: 500 mg

Extemporaneous Preparations

Pyrazinamide suspension can be compounded with simple syrup or 0.5% methylcellulose with simple syrup at a concentration of 100 mg/mL; the suspension is stable for 2 months at 4°C or 25°C when stored in glass or plastic bottles

To prepare pyrazinamide suspension in 0.5% methylcellulose with simple syrup: Crush 200 pyrazinamide 500 mg tablets and mix with a suspension containing 500 mL of 1% methylcellulose and 500 mL simple syrup. Add to this a suspension containing 140 crushed pyrazinamide tablets in 350 mL of 1% methylcellulose and 350 mL of simple syrup to make 1.7 L of suspension containing pyrazinamide 100 mg/mL in 0.5% methylcellulose with simple syrup.

Nahata MC, Morosco RS, and Peritre SP, "Stability of Pyrazinamide in Two Suspensions," *Am J Health-Syst Pharm*, 1995, 52:1558-60.

References

Ad Hoc Committee of the Scientific Assembly on Microbiology, Tuberculosis and Pulmonary Infections, "Treatment of Tuberculosis and Tuberculosis Infection in Adults and Children," *Clin Infect Dis*, 1995, 21:9-27.

American Academy of Pediatrics, Committee on Infectious Diseases, "Chemotherapy for Tuberculosis in Infants and Children," *Pediatrics*, 1992, 89(1):161-5.

"Update: Fatal and Severe Liver Injuries Associated With Rifampin and Pyrazinamide for Latent Tuberculosis Infection, and Revisions in American Thoracic Society/CDC Recommendations - United States, 2001," *MMWR Morb Mortal Wkly Rep*, 2001, 50(34):733-5.

Starke JR, "Multidrug Therapy for Tuberculosis in Children," *Pediatr Infect Dis J*, 1990, 9(11):785-93.

Starke JR and Correa AG, "Management of Mycobacterial Infection and Disease in Children," *Pediatr Infect Dis J*, 1995, 14(6):455-70.

♦ **Pyrazinoic Acid Amide** *see* Pyrazinamide *on page 1350*

♦ **2-Pyridine Aldoxime Methochloride** *see* Pralidoxime *on page 1299*

♦ **Pyridium®** *see* Phenazopyridine *on page 1244*

Pyridostigmine (peer id oh STIG meen)

Medication Safety Issues

Sound-alike/look-alike issues:

Pyridostigmine may be confused with physostigmine

Mestinon® may be confused with Metatensin®

Regonol® may be confused with Reglan®, Renagel®

Related Information

Commonly Used Antidotes for Acute Overdoses *on page 1920*

Overdose and Toxicology *on page 1916*

U.S. Brand Names Mestinon®; Mestinon® Timespan®; Regonol®

Canadian Brand Names Mestinon®; Mestinon®-SR

Index Terms Pyridostigmine Bromide

Therapeutic Category Antidote, Neuromuscular Blocking Agent; Cholinergic Agent

Generic Available Yes: Tablet

Use Symptomatic treatment of myasthenia gravis by improving muscle strength; reversal of effects of nondepolarizing neuromuscular blocking agents; pretreatment for Soman nerve gas exposure (military use only)

Pregnancy Risk Factor B

Lactation Enters breast milk/compatible

Contraindications Hypersensitivity to pyridostigmine, bromides, or any component (see Warnings); GI or GU obstruction

Warnings Overdosage may result in cholinergic crisis, this must be distinguished from myasthenic crisis; adequate facilities should be available for cardiopulmonary resuscitation when testing and adjusting dose for myasthenia gravis; have atropine and epinephrine ready to treat hypersensitivity reactions; neonates of myasthenic mothers may have transient difficulties in swallowing, sucking, and breathing; use of pyridostigmine may be of benefit; use edrophonium test to assess neonate with these symptoms

(Continued)

Pyridostigmine *(Continued)*

Some injections contain benzyl alcohol which may cause allergic reactions in susceptible individuals; syrup contains sodium benzoate; large amounts of benzyl alcohol (≥99 mg/kg/day) have been associated with a potentially fatal toxicity ("gasping syndrome") in neonates; the "gasping syndrome" consists of metabolic acidosis, respiratory distress, gasping respirations, CNS dysfunction (including convulsions, intracranial hemorrhage), hypotension and cardiovascular collapse; use injections containing benzyl alcohol with caution in neonates; *in vitro* and animal studies have shown that benzoate, a metabolite of benzyl alcohol, displaces bilirubin from protein binding sites; avoid use of the syrup in neonates

Pretreatment with pyridostigmine alone will not protect against exposure to Soman nerve gas; its efficacy is dependent upon the rapid use of atropine and pralidoxime after exposure. Discontinue use of pyridostigmine after exposure.

Precautions Use with caution in patients with epilepsy, asthma, bradycardia, hyperthyroidism, arrhythmias, recent coronary occlusion, vagotonia, or peptic ulcer; use with caution and modify dosage in patients with renal disease

Adverse Reactions

Cardiovascular: Bradycardia, hypotension, arrhythmias, A-V block, syncope
Central nervous system: Headache, convulsions, drowsiness, dizziness
Dermatologic: Rash, dry skin
Gastrointestinal: Nausea, vomiting, diarrhea, increased peristalsis, abdominal cramps, dysphagia, salivation
Genitourinary: Urinary frequency, dysmenorrhea
Local: Thrombophlebitis (after I.V. administration)
Neuromuscular & skeletal: Muscle cramps, weakness, myalgia
Ocular: Miosis, lacrimation, diplopia, conjunctival hyperemia
Respiratory: Increased bronchial secretions, bronchospasm, laryngospasm, dyspnea, epistaxis
Miscellaneous: Diaphoresis

Drug Interactions Corticosteroids and magnesium may decrease effect of pyridostigmine; increases effects of depolarizing neuromuscular blocking agents (eg, succinylcholine); decreases the effects of nondepolarizing neuromuscular blocking agents (eg, pancuronium); may prolong neuromuscular blockade associated with aminoglycoside antibiotics; additive effects with beta-blockers; atropine is direct antagonist; additive effects with anticholinesterase drugs

Stability Protect from light; tablets are extremely moisture sensitive; do not remove desiccant and keep bottle closed tightly. Store 30 mg tablets in refrigerator; stable at room temperature for 3 months

Mechanism of Action Competitively inhibits destruction of acetylcholine by acetylcholinesterase which facilitates transmission of impulses across myoneural junction producing generalized cholinergic responses such as miosis, increased tonus of skeletal and intestinal musculature, bronchial and ureteral constriction, bradycardia, and increased salivary and sweat gland production

Pharmacodynamics

Onset of action:
- Oral: 30-45 minutes
- I.M.: <15 minutes
- I.V.: Within 2-5 minutes

Duration:
- Oral: 3-6 hours
- I.M., I.V.: 2-3 hours

Pharmacokinetics

Absorption: Oral: Very poor (10% to 20%) from the GI tract
Distribution: Adults: V_d: 19 ± 12 L
Metabolism: In the liver and at tissue site by cholinesterases
Bioavailability: 10% to 20%
Half-life: Adults: 3 hours
Elimination: Clearance: Adults: 830 mL/minute

Usual Dosage Myasthenia gravis (dosage should be adjusted so patient takes larger doses prior to time of greatest fatigue)

Oral:
- Neonates: 5 mg every 4-6 hours
- Children: 7 mg/kg/day in 5-6 divided doses
- Adults: Initial: 60 mg 3 times/day with maintenance dose ranging from 60 mg to 1.5 g/day (incremental increases every 48 hours or more if needed) or as sustained release tablet (Mestinon® Timespan®) 180-540 mg (1-3 tablets) once or twice daily (the interval between doses should be at least 6 hours)

I.M., I.V.:
- Neonates and Children: 0.05-0.15 mg/kg/dose (maximum single dose: 10 mg)

Adults: 2 mg every 2-3 hours (or 1/30th of oral dose)
Reversal of nondepolarizing neuromuscular blocker: I.V.:
Children: 0.1-0.25 mg/kg/dose preceded by atropine or glycopyrrolate
Adults: 10-20 mg preceded by atropine or glycopyrrolate
Pretreatment for Soman nerve gas exposure: Oral: Adults: 30 mg every 8 hours beginning several hours before exposure; discontinue after exposure to nerve gas (treatment with atropine and pralidoxime are indicated after exposure)

Administration
Parenteral: Administer direct I.V. slowly over 2-4 minutes; patients receiving large parenteral doses should be pretreated with atropine
Oral: Swallow sustained release tablets whole, do not chew or crush

Monitoring Parameters Muscle strength, heart rate, vital capacity

Dosage Forms Excipient information presented when available (limited, particularly for generics); consult specific product labeling.
Injection, solution, as bromide:
Regonol®: 5 mg/mL (2 mL) [contains benzyl alcohol]
Syrup, as bromide:
Mestinon®: 60 mg/5 mL (480 mL) [raspberry flavor; contains alcohol 5%, sodium benzoate]
Tablet, as bromide: 60 mg
Mestinon®: 60 mg
Tablet, sustained release, as bromide:
Mestinon® Timespan®: 180 mg

♦ **Pyridostigmine Bromide** *see* Pyridostigmine *on page 1351*

Pyridoxine (peer i DOKS een)

Medication Safety Issues
Sound-alike/look-alike issues:
Pyridoxine may be confused with paroxetine, pralidoxime, Pyridium®

Related Information
Antiepileptic Drugs *on page 1902*
Commonly Used Antidotes for Acute Overdoses *on page 1920*

U.S. Brand Names Aminoxin® [OTC]

Index Terms Pyridoxine Hydrochloride; Vitamin B_6

Therapeutic Category Antidote, Cycloserine Toxicity; Antidote, Hydrazine Toxicity; Antidote, Mushroom Toxicity; Drug-induced Neuritis, Treatment Agent; Nutritional Supplement; Vitamin, Water Soluble

Generic Available Yes

Use Prevention and treatment of vitamin B_6 deficiency, pyridoxine-dependent seizures in infants; treatment of drug-induced deficiency (eg, isoniazid or hydralazine); treatment of acute intoxication of isoniazid, cycloserine, hydrazine, mushroom (genus *Gyromitra*)

Pregnancy Risk Factor A (C if dose exceeds RDA recommendation)

Lactation Enters breast milk/compatible

Contraindications Hypersensitivity to pyridoxine or any component

Adverse Reactions
Central nervous system: Sensory neuropathy (after chronic administration of large doses), seizures (following I.V. administration of very large doses), headache
Gastrointestinal: Nausea
Hematologic: Decreased serum folic acid concentration
Hepatic: Elevated AST
Local: Burning or stinging at injection site
Neuromuscular & skeletal: Paresthesia
Respiratory: Respiratory distress
Miscellaneous: Allergic reactions have been reported

Drug Interactions Decreases levodopa effectiveness when used without carbidopa; decreases serum levels of phenobarbital and phenytoin

Mechanism of Action Precursor to pyridoxal and pyridoxamine which function as cofactors in the metabolism of proteins, carbohydrates, and fats; also aids in the release of liver and muscle stored glycogen and in the synthesis of GABA (within the CNS) and heme

Pharmacokinetics
Absorption: Readily from the GI tract; primarily in jejunum
Metabolism: Converted to pyridoxal (active form in liver)
Half-life, biologic: 15-20 days
Elimination: By liver metabolism

(Continued)

Pyridoxine *(Continued)*

Usual Dosage

Adequate intake: Oral: Infants:
- <6 months: 0.1 mg (0.01 mg/kg)
- 6-12 months: 0.3 mg (0.03 mg/kg)

Recommended daily allowance: Oral:
- 1-3 years: 0.5 mg
- 4-8 years: 0.6 mg
- 9-13 years: 1 mg
- 14-19 years:
  - Male: 1.3 mg
  - Female: 1.2 mg
- 20-50 years: 1.3 mg
- >50 years:
  - Male: 1.7 mg
  - Female: 1.5 mg

Pyridoxine-dependent seizures: Oral, I.M., I.V.:
- Neonates and Infants: Initial: 10-100 mg; maintenance: Oral: 50-100 mg/day

Dietary deficiency: Oral:
- Children: 5-25 mg/day for 3 weeks, then 1.5-2.5 mg/day in multivitamin product
- Adults: 2.5-10 mg/day until clinical signs are corrected, then 2-5 mg/day (dosage found in multivitamin products)

Drug-induced neuritis (eg, isoniazid, hydralazine, penicillamine, cycloserine): Oral:
- Children:
  - Treatment: 10-50 mg/day
  - Prophylaxis: 1-2 mg/kg/day
- Adults:
  - Cycloserine: Treatment 100-300 mg/day in divided doses
  - Isoniazid or penicillamine: Treatment: 100-200 mg/day for 3 weeks; prophylaxis: 25-100 mg/day

Acute intoxication: Children and Adults:
- Hydrazine: 25 mg/kg: 1/3 dose I.M. and 2/3 dose I.V. infusion over 3 hours
- Isoniazid: Dose equal to isoniazid ingested given as a first dose of 1-4 g I.V., followed by 1 g I.M. every 30 minutes until total dosage completed
- Mushroom ingestion (genus *Gyromitra*): I.V.: 25 mg/kg; repeat as necessary to a maximum total dose of 15-20 g

Administration

Parenteral: Administer slow I.V.

Oral: Administer without regard to meals

Monitoring Parameters When administering large I.V. doses, monitor respiratory rate, heart rate, and blood pressure

Reference Range 30-80 ng/mL

Test Interactions False positive urobilinogen spot test using Ehrlich's reagent

Dosage Forms Excipient information presented when available (limited, particularly for generics); consult specific product labeling.

Capsule, as hydrochloride: 250 mg

Injection, solution, as hydrochloride: 100 mg/mL (1 mL)

Tablet, as hydrochloride: 25 mg, 50 mg, 100 mg, 200 mg, 250 mg, 500 mg

Tablet, enteric coated, as hydrochloride (Aminoxin®): 20 mg

Extemporaneous Preparations A 1 mg/mL oral solution has an expected stability of 30 days when refrigerated when compounded as follows: Withdraw 100 mg (1 mL of a 100 mg/mL injection) from a vial with a needle and syringe, add to 99 mL of simple syrup in an amber bottle; keep in refrigerator

Nahata, MC, Pai VB, and Hipple TF, *Pediatric Drug Formulations*, 5th ed, Cincinnati, OH: Harvey Whitney Books Co, 2004.

◆ **Pyridoxine Hydrochloride** *see* Pyridoxine *on page 1353*

Pyrimethamine (peer i METH a meen)

Medication Safety Issues

Sound-alike/look-alike issues:

Daraprim® may be confused with Dantrium®, Daranide®

U.S. Brand Names Daraprim®

Canadian Brand Names Daraprim®

Therapeutic Category Antimalarial Agent

Generic Available No

Use Used in combination with sulfadiazine for treatment of toxoplasmosis; used in combination with dapsone as primary or secondary prophylaxis for *Pneumocystis carinii* in HIV-infected patients; pyrimethamine has been used for chemoprophylaxis of malaria, however, due to severe adverse reactions and reports of resistance to pyrimethamine, other antimalarial agents are now generally preferred

Pregnancy Risk Factor C

Lactation Enters breast milk/not recommended (AAP rates "compatible")

Contraindications Hypersensitivity to pyrimethamine, chloroguanide, or any component; megaloblastic anemia; resistant malaria and patients with seizure disorders

Precautions Use with caution in patients with impaired renal or hepatic function and in patients with possible folate deficiency

Adverse Reactions

Cardiovascular: Shock
Central nervous system: Seizures, fever, fatigue, ataxia, headache
Dermatologic: Rash, photosensitivity
Endocrine & metabolic: Folic acid deficiency
Gastrointestinal: Anorexia, abdominal cramps, vomiting, atrophic glossitis, diarrhea
Hematologic: Megaloblastic anemia, leukopenia, thrombocytopenia, agranulocytosis, pancytopenia, pulmonary eosinophilia
Neuromuscular & skeletal: Tremor
Renal: Hematuria
Respiratory: Respiratory failure

Drug Interactions Para-aminobenzoic acid, sulfonamides

Mechanism of Action Inhibits parasitic dihydrofolate reductase resulting in inhibition of tetrahydrofolic acid synthesis

Pharmacokinetics

Absorption: Oral: Well absorbed
Distribution: V_d: Adults: 2.9 L/kg; appears in breast milk; distributed to the kidneys, lung, liver, and spleen
Protein binding: 80% to 87%
Half-life: 111 hours (range: 54-148 hours)
Time to peak serum concentration: Within 2-6 hours
Elimination: Pyrimethamine and metabolites are excreted in urine

Usual Dosage Oral:

Toxoplasmosis (with sulfadiazine):

Newborns and Infants: Initial: 2 mg/kg/day divided every 12 hours for 2 days, then 1 mg/kg/day once daily given with sulfadiazine for the first 6 months; next 6 months: 1 mg/kg/day 3 times/week with sulfadiazine; oral folinic acid 5-10 mg 3 times/week should be administered to prevent hematologic toxicity

Children: 2 mg/kg/day divided every 12 hours for 3 days followed by 1 mg/kg/day (maximum: 25 mg/day) once daily or divided twice daily for 4 weeks given with sulfadiazine; oral folinic acid 5-10 mg 3 times/week should be administered to prevent hematologic toxicity

Adults: 50-75 mg/day together with 1-4 g of a sulfonamide plus oral folinic acid 5-10 mg 3 times/week for 1-3 weeks depending on patient's tolerance and response, then reduce dose by 50% and continue for 4-5 weeks **or** 25-50 mg/day for 3-4 weeks

Prophylaxis for first episode of *Toxoplasma gondii*:

Children ≥1 month of age: 1 mg/kg/day once daily with dapsone plus oral folinic acid 5 mg every 3 days

Adolescents and Adults: 50 mg once weekly with dapsone plus oral folinic acid 25 mg once weekly

Prophylaxis for recurrence of *Toxoplasma gondii*:

Children ≥1 month of age: 1 mg/kg/day once daily given with sulfadiazine or clindamycin, plus oral folinic acid 5 mg every 3 days

Adolescents and Adults: 25-75 mg once daily in combination with sulfadiazine or clindamycin, plus oral folinic acid 10-25 mg daily

Prophylaxis for first episode or recurrence of *Pneumocystis carinii*:

Adolescents and Adults: 50-75 mg once weekly in combination with dapsone plus oral folinic acid 25 mg once weekly

Administration Oral: Administer with meals to minimize vomiting

Monitoring Parameters CBC including platelet counts

Patient Information Notify physician if rash, sore throat, pallor, or glossitis occurs. May cause photosensitivity reactions (eg, exposure to sunlight may cause severe sunburn, skin rash, redness, or itching); avoid exposure to sunlight and artificial light sources (sunlamps, tanning booth/bed); wear protective clothing, wide-brimmed hats, sunglasses, and lip sunscreen (SPF ≥15); use a sunscreen [broad-spectrum sunscreen or physical sunscreen (preferred) or sunblock with SPF ≥15]; contact physician if reaction occurs.

Additional Information Folinic acid may be given in a dosage of 3-9 mg/day for 3 days, or 5 mg every 3 days, or as required to reverse symptoms or to prevent hematologic problems due to pyrimethamine-induced folic acid deficiency

(Continued)

Pyrimethamine *(Continued)*

Dosage Forms Excipient information presented when available (limited, particularly for generics); consult specific product labeling.

Tablet: 25 mg

Extemporaneous Preparations Pyrimethamine tablets may be crushed to prepare oral suspensions of the drug in a 1:1 mixture of simple syrup and 1% methylcellulose to yield a suspension with a pyrimethamine concentration of 2 mg/mL; stable for at least 91 days when stored in plastic or glass prescription bottles at 4°C or 25°C

Nahata MC, Morosco RS, and Hipple TF, "Stability of Pyrimethamine in a Liquid Dosage Formulation Stored for Three Months," *Am J Health-Syst Pharm*, 1997, 54:2714-6.

References

"1997 USPHS/IDSA Guidelines for the Prevention of Opportunistic Infections in Persons Infected With Human Immunodeficiency Virus," *MMWR Morb Mortal Wkly Rep*, 1997, 46(RR-12):1-46.

Van Voorhis WC, "Therapy and Prophylaxis of Systemic Protozoan Infections," *Drugs*, 1990, 40(2):176-202.

♦ **Pyrimethamine and Sulfadoxine** *see* Sulfadoxine and Pyrimethamine *on page 1486*
♦ **QDALL® AR** *see* Chlorpheniramine *on page 344*
♦ **Q-Naftate [OTC]** *see* Tolnaftate *on page 1550*
♦ **Quadrivalent Human Papillomavirus Vaccine** *see* Papillomavirus (Types 6, 11, 16, 18) Recombinant Vaccine *on page 1212*
♦ **Quadrivalent Meningococcal Conjugate Vaccine** *see* Meningococcal Polysaccharide (Groups A / C / Y and W-135) Diphtheria Toxoid Conjugate Vaccine *on page 999*
♦ **Quadrivalent Meningococcal Conjugate Vaccine** *see* Meningococcal Polysaccharide Vaccine (Groups A / C / Y and W-135) *on page 1000*
♦ **Qualaquin™** *see* Quinine *on page 1358*
♦ **Quelicin®** *see* Succinylcholine *on page 1479*
♦ **Questran®** *see* Cholestyramine Resin *on page 349*
♦ **Questran® Light** *see* Cholestyramine Resin *on page 349*
♦ **Questran® Light Sugar Free (Can)** *see* Cholestyramine Resin *on page 349*
♦ **Quibron®-T [DSC]** *see* Theophylline *on page 1520*
♦ **Quibron®-T/SR [DSC]** *see* Theophylline *on page 1520*
♦ **Quinalbarbitone Sodium** *see* Secobarbital *on page 1423*
♦ **Quinate® (Can)** *see* Quinidine *on page 1356*

Quinidine (KWIN i deen)

Medication Safety Issues

Sound-alike/look-alike issues:

Quinidine may be confused with clonidine, quinine, Quinora®

Canadian Brand Names Apo-Quinidine®; BioQuin® Durules™; Novo-Quinidin; Quinate®

Index Terms Quinidine Gluconate; Quinidine Polygalacturonate; Quinidine Sulfate

Therapeutic Category Antiarrhythmic Agent, Class I-A

Generic Available Yes

Use Prophylaxis after cardioversion of atrial fibrillation and/or flutter to maintain normal sinus rhythm; also used to prevent reoccurrence of paroxysmal supraventricular tachycardia, paroxysmal A-V junctional rhythm, paroxysmal ventricular tachycardia, paroxysmal atrial fibrillation, and atrial or ventricular premature contractions; also has activity against *Plasmodium falciparum* malaria

Pregnancy Risk Factor C

Lactation Enters breast milk/compatible

Contraindications Hypersensitivity to quinidine, any component, or cinchona derivatives; patients with complete A-V block with an A-V junctional or idioventricular pacemaker; patients with intraventricular conduction defects (marked widening of QRS complex); patients with cardiac glycoside-induced A-V conduction disorders

Warnings May cause syncope, most likely due to ventricular tachycardia or fibrillation; syncope may subside spontaneously, but occasionally may be fatal; discontinue quinidine if syncope occurs

Precautions Use with caution in patients with myocardial depression, sick sinus syndrome, incomplete A-V block, cardiac glycoside intoxication, hepatic and/or renal insufficiency, myasthenia gravis; hemolysis may occur in patients with G-6-PD deficiency; quinidine-induced hepatotoxicity, including granulomatous hepatitis, increased serum AST and alkaline phosphatase concentrations, and jaundice may occur; use with caution in nursing women; adjust dose with severe renal impairment

Adverse Reactions

Cardiovascular: Syncope, hypotension, tachycardia, heart block, ventricular fibrillation, vascular collapse, severe hypotension with rapid I.V. administration

Central nervous system: Fever, headache

Dermatologic: Angioedema, rash; photosensitivity (rare)
Gastrointestinal: GI disturbances, nausea, vomiting, cramps
Hematologic: Blood dyscrasias, thrombotic thrombocytopenic purpura
Hepatic: Elevated AST; elevated alkaline phosphatase, jaundice, granulomatous hepatitis
Respiratory: Respiratory depression
Miscellaneous: Cinchonism (nausea, tinnitus, headache, impaired hearing or vision, vomiting, abdominal pain, vertigo, confusion, delirium, syncope)

Drug Interactions Cytochrome P450 isoenzyme CYP3A3/4 substrate; CYP2D6 (potent) and CYP3A3/4 (weak) isoenzyme inhibitor

Quinidine potentiates nondepolarizing and depolarizing muscle relaxants; diltiazem, verapamil, delavirdine, saquinavir, amiodarone, alkalinizing agents, and cimetidine may increase quinidine serum concentrations; phenobarbital, phenytoin, and rifampin may decrease quinidine serum concentrations. Quinidine may increase plasma concentration of digoxin; closely monitor digoxin concentrations; digoxin dosage may need to be reduced (by one-half) when quinidine is initiated; new steady-state digoxin plasma concentrations occur in 5-7 days. Beta-blockers plus quinidine may increase bradycardia; quinidine may enhance coumarin anticoagulants; potential interaction with ritonavir, concurrent use is not recommended

Food Interactions Excessive intake of fruit juices or vitamin C may decrease urine pH and result in increased clearance of quinidine with decreased serum concentration; alkaline foods may result in increased quinidine serum concentrations; food has a variable effect on absorption of extended release formulation. Grapefruit juice delays absorption of quinidine, decreases quinidine clearance, inhibits cytochrome P450 CYP3A4 mediated metabolism of quinidine to 3-hydroxyquinidine (major metabolite of quinidine), and significantly decreases the AUC of 3-hydroxyquinidine (although the clinical significance of the quinidine-grapefruit juice interaction is unknown, grapefruit juice should be avoided). A decrease in dietary salt intake may increase serum quinidine concentrations.

Stability Do not use discolored parenteral solution

Mechanism of Action Class IA antiarrhythmic with anticholinergic, local anesthetic, and mild negative inotropic effects; depresses phase 0 of the action potential; decreases myocardial excitability, conduction velocity, and myocardial contractility by decreasing sodium influx during depolarization and potassium efflux in repolarization; also reduces calcium transport across cell membrane

Pharmacokinetics

Distribution: V_d: Adults: 2-3.5 L/kg, decreased V_d with CHF, malaria; increased V_d with cirrhosis; crosses the placenta; appears in breast milk
Protein-binding:
- Newborns: 60% to 70%
- Adults: 80% to 90%
- Decreased protein binding with cyanotic congenital heart disease, cirrhosis, or acute MI

Metabolism: Extensive in the liver (50% to 90%) to inactive compounds
Bioavailability:
- Gluconate: 70%
- Sulfate: 80%

Half-life, plasma (increased half-life with cirrhosis and CHF):
- Children: 2.5-6.7 hours
- Adults: 6-8 hours

Elimination: In urine (15% to 25% as unchanged drug)
Dialysis: Slightly dialyzable (5% to 20%) by hemodialysis; not removed by peritoneal dialysis

Usual Dosage Note: Dose expressed in terms of the salt: 267 mg of quinidine gluconate = 200 mg of quinidine sulfate

Children: Test dose (for idiosyncratic reaction, intolerance, syncope, thrombocytopenia) (**sulfate**, oral or **gluconate**, I.M.): 2 mg/kg or 60 mg/m^2
- Oral (**quinidine sulfate**): Usual: 30 mg/kg/day or 900 mg/m^2/day given in 5 daily doses or 6 mg/kg every 4-6 hours; range: 15-60 mg/kg/day in 4-5 divided doses
- I.V. (**quinidine gluconate**): 2-10 mg/kg/dose every 3-6 hours as needed (I.V. route **not** recommended)

Adults: Test dose (for idiosyncratic reaction, intolerance, syncope, thrombocytopenia): 200 mg administered several hours before full dosage
- Oral (**sulfate**): 100-600 mg/dose every 4-6 hours; begin at 200 mg/dose and titrate to desired effect
- Oral (**gluconate**): 324-972 mg every 8-12 hours
- I.M.: 400 mg/dose every 4-6 hours
- I.V.: 200-400 mg/dose diluted and given at a rate ≤10 mg/minute

Dosing adjustment in renal impairment: Children and Adults: Cl_{cr} <10 mL/minute: Administer 75% of normal dose

(Continued)

Quinidine *(Continued)*

Administration

Oral: Administer with water on an empty stomach, but may administer with food or milk to decrease GI upset; best to administer in a consistent manner with regards to meals; avoid administration with grapefruit juice; swallow extended release tablets whole, do not chew or crush

Parenteral: I.V.: Maximum rate of infusion: 10 mg/minute; maximum concentration: 16 mg/mL; I.V. tubing length should be minimized (quinidine may be significantly adsorbed to polyvinyl chloride tubing)

Monitoring Parameters CBC with differential, platelet count, liver and renal function tests, and serum concentrations should be routinely performed during long-term administration

Reference Range Optimal therapeutic level is method dependent

Therapeutic: 2-7 mcg/mL (SI: 6.2-15.4 micromoles/L)

Toxic: >8 mcg/mL (SI: >18 micromoles/L)

Patient Information Notify physician if fever, rash, unusual bruising or bleeding, visual disturbances, or ringing in the ears occurs; avoid grapefruit juice; avoid excessive intake of fruit juices or vitamin C. May rarely cause photosensitivity reactions; avoid exposure to sunlight and artificial light sources (sunlamps, tanning booth/bed); use a sunscreen; contact physician if reaction occurs.

Additional Information Use of extended release products is not recommended in children. Formation of a concretion of tablets or bezoar in the stomach has been reported following tablet ingestion by a 16-month old infant; diagnostic or therapeutic endoscopy may be required in patients with massive overdose and prolonged elevated serum quinidine concentrations

Dosage Forms Excipient information presented when available (limited, particularly for generics); consult specific product labeling.

Injection, solution, as gluconate: 80 mg/mL (10 mL) [equivalent to quinidine base 50 mg/mL]

Tablet, as sulfate: 200 mg, 300 mg

Tablet, extended release, as gluconate: 324 mg [equivalent to quinidine base 202 mg]

Tablet, extended release, as sulfate: 300 mg [equivalent to quinidine base 249 mg]

Extemporaneous Preparations

A 10 mg/mL quinidine sulfate oral liquid preparation made from tablets and 3 different vehicles (cherry syrup, a 1:1 mixture of Ora-Sweet® and Ora-Plus®, or a 1:1 mixture of Ora-Sweet® SF and Ora-Plus®) was stable for 60 days when stored in amber plastic prescription bottles in the dark at room temperature (25°C) or under refrigeration (5°C); Grind six 200 mg tablets in a mortar into a fine powder; add 15 mL of the vehicle and mix well to form a uniform paste; mix while adding the vehicle in geometric proportions to **almost** 120 mL; transfer to a calibrated bottle and qsad to 120 mL; label "shake well" and "protect from light" (Allen 1998).

Allen LV and Erickson MA, "Stability of Bethanechol Chloride, Pyrazinamide, Quinidine Sulfate, Rifampin, and Tetracycline in Extemporaneously Compounded Oral Liquids," *Am J Health Syst Pharm*, 1998, 55(17):1804-9.

References

Pickoff AS, Singh S, and Gelband H, *The Medical Management of Cardiac Arrhythmias in Cardiac Arrhythmias in the Neonate, Infant and Child*, Roberts NK and Gelband H, ed, Norwalk, CT: Appleton-Century-Crofts, 1983.

Szefler SJ, Pieroni DR, Gingell RL, et al, "Rapid Elimination of Quinidine in Pediatric Patients," *Pediatrics*, 1982, 70(3):370-5.

♦ **Quinidine Gluconate** *see* Quinidine *on page 1356*

♦ **Quinidine Polygalacturonate** *see* Quinidine *on page 1356*

♦ **Quinidine Sulfate** *see* Quinidine *on page 1356*

Quinine (KWYE nine)

Medication Safety Issues

Sound-alike/look-alike issues:

Quinine may be confused with quinidine

Related Information

Malaria *on page 1855*

Medications for Which A Single Dose May Be Fatal When Ingested By A Toddler *on page 1932*

U.S. Brand Names Qualaquin™

Canadian Brand Names Apo-Quinine®; Novo-Quinine; Quinine-Odan™

Index Terms Quinine Sulfate

Therapeutic Category Antimalarial Agent; Skeletal Muscle Relaxant, Miscellaneous

Generic Available No

Use Suppression or treatment of chloroquine-resistant *P. falciparum* malaria (inactive against sporozoites, pre-erythrocytic or exoerythrocytic forms of plasmodia) in conjunction with other antimalarial agents; treatment of *Babesia microti* infection in conjunction with clindamycin

Pregnancy Risk Factor C

Lactation Enters breast milk/use caution (AAP rate "compatible")

Contraindications Hypersensitivity to quinine or any component; tinnitus, optic neuritis, G6PD deficiency; history of black water fever; history of thrombocytopenic purpura with previous quinine administration; pregnancy

Precautions Use with caution in patients with clinical conditions or on medications which may prolong the QT interval or cause cardiac arrhythmias (quinine has quinidine-like activity), in patients with myasthenia gravis, and in patients with impaired liver function

Adverse Reactions

Cardiovascular: Flushing of the skin, anginal symptoms, conduction disturbances, ventricular tachycardia, syncope

Central nervous system: Fever, headache, confusion, vertigo, restlessness, seizures, dizziness

Dermatologic: Rash, pruritus, Stevens-Johnson syndrome

Endocrine & metabolic: Hypoglycemia

Gastrointestinal: Nausea, vomiting, epigastric pain, diarrhea

Hematologic: Hemolysis, thrombocytopenia, leukopenia, disseminated intravascular coagulation, thrombocytopenic purpura

Hepatic: Hepatitis

Ocular: Visual disturbances, night blindness, optic atrophy, blurred vision

Otic: Tinnitus, impaired hearing

Respiratory: Dyspnea

Miscellaneous: Hypersensitivity reactions, cinchonism (nausea, tinnitus, headache, impaired hearing or vision, vomiting, abdominal pain, vertigo, confusion, delirium, syncope)

Drug Interactions Cytochrome P450 isoenzyme CYP1A2, CYP2C19, and CYP3A3/4 substrate; CYP2C8/9, CYP2D6 (potent), and CYP3A4 (weak) isoenzyme inhibitor

Quinine may decrease the clearance of digoxin or digitoxin leading to increased plasma concentrations of these cardiac glycosides; cimetidine (prolongs half-life of quinine), aluminum-containing antacids (decreases quinine absorption); quinine may potentiate the effects of neuromuscular blocking agents; oral anticoagulants, urinary alkalinizers (may increase quinine toxicity); mefloquine (additive cardiotoxicity); ritonavir, verapamil, and amiodarone may increase serum quinine concentrations

Stability Protect from light

Mechanism of Action Depresses oxygen uptake and carbohydrate metabolism; intercalates into DNA, disrupting the parasite's replication and transcription; affects calcium distribution within muscle fibers and decreases the excitability of the motor end-plate region

Pharmacokinetics

Absorption: Oral: Readily absorbed, mainly from the upper small intestine

Distribution: Widely distributed to body tissues and fluids including small amounts into bile and CSF; crosses the placenta; excreted into breast milk

V_d (children): 0.8 L/kg

V_d (adults): 1.9 L/kg

Protein binding: 70% to 90%

Metabolism: Primarily in the liver via hydroxylation pathways

Half-life:

Children: 6-12 hours

Adults: 8-14 hours

Time to peak serum concentration: Within 1-3 hours

Elimination: In bile and saliva with <5% excreted unchanged in urine

Dialysis: Not effectively removed by peritoneal dialysis; removed by hemodialysis

Usual Dosage Oral:

Children:

Treatment of chloroquine-resistant malaria: 30 mg/kg/day in divided doses every 8 hours for 3-7 days in conjunction with another agent; maximum dose: 2 g/day

Babesiosis: 25 mg/kg/day, divided every 8 hours for 7-10 days; maximum dose: 650 mg/dose

Adults:

Treatment of chloroquine-resistant malaria: 650 mg every 8 hours for 3-7 days in conjunction with another agent

Suppression of malaria: 325 mg twice daily and continued for 6 weeks after exposure

Babesiosis: 650 mg every 8 hours for 7-10 days

(Continued)

Quinine *(Continued)*

Administration Oral: Do not crush capsule to avoid bitter taste

Monitoring Parameters CBC with platelet count, liver function tests, blood glucose, ophthalmologic examination

Patient Information Report to physician if tinnitus, hearing loss, rash, or visual disturbances occur during therapy

Additional Information Parenteral form of quinine (dihydrochloride) is no longer available from the CDC; quinidine gluconate should be used instead; the FDA has banned over-the-counter (OTC) drug products containing quinine sold for treatment and/or prevention of malaria, as well as, products labeled for treatment or prevention of nocturnal leg cramps

Dosage Forms Excipient information presented when available (limited, particularly for generics); consult specific product labeling. [DSC] = Discontinued product

Capsule, as sulfate: 325 mg [DSC]

Qualaquin™: 324 mg

Tablet, as sulfate: 260 mg [DSC]

References

Schulbe DE, "Quinine Ban Signals Change for Pharmacists, APhA," *Pharmacy Today*, 1995, 1(12):6.

♦ **Quinine-Odan™ (Can)** *see* Quinine *on page 1358*

♦ **Quinine Sulfate** *see* Quinine *on page 1358*

♦ **Quintasa® (Can)** *see* Mesalamine *on page 1011*

Quinupristin/Dalfopristin (kwi NYOO pris tin/dal FOE pris tin)

U.S. Brand Names Synercid®

Canadian Brand Names Synercid®

Index Terms Pristinamycin; RP-59500

Therapeutic Category Antibiotic, Streptogramin

Generic Available No

Use Treatment of serious or life-threatening infections caused by vancomycin-resistant *Enterococcus faecium*; treatment of complicated skin and skin structure infections caused by *Staphylococcus aureus* (methicillin-susceptible and methicillin-resistant strains) or *Streptococcus pyogenes*

Pregnancy Risk Factor B

Lactation Excretion in breast milk unknown/use caution

Contraindications Hypersensitivity to quinupristin, dalfopristin, other streptogramins (pristinamycin or virginiamycin), or to any component

Warnings Quinupristin/dalfopristin inhibit cytochrome P450 3A4 metabolism of cyclosporine, midazolam, nifedipine, and terfenadine. There was a 77% increase in cyclosporine's half-life with a 63% increase in the AUC. Cyclosporine levels should be closely monitored in patients who are receiving quinupristin/dalfopristin therapy concomitantly. Coadministration of quinupristin/dalfopristin with cytochrome P450 3A4 substrates with narrow therapeutic ranges require serum concentration monitoring of these drugs. Concurrent use with astemizole, terfenadine, and cisapride is not recommended. Superinfections and pseudomembranous colitis have been reported with the use of quinupristin/dalfopristin. Resistance to quinupristin/dalfopristin has been reported in a few cases of *Entercoccus faecium* infections.

Precautions Use with caution in patients with hepatic or renal dysfunction; dosage reduction may be necessary in patients with hepatic cirrhosis; may cause pain and phlebitis when infused through a peripheral line; episodes of severe arthralgia and myalgia have been reported which improve with a dose frequency reduction to "q12h" or discontinuation of quinupristin/dalfopristin

Adverse Reactions

Central nervous system: Headache

Dermatologic: Rash, pruritus, urticaria

Hepatic: Elevated AST, ALT, bilirubin

Local: Pain, edema, inflammation at infusion site; thrombophlebitis

Neuromuscular & skeletal: Arthralgia, myalgia

Miscellaneous: Superinfection

Drug Interactions Cytochrome P450 isoenzyme CYP3A4 inhibitor

Quinupristin/dalfopristin may increase plasma concentration of cyclosporine, tacrolimus, astemizole, terfenadine, delavirdine, nevirapine, indinavir, ritonavir, vinca alkaloids, docetaxel, paclitaxel, midazolam, diazepam, dihydropyridines, verapamil, diltiazem, HMG-CoA reductase inhibitors, cisapride, methylprednisolone, carbamazepine, quinidine, lidocaine, disopyramide (see Warnings)

Stability Unopened vials should be stored in a refrigerator at 2°C to 8°C; reconstituted drug is stable for 1 hour at room temperature; infusion bag is stable for 5 hours at room temperature and for 54 hours if refrigerated at 2°C to 8°C; incompatible with NS and heparin; compatible with aztreonam, ciprofloxacin, fluconazole, haloperidol, metoclopramide, morphine, and potassium chloride during Y-site administration

Mechanism of Action Inhibits bacterial protein synthesis by binding to the 50S bacterial ribosomal subunit resulting in peptide chain elongation inhibition and peptidyl transferase inhibition

Pharmacokinetics

Distribution:

V_d: Quinupristin: 0.45 L/kg

V_d: Dalfopristin: 0.24 L/kg

Protein binding:

Quinupristin: 23% to 32%

Dalfopristin: 50% to 56%

Metabolism: Quinupristin is conjugated with glutathione and cysteine to active metabolites; dalfopristin is hydrolyzed to an active metabolite

Half-life:

Quinupristin: 0.85 hour

Dalfopristin: 0.7 hour

Elimination: 75% to 77% excreted in the bile and feces

Usual Dosage Dosage is expressed in terms of combined "mg" of quinupristin plus dalfopristin: I.V.:

Children: Limited information is available; quinupristin/dalfopristin has been used in a limited number of pediatric patients under a compassionate use protocol

Treatment of vancomycin-resistant *Enterococcus faecium* infection: 7.5 mg/kg/dose every 8 hours

Treatment of vancomycin-resistant *Enterococcus faecium* CNS shunt infection: 7.5 mg/kg/dose every 8 hours (plus 1 mg intrathecal dose daily at the time of shunt tap was used in an 8-month old infant for 28 days in one case report; 1 or 2 mg doses every day for 5-33 days have been administered intrathecally in 6 patients)

Treatment of complicated skin and skin structure infection: 7.5 mg/kg/dose every 12 hours for at least 7 days

Adolescents ≥16 years and Adults:

Treatment of vancomycin-resistant *Enterococcus faecium* infection: 7.5 mg/kg/dose every 8 hours

Treatment of complicated skin and skin structure infection: 7.5 mg/kg/dose every 12 hours

Dosage adjustment in hepatic impairment: Dosage adjustment may be necessary, but exact recommendations cannot be made at this time

Administration Parenteral: Reconstitute vial by slowly adding 5 mL D_5W or SWI to make a 100 mg/mL solution; gently swirl the vial contents without shaking to minimize foam formation; further dilute the reconstituted solution with D_5W to a final maximum concentration for administration via peripheral line of 2 mg/mL; maximum concentration for administration via a central line is 5 mg/mL; if an injection site reaction occurs, the dose can be further diluted to a final concentration of <1 mg/mL; administer infusion over 60 minutes; following infusion of quinupristin/dalfopristin, the infusion line should be flushed with D_5W to minimize venous irritation; **DO NOT FLUSH** with saline or heparin solutions due to incompatibility

Monitoring Parameters CBC, liver function test; monitor infusion site closely

Nursing Implications If moderate to severe venous irritation occurs following peripheral quinupristin/dalfopristin administration, consider increasing the infusion volume, changing infusion sites, or establishing central venous access; administration of hydrocortisone or diphenhydramine did not decrease infusion site reactions

Dosage Forms Excipient information presented when available (limited, particularly for generics); consult specific product labeling.

Injection, powder for reconstitution:

500 mg: Quinupristin 150 mg and dalfopristin 350 mg

600 mg: Quinupristin 180 mg and dalfopristin 420 mg

References

Garey KW, Tesoro E, Muggia V, et al, "Cerebrospinal Fluid Concentrations of Quinupristin-Dalfopristin in a Patient With Vancomycin-Resistant *Enterococcus faecium* Ventriculitis," *Pharmacotherapy*, 2001, 21(6):748-50.

Gransden WR, King A, Marossy D, et al, "Quinupristin/Dalfopristin in Neonatal *Enterococcus faecium* Meningitis," *Arch Dis Child Fetal Neonatal Ed*, 1998, 78(3):F235-6.

Gray JW, Darbyshire PJ, Beath SV, et al, "Experience With Quinupristin/Dalfopristin in Treating Infections With Vancomycin-Resistant *Enterococcus faecium* in Children," *Pediatr Infect Dis J*, 2000, 19(3):234-8.

Nachman SA, Verma R, and Egnor M, "Vancomycin-Resistant *Enterococcus faecium* Shunt Infection in an Infant: An Antibiotic Cure," *Microb Drug Resist*, 1995, 1(1):95-6

♦ **Quixin™** *see* Levofloxacin *on page 927*

♦ **QVAR®** *see* Beclomethasone *on page 200*

♦ **RabAvert®** *see* Rabies Virus Vaccine *on page 1364*

Rabeprazole (ra BE pray zole)

Medication Safety Issues
Sound-alike/look-alike issues:
AcipHex® may be confused with Acephen®, Accupril®, Aricept®
Rabeprazole may be confused with aripiprazole

U.S. Brand Names AcipHex®

Canadian Brand Names AcipHex®; Pariet®

Index Terms Pariprazole

Therapeutic Category Gastric Acid Secretion Inhibitor; Gastrointestinal Agent, Gastric or Duodenal Ulcer Treatment; Proton Pump Inhibitor

Generic Available No

Use Treatment and maintenance of erosive or ulcerative gastroesophageal reflux disease (GERD); treatment of duodenal ulcers; treatment of pathological hypersecretory conditions; adjunctive treatment of duodenal ulcers associated with *Helicobacter pylori*

Pregnancy Risk Factor B

Lactation Excretion in breast milk unknown/not recommended

Contraindications Hypersensitivity to rabeprazole, substituted benzimidazole proton pump inhibitors (eg, lansoprazole, omeprazole), or any component

Warnings Symptomatic response to therapy with rabeprazole does not preclude the presence of gastric malignancy. Use of gastric acid inhibitors including proton pump inhibitors and H_2 blockers has been associated with an increased risk for development of acute gastroenteritis and community-acquired pneumonia (Canani, 2006).

Precautions Use with caution in patients with severe hepatic impairment

Adverse Reactions
Cardiovascular: Chest pain, hypertension, MI, syncope, angina, palpitations, bradycardia, tachycardia
Central nervous system: Headache, fever, chills, malaise, migraine, insomnia, anxiety, dizziness, depression, nervousness, somnolence, vertigo, convulsion, abnormal dreams
Dermatologic: Photosensitivity, rash, pruritus, urticaria, alopecia
Endocrine & metabolic: Hyperthyroidism, hypothyroidism, weight gain or loss, gout
Gastrointestinal: Diarrhea, nausea, abdominal pain, vomiting, dyspepsia, flatulence, constipation, dry mouth, eructation, gastroenteritis, melena, anorexia, cholelithiasis, stomatitis, dysphagia, gingivitis, cholecystitis, abnormal stools, colitis, glossitis, pancreatitis, proctitis
Genitourinary: Cystitis, urinary frequency, dysmenorrhea, dysuria, polyuria
Hematologic: Anemia
Neuromuscular & skeletal: Neck rigidity, myalgia, arthritis, leg cramps, bone pain, arthrosis, bursitis, neuropathy, paresthesia, tremor
Ocular: Dry eyes, abnormal vision, glaucoma
Otic: Otitis media, tinnitus
Renal: Renal calculus
Respiratory: Dyspnea, asthma, laryngitis, hyperventilation, hiccup
Miscellaneous: Hypersensitivity reactions

Drug Interactions Cytochrome P450 isoenzyme CYP2C19 and CYP3A3/4 substrate; isoenzyme CYP3A3/4 and CYP2C19 inhibitor
Rabeprazole inhibits oxidative metabolism and may increase or decrease drug absorption due to increased gastric pH values, the full potential related to specific drugs remains to be determined; may decrease absorption of indinavir, ketoconazole, and itraconazole; may increase absorption of digoxin

Food Interactions When administered with a high fat meal, absorption may be delayed; however, the extent of absorption (AUC) is not significantly altered.

Stability Store at room temperature; protect from moisture

Mechanism of Action Suppresses gastric acid secretion by inhibiting the parietal cell membrane enzyme (H^+/K^+)-ATPase or proton pump; demonstrates antimicrobial activity against *Helicobacter pylori*

Pharmacodynamics Onset of action: 1 hour

Pharmacokinetics
Protein binding: 96.3%
Metabolism: Extensive metabolism in the liver by cytochrome isoenzymes CYP3A and CYP2C19 to inactive metabolites; [CYP2C19 exhibits a known genetic polymorphism due to its deficiency in some sub-populations (3% to 5% of Caucasians and 17% to 20% of Asians) which results in slower metabolism]
Bioavailability: 52%
Half-life: Adults: 1-2 hours
Time to peak serum concentration: 2-5 hours
Excretion: 90% in urine

Usual Dosage Oral: Adults:

GERD, ulcers, esophagitis:

Healing of erosive or ulcerative GERD: 20 mg/day for 4-8 weeks; an additional 8 weeks may be considered in patients who have not healed after 8 weeks of treatment

Maintenance of healing of erosive or ulcerative GERD: 20 mg/day

Treatment of symptomatic GERD or duodenal ulcers: 20 mg/day for 4 weeks

Pathological hypersecretory conditions: 60 mg/day to start; titrate dosage based upon the patient's response; doses of 100 mg/day and 60 mg 2 times/day have been administered; treatment courses have continued for up to one year

Active therapy of duodenal ulcers associated with *Helicobacter pylori* (in combination with amoxicillin and clarithromycin): 20 mg twice daily for 7 days

Dosage adjustment in hepatic impairment:

Mild to moderate: No adjustment is necessary

Severe impairment: Use cautiously due to lack of clinical data

Dosage adjustment in renal impairment: No dosage adjustment necessary

Administration Oral: May be administered without regard to food; tablets should be swallowed whole, do not chew, crush, or split. May administer with an antacid.

Patient Information May cause dry mouth and eyes; do not chew or crush tablets; may cause photosensitivity reactions (eg, exposure to sunlight may cause severe sunburn, skin rash, redness, or itching); avoid exposure to sunlight and artificial light sources (sunlamps, tanning booth/bed); wear protective clothing, wide-brimmed hats, sunglasses, and lip sunscreen (SPF ≥15); use a sunscreen [broad-spectrum sunscreen or physical sunscreen (preferred) or sunblock with SPF ≥15]; contact physician if reaction occurs

Dosage Forms Excipient information presented when available (limited, particularly for generics); consult specific product labeling.

Tablet, delayed release, enteric coated, as sodium: 20 mg

References

Canani RB, Cirillo P, Roggero P, et al, "Therapy With Gastric Acidity Inhibitors Increases the Risk of Acute Gastroenteritis and Community-Acquired Pneumonia in Children," *Pediatrics*, 2006, 117(5):e817-20.

Gibbons TE and Gold BD, "The Use of Proton Pump Inhibitors in Children: A Comprehensive Review," *Paediatr Drugs*, 2003, 5(1):25-40.

Rabies Immune Globulin (Human)

(RAY beez i MYUN GLOB yoo lin, HYU man)

U.S. Brand Names HyperRAB™ S/D; Imogam® Rabies-HT

Canadian Brand Names HyperRAB™ S/D; Imogam® Rabies Pasteurized

Index Terms RIG

Therapeutic Category Immune Globulin

Generic Available No

Use Postexposure prophylaxis of persons with suspected rabies exposure who previously have not been vaccinated against rabies; postexposure prophylaxis consists of thorough wound treatment and the administration of rabies vaccine and rabies immune globulin

Pregnancy Risk Factor C

Contraindications Persons who have been previously immunized with rabies vaccine and have a confirmed adequate rabies antibody titer should not receive rabies immune globulin as part of the postexposure regimen

Warnings Since rabies immune globulin is made from human plasma, it may potentially transmit an infectious agent. Screening of donors, testing for presence of viruses, and inactivating/removing viruses reduces this risk.

Precautions Use with caution in patients with a history of allergic reactions to human immunoglobulin preparations or with IgA deficiency. Epinephrine should be available for treatment of anaphylaxis. Use caution in patients with thrombocytopenia or coagulation disorders (I.M. injections may be contraindicated).

Adverse Reactions

Central nervous system: Fever, headache, malaise

Dermatologic: Rash, angioneurotic edema

Local: Soreness, pain, tenderness, stiffness at injection site

Renal: Nephrotic syndrome

Miscellaneous: Anaphylaxis

Drug Interactions Rabies vaccine: Neutralization of the vaccine if rabies immune globulin and vaccine are mixed in the same syringe or injected at the same site; repeat rabies immune globulin doses may suppress active antibody production and interfere with immune response to the vaccine. Live vaccines (MMR, varicella): Rabies immune globulin may interfere with immune response to live vaccines (do not

(Continued)

Rabies Immune Globulin (Human) *(Continued)*

administer live vaccines within 4 months after rabies immune globulin dose; revaccination is needed in patients who received live vaccine within 14 days before a rabies immune globulin dose).

Stability Store in refrigerator; do not freeze. Solution that has been frozen should be discarded.

Mechanism of Action Provides immediate antibodies to rabies which neutralize rabies virus and inhibit its spread and infective properties.

Pharmacodynamics

Onset of action: Rabies antibody appears in serum within 24 hours

Peak antibody level: 2-13 days

Pharmacokinetics Half-life: 24 days

Usual Dosage Children and Adults: Local wound infiltration: 20 international units/kg single dose administered as soon as possible after exposure with the first dose of rabies vaccine. If anatomically feasible, the full rabies immune globulin dose should be infiltrated around and into the wound(s); remaining volume should be administered I.M. at a site distant from the vaccine administration site. If rabies vaccine was initiated without rabies immune globulin, rabies immune globulin may be administered through the seventh day after the first vaccine dose. **Do not** administer rabies immune globulin beyond the seventh day.

Administration Do **not** administer I.V. Do not administer vaccine with or at same site as RIG administration.

Wound infiltration: Thoroughly infiltrate in the area around and into the wound(s)

I.M.: Children and Adults: Inject into the gluteal area or anterolateral aspect of the thigh at a site distant from rabies vaccine administration. Children with small muscle mass may require multiple I.M. sites for dose delivery.

Monitoring Parameters Serum rabies antibody titer (if rabies immune globulin is inadvertently administered after the eighth day from the first vaccine dose)

Dosage Forms Excipient information presented when available (limited, particularly for generics); consult specific product labeling.

Injection, solution [preservative free]:

HyperRAB™ S/D: 150 int. units/mL (2 mL, 10 mL) [solvent/detergent treated]

Imogam® Rabies-HT: 150 int. units/mL (2 mL, 10 mL) [heat treated]

References

Willoughby RE Jr and Hammarin AL, "Prophylaxis Against Rabies in Children Exposed to Bats," *Pediatr Infect Dis Jp*, 2005, 24(12):1109-10.

Rabies Virus Vaccine (RAY beez VYE rus vak SEEN)

U.S. Brand Names Imovax® Rabies; RabAvert®

Canadian Brand Names Imovax® Rabies; RabAvert®

Index Terms HDCV; Human Diploid Cell Cultures Rabies Vaccine; PCEC; Purified Chick Embryo Cell

Therapeutic Category Vaccine

Generic Available No

Use

Pre-exposure immunization: Vaccinate persons with greater than usual risk due to occupation or avocation including veterinarians, rangers, animal handlers, certain laboratory workers, and persons living in or visiting countries for longer than 1 month where rabies is a constant threat.

Postexposure prophylaxis: If a bite from a carrier animal is unprovoked or if the animal is not captured and rabies is present in that species and area, administer rabies immune globulin (RIG) and the vaccine as indicated

Pregnancy Risk Factor C

Contraindications

Pre-exposure treatment: Hypersensitivity to any component of the formulation; (Imovax® Rabies contains albumin and neomycin; RabAvert® contains amphotericin B, bovine gelatin, chicken protein, chlortetracycline, and neomycin); developing febrile illness

Postexposure treatment: Life-threatening allergic reactions to rabies vaccine or any components of the formulation (carefully consider a patient's risk of rabies before continuing therapy)

Warnings Immediate treatment for anaphylactic/anaphylactoid reaction should be available during administration of this vaccine. An immune complex reaction characterized by generalized urticaria, arthralgia, arthritis, angioedema, nausea, vomiting, fever, and malaise has been reported 2-21 days following booster doses of HDCV. Immune response may be decreased in immunocompromised patients. Pre-exposure immunization does not eliminate the need for prompt prophylaxis following an exposure but does reduce the postexposure treatment regimen.

Precautions Administer with caution to patients with thrombocytopenia or any coagulation disorder that would be compromised by I.M. injection

Adverse Reactions All serious adverse reactions must be reported to the U.S. Department of Health and Human Services (DHHS) Vaccine Adverse Event Reporting System (VAERS) 1-800-822-7967.

Cardiovascular: Edema

Central nervous system: Dizziness, malaise, encephalomyelitis, transverse myelitis, fever, pain, headache, neuroparalytic reactions, Guillain-Barré syndrome, meningitis, encephalitis

Dermatologic: Urticaria pigmentosa

Gastrointestinal: Nausea, abdominal pain

Local: Local discomfort, pain at injection site, itching, erythema, swelling or pain

Neuromuscular & skeletal: Myalgia, transient paralysis

Miscellaneous: Anaphylaxis

Drug Interactions Decreased effect with immunosuppressive agents, corticosteroids, antimalarial drugs (ie, chloroquine); persons on these drugs should receive RIG (3 doses/1 mL each) by the I.M. route

Stability Store under refrigeration at 2°C to 8°C (36°F to 46°F). Protect from light; do not freeze.

Mechanism of Action Rabies vaccine is an inactivated virus vaccine which promotes immunity by inducing an active immune response. The production of specific antibodies requires about 7-10 days. Rabies immune globulin (RIG) or antirabies serum, equine (ARS) is administered in conjunction with rabies vaccine to provide immune protection until an antibody response can occur.

Pharmacodynamics

Onset of action: I.M.: Rabies antibody: ~7-10 days

Peak effect: ~30-60 days

Duration: ≥1 year

Usual Dosage Children and Adults: I.M.:

Pre-exposure prophylaxis: 1 mL/dose for 3 doses, on days 0, 7, and 21 to 28.

Postexposure prophylaxis: All postexposure treatment should begin with immediate cleansing of the wound with soap and water; immunization should begin as soon as possible after exposure

Persons not previously immunized: Rabies immune globulin (RIG) 20 units/kg body weight, half of this is infiltrated at bite site if possible, and the remainder is administered I.M. along with rabies vaccine: 1 mL/dose for 5 doses, on days 0, 3, 7, 14, 28

Persons who have previously received postexposure prophylaxis with rabies vaccine, received a recommended I.M. pre-exposure series of rabies vaccine or have a previously documented rabies antibody titer considered adequate: 1 mL/dose on days 0 and 3; do not administer RIG

Booster (for occupational or other continuing risk): 1 mL/dose every 2-5 years or as indicated by antibody titer measurements

Administration I.M.: Reconstitute with provided diluent; **not for I.V. or SubQ administration;** administer injections in the deltoid muscle, not the gluteal; for younger children the outer aspect of the thigh may be used

Monitoring Parameters Serum rabies antibody titers are not routinely recommended in postexposure patients unless the patient was immunocompromised; to determine the need for repeat booster treatment, titers may be measured every 6 months to 2 years in persons at high risk for exposure

Nursing Implications Federal law requires that the date of administration, the vaccine manufacturer, lot number of vaccine, and the administering person's name, title, and address be entered into the patient's permanent medical record.

Dosage Forms Injection, powder for reconstitution:

Imovax® Rabies: 2.5 int. units [HDCV; grown in human diploid cell culture; contains albumin <100 mg, neomycin <150 mcg]

RabAvert®: 2.5 int. units [PCEC; grown in chicken fibroblasts; contains amphotericin <2 ng, chlortetracycline <20 ng, and neomycin <1 mcg]

References

Atkinson WL, Pickering LK, Schwartz B, et al, "General Recommendations on Immunization. Recommendations of the Advisory Committee on Immunization Practices (ACIP) and the American Academy of Family Physicians (AAFP)," *MMWR Recomm Rep*, 2002, 51(RR-2):18.

"Human Rabies Prevention - United States, 1999. Recommendations of the Advisory Committee on Immunization Practices (ACIP)," *MMWR Recomm Rep*, 1999, 48(RR-1):1-21.

♦ **Racepinephrine** *see* Epinephrine *on page 577*

♦ **rAHF** *see* Antihemophilic Factor (Recombinant) *on page 138*

♦ **R-albuterol** *see* Levalbuterol *on page 920*

♦ **RAN™-Atenolol (Can)** *see* Atenolol *on page 170*

♦ **RAN™-Carvedilol (Can)** *see* Carvedilol *on page 293*

♦ **RAN™-Ciprofloxacin (Can)** *see* Ciprofloxacin *on page 357*

- **RAN™-Citalopram (Can)** *see* Citalopram *on page 368*
- **Raniclor™** *see* Cefaclor *on page 301*

Ranitidine (ra NI ti deen)

Medication Safety Issues

Sound-alike/look-alike issues:

Ranitidine may be confused with amantadine, rimantadine

Zantac® may be confused with Xanax®, Zarontin®, Zofran®, Zyrtec®

International issues:

Antagon®: Brand name for astemizole in Mexico; brand name for ganirelix in the U.S.

U.S. Brand Names Zantac®; Zantac 75® [OTC]; Zantac 150™ [OTC]; Zantac® EFFERdose®

Canadian Brand Names Alti-Ranitidine; Apo-Ranitidine®; BCI-Ranitidine; CO Ranitidine; Gen-Ranidine; Novo-Ranidine; Nu-Ranit; PMS-Ranitidine; Ranitidine Injection, USP; Rhoxal-ranitidine; Sandoz-Ranitidine; Zantac®; Zantac 75®

Index Terms Ranitidine Hydrochloride

Therapeutic Category Gastrointestinal Agent, Gastric or Duodenal Ulcer Treatment; Histamine H_2 Antagonist

Generic Available Yes: Excludes effervescent tablet

Use Short-term treatment of active duodenal ulcers and benign gastric ulcers; long-term prophylaxis of duodenal ulcer and gastric hypersecretory states; gastroesophageal reflux disease (GERD); recurrent postoperative ulcer; treatment and prophylaxis of erosive esophagitis; upper GI bleeding, prevention of acid-aspiration pneumonitis during surgery, and prevention of stress-induced ulcers; over-the-counter (OTC) formulation for use in the relief of heartburn, acid indigestion, and sour stomach

Pregnancy Risk Factor B

Lactation Enters breast milk/use caution

Contraindications Hypersensitivity to ranitidine or any component or other H_2 antagonists; patients with history of acute porphyria (may precipitate an acute attack)

Warnings Use of gastric acid inhibitors including proton pump inhibitors and H_2 blockers has been associated with an increased risk for development of acute gastroenteritis and community-acquired pneumonia (Canani, 2006). A large epidemiological study has suggested an increased risk for developing pneumonia in patients receiving H_2 receptor antagonists; however, a causal relationship with ranitidine has not been demonstrated. Rapid I.V. administration of ranitidine has been associated with bradycardia, particularly in patients predisposed to cardiac rhythm disturbances.

Zantac® EFFERdose® tablets and granules contain sodium benzoate; benzoic acid (benzoate) is a metabolite of benzyl alcohol; large amounts of benzyl alcohol (≥99 mg/kg/day) have been associated with a potentially fatal toxicity ("gasping syndrome") in neonates; *in vitro* and animal studies have shown that benzoate displaces bilirubin from protein binding sites; avoid use in neonates

Precautions Use with caution in patients with liver and renal impairment; dosage modification required in patients with renal impairment. Zantac® 150 EFFERdose® tablets and Zantac® 150 EFFERdose® granules contain phenylalanine; use with caution in patients with phenylketonuria.

Adverse Reactions

Cardiovascular: Bradycardia, tachycardia, vasculitis (rare)

Central nervous system: Dizziness, sedation, malaise, mental confusion, headache, hallucinations, anxiety

Dermatologic: Rash, alopecia (rare), erythema multiforme (rare)

Endocrine & metabolic: Gynecomastia

Gastrointestinal: Constipation, nausea, vomiting, abdominal discomfort, pancreatitis (rare)

Hematologic: Thrombocytopenia, aplastic anemia (rare), granulocytopenia, leukopenia

Hepatic: Hepatitis

Local: Transient pain at injection site

Neuromuscular & skeletal: Arthralgias

Renal: Elevated serum creatinine

Respiratory: Pneumonia (causal relationship not established; see Warnings)

Drug Interactions Cytochrome P450 isoenzyme CYP2D6 and 3A3/4 inhibitor

Variable effects on warfarin; antacids may decrease absorption of ranitidine; ranitidine decreases the absorption of ketoconazole, itraconazole, atazanavir, cefuroxime, and cefpodoxime (separate administration times by at least 2 hours)

Stability Protect injection from light; stable for 48 hours at room temperature or 30 days when frozen in D_5W or NS; stable for 24 hours in TPN solutions; stable for 24 hours in 3-in-1 total nutrient admixture

Mechanism of Action Competitive inhibition of histamine at H_2-receptors of the gastric parietal cells, which inhibits gastric acid secretion

Pharmacokinetics

Distribution: Minimally penetrates the blood-brain barrier; breast milk to plasma ratio: 1.9-6.7
- V_d:
  - Children: 1-1.3 L/kg
  - Adults: 1.4 L/kg

Protein binding: 15%

Metabolism: In the liver

Bioavailability:
- Oral: ~50%
- I.M.: 90% to 100%

Half-life:
- Neonates (receiving ECMO): 6.6 hours
- Infants: 3.5 hours
- Children 3.5-16 years: 1.8-2 hours
- Adults:
  - Normal renal and hepatic function: 2-2.5 hours
  - Decreased renal function (Cl_{cr} 25-35 mL/minute): 4.8 hours

Time to peak serum concentration:
- Oral: 1-3 hours
- I.M.: 15 minutes

Elimination: 30% (oral) or 70% (I.V.) eliminated as unchanged drug in the urine and in feces

Dialysis: Hemodialysis: Slightly dialyzable (5% to 20%)

Usual Dosage

Premature and Term Infants <2 weeks:
- Oral: 2 mg/kg/day divided every 12 hours
- I.V.: 1.5 mg/kg/dose as loading dose, then 12 hours later maintenance dose of 1.5-2 mg/kg/day divided every 12 hours
- Continuous infusion: 1.5 mg/kg/dose as loading dose followed by 0.04-0.08 mg/kg/hour infusion (or 1-2 mg/kg/day)

Children ≥1 month to 16 years:
- Gastric/duodenal ulcer:
  - Oral:
    - Treatment: 2-4 mg/kg/day divided twice daily; maximum: 300 mg/day
    - Maintenance: 2-4 mg/kg/day divided twice daily; maximum: 150 mg/day
  - I.V.: 2-4 mg/kg/day divided every 6-8 hours; maximum: 200 mg/day
- GERD and erosive esophagitis:
  - Oral: 4-10 mg/kg/day divided twice daily; maximum: GERD: 300 mg/day; erosive esophagitis: 600 mg/day
  - I.V.: 2-4 mg/kg/day divided every 6-8 hours; maximum: 200 mg/day **or as an alternative**
  - Continuous infusion: Initial: 1 mg/kg/dose for one dose followed by infusion of 0.08-0.17 mg/kg/hour or 2-4 mg/kg/day

Children ≥16 years and Adults:
- Treatment of duodenal or gastric ulcers, GERD, maintenance of erosive esophagitis: Oral: 150 mg/dose twice daily or 300 mg at bedtime
- Prophylaxis of recurrent duodenal ulcer: Oral: 150 mg at bedtime
- Gastric hypersecretory conditions:
  - Oral: 150 mg twice daily; maximum: 600 mg/day
  - I.M., I.V.: 50 mg/dose every 6-8 hours (dose not to exceed 400 mg/day)
  - Continuous I.V. infusion: Initial 50 mg I.V. followed by 6.25 mg/hour titrated to gastric pH >4.0 for prophylaxis or >7.0 for treatment; **continuous I.V. infusion is preferred in patients with active bleeding**
- Erosive esophagitis: Oral: 150 mg 4 times/day

Pathologic hypersecretory conditions (eg, Zollinger-Ellison syndrome):
- Continuous I.V. infusion: Initial 50 mg I.V. followed by 1 mg/kg/hour infusion; titrate dosage in 0.5 mg/kg/hour increments to maintain gastric acid output at <10 mEq/hour; doses up to 2.5 mg/kg/hour (220 mg/hour) have been used
- Oral: 150 mg twice daily; more frequent administration may be indicated depending upon response; doses up to 6.3 g/day have been used in severe cases

Relief of heartburn, acid indigestion, sour stomach (OTC use): Oral: 75 mg 30-60 minutes before eating; no more than 2 tablets/day

Dosing adjustment in renal impairment:
- Children and Adults (Aronoff, 1999):
- Cl_{cr} 10-50 mL/minute: Reduce dose to 50% of dose recommended for indication

(Continued)

Ranitidine *(Continued)*

Cl_{cr} <10 mL/minute: Reduce dose to 25% of dose recommended for indication or as an alternative per manufacturer's recommendations:

Adults: Cl_{cr} <50 mL/minute:

Oral: 150 mg every 24 hours; adjust dose cautiously if needed

I.V.: 50 mg every 18-24 hours; adjust dose cautiously if needed

Hemodialysis: Adjust dose schedule to administer dose at the end of dialysis

Administration

Oral: Administer with meals and at bedtime; dissolve 25 mg EFFERdose® tablet in 5 mL of water until completely dissolved; dissolve 150 mg EFFERdose® tablet or granules in 6-8 ounces of water before administration

Parenteral: Intermittent I.V. infusion preferred over direct injection to decrease risk of bradycardia; for intermittent infusion, infuse over 15-30 minutes, at a usual concentration of 0.5 mg/mL; for direct I.V. injection, administer over a period of at least 5 minutes, not to exceed 10 mg/minute (4 mL/minute) at a final concentration not to exceed 2.5 mg/mL; For I.M., administer undiluted (25 mg/mL)

Monitoring Parameters AST, ALT, serum creatinine; when used to prevent stress-related GI bleeding, measure the intragastric pH and try to maintain pH >4; gastric acid secretion (<10 mEq/hour)

Reference Range Serum level necessary to inhibit basal acid secretion:

Children: 90% suppression: 40-60 ng/mL

Adults: 50% suppression: 36-94 ng/mL

Test Interactions False-positive urine protein using Multistix®; gastric acid secretion test, skin test allergen extracts

Patient Information Avoid excessive amounts of coffee and aspirin; when self-medicating, if symptoms of heartburn, acid indigestion, or sour stomach persist after 2 weeks of continuous use of the drug, consult a clinician.

Additional Information Causes fewer CNS adverse reactions and drug interactions compared to cimetidine; safety and efficacy of full-dose therapy extending beyond 8 weeks have not been determined; Zantac® EFFERdose® 150 mg tablets and granules contain 7.55 mEq sodium

Dosage Forms Excipient information presented when available (limited, particularly for generics); consult specific product labeling.

Capsule 150 mg, 300 mg

Infusion [premixed in NaCl 0.45%; preservative free]:

Zantac®: 50 mg (50 mL)

Injection, solution: 25 mg/mL (2 mL, 6 mL)

Zantac®: 25 mg/mL (2 mL, 6 mL, 40 mL) [contains phenol 0.5% as preservative]

Syrup: 15 mg/mL (10 mL) [contains alcohol 7.5%; peppermint flavor]

Zantac®: 15 mg/mL (473 mL) [contains alcohol 7.5%; peppermint flavor]

Tablet: 75 mg [OTC], 150 mg, 300 mg

Zantac®: 150 mg, 300 mg

Zantac 75®: 75 mg

Zantac 150™: 150 mg

Tablet, effervescent:

Zantac® EFFERdose®: 25 mg [contains sodium 1.33 mEq/tablet, phenylalanine 2.81 mg/tablet, and sodium benzoate]; 150 mg [contains sodium 7.96 mEq/tablet, phenylalanine 16.84 mg/tablet, and sodium benzoate]

References

Blumer JL, Rothstein FC, Kaplan BS, et al, "Pharmacokinetic Determination of Ranitidine Pharmacodynamics in Pediatric Ulcer Disease," *J Pediatr*, 1985, 107(2):301-6.

Canani RB, Cirillo P, Roggero P, et al, "Therapy With Gastric Acidity Inhibitors Increases the Risk of Acute Gastroenteritis and Community-Acquired Pneumonia in Children," *Pediatrics*, 2006, 117(5):e817-20.

Drug Prescribing in Renal Failure: Dosing Guidelines for Adults, 4th ed, Aronoff GR, et al, eds, Philadelphia, PA: American College of Physicians, 1999, 71.

Eddleston JM, Booker PD, and Green JR, "Use of Ranitidine in Children Undergoing Cardiopulmonary Bypass," *Crit Care Med*, 1989, 17(1):26-9.

Fontana M, Massironi E, Rossi A, et al, "Ranitidine Pharmacokinetics in Newborn Infants," *Arch Dis Child*, 1993, 68(5 Spec No):602-3.

Lopez-Herce J, Albajara L, Codoceo R, et al, "Ranitidine Prophylaxis in Acute Gastric Mucosal Damage in Critically Ill Pediatric Patients," *Crit Care Med*, 1988, 16(6):591-93.

Morris DL, Markham SJ, Beechey A, et al, "Ranitidine-Bolus or Infusion Prophylaxis for Stress Ulcer," *Crit Care Med*, 1988, 16(3):229-32.

Roberts CJ, "Clinical Pharmacokinetics of Ranitidine," *Clin Pharmacokinet*, 1984, 9(3):211-21.

♦ **Ranitidine Hydrochloride** *see* Ranitidine *on page 1366*

♦ **Ranitidine Injection, USP (Can)** *see* Ranitidine *on page 1366*

♦ **RAN™-Lovastatin (Can)** *see* Lovastatin *on page 964*

♦ **RAN™-Metformin (Can)** *see* Metformin *on page 1016*

♦ **Rapamune®** *see* Sirolimus *on page 1444*

♦ **Rapamycin** *see* Sirolimus *on page 1444*

♦ **Raphon [OTC]** *see* Epinephrine *on page 577*

Rasburicase (ras BYOOR i kayse)

U.S. Brand Names Elitek™

Canadian Brand Names Fasturtec®

Index Terms NSC-721631; Urate Oxidase

Therapeutic Category Uric Acid Lowering Agent

Generic Available No

Use Initial management of plasma uric acid levels in pediatric patients with leukemia, lymphoma, and solid tumor malignancies who are receiving anticancer therapy expected to result in tumor lysis and subsequent elevation of plasma uric acid; management of malignancy-associated hyperuricemia in adults (unlabeled use)

Pregnancy Risk Factor C

Lactation Excretion in breast milk unknown/not recommended

Contraindications Hypersensitivity to rasburicase (see Warnings) or any component; patients with G-6-PD deficiency

Warnings Rasburicase may cause severe allergic reactions, including anaphylaxis at any time during the course of therapy including with the first dose; **discontinue immediately and permanently** in any patient exhibiting signs and symptoms of severe allergy, including chest pain, dyspnea, hypotension, and/or urticaria; rasburicase is immunogenic and can elicit antibodies that inhibit its activity (time to detection of antibodies after exposure to rasburicase varied from 1-6 weeks in normal, healthy volunteers); due to the potential for developing hypersensitivity reactions, rasburicase is indicated only for a single course of treatment.

Because hydrogen peroxide is one of the major byproducts of the conversion of uric acid to allantoin, rasburicase may cause severe hemolytic reactions in patients with G-6-PD deficiency (eg, African or Mediterranean ancestry); patients at high risk for G-6-PD deficiency should be screened prior to treatment with rasburicase; **discontinue treatment immediately and permanently** in any patient developing hemolysis; rasburicase has been associated with methemoglobinemia; **discontinue treatment immediately** in any patient developing methemoglobinemia

Precautions Rasburicase may interfere with uric acid measurements (see Test Interactions); patients receiving rasburicase should receive I.V. hydration as appropriate for the management of tumor lysis syndrome

Adverse Reactions Children <2 years of age may experience a higher frequency of adverse effects, particularly vomiting, diarrhea, fever, and rash

Cardiovascular: Arrhythmias, CHF, cardiac arrest, chest pain, cyanosis, flushing, MI, thrombosis, cerebrovascular disorder

Central nervous system: Fever, seizures, headache

Dermatologic: Rash, cellulitis

Gastrointestinal: Mucositis, diarrhea, ileus, intestinal obstruction, nausea, abdominal pain, constipation, vomiting

Hematologic: Hemolysis (see Warnings), neutropenia, pancytopenia, methemoglobinemia (see Warnings)

Neuromuscular & skeletal: Paresthesia

Ophthalmic: Retinal hemorrhages

Renal: Acute renal failure

Respiratory: Respiratory distress, bronchospasm, pulmonary edema, pulmonary hypertension

Miscellaneous: Severe hypersensitivity reactions, including anaphylaxis (see Warnings), sepsis

Drug Interactions None have as yet been identified

Stability Store rasburicase and diluent in the refrigerator; protect from light and do not freeze; reconstituted solution and final dilution (see Administration) are stable refrigerated, but must be used within 24 hours due to the lack of a preservative

Mechanism of Action Rasburicase is a recombinant urate-oxidase enzyme that catalyzes the enzymatic oxidation of uric acid into an inactive and soluble metabolite, allantoin; it does not inhibit the formation of uric acid

Pharmacokinetics

Distribution: V_d: Children: 110-127 mL/kg

Half-life: Children: 18 hours

Usual Dosage I.V.:

Children: 0.15-0.2 mg/kg/dose once daily for up to 5 days (manufacturer-recommended duration); begin chemotherapy 4-24 hours after the first dose

Note: Limited data suggest that a single prechemotherapy dose (versus multiple-day administration) may be sufficiently efficacious. Monitoring electrolytes, hydration status, and uric acid concentrations are necessary to identify the need for additional doses. Other clinical manifestations of tumor lysis syndrome (eg, hyperphosphatemia, hypocalcemia, and hyperkalemia) may occur.

(Continued)

Rasburicase *(Continued)*

Adults (unlabeled use): Management of malignancy-associated hyperuricemia: 0.2 mg/kg/day once daily for 3-7 days, beginning the day before or day of chemotherapy **or** 0.15-0.2 mg/kg as a single dose, repeated if needed based upon the uric acid level **or** 3-6 mg as a single dose, repeated (1.5-6 mg) if needed based upon the uric acid level

Administration I.V.: Dilute each vial with 1 mL of provided diluent; gently swirl, do not shake; further dilute desired dose in NS to a final volume of 50 mL; infuse over 30 minutes, do not bolus; do not filter or mix with other medications; chemotherapy may be initiated 4-24 hours after the first dose of rasburicase

Monitoring Parameters Uric acid (See Test Interactions); BUN, serum creatinine, phosphorus, urine output, CBC with differential

Test Interactions Rasburicase will cause enzymatic degradation of the uric acid within blood samples when left at room temperature, resulting in spuriously low uric acid levels; to avoid this interaction, blood must be collected into prechilled tubes containing heparin anticoagulant and immediately immersed and maintained in an ice water bath; plasma samples should be assayed within 4 hours of collection

Dosage Forms Excipient information presented when available (limited, particularly for generics); consult specific product labeling.

Injection, powder for reconstitution:

Elitek™: 1.5 mg [packaged with three 1 mL ampuls of diluent]; 7.5 mg [packaged with 5 mL of diluent]

References

Goldman SC, Holcenberg JS, Finklestein JZ, et al, "A Randomized Comparison Between Rasburicase and Allopurinol in Children With Lymphoma or Leukemia at High Risk for Tumor Lysis," *Blood*, 2001, 97(10):2998-3003.

Pui CH, Mahmoud HH, Wiley JM, et al, "Recombinant Urate Oxidase for the Prophylaxis or Treatment of Hyperuricemia in Patients With Leukemia or Lymphoma," *J Clin Oncol*, 2001, 19(3):697-704.

- **rATG** *see* Antithymocyte Globulin (Rabbit) *on page 147*
- **ratio-Aclavulanate (Can)** *see* Amoxicillin and Clavulanic Acid *on page 115*
- **ratio-Acyclovir (Can)** *see* Acyclovir *on page 54*
- **ratio-Azithromycin (Can)** *see* Azithromycin *on page 191*
- **ratio-Brimonidine (Can)** *see* Brimonidine *on page 231*
- **ratio-Carvedilol (Can)** *see* Carvedilol *on page 293*
- **ratio-Cefuroxime (Can)** *see* Cefuroxime *on page 322*
- **ratio-Ciprofloxacin (Can)** *see* Ciprofloxacin *on page 357*
- **ratio-Citalopram (Can)** *see* Citalopram *on page 368*
- **ratio-Clarithromycin (Can)** *see* Clarithromycin *on page 375*
- **ratio-Diltiazem CD (Can)** *see* Diltiazem *on page 503*
- **ratio-Emtec (Can)** *see* Acetaminophen and Codeine *on page 46*
- **ratio-Famotidine (Can)** *see* Famotidine *on page 638*
- **ratio-Glyburide (Can)** *see* GlyBURIDE *on page 734*
- **ratio-Inspra-Sal (Can)** *see* Albuterol *on page 66*
- **ratio-Ketorolac (Can)** *see* Ketorolac *on page 889*
- **ratio-Lamotrigine (Can)** *see* Lamotrigine *on page 906*
- **ratio-Lenoltec (Can)** *see* Acetaminophen and Codeine *on page 46*
- **ratio-Lovastatin (Can)** *see* Lovastatin *on page 964*
- **ratio-Metformin (Can)** *see* Metformin *on page 1016*
- **ratio-Methotrexate (Can)** *see* Methotrexate *on page 1027*
- **ratio-Mometasone (Can)** *see* Mometasone Furoate *on page 1076*
- **ratio-Morphine SR (Can)** *see* Morphine Sulfate *on page 1082*
- **Ratio-Orciprenaline® (Can)** *see* Metaproterenol *on page 1014*
- **ratio-Paroxetine (Can)** *see* Paroxetine *on page 1218*
- **ratio-Pentoxifylline (Can)** *see* Pentoxifylline *on page 1241*
- **ratio-Pravastatin (Can)** *see* Pravastatin *on page 1300*
- **ratio-Salbutamol (Can)** *see* Albuterol *on page 66*
- **ratio-Sertraline (Can)** *see* Sertraline *on page 1429*
- **ratio-Simvastatin (Can)** *see* Simvastatin *on page 1441*
- **ratio-Sumatriptan (Can)** *see* Sumatriptan *on page 1495*
- **ratio-Theo-Bronc (Can)** *see* Theophylline *on page 1520*
- **ratio-Topiramate (Can)** *see* Topiramate *on page 1551*
- **ratio-Trazodone (Can)** *see* Trazodone *on page 1564*
- **Reactine™ (Can)** *see* Cetirizine *on page 327*
- **ReAzo [OTC]** *see* Phenazopyridine *on page 1244*
- **Rebetol®** *see* Ribavirin *on page 1378*

Remifentanil (rem i FEN ta nil)

Medication Safety Issues
Sound-alike/look-alike issues:
Remifentanil may be confused with alfentanil

U.S. Brand Names Ultiva®

Canadian Brand Names Ultiva®

Index Terms GI87084B

Therapeutic Category Analgesic, Narcotic; General Anesthetic

Generic Available No

Use Analgesic for use during the induction and maintenance of general anesthesia; for continued analgesia into the immediate postoperative period; as the analgesic component of monitored anesthesia

Restrictions C-II

Pregnancy Risk Factor C

Lactation Excretion in breast milk unknown/use caution

Contraindications Hypersensitivity to remifentanil, fentanyl or fentanyl analogs, or any component; **not for intrathecal or epidural administration,** due to the presence of glycine in the formulation

Warnings Remifentanil is not recommended as the sole agent in general anesthesia, because the loss of consciousness cannot be assured and due to the high incidence of apnea, hypotension, tachycardia, and muscle rigidity; it should be administered by individuals specifically trained in the use of anesthetic agents and should not be used in diagnostic or therapeutic procedures outside the monitored anesthesia setting; resuscitative and intubation equipment should be readily available; monitor vital signs and oxygenation continuously during administration.

Rapid I.V. infusion (single doses of >1mcg/kg administered over 30-60 seconds or infusion rates >0.1mcg/kg/minute) may result in skeletal muscle and chest wall rigidity; administer slowly. Interruption of an infusion will result in offset of effects within 5-10 minutes; the discontinuation of remifentanil infusion should be preceded by the establishment of adequate postoperative analgesia orders, especially for patients in whom postoperative pain is anticipated

Precautions Use with caution in the morbidly obese

Adverse Reactions
Cardiovascular: Hypotension (dose dependent), bradycardia (dose dependent), tachycardia, hypertension, asystole, arrhythmias, heart block, syncope, CPK-MB increased
Central nervous system: Dizziness, headache, agitation, fever, hallucinations, anxiety, seizure, amnesia
Dermatologic: Pruritus, erythema, rash
Endocrine & metabolic: Hyperglycemia, electrolyte disorders
Gastrointestinal: Nausea, vomiting, constipation, abdominal discomfort, xerostomia, GERD, dysphagia, diarrhea, heartburn
(Continued)

Remifentanil *(Continued)*

Hematologic: Thrombocytopenia, anemia, leukocytosis, lymphopenia

Neuromuscular & skeletal: Muscle rigidity (dose and rate of infusion dependent), tremors

Ocular: Visual disturbances, nystagmus

Respiratory: Respiratory depression, apnea, hypoxia, cough, bronchospasm, stridor, pleural effusion, pulmonary edema

Miscellaneous: Shivering, postoperative pain, anaphylactic/anaphylactoid reactions

Drug Interactions Additive respiratory depression with CNS depressants, alcohol, phenothiazines, and centrally-acting muscle relaxants (dantrolene); synergistic with other anesthetics, may need to decrease thiopental, propofol, isoflurane, and midazolam by up to 75%; the herbal medicine St John's wort (*Hypericum perforatum*) may increase sedation

Stability Prior to reconstitution, store at 2°C to 25°C (36°F to 77°F). Stable for 24 hours at room temperature after reconstitution and further dilution to concentrations of 20-250 mcg/mL in D_5LR, D_5NS, D_5W, 1/2NS, NS, (4 hours if diluted with LR).

Y-site administration: Compatible: Acyclovir, alfentanil, amikacin, aminophylline, ampicillin, ampicillin/sulbactam, aztreonam, bretylium, bumetanide, buprenorphine, butorphanol, calcium gluconate, cefazolin, cefotaxime, cefotetan, cefoxitin, ceftazidime, ceftizoxime, ceftriaxone, cefuroxime, cimetidine, ciprofloxacin, cisatracurium, clindamycin, dexamethasone sodium phosphate, digoxin, diphenhydramine, dobutamine, dopamine, doxycycline, droperidol, enalaprilat, epinephrine, esmolol, famotidine, fentanyl, fluconazole, furosemide, ganciclovir gatifloxacin, gentamicin, haloperidol, heparin, hydrocortisone sodium succinate, hydromorphone, hydroxyzine, imipenem/cilastatin, inamrinone, isoproterenol, ketorolac, lidocaine, linezolid, lorazepam, magnesium sulfate, mannitol, meperidine, methylprednisolone sodium succinate, metoclopramide, metronidazole, midazolam, minocycline, morphine, nalbuphine, netilmicin, nitroglycerin, norepinephrine, ofloxacin, ondansetron, phenylephrine, piperacillin, piperacillin/tazobactam, potassium chloride, procainamide, prochlorperazine, propofol, promethazine, ranitidine, sodium bicarbonate, sufentanil, theophylline, thiopental, ticarcillin, ticarcillin/clavulanate potassium, tobramycin, trimethoprim/sulfamethoxazole, vancomycin, zidovudine.

Mechanism of Action Binds with stereospecific mu-opioid receptors at many sites within the CNS, increases pain threshold, alters pain reception, inhibits ascending pain pathways

Pharmacodynamics

Onset of action: 1-3 minutes

Maximum effect: 3-5 minutes

Duration: 3-10 minutes

Pharmacokinetics

Distribution: V_d:

Neonates <2 months: 452 ± 144 mL/kg

Children 2-6 years: 240 mL/kg

Children 7-12 years: 249 mL/kg

Adolescents: 223 ± 30.6 mL/kg

Adults: 100-176 mL/kg

Protein binding: ~70% (primarily $alpha_1$ acid glycoprotein)

Metabolism: Rapid via blood and tissue esterases; not metabolized by plasma cholinesterase (pseudocholinesterase) and is not appreciably metabolized by the liver

Half-life (dose dependent): Terminal: 10-20 minutes; effective: 3-10 minutes

Elimination: Clearance:

Neonates <2 months of age: 90.5 ± 36.8 mL/minute/kg

Adolescents: 57.2 ± 21.2 mL/minute/kg

Adults: 41.2 mL/minute/kg

Usual Dosage I.V. continuous infusion: Dose should be based on ideal body weight (IBW) in obese patients (>30% over IBW).

Children birth to 2 months: Maintenance of anesthesia with nitrous oxide (70%): 0.4 mcg/kg/minute (range: 0.4-1 mcg/kg/minute); supplemental bolus dose of 1 mcg/kg may be administered, smaller bolus dose may be required with potent inhalation agents, potent neuraxial anesthesia, significant comorbidities, significant fluid shifts, or without atropine pretreatment. Clearance in neonates is highly variable; dose should be carefully titrated.

Children 1-12 years: Maintenance of anesthesia with halothane, sevoflurane, or isoflurane: 0.25 mcg/kg/minute (range 0.05-1.3 mcg/kg/minute); supplemental bolus dose of 1 mcg/kg may be administered every 2-5 minutes. Consider increasing concomitant anesthetics with infusion rate >1 mcg/kg/minute. Infusion rate can be titrated upward in increments up to 50% or titrated downward in decrements of 25% to 50%. May titrate every 2-5 minutes.

Adults:

Induction of anesthesia: 0.5-1 mcg/kg/minute; if endotracheal intubation is to occur in <8 minutes, an initial dose of 1 mcg/kg may be given over 30-60 seconds; in coronary bypass surgery: 1 mcg/kg/minute

Maintenance of anesthesia: **Note:** Supplemental bolus dose of 1 mcg/kg may be administered every 2-5 minutes. Consider increasing concomitant anesthetics with infusion rate >1 mcg/kg/minute. Infusion rate can be titrated upward in increments of 25% to 100% or downward in decrements of 25% to 50%. May titrate every 2-5 minutes.

With nitrous oxide (66%): 0.4 mcg/kg/minute (range: 0.1-2 mcg/kg/minute)

With isoflurane: 0.25 mcg/kg/minute (range: 0.05-2 mcg/kg/minute)

With propofol: 0.25 mcg/kg/minute (range: 0.05-2 mcg/kg/minute)

Coronary bypass surgery: 1 mcg/kg/minute (range: 0.125-4 mcg/kg/minute); supplemental dose: 0.5-1 mcg/kg

Continuation as an analgesic in immediate postoperative period: 0.1 mcg/kg/minute (range: 0.025-0.2 mcg/kg/minute). Infusion rate may be adjusted every 5 minutes in increments of 0.025 mcg/kg/minute. Bolus doses are not recommended. Infusion rates >0.2 mcg/kg/minute are associated with respiratory depression.

Coronary bypass surgery, continuation as an analgesic into the ICU: 1 mcg/kg/minute (range: 0.05-1 mcg/kg/minute)

Analgesic component of monitored anesthesia care: **Note:** Supplemental oxygen is recommended:

Single I.V. dose given 90 seconds prior to local anesthetic:

Remifentanil alone: 1 mcg/kg over 30-60 seconds

With midazolam: 0.5 mcg/kg over 30-60 seconds

Continuous infusion beginning 5 minutes prior to local anesthetic:

Remifentanil alone: 0.1 mcg/kg/minute

With midazolam: 0.05 mcg/kg/minute

Continuous infusion given after local anesthetic:

Remifentanil alone: 0.05 mcg/kg/minute (range: 0.025-0.2 mcg/kg/minute)

With midazolam: 0.025 mcg/kg/minute (range: 0.025-0.2 mcg/kg/minute)

Note: Following local or anesthetic block, infusion rate should be decreased to 0.05 mcg/kg/minute; rate adjustments of 0.025 mcg/kg/minute may be done at 5-minute intervals

Mechanically-ventilated patients: Acute pain (moderate-to-severe) (unlabeled use): 0.6-15 mcg/kg/hour

Administration I.V.: Prepare solution by adding 1 mL of diluent per 1 mg of remifentanil. Shake well. Further dilute to a final concentration of 20, 25, 50, or 250 mcg/mL in compatible I.V. solution (see Stability). An infusion device should be used to administer continuous infusions. During the maintenance of general anesthesia, I.V. boluses ≤1 mcg/kg may be administered over 30-60 seconds; for doses >1 mcg/kg, administer over >60 seconds (to reduce the potential to develop skeletal muscle and chest wall rigidity). Injections should be given into I.V. tubing close to the venous cannula; tubing should be cleared after treatment to prevent residual effects when other fluids are administered through the same I.V. line.

Monitoring Parameters Respiratory and cardiovascular status, blood pressure, heart rate

Dosage Forms Excipient information presented when available (limited, particularly for generics); consult specific product labeling.

Injection, powder for reconstitution: 1 mg, 2 mg, 5 mg [contains glycine 15 mg]

References

"Clinical Practice Guidelines for the Sustained Use of Sedatives and Analgesics in the Critically Ill Adult. Task Force of the American College of Critical Care Medicine (ACCM) of the Society of Critical Care Medicine (SCCM), American Society of Health-System Pharmacists (ASHP), American College of Chest Physicians," *Am J Health Syst Pharm*, 2002, 59(2):150-78.

Scott LJ and Perry CM, "Remifentanil: A Review of Its Use During the Induction and Maintenance of General Anaesthesia," *Drugs*, 2005, 65(13):1793-823.

♦ **Renagel®** *see* Sevelamer *on page 1433*

♦ **Renova®** *see* Tretinoin *on page 1567*

♦ **Resectisol®** *see* Mannitol *on page 979*

♦ **Respa-DM®** *see* Guaifenesin and Dextromethorphan *on page 748*

♦ **Restasis®** *see* CycloSPORINE *on page 422*

♦ **Retin-A®** *see* Tretinoin *on page 1567*

♦ **Retin-A® Micro** *see* Tretinoin *on page 1567*

♦ **Retinoic Acid** *see* Tretinoin *on page 1567*

♦ **Retinova® (Can)** *see* Tretinoin *on page 1567*

♦ **Retisert™** *see* Fluocinolone *on page 672*

♦ **Retrovir®** *see* Zidovudine *on page 1637*

♦ **Revatio™** *see* Sildenafil *on page 1435*

♦ **Reversol®** *see* Edrophonium *on page 556*

Rh$_o$(D) Immune Globulin (ar aych oh (dee) i MYUN GLOB yoo lin)

U.S. Brand Names HyperRHO™ S/D Full Dose; HyperRHO™ S/D Mini Dose; MICRhoGAM®; RhoGAM®; Rhophylac®; WinRho® SDF

Canadian Brand Names WinRho® SDF

Index Terms RhIG; Rho(D) Immune Globulin (Human); RhoIGIV; RhoIVIM

Therapeutic Category Immune Globulin

Generic Available No

Use

Suppression of Rh isoimmunization: Use in the following situations when an Rh$_o$(D)-negative individual is exposed to Rh$_o$(D)-positive blood: During delivery of an Rh$_o$(D)-positive infant; abortion; amniocentesis; chorionic villus sampling; ruptured tubal pregnancy; abdominal trauma; transplacental hemorrhage. Used when the mother is Rh$_o$(D) negative, the father of the child is either Rh$_o$(D) positive or Rh$_o$(D) unknown, the baby is either Rh$_o$(D) positive or Rh$_o$(D) unknown.

Transfusion: Suppression of Rh isoimmunization in Rh$_o$(D)-negative female children and female adults in their childbearing years transfused with Rh$_o$(D) antigen-positive RBCs or blood components containing Rh$_o$(D) antigen-positive RBCs

Treatment of idiopathic thrombocytopenic purpura (ITP): **WinRho® SDF only:** Used in the following nonsplenectomized Rh$_o$(D) positive individuals: Children with acute or chronic ITP, adults with chronic ITP, children and adults with ITP secondary to HIV infection

Pregnancy Risk Factor C

Lactation Does not enter breast milk

Contraindications Hypersensitivity to immune globulin, thimerosal (RhoGAM® formulation) or any component; IgA deficiency; Rh$_o$(D)-positive mother or pregnant woman; transfusion of Rh$_o$(D)-positive blood in previous 3 months; prior sensitization to Rh$_o$(D); mothers whose Rh group or immune status is uncertain

Warnings Rare postmarketing reports of severe, sometimes fatal, intravascular hemolysis including DIC; symptoms including back pain, shaking chills, fever, and discolored urine have occurred in most cases within 4 hours of administration. Serious complications of intravascular hemolysis (anemia, ARF, or DIC) have in some cases been fatal.

Use only WinRho® SDF when treating ITP; when treating ITP, a decrease in hemoglobin concentration as a result of destruction of Rh$_o$(D)-positive red blood cells can be expected; reduce WinRho® SDF dosage in ITP patients with Hgb <10 g/dL (see Usual Dosage) to minimize the risk of increasing the severity of anemia. These patients should be monitored for signs and/or symptoms of intravascular hemolysis, clinically compromising anemia, and renal insufficiency

When used to suppress Rh isoimmunization, the drug is administered to the mother **not** the infant; anaphylactic hypersensitivity reactions can occur; studies indicate that there is no discernible risk of transmitting HIV or hepatitis B; not intended for use as immunoglobulin replacement therapy for immune deficiency syndromes

Precautions Use with caution in patients with thrombocytopenia or bleeding disorders or in patients with hemoglobin concentrations <8 g/dL; may cause false-positive glucose levels (see Test Interactions)

Adverse Reactions

Cardiovascular: Hypotension, pallor, tachycardia, vasodilation (I.V. formulation), hypertension

Central nervous system: Fever, headache, chills, dizziness, somnolence, lethargy, malaise

Dermatologic: Rash, pruritus

Gastrointestinal: Abdominal pain, diarrhea, splenomegaly, nausea, vomiting

Genitourinary: Hemoglobinuria

Hematologic: Decreased hemoglobin (hemoglobin decrease >2 g/dL in 5% to 10% of ITP patients), intravascular hemolysis (rare; see Warnings), DIC (rare; see Warnings)

Hepatic: Elevated bilirubin, elevated LDH

Local: Discomfort and swelling at injection site

Neuromuscular & skeletal: Back pain, myalgia, hyperkinesia, arthralgia, weakness, hyperkinesia

Renal: Acute renal failure (rare; see Warnings)

Miscellaneous: Hypersensitivity reactions, diaphoresis

Drug Interactions May interfere with the immune response to live virus vaccines (allow 3 months after administration of vaccine)

Stability Refrigerate, do not freeze; RhoGAM® and BayRho-D® are stable for up to 30 days at room temperature

Mechanism of Action The Rh_o(D) antigen is responsible for most cases of Rh sensitization, which occurs when Rh-positive fetal RBCs enter the maternal circulation of an Rh-negative woman. Injection of anti-D globulin results in opsonization of the fetal RBCs, which are then phagocytized in the spleen, preventing immunization of the mother. Injection of anti-D into an Rh-positive patient with ITP coats the patient's own D-positive RBCs with antibody and, as they are cleared by the spleen, they saturate the capacity of the spleen to clear antibody-coated cells, sparing antibody-coated platelets. Other proposed mechanisms involve the generation of cytokines following the interaction between antibody-coated RBCs and macrophages.

Rh_oD Immune Globulin Dosage in Pregnancy and Obstetrical Conditions

Condition	WinRho® SDF Dosage I.V. or I.M.	BayRho-D® or RhoGAM® Dosage I.M.	Rhophylac® Dosage I.V. or I.M
Pregnancy	300 mcg (1500 international units) at 28 weeks gestation; repeat every 12 weeks throughout pregnancy	300 mcg at 28 weeks and following delivery, preferably within 72 hours of delivery	300 mcg at 28-30 weeks of gestation
Postpartum (if newborn Rh-positive)	120 mcg (600 international units) as soon as possible, preferably <72 hours, after delivery; if baby's Rh status is not known by 72 hours administer as soon as possible up to 28 days after delivery	300 mcg as soon as possible, preferably within 72 hours of delivery	300 mcg within 72 hours of delivery
Threatened abortion at any time	300 mcg (1500 international units) as soon as possible within 72 hours	300 mcg as soon as possible	300 mcg as soon as possible
Amniocentesis and chronic villus sampling	Before 34 weeks gestation: 300 mcg (1500 international units) administered immediately; repeat every 12 weeks throughout pregnancy After 34 weeks gestation: 120 mcg (600 international units) administered immediately or within 72 hours	At 15-18 weeks gestation or during the 3rd trimester: 300 mcg; if given between 13-18 weeks, repeat at 26-28 weeks and within 72 hours of delivery	300 mcg as soon as possible
Abortion, miscarriage, termination of ectopic pregnancy	After 34 weeks gestation: 120 mcg (600 international units) administered immediately or within 72 hours	<13 weeks gestation: 50 mcg ≥13 weeks gestation: 300 mcg administered immediately or within 72 hours	300 mcg as soon as possible
Abdominal trauma, manipulation	After 34 weeks gestation: 120 mcg (600 international units) administered immediately or within 72 hours	During the 2nd or 3rd trimester: 300 mcg; if given between 13-18 weeks, repeat at 26-28 weeks and within 72 hours of delivery	300 mcg as soon as possible

Pharmacodynamics

Onset of action:

Rh isoimmunization: I.V.: 8 hours

ITP: I.V.: 1-2 days

Maximum effect: ITP: 7-14 days

Duration:

ITP (single dose): I.V.: 30 days

Passive anti-Rh_o(D) antibodies (after 120 mcg dose): I.V.: 6 weeks

Pharmacokinetics

Distribution: Appears in breast milk, however, not absorbed by the nursing infant

(Continued)

$Rh_o(D)$ Immune Globulin *(Continued)*

Half-life, elimination:
- I.M.: 18-30 days
- I.V.: 16-24 days

Time to peak serum concentration:
- I.M.: 5-10 days
- I.V.: 2 hours

Usual Dosage

ITP: Children and Adults: **WinRho® SDF only:**

Initial:
- Hemoglobin ≥10 g/dL: 50 mcg/kg (250 international units/kg) as single dose or divided into 2 doses given on separate days
- Hemoglobin <10 g/dL: 25-40 mcg/kg (125-200 international units/kg) as single dose or divided into 2 doses given on separate days
- Hemoglobin <8 g/dL: Use with caution (see Warnings and Precautions)

Maintenance (usage dependent upon clinical response, platelet count, hemoglobin, red blood cell counts, and reticulocyte levels)

Response to initial dose: 25-60 mcg/kg (125-300 international units/kg) as single dose

Nonresponse to initial therapy:
- Hemoglobin >10 g/dL: 50-60 mcg/kg (250-300 international units/kg) as single dose
- Hemoglobin 8-10 g/dL: 25-40 mcg/kg (125-200 international units/kg) as single dose
- Hemoglobin <8 g/dL: Use with caution (see Warnings and Precautions)

Suppression of RH isoimmunization: **Adult female:** I.V., I.M.: See table on previous page.

Note: One "full dose" (300 mcg) provides enough antibody to prevent Rh sensitization if the volume of fetal RBCs entering the maternal circulation is ≤15 mL. When >15 mL is suspected, a fetal red cell count should be performed to determine the appropriate dose.

Treatment of exposure to incompatible blood transfusion or massive fetal hemorrhage, within 72 hours of event:

WinRho® SDF: Children and Adults:

Exposed to $Rh_o(D)$ positive whole blood:
- I.M.: 12 mcg (60 international units)/mL blood; administer in 1200 mcg (6000 international units) aliquots every 12 hours until the total calculated dose is administered
- I.V.: 9 mcg (45 international units)/mL blood; administer in 600 mcg (3000 international units) aliquots every 8 hours until the total calculated dose is administered

Exposed to $Rh_o(D)$ positive red blood cells:
- I.M.: 24 mcg (120 international units)/mL cells administer in 1200 mcg (6000 international units) aliquots every 12 hours until the total calculated dose is administered
- I.V.: 18 mcg (90 international units)/mL cells; administer in 600 mcg (3000 international units) aliquots every 8 hours until the total calculated dose is administered

BayRho-D®, RhoGAM®: Adults: I.M.: Multiply the volume of Rh-positive whole blood administered by the hematocrit of the donor unit to equal the volume of RBCs transfused. The volume of RBCs is then divided by 15 mL, resulting in the number of 300 mcg doses to administer. If the dose calculated results in a fraction, round up to the next higher whole 300 mcg dose.

Rhophylac®: Adults: I.M., I.V.: 100 international units (20 mcg) per 2 mL transfused blood or per 1 mL erythrocyte concentrate

Administration Parenteral: WinRho® SDF and Rhophylac® are the only immune globulin products available that can be administered both I.M. and I.V.; however, **for the treatment of ITP, only WinRho SDF® is approved for use and it must be administered I.V.**

I.M.: Administer into the deltoid muscle of upper arm or the anterolateral aspect of the upper thigh; the gluteal region is not recommended for routine administration due to the potential risk of sciatic nerve injury; if gluteal area is used, administer only in the upper, outer quadrant. The total volume can be given in divided doses at different sites at one time or may be divided and given at intervals provided the total dosage is given within 72 hours of the fetomaternal hemorrhage or transfusion

WinRho® SDF: Reconstitute 120 mcg and 300 mcg vials with 1.25 mL NS and the 100 mcg vial with 8.5 mL NS; gently swirl vial; do not shake

I.V.: WinRho® SDF, Rhophylac®: Infuse without further dilution over 3-5 minutes

Monitoring Parameters ITP: Signs and symptoms of intravascular hemolysis, CBC, reticulocytes, UA, renal function, platelets, liver function, DIC-specific tests (eg, FSP, fibrin degradation products, or D-dimer) if applicable

Test Interactions Maltose, present in liquid formulation of RH_o(D) immune globulin, may cause falsely elevated glucose when using glucose dehydrogenase pyrroloquinolinequinone (GDH-PQQ) or glucose-dye-oxidoreductase methods.

Patient Information Report symptoms of intravascular hemolysis (eg, back pain, shaking chills, fever, discolored urine, decreased urination, sudden weight gain, fluid retention, and shortness of breath) to your healthcare provider immediately.

Additional Information WinRho® SDF 1 mcg = 5 international units

Treatment of ITP in Rh-positive patients with an intact spleen appears to be about as effective as IVIG.

Dosage Forms Excipient information presented when available (limited, particularly for generics); consult specific product labeling.

Injection, solution [preservative free]:

HyperRHO™ S/D Full Dose, RhoGAM®: 300 mcg [for I.M. use only]

HyperRHO™ S/D Mini Dose, MICRhoGAM®: 50 mcg [for I.M. use only]

Rhophylac®: 300 mcg/2 mL (2 mL) [1500 int. units; for I.M. or I.V. use; contains human albumin]

WinRho® SDF:

120 mcg/~0.5 mL (~0.5 mL) [600 int. units; contains maltose and polysorbate 80; for I.M. or I.V. use]

300 mcg/~1.3 mL (~1.3 mL) [1500 int. units; contains maltose and polysorbate 80; for I.M. or I.V. use]

500 mcg/~2.2 mL (~2.2 mL) [2500 int. units; contains maltose and polysorbate 80; for I.M. or I.V. use]

1000 mcg/~4.4 mL (~4.4 mL) [5000 int. units; contains maltose and polysorbate 80; for I.M. or I.V. use]

3000 mcg/~13 mL (~13 mL) [15,000 int. units; contains maltose and polysorbate 80; for I.M. or I.V. use]

References

Gaines AR, "Acute Onset Hemoglobinemia and/or Hemoglobinuria and Sequelae Following Rh(o)(D) Immune Globulin Intravenous Administration in Immune Thrombocytopenic Purpura Patients," *Blood*, 2000, 95(8):2523-9.

♦ **RhoGAM®** *see* Rh_o(D) Immune Globulin *on page 1374*
♦ **RhoIGIV** *see* Rh_o(D) Immune Globulin *on page 1374*
♦ **RhoIVIM** *see* Rh_o(D) Immune Globulin *on page 1374*
♦ **Rho®-Loperamine (Can)** *see* Loperamide *on page 952*
♦ **Rho®-Metformin (Can)** *see* Metformin *on page 1016*
♦ **Rho®-Nitro (Can)** *see* Nitroglycerin *on page 1141*
♦ **Rhophylac®** *see* Rh_o(D) Immune Globulin *on page 1374*
♦ **Rho®-Sotalol (Can)** *see* Sotalol *on page 1463*
♦ **Rhoxal-amiodarone (Can)** *see* Amiodarone *on page 100*
♦ **Rhoxal-atenolol (Can)** *see* Atenolol *on page 170*
♦ **Rhoxal-ciprofloxacin (Can)** *see* Ciprofloxacin *on page 357*
♦ **Rhoxal-citalopram (Can)** *see* Citalopram *on page 368*
♦ **Rhoxal-cyclosporine (Can)** *see* CycloSPORINE *on page 422*
♦ **Rhoxal-diltiazem CD (Can)** *see* Diltiazem *on page 503*
♦ **Rhoxal-diltiazem SR (Can)** *see* Diltiazem *on page 503*
♦ **Rhoxal-diltiazem T (Can)** *see* Diltiazem *on page 503*
♦ **Rhoxal-fluoxetine (Can)** *see* Fluoxetine *on page 681*
♦ **Rhoxal-fluvoxamine (Can)** *see* Fluvoxamine *on page 697*
♦ **Rhoxal-minocycline (Can)** *see* Minocycline *on page 1066*
♦ **Rhoxal-pamidronate (Can)** *see* Pamidronate *on page 1200*
♦ **Rhoxal-paroxetine (Can)** *see* Paroxetine *on page 1218*
♦ **Rhoxal-ranitidine (Can)** *see* Ranitidine *on page 1366*
♦ **Rhoxal-salbutamol (Can)** *see* Albuterol *on page 66*
♦ **Rhoxal-sertraline (Can)** *see* Sertraline *on page 1429*
♦ **Rhoxal-sumatriptan (Can)** *see* Sumatriptan *on page 1495*
♦ **Rhoxal-topiramate (Can)** *see* Topiramate *on page 1551*
♦ **Rhoxal-valproic (Can)** *see* Valproic Acid and Derivatives *on page 1592*
♦ ***r*HuEPO-α** *see* Epoetin Alfa *on page 580*
♦ **rhuMAb-E25** *see* Omalizumab *on page 1165*
♦ **RibaPak™** *see* Ribavirin *on page 1378*
♦ **Ribasphere™** *see* Ribavirin *on page 1378*

Ribavirin (rye ba VYE rin)

Medication Safety Issues

Sound-alike/look-alike issues:

Ribavirin may be confused with riboflavin

U.S. Brand Names Copegus®; Rebetol®; RibaPak™; Ribasphere™; Virazole®

Canadian Brand Names Virazole®

Index Terms RTCA; Tribavirin

Therapeutic Category Antiviral Agent, Inhalation Therapy

Generic Available Yes: Capsule, tablet

Use

Inhalation: Treatment of patients with RSV infections; specially indicated for treatment of severe lower respiratory tract RSV infections in patients with an underlying compromising condition (prematurity, BPD and other chronic lung conditions, congenital heart disease, immunodeficiency, immunosuppression), and recent transplant recipients; may also be used in other viral infections including influenza A and B and adenovirus

Oral solution: Used in combination with interferon alfa-2b, recombinant injection for the treatment of chronic hepatitic C in patients ≥3 years of age with compensated liver disease who were previously untreated with alpha interferon or patients ≥18 years of age who have relapsed after alpha interferon therapy

Oral capsule: Used in combination with interferon alfa-2b, recombinant injection for the treatment of chronic hepatitis C in patients with compensated liver disease who have relapsed after alpha interferon therapy or were previously untreated with alpha interferon; or used in combination with peginterferon alfa-2b, recombinant injection for the treatment of chronic hepatitis C in patients with compensated liver disease who were previously untreated with alpha interferon

Oral tablet: Used in combination with peginterferon alfa-2a, recombinant injection for the treatment of chronic hepatitis C in patients with compensated liver disease who were previously untreated with alpha interferon

Medication Guide An FDA-approved patient medication guide, which is available with the product information and at http://www.fda.gov/cder/Offices/ODS/medication_guides.htm, must be dispensed with this medication for each new outpatient prescription and refill.

Pregnancy Risk Factor X

Lactation Excretion in breast milk unknown/not recommended

Contraindications Hypersensitivity to ribavirin or any component; pregnancy

Additional contraindications for oral formulation: Men whose female partners are pregnant; patients with hemoglobinopathies (ie, thalassemia major, sickle cell anemia); autoimmune hepatitis; as monotherapy for treatment of chronic hepatitis C; pancreatitis; patients with significant or unstable cardiac disease; Cl_{cr} <50 mL/minute; coadministration with didanosine (cases of fatal hepatic failure, peripheral neuropathy, pancreatitis, and hyperlactatemia/lactic acidosis have been reported; see Drug Interactions)

Additional contraindications for ribavirin tablet used in combination with peginterferon alfa-2a: Hepatic impairment (Child-Pugh score >6; class B or C) in cirrhotic chronic hepatitis C monoinfected patients before or during treatment; hepatic impairment (Child-Pugh score ≥6) in cirrhotic chronic hepatitis C patients coinfected with HIV before or during treatment

Warnings Ribavirin is potentially mutagenic, tumor-promoting, and gonadotoxic; ribavirin may cause birth defects and/or death of the exposed fetus. A primary adverse effect of oral ribavirin is hemolytic anemia which may worsen cardiac disease and lead to myocardial infarction. The anemia usually occurs within 1-2 weeks of therapy initiation. Closely monitor hemoglobin or hematocrit pretreatment and during the first 4 weeks of therapy. Patients with underlying cardiac disease should have an ECG performed prior to initiation of oral ribavirin therapy. Severe depression and suicidal ideation have occurred during ribavirin/pegylated interferon alfa-2a therapy (avoid use in patients with a history of depression or psychiatric disorder).

Ribavirin oral solution contains sodium benzoate; benzoic acid (benzoate) is a metabolite of benzyl alcohol; large amounts of benzyl alcohol (≥99 mg/kg/day) have been associated with a potentially fatal toxicity ("gasping syndrome") in neonates; the "gasping syndrome" consists of metabolic acidosis, respiratory distress, gasping respirations, CNS dysfunction (including convulsions, intracranial hemorrhage), hypotension and cardiovascular collapse; avoid use of ribavirin products containing sodium benzoate in neonates; *in vitro* and animal studies have shown that benzoate displaces bilirubin from protein binding sites

Precautions

Inhalation: Use with caution in patients requiring assisted ventilation because precipitation of the drug in the respiratory equipment may interfere with safe and effective patient ventilation; carefully monitor patients with COPD and asthma for deterioration of respiratory function

Oral: Use with caution in patients with pre-existing cardiac disease, patients with evidence of pulmonary infiltrates or pulmonary function impairment (closely monitor), or patients with sarcoidosis (may exacerbate sarcoidosis)

Adverse Reactions

Inhalation:

Cardiovascular: Hypotension, cardiac arrest

Central nervous system: Headache

Dermatologic: Rash, skin irritation

Hematologic: Anemia

Ocular: Conjunctivitis

Respiratory: Mild bronchospasm, worsening of respiratory function, nasal and throat irritation

Oral (documented adverse reactions while receiving combination therapy with interferon alfa-2b):

Cardiovascular: MI, chest pain, arrhythmia

Central nervous system: Depression, suicidal ideation, fever, emotional lability, insomnia, irritability, impaired concentration, headache, fatigue, dizziness, asthenia

Dermatologic: Rash, alopecia, pruritus, urticaria, angioedema

Endocrine & metabolic: Diabetes

Gastrointestinal: Nausea, anorexia, dyspepsia, vomiting, bloody diarrhea, taste perversion, pancreatitis, GI bleeding

Hematologic: Hemolytic anemia (maximum decrease in hemoglobin usually occurs during the first 8 weeks of ribavirin therapy), neutropenia, leukopenia, thrombocytopenia

Hepatic: Hepatic failure

Neuromuscular & skeletal: Myalgia, arthralgia, weakness, pain, peripheral neuropathy

Respiratory: Dyspnea, cough, pharyngitis, nasal congestion, sinusitis, pulmonary infiltrates

Miscellaneous: Flu-like symptoms, anaphylaxis, bacterial infection, autoimmune disorders

Note: Fever, anemia, vomiting, emotional lability, and suicidal ideation occurred more frequently in pediatric patients receiving oral ribavirin with interferon alfa compared to adults.

Drug Interactions Ribavirin antagonizes the antiviral activity of zidovudine and stavudine against HIV; ribavirin and nucleoside analogues adefovir, didanosine, lamivudine, stavudine, zalcitabine, or zidovudine (may increase risk of developing lactic acidosis); ribavirin reduces phosphorylation of lamivudine, stavudine, and zidovudine; ribavirin increases didanosine levels (see Contraindications)

Food Interactions Fatty meal increases bioavailability of oral ribavirin.

Stability

Inhalation: Reconstituted solution is stable for 24 hours at room temperature; do not mix with other aerosolized medications

Oral: Store capsules, tablets, and solution at room temperature; oral solution may also be refrigerated

Mechanism of Action Inhibits replication of RNA and DNA viruses; inhibits influenza virus RNA polymerase activity and interferes with the expression of messenger RNA resulting in inhibition of viral protein synthesis

Pharmacokinetics

Absorption: Inhalation: Systemically absorbed from the respiratory tract following nasal and oral inhalation; absorption is dependent upon respiratory factors and method of drug delivery; maximal absorption occurs with the use of the aerosol generator via an endotracheal tube

Distribution: Highest concentrations are found in the respiratory tract and erythrocytes; with chronic oral administration, ribavirin distributes slowly into CSF

Metabolism: Occurs intracellularly and may be necessary for drug action; metabolized by the liver to deribosylated ribavirin (active metabolite)

Bioavailability: Oral: 64%

Half-life:

Respiratory tract secretions: ~2 hours

Plasma:

Children: Inhalation: 6.5-11 hours

(Continued)

Ribavirin *(Continued)*

Adults: Oral: 24-36 hours after a single dose; half-life is much longer in the erythrocyte (16-40 days), which can be used as a marker for intracellular metabolism; terminal half-life after multiple doses is 151 hours

Time to peak serum concentration: Aerosol inhalation: At the end of the inhalation period

Oral capsule: 3 hours

Tablet: 2 hours

Elimination: Hepatic metabolism is the major route of elimination with 40% of the drug cleared renally as unchanged drug and metabolites

Usual Dosage

Infants, Children, and Adults: Aerosol inhalation:

Use with Viratek® small particle aerosol generator (SPAG-2) at a concentration of 20 mg/mL (6 g reconstituted with 300 mL of sterile water without preservatives); 6 g ribavirin vial has also been diluted with 300 mL of sterile NS solution rather than sterile water to achieve a near isotonic solution.

Note: Dose actually delivered to the patient will depend on patient's minute ventilation

Continuous aerosolization: 12-18 hours/day for 3 days, or up to 7 days in length

Intermittent aerosolization (high-dose, short-duration aerosol): 2 g over 2 hours 3 times/day at a concentration of 60 mg/mL (6 g reconstituted with 100 mL of sterile water without preservatives) in **non-mechanically ventilated** patients for 3-7 days has been used to permit easier accessibility for patient care and limit environmental exposure of healthcare worker. Due to apparent increased potential for crystallization of the high-dose 60 mg/mL solution around areas of turbulent flow such as bends in tubing or connector pieces, use of high-dose therapy in individuals with an endotracheal tube in place is **not** recommended.

Children ≥3 years: Chronic hepatitis C (in combination with interferon alfa-2b):

Oral capsule or solution: 15 mg/kg/day in 2 divided doses (morning and evening)

25-36 kg: 200 mg twice daily

37-49 kg: 200 mg in morning and 400 mg in evening

50-61 kg: 400 mg twice daily

>61 kg: See Adult dosing

Adults:

Oral capsule:

Chronic hepatitis C (in combination with interferon alfa-2b):

≤75 kg: 400 mg in morning and 600 mg in evening

>75 kg: 600 mg twice daily

Chronic hepatitis C (in combination with peginterferon alfa-2b): 400 mg twice daily

Oral tablet:

Chronic hepatitis C, genotype 1,4 (in combination with peginterferon alfa-2a):

<75 kg: 500 mg twice daily for 48 weeks

≥75 kg: 600 mg twice daily for 48 weeks

Chronic hepatitis C, genotype 2,3 (in combination with peginterferon alfa-2a): 400 mg twice daily for 24 weeks

Chronic hepatitis C in HIV coinfected patient (in combination with peginterferon alfa-2a): 400 mg twice daily for 48 weeks, regardless of genotype

Dosage adjustment in renal impairment: Cl_{cr} <50 mL/minute: Oral route is contraindicated

Dosage adjustment for toxicity: Oral:

Patient without cardiac toxicity:

Hemoglobin <10 g/dL but ≥8.5 g/dL:

Children: 7.5 mg/kg once daily

Adults:

Capsule or solution: 600 mg once daily

Tablet: 200 mg in morning and 400 mg in evening

Hemoglobin <8.5 g/dL: Permanently discontinue treatment

Patient with cardiac toxicity:

≥2 g/dL decrease in hemoglobin during any 4-week period during treatment:

Children: 7.5 mg/kg once daily

Adults:

Capsule or solution: 600 mg once daily

Tablet: 200 mg in morning and 400 mg in evening

Hemoglobin <12 g/dL after 4 weeks of reduced dose: Permanently discontinue treatment

Administration

Inhalation: Ribavirin should be administered in well-ventilated rooms (at least 6 air changes/hour)

Mechanically ventilated patients: Ribavirin can potentially be deposited in the ventilator delivery system depending on temperature, humidity, and electrostatic forces; this deposition can lead to malfunction or obstruction of the expiratory valve, resulting in inadvertently high positive end-expiratory pressures. The use of one-way valves in the inspiratory lines, a breathing circuit filter in the expiratory line, and frequent monitoring and filter replacement have been effective in preventing these problems.

Oral: Administer concurrently with interferon alfa injection. Capsule should not be opened, crushed, chewed, or broken. Use oral solution in children ≤5 years of age, those ≤25 kg, or those who cannot swallow capsules.

Capsule or solution in combination with interferon alfa-2b: May be administered with or without food

Capsule in combination with peginterferon alfa-2b: Administer with food

Tablet: Administer with food

Monitoring Parameters

Inhalation: Respiratory function, hemoglobin, reticulocyte count, CBC, I & O

Oral: Hemoglobin, hematocrit, CBC with differential, platelet count, liver function tests, EKG, pregnancy test (for women of childbearing potential), HCV-RNA after 24 weeks of therapy, TSH

Patient Information Oral: Read the patient Medication Guide that you receive with each prescription and refill of ribavirin. Avoid pregnancy in female patients and female partners of male patients during therapy by using 2 effective forms of contraception; continue contraceptive measures for at least 6 months after therapy completion. Negative pregnancy test is required before therapy initiation, monthly thereafter during treatment and for 6 months after treatment ends. Avoid alcohol. May cause dizziness, somnolence, fatigue, or impaired concentration decreasing ability to perform activities requiring mental alertness or physical coordination. Inform physician if you feel tired, dizzy, have chest pain, or shortness of breath; hives; suicidal ideation, depression, or a feeling of loss of contact with reality; severe stomach pain or bloody diarrhea; bruising or bleeding. If pregnancy occurs, inform physician immediately.

Nursing Implications Healthcare workers who are pregnant or who may become pregnant should be advised of the potential risks of exposure and counseled about risk reduction strategies including alternate job responsibilities; limit contact by visitors with patients receiving ribavirin; ribavirin may adsorb to contact lenses

Additional Information RSV season is usually December to April; viral shedding period for RSV is usually 3-8 days

Dosage Forms Excipient information presented when available (limited, particularly for generics); consult specific product labeling.

Capsule: 200 mg

Rebetol®, Ribasphere™: 200 mg

Powder for solution, inhalation [for aerosol administration]:

Virazole®: 6 g [reconstituted product provides 20 mg/mL]

Solution, oral:

Rebetol®: 40 mg/mL (100 mL) [contains sodium benzoate; bubble-gum flavor]

Tablet: 200 mg

Copegus®: 200 mg

Tablet [dose pack]:

RibaPak™: 400 mg (14s), 600 mg (14s)

References

American Academy of Pediatrics Committee on Infectious Diseases, "Reassessment of the Indications for Ribavirin Therapy in Respiratory Syncytial Virus Infections," *Pediatrics*, 1996, 97(1):137-40.

Englund JA, Piedra PA, Ahn Y-M, et al, "High-Dose, Short-Duration Ribavirin Aerosol Therapy Compared With Standard Ribavirin Therapy in Children With Suspected Respiratory Syncytial Virus Infection," *J Pediatr*, 1994, 125:635-41.

Janai HK, Marks MI, Zaleska M, et al, "Ribavirin: Adverse Drug Reactions 1986 to 1988," *Pediatr Infect Dis J*, 1990, 9(3):209-11.

Meert KL, Sarnaik AP, Gelmini MJ, et al, "Aerosolized Ribavirin in Mechanically Ventilated Children With Respiratory Syncytial Virus Lower Respiratory Tract Disease: A Prospective, Double-Blind, Randomized Trial," *Crit Care Med*, 1994, 22(4):566-72.

"NIH Consensus Statement on Management of Hepatitis C: 2002," *NIH Consens State Sci Statements*, 2002, 19(3):1-46.

Smith DW, Frankel LR, Mathers LH, et al, "A Controlled Trial of Aerosolized Ribavirin in Infants Receiving Mechanical Ventilation for Severe Respiratory Syncytial Virus Infection," *N Engl J Med*, 1991, 325(1):24-9.

Wirth S, Lang T, Gehring S, et al, "Recombinant Alfa-Interferon Plus Ribavirin Therapy in Children and Adolescents With Chronic Hepatitis C," *Hepatology*, 2002, 36(5):1280-4.

♦ **Ribo-100** *see* Riboflavin *on page 1382*

Riboflavin (RYE boe flay vin)

Medication Safety Issues
Sound-alike/look-alike issues:
Riboflavin may be confused with ribavirin
U.S. Brand Names Ribo-100
Index Terms Lactoflavin; Vitamin B_2; Vitamin G
Therapeutic Category Nutritional Supplement; Vitamin, Water Soluble
Generic Available Yes
Use Prevention of riboflavin deficiency and treatment of ariboflavinosis; microcytic anemia associated with glutathione reductase deficiency
Pregnancy Risk Factor A (C if dose exceeds RDA recommendation)
Lactation Enters breast milk/compatible
Contraindications Hypersensitivity to riboflavin or any component
Adverse Reactions Genitourinary: Discoloration of urine (bright yellow) with large doses
Drug Interactions Probenecid
Food Interactions Food increases the extent of GI absorption
Stability Protect from light
Mechanism of Action Converted to coenzymes which act as hydrogen-carrier molecules, which are necessary for normal tissue respiration; also needed for activation of pyridoxine and conversion of tryptophan to niacin
Pharmacokinetics
Absorption: Readily via GI tract; GI absorption is decreased in patients with hepatitis, cirrhosis, or biliary obstruction
Metabolism: Metabolic fate unknown
Half-life, biologic: 66-84 minutes
Elimination: 9% eliminated unchanged in urine
Usual Dosage Oral:
Riboflavin deficiency:
Children: 3-10 mg/day in divided doses
Adults: 5-30 mg/day in divided doses
Adequate intake: Infants:
<6 months: 0.3 mg (0.04 mg/kg)
6-12 months: 0.4 mg (0.04 mg/kg)
Recommended daily allowance (RDA):
Children:
1-3 years: 0.5 mg
4-8 years: 0.6 mg
9-13 years: 0.9 mg
14-18 years:
Male: 1.3 mg
Female: 1 mg
19-70 years:
Male: 1.3 mg
Female: 1.1 mg
Microcytic anemia associated with glutathione reductase deficiency: Adults: 10 mg daily for 10 days
Administration Oral: Administer with food
Monitoring Parameters CBC and reticulocyte counts (if anemic when treating deficiency)
Test Interactions Large doses may interfere with urinalysis based on spectrometry; may cause false elevations in fluorometric determinations of catecholamines and urobilinogen
Patient Information Large doses may cause bright yellow urine
Dosage Forms Excipient information presented when available (limited, particularly for generics); consult specific product labeling.
Tablet: 25 mg, 50 mg, 100 mg
Ribo-100: 100 mg

♦ **Rid-A-Pain Dental Drops [OTC]** *see* Benzocaine *on page 204*
♦ **Ridaura®** *see* Auranofin *on page 185*
♦ **Rid® Spray [OTC]** *see* Permethrin *on page 1243*

Rifabutin (rif a BYOO tin)

Medication Safety Issues
Sound-alike/look-alike issues:
Rifabutin may be confused with rifampin

U.S. Brand Names Mycobutin®

Canadian Brand Names Mycobutin®

Index Terms Ansamycin

Therapeutic Category Antibiotic, Miscellaneous; Antitubercular Agent

Generic Available No

Use Prevention of disseminated *Mycobacterium avium* complex (MAC) in patients with advanced HIV infection; utilized in multiple drug regimens for treatment of MAC

Pregnancy Risk Factor B

Lactation Excretion in breast milk unknown

Contraindications Hypersensitivity to rifabutin, any component, or other rifamycin; rifabutin is contraindicated in patients with a WBC <1000/mm^3 or a platelet count <50,000 mm^3; coadministration of rifabutin with delavirdine or ritonavir (see Drug Interactions)

Warnings Rifabutin as a single agent must not be administered to patients with active tuberculosis since its use may lead to the development of tuberculosis that is resistant to both rifabutin and rifampin; rifabutin should be discontinued in patients with AST >500 international units/L or if total bilirubin is >3 mg/dL. Tiny, asymptomatic peripheral and central corneal deposits have been observed during routine ophthalmologic exams in HIV-positive patients receiving rifabutin.

Precautions Use with caution in patients with liver or renal impairment; modify dose in patients with Cl_{cr} <30 mL/minute. Rifabutin is a CYP3A3/4 isoenzyme inducer which may reduce the plasma concentrations of itraconazole, clarithromycin, and saquinavir. CYP3A3/4 isoenzyme inhibitors such as fluconazole and clarithromycin may elevate levels of rifabutin increasing the risk of adverse reactions. Monitor patients, and in some cases, reduce the rifabutin dose when coadministered with fluconazole or clarithromycin (see Drug Interactions).

Adverse Reactions

Central nervous system: Fever, headache, seizures, confusion, insomnia

Dermatologic: Rash, staining of skin (brown-orange)

Gastrointestinal: Abdominal pain, diarrhea, dyspepsia, nausea, anorexia, vomiting, dysgeusia, flatulence

Genitourinary: Discoloration of urine (brown-orange)

Hematologic: Thrombocytopenia, anemia, leukopenia, neutropenia

Hepatic: Elevated liver enzymes

Neuromuscular & skeletal: Arthralgia, myositis

Ocular: Uveitis, corneal deposits

Miscellaneous: Discoloration of body fluids (brown-orange)

Drug Interactions Cytochrome P450 isoenzyme CYP3A3/4 inducer

May decrease the serum concentration or effect of dapsone, verapamil, methadone, ketoconazole, digoxin, theophylline, barbiturates, itraconazole, clarithromycin, protease inhibitors, non-nucleoside reverse transcriptase inhibitors, anticoagulants, corticosteroids, zidovudine, cyclosporine, quinidine, and oral contraceptives (alternative form of contraception should be considered); indinavir and ritonavir increase rifabutin concentrations (decrease daily rifabutin dose by 50% if given with indinavir or nelfinavir; decrease rifabutin adult dose to 150 mg 2-3 times per week if given with ritonavir); protease inhibitors, erythromycin, clarithromycin, delavirdine, ketoconazole, fluconazole, and itraconazole may increase serum concentration of rifabutin

Food Interactions High-fat meal may decrease the rate but not the extent of absorption

Mechanism of Action Inhibits DNA-dependent RNA polymerase at the beta subunit which prevents chain initiation

Pharmacokinetics

Absorption: Oral: Readily absorbed

Distribution: To body tissues including the lungs, liver, spleen, eyes, and kidneys

V_d: Adults: 9.3 ± 1.5 L/kg

Protein binding: 85%

Metabolism: To active and inactive metabolites

Bioavailability: Adults: 20% in HIV patients

Half-life, terminal: Adults: 45 hours (range: 16-69 hours)

Time to peak serum concentration: 2-4 hours

Elimination: Renal and biliary clearance of unchanged drug is 10%; 30% excreted in feces

Usual Dosage Oral:

Children: Efficacy and safety of rifabutin have not been established in children; a limited number of HIV-positive children with MAC (n=22) have been given rifabutin for MAC prophylaxis; dosages of up to 75 mg/day have been given to children <4 years of age (~5-6 mg/kg/day)

Infants and Children: Prophylaxis for first episode of MAC in HIV-infected patients:

Children <6 years: 5 mg/kg once daily

(Continued)

Rifabutin *(Continued)*

Children ≥6 years: 300 mg once daily

Infants and Children: Prophylaxis for recurrence of MAC in HIV-infected patients: 5 mg/kg (maximum dose: 300 mg) once daily in combination with clarithromycin

Adolescents and Adults:

Prophylaxis for first episode of MAC in HIV-infected patient: 300 mg once daily; for patients who experience GI upset, rifabutin can be administered 150 mg twice daily with food

Prophylaxis for recurrence of MAC in HIV-infected patient: 300 mg once daily as a component of a multiple drug regimen

Dosage adjustment in renal impairment: Cl_{cr} <30 mL/minute: Reduce dose by 50%

Administration Oral: May administer with or without food or mix with applesauce; administer with food to decrease GI upset

Monitoring Parameters Periodic liver function tests, CBC with differential, platelet count, hemoglobin, hematocrit, ophthalmologic exam

Patient Information May discolor skin, urine, tears, perspiration, or other body fluids to a brown-orange color; soft contact lenses may be permanently stained. Notify physician of any severe flu-like symptoms, nausea, vomiting, dark urine, unusual bleeding or bruising, or any eye problems

Dosage Forms Excipient information presented when available (limited, particularly for generics); consult specific product labeling.

Capsule: 150 mg

Extemporaneous Preparations A 20 mg/mL rifabutin suspension is made by placing the powder from eight 150 mg rifabutin capsules into a glass mortar, levigating with 20 mL of a 1:1 vehicle of Ora-Sweet® and Ora-Plus® and triturating the mixture to make a paste. Additional vehicle is added in geometric proportion levigating until a uniform mixture is obtained; qsad to 60 mL with vehicle. Stable for 12 weeks at 4°C, 25°C, 30°C, and 40°C. Label "shake well before using."

Haslam JL, Egodage KL, Chen Y, et al, "Stability of Rifabutin in Two Extemporaneously Compounded Oral Liquids," *Am J Health Syst Pharm*, 1999, 56(4):333-6.

References

Kaplan JE, Masur H, and Holmes KK, "Guidelines for Preventing Opportunistic Infections Among HIV-Infected Persons - 2002 Recommendations of the USPHS and IDSA," *MMWR*, 2002, 51(RR-8):1-46.

Krause PJ, Hight DW, Schwartz AN, et al, "Successful Management of *Mycobacterium intracellulare* Pneumonia in a Child," *Pediatr Infect Dis*, 1986, 5(2):269-71.

Levin RH and Bolinger AM, "Treatment of Nontuberculous Mycobacterial Infections in Pediatric Patients," *Clin Pharm*, 1988, 7(7):545-51.

Starke JR and Correa AG, "Management of Mycobacterial Infection and Disease in Children," *Pediatr Infect Dis J*, 1995, 14(6):455-70.

♦ **Rifadin®** *see* Rifampin *on page 1384*

♦ **Rifampicin** *see* Rifampin *on page 1384*

Rifampin (RIF am pin)

Medication Safety Issues

Sound-alike/look-alike issues:

Rifampin may be confused with rifabutin, Rifamate®, rifapentine, rifaximin

Rifadin® may be confused with Ritalin®

U.S. Brand Names Rifadin®

Canadian Brand Names Rifadin®; Rofact™

Index Terms Rifampicin

Therapeutic Category Antibiotic, Miscellaneous; Antitubercular Agent

Generic Available Yes

Use Used in combination with other antitubercular drugs for the treatment of active tuberculosis; elimination of meningococci from asymptomatic carriers; prophylaxis in contacts of patients with *Haemophilus influenzae* type B infection; used in combination with other anti-infectives in the treatment of staphylococcal infections

Pregnancy Risk Factor C

Lactation Enters breast milk/not recommended (AAP rates "compatible")

Contraindications Hypersensitivity to rifampin, rifamycins, or any component; concurrent use with amprenavir

Warnings Two month rifampin-pyrazinamide regimen for the treatment of latent tuberculosis infection (LTBI) has been associated with severe and fatal liver injuries. The IDSA and CDC now recommend that this regimen should not generally be used in patients with LTBI.

Precautions Use with caution in patients with liver impairment, patients receiving concurrent medications associated with liver injury (particularly with pyrazinamide), or in patients with a history of alcoholism; modification of dosage should be considered in patients with severe liver impairment

Adverse Reactions

Central nervous system: Drowsiness, fatigue, confusion, ataxia, fever, headache, dizziness

Dermatologic: Rash, pruritus, urticaria

Gastrointestinal: Nausea, vomiting, diarrhea, stomatitis, anorexia

Hematologic: Eosinophilia, blood dyscrasias (leukopenia, thrombocytopenia), hemolytic anemia

Hepatic: Hepatitis, cholestatic jaundice, elevated liver enzymes

Local: Irritation at the I.V. site

Neuromuscular & skeletal: Myalgias, arthralgia, weakness

Renal: Renal failure, interstitial nephritis

Miscellaneous: Flu-like syndrome; discoloration of body fluids (red-orange)

Drug Interactions Cytochrome P450 isoenzyme CYP3A3/4 substrate; isoenzyme CYP1A2, CYP2C9, CYP2C18, CYP2C19, CYP3A3/4, and CYP3A5-7 inducer

Rifampin induces liver enzymes which may decrease the plasma concentration of the following drugs: verapamil, diltiazem, nifedipine, methadone, digoxin, cyclosporine, tacrolimus, benzodiazepines, corticosteroids, oral anticoagulants, theophylline, barbiturates, chloramphenicol, ketoconazole, oral contraceptives (alternate form of contraception should be considered), protease inhibitors, non-nucleoside reverse transcriptase inhibitors, and quinidine; halothane, pyrazinamide, or isoniazid (additive hepatotoxic effects)

Food Interactions Food may delay and reduce the amount of rifampin absorbed

Stability Reconstituted I.V. solution is stable for 24 hours at room temperature; once the reconstituted rifampin I.V. solution is further diluted, it is stable for 4 hours in D_5W and up to 24 hours in NS. However, 11% to 13% rifampin decomposition has been reported to occur in 24 hours for solutions diluted in NS. Administer rifampin I.V. solution within 4 hours after preparation to avoid potential for precipitation and decomposition beyond this period.

Mechanism of Action Inhibits bacterial RNA synthesis by binding to the beta subunit of DNA-dependent RNA polymerase, blocking RNA transcription

Pharmacokinetics

Absorption: Oral: Well absorbed

Distribution: Highly lipophilic; crosses the blood-brain barrier and is widely distributed into body tissues and fluids such as the liver, lungs, gallbladder, bile, tears, and breast milk; distributes into CSF when meninges are inflamed

Protein binding: 80%

Metabolism: Undergoes enterohepatic recycling; metabolized in the liver to a deacetylated metabolite (active)

Half-life: 3-4 hours, prolonged with hepatic impairment

Time to peak serum concentration: Oral: Within 2-4 hours

Elimination: Principally in feces (60% to 65%) and urine (~30%)

Dialysis: Plasma rifampin concentrations are not significantly affected by hemodialysis or peritoneal dialysis

Usual Dosage Oral (I.V. infusion dose is the same as for the oral route):

Tuberculosis:

Infants and Children: 10-20 mg/kg/day in divided doses every 12-24 hours

Adults: 10 mg/kg/day administered once daily; maximum dose: 600 mg/day

American Thoracic Society and CDC currently recommend twice weekly therapy as part of a short-course regimen which follows 1-2 months of daily treatment of uncomplicated pulmonary tuberculosis in the compliant patient

Children: 10-20 mg/kg/dose (up to 600 mg) twice weekly under supervision to ensure compliance

Adults: 10 mg/kg (up to 600 mg) twice weekly

H. influenzae prophylaxis:

Neonates <1 month: 10 mg/kg/day every 24 hours for 4 days

Infants and Children: 20 mg/kg/day every 24 hours for 4 days, not to exceed 600 mg/dose

Adults: 600 mg every 24 hours for 4 days

Meningococcal prophylaxis:

<1 month: 10 mg/kg/day in divided doses every 12 hours for 2 days

Infants and Children: 20 mg/kg/day in divided doses every 12 hours for 2 days, not to exceed 600 mg/dose

Adults: 600 mg every 12 hours for 2 days

Nasal carriers of *Staphylococcus aureus*:

Children: 15 mg/kg/day divided every 12 hours for 5-10 days in combination with other antibiotics

Adults: 600 mg once daily for 5-10 days in combination with other antibiotics

Synergy for *Staphylococcus aureus* infections:

Neonates: 5-20 mg/kg/day in divided doses every 12 hours with other antibiotics

Adults: 300-600 mg twice daily with other antibiotics

(Continued)

Rifampin *(Continued)*

Administration

Oral: Administer 1 hour before or 2 hours after a meal on an empty stomach; may administer with food to decrease GI distress; may mix contents of capsule with applesauce or jelly

Parenteral: Do not administer I.M. or SubQ; administer I.V. preparation once daily by slow I.V. infusion over 30 minutes to 3 hours at a final concentration not to exceed 6 mg/mL

Monitoring Parameters Periodic monitoring of liver function (AST, ALT); bilirubin, CBC, platelet count

Test Interactions Positive Coombs' reaction [direct], rifampin inhibits standard assay's ability to measure serum folate and vitamin B_{12}

Patient Information May discolor urine, tears, sweat, or other body fluids to a red-orange color; soft contact lenses may be permanently stained. Notify physician of any severe or persistent flu-like symptoms, nausea, vomiting, dark urine, or unusual bleeding or bruising

Nursing Implications The compounded oral suspension must be shaken well before using. Extravasation may cause local irritation and inflammation.

Dosage Forms Excipient information presented when available (limited, particularly for generics); consult specific product labeling.

Capsule: 150 mg, 300 mg

Injection, powder for reconstitution: 600 mg

Extemporaneous Preparations Rifampin oral suspension can be compounded with simple syrup or wild cherry syrup at a concentration of 10 mg/mL; the suspension is stable for 4 weeks at room temperature or in a refrigerator when stored in a glass amber prescription bottle. However, there are some experts who do not recommend using rifampin syrup formulated from capsules due to conflicting reports indicating that the product is unstable (14.5% to 68% of labeled potency after preparation). It may be preferable to perform trituration, rather than simple mixing in syrup when preparing rifampin oral suspension.

Nahata MC, Morosco RS, and Hipple TF, "Effect of Preparation Method and Storage on Rifampin Concentration in Suspensions," *Ann Pharmacother*, 1994, 28(2):182-5.

References

American Academy of Pediatrics Committee on Infectious Diseases, "Chemotherapy for Tuberculosis in Infants and Children," *Pediatrics*, 1992, 89(1):161-5.

Starke JR, "Modern Approach to the Diagnosis and Treatment of Tuberculosis in Children," *Pediatr Clin North Am*, 1988, 35(3):441-64.

Starke JR, "Multidrug Therapy for Tuberculosis in Children," *Pediatr Infect Dis J*, 1990, 9(11):785-93.

Tan TQ, Mason EO Jr, Ou CN, et al, "Use of Intravenous Rifampin in Neonates With Persistent Staphylococcal Bacteremia," *Antimicrob Agents Chemother*, 1993, 37(11):2401-6.

♦ **rIFN-A** *see* Interferon Alfa-2a *on page 854*

♦ **RIG** *see* Rabies Immune Globulin (Human) *on page 1363*

♦ **rIL-11** *see* Oprelvekin *on page 1174*

Rimantadine (ri MAN ta deen)

Medication Safety Issues

Sound-alike/look-alike issues:

Rimantadine may be confused with amantadine, ranitidine, Rimactane®

Flumadine® may be confused with fludarabine, flunisolide, flutamide

U.S. Brand Names Flumadine®

Canadian Brand Names Flumadine®

Index Terms Rimantadine Hydrochloride

Therapeutic Category Antiviral Agent, Oral

Generic Available Yes: Tablet

Use Prophylaxis and treatment of influenza A viral infection (see Warnings)

Pregnancy Risk Factor C

Lactation Excretion in breast milk unknown/ not recommended

Contraindications Hypersensitivity to rimantadine, amantadine, or any component

Warnings Resistance of influenza A virus to rimantadine may develop spontaneously or rapidly during treatment; cross-resistance between amantadine and rimantadine occurs; a high frequency of resistance to rimantadine and amantadine was found among influenza A viruses tested during the 2005-06 influenza season in the United States; this prompted the CDC (in January 2006) to recommend that neither rimantadine nor amantadine be used for the prophylaxis or treatment of influenza A infections in the United States for the rest of the 2005-06 influenza season; oseltamivir or zanamivir should be used, if an antiviral medication is needed

Precautions Use with caution in patients with liver disease, epilepsy, history of recurrent eczematoid dermatitis, uncontrolled psychosis, severe psychoneurosis, and in patients receiving CNS stimulant drugs; modify dosage in patients with renal impairment, severe hepatic dysfunction, or active seizure disorder; use in patients <1 year of age has not been adequately assessed

Adverse Reactions

Cardiovascular: Orthostatic hypotension, edema

Central nervous system: Dizziness, confusion, headache, insomnia, difficulty in concentrating, anxiety, restlessness, irritability, hallucinations; CNS adverse effects are less than with amantadine

Gastrointestinal: Nausea, vomiting, xerostomia

Genitourinary: Urinary retention

Drug Interactions Anticholinergic agents, CNS stimulants may possibly increase adverse effects

Food Interactions Food does not affect rate or extent of absorption

Mechanism of Action Blocks the uncoating of influenza A viral RNA and prevents penetration of the virus into host cell; inhibits M_2 protein in the assembly of progeny virions

Pharmacokinetics

Absorption: Oral: Well absorbed

Distribution: Adults: 17-25 L/kg

Protein binding: ~40%

Metabolism: Extensively in the liver via hydroxylation and glucuronidation

Half-life:

- Children 4-8 years: 13-38 hours
- Adults: 24-36 hours

Elimination: <25% excreted unchanged in the urine

Dialysis: Hemodialysis: Negligible effect

Usual Dosage Oral: **Note:** Dosages for prophylaxis and treatment are the same; rimantadine is FDA-approved for prophylaxis in children and adults, and for treatment only in adults; however, it is considered appropriate by certain experts for treatment in children (see AAP, 2000). See Additional Information for duration of therapy.

Children 1-9 years and Children ≥10 years who weigh <40 kg: 5 mg/kg/day in 1-2 divided doses; maximum dose: 150 mg/day

Children ≥10 years who weigh ≥40 kg and Adults: 100 mg twice daily

Dosage adjustment in renal impairment:

- Cl_{cr} >10 mL/minute: Dose adjustment not required
- Cl_{cr} ≤10 mL/minute: Adults: 100 mg/day

Dosage adjustment in hepatic impairment: Severe dysfunction: Adults: 100 mg/day

Administration Oral: May administer with food

Patient Information May cause dizziness or confusion and impair ability to perform activities requiring mental alertness or physical coordination; may cause dry mouth

Additional Information Not active against influenza B; treatment or prophylaxis in immunosuppressed patients has not been fully evaluated

- Duration of treatment: 5-7 days; optimal duration not established
- Duration of prophylactic therapy: For at least 10 days after known exposure; usually for 6-8 weeks during influenza A season or local outbreak (or until vaccine produces sufficient antibody titers)
- Duration of fever and other symptoms can be reduced if rimantadine therapy is started within the first 48 hours of influenza A illness

During an outbreak of influenza, administer rimantadine prophylaxis for 2-3 weeks after influenza vaccination until vaccine antibody titers are sufficient to provide protection

Dosage Forms Excipient information presented when available (limited, particularly for generics); consult specific product labeling.

Syrup, as hydrochloride:

- Flumadine®: 50 mg/5 mL (240 mL) [raspberry flavor]

Tablet, as hydrochloride: 100 mg

- Flumadine®: 100 mg

References

American Academy of Pediatrics, "Influenza," Red Book®: 2000 Report of the Committee on Infectious Diseases, 25th ed, Pickering LK, ed, Elk Grove Village, IL: American Academy of Pediatrics, 2000, 354.

♦ **Rimantadine Hydrochloride** *see* Rimantadine *on page 1386*
♦ **Riomet™** *see* Metformin *on page 1016*
♦ **Riphenidate (Can)** *see* Methylphenidate *on page 1034*
♦ **Risperdal®** *see* Risperidone *on page 1388*
♦ **Risperdal M-Tab** *see* Risperidone *on page 1388*
♦ **Risperdal® M-Tab®** *see* Risperidone *on page 1388*

♦ **Risperdal® Consta®** *see* Risperidone *on page 1388*

Risperidone (ris PER i done)

Medication Safety Issues

Sound-alike/look-alike issues:

Risperidone may be confused with reserpine

Risperdal® may be confused with lisinopril, reserpine

U.S. Brand Names Risperdal®; Risperdal® Consta®; Risperdal® M-Tab®

Canadian Brand Names Apo-Risperidone®; PMS-Risperidone ODT; Risperdal®; Risperdal® Consta®; Risperdal® M-Tab®; Sandoz Risperidone

Index Terms Risperdal M-Tab

Therapeutic Category Antipsychotic Agent, Atypical; Antipsychotic Agent, Benzisoxazole

Generic Available No

Use

Oral: Management of schizophrenia; treatment of acute mania or mixed episodes associated with bipolar I disorder (as monotherapy or in combination with lithium or valproate); treatment of irritability (including aggression, temper tantrums, self-injurious behavior, and quickly changing moods) associated with autistic disorder in children and adolescents; has also been used to treat Tourette's syndrome and aggressive behavior in patients with other pervasive developmental disorders or psychiatric diagnoses

I.M.: Management of schizophrenia in adults

Pregnancy Risk Factor C

Lactation Enters breast milk/not recommended

Contraindications Hypersensitivity to risperidone or any component (see Warnings)

Warnings May cause neuroleptic malignant syndrome (symptoms include hyperpyrexia, altered mental status, muscle rigidity, autonomic instability, acute renal failure, rhabdomyolysis, and elevated CPK). May cause extrapyramidal reactions, including pseudoparkinsonism, acute dystonic reactions, akathisia, and tardive dyskinesia (risk of these reactions is low relative to other neuroleptics, and is dose-dependent; to decrease risk of tardive dyskinesia: use smallest dose and shortest duration possible; evaluate continued need periodically). May cause hyperglycemia, which may be severe and include potentially fatal ketoacidosis or hyperosmolar coma; use with caution and monitor glucose closely in patients with diabetes mellitus (or with risk factors such as family history or obesity); measure fasting blood glucose at the beginning of therapy and periodically during therapy in these patients; monitor for symptoms of hyperglycemia in all patients treated with risperidone; measure fasting blood glucose in patients who develop symptoms. May alter cardiac conduction (low risk relative to other neuroleptics); life-threatening arrhythmias have occurred with therapeutic doses of neuroleptics. An increased risk of death has been reported with risperidone use in elderly patients with dementia-related psychosis; most deaths seemed to be cardiovascular (eg, sudden death, heart failure) or infectious (eg, pneumonia) in nature; use of furosemide was associated with a higher risk of mortality

Oral solution contains benzoic acid; benzoic acid (benzoate) is a metabolite of benzyl alcohol; large amounts of benzyl alcohol (≥99 mg/kg/day) have been associated with a potentially fatal toxicity ("gasping syndrome") in neonates; avoid use of risperidone products containing benzoic acid in neonates; *in vitro* and animal studies have shown that benzoate displaces bilirubin from protein binding sites

Precautions Use with caution and decrease the dose in patients with renal or hepatic impairment. Use with caution in patients with breast cancer or other prolactin-dependent tumors; risperidone elevates prolactin levels to a greater degree than other antipsychotic agents; high levels of prolactin may reduce pituitary gonadotropin secretion; galactorrhea, amenorrhea, gynecomastia, impotence, decreased bone density may occur. Use with caution in children and adolescents; adverse effects due to elevated prolactin levels have been observed; long-term effects on growth or sexual maturation have not been evaluated; risperidone may cause a higher than normal weight gain in children; monitor growth in pediatric patients receiving risperidone and compare weight gain to standard growth curves; risperidone use in pediatric patients may cause somnolence (at a higher incidence than in adults) or tardive dyskinesia (0.1%). Safety and efficacy have not been established in pediatric patients <5 years of age with autistic disorder or in pediatric patients with psychiatric or behavioral disorders other than autism.

Use with caution in patients with seizure disorders (seizures have been rarely reported), concomitant illnesses that may effect hepatic metabolism or hemodynamic responses (eg, unstable cardiac disease, recent MI), Parkinson's disease or dementia with Lewy Bodies (an increased sensitivity to antipsychotic medications has been reported), in suicidal patients, and in those at risk of aspiration pneumonia (esophageal dysmotility and aspiration have been associated with antipsychotic agents). May cause orthostatic hypotension with resultant dizziness, tachycardia, or syncope (especially during initial dose titration); use with caution in patients with cardiovascular disease (conduction abnormalities, heart failure, past MI, or myocardia ischemia), cerebrovascular disease, dehydration, hypovolemia, or other conditions which may predispose patients to hypotension; may cause hypotension when used with antihypertensive agents. May cause somnolence (dose-related), priapism (rarely), alteration of temperature regulation (use with caution in patients exposed to temperature extremes); may mask diseases or toxicity of other drugs due to antiemetic effects

Orally-disintegrating tablets contain aspartame which is metabolized to phenylalanine and must be avoided (or used with caution) in patients with phenylketonuria

Adverse Reactions Note: Unless otherwise noted, frequency of adverse effects is reported for the oral formulation in adults; incidences given for children are from studies in children and adolescents

Cardiovascular: Hypotension (especially orthostatic), tachycardia (adults 3% to 5%; children 7%), chest pain, hypertension, syncope (incidence: Oral: 0.2%; I.M.: 0.8%)

Central nervous system: Somnolence (adults 3% to 28%; children 67%), fatigue (adults 4%; children 42%), extrapyramidal symptoms (dose dependent; adults 17% to 34%; children 28%), dystonia (adults 18%; children 12%), confusion (children 5%), dizziness (adults 4% to 11%; children 9%), automatism (children 7%), pseudoparkinsonism (adults 6%; children 7%), insomnia (23% to 26%), agitation (8% to 26%), anxiety (4% to 20%), headache (12% to 14%), restlessness, tardive dyskinesia (children 0.1%), akathisia (16%), hypoesthesia (2%), hallucinations, mania (8%), increased dreaming (≥5%), prolonged sleep (≥5%), pain (5%), fever (2% to 3%), aggressiveness (1% to 3%), impaired concentration (2%), nervousness, increased sleep duration, neuroleptic malignant syndrome, altered central temperature regulation, seizures (0.3%)

Dermatologic: Rash (2% to 5%), dry skin (2% to 4%), acne (2%), pruritus (2%), seborrhea (up to 1%), pigmentation increased, photosensitivity

Endocrine & metabolic: Weight gain (adults 2% to 18%; children 5%; **Note:** After 12 months of risperidone therapy, children gained a mean of 7.5 kg which was higher than the expected normal weight gain of 3-3.5 kg/year adjusted for age), increased appetite (children 49%), elevated serum prolactin, amenorrhea, galactorrhea (children 1%), gynecomastia (children 2%), sexual dysfunction, hyperglycemia

Gastrointestinal: Increased salivation (adults up to 5%; children 22%), constipation (adults 7% to 13%; children 21%), nausea (4% to 11%), xerostomia (adults 3% to ≥5%; children 13%), dyspepsia (5% to 11%), vomiting (5% to 7%), abdominal pain (1% to 4%), anorexia, diarrhea (≥5%), toothache

Genitourinary: Polyuria, polydypsia, nocturnal enuresis, priapism (rare)

Hematologic: Anemia (I.M. ≥1%)

Hepatic: Elevated transaminases (I.M. ≥1%), hepatotoxicity (rare) (see Kumra, 1997 and McDougle, 2000)

Local: I.M.: Pain, redness, swelling at injection site

Neuromuscular & skeletal: Tremor (Children 12%), dyskinesia (children 7%), arthralgia (2% to 3%), myalgia (5%), skeletal pain, back pain

Ocular: Abnormal vision (1% to 6%), accommodation disturbances (≥5%)

Respiratory: Upper respiratory tract infection (adults 3%; children 34%), rhinitis (3% to 10%), coughing (2% to 3%), pharyngitis (2% to 3%), sinusitis (1% to 4%), dyspnea (up to 1%)

Drug Interactions Cytochrome P450 isoenzyme CYP2D6 and CYP3A4 substrate; isoenzyme CYP2D6 inhibitor (weak)

Risperidone may enhance the hypotensive effects of antihypertensive agents; may antagonize the effects of levodopa and dopamine agonists; CNS depressants, alcohol may potentiate the adverse effects of risperidone; the herbal medicine St John's wort (*Hypericum perforatum*), may increase serious side effects (its use is **not** recommended)

Use with valproic acid may result in generalized edema (case report); risperidone may increase peak plasma concentrations of valproic acid. Carbamazepine and other enzyme inducers (eg, rifampin, phenobarbital, phenytoin) may decrease serum concentrations of risperidone and its active metabolite (9-hydroxyrisperidone) and reduce efficacy (the dose of risperidone may need to be adjusted when enzyme inducers are added or discontinued). Drugs that inhibit cytochrome P450 CYP2D6 may inhibit the metabolism of risperidone (monitor for increased effect or toxicity); clozapine may decrease the clearance of risperidone; fluoxetine may increase the serum concentration of risperidone (dosage adjustment of risperidone is needed); paroxetine may increase serum concentrations of risperidone and decrease concentrations of 9-hydroxyrisperidone (dosage adjustment of risperidone is needed);

(Continued)

Risperidone *(Continued)*

venlafaxine may increase serum concentrations of risperidone, but does not significantly alter the disposition of the total active moiety [risperidone plus 9-hydroxyrisperidone (active metabolite)]. Cimetidine may increase the bioavailability of risperidone by 64% but does not affect the AUC of the active moiety; ranitidine may increase the bioavailability of risperidone and increase the AUC of the active moiety by 20%.

Food Interactions Food does not affect rate or extent of oral absorption; oral solution is not compatible with cola or tea

Stability Store at controlled room temperature 15°C to 25°C (59°F to 77°F); protect from light; protect tablets from moisture; protect oral solution from freezing; do not store orally-disintegrating tablets once removed from blister unit

Injection: Store undiluted vials and diluent at 2°C to 8°C (36°F to 46°F); protect from light; may store at room temperature ≤77°F (25°C) for ≤7 days prior to reconstitution; reconstituted suspension must be used within 6 hours

Mechanism of Action Atypical antipsychotic (benzisoxazole derivative); highly potent serotonin and dopamine receptor antagonist; binds to 5-HT_2-receptors in the CNS and in the periphery with a very high affinity; binds to dopamine-D_2 receptors, but with less affinity (~20 times lower). The addition of serotonin antagonism to dopamine antagonism (classic neuroleptic mechanism) is thought to improve negative symptoms of psychoses and reduce the incidence of extrapyramidal side effects. $Alpha_1$, $alpha_2$ adrenergic, and histaminergic receptors are also antagonized with high affinity. Risperidone has low to moderate affinity for 5-HT_{1C}, 5-HT_{1D}, and 5-HT_{1A} receptors, weak affinity for D_1 and no affinity for cholinergic muscarinic or $beta_1$ and $beta_2$ receptors

Pharmacokinetics Note: Following oral administration, the pharmacokinetics of risperidone and 9-hydroxyrisperidone in children were found to be similar to values in adults (after adjusting for differences in body weight).

Absorption:

Oral: Well absorbed

I.M.: Initial: <1% of dose released from microspheres; main release starts at ≥3 weeks; release is maintained from 4-6 weeks; release ends by 7 weeks

Distribution: Distributes into breast milk; breast milk to plasma ratio (n=1): Risperidone: 0.42; 9-hydroxyrisperidone: 0.24 (Hill, 2000)

V_d: Risperidone: Adults: 1-2 L/kg

Protein binding: Risperidone: ~90%, plasma protein binding increases with increasing concentrations of $alpha_1$-acid glycoprotein; 9-hydroxyrisperidone: 77%; **Note:** Risperidone free fraction may be increased by ~35% in patients with hepatic impairment due to decreased concentrations of albumin and $alpha_1$-acid glycoprotein

Metabolism: Extensive in the liver via cytochrome P450 CYP2D6 to 9-hydroxyrisperidone (major active metabolite); also undergoes N-dealkylation (minor pathway); **Note:** 9-hydroxyrisperidone is the predominant circulating form and is approximately equal to risperidone in receptor binding activity; clinical effects are from combined concentrations of risperidone and 9-hydroxyrisperidone; clinically important differences between CYP2D6 poor and extensive metabolizers are not expected (pharmacokinetics of the sum of risperidone and 9-hydroxyrisperidone were similar in poor and extensive metabolizers)

Bioavailability: Oral: 70%; tablet (relative to solution): 94%; **Note:** Orally-disintegrating tablets are bioequivalent to regular tablets.

Half-life (apparent): Adults:

Oral:

Risperidone: Extensive metabolizers: 3 hours; poor metabolizers: 20 hours

9-hydroxyrisperidone: Extensive metabolizers: 21 hours; poor metabolizers: 30 hours

Sum of risperidone and 9-hydroxyrisperidone: Overall mean: 20 hours

I.M.: 3-6 days (due to extended release of drug from microspheres and subsequent absorption)

Time to peak serum concentration: Oral: Solution or tablet:

Risperidone: 1 hour

9-hydroxyrisperidone: Extensive metabolizers: 3 hours; poor metabolizers: 17 hours

Elimination: Excreted as risperidone and metabolites in urine (70%) and feces (14%)

Clearance: Moderate to severe renal impairment (sum of risperidone and 9-hydroxyrisperidone): Decreased by 60%

Usual Dosage

Children and Adolescents: Limited information is available: Oral:

Autism: Treatment of irritability associated with autistic disorder, including aggression, temper tantrums, self-injurious behavior, and quickly changing moods:

Children ≥5 years and Adolescents: Manufacturer's recommendation: **Note:** Individualize dose according to patient response and tolerability:

<15 kg: Use with caution; specific dosing recommendations not available

<20 kg: Initial: 0.25 mg/day; after ≥4 days may increase dose to 0.5 mg/day; maintain this dose for ≥14 days. In patients not achieving sufficient clinical response, may increase dose in increments of 0.25 mg/day at ≥2-week intervals. Therapeutic effect reached plateau at 1 mg/day in clinical trials. Following clinical response, consider gradually decreasing dose to lowest effective dose. May be administered once daily or in divided doses twice daily.

≥20 kg: Initial: 0.5 mg/day; after ≥4 days may increase dose to 1 mg/day; maintain this dose for ≥14 days. In patients not achieving sufficient clinical response, may increase dose in increments of 0.5 mg/day at ≥2-week intervals. Therapeutic effect reached plateau at 2.5 mg/day (3 mg/day in children >45 kg) in clinical trials. Following clinical response, consider gradually decreasing to lowest effective dose. May be administered once daily or in divided doses twice daily.

Note: See Additional Information for detailed information concerning doses used in studies to treat aggressive behavior and serious behavioral problems in pediatric patients with autism, pervasive developmental disorders, and other various psychiatric diagnoses.

Bipolar disorder: In a retrospective chart review, 28 patients 4-17 years of age (mean: 10.4 ± 3.8 years) were treated for bipolar disorder; risperidone doses were titrated as needed; optimal mean dose: 1.7 ± 1.3 mg/day; 82% of patients showed improvement in their manic and aggressive symptoms (Frazier 1999). Further studies are needed.

Schizophrenia: In a prospective, open-labeled pilot study, 10 patients 11-18 years of age (mean: 15.1 years) were treated for schizophrenia with initial doses of 1 mg twice daily; doses were increased as needed by 1 mg/day increments every 2 days up to a maximum of 10 mg/day and given twice daily; final dose: Range: 4-10 mg/day (0.05-0.17 mg/kg/day); mean: 6.6 mg/day (0.095 mg/kg/day) (Armenteros, 1997). In a retrospective study, 16 patients 9-20 years of age (mean 14.9 ± 2.73 years) were treated for psychotic disorders (13 with schizophrenia) with initial doses of 1 mg twice daily; doses were increased as needed by 1 mg increments every 3-4 days; optimal dose: 2-10 mg/day (mean 5.9 ± 2.8 mg/day) divided and given in 2-3 doses/day; 15 of 16 patients responded (Grcevich, 1996). Further studies are needed.

Tourette's syndrome: In a multicenter, double-blind, parallel-group comparative study, 50 patients 11-50 years of age were treated for Tourette's syndrome with risperidone (n=26; median age: 20 years; 10 patients <18 years of age) versus pimozide (n=24); a fixed-dose titration of risperidone from 0.5 mg/day to 2 mg/day was used for the first week of therapy; this was followed by a flexible dosing period of 7 weeks; doses were increased by ≤1 mg/week up to a maximum of 6 mg/day and were given once daily; final dose: 0.5-6 mg/day (mean: 3.8 mg/day); both drugs significantly improved tics; although there was no difference in efficacy between drugs, risperidone was better tolerated; the authors suggest that the average dose in this study is high compared to their clinical experience and that the fixed-dose titration during the first week may have been too rapid; a slower dosing schedule and lower long-term doses (eg, 1-2 mg/day) may be needed (Bruggeman, 2001).

Seven patients 11-16 years of age (mean: 12.9 ± 1.9 years) were treated in a prospective open-labeled trial for chronic tic disorders (5 with Tourette's syndrome) with initial doses of 0.5 mg at bedtime; doses were increased in 5 of the 7 patients by 0.5 mg/day increments every 5 days as tolerated to a maximum of 2.5 mg/day and given in twice daily doses (doses were increased more rapidly in 2 patients); final dose: 1-2.5 mg/day; a decrease in tic severity was seen in all patients; the authors recommend initial doses of 0.5 mg/day and increases of 0.5 mg/day every 5-7 days (Lombroso, 1995). In a retrospective review, 28 patients 5-18 years of age (mean 11.1 ± 3.6 years) with Tourette's syndrome and aggressive behavior were treated with risperidone; final dose: 0.5-9 mg/day (mean: 2 mg/day); a decrease in aggression scores occurred in 22 of 28 patients (78.5%); frequency and severity of tics were decreased in 17 patients (61.7%) (Sandor, 2000). Further studies are needed.

Adults: Oral: **Note:** Patients predisposed to hypotension or in whom hypotension would be a risk, and debilitated patients should use the dose listed below for renal or hepatic impairment; monitor carefully; debilitated patients should receive twice daily dosing for 2-3 days at the target dose before switching to once daily dosing.

(Continued)

Risperidone *(Continued)*

Schizophrenia: Initial: 1 mg twice daily; increase (as tolerated) in increments of 1 mg twice daily on day 2 and 3, to a target dose of 3 mg twice daily by day 3; slower titration may be required in some patients; doses up to 8 mg once daily have also been shown to be safe and effective; if needed, further changes may be made at intervals of ≥7 days, in small increments or decrements of 1-2 mg; maximal effect: 4-8 mg/day; for twice daily dosing, doses >6 mg/day did not appear to be more effective than lower doses and were associated with more adverse effects (eg, extrapyramidal symptoms); doses >3 mg twice daily are generally not recommended; safety of doses >16 mg/day has not been assessed. Use lowest effective dose; reassess periodically for continued need.

Maintenance therapy: A long-term controlled trial in patients who were clinically stable for at least 4 weeks on antipsychotic medication used initial risperidone doses of 1 mg once daily; doses were increased to 2 mg once daily on day 2, and to a target dose of 4 mg once daily on day 3; maximum dose: 8 mg/day; patients were observed for relapse for 1-2 years; risperidone patients had a significantly longer time to relapse versus the comparator drug

Bipolar mania: Initial: 2-3 mg/dose once daily; adjust dose as needed, by 1 mg/day increments at intervals ≥24 hours; dosing range: 1-6 mg/day

Adults: I.M.: **Schizophrenia:** 25 mg every 2 weeks; some patients may benefit from larger doses; maximum dose: 50 mg every 2 weeks; do **not** increase dose more often than every 4 weeks

Note: Oral risperidone (or other antipsychotic) should be administered with the initial I.M. injection and continued for 3 weeks (then discontinued) to maintain adequate therapeutic plasma concentrations before the main release phase of risperidone from the injection site (see Pharmacokinetics, Absorption). When switching from depot administration to short-acting formulation, administer short-acting agent in place of the next regularly-scheduled depot injection.

Dosing adjustment in renal or hepatic impairment: Adults: Oral: Initial: 0.5 mg twice daily; increase (as tolerated) in increments of ≤0.5 mg twice daily; increases above 1.5 mg twice daily should be made at intervals of ≥7 days; slower titration may be required in some patients

Administration

Oral: May be administered without regard to meals.

Oral solution: May mix with water, coffee, orange juice, or low-fat milk; do not mix with cola or tea

Orally-disintegrating tablets: Do not remove tablet from blister pack until ready to administer; do not push tablet through foil (tablet may become damaged); peel back foil to expose tablet; use dry hands to remove tablet and place immediately on tongue; tablet will dissolve within seconds and may be swallowed with or without liquid; do not split or chew tablet

I.M.: Before reconstitution, bring injection and diluent to room temperature; reconstitute with provided diluent only; shake vial vigorously for a minimum of 10 seconds to properly mix; suspension should appear thick, milky, and uniform; use immediately (or within 6 hours of reconstitution); if suspension settles prior to use, shake vigorously to resuspend

Adults: Administer I.M. into the upper-outer quadrant of the gluteal area; **do not administer I.V.;** alternate injection site between two buttocks; do not combine 2 different dosage strengths into one single administration; administer with needle provided; do not substitute any components of the dose pack

Monitoring Parameters Orthostatic blood pressure and heart rate, especially during dosage titration; weight and growth, especially in children; liver enzymes in children (especially obese children or those who are rapidly gaining weight while receiving therapy); lipid profile; serum glucose; fasting blood glucose at the beginning of therapy and periodically in patients with diabetes mellitus (or with risk factors such as family history or obesity); fasting blood glucose in patients who develop symptoms of hyperglycemia

Patient Information May cause dizziness or drowsiness and impair ability to perform activities requiring mental alertness or physical coordination; may cause dry mouth; may cause postural hypotension, especially during initial dose titration (use caution when changing position from lying or sitting to standing). May cause photosensitivity reactions (eg, exposure to sunlight may cause severe sunburn, skin rash, redness, or itching); avoid exposure to sunlight and artificial light sources (sunlamps, tanning booth/bed); wear protective clothing, wide-brimmed hats, sunglasses, and lip sunscreen (SPF ≥15); use a sunscreen [broad-spectrum sunscreen or physical sunscreen (preferred) or sunblock with SPF ≥15]; contact physician if reaction occurs. Report the use of other medications, nonprescription medications and herbal or natural products to your physician and pharmacist; avoid alcohol and the herbal medicine, St John's wort. Report persistent CNS effects (eg, trembling fingers, altered gait or balance, excessive sedation, seizures, unusual muscle or skeletal movements), rapid heartbeat, palpitations, severe dizziness, fainting, swelling or pain in breasts (male and female), altered menstrual pattern, changes in urinary patterns, vision changes, skin rash, difficulty breathing, or worsening of condition to your physician

Nursing Implications May need to assist patient in rising slowly from lying or sitting to standing position [orthostatic blood pressure changes, tachycardia and syncope (rare) may occur (see Warnings and Monitoring Parameters)]

Additional Information Long-term usefulness of risperidone should be periodically re-evaluated in patients receiving the drug for extended periods of time. Risperdal® Consta® is a long-acting injection comprised of an extended release microsphere formulation; prior to injection, the microspheres are suspended in the provided diluent; the small polymeric microspheres degrade slowly, releasing the medication at a controlled rate (see Pharmacokinetics, Absorption). Lactating women receiving oral risperidone should **not** breast-feed an infant; lactating women receiving I.M. risperidone should **not** breast-feed an infant during therapy and for at least 12 weeks after her last injection.

Additional detailed risperidone dosing information for Children and Adolescents: Oral:

Aggressive behavior in patients with various psychiatric diagnoses: In a randomized, double-blind, placebo-controlled study, 10 patients 6-14 years of age (mean: 9.2 ± 2.9 years) with conduct disorder and prominent aggressive behavior received risperidone in the following doses: Patients <50 kg: Initial: 0.25 mg once daily; doses were increased as needed by 0.25 mg/day increments each week to a maximum of 1.5 mg/day; patients ≥50 kg: Initial: 0.5 mg once daily; doses were increased as needed by 0.5 mg/day increments each week to a maximum of 3 mg/day; doses were given once daily in the morning; 6 of 10 patients completed the 10-week study; final dose: 0.75-1.5 mg/day; mean: 0.028 ± 0.004 mg/kg/day; risperidone was more effective than placebo in decreasing aggressive behavior (Findling, 2000). In another randomized, double-blind, placebo-controlled study, 19 adolescents (mean age: 14 ± 1.5 years; 7 with borderline IQ and 6 with mild mental retardation) who were hospitalized for treatment of psychiatric disorders associated with aggressive behavior, received initial risperidone doses of 0.5 mg twice daily; doses were increased as needed by 1 mg/day increments up to a planned maximum of 5 mg twice daily; final doses: Range: 1.5-4 mg/day (0.019-0.08 mg/kg/day); mean: 2.9 mg/day (0.044 mg/kg/day); risperidone was more effective than placebo in decreasing aggressive behavior; although the initial dose was well tolerated by all patients, the authors recommend the following initial doses for clinical practice: Patients <25 kg: 0.25 mg/day; patients ≥25 kg: 0.5 mg/day (Buitelaar, 2001).

In an open trial, 26 patients 10-18 years of age (mean: 15 ± 1.9 years) with a borderline IQ (n=19) or mild mental retardation (n=5), who were hospitalized for treatment of psychiatric disorders associated with aggressive behavior, received initial risperidone doses of 0.5 mg/day; doses were increased by 0.5-1 mg/day increments every 3 days up to a planned maximum of 6 mg/day and given in twice daily doses; final dose: 0.5-4 mg/day; mean: 2.1 ± 1 mg/day; a marked reduction in aggressive behavior was observed in 14 of 26 patients (54%); **Note:** Four subjects who discontinued therapy after 8 weeks received higher doses (mean: 3.3 ± 1 mg/day) than those who continued on medication (mean: 1.9 ± 0.9 mg/day) (Buitelaar, 2000). Eleven patients 5.5-16 years of age (mean: 9.8 years) with mood disorders and aggressive behavior received risperidone in titrated doses in an open trial; final dose: 0.75-2.5 mg/day given in 2-3 divided doses; a decrease in aggressive behavior was observed in 8 of 11 patients (Schreier, 1998).

Autism and pervasive developmental disorders (PDDs): A recent multicenter double-blind, placebo-controlled trial in patients 5-17 years of age (mean: 8.8 ± 2.7 years) with autism and serious behavioral problems demonstrated the short-term efficacy of risperidone for the treatment of aggression, tantrums, or self-injurious behavior. The following doses were used: Children 15-20 kg: Initial: 0.25 mg/day. Children 20-45 kg: Initial: 0.5 mg at bedtime on days 1-3 and 0.5 mg twice daily on day 4; dose was gradually increased in 0.5 mg increments to a maximum dose of 2.5 mg/day (given as 1 mg in the morning and 1.5 mg at bedtime) by day 29. Children >45 kg: A "slightly accelerated dose schedule" was used; maximum dose: 3.5 mg/day (given as 1.5 mg in the morning and 2 mg at bedtime). Doses were titrated to effect; mean effective dose: 1.8 ± 0.7 mg/day (range: 0.5-3.5 mg/day). **Note:** This study did **not** identify the minimal effective dose (McCraken, 2002).

In an open-labeled prospective study, 10 boys 4.5-10.8 years of age (mean: 7.2 ± 2.2 years) with autistic disorder were started on risperidone 0.5 mg/day; doses were titrated as needed by increments of ≤0.5 mg/day at intervals of ≥7 days; final dose (at 12 weeks): Range: 1-2.5 mg/day (0.03-0.08 mg/kg/day); mean: 1.3 ± 0.5 mg/day (0.05 ± 0.2 mg/kg/day); 8 of 10 children responded (Nicolson,

(Continued)

Risperidone *(Continued)*

1998). In an open clinical trial, 6 children 5-9 years of age (mean: 7.33 years) with autistic disorder were started on risperidone monotherapy 0.25 mg at bedtime; doses were titrated as needed by 0.25 mg increments at intervals of ≥7 days and dosed twice daily; final doses (at week 8): Range: 0.75-1.5 mg/day (0.03-0.06 mg/kg/day); mean: 1.1 mg (0.04 mg/kg/day); improvement was noted in all 6 patients (Findling, 1997).

In a prospective open-labeled study, 18 patients 5-18 years of age (mean 10.2 ± 3.7 years) were treated for PDDs (11 with autistic disorder) with initial doses of 0.5 mg at night; doses were increased as needed by 0.5 mg/day increments every week and dosed twice daily; optimal dose: 1-4 mg/day (mean: 1.8 ± 1 mg/day); 12 of 18 patients responded (McDougle, 1997). Fourteen patients 9-17 years of age (mean: 12.7 ± 4 years) were treated in an open case series, for PDDs (4 with autistic disorder) with initial doses of 0.25 mg twice daily; doses were increased as needed by 0.25 mg/day increments every 5-7 days; optimal dose: 0.75-1.5 mg/day given in divided doses; 13 of 14 patients showed a beneficial response (Fisman, 1996). In an open trial, 6 patients 7-14 years of age (mean: 10.7 ± 3.3 years) were treated for PDDs (5 with autistic disorder; all 6 with severe behavioral problems) with initial doses of 0.5 mg once or twice daily; doses were increased as needed by 0.5 mg/day increments every few days; optimal dose: 1-6 mg/day (mean 2.7 ± 2.2 mg/day); significant benefit was seen in 5 of the 6 patients (Perry, 1997). Twenty patients (age: 8-17 years) with developmental disorders refractory to previous psychotropic agents were treated in an open clinical trial with risperidone; doses were increased as needed slowly over several weeks; final doses (n=20): 1.5-10 mg/day; responders (n=13): 1-4 mg/day; nonresponders: 4.5-10 mg/day (Hardan, 1996). Further studies are needed.

Dosage Forms Excipient information presented when available (limited, particularly for generics); consult specific product labeling.

Injection, microspheres for reconstitution, extended release:

Risperdal® Consta®: 25 mg, 37.5 mg, 50 mg [supplied in a dose-pack containing vial with active ingredient in microsphere formulation, prefilled syringe with diluent, needle-free vial access device, and safety needle]

Solution, oral:

Risperdal®: 1 mg/mL (30 mL) [contains benzoic acid]

Tablet:

Risperdal®: 0.25 mg, 0.5 mg, 1 mg, 2 mg, 3 mg, 4 mg

Tablet, orally disintegrating:

Risperdal® M-Tabs®: 0.5 mg [contains phenylalanine 0.14 mg]; 1 mg [contains phenylalanine 0.28 mg]; 2 mg [contains phenylalanine 0.42 mg]; 3 mg [contains phenylalanine 0.63 mg]; 4 mg [contains phenylalanine 0.84 mg]

References

American Diabetes Association, American Psychiatric Association, American Association of Clinical Endocrinologists, and North American Association for the Study of Obesity, "Consensus Development Conference on Antipsychotic Drugs and Obesity and Diabetes," *Diabetes Care*, 2004, 27(2):596-601.

Armenteros JL, Whitaker AH, Welikson M, et al, "Risperidone in Adolescents With Schizophrenia: An Open Pilot Study," *J Am Acad Child Adolesc Psychiatry*, 1997, 36(5):694-700.

Bruggeman R, van der Linden C, Buitelaar JK, et al, "Risperidone Versus Pimozide in Tourette's Disorder: A Comparative Double-Blind Parallel-Group Study," *J Clin Psychiatry*, 2001, 62(1):50-6.

Buitelaar JK, "Open-Label Treatment With Risperidone of 26 Psychiatrically-Hospitalized Children and Adolescents With Mixed Diagnoses and Aggressive Behavior," *J Child Adolesc Psychopharmacol*, 2000, 10(1):19-26.

Buitelaar JK, van der Gaag RJ, Cohen-Kettenis P, et al, "A Randomized Controlled Trial of Risperidone in the Treatment of Aggression in Hospitalized Adolescents With Subaverage Cognitive Abilities," *J Clin Psychiatry*, 2001, 62(4):239-48.

Findling RL, Maxwell K, and Wiznitzer M, "An Open Clinical Trial of Risperidone Monotherapy in Young Children With Autistic Disorder," *Psychopharmacol Bull*, 1997, 33(1):155-9.

Findling RL, McNamara NK, Branicky LA, et al, "A Double-Blind Pilot Study of Risperidone in the Treatment of Conduct Disorder," *J Am Acad Child Adolesc Psychiatry*, 2000, 39(4):509-16.

Fisman S and Steele M, "Use of Risperidone in Pervasive Developmental Disorders: A Case Series," *J Child Adolesc Psychopharmacol*, 1996, 6(3):177-90.

Frazier JA, Meyer MC, Biederman J, et al, "Risperidone Treatment for Juvenile Bipolar Disorder: A Retrospective Chart Review," *J Am Acad Child Adolesc Psychiatry*, 1999, 38(8):960-5.

Grcevich SJ, Findling RL, Rowane WA, et al, "Risperidone in the Treatment of Children and Adolescents With Schizophrenia: A Retrospective Study," *J Child Adolesc Psychopharmacol*, 1996, 6(4):251-7.

Hardan A, Johnson K, Johnson C, et al, "Case Study: Risperidone Treatment of Children and Adolescents With Developmental Disorders," *J Am Acad Child Adolesc Psychiatry*, 1996, 35(11):1551-6.

Hill RC, McIvor RJ, Wojnar-Horton RE, et al, "Risperidone Distribution and Excretion Into Human Milk: Case Report and Estimated Infant Exposure During Breast-Feeding," *J Clin Psychopharmacol*, 2000, 20(2):285-6.

Kumra S, Herion D, Jacobsen LK, et al, "Case Study: Risperidone-Induced Hepatotoxicity in Pediatric Patients," *J Am Acad Child Adolesc Psychiatry*, 1997, 36(5):701-5.

Lombroso PJ, Scahill L, King RA, et al, "Risperidone Treatment of Children and Adolescents With Chronic Tic Disorders: A Preliminary Report," *J Am Acad Child Adolesc Psychiatry*, 1995, 34(9):1147-52.

McCracken JT, McGough J, Shah B, et al, "Risperidone in Children With Autism and Serious Behavioral Problems," *N Engl J Med*, 2002, 347(5):314-21.

McDougle CJ, Holmes JP, Bronson MR, et al, "Risperidone Treatment of Children and Adolescents With Pervasive Developmental Disorders: A Prospective Open-Label Study," *J Am Acad Child Adolesc Psychiatry*, 1997, 36(5):685-93.

McDougle CJ, Scahill L, McCracken JT, et al, "Research Units on Pediatric Psychopharmacology (RUPP) Autism Network. Background and Rationale for an Initial Controlled Study of Risperidone," *Child Adolesc Psychiatr Clin N Am*, 2000, 9(1):201-24.

Nicolson R, Awad G, and Sloman L, "An Open Trial of Risperidone in Young Autistic Children," *J Am Acad Child Adolesc Psychiatry*, 1998, 37(4):372-6.

Perry R, Pataki C, Munoz-Silva DM, et al, "Risperidone in Children and Adolescents With Pervasive Developmental Disorder: Pilot Trial and Follow-Up," *J Child Adolesc Psychopharmacol*, 1997, 7(3):167-79.

Sandor P and Stephens RJ, "Risperidone Treatment of Aggressive Behavior in Children With Tourette Syndrome," *J Clin Psychopharmacol*, 2000, 20(6):710-2.

Schreier HA, "Risperidone for Young Children With Mood Disorders and Aggressive Behavior," *J Child Adolesc Psychopharmacol*, 1998, 8(1):49-59.

♦ **Ritalin®** *see* Methylphenidate *on page 1034*

♦ **Ritalin® LA** *see* Methylphenidate *on page 1034*

♦ **Ritalin-SR®** *see* Methylphenidate *on page 1034*

♦ **Ritalin® SR (Can)** *see* Methylphenidate *on page 1034*

Ritonavir (rit ON uh veer)

Medication Safety Issues

Sound-alike/look-alike issues:

Ritonavir may be confused with Retrovir®

Norvir® may be confused with Norvasc®

Related Information

Adult and Adolescent HIV *on page 1821*

Pediatric HIV *on page 1816*

Perinatal HIV *on page 1831*

U.S. Brand Names Norvir®

Canadian Brand Names Norvir®; Norvir® SEC

Therapeutic Category Antiretroviral Agent; HIV Agents (Anti-HIV Agents); Protease Inhibitor

Generic Available No

Use Treatment of HIV infection in combination with other antiretroviral agents. (**Note:** HIV regimens consisting of **three** antiretroviral agents are strongly recommended)

Pregnancy Risk Factor B

Lactation Excretion in breast milk unknown/contraindicated

Contraindications Hypersensitivity to ritonavir or any component; concurrent therapy with alfuzosin, amiodarone, astemizole, bepridil, cisapride, dihydroergotamine, ergotamine, ergonovine, methylergonovine, flecainide, pimozide, propafenone, quinidine, terfenadine, midazolam, triazolam; concurrent therapy with voriconazole when using therapeutic doses of ritonavir (see Drug Interactions)

Warnings Ritonavir is a potent CYP3A enzyme inhibitor that interacts with numerous drugs. Due to potential serious and/or life-threatening drug interactions, some drugs are contraindicated (see Contraindications and Drug Interactions). Concurrent use with St John's wort or certain cholesterol-lowering agents (lovastatin, simvastatin) is **not** recommended. Alteration of dose or serum concentration monitoring may be required with other medications (see Drug Interactions).

Potentially fatal pancreatitis may occur; advanced HIV disease and elevated serum triglycerides may place patient at increased risk; discontinue ritonavir in patients with pancreatitis. Hepatic reactions, including elevated liver enzymes, hepatitis, and jaundice may occur; coinfection with hepatitis B or C may increase risk; hepatic dysfunction with fatalities has also been reported. Significant elevations of serum triglycerides and cholesterol may occur (monitor and manage appropriately). Allergic reactions may also occur (see Adverse Reactions).

New onset diabetes mellitus, exacerbation of diabetes, and hyperglycemia have been reported in HIV-infected patients receiving protease inhibitors.

Precautions Use with caution in patients with hepatic insufficiency, elevated liver enzymes, or hepatitis. Spontaneous bleeding episodes have been reported in patients with hemophilia type A and B receiving protease inhibitors. Fat redistribution and accumulation [ie, central obesity, peripheral wasting, facial wasting, breast enlargement, dorsocervical fat enlargement (buffalo hump), and cushingoid appearance] have been observed in patients receiving antiretroviral agents (causal relationship not established). Immune reconstitution syndrome (an acute inflammatory response to residual or indolent opportunistic infections) may occur in HIV patients during initial treatment with combination antiretroviral agents, including ritonavir; this syndrome may require further patient assessment and therapy. Ritonavir oral solution contains 43% alcohol by volume; accidental ingestion could result in alcohol-related

(Continued)

Ritonavir *(Continued)*

toxicity. Safety and efficacy of ritonavir in patients <1 month of age have not been established.

Adverse Reactions Note: In pediatric clinical trials, adverse event profiles were similar to adults.

Central nervous system: Headache, confusion

Endocrine & metabolic: Elevated triglycerides and cholesterol, elevated creatine phosphokinase; rare: hyperglycemia, diabetes, ketoacidosis; fat redistribution and accumulation (see Precautions)

Gastrointestinal: Nausea, vomiting, diarrhea, taste perversion, abdominal pain, anorexia, pancreatitis

Hematologic: Rare: Spontaneous bleeding episodes in hemophiliacs

Hepatic: Elevated liver enzymes, hepatitis (may be life-threatening in rare cases)

Neuromuscular & skeletal: Circumoral and peripheral paresthesias, weakness

Miscellaneous: Allergic reaction (urticaria, rash, bronchospasm, angioedema); immune reconstitution syndrome (see Precautions)

Drug Interactions Cytochrome P450 isoenzyme CYP1A2, CYP2B6, CYP2D6, and CYP3A3/4 substrate; isoenzyme CYP1A2, CYP2C9, and CYP3A4 inducer; isoenzyme CYP2C9, CYP2C19, CYP2D6, CYP2E1, and CYP3A3/4 inhibitor; also induces glucuronidation

Ritonavir may inhibit the metabolism of the following drugs and cause serious or life-threatening adverse effects: Alfuzosin, amiodarone, astemizole, bepridil, cisapride, dihydroergotamine, ergonovine, ergotamine, flecainide, methylergonovine, midazolam, pimozide, propafenone, quinidine, terfenadine, and triazolam (concurrent therapy with these drugs and indinavir is contraindicated). Ritonavir may significantly decrease serum concentrations of voriconazole [use of voriconazole is contraindicated when using therapeutic doses of ritonavir; use of voriconazole with low-dose ritonavir (booster doses) should be avoided, unless benefits outweigh risks of reduced voriconazole levels].

Ritonavir increases serum concentrations or toxic effects of: Meperidine (normeperidine concentrations are increased; long-term use or increased doses of meperidine are not recommended); warfarin (monitor anticoagulant effect); desipramine (use reduced dose of desipramine; monitor serum concentrations); trazodone (use reduced dose of trazodone); ketoconazole (high dose ketoconazole is not recommended); clarithromycin (decrease clarithromycin dosage in patients with renal impairment); rifabutin and rifabutin metabolite (rifabutin dose should be decreased by at least 75% of the normal dose; further reduction in dosage may be needed; monitor closely for adverse effects); cholesterol-lowering agents (increased risk of myopathy and rhabdomyolysis; concurrent use of lovastatin or simvastatin is **not** recommended; use lowest possible dose of atorvastatin and carefully monitor patient; consider use of pravastatin or fluvastatin for concurrent use with ritonavir); sildenafil or other phosphodiesterase-5 (PDE-5) enzyme inhibitors (use decreased dose of sildenafil or other PDE-5 enzyme inhibitor). Ritonavir significantly increases fluticasone serum concentrations and may result in systemic corticosteroid effects (eg, Cushing's syndrome and adrenal suppression); concurrent use of ritonavir and fluticasone is not recommended unless benefits outweigh risks. Ritonavir increases serum concentrations of indinavir and saquinavir (dosage adjustment is recommended).

Ritonavir may increase the serum concentration or adverse effects of the following drugs (use with caution; a reduced dose of these drugs may be needed; monitor therapeutic serum drug concentrations of these agents, if available): Atorvastatin, bupropion, buspirone, carbamazepine, clonazepam, clorazepate, cyclosporine, diazepam, digoxin, diltiazem, disopyramide, dexamethasone, dronabinol, estazolam, ethosuximide, flurazepam, itraconazole, lidocaine, methamphetamine, metoprolol, mexiletine, nefazodone, nifedipine, perphenazine, prednisone, propoxyphene, quinine, risperidone, sirolimus, SSRIs, tacrolimus, TCAs, thioridazine, timolol, tramadol, verapamil, zolpidem.

Ritonavir significantly decreases serum concentrations of theophylline (monitor theophylline levels; increased theophylline dose may be needed); methadone (increased methadone dose may be required); ethinyl estradiol, oral or transdermal contraceptives (use additional or alternative contraceptive measures). Ritonavir may decrease concentrations of phenytoin, valproic acid, lamotrigine, atovaquone (use with caution; an increased dose of these drugs may be needed).

The herbal medicine St John's wort (*Hypericum perforatum*) may significantly decrease concentrations of ritonavir and lead to treatment failure; concurrent use is **not** recommended. Rifampin significantly reduces ritonavir concentrations and may lead to treatment failure (consider alternative antimycobacterial agent, such as rifabutin). The combined use of saquinavir plus ritonavir and rifampin significantly increases the risk of severe hepatotoxicity (avoid use). Delavirdine may significantly increase ritonavir serum concentrations (appropriate doses not established).

Ritonavir formulations contain alcohol and may produce disulfiram-like reaction when coadministered with disulfiram or metronidazole. Use of ritonavir with fluoxetine may result in serotonin syndrome. Coadministration with didanosine will result in a 13% decrease in didanosine AUC (doses of didanosine and ritonavir should be spaced 2.5 hours apart).

Stability Avoid exposure to excessive heat or cold

Capsules: Refrigerate; stable for 30 days at room temperature <77°F (25°C); protect from light

Oral solution: Dispense and store in original container; store at room temperature; do not refrigerate; keep bottle tightly closed; use by product expiration date (limited shelf life of 6 months)

Mechanism of Action A protease inhibitor which acts on an enzyme (protease) late in the HIV replication process after the virus has entered into the cell's nucleus; ritonavir binds to the protease activity site and inhibits the activity of the enzyme, thus preventing cleavage of viral polyprotein precursors (gag-pol protein precursors) into individual functional proteins found in infectious HIV; this results in the formation of immature, noninfectious viral particles

Pharmacokinetics

Absorption: Well absorbed

Distribution: High concentrations in serum and lymph nodes

Protein binding: 98% to 99%

Metabolism: In the liver by cytochrome P450 isoenzyme CYP3A and (to a lesser extent) CYP2D6; five metabolites have been identified; the major metabolite (M-2), an isopropylthiazole oxidation metabolite, is active at a level similar to ritonavir, but is found in low concentrations in the plasma

Half-life:

Children: 2-4 hours

Adults: 3-5 hours

Time to peak serum concentration: 2-4 hours

Elimination: Renal clearance is negligible; 3.5% of dose is excreted as unchanged drug in the urine; 34% excreted as unchanged drug in the feces

Clearance: Pediatric patients: 1.5 to 1.7 times faster than adults

Usual Dosage Oral (use in combination with other antiretroviral agents):

Neonates: Not approved for use; further studies are needed

Infants >1 month and Children: Initial: 250 mg/m^2/dose twice daily (every 12 hours); titrate upward at 2-3 day intervals by 50 mg/m^2/dose twice daily increments to 350-400 mg/m^2/dose twice daily; maximum dose: 600 mg/dose twice daily; **Note:** Patients who do not tolerate 400 mg/m^2 twice daily (due to adverse effects) may be treated with the highest tolerated dose; however, an alternative antiretroviral agent should be considered. Serum concentrations comparable to those seen in adults receiving standard doses were obtained in children >2 years of age who received 350-400 mg/m^2 twice daily. In younger patients (1 month to 2 years of age), who received 350 or 450 mg/m^2/dose twice daily, ritonavir AUCs were 16% lower and trough concentrations were 60% lower than those observed in adults receiving standard doses; higher ritonavir AUCs were not observed with the 450 mg/m^2/dose twice daily compared to the 350 mg/m^2/dose twice daily dosing.

Adolescents and Adults: 600 mg twice daily; may use a dose titration schedule to reduce adverse events (nausea/vomiting) by initiating therapy at 300 mg twice daily; increase dose at 2-3 day intervals by 100 mg twice daily increments up to a maximum dose of 600 mg twice daily

Adults:

Concomitant therapy with saquinavir: Ritonavir 400 mg twice daily with saquinavir 400 mg twice daily; **Note:** Although the optimum dose of ritonavir with saquinavir has not be established, ritonavir 400 mg twice daily was better tolerated than 600 mg twice daily with saquinavir

Pharmacokinetic enhancer ("booster doses" of ritonavir): Ritonavir is used at lower doses to increase the serum concentrations of other protease inhibitors; usual dose: 100 mg twice daily or 200 mg once daily; range: 100-400 mg twice daily has been used in combination with other protease inhibitors; see monographs for individual protease inhibitors for recommended doses. **Note:** Appropriate pediatric "booster doses" of ritonavir have not been established.

Dosage adjustment in renal impairment: No adjustment recommended (renal clearance is negligible)

Dosage adjustment in hepatic impairment:

Mild to moderate hepatic impairment: No adjustment recommended; lower ritonavir serum concentrations have been reported in patients with moderate hepatic impairment (use with caution; monitor closely for adequate response)

(Continued)

Ritonavir *(Continued)*

Severe hepatic impairment: Use with caution; pharmacokinetics of ritonavir has not been studied in these patients

Administration Administer with food to increase absorption; consider reserving liquid formulation for use in patients receiving tube feeding due to its bad taste. Shake liquid well before use. May mix liquid formulation with milk, chocolate milk, vanilla or chocolate pudding or ice cream, or a liquid nutritional supplement. Other techniques used to increase tolerance in children include dulling the taste buds by chewing ice, giving popsicles or spoonfuls or partially frozen orange or grape juice concentrates before administration of ritonavir; coating the mouth with peanut butter to eat before the dose; administration of strong-tasting foods such as maple syrup, cheese, or strong-flavored chewing gum immediately after a dose.

Monitoring Parameters Liver function tests, blood glucose levels, serum triglycerides, cholesterol, CPK, uric acid, CD4 cell count, plasma levels of HIV RNA

Patient Information Ritonavir is not a cure for HIV. Some medicines should not be taken with ritonavir; report the use of other medications, nonprescription medications, and herbal or natural products to your physician and pharmacist; avoid the herbal medicine St John's wort. Take ritonavir every day as prescribed; do not change dose or discontinue without physician's advice; if dose is missed, take it as soon as possible, then return to normal dosing schedule; if a dose is skipped, do not double the next dose. Notify physician if you have an increase in thirst and/or frequent urination, nausea, vomiting, or abdominal pain

HIV medications may cause changes in body fat, including an increase in fat in the upper back and neck, breasts, and trunk; a loss of fat from the face, arms, and legs may also occur.

Nursing Implications Ritonavir is started at lower initial doses and titrated upwards to minimize nausea and vomiting.

Dosage Forms Excipient information presented when available (limited, particularly for generics); consult specific product labeling.

Capsule: 100 mg [contains ethanol and polyoxyl 35 castor oil]

Solution: 80 mg/mL (240 mL) [contains ethanol and polyoxyl 35 castor oil; peppermint and caramel flavor]

References

Briars LA, Hilao JJ, and Kraus DM, "A Review of Pediatric Human Immunodeficiency Virus Infection," *Journal of Pharmacy Practice*, 2004, 17(6):407-31.

Danner SA, Carr A, Leonard JM, et al, "A Short-Term Study of the Safety, Pharmacokinetics, and Efficacy of Ritonavir, an Inhibitor of HIV-1 Protease. European-Australian Collaborative Ritonavir Study Group," *N Engl J Med*, 1995, 333(23):1528-33.

DeSilva KE, Le Flore DB, Marston BJ, et al, "Serotonin Syndrome in HIV-Infected Individuals Receiving Antiretroviral Therapy and Fluoxetine," *AIDS*, 2001, 15(10)1281-5.

Gatti G, Pontali E, Boni S, et al, "The Relationship Between Ritonavir Plasma Trough Concentration and Virological and Immunological Response in HIV-Infected Children," *HIV Med*, 2002, 3(2):125-8.

Mueller BU, Nelson RP Jr, Sleasman J, et al, "A Phase I/II Study of the Protease Inhibitor Ritonavir in Children With Human Immunodeficiency Virus Infection," *Pediatrics*, 1998, 101(3 Pt 1):335-43.

Nachman SA, Lindsey JC, Pelton S, et al, "Growth in Human Immunodeficiency Virus-Infected Children Receiving Ritonavir-Containing Antiretroviral Therapy," *Arch Pediatr Adolesc Med*, 2002, 156(5):497-503.

Nachman SA, Stanley K, Yogev R, et al, "Nucleoside Analogs Plus Ritonavir in Stable Antiretroviral Therapy-Experienced HIV-Infected Children: A Randomized Controlled Trial. Pediatric AIDS Clinical Trials Group 338 Study Team," *JAMA*, 2000, 283(4):492-8.

Panel on Clinical Practices for Treatment of HIV Infection, "Guidelines for the Use of Antiretroviral Agents in HIV-Infected Adults and Adolescents," October 10, 2006, http://www.aidsinfo.nih.gov.

Working Group on Antiretroviral Therapy and Medical Management of HIV-Infected Children, "Guidelines for the Use of Antiretroviral Agents in Pediatric HIV Infection," October 26, 2006, http://www.aidsinfo.nih.gov.

♦ **Ritonavir and Lopinavir** *see* Lopinavir and Ritonavir *on page 954*

♦ **Rituxan®** *see* Rituximab *on page 1398*

Rituximab (ri TUK si mab)

Medication Safety Issues

Sound-alike/look-alike issues:

Rituxan® may be confused with Remicade®

Rituximab may be confused with infliximab

High alert medication: The Institute for Safe Medication Practices (ISMP) includes this medication among its list of drugs which have a heightened risk of causing significant patient harm when used in error.

The rituximab dose for rheumatoid arthritis is a flat dose (1000 mg) and is not based on body surface area (BSA).

U.S. Brand Names Rituxan®

Canadian Brand Names Rituxan®

Index Terms Anti-CD20 Monoclonal Antibody; C2B8; C2B8 Monoclonal Antibody; IDEC-C2B8; NSC-687451; Pan-B Antibody

Therapeutic Category Antineoplastic Agent, Monoclonal Antibody; Monoclonal Antibody

Generic Available No

Use Treatment of relapsed or refractory low-grade or follicular, CD20 positive, B-cell non-Hodgkin's lymphoma; first-line treatment of diffuse large B-cell, CD20-positive, non-Hodgkin's lymphoma in combination with CHOP or other anthracycline-based chemotherapy regimen; systemic autoimmune disorders (ie, autoimmune hemolytic anemia); post-transplant lymphoproliferative disorder (PTLD); rheumatoid arthritis

Pregnancy Risk Factor C

Lactation Excretion in breast milk unknown/not recommended

Contraindications Hypersensitivity to rituximab, murine proteins, or any component; breast-feeding

Warnings Two deaths have been reported in patients being treated with rituximab for systemic lupus erythematosus (SLE). Cause of death was due to progressive multifocal leukoencephalopathy (PML) that is caused by reactivated JC virus which is present in ~80% of adults. Patients who develop new neurological signs or symptoms should be evaluated for PML.

Fatal infusion reactions which may include hypotension, angioedema, hypoxia, bronchospasm, pulmonary infiltrates, acute respiratory distress syndrome, MI, ventricular fibrillation, and cardiogenic shock have occurred within 24 hours of rituximab administration. Eighty percent of these reactions occurred during the first infusion with time to onset of 30-120 minutes. Fatal infusion reactions were more frequently associated with female gender, pulmonary infiltrates, CLL, or mantle cell lymphoma. Close monitoring required during first and subsequent infusions of patients with pre-existing cardiac and pulmonary conditions, patients with prior cardiopulmonary adverse events, and those with high levels of circulating malignant cells ($\geq$25,000/mm^3). In the event of a severe reaction, interrupt the rituximab infusion and institute supportive care measures (eg, I.V. fluids, vasopressors, oxygen, bronchodilators, diphenhydramine and acetaminophen). When symptoms completely resolve, may resume rituximab at a 50% reduction from the previous infusion rate. Discontinue rituximab in the event of serious or life-threatening cardiac arrhythmias.

Tumor lysis syndrome which may include hyperkalemia, hypocalcemia, hyperuricemia, hyperphosphatemia, and acute renal failure requiring dialysis has been reported within 12-24 hours after the first rituximab infusion. Prophylaxis for tumor lysis syndrome should be considered for patients at risk (patients with high tumor burden or with high numbers of circulating malignant cells). Severe mucocutaneous reactions which include paraneoplastic pemphigus, Stevens-Johnson syndrome, lichenoid dermatitis, vesiculobullous dermatitis, and toxic epidermal necrolysis have been reported to occur 1-13 weeks following rituximab exposure. Bowel obstruction and perforation have been reported; complaints of abdominal pain should be evaluated.

Postmarketing reports of hepatitis B virus (HBV) reactivation with fulminant hepatitis, hepatic failure, and death have occurred ~4 months after the initiation of rituximab in some patients with hematologic malignancies. Prior to initiating rituximab, screen patients for HBV infection. Monitor carriers of hepatitis B for clinical and laboratory signs of active HBV infection and hepatitis during and for several months following rituximab therapy. Discontinue rituximab and initiate appropriate antiviral therapy in patients who develop viral hepatitis.

Precautions Use with caution in patients with pre-existing cardiac or pulmonary conditions, renal impairment, and patients at risk for developing tumor lysis syndrome.

Adverse Reactions

Cardiovascular: Hypotension, angina, arrhythmia, MI, peripheral edema, flushing, syncope, cardiogenic shock

Central nervous system: Fever, chills, headache, dizziness, anxiety

Dermatologic: Angioedema, pruritus, rash, urticaria, Stevens-Johnson syndrome, toxic epidermal necrolysis

Endocrine & metabolic: Hyperglycemia, tumor lysis syndrome

Gastrointestinal: Nausea, vomiting, abdominal pain, diarrhea, bowel obstruction and perforation

Hematologic: Lymphopenia, leukopenia, thrombocytopenia, neutropenia (up to 30 days after last dose), aplastic anemia, hemolytic anemia

Hepatic: Hepatitis

Local: Pain at injection site

Neuromuscular & skeletal: Myalgia, asthenia, arthralgia

Renal: Acute renal failure

(Continued)

Rituximab *(Continued)*

Respiratory: Bronchospasm, dyspnea, rhinitis, throat irritation, cough, pneumonitis, bronchiolitis obliterans, sinusitis

Miscellaneous: Immunosuppression, infection, hepatitis B virus reactivation, anaphylaxis, infusion related reaction (fever, chills, rigors occur in 80% of patients after first infusion, decreasing to 40% in subsequent infusions), lupus-like syndrome, serum sickness

Drug Interactions Concurrent administration of cisplatin may result in severe renal toxicity; live vaccines (unknown whether secondary transmission of infection from live vaccines can occur)

Stability Store vials in refrigerator at 2°C to 8°C; do not freeze or shake; protect vials from direct sunlight; dilution of rituximab to a final concentration of 1-4 mg/mL in NS or D_5W is stable for 24 hours if refrigerated or stored at room temperature

Mechanism of Action Rituximab is a monoclonal antibody directed against the CD20 antigen on B-lymphocytes. Rituximab binds to the antigen on the cell surface, activating complement-dependent cytotoxicity; binds to human Fc receptors mediating cell killing through an antibody-dependent cellular toxicity.

Pharmacodynamics Duration: B-cell recovery begins ~6 months following completion of treatment

Pharmacokinetics

Distribution: Binds to lymphoid cells in the thymus, spleen, and B lymphocytes in peripheral blood and lymph nodes

Half-life:

Cancer: Range in half-life may reflect variable tumor burden among patients and changes in CD20 positive B-cell population with repeat doses:

1st infusion: 76.3 hours (range: 31.5-152.6 hours)

4th infusion: 205.8 hours (range: 83.9-407 hours)

Rheumatoid arthritis: 19 days

Usual Dosage Refer to individual protocols

Children and Adults: I.V. infusion:

CD20 positive B-cell, non-Hodgkin's lymphoma: Initial: 375 mg/m² once weekly for 4-8 doses as single drug therapy or in combination with CHOP (cyclophosphamide, doxorubicin, vincristine, and prednisone)

Retreatment (patients who subsequently develop progressive disease may receive an additional course): 375 mg/m² once weekly for 4 doses or retreatment for refractory cases: 375 mg/m² once weekly for 4 doses given every 6 months for up to 2 years

Refractory CD20 positive non-Hodgkin's lymphoma or B-cell ALL: 375 mg/m² on days 1 and 3 in combination with ifosfamide with mesna, carboplatin and etoposide (ICE)

Relapsed or refractory low-grade, follicular or transformed B-cell non-Hodgkin's lymphoma: Radioimmunotherapy with Ibritumomab: 250 mg/m² infused within 4 hours prior to administration of indium ibritumomab; 7-9 days later, 250 mg/m² infused within 4 hours prior to yttrium Y90 ibritumomab

Post-transplant lymphoproliferative disorder: 375 mg/m² once weekly for 3-4 doses

Autoimmune hemolytic anemia: 375 mg/m² once weekly for 3-6 doses

Adults: Rheumatoid arthritis: 1000 mg on days 1 and 15; premedication with a corticosteroid (eg, methylprednisolone 100 mg I.V.) prior to each rituximab dose is recommended.

Administration DO NOT ADMINISTER UNDILUTED NOR as an I.V. Push or rapid injection: I.V. infusion: Administer first infusion at an initial rate of 50 mg/hour at a final concentration for administration of 1-4 mg/mL in NS or D_5W. If no hypersensitivity or infusion-related reactions occur, increase infusion rate in 50 mg/hour increments every 30 minutes to a maximum infusion rate of 400 mg/hour as tolerated. Subsequent rituximab doses can be administered at an initial rate of 100 mg/hour and increased by 100 mg/hour increments at 30 minute intervals to a maximum infusion rate of 400 mg/hour. If hypersensitivity or infusion-related reactions occur, slow or interrupt the infusion. If symptoms completely resolve, resume infusion at ½ the previous rate.

Monitoring Parameters Vital signs, CBC and platelet counts, serum electrolytes, renal function tests, liver function tests, fluid balance; cardiac monitoring for patients with pre-existing cardiac condition; peripheral CD20+ cells; human antimurine antibody and human antichimeric antibody titers

Reference Range Peripheral CD20+ cells: High pretreatment level (500-1600 cells/microliter) may indicate risk for severe infusion reactions

Patient Information Notify physician if fever, sore throat, rash, dizziness, chest pain, abdominal pain, yellowing of skin or eyes, feeling of weakness, bruising, bleeding, or shortness of breath occurs. Advise individuals of childbearing potential to use effective contraceptive methods and avoid becoming pregnant during and for 12 months following treatment with rituximab.

Nursing Implications Maintain adequate patient hydration during therapy unless instructed to restrict fluid intake. Hold antihypertensive medications for 12 hours prior to infusion; patient may need to be premedicated with acetaminophen and diphenhydramine prior to each dose to prevent infusion-related reactions. Epinephrine, diphenhydramine, and corticosteroids should be available for immediate use in case of a hypersensitivity reaction.

Dosage Forms Excipient information presented when available (limited, particularly for generics); consult specific product labeling.

Injection, solution [preservative free]:

Rituxan®: 10 mg/mL (10 mL, 50 mL) [contains polysorbate 80]

References

Edwards JC, Szczepanski L, Szechinski J, et al, "Efficacy of B-Cell-Targeted Therapy With Rituximab in Patients With Rheumatoid Arthritis," *N Engl J Med*, 2004, 350(25):2572-81.

Serinet MO, Jacquenin E, Habes D, et al, "Anti-CD20 Monoclonal Antibody (Rituximab) Treatment for Epstein-Barr Virus-Associated, B-Cell Lymphoproliferative Disease in Pediatric Liver Transplant Recipients," *J Ped Gastroenterology & Nutrition*, 2002, 34(4):389-93.

Wang J, Wiley JM, Luddy R, et al, "Chronic Immune Thrombocytopenic Purpura in Children: Assessment of Rituximab Treatment," *J Pediatr*, 2005, 146(2):217-21.

Zecca M, Nobili B, Ramenghi U, et al, "Rituximab for the Treatment of Refractory Autoimmune Hemolytic Anemia in Children," *Blood*, 2003, 101(10):3857-61.

♦ **Riva-Atenolol (Can)** *see* Atenolol *on page 170*
♦ **Riva-Clindamycin (Can)** *see* Clindamycin *on page 379*
♦ **Riva-Diclofenac (Can)** *see* Diclofenac *on page 486*
♦ **Riva-Diclofenac-K (Can)** *see* Diclofenac *on page 486*
♦ **Riva-Dicyclomine (Can)** *see* Dicyclomine *on page 490*
♦ **Riva-Famotidine (Can)** *see* Famotidine *on page 638*
♦ **Riva-Fluconazole (Can)** *see* Fluconazole *on page 660*
♦ **Riva-Loperamine (Can)** *see* Loperamide *on page 952*
♦ **Riva-Lorazepam (Can)** *see* Lorazepam *on page 962*
♦ **Riva-Lovastatin (Can)** *see* Lovastatin *on page 964*
♦ **Riva-Naproxen (Can)** *see* Naproxen *on page 1108*
♦ **Rivanase AQ (Can)** *see* Beclomethasone *on page 200*
♦ **Riva-Pravastatin (Can)** *see* Pravastatin *on page 1300*
♦ **Riva-Simvastatin (Can)** *see* Simvastatin *on page 1441*
♦ **Riva-Sotalol (Can)** *see* Sotalol *on page 1463*
♦ **Riva-Sumatriptan (Can)** *see* Sumatriptan *on page 1495*
♦ **Riva-Verapamil SR (Can)** *see* Verapamil *on page 1611*
♦ **Rivotril® (Can)** *see* Clonazepam *on page 387*
♦ **rLFN-α2** *see* Interferon Alfa-2b *on page 856*
♦ **RMS®** *see* Morphine Sulfate *on page 1082*
♦ **Robafen® AC** *see* Guaifenesin and Codeine *on page 746*
♦ **Robafen DM [OTC]** *see* Guaifenesin and Dextromethorphan *on page 748*
♦ **Robafen DM Clear [OTC]** *see* Guaifenesin and Dextromethorphan *on page 748*
♦ **Robaxin®** *see* Methocarbamol *on page 1024*
♦ **Robidrine® (Can)** *see* Pseudoephedrine *on page 1344*
♦ **Robinul®** *see* Glycopyrrolate *on page 738*
♦ **Robinul® Forte** *see* Glycopyrrolate *on page 738*
♦ **Robitussin® [OTC]** *see* Guaifenesin *on page 745*
♦ **Robitussin® (Can)** *see* Guaifenesin *on page 745*
♦ **Robitussin® Cough and Congestion [OTC]** *see* Guaifenesin and Dextromethorphan *on page 748*
♦ **Robitussin® CoughGels™ [OTC]** *see* Dextromethorphan *on page 477*
♦ **Robitussin® DM [OTC]** *see* Guaifenesin and Dextromethorphan *on page 748*
♦ **Robitussin® DM (Can)** *see* Guaifenesin and Dextromethorphan *on page 748*
♦ **Robitussin® DM Infant [OTC]** *see* Guaifenesin and Dextromethorphan *on page 748*
♦ **Robitussin® Maximum Strength Cough [OTC]** *see* Dextromethorphan *on page 477*
♦ **Robitussin® Pediatric Cough [OTC]** *see* Dextromethorphan *on page 477*
♦ **Robitussin® Sugar Free Cough [OTC]** *see* Guaifenesin and Dextromethorphan *on page 748*
♦ **Rocaltrol®** *see* Calcitriol *on page 259*
♦ **Rocephin®** *see* Ceftriaxone *on page 320*

Rocuronium (roe kyoor OH nee um)

Medication Safety Issues

Sound-alike/look-alike issues:

Zemuron® may be confused with Remeron®

High alert medication: The Institute for Safe Medication Practices (ISMP) includes this medication among its list of drugs which have a heightened risk of causing significant patient harm when used in error.

U.S. Brand Names Zemuron®

Canadian Brand Names Zemuron®

Index Terms ORG 946; Rocuronium Bromide

Therapeutic Category Neuromuscular Blocker Agent, Nondepolarizing; Skeletal Muscle Relaxant, Paralytic

Generic Available No

Use Produces skeletal muscle relaxation during surgery after induction of general anesthesia, increases pulmonary compliance during assisted mechanical respiration, facilitates endotracheal intubation

Pregnancy Risk Factor C

Lactation Excretion in breast milk unknown/use caution

Contraindications Hypersensitivity to rocuronium or any component

Warnings Dosage adjustment needed in patients with severe hepatic disease; ventilation must be supported during neuromuscular blockade; rocuronium should only be used by individuals who are experienced in the maintenance of an adequate airway and respiratory support

Precautions Many clinical conditions may potentiate or antagonize neuromuscular blockade, see table on next page.

Increased sensitivity in patients with myasthenia gravis, Eaton-Lambert syndrome; resistance to neuromuscular blockade in burn patients (>30% of body) for period of 5-70 days postinjury; resistance to neuromuscular blockade in patients with muscle trauma, denervation, immobilization, infection

Adverse Reactions Most frequent adverse reactions are associated with prolongation of its pharmacologic actions

Cardiovascular: Hypotension, hypertension, arrhythmias, tachycardia

Dermatologic: Rash, pruritus

Gastrointestinal: Vomiting

Potential Drug Interactions

Potentiation	Antagonism
Inhalation anesthetics	Calcium
Desflurane, sevoflurane, enflurane and isoflurane > halothane > nitrous oxide	Carbamazepine
	Phenytoin
	Steroids (chronic administration)
Antibiotics	Theophylline
Aminoglycosides, polymyxins, clindamycin, vancomycin, tetracycline	Anticholinesterases[1]
	Neostigmine, pyridostigmine, edrophonium, echothiophate ophthalmic solution
Magnesium	
Antiarrhythmics	
Quinidine, procainamide, bretylium, and possibly lidocaine	Caffeine
	Azathioprine
Diuretics	
Furosemide, mannitol, thiazides	
Amphotericin B (secondary to hypokalemia)	
Local anesthetics	
Dantrolene (directly depresses skeletal muscle)	
Beta blockers	
Calcium channel blockers	
Ketamine	
Lithium	
Succinylcholine (when administered prior to nondepolarizing neuromuscular-blocking agent)	
Cyclosporine	

[1]Can prolong the effects of acetylcholine

Local: Injection site edema
Neuromuscular & skeletal: Muscle weakness
Respiratory: Bronchospasm
Miscellaneous: Hiccups, hypersensitivity reactions including anaphylaxis

Clinical Conditions Affecting Neuromuscular Blockade

Potentiation	Antagonism
Electrolyte abnormalities	Alkalosis
Severe hyponatremia	Hypercalcemia
Severe hypocalcemia	Demyelinating lesions
Severe hypokalemia	Peripheral neuropathies
Hypermagnesemia	Diabetes mellitus
Neuromuscular diseases	
Acidosis	
Acute intermittent porphyria	
Renal failure	
Hepatic failure	

Drug Interactions See table on previous page.

Stability Refrigerate; unopened vials are stable 60 days at room temperature; open vials are stable for 30 days at room temperature; compatible with NS and D_5W; do not mix with alkaline solutions

Mechanism of Action Nondepolarizing neuromuscular blocking agent which blocks neural transmission at the myoneural junction by binding with cholinergic receptor sites

Pharmacodynamics

Maximum effect:
- Children: 30 seconds to 1 minute
- Adults: 1-3.7 minutes

Duration:
- Children:
  - 3-12 months: 40 minutes
  - 1-12 years: 26-30 minutes
- Adults: 20-94 minutes (dose-related) (most prolonged in elderly ≥65 years of age)

Pharmacokinetics

Distribution: V_d:
- Children: 0.21-0.3 L/kg
- Adults: 0.22-0.26 L/kg
  - Hepatic dysfunction: 0.53 L/kg
  - Renal dysfunction: 0.34 L/kg

Protein binding: ~30%

Half-life:
- Alpha elimination: 1-2 minutes
- Beta elimination:
  - Children:
    - 3-12 months: 1.3 ± 0.5 hours
    - 1 to <3 years: 1.1 ± 0.7 hours
    - 3 to <8 years: 0.8 ± 0.3 hours
  - Adults: 1.4-2.4 hours
  - Hepatic dysfunction: 4.3 hours
  - Renal dysfunction: 2.4 hours

Elimination: Primarily biliary excretion (70%); up to 30% of dose excreted unchanged in urine
- Clearance: Children:
  - 3 to <12 months: 0.35 L/kg/hour
  - 1 to <3 years: 0.32 L/kg/hour
  - 3 to <8 years: 0.44 L/kg/hour

Usual Dosage I.V. (dosage based upon actual body weight even if the patient is obese):

Infants: 0.5 mg/kg/dose repeat every 20-30 minutes as needed

Children: Initial: 0.6 mg/kg/dose with repeat doses of 0.075-0.125 mg/kg every 20-30 minutes as determined by clinical response

Adolescents and Adults:
- Rapid sequence intubation: 0.6-1.2 mg/kg
- Tracheal intubation: 0.6 mg/kg with repeated doses of 0.1-0.2 mg/kg every 20-30 minutes as determined by clinical response

Children and Adults: Continuous infusion: 10-12 mcg/kg/minute (effective range reported to be 4-16 mcg/kg/minute)

(Continued)

Rocuronium *(Continued)*

Note: While I.V. administration is preferred, I.M. administration in single doses of 1 mg/kg (infants) and 1.8 mg/kg (children) has been used successfully (Kaplan, 1999).

Administration Parenteral: May be administered undiluted by rapid I.V. injection; for continuous infusion, dilute with NS, D_5W, or LR to a concentration of 0.5-1 mg/mL

Monitoring Parameters Peripheral nerve stimulator measuring twitch response, heart rate, blood pressure, assisted ventilation status

Nursing Implications Does not alter the patient's state of consciousness; addition of sedation and analgesia are recommended

Dosage Forms Excipient information presented when available (limited, particularly for generics); consult specific product labeling.

Injection, solution, as bromide: 10 mg/mL (5 mL, 10 mL)

References

Kaplan RF, Uejima T, Lobel G, et al, "Intramuscular Rocuronium in Infants and Children: A Multicenter Study to Evaluate Tracheal Intubating Conditions, Onset, and Duration of Action," *Anesthesiology*, 1999, 91(3):633-8.

Martin LD, Bratton SL, and O'Rourke PP, "Clinical Uses and Controversies of Neuromuscular Blocking Agents in Infants and Children," *Crit Care Med*, 1999, 27(7):1358-68.

Reynolds LM, Lau M, Brown R, et al, "Bioavailability of Intramuscular Rocuronium in Infants and Children," *Anesthesiology*, 1997, 87(5):1096-105.

Willets LS, "Rocuronium for Tracheal Intubation," *Ped Pharmacotherapy*, 2000, 6(10):1-6.

- ♦ **Rocuronium Bromide** *see* Rocuronium *on page 1402*
- ♦ **Rofact™ (Can)** *see* Rifampin *on page 1384*
- ♦ **Roferon®-A** *see* Interferon Alfa-2a *on page 854*
- ♦ **Rogaine® (Can)** *see* Minoxidil *on page 1068*
- ♦ **Rogaine® Extra Strength for Men [OTC]** *see* Minoxidil *on page 1068*
- ♦ **Rogaine® for Men [OTC]** *see* Minoxidil *on page 1068*
- ♦ **Rogaine® for Women [OTC]** *see* Minoxidil *on page 1068*
- ♦ **Rogitine® (Can)** *see* Phentolamine *on page 1248*
- ♦ **Rolaids® Softchews [OTC]** *see* Calcium Carbonate *on page 264*
- ♦ **Rolaids® Softchews [OTC]** *see* Calcium Supplements *on page 272*
- ♦ **Romazicon®** *see* Flumazenil *on page 667*
- ♦ **Romilar® AC** *see* Guaifenesin and Codeine *on page 746*
- ♦ **Romycin®** *see* Erythromycin *on page 595*

Ropivacaine (roe PIV a kane)

Medication Safety Issues

Sound-alike/look-alike issues:

Ropivacaine may be confused with bupivacaine, ropinirole

U.S. Brand Names Naropin®

Canadian Brand Names Naropin®

Index Terms Ropivacaine Hydrochloride

Therapeutic Category Local Anesthetic, Injectable

Generic Available No

Use Production of local or regional anesthesia for surgery, obstetrical procedures, and for acute pain management: peripheral nerve block, local infiltration, sympathetic block, caudal or epidural block

Pregnancy Risk Factor B

Lactation Excretion in breast milk unknown/use caution

Contraindications Hypersensitivity to ropivacaine hydrochloride, any anesthetic of the amide type (eg, bupivacaine, lidocaine, mepivacaine), or any component; not recommended for I.V. regional anesthesia (Bier block)

Warnings Convulsions and cardiac arrhythmias, due to systemic toxicity leading to cardiac arrest have been reported, presumably following unintentional I.V. injection; should be administered in small incremental doses; not for use in emergency situations when rapid onset of surgical anesthesia is necessary; not for use for the production of obstetrical paracervical block anesthesia, retrobulbar block, or spinal anesthesia (subarachnoid block); unlike other local anesthetics, administration with epinephrine does not affect onset, duration of action, or the systemic absorption of ropivacaine. Supraclavicular brachial plexus blocks may be associated with a higher frequency of serious adverse effects; major peripheral nerve blocks, often close to large blood vessels pose an increased risk of intravenous systemic absorption due to the proximity and large volume of dosage.

Precautions Use with caution in patients with liver disease, impaired cardiovascular function, particularly CHF, hypotension, hypovolemia, heart block, and neurological or psychiatric disorders. Patients treated with class III antiarrhythmics may be at increased risk for additive cardiac effects and should be monitored closely (consider ECG monitoring). For epidural use, it is recommended that a test dose of either a local anesthetic with rapid onset alone or in combination with epinephrine be administered prior to ropivacaine to detect unintentional intravascular or intrathecal injection which would result in systemic toxicity (CNS or cardiovascular)

Adverse Reactions

Cardiovascular: Cardiac arrest, hypotension, bradycardia, fetal bradycardia (during epidural anesthesia for cesarean section), arrhythmias, hypertension, tachycardia, chest pain

Central nervous system: Headache, restlessness, anxiety, agitation, lightheadedness, dizziness, tinnitus, seizures, fever, incoherent speech, depression, drowsiness

Dermatologic: Pruritus, rash

Endocrine & metabolic: Hypomagnesemia, hypokalemia

Gastrointestinal: Nausea, vomiting, fecal incontinence, tenesmus

Genitourinary: Urinary retention

Hepatic: Jaundice

Local: Pain at injection site

Neuromuscular & skeletal: Weakness, back pain, paresthesia (particularly of the mouth and lips), tremors, twitching

Ocular: Vision abnormalities

Otic: Tinnitus

Respiratory: Dyspnea, rhinitis

Miscellaneous: Shivering, chills, rigor, fetal disorders including tachycardia, fetal distress, jaundice, tachypnea, fever, and vomiting

Drug Interactions Cytochrome P450 isoenzyme CYP1A2 (major), CYP2D6 (minor), and CYP3A4 (minor) substrate (may be major in cases of CYP1A2 inhibition/deficiency)

Fluvoxamine decreases ropivacaine clearance; class III antiarrhythmics may have additive effects (see Precautions); CYP1A2 inhibitors (eg, ketoconazole, amiodarone, and quinolone antibiotics) and propofol may increase effect

Stability Store at controlled room temperature; preservative-free, discard promptly after use; do not mix with alkaline solutions as precipitation will occur

Mechanism of Action Blocks both the initiation and conduction of nerve impulses by decreasing the neuronal membrane's permeability to sodium ions, which results in inhibition of depolarization with resultant blockade of conduction

Pharmacodynamics

Onset of anesthetic action (dependent on dose and route of administration):
- Epidural block (100-200 mg): T10 sensory block: 10 minutes (range: 5-13 minutes)
- Epidural block, Cesarean section (up to 150 mg): T6 sensory block: 11-26 minutes

Duration (dependent upon dose and route of administration):
- Epidural block (100-200 mg): 4 hours (range: 3-5 hours)
- Epidural block, Cesarean section (up to 150 mg):
  - Sensory block: 1.7-3.2 hours
  - Motor block: 1.4-2.9 hours

Pharmacokinetics

Absorption: Well absorbed systemically in a biphasic manner following epidural administration; addition of epinephrine has no affect on the absorption of ropivacaine

Distribution: Distributes into breast milk
- V_d (after intravascular infusion):
  - Children: 2.1-4.2 L/kg
  - Adults: 41 ± 7 L

Protein binding: 94%

Metabolism: In the liver via cytochrome P450 isoenzyme, predominantly CYP1A2 and CYP3A4 (10 metabolites with 2 active)

Bioavailability: 87% to 98% (epidural)

Half-life:
- Epidural: Terminal phase:
  - Children: 4.9 hours (range: 3-6.7 hours)
  - Adults: 4.2 ± 1 hour
- I.V.: Adults: 1.9 ± 0.5 hours

Time to peak serum concentration (dose and route dependent):
- Caudal (children): 0.33-2.05 hours
- Cesarean section: 14-65 minutes
- Epidural (adults): 17-97 minutes

Elimination: 1% to 2% excreted unchanged in urine

Usual Dosage Dose varies with procedure, depth of anesthesia, vascularity of tissues, duration of anesthesia,and condition of patient

Caudal block: Children (limited data): 2 mg/kg

Epidural block (other than caudal block): Children: 1.7 mg/kg

(Continued)

Ropivacaine *(Continued)*

Lumbar epidural surgery: Adults: 75-150 mg (15-30 mL 0.5%); maximum: 200 mg (40 mL 0.5%)
Lumbar epidural Cesarean section: Adults: 100-150 mg (20-30 mL 0.5% **or** 15-20 mL 0.75%)
Thoracic epidural surgery: Adults: 25-75 mg (5-15 mL 0.5%)
Epidural continuous infusion:
Children 4 months to 7 years (limited data) (Hansen, 2000): 1 mg/kg loading dose followed by 0.4 mg/kg/hour continuous **epidural** infusion
Adults: 10-14 mg loading dose (5-7 mL 0.2%) followed by 12-28 mg/hour (6-14 mL/hour 0.2%) continuous **epidural** infusion
Major nerve block (eg, brachial plexus block): Adults: 75-300 mg (10-40 mL 0.75%)
Minor nerve block and infiltration: Adults: 5-200 mg (1-40 mL 0.5%)

Administration Parenteral: Administer in small incremental doses; when using continuous intermittent catheter techniques, use frequent aspirations before and during the injection to avoid intravascular injection

Monitoring Parameters After epidural or subarachnoid administration: Blood pressure, heart rate, respiration, signs of CNS toxicity (lightheadedness, dizziness, tinnitus, restlessness, tremors, twitching, drowsiness, circumoral paresthesia)

Patient Information Temporary loss of sensation and motor activity in the anesthetized part of the body may occur following proper administration of lumbar epidural anesthesia.

Dosage Forms Excipient information presented when available (limited, particularly for generics); consult specific product labeling.
Infusion, as hydrochloride:
Naropin®: 2 mg/mL (100 mL, 200 mL)
Injection, solution, as hydrochloride [preservative free]:
Naropin®: 2 mg/mL (10 mL, 20 mL); 5 mg/mL (20 mL, 30 mL); 7.5 mg/mL (20 mL); 10 mg/mL (10 mL, 20 mL)

References

Hansen TG, Ilett KF, Lim SI, et al, "Pharmacokinetics and Clinical Efficacy of Long-Term Epidural Ropivacaine Infusion in Children," *Br J Anaesth*, 2000, 85(3):347-53.
Hansen TG, Ilett KF, Reid C, et al, "Caudal Ropivacaine in Infants: Population Pharmacokinetics and Plasma Concentrations," *Anesthesiology*, 2001, 94(4):579-84.
Lonnqvist PA, Westrin P, Larsson BA, et al, "Ropivacaine Pharmacokinetics After Caudal Block in 1-8 Year Old Children," *Br J Anaesth*, 2000, 85(4):506-11.
Wulf H, Peters C, and Behnke H, "The Pharmacokinetics of Caudal Ropivacaine 0.2% in Children. A Study of Infants Aged Less Than 1 Year and Toddlers Aged 1-5 Years Undergoing Inguinal Hernia Repair," *Anaesthesia*, 2000, 55(8):757-60.

♦ **Ropivacaine Hydrochloride** *see* Ropivacaine *on page 1404*

Rosiglitazone (ROSE i gli ta zone)

Medication Safety Issues
Sound-alike/look-alike issues:
Avandia® may be confused with Avalide®, Coumadin®, Prandin®
International issues:
Avandia® may be confused with Avanza® which is a brand name for mirtazapine in Australia

U.S. Brand Names Avandia®

Canadian Brand Names Avandia®

Therapeutic Category Antidiabetic Agent, Oral; Antidiabetic Agent, Thiazolidinedione

Generic Available No

Use Type 2 diabetes mellitus (noninsulin-dependent, NIDDM) when diet and exercise alone do not result in adequate glycemic control; may be used in combination with metformin, sulfonylurea, or insulin

Pregnancy Risk Factor C

Lactation Excretion in breast milk unknown/not recommended

Contraindications Hypersensitivity to rosiglitazone or any component; moderate to severe liver disease (transaminases >2.5 times the upper limit of normal at baseline); patients who experienced jaundice during troglitazone therapy; type 1 diabetes mellitus; diabetic ketoacidosis

Warnings Used alone or in combination with insulin, rosiglitazone can cause fluid retention which can exacerbate or lead to CHF; patients should be closely monitored for signs and symptoms of CHF; discontinue use if any deterioration of cardiac function occurs; avoid use in patients with NYHA class 3 or 4 heart failure

A dose-related weight gain has been reported with rosiglitazone which may be due to a combination of fluid retention and fat accumulation over time; a more rapid onset of weight gain may be suggestive of excessive edema and heart failure; idiosyncratic hepatotoxicity has been reported with another thiazolidinedione agent (troglitazone); two cases of hepatocellular injury (Forman, et al and Al-Salman, 2000) have been reported occurring within 2-3 weeks after initiation of rosiglitazone therapy; LFTs in these patients revealed severe hepatocellular injury which responded with rapid improvement of liver function and resolution of symptoms upon discontinuation of rosiglitazone; monitoring should include periodic determinations of liver function

Precautions Use with extreme caution in patients with heart failure or edema (see Warnings); use with caution in patients with elevated transaminases (AST or ALT) and in patients with anemia or depressed leukocyte counts (may reduce hemoglobin, hematocrit, and/or WBC); may induce ovulation in premenopausal anovulatory women; adequate contraception in premenopausal women is recommended

Adverse Reactions

Cardiovascular: Edema, CHF

Central nervous system: Headache, fatigue

Endocrine & metabolic: Weight gain, elevated total LDL and HDL cholesterol, hyperglycemia, hypoglycemia, ovulation

Gastrointestinal: Diarrhea

Hematologic: Anemia

Hepatic: Elevated transaminases, elevated bilirubin

Neuromuscular & skeletal: Back pain

Respiratory: Upper respiratory tract infection, sinusitis

Miscellaneous: Injury

Drug Interactions Cytochrome P450 isoenzyme CYP2C8 substrate; isoenzyme CYP2C9 (minor)

Gemfibrozil may increase rosiglitazone AUC; decrease rosiglitazone dose if used with gemfibrozil; rifampin may decrease rosiglitazone AUC

Food Interactions Peak concentrations are lower by 28% and delayed when administered with food; these effects are not believed to be clinically significant

Mechanism of Action Thiazolidinedione antidiabetic agent that lowers blood glucose by improving target cell response to insulin, without increasing pancreatic insulin secretion; this mechanism of action is dependent on the presence of insulin for activity

Pharmacodynamics Maximum effect: Up to 12 weeks

Pharmacokinetics

Distribution: V_{dss} (apparent): Adults: 17.6 L

Protein binding: Adults: 99%

Metabolism: Hepatic (99%), metabolism by cytochrome P450 isoenzyme CYP2C8, minor metabolism via CYP2C9

Bioavailability: 99%

Half-life: 3-4 hours

Time to peak serum concentration: 1 hour

Elimination: As metabolites, in urine (64%) and feces (23%)

Usual Dosage Adults: Oral: All patients should be initiated at the lowest recommended dose:

Monotherapy: Initial: 4 mg in single or divided doses twice daily; after 8-12 weeks of treatment the dosage may be increased to 8 mg daily in single or divided doses twice daily. **Note:** When changing patients from troglitazone to rosiglitazone, a 1-week washout is recommended before initiating therapy with rosiglitazone

Combination therapy: When adding rosiglitazone to existing therapy, continue current dose(s) of previous agents:

With sulfonylureas: Initial: 4 mg daily as a single daily dose or in divided doses twice daily; dose of sulfonylurea should be reduced if the patient reports hypoglycemia. Doses of rosiglitazone >4 mg/day are not indicated in combination with sulfonylureas.

With metformin: Initial: 4 mg daily as a single daily dose or in divided doses twice daily. If response is inadequate after 12 weeks of treatment, the dosage may be increased to 8 mg daily as a single daily dose or in divided doses twice daily. It is unlikely that the dose of metformin will need to be reduced due to hypoglycemia

With insulin: Initial: 4 mg daily as a single daily dose or in divided doses twice daily. Dose of insulin should be reduced by 10% to 25% if the patient reports hypoglycemia or if the plasma glucose falls to <100 mg/dL. Doses of rosiglitazone >4 mg/day are not indicated in combination with insulin.

Dosage adjustment in renal impairment: No dosage adjustment is required

Dosage comment in hepatic impairment: Clearance is significantly lower in hepatic impairment. Therapy should not be initiated if the patient exhibits active liver disease with increased transaminases (>2.5 times the upper limit of normal) at baseline (see Contraindications and Warnings)

Administration Oral: May be taken without regard to meals

Monitoring Parameters Signs and symptoms of hypoglycemia, fluid retention, or heart failure, fasting blood glucose, hemoglobin A_{1c}; liver enzymes: baseline, every 2

(Continued)

Rosiglitazone *(Continued)*

months for the first 12 months of therapy, and periodically thereafter; patients with an elevation in ALT >3 times the upper limit of normal should be rechecked as soon as possible; if the ALT levels remain >3 times the upper limit of normal, therapy with rosiglitazone should be discontinued

Reference Range Target range:

Blood glucose: Fasting and preprandial: 80-120 mg/dL; bedtime: 100-140 mg/dL

Glycosylated hemoglobin (hemoglobin A_{1c}): <7%

Patient Information Follow directions of prescriber; if dose is missed at the usual meal, take it with next meal; do not double dose if daily dose is missed completely; more frequent monitoring is required during periods of stress, trauma, surgery, pregnancy, increased activity, or exercise; avoid alcohol; report an unusually rapid increase in weight, edema, or shortness of breath immediately to your physician; also report chest pain, rapid heartbeat or palpitations, abdominal pain, fever, rash, hypoglycemic reactions, yellowing of skin or eyes, dark urine or light stool, or unusual fatigue or nausea/vomiting.

Dosage Forms Excipient information presented when available (limited, particularly for generics); consult specific product labeling.

Tablet:

Avandia®: 2 mg, 4 mg, 8 mg

References

Al-Salman J, Arjomand H, Kemp DG, et al, "Hepatocellular Injury in a Patient Receiving Rosiglitazone. A Case Report," *Ann Intern Med*, 2000, 132(2):121-4.

DeFronzo RA, "Pharmacologic Therapy for Type 2 Diabetes Mellitus," *Ann Intern Med*, 1999, 131(4):281-303.

Forman LM, Simmons DA, and Diamond RH, "Hepatic Failure in a Patient Taking Rosiglitazone," *Ann Intern Med*, 2000, 132(2):118-21.

♦ **Rosula® NS** *see* Sulfacetamide *on page 1483*

♦ **RotaTeq®** *see* Rotavirus Vaccine (Live/Pentavalent) *on page 1408*

Rotavirus Vaccine (Live/Pentavalent)

(ROE ta vye us vak SEEN live pen ta VAY lent)

U.S. Brand Names RotaTeq®

Index Terms Pentavalent Human-Bovine Reassortant Rotavirus Vaccine; Rotavirus Vaccine, Pentavalent

Therapeutic Category Vaccine

Generic Available No

Use Immunization to prevent rotavirus gastroenteritis caused by serotypes G1, G2, G3, and G4.

Lactation Infants receiving vaccine may be breast-fed.

Contraindications Hypersensitivity to rotavirus vaccine or any component

Warnings Rotavirus vaccine should not be administered to infants with acute, moderate-to-severe gastroenteritis until the condition improves. Rotavirus vaccine administration may be delayed in patients with febrile illness except when the physician decides that withholding the vaccine entails a greater risk. Patients with mild low-grade fever (<38.1°C) or mild upper respiratory infection may receive vaccine. Information is not available for use of rotavirus vaccine in postexposure prophylaxis. Live virus vaccines may be transmitted to nonvaccinated contacts. Postmarketing cases of intussusception associated with RotaTeq® vaccine administration have been reported.

Precautions Use with caution in infants with a history of gastrointestinal disorders (eg, active acute gastrointestinal disorders, chronic diarrhea, failure to thrive, history of congenital abdominal disorders, abdominal surgery and intussusception), infants with immunodeficient close contacts, such as immunocompromised individuals with malignancies or individuals receiving immunosuppressive therapy. No safety or efficacy data available for administration of rotavirus vaccine to immunodeficient or immunocompromised infants, infants receiving immunosuppressive therapy, or infants who have received blood products within 42 days of vaccination. Rotavirus vaccine administration should be deferred for 42 days after receipt of an antibody-containing product. However, if deferral causes first dose of vaccine to be scheduled at ≥13 weeks of age, a shorter deferral interval should be used.

Adverse Reactions All serious adverse reactions must be reported to the U.S. Department of Health and Human Services (DHHS) Vaccine Adverse Event Reporting System (VAERS) 1-800-822-7967 or report online to www.vaers.hhs.gov.

Central nervous system: Fever, irritability

Gastrointestinal: Gastroenteritis, vomiting, diarrhea, intussusception

Genitourinary: Urinary tract infection

Otic: Otitis media

Respiratory: Bronchiolitis, pneumonia, bronchospasm, nasopharyngitis

Drug Interactions Radiation, immunosuppressive therapy (eg, antimetabolites, alkylating agents, cytotoxic drugs, and corticosteroids used in doses greater than physiologic doses) may decrease the immune response to vaccines

Stability Refrigerate; protect from light. Do not dilute. Administer rotavirus vaccine as soon as possible once removed from refrigerator.

Mechanism of Action Live viral vaccine that replicates in the small intestine and induces active immunity

Usual Dosage Oral: Infants: 2 mL per dose

Recommended schedule: A three-dose series at 2, 4, and 6 months of age. Initial dose should be administered at 6-12 weeks of age; subsequent two doses administered at 4-10 week intervals (final third dose should not be given after 32 weeks of age)

Administration Oral: **Not for injection.** Clear fluid from the dispensing tip by holding dosing tube vertically and tapping cap; puncture dispensing tip by screwing cap clockwise; remove cap by turning counterclockwise; gently squeeze liquid dose into infant's mouth toward the inner cheek until dosing tube is empty. If an incomplete dose is given (eg, infants spits or regurgitates dose), do not administer replacement dose. The infant can continue to receive any remaining doses of the series at the designated time interval. Do not mix or dilute vaccine with any other vaccine or solution.

Patient Information Infants living in households with pregnant women may be vaccinated. Inform healthcare provider if there has been a previous reaction to rotavirus vaccine. Advise parents to contact the child's physician immediately if stomach pain, vomiting, diarrhea, blood in stool, or change in bowel movements occur after RotaTeq® vaccine administration.

Nursing Implications

Discard empty tube and cap in approved biological waste container. Federal law requires that the date of administration, the vaccine manufacturer, lot number of vaccine, and the administering person's name, title, and address be entered into the patient's permanent medical record.

Additional Information Diphtheria and tetanus antigens in DTaP, HIB, IPV, hepatitis B vaccine, and pneumococcal conjugate vaccine may be given concurrently with rotavirus vaccine. Insufficient data is currently available to confirm lack of interference between pentavalent rotavirus vaccine and childhood vaccines to prevent pertussis.

In the United States, rotavirus outbreaks occur from late fall to early spring. In the Southwest, the peak rotavirus season is November through December; the peak epidemic travels across the United States from west to east terminating in April through May in the Northeast.

Dosage Forms Excipient information presented when available (limited, particularly for generics); consult specific product labeling.

Suspension, oral [preservative free]:

RotaTeq®: G1 ≥2.2 10^6 infectious units, G2 ≥2.8 10^6 infectious units, G3 ≥2.2 10^6 infectious units, G4 ≥2.0 10^6 infectious units, and P1 [8] ≥2.3 10^6 infectious units (2 mL) [bovine and human derived; available in a prefilled, ready-to-use dosing tube]

References

American Academy of Pediatrics Committee on Infectious Diseases, "Prevention of Rotavirus Disease: Guidelines for Use of Rotavirus Vaccine," *Pediatrics*, 2007, 119(1):171-82.

Parashar UD, Alexander JP, and Glass RI, "Prevention of Rotavirus Gastroenteritis Among Infants and Children. Recommendations of the Advisory Committee on Immunization Practices (ACIP)," *MMWR Recomm Rep*, 2006, 55(RR-12):1-13.

Vesikari T, Matson DO, Dennehy P, et al, "Safety and Efficacy of a Pentavalent Human-Bovine (WC3) Reassortant Rotavirus Vaccine," *N Engl J Med*, 2006, 354(1):23-33.

♦ **Rotavirus Vaccine, Pentavalent** *see* Rotavirus Vaccine (Live/Pentavalent) *on page 1408*

♦ **Rowasa®** *see* Mesalamine *on page 1011*

♦ **Roxanol™** *see* Morphine Sulfate *on page 1082*

♦ **Roxicet™** *see* Oxycodone and Acetaminophen *on page 1191*

♦ **Roxicet™ 5/500** *see* Oxycodone and Acetaminophen *on page 1191*

♦ **Roxicodone®** *see* Oxycodone *on page 1189*

♦ **Roychlor® (Can)** *see* Potassium Chloride *on page 1287*

♦ **RP-59500** *see* Quinupristin/Dalfopristin *on page 1360*

♦ **RS-25259** *see* Palonosetron *on page 1199*

♦ **RS-25259-197** *see* Palonosetron *on page 1199*

♦ **RTCA** *see* Ribavirin *on page 1378*

♦ **Rubella, Measles and Mumps Vaccines, Combined** *see* Measles, Mumps, and Rubella Vaccines (Combined) *on page 980*

♦ **Rubella, Varicella, Measles, and Mumps Vaccine** *see* Measles, Mumps, Rubella, and Varicella Virus Vaccine *on page 982*

Rubella Virus Vaccine (Live) (rue BEL a VYE rus vak SEEN, live)

Medication Safety Issues
Sound-alike/look-alike issues:
Meruvax® II may be confused with Attenuvax®

Related Information
Immunization Guidelines *on page 1837*

U.S. Brand Names Meruvax® II

Index Terms German Measles Vaccine

Therapeutic Category Vaccine

Generic Available No

Use Selective active immunization against rubella

Pregnancy Risk Factor C

Lactation Enters breast milk/use caution

Contraindications Hypersensitivity to gelatin or any other component of the vaccine; history of anaphylactic reactions to neomycin; individuals with blood dyscrasias, leukemia, lymphomas, or other malignant neoplasms affecting the bone marrow or lymphatic systems; concurrent immunosuppressive therapy; primary and acquired immunodeficiency states; family history of congenital or hereditary immunodeficiency; active/untreated tuberculosis; current febrile illness or active febrile infection; pregnancy

Warnings Women who are pregnant when vaccinated or who become pregnant within 28 days of vaccination should be counseled on the theoretical risks to the fetus. Immediate treatment for anaphylactic/anaphylactoid reaction should be available during vaccine use. Defer vaccination at least 3 months after receiving blood and plasma transfusions or immune globulin (See Appendix Immunization Guidelines, "Suggested Intervals Between Administration of Immune Globulin Preparations for Various Indications and Measles Immunization").

Children with HIV infection, who are asymptomatic and not immunosuppressed may be vaccinated. Patients with minor illnesses (diarrhea, mild upper respiratory tract infection with or without low-grade fever or other illnesses with low-grade fever) may receive vaccine.

Precautions Use with caution in patients with thrombocytopenia and those who develop thrombocytopenia after first dose; thrombocytopenia may worsen; excretion of small amounts of the live attenuated rubella virus from the nose or throat occurs 7-28 days after vaccination; however, transmission to a susceptible individual is not considered a significant risk.

Adverse Reactions All serious adverse reactions must be reported to the U.S. Department of Health and Human Services (DHHS) Vaccine Adverse Event Reporting System (VAERS) 1-800-822-7967.

Cardiovascular: Syncope, vasculitis

Central nervous system: Dizziness, encephalitis, fever, Guillain-Barré syndrome, headache, irritability, malaise, polyneuritis, polyneuropathy

Dermatologic: Angioneurotic edema, erythema multiforme, purpura, rash, Stevens-Johnson syndrome, urticaria

Gastrointestinal: Diarrhea, nausea, sore throat, vomiting

Hematologic: Leukocytosis, thrombocytopenia

Local: Injection site reactions which include burning, induration, pain, redness, stinging, wheal, and flare

Neuromuscular & skeletal: Arthralgia/arthritis (variable; highest rates in women, 12% to 26% versus children, up to 3%), myalgia, paresthesia

Ocular: Conjunctivitis, optic neuritis, papillitis, retrobulbar neuritis

Otic: Nerve deafness, otitis media

Respiratory: Bronchial spasm, cough, rhinitis

Miscellaneous: Anaphylactoid reactions, anaphylaxis, regional lymphadenopathy

Drug Interactions Immunosuppressant medications may decrease the effect of the vaccine and increase the risk of rubella disease in individuals who are receiving immunosuppressant drugs. In patients receiving high doses of systemic corticosteroids for ≥14 days, wait at least 1 month between discontinuing steroid therapy and administering immunization. Immune globulin, whole blood, and plasma may compromise the response to the vaccine; defer vaccination at least 3 months after receiving blood and plasma transfusions or immune globulin (See Appendix Immunization Guidelines, "Suggested Intervals Between Administration of Immune Globulin Preparations for Various Indications and Measles Immunization")

Stability Refrigerate, discard reconstituted vaccine after 8 hours; store at 2°C to 8°C (36°F to 46°F); ship vaccine at 10°C; may use dry ice; protect from light.

Mechanism of Action Rubella vaccine is a live attenuated vaccine that contains the Wistar Institute RA 27/3 strain, which is adapted to and propagated in human diploid cell culture. Promotes active immunity by inducing rubella hemagglutination-inhibiting antibodies.

Pharmacodynamics Onset of action: Antibodies to vaccine: 2-4 weeks

Pharmacokinetics Distribution: Rubella virus distributes into breast milk. Infants of recently immunized mothers may show serologic evidence of infection; however, severe disease is not expected.

Usual Dosage SubQ: 0.5 mL

Infants and Children: First dose at 12-15 months of age and a second dose 4-6 years of age

Adults: One dose for women of childbearing age whose immunization history is unreliable, young adults who work in or congregate in hospitals, colleges, or military bases, and susceptible travelers

Note: MMR (trivalent vaccine for measles, mumps, and rubella) is the vaccine of choice if recipients are likely to be susceptible to measles and/or mumps as well as to rubella.

Administration Reconstitute only with provided diluent and agitate to mix thoroughly; administer subcutaneously into the antereolateral aspect of the thigh or the outer aspect of upper arm; avoid injection into blood vessel; **not for I.V. administration**

Test Interactions May depress tuberculin skin test sensitivity

Patient Information This medication is only given by subcutaneous injection. You may experience burning or stinging at the injection site; joint pain usually occurs 1-10 weeks after vaccination and persists 1-3 days. Notify your healthcare provider immediately if these effects continue or are severe, or for a high fever, seizures or allergic reaction (respiratory difficulty, hives, weakness, dizziness, fast heartbeat). Not to be used during pregnancy; do not get pregnant for 28 days after getting the vaccine. Pregnant women should wait until after giving birth to get the vaccine. Consult healthcare provider if breast-feeding.

Nursing Implications Federal law requires that the date of administration, the vaccine manufacturer, lot number of vaccine, and the administering person's name, title, and address be entered into the patient's permanent record.

Additional Information Live attenuated virus vaccine. Using separate sites and syringes, rubella virus vaccine may be administered concurrently with DTaP, *Haemophilus* b conjugate vaccine (PedvaxHIB®), or hepatitis B vaccine. Unless otherwise specified, rubella virus vaccine should be given 1 month before or 1 month after other live viral vaccines. Rubella virus vaccine and varicella virus vaccine may be administered together (using separate sites and syringes); however, if vaccines are not administered simultaneously, doses should be separated by at least 30 days.

Dosage Forms Excipient information presented when available (limited, particularly for generics); consult specific product labeling.

Injection, powder for reconstitution [preservative free]:

Meruvax® II: ≥1000 $TCID_{50}$ (Wistar RA 27/3 Strain) [contains gelatin, human albumin, sorbitol, sucrose, and neomycin]

References

American Academy of Pediatrics Committee on Infectious Diseases, "Recommended Immunization Schedules for Children and Adolescents - United States, 2007," *Pediatrics*, 2007, 119(1):207-8.

Centers for Disease Control, "Recommended Adult Immunization Schedule by Age Group and Medical Conditions, United States, 2003-2004," available at www.cdc.gov.

"Revised ACIP Recommendation for Avoiding Pregnancy After Receiving a Rubella-Containing Vaccine," *MMWR Morb Mortal Wkly Rep*, 2001, 50(49):1117.

"Simultaneous Administration of Varicella Vaccine and Other Recommended Childhood Vaccines - United States, 1995-1999," *MMWR Morb Mortal Wkly Rep*, 2001, 50(47):1058-61.

- **Rubeola Vaccine** *see* Measles Virus Vaccine (Live) *on page 984*
- **Rubex® [DSC]** *see* DOXOrubicin *on page 540*
- **Rubidomycin Hydrochloride** *see* DAUNOrubicin *on page 447*
- **Rulox [OTC]** *see* Antacid Preparations *on page 132*
- **Rulox No. 1 [DSC]** *see* Antacid Preparations *on page 132*
- **Rum-K®** *see* Potassium Chloride *on page 1287*
- **Rylosol (Can)** *see* Sotalol *on page 1463*
- **Rythmodan® (Can)** *see* Disopyramide *on page 523*
- **Rythmodan®-LA (Can)** *see* Disopyramide *on page 523*
- **S2® [OTC]** *see* Epinephrine *on page 577*
- **SAB-Dimenhydrinate (Can)** *see* DimenhyDRINATE *on page 507*
- **SAB-Gentamicin (Can)** *see* Gentamicin *on page 726*
- **Sab-Prenase (Can)** *see* PrednisoLONE *on page 1304*
- **SAB-Trifluridine (Can)** *see* Trifluridine *on page 1575*

Sacrosidase (sak RO se dase)

U.S. Brand Names Sucraid®
Canadian Brand Names Sucraid®
Therapeutic Category Sucrase Deficiency, Treatment Agent
Generic Available No
Use Oral replacement therapy in congenital sucrase-isomaltase deficiency (CSID)
Pregnancy Risk Factor C
Lactation Enters breast milk/compatible
Contraindications Hypersensitivity to sacrosidase or any component, yeast and yeast products and glycerol
Warnings Hypersensitivity reactions to sacrosidase, including bronchospasm, have been reported; administer initial doses in a setting where acute hypersensitivity reactions may be treated within a few minutes; skin testing may be performed prior to administration to potentially identify patients at risk for hypersensitivity reactions.
Precautions Use with caution in CSID patients with diabetes mellitus, as Sucraid® will improve absorption of the products of sucrose hydrolysis (glucose and fructose); diet and/or insulin dosage may need to be adjusted
Adverse Reactions
Central nervous system: Insomnia, headache, nervousness
Endocrine & metabolic: Dehydration
Gastrointestinal: Abdominal pain, vomiting, nausea, diarrhea, constipation
Respiratory: Bronchospasm
Miscellaneous: Hypersensitivity reactions (see Warnings)
Drug Interactions None as yet have been identified
Food Interactions May be inactivated or denatured if administered with fruit juice, warm or hot food or liquids; since isomaltase deficiency is not affected by sacrosidase, adherence to a low-starch diet may be required to decrease symptomatology
Stability Refrigerate at 4°C to 8°C (36°F to 46°F); protect from light; discard 4 weeks after opening
Mechanism of Action Sacrosidase is a naturally occurring GI enzyme which breaks down the disaccharide sucrose into its monosaccharide components; this hydrolysis is necessary to allow absorption of these nutrients
Pharmacokinetics Metabolism: Sacrosidase is metabolized in the GI tract to individual amino acids which are systemically absorbed
Usual Dosage Oral:
Infants and Children ≤15 kg: 8500 international units (1 mL) per meal or snack
Children >15 kg and Adults: 17,000 international units (2 mL) per meal or snack
Administration Oral: Dilute in 2-4 ounces of water, milk, or formula; approximately 1/2 of the dose may be taken before, and the remainder of the dose at the completion of, each meal or snack; do not administer with fruit juices, warm or hot food or liquids (see Food Interactions)
Monitoring Parameters Breath hydrogen test, oral sucrose tolerance test, urinary disaccharides, intestinal disaccharidases (measured from small bowel biopsy)
CSID symptomatology: Diarrhea, abdominal pain, gas and bloating
Additional Information 1 mL = 22 drops from sacrosidase container tip
Dosage Forms Excipient information presented when available (limited, particularly for generics); consult specific product labeling.
Solution, oral: 8500 int. units per mL (118 mL)
References

Treem WR, McAdams L, Stanford L, et al, "Sacrosidase Therapy for Congenital Sucrose-Isomaltase Deficiency," *J Pediatr Gastroenterol Nutr*, 1999, 28(2):137-42.

Salicylic Acid (sal i SIL ik AS id)

Medication Safety Issues

Transdermal patch may contain conducting metal (eg, aluminum); remove patch prior to MRI.

U.S. Brand Names Compound W® [OTC]; Compound W® One Step Wart Remover [OTC]; DHS™ Sal [OTC]; Dr. Scholl's® Callus Remover [OTC]; Dr. Scholl's® Clear Away [OTC]; DuoFilm® [OTC]; DuoPlant® [DSC] [OTC]; Freezone® [OTC]; Fung-O® [OTC]; Gordofilm® [OTC]; Hydrisalic™ [OTC]; Ionil® [OTC]; Ionil® Plus [OTC]; Keralyt® [OTC]; LupiCare™ Dandruff [OTC]; LupiCare™ II Psoriasis [OTC]; LupiCare™ Psoriasis [OTC]; Mediplast® [OTC]; MG217 Sal-Acid® [OTC]; Mosco® Corn and Callus Remover [OTC]; NeoCeuticals™ Acne Spot Treatment [OTC]; Neutrogena® Acne Wash [OTC]; Neutrogena® Body Clear™ [OTC]; Neutrogena® Clear Pore [OTC]; Neutrogena® Clear Pore Shine Control [OTC]; Neutrogena® Healthy Scalp [OTC]; Neutrogena® Maximum Strength T/Sal® [OTC]; Neutrogena® On The Spot® Acne Patch [OTC]; Occlusal®-HP [OTC]; Oxy Balance® [OTC]; Oxy Balance® Deep Pore [OTC]; Palmer's® Skin Success Acne Cleanser [OTC]; Pedisilk® [OTC]; Propa pH [OTC]; SalAc® [OTC]; Sal-Acid® [OTC]; Salactic® [OTC]; Sal-Plant® [OTC]; Stri-dex® [OTC]; Stri-dex® Body Focus [OTC]; Stri-dex® Facewipes To Go™ [OTC]; Stri-dex® Maximum Strength [OTC]; Tinamed® [OTC]; Tiseb® [OTC]; Trans-Ver-Sal® [OTC]; Wart-Off® Maximum Strength [OTC]; Zapzyt® Acne Wash [OTC]; Zapzyt® Pore Treatment [OTC]

Canadian Brand Names Duofilm®; Duoforte® 27; Occlusal™-HP; Sebcur®; Soluver®; Soluver® Plus; Trans-Plantar®; Trans-Ver-Sal®

Therapeutic Category Keratolytic Agent

Generic Available Yes: Gel, soap

Use Topically for its keratolytic effect in controlling seborrheic dermatitis or psoriasis of body and scalp, dandruff, and other scaling dermatoses; to remove warts, corns, calluses; also used in the treatment of acne

Pregnancy Risk Factor C

Contraindications Hypersensitivity to salicylic acid or any component (see Warnings); children <2 years of age

Warnings Should not be used systemically due to severe irritating effect on GI mucosa; prolonged use over large areas, especially in children, may result in salicylate toxicity; do not apply on irritated, reddened, or infected skin; do not use on moles, birthmarks, warts with hair growing from them, or genital warts; topical liquid may contain tartrazine which may cause allergic reactions in susceptible individuals

Precautions For external use only; avoid contact with eyes, face, and other mucous membranes

Adverse Reactions

Dermatologic: Facial scarring, erythema, scaling

Local: Irritation, burning

Mechanism of Action Produces desquamation of hyperkeratotic epithelium; increases hydration of the stratum corneum causing the skin to swell, soften, and desquamate

Pharmacokinetics

Absorption: Topical: Readily absorbed

Time to peak serum concentration: Within 5 hours when applied with an occlusive dressing

Elimination: Salicyluric acid (52%), salicylate glucuronides (42%), and salicylic acid (6%) are the major metabolites identified in urine after percutaneous absorption

Usual Dosage Children ≥2 years and Adults: Topical:

Lotion, cream, gel: Apply a thin layer to the affected area once or twice daily

Plaster: Cut to size that covers the corn or callus, apply and leave in place for 48 hours; do not exceed 5 applications over a 14-day period

Shampoo: Initial: Use daily or every other day; apply to wet hair and massage vigorously into the scalp; rinse hair thoroughly after shampooing; 1-2 treatments/week will usually maintain control

Solution: Apply a thin layer directly to wart using brush applicator once daily as directed for 1 week or until the wart is removed

Administration Topical: For external use only; when applying in concentrations >10%, protect surrounding normal tissue with petrolatum

Monitoring Parameters Signs and symptoms of salicylate toxicity: Nausea, vomiting, dizziness, tinnitus, loss of hearing, lethargy, diarrhea, psychic disturbances

Nursing Implications For warts: Before applying product, soak area in warm water for 5 minutes; dry area thoroughly, then apply medication

Dosage Forms Excipient information presented when available (limited, particularly for generics); consult specific product labeling. [DSC] = Discontinued product

(Continued)

Salicylic Acid *(Continued)*

Cream:
- LupiCare™ Dandruff, LupiCare™ Psoriasis: 2.5% (120 g, 240 g) [contains alcohol]
- LupiCare™ II Psoriasis: 2.5% (60 g, 240 g) [contains alcohol]
- Neutrogena® Acne Wash: 2% (200 mL) [contains alcohol]

Cloths (Neutrogena® Acne Wash): 2% (30s) [disposable cloths]

Foam:
- Neutrogena® Acne Wash: 2% (150 mL) [foaming cleanser]
- SalAc®: 2% (100 g)

Gel: 17% (15 g)
- Compound W®: 17% (7 g) [contains alcohol]
- DuoPlant® [DSC]: 17% (15 g)
- Hydrisalic™: 6% (28 g) [contains alcohol and propylene glycol]
- Keralyt®: 6% (30 g) [contains alcohol and propylene glycol]
- NeoCeuticals™ Acne Spot Treatment: 2% (15 g) [contains alcohol]
- Neutrogena® Clear Pore: 2% (60 g) [contains alcohol]
- Neutrogena® Clear Pore Shine Control: 0.5% (10 g)
- Oxy Balance®: 2% (240 mL) [shower gel]
- Sal-Plant®: 17% (14 g) [contains alcohol]
- Stri-dex® Body Focus™: 2% (300 mL)
- Zapzyt® Acne Wash: 2% (190 g) [alcohol free]
- Zapzyt® Pore Treatment: 2% (23 g) [alcohol free]

Liquid, topical:
- Compound W®: 17% (9 mL) [contains alcohol]
- DuoFilm®: 17% (15 mL) [contains alcohol]
- Freezone®: 17.6% (9.3 mL) [contains alcohol]
- Fung-O®: 17% (15 mL)
- Gordofilm®: 16.7% (15 mL)
- Mosco® Corn and Callus Remover: 17.6% (10 mL)
- NeoCeuticals™ Acne Spot Treatment: 2% (60 mL) [contains alcohol]
- Neutrogena® Acne Wash: 2% (180 mL) [contains tartrazine]
- Neutrogena® Body Clear™ [body scrub with microbeads]: 2% (250 mL) [contains tartrazine]
- Neutrogena® Body Clear™ [body wash]: 2% (250 mL) [contains tartrazine]
- Occlusal®-HP: 17% (10 mL)
- Palmer's® Skin Success Acne Cleanser: 0.5% (240 mL)
- Pedisilk®: 17% (15 mL)
- Propa pH: 2% (80 mL) [alcohol free; contains aloe vera]
- SalAc®: 2% (180 mL)
- Salactic®: 17% (15 mL) [contains alcohol]
- Tinamed®: 17% (15 mL)
- Wart-Off®: 17% (13 mL) [contains alcohol]

Ointment (MG217 Sal-Acid®): 3% (56 g) [contains vitamin E]

Pads:
- Oxy Balance®, Oxy Balance® Deep Pore: 0.5% (55s, 90s) [contains alcohol]
- Stri-dex®: 0.5% (55s)
- Stri-dex® Facewipes To Go™: 0.5% (32s) [contains alcohol]
- Stri-dex® Maximum Strength: 2% (32s, 55s, 90s)

Patch, transdermal:
- Compound W® One Step Wart Remover: 40% (12s, 14s)
- Dr. Scholl's® Callus Remover: 40% (4s)
- Dr. Scholl's® Clear Away: 40% (14s, 16s, 18s, 24s)
- DuoFilm®: 40% (18s)
- Neutrogena® On The Spot® Acne Patch: 2% (27s)
- Trans-Ver-Sal®: 15% [6 mm PediaPatch, 12 mm AdultPatch, 20 mm PlantarPatch] (10s, 12s, 15s, 25s, 40s)

Plaster:
- Mediplast®: 40% (25s)
- Sal-Acid®: 40% (14s)
- Tinamed®: 40% (24s)

Shampoo:
- DHS™ Sal: 3% (120 mL)
- Ionil®: 2% (240 mL, 480 mL, 960 mL)
- Ionil® Plus: 2% (240 mL) [conditioning shampoo]
- LupiCare™ Dandruff, LupiCare™ Psoriasis: 2% (120 mL, 240 mL)
- Neutrogena® Healthy Scalp: 1.8% (90 mL, 180 mL)
- Neutrogena® Maximum Strength T/Sal®: 3% (135 mL)
- Tiseb®: 2% (240 mL)

Soap: 2% (114 g)

♦ **Salicylic Acid and Sulfur** *see* Sulfur and Salicylic Acid *on page 1493*

- **SalineX® [OTC]** *see* Sodium Chloride *on page 1450*
- **Salk Vaccine** *see* Poliovirus Vaccine (Inactivated) *on page 1275*

Salmeterol (sal ME te role)

Medication Safety Issues

Sound-alike/look-alike issues:

Salmeterol may be confused with Salbutamol

Serevent® may be confused with Serentil®

Related Information

Asthma *on page 1904*

U.S. Brand Names Serevent® Diskus®

Canadian Brand Names Serevent®

Index Terms Salmeterol Xinafoate

Therapeutic Category Adrenergic Agonist Agent; Antiasthmatic; $Beta_2$-Adrenergic Agonist Agent; Bronchodilator

Generic Available No

Use Maintenance treatment of asthma; prevention of bronchospasm in patients with reversible obstructive airway disease; prevention of exercise-induced bronchospasm

Medication Guide An FDA-approved patient medication guide, which is available with the product information and at http://www.fda.gov/cder/Offices/ODS/medication_guides.htm, must be dispensed with this medication for each new outpatient prescription and refill.

Pregnancy Risk Factor C

Lactation Enters breast milk/use caution

Contraindications Hypersensitivity to salmeterol, adrenergic amines, or any component

Warnings Cardiovascular effects are not common with salmeterol when used in recommended doses. Salmeterol is not meant to relieve acute asthmatic symptoms. Acute episodes should be treated with short-acting $beta_2$ agonist. Do not increase the frequency of salmeterol use. Paroxysmal bronchospasm (which can be fatal) has been reported with this and other inhaled agents. If this occurs, discontinue treatment; most commonly occurs with first use of a new canister or vial

Long-acting $beta_2$ adrenergic agents (eg, salmeterol) have been associated with an increased risk of asthma-related death. Salmeterol should only be prescribed in patients not adequately controlled on other asthma-controller medications or whose disease severity clearly warrants treatment with two maintenance therapies. A medication guide is available to provide information to patients covering the risk of use.

Precautions Use with caution in patients with cardiovascular disorders (especially coronary artery insufficiency, cardiac arrhythmias, and hypertension), hepatic impairment, convulsive disorders, thyrotoxicosis, or others who are sensitive to the effects of sympathomimetic amines

Adverse Reactions

Cardiovascular: Prolonged QT_c interval (large doses), tachycardia, palpitations, arrhythmias, angioedema, hypertension

Central nervous system: Dizziness, headache, nervousness, hyperactivity, insomnia, malaise

Dermatologic: Rash, pruritus, urticaria

Endocrine & metabolic: Hypokalemia

Gastrointestinal: GI upset, diarrhea, nausea, oropharyngeal irritation

Neuromuscular & skeletal: Joint and back pain, tremors, muscle cramps

Respiratory: Respiratory arrest, cough, pharyngitis, nasal and sinus congestion, rhinitis, paradoxical bronchospasm (see Warnings)

Miscellaneous: Hypersensitivity reactions including anaphylaxis in patients with milk allergy (very rare; noted in postmarketing case reports), tachyphylaxis

Drug Interactions Cytochrome P450 isoenzyme CYP3A3/4 substrate (major)

Additive effects with beta-adrenergic agents; MAO inhibitors and tricyclic antidepressants potentiate cardiovascular effects (wait 2 weeks after discontinuation of these agents before initiating salmeterol therapy); beta-blocking agents antagonize effects; increased potassium losses with diuretics

Stability Store at controlled room temperature in a dry place; stable for 6 weeks after protective foil is removed

Mechanism of Action Relaxes bronchial smooth muscle by selective action on $beta_2$-receptors with little effect on heart rate

Pharmacodynamics

Onset of action: 20 minutes to 2 hours

Maximum effect: 2-5 hours

Duration: Up to 12 hours

(Continued)

Salmeterol *(Continued)*

Pharmacokinetics

Protein binding: 96%

Metabolism: Extensive via hydroxylation

Half-life: 2-5 hours

Elimination: 60% in feces and 25% in urine over a 7-day period

Usual Dosage Children >4 years and Adults:

Maintenance and prevention of asthma, COPD: Inhalation, oral: 50 mcg (1 actuation/puff) twice daily, 12 hours apart

Prevention of exercise-induced asthma: Inhalation: 50 mcg (1 inhalation/puff) 30 minutes prior to exercise; additional doses should not be used for 12 hours; patients who are using salmeterol twice daily should **not** use an additional salmeterol dose prior to exercise; if twice daily use is not effective during exercise, consider other appropriate therapy

Administration Inhalation: May not be used with a spacer

Monitoring Parameters Pulmonary function tests

Patient Information Do not use to treat acute symptoms; do not exceed the prescribed dose of salmeterol; do not stop using inhaled or oral corticosteroids without medical advice even if feeling better; do not exhale into the Diskus®; do not wash the mouthpiece or any part of the diskus; keep it dry; never attempt to take Diskus® apart

Additional Information When salmeterol is initiated in patients previously receiving a short-acting beta agonist, instruct the patient to discontinue the regular use of the short-acting beta agonist and to utilize the shorter-acting agent for symptomatic or acute episodes only.

Dosage Forms Excipient information presented when available (limited, particularly for generics); consult specific product labeling.

Powder for oral inhalation: 50 mcg (28s, 60s) [delivers 50 mcg/inhalation; contains lactose]

References

Meyer JM, Wenzel CL, and Kradjan WA, "Salmeterol: A Novel, Long-Acting Beta$_2$-Agonist," *Ann Pharmacother*, 1993, 27(12):1478-87.

"National Asthma Education and Prevention Program. Expert Panel Report: Guidelines for the Diagnosis and Management of Asthma Update on Selected Topics--2002," *J Allergy Clin Immunol*, 2002, 110(5 Suppl):S141-219.

♦ **Salmeterol and Fluticasone** *see* Fluticasone and Salmeterol *on page 694*
♦ **Salmeterol Xinafoate** *see* Salmeterol *on page 1415*
♦ **Salofalk® (Can)** *see* Mesalamine *on page 1011*
♦ **Sal-Plant® [OTC]** *see* Salicylic Acid *on page 1413*
♦ **Salt** *see* Sodium Chloride *on page 1450*
♦ **Salt Poor Albumin** *see* Albumin *on page 64*
♦ **Sal-Tropine™** *see* Atropine *on page 181*
♦ **Sandimmune®** *see* CycloSPORINE *on page 422*
♦ **Sandimmune® I.V. (Can)** *see* CycloSPORINE *on page 422*
♦ **Sandostatin®** *see* Octreotide Acetate *on page 1157*
♦ **Sandostatin LAR®** *see* Octreotide Acetate *on page 1157*
♦ **Sandoz-Amiodarone (Can)** *see* Amiodarone *on page 100*
♦ **Sandoz-Atenolol (Can)** *see* Atenolol *on page 170*
♦ **Sandoz-Azithromycin (Can)** *see* Azithromycin *on page 191*
♦ **Sandoz-Ciprofloxacin (Can)** *see* Ciprofloxacin *on page 357*
♦ **Sandoz-Citalopram (Can)** *see* Citalopram *on page 368*
♦ **Sandoz-Clonazepam (Can)** *see* Clonazepam *on page 387*
♦ **Sandoz-Cyclosporine (Can)** *see* CycloSPORINE *on page 422*
♦ **Sandoz-Diltiazem CD (Can)** *see* Diltiazem *on page 503*
♦ **Sandoz-Diltiazem T (Can)** *see* Diltiazem *on page 503*
♦ **Sandoz-Estradiol Derm 50 (Can)** *see* Estradiol *on page 605*
♦ **Sandoz-Estradiol Derm 75 (Can)** *see* Estradiol *on page 605*
♦ **Sandoz-Estradiol Derm 100 (Can)** *see* Estradiol *on page 605*
♦ **Sandoz-Fluoxetine (Can)** *see* Fluoxetine *on page 681*
♦ **Sandoz-Fluvoxamine (Can)** *see* Fluvoxamine *on page 697*
♦ **Sandoz-Glyburide (Can)** *see* GlyBURIDE *on page 734*
♦ **Sandoz-Levobunolol (Can)** *see* Levobunolol *on page 925*
♦ **Sandoz-Lovastatin (Can)** *see* Lovastatin *on page 964*
♦ **Sandoz-Metformin FC (Can)** *see* Metformin *on page 1016*
♦ **Sandoz-Metoprolol (Can)** *see* Metoprolol *on page 1046*
♦ **Sandoz-Minocycline (Can)** *see* Minocycline *on page 1066*

Saquinavir (sa KWIN a veer)

Medication Safety Issues

Sound-alike/look-alike issues:

Saquinavir may be confused with Sinequan®

Fortovase® may be confused with Invirase®

Invirase® may be confused with Fortovase®

Related Information

Adult and Adolescent HIV *on pago 1821*

Pediatric HIV *on page 1816*

Perinatal HIV *on page 1831*

U.S. Brand Names Fortovase® [DSC]; Invirase®

Canadian Brand Names Fortovase®; Invirase®

Index Terms Saquinavir Mesylate

Therapeutic Category Antiretroviral Agent; HIV Agents (Anti-HIV Agents); Protease Inhibitor

Generic Available No

Use Treatment of HIV infection in combination with other antiretroviral agents; (**Note:** HIV regimens consisting of **three** antiretroviral agents are strongly recommended; due to its low bioavailability, Invirase® should be used only in combination regimens that include ritonavir "booster doses" so that adequate plasma saquinavir levels are attained); postexposure chemoprophylaxis following occupational exposure to HIV

Pregnancy Risk Factor B

Lactation Excretion in breast milk unknown/contraindicated

Contraindications Hypersensitivity to saquinavir or any component; patients with severe hepatic impairment; concurrent therapy with amiodarone, astemizole, bepridil, cisapride, dihydroergotamine, ergonovine, ergotamine, flecainide, methylergonovine, midazolam, pimozide, propafenone, quinidine, rifampin, terfenadine, triazolam

Warnings Saquinavir is a potent CYP3A4 isoenzyme inhibitor that interacts with numerous drugs. Due to potential serious and/or life-threatening drug interactions, some drugs are contraindicated (see Contraindications and Drug Interactions). Concurrent use with St John's wort, garlic capsules, or certain cholesterol-lowering agents (lovastatin, simvastatin) is **not** recommended. Alteration of dose or serum concentration monitoring may be required with other medications (see Drug Interactions).

Spontaneous bleeding episodes have been reported in patients with hemophilia receiving an HIV protease inhibitor. New onset diabetes mellitus, exacerbation of diabetes and hyperglycemia have been reported in HIV-infected patients receiving protease inhibitors. Significant elevations of serum triglycerides and cholesterol may occur (monitor and manage appropriately).

Precautions Use with caution in patients with hepatic impairment; elevated saquinavir levels, elevated liver enzymes, or worsening liver disease may occur. Fat redistribution and accumulation [ie, central obesity, peripheral wasting, facial wasting, breast enlargement, dorsocervical fat enlargement (buffalo hump), and cushingoid appearance] have been observed in patients receiving antiretroviral agents (causal relationship not established).

Adverse Reactions

Central nervous system: Confusion, ataxia, headache, dizziness, seizures, fever, hallucinations, asthenia, agitation, fatigue

Dermatologic: Rash, photosensitivity, acne

Endocrine & metabolic: Hypoglycemia, elevated creatine phosphokinase; rare: hyperglycemia, diabetes, ketoacidosis; fat redistribution (see Precautions)

Gastrointestinal: Diarrhea, abdominal discomfort, nausea, vomiting, stomatitis

(Continued)

Saquinavir *(Continued)*

Hematologic: Hemolytic anemia, pancytopenia, thrombocytopenia, microhemorrhages; rare: spontaneous bleeding episodes in hemophiliacs

Hepatic: Elevated ALT, AST, bilirubin, and amylase; worsening of chronic liver disease

Neuromuscular & skeletal: Parethesias, peripheral neuropathy, tremor, arthralgia

Respiratory: Cough

Drug Interactions Cytochrome P450 isoenzyme CYP3A3/4 substrate and inhibitor; p-glycoprotein substrate

Saquinavir may inhibit the metabolism of the following drugs and cause serious or life-threatening adverse effects: Amiodarone, astemizole, bepridil, cisapride, dihydroergotamine, ergonovine, ergotamine, flecainide, methylergonovine, midazolam, pimozide, propafenone, quinidine, terfenadine, and triazolam (concurrent therapy with these drugs and indinavir is contraindicated). Saquinavir may increase the toxic effects of amitriptyline, imipramine, lidocaine, cyclosporine, tacrolimus, sirolimus (serum concentration monitoring of these drugs is necessary). Saquinavir may increase serum concentrations or toxicity of calcium channel blockers; benzodiazepines; cholesterol-lowering agents (increased risk of myopathy and rhabdomyolysis; concurrent use of lovastatin or simvastatin is **not** recommended; use lowest possible dose of atorvastatin and carefully monitor patient; consider use of pravastatin, fluvastatin or rosuvastatin for concurrent use with saquinavir); sildenafil or other phosphodiesterase-5 (PDE-5) enzyme inhibitors (use decreased dose of sildenafil or other PDE-5 enzyme inhibitor); warfarin (monitor INR); clarithromycin (decrease clarithromycin dosage in patients with renal impairment); rifabutin (appropriate doses not established); dapsone, disopyramide, quinine, carbamazepine, fentanyl, alfentanil (use with caution; monitor closely). Concomitant use of saquinavir and nelfinavir increases serum concentrations of both drugs.

Saquinavir significantly decreases serum concentrations of methadone (increased methadone dose may be required); ethinyl estradiol (use additional or alternative contraceptive measures). Concomitant use of saquinavir with efavirenz or nevirapine may decrease serum concentrations of both drugs (appropriate doses not established).

The herbal medicine St John's wort (*Hypericum perforatum*) may significantly decrease concentrations of saquinavir and lead to treatment failure (concurrent use is **not** recommended). Garlic capsules may decrease saquinavir serum concentrations (concurrent use is **not** recommended). Use of rifampin is contraindicated with saquinavir; rifampin significantly reduces saquinavir concentrations and may lead to treatment failure; use of rifampin with ritonavir-boosted saquinavir resulted in significant hepatocellular toxicity. Enzyme inducing drugs, such as carbamazepine, dexamethasone, phenobarbital, phenytoin, may decrease indinavir concentrations (use with caution).

Delavirdine, indinavir, ritonavir, lopinavir/ritonavir, ketoconazole, itraconazole may increase saquinavir serum concentrations.

Food Interactions Presence of a high fat meal maximizes bioavailability of saquinavir; grapefruit juice may increase saquinavir levels

Stability

Fortovase® capsules: Store in refrigerator; stable for 3 months if stored at room temperature

Invirase® capsules and tablets: Store at room temperature in tightly closed bottles

Mechanism of Action A protease inhibitor which acts on an enzyme (protease) late in the HIV replication process after the virus has entered into the cell's nucleus; saquinavir binds to the protease activity site and inhibits the activity of the enzyme, thus preventing cleavage of viral polyprotein precursors (gag-pol protein precursors) into individual functional proteins found in infectious HIV; this results in the formation of immature, noninfectious viral particles

Pharmacokinetics

Distribution: CSF concentration is negligible when compared to concentrations from matched plasma samples; partitions into tissues

V_d: Adults: 700 L

Protein binding: 98%

Metabolism: Extensive first-pass effect; hepatic metabolism by cytochrome P450 3A system to inactive mono- and dihydroxylated metabolites

Bioavailability:

Invirase® capsules: 4% (increased in the presence of food); bioavailability of Invirase® capsules and tablets are similar when administered with low dose ritonavir (ie, booster doses of ritonavir); bioavailability of Invirase® combined with ritonavir booster does is ≥ Fortovase®

Fortovase®: Relative to Invirase®: 331%

Half-life: Adults: 13 hours

Elimination: 88% of dose eliminated in feces; 1% excreted in urine

Clearance: Children: Significantly higher than adults

Usual Dosage Oral (use in combination with other antiretroviral agents): **Note:** Invirase® and Fortovase® are not bioequivalent and cannot be used interchangeably. Due to its greater bioavailability, Fortovase® is the recommended formulation when saquinavir is the sole protease inhibitor in an antiretroviral regimen. Invirase® should be used only in regimens that include ritonavir "booster doses" so that adequate saquinavir serum concentrations are attained. **Note:** Fortovase® has recently been discontinued because ritonavir-boosted Invirase® tablet containing regimens result in fewer gastrointestinal side effects and a lower pill burden compared to ritonavir-boosted Fortovase® regimens.

Neonates and Infants: Not approved for use; appropriate dose is unknown.

Children: Not approved for use; Fortovase® 50 mg/kg/dose every 8 hours did **not** provide adequate saquinavir serum concentrations in children; ongoing studies are evaluating saquinavir in combination with ritonavir, nelfinavir, or lopinavir/ritonavir; do **not** use saquinavir as sole protease inhibitor in pediatric patients ≤16 years of age

Adolescents >16 years and Adults:

Unboosted regimen (ie, regimen **without** ritonavir):

Fortovase®: 1200 mg 3 times/day

Invirase®: Not recommended; do **not** use without ritonavir booster doses

Ritonavir boosted regimen: **Note:** Take ritonavir at the same time as saquinavir

Fortovase® or Invirase®: 1000 mg twice daily with ritonavir 100 mg twice daily

Lopinavir/ritonavir boosted regimen: Fortovase® or Invirase®: 1000 mg twice daily with lopinavir 400 mg/ritonavir 100 mg twice daily

Administration Oral: Administer within 2 hours after a full meal to increase absorption; avoid taking saquinavir with grapefruit juice

Monitoring Parameters Liver function tests, cholesterol and triglyceride levels, blood glucose levels, CD4 cell count, plasma levels of HIV RNA

Patient Information Saquinavir is not a cure for HIV infection. Notify physician if numbness, tingling, persistent severe abdominal pain, nausea, or vomiting occurs. Some medicines should not be taken with saquinavir; report the use of other medications, nonprescription medications, and herbal or natural products to your physician and pharmacist; avoid the herbal medicine St John's wort and garlic capsules. Take saquinavir every day as prescribed; do not change dose or discontinue without physician's advice; if a dose is missed, take it as soon as possible, then return to normal dosing schedule; if a dose is skipped, do not double the next dose. May cause photosensitivity reactions (eg, exposure to sunlight may cause severe sunburn, skin rash, redness, or itching); avoid exposure to sunlight and artificial light sources (sunlamps, tanning booth/bed); wear protective clothing, wide-brimmed hats, sunglasses, and lip sunscreen (SPF ≥15); use a sunscreen [broad-spectrum sunscreen or physical sunscreen (preferred) or sunblock with SPF ≥15]; contact physician if reaction occurs.

HIV medications may cause changes in body fat, including an increase in fat in the upper back and neck, breasts, and trunk; a loss of fat from the face, arms, and legs may also occur.

Dosage Forms Excipient information presented when available (limited, particularly for generics); consult specific product labeling. **Note:** Strength expressed as base; [DSC] = Discontinued product

Capsule, as mesylate:

Invirase®: 200 mg [contains lactose 63.3 mg/capsule]

Capsule, soft gelatin, as base:

Fortovase®: 200 mg [DSC]

Tablet, as mesylate:

Invirase®: 500 mg

References

Briars LA, Hilao JJ, and Kraus DM, "A Review of Pediatric Human Immunodeficiency Virus Infection," *Journal of Pharmacy Practice*, 2004, 17(6):407-31.

Collier AC, Coombs RW, Schoenfeld DA, et al, "Treatment of Human Immunodeficiency Virus Infection With Saquinavir, Zidovudine, and Zalcitabine," *N Engl J Med*, 1996, 334(16):1011-7.

Mueller BU, "Antiviral Chemotherapy," *Curr Opin Pediatr*, 1997, 9(2):178-83.

Panel on Clinical Practices for Treatment of HIV Infection, "Guidelines for the Use of Antiretroviral Agents in HIV-Infected Adults and Adolescents," October 10, 2006, http://www.aidsinfo.nih.gov.

Working Group on Antiretroviral Therapy and Medical Management of HIV-Infected Children, "Guidelines for the Use of Antiretroviral Agents in Pediatric HIV Infection," October 26, 2006, http://www.aidsinfo.nih.gov.

♦ **Saquinavir Mesylate** *see* Saquinavir *on page 1417*

♦ **Sarafem®** *see* Fluoxetine *on page 681*

Sargramostim (sar GRAM oh stim)

Medication Safety Issues

Sound-alike/look-alike issues:

Leukine® may be confused with Leukeran®

Related Information

Compatibility of Chemotherapy and Related Supportive Care Medications *on page 1777*

U.S. Brand Names Leukine®

Canadian Brand Names Leukine®

Index Terms GM-CSF; Granulocyte-Macrophage Colony Stimulating Factor; NSC-613795; rGM-CSF

Therapeutic Category Colony-Stimulating Factor

Generic Available No

Use Accelerates myeloid recovery in patients undergoing autologous or allogeneic BMT; mobilize hematopoietic progenitor cells into peripheral blood for collection by leukapheresis; accelerate myeloid engraftment following autologous peripheral blood progenitor cell transplantation; increase neutrophil counts in patients with malignancies receiving myelosuppressive chemotherapy; increase leukocyte counts in patients with severe aplastic anemia; neonatal neutropenia

Pregnancy Risk Factor C

Lactation Excretion in breast milk unknown/use caution

Contraindications Hypersensitivity to GM-CSF, yeast-derived products, or any component (see Warnings); excessive leukemic myeloid blasts in bone marrow or peripheral blood ≥10%; history of idiopathic thrombocytopenic purpura

Warnings Injection solution contains benzyl alcohol which may cause allergic reactions in susceptible individuals; large amounts of benzyl alcohol (≥99 mg/kg/day) have been associated with a potentially fatal toxicity ("gasping syndrome") in neonates; the "gasping syndrome" consists of metabolic acidosis, respiratory distress, gasping respirations, CNS dysfunction (including convulsions, intracranial hemorrhage), hypotension and cardiovascular collapse; use sargramostim injection products containing benzyl alcohol with caution in neonates; *in vitro* and animal studies have shown that benzoate, a metabolite of benzyl alcohol, displaces bilirubin from protein binding sites

Precautions Use with caution in patients with autoimmune or chronic inflammatory disease, hypertension, cardiovascular disease, pulmonary disease, or renal or hepatic impairment

Rapid increase in peripheral blood counts: If ANC is >20,000/mm^3 or platelets >500,000/mm^3, decrease dose by 50% or discontinue drug (counts will fall to normal within 3-7 days after discontinuing drug)

Growth factor potential: Caution with myeloid malignancies; do **not** administer within 24 hours prior to or after chemotherapy or 12 hours prior to or after radiation therapy

Adverse Reactions

Cardiovascular: Hypotension, tachycardia, flushing, pericardial effusion, fluid retention, venous thrombosis

Central nervous system: Malaise, fever, headache, chills

Dermatologic: Rash

Endocrine & metabolic: Polydipsia

Gastrointestinal: Nausea, vomiting, diarrhea, stomatitis, GI hemorrhage

Hepatic: Elevated liver function tests

Neuromuscular & skeletal: Bone pain, myalgia, rigors, weakness

Respiratory: Dyspnea

Miscellaneous: "First dose" reaction (fever, hypotension, tachycardia, rigors, flushing, nausea, vomiting, dyspnea)

Drug Interactions Lithium and corticosteroids may potentiate myeloproliferative effects of sargramostim

Stability Store vial in the refrigerator; stable after reconstitution for 6 hours at room temperature; use only NS to prepare I.V. infusion solution; GM-CSF at a concentration ≥10 mcg/mL is compatible with TPN during Y-site administration

Mechanism of Action Stimulates proliferation, differentiation and functional activity of neutrophils, eosinophils, monocytes and macrophages

Pharmacodynamics

Onset of action: Increase in WBC in 7-14 days

Duration: WBC will return to baseline within 1 week after discontinuing drug

Pharmacokinetics

Half-life: 2 hours

Time to peak serum concentration: SubQ: Within 3 hours

Usual Dosage I.V., SubQ:

Neonates: 10 mcg/kg/day once daily for 5 days has been administered to preterm neonates at high risk of both neutropenia and sepsis

Children (no dosing for children has been FDA approved): 250 mcg/m^2/day once daily for 21 days to begin 2-4 hours after the marrow infusion on day 0 of BMT or not less than 24 hours after chemotherapy. If significant adverse effects or "first dose" reaction is seen at this dose, discontinue the drug until toxicity resolves, then restart at a reduced dose of 125 mcg/m^2/day

Aplastic anemia: 8-32 mcg/kg/day once daily

Cancer chemotherapy recovery: 3-15 mcg/kg/day once daily for 14-21 days; maximum dose: 30 mcg/kg/day or 1500 mcg/m^2/day

Adults: 250 mcg/m^2/day once daily for 21 days to begin 2-4 hours after BMT, or not less than 24 hours after chemotherapy (to minimize first dose reaction, start with low doses and increase gradually)

Aplastic anemia: 15-480 mcg/m^2 once daily

Cancer chemotherapy recovery: 3-15 mcg/kg/day once daily for 10 days

Administration Parenteral:

I.V.: Administer as a 30-minute, 2-hour, or 6-hour I.V. infusion or by continuous I.V. infusion. Do not shake solution to avoid foaming. Dilute in NS; if the final concentration of GM-CSF in NS is <10 mcg/mL, then add 1 mg albumin per mL of I.V. fluid. Albumin acts as a carrier molecule to prevent drug adsorption to the I.V. tubing. Albumin should be added to NS prior to addition of GM-CSF.

SubQ: Reconstituted 250 mcg/mL or 500 mcg/mL solution may be administered without further dilution; rotate injection sites

Monitoring Parameters CBC with differential, platelets; renal/liver function tests, especially with previous dysfunction; vital signs, weight; pulmonary function

Reference Range Excessive leukocytosis (WBC >50,000 cells/mm^3, ANC >20,000 cells/mm^3)

Patient Information Possible bone pain may occur

Nursing Implications Can premedicate with analgesics and antipyretics; control bone pain with non-narcotic analgesics

Additional Information Produced by recombinant DNA technology using a yeast-derived expression system

Dosage Forms Excipient information presented when available (limited, particularly for generics); consult specific product labeling.

Injection, powder for reconstitution:

Leukine®: 250 mcg [contains mannitol 40 mg/mL and sucrose 10 mg/mL]

Injection, solution:

Leukine®: 500 mcg/mL (1 mL) [contains benzyl alcohol, disodium edetate, mannitol 40 mg/mL, and sucrose 10 mg/mL]

References

Carr R, Modi N, Dore CJ, et al, "A Randomized, Controlled Trial of Prophylactic Granulocyte-Macrophage Colony-Stimulating Factor in Human Newborns Less Than 32 Weeks Gestation," *Pediatrics*, 1999, 103(4 Pt 1):796-802.

Lieschke GJ and Burgess AW, "Granulocyte Colony-Stimulating Factor and Granulocyte-Macrophage Colony-Stimulating Factor," (1) *N Engl J Med*, 1992, 327(1):28-35.

Lieschke GJ and Burgess AW, "Granulocyte Colony-Stimulating Factor and Granulocyte-Macrophage Colony-Stimulating Factor," (2) *N Engl J Med*, 1992, 327(2):99-106.

Stute N, Furman WL, Schell M, et al, "Pharmacokinetics of Recombinant Human Granulocyte - Macrophage Colony - Stimulating Factor in Children After Intravenous and Subcutaneous Administration," *J Pharm Sci*, 1995, 84(7):824-8.

Trissel LA, Bready BB, Kwan JW, et al, "Visual Compatibility of Sargramostim With Selected Antineoplastic Agents, Anti-infectives, or Other Drugs During Simulated Y-Site Injection," *Am J Hosp Pharm*, 1992, 49(2):402-6.

- **Sarna® HC (Can)** *see* Hydrocortisone *on page 781*
- **Sarnol®-HC [OTC]** *see* Hydrocortisone *on page 781*
- **SC 33428** *see* Idarubicin *on page 808*
- **SCH 56592** *see* Posaconazole *on page 1281*
- **Scopace™** *see* Scopolamine *on page 1421*

Scopolamine (skoe POL a meen)

Medication Safety Issues

Transdermal patch may contain conducting metal (eg, aluminum); remove patch prior to MRI.

Related Information

Overdose and Toxicology *on page 1916*

U.S. Brand Names Isopto® Hyoscine; Maldemar™; Scopace™; Transderm Scōp®

Canadian Brand Names Buscopan®; Transderm-V®

Index Terms Hyoscine Butylbromide; Hyoscine Hydrobromide; Scopolamine Base; Scopolamine Butylbromide; Scopolamine Hydrobromide

(Continued)

Scopolamine *(Continued)*

Therapeutic Category Anticholinergic Agent; Anticholinergic Agent, Ophthalmic; Anticholinergic Agent, Transdermal; Ophthalmic Agent, Mydriatic

Generic Available Yes: Injection

Use Preoperative medication to produce amnesia and decrease salivary and respiratory secretions; to produce cycloplegia and mydriasis (ophthalmic formulation); treatment of iridocyclitis (ophthalmic formulation); prevention of motion sickness (oral and transdermal formulations) and prevention of postoperative nausea and vomiting (transdermal formulation)

Pregnancy Risk Factor C

Lactation Enters breast milk/use caution (AAP rates "compatible")

Contraindications Hypersensitivity to scopolamine or any component; patients hypersensitive to belladonna or barbiturates may be hypersensitive to scopolamine; narrow-angle glaucoma, GI or GU obstruction, thyrotoxicosis, tachycardia secondary to cardiac insufficiency, paralytic ileus, myasthenia gravis

Warnings Drug withdrawal symptoms such as nausea, vomiting, headache, dizziness, and equilibrium disturbance have been reported following removal of transdermal system, primarily in patients using the system for more than 3 days

Precautions Use with caution with hepatic or renal dysfunction since adverse CNS effects occur more often in these patients; use with caution in infants and children since they may be more susceptible to adverse effects of scopolamine; use with caution in patients with cardiac disease, seizures, or psychoses

Adverse Reactions

Cardiovascular: Tachycardia, palpitations

Central nervous system: Disorientation, drowsiness, hallucinations, confusion, psychosis, delirium, excitement, restlessness, dizziness

Gastrointestinal: Xerostomia, constipation, nausea, vomiting, dysphagia, dysgeusia

Genitourinary: Urinary retention

Ocular: Blurred vision, cycloplegia, mydriasis, photophobia, elevated intraocular pressure

Miscellaneous: Anaphylaxis, allergic reactions

Note: Systemic adverse effects have been reported with both the topical and ophthalmic preparations

Drug Interactions Additive adverse effects with other anticholinergic agents and amantadine; GI absorption of the following drugs may be affected: acetaminophen, levodopa, ketoconazole, digoxin (tablets only), riboflavin, KCl wax-matrix preparations; additive CNS effects with other CNS depressants, alcohol

Stability Physically compatible when mixed in the same syringe with atropine, butorphanol, chlorpromazine, dimenhydrinate, diphenhydramine, droperidol, fentanyl, glycopyrrolate, hydromorphone, hydroxyzine, meperidine, metoclopramide, morphine, pentazocine, pentobarbital, perphenazine, prochlorperazine, promazine, promethazine, or thiopental

Mechanism of Action Blocks the action of acetylcholine at parasympathetic sites in smooth muscle, secretory glands and the CNS, resulting in anticholinergic activity (inhibition of secretion of saliva and sweat, decreased GI motility and secretions, dilated pupils, increased heart rate, drowsiness, depressed motor function); antagonizes histamine and serotonin

Pharmacodynamics

Onset of action:
- Oral, I.M.: 30 minutes to 1 hour
- I.V.: 10 minutes
- Transdermal: 4 hours

Duration:
- Oral, I.M.: 4-6 hours
- I.V.: 2 hours
- Transdermal: 72 hours

Pharmacokinetics

Absorption: Well absorbed by all routes of administration

Metabolism: In the liver

Half-life: 9.5 hours

Excretion: <5% excreted unchanged in the urine

Usual Dosage

Preoperatively and antiemetic:

I.M., I.V., SubQ:

Children: 6 mcg/kg/dose (maximum dose: 0.3 mg/dose); may be repeated every 6-8 hours

Adults: 0.3-0.65 mg; may be repeated 3-4 times/day

Transdermal: Adults: Apply 1 disc behind the ear the evening before surgery; if prior to cesarean section, apply 1 hour prior to minimize exposure to infant

Motion sickness:

Oral: Children >12 years and Adults: 1-2 tablets 1 hour prior to exposure; may repeat after 8 hours of continued exposure

Transdermal: Children >12 years and Adults: Apply 1 disc behind the ear at least 4 hours prior to exposure every 3 days as needed

Ophthalmic:

Refraction:

Children: Instill 1 drop of 0.25% to eye(s) twice daily for 2 days before procedure

Adults: Instill 1-2 drops of 0.25% to eye(s) 1 hour before procedure

Iridocyclitis:

Children: Instill 1 drop of 0.25% to eye(s) up to 3 times/day

Adults: Instill 1-2 drops of 0.25% to eye(s) up to 3 times/day

Administration

Oral: May be administered without regard to food

Parenteral: I.V.: Dilute with an equal volume of SWI and administer by direct I.V. injection over 2-3 minutes

Transdermal: Apply patch to hairless area behind one ear; wash hands before and after application; if becomes dislodged, replace with fresh patch; if usage >72 hours, replace with new patch (see Usual Dosage for time of administration)

Ophthalmic: Instill drops to conjunctival sac of affected eye(s); avoid contact of bottle tip with skin or eye; finger pressure should be applied to lacrimal sac during and for 1-2 minutes after instillation to decrease risk of absorption and systemic reactions

Patient Information May cause drowsiness and impair ability to perform activities requiring mental alertness or physical coordination; may cause dry mouth; avoid alcohol; wash hands thoroughly with soap and water after handling the patch as dilation of pupils and blurred vision may occur if contact with eye; dispose of patches properly to avoid contact with children or pets; remove patch immediately if experiencing difficulty urinating or pain and reddening of eyes accompanied by dilated pupils

Additional Information Transdermal disc is programmed to deliver *in vivo* 0.5 mg over 3 days

Dosage Forms Excipient information presented when available (limited, particularly for generics); consult specific product labeling. [CAN] = Canadian brand name

Injection, solution, as hydrobromide: 0.4 mg/mL (1 mL)

Injection, solution, as hyoscine-N-butylbromide:

Buscopan® [CAN]: 20 mg/mL [not available in U.S.]

Solution, ophthalmic, as hydrobromide:

Isopto® Hyoscine: 0.25% (5 mL, 15 mL) [contains benzalkonium chloride]

Tablet, as hyoscine-N-butylbromide:

Buscopan® [CAN]: 10 mg [not available in U.S.]

Tablet, soluble, as hydrobromide:

Maldemar™, Scopace™: 0.4 mg

Transdermal system:

Transderm Scōp®: 1.5 mg (4s, 10s, 24s) [releases ~1 mg over 72 hours]

- ♦ **Scopolamine Base** *see* Scopolamine *on page 1421*
- ♦ **Scopolamine Butylbromide** *see* Scopolamine *on page 1421*
- ♦ **Scopolamine Hydrobromide** *see* Scopolamine *on page 1421*
- ♦ **Scopolamine, Hyoscyamine, Atropine, and Phenobarbital** *see* Hyoscyamine, Atropine, Scopolamine, and Phenobarbital *on page 800*
- ♦ **Scot-Tussin DM® Cough Chasers [OTC]** *see* Dextromethorphan *on page 477*
- ♦ **Scot-Tussin® Expectorant [OTC]** *see* Guaifenesin *on page 745*
- ♦ **Scot-Tussin® Senior [OTC]** *see* Guaifenesin and Dextromethorphan *on page 748*
- ♦ **SDZ ASM 981** *see* Pimecrolimus *on page 1262*
- ♦ **Seba-Gel™** *see* Benzoyl Peroxide *on page 207*
- ♦ **Sebcur® (Can)** *see* Salicylic Acid *on page 1413*

Secobarbital (see koe BAR bi tal)

Medication Safety Issues

Sound-alike/look-alike issues:

Seconal® may be confused with Sectral®

Related Information

Laboratory Detection of Drugs in Urine *on page 1928*

U.S. Brand Names Seconal®

Index Terms Quinalbarbitone Sodium; Secobarbital Sodium

Therapeutic Category Barbiturate; Hypnotic; Sedative

Generic Available No

Use Short-term treatment of insomnia; preanesthetic agent

(Continued)

Secobarbital *(Continued)*

Restrictions C-II

Pregnancy Risk Factor D

Lactation Enters breast milk/use caution (AAP rates "compatible")

Contraindications Hypersensitivity to secobarbital or any component; pre-existing CNS depression, severe uncontrolled pain, porphyria, severe respiratory disease with dyspnea or obstruction

Warnings Hypersensitivity reactions including anaphylaxis and angioedema may occur. Hazardous sleep-related activities, such as sleep-driving (driving while not fully awake without any recollection of driving), preparing and eating food, and making phone calls while asleep have also been reported. Effects with other sedative drugs or ethanol may be potentiated.

Precautions Use with caution in patients with hypovolemic shock, CHF, hepatic impairment, respiratory dysfunction or depression, previous addiction to the sedative/hypnotic group, chronic or acute pain, renal dysfunction; tolerance or psychological and physical dependence may occur with prolonged use; abrupt discontinuation after prolonged use may result in withdrawal symptoms

Adverse Reactions

Cardiovascular: Hypotension, cardiac arrhythmias, bradycardia

Central nervous system: Dizziness, lightheadedness, drowsiness, "hangover" effect, lethargy, impaired judgment, CNS depression or paradoxical excitation, hypothermia, nightmares, hallucinations

Dermatologic: Rash, exfoliative dermatitis, Stevens-Johnson syndrome

Gastrointestinal: Nausea, vomiting, constipation

Hematologic: Megaloblastic anemia, thrombocytopenia, agranulocytosis

Respiratory: Respiratory depression, apnea

Miscellaneous: Psychological and physical dependence with prolonged use; hypersensitivity reactions, anaphylaxis, angioedema; hazardous sleep-related activities (see Warnings)

Drug Interactions Cytochrome P450 isoenzyme CYP2A6, CYP2C9, and CYP3A3/4 inducer

Barbiturates are enzyme inducers (monitor patients closely for decreased effect of concomitantly administered medications or increased effect when barbiturates are discontinued)

Secobarbital may decrease the serum concentration or effect of ethosuximide, warfarin, oral contraceptives, chloramphenicol, griseofulvin, doxycycline, beta-blockers, cyclophosphamide, theophylline, corticosteroids, tricyclic antidepressants, quinidine, haloperidol, and phenothiazines. Secobarbital given with other CNS depressants may increase CNS and respiratory depression. Chloramphenicol, valproic acid, and chlorpropamide may inhibit the metabolism of secobarbital with a resultant increase in secobarbital serum concentration.

Food Interactions High doses of pyridoxine may decrease drug effect; barbiturates may increase the metabolism of vitamins D and K

Mechanism of Action Depresses CNS activity by binding to barbiturate site at GABA-receptor complex enhancing GABA activity; depresses reticular activating system; higher doses may be gabamimetic

Pharmacodynamics

Onset of action: Hypnosis: Oral: 15-30 minutes

Duration: Hypnosis: Oral: 3-4 hours with 100 mg dose

Pharmacokinetics

Absorption: Oral: Well absorbed (90%)

Distribution: V_d: Adult: 1.5 L/kg; crosses the placenta; appears in breast milk

Protein binding: 45% to 60%

Metabolism: In the liver by the microsomal enzyme system

Half-life:

- Children: 2-13 years: 2.7-13.5 hours
- Adults: 15-40 hours; mean 28 hours

Time to peak serum concentration: Oral: Within 2-4 hours

Elimination: Renally as inactive metabolites and small amounts as unchanged drug

Dialysis: Hemodialysis: Slightly dialyzable (5% to 20%)

Usual Dosage Oral:

Children:

- Preoperative sedation: 2-6 mg/kg (maximum dose: 100 mg/dose) 1-2 hours before procedure
- Sedation: 6 mg/kg/day divided every 8 hours

Adults:

- Hypnotic: Usual: 100 mg/dose at bedtime; range 100-200 mg/dose
- Preoperative sedation: 100-300 mg 1-2 hours before procedure

Monitoring Parameters Blood pressure, heart rate, respiratory rate, pulse oximetry, CNS status

Patient Information Avoid alcohol and other CNS depressants. May be habit-forming; avoid abrupt discontinuation after prolonged use. May cause dizziness or drowsiness and impair ability to perform activities requiring mental alertness or physical coordination. May cause hypersensitivity reactions. May cause hazardous sleep-related activities (ie, driving, preparing and eating foods, and making phone calls while not fully awake).

Additional Information Effectiveness for insomnia decreases greatly after 2 weeks of use; alkalinization of urine does not significantly increase excretion; withdraw slowly over 5-6 days after prolonged use to avoid sleep disturbances and rapid eye movement (REM) rebound

In March 2007, the FDA requested that all manufacturers of sedative-hypnotic drug products, including Seconal® (secobarbital), revise the labeling to include a greater emphasis on the risks of adverse events. The events include severe hypersensitivity reactions including anaphylaxis and/or angioedema, as well as hazardous sleep-related activities (eg, sleep-driving - driving while not fully awake after consumption of sedative-hypnotic drug, with no recollection of the event). Other activities may include preparing and ingesting food, and the use of the telephone, while asleep. These events may occur at any time during therapy including with the first dose administered.

Manufacturers must provide written notification to healthcare providers regarding the new warnings. In addition, manufacturers are to develop "Patient Medication Guides" designed to educate consumers about the potential risks and to advise them of precautionary measures that can be taken. This advice will contain recommendations on correct utilization of the medication as well as the avoidance of the consumption of ethanol and/or other CNS-depressant agents. The FDA is also recommending manufacturers conduct studies evaluating the frequencies of sleep-driving (and other sleep-related behaviors) with the individual products.

Patients should be instructed not to discontinue these medications without first speaking with their healthcare provider. Patients should also be informed of the potential for an allergic reaction, the signs and symptoms of anaphylaxis, and the appropriate emergency self-treatment of an anaphylactic reaction.

Additional information on the sedative-hypnotic products and sleep disorders is available at http://www.fda.gov/cder/drug/infopage/sedative_hypnotics/default.htm

Dosage Forms Excipient information presented when available (limited, particularly for generics); consult specific product labeling.

Capsule, as sodium: 100 mg

References

Levine HL, Cohen ME, Duffner PK, et al, "Rectal Absorption and Disposition of Secobarbital in Epileptic Children," *Pediatr Pharmacol (New York)*, 1982, 2(1):33-8.

Nahata MC, Starling S, and Edwards RC, "Prolonged Sedation Associated With Secobarbital in Newborn Infants Receiving Ventilatory Support," *Am J Perinatol*, 1991, 8(1):35-6.

Wolfert RR and Cox RM, "Room Temperature Stability of Drug Products Labeled for Refrigerated Storage," *Am J Hosp Pharm*, 1975, 32(6):585-7.

♦ **Secobarbital Sodium** *see* Secobarbital *on page 1423*

♦ **Seconal®** *see* Secobarbital *on page 1423*

♦ **SecreFlo™** *see* Secretin *on page 1425*

Secretin (SEE kre tin)

U.S. Brand Names ChiRhoStim™; SecreFlo™

Index Terms Secretin, Human; Secretin, Porcine

Therapeutic Category Diagnostic Agent, Gastrinoma (Zollinger-Ellison Syndrome); Diagnostic Agent, Pancreatic Exocrine Insufficiency

Generic Available No

Use Diagnosis of gastrinoma (Zollinger-Ellison syndrome) and diagnosis of pancreatic exocrine dysfunction (chronic pancreatitis); facilitation of endoscopic retrograde cholangiopancreatography (ERCP) visualization

Pregnancy Risk Factor C

Lactation Excretion in breast milk unknown/use caution

Contraindications Hypersensitivity to secretin or any component; do not give to patients with acute pancreatitis until attack has subsided

Precautions Administer an I.V. test dose of 0.2 mcg (0.1 mL) particularly in patients with a history of hypersensitivity, allergy or asthma; use with caution in patients who are highly nervous or have an excessive gag reflex; patients receiving anticholinergics, patients who have had a vagotomy, or patients with inflammatory bowel disease may have a reduced response to secretin; patients with alcoholic or other liver diseases may have an increased response to secretin

Adverse Reactions

Cardiovascular: Hypotension, bradycardia (mild), flushing, tachycardia

(Continued)

Secretin *(Continued)*

Central nervous system: Headache, fever, anxiety, faintness, sedation
Gastrointestinal: Abdominal discomfort and cramps, vomiting, diarrhea, nausea, increased oral secretions
Neuromuscular & skeletal: Tingling in legs
Respiratory: Transient decrease in oxygen saturation, respiratory distress
Miscellaneous: Hypersensitivity reactions, diaphoresis

Drug Interactions Anticholinergics may reduce response to secretin

Stability Store in freezer (-20°C); SecreFlo™ should be used immediately after reconstitution; human secretin is also stable for 1 year refrigerated and 6 months at room temperature

Mechanism of Action Secretin is a naturally-occurring hormone secreted by cells in the duodenal and upper jejunal mucosa which increases the volume and bicarbonate content of pancreatic juice; when used as a diagnostic agent, synthetic porcine secretin stimulates an increase in gastrin release in patients with Zollinger-Ellison syndrome when compared with normal patients; gastrin bicarbonate concentration is reduced in patients with chronic pancreatitis when compared with a normal patient's response to secretin

Pharmacodynamics
Maximum output of pancreatic secretions: Within 30 minutes
Duration: At least 2 hours

Pharmacokinetics
Distribution: V_d: Porcine formulation: 2 L (approximately); human formulation: 2.7 L
Protein binding: 40%
Inactivated by proteolytic enzymes if administered orally
Metabolism: Metabolic fate is thought to be hydrolysis to smaller peptides
Half-life: Porcine formulation: 27 minutes; human formulation: 45 minutes
Elimination: Clearance: Porcine formulation: 487 ± 136 mL/minute; human formulation: 580.9 ± 51.3 mL/minute

Usual Dosage Children and Adults: I.V.:
Diagnostic agent for pancreatic function: 0.2 mcg/kg as single dose
Diagnostic agent for gastrinoma (Zollinger-Ellison): 0.4 mcg/kg as single dose
Facilitation of ERCP visualization: 0.2 mcg/kg as a single dose

Administration Parenteral: Reconstitute with 8 mL of NS resulting in a 2 mcg/mL solution; shake vigorously to ensure dissolution; use immediately by direct I.V. injection slowly over 1 minute

Monitoring Parameters Peak bicarbonate concentration of duodenal fluid aspirate (chronic pancreatitis); serum gastrin (gastrinoma)

Reference Range
Peak gastric bicarbonate concentration:
- Normal: 94-134 mEq/L
- Chronic pancreatitis: <80 mEq/L
- Severe pancreatitis: <50 mEq/L

Serum gastrin:
- Normal: ≤110 pg/mL
- Gastrinoma: >110 pg/mL

Nursing Implications Patients should fast at least 12 hours before testing for Zollinger-Ellison syndrome

Additional Information SecreFlo™ is available currently as an orphan drug by contacting the manufacturer Repligen; a double-blind crossover study of secretin 0.2 clinical units/kg versus placebo in 56 autistic children revealed no significant differences between the 2 groups (1 clinical unit is equivalent to 0.2 mcg) (Owley, 2001)

Dosage Forms Excipient information presented when available (limited, particularly for generics); consult specific product labeling.
Injection, powder for reconstitution [human]:
- ChiRhoStim™: 16 mcg

Injection, powder for reconstitution [porcine]:
- SecreFlo™: 16 mcg

References

Owley T, McMahon W, Cook EH, et al, "Multisite, Double-Blind, Placebo-Controlled Trial of Porcine Secretin in Autism," *J Am Acad Child Adolesc Psychiatry*, 2001, 40(11):1293-9.

♦ **Secretin, Human** *see* Secretin *on page 1425*
♦ **Secretin, Porcine** *see* Secretin *on page 1425*
♦ **Secura® Antifungal [OTC]** *see* Miconazole *on page 1056*
♦ **Selax® (Can)** *see* Docusate *on page 526*
♦ **Selenium** *see* Trace Metals *on page 1558*

Selenium Sulfide (se LEE nee um SUL fide)

U.S. Brand Names Exsel® [DSC]; Head & Shoulders® Intensive Treatment [OTC]; Selsun®; Selsun Blue® 2-in-1 Treatment [OTC]; Selsun Blue® Balanced Treatment [OTC]; Selsun Blue® Medicated Treatment [OTC]; Selsun Blue® Moisturizing Treatment [OTC]

Canadian Brand Names Versel®

Therapeutic Category Antiseborrheic Agent, Topical; Shampoos

Generic Available Yes

Use To treat itching and flaking of the scalp associated with dandruff; to control scalp seborrheic dermatitis; treatment of tinea versicolor

Pregnancy Risk Factor C

Contraindications Hypersensitivity to selenium or any component

Warnings Safety in infants has not been established; avoid use in children <2 years of age

Precautions Do not use on damaged skin to avoid any systemic toxicity

Adverse Reactions

Central nervous system: Lethargy

Dermatologic: Alopecia, discoloration of hair

Gastrointestinal: Vomiting following long-term use on damaged skin, abdominal pain, garlic breath

Local: Local irritation

Neuromuscular & skeletal: Tremor

Miscellaneous: Perspiration

Mechanism of Action May block the enzymes involved in growth of epithelial tissue

Pharmacokinetics Absorption: Not absorbed topically through intact skin, but can be absorbed topically through damaged skin

Usual Dosage Children ≥ 2 years and Adults: Topical:

Dandruff, seborrhea: Massage 5-10 mL into wet scalp, leave on scalp 2-3 minutes, rinse thoroughly and repeat application; alternatively, 5-10 mL of shampoo is applied and allowed to remain on scalp for 5-10 minutes before being rinsed off thoroughly without a repeat application; shampoo twice weekly for 2 weeks initially, then use once every 1-4 weeks as indicated depending upon control

Tinea versicolor: Apply the 2.5% lotion in a thin layer covering the body surface from the face to the knees; leave on skin for 30 minutes, then rinse thoroughly; apply every day for 7 days; then follow with monthly applications for 3 months to prevent recurrences

Administration Topical: For external use only; avoid contact with eyes or acutely inflamed skin

Patient Information Remove all jewelry before using the lotion; wash hands thoroughly following application of the lotion; may discolor hair

Dosage Forms Excipient information presented when available (limited, particularly for generics); consult specific product labeling. [DSC] = Discontinued product

Lotion, topical: 2.5% (120 mL)

Shampoo, topical: 1% (210 mL)

Exsel® [DSC], Selsun®: 2.5% (120 mL)

Head & Shoulders® Intensive Treatment: 1% (400 mL)

Selsun Blue® Balanced Treatment, Selsun Blue® Medicated Treatment, Selsun Blue® Moisturizing Treatment, Selsun Blue® 2-in-1 Treatment: 1% (120 mL, 210 mL, 330 mL)

References

Lester RS, "Topical Formulary for the Pediatrician," *Pediatr Clin North Am*, 1983, 30(4):749-65.

- **Selepen®** *see* Trace Metals *on page 1558*
- **Selsun®** *see* Selenium Sulfide *on page 1427*
- **Selsun Blue® 2-in-1 Treatment [OTC]** *see* Selenium Sulfide *on page 1427*
- **Selsun Blue® Balanced Treatment [OTC]** *see* Selenium Sulfide *on page 1427*
- **Selsun Blue® Medicated Treatment [OTC]** *see* Selenium Sulfide *on page 1427*
- **Selsun Blue® Moisturizing Treatment [OTC]** *see* Selenium Sulfide *on page 1427*
- **Senexon [OTC]** *see* Senna *on page 1427*

Senna (SEN na)

Medication Safety Issues

Sound-alike/look-alike issues:

Senexon® may be confused with Cenestin®

Senokot® may be confused with Depakote®

U.S. Brand Names Black-Draught Tablets [OTC]; Evac-U-Gen [OTC]; ex-lax® [OTC]; ex-lax® Maximum Strength [OTC]; Fletcher's® [OTC]; Perdiem® Overnight Relief

(Continued)

Senna *(Continued)*

[OTC]; Senexon [OTC]; Senna-Gen® [OTC]; Sennatural™ [OTC]; Senokot® [OTC]; SenokotXTRA® [OTC]; Uni-Senna [OTC]

Therapeutic Category Laxative, Stimulant

Generic Available Yes

Use Short-term treatment of constipation; evacuate the colon for bowel or rectal examinations

Pregnancy Risk Factor C

Contraindications Hypersensitivity to senna or any component; nausea and vomiting; undiagnosed abdominal pain, appendicitis, intestinal obstruction or perforation

Warnings Concentrated liquid contains sodium benzoate which may cause allergic reactions in susceptible individuals; use products containing sodium benzoate with caution in neonates; *in vitro* and animal studies have shown that benzoate displaces bilirubin from protein binding sites

Precautions Avoid prolonged use (>1 week); chronic use may lead to dependency, fluid and electrolyte imbalance, vitamin and mineral deficiencies

Adverse Reactions

Endocrine & metabolic: Electrolyte and fluid imbalance

Gastrointestinal: Nausea, vomiting, diarrhea, abdominal cramps, perianal irritation, discoloration of feces

Genitourinary: Discoloration of urine

Drug Interactions Docusate may enhance the absorption of senna

Mechanism of Action Active metabolite (aglycone) acts as a local irritant on the colon, stimulates Auerbach's plexus to produce peristalsis

Pharmacodynamics Onset of action:

Oral: Within 6-24 hours

Rectal: Evacuation occurs in 30 minutes to 2 hours

Pharmacokinetics

Metabolism: In the liver

Elimination: In the feces (via bile) and in urine

Usual Dosage Oral:

Constipation:

- Infants 1 month to 2 years: Syrup: 1.25-2.5 mL (2.2-4.4 mg sennosides) at bedtime, not to exceed 5 mL (8.8 mg sennosides)/day
- Children:
  - Syrup:
    - 2 to <6 years: 2.5-3.75 mL (4.4-6.6 mg sennosides) at bedtime, not to exceed 3.75 mL (6.6 mg sennosides) twice daily
    - 6-12 years: 5-7.5 mL (8.8-13.2 mg sennosides) at bedtime, not to exceed 7.5 mL (13.2 mg sennosides) twice daily
  - Tablet:
    - 2 to <6 years: ½ tablet (4.3 mg sennosides) at bedtime, not to exceed 1 tablet (8.6 mg sennosides) twice daily
    - 6-12 years: 1 tablet (8.6 mg sennosides) at bedtime, not to exceed 2 tablets (17.2 mg sennosides) twice daily
- Children ≥12 years and Adults:
  - Syrup: 10-15 mL (17.6-26.4 mg sennosides) at bedtime, not to exceed 15 mL (26.4 mg sennosides) twice daily
  - Tablet: 2 tablets (17.2 mg sennosides) at bedtime, not to exceed 4 tablets (34.4 mg sennosides) twice daily

Bowel evacuation: Children ≥12 years and Adults: 130 mg sennosides (X-Prep® 75 mL) between 2:00 PM to 4:00 PM on the day prior to procedure

Administration Oral: Administer with water; syrup can be taken with juice or milk or mixed with ice cream to mask taste.

Monitoring Parameters I & O, frequency of bowel movements, serum electrolytes if severe diarrhea occurs

Patient Information May discolor urine or feces; drink plenty of fluids

Dosage Forms Excipient information presented when available (limited, particularly for generics); consult specific product labeling.

Liquid:

- Senexon: Sennosides 8.8 mg/5 mL (240 mL)

Liquid [concentrate]:

- Fletcher's®: Senna concentrate 33.3 mg/mL (75 mL) [alcohol free; contains sodium benzoate; root beer flavor]

Syrup: Sennosides 8.8 mg/5 mL (240 mL)

Tablet: Sennosides 8.6 mg

- ex-lax®: Sennosides USP 15 mg
- ex-lax® Maximum Strength: Sennosides USP 25 mg

Perdiem® Overnight Relief: Sennosides USP 15 mg
Sennatural™, Senokot®, Senexon®, Senna-Gen®, Uni-Senna: Sennosides 8.6 mg
SenokotXTRA®: Sennosides 17 mg

Tablet, chewable:
Black-Draught™: Sennosides 10 mg
ex-lax®: Sennosides USP 15 mg [chocolate flavor]
Evac-U-Gen: Sennosides 10 mg

References

Perkin JM, "Constipation in Childhood: A Controlled Comparison Between Lactulose and Standardized Senna," *Curr Med Res Opin*, 1977, 4(8):540-3.

- **Senna and Docusate** *see* Docusate and Senna *on page 527*
- **Senna-Gen® [OTC]** *see* Senna *on page 1427*
- **Senna-S** *see* Docusate and Senna *on page 527*
- **Sennatural™ [OTC]** *see* Senna *on page 1427*
- **Senokot® [OTC]** *see* Senna *on page 1427*
- **Senokot-S® [OTC]** *see* Docusate and Senna *on page 527*
- **SenokotXTRA® [OTC]** *see* Senna *on page 1427*
- **SenoSol™-SS [OTC]** *see* Docusate and Senna *on page 527*
- **Sensorcaine®** *see* Bupivacaine *on page 244*
- **Sensorcaine®-MPF** *see* Bupivacaine *on page 244*
- **Sensorcaine®-MPF Spinal** *see* Bupivacaine *on page 244*
- **Septra®** *see* Sulfamethoxazole and Trimethoprim *on page 1487*
- **Septra® DS** *see* Sulfamethoxazole and Trimethoprim *on page 1487*
- **Septra® Injection (Can)** *see* Sulfamethoxazole and Trimethoprim *on page 1487*
- **Serevent® (Can)** *see* Salmeterol *on page 1415*
- **Serevent® Diskus®** *see* Salmeterol *on page 1415*
- **Seromycin®** *see* CycloSERINE *on page 421*
- **Serostim®** *see* Human Growth Hormone *on page 769*

Sertraline (SER tra leen)

Medication Safety Issues

Sound-alike/look-alike issues:
Sertraline may be confused with selegiline, Serentil®
Zoloft® may be confused with Zocor®

Related Information

Antidepressant Agents *on page 1681*

U.S. Brand Names Zoloft®

Canadian Brand Names Apo-Sertraline®; Gen-Sertraline; GMD-Sertraline; Novo-Sertraline; Nu-Sertraline; PMS-Sertraline; ratio-Sertraline; Rhoxal-sertraline; Sandoz-Sertraline; Zoloft®

Index Terms Sertraline Hydrochloride

Therapeutic Category Antidepressant, Selective Serotonin Reuptake Inhibitor (SSRI)

Generic Available Yes

Use Treatment of major depression, obsessive-compulsive disorder, panic disorder (with or without agoraphobia), post-traumatic stress disorder, premenstrual dysphoric disorder, social anxiety disorder

Medication Guide An FDA-approved patient medication guide, which is available with the product information and at http://www.fda.gov/cder/Offices/ODS/medication_guides.htm, must be dispensed with this medication for each new outpatient prescription and refill.

Pregnancy Risk Factor C

Lactation Enters breast milk/not recommended (AAP rates "of concern")

Contraindications Hypersensitivity to sertraline or any component; use of MAO inhibitors within 14 days (potentially fatal reactions may occur, see Drug Interactions); concurrent use of pimozide; oral concentrate is contraindicated in patients receiving disulfiram (contains 12% alcohol)

Warnings Safety and efficacy in pediatric patients ≥6 years of age have been established only for the treatment of obsessive compulsive disorder; sertraline is not approved for the treatment of depression in pediatric patients. Clinical worsening of depression or suicidal ideation and behavior may occur in children and adults with major depressive disorder. In clinical trials, antidepressants increased the risk of suicidal thinking and behavior (suicidality) in children, adolescents, and young adults (18-24 years of age) with major depressive disorder and other psychiatric disorders. This risk must be considered before prescribing antidepressants for any clinical use. (Continued)

Sertraline *(Continued)*

Short-term studies did **not** show an increased risk of suicidality with antidepressant use in patients >24 years of age and showed a decreased risk in patients ≥65 years.

Patients of all ages who are treated with antidepressants for any indication require appropriate monitoring and close observation for clinical worsening of depression, suicidality, and unusual changes in behavior, especially during the first few months after antidepressant initiation or when the dose is adjusted. Family members and caregivers should be instructed to closely observe the patient (ie, daily) and communicate condition with healthcare provider. Patients should also be monitored for associated behaviors (eg, anxiety, agitation, panic attacks, insomnia, irritability, hostility, aggressiveness, impulsivity, akathisia, hypomania, mania) which may increase the risk for worsening depression or suicidality. Worsening depression or emergence of suicidality (or associated behaviors listed above) that is abrupt in onset, severe, or not part of the presenting symptoms, may require discontinuation or modification of drug therapy.

Avoid abrupt discontinuation; discontinuation symptoms (including agitation, dysphoria, anxiety, confusion, dizziness, hypomania, nightmares, and other symptoms) may occur if therapy is abruptly discontinued or dose reduced; taper the dose to minimize risks of discontinuation symptoms; if intolerable symptoms occur following a decrease in dosage or upon discontinuation of therapy, consider resuming the previous dose with a more gradual taper. To reduce risk of intentional overdose, write prescriptions for the smallest quantity consistent with good patient care. Screen individuals for bipolar disorder prior to treatment (using antidepressants alone may induce manic episodes in patients with this condition). Potentially fatal serotonin syndrome may occur when SSRIs are used in combination with serotonergic drugs (eg, triptans) or drugs that impair the metabolism of serotonin (eg, MAO inhibitors); see Drug Interactions.

Dropper for oral concentrate contains natural rubber latex which may cause allergic reactions in susceptible individuals; avoid use in patients with allergy to latex.

Precautions Use with caution in patients with seizure disorders, concomitant illnesses that may effect hepatic metabolism or hemodynamic responses (eg, unstable cardiac disease, recent MI), and in suicidal patients; use with caution and decrease dose in patients with hepatic dysfunction; may result in hyponatremia, SIADH, significant weight loss (monitor weight and growth in pediatric patients), decrease in serum uric acid (mild uricosuric effect, use with caution in patient at risk of uric acid nephropathy), activation of mania/hypomania, or abnormal bleeding; SSRIs may increase risk of bleeding (eg, upper GI bleeding) especially in patients receiving nonselective NSAIDs, aspirin, or other drugs that affect coagulation. Use with caution during late third trimester of pregnancy [newborns may experience adverse effects or withdrawal symptoms (consider risk and benefits); see Additional Information; exposure to SSRIs late in pregnancy may also be associated with an increased risk for persistent pulmonary hypertension of the newborn (see Chambers, 2006)].

Adverse Reactions

Central nervous system: Agitation, dizziness, headache, insomnia, nervousness, fatigue, somnolence, fever, impaired concentration, activation of mania or hypomania, emotional lability, aggressive reaction, abnormal thinking, seizures, hyperkinesia; suicidal thinking and behavior (see Warnings)

Note: SSRI-associated behavioral activation (ie, restlessness, hyperkinesis, hyperactivity, agitation) is 2- to 3-fold more prevalent in children compared to adolescents; it is more prevalent in adolescents compared to adults. Somnolence (including sedation and drowsiness) is more common in adults compared to children and adolescents (see Safer, 2006).

Dermatologic: Rash

Endocrine & metabolic: Weight loss; SIADH, hyponatremia (volume-depleted patients); decreased serum uric acid, sexual dysfunction, decreased libido; weight gain has also been reported

Gastrointestinal: Nausea, vomiting, diarrhea, loose stools, xerostomia, constipation, anorexia, dyspepsia

Note: SSRI-associated vomiting is 2- to 3-fold more prevalent in children compared to adolescents; it is more prevalent in adolescents compared to adults.

Genitourinary: Urinary incontinence

Hematologic: Altered platelet function, purpura

Neuromuscular & skeletal: Tremor, paresthesia, hyperkinesia, twitching, malaise

Ocular: Abnormal vision

Respiratory: Epistaxis

Miscellaneous: Diaphoresis; withdrawal symptoms following abrupt discontinuation (see Warnings)

Drug Interactions Cytochrome P450 isoenzyme CYP3A3/4 and CYP2D6 (minor) substrate; isoenzyme CYP2C9, CYP2C19, and CYP3A3/4 inhibitor; weak inhibitor of CYP1A2 and CYP2D6

Use within 2 weeks of MAO inhibitors may result in fever, tremors, rigidity, myoclonus, autonomic instability, rapid fluctuations in vital signs, irritability, confusion, extreme agitation, delirium, and coma (use of sertraline within 14 days of MAO inhibitors is contraindicated); sertraline may increase serum concentrations of pimozide by ~40% and potentially cause serious adverse effects (concurrent use of pimozide and sertraline is contraindicated); sertraline may displace highly protein bound drugs and cause adverse effects; may increase risk of bleeding in patients receiving nonselective NSAIDs, aspirin, or other drugs that affect coagulation; may increase prothrombin time in patients receiving warfarin; use with sumatriptan may cause weakness, incoordination, and hyper-reflexia; although lithium levels were not significantly affected in one study, monitoring of lithium levels and appropriate dosage adjustments is recommended in patients initiating sertraline therapy. Tryptophan (which can be metabolized to serotonin) and the herbal medicine St John's wort (*Hypericum perforatum*) may increase serious side effects; use of these agents is **not recommended.**

Sertraline may decrease the metabolism of tricyclic antidepressants, tolbutamide, diazepam, flecainide, phenytoin, propafenone, and other drugs metabolized by CYP enzymes (monitoring of serum drug concentrations and dosage reduction of these agents may be required); **Note:** One study suggests that chronic therapy with sertraline does not cause clinically important inhibition of phenytoin metabolism; however, monitoring of phenytoin serum drug concentrations with appropriate dosage adjustments is recommended. The effect of sertraline on valproate serum concentrations is unknown (monitor valproate serum levels and adjust dose as appropriate). Cimetidine may increase sertraline concentrations. The following drugs may increase the risk of serotonin syndrome if given with selective serotonin reuptake inhibitors: Amitriptyline, amphetamines, buspirone, dihydroergotamine, erythromycin, fentanyl, meperidine, nefazodone, ritonavir, sumatriptan, sympathomimetics, tramadol

Food Interactions Tryptophan supplements may increase serious side effects; its use is **not recommended**. Grapefruit juice may significantly increase sertraline serum concentrations

Tablets: Food may slightly increase AUC, increase peak concentrations by 25% and shorten the time to peak plasma concentrations

Oral concentrate: Food may prolong the rate, but does not effect the extent of absorption

Stability Store at room temperature

Mechanism of Action Selective inhibitor of CNS neuronal serotonin uptake; minimal effects on reuptake of norepinephrine or dopamine; does not significantly bind to alpha-adrenergic, benzodiazepine, cholinergic, dopamine, GABA, histamine, or serotonin receptors; may therefore be useful in patients at risk from sedation, hypotension and anticholinergic effects of tricyclic antidepressants; does not inhibit monoamine oxidase

Pharmacodynamics Maximum effect may take several weeks

Pharmacokinetics

Protein binding: 98%

Metabolism: Significant first pass effect; undergoes N-demethylation to N-desmethylsertraline (significantly less active than sertraline); both parent and metabolite undergo oxidative deamination, followed by reduction, hydroxylation and conjugation with glucuronide (**Note:** Children 6-17 years may metabolize sertraline slightly better than adults, as pediatric AUCs and peak concentrations were 22% lower than adults when adjusted for weight; however, lower doses are recommended for younger pediatric patients to avoid excessive drug levels)

Bioavailability: Tablets approximately equal to oral solution

Half-life: Parent: Mean: 26 hours; metabolite (N-desmethylsertraline): 62-104 hours
- Children: 6-12 years: Mean: 26.2 hours
- Children: 13-17 years: Mean: 27.8 hours
- Adults: 18-45 years: Mean: 27.2 hours

Elimination: 40% to 45% of dose eliminated in urine (none as unchanged drug); 40% to 45% eliminated in feces (12% to 14% as unchanged drug)
- Clearance: May be decreased in patients with hepatic impairment

Dialysis: Not likely to remove significant amount of drug due to large V_d

Usual Dosage Oral: (**Note:** See Additional Information)

Children 6-12 years:

Depression: **Note:** Not FDA approved; see Warnings: Initial: 12.5-25 mg once daily; titrate dose upwards if clinically needed; may increase by 25-50 mg/day increments at intervals of at least 1 week; mean final dose in 21 children (8-18 years of age) was 100 ± 53 mg or 1.6 mg/kg/day (n=11); range: 25-200 mg/day; maximum dose: 200 mg/day (see Tierney, 1995 and Dopheide, 2006); avoid excessive dosing

(Continued)

Sertraline *(Continued)*

Obsessive-compulsive disorder: Initial: 25 mg once daily; titrate dose upwards if clinically needed; increase by 25-50 mg/day increments at intervals of at least 1 week; range: 25-200 mg/day; maximum dose: 200 mg/day; avoid excessive dosing

Adolescents 13-17 years:

Depression: Initial 25-50 mg once daily; titrate dose upwards if clinically needed; may increase by 50 mg/day increments at intervals of at least 1 week; mean final dose in 13 adolescents was 110 ± 50 mg or about 2 mg/kg/day (see McConville, 1996); in another study using a slower titration, the mean dose at week 6 was 93 mg (n=41) and at week 10 was 127 mg (n=34) (see Ambrosini, 1999); range: 25-200 mg/day; maximum dose: 200 mg/day (see Dopheide, 2006).

Obsessive-compulsive disorder: Initial: 50 mg once daily; titrate dose upwards if clinically needed; increase by 50 mg/day increments at intervals of at least 1 week; range: 25-200 mg/day; maximum dose: 200 mg/day

Adults:

Depression and obsessive-compulsive disorder: Initial: 50 mg once daily; titrate dose upwards if clinically needed; increase by 50 mg/day increments at intervals of at least 1 week; range: 50-200 mg/day; maximum dose: 200 mg/day

Panic disorder, post-traumatic stress disorder, and social anxiety disorder: Initial: 25 mg once daily; increase dose after 1 week to 50 mg once daily; titrate dose further if clinically needed; increase by 50 mg/day increments at intervals of at least 1 week; range: 50-200 mg/day; maximum dose: 200 mg/day

Premenstrual dysphoric disorder: Initial: 50 mg/day given daily throughout the menstrual cycle **or** only during the luteal phase of the menstrual cycle (depending on assessment of physician); may increase if needed by 50 mg increments per menstrual cycle; maximum dose when using daily dosing throughout the menstrual cycle: 150 mg/day; maximum dose when dosing only during the luteal phase of the menstrual cycle: 100 mg/day. **Note:** If using a 100 mg/day dose with luteal phase dosing, use a 50 mg/day titration step for 3 days at the beginning of each luteal phase dosing period.

Dosing adjustment in renal impairment: None needed

Dosing adjustment in hepatic impairment: Use with caution and in reduced doses

Administration Oral: May be administered without regard to food; avoid administration with grapefruit juice; administer once daily dosage in morning or evening. Must dilute oral concentrate before use; measure dose with dropper provided and mix with 4 ounces of water, orange juice, lemonade, ginger ale, or lemon/lime soda; do not mix with other liquids; take dose immediately after mixing, do not mix ahead of time; sometimes a slight haze may be seen after mixing (this is normal)

Monitoring Parameters Weight and growth in children if long-term therapy; uric acid, CBC, liver function, serum sodium, urine output. Monitor patient periodically for symptom resolution; monitor for worsening depression, suicidality, and associated behaviors (especially at the beginning of therapy or when doses are increased or decreased; see Warnings)

Patient Information Read the Patient Medication Guide that you receive with each prescription and refill of sertraline. An increased risk of suicidal thinking and behavior has been reported with the use of antidepressants in children, adolescents, and young adults (18-24 years of age). Notify physician if you feel depressed, have thoughts of suicide, or become more agitated or irritable (see Warnings). May cause dizziness or drowsiness and impair ability to perform activities requiring mental alertness or physical coordination; may cause dry mouth. Take as directed; do not alter dose or frequency without consulting prescriber; avoid abrupt discontinuation. Some medicines should not be taken with sertraline or should not be taken for a while after sertraline has been discontinued; report the use of other medications, nonprescription medications, and herbal or natural products to your physician and pharmacist; avoid alcohol, grapefruit juice, tryptophan supplements, and the herbal medicine St John's wort; avoid aspirin, NSAIDs, or other drugs that affect coagulation (may increase risks of bleeding).

Nursing Implications If patient experiences somnolence, administer dose at bedtime; if patient experiences insomnia, administer dose in morning. Assess other medications patient may be taking for possible interaction (especially MAO inhibitors, P450 inhibitors, and other CNS active agents). Assess mental status for depression, suicidal ideation, anxiety, social functioning, mania, or panic attack.

Additional Information Two larger studies of children and adolescents with depression and obsessive-compulsive disorder utilized a forced upward dosage titration of sertraline to 200 mg/day; these studies conclude that the adult dosage titration regimen can be used in children ≥6 years and adolescents (see Alderman, 1998 and March, 1998); however, other studies in adults (see Fabre, 1995) demonstrate that lower sertraline doses (50 mg/day) are as effective as higher doses with fewer adverse effects and discontinuations of therapy. Further studies are needed in pediatric patients to identify optimal doses; clinically, doses should be individually titrated based on patient response and adverse effects.

A recent report (Lake, 2000) describes 5 children (age 8-15 years) who developed epistaxis (n=4) or bruising (n=1) while receiving sertraline therapy. Another recent report describes the SSRI discontinuation syndrome in 6 children; the syndrome was similar to that reported in adults (see Diler, 2002). Due to limited long-term studies, the clinical usefulness of sertraline should be periodically re-evaluated in patients receiving the drug for extended intervals; effects of long term use of sertraline on pediatric growth, development, and maturation have not been directly assessed.

Neonates born to women receiving SSRIs late during the third trimester may experience respiratory distress, apnea, cyanosis, temperature instability, vomiting, feeding difficulty, hypoglycemia, constant crying, irritability, hypotonia, hypertonia, hyper-reflexia, tremor, jitteriness, and seizures; these symptoms may be due to a direct toxic effect, withdrawal syndrome, or (in some cases) serotonin syndrome. Withdrawal symptoms occur in 30% of neonates exposed to SSRIs *in utero*; monitor newborns for at least 48 hours after birth; long-term effects of *in utero* exposure to SSRIs are unknown (see Levinson-Castiel, 2006).

Dosage Forms Excipient information presented when available (limited, particularly for generics); consult specific product labeling.

Solution, oral [concentrate]: 20 mg/mL (60 mL)

Zoloft®: 20 mg/mL (60 mL) [contains alcohol 12%; dropper contains dry natural rubber]

Tablet: 25 mg, 50 mg, 100 mg

Zoloft®: 25 mg, 50 mg, 100 mg

References

Alderman J, Wolkow R, Chung M, et al, "Sertraline Treatment of Children and Adolescents With Obsessive-Compulsive Disorder or Depression: Pharmacokinetics, Tolerability, and Efficacy," *J Am Acad Child Adolesc Psychiatry*, 1998, 37(4):386-94.

Ambrosini PJ, Wagner KD, Biederman J, et al, "Multicenter Open-Label Sertraline Study in Adolescent Outpatients With Major Depression," *J Am Acad Child Adolesc Psychiatry*, 1999, 38(5):566-72.

Chambers CD, Hernandez-Diaz S, Van Marter LJ, et al, "Selective Serotonin-Reuptake Inhibitors and Risk of Persistent Pulmonary Hypertension of the Newborn," *N Engl J Med*, 2006, 354(6):579-87.

Diler R and Avci A, "Selective Serotonin Reuptake Inhibitor Discontinuation Syndrome in Children: Six Case Reports," *Current Therapeutic Research*, 2002, 63(3):188-97.

Dopheide JA, "Recognizing and Treating Depression in Children and Adolescents," *Am J Health Syst Pharm*, 2006, 63(3):233-43.

Fabre LF, Abuzzahab FS, Amin M, et al, "Sertraline Safety and Efficacy in Major Depression: A Double-Blind Fixed-Dose Comparison With Placebo," *Biol Psychiatry*, 1995, 38(9):592-602.

Findling RL, Reed MD, and Blumer JL, "Pharmacological Treatment of Depression in Children and Adolescents," *Paediatr Drugs*, 1999, 1(3):161-82.

Lake MB, Birmaher B, Wassick S, et al, "Bleeding and Selective Serotonin Reuptake Inhibitors in Childhood and Adolescence," *J Child Adolesc Psychopharmacol*, 2000, 10(1):35-8.

Levinson-Castiel R, Merlob P, Linder N, et al, "Neonatal Abstinence Syndrome After *in utero* Exposure to Selective Serotonin Reuptake Inhibitors in Term Infants," *Arch Pediatr Adolesc Med*, 2006, 160(2):173-6.

March JS, Biederman J, Wolkow R, et al, "Sertraline in Children and Adolescents With Obsessive-Compulsive Disorder: A Multicenter Randomized Controlled Trial," *JAMA*, 1998, 280(20):1752-6.

McConville BJ, Minnery KL, Sorter MT, et al, "An Open Study of the Effects of Sertraline on Adolescent Major Depression," *J Child Adolesc Psychopharmacol*, 1996, 6(1):41-51.

Safer DJ and Zito JM, "Treatment Emergent Adverse Effects of Selective Serotonin Reuptake Inhibitors by Age Group: Children vs. Adolescents," *J Child Adolesc Psychopharmacol*, 2006, 16(1/2):159-69.

Sharp SC and Hellings JA, "Efficacy and Safety of Selective Serotonin Reuptake Inhibitors in the Treatment of Depression in Children and Adolescents: Practitioner Review," *Clin Drug Investig*, 2006, 26(5):247-55.

Thomsen PH, "Obsessive-Compulsive Disorder: Pharmacological Treatment," *Eur Child Adolesc Psychiatry*, 2000, 9 Suppl 1:I76-84.

Tierney E, Joshi PT, Llinas JF, et al, "Sertraline for Major Depression in Children and Adolescents: Preliminary Clinical Experience," *J Child Adolesc Psychopharmacol*, 1995; 5(1):13-27.

Wagner KD, "Pharmacotherapy for Major Depression in Children and Adolescents," *Prog Neuropsychopharmacol Biol Psychiatry*, 2005, 29(5):819-26.

- ♦ **Sertraline Hydrochloride** *see* Sertraline *on page 1429*
- ♦ **Serutan® [OTC]** *see* Psyllium *on page 1347*

Sevelamer (se VEL a mer)

Medication Safety Issues

Sound-alike/look-alike issues:

Renagel® may be confused with Reglan®, Regonol®

U.S. Brand Names Renagel®

Canadian Brand Names Renagel®

Index Terms Sevelamer Hydrochloride

Therapeutic Category Phosphate Binder

Generic Available No

Use Reduction of serum phosphorus in patients with chronic kidney disease on hemodialysis

Pregnancy Risk Factor C

Lactation Excretion in breast milk unknown/use caution (not absorbed systemically but may alter maternal nutrition)

(Continued)

Sevelamer *(Continued)*

Contraindications Hypersensitivity to sevelamer or any component; hypophosphatemia, bowel obstruction

Warnings In preclinical animal studies, sevelamer (at doses of 6-100 times the recommended human dose) reduced the levels of vitamin D, E, K, and folic acid; no evidence of decreased vitamin levels has been shown in human trials, however, most patients were receiving vitamin supplements

Precautions Use with caution in patients with GI disorders including dysphagia, swallowing disorders, severe GI motility disorders, or major GI surgery

Adverse Reactions

Cardiovascular: Hypertension, hypotension, thrombosis
Central nervous system: Headache
Dermatologic: Pruritus
Endocrine & metabolic: Hypercalcemia, metabolic acidosis
Gastrointestinal: Diarrhea, dyspepsia, vomiting, constipation, flatulence, nausea
Neuromuscular & skeletal: Pain
Respiratory: Cough

Drug Interactions Decreases bioavailability of ciprofloxacin by 50%; sevelamer has the potential to bind to other medications in the GI tract and limit their absorption; separate administration of sevelamer with other medications by at least 1 hour prior or 3 hours after a sevelamer dose. No interactions have been seen with digoxin, warfarin, enalapril, or metoprolol.

Stability Store in room temperature.

Mechanism of Action Sevelamer is a cationic polymeric compound that binds phosphate in the intestinal lumen, limiting absorption and decreasing serum phosphate concentrations without altering calcium, aluminum, or bicarbonate concentrations. It may also lower low-density lipoprotein (LDL) and total serum cholesterol levels.

Pharmacokinetics

Absorption: Not systemically absorbed
Elimination: Feces 100%

Usual Dosage Oral:

Children: In a small pilot study of 17 pediatric patients aged 11.8 ± 3.7 years on hemodialysis (n=3) or peritoneal dialysis (n=14), initial doses of 121 ± 50 mg/kg (4.5±5 g/day) were used. Doses were adjusted based on the serum phosphorus with final doses of 163 ± 46 mg/kg (6.7 ± 2.4 g/day) without any adverse effects (Mahdavi, 2003).

Adults (not taking another phosphate binder, eg, calcium acetate): 800-1600 mg with each meal; the initial dose may be based on the serum phosphorus: See table:

Serum Phosphorus (mg/dL)	Initial Sevelamer Dose (mg)[1]
>5.5 and <7.5	800
≥7.5 and <9	1200-1600
≥9	1600

[1] Administered 3 times/day

Adjust the daily dosage by 1 tablet or capsule per meal at 2-week intervals depending upon the serum phosphorus. The manufacturer recommends the following titration schedule:

Serum Phosphorus (mg/dL)	Sevelamer Dosage Adjustment
>5.5	Increase by 1 tablet per meal at 2-week intervals
3.5-5.5	Maintain current dose
<3	Decrease by 1 tablet per meal

Patients changing from calcium acetate to sevelamer may use the following conversions:

Calcium Acetate Dosage (mg)	Initial Sevelamer Dose (mg)[1]
667 (1 tablet)	800
1334 (2 tablets)	1200
2001 (3 tablets)	2000

[1]Administer 3 times/day

Administration Oral: Administer with meals, at least 1 hour before or 3 hours after other medications; because the contents will expand with water, swallow capsules/tablets whole, do not chew, crush, or open capsules.

Monitoring Parameters Serum electrolytes

Dosage Forms Excipient information presented when available (limited, particularly for generics); consult specific product labeling.

Tablet, as hydrochloride: 400 mg, 800 mg

References

Mahdavi H, Kuizon BD, Gales B, et al, "Sevelamer Hydrochloride: An Effective Phosphate Binder in Dialyzed Children," *Pediatr Nephrol*, 2003, 18(12):1260-4.

- ♦ **Sevelamer Hydrochloride** *see* Sevelamer *on page 1433*
- ♦ **Shohl's Solution, Modified** *see* Citrate and Citric Acid *on page 372*
- ♦ **Silace [OTC]** *see* Docusate *on page 526*
- ♦ **Siladryl® Allergy [OTC]** *see* DiphenhydrAMINE *on page 509*
- ♦ **Silafed® [OTC]** *see* Triprolidine and Pseudoephedrine *on page 1580*
- ♦ **Silapap® Children's [OTC]** *see* Acetaminophen *on page 42*
- ♦ **Sildec [DSC]** *see* Carbinoxamine and Pseudoephedrine *on page 286*
- ♦ **Sildec Syrup** *see* Brompheniramine and Pseudoephedrine *on page 235*

Sildenafil (sil DEN a fil)

Medication Safety Issues

Sound-alike/look-alike issues:

Viagra® may be confused with Allegra®, Vaniqa™

U.S. Brand Names GD-Sildenafil; Revatio™; Viagra®

Canadian Brand Names Viagra®

Index Terms UK92480

Therapeutic Category Phosphodiesterase Type-5 (PDE5) Inhibitor

Generic Available No

Use Treatment of pulmonary arterial hypertension (PAH) (Revatio™); primary pulmonary hypertension; persistent pulmonary hypertension of the newborn (PPHN) refractory to treatment with inhaled nitric oxide; to facilitate weaning from nitric oxide (ie, to attenuate rebound effects after discontinuing inhaled nitric oxide); secondary pulmonary hypertension following cardiac surgery; treatment of erectile dysfunction in adult males (Viagra®)

Pregnancy Risk Factor B

Lactation Excretion in breast milk unknown/use caution

Contraindications Hypersensitivity to sildenafil or any component; concurrent use of organic nitrates (eg, nitroglycerin) in any form (potentiates the hypotensive effects)

Warnings Decreases in blood pressure may occur due to vasodilator effects; the cardiovascular status of the patient should be considered prior to initiating treatment; certain patients may be adversely affected by vasodilator effects (eg, patients with resting hypotension, fluid depletion, severe left ventricular outflow obstruction, or autonomic dysfunction). Sildenafil is not recommended for use in patients with pulmonary veno-occlusive disease; consider diagnosis of pulmonary veno-occlusive disease in patients who develop pulmonary edema when receiving sildenafil. Sildenafil may cause transient dose-related impairment of blue/green color discrimination.

Additional warnings for patients treated for erectile dysfunction: Rare cases of sudden vision loss attributed to nonarteritic ischemic optic neuropathy (NAION) have been reported with the use of phosphodiesterase type-5 (PDE5) inhibitors when used for the treatment of male erectile dysfunction; NAION is a condition where blood flow is blocked to the optic nerve. NAION is more common in individuals with heart disease, diabetes, hypertension, certain eye problems, smokers, or those >50 years of age. Vision loss in one eye has been reported in some men after taking PDE5 inhibitors. It is not known if PDE5 inhibitors cause this condition or if other related factors are responsible. Patients taking a PDE5 inhibitor and who experience vision loss should stop taking the drug and notify a healthcare provider immediately.

A degree of cardiac risk is associated with sexual activity in patients with pre-existing cardiovascular disease; sildenafil should not generally be used to treat erectile dysfunction in men with underlying cardiovascular disease which would deem sexual activity inadvisable. Prolonged or painful erections may occur; patients should seek immediate medical assistance if erection lasts >4 hours; permanent damage to the penis may occur without immediate treatment. The safety and efficacy of sildenafil with other treatments for erectile dysfunction have not been established; concurrent use is not recommended.

Precautions Use with caution in patients with resting hypotension or hypertension; cardiovascular disease, including cardiac failure, unstable angina, or a recent history (within the last 6 months) of MI, stroke, or life-threatening arrhythmia; patients with retinitis pigmentosa (subpopulation of these patients have a retinal phosphodiesterase disorder); patients receiving concurrent bosentan (efficacy has not been evaluated; bosentan decreases sildenafil serum concentrations); patients receiving alpha-blockers or other antihypertensive agents (additive hypotensive effects; symptomatic hypotension may occur).

Use with caution in patients with anatomical deformation of the penis (angulation, cavernosal fibrosis, Peyronie's disease); conditions which may predispose patients to priapism (sickle cell anemia, multiple myeloma, leukemia). Epistaxis may occur and

(Continued)

Sildenafil *(Continued)*

at a higher incidence in patients with pulmonary arterial hypertension due to connective tissue disorders or in patients receiving concurrent oral vitamin K antagonists. Safety of sildenafil is not known in patients with bleeding disorders or with active peptic ulcer disease. Safety and efficacy in pediatric patients have not been established.

Adverse Reactions Note: Adverse effects such as flushing, diarrhea, myalgia, and visual disturbances may be increased with higher doses (eg, adult doses >100 mg/24 hours).

Cardiovascular: Flushing, hypotension, tachycardia, MI, ventricular arrhythmia, cerebrovascular hemorrhage, pulmonary hemorrhage

Central nervous system: Headache, insomnia, pyrexia, dizziness, seizure, anxiety

Dermatologic: Erythema, rash

Gastrointestinal: Nausea, diarrhea, dyspepsia, gastritis

Genitourinary: Prolonged erection, priapism, hematuria, urinary tract infection

Hematologic: Platelet dysfunction (*in vitro* study with human platelets indicates that sildenafil potentiates the antiaggregatory effect of nitric oxide)

Neuromuscular & skeletal: Myalgia, paresthesia

Ocular: Blurred vision, increased sensitivity to light, change in color vision; nonarteritic ischemic optic neuropathy (NAION; see Warnings); retinopathy of prematurity (1 possible case reported after treatment with IV sildenafil; see Marsh, 2004 and Pierce, 2005)

Respiratory: Epistaxis, dyspnea, rhinitis, sinusitis, nasal congestion

Drug Interactions Cytochrome P450 isoenzyme CYP2C8/9 (minor) and CYP3A4 (major) substrate; isoenzyme CYP1A2 (weak), CYP2C8/9 (weak), CYP2C19 (weak), CYP2D6 (weak), CYP2E1 (weak), and CYP3A4 (weak) inhibitor

Sildenafil potentiates the hypotensive effects of nitrates (severe, potentially fatal, hypotensive responses may occur; concurrent use is contraindicated); concomitant use with alpha-blockers may lead to hypotension (patients receiving alpha-blocker therapy must demonstrate hemodynamic stability prior to initiation of PDE-5 inhibitors; use lowest dose of sildenafil when initiating therapy; use lowest dose of alpha-blocker when initiating in patients receiving PDE-5 inhibitors); sildenafil potentiates the effect of other antihypertensives. Concurrent use with heparin may have an additive effect on bleeding time. Use of sildenafil with vitamin K antagonists may increase risk of bleeding (primarily epistaxis).

Concurrent use of sildenafil with CYP3A4 substrates, or the combination of CYP3A4 substrates plus beta-blockers, may reduce sildenafil clearance and/or increase its oral bioavailability. Cytochrome P450 CYP3A4 inhibitors (eg, azole antifungals, cimetidine, ciprofloxacin, clarithromycin, erythromycin, nicardipine, propofol, protease inhibitors, quinidine, and verapamil) may increase the serum concentrations or effects of sildenafil. Concurrent use with potent CYP3A4 inhibitors (eg, ketoconazole, itraconazole, ritonavir) significantly increase sildenafil serum concentrations; concurrent use of these agents and Revatio™ is not recommended; dosage reduction of Viagra® is recommended if used concurrently with ketoconazole, itraconazole, erythromycin, saquinavir, or ritonavir (see Usual Dosage).

Bosentan decreases serum concentrations of sildenafil; sildenafil increases serum concentrations of bosentan. Efavirenz, carbamazepine, phenobarbital, phenytoin, rifampin, and the herbal medicine St John's wort (*Hypericum perforatum*) may decrease serum concentrations of sildenafil; serum concentrations of these agents may also be altered; dosage adjustments may be needed.

Food Interactions A high fat meal decreases the rate of absorption and peak concentration. Grapefruit juice may increase serum concentrations or toxicity of sildenafil (avoid concurrent use).

Stability Store tablets at controlled room temperature.

Mechanism of Action Selective phosphodiesterase-type 5 (PDE-5) inhibitor. PDE-5 is found in the pulmonary vascular smooth muscle, vascular and visceral smooth muscle, corpus cavernosum, and platelets. PDE-5 is responsible for the degradation of cyclic guanosine monophosphate (cGMP). Normally, nitric oxide (NO) activates the enzyme guanylate cyclase, which increases the levels of cGMP; cGMP produces smooth muscle relaxation. Inhibition of PDE-5 by sildenafil increases the cellular levels of cGMP.

Increased levels of cGMP potentiate vascular smooth muscle relaxation, particularly in the lung where PDE5 is found in high concentrations. In patients with pulmonary arterial hypertension, sildenafil causes vasodilation in the pulmonary vasculature and, to a lesser extent, in the systemic circulation. Clinically, the drug decreases pulmonary arterial pressure and increases exercise capacity in these patients.

In patients with erectile dysfunction, sildenafil does not directly cause penile erections, but affects the response to sexual stimulation. Normally, NO is released in the corpus cavernosum during sexual stimulation. NO then activates the enzyme guanylate cyclase, which increases the levels of cGMP; cGMP produces smooth muscle relaxation and allows an inflow of blood to the corpus cavernosum producing an erection. Sildenafil enhances the effect of NO by inhibiting PDE-5 and increasing the levels of cGMP in the corpus cavernosum. At recommended doses, sildenafil has no effect on erection in the absence of sexual stimulation.

Pharmacokinetics

Absorption: Oral: Rapid; slower with a high-fat meal

Distribution: Distributes into tissues

V_{dss}: Adults: 105 L

Protein binding: 96%

Metabolism: Via the liver via cytochrome P450 isoenzyme CYP3A4 (major route) and CYP2C9 (minor route). Major metabolite is formed via N-desmethylation pathway and has 50% of the activity as sildenafil.

Bioavailability: Oral: 40% (may be higher in patients with PAH compared to healthy volunteers)

Half-life: Sildenafil: 4 hours; active N-desmethyl metabolite: 4 hours

Time to peak serum concentration: Oral: Fasting: 30-120 minutes (median 60 minutes); delayed by 60 minutes with a high-fat meal

Elimination: Excreted as metabolites; 80% of dose excreted in feces, 13% in urine

Clearance: Decreased in patients with hepatic cirrhosis or severe renal impairment; clearance may be lower in patients with PAH compared to normal volunteers

Dialysis: Not likely to be beneficial due to high protein binding

Usual Dosage Oral: **Note:** Limited pediatric information exists; most pediatric literature consists of case reports or small studies; further studies are needed.

Neonates: Pulmonary hypertension: A wide range of doses has been reported: Initial: 0.3 mg/kg/dose every 8-12 hours; doses of 0.25-1 mg/kg/dose every 6-12 hours have been used; **Note:** Individual doses of 0.3 mg/kg/dose given only one time have been used in select patients to facilitate weaning from inhaled nitric oxide (see Atz, 1999).

One randomized placebo controlled study of 13 neonates (>35.5 weeks GA and <3 days old) with severe PPHN and an oxygenation index (OI) of >25 received placebo (n=6) or sildenafil (n=7) at initial doses of 1 mg/kg every 6 hours; **Note:** OI = (fraction of inspired oxygen x mean airway pressure) / PaO_2; the sildenafil dose was doubled if the OI did not improve and the mean blood pressure remained stable; therapy was discontinued if the OI became <20 or the patient received a maximum of 8 doses; 5 of 7 neonates received 1 mg/kg every 6 hours for all doses; 2 neonates required a dosage increase to 2 mg/kg every 6 hours; overall, 2 patients required 6 doses and 5 patients required 7 doses; the median total amount of sildenafil was 7 mg/kg/course of therapy (see Baquero, 2006).

Infants and Children: Pulmonary hypertension: A wide range of doses has been reported: Initial: 0.25-0.5 mg/kg/dose every 4-8 hours; increase if needed and if tolerated to 1 mg/kg/dose every 4-8 hours; doses as high as 2 mg/kg/dose every 4 hours have been used in several case reports (see Karatza 2004, Karatza 2005).

One 12 month, open-label, pilot study of sildenafil in 14 children, 5-18 years of age (median 9.8 years) used initial doses of 0.25 mg/kg/dose given 4 times daily for 2 doses; if this dose was tolerated, it was increased to 0.5 mg/kg/dose given 4 times daily; doses were adjusted so that easily divisible fractions of the commercially available tablets could be administered; the first 4 doses were administered in the hospital; at 12 months, the median dose was 0.5 mg/kg/dose (range: 0.3-1 mg/kg/dose) given 4 times daily (see Humpl, 2005).

Adults:

Erectile dysfunction (Viagra®): Usual: 50 mg taken as needed, ~1 hour before sexual activity (dose may be taken 30 minutes to 4 hours before sexual activity). Based on effectiveness and tolerance, may increase dose to a maximum of 100 mg or decrease to 25 mg. Maximum recommended dosing frequency: Once daily

Pulmonary arterial hypertension (Revatio™): 20 mg 3 times/day; no evidence for additional efficacy was observed with higher doses; treatment with higher doses is not recommended

Dosage adjustment in hepatic impairment: Adults:

Revatio™:

Mild to moderate hepatic impairment (Child Pugh class A and B): No dosage adjustment needed

Severe hepatic impairment (Child Pugh class C): Has not been studied

Viagra®: Cirrhosis: Starting dose of 25 mg should be considered

Dosage adjustment in renal impairment: Adults:

Revatio™: No dosage adjustments needed

Viagra®: Severe renal impairment (creatinine clearance <30 mL/minute): Starting dose of 25 mg should be considered

Dosage considerations for patients taking alpha blockers: Adults: Viagra®: Initial: 25 mg

(Continued)

Sildenafil *(Continued)*

Dosage adjustment for concomitant use of potent CYP34A inhibitors: Adults:

Revatio™:

Erythromycin, saquinavir: No dosage adjustment needed

Bosentan, barbiturates, carbamazepine, efavirenz, nevirapine, phenytoin, rifabutin, rifampin: Dosage adjustments may be needed; specific guidelines are not available; see Drug Interactions

Itraconazole, ketoconazole, ritonavir: Use is not recommended

Viagra®:

Erythromycin, itraconazole, ketoconazole, saquinavir: Starting dose of 25 mg should be considered

Ritonavir: Maximum: 25 mg every 48 hours

Administration Oral:

Revatio™: Administer doses at least 4-6 hours apart; may be administered without regard to meals

Viagra®: Administer dose ~1 hour before sexual activity (may be administered 30 minutes to 4 hours before sexual activity).

Monitoring Parameters Heart rate, blood pressure, oxygen saturation, PaO_2

Patient Information Do not take nitroglycerin or other nitrate medications while using sildenafil (serious side effects may occur). Avoid grapefruit juice and the herbal medicine, St John's wort. Certain other medications should not be taken with sildenafil or may require a dosage adjustment of sildenafil; report the use of other medications, nonprescription medications, and herbal or natural products to your physician and pharmacist.

Headache, flushing, or abnormal vision (color changes, blurred or increased sensitivity to light) may occur; use caution when driving at night or in poorly lit environments. Seek immediate medical attention if a sudden vision loss in one or both eyes occurs. Report immediately acute allergic reactions; chest pain or palpitations; persistent dizziness; signs of urinary tract infection; skin rash; respiratory difficulty; genital swelling; or other adverse reactions.

Do not combine sildenafil with other approaches to treating erectile dysfunction without consulting prescriber. If erection lasts longer than 4 hours, contact prescriber immediately; permanent damage to the penis can occur. **Note:** Sildenafil provides no protection against sexually-transmitted diseases, including HIV.

Nursing Implications Do not administer sildenafil to patients receiving nitroglycerin or other organic nitrates; be aware of other drug interactions. Instruct patient to seek immediate medical attention if a sudden loss of vision occurs in one or both eyes, or if erection lasts longer than 4 hours.

Additional Information Sildenafil is ~10 times more selective for PDE-5 as compared to PDE-6. PDE-6 is found in the retina and is involved in phototransduction. At higher plasma levels, inhibition of PDE-6 may occur and may account for the abnormalities in color vision noted in some patients.

Dosage Forms Excipient information presented when available (limited, particularly for generics); consult specific product labeling. Available as sildenafil citrate; mg strength refers to sildenafil.

Tablet:

Revatio™: 20 mg

Viagra®: 25 mg, 50 mg, 100 mg

Extemporaneous Preparations A 2.5 mg/mL oral suspension made from sildenafil citrate (Viagra®) and 2 different vehicles (a 1:1 mixture of Ora-Sweet® and Ora-Plus® or a 1:1 mixture of methylcellulose 1% and Simple Syrup, NF) was stable for 91 days when stored in amber plastic prescription bottles at room temperature (25°C) or under refrigeration (5°C); grind thirty 25 mg tablets in a mortar into a fine powder; add a small amount of the vehicle and mix well to form a uniform paste; mix while adding the vehicle in geometric proportions to almost 300 mL; transfer to a graduated cylinder and qsad with vehicle to 300 mL while mixing; place in amber plastic prescription bottles; label "shake well."

Nahata MC, Morosco RS, and Brady M, "Extemporaneous Sildenafil Citrate Oral Suspensions for the Treatment of Pulmonary Hypertension in Children," *Am J Health Syst Pharm*, 2006, 63(3):254-7.

References

Atz AM and Wessel DL, "Sildenafil Ameliorates Effects of Inhaled Nitric Oxide Withdrawal," *Anesthesiology*, 1999, 91(1):307-10.

Baquero H, Soliz A, Neira F, et al, "Oral Sildenafil in Infants With Persistent Pulmonary Hypertension of the Newborn: A Pilot Randomized Blinded Study," *Pediatrics*, 2006, 117(4):1077-83.

Carroll WD and Dhillon R, "Sildenafil as a Treatment for Pulmonary Hypertension," *Arch Dis Child*, 2003, 88(9):827-8.

Erickson S, Reyes J, Bohn D, et al, "Sildenafil (Viagra) in Childhood and Neonatal Pulmonary Hypertension," *J Am Coll Cardiol*, 2002, 39(Suppl):S402.

Humpl T, Reyes JT, Holtby H, et al, "Beneficial Effect of Oral Sildenafil Therapy on Childhood Pulmonary Arterial Hypertension: Twelve-Month Clinical Trial of a Single-Drug, Open-Label, Pilot Study," *Circulation*, 2005, 111(24):3274-80.

Karatza AA, Bush A, and Magee AG, "Safety and Efficacy of Sildenafil Therapy in Children With Pulmonary Hypertension," *Int J Cardiol*, 2005, 100(2):267-73.

Karatza AA, Narang I, Rosenthal M, et al, "Treatment of Primary Pulmonary Hypertension With Oral Sildenafil," *Respiration*, 2004, 71(2):192-4.

Kothari SS and Duggal B, "Chronic Oral Sildenafil Therapy in Severe Pulmonary Artery Hypertension," *Indian Heart J*, 2002, 54(4):404-9.

Marsh CS, Marden B, and Newsom R, "Severe Retinopathy of Prematurity (ROP) in a Premature Baby Treated With Sildenafil Acetate (Viagra) for Pulmonary Hypertension," *Br J Ophthalmol*, 2004, 88(2):306-7.

Pierce CM, Petros AJ, and Fielder AR, "No Evidence for Severe Retinopathy of Prematurity Following Sildenafil," *Br J Ophthalmol*, 2005, 89(2):250.

- **Silexin [OTC]** *see* Guaifenesin and Dextromethorphan *on page 748*
- **Silfedrine Children's [OTC]** *see* Pseudoephedrine *on page 1344*
- **Silphen® [OTC]** *see* DiphenhydrAMINE *on page 509*
- **Silphen DM® [OTC]** *see* Dextromethorphan *on page 477*
- **Siltussin DAS [OTC]** *see* Guaifenesin *on page 745*
- **Siltussin DM [OTC]** *see* Guaifenesin and Dextromethorphan *on page 748*
- **Siltussin DM DAS [OTC]** *see* Guaifenesin and Dextromethorphan *on page 748*
- **Siltussin SA [OTC]** *see* Guaifenesin *on page 745*
- **Silvadene®** *see* Silver Sulfadiazine *on page 1439*

Silver Nitrate (SIL ver NYE trate)

Index Terms $AgNO_3$

Therapeutic Category Ophthalmic Agent, Miscellaneous; Topical Skin Product

Generic Available Yes

Use Cauterization of wounds and sluggish ulcers, removal of granulation tissue and warts

Pregnancy Risk Factor C

Contraindications Hypersensitivity to silver nitrate or any component; not for use on broken skin or cuts

Warnings Do not use applicator sticks on the eyes

Adverse Reactions

Dermatologic: Staining of the skin
Hematologic: Methemoglobinemia
Local: Burning and skin irritation
Ocular: Cauterization of the cornea, blindness, chemical conjunctivitis

Stability Store applicator sticks in a dry place since moisture causes the oxidized film to dissolve; protect from light

Mechanism of Action Free silver ions precipitate bacterial proteins by combining with chloride in tissue forming silver chloride; coagulates cellular protein to form an eschar

Pharmacokinetics Absorption: Not readily absorbed from mucous membranes

Usual Dosage Children and Adults:

Sticks: Apply to mucous membranes and other moist skin surfaces only on area to be treated 2-3 times/week for 2-3 weeks

Topical solution: Apply a cotton applicator dipped in solution on the affected area 2-3 times/week for 2-3 weeks

Monitoring Parameters With prolonged use, monitor methemoglobin levels

Patient Information Discontinue topical preparation if redness or irritation develop; silver nitrate solution may stain skin

Nursing Implications Silver nitrate solutions stain skin and utensils

Dosage Forms Excipient information presented when available (limited, particularly for generics); consult specific product labeling.

Applicator sticks, topical: Silver nitrate 75% and potassium nitrate 25% (6", 12", 18")
Solution, topical: 10% (30 mL); 25% (30 mL); 50% (30 mL)

References

Cushing AH and Smith S, "Methemoglobinemia With Silver Nitrate Therapy of a Burn: Report of a Case," *J Pediatr*, 1969, 74(4):613-5.

Silver Sulfadiazine (SIL ver sul fa DYE a zeen)

U.S. Brand Names Silvadene®; SSD®; SSD® AF; Thermazene®

Canadian Brand Names Flamazine®

Therapeutic Category Antibiotic, Topical

Generic Available Yes

(Continued)

Silver Sulfadiazine *(Continued)*

Use Adjunct in the prevention and treatment of infection in second and third degree burns

Pregnancy Risk Factor C

Lactation For external use

Contraindications Hypersensitivity to silver sulfadiazine or any component; premature infants or neonates <2 months of age since sulfas may displace bilirubin from protein binding sites and cause kernicterus

Precautions Use with caution in patients with G-6-PD deficiency and renal impairment; sulfadiazine may accumulate in patients with impaired hepatic or renal function

Adverse Reactions

Dermatologic: Itching, rash, erythema multiforme, discoloration of skin

Hematologic: Hemolytic anemia, leukopenia, agranulocytosis, aplastic anemia, thrombocytopenia

Hepatic: Hepatitis

Local: Pain, burning

Renal: Interstitial nephritis

Miscellaneous: Serum hyperosmolality (due to propylene glycol component in the cream), hypersensitivity reactions to sulfas

Drug Interactions Topical proteolytic enzymes (silver may inactivate enzymes)

Stability Discard if cream is darkened (reacts with heavy metals resulting in release of silver)

Mechanism of Action Acts upon the bacterial cell wall and cell membrane

Pharmacokinetics

Absorption: Significant percutaneous absorption of sulfadiazine can occur especially when applied to extensive burns

Half-life: 10 hours and is prolonged in patients with renal insufficiency

Time to peak serum concentration: Within 3-11 days of continuous topical therapy

Elimination: ~50% excreted unchanged in urine

Usual Dosage Children and Adults: Topical: Apply once or twice daily with a sterile gloved hand; apply to a thickness of $^1/_{16}$"; burned area should be covered with cream at all times

Administration Topical: Apply to cleansed, debrided burned areas

Monitoring Parameters Serum electrolytes, UA, renal function test, CBC in patients with extensive burns on long-term treatment

Patient Information For external use only; may discolor skin

Additional Information Contains methylparaben

Dosage Forms Excipient information presented when available (limited, particularly for generics); consult specific product labeling.

Cream, topical: 1% (25 g, 50 g, 85 g, 400 g)

Silvadene®, Thermazene®: 1% (20 g, 50 g, 85 g, 400 g, 1000 g)

SSD®: 1% (25 g, 50 g, 85 g, 400 g)

SSD® AF: 1% (50 g, 400 g)

References

Kulick MI, Wong R, Okarma TB, et al, "Prospective Study of Side Effects Associated With the Use of Silver Sulfadiazine in Severely Burned Patients," *Ann Plast Surg*, 1985, 14(5):407-18.

Lockhart SP, Rushworth A, Azmy AA, et al, "Topical Silver Sulfadiazine: Side Effects and Urinary Excretion," *Burns Incl Therm Inj*, 1983, 10(1):9-12.

Simethicone (sye METH i kone)

Medication Safety Issues

Sound-alike/look-alike issues:

Simethicone may be confused with cimetidine

Mylanta® may be confused with Mynatal®

Mylicon® may be confused with Modicon®, Myleran®

Phazyme® may be confused with Pherazine®

U.S. Brand Names Equalizer Gas Relief [OTC]; GasAid [OTC]; Gas-X® [OTC]; Gas-X® Extra Strength [OTC]; Gas-X® Maximum Strength [OTC]; Genasyme® [OTC]; Infantaire Gas Drops [OTC]; Mylanta® Gas [OTC]; Mylanta® Gas Maximum Strength [OTC]; Mylicon® Infants [OTC]; Phazyme® Quick Dissolve [OTC]; Phazyme® Ultra Strength [OTC]

Canadian Brand Names Ovol®; Phazyme™

Index Terms Activated Dimethicone; Activated Methylpolysiloxane

Therapeutic Category Antiflatulent

Generic Available Yes

Use Relieve flatulence, functional gastric bloating, and postoperative gas pains

Pregnancy Risk Factor C

Contraindications Hypersensitivity to simethicone or any component

Warnings Mylicon® Infant drops contain sodium benzoate; benzoic acid (benzoate) is a metabolite of benzyl alcohol; large amounts of benzyl alcohol (≥99 mg/kg/day) have been associated with a potentially fatal toxicity ("gasping syndrome") in neonates; *in vitro* and animal studies have shown that benzoate displaces bilirubin from protein binding sites; avoid use of Mylicon® Infant drops in neonates.

Precautions Phazyme® Quick Dissolve contains phenylalanine; avoid use or use with caution in phenylketonurics

Food Interactions Avoid gas-forming foods

Mechanism of Action Spreads on surface of aqueous liquids forming a film of low surface tension which collapses foam bubbles; allows mucous-surrounded gas bubbles to coalesce and be expelled

Pharmacokinetics Elimination: In feces

Usual Dosage Oral:

Infants and Children <2 years: 20 mg 4 times/day

Children 2-12 years: 40 mg 4 times/day

Children >12 years and Adults: 40-250 mg after meals and at bedtime as needed, not to exceed 500 mg/day

Administration Oral: Administer after meals or at bedtime; chew tablets thoroughly before swallowing; mix with water, infant formula or other liquids

Patient Information Avoid carbonated beverages

Dosage Forms Excipient information presented when available (limited, particularly for generics); consult specific product labeling.

Softgels: 125 mg

GasAid, Gas-X® Extra Strength, Mylanta® Gas Maximum Strength: 125 mg

Gas-X® Maximum Strength: 166 mg

Phazyme® Ultra Strength: 180 mg

Suspension, oral drops: 40 mg/0.6 mL (30 mL)

Equalizer Gas Relief, Genasyme®, Infantaire Gas: 40 mg/0.6 mL (30 mL)

Mylicon® Infants: 40 mg/0.6 mL (15 mL, 30 mL) [alcohol free; contains sodium benzoate; available in a nonstaining formula]

Tablet, chewable: 80 mg, 125 mg

Gas-X®: 80 mg [sodium free; peppermint crème or cherry crème flavor]

Gas-X® Extra Strength: 125 mg [peppermint crème or cherry crème flavor]

Genasyme®: 80 mg

Mylanta® Gas: 80 mg [mint flavor]

Mylanta® Gas Maximum Strength: 125 mg [cherry and mint flavors]

Phazyme® Quick Dissolve: 125 mg [contains phenylalanine 0.4 mg per tablet; mint flavor]

- **Simply Cough® [OTC] [DSC]** *see* Dextromethorphan *on page 477*
- **Simply Saline® [OTC]** *see* Sodium Chloride *on page 1450*
- **Simply Saline® Baby [OTC]** *see* Sodium Chloride *on page 1450*
- **Simply Saline® Nasal Moist® [OTC]** *see* Sodium Chloride *on page 1450*
- **Simply Sleep® [OTC]** *see* DiphenhydrAMINE *on page 509*
- **Simply Sleep® (Can)** *see* DiphenhydrAMINE *on page 509*
- **Simply Stuffy™ [OTC] [DSC]** *see* Pseudoephedrine *on page 1344*
- **Simuc-DM** *see* Guaifenesin and Dextromethorphan *on page 748*

Simvastatin (SIM va stat in)

Medication Safety Issues

Sound-alike/look-alike issues:

Zocor® may be confused with Cozaar®, Yocon®, Zoloft®

International issues:

Cardin® [Poland] may be confused with Cardene® which is a brand name for nicardipine in the U.S.

Cardin® [Poland] may be confused with Cardem® which is a brand name for celiprolol in Spain

U.S. Brand Names Zocor®

Canadian Brand Names Apo-Simvastatin®; BCI-Simvastatin; CO Simvastatin; Gen-Simvastatin; Novo-Simvastatin; PMS-Simvastatin; ratio-Simvastatin; Riva-Simvastatin; Sandoz-Simvastatin; Taro-Simvastatin; Zocor®

Therapeutic Category Antilipemic Agent; HMG-CoA Reductase Inhibitor

Generic Available Yes

Use Hyperlipidemia: Adjunct to dietary therapy to decrease elevated serum total and low density lipoprotein cholesterol (LDL-C), apolipoprotein B (apo-B), and triglyceride levels, and to increase high density lipoprotein cholesterol (HDL-C) in patients with primary hypercholesterolemia (heterozygous, familial and nonfamilial) and mixed (Continued)

Simvastatin *(Continued)*

dyslipidemia (Fredrickson types IIa and IIb); treatment of homozygous familial hypercholesterolemia; treatment of isolated hypertriglyceridemia (Fredrickson type IV) and type III hyperlipoproteinemia

Primary prevention of cardiovascular disease in high risk patients; risk factors include: Age ≥55 years, smoking, hypertension, low HDL-C or family history of early coronary heart disease

Pregnancy Risk Factor X

Lactation Excretion in breast milk unknown/contraindicated

Contraindications Hypersensitivity to simvastatin or any component; active liver disease; unexplained persistent elevations of serum transaminases; pregnancy

Warnings Rhabdomyolysis with or without acute renal failure secondary to myoglobinuria has occurred rarely. Risk is increased with increasing doses (0.02% at 20 mg, 0.08% at 40 mg, and 0.53% at 80 mg) and with concurrent use of amiodarone, clarithromycin, danazol, diltiazem, fluvoxamine, indinavir, nefazodone, nelfinavir, ritonavir, verapamil, troleandomycin, cyclosporine, fibric acid derivatives, erythromycin, niacin, or azole antifungals. Assess the risk versus benefit before combining any of these medications with simvastatin. A lowered dosage of simvastatin is recommended when used with these medications (see Usual Dosage). Advise patients to promptly report any unexplained muscle pain, tenderness, or weakness. Temporarily discontinue simvastatin in any patient experiencing an acute or serious condition predisposing to renal failure due to the potential risk of developing rhabdomyolysis.

Precautions Persistent increases in serum transaminases have occurred; liver function must be monitored by laboratory assessment at the initiation of therapy and periodically thereafter for the first year of treatment or until one year after the last elevation in dose. Patients titrated to the 80 mg dose should receive an additional test at 3 months of therapy. Use with caution in patients who consume substantial quantities of alcohol or have a previous history of liver disease. Use with caution in patients with diabetes mellitus and renal impairment (may be at increased risk for developing rhabdomyolysis)

Adverse Reactions

Cardiovascular: Angina, transient symptomatic hypotension, sinus tachycardia

Central nervous system: Dizziness, headache, vertigo, fatigue, insomnia, depression, tremor, memory loss, psychic disturbances, anxiety

Dermatologic: Eczema, pruritus, rash, lichen planus, photosensitivity, alopecia, Stevens-Johnson syndrome, skin discoloration, dry skin

Endocrine & metabolic: Gynecomastia, thyroid function abnormalities

Gastrointestinal: Constipation, dyspepsia, flatulence, abdominal pain, diarrhea, nausea, pancreatitis

Hematologic: Thrombocytopenia

Hepatic: Elevated serum transaminases, hepatitis (including chronic active hepatitis), cholestatic jaundice

Neuromuscular & skeletal: Elevated CPK, myalgia, muscle cramps, myopathy, peripheral neuropathy, paresthesias, rhabdomyolysis, arthralgias, dysfunction of certain cranial nerves (including alteration of taste, impairment of extraocular movement, and facial paresis)

Ocular: Cataracts, ophthalmoplegia, diplopia

Renal: Acute renal failure

Respiratory: Upper respiratory infections

Miscellaneous: Hypersensitivity syndrome (including one or more of the following features: Anaphylaxis, angioedema, lupus erythematous-like syndrome, polymyalgia rheumatica, dermatomyositis, vasculitis, purpura, leukopenia, hemolytic anemia, erythema multiforme, toxic epidermal necrolysis)

Drug Interactions Cytochrome P450 isoenzyme CYP3A3/4 enzyme substrate

Plasma concentrations may be decreased when given with magnesium-aluminum hydroxide containing antacids; cholestyramine reduces absorption; clofibrate, fenofibrate, gemfibrozil, niacin (≥1 g/day), amiodarone, and cyclosporine may increase the risk of myopathy and rhabdomyolysis (see Warnings); CYP3A3/4 inhibitors (clarithromycin, cyclosporine, danazol, diltiazem, fluconazole, fluvoxamine, erythromycin, indinavir, itraconazole, ketoconazole, telithromycin, miconazole, nefazodone, nelfinavir, ritonavir, saquinavir, indinavir, amprenavir, troleandomycin, and verapamil) increase simvastatin blood levels and may increase the risk of simvastatin-induced myopathy and rhabdomyolysis (see Warnings); simvastatin increases the hypoprothrombinemic response to warfarin; may increase digoxin serum level

Food Interactions Simvastatin serum concentration may be increased when taken with large quantities (>1 quart/day) of grapefruit juice; avoid concurrent use

Stability Tablets should be stored in well closed containers at temperatures between 5°C to 30°C (41°F to 86°F)

Mechanism of Action Simvastatin is a methylated derivative of lovastatin that acts by competitively inhibiting 3-hydroxy-3-methylglutaryl-coenzyme A (HMG-CoA) reductase, the enzyme that catalyzes the rate-limiting step in cholesterol biosynthesis

Pharmacodynamics

Onset of action: >3 days

Maximum effect: After 2 weeks

LDL-C reduction: 20-40 mg/day: 35% to 41% (for each doubling of this dose, LDL-C is lowered ~6%)

Average HDL-C increase: 5% to 15%

Average triglyceride reduction: 7% to 30%

Pharmacokinetics

Absorption: Oral: Although 85% is absorbed following administration, <5% reaches the general circulation due to an extensive first-pass effect

Time to peak serum concentration: 1.3-2.4 hours

Protein binding: ~95%

Elimination: 13% excreted in urine and 60% in feces

Usual Dosage Oral:

Hyperlipidemia: Limited data in 32 children (<17 years of age) enrolled in compassionate use study (Ducobu, 1992):

Children <10 years: 5 mg once daily in the evening increasing to 10 mg once daily after 4 weeks and to 20 mg once daily after 8 weeks as tolerated

Children ≥10 years: 10 mg once daily in the evening increasing to 20 mg once daily after 6 weeks and to 40 mg once daily after 12 weeks as tolerated

Adults:

Initial: 20 mg once daily in the evening; patients who require only a moderate reduction of LDL-C may be started at 10 mg once daily; patients who require a reduction of >45% in LDL-C may be started at 40 mg once daily

Maintenance: Recommended dosage range: 5-80 mg/day as a single dose in the evening; doses should be adjusted at intervals of at least 4 weeks

Heterozygous familial hypercholesterolemia: Adolescents 10-17 years: 10 mg once daily in the evening; increase in intervals of 4 weeks or more to a maximum of 40 mg/day

Homozygous familial hypercholesterolemia: Adults: 40 mg in the evening or 80 mg/day in 3 divided doses of 20 mg, 20 mg, and an evening dose of 40 mg.

Dosage adjustment in patients who are concomitantly receiving cyclosporine or danazol: Adults: Initial: 5 mg, not to exceed 10 mg/day

Dosage adjustment in patients receiving concomitant fibrates or niacin: Adults: Dose should not exceed 10 mg/day

Dosage adjustment in patients receiving concomitant amiodarone or verapamil: Adults: Dose should not exceed 20 mg/day

Dosing adjustment in renal impairment: Adults: Because simvastatin does not undergo significant renal excretion, modification of dose should only be necessary in patients with severe renal impairment: Cl_{cr} <10 mL/minute: Initial: 5 mg/day

Administration Oral: May be taken without regard to meals. Administration with the evening meal or at bedtime has been associated with somewhat greater LDL-C reduction

Monitoring Parameters Serum cholesterol (total and fractionated), CPK; liver function tests (see Precautions)

Reference Range Hypercholesterolemia as defined by serum cholesterol, LDL-C, and TG concentrations: See table below; Desired: HDL-C <40 mg/dL

Classification of Blood Cholesterol, LDL-C, and Triglyceride Concentrations[1]

Classification	Cholesterol (mg/dL)		LDL-C (mg/dL)		Triglycerides (mg/dL)
	Children	Adults	Children	Adults	Adults
Acceptable/optimal	<170	<200	<110	<100	<150
Above optimal	†	†	†	100-129	†
Borderline high	170-199	200-239	110-129	130-159	150-199
High	≥200	≥240	≥130	160-189	200-499
Very high	†	†	†	≥190	≥500

[1]Adapted from American Academy of Pediatrics Committee on Nutrition, "Cholesterol in Childhood," *Pediatrics*, 1998, 101(1 Pt 1):141-7 and "Third Report of the National Cholesterol Education Program Expert Panel on Detection, Evaluation, and Treatment of High Blood Cholesterol in Adults (Adult Treatment Panel III)," May 2001, www.nhlbi.nih.gov/guidelines/cholesterol.

†Lack of specific type of classification in either pediatric or adult recommendations.

Patient Information May rarely cause photosensitivity reactions (eg, exposure to sunlight may cause severe sunburn, skin rash, redness, or itching); avoid direct exposure to sunlight. Report severe and unresolved gastric upset, any vision changes, muscle pain and weakness, changes in color of urine or stool, yellowing of

(Continued)

Simvastatin *(Continued)*

skin or eyes, and any unusual bruising. Female patients of childbearing age must be counseled to use 2 effective forms of contraception simultaneously, unless absolute abstinence is the chosen method; this drug may cause severe fetal defects.

Additional Information The current recommendation for treatment of hypercholesterolemia in children is limited to children ≥10 years of age who, after a 6-month to 1-year trial of diet therapy, continue to have LDL-C concentrations ≥190 mg/dL alone, or LDL-C concentrations ≥160 mg/dL and a family history of premature coronary artery disease or two or more other coronary artery disease risk factors (AAP Committee on Nutrition, 1998). For each 1% lowering in LDL-C, the relative risk for major cardiovascular events is reduced by approximately 1%. For more specific risk assessment and treatment recommendations for adults, see NCEP ATPIII.

Dosage Forms Excipient information presented when available (limited, particularly for generics); consult specific product labeling.

Tablet: 5 mg, 10 mg, 20 mg, 40 mg

Zocor®: 5 mg, 10 mg, 20 mg, 40 mg, 80 mg

References

American Academy of Pediatrics Committee on Nutrition, "Cholesterol in Childhood," *Pediatrics*, 1998, 101(1 Pt 1):141-7.

American Academy of Pediatrics, "National Cholesterol Education Program: Report of the Expert Panel on Blood Cholesterol Levels in Children and Adolescents," *Pediatrics*, 1992, 89(3 Pt 2):525-84.

DeJongh S, et al, "Efficacy, Safety, and Tolerability of Simvastatin in Children With Familial Hypercholesterolemia," *Clin Drug Invest*, 2002, 22(8): 533-40.

Ducobu J, Brasseur D, Chaudron JM, et al, "Simvastatin Use in Children," *Lancet*, 1992, 339(8807):1488.

Duplaga BA, "Treatment of Childhood Hypercholesterolemia With HMG-CoA Reductase Inhibitors," *Ann Pharmacother*, 1999, 33(11):1224-7.

Grundy SM, Cleeman JI, Merz CN, et al, "Implications of Recent Clinical Trials for the National Cholesterol Education Program Adult Treatment Panel III Guidelines," *Circulation*, 2004, 110(2):227-39.

"Third Report of the National Cholesterol Education Program Expert Panel on Detection, Evaluation, and Treatment of High Blood Cholesterol in Adults (Adult Treatment Panel III)," May 2001, www.nhlbi.nih.gov/guidelines/cholesterol.

♦ **Sinequan® [DSC]** *see* Doxepin *on page 537*

♦ **Sinequan® (Can)** *see* Doxepin *on page 537*

♦ **Singulair®** *see* Montelukast *on page 1080*

Sirolimus (sir OH li mus)

Medication Safety Issues

Sound-alike/look-alike issues:

Sirolimus may be confused with temsirolimus

U.S. Brand Names Rapamune®

Canadian Brand Names Rapamune®

Index Terms Rapamycin

Therapeutic Category Immunosuppressant Agent

Generic Available No

Use Rescue agent for acute and chronic organ rejection (rescue due to calcineurin toxicity or to treat resistant acute or chronic rejection despite calcineurin inhibitor therapy); primary immunosuppression after kidney, heart, liver, lung, or intestinal transplantation (given in conjunction with a calcineurin inhibitor, as a substitute for a calcineurin inhibitor to reduce side effects, or to eliminate steroid use); GVHD prophylaxis in BMT or hematopoietic stem cell transplant patients

Pregnancy Risk Factor C

Lactation Excretion in breast milk unknown/not recommended

Contraindications Hypersensitivity to sirolimus, its derivatives, or any component. Concurrent use with strong inhibitors of CYP3A4 and/or p-glycoprotein (ie, ketoconazole, voriconazole, itraconazole, telithromycin, or clarithromycin) or strong inducers of CYP3A4 and/or p-glycoprotein (rifampin or rifabutin) is not recommended.

Warnings Immunosuppression with sirolimus may result in increased susceptibility to infection and the possible development of lymphoma or other malignancies, particularly of the skin. Hypersensitivity reactions and anaphylaxis have been reported following administration of sirolimus. Cases of fatal bronchial anastomotic dehiscence have been reported in lung transplant patients who received sirolimus in combination with other immunosuppressants. Hepatic artery thrombosis, graft loss, and death have been reported in liver transplant patients who received sirolimus in combination with other immunosuppressants.

Precautions

Use with caution in patients with hyperlipidemia (sirolimus may increase serum cholesterol and triglycerides), renal impairment, or when used concurrently with medications which alter renal function (sirolimus may decrease GFR and increase serum creatinine). Delay use of sirolimus until after the perioperative period due to increased chance of surgical complications from impaired wound and tissue healing. Antimicrobial prophylaxis for *Pneumocystis carinii* pneumonia should be administered for 1 year following transplantation; CMV prophylaxis is recommended for 3 months after transplantation.

Adverse Reactions

Cardiovascular: Hypertension, peripheral edema, edema, chest pain, CHF, postural hypotension, syncope, thrombosis, venous thromboembolism, atrial fibrillation, thrombotic microangiopathy, hepatic artery thrombosis

Central nervous system: Fever, chills, headache, pain, insomnia, anxiety, confusion, depression, emotional lability, somnolence, dizziness

Dermatologic: Acne, hirsutism, pruritus, rash, skin hypertrophy, ecchymosis

Endocrine & metabolic: Hypercholesterolemia, hypophosphatemia, hypertriglyceridemia, hypokalemia, Cushing's syndrome, diabetes mellitus, hypercalcemia, hyperkalemia, hyperglycemia, hyperphosphatemia, hypocalcemia, hypoglycemia, hypomagnesemia, hyponatremia

Gastrointestinal: Abdominal pain, nausea, vomiting, diarrhea, constipation, dyspepsia, weight gain, esophagitis, gastritis, gingival hyperplasia, ileus, aphthous ulcers

Genitourinary: Urinary tract infection, impotence

Hematologic: Anemia, thrombocytopenia, hemolytic-uremic syndrome, hemorrhage, leukopenia, neutropenia

Hepatic: Elevated AST, ALT

Renal: Hemolytic uremic syndrome, elevated serum creatinine

Respiratory: Interstitial pneumonitis, bronchial anastomotic dehiscence, pulmonary fibrosis

Miscellaneous: Sepsis, interference with wound and tissue healing, lymphocele, anaphylaxis

Drug Interactions Cytochrome P450 isoenzyme CYP3A4 substrate; CYP3A4 inhibitor (weak); p-glycoprotein substrate

Cyclosporine increases sirolimus levels during concurrent therapy and cyclosporine levels may be increased [sirolimus should be taken 4 hours after cyclosporine (modified) oral solution or capsules]; rifampin, phenobarbital, carbamazepine, rifabutin, phenytoin, and the herbal medicine St John's wort (*Hypericum perforatum*) may decrease sirolimus levels; sirolimus may potentiate nephrotoxicity induced by calcineurin inhibitors; additive effect on leukopenia when used with clozapine or carbamazepine; diltiazem, azole antifungals, ciprofloxacin, clarithromycin, doxycycline, erythromycin, telithromycin, isoniazid, diclofenac, imatinib, nicardipine, propofol, protease inhibitors, quinidine, verapamil, and nefazodone may increase serum levels of sirolimus (avoid concurrent use). Vaccination may be less effective (use of live vaccines should be avoided during sirolimus therapy).

Food Interactions Avoid administration with grapefruit juice (may reduce metabolism of sirolimus); ingestion with a high fat meal decreases peak concentration but increases AUC by 35% (take sirolimus consistently either with or without food to minimize variability)

Stability Store tablet at room temperature and protect from light. Refrigerate oral solution and protect from light; store oral solution in original container and use contents within one month after opening. Oral solution bottle may be stored at room temperature for a short period of time not to exceed 15 days; amber syringe containing solution may be stored at room temperature or in the refrigerator for a maximum of 24 hours.

Mechanism of Action Sirolimus reduces T-cell activation by inhibiting cytokine-induced signal transduction pathways resulting in the suppression of IL-2 or IL-4 driven T-cell proliferation. Sirolimus inhibits antibody production.

Pharmacokinetics

Absorption: Rapid

Distribution: V_{dss}: Adults: 12 ± 8 L/kg

Protein binding: 92%

Metabolism: By liver and intestinal cytochrome P450 enzyme CYP3A4; undergoes counter-transport from enterocytes of the small intestine into the gut lumen by the p-glycoprotein drug efflux pump; metabolized by O-demethylation and/or hydroxylation

Bioavailability: Oral solution: 14%; tablet: 18%

Half-life, elimination:

Children: 13.7 ± 6.2 hours

Adults: 62 ± 16 hours

Time to peak serum concentration: 1-2.5 hours

Elimination: Primarily eliminated via feces (91%) and urine (2.2%)

Usual Dosage Oral: **Note:** Sirolimus tablets and oral solution are not bioequivalent due to differences in absorption; however, clinical equivalence has been demonstrated at the 2 mg dose level

(Continued)

Sirolimus *(Continued)*

Children ≥13 years of age and <40 kg: Loading dose: 3 mg/m^2 on day 1; initial maintenance dose: 1 mg/m^2/day divided every 12 hours or once daily; adjust dose to achieve target sirolimus trough blood concentration

Adults >40 kg: Loading dose: 6 mg on day 1; maintenance dose: 2 mg once daily

Intestinal transplant: Initial loading dose: 2-3 mg/m^2; maintenance dose: 1 mg/m^2 once daily to achieve blood levels of 8-10 ng/mL

Dosage adjustment in renal impairment: No dosage adjustment necessary

Dosage adjustment in hepatic impairment: Reduce maintenance dose by 33%; loading dose does not require adjustment

Administration May be taken with or without meals, but take medication consistently with respect to meals to minimize absorption variability

Oral solution: Use amber oral syringe to withdraw solution from the bottle. Empty dose from syringe into a cup and mix with at least 2 ounces of water or orange juice. No other liquids should be used for dilution. Patient should drink the diluted sirolimus solution immediately. Then refill cup with an additional 4 ounces of water or orange juice; stir contents vigorously and have patient drink solution at once.

Monitoring Parameters Whole blood sirolimus trough concentration, serum cholesterol and triglycerides, serum creatinine; blood pressure, CBC with differential, hemoglobin, platelet count

Reference Range Trough levels correlate with AUC; trough levels >15 ng/mL appear to be associated with a greater risk of thrombocytopenia and hyperlipidemia; trough levels <6 ng/mL appear to be associated with an increased incidence of acute rejection

Target serum trough concentrations: 6-15 ng/mL

Patient Information Due to the increased risk for skin cancer, avoid exposure to sunlight and artificial light sources (sunlamps, tanning booth/bed); wear protective clothing, wide-brimmed hats, sunglasses, and lip sunscreen (SPF ≥15); use a sunscreen [broad-spectrum sunscreen or physical sunscreen (preferred) or sunblock with SPF ≥15]. Advise women of childbearing potential to avoid becoming pregnant; use effective contraception prior to starting sirolimus therapy, during therapy and for 12 weeks after sirolimus has been stopped.

Dosage Forms Excipient information presented when available (limited, particularly for generics); consult specific product labeling.

Solution, oral [bottle]:

Rapamune®: 1 mg/mL (60 mL) [contains ethanol 1.5% to 2.5%; packaged with oral syringes and a carrying case]

Tablet:

Rapamune®: 1 mg, 2 mg

References

Ettenger RB and Grimm EM, "Safety and Efficacy of TOR Inhibitors in Pediatric Renal Transplant Recipients," *Am J Kidney Dis*, 2001, 38(4 Suppl 2):S22-8.

Gupta P, Kaufman S, and Fishbein TM, "Sirolimus for Solid Organ Transplantation in Children," Pediatr Transplant, 2005, 9(3):269-76.

Schubert M, Venkataramanan R, Holt DW, et al, "Pharmacokinetics of Sirolimus and Tacrolimus in Pediatric Transplant Patients," *Am J Transplant*, 2004, 4(5):767-73.

♦ **SK** *see* Streptokinase *on page 1474*

♦ **SK and F 104864** *see* Topotecan *on page 1554*

♦ **Skeeter Stik [OTC]** *see* Benzocaine *on page 204*

♦ **SKF 104864** *see* Topotecan *on page 1554*

♦ **SKF 104864-A** *see* Topotecan *on page 1554*

♦ **Sleep-ettes D [OTC]** *see* DiphenhydrAMINE *on page 509*

♦ **Sleepinal® [OTC]** *see* DiphenhydrAMINE *on page 509*

♦ **Slo-Niacin® [OTC]** *see* Niacin *on page 1127*

♦ **Slo-Pot (Can)** *see* Potassium Chloride *on page 1287*

♦ **Slow FE® [OTC]** *see* Iron Supplements (Oral/Enteral) *on page 868*

♦ **Slow-K® (Can)** *see* Potassium Chloride *on page 1287*

♦ **Slow-Mag® [OTC]** *see* Magnesium Chloride *on page 969*

♦ **Slow-Mag® [OTC]** *see* Magnesium Supplements *on page 976*

♦ **SM-7338** *see* Meropenem *on page 1009*

♦ **SMZ-TMP** *see* Sulfamethoxazole and Trimethoprim *on page 1487*

♦ **Snake (Pit Vipers) Antivenin** *see Crotalidae* Polyvalent Antivenin (Equine) *on page 409*

♦ **Sodium 2-Mercaptoethane Sulfonate** *see* Mesna *on page 1013*

♦ **Sodium *L*-Triiodothyronine** *see* Liothyronine *on page 943*

Sodium Acetate (SOW dee um AS e tate)

Therapeutic Category Alkalinizing Agent, Parenteral; Electrolyte Supplement, Parenteral; Sodium Salt

Generic Available Yes

Use Sodium salt replacement; correction of acidosis through conversion of acetate to bicarbonate

Pregnancy Risk Factor C

Contraindications Hypersensitivity to sodium acetate or any component; alkalosis, hypocalcemia, edema, cirrhosis, excessive chloride losses, hypernatremia

Warnings Avoid extravasation

Precautions Use with caution in patients with hepatic failure, CHF or other sodium-retaining conditions

Adverse Reactions

Cardiovascular: Thrombosis, hypervolemia, edema, cerebral hemorrhage

Endocrine & metabolic: Hypernatremia, hypokalemic metabolic alkalosis, hypocalcemia

Local: Extravasant, local cellulitis

Respiratory: Pulmonary edema

Stability Protect from light, heat, and from freezing; **incompatible** with acids, acidic salts, catecholamines, atropine

Mechanism of Action Sodium is the principal extracellular cation; functions in fluid and electrolyte balance, osmotic pressure control, and water distribution; acetate is metabolized to bicarbonate which neutralizes hydrogen ion concentration and raises blood and urinary pH

Usual Dosage Sodium acetate is metabolized to bicarbonate on an equimolar basis outside the liver; administer in large volume I.V. fluids as a sodium source. Dosage is dependent upon the clinical condition, fluid, electrolytes and acid-base balance of the patient.

Maintenance sodium requirements: I.V.:

- Neonates, Infants, and Children: 3-4 mEq/kg/day; maximum dose: 100-150 mEq/day
- Adults: 154 mEq/day

Metabolic acidosis: If sodium acetate is desired over sodium bicarbonate, the amount of acetate may be dosed utilizing the equation found in the sodium bicarbonate monograph as each mEq acetate is converted to a mEq of HCO_3; see Sodium Bicarbonate *on page 1448*

Administration Parenteral: Must be diluted prior to I.V. administration; infuse hypertonic solutions (>154 mEq/L) via a central line; maximum rate of administration: 1 mEq/kg/hour

Monitoring Parameters Serum electrolytes including calcium, arterial blood gases (if indicated)

Additional Information Sodium and acetate content of 1 g: 7.3 mEq

Dosage Forms Excipient information presented when available (limited, particularly for generics); consult specific product labeling.

Injection, solution: 2 mEq/mL (20 mL, 50 mL, 100 mL); 4 mEq/mL (50 mL, 100 mL)

♦ **Sodium Acid Carbonate** *see* Sodium Bicarbonate *on page 1448*

Sodium Benzoate (SOW dee um BENZ oh ate)

Therapeutic Category Ammonium Detoxicant; Hyperammonemia Agent; Urea Cycle Disorder (UCD) Treatment Agent

Use Adjunctive therapy for the prevention and treatment of hyperammonemia due to suspected or proven urea cycle disorders

Precautions Use with caution in patients with Reye's syndrome, propionic or methylmalonic acidemia. *In vitro* and animal studies have shown that benzoate, a metabolite of benzyl alcohol, displaces bilirubin from protein binding sites; use cautiously in neonates, particularly those with hyperbilirubinemia.

Adverse Reactions

Endocrine & metabolic: Metabolic acidosis

Gastrointestinal: Nausea, vomiting

Mechanism of Action Assists in lowering serum ammonia levels by activation of a nonurea cycle pathway (the benzoate-hippurate pathway); ammonia in the presence of benzoate will conjugate with glycine to form hippurate which is excreted by the kidney

Pharmacokinetics

Half-life: 0.75-7.4 hours

(Continued)

Sodium Benzoate *(Continued)*

Elimination: Clearance is largely attributable to metabolism with urinary excretion of hippurate, the major metabolite

Usual Dosage Investigational use (not FDA approved): Oral, I.V.:

Infants and Children: 0.25 g/kg bolus followed by 0.25 g/kg/day as continuous infusion or divided every 6-8 hours

Adolescents and Adults: Initial 5.5 g/m^2 bolus followed by 5.5 g/m^2/day as continuous I.V. infusion or divided every 6-8 hours

Administration Not available commercially

Oral: Must be compounded using chemical powder

I.V.: I.V. solutions must also be compounded and tested for sterility and pyrogenicity prior to use; infuse bolus (with sodium phenylacetate) over 90 minutes in 25-35 mL/kg $D_{10}W$

Monitoring Parameters Plasma ammonia and amino acids

Additional Information Used to treat urea cycle enzyme deficiency in combination with arginine; a maximum of 1 mole nitrogen is removed for every 1 mole of benzoate administered

Dosage Forms Excipient information presented when available (limited, particularly for generics); consult specific product labeling.

Powder: 454 g

References

Batshaw ML, "Hyperammonemia," *Curr Probl Pediatr*, 1984, 14(11):1-69.

Batshaw ML and Brusilow SW, "Treatment of Hyperammonemic Coma Caused by Inborn Errors of Urea Synthesis," *J Pediatr*, 1980, 97(6):893-900.

Batshaw ML, MacArthur RB, and Tuchman M, "Alternative Pathway Therapy for Urea Cycle Disorders: Twenty Years Later," *J Pediatr*, 2001, 138(1 Suppl):S46-54.

Green TP, Marchessault RP, and Freese DK, "Disposition of Sodium Benzoate in Newborn Infants With Hyperammonemia," *J Pediatr*, 1983, 102(5):785-90.

Maestri NE, Hauser ER, Bartholomew D, et al, "Prospective Treatment of Urea Cycle Disorders," *J Pediatr*, 1991, 119(6):923-8.

Summar M, "Current Strategies for the Management of Neonatal Urea Cycle Disorders," *J Pediatr*, 2001, 138(1 Suppl):S30-9.

♦ **Sodium Benzoate and Caffeine** *see* Caffeine *on page 255*

♦ **Sodium Benzoate and Sodium Phenylacetate** *see* Sodium Phenylacetate and Sodium Benzoate *on page 1453*

Sodium Bicarbonate (SOW dee um bye KAR bun ate)

Related Information

Adult ACLS Algorithms *on page 1660*

Antacid Preparations *on page 132*

Commonly Used Antidotes for Acute Overdoses *on page 1920*

CPR Pediatric Drug Dosages *on page 1650*

U.S. Brand Names Brioschi® [OTC]; Neut®

Index Terms Baking Soda; $NaHCO_3$; Sodium Acid Carbonate; Sodium Hydrogen Carbonate

Therapeutic Category Alkalinizing Agent, Oral; Alkalinizing Agent, Parenteral; Antacid; Electrolyte Supplement, Oral; Electrolyte Supplement, Parenteral; Sodium Salt

Generic Available Yes

Use Management of metabolic acidosis; antacid; alkalinization of urine; stabilization of acid base status in cardiac arrest (see Warnings) and treatment of life-threatening hyperkalemia

Pregnancy Risk Factor C

Lactation Enters breast milk/compatible

Contraindications Hypersensitivity to sodium bicarbonate or any component; alkalosis, hypocalcemia, hypernatremia; unknown abdominal pain, inadequate ventilation during cardiopulmonary resuscitation; excessive chloride losses

Warnings Avoid extravasation, tissue necrosis can occur due to the hypertonicity of $NaHCO_3$; use of I.V. $NaHCO_3$ should be reserved for documented metabolic acidosis and for life-threatening hyperkalemia; routine use in cardiac arrest is not recommended; patient should be adequately ventilated before administering in cardiac arrest; administration of excessive amounts of sodium bicarbonate may result in metabolic alkalosis which decreases the delivery of oxygen to tissues; monitor use closely

Precautions Use with caution in patients with CHF or other sodium-retaining conditions, renal insufficiency

Adverse Reactions

Cardiovascular: Edema, cerebral hemorrhage (especially with rapid injection of the hyperosmotic $NaHCO_3$ solution in infants)

Central nervous system: Tetany, intracranial acidosis
Endocrine & metabolic: Metabolic alkalosis, hypernatremia, hypokalemia, hypocalcemia, hyperosmolality
Gastrointestinal: Gastric distention, flatulence may occur with oral administration
Local: Tissue necrosis, ulceration after I.V. extravasation
Respiratory: Pulmonary edema

Drug Interactions Chlorpropamide, lithium, methotrexate, salicylates, and tetracycline have increased renal clearance with alkaline urine; anorexiants, flecainide, mecamylamine, quinidine, and sympathomimetics have decreased renal clearance with alkaline urine; concurrent doses with iron may decrease iron absorption

Stability Do not mix $NaHCO_3$ with calcium salts, catecholamines, atropine

Mechanism of Action Dissociates to provide bicarbonate ion which neutralizes hydrogen ion concentration and raises blood and urinary pH

Pharmacodynamics
Onset of action:
Oral, as antacid: 15 minutes
I.V.: Rapid
Duration:
Oral: 1-3 hours
I.V.: 8-10 minutes

Pharmacokinetics
Absorption: Oral: Well absorbed
Elimination: Reabsorbed by kidney and <1% is excreted in urine

Usual Dosage
Cardiac arrest: See Warnings; patient should be adequately ventilated before administering $NaHCO_3$
Infants: 1 mEq/kg slow IVP initially; may repeat with 0.5 mEq/kg in 10 minutes one time, or as indicated by the patient's acid-base status
Children and Adults: 1 mEq/kg IVP initially; may repeat with 0.5 mEq/kg in 10 minutes one time, or as indicated by the patient's acid-base status
Metabolic acidosis: Dosage should be based on the following formula if blood gases and pH measurements are available:
Neonates, Infants and Children: HCO_3^-(mEq) = 0.3 x weight (kg) x base deficit (mEq/L) **or** HCO_3^-(mEq) = 0.5 x weight (kg) x [24 - serum HCO_3^-(mEq/L)]
Adults: HCO_3^-(mEq) = 0.2 x weight (kg) x base deficit (mEq/L) **or** HCO_3^-(mEq) = 0.5 x weight (kg) x [24 - serum HCO_3^-(mEq/L)]
If acid-base status is not available: Dose for older Children and Adults: 2-5 mEq/kg I.V. infusion over 4-8 hours; subsequent doses should be based on patient's acid-base status
Prevention of hyperuricemia secondary to tumor lysis syndrome (urinary alkalinization) (refer to individual protocols):
Infants and Children:
I.V.: 120-200 mEq/m^2/day diluted in maintenance I.V. fluids of 3000 mL/m^2/day; titrate to maintain urine pH between 6-7
Oral: 12 g/m^2/day divided into 4 doses; titrate to maintain urine pH between 6-7
Chronic renal failure: Oral: Initiate when plasma HCO_3^- <15 mEq/L:
Children: 1-3 mEq/kg/day in divided doses
Adults: 20-36 mEq/day in divided doses
Renal tubular acidosis: Oral:
Distal:
Children: 2-3 mEq/kg/day in divided doses
Adults: 0.5-2 mEq/kg/day given in 4-5 divided doses
Proximal: Children and Adults: Initial: 5-10 mEq/kg/day in divided doses; maintenance: Increase as required to maintain serum bicarbonate in the normal range
Urine alkalinization: Oral:
Children: 1-10 mEq (84-840 mg)/kg/day in divided doses; dose should be titrated to desired urinary pH
Adults: 48 mEq (4 g) initially, then 12-24 mEq (1-2 g) every 4 hours; dose should be titrated to desired urinary pH; doses up to 16 g/day have been used
Antacid: Oral: Adults: 325 mg to 2 grams 1-4 times/day

Administration
Oral: Administer 1-3 hours after meals
Parenteral: For direct I.V. administration: in neonates and infants, use the 0.5 mEq/mL solution or dilute the 1 mEq/mL solution 1:1 with **SWI**; in children and adults, the 1 mEq/mL solution may be used; administer slowly (maximum rate in neonates and infants: 10 mEq/minute); for infusion, dilute to a maximum concentration of 0.5 mEq/mL in dextrose solution and infuse over 2 hours (maximum rate of administration: 1 mEq/kg/hour)

Monitoring Parameters Serum electrolytes including calcium, urinary pH, arterial blood gases (if indicated)
(Continued)

Sodium Bicarbonate *(Continued)*

Additional Information 1 mEq $NaHCO_3$ is equivalent to 84 mg; each g of $NaHCO_3$ provides 12 mEq each of sodium and bicarbonate ions; the osmolarity of 0.5 mEq/mL is 1000 mOsm/L and 1 mEq/mL is 2000 mOsm/L

Dosage Forms Excipient information presented when available (limited, particularly for generics); consult specific product labeling.

Granules, effervescent (Brioschi®): 2.69 g/packet (6 g) [unit-dose packets; contains sodium 770 mg/packet; lemon flavor]; 2.69 g/capful (120 g, 240 g) [contains sodium 770 mg/capful; lemon flavor]

Infusion [premixed in sterile water]: 5% (500 mL)

Injection, solution:

- 4.2% [42 mg/mL = 5 mEq/10 mL] (10 mL)
- 7.5% [75 mg/mL = 8.92 mEq/10 mL] (50 mL)
- 8.4% [84 mg/mL = 10 mEq/10 mL] (10 mL, 50 mL)
- Neut®: 4% [40 mg/mL = 2.4 mEq/5 mL] (5 mL)

Powder: Sodium bicarbonate USP (120 g, 480 g) [contains sodium 30 mEq per ½ teaspoon]

Tablet: 325 mg [3.8 mEq]; 650 mg [7.6 mEq]

Sodium Chloride (SOW dee um KLOR ide)

Medication Safety Issues

Per JCAHO recommendations, concentrated electrolyte solutions (eg, NaCl >0.9%) should not be available in patient care areas.

High alert medication: The Institute for Safe Medication Practices (ISMP) includes this medication (I.V. formulation) among its list of drugs which have a heightened risk of causing significant patient harm when used in error.

U.S. Brand Names Altachlore [OTC]; Altamist [OTC]; Ayr® Baby Saline [OTC]; Ayr® Saline [OTC]; Ayr® Saline No-Drip [OTC]; Breathe Right® Saline [OTC]; Broncho Saline® [OTC] [DSC]; Deep Sea [OTC]; Entsol® [OTC]; Muro 128® [OTC]; Mycinaire™ [OTC]; NaSal™ [OTC]; Nasal Moist® [OTC]; Na-Zone® [OTC]; Ocean® [OTC]; Oceant® for Kids [OTC]; Pretz® [OTC]; SalineX® [OTC]; Simply Saline® [OTC]; Simply Saline® Baby [OTC]; Simply Saline® Nasal Moist® [OTC]; Syrex; 4-Way® Saline Moisturizing Mist [OTC]; Wound Wash Saline™ [OTC]

Index Terms NaCl; Normal Saline; Salt

Therapeutic Category Electrolyte Supplement, Oral; Electrolyte Supplement, Parenteral; Lubricant, Ocular; Sodium Salt

Generic Available Yes

Use Prevention of muscle cramps and heat prostration; restoration of sodium ion in hyponatremia; restores moisture to nasal membranes; reduction of corneal edema; source of electrolytes and water for expansion of the extracellular fluid compartment

Pregnancy Risk Factor C

Contraindications Hypersensitivity to sodium chloride or any component; hypertonic uterus, hypernatremia, fluid retention

Warnings Sodium toxicity is almost exclusively related to how fast a sodium deficit is corrected; both rate and magnitude of correction are extremely important

Precautions Use with caution in patients with CHF, renal insufficiency, cirrhosis, hypertension

Adverse Reactions

Cardiovascular: Edema, thrombosis, hypervolemia

Endocrine & metabolic: Hypernatremia, dilution of serum electrolytes, overhydration

Gastrointestinal: Nausea, vomiting (oral use)

Local: Phlebitis (with concentrations >0.9%)

Respiratory: Pulmonary edema

Mechanism of Action Principal extracellular cation; functions in fluid and electrolyte balance, osmotic pressure control and water distribution

Pharmacokinetics

Absorption: Oral, I.V.: Rapid

Distribution: Widely distributed

Elimination: Mainly in urine but also in sweat, tears, and saliva

Usual Dosage Dosage depends upon clinical condition, fluid, electrolyte and acid-base balance of patient; hypertonic solutions (>0.9%) should only be used for the initial treatment of acute serious symptomatic hyponatremia; see Fluid and Electrolyte Requirements in Children *on page 1751*

Maintenance sodium requirements: Oral, I.V.:

- Premature neonates: 2-8 mEq/kg/day
- Term neonates: 1-4 mEq/kg/day
- Infants and Children: 3-4 mEq/kg/day; maximum dose: 100-150 mEq/day
- Adults: 154 mEq/day

Nasal: Children and Adults: Use as often as needed
Heat cramps: Adults: Oral: 0.5-1 g, up to 5-10 times/day (5 g/day maximum)
Ophthalmic, ointment: Children and Adults: Apply once daily or more often as needed
To correct acute, serious hyponatremia: mEq sodium = [desired sodium (mEq/L) - actual sodium (mEq/L)] x 0.6 x wt (kg); for acute correction use 125 mEq/L as the desired serum sodium; acutely correct serum sodium in 5 mEq/L/dose increments; more gradual correction in increments of 10 mEq/L/day is indicated in the asymptomatic patient

Administration
Nasal: Spray into 1 nostril while gently occluding other
Ophthalmic: Apply to affected eye(s); avoid contact of bottle tip with eye or skin
Oral: Administer with full glass of water
Parenteral: Infuse hypertonic solutions (>0.9% saline) via central line only; maximum rate of administration: 1 mEq/kg/hour

Monitoring Parameters Serum sodium, chloride, I & O, weight

Reference Range Serum/plasma sodium levels:
Premature neonates: 132-140 mEq/L
Full-term neonates: 133-142 mEq/L
Infants ≥2 months to Adults: 135-145 mEq/L

Nursing Implications Bacteriostatic NS should not be used for diluting or reconstituting drugs for administration in neonates

Additional Information Normal saline (0.9%) = 154 mEq/L; 3% NaCl = 513 mEq/L; 5% NaCl = 855 mEq/L

Dosage Forms Excipient information presented when available (limited, particularly for generics); consult specific product labeling. [DSC] = Discontinued product
Gel, intranasal:
Ayr® Saline No-Drip: 0.5% (22 mL) [spray gel; contains benzalkonium chloride, benzyl alcohol and soybean oil]
Ayr® Saline: 0.5% (14 g) [contains soybean oil]
Entsol®: 3% (20 g) [contains aloe, benzalkonium chloride, and vitamin E]
Simply Saline® Nasal Moist®: 0.65% (30 g)
Injection, solution [preservative free]: 0.9% (2 mL, 5 mL, 10 mL, 20 mL, 100 mL)
Injection, solution [preservative free, prefilled I.V. flush syringe]: 0.9% (2 mL, 2.5 mL, 3 mL, 5 mL, 10 mL)
Injection, solution: 0.45% (25 mL, 50 mL, 100 mL, 250 mL, 500 mL, 1000 mL); 0.9% (3 mL, 5 mL, 10 mL, 20 mL, 25 mL, 30 mL, 50 mL, 100 mL, 150 mL, 250 mL, 500 mL, 1000 mL); 3% (500 mL); 5% (500 mL)
Syrex: 0.9% (2.5 mL, 5 mL, 10 mL) [prefilled syringe]
Injection, solution [bacteriostatic]: 0.9% (10 mL, 20 mL, 30 mL) [contains benzyl alcohol]
Injection, solution [concentrate]: 14.6% (2.5 mEq/mL) (20 mL, 40 mL); 23.4% (4 mEq/mL) (30 mL, 100 mL, 200 mL, 250 mL)
Ointment, ophthalmic: 5% (3.5 g)
Altachlore, Muro 128®: 5% (3.5 g)
Powder for nasal solution (Entsol®): 3% (10.5 g)
Solution for inhalation: 0.45% (3 mL, 5 mL); 0.9% (3 mL, 5 mL, 15 mL); 3% (15 mL); 10% (15 mL)
Broncho® Saline: 0.9% (90 mL, 240 mL) [for dilution of bronchodilator solutions] [DSC]
Solution, intranasal: 0.65% (45 mL)
Altamist: 0.65% (60 mL) [spray; contains benzalkonium chloride]
Ayr® Baby Saline: 0.65% (30 mL) [spray/drops; contains benzalkonium chloride]
Ayr® Saline: 0.65% (50 mL) [drops; contains benzalkonium chloride]
Ayr® Saline: 0.65% (50 mL) [mist, contains benzalkonium chloride]
Breathe Right® Saline: 0.65% (44 mL) [spray; contains benzalkonium chloride]
Deep Sea: 0.65% (45 mL) [spray; contains benzalkonium chloride]
Entsol® Mist: 3% (30 mL) [spray; contains benzalkonium chloride]
Entsol® [preservative free]: 3% (100 mL) [spray]
Entsol® [preservative free]: 3% (240 mL) [nasal wash]
Mycinaire™: 0.65% (30 mL) [mist; contains benzalkonium chloride]
Na-Zone®: 0.65% (60 mL) [spray; contains benzalkonium chloride]
NaSal™: 0.65% (15 mL) [drops; contains benzalkonium chloride], (30 mL) [spray; contains benzalkonium chloride]
Nasal Moist®: 0.65% (45 mL) [spray]
Ocean®: 0.65% (45 mL) [mist/spray/drops; contains benzalkonium chloride]; (473 mL) [refill bottle; contains benzalkonium chloride]
Ocean® for Kids: 0.65% (37.5 mL) [drops/spray/stream; contains benzalkonium chloride]
Pretz®: 0.75% (50 mL) [spray; contains benzalkonium chloride and yerba santa]; (240 mL) [irrigation; contains benzalkonium chloride and yerba santa]; (960 mL) [refill bottle; contains benzalkonium chloride and yerba santa]

(Continued)

Sodium Chloride *(Continued)*

SalineX®: 0.4% (15 mL) [drops]; (50 mL) [spray]
Simply Saline®: 0.9% (44 mL, 90 mL) [mist]
Simply Saline® Baby: 0.9% (45 mL) [mist]
4-Way® Saline Moisturizing Mist: 0.74% (30 mL) [alcohol free; contains benzalkonium chloride, eucalyptol, and menthol]

Solution for irrigation: 0.45% (1500 mL, 2000 mL); 0.9% (250 mL, 500 mL, 1000 mL, 1500 mL, 2000 mL, 3000 mL, 4000 mL, 5000 mL)
Wound Wash Saline™: 0.9% (90 mL, 210 mL)

Solution, ophthalmic: 5% (15 mL)
Altachlore: 5% (15 mL, 30 mL)
Muro 128®: 2% (15 mL); 5% (15 mL, 30 mL)

- ♦ **Sodium Edetate** *see* Edetate Disodium *on page 555*
- ♦ **Sodium Etidronate** *see* Etidronate Disodium *on page 622*
- ♦ **Sodium Ferric Gluconate** *see* Iron Supplements (Parenteral) *on page 870*
- ♦ **Sodium Fluoride** *see* Fluoride *on page 675*
- ♦ **Sodium Hydrogen Carbonate** *see* Sodium Bicarbonate *on page 1448*
- ♦ **Sodium Hyposulfate** *see* Sodium Thiosulfate *on page 1461*
- ♦ **Sodium Nafcillin** *see* Nafcillin *on page 1099*

Sodium Nitrite, Sodium Thiosulfate, and Amyl Nitrite

(AM il NYE trate, SOW dee um NYE trate, & SOW dee um thye oh SUL fate)

Related Information
Commonly Used Antidotes for Acute Overdoses *on page 1920*

U.S. Brand Names Cyanide Antidote Package

Index Terms Amyl Nitrite,Sodium Thiosulfate, and Sodium Nitrite; Cyanide Antidote Kit; Sodium Thiosulfate, Sodium Nitrite, and Amyl Nitrite

Therapeutic Category Antidote, Cyanide

Generic Available No

Use Treatment agents for cyanide poisoning

Pregnancy Risk Factor Sodium thiosulfate, sodium nitrite, and amyl nitrite: C

Contraindications Hypersensitivity to amyl nitrite, sodium nitrite, sodium thiosulfate, or any component

Warnings Excessive methemoglobin results when sodium nitrite dosage is exceeded; use only enough sodium nitrite to achieve a satisfactory clinical response; avoid methemoglobin levels >30%; patients with malignancy and G6PD deficiency have increased sensitivity to the methemoglobin-generating activities of sodium nitrite

Precautions When cyanide poisoning is related to smoke inhalation, if possible, the patient should be at pressure in a hyperbaric chamber before the kit is administered; the methemoglobin initially produced by sodium nitrite injection may otherwise exacerbate concomitant carbon monoxide poisoning that has already severely diminished oxygen-carrying capacity in red cells

Adverse Reactions Reactions listed are those of sodium nitrite; see individual monographs for Amyl Nitrite *on page 130* and Sodium Thiosulfate *on page 1461*
Cardiovascular: Tachycardia, syncope, cyanosis, hypotension (associated with rapid infusion), flushing
Central nervous system: Dizziness, headache
Gastrointestinal: Nausea, vomiting
Miscellaneous: Methemoglobin formation

Drug Interactions Sodium nitrite antagonizes acetylcholine, epinephrine, and histamine effects; sodium nitrite potentiates hypotensive effects and/or anticholinergic effects of tricyclic antidepressants, antihistamines, and meperidine and related CNS depressants; also see Amyl Nitrite *on page 130*

Stability Sodium nitrite is stable at room temperature; do not mix with other medications; see individual monographs Amyl Nitrite *on page 130* and Sodium Thiosulfate *on page 1461*

Mechanism of Action Amyl nitrite and sodium nitrite promote the formation of methemoglobin which binds with cyanide to form cyanomethemoglobin (nontoxic); sodium thiosulfate, by providing an extra sulfur group to the enzyme rhodanese, increases the rate of detoxification of cyanide

Usual Dosage Administer in sequential order:
Amyl nitrite: Infants, Children, and Adults: Inhale vapors from 1 ampul continuously for 15-30 seconds, followed by a rest for 15 seconds (this interrupted schedule is important because continuous use of amyl nitrite may prevent adequate oxygenation); reapply until sodium nitrite can be administered
Sodium nitrite: I.V.:
Infants and Children ≤25 kg: See table on next page.

Variation of Sodium Nitrite and Sodium Thiosulfate Dose With Hemoglobin Concentration[1]

Hemoglobin (g/dL)	Initial Dose Sodium Nitrite (mg/kg)	Initial Dose Sodium Nitrite 3% (mL/kg)	Initial Dose Sodium Thiosulfate 25% (mL/kg)
7	5.8	0.19	0.95
8	6.6	0.22	1.10
9	7.5	0.25	1.25
10	8.3	0.27	1.35
11	9.1	0.30	1.50
12	10.0	0.33	1.65
13	10.8	0.36	1.80
14	11.6	0.39	1.95

[1]Adapted from Berlin DM Jr, "The Treatment of Cyanide Poisoning in Children," *Pediatrics*, 1970, 46:793.

Follow immediately with sodium thiosulfate

Children >25 kg, Adolescents, and Adults: 300 mg; follow immediately with sodium thiosulfate

Sodium thiosulfate: I.V.:

Infants and Children ≤25 kg: See table

Children >25 kg, Adolescents, and Adults: 12.5 g

Patients should be watched for at least 24-48 hours; if signs of poisoning reappear, injection of both sodium nitrite and sodium thiosulfate should be repeated, but each in ½ of the original dose; even if the patient is asymptomatic, repeat ½ doses of both sodium nitrite and sodium thiosulfate may be given for prophylactic purposes 2 hours after the first injection

Administration

Inhalation: **Amyl nitrite:** Crush ampul in cloth and hold under patient's nares for 15-30 seconds; remove for 15 seconds; repeat

Parenteral: I.V.:

Sodium nitrite: Administer undiluted at a rate of 2.5-5 mL/minute

Sodium thiosulfate: Administer undiluted over at least 10 minutes; rapid administration may cause hypotension

Monitoring Parameters Blood cyanide levels, methemoglobin levels, arterial blood gases, oxygen saturation, vital signs

Reference Range Symptoms associated with blood cyanide levels:

Flushing and tachycardia: 0.5-1 mcg/mL

Obtundation: 1-2.5 mcg/mL

Coma and respiratory depression: >2.5 mcg/mL

Death: >3 mcg/mL

Dosage Forms Excipient information presented when available (limited, particularly for generics); consult specific product labeling.

Kit [each kit contains] (Cyanide Antidote Package):

Injection, solution:

Sodium nitrite 300 mg/10 mL (2)

Sodium thiosulfate 12.5 g/50 mL (2)

Inhalant: Amyl nitrite 0.3 mL (12)

[kit also includes disposable syringes, stomach tube, tourniquet, and instructions]

- **Sodium Nitroferricyanide** *see* Nitroprusside *on page 1143*
- **Sodium Nitroprusside** *see* Nitroprusside *on page 1143*

Sodium Phenylacetate and Sodium Benzoate

(SOW dee um fen il AS e tate & SOW dee um BENZ oh ate)

U.S. Brand Names Ammonul®

Index Terms NAPA and NABZ; Sodium Benzoate and Sodium Phenylacetate

Therapeutic Category Ammonium Detoxicant; Hyperammonemia Agent; Urea Cycle Disorder (UCD) Treatment Agent

Generic Available No

Use Adjunct to treatment of acute hyperammonemia and encephalopathy in patients with urea cycle disorders involving partial or complete deficiencies of carbamyl-phosphate synthetase (CPS), ornithine transcarbamoylase (OTC), argininosuccinate lysase (ASL), or argininosuccinate synthetase (ASS); for use with hemodialysis in acute neonatal hyperammonemic coma, moderate-to-severe hyperammonemic encephalopathy and hyperammonemia which fails to respond to initial therapy

Pregnancy Risk Factor C

(Continued)

Sodium Phenylacetate and Sodium Benzoate *(Continued)*

Lactation Excretion in breast milk unknown/use caution

Contraindications Hypersensitivity to sodium phenylacetate, sodium benzoate, or any component of the formulation

Warnings Severity of hyperammonemia may require hemodialysis, as well as nutritional management and medical support; due to enhanced potassium excretion, monitor potassium level closely; potential tissue extravasant which may result in skin necrosis, administer only through central I.V. line. Repeat loading doses are not indicated due to prolonged plasma levels noted in pharmacokinetic studies.

Precautions Due to high sodium content use with caution in patients with congestive heart failure, renal or hepatic dysfunction, or sodium retention associated with edema; maintain caloric intake at 80 cal/kg/day

Adverse Reactions Patients ≤30 days of age reported more blood, lymphatic system, and vascular disorders; patients >30 days of age reported more gastrointestinal disorders.

Cardiovascular: Hypotension, edema, cardiac arrest, cardiomyopathy, chest pain, hypertension

Central nervous system: Fever, agitation, coma, acute psychosis, confusion, hallucinations, ataxia, increased intracranial pressure

Dermatologic: Pruritus, maculo-papular rash, urticaria, hemangioma

Endocrine & metabolic: Hyperglycemia, hypoglycemia, hypokalemia, hyperammonemia, metabolic acidosis, hypocalcemia, hypernatremia

Gastrointestinal: Vomiting, diarrhea, nausea, GI hemorrhage

Genitourinary: Urinary tract infection, urinary retention, renal failure, anuria

Hematologic: Anemia, DIC, thrombocytopenia, thrombosis, pancytopenia

Hepatic: Hepatotoxicity, jaundice, cholestasis

Local: Injection site reaction, extravasation, skin necrosis

Neuromuscular & skeletal: Areflexia, weakness, tremor, clonus

Ophthalmic: Blindness

Respiratory: Respiratory distress, dyspnea, ARDS, pneumonia, pulmonary edema, pulmonary hemorrhage, hyperventilation, pneumothorax

Drug Interactions Probenecid and penicillin antibiotics may decreased renal excretion; valproic acid may reduce effectiveness by increasing ammonia level

Stability Prior to dilution, store at room temperature of 25°C (77°F). Following dilution in $D_{10}W$, solution for infusion may be stored at room temperature for up to 24 hours. Stable when mixed with arginine HCl 10% injection

Mechanism of Action Sodium phenylacetate and sodium benzoate provide alternate pathways for the removal of ammonia through the formation of their metabolites. One mole of sodium phenylacetate removes two moles of nitrogen; one mole of sodium benzoate removes one mole of nitrogen.

Pharmacokinetics

Metabolism: Hepatic and renal; sodium phenylacetate conjugates with glutamine, forming the active metabolite, phenylacetylglutamine (PAG); sodium benzoate combines with glycine to form the active metabolite hippuric acid (HIP)

Excretion: Urine

Usual Dosage IV: Administer as a loading dose over 90-120 minutes, followed by an equivalent dose as a maintenance infusion over 24 hours. Arginine HCl is administered concomitantly. Dosage based on weight and specific enzyme deficiency; therapy should continue until ammonia levels are in normal range. Do not repeat loading dose.

Infants and Children ≤20 kg:

CPS and OTC deficiency: Ammonul® 2.5 mL/kg and arginine 10% 2 mL/kg (provides sodium phenylacetate 250 mg/kg, sodium benzoate 250 mg/kg, and arginine hydrochloride 200 mg/kg)

ASS and ASL deficiency: Ammonul® 2.5 mL/kg and arginine 10% 6 mL/kg (provides sodium phenylacetate 250 mg/kg, sodium benzoate 250 mg/kg, and arginine hydrochloride 600 mg/kg)

Note: Pending a specific diagnosis in infants, the bolus and maintenance dose of arginine should be 6 mL/kg. If ASS or ASL are excluded as diagnostic possibilities, reduce dose of arginine to 2 mL/kg/day.

Children >20 kg:

CPS and OTC deficiency: Ammonul® 55 mL/m^2 and arginine 10% 2 mL/kg (provides sodium phenylacetate 5.5 g/m^2, sodium benzoate 5.5 g/m^2, and arginine hydrochloride 200 mg/kg)

ASS and ASL deficiency: Ammonul® 55 mL/m^2 and arginine 10% 6 mL/kg (provides sodium phenylacetate 5.5 g/m^2, sodium benzoate 5.5 g/m^2, and arginine hydrochloride 600 mg/kg)

Dosage adjustment in renal impairment: Use with caution; monitor closely

Dialysis: Ammonia clearance is ~10 times greater with hemodialysis than by peritoneal dialysis or hemofiltration. Exchange transfusion is ineffective.

Dosage adjustment in hepatic impairment: Use with caution

Administration I.V.: Must be administered via central line; administration via peripheral line may cause burns. Dilute in $D_{10}W$ at ≥25 mL/kg prior to administration. May mix with arginine HCl. In case of extravasation, discontinue infusion and resume at new injection site.

Monitoring Parameters Neurologic status, plasma ammonia, plasma glutamine, clinical response, serum electrolytes (potassium or bicarbonate supplementation may be required), acid-base balance, infusion site

Reference Range Long-term target levels (may not be appropriate for every patient):

Plasma ammonia: <40 µmol/L

Plasma glutamine: <1000 µmol/L

Normal plasma levels of alanine, glycine, lysine, arginine (except in arginase deficiency); normal urinary orotate excretion; normal plasma protein concentration

Nursing Implications Extravasation may cause skin necrosis; administer through central line only. Treatment of extravasation may include aspiration of residual mediation from catheter, limb elevation, intermittent cooling with cold packs. Due to its lingering odor, exercise care in mixing to minimize contact with skin and clothing.

Additional Information Ucephan® (sodium phenylacetate and sodium benzoate), was previously available as an oral liquid for chronic treatment of urea cycle disorders. Although no longer commercially available, this combination may be compounded for patients not responsive to or tolerant of other treatments.

Dosage Forms Excipient information presented when available (limited, particularly for generics); consult specific product labeling.

Injection, solution: Sodium phenylacetate 100 mg and sodium benzoate 100 mg per mL (50 mL)

References

Batshaw ML, MacArthur RB, and Tuchman M, "Alternative Pathway Therapy for Urea Cycle Disorders: Twenty Years Later," *J Pediatr*, 2001, 138(1 Suppl):46-54.

Berry GT and Steiner RD, "Long-Term Management of Patients With Urea Cycle Disorders," *J Pediatr*, 2001, 138(1 Suppl):56-60.

Brusilow SW, Danney M, Waber LJ, et al, "Treatment of Episodic Hyperammonemia in Children With Inborn Errors of Urea Synthesis," *N Engl J Med*, 1984, 310(25):1630-4.

"Consensus Statement From a Conference for the Management of Patients With Urea Cycle Disorders. Urea Cycle Disorders Conference Group," *J Pediatr*, 2001, 138(1 Suppl):1-5.

Gutteridge C and Kuhn RJ, "Compatibility of 10% Sodium Benzoate Plus 10% Sodium Phenylacetate With Various Flavored Vehicles," *Am J Hosp Pharm*, 1994, 51(19):2508, 2510.

Sodium Phenylbutyrate (SOW dee um fen il BYOO ti rate)

U.S. Brand Names Buphenyl®

Index Terms Ammonapse

Therapeutic Category Ammonium Detoxicant; Hyperammonemia Agent; Urea Cycle Disorder (UCD) Treatment Agent

Generic Available No

Use Adjunctive therapy in the chronic management of patients with urea cycle disorder involving deficiencies of carbamoylphosphate synthetase, ornithine transcarbamylase, or argininosuccinic acid synthetase; provides an alternative pathway for waste nitrogen excretion

Pregnancy Risk Factor C

Lactation Excretion in breast milk unknown

Contraindications Hypersensitivity to phenylbutyrate, or any component; patients with severe hypertension, heart failure or renal dysfunction; **phenylbutyrate is not indicated in the treatment of acute hyperammonemia**

Precautions Use cautiously in patients with renal or hepatic dysfunction and in patients who must maintain a low sodium diet as each gram of drug contains 125 mg sodium

Adverse Reactions

Cardiovascular: Edema, arrhythmias, syncope

Central nervous system: Headache, depression

Dermatologic: Rash

Endocrine & metabolic: Amenorrhea, menstrual dysfunction, acidosis, alkalosis, hyperchloremia, hyperuricemia, hypokalemia, hypernatremia, hyperphosphatemia, weight gain

Gastrointestinal: Anorexia, abnormal taste, abdominal pain, nausea, vomiting, gastritis; rare: peptic ulcer, rectal bleeding, pancreatitis

Hematologic: Anemia, leukopenia, leukocytosis, thrombocytopenia, aplastic anemia

Hepatic: Hypoalbuminemia, elevated liver enzymes, elevated bilirubin

Renal: Renal tubular acidosis

Miscellaneous: Offensive body odor

(Continued)

Sodium Phenylbutyrate *(Continued)*

Drug Interactions Haloperidol, valproic acid and corticosteroids increase ammonia concentrations and may decrease effectiveness of sodium phenylbutyrate; probenecid may decrease urinary excretion

Food Interactions Avoid mixing with acidic-type beverages (eg, colas, lemonade, grape juice) since drug may precipitate

Stability Store at room temperature (59°F to 86°F); after opening, containers should be kept tightly closed

Mechanism of Action Sodium phenylbutyrate is a prodrug that, when given orally, is rapidly converted to phenylacetate. Phenylacetate is conjugated with glutamine to form the active compound phenylacetyglutamine. Phenylacetyglutamine serves as a substitute for urea and is excreted in the urine carrying with it 2 moles nitrogen (equivalent to urea) per mole of phenylacetyglutamine thus assisting in the clearance of nitrogenous waste in patients with urea cycle disorders.

Pharmacokinetics

Distribution: V_d: 0.2 L/kg

Metabolism: conjugation to phenylacetylglutamine (active form); undergoes nonlinear Michaelis-Menten elimination kinetics

Half-life: 0.8 hours (parent compound); 1.2 hours (phenylacetate)

Time to peak serum concentration:

Powder: 1 hour

Tablet: 1.35 hours

Elimination: 80% of metabolite excreted in urine in 24 hours

Usual Dosage Oral:

Neonates, Infants, and Children <20 kg: 450-600 mg/kg/day divided four to six times daily; maximum daily dose 20 g/day

Children >20 kg and Adults: 9.9-13 g/m^2/day, divided four to six times daily; maximum daily dose 20 g/day

Administration Oral: Administer with meals or feedings; mix powder with food or drink; avoid mixing with acidic beverages (eg, most fruit juices or colas)

Monitoring Parameters Plasma ammonia and glutamine concentrations, serum electrolytes, proteins, hepatic and renal function tests, physical signs/symptoms of hyperammonemia (ie, lethargy, ataxia, confusion, vomiting, seizures, and memory impairment)

Patient Information It is important to follow the dietary restrictions required when treating this disorder, the medication must be taken in strict accordance with the prescribed regimen; avoid altering the dosage without the prescriber's knowledge; the powder formulation has a very salty taste

Additional Information Teaspoon and tablespoon measuring devices are provided with the powder; each 1 g powder contains 0.94 g sodium phenylbutyrate = 125 mg sodium; each tablet contains 0.5 g sodium phenylbutyrate = 62 mg sodium

Dosage Forms Excipient information presented when available (limited, particularly for generics); consult specific product labeling.

Powder, for oral solution: 3 g/level teaspoon (250 g) [contains sodium 125 mg/g; packaged with measuring device]

Tablet: 500 mg [contains sodium 124 mg/g]

References

Batshaw ML, MacArthur RB, and Tuchman M, "Alternative Pathway Therapy for Urea Cycle Disorders: Twenty Years Later," *J Pediatr*, 2001, 138(1 Suppl):S46-S55.

Berry GT and Steiner RD, "Long-Term Management of Patients With Urea Cycle Disorders," *J Pediatr*, 2001, 138(1 Suppl):S56-60.

Brusilow SW, "Phenylacetylglutamine May Replace Urea as a Vehicle for Waste Nitrogen Excretion," *Pediatr Res*, 1991, 29(2):147-50.

Maestri NE, Brusilow SW, Clissold DB, et al, "Long-Term Treatment of Girls With Ornithine Transcarbamylase Deficiency," *N Engl J Med*, 1996, 335(12):855-9.

♦ **Sodium Phosphate and Potassium Phosphate** *see* Potassium Phosphate and Sodium Phosphate *on page 1296*

Sodium Phosphate (SOW dee um FOS fates)

Medication Safety Issues

Sound-alike/look-alike issues:

Visicol® may be confused with VESIcare®

Enemas and oral solution are available in pediatric and adult sizes; prescribe by "volume" not by "bottle."

U.S. Brand Names Fleet® Accu-Prep® [OTC]; Fleet® Enema [OTC]; Fleet® Phospho-Soda® [OTC]; OsmoPrep™; Visicol®

Canadian Brand Names Fleet Enema®; Fleet® Phospho-Soda® Oral Laxative

Therapeutic Category Electrolyte Supplement, Oral; Electrolyte Supplement, Parenteral; Laxative, Saline; Sodium Salt

Generic Available Yes: Enema, injection

Use Treatment and prevention of hypophosphatemia; short-term treatment of constipation (oral/rectal); evacuation of the colon for rectal and bowel exams; source of phosphate in large volume I.V. fluids

Pregnancy Risk Factor C

Lactation Use caution in nursing women.

Contraindications Hypersensitivity to phosphate (salts) or any component; hyperphosphatemia, hypocalcemia, hypomagnesemia, hypernatremia, severe renal impairment, severe tissue trauma, heat cramps, CHF, abdominal pain (rectal forms), fecal impaction (rectal forms)

Warnings Use of >45 mL/day oral sodium phosphate solution as a bowel preparation in adults has been associated with significant electrolyte changes resulting in symptomatic dehydration, renal failure, metabolic acidosis, tetany, and death; consider obtaining baseline and post-treatment electrolytes in patients receiving >45 mL/day of sodium phosphate solution

Precautions

Use with caution in patients with renal impairment, patients with adrenal insufficiency, cirrhosis

Adverse Reactions Cardiovascular: Hypotension, cardiac arrhythmias, edema

Central nervous system: Mental confusion, seizures, dizziness, headache

Endocrine & metabolic: Hyperphosphatemia, hypocalcemia, hypernatremia, hypomagnesemia

Gastrointestinal: Nausea, vomiting, diarrhea, flatulence (oral use)

Local: Phlebitis (parenteral forms)

Neuromuscular & skeletal: Paresthesia, bone and joint pain, arthralgia, weakness, muscle cramps, tetany

Renal: Acute renal failure

Clinical manifestations of hypophosphatemia by systems:

Neuromuscular: Muscle weakness, anorexia, tremor, paresthesia, convulsions, coma, hyporeflexia, irritability, numbness, abnormal EEG, cardiomyopathy, respiratory failure, inability to wean from ventilator

Hematologic: Rhabdomyolysis, hemolytic anemia, decreased oxygen release, decreased chemotaxis, decreased phagocytosis, decreased platelet survival, myoglobinuria, thrombocytopenia

Skeletal: Osteomalacia, joint arthralgias, pathologic fractures

Drug Interactions Do not give orally at the same time as aluminum and magnesium-containing antacids or sucralfate which can act as phosphate binders.

Food Interactions

Avoid giving with oxalate (ie, berries, nuts, chocolate, beans, celery, tomatoes) or phytate-containing foods (ie, bran, whole wheat).

Stability Phosphate salts may precipitate when mixed with calcium salts; solubility is improved in parenteral nutrition solutions which contain amino acids; check with a pharmacist to determine compatibility

Mechanism of Action Phosphorus is an essential mineral that is usually found in nature combined with oxygen as phosphate. It participates in bone deposition, calcium metabolism, as part of molecules that regulate many coenzymes, steps in the clotting cascade, and functions of the immune system. It is a component of the lipid bilayer of cell membranes in the form of phospholipids and of other intracellular compounds like nucleic acids and nucleoproteins. It acts as a buffer for the maintenance of plasma and urinary pH. When administered orally or rectally as a laxative, it exerts osmotic effect in the small intestine by drawing water into the lumen of the gut, producing distension, promoting peristalsis, and evacuation of the bowel.

Pharmacodynamics Onset of action (catharsis):

Oral: 3-6 hours

Rectal: 2-5 minutes

Phosphorus - Recommended Daily Allowance (RDA) and Estimated Average Requirement (EAR)

Age	RDA (mmol/day)	EAR (mmol/day)
0-6 mo	—	3.2[1]
7-12 mo	—	8.9[1]
1-3 y	14.8	12.3
4-8 y	16.1	13.1
9-18 y	40.3	34
19-30 y	22.6	18.7

[1]Adequate intake (AI)

(Continued)

Sodium Phosphate *(Continued)*

Pharmacokinetics

Absorption: Oral: 1% to 20%

Elimination: Oral forms excreted in feces; I.V. forms are excreted in the urine with over 80% to 90% of dose reabsorbed by the kidney

Usual Dosage Note: Consider the contribution of sodium when determining the appropriate phosphate replacement.

Phosphorus: Oral: See table on previous page.

Hypophosphatemia: Hypophosphatemia does not necessarily equate with phosphate depletion. Hypophosphatemia may occur in the presence of low, normal, or high total body phosphate and conversely, phosphate depletion may exist with normal, low, or elevated levels of serum phosphate (Gaasbeek, 2005). It is difficult to provide concrete guidelines for the treatment of severe hypophosphatemia because the extent of total body deficits and response to therapy are difficult to predict. Aggressive doses of phosphate may result in a transient serum elevation followed by redistribution into intracellular compartments or bone tissue. Various regimens for replacement of phosphate in adults have been studied. The regimens below have only been studied in adult patients; however, many institutions have used them in children safely and successfully.

I.V. doses may be incorporated into the patient's maintenance I.V. fluids; intermittent I.V. infusion should be reserved for severe depletion situations. **Note:** Doses listed as mmol of **phosphate** (see also Additional Information).

Intermittent I.V. infusion: It is recommended that repletion of severe hypophosphatemia be done I.V. because large doses of oral phosphate may cause diarrhea and intestinal absorption may be unreliable.

Children and Adults: **Note:** There are no prospective studies of parenteral phosphate replacement in children. The following weight-based guidelines for adult dosing may be cautiously employed in pediatric patients. Guidelines differ based on degree of illness, use of TPN, and severity of hypophosphatemia.

General replacement guidelines (Lentz, 1978): **Note:** The initial dose may be increased by 25% to 50% if the patient is symptomatic secondary to hypophosphatemia and lowered by 25% to 50% if the patient is hypercalcemic.

Low dose: 0.08 mmol/kg over 6 hours; use if losses are recent and uncomplicated

Intermediate dose: 0.16-0.24 mmol/kg over 4-6 hours; use if serum phosphorus level 0.5-1 mg/dL (0.16-0.32 mmol/L)

High dose: 0.36 mmol/kg over 6 hours; use if serum phosphorus <0.5 mg/dL (<0.16 mmol/L)

Patients receiving TPN (Clark, 1995):

Low dose: 0.16 mmol/kg over 4-6 hours; use if serum phosphorus level 2.3-3 mg/dL (0.73- 0.96 mmol/L)

Intermediate dose: 0.32 mmol/kg over 4-6 hours; use if serum phosphorus level 1.6-2.2 mg/dL (0.51-0.72 mmol/L)

High dose: 0.64 mmol/kg over 8-12 hours; use if serum phosphorus <1.5 mg/dL (< 0.5 mmol/L)

Critically ill adult trauma patients receiving TPN (Brown, 2006):

Low dose: 0.32 mmol/kg over 4-6 hours; use if serum phosphorus level 2.3-3 mg/dL (0.73-0.96 mmol/L)

Intermediate dose: 0.64 mmol/kg over 4-6 hours; use if serum phosphorus level 1.6-2.2 mg/dL (0.51-0.72 mmol/L)

High dose: 1 mmol/kg over 8-12 hours; use if serum phosphorus <1.5 mg/dL (< 0.5 mmol/L)

Alternative method in critically ill patients (Kingston, 1985):

Low dose: 0.25 mmol/kg over 4 hours; use if serum phosphorus level 0.5-1 mg/dL (0.16-0.32 mmol/L)

Moderate dose: 0.5 mmol/kg over 4 hours; use if serum phosphorus level <0.5 mg/dL (<0.16 mmol/L)

Adults: 15 mmol/dose over 2 hours; use if serum phosphorus <2 mg/dL (0.65 mmol/L); may repeat in 6- to 8-hour intervals if repeat serum phosphorus (at least 6 hours postdose) <2 mg/dL (0.65 mmol/L); not to exceed 45 mmol/24 hours (Rosen, 1995)

Maintenance:

I.V.:

Neonates: 0.8-1.5 mmol/kg/day

Infants and Children <25 kg: 0.5-1.5 mmol/kg/day

Children 25-45 kg: 0.5-1 mmol/kg/day

Oral: 2-3 mmol/kg/day in divided doses (including dietary intake: See Additional Information)

Adults:

I.V.: 50-70 mmol/day

Oral: 50-150 mmol/day in divided doses (including dietary intake; see Additional Information)

Laxative:

Oral:

Fleet® Phospho-Soda®: Oral:

Children 5-9 years: 5 mL as a single dose

Children 10-12 years: 10 mL as a single dose

Children ≥12 years and Adults: 20-30 mL as a single dose

Visicol®: Oral: Must be administered with a full glass of water

Children 5-9 years: 2-4 tablets (~0.9-1.8 g dibasic sodium phosphate and 2.4-4.8 g monobasic sodium phosphate) daily as a single dose

Children 10-11 years: 4-9 tablets (~1.8-3.6 g dibasic sodium phosphate and 4.8-9.6 g monobasic sodium phosphate) daily as a single dose

Children ≥12 years and Adults: 9-20 tablets (~3.6-8.1 g dibasic sodium phosphate and 9.6-21.6 g monobasic sodium phosphate) daily as a single dose

Adults ≥18 years: Prior to colonoscopy per manufacturer: The night before the procedure: 4 tablets every 15 minutes until a total dose of 20 tablets; repeat 3-5 hours **before** the procedure with 4 tablets every 15 minutes until a total dose of 40 tablets has been administered

Rectal: Fleet® Enema:

Children 2-11 years: Contents of one 2.25 oz pediatric enema as a single dose, may repeat

Children ≥12 years and Adults: Contents of one 4.5 oz enema as a single dose, may repeat

Administration

Oral: Administer with food to reduce the risk of diarrhea; contents of 1 packet should be diluted in 75 mL water before administration; administer tablets with a full glass of water; maintain adequate fluid intake; dilute oral solution with an equal volume of cool water

Parenteral: For intermittent I.V. infusion: Peripheral line: Dilute to a maximum concentration of 0.05 mmol/mL; Central line: Dilute to a maximum concentration of 0.12 mmol/mL (maximum concentrations were determined with consideration for maximum sodium concentration); maximum rate of infusion: 0.06 mmol/kg/hour; do **not** infuse with calcium-containing I.V. fluids

Monitoring Parameters

Serum sodium, calcium, phosphorus, renal function, reflexes, stool output (laxative use)

Reference Range Note: There is a diurnal variation with the nadir at 1100, plateau at 1600, and peak in the early evening (Gaasbeek, 2005); 1 mmol/L phosphate = 3.1mg/dL phosphorus

Newborns: 4.2-9 mg/dL phosphorus (1.36-2.91 mmol/L phosphate)

6 weeks to 18 months: 3.8-6.7 mg/dL phosphorus (1.23-2.16 mmol/L phosphate)

18 months to 3 years: 2.9-5.9 mg/dL phosphorus (0.94-1.91 mmol/L phosphate)

3-15 years: 3.6-5.6 mg/dL phosphorus (1.16-1.81 mmol/L phosphate)

>15 years: 2.5-5 mg/dL phosphorus (0.81-1.62 mmol/L phosphate)

Hypophosphatemia:

Moderate: 1-2 mg/dL phosphorus (0.32-0.65 mmol/L phosphate)

Severe: <1 mg/dL phosphorus (<0.32 mmol/L phosphate)

Additional Information Each mmol of phosphate contains 31 mg elemental phosphorus; 1 mmol/L phosphate = 3.1 mg/dL phosphorus; cow's milk is a good source of phosphate with 1 mg elemental (0.032 mmol) elemental phosphate per mL

With orders for I.V. phosphate, there is considerable confusion associated with the use of millimoles (mmol) versus milliequivalents (mEq) to express the phosphate requirement. Because inorganic phosphate exists as monobasic and dibasic anions, with the mixture of valences dependent on pH, ordering by mEq amounts is unreliable and may lead to large dosing errors. In addition, I.V. phosphate is available in the sodium and potassium salt; therefore, the content of these cations must be considered when ordering phosphate. The most reliable method of ordering I.V. phosphate is by millimoles, then specifying the potassium or sodium salt.

Dosage Forms Excipient information presented when available (limited, particularly for generics); consult specific product labeling.

Kit:

Fleet® Accu-Prep®:

Solution, oral (Fleet® Phosph-Soda®): Monobasic sodium phosphate monohydrate 2.4 g and dibasic sodium phosphate heptahydrate 0.9 g per 5 mL (15 mL) [contains contains sodium 556 mg/5 mL, phosphate 62.25 mEq/5 mL and

(Continued)

Sodium Phosphate *(Continued)*

sodium benzoate; kit contains six 15 mL unit-dose containers (equal to two 45 mL doses)]

Pads, anorectal (Fleet® Relief™): Pramoxine hydrochloride 1% and glycerin 12% (4s)

Injection, solution [preservative free]: Phosphorus 3 mmol and sodium 4 mEq per mL (5 mL, 15 mL, 50 mL)

Solution, oral:

Fleet® Phospho-Soda®: Monobasic sodium phosphate monohydrate 2.4 g and dibasic sodium phosphate heptahydrate 0.9 g per 5 mL (45 mL) [sugar free; contains sodium 556 mg/5 mL, sodium benzoate, and phosphate 62.25 mEq/5 mL; unflavored or ginger-lemon flavor]

Solution, rectal [enema]: Monobasic sodium phosphate 19 g and dibasic sodium phosphate 7 g per 118 mL delivered dose (135 mL)

Fleet® Enema: Monobasic sodium phosphate 19 g and dibasic sodium phosphate 7 g per 118 mL delivered dose (135 mL)

Fleet® Enema for Children: Monobasic sodium phosphate 9.5 g and dibasic sodium phosphate 3.5 g per 59 mL delivered dose (68 mL)

Tablet, oral:

OsmoPrep™: Sodium phosphate monobasic monohydrate 1.102 g and sodium phosphate dibasic anhydrous 0.398 g [sodium phosphate 1.5 g per tablet; gluten free]

Visicol®: Sodium phosphate monobasic monohydrate 1.102 g and sodium phosphate dibasic anhydrous 0.398 g [sodium phosphate 1.5 g per tablet]

References

Brown KA, Dickerson RN, Morgan LM, et al, "A New Graduated Dosing Regimen for Phosphorus Replacement in Patients Receiving Nutrition Support," *JPEN*, 2006, 30(3):209-14.

Clark CL, Sacks GS, Dickerson RN, et al, "Treatment of Hypophosphatemia in Patients Receiving Specialized Nutrition Support Using a Graduated Dosing Scheme: Results From a Prospective Clinical Trial," *Crit Care Med*, 1995, 23(9):1504-11.

"Dietary Reference Intakes for Calcium, Phosphorus, Magnesium, Vitamin D, and Fluoride. Standing Committee on the Scientific Evaluation of Dietary Reference Intakes, Food and Nutrition Board, Institute of Medicine," National Academy of Sciences, Washington, DC: National Academy Press, 1997.

Gaasbeek A and Meinders AE, "Hypophosphatemia: An Update on Its Etiology and Treatment", *Am J Med*, 2005, 118(10):1094-101.

Kingston M and Al-Siba'i MB, "Treatment of Severe Hypophosphatemia," *Crit Care Med*, 1985, 13(1):16-8

Lentz RD, Brown BM, and Kjellstrand CM, "Treatment of Severe Hypophosphatemia," *Ann Intern Med*, 1978, 89(6):941-4.

Lloyd CW and Johnson CE, "Management of Hypophosphatemia," *Clin Pharm*, 1988, 7(2):123-8.

Rosen GH, Boullata JI, O'Rangers EA, et al, "Intravenous Phosphate Repletion Regimen for Critically Ill Patients With Moderate Hypophosphatemia," *Crit Care Med*, 1995, 23(7):1204-10.

Sodium Polystyrene Sulfonate

(SOW dee um pol ee STYE reen SUL fon ate)

Medication Safety Issues

Sound-alike/look-alike issues:

Kayexalate® may be confused with Kaopectate®

Always prescribe either one-time doses or as a specific number of doses (eg, 15 g q6h x 2 doses). Scheduled doses with no dosage limit could be given for days leading to dangerous hypokalemia.

International issues:

Kionex™ may be confused with Kinex® which is a brand name for biperiden in Mexico

U.S. Brand Names Kayexalate®; Kionex™; SPS®

Canadian Brand Names Kayexalate®; PMS-Sodium Polystyrene Sulfonate

Therapeutic Category Antidote, Hyperkalemia

Generic Available Yes

Use Treatment of hyperkalemia

Pregnancy Risk Factor C

Lactation Excretion in breast milk unknown/use caution

Contraindications Hypersensitivity to sodium polystyrene sulfonate or any component; hypernatremia; hypokalemia; intestinal obstruction or perforation (oral use)

Warnings Treatment with this drug alone may be insufficient to rapidly correct severe hyperkalemia; other more rapidly effective appropriate measures should be used; enema will reduce the serum potassium faster than oral administration, but the oral route will result in a greater reduction over several hours; systemic alkalosis has been reported when administered in conjunction with nonabsorbable cation-donating antacids and laxatives such as magnesium hydroxide and aluminum carbonate. Intestinal obstructions due to concretions of aluminum hydroxide have been reported when administered with sodium polystyrene sulfonate.

Precautions Use with caution in patients with severe CHF, hypertension, or edema; small amounts of magnesium and calcium may also be lost in binding

Adverse Reactions

Endocrine & metabolic: Hypokalemia, hypocalcemia, hypomagnesemia, hypernatremia

Gastrointestinal: Anorexia, nausea, vomiting, constipation, intestinal colonic necrosis (rare), diarrhea

Drug Interactions Cation-donating antacids (such as magnesium hydroxide or calcium carbonate) (see Warnings)

Food Interactions Never mix in orange juice

Stability Store at room temperature; suspensions made from powder should be freshly prepared and used within 24 hours of preparation

Mechanism of Action Removes potassium by exchanging sodium ions for potassium ions in the intestine before the resin is passed from the body

Pharmacodynamics Onset of action: Within 2-24 hours

Pharmacokinetics Elimination: Remains in the GI tract to be completely excreted in the feces (primarily as potassium polystyrene sulfonate)

Usual Dosage

Children:

Oral: 1 g/kg/dose every 6 hours

Rectal: 1 g/kg/dose every 2-6 hours

Adults:

Oral: 15 g 1-4 times/day

Rectal: 30-50 g every 6 hours

Administration

Oral or NG: Shake commercially available suspension well before use; when using powder, dilute in 3-4 mL fluid per g of resin; 10% sorbitol, water, or syrup may be used as diluent

Enema: Shake commercially available suspension well before use; when using powder, dilute in water or 25% sorbitol at a concentration of 0.3-0.5 g/mL; retain enema in colon for at least 30-60 minutes or several hours, if possible

Monitoring Parameters Serum sodium, potassium, calcium, magnesium, EKG (if applicable)

Additional Information 1 g of resin binds ~1 mEq of potassium; 4.1 mEq sodium per g of powder; 1 level teaspoon contains 3.5 g polystyrene sulfonate

Dosage Forms Excipient information presented when available (limited, particularly for generics); consult specific product labeling.

Powder for suspension, oral/rectal:

Kayexalate®: 15 g/4 level teaspoons (480 g) [contains sodium 100 mg (4.1 mEq)/g]

Kionex™: 15 g/4 level teaspoons (454 g) [contains sodium 100 mg (4.1 mEq)/g]

Suspension, oral/rectal: 15 g/60 mL (60 mL, 120 mL, 200 mL, 500 mL) [contains sodium 1500 mg (65 mEq)/60 mL, sorbitol, and alcohol 0.1%; cherry/caramel flavor]

SPS®: 15 g/60 mL (60 mL, 120 mL, 480 mL) [contains alcohol 0.3%, sodium 1500 mg (65 mEq)/60 mL, and sorbitol; cherry flavor]

♦ **Sodium Sulfacetamide** *see* Sulfacetamide *on page 1483*

Sodium Thiosulfate (SOW dee um thye oh SUL fate)

U.S. Brand Names Versiclear™

Index Terms Disodium Thiosulfate Pentahydrate; Pentahydrate; Sodium Hyposulfate; Sodium Thiosulphate; Thiosulfuric Acid Disodium Salt

Therapeutic Category Antidote, Cisplatin; Antidote, Cyanide; Antidote, Extravasation; Antifungal Agent, Topical

Generic Available Yes: Injection

Use

Parenteral: Used alone or with sodium nitrite or amyl nitrite in cyanide poisoning; reduce the risk of nephrotoxicity associated with cisplatin therapy; local infiltration (in diluted form) of selected chemotherapy extravasation

Topical: Treatment of tinea versicolor, acne

Pregnancy Risk Factor C

Contraindications Hypersensitivity to sodium thiosulfate or any component

Precautions Discontinue if irritation or sensitivity occurs; rapid I.V. infusion has caused transient hypotension and EKG changes in dogs

Adverse Reactions

Cardiovascular: Hypotension

Central nervous system: Coma, CNS depression secondary to thiocyanate intoxication, psychosis, confusion

Dermatologic: Contact dermatitis

(Continued)

Sodium Thiosulfate *(Continued)*

Local: Local irritation
Neuromuscular & skeletal: Weakness
Otic: Tinnitus

Stability Stable diluted in NS or D_5W at concentrations of 1.5% and 9.76% sodium thiosulfate for 24 hours

Mechanism of Action

Prevention of cyanide toxicity: By providing an extra sulfur group to the enzyme rhodanase, it increases the rate of detoxification of cyanide

Prevention of cisplatin nephrotoxicity: Complexes with cisplatin to form a compound that is nontoxic to either normal or cancerous cells

Pharmacokinetics

Half-life, elimination: 0.65 hours

Elimination: 28.5% excreted unchanged in the urine

Usual Dosage

Cyanide and nitroprusside antidote: I.V.: See Usual Dosage in Sodium Nitrite, Sodium Thiosulfate, and Amyl Nitrite *on page 1452*

Prevention of cisplatin nephrotoxicity: Adults: I.V.: 12 g over 6 hours in association with cisplatin **or** 9 g/m^2 I.V. bolus then 1.2 g/m^2/hour for 6 hours; should be administered before or during cisplatin administration

Chemotherapy infiltration: Children and Adults: Dilute 10% sodium thiosulfate 4-8 mL with 6 mL SWI to make $^1/_6$ to $^1/_3$ molar solution; as local infiltration for the following chemotherapy agents:

Mechlorethamine: Use 2 mL for each mg infiltrated

Cis-platinum: 2 mL for each 100 mg infiltrated; use only for large infiltrates (>20 mL) and concentrations >0.5 mg/mL of cis-platinum

Topical use (antifungal, acne): Children and Adults: 25% solution: Apply thin film twice daily to affected areas for several weeks to months

Administration

Parenteral: I.V.: Inject slowly, over at least 10 minutes; rapid administration may cause hypotension

Topical: Do not apply topically to or near eyes; thoroughly cleanse and dry affects areas prior to application

Dosage Forms Excipient information presented when available (limited, particularly for generics); consult specific product labeling.

Injection, solution [preservative free]: 100 mg/mL (10 mL); 250 mg/mL (50 mL)

Lotion: Sodium thiosulfate 25% and salicylic acid 1% (120 mL) [contains isopropyl alcohol 10%]

References

Hall AH and Rumack BH, "Hydroxocobalamin/Sodium Thiosulfate as a Cyanide Antidote," *J Emerg Med*, 1987, 5(2):115-21.

Naughton M, "Acute Cyanide Poisoning," *Anaesth Intensive Care*, 1974, 2(4):351-6.

♦ **Sodium Thiosulfate, Sodium Nitrite, and Amyl Nitrite** *see* Sodium Nitrite, Sodium Thiosulfate, and Amyl Nitrite *on page 1452*
♦ **Sodium Thiosulphate** *see* Sodium Thiosulfate *on page 1461*
♦ **Soflax™ (Can)** *see* Docusate *on page 526*
♦ **Solaraze®** *see* Diclofenac *on page 486*
♦ **Solarcaine® Aloe Extra Burn Relief [OTC]** *see* Lidocaine *on page 933*
♦ **Solodyn™** *see* Minocycline *on page 1066*
♦ **Solu-Cortef®** *see* Hydrocortisone *on page 781*
♦ **Solugel® (Can)** *see* Benzoyl Peroxide *on page 207*
♦ **Solu-Medrol®** *see* MethylPREDNISolone *on page 1039*
♦ **Soluver® (Can)** *see* Salicylic Acid *on page 1413*
♦ **Soluver® Plus (Can)** *see* Salicylic Acid *on page 1413*
♦ **Somatrem** *see* Human Growth Hormone *on page 769*
♦ **Sominex® [OTC]** *see* DiphenhydrAMINE *on page 509*
♦ **Sominex® Maximum Strength [OTC]** *see* DiphenhydrAMINE *on page 509*
♦ **Somnote™** *see* Chloral Hydrate *on page 331*
♦ **Som Pam (Can)** *see* Flurazepam *on page 686*

Sorbitol (SOR bi tole)

Therapeutic Category Laxative, Hyperosmolar; Laxative, Osmotic

Generic Available Yes

Use Humectant; sweetening agent; hyperosmotic laxative; facilitates the passage of sodium polystyrene sulfonate or a charcoal-toxin complex through the intestinal tract

Lactation Excretion in breast milk unknown

Contraindications Anuria

Adverse Reactions

Endocrine & metabolic: Fluid and electrolyte losses, lactic acidosis

Gastrointestinal: Diarrhea, abdominal distress, nausea, vomiting

Mechanism of Action A polyalcoholic sugar with osmotic cathartic actions

Pharmacodynamics

Onset of action: Oral: Mean time to first stool in patients receiving a charcoal-sorbitol slurry:

- Children (ingestions):
  - 6.4 hours (dose: 1.5 g/kg in 4 patients)
  - 8.48 hours (dose: 2 g/kg in 33 patients)
- Adults:
  - Nonpoisoned volunteers: 1.6 hours (dose: 2 g/kg)
  - Ingestion: 7.2 hours (14 adults; dose not specified)

Pharmacokinetics

Absorption: Oral, rectal: Poor

Metabolism: Mainly in the liver to fructose

Usual Dosage Hyperosmotic laxative (as single dose, at infrequent intervals):

Children 2-11 years:

- Oral: 2 mL/kg (as 70% solution)
- Rectal enema: 30-60 mL as 25% to 30% solution

Children ≥12 years and Adults:

- Oral: 30-150 mL (as 70% solution)
- Rectal enema: 120 mL as 25% to 30% solution
- Adjunct to sodium polystyrene sulfonate: 15 mL as 70% solution orally until diarrhea occurs (10-20 mL/2 hours) or 20-100 mL as an oral vehicle for the sodium polystyrene sulfonate resin

When administered with charcoal: Oral:

- Children: 4.3 mL/kg of 35% sorbitol with 1 g/kg of activated charcoal or maximum dose: 2 g/kg sorbitol with activated charcoal
- Adults: 4.3 mL/kg of 70% sorbitol with 1 g/kg of activated charcoal

Monitoring Parameters Serum electrolytes, I & O

Dosage Forms Excipient information presented when available (limited, particularly for generics); consult specific product labeling.

Solution, genitourinary irrigation: 3% (3000 mL, 5000 mL); 3.3% (2000 mL, 4000 mL)

Solution, oral: 70% (30 mL, 480 mL, 3840 mL)

References

Charney EB and Bodurtha JN, "Intractable Diarrhea Associated With the Use of Sorbitol," *J Pediatr*, 1981, 98:157-8.

James LP, Nichols MH, and King WD, "A Comparison of Cathartics in Pediatric Ingestions," *Pediatrics*, 1995, 96(2 Pt 1):235-8.

Kumar A, Weatherly MR, and Beaman DC, "Sweeteners, Flavorings, and Dyes in Antibiotic Preparations," *Pediatrics*, 1991, 87(3):352-60.

♦ **Sorine®** *see* Sotalol *on page 1463*

♦ **Sotacor® (Can)** *see* Sotalol *on page 1463*

Sotalol (SOE ta lol)

Medication Safety Issues

Sound-alike/look-alike issues:

- Sotalol may be confused with Stadol®
- Betapace® may be confused with Betapace AF®
- Betapace AF® may be confused with Betapace®

Related Information

Adult ACLS Algorithms *on page 1660*

U.S. Brand Names Betapace®; Betapace AF®; Sorine®

Canadian Brand Names Alti-Sotalol; Apo-Sotalol®; Betapace AF®; CO Sotalol; Gen-Sotalol; Lin-Sotalol; Novo-Sotalol; Nu-Sotalol; PMS-Sotalol; Rho®-Sotalol; Riva-Sotalol; Rylosol; Sotacor®

Index Terms Sotalol Hydrochloride

Therapeutic Category Antiarrhythmic Agent, Class II; Antiarrhythmic Agent, Class III; Beta-Adrenergic Blocker

Generic Available Yes

Use

Betapace®, Sorine™, generic: Treatment of life-threatening ventricular arrhythmias (eg, sustained ventricular tachycardia)

Betapace AF™: Maintenance of normal sinus rhythm in patients who have highly symptomatic atrial fibrillation and atrial flutter, but who are currently in normal sinus rhythm [not usually for use in patients with paroxysmal atrial fibrillation/flutter that is easily reversed (eg, by Valsalva maneuver)]

(Continued)

Sotalol *(Continued)*

Note: Do not substitute Betapace AF™ for other products (and vice versa); significant differences in FDA approved labeling exist [eg, dosage and administration, safety information and patient package insert (Betapace AF™ labeling contains a patient package insert specific for atrial fibrillation/flutter)]

Pregnancy Risk Factor B

Lactation Enters breast milk/use caution (AAP rates "compatible")

Contraindications Hypersensitivity to sotalol or any component; sinus bradycardia; heart block greater than first degree (except in patients with a functioning artificial pacemaker); congenital or acquired long QT syndromes; uncontrolled CHF; cardiogenic shock; asthma. Betapace AF™ is also contraindicated in patients with sick sinus syndrome (except in patients with a functioning artificial pacemaker), a baseline QT interval >450 msec, hypokalemia (serum potassium <4 mEq/L), or significantly reduced renal function (Cl_{cr} <40 mL/minute).

Warnings Initiation, reinitiation, and dosage increases of sotalol must occur in a hospital facility that can provide continuous EKG monitoring, recognition and treatment of life-threatening arrhythmias, and CPR. Patients must be monitored with continuous EKG for a minimum of 3 days (on their maintenance dose). Use with caution and adjust the dose in patients with renal impairment; creatinine clearance must be calculated prior to dosing.

May cause serious and life-threatening proarrhythmias [may cause or worsen ventricular arrhythmias (eg, sustained ventricular tachycardia, torsade de pointes, ventricular fibrillation)]; risk factors for torsade de pointes include: Higher sotalol doses, presence of sustained VT, female gender, excessive prolongation of the QT_c interval, history of CHF or cardiomegaly, decreased renal function, hypokalemia, hypomagnesemia, and bradycardia; monitor EKG for proarrhythmic effects; adjust dose to prevent QT_c prolongation; correct electrolyte imbalances (especially hypokalemia and hypomagnesemia) before initiating sotalol

Bradycardia and heart block may occur; consider pre-existing conditions such as sick sinus syndrome before initiating; may cause or worsen CHF (use with caution in patients with compensated CHF); use with caution and titrate dose carefully within the first 2 weeks post-MI (experience is limited); use with caution in patients with peripheral vascular disease (may aggravate arterial insufficiency); concomitant use with other drugs that prolong the QT interval or prolong refractoriness is not recommended (see Drug Interactions)

Exacerbation of angina, arrhythmias, and in some cases MI may occur following abrupt discontinuation of beta-blockers; avoid abrupt discontinuation, wean slowly, monitor for signs and symptoms of ischemia. Beta-blockers should generally be avoided in patients with bronchospastic disease; if administered, use the lowest possible dose and monitor patients carefully. Patients receiving beta-blockers, who have a history of anaphylactic reactions, may be more reactive to a repeated allergen challenge and may not be responsive to the usual epinephrine doses used to treat an allergic reaction. Beta-blockers may block hypoglycemia-induced tachycardia and blood pressure changes; use with caution in patients with diabetes mellitus. May mask signs of thyrotoxicosis. Use caution with anesthetic agents that decrease myocardial function.

Precautions Use with caution in patients receiving calcium channel blockers (see Drug Interactions)

Adverse Reactions

Cardiovascular: Bradycardia, chest pain, palpitations, CHF, peripheral vascular disorders, edema, abnormal EKG, proarrhythmias, QT interval prolongation, torsade de pointes, heart block, hypotension, syncope, sinus pauses

Central nervous system: Fatigue, dizziness, lightheadedness, confusion, anxiety, headache, insomnia, depression, mood change

Dermatologic: Rash

Endocrine & metabolic: Weight change, sexual dysfunction; hyperglycemia in diabetic patients

Gastrointestinal: Diarrhea, nausea, vomiting, dyspepsia, abdominal pain, abdominal distention, flatulence, appetite disorder

Hematologic: Bleeding

Neuromuscular & skeletal: Weakness, paresthesia, extremity pain, back pain

Ocular: Vision problems

Respiratory: Dyspnea, upper respiratory tract problems, cough, asthma

Miscellaneous: Sweating

Drug Interactions Drugs that prolong the QT interval (eg, class I and class III antiarrhythmics, phenothiazines, TCAs, astemizole, bepridil, and certain quinolone and oral macrolide antibiotics) may increase adverse cardiac effects (concomitant use of these drugs is not recommended); class I or III antiarrhythmics should be withheld for ≥3 half-lives prior to starting sotalol; in clinical studies, sotalol was not given to patients who were treated with oral amiodarone for >1 month in the previous 3 months; do not initiate sotalol after discontinuation of amiodarone until the QT interval is normalized; concomitant use with drugs that prolong refractoriness [class Ia (eg, disopyramide, quinidine, procainamide) and other class III (eg, amiodarone) antiarrhythmics] is not recommended; use with other beta-blockers may potentiate cardiovascular effects; calcium channel blockers may have additive effects on AV conduction, ventricular function, or blood pressure (use with caution)

Catecholamine-depleting drugs, such as reserpine, may have additive effects (hypotension, bradycardia); abrupt withdrawal of clonidine while receiving beta-blockers may result in an exaggerated hypertensive crisis; myocardial depressant general anesthetics may have additive effects with beta-blockers. Concomitant administration of magnesium- and aluminum-containing antacids will significantly decrease the oral absorption of sotalol (administer antacids 2 hours after sotalol); bronchodilation effects of $beta_2$-adrenergic agonists may be antagonized by sotalol (increased doses of $beta_2$ agonists may be needed)

Food Interactions Food decreases oral absorption by ~20% compared to fasting

Stability Store at controlled room temperature 25°C (77°F); dispense in tight, light-resistant container

Mechanism of Action Beta-blocker with both class II antiarrhythmic (beta-adrenergic blockade) and class III antiarrhythmic (prolongation of the cardiac action potential duration) properties; does not possess partial agonist or membrane stabilizing activity. Class II effects: Nonselective beta-blockade; competitively blocks response to $beta_1$- and $beta_2$-adrenergic stimulation; decreases heart rate and AV nodal conduction; increases AV nodal refractoriness. Class III effects: Prolongs atrial and ventricular monophasic action potentials; prolongs the effective refractory period of atrial muscle, ventricular muscle, and AV accessory pathways (if present) in both antegrade and retrograde directions. Significant beta-blocking effects may be seen at lower doses (children: ≥90 mg/m²/day; adults: 25 mg); class III electrophysiologic effects are seen at higher doses (children: 210 mg/m²/day; adults: ≥160 mg/day). Sotalol is available as a racemic mixture; both isomers (d- and l-sotalol) have similar class III antiarrhythmic effects; the l-isomer is responsible for almost all of the beta-adrenergic blocking activity

Pharmacokinetics

Distribution: Poor penetration across blood-brain barrier; distributes into breast milk; breast milk to plasma ratio: 2.2-8.8 (mean: 5.4) (O'Hare, 1980)

Protein binding: Sotalol is not protein bound

Metabolism: Sotalol is not metabolized

Bioavailability: Oral: 90% to 100%

Half-life (mean):

- Neonates ≤1 month: 8.4 hours
- Infants and children >1 month to 24 months: 7.4 hours
- Children >2 years to <7 years: 9.1 hours
- Children 7-12 years: 9.2 hours
- Adults: 12 hours
- Adults with renal failure (anuric): Up to 69 hours

Time to peak serum concentration:

- Children 4 days to 12 years: Mean: 2-3 hours
- Adults: 2.5-4 hours

Elimination: Primarily as unchanged drug via the kidney

Clearance (apparent):

- Neonates ≤1 month: 11 mL/minute
- Infants and children >1 month to 24 months: 32 mL/minute
- Children >2 years to <7 years: 63 mL/minute
- Children 7-12 years: 95 mL/minute

Dialysis: Partially removed by hemodialysis; partial rebound in serum concentrations may occur following dialysis

Usual Dosage Oral: **Note:** Dosage must be adjusted to individual response and tolerance; doses should be initiated or increased in a hospital facility that can provide continuous EKG monitoring, recognition and treatment of life-threatening arrhythmias, and CPR (see Warnings):

Neonates, Infants, and Children: **Note:** Safety and efficacy in pediatric patients have not been established; manufacturer's dosing recommendations are based on doses per m² (that are equivalent to the doses recommended in adults) and on pediatric pharmacokinetic and pharmacodynamic studies (see Saul, 2001 and Saul, 2001a). BSA, rather than body weight, better predicted apparent clearance of sotalol; however, for a given dose per m², a larger drug exposure (larger AUC) and greater pharmacologic effects were observed in smaller subjects (ie, those with BSA <0.33 m² versus those with BSA ≥0.33 m²). For infants and children ≤2 years of age, the manufacturer recommends a dosage reduction based on an age factor determined from a graph (see next page).

(Continued)

Sotalol *(Continued)*

Manufacturer's recommendations: **Note:** Use with extreme caution if QT_c is >500 msec while receiving sotalol; reduce the dose or discontinue drug if QT_c >550 msec

Neonates, infants, and children ≤2 years: The pediatric dosage listed below must be reduced by an age-related factor that is obtained from the graph (see graph). First, obtain the patient's age in months; use the graph to determine where the patient's age (on the logarithmic scale) intersects the age factor curve; read the age factor from the Y-axis; then multiply the age factor by the pediatric dose listed below (ie, the dose for children >2 years); this will result in the proper reduction in dose for age. For example, the age factor for an infant 1 month of age is 0.68, so the initial dosage would be (0.68 x 30 mg/m²/dose) = 20 mg/m²/dose given 3 times daily. Similar calculations should be made for dosage titrations; increase dosage gradually, if needed; allow adequate time between dosage increments to achieve new steady-state and to monitor clinical response, heart rate and QT_c intervals; half-life is prolonged with decreasing age (<2 years), so time to reach new steady-state will increase; for example, the time to reach steady-state in a neonate may be ≥1 week

Sotalol: Age Factor Nomogram for Patients ≤2 Years of Age

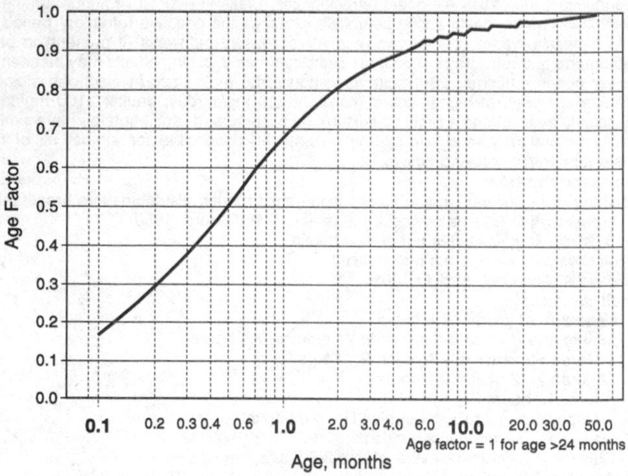

Adapted from U.S. Food and Drug Administration.
http://www.fda.gov/cder/foi/label/2001/2115s3lbl.PDF

Children >2 years: Initial: 30 mg/m²/dose given 3 times daily; increase dosage gradually if needed; allow at least 36 hours between dosage increments to achieve new steady-state and to monitor clinical response, heart rate, and QT_c intervals; may increase gradually to a maximum of 60 mg/m²/dose given 3 times daily

Alternative pediatric dosing: Initial: 2 mg/kg/day divided in 2-3 doses/day; if needed, increase dosage gradually by 1-2 mg/kg/day increments, allow 3 days between dosage increments to achieve new steady-state and to monitor clinical response, heart rate and QT_c intervals; maximum: 8 mg/kg/day (Pfammatter, 1997); do not exceed adult doses; **Note:** Although clinical studies have not assessed the relationship between mg/kg/day doses and age, it appears that the mean effective mg/kg/day dose for infants is less than in older children (see Tipple, 1991; Maragnes, 1992; Colloridi, 1992; Pfammatter, 1995; Beaufort-Krol, 1997).

Adults:

Ventricular arrhythmias (Betapace®, Sorine™, generic) (**Note:** Use with extreme caution if QT_c is >500 msec while receiving sotalol; reduce the dose or discontinue drug if QT_c >550 msec):

Initial: 80 mg twice daily; increase dosage gradually if needed; allow 3 days between dosage increments to achieve new steady-state and to determine maximum effects on QT interval; may increase gradually to 240-320 mg/day in 2 divided doses; usual effective dose: 160-320 mg/day given in 2-3 divided doses; **Note:** Doses as high as 480-640 mg/day may be required in some patients with life-threatening refractory ventricular arrhythmias; however, potential benefit must outweigh increased risk of adverse effects (eg, proarrhythmias).

Atrial fibrillation or atrial flutter (Betapace AF™): [**Note:** If baseline QT interval is >450 msec, do not initiate therapy (see Contraindications). During initiation and dose titration, if the QT interval is ≥500 msec, reduce the dose or discontinue the drug. During maintenance therapy, monitor the QT interval regularly; if the QT interval is ≥520 msec, reduce the dose or discontinue the drug]:

Initial: 80 mg twice daily; increase dosage gradually after 3 days, if needed [ie, if frequency of relapses of atrial fibrillation/flutter is not reduced and the dose is tolerated without excessive QT prolongation (ie, if QT interval is <520 msec)]; allow 3 days between dosage increments to achieve new steady-state and to determine maximum effects on QT interval; reduce the dose or discontinue the drug if the QT interval is ≥500 msec; dose may be increased to 120 mg twice daily (usual effective dose); the dosage may be further increased to 160 mg twice daily if response is inadequate and the dose is tolerated without excessive QT prolongation; maximum dose: 160 mg twice daily.

Dosing adjustment in renal impairment:

Children: Dosing in children with renal impairment has not been investigated; use lower doses or increased dosing intervals; closely monitor clinical response, heart rate and QT_c interval; allow adequate time between dosage increments to achieve new steady-state, since half-life will be prolonged with renal impairment

Adults: Administer the initial dose (ie, 80 mg) and subsequent doses at the following intervals:

Ventricular arrhythmias (Betapace®, Sorine™, generic):

- Cl_{cr} >60 mL/minute: Administer every 12 hours
- Cl_{cr} 30-59 mL/minute: Administer every 24 hours
- Cl_{cr} 10-29 mL/minute: Administer every 36-48 hours
- Cl_{cr} <10 mL/minute: Individualize dose

Atrial fibrillation/flutter (Betapace AF™):

- Cl_{cr} >60 mL/minute: Administer every 12 hours
- Cl_{cr} 40-60 mL/minute: Administer every 24 hours
- Cl_{cr} <40 mL/minute: Use is contraindicated (per product labeling)

Note: Due to the prolonged half-life in patients with renal dysfunction, allow at least 5-6 doses (at the above recommended interval) between dosage increments to achieve a new steady-state and to monitor QT intervals

Dosing adjustment in hepatic impairment: Not needed

Administration May be administered without regard to meals, but should be administered at the same time each day

Monitoring Parameters Continuous EKG for a minimum of 3 days with initiation of therapy or dosage increase, QT interval, heart rate, renal function, serum potassium and magnesium

Betapace AF™: In addition, during initiation and dosage titration, monitor the QT interval 2-4 hours after each dose

Test Interactions May falsely elevate urinary metanephrine values when fluorimetric or photometric methods are used; does not interact with HPLC assay with solid phase extraction for determination of urinary catecholamines

Patient Information Take sotalol every day as prescribed; do not change dose or discontinue without physician's advice; if a dose is missed, do not double the next dose, take the next dose at the usual time. Avoid abrupt discontinuation; if sotalol is to be discontinued, physician will advise how to slowly taper the dose over 1-2 weeks. May cause drowsiness and impair ability to perform activities requiring mental alertness or physical coordination. Regular cardiac checkups, EKGs, and blood tests will be needed while taking this medication. Report the use of other medications, nonprescription medications, and herbal or natural products to your physician and pharmacist; do not start new medications without checking with your physician and pharmacist; tell your dentist and physician that you are taking sotalol before you have dental surgery or an operation (sotalol may interact with certain anesthetic agents). Report fast heartbeats, dizziness, or fainting immediately to your physician or go to an emergency room (these may be signs of an abnormal heartbeat); report severe diarrhea, unusual sweating, vomiting, increased thirst, or decreased appetite immediately to your physician (these may be things that make an abnormal heartbeat more likely to occur); report chest pain, fast heartbeat, swelling of ankles or legs, difficulty breathing or unusual cough to your physician (these may be serious side effects of the medication).

Nursing Implications Be prepared to recognize and treat cardiac arrhythmias; lidocaine and other resuscitative measures should be available (see Warnings)

(Continued)

Sotalol *(Continued)*

Additional Information Betapace AF™: Do not discharge patients from the hospital within 12 hours of electrical or pharmacological conversion from atrial fibrillation/flutter to normal sinus rhythm.

Dosage Forms Excipient information presented when available (limited, particularly for generics); consult specific product labeling.

Tablet, as hydrochloride: 80 mg, 80 mg [AF], 120 mg, 120 mg [AF], 160 mg, 160 mg [AF], 240 mg

Betapace® [light blue]: 80 mg, 120 mg, 160 mg, 240 mg

Betapace AF® [white]: 80 mg, 120 mg, 160 mg

Sorine® [white]: 80 mg, 120 mg, 160 mg, 240 mg

Extemporaneous Preparations A 5 mg/mL syrup of sotalol hydrochloride made from Betapace® or Betapace AF™ tablets and Simple Syrup containing 0.1% sodium benzoate (Syrup, NF) is stable for 3 months when stored at controlled room temperature (15°C to 30°C; 59°F to 86°F) and ambient humidity; place 120 mL of Syrup, NF into a 6 ounce amber plastic (polyethylene terephthalate) prescription bottle; add five Betapace® or Betapace AF™ 120 mg tablets; shake the bottle to wet the tablets; allow tablets to hydrate for at least 2 hours; then shake intermittently over ≥2 hours until the tablets are completely disintegrated; a dispersion of fine particles (water-insoluble inactive ingredients) in syrup should be obtained (**Note:** To simplify the disintegration process, tablets can hydrate overnight; tablets may also be crushed, carefully transferred into the bottle and shaken well until a dispersion of fine particles in syrup is obtained); label "shake well" [Betapace® and Betapace AF™ tablets (package inserts), 2001].

A 5 mg/mL liquid formulation of sotalol hydrochloride made from 160 mg tablets [Sotocor® (from Canada)] and a suspending vehicle (300 mL of Simple Syrup and 700 mL of a methylcellulose 1% gel containing sodium benzoate) was stable and had no evidence of microbial growth for 8 weeks when stored in amber glass bottles under refrigeration (4°C); **Note:** Microbial growth was observed in samples stored at room temperature; to prepare the methylcellulose 1% gel and the suspending vehicle, see reference; label "shake well" and "refrigerate" (Dupuis, 1988).

Betapace® and Betapace AF™ (package inserts), Wayne, NJ: Berlex Laboratories; 2001

Dupuis LL, James G, and Bacola G, "Stability of Sotalol Hydrochloride Oral Liquid Formulation," *Canadian Journal of Hospital Pharmacy*, 1988, 41(3):121-3.

References

Beaufort-Krol GC and Bink-Boelkens MT, "Effectiveness of Sotalol for Atrial Flutter in Children After Surgery for Congenital Heart Disease," *Am J Cardiol*, 1997, 79(1):92-4.

Colloridi V, Perri C, Ventriglia F, et al, "Oral Sotalol in Pediatric Atrial Ectopic Tachycardia," *Am Heart J*, 1992, 123(1):254-6.

Maragnes P, Tipple M, and Fournier A, "Effectiveness of Oral Sotalol for Treatment of Pediatric Arrhythmias," *Am J Cardiol*, 1992, 69(8):751-4.

O'Hare MF, Murnaghan GA, Russell CJ, et al, "Sotalol as a Hypotensive Agent in Pregnancy," *Br J Obstet Gynaecol*, 1980, 87(9):814-20.

Pfammatter JP and Paul T, "New Antiarrhythmic Drug in Pediatric Use: Sotalol," *Pediatr Cardiol*, 1997, 18(1):28-34.

Pfammatter JP, Paul T, Lehmann C, et al, "Efficacy and Proarrhythmia of Oral Sotalol in Pediatric Patients," *J Am Coll Cardiol*, 1995, 26(4):1002-7.

Saul JP, Ross B, Schaffer MS, et al, "Pharmacokinetics and Pharmacodynamics of Sotalol in a Pediatric Population With Supraventricular and Ventricular Tachyarrhythmia," *Clin Pharmacol Ther*, 2001, 69(3):145-57.

Saul JP, Schaffer MS, Karpawich PP, et al, "Single-Dose Pharmacokinetics of Sotalol in a Pediatric Population With Supraventricular and/or Ventricular Tachyarrhythmia," *J Clin Pharmacol*, 2001a, 41(1):35-43.

Tanel RE, Walsh EP, Lulu JA, et al, "Sotalol for Refractory Arrhythmias in Pediatric and Young Adult Patients: Initial Efficacy and Long-Term Outcome," *Am Heart J*, 1995, 130(4):791-7.

Tipple M and Sandor G, "Efficacy and Safety of Oral Sotalol in Early Infancy," *Pacing Clin Electrophysiol*, 1991, 14(11 Pt 2):2062-5.

- ♦ **Sotalol Hydrochloride** *see* Sotalol *on page 1463*
- ♦ **Sotret**® *see* Isotretinoin *on page 876*
- ♦ **SPA** *see* Albumin *on page 64*
- ♦ **Spacol [DSC]** *see* Hyoscyamine *on page 798*
- ♦ **Spacol T/S [DSC]** *see* Hyoscyamine *on page 798*
- ♦ **SPD417** *see* Carbamazepine *on page 279*
- ♦ **Spectazole**® *see* Econazole *on page 553*
- ♦ **Spectazole™ (Can)** *see* Econazole *on page 553*
- ♦ **Spiriva**® *see* Tiotropium *on page 1544*

Spironolactone (speer on oh LAK tone)

Medication Safety Issues
Sound-alike/look-alike issues:
Aldactone® may be confused with Aldactazide®
International issues:
Aldactone®: Brand name for potassium canrenoate in Austria, Czech Republic, Germany, and Hungary

Related Information
Antihypertensive Agents by Class *on page 1678*

U.S. Brand Names Aldactone®

Canadian Brand Names Aldactone®; Novo-Spiroton

Therapeutic Category Antihypertensive Agent; Diuretic, Potassium Sparing

Generic Available Yes

Use Management of edema associated with CHF, cirrhosis of the liver accompanied by edema or ascites, and nephrotic syndrome; treatment of essential hypertension, primary hyperaldosteronism, hypokalemia, and hirsutism

Pregnancy Risk Factor C

Lactation Enters breast milk/not recommended (AAP rates "compatible")

Contraindications Hypersensitivity to spironolactone or any component; renal failure, anuria, hyperkalemia

Warnings Spironolactone has been shown to be tumorigenic in toxicity studies using 25-250 times the usual human dose in rats; use in combination with ACE inhibitors, potassium, and NSAIDs may result in severe hyperkalemia; monitor potassium levels closely; in CHF, potassium levels and renal function should be checked in 3 days and 1 week after beginning therapy, then every 2-4 weeks for 3-12 months, then every 3-6 months

Precautions Use with caution in patients with dehydration, hyponatremia, impaired renal clearance (Cl_{cr} <50 mL/minute) or hepatic dysfunction; patients receiving other potassium-sparing diuretics or potassium supplements

Adverse Reactions
Cardiovascular: Arrhythmia
Central nervous system: Lethargy, headache, mental confusion, fever, ataxia
Dermatologic: Rash, urticaria
Endocrine & metabolic: Hyperkalemia, dehydration, hyponatremia, hyperchloremic metabolic acidosis, postmenopausal bleeding, amenorrhea, gynecomastia (in males); breast tenderness, deepening of voice, and increased hair growth (in females)
Gastrointestinal: Anorexia, nausea, vomiting, diarrhea, gastritis, cramping, gastric bleeding
Genitourinary: Dysuria
Hematologic: Agranulocytosis
Neuromuscular & skeletal: Weakness, numbness or paresthesia in hands, feet or lips, lower back or side pain
Renal: Decreased renal function (including renal failure)
Respiratory: Cough, shortness of breath, dyspnea, hoarseness

Drug Interactions Potassium, other potassium-sparing diuretics, NSAIDs, and ACE inhibitors (eg, captopril) may additively increase the serum potassium; may decrease digoxin clearance and attenuate its inotropic effect; decreased hypoprothrombinemic effect of oral anticoagulants; decreases vascular response to norepinephrine; salicylates may interfere with natriuretic action of spironolactone

Food Interactions Avoid natural licorice (causes sodium and water retention and increases potassium loss) and salt substitutes; avoid diets high in potassium

Mechanism of Action Competes with aldosterone for receptor sites in the distal renal tubules, increasing sodium chloride and water excretion while conserving potassium and hydrogen ions; may block the effect of aldosterone on arteriolar smooth muscle as well

Pharmacokinetics
Distribution: V_d: Breast milk to plasma ratio: 0.51-0.72
Protein binding: 91% to 98%
Metabolism: In the liver to multiple metabolites, including canrenone (active)
Half-life:
Spironolactone: 78-84 minutes
Canrenone: 13-24 hours
Time to peak serum concentration: Within 1-3 hours (primarily as the active metabolite)
Elimination: Urinary and biliary

Usual Dosage Oral:
Neonates: Diuretic: 1-3 mg/kg/day every 12-24 hours
(Continued)

Spironolactone *(Continued)*

Children:

Diuretic, hypertension: 1-3.3 mg/kg/day or 60 mg/m²/day in divided doses every 6-12 hours; not to exceed 100 mg/day

Diagnosis of primary aldosteronism: 100-400 mg/m²/day in 1-2 divided doses

Adults:

Edema, hypokalemia: 25-200 mg/day in 1-2 divided doses

Hypertension (JCN 7): 25-50 mg/day divided once or twice daily

Diagnosis of primary aldosteronism: 100-400 mg/day in 1-2 divided doses

Acne in women: 25-200 mg once daily

Hirsutism in women: 50-200 mg/day in 1-2 divided doses

CHF: Patients with severe heart failure already using an ACE inhibitor and a loop diuretic ± digoxin: 12.5-25 mg/day, increase or reduce depending on individual response and evidence of hyperkalemia; maximum daily dose: 50 mg

Dosing interval in renal impairment:

Cl_{cr} 10-50 mL/minute: Administer every 12-24 hours

Cl_{cr} <10 mL/minute: Avoid use

Administration Oral: Administer with food

Monitoring Parameters Serum potassium, sodium, and renal function

Test Interactions May cause false elevation in serum digoxin concentrations measured by RIA

Patient Information May cause drowsiness and impair ability to perform activities requiring mental alertness or physical coordination

Dosage Forms Excipient information presented when available (limited, particularly for generics); consult specific product labeling.

Tablet: 25 mg, 50 mg, 100 mg

Extemporaneous Preparations

A 1 mg/mL suspension may be compounded by crushing ten 25 mg tablets, add a small amount of water and soak for 5 minutes; add 50 mL 1.5% carboxymethylcellulose, 100 mL syrup NF, and mix; use a sufficient quantity of purified water to a total volume of 250 mL; stable at room temperature or refrigerated for 3 months (Nahata, 1993)

A 2.5 mg/mL suspension may be made by crushing twelve 25 mg tablets, levigating with a small amount of distilled water or glycerin; dilute with cherry syrup to make a final volume of 120 mL; stable 28 days when refrigerated (Mathur, 1989)

A 5 mg/mL suspension may be made by crushing twenty-four 25 mg tablets, levigating with a small amount of distilled water or glycerin; dilute with cherry syrup to a total volume of 120 mL; stable 28 days refrigerated (Mathur, 1989)

A 25 mg/mL suspension may be made by crushing one-hundred twenty (120) 25 mg tablets, add in geometric proportions a 1:1 mixture of Ora-Sweet® and Ora-Plus® or Ora-Sweet® SF and Ora-Plus® to a total volume of 120 mL; stable 60 days refrigerated stored in amber bottles; shake well (Allen, 1996)

Allen LV and Erickson MA, "Stability of Labetalol Hydrochloride, Metoprolol Tartrate, Verapamil Hydrochloride, and Spironolactone With Hydrochlorothiazide in Extemporaneously Compounded Oral Liquids," *Am J Health Syst Pharm*, 1996, 53(19):2304-9.

Mathur LK and Wickman A, "Stability of Extemporaneously Compounded Spironolactone Suspensions," *Am J Hosp Pharm*, 1989, 46(10):2040-2.

Nahata MC, Morosco RS, and Hipple TF, "Stability of Spironolactone in an Extemporaneously Prepared Suspension at Two Temperatures," *Ann Pharmacother*, 1993, 27:1198-9.

References

Chobanian AV, Bakris GL, Black HR, et al, "The Seventh Report of the Joint National Committee on Prevention, Detection, Evaluation, and Treatment of High Blood Pressure: The JNC 7 Report," *JAMA*, 2003, 289(19):2560-72.

Hunt SA, Abraham WT, Chin MH, et al, "ACC/AHA 2005 Guideline Update for the Diagnosis and Management of Chronic Heart Failure in the Adult-Summary Article: A Report of the American College of Cardiology/American Heart Association Task Force on Practice Guidelines (Writing Committee to Update the 2001 Guidelines for the Evaluation and Management of Heart Failure)," *J Am Coll Cardiol*, 2005, 46(6):1116-43.

National High Blood Pressure Education Program Working Group on High Blood Pressure in Children and Adolescents, "The Fourth Report on the Diagnosis, Evaluation, and Treatment of High Blood Pressure in Children and Adolescents," *Pediatrics*, 2004, 114(2 Suppl):555-76.

van der Vorst MM, Kist JE, van der Heijden AJ, et al, "Diuretics in Pediatrics: Current Knowledge and Future Prospects," *Paediatr Drugs*, 2006, 8(4):245-64.

♦ **Spironolactone and Hydrochlorothiazide** *see* Hydrochlorothiazide and Spironolactone *on page 778*

♦ **Sporanox®** *see* Itraconazole *on page 881*

♦ **SPS®** *see* Sodium Polystyrene Sulfonate *on page 1460*

♦ **SSD®** *see* Silver Sulfadiazine *on page 1439*

♦ **SSD® AF** *see* Silver Sulfadiazine *on page 1439*

♦ **SSKI®** *see* Potassium Iodide *on page 1290*
♦ **Stagesic®** *see* Hydrocodone and Acetaminophen *on page 779*
♦ **Stanazol** *see* Stanozolol *on page 1471*
♦ **StanGard®** *see* Fluoride *on page 675*
♦ **StanGard® Perio** *see* Fluoride *on page 675*
♦ **Stannous Fluoride** *see* Fluoride *on page 675*

Stanozolol (stan OH zoe lole)

U.S. Brand Names Winstrol®

Index Terms Androstanazole; Stanazol

Therapeutic Category Androgen, Anabolic Steroid

Generic Available No

Use Prophylaxis to decrease the frequency and severity of angioedema attacks

Restrictions C-III

Pregnancy Risk Factor X

Lactation Enters breast milk/contraindicated

Contraindications Hypersensitivity to stanozolol or any component; pregnancy; male patients with carcinoma of breast or prostate; female patients with carcinoma of the breast and hypercalcemia; nephrosis

Warnings Stanozolol is a prophylactic agent and is not effective in controlling an acute attack of angioedema. Use has been associated with peliosis hepatitis (a condition where liver and sometimes splenic tissue is replaced with blood-filled cysts) and liver cell tumors; these conditions may be complicatod by acute, potentially life-threatening intra-abdominal hemorrhage and liver failure; monitor liver function. May increase risk of atherosclerosis and CAD due to decreased HDL and possible increase LDL. May cause virilization (deepening of the voice, hirsutism, acne, clitoromegaly, and menstrual irregularities) in women; discontinue therapy when virilization is mild to prevent irreversible effects. Stanozolol has not been shown to be safe and effective for the enhancement of athletic performance.

May accelerate bone maturation without producing compensating gain in linear growth; perform radiographic examination of the hand and wrist every 6 months to determine the rate of bone maturation (when using in prepubertal children). Exposure to stanozolol *in utero* may result in androgenic effects on the female fetus; clitoral hypertrophy, labial fusion, urogenital sinus defect, vaginal atresia, and ambiguous genitalia; a sensitive test capable of determining early pregnancy is recommended immediately prior to initiation of therapy; nonhormonal method of contraception should be used during treatment if indicated. Considering the relatively infrequent attacks of angioedema in childhood and the risk of significant toxicities of stanzolol, long term prophylactic use in children is generally not recommended.

Precautions Use with caution in patients with cardiac, renal, or hepatic disease. May cause fluid retention; may alter insulin or oral hypoglycemic drug dosages in diabetic patients. May cause hypercalcemia in breast cancer patients. Decreases levels of thyroxine-binding globulin resulting in decreased total T4 serums levels and increased resin uptake of T3 and T4. Free thyroid hormone levels remain unchanged and there is no clinical evidence of thyroid dysfunction.

Adverse Reactions

Cardiovascular: Edema, MI

Central nervous system: Habituation, excitation, insomnia, depression

Dermatologic: Mild hirsutism, hair loss, acne, oily skin

Endocrine & metabolic: Decreased glucose tolerance, gynecomastia, menstrual irregularities, weight gain

Gastrointestinal: Nausea, vomiting, diarrhea

Genitourinary:

- Prepubertal males: Penile enlargement and increased frequency of erections
- Postpubertal males: Inhibition of testicular function, testicular atrophy, oligospermia, impotence, chronic priapism, epididymitis, bladder irritability
- Women: Clitoral enlargement
- Both Sexes: Increased or decreased libido

Hepatic: Peliosis hepatis, liver tumors, cholestatic jaundice, elevated liver enzymes, hypertriglyceridemia, increased LDL, decreased HDL, suppression of clotting factors (Factors II, VII, and X)

Neuromuscular & skeletal: Premature epiphyses closure (pediatric use)

Drug Interactions Nandrolone may potentiate the effects of oral anticoagulants, insulins, and oral hypoglycemic agents.

Stability Store at room temperature.

Mechanism of Action Angioedema is a disorder characterized by attacks of facial swelling, and also swelling of extremities, genitalia, bowel wall, and upper respiratory tract. Stanozolol is an anabolic steroid (synthetic derivative of testosterone) that

(Continued)

Stanozolol *(Continued)*

suppresses gonadotropic functions of the pituitary. Stanzolol acts prophylactically to decrease the frequency and severity of hereditary angioedema attacks by increasing circulating levels of C1 esterase inhibitor (C1 INH) which is either deficient or nonfunctional in hereditary angioedema.

Pharmacokinetics

Metabolism: Hepatic

Elimination: Urine (90%); feces (6%)

Usual Dosage

Children: Generally not recommended due to infrequency of angioedema attacks and relative risk of toxicity with long term use

Children <6 years: 1 mg daily

Children 6-12 years: 2 mg daily

Adults: Initial: 2 mg 3 times/day; may increase up to 4 mg 4 times/day for up to the first 5 days of therapy. **Note:** In young women who may be particularly susceptible to virilization, 2 mg twice daily may be used

Maintenance: Decrease the dosage at intervals of 1-2 months as tolerated to a dosage of 2 mg/day; some patients may only require 2 mg every other day

Dosing adjustment in hepatic impairment: Not recommended for patients with severe liver dysfunction

Administration Oral: Administer without regard to food

Monitoring Parameters Liver function tests, serum glucose (if diabetic), HDL and LDL cholesterol, androgenic effects, severity and frequency of angioedema attacks

Patient Information Report any prodromal symptoms of hepatitis (fatigue, weakness, nausea, vomiting, dark urine, or yellowing of eyes); avoid becoming pregnant while taking this medicine and for several months after stopping; use an effective form of birth control. This medication may alter hypoglycemic requirements; diabetics should monitor serum glucose closely.

Dosage Forms Excipient information presented when available (limited, particularly for generics); consult specific product labeling.

Tablet: 2 mg

♦ **Statex® (Can)** *see* Morphine Sulfate *on page 1082*

Stavudine (STAV yoo deen)

Medication Safety Issues

Sound-alike/look-alike issues:

Zerit® may be confused with Ziac®

Related Information

Adult and Adolescent HIV *on page 1821*

Pediatric HIV *on page 1816*

Perinatal HIV *on page 1831*

U.S. Brand Names Zerit®

Canadian Brand Names Zerit®

Index Terms d4T; 2',3'-didehydro-3'-deoxythymidine

Therapeutic Category Antiretroviral Agent; HIV Agents (Anti-HIV Agents); Nucleoside Reverse Transcriptase Inhibitor (NRTI)

Generic Available No

Use Treatment of HIV infection in combination with other antiretroviral agents. (**Note:** HIV regimens consisting of **three** antiretroviral agents are strongly recommended)

Pregnancy Risk Factor C

Lactation Excretion in breast milk unknown/contraindicated

Contraindications Hypersensitivity to stavudine or any component

Warnings The major clinical toxicity of stavudine is peripheral neuropathy which has occurred in 15% to 21% of patients in controlled trials. Lactic acidosis and severe hepatomegaly with steatosis is a rare but potentially life-threatening toxicity associated with the use of NRTIs; it may be more common with antiretroviral regimens containing stavudine. Risk may be increased in obesity, prolonged nucleoside exposure, or in female patients. Increased risk of hepatotoxicity also occurs with combined use of stavudine, didanosine, and hydroxyurea versus stavudine alone. Fatal lactic acidosis has occurred in pregnant women who received stavudine plus didanosine with other antiretroviral agents; use stavudine plus didanosine with caution during pregnancy and only if benefit clearly outweighs risks. Severe motor weakness (resembling Guillain-Barré syndrome) has been reported, usually in association with lactic acidosis. Manufacturer recommends prompt suspension of all antiretroviral therapy in suspected cases of symptomatic hyperlactatemia, lactic acidosis (with or without neuromuscular weakness), or pronounced hepatotoxicity (see also Additional

Information). Fatal and nonfatal pancreatitis has occurred during combination therapy which included stavudine plus didanosine with or without hydroxyurea.

Precautions Fat redistribution and accumulation [ie, central obesity, peripheral wasting, facial wasting, breast enlargement, dorsocervical fat enlargement (buffalo hump), and cushingoid appearance] have been observed in patients receiving antiretroviral agents (causal relationship not established). Use with caution in patients with a history of peripheral neuropathy, or hepatic or renal impairment; dosage adjustment required in patients with impaired renal function

Adverse Reactions

Central nervous system: Headache, fever, insomnia, malaise, dizziness, nervousness, increased energy, mania

Dermatologic: Rash, pruritus

Endocrine & metabolic: Lactic acidosis, fat redistribution and accumulation (see Precautions)

Gastrointestinal: Abdominal pain, diarrhea, nausea, vomiting, anorexia, pancreatitis

Hematologic: Anemia, leukopenia, thrombocytopenia

Hepatic: Elevated AST and ALT, hepatomegaly, hepatic steatosis, hepatitis, elevated bilirubin

Neuromuscular & skeletal: Peripheral neuropathy (tingling, burning, pain, numbness of hands or feet), motor weakness (may resemble Guillain-Barré syndrome), myalgia

Otic: Ear pain

Respiratory: Rhinitis, cough

Drug Interactions Drugs associated with peripheral neuropathy (chloramphenicol, cisplatin, dapsone, ethionamide, gold, hydralazine, iodoquinol, isoniazid, lithium, metronidazole, nitrofurantoin, pentamidine, phenytoin, ribavirin, vincristine) may increase risk for stavudine peripheral neuropathy; drugs that decrease renal function could decrease clearance of stavudine; stavudine should not be administered in combination with zidovudine (poor antiretroviral effect; zidovudine competitively inhibits intracellular phosphorylation of stavudine); phosphorylation of stavudine is also inhibited by doxorubicin and ribavirin (use with caution); concurrent use with didanosine with or without hydroxyurea may increase risk of pancreatitis, peripheral neuropathy, and liver function abnormalities; concurrent use with didanosine and hydroxyurea may increase risk of fatal pancreatitis and hepatotoxicity; methadone may decrease stavudine levels by 27% (no dosage adjustment needed)

Stability

Capsules: Store in tightly closed containers at room temperature

Oral solution: Reconstitute powder for oral solution according to manufacturer's instructions; dispense in original container; keep refrigerated; solution is stable for 30 days

Mechanism of Action Antiviral activity is dependent on intracellular conversion of stavudine to the active metabolite d4-triphosphate; Inhibits replication of retroviruses by competing with thymidine triphosphate for viral RNA-directed DNA polymerase and incorporation into viral DNA

Pharmacokinetics

Absorption: Rapid

Distribution: Penetrates into the CSF achieving 16% to 97% (mean: 59%) of concomitant plasma concentrations; distributes into extravascular spaces and equally between RBCs and plasma

V_d:
- Children: 0.73 ± 0.32 L/kg
- Adults: 46 ± 21 L

Protein binding: Negligible

Metabolism: Converted intracellularly to active triphosphate form

Bioavailability: Capsule and solution are bioequivalent
- Children: 77%
- Adults: 86%

Half-life, elimination:
- Newborns (at birth): 5.3 ± 2 hours
- Neonates 14-28 days old: 1.6 ± 0.3 hours
- Infants 5 weeks to Children 15 years: 0.9 ± 0.3 hours
- Adults: 1.6 ± 0.2 hours
- **Note:** Half-life is prolonged with renal dysfunction

Time to peak serum concentration: Within 1 hour

Elimination: 24% to 57% is excreted unchanged in the urine; undergoes glomerular filtration and active tubular secretion

Dialysis: 31 ± 5% of the dose is removed by hemodialysis; hemodialysis clearance (n=12) (mean ± SD): 120 ± 18 mL/minute

Usual Dosage Oral (use in combination with other antiretroviral agents):

Neonates 0-13 days old: 0.5 mg/kg/dose every 12 hours

(Continued)

Stavudine *(Continued)*

Neonates ≥14 days old, Infants, and Children <30 kg: 1 mg/kg/dose every 12 hours; maximum: 30 mg every 12 hours

Children, Adolescents, and Adults:

30-59 kg: 30 mg every 12 hours

≥60 kg: 40 mg every 12 hours

Dosing adjustment in renal impairment:

Cl_{cr} 26-50 mL/minute: Decrease dose by 50% (eg, ≥60 kg: administer 20 mg every 12 hours)

Cl_{cr} <10-25 mL/minute: Decrease dose by 75% (eg, ≥60 kg: administer 20 mg every 24 hours)

Dosing adjustment in hepatic impairment: no data

Administration Oral: Administer with or without food; shake solution well before using

Monitoring Parameters Periodic CBC with differential, hemoglobin, renal function, liver enzymes, serum amylase and lipase, CD4 cell count, HIV RNA plasma levels, signs/symptoms of peripheral neuropathy

Patient Information Stavudine is not a cure for HIV. Take stavudine every day as prescribed; do not change dose or discontinue without physician's advice. If a dose is missed, take it as soon as possible, then return to normal dosing schedule; if a dose is skipped, do **not** double the next dose. Avoid alcohol. Notify physician if tingling, burning, pain, numbness of hands or feet, unexplained weight loss, abdominal discomfort, nausea, vomiting, fatigue, dyspnea, or motor weakness occurs

HIV medications may cause changes in body fat, including an increase in fat in the upper back and neck, breasts, and trunk; a loss of fat from the face, arms, and legs may also occur.

Additional Information Signs and symptoms of symptomatic hyperlactemia or lactic acidosis syndrome may include generalized fatigue, GI symptoms (nausea, vomiting, abdominal pain, unexplained weight loss), respiratory symptoms (tachypnea, dyspnea), or neurologic symptoms (motor weakness, Guillain-Barré type syndrome)

Dosage Forms Excipient information presented when available (limited, particularly for generics); consult specific product labeling.

Capsule: 15 mg, 20 mg, 30 mg, 40 mg

Powder, for oral solution: 1 mg/mL (200 mL) [dye free; fruit flavor]

References

Briars LA, Hilao JJ, and Kraus DM, "A Review of Pediatric Human Immunodeficiency Virus Infection," *Journal of Pharmacy Practice*, 2004, 17(6):407-31.

Kline MW, Dunkle LM, Church JA, et al, "A Phase I/II Evaluation of Stavudine (d4T) in Children With Human Immunodeficiency Virus Infection," *Pediatrics*, 1995, 96(2 Pt 1):247-52.

Panel on Clinical Practices for Treatment of HIV Infection, "Guidelines for the Use of Antiretroviral Agents in HIV-Infected Adults and Adolescents," October 10, 2006, http://www.aidsinfo.nih.gov.

Working Group on Antiretroviral Therapy and Medical Management of HIV-Infected Children, "Guidelines for the Use of Antiretroviral Agents in Pediatric HIV Infection," October 26, 2006, http://www.aidsinfo.nih.gov.

♦ **Stemetil® (Can)** *see* Prochlorperazine *on page 1321*
♦ **Sterapred®** *see* PredniSONE *on page 1308*
♦ **Sterapred® DS** *see* PredniSONE *on page 1308*
♦ **Stimate™** *see* Desmopressin *on page 459*
♦ **Sting-Kill [OTC]** *see* Benzocaine *on page 204*
♦ **St. Joseph® Adult Aspirin [OTC]** *see* Aspirin *on page 163*
♦ **Stop®** *see* Fluoride *on page 675*
♦ **Strattera®** *see* Atomoxetine *on page 172*
♦ **Streptase®** *see* Streptokinase *on page 1474*

Streptokinase (strep toe KYE nase)

Medication Safety Issues

High alert medication: The Institute for Safe Medication Practices (ISMP) includes this medication (I.V.) among its list of drugs which have a heightened risk of causing significant patient harm when used in error.

Related Information

Antithrombotic Therapy in Children *on page 1804*

U.S. Brand Names Streptase®

Canadian Brand Names Streptase®

Index Terms SK

Therapeutic Category Thrombolytic Agent; Thrombotic Occlusion (Central Venous Catheter), Treatment Agent

Generic Available No

Use Thrombolytic agent used in treatment of recent severe or massive deep vein thrombosis, pulmonary emboli, MI, arterial thrombosis or embolism, and occluded arteriovenous cannulas

Pregnancy Risk Factor C

Lactation Excretion in breast milk unknown

Contraindications Hypersensitivity to streptokinase or any component; recent streptococcal infection; any internal bleeding; CVA or intracranial or intraspinal surgery (within 2 months); severe uncontrolled hypertension; brain carcinoma

Warnings Bleeding may occur; avoid I.M. injections

Precautions Relative contraindications: major surgery within the last 10 days, GI bleeding, recent trauma, severe hypertension

Adverse Reactions

Cardiovascular: Hypotension, arrhythmias, flushing
Central nervous system: Fever
Dermatologic: Itching, urticaria, angioneurotic edema
Hematologic: Surface bleeding, internal bleeding, cerebral hemorrhage
Neuromuscular & skeletal: Musculoskeletal pain
Respiratory: Bronchospasm

Drug Interactions Anticoagulants, antiplatelet agents, antifibrinolytic agents

Stability Store unopened vials at room temperature; store reconstituted solutions in refrigerator and use within 24 hours

Mechanism of Action Promotes thrombolysis; activates the conversion of plasminogen to plasmin by forming a complex, exposing plasminogen-activating site, and cleaving a peptide bond that converts plasminogen to plasmin; plasmin degrades fibrin, fibrinogen and other procoagulant proteins into soluble fragments; effective both outside and within the formed thrombus/embolus

Pharmacodynamics

Onset of action: Activation of plasminogen: Almost immediate
Duration:
- Fibrinolytic effects: Only a few hours
- Anticoagulant effects: 12-24 hours

Pharmacokinetics

Half-life, biologic: 83 minutes
Elimination: By circulating antibodies and via the reticuloendothelial system

Usual Dosage

Children: Safety and efficacy not established
- Thromboses: I.V.: *Chest*, 2001 recommendations: Initial (loading dose): 2000 units/kg followed by 2000 units/kg/hour for 6-12 hours; some patients may require longer or shorter courses of treatment; dose should be individualized based on response
- Clotted catheter: **Note**: **Not recommended** due to possibility of allergic reactions with repeated doses: 10,000-25,000 units diluted in NS to a final volume equivalent to catheter volume; instill into catheter and leave in place for 1 hour, then aspirate contents out of catheter and flush catheter with NS

Adults:
- Thromboses: I.V.: 250,000 units to start, then 100,000 units/hour for 24-72 hours depending on location
- Cannula occlusion: **Note:** Not recommended due to possibility of allergic reactions with repeated doses: 250,000 units into cannula, clamp for 2 hours, then aspirate contents out of catheter and flush with NS; **Note:** Serious adverse effects (hypersensitivity reactions, hypotension, apnea, and bleeding), some of which were life-threatening, have been reported with this use and dose; lower doses of 3000 units/hour for 12-24 hours infused into each lumen have been successfully used (see Phelps, 2001)

Administration Parenteral: I.V.: Dilute in NS (preferred) or D_5W; maximum concentration: 1.5 million units/50 mL

Monitoring Parameters For systemic therapy: Blood pressure, thrombin clotting time, PTT, APTT, fibrinogen level, fibrin/fibrinogen degradation products, D-dimers, platelet count, hemoglobin, hematocrit, signs of bleeding

Nursing Implications For intravenous or intracoronary use only; avoid I.M. injections

Additional Information Best results are realized if used within 5-6 hours of MI; antibodies to streptokinase remain for 3-6 months after initial dose, use another thrombolytic enzyme (ie, urokinase) if repeat thrombolytic therapy is indicated

Failure of thrombolytic agents in newborns/neonates may occur due to the low plasminogen concentrations (~50% to 70% of adult levels); streptokinase- induced clot lysis may be more impaired than urokinase or TPA in these patients; supplementing plasminogen (via administration of fresh frozen plasma) may possibly help

Dosage Forms Excipient information presented when available (limited, particularly for generics); consult specific product labeling. [DSC] = Discontinued product

(Continued)

Streptokinase *(Continued)*

Injection, powder for reconstitution: 250,000 international units; 750,000 international units; 1,500,000 international units [DSC]

References

Andrew M, Brooker L, Leaker M, et al,"Fibrin Clot Lysis by Thrombolytic Agents Is Impaired in Newborns Due to a Low Plasminogen Concentration," *Thromb Haemost*, 1992, 68(3):325-30.

Kothari SS, Varma S, and Wasir HS, "Thrombolytic Therapy in Infants and Children," *Am Heart J*, 1994, 127(3):651-7.

Monagle P, Michelson AD, Bovill E, et al, "Antithrombotic Therapy in Children," *Chest*, 2001, 119:344S-70S.

Nowak-Göttl U, Auberger K, Halimeh S, et al, "Thrombolysis in Newborns and Infants," *Thromb Haemost*, 1999, 82(Suppl 1):112-6.

Phelps KC and Verazino KC, "Alternatives to Urokinase for the Management of Central Venous Catheter Occlusion," *Hospital Pharmacy*, 2001, 36(3): 265-74.

Streptomycin (strep toe MYE sin)

Medication Safety Issues

Sound-alike/look-alike issues:

Streptomycin may be confused with streptozocin

Related Information

Overdose and Toxicology *on page 1916*

Index Terms Streptomycin Sulfate

Therapeutic Category Antibiotic, Aminoglycoside; Antitubercular Agent

Generic Available Yes

Use Combination therapy of active tuberculosis; used in combination with other agents for treatment of streptococcal or enterococcal endocarditis, mycobacterial infections, plague, tularemia, and brucellosis

Pregnancy Risk Factor D

Lactation Enters breast milk/compatible

Contraindications Hypersensitivity to streptomycin or any component

Warnings Aminoglycosides are associated with significant nephrotoxicity or ototoxicity; the ototoxicity is directly proportional to the amount of drug given and the duration of treatment; tinnitus or vertigo are indications of vestibular injury and impending bilateral irreversible deafness; renal damage is usually reversible

Precautions Use with caution in patients with pre-existing vertigo, tinnitus, hearing loss, neuromuscular disorders, or renal impairment; modify dosage in patients with renal impairment

Adverse Reactions

Cardiovascular: Myocarditis, cardiovascular collapse

Central nervous system: Dizziness, vertigo, headache, ataxia

Dermatologic: Toxic epidermal necrolysis

Gastrointestinal: Vomiting

Hematologic: Bone marrow suppression

Neuromuscular & skeletal: Neuromuscular blockade

Otic: Ototoxicity, hearing loss

Renal: Nephrotoxicity

Miscellaneous: Hypersensitivity reactions, serum sickness

Drug Interactions Additive nephrotoxicity with acyclovir, amphotericin B, cisplatin, vancomycin; additive ototoxicity with ethacrynic acid, furosemide, urea, mannitol; potentiates neuromuscular blocking action of succinylcholine, tubocurarine

Stability Streptomycin injection should be stored in the refrigerator

Mechanism of Action Inhibits bacterial protein synthesis by binding directly to the 30S ribosomal subunits causing faulty peptide sequence to form in the protein chain

Pharmacokinetics

Distribution: Distributes into most body tissues and fluids except the brain; small amounts enter the CSF only with inflamed meninges; crosses the placenta; small amounts appear in breast milk

Protein binding: 34%

Half-life (prolonged with renal impairment):

Newborns: 4-10 hours

Adults: 2-4.7 hours

Time to peak serum concentration: I.M.: Within 1-2 hours

Elimination: 30% to 90% of dose excreted as unchanged drug in urine, with small amount (1%) excreted in bile, saliva, sweat, and tears

Usual Dosage I.M. (I.V. in patients who cannot tolerate I.M. injections):

Newborns: 10-20 mg/kg/day once daily

Infants: 20-30 mg/kg/day in divided doses every 12 hours

Children:

Tuberculosis: 20-40 mg/kg/day once daily, not to exceed 1 g/day; **or** 20-40 mg/kg/dose twice weekly under direct observation, not to exceed 1.5 g/dose; usually discontinued after 2-3 months of therapy or as soon as isoniazid and rifampin susceptibility is established

Other infections: 20-40 mg/kg/day in combination with other antibiotics divided every 6-12 hours

Plague: 30 mg/kg/day divided every 8-12 hours

Adults:

Tuberculosis: 15 mg/kg/day once daily, not to exceed 1 g/day; **or** 25-30 mg/kg/dose twice weekly under direct observation, not to exceed 1.5 g/dose

Enterococcal endocarditis: 1 g every 12 hours for 2 weeks, then 500 mg every 12 hours for 4 weeks in combination with penicillin

Streptococcal endocarditis: 1 g every 12 hours for 1 week, then 500 mg every 12 hours for 1 week

Tularemia: 1-2 g/day in divided doses for 7-10 days or until patient is afebrile for 5-7 days

Plague: 2 g/day in divided doses until the patient is afebrile for at least 3 days

Dosing adjustment in renal impairment:

Cl_{cr} 50-80 mL/minute: Administer 7.5 mg/kg/dose every 24 hours

Cl_{cr} 10-50 mL/minute: Administer 7.5 mg/kg/dose every 24-72 hours

Cl_{cr} <10 mL/minute: Administer 7.5 mg/kg/dose every 72-96 hours

Administration Parenteral:

I.M.: Inject deep I.M. into a large muscle mass; administer at a concentration not to exceed 500 mg/mL; rotate injection sites

I.V.: I.V. infusion through a peripheral or central line; 12-15 mg/kg/dose is diluted in 100 mL of NS; infuse over 30-60 minutes

Monitoring Parameters Hearing (audiogram), BUN, creatinine; serum concentration of the drug should be monitored in patients with renal impairment; eighth cranial nerve damage is usually preceded by high-pitched tinnitus, roaring noises, sense of fullness in ears, or impaired hearing and may persist for weeks after drug is discontinued

Reference Range Therapeutic serum concentrations: Peak: 15-40 mcg/mL; trough: <5 mcg/mL

Test Interactions False-positive urine glucose with Benedict's solution

Additional Information For use by patients with active tuberculosis that is resistant to isoniazid and rifampin or patients with active tuberculosis in areas where resistance is common and whose drug susceptibility is not yet known. Pfizer will distribute streptomycin directly to physicians and health clinics at no charge. Call Pfizer at 1-800-254-4445.

Dosage Forms Excipient information presented when available (limited, particularly for generics); consult specific product labeling.

Injection, powder for reconstitution: 1 g

References

Ad Hoc Committee of the Scientific Assembly on Microbiology, Tuberculosis, and Pulmonary Infections, "Treatment of Tuberculosis and Tuberculosis Infection in Adults and Children," *Clin Infect Dis*, 1995, 21:9-27.

American Academy of Pediatrics Committee on Infectious Diseases, "Chemotherapy for Tuberculosis in Infants and Children," *Pediatrics* 1992, 89(1):161-5.

Arguedas AG and Wehrle PP, "New Concepts for Antimicrobial Use in Central Nervous System Infections," *Semin Pediatr Infect Dis*, 1991, 2(1):36-42.

Lorin MI, Hsu KH, and Jacob SC, "Treatment of Tuberculosis in Children," *Pediatr Clin North Am*, 1983, 30(2):333-48.

- **Streptomycin Sulfate** *see* Streptomycin *on page 1476*
- **Striant®** *see* Testosterone *on page 1511*
- **Stri-dex® [OTC]** *see* Salicylic Acid *on page 1413*
- **Stri-dex® Body Focus [OTC]** *see* Salicylic Acid *on page 1413*
- **Stri-dex® Facewipes To Go™ [OTC]** *see* Salicylic Acid *on page 1413*
- **Stri-dex® Maximum Strength [OTC]** *see* Salicylic Acid *on page 1413*
- **Strifon Forte® (Can)** *see* Chlorzoxazone *on page 348*
- **Strong Iodine Solution** *see* Potassium Iodide and Iodine *on page 1292*
- **Sublimaze®** *see* Fentanyl *on page 644*
- **Suboxone®** *see* Buprenorphine and Naloxone *on page 249*
- **Subutex®** *see* Buprenorphine *on page 246*

Succimer (SUKS i mer)

Related Information

Commonly Used Antidotes for Acute Overdoses *on page 1920*

U.S. Brand Names Chemet®

Canadian Brand Names Chemet®

(Continued)

Succimer *(Continued)*

Index Terms DMSA

Therapeutic Category Antidote, Lead Toxicity; Chelating Agent, Oral

Generic Available No

Use Treatment of lead poisoning in children with blood levels >45 mcg/dL; not indicated for prophylaxis of lead poisoning in a lead-containing environment

Pregnancy Risk Factor C

Contraindications Hypersensitivity to succimer or any component

Warnings Elevated blood lead levels and associated symptoms may return rapidly after discontinuation due to redistribution of lead from bone stores to soft tissues and blood; monitor blood lead levels for "rebound" after therapy; mild to moderate neutropenia has been reported; monitor CBC with differential prior to and during therapy; discontinue treatment if ANC <1200/microliter

Precautions Use with caution in patients with renal or hepatic impairment; adequate hydration should be maintained during therapy

Adverse Reactions The most common events attributable to succimer have been observed in about 10% of patients treated

Central nervous system: Headache, fatigue, dizziness

Dermatologic: Rash, pruritus

Gastrointestinal: Nausea, vomiting, diarrhea, appetite loss, metallic taste, hemorrhoidal symptoms, sulfurous odor to breath, sore throat

Hematologic: Thrombocytosis, eosinophilia, reversible neutropenia

Hepatic: Transiently elevated AST, ALT, alkaline phosphatase, and serum cholesterol

Neuromuscular & skeletal: Paresthesia, sensorimotor neuropathy, back, rib, kneecap, and leg pains

Ocular: Watery eyes, cloudy film in eye

Renal: Sulfurous odor to urine, decreased urination, proteinuria

Respiratory: Rhinorrhea, nasal congestion

Miscellaneous: Flu-like symptoms, mucocutaneous hypersensitivity reactions (with repeat administration)

Drug Interactions Not recommended to be used concomitantly with edetate calcium disodium or penicillamine

Mechanism of Action Forms stable water-soluble complexes with lead resulting in increased urinary excretion; also chelates other toxic heavy metals such as arsenic and mercury

Pharmacokinetics

Absorption: Oral: Rapid, variable

Metabolism: Extensive to mixed succimer-cysteine disulfides

Half-life, elimination: 2 days

Time to peak serum concentration: ~1-2 hours

Elimination: ~25% in urine with peak urinary excretion occurring between 2-4 hours after dosing; of the total amount of succimer eliminated in urine, 90% is eliminated as mixed succimer-cysteine disulfide conjugates; 10% is excreted unchanged; fecal excretion of succimer probably represents unabsorbed drug

Dialysis: Succimer is dialyzable but lead chelates are not

Usual Dosage Children and Adults: Oral: 10 mg/kg/dose (or 350 mg/m^2/dose) every 8 hours for 5 days followed by 10 mg/kg/dose (or 350 mg/m^2/dose) every 12 hours for 14 days

Note: Concomitant iron therapy has been reported in a small number of children without the formation of a toxic complex with iron (as seen with dimercaprol); courses of therapy may be repeated if indicated by weekly monitoring of blood lead levels; lead levels should be stabilized to <15 mcg/dL; 2 weeks between courses is recommended unless more timely treatment is indicated by lead levels; patients who have received calcium disodium EDTA with or without BAL may be treated with succimer after at least 4 weeks have passed since treatment

Dosing adjustment in renal/hepatic impairment: Administer with caution and monitor closely

Administration Oral: Ensure adequate patient hydration; for patients who cannot swallow the capsule, sprinkle the medicated beads on a small amount of soft food or administer with a fruit juice to mask the odor

Monitoring Parameters Blood lead levels; liver enzymes and CBC with differential (prior to therapy and weekly during therapy)

Test Interactions Falsely decreased CPK; false-positive urine ketones with Ketostix®, falsely decreased uric acid measurements

Dosage Forms Excipient information presented when available (limited, particularly for generics); consult specific product labeling.

Capsule: 100 mg

References

Mann KV and Travers JD, "Succimer, An Oral Lead Chelator," *Clin Pharm*, 1991, 10(12):914-22.

Succinylcholine (suks in il KOE leen)

Medication Safety Issues

High alert medication: The Institute for Safe Medication Practices (ISMP) includes this medication among its list of drugs which have a heightened risk of causing significant patient harm when used in error.

U.S. Brand Names Quelicin®

Canadian Brand Names Quelicin®

Index Terms Succinylcholine Chloride; Suxamethonium Chloride

Therapeutic Category Neuromuscular Blocker Agent, Depolarizing; Skeletal Muscle Relaxant, Paralytic

Generic Available No

Use Used to produce skeletal muscle relaxation in procedures of short duration such as endotracheal intubation or endoscopic exams

Pregnancy Risk Factor C

Lactation Excretion in breast milk unknown/use caution

Contraindications Hypersensitivity to succinylcholine chloride or any component; history of decreased concentration and/or decreased activity of plasma pseudocholinesterase; malignant hyperthermia; myopathies associated with elevated serum creatinine values; narrow-angle glaucoma; penetrating eye injuries

Warnings Malignant hyperthermia may be triggered by succinylcholine use; monitor closely for signs/symptoms; avoid use in patients with serum potassium >5.5 mEq/L; if sudden cardiac arrest occurs immediately after administration of succinylcholine, consider hyperkalemia as potential etiology and manage accordingly

Precautions As rare reports of acute rhabdomyolysis with hyperkalemia followed by ventricular dysrhythmias, cardiac arrest, and death have been reported in children with undiagnosed skeletal muscle myopathy, use with caution in patients recovering from severe trauma; use with caution in patients with pre-existing hyperkalemia, paraplegia, extensive or severe burns, extensive denervation of skeletal muscle because of disease or injury to the CNS or with degenerative or dystrophic neuromuscular disease

Adverse Reactions

Cardiovascular: Bradycardia, hypotension, cardiac arrhythmias, flushing, cardiac arrest, hypertension, tachycardia

Central nervous system: Malignant hyperthermia

Dermatologic: Rash

Endocrine & metabolic: Hyperkalemia, myoglobinemia

Gastrointestinal: Elevated intragastric pressure, salivation

Neuromuscular & skeletal: Myalgia due to muscle fasciculations, muscle weakness

Ocular: Elevated intraocular pressure

Renal: Myoglobinuria

Respiratory: Apnea, bronchospasm, respiratory depression

Drug Interactions Decreased neuromuscular blockade with diazepam; increased neuromuscular blockade with promazine, cyclophosphamide, oral contraceptives, glucocorticoids, MAO inhibitors, oxytocin, phenothiazines, quinidine, beta-blocking agents, procainamide, lidocaine, lithium, trimethaphan, furosemide, magnesium, chloroquine, acetylcholine, anticholinesterases, amphotericin B, and thiazide diuretics (due to electrolyte imbalances); cyclophosphamide, aminoglycosides, clindamycin may increase bradycardia; narcotic analgesics and inhalation anesthetics may increase the risk of sinus arrest; increased arrhythmias with digoxin (due to potassium changes)

Stability Injection is incompatible with alkaline solutions; store in refrigerator; stability at room temperature is product specific; check with each manufacturer

Mechanism of Action Acts similarly to acetylcholine, produces depolarization of the motor endplate at the myoneural junction which causes sustained flaccid skeletal muscle paralysis

Pharmacodynamics

I.M.:

Onset of action: 2-3 minutes

Duration: 10-30 minutes

I.V.:

Onset of action: Within 30-60 seconds

Duration: ~4-6 minutes

Pharmacokinetics

Metabolism: Succinylcholine is rapidly hydrolyzed by plasma pseudocholinesterase

Elimination: 10% excreted unchanged in urine

(Continued)

Succinylcholine *(Continued)*

Usual Dosage
Children:
I.M.: 2.5-4 mg/kg (maximum dose: 150 mg)
I.V.: Initial: 1-2 mg/kg (maximum dose: 150 mg); maintenance: 0.3-0.6 mg/kg every 5-10 minutes as needed; because of the risk of malignant hyperthermia, use of continuous infusions is **not** recommended in infants and children
Adults: I.M., I.V.: 0.6 mg/kg (range: 0.3-1.1 mg/kg), up to 150 mg total dose; maintenance: 0.04-0.07 mg/kg every 5-10 minutes as needed
Continuous infusion: 2.5 mg/minute (range: 0.5-10 mg/minute)
Note: Pretreatment with atropine may reduce occurrence of bradycardia
Dosing adjustment in hepatic impairment: Dose should be decreased in patients with severe liver disease

Administration Parenteral: I.V.: May be administered by rapid I.V. injection without further dilution; continuous infusion: Dilute 1-2 mg/mL in NS or D_5W; I.M.: Injection should be made deeply

Monitoring Parameters Heart rate, serum potassium, assisted ventilator status, peripheral nerve stimulator measuring twitch response

Dosage Forms Excipient information presented when available (limited, particularly for generics); consult specific product labeling.
Injection, solution, as chloride: 20 mg/mL (5 mL, 10 mL); 50 mg/mL (10 mL); 100 mg/mL (10 mL)

♦ **Succinylcholine Chloride** *see* Succinylcholine *on page 1479*
♦ **Sucraid®** *see* Sacrosidase *on page 1412*

Sucralfate (soo KRAL fate)

Medication Safety Issues
Sound-alike/look-alike issues:
Sucralfate may be confused with salsalate
Carafate® may be confused with Cafergot®

U.S. Brand Names Carafate®

Canadian Brand Names Novo-Sucralate; Nu-Sucralate; PMS-Sucralate; Sulcrate®; Sulcrate® Suspension Plus

Index Terms Aluminum Sucrose Sulfate, Basic

Therapeutic Category Gastrointestinal Agent, Gastric or Duodenal Ulcer Treatment

Generic Available Yes

Use Short-term management of duodenal ulcers
Unlabeled use: Gastric ulcers; suspension may be used topically for treatment of stomatitis due to cancer chemotherapy or other causes of esophageal, gastric, and rectal erosions; treatment of NSAID mucosal damage; prevention of stress ulcers

Pregnancy Risk Factor B

Lactation Enters breast milk/compatible

Contraindications Hypersensitivity to sucralfate or any component

Warnings Because of the potential for sucralfate to alter the absorption of some drugs, separate administration times (administer other medications 2 hours before or after sucralfate) should be considered when alterations in bioavailability are believed to be critical

Precautions Use with caution in renal failure due to accumulation of aluminum

Adverse Reactions
Cardiovascular: Facial edema
Central nervous system: Dizziness, sleepiness, vertigo, headache
Dermatologic: Rash, pruritus, angioedema
Gastrointestinal: Constipation, diarrhea, nausea, gastric discomfort, indigestion, xerostomia, flatulence
Neuromuscular & skeletal: Back pain
Respiratory: Laryngospasm, rhinitis, respiratory difficulty

Drug Interactions Absorption of cimetidine colistin, digoxin, gentamicin, ketoconazole, L-thyroxine, phenytoin, quinidine, quinolones, ranitidine, sodium and potassium phosphate salts, tetracycline, and sustained release theophylline may be decreased (separate administration by 2 hours); aluminum-containing antacids may increase total body burden of aluminum; antacids, cimetidine, and ranitidine when administered concomitantly may decrease sucralfate's activity (gastric acidity is required for sucralfate to form its protective barrier)

Food Interactions Interferes with absorption of vitamin A, vitamin D, vitamin E, and vitamin K

Mechanism of Action Aluminum salt of sulfated sucrose which in the presence of acid pH (gastric acid) forms a complex, paste-like substance that adheres to the damaged mucosal area. This selectively forms a protective coating that protects the lining against peptic acid, pepsin, and bile salts.

Pharmacodynamics GI protection effect:

Acid neutralizing capacity: 14-17 mEq/1 g dose of sucralfate

Onset of action: 1-2 hours

Duration: Up to 6 hours

Pharmacokinetics

Absorption: Oral: <5%

Metabolism: Not metabolized

Elimination: 90% excreted in stool; small amounts that are absorbed are excreted in the urine as unchanged compounds

Usual Dosage Oral:

Children: Dose not established; doses of 40-80 mg/kg/day divided every 6 hours have been used

Stomatitis: 5-10 mL (1 g/10 mL); swish and spit or swish and swallow 4 times/day

Adults:

Stress ulcer prophylaxis: 1 g 4 times/day

Stress ulcer treatment: 1 g every 4 hours

Duodenal ulcer:

Treatment: 1 g 4 times/day for 4-8 weeks, or alternatively 2 g twice daily; treatment is recommended for 4-8 weeks in adults

Maintenance: Prophylaxis: 1 g twice daily

Stomatitis: 1 g/10 mL suspension, swish and spit or swish and swallow 4 times/day

Proctitis: Rectal enema: 2 g/20 mL once or twice daily

Dosage comment in renal impairment: Aluminum salt is minimally absorbed (<5%), however, may accumulate in renal failure

Administration

Oral: Administer on an empty stomach 1 hour before meals and at bedtime (see Warnings); tablet may be broken or dissolved in water before ingestion; do not administer antacids within 30 minutes of administration; shake suspension well before use

Rectal: May administer oral suspension as rectal enema; shake suspension well before use

Patient Information May cause dry mouth; separate times of administration with other medications (see Drug Interactions) by at least 2 hours

Additional Information There is approximately 14-16 mEq acid neutralizing capacity per 1 g sucralfate

Dosage Forms Excipient information presented when available (limited, particularly for generics); consult specific product labeling.

Suspension, oral: 1 g/10 mL (10 mL)

Carafate®: 1 g/10 mL (420 mL)

Tablet: 1 g

Carafate®: 1 g

References

Melko GP, Turco TF, Phelan TF, et al, "Treatment of Radiation-Induced Proctitis With Sucralfate Enemas," *Ann Pharmacother*, 1999, 33(12):1274-6.

- **Sucrets® [OTC]** *see* Dyclonine *on page 551*
- **Sudafed® 12 Hour [OTC]** *see* Pseudoephedrine *on page 1344*
- **Sudafed® 24 Hour [OTC]** *see* Pseudoephedrine *on page 1344*
- **Sudafed® Children's [OTC]** *see* Pseudoephedrine *on page 1344*
- **Sudafed® Decongestant (Can)** *see* Pseudoephedrine *on page 1344*
- **Sudafed® Maximum Strength Nasal Decongestant [OTC]** *see* Pseudoephedrine *on page 1344*
- **Sudafed® Maximum Strength Sinus Nighttime [OTC] [DSC]** *see* Triprolidine and Pseudoephedrine *on page 1580*
- **Sudafed PE™ [OTC]** *see* Phenylephrine *on page 1250*
- **Sudafed® Sinus Advance (Can)** *see* Pseudoephedrine and Ibuprofen *on page 1346*
- **Sudodrin [OTC]** *see* Pseudoephedrine *on page 1344*
- **SudoGest [OTC]** *see* Pseudoephedrine *on page 1344*
- **Sudo-Tab® [OTC]** *see* Pseudoephedrine *on page 1344*
- **Sufenta®** *see* Sufentanil *on page 1481*

Sufentanil (soo FEN ta nil)

Medication Safety Issues

Sound-alike/look-alike issues:

Sufentanil may be confused with alfentanil, fentanyl

Sufenta® may be confused with Alfenta®, Sudafed®, Survanta®

(Continued)

Sufentanil *(Continued)*

Related Information
Overdose and Toxicology *on page 1916*

U.S. Brand Names Sufenta®

Canadian Brand Names Sufenta®; Sufentanil Citrate Injection, USP

Index Terms Sufentanil Citrate

Therapeutic Category Analgesic, Narcotic; General Anesthetic

Generic Available Yes

Use Analgesia; analgesia adjunct; anesthetic agent

Restrictions C-II

Pregnancy Risk Factor C

Contraindications Hypersensitivity to sufentanil or any component; increased intracranial pressure; severe respiratory depression

Warnings May cause severe respiratory depression; rapid I.V. infusion may result in skeletal muscle and chest wall rigidity, impaired ventilation, respiratory distress, apnea, bronchoconstriction, laryngospasm, arrest; inject slowly over 3-5 minutes; nondepolarizing skeletal muscle relaxant may be required; abrupt discontinuation after prolonged use may result in withdrawal symptoms

Precautions Use with caution in patients with head injuries, hepatic impairment, pulmonary disease, or with use of MAO inhibitors within past 14 days; sufentanil shares the toxic potential of opiate agonists, precautions of opiate agonist therapy should be observed

Adverse Reactions
Cardiovascular: Bradycardia, hypotension, peripheral vasodilation
Central nervous system: CNS depression, drowsiness, dizziness, sedation
Dermatologic: Erythema, pruritus, rash
Endocrine & metabolic: ADH release
Gastrointestinal: Nausea, vomiting, constipation, biliary tract spasm
Genitourinary: Urinary tract spasm
Neuromuscular & skeletal: Skeletal and thoracic muscle rigidity, especially after rapid I.V. administration
Ocular: Miosis, blurred vision
Respiratory: Respiratory depression, apnea
Miscellaneous: Physical and psychological dependence with prolonged use

Drug Interactions Cytochrome P450 isoenzyme CYP3A3/4 substrate
CNS depressants, phenothiazines, MAO inhibitors, tricyclic antidepressants may potentiate adverse effects of opiates; beta-blocker therapy may potentiate sufentanil bradycardia

Mechanism of Action Binds with stereospecific receptors at many sites within the CNS, increases pain threshold, alters pain reception, inhibits ascending pain pathways; ultra short-acting narcotic

Pharmacodynamics
Onset of action: 1-3 minutes
Duration: Dose dependent; anesthesia adjunct doses: 5 minutes

Pharmacokinetics
Distribution: V_{dss}:
- Children 2-8 years: 2.9 ± 0.6 L/kg
- Adults: 1.7 ± 0.2 L/kg

Protein binding (alpha$_1$-acid glycoprotein):
- Neonates: 79%
- Adults:
  - Male: 93%
  - Postpartum women: 91%

Metabolism: Primarily by the liver via demethylation and dealkylation
Half-life, elimination:
- Neonates: 382-1162 minutes
- Children 2-8 years: 97 ± 42 minutes
- Adolescents 10-15 years: 76 ± 33 minutes
- Adults: 164 ± 22 minutes

Elimination: ~2% excreted unchanged in the urine; 80% of dose excreted in urine (mostly as metabolites) within 24 hours
Clearance:
- Children 2-8 years: 30.5 ± 8.8 mL/minute/kg
- Adolescents: 12.8 ± 12 mL/minute/kg
- Adults: 12.7 ± 0.8 mL/minute/kg

Usual Dosage Doses should be titrated to appropriate effects; wide range of doses, dependent upon desired degree of analgesia or anesthesia; use lean body weight to dose patients who are >20% above ideal body weight

Children <12 years: Anesthesia: I.V.: Initial: 10-25 mcg/kg; maintenance: Up to 25-50 mcg as needed

Adults: I.V.:

Adjunct to general anesthesia:

Low dose: Initial: 0.5-1 mcg/kg; maintenance: 10-25 mcg as needed

Moderate dose: Initial: 2-8 mcg/kg; maintenance: 10-50 mcg as needed

Anesthesia: Initial: 8-30 mcg/kg; maintenance: 10-50 mcg as needed

Administration Parenteral: I.V.: Slow I.V. injection or by infusion

Monitoring Parameters Respiratory rate, blood pressure, heart rate, oxygen saturation, neurological status (for degree of analgesia/anesthesia)

Patient Information May be habit-forming; avoid abrupt discontinuation after prolonged use

Nursing Implications Patient may develop rebound respiratory depression postoperatively

Dosage Forms Excipient information presented when available (limited, particularly for generics); consult specific product labeling. Available as sufentanil citrate; mg strength refers to sufentanil.

Injection, solution [preservative free]: 50 mcg/mL (1 mL, 2 mL, 5 mL)

References

Guay J, Gaudreault P, Tang A, et al, "Pharmacokinetics of Sufentanil in Normal Children," *Can J Anaesth*, 1992, 39(1):14-20.

Seguin JH, Erenberg A, and Leff RD, "Safety and Efficacy of Sufentanil Therapy in the Ventilated Infant," *Neonatal Netw*, 1994, 13(4):37-40.

♦ **Sufentanil Citrate** *see* Sufentanil *on page 1481*

♦ **Sufentanil Citrate Injection, USP (Can)** *see* Sufentanil *on page 1481*

♦ **Sulbactam and Ampicillin** *see* Ampicillin and Sulbactam *on page 125*

♦ **Sulcrate® (Can)** *see* Sucralfate *on page 1480*

♦ **Sulcrate® Suspension Plus (Can)** *see* Sucralfate *on page 1480*

Sulfacetamide (sul fa SEE ta mide)

Medication Safety Issues

Sound-alike/look-alike issues:

Bleph®-10 may be confused with Blephamide®

Klaron® may be confused with Klor-Con®

U.S. Brand Names Bleph®-10; Carmol® Scalp; Klaron®; Mexar™ Wash; Ovace®; Ovace® Wash; Rosula® NS

Canadian Brand Names Cetamide™; Diosulf™

Index Terms Sodium Sulfacetamide; Sulfacetamide Sodium

Therapeutic Category Antibiotic, Ophthalmic; Antibiotic, Sulfonamide Derivative

Generic Available Yes: Ointment, solution, suspension

Use

Ophthalmic: Treatment and prophylaxis of conjunctivitis, corneal ulcers, and other superficial ocular infections due to susceptible organisms

Dermatologic: Scaling dermatosis (seborrheic); bacterial infections of the skin due to organisms susceptible to sulfonamides; acne vulgaris

Pregnancy Risk Factor C

Lactation Excretion in breast milk unknown/use caution

Contraindications Hypersensitivity to sulfacetamide, any component (see Warnings), or sulfonamides; infants <2 months of age; epithelial herpes simplex keratitis, vaccinia, varicella, and other viral diseases of the cornea and conjunctiva; fungal diseases of the ocular structures

Warnings Antibacterial activity may be decreased in the presence of purulent exudates containing para-aminobenzoic acid (PABA); nonsusceptible organisms such as fungi may proliferate with prolonged or repeated use of sulfonamide preparations; hemolysis may occur in patients with G-6-PD deficiency. Hypersensitivity reactions may occur when a sulfonamide is readministered, irrespective of the route of administration. Stevens-Johnson syndrome has been reported following the use of sulfacetamide topically. At the first sign of hypersensitivity, skin rash, or other reactions, inform physician and discontinue use. Some products contain sulfites which may cause allergic reactions in susceptible individuals

Precautions Use with caution in patients with severe dry eye or G-6-PD deficiency

Adverse Reactions

Central nervous system: Headache, fever

Dermatologic: Stevens-Johnson syndrome, exfoliative dermatitis, toxic epidermal necrolysis, rash, photosensitivity, erythema, pruritus, scaling of the skin

Hematologic: Bone marrow suppression

Local: Irritation, stinging and burning (especially with 30% solution), itching

(Continued)

Sulfacetamide *(Continued)*

Ocular: Blurred vision, transient epithelial keratitis, reactive hyperemia, conjunctival edema

Miscellaneous: Hypersensitivity reactions, syndrome resembling systemic lupus erythematosus

Drug Interactions Silver, gentamicin (antagonism)

Stability Protect from light; discolored or cloudy solutions should not be used; incompatible with silver and zinc sulfate; sulfacetamide is inactivated by blood or purulent exudates

Mechanism of Action Interferes with bacterial growth by inhibiting bacterial folic acid synthesis through competitive antagonism of PABA

Pharmacodynamics Onset of action: Improvement of conjunctivitis is usually seen within 3-6 days

Pharmacokinetics

Distribution: Excreted in breast milk

Half-life: 7-13 hours

Elimination: When absorbed, excreted primarily in urine as unchanged drug

Usual Dosage Children >2 months and Adults:

Ophthalmic:

Ointment: Apply to lower conjunctival sac 1-4 times/day and at bedtime or apply ½" to 1" into the conjunctival sac at night in conjunction with the use of drops during the day

Solution: Instill 1-2 drops into the lower conjunctival sac every 1-3 hours according to severity of infection during the waking hours and less frequently at night; increase dosing interval as condition responds. Usual duration of treatment: 7-10 days

Topical: Children and Adults:

Lotion: Apply to affected areas twice daily

Scalp lotion: Apply at bedtime. For severe cases with crusting, heavy scaling and inflammation, apply twice daily. Once eruption subsides, apply once or twice weekly or every other week to prevent reoccurrence.

Wash: Wash affected areas twice daily. If skin dryness occurs, use less frequently.

Medicated pads: Gently apply to affected areas 1-2 times/day

Administration

Ophthalmic: Avoid contact of tube or bottle tip with skin or eye; solution: Apply finger pressure to lacrimal sac during and for 1-2 minutes after instillation to decrease risk of absorption and systemic effects

Topical: For external use only

Lotion: Shake lotion well before using; apply a thin film to affected area.

Scalp lotion: Wash hair and scalp prior to application. Part hair a section at a time and apply a small quantity of lotion. Completely moisten scalp and gently rub in lotion with the fingertips. Then brush hair thoroughly for 2-3 minutes.

Wash: Wet skin and apply wash liberally to areas to be cleansed. Massage gently into skin working into a lather; rinse thoroughly and pat dry.

Monitoring Parameters Response to therapy

Patient Information Eye drops may burn and sting when first instilled; may cause sensitivity to bright light.

Dosage Forms Excipient information presented when available (limited, particularly for generics); consult specific product labeling.

Cream, topical, as sodium:

Ovace®: 10% (30 g, 60 g)

Foam, topical, as sodium:

Ovace®: 10% (50 g, 100 g)

Gel, topical, as sodium:

Ovace®: 10% (30 g, 60 g)

Lotion, as sodium:

Carmol® Scalp: 10% (85 g) [contains urea 10%]

Klaron®: 10% (120 mL) [contains sodium metabisulfite]

Ovace® Wash: 10% (180 mL, 360 mL)

Ointment, ophthalmic, as sodium: 10% (3.5 g)

Pad, topical:

Rosula® NS: 10% (30s) [contains urea 10%]

Soap, topical:

Mexar™ Wash: 10% (170 mL)

Solution, ophthalmic, as sodium: 10% (15 mL)

Bleph®-10: 10% (5 mL) [contains benzalkonium chloride]

Suspension, topical: 10% (118 mL)

References

Lohr JA, Austin RD, Grossman M, et al, "Comparison of Three Topical Antimicrobials for Acute Bacterial Conjunctivitis," *Pediatr Infect Dis J*, 1988, 7(9):626-9.

♦ **Sulfacetamide Sodium** *see* Sulfacetamide *on page 1483*

SulfaDIAZINE (sul fa DYE a zeen)

Medication Safety Issues
Sound-alike/look-alike issues:
SulfaDIAZINE may be confused with sulfasalazine, sulfiSOXAZOLE

Therapeutic Category Antibiotic, Sulfonamide Derivative

Generic Available Yes

Use Adjunctive treatment in toxoplasmosis; treatment of urinary tract infections and nocardiosis; rheumatic fever prophylaxis in penicillin-allergic patient; uncomplicated attack of malaria

Pregnancy Risk Factor B (D at term)

Lactation Enters breast milk/contraindicated

Contraindications Hypersensitivity to any sulfa drug or any component; porphyria; infants <2 months of age due to competition with bilirubin for protein-binding sites (unless indicated for the treatment of congenital toxoplasmosis); pregnant women during third trimester

Precautions Use with caution in patients with impaired hepatic function or impaired renal function, urinary obstruction, blood dyscrasia, G-6-PD deficiency; dosage modification required in patients with renal impairment

Adverse Reactions
Cardiovascular: Vasculitis
Central nervous system: Dizziness, fever, headache
Dermatologic: Rash, exfoliative dermatitis, Stevens-Johnson syndrome, photosensitivity, urticaria
Gastrointestinal: Nausea, vomiting, abdominal pain
Genitourinary: Crystalluria
Hematologic: Granulocytopenia, leukopenia, thrombocytopenia, aplastic anemia, hemolytic anemia
Hepatic: Jaundice, hepatitis
Renal: Acute nephropathy, hematuria
Miscellaneous: Serum sickness-like reactions

Drug Interactions PABA, procaine; tetracaine antagonizes antibacterial action of sulfonamides; paraldehyde increases potential for crystalluria; displaces agents from protein binding sites: coumarin anticoagulants increase bleeding, methotrexate increases toxicity, sulfonylurea antidiabetic agents (hypoglycemia)

Food Interactions Supplemental folinic acid should be administered to reverse symptoms or prevent problems due to folic acid deficiency; avoid large quantities of vitamin C or acidifying agents (cranberry juice) to prevent crystalluria

Stability Protect from light

Mechanism of Action Interferes with bacterial growth by inhibiting bacterial folic acid synthesis through competitive antagonism of PABA

Pharmacokinetics
Absorption: Oral: Well absorbed
Distribution: Excreted in breast milk; diffuses into CSF with higher concentrations reached when meninges are inflamed; distributed into most body tissues
Protein binding: 32% to 56%
Metabolism: Metabolized by N-acetylation
Half-life: 10 hours
Time to peak serum concentration: Within 4 hours
Elimination: In urine as metabolites (15% to 40%) and as unchanged drug (43% to 60%)

Usual Dosage Oral:
Congenital toxoplasmosis: Newborns: 100 mg/kg/day divided every 12 hours for 12 months in conjunction with pyrimethamine 1 mg/kg/day once daily and supplemental folinic acid 5 mg every 3 days for first 6 months, then pyrimethamine 1 mg/kg/day 3 times/week and folinic acid 10 mg 3 times/week for the next 6 months
Toxoplasmosis:
Children: 120-200 mg/kg/day divided every 6 hours in conjunction with pyrimethamine 2 mg/kg/day divided every 12 hours for 3 days followed by 1 mg/kg/day once daily (maximum dose: 25 mg/day) with supplemental folinic acid 5-10 mg every 3 days
Adults: 2-8 g/day divided every 6 hours in conjunction with pyrimethamine 25 mg/day and with supplemental folinic acid 5-10 mg every 3 days
Prophylaxis of recurrent rheumatic fever:
≤30 kg: 500 mg once daily
>30 kg: 1 g once daily

Administration Oral: Administer with water on an empty stomach

Monitoring Parameters CBC, renal function tests, urinalysis

(Continued)

SulfaDIAZINE *(Continued)*

Patient Information Drink plenty of fluids; limit alcohol; notify physician if rash, sore throat, fever, arthralgia, shortness of breath, or jaundice occurs. May cause photosensitivity reactions (eg, exposure to sunlight may cause severe sunburn, skin rash, redness, or itching); avoid exposure to sunlight and artificial light sources (sunlamps, tanning booth/bed); wear protective clothing, wide-brimmed hats, sunglasses, and lip sunscreen (SPF ≥15); use a sunscreen [broad-spectrum sunscreen or physical sunscreen (preferred) or sunblock with SPF ≥15]; contact physician if reaction occurs.

Dosage Forms Excipient information presented when available (limited, particularly for generics); consult specific product labeling.

Tablet: 500 mg

Extemporaneous Preparations Tablets may be crushed to prepare oral suspension of the drug in water or with a sucrose-containing solution; aqueous suspension with concentrations of 100 mg/mL should be stored in the refrigerator and used within 7 days

References

Frenkel JK, "Toxoplasmosis," *Pediatr Clin North Am*, 1985, 32(4):917-32.

Sulfadoxine and Pyrimethamine

(sul fa DOKS een & peer i METH a meen)

U.S. Brand Names Fansidar®

Index Terms Pyrimethamine and Sulfadoxine

Therapeutic Category Antimalarial Agent

Generic Available No

Use Treatment of *Plasmodium falciparum* malaria in patients in whom chloroquine resistance is suspected; malaria prophylaxis for travelers to areas where chloroquine-resistant malaria is endemic

Pregnancy Risk Factor C

Contraindications Hypersensitivity to any sulfa drug, pyrimethamine, or any component; porphyria, megaloblastic anemia, severe renal insufficiency; children <2 months of age due to competition with bilirubin for protein binding sites; pregnant women at term; do not use for treatment of malaria acquired in Southeast Asia or the Amazon Basin since resistance to sulfadoxine and pyrimethamine has been reported

Warnings Fatalities associated with sulfonamides, although rare, have occurred due to severe reactions including Stevens-Johnson syndrome, toxic epidermal necrolysis, hepatic necrosis, agranulocytosis, aplastic anemia and other blood dyscrasias; discontinue use at first sign of rash or any sign of adverse reaction; hemolysis may occur in patients with G-6-PD deficiency

Precautions Use with caution in patients with renal or hepatic impairment, patients with possible folate deficiency, patients with bronchial asthma, and patients with seizure disorders

Adverse Reactions

Cardiovascular: Vasculitis

Central nervous system: Seizures, headache, insomnia, ataxia, fatigue, hyperesthesia

Dermatologic: Erythema multiforme, Stevens-Johnson syndrome, toxic epidermal necrolysis, rash, photosensitivity, urticaria, pruritus

Endocrine & metabolic: Folic acid deficiency

Gastrointestinal: Anorexia, vomiting, gastritis, glossitis, diarrhea, abdominal cramps

Hematologic: Megaloblastic anemia, leukopenia, thrombocytopenia, pancytopenia, agranulocytosis, pulmonary eosinophilia

Hepatic: Hepatic necrosis; jaundice; elevated ALT, AST

Neuromuscular & skeletal: Tremor

Respiratory: Respiratory failure

Drug Interactions Para-aminobenzoic acid, folic acid

Stability Protect from light

Mechanism of Action Sulfadoxine interferes with bacterial folic acid synthesis and growth via competitive inhibition of para-aminiobenzoic acid; pyrimethamine inhibits microbial dihydrofolate reductase, resulting in inhibition of tetrahydrofolic acid synthesis

Pharmacokinetics

Absorption: Oral: Well absorbed

Distribution: Excreted in breast milk; pyrimethamine is distributed to kidneys, lungs, liver, and spleen; sulfadoxine is widely distributed in the body

Protein binding:

- Pyrimethamine: 80% to 87%
- Sulfadoxine: 90% to 95%

Half-life:
Pyrimethamine: 111 hours
Sulfadoxine: 169 hours
Time to peak serum concentration: Within 2-8 hours
Elimination: In urine as parent compounds and several unidentified metabolites

Usual Dosage Children ≥ 2 months and Adults: Oral:
Treatment of acute attack of malaria: A single dose of the following number of Fansidar® tablets is used in sequence with quinine on last day of quinine therapy:
2-11 months: 1/4 tablet
1-3 years: 1/2 tablet
4-8 years: 1 tablet
9-14 years: 2 tablets
>14 years: 3 tablets
Adults: 3 tablets on last day of quinine therapy
Malaria prophylaxis (for areas where chloroquine-resistant *P. falciparum* exists):
Short-term travel (≤3 weeks): Travelers should carry pyrimethamine-sulfadoxine for use as presumptive self-treatment if a febrile illness develops while taking chloroquine for prophylaxis. Take single dose in the event of febrile illness when medical attention is not immediately available:
2-11 months: 1/4 tablet
1-3 years: 1/2 tablet
4-8 years: 1 tablet
9-14 years: 2 tablets
>14 years and Adults: 3 tablets

Administration Oral: Administer with meals

Monitoring Parameters Liver function tests, CBC including platelet counts, renal function tests and urinalysis should be performed periodically

Patient Information Drink plenty of fluids; notify physician if rash, sore throat, pallor, glossitis, fever, arthralgia, cough, shortness of breath, or jaundice occurs; limit alcohol. May cause photosensitivity reactions (eg, exposure to sunlight may cause severe sunburn, skin rash, redness, or itching); avoid exposure to sunlight and artificial light sources (sunlamps, tanning booth/bed); wear protective clothing, wide-brimmed hats, sunglasses, and lip sunscreen (SPF ≥15); use a sunscreen [broad-spectrum sunscreen or physical sunscreen (preferred) or sunblock with SPF ≥15]; contact physician if reaction occurs.

Additional Information Leucovorin should be administered to reverse signs and symptoms of folic acid deficiency

Dosage Forms Excipient information presented when available (limited, particularly for generics); consult specific product labeling.
Tablet: Sulfadoxine 500 mg and pyrimethamine 25 mg

References

Lynk A and Gold R, "Review of 40 Children With Imported Malaria," *Pediatr Infect Dis J*, 1989, 8(11):745-50.
Randall G and Seidel JS, "Malaria," *Pediatr Clin North Am*, 1985, 32(4):893-916.

Sulfamethoxazole and Trimethoprim

(sul fa meth OKS a zole & trye METH oh prim)

Medication Safety Issues
Sound-alike/look-alike issues:
Bactrim™ may be confused with bacitracin, Bactine®
Co-trimoxazole may be confused with clotrimazole
Septra® may be confused with Ceptaz®, Sectral®, Septa®

U.S. Brand Names Bactrim™; Bactrim™ DS; Septra®; Septra® DS

Canadian Brand Names Apo-Sulfatrim®; Apo-Sulfatrim® DS; Apo-Sulfatrim® Pediatric; Novo-Trimel; Novo-Trimel D.S.; Nu-Cotrimox; Septra® Injection

Index Terms Co-Trimoxazole; SMZ-TMP; Sulfatrim; TMP-SMZ; Trimethoprim and Sulfamethoxazole

Therapeutic Category Antibiotic, Sulfonamide Derivative

Generic Available Yes

Use Treatment of urinary tract infections caused by susceptible *E. coli*, *Klebsiella*, *Enterobacter*, *Proteus mirabilis*, *Proteus* (indole positive); acute otitis media due to amoxicillin-resistant *H. influenzae*, *S. pneumoniae*, and *M. catarrhalis*; acute exacerbations of chronic bronchitis; prophylaxis and treatment of *Pneumocystis carinii* pneumonitis (PCP); treatment of susceptible shigellosis, typhoid fever, *Nocardia asteroides* infection, and *Xanthomonas maltophilia* infection; the I.V. preparation is used for treatment of *Pneumocystis carinii* pneumonitis, *Shigella*, and severe urinary tract infections

Pregnancy Risk Factor C

Lactation Enters breast milk/contraindicated (AAP rates "compatible with restrictions")
(Continued)

Sulfamethoxazole and Trimethoprim *(Continued)*

Contraindications Hypersensitivity to any sulfa drug, trimethoprim, or any component (see Warnings); porphyria; megaloblastic anemia due to folate deficiency; infants <2 months of age (for exception, see Additional Information)

Warnings Fatalities associated with sulfonamides, although rare, have occurred due to severe reactions including Stevens-Johnson syndrome, toxic epidermal necrolysis, hepatic necrosis, agranulocytosis, aplastic anemia, and other blood dyscrasias; discontinue use at first sign of rash or any sign of adverse reaction

Oral suspension and tablets may contain sodium benzoate; injection contains propylene glycol, benzyl alcohol, and sodium metabisulfites; propylene glycol may be toxic to newborns in high doses; sodium benzoate, benzyl alcohol and sodium metabisulfites may cause allergic reactions in susceptible individuals; large amounts of benzyl alcohol (≥99 mg/kg/day) have been associated with a potentially fatal toxicity ("gasping syndrome") in neonates; the "gasping syndrome" consists of metabolic acidosis, respiratory distress, gasping respirations, CNS dysfunction (including convulsions, intracranial hemorrhage), hypotension and cardiovascular collapse; use products containing benzyl alcohol with caution in neonates; *in vitro* and animal studies have shown that benzoate, a metabolite of benzyl alcohol, displaces bilirubin from protein binding sites

Precautions Use with caution in patients with G-6-PD deficiency, impaired renal or hepatic function; adjust dosage in patients with renal impairment

Adverse Reactions

Cardiovascular: Allergic myocarditis, hypotension

Central nervous system: Confusion, depression, hallucinations, seizures, fever, ataxia, kernicterus in neonates, aseptic meningitis, headache, insomnia

Dermatologic: Rash (more common in patients taking large dosages or in patients with AIDS), erythema multiforme, epidermal necrolysis, Stevens-Johnson syndrome, pruritus, urticaria

Endocrine & metabolic: Hyperkalemia

Gastrointestinal: Nausea, vomiting, glossitis, stomatitis, diarrhea, pseudomembranous colitis, pancreatitis, splenomegaly, anorexia

Hematologic: Thrombocytopenia, megaloblastic anemia, granulocytopenia, aplastic anemia, hemolysis (with G-6-PD deficiency)

Hepatic: Hepatitis, cholestatic jaundice

Local: Local irritation, pain, phlebitis

Neuromuscular & skeletal: Arthralgia, myalgia, rhabdomyolysis

Renal: Interstitial nephritis, renal tubular acidosis

Respiratory: Shortness of breath, cough, pulmonary infiltrates

Miscellaneous: Serum sickness, angioedema

Drug Interactions Cytochrome P450 isoenzyme CYP2C9 inhibitor

Sulfamethoxazole and trimethoprim decreases the clearance of warfarin; methotrexate (displaced from protein binding sites); increases the effect of sulfonylureas, phenytoin, digoxin, and thiopental; decreases serum cyclosporine concentrations

Stability Do not refrigerate concentrate for injection; protect from light. For I.V. administration, a 1:25 dilution in D_5W (5 mL drug to 125 mL D_5W) is stable for 6 hours or a 1:20 dilution in D_5W (5 mL drug to 100 mL D_5W) is stable for 4 hours at room temperature; in patients who require fluid restriction, 1:15 dilution (5 mL drug to 75 mL D_5W) is stable for 2 hours. 1:10 highly concentrated admixture (5 mL drug to 50 mL D_5W) may precipitate in 1-2 hours; do not mix with other drugs or solutions.

Mechanism of Action Sulfamethoxazole interferes with bacterial folic acid synthesis and growth via inhibition of dihydrofolic acid formation from para-aminobenzoic acid; trimethoprim inhibits dihydrofolic acid reduction to tetrahydrofolate resulting in sequential inhibition of enzymes of the folic acid pathway

Pharmacokinetics

Absorption: Oral: Almost completely (90% to 100%)

Distribution: Crosses the placenta; distributes into breast milk, joint fluid, sputum, middle ear fluid, bile, and CSF

Protein binding:

- TMP: 45%
- SMX: 68%

Metabolism:

- TMP: Metabolized to oxide and hydroxylated metabolites
- SMX: N-acetylated and glucuronidated

Half-life:

- TMP: 6-11 hours, prolonged in renal failure
- SMX: 9-12 hours, prolonged in renal failure

Time to peak serum concentration: Oral: Within 1-4 hours

Elimination: Both excreted in urine as metabolites and unchanged drug

Usual Dosage Oral, I.V. **(dosage recommendations are based on the trimethoprim (TMP) component):**

Children >2 months and Adults:

Mild-moderate infections: 6-12 mg TMP/kg/day in divided doses every 12 hours

Serious infection/*Pneumocystis*: 15-20 mg TMP/kg/day in divided doses every 6-8 hours

Prophylaxis of *Pneumocystis* (see **Note** in Additional Information): 150 mg TMP/m^2/day in divided doses every 12 hours 3 days/week on consecutive days; acceptable alternative dosage schedules include 150 mg TMP/m^2/day as a single daily dose 3 times/week on consecutive days or 150 mg TMP/m^2/day in divided doses every 12 hours administered 7 days/week, or 150 mg TMP/m^2/day in divided doses every 12 hours administered 3 times/week on alternate days; dose should not exceed 320 mg trimethoprim and 1600 mg sulfamethoxazole/day

Urinary tract infection prophylaxis: 2 mg TMP/kg/dose daily or 5 mg TMP/kg/dose twice weekly

Adults:

Urinary tract infection/chronic bronchitis: 1 double strength tablet every 12 hours for 10-14 days

Prophylaxis of *Pneumocystis*: One double-strength tablet daily or an acceptable alternative is 1 single-strength tablet daily

Dosing adjustment in renal impairment (frequency may need to be adjusted):

Cl_{cr} 15-30 mL/minute: Reduce dose by 50%

Cl_{cr} <15 mL/minute: Not recommended

Administration

Oral: May administer with water on an empty stomach; shake suspension well before use

Parenteral: **Do not administer I.M.**

I.V. infusion: Inspect solution for evidence of cloudiness or precipitation prior to administration; infuse I.V. sulfamethoxazole and trimethoprim over 60-90 minutes; must be further diluted 1:25 (5 mL drug to 125 mL diluent, ie, D_5W); in patients who require fluid restriction, a 1:15 dilution (5 mL drug to 75 mL diluent, ie, D_5W) or a 1:10 dilution (5 mL drug to 50 mL diluent, ie, D_5W) may be administered; see Stability

Monitoring Parameters CBC, renal function test, liver function test, urinalysis; observe for change in bowel frequency

Patient Information Maintain adequate fluid intake

Additional Information Note: Guidelines for prophylaxis of *Pneumocystis carinii* pneumonia: Initiate PCP prophylaxis in the following patients: Children born to HIV-infected mothers should be given prophylaxis with TMP/SMZ beginning at 4-6 weeks of age and continue through the first year of life or until HIV infection has been reasonably excluded; children 1-5 years of age with CD4+ count <500 or CD4+ percentage <15%; children 6-12 years of age with CD4+ count <200 or CD4+ percentage <15%; adolescents and adults with CD4+ count <200 or oropharyngeal candidiasis. Folinic acid should be given if bone marrow suppression occurs.

Dosage Forms Excipient information presented when available (limited, particularly for generics); consult specific product labeling. **Note:** The 5:1 ratio (SMX:TMP) remains constant in all dosage forms.

Injection, solution: Sulfamethoxazole 80 mg and trimethoprim 16 mg per mL (5 mL, 10 mL, 30 mL)

Suspension, oral: Sulfamethoxazole 200 mg and trimethoprim 40 mg per 5 mL (480 mL)

Tablet: Sulfamethoxazole 400 mg and trimethoprim 80 mg

Bactrim™: Sulfamethoxazole 400 mg and trimethoprim 80 mg

Septra®: Sulfamethoxazole 400 mg and trimethoprim 80 mg

Tablet, double strength: Sulfamethoxazole 800 mg and trimethoprim 160 mg

Bactrim™ DS: Sulfamethoxazole 800 mg and trimethoprim 160 mg

Septra® DS: Sulfamethoxazole 800 mg and trimethoprim 160 mg

References

Jarosinki PF, Kennedy PE, and Gallelli JF, "Stability of Concentrated Trimethoprim-Sulfamethoxazole Admixtures," *AJHP*, 1989, 46(4):732-7.

Hughes WT, "*Pneumocystis carinii* Pneumonia: New Approaches to Diagnosis, Treatment, and Prevention," *Pediatr Infect Dis J*, 1991, 10(5):391-9.

"1999 USPHS/IDSA Guidelines for the Prevention of Opportunistic Infections in Persons Infected With Human Immunodeficiency Virus. USPHS/IDSA Prevention of Opportunistic Infections Working Group," *MMWR Morb Mortal Wkly Rep*, 1999, 48(RR-10):1-66.

♦ **Sulfamylon®** *see* Mafenide *on page 968*

Sulfasalazine (sul fa SAL a zeen)

Medication Safety Issues
Sound-alike/look-alike issues:
Sulfasalazine may be confused with salsalate, sulfaDIAZINE, sulfiSOXAZOLE
Azulfidine® may be confused with Augmentin®, azathioprine

U.S. Brand Names Azulfidine®; Azulfidine® EN-tabs®; Sulfazine; Sulfazine EC

Canadian Brand Names Alti-Sulfasalazine; Salazopyrin®; Salazopyrin En-Tabs®

Index Terms Salicylazosulfapyridine

Therapeutic Category 5-Aminosalicylic Acid Derivative; Anti-inflammatory Agent

Generic Available Yes

Use Management of ulcerative colitis; treatment of active Crohn's disease and juvenile rheumatoid arthritis

Pregnancy Risk Factor B (D at term)

Lactation Enters breast milk/use caution (AAP recommends use "with caution")

Contraindications Hypersensitivity to sulfasalazine, sulfa drugs, or any component; porphyria, GI or GU obstruction; hypersensitivity to salicylates; children <2 years of age

Precautions Use with caution in patients with renal impairment, G-6-PD deficiency, blood dyscrasias, or bronchial asthma

Adverse Reactions Incidence of adverse effects increase with dosage >4 g/day and in slow acetylators of sulfapyridine
Cardiovascular: Vasculitis
Central nervous system: Headache, fever, convulsions, vertigo, malaise, mood changes
Dermatologic: Rash, toxic epidermal necrolysis, urticaria, Stevens-Johnson syndrome, photosensitivity, staining of skin (orange-yellow)
Gastrointestinal: Nausea, vomiting, diarrhea, pancreatitis, anorexia
Genitourinary: Crystalluria, infertility (oligospermia), discoloration of urine (orange-yellow)
Hematologic: Hemolytic anemia, agranulocytosis, neutropenia, leukopenia
Hepatic: Elevated liver enzymes, jaundice, cholestatic jaundice, cirrhosis, liver necrosis/failure
Otic: Tinnitus
Renal: Nephrotoxicity
Respiratory: Fibrosing alveolitis, pulmonary eosinophilia
Miscellaneous: Serum sickness-like reaction

Drug Interactions
Decreased effect of iron, digoxin, folic acid, and PABA or PABA metabolites of drugs (ie, procaine, proparacaine, tetracaine)
Increased effect of oral anticoagulants, methotrexate, and oral hypoglycemic agents (as with other sulfa drugs)

Food Interactions Need to increase dietary intake of iron; since sulfasalazine impairs folate absorption, consider providing 1 mg/day folate supplement

Mechanism of Action Acts locally in the colon to decrease the inflammatory response and interfere with secretion by inhibiting prostaglandin synthesis; therapeutic effect may result from antibacterial action with change in intestinal flora

Pharmacodynamics Onset of action:
JRA: Minimum trial of 3 months is necessary
Ulcerative colitis: >3-4 weeks

Pharmacokinetics
Absorption: Oral: 10% to 15% as unchanged drug from the small intestine; upon administration, the drug is split into sulfapyridine and 5-aminosalicylic acid (5-ASA) in the colon
Distribution: Breast milk to plasma ratio: 0.09-0.17
Metabolism: Both components are metabolized in the liver; slow acetylators have higher plasma sulfapyridine concentrations
Half-life:
- Sulfasalazine:
  - Single dose: 5.7 hours
  - Multiple doses: 7.6 hours
- Sulfapyridine:
  - Single dose: 8.4 hours
  - Multiple doses: 10.4 hours

Time to peak serum concentration:
- Serum sulfasalazine: Within 1.5-6 hours
- Serum sulfapyridine (active metabolite): Within 6-24 hours

Elimination: Primarily in urine (as unchanged drug, components, and acetylated metabolites); small amounts appear in feces

Usual Dosage Oral:

Children ≥2 years:

Ulcerative colitis:

Mild exacerbation: 40-50 mg/kg/day divided every 6 hours

Moderate-severe exacerbation: 50-75 mg/kg/day divided every 4-6 hours, not to exceed 6 g/day

Maintenance dose: 30-50 mg/kg/day divided every 4-8 hours; not to exceed 2 g/day

Juvenile rheumatoid arthritis (JRA): Initial: 10 mg/kg/day; increase weekly by 10 mg/kg/day; usual dose: 30-50 mg/kg/day in 2 divided doses; maximum dose: 2 g/day

Adults: 1 g 3-4 times/day divided every 4-6 hours, not to exceed 6 g/day; maintenance: 2 g/day divided every 6-12 hours

Administration Oral: Administer after meals or with food; do not administer with antacids

Monitoring Parameters Stool frequency, hematocrit, reticulocyte count, CBC, urinalysis, renal function tests, liver function tests

Patient Information Maintain adequate fluid intake; may cause orange-yellow discoloration of urine and skin; may stain soft contact lenses yellow. May cause photosensitivity reactions (eg, exposure to sunlight may cause severe sunburn, skin rash, redness, or itching); avoid exposure to sunlight and artificial light sources (sunlamps, tanning booth/bed); wear protective clothing, wide-brimmed hats, sunglasses, and lip sunscreen (SPF ≥15); use a sunscreen [broad-spectrum sunscreen or physical sunscreen (preferred) or sunblock with SPF ≥15]; contact physician if reaction occurs.

Additional Information Good response to sulfasalazine for JRA is most likely to occur in HLA B27-positive boys who are older than 9 years of age at onset of arthritis

Dosage Forms Excipient information presented when available (limited, particularly for generics); consult specific product labeling.

Tablet: 500 mg

Azulfidine®, Sulfazine: 500 mg

Tablet, delayed release, enteric coated: 500 mg

Azulfidine® EN-tabs®, Sulfazine EC: 500 mg

References

American College of Rheumatology Ad Hoc Committee on Clinical Guidelines, "Guidelines for the Management of Rheumatoid Arthritis," *Arthritis Rheum*, 1996, 39(5):713-22.

Giannini EH and Cawkwell GD, "Drug Treatment in Children With Juvenile Rheumatoid Arthritis," *Pediatr Clin North Am*, 1995, 42(5):1099-125.

Kirschner BS, "Inflammatory Bowel Disease in Children," *Pediatr Clin North Am*, 1988, 35(1):189-208.

♦ **Sulfatrim** *see* Sulfamethoxazole and Trimethoprim *on page 1487*

♦ **Sulfazine** *see* Sulfasalazine *on page 1490*

♦ **Sulfazine EC** *see* Sulfasalazine *on page 1490*

SulfiSOXAZOLE (sul fi SOKS a zole)

Medication Safety Issues

Sound-alike/look-alike issues:

SulfiSOXAZOLE may be confused with sulfaDIAZINE, sulfamethoxazole, sulfasalazine

Gantrisin® may be confused with Gastrosed™

U.S. Brand Names Gantrisin®

Canadian Brand Names Novo-Soxazole; Sulfizole®

Index Terms Sulfisoxazole Acetyl; Sulphafurazole

Therapeutic Category Antibiotic, Sulfonamide Derivative

Generic Available Yes: Tablet

Use Treatment of uncomplicated urinary tract infections, otitis media, *Chlamydia*; nocardiosis; treatment of acute pelvic inflammatory disease in prepubertal children

Pregnancy Risk Factor B (D at term)

Lactation Enters breast milk/compatible

Contraindications Hypersensitivity to any sulfa drug or any component; porphyria; infants <2 months of age (sulfas compete with bilirubin for protein binding sites which may result in kernicterus in newborns); patients with urinary obstruction; pregnant women during third trimester; nursing mothers

Precautions Use with caution in patients with G-6-PD deficiency (hemolysis may occur), hepatic or renal impairment; dosage modification required in patients with renal impairment; risk of crystalluria should be considered in patients with impaired renal function

Adverse Reactions

Cardiovascular: Vasculitis

Central nervous system: Dizziness, headache, fever, vertigo, disorientation

(Continued)

SulfiSOXAZOLE *(Continued)*

Dermatologic: Rash, Stevens-Johnson syndrome, photosensitivity, exfoliative dermatitis
Gastrointestinal: Nausea, vomiting, anorexia, stomatitis, pseudomembranous colitis
Genitourinary: Crystalluria (rare)
Hematologic: Thrombocytopenia, leukopenia, agranulocytosis, aplastic anemia, hemolytic anemia, neutropenia
Hepatic: Jaundice, hepatitis
Renal: Nephrotoxicity
Miscellaneous: Hypersensitivity reactions

Drug Interactions Methotrexate, tolbutamide, chlorpropamide, oral anticoagulants (displaced from protein binding sites); PABA (antagonizes the antibacterial activity of sulfas); thiopental (competes for plasma protein binding)

Food Interactions Interferes with folate absorption

Stability Protect from light

Mechanism of Action Interferes with bacterial growth by inhibiting bacterial folic acid synthesis through competitive antagonism of PABA

Pharmacokinetics

Absorption: Sulfisoxazole acetyl is hydrolyzed in the GI tract to sulfisoxazole which is readily absorbed
Distribution: Crosses the placenta; excreted into breast milk; distributes into extracellular space; CSF concentration ranges from 8% to 57% of blood concentration in patients with normal meninges
Protein binding: 85% to 88%
Metabolism: In the liver by acetylation and glucuronide conjugation to inactive compounds
Half-life: 4-8 hours, prolonged with renal impairment
Time to peak serum concentration: Within 2-4 hours
Elimination: Primarily in urine (95% within 24 hours), 40% to 60% as unchanged drug
Dialysis: >50% removed by hemodialysis

Usual Dosage

Infants ≥2 months and Children: Oral: Initial: 75 mg/kg for 1 dose, followed by 120-150 mg/kg/day in divided doses every 4-6 hours; not to exceed 6 g/day
Pelvic inflammatory disease: 100 mg/kg/day in divided doses every 6 hours; used in combination with ceftriaxone
Chlamydia trachomatis: 100 mg/kg/day divided every 6 hours; maximum dose: 2 g/day
Prophylaxis of UTI: 10-20 mg/kg/day divided every 12 hours
Prophylaxis of recurrent acute otitis media: 35-75 mg/kg/day once daily at bedtime
Adults: Oral: 2-4 g stat, followed by 4-8 g/day in divided doses every 4-6 hours
Children and Adults: Ophthalmic: Solution: Instill 1-2 drops to conjunctiva of affected eye every 2-3 hours

Dosing interval in renal impairment:
Cl_{cr} 10-50 mL/minutes: Administer every 8-12 hours
Cl_{cr} <10 mL/minute: Administer every 12-24 hours

Administration

Ophthalmic: Avoid contact of bottle tip with skin or eye; apply finger pressure to lacrimal sac during and for 1-2 minutes after instillation of drops to decrease risk of absorption and systemic effects
Oral: Administer with a glass of water on an empty stomach; shake suspension well before use

Monitoring Parameters CBC, urinalysis, renal function tests

Test Interactions False-positive protein in urine; false-positive urine glucose with Clinitest®

Patient Information Report to physician any sore throat, mouth sores, rash, unusual bleeding, or fever; limit alcohol. May cause photosensitivity reactions (eg, exposure to sunlight may cause severe sunburn, skin rash, redness, or itching); avoid exposure to sunlight and artificial light sources (sunlamps, tanning booth/bed); wear protective clothing, wide-brimmed hats, sunglasses, and lip sunscreen (SPF ≥15); use a sunscreen [broad-spectrum sunscreen or physical sunscreen (preferred) or sunblock with SPF ≥15]; contact physician if reaction occurs.

Nursing Implications Maintain adequate patient fluid intake

Dosage Forms Excipient information presented when available (limited, particularly for generics); consult specific product labeling.

Suspension, oral, pediatric, as acetyl (Gantrisin®): 500 mg/5 mL (480 mL) [contains alcohol 0.3%; raspberry flavor]
Tablet: 500 mg

References

Erramouspe J and Heyneman CA, "Treatment and Prevention of Otitis Media," *Ann Pharmacother*, 2000, 34(12):1452-68.

Klein JO, "Protecting the Therapeutic Advantage of Antimicrobial Agents Used for Otitis Media," *Pediatr Infect Dis J*, 1998, 17(6):571-5.

"Practice Parameter: The Diagnosis, Treatment, and Evaluation of the Initial Urinary Tract Infection in Febrile Infants and Young Children. American Academy of Pediatrics. Committee on Quality Improvement. Subcommittee on Urinary Tract Infection," *Pediatrics*, 1999, 103(4 Pt 1):843-52.

Thoene DE and Johnson CE, "Pharmacotherapy of Otitis Media," *Pharmacotherapy*, 1991, 11(3):212-21.

♦ **Sulfisoxazole Acetyl** *see* SulfiSOXAZOLE *on page 1491*

♦ **Sulfisoxazole and Erythromycin** *see* Erythromycin and Sulfisoxazole *on page 599*

♦ **Sulfizole® (Can)** *see* SulfiSOXAZOLE *on page 1491*

Sulfur and Salicylic Acid (SUL fur & sal i SIL ik AS id)

Index Terms Salicylic Acid and Sulfur

Therapeutic Category Antiseborrheic Agent, Topical

Use Therapeutic shampoo for dandruff and seborrheal dermatitis; acne skin cleanser

Contraindications Hypersensitivity to sulfur, salicylic acid, or any component

Warnings For external use only; avoid contact with eyes; discontinue use if skin irritation develops

Precautions Infants are more sensitive to sulfur than adults; do not use in children <2 years of age

Adverse Reactions Topical preparations containing 2% to 5% sulfur generally are well tolerated; concentration >15% is very irritating to the skin; higher concentrations (eg, 10% or higher) may cause systemic toxicity

Cardiovascular: Collapse (with sulfur concentration >10%)
Central nervous system: Dizziness, headache
Gastrointestinal: Vomiting
Local: Irritation
Neuromuscular & skeletal: Muscle cramps

Stability Preparations containing sulfur may react with metals including silver and copper, resulting in discoloration of the metal

Mechanism of Action Salicylic acid works synergistically with sulfur in its keratolytic action to break down keratin and promote skin peeling

Pharmacokinetics Absorption: 1% of topically applied sulfur is absorbed; sulfur is reduced to hydrogen sulfide

Usual Dosage Children ≥2 years and Adults: Topical:

Shampoo: Initial: Massage onto wet scalp; leave lather on scalp for 5 minutes, rinse, repeat application, then rinse thoroughly; use daily or every other day; 1-2 treatments/week will usually maintain control

Soap: Use daily or every other day

Administration Topical: Avoid contact with the eyes; for external use only

Patient Information Contact physician if condition worsens or rash or irritation develops

Dosage Forms

Cake: Sulfur 2% and salicylic acid 2% (123 g)
Cleanser: Sulfur 2% and salicylic acid 1.5% (60 mL, 120 mL)
Shampoo: Micropulverized sulfur 2% and salicylic acid 2% (120 mL, 240 mL)
Soap: Micropulverized sulfur 2% and salicylic acid 2% (113 g)
Wash: Sulfur 1.6% and salicylic acid 1.6% (75 mL)

Sulindac (sul IN dak)

Medication Safety Issues

Sound-alike/look-alike issues:

Clinoril® may be confused with Cleocin®, Clozaril®, Oruvail®

Related Information

Overdose and Toxicology *on page 1916*

U.S. Brand Names Clinoril®

Canadian Brand Names Apo-Sulin®; Novo-Sundac; Nu-Sundac

Therapeutic Category Analgesic, Non-narcotic; Anti-inflammatory Agent; Nonsteroidal Anti-inflammatory Drug (NSAID), Oral

Generic Available Yes

Use Management of inflammatory disease, rheumatoid disorders; acute gouty arthritis

Medication Guide An FDA-approved patient medication guide, which is available with the product information and at http://www.fda.gov/cder/Offices/ODS/medication_guides.htm, must be dispensed with this medication for each new outpatient prescription and refill.

Pregnancy Risk Factor C (D if used in the 3rd trimester or near delivery)

Lactation Excretion in breast milk unknown/not recommended

(Continued)

Sulindac *(Continued)*

Contraindications Hypersensitivity to sulindac, any component, aspirin, or other NSAIDs; active GI bleeding, ulcer disease; patients who have acute asthmatic attacks, urticaria, or rhinitis that are precipitated by aspirin or other NSAIDs; patients with the "aspirin triad" [asthma, rhinitis (with or without nasal polyps), and aspirin intolerance] (fatal asthmatic and anaphylactoid reactions may occur in these patients)

Warnings In April 2005, the FDA announced product labeling changes for all NSAIDs, including COX-2 selective and OTC medications; although revised product labeling is currently not available for all products, sample labeling and a template of the required medication guide are now available. Labels for prescription nonselective NSAIDs will contain a contraindication for use in patients who have recently undergone coronary artery bypass graft (CABG) surgery and a boxed warning concerning the potential for increased risk of cardiovascular (CV) events and GI bleeding associated with NSAID use. Patients at increased risk of adverse events include patients immediately post-operative from CABG surgery, and those with existing CAD, CVD, or history of TIA or stomach ulcers. Prescribers are encouraged to use the lowest effective NSAID dose for the shortest time based on individual patient treatment goals. Medication guides will be required for all prescription products. Complete details for the labeling update can be found on the following FDA website: http://www.fda.gov/medwatch/SAFETY/2005/safety05.htm#NSAID.

Precautions Use with caution in patients with peptic ulcer disease, GI bleeding, bleeding abnormalities, impaired renal or hepatic function, CHF, hypertension, and patients receiving anticoagulants

Adverse Reactions

Cardiovascular: Edema

Central nervous system: Dizziness, nervousness, headache

Dermatologic: Rash, pruritus

Gastrointestinal: Abdominal pain; GI bleeding, ulcer, perforation; nausea; vomiting; diarrhea; constipation

Hematologic: Thrombocytopenia, agranulocytosis, inhibition of platelet aggregation, bone marrow suppression

Hepatic: Hepatitis

Otic: Tinnitus

Renal: Renal impairment

Respiratory: Bronchospasm

Drug Interactions Cytochrome P450 isoenzyme CYP2C9 inhibitor

Sulindac may potentiate effects of warfarin; probenecid may increase serum concentration of sulindac; dimethyl sulfoxide or ASA may decrease sulindac serum concentration; sulindac may increase methotrexate serum concentrations and may increase cyclosporin nephrotoxicity; potassium supplements and other GI irritants may increase GI adverse effects; effects of antihypertensive agents, furosemide, thiazides may be decreased; drug interactions similar to other NSAIDs may also occur

Food Interactions Food may decrease rate and extent of absorption

Mechanism of Action Inhibits prostaglandin synthesis by decreasing the activity of the enzyme, cyclooxygenase, which results in decreased formation of prostaglandin precursors

Usual Dosage Oral:

Children: Limited information exists; some centers use the following: 2-4 mg/kg/day in 2 divided doses; maximum: 6 mg/kg/day; do not exceed 400 mg/day (Skeith, 1991; Giannini, 1995)

Adults: 150-200 mg twice daily; not to exceed 400 mg/day

Administration Oral: Administer with food or milk to decrease GI upset

Monitoring Parameters Liver enzymes, BUN, serum creatinine, CBC with differential, platelet count; periodic ophthalmologic exams with chronic use

Patient Information Avoid alcohol; may cause dizziness; do not take with aspirin

Dosage Forms Excipient information presented when available (limited, particularly for generics); consult specific product labeling.

Tablet: 150 mg, 200 mg

Clinoril®: 200 mg

References

Giannini EH and Cawkwell GD, "Drug Treatment in Children With Juvenile Rheumatoid Arthritis. Past, Present, and Future," *Pediatr Clin North Am*, 1995, 42(5):1099-125.

Skeith KJ and Jamali F, "Clinical Pharmacokinetics of Drugs Used in Juvenile Arthritis," *Clin Pharmacokinet*, 1991, 21(2):129-49.

♦ **Sulphafurazole** *see* SulfiSOXAZOLE *on page 1491*

Sumatriptan (SOO ma trip tan)

Medication Safety Issues

Sound-alike/look-alike issues:

Sumatriptan may be confused with somatropin, zolmitriptan

International issues:

Imitrex® may be confused with Nitrex® which is a brand name for isosorbide mononitrate in Italy

Related Information

Serotonin Syndrome *on page 1955*

U.S. Brand Names Imitrex®

Canadian Brand Names Apo-Sumatriptan®; CO Sumatriptan; Dom-Sumatriptan; Gen-Sumatriptan; Imitrex®; Imitrex® DF; Imitrex® Nasal Spray; Novo-Sumatriptan; PHL-Sumatriptan; PMS-Sumatriptan; ratio-Sumatriptan; Rhoxal-sumatriptan; Riva-Sumatriptan; Sandoz-Sumatriptan; Sumatryx

Index Terms Sumatriptan Succinate

Therapeutic Category Antimigraine Agent

Generic Available No

Use

Injection, intranasal, and tablets: Acute treatment of migraine with or without aura

Injection: Acute treatment of cluster headaches

Pregnancy Risk Factor C

Lactation Enters breast milk/use caution (AAP rates "compatible")

Contraindications Hypersensitivity to sumatriptan or any component; I.V. administration (coronary vasospasm may occur); ischemic heart disease, Prinzmetal angina, cerebrovascular or peripheral vascular syndromes (eg, stroke, TIA, ischemic bowel disease), severe hepatic impairment, patients with signs or symptoms of ischemic heart disease, MI, silent MI, uncontrolled hypertension; concomitant use of ergotamine derivatives (within last 24 hours), vasoconstrictive drugs, methysergide, or MAO inhibitors; use of MAO inhibitors within past 2 weeks; management of hemiplegic or basilar migraine

Warnings Life-threatening or fatal hypersensitivity reactions may occur; rarely, serious coronary events including acute MI, life-threatening arrhythmias, and death, may occur; avoid use in patients with risk factors for coronary artery disease, unless cardiovascular disease can be ruled out; consider administering first dose under close supervision to patients at high risk for coronary disease; EKG should be performed if angina-like symptoms occur; periodically evaluate cardiovascular system in patients with risk factors for coronary artery disease

Precautions Temporary increases in peripheral vascular resistance and blood pressure may occur; use with caution in patients with impaired hepatic or renal function, history of seizure disorder or conditions associated with a decrease in the seizure threshold; cross-hypersensitivity to sulfonamides is possible; other potentially serious neurological conditions should be ruled out prior to acute migraine therapy; sumatriptan (given at five times the maximum oral single dose) has caused corneal opacities in dogs; other animal studies suggest it may bind to the melanin of the eye; human studies are not available

Serious adverse effects, such as MI, stroke, visual loss, and death have been reported in pediatric patients after sumatriptan use by the oral, intranasal, and/or SubQ route; frequency of such adverse effects cannot currently be determined, thus the use of sumatriptan in patients <18 years of age is not recommended.

Adverse Reactions

Cardiovascular: Hypertension; flushing; chest tightness, pressure, pain; coronary artery vasospasm; vascular ischemia; colonic ischemia; rarely: acute MI, life-threatening arrhythmias

Central nervous system: Dizziness, drowsiness, headache; seizures (rare)

Gastrointestinal: Nausea, vomiting, abdominal discomfort; bad or unusual taste (with intranasal use)

Local: Injection site reaction (59%), pain, redness at injection site

Neuromuscular & skeletal: Weakness, myalgia, neck pain with stiffness

Miscellaneous: Atypical sensations of tingling, heat, flushing, burning, heaviness, pressure, tightness, numbness; jaw, mouth, tongue discomfort; diaphoresis; rarely: hypersensitivity reactions (potentially fatal anaphylaxis or anaphylactoid reactions)

Drug Interactions Use with ergot-containing drugs may result in prolonged vasospasm reactions; vasoconstrictive drugs; methysergide; MAO inhibitors (MAO inhibitors may significantly increase sumatriptan serum concentrations; use of MAO inhibitors is contraindicated); selective serotonin reuptake inhibitors (may cause weakness, incoordination, hyper-reflexia; monitor patients carefully)

Food Interactions Food slightly delays the rate but not the extent of oral absorption

Stability Store at 2°C to 20°C (36°F to 86°F); protect from light

(Continued)

Sumatriptan *(Continued)*

Mechanism of Action Selective agonist for serotonin (5-HT_1) receptor in cranial arteries; causes vasoconstriction and reduces sterile inflammation associated with antidromic neuronal transmission correlating with relief of migraine

Pharmacodynamics Migraine pain relief:

Onset of action:

Oral: 1-1.5 hours

SubQ: 10 minutes to 2 hours

Maximum effect: Oral: 2-4 hours

Pharmacokinetics

Distribution: Adults:

V_d (central): 50 L;

V_d (apparent): 2.4 L/kg

Protein binding: 14% to 21%

Metabolism: In the liver to an indole acetic acid metabolite (inactive) which then undergoes ester glucuronide conjugation; may be metabolized by monoamine oxidase (MAO)

Bioavailability:

Oral: ~15%; may be significantly increased with liver disease

Intranasal: 17% (compared to SubQ)

SubQ: 97%

Half-life:

Distribution: 15 minutes

Terminal: 2 hours; range: 1-4 hours

Time to peak serum concentration:

Oral: Healthy adults: 2 hours; during migraine attacks: 2.5 hours

SubQ: Range: 5-20 minutes; mean: 12 minutes

Elimination: 60% of an oral dose is renally excreted (primarily as metabolites), 40% is eliminated via the feces, and only 3% as unchanged drug; 42% of an intranasal dose is excreted as the indole acetic acid metabolite with 3% excreted in the urine unchanged; 22% of a SubQ dose is excreted in urine unchanged and 38% as the indole acetic acid metabolite

Usual Dosage

Children and Adolescents <18 years: Use not recommended (see Precautions):

Intranasal: Efficacy of intranasal sumatriptan was **not** established in 2 controlled clinical trials in migraine patients 12-17 years of age (n=1248) with doses of 5-20 mg; adverse events were similar to adults (see also Additional Information)

Oral: Efficacy of oral sumatriptan was **not** established in placebo-controlled trials in patients 12-17 years of age (n=701) with doses of 25-100 mg; adverse events were similar to adults; frequency of adverse events was dose- and age-dependent (increased frequency of adverse events in younger patients); postmarketing reports include the occurrence of MI in a 14-year-old male after oral sumatriptan with symptoms occurring within 1 day of drug use

SubQ: An open-labeled prospective trial in 17 children 6-16 years of age with juvenile migraine used SubQ doses of 6 mg in 15 children 30-70 kg, and 3 mg/dose in two children who weighed 22 kg and 30 kg (MacDonald, 1994); additional studies are needed

Adults:

Intranasal: Initial single dose: 5 mg, 10 mg, or 20 mg administered in one nostril, given as soon as possible after the onset of migraine; 10 mg dose may be administered as 5 mg in each nostril; may repeat after 2 hours; maximum: 40 mg/day

Oral: Initial single dose: 25 mg given as soon as possible after the onset of a migraine; range: 25-100 mg/dose; maximum single dose: 100 mg; may repeat after 2 hours; maximum: 200 mg/day

SubQ: 6 mg given as soon as possible after the onset of a migraine; a second injection (≤6 mg) may be administered at least 1 hour after the initial dose; maximum dose: 12 mg/24 hours

Dosing adjustment in hepatic dysfunction: Adults: Oral: Maximum single dose: 50 mg

Administration

Intranasal: Each nasal spray unit is preloaded with 1 dose; **do not** test the spray unit before use; remove unit from plastic pack when ready to use; while sitting down, gently blow nose to clear nasal passages; keep head upright and close one nostril gently with index finger; hold container with other hand, with thumb supporting bottom and index and middle fingers on either side of nozzle; insert nozzle into nostril about ½ inch; close mouth; take a breath through nose while releasing spray into nostril by pressing firmly on blue plunger; remove nozzle from nostril; keep head level for 10-20 seconds and gently breathe in through nose and out through mouth; **do not breathe deeply**

Oral: Administer with fluids

Parenteral: SubQ use only; do **not** administer I.M.; do **not** administer I.V. (may cause coronary vasospasm)

Patient Information If pain or tightness in chest or throat occurs, notify physician; females should avoid pregnancy; pain at injection site lasts <1 hour

Additional Information Safety of treating >4 headaches per month is not established; sumatriptan is **not** indicated for migraine prophylaxis

A randomized, double-blind, placebo-controlled, single-attack study in adolescent migraine patients (12-17 years of age) used sumatriptan nasal spray in doses of 5 mg (n=128), 10 mg (n=133), and 20 mg (n=118). Compared to placebo, the percent of patients with headache relief (reduction in headache pain) at 1 hour postdose was significantly greater for the 10 mg and 20 mg group and at 2 hours postdose was significantly greater for the 5 mg group. The percent of patients with **complete** headache relief at 2 hours was significantly greater for the 20 mg group. Younger patients (12-14 years of age) had higher efficacy rates at lower doses, but patients 15-17 years of age had the highest efficacy with the 20 mg doses (Winner, 2000); a small retrospective review of 10 younger children, 5-12 years of age (mean: 9.9 years) used intranasal doses of 5 mg (n=2) or 20 mg (n=8) to treat 57 headaches; 82.5% of headaches responded to sumatriptan (Hershey, 2001); additional studies are needed

Dosage Forms Excipient information presented when available (limited, particularly for generics); consult specific product labeling. **Note:** Strength expressed as sumatriptan base

Injection, solution, as succinate: 8 mg/mL (0.5 mL) [disposable cartridge for use with STATdose System®]; 12 mg/mL (0.5 mL) [disposable cartridge for use with STATdose System® or vial]

Solution, intranasal spray: 5 mg (100 µL unit dose spray device); 20 mg (100 µL unit dose spray device)

Tablet, as succinate: 25 mg, 50 mg, 100 mg

Extemporaneous Preparations A 5 mg/mL oral liquid preparation made from tablets and 3 different vehicles (Ora-Sweet®, Ora-Sweet® SF, or Syrpalta® syrups) was stable for 21 days when stored in amber glass bottles in the dark under refrigeration (4°C); **Note:** Preparations with Ora-Sweet® and Ora-Sweet® SF used Ora-Plus® as a suspending vehicle; grind nine 100 mg tablets in a mortar into a fine powder; add 40 mL of Ora-Plus® Suspending Vehicle, 5 mL at a time, and mix thoroughly between each addition; **Note:** The suspending vehicle helps to facilitate dispersion of the tablets and is used only if Ora-Sweet® or Ora-Sweet® SF is the vehicle to be used (ie, suspending vehicle is not used if preparation uses Syrpalta® syrup as the vehicle); transfer to a calibrated amber glass bottle; rinse mortar and pestle 5 times with 10 mL of Ora-Plus® suspension vehicle pouring into bottle each time; qsad with appropriate syrup (Ora-Sweet® or Ora-Sweet® SF) to 180 mL; label "shake well," "refrigerate," and "protect from light"; (**Note:** This study also tested microbial growth on days 0 and 28; no growth of bacteria or fungus occurred) (Fish, 1997)

Fish DN, Beall HD, Goodwin SD, et al, "Stability of Sumatriptan Succinate in Extemporaneously Prepared Oral Liquids," *Am J Health Syst Pharm*, 1997, 54(14):1619-22.

References

Hershey AD, Powers SW, LeCates S, et al, "Effectiveness of Nasal Sumatriptan in 5- to 12-Year-Old Children," *Headache*, 2001, 41(7):693-7.

MacDonald JT, "Treatment of Juvenile Migraine With Subcutaneous Sumatriptan," *Headache*, 1994, 34(10):581-2.

Scott AK, "Sumatriptan Clinical Pharmacokinetics," *Clin Pharmacokinet*, 1994, 27(5):337-44.

Winner P, Rothner AD, Saper J, et al, "A Randomized, Double-Blind, Placebo-Controlled Study of Sumatriptan Nasal Spray in the Treatment of Acute Migraine in Adolescents," *Pediatrics*, 2000, 106(5):989-97.

♦ **Sumatriptan Succinate** *see* Sumatriptan *on page 1495*

♦ **Sumatryx (Can)** *see* Sumatriptan *on page 1495*

♦ **Summer's Eve® SpecialCare™ Medicated Anti-Itch Cream [OTC]** *see* Hydrocortisone *on page 781*

♦ **Sumycin® [DSC]** *see* Tetracycline *on page 1518*

♦ **Superdophilus® [OTC]** *see Lactobacillus acidophilus* and *Lactobacillus bulgaricus on page 898*

♦ **Supeudol® (Can)** *see* Oxycodone *on page 1189*

♦ **Suprax®** *see* Cefixime *on page 308*

♦ **Surfak® [OTC]** *see* Docusate *on page 526*

♦ **Survanta®** *see* Beractant *on page 210*

♦ **Sustiva®** *see* Efavirenz *on page 558*

♦ **Su-Tuss DM** *see* Guaifenesin and Dextromethorphan *on page 748*

♦ **Suxamethonium Chloride** *see* Succinylcholine *on page 1479*

♦ **Symax SL** *see* Hyoscyamine *on page 798*

♦ **Symax SR** *see* Hyoscyamine *on page 798*

- ♦ **Symmetrel®** *see* Amantadine *on page 89*
- ♦ **Synacthen** *see* Cosyntropin *on page 405*
- ♦ **Synagis®** *see* Palivizumab *on page 1198*
- ♦ **Synalar®** *see* Fluocinolone *on page 672*
- ♦ **Syn-Diltiazem® (Can)** *see* Diltiazem *on page 503*
- ♦ **Synercid®** *see* Quinupristin/Dalfopristin *on page 1360*
- ♦ **Synthroid®** *see* Levothyroxine *on page 930*
- ♦ **Syrex** *see* Sodium Chloride *on page 1450*
- ♦ **Syrup of Ipecac** *see* Ipecac Syrup *on page 862*
- ♦ **T_3 Sodium (error-prone abbreviation)** *see* Liothyronine *on page 943*
- ♦ **T_4** *see* Levothyroxine *on page 930*
- ♦ **T-20** *see* Enfuvirtide *on page 569*
- ♦ **642® Tablet (Can)** *see* Propoxyphene *on page 1334*
- ♦ **Tabloid®** *see* Thioguanine *on page 1527*

Tacrolimus (ta KROE li mus)

Medication Safety Issues

Sound-alike/look-alike issues:

Prograf® may be confused with Gengraf®

U.S. Brand Names Prograf®; Protopic®

Canadian Brand Names Prograf®; Protopic®

Index Terms FK506

Therapeutic Category Immunosuppressant Agent

Generic Available No

Use

Oral/injection: Immunosuppressant used with corticosteroids to prevent graft versus host disease in patients who have received organ transplants and are not responding to cyclosporine

Topical: Second-line agent for short-term and intermittent treatment of moderate to severe atopic dermatitis in nonimmunocompromised patients not responsive to conventional therapy or when conventional therapy is not appropriate

Medication Guide An FDA-approved patient medication guide, which is available with the product information and at http://www.fda.gov/cder/Offices/ODS/medication_guides.htm, must be dispensed with this medication for each new outpatient prescription and refill.

Pregnancy Risk Factor C

Lactation Enters breast milk/contraindicated

Contraindications Hypersensitivity to tacrolimus, polyoxyl 60 hydrogenated castor oil, or any component

Warnings Avoid use with other immunosuppressants; immunosuppression with tacrolimus may result in increased susceptibility to infection and the possible development of lymphoma; insulin-dependent post-transplant diabetes mellitus was reported in 11% to 20% of transplant patients; risk increases in African-American and Hispanic kidney transplant patients. Neurotoxicity and nephrotoxicity have been reported especially when used in high doses. To avoid excess nephrotoxicity, do not administer simultaneously with cyclosporine. Adequate airway, supportive measures, and agents for treating anaphylaxis should be available when tacrolimus is administered I.V.

Precautions Use with caution and modify dosage in patients with hepatic or renal impairment

Adverse Reactions

Cardiovascular: Hypertension, hypotension, peripheral edema, chest pain, myocardial hypertrophy, angina pectoris, palpitations, CHF, arrhythmias, hypertrophic obstructive cardiomyopathy, thrombosis

Central nervous system: Encephalopathy, headache, hallucinations, agitation, pain, fever, seizures, altered mental status, insomnia, dizziness, depression

Dermatologic: Pruritus, rash, Stevens-Johnson syndrome, photosensitivity, skin cancer

Endocrine & metabolic: Hyperkalemia, hyperglycemia, hypomagnesemia, hypophosphatemia, hypercalcemia, hypercholesterolemia, Cushing's syndrome

Gastrointestinal: Diarrhea, nausea, vomiting, constipation, dyspepsia, pancreatitis, GI hemorrhage

Genitourinary: Dysuria, hematuria, albuminuria, nocturia, cystitis, oliguria

Hematologic: Anemia, thrombocytopenia, leukocytosis, eosinophilia

Hepatic: Hepatotoxicity; elevated AST, ALT, and LDH

Neuromuscular & skeletal: Tremor, paresthesia, back pain, arthralgia, myalgia

Ocular: Abnormal vision

Otic: Tinnitus, deafness

Renal: Nephrotoxicity, elevated BUN and serum creatinine, oliguria

Respiratory: Pleural effusion, respiratory distress, cough

Miscellaneous: Increased susceptibility to infections, lymphoproliferative disorders, anaphylaxis (may be due to polyoxyl 60 hydrogenated castor oil injectable vehicle), hemolytic-uremic syndrome

Topical:

Cardiovascular: Peripheral edema

Central nervous system: Headache, fever, hyperesthesia, pain

Dermatologic: Skin burning, pruritus, erythema, acne, urticaria, rash, skin cancer

Endocrine & metabolic: Dysmenorrhea

Gastrointestinal: Diarrhea, abdominal pain, nausea

Respiratory: Cough, rhinitis

Miscellaneous: Lymphoma

Drug Interactions Cytochrome P450 isoenzyme CYP3A3/4 substrate

Diltiazem, verapamil, nifedipine, fluconazole, itraconazole, ketoconazole, cimetidine, clarithromycin, erythromycin, methylprednisolone, omeprazole, nefazodone, cisapride, protease inhibitors, metoclopramide, cyclosporine, and oral clotrimazole increase tacrolimus serum concentrations; antacids, cholestyramine, sodium polystyrene sulfonate, carbamazepine, phenobarbital, primidone, phenytoin, rifabutin, rifampin, and St John's wort decrease tacrolimus serum concentrations; additive nephrotoxicity when used with NSAIDs, cisplatin, nephrotoxic antibiotics, amphotericin B, or cyclosporine

Food Interactions Food reduces the rate and extent of absorption by ~27%; grapefruit juice may increase tacrolimus blood concentration

Stability Reconstitution: Stable for 24 hours when mixed in D_5W or NS in glass or polyolefin containers; 24-hour stability in plastic syringes stored at 24°C; no need to protect from light; do not store in polyvinyl chloride containers since the polyoxyl 60 hydrogenated castor oil injectable vehicle may leach phthalates from polyvinyl chloride containers; polyvinyl-containing administration sets adsorb drug and may lead to a lower dose being delivered to the patient; tacrolimus is unstable in alkaline media; do not mix with acyclovir or ganciclovir

Mechanism of Action Binds to an intracellular protein forming a complex which inhibits phosphatase activity of calcineurin resulting in the inhibition of T-cell activation

Pharmacokinetics

Absorption: Erratic and incomplete oral absorption (5% to 67%)

Distribution: Distributes to erythrocytes, breast milk, lung, kidneys, pancreas, liver, placenta, heart, and spleen; V_d: 5-65 L/kg (V_d is increased in pediatric patients versus adults)

Protein binding: 99% to alpha-acid glycoprotein (some binding to albumin)

Metabolism: Hepatic metabolism through the cytochrome P450 system (CYP3A) to eight possible metabolites (major metabolite: 31-demethyl tacrolimus has same activity as tacrolimus *in vitro*)

Bioavailability:

Oral:

Children: 10% to 52%

Adults: 7% to 28%

Topical: <0.5%

Half-life, elimination: 3.5-40.5 hours (mean: 8.7 hours)

Time to peak serum concentration: Oral: 1-4 hours

Elimination: Primarily in bile; <1% excreted unchanged in urine

Clearance: 7-103 mL/minute/kg (average: 30 mL/minute/kg); clearance may be higher in children

Usual Dosage

Children:

Oral: 0.15-0.4 mg/kg/day divided every 12 hours; children generally require higher maintenance dosages on a mg/kg basis than adults

Liver transplant: Initial: 0.15-0.2 mg/kg/day divided every 12 hours

I.V. continuous infusion: 0.03-0.15 mg/kg/day

Children ≥2 years: Topical: Moderate to severe atopic dermatitis: Apply 0.03% ointment to affected area twice daily; continue applications for 1 week after symptoms have cleared

Adults:

Oral: 0.15-0.3 mg/kg/day divided every 12 hours

Liver transplant: Initial: 0.1-0.15 mg/kg/day divided every 12 hours

Kidney transplant: Initial: 0.2 mg/kg/day divided every 12 hours

I.V. continuous infusion: 0.03-0.1 mg/kg/day

(Continued)

Tacrolimus *(Continued)*

Dosing adjustment in renal or hepatic impairment: Patients with renal or hepatic impairment should receive the lowest dose in the recommended dosage range; further reductions in dose below these ranges may be required

Hemodialysis: Not removed by hemodialysis

Administration

Oral: Administer on an empty stomach; use oral syringe or glass container (not plastic or foam cup) when administering this medication; do not administer with grapefruit juice; do not administer within 2 hours before or after antacids

Parenteral: May administer by I.V. continuous infusion; I.V. concentrate for injection must be diluted to 0.004-0.02 mg/mL in NS or D_5W prior to administration; PVC-free administration tubing should be used to minimize the potential for significant drug absorption onto the tubing; begin no sooner than 6-hours post-transplant; continue only until oral medication can be tolerated

Topical: For external use only; do not cover with occlusive dressings; apply thin layer and rub ointment in gently and completely onto clean, dry skin

Monitoring Parameters Liver enzymes, BUN, serum creatinine, glucose, potassium, magnesium, phosphorus, blood tacrolimus concentrations, CBC with differential; blood pressure, neurologic status, EKG

Reference Range Limited data correlating serum level to therapeutic efficacy/toxicity:

Trough (whole blood ELISA): 5-20 ng/mL

Trough (HPLC): 0.5-1.5 ng/mL

Patient Information Administer dose at the same time each day; you will be susceptible to infection (avoid crowds and people with infections); notify physician if you develop increased urination, thirst, chest pain, acute headache or dizziness, symptoms of respiratory infection, rash, unusual bruising or bleeding. May cause photosensitivity reactions (eg, exposure to sunlight may cause severe sunburn, skin rash, redness, or itching); avoid exposure to sunlight and artificial light sources (sunlamps, tanning booth/bed); wear protective clothing, wide-brimmed hats, sunglasses, and lip sunscreen (SPF ≥15); use a sunscreen [broad-spectrum sunscreen or physical sunscreen (preferred) or sunblock with SPF ≥15]; contact physician if reaction occurs.

Nursing Implications Patients receiving I.V. tacrolimus should be under continuous observation for at least the first 30 minutes following dosage initiation; adequate airway, supportive measures, and agents for treating anaphylaxis should be available when tacrolimus is administered I.V.

Additional Information Tacrolimus should be initiated no sooner than 6 hours after transplant; convert I.V. tacrolimus to oral form as soon as possible or within 2-3 days (the oral formulation should be started 8-12 hours after stopping the I.V. infusion); when switching a patient from cyclosporine to tacrolimus, allow at least 24 hours after discontinuing cyclosporine before initiating tacrolimus therapy to minimize the risk of nephrotoxicity

Additional dosing considerations:

Switch from I.V. to oral therapy: Approximately three-fold increase in dose compared to I.V.

Pediatric patients: Approximately two times higher dose compared to adults

Dosage Forms Excipient information presented when available (limited, particularly for generics); consult specific product labeling.

Capsule (Prograf®): 0.5 mg, 1 mg, 5 mg

Injection, solution (Prograf®): 5 mg/mL (1 mL) [contains dehydrated alcohol 80% and polyoxyl 60 hydrogenated castor oil]

Ointment, topical (Protopic®): 0.03% (30 g, 60 g, 100 g); 0.1% (30 g, 60 g, 100 g)

Extemporaneous Preparations A 0.5 mg/mL suspension has been prepared by mixing the contents of six 5 mg tacrolimus capsules with equal amounts of Ora-Plus® and Simple Syrup, NF to make a final volume of 60 mL. When compounding tacrolimus oral suspension, protect hands with latex gloves. The suspension is stable for 56 days when stored at room temperature in either glass or plastic amber prescription bottles. Label "shake well before using."

Jacobson PA, Johnson CE, West NJ, et al, "Stability of Tacrolimus in an Extemporaneously Compounded Oral Liquid," *Am J Health Sys Pharm*, 1997, 54(2):178-80.

References

Asante-Korang A, Boyle GJ, Webber SA, et al, "Experience of FK506 Immune Suppression in Pediatric Heart Transplantation: A Study of Long-Term Adverse Effects," *J Heart Lung Transplant*, 1996, 15(4):415-22.

McDiarmid SV, Colonna JO, Shaked A, et al, "Differences in Oral FK506 Dose Requirements Between Adults and Pediatric Liver Transplant Patients," *Transplantation*, 1993, 55(6):1328-32.

Menegaux F, Keeffe EB, Andrews BT, et al, "Neurological Complications of Liver Transplantation in Adult Versus Pediatric Patients," *Transplantation*, 1994, 58(4):447-50.

♦ **Tagamet® [DSC]** *see* Cimetidine *on page 355*

♦ **Tagamet® HB (Can)** *see* Cimetidine *on page 355*

- ♦ **Tagamet® HB 200 [OTC]** *see* Cimetidine *on page 355*
- ♦ **Talwin®** *see* Pentazocine *on page 1237*
- ♦ **Talwin® NX** *see* Pentazocine *on page 1237*
- ♦ **Tambocor™** *see* Flecainide *on page 657*
- ♦ **Tamiflu®** *see* Oseltamivir *on page 1176*
- ♦ **Tanac® [OTC]** *see* Benzocaine *on page 204*
- ♦ **Tanta-Orciprenaline® (Can)** *see* Metaproterenol *on page 1014*
- ♦ **TAP-144** *see* Leuprolide *on page 918*
- ♦ **Tapazole®** *see* Methimazole *on page 1022*
- ♦ **Targel® (Can)** *see* Coal Tar *on page 394*
- ♦ **Taro-Carbamazepine Chewable (Can)** *see* Carbamazepine *on page 279*
- ♦ **Taro-Ciprofloxacin (Can)** *see* Ciprofloxacin *on page 357*
- ♦ **Taro-Clindamycin (Can)** *see* Clindamycin *on page 379*
- ♦ **Taro-Clobetasol (Can)** *see* Clobetasol *on page 383*
- ♦ **Taro-Mometasone (Can)** *see* Mometasone Furoate *on page 1076*
- ♦ **Taro-Simvastatin (Can)** *see* Simvastatin *on page 1441*
- ♦ **Taro-Sone® (Can)** *see* Betamethasone *on page 212*
- ♦ **Taro-Warfarin (Can)** *see* Warfarin *on page 1626*
- ♦ **Tavist® Allergy [OTC]** *see* Clemastine *on page 378*
- ♦ **Tavist® ND [OTC]** *see* Loratadine *on page 959*
- ♦ **Taxol®** *see* Paclitaxel *on page 1196*

Tazarotene (taz AR oh teen)

U.S. Brand Names Avage™; Tazorac®

Canadian Brand Names Tazorac®

Therapeutic Category Acne Products; Keratolytic Agent

Generic Available No

Use Topical treatment of facial acne vulgaris; topical treatment of stable plaque psoriasis of up to 20% body surface area involvement; mitigation (palliation) of facial skin wrinkling, facial mottled hyper/hypopigmentation, and benign facial lentigines

Pregnancy Risk Factor X

Lactation Excretion in breast milk unknown/use caution

Contraindications Hypersensitivity to tazarotene, other retinoids, or vitamin A derivatives (eg, isotretinoin, tretinoin), or any component; pregnancy; use in women of childbearing potential who are unable to comply with birth control requirements; sunburn

Warnings Retinoids should not be used on eczematous skin as they may cause severe irritation; may cause photosensitivity; avoid excessive exposure to sunlight or sunlamps; women of childbearing potential should use adequate birth control measures; a negative pregnancy test within 2 weeks prior to beginning treatment is recommended; begin treatment during a normal menstrual period

Precautions Administer with caution to patients receiving medications known to be photosensitizing (see Drug Interactions) as they may potentiate photosensitivity reactions

Adverse Reactions Dermatologic: Pruritus, burning/stinging, erythema, worsening of psoriasis, irritation, skin pain, rash, desquamation, irritant contact dermatitis, skin inflammation, dry skin, skin fissures, localized edema, skin discoloration

Drug Interactions Photosensitizing medications (thiazides, tetracyclines, fluoroquinolones, phenothiazines, sulfonamides) may increase risk of photosensitivity reactions; medications with strong drying effects (sulfur, benzoyl peroxide, salicylic acid, resorcinol) which may potentiate adverse skin effects

Stability Store at room temperature

Mechanism of Action A retinoid prodrug which is converted to its active form by rapid de-esterification; its mechanism of action for treatment of acne and psoriasis is not well defined

Pharmacodynamics

Onset of action: Psoriasis: 1 week

Duration: Psoriasis: Up to 12 weeks after discontinuation when initially treated for 2-3 months (duration may be less if initial treatment was shorter)

Pharmacokinetics

Absorption (without occlusion): Adults: Psoriatic patients: <1%; normal controls: <5%

Protein binding: Metabolite: >99%

Metabolism: Following topical application, undergoes esterase hydrolysis to form its active metabolite, AGN 190299

Half-life: Metabolite: 18 hours

Excretion: Urine and feces as metabolites

(Continued)

Tazarotene *(Continued)*

Usual Dosage Topical:

Acne vulgaris: Children ≥12 years and Adults: Tazorac®: 0.1% cream or gel applied as a thin film (2 mg/cm^2) to affected areas once daily in the evening

Psoriasis: Children ≥12 years and Adults: Tazorac®: 0.05% to 0.1% cream or gel applied as a thin film (2 mg/cm^2) to affected area once daily in the evening; apply to no more than 20% of the body surface area

Palliation of fine facial wrinkles, facial mottled hyper/hypopigmentation, benign facial lentigines: Adolescents ≥17 years and Adults: Avage™: Apply a pea-sized amount once daily at bedtime; lightly cover entire face including eyelids if desired

Administration Topical: Apply thin film to affected areas; avoid eyes and mouth; skin should be dry before applying

Monitoring Parameters Disease severity in plaque psoriasis (reduction in erythema, scaling, induration); pregnancy test prior to treatment of females of childbearing age

Patient Information May cause photosensitivity reactions (eg, exposure to sunlight may cause severe sunburn, skin rash, redness, or itching); avoid exposure to sunlight and artificial light sources (sunlamps, tanning booth/bed); wear protective clothing, wide-brimmed hats, sunglasses, and lip sunscreen (SPF ≥15); use a sunscreen [broad-spectrum sunscreen or physical sunscreen(preferred) or sunblock with SPF ≥15]; contact physician if reaction occurs. Avoid washing face more frequently than 2-3 times/day; avoid using topical preparations with high alcoholic content during treatment period.

Dosage Forms Excipient information presented when available (limited, particularly for generics); consult specific product labeling.

Cream:

Avage™: 0.1% (30 g) [contains benzyl alcohol]

Tazorac®: 0.05% (30 g, 60 g); 0.1% (30 g, 60 g) [contains benzyl alcohol]

Gel (Tazorac®): 0.05% (30 g, 100 g); 0.1% (30 g, 100 g) [contains benzyl alcohol]

- ♦ **Tazicef®** *see* Ceftazidime *on page 317*
- ♦ **Tazobactam and Piperacillin** *see* Piperacillin and Tazobactam *on page 1264*
- ♦ **Tazocin® (Can)** *see* Piperacillin and Tazobactam *on page 1264*
- ♦ **Tazorac®** *see* Tazarotene *on page 1501*
- ♦ **Taztia XT™** *see* Diltiazem *on page 503*
- ♦ **3TC** *see* Lamivudine *on page 901*
- ♦ **3TC® (Can)** *see* Lamivudine *on page 901*
- ♦ **3TC, Abacavir, and AZT** *see* Abacavir, Lamivudine, and Zidovudine *on page 38*
- ♦ **3TC, Abacavir, and ZDV** *see* Abacavir, Lamivudine, and Zidovudine *on page 38*
- ♦ **3TC, Abacavir, and Zidovudine** *see* Abacavir, Lamivudine, and Zidovudine *on page 38*
- ♦ **3TC, ABC, and AZT** *see* Abacavir, Lamivudine, and Zidovudine *on page 38*
- ♦ **3TC, ABC, and ZDV** *see* Abacavir, Lamivudine, and Zidovudine *on page 38*
- ♦ **3TC and Abacavir** *see* Abacavir and Lamivudine *on page 35*
- ♦ **3TC and ABC** *see* Abacavir and Lamivudine *on page 35*
- ♦ **3TC and AZT** *see* Lamivudine and Zidovudine *on page 904*
- ♦ **3TC and ZDV** *see* Lamivudine and Zidovudine *on page 904*
- ♦ **T-Cell Growth Factor** *see* Aldesleukin *on page 70*
- ♦ **TCGF** *see* Aldesleukin *on page 70*
- ♦ **TCN** *see* Tetracycline *on page 1518*
- ♦ **Td** *see* Diphtheria and Tetanus Toxoid *on page 514*
- ♦ **Td Adsorbed (Can)** *see* Diphtheria and Tetanus Toxoid *on page 514*
- ♦ **Tdap** *see* Diphtheria, Tetanus Toxoids, and Acellular Pertussis Vaccine *on page 517*
- ♦ **TDF** *see* Tenofovir *on page 1506*
- ♦ **Tebrazid™ (Can)** *see* Pyrazinamide *on page 1350*
- ♦ **Tegretol®** *see* Carbamazepine *on page 279*
- ♦ **Tegretol®-XR** *see* Carbamazepine *on page 279*
- ♦ **Teldrin® HBP [OTC]** *see* Chlorpheniramine *on page 344*
- ♦ **Telzir® (Can)** *see* Fosamprenavir *on page 705*
- ♦ **Temodal® (Can)** *see* Temozolomide *on page 1503*
- ♦ **Temodar®** *see* Temozolomide *on page 1503*
- ♦ **Temovate®** *see* Clobetasol *on page 383*
- ♦ **Temovate E®** *see* Clobetasol *on page 383*

Temozolomide (te mo ZOLE oh mide)

Medication Safety Issues

High alert medication: The Institute for Safe Medication Practices (ISMP) includes this medication among its list of drugs which have a heightened risk of causing significant patient harm when used in error.

U.S. Brand Names Temodar®

Canadian Brand Names Temodal®; Temodar®

Index Terms NSC-362856; TMZ

Therapeutic Category Antineoplastic Agent, Alkylating Agent

Generic Available No

Use Treatment of refractory anaplastic astrocytoma with relapse after initial therapy with a nitrosourea and procarbazine; active against primary and recurrent grade 3 and 4 gliomas and metastatic melanoma

Pregnancy Risk Factor D

Lactation Excretion in breast milk unknown/not recommended

Contraindications Hypersensitivity to temozolomide, dacarbazine, or any component; pregnancy

Warnings The FDA currently recommends that procedures for proper handling and disposal of antineoplastic agents be considered. Thrombocytopenia and neutropenia are dose-limiting toxicities which occur late in the treatment cycle and usually resolve within 14 days; prior to therapy initiation patients must have an absolute neutrophil count (ANC) $\geq 1.5 \times 10^9$ and a platelet count $\geq 100 \times 10^9$/L; obtain a CBC on day 22 and weekly until the ANC $>1.5 \times 10^9$ and platelet count $>100 \times 10^9$; may cause fetal harm so pregnancy should be avoided during therapy

Precautions Use with caution in patients with severe renal or hepatic impairment; since it is unknown whether temozolomide is excreted in breast milk, patients receiving temozolomide should discontinue nursing

Adverse Reactions

Cardiovascular: Peripheral edema, thromboembolism

Central nervous system: Headache, dizziness, fatigue, anxiety, confusion, depression, amnesia, insomnia, convulsions, hemiparesis, lethargy, fever

Dermatologic: Rash, pruritus, alopecia, erythema multiforme (rare)

Gastrointestinal: Nausea, vomiting, anorexia, diarrhea, abdominal pain, constipation, mucositis, dysphagia

Genitourinary: Urinary tract infection, urinary frequency

Hematologic: Thrombocytopenia, leukopenia, anemia, lymphopenia, neutropenia

Hepatic: Hepatotoxicity, elevated liver enzymes

Neuromuscular & skeletal: Myalgia, ataxia

Ocular: Diplopia, visual changes

Miscellaneous: Secondary tumors or malignancy, anaphylaxis (rare), opportunistic infections

Drug Interactions Valproic acid may decrease temozolomide clearance by 5%

Food Interactions Food reduces the rate and extent of absorption

Stability Store capsules at room temperature.

Mechanism of Action Prodrug which is hydrolyzed to MTIC and exerts its effect by site-specific DNA cross-linking resulting from the methylation of the O^6 and N^7 positions of guanine.

Pharmacokinetics

Absorption: Oral: Rapidly and completely absorbed

Distribution: Penetrates CNS at ~30% of plasma levels

V_d: Adults: 17-28 L/m^2

Protein binding: 14%

Bioavailability: 100%

Metabolism: At a neutral or alkaline pH, hydrolyzes to active MTIC (3-methyl-(triazen-1-yl) imidazole-4-carboxamide) and temozolomide acid metabolite; MTIC is further metabolized to 5-amino-imidazole-4-carboxamide (AIC) and methylhydrazine (active alkylating agent)

Half-life:

Children: 1.7 hours

Adults: 1.6-1.8 hours

Time to peak serum concentration: Oral: 1 hour; 2.3 hours after high fat meal

Elimination: <1% excreted in feces; 5% to 7% of unchanged temozolomide excreted renally

Clearance: 5.5 L/hour/m^2; women have a ~5% lower clearance than men (adjusted for body surface area); children 3-17 years have similar temozolomide clearance as adults

Usual Dosage Oral (refer to individual protocols):

Children: 160-200 mg/m^2 once daily for 5 days every 28 days

(Continued)

Temozolomide *(Continued)*

In a Phase I study to determine the maximum tolerated dose of temozolomide in pediatric solid tumor patients with prior craniospinal irradiation (CSI) therapy and those without prior CSI (n=53; age range: 1-19 years), 100-240 mg/m²/day was administered; the maximum tolerated dose was 215 mg/m²/day for 5 days in patients without prior CSI and 180 mg/m²/day for 5 days in patients with prior CSI with subsequent courses to begin on day 28 (Nicholson, 1998)

Adults: Initial: 150 mg/m²/day for 5 consecutive days of a 28-day cycle; subsequent doses are adjusted based on nadir platelet count and ANC during the previous cycle (day 22) and ANC and platelet count on day 29; treatment cycle should be held until ANC >1500/microliter and platelet count >100,000/microliter

Minimum dose: 100 mg/m²/day once daily for 5 days every 4 weeks; maintenance dose: 200 mg/m²/day once daily for 5 days every 4 weeks; treatment can be continued until there is disease progression, but optimum duration of therapy is unknown

Dose modification:

If ANC <1000/microliter or the platelet count is <50,000/microliter, postpone therapy until ANC >1500/microliter and platelet count >100,000/microliter; reduce dose by 50 mg/m² for subsequent cycle.

If ANC 1000-1500/microliter or platelets 50,000-100,000/microliter, postpone therapy until ANC >1500/microliter and platelet count >100,000/microliter; maintain initial dose.

If ANC >1500/microliter and platelet count >100,000/microliter, increase dose to, or maintain dose at 200 mg/m²/day for 5 days for subsequent cycle.

Administration Oral: Swallow capsule intact with a glass of water; do not chew; if patient is unable to swallow capsule, open capsule and dissolve in apple juice or applesauce taking precautions to avoid exposure to the cytotoxic agent; administer on an empty stomach to reduce the incidence of nausea and vomiting; may administer with food as long as food intake and administration time are performed in a consistent manner to ensure consistent bioavailability; bedtime administration may be preferred

Monitoring Parameters CBC with ANC (absolute neutrophil count) and platelet count

Patient Information Instruct patient to take all the capsules in a single dose package for that day of the cycle (each day's dose is packaged separately); advise women and men to avoid pregnancy

Nursing Implications Avoid opening capsules; if capsules are accidentally opened, avoid inhalation or contact with skin or mucous membranes

Additional Information To minimize the risk of a wrong dose error, each day's dose should be packaged separately and labeled as day 1, day 2, day 3, day 4, and day 5.

Dosage Forms Excipient information presented when available (limited, particularly for generics); consult specific product labeling.

Capsule:

Temodar®: 5 mg, 20 mg, 100 mg, 140 mg, 180 mg, 250 mg

References

Friedman HS, Kerby T, and Calvert H, "Temozolomide and Treatment of Malignant Glioma," *Clin Cancer Res*, 2000, 6(7):2585-97.

Loh KC, Willert J, Meltzer H, et al, "Temozolomide and Radiation for Aggressive Pediatric Central Nervous System Malignancies," *J Pediatr Hematol Oncol*, 2005, 27(5):254-8.

Middleton MR, Grob JJ, Aaronson N, et al, "Randomized Phase III Study of Temozolomide Versus Dacarbazine in the Treatment of Patients With Advanced Metastatic Malignant Melanoma," *J Clin Oncol*, 2000, 18(1):158-66.

Nicholson HS, Krailo M, Ames MM, et al, "Phase I Study of Temozolomide in Children and Adolescents With Recurrent Solid Tumors: A Report From the Children's Cancer Group," *J Clin Oncol*, 1998, 16(9):3037-43.

♦ **Tempra® (Can)** *see* Acetaminophen *on page 42*

Teniposide (ten i POE side)

Medication Safety Issues

Sound-alike/look-alike issues:

Teniposide may be confused with etoposide

High alert medication: The Institute for Safe Medication Practices (ISMP) includes this medication among its list of drugs which have a heightened risk of causing significant patient harm when used in error.

U.S. Brand Names Vumon®

Canadian Brand Names Vumon®

Index Terms EPT; VM-26

Therapeutic Category Antineoplastic Agent, Miscellaneous

Generic Available No

Use Treatment of acute lymphoblastic leukemia refractory to induction with other therapy; treatment of neuroblastoma, small cell lung cancer, non-Hodgkin's lymphoma

Pregnancy Risk Factor D

Lactation Not recommended

Contraindications Hypersensitivity to teniposide, polyoxyethylated castor oil, or any component

Warnings The FDA currently recommends that procedures for proper handling and disposal of antineoplastic agents be considered. Teniposide should be administered under the supervision of a physician experienced in the use of cancer chemotherapy agents. Severe, dose-related myelosuppression with resulting infection or bleeding may occur. Hypersensitivity reactions, including anaphylaxis-like reactions have been reported with initial dosing or with repeated dosing; risk for hypersensitivity reactions appears to increase with previous reactions and in patients with neuroblastoma or brain tumors; medications for treatment of hypersensitivity reactions (epinephrine, I.V. fluids, corticosteroids, and antihistamines) must be readily available for use in case of a reaction.

Teniposide injection contains benzyl alcohol which may cause allergic reactions in susceptible individuals; large amounts of benzyl alcohol (≥99 mg/kg/day) have been associated with a potentially fatal toxicity ("gasping syndrome") in neonates; use teniposide injection with caution in neonates. The injection contains polyoxyl 35 castor oil which may cause hypotension and increase the frequency of hypersensitivity reactions. If hypotension occurs during administration, discontinue infusion and administer I.V. fluids and supportive therapy as needed. The teniposide formulation contains ~43% alcohol and may contribute to adverse effects such as CNS depression, somnolence, lethargy, hypotension, and metabolic acidosis. Teniposide may cause local tissue necrosis or thrombophlebitis if extravasation occurs. Teniposide is a potential carcinogen; may cause fetal harm when administered to pregnant women; may induce a secondary leukemia.

Precautions Use with caution in patients with hepatic impairment; use with caution and adjust dosage in patients with Down's syndrome who may be more sensitive to myelosuppressive effects of teniposide

Adverse Reactions

Cardiovascular: Hypotension (associated with rapid infusions <30 minutes), hypertension, tachycardia, flushing

Central nervous system: Somnolence, chills, fever, lethargy

Dermatologic: Alopecia, rash

Endocrine & metabolic: Metabolic acidosis

Gastrointestinal: Mucositis, diarrhea, nausea, vomiting, anorexia

Hematologic: Myelosuppression, leukopenia, neutropenia, thrombocytopenia, anemia

Hepatic: Hepatic impairment

Local: Thrombophlebitis, tissue necrosis upon extravasation

Neuromuscular & skeletal: Peripheral neuropathy

Renal: Renal impairment

Respiratory: Dyspnea, bronchospasm

Miscellaneous: Anaphylactoid reactions, secondary leukemia

Drug Interactions Cytochrome P450 CYP3A4 substrate; CYP2C9, CYP3A4 inhibitor

Concomitant administration with sodium salicylate, sulfamethizole, and tolbutamide may displace teniposide from protein-binding sites causing substantial increases in free drug levels and potential for increased toxicity. May increase toxicity of methotrexate. Concurrent use with vincristine may increase the incidence of peripheral neuropathy. CYP3A4 inhibitors (azole antifungals, clarithromycin, diclofenac, doxycycline, erythromycin, imatinib, isoniazid, nefazodone, nicardipine, propofol, protease inhibitors, quinidine, telithromycin, and verapamil) may increase the levels of teniposide, CYP3A4 inducers (aminoglutethimide, carbamazepine, nafcillin, nevirapine, phenobarbital, phenytoin, fosphenytoin, and rifampin) may decrease the levels of teniposide. The herbal medicine St John's wort (*Hypericum perforatum*) may decrease teniposide levels. Live vaccines may increase risk of infection (avoid vaccination during therapy).

Stability Store ampuls in refrigerator. Diluted solutions are stable at room temperature for up to 24 hours after preparation. Solutions should be prepared in non-DEHP-containing containers such as glass or polyolefin containers. Use of polyvinyl chloride (PVC) containers is not recommended.

Mechanism of Action Type II topoisomerase inhibitor that induces single-stranded DNA breaks, double-stranded DNA breaks, and DNA-protein cross-links; induces late S phase or early G2-phase arrest resulting in inhibition of DNA synthesis

Pharmacokinetics

Distribution: Mainly into liver, kidneys, small intestine, and adrenals; limited distribution into CSF <1%

Children: V_d: 3-10 L/m^2

(Continued)

Teniposide *(Continued)*

Adults: V_d: 7.5-30 L/m^2

Protein binding: >99%

Metabolism: In liver

Half-life: 5 hours

Elimination: 0% to 10% excreted in feces; 21% excreted unchanged in urine

Usual Dosage I.V.: Refer to individual protocols.

Children: 130 mg/m^2/week, increasing to 150 mg/m^2/week after 3 weeks and up to 180 mg/m^2/week after 6 weeks

Acute lymphoblastic leukemia (ALL): 165 mg/m^2 twice weekly for 8-9 doses or 250 mg/m^2 weekly for 4-8 weeks

Dosing adjustment in renal or hepatic impairment: No specific recommendation (insufficient data). Dose adjustments may be necessary in patient with significant renal or hepatic impairment.

Dosing adjustment in Down's syndrome patients: Reduce initial dose (50% of the usual dose for the first course of therapy)

Administration Parenteral: I.V. infusion: Do not administer by rapid I.V. injection. Administer by I.V. infusion over at least 30-60 minutes to minimize the risk of hypotensive reactions; administer at a final concentration of 0.1, 0.2, 0.4, or 1 mg/mL diluted in D_5W or NS. Inspect infusion solution for particulate matter since precipitation may occur at any concentration. Administer 1 mg/mL solutions within 4 hours of preparation to reduce the potential for precipitation.

Monitoring Parameters Vital signs (blood pressure), CBC with differential, hemoglobin, platelet count, renal and hepatic function tests; observe for possible hypersensitivity reactions. Inspect solution and tubing for precipitation before and during infusion.

Patient Information Notify physician if fever, sore throat, painful/burning urination, bleeding problems, tiredness or weakness, skin rash, pain or numbness in extremities, or shortness of breath occur. Advise women of childbearing potential to avoid becoming pregnant while receiving teniposide.

Nursing Implications Agents for treating hypotension or anaphylactoid reactions should be present when I.V. teniposide is being administered; avoid extravasation.

Dosage Forms Excipient information presented when available (limited, particularly for generics); consult specific product labeling.

Injection, solution: 10 mg/mL (5 mL) [contains benzyl alcohol, dehydrated alcohol, and polyoxyethylated castor oil]

References

Clark PI and Slevin ML, "The Clinical Pharmacology of Etoposide and Teniposide," *Clin Pharmacokinet*, 1987, 12(4):223-52.

Sinkule JA, Stewart CF, Crom WR, et al, "Teniposide (VM26) Disposition in Children With Leukemia," *Cancer Res*, 1984, 44(3):1235-7.

Tenofovir (te NOE fo veer)

Related Information

Adult and Adolescent HIV *on page 1821*

Pediatric HIV *on page 1816*

Perinatal HIV *on page 1831*

U.S. Brand Names Viread®

Canadian Brand Names Viread®

Index Terms PMPA; TDF; Tenofovir Disoproxil Fumarate

Therapeutic Category Antiretroviral Agent; HIV Agents (Anti-HIV Agents); Nucleotide Reverse Transcriptase Inhibitor (NRTI)

Generic Available No

Use Treatment of HIV-1 infection in combination with other antiretroviral agents. (**Note:** HIV regimens consisting of **three** antiretroviral agents are strongly recommended)

Pregnancy Risk Factor B

Lactation Excretion in breast milk unknown/contraindicated

Contraindications Hypersensitivity to tenofovir or any component

Warnings Cases of lactic acidosis, severe hepatomegaly with steatosis and death have been reported in patients receiving nucleoside analogues; most of these cases have been in women; prolonged nucleoside use, obesity, and prior liver disease may be risk factors; use with extreme caution in patients with other risk factors for liver disease; discontinue therapy in patients who develop laboratory or clinical evidence of lactic acidosis or pronounced hepatotoxicity. Use with caution and adjust dose in patients with renal dysfunction (Cl_{cr} <50 mL/minute); renal dysfunction, including acute renal failure and Fanconi syndrome (renal tubular injury with severe hypophosphatemia) may occur (especially in patients with renal disease, underlying systemic disease, or those taking nephrotoxic medications); adults with a low body weight and those taking medications that increase tenofovir serum concentration may also be at increased risk for tenofovir-associated nephrotoxicity; avoid tenofovir in patients with concomitant or recent use of nephrotoxic agents; cases of nephrotoxicity have been reported in adolescents receiving tenofovir-containing regimens; evaluate and monitor renal function in all patients receiving tenofovir (regardless of age).

Safety and efficacy of tenofovir during coinfection of HIV and hepatitis B virus (HBV) have not been established; severe acute exacerbations of HBV have occurred after tenofovir discontinuation; follow hepatic function of coinfected patients closely (clinically and with laboratory tests) for at least several months after discontinuing tenofovir therapy. Immune reconstitution syndrome (an acute inflammatory response to residual or indolent opportunistic infections) may occur in HIV patients during initial treatment with combination antiretroviral agents including tenofovir; this syndrome may require further patient assessment and therapy.

Precautions Significant drug interactions may occur (see Drug Interactions); use with caution in patients with hepatic impairment; fat redistribution and accumulation [ie, central obesity, peripheral wasting, facial wasting, breast enlargement, dorsocervical fat enlargement (buffalo hump), and cushingoid appearance] have been observed in patients receiving antiretroviral agents (causal relationship not established). Bone toxicity (osteomalacia and reduced bone mineral density) may occur; long term effects in humans are not known (see also Adverse Reactions); monitor for potential bone toxicities during therapy; supplementation with calcium and vitamin D may be beneficial (but has not been studied).

Adverse Reactions

Central nervous system: Headache, dizziness, fever, depression, insomnia, anxiety

Dermatologic: Rash

Endocrine & metabolic: Hypophosphatemia, lactic acidosis, weight loss, fat redistribution and accumulation (see Precautions)

Gastrointestinal: Nausea, diarrhea, vomiting, dyspepsia, abdominal pain, flatulence, anorexia, pancreatitis

Hepatic: Elevated liver enzymes

Neuromuscular & skeletal: Asthenia, peripheral neuropathy, arthralgia, myalgia, reduction in bone mineral density, osteomalacia, elevations in biochemical markers of bone metabolism (eg, serum bone-specific alkaline phosphatase); **Note:** A significant decrease in lumbar spine bone mineral density (>6%) was reported in 5 of 15 pediatric patients who received a tenofovir-containing regimen for 48 weeks. No orthopedic fractures occurred, but 2 patients required discontinuation of tenofovir. All 5 patients with a decrease in bone mineral density were virologic responders and prepubertal (Tanner Stage 1). This study found a moderately strong correlation between decreases in bone mineral density z scores at week 48 and age at baseline. No correlation between decreases in bone mineral density z scores and tenofovir dose or pharmacokinetics was observed. The authors conclude that bone mineral density loss may limit the usefulness of tenofovir in prepubertal children (see Hazra, 2005).

Renal: Renal impairment, elevated serum creatinine, acute renal failure, Fanconi syndrome, acute tubular necrosis

Respiratory: Dyspnea

Miscellaneous: Sweating, immune reconstitution syndrome (see Warnings)

Drug Interactions Cytochrome P450 isoenzyme CYP1A2 inhibitor (minor)

Tenofovir significantly increases didanosine peak concentrations and AUC, potentially increasing didanosine-related adverse effects, such as pancreatitis, hyperglycemia, lactic acidosis, and peripheral neuropathy; some patients have experienced decreased CD4 cell counts and/or decreased virologic response; use didanosine with great caution and reduce the dose in patients receiving tenofovir; monitor patients closely; discontinue didanosine if adverse effects/toxicity develop. Tenofovir significantly decreases atazanavir serum concentrations and may result in a loss or lack of virologic response and possible resistance to atazanavir (booster doses of ritonavir are required for patients receiving atazanavir and tenofovir); tenofovir may decrease peak serum concentrations of lamivudine by 24% and indinavir by 11%; tenofovir may decrease peak concentrations and AUC of lopinavir and ritonavir. Indinavir may increase tenofovir peak concentrations by 14%; lopinavir/ritonavir and atazanavir may increase tenofovir serum concentrations and adverse effects (monitor patients; discontinue tenofovir if significant adverse effects occur). Drugs that are excreted by active tubular secretion (eg, acyclovir, adefovir, cidofovir, ganciclovir, valacyclovir, valganciclovir) may compete with tenofovir for elimination and may result in an increase in serum concentrations of tenofovir or these coadministered drugs (monitor for dose-related toxicities); drugs that impair renal function may decrease the renal elimination of tenofovir and result in increased tenofovir serum concentrations

Food Interactions A high-fat meal increases oral bioavailability (AUC) by 40% and increases peak serum concentrations by 14%; a light meal had no significant effect

(Continued)

Tenofovir *(Continued)*

on tenofovir pharmacokinetics compared to administration while fasting; food delays the time to peak concentrations by 1 hour

Mechanism of Action Tenofovir disoproxil fumarate (TDF) is a prodrug of tenofovir; *in vivo*, TDF undergoes diester hydrolysis to tenofovir; tenofovir is an acyclic nucleoside phosphate (nucleotide) analog of adenosine 5'-monophosphate; tenofovir undergoes phosphorylation by cellular enzymes to the active tenofovir diphosphate, which serves as an alternative substrate to deoxyadenosine 5'-triphosphate, a natural substrate for cellular DNA polymerase and reverse transcriptase; tenofovir diphosphate inhibits HIV viral reverse transcriptase by competing with natural deoxyadenosine 5'-triphosphate and by becoming incorporated into viral DNA causing chain termination. **Note:** Tenofovir also has activity against the hepatitis B virus (studies are ongoing).

Pharmacokinetics

Distribution: Mean V_d: Adults: 1.2-1.3 L/kg

Protein binding: Minimal (7.2% to serum proteins)

Metabolism: Not metabolized by CYP isoenzymes; tenofovir disoproxil fumarate (a prodrug) undergoes diester hydrolysis to tenofovir; tenofovir undergoes phosphorylation to the active tenofovir diphosphate

Bioavailability: 25% (fasting); high-fat meals will increase AUC by 40%

Half-life: Adults: Serum: 17 hours; intracellular: 10-50 hours

Time to peak serum concentration: Fasting: 1 hour

Elimination: Excreted via glomerular filtration and active tubular secretion; after I.V. administration: 70% to 80% is excreted in the urine as unchanged drug within 72 hours; after multiple oral doses (administered with food): 32% ± 10% is excreted in the urine within 24 hours

Clearance: Total body clearance is decreased in patients with renal impairment

Dialysis:

Hemodialysis: Efficiently removes tenofovir; 4 hours of hemodialysis removed ~10% of a single 300 mg dose

Peritoneal dialysis: Effects unknown

Usual Dosage Oral (use in combination with other antiretroviral agents):

Neonates and Infants: Not approved for use; dose is unknown

Children: Clinical trials previously excluded patients <18 years of age; current pediatric studies are assessing the following doses using investigational formulations:

Children 2-8 years: 8 mg/kg/dose once daily; maximum: 300 mg/day

Children >8 years: Median dose: 210 mg/m^2/dose once daily; maximum: 300 mg/day

Note: A phase III study in children >8 years of age will use a dose of 175 mg/m^2 once daily. This target dose was used in a pharmacokinetic study of 18 children 6.2-16.2 years of age (mean ± SD: 12 ± 2.5 years of age). The actual dose administered was 208 mg/m^2 (range: 161-256 mg/m^2) once daily, due to constraints of using a 75 mg investigational tablet. Tenofovir exposure at steady state in 16 subjects receiving combination antiretroviral therapy [that included a protease inhibitor plus low-dose ritonavir ("Booster doses")] approached values observed in adult patients treated with tenofovir disoproxil fumarate 300 mg once daily (see Hazra, 2004). Further pediatric studies are needed.

Adolescents ≥18 years and Adults: 300 mg once daily

Adults:

Coadministration with atazanavir: Tenofovir 300 mg is recommended to be given with atazanavir 300 mg plus ritonavir 100 mg (all as a single daily dose); administer with food; do **not** use tenofovir and atazanavir without booster doses of ritonavir (see Drug Interactions)

Coadministration with didanosine: Reduce dose of didanosine when used in combination with tenofovir; use didanosine delayed release capsule formulation (Videx EC®):

Adults <60 kg: Videx EC® 200 mg once daily with tenofovir 300 mg once daily

Adults ≥60 kg: Videx EC® 250 mg once daily with tenofovir 300 mg once daily

Dosing adjustment in renal impairment: Adolescents ≥18 years and Adults: Oral:

Note: Closely monitor clinical response and renal function in these patients (clinical effectiveness and safety of these guidelines have not been evaluated)

Cl_{cr} 30-49 mL/minute: 300 mg every 48 hours

Cl_{cr} 10-29 mL/minute: 300 mg twice weekly

Cl_{cr} <10 mL/minute without dialysis: No dosing recommendation available

Hemodialysis: 300 mg every 7 days or after a total of ~12 hours of dialysis (eg, once weekly with 3 hemodialysis sessions of ~4 hours in length); administer dose after completion of dialysis

Dosing adjustment in hepatic impairment: No dosage adjustment required

Administration May be administered without regard to meals

Monitoring Parameters CBC with differential, hemoglobin, MCV, reticulocyte count, liver enzymes, bilirubin, CD4 cell count, HIV RNA plasma levels, renal and hepatic function tests. Monitor for potential bone and renal abnormalities; monitor for alterations in S_{cr} and serum phosphorus in patients at risk or with a history of renal dysfunction and patients receiving concurrent nephrotoxic agents. In patients coinfected with HBV, monitor hepatic function closely (clinically and with laboratory tests) for at least several months after discontinuing tenofovir therapy (see Warnings).

Patient Information Tenofovir is not a cure for HIV; take tenofovir every day as prescribed; do not change dose or discontinue without physician's advice; if a dose is missed, take it as soon as possible, then return to normal dosing schedule; if a dose is skipped, do **not** double the next dose; report the use of other medications, nonprescription medications and herbal or natural products to your physician and pharmacist; long-term effects are not known; notify physician if persistent severe abdominal pain, nausea, or vomiting occurs

HIV medications may cause changes in body fat, including an increase in fat in the upper back and neck, breasts, and trunk; a loss of fat from the face, arms, and legs may also occur.

Additional Information A powder formulation is in development; 75 mg investigational tablets are currently being studied in children.

Long term studies demonstrating a decrease of clinical progression of HIV in patients receiving tenofovir are needed. Consider tenofovir in patients with HIV strains that would be susceptible as assessed by treatment history or laboratory tests. Mutation of reverse transcriptase at the 65 codon (K65R mutation) confers *in vitro* resistance to tenofovir; the K65R mutation is selected in some patients after treatment with didanosine, zalcitabine, or abacavir; thus, cross-resistance may occur. Multiple nucleoside mutations with a T69S double insertion showed decreased *in vitro* susceptibility to tenofovir; patients with HIV strains that had ≥3 zidovudine-associated mutations that included M41L or L210W showed decreased responses to tenofovir (but these responses were still better than placebo); patients with mutations at K65R, or L74V without zidovudine-associated mutations seemed to have a decreased response to tenofovir

A high rate of early virologic failure in therapy-naive adult HIV patients has been observed with the once-daily three-drug combination therapy of didanosine enteric-coated beadlets (Videx® EC), lamivudine, and tenofovir and the once-daily three-drug combination therapy of abacavir, lamivudine, and tenofovir. These combinations should not be used as a new treatment regimen for naive or pretreated patients. Any patient currently receiving either of these regimens should be closely monitored for virologic failure and considered for treatment modification. Early virologic failure was also observed in therapy-naive adult HIV patients treated with tenofovir, didanosine enteric-coated beadlets (Videx® EC) and either efavirenz or nevirapine; rapid emergence of resistant mutations has also been reported with this combination; the combination of tenofovir, didanosine, and any non-nucleoside reverse transcriptase inhibitor is **not** recommended as initial antiretroviral therapy.

Dosage Forms Excipient information presented when available (limited, particularly for generics); consult specific product labeling.

Tablet, as disoproxil fumarate: 300 mg [equivalent to 245 mg tenofovir disoproxil]

References

Briars LA, Hilao JJ, and Kraus DM, "A Review of Pediatric Human Immunodeficiency Virus Infection," *Journal of Pharmacy Practice*, 2004, 17(6):407-31.

Center for Disease Control and Prevention, "Guidelines for Using Antiretroviral Agents Among HIV-Infected Adults and Adolescents. Recommendations of the Panel on Clinical Practices for Treatment of HIV," *MMWR*, 2002, 51(RR-7):1-55.

Deeks SG, Barditch-Crovo P, Lietman PS, et al, "Safety, Pharmacokinetics, and Antiretroviral Activity of Intravenous 9-[2-(R)-(Phosphonomethoxy)propyl]adenine, a Novel Anti-human Immunodeficiency Virus (HIV) Therapy, in HIV-Infected Adults," *Antimicrob Agents Chemother*, 1998, 42(9):2380-4.

Hazra R, Balis FM, Tullio AN, et al, "Single-Dose and Steady-State Pharmacokinetics of Tenofovir Disoproxil Fumarate in Human Immunodeficiency Virus-Infected Children," *Antimicrob Agents Chemother*, 2004, 48(1):124-9.

Hazra R, Gafni RI, Maldarelli F, et al, "Tenofovir Disoproxil Fumarate and an Optimized Background Regimen of Antiretroviral Agents as Salvage Therapy for Pediatric HIV Infection," *Pediatrics*, 2005, 116(6):e846-54.

Morris JL and Kraus DM, "New Antiretroviral Therapies for Pediatric HIV Infection," *J Pediatr Pharmacol Ther*, 2005, 10:215-47.

Panel on Clinical Practices for Treatment of HIV Infection. "Guidelines for the Use of Antiretroviral Agents in HIV-Infected Adults and Adolescents," October 10, 2006, http://www.aidsinfo.nih.gov.

Robbins BL, Srinivas RV, Kim C, et al, "Anti-human Immunodeficiency Virus Activity and Cellular Metabolism of a Potential Prodrug of the Acyclic Nucleoside Phosphonate 9-R-(2-phosphonomethoxypropyl)adenine (PMPA), Bis(Isopropyloxymethyl-carbonyl)PMPA," *Antimicrob Agents Chemother*, 1998, 42(3):612-7.

Srinivas RV and Fridland A, "Antiviral Activities of 9-R-2-Phosphonomethoxypropyl adenine (PMPA) and Bis(Isopropyloxymethylcarbonyl)PMPA Against Various Drug-Resistant Human Immunodeficiency Virus Strains," *Antimicrob Agents Chemother*, 1998, 42(6):1484-7.

Working Group on Antiretroviral Therapy and Medical Management of HIV-Infected Children, "Guidelines for the Use of Antiretroviral Agents in Pediatric HIV Infection," October 26, 2006, http://www.aidsinfo.nih.gov.

(Continued)

Tenofovir *(Continued)*

Working Group on Antiretroviral Therapy and Medical Management of HIV-Infected Children, "Guidelines for the Use of Antiretroviral Agents in Pediatric HIV Infection. Supplement I: Pediatric Antiretroviral Drug Information," October 26, 2006, http://www.aidsinfo.nih.gov.

♦ **Tenofovir Disoproxil Fumarate** *see* Tenofovir *on page 1506*
♦ **Tenolin (Can)** *see* Atenolol *on page 170*
♦ **Tenormin®** *see* Atenolol *on page 170*
♦ **Tensilon® (Can)** *see* Edrophonium *on page 556*
♦ **Tera-Gel™ [OTC]** *see* Coal Tar *on page 394*

Terbutaline (ter BYOO ta leen)

Medication Safety Issues
Sound-alike/look-alike issues:
Terbutaline may be confused with terbinafine, TOLBUTamide

Related Information
Asthma *on page 1904*

Canadian Brand Names Bricanyl®

Index Terms Brethaire [DSC]; Bricanyl [DSC]

Therapeutic Category Adrenergic Agonist Agent; Antiasthmatic; Beta$_2$-Adrenergic Agonist Agent; Bronchodilator; Sympathomimetic; Tocolytic Agent

Generic Available Yes

Use Bronchodilator for relief of reversible bronchospasm in patients with asthma, bronchitis, and emphysema

Pregnancy Risk Factor B

Lactation Enters breast milk/compatible

Contraindications Hypersensitivity to terbutaline, other sympathomimetic amines, or any component

Warnings Paradoxical bronchoconstriction may occur with excessive use; if it occurs, discontinue terbutaline immediately

Precautions Use with caution in patients with diabetes mellitus, hypertension, hyperthyroidism, history of seizures, or cardiac disease; excessive or prolonged use may lead to tolerance

Adverse Reactions
Cardiovascular: Tachycardia, hypertension, arrhythmias, flushing, prolonged QT_c interval, elevated CPK isoenzyme
Central nervous system: Drowsiness, headache, nervousness, seizures, dizziness
Endocrine & metabolic: Hyperglycemia, hypokalemia
Gastrointestinal: Nausea, vomiting, dysgeusia
Neuromuscular & skeletal: Tremor
Otic: Tinnitus
Respiratory: Dyspnea, bronchospasm (with excessive use), pharyngitis, dry throat, chest tightness
Miscellaneous: Diaphoresis

Drug Interactions Additive effects with other sympathomimetics; increased pressor response with methyldopa, MAO inhibitors, oxytocic drugs, and tricyclic antidepressants

Mechanism of Action Relaxes bronchial smooth muscle and muscles of peripheral vasculature by action on beta$_2$-receptors with less effect on heart rate

Pharmacodynamics
Onset of action:
Oral: 30 minutes
Oral inhalation: 5-30 minutes
SubQ: 6-15 minutes
Duration:
Oral: 4-8 hours
Oral inhalation: 3-6 hours
SubQ: 1.5-4 hours

Pharmacokinetics
Absorption: 33% to 50%
Distribution: Breast milk to plasma ratio: <2.9
Metabolism: Possible first-pass metabolism after oral use
Half-life: 5.7 hours (range: 2.9-14 hours)
Time to peak serum concentration: SubQ: 0.5 hours
Elimination: Primarily (60%) unchanged in urine after parenteral use

Usual Dosage

Children <12 years:

Oral: Initial: 0.05 mg/kg/dose every 8 hours, increase gradually, up to 0.15 mg/kg/dose; maximum daily dose: 5 mg

SubQ: 0.005-0.01 mg/kg/dose to a maximum of 0.4 mg/dose every 15-20 minutes for 3 doses; may repeat every 2-6 hours as needed

Note: Continuous I.V. infusion has been used successfully in children with asthma; a 2-10 mcg/kg loading dose followed by an 0.08-0.4 mcg/kg/minute continuous infusion; depending upon the clinical response, the dosage may require titration in increments of 0.1-0.2 mcg/kg/minute every 30 minutes; doses as high as 10 mcg/kg/minute have been used.

Children ≥12 years and Adults:

Oral: 2.5-5 mg/dose every 6-8 hours; maximum daily dose:

12-15 years: 7.5 mg

>15 years: 15 mg

SubQ: 0.25 mg/dose repeated in 20 minutes for 3 doses; a total dose of 0.75 mg should not be exceeded

Nebulization: Children and Adults: 0.01-0.03 mL/kg (1 mg = 1 mL using injection); minimum dose: 0.1 mL; maximum dose: 2.5 mL every 4-6 hours

Administration

Oral: May administer without regard to food

Parenteral: May administer undiluted, direct I.V. over 5-10 minutes; for continuous infusion, dilute to a maximum concentration of 1 mg/mL in D_5W or NS

Inhalation: Nebulization: Dilute dose with 1-2 mL NS

Monitoring Parameters Heart rate, blood pressure, respiratory rate, serum potassium, arterial or capillary blood gases (if applicable)

Dosage Forms Excipient information presented when available (limited, particularly for generics); consult specific product labeling. [CAN] = Canadian brand name

Injection, solution, as sulfate: 1 mg/mL (1 mL)

Powder for oral inhalation:

Bricanyl® Turbuhaler [CAN]: 500 mcg/actuation [50 or 200 metered actuations] [not available in U.S.]

Tablet, as sulfate: 2.5 mg, 5 mg

Extemporaneous Preparations A 1 mg/mL suspension made from terbutaline tablets in simple syrup NF is stable 30 days when refrigerated

Horner RK and Johnson CE, "Stability of An Extemporaneously Compounded Terbutaline Sulfate Oral Liquid," *Am J Hosp Pharm*, 1991, 48(2):293-5.

References

Bohn D, Kalloghlian A, Jenkins J, et al, "Intravenous Salbutamol in the Treatment of Status Asthmaticus in Children," *Crit Care Med*, 1984, 12(10):892-6.

Canny GJ and Levison H, "Aerosols - Therapeutic Use and Delivery in Childhood Asthma," *Ann Allergy*, 1988, 60(1):11-9.

Fuglsang G, Pedersen S, and Borgstrom L, "Dose-Response Relationships of I.V. Administered Terbutaline in Children With Asthma," *J Pediatr*, 1989, 114(2):315-20.

Goldenhersh N and Rachelefsky GS, "Childhood Asthma: Management," *Pediatr Rev*, 1989, 10(9):259-67.

Expert Panel Report 2, "Guidelines for the Diagnosis and Management of Asthma," *Clinical Practice Guidelines*, National Institutes of Health, National Heart, Lung, and Blood Institute, NIH Publication No. 94-4051, April, 1997.

"National Asthma Education and Prevention Program. Expert Panel Report: Guidelines for the Diagnosis and Management of Asthma Update on Selected Topics--2002," *J Allergy Clin Immunol*, 2002, 110(5 Suppl):S141-219.

Rachelefsky GS and Siegel SC, "Asthma in Infants and Children - Treatment of Childhood Asthma: Part II," *J Allergy Clin Immunol*, 1985, 76(3):409-25.

Tipton WR and Nelson HS, "Frequent Parenteral Terbutaline in the Treatment of Status Asthmaticus in Children," *Ann Allergy*, 1987, 58(4):252-6.

♦ **TESPA** *see* Thiotepa *on page 1532*

♦ **Testim**® *see* Testosterone *on page 1511*

♦ **Testopel**® *see* Testosterone *on page 1511*

Testosterone (tes TOS ter one)

Medication Safety Issues

Sound-alike/look-alike issues:

Testosterone may be confused with testolactone

Testoderm® may be confused with Estraderm®

Transdermal patch may contain conducting metal (eg, aluminum); remove patch prior to MRI.

U.S. Brand Names Androderm®; AndroGel®; Delatestryl®; Depo®-Testosterone; First® Testosterone; First® Testosterone MC; Striant®; Testim®; Testopel®

Canadian Brand Names Andriol®; Androderm®; AndroGel®; Andropository; Delatestryl®; Depotest® 100; Everone® 200; Virilon® IM

(Continued)

Testosterone *(Continued)*

Index Terms Testosterone Cypionate; Testosterone Enanthate

Therapeutic Category Androgen

Generic Available Yes: Injection

Use Testosterone replacement therapy in males for conditions associated with a deficiency or absence of endogenous testosterone; primary hypogonadism (congenital or acquired) and hypogonadotropic hypogonadism (congenital or acquired)

Restrictions C-III

Pregnancy Risk Factor X

Lactation Enters breast milk/not recommended

Contraindications Hypersensitivity to testosterone or any component including testosterone USP that is chemically synthesized from soy (see Warnings); severe renal, hepatic, or cardiac disease; male patients with prostatic or breast cancer, hypercalcemia, pregnancy; use in women

Warnings May accelerate bone maturation without producing compensating gain in linear growth; perform radiographic examination of the hand and wrist every 6 months to determine the rate of bone maturation (when using in prepubertal children). Depo®-Testosterone contains benzyl alcohol which may cause allergic reactions in susceptible individuals; large amounts of benzyl alcohol (≥99 mg/kg/day) have been associated with a potentially fatal toxicity ("gasping syndrome") in neonates; the "gasping syndrome" consists of metabolic acidosis, respiratory distress, gasping respirations, CNS dysfunction (including convulsions, intracranial hemorrhage), hypotension and cardiovascular collapse; *in vitro* and animal studies have shown that benzoate, a metabolite of benzyl alcohol, displaces bilirubin from protein binding sites; avoid use of Depo®-Testosterone in neonates. In the event that unwashed or unclothed skin of a pregnant woman comes in direct contact with testosterone gel, wash with soap and water. Long-term therapy has been associated with serious hepatic adverse effects (hepatitis, hepatic neoplasms, cholestatic hepatitis, jaundice).

Precautions Use with caution in patients with hepatic, cardiac, or renal dysfunction; virilization of female sexual partners has been reported with male use of topical testosterone; may decrease blood glucose and insulin requirements in diabetics; may cause fluid retention; use with caution in patients with mild to moderate cardiovascular disease or other edematous conditions; use in hypogonadal men may potentiate sleep apnea especially those with risk factors such as obesity or chronic lung disease; long-term effects on gum safety when using the buccal formulation are not available; instruct patients to regularly inspect gum region where buccal formulation has been applied

Adverse Reactions

Cardiovascular: Flushing, edema, hypertension, tachycardia

Central nervous system: Excitation, aggressive behavior, sleeplessness, anxiety, mental depression, headache, nervousness

Dermatologic: Acne, hirsutism, urticaria

Endocrine & metabolic: Gynecomastia, hypercalcemia, hypoglycemia, elevated serum cholesterol, hyperlipemia, hyponatremia, increased or decreased libido, breast pain

Gastrointestinal: Nausea, abdominal pain, diarrhea; gum or mouth irritation or pain, bitter taste, gum edema, taste perversion (buccal formulation)

Genitourinary: Epididymitis, priapism, bladder irritability

Hematologic: Leukopenia, suppression of clotting factors, polycythemia

Hepatic: Cholestatic hepatitis, peliosis hepatitis, hepatocellular carcinoma (high doses), elevated liver function tests

Local: Inflammation and itching at injection site

Neuromuscular & skeletal: Myalgia

Respiratory: Sleep apnea

Drug Interactions Cytochrome P450 isoenzyme CYP3A3/4 and CYP3A5-7 substrate

Potentiates effects of oral anticoagulants; increases propranolol clearance; increases oxyphenbutazone serum level; may enhance the serum concentration and hepatotoxic effects of cyclosporine; avoid concurrent use, monitor closely; may decrease blood glucose and insulin requirements in diabetics; the herbal medicine St John's wort (*Hypericum perforatum*) may decrease testosterone serum levels

Stability Store at room temperature; protect from light; drug reservoirs for transdermals may burst due to excessive pressure or heat; do not store transdermal formulations outside of protective pouches

Mechanism of Action Principal endogenous androgen responsible for promoting the growth and development of the male sex organs and maintaining secondary sex characteristics in androgen-deficient males

Pharmacodynamics Duration: Based upon the route of administration and the specific testosterone ester used; the cypionate and enanthate esters have the longest duration, up to 2-4 weeks after I.M. administration; pellets 3-4 months; gel: 24-48 hours

Pharmacokinetics

Absorption: Transdermal gel: 10%

Protein binding: 98%

Metabolism: In the liver to various 17-keto steroids; major active metabolites are estradiol and dihydrotestosterone

Half-life: Cypionate: I.M.: 8 days

Time to peak serum concentration: Buccal: 10-12 hours

Elimination: 90% excreted in urine as metabolites

Usual Dosage

Children: I.M.:

Male hypogonadism: Testosterone cypionate or enanthate: Dosage and duration of therapy depends upon age, sex, diagnosis, patient's response to therapy, and appearance of adverse effects; in general total doses >400 mg/month are not required due to the prolonged action of the drug

Initiation of pubertal growth: 40-50 mg/m^2/dose monthly until the growth rate falls to prepubertal levels

Terminal growth phase: 100 mg/m^2/dose monthly until growth ceases

Maintenance virilizing dose: 100 mg/m^2/dose twice monthly

Delayed puberty: 40-50 mg/m^2/dose monthly for 6 months or per manufacturer: 50-200 mg every 2-4 weeks

Adults: Hypogonadism:

Buccal (Striant™): Apply one mucoadhesive dose (30 mg) twice daily every 12 hours in the morning and evening

Testosterone cypionate or enanthate: I.M.: 50-400 mg every 2-4 weeks

Transdermal: Androderm®: 5 mg/day initially (as one 5 mg or two 2.5 mg systems applied at night); adjust dosage in 3-4 weeks depending upon testosterone level to a maximum of 7.5 mg/day

Testosterone pellets: SubQ: Dosage depends on the minimum daily requirements of testosterone propionate [each 25 mg testosterone propionate weekly equals 150 mg (2 pellets)]; usual dose (testosterone pellets): 150-450 mg (2-6 pellets) every 3 months

AndroGel®: Transdermal gel or metered dose pump: Males >18 years: Initial: 5 g applied once daily (preferably in the morning); may increase as needed to a maximum of 10 g once daily

Adults: Postpubertal cryptorchism: Testosterone or testosterone propionate: I.M.: 10-25 mg 2-3 times/week

Administration

Buccal: Striant™: One mucoadhesive for buccal application (buccal system) should be applied to a comfortable area above the incisor tooth. Apply flat side of system to gum. Rotate to alternate sides of mouth with each application. Hold buccal system firmly in place for 30 seconds to ensure adhesion. The buccal system should adhere to gum for 12 hours. If the buccal system falls out, replace with a new system. If the system falls out within 4 hours of next dose, the new buccal system should remain in place until the time of the following scheduled dose. System will soften and mold to shape of gum as it absorbs moisture from mouth. Do not chew or swallow the buccal system; check to ensure buccal system is in place following toothbrushing, use of mouthwash, and consumption of food or beverages. The buccal system will not dissolve; gently remove by sliding downwards from gum; avoid scratching gum.

Parenteral: Administer deep I.M.; not for I.V. administration; pellets only are for SubQ administration

Topical:

Androderm®: The adhesive side of system should be applied to clean, dry area of the skin on the back, abdomen, upper arms or thighs at night; avoid application over boney prominences or on a part of the body that may be subject to prolonged pressure; **do not apply to the scrotum**; rotate sites every 7 days

AndroGel®: Apply AndroGel® to clean, dry, intact skin of the shoulder and upper arms and/or abdomen. Upon opening the packet(s), the entire contents should be squeezed into the palm of the hand and immediately applied to the application site(s). Application sites should be allowed to dry for a few minutes prior to dressing. Hands should be washed with soap and water after application. Wait at least 1 hour, preferably 5-6 hours, after application before showering or swimming. **Do not apply AndroGel® to the genitals**

Androgel® metered dose pump: Apply topically as described for Androgel®; each actuation delivers 1.25 g of testosterone (4 actuations = 5 g; 6 actuations = 7.5 g; 8 actuations = 10 g); pump must be primed prior to initial use by fully depressing pump mechanism 3 times and discarding any portion delivered; each actuation may be applied individually or all at the same time.

(Continued)

Testosterone *(Continued)*

Monitoring Parameters Periodic liver function tests, radiologic examination of wrist and hand every 6 months (when using in prepubertal children); hemoglobin, hematocrit, serum electrolytes, HDL cholesterol, prostate-specific antigen (PSA); testosterone level; (when using buccal formulation, measure testosterone level prior to morning dose and when using the transdermal formulation, in the morning following application the night before), measure testosterone level 4-12 weeks after initiating treatment

Reference Range Normal physiologic: Male:

Testosterone, urine: 100-1500 ng/24 hours

Testosterone, serum: 300-1050 ng/dL

Patient Information See Administration. Notify healthcare provider if penile erections are too frequent or prolonged, if nausea, vomiting, yellow skin (jaundice), ankle swelling, or breathing problems develop and in particular if sleeping or difficulty with urination occurs; if using buccal formulation, regularly inspect gum region where it is applied; gum irritation or tenderness should resolve in 1-14 days; notify healthcare provider if persists beyond this time

Nursing Implications 0.1% triamcinolone cream may be applied to skin under Androderm® to decrease irritation; do not use ointment formulations for pretreatment; they may significantly reduce testosterone absorption

Additional Information Testosterone 5% cream, not available commercially (must be compounded), has been effective in the treatment of microphallus when applied topically for 21 days

Dosage Forms Excipient information presented when available (limited, particularly for generics); consult specific product labeling. [CAN] = Canadian brand name

Capsule, gelatin, as undecanoate:

Andriol™ [CAN]: 40 mg (10s) [not available in U.S.]

Gel, topical:

AndroGel®:

1.25 g/actuation (75 g) [1% metered-dose pump; delivers 5 g/4 actuations; provides 60 1.25 g actuations; contains ethanol; may be chemically synthesized from soy]

2.5 g (30s) [1% unit dose packets; contains ethanol; may be chemically synthesized from soy]

5 g (30s) [1% unit dose packets; contains ethanol; may be chemically synthesized from soy]

Testim®: 5 g (30s) [1% unit-dose tube; contains ethanol; may be chemically synthesized from soy]

Injection, in oil, as cypionate: 200 mg/mL (10 mL)

Depo®-Testosterone: 100 mg/mL (10 mL); 200 mg/mL (1 mL, 10 mL) [contains benzyl alcohol, benzyl benzoate, and cottonseed oil]

Injection, in oil, as enanthate: 200 mg/mL (5 mL)

Delatestryl®: 200 mg/mL (1 mL) [prefilled syringe; contains sesame oil]; (5 mL) [multidose vial; contains sesame oil]

Kit [for prescription compounding testosterone 2%; kits also contain mixing jar and stirrer]:

First® Testosterone:

Injection, in oil: Testosterone propionate 100 mg/mL (12 mL) [contains sesame oil and benzyl alcohol]

Ointment: White petroleum (48 g)

First® Testosterone MC:

Injection, in oil: Testosterone propionate 100 mg/mL (12 mL) [contains sesame oil and benzyl alcohol]

Cream: Moisturizing cream (48 g)

Mucoadhesive, for buccal application [buccal system]:

Striant®: 30 mg (10s) [may be chemically synthesized from soy]

Pellet, for subcutaneous implantation:

Testopel®: 75 mg

Transdermal system, topical:

Androderm®: 2.5 mg/day (60s) [contains ethanol]; 5 mg/day (30s) [contains ethanol]

- **Testosterone Cypionate** *see* Testosterone *on page 1511*
- **Testosterone Enanthate** *see* Testosterone *on page 1511*
- **Tetanus and Diphtheria Toxoid** *see* Diphtheria and Tetanus Toxoid *on page 514*

Tetanus Immune Globulin (Human)

(TET a nus i MYUN GLOB yoo lin HYU man)

Related Information

Immunization Guidelines *on page 1837*

U.S. Brand Names HyperTET™ S/D

Canadian Brand Names HyperTET™ S/D

Index Terms TIG

Therapeutic Category Immune Globulin

Generic Available No

Use Prophylaxis for tetanus following injury in patients whose immunization for tetanus is incomplete or uncertain

Pregnancy Risk Factor C

Contraindications Hypersensitivity to tetanus immune globulin, thimerosal, or any component

Warnings As a product of human plasma, this product may potentially transmit infectious agents such as viruses; screening of donors, as well as testing and/or inactivation of certain viruses has reduced this risk. Although extremely rare, severe hypersensitivity reactions including anaphylaxis may occur; epinephrine and other anaphylactic treatment agents should be readily available. Not for I.V. administration; serious systemic reactions including hypotension have occurred with inadvertent I.V. administration

Precautions Administer with caution to patients with thrombocytopenia or any coagulation disorder that would be compromised by I.M. injection; administer with caution in patients with IgA deficiency or a prior history of systemic allergic reactions following the administration of human immunoglobulin preparations

Adverse Reactions

Central nervous system: Fever (mild)
Dermatologic: Urticaria, angioedema
Local: Pain, tenderness, erythema at injection site
Neuromuscular & skeletal: Muscle stiffness
Renal: Nephrotic syndrome (rare)
Miscellaneous: Anaphylaxis reaction (rare)

Drug Interactions Antibodies in immune globulin may interfere with the response to live viral vaccines (eg, MMR, varicella); delay administration of these vaccines for approximately 3 months following immune globulin administration

Stability Refrigerate; do not freeze

Mechanism of Action Passive immunity toward tetanus

Pharmacodynamics

A single dose may provide protection for up to 14 weeks

Pharmacokinetics Absorption: Well absorbed

Time to peak serum concentration: 2 days

Usual Dosage I.M.:

Prophylaxis of tetanus:

- Children <7 years: 4 units/kg as a single dose; some experts recommend administering 250 units regardless of weight or age
- Children ≥7 years and Adults: 250 units as a single dose; may be increased to 500 units if there has been a delay in initiating prophylaxis or when the wound is considered very tetanus prone

Tetanus Immune Globulin (TIG) and/or Tetanus Toxoid (Td) Wound Management

Number of Prior Tetanus Toxoid Doses	Clean, Minor Wounds		All Other Wounds	
	DT or Td[1]	TIG[2]	DT or Td[1]	TIG[2]
Unknown or <3	Yes	No	Yes	Yes
≥3[3]	No[4]	No	No[5]	No

[1]Use of combined antigen immunization (DT, Td, or DTaP) is preferred). Use tetanus and diphtheria toxoids formulation based upon age; use pediatric preparations (DT or DTaP) if the patient is <7 years old and Td if ≥7 years

[2]Tetanus immune globulin.

[3]If only three doses of fluid tetanus toxoid have been received, a fourth dose of toxoid, preferably an adsorbed toxoid, should be given.

[4]Yes, if >10 years since last dose.

[5]Yes, if >5 years since last dose.

Adapted from Report of the Committee on Infectious Diseases, American Academy of Pediatrics, Elk Grove Village, IL: American Academy of Pediatrics, 1986.

(Continued)

Tetanus Immune Globulin (Human) *(Continued)*

Note: Additional doses of TIG can be given at 4-week intervals in situations where the risk of tetanus infection persists

Treatment of tetanus:

Neonates: 500 units

Children and Adults: 3000-6000 units

Administration I.M.: Administer into lateral aspect of midthigh or deltoid muscle of upper arm; **not for I.V. administration.** When administered for treatment of tetanus, may be infiltrated locally around the wound site. Do not administer tetanus toxoid and TIG in same syringe (toxoid will be neutralized); tetanus toxoid may be administered at the same time at a separate site

Dosage Forms Excipient information presented when available (limited, particularly for generics); consult specific product labeling.

Injection, solution [preservative free]:

HyperTET™ S/D: 250 units/mL (1 mL) [prefilled syringe]

Tetanus Toxoid (Adsorbed) (TET a nus TOKS oyd, ad SORBED)

Medication Safety Issues

Sound-alike/look-alike issues:

Tetanus toxoid products may be confused with influenza virus vaccine and tuberculin products. Medication errors have occurred when tetanus toxoid products have been inadvertently administered instead of tuberculin skin tests (PPD) and influenza virus vaccine. These products are refrigerated and often stored in close proximity to each other.

Related Information

Immunization Guidelines *on page 1837*

Index Terms Tetanus Toxoid Plain

Therapeutic Category Vaccine

Generic Available No

Use Indicated as booster dose in the active immunization against tetanus in children >7 years or adults when combined antigen preparations are not indicated

Pregnancy Risk Factor C

Contraindications Hypersensitivity to tetanus toxoid or any component of the formulation

Warnings Patients with a history of severe local reaction (Arthus-type) or temperature of >39.4°C (103°F) following a previous dose should not be given further routine or emergency doses of tetanus toxoid more frequently than every 10 years. Guillain-Barré syndrome occurring within 6 weeks of tetanus toxoid vaccination has been reported. Defer administration during moderate or severe illness (with or without fever). Immune response may be decreased in immunocompromised patients; may be used in patients with HIV infection. Contains thimerosal; vial stopper contains natural latex rubber. Safety and efficacy in children <6 weeks of age have not been established; this product is not indicated for use in children <7 years of age; see diphtheria, pertussis, and tetanus vaccine and diphtheria and tetanus vaccine

Precautions Administer with caution to patients with thrombocytopenia or any coagulation disorder that would be compromised by I.M. injection; if the patient receives antihemophilia or other similar therapy, I.M. injection can be scheduled shortly after such therapy is administered; immediate treatment for anaphylactoid or acute hypersensitivity reactions should be available during vaccine use

Adverse Reactions All serious adverse reactions must be reported to the U.S. Department of Health and Human Services (DHHS) Vaccine Adverse Event Reporting System (VAERS) 1-800-822-7967.

Cardiovascular: Hypotension

Central nervous system: Brachial neuritis, fever, malaise

Dermatologic: Rash, urticaria

Gastrointestinal: Nausea

Local: Edema, induration (with or without tenderness), redness, warmth

Neuromuscular & skeletal: Arthralgia, Guillain-Barré syndrome, brachial neuritis

Miscellaneous: Anaphylaxis, Arthus-type hypersensitivity reactions (severe local reaction developing 2-8 hours following injection)

Drug Interactions Immunosuppressant medications or therapies (antimetabolites, alkylating agents, cytotoxic drugs, corticosteroids, irradiation): The effect of the vaccine may be decreased; consider deferring vaccination for 3 months after immunosuppressant therapy is discontinued

Stability Refrigerate 2°C to 8°C (35°F to 46°F). Do not freeze.

Mechanism of Action Tetanus toxoid preparations contain the toxin produced by virulent tetanus bacilli (detoxified growth products of *Clostridium tetani*). The toxin has been modified by treatment with formaldehyde so that is has lost toxicity but still retains ability to act as antigen and produce active immunity.

Usual Dosage

Primary immunization: Not indicated for this use; combined antigen vaccines are recommended

Booster doses: I.M.: 0.5 mL every 10 years

Tetanus prophylaxis in wound management: Use of tetanus toxoid and/or tetanus immune globulin (TIG) depends upon the number of prior tetanus toxoid doses and type of wound: See table.

Tetanus Immune Globulin (TIG) and/or Tetanus Toxoid (Td) Wound Management

Number of Prior Tetanus Toxoid Doses	Clean, Minor Wounds		All Other Wounds	
	DT or Td[1]	TIG[2]	DT or Td[1]	TIG[2]
Unknown or <3	Yes	No	Yes	Yes
≥3[3]	No[4]	No	No[5]	No

[1]Use of combined antigen immunization (DT, Td, or DTaP) is preferred). Use tetanus and diphtheria toxoids formulation based upon age; use pediatric preparations (DT or DTaP) if the patient is <7 years old and Td if ≥7 years

[2]Tetanus immune globulin.

[3]If only three doses of fluid tetanus toxoid have been received, a fourth dose of toxoid, preferably an adsorbed toxoid, should be given.

[4]Yes, if >10 years since last dose.

[5]Yes, if >5 years since last dose.

Adapted from Report of the Committee on Infectious Diseases, American Academy of Pediatrics, Elk Grove Village, IL: American Academy of Pediatrics, 1986.

Administration I.M. Shake well prior to use. Administer into lateral aspect of midthigh or deltoid muscle of upper arm; **not for I.V. or SubQ administration**

Patient Information May experience mild fever or soreness, swelling, and redness/ knot at the injection site usually lasting 1-2 days

Nursing Implications Federal law requires that the date of administration, the vaccine manufacturer, lot number of vaccine, and the administering person's name, title, and address be entered into the patient's permanent medical record.

Dosage Forms Excipient information presented when available (limited, particularly for generics); consult specific product labeling.

Injection, suspension: Tetanus 5 Lf units per 0.5 mL (0.5 mL) [contains trace amounts of thimerosal]; (5 mL) [contains thimerosal; vial stopper contains latex]

References

American Academy of Pediatrics Committee on Infectious Diseases, "Recommended Childhood and Adolescent Immunization Schedule - United States, January-June 2004," *Pediatrics*, 2004, 113(1 Pt 1):142-3.

Atkinson WL, Pickering LK, Schwartz B, et al, "General Recommendations on Immunization. Recommendations of the Advisory Committee on Immunization Practices (ACIP) and the American Academy of Family Physicians (AAFP)," *MMWR Recomm Rep*, 2002, 51(RR-2):18.

Centers for Disease Control, "Recommended Adult Immunization Schedule, October 2004-September 2005," available at www.cdc.gov.

♦ **Tetanus Toxoid Plain** *see* Tetanus Toxoid (Adsorbed) *on page 1516*

♦ **Tetanus Toxoid, Reduced Diphtheria Toxoid, and Acellular Pertussis, Adsorbed** *see* Diphtheria, Tetanus Toxoids, and Acellular Pertussis Vaccine *on page 517*

Tetracaine (TET ra kane)

U.S. Brand Names Pontocaine®; Pontocaine® Niphanoid®

Canadian Brand Names Ametop™; Pontocaine®

Index Terms Amethocaine Hydrochloride; Tetracaine Hydrochloride

Therapeutic Category Analgesic, Topical; Local Anesthetic, Injectable; Local Anesthetic, Ophthalmic; Local Anesthetic, Oral; Local Anesthetic, Topical

Generic Available Yes: Ophthalmic solution, solution for injection

Use Local anesthesia in the eye for various diagnostic and examination purposes; spinal anesthesia; local anesthesia for mucous membranes

Pregnancy Risk Factor C

Lactation Excretion in breast milk unknown/use caution

Contraindications Hypersensitivity to tetracaine or any component (see Warnings); patients with liver disease; CNS disease, meningitis (if used for epidural or spinal anesthesia); myasthenia gravis, impaired cardiac conduction; eye infection (ophthalmic) formulation

Warnings Parenteral form may contain sulfites which may cause allergic reactions in susceptible individuals

(Continued)

Tetracaine *(Continued)*

Precautions Use with caution in patients with cardiac disease and hyperthyroidism

Adverse Reactions

Cardiovascular: Cardiac arrest, bradycardia, myocardial depression, cardiac arrhythmias, hypotension

Central nervous system: Anxiety, apprehension, nervousness, disorientation, seizures, drowsiness, unconsciousness

Dermatologic: Urticaria

Gastrointestinal: Nausea, vomiting

Local: Stinging, burning at injection site

Ocular: Lacrimation, photophobia, corneal epithelial erosion, keratitis, corneal opacification, miosis

Otic: Tinnitus

Respiratory: Respiratory arrest

Drug Interactions Inhibits sulfonamide activity; enhances CNS depression of other CNS depressants

Mechanism of Action Blocks both the generation and conduction of sensory, motor, and autonomic nerve fibers by decreasing the neuronal membrane's permeability to sodium ions, which results in decreasing the rate of depolarization of the nerve membrane

Pharmacodynamics

Onset of action:

- Ophthalmic instillation: Anesthetic effects occur within 60 seconds
- Topical: Within 3 minutes when applied to mucous membranes

Duration: 1.5-3 hours

Pharmacokinetics

Metabolism: By the liver

Elimination: Metabolites are renally excreted

Usual Dosage

Children: Safety and efficacy have not been established

Adults:

- Cream: Apply to affected area as needed
- Injection: Dosage varies with the anesthetic procedure, the degree of anesthesia required, and the individual patient response; it is administered by subarachnoid injection for spinal anesthesia. High, medium, low, or saddle blocks use 0.2% or 0.3% solution. Prolonged effect (2-3 hours): Use 1% solution (a 1% solution should be diluted with an equal volume of CSF before administration)
  - Perineal anesthesia: 5 mg
  - Perineal and lower extremities: 10 mg
  - Anesthesia extending up to the costal margin: 15-20 mg
  - Low spinal anesthesia (saddle block): 2-5 mg
- Ophthalmic: Solution: Instill 1-2 drops
- Topical solution (mucous membranes): Apply 2% solution as needed; do not exceed 20 mg (1 mL) per application

Administration

Ophthalmic: Apply drops to conjunctiva of affected eye(s); avoid contact of bottle tip with skin or eye; finger pressure should be applied to lacrimal sac during and for 1-2 minutes after instillation to decrease risk of absorption and systemic reactions

Parenteral: Subarachnoid administration by experienced individuals only

Patient Information Do not touch or rub eye until anesthesia (if ophthalmic) has worn off

Nursing Implications Not for prolonged use topically

Dosage Forms Excipient information presented when available (limited, particularly for generics); consult specific product labeling.

Injection, solution, as hydrochloride [preservative free] (Pontocaine®): 1% [10 mg/mL] (2 mL) [contains sodium bisulfite]

Injection, powder for reconstitution, as hydrochloride [preservative free] (Pontocaine® Niphanoid®): 20 mg

Solution, ophthalmic, as hydrochloride: 0.5% [5 mg/mL] (15 mL)

Solution, topical, as hydrochloride (Pontocaine®): 2% [20 mg/mL] (30 mL, 118 mL) [for rhinolaryngology]

♦ **Tetracaine Hydrochloride** *see* Tetracaine *on page 1517*

♦ **Tetracosactide** *see* Cosyntropin *on page 405*

Tetracycline (tet ra SYE kleen)

Medication Safety Issues

Sound-alike/look-alike issues:

- Tetracycline may be confused with tetradecyl sulfate

Achromycin may be confused with actinomycin, Adriamycin PFS®

Related Information

Malaria *on page 1855*

U.S. Brand Names Sumycin® [DSC]

Canadian Brand Names Apo-Tetra®; Nu-Tetra

Index Terms Achromycin; TCN; Tetracycline Hydrochloride

Therapeutic Category Acne Products; Antibiotic, Ophthalmic; Antibiotic, Tetracycline Derivative; Antibiotic, Topical

Generic Available Yes: Capsule

Use

Children, Adolescents and Adults: Treatment of Rocky Mountain spotted fever caused by susceptible *Rickettsia* or brucellosis

Adolescents and Adults: Presumptive treatment of chlamydial infection in patients with gonorrhea

Children >8 years, Adolescents and Adults: Treatment of moderate to severe inflammatory acne vulgaris, Lyme disease, mycoplasmal disease or *Legionella*

Pregnancy Risk Factor D; B (topical)

Lactation Enters breast milk/not recommended (AAP rates "compatible")

Contraindications Hypersensitivity to tetracycline or any component; pregnancy; children ≤8 years; use of tetracyclines during tooth development may cause permanent discoloration of the teeth, enamel hypoplasia and retardation of skeletal development and bone growth with risk being greatest for children <4 years and in those receiving high doses

Warnings Photosensitivity reaction may occur with this drug; avoid prolonged exposure to sunlight or tanning equipment; prolonged use may result in superinfection

Precautions Use with caution in patients with renal and liver impairment; dosage modification required in patients with renal impairment

Adverse Reactions

Central nervous system: Pseudotumor cerebri, fever

Dermatologic: Rash, exfoliative dermatitis, photosensitivity, angioedema, discoloration of nails

Gastrointestinal: Nausea, vomiting, diarrhea, stomatitis, glossitis, antibiotic-associated pseudomembranous colitis, esophagitis, oral candidiasis

Hematologic: Hemolytic anemia

Hepatic: Hepatotoxicity

Neuromuscular & skeletal: Injury to growing bones and teeth

Renal: Renal damage, Fanconi-like syndrome

Respiratory: Pulmonary infiltrates with eosinophilia

Miscellaneous: Hypersensitivity reactions, candidal superinfection

Drug Interactions Calcium-, magnesium- or aluminum-containing antacids; iron, zinc; kaolin-, pectin-, or bismuth-containing antidiarrheals decrease tetracycline absorption. Tetracycline enhances the hypoprothrombinemic effect of warfarin; methoxyflurane increases chance of nephrotoxicity; concomitant use with isotretinoin has been associated with cases of pseudotumor cerebri

Food Interactions Tetracyclines decrease absorption of magnesium, zinc, calcium, dairy products, iron, and amino acids; calcium, dairy products, iron supplements decrease tetracycline absorption

Stability Protect from light; outdated tetracyclines have caused a Fanconi-like syndrome

Mechanism of Action Inhibits bacterial protein synthesis by binding to the 30S and possibly the 50S ribosomal subunit(s) of susceptible bacteria preventing additions of amino acids to the growing peptide chain; may also cause alterations in the cytoplasmic membrane

Pharmacokinetics

Distribution: Widely distributed to most body fluids and tissues including ascitic, synovial and pleural fluids; bronchial secretions; appears in breast milk; poor penetration into CSF

Absorption:

Oral: 75%

I.M.: Poor, with less than 60% of dose absorbed

Protein binding: 30% to 60%

Half-life: 6-12 hours with normal renal function and is prolonged with renal impairment

Time to peak serum concentration: Within 2-4 hours

Elimination: Primary route is the kidney, with 60% of a dose excreted as unchanged drug in urine, small amounts appear in bile

Dialysis: Slightly dialyzable (5% to 20%)

Usual Dosage

Children >8 years: Oral: 25-50 mg/kg/day in divided doses every 6 hours; not to exceed 3 g/day

(Continued)

Tetracycline *(Continued)*

Adolescents and Adults:

Oral: 250-500 mg/dose every 6-12 hours

Topical: Ointment: Apply small amount of ointment to cleansed area 2-3 times daily

Dosing adjustment in renal impairment:

Cl_{cr} 50-80 mL/minute: Administer every 8-12 hours

Cl_{cr} 10-50 mL/minute: Administer every 12-24 hours

Cl_{cr} <10 mL/minute: Administer every 24 hours

Administration

Oral: Administer 1 hour before or 2 hours after meals with adequate amounts of fluid; avoid taking antacids, calcium, iron, dairy products, or milk formulas within 3 hours of tetracyclines

Topical: Small amount of ointment should be applied to cleansed affected area.

Monitoring Parameters Renal, hepatic, and hematologic function tests

Test Interactions False-negative urine glucose with Clinistix®

Patient Information May discolor nails. May cause photosensitivity reactions (eg, exposure to sunlight may cause severe sunburn, skin rash, redness, or itching); avoid exposure to sunlight and artificial light sources (sunlamps, tanning booth/bed); wear protective clothing, wide-brimmed hats, sunglasses, and lip sunscreen (SPF ≥15); use a sunscreen [broad-spectrum sunscreen or physical sunscreen (preferred) or sunblock with SPF ≥15]; contact physician if reaction occurs.

Dosage Forms Excipient information presented when available (limited, particularly for generics); consult specific product labeling.

Capsule, as hydrochloride: 250 mg, 500 mg

Suspension, oral, as hydrochloride:

Sumycin®: 125 mg/5 mL (480 mL) [contains sodium benzoate and sodium metabisulfite; fruit flavor] [DSC]

Tablet, as hydrochloride:

Sumycin®: 250 mg, 500 mg [DSC]

References

American Academy of Pediatrics. Committee on Drugs. "Requiem for Tetracyclines," *Pediatrics*, 1975, 55(1):142-3.

- ♦ **Tetracycline Hydrochloride** *see* Tetracycline *on page 1518*
- ♦ **Tetrahydrocannabinol** *see* Dronabinol *on page 546*
- ♦ **Tev-Tropin®** *see* Human Growth Hormone *on page 769*
- ♦ **Texacort®** *see* Hydrocortisone *on page 781*
- ♦ **TG** *see* Thioguanine *on page 1527*
- ♦ **6-TG (error-prone abbreviation)** *see* Thioguanine *on page 1527*
- ♦ **THAM®** *see* Tromethamine *on page 1581*
- ♦ **THC** *see* Dronabinol *on page 546*
- ♦ **Theo-24®** *see* Theophylline *on page 1520*
- ♦ **TheoCap™** *see* Theophylline *on page 1520*
- ♦ **Theochron®** *see* Theophylline *on page 1520*
- ♦ **Theochron® SR (Can)** *see* Theophylline *on page 1520*
- ♦ **Theolair™ (Can)** *see* Theophylline *on page 1520*

Theophylline (thee OF i lin)

Medication Safety Issues

Sound-alike/look-alike issues:

Theolair™ may be confused with Thiola®, Thyrolar®

Related Information

Asthma *on page 1904*

Blood Level Sampling Time Guidelines *on page 1914*

Medications for Which A Single Dose May Be Fatal When Ingested By A Toddler *on page 1932*

Overdose and Toxicology *on page 1916*

U.S. Brand Names Elixophyllin®; Quibron®-T [DSC]; Quibron®-T/SR [DSC]; Theo-24®; TheoCap™; Theochron®; Uniphyl®

Canadian Brand Names Apo-Theo LA®; Novo-Theophyl SR; PMS-Theophylline; Pulmophylline; ratio-Theo-Bronc; Theochron® SR; Theolair™; Uniphyl® SRT

Index Terms Theophylline Anhydrous

Therapeutic Category Antiasthmatic; Bronchodilator; Respiratory Stimulant; Theophylline Derivative

Generic Available Yes: Extended release capsule and tablet, infusion

Use Treatment of symptoms and reversible airway obstruction due to chronic asthma, chronic bronchitis, or COPD; treatment of idiopathic apnea of prematurity in neonates

Pregnancy Risk Factor C

Lactation Enters breast milk/compatible (AAP rates "compatible")

Contraindications Hypersensitivity to theophylline or any component

Warnings If a patient develops signs and symptoms of theophylline toxicity (eg, persistent, repetitive vomiting), a serum theophylline level should be measured and subsequent doses held; due to potential saturation of theophylline clearance at serum levels within or (in some patients) less than the therapeutic range, dosage adjustments should be made in small increments (maximum dosage adjustment: 25%); due to wide interpatient variability, theophylline serum level measurements must be used to optimize therapy and prevent serious toxicity

Precautions Use with caution in patients with peptic ulcer, hyperthyroidism, seizure disorders, hypertension, and patients with cardiac arrhythmias (excluding bradyarrhythmias)

Adverse Reactions See table.

Theophylline Serum Levels (micrograms/mL)[1]	Adverse Reactions
15-25	GI upset, GE reflux, diarrhea, nausea, vomiting, abdominal pain, nervousness, headache, insomnia, agitation, dizziness, muscle cramp, tremor
25-35	Tachycardia, occasional PVC
>35	Ventricular tachycardia, frequent PVC, seizure

[1]Adverse effects do not necessarily occur according to serum levels. Arrhythmia and seizure can occur without seeing the other adverse effects.

Drug Interactions Cytochrome P450 isoenzyme CYP1A2, CYP2E1, and CYP3A3/4 substrate

Decreases adenosine, esmolol, benzodiazepine, and pancuronium effects; increases lithium clearance; increases CNS side effects with ephedrine; increases risk of cardiac arrhythmias with halothane; decreases zafirlukast serum levels; for medications which alter theophylline clearance, see tables below and on next page.

Clinical Factors Reported to Affect Theophylline Clearance

Decreased Theophylline Level	Increased Theophylline Level
Smoking (cigarettes, marijuana)	Acute pulmonary edema
High protein/low carbohydrate diet	Cessation of smoking (after chronic use)
Charcoal broiled beef	Cor pulmonale
	Congestive heart failure
	Hypothyroidism
	Fever (≥102° for 24 hours or more, or lesser temperature elevations for longer periods)
	Hepatic cirrhosis/acute hepatitis
	Renal failure in infants <3 mo of age
	Sepsis with multisystem organ failure
	Shock
	Viral illness

Food Interactions Food does not appreciably affect the absorption of liquid, fast-release products and most sustained release products; however, food may induce a sudden release (dose-dumping) of once-daily sustained release products resulting in an increase in serum drug levels and potential toxicity; avoid excessive

(Continued)

Theophylline *(Continued)*

amounts of caffeine; avoid extremes of dietary protein and carbohydrate intake; limit charcoal-broiled foods and caffeinated beverages

Medications Affecting Theophylline Clearance Resulting in Either Increased or Decreased Serum Levels

Decreased Theophylline Level	Increased Theophylline Level
Aminoglutethimide Carbamazepine Isoproterenol (I.V.) Isoniazid[1] Ketoconazole Loop diuretics[1] Nevirapine Phenobarbital Phenytoin Rifampin Ritonavir Sulfinpyrazone Sympathomimetics	Alcohol Allopurinol (>600 mg/day) Beta-blockers Calcium channel blockers Cimetidine Ciprofloxacin Clarithromycin Corticosteroids Disulfiram Ephedrine Erythromycin Esmolol Influenza virus vaccine Interferon, human recombinant alpha 2-a and 2-b Isoniazid[1] Loop diuretics[1] Methotrexate Mexiletine Oral contraceptives Propafenone Propranolol Tacrine Thiabendazole Thyroid hormones Troleandomycin (TAO®) Verapamil Zileuton

[1]Both increased and decreased theophylline levels have been reported.

Mechanism of Action Competitively inhibits two isoenzymes of the enzyme phosphodiesterase resulting in increased levels of cyclic adenine monophosphate (cAMP) which may be responsible for most of theophylline's effects; effects on the myocardium and neuromuscular transmission may be due to the intracellular translocation of ionized calcium; overall, theophylline produces the following effects: relaxation of the smooth muscle of the respiratory tract, suppression of the response of airways to stimuli, increases the force of contraction of diaphragmatic muscles; pulmonary, coronary, and renal artery dilation; CNS stimulation, diuresis, stimulation of catecholamine release, gastric acid secretion, and relaxation of biliary and GI smooth muscle

Pharmacokinetics

Absorption: Oral: Rapid and complete with up to 100% absorption depending upon the formulation used

Distribution: V_d: 0.45 L/kg; distributes into breast milk; breast milk to plasma ratio: 0.67; crosses the placenta and into the CSF

Protein binding: 40%; decreased protein binding in neonates (due to a greater percentage of fetal albumin), hepatic cirrhosis, uncorrected acidemia, women in third trimester of pregnancy, and geriatric patients

Metabolism: In the liver by demethylation and oxidation; theophylline is metabolized to caffeine (active); in neonates this theophylline-derived caffeine accumulates (due to decreased hepatic metabolism) and significant concentrations of caffeine may occur; a substantial decrease in serum caffeine concentrations occurs after 40 weeks postconceptional age

Half-life: See table.

Theophylline Clearance and Half-Life With Respect to Age and Altered Physiological States[1]

Patient Group	Mean Clearance (mL/kg/min)	Mean Half-life (h)
Premature infants		
postnatal age 3-15 d	0.29	30
postnatal age 25-57 d	0.64	20
Term infants		
postnatal age 1-2 d	Not reported[2]	25
postnatal age 3-30 wk[3]	Not reported[2]	11
Children		
1-4 y	1.7	3.4
4-12 y	1.6	Not reported[2]
13-15 y	0.9	Not reported[2]
16-17 y	1.4	3.7 (range: 1.5-5.9)
Adults		
16-60 (nonsmoking)	0.65	8.2
>60 y (nonsmoking, healthy)	0.41	9.8
Acute pulmonary edema	0.33	19
Cystic fibrosis (14-28 y)	1.25	6
Liver disease		
acute hepatitis	0.35	19.2
cholestasis	0.65	14.4
cirrhosis	0.31	32
Sepsis with multiorgan failure	0.46	18.8
Hypothyroid	0.38	11.6
Hyperthyroid	0.8	4.5
COPD >60 y, nonsmoking >1 y	0.54	11

[1]From Hendeles L, 1995

[2]Either not reported or not reported in a comparable format

[3]Maturation of clearance in premature infants and term infants is most closely related to postconceptional age (PCA); adult clearance values are reached at approximately 55 weeks PCA and higher pediatric values at approximately 60 weeks PCA (Kraus, 1993).

Elimination: In urine; children >3 months and adults excrete 10% in urine as unchanged drug; neonates excrete approximately 50% of the dose unchanged in urine

Usual Dosage Oral (see Aminophylline *on page 98* for I.V. doses):

Loading dose:

Neonates: Apnea of prematurity: 4 mg/kg/dose

Infants and Children: Treatment of acute bronchospasm: (to achieve a serum level of about 10 mcg/mL; loading doses should be given using a rapidly absorbed oral product **not** a sustained release product):

If no theophylline has been administered in the previous 24 hours: 5 mg/kg theophylline

If theophylline has been administered in the previous 24 hours: 2.5 mg/kg theophylline may be given in emergencies when serum levels are not available

A modified loading dose (mg/kg) may be calculated (when the serum level is known) by: [Blood level desired - blood level measured] divided by 2 (for every 1 mg/kg theophylline given, the blood level will rise by approximately 2 mcg/mL)

Maintenance dose: See table on next page.

These recommendations, based on mean clearance rates for age or risk factors, were calculated to achieve a serum level of 10 mcg/mL (5 mcg/mL for newborns with apnea/bradycardia). In newborns and infants, a fast-release oral product can be used. The total daily dose can be divided every 12 hours in newborns and

(Continued)

Theophylline *(Continued)*

Maintenance Dose for Acute Symptoms

Population Group	Oral Theophylline (mg/kg/day)
Premature infant or newborn to 6 wk (for apnea/ bradycardia)	4[1]
6 wk to 6 mo	10[1]
Infants 6 mo to 1 y	12-18[1]
Children 1-9 y	20-24
Children 9-12 y, adolescent daily smokers of cigarettes or marijuana, and otherwise healthy adult smokers <50 y	16
Adolescents 12-16 y (nonsmokers)	13
Otherwise healthy nonsmoking adults (including elderly patients)	10 (not to exceed 900 mg/ day)
Cardiac decompensation, cor pulmonale, and/or liver dysfunction	5 (not to exceed 400 mg/ day)
[1]**Alternative dosing regimen for full-term infants <1 year of age:** Total daily dose (mg) = [(0.2 x age in weeks) + 5] x weight (kg); Postnatal Age <26 weeks: Total daily dose divided every 8 hours; Postnatal Age >26 weeks: Total daily dose divided every 6 hours	

every 6-8 hours in infants. In children and healthy adults, a slow-release product can be used. The total daily dose can be divided every 8-12 hours.

Use ideal body weight for obese patients

Dose should be further adjusted based on serum levels. Guidelines for drawing theophylline serum levels are shown in the table.

Guidelines for Drawing Theophylline Serum Levels

Dosage Form	Time to Draw Level[1]
I.V. bolus	30 min after end of 30-min infusion
I.V. continuous infusion	12-24 h after initiation of infusion
P.O. liquid, fast-release formulation	Peak: 1 h postdose after at least 1 day of therapy Trough: Just before a dose after at least 1 day of therapy

[1]The time to achieve steady-state serum levels is prolonged in patients with longer half-lives (eg, premature neonates, infants, and adults with cardiac or liver failure (see theophylline half-life table). In these patients, serum theophylline levels should be drawn after 48-72 hours of therapy; serum levels may need to be done prior to steady-state to assess the patient's current progress or evaluate potential toxicity.

Administration

Oral: Sustained release preparations should be administered with a full glass of water, whole or cut by half only; do not crush; sustained release capsule forms may be opened and sprinkled on soft foods; do not chew or crush beads

Parenteral: Premade I.V. infusion bags for continuous infusion usage; rate of infusion dependent upon dosage; loading doses using I.V. infusion should be administered over 20-30 minutes

Monitoring Parameters Respiratory rate, heart rate, serum theophylline level, arterial or capillary blood gases (if applicable); number and severity of apnea spells (apnea of prematurity)

Reference Range

Therapeutic levels:

Asthma: 10-15 mcg/mL (peak level)

Apnea of prematurity: 6-14 mcg/mL

Toxic concentration: >20 mcg/mL

Test Interactions May elevate uric acid levels

Patient Information Contact physician whenever nausea, vomiting, persistent headache, or irregular heartbeats occur; notify physician if a new illness develops (especially if high fevers); do not alter time, dose, or frequency of administration without physician knowledge; avoid drinking or eating of large quantities of caffeine-containing beverages or food

Additional Information Due to improved theophylline clearance during the first year of life, serum concentration determinations and dosage adjustments may be needed to optimize therapy

Dosage Forms Excipient information presented when available (limited, particularly for generics); consult specific product labeling.

Capsule, extended release: 100 mg, 125 mg, 200 mg, 300 mg
- TheoCap™: 125 mg, 200 mg, 300 mg [12 hour]
- Theo-24®: 100 mg, 200 mg, 300 mg, 400 mg [24 hours]

Elixir:
- Elixophyllin®: 80 mg/15 mL (480 mL) [contains alcohol 20%; fruit flavor]

Infusion [premixed in D_5W]: 200 mg (50 mL, 100 mL); 400 mg (100 mL, 250 mL, 500 mL); 800 mg (250 mL, 500 mL, 1000 mL)

Tablet, controlled release:
- Uniphyl®: 400 mg, 600 mg [24 hours; contains cetostearyl alcohol]

Tablet, extended release: 100 mg, 200 mg, 300 mg, 450 mg
- Theochron®: 100 mg, 200 mg, 300 mg, 450 mg [12-24 hours]

Tablet, immediate release:
- Quibron®-T: 300 mg [DSC]

Tablet, sustained release:
- Quibron®-T/SR: 300 mg [8-12 hours] [DSC]

References

Bhatt-Mehta V and Schumacher RE, "Treatment of Apnea of Prematurity," *Paediatr Drugs*, 2003, 5(3):195-210.

Hendeles L, Jenkins J, and Temple R, "Revised FDA Labeling Guideline for Theophylline Oral Dosage Forms," *Pharmacotherapy*, 1995, 15(4):409-427.

Kearney TE, Manoguerra AS, Curtis GP, et al, "Theophylline Toxicity and the Beta-Adrenergic System," *Ann Intern Med*, 1985, 102(6):766-9.

Kraus DM, Fischer JH, Reitz SJ, et al, "Alterations in Theophylline Metabolism During the First Year of Life," *Clin Pharmacol Ther*, 1993, 54(4):351-9.

"National Asthma Education and Prevention Program. Expert Panel Report: Guidelines for the Diagnosis and Management of Asthma Update on Selected Topics--2002," *J Allergy Clin Immunol*, 2002, 110(5 Suppl):S141-219.

Upton RA, "Pharmacokinetic Interactions Between Theophylline and Other Medication (Part I)," *Clin Pharmacokinet*, 1991, 20(1):66-80.

- **Theophylline Anhydrous** *see* Theophylline *on page 1520*
- **Theophylline Ethylenediamine** *see* Aminophylline *on page 98*
- **Thera-Flur-N®** *see* Fluoride *on page 675*
- **Thermazene®** *see* Silver Sulfadiazine *on page 1439*

Thiabendazole (thye a BEN da zole)

U.S. Brand Names Mintezol®

Index Terms Tiabendazole

Therapeutic Category Anthelmintic

Generic Available No

Use Treatment of strongyloidiasis, cutaneous larva migrans, visceral larva migrans, dracunculosis, trichinosis, and mixed helminthic infections

Pregnancy Risk Factor C

Lactation Excretion in breast milk unknown/not recommended

Contraindications Hypersensitivity to thiabendazole or any component; pregnancy. Contraindicated as prophylactic treatment for pinworm infestation.

Warnings Abnormal sensation in eyes, blurred vision, xanthopsia, drying of mucous membranes, and Sicca syndrome have been reported in patients receiving thiabendazole; ocular adverse effect may persist beyond one year in some cases

Precautions Use with caution in patients with renal or hepatic impairment, malnutrition, anemia, or dehydration

Adverse Reactions

Cardiovascular: Flushing, hypotension, bradycardia

Central nervous system: Dizziness, drowsiness, vertigo, seizures, fever, malaise, headache, chills, hallucinations

Dermatologic: Rash, Stevens-Johnson syndrome, erythema multiforme, pruritus

Endocrine & metabolic: Hyperglycemia

Gastrointestinal: Nausea, vomiting, diarrhea, anorexia, abdominal pain

Genitourinary: Malodor of the urine

Hematologic: Leukopenia

Hepatic: Hepatotoxicity, jaundice, cholestasis

Neuromuscular & skeletal: Paresthesia, numbness

Ocular: Blurred vision, Sicca syndrome

Otic: Tinnitus

Renal: Nephrotoxicity, hematuria

Miscellaneous: Hypersensitivity reactions, lymphadenopathy

(Continued)

Thiabendazole *(Continued)*

Drug Interactions Increases serum theophylline concentrations (monitor serum theophylline level in patients receiving both drugs concomitantly)

Mechanism of Action Inhibits helminth-specific mitochondrial fumarate reductase

Pharmacokinetics

Absorption: From the GI tract and through the skin

Metabolism: Extensive in the liver via hydroxylation and conjugation with sulfuric and/or glucuronic acid

Time to peak serum concentration: Within 1-2 hours

Elimination: In feces (5%) and urine (87%), primarily as conjugated metabolites

Usual Dosage

Oral:

Children and Adults: 50 mg/kg/day divided every 12 hours (maximum dose: 3 g/day)

Strongyloidiasis: For 2 consecutive days (5 days or longer for disseminated disease)

Cutaneous larva migrans: For 2-5 consecutive days

Visceral larva migrans: For 5-7 consecutive days

Trichinosis: For 2-4 consecutive days

Angiostrongylosis: 50-75 mg/kg/day divided every 8-12 hours for 3 days

Dracunculosis: 50-75 mg/kg/day divided every 12 hours for 3 days

Topical: Cutaneous larva migrans: Instead of oral therapy, thiabendazole 10% to 15% suspension or a 10% ointment in white petrolatum has been applied topically to lesions 4-6 times/day

Administration Oral: Administer after meals; chew tablet well before swallowing

Monitoring Parameters Periodic renal and hepatic function tests, serum glucose

Patient Information May cause drowsiness and impair ability to perform activities requiring mental alertness or physical coordination

Nursing Implications Purgation is not required prior to use

Dosage Forms Excipient information presented when available (limited, particularly for generics); consult specific product labeling. [DSC] = Discontinued product

Suspension, oral: 500 mg/5 mL (120 mL) [DSC]

Tablet, chewable: 500 mg [orange flavor]

References

Walden J, "Parasitic Diseases. Other Roundworms. *Trichuris*, Hookworm, and *Strongyloides*," *Prim Care*, 1991, 18(1):53-74.

Zygmunt DJ, "*Strongyloides stearcoralis*," *Infect Control Hosp Epidemiol*, 1990, 11(9):495-7.

♦ **Thiamazole** *see* Methimazole *on page 1022*

♦ **Thiamin** *see* Thiamine *on page 1526*

Thiamine (THYE a min)

Medication Safety Issues

Sound-alike/look-alike issues:

Thiamine may be confused with Tenormin®, Thorazine®

International issues:

Doxal® [Brazil] may be confused with Doxil® which is a brand name for doxorubicin in the U.S.

Doxal® [Brazil]: Brand name for doxycycline in Austria; brand name for pyridoxine in Brazil; brand name for doxepin in Finland

Canadian Brand Names Betaxin®

Index Terms Aneurine Hydrochloride; Thiamin; Thiamine Hydrochloride; Thiaminium Chloride Hydrochloride; Vitamin B_1

Therapeutic Category Nutritional Supplement; Vitamin, Water Soluble

Generic Available Yes

Use Treatment of thiamine deficiency including beriberi, Wernicke's encephalopathy syndrome, and peripheral neuritis associated with pellagra; alcoholic patients with altered sensorium; various genetic metabolic disorders

Pregnancy Risk Factor A (C if dose exceeds RDA recommendation)

Lactation Enters breast milk/use caution (AAP rates "compatible")

Contraindications Hypersensitivity to thiamine or any component

Warnings Large doses should be given in divided doses for better oral absorption

Precautions Use parenteral route cautiously, see Adverse Reactions

Adverse Reactions

Cardiovascular: Cardiovascular collapse and death (primarily following repeated I.V. administration), warmth

Dermatologic: Rash, angioedema

Genitourinary: Discoloration of urine (bright yellow) with large doses

Neuromuscular & skeletal: Paresthesia

Drug Interactions I.V. dextrose solutions increase thiamine requirement; thiamine may enhance the effects of neuromuscular blocking agents

Food Interactions High carbohydrate diets may increase thiamine requirement

Stability Unstable with alkaline or neutral solutions

Mechanism of Action An essential coenzyme in carbohydrate metabolism; combines with adenosine triphosphate to form thiamine pyrophosphate

Pharmacokinetics

Absorption:

Oral: Poor

I.M.: Rapid and complete

Metabolism: In the liver

Elimination: Renally as unchanged drug only after body storage sites become saturated

Usual Dosage

Adequate intake: Oral: Infants:

<6 months: 0.2 mg (0.03 mg/kg)

6-12 months: 0.3 mg (0.03 mg/kg)

Recommended daily allowance (RDA): Oral:

1-3 years: 0.5 mg

4-8 years: 0.6 mg

9-13 years: 0.9 mg

14-18 years:

Male: 1.2 mg

Female: 1 mg

≥19 years:

Male: 1.2 mg

Female: 1.1 mg

Dietary supplement (depends on caloric or carbohydrate content of the diet)

Oral:

Infants: 0.3-0.5 mg/day

Children: 0.5-1 mg/day

Adults: 1-2 mg/day

Note: The above doses can be found in multivitamin preparations

Thiamine deficiency (beriberi):

Children: 10-25 mg/dose I.M. or I.V. daily (if critically ill), or 10-50 mg/dose orally every day for 2 weeks, then 5-10 mg/dose orally daily for 1 month

Adults: 5-30 mg/dose I.M. or I.V. 3 times/day (if critically ill); then orally 5-30 mg/day in single or divided doses 3 times/day for 1 month

Wernicke's encephalopathy: Adults: Initial: 100 mg I.V., then 50-100 mg/day I.M. or I.V. until consuming a regular, balanced diet

Metabolic disorders: Oral: Adults: 10-20 mg/day (dosages up to 4 g/day in divided doses have been used)

Administration

Oral: May administer with or without food

Parenteral: Administer by slow I.V. injection or I.M.

Reference Range Normal values: 1.6-4 mg/dL

Test Interactions False-positive for uric acid using the phosphotungstate method and for urobilinogen using the Ehrlich's reagent; large doses may interfere with the spectrophotometric determination of serum theophylline concentration

Patient Information May color urine bright yellow

Additional Information Dietary sources include legumes, pork, beef, whole grains, yeast, fresh vegetables; a deficiency state can occur in as little as 3 weeks following total dietary absence

Dosage Forms Excipient information presented when available (limited, particularly for generics); consult specific product labeling.

Injection, solution, as hydrochloride: 100 mg/mL (2 mL)

Tablet, as hydrochloride: 50 mg, 100 mg, 250 mg, 500 mg

♦ **Thiamine Hydrochloride** *see* Thiamine *on page 1526*

♦ **Thiaminium Chloride Hydrochloride** *see* Thiamine *on page 1526*

Thioguanine (thye oh GWAH neen)

Medication Safety Issues

High alert medication: The Institute for Safe Medication Practices (ISMP) includes this medication among its list of drugs which have a heightened risk of causing significant patient harm when used in error.

6-thioguanine and 6-TG are error-prone abbreviations (associated with six-fold overdoses of thioguanine)

(Continued)

Thioguanine *(Continued)*

Related Information

Emetogenic Potential of Single Chemotherapeutic Agents *on page 1776*

U.S. Brand Names Tabloid®

Canadian Brand Names Lanvis®

Index Terms 2-Amino-6-Mercaptopurine; NSC-752; TG; 6-TG (error-prone abbreviation); 6-Thioguanine (error-prone abbreviation); Tioguanine

Therapeutic Category Antineoplastic Agent, Antimetabolite

Generic Available No

Use Remission induction and remission consolidation treatment of acute myelogenous (nonlymphocytic) leukemia; treatment of chronic myelogenous leukemia and acute lymphocytic leukemia; **Note:** Response to thioguanine depends upon patient age (younger patients do better than older) and whether use is in a previously treated or untreated patient

Pregnancy Risk Factor D

Lactation Excretion in breast milk unknown

Contraindications Hypersensitivity to thioguanine or any component; pregnancy; history of previous therapy resistance with thioguanine and in patients resistant to mercaptopurine (usual to find cross-resistance between thioguanine and mercaptopurine)

Warnings The FDA currently recommends that procedures for proper handling and disposal of antineoplastic agents be considered; thioguanine is potentially carcinogenic and teratogenic. Liver toxicity associated with vascular endothelial damage has been reported in patients receiving long-term thioguanine maintenance therapy. The liver toxicity is particularly prevalent in children receiving maintenance therapy for acute lymphoblastic leukemia and in males; liver toxicity usually presents as the clinical syndrome of hepatic veno-occlusive disease or portal hypertension. Discontinue thioguanine therapy in patients with signs and symptoms of liver toxicity.

Precautions Use with caution and reduce dose of thioguanine in patients with renal or hepatic impairment. Substantial dosage reductions may be required in patients with an inherited deficiency of the enzyme thiopurine methyltransferase (TPMT).

Adverse Reactions

Central nervous system: Neurotoxicity, headache

Dermatologic: Skin rash, photosensitivity, staining of skin or eyes (yellow)

Endocrine & metabolic: Hyperuricemia

Gastrointestinal: Mild nausea or vomiting, anorexia, stomatitis, diarrhea, intestinal necrosis and perforation, splenomegaly

Hematologic: Myelosuppression (leukopenia, granulocytopenia, thrombocytopenia, anemia)

Hepatic: Hepatitis, jaundice, veno-occlusive hepatic disease, hyperbilirubinemia, ascites, portal hypertension, elevated liver transaminases

Neuromuscular & skeletal: Unsteady gait

Drug Interactions Busulfan (thioguanine increases busulfan toxicity); olsalazine, mesalamine, and sulfasalazine may inhibit TPMT (increases bone marrow suppression)

Food Interactions Enhanced absorption if administered between meals

Stability Store at room temperature in a dry location.

Mechanism of Action Purine analog that is incorporated into DNA and RNA resulting in the inhibition of synthesis and utilization of purine nucleotides

Pharmacokinetics

Absorption: Oral: 30% (variable and incomplete)

Distribution: Crosses the placenta; does not appear to cross into CSF

Metabolism: Rapid and extensive hepatic metabolism by methylation of thioguanine to 2-amino-6-methylthioguanine (active) and inactive compounds

Half-life, terminal: 11 hours

Time to peak serum concentration: Within 8-12 hours

Elimination: Metabolites excreted in urine

Usual Dosage Oral (refer to individual protocols):

Infants <3 years: Combination drug therapy for ANLL: 3.3 mg/kg/day in divided doses twice daily for 4 days

Children and Adults:

Single agent chemotherapy for ANLL: 2-3 mg/kg/day once daily calculated to nearest 20 mg

Induction of remission in patients with acute leukemia (combination therapy): 75-200 mg/m^2/day in 1-2 divided doses for 5-7 days or until remission is attained

Note: Lower dose maintenance therapy is no longer recommended in the U.S. Instead, shorter period induction and consolidation therapy at higher doses is employed.

Administration Oral: Administer between meals on an empty stomach

Monitoring Parameters CBC with (differential, platelet count), liver function tests (serum transaminases, alkaline phosphatase, bilirubin), hemoglobin, hematocrit, serum uric acid; testing for thiopurine methyltransferase (TPMT) deficiency; clinical signs of portal hypertension or veno-occlusive disease

Patient Information Notify physician if fever, sore throat, bleeding, bruising, nausea, vomiting, yellow discoloration of skin or eyes, or leg swelling occurs. May cause photosensitivity reactions (eg, exposure to sunlight may cause severe sunburn, skin rash, redness, or itching); avoid exposure to sunlight and artificial light sources (sunlamps, tanning booth/bed); wear protective clothing, wide-brimmed hats, sunglasses, and lip sunscreen (SPF ≥15); use a sunscreen [broad-spectrum sunscreen or physical sunscreen (preferred) or sunblock with SPF ≥15]; contact physician if reaction occurs. Women of childbearing potential should be advised to avoid becoming pregnant.

Nursing Implications Ensure adequate patient hydration, alkalinization of the urine, and/or administration of allopurinol to prevent hyperuricemia

Additional Information Myelosuppressive effects:

WBC: Moderate
Platelets: Moderate
Onset (days): 7-10
Nadir (days): 14
Recovery (days): 21

Dosage Forms Excipient information presented when available (limited, particularly for generics); consult specific product labeling.

Tablet [scored]:
Tabloid®: 40 mg

Extemporaneous Preparations A 20 mg/mL oral suspension can be made by crushing fifteen 40 mg tablets in a mortar. Add 10 mL of methylcellulose 1% in small amounts and mix. Transfer to a graduate and add a sufficient quantity of syrup to make 30 mL. Stable for 60 days at room temperature. Label "shake well."

Nahata MC and Hipple TF, *Pediatric Drug Formulations*, 4th ed, Cincinnati, OH: Harvey Whitney Books Co, 2000.

References

Broxson EH, Dole M, Wong R, et al, "Portal Hypertension Develops in a Subset of Children With Standard Risk Acute Lymphoblastic Leukemia Treated With Oral 6-Thioguanine During Maintenance Therapy," *Pediatr Blood Cancer*, 2005, 44(3):226-31.

Culbert SJ, Shuster JJ, Land VJ, et al, "Remission Induction and Continuation Therapy in Children With Their First Relapse of Acute Lymphoid Leukemia: A Pediatric Oncology Group Study," *Cancer*, 1991, 67(1):37-42.

Steuber CP, Civin C, Krischer J, et al, "A Comparison of Induction and Maintenance Therapy for Acute Nonlymphocytic Leukemia in Childhood: Results of a Pediatric Oncology Group Study," *J Clin Oncol*, 1991, 9(2):247-58.

♦ **6-Thioguanine (error-prone abbreviation)** *see* Thioguanine *on page 1527*

Thiopental (thye oh PEN tal)

Related Information

Preprocedure Sedatives in Children *on page 1895*

U.S. Brand Names Pentothal®

Canadian Brand Names Pentothal®

Index Terms Thiopental Sodium

Therapeutic Category Anticonvulsant, Barbiturate; Barbiturate; General Anesthetic; Hypnotic; Sedative

Generic Available No

Use Induction of anesthesia; adjunct for intubation in head injury patients; control of convulsive states; treatment of elevated intracranial pressure

Restrictions C-III

Pregnancy Risk Factor C

Contraindications Hypersensitivity to thiopental, pentobarbital, any component, or other barbiturates; porphyria (variegate or acute intermittent)

Precautions Use with caution in patients with asthma or pharyngeal infections because cough, laryngospasm, or bronchospasms may occur; use with caution in patients with hypotension, severe cardiovascular disease, hepatic or renal dysfunction; avoid extravasation or intra-arterial injection which may cause necrosis due to pH of 10.6; ensure patient has intravenous access

Adverse Reactions

Cardiovascular: Decreased cardiac output, hypotension
Local: Necrosis with I.V. extravasation
Renal: Decreased urine output
Respiratory: Cough, laryngospasm, bronchospasm, respiratory depression, apnea
Miscellaneous: Anaphylaxis
(Continued)

Thiopental *(Continued)*

Drug Interactions Barbiturates are enzyme inducers (monitor patients closely for decreased effect of concomitantly administered medications or increased effect when barbiturates are discontinued); CNS depressants

Stability Solutions are alkaline and incompatible with drugs with acidic pH, such as succinylcholine, atropine sulfate

Mechanism of Action Ultra-short-acting barbiturate; depresses CNS activity by binding to barbiturate site at GABA-receptor complex enhancing GABA activity; depresses reticular activating system; higher doses may be gabamimetic

Pharmacodynamics Anesthesia effects:

Onset of action: I.V.: 30-60 seconds

Duration: 5-30 minutes

Pharmacokinetics

Distribution: V_d: Adults: 1.4 L/kg

Protein binding: 72% to 86%

Metabolism: In the liver primarily to inactive metabolites but pentobarbital is also formed

Half-life, adults: 3-11.5 hours (shorter half-life in children)

Usual Dosage

Induction anesthesia: I.V.:
- Neonates: 3-4 mg/kg
- Infants: 5-8 mg/kg
- Children 1-12 years: 5-6 mg/kg
- Children >12 years and Adults: 3-5 mg/kg

Maintenance anesthesia: I.V.:
- Children: 1 mg/kg as needed
- Adults: 25-100 mg as needed

Increased intracranial pressure: Children: I.V.: 1.5-5 mg/kg/dose; repeat as needed to control intracranial pressure; larger doses (30 mg/kg) to induce coma after hypoxic-ischemic injury do not appear to improve neurologic outcome

Seizures: I.V.:
- Children: 2-3 mg/kg/dose, repeat as needed
- Adults: 75-250 mg/dose, repeat as needed

Sedation: Rectal:
- Children: 5-10 mg/kg/dose
- Adults: 3-4 g/dose

Administration Parenteral: Avoid rapid I.V. injection (may cause hypotension or decreased cardiac output); may administer by intermittent infusion over 10-60 minutes at a maximum concentration of 50 mg/mL

Monitoring Parameters Respiratory rate, heart rate, blood pressure

Reference Range

Therapeutic:
- Hypnotic: 1-5 mcg/mL (SI: 4.1-20.7 micromoles/L)
- Coma: 30-100 mcg/mL (SI: 124-413 micromoles/L)
- Anesthesia: 7-130 mcg/mL (SI: 29-536 micromoles/L)

Nursing Implications Avoid extravasation, necrosis may occur

Additional Information Accumulation may occur with chronic dosing due to lipid solubility; prolonged recovery occurs due to redistribution of thiopental from fat stores; therefore, thiopental is usually not used for procedures lasting >15-20 minutes; sodium content, injection: 4.9 mEq/g

Dosage Forms Excipient information presented when available (limited, particularly for generics); consult specific product labeling.

Injection, powder for reconstitution, as sodium: 250 mg, 400 mg, 500 mg, 1 g

- **Thiopental Sodium** *see* Thiopental *on page 1529*
- **Thiophosphoramide** *see* Thiotepa *on page 1532*

Thioridazine (thye oh RID a zeen)

Medication Safety Issues

Sound-alike/look-alike issues:
- Thioridazine may be confused with thiothixene, Thorazine®
- Mellaril® may be confused with Elavil®, Mebaral®

Related Information

Medications for Which A Single Dose May Be Fatal When Ingested By A Toddler *on page 1932*

Overdose and Toxicology *on page 1916*

Canadian Brand Names Mellaril®

Index Terms Thioridazine Hydrochloride

Therapeutic Category Antipsychotic Agent; Phenothiazine Derivative

Generic Available Yes

Use Due to prolongation of the QT_c interval (see Warnings), thioridazine is currently indicated only for the treatment of refractory schizophrenic patients; in the past, the drug had been used for management of psychotic disorders; depressive neurosis; dementia in elderly; severe behavioral problems in children

Pregnancy Risk Factor C

Lactation Excretion in breast milk unknown/not recommended

Contraindications Hypersensitivity to thioridazine or any component; cross-sensitivity to other phenothiazines may exist; concurrent therapy with propranolol, pindolol, fluvoxamine, fluoxetine, paroxetine, drugs that inhibit cytochrome P450 isoenzyme CYP2D6, drugs that prolong the QT_c interval, and patients with reduced levels of CYP2D6, a history of cardiac arrhythmias, congenital long QT syndrome, or a QT_c interval >450 msec (adults); severe CNS depression; avoid use in patients with narrow-angle glaucoma, blood dyscrasias, severe liver or cardiac disease

Warnings Prolongation of the QT_c interval may occur and may be associated with torsade de pointes arrhythmias and sudden death; tablets may contain sodium benzoate; benzoic acid (benzoate) is a metabolite of benzyl alcohol; large amounts of benzyl alcohol (≥99 mg/kg/day) have been associated with a potentially fatal toxicity ("gasping syndrome") in neonates; avoid use of thioridazine products containing sodium benzoate in neonates; *in vitro* and animal studies have shown that benzoate displaces bilirubin from protein binding sites

Precautions Use with caution in patients with severe cardiovascular disorder or seizures

Adverse Reactions Sedation and anticholinergic effects are more pronounced than extrapyramidal effects; EKG changes and retinal pigmentation are more common than with chlorpromazine

Cardiovascular: Hypotension, orthostatic hypotension, tachycardia, arrhythmias

Central nervous system: Sedation, drowsiness, restlessness, anxiety, extrapyramidal reactions, pseudoparkinsonian signs and symptoms, tardive dyskinesia, neuroleptic malignant syndrome, seizures, altered central temperature regulation

Dermatologic: Hyperpigmentation, pruritus, rash, contact dermatitis, photosensitivity (rare)

Endocrine & metabolic: Amenorrhea, galactorrhea, gynecomastia, weight gain

Gastrointestinal: GI upset, xerostomia, constipation

Genitourinary: Urinary retention

Hematologic: Agranulocytosis, leukopenia (usually in patients with large doses for prolonged periods)

Hepatic: Cholestatic jaundice

Ocular: Retinal pigmentation (usually in patients receiving larger than recommended doses), blurred vision, brownish coloring of vision, decreased night vision, decreased visual acuity (may be irreversible)

Miscellaneous: Anaphylactoid reactions

Drug Interactions Cytochrome P450 isoenzyme CYP1A2 and CYP2D6 substrate; CYP2D6 isoenzyme inhibitor

Additive effects with alcohol and other CNS depressants; concurrent use with lithium has caused acute encephalopathy-like syndrome (rare); increased cardiac arrhythmias with tricyclic antidepressants; epinephrine may cause hypotension; drugs that inhibit the metabolism of thioridazine (eg, fluoxetine, fluvoxamine, paroxetine) or drugs that prolong the QT_c interval may increase the risk of serious adverse effects, such as QT_c prolongation, serious ventricular arrhythmias (eg, torsade de pointes) and sudden death (such drugs are contraindicated; see Contraindications); mixing liquid thioridazine with carbamazepine suspension will result in precipitation of an orange rubbery mass (see also Contraindications)

Food Interactions May increase dietary requirements for riboflavin; liquid thioridazine formulations may precipitate with enteral formulas

Mechanism of Action Blocks postsynaptic mesolimbic dopaminergic receptors in the brain; exhibits a strong alpha-adrenergic blocking effect and depresses the release of hypothalamic and hypophyseal hormones

Pharmacokinetics

Protein binding: 99%

Metabolism: In the liver to active and inactive metabolites

Bioavailability: 25% to 33%

Half-life: Adults: 9-30 hours

Dialysis: Not dialyzable: (0% to 5%)

Usual Dosage Oral:

Children >2 years: Initial: 0.5 mg/kg/day in 2-3 divided doses; range: 0.5-3 mg/kg/day; usual: 1 mg/kg/day in 2-3 divided doses; maximum dose: 3 mg/kg/day

(Continued)

Thioridazine *(Continued)*

Behavior problems: Initial: 10 mg 2-3 times/day, increase gradually
Severe psychoses: Initial: 25 mg 2-3 times/day, increase gradually

Children >12 years and Adults:

Schizophrenia/psychoses: Initial: 25-100 mg 3 times/day with gradual increments as needed and tolerated; maximum daily dose: 800 mg/day in 2-4 divided doses; maintenance: 10-200 mg/dose 2-4 times/day

Depressive disorders, dementia: Initial: 25 mg 3 times/day; maintenance dose: 20-200 mg/day

Administration Oral: Administer with water, food, or milk to decrease GI upset; dilute the oral concentrate with water or juice before administration; do not administer liquid thioridazine simultaneously with carbamazepine suspension (see Drug Interactions); do not mix liquid thioridazine with enteric formulas (see Food Interactions)

Monitoring Parameters Baseline and periodic EKG and serum potassium; periodic eye exam, CBC with differential, blood pressure, liver enzyme tests

Test Interactions False-positives for phenylketonuria, urinary amylase, uroporphyrins, urobilinogen

Patient Information Avoid alcohol; may cause drowsiness and impair ability to perform activities requiring mental alertness or physical coordination; may cause dry mouth; avoid skin contact with oral liquid preparations, may cause contact dermatitis; do not discontinue or alter dose without physician approval. May rarely cause photosensitivity reactions; avoid exposure to sunlight and artificial light sources (sunlamps, tanning booth/bed); use a sunscreen; contact physician if reaction occurs

Additional Information In cases of overdoses, cardiovascular monitoring and continuous EKG monitoring should be performed; avoid drugs (such as quinidine, disopyramide, and procainamide) that may further prolong the QT interval

Note: All Mellaril® (brand name) products have been discontinued; Mellaril® suspension was discontinued October, 2000; oral concentrate 100 mg/mL was discontinued March 2001; tablets and 30 mg/mL oral concentrate were discontinued in January 2002.

Dosage Forms Excipient information presented when available (limited, particularly for generics); consult specific product labeling.

Tablet, as hydrochloride: 10 mg, 15 mg, 25 mg, 50 mg, 100 mg, 150 mg, 200 mg

References

Aman MG, Marks RE, Turbott SH, et al, "Clinical Effects of Methylphenidate and Thioridazine in Intellectually Subaverage Children," *J Am Acad Child Adolesc Psychiatry*, 1991, 30(2):246-56.

♦ **Thioridazine Hydrochloride** *see* Thioridazine *on page 1530*

♦ **Thiosulfuric Acid Disodium Salt** *see* Sodium Thiosulfate *on page 1461*

Thiotepa (thye oh TEP a)

Medication Safety Issues

High alert medication: The Institute for Safe Medication Practices (ISMP) includes this medication among its list of drugs which have a heightened risk of causing significant patient harm when used in error.

Related Information

Compatibility of Chemotherapy and Related Supportive Care Medications *on page 1777*

Emetogenic Potential of Single Chemotherapeutic Agents *on page 1776*

Index Terms TESPA; Thiophosphoramide; Triethylenethiophosphoramide; TSPA

Therapeutic Category Antineoplastic Agent, Alkylating Agent

Generic Available Yes

Use Treatment of superficial tumors of the bladder; palliative treatment of adenocarcinoma of breast or ovary; lymphomas and sarcomas; meningeal neoplasms; control of pleural, pericardial or peritoneal effusions caused by metastatic tumors; high-dose regimens with autologous bone marrow transplantation

Pregnancy Risk Factor D

Lactation Enters breast milk/not recommended

Contraindications Hypersensitivity to thiotepa or any component; severe myelosuppression with leukocyte count <3000/mm^3 or platelet count <150,000 mm^3; pregnancy

Warnings The FDA currently recommends that procedures for proper handling and disposal of antineoplastic agents be considered. The drug is potentially mutagenic, carcinogenic, teratogenic, and may cause fertility impairment. Death due to bone marrow depression has been reported after intravesical administration. Death due to sepsis and hemorrhage as a result of thiotepa administration has also been reported.

Precautions Reduce dosage in patients with hepatic, renal, or bone marrow dysfunction

Adverse Reactions

Central nervous system: Dizziness, fever, headache, confusion, fatigue, somnolence

Dermatologic: Alopecia, rash, pruritus, hyperpigmentation of skin with high-dose therapy, contact dermatitis, urticaria

Endocrine & metabolic: Amenorrhea, hyperuricemia, azoospermia

Gastrointestinal: Nausea, vomiting, stomatitis, esophagitis, anorexia, abdominal pain, mucositis

Genitourinary: Rarely hemorrhagic cystitis, urinary retention

Hematologic: Leukopenia (nadir: 7-10 days), anemia, thrombocytopenia (nadir: 3 weeks), granulocytopenia

Hepatic: Elevated liver transaminase and bilirubin (high-dose therapy)

Local: Pain at injection site

Ocular: Conjunctivitis, blurred vision

Renal: Hematuria

Respiratory: Laryngeal edema, wheezing

Miscellaneous: Anaphylaxis

Drug Interactions Cytochrome P450 isoenzyme CYP2B6 inhibitor

Succinylcholine (thiotepa inhibits pseudocholinesterase activity; prolongs muscular paralysis); other alkylating agents such as nitrogen mustard or cyclophosphamide (intensifies toxicity)

Stability Refrigerate, protect from light; the reconstituted 10 mg/mL solution is chemically stable for 5 days when stored in the refrigerator; since it contains no preservatives use within 8 hours; unstable in acid medium. Thiotepa is stable for 24 hours at a concentration of 1-5 mg/mL in NS when stored at room temperature; at 0.5 mg/mL, thiotepa is stable for 8 hours at room temperature; stability decreases significantly at concentrations <0.5 mg/mL (1 hour).

Mechanism of Action Polyfunctional alkylating agent that reacts with DNA phosphate groups to produce cross-linking of DNA strands leading to inhibition of DNA, RNA, and protein synthesis

Pharmacokinetics

Absorption: Variable absorption through serous membranes and from I.M. injection sites; bladder mucosa: 10% to 100% and is increased with mucosal inflammation or tumor infiltration

Distribution: V_{dss}: 0.7-1.6 L/kg; distributes into CSF

Protein binding: 8% to 13%

Metabolism: In the liver via oxidative desulfuration (cytochrome P450 microsomal enzyme system) primarily to TEPA (active metabolite)

Half-life, terminal:

- Thiotepa: 109 minutes (51.6-212 minutes) with dose-dependent clearance
- TEPA: 10-21 hours

Elimination: Very little thiotepa or active metabolite are excreted unchanged in urine (1.5% of thiotepa dose)

Usual Dosage Refer to individual protocols

Children:

- I.V.: Sarcomas: 25-65 mg/m^2 as a single dose every 3-4 weeks
  - High-dose thiotepa with ABMT: One regimen uses 300 mg/m^2/dose over 3 hours; repeat every 24 hours for a total of 3 doses; maximum tolerated dose over 3 days: 900-1125 mg/m^2
- Intrathecal: 5-11.5 mg/m^2 per dose weekly for 2-7 doses

Adults:

- I.V.: 0.3-0.4 mg/kg at 1- to 4-week intervals or 0.2 mg/kg (6 mg/m^2)/day for 4-5 days, repeat at 2- to 4-week intervals; continuous infusion: 15-35 mg/m^2 over 48 hours
- Intracavitary: 0.6-0.8 mg/kg; dose should not be repeated more frequently than at a 1 week interval

Administration

Bladder instillation: Prepare with 30-60 mg diluted in 30-60 mL sterile water and instill by catheter and retain for 2 hours

Intrapleural or pericardial: Dose is further diluted to a volume of 10-20 mL in NS or D_5W

Intraperitoneal: Administration requires dilution in larger volumes (up to 2 L)

Intrathecal: Reconstitute drug with SWI then dilute to a final concentration of 1 mg/mL with NS

I.V.: Filter through a 0.22 micron filter (Millex-GS or Gelman Sterile Acrodisc®) prior to administration; administer direct I.V. over 5 minutes at a final concentration of about 10 mg/mL; administer I.V. intermittent or continuous infusion at a final concentration for administration of 1 mg/mL (thiotepa may be further diluted in D_5W, NS, or LR)

Monitoring Parameters CBC with differential and platelet count, uric acid, urinalysis, renal and hepatic function tests

Patient Information Notify physician if fever, sore throat, urine color change, bleeding, or bruising occurs. Patients of childbearing potential should avoid becoming

(Continued)

Thiotepa *(Continued)*

pregnant while on thiotepa therapy. Effective contraception should be used if either the patient or partner is of childbearing potential.

Nursing Implications Wear protective gloves during handling of thiotepa solution; if thiotepa solution comes in contact with skin or mucosa, the affected area should be washed with soap and water immediately or affected mucosa should be rinsed thoroughly with water.

Additional Information Myelosuppressive effects:

WBC: Moderate
Platelets: Severe
Onset (days): 7-10
Nadir (days): 14-20
Recovery (days): 28

Dosage Forms Excipient information presented when available (limited, particularly for generics); consult specific product labeling.

Injection, powder for reconstitution: 15 mg, 30 mg

References

Fagioli F, Biasin E, Mastrodicasa L, et al, "High-Dose Thiotepa and Etoposide in Children With Poor-Prognosis Brain Tumors," *Cancer*, 2004, 100(10):2215-21.

Fisher PG, Kadan-Lottick NS, and Korones DN, "Intrathecal Thiotepa: Reappraisal of an Established Therapy," *J Pediatr Hematol Oncol*, 2002, 24(4):274-8.

Grovas AC, Boyett JM, Lindsley K, et al, "Regimen-Related Toxicity of Myeloablative Chemotherapy With BCNU, Thiotepa, and Etoposide Followed by Autologous Stem Cell Rescue for Children With Newly Diagnosed Glioblastoma Multiforme: Report From the Children's Cancer Group," *Med Pediatr Oncol*, 1999, 33(2):83-7.

Heideman R, Cole D, Balis F, et al, "Phase I and Pharmacokinetic Evaluation of Thiotepa in the Cerebrospinal Fluid and Plasma of Pediatric Patients: Evidence for Dose-Dependent Plasma Clearance of Thiotepa," *Cancer Res*, 1989, 49(3):736-41.

Herzig GP, "Phase I-II Studies of High-Dose Thiotepa and Autologous BMT in Patients With Refractory Malignancies," *Adv Cancer Chemotherapy*, 1987, 17-29 (proceedings of a symposium, Oct 1986)

Saarinen UM, Hovi L, and Makipern CA, "High Dose Thiotepa With Autologous Bone Marrow Rescue in Pediatric Solid Tumors," *Proc Am Soc Clin Oncol*, 1989, 8:303.

Thiothixene (thye oh THIKS een)

Medication Safety Issues

Sound-alike/look-alike issues:

Thiothixene may be confused with thioridazine
Navane® may be confused with Norvasc®, Nubain®

Related Information

Overdose and Toxicology *on page 1916*

U.S. Brand Names Navane®

Canadian Brand Names Navane®

Index Terms Tiotixene

Therapeutic Category Antipsychotic Agent; Phenothiazine Derivative

Generic Available Yes

Use Management of schizophrenia; also used for management of psychotic disorders

Pregnancy Risk Factor C

Lactation Excretion in breast milk unknown/not recommended

Contraindications Hypersensitivity to thiothixene or any component; cross-sensitivity with other phenothiazines may exist; patients with CNS depression, comatose states, circulatory collapse, or blood dyscrasias; avoid use in patients with narrow-angle glaucoma, bone marrow suppression, severe liver or cardiac disease

Warnings Tardive dyskinesias and neuroleptic malignant syndrome may occur

Precautions Use with caution in patients with cardiovascular disease or seizures

Adverse Reactions Sedation and extrapyramidal effects occur more often

Cardiovascular: Hypotension (especially with parenteral use), orthostatic hypotension, tachycardia, arrhythmias

Central nervous system: Sedation, drowsiness, restlessness, anxiety, insomnia, extrapyramidal reactions, tardive dyskinesia, neuroleptic malignant syndrome, seizures, altered central temperature regulation

Dermatologic: Rash, photosensitivity

Endocrine & metabolic: Amenorrhea, galactorrhea, gynecomastia, weight gain

Gastrointestinal: GI upset, xerostomia, constipation

Genitourinary: Urinary retention

Hematologic: Agranulocytosis, leukopenia

Ocular: Retinal pigmentation, blurred vision

Drug Interactions Cytochrome P450 isoenzyme CYP1A2 substrate

Alcohol, other CNS depressants, or anticholinergics may increase adverse effects; antihypertensive agents may produce additive hypotensive effect (monitor blood pressure); hepatic enzyme inducers (eg, carbamazepine) may significantly increase thiothixene clearance and decrease effectiveness (monitor closely)

Food Interactions May cause increase in dietary riboflavin requirements

Mechanism of Action Elicits antipsychotic activity by postsynaptic blockade of CNS dopamine receptors resulting in inhibition of dopamine-mediated effects; also has alpha-adrenergic blocking activity

Usual Dosage Oral:

Children ≤12 years: Dose not well established (use not recommended); 0.25 mg/kg/day in divided doses

Children >12 years and Adults: Initial: 2 mg 3 times/day, up to 20-30 mg/day; maximum dose: 60 mg/day

Administration Oral: Administer with food or water

Monitoring Parameters Periodic eye exam, CBC with differential, blood pressure, liver enzyme tests

Patient Information Avoid alcohol; limit caffeine; may cause drowsiness and impair ability to perform activities requiring mental alertness or physical coordination; may cause dry mouth. May cause photosensitivity reactions (eg, exposure to sunlight may cause severe sunburn, skin rash, redness, or itching); avoid exposure to sunlight and artificial light sources (sunlamps, tanning booth/bed); wear protective clothing, wide-brimmed hats, sunglasses, and lip sunscreen (SPF ≥15); use a sunscreen [broad-spectrum sunscreen or physical sunscreen (preferred) or sunblock with SPF ≥15]; contact physician if reaction occurs.

Dosage Forms Excipient information presented when available (limited, particularly for generics); consult specific product labeling. [DSC] = Discontinued product

Capsule: 1 mg, 2 mg, 5 mg, 10 mg

Navane®: 1 mg [DSC], 2 mg, 5 mg, 10 mg, 20 mg

References

Wiener JM, "Psychopharmacology in Childhood Disorders," *Psychiatr Clin North Am*, 1984, 7(4):831-43.

♦ **Thorets [OTC]** *see* Benzocaine *on page 204*

♦ **Thrombin-JMI®** *see* Thrombin (Topical) *on page 1535*

Thrombin (Topical) (THROM bin, TOP i kal)

U.S. Brand Names Thrombin-JMI®

Therapeutic Category Hemostatic Agent

Generic Available No

Use Hemostasis whenever minor bleeding from capillaries and small venules is accessible

Pregnancy Risk Factor C

Contraindications Hypersensitivity to thrombin, any component, or material of bovine origin

Warnings For topical use only - do not inject; injection may result in extensive intravascular clotting and death. Use of topical thrombin has been associated with abnormalities in hemostasis ranging from asymptomatic alterations in PT and PTT to severe bleeding or thrombosis which have rarely been fatal. These hemostatic effects may be related to formation of antibodies against bovine thrombin and/or factor V which in some cases may cross react with human factor V resulting in factor V deficiency; patients with antibodies to bovine thrombin should not receive topical thrombin again

Adverse Reactions

Central nervous system: Fever

Miscellaneous: Allergic reactions

Stability Following reconstitution, use immediately; stable 3 hours refrigerated; stable frozen (reconstituted) for 48 hours

Mechanism of Action Catalyzes the conversion of fibrinogen to fibrin

Usual Dosage Topical: Apply powder directly to the site of bleeding or on oozing surfaces or use 1000-2000 units/mL of solution where bleeding is profuse; use 100 units/mL for bleeding from skin or mucosal surfaces

Administration Not for injection

Topical: May be applied directly as a powder or as reconstituted solution; the most effective hemostasis results when the thrombin mixes freely with blood as it appears; use sterile water or NS to reconstitute powder to 1000-2000 units/mL concentration; for profuse bleeding, 1000 units/mL may be required; for use in dental extractions, plastic surgery, or skin grafting 100 units/mL is frequently used. The recipient surface should be sponged (not wiped) free of blood before application; do not sponge **treated** surfaces to assure that clot remains securely in place

Additional Information One unit is amount required to clot 1 mL of standardized fibrinogen solution in 15 seconds

Dosage Forms Excipient information presented when available (limited, particularly for generics); consult specific product labeling.

(Continued)

Thrombin (Topical) *(Continued)*

Powder for reconstitution, topical:
Thrombin-JMI®: 5000 units, 20,000 units [packaged with diluent]
Thrombin-JMI® Spray Kit: 20,000 units [packaged with diluent and spray pump]
Thrombin-JMI® Syringe Spray Kit: 20,000 units [packaged with diluent, spray tip, and syringe]

- **Thymocyte Stimulating Factor** *see* Aldesleukin *on page 70*
- **Thymoglobulin®** *see* Antithymocyte Globulin (Rabbit) *on page 147*
- **Thyrel® TRH [DSC]** *see* Protirelin *on page 1343*
- **ThyroSafe™ [OTC]** *see* Potassium Iodide *on page 1290*
- **ThyroShield™ [OTC]** *see* Potassium Iodide *on page 1290*
- **Thyrotropin Releasing Hormone** *see* Protirelin *on page 1343*
- **Tiabendazole** *see* Thiabendazole *on page 1525*

Tiagabine (tye AG a bene)

Medication Safety Issues
Sound-alike/look-alike issues:
Tiagabine may be confused with tizanidine

U.S. Brand Names Gabitril®

Canadian Brand Names Gabitril®

Index Terms Tiagabine Hydrochloride

Therapeutic Category Anticonvulsant, Miscellaneous

Generic Available No

Use Adjunctive therapy of partial epilepsy

Pregnancy Risk Factor C

Lactation Enters breast milk/not recommended

Contraindications Hypersensitivity to tiagabine or any component

Warnings Current tiagabine dosing recommendations are based on studies in which most patients also received enzyme-inducing AEDs. Use of recommended tiagabine doses in patients **not** receiving enzyme-inducing AEDs may result in serum concentrations more than twice that of patients receiving enzyme-inducing AEDs. Use with caution and decrease the dose in patients who are **not** receiving enzyme-inducing AEDs; a slower titration of the drug may also be required in these patients.

New-onset seizures and status epilepticus have been reported with tiagabine use (for unlabeled indications) in patients without epilepsy. Higher doses may be a risk factor, but seizures have occurred in patients taking doses as low as 4 mg/day. Seizures have also occurred shortly after a dosage increase. In most cases, patients were also receiving concomitant medications that are thought to lower the seizure threshold (eg, antidepressants, antipsychotics, stimulants, narcotics). Discontinue tiagabine and evaluate patients for an underlying seizure disorder in nonepileptic patients who develop seizures while receiving tiagabine.

When used to treat epilepsy, do not abruptly discontinue therapy; withdraw gradually to lessen chance for increased seizure frequency (unless a more rapid withdrawal is required due to safety concerns). Cognitive and neuropsychiatric adverse effects may occur (see Adverse Reactions). Exacerbation of EEG abnormalities associated with CNS adverse events (cognitive and neuropsychiatric) may occur in patients with an EEG history of spike and wave discharges and may require dosage adjustment. Nonconvulsant status epilepticus has also been reported and may respond to dosage reduction or discontinuation. Seizures and status epilepticus may also occur with tiagabine overdose.

Precautions Use with caution in patients with hepatic impairment. Possible long-term ophthalmologic effects exist (more studies are needed). Use with caution with alcohol or other CNS depressants. Safety and effectiveness have not been established in children <12 years of age or for any indication other than as adjunctive therapy for partial seizures.

Adverse Reactions
Central nervous system: Impaired concentration, speech/language problems, confusion, somnolence, fatigue, dizziness, nervousness, depression, ataxia, insomnia, emotional lability, headache
Gastrointestinal: Nausea, abdominal pain, diarrhea
Neuromuscular & skeletal: Asthenia, tremor

Drug Interactions Cytochrome P450 isoenzyme CYP3A substrate, may also be metabolized by CYP1A2, 2D6, or 2C19

Tiagabine may decrease valproic acid concentrations by ~10%; carbamazepine, phenytoin, primidone, and phenobarbital may increase tiagabine clearance by 60%;

naproxen, salicylates, and valproic acid may decrease tiagabine protein binding and increase tiagabine free concentrations; other interactions with drugs that are highly protein bound may also occur

Food Interactions Food may decrease the rate but not the extent of absorption

Stability Protect from moisture and light; store at room temperature

Mechanism of Action Exact mechanism unknown; thought to potentiate the action of GABA (an inhibitory neurotransmitter) by selectively binding to the GABA uptake carrier and blocking GABA uptake into presynaptic neurons. This allows more GABA to be available at its site of action to bind to postsynaptic neuronal receptors.

Pharmacokinetics

Absorption: Rapid and nearly complete (>95%)

Distribution: Mean V_d:

Children 3-10 years: 2.4 L/kg

Adults: 1.3-1.6 L/kg

Note: V_d values are more similar between children and adults when expressed as L/m² (see Gustavson, 1997)

Protein binding: 96%, mainly to albumin and alpha₁-acid glycoprotein

Metabolism: Extensive in the liver via oxidation and glucuronidation; undergoes enterohepatic recirculation

Bioavailability: Oral: 90%

Diurnal effect: Trough concentrations and AUC are lower in the evening versus morning

Half-life:

Children 3-10 years: Mean: 5.7 hours (range: 2-10 hours)

Children 3-10 years receiving enzyme-inducing AEDs: Mean: 3.2 hours (range: 2-7.8 hours)

Adults (normal volunteers): 7-9 hours

Adult patients receiving enzyme-inducing AEDs: 2-5 hours

Time to peak serum concentration: Fasting state: ~45 minutes

Elimination: ~2% excreted unchanged in urine; 25% excreted in urine and 63% excreted in feces as metabolites

Clearance:

Children 3-10 years: 4.2 ± 1.6 mL/minute/kg

Children 3-10 years receiving enzyme-inducing AEDs: 8.6 ± 3.3 mL/minute/kg

Adults (normal volunteers): 109 mL/minute

Adult patients: 1.9 ± 0.5 mL/minute/kg

Adult patients receiving enzyme-inducing AEDs: 6.3 ± 3.5 mL/minute/kg

Note: Clearance values are more similar between children and adults when expressed as mL/minute/m² (see Gustavson, 1997)

Hepatic impairment: Clearance of unbound drug is decreased by 60%

Usual Dosage Oral: **Note:** Doses were determined in patients receiving enzyme-inducing AEDs; use of these doses in patients **not** receiving enzyme-inducing AEDs may result in serum concentrations more than twice those of patients receiving enzyme-inducing AEDS; **lower doses are required in patients not receiving enzyme-inducing agents;** a slower titration may also be necessary in these patients. Consider tiagabine dosage adjustment if enzyme-inducing agent is added, discontinued, or dose is changed. Do **not** use loading doses of tiagabine in any patient; do **not** use a rapid dosage escalation or increase the dose in large increments.

Children <12 years: Only limited preliminary information is available; dosing guidelines are not established (see Adkins, 1998 and Pellock, 1999)

Children 12-18 years: Initial: 4 mg once daily for 1 week, then 8 mg/day given in 2 divided doses for 1 week, then increase weekly by 4-8 mg/day; administer in 2-4 divided doses per day; titrate dose to response; maximum dose: 32 mg/day (doses >32 mg/day have been used in select adolescent patients for short periods of time)

Adults: Initial: 4 mg once daily for 1 week, then increase weekly by 4-8 mg/day; administer in 2-4 divided doses per day; titrate dose to response; usual maintenance: 32-56 mg/day in 2-4 divided doses; maximum dose: 56 mg/day. **Note:** Twice daily dosing may not be well tolerated and dosing 3 times/day is the currently favored dosing frequency (see Kalviainen, 1998).

Dosing adjustment in renal impairment: None needed

Dosing adjustment in hepatic impairment: Reduced doses and longer dosing intervals may be required

Administration Oral: Administer with food (to avoid rapid increase in plasma concentrations and adverse CNS effects)

Monitoring Parameters Seizure frequency, duration, and severity

Reference Range Not established

Patient Information May cause dizziness or drowsiness and impair ability to perform activities requiring mental alertness or physical coordination. If a dose is missed, do

(Continued)

Tiagabine *(Continued)*

not increase or double the next dose; if multiple doses are missed, contact your healthcare provider for possible retitration of the dose as clinically needed.

Additional Information Population pharmacokinetic analysis suggests that tiagabine may be administered at similar doses without adjustment for age, gender, or body weight in epilepsy patients ≥11 years of age (see Samara, 1998)

Dosage Forms Excipient information presented when available (limited, particularly for generics); consult specific product labeling.

Tablet, as hydrochloride:

Gabitril®: 2 mg, 4 mg, 12 mg, 16 mg

Extemporaneous Preparations

A 1 mg/mL tiagabine hydrochloride oral suspension made from tablets and a 1:1 mixture of Ora-Sweet® and Ora-Plus® was stable for 10 weeks when stored at room temperature (25°C) or for 13 weeks when stored under refrigeration (4°C) in amber plastic prescription bottles (Nahata, 2003). Grind ten 12 mg tablets in a mortar into a fine powder; add a small amount of the vehicle and mix well to form a uniform paste; mix while adding the vehicle in geometric proportions to **almost** 120 mL; transfer to a graduate; rinse the mortar with the vehicle and transfer to the graduate; qsad with vehicle to make 120 mL; label "shake well" and "refrigerate" (Nahata, 2004).

A 1 mg/mL suspension made from tablets and a 6:1 mixture of simple syrup, NF and 1% methylcellulose was stable for 6 weeks when stored at room temperature (25°C) and for 13 weeks when stored under refrigeration (4°C) in amber prescription bottles (Nahata, 2003). Grind ten 12 mg tablets in a mortar into a fine powder; add 17 mL of 1% methylcellulose gel and mix well to obtain a uniform paste; mix while adding simple syrup, NF in geometric proportions to **almost** 120 mL; transfer to a graduate; rinse the mortar with syrup and transfer to the graduate; qsad with syrup to 120 mL; label "shake well" and "refrigerate" (Nahata, 2004).

Nahata MC and Morosco RS, "Stability of Tiagabine in Two Oral Liquid Vehicles," *Am J Health-Syst Pharm*, 2003, 60: 75-77.

Nahata MC, Pai VB, and Hipple TF, *Pediatric Drug Formulations*, 5th ed, Cincinnati, OH: Harvey Whitney Books Co, 2004.

References

Adkins JC and Noble S, "Tiagabine. A Review of Its Pharmacodynamic and Pharmacokinetic Properties and Therapeutic Potential in the Management of Epilepsy," *Drugs*, 1998, 55(3):437-60.

Gustavson LE, Boellner SW, Granneman GR, et al, "A Single-Dose Study to Define Tiagabine Pharmacokinetics in Pediatric Patients With Complex Partial Seizures," *Neurology*, 1997, 48(4):1032-7.

Kalviainen R, Brodie MJ, Duncan J, et al, "A Double-Blind, Placebo-Controlled Trial of Tiagabine Given Three-Times Daily as Add-On Therapy for Refractory Partial Seizures. Northern European Tiagabine Study Group," *Epilepsy Res*, 1998, 30(1):31-40.

Leach JP and Brodie MJ, "Tiagabine," *Lancet*, 1998, 351(9097):203-7.

Pellock JM, "Managing Pediatric Epilepsy Syndromes With New Antiepileptic Drugs," *Pediatrics*, 1999, 104(5 Pt 1):1106-16.

Samara EE, Gustavson LE, El-Shourbagy T, et al, "Population Analysis of the Pharmacokinetics of Tiagabine in Patients With Epilepsy," *Epilespy*, 1998, 39(8):868-73.

♦ **Tiagabine Hydrochloride** *see* Tiagabine *on page 1536*
♦ **Tiamol® (Can)** *see* Fluocinonide *on page 674*
♦ **Tiazac®** *see* Diltiazem *on page 503*
♦ **Tiazac® XC (Can)** *see* Diltiazem *on page 503*
♦ **Ticar®** *see* Ticarcillin *on page 1538*

Ticarcillin (tye kar SIL in)

Medication Safety Issues

Sound-alike/look-alike issues:

Ticar® may be confused with Tigan®

U.S. Brand Names Ticar®

Index Terms Ticarcillin Disodium

Therapeutic Category Antibiotic, Penicillin (Antipseudomonal)

Generic Available No

Use Treatment of infections such as septicemia, acute and chronic respiratory tract infections, skin and soft tissue infections, and urinary tract infections due to susceptible strains of *Pseudomonas*, *Proteus*, *Escherichia coli*, and *Enterobacter*

Pregnancy Risk Factor B

Lactation Enters breast milk/compatible

Contraindications Hypersensitivity to ticarcillin, any component, or penicillins

Warnings Prolonged use may result in superinfection

Precautions Use with caution in patients with CHF due to ticarcillin's high sodium content; dosage modification required in patients with impaired renal and/or hepatic function

Adverse Reactions

Central nervous system: Seizures, headache, fever
Dermatologic: Rash
Endocrine & metabolic: Hypernatremia, hypokalemia, metabolic alkalosis
Gastrointestinal: Diarrhea, pseudomembranous colitis, stomatitis, nausea
Genitourinary: Cystitis, hematuria
Hematologic: Inhibition of platelet aggregation, leukopenia, neutropenia, eosinophilia, prolonged prothrombin time, bleeding diathesis, hemolytic anemia, decreased hemoglobin and hematocrit
Hepatic: Elevated AST and ALT, hepatitis
Local: Phlebitis
Renal: Elevated BUN, elevated serum creatinine
Miscellaneous: Hypersensitivity reactions including anaphylaxis; superinfection

Drug Interactions Aminoglycosides (antibacterial activity is synergistic), probenecid (increases serum concentration of ticarcillin); may alter renal elimination of lithium

Stability Reconstituted ticarcillin solution 200-300 mg/mL is stable for 24 hours at room temperature or 72 hours when refrigerated; incompatible with aminoglycosides

Mechanism of Action Inhibits bacterial cell wall synthesis by binding to one or more of the penicillin-binding proteins; inhibits the final transpeptidation step of peptidoglycan synthesis in bacterial cell walls

Pharmacokinetics

Absorption: I.M.: 86%
Distribution: V_d: Neonates: 0.42-0.76 L/kg; distributed into breast milk at low concentrations; attains high concentrations in bile; minimal concentrations attained in CSF with uninflamed meninges
Protein binding: 45% to 65%
Metabolism: 10%
Half-life, adults: 1-1.3 hours, prolonged with renal impairment and/or hepatic impairment
- Neonates:
  - <1 week: 3.5-5.6 hours
  - 1-8 weeks: 1.3-2.2 hours
- Children 5-13 years: 0.9 hours

Time to peak serum concentration: I.M.: Within 30-75 minutes
Elimination: Almost entirely in urine as unchanged drug and its metabolites with small amounts excreted in feces (3.5%)
Dialysis: Moderately dialyzable (20% to 50%)

Usual Dosage Ticarcillin is generally only given I.M. for the treatment of uncomplicated urinary tract infections

Neonates: I.V.:
- Postnatal age ≤7 days:
  - ≤2000 g: 150 mg/kg/day in divided doses every 12 hours
  - >2000 g: 225 mg/kg/day in divided doses every 8 hours
- Postnatal age >7 days:
  - <1200 g: 150 mg/kg/day in divided doses every 12 hours
  - 1200-2000 g: 225 mg/kg/day in divided doses every 8 hours
  - >2000 g: 300 mg/kg/day in divided doses every 6-8 hours

Infants and Children:
- I.M.: 50-100 mg/kg/day in divided doses every 6-8 hours
- I.V.: 200-300 mg/kg/day in divided doses every 4-6 hours; doses as high as 400 mg/kg/day divided every 4-6 hours have been used in acute pulmonary exacerbations of cystic fibrosis
- Maximum dose: 24 g/day

Adults:
- I.M.: 1 g every 6 hours
- I.V.: 1-4 g every 4-6 hours; maximum dose: 24 g/day

Dosing interval in renal impairment:
- Cl_{cr} 10-30 mL/minute: Administer every 8 hours
- Cl_{cr} <10 mL/minute: Administer every 12 hours

Administration Parenteral:

I.M.: Reconstitute each gram of ticarcillin with 2 mL SWI or 1% lidocaine hydrochloride injection (without epinephrine) to make a 385 mg/mL solution; administer by deep I.M. injection into a large muscle mass
I.V.: Ticarcillin may be administered I.V. push over 10-20 minutes or by I.V. intermittent infusion over 30-120 minutes at a final concentration not to exceed 100 mg/mL; concentrations ≤50 mg/mL are preferred for peripheral intermittent infusions to avoid vein irritation; if the patient is on concurrent aminoglycoside therapy, separate ticarcillin administration from the aminoglycoside by at least 30-60 minutes

Monitoring Parameters Serum electrolytes, bleeding time, and periodic tests of renal, hepatic, and hematologic function

(Continued)

Ticarcillin *(Continued)*

Test Interactions False-positive urinary or serum protein, positive Coombs' [direct]

Additional Information Sodium content of 1 g: 5.2-6.5 mEq

Dosage Forms Excipient information presented when available (limited, particularly for generics); consult specific product labeling.

Injection, powder for reconstitution, as disodium: 3 g

References

Brogden RN, Heel RC, Speight TM, et al, "Ticarcillin: A Review of Its Pharmacological Properties and Therapeutic Efficacy," *Drugs*, 1980, 20(5):325-52.

Nelson JD, Kusmiesz H, Shelton S, et al, "Clinical Pharmacology and Efficacy of Ticarcillin in Infants and Children," *Pediatrics*, 1978, 61(6):858-63.

Ticarcillin and Clavulanate Potassium

(tye kar SIL in & klav yoo LAN ate poe TASS ee um)

U.S. Brand Names Timentin®

Canadian Brand Names Timentin®

Index Terms Ticarcillin and Clavulanic Acid

Therapeutic Category Antibiotic, Beta-lactam and Beta-lactamase Combination; Antibiotic, Penicillin (Antipseudomonal)

Generic Available No

Use Treatment of infections caused by susceptible organisms involving the lower respiratory tract, urinary tract, skin and skin structures, bone and joint, and septicemia. Clavulanate expands activity of ticarcillin to include beta-lactamase producing strains of *S. aureus, H. influenzae, Moraxella catarrhalis, B. fragilis, Klebsiella*, and *Proteus* species

Pregnancy Risk Factor B

Lactation Enters breast milk (other penicillins are compatible with breast-feeding)/use caution

Contraindications Hypersensitivity to ticarcillin, clavulanate, or penicillin

Warnings Abnormal platelet aggregation and prolonged bleeding have been reported in patients with renal impairment receiving high doses; prolonged use may result in superinfection

Precautions Use with caution and modify dosage in patients with renal impairment; use with caution in patients with CHF due to high sodium content of the formulation

Adverse Reactions

Central nervous system: Seizures, headache, fever

Dermatologic: Rash, erythema multiforme, toxic epidermal necrolysis, Stevens-Johnson syndrome

Endocrine & metabolic: Hypernatremia, hypokalemia, metabolic alkalosis

Gastrointestinal: Diarrhea, stomatitis, nausea, pseudomembranous colitis

Genitourinary: Cystitis, hematuria

Hematologic: Eosinophilia, leukopenia, decreased hemoglobin and hematocrit, inhibition of platelet aggregation, prolongation of bleeding time, neutropenia, hemolytic anemia

Hepatic: Elevated ALT and AST, hepatitis

Local: Thrombophlebitis

Renal: Elevated BUN, elevated serum creatinine

Miscellaneous: Hypersensitivity reactions including anaphylaxis; superinfection

Drug Interactions Aminoglycosides (antibacterial activity is synergistic), probenecid (increases serum concentration of ticarcillin)

Stability Reconstituted 200 mg/mL solution is stable for 6 hours at room temperature and 72 hours when refrigerated; darkening of drug indicates loss of potency of clavulanate potassium; incompatible with sodium bicarbonate and aminoglycosides

Mechanism of Action Ticarcillin inhibits bacterial cell wall synthesis by binding to one or more of the penicillin-binding proteins; inhibits the final transpeptidation step of peptidoglycan synthesis in bacterial cell walls; clavulanic acid inhibits degradation of ticarcillin by binding to beta-lactamases

Pharmacokinetics

Distribution: Ticarcillin is distributed into tissue, interstitial fluid, pleural fluid, bile, and breast milk; low concentrations of ticarcillin distribute into the CSF but increase when meninges are inflamed

V_{dss} ticarcillin: 0.22 L/kg

V_{dss} clavulanic acid: 0.4 L/kg

Protein binding:

Ticarcillin: 45% to 65%

Clavulanic acid: 9% to 30%

Metabolism: Clavulanic acid is metabolized in the liver

Half-life: In patients with normal renal function

Neonates:
- Clavulanic acid: 1.9 hours
- Ticarcillin: 4.4 hours

Children (1 month to 9.3 years):
- Clavulanic acid: 54 minutes
- Ticarcillin: 66 minutes

Adults:
- Clavulanic acid: 66-90 minutes
- Ticarcillin: 66-72 minutes
- Clavulanic acid does not affect the clearance of ticarcillin

Elimination:
- Children: 71% of the ticarcillin and 50% of the clavulanic acid dose are excreted unchanged in the urine over 4 hours
- Adults: 45% of clavulanate is excreted unchanged in urine, whereas 60% to 90% of ticarcillin is excreted unchanged in urine

Dialysis: Removed by hemodialysis

Usual Dosage I.V.: (**Note:** Timentin® (ticarcillin/clavulanate) is a combination product; each 3.1 g vial contains 3 g ticarcillin disodium and 0.1 g clavulanic acid. Dosage recommendations are based on **ticarcillin** component):

Term neonates and Infants <3 months: 200-300 mg ticarcillin component/kg/day divided every 6-8 hours

Infants ≥3 months and Children:
- Mild to moderate infection: 200 mg ticarcillin component/kg/day divided every 6 hours
- Severe infections that occur outside the CNS: 300 mg ticarcillin component/kg/day in divided doses every 4-6 hours; maximum dose: 400 mg/kg/day not to exceed 18-24 g/day

Adults: 3 g ticarcillin component every 4-6 hours; maximum dose: 18-24 g/day
- Urinary tract infections: 3 g ticarcillin component every 6-8 hours

Dosing interval in renal impairment:
- Cl_{cr} 10-30 mL/minute: Administer every 8 hours
- Cl_{cr} <10 mL/minute: Administer every 12 hours

Dosing interval in hepatic impairment and a Cl_{cr} <10 mL/minute: Administer every 24 hours

Administration Parenteral: Administer by I.V. intermittent infusion over 30 minutes; final concentration for administration should not exceed 100 mg/mL of ticarcillin; however, concentrations ≤50 mg/mL are preferred; if the patient is on concurrent aminoglycoside therapy, separate ticarcillin and clavulanate potassium administration from the aminoglycoside by at least 30-60 minutes

Monitoring Parameters Serum electrolytes, periodic renal, hepatic and hematologic function tests

Test Interactions Positive Coombs' [direct], false-positive urinary and serum proteins

Additional Information
- Sodium content of 1 g: 4.75 mEq
- Potassium content of 1 g: 0.15 mEq

Dosage Forms Excipient information presented when available (limited, particularly for generics); consult specific product labeling.
- Infusion [premixed, frozen]: Ticarcillin 3 g and clavulanic acid 0.1 g (100 mL) [contains sodium 4.51 mEq and potassium 0.15 mEq per g]
- Injection, powder for reconstitution: Ticarcillin 3 g and clavulanic acid 0.1 g (3.1 g, 31 g) [contains sodium 4.51 mEq and potassium 0.15 mEq per g]

References

Begue P, Quiniou F, Quinet B, "Efficacy and Pharmacokinetics of Timentin® in Paediatric Infections," *J Antimicrob Chemother*, 1986, 17(Suppl C):81-91.

Reed MD, Yamashita TS, and Blumer JL, "Pharmacokinetic-Based Ticarcillin/Clavulanic Acid Dose Recommendations for Infants and Children," *J Clin Pharmacol*, 1995, 35(7):658-65.

Stutman HR and Marks MI, "Review of Pediatric Antimicrobial Therapies," *Semin Pediatr Infect Dis*, 1991, 2:3-17.

♦ **Ticarcillin and Clavulanic Acid** *see* Ticarcillin and Clavulanate Potassium *on page 1540*

♦ **Ticarcillin Disodium** *see* Ticarcillin *on page 1538*

♦ **TIG** *see* Tetanus Immune Globulin (Human) *on page 1515*

♦ **Tigan®** *see* Trimethobenzamide *on page 1576*

♦ **Tilade®** *see* Nedocromil *on page 1112*

♦ **Tim-AK (Can)** *see* Timolol *on page 1542*

♦ **Time-C [OTC]** *see* Ascorbic Acid *on page 159*

♦ **Time-C-Bio [OTC]** *see* Ascorbic Acid *on page 159*

♦ **Timentin®** *see* Ticarcillin and Clavulanate Potassium *on page 1540*

Timolol (TYE moe lole)

Medication Safety Issues

Sound-alike/look-alike issues:

Timolol may be confused with atenolol, Tylenol®

Timoptic® may be confused with Talacen®, Viroptic®

Bottle cap color change:

Timoptic®: Both the 0.25% and 0.5% strengths are now packaged in bottles with yellow caps; previously, the color of the cap on the product corresponded to different strengths.

International issues:

Betimol® may be confused with Betanol® which is a brand name for metipranolol in Monaco

Related Information

Antihypertensive Agents by Class *on page 1678*

Overdose and Toxicology *on page 1916*

U.S. Brand Names Betimol®; Blocadren®; Istalol™; Timoptic®; Timoptic® in OcuDose®; Timoptic-XE®

Canadian Brand Names Alti-Timolol; Apo-Timol®; Apo-Timop®; Gen-Timolol; Nu-Timolol; Phoxal-timolol; PMS-Timolol; Sandoz-Timolol; Tim-AK; Timoptic®; Timoptic-XE®

Index Terms Timolol Hemihydrate; Timolol Maleate

Therapeutic Category Antihypertensive Agent; Antimigraine Agent; Beta-Adrenergic Blocker; Beta-Adrenergic Blocker, Ophthalmic

Generic Available Yes: Excludes hemihydrate ophthalmic solutions

Use

Ophthalmic: Treatment of elevated intraocular pressure such as glaucoma or ocular hypertension

Oral: Treatment of hypertension and angina; prevention of MI and migraine headaches

Pregnancy Risk Factor C

Lactation Enters breast milk/use caution (AAP rates "compatible")

Contraindications Hypersensitivity to timolol or any component; uncompensated CHF, cardiogenic shock, bradycardia or heart block, bronchial asthma, severe chronic obstructive pulmonary disease or history of asthma, CHF or bradycardia

Warnings In patients with angina pectoris, exacerbation of angina and, in some cases, MI occurred following abrupt discontinuation of therapy; severe CNS, cardiovascular and respiratory adverse effects have been seen following ophthalmic use; timolol decreases the ability of the heart to respond to reflex adrenergic stimuli and may increase the risk of general anesthesia and surgical procedures; timolol may mask clinical signs of hyperthyroidism (exacerbation of symptoms of hyperthyroidism, including thyroid storm, may occur following abrupt discontinuation)

Precautions Similar to other beta-blockers; use with caution in patients with decreased renal or hepatic function (dosage adjustment required); use with a miotic in angle-closure or narrow-angle glaucoma; use with caution in patients with diabetes mellitus, may block hypoglycemia-induced tachycardia and blood pressure changes

Adverse Reactions

Cardiovascular: Bradycardia, arrhythmia, hypotension, syncope; hypertension after ophthalmic use

Central nervous system: Dizziness, headache

Dermatologic: Rash

Gastrointestinal: Diarrhea, nausea

Local (ocular): Burning, stinging, irritation, itching, conjunctivitis, keratitis, visual disturbances, blurred vision, cataract, decreased visual acuity

Respiratory: Bronchospasm, dyspnea

Miscellaneous: Hypersensitivity reactions, anaphylaxis

Drug Interactions Cytochrome P450 isoenzyme CYP2D6 substrate

Verapamil, nifedipine, diltiazem, digitalis, quinidine may increase adverse cardiac effects; NSAIDs may decrease antihypertensive effects of timolol; patients receiving beta blockers, who have a history of anaphylactic reactions, may be more reactive to a repeated allergen challenge and may not be responsive to the usual epinephrine doses used to treat an allergic reaction; abrupt withdrawal of clonidine while receiving beta-blockers may result in an exaggerated hypertensive crisis; drug interactions similar to other beta-blockers may occur

Stability Ophthalmic: Store at room temperature; do not freeze; protect from light

Timpotic® OcuDose®: Store in protective foil wrap; use within 1 month after opening foil package

Mechanism of Action Blocks both beta$_1$- and beta$_2$-adrenergic receptors; reduces intraocular pressure by reducing aqueous humor production or possibly outflow;

reduces blood pressure by blocking adrenergic receptors and decreasing sympathetic outflow; produces negative chronotropic and negative inotropic activity

Pharmacodynamics

Hypotensive effects: Oral:
- Onset of action: Within 15-45 minutes
- Maximum effect: 30-150 minutes
- Duration: 4 hours

Intraocular pressure reduction: Ophthalmic:
- Onset of action: Within 30 minutes
- Maximum effect: 1-2 hours
- Duration: 24 hours

Pharmacokinetics

Distribution: Oral and Ophthalmic: Distributes into human breast milk
Protein binding: <10%
Metabolism: Extensively in the liver, extensive first-pass effect
Bioavailability: Oral: ~60%
Half-life: Adults: 2-4 hours; prolonged with reduced renal function
Elimination: Urinary excretion (15% to 20% as unchanged drug)
Dialysis: Not readily dialyzable

Usual Dosage

Ophthalmic:
- Gel (Timoptic-XE®): Adults: 0.25% or 0.5% gel, instill 1 drop once daily; do not exceed 1 drop once daily of 0.5% gel
- Solution (Timoptic®): Children and Adults: Initial: 0.25% solution, instill 1 drop twice daily; increase to 0.5% solution if response not adequate; decrease to 1 drop/day if controlled; do not exceed 1 drop twice daily of 0.5% solution (see Additional Information)
- Solution (Istalol™): Adults: Initial: 0.5% solution: Instill 1 drop once daily in the morning

Oral:
- Children: No information regarding pediatric dose is currently available in literature
- Adults:
  - Hypertension: Initial: 10 mg twice daily, increase gradually every 7 days, usual dosage: 20-40 mg/day in 2 divided doses; maximum dose: 60 mg/day; usual dosage range (JNC 7): 20-40 mg/day in 2 divided doses
  - Prevention of MI: 10 mg twice daily initiated within 1-4 weeks after infarction
  - Migraine headache: Initial: 10 mg twice daily, increase to maximum of 30 mg/day

Administration

Ophthalmic: Apply gentle pressure to lacrimal sac during and immediately following instillation (1 minute) or instruct patient to gently close eyelid after administration, to decrease systemic absorption of ophthalmic drops; avoid contact of bottle tip with skin or eye. Remove contact lenses prior to administration (ophthalmic solution contains benzalkonium chloride which may adsorb to soft contact lenses); lenses may be inserted 15 minutes after administration. Gel: Invert container, shake once before use; administer other topical ophthalmic medications at least 10 minutes before Timoptic-XE®

Oral: May be administered without regard to food

Monitoring Parameters Heart rate, blood pressure; liver enzymes, BUN, serum creatinine with long-term oral use; monitor IOP with ophthalmic use; monitor respiratory rate, CNS status, and cardiovascular status with ophthalmic use in patients at risk for adverse effects (eg, asthmatics, CHF patients, etc)

Patient Information Potential visual disturbances from ophthalmic use may impair ability to perform hazardous duties such as driving or operating machinery

Nursing Implications Discontinue medication if breathing difficulty occurs

Additional Information Ophthalmic: Use lowest effective dose in pediatric patients. Children had higher plasma concentrations vs adults following ophthalmic use; some achieved therapeutic levels; this may result in increased adverse systemic effects. The concurrent use of 2 ophthalmic beta blockers is not recommended.

Dosage Forms Excipient information presented when available (limited, particularly for generics); consult specific product labeling.

Note: Unless otherwise specified, strength expressed as base.

Gel-forming solution, ophthalmic, as maleate: 0.25% (5 mL); 0.5% (2.5 mL, 5 mL)
- Timoptic-XE®: 0.25% (5 mL); 0.5% (5 mL)

Solution, ophthalmic, as hemihydrate:
- Betimol®: 0.25% (5 mL, 10 mL, 15 mL); 0.5% (5 mL, 10 mL, 15 mL) [contains benzalkonium chloride]

Solution, ophthalmic, as maleate: 0.25% (5 mL, 10 mL, 15 mL); 0.5% (5 mL, 10 mL, 15 mL) [contains benzalkonium chloride]
- Istalol™: 0.5% (10 mL) [contains benzalkonium chloride and potassium sorbate]
- Timoptic®: 0.25% (5 mL); 0.5% (5 mL, 10 mL) [contains benzalkonium chloride]

(Continued)

Timolol *(Continued)*

Solution, ophthalmic, as maleate [preservative free]:
Timoptic® in OcuDose®: 0.25% (0.2 mL); 0.5% (0.2 mL) [single use]
Tablet, as maleate: 5 mg, 10 mg, 20 mg [strength expressed as salt]
Blocadren®: 20 mg [strength expressed as salt]

References

Chobanian AV, Bakris GL, Black HR, et al, "The Seventh Report of the Joint National Committee on Prevention, Detection, Evaluation, and Treatment of High Blood Pressure: The JNC 7 report," *JAMA*, 2003, 289(19):2560-72.

Hoskins HD, Hetherington J Jr, Magee SD, et al, "Clinical Experience With Timolol in Childhood Glaucoma," *Arch Ophthalmol*, 1985, 103(8):1163-5.

Passo MS, Palmer EA, and Van Buskirk EM, "Plasma Timolol in Glaucoma Patients," *Ophthalmology*, 1984, 91(11):1361-3.

- **Timolol Hemihydrate** *see* Timolol *on page 1542*
- **Timolol Maleate** *see* Timolol *on page 1542*
- **Timoptic®** *see* Timolol *on page 1542*
- **Timoptic® in OcuDose®** *see* Timolol *on page 1542*
- **Timoptic-XE®** *see* Timolol *on page 1542*
- **Tinactin® Antifungal [OTC]** *see* Tolnaftate *on page 1550*
- **Tinactin® Antifungal Jock Itch [OTC]** *see* Tolnaftate *on page 1550*
- **Tinaderm [OTC]** *see* Tolnaftate *on page 1550*
- **Tinamed® [OTC]** *see* Salicylic Acid *on page 1413*
- **Ting® Cream [OTC]** *see* Tolnaftate *on page 1550*
- **Ting® Spray Liquid [OTC]** *see* Tolnaftate *on page 1550*
- **Tioguanine** *see* Thioguanine *on page 1527*
- **Tiotixene** *see* Thiothixene *on page 1534*

Tiotropium (ty oh TRO pee um)

Medication Safety Issues

Sound-alike/look-alike issues:
Spiriva® may be confused with Inspra™
Spiriva® capsules for inhalation are for administration via HandiHaler® device and are not for oral use

U.S. Brand Names Spiriva®

Canadian Brand Names Spiriva®

Index Terms Tiotropium Bromide Monohydrate

Therapeutic Category Antiasthmatic; Anticholinergic Agent; Bronchodilator

Generic Available No

Use Maintenance treatment of bronchospasm associated with COPD including chronic bronchitis and emphysema

Pregnancy Risk Factor C

Lactation Excretion in breast milk unknown/use caution

Contraindications Hypersensitivity to tiotropium, ipratropium, or any component of the formulation (contains lactose); not for use as an acute ("rescue") bronchodilator

Warnings Not indicated for the initial treatment of acute episodes of bronchospasm. Immediate hypersensitivity reactions including angioedema may occur. May cause paradoxical bronchospasm. Safety and efficacy have not been established in pediatric patients.

Precautions Use with caution in patients with myasthenia gravis, narrow-angle glaucoma, prostatic hyperplasia, or bladder neck obstruction; use with caution and monitor use closely in patients with moderate to severe renal impairment. Avoid inadvertent instillation of powder into the eyes. Explain administration carefully; capsules are not for oral use and must only be administered using HandiHaler® inhalation device.

Adverse Reactions

Cardiovascular: Angina, edema, tachycardia
Central nervous system: Depression
Dermatologic: Rash, pruritus, urticaria
Endocrine & metabolic: Hypercholesterolemia, hyperglycemia
Gastrointestinal: Xerostomia, dyspepsia, abdominal pain, constipation, vomiting, reflux, ulcerative stomatitis
Genitourinary: Urinary tract infection, urinary retention
Neuromuscular & skeletal: Myalgia, leg pain, skeletal pain, paresthesia
Ocular: Cataract, blurred vision, pupil dilation (powder contact with eyes), glaucoma
Respiratory: Upper respiratory tract infection, sinusitis, pharyngitis, rhinitis, epistaxis, dysphonia, laryngitis, paradoxical bronchospasm

Miscellaneous: Infection, moniliasis, allergic reaction, herpes zoster, hypersensitivity reactions

Drug Interactions Cytochrome P450 isoenzyme CYP2D6 and CYP3A4 substrate (minor)

Increased toxicity with anticholinergics or medications with anticholinergic properties

Stability Store between 15°C and 25°C. Do not store capsules in HandiHaler® device. Capsules should be stored in the blister pack and only removed immediately before use. After first capsule in the strip is used, the 2 remaining capsules should be used over the next 2 days.

Mechanism of Action Blocks the action of acetylcholine at parasympathetic sites in bronchial smooth muscle causing bronchodilation

Pharmacokinetics

Absorption: Poorly absorbed from GI tract; systemic absorption may occur from lung
Distribution: V_d: 32 L/kg
Protein binding: 72%
Metabolism: Hepatic (minimal), via CYP2D6 and CYP3A4
Bioavailability: Absolute: 19.5%
Half-life: 5-6 days
Time to peak serum concentration: 5 minutes (following inhalation)
Elimination: Urine (74% as unchanged drug)

Usual Dosage Inhalation: Adults: Contents of 1 capsule (18 mcg) inhaled once daily using HandiHaler® device (see Administration)

Dosage adjustment in renal impairment: Plasma concentrations increase in renal impairment. Use caution; no specific dosage adjustment recommended.

Administration Inhalation: **Not for oral use.** Remove capsule from foil blister immediately before use. Place capsule in the capsule-chamber in the base of the HandiHaler® Inhaler. Must only use the HandiHaler® Inhaler. Close mouthpiece until a click is heard, leaving dustcap open. Exhale fully. Do not exhale into inhaler. Tilt head slightly back and inhale (rapidly, steadily, and deeply); the capsule vibration may be heard within the device. Hold breath as long as possible. If any powder remains in capsule, exhale and inhale again. Repeat until capsule is empty. Throw away empty capsule; do not leave in inhaler. Do not use a spacer with the HandiHaler® Inhaler. Always keep capsules and inhaler dry.

Delivery of dose: Instruct patient to place mouthpiece gently between teeth, closing lips around inhaler. Instruct patient to inhale deeply and hold breath for 5-10 seconds. The amount of drug delivered is small, and the individual will not sense the medication as it is inhaled. Remove mouthpiece prior to exhalation. Patient should not breathe out through the mouthpiece. After use of the inhaler, patient should rinse mouth/oropharynx with water and spit out rinse solution.

Monitoring Parameters FEV_1, peak flow (or other pulmonary function studies)

Patient Information Use inhaler and medication as instructed - once daily, at same time each day. Do not use more often than prescribed. Do not use as an acute "rescue" bronchodilator. Report swelling of face, mouth, or tongue; skin rash; chest pain or palpitations; persistent gastrointestinal effects; muscle or skeletal pain or weakness; change in vision; respiratory changes, sore throat, or flu-like symptoms. May cause dry mouth.

Dosage Forms Excipient information presented when available (limited, particularly for generics); consult specific product labeling.

Powder for oral inhalation [capsule]:

Spiriva®: 18 mcg/capsule (5s, 30s) [contains lactose; packaged with HandiHaler® device]

- ♦ **Tiotropium Bromide Monohydrate** *see* Tiotropium *on page 1544*
- ♦ **Tiseb® [OTC]** *see* Salicylic Acid *on page 1413*
- ♦ **Titralac™ [OTC]** *see* Calcium Carbonate *on page 264*
- ♦ **Titralac® [OTC]** *see* Calcium Supplements *on page 272*
- ♦ **Titralac® Extra Strength [OTC]** *see* Calcium Supplements *on page 272*
- ♦ **TMP** *see* Trimethoprim *on page 1578*
- ♦ **TMP-SMZ** *see* Sulfamethoxazole and Trimethoprim *on page 1487*
- ♦ **TMZ** *see* Temozolomide *on page 1503*
- ♦ **TOBI®** *see* Tobramycin *on page 1545*

Tobramycin (toe bra MYE sin)

Medication Safety Issues

Sound-alike/look-alike issues:

Tobramycin may be confused with Trobicin®
AKTob® may be confused with AK-Trol®
Nebcin® may be confused with Inapsine®, Naprosyn®, Nubain®

(Continued)

Tobramycin *(Continued)*

Tobrex® may be confused with TobraDex®

Related Information

Blood Level Sampling Time Guidelines *on page 1914*

Overdose and Toxicology *on page 1916*

U.S. Brand Names AKTob®; TOBI®; Tobrex®

Canadian Brand Names PMS-Tobramycin; Sandoz-Tobramycin; TOBI®; Tobramycin Injection, USP; Tobrex®

Index Terms Tobramycin Sulfate

Therapeutic Category Antibiotic, Aminoglycoside; Antibiotic, Ophthalmic

Generic Available Yes: Excludes ophthalmic ointment, solution for nebulization

Use Treatment of documented or suspected infections caused by susceptible gram-negative bacilli including *Pseudomonas aeruginosa*; nonpseudomonal enteric bacillus infection which is more sensitive to tobramycin than gentamicin based on susceptibility tests; susceptible organisms in lower respiratory tract infections, septicemia; intra-abdominal, skin, bone, and urinary tract infections; empiric therapy in cystic fibrosis and immunocompromised patients; used topically to treat superficial ophthalmic infections caused by susceptible bacteria; inhalation therapy management of cystic fibrosis patients with *P. aeruginosa*

Pregnancy Risk Factor D (injection, inhalation); B (ophthalmic)

Lactation Enters breast milk/not recommended

Contraindications Hypersensitivity to tobramycin, any component (see Warnings), or aminoglycosides

Warnings I.M., I.V.: Aminoglycosides are associated with significant nephrotoxicity or ototoxicity; the ototoxicity is directly proportional to the amount of drug given and the duration of treatment; tinnitus, vertigo, ataxia, or dizziness are indications of vestibular injury and impending irreversible bilateral deafness; renal damage is usually reversible. Some formulations contain sulfites which may cause allergic reactions in susceptible individuals; transient tinnitus and hearing loss have been reported in tobramycin inhalation-treated patients; bronchospasm can occur with inhalation of tobramycin. Prolonged use may result in superinfection. Aminoglycosides can cause fetal harm when administered to a pregnant woman; aminoglycosides have been associated with several reports of total, irreversible, bilateral congenital deafness in pediatric patients exposed *in utero*

Precautions Use with caution in patients with renal impairment, pre-existing auditory or vestibular impairment, patients receiving anesthetics or neuromuscular blocking agents, and in patients with neuromuscular disorders; dosage modification required in patients with impaired renal function

Adverse Reactions

Central nervous system: Vertigo, gait instability, fever, ataxia, dizziness, headache

Dermatologic: Allergic contact dermatitis, rash

Endocrine & metabolic: Hypomagnesemia

Gastrointestinal: Nausea, vomiting

Hematologic: Granulocytopenia, thrombocytopenia, eosinophilia

Hepatic: Elevated AST and ALT

Local: Thrombophlebitis

Neuromuscular & skeletal: Neuromuscular blockade, paresthesia, tremor, weakness

Ocular: Ophthalmic use: Lacrimation, itching, edema of the eyelid, keratitis

Otic: Ototoxicity (may be associated with high serum aminoglycoside concentrations persisting for prolonged periods or with high peak serum concentrations following rapid I.V. bolus administration) with tinnitus, hearing loss; early toxicity usually affects high-pitched sound

Renal: Nephrotoxicity (high trough levels) with proteinuria, reduction in glomerular filtration rate, elevated serum creatinine, decrease in urine specific gravity, casts in urine and possible electrolyte wasting

Respiratory: With inhalation therapy: Voice alteration, bronchospasm, dyspnea, increased cough, pharyngitis, hoarseness

Drug Interactions Increased toxicity: Concurrent use of amphotericin B, cephalosporins, penicillins, loop diuretics, urea, mannitol, vancomycin, cisplatin, indomethacin; potentiates effect of neuromuscular blocking agents and botulinum toxin

Stability Incompatible with penicillins, cephalosporins, heparin

Inhalation solution: Store in refrigerator; upon removal from the refrigerator, the solution may be stored at room temperature for up to 28 days; do not use solution if it is cloudy or contains particles; a darkened yellow solution does not indicate loss of potency; protect from intense light; incompatible with dornase alfa (may precipitate)

Mechanism of Action Inhibits cellular initiation of bacterial protein synthesis by binding to 30S and 50S ribosomal subunits resulting in a defective bacterial cell membrane

Pharmacokinetics

Absorption:

Oral: Poor

I.M.: Rapid and complete

Inhalation: Low systemic bioavailability although peak tobramycin serum concentration 1 hour after inhalation ranges between 0.95-1.05 mg/mL

Distribution: Crosses the placenta; distributes primarily in the extracellular fluid volume; poor penetration into the CSF and into bronchial secretions; drug accumulates in the renal cortex; small amounts distribute into bile, sputum, saliva, tears, and breast milk

V_d: Increased by fever, edema, ascites, fluid overload, and in neonates; V_d is decreased in patients with dehydration

Neonates: 0.45 ± 0.1 L/kg

Infants: 0.4 ± 0.1 L/kg

Children: 0.35 ± 0.15 L/kg

Adolescents: 0.3 ± 0.1 L/kg

Adults: 0.2-0.3 L/kg

Protein binding: <30%

Half-life:

Neonates:

≤1200 g: 11 hours

>1200 g: 2-9 hours

Infants: 4 ± 1 hour

Children: 2 ± 1 hour

Adolescents: 1.5 ± 1 hour

Adults with normal renal function: 2-3 hours, directly dependent upon glomerular filtration rate; impaired renal function: 5-70 hours

Time to peak serum concentration:

I.M.: Within 30-60 minutes

I.V.: 30 minutes after a 30-minute infusion

Elimination: With normal renal function, ~90% to 95% of dose excreted in urine within 24 hours

Dialysis: Dialyzable (50% to 100%)

Usual Dosage Dosage should be based on an estimate of ideal body weight except in neonates (neonatal dosage should be based on actual weight unless the patient has hydrocephalus or hydrops fetalis)

Neonates: I.M., I.V.:

Preterm neonates <1000 g: 3.5 mg/kg/dose every 24 hours

0-4 weeks, <1200 g: 2.5 mg/kg/dose every 18 hours

Postnatal age ≤7 days:

1200-2000 g: 2.5 mg/kg/dose every 12 hours

>2000 g: 2.5 mg/kg/dose every 12 hours

Postnatal age >7 days:

1200-2000 g: 2.5 mg/kg/dose every 8-12 hours

>2000 g: 2.5 mg/kg/dose every 8 hours

Infants and Children <5 years: I.M., I.V.: 2.5 mg/kg/dose every 8 hours*

Pulmonary infection in cystic fibrosis: 2.5-3.3 mg/kg/dose every 6-8 hours

Patients on hemodialysis: 1.25-1.75 mg/kg/dose postdialysis

Children ≥5 years: I.M., I.V.: 2-2.5 mg/kg/dose every 8 hours*

Pulmonary infection in cystic fibrosis: 2.5-3.3 mg/kg/dose every 6-8 hours

Patients on hemodialysis: 1.25-1.75 mg/kg/dose postdialysis

***Note:** Some patients may require larger or more frequent doses if serum levels document the need (ie, cystic fibrosis, patients undergoing continuous hemofiltration, patients with major burns, or febrile granulocytopenic patients); modify dose based on individual patient requirements as determined by renal function, serum drug concentrations, and patient-specific clinical parameters.

Children ≥2 months and Adults: Ophthalmic:

Ointment: Apply 0.5" ribbon into the affected eye 2-3 times/day; for severe infections, apply ointment every 3-4 hours

Solution:

Mild to moderate infections: Instill 1-2 drops every 4 hours

Severe infections: instill 2 drops every 30-60 minutes initially, then reduce to less frequent intervals

Inhalation: Cystic fibrosis:

Standard aerosolized tobramycin:

Children: 40-80 mg 2-3 times/day

Adults: 60-80 mg 3 times/day

High dose regimen: Children ≥6 years and Adults: 300 mg every 12 hours (do not administer doses less than 6 hours apart); administer in repeated cycles of 28 days on drug followed by 28 days off drug

(Continued)

Tobramycin *(Continued)*

Adults: I.M., I.V.: 3-6 mg/kg/day in 3 divided doses; studies of once daily dosing have used I.V. doses of 4-6.6 mg/kg once daily

Patients on hemodialysis: 0.5-0.7 mg/kg/dose postdialysis

Dosing in Renal Impairment:

Children and Adults: 2.5 mg/kg (2-3 serum level measurements should be obtained after the initial dose to measure the half-life in order to determine the frequency of subsequent doses)

Administration

Inhalation (high-dose regimen): Use a PARI LC Plus™ reusable nebulizer and a DeVilbiss Pulmo-Aide® air compressor for administration of tobramycin by inhalation; patient should be sitting or standing upright and breathing normally through the mouthpiece of the nebulizer. Nebulizer treatment period is usually over 15 minutes.

Ophthalmic: Avoid contact of tube or bottle tip with skin or eye; apply finger pressure to lacrimal sac during and for 1-2 minutes after instillation of drops to decrease risk of absorption and systemic effects

Parenteral: Administer by I.M., I.V. slow intermittent infusion over 30-60 minutes or by direct injection over 15 minutes; final I.V. concentration for administration should not exceed 10 mg/mL; administer other antibiotics such as penicillins and cephalosporins at least 1 hour before or after tobramycin

Monitoring Parameters Urinalysis, urine output, BUN, serum creatinine, peak and trough serum tobramycin levels; be alert to ototoxicity, audiograms

Not all pediatric patients who receive aminoglycosides require monitoring of serum aminoglycoside concentrations. Indications for use of aminoglycoside serum concentration monitoring include:

- Treatment course >5 days
- Patients with decreased or changing renal function
- Patients with a poor therapeutic response
- Infants <3 months of age
- Atypical body constituency (obesity, expanded extracellular fluid volume)
- Clinical need for higher doses or shorter intervals (cystic fibrosis, burns, endocarditis, meningitis, relatively resistant organism)
- Patients on hemodialysis or chronic ambulatory peritoneal dialysis
- Signs of nephrotoxicity or ototoxicity
- Concomitant use of other nephrotoxic agents

Patients on high-dose aerosolized tobramycin: Peak tobramycin level obtained 1 hour following inhalation to identify patients who are significant absorbers

Reference Range

Peak: 4-12 mcg/mL; peak values are 2-3 times greater with once daily dosing regimens

Trough: 0.5-2 mcg/mL

Test Interactions Aminoglycoside serum levels measured in blood taken from Silastic® central line catheters can sometimes give falsely high readings

Patient Information Report any dizziness or sensation of ringing or fullness in ears to the physician

Nursing Implications Obtain serum concentration after the third dose except in neonates or patients with rapidly changing renal function in whom levels need to be measured sooner; peak tobramycin serum concentrations are drawn 30 minutes after the end of a 30-minute infusion, immediately on completion of a 1-hour I.V. infusion or 1 hour after an intramuscular injection; the trough is drawn just before the next dose; provide optimal patient hydration and perfusion

Dosage Forms Excipient information presented when available (limited, particularly for generics); consult specific product labeling.

Infusion [premixed in NS]: 60 mg (50 mL); 80 mg (100 mL)

Injection, powder for reconstitution: 1.2 g

Injection, solution: 10 mg/mL (2 mL, 8 mL); 40 mg/mL (2 mL, 30 mL, 50 mL) [may contain sodium metabisulfite]

Ointment, ophthalmic (Tobrex®): 0.3% (3.5 g)

Solution for nebulization [preservative free] (TOBI®): 60 mg/mL (5 mL)

Solution, ophthalmic (AKTob®, Tobrex®): 0.3% (5 mL) [contains benzalkonium chloride]

References

Gilbert DN, "Once-Daily Aminoglycoside Therapy," *Antimicrob Agents Chemother*, 1991, 35(3):399-405.

Green TP, Mirkin BL, Peterson PK, et al, "Tobramycin Serum Level Monitoring in Young Patients With Normal Renal Function," *Clin Pharmacokinet*, 1984, 9(5):457-68.

Nahata MC, Powell DA, Durrell DE, et al, "Effect of Gestational Age and Birth Weight on Tobramycin Kinetics in Newborn Infants," *J Antimicrob Chemother*, 1984, 14(1):59-65.

Ramsey BW, Burns J, Smith A, et al, "Safety and Efficacy of Tobramycin for Inhalation in Patients With Cystic Fibrosis: The Results of Two Phase III Placebo Controlled Clinical Trials," *Pediatr Pulmonol*, 1997, (Suppl 14):137-8, S10.3.

Ramsey BW, Dorkin HL, Eisenberg JD, et al, "Efficacy of Aerosolized Tobramycin in Patients With Cystic Fibrosis," *N Engl J Med*, 1993, 328(24):1740-6.

Shaw PK, Braun TL, Liebergen A, et al, "Aerosolized Tobramycin Pharmacokinetics in Cystic Fibrosis Patients," *J Pediatr Pharm Pract*, 1997, 2(1):23-6.

- ♦ **Tobramycin Injection, USP (Can)** *see* Tobramycin *on page 1545*
- ♦ **Tobramycin Sulfate** *see* Tobramycin *on page 1545*
- ♦ **Tobrex®** *see* Tobramycin *on page 1545*
- ♦ **Tofranil®** *see* Imipramine *on page 815*
- ♦ **Tofranil-PM®** *see* Imipramine *on page 815*
- ♦ **Tolectin®** *see* Tolmetin *on page 1549*

Tolmetin (TOLE met in)

Related Information
Overdose and Toxicology *on page 1916*

U.S. Brand Names Tolectin®

Index Terms Tolmetin Sodium

Therapeutic Category Analgesic, Non-narcotic; Nonsteroidal Anti-inflammatory Drug (NSAID), Oral

Generic Available Yes

Use Treatment of inflammatory and rheumatoid disorders, including juvenile rheumatoid arthritis

Medication Guide An FDA-approved patient medication guide, which is available with the product information and at http://www.fda.gov/cder/Offices/ODS/medication_guides.htm, must be dispensed with this medication for each new outpatient prescription and refill.

Pregnancy Risk Factor C (D if used in the 3rd trimester or near delivery)

Lactation Enters breast milk/not recommended (AAP rates "compatible")

Contraindications Hypersensitivity to tolmetin, any component, aspirin, or other NSAIDs; active GI bleeding, ulcer disease; patients with the "aspirin triad" [asthma, rhinitis (with or without nasal polyps), and aspirin intolerance] (fatal asthmatic and anaphylactoid reactions may occur in these patients)

Warnings In April 2005, the FDA announced product labeling changes for all NSAIDs, including COX-2 selective and OTC medications; although revised product labeling is currently not available for all products, sample labeling and a template of the required medication guide are now available. Labels for prescription nonselective NSAIDs will contain a contraindication for use in patients who have recently undergone coronary artery bypass graft (CABG) surgery and a boxed warning concerning the potential for increased risk of cardiovascular (CV) events and GI bleeding associated with NSAID use. Patients at increased risk of adverse events include patients immediately postoperative from CABG surgery, and those with existing CAD, CVD, or history of TIA or stomach ulcers. Prescribers are encouraged to use the lowest effective NSAID dose for the shortest time based on individual patient treatment goals. Medication guides will be required for all prescription products. Complete details for the labeling update can be found on the following FDA website: http://www.fda.gov/medwatch/SAFETY/2005/safety05.htm#NSAID.

Precautions Use with caution in patients with upper GI disease, impaired renal function, CHF, hypertension, and patients receiving anticoagulants; although rare, anaphylactoid reactions occur more commonly with tolmetin than other NSAIDs

Adverse Reactions
Cardiovascular: Edema
Central nervous system: Dizziness, nervousness, drowsiness, headache
Dermatologic: Rash, urticaria
Gastrointestinal: Nausea, abdominal pain, dyspepsia, diarrhea, constipation; GI bleeding, ulcer, perforation
Hematologic: Anemia, leukopenia, prolongation of bleeding time
Hepatic: Hepatitis
Otic: Tinnitus
Renal: Acute renal failure, renal dysfunction

Drug Interactions Tolmetin may potentiate the effects of warfarin and may increase prothrombin time and bleeding; aspirin may decrease tolmetin serum concentration; tolmetin may increase serum concentrations of methotrexate; tolmetin may decrease antihypertensive effects of ACE inhibitors or angiotensin II antagonists; drug interactions similar to other NSAIDs may also occur

Food Interactions Food or milk may decrease the extent of oral absorption

Mechanism of Action Inhibits prostaglandin synthesis by decreasing the activity of the enzyme, cyclooxygenase, which results in decreased formation of prostaglandin precursors

(Continued)

Tolmetin *(Continued)*

Pharmacokinetics

Absorption: Oral: Well absorbed
Protein binding: 99%
Metabolism: In the liver via oxidation and conjugation
Half-life, elimination: 5 hours
Time to peak serum concentration: Within 30-60 minutes
Elimination: Excreted in the urine as metabolites or conjugates

Usual Dosage Oral:

Children ≥2 years:
Anti-inflammatory: Initial: 20 mg/kg/day in 3-4 divided doses, then 15-30 mg/kg/day in 3-4 divided doses; maximum dose: 30 mg/kg/day in 4 divided doses; do not exceed 1800 mg/day
Analgesic: 5-7 mg/kg/dose every 6-8 hours
Adults: 400 mg 3 times/day; usual dose: 600 mg to 1.8 g/day; maximum dose: 2 g/day

Administration Oral: May administer with food, milk, or antacids to decrease GI adverse effects

Monitoring Parameters CBC with differential, liver enzymes, occult blood loss, BUN, serum creatinine; periodic ophthalmologic exams

Patient Information Avoid alcohol; may cause dizziness or drowsiness and impair ability to perform activities requiring mental alertness or physical coordination

Dosage Forms Excipient information presented when available (limited, particularly for generics); consult specific product labeling. Available as tolmetin sodium; mg strength refers to tolmetin.

Capsule: 400 mg
Tablet: 200 mg, 600 mg
Tolectin®: 600 mg [contains sodium 54 mg (2.35 mEq)]

References

Berde C, Ablin A, Glazer J, et al, "American Academy of Pediatrics Report of the Subcommittee on Disease-Related Pain in Childhood Cancer," *Pediatrics*, 1990, 86(5 Pt 2):818-25.
Giannini EH and Cawkwell GD, "Drug Treatment in Children With Juvenile Rheumatoid Arthritis. Past, Present, and Future," *Pediatr Clin North Am*, 1995, 42(5):1099-125.
Hollingworth P, "The Use of Non-Steroidal Anti-inflammatory Drugs in Paediatric Rheumatic Diseases," *Br J Rheumatol*, 1993, 32(1):73-7.
Rose CD and Doughty RA, "Pharmacological Management of Juvenile Rheumatoid Arthritis," *Drugs*, 1992, 43(6):849-63.

♦ **Tolmetin Sodium** *see* Tolmetin *on page 1549*

Tolnaftate (tole NAF tate)

Medication Safety Issues

Sound-alike/look-alike issues:
Tolnaftate may be confused with Tornalate®
Tinactin® may be confused with Talacen®

U.S. Brand Names Blis-To-Sol® [OTC]; Fungi-Guard [OTC]; Gold Bond® Antifungal [OTC] [DSC]; Mycocide® NS [OTC]; Podactin Powder [OTC]; Q-Naftate [OTC]; Tinactin® Antifungal [OTC]; Tinactin® Antifungal Jock Itch [OTC]; Tinaderm [OTC]; Ting® Cream [OTC]; Ting® Spray Liquid [OTC]

Canadian Brand Names Pitrex

Therapeutic Category Antifungal Agent, Topical

Generic Available Yes: Cream, powder, solution

Use Treatment of tinea pedis, tinea cruris, tinea corporis, tinea manuum caused by *Trichophyton rubrum, T. mentagrophytes, T. tonsurans, M. canis, M. audouinii*, and *E. floccosum*; also effective in the treatment of tinea versicolor infections due to *Malassezia furfur*

Pregnancy Risk Factor C

Contraindications Hypersensitivity to tolnaftate or any component; nail and scalp infections

Adverse Reactions

Dermatologic: Pruritus, contact dermatitis
Local: Irritation, stinging
Miscellaneous: Hypersensitivity reaction, sensitization to butylated hydroxytoluene component of cream, solution, and aerosol powder

Mechanism of Action Distorts the hyphae and stunts mycelial growth in susceptible fungi

Pharmacodynamics Onset of action: Response may be seen 24-72 hours after initiation of therapy

Usual Dosage Children and Adults: Topical: Apply 1-3 drops of solution or a small amount of cream or powder and rub into the affected areas 2-3 times/day for 2-4 weeks

Administration Topical: Wash and dry affected area before drug application; avoid contact with eyes

Monitoring Parameters Resolution of skin infection

Patient Information Avoid contact with the eyes; apply to clean dry area; consult the physician if a skin irritation develops or if the skin infection worsens or does not improve after 10 days of therapy

Additional Information Usually not effective alone for the treatment of infections involving hair follicles or nails

Dosage Forms Excipient information presented when available (limited, particularly for generics); consult specific product labeling. [DSC] = Discontinued product

Aerosol, liquid, topical:
- Tinactin® Antifungal: 1% (60 mL, 150 mL) [contains alcohol]
- Ting®: 1% (90 mL)

Aerosol, powder, topical:
- Tinactin® Antifungal: 1% (133 g) [contains alcohol]
- Tinactin® Antifungal Jock Itch: 1% (100 g, 133 g) [contains alcohol]

Cream, topical: 1% (15 g, 30 g)
- Fungi-Guard, Tinactin® Antifungal Jock Itch, Ting®: 1% (15 g)
- Q-Naftate, Tinactin® Antifungal: 1% (15 g, 30 g)

Liquid, topical:
- Blis-To-Sol®: 1% (30 mL, 55 mL)
- Fungi-Guard: 1% (30 mL) [contains vitamin E and aloe; brush applicator provided]

Powder, topical: 1% (45 g)
- Podactin: 1% (45 g)
- Tinactin® Antifungal: 1% (108 g)

Solution, topical: 1% (10 mL)
- Mycocide® NS: 1% (30 mL)
- Tinaderm: 1% (10 mL)

Swab, topical [liquid-filled swabstick]:
- Gold Bond® Antifungal: 1% (24s) [DSC]

♦ **Tomoxetine** *see* Atomoxetine *on page 172*
♦ **Topamax®** *see* Topiramate *on page 1551*
♦ **Topicaine® [OTC]** *see* Lidocaine *on page 933*
♦ **Topilene® (Can)** *see* Betamethasone *on page 212*

Topiramate (toe PYE ra mate)

Medication Safety Issues

Sound-alike/look-alike issues:
- Topamax® may be confused with Tegretol®, Tegretol®-XR, Toprol-XL®

Related Information

Antiepileptic Drugs *on page 1902*

U.S. Brand Names Topamax®

Canadian Brand Names Dom-Topiramate; Gen-Topiramate; Novo-Topiramate; PHL-Topiramate; PMS-Topiramate; ratio-Topiramate; Rhoxal-topiramate; Sandoz-Topiramate; Topamax®

Therapeutic Category Anticonvulsant, Miscellaneous

Generic Available No

Use Initial monotherapy of primary generalized tonic-clonic seizures or partial onset seizures in children ≥10 years of age and adults. Adjunctive treatment of primary generalized tonic-clonic seizures or partial onset seizures in children 2-16 years of age and adults; adjunctive treatment of seizures associated with Lennox-Gastaut syndrome in patients ≥2 years of age; prophylaxis of migraine headache in adults; may potentially be useful in infantile spasms

Pregnancy Risk Factor C

Lactation Enters breast milk/not recommended

Contraindications Hypersensitivity to topiramate or any component

Warnings Hyperchloremic metabolic acidosis may occur in patients receiving topiramate. Topiramate may decrease serum bicarbonate concentrations, due to inhibition of carbonic anhydrase and increased renal bicarbonate loss. In pediatric clinical trials for adjunctive treatment of seizures, persistent decreases in serum bicarbonate occurred in 67% of patients receiving topiramate (versus 10% of those receiving placebo). Markedly low serum bicarbonate values were reported in 11% of pediatric patients receiving topiramate (versus 0% of those receiving placebo). In pediatric monotherapy trials, persistent decreases in serum bicarbonate occurred in 7% of patients receiving 50 mg/day and 20% of patients receiving 400 mg/day. Markedly low serum bicarbonate values were reported in 4% of pediatric patients receiving topiramate monotherapy. The risk of topiramate-induced metabolic acidosis may be increased in patients with predisposing conditions (eg, diarrhea, status epilepticus,
(Continued)

Topiramate *(Continued)*

renal dysfunction, severe respiratory disorders, ketogenic diet, surgery) or concurrent treatment with other drugs that may cause acidosis.

Serum bicarbonate should be monitored at baseline and periodically during topiramate therapy. Patients should also be monitored for symptoms of metabolic acidosis (eg, hyperventilation, fatigue, anorexia, stupor, cardiac arrhythmias) and for potential complications of chronic acidosis (eg, nephrolithiasis, rickets, and reduced growth rates). Dose reduction or discontinuation (by tapering the dose) should be considered in patients with persistent or severe metabolic acidosis. If treatment is continued, alkali supplementation should be considered.

An ocular syndrome (characterized by secondary acute angle closure glaucoma and acute myopia) has been reported in adult and pediatric patients. Symptoms generally occur within 1 month of treatment initiation and include an acute decrease in visual acuity and/or ocular pain. Ophthalmologic findings may include increased IOP, anterior chamber shallowing, ocular hyperemia, mydriasis, and supracilliary effusion with anterior displacement of lens and iris. Patients experiencing blurred vision and/or eye pain should contact their physician immediately. Primary treatment of this syndrome is discontinuation of topiramate as soon as possible, based on physician judgment. If left untreated, this syndrome may cause serious damage to the eye, including permanent vision loss.

Rare, but significant, reports of oligohydrosis (decreased sweating) and hyperthermia have occurred in patients receiving topiramate. Most cases occurred in children, and were associated with vigorous exercise and/or high environmental temperatures. Due to the potential for serious sequelae, the use of preventative strategies (hydration before and during exercise or exposure to warm temperatures) is recommended. Monitor patients, especially pediatric patients, for decreased sweating and hyperthermia, especially in warm or hot weather. Use topiramate with caution in patients receiving drugs that predispose to heat-related disorders (eg, anticholinergic agents, carbonic anhydrase inhibitors).

Do not abruptly discontinue therapy, withdraw gradually to lessen chance for increased seizure frequency. CNS adverse effects are common (see Adverse Reactions); nephrolithiasis (kidney stones) or paresthesia (usually tingling of extremities) may occur; avoid use with alcohol, CNS depressants, or carbonic anhydrase inhibitors (see Drug Interactions); avoid use of ketogenic diet (may increase risk of nephrolithiasis)

Precautions Use with caution and decrease the dose in patients with renal dysfunction; use with caution in patients allergic to sulfa drugs and in patients with hepatic impairment. Concurrent use with valproic acid may result in hyperammonemia with or without encephalopathy; use with caution in patients with inborn errors of metabolism or decreased hepatic mitochondrial activity; these patients may be at increased risk.

Adverse Reactions

Central nervous system: Ataxia, difficulty in concentrating, dizziness, memory difficulties, fatigue, nervousness, somnolence, psychomotor slowing, speech/language problems, confusion, depression, mood problems, anxiety, cognitive problems; fever, irritability, and sleep disturbances (reported in children); **Note:** Somnolence and fatigue are the most common neuropsychiatric adverse effects in children

Dermatologic: Alopecia, rash, pruritus, acne

Endocrine & metabolic: Weight loss; decreased serum bicarbonate, hyperchloremic metabolic acidosis (non-anion gap) (see Warnings); dehydration

Gastrointestinal: Anorexia, nausea, diarrhea

Hematologic: Purpura

Neuromuscular & skeletal: Paresthesia, tremor

Ocular: Nystagmus, diplopia, abnormal vision, ocular syndrome (see Warnings)

Otic: Tinnitus

Renal: Nephrolithiasis

Respiratory: Epistaxis

Miscellaneous: Oligohydrosis (decreased sweating) and hyperthermia [pediatric patients may be at increased risk (see Warnings)]

Drug Interactions Cytochrome P450 isoenzyme CYP2C19 substrate and inhibitor

Phenytoin and carbamazepine may significantly decrease topiramate serum concentrations (topiramate dosage increase may be needed); valproic acid may decrease topiramate concentrations; lamotrigine and hydrochlorothiazide may increase topiramate concentrations; topiramate may decrease serum concentrations of valproic acid, digoxin, lithium, risperidone, and ethinyl estradiol (may decrease the efficacy of oral contraceptives); alcohol or other CNS depressants may increase adverse CNS effects; carbonic anhydrase inhibitors may increase the risk of nephrolithiasis or paresthesia; topiramate may increase phenytoin serum concentrations by 25% in some patients; topiramate may increase serum concentrations of amitriptyline; coadministration with drugs that predispose patients to heat-related disorders (eg, anticholinergic agents, carbonic anhydrase inhibitors) may increase the risk of hyperthermia (see Warnings); coadministration with valproic acid may result in hyperammonemia with or without encephalopathy (see Precautions)

Food Interactions Food may decrease the rate but not the extent of absorption

Stability Protect from moisture; store at room temperature

Mechanism of Action Exact mechanism unknown; efficacy for epilepsy and migraine prophylaxis may be due to blockade of voltage-dependent sodium channels, potentiation of GABA (an inhibitory neurotransmitter) and antagonism of kainate activation of glutamate (an excitatory amino acid) subtype receptors; also inhibits carbonic anhydrase (minor effect)

Pharmacokinetics Note: Sprinkle capsule is bioequivalent to tablet

Absorption: Rapid

Distribution: Distributes extensively into breast milk

V_d: Adults: 0.6-0.8 L/kg

Protein binding: 15% to 41%; percent protein bound decreases as blood concentrations increase

Metabolism: Minor amounts metabolized in liver via hydroxylation, hydrolysis, and glucuronidation; percentage of dose metabolized in liver and clearance are increased in patients receiving enzyme inducers

Bioavailability: Tablet: 80% (relative to a prepared solution)

Half-life:

Adults: 19-23 hours (mean 21 hours)

Adults with renal impairment: 59 ± 11 hours (n=7)

Time to peak serum concentration: 2 hours; range: 1.4-4.3 hours

Elimination: 70% of dose excreted unchanged in urine; may undergo renal tubular reabsorption

Clearance:

Children 4-17 years: ~50% higher than adults (per kg)

Adults: 20-30 mL/minute

Renal impairment: Reduced

Hepatic impairment: May be reduced

Dialysis: Significantly hemodialyzed; dialysis clearance: 120 mL/minute (4-6 times higher than in adults with normal renal function); supplemental doses may be required

Usual Dosage Oral:

Anticonvulsant, adjunctive therapy:

Children 2-16 years:

Partial onset seizures or Lennox-Gastaut syndrome: Initial: 1-3 mg/kg/day (maximum: 25 mg) given nightly for 1 week; increase at 1- to 2-week intervals by 1-3 mg/kg/day given in 2 divided doses; titrate dose to response; usual maintenance: 5-9 mg/kg/day given in 2 divided doses

Primary generalized tonic-clonic seizures: Use initial dose as listed above, but use slower initial titration rate; titrate to 6 mg/kg/day by the end of 8 weeks

Adolescents ≥17 years and Adults:

Partial onset seizures: Initial: 25-50 mg/day given daily for 1 week; increase at weekly intervals by 25-50 mg/day; give in 2 divided doses; titrate dose to response; usual maintenance: 100-200 mg twice daily; maximum dose: 1600 mg/day

Primary generalized tonic-clonic seizures: Use initial dose as listed above, but use slower initial titration rate; give in 2 divided doses; titrate upwards to recommended dose by the end of 8 weeks; usual maintenance: 200 mg twice daily; maximum dose: 1600 mg/day

Anticonvulsant, monotherapy: Partial onset seizures or primary generalized tonic-clonic seizures: Children ≥10 years and Adults: Initial: 25 mg twice daily; increase at weekly intervals by 50 mg/day up to a dose of 100 mg twice daily (week 4 dose); thereafter, may further increase at weekly intervals by 100 mg/day up to the recommended maximum dose of 200 mg twice daily

Migraine prophylaxis: Adults: Initial: 25 mg/day; increase at weekly intervals by 25 mg/day; give in 2 divided doses; titrate dose to response; recommended dose: 50 mg twice daily; **Note:** A randomized controlled trial that included adolescent patients, titrated doses based on response, up to a maximum dose of 100 mg twice daily (see Brandes, 2004)

Dosing adjustment in renal impairment: Cl_{cr} <70 mL/minute/1.73 m^2: Administer 50% of the usual dose; titrate more slowly due to prolonged half-life; supplemental doses may be required in patients undergoing hemodialysis (see Pharmacokinetics)

Dosing adjustment in hepatic impairment: Carefully adjust dose as plasma concentrations may be increased if normal dosing is used

(Continued)

Topiramate *(Continued)*

Administration May be administered without regard to food; broken tablets have a bitter taste; tablets may be crushed, mixed with water, and administered immediately. Swallow sprinkle capsules whole or open and sprinkle contents on small amount of soft food (eg, 1 teaspoonful of applesauce); swallow sprinkle/food mixture immediately; do not chew; do not store for later use; drink fluids after dose to make sure mixture is completely swallowed

Monitoring Parameters Frequency, duration, and severity of seizure episodes or migraine headaches; renal function; monitor serum electrolytes including baseline and periodic serum bicarbonate, symptoms of metabolic acidosis (see Warnings), complications of chronic acidosis (eg, nephrolithiasis, rickets, and reduced growth rates); monitor body temperature and for decreased sweating, especially in warm or hot weather; monitor serum ammonia concentration in patients with unexplained lethargy, vomiting, or mental status changes

Reference Range Not applicable; plasma topiramate concentrations have not been shown to correlate with clinical efficacy

Patient Information Contact physician immediately if blurred vision or eye pain occur; ensure adequate fluid intake to avoid kidney stone formation and to help prevent dehydration and hyperthermia before and during exercise or exposure to warm temperatures; may cause dizziness or drowsiness and impair ability to perform activities requiring mental alertness or physical coordination; avoid alcohol

Dosage Forms Excipient information presented when available (limited, particularly for generics); consult specific product labeling.

Capsule, sprinkle: 15 mg, 25 mg

Tablet: 25 mg, 50 mg, 100 mg, 200 mg

Extemporaneous Preparations A 6 mg/mL topiramate oral suspension made from tablets and 2 different vehicles (a 1:1 mixture of Ora-Sweet® and Ora-Plus®, or a mixture of Simple Syrup, NF and methylcellulose 1% with parabens) was stable for 90 days when stored in plastic prescription bottles under refrigeration (preferred) or at room temperature; grind six 100 mg tablets in a mortar into a fine powder; add a small amount of methylcellulose gel and mix well to form a uniform paste (**Note:** Use a small amount of methylcellulose gel when using the 1:1 Ora-Sweet® and Ora-Plus® mixture as the vehicle; use 10 mL of methylcellulose 1% with parabens when using Simple Syrup, NF as the vehicle); mix while adding the vehicle in geometric proportions to **almost** 100 mL; transfer to a graduate; rinse the mortar with the vehicle and transfer to the graduate; qsad with vehicle to make 100 mL; label "shake well" and "refrigerate" (Nahata, 2004).

Nahata MC, Pai VB, and Hipple TF, *Pediatric Drug Formulations*, 5th ed, Cincinnati, OH: Harvey Whitney Books Co, 2004.

References

Brandes JL, Saper JR, Diamond M, et al, "Topiramate for Migraine Prevention: A Randomized Controlled Trial," *JAMA*, 2004, 291(8):965-73.

Doose DR, Walker SA, Gisclon LG, et al, "Single-Dose Pharmacokinetics and Effect of Food on the Bioavailability of Topiramate, a Novel Antiepileptic Drug," *J Clin Pharmacol*, 1996, 36(10):884-91.

Glauser TA, "Preliminary Observations on Topiramate in Pediatric Epilepsies," *Epilepsia*, 1997, 38(Suppl 1):S37-41.

Glauser TA, "Topiramate Use in Pediatric Patients," *Can J Neurol Sci*, 1998, 25(3):S8-12.

Glauser TA, Clark PO, and Strawsburg R, "A Pilot Study of Topiramate in the Treatment of Infantile Spasms," *Epilepsia*, 1998, 39(12):1324-8.

Hershey AD, Powers SW, Vockell AL, et al, "Effectiveness of Topiramate in the Prevention of Childhood Headaches," *Headache*, 2002, 42(8):810-8.

Pellock JM, "Managing Pediatric Epilepsy Syndromes With New Antiepileptic Drugs," *Pediatrics*, 1999, 104(5 Pt 1):1106-16.

Sachdeo RC, "Topiramate. Clinical Profile in Epilepsy," *Clin Pharmacokinet*, 1998, 34(5):335-46.

♦ **Topisone® (Can)** *see* Betamethasone *on page 212*

♦ **TOPO** *see* Topotecan *on page 1554*

♦ **Toposar®** *see* Etoposide *on page 625*

Topotecan (toe poe TEE kan)

Medication Safety Issues

Sound-alike/look-alike issues:

Hycamtin® may be confused with Hycomine®

High alert medication: The Institute for Safe Medication Practices (ISMP) includes this medication among its list of drugs which have a heightened risk of causing significant patient harm when used in error.

U.S. Brand Names Hycamtin®

Canadian Brand Names Hycamtin®

Index Terms Hycamptamine; NSC-609699; SK and F 104864; SKF 104864; SKF 104864-A; TOPO; Topotecan Hydrochloride; TPT

Therapeutic Category Antineoplastic Agent, Topoisomerase Inhibitor

Generic Available No

Use Treatment of ovarian cancer after failure of first-line chemotherapy; second-line treatment of small cell lung cancer; pediatric solid tumors including rhabdomyosarcoma, osteosarcoma, ependymoma, and neuroblastoma; pediatric leukemia

Pregnancy Risk Factor D

Lactation Excretion in breast milk unknown/contraindicated

Contraindications Hypersensitivity to topotecan or any component; severe bone marrow depression (patients with baseline neutrophil counts <1,500 cells/mm^3 and platelet count <100,000/mm^3); pregnancy; breast-feeding

Warnings The FDA currently recommends that procedures for proper handling and disposal of antineoplastic agents be considered. Neutropenia is the dose-limiting toxicity of topotecan; neutropenia may be severe and potentially fatal.

Precautions Use caution in patients with renal or hepatic impairment; modify dosage in patients with renal impairment

Adverse Reactions

Cardiovascular: Hypotension

Central nervous system: Fatigue, fever, pain, asthenia, headache

Dermatologic: Alopecia, rash, pruritus, angioedema

Genitourinary: Hematuria

Gastrointestinal: Nausea, vomiting, diarrhea, constipation, abdominal pain, mucositis, anorexia

Hematologic: Leukopenia, neutropenia, thrombocytopenia, decreased fibrinogen level, anemia

Hepatic: Elevated liver enzymes, elevated bilirubin and alkaline phosphatase

Local: Erythema, bruising

Neuromuscular & skeletal: Paresthesia

Respiratory: Dyspnea, cough

Miscellaneous: Anaphylactoid reactions, sepsis

Drug Interactions Concurrent administration of G-CSF and topotecan results in severe, prolonged neutropenia (G-CSF therapy should not be initiated until 24 hours after completion of topotecan); concurrent cisplatin or carboplatin with topotecan therapy results in greater myelosuppression

Stability Store intact vial containing lyophilized powder at room temperature; protect from light; reconstituted solution is stable for 24 hours at room temperature or up to 7 days if refrigerated; if topotecan is further diluted in D_5W or NS, it is stable for 24 hours at room temperature or up to 7 days under refrigeration. Do **not** dilute in alkaline solutions.

Mechanism of Action Topoisomerase I inhibitor which stabilizes the covalent complex between topoisomerase I and DNA preventing religation of DNA single-strand breaks resulting in interference with DNA replication, RNA transcription, and DNA repair.

Pharmacokinetics

Distribution: V_d: Adults: 87.3 L/m^2; distributes into CSF

Protein binding: 35%

Metabolism: Undergoes pH dependent hydrolysis of its lactone moiety to yield a relatively inactive open-ring hydroxy acid form in plasma; N-demethylated metabolite formed in the liver

Bioavailability: Oral: 30% to 44%

Half-life: 2-3 hours; 5 hours with renal impairment

Elimination: 30% to 39% of a dose is excreted in urine; remaining drug is excreted in stool via biliary excretion

Clearance: Topotecan plasma clearance is 24% higher in males than in female patients

Children:

No previous radiation therapy and no bone marrow involvement: 12.2 ± 3.5 L/hour/m^2 (range: 6.8-17.4 L/hour/m^2)

Previous radiation without bone marrow involvement: 9.8 ± 4.1 L/hour/m^2 (range: 4.8-17.4 L/hour/m^2)

Adults: 6.5-30 L/hour/m^2

Usual Dosage Refer to Individual Protocols:

Children: I.V.:

Pediatric solid tumors: 1 mg/m^2/day (range: 0.75-1.9 mg/m^2/day) for 3 days as a continuous infusion, repeated every 3 weeks

Single-agent therapy for refractory solid tumors or hematologic malignancies: 2.4 mg/m^2/day once daily for 5 days of a 21 day course.

Combination therapy for solid tumors: 0.75 mg/m^2/dose once daily for 5 days every 21 days in combination with cyclophosphamide.

(Continued)

Topotecan *(Continued)*

Adults:

I.V.: Intermittent infusion: 1.5 mg/m²/day once daily for 5 days followed by a 16 day rest period; repeat course every 21 days for 4 courses. If neutrophil count falls to <500/mm³ or if platelets decrease to <25,000 cells/mm³, reduce dose by 0.25 mg/m² for subsequent courses. Alternatively for severe neutropenia, administer G-CSF 24 hours after completion of topotecan infusion following subsequent courses

I.V. continuous infusion: 0.2-0.7mg/m²/day for 7-21 days

Dosing adjustment in renal impairment:

Cl_{cr} 20-39 mL/minute: Reduce dosage by 50% or by 0.75 mg/m²/dose

Cl_{cr} <20 mL/minute: Insufficient data available to recommend dosage adjustment guidelines

Administration Parenteral: May administer by intermittent infusion over 30 minutes or by continuous infusion at a final concentration not to exceed 0.5 mg/mL in D_5W or NS.

Monitoring Parameters CBC with differential and platelet count; renal and hepatic function tests; blood pressure during infusion

Patient Information Inform physician of persistent fever, chills, bruising, bleeding, yellowing of eyes or skin, or pain at infusion site. Avoid alcohol; may cause fatigue and impair ability to perform activities requiring mental alertness or physical coordination. Topotecan may cause birth defects; contraceptive measures are recommended during therapy.

Nursing Implications Care should be taken to avoid extravasation. Extravasation of topotecan has been associated with local reactions such as erythema and bruising. If a topotecan solution comes in contact with skin or mucous membranes, wash skin immediately and thoroughly with soap and water; flush mucosa thoroughly with water.

Additional Information

Myelosuppressive effects:

WBC (nadir): 8-11 days; recovery: 21 days

Neutrophils (nadir): 12 days

Platelets (nadir): 15 days

Dosage Forms Excipient information presented when available (limited, particularly for generics); consult specific product labeling.

Injection, powder for reconstitution, as hydrochloride:

Hycamtin®: 4 mg [base]

References

Furman WL, Stewart CF, Kirstein M, et al, "Protracted Intermittent Schedule of Topotecan in Children With Refractory Acute Leukemia: A Pediatric Oncology Group Study," *J of Clin Oncology*, 2002, 20(6):1617-24.

Santana VM, Zamboni WC, Kirstein MN, et al, "A Pilot Study of Protracted Topotecan Dosing Using a Pharmacokinetically Guided Dosing Approach in Children With Solid Tumors," *Clin Cancer Res*, 2003, 9(2):633-40.

Saylors RL 3rd, Stine KC, Sullivan J, et al, "Cyclophosphamide Plus Topotecan in Children With Recurrent or Refractory Solid Tumors: A Pediatric Oncology Group Phase II Study," *J Clin Oncol*, 2001, 19(15):3463-9.

Walterhouse DO, Lyden ER, Breitfeld PP, et al, "Efficacy of Topotecan and Cyclophosphamide Given in a Phase II Window Trial in Children With Newly Diagnosed Metastatic Rhabdomyosarcoma: A Children's Oncology Group Study," *J Clin Oncol*, 2004, 22(8):1398-403.

Wells RJ, Reid JM, Ames MM, et al, "Phase I Trial of Cisplatin and Topotecan in Children With Recurrent Solid Tumors: Children's Cancer Group Study 0942," *J Pediatr Hematol Oncol*, 2002, 24(2):89-93.

◆ **Topotecan Hydrochloride** *see* Topotecan *on page 1554*
◆ **Toprol-XL®** *see* Metoprolol *on page 1046*
◆ **Topsyn® (Can)** *see* Fluocinonide *on page 674*
◆ **Toradol®** *see* Ketorolac *on page 889*
◆ **Toradol® IM (Can)** *see* Ketorolac *on page 889*

Torsemide (TOR se mide)

Medication Safety Issues

Sound-alike/look-alike issues:

Torsemide may be confused with furosemide

Demadex® may be confused with Denorex®

Related Information

Antihypertensive Agents by Class *on page 1678*

U.S. Brand Names Demadex®

Therapeutic Category Antihypertensive Agent; Diuretic, Loop

Generic Available Yes: Tablet

Use Management of edema associated with CHF and hepatic or renal disease; used alone or in combination with antihypertensives in treatment of hypertension

Pregnancy Risk Factor B

Lactation Excretion in breast milk unknown/use caution

Contraindications Hypersensitivity to torsemide, any component, or other sulfonylureas; anuria

Warnings Loop diuretics are potent diuretics, excess amounts can lead to profound diuresis with fluid and electrolyte loss; close medical supervision and dose evaluation is required

Adverse Reactions

Cardiovascular: Orthostatic hypotension, EKG abnormality, chest pain, atrial fibrillation, ventricular tachycardia, syncope

Central nervous system: Headache, dizziness, insomnia, nervousness

Dermatologic: Rash, photosensitivity

Endocrine & metabolic: Hyponatremia, hypokalemia, hypochloremia, alkalosis, hypocalcemia, dehydration, hyperuricemia, gout

Gastrointestinal: Diarrhea, nausea, constipation, dyspepsia, GI hemorrhage, stomach cramps, pancreatitis

Genitourinary: Excessive urination

Hematologic: Agranulocytosis, anemia

Neuromuscular & skeletal: Myalgia, arthralgia, weakness

Otic: Ototoxicity

Renal: Prerenal azotemia, interstitial nephritis, nephrocalcinosis

Drug Interactions Cytochrome P450 isoenzyme CYP2C9 substrate

Increased risk of ototoxicity with aminoglycosides and cis-platinum; increased anticoagulant effects of warfarin; increased risk of digoxin toxicity when used alone or combined with other medications which cause increased potassium losses (eg, corticosteroids, amphotericin B); decreased glucose tolerance which may result in increased requirements of sulfonylureas and other antidiabetic agents; decreased diuretic effects of torsemide when combined with NSAIDs; increased lithium serum levels; increased salicylate levels with potential toxicity (with high dose salicylates)

Stability Stable for 24 hours at room temperature when mixed with D_5W or NS

Mechanism of Action Inhibits reabsorption of sodium and chloride in the ascending loop of Henle and distal renal tubule, interfering with the chloride-binding cotransport system, thus causing increased excretion of water, sodium, chloride, magnesium, and calcium

Pharmacodynamics

Onset of action:

Oral: 60 minutes

I.V.: 10 minutes

Maximum effect:

Oral: 60-120 minutes

I.V.: Within 60 minutes

Duration: Oral, I.V.: 6-8 hours

Pharmacokinetics

Absorption: Oral: Rapid

Distribution: V_d: 12-15 L (adults)

Protein binding: Plasma: ~97% to 99%

Metabolism: Hepatic by cytochrome P450, 80%

Bioavailability: 80% to 90%

Half-life: 3.5 hours (range 2-4 hours); 7-8 hours in cirrhosis (dose modification appears unnecessary)

Time to peak serum concentration: Oral: 1 hour

Elimination: 20% eliminated unchanged in urine

Usual Dosage Adults: Oral, I.V.:

Edema: 10-20 mg once daily; titrate upward as needed (maximum dose: 200 mg/day)

Hepatic cirrhosis: 5-10 mg once daily

Hypertension: Initial: 5 mg once daily; increase to 10 mg if ineffective after 4-6 weeks of therapy

Administration

Oral: May be administered with food or milk

Parenteral: May be administered undiluted direct I.V. over 3-5 minutes

Monitoring Parameters Renal function, serum electrolytes, fluid balance, blood pressure, body weight

Patient Information Rise slowly from a lying or sitting position to minimize dizziness, lightheadedness or fainting; also use extra care when exercising, standing for long periods of time. Take last dose of day early in the evening to prevent nocturia. May cause photosensitivity reactions (eg, exposure to sunlight may cause severe sunburn, skin rash, redness, or itching); avoid exposure to sunlight and artificial light sources (sunlamps, tanning booth/bed); wear protective clothing, wide-brimmed hats, sunglasses, and lip sunscreen (SPF ≥15); use a sunscreen [broad-spectrum sunscreen or physical sunscreen (preferred) or sunblock with SPF ≥15]; contact physician if reaction occurs.

(Continued)

Torsemide *(Continued)*

Additional Information 10-20 mg torsemide is approximately equivalent to:
Furosemide 40 mg
Bumetanide 1 mg

Dosage Forms Excipient information presented when available (limited, particularly for generics); consult specific product labeling.
Injection, solution: 10 mg/mL (2 mL, 5 mL)
Tablet: 5 mg, 10 mg, 20 mg, 100 mg

References

Chobanian AV, Bakris GL, Black HR, et al, "The Seventh Report of the Joint National Committee on Prevention, Detection, Evaluation, and Treatment of High Blood Pressure: The JNC 7 Report," *JAMA*, 2003, 289(19):2560-72.

- **Touro® Allergy** *see* Brompheniramine and Pseudoephedrine *on page 235*
- **Touro® DM** *see* Guaifenesin and Dextromethorphan *on page 748*
- **tPA** *see* Alteplase *on page 83*
- **TPT** *see* Topotecan *on page 1554*
- **Trace Elements** *see* Trace Metals *on page 1558*

Trace Metals (trase MET als)

Related Information
Parenteral Nutrition (PN) *on page 1755*

U.S. Brand Names Iodopen®; Molypen®; M.T.E.-4®; M.T.E.-5®; M.T.E.-6®; M.T.E.-7®; Multitrace™-4; Multitrace™-4 Neonatal; Multitrace™-4 Pediatric; Multitrace™-5; Neotrace-4®; Pedtrace-4®; P.T.E.-4®; P.T.E.-5®; Selepen®

Index Terms Ammonium Molybdate; Chromium Chloride; Copper Sulfate; Cupric Chloride; Iodine Sodium; Manganese Chloride; Manganese Sulfate; Multiple Trace Metals; Neonatal Trace Metals; Selenium; Trace Elements; Zinc Chloride; Zinc Sulfate

Therapeutic Category Mineral, Parenteral; Trace Element, Multiple, Neonatal; Trace Element, Parenteral

Generic Available Yes

Use Prevent and correct trace metal deficiencies

Pregnancy Risk Factor C

Contraindications Hypersensitivity to a specific trace metal or component of the trace metal solution (see Warnings); do not give by direct injection because of potential for phlebitis, tissue irritation, and potential to increase renal loss of minerals from a bolus injection

Warnings Metals may accumulate in conditions of renal failure or biliary obstruction; consider reduction in dosage or deletion of copper and manganese in patients with biliary obstruction; avoid copper use in patients with Wilson's disease; administration of copper in the absence of zinc or zinc in the absence of copper may cause decreases in their respective plasma levels; molybdenum promotes the utilization of copper and increases its excretion; excessive amounts of molybdenum may produce copper deficiency; multiple trace metal solutions present a risk of overdosage when the need for one trace element is appreciably higher than for others in the formulation; utilization of individual trace metal solutions may be needed. Consider reduction in dosage or deletion of selenium and chromium in patients with renal dysfunction.

Some products contain benzyl alcohol which may cause allergic reactions in susceptible individuals; large amounts of benzyl alcohol (≥99 mg/kg/day) have been associated with a potentially fatal toxicity ("gasping syndrome") in neonates; the "gasping syndrome" consists of metabolic acidosis, respiratory distress, gasping respirations, CNS dysfunction (including convulsions, intracranial hemorrhage), hypotension and cardiovascular collapse; *in vitro* and animal studies have shown that benzoate, a metabolite of benzyl alcohol, displaces bilirubin from protein-binding sites; use benzyl alcohol-containing products with caution in neonates.

Precautions Chromic chloride contains aluminum which may accumulate with prolonged use, particularly in patients with decreased renal function; use cautiously in neonates and other patients with decreased renal function

Adverse Reactions The following describe the symptomatology associated with excess trace metals:

Chromium: Nausea, vomiting, GI ulcers, renal and hepatic dysfunction, convulsions, coma

Copper: Prostration, behavioral changes, diarrhea, progressive marasmus, hypotonia, photophobia, hepatic dysfunction, peripheral edema

Manganese: Irritability, speech disturbances, abnormal gait, headache, anorexia, apathy, impotence, cholestatic jaundice, movement disorders

Molybdenum: Gout-like syndrome with elevated blood levels of uric acid and xanthine oxidase

Selenium: Alopecia, weak nails, dermatitis, dental defects, GI disorders, nervousness, mental depression, metallic taste, garlic odor of breath and sweat

Zinc: Profuse diaphoresis, decreased consciousness, blurred vision, tachycardia, hypothermia

Mechanism of Action

Chromium: Part of glucose tolerance factor, an essential activator of insulin-mediated reactions; helps maintain normal glucose metabolism and peripheral nerve function

Copper: Cofactor for serum ceruloplasmin, helps maintain normal rates of red and white cell formation

Manganese: Activator for several enzymes including manganese-dependent superoxide dismutase and pyruvate carboxylase; activates glycosyl transferases involved in mucopolysaccharide synthesis

Molybdenum: Constituent of the enzymes xanthine oxidase, sulfite oxidase, and aldehyde oxidase

Selenium: Part of glutathione peroxidase which protects cell components from oxidative damage due to peroxides produced in cellular metabolism

Zinc: A cofactor for >70 different enzymes; facilitates wound healing, helps maintain normal growth rates, normal skin hydration, and the senses of taste and smell

Pharmacokinetics

Chromium: 10% to 20% oral absorption; excretion primarily via kidneys and bile

Copper: 30% oral absorption; 80% elimination via bile; intestinal wall 16% and urine 4%

Manganese: 10% oral absorption; excretion primarily via bile; ancillary routes via pancreatic secretions or reabsorption into the intestinal lumen occur during periods of biliary obstruction

Molybdenum: 30% to 70% oral absorption; primarily renal excretion; some biliary excretion associated with an enterohepatic cycle

Selenium: Very poor oral absorption; 75% excretion via kidneys, remainder via feces, lung, and skin

Zinc: 20% to 30% oral absorption; 90% excretion in stools, remainder via urine and perspiration

Usual Dosage See table.

Trace Mineral Daily Requirements[1]

	Infants	Children (≥3 mo to ≤5 y)	Older Children, Adolescents, and Adults
Chromium[2]	0.2 mcg/kg	0.14-0.2 mcg/kg (max: 5 mcg)	10-15 mcg
Copper[3]	20 mcg/kg	20 mcg/kg (max: 300 mcg)	0.3-0.5 mg
Iodide[4]	1 mcg/kg	1 mcg/kg	1 mcg/kg
Manganese[3]	1 mcg/kg	2-10 mcg/kg (max: 50 mcg)	60-150 mcg
Selenium[2,5]	2-3 mcg/kg	2-3 mcg/kg (max: 30 mcg)	20-60 mcg
Zinc	400 mcg/kg (preterm) 300 mcg/kg (term <3 mo)	100 mcg/kg (max: 5 mg)	2.5-5 mg

[1]Recommended intakes of trace elements cannot be achieved through the use of a commercially available combination trace element product. Only through the use of individualized trace element products can recommended intakes be achieved.

[2]Omit in patients with renal dysfunction.

[3]Omit in patients with impaired biliary excretion or cholestatic liver disease.

[4]Percutaneous absorption from protein-bound iodine may be adequate.

[5]Indicated for use in long-term parenteral nutrition patients.

Administration Parenteral: Must be diluted prior to use and infused as component of parenteral nutrition or parenteral solutions

Reference Range

Chromium: 0.18-0.47 ng/mL (SI: 35-90 nmol/L); some laboratories report much higher

*Copper: ~0.7-1.5 mcg/mL (SI: 11-24 micromoles/L); levels are higher in pregnant women and children

Manganese: 18-30 mcg/dL (SI: 2.3-3.8 micromoles/L)

Selenium: 95-165 ng/mL (SI: 120-209 nmol/L)

Zinc: 70-120 mcg/dL (SI: 10-18.4 micromoles/L)

*May not be a meaningful measurement of body stores

(Continued)

Trace Metals *(Continued)*

Additional Information Persistent diarrhea or excessive GI fluid losses from ostomy sites may grossly increase zinc losses

Dosage Forms Excipient information presented when available (limited, particularly for generics); consult specific product labeling.

Injection, solution [combination products]:

M.T.E.-4®: Chromium 4 mcg, copper 0.4 mg, manganese 0.1 mg, and zinc 1 mg per mL (3 mL, 10 mL, 30 mL) [30 mL contains benzyl alcohol]

M.T.E.-4® Concentrate: Chromium 10 mcg, copper 1 mg, manganese 0.5 mg, and zinc 5 mg per mL (1 mL, 10 mL) [10 mL contains benzyl alcohol]

M.T.E.-5® [preservative free]: Chromium 4 mcg, copper 0.4 mg, manganese 0.1 mg, selenium 20 mcg, and zinc 1 mg per mL (10 mL)

M.T.E.-5® Concentrate: Chromium 10 mcg, copper 1 mg, manganese 0.5 mg, selenium 60 mcg, and zinc 5 mg per mL (1 mL, 10 mL) [10 mL contains benzyl alcohol]

M.T.E.-6® [preservative free]: Chromium 4 mcg, copper 0.4 mg, iodide 25 mcg, manganese 0.1 mg, selenium 20 mcg, and zinc 1 mg per mL (10 mL)

M.T.E.-6® Concentrate: Chromium 10 mcg, copper 1 mg, iodide 75 mcg, manganese 0.5 mg, selenium 60 mcg, and zinc 5 mg per mL (10 mL) [contains benzyl alcohol]

M.T.E.-7® [preservative free]: Chromium 4 mcg, copper 0.4 mg, iodide 25 mcg, manganese 0.1 mg, molybdenum 25 mcg, selenium 20 mcg, and zinc 1 mg per mL (10 mL)

Multitrace™-4: Chromium 4 mcg, copper 0.4 mg, manganese 0.1 mg, and zinc 1 mg per mL (10 mL) [contains benzyl alcohol]

Multitrace™-4 Neonatal: Chromium 0.85 mcg, copper 0.1 mg, manganese 0.025 mg, and zinc 1.5 mg per mL (2 mL)

Multitrace™-4 Pediatric: Chromium 1 mcg, copper 0.1 mg, manganese 0.025 mg, and zinc 1 mg per mL (3 mL)

Multitrace™-4 Concentrate: Chromium 10 mcg, copper 1 mg, manganese 0.5 mg, and zinc 5 mg per mL (1 mL, 10 mL) [10 mL contains benzyl alcohol]

Multitrace™-5: Chromium 4 mcg, copper 0.4 mg, manganese 0.1 mg, selenium 20 mcg, and zinc 1 mg per mL (10 mL) [contains benzyl alcohol]

Multitrace™-5 Concentrate: Chromium 10 mcg, copper 1 mg, manganese 0.5 mg, selenium 60 mcg, and zinc 5 mg per mL (1 mL, 10 mL) [10 mL contains benzyl alcohol]

Neotrace-4® [preservative free]: Chromium 0.85 mcg, copper 0.1 mg, manganese 0.025 mg, and zinc 1.5 mg per mL (2 mL)

Pedtrace-4® [preservative free]: Chromium 0.85 mcg, copper 0.1 mg, manganese 0.025 mg, and zinc 0.5 mg per mL (3 mL, 10 mL)

P.T.E.-4® [preservative free]: Chromium 1 mcg, copper 0.1 mg, manganese 0.025 mg, and zinc 1 mg per mL (3 mL)

P.T.E.-5® [preservative free]: Chromium 1 mcg, copper 0.1 mg, manganese 0.025 mg, selenium 15 mcg, and zinc 1 mg per mL (3 mL)

Trace elements pediatric: Chromium 1 mcg, copper 0.1 mg, manganese 0.03 mg, and zinc 0.5 mg per mL (10 mL) [contains benzyl alcohol]

Injection, solution [elemental equivalence]:

Chromium, as chromic chloride (hexahydrate) [preservative free]: 0.0205 mg/mL [0.004 mg/mL] (10 mL)

Copper, as cupric chloride: 1.07 mg/mL [0.4 mg/mL] (10 mL)

Iodine, as iodine sodium (Iodopen®): 0.118 mg/mL [0.1 mg/mL] (10 mL)

Manganese:

As chloride: 0.36 mg/mL [0.1 mg/mL] (10 mL)

As sulfate [preservative free]: 0.31 mg/mL [0.1 mg/mL] (10 mL)

Molybdenum, as ammonium molybdate (tetrahydrate) (Molypen®): 46 mcg/mL [25 mcg/mL] (10 mL)

Selenium, as selenious acid: 0.0654 mg/mL [0.04 mg/mL] (10 mL)

Selepen®: 0.0654 mg/mL [0.04 mg/mL] (10 mL, 30 mL) [30 mL contains benzyl alcohol]

Zinc:

As chloride: 2.09 mg/mL [1 mg/mL] (10 mL, 50 mL)

As sulfate, anhydrous [preservative free]: 2.46 mg/mL [1 mg/mL] (10 mL)

As sulfate, anhydrous, concentrate [preservative free]: 12.32 mg/mL [5 mg/mL] (5 mL)

References

Dahlstrom KA, Ament ME, Medhin MG, et al, "Serum Trace Elements in Children Receiving Long-Term Parenteral Nutrition," *J Pediatr*, 1986, 109(4):625-30.

Fell JM, Reynolds AP, Meadows N, et al, "Manganese Toxicity in Children Receiving Long-Term Parenteral Nutrition," *Lancet*, 1996, 347(9010):1218-21.

Greene HL, Hambridge KM, Schanler R, et al, "Guidelines for the Use of Vitamins, Trace Elements, Calcium, Magnesium and Phosphorus in Infants and Children Receiving Total Parenteral Nutrition: Report of the Subcommittee on Pediatric Nutrient Requirements From the Committee on Clinical Practice Issues of The American Society for Clinical Nutrition," *Am J Clin Nutr*, 1988, 48(5):1324-42.
"Guidelines for the Use of Parenteral and Enteral Nutrition in Adult and Pediatric Patients. ASPEN Board of Directors and The Clinical Guidelines Task Force," *JPEN J Parenter Enteral Nutr*, 2002, 26(1 Suppl):1-138SA.
Litov RE, and Combs GF Jr, "Selenium in Pediatric Nutrition," *Pediatrics*, 1991, 87(3):339-51.

♦ **Tracleer®** *see* Bosentan *on page 222*

Tramadol (TRA ma dole)

Medication Safety Issues

Sound-alike/look-alike issues:

Tramadol may be confused with Toradol®, Trandate®, Voltaren®

Ultram® may be confused with Ultane®, Voltaren®

International issues:

Theradol® [Netherlands] may be confused with Foradil® which is a brand name for formoterol in the U.S.

Theradol® [Netherlands] may be confused with Terazol® which is a brand name for terconazole in the U.S.

Theradol® [Netherlands] may be confused with Toradol® which is a brand name for ketorolac in the U.S.

U.S. Brand Names Ultram®; Ultram® ER

Canadian Brand Names Ultram®; Zytram® XL

Index Terms Tramadol Hydrochloride

Therapeutic Category Analgesic, Nonopioid

Generic Available Yes: Excludes extended release tablet

Use Relief of moderate to moderately-severe acute or chronic pain, including postoperative, cancer, neuropathic, low back pain, and pain associated with orthopedic disorders

Pregnancy Risk Factor C

Lactation Enters breast milk/contraindicated

Contraindications Hypersensitivity to tramadol, opioids, or any component; opioid-dependent patients; acute intoxication with alcohol, hypnotics, centrally-acting analgesics, opioids, or psychotropic drugs

Tramadol extended release tablets: Patients with severe renal impairment (Cl_{cr} <30 mL/minute) or severe hepatic impairment (Child-Pugh Class C) since the extended release dosage form does not permit dosing flexibility required in this patient population

Warnings Should only be used with **EXTREME** caution in patients receiving MAO inhibitors. Not recommended for use during pregnancy or in nursing mothers. Tolerance or drug dependence may result from extended use (withdrawal symptoms have been reported); abrupt discontinuation should be avoided. Tapering of dose at the time of discontinuation reduces the risk of withdrawal symptoms.

Precautions Use with caution and reduce dosage when administered to patients receiving other CNS depressants (may cause CNS depression and/or respiratory depression when combined with other CNS depressants). Use with caution in patients with a history or with an increased risk of seizures (head trauma, metabolic disorders, CNS infection, malignancy, or drug withdrawal). An increased risk of seizures may occur in patients receiving serotonin reuptake inhibitors (SSRIs) or anorectics, tricyclic antidepressants, cyclobenzaprine, promethazine, neuroleptics, MAO inhibitors, or drugs which lower seizure threshold. Concurrent use of tramadol with SSRIs increases the risk of serotonin syndrome. Use with caution in patients with increased intracranial pressure or head injury. Use with caution and reduce dosage in patients with liver disease, renal impairment, myxedema, hypothyroidism, or hypoadrenalism. Avoid use in patients who are suicidal or addiction prone.

Adverse Reactions

Cardiovascular: Vasodilation, syncope, tachycardia, flushing, chest pain

Central nervous system: Dizziness, headache, somnolence, vertigo, agitation, anxiety, confusion, seizure, emotional lability, euphoria, hallucinations, malaise, nervousness, sleep disorder, amnesia, depression, suicidal tendency, fever

Dermatologic: Pruritus, rash, angioedema, Stevens-Johnson syndrome, toxic epidermal necrolysis

Endocrine & metabolic: Menopausal symptoms

Gastrointestinal: Constipation, nausea, abdominal pain, anorexia, diarrhea, dry mouth, dyspepsia, vomiting, GI bleeding

Genitourinary: Urinary frequency, urinary retention

Hepatic: Liver failure, hepatitis, cholelithiasis

Neuromuscular & skeletal: Tremor, impaired coordination, hypertonia, spasticity, weakness, arthralgia

(Continued)

Tramadol *(Continued)*

Ocular: Miosis, visual disturbance
Renal: Elevated serum creatinine
Respiratory: Bronchospasm, dyspnea, respiratory depression
Miscellaneous: Diaphoresis, anaphylaxis, withdrawal syndrome

Drug Interactions Cytochrome P450 isoenzyme CYP2D6 (major) and 3A4 (minor) substrate

Amphetamines, linezolid, MAO inhibitors, tricyclic antidepressants, and SSRIs may increase risk of seizures; naloxone may increase risk of seizures in tramadol overdose. Neuroleptic agents and opioids may increase risk of seizures and have additive CNS depressant effects. Cimetidine increases the half-life of tramadol by 20% to 25%. Quinidine and other CYP2D6 inhibitors may increase tramadol levels. Alcohol, St John's wort (*Hypericum perforatum*) may increase CNS depression. Tramadol may prolong INR and PT in patients receiving warfarin.

CYP2D6 inhibitors (ie, chlorpromazine, delavirdine, fluoxetine, miconazole, paroxetine, pergolide, quinidine, quinine, ritonavir) may decrease effects of tramadol; carbamazepine may decrease analgesic efficacy of tramadol (half-life decreases 33% to 50%) and may increase risk of seizures in patients requiring anticonvulsants (avoid concurrent use with carbamazepine).

Stability Store tablets at room temperature.

Mechanism of Action Tramadol and its O-desmethyl metabolite bind to μ-opiate receptors in the CNS causing inhibition of ascending pain pathways, altering the perception of and response to pain; inhibits the reuptake of norepinephrine and serotonin which also modifies the ascending pain pathway

Pharmacodynamics Immediate release formulation:
Onset of action: ~1 hour
Maximum effect: 2-4 hours
Duration: 3-6 hours

Pharmacokinetics
Absorption: Rapid and complete
Distribution: Crosses the placenta; distributes to breast milk
V_d: 2.5-3 L/kg
Protein binding: 20%
Metabolism: Primarily hepatic via demethylation, glucuronidation, and sulfation; active metabolite formed by CYP2D6
Bioavailability: Immediate release: 75%; extended release: 85% to 90% as compared to the immediate-release dosage form
Half-life:
Tramadol: ~6-8 hours
Active metabolite: 7-9 hours (prolonged in hepatic or renal impairment)
Time to peak serum concentration: Immediate release: 2 hours; extended release: 12 hours
Elimination: Excreted in urine as unchanged drug (30%) and metabolites (60%)
Dialysis: <7% removed in a 4-hour hemodialysis period

Usual Dosage Oral:
Immediate release formulation:
Children: 1-2 mg/kg/dose every 4-6 hours; maximum: 400 mg/day
Adolescents and Adults: 50-100 mg every 4-6 hours; maximum: 400 mg/day
For patients not requiring rapid onset of effect, tolerability to adverse effects may be improved by initiating therapy at 25 mg/day and titrating dose by 25 mg every 3 days until 25 mg 4 times/day is reached. Dose may then be increased by 50 mg every 3 days as tolerated to reach 50 mg 4 times/day.
Extended release formulation: Adults ≥18 years: 100 mg once daily; titrate by 100 mg increments every 5 days if needed for pain relief; maximum: 300 mg/day

Dosing adjustment in hepatic impairment:
Immediate release formulation: Adults: Cirrhosis: Recommended dose: 50 mg every 12 hours
Extended release formulation: Do not use in patients with severe (Child-Pugh Class C) hepatic impairment

Dosing adjustment in renal impairment:
Immediate release formulation: Adults: Cl_{cr} <30 mL/minute: Administer 50-100 mg dose every 12 hours (maximum: 200 mg/day)
Extended release formulation: Do not use in patients with Cl_{cr} <30 mL/minute

Administration Oral: May administer with or without food, but it is recommended that it be administered in a consistent manner. Do not crush, cut, or chew extended release tablet.

Monitoring Parameters Pain relief, respiratory rate, blood pressure, and pulse; signs of tolerance, oversedation, or withdrawal; renal and hepatic function

Patient Information Avoid alcohol and medications such as sedatives, hypnotics, or other narcotic-containing preparations; may cause drowsiness and impair ability to perform activities requiring mental alertness or physical coordination; may be habit-forming; avoid abrupt discontinuation after prolonged use

Dosage Forms Excipient information presented when available (limited, particularly for generics); consult specific product labeling. [CAN] = Canadian brand name

Tablet, as hydrochloride: 50 mg

Ultram®: 50 mg

Tablet, extended release, as hydrochloride:

Ultram® ER: 100 mg, 200 mg, 300 mg

Zytram® XL [CAN]: 150 mg, 200 mg, 300 mg, 400 mg [not available in the U.S.]

Extemporaneous Preparations A 5 mg/mL oral liquid may be made by crushing six 50 mg tramadol tablets; add 30 mL of Oral-Plus® with 30 mL of strawberry syrup or Ora-Sweet® SF to total volume of 60 mL. Label "shake well before use"; stable for 90 days when stored at 3°C to 5°C or 23°C to 25°C.

Wagner DS, Johnson CE, Cichon-Hensley BK, et al, "Stability of Oral Liquid Preparations of Tramadol in Strawberry Syrup and a Sugar-Free Vehicle," *Am J Health Syst Pharm*, 2003, 60(12):1268-70.

References

Rose JB, Finkel JC, Arquedas-Mohs A, et al, "Oral Tramadol for the Treatment of Pain of 7-30 Days' Duration in Children," *Anesth Analg*, 2003, 96(1):78-81.

♦ **Tramadol Hydrochloride** *see* Tramadol *on page 1561*

♦ **Trandate®** *see* Labetalol *on page 895*

Tranexamic Acid (tran eks AM ik AS id)

Medication Safety Issues

Sound-alike/look-alike issues:

Cyklokapron® may be confused with cycloSPORINE

U.S. Brand Names Cyklokapron®

Canadian Brand Names Cyklokapron®; Tranexamic Acid Injection BP

Index Terms AMCA; CL-65336; transAMCA

Therapeutic Category Antihemophilic Agent

Generic Available No

Use Prevention of excessive bleeding after tonsillectomy; short-term use (2-8 days) in hemophilia patients during and following tooth extraction; primary menorrhagia; prevention of GI hemorrhage and hemorrhage following ocular trauma; recurrent epistaxis; hereditary angioneurotic edema

Pregnancy Risk Factor B

Lactation Enters breast milk/use caution

Contraindications Hypersensitivity to tranexamic acid or any component; subarachnoid hemorrhage; acquired defective color vision, active intravascular clotting process

Warnings Patients receiving therapy for a long duration should have baseline and frequent ophthalmologic exams; do not administer concomitantly with factor IX complex concentrates or anti-inhibitor coagulant concentrates due to increased risk of thrombosis

Precautions Dosage modification required in patients with renal impairment; use with caution in patients with cardiovascular, renal, cerebrovascular disease, or transurethral prostatectomy

Adverse Reactions

Cardiovascular: Hypotension (with rapid I.V. administration), thromboembolic events (eg, deep vein thrombosis, pulmonary embolism, acute cortical necrosis)

Central nervous system: Cerebral ischemia and infarction (when used in the treatment of subarachnoid hemorrhage), headache, hydrocephalus, giddiness

Gastrointestinal: Nausea, diarrhea, vomiting

Hematologic: Thrombocytopenia, coagulation defects, abnormal bleeding times

Ocular: Visual abnormalities (focal areas of retinal degeneration have been seen in animals), central venous stasis retinopathy

Drug Interactions Chlorpromazine

Stability Incompatible with solutions containing penicillin; compatible with dextrose, saline, and electrolyte solutions

Mechanism of Action Forms a reversible complex that displaces plasminogen from fibrin resulting in inhibition of fibrinolysis; it also inhibits the proteolytic activity of plasmin

Pharmacokinetics

Distribution: Breast milk levels are 1% of serum; CSF levels are 10% of plasma

V_d: Adults: 9-12 L

Protein binding: 3%

Bioavailability:

Oral: 33% to 35%

I.M.: 100%

(Continued)

Tranexamic Acid *(Continued)*

Half-life: 2 hours
Time to peak serum concentration:
Oral: 3 hours
I.M.: 1 hour
I.V.: 5 minutes
Elimination: Elimination characteristics differ by route of administration: after I.V. administration 95% excreted as unchanged drug in urine vs 39% after oral administration

Usual Dosage Dental extraction in hemophiliacs: Children and Adults: 10 mg/kg I.V. immediately before surgery, then 25 mg/kg/dose orally 3-4 times/day for 2-8 days

Alternatives:
I.V.: 10 mg/kg/dose 3-4 times/day (if unable to take orally)
Oral: 25 mg/kg/dose 3-4 times/day beginning 1 day prior to surgery
Menorrhagia: Oral: Adolescents and Adults: 1-1.5 g (12-25 mg/kg/dose) 3-4 times daily for 3-4 days
Adults: Oral:
Epistaxis: 1.5 g 3 times/day
Ocular trauma: 1 g 3 times/day
Dosing adjustment in renal impairment: Adults: See table.

Tranxemic Acid Dosage Adjustments in Renal Impairment (Adult Data)

Serum Creatinine (mg/dL)	I.V. dose	Oral dose
1.36-2.83	10 mg/kg twice daily	15 mg/kg twice daily
>2.83-5.66	10 mg/kg once daily	15 mg/kg once daily
>5.66	10 mg/kg every 48 h or 5 mg/kg every 24 h	15 mg/kg every 48 h or 7.5 mg/kg every 24 h

Administration
Parenteral: May be administered by direct I.V. injection at a maximum rate of 100 mg/minute (1 mL/minute)
Oral: May be administered with food

Monitoring Parameters Ophthalmologic exams (baseline and at regular intervals) of chronic therapy

Reference Range 5-10 mcg/mL is required to decrease fibrinolysis

Additional Information Tablets available in U.S. only for individual patients by contacting manufacturer (Pharmacia) directly.

Dosage Forms Excipient information presented when available (limited, particularly for generics); consult specific product labeling.
Injection, solution: 100 mg/mL (10 mL)
Tablet: 500 mg [Not marketed in U.S.; available from manufacturer for select cases]

- **Tranexamic Acid Injection BP (Can)** *see* Tranexamic Acid *on page 1563*
- **transAMCA** *see* Tranexamic Acid *on page 1563*
- **Transderm-V® (Can)** *see* Scopolamine *on page 1421*
- **Transderm-Nitro® (Can)** *see* Nitroglycerin *on page 1141*
- **Transderm Scōp®** *see* Scopolamine *on page 1421*
- **Trans-Plantar® (Can)** *see* Salicylic Acid *on page 1413*
- ***trans*-Retinoic Acid** *see* Tretinoin *on page 1567*
- **Trans-Ver-Sal® [OTC]** *see* Salicylic Acid *on page 1413*
- **Trans-Ver-Sal® (Can)** *see* Salicylic Acid *on page 1413*
- **Tranxene® SD™** *see* Clorazepate *on page 391*
- **Tranxene® SD™-Half Strength** *see* Clorazepate *on page 391*
- **Tranxene T-Tab®** *see* Clorazepate *on page 391*
- **Tranxene® T-Tab®** *see* Clorazepate *on page 391*
- **Trasylol®** *see* Aprotinin *on page 155*

Trazodone (TRAZ oh done)

Medication Safety Issues
Sound-alike/look-alike issues:
Desyrel® may be confused with Demerol®, Delsym®, Zestril®

International issues:

Desyrel® may be confused with Deseril® which is a brand name for methysergide in multiple international markets

Related Information

Antidepressant Agents *on page 1681*

Serotonin Syndrome *on page 1955*

U.S. Brand Names Desyrel® [DSC]

Canadian Brand Names Alti-Trazodone; Apo-Trazodone®; Apo-Trazodone D®; Desyrel®; Gen-Trazodone; Novo-Trazodone; Nu-Trazodone; PMS-Trazodone; ratio-Trazodone; Trazorel®

Index Terms Trazodone Hydrochloride

Therapeutic Category Antidepressant

Generic Available Yes

Use Treatment of depression

Medication Guide An FDA-approved patient medication guide, which is available with the product information and at http://www.fda.gov/cder/Offices/ODS/medication_guides.htm, must be dispensed with this medication for each new outpatient prescription and refill.

Pregnancy Risk Factor C

Lactation Enters breast milk/use caution (AAP rates "of concern")

Contraindications Hypersensitivity to trazodone or any component

Warnings Trazodone is not approved for use in pediatric patients. Clinical worsening of depression or suicidal ideation and behavior may occur in children and adults with major depressive disorder. In clinical trials, antidepressants increased the risk of suicidal thinking and behavior (suicidality) in children, adolescents, and young adults (18-24 years of age) with major depressive disorder and other psychiatric disorders. This risk must be considered before prescribing antidepressants for any clinical use. Short-term studies did **not** show an increased risk of suicidality with antidepressant use in patients >24 years of age and showed a decreased risk in patients ≥65 years.

Patients of all ages who are treated with antidepressants for any indication require appropriate monitoring and close observation for clinical worsening of depression, suicidality, and unusual changes in behavior, especially during the first few months after antidepressant initiation or when the dose is adjusted. Family members and caregivers should be instructed to closely observe the patient (ie, daily) and communicate condition with healthcare provider. Patients should also be monitored for associated behaviors (eg, anxiety, agitation, panic attacks, insomnia, irritability, hostility, aggressiveness, impulsivity, akathisia, hypomania, mania) which may increase the risk for worsening depression or suicidality. Worsening depression or emergence of suicidality (or associated behaviors listed above) that is abrupt in onset, severe, or not part of the presenting symptoms, may require discontinuation or modification of drug therapy.

To reduce risk of intentional overdose, write prescriptions for the smallest quantity consistent with good patient care. Screen individuals for bipolar disorder prior to treatment (using antidepressants alone may induce manic episodes in patients with this condition).

Monitor closely and use with extreme caution in patients with cardiac disease or arrhythmias; not recommended for use during post-MI initial recovery phase. Trazodone may cause prolonged priapism requiring surgical intervention; discontinue use immediately if prolonged or inappropriate erections occur.

Precautions Hypotension and syncope may occur; use with caution in patients receiving antihypertensive agents. Discontinue use prior to elective surgery (unknown interactions with general anesthetics may exist).

Adverse Reactions Possesses fewer anticholinergic and cardiac adverse effects than tricyclic antidepressants

Cardiovascular: Postural hypotension (5%), arrhythmias, syncope

Central nervous system: Drowsiness (20% to 50%), sedation, dizziness, insomnia, confusion, agitation, seizures, extrapyramidal reactions, headache; suicidal thinking and behavior (see Warnings)

Gastrointestinal: Xerostomia, constipation, nausea, vomiting

Genitourinary: Prolonged priapism (1:6000), urinary retention (rare)

Hepatic: Hepatitis

Neuromuscular & skeletal: Weakness

Ocular: Blurred vision (15% to 30%)

Drug Interactions Cytochrome P450 isoenzyme CYP2D6 (minor) and CYP3A3/4 (major) substrate

May enhance the adverse effects of antihypertensive agents (eg, hypotension, syncope); may antagonize the antihypertensive effects of clonidine and methyldopa; may increase the serum concentrations of phenytoin or digoxin; effects may

(Continued)

Trazodone *(Continued)*

be additive with other CNS depressants, alcohol; fluoxetine may increase trazodone serum concentrations; interaction with MAO inhibitors may occur (eg, precipitation of serotonin syndrome) (use with extreme caution in patients with concurrent or recent MAO inhibitor therapy)

Potent CYP3A4 inhibitors (eg, ritonavir, indinavir, ketoconazole, itraconazole, nefazodone) may significantly increase trazodone serum concentrations and the potential for adverse effects (eg, nausea, hypotension, and syncope) (consider trazodone dosage decrease); CYP3A4 enzyme inducers (eg, carbamazepine) may significantly decrease trazodone serum concentrations (monitor patients closely; consider trazodone dosage increase)

Food Interactions Food may decrease the rate but increase the extent of absorption

Stability Store tablets at room temperature; avoid temperatures >104°F (40°C); dispense in tight, light-resistant container

Mechanism of Action Inhibits reuptake of serotonin; minimal or no effect on reuptake of norepinephrine or dopamine; possesses little if any anticholinergic effects; alpha-adrenergic blockade thought to be responsible for orthostatic hypotension and dry mouth

Pharmacodynamics Maximum antidepressant effect: 2-4 weeks

Pharmacokinetics

Protein binding: 85% to 95%

Metabolism: In the liver via hydroxylation and oxidation; metabolized by cytochrome P450 isoenzyme CYP3A4 to active metabolite, m-chlorophenylpiperazine (mCPP)

Half-life, elimination: 5-9 hours, prolonged in obese patients

Time to peak serum concentration:

Administration on empty stomach: 1 hour

Administration with food: 2 hours

Elimination: Primarily in urine (74%) with ~21% excreted in feces

Usual Dosage Oral: **Note:** Not FDA approved for the treatment of depression in pediatric patients (see Warnings)

Children 6-18 years: Initial: 1.5-2 mg/kg/day in divided doses; increase gradually every 3-4 days as needed; maximum dose: 6 mg/kg/day in 3 divided doses

Adolescents: Initial: 25-50 mg/day; increase to 100-150 mg/day in divided doses

Adults: Initial: 150 mg/day in 3 divided doses (may increase by 50 mg/day every 3-7 days); maximum dose: 600 mg/day

Administration Oral: Administer after meals or a snack to decrease lightheadedness, sedation, and postural hypotension

Monitoring Parameters Blood pressure, mental status, liver enzymes. Monitor patient periodically for symptom resolution; monitor for worsening depression, suicidality, and associated behaviors (especially at the beginning of therapy or when doses are increased or decreased; see Warnings).

Reference Range

Therapeutic: 0.5-2.5 mcg/mL (SI: 1-6 micromoles/L)

Potentially toxic: >2.5 mcg/mL (SI: >6 micromoles/L)

Toxic: >4 mcg/mL (SI: >10 micromoles/L)

Patient Information Read the patient Medication Guide that you receive with each prescription and refill of trazodone. An increased risk of suicidal thinking and behavior has been reported with the use of antidepressants in children, adolescents, and young adults (18-24 years of age). Notify physician if you feel more depressed, have thoughts of suicide, or become more agitated or irritable (see Warnings). Avoid alcohol; may cause drowsiness and impair ability to perform activities requiring mental alertness or physical coordination; may cause dry mouth; discontinue use and consult physician immediately if prolonged or inappropriate erections occur

Additional Information Mean doses of ~5 mg/kg/day were used in 22 children 5-12 years of age to treat severe behavioral disorders (Zubieta, 1992). Doses of 1 mg/kg/day given in 3 divided doses were used for migraine prophylaxis in 40 patients 7-18 years of age (Battistella, 1993). Further studies are needed before trazodone can be recommended in children for these indications.

Dosage Forms Excipient information presented when available (limited, particularly for generics); consult specific product labeling. [DSC] = Discontinued product

Tablet: 50 mg, 100 mg, 150 mg, 300 mg

Desyrel®: 50 mg, 100 mg, 150 mg, 300 mg [DSC]

References

Battistella PA, Ruffilli R, Cernetti R, et al, "A Placebo-Controlled Crossover Trial Using Trazodone in Pediatric Migraine," *Headache*, 1993, 33(1):36-9.

Zubieta JK and Alessi NE, "Acute and Chronic Administration of Trazodone in the Treatment of Disruptive Behavior Disorders in Children," *J Clin Psychopharmacol*, 1992, 12(5):346-51.

- **Trazodone Hydrochloride** *see* Trazodone *on page 1564*
- **Trazorel® (Can)** *see* Trazodone *on page 1564*
- **Trecator®** *see* Ethionamide *on page 617*

♦ **Trental®** *see* Pentoxifylline *on page 1241*

Tretinoin (TRET i noyn)

Medication Safety Issues
Sound-alike/look-alike issues:
Tretinoin may be confused with trientine
International issues:
Renova® may be confused with Remov® which is a brand name for nimesulide in Italy

U.S. Brand Names Avita®; Renova®; Retin-A®; Retin-A® Micro

Canadian Brand Names Rejuva-A®; Retin-A®; Retin-A® Micro; Retinova®

Index Terms Retinoic Acid; *trans*-Retinoic Acid; Vitamin A Acid

Therapeutic Category Acne Products; Retinoic Acid Derivative; Vitamin, Topical

Generic Available Yes: Cream, gel

Use Treatment of acne vulgaris, photodamaged skin, and some skin cancers

Pregnancy Risk Factor C

Lactation Enters breast milk/compatible

Contraindications Hypersensitivity to tretinoin or any component; sunburn

Warnings Avoid contact with abraded skin, mucous membranes, eyes, mouth, angles of the nose; avoid excessive exposure to sunlight or sunlamps

Precautions Use with caution in patients with eczema

Adverse Reactions
Cardiovascular: Edema
Dermatologic: Excessive dryness, erythema, scaling of the skin, hyperpigmentation or hypopigmentation, photosensitivity, initial acne flare-up
Local: Stinging, blistering

Drug Interactions Sulfur, benzoyl peroxide, salicylic acid, and resorcinol potentiate adverse reactions seen with tretinoin

Food Interactions Avoid excessive intake of vitamin A

Mechanism of Action Keratinocytes in the sebaceous follicle become less adherent which allows for easy removal; inhibits microcomedone formation and eliminates lesions already present

Pharmacodynamics
Onset of action: 2-3 weeks
Maximum effect: May require 6 weeks or longer

Pharmacokinetics
Absorption: Topical: Minimum absorption
Metabolism: In the liver
Elimination: In bile and urine

Usual Dosage Children >12 years and Adults: Topical: Begin therapy with a weaker formulation of tretinoin (0.025% cream or 0.01% gel) and increase the concentration as tolerated; apply once daily before retiring or on alternate days; if stinging or irritation develop, decrease frequency of application

Administration Topical: Apply to dry skin (wait at least 15-30 minutes to apply after cleansing); avoid contact with eyes, mucous membranes, mouth, or open wounds

Patient Information May cause photosensitivity reactions (eg, exposure to sunlight may cause severe sunburn, skin rash, redness, or itching); avoid exposure to sunlight and artificial light sources (sunlamps, tanning booth/bed); wear protective clothing, wide-brimmed hats, sunglasses, and lip sunscreen (SPF ≥15); use a sunscreen [broad-spectrum sunscreen or physical sunscreen (preferred) or sunblock with SPF ≥15]; contact physician if reaction occurs. Avoid washing face more frequently than 2-3 times/day; avoid using topical preparations with high alcoholic content during treatment period.

Additional Information Liquid preparation generally is more irritating

Dosage Forms [DSC] = Discontinued product
Cream, topical: 0.025% (20 g, 45 g); 0.05% (20 g, 45 g); 0.1% (20 g, 45 g)
Avita®: 0.025% (20 g, 45 g)
Renova®: 0.02% (40 g); 0.05% (40 g, 60 g) [DSC]
Retin-A®: 0.025% (20 g, 45 g); 0.05% (20 g, 45 g); 0.1% (20 g, 45 g)
Gel, topical: 0.025% (15 g, 45 g)
Avita®: 0.025% (20 g, 45 g) [contains ethanol 83%]
Retin-A®: 0.01% (15 g, 45 g); 0.025% (15 g, 45 g) [contains alcohol 90%]
Retin-A® Micro [microsphere gel]: 0.04% (20 g, 45 g); 0.1% (20 g, 45 g) [contains benzyl alcohol]
Liquid, topical (Retin-A®): 0.05% (28 mL) [contains alcohol 55%] [DSC]

References
Winston MH, Shalita AR, "Acne Vulgaris, Pathogenesis and Treatment," *Pediatr Clin North Am*, 1991, 38(4):889-903.

♦ **Trexall™** *see* Methotrexate *on page 1027*
♦ **TRH** *see* Protirelin *on page 1343*
♦ **Triaderm (Can)** *see* Triamcinolone *on page 1568*

Triamcinolone (trye am SIN oh lone)

Medication Safety Issues
Sound-alike/look-alike issues:
Kenalog® may be confused with Ketalar®
Nasacort® may be confused with NasalCrom®

TAC (occasional abbreviation for triamcinolone) is an error-prone abbreviation (mistaken as tetracaine-adrenaline-cocaine)

Related Information
Asthma *on page 1904*
Corticosteroids, Topical: Guidelines for Selection and Use *on page 1686*

U.S. Brand Names Aristocort® [DSC]; Aristocort® A [DSC]; Aristospan®; Azmacort®; Kenalog®; Kenalog-10®; Kenalog-40®; Nasacort® AQ; Triderm®; Tri-Nasal®

Canadian Brand Names Aristospan®; Kenalog®; Kenalog® in Orabase; Nasacort® AQ; Oracort; Triaderm; Trinasal®

Index Terms Triamcinolone Acetonide, Aerosol; Triamcinolone Acetonide, Parenteral; Triamcinolone Diacetate, Oral; Triamcinolone Diacetate, Parenteral; Triamcinolone Hexacetonide; Triamcinolone, Oral

Therapeutic Category Adrenal Corticosteroid; Anti-inflammatory Agent; Antiasthmatic; Corticosteroid, Inhalant (Oral); Corticosteroid, Intranasal; Corticosteroid, Systemic; Corticosteroid, Topical; Glucocorticoid

Generic Available Yes: Cream, lotion, ointment, paste

Use
Oral inhalation: Long-term (chronic) control of persistent bronchial asthma; **NOT** indicated for the relief of acute bronchospasm. Also used to help reduce or discontinue oral corticosteroid therapy for asthma.
Intralesional (injectable suspension): Alopecia areata; discoid lupus erythematosus; infiltrated, inflammatory lesions associated with granuloma annulare, lichen planus, neurodermatitis, and psoriatic plaques; keloids; necrobiosis lipoidica diabeticorum; possibly helpful in cystic tumors of an aponeurosis or tendon (ganglia)
Intranasal: Management of seasonal and perennial allergic rhinitis
Systemic: Immunosuppression; relief of severe inflammation
Topical: Relief of inflammation and pruritus associated with corticosteroid-responsive dermatoses
Topical (dental paste): Adjunctive treatment and temporary relief of symptoms related to oral inflammatory lesions and ulcerative lesions due to trauma

Pregnancy Risk Factor C

Lactation Excretion in breast milk unknown/use caution

Contraindications Hypersensitivity to triamcinolone or any component (see Warnings); primary treatment of status asthmaticus; systemic fungal infections; serious infections (except septic shock or tuberculous meningitis). Topical: Contraindicated with local fungal, viral, or bacterial infections. I.M.: Contraindicated with idiopathic thrombocytopenic purpura

Warnings Fatalities have occurred due to adrenal insufficiency in asthmatic patients during and after switching from systemic corticosteroids to aerosol steroids; several months may be required for full recovery of hypothalamic-pituitary-adrenal (HPA) function; patients receiving higher doses of systemic corticosteroids (eg, adults receiving ≥20 mg of prednisone per day) may be at greater risk; during this period of HPA suppression, aerosol steroids do **not** provide the systemic glucocorticoid or mineralocorticoid activity needed to treat patients requiring stress doses (ie, patients with major stress such as trauma, surgery, infections, or other conditions associated with severe electrolyte loss). When used at high doses or for a prolonged time, hypocorticism and HPA suppression (including adrenal crisis) may occur; use with inhaled or systemic corticosteroids (even alternate-day dosing) may increase risk of HPA suppression; withdrawal and discontinuation of corticosteroids should be done carefully; patients with HPA axis suppression may require doses of systemic glucocorticosteroids prior to, during, and after unusual stress (eg, surgery). Immunosuppression may occur; patients may be more susceptible to infections; avoid exposure to chickenpox and measles. Switching patients from systemic corticosteroids to aerosol steroids may unmask allergic conditions previously treated by the systemic steroid. Bronchospasm may occur after use of inhaled asthma medications (see Additional Information).

Injection contains and cream may contain benzyl alcohol which may cause allergic reactions in susceptible individuals; large amounts of benzyl alcohol (≥99 mg/kg/day) have been associated with a potentially fatal toxicity ("gasping syndrome") in neonates; the "gasping syndrome" consists of metabolic acidosis, respiratory distress, gasping respirations, CNS dysfunction (including convulsions, intracranial hemorrhage), hypotension and cardiovascular collapse; avoid use of triamcinolone products containing benzyl alcohol or sodium benzoate in neonates; *in vitro* and animal studies have shown that benzoate displaces bilirubin from protein binding sites

Precautions Avoid using higher than recommended doses; suppression of HPA axis function, suppression of linear growth (ie, reduction of growth velocity), reduced bone mineral density, hypercorticism (Cushing's syndrome), hyperglycemia, or glucosuria may occur; titrate to lowest effective dose. Use with extreme caution in patients with respiratory tuberculosis, untreated systemic infections, or ocular herpes simplex. Use with caution in patients with thyroid dysfunction, peptic ulcer disease, osteoporosis, myasthenia gravis, hypertension, CHF, nonspecific ulcerative colitis, thromboembolic disorders, renal dysfunction, recent MI (left ventricular free wall rupture has been reported).

Adverse Reactions

Cardiovascular: Edema, hypertension, CHF

Central nervous system: Fatigue, dizziness, malaise, insomnia, depression, euphoria

Dermatologic: Itching, hypertrichosis, skin atrophy, hyperpigmentation, hypopigmentation, acne

Endocrine & metabolic: HPA suppression, Cushing's syndrome, growth suppression, sodium and water retention, glucose intolerance, hypokalemia

Gastrointestinal: Oral candidiasis, dry throat, xerostomia, peptic ulcer, nausea, vomiting

Local: Burning, sterile abscesses

Neuromuscular & skeletal: Muscle weakness, osteoporosis, decreased bone mineral density

Ocular: Cataracts, elevated IOP, glaucoma

Respiratory: Hoarseness, wheezing, cough; anaphylactoid reactions (rare)

Drug Interactions Cytochrome P450 isoenzyme CYP3A3/4 inducer

Barbiturates, phenytoin, rifampin increase the metabolism of triamcinolone; salicylates; NSAIDs, caffeine and alcohol may increase risk of GI ulcer; live virus vaccines (increase risk of viral infection); vaccines may have decreased effects

Food Interactions Systemic use of corticosteroids may require a diet with increased potassium, vitamins A, B_6, C, D, folate, calcium, zinc, and phosphorus and decreased sodium

Mechanism of Action Controls the rate of protein synthesis, depresses the migration of polymorphonuclear leukocytes and fibroblasts, reverses capillary permeability, and stabilizes lysosomal membranes at the cellular level to prevent or control inflammation

Pharmacokinetics

Half-life: 88 minutes

Time to peak serum concentration: I.M.: Within 8-10 hours

Usual Dosage

I.M. (as acetonide or hexacetonide): Children: 6-12 years: 0.03-0.2 mg/kg at 1- to 7-day intervals

Intra-articular (as hexacetonide): Children >12 years and Adults: 2-20 mg every 3-4 weeks

Intra-articular, intrabursal, or tendon-sheath injection: Children: 6-12 years: 2.5-15 mg, repeat as needed

Intra-articular, intrasynovial, intralesional (as acetonide): Children >12 years and Adults: 2.5-40 mg, repeat as needed when signs and symptoms recur

Intralesional, sublesional (as acetonide): Children >12 years and Adults: Up to 1 mg per injection site and may be repeated 1 or more times weekly; multiple sites may be injected if they are 1 cm or more apart, not to exceed 30 mg

Intranasal:

Nasacort® AQ: Children >12 years and Adults: Initial: 2 sprays in each nostril once daily; titrate to lowest effective dose once symptoms are controlled; usual maintenance dose: 1 spray in each nostril once daily

Tri-Nasal®: Children >12 years and Adults: Initial: 2 sprays in each nostril once daily; may increase to maximum dose of 4 sprays in each nostril once daily or 2 sprays in each nostril twice daily; may initiate at maximum doses if faster relief of symptoms is required; titrate to lowest effective dose once symptoms are controlled

Oral: Children >12 years and Adults: 4-100 mg/day in 1-4 divided doses

Oral inhalation: Doses should be titrated to the lowest effective dose once asthma is controlled; maintenance doses may be given twice daily. Manufacturer recommendation:

Children: 6-12 years: 1-2 puffs given 3-4 times/day; maximum dose: 12 puffs/day

Children >12 years and Adults: 2 puffs given 3-4 times/day; for severe asthma: 12-16 puffs/day divided into 3-4 doses/day; maximum dose: 16 puffs/day

(Continued)

Triamcinolone *(Continued)*

NIH Asthma Guidelines (NAEPP, 2002; NIH, 1997) [give in divided doses 3-4 times/day]:
Children ≤12 years:
"Low" dose: 400-800 mcg/day (4-8 puffs/day)
"Medium" dose: 800-1200 mcg/day (8-12 puffs/day)
"High" dose: >1200 mcg/day (>12 puffs/day)
Children >12 years and Adults:
"Low" dose: 400-1000 mcg/day (4-10 puffs/day)
"Medium" dose: 1000-2000 mcg/day (10-20 puffs/day)
"High" dose: >2000 mcg/day (>20 puffs/day)

Topical: Children and Adults: Apply a thin film 2-3 times/day

Topical (dental): Adults: Press a small amount (~1/4 inch) to the lesion until a thin film develops; some lesions may require a larger quantity; apply once daily at bedtime; more severe lesions may require application 2-3 times/day (preferably after meals)

Administration

Oral: May administer with meals to decrease GI upset

Oral inhalant: Shake canister well before use; use a spacer device for children <8 years of age; do not spray in eyes

Intranasal: Shake container well before use; clear nasal passages by blowing nose prior to use; do not spray in eyes

Parenteral: Avoid SubQ use; **do not inject I.V.**; acetonide or hexacetonide may be administered I.M.; see Usual Dosage for other parenteral routes of administration

Topical: Apply sparingly to affected area, gently rub in until disappears; avoid application on face; do not occlude area unless directed; do not use on open skin; avoid contact with eyes

Topical (dental): Apply sparingly; do not rub in; spreading the paste may result in a granular, gritty sensation and crumbling; apply at bedtime to allow contact of the medication with the lesion overnight.

Monitoring Parameters Oral inhalation: Check mucus membranes for signs of fungal infection; monitor growth in pediatric patients. Assess HPA suppression in patients using potent topical steroids applied to a large surface area or to areas under occlusion. Monitor IOP with therapy >6 weeks. Monitor blood pressure and for clinical presence of adverse effects.

Patient Information Notify physician if condition being treated persists or worsens; do not decrease dose or discontinue without physician approval; avoid exposure to chicken pox or measles, if exposed seek medical advice without delay; may cause dry mouth; avoid alcohol

Oral inhalant: Rinse mouth with water without swallowing to decrease chance of oral candidiasis; report sore mouth or mouth lesions to physician

Nursing Implications Once daily oral doses should be given in the morning

Additional Information Oral inhalation: If bronchospasm with wheezing occurs after use, a fast-acting bronchodilator may be used; discontinue orally inhaled corticosteroid and initiate alternative chronic therapy.

Dosage Forms Excipient information presented when available (limited, particularly for generics); consult specific product labeling. [DSC] = Discontinued product

Aerosol for oral inhalation, as acetonide:
Azmacort®: 100 mcg per actuation (20 g) [240 actuations]

Aerosol, topical, as acetonide:
Kenalog®: 0.2 mg/2-second spray (63 g)

Cream, as acetonide: 0.025% (15 g, 80 g, 454 g); 0.1% (15 g, 80 g, 454 g, 2270 g); 0.5% (15 g)
Aristocort® A: 0.025% (15 g, 60 g); 0.1% (15 g, 60 g); 0.5% (15 g) [DSC]
Triderm®: 0.1% (30 g, 85 g)

Injection, suspension, as acetonide:
Kenalog-10®: 10 mg/mL (5 mL) [contains benzyl alcohol; not for I.V. or I.M. use]
Kenalog-40®: 40 mg/mL (1 mL, 5 mL, 10 mL) [contains benzyl alcohol; not for I.V. or intradermal use]

Injection, suspension, as hexacetonide:
Aristospan®: 5 mg/mL (5 mL); 20 mg/mL (1 mL, 5 mL) [contains benzyl alcohol; not for I.V. use]

Lotion, as acetonide: 0.025% (60 mL); 0.1% (60 mL)

Ointment, topical, as acetonide: 0.025% (15 g, 80 g, 454 g); 0.1% (15 g, 80 g, 454 g); 0.5% (15 g)
Aristocort® A: 0.1% (15 g, 60 g) [DSC]

Paste, oral, topical, as acetonide: 0.1% (5 g)

Solution, intranasal, as acetonide [spray]:
Tri-Nasal®: 50 mcg/inhalation (15 mL) [120 actuations]

Suspension, intranasal, as acetonide [spray]:
Nasacort® AQ: 55 mcg/inhalation (16.5 g) [120 actuations]

Tablet:
Aristocort®: 4 mg [DSC]

References

Expert Panel Report 2, "Guidelines for the Diagnosis and Management of Asthma," *Clinical Practice Guidelines*, National Institutes of Health, National Heart, Lung, and Blood Institute, NIH Publication No. 94-4051, April, 1997.
"National Asthma Education and Prevention Program. Expert Panel Report: Guidelines for the Diagnosis and Management of Asthma Update on Selected Topics--2002," *J Allergy Clin Immunol*, 2002, 110(5 Suppl):S141-219.

♦ **Triamcinolone Acetonide, Aerosol** *see* Triamcinolone *on page 1568*
♦ **Triamcinolone Acetonide, Parenteral** *see* Triamcinolone *on page 1568*
♦ **Triamcinolone Diacetate, Oral** *see* Triamcinolone *on page 1568*
♦ **Triamcinolone Diacetate, Parenteral** *see* Triamcinolone *on page 1568*
♦ **Triamcinolone Hexacetonide** *see* Triamcinolone *on page 1568*
♦ **Triamcinolone, Oral** *see* Triamcinolone *on page 1568*
♦ **Triaminic® Allerchews™ [OTC]** *see* Loratadine *on page 959*
♦ **Triaminic® Thin Strips™ Cough and Runny Nose [OTC]** *see* DiphenhydrAMINE *on page 509*
♦ **Triaminic® Thin Strips™ Long Acting Cough [OTC]** *see* Dextromethorphan *on page 477*

Triamterene (trye AM ter een)

Medication Safety Issues
Sound-alike/look-alike issues:
Triamterene may be confused with trimipramine
Dyrenium® may be confused with Pyridium®

Related Information
Antihypertensive Agents by Class *on page 1670*

U.S. Brand Names Dyrenium®

Therapeutic Category Antihypertensive Agent; Diuretic, Potassium Sparing

Generic Available No

Use Used alone or in combination with other diuretics to treat edema and hypertension; decreases potassium excretion caused by kaliuretic diuretics

Pregnancy Risk Factor B

Lactation Excretion in breast milk unknown

Contraindications Hypersensitivity to triamterene or any component; severe renal or hepatic impairment, hyperkalemia

Precautions Use with caution in patients with impaired hepatic or renal function, history of renal calculi, diabetes mellitus; patients receiving other potassium-sparing diuretics or potassium supplements

Adverse Reactions
Cardiovascular: Hypotension
Central nervous system: Dizziness, headache
Endocrine & metabolic: Hyperkalemia, hyponatremia, hypomagnesemia, hyperchloremia, hyperuricemia, metabolic acidosis
Dermatologic: Photosensitivity
Gastrointestinal: Nausea, vomiting, diarrhea, xerostomia
Genitourinary: Slight alkalinization of urine
Hematologic: Blood dyscrasias, thrombocytopenia, megaloblastic anemia
Hepatic: Abnormal liver function
Neuromuscular & skeletal: Muscle cramps, weakness
Renal: Prerenal azotemia, nephrolithiasis (rare), reversible acute renal failure
Miscellaneous: Allergic reactions have been reported

Drug Interactions Increased risk of hyperkalemia if given together with other potassium-sparing diuretics (ie, spironolactone); may increase risk of hyperkalemia with ACE inhibitors, (ie, captopril, enalapril); concomitant administration of triamterene and indomethacin may increase nephrotoxicity; increased risk of hyperkalemia with potassium-containing preparations; may increase lithium toxicity by decreasing lithium clearance; may increase amantadine toxicity possibly by decreasing its renal excretion

Food Interactions Avoid salt substitutes and diets with increased potassium

Mechanism of Action Interferes with potassium/sodium exchange (active transport) in the distal tubule, cortical collecting tubule and collecting duct by inhibiting sodium, potassium-ATPase; decreases calcium excretion; increases magnesium loss

Pharmacodynamics
Onset of action: Diuresis occurs within 2-4 hours
Duration: 7-9 hours
Note: Maximum therapeutic effect may not occur until after several days of therapy

(Continued)

Triamterene *(Continued)*

Pharmacokinetics

Absorption: Oral: Unreliably absorbed
Metabolism: Hepatic conjugation
Half-life: 100-150 minutes
Elimination: 21% excreted unchanged in urine

Usual Dosage Oral:

Children: 1-2 mg/kg/day in 1-2 divided doses; maximum dose: 3-4 mg/kg/day and not to exceed 300 mg/day

Adults: 100-300 mg/day in 1-2 divided doses; usual dosage range (JNC 7): 50-100 mg/day

Dosage adjustment in renal impairment: Cl_{cr} <10 mL/minute: Avoid use

Dosage adjustment in hepatic impairment: Dose reduction is recommended in patients with cirrhosis

Administration Oral: Administer with food to avoid GI upset

Monitoring Parameters Electrolytes (sodium, potassium, magnesium, HCO_3, chloride), CBC, BUN, creatinine, platelets

Test Interactions Interferes with fluorometric assay of quinidine

Patient Information May cause dry mouth. May cause photosensitivity reactions (eg, exposure to sunlight may cause severe sunburn, skin rash, redness, or itching); avoid exposure to sunlight and artificial light sources (sunlamps, tanning booth/bed); wear protective clothing, wide-brimmed hats, sunglasses, and lip sunscreen (SPF ≥15); use a sunscreen [broad-spectrum sunscreen or physical sunscreen (preferred) or sunblock with SPF ≥15]; contact physician if reaction occurs.

Additional Information Abrupt discontinuation of therapy may result in rebound kaliuresis; taper off gradually

Dosage Forms Excipient information presented when available (limited, particularly for generics); consult specific product labeling.

Capsule: 50 mg, 100 mg [contains benzyl alcohol]

References

Chobanian AV, Bakris GL, Black HR, et al, "The Seventh Report of the Joint National Committee on Prevention, Detection, Evaluation, and Treatment of High Blood Pressure: The JNC 7 Report.," *JAMA*, 2003, 289(19):2560-72.

National High Blood Pressure Education Program Working Group on High Blood Pressure in Children and Adolescents, "The Fourth Report on the Diagnosis, Evaluation, and Treatment of High Blood Pressure in Children and Adolescents," *Pediatrics*, 2004, 114(2 Suppl):555-76.

van der Vorst MM, Kist JE, van der Heijden AJ, et al, "Diuretics in Pediatrics: Current Knowledge and Future Prospects," *Paediatr Drugs*, 2006, 8(4):245-64.

◆ **Triatec-8 (Can)** *see* Acetaminophen and Codeine *on page 46*
◆ **Triatec-8 Strong (Can)** *see* Acetaminophen and Codeine *on page 46*
◆ **Triatec-30 (Can)** *see* Acetaminophen and Codeine *on page 46*
◆ **Triaz®** *see* Benzoyl Peroxide *on page 207*
◆ **Triaz® Cleanser** *see* Benzoyl Peroxide *on page 207*

Triazolam (trye AY zoe lam)

Medication Safety Issues

Sound-alike/look-alike issues:
Triazolam may be confused with alprazolam
Halcion® may be confused with halcinonide, Haldol®

Related Information

Overdose and Toxicology *on page 1916*

U.S. Brand Names Halcion® [DSC]

Canadian Brand Names Apo-Triazo®; Gen-Triazolam; Halcion®

Therapeutic Category Benzodiazepine; Hypnotic; Sedative

Generic Available Yes

Use Short-term treatment of insomnia

Restrictions C-IV

Pregnancy Risk Factor X

Lactation Excretion in breast milk unknown/not recommended

Contraindications Hypersensitivity to triazolam or any component; cross-sensitivity with other benzodiazepines may occur; severe uncontrolled pain; pre-existing CNS depression; narrow-angle glaucoma; pregnancy; concomitant use with ketoconazole, itraconazole, or nefazodone (see Drug Interactions)

Warnings Evaluate patient carefully for medical or psychiatric causes of insomnia prior to initiation of drug treatment; failure of triazolam to treat insomnia (after 7-10 days of therapy), a worsening of insomnia, or the emergence of behavioral changes or thinking abnormalities, may indicate a medical or psychiatric illness requiring evaluation; these effects also have been reported with triazolam use. Due to possible adverse effects, use lowest effective dose. Abrupt discontinuation after prolonged use may result in withdrawal symptoms or rebound insomnia. Triazolam is a substrate of cytochrome P450 isoenzyme CYP3A4; serious drug interactions may occur (see Drug Interactions).

Hypersensitivity reactions including anaphylaxis and angioedema may occur. Hazardous sleep-related activities, such as sleep-driving (driving while not fully awake without any recollection of driving), preparing and eating food, and making phone calls while asleep have also been reported. Effects with other sedative drugs or ethanol may be potentiated.

Precautions Use with caution in patients with depression, renal or hepatic dysfunction, chronic pulmonary insufficiency, or sleep apnea; use in lactating women is not recommended

Adverse Reactions

Central nervous system: Drowsiness, anterograde amnesia, confusion, bizarre behavior, agitation, dizziness, hallucinations, nightmares, headache, ataxia

Gastrointestinal: Xerostomia, nausea, vomiting

Hepatic: Cholestatic jaundice

Miscellaneous: Physical and psychological dependence; hypersensitivity reactions, anaphylaxis, angioedema; hazardous sleep-related activities (see Warnings)

Drug Interactions Cytochrome P450 isoenzyme CYP3A3/4 and CYP3A5-7 substrate

CNS depressants, alcohol may increase CNS adverse effects. P450 enzyme inhibitors (eg, cimetidine, erythromycin) may increase and enzyme inducers may decrease serum concentrations of triazolam. Protease inhibitors (atazanavir, indinavir, lopinavir, nelfinavir, ritonavir, saquinavir) and delavirdine may potentially decrease triazolam's metabolism and increase triazolam serum concentrations; concurrent use of triazolam with protease inhibitors or delavirdine is not recommended. Ketoconazole, itraconazole, nefazodone, may significantly increase intensity and duration of triazolam effects (use of these agents is contraindicated). Ranitidine and oral contraceptive agents may increase triazolam serum concentrations.

Food Interactions Food may decrease the rate, but not the extent of absorption; grapefruit juice significantly increases the bioavailability of oral triazolam

Mechanism of Action Depresses all levels of the CNS, including the limbic and reticular formation, by binding to the benzodiazepine site on the gamma-aminobutyric acid (GABA) receptor complex and modulating GABA, which is a major inhibitory neurotransmitter in the brain

Pharmacodynamics Hypnotic effects:

Onset of action: Within 15-30 minutes

Duration: 6-7 hours

Pharmacokinetics

Distribution: Drug and metabolites distribute into breast milk

V_d: Adults: 0.8-1.8 L/kg

Protein binding: 89%

Metabolism: Extensive in the liver; primary metabolites are conjugated glucuronides

Half-life: Adults: 1.5-5.5 hours

Time to peak serum concentration: Within 2 hours

Elimination: In urine as unchanged drug (minor amounts) and metabolites

Usual Dosage Oral:

Children <18 years: Dosage not established; investigational doses of 0.02 mg/kg given as an elixir have been used in children (n=20) for sedation prior to dental procedures; further studies are needed before this dose can be recommended

Adolescents ≥18 years and Adults: Usual: 0.125-0.25 mg at bedtime; dose may be increased to 0.5 mg at bedtime in patients who do not respond to lower doses; maximum dose: 0.5 mg/day

Administration Oral: Administer dose in bed, since onset of hypnotic effect is rapid; do not administer with grapefruit juice

Monitoring Parameters Liver enzymes with prolonged use

Patient Information Avoid alcohol, other CNS depressants, and grapefruit juice. May be habit-forming; avoid abrupt discontinuation with prolonged use. May cause drowsiness and impair ability to perform activities requiring mental alertness or physical coordination. Take dose in bed at bedtime. May also cause daytime drowsiness. May cause dry mouth. May cause hypersensitivity reactions. May cause hazardous sleep-related activities (ie, driving, preparing and eating foods, and making phone calls while not fully awake).

Additional Information Onset of action is rapid; patient should be in bed when taking medication

In March 2007, the FDA requested that all manufacturers of sedative-hypnotic drug products, including Halcion® (triazolam), revise the labeling to include a greater emphasis on the risks of adverse events. The events include severe hypersensitivity

(Continued)

Triazolam *(Continued)*

reactions including anaphylaxis and/or angioedema, as well as hazardous sleep-related activities (eg, sleep-driving - driving while not fully awake after consumption of sedative-hypnotic drug, with no recollection of the event). Other activities may include preparing and ingesting food, and the use of the telephone, while asleep. These events may occur at any time during therapy including with the first dose administered.

Manufacturers must provide written notification to healthcare providers regarding the new warnings. In addition, manufacturers are to develop "Patient Medication Guides" designed to educate consumers about the potential risks and to advise them of precautionary measures that can be taken. This advice will contain recommendations on correct utilization of the medication as well as the avoidance of the consumption of ethanol and/or other CNS-depressant agents. The FDA is also recommending manufacturers conduct studies evaluating the frequencies of sleep-driving (and other sleep-related behaviors) with the individual products.

Patients should be instructed not to discontinue these medications without first speaking with their healthcare provider. Patients should also be informed of the potential for an allergic reaction, the signs and symptoms of anaphylaxis, and the appropriate emergency self-treatment of an anaphylactic reaction.

Additional information on the sedative-hypnotic products and sleep disorders is available at http://www.fda.gov/cder/drug/infopage/sedative_hypnotics/default.htm

Dosage Forms Excipient information presented when available (limited, particularly for generics); consult specific product labeling.

Tablet: 0.125 mg, 0.25 mg

Halcion®: 0.125 mg, 0.25 mg [DSC]

References

Meyer ML, Mourino AP, and Farrington FH, "Comparison of Triazolam to a Chloral Hydrate/Hydroxyzine Combination in the Sedation of Pediatric Dental Patients," *Pediatr Dent*, 1990, 12(5):283-7.

♦ **Tribavirin** *see* Ribavirin *on page 1378*
♦ **Tricalcium Phosphate** *see* Calcium Phosphate, Tribasic *on page 271*
♦ **Trichloroacetaldehyde Monohydrate** *see* Chloral Hydrate *on page 331*
♦ **Tricosal** *see* Choline Magnesium Trisalicylate *on page 350*
♦ **Triderm®** *see* Triamcinolone *on page 1568*

Triethanolamine Polypeptide Oleate-Condensate

(trye eth a NOLE a meen pol i PEP tide OH lee ate-KON den sate)

U.S. Brand Names Cerumenex® [DSC]

Canadian Brand Names Cerumenex®

Therapeutic Category Otic Agent, Cerumenolytic

Generic Available No

Use Removal of ear wax (cerumen)

Pregnancy Risk Factor C

Contraindications Hypersensitivity to triethanolamine polypeptide oleate-condensate or any component; perforated tympanic membrane or otitis media

Warnings Discontinue if sensitization or irritation occurs

Precautions Avoid undue exposure to skin during administration and the flushing out of ear canal; exposure of ear canal to otic solution should be limited to 15-30 minutes

Adverse Reactions Local: Localized dermatitis, mild erythema and pruritus, severe eczematoid reactions involving the external ear and periauricular tissue

Mechanism of Action Emulsifies and disperses accumulated cerumen for easier removal

Pharmacodynamics Onset of action: Produces slight disintegration of very hard ear wax by 24 hours

Usual Dosage Children and Adults: Otic: Fill ear canal, insert cotton plug; allow to remain 15-30 minutes; flush ear with lukewarm water as a single treatment; if a second application is needed for unusually hard impactions, repeat the procedure

Monitoring Parameters Evaluate hearing before and after instillation of medication

Patient Information For external use in the ear only; warm to body temperature before using to improve effect

Nursing Implications Avoid undue exposure of the drug to the peridural skin

Dosage Forms Excipient information presented when available (limited, particularly for generics); consult specific product labeling. [DSC] = Discontinued product

Solution, otic: 10% (6 mL, 12 mL) [DSC]

References

Mehta AK, "An *In Vitro* Comparison of the Disintegration of Human Ear Wax by Five Cerumenolytics Commonly Used in General Practice," *Br J Clin Pract*, 1985, 39(5):200-3.

♦ **Triethylenethiophosphoramide** *see* Thiotepa *on page 1532*

♦ **Trifluorothymidine** *see* Trifluridine *on page 1575*

Trifluridine (trye FLURE i deen)

Medication Safety Issues

Sound-alike/look-alike issues:

Viroptic® may be confused with Timoptic®

U.S. Brand Names Viroptic®

Canadian Brand Names SAB-Trifluridine; Sandoz-Trifluridine; Viroptic®

Index Terms F_3T; Trifluorothymidine

Therapeutic Category Antiviral Agent, Ophthalmic

Generic Available Yes

Use Treatment of primary keratoconjunctivitis and recurrent epithelial keratitis caused by herpes simplex virus types I and II

Pregnancy Risk Factor C

Lactation Excretion in breast milk unknown

Contraindications Hypersensitivity to trifluridine or any component

Adverse Reactions

Cardiovascular: Hyperemia

Local: Burning, stinging

Ocular: Palpebral edema, epithelial keratopathy, keratitis, stromal edema, elevated intraocular pressure

Miscellaneous: Hypersensitivity reactions

Stability Store in refrigerator; storage at room temperature may result in a solution with altered pH which could result in ocular discomfort upon administration and/or decreased potency

Mechanism of Action Interferes with viral replication by incorporating into viral DNA in place of thymidine, inhibiting thymidylate synthetase resulting in the formation of defective proteins

Pharmacodynamics Onset of action: Response to treatment occurs within 2-7 days; epithelial healing is complete in 1-2 weeks

Pharmacokinetics Absorption: Ophthalmic: Systemic absorption is negligible, while corneal penetration is adequate

Usual Dosage Children and Adults: Ophthalmic: Instill 1 drop into affected eye every 2 hours while awake, to a maximum of 9 drops/day, until re-epithelialization of corneal ulcer occurs; then use 1 drop every 4 hours for another 7 days; do **not** exceed 21 days of treatment

Administration Ophthalmic: Avoid contact of bottle tip with skin or eye; instill drops onto the cornea of the affected eye(s); apply finger pressure to lacrimal sac during and for 1-2 minutes after instillation to decrease risk of absorption and systemic effects

Monitoring Parameters Ophthalmologic exam (test for corneal staining with fluorescein or rose Bengal)

Additional Information Found to be effective in 138 of 150 patients unresponsive or intolerant to idoxuridine or vidarabine

Dosage Forms Excipient information presented when available (limited, particularly for generics); consult specific product labeling.

Solution, ophthalmic: 1% (7.5 mL)

♦ **Triglycerides, Medium Chain** *see* Medium Chain Triglycerides *on page 989*

Trihexyphenidyl (trye heks ee FEN i dil)

Medication Safety Issues

Sound-alike/look-alike issues:

Trihexyphenidyl may be confused with trifluoperazine

Artane may be confused with Altace®, Anturane®, Aramine®

Related Information

Overdose and Toxicology *on page 1916*

Canadian Brand Names Apo-Trihex®

Index Terms Artane; Benzhexol Hydrochloride; Trihexyphenidyl Hydrochloride

Therapeutic Category Anti-Parkinson's Agent; Anticholinergic Agent; Antidote, Drug-induced Dystonic Reactions

Generic Available Yes

Use Adjunctive treatment of Parkinson's disease; also used in treatment of drug-induced extrapyramidal effects and acute dystonic reactions

Pregnancy Risk Factor C

Lactation Excretion in breast milk unknown/use caution

(Continued)

Trihexyphenidyl *(Continued)*

Contraindications Hypersensitivity to trihexyphenidyl or any component; children younger than 3 years of age; patients with narrow-angle glaucoma, GI or GU obstruction; myasthenia gravis, achalasia

Precautions Use with caution in patients with hyperthyroidism, renal or hepatic dysfunction, hypertension, hiatal hernia, tachycardia, cardiac arrhythmias, peptic ulcer, esophageal reflux; use with caution in hot weather or during exercise

Adverse Reactions

Cardiovascular: Tachycardia

Central nervous system: Dizziness, nervousness, drowsiness, agitation, delirium, headache

Dermatologic: Rash

Gastrointestinal: Xerostomia, nausea, constipation

Genitourinary: Urinary hesitancy or retention

Neuromuscular & skeletal: Weakness

Ocular: Blurred vision, mydriasis, elevated intraocular tension

Drug Interactions May increase gastric degradation of levodopa and decrease the amount of levodopa absorbed by delaying gastric emptying; antagonizes the therapeutic effects of cholinergic agents (tacrine, donepezil) and neuroleptics; increases central and/or peripheral anticholinergic effects when administered with amantadine, rimantadine, narcotic analgesics, phenothiazines and other antipsychotics (especially with high anticholinergic activity), tricyclic antidepressants, quinidine and some other antiarrhythmics, and antihistamines

Mechanism of Action Presumed to act by blocking excess acetylcholine at cerebral synapses; many of its effects are due to its pharmacologic similarities with atropine

Pharmacodynamics

Onset of action: 1 hour

Maximum effect: 2-3 hours

Duration: 6-12 hours

Pharmacokinetics

Metabolism: Metabolic fate undetermined

Bioavailability: 100%

Half-life: 5.6-10.2 hours

Elimination: Some urinary excretion

Usual Dosage Adults: Oral:

Extrapyramidal: 5-15 mg/day in 3-4 divided doses

Parkinsonism: 1 mg daily; increase by 2 mg increments every 3-5 days to 6-10 mg/day (maximum daily dosage: 12-15 mg); doses >10 mg/day should be divided into 3-4 doses

Administration Oral: Administer with food or water to decrease GI irritation

Monitoring Parameters Intraocular pressure monitoring (baseline and at regular intervals)

Patient Information May cause drowsiness and impair ability to perform activities requiring mental alertness or physical coordination; may cause dry mouth

Dosage Forms Excipient information presented when available (limited, particularly for generics); consult specific product labeling.

Elixir, as hydrochloride: 2 mg/5 mL (480 mL)

Tablet, as hydrochloride: 2 mg, 5 mg

♦ **Trihexyphenidyl Hydrochloride** *see* Trihexyphenidyl *on page 1575*

♦ **TriHIBit®** *see* Diphtheria, Tetanus Toxoids, and Acellular Pertussis Vaccine and *Haemophilus influenzae* b Conjugate Vaccine *on page 519*

♦ **Trikacide (Can)** *see* Metronidazole *on page 1049*

♦ **Trileptal®** *see* Oxcarbazepine *on page 1184*

♦ **Trilisate® [DSC]** *see* Choline Magnesium Trisalicylate *on page 350*

♦ **TriLyte™** *see* Polyethylene Glycol-Electrolyte Solution *on page 1277*

Trimethobenzamide (trye meth oh BEN za mide)

Medication Safety Issues

Sound-alike/look-alike issues:

Tigan® may be confused with Tiazac®, Ticar®

Related Information

Compatibility of Medications Mixed in A Syringe *on page 1941*

U.S. Brand Names Tigan®

Canadian Brand Names Tigan®

Index Terms Trimethobenzamide Hydrochloride

Therapeutic Category Antiemetic

Generic Available Yes: Injection

Use Treatment of nausea and vomiting

Pregnancy Risk Factor C

Lactation Excretion in breast milk unknown

Contraindications Hypersensitivity to trimethobenzamide or any component; injection is contraindicated in children

Precautions Use cautiously in infants and children; may mask emesis due to Reye's syndrome or mimic CNS effects of Reye's syndrome in patients with emesis of other etiologies. May cause extrapyramidal symptoms (EPS) which may be confused with CNS symptoms of primary disease responsible for emesis. Risk of adverse effects (eg, EPS, seizure) may be increased in patients with acute febrile illness, dehydration, or electrolyte imbalance; use with caution.

Adverse Reactions

Cardiovascular: Hypotension (especially after I.M. use)

Central nervous system: Drowsiness, sedation, extrapyramidal symptoms, dizziness, seizures, coma, depression, opisthotonos

Dermatologic: Hypersensitivity skin reactions

Gastrointestinal: Diarrhea

Hematologic: Blood dyscrasias

Hepatic: Jaundice

Local: Pain, stinging, burning at I.M. injection site

Ocular: Blurred vision

Stability Store at room temperature.

Mechanism of Action Acts centrally to inhibit stimulation of the medullary chemoreceptor trigger zone

Pharmacodynamics

Onset of action:

Oral: 10-40 minutes

I.M.: 15-35 minutes

Duration:

Oral: 3-4 hours

I.M.: 2-3 hours

Pharmacokinetics

Metabolism: Not well determined

Bioavailability: Oral dose is ~60% of I.M. dose

Half-life: Adults: 7-9 hours

Time to peak serum concentration:

I.V.: ~30 minutes

Oral: 45 minutes

Elimination: 20% excreted unchanged in urine in 24 hours

Usual Dosage

Children:

Oral: 15-20 mg/kg/day (400-500 mg/m^2/day) divided into 3-4 doses; **or as an alternative**

<13.6 kg (30 lbs): 100 mg 3-4 times/day

13.6-40 kg (30-90 lbs): 100-200 mg 3-4 times/day

>40 kg: 300 mg 3-4 times/day

I.M.: Not recommended

Adults:

Oral: 300 mg 3-4 times/day

I.M.: 200 mg 3-4 times/day

Administration

Oral: May administer without regard to food

Parenteral: I.M. use only by deep injection into upper outer quadrant of gluteal region; **not** for I.V. use

Patient Information May cause drowsiness and impair ability to perform activities requiring mental alertness or physical coordination

Additional Information Note: Less effective than phenothiazines but may be associated with fewer side effects

Dosage Forms Excipient information presented when available (limited, particularly for generics); consult specific product labeling.

Capsule, as hydrochloride:

Tigan®: 300 mg

Injection, solution, as hydrochloride: 100 mg/mL (2 mL)

Tigan®: 100 mg/mL (2 mL [preservative free], 20 mL)

♦ **Trimethobenzamide Hydrochloride** *see* Trimethobenzamide *on page 1576*

Trimethoprim (trye METH oh prim)

Medication Safety Issues

Sound-alike/look-alike issues:

Trimethoprim may be confused with trimethaphan

Proloprim® may be confused with Prolixin®, Protropin®

Related Information

Blood Level Sampling Time Guidelines *on page 1914*

U.S. Brand Names Primsol®; Proloprim®

Canadian Brand Names Apo-Trimethoprim®

Index Terms TMP

Therapeutic Category Antibiotic, Miscellaneous

Generic Available Yes: Tablet

Use Treatment of urinary tract infections caused by susceptible *Escherichia coli*, *Proteus mirabilis*, *Klebsiella pneumoniae*, *Enterobacter* species, and coagulase-negative *Staphylococcus* (including *S. saprophyticus*); prophylaxis of urinary tract infections; in combination with other agents for treatment of *Pneumocystis carinii* pneumonia; treatment of otitis media caused by susceptible *Streptococcus pneumoniae* and *Haemophilus influenzae* (not indicated for *Moraxella catarrhalis* due to consistent resistance); not indicated for prolonged administration or prophylaxis of otitis media

Pregnancy Risk Factor C

Lactation Enters breast milk/use caution (AAP rates "compatible")

Contraindications Hypersensitivity to trimethoprim or any component; megaloblastic anemia due to folate deficiency

Warnings May cause folate deficiencies with subsequent bone marrow suppression and blood dyscrasias; monitor patients for fever, sore throat, purpura, or pallor; discontinue trimethoprim if bone marrow depression occurs; leucovorin (folinic acid) may be needed to restore normal hematopoiesis

Oral solution contains propylene glycol and sodium benzoate; benzoic acid (benzoate) is a metabolite of benzyl alcohol; large amounts of benzyl alcohol (≥99 mg/kg/day) have been associated with a potentially fatal toxicity ("gasping syndrome") in neonates; the "gasping syndrome" consists of metabolic acidosis, respiratory distress, gasping respirations, CNS dysfunction (including convulsions, intracranial hemorrhage), hypotension and cardiovascular collapse; avoid use of trimethoprim products containing sodium benzoate in neonates; *in vitro* and animal studies have shown that benzoate displaces bilirubin from protein binding sites

Precautions Use with caution in patients with impaired renal or hepatic function or with possible folate deficiency; decrease dose in patients with renal dysfunction; safety is not established in infants <2 months of age; effectiveness for treatment of acute otitis media is not established in infants <6 months of age

Adverse Reactions

Central nervous system: Fever, headache, aseptic meningitis (rare)

Dermatologic: Rash, pruritus, phototoxic skin eruptions, exfoliative dermatitis (rare), erythema multiforme (rare), Stevens-Johnson syndrome (rare), toxic epidermal necrolysis (rare)

Endocrine & metabolic: Hyperkalemia, hyponatremia

Hematologic: Megaloblastic anemia, neutropenia, leukopenia, thrombocytopenia, methemoglobinemia

Hepatic: Elevated liver enzymes, cholestatic jaundice

Gastrointestinal: Nausea, vomiting, epigastric distress, glossitis

Renal: Elevated BUN and serum creatinine

Miscellaneous: Anaphylaxis, hypersensitivity reactions

Drug Interactions Cytochrome P450 isoenzyme CYP2C8 and CYP2C9 inhibitor

Use with other folate antagonists (methotrexate, pyrimethamine) may increase risk of megaloblastic anemia; trimethoprim may decrease the metabolism of phenytoin resulting in increased phenytoin serum concentrations; cyclosporine, dapsone, procainamide, rifampin, warfarin

Food Interactions May cause folic acid deficiency, supplements may be needed

Stability Store tablets and solution at 15°C to 25°C (59°F to 77°F); protect from light

Mechanism of Action Binds to the enzyme dihydrofolate reductase in bacteria and inhibits conversion of dihydrofolic acid to tetrahydrofolate (functional form of folic acid). This results in depletion of folic acid, interference with bacterial biosynthesis of nucleic acids and protein production, and inhibition of microbial growth.

Pharmacokinetics

Absorption: Oral: Readily and extensively absorbed (90% to 100%)

Distribution: Penetrates into middle ear fluid with a mean peak middle ear fluid concentration in children 1-12 years of 2 mcg/mL after a single 4 mg/kg dose; crosses the placenta; excreted in breast milk

V_d:
Newborns: ~2.7 L/kg
Infants: 1.5 L/kg
Children 1-10 years: ~1 L/kg
Adults: 1.3-1.8 L/kg
Protein binding: 42% to 46%
Metabolism: Partially (10% to 20%) metabolized in the liver via demethylation, oxidation, and hydroxylation
Bioavailability: Similar for tablets and solution
Half-life (prolonged in renal dysfunction):
Newborns: ~19 hours
Infants 2 months to 1 year: 3-6 hours; mean: 4.6 hours
Children 1-10 years: 3-5.5 hours
Adults, normal renal function: 8-11 hours
Adults, anuric: 20-50 hours
Time to peak serum concentration: Within 1-4 hours
Elimination: Significantly excreted in urine (60% to 80%) as unchanged drug via glomerular filtration and tubular secretion; increased renal excretion with acidic urine
Dialysis: Moderately dialyzable (20% to 50%)

Usual Dosage Oral:
Infants ≥6 months and Children: Acute otitis media: 10 mg/kg/day in divided doses every 12 hours for 10 days
Infants and Children <12 years: Urinary tract infection: Treatment: 4-6 mg/kg/day in divided doses every 12 hours for 10 days
Children ≥12 years and Adults:
Urinary tract infection: Treatment: 100 mg every 12 hours or 200 mg every 24 hours for 10 days
Prophylaxis: 100 mg once daily
Pneumocystis carinii pneumonia treatment (given with dapsone): 15-20 mg/kg/day in 4 divided doses for 21 days
Dosing adjustment in renal impairment:
Cl_{cr} 15-30 mL/minute: Administer 50% of normal dose
Cl_{cr} <15 mL/minute: Avoid use

Administration Oral: Administer on an empty stomach; may administer with milk or food if GI upset occurs

Monitoring Parameters CBC with differential, platelet count, liver enzyme tests, bilirubin, serum creatinine and BUN

Reference Range Therapeutic:
Peak: 5-15 mg/L
Trough: 2-8 mg/L

Test Interactions May falsely increase creatinine determination measured by the Jaffé alkaline picrate assay; may interfere with determination of serum methotrexate when measured by methods that use a bacterial dihydrofolate reductase as the binding protein (eg, the competitive binding protein technique); does **not** interfere with RIA for methotrexate

Patient Information Report any skin rash, persistent or severe fatigue, fever, sore throat, or unusual bleeding or bruising; complete full course of therapy

Additional Information Not effective versus *Pseudomonas* or *B. fragilis*; discontinue if bone marrow suppression occurs

Dosage Forms Excipient information presented when available (limited, particularly for generics); consult specific product labeling. [DSC] = Discontinued product
Solution, oral (Primsol®): 50 mg (base)/5 mL (480 mL) [contains sodium benzoate; bubble gum flavor]
Tablet: 100 mg
Proloprim®: 100 mg, 200 mg [DSC]

References

Hoppu K, "Age Differences in Trimethoprim Pharmacokinetics: Need for Revised Dosing in Children?" *Clin Pharmacol Ther*, 1987, 41(3):336-43.
Hoppu K, Koskimies O, and Vilska J, "Trimethoprim in the Treatment of Acute Urinary Tract Infections in Children," *Int J Clin Pharmacol Ther Toxicol*, 1988, 26(2):65-8.
Leff RD, Cho CT, and Reed MD, "Safety and Efficacy of Trimethoprim Hydrochloride Solution for the Treatment of Children With Otitis Media," *Journal of Pediatric Pharmacy Practice*, 1998, 3(1): 33-9.

♦ **Trimethoprim and Sulfamethoxazole** *see* Sulfamethoxazole and Trimethoprim *on page 1487*
♦ **Tri-Nasal®** *see* Triamcinolone *on page 1568*
♦ **Trinasal® (Can)** *see* Triamcinolone *on page 1568*
♦ **Trinipatch® 0.2 (Can)** *see* Nitroglycerin *on page 1141*
♦ **Trinipatch® 0.4 (Can)** *see* Nitroglycerin *on page 1141*
♦ **Trinipatch® 0.6 (Can)** *see* Nitroglycerin *on page 1141*

- **Triostat®** *see* Liothyronine *on page 943*
- **Tripedia®** *see* Diphtheria, Tetanus Toxoids, and Acellular Pertussis Vaccine *on page 517*
- **Triple Antibiotic** *see* Neomycin, Polymyxin B, and Bacitracin *on page 1121*

Triprolidine and Pseudoephedrine

(trye PROE li deen & soo doe e FED rin)

Medication Safety Issues
Sound-alike/look-alike issues:
Aprodine® may be confused with Aphrodyne®

Related Information
OTC Cough and Cold Preparations, Pediatric *on page 1706*
Overdose and Toxicology *on page 1916*

U.S. Brand Names Actifed® Cold and Allergy [OTC] [DSC]; Allerfrim® [OTC]; Aprodine® [OTC]; Genac® [OTC]; Silafed® [OTC]; Sudafed® Maximum Strength Sinus Nighttime [OTC] [DSC]; Tri-Sudo® [OTC] [DSC]; Zymine®-D

Canadian Brand Names Actifed®

Index Terms Pseudoephedrine and Triprolidine

Therapeutic Category Antihistamine/Decongestant Combination; Sympathomimetic

Generic Available Yes

Use Temporary relief of nasal congestion, running nose, sneezing, itching of nose or throat and itchy, watery eyes due to common cold, hay fever or other upper respiratory allergies

Pregnancy Risk Factor C

Contraindications Hypersensitivity to triprolidine, pseudoephedrine, or any component; severe hypertension or coronary artery disease; MAO inhibitor therapy, GI or GU obstruction, narrow-angle glaucoma

Warnings Not recommended for use in children <4 months of age

Precautions Use with caution in patients with mild to moderate high blood pressure, heart disease, diabetes mellitus, asthma, thyroid disease, or prostatic hypertrophy

Adverse Reactions
Cardiovascular: Hypertension, tachycardia
Central nervous system: Sedation, CNS stimulation, headache
Gastrointestinal: Nausea, vomiting, xerostomia, anorexia

Drug Interactions MAO inhibitors, beta-blocking agents, other sympathomimetics, methyldopa, reserpine, alpha-blocking agents, CNS depressants

Usual Dosage Oral:
Children: May dose according to **pseudoephedrine** component: 4 mg/kg/day in divided doses 3-4 times/day **or**
4 months to 2 years: 1.25 mL 3-4 times/day
2-4 years: 2.5 mL 3-4 times/day
4-6 years: 3.75 mL 3-4 times/day
6-12 years: 5 mL or ½ tablet 3-4 times/day
Children >12 years and Adults: 10 mL or 1 tablet 3-4 times/day

Administration Oral: Administer with food or milk to decrease GI irritation

Patient Information May cause drowsiness and impair ability to perform activities requiring mental alertness or physical coordination; may cause dry mouth

Dosage Forms Excipient information presented when available (limited, particularly for generics); consult specific product labeling. [DSC] = Discontinued product
Liquid:
Zymine®-D: Triprolidine hydrochloride 1.25 mg and pseudoephedrine hydrochloride 45 mg per 5 mL (480 mL)
Syrup: Triprolidine hydrochloride 1.25 mg and pseudoephedrine hydrochloride 30 mg per 5 mL (120 mL)
Allerfrim®: Triprolidine hydrochloride 1.25 mg and pseudoephedrine hydrochloride 30 mg per 5 mL (120 mL, 480 mL) [contains sodium benzoate]
Aprodine®: Triprolidine hydrochloride 1.25 mg and pseudoephedrine hydrochloride 30 mg per 5 mL (120 mL)
Silafed®: Triprolidine hydrochloride 1.25 mg and pseudoephedrine hydrochloride 30 mg per 5 mL (120 mL, 240 mL)
Tablet:
Actifed® Cold and Allergy [DSC], Allerfrim® [DSC], Aprodine®, Genac®, Sudafed® Maximum Strength Sinus Nighttime, Tri-Sudo® [DSC]: Triprolidine hydrochloride 2.5 mg and pseudoephedrine hydrochloride 60 mg

- **TripTone® [OTC] [DSC]** *see* DimenhyDRINATE *on page 507*
- **Tris Buffer** *see* Tromethamine *on page 1581*
- **Tris(hydroxymethyl)aminomethane** *see* Tromethamine *on page 1581*

- **Tri-Sudo® [OTC] [DSC]** *see* Triprolidine and Pseudoephedrine *on page 1580*
- **Trivagizole-3® (Can)** *see* Clotrimazole *on page 393*
- **Trivalent Inactivated Influenza Vaccine (TIV)** *see* Influenza Virus Vaccine (Inactivated) *on page 833*
- **Trizivir®** *see* Abacavir, Lamivudine, and Zidovudine *on page 38*
- **Trocaine® [OTC]** *see* Benzocaine *on page 204*

Tromethamine (troe METH a meen)

Medication Safety Issues

Sound-alike/look-alike issues:

Tromethamine may be confused with TrophAmine®

U.S. Brand Names THAM®

Index Terms Tris Buffer; Tris(hydroxymethyl)aminomethane

Therapeutic Category Alkalinizing Agent, Parenteral

Generic Available No

Use Correction of metabolic acidosis associated with cardiac bypass surgery or cardiac arrest; to correct excess acidity of stored blood that is preserved with acid citrate dextrose (ACD); to prime the pump-oxygenator during cardiac bypass surgery; indicated in severe metabolic acidosis in patients in whom sodium or carbon dioxide elimination is restricted [eg, infants needing alkalinization after receiving maximum sodium bicarbonate (8-10 mEq/kg/24 hours)]

Pregnancy Risk Factor C

Lactation Excretion in breast milk unknown/use caution

Contraindications Hypersensitivity to tromethamine or any component; uremia or anuria; chronic respiratory acidosis (neonates); salicylate intoxication (neonates)

Warnings Avoid infusion via low-lying umbilical venous catheters due to associated risk of hepatocellular necrosis; severe local tissue necrosis and sloughing may occur if solution extravasates; administer via central line or large vein slowly. Due to tromethamine's greater osmotic effects, use of sodium bicarbonate for the treatment of acidotic neonates and infants with RDS may be preferred; rapid I.V. infusion and overdosage may cause prolonged hypoglycemia. Monitor pH carefully as large doses may increase blood pH greater than normal which may result in depressed respiration.

Precautions Reduce dose and monitor pH and serum potassium carefully in renal impairment.

Adverse Reactions

Cardiovascular: Venospasm

Central nervous system: Fever

Endocrine & metabolic: Hyperosmolality of serum, hyperkalemia, hypoglycemia (rapid administration and use in neonates)

Hepatic: Liver cell destruction from direct contact with tromethamine, hemorrhagic hepatic necrosis (when administered through umbilical vein at concentrations ≥1.2 M)

Local: Tissue irritation, necrosis with extravasation

Respiratory: Respiratory depression, apnea

Stability Store at room temperature; protect from freezing

Mechanism of Action Acts as a proton acceptor, which combines with hydrogen ions to form bicarbonate and buffer to correct acidosis; buffers both metabolic and respiratory acids, limiting carbon dioxide generation; also acts as an osmotic diuretic

Pharmacokinetics 30% of dose is not ionized; rapidly eliminated by kidneys

Usual Dosage I.V.: Dose depends on severity and progression of acidosis:

Neonates: Manufacturer's recommendation: 1 mL/kg for each pH unit below 7.4; additional doses to be determined by changes in PaO_2, pH, and pCO_2

Infants, Children, and Adults:

Empiric dosage based upon base deficit: Tromethamine mL of 0.3 M solution = body weight (kg) x base deficit (mEq/L) x 1.1*; maximum: 500 mg/kg/dose = 13.9 mL/kg/dose using 0.3 M solution

*Factor of 1.1 accounts for an approximate reduction of 10% in buffering capacity due to the presence of sufficient acetic acid to lower the pH of the 0.3 M solution to approximately 8.6

Metabolic acidosis with cardiac arrest: Tromethamine mL of 0.3 M solution: 3.5-6 mL/kg/dose (126-216 mg/kg/dose); maximum: 500 mg/kg/dose = 13.9 mL/kg/dose

Metabolic acidosis with cardiac arrest: Direct instillation to ventricle: Adults: Tromethamine 0.3 M solution: 2-6 g (62-185 mL); do not inject into cardiac muscle

(Continued)

Tromethamine *(Continued)*

Excess acidity of acid citrate dextrose priming blood: Tromethamine mL of 0.3 M solution: 15-77 mL added to each 500 mL of ACD blood used for priming the pump-oxygenator

Acidosis during cardiac bypass surgery: Tromethamine mL of 0.3 M solution: 9 mL/kg (324 mg/kg/dose); maximum: 1000 mL (36 g) as single dose dose in severe cases and not to exceed 500 mg/kg over a period of 1 hour (eg, for 70 kg patient, not to exceed 35 g/hour)

Administration Parenteral: Maximum concentration: 0.3 molar; infuse slowly over at least 1 hour or 3-16 mL/kg/hour up to 33-40 mL/kg/day; administer into a central venous line and avoid administration into low-lying umbilical venous lines

Monitoring Parameters Serum electrolytes, arterial blood gases, serum pH, blood sugar, EKG monitoring, renal function tests

Additional Information 1 mM = 120 mg = 3.3 mL = 1 mEq of THAM®

Dosage Forms Excipient information presented when available (limited, particularly for generics); consult specific product labeling.

Injection, solution:

THAM®: 18 g [0.3 molar] (500 mL)

- **Tronolane® Suppository [OTC]** *see* Phenylephrine *on page 1250*
- **Tropicacyl®** *see* Tropicamide *on page 1582*

Tropicamide (troe PIK a mide)

U.S. Brand Names Mydral™; Mydriacyl®; Tropicacyl®

Canadian Brand Names Diotrope®; Mydriacyl®

Index Terms Bistropamide

Therapeutic Category Ophthalmic Agent, Mydriatic

Generic Available Yes

Use Short-acting mydriatic used in diagnostic procedures; as well as preoperatively and postoperatively; treatment of some cases of acute iritis, iridocyclitis, and keratitis

Pregnancy Risk Factor C

Contraindications Hypersensitivity to tropicamide or any component; glaucoma, adhesions between the iris and the lens

Warnings Tropicamide may cause an increase in intraocular pressure

Precautions Use with caution in infants and children since tropicamide may cause potentially dangerous CNS disturbances and psychotic reactions

Adverse Reactions

Cardiovascular: Tachycardia, flushing

Central nervous system: Parasympathetic stimulation, drowsiness, headache, behavioral disturbances, psychotic reactions

Gastrointestinal: Xerostomia

Local: Transient stinging

Ocular: Blurred vision, photophobia, elevated intraocular pressure, follicular conjunctivitis

Miscellaneous: Allergic reactions

Stability Store at room temperature; do not refrigerate

Mechanism of Action Prevents the sphincter muscle of the iris and the muscle of the ciliary body from responding to cholinergic stimulation producing pupillary dilation and paralysis of accommodation

Pharmacodynamics

Maximum mydriatic effect: ~20-40 minutes

Duration: ~6-7 hours

Maximum cycloplegic effect:

Peak: 20-35 minutes

Duration: <6 hours

Usual Dosage Children and Adults: Ophthalmic:

Cycloplegia: Instill 1-2 drops (1%); may repeat in 5 minutes. The exam must be performed within 30 minutes after the repeat dose; if the patient is not examined within 20-30 minutes, instill an additional drop. Concentrations <1% are inadequate for producing satisfactory cycloplegia.

Mydriasis: Instill 1-2 drops (0.5%) 15-20 minutes before exam; may repeat every 30 minutes as needed

Administration Ophthalmic: To minimize systemic absorption, apply finger pressure on the lacrimal sac for 1-2 minutes following instillation of the ophthalmic solution; avoid contact of bottle tip with skin or eye

Patient Information May cause blurred vision; do not drive or engage in hazardous activities while the pupils are dilated; may cause sensitivity to light; may cause dry mouth

Dosage Forms Excipient information presented when available (limited, particularly for generics); consult specific product labeling.

Solution, ophthalmic: 0.5% (15 mL); 1% (2 mL, 15 mL) [contains benzalkonium chloride]

Mydriacyl®: 1% (3 mL, 15 mL) [contains benzalkonium chloride]

Mydral™, Tropicacyl®: 0.5% (15 mL); 1% (15 mL) [contains benzalkonium chloride]

References

Caputo AR and Schnitzer RE, "Systemic Response to Mydriatic Eyedrops in Neonates: Mydriatics in Neonates," *J Pediatr Ophthalmol Strabismus*, 1978, 15(2):109-22.

- **Trusopt®** *see* Dorzolamide *on page 532*
- **TSPA** *see* Thiotepa *on page 1532*
- **Tucks® Anti-Itch [OTC]** *see* Hydrocortisone *on page 781*
- **Tums® [OTC]** *see* Calcium Carbonate *on page 264*
- **Tums® [OTC]** *see* Calcium Supplements *on page 272*
- **Tums® E-X [OTC]** *see* Calcium Carbonate *on page 264*
- **Tums® E-X [OTC]** *see* Calcium Supplements *on page 272*
- **Tums® Extra Strength Sugar Free [OTC]** *see* Calcium Carbonate *on page 264*
- **Tums® Extra Strength Sugar Free [OTC]** *see* Calcium Supplements *on page 272*
- **Tums® Smoothies™ [OTC]** *see* Calcium Carbonate *on page 264*
- **Tums® Smoothies™ [OTC]** *see* Calcium Supplements *on page 272*
- **Tums® Ultra [OTC]** *see* Calcium Carbonate *on page 264*
- **Tums® Ultra® [OTC]** *see* Calcium Supplements *on page 272*
- **Tur-bi-kal® [OTC]** *see* Phenylephrine *on page 1250*
- **Tussi-Organidin® DM NR** *see* Guaifenesin and Dextromethorphan *on page 748*
- **Tussi-Organidin® DM-S NR** *see* Guaifenesin and Dextromethorphan *on page 748*
- **Tussi-Organidin® NR** *see* Guaifenesin and Codeine *on page 746*
- **Tussi-Organidin® S-NR** *see* Guaifenesin and Codeine *on page 746*
- **Twelve Resin-K** *see* Cyanocobalamin *on page 413*
- **Twilite® [OTC]** *see* DiphenhydrAMINE *on page 509*
- **Twinject™** *see* Epinephrine *on page 577*
- **Ty21a Vaccine** *see* Typhoid Vaccine *on page 1583*
- **Tycolene [OTC]** *see* Acetaminophen *on page 42*
- **Tycolene Maximum Strength [OTC]** *see* Acetaminophen *on page 42*
- **Tylenol® [OTC]** *see* Acetaminophen *on page 42*
- **Tylenol® (Can)** *see* Acetaminophen *on page 42*
- **Tylenol® 8 Hour [OTC]** *see* Acetaminophen *on page 42*
- **Tylenol® Arthritis Pain [OTC]** *see* Acetaminophen *on page 42*
- **Tylenol® Children's [OTC]** *see* Acetaminophen *on page 42*
- **Tylenol® Children's with Flavor Creator [OTC]** *see* Acetaminophen *on page 42*
- **Tylenol Elixir with Codeine (Can)** *see* Acetaminophen and Codeine *on page 46*
- **Tylenol® Extra Strength [OTC]** *see* Acetaminophen *on page 42*
- **Tylenol® Infants [OTC]** *see* Acetaminophen *on page 42*
- **Tylenol® Junior [OTC]** *see* Acetaminophen *on page 42*
- **Tylenol No. 1 (Can)** *see* Acetaminophen and Codeine *on page 46*
- **Tylenol No. 1 Forte (Can)** *see* Acetaminophen and Codeine *on page 46*
- **Tylenol No. 2 with Codeine (Can)** *see* Acetaminophen and Codeine *on page 46*
- **Tylenol No. 3 with Codeine (Can)** *see* Acetaminophen and Codeine *on page 46*
- **Tylenol No. 4 with Codeine (Can)** *see* Acetaminophen and Codeine *on page 46*
- **Tylenol® With Codeine** *see* Acetaminophen and Codeine *on page 46*
- **Tylox®** *see* Oxycodone and Acetaminophen *on page 1191*
- **Typhim Vi®** *see* Typhoid Vaccine *on page 1583*

Typhoid Vaccine (TYE foid vak SEEN)

Related Information

Immunization Guidelines *on page 1837*

U.S. Brand Names Typhim Vi®; Vivotif®

Index Terms Ty21a Vaccine; Typhoid Vaccine Live Oral Ty21a; Vi Vaccine

Therapeutic Category Vaccine

Generic Available No

Use Immunization to prevent disease from exposure to *Salmonella typhi*; use is not routinely recommended in the U.S. but is reserved for selected individuals who are either traveling to an area in which there is a recognized risk of exposure to *S. typhi*, who have intimate exposure (eg, household contact) to a *S. typhi* carrier, or who work frequently with *S. typhi* in laboratory settings

(Continued)

Typhoid Vaccine *(Continued)*

Parenteral: Typhim Vi®: Approved for use in children ≥2 years and adults

Oral: Live attenuated Ty21a vaccine (Vivotif Berna®): Approved for use in children ≥6 years and adults

Pregnancy Risk Factor C

Lactation Excretion in breast milk unknown/use caution

Contraindications Hypersensitivity to the vaccine or any component; individuals with blood dyscrasias, leukemia, lymphomas, or other malignant neoplasms affecting the bone marrow or lymphatic systems; concurrent immunosuppressive therapy; primary and acquired immunodeficiency states; family history of congenital or hereditary immunodeficiency; current febrile illness or active febrile infection, oral formulation only: Acute GI illness, persistent diarrhea or vomiting, concurrent systemic antibiotics

Warnings Not all recipients of typhoid vaccine will be fully protected against typhoid fever; demonstrated efficacy ranges from 50% to 80%. Travelers should take all necessary precautions to avoid contact or ingestion of potentially contaminated food or water sources. Unless a complete immunization schedule with oral live attenuated Ty21a vaccine (Vivotif Berna®) is followed, an optimum immune response may not be achieved. Vivotif Berna® should not be administered to immunocompromised persons, including those known to be infected with HIV. Parenteral inactivated vaccine may be an alternative for these individuals.

Precautions Administer Typhim Vi® with caution to patients with thrombocytopenia or any coagulation disorder that would be compromised by I.M. injection.

Adverse Reactions All serious adverse reactions must be reported to the U.S. Department of Health and Human Services (DHHS) Vaccine Adverse Event Reporting System (VAERS) 1-800-822-7967.

Injection: Typhim Vi®:

Cardiovascular: Hypotension

Central nervous system: Headache (20%), fever, malaise (4% to 24%)

Gastrointestinal: Nausea, diarrhea, vomiting

Local at injection site: Erythema, pain (27% to 41%), tenderness (98%), induration (5% to 15%)

Neuromuscular & skeletal: Myalgia

Miscellaneous: Allergic reactions

Oral: Vivotif Berna®:

Central nervous system: Headache (4.8%), fever (3.3%)

Dermatologic: Rash, urticaria

Gastrointestinal: Abdominal pain (6.4%), diarrhea (2.9%), nausea, vomiting

Miscellaneous: Anaphylactic reaction

Drug Interactions Antibiotics (systemic) may decrease the effect of oral live attenuated Ty21a vaccine (Vivotif Berna®); delay vaccine administration for at least 24 hours after administration of any systemic antibiotic; antimalarial drug, proguanil (not approved for use in the U.S.) should not be administered with Vivotif Berna® as it may decrease the response to Vivotif Berna®; separate administration by at least 10 days (other antimalarials, chloroquine and mefloquine, may be administered concomitantly)

Stability Refrigerate at 2°C to 8°C (35°F to 46°F); do not freeze

Mechanism of Action Each vaccine formulation promotes immunity to disease caused by *Salmonella typhi.* I.M. formulation (Typhim Vi®) is an inactivated vaccine which contains the cell surface Vi polysaccharide extracted from *Salmonella enterica serovar typhi, S typhi* Ty2 strain. Oral formulation (Vivotif Berna®) is a live attenuated virus vaccine which confers immunity by provoking a local immune response in the intestinal tract.

Pharmacokinetics

Onset of action: Immunity to *Salmonella typhi*: Oral: ~1 week; I.M.: ~2 weeks

Duration: Immunity: Oral: ~5 years; Parenteral: ~3 years

Usual Dosage Immunization:

Oral (Vivotif Berna®): Children ≥6 years and Adults:

Primary immunization: One capsule on alternate days (day 1, 3, 5, and 7) for a total of 4 doses; all doses should be completed at least 1 week prior to potential exposure

Reimmunization: Repeat full course of primary immunization every 5 years

I.M. (Typhim Vi®): Children ≥2 years and Adults:

Primary immunization: 0.5 mL given at least 2 weeks prior to expected exposure

Reimmunization: 0.5 mL; optimal schedule has not been established; a single dose every 2 years is currently recommended for repeated or continued exposure

Note: There is no data concerning using one vaccine (oral vs. I.M.) as a booster after primary immunization with the other vaccine.

Administration

Parenteral: Administer by I.M. injection into the anterolateral aspect of the thigh or arm; **not for I.V. or SubQ administration**

Oral: Oral capsule should be taken 1 hour before a meal with cold or lukewarm drink on alternate days (days 1, 3, 5, and 7); swallow capsule whole, do not chew

Nursing Implications Federal law requires that the date of administration, the vaccine manufacturer, lot number of vaccine, and the administering person's name, title, and address be entered into the patient's permanent medical record.

Dosage Forms Excipient information presented when available (limited, particularly for generics); consult specific product labeling.

Capsule, enteric coated:

Vivotif®: Viable *S. typhi* Ty21a 2-6 x 10^9 colony-forming units and nonviable *S. typhi* Ty21a 5-50 x 10^9 bacterial cells [contains lactose and sucrose]

Injection, solution:

Typhim Vi®: Purified Vi capsular polysaccharide 25 mcg/0.5 mL (0.5 mL, 10 mL) [derived from *S. typhi* Ty2 strain]

References

Centers for Disease Control, "Recommendations of the Advisory Committee on Immunization Practices (ACIP): General Recommendations on Immunization," *MMWR Recomm Rep*, 1994, 43(RR-1):23.

Red Book: 2006 Report of the Committee on Infectious Diseases, 27th ed, Pickering LK,ed, Elk Grove Village, IL: American Academy of Pediatrics, 2006.

♦ **Typhoid Vaccine Live Oral Ty21a** *see* Typhoid Vaccine *on page 1583*
♦ **506U78** *see* Nelarabine *on page 1113*
♦ **UCB-P071** *see* Cetirizine *on page 327*
♦ **UK92480** *see* Sildenafil *on page 1435*
♦ **UK109496** *see* Voriconazole *on page 1622*
♦ **Ulcidine (Can)** *see* Famotidine *on page 638*
♦ **Ultiva®** *see* Remifentanil *on page 1371*
♦ **Ultracaps MT** *see* Pancrelipase *on page 1203*
♦ **Ultram®** *see* Tramadol *on page 1561*
♦ **Ultram® ER** *see* Tramadol *on page 1561*
♦ **Ultraprin [OTC]** *see* Ibuprofen *on page 802*
♦ **Ultrase®** *see* Pancrelipase *on page 1203*
♦ **Ultrase® MT** *see* Pancrelipase *on page 1203*
♦ **Ultravate®** *see* Halobetasol *on page 753*
♦ **Unasyn®** *see* Ampicillin and Sulbactam *on page 125*

Undecylenic Acid and Derivatives

(un de sil EN ik AS id & dah RIV ah tivs)

U.S. Brand Names Fungi-Nail® [OTC]

Index Terms Zinc Undecylenate

Therapeutic Category Antifungal Agent, Topical

Generic Available No

Use Treatment of athlete's foot (tinea pedis), ringworm (except nails and scalp), prickly heat, jock itch (tinea cruris), diaper rash, and other minor skin irritations due to superficial dermatophytes

Contraindications Hypersensitivity to undecylenic acid and derivatives or any component; fungal infections of the scalp or nails

Warnings Do not apply to blistered, raw, or oozing areas of skin or over deep wounds or puncture wounds

Adverse Reactions

Dermatologic: Rash

Local: Skin irritation, stinging, sensitization

Mechanism of Action Undecylenic acid is a fatty acid with fungistatic activity that retards proliferation of the fungus by altering the conditions of growth; zinc undecylenate provides an astringent action that aids in the reduction of inflammation and irritation

Pharmacodynamics Onset of action: Improvement in erythema and pruritus may be seen within 1 week after initiation of therapy

Usual Dosage Children and Adults: Topical: Apply as needed twice daily for 2-4 weeks

Administration Topical: Clean and dry the affected area before topical application; if the solution is sprayed or applied onto the affected area, allow area to air dry; ointment or cream should be applied at night, the powder may be applied during the day or used alone when a drying effect is needed

Monitoring Parameters Resolution of skin infection

Patient Information For external use only; avoid contact with the eye; do not inhale the powder

Dosage Forms Excipient information presented when available (limited, particularly for generics); consult specific product labeling.

Solution, topical: Undecylenic acid 25% (29.57 mL)

- **Unipen® (Can)** *see* Nafcillin *on page 1099*
- **Uniphyl®** *see* Theophylline *on page 1520*
- **Uniphyl® SRT (Can)** *see* Theophylline *on page 1520*
- **Uni-Senna [OTC]** *see* Senna *on page 1427*
- **Unisom® Maximum Strength SleepGels® [OTC]** *see* DiphenhydrAMINE *on page 509*
- **Unithroid®** *see* Levothyroxine *on page 930*
- **Urasal® (Can)** *see* Methenamine *on page 1021*
- **Urate Oxidase** *see* Rasburicase *on page 1369*
- **Urea Peroxide** *see* Carbamide Peroxide *on page 283*
- **Urecholine®** *see* Bethanechol *on page 215*
- **Urex®** *see* Methenamine *on page 1021*
- **Uristat® [OTC]** *see* Phenazopyridine *on page 1244*
- **Uro-KP-Neutral®** *see* Potassium Phosphate and Sodium Phosphate *on page 1296*
- **Urolene Blue®** *see* Methylene Blue *on page 1033*
- **Uro-Mag® [OTC]** *see* Magnesium Oxide *on page 973*
- **Uro-Mag® [OTC]** *see* Magnesium Supplements *on page 976*
- **Uromax® (Can)** *see* Oxybutynin *on page 1187*
- **Uromitexan (Can)** *see* Mesna *on page 1013*
- **Urso® (Can)** *see* Ursodiol *on page 1586*
- **Urso 250™** *see* Ursodiol *on page 1586*
- **Ursodeoxycholic Acid** *see* Ursodiol *on page 1586*

Ursodiol (ER soe dye ole)

U.S. Brand Names Actigall®; Urso 250™; Urso Forte™

Canadian Brand Names Urso®; Urso® DS

Index Terms Ursodeoxycholic Acid

Therapeutic Category Gallstone Dissolution Agent

Generic Available Yes: Capsule

Use Gallbladder stone dissolution; prevention of gallstone formation (obese patients experiencing rapid weight loss); primary biliary cirrhosis (Urso®)

Unlabeled use: facilitate bile excretion in infants with biliary atresia; treatment of cholestasis secondary to PN; improve the hepatic metabolism of essential fatty acids in patients with cystic fibrosis

Pregnancy Risk Factor B

Lactation Excretion in breast milk unknown/use caution

Contraindications Hypersensitivity to ursodiol, bile acids, or any component; not to be used with calcified cholesterol stones, radiopaque stones, bile pigment stones, or stones larger than 20 mm in diameter; patients with compelling reasons for cholecystectomy (eg, unremitting acute cholecystitis, cholangitis, biliary obstruction)

Warnings Gallbladder stone dissolution may take several months of therapy; complete dissolution may not occur and recurrence of stones within 5 years has been observed in 50% of patients

Precautions Use with caution in patients with a nonvisualizing gallbladder and those with chronic liver disease

Adverse Reactions

Central nervous system: Headache, fatigue, anxiety, depression, sleep disorder

Dermatologic: Rash, pruritus, hair thinning

Gastrointestinal: Diarrhea, biliary pain, constipation, stomatitis, flatulence, nausea, vomiting, abdominal pain

Hepatic: Elevated liver enzymes

Neuromuscular & skeletal: Arthralgias, myalgia, back pain

Respiratory: Cough, rhinitis

Drug Interactions Decreased effect with aluminum-containing antacids, cholestyramine, colestipol, clofibrate, oral contraceptives (estrogens), activated charcoal

Stability Store at room temperature

Mechanism of Action Decreases the cholesterol content of bile and bile stones by reducing the secretion of cholesterol from the liver and the fractional reabsorption of cholesterol by the intestines; mechanism of action in primary biliary cirrhosis is not clearly defined

Pharmacokinetics

Absorption: 90%

Protein binding: 70%

Metabolism: Undergoes extensive enterohepatic recycling; following hepatic conjugation and biliary secretion, the drug is hydrolyzed to active ursodiol, where it is recycled or transformed to lithocholic acid by colonic microbial flora; during chronic administration, ursodiol becomes a major biliary and plasma bile acid constituting 30% to 50% of biliary and plasma bile acids

Half-life: 100 hours

Elimination: In feces via bile

Usual Dosage Oral:

Biliary atresia: Infants: 10-15 mg/kg/day once daily

Improvement in the hepatic metabolism of essential fatty acids in cystic fibrosis: Children: 30 mg/kg/day in 2 divided doses

TPN-induced cholestasis: Infants and Children: 30 mg/kg/day in 3 divided doses

Gallstone dissolution: Adults: 8-10 mg/kg/day in 2-3 divided doses; maintenance therapy: 250 mg/day at bedtime for 6 months to 1 year; use beyond 24 months is not established

Gallstone prevention: Adults: 300 mg twice daily

Primary biliary cirrhosis: Adults: 13-15 mg/kg/day in 4 divided doses

Administration Oral: Administer with food or, if a single dosage, at bedtime

Monitoring Parameters ALT, AST, sonogram, oral cholecystogram before therapy and every 6 months during therapy; obtain ultrasound images of gallbladder at 6-month intervals for the first year of therapy

Patient Information Frequent blood work necessary to follow drug effects; report any persistent nausea, vomiting, abdominal pain

Additional Information 30% to 50% of patients have stone recurrence after dissolution

Dosage Forms Excipient information presented when available (limited, particularly for generics); consult specific product labeling.

Capsule (Actigall®): 300 mg

Tablet:

Urso 250™: 250 mg

Urso Forte™: 500 mg

Extemporaneous Preparations

A 20 mg/mL ursodiol suspension may be made by opening seventeen 300 mg capsules; add in geometric proportions a 1:1 mixture of Ora-Sweet®:Ora-Plus® or 1% methylcellulose:syrup NF to a total volume of 255 mL; stable 91 days refrigerated. (Nahata, 1999)

A 25 mg/mL ursodiol suspension may be made by opening ten 300 mg capsules; mix with 10 mL Glycerin, USP until smooth mixture is obtained. Add 60 mL Ora-Plus® and continue to levigate until a smooth mixture is achieved. Transfer mixture to a light-resistant bottle; add a small amount of Orange Syrup, NF to wash remaining drug from the mortar to bottle. Add additional syrup to make final volume of 120 mL. Label "shake well"; stable 60 days at room temperature or refrigerated. (Mallett MS)

A 50 mg/mL ursodiol suspension may be made by crushing twelve 250 mg tablets, add 30 mL Ora-Plus® and 30 mL either strawberry syrup or Ora-Sweet® SF; final volume 60 mL. Stable 90 days refrigerated (Johnson, 2002)

A 60 mg/mL ursodiol suspension may be made in a similar method by opening twelve 300 mg capsules and wetting with sufficient glycerin and triturating to make a fine paste; gradually add simple syrup to make a final volume of 60 mL. Label "shake well"; stable 35 days in refrigerator. (Johnson, 1995)

Johnson CE and Nesbitt J, "Stability of Ursodiol in an Extemporaneously Compounded Oral Liquid," *Am J Health Syst Pharm*, 1995, 52(16):1798-800.

Johnson CE and Streetman DD, "Stability of Oral Suspension of Ursodiol Made From Tablets," *Am J Health Syst Pharm*, 2002, 59(4):361-3.

Mallett MS, Hagan RL, and Peters DA, "Stability of Ursodiol 25 mg/mL in an Extemporaneously Prepared Oral Liquid," *Am J Health-Syst Pharm*, 1997, 54(12):1401-4.

Nahata MC, Morosco RS, and Hipple TF, "Stability of Ursodiol in Two Extemporaneously Prepared Oral Suspensions," *J Appl Ther Res*, 1999, 3:221-4.

References

Colombo C, Setchell KD, Podda M, et al, "Effect of Ursodeoxycholic Acid Therapy for Liver Disease Associated With Cystic Fibrosis," *J Pediatr*, 1990, 117(3):482-9.

Lepage G, Paradis K, Lacaille F, et al, "Ursodeoxycholic Acid Improves the Hepatic Metabolism of Essential Fatty Acids and Retinol in Children With Cystic Fibrosis," *J Pediatr*, 1997, 130(1)52-8.

Spagnuolo MI, Iorio R, Vegnente A, et al, "Ursodeoxycholic Acid for Treatment of Cholestasis in Children on Long-Term Total Parenteral Nutrition - A Pilot Study," *Gastroenterology*, 1996, 111(3):716-9.

Ullrich D, Rating D, Schroter W, et al, "Treatment With Ursodeoxycholic Acid Renders Children With Biliary Atresia Suitable for Liver Transplantation," *Lancet*, 1987, 2(8571):1324.

♦ **Urso® DS (Can)** *see* Ursodiol *on page 1586*

♦ **Urso Forte™** *see* Ursodiol *on page 1586*

♦ **UTI Relief® [OTC]** *see* Phenazopyridine *on page 1244*

♦ **Vagifem®** *see* Estradiol *on page 605*

Valacyclovir (val ay SYE kloe veer)

Medication Safety Issues
Sound-alike/look-alike issues:
Valtrex® may be confused with Valcyte™
Valacyclovir may be confused with valganciclovir

U.S. Brand Names Valtrex®

Canadian Brand Names Valtrex®

Index Terms Valacyclovir Hydrochloride

Therapeutic Category Antiviral Agent, Oral

Generic Available No

Use Treatment of herpes zoster (shingles) in immunocompetent patients; treatment of initial and recurrent episodes of genital herpes; suppression of recurrent genital herpes and reduction of heterosexual transmission of genital herpes in immunocompetent patients; suppression of genital herpes in HIV-infected individuals; treatment of herpes labialis (cold sores); used investigationally for prevention and treatment of herpes infections in both immunocompromised and immunocompetent patients

Pregnancy Risk Factor B

Lactation Enters breast milk/use caution

Contraindications Hypersensitivity to valacyclovir, acyclovir, or any component

Warnings Cases of thrombotic thrombocytopenic purpura/hemolytic uremic syndrome (TTP/HUS) occurring in patients who received a bone marrow transplant, renal transplant, or had advanced HIV disease while taking valacyclovir doses of 8 g/day have been reported. In the presence of metabolic activation to acyclovir, valacyclovir was mutagenic in mice.

Precautions Use with caution in patients with renal impairment or patients receiving concomitant nephrotoxic drugs; modify dose in patients with renal impairment.

Adverse Reactions
Cardiovascular: Hypertension, tachycardia, facial edema
Central nervous system: Headache, dizziness, depression, agitation, confusion, psychosis, hallucinations, seizures, ataxia, tremors
Dermatologic: Erythema multiforme, rash, pruritus, alopecia, photosensitivity
Endocrine & metabolic: Dysmenorrhea
Gastrointestinal: Nausea, vomiting
Hematologic: Thrombocytopenia, leukopenia, aplastic anemia, TTP/HUS
Hepatic: Elevated AST, hepatitis
Neuromuscular & skeletal: Arthralgia
Ocular: Visual disturbances
Renal: Elevated creatinine, renal failure
Miscellaneous: Anaphylaxis

Drug Interactions Probenecid, cimetidine may increase plasma concentrations of acyclovir.

Food Interactions Food does not appear to affect absorption.

Stability Store at room temperature.

Mechanism of Action Valacyclovir is rapidly converted to acyclovir by intestinal and hepatic metabolism. Thymidine kinase converts acyclovir to acyclovir monophosphate; it is further phosphorylated by cellular enzymes to acyclovir triphosphate which inhibits DNA synthesis and viral replication by competing with deoxyguanosine triphosphate for viral DNA polymerase and being incorporated into viral DNA.

Pharmacokinetics
Absorption: Rapid
Distribution: Acyclovir is widely distributed throughout the body including brain, kidney, lungs, liver, spleen, muscle, uterus, vagina, and CSF; CSF acyclovir concentration is 50% of serum concentration; crosses the placenta; excreted into breast milk
Protein binding: 13.5% to 17.9%
Metabolism: Valacyclovir is converted to acyclovir and L-valine by first-pass intestinal and/or hepatic metabolism; acyclovir is metabolized to a small extent by aldehyde oxidase, alcohol, and aldehyde dehydrogenase to inactive metabolites
Bioavailability: ~45% to 50%
Half-life:
Normal renal function:
Acyclovir:
Children: 2-3 hours
Adults: 2-3.5 hours
Valacyclovir: Adults: ~30 minutes
End-stage renal disease: Acyclovir: 14-20 hours
Time to peak serum concentration: 1.5 hours

Elimination: 88% as acyclovir in the urine. **Note:** Following oral radiolabeled valacyclovir administration, 46% of the label is eliminated in feces and 47% is eliminated in urine.

Dialysis: 33% removed during 4-hour hemodialysis session; administer dose postdialysis

Usual Dosage Oral:

Children: Limited information available.

Immunocompromised children at risk for HSV or VZV infection: One study assessing steady-state pharmacokinetics of multiple oral dose valacyclovir in immunocompromised children with normal renal function (n=28, 5-12 years of age) determined a comparable valacyclovir dosing regimen to I.V. acyclovir 250 mg/m^2 3 times/day using linear regression analysis of valacyclovir doses (mg/kg) versus acyclovir AUC over a steady-state dosing interval; a valacyclovir dosing regimen corresponding to an oral acyclovir dose of 20 mg/kg 4 or 5 times/day was also proposed (Nadal, 2002).

30 mg/kg/dose 3 times/day (corresponds to I.V. acyclovir 250 mg/m^2 or 10 mg/kg/dose 3 times/day)

20 mg/kg/dose 3 times/day (corresponds to oral acyclovir 20 mg/kg 4 or 5 times/day)

Adolescents and Adults:

Herpes labialis (cold sores): 2 g every 12 hours for 1 day

Genital herpes:

Initial episode: 1 g twice daily for 7-10 days

Recurrent episodes: Initiate within 1 day of lesion onset or first sign/symptom of an episode:

Immunocompetent patients: 500 mg twice daily for 3 days or 1 g once daily for 5 days

HIV-infected patients: 1 g 2 times/day for 5-10 days

Reduction of transmission (source partner): 500 mg once daily

Suppressive therapy:

Immunocompetent patients: 1 g once daily (500 mg once daily in patients with <9 recurrences per year)

HIV-infected patients (CD4 ≥100 cells/mm^3): 500 mg twice daily

Adults: Herpes zoster (shingles): 1g 3 times/day for 7 days

Dosing interval in renal impairment:

Herpes labialis: Adolescents and Adults:

Cl_{cr} 30-49 mL/minute: 1 g every 12 hours for 2 doses

Cl_{cr} 10-29 mL/minute: 500 mg every 12 hours for 2 doses

Cl_{cr} <10 mL/minute: 500 mg as a single dose

Herpes zoster: Adults:

Cl_{cr} 30-49 mL/minute: 1 g every 12 hours

Cl_{cr} 10-29 mL/minute: 1 g every 24 hours

Cl_{cr} <10 mL/minute: 500 mg every 24 hours

Genital herpes: Adolescents and Adults:

Initial episode:

Cl_{cr} 10-29 mL/minute: 1 g every 24 hours

Cl_{cr} <10 mL/minute: 500 mg every 24 hours

Recurrent episode: Cl_{cr} <10-29 mL/minute: 500 mg every 24 hours

Suppressive therapy: Cl_{cr} <10-29 mL/minute:

For usual dose of 1 g every 24 hours, decrease dose to 500 mg every 24 hours

For usual dose of 500 mg every 24 hours, decrease dose to 500 mg every 48 hours

HIV-infected patients: 500 mg every 24 hours

Administration Oral: May administer with or without food

Monitoring Parameters Urinalysis, BUN, serum creatinine, liver enzymes, CBC

Patient Information Report any rash, headache, nausea, vomiting, problems with vision, behavioral changes, unusual bleeding or bruising, or blood in urine or stool.

Dosage Forms Excipient information presented when available (limited, particularly for generics); consult specific product labeling.

Caplet: 500 mg, 1000 mg

Extemporaneous Preparations A 50 mg/mL oral suspension can be prepared using 2 different vehicles (Ora-Sweet® or Ora-Sweet SF®); crush eighteen 500 mg valacyclovir hydrochloride caplets into a fine powder in a mortar; add 40 mL of the vehicle, 5 mL at a time and mix thoroughly; transfer to a 180 mL amber glass bottle; rinse mortar with 10 mL of vehicle and transfer into bottle; repeat rinsing process for a total of five rinses, 10 mL each; qsad with vehicle to 180 mL; suspension is stable for 21 days when stored in an amber glass bottle under refrigeration (4°C); label "shake well" and "refrigerate".

Fish DN, Vidaurri VA, and Deeter RG. "Stability of Valacyclovir Hydrochloride in Extemporaneously Prepared Oral Liquids," *Am J Health Syst Pharm*, 1999, 56(19):1957-60.

(Continued)

Valacyclovir *(Continued)*

References

Nadal D, Leverger G, Sokal EM, et al, "An Investigation of the Steady-State Pharmacokinetics of Oral Valacyclovir in Immunocompromised Children," *J Infect Dis*, 2002, 186(Suppl 1):S123-30.
Simon MW, Fish DN, and Deeter RG, "Pharmacokinetics and Safety of Valaciclovir in Children With Epstein-Barr Virus Illness," *Drugs R D*, 2002, 3(6):365-73.

- **Valacyclovir Hydrochloride** *see* Valacyclovir *on page 1588*
- **Valcyte™** *see* Valganciclovir *on page 1590*
- **23-Valent Pneumococcal Polysaccharide Vaccine** *see* Pneumococcal Polysaccharide Vaccine (Polyvalent) *on page 1273*

Valganciclovir (val gan SYE kloh veer)

Medication Safety Issues
Sound-alike/look-alike issues:
Valcyte™ may be confused with Valium®, Valtrex®
Valganciclovir may be confused with valacyclovir

U.S. Brand Names Valcyte™

Canadian Brand Names Valcyte™

Index Terms Valganciclovir Hydrochloride

Therapeutic Category Antiviral Agent

Generic Available No

Use Treatment of cytomegalovirus (CMV) retinitis in patients with acquired immunodeficiency syndrome (AIDS); prevention of CMV disease in high-risk patients (donor CMV positive/recipient CMV negative) undergoing BMT, kidney, heart, or kidney/pancreas transplantation

Pregnancy Risk Factor C

Lactation Excretion in breast milk unknown/contraindicated

Contraindications Hypersensitivity to valganciclovir, ganciclovir, acyclovir, or any component; absolute neutrophil count <500/mm^3; platelet count <25,000/mm^3; hemoglobin <8 g/dL; not indicated for use in liver transplant patients (higher incidence of tissue-invasive CMV relative to oral ganciclovir was observed in trials)

Warnings Valganciclovir is converted to ganciclovir and shares its reproductive toxicity. Ganciclovir may adversely affect spermatogenesis and fertility. Due to its mutagenic potential, contraceptive precautions for female and male patients need to be followed during and for at least 90 days after therapy with this drug. Severe bone marrow depression, leukopenia, neutropenia, pancytopenia, thrombocytopenia, and aplastic anemia have been reported in patients receiving valganciclovir.

Precautions Use with caution in patients with pre-existing bone marrow suppression, cytopenias, or in those patients receiving myelosuppressive drugs or irradiation; adjust dose or interrupt valganciclovir therapy in patients with neutropenia and/or thrombocytopenia. Use with caution and modify dosage in patients with impaired renal function.

Adverse Reactions
Central nervous system: Fever, headache, insomnia, seizure, psychosis, hallucinations, confusion, agitation
Gastrointestinal: Diarrhea, nausea, vomiting, abdominal pain
Hematologic: Granulocytopenia, leukopenia, neutropenia, anemia, thrombocytopenia, pancytopenia, aplastic anemia, bleeding
Neuromuscular & skeletal: Peripheral neuropathy, paresthesia, tremors
Ocular: Retinal detachment
Renal: Decreased renal function, elevated serum creatinine
Miscellaneous: Infections, including sepsis; allergic reactions

Drug Interactions Immunosuppressive agents may increase hematologic toxicity; valganciclovir may increase seizure potential of imipenem/cilastatin; zidovudine (pancytopenia); may increase blood levels of zidovudine and didanosine; zidovudine may decrease ganciclovir levels; nephrotoxic drugs (ie, amphotericin, cyclosporine, tacrolimus) may have additive nephrotoxicity with ganciclovir; probenecid may decrease renal clearance of ganciclovir; didanosine may decrease blood levels of ganciclovir

Food Interactions High fat meal may increase AUC by 30%.

Stability Store tablets at room temperature.

Mechanism of Action Valganciclovir is rapidly converted to ganciclovir in the body. The bioavailability of ganciclovir from valganciclovir is increased 10-fold compared to oral ganciclovir. A dose of 900 mg achieved systemic ganciclovir exposure comparable to that achieved with the recommended 5 mg/kg doses of intravenous ganciclovir. Ganciclovir is phosphorylated to a substrate which competitively inhibits the binding of deoxyguanosine triphosphate to DNA polymerase resulting in inhibition of viral DNA synthesis.

Pharmacokinetics

Absorption: Well absorbed

Distribution: Ganciclovir: V_d: 15.26 L/1.73 m^2; distributes to most body fluids, tissues, and organs including CSF, ocular tissue, and brain

Protein binding: 1% to 2%

Metabolism: Prodrug converted to ganciclovir by intestinal mucosal cells and hepatocytes

Bioavailability: 60% (with food)

Half-life elimination: Ganciclovir: 4.08 hours; prolonged with renal impairment (up to 68 hours with severe renal impairment)

Elimination: Majority (80% to 90%) excreted as ganciclovir in the urine

Dialysis: 50% removed by a 4-hour hemodialysis

Usual Dosage Note: Valganciclovir tablets and ganciclovir capsules cannot be substituted on a mg per mg basis since they are **NOT BIOEQUIVALENT.**

Oral:

Children: Minimal information available; one center used the following for prevention of CMV disease following transplantation: 15-18 mg/kg/day for the first 100 days post-liver transplant in patients considered low-risk for CMV disease (see Clark, 2004)

Adolescents and Adults:

CMV retinitis:

Induction: 900 mg twice daily for 21 days

Maintenance: Following induction treatment or for patients with inactive CMV retinitis who require maintenance therapy: 900 mg once daily

Prevention of CMV disease following transplantation: 900 mg once daily beginning within 10 days of transplantation; continue therapy until 100 days post-transplantation

Dosage adjustment in renal impairment: Adults:

Induction dose:

Cl_{cr} 40-59 mL/minute: 450 mg twice daily

Cl_{cr} 25-39 mL/minute: 450 mg once daily

Cl_{cr} 10-24 mL/minute: 450 mg every 2 days

Maintenance dose:

Cl_{cr} 40-59 mL/minute: 450 mg once daily

Cl_{cr} 25-39 mL/minute: 450 mg every 2 days

Cl_{cr} 10-24 mL/minute: 450 mg twice weekly

Note: Valganciclovir is not recommended in patients receiving hemodialysis. For patients on hemodialysis (Cl_{cr} <10 mL/minute), it is recommended that ganciclovir be used instead of valganciclovir with dose adjusted as specified for ganciclovir.

Administration Oral: Administer with meals.

Monitoring Parameters Retinal exam at least every 4-6 weeks; CBC with differential, platelet count, serum creatinine

Patient Information Valganciclovir is not a cure for CMV retinitis. Regular follow-up ophthalmologic exams are necessary. For oral administration, take with food and maintain adequate fluid hydration. Swallow tablets whole; do not break or crush. Avoid handling broken or crushed tablets. Wash area thoroughly if contact occurs. Report fever, chills, unusual bleeding or bruising, infection, or unhealed sores or white plaques in mouth. Male and female patients need to follow contraceptive precautions during and for at least 3 months after therapy with valganciclovir.

Nursing Implications Consideration should be given to handling and disposal of valganciclovir according to guidelines issued for antineoplastic agents. Avoid direct contact of skin or mucous membranes with broken or crushed tablets.

Dosage Forms Excipient information presented when available (limited, particularly for generics); consult specific product labeling.

Tablet, as hydrochloride: 450 mg [valganciclovir hydrochloride 496.3 mg equivalent to valganciclovir 450 mg]

Extemporaneous Preparations A 60 mg/mL oral liquid preparation made from valganciclovir 450 mg tablets and a 1:1 mixture of Ora-Sweet® and Ora-Plus® was stable for 35 days when stored in an amber glass bottle under refrigeration at 4°C; grind sixteen 450 mg tablets in a mortar into a fine powder; add 10 mL of the vehicle in 1 mL increments and triturate to a paste; mix while adding the vehicle in geometric proportions to almost 120 mL. Pour the resulting mixture into a 120 mL amber glass bottle; rinse mortar with vehicle and transfer to bottle; qsad with vehicle to 120 mL; label "shake well" and "refrigerate".

Henkin CC, Griener JC, and Ten Eick AP, "Stability of Valganciclovir in Extemporaneously Compounded Liquid Formulations," *Am J Health-Syst Pharm*, 2003, 60:687-90.

References

Burri M, Wiltshire H, Kahlert C, et al, "Oral Valganciclovir in Children: Single Dose Pharmacokinetics in a Six-Year-Old Girl," *Pediatr Infect Dis J*, 2004, 23(3):263-6.

(Continued)

Valganciclovir *(Continued)*

Clark BS, Chang IF, Karpen SJ, et al, "Valganciclovir for the Prophylaxis of Cytomegalovirus Disease in Pediatric Liver Transplant Recipients," *Transplantation*, 2004, 77(9):1480.

Peyriere H, Jeziorsky E, Jalabert A, et al, "Neurotoxicity Related to Valganciclovir in a Child With Impaired Renal Function: Usefulness of Therapeutic Drug Monitoring," Ann Pharmacother, 2006, 40(1):143-6.

◆ **Valganciclovir Hydrochloride** *see* Valganciclovir *on page 1590*
◆ **Valisone® Scalp Lotion (Can)** *see* Betamethasone *on page 212*
◆ **Valium®** *see* Diazepam *on page 481*
◆ **Valorin [OTC]** *see* Acetaminophen *on page 42*
◆ **Valorin Extra [OTC]** *see* Acetaminophen *on page 42*
◆ **Valproate Semisodium** *see* Valproic Acid and Derivatives *on page 1592*
◆ **Valproate Sodium** *see* Valproic Acid and Derivatives *on page 1592*
◆ **Valproic Acid** *see* Valproic Acid and Derivatives *on page 1592*

Valproic Acid and Derivatives (val PROE ik AS id & dah RIV ah tivs)

Medication Safety Issues
Sound-alike/look-alike issues:
Depakene® may be confused with Depakote®
Depakote® may be confused with Depakene®, Depakote® ER, Senokot®

Related Information
Antiepileptic Drugs *on page 1902*
Blood Level Sampling Time Guidelines *on page 1914*
Febrile Seizures *on page 1898*
Serotonin Syndrome *on page 1955*

U.S. Brand Names Depacon®; Depakene®; Depakote®; Depakote® ER; Depakote® Sprinkle

Canadian Brand Names Alti-Divalproex; Apo-Divalproex®; Apo-Valproic®; Depakene®; Epival® I.V.; Gen-Divalproex; Novo-Divalproex; Nu-Divalproex; PMS-Valproic Acid; PMS-Valproic Acid E.C.; Rhoxal-valproic; Sandoz-Valproic

Index Terms Dipropylacetic Acid; Divalproex Sodium; DPA; 2-Propylpentanoic Acid; 2-Propylvaleric Acid; Valproate Semisodium; Valproate Sodium; Valproic Acid; VPA

Therapeutic Category Anticonvulsant, Miscellaneous; Infantile Spasms, Treatment

Generic Available Yes: Capsule (excluding sprinkle), injection, syrup

Use All products: Monotherapy and adjunctive therapy in the treatment of patients with complex partial seizures; monotherapy and adjunctive therapy of simple and complex absence seizures; adjunctive therapy in patients with multiple seizure types that include absence seizures; has also been used to treat mixed seizure types, myoclonic and generalized tonic-clonic (grand mal) seizures; may be effective in infantile spasms. **Note:** I.V. formulation is indicated for patients in whom oral administration of valproate is temporarily not feasible; has also been used in patients with absence status epileptics.

Divalproex sodium delayed-release tablets (Depakote®) are also indicated in adults for the treatment of manic episodes of bipolar disorders and the prevention of migraine headaches. Divalproex extended-release tablets (Depakote®-ER) are also indicated in adults for the treatment of acute manic or mixed episodes associated with bipolar disorder and for the prevention of migraine headaches.

Pregnancy Risk Factor D

Lactation Enters breast milk/not recommended (AAP considers "compatible")

Contraindications Hypersensitivity to valproic acid or derivatives or any component; hepatic disease or significant hepatic dysfunction; urea cycle disorders

Warnings Hepatic failure resulting in death may occur; children <2 years of age (especially those on polytherapy, with congenital metabolic disorders, with seizure disorders and mental retardation, or with organic brain disease) are at considerable risk; monitor patients closely for appearance of malaise, loss of seizure control, weakness, facial edema, anorexia, jaundice and vomiting; hepatotoxicity has been reported after 3 days to 6 months of therapy; discontinue valproate if hepatotoxicity occurs. Pancreatitis resulting in death may occur; pancreatitis may be hemorrhagic and rapidly progress to death; onset has occurred shortly after starting therapy and after several years of treatment; monitor patients closely for nausea, vomiting, anorexia, and abdominal pain and evaluate promptly; discontinue valproate if pancreatitis occurs. Dose-related thrombocytopenia may occur. I.V. valproate is not recommended for the prophylaxis of post-traumatic seizures in patients with acute head trauma

Hyperammonemic encephalopathy, which was sometimes fatal, has been reported following initiation of valproate therapy in patients with known or suspected urea cycle disorders (UCD) (particularly ornithine transcarbamylase deficiency). Before valproate therapy is started, evaluation for UCD should be considered in patients with

1) a history of unexplained coma or encephalopathy, encephalopathy associated with a protein load, unexplained mental retardation, pregnancy-related encephalopathy, postpartum encephalopathy, or history of increased plasma ammonia or glutamine; 2) cyclical vomiting and lethargy, episodic extreme irritability, ataxia, low BUN, or protein avoidance; 3) family history of UCD or family history of unexplained infant deaths (especially males); 4) other signs and symptoms of UCD. Patients who develop symptoms of hyperammonemic encephalopathy during therapy with valproate should receive prompt treatment; valproate therapy should be discontinued, and patients should be evaluated for UCD.

Congenital malformations such as neural tube defects (eg, spina bifida), craniofacial defects, cardiovascular malformations, and anomalies of other body systems may occur. Use in women of childbearing potential requires that benefits of use in mother be weighed against the potential risk to fetus, especially when used for conditions not associated with permanent injury or risk of death (eg, migraine). Maternal use of valproate during pregnancy may result in clotting abnormalities or hepatic failure in the newborn.

Precautions Hyperammonemia may occur, even in the absence of liver enzyme abnormalities; asymptomatic elevations of ammonia require continued monitoring; discontinuation of valproate should be considered if elevations persist. Hyperammonemic encephalopathy should be considered in patients with unexplained lethargy, vomiting, or changes in mental status and serum ammonia should be measured; valproate should be discontinued in symptomatic patients with elevated serum ammonia; hyperammonemia should be treated and patients should be evaluated for UCD. Concurrent use of valproic acid with topiramate may result in hyperammonemia with or without encephalopathy; use with caution in patients with inborn errors of metabolism or decreased hepatic mitochondrial activity; these patients may be at increased risk.

Multiorgan hypersensitivity reactions have been rarely reported in adults and pediatric patients in association with initiation of valproic acid use; at least one death has been reported; patient may present with fever and rash in association with symptoms of organ system dysfunction [eg, lymphadenopathy, hepatitis, abnormalities in liver function tests, hematologic abnormalities (eosinophilia, neutropenia, thrombocytopenia), pruritus, oliguria, nephritis, arthralgia, asthenia]; valproate should be discontinued in patients suspected of having multiorgan hypersensitivity reactions.

Valproate may stimulate the replication of HIV and CMV *in vitro*; clinical effects are unknown. CNS depression may occur with valproic acid use. Patients must be cautioned about performing tasks which require mental alertness (operating machinery or driving). Effects with other sedative drugs or ethanol may be potentiated. Anticonvulsants should not be discontinued abruptly because of the possibility of increasing seizure frequency; valproic acid should be withdrawn gradually to minimize the potential of increased seizure frequency, unless safety concerns require a more rapid withdrawal. Patients treated for bipolar disorder should be monitored closely for clinical worsening or suicidality; prescriptions should be written for the smallest quantity consistent with good patient care.

Adverse Reactions

Cardiovascular: Chest pain, hypertension, palpitation, peripheral edema, tachycardia

Central nervous system: Drowsiness, somnolence, irritability, confusion, restlessness, nervousness, hyperactivity, malaise, headache, ataxia, dizziness, abnormal dreams, amnesia, anxiety, abnormal coordination, depression, personality disorder; hyperammonemic encephalopathy (in patients with UCD; see Warnings)

Dermatologic: Alopecia, erythema multiforme, bruising, dry skin, petechia, pruritus, rash

Endocrine & metabolic: Hyperammonemia, impaired fatty-acid oxidation, carnitine deficiency, weight gain, amenorrhea, dysmenorrhea

Gastrointestinal: Nausea, vomiting, diarrhea, dyspepsia, constipation, abdominal pain, anorexia, increase appetite, eructation, flatulence, hematemesis, pancreatitis (potentially fatal), taste perversion (I.V.)

Genitourinary: Urinary frequency, urinary incontinence, vaginitis

Hematologic: Thrombocytopenia [risk increases significantly with serum levels ≥110 mcg/mL (females) or ≥135 mcg/mL (males)], prolongation of bleeding time

Hepatic: Transiently elevated liver enzymes, liver failure (can be fatal; see Warnings)

Local: I.V.: Pain and local reaction at injection site

Neuromuscular & skeletal: Tremor, asthenia, abnormal gait, arthralgia, back pain, hypertonia, leg cramps, myalgia, myasthenia, paresthesia, twitching

Ocular: Diplopia, blurred vision, nystagmus

Otic: Deafness, otitis media, tinnitus

Respiratory: Cough increased, dyspnea, epistaxis, pharyngitis, pneumonia, sinusitis

Miscellaneous: Multiorgan hypersensitivity reactions (rare, but potentially fatal; see Precautions)

(Continued)

Valproic Acid and Derivatives *(Continued)*

Drug Interactions Cytochrome P450 isoenzyme CYP2C19 substrate; CYP2C9 and CYP2D6 isoenzyme inhibitor, CYP3A3/4 isoenzyme inhibitor (weak)

Valproic acid may displace phenytoin and diazepam from protein binding sites. Aspirin may displace valproic acid from protein binding sites which may result in toxicity. Valproic acid may significantly increase phenobarbital serum concentrations in patients receiving phenobarbital or primidone. Valproic acid may increase zidovudine, amitriptyline, or nortriptyline concentrations; valproic acid may inhibit the metabolism of lamotrigine and phenytoin. Phenobarbital, primidone, phenytoin, carbamazepine, and meropenem may decrease serum levels of valproic acid; felbamate may increase plasma concentrations of valproic acid; antacids may increase the oral absorption of valproic acid. Use with lamotrigine may increase risk of lamotrigine-associated skin rash, including Stevens-Johnson syndrome and toxic epidermal necrolysis. Use with risperidone may result in generalized edema (case report). Concomitant use with clonazepam may induce absence status. Concomitant use with topiramate may result in hyperammonemia with or without encephalopathy (see Precautions).

Food Interactions Dietary carnitine requirements may be increased; food may decrease the rate but not the extent of absorption

Stability

Depakote® tablets and Depakene® solution: Store below 30°C (86°F)

Depakote® Sprinkles: Store below 25°C (77°F)

Depakote® ER: Store at controlled room temperature of 25°C (77°F); excursions permitted to 15°C to 30°C (59°F to 86°F)

Depakene® capsule: Store at 15°C to 25°C (59°F to 77°F)

Depacon® injection: Store vials at controlled room temperature of 15°C to 30°C (59°F to 86°F). Stable for at least 24 hours at room temperature when diluted in D_5W, NS, or LR and stored in glass or polyvinyl chloride bags. Discard unused portion of vial (does not contain preservative).

Mechanism of Action Causes increased availability of gamma-aminobutyric acid (GABA), an inhibitory neurotransmitter, to brain neurons or may enhance the action of GABA or mimic its action at postsynaptic receptor sites

Pharmacokinetics

Protein binding: 80% to 90% (dose dependent); decreased protein binding in neonates and patients with renal impairment or chronic hepatic disease

Distribution: Distributes into CSF at concentrations similar to unbound concentration in plasma (ie, ~10% of total plasma concentration)

Metabolism: Extensive in liver via glucuronide conjugation and oxidation

Bioavailability: Oral (all products except Depakote®-ER): Equivalent to I.V.; **Depakote®-ER tablets are not bioequivalent to Depakote® delayed release tablets**; mean bioavailability of Depakote®-ER tablets is 81% to 89%, relative to Depakote® delayed release tablets; recent studies in adults show that when Depakote®-ER is administered in doses 8% to 20% higher than the total daily dose of Depakote®, then the 2 products are bioequivalent. In patients 10-17 years of age, once-daily administration of Depakote®-ER produced valproic acid plasma concentration-time profiles similar to adults.

Half-life: Increased with liver disease

- Newborns (exposed to VPA *in utero*): 30-60 hours
- Newborns 1st week of life: 40-45 hours
- Newborns <10 days: 10-67 hours
- Children >2 months: 7-13 hours
- Children 2-14 years: Mean: 9 hours; range: 3.5-20 hours
- Adults: 8-17 hours

Time to peak serum concentration:

- Oral: 1-4 hours; divalproex (enteric coated): 3-5 hours
- I.V.: At the end of the infusion

Elimination: 2% to 3% excreted unchanged in urine; faster clearance in children who receive other antiepileptic drugs and those who are younger; age and polytherapy explain 80% of interpatient variability in total clearance; children >10 years of age have pharmacokinetic parameters similar to adults

Usual Dosage Note: Use of Depakote®-ER in pediatric patients <10 years of age is not recommended; do not confuse Depakote®-ER with Depakote®. **Erroneous substitution of Depakote® (delayed release tablets) for Depakote®-ER has resulted in toxicities; only Depakote®-ER is intended for once daily administration.**

Seizures: Children and Adults:

Oral: Initial: 10-15 mg/kg/day in 1-3 divided doses; increase by 5-10 mg/kg/day at weekly intervals until therapeutic levels are achieved; maintenance: 30-60 mg/kg/day in 2-3 divided doses; Depakote® and Depakote® Sprinkle can be given twice daily

Note: Children receiving more than 1 anticonvulsant (ie, polytherapy) may require doses up to 100 mg/kg/day in 3-4 divided doses. Due to differences in bioavailability, children ≥10 years of age and adult epilepsy patients receiving Depakote® may be switched to Depakote®-ER by using a once-daily Depakote®-ER dose that is 8% to 20% higher than the total daily dose of Depakote® (see Depakote®-ER package insert for details)

I.V.: Total daily I.V. dose is equivalent to the total daily oral dose, however, I.V. dose should be divided with a frequency of every 6 hours; if I.V. form is administered 2-3 times/day, close monitoring of trough levels is recommended; switch patients to oral product as soon as clinically possible (I.V. use has not been studied for >14 days)

Rectal: Dilute syrup 1:1 with water for use as a retention enema; loading dose: 17-20 mg/kg one time; maintenance: 10-15 mg/kg/dose every 8 hours

Prophylaxis of migraine headaches: Adults: Oral:

Depakote®: Initial: 250 mg twice daily; increase dose based on patient response; maximum dose: 1000 mg/day

Depakote®-ER: Initial: 500 mg once daily for 7 days; may increase if needed to 1000 mg once daily; range: 500-1000 mg/day; dose should be individualized; if smaller dosage adjustments are needed, use Depakote® delayed release tablets; may initiate treatment with lower dose of Depakote® delayed release tablet in patients who have GI upset

Mania: Adults: Oral:

Depakote®: Initial: 750 mg/day in divided doses; adjust dose as rapidly as possible to desired clinical effect or plasma concentration; maximum recommended dose: 60 mg/kg/day

Depakote®-ER: Initial 25 mg/kg/day given once daily; increase dose rapidly to achieve lowest therapeutic dose (based on clinical effects) or target range of serum concentrations; maximum recommended dose: 60 mg/kg/day

Dosing adjustment in renal impairment: Cl_{cr} <10 mL/minute: No dosage adjustment is needed for patients on hemodialysis (unbound clearance of valproate is reduced (27%) in these patients, but hemodialysis reduces valproate concentrations by ~20%). Protein binding is reduced in patients with renal impairment; monitoring only total valproate serum concentrations may be misleading.

Dosing adjustment in hepatic impairment: Valproic acid is contraindicated in patients with hepatic disease or significant hepatic dysfunction. Potentially fatal hepatotoxicity may occur with valproic acid use (see Warnings). Clearance is decreased in patients with liver impairment. Hepatic disease is also associated with decreased albumin concentrations and 2- to 2.6-fold increase in the unbound fraction of valproate. Free concentrations of valproate may be elevated while total concentrations appear normal.

Administration

Oral: May administer with food to decrease adverse GI effects. Do not administer with carbonated drinks; do not administer tablet with milk. May mix contents of Depakote® Sprinkle capsule with semisolid food (eg, applesauce, pudding, mashed potatoes) and swallow immediately; do not crush or chew sprinkle beads; do not store drug food mixture for later use. Swallow delayed release and extended release tablets whole; do not crush, break, or chew.

I.V.: Dilute dose with at least 50 mL of D_5W, NS, or LR; infuse over 60 minutes; maximum infusion rate: 20 mg/minute; **Note:** Rapid infusions may be associated with an increase in adverse effects; a limited number of patients have received infusions of ≤15 mg/kg administered over 5-10 minutes (1.5-3 mg/kg/minute); patients generally tolerated these faster infusion rates, but the study was not designed to directly compare adverse effects with the recommended 1 hour infusion rate, or to assess efficacy.

Monitoring Parameters Liver enzymes, bilirubin, serum ammonia, CBC with platelets, serum concentrations, PT/PTT (especially prior to surgery)

Reference Range

Epilepsy:

Therapeutic: 50-100 mcg/mL (SI: 350-690 micromoles/L)

Toxic: >100-150 mcg/mL (SI: >690-1040 micromoles/L)

Seizure control may improve at levels >100 mcg/mL (SI: >690 micromoles/L), but toxicity may occur

Mania: Therapeutic trough: 50-125 mcg/mL (SI: 350-860 micromoles/L)

Test Interactions False-positive result for urine ketones; altered thyroid function tests

Patient Information Avoid alcohol. May cause drowsiness and impair ability to perform activities requiring mental alertness and physical coordination. Notify physician if nausea, vomiting, unexplained lethargy, change in mental status, general feeling of weakness, loss of appetite, abdominal pain, yellow skin, bleeding, or easy bruising occur. Report fever associated with rash, swelling, or other organ system involvement immediately to physician.

(Continued)

Valproic Acid and Derivatives *(Continued)*

Nursing Implications Instruct patients/parents to report signs or symptoms of hepatotoxicity, pancreatitis, hyperammonemic encephalopathy, and multiorgan hypersensitivity reactions (see Warnings and Precautions). GI side effects of divalproex may be less than valproic acid

Additional Information A valproic acid associated Reye's-like syndrome has been reported (see Hilmas, 2000). Acute intoxications: Naloxone may reverse the CNS depressant effects but may also block the action of other anticonvulsants; carnitine may reduce the ammonia level; multiple dosing of activated charcoal can enhance elimination.

Routine prophylactic use of carnitine in children receiving valproic acid to avoid carnitine deficiency and hepatotoxicity is probably not indicated (Freeman, 1994); a case of fatal hepatotoxic reaction has been reported in a child receiving valproic acid despite carnitine supplementation (Murphy, 1993)

Sodium content of valproate sodium syrup: 5 mL = 23 mg (1 mEq of sodium). Safety of I.V. form has not been well studied in children <2 years of age. Long-term usefulness of Depakote®-ER for the treatment of mania should be periodically re-evaluated in patients receiving the drug for extended periods of time (>3 weeks).

Dosage Forms Excipient information presented when available (limited, particularly for generics); consult specific product labeling. **Note:** Strength expressed as valproic acid

Capsule, as valproic acid: 250 mg
- Depakene®: 250 mg

Capsule, sprinkles, as divalproex sodium:
- Depakote® Sprinkle: 125 mg

Injection, solution, as valproate sodium: 100 mg/mL (5 mL)
- Depacon®: 100 mg/mL (5 mL) [contains edetate disodium]

Syrup, as valproic acid: 250 mg/5 mL (5 mL, 480 mL)
- Depakene®: 250 mg/5 mL (480 mL)

Tablet, delayed release, as divalproex sodium:
- Depakote®: 125 mg, 250 mg, 500 mg

Tablet, extended release, as divalproex sodium:
- Depakote® ER: 250 mg, 500 mg

References

Cloyd JC, Fischer JH, Kriel RL, et al, "Valproic Acid Pharmacokinetics in Children. IV. Effects of Age and Antiepileptic Drugs on Protein Binding and Intrinsic Clearance," *Clin Pharmacol Ther*, 1993, 53(1):22-9.

Cloyd JC, Kriel RL, Fischer JH, et al, "Pharmacokinetics of Valproic Acid in Children: I. Multiple Antiepileptic Drug Therapy," *Neurology*, 1983, 33(2):185-91.

Dreifuss FE, Santilli N, Langer DH, et al, "Valproic Acid Hepatic Fatalities: A Retrospective Review," *Neurology*, 1987, 37(3):379-85.

Freeman JM, Vining EP, Cost S, et al, "Does Carnitine Administration Improve the Symptoms Attributed to Anticonvulsant Medications?: A Double-Blinded, Crossover Study," *Pediatrics*, 1994, 93(6 Pt 1):893-5.

Hilmas E and Lee CK, "Valproic Acid-Related Reye's-Like Syndrome," *The Journal of Pediatric Pharmacy Practice*, 2000, 5(3):149-55.

Murphy JV, Groover RV and Hodge C, "Hepatotoxic Effects in a Child Receiving Valproate and Carnitine," *J Pediatr*, 1993, 123(2):318-20.

♦ **Valtrex®** *see* Valacyclovir *on page 1588*

♦ **Vanceril® AEM (Can)** *see* Beclomethasone *on page 200*

♦ **Vancocin®** *see* Vancomycin *on page 1596*

Vancomycin (van koe MYE sin)

Medication Safety Issues

Sound-alike/look-alike issues:
- I.V. vancomycin may be confused with Invanz®
- Vancomycin may be confused with vecuronium

Related Information

Blood Level Sampling Time Guidelines *on page 1914*

Compatibility of Chemotherapy and Related Supportive Care Medications *on page 1777*

Endocarditis Prophylaxis *on page 1812*

U.S. Brand Names Vancocin®

Canadian Brand Names Vancocin®

Index Terms Vancomycin Hydrochloride

Therapeutic Category Antibiotic, Miscellaneous

Generic Available Yes: Injection

Use

Parenteral: Treatment of patients with the following infections or conditions: Infections due to documented or suspected methicillin-resistant *S. aureus* or beta-lactam resistant coagulase negative *Staphylococcus*; serious or life-threatening infections (ie, endocarditis, meningitis, osteomyelitis) due to documented or suspected staphylococcal or streptococcal infections in patients who are allergic to penicillins and/or cephalosporins; empiric therapy of infections associated with central lines, VP shunts, hemodialysis shunts, vascular grafts, prosthetic heart valves

Oral: Treatment of staphylococcal enterocolitis or for antibiotic-associated pseudomembranous colitis produced by *C. difficile*

Pregnancy Risk Factor C

Lactation Enters breast milk/use caution

Contraindications Hypersensitivity to vancomycin or any component; avoid in patients with previous hearing loss

Warnings Use may result in superinfection

Precautions Use with caution in patients with renal impairment or those receiving other nephrotoxic or ototoxic drugs; dosage modification required in patients with impaired renal function

Adverse Reactions Rapid infusion associated with red neck or red man syndrome: Erythema multiforme-like reaction with intense pruritus, tachycardia, hypotension, rash involving face, neck, upper trunk, back and upper arms; red man or red neck syndrome usually develops during a rapid infusion of vancomycin or with doses ≥15-20 mg/kg/hour; reaction usually dissipates in 30-60 minutes

Cardiovascular: Cardiac arrest
Central nervous system: Fever, chills
Dermatologic: Red neck or red man syndrome, urticaria, macular skin rash
Gastrointestinal: Nausea
Hematologic: Neutropenia, eosinophilia
Local: Phlebitis
Neuromuscular & skeletal: Lower back pain
Otic: Ototoxicity associated with prolonged serum concentration >40 mcg/mL
Renal: Nephrotoxicity (higher incidence with trough concentrations >10 mcg/mL)
Miscellaneous: Hypersensitivity reactions

Drug Interactions Anesthetic agents (erythema, hypotension, hypothermia, and facial flushing); concurrent ototoxic or nephrotoxic drugs including loop diuretics, cisplatin, and aminoglycosides

Stability After the oral or parenteral solution is reconstituted, refrigerate and use within 2 weeks; incompatible with heparin, phenobarbital, and ceftazidime

Mechanism of Action Inhibits bacterial cell wall synthesis; alters bacterial-cell-membrane permeability; blocks glycopeptide polymerization of the phosphodisaccharide-pentapeptide complex in the second stage of cell wall synthesis by binding tightly to D-alanyl-D-alanine portion of cell wall precursor

Pharmacokinetics

Absorption:
- Oral: Poor
- I.M.: Erratic
- Intraperitoneal administration can result in 38% systemic absorption

Distribution: Widely distributed in body tissues and fluids including pericardial, pleural, ascites, and synovial fluids; low concentration in CSF if meninges are inflamed

Protein binding: 55%

Metabolism: <3%

Half-life, biphasic: Prolonged significantly with reduced renal function
- Terminal:
  - Newborns: 6-10 hours
  - 3 months to 4 years: 4 hours
  - >3 years: 2.2-3 hours
  - Adults: 5-8 hours

Elimination: Primarily via glomerular filtration; excreted as unchanged drug in the urine (80% to 90%); oral doses are excreted primarily in the feces; presence of malignancy in children is associated with an increase in vancomycin clearance

Dialysis: Not dialyzable (0% to 5%)

Usual Dosage Initial dosage recommendation:

Neonates: I.V.:
- Postnatal age ≤7 days:
  - <1200 g: 15 mg/kg/day given every 24 hours
  - 1200-2000 g: 10-15 mg/kg/dose given every 12-18 hours
  - >2000 g: 10-15 mg/kg/dose given every 8-12 hours
- Postnatal age >7 days:
  - <1200 g: 15 mg/kg/day given every 24 hours
  - 1200-2000 g: 10-15 mg/kg/dose given every 8-12 hours
  - >2000 g: 15-20 mg/kg/dose given every 8 hours

Infants >1 month and Children: I.V.: 40 mg/kg/day in divided doses every 6-8 hours

(Continued)

Vancomycin *(Continued)*

Nonobese pediatric cancer patients with normal renal function (n=28, age range: 9 months to 13 years): initial dosage regimen of 60 mg/kg/day divided every 6 hours has been recommended

Staphylococcal CNS infection: I.V.: 60 mg/kg/day in divided doses every 6 hours; maximum dose: 1 g/dose

Adults (with normal renal function): I.V.: 0.5 g every 6 hours or 1 g every 12 hours; maximum dose: 4 g/day

Dosing interval in renal impairment:

Cl_{cr} >90 mL/minute: Administer normal dose every 6 hours

Cl_{cr} 70-89 mL/minute: Administer normal dose every 8 hours

Cl_{cr} 46-69 mL/minute: Administer normal dose every 12 hours

Cl_{cr} 30-45 mL/minute: Administer normal dose every 18 hours

Cl_{cr} 15-29 mL/minute: Administer normal dose every 24 hours

Renal dysfunction, end-stage renal disease, or on dialysis: 10-20 mg/kg; subsequent dosages and frequency of administration are best determined by measurement of serum levels and assessment of renal insufficiency

Intrathecal/intraventricular:

Neonates: 5-10 mg/day

Children: 5-20 mg/day

Adults: 20 mg/day

Oral (antibiotic-associated pseudomembraneous colitis: Metronidazole is the drug of initial choice per 2000 Red Book recommendations):

Children: 40 mg/kg/day in divided doses every 6 hours for 7-10 days; not to exceed 2 g/day

Adults: 0.5-2 g/day in divided doses every 6-8 hours

Prophylaxis of endocarditis in penicillin allergic patients: I.V.:

GI or genitourinary procedures:

Children: 20 mg/kg 1 hour prior to the procedure **plus** gentamicin 1.5 mg/kg 30 minutes prior to the procedure

Adults: 1 g 1 hour prior to the procedure **plus** gentamicin 1.5 mg/kg (maximum dose: 120 mg) 30 minutes prior to the procedure

Administration

Oral: May further dilute the appropriate oral solution dose in water or with a flavoring syrup to improve the taste

Parenteral: Administer vancomycin by I.V. intermittent infusion over 60 minutes at a final concentration not to exceed 5 mg/mL; if a maculopapular rash appears on face, neck, trunk, and upper extremities, slow the infusion rate to administer dose over 1½ to 2 hours and increase the dilution volume; the reaction usually dissipates in 30-60 minutes; administration of antihistamines just before the infusion may also prevent or minimize this reaction

Intrathecal/Intraventricular: Dilute in NS without preservatives to a final concentration between 2-5 mg/mL

Monitoring Parameters Periodic renal function tests, urinalysis, serum vancomycin concentrations, WBC; audiogram (in patients who concurrently receive ototoxic chemotherapy)

Reference Range

Peak: 25-40 mcg/mL

Trough: 5-10 mcg/mL

Patient Information Report pain at infusion site; dizziness, fullness or ringing in ears with I.V. use

Nursing Implications Do not administer I.M.; peak levels are drawn 30 minutes to 1 hour after the completion of a 1-hour infusion; troughs are obtained just before the next dose

Dosage Forms Excipient information presented when available (limited, particularly for generics); consult specific product labeling.

Capsule (Vancocin®): 125 mg, 250 mg

Infusion [premixed in iso-osmotic dextrose] (Vancocin®): 500 mg (100 mL); 1 g (200 mL)

Injection, powder for reconstitution: 500 mg, 1 g, 5 g, 10 g

References

American Academy of Pediatrics Committee on Infectious Diseases, "Treatment of Bacterial Meningitis," *Pediatrics*, 1988, 81(6):904-7.

Chang D, "Influence of Malignancy on the Pharmacokinetics of Vancomycin in Infants and Children," *Pediatr Infect Dis J*, 1995, 14(8):667-73.

Chang D, Liem L, and Malogolowkin M, "A Prospective Study of Vancomycin Pharmacokinetics and Dosage Requirements in Pediatric Cancer Patients," *Pediatr Infect Dis J*, 1994, 13(11):969-74.

Leonard MB, Koren G, Stevenson DK, et al, "Vancomycin Pharmacokinetics in Very Low Birth Weight Neonates," *Pediatr Infect Dis J*, 1989, 8(5):282-6.

Matzke GR, Zhanel GG, and Guay DRP, "Clinical Pharmacokinetics of Vancomycin," *Clin Pharmacokinet*, 1986, 11(4):257-82.

Rodvold KA, Everett JA, Pryka RD, and Kraus DM, "Pharmacokinetics and Administration Regimens of Vancomycin in Neonates, Infants and Children," *Clin Pharmacokinet*, 1997, 33(1):32-51.
Rybak MJ, Albrecht LM, Boike SC, et al, "Nephrotoxicity of Vancomycin, Alone and With an Aminoglycoside," *J Antimicrob Chemother*, 1990, 25(4):679-87.

♦ **Vancomycin Hydrochloride** *see* Vancomycin *on page 1596*
♦ **Vandazole™** *see* Metronidazole *on page 1049*
♦ **Vanos™** *see* Fluocinonide *on page 674*
♦ **Vantin®** *see* Cefpodoxime *on page 314*
♦ **VAQTA®** *see* Hepatitis A Vaccine *on page 761*
♦ **Varicella, Measles, Mumps, and Rubella Vaccine** *see* Measles, Mumps, Rubella, and Varicella Virus Vaccine *on page 982*

Varicella Virus Vaccine (var i SEL a VYE rus vak SEEN)

Medication Safety Issues

Sound-alike/look-alike issues:

Varicella virus vaccine has been given in error (instead of the indicated varicella immune globulin) to pregnant women exposed to varicella.

Both varicella vaccine and zoster vaccine are live, attenuated strains of varicella-zoster virus. Their indications, dosing, and composition are distinct. Varicella is indicated in children to prevent chickenpox, while zoster vaccine is indicated in older individuals to prevent reactivation of the virus which causes shingles. Zoster vaccine is **not** a substitute for varicella vaccine and should not be used in children.

Related Information

Immunization Guidelines *on page 1837*

U.S. Brand Names Varivax®

Canadian Brand Names Varilrix®; Varivax® III

Index Terms Chickenpox Vaccine; Varicella-Zoster Virus (VZV) Vaccine (Varicella); VZV Vaccine (Varicella)

Therapeutic Category Vaccine

Generic Available No

Use Immunization against varicella in children ≥12 months of age and adults

Pregnancy Risk Factor C

Lactation Excretion in breast milk unknown/use caution

Contraindications Hypersensitivity to any component of the vaccine, including gelatin; a history of anaphylactoid reaction to neomycin; individuals with blood dyscrasias, leukemia, lymphomas, or other malignant neoplasms affecting the bone marrow or lymphatic systems; those receiving immunosuppressive therapy; primary and acquired immunodeficiency states including those who are immunosuppressed in association with HIV; a family history of congenital or hereditary immunodeficiency; active untreated tuberculosis; current febrile illness; pregnancy

Warnings Immediate treatment for anaphylactoid reaction should be available during vaccine use; salicylates should be avoided for 6 weeks after vaccination; defer vaccination at least 3 months after receiving blood and plasma transfusions or immune globulin (See Appendix Immunization Guidelines, "Suggested Intervals Between Administration of Immune Globulin Preparations for Various Indications and Measles Immunization"); vaccinated individuals should not have close association with susceptible high risk individuals (newborns, pregnant women, immunocompromised persons) for 6 weeks following vaccination. Children with HIV infection, who are asymptomatic and not immunosuppressed (CDC immunologic category 1) may receive varicella vaccine at 12-15 months of age or older.

Adverse Reactions **All serious adverse reactions must be reported to the U.S. Department of Health and Human Services (DHHS) Vaccine Adverse Event Reporting System (VAERS) 1-800-822-7967.**

Central nervous system: Fever (10% to 15%), chills, fatigue, headache, irritability, malaise, nervousness, sleep disturbance, febrile and nonfebrile seizures, ataxia, Bell's palsy, cerebrovascular accident, dizziness, encephalitis

Dermatologic: Generalized varicella-like rash (4% to 5%), contact rash, dermatitis, diaper rash, dry skin, eczema, heat rash, itching, cellulites, erythema multiforme, Henoch-Schönlein purpura, impetigo, Stevens-Johnson syndrome, secondary skin infections

Gastrointestinal: Abdominal pain, appetite decreased, cold/canker sore, constipation, nausea, vomiting, diarrhea

Hematologic: Lymphadenopathy, thrombocytopenia

Local: Injection site reaction (19% to 24%), varicella-like rash at the injection site (3%)

Neuromuscular & skeletal: Arthralgia, myalgia, stiff neck, paresthesia, Guillain-Barré syndrome, transverse myelitis

Ophthalmic: Eye complaints

Otic: Otitis

(Continued)

Varicella Virus Vaccine *(Continued)*

Respiratory: Cough, lower and upper respiratory illness, pneumonitis, pharyngitis

Miscellaneous: Allergic reactions, teething, herpes zoster

Drug Interactions Salicylates may increase the risk of Reye's following varicella vaccination; avoid use of salicylates for 6 weeks following vaccination. Immunosuppressant medications may decrease the effectiveness of the vaccine and increase the risk of varicella disease in these patients; avoid high doses of systemic corticosteroids for ≥14 days, wait at least 1 month between discontinuing steroid therapy and administering vaccine. Immune globulin (including varicella zoster immune globulin) may decrease effectiveness of vaccine; do not administer together; vaccination should be deferred for at least 3 months following immune globulin administration (See Appendix Immunization Guidelines, "Suggested Intervals Between Administration of Immune Globulin Preparations for Various Indications and Measles Immunization")

Stability Powder stable refrigerated for 18 months; may also be frozen. If transferred to refrigerator from freezer, do not refreeze. Protect from light; store diluent separately at room temperature or in refrigerator. Discard reconstituted vaccine if not used within 30 minutes; do not freeze reconstituted vaccine.

Mechanism of Action As a live, attenuated vaccine, varicella virus vaccine offers active immunity to disease caused by the varicella-zoster virus

Pharmacodynamics Onset of action: Seroconversion: ~4-6 weeks

Usual Dosage SubQ:

Children: Initial dose: Minimum age 12 months: 0.5 mL

Booster dose: 4-6 years: 0.5 mL (second dose may be administered prior to age 4-6 years if >3 months since initial dose and both doses are administered at age >12 months. If second dose was administered >28 days following the first dose, the second dose does not need to be repeated.

Children 7-13 years: Initial 0.5 mL followed by second dose at least 3 months later; do not repeat the second dose if administered >28 days following the first dose

Children >13 years to Adult: 0.5 mL followed by a second dose at least 4 weeks later

Administration Use 0.7 mL of the provided diluent to reconstitute vaccine. Gently agitate to mix thoroughly. Total volume of reconstituted vaccine will be ~0.5 mL. Inject into the outer aspect of the upper arm or anterolateral aspect of the thigh; **not for I.V. or I.M. administration.**

Monitoring Parameters Rash, fever

Patient Information Report any adverse reactions to your healthcare provider or Vaccine Adverse Event Reporting System (1-800-822-7967); avoid pregnancy for 3 months following vaccination; avoid salicylates for 6 weeks after vaccination; avoid close association with susceptible high risk individuals following vaccination

Nursing Implications Federal law requires that the date of administration, the vaccine manufacturer, lot number of vaccine, and the administering person's name, title and address be entered into the patient's permanent medical record.

Dosage Forms Excipient information presented when available (limited, particularly for generics); consult specific product labeling. [CAN] = Canadian brand name

Injection, powder for reconstitution [preservative free]:

Varivax®: 1350 plaque-forming units (PFU) [contains gelatin and trace amounts of neomycin; packaged with diluent]

Varivax® III [CAN]: 1350 plaque-forming units (PFU) [contains gelatin and trace amounts of neomycin; packaged with diluent; not available in U.S.]

Injection, powder for reconstitution (Valrilix® [CAN]): $10^{3.3}$ plaque-forming units (PFU) [contains albumin and gelatin; packaged with diluent; not available in U.S.]

References

American Academy of Pediatrics Committee on Infectious Diseases, "Recommended Immunization Schedules for Children and Adolescents - United States, 2007," *Pediatrics*, 2007, 119(1):207-8.

Centers for Disease Control, "Recommended Adult Immunization Schedule by Age Group and Medical Conditions, United States, 2003-2004," available at www.cdc.gov.

Kuter BJ, Weibel RE, Guess HA, et al, "Oka/Merck Varicella Vaccine in Healthy Children: Final Report of a 2-Year Efficacy Study and 7-Year Follow-Up Studies," *Vaccine*, 1991, 9(9):643-7.

US Public Health Service (USPHS), Infectious Diseases Society of America (IDSA), USPHS/IDSA Prevention of Opportunistic Infections Working Group, "2001 USPHS/IDSA Guidelines for the Prevention of Opportunistic Infections in Persons Infected With Human Immunodeficiency Virus," *HIV Clin Trials*, 2001, 2(6):493-554.

Varicella-Zoster Immune Globulin (Human) [DSC]

(var i SEL a- ZOS ter i MYUN GLOB yoo lin HYU man)

Related Information

Immunization Guidelines *on page 1837*

Index Terms VZIG
Therapeutic Category Immune Globulin
Generic Available No
Use Provide passive immunity to susceptible, immunocompromised patients after exposure to varicella.

Restrict administration to those patients meeting the following criteria:

Neoplastic disease (eg, leukemia or lymphoma)
Congenital or acquired immunodeficiency
Immunosuppressive therapy with steroids, antineoplastic agents, radiation, or other immunosuppressive treatment regimens
Newborn of mother who had onset of chickenpox within 5 days before delivery or within 48 hours after delivery
Premature (≥28 weeks gestation) whose mother has no history of chickenpox
Premature (<28 weeks gestation or ≤1000 g) regardless of maternal history

One of the following types of exposure to varicella or zoster may warrant VZIG administration in a susceptible patient:

Continuous household contact
Playmate contact (>1 hour play indoors)
Hospital contact (in same 2-4 bed room or adjacent beds in a large ward or prolonged face-to-face contact with an infectious staff member or patient)
Immunocompromised adolescents and adults and to other older patients on an individual basis

Note: Age is the most important risk factor for reactivation of varicella zoster; persons <50 years of age have incidence of 2.5 cases per 1000, whereas those 60-79 have 6.5 cases per 1000 and those >80 years have 10 cases per 1000.

Pregnancy Risk Factor C
Contraindications Hypersensitivity to VZIG, immune globulin, or any component; patients with IgA deficiency. Not for prophylactic use in immunodeficient patients with history of varicella, unless patient's immunosuppression is associated with bone marrow transplantation; not recommended for nonimmunodeficient patients, including pregnant women, because the severity of chickenpox is much less than in immunosuppressed patients; patients receiving monthly treatments of high-dose intravenous immunoglobulins (100-400 mg/kg) are likely to be protected and probably do not require VZIG if the last dose of IVIG was given in the 3 weeks before exposure. Do not administer to patients with thrombocytopenia or coagulopathies.
Warnings VZIG is not indicated for prophylaxis or therapy of normal adults who are exposed to or who develop varicella; not indicated for treatment of herpes zoster
Precautions Use of VZIG in patients with a bleeding diathesis should be avoided
Adverse Reactions

Central nervous system: Fever, headache, chills, malaise
Dermatologic: Rash, angioedema
Gastrointestinal: Emesis
Local effects: Pain, redness, swelling
Neuromuscular & skeletal: Myalgia
Miscellaneous: Hypersensitivity reactions, anaphylaxis

Drug Interactions Live virus vaccines (MMR, varicella): VZIG may interfere with the immune response; do not administer live virus vaccines within 5 months of VZIG administration
Stability Refrigerate; do not freeze
Mechanism of Action The varicella-zoster antibody present in VZIG provides passive immunity to susceptible immunodeficient patients exposed to the varicella-zoster virus by neutralizing the virus.
Pharmacodynamics Duration: 3 weeks
Usual Dosage Children and Adults: I.M.: Most effective if administered within 48-96 hours after exposure: 125 units/10 kg; maximum dose: 625 units; minimum dose: 125 units; do not give fractional doses

VZIG Dose Based on Patient Weight:

<10 kg: 125 units = 1 x 125 unit vial
10.1-20 kg: 250 units = 2 x 125 unit vials
20.1-30 kg: 375 units = 3 x 125 unit vials
30.1-40 kg: 500 units = 4 x 125 unit vials
>40 kg: 625 units = 5 x 125 unit vials or 1 x 625 unit vial

Note: High-risk, susceptible patients who are re-exposed more than 3 weeks after a prior dose of VZIG should receive another full dose; there is no evidence VZIG modifies established varicella-zoster infections

Administration Parenteral: I.M.: **DO NOT ADMINISTER I.V.** For infants and small children, administer I.M. into the anterolateral aspect of the thigh. For adults and older children, administer I.M. into the deltoid muscle or the anterolateral aspect of the thigh. For adults who require large dose volumes, may administer by deep I.M.
(Continued)

Varicella-Zoster Immune Globulin (Human) [DSC] *(Continued)*

injection into the upper, outer quadrant of the gluteal muscle. For patients ≤10 kg, administer 1.25 mL at a single site; for patients >10 kg, give no more than 2.5 mL at a single injection site.

Test Interactions False positive serologic test for immunity to varicella-zoster virus (false positive can occur for 2 months after VZIG administration)

Additional Information An acceptable alternative to VZIG prophylaxis is to treat varicella, if it occurs, with high-dose I.V. acyclovir. In susceptible children and adults for whom the varicella vaccine is not contraindicated, live varicella virus vaccine can be given within 3 to 5 days after exposure to prevent or modify infection severity. There is no evidence VZIG modifies established varicella-zoster infections.

Varicella-zoster immune globulin (VZIG) was discontinued by the manufacturer. An investigational product (VariZIG) is available under the product's IND application. Investigational Review Board (IRB) approval for this agent should be in place before accessing this product. Eligible patients include pregnant women, immunocompromised patients, neonates, or premature infants in selected situations. Inventory for anticipated patients may be obtained by contacting FFF Enterprises at 800-843-7477 and faxing a release form. The release form can be accessed from the CDC at http://www.cdc.gov/mmwr/preview/mmwrhtml/mm55e224a1.htm.

Dosage Forms Excipient information presented when available (limited, particularly for generics); consult specific product labeling.

Injection, solution [preservative free]: 125 units (1.25 mL); 625 units (6.25 mL) [DSC]

References

Centers for Disease Control and Prevention (CDC), "Prevention of Varicella: Recommendations of the Advisory Committee on Immunization Practices (ACIP), Centers for Disease Control and Prevention," *MMWR*, 1996, 45(RR-11):1-36.

Centers for Disease Control and Prevention 9CDC, "Prevention of Varicella Update: Recommendations of the Advisory Committee on Immunization Practices (ACIP)," *MMWR*, 1999, 48(RR-6):1-5.

♦ **Varicella-Zoster Virus (VZV) Vaccine (Varicella)** *see* Varicella Virus Vaccine *on page 1599*

♦ **Varilrix® (Can)** *see* Varicella Virus Vaccine *on page 1599*

♦ **Varivax®** *see* Varicella Virus Vaccine *on page 1599*

♦ **Varivax® III (Can)** *see* Varicella Virus Vaccine *on page 1599*

♦ **Vasocon® (Can)** *see* Naphazoline *on page 1106*

Vasopressin (vay soe PRES in)

Medication Safety Issues

Sound-alike/look-alike issues:

Pitressin® may be confused with Pitocin®

Related Information

Adult ACLS Algorithms *on page 1660*

U.S. Brand Names Pitressin®

Canadian Brand Names Pressyn®; Pressyn® AR

Index Terms ADH; Antidiuretic Hormone; 8-Arginine Vasopressin

Therapeutic Category Antidiuretic Hormone Analog; Hormone, Posterior Pituitary

Generic Available Yes

Use Treatment of diabetes insipidus; prevention and treatment of postoperative abdominal distention; differential diagnosis of diabetes insipidus; adjunct in the treatment of acute massive hemorrhage of GI tract or esophageal varices; treatment of pulseless arrest, ventricular fibrillation or tachycardia, asystole/pulseless electrical activity, and vasodilator shock with hypotension unresponsive to fluid resuscitation or exogenous catecholamines

Pregnancy Risk Factor B

Lactation Enters breast milk/use caution

Contraindications Hypersensitivity to vasopressin or any component

Warnings I.V. infiltration may lead to severe vasoconstriction and localized tissue necrosis

Precautions Use with caution in patients with seizure disorders, migraine, asthma, vascular disease, renal disease, cardiac disease, goiter with cardiac complications, arteriosclerosis, chronic nephritis with nitrogen retention; an increased risk of cardiac arrest has been reported in adults receiving I.V. infusions at rates >0.05 units/minute

Adverse Reactions

Cardiovascular: Circumoral pallor; with high doses: hypertension, bradycardia, arrhythmias, venous thrombosis, vasoconstriction, angina, heart block, cardiac arrest, distal limb ischemia (I.V. infusion rates >10 units/hour)

Central nervous system: Vertigo, fever, headache

Dermatologic: Urticaria
Endocrine & metabolic: Water intoxication, hyponatremia
Gastrointestinal: Abdominal cramps, nausea, vomiting, flatus, diarrhea
Local: Skin necrosis (after extravasation of I.V. infiltration)
Neuromuscular & skeletal: Tremor
Respiratory: Wheezing, bronchoconstriction
Miscellaneous: Diaphoresis

Drug Interactions

Decreased antidiuretic activity: Lithium, demeclocycline, large doses of epinephrine, heparin (therapeutic doses), alcohol

Increased antidiuretic activity: Chlorpropamide, carbamazepine, phenformin, tricyclic antidepressants, clofibrate, fludrocortisone

Mechanism of Action Endogenous hormone released by the posterior pituitary gland in response to increases in plasma osmolarity or as a baroreflex in response to decreased blood pressure and/or blood volume; increases cyclic adenosine monophosphate (cAMP) which increases water permeability at the distal convoluted tubule and collecting duct resulting in decreased urine volume and increased urine osmolality; causes peristalsis by directly stimulating the smooth muscle in the GI tract (in doses greater than those required for its antidiuretic action); causes vasoconstriction (primarily of capillaries and small arterioles); directly stimulates receptors in pituitary gland resulting in increased ACTH production; may restore catecholamine sensitivity

Pharmacodynamics I.M., SubQ:

Onset of action: 1 hour
Duration: 2-8 hours

Pharmacokinetics Destroyed by trypsin in GI tract, must be administered parenterally

Metabolism: Most of dose is rapidly metabolized in liver and kidney
Half-life: 10-35 minutes

Usual Dosage

Diabetes insipidus:

I.M., SubQ: (Highly variable dosage; titrate dosage based upon serum and urine sodium and osmolality in addition to fluid balance and urine output)

Children: 2.5-10 units 2-4 times/day
Adults: 5-10 units 2-4 times/day as needed (range: 5-60 units/day)

Continuous infusion: Children and Adults: Initial: 0.5 milliunit/kg/hour (0.0005 unit/kg/hour); double dosage as needed every 30 minutes to a maximum of 10 milliunit/kg/hour (0.01 units/kg/hour)

Abdominal distention: Adults: I.M.: 5 units initially, then repeated every 3-4 hours; dosage may be increased to 10 units if necessary

Pulseless arrest, ventricular fibrillation, or tachycardia:

Children: I.V.: Very limited case reports: 0.4 units/kg after traditional resuscitation methods and at least 2 doses of epinephrine have been used. (The American Heart Association does not recommend this use as there is insufficient evidence as yet.)

Adults: I.V., I.O.: 40 units as a single dose only (see Adult ACLS Algorithms *on page 1660*) (**Note:** May also be administered intratracheal at dose 2-2.5 times the I.V. dose)

GI hemorrhage: I.V. continuous infusion (may also be infused directly into the superior mesenteric artery):

Children: Initial: 0.002-0.005 units/kg/minute; titrate dose as needed; maximum dose: 0.01 units/kg/minute;

or as an alternative: Initial: 0.1 units/minute; increase by 0.05 units/minute to a maximum of:

<5 years: 0.2 units/minute
5-12 years: 0.3 units/minute
>12 years: 0.4 units/minute

If bleeding stops for 12 hours, then taper off over 24-48 hours

Adults: Initial: I.V.: 0.2-0.4 unit/minute, then titrate dose as needed (maximum dose: 0.9 units/minute); if bleeding stops, continue at same dose for 12 hours, taper off over 24-48 hours

Vasodilatory shock with hypotension unresponsive to fluid resuscitation and exogenous catecholamines: **Note:** Optimal dosage has not been clearly established in any patient population: I.V.:

Infants and Children: Limited study in 11 infants and children treated for profound hypotension following cardiac surgery: Initial: 0.0003-0.002 units/kg/minute (0.018-0.12 units/kg/hour); titrate to effect (Rosenzweig, 1999)

Adults: Initial: 0.01-0.1 units/minute; titrate to effect (doses >0.05 units/minute have been associated with increased risk of cardiac arrest in some patients)

Note: Abrupt discontinuation of infusion may result in hypotension; to discontinue gradually taper infusion

Dosing adjustment in hepatic impairment: Some patients with cirrhosis respond to much lower doses

(Continued)

Vasopressin *(Continued)*

Administration Parenteral:

I.V.: Continuous infusion: Dilute in NS or D_5W to a final concentration of 0.1-1 unit/mL; see Usual Dosage for rate of infusion; infusion through central line is strongly recommended

I.M.: Administer without further dilution

Intratracheal: Administer then flush with 5-10 mL NS followed by several manual ventilations

Monitoring Parameters Fluid intake and output, urine specific gravity, urine and serum osmolality, serum and urine sodium; hemoglobin and hematocrit (GI bleeding)

Reference Range Vasopressin levels:

Basal: <4 pg/mL

Water deprivation: 10 pg/mL

Shock: 100-1000 pg/mL (biphasic response)

Patient Information Avoid alcohol

Nursing Implications Monitor injection site closely (I.V. infusion) to identify early signs of decreased perfusion

Dosage Forms Excipient information presented when available (limited, particularly for generics); consult specific product labeling.

Injection, solution: 20 units/mL (0.5 mL, 1 mL, 10 mL)

Pitressin®: 20 units/mL (1 mL)

References

"2005 American Heart Association Guidelines for Cardiopulmonary Resuscitation and Emergency Cardiovascular Care," *Circulation*, 2005, 112(24 Suppl): 1-211.

"2005 American Heart Association (AHA) Guidelines for Cardiopulmonary Resuscitation (CPR) and Emergency Cardiovascular Care (ECC) of Pediatric and Neonatal Patients: Pediatric Advanced Life Support," *Pediatrics*, 2006, 117(5):1005-28.

Hodges BM and Fraser G, "Vasopressin for Vasodilatory Shock," *Hosp Pharm*, 2002, 37(11):1149-57.

Koshman SL, Zed PJ, and Abu-Laban RB, "Vasopressin in Cardiac Arrest," *Ann Pharmacother*, 2005, 39(10):1687-92.

Liedel JL, et al, "The Successful Use of Vasopressin in Children With Hypotension," *Crit Care Med*, 2001, 29(12):A63.

Mann K, Berg RA, and Nadkarni V, "Beneficial Effects of Vasopressin in Prolonged Pediatric Cardiac Arrest: A Case Series," *Resuscitation*, 2002, 52(2): 149-56.

Rosenzweig EB, Starc TJ, Chen JM, et al, "Intravenous Arginine-Vasopressin in Children With Vasodilatory Shock After Cardiac Surgery," *Circulation*, 1999, 100(19 Suppl):II182-6.

Tuggle DW, Bennett KG, Scott J, et al, "Intravenous Vasopressin and Gastrointestinal Hemorrhage in Children," *J Pediatr Surg*, 1988, 23(7):627-9.

♦ **Vasotec®** *see* Enalapril/Enalaprilat *on page 565*

♦ **VCR** *see* VinCRIStine *on page 1617*

Vecuronium (ve KYOO roe nee um)

Medication Safety Issues

Sound-alike/look-alike issues:

Vecuronium may be confused with vancomycin

Norcuron® may be confused with Narcan®

High alert medication: The Institute for Safe Medication Practices (ISMP) includes this medication among its list of drugs which have a heightened risk of causing significant patient harm when used in error.

U.S. Brand Names Norcuron® [DSC]

Canadian Brand Names Norcuron®

Index Terms ORG NC 45

Therapeutic Category Neuromuscular Blocker Agent, Nondepolarizing; Skeletal Muscle Relaxant, Paralytic

Generic Available Yes

Use Adjunct to anesthesia, to facilitate endotracheal intubation, and provide skeletal muscle relaxation during surgery or mechanical ventilation

Pregnancy Risk Factor C

Lactation Excretion in breast milk unknown/use caution

Contraindications Hypersensitivity to vecuronium or any component (see Warnings)

Warnings Ventilation must be supported during neuromuscular blockade; use only by individuals who are experienced in the maintenance of an adequate airway and respiratory support. Commercially supplied diluent contains benzyl alcohol which may cause allergic reactions in susceptible individuals; large amounts of benzyl alcohol (≥99 mg/kg/day) have been associated with a potentially fatal toxicity ("gasping syndrome") in neonates; the "gasping syndrome" consists of metabolic acidosis, respiratory distress, gasping respirations, CNS dysfunction (including convulsions, intracranial hemorrhage), hypotension and cardiovascular collapse; *in vitro* and animal studies have shown that benzoate, a metabolite of benzyl alcohol, displaces bilirubin from protein binding sites; avoid use of benzyl alcohol containing diluent in neonates; SWI may be used for reconstitution in neonates

Precautions Use with caution in patients with hepatic impairment, neuromuscular disease, myasthenia gravis; many clinical conditions may potentiate or antagonize neuromuscular blockade, see table.

Clinical Conditions Affecting Neuromuscular Blockade

Potentiation	Antagonism
Electrolyte abnormalities	Alkalosis
Severe hyponatremia	Hypercalcemia
Severe hypocalcemia	Demyelinating lesions
Severe hypokalemia	Peripheral neuropathies
Hypermagnesemia	Diabetes mellitus
Neuromuscular diseases	
Acidosis	
Acute intermittent porphyria	
Renal failure	
Hepatic failure	

Adverse Reactions Most frequent reactions are associated with prolongation of its pharmacologic effect

Cardiovascular: Arrhythmias, tachycardia, hypotension, hypertension

Dermatologic: Urticaria, rash

Neuromuscular & skeletal: Muscle weakness

Respiratory: Respiratory insufficiency, bronchospasm, apnea

Drug Interactions See table.

Potential Drug Interactions

Potentiation	Antagonism
Inhalation anesthetics	Calcium
Desflurane, sevoflurane, enflurane and isoflurane > halothane > nitrous oxide	Carbamazepine
	Phenytoin
	Steroids (chronic administration)
Antibiotics	Theophylline
Aminoglycosides, polymyxins, clindamycin, vancomycin, tetracycline	Anticholinesterases[1]
	Neostigmine, pyridostigmine, edrophonium, echothiophate ophthalmic solution
Magnesium	
Antiarrhythmics	
Quinidine, procainamide, bretylium, and possibly lidocaine	Caffeine
	Azathioprine
Diuretics	
Furosemide, mannitol, thiazides	
Amphotericin B (secondary to hypokalemia)	
Local anesthetics	
Dantrolene (directly depresses skeletal muscle)	
Beta blockers	
Calcium channel blockers	
Ketamine	
Lithium	
Succinylcholine (when administered prior to nondepolarizing neuromuscular-blocking agent)	
Cyclosporine	

[1]Can prolong the effects of acetylcholine

Stability Stable for 5 days at room temperature when reconstituted with bacteriostatic water; stable for 24 hours at room temperature when reconstituted with preservative free SWI or other compatible I.V. fluid (dextrose, NS, or LR) (avoid preservatives in neonates); do not mix with alkaline drugs

Mechanism of Action Nondepolarizing neuromuscular blocker which blocks acetylcholine from binding to receptors on motor endplate thus inhibiting depolarization

Pharmacodynamics

Onset of action: Within 1-3 minutes

(Continued)

Vecuronium *(Continued)*

Duration (dose dependent): 30-40 minutes

Pharmacokinetics

Distribution: V_d:

Infants: 0.36 L/kg

Children: 0.2 L/kg

Adults: 0.27 L/kg

Protein binding: 60% to 80%

Half-life, distribution: Adults: 4 minutes

Half-life, elimination:

Infants: 65 minutes

Children: 41 minutes

Adults: 65-75 minutes

Elimination: Vecuronium bromide and its metabolite(s) appear to be excreted principally in feces via biliary elimination (50%); the drug and its metabolite(s) are also excreted in urine (25%); the rate of elimination is appreciably reduced with hepatic dysfunction but not with renal dysfunction

Usual Dosage I.V.:

Neonates: 0.1 mg/kg/dose; maintenance: 0.03-0.15 mg/kg/dose every 1-2 hours as needed

Infants >7 weeks to 1 year: 0.1 mg/kg/dose; repeat every hour as needed; may be administered as a continuous infusion at 1-1.5 mcg/kg/minute (0.06-0.09 mg/kg/hour)

Children >1 year: 0.1 mg/kg/dose; repeat every hour as needed; may be administered as a continuous infusion at 1.5-2.5 mcg/kg/minute (0.09-0.15 mg/kg/hour)

Adults: 0.1 mg/kg/dose; repeat every hour as needed; may be administered as a continuous infusion at 1.5-2 mcg/kg/minute (0.09-0.12 mg/kg/hour)

Dosing adjustment in hepatic impairment: Dose reductions are necessary in patients with cirrhosis or cholestasis

Administration Parenteral: I.V.: Dilute vial to a maximum concentration of 2 mg/mL and administer by rapid direct injection; for continuous infusion, dilute to a maximum concentration of 1 mg/mL in D_5W, NS, or LR; use SWI instead of provided diluent (contains benzyl alcohol) in neonates (see Warnings)

Monitoring Parameters Assisted ventilation status, heart rate, blood pressure, peripheral nerve stimulator measuring twitch response

Nursing Implications Does not alter the patient's state of consciousness; addition of sedation and analgesia is recommended

Additional Information Produces minimal, if any, histamine release

Dosage Forms Excipient information presented when available (limited, particularly for generics); consult specific product labeling.

Injection, powder for reconstitution, as bromide: 10 mg, 20 mg [may be supplied with diluent containing benzyl alcohol]

References

Martin LD, Bratton SL, and O'Rourke PP, "Clinical Uses and Controversies of Neuromuscular Blocking Agents in Infants and Children," *Crit Care Med*, 1999, 27(7):1358-68.

♦ **Veg-Pancreatin 4X [OTC]** *see* Pancreatin *on page 1202*

♦ **Velosef®** *see* Cephradine *on page 325*

Venlafaxine (VEN la faks een)

Related Information

Antidepressant Agents *on page 1681*

U.S. Brand Names Effexor®; Effexor® XR

Canadian Brand Names Effexor® XR; Novo-Venlafaxine XR

Therapeutic Category Antidepressant, Serotonin/Norepinephrine Reuptake Inhibitor

Generic Available Yes: Tablet

Use Treatment of depression, generalized anxiety disorder, social anxiety disorder (social phobia), panic disorder; prevention of recurrences/relapses of depression; has also been used to treat ADHD and autism in children and obsessive-compulsive disorder and chronic fatigue syndrome in adults

Medication Guide An FDA-approved patient medication guide, which is available with the product information and at http://www.fda.gov/cder/Offices/ODS/medication_guides.htm, must be dispensed with this medication for each new outpatient prescription and refill.

Pregnancy Risk Factor C

Lactation Enters breast milk/not recommended

Contraindications Hypersensitivity to venlafaxine or any component; use of MAO inhibitors within 14 days (potentially fatal reactions may occur, see Drug Interactions); do not initiate MAO inhibitor within 7 days of discontinuing venlafaxine

Warnings Venlafaxine is not approved for use in pediatric patients. Clinical worsening of depression or suicidal ideation and behavior may occur in children and adults with major depressive disorder. In clinical trials, antidepressants increased the risk of suicidal thinking and behavior (suicidality) in children, adolescents, and young adults (18-24 years of age) with major depressive disorder and other psychiatric disorders. This risk must be considered before prescribing antidepressants for any clinical use. Short-term studies did **not** show an increased risk of suicidality with antidepressant use in patients >24 years of age and showed a decreased risk in patients ≥65 years.

Patients of all ages who are treated with antidepressants for any indication require appropriate monitoring and close observation for clinical worsening of depression, suicidality, and unusual changes in behavior, especially during the first few months after antidepressant initiation or when the dose is adjusted. Family members and caregivers should be instructed to closely observe the patient (ie, daily) and communicate condition with healthcare provider. Patients should also be monitored for associated behaviors (eg, anxiety, agitation, panic attacks, insomnia, irritability, hostility, aggressiveness, impulsivity, akathisia, hypomania, mania) which may increase the risk for worsening depression or suicidality. Worsening depression or emergence of suicidality (or associated behaviors listed above) that is abrupt in onset, severe, or not part of the presenting symptoms, may require discontinuation or modification of drug therapy.

Avoid abrupt discontinuation; discontinuation symptoms (including agitation, dysphoria, anxiety, confusion, dizziness, hypomania, nightmares, and other symptoms) may occur if therapy is abruptly discontinued or dose reduced; risk of discontinuation symptoms may be increased at higher doses and with longer duration of therapy; to discontinue therapy in patients receiving venlafaxine for >1 week, taper the dose to minimize risks of discontinuation symptoms; to discontinue therapy in patients receiving venlafaxine for ≥6 weeks, taper the dose gradually over at least 2 weeks; **Note:** Clinical trials of Effexor® XR tapered the daily dose slowly at 1 week intervals by increments of 75 mg; if intolerable symptoms occur following a decrease in dosage or upon discontinuation of therapy, consider resuming the previous dose with a more gradual taper. To reduce risk of intentional overdose, write prescriptions for the smallest quantity consistent with good patient care.

Screen individuals for bipolar disorder prior to treatment (using antidepressants alone may induce manic episodes in patients with this condition). Venlafaxine may cause sustained increase in blood pressure (dose dependent; monitor blood pressure; dose reduction or discontinuation may be needed). Serious adverse reactions may occur when venlafaxine is used in combination with serotonergic drugs (eg, triptans) or drugs that impair the metabolism of serotonin (eg, MAO inhibitors); see Drug Interactions.

Precautions Use with caution and decrease the dose in patients with renal or hepatic impairment. Use with caution in patients with seizure disorders (seizures have been reported; discontinue if seizures occur), concomitant illnesses that may affect hepatic metabolism or hemodynamic responses (eg, unstable cardiac disease, recent MI), history of mania (may activate mania or hypomania), in suicidal patients, children, or during breast-feeding in lactating women; use with caution during late third trimester of pregnancy [newborns may experience adverse effects or venlafaxine withdrawal symptoms (consider risks and benefits); see Additional Information]. Use with caution in patients receiving diuretics or those who are volume-depleted (may cause hyponatremia or SIADH); may cause mydriasis (use with caution and closely monitor patients with increased IOP or those at risk of acute narrow-angle glaucoma). May cause anxiety, nervousness, and insomnia. May cause anorexia and significant weight loss (use with caution in patients where weight loss is undesirable); may adversely affect weight and height in children (monitor closely in pediatric patients; weight loss in pediatric patients was not limited to those with venlafaxine-associated anorexia; reduction in growth rate, as assessed by height, was greater in children <12 years of age than in adolescents). May cause abnormal bleeding (eg, ecchymosis; use with caution in patients with abnormal platelet function); may cause tachycardia [use with caution in patients with underlying medical conditions (eg, recent MI, heart failure, hyperthyroidism) that may worsen with tachycardia, especially at doses >200 mg/day in adults]. In adult studies of depression, Effexor® XR was associated with an increase in QT_c interval of 4.7 msec from baseline (versus a 1.9 msec decrease for placebo); clinical significance of this effect is not known.

Adverse Reactions

Cardiovascular system: Vasodilation, hypertension (dose-related), tachycardia, chest pain, postural hypotension

Central nervous system: Headache, somnolence, dizziness, insomnia, nervousness, anxiety, abnormal dreams, yawning, agitation, confusion, abnormal thinking, depersonalization, depression, manic reaction (0.5%), seizures (0.3%); suicidal thinking and behavior (see Warnings); **Note:** Increased hyperactivity (behavioral activation) was observed in several children treated for ADHD (see Olvera, 1996)

(Continued)

Venlafaxine *(Continued)*

Dermatologic: Rash, pruritus

Endocrine & metabolic: Anorexia, weight loss (dose-related), hyponatremia, SIADH, hypercholesterolemia

Gastrointestinal: Nausea, xerostomia, constipation, diarrhea, vomiting, dyspepsia, flatulence, altered taste, abdominal pain

Genitourinary: Sexual dysfunction, urinary frequency, impaired urination, urinary retention; priapism (case report in an adolescent patient; see Samuel, 2000)

Hematologic: Abnormal bleeding, ecchymosis

Neuromuscular & skeletal: Asthenia, tremor, hypertonia, twitching, paresthesia

Ocular: Blurred vision, mydriasis

Otic: Tinnitus

Miscellaneous: Diaphoresis, chills; withdrawal symptoms following abrupt discontinuation (see Warnings)

Drug Interactions Cytochrome P450 isoenzyme CYP2D6 (O-desmethylation), CYP2E1, and CYP3A3/4 (N-demethylation) enzyme substrate; CYP2D6 enzyme inhibitor (weak)

Use within 2 weeks of MAO inhibitors or use of MAO inhibitors within 7 days of discontinuing venlafaxine may result in hyperthermia (with features similar to neuroleptic malignant syndrome), tremors, myoclonus, nausea, vomiting, diaphoresis, flushing, dizziness, seizures, and death (see Contraindications). Concurrent use with buspirone, meperidine, TCAs, SSRIs, lithium, or serotonin agonists (eg, sumatriptan) may result in serotonin syndrome (concurrent use is best avoided). Tryptophan (which can be metabolized to serotonin) and the herbal medicine St John's wort (*Hypericum perforatum*), may increase serious side effects; use of these agents is **not** recommended.

Venlafaxine significantly increases haloperidol serum concentrations (increases AUC by 70%); may increase clozapine concentrations and result in adverse effects (eg, seizures); may increase PT, PTT, or INR in patients receiving warfarin. Concurrent use with imipramine may increase serum concentrations of desipramine and 2-OH-desipramine (metabolites of imipramine). Venlafaxine may increase serum concentrations of risperidone, but does not significantly alter the disposition of the total active moiety [risperidone plus 9-hydroxyrisperidone (active metabolite)]. **Note:** Interactions of venlafaxine with other CNS agents have not been evaluated (use such drugs with caution). Venlafaxine may decrease indinavir AUC by 28% and peak serum concentrations by 36%.

Drugs that inhibit cytochrome P450 CYP2D6, CYP2E1, or CYP3A4 may inhibit the metabolism of venlafaxine (monitor for increased effect or toxicity). Cimetidine increased venlafaxine serum concentrations, but did not affect ODV (active metabolite) concentrations; no dosage adjustment is needed for most patients; however, this interaction may be more pronounced in patients with hepatic dysfunction or hypertension (use with caution and monitor in these patients). Diphenhydramine may increase venlafaxine serum concentrations. Enzyme inducers may increase the metabolism of venlafaxine, reducing its effectiveness.

Food Interactions Food does not affect bioavailability of venlafaxine or ODV (active metabolite); tryptophan supplements may increase serious side effects; its use is **not recommended**

Stability Tablets and capsules: Store at controlled room temperature, 20°C to 25°C (68°F to 77°F); Effexor® tablets: Store in a dry place, dispense in a tight container; Effexor® XR 37.5 mg capsules: Protect from light and dispense in light resistant container

Mechanism of Action Venlafaxine and o-desmethylvenlafaxine (ODV) are potent inhibitors of CNS neuronal serotonin and norepinephrine reuptake and weak inhibitors of dopamine reuptake; venlafaxine and ODV do not significantly bind to alpha-adrenergic, histamine, or muscarinic cholinergic receptors (may therefore be useful in patients at risk from sedation, hypotension and anticholinergic effects of tricyclic antidepressants); venlafaxine and ODV do not inhibit monoamine oxidase

Pharmacokinetics

Absorption: Oral: ≥92%

Distribution: Distributes into breast milk; breast milk to plasma ratio: Venlafaxine: 2.8-4.8 (mean 4.1); ODV: 2.8-3.8 (mean 3.1) (Ilett, 1998)

Mean V_d (apparent): Adults:

Venlafaxine: 7.5 ± 3.7 L/kg

ODV: 5.7 ± 1.8 L/kg

Protein binding: Venlafaxine: 27%; ODV: 30%

Metabolism: Extensive in the liver, primarily via cytochrome P450 CYP2D6 to o-desmethylvenlafaxine (ODV; active metabolite); also metabolized to N-desmethylvenlafaxine, N,O-desmethylvenlafaxine, and other minor metabolites. **Note:** Clinically important differences between CYP2D6 poor and extensive metabolizers is not expected (sum of venlafaxine and ODV serum concentrations is similar in poor and extensive metabolizers; ODV is approximately equal in activity and potency to venlafaxine)

Bioavailability: Oral: 45%

Half-life:

Adults: Venlafaxine: 5 ± 2 hours; ODV: 11 ± 2 hours

Adults with cirrhosis: Venlafaxine: Half-life prolonged by ~30%; ODV: Half-life prolonged by ~60%

Adults with renal impairment (GFR: 10-70 mL/minute): Venlafaxine: Half-life prolonged by ~50%; ODV: Half-life prolonged by ~40%

Adults on dialysis: Venlafaxine: Half-life prolonged by ~180%; ODV: Half-life prolonged by 142%

Time to peak serum concentration:

Immediate release: Venlafaxine: 2 hours; ODV: 3 hours

Extended release: Venlafaxine: 5.5 hours; ODV: 9 hours

Elimination: ~87% of dose is excreted in urine within 48 hours; 5% as unchanged drug, 29% as unconjugated ODV, 26% as conjugated ODV, and 27% as other minor metabolites

Clearance:

Adults with cirrhosis: Venlafaxine: Clearance is decreased by ~50%; ODV: Clearance is decreased by ~30%

Adults with more severe cirrhosis: Venlafaxine: Clearance is decreased by ~90%

Adults with renal impairment (GFR: 10-70 mL/minute): Venlafaxine: Clearance is decreased by ~24%; ODV: Clearance unchanged versus normal subjects

Adults on dialysis: Venlafaxine: Clearance decreased by ~57%; ODV: Clearance decreased by ~56%

Dialysis: Not likely to significantly remove drug due to large volume of distribution

Usual Dosage Oral:

Children and Adolescents: Note: Not FDA approved; see Warnings. Limited information is available.

ADHD: One open-label clinical trial and one case report are available; 16 children and adolescents (8-16 years of age; mean: 11.6 ± 2.3 years) were enrolled in a 5-week open trial of venlafaxine; doses were initiated at 12.5 mg/day for the first week; for children <40 kg, the daily dose was increased (if tolerated) by 12.5 mg each week to a maximum of 50 mg/day divided in 2 doses; for patients ≥40 kg, the daily dose was increased (if tolerated) by 25 mg each week to a maximum of 75 mg/day divided in 3 doses; mean dose: 60 mg/day (1.4 mg/kg/day) in 2-3 divided doses; 10 patients completed the study [2 were lost to follow-up; 5 discontinued therapy due to adverse effects (4 had an increase in hyperactivity; 1 had severe nausea)]; venlafaxine decreased behavioral symptoms (but not cognitive symptoms) in 7 of 16 subjects (44%) (Olvera, 1996). An initial dose of 37.5 mg given 3 times/day was used in an 11-year-old female with ADHD; the dose was slowly titrated to 100 mg given 3 times/day; after 6 weeks the patient showed moderate to marked improvement in symptoms, but developed hypertension; the dose was then decreased to 75 mg given 3 times/day with normalization of blood pressure (Pleak, 1995). Further studies are needed.

Autism: One retrospective report is available; 10 patients (3-21 years of age; mean 10.5 ± 5.6 years) with autism spectrum disorders (autism, Asperger's syndrome, and pervasive developmental disorders not otherwise specified) received initial doses of 12.5 mg/day administered once daily at breakfast; doses were gradually titrated based on clinical response and side effects; mean final dose: 24.4 mg/day; range: 6.25-50 mg/day; 6 of the 10 patients were sustained-treatment responders (Hollander, 2000). Further studies are needed.

Depression: **Note:** Due to the lack of demonstrated efficacy and concerns about an increased risk for suicidal behavior, venlafaxine should be reserved for pediatric patients with major depression who do not respond to fluoxetine or sertraline (see Dopheide, 2006).

One double-blind, placebo-controlled, 6-week study is available; 33 children and adolescents (8-17 years of age) with major depression completed the trial (16 received venlafaxine; **Note:** One patient who did not complete the study, discontinued venlafaxine due to development of a manic episode requiring hospitalization and lithium therapy); immediate release venlafaxine was used; for children 8-12 years, doses were initiated at 12.5 mg once daily for 3 days, then increased to 12.5 mg twice daily for 3 days, then increased to 12.5 mg given 3 times/day for the rest of the study; for adolescents 13-17 years, doses were initiated at 25 mg once daily for 3 days, then increased to 25 mg twice daily for 3 days, then increased to 25 mg given 3 times/day for the rest of the study; both venlafaxine and placebo patients improved over time; however, no significant difference in symptoms was noted between groups (ie, venlafaxine did not have a significant effect on symptoms or specific behaviors); the

(Continued)

Venlafaxine *(Continued)*

authors suggest this lack of efficacy may be due to the low doses used and short duration of treatment (Mandoki, 1997).

A large multicenter double-blind, placebo-controlled study of venlafaxine-ER in children and adolescents 7-17 years of age with major depression is ongoing; this study is using higher doses; initial: 37.5 mg/day for 1 week; with increases to 75 mg/day for weeks 2-8; results are not yet available (see Weller, 2000). One report of two 16-year-old patients used higher doses of venlafaxine (final doses: 112.5 mg/day and 150 mg/day) in combination with lithium to successfully treat major depression (see Walter, 1998). Further studies are needed.

Adults:

Immediate release: Depression: Initial: 75 mg/day in 2-3 divided doses; dose may be increased (if needed) by increments of up to 75 mg/day at intervals of ≥4 days as tolerated, up to 225 mg/day. **Note:** Doses >225 mg/day for outpatients (moderately depressed patients) were not more effective; more severely depressed patients may require 350 mg/day; maximum: 375 mg/day in 3 divided doses

Extended release:

Depression: Initial: Usual: 75 mg/day; may start with 37.5 mg/day for 4-7 days to allow patient to adjust to medication, then increase to 75 mg/day; dose may be increased (if needed) by increments of up to 75 mg/day at intervals of ≥4 days as tolerated, up to a maximum of 225 mg/day. **Note:** Although higher doses of the immediate release tablets have been used in more severely depressed inpatients (see above), experience with extended release capsule in doses >225 mg/day is very limited

Generalized anxiety disorder and social anxiety disorder: 75 mg/day; may start with 37.5 mg/day for 4-7 days to allow patient to adjust to medication, then increase to 75 mg/day. **Note:** Although a dose-response relationship has not been clearly established, certain patients may benefit from doses >75 mg/day; dose may be increased (if needed) by increments of up to 75 mg/day at intervals of ≥4 days as tolerated, up to a maximum of 225 mg/day

Panic disorder: Initial: 37.5 mg once daily for 7 days; may increase to 75 mg daily; dose may be increased further (if needed) by increments of up to75 mg/day at intervals of ≥7 days; maximum dose: 225 mg/day

Dosing adjustment in renal impairment: Adults: GFR 10-70 mL/minute: Decrease total daily dose by 25% to 50%

Dosing adjustment in patients on dialysis: Decrease total daily dose by 50%; withhold dose until completion of dialysis treatment; further individualization of dose may be needed

Dosing adjustment in hepatic impairment: Moderate hepatic impairment: Decrease total daily dose by 50%; further individualization of dose may be needed

Administration

Immediate release tablet: Administer with food

Extended release capsule: Administer with food once daily at about the same time each day; swallow whole with fluid; do not crush, chew, divide, or place in water; capsule may be opened and entire contents sprinkled on spoonful of applesauce; swallow drug/food mixture immediately. Do not store for future use; do not chew contents (ie, pellets) of capsule; follow drug/food mixture with water to ensure complete swallowing of pellets.

Monitoring Parameters Monitor blood pressure regularly, especially in patients with high baseline blood pressure; monitor renal and hepatic function (for possible dose reductions), heart rate, weight, height, serum cholesterol and sodium. Monitor patient periodically for symptom resolution; monitor for worsening depression, suicidality, and associated behaviors (especially at the beginning of therapy or when doses are increased or decreased; see Warnings)

Patient Information Read the Patient Medication Guide that you receive with each prescription and refill of venlafaxine. An increased risk of suicidal thinking and behavior has been reported with the use of antidepressants in children, adolescents, and young adults (18-24 years of age). Notify physician if you feel more depressed, have thoughts of suicide, or become more agitated or irritable (see Warnings). May cause dizziness or drowsiness and impair ability to perform activities requiring mental alertness or physical coordination; may cause dry mouth; report the use of other medications, nonprescription medications, and herbal or natural products to your physician and pharmacist; avoid alcohol, tryptophan supplements, and the herbal medicine, St John's wort; report skin rashes, hives, or allergic reactions to your physician. Take as directed; do not alter dose or frequency without consulting prescriber, avoid abrupt discontinuation.

Nursing Implications Mean increases in heart rate of 4 beats/minute and 8.5 beats/minute have been reported; when discontinuing therapy, dose must be tapered to minimize risk of discontinuation symptoms (see Precautions). Assess mental status for depression, suicidal ideation, anxiety, social functioning, mania, or panic attack.

Additional Information Drug release from extended release capsules is not pH dependent (it is controlled by diffusion through the coating membrane on the spheroids); patients with depression who are receiving Effexor® may be switched to Effexor® XR using the nearest mg/day equivalent dose (dosing may need further individualization)

Long-term usefulness of venlafaxine should be periodically re-evaluated in patients receiving the drug for extended periods of time. Neonates born to women receiving venlafaxine, other SNRIs (serotonin and norepinephrine reuptake inhibitors), and SSRIs late during the third trimester may experience respiratory distress, apnea, cyanosis, temperature instability, vomiting, feeding difficulty, hypoglycemia, constant crying, irritability, hypotonia, hypertonia, hyper-reflexia, tremor, jitteriness, and seizures; these symptoms may be due to a direct toxic effect, withdrawal syndrome, or (in some cases) serotonin syndrome. Withdrawal symptoms occur in 30% of neonates exposed to SSRIs and SNRIs *in utero*; monitor newborns for at least 48 hours after birth; long-term effects of *in utero* exposure to SSRIs and SNRIs are unknown (see Levinson-Castiel, 2006).

Dosage Forms Excipient information presented when available (limited, particularly for generics); consult specific product labeling. Available as venlafaxine hydrochloride; mg strength refers to venlafaxine.

Capsule, extended release:
  Effexor® XR: 37.5 mg, 75 mg, 150 mg

Tablet: 25 mg, 37.5 mg, 50 mg, 75 mg, 100 mg
  Effexor®: 25 mg, 37.5 mg, 50 mg, 75 mg, 100 mg

References

Dopheide JA, "Recognizing and Treating Depression in Children and Adolescents," *Am J Health Syst Pharm*, 2006, 63(3):233-43.

Emslie GJ, Yeung PP, and Kunz NR, "Long-Term, Open-Label Venlafaxine Extended-Release Treatment in Children and Adolescents With Major Depressive Disorder," *CNS Spectr*, 2007, 12(3):223-33.

Hollander E, Kaplan A, Cartwright C, et al, "Venlafaxine in Children, Adolescents, and Young Adults With Autism Spectrum Disorders: An Open Retrospective Clinical Report," *J Child Neurol*, 2000, 15(2):132-5.

Ilett KF, Hackett LP, Dusci LJ, et al, "Distribution and Excretion of Venlafaxine and O-Desmethylvenlafaxine in Human Milk," *Br J Clin Pharmacol*, 1998, 45(5):459-62.

Lessard E, Yessine MA, Hamelin BA, et al, "Diphenhydramine Alters the Disposition of Venlafaxine Through Inhibition of CYP2D6 Activity in Humans," *J Clin Psychopharmacol*, 2001, 21(2):175-84.

Levinson-Castiel R, Merlob P, Linder N, et al, "Neonatal Abstinence Syndrome After *in utero* Exposure to Selective Serotonin Reuptake Inhibitors in Term Infants," *Arch Pediatr Adolesc Med*, 2006, 160(2):173-6.

Mandoki MW, Tapia MR, Tapia MA, et al, "Venlafaxine in the Treatment of Children and Adolescents With Major Depression," *Psychopharmacol Bull*, 1997, 33(1):149-54.

Olvera RL, Pliszka SR, Luh J, et al, "An Open Trial of Venlafaxine in the Treatment of Attention-Deficit/Hyperactivity Disorder in Children and Adolescents," *J Child Adolesc Psychopharmacol*, 1996, 6(4):241-50.

Pleak RR and Gormly LJ, "Effects of Venlafaxine Treatment for ADHD in a Child," *Am J Psychiatry*, 1995, 152(7):1099.

Samuel RZ, "Priapism Associated With Venlafaxine Use," *J Am Acad Child Adolesc Psychiatry*, 2000, 39(1):16-7.

Walter G, Lyndon B, and Kubb R, "Lithium Augmentation of Venlafaxine in Adolescent Major Depression," *Aust N Z J Psychiatry* 1998, 32(3):457-9.

Weller EB, Weller RA, and Davis GP, "Use of Venlafaxine in Children and Adolescents: A Review of Current Literature," *Depress Anxiety*, 2000, 12(Suppl 1):85-9.

♦ **Venofer®** *see* Iron Supplements (Parenteral) *on page 870*
♦ **Ventolin® (Can)** *see* Albuterol *on page 66*
♦ **Ventolin® Diskus (Can)** *see* Albuterol *on page 66*
♦ **Ventolin® HFA** *see* Albuterol *on page 66*
♦ **Ventrodisk (Can)** *see* Albuterol *on page 66*
♦ **VePesid®** *see* Etoposide *on page 625*
♦ **Veracolate [OTC]** *see* Bisacodyl *on page 217*

Verapamil (ver AP a mil)

Medication Safety Issues

Sound-alike/look-alike issues:
  Verapamil may be confused with Verelan®
  Calan® may be confused with Colace®
  Covera-HS® may be confused with Provera®
  Isoptin® may be confused with Isopto® Tears
  Verelan® may be confused with verapamil, Virilon®, Voltaren®

Significant differences exist between oral and I.V. dosing. Use caution when converting from one route of administration to another.

International issues:
  Calan®: Brand name for vinpocetine in Japan

(Continued)

Verapamil *(Continued)*

Related Information

Antihypertensive Agents by Class *on page 1678*

Medications for Which A Single Dose May Be Fatal When Ingested By A Toddler *on page 1932*

U.S. Brand Names Calan®; Calan® SR; Covera-HS®; Isoptin® SR; Verelan®; Verelan® PM

Canadian Brand Names Alti-Verapamil; Apo-Verap®; Apo-Verap® SR; Calan®; Chronovera®; Covera®; Covera-HS®; Gen-Verapamil; Gen-Verapamil SR; Isoptin® SR; Novo-Veramil SR; Nu-Verap; Riva-Verapamil SR; Verapamil Hydrochloride Injection, USP

Index Terms Iproveratril Hydrochloride; Verapamil Hydrochloride

Therapeutic Category Antianginal Agent; Antiarrhythmic Agent, Class IV; Antihypertensive Agent; Calcium Channel Blocker

Generic Available Yes: Excludes controlled onset products

Use Orally for the treatment of angina and hypertension; I.V. for supraventricular tachyarrhythmias (PSVT, atrial fibrillation, atrial flutter)

Pregnancy Risk Factor C

Lactation Enters breast milk (small amounts)/not recommended

Contraindications Hypersensitivity to verapamil or any component; sinus bradycardia; advanced heart block; ventricular tachycardia; cardiogenic shock; atrial fibrillation or flutter associated with accessory conduction pathways

Warnings Avoid I.V. use in neonates and young infants due to severe apnea, bradycardia, hypotensive reactions, and cardiac arrest; I.V. use is discouraged in children due to hypotension and myocardial depression; monitor EKG and blood pressure closely in patients receiving I.V. therapy; have I.V. calcium chloride 10 mg/kg available at bedside to treat hypotension. I.V. administration, hypertrophic cardiomyopathy, sick sinus syndrome, moderate to severe CHF, concomitant therapy with beta-blockers or digoxin can all increase the incidence of adverse effects.

Precautions Use with caution in patients with sick sinus syndrome, severe left ventricular dysfunction, hepatic or renal impairment, hypertrophic cardiomyopathy (especially obstructive), concomitant therapy with beta-blockers or digoxin; reduce dose in patients with severe renal dysfunction; verapamil may decrease neuromuscular transmission in patients with Duchenne's muscular dystrophy and may worsen myasthenia gravis (use with caution in these patients; verapamil dosage reduction may be needed)

Adverse Reactions

Cardiovascular: Hypotension, bradycardia; first, second, or third degree A-V block, worsening heart failure

Central nervous system: Dizziness, fatigue, seizures (occasionally with I.V. use), headache

Gastrointestinal: Constipation, nausea, abdominal discomfort

Hepatic: Elevated hepatic enzymes

Otic: Tinnitus

Respiratory: May precipitate insufficiency of respiratory muscle function in Duchenne muscular dystrophy

Drug Interactions Cytochrome P450 isoenzyme CYP1A2, CYP2C8 (minor), CYP2C9 (minor), CYP2C18 (minor), and CYP3A3/4 substrate; CYP3A3/4 isoenzyme inhibitor

Increased cardiovascular adverse effects with beta-adrenergic blocking agents, digoxin, quinidine, and disopyramide. Verapamil may increase serum concentrations of caffeine, ethanol, digoxin, quinidine, carbamazepine, and cyclosporine necessitating a decrease in dosage. Combined use of verapamil with lovastatin or simvastatin may result in an increased risk of myopathy or rhabdomyolysis (dosage reduction of lovastatin and simvastatin is recommended); phenobarbital and rifampin may decrease verapamil serum concentrations by increasing hepatic metabolism. Enzyme inhibitors (eg, erythromycin, ritonavir) may increase verapamil serum concentration. Use with aspirin may increase bleeding time. Verapamil may prolong recovery from vecuronium. Avoid combination with disopyramide, discontinue disopyramide 48 hours before starting therapy, do not restart until 24 hours after verapamil has been discontinued. Verapamil may increase, decrease, or have no effect on lithium serum concentrations (monitor patients carefully).

Food Interactions Grapefruit juice may increase verapamil serum concentrations

Calan® SR and Isoptin® SR: Food may decrease bioavailability, but produces a narrow peak to trough ratio

Covera-HS®: A high fat meal does not affect absorption

Verelan®: Food does not affect rate or extent of absorption

Verelan® PM: A high fat meal slightly affects the rate, but not the extent of absorption

Stability Store injection at room temperature; protect from heat and from freezing; use only clear solutions; compatible in solutions of pH of 3-6, but may precipitate in solutions having a pH ≥6

Mechanism of Action Inhibits calcium ions from entering the "slow channels" or select voltage-sensitive areas of vascular smooth muscle and myocardium during depolarization; produces a relaxation of coronary vascular smooth muscle and coronary vasodilation; increases myocardial oxygen delivery in patients with vasospastic angina

Pharmacodynamics

Maximum effect:

Oral (nonsustained tablets): 2 hours

I.V.: 1-5 minutes

Duration:

Oral: 6-8 hours

I.V.: 10-20 minutes

Pharmacokinetics

Protein binding:

Neonates: ~60%

Adults: 90%

Metabolism: Extensive first-pass effect, metabolized in the liver to several inactive dealkylated metabolites; major metabolite is norverapamil which possesses weak hemodynamic effects

Bioavailability: Oral: 20% to 30%

Half-life:

Infants: 4.4-6.9 hours

Adults (single dose): 2-8 hours, increased up to 12 hours with multiple dosing

Increased half-life with hepatic cirrhosis

Elimination: 70% of dose excreted in urine (3% to 4% as unchanged drug), and 16% in feces

Usual Dosage

Infants <1 year: I.V.: **Not recommended** (see Warnings); administer with continuous EKG monitoring, have I.V. calcium available at bedside: 0.1-0.2 mg/kg (usual: 0.75-2 mg/dose) may repeat dose in 30 minutes if adequate response not achieved

Children 1-16 years: I.V.: 0.1-0.3 mg/kg/dose (**Note:** PALS 2000 guidelines recommend 0.1 mg/kg); maximum dose: 5 mg/dose; may repeat dose in 30 minutes if adequate response not achieved; maximum for second dose: 10 mg/dose

Children: Oral (dose not well established):

4-8 mg/kg/day in 3 divided doses

or

1-5 years: 40-80 mg every 8 hours

>5 years: 80 mg every 6-8 hours

Note: A mean daily dose of ~5 mg/kg/day (range: 2.3-8.1 mg/kg/day) was used in 22 children 15 days to 17 years of age receiving chronic oral therapy for SVT (n=20) or hypertrophic cardiomyopathy (n=2) (Piovan, 1995)

Adults:

Oral: 240-480 mg/24 hours divided 3-4 times/day or divided 1-2 times/day for sustained release products or given once daily for extended release product (see Administration); usual dosage range for hypertension (JNC 7): Immediate release: 80-320 mg/day in 2 divided doses; sustained release: 120-360 mg/day in 1-2 divided doses; extended release: 120-360 mg once daily at bedtime

I.V. (ACLS 2000 guidelines): PSVT (narrow complex, unresponsive to vagal maneuvers and adenosine, in patients with preserved cardiac function): Initial: 2.5-5 mg; if no response in 15-30 minutes and no adverse effects seen, give 5-10 mg every 15-30 minutes to a maximum total dose of 20 mg

I.V.: 5-10 mg (0.075-0.15 mg/kg); may repeat 10 mg (0.15 mg/kg) 15-30 minutes after the initial dose if needed and if patient tolerated initial dose

I.V. continuous infusion: Loading dose: 5-10 mg; may repeat in 30 minutes if adequate response is not achieved; follow with continuous infusion: 5 mg/hour; titrate dose to ventricular rate; usual: 5-10 mg/hour; range: 4-24 mg/hour. **Note**: Previously recommended doses of 0.005 mg/kg/minute (5 mcg/kg/minute) will result in doses of ~20 mg/hour and may produce adverse effects such as hypotension; lower infusion rates (5-10 mg/hour) are effective in most adult patients.

Dosing adjustment in renal impairment: Children and Adults: Cl_{cr} <10 mL/minute: Administer 50% to 75% of normal dose

Administration

Oral: Do not administer with grapefruit juice; nonsustained-release tablets can be administered with or without food; swallow extended and sustained released preparations whole, do not chew or crush; administer Calan® SR and Isoptin® SR with food on a once daily or twice daily schedule; administer Covera-HS® and Verelan® PM once daily at bedtime. Administer Verelan® (sustained release capsules) once

(Continued)

Verapamil *(Continued)*

daily in the morning; capsule may be opened and contents sprinkled on a spoonful of applesauce; swallow immediately, do not chew; do not store for future use; follow with water to ensure complete swallowing of capsule pellets; do not divide capsule

Parenteral:

I.V.: Infuse I.V. dose over 2-3 minutes; infuse I.V. over 3-4 minutes if blood pressure is in the lower range of normal: Maximum concentration: 2.5 mg/mL

I.V. continuous infusion: Final concentration for administration: 0.5-2.5 mg/mL

Monitoring Parameters EKG, blood pressure, heart rate; hepatic enzymes with long-term use

Patient Information Avoid alcohol and grapefruit juice; limit caffeine; insoluble shell of extended release tablet (eg, Covera-HS®) may appear in the stool (this is normal)

Dosage Forms Excipient information presented when available (limited, particularly for generics); consult specific product labeling.

Caplet, sustained release: 120 mg, 180 mg, 240 mg
  Calan® SR: 120 mg, 180 mg, 240 mg
Capsule, extended release, controlled onset, as hydrochloride:
  Verelan® PM: 100 mg, 200 mg, 300 mg
Capsule, sustained release, as hydrochloride: 120 mg, 180 mg, 240 mg, 360 mg
  Verelan®: 120 mg, 180 mg, 240 mg, 360 mg
Injection, solution, as hydrochloride: 2.5 mg/mL (2 mL, 4 mL)
Tablet, as hydrochloride: 80 mg, 120 mg
  Calan®: 40 mg, 80 mg, 120 mg
Tablet, extended release: 120 mg, 180 mg, 240 mg
Tablet, extended release, controlled onset, as hydrochloride:
  Covera-HS®: 180 mg, 240 mg
Tablet, sustained release, as hydrochloride: 120 mg, 180 mg, 240 mg
  Isoptin® SR: 120 mg, 180 mg, 240 mg

Extemporaneous Preparations

A 50 mg/mL oral suspension may be made using twenty 80 mg verapamil tablets (regular, not sustained release), 3 mL of purified water USP, 8 mL of methylcellulose 1% and simple syrup qs ad to 32 mL; stability is 91 days under refrigeration; shake well before use (Nahata, 2000)

A 50 mg/mL oral liquid preparation made from tablets (regular, not sustained release) and 3 different vehicles (cherry syrup, a 1:1 mixture of Ora-Sweet® and Ora-Plus®, or a 1:1 mixture of Ora-Sweet® SF and Ora-Plus®) was stable for 60 days when stored in amber plastic prescription bottles in the dark at room temperature (25°C) or under refrigeration (5°C); grind seventy-five 80 mg tablets in a mortar into a fine powder; add 40 mL of the vehicle and mix well to form a uniform paste; mix while adding the vehicle in geometric proportions to **almost** 120 mL; transfer to a calibrated bottle and qsad with vehicle to make 120 mL; label "shake well" and "protect from light" (Allen, 1996).

Allen LV and Erickson MA, "Stability of Labetalol Hydrochloride, Metoprolol Tartrate, Verapamil Hydrochloride, and Spironolactone With Hydrochlorothiazide in Extemporaneously Compounded Oral Liquids," *Am J Health Syst Pharm*, 1996, 53(19):2304-9.

Nahata MC and Hipple TF, *Pediatric Drug Formulations*, 4th ed, Cincinnati, OH: Harvey Whitney Books Co, 2000.

References

Barbarash RA, Bauman JL, Lukazewski AA, et al, "Verapamil Infusions in the Treatment of Atrial Tachyarrhythmias," *Crit Care Med*, 1986, 14(10):886-8.

Chobanian AV, Bakris GL, Black HR, et al, "The Seventh Report of the Joint National Committee on Prevention, Detection, Evaluation, and Treatment of High Blood Pressure: The JNC 7 report," *JAMA*, 2003, 289(19):2560-72.

"Guidelines 2000 for Cardiopulmonary Resuscitation and Emergency Cardiovascular Care, Part 6: Advanced Cardiovascular Life Support, The American Heart Association in Collaboration With the International Liaison Committee on Resuscitation," *Circulation*, 2000, 102(8 Suppl):I86-171.

"Guidelines 2000 for Cardiopulmonary Resuscitation and Emergency Cardiovascular Care, Part 10: Pediatric Advanced Life Support, The American Heart Association in Collaboration With the International Liaison Committee on Resuscitation," *Circulation*, 2000, 102(8 Suppl): I291-342.

Piovan D, Padrini R, Svalato Moreolo G, et al, "Verapamil and Norverapamil Plasma Levels in Infants and Children During Chronic Oral Treatment," *Ther Drug Monit*, 1995, 17(1):60-7.

Sapire DW, O'Riordan AC, and Black IF, "Safety and Efficacy of Short- and Long-Term Verapamil Therapy in Children With Tachycardia," *Am J Cardiol*, 1981, 48(6):1091-7.

Shakibi JG, "Arrhythmias in Infants and Children," *Pediatrician*, 1981, 10(1-3):117-22.

- ♦ **Verapamil Hydrochloride** *see* Verapamil *on page 1611*
- ♦ **Verapamil Hydrochloride Injection, USP (Can)** *see* Verapamil *on page 1611*
- ♦ **Verelan®** *see* Verapamil *on page 1611*
- ♦ **Verelan® PM** *see* Verapamil *on page 1611*
- ♦ **Vermox® [DSC]** *see* Mebendazole *on page 986*
- ♦ **Vermox® (Can)** *see* Mebendazole *on page 986*
- ♦ **Versed** *see* Midazolam *on page 1058*

- ♦ **Versel® (Can)** *see* Selenium Sulfide *on page 1427*
- ♦ **Versiclear™** *see* Sodium Thiosulfate *on page 1461*
- ♦ **VFEND®** *see* Voriconazole *on page 1622*
- ♦ **Viadur®** *see* Leuprolide *on page 918*
- ♦ **Viagra®** *see* Sildenafil *on page 1435*
- ♦ **Vibramycin®** *see* Doxycycline *on page 543*
- ♦ **Vibra-Tabs®** *see* Doxycycline *on page 543*
- ♦ **Vicks® 44® Cough Relief [OTC]** *see* Dextromethorphan *on page 477*
- ♦ **Vicks® 44E [OTC]** *see* Guaifenesin and Dextromethorphan *on page 748*
- ♦ **Vicks® Casero™ Chest Congestion Relief [OTC]** *see* Guaifenesin *on page 745*
- ♦ **Vicks® Pediatric Formula 44E [OTC]** *see* Guaifenesin and Dextromethorphan *on page 748*
- ♦ **Vicks Sinex® 12 Hour [OTC]** *see* Oxymetazoline *on page 1194*
- ♦ **Vicks Sinex® 12 Hour Ultrafine Mist [OTC]** *see* Oxymetazoline *on page 1194*
- ♦ **Vicks® Sinex® Nasal Spray [OTC]** *see* Phenylephrine *on page 1250*
- ♦ **Vicks® Sinex® UltraFine Mist [OTC]** *see* Phenylephrine *on page 1250*
- ♦ **Vicks® Vitamin C [OTC]** *see* Ascorbic Acid *on page 159*
- ♦ **Vicodin®** *see* Hydrocodone and Acetaminophen *on page 779*
- ♦ **Vicodin® ES** *see* Hydrocodone and Acetaminophen *on page 779*
- ♦ **Vicodin® HP** *see* Hydrocodone and Acetaminophen *on page 779*
- ♦ **Videx®** *see* Didanosine *on page 491*
- ♦ **Videx® EC** *see* Didanosine *on page 491*

VinBLAStine (vin BLAS teen)

Medication Safety Issues

Sound-alike/look-alike issues:

VinBLAStine may be confused with vinCRIStine, vinorelbine

High alert medication: The Institute for Safe Medication Practices (ISMP) includes this medication among its list of drugs which have a heightened risk of causing significant patient harm when used in error.

Note: Must be dispensed in overwrap which bears the statement **"Do not remove covering until the moment of injection. Fatal if given intrathecally. For I.V. use only."** Syringes should be labeled: **"Fatal if given intrathecally. For I.V. use only."**

Related Information

Compatibility of Chemotherapy and Related Supportive Care Medications *on page 1777*

Emetogenic Potential of Single Chemotherapeutic Agents *on page 1776*

Extravasation Treatment *on page 1726*

Index Terms NSC-49842; Vinblastine Sulfate; VLB

Therapeutic Category Antineoplastic Agent, Mitotic Inhibitor

Generic Available Yes

Use Palliative treatment of Hodgkin's disease; advanced testicular germinal-cell cancers; non-Hodgkin's lymphoma, histiocytosis, and choriocarcinoma

Pregnancy Risk Factor D

Lactation Enters breast milk/not recommended

Contraindications Hypersensitivity to vinblastine or any component (see Warnings); severe leukopenia

Warnings The FDA currently recommends that procedures for proper handling and disposal of antineoplastic agents be considered; vinblastine may cause fetal toxicity when administered to pregnant women; for I.V. use only; **intrathecal administration may result in death**

Injection (solution) contains benzyl alcohol which may cause allergic reactions in susceptible individuals; large amounts of benzyl alcohol (≥99 mg/kg/day) have been associated with a potentially fatal toxicity ("gasping syndrome") in neonates; the "gasping syndrome" consists of metabolic acidosis, respiratory distress, gasping respirations, CNS dysfunction (including convulsions, intracranial hemorrhage), hypotension and cardiovascular collapse; avoid use of vinblastine products containing benzyl alcohol in neonates; *in vitro* and animal studies have shown that benzoate, a metabolite of benzyl alcohol, displaces bilirubin from protein binding sites

Precautions Avoid extravasation; dosage modification required in patients with impaired liver function or neurotoxicity; dosage should be reduced in patients with recent exposure to radiation therapy or chemotherapy

Adverse Reactions

Cardiovascular: Tachycardia, orthostatic hypotension

(Continued)

VinBLAStine *(Continued)*

Central nervous system: Depression, malaise, seizures, headache
Dermatologic: Rashes, mild alopecia, photosensitivity
Endocrine & metabolic: Hyperuricemia
Gastrointestinal: Nausea, hemorrhagic enterocolitis, vomiting, constipation, abdominal pain, paralytic ileus, stomatitis
Genitourinary: Urinary retention
Hematologic: Myelosuppression: Leukopenia (nadir: 4-10 days), thrombocytopenia
Local: Severe tissue burn if infiltrated
Neuromuscular & skeletal: Jaw pain, myalgia, peripheral neuropathy, paresthesia

Drug Interactions Cytochrome P450 isoenzyme CYP3A3/4 and CYP3A5-7 substrate; isoenzyme CYP2D6 inhibitor

Concomitant administration with mitomycin has resulted in severe bronchospasm and shortness of breath; may decrease serum phenytoin concentrations

Stability Store in refrigerator; 1 mg/mL solutions prepared with preserved NS injection is stable for 30 days when refrigerated and protected from light. **Note:** Vinblastine must be dispensed in overwrap which bears the statement "Do not remove covering until the moment of injection. Fatal if given intrathecally. For I.V. use only."

Mechanism of Action Binds to microtubular protein of the mitotic spindle causing metaphase arrest

Pharmacokinetics

Distribution: Poor penetration into CSF; rapidly distributed into body tissues; V_{dss}: 27.3 L/kg
Protein binding: 75%
Metabolism: Extensive in the liver to a more active metabolite
Half-life, terminal: 24 hours
Elimination: Biliary excretion (95%)

Usual Dosage Vinblastine may be administered at intervals of every 7 days or greater and only after leukocyte count has returned to at least 4000/mm^3; maintenance therapy should be titrated according to leukocyte count

I.V. (refer to individual protocols):

Children:

Hodgkin's disease: 2.5-6 mg/m^2/day once every 1-2 weeks for 3-6 weeks; maximum weekly dose: 12.5 mg/m^2
Histiocytosis: 0.4 mg/kg once ever 7-10 days
Germ cell tumor: 0.2 mg/kg on days 1 and 2 of cycle every 3 weeks times 4 cycles

Adults: 3.7-18.5 mg/m^2/day every 7-10 days or 0.1-0.5 mg/kg/day once weekly or 1.4-1.8 mg/m^2/day for 5 days given as an I.V. continuous infusion

Dosing adjustment in hepatic impairment: Children and Adults: Direct serum bilirubin concentration >3 mg/dL: Reduce dose 50%

Administration Parenteral: **Do not administer intrathecally, death may occur**; do not administer I.M. or SubQ since the drug is very irritating; may be administered IVP directly into the vein or through a Y-site of a freely running I.V. over a 1-minute period at a concentration for administration of 1 mg/mL; I.V. continuous infusion: Each day's dose may be diluted in 1000 mL of D_5W or NS; administer over 24 hours

Monitoring Parameters CBC with differential and platelet count, serum uric acid, hepatic function tests

Patient Information Report to physician any fever, sore throat, bleeding, or bruising; avoid contact with the eyes since the drug is very irritating and corneal ulceration may result. May cause photosensitivity reactions (eg, exposure to sunlight may cause severe sunburn, skin rash, redness, or itching); avoid exposure to sunlight and artificial light sources (sunlamps, tanning booth/bed); wear protective clothing, wide-brimmed hats, sunglasses, and lip sunscreen (SPF ≥15); use a sunscreen [broad-spectrum sunscreen or physical sunscreen (preferred) or sunblock with SPF ≥15]; contact physician if reaction occurs.

Nursing Implications Maintain adequate hydration. Allopurinol may be given to prevent uric acid nephropathy; stool softeners may be helpful in preventing constipation; vinblastine is a tissue irritant and can cause sloughing upon extravasation; check vein patency before drug administration; care should be taken to avoid extravasation. If extravasation occurs, local injection of hyaluronidase into the leading edge of the extravasation site and a warm compress can be used for treatment; apply warm pack immediately for 30-60 minutes, then alternate off/on every 15 minutes for 1 day. Refer to Extravasation Treatment *on page 1726*.

Additional Information Myelosuppressive effects:

Nadir (days): 4-10
Recovery (days): 7-14

Dosage Forms Excipient information presented when available (limited, particularly for generics); consult specific product labeling.

Injection, powder for reconstitution, as sulfate: 10 mg
Injection, solution, as sulfate: 1 mg/mL (10 mL) [contains benzyl alcohol]

References

Balis FM, Holcenberg JS and Bleyer WA, "Clinical Pharmacokinetics of Commonly Used Anticancer Drugs," *Clin Pharmacokinet*, 1983, 8(3):202-32.
Crom WR, Glynn-Barnhart AM, Rodman JH, et al, "Pharmacokinetics of Anticancer Drugs in Children," *Clin Pharmacokinet*, 1987, 12(3):168-213.
Tannock I, Ehrlichman C, Perrault D, et al, "Failure of 5-Day Vinblastine Infusion in the Treatment of Patients With Advanced Refractory Breast Cancer," *Cancer Treat Rep*, 1982, 66(9):1783-4.
Yap HY, Blumenschein GR, Keating MJ, et al, "Vinblastine Given as a Continuous 5-Day Infusion in the Treatment of Refractory Breast Cancer," *Cancer Treat Rep*, 1980, 64(2-3):279-83.

♦ **Vinblastine Sulfate** *see* VinBLAStine *on page 1615*
♦ **Vincasar PFS®** *see* VinCRIStine *on page 1617*
♦ **Vincasar® PFS® (Can)** *see* VinCRIStine *on page 1617*

VinCRIStine (vin KRIS teen)

Medication Safety Issues

Sound-alike/look-alike issues:
VinCRIStine may be confused with vinBLAStine
Oncovin® may be confused with Ancobon®

High alert medication: The Institute for Safe Medication Practices (ISMP) includes this medication among its list of drugs which have a heightened risk of causing significant patient harm when used in error.

To prevent fatal inadvertent intrathecal injection, it is recommended that all doses be dispensed in a small minibag. When dispensing vincristine in a syringe, vincristine must be packaged in the manufacturer-provided overwrap which bears the statement **"Do not remove covering until the moment of injection. For intravenous use only. Fatal if given intrathecally."**

Related Information

Compatibility of Chemotherapy and Related Supportive Care Medications *on page 1777*
Emetogenic Potential of Single Chemotherapeutic Agents *on page 1776*
Extravasation Treatment *on page 1726*

U.S. Brand Names Vincasar PFS®

Canadian Brand Names Vincasar® PFS®

Index Terms LCR; Leurocristine Sulfate; NSC-67574; VCR; Vincristine Sulfate

Therapeutic Category Antineoplastic Agent, Mitotic Inhibitor

Generic Available Yes

Use Treatment of leukemias, Hodgkin's disease, neuroblastoma, malignant lymphomas, Wilms' tumor, and rhabdomyosarcoma

Pregnancy Risk Factor D

Lactation Enters breast milk/not recommended

Contraindications Hypersensitivity to vincristine or any component; patients with demyelinating form of Charcot-Marie-Tooth syndrome

Warnings The FDA currently recommends that procedures for proper handling and disposal of antineoplastic agents be considered; vincristine may cause fetal toxicity when administered to pregnant women; for I.V. use only; **intrathecal administration may result in death.**

Precautions Dosage modification required in patients with impaired hepatic function, patients receiving other neurotoxic drugs, or patients with pre-existing neuromuscular disease; avoid extravasation

Adverse Reactions

Cardiovascular: Orthostatic hypotension
Central nervous system: Neurotoxicity, seizures, CNS depression, cranial nerve paralysis, headache, confusion
Dermatologic: Alopecia, rash
Endocrine & metabolic: Hyperuricemia, SIADH
Gastrointestinal: Constipation, paralytic ileus, nausea, vomiting, diarrhea, stomatitis
Local: Pain, cellulitis and tissue necrosis if infiltrated, phlebitis
Neuromuscular & skeletal: Jaw pain, leg pain, myalgia, numbness, motor difficulties, paresthesia of the fingers and toes (stocking glove sensation), cramping, weakness, and "foot drop" or "wrist drop"
Ocular: Extraocular muscle paresis, photophobia
Respiratory: Dyspnea

Drug Interactions Cytochrome P450 isoenzyme CYP3A3/4 and CYP3A5-7 substrate; isoenzyme CYP2D6 inhibitor

Asparaginase may decrease vincristine clearance; acute pulmonary reactions may occur with concomitant use of mitomycin C; concurrent administration with itraconazole may result in an increased severity of neuromuscular side effects.
(Continued)

VinCRIStine *(Continued)*

CYP3A4 inhibitors (ie, azole antifungals, ciprofloxacin, clarithromycin, diclofenac, doxycycline, erythromycin, imatinib, isoniazid, nefazodone, nicardipine, propofol, protease inhibitors, quinidine, and verapamil) may decrease vincristine metabolism.

Stability Store in refrigerator; injectable solution is stable for 1 month at room temperature. **Note:** Vincristine must be dispensed in overwrap which bears the statement "Do not remove covering until the moment of injection. Fatal if given intrathecally. For I.V. use only."

Mechanism of Action Binds to microtubular protein of the mitotic spindle causing metaphase arrest

Pharmacokinetics

Distribution: Poor penetration into the CSF; V_{dss}: 120 L/m^2

Protein binding: 75%

Metabolism: Extensive in the liver

Half-life, terminal: 24 hours

Elimination: Primarily in bile (~80%)

Clearance:

Infants: Vincristine clearance is more closely related to body weight than to body surface area

Children 2-18 years: 482 mL/minute/m^2 (faster clearance in children <10 years of age than in adolescents)

Usual Dosage I.V. (refer to individual protocols):

Children ≤10 kg or BSA <1 m^2: Initial therapy: 0.05 mg/kg once weekly then titrate dose; maximum single dose: 2 mg

Children >10 kg or BSA ≥1 m^2: 1-2 mg/m^2, may repeat once weekly for 3-6 weeks; maximum single dose: 2 mg

Neuroblastoma: I.V. continuous infusion with doxorubicin: 1 mg/m^2/day for 72 hours

Adults: 0.4-1.4 mg/m^2 up to 2 mg; may repeat every week

Dosing adjustment in hepatic impairment: Children and Adults: Direct serum bilirubin concentration >3 mg/dL: Dosage reduction of 50% is recommended

Administration Parenteral: **Do not administer intrathecally, death may occur**; do not administer I.M. or SubQ since the drug is very irritating; I.V.: Vincristine is administered IVP or through a Y-site of a freely running I.V. over a period of 1 minute at a concentration for administration of 1 mg/mL; may administer as a dilute I.V. infusion

Monitoring Parameters Serum electrolytes (sodium), hepatic function tests, neurologic examination, CBC, hemoglobin, serum uric acid

Patient Information Stool softener should be used for constipation prophylaxis; report to physician any fever, sore throat, bleeding, bruising, or shortness of breath

Nursing Implications Maintain adequate hydration. Allopurinol may be given to prevent uric acid nephropathy; vincristine is a tissue irritant; care should be taken to avoid extravasation. If extravasation occurs, local injection of hyaluronidase into the leading edge of the extravasation site and a warm compress can be used for treatment; apply warm pack immediately for 30-60 minutes, then alternate off/on every 15 minutes for 1 day; refer to Extravasation Treatment *on page 1726*. Avoid contact with the eye since vincristine is very irritating.

Additional Information Ten times the usual recommended dose of vincristine in children < 13 years of age have been lethal; 3-4 mg/m^2 doses can be expected to produce severe toxic manifestations. Treatment is supportive and symptomatic including fluid restriction and diuretics to prevent adverse effects from SIADH. Use of leucovorin may be helpful in treating vincristine overdose.

Dosage Forms Excipient information presented when available (limited, particularly for generics); consult specific product labeling.

Injection, solution, as sulfate: 1 mg/mL (1 mL, 2 mL)

References

Crom WR, deGraaf SS, Synold T, et al, "Pharmacokinetics of Vincristine in Children and Adolescents With Acute Lymphocytic Leukemia," *J Pediatr*, 1994, 125(4):642-9.

Woods WG, O'Leary M, and Nesbit ME, "Life-Threatening Neuropathy and Hepatotoxicity in Infants During Induction Therapy for Acute Lymphoblastic Leukemia," *J Pediatr*, 1981, 98(4):642-5.

♦ **Vincristine Sulfate** *see* VinCRIStine *on page 1617*
♦ **Viokase®** *see* Pancrelipase *on page 1203*
♦ **Viosterol** *see* Ergocalciferol *on page 588*
♦ **Viracept®** *see* Nelfinavir *on page 1114*
♦ **Viramune®** *see* Nevirapine *on page 1124*
♦ **Virazole®** *see* Ribavirin *on page 1378*
♦ **Viread®** *see* Tenofovir *on page 1506*
♦ **Virilon® IM (Can)** *see* Testosterone *on page 1511*
♦ **Viroptic®** *see* Trifluridine *on page 1575*
♦ **Visicol®** *see* Sodium Phosphate *on page 1456*
♦ **Visine® L.R. [OTC]** *see* Oxymetazoline *on page 1194*

◆ **Visipaque™** *see* Iodixanol *on page 860*
◆ **Vistaril®** *see* HydrOXYzine *on page 796*
◆ **Vistide®** *see* Cidofovir *on page 353*
◆ **Vita-C® [OTC]** *see* Ascorbic Acid *on page 159*
◆ **Vitamin C** *see* Ascorbic Acid *on page 159*
◆ **Vitamin D_2** *see* Ergocalciferol *on page 588*

Vitamin A (VYE ta min aye)

Medication Safety Issues

Sound-alike/look-alike issues:

Aquasol® may be confused with Anusol®

U.S. Brand Names Aquasol A®; Palmitate-A® [OTC]

Index Terms Oleovitamin A

Therapeutic Category Nutritional Supplement; Vitamin, Fat Soluble

Generic Available Yes: Capsule

Use Treatment and prevention of vitamin A deficiency; supplementation in children 6 months to 2 years with measles

Pregnancy Risk Factor A (X if dose exceeds RDA recommendation)

Lactation Enters breast milk/compatible at normal daily doses

Contraindications Hypersensitivity to vitamin A or any component; hypervitaminosis A; pregnancy (dose exceeding RDA)

Warnings Patients receiving >25,000 units/day should be closely monitored for toxicity; polysorbates contained in parenteral vitamin A have been associated with thrombocytopenia, renal dysfunction, hepatomegaly, cholestasis, ascites, hypotension, and metabolic acidosis when administered to neonates (E-Ferol syndrome); avoid use in neonates

Adverse Reactions Seen only with doses exceeding physiologic replacement

Central nervous system: Irritability, drowsiness, vertigo, delirium, headache, coma, elevated intracranial pressure

Dermatologic: Erythema, peeling skin

Gastrointestinal: Vomiting, diarrhea

Ocular: Visual disturbances, papilledema

Drug Interactions Cholestyramine decreases absorption of vitamin A; neomycin and mineral oil may also interfere with vitamin A absorption; retinoids may have additive adverse effects; enhances hypoprothrombinemic effects of warfarin

Stability Protect injectable preparation from light

Mechanism of Action Needed for bone development, growth, visual adaptation to darkness, testicular and ovarian function, and as a cofactor in many biochemical processes

Pharmacokinetics

Absorption: Vitamin A in dosages **not** exceeding physiologic replacement is well absorbed after oral administration; water miscible preparations are absorbed more rapidly than oil preparations; large oral doses, conditions of fat malabsorption, low protein intake, or hepatic or pancreatic disease reduce oral absorption

Metabolism: Conjugated with glucuronide, undergoes enterohepatic circulation

Elimination: In feces via biliary elimination

Usual Dosage

Recommended daily allowance (RDA): Oral:

- <1 year: 375 mcg* (1250 units)
- 1-3 years: 400 mcg* (1330 units)
- 4-6 years: 500 mcg* (1670 units)
- 7-10 years: 700 mcg* (2330 units)
- >10 years: Female: 800 mcg* (2670 units); Male: 1000 mcg* (3330 units)

***mcg retinol equivalent (0.3 mcg retinol = 1 unit vitamin A)**

Daily dietary supplement: Oral:

Infants up to 6 months: 1500 units

Children:

- 6 months to 3 years: 1500-2000 units
- 4-6 years: 2500 units
- 7-10 years: 3300-3500 units

Children >10 years and Adults: 4000-5000 units

Vitamin A supplementation in measles (recommendation of the World Health Organization): Children: Oral: Give as a single dose; repeat the next day and at 4 weeks for children with ophthalmologic evidence of vitamin A deficiency:

6 months to 1 year: 100,000 units

>1 year: 200,000 units

Note: Use of vitamin A in measles is recommended only for patients 6 months to 2 years of age hospitalized with measles and its complications **or** patients >6

(Continued)

Vitamin A *(Continued)*

months of age who have any of the following risk factors and who are not already receiving vitamin A: immunodeficiency, ophthalmologic evidence of vitamin A deficiency including night blindness, Bitot's spots or evidence of xerophthalmia, impaired intestinal absorption, moderate to severe malnutrition including that associated with eating disorders, or recent immigration from areas where high mortality rates from measles have been observed

Note: Monitor patients closely; dosages >25,000 units/day have been associated with toxicity

Vitamin A deficiency (varying recommendations available):

Severe deficiency with xerophthalmia:

Infants: I.M.: 7500-15,000 units/day followed by oral 5000-10,000 units/day for 10 days

Children 1-8 years: Oral: 5000 units/kg/day for 5 days then 5000-10,000 units/day for 2 months; I.M.: 17,500-35,000 units/day for 10 days

Children >8 years and Adults: Oral: 500,000 units/day for 3 days, then 50,000 units/day for 14 days; then 10,000-20,000 units/day for 2 months; I.M.: 100,000 units/day for 3 days; then 50,000 units/day for 14 days

Prophylactic therapy for children at risk for developing deficiency: Oral: Given every 4-6 months:

Infants ≤1 year: 100,000 units

Children >1 year: 200,000 units

Malabsorption syndrome (prophylaxis): Children >8 years and Adults: Oral: 10,000-50,000 units/day of water miscible product

Administration

Oral: Administer with food or milk

Parenteral: I.M. only

Additional Information 1 USP vitamin A unit = 0.3 mcg of all-*trans* isomer of retinol; 1 RE (retinol equivalent) = 1 mcg of all-*trans*-retinol

Dosage Forms Excipient information presented when available (limited, particularly for generics); consult specific product labeling.

Capsule [softgel]: 10,000 units; 25,000 units

Injection, solution (Aquasol A®): 50,000 units/mL (2 mL) [contains polysorbate 80]

Tablet (Palmitate-A®): 5000 units, 15,000 units

References

Committee on Infectious Diseases, "Vitamin A in the Treatment of Measles," *Pediatrics*, 1993, 91(5):1014-5.

DeMaeyer EM, "The WHO Programme of Prevention and Control of Vitamin A Deficiency, Xerophthalmia, and Nutritional Blindness," *Nutr Health*, 1986, 4(2):105-12.

Hussey GD and Klein M, "A Randomized, Controlled Trial of Vitamin A in Children With Severe Measles," *N Engl J Med*, 1990, 323(3):160-4.

- **Vitamin A Acid** *see* Tretinoin *on page 1567*
- **Vitamin B_1** *see* Thiamine *on page 1526*
- **Vitamin B_2** *see* Riboflavin *on page 1382*
- **Vitamin B_3** *see* Niacin *on page 1127*
- **Vitamin B_6** *see* Pyridoxine *on page 1353*
- **Vitamin B_{12}** *see* Cyanocobalamin *on page 413*
- **Vitamin B_{12a}** *see* Hydroxocobalamin *on page 790*
- **Vitamin Bw** *see* Biotin *on page 217*

Vitamin E (VYE ta min ee)

Medication Safety Issues

Sound-alike/look-alike issues:

Aquasol E® may be confused with Anusol®

U.S. Brand Names Alph-E [OTC]; Alph-E-Mixed [OTC]; Aquasol E® [OTC]; Aquavit-E [OTC]; d-Alpha-Gems™ [OTC]; E-Gems® [OTC]; E-Gems Elite® [OTC]; E-Gems Plus® [OTC]; Ester-E™ [OTC]; Gamma E-Gems® [OTC]; Gamma-E Plus [OTC]; High Gamma Vitamin E Complete™ [OTC]; Key-E® [OTC]; Key-E® Kaps [OTC]

Index Terms *d*-Alpha Tocopherol; *dl*-Alpha Tocopherol

Therapeutic Category Nutritional Supplement; Vitamin, Fat Soluble; Vitamin, Topical

Generic Available Yes

Use Prevention and treatment of vitamin E deficiency

Pregnancy Risk Factor A (C if dose exceeds RDA recommendation)

Lactation Enters breast milk/compatible

Contraindications Hypersensitivity to vitamin E or any component

Warnings Necrotizing enterocolitis has been associated with oral administration of large dosages (eg, >200 units/day) of a hyperosmolar vitamin E preparation in low birth weight infants

Adverse Reactions

Central nervous system: Headache

Dermatologic: Rash

Endocrine & metabolic: Gonadal dysfunction; decreased serum thyroxine and triiodothyronine; elevated cholesterol and triglycerides

Gastrointestinal: Nausea, diarrhea, intestinal cramps, necrotizing enterocolitis (see Warnings)

Neuromuscular & skeletal: Weakness

Ocular: Blurred vision

Renal: Creatinuria and elevated serum creatinine kinase; elevated urinary estrogens and androgens

Drug Interactions Iron, mineral oil, warfarin

Mechanism of Action Antioxidant which prevents oxidation of vitamin A and C; protects polyunsaturated fatty acids in membranes from attack by free radicals and protects red blood cells against hemolysis by oxidizing agents

Pharmacokinetics

Absorption: Oral: Depends upon the presence of bile; absorption is reduced in conditions of malabsorption, in low birth weight premature infants, and as dosage increases; water miscible preparations are better absorbed than oil preparations

Metabolism: In the liver to glucuronides

Elimination: Primarily in bile

Usual Dosage 1 unit vitamin E = 1 mg *dl*-alpha-tocopherol acetate. Oral:

Vitamin E - Recommended Daily Allowance (RDA) and Estimated Average Requirement (EAR)

Age	RDA (mg/day)	EAR (mg/day)
0-6 mo	-	4 (6 units)
7-12 mo	-	6 (9 units)
1-3 y	6 (9 units)	5 (7.5 units)
4-8 y	7 (10.5 units)	6 (9 units)
9-13 y	11 (16.5 units)	9 (13.5 units)
≥14 y	15 (22.5 units)	12 (18 units)

Vitamin E deficiency:

Neonates, premature, low birth weight: 25-50 units/day results in normal levels within 1 week

Children (with malabsorption syndrome): 1 unit/kg/day of water miscible vitamin E (to raise plasma tocopherol concentrations to the normal range within 2 months and to maintain normal plasma concentrations)

Adults: 60-75 units/day

Prevention of vitamin E deficiency:

Neonates:

Low birth weight: 5 units/day

Full-term: 5 units/L of formula ingested

Adults: 30 units/day

Prevention of retinopathy of prematurity or BPD secondary to O_2 therapy: Neonates and Infants: (American Academy of Pediatrics considers this use investigational and routine use is not recommended): 15-30 units/kg/day to maintain plasma levels between 1.5-2 mcg/mL (may need as high as 100 units/kg/day)

Cystic fibrosis, beta-thalassemia, sickle cell anemia may require higher daily maintenance doses: Infants, Children, and Adolescents:

Cystic fibrosis: 100-400 units/day

Beta-thalassemia: 750 units/day

Sickle cell: 450 units/day

Topical: Apply a thin layer over affected area

Administration Oral: May administer with or without food

Monitoring Parameters Plasma tocopherol concentrations

Reference Range Plasma tocopherol: 6-14 mcg/mL

Dosage Forms Excipient information presented when available (limited, particularly for generics); consult specific product labeling.

Capsule: 400 int. units, 1000 int. units

Key-E® Kaps: 200 int. units, 400 int. units

Capsule, softgel: 200 int. units, 400 int. units, 600 int. units, 1000 int. units

Alph-E: 200 int. units, 400 int. units

Alph-E-Mixed: 200 int. units [contains mixed tocopherols]; 400 int. units [contains mixed tocopherols], 1000 int. units [sugar free; contains mixed tocopherols]

Aqua Gem E®: 200 units, 400 units

(Continued)

Vitamin E *(Continued)*

d-Alpha-Gems™: 400 int. units [derived from soybean oil]
E-Gems®: 30 int. units, 100 int. units, 200 int. units, 400 int. units, 600 int. units, 800 int. units, 1000 int. units, 1200 int. units [derived from soybean oil]
E-Gems Plus®: 200 int. units, 400 int. units, 800 int. units [contains mixed tocopherols]
E-Gems Elite®: 400 int. units [contains mixed tocopherols]
Ester-E™: 400 int. units
Gamma E-Gems®: 90 int. units [also contains mixed tocopherols]
Gamma-E Plus: 200 int. units [contains soybean oil]
High Gamma Vitamin E Complete™: 200 int. units [contains soybean oil, mixed tocopherols]
Cream: 50 int. units/g (60 g), 100 int. units/g (60 g), 1000 int. units/120 g (120 g), 30,000 int. units/57 g (57 g)
Key-E®: 30 int. units/g (60 g, 120 g, 600 g)
Lip balm (E-Gem® Lip Care): 1000 int. units/tube [contains vitamin A and aloe]
Oil, oral/topical: 100 int. units/0.25 mL (60 mL, 75 mL); 1150 units/0.25 mL (30 mL, 60 mL, 120 mL); 28,000 int. units/30 mL (30 mL)
Alph-E: 28,000 int. units/30 mL (30 mL) [topical]
E-Gems®: 100 units/10 drops (15 mL, 60 mL)
Ointment, topical (Key-E®): 30 units/g (60 g, 120 g, 480 g)
Powder (Key-E®): 700 int. units per 1/4 teaspoon (15 g, 75 g, 1000 g) [derived from soybean oil]
Solution, oral drops: 15 int. units/0.3 mL (30 mL)
Aquasol E®: 15 int. units/0.3 mL (12 mL, 30 mL) [latex free]
Aquavit-E: 15 int. units/0.3 mL (30 mL) [butterscotch flavor]
Suppository, rectal/vaginal (Key-E®): 30 int. units (12s, 24s) [contains coconut oil]
Tablet: 100 int. units, 200 int. units, 400 int. units, 500 int. units
Key-E®: 200 int. units, 400 int. units

References

American Academy of Pediatrics Committee on Fetus and Newborn, "Vitamin E and the Prevention of Retinopathy of Prematurity," *Pediatrics*, 1985, 76(2):315-6.

- **Vitamin G** *see* Riboflavin *on page 1382*
- **Vitamin H** *see* Biotin *on page 217*
- **Vitamin K_1** *see* Phytonadione *on page 1258*
- **Vitrase®** *see* Hyaluronidase *on page 774*
- **Vitrasert®** *see* Ganciclovir *on page 719*
- **Vi Vaccine** *see* Typhoid Vaccine *on page 1583*
- **Vivarin® [OTC]** *see* Caffeine *on page 255*
- **Vivelle®** *see* Estradiol *on page 605*
- **Vivelle-Dot®** *see* Estradiol *on page 605*
- **Vivotif®** *see* Typhoid Vaccine *on page 1583*
- **VLB** *see* VinBLAStine *on page 1615*
- **VM-26** *see* Teniposide *on page 1504*
- **Voltaren®** *see* Diclofenac *on page 486*
- **Voltaren Ophtha® (Can)** *see* Diclofenac *on page 486*
- **Voltaren Ophthalmic®** *see* Diclofenac *on page 486*
- **Voltaren Rapide® (Can)** *see* Diclofenac *on page 486*
- **Voltaren®-XR** *see* Diclofenac *on page 486*
- **Voluven® (Can)** *see* Hetastarch *on page 766*

Voriconazole (vor i KOE na zole)

Related Information
Assessment of Liver Function *on page 1810*
U.S. Brand Names VFEND®
Canadian Brand Names VFEND®
Index Terms UK109496
Therapeutic Category Antifungal Agent, Systemic; Antifungal Agent, Triazole
Generic Available No
Use Treatment of invasive aspergillosis, especially in immunocompromised patients; treatment of candidemia in non-neutropenic patients; deep tissue *Candida* infections; esophageal candidiasis; treatment of serious fungal infections caused by *Scedosporium apiospermum* or *Fusarium* spp (including *Fusarium solanae*) in patients intolerant of, or refractory to, conventional antifungal therapy
Pregnancy Risk Factor D
Lactation Excretion in breast milk unknown/not recommended

Contraindications Hypersensitivity to voriconazole or any component; concurrent therapy with rifampin, carbamazepine, phenobarbital, mephobarbital, sirolimus, terfenadine, astemizole, cisapride, pimozide, ritonavir, efavirenz, quinidine, ergot alkaloids, or rifabutin (see Drug Interactions).

Warnings Serious hepatic reactions including hepatitis, cholestasis, fulminant hepatic failure, and death have been reported. Liver function test abnormalities may be associated with higher plasma drug concentrations and/or doses; dosage adjustment or discontinuation of therapy may be required. Visual changes such as blurred vision, photophobia, changes in visual acuity and color have been reported in 30% of patients in clinical trials. Patients should be warned to avoid tasks which depend on vision, including operating machinery or driving; the effect on vision with long-term administration (beyond 28 days) is unknown and should be monitored. Torsade de pointes and QT interval prolongation have been reported in patients taking voriconazole. Administer with caution to patients with proarrhythmic conditions. If used during pregnancy, the patient should be informed that voriconazole may cause fetal harm. Voriconazole tablets contain lactose; avoid use in patients with rare hereditary problems of galactose intolerance, Lapp lactase deficiency, or glucose-galactose malabsorption. Voriconazole oral suspension contains sucrose; avoid use in patients with rare hereditary problems of fructose intolerance, sucrose-isomaltase deficiency or glucose-galactose malabsorption.

Voriconazole is metabolized by cytochrome P450 enzymes resulting in interactions with other drugs. Due to potential serious and/or life-threatening drug interactions, some drugs are contraindicated (see Contraindications and Drug Interactions).

Voriconazole oral suspension contains sodium benzoate; benzoic acid (benzoate) is a metabolite of benzyl alcohol; large amounts of benzyl alcohol (≥99 mg/kg/day) have been associated with a potentially fatal toxicity ("gasping syndrome") in neonates; the "gasping syndrome" consists of metabolic acidosis, respiratory distress, gasping respirations, CNS dysfunction (including convulsions, intracranial hemorrhage), hypotension and cardiovascular collapse; use voriconazole oral suspension containing sodium benzoate with caution in neonates; *in vitro* and animal studies have shown that benzoate displaces bilirubin from protein binding sites

Precautions Use caution in patients with hypersensitivity to other azole antifungal agents since cross-reaction may occur but has not been established; use with caution in patients with severe renal or hepatic impairment; modify dosage in patients with mild to moderate hepatic cirrhosis (Child-Pugh class A and B); avoid administration of voriconazole injection in patients with Cl_{cr} <50 mL/minute since I.V. formulation contains sulfobutyl ether beta-cyclodextrin (SBECD) which may accumulate in renal insufficiency

Adverse Reactions

Cardiovascular: Arrhythmias, peripheral edema, tachycardia, hypertension, hypotension, vasodilation, QT interval prolongation, torsade de pointes (rare)

Central nervous system: Headache, dizziness, fatigue, anxiety, confusion, depression, amnesia, insomnia, convulsions, hemiparesis, lethargy, fever, chills, hallucinations

Dermatologic: Rash, pruritus, alopecia; photosensitivity (occurs more frequently with long-term treatment), Stevens-Johnson syndrome (rare), toxic epidermal necrolysis (rare), erythema multiforme (rare)

Endocrine & metabolic: Hypokalemia, hypomagnesemia

Gastrointestinal: Nausea, vomiting, anorexia, diarrhea, abdominal pain, constipation, mucositis, dysphagia, xerostomia, GI hemorrhage, pancreatitis

Genitourinary: Urinary tract infection, urinary retention, hemorrhagic cystitis

Hematologic: Thrombocytopenia, leukopenia, anemia, lymphopenia

Hepatic: Elevated ALT, AST, alkaline phosphatase, and bilirubin; cholestatic jaundice, hepatitis, fulminant hepatic failure

Neuromuscular & skeletal: Myalgia, ataxia

Ocular: Photophobia, visual changes, color vision change, blurred vision (visual disturbance is reversible; incidence is dose-related; onset after 1st-2nd dose)

Renal: Elevated creatinine, acute renal failure

Respiratory: Cough, dyspnea

Miscellaneous: Anaphylaxis, anaphylactoid-type reaction (flushing, fever, sweating, tachycardia, chest tightness, dyspnea, faintness, nausea, pruritus and rash) may appear immediately after initiating the I.V. infusion

Drug Interactions Cytochrome P450 isoenzyme CYP2C9, CYP2C19, and CYP3A4 (minor) substrate; isoenzyme CYP2C9, CYP2C19, and CYP3A3/4 (minor) inhibitor.

May increase plasma levels of lovastatin, midazolam, triazolam, alprazolam, phenytoin, calcium channel blockers, sulfonylureas, saquinavir, amprenavir, nelfinavir, omeprazole, and vinca alkaloids; saquinavir, amprenavir, and delavirdine may inhibit voriconazole metabolism; rifabutin may decrease voriconazole serum concentrations and voriconazole may increase rifabutin serum levels (coadministration of rifabutin with voriconazole is contraindicated; see Warnings); efavirenz may decrease

(Continued)

Voriconazole *(Continued)*

voriconazole serum concentrations and voriconazole may increase efavirenz serum levels (coadministration of efavirenz with voriconazole is contraindicated; see Warnings); increases plasma concentration of sirolimus, terfenadine, astemizole, cisapride, pimozide, ergot alkaloids, and quinidine (coadministration with voriconazole is contraindicated; see Warnings); increases prothrombin time with warfarin (monitor anticoagulation tests); increases plasma cyclosporine and tacrolimus levels (reduce cyclosporine dose to ½ of the starting dose; reduce tacrolimus dose to ⅓ of the starting dose; monitor blood levels); phenytoin decreases voriconazole serum concentrations (adjust voriconazole dose and monitor phenytoin levels); synergistic with caspofungin; rifampin, carbamazepine, ritonavir, efavirenz, phenobarbital, and mephobarbital reduce voriconazole serum concentrations (coadministration with voriconazole is contraindicated; see Warnings); delavirdine may inhibit voriconazole metabolism; voriconazole may inhibit delavirdine metabolism

Food Interactions High fat meals reduce the extent of absorption by 24% for tablets and 37% for the oral suspension; avoid grapefruit juice (may increase voriconazole serum levels)

Stability Store tablets and unreconstituted vials at room temperature; store powder for oral suspension in refrigerator before reconstitution; protect from light. Reconstituted oral suspension is stable for 14 days at room temperature. Do not refrigerate or freeze oral suspension. Reconstituted 10 mg/mL I.V. solution should be used immediately after preparation since it contains no preservative. If not used immediately, the solution is stable for 24 hours at 2°C to 8°C. The reconstituted I.V. solution can be further diluted with NS, D_5W, LR, D_5WLR, D_5W with 20 mEq KCl/liter, D_5W½NS, D_5WNS, or ½NS; voriconazole is incompatible with TPN, blood products, sodium bicarbonate, and electrolyte supplement infusions.

Mechanism of Action Inhibits fungal cytochrome P450-dependent 14a-sterol demethylase, an essential enzyme in ergosterol biosynthesis resulting in the inhibition of fungal cell membrane formation

Pharmacokinetics

Absorption: Oral: Rapid and complete

Distribution: Extensive tissue distribution

V_d: Adults: 4.6 L/kg

Protein binding: 58%

Metabolism: Metabolized by cytochrome P450 enzymes CYP2C19, CYP2C9, and CYP3A4 to voriconazole N-oxide (minimal antifungal activity); CYP2C19 is significantly involved in metabolism of voriconazole; CYP2C19 exhibits genetic polymorphism (15% to 20% Asians may be poor metabolizers of voriconazole; 3% to 5% Caucasians and African Americans may be poor metabolizers)

Bioavailability: 96%

Half-life: Terminal (dose-dependent): Adults: 6-9 hours

Time to peak serum concentration: Oral: 1-2 hours

Elimination: <2% excreted unchanged in urine

Usual Dosage

I.V.:

Children 2-11 years:

Loading dose: 6 mg/kg/dose every 12 hours for 2 doses on day 1

Maintenance dose: 4 mg/kg/dose every 12 hours (achieves exposure that approximates the adult maintenance dose of 3 mg/kg every 12 hours)

Children ≥12 years and Adults:

Loading dose: 6 mg/kg/dose every 12 hours for 2 doses on day 1

Maintenance dose: Invasive aspergillosis, other serious fungal infections, and deep tissue *Candida* infections: 4 mg/kg/dose every 12 hours

If patient is unable to tolerate I.V. therapy, reduce the dose to 3 mg/kg/dose every 12 hours.

Maintenance dose: Candidemia: 3 mg/kg/dose every 12 hours

Oral:

Patients <40 kg:

Invasive aspergillosis, other serious fungal infection, candidemia, or deep tissue *Candida* infections: Maintenance dose: 100 mg every 12 hours

If patient response is inadequate, increase dose to 150 mg every 12 hours

If patient is unable to tolerate oral dose, decrease dose by 50 mg decrement to a minimum of 100 mg every 12 hours

Esophageal candidiasis: 100 mg every 12 hours for a minimum of 14 days and for at least 7 days following symptom resolution

Note: Limited information is currently available in the literature regarding oral voriconazole use in pediatric patients; some centers have used initial maintenance doses of 3-5 mg/kg/dose every 12 hours in patients <25 kg

Patients ≥40 kg:

Invasive aspergillosis, other serious fungal infection, candidemia, or deep tissue *Candida* infections: Maintenance dose: 200 mg every 12 hours

If patient response is inadequate, increase dose to 300 mg every 12 hours

If patient is unable to tolerate oral dose, decrease dose by 50 mg decrement to a minimum of 200 mg every 12 hours

Esophageal candidiasis: 200 mg every 12 hours for a minimum of 14 days and for at least 7 days following symptom resolution

Dosing adjustment for patients on concurrent phenytoin therapy:

I.V.: Increase voriconazole maintenance dose from 4 mg/kg/dose to 5 mg/kg/dose every 12 hours

Oral:

<40 kg: Increase voriconazole maintenance dose from 100 mg to 200 mg every 12 hours

≥40 kg: Increase voriconazole maintenance dose from 200 mg to 400 mg every 12 hours

Dosing adjustment in renal impairment:

Oral: No adjustment is necessary

I.V.: Cl_{cr} <50 mL/minute: Switch patient to oral voriconazole (parenteral formulation contains the excipient sulfobutyl ether beta-cyclodextrin sodium which accumulates in patients with renal impairment)

Dialysis: No dosage adjustment needed after 4-hour hemodialysis session

Dosing adjustment in hepatic impairment:

Child-Pugh Class A and B: Use standard loading dose regimen; decrease maintenance dose by 50%

Child-Pugh Class C: Not recommended for use unless benefit outweighs the risk

Administration Correct any electrolyte disturbances such as hypokalemia, hypomagnesemia, or hypocalcemia prior to starting voriconazole therapy

Oral: Administer at least one hour before or one hour after a meal; shake suspension for approximately 10 seconds before use; do not mix suspension with other medications, flavoring agents, or other fluids

Parenteral: I.V.: **Do not administer I.V. push;** voriconazole must be administered by I.V. infusion over 1-2 hours at a rate not to exceed 3 mg/kg/hour; final concentration for administration should be 0.5-5 mg/mL

Monitoring Parameters Serum electrolytes, periodic renal function tests (particularly serum creatinine), hepatic function tests, and bilirubin; monitor visual activity, visual field, and color perception; EKG in select patients

Patient Information Avoid drinking grapefruit juice while taking voriconazole. Avoid driving at night or performing hazardous tasks while taking voriconazole; it may cause blurred vision and/or photophobia. May cause photosensitivity reactions (eg, exposure to sunlight may cause severe sunburn, skin rash, redness, or itching); avoid exposure to sunlight and artificial light sources (sunlamps, tanning booth/bed); wear protective clothing, wide-brimmed hats, sunglasses, and lip sunscreen (SPF ≥15); use a sunscreen [broad-spectrum sunscreen or physical sunscreen (preferred) or sunblock with SPF ≥15]; contact physician if reaction occurs. Women of childbearing age should use effective contraception during treatment to avoid pregnancy.

Nursing Implications Stop voriconazole infusion if anaphylactoid-type reaction occurs

Dosage Forms Excipient information presented when available (limited, particularly for generics); consult specific product labeling.

Injection, powder for reconstitution: 200 mg [contains SBECD 3200 mg]

Powder for oral suspension: 200 mg/5 mL (70 mL) [contains sodium benzoate and sucrose; orange flavor]

Tablet: 50 mg, 200 mg [contains lactose]

References

Romero AJ, Pogamp PL, Nilsson LG, et al, "Effect of Voriconazole on the Pharmacokinetics of Cyclosporine in Renal Transplant Patients," *Clin Pharmacol Ther*, 2002, 71(4):226-34.

Walsh TJ, Karlsson MO, Driscoll T, et al, "Pharmacokinetics and Safety of Intravenous Voriconazole in Children After Single- or Multiple-Dose Administration," *Antimicrob Agents Chemother*, 2004, 48(6):2166-72.

Walsh TJ, Lutsar I, Driscoll T, et al, "Voriconazole in the Treatment of Aspergillosis, Scedosporiosis and Other Invasive Fungal Infections in Children," *Pediatr Infect Dis J*, 2002, 21(3):240-8.

Walsh TJ, Pappas P, Winston DJ, et al, "Voriconazole Compared With Liposomal Amphotericin B for Empirical Antifungal Therapy in Patients With Neutropenia and Persistent Fever," *N Engl J Med*, 2002, 346(4):225-34.

♦ **VoSpire ER®** *see* Albuterol *on page 66*

♦ **VP-16** *see* Etoposide *on page 625*

♦ **VP-16-213** *see* Etoposide *on page 625*

♦ **VPA** *see* Valproic Acid and Derivatives *on page 1592*

♦ **Vumon®** *see* Teniposide *on page 1504*

♦ **Vytorin®** *see* Ezetimibe and Simvastatin *on page 629*

◆ **VZIG** *see* Varicella-Zoster Immune Globulin (Human) [DSC] *on page 1600*
◆ **VZV Vaccine (Varicella)** *see* Varicella Virus Vaccine *on page 1599*

Warfarin (WAR far in)

Medication Safety Issues
Sound-alike/look-alike issues:
Coumadin® may be confused with Avandia®, Cardura®, Compazine®, Kemadrin®
High alert medication: The Institute for Safe Medication Practices (ISMP) includes this medication among its list of drugs which have a heightened risk of causing significant patient harm when used in error.

Related Information
Antithrombotic Therapy in Children *on page 1804*
Commonly Used Antidotes for Acute Overdoses *on page 1920*
Overdose and Toxicology *on page 1916*

U.S. Brand Names Coumadin®; Jantoven™

Canadian Brand Names Apo-Warfarin®; Coumadin®; Gen-Warfarin; Novo-Warfarin; Taro-Warfarin

Index Terms Warfarin Sodium

Therapeutic Category Anticoagulant

Generic Available Yes: Tablet

Use Prophylaxis and treatment of venous thrombosis, pulmonary embolism, and thromboembolic disorders; prevention and treatment of arterial thromboembolism in patients with prosthetic heart valves or atrial fibrillation; prevention of death, recurrent MI, and thromboembolic events such as systemic embolization or stroke after MI

Medication Guide An FDA-approved patient medication guide, which is available with the product information and at http://www.fda.gov/cder/Offices/ODS/medication_guides.htm, must be dispensed with this medication for each new outpatient prescription and refill.

Pregnancy Risk Factor X

Lactation Does not enter breast milk, only metabolites are excreted (AAP rates "compatible")

Contraindications Hypersensitivity to warfarin or any component; severe liver or kidney disease; hemorrhagic tendencies or blood dyscrasias; recent or contemplated surgery of the CNS, eye, or traumatic surgery with large open wounds; active ulceration or overt bleeding of GI, GU, or respiratory tracts, cerebrovascular hemorrhage, cerebral aneurysms, dissecting aortic aneurysms, pericarditis and pericardial effusions, bacterial endocarditis; uncontrolled bleeding; spinal puncture; major regional or lumbar block anesthesia; neurosurgical procedures; malignant hypertension; pregnancy, threatened abortion, eclampsia, pre-eclampsia; inadequate laboratory facilities; unsupervised patients with senility, alcoholism, or psychoses or other lack of patient cooperation

Warnings Serious and potentially fatal hemorrhage hemorrhage may occur. Bleeding is more likely during initiation of treatment and with higher doses. Risk factors for bleeding include high intensity anticoagulation (INR >4), age (>65 years), highly variable INRs, history of GI bleeding, hypertension, cerebrovascular disease, serious heart disease, anemia, severe diabetes, malignancy, trauma, renal insufficiency, polycythemia vera, vasculitis, open wound, history of PUD, indwelling catheters, menstruating and postpartum women, drug-drug interactions, and long duration of therapy. Dosage must be individualized for each patient (see Precautions). Patients must be instructed to report bleeding, accidents, or falls as well as any new or discontinued medications, herbal, or alternative products used, or significant changes in smoking or dietary habits.

Necrosis and/or gangrene of the skin and other tissues may occur (rarely) due to early hypercoagulability; risk is increased in patients with protein C deficiency; tissue debridement or amputation may be required; permanent disability or death has been reported; discontinue warfarin if warfarin-associated necrosis occurs; consider heparin for anticoagulation. Systemic cholesterol microemboli (eg, "purple toes syndrome") and atheroemboli may occur.

May cause hypersensitivity reactions, including anaphylaxis; use with caution in patients with anaphylactic disorders. Concomitant use with vitamin K may decrease anticoagulant effect; monitor carefully. Concomitant use with ethacrynic acid, indomethacin, NSAIDs, phenylbutazone, or aspirin increases warfarin's anticoagulant effect and may cause severe GI irritation (see Drug Interactions). Oral anticoagulant therapy is usually avoided in neonates due to a greater potential risk of bleeding (see Monagle, 2001).

Precautions Do not switch brands once desired therapeutic response has been achieved. Use with caution in patients with acute infection or active tuberculosis (antibiotics and fever may alter the response to warfarin), prolonged dietary insufficiencies (vitamin K deficiency), diabetes mellitus, thyroid disease, moderate-to-severe renal or hepatic impairment, ovulating women (may be at risk of developing ovarian hemorrhage at the time of ovulation) or heparin-induced thrombocytopenia with deep vein thrombosis (limb ischemia, necrosis, and gangrene have occurred when warfarin was started or continued after heparin was stopped; warfarin monotherapy is contraindicated in the initial treatment of active HIT; warfarin initially inhibits the synthesis of protein C, potentially accelerating the underlying active thrombotic process). Use with caution in patients with or at risk for hemorrhage, necrosis, or gangrene. Use care in the selection of patients appropriate for this treatment; ensure patient cooperation especially from the alcoholic, illicit drug user, demented, or psychotic patient. Safety and efficacy have not been established in children.

Periodic monitoring of INR (preferred) or prothrombin time is essential. A large number of factors (alone or in combination), including changes in diet, medications, and herbal remedies, may influence the patient's response to warfarin; monitor patients more closely when these factors change.

Adverse Reactions Bleeding is the major adverse effect of warfarin. Hemorrhage may occur at virtually any site. Risk is dependent on multiple variables, including the intensity of anticoagulation and patient susceptibility.

Cardiovascular: Angina, edema, hemorrhagic shock, hypotension, pallor, syncope, vasculitis

Central nervous system: Fever, fatigue, asthenia, dizziness, headache, lethargy, pain, stroke

Dermatologic: Skin lesions, rash, dermatitis, bullous eruptions, pruritus, urticaria, skin necrosis; gangrene of skin; hair loss (rare in children)

Gastrointestinal: Anorexia, nausea, vomiting, diarrhea, abdominal cramps, abdominal pain, flatulence, bloating, GI bleeding, mouth ulcers, taste disturbance

Genitourinary: Hematuria, priapism

Hematologic: Hemorrhage, agranulocytosis, anemia, leukopenia, retroperitoneal hematoma; unrecognized bleeding sites (eg, colon cancer) may be uncovered by anticoagulation

Hepatic: Hepatitis, elevated liver enzymes, cholestatic hepatic injury, jaundice

Neuromuscular & skeletal: Osteoporosis, paresthesia, weakness

Respiratory: Hemoptysis, epistaxis, pulmonary hemorrhage; tracheal calcification (rare in children)

Miscellaneous: Systemic cholesterol microembolization ("purple toes syndrome"), hypersensitivity reactions, anaphylaxis

Drug Interactions Cytochrome P450 isoenzyme CYP1A2 substrate (minor), CYP2C8, CYP2C9, CYP2C18, CYP2C19, and CYP3A3/4 isoenzyme substrate; CYP2C9 and CYP2C19 isoenzyme inhibitor

Alcohol, alteplase, amiodarone, anabolic steroids, aspirin, amoxicillin, barbiturates, carbamazepine, cefaclor, chloral hydrate, chloramphenicol, chlordiazepoxide, cholestyramine, cimetidine, clofibrate, cloxacillin, disulfiram, erythromycin, fluconazole, griseofulvin, isoniazid, ketoconazole, metronidazole, miconazole (systemic or intravaginal use), nafcillin, omeprazole, phenylbutazone, phenytoin, phenobarbital, piroxicam, prednisone, propranolol, proton pump inhibitors, ranitidine, rifampin, salicylates, streptokinase, sucralfate, sulfamethoxazole and trimethoprim, sulfonamides, urokinase, vitamin K, zafirlukast, zileuton. Ritonavir and delavirdine may decrease warfarin metabolism; concurrent use of delavirdine and warfarin is not recommended; suspected drug interaction with nevirapine (monitor closely)

Herbal remedies such as bromelains, danshen, dong quai, garlic, ginkgo biloba, and ginseng may increase the effects of warfarin; coenzyme Q_{10} (ubidecarenone) and St John's wort (*Hypericum perforatum*) may decrease the effects of Coumadin®.

Food Interactions Vitamin K can reverse the anticoagulation effects of warfarin; large amounts of food high in vitamin K (such as beef liver, pork liver, green tea, and green leafy vegetables) may reverse warfarin, decrease prothrombin time, and lead to therapeutic failure. Patients should not change dietary habits once stabilized on warfarin therapy. A balanced diet with a consistent intake of vitamin K is essential. Avoid large amounts of alfalfa, asparagus, broccoli, brussel sprouts, cabbage, cauliflower, green teas, kale, lettuce, spinach, turnip greens, watercress. Avoid enteral feeds high in vitamin K. **Note:** Breast-fed infants may be more sensitive to warfarin due to low amounts of vitamin K in breast milk.

High doses of vitamin A, E, or C may alter PT; use caution with fish oils or omega 3 fatty acids; avoid fried or boiled onions as they may increase drug effect by increasing fibrinolytic activity; avoid herbal teas and remedies such as tonka beans, melilot, and woodruff as they contain natural coumarins and will increase effect of warfarin; avoid large amounts of liver, avocado, soy protein, soybean oil, papain.

Cranberry juice or other cranberry products may increase the INR in patients receiving warfarin and cause severe bleeding (flavonoids found in cranberries may inhibit cytochrome P450 isoenzyme CYP2C9 and reduce the metabolism of warfarin)

Stability

Tablets: Store at controlled room temperature of 15°C to 30°C (59°F to 86°F). Protect from light. Dispense in tight, light-resistant container.

Injection: Store unopened vials in box at controlled room temperature of 15°C to 30°C

(Continued)

Warfarin *(Continued)*

(59°F to 86°F). Protect from light. After reconstitution, store at controlled room temperature and use within 4 hours after reconstitution. Do not refrigerate. Discard unused portion (does not contain preservative). Reconstituted solution is stable in D_5LR, $D_5½NS$, D_5NS, D_5W, $D_{10}W$; **variable stability (consult detailed reference)** in LR, NS.

Mechanism of Action Interferes with hepatic synthesis of vitamin K-dependent coagulation factors (II, VII, IX, X)

Pharmacodynamics Anticoagulation effects:

Onset of action: Within 36-72 hours

Maximum effect: Within 5-7 days

Pharmacokinetics

Absorption: Oral: Rapid

Distribution: Adults: V_d: 0.14 L/kg

Protein binding: 99%

Metabolism: Hepatic, primarily via CYP2C9; minor pathways include CYP2C19, 1A2, and 3A4

Half-life, elimination: Adults: 20-60 hours; mean: 40 hours; highly variable among individuals

Usual Dosage Note: Dosing must be individualized.

Oral:

Infants and Children: **To maintain an International Normalized Ratio (INR) between 2-3**:

Initial loading dose on day 1 (if baseline INR is 1-1.3): 0.2 mg/kg (maximum dose: 10 mg); use initial loading dose of 0.1 mg/kg if patient has liver dysfunction or has undergone a Fontan procedure (see Streif, 1999)

Loading dose for days 2-4: doses are dependent upon patient's INR

- if INR is 1.1-1.3, repeat the initial loading dose
- if INR is 1.4-1.9, give 50% of the initial loading dose
- if INR is 2-3, give 50% of the initial loading dose
- if INR is 3.1-3.5, give 25% of the initial loading dose
- if INR is >3.5, hold the drug until INR <3.5, then restart using maintenance dose guidelines immediately below

Maintenance dose guidelines for day 5 of therapy and beyond: Doses are dependent upon patient's INR

- if INR is 1.1-1.4, increase dose by 20% of previous dose
- if INR is 1.5-1.9, increase dose by 10% of previous dose
- if INR is 2-3, do not change the dose
- if INR is 3.1-3.5, decrease dose by 10% of previous dose
- if INR is >3.5, hold the drug and check INR daily until INR <3.5, then restart at 20% less than the previous dose

Usual maintenance dose: ~0.1 mg/kg/day; range: 0.05-0.34 mg/kg/day; the dose in mg/kg/day is inversely related to age. In the largest pediatric study (n=319; Streif, 1999), infants <12 months of age required a mean dose of 0.33 mg/kg/day, but children 13-18 years required a mean dose of 0.09 mg/kg/day; a target INR of 2-3 was used for a majority of these patients (75% of warfarin courses). Overall, children required a mean dose of 0.16 mg/kg/day to achieve a target INR of 2-3. In another study (Andrew, 1994), to attain an INR of 1.3-1.8, infants <12 months (n=2) required 0.24 and 0.27 mg/kg/day, but children >1 year required a mean of 0.08 mg/kg/day (range: 0.03-0.17 mg/kg/day). Consistent anticoagulation may be difficult to maintain in children <5 years of age. Children receiving phenobarbital, carbamazepine, or enteral nutrition may require higher maintenance doses (see Streif, 1999).

Adults: **Note:** Initial dosing must be individualized. Consider patient factors (hepatic function, cardiac function, age, nutritional status, concurrent therapy, risk of bleeding) in addition to prior dose response (if available) and the clinical situation. Initial dose: 5-10 mg daily for 2 days, then adjust dose according to results of INR or PT; usual maintenance dose ranges from 2-10 mg daily; individual patients may require loading and maintenance doses outside these general guidelines.

Note: Lower starting doses may be required for patients with hepatic impairment, poor nutrition, CHF, elderly, high risk of bleeding, or patients who are debilitated. Higher initial doses may be reasonable in selected patients (ie, receiving enzyme-inducing agents and with low risk of bleeding).

I.V.: (For patients who cannot take oral form): I.V. dose is equal to oral dose

Dosing adjustment in renal disease: No adjustment required; however, patients with renal failure have an increased risk of bleeding complications. Monitor closely.

Dosing adjustment in hepatic disease: Monitor effect at usual doses; the response to oral anticoagulants may be markedly enhanced in obstructive jaundice (due to reduced vitamin K absorption) and also in hepatitis and cirrhosis (due to decreased production of vitamin K-dependent clotting factors); INR should be closely monitored

Administration

Oral: May administer on an empty or full stomach. Take at the same time each day.

Parenteral: For I.V. use only; do not administer I.M. Reconstitute 5 mg vial with 2.7 mL SWI to produce 2 mg/mL solution. Administer by slow I.V. injection over 1-2 minutes into peripheral vein

Monitoring Parameters INR (preferred) or prothrombin time; hemoglobin, hematocrit, signs and symptoms of bleeding

Reference Range The INR is now the standard test used to monitor warfarin anticoagulation; the desired INR is based upon indication; due to the lack of pediatric clinical trials assessing optimal INR ranges and clinical outcomes, the desired INR ranges for children are extrapolated from adult studies; the optimal therapeutic INR ranges may possibly be lower in children versus adults. Further pediatric studies are needed (see Monagle, 2004). **Note:** If INR is not available, prothrombin time should be 1½ to 2 times the control.

Warfarin levels are not used for monitoring degree of anticoagulation. They may be useful if a patient with unexplained coagulopathy is using the drug surreptitiously or if it is unclear whether clinical resistance is due to true drug resistance or lack of drug intake.

Normal prothrombin time (PT): 10.9-12.9 seconds. Healthy premature newborns have prolonged coagulation test screening results (eg, PT, aPTT, TT) which return to normal adult values at approximately 6 months of age. However, healthy premature newborns (ie, those not receiving antithrombotic agents), do not develop spontaneous hemorrhage or thrombotic complications because of a balance between procoagulants and inhibitors.

Targeted INR and Ranges for Children, Based on Indication
See "Antithrombotic Therapy in Children" in the Appendix for timing of initiation, duration of therapy, and adjunct antithrombotic and antiplatelet therapy.

Indication	Targeted INR	Targeted INR Range
Systemic venous thromboembolism (children >2 months of age)	2.5	2.0-3.0
Central venous line-related thrombosis, initial 3 months of therapy	2.5	2.0-3.0
Central venous line-related thrombosis after first 3 months of warfarin therapy (**Note:** This is a prophylactic dose)		1.5-1.8
Central venous line, long-term home TPN (prophylactic dose)		2.0-2.5
Primary prophylaxis following Fontan procedure	2.5	2.0-3.0
Primary prophylaxis for dilated cardiomyopathy	2.5	2.0-3.0
Primary prophylaxis for biological prosthetic heart valves in children (follow adult guidelines in table below)		
Primary prophylaxis for mechanical prosthetic heart valves in children (follow adult guidelines in table below)		
Kawasaki disease with giant aneurysm	2.5	2.0-3.0
Cerebral sinovenous thrombosis	2.5	2.0-3.0

Targeted INR and Ranges for Adults, Based on Indication

Indication	Targeted INR	Targeted INR Range
Acute myocardial infarction (high risk)	2.5	2.0-3.0[1,2,3]
Atrial fibrillation	2.5	2.0-3.0
St Jude Medical bileaflet mechanical aortic valve	2.5	2.0-3.0
Bileaflet or tilting disk mechanical mitral valve	3	2.5-3.5
Caged ball or caged disk mechanical valve	3	2.5-3.5[1]
Mechanical prosthetic valve with systemic embolism despite adequate anticoagulation	3	2.5-3.5[1]
Carbomedics bileaflet/Medtronic Hall tilting disk mechanical aortic valve (NSR, Nl LA size)	2.5	2.0-3.0
Mechanical valve and risk factors (atrial fibrillation, MI, left atrial enlargement, low EF, endocardial damage)	3	2.5-3.5[1]
Bioprosthetic mitral valve	2.5	2.0-3.0[2]
Bioprosthetic aortic valve	2.5	2.0-3.0[2] (or aspirin 81 mg/day)
Bioprosthetic mitral or aortic valve with atrial fibrillation	2.5	2.0-3.0
Rheumatic mitral valve disease and NSR (left atrial diameter >5.5 cm)	2.5	2.0-3.0
Venous thromboembolism	2.5	2.0-3.0
Lupus inhibitor (no other risk factors)	2.5	2.0-3.0
Lupus inhibitor and recurrent thromboembolism	3	2.5-3.5

[1]Combine with aspirin 81 mg/day

[2]Maintain anticoagulation for 3 months

[3]High-risk includes a large anterior MI, significant heart failure, intracardiac thrombus, thromboembolism

(Continued)

Warfarin *(Continued)*

Patient Information Read the patient Medication Guide that you receive with each prescription and refill of warfarin. Take exactly as directed; if a dose is missed, take it as soon as possible, then return to normal dosing schedule; if a dose is skipped, do **not** double the next dose. Follow diet and activity as recommended by prescriber; check with prescriber before changing diet. Do not make major changes in your dietary intake of vitamin K (green leafy vegetables). Avoid alcohol, cranberry juice, and cranberry products; limit caffeine. Report any signs of bleeding to physician at once (eg, nosebleeds, bleeding gums, prolonged bleeding from a cut, heavier than normal menstrual or vaginal bleeding, coughing up blood, vomiting blood or coffee ground-like material, pink or dark brown urine, red or black tar-like stools, unusual bruising, headaches, dizziness, weakness, pain, swelling, or discomfort). Avoid hazardous activities; use soft toothbrush; carry Medi-Alert® ID identifying drug use. Be aware of other drugs, foods, and herbal remedies to avoid. Report the use of other medications, nonprescription medications, and herbal or natural products to your physician and pharmacist. Do not take any new medication during therapy unless approved by prescriber. Report adverse effects such as skin rash or irritation, unusual fever, persistent nausea or GI upset, pain in joints or back, or unhealed wounds.

Nursing Implications Be aware of drug interactions, interactions with herbal remedies, and foods that contain vitamin K which can alter anticoagulant effects. Avoid I.M. injections of all drugs in patients receiving warfarin.

Additional Information Overdoses of warfarin may be treated with vitamin K, to reverse warfarin's anticoagulation effect

Dosage Forms Excipient information presented when available (limited, particularly for generics); consult specific product labeling.

Injection, powder for reconstitution, as sodium:
  Coumadin®: 5 mg

Tablet, as sodium: 1 mg, 2 mg, 2.5 mg, 3 mg, 4 mg, 5 mg, 6 mg, 7.5 mg, 10 mg
  Coumadin®, Jantoven™: 1 mg, 2 mg, 2.5 mg, 3 mg, 4 mg, 5 mg, 6 mg, 7.5 mg, 10 mg

References

Andrew M, Marzinotto V, Brooker LA, et al, "Oral Anticoagulation Therapy in Pediatric Patients: A Prospective Study," *Thromb Haemost*, 1994, 71(3):265-9.

Ansell J, Hirsh J, Poller L, et al, "The Pharmacology and Management of the Vitamin K Antagonists: The Seventh ACCP Conference on Antithrombotic and Thrombolytic Therapy," *Chest*, 2004, 126(3 Suppl):204S-33S.

Arepally GM and Ortel TL, "Clinical Practice. Heparin-Induced Thrombocytopenia," *N Engl J Med*, 2006, 355(8):809-17

David M and Andrew M, "Venous Thromboembolic Complications in Children," *J Pediatr*, 1993, 123(3):337-46.

Fihn SD "Aiming for Safe Anticoagulation," *N Engl J Med*, 1995, 333(1):54-5.

Hirsh J, Dalen JE, Anderson DR, et al, "Oral Anticoagulants. Mechanism of Action, Clinical Effectiveness, and Optimal Therapeutic Range," *Chest*, 2001, 119:8S-21S.

Monagle P, Chan A, Massicotte P, et al, "Antithrombotic Therapy in Children: The Seventh ACCP Conference on Antithrombotic and Thrombolytic Therapy," *Chest*, 2004, 126(3 Suppl):645S-87S.

Monagle P, Michelson AD, Bovill E, et al, "Antithrombotic Therapy in Children," *Chest*, 2001, 119:344S-70S.

Salem DN, Stein PD, Al-Ahmad A, et al, "Antithrombotic Therapy in Valvular Heart Disease - Native and Prosthetic: The Seventh ACCP Conference on Antithrombotic and Thrombolytic Therapy," *Chest*, 2004, 126(3 Suppl):457S-82S.

Streif W, Andrew M, Marzinotto V, et al, "Analysis of Warfarin Therapy in Pediatric Patients: A Prospective Cohort Study of 319 Patients," *Blood*, 1999, 94(9):3007-14.

Suvarna R, Pirmohamed M, and Henderson L, "Possible Interaction Between Warfarin and Cranberry Juice," *BMJ*, 2003, 327(7429):1454.

Wells PS, Holbrook AM, Crowther NR, et al, "Interactions of Warfarin With Drugs and Food," *Ann Intern Med*, 1994, 121(9):676-83.

♦ **Warfarin Sodium** *see* Warfarin *on page 1626*

♦ **Wart-Off® Maximum Strength [OTC]** *see* Salicylic Acid *on page 1413*

♦ **4-Way® 12 Hour [OTC]** *see* Oxymetazoline *on page 1194*

♦ **4 Way® Fast Acting [OTC]** *see* Phenylephrine *on page 1250*

♦ **4-Way® Saline Moisturizing Mist [OTC]** *see* Sodium Chloride *on page 1450*

♦ **Westcort®** *see* Hydrocortisone *on page 781*

♦ **White Mineral Oil** *see* Mineral Oil *on page 1065*

♦ **Winpred™ (Can)** *see* PredniSONE *on page 1308*

♦ **WinRho® SDF** *see* Rh_o(D) Immune Globulin *on page 1374*

♦ **Winstrol®** *see* Stanozolol *on page 1471*

♦ **Wound Wash Saline™ [OTC]** *see* Sodium Chloride *on page 1450*

♦ **WR-2721** *see* Amifostine *on page 91*

♦ **WR-139007** *see* Dacarbazine *on page 433*

♦ **WR-139013** *see* Chlorambucil *on page 333*

- ♦ **WR-139021** *see* Carmustine *on page 290*
- ♦ **Wycillin [DSC]** *see* Penicillin G Procaine *on page 1233*
- ♦ **Xanax®** *see* Alprazolam *on page 79*
- ♦ **Xanax TS™ (Can)** *see* Alprazolam *on page 79*
- ♦ **Xanax XR®** *see* Alprazolam *on page 79*
- ♦ **Xigris®** *see* Drotrecogin Alfa (Activated) *on page 549*
- ♦ **Xodol®** *see* Hydrocodone and Acetaminophen *on page 779*
- ♦ **Xolair®** *see* Omalizumab *on page 1165*
- ♦ **Xolegel™** *see* Ketoconazole *on page 887*
- ♦ **Xopenex®** *see* Levalbuterol *on page 920*
- ♦ **Xopenex HFA™** *see* Levalbuterol *on page 920*
- ♦ **XPECT™ [OTC]** *see* Guaifenesin *on page 745*
- ♦ **Xylocaine®** *see* Lidocaine *on page 933*
- ♦ **Xylocaine® MPF** *see* Lidocaine *on page 933*
- ♦ **Xylocaine® MPF With Epinephrine** *see* Lidocaine and Epinephrine *on page 936*
- ♦ **Xylocaine® Viscous** *see* Lidocaine *on page 933*
- ♦ **Xylocaine® With Epinephrine** *see* Lidocaine and Epinephrine *on page 936*
- ♦ **Xylocard® (Can)** *see* Lidocaine *on page 933*

Yellow Fever Vaccine (YEL oh FEE ver vak SEEN)

U.S. Brand Names YF-VAX®

Canadian Brand Names YF-VAX®

Therapeutic Category Vaccine

Generic Available No

Use To provide active immunity to yellow fever virus to children ≥ 9 months of age and adults, who are either traveling or living in areas where yellow fever infection exists

Pregnancy Risk Factor C

Lactation Excretion in breast milk unknown/use caution

Contraindications Hypersensitivity to the vaccine, egg or chick embryo protein, or any component; individuals with blood dyscrasias, leukemia, lymphomas, or other malignant neoplasms affecting the bone marrow or lymphatic systems; concurrent immunosuppressive therapy; primary and acquired immunodeficiency states including those who are immunosuppressed in association with HIV; family history of congenital or hereditary immunodeficiency; children <4 months of age

Warnings Not for use in patients who are immunosuppressed due to an increased risk of encephalitis with yellow fever vaccine administration; consider delaying travel or obtaining a waiver letter. Patients on low-dose or short-term corticosteroids, or with asymptomatic HIV infection are not considered immunosuppressed and may receive the vaccine. Chicken embryos are used in the manufacture of this vaccine; use caution in patients with immediate-type hypersensitivity reactions to eggs; immediate treatment for anaphylactic reactions should be available during vaccine use.

Avoid use in infants <9 months and pregnant women unless travel to high-risk areas are unavoidable; use in infants <4 months of age is contraindicated due to risk of encephalitis. The decision to use in children between 4-9 months of age must weigh the risks of exposure to the virus with the theoretic risks of vaccine-associated encephalitis (*Red Book*, 2006). Advice regarding use of this vaccine can be obtained from the Division of Vector-Borne Infectious Diseases of the CDC (see Additional Information).

Precautions Use with caution in patients with thymic disorders including myasthenia gravis, thymoma, or prior thymectomy and adults >65 years of age due to an increased risk of vaccine-associated viscerotropic disease (multisystem organ failure).

Adverse Reactions All serious adverse reactions must be reported to the U.S. Department of Health and Human Services (DHHS) Vaccine Adverse Event Reporting System (VAERS) 1-800-822-7967.

Frequency not defined (adverse reactions may be increased in patients <9 months or ≥65 years of age)

Central nervous system: Headache, myalgia, fever (incidence of these reactions have been reported to be as low as <5% and as high as 10% to 30% depending on the study), vaccine-associated neurotropic disease (postvaccinal encephalitis; rare)

Local: Injection site reactions (edema, erythema, pain)

Neuromuscular & skeletal: Weakness

Miscellaneous: Hypersensitivity (immediate), viscerotropic disease (multiple organ system failure; rare)

(Continued)

Yellow Fever Vaccine *(Continued)*

Drug Interactions Immunosuppressive agents: Decreased effect of live vaccines may occur.

Stability Stable refrigerated; do not freeze. Must be used within 60 minutes of reconstitution.

Mechanism of Action
A live, attenuated virus vaccine; offers active immunity to disease caused by yellow fever virus

Pharmacodynamics Onset of action: Seroconversion: 10-14 days

Usual Dosage Children ≥9 months and Adults: SubQ: One dose (0.5 mL) ≥10 days before travel; Booster: Repeat same dosage every 10 years if at continued risk of exposure.

Administration Parenteral: Use entire contents of provided diluent to reconstitute vaccine. Gently swirl until a uniform suspension forms; swirl well before withdrawing dose. Avoid vigorous shaking to prevent foaming of suspension. Use within 60 minutes following reconstitution; keep suspension refrigerated until used. Administer by SubQ injection into the anterolateral aspect of the thigh or arm; **not for I.V. administration**

Monitoring Parameters Monitor for adverse effects up to 10 days after vaccination.

Patient Information Immunity develops by the tenth day and **WHO** requires revaccination every 10 years to maintain travelers' vaccination certificates.

Nursing Implications Federal law requires that the date of administration, the vaccine manufacturer, lot number of vaccine, and the administering person's name, title, and address be entered into the patient's permanent medical record.

Additional Information A desensitization procedure is available for persons with severe egg sensitivity. Consult manufacturer's labeling for details. Some countries require a valid international Certification of Vaccination showing receipt of vaccine. The WHO requires revaccination every 10 years to maintain traveler's vaccination certificate. Current requirements and recommendations for immunization related to travel destination can be obtained from the CDC Travelers' Health Web site (www.cdc.gov/travel).

The following CDC agencies may be contacted if serologic testing is needed or for advice when administering yellow fever vaccine to pregnant women, children < 9 months, or patients with altered immune status:
Division of Vector-Borne Infectious Diseases: 970-221-6400
Division of Global Migration and Quarantine: 404-498-1600

Dosage Forms Excipient information presented when available (limited, particularly for generics); consult specific product labeling.

Injection, powder for reconstitution [17D-204 strain]: ≥4.74 Log_{10} plaque-forming units (PFU) per 0.5 mL dose [single-dose or 5-dose vial; produced in chicken embryos; packaged with diluent; vial stopper contains latex]

References

Centers for Disease Control and Prevention, "General Recommendations on Immunization. Recommendations of the Advisory Committee on Immunization Practices (ACIP) and the American Academy of Family Physicians (AAFP)," *MMMR Recomm Rep*, 2002, 51(R-2):1-35.

Centers for Disease Control and Prevention, "Guidelines for Preventing Opportunistic Infections Among Hematopoietic Stem Cell Transplant Recipients. Recommendations of CDC, the Infectious Disease Society of America, and the American Society of Blood and Marrow Transplantation," *MMWR Recomm Rep*, 2004, 49(RR-10):89-90.

Centers for Disease Control and Prevention, "Yellow Fever Vaccine. Recommendations of the Advisory Committee on Immunization Practices (ACIP)," *MMMR Recomm Rep*, 2002, 51(R-2):1-11.

Red Book: 2006 Report of the Committee on Infectious Diseases, 27th ed, Pickering LK, ed, Elk Grove Village, IL: American Academy of Pediatrics, 2006, 101 and 216.

♦ **YF-VAX®** *see* Yellow Fever Vaccine *on page 1631*
♦ **YM-08310** *see* Amifostine *on page 91*
♦ **Yodoxin®** *see* Iodoquinol *on page 862*
♦ **Z4942** *see* Ifosfamide *on page 810*
♦ **Zaditen® (Can)** *see* Ketotifen *on page 893*
♦ **Zaditor® [OTC]** *see* Ketotifen *on page 893*

Zafirlukast (za FIR loo kast)

Medication Safety Issues
Sound-alike/look-alike issues:
Accolate® may be confused with Accupril®, Accutane®, Aclovate®

Related Information
Asthma *on page 1904*

U.S. Brand Names Accolate®

Canadian Brand Names Accolate®

Index Terms ICI-204,219

Therapeutic Category Antiasthmatic; Leukotriene Receptor Antagonist

Generic Available No

Use Prophylaxis and chronic treatment of asthma

Pregnancy Risk Factor B

Lactation Enters breast milk/contraindicated

Contraindications Hypersensitivity to zafirlukast or any component

Warnings Zafirlukast is not indicated for use in the reversal of bronchospasm in acute asthma attacks, including status asthmaticus. Therapy with zafirlukast can be continued during acute exacerbations of asthma. An increased proportion of zafirlukast patients (>55 years of age) reported infections as compared to placebo-treated patients; these infections were mostly mild or moderate in intensity, predominantly affected the respiratory tract, were dose-proportional to the total milligrams of zafirlukast exposure, and associated with coadministration of inhaled corticosteroids.

Hepatic adverse events (including hepatitis, hyperbilirubinemia, and hepatic failure) have been reported. Female patients may be at greater risk. Discontinue **immediately** if liver dysfunction is suspected. Periodic testing of liver function may be considered (early detection is generally believed to improve the likelihood of recovery). If hepatic dysfunction is suspected (due to clinical signs/symptoms) liver function tests should be measured immediately. Do not resume or restart if hepatic function tests are consistent with dysfunction.

Rare cases of eosinophilic vasculitis (Churg-Strauss) have been reported in patients receiving zafirlukast (usually, but not always, associated with reduction in concurrent steroid dosage). No causal relationship established.

Precautions Use with caution in patients receiving warfarin (see Drug Interactions) and patients with liver disease; dosage reduction in patients with hepatic impairment may be needed; discontinue therapy if liver dysfunction occurs; where no other attributable cause of liver dysfunction is identified, do not resume zafirlukast therapy

Adverse Reactions

Central nervous system: Headache, dizziness, pain, fever, asthenia
Dermatologic: Vasculitic rash (rare)
Gastrointestinal: Nausea, diarrhea, abdominal pain, vomiting, dyspepsia, xerostomia
Hematologic: Systemic eosinophilic vasculitis (rare), agranulocytosis
Hepatic: Elevated liver enzymes, hepatitis, hyperbilirubinemia, hepatic failure
Neuromuscular & skeletal: Myalgia, weakness, arthralgia
Respiratory: Rhinitis, pharyngitis
Miscellaneous: Infections (primarily respiratory), hypersensitivity reactions

Drug Interactions Cytochrome P450 isoenzyme CYP2C9 substrate; CYP2C9 and CYP3A3/4 isoenzyme inhibitor

Erythromycin, terfenadine, and theophylline decrease zafirlukast serum levels; aspirin increases plasma levels of zafirlukast; coadministration of zafirlukast with warfarin results in a clinically significant increase in prothrombin time (PT)

Food Interactions Food decreases zafirlukast absorption by 40%

Stability Store tablets at controlled room temperature; protect from light and moisture; dispense in original airtight container

Mechanism of Action Zafirlukast is a selective and competitive leukotriene-receptor antagonist (LTRA) of cysteinyl leukotrienes C_4 (LTC_4), D_4 (LTD_4), and E_4 (LTE_4). This activity produces inhibition of the effects of these leukotrienes on bronchial smooth muscle resulting in the attenuation of bronchoconstriction and decreased vascular permeability, mucosal edema, and mucus production.

Pharmacodynamics Asthma symptom improvement:
Maximum effect: 2-6 weeks
Duration: 12 hours

Pharmacokinetics

Absorption: Rapid
Distribution: Extensively excreted into breast milk; breast milk to plasma ratio: 0.15
  V_d: Adults: 70 L
Protein binding: 99%, predominantly albumin
Metabolism: Extensively metabolized by liver via cytochrome P450 isoenzyme CYP2C9 pathway
Half-life, elimination: Adults: 10 hours (range: 8-16 hours)
Time to peak serum concentration: 3 hours
Elimination: Fecal (90%) and urine (10%)
  Clearance:
    Children 5-6 years: 9.2 L/hour
    Children 7-11 years: 11.4 L/hour
    Adults: 20 L/hour

Usual Dosage Oral:
Children 5-11 years: 10 mg twice daily
Children ≥12 years and Adults: 20 mg twice daily
(Continued)

Zafirlukast *(Continued)*

Dosing adjustment in hepatic impairment: In patients with hepatic impairment (ie, biopsy-proven cirrhosis), there is a 50% to 60% greater C_{max} and AUC compared to normal subjects; these patients should be monitored closely for adverse effects and dosage reductions made if indicated (see Precautions)

Administration Oral: Administer at least 1 hour before or 2 hours after a meal

Monitoring Parameters Pulmonary function tests (FEV-1, PEF), improvement in asthma symptoms, periodic liver function tests

Reference Range Plasma levels not clinically indicated; plasma zafirlukast serum concentrations exceeding 5 ng/mL at 12-14 hours following oral doses have correlated with activity; mean trough serum levels at doses of 20 mg twice daily were 20 ng/mL

Patient Information Take regularly as prescribed, even during symptom-free periods. Do not use to treat acute episodes of asthma. Do not decrease the dose or stop taking any other asthma medications unless instructed by a physician. May cause dry mouth. Nursing women should not take zafirlukast. Notify healthcare provider if experiencing symptoms of abdominal pain, nausea, fatigue, lethargy, itching, jaundice, flu-like symptoms, or anorexia.

Dosage Forms Excipient information presented when available (limited, particularly for generics); consult specific product labeling.

Tablet: 10 mg, 20 mg

References

"National Asthma Education and Prevention Program. Expert Panel Report: Guidelines for the Diagnosis and Management of Asthma Update on Selected Topics--2002," *J Allergy Clin Immunol*, 2002, 110(5 Suppl):S141-219.

Zalcitabine [DSC] (zal SITE a been)

Related Information

Adult and Adolescent HIV *on page 1821*
Pediatric HIV *on page 1816*
Perinatal HIV *on page 1831*

U.S. Brand Names Hivid® [DSC]

Canadian Brand Names Hivid®

Index Terms ddC; Dideoxycytidine

Therapeutic Category Antiretroviral Agent; HIV Agents (Anti-HIV Agents); Nucleoside Reverse Transcriptase Inhibitor (NRTI)

Generic Available No

Use Treatment of HIV infection in combination with other antiretroviral agents. (**Note:** HIV regimens consisting of **three** antiretroviral agents are strongly recommended)

Pregnancy Risk Factor C

Lactation Excretion in breast milk unknown/contraindicated

Contraindications Hypersensitivity to zalcitabine or any component

Warnings An accumulative dose-related, clinically disabling peripheral neuropathy (treatment-limiting), or fatal pancreatitis may occur; discontinue therapy in patients with symptoms of pancreatitis until pancreatitis can be ruled out; cases of fatal lactic acidosis and severe hepatomegaly with steatosis may occur; hepatic failure and death (which may be related to underlying hepatitis B) have been reported (rare); discontinue therapy in patients with clinical or laboratory signs suggestive of lactic acidosis or hepatotoxicity (eg, steatosis and hepatomegaly even without marked elevations of liver enzymes) or if liver function tests increase to >5 times the upper limit of normal

Precautions Use with extreme caution in patients with pre-existing peripheral neuropathy; avoid use in patients with moderate or severe peripheral neuropathy; use with caution in patients at risk for developing peripheral neuropathy [patients with low CD4 count (<50 cells/mm^2), diabetes mellitus, weight loss, concurrent therapy with other drugs that cause peripheral neuropathy]; zalcitabine may exacerbate existing liver dysfunction in patients with a previous history of liver disease or alcohol abuse; increased liver function tests were observed in patients on zalcitabine therapy; use with caution in patients with hepatic impairment; obtain CBC and clinical chemistry tests prior to and during therapy; obtain serum amylase and triglyceride levels and use with caution in patients with history of pancreatitis, increased amylase, ethanol abuse or patients receiving hyperalimentation; use with caution and adjust dose in patients with renal dysfunction; multiple potentially serious drug interactions exist (see Drug Interactions); fat redistribution and accumulation [ie, central obesity, peripheral wasting, facial wasting, breast enlargement, dorsocervical fat enlargement (buffalo hump), and cushingoid appearance] have been observed in patients receiving antiretroviral agents (causal relationship not established).

Adverse Reactions

Cardiovascular: Chest pain, edema, hypertension, palpitations, syncope, atrial fibrillation, tachycardia, CHF, cardiomyopathy, tachycardia

Central nervous system: Headache, dizziness, fever, malaise, fatigue

Dermatologic: Pruritus, rash (may be erythematous, maculopapular, follicular or other)

Endocrine & metabolic: Lactic acidosis (rare, but potentially fatal), hyperglycemia, hypocalcemia, fat redistribution and accumulation (see Precautions), weight loss

Gastrointestinal: Oral ulcers, nausea, esophageal ulcers, dysphagia, anorexia, abdominal pain, vomiting, diarrhea, constipation, pancreatitis (1.1%; can be fatal)

Hematologic: Leukopenia, absolute neutrophil count alteration, anemia, granulocytosis, neutrophilia, thrombocytopenia

Hepatic: Jaundice, hepatitis; severe hepatomegaly with steatosis (can be fatal)

Neuromuscular & skeletal: Peripheral neuropathy (22% to 35%), myalgia, arthralgia, weakness, foot pain, myositis

Respiratory: Pharyngitis, epistaxis

Miscellaneous: Anaphylactoid reactions, hypersensitivity reactions, night sweats

Drug Interactions Magnesium- and aluminum-containing antacids and metoclopramide may decrease the bioavailability of zalcitabine; amphotericin, foscarnet, probenecid, cimetidine, and aminoglycosides may interfere with the renal elimination of zalcitabine and potentiate the risk of peripheral neuropathy or other zalcitabine toxicities; drugs associated with peripheral neuropathy (chloramphenicol, cisplatin, dapsone, disulfiram, ethionamide, glutethimide, gold, hydralazine, iodoquinol, isoniazid, lithium, metronidazole, nitrofurantoin, pentamidine, phenytoin, ribavirin, and vincristine) may increase the risk for zalcitabine peripheral neuropathy; concomitant use of zalcitabine with didanosine or stavudine is **not** recommended (increased risk of pancreatitis and peripheral neuropathy); lamivudine and zalcitabine may inhibit the intracellular phosphorylation of each other (concurrent use of lamivudine and zalcitabine is **not** recommended); one case of fulminant pancreatitis associated with concomitant zalcitabine and pentamidine use has been reported; if I.V. pentamidine is required to treat *Pneumocystis carinii* pneumonia, treatment with zalcitabine should be interrupted; doxorubicin may decrease zalcitabine phosphorylation to the active metabolite (*in vitro* study; clinical relevance unknown)

Food Interactions Food decreases the rate and extent of absorption (AUC decreased by 14%)

Stability Tablets should be stored in tightly closed bottles at 59°F to 86°F

Mechanism of Action A nucleoside (pyrimidine) analogue that is converted within cells to the active metabolite dideoxycytidine triphosphate (ddCTP) which serves as an alternative substrate to deoxycytidine triphosphate (dCTP), a natural substrate for cellular DNA polymerase and reverse transcriptase; inhibits HIV viral enzyme reverse transcriptase and DNA synthesis causing chain termination

Pharmacokinetics

Distribution: V_{dss}:

Children: 9.3 L/m^2

Adults: 0.53 L/kg

CSF levels are 9% to 37% of serum levels (mean 20%)

Protein binding: Minimal, <4%

Metabolism: Converted intracellularly to active triphosphate form; minimal hepatic metabolism; primary identified metabolite is dideoxyuridine

Bioavailability:

Children: 29% to 100% (mean: 54%)

Adults: >80%

Half-life:

Children: Mean: 1.4 hours

Adults: 1-3 hours (mean: 2 hours)

Adults with Cl_{cr} <55 mL/minute: up to 8.5 hours

Elimination: Primarily renal with 60% of dose excreted unchanged in urine within 24 hours; elimination is prolonged in patients with renal dysfunction

Dialysis: Hemodialysis reduces plasma levels by 50%

Usual Dosage Oral (use in combination with other antiretroviral agents):

Neonates: Not approved for use; dose unknown

Infants and Children <13 years: Not approved for use; investigational: 0.01 mg/kg every 8 hours

Adolescents and Adults: 0.75 mg 3 times/day

Dosing adjustment in severe renal impairment: Adults:

Cl_{cr} 10-40 mL/minute: 0.75 mg every 12 hours

Cl_{cr} <10 mL/minute: 0.75 mg every 24 hours

Administration Oral: May be administered without regard to meals; do not administer concurrently with antacids

(Continued)

Zalcitabine [DSC] *(Continued)*

Monitoring Parameters Renal function, CD4 counts, viral load, CBC with differential, liver enzymes, serum chemistries, serum amylase, triglyceride, signs/symptoms of peripheral neuropathy

Patient Information Avoid alcohol; zalcitabine is not a cure; notify physician if numbness, tingling, persistent severe abdominal pain, nausea, or vomiting occurs; take zalcitabine every day as prescribed; do not change dose or discontinue without physician's advice; if a dose is missed, take it as soon as possible, then return to normal dosing schedule; if a dose is skipped, do **not** double the next dose

HIV medications may cause changes in body fat, including an increase in fat in the upper back and neck, breasts, and trunk; a loss of fat from the face, arms, and legs may also occur.

Additional Information Adverse events may be increased in patients with decreased CD4 cell counts; an oral 0.1 mg/mL zalcitabine raspberry syrup formulation is available on an investigational basis from Roche Pharmaceuticals as part of a U.S. pediatric compassionate use study (NV14610)

Dosage Forms Excipient information presented when available (limited, particularly for generics); consult specific product labeling. [DSC] = Discontinued product

Tablet:

Hivid®: 0.375 mg, 0.75 mg [DSC]

References

Adkins JC, Peters DH, and Faulds D, "Zalcitabine. An Update of Its Pharmacodynamic and Pharmacokinetic Properties and Clinical Efficacy in the Management of HIV Infection," *Drugs*, 1997, 53(6):1054-80.

Bakshi SS, Britto P, Capparelli E, et al, "Evaluation of Pharmacokinetics, Safety, Tolerance, and Activity of Combination of Zalcitabine and Zidovudine in Stable, Zidovudine-Treated Pediatric Patients With Human Immunodeficiency Virus Infection. AIDS Clinical Trials Group Protocol 190 Team," *J Infect Dis*, 1997, 175(5):1039-50.

Briars LA, Hilao JJ, and Kraus DM, "A Review of Pediatric Human Immunodeficiency Virus Infection," *Journal of Pharmacy Practice*, 2004, 17(6):407-31.

Center for Disease Control and Prevention, "Guidelines for Using Antiretroviral Agents Among HIV-Infected Adults and Adolescents. Recommendations of the Panel on Clinical Practices for Treatment of HIV," *MMWR*, 2002, 51(RR-7):1-55.

Chadwick EG, Nazareno LA, Nieuwenhuis TJ, et al, "Phase I Evaluation of Zalcitabine Administered to Human Immunodeficiency Virus-Infected Children," *J Infect Dis*, 1995, 172(6):1475-9.

Panel on Clinical Practices for Treatment of HIV Infection, "Guidelines for the Use of Antiretroviral Agents in HIV-Infected Adults and Adolescents," October 10, 2006, http://www.aidsinfo.nih.gov.

Pizzo PA, Butler K, Balis F, et al, "Dideoxycytidine Alone and in an Alternating Schedule With Zidovudine in Children With Symptomatic Human Immunodeficiency Virus Infection," *J Pediatr*, 1990, 117(5):799-808.

Spector SA, "HIV Therapy Advances. Pediatric Antiretroviral Choices," *AIDS*, 1994, 8(Suppl 3):S15-8.

Spector SA, Blanchard S, Wara DW, et al, "Comparative Trial of Two Dosages of Zalcitabine in Zidovudine-Experienced Children With Advanced Human Immunodeficiency Virus Disease. Pediatric AIDS Clinical Trials Group," *Pediatr Infect Dis J*, 1997, 16(6):623-6.

Working Group on Antiretroviral Therapy and Medical Management of HIV-Infected Children, "Guidelines for the Use of Antiretroviral Agents in Pediatric HIV Infection," October 26, 2006, http://www.aidsinfo.nih.gov.

Working Group on Antiretroviral Therapy and Medical Management of HIV-Infected Children, "Guidelines for the Use of Antiretroviral Agents in Pediatric HIV Infection. Supplement I: Pediatric Antiretroviral Drug Information," October 26, 2006, http://www.aidsinfo.nih.gov.

- **Zantac®** *see* Ranitidine *on page 1366*
- **Zantac 75® [OTC]** *see* Ranitidine *on page 1366*
- **Zantac 75® (Can)** *see* Ranitidine *on page 1366*
- **Zantac 150™ [OTC]** *see* Ranitidine *on page 1366*
- **Zantac® EFFERdose®** *see* Ranitidine *on page 1366*
- **Zapzyt® [OTC]** *see* Benzoyl Peroxide *on page 207*
- **Zapzyt® Acne Wash [OTC]** *see* Salicylic Acid *on page 1413*
- **Zapzyt® Pore Treatment [OTC]** *see* Salicylic Acid *on page 1413*
- **Zarontin®** *see* Ethosuximide *on page 618*
- **Zaroxolyn®** *see* Metolazone *on page 1044*
- **Z-Cof LA™** *see* Guaifenesin and Dextromethorphan *on page 748*
- **ZDV** *see* Zidovudine *on page 1637*
- **ZDV, Abacavir, and 3TC** *see* Abacavir, Lamivudine, and Zidovudine *on page 38*
- **ZDV, Abacavir, and Lamivudine** *see* Abacavir, Lamivudine, and Zidovudine *on page 38*
- **ZDV, ABC, and 3TC** *see* Abacavir, Lamivudine, and Zidovudine *on page 38*
- **ZDV and 3TC** *see* Lamivudine and Zidovudine *on page 904*
- **Zeasorb®-AF [OTC]** *see* Miconazole *on page 1056*
- **Zemplar®** *see* Paricalcitol *on page 1214*
- **Zemuron®** *see* Rocuronium *on page 1402*
- **Zenapax®** *see* Daclizumab *on page 434*
- **Zerit®** *see* Stavudine *on page 1472*
- **Zestril®** *see* Lisinopril *on page 946*

- **Zetar® [OTC]** *see* Coal Tar *on page 394*
- **Zetia™** *see* Ezetimibe *on page 627*
- **Ziagen®** *see* Abacavir *on page 32*

Zidovudine (zye DOE vyoo deen)

Medication Safety Issues

Sound-alike/look-alike issues:

Azidothymidine may be confused with azathioprine, aztreonam

Retrovir® may be confused with ritonavir

AZT is an error-prone abbreviation (mistaken as azathioprine, aztreonam)

Related Information

Adult and Adolescent HIV *on page 1821*

Pediatric HIV *on page 1816*

Perinatal HIV *on page 1831*

U.S. Brand Names Retrovir®

Canadian Brand Names Apo-Zidovudine®; AZT™; Retrovir®

Index Terms Azidothymidine; AZT (error-prone abbreviation); Compound S; ZDV

Therapeutic Category Antiretroviral Agent; HIV Agents (Anti-HIV Agents); Nucleoside Reverse Transcriptase Inhibitor (NRTI)

Generic Available Yes: Tablet

Use Treatment of HIV infection in combination with other antiretroviral agents; (**Note:** HIV regimens consisting of **three** antiretroviral agents are strongly recommended); chemoprophylaxis after occupational exposure to HIV; chemoprophylaxis to reduce perinatal HIV transmission

Pregnancy Risk Factor C

Lactation Enters breast milk/contraindicated

Contraindications Life-threatening hypersensitivity to zidovudine or any component

Warnings Hematologic toxicity including neutropenia and severe anemia requiring transfusions may occur; use with caution in patients with ANC <1000 cells/mm^3 or hemoglobin <9.5 g/dL; discontinue treatment in children with an ANC <500 cells/mm^3 until marrow recovery is observed; use of erythropoietin, filgrastim, or reduced zidovudine dosage may be necessary in some patients; prolonged use of zidovudine may cause myositis and myopathy; zidovudine has been shown to be carcinogenic in rats and mice.

Cases of lactic acidosis, severe hepatomegaly with steatosis, and death have been reported in patients receiving nucleoside analogues; most of these cases have been in women; prolonged nucleoside use, obesity, and prior liver disease may be risk factors; use with extreme caution in patients with other risk factors for liver disease; discontinue therapy in patients who develop laboratory or clinical evidence of lactic acidosis or pronounced hepatotoxicity. Concomitant use of combination antiretroviral therapy with interferon alfa (with or without ribavirin) has resulted in hepatic decompensation (with some fatalities) in patients coinfected with HIV and HCV; monitor patients closely, especially for hepatic decompensation, neutropenia, and anemia; consider discontinuation of zidovudine if needed; consider dose reduction or discontinuation of interferon alfa, ribavirin, or both if clinical toxicities, including hepatic decompensation, worsen.

Syrup contains sodium benzoate; benzoic acid (benzoate) is a metabolite of benzyl alcohol; large amounts of benzyl alcohol (≥99 mg/kg/day) have been associated with a potentially fatal toxicity ("gasping syndrome") in neonates; the "gasping syndrome" consists of metabolic acidosis, respiratory distress, gasping respirations, CNS dysfunction (including convulsions, intracranial hemorrhage), hypotension and cardiovascular collapse; use syrup containing sodium benzoate with caution in neonates; *in vitro* and animal studies have shown that benzoate displaces bilirubin from protein binding sites

Precautions Use with caution in patients with bone marrow compromise or in patients with impaired renal or hepatic function; reduce dosage or interrupt therapy in patients with anemia, granulocytopenia, or myopathy; reduce dosage in patients with severe renal or hepatic impairment. Fat redistribution and accumulation [ie, central obesity, peripheral wasting, facial wasting, breast enlargement, dorsocervical fat enlargement (buffalo hump), and cushingoid appearance] have been observed in patients receiving antiretroviral agents (causal relationship not established). Immune reconstitution syndrome (an acute inflammatory response to residual or indolent opportunistic infections) may occur in HIV patients during initial treatment with combination antiretroviral agents; this syndrome may require further patient assessment and therapy.

Adverse Reactions

Central nervous system: Malaise, dizziness, manic syndrome, seizures, confusion, fever, severe headache, insomnia, asthenia

(Continued)

Zidovudine *(Continued)*

Dermatologic: Rash, pigmentation of nails (blue)

Endocrine & metabolic: Lactic acidosis; fat redistribution and accumulation (see Precautions)

Gastrointestinal: Nausea, diarrhea, vomiting, anorexia

Hematologic: Granulocytopenia, thrombocytopenia, leukopenia, anemia

Hepatic: Cholestatic hepatitis, hepatic steatosis, severe hepatomegaly; elevated serum AST, LDH, and alkaline phosphatase

Neuromuscular & skeletal: Myalgia, tremor, weakness; unusual: myopathy, myositis

Miscellaneous: Immune reconstitution syndrome

Drug Interactions Acyclovir may increase CNS adverse effects of zidovudine. Coadministration with drugs that increase zidovudine serum concentration (acetaminophen, atovaquone, methadone, valproic acid, cimetidine, indomethacin, lorazepam, fluconazole, probenecid, aspirin) may increase toxicity of zidovudine. Flucytosine, ganciclovir, interferon-alpha, pentamidine, and sulfamethoxazole and trimethoprim may increase hematologic side effects. Doxorubicin may reduce the intracellular phosphorylation of zidovudine (*in vitro* data) resulting in an antagonistic effect (avoid concurrent use). Coadministration with phenytoin, rifampin, or rifabutin may increase metabolism of zidovudine. Clarithromycin decreases zidovudine concentration by interfering with its absorption (administer doses 4 hours apart). Do not administer in combination with stavudine (antagonistic antiretroviral effect)

Ribavirin may decrease the intracellular phosphorylation of zidovudine (*in vitro* data); however, one clinical study did not identify a pharmacokinetic or pharmacodynamic interaction. Concomitant use of zidovudine with interferon alfa (with or without ribavirin) in patients coinfected with HIV and HCV, may result in hepatic decompensation which may be fatal (see Warnings).

Food Interactions Food does not significantly affect bioavailability; folate or vitamin B_{12} deficiency increases zidovudine-associated myelosuppression

Stability

I.V.: Store undiluted vials at 15°C to 25°C (59°F to 77°F); protect from light. Dilute with D_5W to a final concentration ≤4 mg/mL. The diluted I.V. solution is physically and chemically stable for 24 hours at room temperature and 48 hours if refrigerated. Administer diluted I.V. solution within 8 hours if stored at room temperature and within 24 hours if refrigerated to minimize the potential for microbial contamination (vials are single-use and do not contain preservative)

Tablets, capsules, syrup: Store at 15°C to 25°C (59°F to 77°F); protect capsules from moisture

Mechanism of Action Zidovudine is a thymidine analog that enters the cell and is phosphorylated by cellular kinases to the active metabolite zidovudine triphosphate which serves as an alternative substrate to deoxythymidine triphosphate for incorporation by reverse transcriptase; inhibits HIV viral polymerases and DNA synthesis

Pharmacokinetics

Absorption: Oral: Well absorbed

Distribution: Crosses the placenta; distributes into breast milk at concentrations similar to plasma; significant penetration into the CSF

CSF/plasma ratio:

Children 3 months to 12 years (n=38): Median: 0.68; range: 0.03-3.25

Adults (n=39): Median: 0.6; range: 0.04-2.62

V_d: Adults: 1.6 L/kg

Protein binding: 25% to 38%

Metabolism: Extensive first-pass effect; metabolized in the liver via glucuronidation to inactive metabolites

Bioavailability: Oral: Similar for tablets, capsules, and syrup

Neonates <14 days: 89%

Infants 14 days to 3 months: 61%

Infants 3 months to Children 12 years: 65%

Adults: 64% ± 10%

Half-life, terminal:

Premature neonate: 6.3 hours

Full-term neonates: 3.1 hours

Infants 14 days to 3 months: 1.9 hours

Infants 3 months to Children 12 years: 1.5 hours

Adults: 0.5-3 hours (mean: 1.1 hours)

Time to peak serum concentration: Within 30-90 minutes

Elimination: Urinary excretion (63% to 95%)

Oral: 72% to 74% of drug excreted in urine as metabolites and 14% to 18% as unchanged drug

I.V.: 45% to 60% excreted in urine as metabolites and 18% to 29% as unchanged drug

Usual Dosage Note: For treatment of HIV infection, use in combination with other antiretroviral agents; used as monotherapy in neonates to prevent perinatal transmission of HIV. The recommended regimen to prevent perinatal transmission of HIV also includes maternal antepartum oral zidovudine and maternal intrapartum I.V. zidovudine (see "Perinatal HIV" section in Appendix for details). Use I.V. route only until oral therapy can be administered.

Premature Infants <35 weeks gestational age (GA) at birth: **Note:** Standard neonatal dose may be excessive in premature infants: Initial:

Oral: 2 mg/kg/dose every 12 hours

I.V.: 1.5 mg/kg/dose every 12 hours

Increase to every 8 hours as follows:

GA at birth <30 weeks: Increase above dose to every 8 hours at 4 weeks of age

GA at birth ≥30 weeks: Increase above dose to every 8 hours at 2 weeks of age

Neonates and Infants <6 weeks:

Oral: 2 mg/kg/dose every 6 hours

I.V.: 1.5 mg/kg/dose every 6 hours

Infants ≥6 weeks and Children:

Oral: 160 mg/m^2/dose every 8 hours; maximum: 200 mg every 8 hours; twice daily dosing is not FDA approved in children, but some investigators use 180-240 mg/m^2/dose every 12 hours to improve compliance; data on this dose in children is limited

I.V. continuous infusion: 20 mg/m^2/hour

I.V. intermittent infusion: 120 mg/m^2/dose every 6 hours

Children >12 years and Adults:

HIV postexposure prophylaxis: 300 mg twice daily or 200 mg 3 times/day (with food) in combination with lamivudine or emtricitabine, with or without a protease inhibitor depending on risk

Treatment of HIV:

Oral: 300 mg twice daily or 200 mg 3 times/day

I.V.: 1 mg/kg/dose administered every 4 hours

Dosage adjustment in renal impairment: Adults: End-stage renal disease patients (Cl_{cr} <15 mL/minute) maintained on hemodialysis or peritoneal dialysis:

Oral: 100 mg every 6-8 hours

I.V.: 1 mg/kg/dose every 6-8 hours

Dosage adjustment in hepatic impairment: Specific recommendations currently unknown; dosage reduction may be required; use with caution; monitor for hematologic toxicities frequently

Dosage adjustment for zidovudine hematologic toxicity: Significant anemia (Hgb <7.5 g/dL or >25% decrease from baseline) and/or significant neutropenia (ANC <750 cells/mm^3 or >50% decrease from baseline): Dose interruption may be required until evidence of bone marrow recovery occurs; once bone marrow recovers, dose may be resumed using appropriate adjunctive therapy (eg, epoetin alfa). Zidovudine dosage reduction may be considered in patients with significant anemia while receiving concomitant medications that significantly increase zidovudine serum concentrations (eg, fluconazole, valproic acid).

Administration

Oral: May be administered without regard to meals; the patient should be in an upright position while taking zidovudine capsules to minimize the risk of esophageal ulceration

Parenteral: Do not administer I.M.; do not administer I.V. push or by rapid infusion; infuse I.V. zidovudine over 1 hour at a final concentration not to exceed 4 mg/mL in D_5W

Monitoring Parameters CBC with differential, hemoglobin, MCV, reticulocyte count, serum creatine kinase, CD4 cell count, HIV RNA plasma levels, renal and hepatic function tests; signs and symptoms of lactic acidosis, pronounced hepatotoxicity, anemia, and bone marrow suppression

Patient Information Zidovudine is not a cure for HIV. Notify physician if muscle weakness, shortness of breath, headache, insomnia, signs of infection, unusual bleeding, or rash occur. Take zidovudine every day as prescribed; do not change dose or discontinue without physician's advice. If a dose is missed, take it as soon as possible, then return to normal dosing schedule; if a dose is skipped, do **not** double the next dose.

HIV medications may cause changes in body fat, including an increase in fat in the upper back and neck, breasts, and trunk; a loss of fat from the face, arms, and legs may also occur.

Additional Information Conversion from oral to I.V. dose: I.V. dose = $^2/_3$ of the oral dose. Zidovudine-associated reduction in Hgb may occur as early as 2-4 weeks after initiation of therapy; onset of neutropenia usually occurs after 6-8 weeks.

Dosage Forms Excipient information presented when available (limited, particularly for generics); consult specific product labeling.

(Continued)

Zidovudine *(Continued)*

Capsule:
Retrovir®: 100 mg
Injection, solution [preservative free]:
Retrovir®: 10 mg/mL (20 mL)
Syrup:
Retrovir®: 50 mg/5 mL (240 mL) [contains sodium benzoate; strawberry flavor]
Tablet: 300 mg
Retrovir®: 300 mg

References

Briars LA, Hilao JJ, and Kraus DM, "A Review of Pediatric Human Immunodeficiency Virus Infection," *Journal of Pharmacy Practice*, 2004, 17(6):407-31.

Mueller BU, Jacobsen F, Butler KM, et al, "Combination Treatment With Azidothymidine and Granulocyte Colony-Stimulating Factor in Children With Human Immunodeficiency Virus Infection," *J Pediatr*, 1992, 121(5 Pt 1):797-802.

Panel on Clinical Practices for Treatment of HIV Infection, "Guidelines for the Use of Antiretroviral Agents in HIV-Infected Adults and Adolescents," October 10, 2006, http://www.aidsinfo.nih.gov.

Perinatal HIV Guidelines Working Group, "Recommendations for the Use of Antiretroviral Drugs in Pregnant HIV-1-Infected Women for Maternal Health and Interventions to Reduce Perinatal HIV-1 Transmission in the United States," October 12, 2006, http://www.aidsinfo.nih.gov.

"Updated U.S. Public Health Service Guidelines for the Management of Occupational Exposures to HIV and Recommendations for Postexposure Prophylaxis," *MMWR Recomm Rep*, 2005, 54(RR-9):1-17.

Volberding PA, Lagakos SW, Koch MA, et al, "Zidovudine in Asymptomatic Human Immunodeficiency Virus Infection. A Controlled Trial in Persons With Fewer Than 500 CD4-Positive Cells Per Cubic Millimeter. The AIDS Clinical Trials Group of the National Institute of Allergy and Infectious Diseases," *N Engl J Med*, 1990, 322(14):941-9.

Working Group on Antiretroviral Therapy and Medical Management of HIV-Infected Children, "Guidelines for the Use of Antiretroviral Agents in Pediatric HIV Infection," October 26, 2006, http://www.aidsinfo.nih.gov.

♦ **Zidovudine, Abacavir, and Lamivudine** *see* Abacavir, Lamivudine, and Zidovudine *on page 38*
♦ **Zidovudine and Lamivudine** *see* Lamivudine and Zidovudine *on page 904*
♦ **Zilactin® (Can)** *see* Lidocaine *on page 933*
♦ **Zilactin-L® [OTC]** *see* Lidocaine *on page 933*
♦ **Zilactin®-B [OTC]** *see* Benzocaine *on page 204*
♦ **Zilactin-B® (Can)** *see* Benzocaine *on page 204*
♦ **Zilactin Baby® (Can)** *see* Benzocaine *on page 204*
♦ **Zilactin Toothache and Gum Pain® [OTC]** *see* Benzocaine *on page 204*
♦ **Zinacef®** *see* Cefuroxime *on page 322*
♦ **Zinc Acetate** *see* Zinc Supplements *on page 1641*
♦ **Zincate®** *see* Zinc Supplements *on page 1641*
♦ **Zinc Carbonate** *see* Zinc Supplements *on page 1641*
♦ **Zinc Chloride** *see* Trace Metals *on page 1558*
♦ **Zinc Chloride** *see* Zinc Supplements *on page 1641*
♦ **Zinc Gluconate** *see* Zinc Supplements *on page 1641*
♦ **Zincofax® (Can)** *see* Zinc Oxide *on page 1640*

Zinc Oxide (zingk OKS ide)

U.S. Brand Names Ammens® Medicated Deodorant [OTC]; Balmex® [OTC]; Boudreaux's® Butt Paste [OTC]; Critic-Aid Skin Care® [OTC]; Desitin® [OTC]; Desitin® Creamy [OTC]

Canadian Brand Names Zincofax®

Index Terms Base Ointment; Lassar's Zinc Paste

Therapeutic Category Topical Skin Product

Generic Available Yes: Ointment

Use Protective coating for mild skin irritations and abrasions; soothing and protective ointment to promote healing of chapped skin, diaper rash

Contraindications Hypersensitivity to zinc oxide or any component

Stability Avoid prolonged storage at temperatures >30°C

Mechanism of Action Mild astringent, protective and weak antiseptic action

Usual Dosage Infants, Children, and Adults: Topical: Apply several times daily to affected area

Administration Topical: For external use only; do not use in the eyes

Patient Information Paste is easily removed with mineral oil

Dosage Forms Excipient information presented when available (limited, particularly for generics); consult specific product labeling.

Cream:
Balmex®: 11.3% (60 g, 120 g, 480 g) [contains aloe and vitamin E]
Ointment, topical: 20% (30 g, 60 g, 454 g); 40% (120 g)

Desitin®: 40% (30 g, 60 g, 90 g, 120 g, 270 g, 480 g) [contains cod liver oil and lanolin]

Desitin® Creamy: 10% (60 g, 120 g)

Paste, topical:

Boudreaux's® Butt Paste: 16% (30 g, 60 g, 120 g, 480 g) [contains castor oil, boric acid, mineral oil, and Peruvian balsam]

Critic-Aid Skin Care®: 20% (71 g, 170 g)

Powder, topical (Ammens® Medicated Deodorant): 9.1% (187.5 g, 330 g) [original and shower fresh scent]

♦ **Zinc Sulfate** *see* Trace Metals *on page 1558*

♦ **Zinc Sulfate** *see* Zinc Supplements *on page 1641*

Zinc Supplements (zink SUP la ments)

U.S. Brand Names Cold-Eeze® [OTC; Galzin™; Orazinc® [OTC]; Zincate®

Index Terms Zinc Acetate; Zinc Carbonate; Zinc Chloride; Zinc Gluconate; Zinc Sulfate

Therapeutic Category Antidote, Copper Toxicity; Mineral, Oral; Mineral, Parenteral

Generic Available Yes

Use Treatment and prevention of zinc deficiency states; may improve wound healing in those who are zinc deficient; maintenance treatment of Wilson's disease (zinc acetate)

Pregnancy Risk Factor C (A for zinc acetate)

Contraindications Hypersensitivity to zinc salts or any component

Warnings Do not administer undiluted by direct injection into a peripheral vein due to potential for phlebitis, tissue irritation, and potential increased renal loss of minerals from a bolus injection; administration of zinc in absence of copper may decrease plasma copper levels; excessive intake in healthy persons may be deleterious as decreases in HDL (high-density lipoproteins) and impairment of immune system function have been reported

Adverse Reactions

Cardiovascular: Hypotension, tachycardia (excessive doses)

Central nervous system: Hypothermia (excessive doses)

Gastrointestinal: Indigestion, nausea, vomiting

Hematologic: Neutropenia, leukopenia

Hepatic: Jaundice (excessive doses)

Ocular: Blurred vision (excessive doses)

Respiratory: Pulmonary edema (excessive doses)

Miscellaneous: Profuse diaphoresis

Drug Interactions Zinc may decrease penicillamine, tetracycline, and quinolone absorption; iron decreases zinc absorption; agents which increase gastric pH, such as H_2 blockers, may decrease zinc absorption

Food Interactions Coffee, foods high in phytate (eg, whole grain cereals & legumes), bran, and dairy products reduce zinc absorption; avoid foods high in calcium or phosphorus

Mechanism of Action A cofactor for more than 70 enzymes which are important to carbohydrate and protein metabolism, zinc helps to maintain normal growth and tissue repair, normal skin hydration, and senses of taste and smell; in Wilson's disease, zinc cation inhibits the absorption of dietary copper by inducing the synthesis of metallothionein, a metal-binding protein present in the intestinal mucosa. This protein binds metals, including copper, forming a nontoxic complex that is not absorbed systematically but excreted in the stool.

Pharmacokinetics

Absorption: pH dependent; poor from GI tract (20% to 30%); solubilized by conversion to zinc chloride in the presence of gastric acid

Distribution: Storage sites are liver and skeletal muscle; serum levels do not adequately reflect whole-body zinc status

Protein binding: 55% bound to albumin; 40% bound to alpha 1-macroglobulin

Elimination: 90% in feces with only traces appearing in urine and perspiration

Usual Dosage Clinical response may not occur for up to 6-8 weeks

RDA: Oral:

Neonates and Infants <12 months: 5 mg **elemental** zinc/day

Children 1-10 years: 10 mg **elemental** zinc/day

Children ≥11 years and Adults: Male: 15 mg **elemental** zinc/day; Female: 12 mg **elemental** zinc/day

Zinc deficiency: Oral:

Infants and Children: 0.5-1 mg **elemental** zinc/kg/day divided 1-3 times/day; larger doses may be needed if impaired intestinal absorption or an excessive loss of zinc (eg, excessive, prolonged diarrhea)

(Continued)

Zinc Supplements *(Continued)*

Adults: 25-50 mg **elemental** zinc/dose (110-220 mg zinc sulfate) 3 times/day

Supplement to parenteral nutrition solutions (clinical response may not occur for up to 6-8 weeks): (See Trace Metals): I.V. (all doses are mcg of **elemental** zinc):

Premature Infants: 400 mcg/kg/day

Term Infants <3 months: 300 mcg/kg/day

Infants ≥3 months and Children ≤5 years: 100 mcg/kg/day (maximum: 5 mg/day)

Children >5 years and Adolescents: 2.5-5 mg/day

Adults:

Stable metabolically: 2.5-4 mg **elemental** zinc/day; catabolic state: Increase by an additional 2 mg/day (eg, 4.5-6 mg **elemental** zinc/day)

Stable with fluid loss from small bowel: Additional 12.2 mg **elemental** zinc/L parenteral nutrition or 17.1 mg **elemental** zinc/kg of stool or ileostomy output

Wound healing: Oral: Adults: 50 mg **elemental** zinc (220 mg zinc sulfate) 3 times daily in patients with low serum zinc levels (<110 mcg/dL)

Maintenance treatment of Wilson's disease: **Zinc acetate:** Dose is in mg elemental zinc:

Children ≥10 years and Pregnant Women: 25 mg 3 times/day

Adults (nonpregnant): 50 mg 3 times/day

Note: Not indicated for initial treatment of Wilson's disease but for maintenance after initial therapy with a chelating agent (approximately 4-6 months)

Administration

Oral: Administer oral formulation with food if GI upset occurs; in patients with Wilson's disease, administer zinc acetate 1 hour before or after meals or beverage (except water); zinc acetate capsules should be swallowed whole; do not open or chew

Parenteral: Dilute as component of daily parenteral nutrition or maintenance fluids; do not give undiluted by direct injection into a peripheral vein due to potential for phlebitis and tissue irritation, and potential to increase renal losses of minerals from a bolus injection

Monitoring Parameters Patients on parenteral nutrition or chronic therapy should have periodic serum copper and serum zinc levels; alkaline phosphatase, taste acuity, mental depression, wound healing (if indicated), growth (if indicated), skin integrity; Wilson's disease: 24-hour urinary copper excretion, neuropsychiatric evaluations, LFTs

Reference Range

Serum: 70-130 mcg/dL

Urinary copper (Wilson's disease patient **not** on chelation therapy): <125 g/24 hours (patients on chelation therapy will have increased urinary copper due to chelated copper)

Patient Information Do not exceed recommended dose

Dosage Forms Excipient information presented when available (limited, particularly for generics); consult specific product labeling.

Zinc acetate:

Capsule (Galzin™): 25 mg elemental zinc, 50 mg elemental zinc

Zinc chloride:

Injection, solution: 1 mg elemental zinc/mL (10 mL, 50 mL)

Zinc, elemental:

Lozenges: 10 mg, 23 mg

Cold-Eeze®: 13.3 mg [bubble gum, citrus, cherry, menthol, and tropical fruit flavors]

Tablet: 30 mg, 60 mg

Zinc gluconate (14.3% zinc):

Tablet: 50 mg [elemental zinc 7 mg]; 100 mg [elemental zinc 14 mg]

Zinc sulfate (23% zinc):

Capsule (Orazinc®, Zincate®): 220 mg [elemental zinc 50 mg]

Injection, solution [preservative free]: 1 mg elemental zinc/mL (10 mL); 5 mg elemental zinc/mL (5 mL)

Tablet (Orazinc®): 110 mg [elemental zinc 25 mg]

References

Anderson LA, Hakojarvi SL, and Boudreaux SK, "Zinc Acetate Treatment in Wilson's Disease," *Ann Pharmacother*, 1998, 32:78-87.

♦ **Zinc Undecylenate** *see* Undecylenic Acid and Derivatives *on page 1585*

♦ **Zinecard®** *see* Dexrazoxane *on page 467*

♦ **Zithromax®** *see* Azithromycin *on page 191*

♦ **Zithromax® TRI-PAK™** *see* Azithromycin *on page 191*

♦ **Zithromax® Z-PAK®** *see* Azithromycin *on page 191*

♦ **Zmax™** *see* Azithromycin *on page 191*

♦ **Zocor®** *see* Simvastatin *on page 1441*

♦ **Zoderm®** *see* Benzoyl Peroxide *on page 207*

- **Zofran®** *see* Ondansetron *on page 1169*
- **Zofran® ODT** *see* Ondansetron *on page 1169*
- **Zoloft®** *see* Sertraline *on page 1429*
- **Zomorph® (Can)** *see* Morphine Sulfate *on page 1082*
- **Zonalon®** *see* Doxepin *on page 537*
- **Zonegran®** *see* Zonisamide *on page 1643*

Zonisamide (zoe NIS a mide)

Related Information

Antiepileptic Drugs *on page 1902*

U.S. Brand Names Zonegran®

Canadian Brand Names Zonegran®

Therapeutic Category Anticonvulsant, Miscellaneous

Generic Available Yes

Use Adjunctive treatment of partial seizures in adolescents >16 years of age and adults with epilepsy; has been used investigationally for the treatment of generalized epilepsies including, generalized tonic-clonic seizures, absence seizures, infantile spasms, myoclonic epilepsies, and Lennox-Gastaut syndrome (see Leppik, 1999 and Oommen, 1999)

Pregnancy Risk Factor C

Lactation Excretion in breast milk unknown/contraindicated

Contraindications Hypersensitivity to zonisamide, sulfonamides, or any component

Warnings Zonisamide is a sulfonamide; although rare, severe, and life-threatening sulfonamide reactions may occur (eg, Stevens-Johnson syndrome, toxic epidermal necrolysis, aplastic anemia, agranulocytosis, other blood dyscrasias, and fulminant hepatic necrosis); discontinue zonisamide in patients with signs of hypersensitivity reaction or other serious reactions; consider discontinuation of zonisamide in any patient who develops a rash or monitor very closely; deaths due to serious rashes have been reported; rashes usually appear within 2-16 weeks of starting therapy.

Oligohydrosis (decreased sweating) and hyperthermia have been reported in 40 pediatric patients; many cases occurred after exposure to elevated environmental temperatures; some cases resulted in heat stroke requiring hospitalization; pediatric patients may be at an increased risk; monitor patients, especially pediatric patients, for decreased sweating and hyperthermia, especially in warm or hot weather; use zonisamide with caution in patients receiving drugs that predispose to heat-related disorders (eg, anticholinergic agents, carbonic anhydrase inhibitors); safety and efficacy in pediatric patients <16 years of age has not been established.

Do not abruptly discontinue therapy; abrupt withdrawal may precipitate seizures; withdraw gradually to lessen chance for increased seizure frequency (unless a more rapid withdrawal is required due to safety concerns). CNS adverse effects may occur including fatigue or somnolence, psychiatric symptoms (eg, depression, psychosis), and cognitive symptoms [difficulty concentrating, speech or language problems (especially word-finding difficulties), and psychomotor slowing]; fatigue and somnolence usually occur within the first month of starting therapy, most commonly at higher doses (eg, in adults at doses of 300-500 mg/day).

Precautions Use with caution in patients with renal or hepatic dysfunction; do not use in patients with Cl_{cr} <50 mL/minute; zonisamide may cause kidney stones (ensure patients have adequate fluid intake); zonisamide may decrease GFR and increase serum creatinine and BUN; discontinue therapy in patients who develop acute renal failure or a persistent significant increase in serum creatinine or BUN

Adverse Reactions

Central nervous system: Somnolence, fatigue, dizziness, headache, agitation, irritability, tiredness, ataxia, confusion, memory impairment, depression, psychosis, difficulty concentrating, speech or language problems (especially word-finding difficulties), psychomotor slowing, insomnia, mental slowing, anxiety, nervousness, tremor, convulsion, hyperesthesia, incoordination; behavior disorders in children have been reported (Kimura, 1994)

Dermatologic: Rash, bruising, pruritus, Stevens-Johnson syndrome (rare), toxic epidermal necrolysis (rare)

Endocrine & metabolic: Weight loss

Gastrointestinal: Anorexia, nausea, diarrhea, abdominal pain, dyspepsia, constipation, xerostomia, taste perversion, vomiting

Hematologic: Aplastic anemia (rare), agranulocytosis (rare), other blood dyscrasias (rare)

Hepatic: Elevated alkaline phosphatase; elevated LDH and transaminases (rare)

Neuromuscular & skeletal: Paresthesia, abnormal gait

Ocular: Diplopia, nystagmus, amblyopia

(Continued)

Zonisamide *(Continued)*

Otic: Tinnitus

Renal: Elevated BUN and serum creatinine

Respiratory: Rhinitis, pharyngitis, increased cough

Miscellaneous: Flu-like syndrome; oligohydrosis and hyperthermia [pediatric patients may be at increased risk (see Warnings)]

Drug Interactions Cytochrome P450 isoenzyme CYP3A4 substrate

Enzyme inducers (eg, carbamazepine, phenobarbital, phenytoin) may increase the metabolism of zonisamide and decrease zonisamide serum concentrations; valproate may decrease the half-life of zonisamide. Lamotrigine may inhibit the clearance of zonisamide and increase zonisamide serum concentrations; enzyme inhibitors may increase zonisamide serum concentrations (monitor for increased effect/toxicity)

Zonisamide does **not** affect serum concentrations of carbamazepine, phenytoin, or valproate. Zonisamide may decrease serum concentrations of the carbamazepine epoxide metabolite in patients receiving carbamazepine. CNS depressants, including alcohol, may increase sedative effects (monitor for increased effect/toxicity).

Food Interactions Food decreases the rate, but not the extent of absorption.

Stability Store at controlled room temperature 25°C (77°C). Protect from moisture and light.

Mechanism of Action Exact mechanism of action is not known; may stabilize neuronal membranes and suppress neuronal hypersynchronization by blocking sodium channels and T-type calcium currents; does not affect GABA activity; possesses weak carbonic anhydrase inhibiting activity, but this in not thought to be a very significant component of its antiepileptic action

Pharmacokinetics

Absorption: Oral: Rapid and complete

Distribution: V_d (apparent): Adults: 1.45 L/kg; highly concentrated in erythrocytes; distributes into breast milk at a transfer rate of 41% to 57% (see Kawada, 2002)

Protein binding: 40%

Metabolism: Hepatic; undergoes acetylation to form N-acetyl zonisamide and reduction via cytochrome P450 isoenzyme CYP3A4 to 2-sulfamoylacetylphenol (SMAP); SMAP then undergoes conjugation with glucuronide

Half-life: Adults: 63 hours (range: 50-68 hours)

Time to peak serum concentration: 2-6 hours

Elimination: Urine: 62% (35% as unchanged drug, 15% as N-acetyl zonisamide, 50% as SMAP glucuronide); feces (3%); **Note:** Of the dose recovered in Japanese patients, 28% is as unchanged drug, 52% is as N-acetyl zonisamide, and 19% is as SMAP glucuronide (Glauser, 2002)

Usual Dosage Oral:

Infants and Children: In a review article of 20 Japanese pediatric studies, the following doses were recommended (see Glauser, 2002): Initial: 1-2 mg/kg/day given in two divided doses/day; increase dose in increments of 0.5-1 mg/kg/day every 2 weeks; usual dose: 5-8 mg/kg/day.

Higher initial and maximum doses have been recommended by others (see Leppik, 1999 and Oommen, 1999): Initial: 2-4 mg/kg/day given in two divided doses/day; titrate dose upwards if needed every 2 weeks; usual dose: 4-8 mg/kg/day; maximum dose: 12 mg/kg/day

Infantile spasms: Several studies used a faster titration of zonisamide to control infantile spasms. Suzuki treated 11 newly diagnosed infants (mean age: ~6 months) with zonisamide monotherapy starting at doses of 3-5 mg/kg/day given in 2 divided doses/day; doses were increased every 4th day until seizures were controlled or a maximum dose of 10 mg/kg/day was attained; 4 of 11 patients responded at doses of 4-5 mg/kg/day (see Suzuki, 1997). Yanai treated 27 newly diagnosed infantile spasm patients with zonisamide add-on or monotherapy starting at doses of 2-4 mg/kg/day given in 2 divided doses/day; doses were increased by 2-5 mg/kg every 2-4 days until seizures were controlled or a maximum of 10-20 mg/kg/day was attained; 9 of 27 patients responded at a mean effective dose of 7.8 mg/kg/day (range: 5-12.5 mg/kg/day); non-responders received doses of 8-20 mg/kg/day (mean: 10.8 mg/kg/day) (see Yania, 1999). Suzuki treated 54 newly diagnosed infants (11 of which were previously reported) with zonisamide monotherapy starting at doses of 3-4 mg/kg/day given in 2 divided doses; doses were increased every 4th day until seizures were controlled or a maximum dose of 10-13 mg/kg/day was attained; 11 of 54 infants responded at a mean effective dose of 7.2 mg/kg/day (range: 4-12 mg/kg/day); the majority of infants who responded did so at a dose of 4-8 mg/kg/day and within 1-2 weeks of starting therapy (see Suzuki, 2001). Further studies are needed.

Adolescents >16 years and Adults: Initial: 100 mg once daily; dose may be increased to 200 mg/day after 2 weeks; further increases in dose should be made in increments of 100 mg/day and only after a minimum of 2 weeks between adjustments;

usual effective dose: 100-600 mg/day. **Note:** There is no evidence of increased benefit with doses >400 mg/day. Steady-state serum concentrations fluctuate 27% with once daily dosing, and 14% with twice daily dosing; patients may benefit from divided doses given twice daily (Leppik, 1999)

Dosage adjustment in renal/hepatic impairment: Slower dosage titration and more frequent monitoring are recommended in patients with renal or hepatic disease. Do not use if Cl_{cr} <50 mL/minute.

Administration May be administered without regard to meals; swallow capsule whole; do not crush, chew, or break capsule

Monitoring Parameters Seizure frequency, duration, and severity; symptoms of CNS adverse effects; skin rash; BUN and serum creatinine; monitor patients, especially pediatric patients, for decreased sweating and hyperthermia, especially in warm or hot weather

Reference Range Monitoring of plasma concentrations may be useful; proposed therapeutic range: 10-20 mcg/mL; patients may benefit from higher concentrations (ie, up to 30 mcg/mL), but concentrations >30 mcg/mL have been associated with adverse effects (see Oommen, 1999 and Leppik, 1999)

Patient Information Inform prescriber if allergic to sulfa drugs (eg, Bactrim®, Septra®); do not abruptly discontinue therapy, an increase in seizure activity may result; may cause drowsiness and impair ability to perform activities that require mental alertness or physical coordination; report excessive drowsiness, unusual thoughts, depression, problems with concentrating or speaking, worsening of seizures, or any skin rashes to physician immediately; avoid alcohol; notify physician immediately if a child taking zonisamide is not sweating as usual or has elevated temperature; drink adequate amount of fluids and report any symptoms of kidney stones (eg, back pain, stomach pain, pain on urination, bloody urine); report any unusual symptoms, such as a bruises, sore throat, fever, or mouth ulcers to physician

Dosage Forms Excipient information presented when available (limited, particularly for generics); consult specific product labeling.

Capsule: 25 mg, 50 mg, 100 mg

Zonegran®: 25 mg, 100 mg

References

Glauser TA and Pellock JM, "Zonisamide in Pediatric Epilepsy: Review of the Japanese Experience," *J Child Neurol*, 2002, 17(2):87-96.

Kawada K, Itoh S, Kusaka T, et al, "Pharmacokinetics of Zonisamide in Perinatal Period," *Brain Dev*, 2002, 24(2):95-7.

Kimura S, "Zonisamide-Induced Behavior Disorder in Two Children," *Epilepsia*, 1994, 35(2):403-5.

Leppik IE, "Zonisamide," *Epilepsia*, 1999, 40(Suppl 5):S23-9.

Oommen KJ and Mathews S, "Zonisamide: A New Antiepileptic Drug," *Clin Neuropharmacol*, 1999, 22(4):192-200.

Suzuki Y, Nagai T, Ono J, et al, "Zonisamide Monotherapy in Newly Diagnosed Infantile Spasms," *Epilepsia*, 1997, 38(9):1035-8.

Suzuki Y, "Zonisamide in West Syndrome," *Brain Dev*, 2001, 23(7):658-61.

Yanai S, Hanai T, and Narazaki O, "Treatment of Infantile Spasms With Zonisamide," *Brain Dev*, 1999, 21(3):157-61.

♦ **Zorbtive®** *see* Human Growth Hormone *on page 769*

♦ **ZORprin®** *see* Aspirin *on page 163*

♦ **Zostrix® [OTC]** *see* Capsaicin *on page 276*

♦ **Zostrix® (Can)** *see* Capsaicin *on page 276*

♦ **Zostrix®-HP [OTC]** *see* Capsaicin *on page 276*

♦ **Zostrix® H.P. (Can)** *see* Capsaicin *on page 276*

♦ **Zosyn®** *see* Piperacillin and Tazobactam *on page 1264*

♦ **Zovirax®** *see* Acyclovir *on page 54*

♦ **Zydone®** *see* Hydrocodone and Acetaminophen *on page 779*

♦ **Zyloprim®** *see* Allopurinol *on page 76*

♦ **Zymine®-D** *see* Triprolidine and Pseudoephedrine *on page 1580*

♦ **Zyrtec®** *see* Cetirizine *on page 327*

♦ **Zytram® XL (Can)** *see* Tramadol *on page 1561*

♦ **Zyvox®** *see* Linezolid *on page 941*

♦ **Zyvoxam® (Can)** *see* Linezolid *on page 941*

APPENDIX TABLE OF CONTENTS

APPENDIX TABLE OF CONTENTS *(Continued)*

Toxicology

Miscellaneous

CPR PEDIATRIC DRUG DOSAGES

Medications for Neonatal Resuscitation

Medication	Dose	Remarks
Epinephrine	I.V.: 0.01-0.03 mg/kg (0.1-0.3 mL/kg, 1:10,000)	I.V. is preferred neonatal route. While obtaining I.V. access, may consider higher doses via E.T.: Up to 0.1 mg/kg (1 mL/kg, 1:10,000), but safety and efficacy of this practice has not been evaluated.
Naloxone	I.V./I.M.: 0.1 mg/kg	E.T. route is not recommended (lack of clinical data in neonates). Avoid use in newborns whose mothers are suspected of long-term exposure to opioids. Monitor neonates closely for recurrent apnea or hypoventilation; additional doses of naloxone may be needed.

Adapted from American Heart Association Emergency Cardiovascular Care Committee, "2005 American Heart Association (AHA) Guidelines for Cardiopulmonary Resuscitation (CPR) and Emergency Cardiovascular Care (ECC), Part 13: Neonatal Resuscitation Guidelines," *Circulation*, 2005, 112(24 Suppl):IV-192.

PALS Medications for Pediatric Resuscitation and Arrhythmias

Medication	Dose	Remarks
Adenosine	0.1 mg/kg (maximum 6 mg) Repeat: 0.2 mg/kg (maximum 12 mg)	Monitor ECG Rapid I.V./I.O. bolus
Amiodarone	I.V./I.O.: 5 mg/kg; repeat up to 15 mg/kg Maximum: 300 mg	Monitor ECG and blood pressure Adjust administration rate to urgency (give more slowly when perfusing rhythm present) Use caution when administering with other drugs that prolong QT (consider expert consultation)
Atropine	I.V./I.O.: 0.02 mg/kg E.T.[1]: 0.03 mg/kg Repeat once if needed Minimum dose: 0.1 mg Maximum single dose: Child: 0.5 mg Adolescent: 1 mg	Higher doses may be used with organophosphate poisoning
Calcium chloride (10%)	I.V./I.O.: 20 mg/kg (0.2 mL/kg)	Slowly Adult dose: 5-10 mL
Epinephrine	I.V./I.O.: 0.01 mg/kg (0.1 mL/kg, 1:10,000) Maximum dose: 1 mg E.T.[1]: 0.1 mg/kg (0.1 mL/kg, 1:1000) Maximum dose: 10 mg	May repeat every 3-5 minutes
Glucose	I.V./I.O.: 0.5-1 g/kg	$D_{10}W$: 5-10 mL/kg $D_{25}W$: 2-4 mL/kg $D_{50}W$: 1-2 mL/kg

PALS Medications for Pediatric Resuscitation and Arrhythmias *(continued)*

Medication	Dose	Remarks
Lidocaine	Bolus I.V./I.O.: 1 mg/kg Maximum dose: 100 mg Infusion: 20-50 mcg/kg/min E.T.[1]: 2-3 mg	
Magnesium sulfate	I.V./I.O.: 25-50 mg/kg over 10-20 minutes; faster in torsade de pointes Maximum dose: 2 g	
Naloxone	<5 y or ≤20 kg: I.V./I.O./E.T.[1]: 0.1 mg/kg ≥5 y or >20 kg: I.V./I.O./E.T.[1]: 2 mg	Use lower doses to reverse respiratory depression associated with therapeutic opioid use (1-15 mcg/kg)
Procainamide	I.V./I.O.: 15 mg/kg over 30-60 minutes Adult dose: I.V. infusion: 20 mg/min up to total maximum dose 17 mg/kg	Monitor ECG and blood pressure Use caution when administering with other drugs that prolong QT (consider expert consultation)
Sodium bicarbonate	I.V./I.O.: 1 mEq/kg/dose slowly	After adequate ventilation

I.V. = intravenous; I.O. = intraosseous; E.T. = endotracheal tube.

[1]Flush with 5 mL of normal saline and follow with 5 ventilations.

Adapted from American Heart Association Emergency Cardiovascular Care Committee, "2005 American Heart Association (AHA) Guidelines for Cardiopulmonary Resuscitation (CPR) and Emergency Cardiovascular Care (ECC), Part 12: Pediatric Advanced Life Support," *Circulation*, 2005, 112(24 Suppl):IV-171.

PALS Medications to Maintain Cardiac Output and for Postresuscitation Stabilization

Medication	Dose Range	Comment
Inamrinone	I.V./I.O.: 0.75-1 mg/kg over 5 minutes; may repeat x 2; then 2-20 mcg/kg/min	Inodilator
Dobutamine	I.V./I.O.: 2-20 mcg/kg/min	Inotrope; vasodilator
Dopamine	I.V./I.O.: 2-20 mcg/kg/min	Inotrope; chronotrope; renal and splanchnic vasodilator in low doses; pressor in high doses
Epinephrine	I.V./I.O.: 0.1-1 mcg/kg/min	Inotrope; chronotrope; vasodilator in low doses; pressor in higher doses
Milrinone	I.V./I.O.: 50-75 mcg/kg over 10-60 minutes, then 0.5-0.75 mcg/kg/min	Inodilator
Norepinephrine	0.1-2 mcg/kg/min	Inotrope; vasopressor
Sodium nitroprusside	1-8 mcg/kg/min	Vasodilator; prepare only in D_5W

I.V. = intravenous; I.O. = intraosseous.

Alternative formula for calculating an infusion:

Infusion rate (mL/h) = [weight (kg) x dose (mcg/kg/min) x 60 (min/h)] / concentration mcg/mL).

Adapted from American Heart Association Emergency Cardiovascular Care Committee, "2005 American Heart Association (AHA) Guidelines for Cardiopulmonary Resuscitation (CPR) and Emergency Cardiovascular Care (ECC)," *Circulation*, 2005, 112(24 Suppl):IV-180.

EMERGENCY PEDIATRIC DRIP CALCULATIONS

A limited number of standard concentrations for emergency medications (eg, vasopressors) is recommended (JCAHO, 2004). When using standardized concentrations, calculate the rate of infusion using the following equation:

$$\text{Rate (mL/h)} = \frac{\text{dose (mcg/kg/min)} \times \text{weight (kg)} \times \text{60 min/h}}{\text{concentration (mcg/mL)}}$$

If a standardized concentration delivers the dose in too low of a volume (eg, <1 mL/hour) then a lower standardized concentration is used. If a standardized concentration delivers the dose in too high of a volume (depending on patient's size and fluid status) then a higher standardized concentration is used. Each center should develop standardized concentrations and guidelines for their own institution.

Some centers use the following pediatric standardized concentrations according to patient weight (see Campbell, 1994):

Standardized Concentrations by Patient Weight

Drug	Patient Weight (kg)	Concentration (mcg/mL)
Dopamine	2-3	200
	4-8	400
	9-15	800
	>15	1600
Epinephrine,	2-3	5
Isoproterenol, or	4-8	10
Norepinephrine	≥9	20

Other centers use the following standardized concentrations depending on both patient weight and dose (Hodding, 2004):

Drug	Standardized Concentrations (mcg/mL)		
Dobutamine	800	1600	3200
Dopamine	800	1600	3200
Epinephrine	8	16	60
Norepinephrine	8	16	60
Isoproterenol	8	16	60

An example of how different standardized concentrations are used for different patient weights and doses for dopamine is given in the following tables. Each table lists the dopamine infusion rate in mL/hour for a specific patient weight (in kg) and dose (in mcg/kg/minute) for a specific standardized concentration. The first table is for dopamine **1600** mcg/mL and the second table is for **800** mcg/mL.

Dopamine Infusion Rate (mL/hour)
According to Patient Weight (kg) and Dose (mcg/kg/minute)
Using Standardized
Concentration of 1600 mcg/mL

Weight (kg)	Dose (mcg/kg/minute)				
	5	7.5	10	15	20
2	0.4*	0.6*	0.8*	1.1	1.5
3	0.6*	0.8*	1.1	1.7	2.3
4	0.8*	1.1	1.5	2.3	3.0
5	0.9*	1.4	1.9	2.8	3.8
7	1.3	2.0	2.6	3.9	5.3
10	1.9	2.8	3.8	5.6	7.5
12	2.3	3.4	4.5	6.8	9.0
14	2.6	3.9	5.3	7.9	10.5
16	3.0	4.5	6.0	9.0	12.0
18	3.4	5.1	6.8	10.1	13.5
20	3.8	5.6	7.5	11.3	15.0
25	4.7	7.0	9.4	14.1	18.8
30	5.6	8.4	11.3	16.9	22.5
35	6.6	9.8	13.1	19.7	26.3
40	7.5	11.3	15.0	22.5	30.0
45	8.4	12.7	16.9	25.3	33.8
50	9.4	14.1	18.8	28.1	37.5

*For rates <1 mL/hour, use 800 mcg/mL concentration

Dopamine Infusion Rate (mL/hour)
According to Patient Weight (kg) and Dose (mcg/kg/minute)
Using Standardized
Concentration of 800 mcg/mL

Weight (kg)	Dose (mcg/kg/minute)				
	5	7.5	10	15	20
2	0.8	1.1	1.5	2.3	3.0
3	1.1	1.7	2.3	3.4	4.5
4	1.5	2.3	3.0	4.5	6.0
5	1.9	2.8	3.8	5.6	7.5

JCAHO and the "Rule of Six"

In its 2004 National Patient Safety Goals (NPSG), the Joint Commission on Accreditation of Healthcare Organizations (JCAHO) required organizations to "standardize and limit the number of drug concentrations available in the organization" to meet patient safety goal # 3 ("Improve the safety of using high-alert medications"). High-alert medications are drugs that possess a great risk of causing significant injury to patients when they are used in error. Emergency medications (eg, vasopressors) qualify as high-alert drugs.

The table at the end of this section uses the "Rule of Six" (the equation in the calculation column) to calculate patient-specific I.V. concentrations of dobutamine, dopamine, epinephrine, and isoproterenol, so that 1 mL/hour will deliver a set mcg/kg/minute dose. For example, application of the "Rule of Six" will calculate the mg amount of dobutamine or dopamine to be added to a 100 mL I.V. solution, so that a rate of 1 mL/hour will deliver 1 mcg/kg/minute.

JCAHO has determined that using the "Rule of Six" or other methods to individualize a concentration of a high-alert drug for a specific patient (ie, use of a nonstandardized concentration) is **not** in compliance with the requirement of the above NPSG goal. [Limiting and standardizing the number of drug concentrations

EMERGENCY PEDIATRIC DRIP CALCULATIONS *(Continued)*

(as opposed to using the "Rule of Six") is thought to be safer and less error prone.] Institutions are required to develop a transition plan to use a limited number of standardized concentrations. Full implementation of the plan was originally required by January 1, 2005, but has been extended to December 31, 2008. Hospitals may request permission to continue to use the "Rule of Six" as an alternative approach to the NPSG requirement during some or all of the interim period. However, ongoing evidence of progress toward full implementation by December 31, 2008 is required.

JCAHO's criteria for institutions to participate in the exceptions process during the transition period include:

- "The exception applies only to neonatal or pediatric acute care services.
- All (emergent and nonemergent) admixtures are prepared only by pharmacy staff in a sterile environment.
- Calculations of the drug solutions are validated during the preparation.
- The labeling of solution concentration and drug per milliliter are clear to all caregivers, and the solution concentration (amount of drug per unit volume of solution) is clearly indicated on the label.
- If the 'Rule of Six' is used in a pediatric setting, but standardized drug concentrations are used in other parts of the hospital, guidance aids are made available to caregivers who may not be familiar with one of these systems.
- If the organization has a Neonatal Intensive Care Unit, the pharmacy is open 24 hours a day to support the admixture service.
- Smart pumps are used. (Smart pumps are designed to recognize prescription errors, dose misinterpretations, and keypad programming errors.)" (See JCAHO, 2005).

Emergency Drips (Using "Rule of Six")

Drug	Dose	Calculation[1]	Rate & Dose
Dobutamine	5-20 mcg/kg/min	6 x body wt (kg) is the mg added to make 100 mL	1 mL/h = 1 mcg/kg/min
Dopamine	2-20 mcg/kg/min	6 x body wt (kg) is the mg added to make 100 mL	1 mL/h = 1 mcg/kg/min
Epinephrine	0.1-1 mcg/kg/min	0.6 x body wt (kg) is the mg added to make 100 mL	1 mL/h = 0.1 mcg/kg/min
Isoproterenol	0.1-1 mcg/kg/min	0.6 x body wt (kg) is the mg added to make 100 mL	1 mL/h = 0.1 mcg/kg/min
Lidocaine	20-50 mcg/kg/min	120 mg in 100 mL of D_5W	1 mL/kg/h = 20 mcg/kg/min

[1]**Note:** Patients ≥40 kg and those requiring fluid restriction may need more concentrated solutions in order to deliver less fluid per hour. In those cases, or as an alternative to the listed calculations above, use the following equation:

$$\text{Rate (mL/h)} = \frac{\text{dose (mcg/kg/min)} \times \text{weight (kg)} \times \text{60 min/h}}{\text{concentration (mcg/mL)}}$$

References

Campbell MM, Taeubel MA, and Kraus DM, "Updated Bedside Charts for Calculating Pediatric Doses of Emergency Medications," *Am J Hosp Pharm*, 1994, 51(17):2147-52.

Hodding JH, Director, Pharmacy Services, Miller Children's Hospital, Long Beach, CA, Personal Correspondence, June 2004.

Joint Commission on Accreditation of Healthcare Organizations, "2004 National Patient Safety Goals, Frequently Asked Questions: Updated 8/30/04," August 30, 2004. Available at http://www.jcaho.org/accredited+organizations/patient+safety/04+npsg/04_npsgs_final2.pdf.

Joint Commission on Accreditation of Healthcare Organizations, "Transition Plan From 'Rule of 6'," JCAHOnline, December 2004/January 2005. Available at http://www.jcaho.org/about+us/news+letters/jcahonline/jo_01_05.htm.

NEONATAL RESUSCITATION ALGORITHM

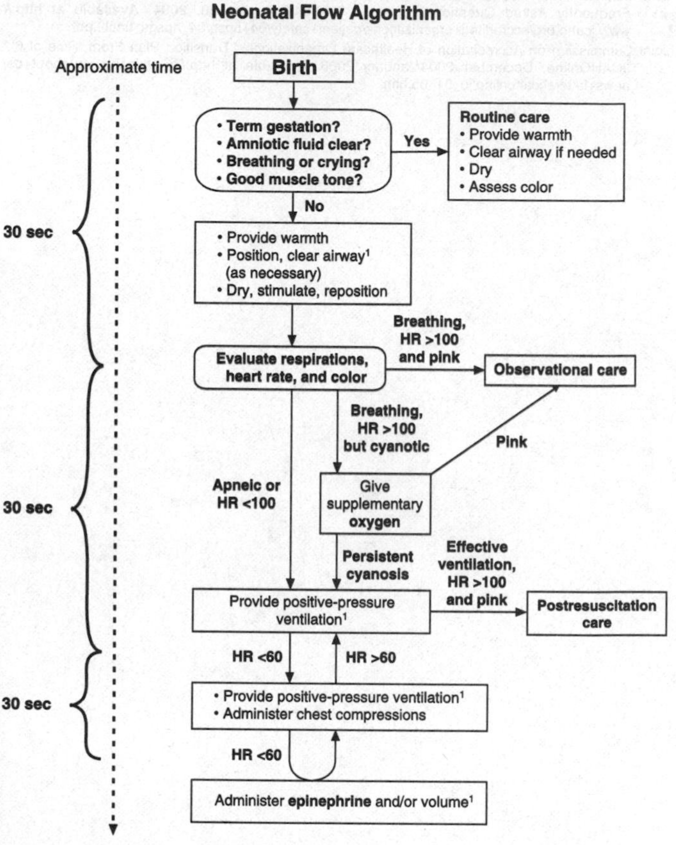

[1]Endotracheal intubation may be considered at several steps.

Epinephrine dose for neonatal resuscitation: I.V.: 0.01-0.03 mg/kg (1:10,000; 0.1-0.3 mL/kg). **Note:** I.V. is the preferred neonatal route. While obtaining I.V. access, one may consider higher doses via E.T.: Up to 0.1 mg/kg (1 mL/kg, 1:10,000), but safety and efficacy of this practice has not been evaluated.

PEDIATRIC ALS ALGORITHMS

PALS Bradycardia Algorithm

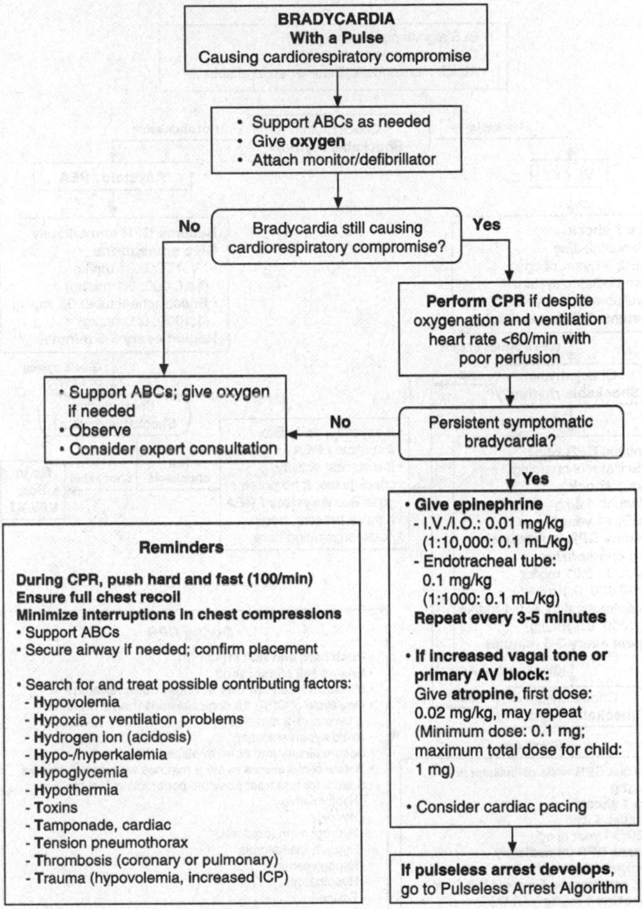

Reproduced With Permission, "2005 American Heart Association Guidelines for Cardiopulmonary Resuscitation and Emergency Cardiovascular Care," ©2005, American Heart Association.

PEDIATRIC ALS ALGORITHMS *(Continued)*

PALS Pulseless Arrest Algorithm

- BLS algorithm: Continue CPR
- Give **oxygen** when available
- Attach monitor/defibrillator when available

Check rhythm
Shockable rhythm?

Shockable → **VF / VT**

Not shockable → **Asystole / PEA**

VF / VT

Give 1 shock
- Manual: 2 J/kg
- AED: >1 year of age
  Use pediatric system if available for 1-8 years of age

Resume CPR immediately

Ⓐ **Give 5 cycles of CPR[1]**

Check rhythm
Shockable rhythm?

No → (go to box below: If asystole…)

Shockable

Continue CPR while defibrillator is charging
Give 1 shock
- Manual: 4 J/kg
- AED: >1 year of age

Resume CPR immediately
Give *epinephrine*
- I.V./I.O.: 0.01 mg/kg
  (1:10,000: 0.1 mL/kg)
- Endotracheal tube: 0.1 mg/kg
  (1:1000: 0.1 mL/kg)

Repeat every 3-5 minutes

Give 5 cycles of CPR[1]

Check rhythm
Shockable rhythm?

No →

Shockable

Continue CPR while defibrillator is charging
Give 1 shock
- Manual: 4 J/kg
- AED: >1 year of age

Resume CPR immediately
Consider **antiarrhythmics**
(eg, **amiodarone** 5 mg/kg I.V./I.O. or **lidocaine** 1 mg/kg I.V./I.O.)
Consider **magnesium** 25-50 mg/kg I.V./I.O., max 2 g for torsade de pointes
After 5 cycles of CPR,[1] go to Box A above

Asystole / PEA

Resume CPR immediately
Give *epinephrine*
- I.V./I.O.: 0.01 mg/kg
  (1:10,000: 0.1 mL/kg)
- Endotracheal tube: 0.1 mg/kg
  (1:1000: 0.1 mL/kg)

Repeat every 3-5 minutes

Give 5 cycles of CPR[1]

Check rhythm
Shockable rhythm?

Not shockable →
- If asystole, go to Box **Asystole / PEA**
- If electrical activity, check pulse. If no pulse, go to Box **Asystole / PEA**
- If pulse present, begin postresuscitation care

Shockable → Go to Box **VF / VT**

During CPR
- **Push hard and fast (100/min)**
- **Ensure full chest recoil**
- **Minimize interruptions in chest compressions**
- One cycle of CPR: 15 compressions then 2 breaths; 5 cycles =1-2 minutes
- Avoid hyperventilation
- Secure airway and confirm placement
- Rotate compressors every 2 minutes with rhythm checks
- Search for and treat possible contributing factors:
  - Hypovolemia
  - Hypoxia
  - Hydrogen ion (acidosis)
  - Hypo-/hyperkalemia
  - Hypoglycemia
  - Hypothermia
  - Toxins
  - Tamponade, cardiac
  - Tension pneumothorax
  - Thrombosis (coronary or pulmonary)
  - Trauma

VF = ventricular fibrillation; VT = ventricular tachycardia; PEA = pulseless electrical activity; AED = automated external defibrillator.

[1]After an advanced airway is placed, rescuers no longer deliver "cycles" of CPR. Give continuous chest compressions without pauses for breaths. Give 8-10 breaths/min. Check rhythm every 2 minutes.

PALS Tachycardia Algorithm With Pulses and Poor Perfusion

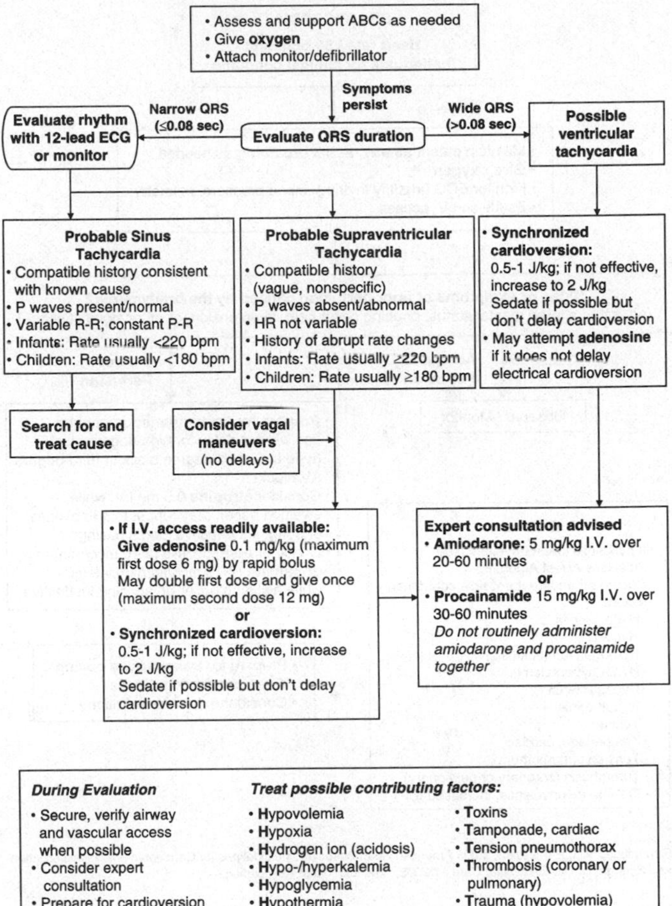

During Evaluation

- Secure, verify airway and vascular access when possible
- Consider expert consultation
- Prepare for cardioversion

Treat possible contributing factors:

- **H**ypovolemia
- **H**ypoxia
- **H**ydrogen ion (acidosis)
- **H**ypo-/hyperkalemia
- **H**ypoglycemia
- **H**ypothermia
- **T**oxins
- **T**amponade, cardiac
- **T**ension pneumothorax
- **T**hrombosis (coronary or pulmonary)
- **T**rauma (hypovolemia)

ADULT ACLS ALGORITHMS

Bradycardia Algorithm

BRADYCARDIA

Heart rate <60 bpm and inadequate for clinical condition

↓

- Maintain patent **airway**; assist **breathing** as needed
- Give **oxygen**
- Monitor ECG (identify thythm), blood pressure, oximetry
- Establish I.V. access

↓

Signs or symptoms of poor perfusion caused by the bradycardia?
(eg, acute altered mental status, ongoing chest pain, hypotension, or other signs of shock)

Adequate Perfusion → Observe / Monitor

Poor Perfusion →

- **Prepare for transcutaneous pacing;** use without delay for high-degree block (type II second-degree block or third-degree AV block)
- Consider **atropine** 0.5 mg I.V. while awaiting pacer. May repeat to a total dose of 3 mg. If ineffective, begin pacing.
- Consider **epinephrine** (2-10 mcg/min) or **dopamine** (2-10 mcg/kg/min) infusion while awaiting pacer or if pacing ineffective

↓

- Prepare for **transvenous pacing**
- Treat contributing causes
- Consider expert consultation

Reminders

- If pulseless arrest develops, *see* Pulseless Arrest Algorithm
- Search for and treat possible contributing factors:
  - **Hypovolemia**
  - **Hypoxia**
  - **Hydrogen ion (acidosis)**
  - **Hypo-/hyperkalemia**
  - **Hypoglycemia**
  - **Hypothermia**
  - **Toxins**
  - **Tamponade, cardiac**
  - **Tension pneumothorax**
  - **Thrombosis (coronary or pulmonary)**
  - **Trauma (hypovolemia, increased ICP)**

ACLS Pulseless Arrest Algorithm

- BLS algorithm: Call for help, give CPR
- Give **oxygen** when available
- Attach monitor/defibrillator when available

Check rhythm — Shockable rhythm?

Shockable → VF / VT

Give 1 shock
- Manual biphasic: Device specific (typically 120-200 J) **Note:** If unknown, use 200 J
- AED: Device specific
- Monophasic: 360 J

Resume CPR immediately

Ⓐ **Give 5 cycles of CPR[1]**

Check rhythm — Shockable rhythm? (**No** → go to box below)

Shockable

Continue CPR while defibrillator is charging
Give 1 shock
- Manual biphasic: Device specific (same as first shock or higher dose) **Note:** If unknown, use 200 J
- AED: Device specific
- Monophasic: 360 J

Resume CPR immediately after the shock. When I.V./I.O. available, give vasopressor during CPR (before or after the shock)
- **Epinephrine** 1 mg I.V./I.O. **Repeat every 3-5 minutes *or***
- May give 1 dose of **vasopressin** 40 units I.V./I.O. to replace first or second dose of **epinephrine**

Give 5 cycles of CPR[1]

Check rhythm — Shockable rhythm? (**No** → go to box below)

Shockable

Continue CPR while defibrillator is charging
Give 1 shock
- Manual biphasic: Device specific (same as first shock or higher dose) **Note:** If unknown, use 200 J
- AED: Device specific
- Monophasic: 360 J

Resume CPR immediately after the shock.
Consider **antiarrhythmics;** give during CPR (before or after the shock) **amiodarone** (300 mg I.V./I.O. once, then consider additional 150 mg I.V./I.O. once) or **lidocaine** (1-1.5 mg/kg first dose, then 0.5-0.75 mg/kg I.V./I.O., maximum 3 doses or 3 mg/kg)
Consider **magnesium,** loading dose 1-2 g I.V./I.O. for torsade de pointes
After 5 cycles of CPR,[1] go to Box A above

No (rhythm not shockable):
- If asystole, go to Box **Asystole / PEA**
- If electrical activity, check pulse. If no pulse, go to Box **Asystole / PEA.**
- If pulse present, begin postresuscitation care

Not shockable → Asystole / PEA

Resume CPR immediately for 5 cycles.
When I.V./I.O. available, give vasopressor.
- **Epinephrine** 1 mg I.V./I.O. **Repeat every 3-5 minutes *or***
- May give 1 dose of **vasopressin** 40 units I.V./I.O. to replace first or second dose of **epinephrine**

Consider **atrophine** 1 mg I.V./I.O. for asystole or slow PEA rate
Repeat every 3-5 min (up to 3 doses)

Give 5 cycles of CPR[1]

Check rhythm — Shockable rhythm?
- **Not shockable** → go to box above (If asystole… / If electrical activity… / If pulse present…)
- **Shockable** → Go to Box **VF / VT**

During CPR
- **Push hard and fast (100/min)**
- **Ensure full chest recoil**
- **Minimize interruptions in chest compressions**
- One cycle of CPR: 30 compressions then 2 breaths; 5 cycles = 2 minutes
- Avoid hyperventilation
- Secure airway and confirm placement
- Rotate compressors every 2 minutes with rhythm checks
- Search for and treat possible contributing factors:
  - Hypovolemia
  - Hypoxia
  - Hydrogen ion (acidosis)
  - Hypo-/hyperkalemia
  - Hypoglycemia
  - Hypothermia
  - Toxins
  - Tamponade, cardiac
  - Tension pneumothorax
  - Thrombosis (coronary or pulmonary)
  - Trauma

[1]After an advanced airway is placed, rescuers no longer deliver "cycles" of CPR. Give continuous chest compressions without pauses for breaths. Give 8-10 breaths/min. Check rhythm every 2 minutes.

VF = ventricular fibrillation; VT = ventricular tachycardia; PEA = pulseless electrical activity; AED = automated external defibrillator.

ADULT ACLS ALGORITHMS *(Continued)*

ACLS Tachycardia Algorithm With Pulses

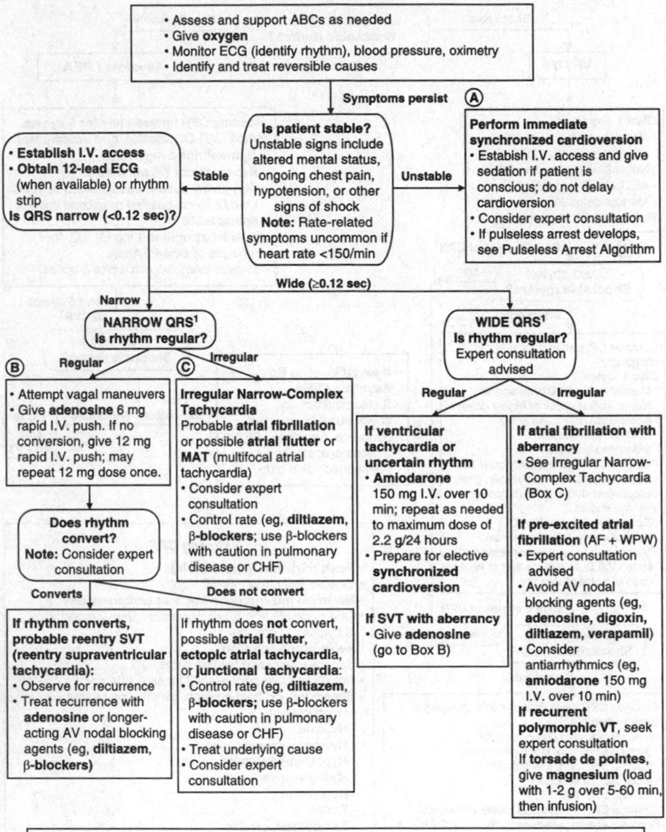

During Evaluation

- Secure, verify airway and vascular access when possible
- Consider expert consultation
- Prepare for cardioversion

Treat possible contributing factors:

- Hypovolemia
- Hypoxia
- Hydrogen ion (acidosis)
- Hypo-/hyperkalemia
- Hypoglycemia
- Hypothermia
- Toxins
- Tamponade, cardiac
- Tension pneumothorax
- Thrombosis (coronary or pulmonary)
- Trauma (hypovolemia)

SVT = supraventricular tachycardia; VT = ventricular tachycardia.

[1]If patient becomes unstable, go to Box A.

NORMAL HEART RATES

Age	Mean Heart Rate (beats/minute)	Heart Rate Range (2nd – 98th percentile)
<1 d	123	93-154
1-2 d	123	91-159
3-6 d	129	91-166
1-3 wk	148	107-182
1-2 mo	149	121-179
3-5 mo	141	106-186
6-11 mo	134	109-169
1-2 y	119	89-151
3-4 y	108	73-137
5-7 y	100	65-133
8-11 y	91	62-130
12-15 y	85	60-119

Adapted from *The Harriet Lane Handbook*, 12th ed, Greene MG, ed, St Louis, MO: Mosby Yearbook, 1991.

Normal QRS Axes (in degrees)

Age	Mean	Range
1 wk – 1 mo	+110	+30 to +180
1–3 mo	+70	+10 to +125
3 mo – 3 y	+60	+10 to +110
>3 y	+60	+20 to +120
Adults	+50	–30 to +105

NORMAL HEART RATES *(Continued)*

INTERVALS AND SEGMENTS OF AN ECG CYCLE

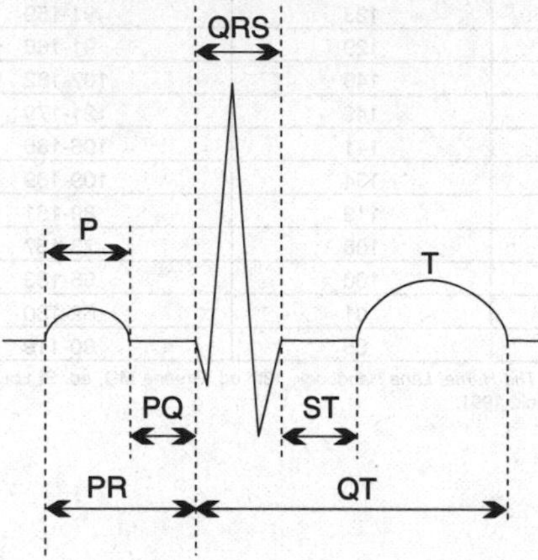

HEXAXIAL REFERENCE SYSTEM

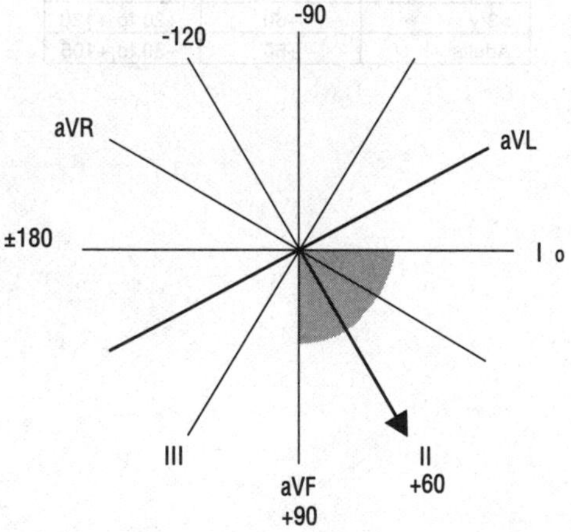

MEASURING PEDIATRIC BLOOD PRESSURE

Figure 1. Determination of Proper Cuff Size, Step 1

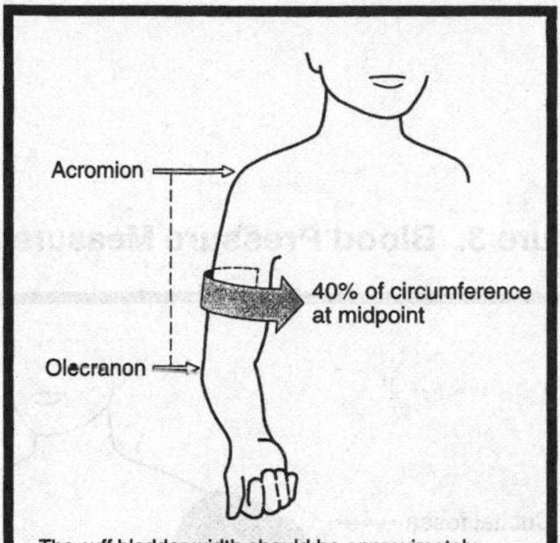

The cuff bladder width should be approximately 40% of the circumference of the arm measured at a point midway between the olecranon and acromion.

Figure 2. Determination of Proper Cuff Size, Step 2

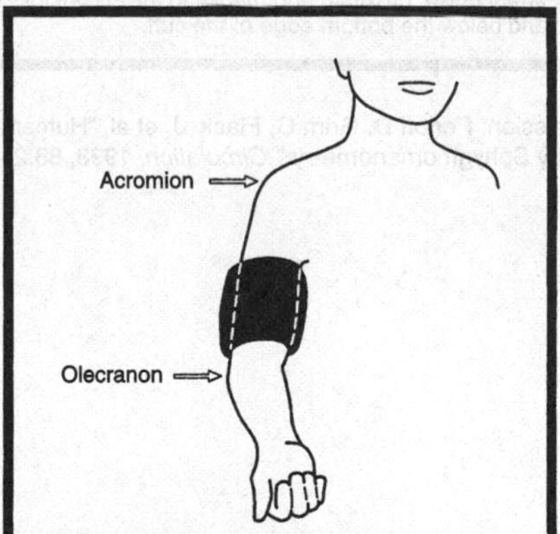

Cuff bladder length should cover 80% to 100% of the circumference of the arm.

MEASURING PEDIATRIC BLOOD PRESSURE *(Continued)*

Figure 3. Blood Pressure Measurement

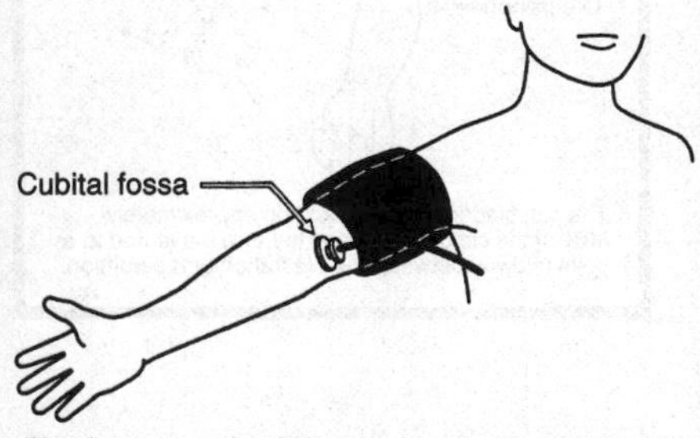

Blood pressure should be measured with cubital fossa at heart level. The arm should be supported. The stethoscope bell is placed over the brachial artery pulse, proximal and medial to the cubital fossa, and below the bottom edge of the cuff.

Used with permission: Perloff D, Grim C, Flack J, et al, "Human Blood Pressure Determination by Sphygmomanometry," *Circulation*, 1993, 88:2460-7.

HYPOTENSION, DEFINITIONS BY AGE GROUP

Hypotension is a *systolic* blood pressure <5th percentile of normal for age, namely:

- <60 mm Hg in term neonates (0-28 days)
- <70 mm Hg in infants (1-12 months)
- <70 mm Hg + (2 x age in years) in children 1-10 years
- <90 mm Hg in children ≥10 years of age

Reference

American Heart Association Emergency Cardiovascular Care Committee, "2005 American Heart Association (AHA) Guidelines for Cardiopulmonary Resuscitation (CPR) and Emergency Cardiovascular Care (ECC)," *Circulation*, 2005, 112(24 Suppl):IV-167.

HYPERTENSION, CLASSIFICATION BY AGE GROUP[1]

Age Group	Significant Hypertension (mm Hg)	Severe Hypertension (mm Hg)
Newborn (7 d)		
systolic BP	≥96	≥106
Newborn (8-30 d)		
systolic BP	≥104	≥110
Infant (<2 y)		
systolic BP	≥112	≥118
diastolic BP	≥74	≥82
Children (3-5 y)		
systolic BP	≥116	≥124
diastolic BP	≥76	≥84
Children (6-9 y)		
systolic BP	≥122	≥130
diastolic BP	≥78	≥86
Children (10-12 y)		
systolic BP	≥126	≥134
diastolic BP	≥82	≥90
Adolescents (13-15 y)		
systolic BP	≥136	≥144
diastolic BP	≥86	≥92
Adolescents (16-18 y)		
systolic BP	≥142	≥150
diastolic BP	≥92	≥98

Adapted from Horan MJ, *Pediatrics*, 1987, 79:1-25.

[1]See also Blood Pressure Measurement, Age Specific Percentiles, and 90th and 95th Percentiles of Blood Pressure by Percentiles of Height.

BLOOD PRESSURE IN PREMATURE INFANTS, NORMAL

(Birth weight 600-1750 g)[1]

Day	600-999 g		1000-1249 g	
	S (± 2SD)	D (± 2SD)	S (± 2SD)	D (± 2SD)
1	37.9 (17.4)	23.2 (10.3)	44 (22.8)	22.5 (13.5)
3	44.9 (15.7)	30.6 (12.3)	48 (15.4)	36.5 (9.6)
7	50 (14.8)	30.4 (12.4)	57 (14)	42.5 (16.5)
14	50.2 (14.8)	37.4 (12)	53 (30)	
28	61 (23.5)	45.8 (27.4)	57 (30)	
Day	**1250-1499 g**		**1500-1750 g**	
	S (± 2SD)	D (± 2SD)	S (± 2SD)	D (± 2SD)
1	48 (18)	27 (12.4)	47 (15.8)	26 (15.6)
3	59 (21.1)	40 (13.7)	51 (18.2)	35 (10)
7	68 (14.8)	40 (11.3)	66 (23)	41 (24)
14	64 (21.2)	36 (24.2)	76 (34.8)	42 (20.3)
28	69 (31.4)	44 (26.2)	73 (5.6)	50 (9.9)

[1]Blood pressure was obtained by the Dinamap method.

S = systolic; D = diastolic; SD = standard deviation.

Modified from Ingelfinger JR, Powers L, and Epstein MF, "Blood Pressure Norms in Low-Weight Infants: Birth Through Four Weeks", *Pediatr Res*, 1983, 17:319A.

BLOOD PRESSURE MEASUREMENTS, AGE-SPECIFIC PERCENTILES

Blood Pressure Measurements: Ages 0-12 Months, BOYS

Korotkoff phase IV (K4) used for diastolic BP. Reproduced with permission from Horan MJ, *Pediatrics*, 1987, 79:11-25.

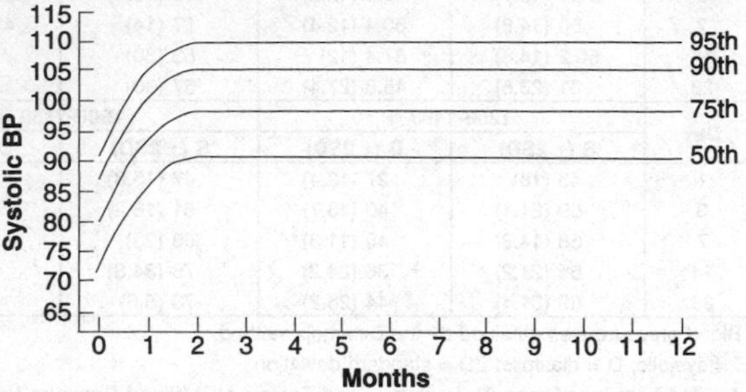

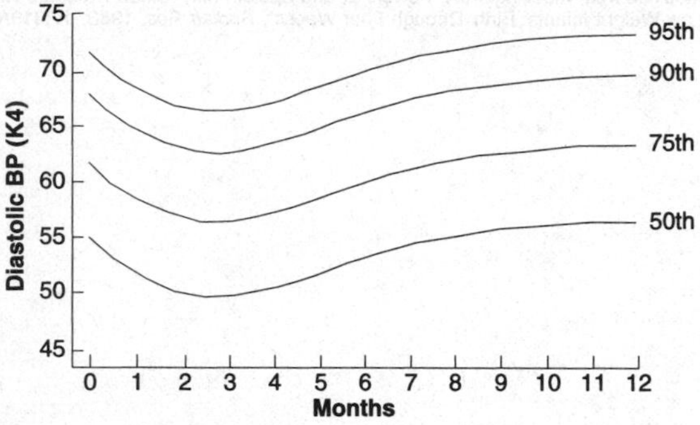

90th Percentile													
Systolic BP	87	101	106	106	106	105	105	105	105	105	105	105	105
Diastolic BP	68	65	63	63	63	65	66	67	68	68	69	69	69
Height cm	51	59	63	66	68	70	72	73	74	76	77	78	80
Weight kg	4	4	5	5	6	7	8	9	9	10	10	11	11

Blood Pressure Measurements: Ages 0-12 Months, GIRLS

Korotkoff phase IV (K4) used for diastolic BP. Reproduced with permission from Horan MJ, *Pediatrics*, 1987, 79:11-25.

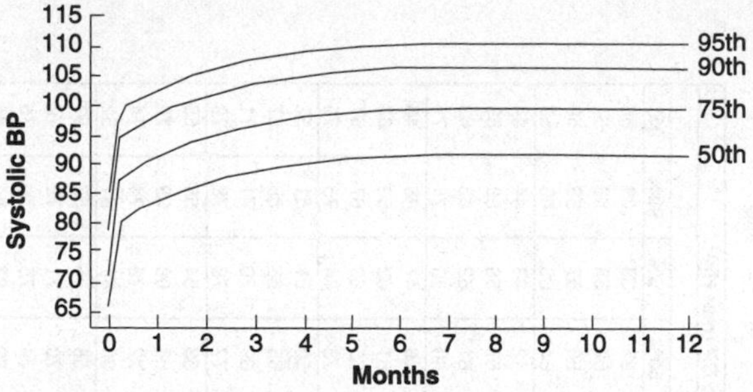

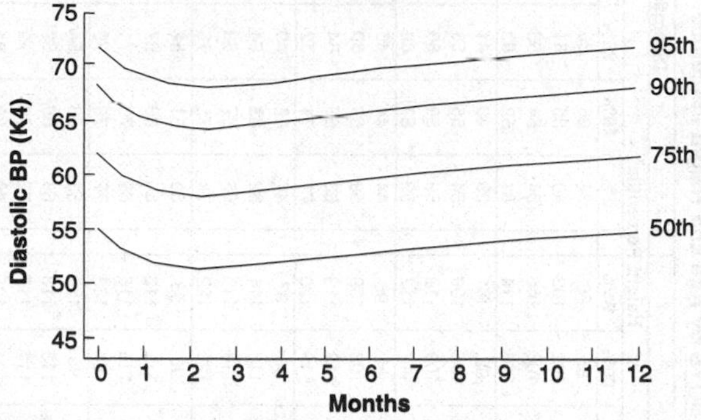

90th Percentile													
Systolic BP	76	98	101	104	105	106	106	106	106	106	106	105	105
Diastolic BP	68	65	64	64	65	65	66	66	66	67	67	67	67
Height cm	54	55	56	58	61	63	66	68	70	72	74	75	77
Weight kg	4	4	4	5	5	6	7	8	9	9	10	10	11

BLOOD PRESSURE MEASUREMENTS, AGE-SPECIFIC PERCENTILES *(Continued)*

Blood Pressure Levels for BOYS by Age and Height Percentile

Age (y)	BP Percentile[1]	Systolic BP (mm Hg)							Diastolic BP (mm Hg)[2]						
		Height Percentile[3]													
		5%	10%	25%	50%	75%	90%	95%	5%	10%	25%	50%	75%	90%	95%
1	50th	80	81	83	85	87	88	89	34	35	36	37	38	39	39
	90th	94	95	97	99	100	102	103	49	50	51	52	53	53	54
	95th	98	99	101	103	104	106	106	54	54	55	56	57	58	58
	99th	105	106	108	110	112	113	114	61	62	63	64	65	66	66
2	50th	84	85	87	88	90	92	92	39	40	41	42	43	44	44
	90th	97	99	100	102	104	105	106	54	55	56	57	58	58	59
	95th	101	102	104	106	108	109	110	59	59	60	61	62	63	63
	99th	109	110	111	113	115	117	117	66	67	68	69	70	71	71
3	50th	86	87	89	91	93	94	95	44	44	45	46	47	48	48
	90th	100	101	103	105	107	108	109	59	59	60	61	62	63	63
	95th	104	105	107	109	110	112	113	63	63	64	65	66	67	67
	99th	111	112	114	116	118	119	120	71	71	72	73	74	75	75
4	50th	88	89	91	93	95	96	97	47	48	49	50	51	51	52
	90th	102	103	105	107	109	110	111	62	63	64	65	66	66	67
	95th	106	107	109	111	112	114	115	66	67	68	69	70	71	71
	99th	113	114	116	118	120	121	122	74	75	76	77	78	78	79
5	50th	90	91	93	95	96	98	98	50	51	52	53	54	55	55
	90th	104	105	106	108	110	111	112	65	66	67	68	69	69	70
	95th	108	109	110	112	114	115	116	69	70	71	72	73	74	74
	99th	115	116	118	120	121	123	123	77	78	79	80	81	81	82
6	50th	91	92	94	96	98	99	100	53	53	54	55	56	57	57
	90th	105	106	108	110	111	113	113	68	68	69	70	71	72	72
	95th	109	110	112	114	115	117	117	72	72	73	74	75	76	76
	99th	116	117	119	121	123	124	125	80	80	81	82	83	84	84

Blood Pressure Levels for BOYS by Age and Height Percentile *(continued)*

Age (y)	BP Percentile[1]	Systolic BP (mm Hg)							Diastolic BP (mm Hg)[2]						
		Height Percentile[3]													
		5%	10%	25%	50%	75%	90%	95%	5%	10%	25%	50%	75%	90%	95%
7	50th	92	94	95	97	99	100	101	55	55	56	57	58	59	59
	90th	106	107	109	111	113	114	115	70	70	71	72	73	74	74
	95th	110	111	113	115	117	118	119	74	74	75	76	77	78	78
	99th	117	118	120	122	124	125	126	82	82	83	84	85	86	86
8	50th	94	95	97	99	100	102	102	56	57	58	59	60	60	61
	90th	107	109	110	112	114	115	116	71	72	72	73	74	75	76
	95th	111	112	114	116	118	119	120	75	76	77	78	79	79	80
	99th	119	120	122	123	125	127	127	83	84	85	86	87	87	88
9	50th	95	96	98	100	102	103	104	57	58	59	60	61	61	62
	90th	109	110	112	114	115	117	118	72	73	74	75	76	76	77
	95th	113	114	116	118	119	121	121	76	77	78	79	80	81	81
	99th	120	121	123	125	127	128	129	84	85	86	87	88	88	89
10	50th	97	98	100	102	103	105	106	58	59	60	61	61	62	63
	90th	111	112	114	115	117	119	119	73	73	74	75	76	77	78
	95th	115	116	117	119	121	122	123	77	78	79	80	81	81	82
	99th	122	123	125	127	128	130	130	85	86	36	88	88	89	90
11	50th	99	100	102	104	105	107	107	59	59	60	61	62	63	63
	90th	113	114	115	117	119	120	121	74	74	75	76	77	78	78
	95th	117	118	119	121	123	124	125	78	78	79	80	81	82	82
	99th	124	125	127	129	130	132	132	86	86	87	88	89	90	90
12	50th	101	102	104	106	108	109	110	59	60	61	62	63	63	64
	90th	115	116	118	120	121	123	123	74	75	75	76	77	78	79
	95th	119	120	122	123	125	127	127	78	79	80	81	82	82	83
	99th	126	127	129	131	133	134	135	86	87	88	89	90	90	91

BLOOD PRESSURE MEASUREMENTS, AGE-SPECIFIC PERCENTILES *(Continued)*

Blood Pressure Levels for BOYS by Age and Height Percentile *(continued)*

Age (y)	BP Percentile[1]	Systolic BP (mm Hg)							Diastolic BP (mm Hg)[2]						
		Height Percentile[3]													
		5%	10%	25%	50%	75%	90%	95%	5%	10%	25%	50%	75%	90%	95%
13	50th	104	105	106	108	110	111	112	60	60	61	62	63	64	64
	90th	117	118	120	122	124	125	126	75	75	76	77	78	79	79
	95th	121	122	124	126	128	129	130	79	79	80	81	82	83	83
	99th	128	130	131	133	135	136	137	87	87	88	89	90	91	91
14	50th	106	107	109	111	113	114	115	60	61	62	63	64	65	65
	90th	120	121	123	125	126	128	128	75	76	77	78	79	79	80
	95th	124	125	127	128	130	132	132	80	80	81	82	83	84	84
	99th	131	132	134	136	138	139	140	87	88	89	90	91	92	92
15	50th	109	110	112	113	115	117	117	61	62	63	64	65	66	66
	90th	122	124	125	127	129	130	131	76	77	78	79	80	80	81
	95th	126	127	129	131	133	134	135	81	81	82	83	84	85	85
	99th	134	135	136	138	140	142	142	88	89	90	91	92	93	93
16	50th	111	112	114	116	118	119	120	63	63	64	65	66	67	67
	90th	125	126	128	130	131	133	134	78	78	79	80	81	82	82
	95th	129	130	132	134	135	137	137	82	83	83	84	85	86	87
	99th	136	137	139	141	143	144	145	90	90	91	92	93	94	94
17	50th	114	115	116	118	120	121	122	65	66	66	67	68	69	70
	90th	127	128	130	132	134	135	136	80	80	81	82	83	84	84
	95th	131	132	134	136	138	139	140	84	85	86	87	87	88	89
	99th	139	140	141	143	145	146	147	92	93	93	94	95	96	97

[1]Blood pressure percentile determined by a single measurement.

[2]Korotkoff phase V (K5) used for diastolic BP.

[3]Height percentile determined by standard growth curves.

Source: National High Blood Pressure Education Program Working Group on High Blood Pressure in Children and Adolescents, "The Fourth Report on the Diagnosis, Evaluation, and Treatment of High Blood Pressure in Children and Adolescents," *Pediatrics*, 2004, 114(2 Suppl 4th Report):555-76.

Blood Pressure Levels for GIRLS by Age and Height Percentile

Age (y)	BP Percentile[1]	Systolic BP (mm Hg)							Diastolic BP (mm Hg)[2]						
		Height Percentile[3]													
		5%	10%	25%	50%	75%	90%	95%	5%	10%	25%	50%	75%	90%	95%
1	50th	83	84	85	86	88	89	90	38	39	39	40	41	41	42
	90th	97	97	98	100	101	102	103	52	53	53	54	55	55	56
	95th	100	101	102	104	105	106	107	56	57	57	58	59	59	60
	99th	108	108	109	111	112	113	114	64	64	65	65	66	67	67
2	50th	85	85	87	88	89	91	91	43	44	44	45	46	46	47
	90th	98	99	100	101	103	104	105	57	58	58	59	60	61	61
	95th	102	103	104	105	107	108	109	61	62	62	63	64	65	65
	99th	109	110	111	112	114	115	116	69	69	70	70	71	72	72
3	50th	86	87	88	89	91	92	93	47	48	48	49	50	50	51
	90th	100	100	102	103	104	106	106	61	62	62	63	64	64	65
	95th	104	104	105	107	108	109	110	65	66	66	67	68	68	69
	99th	111	111	113	114	115	116	117	73	73	74	74	75	76	76
4	50th	88	88	90	91	92	94	94	50	50	51	52	52	53	54
	90th	101	102	103	104	106	107	108	64	64	65	66	67	67	68
	95th	105	106	107	108	110	111	112	68	68	69	70	71	71	72
	99th	112	113	114	115	117	118	119	76	76	76	77	78	79	79
5	50th	89	90	91	93	94	95	96	52	53	53	54	55	55	56
	90th	103	103	105	106	107	109	109	66	67	67	68	69	69	70
	95th	107	107	108	110	111	112	113	70	71	71	72	73	73	74
	99th	114	114	116	117	118	120	120	78	78	79	79	80	81	81
6	50th	91	92	93	94	96	97	98	54	54	55	56	56	57	58
	90th	104	105	106	108	109	110	111	68	68	69	70	70	71	72
	95th	108	109	110	111	113	114	115	72	72	73	74	74	75	76
	99th	115	116	117	119	120	121	122	80	80	80	81	82	83	83

BLOOD PRESSURE MEASUREMENTS, AGE-SPECIFIC PERCENTILES *(Continued)*

Blood Pressure Levels for GIRLS by Age and Height Percentile *(continued)*

Age (y)	BP Percentile[1]	Systolic BP (mm Hg)							Diastolic BP (mm Hg)[2]						
		Height Percentile[3]													
		5%	10%	25%	50%	75%	90%	95%	5%	10%	25%	50%	75%	90%	95%
7	50th	93	93	95	96	97	99	99	55	56	56	57	58	58	59
	90th	106	107	108	109	111	112	113	69	70	70	71	72	72	73
	95th	110	111	112	113	115	116	116	73	74	74	75	76	76	77
	99th	117	118	119	120	122	123	124	81	81	82	82	83	84	84
8	50th	95	95	96	98	99	100	101	57	57	57	58	59	60	60
	90th	108	109	110	111	113	114	114	71	71	71	72	73	74	74
	95th	112	112	114	115	116	118	118	75	75	75	76	77	78	78
	99th	119	120	121	122	123	125	125	82	82	83	83	84	85	86
9	50th	96	97	98	100	101	102	103	58	58	58	59	60	61	61
	90th	110	110	112	113	114	116	116	72	72	72	73	74	75	75
	95th	114	114	115	117	118	119	120	76	76	76	77	78	79	79
	99th	121	121	123	124	125	127	127	83	83	84	84	85	86	87
10	50th	98	99	100	102	103	104	105	59	59	59	60	61	62	62
	90th	112	112	114	115	116	118	118	73	73	73	74	75	76	76
	95th	116	116	117	119	120	121	122	77	77	77	78	79	80	80
	99th	123	123	125	126	127	129	129	84	84	85	86	86	87	88
11	50th	100	101	102	103	105	106	107	60	60	60	61	62	63	63
	90th	114	114	116	117	118	119	120	74	74	74	75	76	77	77
	95th	118	118	119	121	122	123	124	78	78	78	79	80	81	81
	99th	125	125	126	128	129	130	131	85	85	86	87	87	88	89
12	50th	102	103	104	105	107	108	109	61	61	61	62	63	64	64
	90th	116	116	117	119	120	121	122	75	75	75	76	77	78	78
	95th	119	120	121	123	124	125	126	79	79	79	80	81	82	82
	99th	127	127	128	130	131	132	133	86	86	87	88	88	89	90

Blood Pressure Levels for GIRLS by Age and Height Percentile *(continued)*

Age (y)	BP Percentile[1]	Systolic BP (mm Hg)							Diastolic BP (mm Hg)[2]						
		Height Percentile[3]													
		5%	10%	25%	50%	75%	90%	95%	5%	10%	25%	50%	75%	90%	95%
13	50th	104	105	106	107	109	110	110	62	62	62	63	64	65	65
	90th	117	118	119	121	122	123	124	76	76	76	77	78	79	79
	95th	121	122	123	124	126	127	128	80	80	80	81	82	83	83
	99th	128	129	130	132	133	134	135	87	87	88	89	89	90	91
14	50th	106	106	107	109	110	111	112	63	63	63	64	65	66	66
	90th	119	120	121	122	124	125	125	77	77	77	78	79	80	80
	95th	123	123	125	126	127	129	129	81	81	81	82	83	84	84
	99th	130	131	132	133	135	136	136	88	88	89	90	90	91	92
15	50th	107	108	109	110	111	113	113	64	64	64	65	66	67	67
	90th	120	121	122	123	125	126	127	78	78	78	79	80	81	81
	95th	124	125	126	127	129	130	131	82	82	82	83	84	85	85
	99th	131	132	133	134	136	137	138	89	89	90	91	91	92	93
16	50th	108	108	110	111	112	114	114	64	64	65	66	66	67	68
	90th	121	122	123	124	126	127	128	78	78	79	80	81	81	82
	95th	125	126	127	128	130	131	132	82	82	83	84	85	85	86
	99th	132	133	134	135	137	138	139	90	90	90	91	92	93	93
17	50th	108	109	110	111	113	114	115	64	65	65	66	67	67	68
	90th	122	122	123	125	126	127	128	78	79	79	80	81	81	82
	95th	125	126	127	129	130	131	132	82	83	83	84	85	85	86
	99th	133	133	134	136	137	138	139	90	90	91	91	92	93	93

[1]Blood pressure percentile determined by a single measurement.

[2]Korotkoff phase V (K5) used for diastolic BP.

[3]Height percentile determined by standard growth curves.

Source: National High Blood Pressure Education Program Working Group on High Blood Pressure in Children and Adolescents, "The Fourth Report on the Diagnosis, Evaluation, and Treatment of High Blood Pressure in Children and Adolescents," *Pediatrics*, 2004, 114(2 Suppl 4th Report):555-76.

ANTIHYPERTENSIVE AGENTS BY CLASS

Alpha-Adrenergic (Alpha$_1$ and Alpha$_2$) Antagonists
- Phenoxybenzamine
- Phentolamine

Alpha$_1$-Antagonists
- Prazosin

Alpha$_2$-Agonists
- Clonidine
- Methyldopa

Beta (Beta$_1$ and Beta$_2$)-Antagonists
- Nadolol
- Propranolol
- Timolol

Beta$_1$-Antagonists (Selective)
- Atenolol
- Esmolol
- Metoprolol

Mixed Alpha- / Beta-Antagonists
- Carvedilol
- Labetalol

Angiotensin-Converting Enzyme Inhibitors
- Benazepril
- Captopril
- Enalapril/Enalaprilat
- Fosinopril
- Lisinopril

Calcium Channel Blockers
- Amlodipine
- Diltiazem
- Isradipine
- Nicardipine
- Nifedipine
- Verapamil

Diuretics
- Amiloride
- Bumetanide
- Chlorothiazide
- Ethacrynic acid
- Furosemide
- Hydrochlorothiazide
- Metolazone
- Spironolactone
- Torsemide
- Triamterene

Nitrates
- Nitroglycerin

Vasodilators (Direct-Acting)
- Diazoxide
- Hydralazine
- Minoxidil
- Nitroprusside

NEW YORK HEART ASSOCIATION (NYHA) CLASSIFICATION OF FUNCTIONAL CAPACITY OF PATIENTS WITH DISEASES OF THE HEART, 1994 REVISIONS

Class I

Patients with cardiac disease but without resulting limitation of physical activity. Ordinary physical activity does not cause undue fatigue, palpitation, dyspnea, or anginal pain.

Class II

Patients with cardiac disease resulting in slight limitation of physical activity. They are comfortable at rest. Ordinary physical activity results in fatigue, palpitation, dyspnea, or anginal pain.

Class III

Patients with cardiac disease resulting in marked limitation of physical activity. They are comfortable at rest. Less than ordinary activity causes fatigue, palpitation, dyspnea, or anginal pain.

Class IV

Patients with cardiac disease resulting in inability to carry on any physical activity without discomfort. Symptoms of heart failure or the anginal syndrome may be present even at rest. If any physical activity is undertaken, discomfort increases.

Reference

The Criteria Committee of the New York Heart Association, *Nomenclature and Criteria for Diagnosis of Diseases of the Heart and Great Vessels*, 9th ed, Boston, MA: Little, Brown & Co, 1994, 253-6

WORLD HEALTH ORGANIZATION (WHO) FUNCTIONAL CLASSIFICATION OF PULMONARY HYPERTENSION

Class I

Patients with pulmonary hypertension but without resulting limitation of physical activity. Ordinary physical activity does not cause undue dyspnea or fatigue, chest pain, or near syncope.

Class II

Patients with pulmonary hypertension resulting in slight limitation of physical activity. They are comfortable at rest. Ordinary physical activity causes undue dyspnea or fatigue, chest pain, or near syncope.

Class III

Patients with pulmonary hypertension resulting in marked limitation of physical activity. They are comfortable at rest. Less than ordinary activity causes undue dyspnea or fatigue, chest pain, or near syncope.

Class IV

Patients with pulmonary hypertension with inability to carry out any physical activity without symptoms. These patients manifest signs of right heart failure. Dyspnea and/or fatigue may be present even at rest. Discomfort is increased by any physical activity.

Reference

Widlitz A and Barst RJ, "Pulmonary Arterial Hypertension in Children," *Eur Respir J*, 2003, 21(1):155-76.

ANTIDEPRESSANT AGENTS

Comparison of Usual Adult Dosage, Mechanism of Action, and Adverse Effects

Drug	Initial Adult Dose	Usual Adult Dosage (mg/d)	Dosage Forms	Adverse Effects						Comments
				ACH	Drowsiness	Orthostatic Hypotension	Conduction Abnormalities	GI Distress	Weight Gain	
Tricyclic Antidepressants and Related Compounds[1]										
Amitriptyline	25-75 mg qhs	100-300	T, I	4+	4+	3+	3+	1	4+	Also used in chronic pain, migraine, and as a hypnotic; contraindicated with cisapride
Amoxapine	50 mg bid	100-400	T	2+	2+	2+	2+	0	2+	May cause extrapyramidal symptom (EPS)
Clomipramine[2] (Anafranil®)	25-75 mg qhs	100-250	C	4+	4+	2+	3+	1+	4+	Approved for OCD
Desipramine (Norpramin®)	25-75 mg qhs	100-300	T	1+	2+	2+	2+	0	1+	Blood levels useful for therapeutic monitoring
Doxepin (Sinequan®, Zonalon®)	25-75 mg qhs	100-300	C, L	3+	4+	2+	2+	0	4+	
Imipramine (Tofranil®, Tofranil-PM®)	25-75 mg qhs	100-300	T, C	3+	3+	4+	3+	1+	4+	Blood levels useful for therapeutic monitoring
Maprotiline	25-75 mg qhs	100-225	T	2+	3+	2+	2+	0	2+	
Nortriptyline (Pamelor®)	25-50 mg qhs	50-150	C, L	2+	2+	1+	2+	0	1+	Blood levels useful for therapeutic monitoring
Protriptyline (Vivactil®)	15 mg qAM	15-60	T	2+	1+	2+	3+	1+	1+	
Trimipramine (Surmontil®)	25-75 mg qhs	100-300	C	4+	4+	3+	3+	0	4+	

ANTIDEPRESSANT AGENTS *(Continued)*

Comparison of Usual Adult Dosage, Mechanism of Action, and Adverse Effects *(continued)*

Drug	Initial Adult Dose	Usual Adult Dosage (mg/d)	Dosage Forms	Adverse Effects: ACH	Drowsiness	Orthostatic Hypotension	Conduction Abnormalities	GI Distress	Weight Gain	Comments
Selective Serotonin Reuptake Inhibitors[3]										
Citalopram (Celexa™)	20 mg qAM	20-60	T	0	0	0	0	3+[4]	1+	
Escitalopram (Lexapro™)	10 mg qAM	10-20	T	0	0	0	0	3+	1+	S-enantiomer of citalopram
Fluoxetine (Prozac®, Prozac® Weekly™, Sarafem™)	10-20 mg qAM	20-80	C, L, T	0	0	0	0	3+[4]	1+	CYP2B6 and 2D6 inhibitor
Fluvoxamine[2]	50 mg qhs	100-300	T	0	0	0	0	3+[4]	1+	Contraindicated with pimozide, thioridazine, mesoridazine, CYP1A2, 2B6, 2C19, and 3A4 inhibitors
Paroxetine (Paxil®, Paxil® CR™)	10-20 mg qAM	20-50	T, L	1+	1+	0	0	3+[4]	2+	CYP2B6 and 2D6 inhibitor
Sertraline (Zoloft®)	25-50 mg qAM	50-200	T	0	0	0	0	3+[4]	1+	CYP2B6 and 2C19 inhibitor
Dopamine-Reuptake Blocking Compounds										
Bupropion (Wellbutrin®, Wellbutrin SR®, Wellbutrin XL™, Zyban®)	100 mg bid-tid IR[5] 150 mg qAM-bid SR[6]	300-450[7]	T	0	0	0	1+/0	1+	0	Contraindicated with seizures, bulimia, and anorexia; low incidence of sexual dysfunction IR: A 6-h interval between doses preferred SR: An 8-h interval between doses preferred

Comparison of Usual Adult Dosage, Mechanism of Action, and Adverse Effects *(continued)*

Drug	Initial Adult Dose	Usual Adult Dosage (mg/d)	Dosage Forms	Adverse Effects						Comments
				ACH	Drowsiness	Orthostatic Hypotension	Conduction Abnormalities	GI Distress	Weight Gain	
Serotonin / Norepinephrine Reuptake Inhibitors[8]										
Duloxetine (Cymbalta®)	40-60 mg qd	40-60	C	1+	1+	0	1+	3+[4]	0	
Venlafaxine (Effexor®, Effexor® XR)	25 mg bid-tid IR 37.5 mg qd XR	75-375	T	1+	1+	0	1+	3+[4]	0	High-dose is useful to treat refractory depression; frequency of hypertension increases with dosage >225 mg/d
5-HT_2 Receptor Antagonist Properties										
Nefazodone	100 mg bid	300-600	T	1+	1+	2+	1+	1+	0	Contraindicated with carbamazepine, pimozide, astemizole, cisapride, and terfenadine; caution with triazolam and alprazolam; low incidence of sexual dysfunction
Trazodone (Desyrel®)	50 mg tid	150-600	T	0	4+	3+	1+	1+	2+	
Noradrenergic Antagonist										
Mirtazapine (Remeron®, Remeron® SolTab®)	15 mg qhs	15-45	T	1+	3+	1+	1+	0	3+	Dose >15 mg/d less sedating, low incidence of sexual dysfunction

ANTIDEPRESSANT AGENTS *(Continued)*

Comparison of Usual Adult Dosage, Mechanism of Action, and Adverse Effects *(continued)*

Drug	Initial Adult Dose	Usual Adult Dosage (mg/d)	Dosage Forms	Adverse Effects						Comments
				ACH	Drowsiness	Orthostatic Hypotension	Conduction Abnormalities	GI Distress	Weight Gain	
Monoamine Oxidase Inhibitors										
Isocarboxazid (Marplan®)	10 mg tid	10-30	T	2+	2+	2+	1+	1+	2+	Diet must be low in tyramine; contraindicated with sympathomimetics and other antidepressants
Phenelzine (Nardil®)	15 mg tid	15-90	T	2+	2+	2+	0	1+	3+	
Tranylcypromine (Parnate®)	10 mg bid	10-60	T	2+	1+	2+	1+	1+	2+	

ACH = anticholinergic effects (dry mouth, blurred vision, urinary retention, constipation); 0 - 4+ = absent or rare - relatively common. T = tablet, L = liquid, I = injectable, C = capsule; IR = immediate release, SR = sustained release.

[1]**Important note:** A 1-week supply taken all at once in a patient receiving the maximum dose can be fatal.

[2]Not approved by FDA for depression. Approved for OCD.

[3]Flat dose response curve, headache, nausea, and sexual dysfunction are common side effects for SSRIs.

[4]Nausea is usually mild and transient.

[5]IR: 100 mg bid, may be increased to 100 mg tid no sooner than 3 days after beginning therapy.

[6]SR: 150 mg qAM, may be increased to 150 mg bid as early as day 4 of dosing.

[7]To minimize seizure risk, do not exceed IR 150 mg/dose or SR 200 mg/dose.

[8]Do not use with sibutramine; relatively safe in overdose.

CORTICOSTEROIDS, SYSTEMIC

Relative Potencies and Equivalent Doses of Corticosteroids

(Glucocorticoid potency compared to hydrocortisone "mg" for "mg" basis)

Compound	Glucocorticoid Potency	Mineralocorticoid Potency	Equivalent Dose (mg)	Duration[1] of Action
Cortisone Tablet: 25 mg	0.8	++	25	S
Dexamethasone (Dexamethasone Intensol™, DexPak® TaperPak®) Elixir: 0.5 mg/5 mL Injection, solution: 4 mg/mL Intensol: 1 mg/mL Solution: 0.5 mg/5 mL Tablet: 0.5 mg, 0.75 mg, 1 mg, 1.5 mg, 2 mg, 4 mg, 6 mg	25-30	0	0.75	L
Fludrocortisone (Florinef®) Tablet: 0.1 mg	10	+++++		I
Hydrocortisone (Cortef®, Solu-Cortef®) Injection: 100 mg, 250 mg, 500 mg, 1 g Tablet: 5 mg, 10 mg, 20 mg	1	++	20	S
MethylPREDNISolone (Depo-Medrol®, Medrol®, Solu-Medrol®) Injection: 40 mg, 125 mg, 500 mg, 1 g, 2 g Injection, suspension: 20 mg/mL, 40 mg/mL, 80 mg/mL Tablet: 2 mg, 4 mg, 8 mg, 16 mg, 32 mg	5	0	4	I
PrednisoLONE (Orapred®, Pediapred®, Prelone®) Solution: 5 mg/5 mL, 15 mg/5 mL Syrup: 5 mg/5 mL, 15 mg/5 mL Tablet: 5 mg	4	+	5	I
PredniSONE (Prednisone Intensol™, Sterapred®, Sterapred® DS) Intensol: 5 mg/mL Solution: 1 mg/mL Tablet: 1 mg, 2.5 mg, 5 mg, 10 mg, 20 mg, 50 mg	4	+	5	I

[1]S = short, 8-12 hours biologic activity.

I = intermediate, 12-36 hours biologic activity.

L = long, 36-54 hours biologic activity.

Reference

Adapted and updated from Knoben JE, and Anderson PO, *Handbook of Clinical Drug Data*, 6th ed, Drug Intelligence Pub, Inc, 1988.

CORTICOSTEROIDS, TOPICAL: GUIDELINES FOR SELECTION AND USE

The quantity prescribed and the frequency of refills should be monitored to reduce the risk of adrenal suppression. In general, short courses of high-potency agents are preferable to prolonged use of low potency. After control is achieved, control should be maintained with a low potency preparation.

1. Low-to-medium potency agents are usually effective for treating thin, acute, inflammatory skin lesions; whereas, high or super-potent agents are often required for treating chronic, hyperkeratotic, or lichenified lesions.
2. Since the stratum corneum is thin on the face and intertriginous areas, low-potency agents are preferred but a higher potency agent may be used for 2 weeks.
3. Because the palms and soles have a thick stratum corneum, high or super-potent agents are frequently required.
4. **Low potency agents are preferred for infants** and the elderly. Infants have a high body surface area to weight ratio; elderly patients have thin, fragile skin.
5. The vehicle in which the topical corticosteroid is formulated influences the absorption and potency of the drug. Ointment bases are preferred for thick, lichenified lesions; they enhance penetration of the drug. Creams are preferred for acute and subacute dermatoses; they may be used on moist skin areas or intertriginous areas. Solutions, gels, and sprays are preferred for the scalp or for areas where a nonoil-based vehicle is needed.
6. In general, super-potent agents should not be used for longer than 2-3 weeks unless the lesion is limited to a small body area. Medium-to-high potency agents usually cause only rare adverse effects when treatment is limited to 3 months or less, and use on the face and intertriginous areas are avoided. If long-term treatment is needed, intermittent vs continued treatment is recommended.
7. Most preparations are applied once or twice daily. More frequent application may be necessary for the palms or soles because the preparation is easily removed by normal activity and penetration is poor due to a thick stratum corneum. Every-other-day or weekend-only application may be effective for treating some chronic conditions.

Corticosteroids, Topical

The following topical corticosteroid preparations are grouped according to relative anti-inflammatory activity. Preparations in each group are approximately equivalent.

Steroid		Vehicle
Very High Potency		
0.05%	Betamethasone dipropionate, augmented	Ointment, lotion
0.05%	Clobetasol propionate	Cream, foam, gel, lotion, ointment, shampoo, spray
0.05%	Diflorasone diacetate	Ointment
0.05%	Halobetasol propionate	Cream, ointment
High Potency		
0.1%	Amcinonide	Cream, ointment, lotion
0.05%	Betamethasone dipropionate, augmented	Cream
0.05%	Betamethasone dipropionate	Cream, ointment
0.1%	Betamethasone valerate	Ointment
0.05%	Desoximetasone	Gel
0.25%	Desoximetasone	Cream, ointment
0.05%	Diflorasone diacetate	Cream, ointment
0.05%	Fluocinonide	Cream, ointment, gel
0.1%	Halcinonide	Cream, ointment
0.5%	Triamcinolone acetonide	Cream
Intermediate Potency		
0.05%	Betamethasone dipropionate	Lotion
0.1%	Betamethasone valerate	Cream
0.1%	Clocortolone pivalate	Cream
0.05%	Desoximetasone	Cream
0.025%	Fluocinolone acetonide	Cream, ointment
0.05%	Flurandrenolide	Cream, ointment, lotion, tape
0.005%	Fluticasone propionate	Ointment
0.05%	Fluticasone propionate	Cream
0.1%	Hydrocortisone butyrate[1]	Ointment, solution
0.2%	Hydrocortisone valerate[1]	Cream, ointment
0.1%	Mometasone furoate[1]	Cream, ointment, lotion
0.1%	Prednicarbate	Cream, ointment
0.025%	Triamcinolone acetonide	Cream, ointment, lotion
0.1%	Triamcinolone acetonide	Cream, ointment, lotion
Low Potency		
0.05%	Alclometasone dipropionate[1]	Cream, ointment
0.05%	Desonide	Cream
0.01%	Fluocinolone acetonide	Cream, solution
0.5%	Hydrocortisone[1]	Cream, ointment, lotion
0.5%	Hydrocortisone acetate[1]	Cream, ointment
1%	Hydrocortisone acetate[1]	Cream, ointment
1%	Hydrocortisone[1]	Cream, ointment, lotion, solution
2.5%	Hydrocortisone[1]	Cream, ointment, lotion

[1]Not fluorinated.

MULTIVITAMIN PRODUCTS

MULTIVITAMIN PRODUCTS (PARENTERAL)

Product	A (int. units)	B_1 (mg)	B_2 (mg)	B_6 (mg)	B_{12} (mcg)	C (mg)	D (int. units)	E (int. units)	K (mcg)	Additional Information
Formulations for Neonates, Infants, and Children <11 Years of Age										
Infuvite® Pediatric (per 5 mL)	2300	1.2	1.4	1	1	80	400	7	200	Supplied as one 4 mL vial and one 1 mL vial Biotin 20 mcg, folic acid 140 mcg, niacinamide 17 mg, dexpanthenol 5 mg
M.V.I.® Pediatric	2300	1.2	1.4	1	1	80	400	7	200	Biotin 20 mcg, folic acid 140 mcg, niacinamide 17 mg, dexpanthenol 5 mg
Formulations for Children ≥11 Years to Adults										
Infuvite® Adult (per 10 mL)	3300	6	3.6	6	5	200	200	10	150	Supplied as two 5 mL vials Biotin 60 mcg, folic acid 600 mcg, niacinamide 40 mg, dexpanthenol 15 mg
M.V.I.®-12 (per 10 mL)	3300	3	3.6	4	12.5	100	200	10	–	Supplied as two 5 mL vials or a single 2-chambered 10 mL vial Biotin 60 mcg, folic acid 400 mcg, niacinamide 40 mg, dexpanthenol 15 mg

Legend: int. = international.

MULTIVITAMIN PRODUCTS (ORAL / ENTERAL)
Neonatal and Infant Formulations

Product	A (int. units)	B_1 (mg)	B_2 (mg)	B_6 (mg)	B_{12} (mcg)	C (mg)	D (int. units)	E (int. units)	Additional Information
					Drops				
ADEKs (per mL) [OTC]	1500	0.5	0.6	0.6	4	45	400	40	Beta carotene 1 mg, biotin 15 mcg, niacin 6 mg, vitamin K 0.1 mg, Zn 5 mg; alcohol free, dye free (60 mL)
Poly-Vi-Sol® (per mL) [OTC]	1500	0.5	0.6	0.4	2	35	400	5	Niacin 8 mg (50 mL)
Poly-Vi-Sol® With Iron (per mL) [OTC]	1500	0.5	0.6	0.4		35	400	5	Fe 10 mg, niacin 8 mg (50 mL)
Tri-Vi-Sol® (per mL) [OTC]	1500					35	400		Fruit flavor (50 mL)
Tri-Vi-Sol® With Iron (per mL) [OTC]	1500					35	400		Fe 10 mg; fruit flavor (50 mL)
Vi-Daylin® (per mL) [OTC]	1500	0.5	0.6	0.4	1.5	35	400	5	Niacin 8 mg; alcohol <0.5%, sugar free, fruit flavor (50 mL)
Vi-Daylin® + Iron (per mL) [OTC]	1500	0.5	0.6	0.4		35	400	5	Fe 10 mg, niacin 8 mg; alcohol <0.5%, sugar free, fruit flavor (50 mL)
Vi-Daylin® ADC (per mL) [OTC]	1500					35	400		Alcohol <0.5%, sugar free, fruit flavor (50 mL)
Vi-Daylin® ADC + Iron (per mL) [OTC]	1500					35	400		Fe 10 mg; benzoic acid, sugar free, fruit flavor (50 mL)

Legend: Ca = elemental calcium, Cr = chromium, Cu = copper, Fe = elemental iron, int. = international, Mg = magnesium, Mn = manganese, Mo = molybdenum, Zn = zinc.

MULTIVITAMIN PRODUCTS *(Continued)*

MULTIVITAMIN PRODUCTS (ORAL / ENTERAL)
Fluoride-Containing Neonatal and Infant Multivitamin Formulations

Product	A (int. units)	B_1 (mg)	B_2 (mg)	B_6 (mg)	B_{12} (mcg)	C (mg)	D (int. units)	E (int. units)	Additional Information
Drops									
Poly-Vi-Flor® 0.25 mg (per mL)	1500	0.5	0.6	0.4	2	35	400	5	**Fluoride 0.25 mg**, niacin 8 mg; fruit flavor (50 mL)
Poly-Vi-Flor® 0.5 mg (per mL)	1500	0.5	0.6	0.4	2	35	400	5	**Fluoride 0.5 mg**, niacin 8 mg; fruit flavor (50 mL)
Poly-Vi-Flor® With Iron 0.25 mg (per mL)	1500	0.5	0.6	0.4		35	400	5	**Fluoride 0.25 mg**, Fe 10 mg, niacin 8 mg; fruit flavor (50 mL)
Soluvite-F® (per 0.6 mL)	1500					35	400		**Fluoride 0.25 mg**; alcohol free, dye free, orange flavor (57 mL)
Tri-Vi-Flor® 0.25 mg (per mL)	1500					35	400		**Fluoride 0.25 mg**; fruit flavor (50 mL)
Tri-Vi-Flor® With Iron 0.25 mg (per mL)	1500					35	400		**Fluoride 0.25 mg**, Fe 10 mg; fruit flavor (50 mL)
Vi-Daylin®/F (per mL)	1500	0.5	0.6	0.4		35	400	5	**Fluoride 0.25 mg**, niacin 8 mg; alcohol <0.1%, benzoic acid, sugar free, fruit flavor (50 mL)
Vi-Daylin®/F + Iron (per mL)	1500	0.5	0.6	0.4		35	400	5	**Fluoride 0.25 mg**, Fe 10 mg, niacin 8 mg; alcohol <0.1%, benzoic acid, sugar free, fruit flavor (50 mL)
Vi-Daylin®/F ADC (per mL)	1500					35	400		**Fluoride 0.25 mg**; sugar free, fruit flavor (50 mL)
Vi-Daylin®/F ADC + Iron (per mL)	1500					35	400		**Fluoride 0.25 mg**, Fe 10 mg; sugar free, fruit flavor (50 mL)

Legend: Ca = elemental calcium, Cr = chromium, Cu = copper, elemental Fe = iron, int. = international, Mg = magnesium, Mn = manganese, Mo = molybdenum, Zn = zinc.

Pediatric Formulations

Product	A (int. units)	B_1 (mg)	B_2 (mg)	B_6 (mg)	B_{12} (mcg)	C (mg)	D (int. units)	E (int. units)	Additional Information
Drops									
ADEKs [OTC] (per mL)	3170 (50% as beta carotene)	0.5	0.6	0.6	4	45	400	40	Biotin 15 mcg, niacin 6 mg, pantothenic acid 3 mg, vitamin K 0.1 mg, Zn 5 mg; alcohol free, dye free (60 mL)
Poly-Vi-Flor® 0.25 mg (per mL)	1500	0.5	0.6	0.4	2	35	400	5	**Fluoride 0.25 mg**, niacin 8 mg; fruit flavor (50 mL)
Poly-Vi-Flor® 0.5 mg (per mL)	1500	0.5	0.6	0.4	2	35	400	5	**Fluoride 0.5 mg**, niacin 8 mg; fruit flavor (50 mL)
Poly-Vi-Flor® With Iron 0.25 mg (per mL)	1500	0.5	0.6	0.4		35	400	5	**Fluoride 0.25 mg**, iron 10 mg, niacin 8 mg; fruit flavor (50 mL)
Poly-Vi-Sol® [OTC] (per mL)	1500	0.5	0.6	0.4	2	35	400	5	Niacin 8 mg (50 mL)
Poly-Vi-Sol® With Iron [OTC] (per mL)	1500	0.5	0.6	0.4		35	400	5	Iron 10 mg, niacin 8 mg (50 mL)
Soluvite-F® (per 0.6 mL)	1500					35	400		**Fluoride 0.25 mg**; alcohol free, dye free, orange flavor (57 mL)
Tri-Vi-Flor® 0.25 mg (per mL)	1500					35	400		**Fluoride 0.25 mg**; fruit flavor (50 mL)
Tri-Vi-Flor® With Iron 0.25 mg (per mL)	1500					35	400		**Fluoride 0.25 mg**, iron 10 mg; fruit flavor (50 mL)
Tri-Vi-Sol® [OTC] (per mL)	1500					35	400		Fruit flavor (50 mL)
Tri-Vi-Sol® With Iron [OTC] (per mL)	1500					35	400		Iron 10 mg; fruit flavor (50 mL)
Vi-Daylin® [OTC] (per mL) [DSC]	1500	0.5	0.6	0.4	1.5	35	400	5	Niacin 8 mg; alcohol <0.5%, sugar free, fruit flavor (50 mL)
Vi-Daylin® + Iron [OTC] (per mL) [DSC]	1500	0.5	0.6	0.4		35	400	5	Iron 10 mg, niacin 8 mg; alcohol <0.5%, sugar free, fruit flavor (50 mL)
Vi-Daylin® ADC [OTC] (per mL) [DSC]	1500					35	400		Alcohol <0.5%, sugar free, fruit flavor (50 mL)
Vi-Daylin® ADC + Iron [OTC] (per mL) [DSC]	1500					35	400		Iron 10 mg; benzoic acid, sugar free, fruit flavor (50 mL)
Vi-Daylin®/F (per mL) [DSC]	1500	0.5	0.6	0.4		35	400	5	**Fluoride 0.25 mg**, niacin 8 mg; alcohol <0.1%, benzoic acid, sugar free, fruit flavor (50 mL)
Vi-Daylin®/F + Iron (per mL) [DSC]	1500	0.5	0.6	0.4		35	400	5	**Fluoride 0.25 mg**, iron 10 mg, niacin 8 mg; alcohol <0.1%, benzoic acid, sugar free, fruit flavor (50 mL)
Vi-Daylin®/F ADC (per mL) [DSC]	1500					35	400		**Fluoride 0.25 mg**; sugar free, fruit flavor (50 mL)

MULTIVITAMIN PRODUCTS *(Continued)*

Pediatric Formulations *(continued)*

Product	A (int. units)	B_1 (mg)	B_2 (mg)	B_6 (mg)	B_{12} (mcg)	C (mg)	D (int. units)	E (int. units)	Additional Information
Vi-Daylin®/F ADC + Iron (per mL) [DSC]	1500					35	400		**Fluoride 0.25 mg**, iron 10 mg; sugar free, fruit flavor (50 mL)
Gum									
Vitaball®	5000	1.5	1.7	2	6	60	400	30	Biotin 45 mcg, folic acid 400 mcg, niacinamide 20 mg, pantothenic acid 10 mg; bubble gum, cherry, grape, and watermelon (contains tartrazine) flavors
Vitaball® Wild 'N Fruity [OTC]	5000	1.5	1.7	2	6	240	400	30	Biotin 45 mcg, folic acid 400 mcg, niacinamide 20 mg, pantothenic acid 10 mg; berry, lemon (contains tartrazine), orange, and strawberry flavors
Tablet, Chewable									
ADEKs® [OTC]	9000 (60% as beta carotene)	1.2	1.3	1.5	12	60	400	150	Biotin 50 mcg, folic acid 0.2 mg, niacin 10 mg, pantothenic acid 10 mg, vit K 150 mcg, Zn 7.5 mg; dye free
Centrum Kids® Jimmy Neutron™ Complete	5000	1.5	1.7	2	6	60	400	30	Biotin 45 mcg, Ca 108 mg, Cr 20 mcg, Cu 2 mg, Fe 18 mg, folic acid 0.4 mg, iodine 150 mcg, Mg 40 mg, Mn 1 mg, Mo 20 mcg, niacin 20 mg, pantothenic acid 10 mg, phosphorus 50 mg, vitamin K 10 mg, Zn 15 mg; **contains phenylalanine**; cherry, fruit punch, and orange flavors
Centrum Kids® Jimmy Neutron™ Extra C	5000	1.5	1.7	1	5	250	400	15	Ca 108 mg, Cu 0.5 mg, folic aicd 0.3 mg, niacin 13.5 mg, phosphorus 50 mg, sodium 16 mg, Zn 4 mg; **contains phenylalanine**; cherry, fruit punch, and orange flavors
Centrum® Kids Rugrats™ Complete [OTC]	5000	1.5	1.7	2	6	60	400	30	Biotin 45 mcg, Ca 108 mg, Cr 20 mcg, Cu 2 mg, Fe 18 mg, folic acid 0.4 mg, iodine 150 mcg, Mg 40 mg, Mn 1 mg, Mo 20 mcg, niacin 20 mg, pantothenic acid 10 mg, phosphorus 50 mg, vitamin K 10 mg, Zn 15 mg; **contains phenylalanine**; cherry, fruit punch, and orange flavors

Pediatric Formulations *(continued)*

Product	A (int. units)	B_1 (mg)	B_2 (mg)	B_6 (mg)	B_{12} (mcg)	C (mg)	D (int. units)	E (int. units)	Additional Information
Centrum® Kids Rugrats™ Extra C [OTC]	5000	1.5	1.7	1	5	250	400	15	Ca 108 mg, Cu 0.5 mg, folic acid 0.3 mg, niacin 13.5 mg, phosphorus 50 mg, sodium 15 mg, Zn 4 mg; **contains phenylalanine**; cherry, fruit punch, and orange flavors
Centrum® Kids Rugrats™ Extra Calcium [OTC]	5000	1.5	1.7	1	5	60	400	15	Ca 200 mg, Cu 0.5 mg, folic acid 0.3 mg, niacin 13.5 mg, phosphorus 50 mg, Zn 4 mg; **contains phenylalanine**; cherry, fruit punch, and orange flavors
Flintstones® Complete [OTC]	5000	1.5	1.7	2	6	60	400	30	Biotin 40 mcg, Ca 100 mg, Cu 2 mg, Fe 18 mg, folic acid 0.4 mg, iodine 150 mcg, Mg 20 mg, niacin 20 mg, pantothenic acid 10 mg, phosphorus 100 mg, Zn 15 mg; **phenylalanine 4.56 mg**; cherry, grape, and orange flavors
Flintstones® Plus Calcium [OTC]	2500	1.05	1.2	1.05	4.5	60	400	15	Ca 200 mg, folic acid 0.3 mg, niacin 13.5 mg; **phenylalanine <4 mg**; cherry, grape, and orange flavors
Flintstones® Plus Extra C [OTC]	2500	1.05	1.2	1.05	4.5	250	400	15	Folic acid 0.3 mg, niacin 13.5 mg; grape, orange, peach-apricot, raspberry, and strawberry flavors
Flintstones® Plus Iron [OTC]	2500	1.05	1.2	1.05	4.5	60	400	15	Fe 15 mg, folic acid 0.3 mg, niacin 13.5 mg; grape, orange, peach-apricot, raspberry, and strawberry flavors
My First Flintstones® [OTC]	2500	1.05	1.2	1.05	4.5	60	400	15	Folic acid 0.3 mg, niacin 13.5 mg; cherry, grape, and orange flavors
One-A-Day® Kids Bugs Bunny and Friends Complete [OTC]	3000	1.5	1.7	2	6	60	400	30	Biotin 40 mcg, Ca 100 mg, Cu 2 mg, Fe 18 mg, folic acid 0.4 mg, iodine 150 mcg, Mg 20 mg, niacin 15 mg, pantothenic acid 10 mg, phosphorus 100 mg, Zn 12 mg; **contains phenylalanine**; sugar free, fruity flavors
One-A-Day® Kids Bugs Bunny and Friends Plus Extra C [OTC]	2500	1.05	1.2	1.05	4.5	250	400	15	Folic acid 0.3 mg, niacin 13.5 mg, **contains phenylalanine**; sugar free, fruity flavors
One-A-Day® Kids Extreme Sports [OTC]	3000	1.5	1.7	2	6	60	400	30	Biotin 40 mcg, Ca 100 mg, Cu 2 mg, Fe 18 mg, folic acid 0.4 mg, iodine 150 mcg, Mg 20 mg, niacin 15 mg, pantothenic acid 10 mg, phosphorus 100 mg, Zn 12 mg; **contains phenylalanine**

MULTIVITAMIN PRODUCTS *(Continued)*

Pediatric Formulations *(continued)*

Product	A (int. units)	B_1 (mg)	B_2 (mg)	B_6 (mg)	B_{12} (mcg)	C (mg)	D (int. units)	E (int. units)	Additional Information
One-A-Day® Kids Scooby-Doo! Complete [OTC]	3000	1.5	1.7	2	6	60	400	30	Biotin 40 mcg, Ca 100 mg, Cu 2 mg, Fe 18 mg, folic acid 0.4 mg, iodine 150 mcg, Mg 20 mg, niacin 15 mg, pantothenic acid 10 mg, phosphorus 100 mg, Zn 12 mg; **contains phenylalanine**; fruity flavors
One-A-Day® Kids Scooby-Doo! Fizzy Vites [OTC]	1500	0.75	0.85	1	3	170	200	15	Biotin 20 mcg, Ca 50 mg, Cu 1 mg, Fe 9 mg, folic acid 0.2 mg, iodine 75 mcg, Mg 10 mg, niacin 7.5 mg, pantothenic acid 5 mg, phosphorus 50 mg, sodium 20 mg, Zn 6 mg; **contains phenylalanine**; crazy grape, orange pucker, and wild cherry flavors
One-A-Day® Kids Scooby-Doo! Plus Calcium [OTC]	2500	1.05	1.2	1.05	4.5	60	400	15	Ca 200 mg, folic acid 0.3 mg, niacin 13.5 mg; **contains phenylalanine**; fruity flavors
Poly-Vi-Flor® 0.25 mg	2500	1.05	1.2	1.05	4.5	60	400	15	Fluoride 0.25 mg, folic acid 0.3 mg, niacin 13.5 mg; fruity flavor
Poly-Vi-Flor® 0.5 mg	2500	1.05	1.2	1.05	4.5	60	400	15	Fluoride 0.5 mg, folic acid 0.3 mg, niacin 13.5 mg; fruity flavor
Poly-Vi-Flor® 1 mg	2500	1.05	1.2	1.05	4.5	60	400	15	Fluoride 1 mg, folic acid 0.3 mg, niacin 13.5 mg; fruity flavor
Poly-Vi-Flor® 0.25 mg With Iron	2500	1.05	1.2	1.05	4.5	60	400	15	Fluoride 0.25 mg, Cu 1 mg, folic acid 0.3 mg, iron 12 mg, niacin 13.5 mg, Zn 10 mg; fruity flavor
Poly-Vi-Flor® 0.5 mg With Iron	2500	1.05	1.2	1.05	4.5	60	400	15	Fluoride 0.5 mg, Cu 1 mg, folic acid 0.3 mg, iron 12 mg, niacin 13.5 mg, Zn 10 mg; fruity flavor

Ca = calcium, Cr = chromium, Cu = copper, Fe = iron, Mg = magnesium, Mn = manganese, Mo = molybdenum, Zn = zinc.

Prenatal Formulations

Product	A (int. units)	B_1 (mg)	B_2 (mg)	B_6 (mg)	B_{12} (mcg)	C (mg)	D (int. units)	E (int. units)	Additional Information
Caplet									
PreCare® Prenatal		3	3.4	50	12	50	6 mcg	3.5 mg	Ca 250 mg, Cu 2 mg, Fe 40 mg, folic acid 1 mg, Mg 50 mg, Zn 15 mg; dye free
StrongStart™	1000	3	3	20	12	100	400	30	Ca 200 mg, Fe 29 mg, folic acid 1 mg, niacinamide 15 mg, pantothenic acid 7 mg, Zn 20 mg; docusate sodium 25 mg
Capsule									
Chromagen OB®		1.6	1.8	20	12	60	400	30	Ca 200 mg, Cu 2 mg, Fe 28 mg, folic acid 1 mg, Mn 2 mg, niacinamide 5 mg, Zn 25 mg; docusate calcium 25 mg
Prenatal H		10	6	5	15	200			Cu 0.3 mg, Fe 106 mg, folic acid 1 mg, Mg 6.9 mg, Mn 1.3 mg, niacinamide 30 mg, pantothenic acid 10 mg, Zn 18.2 mg
Prenatal U		10	6	5	15	200			Cu 0.8 mg, Fe 106.5 mg, folic acid 1 mg, Mn 1.3 mg, niacinamide 30 mg, pantothenic acid 10 mg
Powder									
Obegyn® (per 4 level tsp/8.25 g)	2500 (as palmatate) 2500 (as beta-carotene)	1.7	2	10	12	120	400	60	Biotin 300 mcg, Ca 455 mg, Cu 2 mg, Fe 18 mg, folic acid 1 mg, iodine 150 mcg, Mg 150 mg, niacin 20 mg, pantothenic acid 10 mg, Zn 25 mg; **phenylalanine 84 mg/8.25 g**; orange flavor (495 g/60 doses)
Tablet									
A-Free Prenatal		2	2	1	2	33.3	133.3	10	Calcium 333.3 mg, biotin 10 mcg, Cu 0.1 mg, Fe 9 mg, folic acid 266.6 mcg, Mg 33.3 mg, Mn 0.1 mg, niacinamide 10 mg, pantothenic acid 5 mg, Zn 7.5 mg
Advanced NatalCare®	2700	3	3.4	20	12	120	400	30	Ca 200 mg, Cu 2 mg, Fe 90 mg, folic acid 1 mg, Mg 30 mg, niacinamide 20 mg, Zn 25 mg; docusate sodium 50 mg
Aminate Fe-90	4000	3	3.4	20	12	120	400	30	Ca 250 mg, Cu 2 mg, Fe 90 mg, folic acid 1 mg, iodine 150 mcg, niacinamide 20 mg, Zn 25 mg; docusate sodium 50 mg

MULTIVITAMIN PRODUCTS *(Continued)*

Prenatal Formulations *(continued)*

Product	A (int. units)	B_1 (mg)	B_2 (mg)	B_6 (mg)	B_{12} (mcg)	C (mg)	D (int. units)	E (int. units)	Additional Information
Cal-Nate™	2700	3	3.4	20		120	400	30	Ca 125 mg, Cu 2 mg, Fe 27 mg, folic acid 1 mg, iodine 150 mcg, niacinamide 20 mg, Zn 25 mg; docusate calcium 50 mg
Citracal® Prenatal Rx	2700	3	3.4	20		120	400	30	Ca 125 mg, Cu 2 mg, Fe 27 mg, folic acid 1 mg, iodine 150 mcg, niacinamide 20 mg, Zn 25 mg; docusate sodium 50 mg
Duet®	3000	1.8	4	25	12	120	400	30	Ca 200 mg, Cu 2 mg, Fe 29 mg, folic acid 1 mg, Mg 25 mg, niacinamide 20 mg, Zn 25 mg
KPN Prenatal	2666.6	2	2	1	2	33.3	133.3	10	Ca 333.3 mg, biotin 10 mcg, Cu 0.1 mg, Fe 9 mg, folic acid 266.6 mcg, Mg 33.3 mg, Mn 0.1 mg, niacinamide 10 mg, pantothenic acid 5 mg, Zn 7.5 mg
NatalCare® GlossTabs™	2700	3	3.4	20	12	120	400	10	Biotin 30 mcg, Ca 200 mg, Cu 2 mg, Fe 90 mg, folic acid 1 mg, Mg 30 mg, niacinamide 20 mg, pantothenic acid 6 mg, Zn 15 mg; docusate sodium 50 mg
NatalCare® PIC	4000	2.43	3	1.64	3	50	400		Ca 125 mg, folic acid 1 mg, niacinamide 10 mg, polysaccharide-iron complex 60 mg, Zn 18 mg
NatalCare® PIC Forte	5000	3	3.4	4	12	80	400	30	Ca 250 mg, Cu 2 mg, folic acid 1 mg, iodine 200 mcg, Mg 10 mg, niacinamide 20 mg, polysaccharide-iron complex 60 mg, Zn 25 mg
NatalCare® Plus	4000	1.84	3	10	12	120	400	22	Ca 200 mg, Cu 2 mg, Fe 27 mg, folic acid 1 mg, niacinamide 20 mg, Zn 25 mg
NatalCare® Rx	2000	0.75	0.8	2	1.25	40	200	7.5	Biotin 15 mcg, Ca 100 mg, Cu 1.5 mg, folate 0.5 mg, Fe 27 mg, Mg 50 mg, niacin 8.5 mg, pantothenic acid 3.75 mg, Zn 12.5 mg
NatalCare® Three	3000	1.8	4	25	12	120	400	22	Ca 200 mg, Cu 2 mg, Fe 28 mg, folic acid 1 mg, Mg 25 mg, niacinamide 20 mg, Zn 25 mg
NataFort®	1000	2	3	10	12	120	400	11	Fe 60 mg, folic acid 1 mg, niacinamide 20 mg
NataTab™ CFe	4000	3	3	3	8	120	400	30	Ca 200 mg, Fe 50 mg, folic acid 1 mg, iodine 150 mcg, niacin 20 mg, Zn 15 mg
NataTab™ FA	4000	3	3	6	8	120	400	30	Ca 200 mg, Fe 29 mg, folic acid 1 mg, iodine 150 mcg, niacin 20 mg, Zn 15 mg

Prenatal Formulations *(continued)*

Product	A (int. units)	B_1 (mg)	B_2 (mg)	B_6 (mg)	B_{12} (mcg)	C (mg)	D (int. units)	E (int. units)	Additional Information
NataTab™ Rx	4000	3	3	3	8	120	400	30	Biotin 30 mcg, Ca 200 mg, Cu 3 mg, Fe 29 mg, folic acid 1 mg, iodine 150 mcg, Mg 100 mg, niacin 20 mg, pantothenic acid 7 mg, Zn 15 mg
Nestabs® CBF	4000	3	3	3	8	120	400	30	Ca 200 mg, Fe 50 mg, folic acid 1 mg, iodine 150 mcg, niacin 20 mg, Zn 15 mg
Nestabs® FA	4000	3	3	3	8	120	400	30	Ca 200 mg, Fe 29 mg, folic acid 1 mg, iodine 150 mcg, niacin 20 mg, Zn 15 mg
Nestabs® RX	4000	3	3	3	8	120	400	30	Biotin 30 mcg, Ca 200 mg, Cu 3 mg, Fe 29 mg, folic acid 1 mg, iodine 150 mcg, Mg 100 mg, niacin 20 mg, pantothenic acid 7 mg, Zn 15 mg
Niferex®-PN	4000	2.43	3	1.64	3	50	400		Ca 125 mg, folic acid 1 mg, niacinamide 10 mg, polysaccharide-iron complex 60 mg, Zn 18 mg
Niferex®-PN Forte	5000	3	3.4	4	12	80	400	30	Ca 250 mg, Cu 2 mg, folic acid 1 mg, iodine 200 mcg, Mg 10 mg, niacinamide 20 mg, polysaccharide-iron complex 60 mg, Zn 25 mg
OB-20	2000	43	0.5	2.5	2	30	100	15	Biotin 37.5 mcg, Ca 125 mg, Cr 6.25 mcg, Fe 12.5 mg, folic acid 2.5 mg, Mg 37.5 mg, Mn 1.25 mg, niacinamide 5 mg, pantothenic acid 2.5 mg, Se 6.25 mcg, Zn 6.2 mg
PreCare® Conceive™		3	3.4	50	12	60		30	Ca 200 mg, Cu 2 mg, Fe 30 mg, folic acid 1 mg, Mg 100 mg, niacinamide 20 mg, Zn 15 mg
Prenatal 1-A-Day	4000	2	3	3	10	100	400	15	Biotin 100 mcg, Ca 200 mg, Cu 2 mg, Fe 27 mg, folic acid 800 mcg, Mg 60 mg, Mn 2 mg, niacinamide 20 mg, pantothenic acid 10 mg, Zn 15 mg
Prenatal AD	2700	3	3.4	12	120	120	400	30	Ca 200 mg, Cu 2 mg, Fe 90 mg, folic acid 1 mg, Mg 30 mg, niacinamide 20 mg, Zn 25 mg; docusate sodium 50 mg
Prenatal MR 90 Fe™	4000	3	3.4	20	12	120	400	30	Ca 250 mg, Cu 2 mg, Fe 90 mg, folic acid 1 mg, iodine 150 mcg, niacinamide 20 mg, Zn 25 mg; docusate sodium 50 mg

MULTIVITAMIN PRODUCTS *(Continued)*

Prenatal Formulations *(continued)*

Product	A (int. units)	B_1 (mg)	B_2 (mg)	B_6 (mg)	B_{12} (mcg)	C (mg)	D (int. units)	E (int. units)	Additional Information
Prenatal MRT with Selenium	5000	3	3.4	10	12	120	400	30	Biotin 30 mcg, Ca 200 mg, Cr 25 mcg, Cu 2 mg, Fe 27 mg, folic acid 1 mg, iodine 150 mcg, Mg 25 mg, Mn 5 mg, Mo 25 mcg, niacinamide 20 mg, pantothenic acid 10 mg, Se 20 mcg, Zn 25 mg
Prenatal Plus	4000	1.8	3	10	12	120	400	22	Ca 200 mg, Cu 2 mg, Fe 27 mg, folic acid 1 mg, niacinamide 20 mg, Zn 25 mg
Prenatal Rx 1	4000	1.5	1.6	4	2.5	80	400	15	Biotin 30 mcg, Ca 200 mg, Cu 3 mg, Fe 60 mg, folic acid 1 mg, Mg 100 mg, niacinamide 17 mg, pantothenic acid 7 mg, Zn 25 mg
Prenatal Z	3000	1.5	1.6	2.2	2.2	70	400	10	Ca 200 mg, Fe 65 mg, folic acid 1 mg, iodine 175 mcg, Mg 100 mg, niacin 17 mg, Zn 15 mg
Prenate Elite™		3	3.4	20	12	120	400	10	Biotin 300 mcg, Ca 200 mg, Cu 2 mg, Fe 90 mg, folate 1 mg, Mg 30 mg, niacinamide 20 mg, pantothenic acid 6 mg, Zn 15 mg; docusate sodium 50 mg
Prenate GT™	2700	3	3.4	20	12	120	400	10	Biotin 30 mcg, Ca 200 mg, Cu 2 mg, Fe 90 mg, folic acid 1 mg, Mg 30 mg, niacinamide 20 mg, pantothenic acid 6 mg, Zn 15 mg; docusate sodium 50 mg
Stuartnatal® Plus 3™ [DSC]	3000	1.8	4	25	12	120	400	22	Ca 200 mg, Cu 2 mg, Fe 28 mg, folic acid 1 mg, Mg 25 mg, niacinamide 20 mg, Zn 25 mg
Stuart Prenatal®	4000	1.8	1.7	2.6	8	120	400	30	Ca 200 mg, Fe 28 mg, folic acid 0.8 mg, niacin 20 mg, Zn 25 mg
Trinate	3000	1.8	4	25	12	120	400	22	Ca 200 mg, Cu 2 mg, Fe 28 mg, folic acid 1 mg, Mg 25 mg, niacin 20 mg, Zn 25 mg
Ultra NatalCare®	2700	3	3.4	20	12	120	400	30	Ca 200 mg, Cu 2 mg, Fe 90 mg, folic acid 1 mg, iodine 150 mcg, niacinamide 20 mg, Zn 25 mg; docusate sodium 50 mg

Prenatal Formulations *(continued)*

Product	A (int. units)	B_1 (mg)	B_2 (mg)	B_6 (mg)	B_{12} (mcg)	C (mg)	D (int. units)	E (int. units)	Additional Information
Tablet, Chewable									
Duet®	3000	1.8	4	25	12	120	400	30	Ca 100 mg, Cu 2 mg, Fe 29 mg, folic acid 1 mg, Mg 25 mg, niacinamide 20 mg, Zn 25 mg; **phenylalanine 15 mg/tablet**
NataChew™	1000	2	3	10	12	120	400	11	Fe 29 mg, folic acid 1 mg, niacinamide 20 mg; peanut extract, wild berry flavor
NutriNate®	1000	2	3	10	12	120	400	11	Fe 29 mg, folic acid 1 mg, niacinamide 20 mg; wild berry flavor
PreCare®				2		50	6 mcg	3.5 mg	Ca 250 mg, Cu 2 mg, Fe 40 mg, folic acid 1 mg, Mg 50 mg, Zn 15 mg
StrongStart™	1000	1	3	20	15	100	400	30	Ca 200 mg, Fe 29 mg, folic acid 1 mg, niacinamide 15 mg, pantothenic acid 7 mg, Zn 20 mg; **phenylalanine 6 mg/tablet**
Combination Package									
Duet™ DHA (tablet)	3000	1.8	4	25	12	120	400	30	Ca 200 mg, Cu 2 mg, Fe 29 mg, folic acid 1 mg, Mg 25 mg, niacinamide 20 mg, Zn 25 mg Packaged with capsules containing Omega-3 fatty acids ≥ DHA 200 mg

Cr = chromium, Cu = copper, Fe = iron, Mg = magnesium, Mn = manganese, Mo = molybdenum, Se = selenium, Zn = zinc.

MULTIVITAMIN PRODUCTS *(Continued)*

Adolescent and Adult Formulations

Product	A (int. units)	B_1 (mg)	B_2 (mg)	B_6 (mg)	B_{12} (mcg)	C (mg)	D (int. units)	E (int. units)	Additional Information
Liquid									
Centrum® (per 15 mL) [OTC]	2500	1.5	1.7	2	6	60	400	30	Biotin 300 mcg, Cr 25 mcg, Fe 9 mg, iodine 150 mcg, Mn 2 mg, Mo 25 mg, niacin 20 mg, pantothenic acid 10 mg, Zn 3 mg; alcohol 5.4%, sodium benzoate (240 mL)
Iberet® (per 5 mL) [OTC]		1.2	1.35	0.925	5.63	33.8			Fe 23.6 mg, niacin 6.8 mg, pantothenic acid 2.4 mg; alcohol (240 mL)
Iberet®-500 (per 5 mL) [OTC]		1.2	1.35	0.925	5.63	125			Fe 23.6 mg, niacin 6.8 mg, pantothenic acid 2.4 mg; alcohol (240 mL)
Vi-Daylin® (per 5 mL) [OTC]	2500	1.05	1.2	1.05	4.5	60	400	15	Niacin 13.5 mg; alcohol <0.5%, benzoic acid; lemon/orange flavor (240 mL, 480 mL)
Vi-Daylin® + Iron (per 5 mL) [OTC]	2500	1.05	1.2	1.05	4.5	60	400	15	Fe 10 mg, niacin 13.5 mg; alcohol <0.5%, benzoic acid; lemon/orange flavor (240 mL, 480 mL)
Caplet									
Theragran-M® Advanced Formula [OTC]	5000	3	3.4	6	12	90	400	60	Biotin 30 mcg, boron 150 mcg, Ca 40 mg, chloride 7.5 mg, Cr 50 mcg, Cu 2 mg, Fe 9 mg, folic acid 0.4 mg, iodine 150 mcg, Mg 100 mg, Mn 2 mg, Mo 75 mcg, niacin 20 mg, nickel 5 mcg, pantothenic acid 10 mg, phosphorus 31 mg, potassium 7.5 mg, Se 70 mcg, silicon 2 mg, tin 10 mcg, vanadium 10 mcg, vitamin K 28 mcg, Zn 15 mg
Capsule									
Vitacon Forte	8000	10	5	2	10	150		50	Folic acid 1 mg, Mg 70 mg, Mn 4 mg, niacinamide 25 mg, Zn 80 mg
Vicon Plus® [OTC]	3400	9.3	4.6	1.5		140		45	Mg 5 mg, Mn 1 mg, niacin 24 mg, pantothenic acid 11 mg, Zn 10 mg

Adolescent and Adult Formulations *(continued)*

Product	A (int. units)	B_1 (mg)	B_2 (mg)	B_6 (mg)	B_{12} (mcg)	C (mg)	D (int. units)	E (int. units)	Additional Information
Tablet									
Centrum® [OTC]	5000	1.5	1.7	2	6	60	400	30	Biotin 30 mcg, boron 150 mcg, Ca 162 mg, chloride 72 mg, Cr 120 mcg, Cu 2 mg, Fe 18 mg, folic acid 0.4 mg, iodine 150 mcg, lutein 250 mcg, Mg 100 mg, Mn 2 mg, Mo 75 mcg, niacin 20 mg, nickel 5 mcg, pantothenic acid 10 mg, phosphorus 109 mg, potassium 80 mg, Se 20 mcg, silicon 2 mg, tin 10 mcg, vanadium 10 mcg, vitamin K 25 mcg, Zn 15 mg
Centrum® Performance™ [OTC]	5000	4.5	5.1	6	18	120	400	60	Biotin 40 mcg, boron 60 mcg, chloride 72 mg, folic acid 0.4 mg, Ca 100 mg, Cr 120 mcg, Cu 2 mg, Fe 18 mg, ginkgo biloba leaf 60 mg, ginseng root 50 mg, iodine 150 mcg, Mg 40 mg, Mn 4 mg, Mo 75 mcg, niacin 40 mg, nickel 5 mcg, pantothenic acid 10 mg, phosphorus 48 mg, potassium 80 mg, Se 70 mcg, silicon 4 mg, tin 10 mcg, vanadium 10 mcg, vitamin K 25 mcg, Zn 15 mg
Iberet®-500 [OTC]		4.96	5.4	3.7	22.5	500			Fe 95 mg (controlled release), niacin 27.2 mg, pantothenic acid 8.28 mg, sodium 65 mg
Iberet-Folic-500® [OTC]		6	6	5	25	500			Fe 105 mg (controlled release), folic acid 0.8 mg, niacinamde 30 mg, pantothenic acid 10 mg
One-A-Day® Active Formula [OTC]	5000	4.5	5.1	6	18	120	400	60	American ginseng 55 mg, biotin 40 mcg, boron 150 mcg, Ca 110 mg, chloride 180 mg, Cr 100 mcg, Cu 2 mg, Fe 9 mg, folic acid 0.4 mg, iodine 150 mcg, Mg 40 mg, Mn 2 mg, Mo 25 mcg, niacin 40 mg, nickel 5 mcg, pantothenic acid 10 mg, phosphorus 48 mg, potassium 200 mg, Se 45 mcg, silicon 6 mg, tin 10 mcg, vanadium 10 mcg, vitamin K 25 mcg, Zn 15 mg
One-A-Day® Essential Formula [OTC]	5000	1.5	1.7	2	6	60	400	30	Folic acid 0.4 mg, niacin 20 mg, pantothenic acid 10 mg

MULTIVITAMIN PRODUCTS *(Continued)*

Adolescent and Adult Formulations *(continued)*

Product	A (int. units)	B_1 (mg)	B_2 (mg)	B_6 (mg)	B_{12} (mcg)	C (mg)	D (int. units)	E (int. units)	Additional Information
One-A-Day® Maximum Formula [OTC]	5000	1.5	1.7	2	6	60	400	30	Biotin 30 mcg, boron 150 mcg, Ca 162 mg, chloride 72 mg, Cr 65 mcg, Cu 2 mg, Fe 18 mg, folic acid 0.4 mg, iodine 150 mcg, Mg 100 mg, Mn 3.5 mg, Mo 160 mcg, niacin 20 mg, nickel 5 mcg, pantothenic acid 10 mg, phosphorus 109 mg, potassium 80 mg, Se 20 mcg, silicon 2 mg, tin 10 mcg, vanadium 10 mcg, vitamin K 25 mcg, Zn 15 mg
One-A-Day® Today [OTC]	3000	1.1	1.7	3	18	75	400	33	Biotin 30 mcg, Ca 240 mg, Cr 120 mcg, Cu 2 mg, folic acid 0.4 mg, Mg 120 mg, Mn 2 mg, niacin 14 mg, pantothenic acid 5 mg, potassium 100 mg, Se 70 mcg, soy extract 10 mg, vitamin K 20 mcg, Zn 15 mg
Tablet, Chewable									
Centrum® [OTC]	5000	1.5	1.7	2	6	60	400	30	Biotin 45 mcg, Ca 108 mg, Cr 20 mcg, Cu 2 mg, Fe 18 mg, folic acid 0.4 mg, iodine 150 mcg, Mg 40 mg, Mn 1 mg, Mo 20 mcg, niacin 20 mg, pantothenic acid 10 mg, Zn 15 mg

Legend: Ca = calcium, Cr = chromium, Cu = copper, Fe = iron, int. = international, Mg = magnesium, Mn = manganese, Mo = molybdenum, Se = selenium, Zn = zinc.

Vitamin B Complex Formulations
Adolescent and Adult

Product	B_1 (mg)	B_2 (mg)	B_6 (mg)	B_{12} (mcg)	C (mg)	E (int. units)	Additional Information
Caplet							
Allbee® with C [OTC]	15	10.2	5		300		Niacinamide 50 mg, pantothenic acid 10 mg
Allbee® C-800 [OTC]	15	17	25	12	800	45	Niacinamide 100 mg, pantothenic acid 25 mg
Allbee® C-800 + Iron [OTC]	15	17	25	12	800	45	Fe 27 mg, folic acid 0.4 mg, niacinamide 100 mg, pantothenic acid 25 mg
Nephronex®	1.5	1.7	10	0.01	50		Biotin 300 mcg, nicotinic acid 20 mg, pantothenic acid 10 mg
Capsule							
Trinsicon® [DSC]				15	75		Fe 110 mg, folic acid 0.5 mg, liver-stomach concentrate (containing intrinsic factor and other vitamin B complex factors) 240 mg
Elixir							
Senilezol (per 30 mL)	2.5	2.5	1	5			Ca 5 mg, Fe 8 mg, niacin 10 mg [contains alcohol 15%]
Liquid							
Apatate® [OTC] (per 5 mL)	15		0.5	25			Cherry flavor (120 mL)
Gevrabon® [OTC] (per 30 mL)	5	2.5	1	1			Choline 10 mg, Fe 15 mg, iodine 100 mcg, Mg 2 mg, Mn 2 mg, niacinamide 60 mg, pantothenic acid 10 mg, Zn 2 mg; alcohol, benzoic acid; sherry wine flavor (480 mL)
Nephronex® (per 5 mL)	1.5	1.7	10	60			Biotin 300 mcg, folic acid 900 mcg, nicotinic acid 20 mg, pantothenic acid 10 mg
Softgel							
Nephrocaps®	1.5	1.7	10	6	100		Biotin 150 mcg, folate 1 mg, niacin 20 mg, pantothenic acid 5 mg
Rhenaphro	1.5	1.7	10	6	100		Biotin 150 mcg, calcium pantothenate 5 mg, folic acid 1 mg, niacinamide 20 mg
Syrup							
Vitafol (per 5 mL)			2	8.34			Fe 100 mg, folic acid 0.25 mg, niacinamide 13.3 mg [contains sodium benzoate; raspberry mint flavor]
Tablet							
DexFol™	1.5	1.5					Biotin 300 mcg, cobalamin 1 mg, folacin 5 mg, niacinamide 20 mg, pantothenic acid 10 mg, pyridoxine 50 mg, vitamin C 60 mg [dye, sugar, and lactose free]
Diatx™	1.5	1.5	50		60		Biotin 300 mcg, cobalamin 1 mg, folacin 5 mg, niacinamide 20 mg, pantothenic acid 10 mg [dye, sugar, and lactose free]
Kobee [OTC]	10	10	10	10			Biotin 10 mcg, choline citrate 10 mg, folic acid 400 mcg, inositol 10 mg, niacinamide 50 mg, PABA 10 mg, pantothenic acid 10 mg

MULTIVITAMIN PRODUCTS *(Continued)*

Vitamin B Complex Formulations
Adolescent and Adult *(continued)*

Product	B_1 (mg)	B_2 (mg)	B_6 (mg)	B_{12} (mcg)	C (mg)	E (int. units)	Additional Information
NephPlex® Rx	1.5	1.7	10	6	60		Biotin 300 mcg, folic acid 1 mg, niacinamide 20 mg, pantothenic acid 10 mg, zinc 12.5 mg
Nephro-Vite®	1.5	1.7	10	6	60		Biotin 300 mcg, folic acid 0.8 mg, niacinamide 20 mg, pantothenic acid 10 mg
Nephro-Vite® Rx	1.5	1.7	10	6	60		Biotin 300 mcg, folic acid 1 mg, niacinamide 20 mg, pantothenic acid 10 mg
Nephron FA®	1.5	1.7	10	6	40		Biotin 300 mcg, docusate sodium 75 mg, ferrous fumarate 200 mg, folic acid 1 mg, pantothenic acid 10 mg
Quin B Strong [OTC]	25	25	25	25			Biotin 25 mcg, folic acid 400 mcg, niacinamide 100 mg, pantothenic acid 25 mg (in a base containing choline citrate, inositol, and PABA)
Rena-Vite [OTC]	1.5	1.7	10	6	60		Biotin 300 mcg, folic acid 800 mcg, niacin 20 mg, pantothenic acid 10 mg
Rena-Vite RX	1.5	1.7	10	6	60		Biotin 300 mcg, folate 1 mg, niacin 20 mg, pantothenic acid 10 mg
Stresstabs® High Potency Advanced [OTC]	10	10	5	12	250	30	Biotin 45 mcg, Ca 70 mg, Cu 3 mg, folic acid 400 mcg, Mg 25 mg, niacinamide 100 mg, pantothenic acid 20 mg, phosphorus 30 mg, Zn 23.9 mg
Stresstabs® High Potency Energy [OTC]	10	10	5	12	300	30	Biotin 45 mcg, Ca 22 mg, Fe 4 mg, folic acid 400 mcg, niacinamide 100 mg, pantothenic acid 20 mg, phosphorus 15 mg
Stresstabs® High Potency Weight [OTC]	10	10	5	12	300	30	Biotin 45 mcg, Ca 44 mg, chromium 200 mcg, folic acid 400 mcg, niacinamide 100 mg, pantothenic acid 20 mg, phosphorus 32 mg
Strovite	15	15	4	5	500		Folic acid 0.5 mg, niacinamide 100 mg, pantothenic acid 18 mg
Super Quints 50 [OTC]	50	50	50	50			Biotin 50 mcg, folic acid 50 mcg, niacinamide 50 mg, pantothenic acid 50 mg (in a base containing choline citrate, glutaminic acid, glutamine, glycine, inositol, lysine, and PABA)
Surbex-T® [OTC]	15	10	5	10	500		Ca 20 mg, niacinamide 100 mg
Z-Bec® [OTC]	15	10.2	10	6	600	45	Niacinamide 100 mg, pantothenic acid 25 mg, Zn 22.5 mg
Tablet, Chewable							
Apatate® [OTC] [DSC]	15		0.5	25			Cherry flavor

Ca = calcium, Cu = copper, Fe = iron, Mg = magnesium, Mn = manganese, Se = selenium, Zn = zinc.

NARCOTIC ANALGESICS COMPARISON

Drug	Onset (min)	Duration (h)	Equianalgesic I.M. Dose (mg)	Equianalgesic P.O. Dose[1] (mg)	Parenteral Oral Ratio	Partial Antagonist
Alfentanil	I.V.: Immediate	<0.25-0.33	ND	—	—	No
Codeine	I.M.: 10-30 P.O.: 30-60	I.M.: 4-6	120	200	1/2-2/3	No
Fentanyl	I.M.: 7-15 I.V.: Immediate	I.M.: 1-2 I.V.: 0.5-1	0.1-0.2	—	—	No
Hydrocodone	P.O.: 10-20	P.O.: 3-6	—	ND	ND	No
Hydromorphone	P.O.: 15-30	P.O.: 4-5	1.5	7.5	1/5	No
Meperidine	P.O. I.M., SubQ: 10-15 I.V.: ≤5	P.O., I.M., SubQ: 2-4 I.V.: 2-3	75-100	300	1/3-1/2	No
Methadone	P.O.: 30-60 I.V.: 10-20	Acute: 4-6 Chronic: >8	Acute: 10 Chronic: 2-4	Acute: 20 Chronic: 2-4	1/2; ratio decreases to 1/1 upon chronic dosing	No
Morphine	P.O.: 15-60 I.V.: ≤5	P.O., I.V., I.M., SubQ: 3-5 Extended release tablets: 8-12	10	Acute: 60 Chronic: 30	1/6; ratio decreases to 1/1.5-2.5 upon chronic dosing	No
Oxycodone	P.O.: 15-30	P.O.: Immediate release: 4-5 controlled release: 12	—	30	—	No
Pentazocine	P.O., I.M., SubQ: 15-30 I.V.: ≤2-3	P.O.: 4-5 I.V., I.M., SubQ: 2-3	50	150	1/3	Yes
Propoxyphene	P.O.: 30-60	P.O.: 4-6	—	HCl salt: 130 Napsylate salt: 200	—	No

[1]Based on acute, short-term use. Chronic administration may alter pharmacokinetics and change parental oral ratio.

ND = no data.

Note: Values are based on adult studies. Duration may be shorter in children due to faster elimination (in general) compared to adults.

OTC COUGH AND COLD PREPARATIONS, PEDIATRIC

Commonly Used Pediatric OTC Cough and Cold Preparations

Brand Name	Type of Preparation
Actifed® Cold & Sinus	Antihistamine/Decongestant
Alavert™	Antihistamine
Alavert™ Allergy and Sinus	Antihistamine/Decongestant
Benadryl-D™ Allergy, Children's	Antihistamine
Benadryl® Allergy & Sinus Children's Elixir	Antihistamine/Decongestant
Benadryl® Allergy & Cold Fastmelt	Antihistamine/Decongestant
Claritin®	Antihistamine
Claritin-D®	Antihistamine/Decongestant
Chlor-Trimeton®	Antihistamine
Delsym®	Antitussive
Dimetapp® Cold & Congestion	Antitussive/Decongestant/Expectorant
Dimetapp® Cold & Allergy	Antihistamine/Decongestant
Dimetapp® Elixir Cold & Allergy, Children's	Antihistamine/Decongestant
Dimetapp® Infant Drops	Decongestant
Dimetapp® Infant Drops Decongestant & Cough	Antitussive/Decongestant
Mucinex® Children's	Expectorant
Mucinex® Children's Cough	Antitussive/Expectorant
Neo-Synephrine® 12-Hour Children's Nose Drops	Decongestant
Neo-Synephrine® Nose Drops/Nasal Spray	Decongestant
Organidin® NR	Expectorant
PediaCare® Decongestant Plus Cough Infant Drops	Antitussive/Decongestant
PediaCare® Infant Decongestant Drops	Decongestant
PediaCare® Long Acting Cough	Antitussive
Robitussin®	Expectorant
Robitussin® Cough & Cold Capsules	Antitussive/Decongestant/Expectorant
Robitussin® Cough & Cold Infant CF Drops	Antitussive/Decongestant/Expectorant
Robitussin® Cold, Cough & Flu Nighttime	Antihistamine/Antitussive/Decongestant
Robitussin® DM	Antitussive/Expectorant
Robitussin® DM Drops	Antitussive/Expectorant
Robitussin® Flu	Antihistamine/Antitussive/Decongestant
Robitussin® Pediatric Cough Syrup	Antitussive
Sudafed® Cold & Cough, Children's	Antitussive/Decongestant
Sudafed® Nasal Decongestant	Decongestant
Sudafed® Nasal Decongestant, Children's	Decongestant
Sudafed® Sinus & Allergy	Antihistamine/Decongestant
Triaminic® Cold & Cough Soft Chews	Antihistamine/Antitussive/Decongestant
Triaminic® Cold Plus Cough	Antihistamine/Antitussive/Decongestant
Triaminic® Cold, Cough, & Fever	Antihistamine/Antitussive/Decongestant
Tylenol® Cold, Children's	Antihistamine/Decongestant
Tylenol® Cold Concentrated Drops, Infants	Decongestant
Tylenol® Cold Plus Cough, Children's	Antihistamine/Antitussive/Decongestant
Tylenol® Flu, Children's	Antihistamine/Antitussive/Decongestant
Tylenol® Sinus, Children's	Decongestant
Vicks® 44e® Cough & Chest Congestion Relief, Pediatric	Antitussive/Expectorant

Content of Commonly Used Pediatric Cough and Cold Preparations

The following chart lists the contents of the more common OTC cough and cold preparations. Products are grouped by preparation type. For specific recommendations, see individual drug monographs.

Brand Name	Generic(s)	Strength	Other Information
Decongestants			
Neo-Synephrine® 12-Hour Children's Nose Drops	Oxymetazoline	0.05%	
Neo-Synephrine® Nose Drops/Nasal Spray	Phenylephrine	0.25% 0.25%-0.5%	≤6 y must be diluted prior to use (see Phenylephrine) >6 to 12 y use 0.25%
PediaCare® Decongestant Infant Drops	Pseudoephedrine	7.5 mg/0.8 mL	–
Sudafed® Nasal Decongestant	Pseudoephedrine	15 mg/5 mL 30 mg/5 mL 15 mg/tab 30 mg/tab 60 mg/tab 120 mg/tab or cap (timed release) 240 mg/tab (timed release)	–
Tylenol® Cold Concentrated Drops, Infants	Pseudoephedrine	15 mg/1.6 mL	Acetaminophen 160 mg/1.6 mL
Tylenol® Sinus, Children's	Pseudoephedrine	15 mg/5 mL 7.5 mg/tab	Acetaminophen 160 mg/5 mL 80 mg/tab
Antihistamines			
Alavert™	Loratadine	10 mg (rapidly disintegrating)	Tablet contains phenylalanine
Benadryl® Allergy Children's	Diphenhydramine	12.5 mg/chew tab 12.5 mg/5 mL	Tablet contains aspartame
Claritin®	Loratadine	5 mg/5 mL 10 mg/tab	–
Chlor-Trimeton®	Chlorpheniramine	4 mg/tab 8 mg/tab 12 mg/tab	–
Expectorants			
Mucinex®	Guaifenesin	600 mg/tab (extended release)	–
Organidin® NR, Robitussin®	Guaifenesin	100 mg/5 mL	–
Antitussives			
Delsym®	Dextromethorphan polistirex	[Equivalent to dextromethorphan HBr 30 mg/5 mL]	Contains sodium 6 mg/5 mL
PediaCare® Long Acting Cough	Dextromethorphan HBr	7.5 mg/0.8 mL drops	–
Robitussin® Pediatric Cough Syrup	Dextromethorphan HBr	7.5 mg/5 mL	–
Antihistamine / Decongestants			
Actifed® Cold & Sinus	Chlorpheniramine Pseudoephedrine	2 mg/tab 30 mg/tab	Acetaminophen 500 mg/tab
Alavert™ Allergy and Sinus	Loratidine Pseudoephedrine	5 mg/tab 120 mg/tab (extended release)	–
Benadryl® Allergy & Cold Fastmelt	Diphenhydramine citrate Pseudoephedrine	19 mg/tab 30 mg/tab	Citrate salt equivalent to 12.5 mg diphenhydramine HCl Phenylalanine 4.6 mg/tab
Benadryl-D™ Allergy & Sinus, Children's	Diphenhydramine Pseudoephedrine	12.5 mg/5 mL 30 mg/5 mL	–

OTC COUGH AND COLD PREPARATIONS, PEDIATRIC *(Continued)*

Brand Name	Generic(s)	Strength	Other Information
Claritin-D®	Loratidine Pseudoephedrine	10 mg/tab 240 mg/tab (extended release)	–
Dimetapp® Cold & Allergy	Chlorpheniramine Phenylephrine	2 mg/tab 5 mg/tab	Acetaminophen 325 mg/tab
Dimetapp® Elixir Cold & Allergy, Children's	Brompheniramine Pseudoephedrine	1 mg/5 mL 15 mg/5 mL	–
Sudafed® Sinus & Allergy	Chlorpheniramine Pseudoephedrine	4 mg/tab 60 mg/tab	–
Tylenol® Cold, Children's	Chlorpheniramine Phenylephrine	1 mg/5 mL 2.5 mg/5 mL	Acetaminophen 160 mg/5 mL
Antitussive / Decongestant			
PediaCare® Decongestant Plus Cough, Infant Drops	Dextromethorphan Pseudoephedrine	2.5 mg/0.8 mL 7.5 mg/0.8 mL	–
Sudafed® Cold & Cough, Children's	Dextromethorphan Pseudoephedrine	5 mg/5 mL 15 mg/5 mL	–
Tylenol® Cold Plus Cough Concentrated Drops, Infants	Dextromethorphan Pseudoephedrine	5 mg/1.6 mL 15 mg/1.6 mL	Acetaminophen 160 mg/1.6 mL
Antitussive / Expectorant			
Mucinex® Children's	Dextromethorphan Guaifenesin	5 mg/5 mL 100 mg/5 mL	–
Robitussin® DM	Dextromethorphan Guaifenesin	10 mg/5 mL 100 mg/5 mL	–
Robitussin® DM Drops	Dextromethorphan Guaifenesin	5 mg/2.5 mL 100 mg/2.5 mL	–
Vicks® 44e® Cough & Chest Congestion Relief, Pediatric	Dextromethorphan Guaifenesin	3.3 mg/5 mL 33 mg/5 mL	–
Antihistamine / Antitussive / Decongestant			
Robitussin® Cold, Cough, & Flu Nighttime	Chlorpheniramine Dextromethorphan Phenylephrine	1 mg/5 mL 5 mg/5 mL 2.5 mg/5 mL	Acetaminophen 160 mg
Triaminic® Cold & Cough Soft Chews	Chlorpheniramine Dextromethorphan Pseudoephedrine	1 mg/chew tab 5 mg/chew tab 15 mg/chew tab	–
Triaminic® Cold, Cough, & Fever	Chlorpheniramine Dextromethorphan Pseudoephedrine	1 mg/5 mL 7.5 mg/5 mL 15 mg/5 mL	Acetaminophen 160 mg
Tylenol® Cold Plus Cough, Children's	Chlorpheniramine Dextromethorphan Pseudoephedrine	1 mg/5 mL 5 mg/5 mL 15 mg/5 mL	Acetaminophen 160 mg/5 mL
Tylenol® Flu, Children's	Chlorpheniramine Dextromethorphan Phenylephrine	1 mg/5 mL 7.5 mg/5 mL 2.5 mg/5 mL	Acetaminophen 160 mg
Antitussive / Decongestant / Expectorant			
Dimetapp® Cold & Congestion	Dextromethorphan Pseudoephedrine Guaifenesin	10 mg/caplet 30 mg/caplet 200 mg/caplet	–
Robitussin® Cough & Cold Infant CF Drops	Dextromethorphan Pseudoephedrine Guaifenesin	5 mg/2.5 mL 15 mg/2.5 mL 100 mg/2.5 mL	–
Robitussin® Cough & Cold Capsules	Dextromethorphan Pseudoephedrine Guaifenesin	10 mg/capsule 30 mg/capsule 200 mg/capsule	–

CONVERSIONS

Apothecary-Metric Exact Equivalents

1 gram (g)	=	15.43 grains	0.1 mg	=	1/600 gr
1 milliliter (mL)	=	16.23 minims	0.12 mg	=	1/500 gr
1 minim	=	0.06 mL	0.15 mg	=	1/400 gr
1 grain (gr)	=	64.8 milligrams	0.2 mg	=	1/300 gr
1 fluid ounce (fl. oz)	=	29.57 mL	0.3 mg	=	1/200 gr
1 pint (pt)	=	473.2 mL	0.4 mg	=	1/150 gr
1 ounce (oz)	=	28.35 grams	0.5 mg	=	1/120 gr
1 pound (lb)	=	453.6 grams	0.6 mg	=	1/100 gr
1 kilogram (kg)	=	2.2 pounds	0.8 mg	=	1/80 gr
1 quart (qt)	=	946.4 mL	1 mg	=	1/65 gr

Apothecary-Metric Approximate Equivalents[1]

Liquids			Solids		
1 teaspoonful	=	5 mL	1/4 grain	=	15 mg
1 tablespoonful	=	15 mL	1/2 grain	=	30 mg
			1 grain	=	60 mg
			1 1/2 grain	=	100 mg
			5 grains	=	300 mg
			10 grains	=	600 mg

[1]Use exact equivalents for compounding and calculations requiring a high degree of accuracy.

Pounds-Kilograms Conversion

1 pound = 0.45359 kilograms
1 kilogram = 2.2 pounds

Temperature Conversion

Celsius to Fahrenheit = (°C x 9/5) + 32 = °F
Fahrenheit to Celsius = (°F - 32) x 5/9 = °C

CYTOCHROME P450 ENZYMES: SUBSTRATES, INHIBITORS, AND INDUCERS

INTRODUCTION

Most drugs are eliminated from the body, at least in part, by being chemically altered to less lipid-soluble products (ie, metabolized), and thus are more likely to be excreted via the kidneys or the bile. Phase I metabolism includes drug hydrolysis, oxidation, and reduction, and results in drugs that are more polar in their chemical structure, while Phase II metabolism involves the attachment of an additional molecule onto the drug (or partially metabolized drug) in order to create an inactive and/or more water soluble compound. Phase II processes include (primarily) glucuronidation, sulfation, glutathione conjugation, acetylation, and methylation.

Virtually any of the Phase I and II enzymes can be inhibited by some xenobiotic or drug. Some of the Phase I and II enzymes can be induced. Inhibition of the activity of metabolic enzymes will result in increased concentrations of the substrate (drug), whereas induction of the activity of metabolic enzymes will result in decreased concentrations of the substrate. For example, the well-documented enzyme-inducing effects of phenobarbital may include a combination of Phase I and II enzymes. Phase II glucuronidation may be increased via induced UDP-glucuronosyltransferase (UGT) activity, whereas Phase I oxidation may be increased via induced cytochrome P450 (CYP) activity. However, for most drugs, the primary route of metabolism (and the primary focus of drug-drug interaction) is Phase I oxidation, and specifically, metabolism.

CYP enzymes may be responsible for the metabolism (at least partial metabolism) of approximately 75% of all drugs, with the CYP3A subfamily responsible for nearly half of this activity. Found throughout plant, animal, and bacterial species, CYP enzymes represent a superfamily of xenobiotic metabolizing proteins. There have been several hundred CYP enzymes identified in nature, each of which has been assigned to a family (1, 2, 3, etc), subfamily (A, B, C, etc), and given a specific enzyme number (1, 2, 3, etc) according to the similarity in amino acid sequence that it shares with other enzymes. Of these many enzymes, only a few are found in humans, and even fewer appear to be involved in the metabolism of xenobiotics (eg, drugs). The key human enzyme subfamilies include CYP1A, CYP2A, CYP2B, CYP2C, CYP2D, CYP2E, and CYP3A.

CYP enzymes are found in the endoplasmic reticulum of cells in a variety of human tissues (eg, skin, kidneys, brain, lungs), but their predominant sites of concentration and activity are the liver and intestine. Though the abundance of CYP enzymes throughout the body is relatively equally distributed among the various subfamilies, the relative contribution to drug metabolism is (in decreasing order of magnitude) CYP3A4 (nearly 50%), CYP2D6 (nearly 25%), CYP2C8/9 (nearly 15%), then CYP1A2, CYP2C19, CYP2A6, and CYP2E1. Owing to their potential for numerous drug-drug interactions, those drugs that are identified in preclinical studies as substrates of CYP3A enzymes are often given a lower priority for continued research and development in favor of drugs that appear to be less affected by (or less likely to affect) this enzyme subfamily.

Each enzyme subfamily possesses unique selectivity toward potential substrates. For example, CYP1A2 preferentially binds medium-sized, planar, lipophilic molecules, while CYP2D6 preferentially binds molecules that possess a basic nitrogen atom. Some CYP subfamilies exhibit polymorphism (ie, multiple allelic variants that manifest differing catalytic properties). The best described polymorphisms involve CYP2C9, CYP2C19, and CYP2D6. Individuals possessing "wild type" gene alleles exhibit normal functioning CYP capacity. Others, however, possess allelic variants that leave the person with a subnormal level of catalytic potential (so called "poor metabolizers"). Poor metabolizers would be more likely to experience toxicity from drugs metabolized by the affected enzymes (or less effects if the enzyme is responsible for converting a prodrug to it's active form as in the case of codeine). The percentage of people classified as poor metabolizers varies by enzyme and population group. As an example, approximately 7% of Caucasians and only about 1% of Orientals appear to be CYP2D6 poor metabolizers.

CYP enzymes can be both inhibited and induced by other drugs, leading to increased or decreased serum concentrations (along with the associated effects), respectively. Induction occurs when a drug causes an increase in the amount of smooth endoplasmic reticulum, secondary to increasing the amount of the affected CYP enzymes in the tissues. This "revving up" of the CYP enzyme system may take several days to reach peak activity, and likewise, may take several days, even months, to return to normal following discontinuation of the inducing agent.

CYP inhibition occurs via several potential mechanisms. Most commonly, a CYP inhibitor competitively (and reversibly) binds to the active site on the enzyme, thus preventing the substrate from binding to the same site, and preventing the substrate from being metabolized. The affinity of an inhibitor for an enzyme may be expressed by an inhibition constant (Ki) or IC50 (defined as the concentration of the inhibitor required to cause 50% inhibition under a given set of conditions). In addition to reversible competition for an enzyme site, drugs may inhibit enzyme activity by binding to sites on the enzyme other than that to which the substrate would bind, and thereby cause a change in the functionality or physical structure of the enzyme. A drug may also bind to the enzyme in an irreversible (ie, "suicide") fashion. In such a case, it is not the concentration of drug at the enzyme site that is important (constantly binding and releasing), but the number of molecules available for binding (once bound, always bound).

Although an inhibitor or inducer may be known to affect a variety of CYP subfamilies, it may only inhibit one or two in a clinically important fashion. Likewise, although a substrate is known to be at least partially metabolized by a variety of CYP enzymes, only one or two enzymes may contribute significantly enough to its overall metabolism to warrant concern when used with potential inducers or inhibitors. Therefore, when attempting to predict the level of risk of using two drugs that may affect each other via altered CYP function, it is important to identify the relative effectiveness of the inhibiting/inducing drug on the CYP subfamilies that significantly contribute to the metabolism of the substrate. The contribution of a specific CYP pathway to substrate metabolism should be considered not only in light of other known CYP pathways, but also other nonoxidative pathways for substrate metabolism (eg, glucuronidation) and transporter proteins (eg, P-glycoprotein) that may affect the presentation of a substrate to a metabolic pathway.

HOW TO USE THE TABLES

The following CYP SUBSTRATES, INHIBITORS, and INDUCERS tables provide a clinically relevant perspective on drugs that are affected by, or affect, cytochrome P450 (CYP) enzymes. Not all human, drug-metabolizing CYP enzymes are specifically (or separately) included in the tables. Some enzymes have been excluded because they do not appear to significantly contribute to the metabolism of marketed drugs (eg, CYP2C18). In the case of CYP3A4, the industry routinely uses this single enzyme designation to represent all enzymes in the CYP3A subfamily. CYP3A7 is present in fetal livers. It is effectively absent from adult livers. CYP3A4 (adult) and CYP3A7 (fetal) appear to share similar properties in their respective hosts. The impact of CYP3A7 in fetal and neonatal drug interactions has not been investigated.

The **CYP Substrates table** contains a list of drugs reported to be metabolized, at least in part, by one or more CYP enzymes. An enzyme that appears to play a clinically significant (major) role in a drug's metabolism is indicated by "●", and an enzyme whose role appears to be clinically insignificant (minor) is indicated by "○". A clinically significant designation is the result of a two-phase review. The first phase considered the contribution of each CYP enzyme to the overall metabolism of the drug. The enzyme pathway was considered potentially clinically relevant if it was responsible for at least 30% of the metabolism of the drug. If so, the drug was subjected to a second phase. The second phase considered the clinical relevance of a substrate's concentration being increased twofold, or decreased by one-half (such as might be observed if combined with an effective CYP inhibitor or inducer, respectively). If either of these changes was considered to present a clinically significant concern, the CYP pathway for the drug was designated "major." If neither change would appear to present a clinically significant concern, or if the CYP enzyme was responsible for a smaller portion of the overall metabolism (ie, <30%), the pathway was designated "minor."

The **CYP Inhibitors table** contains a list of drugs that are reported to inhibit one or more CYP enzymes. Enzymes that are strongly inhibited by a drug are indicated by "●". Enzymes that are moderately inhibited are indicated by "◑". Enzymes that are weakly inhibited are indicated by "○". The designations are the result of a review of published clinical reports, available Ki data, and assessments published by other experts in the field. As it pertains to Ki values set in a ratio with achievable serum drug concentrations ([I]) under normal dosing conditions, the following parameters were employed: [I]/Ki ≥1 = strong; [I]/Ki 0.1-1 = moderate; [I]/Ki <0.1 = weak.

The **CYP Inducers table** contains a list of drugs that are reported to induce one or more CYP enzymes. Enzymes that appear to be effectively induced by a drug are indicated by "●", and enzymes that do not appear to be effectively induced are

CYTOCHROME P450 ENZYMES: SUBSTRATES, INHIBITORS, AND INDUCERS *(Continued)*

indicated by "○". The designations are the result of a review of published clinical reports and assessments published by experts in the field.

In general, clinically significant interactions are more likely to occur between substrates and either inhibitors or inducers of the same enzyme(s), all of which have been indicated by "●". However, these assessments possess a degree of subjectivity, at times based on limited indications regarding the significance of CYP effects of particular agents. An attempt has been made to balance a conservative, clinically-sensitive presentation of the data with a desire to avoid the numbing effect of a "beware of everything" approach. Even so, other potential interactions (ie, those involving enzymes indicated by "○") may warrant consideration in some cases. It is important to note that information related to CYP metabolism of drugs is expanding at a rapid pace, and thus, the contents of this table should only be considered to represent a "snapshot" of the information available at the time of publication.

Selected Readings

Bjornsson TD, Callaghan JT, Einolf HJ, et al, "The Conduct of *in vitro* and *in vivo* Drug-Drug Interaction Studies: A PhRMA Perspective," *J Clin Pharmacol*, 2003, 43(5):443-69.

Drug-Drug Interactions, Rodrigues AD, ed, New York, NY: Marcel Dekker, Inc, 2002.

Levy RH, Thummel KE, Trager WF, et al, eds, *Metabolic Drug Interactions*, Philadelphia, PA: Lippincott Williams & Wilkins, 2000.

Michalets EL, "Update: Clinically Significant Cytochrome P-450 Drug Interactions," *Pharmacotherapy*, 1998, 18(1):84-112.

Thummel KE and Wilkinson GR, "*In vitro* and *in vivo* Drug Interactions Involving Human CYP3A," *Annu Rev Pharmacol Toxicol*, 1998, 38:389-430.

Zhang Y and Benet LZ, "The Gut as a Barrier to Drug Absorption: Combined Role of Cytochrome P450 3A and P-Glycoprotein," *Clin Pharmacokinet*, 2001, 40(3):159-68.

Selected Websites

http://www.gentest.com
http://www.imm.ki.se/CYPalleles
http://medicine.iupui.edu/flockhart
http://www.mhc.com/Cytochromes

CYP Substrates

● = major substrate
○ = minor substrate

Drug	1A2	2A6	2B6	2C8	2C9	2C19	2D6	2E1	3A4
Acenocoumarol	●				●	○			
Acetaminophen	○	○			○		○	○	○
Albendazole	○								○
Albuterol									●
Alfentanil									●
Almotriptan							○		○
Alosetron	○				●				○
Alprazolam									●
Aminophylline	●							○	○
Amiodarone	○			●		○	○		●
Amitriptyline	○		○		○	○	●		○
Amlodipine									●
Amoxapine							●		
Amphetamine							○		
Amprenavir					○				●
Aprepitant	○					○			●
Argatroban									○
Aripiprazole							●		●
Aspirin					○				
Atazanavir									●
Atomoxetine						○	●		
Atorvastatin									●
Azelastine	○					○	○		○
Azithromycin									○
Benzphetamine			○						●
Benztropine							○		
Betaxolol	●						●		

CYP Substrates *(continued)*

Drug	1A2	2A6	2B6	2C8	2C9	2C19	2D6	2E1	3A4
Bexarotene									○
Bezafibrate									○
Bisoprolol							○		●
Bortezomib	○				○	○	○		●
Bosentan					●				●
Brinzolamide									○
Bromazepam									●
Bromocriptine									●
Budesonide									●
Bupivacaine	○					○	○		○
Buprenorphine									●
BuPROPion	○	○	●		○		○	○	○
BusPIRone							○		●
Busulfan									●
Caffeine	●				○		○	○	○
Candesartan					○				
Capsaicin								○	
Captopril							●		
Carbamazepine				○					●
Carisoprodol						●			
Carteolol							○		
Carvedilol	○				●		●	○	○
Celecoxib					●				○
Cerivastatin									●
Cetirizine									○
Cevimeline							○		○
Chlordiazepoxide									●
Chloroquine							●		●
Chlorpheniramine							○		●
ChlorproMAZINE	○						●		○
ChlorproPAMIDE					○				
Chlorzoxazone	○	○					○	●	○
Cilostazol	○					●	○		●
Cinacalcet	○						○		○
Cisapride	○	○	○		○	○			●
Citalopram						●	○		●
Clarithromycin									●
Clobazam						●			●
Clofibrate									○
ClomiPRAMINE	●					●	●		○
Clonazepam									●
Clopidogrel	○								○
Clorazepate									●
Clozapine	●	○			○	○	○		○
Cocaine									●
Codeine[1]							●		○
Colchicine									●
Conivaptan									●
Cyclobenzaprine	●						○		○
Cyclophosphamide[2]		○	●		○	○			●
CycloSPORINE									●
Dacarbazine	●							●	
Dantrolene									●
Dapsone				○	●	○		○	●
Delavirdine							○		●
Desipramine	○						●		
Desogestrel						●			
Dexamethasone									○
Dexmedetomidine		●							
Dextroamphetamine							●		
Dextromethorphan		○			○	○	●	○	○
Diazepam	○		○		○	●			●

CYTOCHROME P450 ENZYMES: SUBSTRATES, INHIBITORS, AND INDUCERS *(Continued)*

CYP Substrates *(continued)*

Drug	1A2	2A6	2B6	2C8	2C9	2C19	2D6	2E1	3A4
Diclofenac	○		○	○	○	○	○		○
Digoxin									○
Dihydrocodeine[1]							●		
Dihydroergotamine									●
Diltiazem					○		○		●
Dirithromycin									○
Disopyramide									●
Disulfiram	○	○	○				○	○	○
Docetaxel									●
Dofetilide									○
Dolasetron					○				○
Domperidone									○
Donepezil							○		○
Dorzolamide					○				○
Doxepin	●						●		●
DOXOrubicin							●		●
Doxycycline									●
Drospirenone									○
Duloxetine	●						●		
Dutasteride									○
Efavirenz			●						●
Eletriptan									●
Enalapril									●
Enflurane								●	
Eplerenone									●
Ergoloid mesylates									●
Ergonovine									●
Ergotamine									●
Erythromycin			○						●
Escitalopram						●			●
Esomeprazole						●			○
Estazolam									○
Estradiol	●	○	○		○	○	○	○	●
Estrogens, conjugated A/synthetic	●	○	○		○	○	○	○	●
Estrogens, conjugated equine	●	○	○		○	○	○	○	●
Estrogens, conjugated esterified	●		○		○			○	●
Estrone	●		○		○			○	●
Estropipate	●		○		○			○	●
Ethinyl estradiol					○				●
Ethosuximide									●
Etonogestrel									○
Etoposide	○							○	●
Exemestane									●
Felbamate								○	●
Felodipine									●
Fenofibrate									○
Fentanyl									●
Fexofenadine									○
Finasteride									○
Flecainide	○						●		
Fluoxetine	○		○		●	○	●	○	○
Fluphenazine							●		
Flurazepam									●
Flurbiprofen					○				
Flutamide	●								●
Fluticasone									●

CYP Substrates *(continued)*

Drug	1A2	2A6	2B6	2C8	2C9	2C19	2D6	2E1	3A4
Fluvastatin					○		○		○
Fluvoxamine	●						●		
Formoterol		○			○	○	○		
Fosamprenavir (as amprenavir)					○				●
Fosphenytoin (as phenytoin)					●	●			○
Frovatriptan	○								
Fulvestrant									○
Galantamine							○		○
Gefitinib									●
Gemfibrozil									○
Glimepiride					●				
GlipiZIDE					●				
Granisetron									○
Guanabenz	●								
Halazepam									○
Haloperidol	○						●		●
Halothane		○	○		○		○	●	○
Hydrocodone[1]							●		
Hydrocortisone									○
Ibuprofen					○	○			
Ifosfamide[3]		○	○	○	○	○			●
Imatinib	○				○	○	○		●
Imipramine	○		○			●	●		○
Imiquimod	○								○
Indinavir							○		●
Indomethacin					○	○			
Irbesartan					○				
Irinotecan			●						●
Isoflurane								●	
Isoniazid								●	
Isosorbide									●
Isosorbide dinitrate									●
Isosorbide mononitrate									●
Isradipine									●
Itraconazole									●
Ivermectin									○
Ketamine			●		●				●
Ketoconazole									●
Labetalol							●		
Lansoprazole					○	●			●
Letrozole		○							●
Levobupivacaine	○								○
Levonorgestrel									●
Lidocaine	○	○	○		○		●		●
Lomustine							●		
Lopinavir									○
Loratadine							○		○
Losartan					●				●
Lovastatin									●
Maprotiline							●		
MedroxyPROGESTERone									●
Mefenamic acid					○				
Mefloquine									●
Meloxicam					○				○
Mephobarbital			○		○	●			
Mestranol[4]					●				●
Methadone					○	○	○		●
Methamphetamine							●		
Methoxsalen		○							
Methsuximide						●			

CYTOCHROME P450 ENZYMES: SUBSTRATES, INHIBITORS, AND INDUCERS *(Continued)*

CYP Substrates *(continued)*

Drug	1A2	2A6	2B6	2C8	2C9	2C19	2D6	2E1	3A4
Methylergonovine									●
Methylphenidate							●		
MethylPREDNISolone									○
Metoclopramide	○						○		
Metoprolol						○	●		
Mexiletine	●						●		
Miconazole									●
Midazolam			○						●
Mifepristone									○
Miglustat									●
Mirtazapine	●				○		●		●
Moclobemide						●	●		
Modafinil									●
Mometasone furoate									○
Montelukast					●				●
Moricizine									●
Morphine sulfate							○		
Naproxen	○				○				
Nateglinide					●				●
Nefazodone							●		●
Nelfinavir					○	●	○		●
Nevirapine			○				○		●
NiCARdipine	○				○		○	○	●
Nicotine	○	○	○		○	○	○	○	○
NIFEdipine							○		●
Nilutamide						●			
Nimodipine									●
Nisoldipine									●
Norelgestromin									○
Norethindrone									●
Norgestrel									●
Nortriptyline	○					○	●		○
Olanzapine	○						○		
Omeprazole		○			○	●	○		○
Ondansetron	○				○		○	○	●
Orphenadrine	○		○				○		○
Oxybutynin									○
Oxycodone[1]							●		
Paclitaxel				●	●				●
Palonosetron	○						○		○
Pantoprazole						●			○
Paroxetine							●		
Pentamidine						●			
Pergolide									●
Perphenazine	○				○	○	●		○
Phencyclidine									●
Phenobarbital					○	●		○	
Phenytoin					●	●			○
Pimecrolimus									○
Pimozide	●								●
Pindolol							●		
Pioglitazone				●					○
Pipotiazine							●		●
Piroxicam					○				
Pravastatin									○
PrednisoLONE									○
PredniSONE									○
Primaquine									●

CYP Substrates *(continued)*

Drug	1A2	2A6	2B6	2C8	2C9	2C19	2D6	2E1	3A4
Procainamide							●		
Progesterone	○	○			○	●	○		●
Proguanil	○					○			○
Promethazine			●				●		
Propafenone	○						●		○
Propofol	○	○	●		●	○	○	○	○
Propranolol	●					○	●		○
Protriptyline							●		
Quazepam									○
Quetiapine							○		●
Quinidine					○			○	●
Quinine	○					○			○
Rabeprazole						●			●
Ranitidine	○					○	○		
Ranolazine							○		●
Repaglinide				●					●
Rifabutin									●
Riluzole	●								
Risperidone							●		○
Ritonavir	○		○				○		●
Rofecoxib					○				
Ropinirole	●								○
Ropivacaine	○		○				○		○
Rosiglitazone				●	○				
Rosuvastatin					○				○
Salmeterol									●
Saquinavir							○		●
Selegiline	○	○	●	○		○	○		○
Sertraline			○		○	●	●		○
Sevoflurane		○	○					●	○
Sibutramine									●
Sildenafil					○				●
Simvastatin									●
Sirolimus									●
Sorafenib									○
Spiramycin									●
Sufentanil									●
SulfaDIAZINE					●			○	○
Sulfamethoxazole					●				○
Sulfinpyrazone					●				○
SulfiSOXAZOLE					●				
Sunitinib									●
Tacrine	●								
Tacrolimus									●
Tamoxifen		○	○		●		●	○	●
Tamsulosin							●		●
Telithromycin	○								●
Temazepam			○		○	○			○
Teniposide									●
Terbinafine	○				○	○			○
Testosterone			○		○	○			○
Tetracycline									●
Theophylline	●				○		○	●	●
Thiabendazole	○								
Thioridazine						○	●		
Thiothixene	●								
Tiagabine									●
Ticlopidine									●
Timolol							●		
Tinidazole									○
Tiotropium							○		○
Tipranavir									●

CYTOCHROME P450 ENZYMES: SUBSTRATES, INHIBITORS, AND INDUCERS *(Continued)*

CYP Substrates *(continued)*

Drug	1A2	2A6	2B6	2C8	2C9	2C19	2D6	2E1	3A4
TOLBUTamide					●	○			
Tolcapone		○							○
Tolterodine					○	○	●		●
Toremifene	○								●
Torsemide				○	●				
Tramadol[1]			○				●		○
Trazodone							○		●
Tretinoin		○	○	●	○				
Triazolam									●
Trifluoperazine	●								
Trimethadione					○	○		●	○
Trimethoprim					●				●
Trimipramine						●	●		●
Troleandomycin									●
Valdecoxib					○				○
Valproic acid		○	○		○	○		○	
Vardenafil									●
Venlafaxine					○	○	●		●
Verapamil	○		○		○			○	●
VinBLAStine							○		●
VinCRIStine									●
Vinorelbine							○		●
Voriconazole					●	●			○
Warfarin	○				●	○			○
Yohimbine							○		
Zafirlukast					●				
Zaleplon									○
Zidovudine		○			○	○			○
Zileuton	○				○				○
Ziprasidone	○								○
Zolmitriptan	○								
Zolpidem	○				○	○	○		●
Zonisamide						○			●
Zopiclone					●				●
Zuclopenthixol							●		

[1]This opioid analgesic is bioactivated *in vivo* via CYP2D6. Inhibiting this enzyme would decrease the effects of the analgesic. The active metabolite might also affect, or be affected by, CYP enzymes.

[2]Cyclophosphamide is bioactivated *in vivo* to acrolein via CYP2B6 and 3A4. Inhibiting these enzymes would decrease the effects of cyclophosphamide.

[3]Ifosfamide is bioactivated *in vivo* to acrolein via CYP3A4. Inhibiting this enzyme would decrease the effects of ifosfamide.

[4]Mestranol is bioactivated *in vivo* to ethinyl estradiol via CYP2C8/9. See Ethinyl Estradiol for additional CYP information.

CYP Inhibitors

● = strong inhibitor
◑ = moderate inhibitor
○ = weak inhibitor

Drug	1A2	2A6	2B6	2C8	2C9	2C19	2D6	2E1	3A4
Acebutolol							○		
Acetaminophen									○
AcetaZOLAMIDE									○
Albendazole	○								
Alosetron	○							○	
Amiodarone	○	◑	○		◑	○	◑		◑
Amitriptyline	○				○	○	○	○	
Amlodipine	◑	○	○	○	○		○		○
Amphetamine							○		
Amprenavir						○			●
Anastrozole	○			○	○				○
Aprepitant					○	○			◑
Atazanavir	○			●	○				●
Atorvastatin									○
Azelastine			○		○	○	○		○
Azithromycin									○
Bepridil							○		
Betamethasone									○
Betaxolol							○		
Biperiden							○		
Bortezomib	○				○	◑	○		○
Bromazepam								○	
Bromocriptine	○								○
Buprenorphine	○	○				○	○		
BuPROPion							○		
Caffeine	●								◑
Candesartan				○	○				
Celecoxib				◑			○		
Cerivastatin									○
Chloramphenicol					○				○
Chloroquine							◑		
Chlorpheniramine							○		
ChlorproMAZINE							●	○	
Chlorzoxazone								○	○
Cholecalciferol					○	○	○		○
Cimetidine	◑				○	◑	◑	○	◑
Cinacalcet							○		
Ciprofloxacin	●								○
Cisapride							○		○
Citalopram	○		○			○	○		
Clarithromycin	○								●
Clemastine							○		○
Clofazimine									○
Clofibrate		○							
ClomiPRAMINE							◑		
Clopidogrel					○				
Clotrimazole	○	○	○	○	○	○	○	○	◑
Clozapine	○				○	○	◑	○	○
Cocaine							●		○
Codeine							○		
Conivaptan									●
Cyclophosphamide									○
CycloSPORINE					○				◑
Danazol									○

CYTOCHROME P450 ENZYMES: SUBSTRATES, INHIBITORS, AND INDUCERS *(Continued)*

CYP Inhibitors *(continued)*

Drug	1A2	2A6	2B6	2C8	2C9	2C19	2D6	2E1	3A4
Delavirdine	○				●	●	●		●
Desipramine		◑	◑				◑	○	◑
Dexmedetomidine	○				○		●		○
Dextromethorphan							○		
Diazepam						○			○
Diclofenac	◑				○			○	○
Dihydroergotamine									○
Diltiazem					○		○		◑
Dimethyl sulfoxide					○	○			
DiphenhydrAMINE							◑		
Disulfiram	○	○	○		○		○	●	○
Docetaxel									○
Dolasetron							○		
DOXOrubicin			◑				○		○
Doxycycline									◑
Drospirenone	○				○	○			○
Duloxetine							◑		
Econazole								○	
Efavirenz					○	○			○
Enoxacin	●								●
Entacapone	○	○			○	○	○	○	○
Eprosartan					○				
Ergotamine									○
Erythromycin	○								◑
Escitalopram							○		
Estradiol	○			○					
Estrogens, conjugated A/synthetic	○								
Estrogens, conjugated equine	○								
Ethinyl estradiol	○		○	○		○			○
Ethotoin						○			
Etoposide					○				○
Felbamate						○			
Felodipine				◑	○		○		○
Fenofibrate		○		◑	◑	○			
Fentanyl									○
Fexofenadine							○		
Flecainide							○		
Fluconazole	○				●	●			◑
Fluoxetine	◑		○		○	◑	●		○
Fluphenazine	○				○		○	○	
Flurazepam								○	
Flurbiprofen					●				
Flutamide	○								
Fluvastatin	○			○	◑		○		○
Fluvoxamine	●		○		○	●	○		○
Fosamprenavir (as amprenavir)						○			●
Gefitinib						○	○		
Gemfibrozil	◑			●	●	●			
Glyburide				○					○
Grapefruit juice									◑
Haloperidol							◑		◑
HydrALAZINE									○
HydrOXYzine							○		

CYP Inhibitors *(continued)*

Drug	1A2	2A6	2B6	2C8	2C9	2C19	2D6	2E1	3A4
Ibuprofen					●				
Ifosfamide									○
Imatinib					○		○		●
Imipramine	○					○	◐	○	
Indinavir					○	○	○		●
Indomethacin					●	○			
Interferon alfa-2a	○								
Interferon alfa-2b	○								
Interferon gamma-1b	○							○	
Irbesartan				◐	◐		○		○
Isoflurane			○						
Isoniazid	○	◐			○	●	◐	◐	●
Isradipine									○
Itraconazole									●
Ketoconazole	●	◐	○	○	●	◐	◐		●
Kotoprofen					○				
Labetalol							○		
Lansoprazole					○	◐	○		○
Leflunomide					○				
Letrozole		●				○			
Lidocaine	●						◐		◐
Lomefloxacin	○								
Lomustine							○		○
Loratadine				○		◐	○		
Losartan	○			◐	◐	○			○
Lovastatin					○		○		○
Mefenamic acid					●				
Mefloquine							○		○
Meloxicam					○				
Mephobarbital						○			
Mestranol	○		○			○			○
Methadone							◐		○
Methimazole	○	○	○		○	○	◐	○	○
Methotrimeprazine							○		
Methoxsalen	●	●			○	○	○	○	○
Methsuximide						○			
Methylphenidate							○		
MethylPREDNISolone				○					○
Metoclopramide							○		
Metoprolol							○		
Metronidazole					○				◐
Metyrapone		○							
Mexiletine	●								
Miconazole	◐	●	○		●	●	●	◐	●
Midazolam				○	○				○
Mifepristone							○		○
Mirtazapine	○								○
Mitoxantrone									○
Moclobemide	○					○	○		
Modafinil	○	○			○	●		○	○
Montelukast				○	○				
Nalidixic acid	○								
Nateglinide					○				
Nefazodone	○		○	○			○		●
Nelfinavir	○		○		○	○	○		●
Nevirapine	○						○		○
NiCARdipine					●	◐	◐		●
Nicotine		○						○	

CYTOCHROME P450 ENZYMES: SUBSTRATES, INHIBITORS, AND INDUCERS *(Continued)*

CYP Inhibitors *(continued)*

Drug	1A2	2A6	2B6	2C8	2C9	2C19	2D6	2E1	3A4
NIFEdipine	◑				○		○		○
Nilutamide						○			
Nisoldipine	○								○
Nizatidine									○
Norfloxacin	●								◑
Nortriptyline							○	○	
Ofloxacin	●								
Olanzapine	○				○	○	○		○
Omeprazole	○				◑	●	○		○
Ondansetron	○				○		○		
Orphenadrine	○	○	○		○	○	○	○	○
Oxcarbazepine						○			
Oxprenolol							○		
Oxybutynin				○			○		○
Pantoprazole					◑				
Paroxetine	○		◑		○	○	●		○
Peginterferon alfa-2a	○								
Peginterferon alfa-2b	○								
Pentamidine					○	○	○		○
Pentoxifylline	○								
Pergolide							●		○
Perphenazine	○						○		
Phencyclidine									○
Pilocarpine		○						○	○
Pimozide						○	○	○	○
Pindolol							○		
Pioglitazone				◑	○	○	◑		
Piroxicam					●				
Pravastatin					○		○		○
Praziquantel							○		
PrednisoLONE									○
Primaquine	●						○		○
Probenecid						○			
Progesterone					○	○			○
Promethazine							○		
Propafenone	○						○		
Propofol	◑				○	◑	○	○	●
Propoxyphene					○		○		○
Propranolol	○						○		
Pyrimethamine					◑		◑		
Quinidine					○		●		●
Quinine				◑	◑		●		○
Quinupristin									○
Rabeprazole				◑		◑	○		○
Ranitidine	○						○		
Ranolazine							○		○
Risperidone							○		○
Ritonavir				●	○	○	●	○	●
Rofecoxib	○								
Ropinirole	○						●		
Rosiglitazone				◑	○	○	○		
Saquinavir					○	○	○		◑
Selegiline	○	○			○	○	○	○	○
Sertraline	○		◑	○	○	◑	◑		◑
Sildenafil	○				○	○	○	○	○

CYP Inhibitors *(continued)*

Drug	1A2	2A6	2B6	2C8	2C9	2C19	2D6	2E1	3A4
Simvastatin				○	○		○		
Sirolimus									○
Sorafenib			○	○					
Sulconazole	○	○			○	○	○	○	○
SulfaDIAZINE					●				
Sulfamethoxazole					◑				
Sulfinpyrazone					◑				
SulfiSOXAZOLE					●				
Tacrine	○								
Tacrolimus									○
Tamoxifen			○	◑	○				○
Telithromycin							○		●
Telmisartan						○			
Teniposide					○				○
Tenofovir	○								
Terbinafine							●		
Testosterone									○
Tetracycline									◑
Theophylline	○								
Thiabendazole	●								
Thioridazine	○				○		◑	○	
Thiotepa			○						
Thiothixene							○		
Ticlopidine	○				○	●	◑	○	○
Timolol							○		
Tioconazole	○	○			○	○	○	○	
Tocainide	○								
TOLBUTamide				○	●				
Tolcapone					○				
Topiramate						○			
Torsemide						○			
Tranylcypromine	◑	●		○	○	◑	◑	○	○
Trazodone							◑		○
Tretinoin					○				
Triazolam				○	○				
Trimethoprim				◑	◑				
Tripelennamine							◑		
Triprolidine							○		
Troleandomycin									◑
Valdecoxib				○	○	○			
Valproic acid					○	○	○		○
Valsartan					○				
Venlafaxine			○				○		○
Verapamil	○				○		○		◑
VinBLAStine							○		○
VinCRIStine									○
Vinorelbine							○		○
Voriconazole					○	○			◑
Warfarin					◑	○			
Yohimbine							○		
Zafirlukast	○			○	◑	○	○		○
Zileuton	◑								
Ziprasidone							○		○

CYTOCHROME P450 ENZYMES: SUBSTRATES, INHIBITORS, AND INDUCERS *(Continued)*

CYP Inducers

● = effectively induced
○ = not effectively induced

Drug	1A2	2A6	2B6	2C8	2C9	2C19	2D6	2E1	3A4
Aminoglutethimide	●					●			●
Amobarbital		●							
Aprepitant					○				○
Bexarotene									○
Bosentan					○				○
Calcitriol									○
Carbamazepine	●		●	●	●	●			●
Clofibrate			○					○	○
Colchicine				○	○			○	○
Cyclophosphamide			○	○	○				
Dexamethasone		○	○	○	○				○
Dicloxacillin									○
Efavirenz (in liver only)			○						○
Estradiol									○
Estrogens, conjugated A/synthetic									○
Estrogens, conjugated equine									○
Exemestane									○
Felbamate									○
Fosphenytoin (as phenytoin)			●	●	●	●			●
Griseofulvin	○			○	○				○
Hydrocortisone									○
Ifosfamide				○	○				
Insulin preparations	○								
Isoniazid (after D/C)								○	
Lansoprazole	○								
MedroxyPROGESTERone									○
Mephobarbital		○							
Metyrapone									○
Modafinil	○		○						○
Moricizine	○								○
Nafcillin									●
Nevirapine			●						●
Norethindrone						○			
Omeprazole	○								
Oxcarbazepine									●
Paclitaxel									○
Pantoprazole	○								○
Pentobarbital		●							●
Phenobarbital	●	●	●	●	●				●
Phenytoin			●	●	●	●			●
Pioglitazone									○
PredniSONE						○			○
Primaquine	○								
Primidone[1]	●		●	●	●				●
Rifabutin									●
Rifampin	●	●	●	●	●	●			●
Rifapentine				●	●				●
Ritonavir (long-term)	○			○	○				○
Rofecoxib									○
Secobarbital		●		●	●				

CYP Inducers *(continued)*

Drug	1A2	2A6	2B6	2C8	2C9	2C19	2D6	2E1	3A4
Sulfinpyrazone									○
Terbinafine									○
Topiramate									○
Tretinoin								○	
Troglitazone									○
Valproic acid		○							

[1]Primidone is partially metabolized to phenobarbital. See Phenobarbital for additional CYP information.

EXTRAVASATION TREATMENT

Medication Extravasated	Cold/Warm Pack	Antidote
	VESICANTS	
Direct Cellular Toxins – Chemotherapeutic Agents		
DNA Intercalators		
Daunorubicin Doxorubicin Epirubicin Idarubicin	Cold	DMSO: Apply to area twice the size of the extravasation; repeat every 6 hours for up to 14 days; allow to air dry; do not cover with dressing
Vinca alkaloids		
Paclitaxel[1] Vinblastine Vincristine Vinorelbine	Warm	*Hyaluronidase 1. Add 1 mL NS to 150 units vial to make 150 units/mL concentration 2. Administer 0.2 mL injection subcutaneously or intradermally into the extravasation site at the leading edge **Note:** Some institutions utilize a 1:10 dilution in infants and children; prepare by mixing 0.1 mL of 150 units/mL solution with 0.9 mL NS in 1 mL syringe to make final concentration = 15 units/mL *Currently unavailable; expected availability late 2004 or early 2005
Alkylating agents		
Cisplatin	Cold	Sodium thiosulfate 1/6 molar solution: mix 4 mL of 10% sodium thiosulfate with 6 mL of sterile water; inject 3-5 mL (use only for large cisplatinum infiltrates >20 mL and when using cisplatinum concentrations >0.5 mg/mL; no data for use in cisplatinum infusions in children)
Mechlorethamine (Nitrogen mustard)		Sodium thiosulfate 1/6 molar solution: mix 4 mL of 10% sodium thiosulfate with 6 mL of sterile water; inject 0.5 mL for each mg mechlorethamine extravasated
Other vesicant chemotherapeutic agents		
Dactinomycin Mitomycin C Mitoxantrone Plicamycin	Cold	None
Ischemic Inducers		
Dobutamine Dopamine Epinephrine Norepinephrine Phenylephrine Vasopressin	None	Phentolamine (Regitine®) Mix 5 mg with 9 mL of NS Inject a small amount of this dilution into extravasated area. Blanching should reverse immediately. Monitor site. If blanching should recur, additional injections of phentolamine may be needed.
Miscellaneous Agents		
Aminophylline Calcium salts Dextrose (>10%) Mannitol (>5%) Phenytoin Contrast media Sodium bicarbonate (8.4%) Sodium chloride (>0.9%) Tetracycline	Cold	Hyaluronidase As described above

Medication Extravasated	Cold/Warm Pack	Antidote
	IRRITANTS	
Arsenic trioxide	Warm	
Bleomycin	Cold	
Carboplatin ≥10 mg/mL	Cold	
Carmustine	Cold	
Cisplatin (concentration <0.5 mg/mL or <20 mL of more concentrated solution)	Cold	
Cyclophosphamide	Cold	Inject 5 mL 1/6 molar sodium thiosulfate (mix 4 mL 10% sodium thriosulfate with 6 mL sterile water)
Dacarbazine	Cold	DMSO as described above
Daunorubicin citrate (liposomal)	Cold	
Dexrazoxane	None	
Docetaxel	Warm	
Doxorubicin, liposomal	Cold	
Etoposide	Warm	Hyaluronidase as described above; use only for large infiltration
Fluorouracil	Cold	
Gemcitabine	Warm	
Gemtuzumab	None	
Ifosfamide	Cold	DMSO as described above
Irinotecan	Cold	
Oxaliplatin	None	Inject 5 mL 1/6 molar sodium thiosulfate (mix 4 mL 10% soldium thiosulfate with 6 mL sterile water)
Teniposide	Warm	Hyaluronidase as described above
Topotecan	Cold	

Note:

Extravasation: The unintentional leakage of pharmacologic and physiologic solutions into the perivascular, subcutaneous, or interstitial space.

Vesicants: Agents that cause redness, pain, and blistering when infiltrated and can progress to ulceration and tissue necrosis.

Irritants: Agents that cause redness at the injection site or along the vein and often include a mild pruritic allergic reaction related to histamine release. These reaction "flares" usually do not require intervention and subside in 30 minutes.

[1]Some references consider agent as an irritant instead of vesicant.

References

Bertelli G, "Prevention and Management of Extravasation of Cytotoxic Drugs, *Drug Saf*, 1995, 12(4):245-55.

Camp-Sorrell D, "Developing Extravasation Protocols and Monitoring Outcomes," *J Intraven Nurs*, 1998, 21(4):232-9.

Cohan RH, Ellis JH, and Garner WL, "Extravasation of Radiographic Contrast Material: Recognition, Prevention, and Treatment", *Radiology*, 1996, 200(3):593-604.

Dorr RT, "Pharmacologic Management of Vesicant Chemotherapy Extravasations," *Cancer Chemotherapy Handbook*, 2nd ed, Norwalk CT: Appleton & Lange, 1994.

Finely RS, et al, *Concepts in Oncology and Therapeutics*, 2nd ed, Bethesda MS: Am Soc Heal Sys Rx, 1998.

Fenchel K and Karthaus M, "Cytotoxic Drug Extravasation," *Antibiot Chemother*, 2000, 50:144-8.

Kassner E, "Evaluation and Treatment of Chemotherapy Extravasation Injuries," *J Pediatr Oncol Nurs*, 2000, 17(3):135-48.

NIH, Standards of Practice: Care of the Patient Receiving I.V. Cytoxic or Biologic Agents, 2001.

Mullin S, Beckwith M, and Tyler L, "Prevention and Management of Antineoplastic Extravasation Injury," *Hosp Pharm*, 2000, 35:57-74.

BURN MANAGEMENT

Modified Lund-Browder Burn Assessment Chart Estimation of Total Body Surface Area of Burn Involvement[1] (% by site and age)

The total body surface area of burn involvement is determined by the sum of the percentages of each site.

Site[2]	0-1 years	1-4 years	5-9 years	10-14 years	15 years	Adult
Head	9.5	8.5	6.5	5.5	4.5	3.5
Neck	0.5	0.5	0.5	0.5	0.5	0.5
Trunk	13	13	13	13	13	13
Upper arm	2	2	2	2	2	2
Forearm	1.5	1.5	1.5	1.5	1.5	1.5
Hand	1.5	1.5	1.5	1.5	1.5	1.5
Perineum	1	1	1	1	1	1
Buttock (each)	2.5	2.5	2.5	2.5	2.5	2.5
Thigh	2.75	3.25	4	4.25	4.5	4.75
Leg	2.5	2.5	2.75	3	3.25	3.5
Foot	1.75	1.75	1.75	1.75	1.75	1.75

[1]Applies only to second- and third-degree burns

[2]Percentage for each site is only for **a single extremity with** anterior **OR** posterior involvement. Percentage should be **doubled if both anterior and posterior** involvement of a single extremity.

Adapted from Coren CV, "Burn Injuries in Children," *Pediatric Annals*, 1987, 16(4):328-39.

Parkland Fluid Replacement Formula

A guideline for replacement of deficits and ongoing losses (**Note:** For infants, maintenance fluids may need to be added to this): Administer 4 mL/kg/% burn of Ringer's lactate (glucose may be added but beware of stress hyperglycemia) over the first 24 hours; half of this total is given over the first 8 hours **calculated from the time of injury**; the remaining half is given over the next 16 hours. The second 24-hour fluid requirements average 50% to 75% of first day's requirement. Concentrations and rates best determined by monitoring weight, serum electrolytes, urine output, NG losses, etc.

Colloid may be added after 18-24 hours (1 g/kg/day of albumin) to maintain serum albumin >2 g/100 mL.

Potassium is generally withheld for the first 48 hours due to the large amount of potassium that is released from damaged tissues. To manage serum electrolytes, monitor urine electrolytes twice weekly and replace calculated urine losses.

ORAL CONTRACEPTIVES

Brand Name	Type	Progestin	Estrogen	Availability
Kariva™ Mircette®	Low Dose 1-21 d 22-23 d 24-28 d	 Desogestrel 0.15 mg — —	 Ethinyl estradiol 20 mcg — Ethinyl estradiol 10 mcg	28
Alesse® Aviane™ Lessina™ Levlite™ Lutera™ Sronyx™	Monophasic	Levonorgestrel 0.1 mg	Ethinyl estradiol 20 mcg	21, 28
Brevicon® Modicon® Necon® 0.5/35 Nortrel™ 0.5/35	Monophasic	Norethindrone 0.5 mg	Ethinyl estradiol 35 mcg	21, 28
Demulen® 1/35 [DSC] Kelnor™ Zovia™ 1/35E	Monophasic	Ethynodiol diacetate 1 mg	Ethinyl estradiol 35 mcg	21, 28
Zovia™ 1/50E	Monophasic	Ethynodiol diacetate 1 mg	Ethinyl estradiol 50 mcg	28
Levlen® Levora® Nordette® Portia™	Monophasic	Levonorgestrel 0.15 mg	Ethinyl estradiol 30 mcg	21, 28
Lo/Ovral® Cryselle™ Low-Ogestrel®	Monophasic	Norgestrel 0.3 mg	Ethinyl estradiol 30 mcg	21, 28
Junel™ 21 1/20 Loestrin 21® 1/20 Microgestin™ 1/20	Monophasic	Norethindrone acetate 1 mg	Ethinyl estradiol 20 mcg	21
Junel™ 21 1.5/30 Loestrin 21® 1.5/30 Microgestin™ 1.5/30	Monophasic	Norethindrone acetate 1.5 mg	Ethinyl estradiol 30 mcg	21
Necon® 1/35 Norinyl® 1+35 Nortrel™ 1/35 Ortho-Novum® 1/35	Monophasic	Norethindrone 1 mg	Ethinyl estradiol 35 mcg	21, 28
Necon® 1/50 Norinyl® 1+50 Ortho-Novum® 1/50	Monophasic	Norethindrone 1 mg	Mestranol 50 mcg	21, 28
Ortho-Cept® Apri® Desogen® Reclipsen™ Solia™	Monophasic	Desogestrel 0.15 mg	Ethinyl estradiol 30 mcg	28
Ortho-Cyclen® MonoNessa™ Previfem™ Sprintec™	Monophasic	Norgestimate 0.25 mg	Ethinyl estradiol 35 mcg	28
Ovcon® 35 Zenchent™	Monophasic	Norethindrone 0.4 mg	Ethinyl estradiol 35 mcg	21, 28
Ovcon® 50	Monophasic	Norethindrone 1 mg	Ethinyl estradiol 50 mcg	28
Ogestrel® 0.5/50	Monophasic	Norgestrel 0.5 mg	Ethinyl estradiol 50 mcg	28
Yaz®	Monophasic	Drospirenone 3 mg	Ethinyl estradiol 20 mcg	28
Yasmin®	Monophasic	Drospirenone 3 mg	Ethinyl estradiol 30 mcg	28
Loestrin® 24 Fe 1/20 Junel™ Fe 1/20 Microgestin™ Fe 1/20	Monophasic / Iron 25-28 d	Norethindrone acetate 1 mg	Ethinyl estradiol 20 mcg	28
Loestrin® Fe 1.5/30 Junel™ Fe 1.5/30 Microgestin™ Fe 1.5/30	Monophasic / Iron 22-28 d	Norethindrone acetate 1.5 mg	Ethinyl estradiol 30 mcg	28
Femcon™ Fe	Monophasic / Iron 22-28 d	Norethindrone 0.4 mg	Ethinyl estradiol 35 mcg	28
Jolessa™ Quasense™ Seasonale®	Monophasic Extended cycle regimen	Levonorgestrel 0.15 mg	Ethinyl estradiol 30 mcg	91
Seasonique™	Biphasic Extended cycle regimen 1-84 85-91	 Levonorgestrel 0.15 mg Levonorgestrel 0.15 mg	 Ethinyl estradiol 30 mcg Ethinyl estradiol 10 mcg	91
Ortho-Novum® 10/11 Necon® 10/11	Biphasic 1-10 d 11-21 d 22-28 d	 Norethindrone 0.5 mg Norethindrone 1 mg Inert	 Ethinyl estradiol 35 mcg Ethinyl estradiol 35 mcg —	21, 28

ORAL CONTRACEPTIVES *(Continued)*

Brand Name	Type	Progestin	Estrogen	Availability
Estrostep® 21	Triphasic			
	1-5 d	Norethindrone acetate 1 mg	Ethinyl estradiol 20 mcg	21
	6-12 d	Norethindrone acetate 1 mg	Ethinyl estradiol 30 mcg	
	13-21 d	Norethindrone acetate 1 mg	Ethinyl estradiol 35 mcg	
Ortho-Novum® 7/7/7 Necon® 7/7/7 Nortrel™ 7/7/7	Triphasic			
	1-7 d	Norethindrone 0.5 mg	Ethinyl estradiol 35 mcg	21, 28
	8-14 d	Norethindrone 0.75 mg	Ethinyl estradiol 35 mcg	
	15-21 d	Norethindrone 1 mg	Ethinyl estradiol 35 mcg	
	22-28 d	Inert	—	
Ortho Tri-Cyclen® TriNessa™ Tri-Previfem™ Tri-Sprintec™	Triphasic			
	1-7 d	Norgestimate 0.18 mg	Ethinyl estradiol 35 mcg	21, 28
	8-14 d	Norgestimate 0.215 mg	Ethinyl estradiol 35 mcg	
	15-21 d	Norgestimate 0.25 mg	Ethinyl estradiol 35 mcg	
	22-28 d	Inert	—	
Ortho Tri-Cyclen® Lo	Triphasic			
	1-7 d	Norgestimate 0.18 mg	Ethinyl estradiol 25 mcg	21, 28
	8-14 d	Norgestimate 0.215 mg	Ethinyl estradiol 25 mcg	
	15-21 d	Norgestimate 0.25 mg	Ethinyl estradiol 25 mcg	
Aranelle™ Leena™ Tri-Norinyl®	Triphasic			
	1-7 d	Norethindrone 0.5 mg	Ethinyl estradiol 35 mcg	28
	8-16 d	Norethindrone 1 mg	Ethinyl estradiol 35 mcg	
	17-21 d	Norethindrone 0.5 mg	Ethinyl estradiol 35 mcg	
	22- 28 d	Inert	—	
Triphasil® Tri-Levlen® Enpresse™ Trivora®	Triphasic			
	1-6 d	Levonorgestrel 0.05 mg	Ethinyl estradiol 30 mcg	21, 28
	7-11 d	Levonorgestrel 0.075 mg	Ethinyl estradiol 40 mcg	
	12-21 d	Levonorgestrel 0.125 mg	Ethinyl estradiol 30 mcg	
	22-28 d	Inert	—	
Velivet™ Cesia™ Cyclessa®	Triphasic			
	1-7 d	Desogestrel 0.1 mg	Ethinyl estradiol 25 mcg	28
	8-14 d	Desogestrel 0.125 mg	Ethinyl estradiol 25 mcg	
	15-21 d	Desogestrel 0.15 mg	Ethinyl estradiol 25 mcg	
	22-28 d	Inert	—	
Estrostep® Fe	Triphasic / Iron 22-28 d			
	1-5 d	Norethindrone acetate 1 mg	Ethinyl estradiol 20 mcg	28
	6-12 d	Norethindrone acetate 1 mg	Ethinyl estradiol 30 mcg	
	13-21 d	Norethindrone acetate 1 mg	Ethinyl estradiol 35 mcg	
Micronor® Camila™ Errin™ Jolivette™ Nora-BE™ Nor-QD®	Progestin only	Norethindrone 0.35 mg	—	28
Ovrette®	Progestin only	Norgestrel 0.075 mg	—	28
Plan B®	Progestin only (emergency contraception)	Levonorestrel 0.75 mg		2
Preven®	Combination (emergency contraception)	Levonorgestrel 0.25 mg	Ethinyl estradiol 50 mcg	4

Monophasic Oral Contraceptives in Order of Decreasing Estrogen Content

Estrogen	Brand Name (Progestin Content)
Mestranol 50 mcg	Necon® 1/50, Norinyl® 1+50, Ortho-Novum® 1/50 **(Norethindrone 1 mg)**
Ethinyl estradiol 50 mcg	Zovia™ 1/50E **(Ethynodiol diacetate 1 mg)**
	Ovcon®-50 **(Norethindrone 1 mg)**
	Ogestrel® 0.5/50 **(Norgestrel 0.5 mg)**
Ethinyl estradiol 35 mcg	Necon® 1/35, Norinyl® 1+35, Nortrel® 1/35, Ortho-Novum® 1/35 **(Norethindrone 1 mg)**
	Brevicon®, Modicon®, Necon® 0.5/35, Nortrel® 0.5/35 **(Norethindrone 0.5 mg)**
	Femcon™ Fe, Ovcon®-35, Zenchent™ **(Norethindrone 0.4 mg)**
	MonoNessa™, Ortho-Cyclen®, Previfem™, Sprintec™ **(Norgestimate 0.25 mg)**
	Demulen® 1/35 [DSC], Kelnor™ 1/35, Zovia™ 1/35E **(Ethynodiol diacetate 1 mg)**
Ethinyl estradiol 30 mcg	Junel™ 21 1.5/30, Junel™ Fe 1.5/30, Loestrin 21® 1.5/30, Loestrin® Fe 1.5/30, Microgestin™ 1.5/30, Microgestin™ Fe 1.5/30 **(Norethindrone acetate 1.5 mg)**
	Cryselle™, Lo/Ovral®, Low-Ogestrel™ **(Norgestrel 0.3 mg)**
	Apri®, Desogen®, Ortho-Cept®, Reclipsen™, Solia™ **(Desogestrel 0.15 mg)**
	Jolessa™, Levlen®, Levora®, Nordette®, Portia™, Quasense™, Seasonale® **(Levonorgestrel 0.15 mg)**
	Yasmin® **(Drospirenone 3 mg)**
Ethinyl estradiol 20 mcg	Alesse®, Aviane™, Lessina™, Levlite™, Lutera™, Sronyx™ **(Levonorgestrel 0.1 mg)**
	Junel™ 21 1/20, Junel™ Fe 1/20, Loestrin 21® 1/20, Loestrin® Fe 1/20, Microgestin™ 1/20, Microgestin™ Fe 1/20 **(Norethindrone acetate 1 mg)**
	Yaz® **(Drospirenone 3 mg)**

Hormonal Effects of Progestins

	Progestin Effect	Estrogen Effect	Antiestrogen Effect	Androgen Effect
Norethynodrel	+1	+3	0	0
Norethindrone	+1	+1 (low dose)	+1 (higher doses)	+2
Norethindrone acetate	+1	+1	+3	+2
Ethynodiol diacetate	+2	+1 (low dose)	+1 (higher doses)	+2
Norgestimate	+3	0	+3	0
Desogestrel	+3	0/+1	+3	0/+1
Norgestrel/ levonorgestrel	+3	0	+2	+3

0 = no effect; +1 = slight effect; +2 = moderate effect; +3 = pronounced effect.

Adapted from *Facts and Comparisons*, St Louis, MO: Facts and Comparisons, Inc, 1996.

Signs / Symptoms of Hormonal Imbalance With Oral Contraceptives

Estrogen Excess	Fluid retention, edema, cyclic weight gain, "bloating," hypertension, breast fullness/tenderness, nausea, migraine headache, melasma, telangiectasia, cervical mucorrhea, and polyposis
Estrogen Deficiency	Increased spotting, early or midcycle breakthrough bleeding, hypomenorrhea
Progestin Excess	Fatigue, lethargy, depression, decreased libido, increased appetite, weight gain, breast regression, monilial vaginitis, hypomenorrhea, hair loss, hirsutism, acne, oily scalp. **Note:** Hair loss, hirsutism, acne, and oily scalp are effects of the androgenic activity of progestins.
Progestin Deficiency	Amenorrhea, late breakthrough bleeding, hypermenorrhea

FLUIDS, ELECTROLYTES, AND NUTRITION

ENTERAL NUTRITIONAL PRODUCT FORMULARY, INFANTS

Milk Based Formulas[1,2]

(Indications: Feeding normal term infants or sick infants without special nutritional requirements)

	Human Milk	Enfamil LIPIL® With Iron	Similac® Advance®
Calories /100 mL	68	68	68
Protein g/100 mL	1	1.42	1.4
Protein source	Mature Term human milk	Nonfat milk whey	Nonfat milk whey protein concentrate
Carbohydrate g/100 mL	7.2	7.4	7.3
Carbohydrate source	Lactose	Lactose	Lactose
Fat g/100 mL	3.91	3.6	3.65
Fat source	Human milk, fat	Palm olein, coconut, soy, and high oleic sunflower oils, single cell oil blend rich in DHA & ARA[3]	High oleic safflower, soy and coconut oils (41:30:28) DHA: 0.15% ARA: 0.40%[3]
Osmolality mOsm/kg H_2O	286		300
Osmolarity mOsm/L		270	270
Sodium mEq/L (mg/L)	7.7 (177)	8 (183)	7.1 (162)
Potassium mEq/L (mg/L)	13.6 (531)	19 (730)	18.2 (710)
Chloride mEq/L (mg/L)	11.9 (422)	12 (430)	12.4 (440)
Calcium mEq/L (mg/L)	13.9 (279)	27 (530)	26.3 (528)
Phosphorus mEq/L (mg/L)	9 (143)	16.4 (360)	18.8 (284)
Iron mg/L	0.27	12.2 (4.7)[4]	12.2 (4.7)[4]

[1]Information based on manufacturer's literature as of 2007 and is subject to change.

[2]To approximate values for the content of a 24, 27, or 30 cal/oz formula (made by dilution of a powder based formulation), multiply the value desired, found in the above 20 cal/oz formula, by the following factors: 1.2 (24 cal/oz), 1.35 (27 cal/oz), or 1.5 (30 cal/oz).

[3]DHA (docosahexaenoic acid) and ARA (arachidonic acid) are fatty acids found naturally in breast milk.

[4]Low iron formulation in parenthesis.

Milk Based Formulas[1]

(Indications: Feeding normal term infants or sick infants without special nutritional requirements)

	Good Start® Supreme	Good Start® Supreme DHA & ARA[2]
Calories /100 mL	67	67
Protein g/100 mL	1.47	1.47
Protein source	Nonfat milk and whey protein concentrate	Whey protein concentrate
Carbohydrate g/100 mL	7.5	7.5
Carbohydrate source	Lactose and corn syrup maltodextrin	Lactose and corn maltodextrin
Fat g/100 mL	3.42	3.42
Fat source	Palm, soy, coconut, high oleic safflower or safflower oils	Palm, soy, coconut, high oleic safflower or sunflower oils, and DHA & ARA[2]
Sodium mEq/L (mg/L)	(181)	8 (181)
Potassium mEq/L (mg/L)	(724)	18.5 (724)
Chloride mEq/L (mg/L)	11.6 (436)	12 (436)
Calcium mEq/L (mg/L)	(449)	21.2 (449)
Phosphorus mEq/L (mg/L)	(255)	15.6 (255)
Iron mg/L	10.1	10.1

[1]Information based on manufacturer's literature as of 2007 and is subject to change.

[2]DHA (docosahexaenoic acid) and ARA (arachidonic acid) are fatty acids found naturally in breast milk.

FLUIDS, ELECTROLYTES, AND NUTRITION *(Continued)*

Milk Based Formulas – Lactose Free[1,2]

(Indications: Feeding normal term infants or sick infants without special nutritional requirements**)**

	Enfamil® LactoFree® LIPIL®[3]	**Similac® Lactose Free Advance®**
Calories /100 mL	68	68
Protein g/100 mL	1.42	1.45
Protein source	Milk protein isolate	Milk protein isolate
Carbohydrate g/100 mL	7.4	7.2
Carbohydrate source	Corn syrup solids	Sucrose and maltodextrin (55:45)
Fat g/100 mL	3.58	3.65
Fat source	Palm olein, coconut, soy, and high oleic sunflower oils, single cell oil blend rich in DHA & ARA[4]	High oleic safflower, soy, and coconut oils (40:30:29) DHA: 0.15% ARA: 0.40%[4]
Osmolality mOsm/kg H_2O	200	200
Osmolarity mOsm/L	182	180
Sodium mEq/L (mg/L)	9 (203)	8.8 (203)
Potassium mEq/L (mg/L)	19 (743)	18.5 (724)
Chloride mEq/L (mg/L)	12.8 (453)	12.4 (440)
Calcium mEq/L (mg/L)	28 (554)	28.3 (568)
Phosphorus mEq/L (mg/L)	(372)	21.6 (379)
Iron mg/L	12.2	12.2

[1]Information based on manufacturer's literature as of 2007 and is subject to change.

[2]To approximate values for the content of a 24, 27, or 30 cal/oz formula (made by dilution of a powder based formulation), multiply the value desired, found in the above 20 cal/oz formula, by the following factors: 1.2 (24 cal/oz), 1.35 (27 cal/oz), or 1.5 (30 cal/oz).

[3]Also available as Enfamil® Gentlease® LIPIL® containing reduced amount of lactose (25%,) corn syrup solids (75%), protein as partially hydrolyzed nonfat milk and whey protein concentrate.

[4]DHA (docosahexaenoic acid) and ARA (arachidonic acid) are fatty acids found naturally in breast milk.

Milk Based Formulas[1]

	Enfamil® A.R. LIPIL®	Enfamil® Next Step® LIPIL®
Calories /100 mL	68	66.7
Protein g/100 mL	1.69	1.73
Protein source	Nonfat milk	Nonfat milk
Carbohydrate g/100 mL	7.4	7
Carbohydrate source	Lactose, rice starch, and maltodextrin	Lactose and corn syrup solids
Fat g/100 mL	3.4	3.53
Fat source	Palm olein, coconut, soy, and high oleic sunflower oils, and DHA & ARA[2]	Palm olein, coconut, soy, and high oleic sunflower oils, and DHA & ARA[2]
Osmolality mOsm/kg H_2O	240	270
Osmolarity mOsm/L	220	240
Sodium mEq/L (mg/L)	11 (270)	10.4 (240)
Potassium mEq/L (mg/L)	18 (730)	22.2 (867)
Chloride mEq/L (mg/L)	14.7 (510)	15 (533)
Calcium mEq/L (mg/L)	26 (530)	64.8 (1300)
Phosphorus mEq/L (mg/L)	22.8 (360)	56 (867)
Iron mg/L	12.2	13.3
Special Uses	Thickened with rice starch for babies who spit up frequently or otherwise need a thickened formula	Infants and toddlers 9-24 months

[1]Information based on manufacturer's literature as of 2007 and is subject to change.

[2]DHA (docosahexaenoic acid) and ARA (arachidonic acid) are fatty acids found naturally in breast milk.

FLUIDS, ELECTROLYTES, AND NUTRITION *(Continued)*

Milk Based Formulas[1]

	Good Start® 2 Supreme DHA & ARA	Similac® 2 Advance®
Calories /100 mL	67	67.6
Protein g/100 mL	1.47	1.4
Protein source	Whey protein concentrate	Nonfat milk, whey
Carbohydrate g/100 mL	7.5	7.17
Carbohydrate source	Corn maltodextrin	Lactose
Fat g/100 mL	3.42	3.71
Fat source	Palm olein, soy, coconut, and high oleic safflower or sunflower oils, and DHA & ARA[2]	High oleic safflower, soy, coconut, and DHA & ARA[2]
Osmolality mOsm/kg H_2O		300
Sodium mEq/L (mg/L)	(181)	7.1 (162)
Potassium mEq/L (mg/L)	(724)	18.2 (710)
Chloride mEq/L (mg/L)	(436)	12.4 (440)
Calcium mEq/L (mg/L)	(1273)	39.8 (798)
Phosphorus mEq/L (mg/L)	(710)	(433)
Iron mg/L	13.4	12.17

[1]Information based on manufacturer's literature as of 2007 and is subject to change.

[2]DHA (docosahexaenoic acid) and ARA (arachidonic acid) are fatty acids found naturally in breast milk.

Soy Formulas[1,2]
(Indications: Lactose deficiency, milk intolerance, or galactosemia)

	Enfamil® ProSobee® LIPIL®	**Similac® Isomil® Advance®**
Calories /100 mL	68	67.6
Protein g/100 mL	1.69	1.66
Protein source	Soy protein isolate L-methionine and taurine	Soy protein isolate L-methionine
Carbohydrate g/100 mL	7.2	6.97
Carbohydrate source	Corn syrup solids	Corn syrup solids and sucrose (80:20)
Fat g/100 mL	3.6	3.69
Fat source	Palm olein, coconut, soy, and high oleic sunflower oils, and DHA & ARA[3]	High oleic safflower, soy and coconut oils, and DHA & ARA[3]
Osmolality mOsm/kg H_2O	200	200
Osmolarity mOsm/L	180	
Sodium mEq/L (mg/L)	10.6 (240)	12.9 (298)
Potassium mEq/L (mg/L)	20.4 (810)	18.7 (730)
Chloride mEq/L (mg/L)	14.5 (540)	11.8 (419)
Calcium mEq/L (mg/L)	35 (710)	35.4 (710)
Phosphorus mEq/L (mg/L)	29.6 (560)	32.9 (507)
Iron mg/L	12.2	12.2

[1]Information based on manufacturer's literature as of 2007 and is subject to change.

[2]To approximate values for the content of a 24, 27, or 30 cal/oz formula (made by dilution of a powder based formulation), multiply the value desired, found in the above 20 cal/oz formula, by the following factors: 1.2 (24 cal/oz), 1.35 (27 cal/oz), or 1.5 (30 cal/oz).

[3]DHA (docosahexaenoic acid) and ARA (arachidonic acid) are fatty acids found naturally in breast milk.

FLUIDS, ELECTROLYTES, AND NUTRITION *(Continued)*

Soy Formulas[1,2]

(Indications: Lactose deficiency, milk intolerance, or galactosemia)

	Enfamil® Next Step® ProSobee® LIPIL®[3]	Similac® Isomil® 2 Advance®[3]
Calories /100 mL	66.7	67.6
Protein g/100 mL	2.2	1.66
Protein source	Soy protein isolate L-methionine	Soy protein isolate L-methionine
Carbohydrate g/100 mL	7.87	6.97
Carbohydrate source	Corn syrup solids	Corn syrup solids and sucrose (80:20)
Fat g/100 mL	2.93	3.69
Fat source	Palm olein, coconut, soy, and high oleic sunflower oils, and 3% DHA & ARA[4]	High oleic safflower, soy, and coconut oils, and DHA & ARA[4]
Osmolality mOsm/kg H_2O	230	200
Osmolarity mOsm/L	200	
Sodium mEq/L (mg/L)	11 (240)	12.9 (298)
Potassium mEq/L (mg/L)	20 (800)	18.7 (730)
Chloride mEq/L (mg/L)	14.5 (533)	11.8 (419)
Calcium mEq/L (mg/L)	64 (1300)	45.5 (913)
Phosphorus mEq/L (mg/L)	56 (867)	39.5 (609)
Iron mg/L	13.3	12.2

[1]Information based on manufacturer's literature as of 2007 and is subject to change.

[2]To approximate values for the content of a 24, 27, or 30 cal/oz formula (made by dilution of a powder based formulation), multiply the value desired, found in the above 20 cal/oz formula, by the following factors: 1.2 (24 cal/oz), 1.35 (27 cal/oz), or 1.5 (30 cal/oz).

[3]Indicated for infants and toddlers 9-24 months.

[4]DHA (docosahexaenoic acid) and ARA (arachidonic acid) are fatty acids found naturally in breast milk.

Soy Formulas[1]

(Indications: Lactose deficiency, milk intolerance, or galactosemia)

	Good Start® Supreme Soy DHA & ARA[2]	Good Start® 2 Supreme Soy DHA & ARA[2]
Calories /100 mL	67	67
Protein g/100 mL	1.68	1.88
Protein source	Soy protein isolate	Soy protein isolate
Carbohydrate g/100 mL	7.44	7.3
Carbohydrate source	Corn maltodextrin sucrose	Corn maltodextrin sucrose
Fat g/100 mL	3.42	3.35
Fat source	Palm olein, soy, coconut, high oleic safflower or sunflower oils, DHA & ARA[2]	Palm olein, soy, coconut, high oleic safflower or sunflower oils, DHA & ARA[2]
Sodium mEq/L (mg/L)	11.8 (268)	11.8 (268)
Potassium mEq/L (mg/L)	20 (777)	20 (777)
Chloride mEq/L (mg/L)	13 (476)	13 (476)
Calcium mEq/L (mg/L)	(704)	63 (1273)
Phosphorus mEq/L (mg/L)	(422)	46 (710)
Iron mg/L	12.1	13.4

[1]Information based on manufacturer's literature as of 2007 and is subject to change.

[2]DHA (docosahexaenoic acid) and ARA (arachidonic acid) are fatty acids found naturally in breast milk.

FLUIDS, ELECTROLYTES, AND NUTRITION *(Continued)*

Soy Formula[1]

(Indications: Dietary management of diarrhea in infants >6 months and toddlers)

	Similac® Isomil® DF
Calories /100 mL	67.6
Protein g/100 mL	1.8
Protein source	Soy protein isolate and L-methionine
Carbohydrate g/100 mL	6.83
Carbohydrate source	Corn syrup and sucrose (80:20)
Fat g/100 mL	3.69
Fat source	Coconut and soy oils
Osmolality mOsm/kg H_2O	240
Sodium mEq/L (mg/L)	12.9 (298)
Potassium mEq/L (mg/L)	18.7 (730)
Chloride mEq/L (mg/L)	11.8 (419)
Calcium mEq/L (mg/L)	35.4 (710)
Phosphorus mEq/L (mg/L)	32.7 (507)
Iron mg/L	12.2

[1]Information based on manufacturer's literature as of 2007 and is subject to change.

Casein Hydrolysate Formulas[1]

(Indication: For infants predisposed to or being treated for hypocalcemia due to hyperphosphatemia whose renal or cardiovascular functions would benefit from lowered mineral levels)

	Similac® PM 60/40
Calories /100 mL	67.6
Protein g/100 mL	1.5
Protein source	Whey and caseinate
Carbohydrate g/100 mL	6.9
Carbohydrate source	Lactose
Fat g/100 mL	3.78
Fat source	Corn, soy and coconut oils (50:12:38)
Osmolality mOsm/kg H_2O	280
Sodium mEq/L (mg/L)	7.1 (162)
Potassium mEq/L (mg/L)	13.8 (541)
Chloride mEq/L (mg/L)	11.3 (399)
Calcium mEq/L (mg/L)	18.9 (379)
Phosphorus mEq/L (mg/L)	12.3 (189)
Iron mg/L	4.73
Special uses	Renal and cardiovascular disease

[1]Information based on manufacturer's literature as of 2007 and is subject to change.

FLUIDS, ELECTROLYTES, AND NUTRITION *(Continued)*

Casein Hydrolysate Formulas[1,2]
(Indication: For infants requiring low molecular weight peptides or amino acids**)**

	Enfamil® Nutramigen® LIPIL®	Enfamil® Pregestimil®	Similac® Alimentum® Advance®
Calories /100 mL	68	68	67.6
Protein g/100 mL	1.89	1.89	1.86
Protein source	Casein hydrolysate, L-cystine, L-tyrosine, and L-tryptophan	Casein hydrolysate, L-cystine, L-tyrosine, and L-tryptophan	Casein hydrolysate, L-cystine, L-tyrosine, and L-tryptophan
Carbohydrate g/100 mL	7	6.9	6.9
Carbohydrate source	Corn syrup solids and modified corn starch; lactose and sucrose free	65% corn syrup solids, 20% dextrose, and 15% modified corn starch; lactose and sucrose free	Sucrose and modified tapioca starch (70:30)
Fat g/100 mL	3.6	3.8	3.75
Fat source	44% palm olein, 19.5% soy, 19.5% coconut, 14.5% high oleic sunflower oils, and 2.5% single cell oil blend rich in DHA & ARA[3]	55% MCT oil, 35% soy oil, and 10% high oleic safflower oil[4]	Safflower, medium chain triglycerides, and soy oilsnn (38:33:28) and DHA & ARA[3]
Osmolality mOsm/kg H_2O	270 (liquid)	280 (liquid)	370
Osmolarity mOsm/L	240 (liquid)	250 (liquid)	
Sodium mEq/L (mg/L)	14 (320)	14 (320)	12.9 (298)
Potassium mEq/L (mg/L)	19 (740)	19 (740)	20.4 (798)
Chloride mEq/L (mg/L)	16.2 (580)	16.2 (580)	15.3 (541)
Calcium mEq/L (mg/L)	32 (640)	39 (780)	35.4 (710)
Phosphorus mEq/L (mg/L)	22.2 (430)	32.6 (510)	32.7 (507)
Iron mg/L	12.2	12.7 (liquid)	12.2
Special uses	Sensitivity to intact proteins, galactosemia	Fat malabsorption or sensitivity to intact proteins; may be used in cystic fibrosis, intractable diarrhea and severe protein calorie malnutrition, short bowel syndrome	Severe food allergies, sensitivity (including colic) to intact proteins, protein maldigestion or fat malabsorption

[1]Information based on manufacturer's literature as of 2007 and is subject to change.

[2]To approximate values for the content of a 24, 27, or 30 cal/oz formula (made by dilution of a powder based formulation), multiply the value desired, found in the above 20 cal/oz formula, by the following factors: 1.2 (24 cal/oz), 1.35 (27 cal/oz), or 1.5 (30 cal/oz).

[3]DHA (docosahexaenoic acid) and ARA (arachidonic acid) are fatty acids found naturally in breast milk.

[4]Powder content varies: 55% MCT oil, 25% soy oil, 10% corn oil, 10% high oleic safflower or sunflower oil

Other Infant and Pediatric Formulas[1] – Special Care
(Indication: Premature infant formulas designed for rapidly growing LBW infants)

	Preterm Human Milk	Enfamil® EnfaCare® LIPIL®	Enfamil® Premature LIPIL®	Similac® Special Care® Advance® 20 With Iron	Similac® Neosure® Advance®
Calories/100 mL	67	74	68	67.6	74.4
Protein g/100 mL	1.41	2.1	2	2.03	2.08
Protein source	Preterm human milk	Nonfat milk and whey protein concentrate	Nonfat milk and whey protein concentrate	Nonfat milk and whey protein concentrate	Nonfat milk and whey protein concentrate
Carbohydrate g/100 mL	6.64	7.7	7.4	6.97	7.51
Carbohydrate source	Lactose	Powder: Corn syrup and lactose Liquid: Maltodextrin and lactose	Corn syrup solids and lactose	Corn syrup solids and lactose (50:50)	Corn syrup solids and lactose (50:50)
Fat g/100 mL	3.89	3.9	3.4	3.67	4.09
Fat source	Preterm human milk	MCT, soy, high oleic vegetable and coconut oils with DHA & ARA[3]	MCT, soy, and high oleic vegetable oils with DHA & ARA[3]	Medium chain triglycerides, soy, and coconut oils (50:30:18.3) with DHA & ARA[3]	Medium chain triglycerides, soy, and coconut oils (24.9:44.7:29) with DHA & ARA[3]
Osmolality mOsm/kg H_2O	290	220 (liquid)	240	235	250
Osmolarity mOsm/L		230	220		
Sodium mEq/L (mg/L)	10.8 (248)	11 (260)	17.1 (390)	12.6 (291)	10.7 (245)
Potassium mEq/L (mg/L)	14.6 (570)	20 (780)	16.7 (660)	22.3 (872)	27 (1056)
Chloride mEq/L (mg/L)	15.6 (550)	16.3 (580)	16.9 (610)	15.5 (548)	15.8 (558)
Calcium mEq/L (mg/L)	12.4 (248)	45 (890)	54.8 (1120)	60.7 (1217)	39 (781)
Phosphorus mEq/L (mg/L)	(128)	31.6 (490)	36.3 (560)	(676)	(463)
Iron mg/L	1.21	13.3	12.2 (3.4)[4]	12.2 (2.5)[4]	13.4

[1]Information based on manufacturer's literature as of 2007 and is subject to change.

[2]To approximate values of 24 cal/oz formulation, multiply the values desired, found in the 20 cal/oz formula by 1.2.

[3]DHA (docosahexaenoic acid) and ARA (arachidonic acid) are fatty acids found naturally in breast milk.

[4]Low iron formulation in parentheses.

FLUIDS, ELECTROLYTES, AND NUTRITION *(Continued)*

Human Milk Fortifiers[1]
(Indication: Add to human milk as a supplement for premature and low birth weight infants**)**

	Enfamil® Human Milk Fortifier	Similac® Human Milk Fortifier	Similac® Natural Care® Advance®[2]
Calories /packet	3.5	3.5	0.812 cal/mL
Protein g/packet	0.28	0.25	2.44 g/100 mL
Protein source	Milk protein isolate and whey protein isolate	Nonfat milk and whey protein concentrate	Nonfat milk and whey protein concentrate
Carbohydrate g/packet	<0.1	0.45	8.36 g/100 mL
Carbohydrate source	Corn syrup solids, lactose	Corn syrup solids	Lactose and corn syrup solids
Fat g/packet	0.25	0.1	4.4 g/100 mL
Fat source	MCT and soy oils	MCT oil	MCT, soy and coconut oils with DHA & ARA[3]
Sodium mEq/packet (mg/packet)	0.19 (4)	0.18 (3.75)	1.5[2] mEq/100 mL (34.9 mg/100 mL)
Potassium mEq/packet (mg/packet)	0.18 (7.25)	0.4 (15.8)	2.68 mEq/100 mL (104.7 mg/100 mL)
Chloride mEq/packet (mg/packet)	0.1 (3.25)	0.28 (9.5)	1.86 mEq/100 mL (65.7 mg/100 mL)
Calcium mEq/packet (mg/packet)	1.1 (22.5)	1.48 (29.3)	8.5 mEq/100 mL (170 mg/100 mL)
Phosphorus mEq/packet (mg/packet)	0.71 (12.5)	0.96 (16.8)	(94.1 mg/100 mL)
Iron mg/packet	0.36	0.1	0.3 mg/100 mL

[1]Information based on manufacturer's literature as of 2007 and is subject to change.

[2]May be mixed with human milk or fed alternatively with human milk to low birth weight infants.

[3]DHA (docosahexaenoic acid) and ARA (arachidonic acid) are fatty acids found naturally in breast milk.

ENTERAL FORMULAS – PEDIATRIC[1]
(A selection of the commonly used enteral feedings for children 1-10 years of age)

	PediaSure®	PediaSure® With Fiber	Peptamen Junior®	Vivonex® Pediatric	Boost®	Carnation Instant Breakfast®[2]	Ensure®	Enfamil® Kindercal® TF
Calories/oz	30	30	30	24	30	35	31	30
Calories/mL	1	1	1.06	0.8	1	1.17	1.06	1.06
Carbohydrate g/100 mL	13.3	13.8	13.8	13	17	16.5	16.7	13.5
Carbohydrate source	Corn maltodextrin, sucrose, dextrose (85:13:2)	Corn maltodextrin, sucrose, dextrose (85:13:2)	Maltodextrin, corn starch	Maltodextrin, modified starch	Sucrose, corn syrup solids	Maltodextrin, sucrose, lactose	Maltodextrin, sucrose, corn syrup	Maltodextrin, sugar, lactose-free
Protein g/100 mL	3	3	3	2.4	4.2	5.4	3.7	3
Protein source	Milk protein concentrate	Milk protein concentrate	Partially hydrolyzed whey protein	L-amino acids	Milk protein concentrate	Nonfat milk	Casein, soy, and whey protein isolates	Milk protein concentrate
Fat g/100 mL	3.97	3.97	3.9	2.4	1.8	3.4	2.5	4.4
Fat source	High oleic safflower, soy, and MCT oils (43:42:16)	High oleic safflower, soy, MCT oils, and lecithin (43:42:16)	MCT, soy, and canola oils, lecithin	MCT and soy oils	Canola, high oleic sunflower, and corn oils	Butterfat	High oleic safflower, corn, and canola oils	Canola, high oleic sunflower, corn, and MCT oils (40:28:20:12)
Osmolality mOsm/kg	335	345	260 unflavored 380 vanilla	360	590-670	661-747; 660 French vanilla	590	345
Sodium mg/100 mL (mEq/100 mL)	38 (1.65)	38 (1.65)	46 (2)	40 (1.7)	55 (2.4)	94 (4.1)	83 (3.6)	37 (1.61)
Potassium mg/100 mL (mEq/100 mL)	131 (3.4)	131 (3.4)	132 (3.4)	120 (3.1)	169 (4.3)	257 (6.6)	154 (3.9)	131 (3.4)
Iron (mg/100 mL)	1.4	1.4	1.4	1	1.9	2	1.9	1.06

[1]Information based on manufacturer's literature as of 2007 and is subject to change.

[2]Mixed with 8 oz whole milk as directed.

FLUIDS, ELECTROLYTES, AND NUTRITION *(Continued)*

ENTERAL FORMULAS – ADOLESCENTS AND ADULTS[1]

	Osmolite®	Osmolite 1.2®	Jevity®
Calories/mL	1.06	1.2	1.06
Carbohydrate g/100 mL	15.1	15.8	15.5
Carbohydrate source	Corn syrup solids	Maltodextrin	Maltodextrin, corn syrup solids, and soy fiber
Protein g/100 mL	3.71	5.55	4.43
Protein source	Caseinate, soy protein isolate	Caseinate, soy protein isolate	Caseinate, soy protein isolate
Fat g/100 mL	3.47	3.93	3.47
Fat source	High oleic safflower, canola, MCT oils, and soy lecithin	High oleic safflower, canola, MCT oils, and soy lecithin	High oleic safflower, canola, MCT oils, and soy lecithin
Osmolality mOsm/kg	300	360	300
Osmolarity mOsm/L	289	465	370
Sodium mg/100 mL (mEq/100 mL)	64 (2.7)	134 (5.8)	93 (4.0)
Potassium mg/100 mL (mEq/100 mL)	102 (2.6)	181 (4.6)	157 (4.0)

[1]Information based on manufacturer's literature as of 2007 and is subject to change.

ENTERAL FORMULAS WITH HIGH CALORIC DENSITY[1]

	Ensure Plus®	Jevity® 1.5 Cal	Isosource® 1.5 Cal	TraumaCal®	Hi-Cal™
Calories/mL	1.5	1.5	1.5	1.5	2
Carbohydrate g/100 mL	20.8	21.6	17	14.4	21.4
Carbohydrate source	Corn syrup solids, maltodextrin, sucrose	Corn maltodextrin and corn syrup solids	Maltodextrin and sucrose	Corn syrup and sucrose	Corn syrup solids
Protein g/100 mL	5.5	6.4	6.8	8.2	8.3
Protein source	Caseinate, soy protein isolate	Caseinate, soy protein isolate	Caseinates	Caseinates	Caseinates
Fat g/100 mL	4.8	5	6.5	6.8	8.8
Fat source	Canola, high oleic safflower and corn oils	High oleic safflower, canola and MCT oils, and soy lecithin	Canola, soy, and MCT oils, and soy lecithin	Soy oil, MCT oil, and soy lecithin	Corn oil and soy lecithin
Osmolality mOsm/kg	680	525	650	560	705
Sodium mg/100 mL (mEq/100 mL)	101 (4.4)	140 (6.09)	129 (5.6)	118 (5.1)	144 (6.3)
Potassium mg/100 mL (mEq/100 mL)	186 (4.7)	215 (5.5)	225 (5.8)	139 (3.6)	242 (6.2)

[1]Information based on manufacturer's literature as of 2007 and is subject to change.

ELEMENTAL ENTERAL FORMULAS – INFANTS / PEDIATRIC[1]

	EleCare® (20 kcal/oz)	EleCare® (30 kcal/oz)	Neocate® Infant (20 kcal/oz)	Neocate® One+ (30 kcal/oz)
Calories/mL	0.676	1.014	0.67	1
Carbohydrate g/100 mL	7.24	10.85	7.84	14.6
Carbohydrate source	Corn syrup solids	Corn syrup solids	Corn syrup solids	Corn syrup solids
Protein g/100 mL	2.04	3.05	2.08	2.5
Protein source	Free amino acids	Free amino acids	Free amino acids	Free amino acids
Fat g/100 mL	3.22	4.83	3.02	3.5
Fat source	High oleic safflower, MCT, soy oils	High oleic safflower, MCT, soy oils	High oleic safflower, coconut, soy oils	Fractionated coconut, canola, high oleic safflower oils
Osmolality mOsm/kg	350	560	375	610
Osmolarity mOsm/L	185	277	—	234
Sodium mg/L (mEq/L)	304 (13.2)	456 (19.9)	250	200
Potassium mg/L (mEq/L)	1014 (25.9)	1522 (38.9)	1039	930
Calcium mg/L (mEq/L)	730 (36.4)	1096 (54.6)	831	620
Phosphorus mg	548	822	624	620
Iron mg	12	18	12.4	7.7

[1]Information based on manufacturer's literature as of 2007 and is subject to change.

ELEMENTAL ENTERAL FORMULAS WITH MODIFIED PROTEIN – ADOLESCENTS AND ADULTS[1]

	Peptamen®	Tolerex®	Vivonex Plus®
Calories/mL	1	1	1
Carbohydrate g/100 mL	12.7	23	19
Carbohydrate source	Maltodextrin, corn starch	Maltodextrin modified corn starch	Maltodextrin, modified starch
Protein g/100 mL	4	2.1	4.5
Protein source	Partially hydrolyzed whey	L-amino acids	L-amino acids
Fat g/100 mL	3.9	0.1	0.67
Fat source	Soy and MCT oils	Safflower oil	Soy oil
Osmolality mOsm/kg	270 unflavored 380 vanilla	550 unflavored 617-678 flavored	650
Sodium mg/100 mL (mEq/100 mL)	56 (2.4)	47 (2)	61 (2.7)
Potassium mg/100 mL (mEq/100 mL)	150 (3.8)	117 (3)	106 (2.7)

[1]Information based on manufacturer's literature as of 2007 and is subject to change.

FLUIDS, ELECTROLYTES, AND NUTRITION *(Continued)*

Portagen®[1]

(Indication: A supplemental nutritional which may be useful in patients with malabsorption and steatorrhea. Not intended as a sole source of nutrition and due to low essential fatty acid content.)

	Portagen®
Calories /100 mL	100
Protein g/100 mL	3.6
Protein source	Caseinates
Carbohydrate g/100 mL	11.8
Carbohydrate source	Corn syrup solids and sucrose
Fat g/100 mL	4.9
Fat source	MCT and corn oils
Osmolality mOsm/kg	230
Sodium mEq/L (mg/L)	24 (560)
Potassium mEq/L (mg/L)	32 (1270)
Chloride mEq/L (mg/L)	24.8 (865)
Calcium mEq/L (mg/L)	48 (960)
Phosphorus mEq/L (mg/L)	40.4 (710)
Iron mg/L	19

[1]Information based on manufacturer's literature as of 2007 and is subject to change.

Nutritional Modules[1]

	Polycose® Liquid	Polycose® Powder	Promod® Powder[2]
Indication	Carbohydrate additive for use as a caloric supplement which is readily mixable in most foods, enteral formulas or beverages without appreciably altering their taste	Carbohydrate additive for use as a caloric supplement which is readily mixable in most foods, enteral formulas or beverages without appreciably altering their taste	Protein supplement which mixes readily in enteral formulas, most foods, or beverages without appreciably altering their taste
Calories	2/mL	3.8/g[3]	4.2/g
Protein (g)	—	—	0.76/g
Protein source	—	—	Whey protein concentrate
Carbohydrate (g)	0.5/mL	0.94/g	<0.1/g
Carbohydrate source	Glucose polymers derived from corn starch	Glucose polymers derived from corn starch	Lactose
Fat (g)	—	—	<0.09/g
Fat source	—	—	Soy lecithin
Osmolality mOsm/kg	900	900 in solution	~1 scoop = 5 g protein (per 6.6 g of powder); contributes about 30 mOsm/kg H_2O to 8 oz beverage
Sodium mEq/L (mg/L)	<0.03/mL (<0.7/mL)	<0.057/g (<1.1/g)	<0.167/g (<3.78/g)
Potassium mEq/L (mg/L)	<0.002/mL (<0.06/mL)	<0.003/g (<0.1/g)	<0.038/g (<6.82/g)
Chloride mEq/L (mg/L)	<0.04/mL (<1.4/mL)	<0.063/g (<2.23/g)	—
Calcium mEq/L (mg/L)	<0.01/mL (<0.2/mL)	<0.015/g (<0.3/g)	<9.85/g)
Phosphorus mEq/L (mg/L)	(<0.03/mL)	(<0.15/g)	(<5/g)
Iron mg/L	—	—	—

[1]These products are not complete formulations and should not be used as a sole source of nutrition.

[2]1 scoop = 6.6 g, 1 tsp = 1.3 g, 1 tbsp = 4 g.

[3]1 tsp (2 g) = 8 calories, 1 tbsp (6 g) = 23 calories, ¼ cup (24 g) = 95 calories.

FLUIDS, ELECTROLYTES, AND NUTRITION *(Continued)*

Nutritional Modules[1]

	Vegetable Oil[2]	Microlipid®	MCT Oil®[3]	Whole Milk
Indication	Inexpensive fat source for calories and essential fatty acids	50% fat emulsion for use as a source of calories or essential fatty acids; it mixes easily and stays in emulsion	Fat supplement for use for patients who cannot efficiently digest and absorb long-chain fats	
Calories	8.3/mL	4.5/mL	7.7/mL	157/8 oz
Protein (g)	—	—	—	8/8 oz
Protein source	—	—	—	82% casein, 18% whey
Carbohydrate (g)	—	—	—	11.5/8 oz
Carbohydrate source	—	—	—	Lactose
Fat (g)	0.93/mL	0.5/mL[4]	0.93/mL	8.2/8 oz
Fat source	Corn, soybean, sunflower or safflower oils[5]	Safflower oil, polyglycerol esters, soy lecithin (high in linoleic acid)	Lipid fraction of coconut oil (consists primarily of C_8 and C_{10} saturated fatty acids)	Butter fat
Osmolality mOsm/kg	—	60	—	285
Sodium mEq/L (mg/L)	—	—	—	5.3/8 oz (120/8 oz)
Potassium mEq/L (mg/L)	—	—	—	9.6/8 oz (377/8 oz)
Chloride mEq/L (mg/L)	—	—	—	7/8 oz (247/8 oz)
Calcium mEq/L (mg/L)	—	—	—	14.9/8 oz (295/8 oz)
Phosphorus mEq/L (mg/L)	—	—	—	14.6/8 oz (230/8 oz)
Iron mg/L	—	—	—	0.12/8 oz

[1]These products are not complete formulations and should not be used as a sole source of nutrition.

[2]1 tbsp = 14 g.

[3]Does not contain essential fatty acids.

[4]1 tbsp = 5.9 g linoleic.

[5]% of linoleic from fat: soybean oil 51%, corn oil 58%, sunflower oil 65%, safflower oil 77%.

FLUID AND ELECTROLYTE REQUIREMENTS IN CHILDREN

Maintenance Fluids (Two methods)

Surface area method (most commonly used in children >10 kg): 1500-2000 mL/m^2/day

Body weight method

<10 kg	100 mL/kg/day
11-20 kg	1000 mL + 50 mL/kg (for each kg >10)
>20 kg	1500 mL + 20 mL/kg (for each kg >20)

Maintenance Electrolytes (See specific electrolyte in Alphabetical Listing of Drugs for more detailed information)

Sodium: 3-4 mEq/kg/day **or** 30-50 mEq/m^2/day
Potassium: 2-3 mEq/kg/day **or** 20-40 mEq/m^2/day

Dehydration Fluid Therapy

Goals of therapy:

- Restore circulatory volume to prevent shock (10% to 15% dehydration)
- Restore combined intracellular and extracellular deficits of water and electrolytes within 24 hours
- Maintain adequate water and electrolytes
- Resolve homeostatic distortions (eg, acidosis)
- Replace ongoing losses

Analysis of the Severity of Dehydration by Physical Signs

Clinical Sign	Mild[1]	Moderate[1]	Severe[1]
Pre-illness body weight	5% loss	10% loss	15% loss
Skin turgor	↓	Tenting	Tenting
Mucous membranes	Dry	Very dry	Parched
Skin color	Pale	Grey	Mottled
Urine output	↓	↓↓	Azotemic
Blood pressure	Normal	Normal, ↓	↓↓
Heart rate	Normal, ↑	↑	↑↑
Fontanelle (<7 mo)	Flat	Soft	Sunken
CNS	Consolable	Irritable	Lethargic/coma

[1]Postpubertal children and adults experience the same symptoms with mild, moderate, and severe dehydration associated with 3%, 6%, and 9% losses in body weight respectively.

Restoration of Circulatory Volume (10% to 15% dehydration estimate)

Fluid boluses of 20 mL/kg using crystalloid (eg, normal saline) or 10 mL/kg colloid (eg, 5% albumin) administered as rapidly as possible; repeat until improved circulation (eg, warm skin, decreased heart rate (towards normal), improved capillary refill time, urine output restored).

Classification of Dehydration (based upon the serum sodium concentration)

Isotonic	130-150 mEq/L
Hypotonic	<130 mEq/L
Hypertonic	>150 mEq/L

FLUID AND ELECTROLYTE REQUIREMENTS IN CHILDREN *(Continued)*

Estimated Water & Electrolyte Deficits in Dehydration
(moderate to severe)

Type of Dehydration	Water (mL/kg)	Na+ (mEq/kg)	K+ (mEq/kg)	Cl^- and HCO_3^- (mEq/kg)
Isotonic	100-150	8-10	8-10	16-20
Hypotonic	50-100	10-14	10-14	20-28
Hypertonic	120-180	2-5	2-5	4-10

Current Pediatric Diagnosis & Treatment, 10th ed, 1991.

Water deficit may also be calculated (in isotonic dehydration):

$$\text{Water deficit (mL)} = \frac{\text{\% dehydration} \times \text{wt (kg)} \times 1000 \text{ g/kg}}{100}$$

Assessment of Water Loss in Relation to Serum Na^+ Concentrations Degree of Dehydration as % Body Weight

Serum Na^+	Mild	Moderate	Severe
Isotonic	5%	10%	15%
Hypotonic (Na^+< 130)	4%	6%	8%
Hypertonic (Na^+ >150)	7%	12%	17%

Example of Fluid Replacement
(assume 10 kg infant with 10% isotonic dehydration)

	Water	Sodium (mEq)	Potassium (mEq)
Maintenance	1000 mL	40	20
Deficit[1]	1000 mL	80	80
Total	2000 mL	120	100

[1]Reduce this total by any fluid boluses given initially.

First 8 hours:

Replace 1/3 maintenance water = 330 mL

Replace 1/2 deficit water = 500 mL

Total 830 mL/8 h = 103 mL/h

Replace 1/2 of Na^+ & K^+ = 60 mEq sodium/803 mL; 50 mEq potassium/803 mL (It is suggested that the maximum potassium initially used is 40 mEq/L and is **not** started until urine output has been established.)

The actual order would appear as: $D_5$1/2NS at 103 mL/hour for 8 hours; add 40 mEq/L KCl after patient voids.

Second 16 hours:

Replace 2/3 maintenance water = 670 mL

Replace 1/2 deficit water = 500 mL

Total 1260 mL/16 h = 79 mL/h

Replace remainder of sodium and potassium.

The actual order would appear as: $D_5$1/3NS with KCl 40 mEq/L at 79 mL/hour for 16 hours. (Use of 1/4NS may be more desirable for convenience.)

Analysis of Ongoing Losses

Electrolyte Composition of Biological Fluids (mEq/L)

Fluid Type	Sodium	Potassium	Chloride	Total HCO_3^-
Stomach	20-120	5-25	90-160	0-5
Duodenal drainage	20-140	3-30	30-120	10-50
Biliary tract	120-160	3-12	70-130	30-50
Small intestine Initial drainage	100-140	4-40	60-100	30-100
Small intestine Established drainage	4-20	4-10	10-100	40-120
Pancreatic	110-160	4-15	30-80	70-130
Diarrheal stool	10-25	10-30	30-120	10-50

Current Pediatric Diagnosis & Treatment, 9th ed, Appleton & Lange, 1987.

Because of the wide range of normal values, specific analyses are suggested in individual cases.

Alterations of Maintenance Fluid Requirements

Fever	Increase maintenance fluids by 5 mL/kg/day for each degree of temperature above 38°C
Hyperventilation	Increase maintenance fluids by 10-60 mL/100 kcal BEE (basal energy expenditure)
Sweating	Increase maintenance fluids by 10-25 mL/100 kcal BEE (basal energy expenditure)
Hyperthyroidism	Variable increase in maintenance fluids: 25%-50%
Renal disease	Monitor and analyze output; adjust therapy accordingly
Renal failure	Maintenance fluids are equal to insensible losses (300 mL/m^3) + urine replacement (mL for mL)
Diarrhea	Increase maintenance fluids on a mL/mL loss basis

Oral Rehydration

Due to the high worldwide incidence of dehydration from infantile diarrhea, effective, inexpensive oral rehydration solutions have been developed. In the U.S., a typical effective solution for rehydration contains 50-60 mEq/L sodium, 20-30 mEq/L potassium, 30 mEq/L bicarbonate or its equivalent, and sufficient chloride to provide electroneutrality. Two percent to 3% glucose facilitates electrolyte absorption and short-term calories. The following table describes the electrolyte/sugar content of commonly used oral rehydration solutions.

FLUID AND ELECTROLYTE REQUIREMENTS IN CHILDREN *(Continued)*

Composition of Frequently Used Oral Electrolyte Replacement Solutions

Solutions	% CHO	Na^+ (mEq/L)	K^+ (mEq/L)	Cl^- (mEq/L)	HCO^- (mEq/L)
Normal saline		154		154	
Ringer's lactate		130	4	109	28
Dextrose 5% in 0.25% NaCl	5% glucose	38		38	
WHO solution	2% glucose or 4% sucrose	90	20	80	30 citrate
WHO solution, modified	2% glucose	55	25	30	50
Rehydralyte®	2.5% glucose	75	20	65	30 citrate
Ricelyte®	3% carbohydrate	50	25	45	34 citrate
Resol®	2% glucose	50	20	50	34 citrate
Rice water	2.5% carbohydrate	90	20	30	80
Pedialyte® (Ross)	2.5% glucose	45	20	35	30 citrate
Pedialyte® Freezer Pops	2.5% glucose	45	20	35	30 citrate
Enfamil Enfalyte®	3% glucose	50	25	45	34 citrate
Kao Lectrolyte	2% glucose	50	20		30 citrate
Naturalyte	2.5% glucose	45	20	35	30 citrate
Oralyte	2.5% glucose	45	20	35	48 citrate
Gatorade®	2.6% glucose, 2% fructose	23.5	<1	17	
Apple juice	3.2% glucose, 1.3% sucrose, 7.5% fructose	<1	25		
Orange juice 1:3 (dilution with water)	1% glucose, 1.2% fructose	<1	50		50 citrate
Grape juice	1.6% glucose, 2.1% fructose	0.2-0.7	8-11		8
One package cherry gelatin dissolved in 4 cups water		24	Needs added K^+		
Coca-Cola®		1.6	<1		13.4 citrate
Pepsi-Coal®		6.5	0.8		
Beef broth		120	10		
Chicken broth		250	8		

Adapted from Aranda-Michel, J and Giannella RA, "Acute Diarrhea" A Practical Review," *Am J of Med,* 1999, 106:670-6.

PARENTERAL NUTRITION (PN)

The following information is intended as a brief overview of the use of PN in infants and children.

Goal: The therapeutic goal of PN in infants and children is both to maintain nutrition status and to achieve balanced somatic growth.

General Indications for Use

PN is the provision of required nutrients by the intravenous route to replenish, optimize, or maintain nutritional status.

Specific Indications

PN of **all** required nutrients (total parenteral nutrition) is indicated in patients for whom it is expected that it would be impossible or dangerous to enterally administer nutrition. PN in combination with enteral nutrition is indicated in patients who are expected to be unable to meet their nutritional needs by the enteral route alone within 5 days. Peripheral PN is indicated only for partial nutritional supplementation or as bridge therapy for patients awaiting central venous access.

1. Patients with an inability to absorb nutrients via the gastrointestinal tract which may include the following: severe diarrhea, short bowel syndrome, developmental anomalies of the GI tract, inflammatory bowel disease, cystic fibrosis, or anatomic or functional loss of GI integrity.
2. Severe malnutrition.
3. Severe catabolic states such as: burns, trauma, or sepsis.
4. Patients undergoing high dose chemotherapy, radiation, and bone marrow transplantation.
5. Patients whose clinical condition may necessitate complete bowel rest (eg, necrotizing enterocolitis, pancreatitis, GI fistulas, or recent GI surgery).
6. Intensive care low-birth-weight infants.
7. Neonatal asphyxia.
8. Meconium ileus.
9. Respiratory distress syndrome (RDS).

Nutritional Assessment

As many as 33% of hospitalized pediatric patients are malnourished and require nutritional therapy. The type of nutritional support indicated depends on the underlying disease, the degree of gastrointestinal function, and the severity of malnutrition. Acutely malnourished patients have an increased risk for serious infection, postoperative complications, and death. Indicators of acute protein-calorie malnutrition include low weight for height, low serum albumin, lymphopenia, decreased body fat folds, and decreased arm muscle area. Nutritional screening may be done by the dietitian. Those patients who are at nutritional risk should receive a complete nutritional assessment.

Nutritional Requirements

Approximate requirements for energy and protein at various ages for normal subjects are listed in the first table at the end of this section. Patients who are severely malnourished or markedly catabolic may require higher levels to achieve catch-up growth or meet increased requirements. Patients who are well-nourished and/or inactive may require less.

During parenteral nutrition, 10% to 16% of calories should be in the form of amino acids to achieve optimal benefit (approximately 2-3 g/kg/day in infants and 1.5-2.5 g/kg/day ideal body weight in older patients). Exceptions include patients with renal or hepatic failure (where less protein is indicated), or in the treatment of severe trauma, head injury, or sepsis (where more protein may be indicated).

PARENTERAL NUTRITION (PN) *(Continued)*

PN ORDERING

Fluid Intake

The patient should be given a total volume of fluid reasonable for his/her age and cardiovascular status. It is generally safe to start with the fluid maintenance level of 1500 mL/m²/day in children (see Fluid and Electrolyte Requirements in Children). The fluid requirements in preterm infants are extremely variable due to much greater insensible water losses from radiant warmers and bili-lights. While the standard fluid maintenance of 100 mL/kg/day may be sufficient for term infants, intakes of up to 150 mL/kg/day may be necessary in the very low birth weight infants. Be sure to consider significant fluid intake from medications or other I.V. fluids and enteral diets in planning the fluids available for PN.

Dextrose

For central PN, dextrose is usually begun with a 10% to 12.5% solution or a solution providing dextrose at no more than 5 mg/kg/minute (in neonates and premature infants). The concentration is advanced, if tolerated, by 2.5% to 5% per day (2-2.5 mg/kg/minute increments in neonates and premature infants) to the desired caloric density, usually 20% to 25% dextrose. Fluid restricted patients often need 30% to 35% dextrose to meet their energy needs. For peripheral PN, 5% to 12.5% dextrose is utilized.

Dextrose calculations:

% Dextrose = dextrose (g)/100 mL

Dextrose calorie value = 3.4 kcal/g

$$\text{Dextrose infusion rate (mg/kg/minute)} = \frac{\text{rate (mL/h)} \times \text{\% dextrose} \times 0.166}{\text{weight (kg)}}$$

$$\text{\% Dextrose desired}^{1} = \frac{\text{desired rate (mg/kg/min)} \times \text{weight (kg)}}{0.166 \times \text{rate (mL/h)}}$$

[1]Do not use dextrose concentrations <5% due to hypotonicity.

Amino Acids

Amino acids may be described as either a "standard" mixture of essential and nonessential amino acids or "specialized" mixtures. Specialized mixtures are intended for use in patients whose physiologic or metabolic needs may not be met with the "standard" amino acid compositions. Examples of specialized solutions include:

TrophAmine®, Aminosyn® PF, PremaSol™	Indicated for use in premature infants and young children due to addition of taurine, L-glutamic acid, L-aspartic acid, increased amounts of histidine, and reduction in amounts of methionine, alanine, phenylalanine, and glycine. Supplementation with a cysteine additive has been recommended.
HepatAmine®	Indicated for treatment in patients with hepatic encephalopathy due to cirrhosis or hepatitis or in patients with liver disease who are intolerant of standard amino acid solutions. Contains higher percentage of branched-chain amino acids and a lower percentage of aromatic amino acids than standard mixtures.
NephrAmine®, Aminosyn® RF	Indicated for use in patients with compromised renal function who are intolerant of standard amino acid solutions. Contains a mixture of essential amino acids and histidine.

Amino acid calculations:

% amino acid = amino acid (g)/100mL

Grams of protein = grams of nitrogen x 6.25

$$\text{\% amino acid desired} = \frac{\text{(g amino acid/kg)} \times \text{weight (kg)} \times 100}{\text{total PN fluid volume (mL)}}$$

Fat Emulsion (FE)

There are three roles for intravenous fat in parenteral nutrition:

1. to provide nonprotein calories
2. to provide essential fatty acids and a "balanced" calorie source
3. to provide calories in catabolic patients with limited ability to excrete CO_2

The FE dosage is increased as tolerated daily (see General Guidelines for Initiation and Advancement for PN following). The maximum fat intake is 4 g/kg/day and no more than 60% of the total daily caloric intake. It is administered as a continuous infusion over 24 hours or at a rate no greater than 0.15-0.2 g/kg/hour via a Y-connector with the dextrose-amino acid I.V. line. In patients receiving cyclic PN, the FE should be administered over the duration of the PN infusion. The triglyceride concentration should be checked before the first infusion and daily as the dose is increased. Subsequently, it should be monitored at least weekly. Triglyceride concentrations should be maintained at <200 mg/dL in neonates, <350 mg/dL in renal patients, and <250 mg/dL in other patients. FE should be used cautiously in neonates with hyperbilirubinemia due to displacement of bilirubin from albumin by the free fatty acids. An increase in free bilirubin may increase the risk of kernicterus. Significant displacement occurs when the free fatty acid to serum albumin molar ratio (FFA/SA) >6. For example, infants with a total bilirubin >8-10 mg/dL (assuming an albumin concentration of 2.5-3 g/dL) should not receive more parenteral FE than required to meet the essential fatty acid requirement of 0.5-1 g/kg/day.

Note: Avoid use of 10% FE in preterm infants because a greater accumulation of plasma lipids occurs due to the greater phospholipid load of the 10% concentration.

Fat emulsion calculations:

20% FE = 20 g fat/100 mL = 2 kcal/mL

$$\text{Desired 20\% FE (mL)} = \frac{\text{(\% total kcal as fat)} \times \text{(total kcal)}}{\text{2 kcal/mL}}$$

or as an alternative

Desired 20% FE (mL) = FE (g/kg) x weight (kg) x 5 mL/g

PARENTERAL NUTRITION (PN) *(Continued)*

General Guidelines for Initiation and Advancement of PN[1]

Age	Initiation and Advancement[2]	Dextrose	Protein (g/kg/d)	Fat (g/kg/d)
Premature infant	Initial	4-6 mg/kg/min	0.5-1.5	0.5
	Daily increase	1-2.5 mg/kg/min	0.5-1	0.5
	Maximum	18 mg/kg/min	2.5-3	3
Term infant - 1 y	Initial	7-9 mg/kg/min	1-1.5	0.5-1
	Daily increase	1-2.5 mg/kg/min	1	0.5-1
	Maximum	21 mg/kg/min	2.5-3	4
Children 1-10 y	Initial dextrose concentration	10%-12.5%	1-1.5	1
	Daily increase	5% increments	1	1
	Maximum	15 mg/kg/min	2-2.5	3
>10 y	Initial dextrose concentration	10%-15%	1-1.5	1
	Daily increase	5% increments	1	1
	Maximum	8.5 mg/kg/min	1.5-2	3

[1]Rate of advancement may be limited by metabolic tolerance (eg, hyperglycemia, azotemia, hypertriglyceridemia)

[2]Timely intervention in premature infants is essential with initiation of dextrose as soon as possible after birth, amino acids within the first 12 hours, and fat emulsion within 24-48 hours of life.

MINERALS, TRACE ELEMENTS, AND VITAMINS

Guideline for Daily Electrolyte Requirements

	Neonates (mEq/kg)	Infants/Children (mEq/kg)	Adolescents
Sodium	2-5[1]	2-6	1-2 mEq/kg
Potassium	2-4	2-4	1-2 mEq/kg
Calcium gluconate[2]	3-4[3]	1-2.5	10-20 mEq/d
Magnesium	0.3-0.5	0.3-0.5	10-30 mEq/d
Phosphate[2]	1-2 mmol/kg[3]	0.5-1 mmol/kg	10-40 mmol/d

[1]Premature infants lose sodium in urine due to the immature resorptive function of kidney and diuretic use. Hyponatremia may lead to poor tissue growth and adverse developmental outcomes. Sodium content in PN may be adjusted to a maximum of 154 mEq/L (NS) to achieve normal sodium serum levels.

[2]Calcium-phosphate stability in parenteral nutrition solutions is dependent upon the pH of the solution, temperature, and relative concentration of each ion. The pH of the solution is primarily dependent upon the amino acid concentration. The higher the percentage amino acids the lower the pH, the more soluble the calcium and phosphate. Individual commercially available amino acid solutions vary significantly with respect to pH lowering potential and consequent calcium phosphate compatibility. See the pharmacist for specific calcium phosphate stability information.

[3]A 1.7:1 calcium to phosphate ratio in PN allows for the highest absolute retention of both minerals and simulates the in utero accretion of calcium and phosphate.

Vitamins

A pediatric parenteral multivitamin product is indicated for children <11 years of age. Children >11 years of age may receive adult multivitamin formulations.

Dosage:

Pediatric MVI:

Neonates: 2 mL/kg/d; maximum 5 mL/d

Infants and children ≤11 y: 5 mL

Children >11 y and adults: Use adult formulation 10 mL/d

Trace Mineral Daily Requirements[1]

	Infants	Children (≥3 mo to ≤5 y)	Older Children and Adolescents
Chromium[2]	0.2 mcg/kg	0.14-0.2 mcg/kg (max: 5 mcg)	10-15 mcg
Copper[3]	20 mcg/kg	20 mcg/kg (max: 300 mcg)	0.3-0.5 mg
Iodide[4]	1 mcg/kg	1 mcg/kg	1 mcg/kg
Manganese[3]	1 mcg/kg	2-10 mcg/kg (max: 50 mcg)	60-150 mcg
Selenium[2,5]	2-3 mcg/kg	2-3 mcg/kg (max: 30 mcg)	20-60 mcg
Zinc	400 mcg/kg (preterm) 300 mcg/kg (term <3 mo)	100 mcg/kg (max: 5 mg)	2.5-5 mg

[1]Recommended intakes of trace elements cannot be achieved through the use of a single pediatric trace element product. Only through the use of individualized trace element products can recommended intakes be achieved.
[2]Omit in patients with renal dysfunction.
[3]Omit in patients with impaired biliary excretion or cholestatic liver disease.
[4]Percutaneous absorption from protein-bound iodine may be adequate.
[5]Indicated for use in long-term parenteral nutrition patients.

These are recommended daily trace mineral requirements. Additional supplementation may be indicated in clinical conditions resulting in excessive losses. For example, additional zinc may be needed in situations of excessive gastrointestinal losses.

Developing the PN Goal Regimen

The purpose of this example is to illustrate the thought process in determining what dextrose and amino acid solution and fat emulsion intake would provide the desired daily fluid calorie and protein goals.

1. Calculate the fluid, protein, and caloric goals. Example:

   Weight = 10 kg
   Fluids = 100 mL/kg/day = 1000 mL
   Calories = 100 kcal/kg/day = 1000 kcal
   Protein = 2.5 g/kg/day = 25 g

2. If fat emulsion (FE) comprises 40% to 60% of the total daily calories, using the above example: 40% of 1000 kcal = 400 kcal.

   400 kcal ÷ 2 kcal/mL (20% FE) = 200 mL

3. To determine the goal dextrose concentration calculate the total daily calories remaining. Example:

   1000 kcal (total daily calories)
   - 400 kcal (daily calories from fats)
   600 kcal (total daily calories remaining)

4. Determine the concentration of dextrose to achieve the total daily calories remaining. Example:

   600 kcal ÷ 3.4 kcal/g x [100 ÷ 800 mL[1]] = 22%

   [1]Total daily fluids desired minus that from fats.

5. Calculate percent amino acid solution to achieve goal protein intake. Example:

   [25 g (total protein) ÷ 800 mL (total fluid)] x 100 = 3.1%

   This patient's goal regimen would be: dextrose 22%, amino acid 3.1%, 800 mL/day plus fat emulsion 20% 200 mL/day.

PARENTERAL NUTRITION (PN) *(Continued)*

Suggested PN Monitoring Guidelines

Parameter	Suggested Frequency Initial/Hospitalized	Suggested Frequency Follow-up/Outpatient
Growth		
Weight	Daily	Daily to q visit
Height/length	Weekly	Weekly to q visit
Body composition (triceps skinfold, bone age)	Initially	Monthly to annually
Metabolic (Serum[1])		
Electrolytes	Twice weekly	Weekly to q visit
BUN/creatinine	Weekly	Weekly to q visit
Acid-base status	Until stable	As indicated
Albumin/prealbumin	Weekly	Weekly to q visit
Glucose	Daily to weekly	Weekly to q visit
Triglyceride	Initially daily	Weekly to q visit
Liver function tests	Weekly	Weekly to q visit
Complete blood count/differential	Weekly	Weekly to q visit
Platelets, PT/PTT	Weekly	As indicated
Iron indices	As indicated	Biannually to annually
Trace elements	As indicated	Annually
Carnitine	As indicated	As indicated
Folate/vitamin B_{12}	As indicated	As indicated
Ammonia	As indicated	As indicated
Bilirubin, direct	Weekly	As indicated
Metabolic (Urine)		
Glucose	Twice daily	Daily to weekly
Ketone	Twice daily	Daily to weekly
Specific gravity	As indicated	As indicated
Urea nitrogen	As indicated	As indicated
Clinical Calculations		
Fluid balance	Daily	As indicated
Projected vs actual intake	Daily	Weekly to q visit
Calorie/protein intake	Daily	As indicated

Frequency depends on clinical condition.

[1]For metabolically unstable patients, need to check more frequently.

Adapted from "Guidelines for the Use of Parenteral and Enteral Nutrition in Adult and Pediatric Patients. ASPEN Board of Directors and The Clinical Guidelines Task Force," *JPEN J Parenter Enteral Nutr*, 2002, 26(1 Suppl):1-138SA.

Nutritional Guidelines for Pediatric Patients

Age	kcal/kg/d	Protein g/kg/d
Preterm neonate	120-140	3-4
Term infant - 1 y	90-120	2-3
1-7 y	75-90	1-1.2
7-12 y	60-75	1-1.2
12-18 y	30-60	0.8-0.9
>18 y	25-30	0.8

PN kcal/mL[1]

Dextrose Concentration						
5%	**10%**	**15%**	**20%**	**25%**	**30%**	**35%**
0.17	0.34	0.51	0.68	0.85	1.02	1.19

Dextrose provides 3.4 kcal/g.

Fat emulsion 10% provides 1.1 kcal/mL.

Fat emulsion 20% provides 2 kcal/mL.

[1]Calories derived from amino acids are not included.

Reference

"Guidelines for the Use of Parenteral and Enteral Nutrition in Adult and Pediatric Patients. ASPEN Board of Directors and The Clinical Guidelines Task Force," *JPEN J Parenter Enteral Nutr*, 2002, 26(1 Suppl):1-138SA.

Pharmacologic considerations of mixing medications with PN solutions include:

- Adsorption — bag, bottle, tubing, filter
- Blood levels
- Site of injection/administration
- Flush
- Amino acid-dextrose concentrations
- pH factors
- Temperature
- Additives in solution
- Heparin dose

GROWTH CHARTS

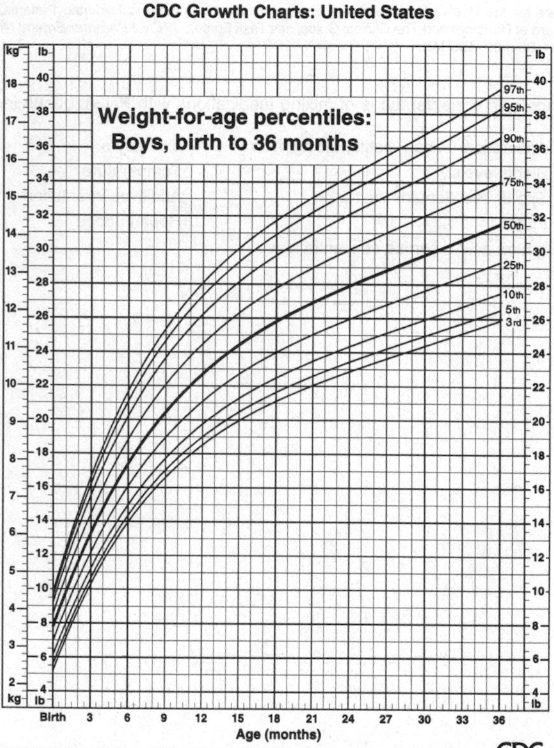

SOURCE: Developed by the National Center for Health Statistics in collaboration with the National Center for Chronic Disease Prevention and Health Promotion (2000). Available at http://www.cdc.gov/growthcharts

CDC Growth Charts: United States

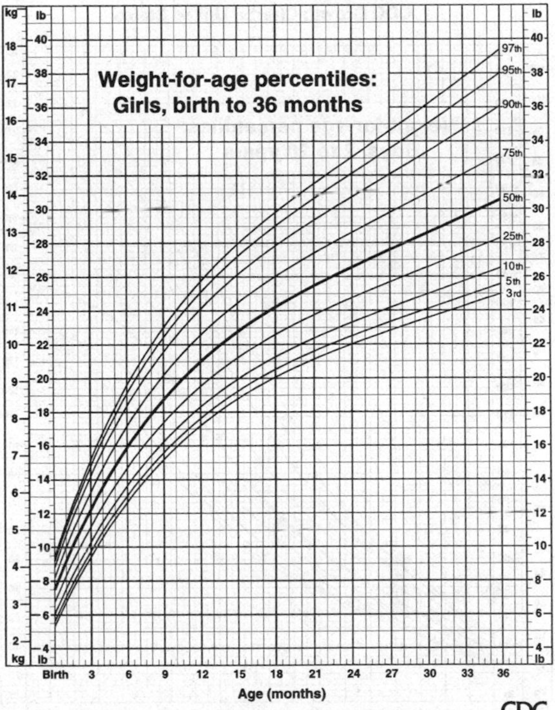

SOURCE: Developed by the National Center for Health Statistics in collaboration with the National Center for Chronic Disease Prevention and Health Promotion (2000).
Available at http://www.cdc.gov/growthcharts

GROWTH CHARTS *(Continued)*

CDC Growth Charts: United States

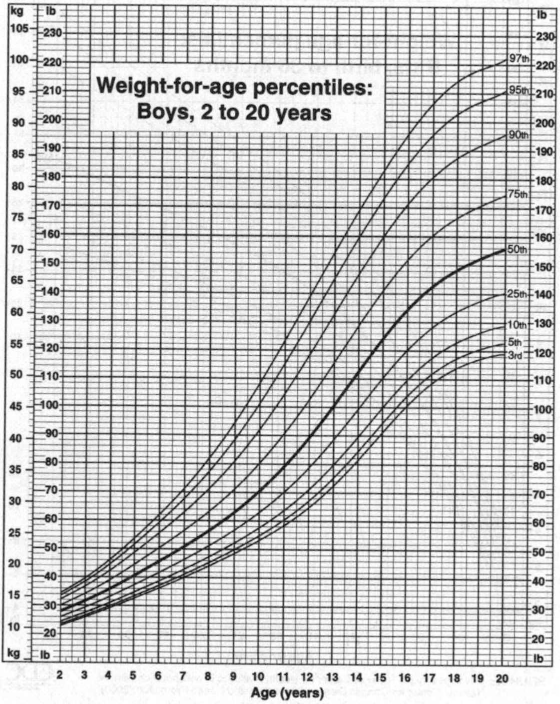

SOURCE: Developed by the National Center for Health Statistics in collaboration with the National Center for Chronic Disease Prevention and Health Promotion (2000).
Available at http://www.cdc.gov/growthcharts

CDC Growth Charts: United States

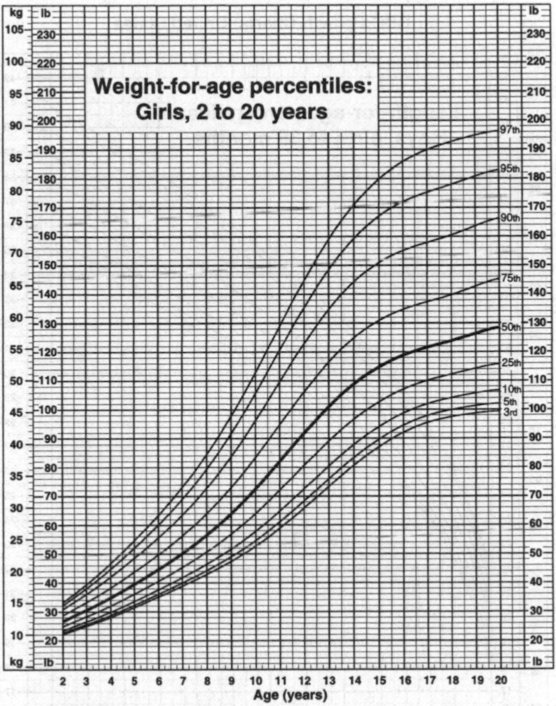

SOURCE: Developed by the National Center for Health Statistics in collaboration with the National Center for Chronic Disease Prevention and Health Promotion (2000).
Available at http://www.cdc.gov/growthcharts

GROWTH CHARTS *(Continued)*

CDC Growth Charts: United States

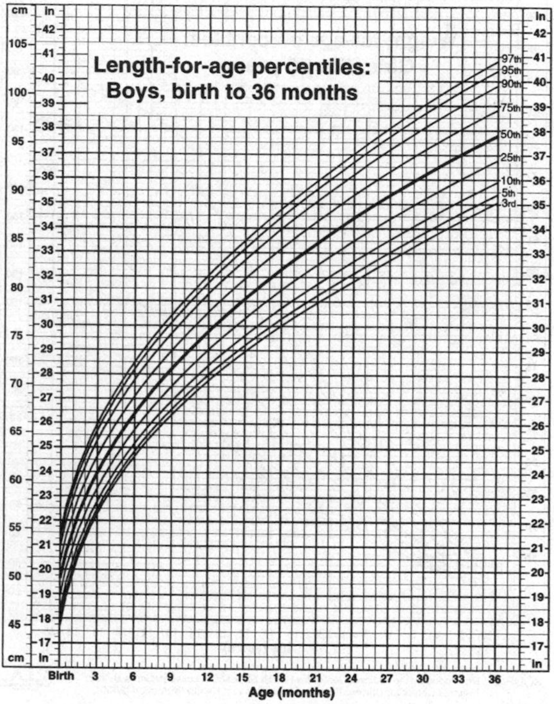

SOURCE: Developed by the National Center for Health Statistics in collaboration with the National Center for Chronic Disease Prevention and Health Promotion (2000).
Available at http://www.cdc.gov/growthcharts

CDC Growth Charts: United States

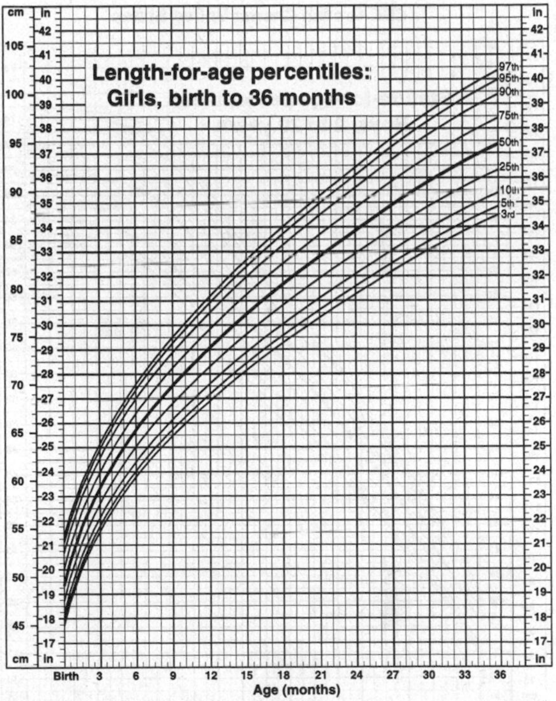

SOURCE: Developed by the National Center for Health Statistics in collaboration with the National Center for Chronic Disease Prevention and Health Promotion (2000).
Available at http://www.cdc.gov/growthcharts

GROWTH CHARTS *(Continued)*

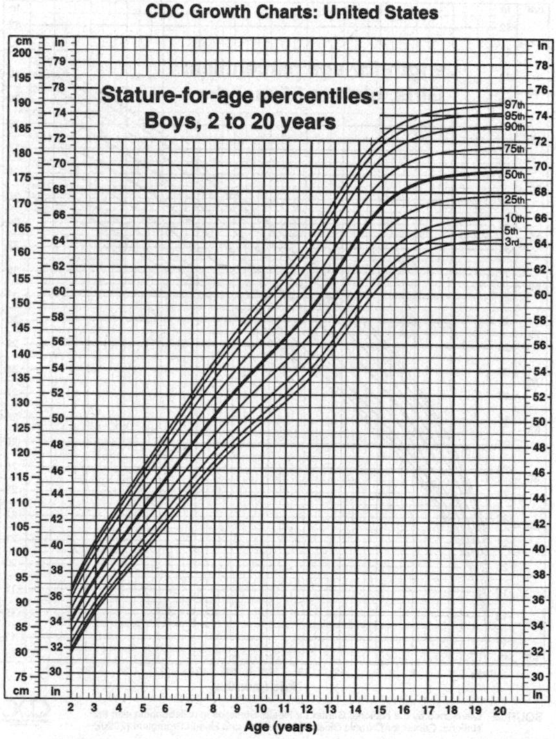

SOURCE: Developed by the National Center for Health Statistics in collaboration with the National Center for Chronic Disease Prevention and Health Promotion (2000). Available at http://www.cdc.gov/growthcharts

CDC Growth Charts: United States

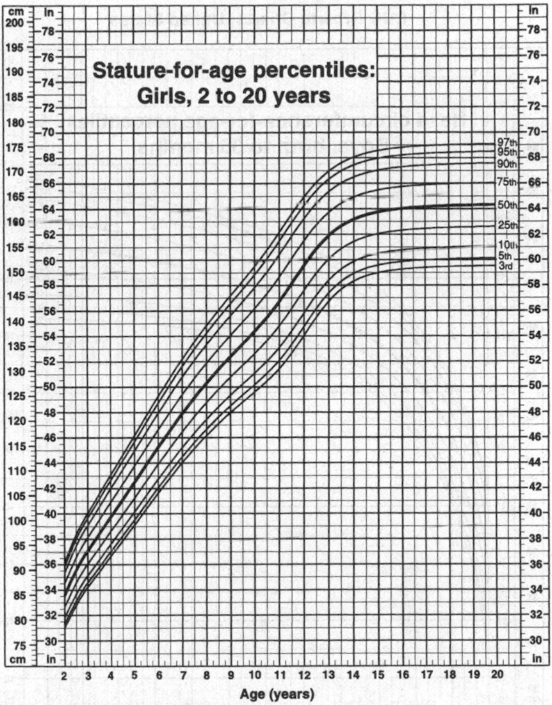

SOURCE: Developed by the National Center for Health Statistics in collaboration with the National Center for Chronic Disease Prevention and Health Promotion (2000).
Available at http://www.cdc.gov/growthcharts

GROWTH CHARTS *(Continued)*

CDC Growth Charts: United States

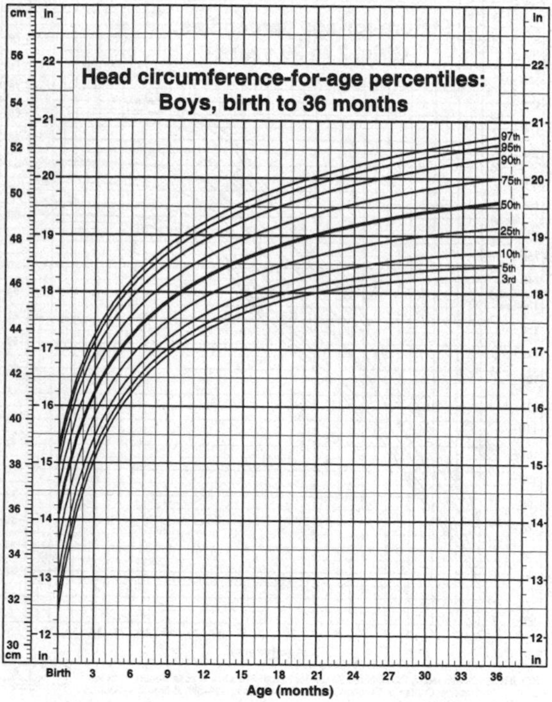

SOURCE: Developed by the National Center for Health Statistics in collaboration with the National Center for Chronic Disease Prevention and Health Promotion (2000). Available at http://www.cdc.gov/growthcharts

CDC Growth Charts: United States

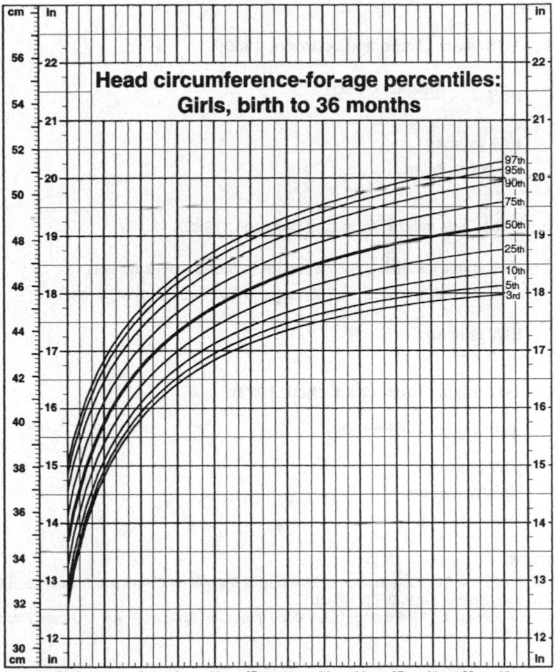

SOURCE: Developed by the National Center for Health Statistics in collaboration with the National Center for Chronic Disease Prevention and Health Promotion (2000).
Available at http://www.cdc.gov/growthcharts

IDEAL BODY WEIGHT CALCULATION

Adults (18 years and older)

IBW (male) = 50 + (2.3 x height in inches over 5 feet)
IBW (female) = 45.5 + (2.3 x height in inches over 5 feet)

IBW is in kg.

Children

a. 1-18 years (Traub and Johnson, 1980)

$$\text{IBW} = \frac{(\text{height}^2 \times 1.65)}{1000}$$

IBW is in kg.
Height is in cm.

b. 5 feet and taller (Traub and Johnson, 1980)

IBW (male) = 39 + (2.27 x height in inches over 5 feet)
IBW (female) = 42.2 + (2.27 x height in inches over 5 feet)

IBW is in kg.

c. 1-17 years (Traub and Kichen, 1983)

$$\text{IBW} = 2.396e^{0.01883\,(\text{height})}$$

IBW is in kg.
Height is in cm.

References

Traub SL and Johnson CE, "Comparison of Methods of Estimating Creatinine Clearance in Children," *Am J Hosp Pharm*, 1980, 37(2):195-201.

Traub SL and Kichen L, "Estimating Ideal Body Mass in Children," *Am J Hosp Pharm*, 1983, 40(1):107-10.

BODY SURFACE AREA OF CHILDREN AND ADULTS

Calculating Body Surface Area in Children

In a child of average size, find weight and corresponding surface area on the boxed scale to the left; or, use the nomogram to the right. Lay a straightedge on the correct height and weight points for the child, then read the intersecting point on the surface area scale.

FOR CHILDREN OF NORMAL HEIGHT AND WEIGHT

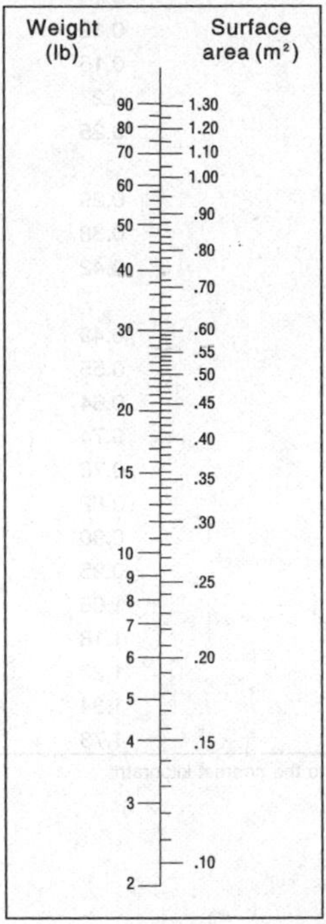

NOMOGRAM

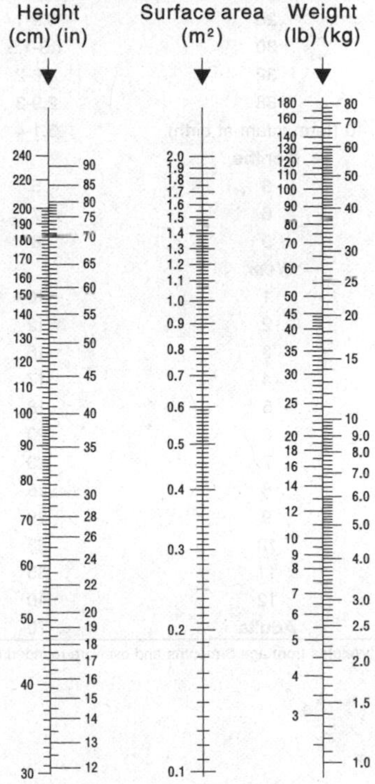

BODY SURFACE AREA FORMULA (Adult and Pediatric)

$$\text{BSA (m}^2\text{)} = \sqrt{\frac{\text{Ht (in)} \times \text{Wt (lb)}}{3131}}$$ or, in metric: $$\text{BSA (m}^2\text{)} = \sqrt{\frac{\text{Ht (cm)} \times \text{Wt (kg)}}{3600}}$$

References

Lam TK and Leung DT, "More on Simplified Calculation of Body Surface Area," *N Engl J Med*, 1988, 318(17):1130 (Letter).

Mosteller RD, "Simplified Calculation of Body Surface Area", *N Engl J Med*, 1987, 317(17):1098 (Letter).

AVERAGE WEIGHTS AND SURFACE AREAS

Average Weight and Surface Area of Preterm Infants, Term Infants, and Children

Age	Average Weight (kg)[1]	Approximate Surface Area (m^2)
Weeks Gestation		
26	0.9-1	0.1
30	1.3-1.5	0.12
32	1.6-2	0.15
38	2.9-3	0.2
40 (term infant at birth)	3.1-4	0.25
Months		
3	5	0.29
6	7	0.38
9	8	0.42
Year		
1	10	0.49
2	12	0.55
3	15	0.64
4	17	0.74
5	18	0.76
6	20	0.82
7	23	0.90
8	25	0.95
9	28	1.06
10	33	1.18
11	35	1.23
12	40	1.34
Adults	70	1.73

[1]Weights from age 3 months and over are rounded off to the nearest kilogram.

PHYSICAL DEVELOPMENT

Weight gain first 6 weeks

20 g/day

Birth weight

regained by day 14
doubles by age 4 mo
triples by age 12 mo
quadruples by age 2 y

Teeth

1st tooth 6-18 mo
teeth = age (mo) − 6 (until 30 mo)

Head circumference

35 cm at birth
44 cm by 6 mo
47 cm by 1 y
1 cm/mo for 1st y
3 cm/mo 2nd y

Length

increases 50% by age 1 y
doubles by age 4 y
triples by age 13 y

Tanner Stages of Sexual Development

Stage	Characteristics	Age at Onset (mean ± SD)
Genital stages: Male		
1	Prepubertal	
2	Scrotum and testes enlarge; skin of scrotum reddens and rugations appear	11.4 ± 1.1 y
3	Penis lengthens; testes enlarge further	12.9 ± 1 y
4	Penis growth continues in length and width; glans develops adult form	13.8 ± 1 y
5	Development completed; adult appearance	14.9 ± 1.1 y
Breast development: Female		
1	Prepubertal	
2	Breast buds appear; areolae enlarge	11.2 ± 1.1 y
3	Elevation of breast contour; areolae enlarge	12.2 ± 1.1 y
4	Areolae and papilla form a secondary mound on breast	13.1 ± 1.2 y
5	Adult form	15.3 ± 1.7 y
Menarche		
Pubic hair: Both sexes		13.5 ± 1 y
1	Prepubertal, no coarse hair	
2	Longer, silky hair appears at base of penis or along labia	F: 11.7 ± 1.2 y M: 12 ± 1 y
3	Hair coarse, kinky, spreads over pubic bone	F: 12.4 ± 1.1 y M: 13.9 ± 1 y
4	Hair of adult quality but not spread to junction of medial thigh with perineum	F: 13 ± 1 y M: 14.4 ± 1.1 y
5	Spread to medial thigh	F: 14.4 ± 1.1 y M: 15.2 ± 1.1 y
6	"Male escutcheon"	Variable if occurs

Maximum growth rate

Male at 14.1±0.9 y
Female at 12.1±0.9 y

EMETOGENIC POTENTIAL OF SINGLE CHEMOTHERAPEUTIC AGENTS

Class I — Low (<10%)

Asparaginase/Pegaspargase
Bleomycin
Busulfan
Chlorambucil (oral)
Cladribine
Corticosteroids
Cyclophosphamide (oral)
Fludarabine
Hydroxyurea
Melphalan (oral)
Mercaptopurine
Methotrexate <50 mg/m^2
Thioguanine (oral)
Vinblastine
Vincristine

Class II — Moderately Low (10% to 30%)

Cytarabine <500 mg/m^2
Doxorubicin ≤20 mg/m^2
Etoposide
Fluorouracil <1000 mg/m^2
Gemcitabine
Interferon-beta
Lomustine
Methotrexate ≥50-250 mg/m^2
Mitomycin <8 mg/m^2
Paclitaxel
Raltitrexed
Thiotepa

Class III — Moderate (30% to 60%)

Amsacrine
Azacitidine
Cyclophosphamide <750 mg/m^2
Cytarabine 500-1000 mg/m^2
Daunorubicin
Docetaxel
Doxorubicin >20 mg to <60 mg/m^2
Epirubicin
Fluorouracil ≥1000 mg/m^2
Idarubicin
Ifosfamide
Irinotecan
Methotrexate >250 mg/m^2 to ≤1000 mg/m^2
Mitomycin ≥8 mg/m^2
Mitoxantrone
Teniposide
Topotecan
Tretinoin
Vinorelbine

Class IV — Moderately High (60% to 90%)

Actinomycin D
Aldesleukin
Carboplatin 200-400 mg/m^2
Carmustine <250 mg
Cisplatin <50 mg/m^2
Cyclophosphamide 750-1500 mg/m^2
Cytarabine >1000 mg/m^2
Dacarbazine <500 mg/m^2
Doxorubicin ≥60 mg/m^2
Melphalan 20-80 mg/m^2
Methotrexate >1000 mg/m^2
Procarbazine (oral)

Class V — High (>90%)

Busulfan (as part of BMT regimen)
Carboplatin >500 mg/m^2
Carmustine ≥250 mg/m^2
Cisplatin ≥50 mg/m^2
Cyclophosphamide ≥1500 mg/m^2
Dacarbazine ≥500 mg/m^2
Mechlorethamine
Melphalan >80 mg/m^2
Pentostatin

COMPATIBILITY OF CHEMOTHERAPY AND RELATED SUPPORTIVE CARE MEDICATIONS

Compatible: The drugs are physically compatible when mixed in the same container or infused through the same I.V. line simultaneously.

Y-site compatible: The drugs are physically compatible when infused through the same I.V. line simultaneously.

Incompatible: The drugs are physically incompatible when mixed in the same container, or infused through the same I.V. line simultaneously.

Variable compatibility: The compatibility of the drugs varies according to the concentration and/or diluent of the drugs. Please refer to the table at the end of this section for more information on variable compatibility.

Abbreviations

AA	Amino acid solution
BNS	Bacteriostatic normal saline
BWI	Bacteriostatic water for injection
D_5W	5% dextrose in water
D_5/NS	5% dextrose in 0.9% sodium chloride
$D_5/^1/_4NS$	5% dextrose in 0.225% sodium chloride
$D_5/^1/_2NS$	5% dextrose in 0.45% sodium chloride
D_5LR	5% dextrose in lactated Ringer's injection
$D_{10}W$	10% dextrose in water
$D_{10}W$/0.01% albumin	10% dextrose in water with 0.01% albumin
$D_{10}W$/0.05% albumin	10% dextrose in water with 0.05% albumin
$D_{10}W$/0.1% albumin	10% dextrose in water with 0.1% albumin
D_{10}/NS	10% dextrose in water in 0.9% sodium chloride
LR	Lactated Ringer's injection
NS	0.9% sodium chloride (normal saline)
SWI	Sterile water for injection
TPN	Total parenteral nutrition solution

COMPATIBILITY OF CHEMOTHERAPY AND RELATED SUPPORTIVE CARE MEDICATIONS *(Continued)*

Reported Compatibilities and Incompatibilities of Parenteral Dosage Forms

Aldesleukin

Compatible:

D_5W
SWI

Y-Site Compatible:

Amikacin
Amphotericin
Calcium gluconate
Cotrimoxazole
Diphenhydramine
Dopamine
Fat emulsion
Fluconazole
Foscarnet
Gentamicin
Heparin
Magnesium sulfate
Metoclopramide
Morphine
Ondansetron
Piperacillin
Potassium chloride
Ranitidine
Thiethylperazine
Ticarcillin
Tobramycin

Incompatible:

Ganciclovir
Heparin
Pentamidine
Prochlorperazine
Promethazine

Amifostine

Compatible:

NS

Y-Site Compatible:

Amikacin
Aminophylline
Ampicillin
Ampicillin/sulbactam
Aztreonam
Bleomycin
Bumetanide
Buprenorphine
Butorphanol
Calcium gluconate
Carboplatin
Carmustine
Cefamandole
Cefepime
Cefotaxime
Cefotetan
Cefoxitin
Ceftazidime
Ceftizoxime
Ceftriaxone
Cefuroxime
Cimetidine
Ciprofloxacin
Clindamycin
Cotrimoxazole
Cyclophosphamide
Cytarabine
Dacarbazine
Dactinomycin
Daunomycin
Dexamethasone
Diphenhydramine
Dobutamine
Dopamine
Doxorubicin
Doxycycline
Droperidol
Enalaprilat
Etoposide
Famotidine
Floxuridine
Fluconazole
Fludarabine
Fluorouracil
Furosemide
Gallium nitrate
Gemcitabine
Gentamicin
Granisetron
Haloperidol
Heparin
Hydrocortisone sodium phosphate
Hydrocortisone sodium succinate
Hydromorphone
Idarubicin
Ifosfamide
Imipenem/cilastatin
Leucovorin
Lorazepam
Magnesium sulfate
Mannitol
Mechlorethamine
Meperidine
Mesna
Methotrexate
Methylprednisolone
Metoclopramide
Metronidazole
Mezlocillin
Mitomycin
Mitoxantrone
Morphine
Nalbuphine
Netilmicin
Ondansetron
Piperacillin
Plicamycin
Potassium chloride
Promethazine
Ranitidine
Sodium bicarbonate
Streptozocin
Teniposide
Thiotepa
Ticarcillin
Ticarcillin/clavulanate
Tobramycin
Trimetrexate
Vancomycin
Vinblastine
Vincristine

Incompatible:

Acyclovir
Amphotericin
Chlorpromazine
Cisplatin
Ganciclovir
Hydroxyzine
Minocycline
Prochlorperazine

Asparaginase

Compatible:

D_5W
NS
SWI

Y-Site Compatible:

Methotrexate
Sodium bicarbonate

Bleomycin

Compatible:

BNS
BWI
SWI
Amikacin
Amsacrine
Ceftazidime
Cephapirin
Cimetidine
Dacarbazine
Dexamethasone
Diphenhydramine
Droperidol
Fluorouracil
Furosemide
Gentamicin
Heparin
Hydrocortisone sodium phosphate
Leucovorin
Metoclopramide
Phenytoin
Streptomycin
Tobramycin
Vinblastine
Vincristine

Y-Site Compatible:

Allopurinol
Amifostine
Aztreonam
Cefepime
Cisplatin
Cyclophosphamide
Doxorubicin
Doxorubicin, liposomal
Filgrastim
Fludarabine
Gemcitabine
Methotrexate
Mitomycin
Ondansetron
Paclitaxel
Piperacillin
Sargramostim
Teniposide
Thiotepa
Vinorelbine

Incompatible:

Aminophylline
Ascorbic acid
Cefazolin
Cephalothin
Diazepam
Doxapram
Hydrocortisone sodium succinate
Nafcillin
Penicillin G
Terbutaline

Variable Compatibility:

D_5W
NS

Busulfan

Compatible:

D_5W
NS

Carboplatin

Compatible:

D_5W
SWI
Etoposide
Floxuridine
Ifosfamide

Y-Site Compatible:

Allopurinol
Amifostine
Aztreonam
Cefazolin
Doxorubicin, liposomal
Filgrastim
Fludarabine
Gemcitabine
Granisetron
Ondansetron
Piperacillin
Piperacillin/tazobactam
Propofol
Sargramostim
Teniposide
Thiotepa
TPN
Vinorelbine

Incompatible:

Fluorouracil
Mesna
Sodium bicarbonate

Variable Compatibility:

D_5/NS
$D_5/^1/_4$NS
$D_5/^1/_2$NS
NS

COMPATIBILITY OF CHEMOTHERAPY AND RELATED SUPPORTIVE CARE MEDICATIONS *(Continued)*

Carmustine

Compatible:

- D_5W
- NS
- SWI
- Dacarbazine

Y-Site Compatible:

- Amifostine
- Aztreonam
- Cefepime
- Filgrastim
- Fludarabine
- Gemcitabine
- Ondansetron
- Piperacillin
- Piperacillin/tazobactam
- Sargramostim
- Teniposide
- Thiotepa
- Vinorelbine

Incompatible:

- Allopurinol
- Sodium bicarbonate

Cisplatin

Compatible:

- D_5/NS
- $D_5/\frac{1}{4}NS$
- $D_5/\frac{1}{2}NS$
- NS
- Cefazolin
- Cephalothin
- Cyclophosphamide
- Floxuridine
- Hydroxyzine
- Hydroxyurea
- Ifosfamide
- Leucovorin
- Mannitol
- Mechlorethamine
- Ondansetron

Y-Site Compatible:

- Allopurinol
- Aztreonam
- Bleomycin
- Bumetanide
- Chlorpromazine
- Cimetidine
- Dexamethasone
- Diphenhydramine
- Doxapram
- Doxorubicin
- Doxorubicin, liposomal
- Droperidol
- Famotidine
- Filgrastim
- Fludarabine
- Fluorouracil
- Furosemide
- Ganciclovir
- Gemcitabine
- Granisetron
- Heparin
- Hydromorphone
- Lorazepam
- Methotrexate
- Methylprednisolone
- Metoclopramide
- Mitomycin
- Morphine
- Paclitaxel
- Potassium chloride
- Prochlorperazine
- Promethazine
- Propofol
- Ranitidine
- Sargramostim
- Teniposide
- Thiotepa
- Vinorelbine

Incompatible:

- Amifostine
- Amsacrine
- Cefepime
- Gallium nitrate
- Mesna
- Oxacillin
- Piperacillin
- Piperacillin/tazobactam
- Sodium bicarbonate

Variable Compatibility:

- D_5W
- SWI
- Etoposide

Cladribine

Compatible:

- NS

Cyclophosphamide

Compatible:

- D_5W
- D_5/NS
- D_5/LR
- NS
- LR
- SWI
- AA 4.25%/$D_{25}W$
- Cisplatin
- Dacarbazine
- Etoposide
- Fluorouracil
- Hydroxyzine
- Mesna
- Methotrexate
- Mitoxantrone
- Ondansetron

Y-Site Compatible:

- Allopurinol
- Amifostine
- Amikacin
- Ampicillin
- Azlocillin
- Aztreonam
- Bleomycin
- Cefamandole
- Cefazolin
- Cefepime
- Cefoperazone
- Cefotaxime
- Cefoxitin
- Ceftriaxone
- Cephalothin
- Cephapirin
- Chloramphenicol
- Chlorpromazine
- Cimetidine
- Clindamycin
- Cotrimoxazole
- Dexamethasone
- Diphenhydramine
- Doxapram
- Doxorubicin
- Doxorubicin, liposomal
- Doxycycline
- Droperidol
- Erythromycin
- Famotidine
- Filgrastim
- Fludarabine
- Furosemide
- Gallium nitrate
- Ganciclovir
- Gemcitabine
- Gentamicin
- Granisetron
- Heparin
- Hydromorphone
- Idarubicin
- Kanamycin

Leucovorin
Lorazepam
Methylprednisolone
Metoclopramide
Metronidazole
Mezlocillin
Minocycline
Mitomycin
Morphine
Moxalactam
Nafcillin
Oxacillin
Paclitaxel
Penicillin G
Piperacillin
Piperacillin/tazobactam
Prochlorperazine
Promethazine
Propofol
Ranitidine
Sargramostim
Sodium bicarbonate
Teniposide
Thiotepa
Ticarcillin
Ticarcillin/clavulanate
Tobramycin
TPN
Vancomycin
Vinblastine
Vincristine
Vinorelbine

Cytarabine

Compatible:

BNS
BWI
D_5W
D_5/NS
$D_5/{}^1/_4NS$
$D_5/{}^1/_2NS$
D_5/LR
D_{10}/NS
NS
LR
AA 4.25%/$D_{25}W$
Corticotropin
Dacarbazine
Daunomycin
Etoposide
Hydroxyzine
Hydroxyurea
Lincomycin
Mitoxantrone
Ondansetron
Potassium chloride
Prednisolone
Sodium bicarbonate
Vincristine

Y-Site Compatible:

Amifostine
Amsacrine
Aztreonam
Cefepime
Chlorpromazine
Cimetidine
Dexamethasone
Diphenhydramine
Doxorubicin, liposomal
Droperidol
Famotidine
Filgrastim
Fludarabine
Furosemide
Gemcitabine
Granisetron
Heparin
Idarubicin
Lorazepam
Metoclopramide
Morphine
Paclitaxel
Piperacillin
Piperacillin/tazobactam
Prochlorperazine
Promethazine
Propofol
Ranitidine
Sargramostim
Teniposide
Thiotepa
TPN
Vinorelbine

Incompatible:

Allopurinol
Ceftazidime
Fluorouracil
Gallium nitrate
Ganciclovir
Insulin
Nafcillin
Oxacillin
Penicillin G

Variable Compatibility:

Cephalothin
Gentamicin
Hydrocortisone sodium phosphate
Methylprednisolone

Dacarbazine

Compatible:

NS
SWI
Bleomycin
Carmustine
Cimetidine
Cyclophosphamide
Cytarabine
Dactinomycin
Doxorubicin
Fluorouracil
Mercaptopurine
Methotrexate
Ondansetron
Vinblastine

Y-Site Compatible:

Amifostine
Aztreonam
Doxorubicin, liposomal
Filgrastim
Fludarabine
Granisetron
Hydrocortisone sodium phosphate
Lidocaine
Paclitaxel
Sargramostim
Teniposide
Thiotepa
Vinorelbine

Incompatible:

D_5W
Allopurinol
Cefepime
Hydrocortisone sodium succinate
Piperacillin
Piperacillin/tazobactam

Variable Compatibility:

Heparin

Dactinomycin

Compatible:

D_5W
NS
SWI
Dacarbazine

Y-Site Compatible:

Allopurinol
Amifostine
Aztreonam
Cefepime
Fludarabine
Gemcitabine
Ondansetron
Sargramostim
Teniposide
Thiotepa
Vinorelbine

COMPATIBILITY OF CHEMOTHERAPY AND RELATED SUPPORTIVE CARE MEDICATIONS *(Continued)*

Incompatible:

- BNS
- BWI
- Filgrastim

Daunomycin

Compatible:

- D_5W
- NS
- LR
- SWI
- Cytarabine
- Etoposide
- Hydrocortisone sodium succinate

Y-Site Compatible:

- Amifostine
- Filgrastim
- Gemcitabine
- Methotrexate
- Ondansetron
- Sodium bicarbonate
- Teniposide
- Thiotepa
- Vinorelbine

Incompatible:

- Allopurinol
- Aztreonam
- Cefepime
- Dexamethasone
- Fludarabine
- Piperacillin
- Piperacillin/tazobactam

Dexrazoxane

Compatible:

- D_5W

Y-Site Compatible:

- Gemcitabine

Diphenhydramine

Compatible:

- Amikacin
- Aminophylline
- Ascorbic acid
- Atropine
- Bleomycin
- Butorphanol
- Cephapirin
- Chlorpromazine
- Cimetidine
- Colistimethate
- Dimenhydrinate
- Droperidol
- Erythromycin
- Fentanyl
- Fluphenazine
- Glycopyrrolate
- Hydrocortisone sodium succinate
- Hydromorphone
- Hydroxyzine
- Lidocaine
- Meperidine
- Methicillin
- Methyldopate
- Metoclopramide
- Midazolam
- Morphine
- Nalbuphine
- Nafcillin
- Netilmicin
- Penicillin G (sodium and potassium)
- Pentazocine
- Perphenazine
- Prochlorperazine
- Promazine
- Promethazine
- Ranitidine
- Scopolamine
- Sufentanil
- Thiothixene
- Polymyxin B
- Vitamin B complex with C

Y-Site Compatible:

- Acyclovir
- Aldesleukin
- Amifostine
- Amsacrine
- Aztreonam
- Ciprofloxacin
- Cisplatin
- Cyclophosphamide
- Cytarabine
- Doxorubicin
- Filgrastim
- Fluconazole
- Fludarabine
- Gallium nitrate
- Gemcitabine
- Granisetron
- Heparin
- Idarubicin
- Melphalan
- Meperidine
- Methotrexate
- Ondansetron
- Paclitaxel
- Piperacillin/tazobactam
- Potassium chloride
- Sargramostim
- Tacrolimus
- Teniposide
- Thiotepa
- Vinorelbine

Incompatible:

Allopurinol
Amobarbital
Amphotericin
Cefepime
Cephalothin
Dexamethasone
Foscarnet
Haloperidol
Pentobarbital
Secobarbital
Thiopental

Variable Compatibility:

Diatrizoate
Iodipamide

Docetaxel

Compatible:

D_5W
NS

Y-Site Compatible:

Gemcitabine

Incompatible:

Doxorubicin, liposomal

Doxorubicin

Compatible:

D_5W
NS
LR
Dacarbazine
Ondansetron
Vincristine

Y-Site Compatible:

Amifostine
Aztreonam
Bleomycin
Chlorpromazine
Cimetidine
Cisplatin
Cyclophosphamide
Dexamethasone
Diphenhydramine
Famotidine
Filgrastim
Fludarabine
Gemcitabine
Granisetron
Hydromorphone
Leucovorin
Lorazepam
Methotrexate
Methylprednisolone
Metoclopramide
Mitomycin
Morphine
Paclitaxel
Prochlorperazine
Promethazine
Propofol
Ranitidine
Sargramostim
Sodium bicarbonate
Teniposide
Thiotepa
Vinorelbine

Incompatible:

Allopurinol
Aminophylline
Cefepime
Cephalothin
Diazepam
Furosemide
Gallium nitrate
Ganciclovir
Heparin
Hydrocortisone sodium succinate
Piperacillin/tazobactam
TPN
Paclitaxel
Tobramycin

Variable Compatibility:

Fluorouracil
Vinblastine

Doxorubicin, Liposomal

Compatible:

D_5W

Y-Site Compatible:

Allopurinol
Aldesleukin
Aminophylline
Ampicillin
Aztreonam
Bleomycin
Calcium chloride
Calcium gluconate
Cefazolin
Cefepime
Cefoperazone
Cefoxitin
Ceftizoxime
Ceftriaxone
Chlorpromazine
Cimetidine
Ciprofloxacin
Cisplatin
Clindamycin
Cotrimoxazole
Cyclophosphamide
Cytarabine
Dacarbazine
Dexamethasone
Diphenhydramine
Dobutamine
Dopamine
Droperidol
Enalaprilat
Etoposide
Famotidine
Fluconazole
Fluorouracil
Furosemide
Ganciclovir
Gentamicin
Granisetron
Haloperidol
Heparin
Hydrocortisone sodium succinate
Hydromorphone
Ifosfamide
Leucovorin
Lorazepam
Magnesium sulfate
Mesna
Methotrexate
Methylprednisolone
Metronidazole
Mezlocillin
Netilmicin
Ondansetron
Piperacillin
Potassium chloride
Prochlorperazine
Ranitidine
Ticarcillin
Ticarcillin/clavulanate
Tobramycin
Vancomycin
Vinblastine
Vincristine
Vinorelbine

COMPATIBILITY OF CHEMOTHERAPY AND RELATED SUPPORTIVE CARE MEDICATIONS *(Continued)*

Incompatible:

- Amphotericin
- Buprenorphine
- Ceftazidime
- Docetaxel
- Gallium nitrate
- Hydroxyzine
- Mannitol
- Meperidine
- Metoclopramide
- Miconazole
- Mitoxantrone
- Morphine
- Ofloxacin
- Piperacillin/tazobactam
- Promethazine
- Sodium bicarbonate

Droperidol

Compatible:

- Atropine
- Bleomycin
- Butorphanol
- Chlorpromazine
- Cimetidine
- Cisplatin
- Cyclophosphamide
- Dimenhydrinate
- Diphenhydramine
- Doxorubicin
- Fentanyl
- Glycopyrrolate
- Hydroxyzine
- Meperidine
- Metoclopramide
- Midazolam
- Mitomycin
- Morphine
- Nalbuphine
- Pentazocine
- Perphenazine
- Prochlorperazine
- Promazine
- Promethazine
- Scopolamine
- Vinblastine
- Vincristine

Y-Site Compatible:

- Amifostine
- Aztreonam
- Filgrastim
- Fluconazole
- Fludarabine
- Gemcitabine
- Hydrocortisone sodium succinate
- Idarubicin
- Melphalan
- Ondansetron
- Paclitaxel
- Potassium chloride
- Sargramostim
- Teniposide
- Thiotepa
- Vinorelbine
- Vitamin B complex with C

Incompatible:

- Allopurinol
- Cefepime
- Fluorouracil
- Foscarnet
- Furosemide
- Heparin
- Leucovorin
- Methotrexate
- Nafcillin
- Pentobarbital
- Piperacillin/tazobactam

Erythropoietin

Compatible:

- BNS
- D_{10}/0.05% albumin
- D_{10}/0.1% albumin

Incompatible:

- $D_{10}W$
- D_{10}/0.01% albumin
- NS
- SWI

Etoposide

Compatible:

- D_5W
- NS
- LR
- Carboplatin
- Cyclophosphamide
- Cytarabine
- Daunomycin
- Floxuridine
- Fluorouracil
- Hydroxyzine
- Ifosfamide
- Ondansetron

Y-Site Compatible:

- Allopurinol
- Amifostine
- Aztreonam
- Doxorubicin, liposomal
- Fludarabine
- Gemcitabine
- Granisetron
- Haloperidol
- Methotrexate
- Paclitaxel
- Piperacillin
- Piperacillin/tazobactam
- Sargramostim
- Sodium bicarbonate
- Teniposide
- Vinorelbine

Incompatible:

- Cefoperazone
- Ceftazidime
- Cefepime
- Filgrastim
- Gallium nitrate
- Idarubicin

Variable Compatibility:

- Cisplatin
- Mannitol
- Potassium chloride

Filgrastim

Compatible:

- D_5W
- SWI

Y-Site Compatible:

- Acyclovir
- Allopurinol
- Amikacin
- Aminophylline
- Ampicillin
- Ampicillin/sulbactam
- Aztreonam
- Bleomycin
- Bumetanide
- Buprenorphine
- Butorphanol
- Calcium gluconate
- Carboplatin
- Carmustine
- Cefazolin
- Cefotetan
- Ceftazidime
- Chlorpromazine
- Cimetidine
- Cisplatin
- Cotrimoxazole
- Cyclophosphamide
- Cytarabine
- Dacarbazine
- Daunomycin
- Dexamethasone
- Diphenhydramine
- Doxorubicin
- Doxycycline
- Droperidol
- Enalaprilat
- Fat emulsion
- Floxuridine
- Fluconazole
- Fludarabine
- Gallium nitrate
- Ganciclovir
- Gentamicin
- Haloperidol
- Hydrocortisone sodium phosphate
- Hydrocortisone sodium succinate
- Hydromorphone
- Hydroxyzine
- Idarubicin
- Ifosfamide
- Imipenem/cilastatin
- Leucovorin
- Lorazepam
- Mechlorethamine
- Meperidine
- Mesna
- Methotrexate
- Metoclopramide
- Miconazole
- Minocycline
- Mitoxantrone
- Morphine
- Nalbuphine
- Netilmicin
- Ondansetron
- Plicamycin
- Potassium chloride
- Promethazine
- Ranitidine
- Sodium bicarbonate
- Streptozocin
- Ticarcillin
- Ticarcillin/clavulanate
- Tobramycin
- Vancomycin
- Vinblastine
- Vincristine
- Vinorelbine

Incompatible:

- NS
- Amphotericin
- Amsacrine
- Cefepime
- Cefonicid
- Cefoperazone
- Cefotaxime
- Cefoxitin
- Ceftizoxime
- Ceftriaxone
- Cefuroxime
- Dactinomycin
- Etoposide
- Fluorouracil
- Furosemide
- Heparin
- Mannitol
- Methylprednisolone
- Metronidazole
- Mezlocillin
- Mitomycin
- Piperacillin
- Prochlorperazine
- Thiotepa

Floxuridine

Compatible:

- D_5W
- NS
- SWI
- Carboplatin
- Cisplatin
- Etoposide
- Fluorouracil
- Heparin
- Leucovorin

Y-Site Compatible:

- Amifostine
- Aztreonam
- Filgrastim
- Fludarabine
- Gemcitabine
- Ondansetron
- Paclitaxel
- Piperacillin/tazobactam
- Sargramostim
- Teniposide
- Thiotepa
- Vinorelbine

Incompatible:

- Allopurinol
- Cefepime

Fludarabine

Compatible:

- D_5W
- NS
- SWI

Y-Site Compatible:

- Allopurinol
- Amifostine
- Amikacin
- Aminophylline
- Ampicillin
- Ampicillin/sulbactam
- Amsacrine
- Aztreonam
- Bleomycin
- Butorphanol
- Carboplatin
- Carmustine
- Cefazolin
- Cefepime
- Cefoperazone
- Cefotaxime
- Cefotetan
- Ceftazidime
- Ceftizoxime
- Ceftriaxone
- Cefuroxime
- Cimetidine
- Cisplatin
- Cotrimoxazole
- Cyclophosphamide
- Cytarabine
- Dacarbazine
- Dactinomycin
- Dexamethasone
- Diphenhydramine
- Doxorubicin
- Doxycycline
- Droperidol
- Etoposide
- Famotidine
- Filgrastim
- Floxuridine
- Fluconazole
- Fluorouracil
- Furosemide
- Gemcitabine
- Gentamicin
- Haloperidol
- Heparin
- Hydrocortisone sodium phosphate
- Hydrocortisone sodium succinate
- Hydromorphone
- Ifosfamide
- Imipenem/cilastatin
- Lorazepam
- Magnesium sulfate
- Mannitol
- Mechlorethamine
- Meperidine
- Mesna

COMPATIBILITY OF CHEMOTHERAPY AND RELATED SUPPORTIVE CARE MEDICATIONS *(Continued)*

Methotrexate
Methylprednisolone
Metoclopramide
Mezlocillin
Minocycline
Mitoxantrone
Morphine
Multivitamins
Nalbuphine
Netilmicin
Ondansetron
Pentostatin
Piperacillin
Piperacillin/tazobactam
Potassium chloride
Promethazine
Ranitidine
Sodium bicarbonate
Teniposide
Tetracycline
Ticarcillin
Ticarcillin/clavulanate
Tobramycin
Vancomycin
Vinblastine
Vincristine
Vinorelbine

Incompatible:

Acyclovir
Amphotericin
Chlorpromazine
Daunomycin
Ganciclovir
Hydroxyzine
Miconazole
Prochlorperazine

Fluorouracil

Compatible:

D_5W
D_5/LR
NS
Bleomycin
Cephalothin
Cyclophosphamide
Dacarbazine
Etoposide
Floxuridine
Ifosfamide
Magnesium sulfate
Methotrexate
Mitoxantrone
Prednisolone
Vincristine

Y-Site Compatible:

Allopurinol
Amifostine
Aztreonam
Cefepime
Cisplatin
Doxorubicin, liposomal
Fludarabine
Furosemide
Gemcitabine
Granisetron
Heparin
Hydrocortisone sodium succinate
Mannitol
Metochlopramide
Mitomycin
Paclitaxel
Piperacillin
Piperacillin/tazobactam
Potassium chloride
Propofol
Sargramostim
Teniposide
Thiotepa
Vinblastine
Vitamin B complex

Incompatible:

Carboplatin
Cytarabine
Diazepam
Droperidol
Epirubicin
Filgrastim
Gallium nitrate
Ondansetron
TPN
Vinorelbine

Variable Compatibility:

Doxorubicin
Leucovorin

Gemcitabine

Compatible:

NS

Y-Site Compatible:

Amifostine
Amikacin
Aminophylline
Ampicillin
Ampicillin/sulbactam
Aztreonam
Bleomycin
Bumetanide
Buprenorphine
Butorphanol
Calcium gluconate
Carboplatin
Carmustine
Cefazolin
Cefonicid
Cefotetan
Cefoxitin
Ceftazidime
Ceftizoxime
Ceftriaxone
Cefuroxime
Chlorpromazine
Cimetidine
Ciprofloxacin
Cisplatin
Clindamycin
Cyclophosphamide
Cytarabine
Dactinomycin
Daunomycin
Dexamethasone
Dexrazoxane
Diphenhydramine
Dobutamine
Docetaxel
Dopamine
Doxorubicin
Doxycycline
Droperidol
Enalaprilat
Etoposide
Etoposide phosphate
Famotidine
Floxuridine
Fludarabine
Fluorouracil
Fluconazole
Gallium nitrate
Gentamicin
Granisetron
Haloperidol
Heparin
Hydrocortisone sodium phosphate
Hydrocortisone sodium succinate
Hydromorphone
Hydroxyzine
Idarubicin
Ifosfamide
Leucovorin
Lorazepam
Mannitol
Meperidine
Mesna
Metoclopramide
Metronidazole
Miconazole
Minocycline
Mitoxantrone
Morphine
Nalbuphine
Netilmicin
Ofloxacin
Ondansetron
Paclitaxel
Plicamycin
Potassium chloride
Promethazine
Ranitidine
Sodium bicarbonate
Streptozocin
Teniposide
Thiotepa
Ticarcillin
Ticarcillin/clavulanate
Tobramycin

Topotecan
Trimethoprim
Vancomycin
Vinblastine
Vincristine
Vinorelbine
Zidovudine

Incompatible:

Acyclovir
Amphotericin
Cefoperazone
Cefotaxime
Furosemide
Ganciclovir
Imipenem/cilastatin
Irinotecan
Methotrexate
Methylprednisolone
Mezlocillin
Mitomycin
Piperacillin
Piperacillin/tazobactam
Prochlorperazine

Haloperidol

Compatible:

Hydromorphone
Sufentanil

Y-Site Compatible:

Amifostine
Amsacrine
Aztreonam
Cimetidine
Dobutamine
Dopamine
Famotidine
Filgrastim
Fludarabine
Gemcitabine
Lidocaine
Lorazepam
Melphalan
Midazolam
Nitroglycerin
Norepinephrine bitartrate
Ondansetron
Paclitaxel
Phenylephrine
Tacrolimus
Teniposide
Theophylline
Thiotepa
TPN
Vinorelbine

Incompatible:

Allopurinol
Cefepime
Diphenhydramine
Fluconazole
Foscarnet
Gallium nitrate
Heparin
Hydroxyzine
Ketorolac
Piperacillin/tazobactam
Sargramostim

Variable Compatibility:

Benztropine
Cyclizine
Diamorphine
Sodium nitroprusside

Heparin

Compatible:

Aminophylline
Amphotericin
Ascorbic acid
Bleomycin
Calcium gluconate
Cefepime
Cephapirin
Chloramphenicol
Cibenzoline
Clindamycin
Cloxacillin
Colistimethate
Dimenhydrinate
Dopamine
Enalaprilat
Erythromycin
Esmolol
Floxacillin
Fluconazole
Flumazenil
Furosemide
Isoproterenol
Lidocaine
Lincomycin
Methyldopate
Methylprednisolone
Metronidazole
Nafcillin
Norepinephrine
Octreotide
Potassium chloride
Prednisolone
Promazine
Ranitidine
Sodium bicarbonate
Verapamil
Vitamin B complex with C

Y-Site Compatible:

Acyclovir
Aldesleukin
Allopurinol
Amifostine
Ampicillin
Ampicillin/sulbactam
Atracurium
Atropine
Aztreonam
Betamethasone sodium phosphate
Cefazolin
Cefotetan
Ceftazidime
Ceftriaxone
Cephalothin
Chlordiazepoxide
Chlorpromazine
Cimetidine
Cisplatin
Cyanocobalamin
Cyclophosphamide
Cytarabine
Digoxin
Diphenhydramine
Edrophonium
Epinephrine
Erythromycin
Esmolol
Estrogens, conjugated
Ethacrynate
Famotidine
Fentanyl
Fludarabine
Fluorouracil
Foscarnet
Gallium nitrate
Gemcitabine
Hydralazine
Hydrocortisone sodium succinate
Insulin
Kanamycin
Leucovorin
Lorazepam
Magnesium sulfate
Melphalan
Menadiol sodium diphosphate
Methicillin
Methotrexate
Methoxamine
Methyldopate
Metoclopramide
Metronidazole
Midazolam
Minocycline
Mitomycin
Morphine
Neostigmine
Nitroglycerin
Ondansetron
Oxacillin
Oxytocin
Paclitaxel
Pancuronium
Penicillin G potassium
Pentazocine
Phytonadione
Piperacillin
Piperacillin/tazobactam
Procainamide
Prochlorperazine
Propranolol
Pyridostigmine
Sargramostim
Scopolamine
Sodium nitroprusside
Streptokinase
Succinylcholine
Tacrolimus
Teniposide
Theophylline
Thiotepa

COMPATIBILITY OF CHEMOTHERAPY AND RELATED SUPPORTIVE CARE MEDICATIONS *(Continued)*

- Ticarcillin
- Ticarcillin/clavulanate
- TPN
- Trimethobenzamide
- Trimethaphan
- Vercuronium
- Vinblastine
- Vincristine
- Vinorelbine
- Zidovudine

Incompatible:

- Alteplase
- Amikacin
- Amiodarone
- Amsacrine
- Ciprofloxacin
- Codeine phosphate
- Daunomycin
- Diazepam
- Dobutamine
- Doxorubicin
- Doxycycline
- Ergotamine
- Filgrastim
- Gentamicin
- Haloperidol
- Hyaluronidase
- Idarubicin
- Labetatol
- Levorphanol
- Methadone
- Methotrimeprazine
- Phenytoin
- Polymyxin B
- Streptomycin
- Tobramycin
- Triflupromazine

Variable Compatibility:

- Cephalothin
- Dacarbazine
- Diltiazem
- Droperidol
- Hydrocortisone sodium succinate
- Methylprednisolone
- Penicillin G sodium
- Promethazine
- Quinidine gluconate
- Vancomycin

Hydroxyzine

Compatible:

- Atropine
- Benzquinamide
- Bupivacaine
- Butorphanol
- Chlorpromazine
- Cimetidine
- Cisplatin
- Codeine
- Cyclophosphamide
- Cytarabine
- Diphenhydramine
- Doxapram
- Droperidol
- Etoposide
- Fentanyl
- Fluphenazine
- Glycopyrrolate
- Hydromorphone
- Lidocaine
- Meperidine
- Methotrimeprazine
- Metoclopramide
- Midazolam
- Morphine
- Nalbuphine
- Oxymorphone
- Pentazocine
- Mesna
- Methotrexate
- Nafcillin
- Perphenazine
- Procaine
- Prochlorperazine
- Promazine
- Promethazine
- Scopolamine
- Sufentanil
- Thiothixene

Y-Site Compatible:

- Aztreonam
- Ciprofloxacin
- Filgrastim
- Foscarnet
- Gemcitabine
- Melphalan
- Ondansetron
- Sufentanil
- Teniposide
- Thiotepa
- Vinorelbine

Incompatible:

- Allopurinol
- Amifostine
- Aminophylline
- Amobarbital
- Cefepime
- Chloramphenicol
- Diphenhydramine
- Fluconazole
- Fludarabine
- Haloperidol
- Ketorolac
- Paclitaxel
- Penicillin G (sodium and potassium)
- Pentobarbital
- Phenobarbital
- Piperacillin/tazobactam
- Ranitidine
- Sargramostim

Idarubicin

Compatible:

- D_5W
- D_5/NS
- NS
- LR

Y-Site Compatible:

- Amifostine
- Amikacin
- Aztreonam
- Ciprofloxacin
- Cyclophosphamide
- Cytarabine
- Diphenhydramine
- Droperidol
- Erythromycin
- Filgrastim
- Gemcitabine
- Imipenem/cilastatin
- Magnesium sulfate
- Mannitol
- Metoclopramide
- Potassium chloride
- Ranitidine
- Sargramostim
- Thiotepa
- Vinorelbine

Incompatible:

- Acyclovir
- Allopurinol
- Ampicillin/sulbactam
- Cefazolin
- Cefepime
- Ceftazidime
- Dexamethasone
- Etoposide
- Furosemide
- Gentamicin
- Heparin
- Hydrocortisone sodium succinate
- Lorazepam
- Meperidine
- Methotrexate
- Mezlocillin
- Piperacillin/tazobactam
- Sodium bicarbonate
- Teniposide
- Vancomycin
- Vincristine

Ifosfamide

Compatible:

- D_5W
- D_5/NS
- $D_5/^1/_4NS$
- D_5/LR
- NS
- LR
- SWI
- Carboplatin
- Cisplatin
- Etoposide
- Fluorouracil

Y-Site Compatible:

- Allopurinol
- Amifostine
- Aztreonam
- Doxorubicin, liposomal
- Filgrastim
- Fludarabine
- Gallium nitrate
- Gemcitabine
- Granisetron
- Ondansetron
- Paclitaxel
- Piperacillin
- Piperacillin/tazobactam
- Propofol
- Sargramostim
- Sodium bicarbonate
- Teniposide
- Thiotepa
- TPN
- Vinorelbine

Incompatible:

- Cefepime
- Methotrexate

Variable Compatibility:

- Epirubicin
- Mesna

Irinotecan

Compatible:

- D_5W

Incompatible:

- Gemcitabine

Leucovorin

Compatible:

- BWI
- D_5W
- D_{10}/NS
- NS
- LR
- SWI
- Bleomycin
- Cisplatin
- Floxuridine

Y-Site Compatible:

- Amifostine
- Aztreonam
- Cefepime
- Cyclophosphamide
- Doxorubicin
- Doxorubicin, liposomal
- Filgrastim
- Fluconazole
- Furosemide
- Gemcitabine
- Heparin
- Methotrexate
- Metoclopramide
- Mitomycin
- Piperacillin
- Piperacillin/tazobactam
- Sodium bicarbonate
- Tacrolimus
- Teniposide
- Thiotepa
- TPN
- Vinblastine
- Vincristine

Incompatible:

- Droperidol
- Foscarnet
- Trimetrexate

Variable Compatibility:

- Fluorouracil

Lorazepam

Compatible:

- Cimetidine
- Hydromorphone

Y-Site Compatible:

- Acyclovir
- Albumin
- Amifostine
- Amikacin
- Amoxicillin
- Amoxicillin/clavulanate
- Amsacrine
- Atracurium
- Bumetanide
- Cefepime
- Cefotaxime
- Ciprofloxacin
- Cisplatin
- Cotrimoxazole
- Cyclophosphamide
- Cytarabine
- Dexamethasone
- Diltiazem
- Doxorubicin
- Erythromycin
- Etomidate
- Fentanyl
- Filgrastim
- Fluconazole
- Fludarabine
- Furosemide
- Gemcitabine
- Gentamicin
- Granisetron
- Haloperidol
- Heparin
- Hydrocortisone sodium succinate
- Kantaserin
- Melphalan
- Methotrexate
- Metronidazole
- Morphine
- Paclitaxel
- Pancuronium
- Piperacillin
- Piperacillin/tazobactam
- Potassium chloride
- Ranitidine
- Tacrolimus
- Teniposide
- Thiotepa
- Vancomycin
- Vercuronium
- Vinorelbine
- Zidovudine

COMPATIBILITY OF CHEMOTHERAPY AND RELATED SUPPORTIVE CARE MEDICATIONS *(Continued)*

Incompatible:

Aldesleukin
Aztreonam
Buprenorphine
Floxacillin
Gallium nitrate
Idarubicin
Imipenem/cilastatin
Ondansetron
Sargramostim
Sufentanil
Thiopental

Variable Compatibility:

Foscarnet

Mechlorethamine

Compatible:

NS
SWI

Y-Site Compatible:

Amifostine
Aztreonam
Filgrastim
Fludarabine
Granisetron
Ondansetron
Sargramostim
Teniposide
Vinorelbine

Incompatible:

D_5W
Allopurinol
Cefepime
Methohexital

Melphalan

Compatible:

NS

Y-Site Compatible:

Acyclovir
Amikacin
Aminophylline
Ampicillin
Aztreonam
Bleomycin
Bumetanide
Buprenorphine
Butorphanol
Calcium gluconate
Carboplatin
Carmustine
Cefazolin
Cefepime
Cefoperazone
Cefotaxime
Cefotetan
Ceftazidime
Ceftriaxone
Cefuroxime
Cimetidine
Cisplatin
Cotrimoxazole
Cyclophosphamide
Cytarabine
Dacarbazine
Dactinomycin
Daunomycin
Diazepam
Doxorubicin
Doxycycline
Droperidol
Enalaprilat
Etoposide
Famotidine
Filgrastim
Floxuridine
Fluconazole
Fludarabine
Fluorouracil
Furosemide
Gallium nitrate
Ganciclovir
Gentamicin
Haloperidol
Heparin
Hydrocortisone sodium phosphate
Hydrocortisone sodium succinate
Hydromorphone
Hydroxyzine
Idarubicin
Ifosfamide
Imipenem/cilastatin
Lorazepam
Mannitol
Mechlorethamine
Meperidine
Mesna
Methotrexate
Methylprednisolone
Metoclopramide
Metronidazole
Miconazole
Minocycline
Mitomycin
Mitoxantrone
Morphine
Nalbuphine
Netilmicin
Ondansetron
Pentostatin
Piperacillin
Plicamycin
Potassium chloride
Prochlorperazine
Promethazine
Ranitidine
Sodium bicarbonate
Streptozocin
Teniposide
Thiotepa
Ticarcillin
Ticarcillin/clavulanate
Tobramycin
Vancomycin
Vinblastine
Vincristine
Vinorelbine

Incompatible:

D_5W
LR
SWI
Amphotericin
Chlorpromazine

Mesna

Compatible:

- BWI
- D_5W
- NS
- LR
- Cyclophosphamide
- Hydroxyzine
- Ifosfamide

Y-Site Compatible:

- Allopurinol
- Amifostine
- Aztreonam
- Cefepime
- Doxorubicin, liposomal
- Filgrastim
- Fludarabine
- Gallium nitrate
- Gemcitabine
- Granisetron
- Methotrexate
- Ondansetron
- Paclitaxel
- Piperacillin/tazobactam
- Sargramostim
- Sodium acetate
- Teniposide
- Thiotepa
- TPN
- Vinorelbine

Incompatible:

- Carboplatin
- Cisplatin
- Chlorpromazine

Methadone

Incompatible:

- Aminophylline
- Ammonium chloride
- Amobarbital
- Chlorothiazide
- Phenytoin
- Heparin
- Methicillin
- Nitrofurantoin
- Pentobarbital
- Sodium bicarbonate
- Thiopental

Methotrexate

Compatible:

- D_5W
- NS
- LR
- SWI
- Amino acid 4.25%/$D_{25}W$
- Cephalothin
- Cyclophosphamide
- Cytarabine
- Dacarbazine
- Fluorouracil
- Hydroxyzine
- Imipenem/cilastatin
- Mercaptopurine
- Ondansetron
- Sodium bicarbonate
- Vincristine

Y-Site Compatible:

- Allopurinol
- Amifostine
- Asparaginase
- Aztreonam
- Bleomycin
- Cefepime
- Ceftriaxone
- Cimetidine
- Cisplatin
- Daunomycin
- Dexchlorpheniramine
- Diphenhydramine
- Doxapram
- Doxorubicin
- Doxorubicin, liposomal
- Etoposide
- Famotidine
- Filgrastim
- Fludarabine
- Furosemide
- Gallium nitrate
- Ganciclovir
- Granisetron
- Heparin
- Hydromorphone
- Leucovorin
- Lorazepam
- Mesna
- Methylprednisolone
- Mitomycin
- Morphine
- Oxacillin
- Paclitaxel
- Piperacillin/tazobactam
- Prochlorperazine
- Ranitidine
- Sargramostim
- Teniposide
- Thiotepa
- Vinblastine
- Vindesine
- Vinorelbine

Incompatible:

- Dexamethasone
- Gemcitabine
- Idarubicin
- Ifosfamide
- Midazolam
- Nalbuphine
- Prednisolone
- Promethazine
- Propofol
- TPN

Variable Compatibility:

- Droperidol
- Metoclopramide
- Vancomycin

COMPATIBILITY OF CHEMOTHERAPY AND RELATED SUPPORTIVE CARE MEDICATIONS *(Continued)*

Metoclopramide

Compatible:

- D_5W
- NS
- Clindamycin
- Mannitol
- Multivitamins
- Potassium acetate
- Potassium chloride
- Potassium phosphate
- Verapamil
- TPN

Y-Site Compatible:

- Acyclovir
- Aldesleukin
- Amifostine
- Aztreonam
- Bleomycin
- Ciprofloxacin
- Cisplatin
- Cyclophosphamide
- Cytarabine
- Diltiazem
- Doxorubicin
- Droperidol
- Famotidine
- Filgrastim
- Fluconazole
- Fludarabine
- Fluorouracil
- Foscarnet
- Gallium nitrate
- Gemcitabine
- Heparin
- Idarubicin
- Leucovorin
- Melphalan
- Meperidine
- Methotrexate
- Mitomycin
- Morphine
- Ondansetron
- Paclitaxel
- Piperacillin/tazobactam
- Sargramostim
- Sufentanil
- Tacrolimus
- Teniposide
- Thiotepa
- Vinblastine
- Vincristine
- Vinorelbine
- Zidovudine

Incompatible:

- Allopurinol
- Ampicillin
- Calcium gluconate
- Cefepime
- Cephalothin
- Chloramphenicol
- Dexamethasone
- Erythromycin
- Floxacillin
- Furosemide
- Penicillin G potassium
- Sodium bicarbonate

Metronidazole

Compatible:

- Amikacin
- Aminophylline
- Cefazolin
- Cefotaxime
- Cefotetan
- Cefoxitin
- Ceftazidime
- Ceftizoxime
- Ceftriaxone
- Cefuroxime
- Cephalothin
- Chloramphenicol
- Ciprofloxacin
- Clindamycin
- Disopyramide
- Floxacillin
- Fluconazole
- Gentamicin
- Heparin
- Hydrocortisone
- Moxalactam
- Multielectrolyte concentrate
- Multivitamins
- Netilmicin
- Penicillin G potassium
- Tobramycin

Y-Site Compatible:

- Acyclovir
- Allopurinol
- Amifostine
- Cefepime
- Cyclophosphamide
- Diltiazem
- Enalaprilat
- Esmolol
- Fluconazole
- Foscarnet
- Gemcitabine
- Heparin
- Hydromorphone
- Labetatol
- Lorazepam
- Magnesium sulfate
- Melphalan
- Meperidine
- Midazolam
- Morphine
- Perphenazine
- Piperacillin/tazobactam
- Sargramostim
- Tacrolimus
- Teniposide
- Theophylline
- Thiotepa
- TPN
- Vinorelbine

Incompatible:

- Aztreonam
- Dopamine
- Filgrastim

Variable Compatibility:

- Ampicillin
- Cefamandole

Mitomycin

Compatible:

NS
LR
Dexamethasone
Hydrocortisone sodium succinate

Y-Site Compatible:

Allopurinol
Amifostine
Bleomycin
Cisplatin
Cyclophosphamide
Doxorubicin
Droperidol
Fluorouracil
Furosemide
Leucovorin
Methotrexate
Metoclopramide
Ondansetron
Teniposide
Thiotepa
Vinblastine
Vincristine

Incompatible:

Aztreonam
Cefepime
Filgrastim
Gemcitabine
Piperacillin/tazobactam
Sargramostim
Vinorelbine

Variable Compatibility:

D_5W
SWI
Heparin

Mitoxantrone

Compatible:

D_5W
D_5/NS
NS
Cyclophosphamide
Cytarabine
Fluorouracil
Potassium chloride

Y-Site Compatible:

Allopurinol
Amifostine
Filgrastim
Fludarabine
Gemcitabine
Ondansetron
Sargramostim
Teniposide
Thiotepa
Vinorelbine

Incompatible:

Aztreonam
Cefepime
Doxorubicin, liposomal
Heparin
Paclitaxel
Piperacillin
Piperacillin/tazobactam
Propofol

Variable Compatibility:

Hydrocortisone sodium phosphate
Hydrocortisone sodium succinate
TPN

Ondansetron

Compatible:

D_5W
NS
LR
Cisplatin
Cyclophosphamide
Cytarabine
Dacarbazine
Dexamethasone
Doxorubicin
Etoposide
Fluconazole
Hydrocortisone sodium succinate
Mannitol
Meperidine
Methotrexate
Morphine
Ranitidine

Y-Site Compatible:

Aldesleukin
Amifostine
Amikacin
Aztreonam
Bleomycin
Carboplatin
Carmustine
Cefazolin
Cefotaxime
Cefoxitin
Ceftazidime
Ceftizoxime
Cefuroxime
Chlorpromazine
Cimetidine
Dactinomycin
Daunomycin
Diphenhydramine
Doxorubicin, liposomal
Doxycycline
Droperidol
Famotidine
Filgrastim
Floxuridine
Fludarabine
Gallium nitrate
Gemcitabine
Gentamicin
Haloperidol
Heparin
Hydrocortisone sodium phosphate
Hydromorphone
Hydroxyzine
Ifosfamide
Imipenem/cilastatin
Magnesium sulfate
Mechlorethamine
Mesna
Metoclopramide
Miconazole
Mitomycin
Mitoxantrone
Paclitaxel
Pentostatin
Piperacillin/tazobactam
Potassium chloride
Prochlorperazine
Promethazine
Sodium acetate
Streptozocin
Teniposide
Thiotepa
Ticarcillin
Ticarcillin/clavulanate
TPN
Vancomycin
Vinblastine
Vincristine
Vinorelbine

COMPATIBILITY OF CHEMOTHERAPY AND RELATED SUPPORTIVE CARE MEDICATIONS *(Continued)*

Incompatible:

Acyclovir
Allopurinol
Aminophylline
Amphotericin
Ampicillin
Ampicillin/sulbactam
Amsacrine
Cefepime
Cefoperazone
Furosemide
Ganciclovir
Lorazepam
Methylprednisolone
Mezlocillin
Piperacillin
Sargramostim
Sodium bicarbonate

Variable Compatibility:

Fluorouracil

Paclitaxel

Compatible:

NS

Y-Site Compatible:

Acyclovir
Amikacin
Aminophylline
Ampicillin/sulbactam
Bleomycin
Butorphanol
Calcium chloride
Carboplatin
Cefepime
Cefotetan
Ceftazidime
Cefuroxime
Cimetidine
Cyclophosphamide
Cytarabine
Dacarbazine
Dexamethasone
Diphenhydramine
Doxorubicin
Droperidol
Etoposide
Famotidine
Floxuridine
Fluconazole
Fluorouracil
Furosemide
Ganciclovir
Gemcitabine
Gentamicin
Granisetron
Haloperidol
Heparin
Hydrocortisone sodium phosphate
Hydrocortisone sodium succinate
Hydromorphone
Ifosfamide
Lorazepam
Magnesium sulfate
Mannitol
Meperidine
Mesna
Methotrexate
Metoclopramide
Morphine
Nalbuphine
Ondansetron
Pentostatin
Potassium chloride
Prochlorperazine
Propofol
Ranitidine
Sodium bicarbonate
Thiotepa
TPN
Vancomycin
Vinblastine
Vincristine

Incompatible:

Amphotericin
Chlorpromazine
Doxorubicin, liposomal
Hydroxyzine
Methylprednisolone
Mitoxantrone

Variable Compatibility:

D_5W
Cisplatin

Pentostatin

Compatible:

NS
LR

Y-Site Compatible:

Fludarabine
Ondansetron
Paclitaxel
Sargramostim

Variable Compatibility:

D_5W

Phytonadione

Compatible:

- Amikacin
- Calcium gluceptate
- Cefapirin
- Chloramphenicol
- Cimetidine
- Netilmicin
- Doxapram
- Sodium bicarbonate
- TPN

Y-Site Compatible:

- Ampicillin
- Epinephrine
- Famotidine
- Heparin
- Hydrocortisone sodium succinate
- Potassium chloride
- Tolazoline
- Vitamin B complex with C

Incompatible:

- Dobutamine
- Ranitidine

Plicamycin

Compatible:

- D_5W
- NS
- SWI
- Piperacillin

Y-Site Compatible:

- Allopurinol
- Amifostine
- Aztreonam
- Filgrastim
- Gemcitabine
- Piperacillin/tazobactam
- Teniposide
- Vinorelbine

Incompatible:

- Cefonicid

Prochlorperazine

Compatible:

- Amikacin
- Ascorbic acid
- Dexamethasone
- Dimenhydrinate
- Erythromycin
- Ethacrinate
- Lidocaine
- Nafcillin
- Sodium bicarbonate
- Vitamin B complex with C

Y-Site Compatible:

- Amsacrine
- Cisplatin
- Cyclophosphamide
- Cytarabine
- Doxorubicin
- Fluconazole
- Heparin
- Hydrocortisone sodium succinate
- Melphalan
- Methotrexate
- Ondansetron
- Paclitaxel
- Potassium chloride
- Sargramostim
- Sufentanil
- Teniposide
- Thiotepa
- Vinorelbine

Incompatible:

- Aldesleukin
- Allopurinol
- Amifostine
- Aminophylline
- Amphotericin
- Ampicillin
- Aztreonam
- Calcium gluceptate
- Cefepime
- Cephalothin
- Chloramphenicol
- Floxacillin
- Fludarabine
- Foscarnet
- Filgrastim
- Furosemide
- Gallium nitrate
- Gemcitabine
- Methohexital
- Penicillin G sodium
- Piperacillin/tazobactam
- Phenobarbital
- Thiopental

Variable Compatibility:

- Calcium gluconate
- Penicillin G potassium

COMPATIBILITY OF CHEMOTHERAPY AND RELATED SUPPORTIVE CARE MEDICATIONS *(Continued)*

Promethazine

Compatible:

- Amikacin
- Ascorbic acid
- Chloroquine
- Netilmicin
- Vitamin B complex with C

Y-Site Compatible:

- Amifostine
- Amsacrine
- Aztreonam
- Ciprofloxacin
- Cisplatin
- Cyclophosphamide
- Cytarabine
- Doxorubicin
- Filgrastim
- Fluconazole
- Fludarabine
- Gemcitabine
- Melphalan
- Ondansetron
- Sargramostim
- Teniposide
- Thiotepa
- Vinorelbine

Incompatible:

- Aldesleukin
- Allopurinol
- Aminophylline
- Cefepime
- Cefoperazone
- Cefotetan
- Ceftizoxime
- Chloramphenicol
- Chlorothiazide
- Floxacillin
- Foscarnet
- Furosemide
- Heparin
- Hydrocortisone sodium succinate
- Methicillin
- Methohexital
- Methotrexate
- Penicillin G (sodium and potassium)
- Pentobarbital
- Piperacillin/tazobactam
- Thiopental

Variable Compatibility:

- Potassium chloride

Sargramostim

Compatible:

- BWI
- D_5W
- NS
- SWI

Y-Site Compatible:

- Allopurinol
- Amikacin
- Aminophylline
- Aztreonam
- Bleomycin
- Butorphanol
- Calcium gluconate
- Carboplatin
- Carmustine
- Cefazolin
- Cefepime
- Cefotetan
- Cefoxitin
- Ceftizoxime
- Ceftriaxone
- Cefuroxime
- Cimetidine
- Cisplatin
- Cotrimoxazole
- Cyclophosphamide
- Cyclosporine
- Cytarabine
- Dacarbazine
- Dactinomycin
- Dexamethasone
- Diphenhydramine
- Dobutamine
- Doxorubicin
- Doxycycline
- Droperidol
- Etoposide
- Famotidine
- Fentanyl
- Floxuridine
- Fluconazole
- Fluorouracil
- Furosemide
- Gentamicin
- Heparin
- Human immune globulin
- Idarubicin
- Ifosfamide
- Magnesium sulfate
- Mannitol
- Mechlorethamine
- Meperidine
- Mesna
- Methotrexate
- Metoclopramide
- Metronidazole
- Mezlocillin
- Miconazole
- Minocycline
- Mitoxantrone
- Netilmicin
- Pentostatin
- Piperacillin/tazobactam
- Potassium chloride
- Prochlorperazine
- Promethazine
- Ranitidine
- Teniposide
- Ticarcillin
- Ticarcillin/clavulanate
- Vinblastine
- Vincristine

Incompatible:

- Acyclovir
- Ampicillin
- Ampicillin/sulbactam
- Cefonicid
- Cefoperazone
- Chlorpromazine
- Ganciclovir
- Haloperidol
- Hydrocortisone sodium phosphate
- Hydrocortisone sodium succinate
- Hydromorphone
- Hydroxyzine
- Imipenem/cilastatin
- Methylprednisolone
- Mitomycin
- Morphine
- Nalbuphine
- Ondansetron
- Piperacillin
- Sodium bicarbonate
- Tobramycin

Variable Compatibility:

- Amphotericin
- Amsacrine
- Ceftazidime
- Vancomycin

Streptozocin

Compatible:

- D_5W
- NS
- SWI

Y-Site Compatible:

- Filgrastim
- Gemcitabine
- Granisetron
- Ondansetron
- Teniposide
- Thiotepa
- Vinorelbine

Incompatible:

- Allopurinol
- Aztreonam
- Cefepime
- Piperacillin
- Piperacillin/tazobactam

Teniposide

Compatible:

- D_5W
- NS
- LR

Y-Site Compatible:

- Acyclovir
- Allopurinol
- Amifostine
- Amikacin
- Aminophylline
- Amphotericin
- Ampicillin
- Ampicillin/sulbactam
- Aztreonam
- Bleomycin
- Bumetanide
- Buprenorphine
- Butorphanol
- Calcium gluconate
- Carboplatin
- Carmustine
- Cefazolin
- Cefonicid
- Cefoperazone
- Cefotaxime
- Cefotetan
- Cefoxitin
- Ceftazidime
- Ceftizoxime
- Ceftriaxone
- Cefuroxime
- Chlorpromazine
- Cimetidine
- Cisplatin
- Corticotropin
- Cotrimoxazole
- Cyclophosphamide
- Cytarabine
- Dacarbazine
- Dactinomycin
- Daunomycin
- Dexamethasone
- Diphenhydramine
- Doxorubicin
- Doxycycline
- Droperidol
- Enalaprilat
- Etoposide
- Famotidine
- Floxuridine
- Fluconazole
- Fludarabine
- Fluorouracil
- Furosemide
- Gallium nitrate
- Ganciclovir
- Gemcitabine
- Gentamicin
- Haloperidol
- Heparin
- Hydrocortisone sodium phosphate
- Hydrocortisone sodium succinate
- Hydromorphone
- Hydroxyzine
- Ifosfamide
- Imipenem/cilastatin
- Leucovorin
- Lorazepam
- Mannitol
- Mechlorethamine
- Meperidine
- Mesna
- Methotrexate
- Methylprednisolone
- Metoclopramide
- Metronidazole
- Mezlocillin
- Miconazole
- Midazolam
- Mitomycin
- Mitoxantrone
- Morphine
- Nalbuphine
- Netilmicin
- Ondansetron
- Piperacillin
- Plicamycin
- Potassium chloride
- Prochlorperazine
- Promethazine
- Ranitidine
- Sargramostim
- Sodium bicarbonate
- Streptozocin
- Thiotepa
- Ticarcillin
- Ticarcillin/clavulanate
- Tobramycin
- Vancomycin
- Vinblastine
- Vincristine
- Vinorelbine

Incompatible:

- Idarubicin

COMPATIBILITY OF CHEMOTHERAPY AND RELATED SUPPORTIVE CARE MEDICATIONS *(Continued)*

Thiethylperazine

Compatible:

NS
Butorphanol
Hydromorphone
Midazolam
Ranitidine

Y-Site Compatible:

Aldesleukin

Incompatible:

Ketorolac
Perphenazine

Variable Compatibility:

Nalbuphine

Thiotepa

Compatible:

NS
SWI

Y-Site Compatible:

Acyclovir
Allopurinol
Amifostine
Amikacin
Aminophylline
Amphotericin
Ampicillin
Ampicillin/sulbactam
Aztreonam
Bleomycin
Bumetanide
Buprenorphine
Butorphanol
Calcium gluconate
Carboplatin
Carmustine
Cefazolin
Cefepime
Cefonicid
Cefoperazone
Cefotaxime
Cefotetan
Cefoxitin
Ceftazidime
Ceftizoxime
Ceftriaxone
Cefuroxime
Chlorpromazine
Cimetidine
Ciprofloxacin
Cotrimoxazole
Cyclophosphamide
Cytarabine
Dacarbazine
Dactinomycin
Daunomycin
Dexamethasone
Diphenhydramine
Dobutamine
Dopamine
Doxorubicin
Doxycycline
Droperidol
Enalaprilat
Etoposide
Famotidine
Floxuridine
Fluconazole
Fludarabine
Fluorouracil
Furosemide
Gallium nitrate
Ganciclovir
Gemcitabine
Gentamicin
Granisetron
Haloperidol
Heparin
Hydrocortisone sodium phosphate
Hydrocortisone sodium succinate
Hydromorphone
Hydroxyzine
Idarubicin
Ifosfamide
Imipenem/cilastatin
Leucovorin
Lorazepam
Magnesium sulfate
Mannitol
Meperidine
Mesna
Methotrexate
Methylprednisolone
Metoclopramide
Metronidazole
Mezlocillin
Miconazole
Mitomycin
Mitoxantrone
Morphine
Nalbuphine
Netilmicin
Ofloxacin
Ondansetron
Paclitaxel
Piperacillin
Piperacillin/tazobactam
Plicamycin
Potassium chloride
Prochlorperazine
Promethazine
Ranitidine
Sodium bicarbonate
Streptozocin
Teniposide
Ticarcillin
Ticarcillin/clavulanate
Tobramycin
TPN
Vancomycin
Vinblastine
Vincristine

Incompatible:

Cisplatin
Filgrastim
Minocycline

Topotecan

Compatible:

D_5W
NS
LR

Y-Site Compatible:

Gemcitabine

Trimetrexate

Compatible:

D_5W

Y-Site Compatible:

Amifostine

Incompatible:

BNS
D_5/NS
$D_5/{}^1/_4NS$
$D_5/{}^1/_2NS$
D_5/LR
D_{10}/NS
NS
LR
Calcium chloride
Chloride ion
Leucovorin
Potassium chloride

Vinblastine

Compatible:

BNS
D_5W
NS
LR
Bleomycin
Dacarbazine

Y-Site Compatible:

Allopurinol
Amifostine
Aztreonam
Cisplatin
Cyclophosphamide
Doxorubicin, liposomal
Droperidol
Filgrastim
Fludarabine
Fluorouracil
Gemcitabine
Leucovorin
Methotrexate
Metoclopramide
Mitomycin
Ondansetron
Paclitaxel
Piperacillin
Piperacillin/tazobactam
Sargramostim
Teniposide
Vincristine
Vinorelbine

Incompatible:

Cefazolin
Furosemide

Variable Compatibility:

Doxorubicin
Heparin

Vincristine

Compatible:

D_5W
NS
LR
Bleomycin
Cytarabine
Doxorubicin
Fluorouracil
Methotrexate

Y-Site Compatible:

Allopurinol
Amifostine
Aztreonam
Cisplatin
Cyclophosphamide
Doxapram
Doxorubicin, liposomal
Droperidol
Filgrastim
Fludarabine
Gemcitabine
Granisetron
Heparin
Leucovorin
Metoclopramide
Mitomycin
Ondansetron
Paclitaxel
Piperacillin/tazobactam
Sargramostim
Teniposide
Vinblastine
Vinorelbine

Incompatible:

Cefepime
Furosemide
Idarubicin
Sodium bicarbonate

COMPATIBILITY OF CHEMOTHERAPY AND RELATED SUPPORTIVE CARE MEDICATIONS *(Continued)*

Vinorelbine

Compatible:

- D_5W
- $D_5/{}^1/_2NS$
- NS
- LR

Y-Site Compatible:

- Amikacin
- Aztreonam
- Bleomycin
- Bumetanide
- Buprenorphine
- Butorphanol
- Calcium gluconate
- Carboplatin
- Carmustine
- Cefotaxime
- Ceftazidime
- Ceftizoxime
- Chlorpromazine
- Cimetidine
- Cisplatin
- Cyclophosphamide
- Cytarabine
- Dacarbazine
- Dactinomycin
- Daunomycin
- Dexamethasone
- Diphenhydramine
- Doxorubicin
- Doxorubicin, liposomal
- Doxycycline
- Droperidol
- Enalaprilat
- Etoposide
- Famotidine
- Filgrastim
- Fluconazole
- Fludarabine
- Fluorouracil
- Gallium nitrate
- Gemcitabine
- Gentamicin
- Haloperidol
- Heparin
- Hydrocortisone sodium phosphate
- Hydrocortisone sodium succinate
- Hydromorphone
- Hydroxyzine
- Idarubicin
- Ifosfamide
- Imipenem/cilastatin
- Lorazepam
- Mannitol
- Mechlorethamine
- Meperidine
- Mesna
- Methotrexate
- Metoclopramide
- Metronidazole
- Minocycline
- Mitoxantrone
- Morphine
- Nalbuphine
- Netilmicin
- Ondansetron
- Plicamycin
- Streptozocin
- Teniposide
- Ticarcillin
- Ticarcillin/clavulanate
- Tobramycin
- Vinblastine
- Vincristine
- Vindesine

Incompatible:

- Acyclovir
- Allopurinol
- Aminophylline
- Amphotericin
- Ampicillin
- Cefazolin
- Cefoperazone
- Cefotetan
- Ceftriaxone
- Cefuroxime
- Cotrimoxazole
- Fluorouracil
- Furosemide
- Ganciclovir
- Methylprednisolone
- Mitomycin
- Sodium bicarbonate
- Thiotepa

Drug	Variable Compatibility
Carboplatin	Solutions in saline are less stable than in dextrose.
Carmustine	Solutions should be dispensed in glass and protected from light. Solutions are stable for <8 hours under most circumstances.
Cisplatin	Must have a chloride concentration of at least 0.2% in the final solution. The commercial product has a NS concentration. Etoposide + mannitol + potassium chloride in normal saline precipitates within 24 hours; when in $D_5/^1/_2NS$, it is stable for 24 hours.
Dacarbazine	Heparin 100 units/mL with dacarbazine 25 mg/mL is **incompatible.** Heparin 100 units/mL with dacarbazine 10 mg/mL is **compatible.**
Filgrastim	Gentamicin is reported to be physically **compatible** for Y-site injection, but with a decrease in biologic activity. Imipenem/cilastatin with filgrastim 40 mcg/mL is reported to be physically **compatible** for Y-site injection, but with a decrease in biologic activity.
Fluorouracil	Doxorubicin 2 mg/mL with fluorouracil 50 mg/mL is **compatible** for 13 minutes. Doxorubicin 0.5-1 mg/mL with fluorouracil 50 mg/mL is **incompatible**. Fluorouracil with doxorubicin is **Y-site compatible.** Variable compatibility with leucovorin.
Mesna	**Compatible** with ifosfamide. **Incompatible** with ifosfamide and epinephrine.
Leucovorin	Variable compatibility with fluorouracil.
Mitomycin	Mitomycin 50 mg/L in NS has a color change and 10% loss of drug concentration in 12 hours. Mitomycin 1 g/L in SWI precipitates in 24 hours under refrigeration. Other temperatures and concentrations are reported to be stable. Mitomycin in D_5W is **incompatible** in 20 mg/L; **compatible** in 40 mg/L. Mitomycin 500 mg/L with heparin 33,300 units/L in NS is **compatible.** PVC containers of mitomycin 167 mg/L with heparin 33,300 units/L in NS is **compatible.** Glass containers of mitomycin 167 mg/L with heparin 33,300 units/L in NS are **incompatible.**
Pentostatin	Pentostatin 20 mg/mL in D_5W at room temperature: a 2% loss of drug in 24 hours; 8% to 10% loss in 48 hours; and a 10% loss in 54 hours. Under refrigeration, there is no loss in 96 hours. There is a 10% loss in 23 hours at room temperature of pentostatin 2 mg/mL in D_5W
Sargramostim	Amphotericin B 0.6 mg/mL in D_5W with sargramostim 10 mcg/mL in NS forms immediate precipitate. Amphotericin B 0.6 mg/mL in D_5W with sargramostim 10 mcg/mL in D_5W is **Y-site compatible**. Amsacrine with sargramostim in NS forms immediate precipitate. Amsacrine with sargramostim in D_5W is **Y-site compatible**. Ceftazidime 40 mg/mL in NS with sargramostim 10 mcg/mL in NS is **incompatible**, with particle formation within 4 hours. Ceftazidime 40 mg/mL with sargramostim 6 or 15 mcg/mL is **compatible** for 2 hours (Y-site **compatible**). Vancomycin 20 mg/mL and sargramostim 6 mcg/mL is **incompatible.** Vancomycin 10 mg/mL and sargramostim 10 mcg/mL is **Y-site compatible**. Vancomycin 20 mg/mL and sargramostim 15 mcg/mL is **Y-site compatible.**
Vancomycin	Vancomycin 5 mg/mL with methotrexate 30 mg/mL is **compatible** for 2 hours, precipitates within 4 hours. Other concentrations tested were **compatible** for 1 hour. Vancomycin with methotrexate is **Y-site compatible.**
Vinblastine	In various volumes, doxorubicin 2 mg/mL with vinblastine 1 mg/mL yields erratic assay results. Vinblastine with doxorubicin is **Y-site compatible**. Heparin 200 units/mL with vinblastine 1 mg/mL is **incompatible** in a syringe for 13 minutes. Heparin 500 units/mL with vinblastine 0.5 mg/mL is **compatible** in a syringe for 13 minutes.

COMPATIBILITY OF CHEMOTHERAPY AND RELATED SUPPORTIVE CARE MEDICATIONS *(Continued)*

Suggested Readings

Hall PD, Yui D, Lyons S, et al, "Compatibility of Filgrastim With Selected Antimicrobial Drugs During Simulated Y-Site Administration," *Am J Health-System Pharm*, 1997, 54:184-9.

McGuire TR, Narducci WA, and Fox JL, "Compatibility and Stability of Ondansetron Hydrochloride, Dexamethasone and Lorazepam in Injectable Solutions," *Am J Health-System Pharm*, 1993, 50:1410-4.

Najari Z and Rucho WJ, "Compatibility of Commonly Used Bone Marrow Drugs During Y-Site Delivery," *Am J Health-System Pharm*, 1997, 54:181-4.

Trissel LA, Chandler SW, and Folstad JT, "Visual Compatibility of Amsacrine With Selected Drugs During Simulated Y-Site Injection," *Am J Hospital Pharm*, 1990, 47:2525-8.

Trissel LA, Bready BB, Kwan JW, et al, "Visual Compatibility of Sargramostim With Selected Antineoplastic Agents, Anti-infectives, or Other Drugs During Simulated Y-Site Injection," *Am J Hospital Pharm*, 1992, 49:402-6.

Trissel LA and Martinez JF, "Physical Compatibility of Melphalan With Selected Drugs During Simulated Y-Site Administration," *Am J Hospital Pharm*, 1993, 50:2359-63.

Trissel LA and Martinez JF, Visual, "Turbidimetric and Particle-Content Assessment of Compatibility of Vinorelbine Tartrate With Selected Drugs During Simulated Y-Site Injection," *Am J Hospital Pharm*, 1994, 51:495-9.

Trissel LA and Martinez JF, "Physical Compatibility of Allopurinol Sodium With Selected Drugs During Simulated Y-Site Administration," *Am J Hospital Pharm*, 1994, 51:1792-9.

Trissel LA and Martinez JF, "Compatibility of Filgrastim With Selected Drugs During Simulated Y-Site Administration," *Am J Hospital Pharm*, 1994, 51:1907-13.

Trissel LA and Martinez JF, "Screening Teniposide For Y-Site Compatibility," *Hospital Pharm*, 1994, 29:1010, 1012-4, 1017.

Trissel LA, *Handbook on Injectable Drugs*, 9th Ed. Bethesda, MD: *Am Society Health-Systems Pharmacists*, 1996.

Trissel LA, *Supplement to Handbook on Injectable Drugs*, 9th Ed. Bethesda, MD: *Am Society of Health-Systems Pharmacists*, 1997.

Trissel LA, Gilbert DL, and Martinez JF, "Compatibility of Granisetron Hydrochloride With Selected Drugs During Simulated Y-Site Administration," *Am J Health-System Pharm*, 1997, 54:56-60.

Trissel LA, Gilbert DL, and Martinez JF, "Compatibility of Propofol With Selected Drugs During Simulated Y-Site Administration," *Am J Health-System Pharm*, 1997, 54:1287-92.

Trissel LA, Gilbert DL, Martinez JF, et al, "Compatibility of Parenteral Nutrient Solutions With Selected Drugs During Simulated Y-Site Administration," *Am J Health-System Pharm*, 1997, 54:1295-300.

Trissel LA, Gilbert DL, and Martinez JF, "Compatibility of Doxorubicin Hydrochloride Liposome With Selected Other Drugs During Simulated Y-Site Administration," *Am J Health-System Pharm*, 1997; 54:2708-13.

Trissel LA, Martinez JF, and Gilbert DL, "Compatibility of Gemcitabine Hydrochloride With 107 Selected Drugs During Simulated Y-Site Administration," *J Am Pharmaceutical Association*, 1999, 39 (4):514-18.

Zhang Y, Xu QA, Trissel LA, et al, "Compatibility and Stability of Paclitaxel Combined With Cisplatin and With Carboplatin in Infusion Solutions," *Ann Pharmacother*, 1997, 31 (12):1465-70.

TUMOR LYSIS SYNDROME, MANAGEMENT

Tumor lysis syndrome (TLS) may be seen with any tumor that is undergoing rapid cell turnover as a result of high growth fraction or high cell death due to therapy. It occurs most often in Burkitt's lymphoma and T-cell ALL, both of which have large tumor burdens and high sensitivity to chemotherapy. Acute lysis of tumor cells results in the rapid release of potassium, phosphates, and nucleic acids into the circulation. Hypocalcemia, hyperuricemia, and renal failure may result. Secondary acute precipitation of calcium and urates in the kidney, tumor infiltration of the kidney, obstructive uropathy, and dehydration may increase the primary metabolic disturbances. The following chart reviews the management of TLS.

Therapy	Infants & Children	Adolescents & Adults
Hydration (patients typically present with dehydration; I.V. fluids should be started immediately)	3000-6000 mL/m^2/day D_5W 1/4 NS (+ sodium bicarbonate) Maintain urine output at ≥1 mL/kg/hour Maintain urine specific gravity at ≤1.010 Strict monitoring of I & O	3000-6000 mL/m^2/day D_5W 1/4 NS (+ sodium bicarbonate) Maintain urine output at 100-150 mL/hour Maintain urine specific gravity at ≤1.010 Strict monitoring of I & O
Alkalinization	50-100 mEq/L sodium bicarbonate in I.V. fluid Maintain urine pH at 7.0-7.5 Reduce bicarbonate if serum bicarbonate >30 mEq/L or urine pH >7.5	50-100 mEq/L sodium bicarbonate in I.V. fluid Maintain urine pH at 7.0-7.5 Reduce bicarbonate if serum bicarbonate >30 mEq/L or urine pH >7.5
Uric acid reduction	Allopurinol: I.V., oral: 200-400 mg/m^2/day in 1-3 divided doses (maximum: 600 mg/day) Urate oxidase: I.V. (investigational, see protocol): 0.2 mg/kg/dose once or twice daily	Allopurinol: I.V.: 200-400 mg/m^2/day in 1-3 divided doses (maximum: 600 mg/day) Oral: 600-800 mg/day in 1-2 doses
Diuretics (avoid if hypovolemic)	Furosemide: I.V.: 1 mg/kg/dose as needed Mannitol: I.V.: 0.25-0.5 g/kg/dose as needed	Furosemide: I.V.: 20-40 mg/dose as needed Mannitol: I.V.: 0.25-0.5 g/kg/dose as needed
Phosphate reduction	Aluminum hydroxide: Oral: 50 mg/kg/dose every 8 hours	Aluminum hydroxide: Oral: 30-40 mL/dose every 6-8 hours
Dialysis indications (peritoneal dialysis is much less efficient for reducing uric acid than other modalities, and is contraindicated in patients with abdominal tumors.)	Potassium level >6 mEq/L Uric acid level >10 mg/dL Creatinine >10 times normal Uremia Phosphorus >10 mg/dL or rapidly rising Symptomatic hypocalcemia Severe, unmanageable hypertension Volume overload	

Kelly KM and Lange B, "Oncologic Emergencies," *Pediatr Clin North Am*, 1997, 44(4):809-30.

ANTITHROMBOTIC THERAPY IN CHILDREN

Recommendations From the Seventh American College of Chest Physicians (ACCP) Conference on Antithrombotic and Thrombolytic Therapy

Used with permission from Monagle P, Chan A, Massicotte P, et al, "Antithrombotic Therapy in Children: The Seventh ACCP Conference on Antithrombotic and Thrombolytic Therapy," *Chest*, 2004, 126(3 Suppl):645S-687S.

Abbreviations: ADP = adenosine diphosphate; AIS = arterial ischemic stroke; aPTT = activated partial thromboplastin time; AT = antithrombin; BT = Blalock-Taussig; CC = cardiac catheterization; CHD = congenital heart disease; CI = confidence interval; CSVT = cerebral sinovenous thrombosis; CVL = central venous line; DVT = deep venous thrombosis; FFP = fresh-frozen plasma; FXa = factor Xa; GP = glycoprotein; HIT = heparin-induced thrombocytopenia; ICH = intracranial hemorrhage; INR = international normalized ratio; IVC = inferior vena cava; LMWH = low-molecular-weight heparin; MRV = magnetic resonance venography; PC = protein C; PE = pulmonary embolism; PICU = pediatric ICU; PS = protein S; PTS = post-thrombotic syndrome; RCT = randomized controlled trial; RR = relative risk; RVT = renal vein thrombosis; SK = streptokinase; SVT = sinovenous thrombosis; TE = thromboembolic event; tPA = tissue plasminogen activator; TPN = total parenteral nutrition; UAC = umbilical arterial catheter; UFH = unfractionated heparin; UK = urokinase; UVC = umbilical vein catheter; VKA = vitamin K antagonist; VTE = venous thromboembolism

1.1 Venous Thromboembolism

Neonates with VTE

1.1.1. ACCP suggests treatment with either UFH or LMWH, or radiographic monitoring and anticoagulation therapy if extension occurs (Grade 2C).

1.1.2. ACCP suggests that if clinicians elect treatment with anticoagulation therapy, they administer UFH or LMWH, and subsequently administer LMWH for 10 days to 3 months (Grade 2C).

1.1.3. ACCP suggests that clinicians adjust the dose of UFH to prolong the aPTT corresponding to an anti-FXa level of 0.35-0.7 units/mL (Grade 2C).

1.1.4. ACCP suggests that clinicians adjust the dose of LMWH to achieve an anti-FXa level of 0.5-1.0 unit/mL (Grade 2C).

1.1.5. ACCP suggests that if the thrombus extends following the discontinuation of heparin therapy, clinicians administer VKAs or extended LMWH therapy (Grade 2C).

1.1.6. ACCP suggests that clinicians **not** use thrombolytic therapy for the treatment of VTEs in neonates unless there is major vessel occlusion that is causing the critical compromise of organs or limbs (Grade 2C). If thrombolytic therapy is used, ACCP suggests supplementation with plasminogen (ie, FFP) immediately prior to thrombolysis (Grade 2C).

1.1.7. ACCP suggests that, in general, clinicians should remove either CVLs or UVCs that are *in situ*. However, if either CVLs or UVCs are still in place at the completion of the above therapy, ACCP suggests prophylactic dosing with LMWH to prevent recurrent VTEs until such time as the CVL or UVC is removed (both Grade 2C).

1.2. Systemic Venous Thromboembolic Disease in Children

First TE for children (>2 months of age)

1.2.1. ACCP recommends treatment with I.V. heparin sufficient to prolong the aPTT to a range that corresponds to an anti-FXa level of 0.35-0.7 units/mL or with LMWH sufficient to achieve an anti-FXa level of 0.5-1.0 unit/mL 4 h after an injection (Grade 1C+).

1.2.2. ACCP recommends initial treatment with heparin or LMWH for 5-10 days (Grade 1C+). For patients in whom subsequent VKAs will be used, ACCP recommends beginning oral therapy as early as day 1 and discontinuing heparin/ LMWH therapy on day 6 if the INR is in the therapeutic range on two consecutive days (Grade 1C+). For massive PEs or extensive DVT, ACCP recommends a longer period of heparin or LMWH therapy (Grade 1C+).

1.2.3. ACCP suggests continuing anticoagulant therapy for idiopathic TEs for at least 6 months using VKAs to achieve a target INR of 2.5 (INR range, 2.0-3.0) or, alternatively, LMWH to maintain an anti-FXa level of 0.5-1.0 unit/mL (Grade 2C). *Underlying values and preferences:* The suggestion to administer anticoagulation therapy to children with idiopathic DVT for at least 6 months rather than on a lifelong basis places a relatively high value on the avoidance of the known risk of bleeding secondary to anticoagulant therapy in young active adults, and less importance on the unknown risk of recurrence in the absence of an ongoing clinical precipitating factor.

1.2.4. ACCP suggests that for secondary TEs anticoagulant therapy be continued for at least 3 months using VKAs to achieve a target INR of 2.5 (INR range, 2.0-3.0) or, alternatively, using LMWH to maintain an anti-FXa level of 0.5-1.0 unit/mL (Grade 2C).

1.2.5. ACCP suggests that, in the presence of ongoing risk factors such as active nephrotic syndrome, ongoing asparaginase therapy, or administration of a lupus anticoagulant, anticoagulant therapy in either therapeutic or prophylactic doses continue until the risk factor has resolved (Grade 2C).

1.2.6. ACCP suggests that clinicians **not** use thrombolytic therapy routinely for the treatment of venous TE in children (Grade 2C). Treatment needs to be individualized, and based on the size and location of the thrombus, and the degree of organ compromise. If thrombolytic therapy is used, in the presence of physiologic or pathologic deficiencies of plasminogen, ACCP suggests supplementation with plasminogen (ie, FFP) (Grade 2C).

Recurrent idiopathic TEs in children

1.2.7. ACCP recommends indefinite therapy with either therapeutic or prophylactic doses of VKAs (Grade 1C+). ACCP suggests LMWH therapy as an alternative if VKA therapy is too difficult (Grade 2C).

Recurrent secondary TEs in children

1.2.8. ACCP suggests that, following the initial 3 months of therapy, anticoagulation therapy be continued for at least a further 3 months or until removal of any precipitating factors (Grade 2C).

CVL-related thrombosis

There are two aspects to the management of CVL-related thrombosis. First, management of the CVL itself and, second, anticoagulation therapy.

1.2.9. ACCP suggests that if the CVL is no longer required, or is nonfunctioning, it be removed (Grade 2C). ACCP suggests at least 3-5 days of anticoagulation therapy prior to its removal. If CVL access is required and the CVL involved is still functioning, ACCP suggests that the CVL remain *in situ* (Grade 2C). Anticoagulation therapy should be administered as described in recommendations 1.2.1-1.2.6.

1.2.10. For children with a first CVL-related DVT after the initial 3 months of therapy, ACCP suggests that prophylactic doses of VKAs (INR range, 1.5-1.8) or LMWH (anti-FXa level range, 0.1- 0.3) be administered until the CVL is removed (Grade 2C).

1.2.11. For children with recurrent CVL-related TEs after the initial 3 months of therapy, ACCP suggests prophylactic doses of VKAs (INR range, 1.5-1.8) or LMWH (anti-FXa level range, 0.1-0.3) be continued until the removal of the CVL. If the recurrence occurs while children are receiving prophylactic therapy, ACCP suggests continuing therapeutic doses until the CVL is removed or for a minimum of 3 months (Grade 2C).

ANTITHROMBOTIC THERAPY IN CHILDREN *(Continued)*

1.3 Renal Vein Thrombosis

1.3.1. For unilateral RVT in the absence of uremia, and in the absence of extension into the IVC, ACCP suggests supportive care with careful monitoring of the RVT for extension (Grade 2C). Alternatively, ACCP suggests anticoagulation therapy with UFH or LMWH (Grade 2C).

1.3.2. For unilateral RVT that does extend into the IVC, ACCP suggests anticoagulation therapy with UFH or LMWH for 6 weeks to 3 months (Grade 2C). *Remark:* The therapeutic range is the same as that for the treatment of venous thrombosis.

1.3.3. For bilateral RVT with various degrees of renal failure, ACCP suggests therapy with UFH (and not LMWH) and thrombolytic therapy (Grade 2C).

1.4 Central Venous Line Prophylaxis

1.4.1. For children With CVLs, ACCP recommends **against** routine primary prophylaxis (Grade 1B).

1.4.2. For children receiving long-term home TPN, ACCP suggests antithrombotic prophylaxis. ACCP suggests continuous therapy with VKAs (target INR, 2-2.5) or, alternatively, for the first 3 months after each CVL is inserted (all Grade 2C). *Remark:* The optimal drug and dose are unknown.

1.5 Primary Prophylaxis for BT Shunts in Neonates

1.5.1. For neonates having BT shunts, ACCP suggests therapy with intraoperative heparin followed by either aspirin (5 mg/kg/d) or no further anticoagulant therapy (Grade 2C).

1.6 Primary Prophylaxis for Stage 1 Norwood Procedures in Neonates

1.6.1. For patients who have undergone the Norwood procedure, ACCP suggests heparin therapy immediately after the procedure (Grade 2C).

1.8 Primary Prophylaxis for Fontan Surgery in Children

1.8.1. For children after Fontan surgery, ACCP suggests therapy with aspirin (5 mg/kg/d) or therapeutic heparin followed by VKAs to achieve a target INR of 2.5 (INR range, 2-3) (Grade 2C). *Remark:* The optimal duration of therapy is unknown. Whether patients with fenestrations require more intensive therapy until fenestration closure is unknown.

1.9 Primary Prophylaxis for Endovascular Stents in Children

1.9.1. For children having endovascular stents inserted, ACCP suggests the administration of heparin perioperatively (Grade 2C).

1.10 Primary Prophylaxis for Dilated Cardiomyopathy in Neonates and Children

1.10.1. For children with cardiomyopathy, ACCP suggests that they receive therapy with VKAs to achieve a target INR of 2.5 (INR range, 2-3) commencing no later than at the time of their activation on a cardiac transplant waiting list (Grade 2C). *Underlying values and preferences:* ACCP's suggestion for the administration of VKAs places a high value on avoiding thrombotic complications, and a relatively low value on avoiding the inconvenience, discomfort, and limitations of anticoagulant monitoring in children who have a potentially curative therapy (for their cardiomyopathy) available to them.

1.11 Primary Prophylaxis for Biological Prosthetic Heart Valves in Children

1.11.1. For children with biological prosthetic heart valves, ACCP recommends treatment according to the adult guidelines (Grade 1C+).

1.12 Primary Prophylaxis for Mechanical Prosthetic Heart Valves in Children

1.12.1. For children with mechanical prosthetic heart valves, ACCP recommends the administration of VKAs following adult guidelines (Grade 1C+).

1.12.2. In children in whom additional antithrombotic therapy is required due to lack of response to therapy with VKAs or a contraindication to therapy with full-dose VKAs, ACCP suggests adding therapy with aspirin (6-20 mg/kg/d) (Grade 2C).

1.14 Thromboprophylaxis for Cardiac Catheterization in Neonates and Children

1.14.1. For neonates and children requiring CC via an artery, ACCP recommends I.V. heparin prophylaxis (Grade 1A).

1.14.2. ACCP suggests the use of heparin doses of 100-150 units/kg as a bolus. Further doses may be required in prolonged procedures (both Grade 2B).

1.14.3. For prophylaxis for CC, ACCP recommends **against** aspirin therapy (Grade 1B).

1.15 Femoral Artery Thrombosis Following Cardiac Catheterization

1.15.1. For children or neonates with a femoral artery thrombosis, ACCP recommends therapeutic doses of I.V. heparin (Grade 1C). ACCP suggests treatment for at least 5-7 days (Grade 2C). *Remark:* The optimal duration of therapy is unknown.

1.15.2. For children or neonates with limb-threatening or organ-threatening (via proximal extension) femoral artery thrombosis who fail to respond to initial heparin therapy, and who have no known contraindications, ACCP recommends the administration of thrombolytic therapy (Grade 1C).

1.15.3. For children with femoral artery thrombosis in selected cases, ACCP suggests surgical intervention, in particular when there is a contraindication to thrombolytic therapy, or when organ or limb death is imminent (Grade 2C).

1.16 Peripheral Artery Thrombosis

1.16.1. For neonates and children with peripheral arterial catheters *in situ*, ACCP recommends the administration of low-dose heparin through the catheter, preferably by continuous infusion, to prolong the catheter patency (Grade 1A).

1.16.2. For children with a peripheral arterial catheter-related TE, ACCP suggests the immediate removal of the catheter (Grade 2C). ACCP suggests subsequent anticoagulation therapy with or without thrombolysis, depending on the clinical situation (Grade 2C).

1.18 Aortic Thrombosis Secondary to UACs in Neonates

1.18.1. For neonates with UACs, ACCP suggests therapy with low-dose heparin infusion (1-5 units/h) (Grade 2A).

1.18.2. ACCP suggests that aortic thrombosis secondary to UACs be managed by the same principles as those for femoral artery thrombosis secondary to cardiac catheters. If there is evidence of renal failure, then urgent restoration of renal blood flow is required, and ACCP suggests thrombolysis or thrombectomy (all Grade 2C).

1.19 Spontaneous Aortic Thrombosis in Neonates

1.19.1. For children experiencing spontaneous aortic thrombosis with evidence of renal ischemia, ACCP suggests urgent, aggressive use of thrombolytic or surgical therapy, supported by anticoagulation therapy with heparin or LMWH (Grade 2C).

1.20 Kawasaki Disease in Children

1.20.1. ACCP recommends aspirin therapy in high doses (ie, 80-100 mg/kg/d during the acute phase, for up to 14 days) as an anti-inflammatory agent, then in lower doses (ie, 3- 5 mg/kg/d for ≥7 weeks) as an antiplatelet agent (Grade 1C+).

1.20.2. ACCP recommends therapy with I.V. gammaglobulin (2 g/kg as a single dose) within 10 days of the onset of symptoms (Grade 1A).

1.21 Anticoagulation Therapy for Kawasaki Disease in Children With Giant Aneurysms

1.21.1. In children with giant coronary aneurysms following Kawasaki disease, ACCP suggests therapy with warfarin (target INR, 2.5; INR range, 2.0-3.0) in addition to low-dose aspirin (Grade 2C).

ANTITHROMBOTIC THERAPY IN CHILDREN *(Continued)*

1.22 Sinovenous Thrombosis in Neonates

1.22.1. For neonates with CSVT, without large ischemic infarctions or ICH, ACCP suggests initial treatment with either UFH or LMWH followed by treatment with LMWH for 3 months (Grade 2C).

1.22.2. For neonates with CSVT, with large ischemic infarctions or ICH, ACCP suggests radiographic monitoring and the commencement of anticoagulation therapy if extension occurs (Grade 2C).

1.23 Sinovenous Thrombosis in Children

1.23.1. For children with CSVT, ACCP suggests treatment for 5-7 days with either UFH or LMWH followed by treatment with LMWH or VKAs (target INR, 2.5; INR range, 2.0-3.0) for 3-6 months even in the presence of a localized hemorrhagic infarction (Grade 2C).

1.24 Arterial Ischemic Stroke in Neonates

1.24.1. For neonates with noncardioembolic AIS, ACCP suggests that clinicians do **not** use anticoagulation or aspirin therapy (Grade 2C).

1.24.2. For neonates with cardioembolic AIS, ACCP suggests anticoagulation therapy with either UFH or LMWH for 3 months (Grade 2C).

1.25 Arterial Ischemic Stroke in Children

1.25.1. For children with AIS, ACCP suggests treatment with UFH or LMWH for 5-7 days and until cardioembolic stroke or vascular dissection has been excluded (Grade 2C).

1.25.2. For children with AIS and cardioembolic stroke or vascular dissection, ACCP suggests treatment for 5-7 days with UFH or LMWH followed by treatment with LMWH or VKAs for 3-6 months (Grade 2C).

1.25.3. For all children with AIS, ACCP suggests treatment with 2-5 mg/kg/d aspirin after anticoagulation therapy has been discontinued (Grade 2C).

1.25.4. For children with sickle cell disease who are >2 years of age, ACCP recommends screening for stroke using transcranial Doppler imaging. If transcranial Doppler imaging is unavailable, ACCP recommends intermittent screening with MRI (Grade 1C).

1.25.5. For children with sickle cell disease who have ischemic stroke, ACCP recommends therapy with I.V. hydration and exchange transfusion to reduce hemoglobin S levels to <30% of total hemoglobin (Grade 1C).

1.25.6. For children with sickle cell disease who have ischemic stroke, after an initial exchange transfusion ACCP suggests a long-term transfusion program (Grade 2C).

1.26 Purpura Fulminans

1.26.1. For neonates with homozygous PC deficiency, ACCP recommends the administration of either 10-20 mL/kg FFP every 12 h or PC concentrate, when available, at a concentration of 20-60 units/kg until the clinical lesions resolve (Grade 1C+).

1.26.2. ACCP suggests long-term treatment with VKAs (Grade 2C), LMWH (Grade 2C), PC replacement (Grade 1C+), or liver transplantation (Grade 2C).

[1]The ACCP Consensus Conference on Antithrombotic Therapy uses grades of recommendations that are based on clarity of benefits versus risks of treatment (1 = clear risk/benefit, strong recommendation; 2 = unclear risk/benefit, weaker recommendation) and quality of the research methodology supporting the underlying evidence (A = randomized trials with consistent results; B = randomized trials with inconsistent results or with major weaknesses in methodology; C = observational studies and generalizations of randomized trials to another group of patients; C+ = observational studies with overwhelmingly compelling results or secure generalizations of randomized trials). The highest rating (1A) implies a strong recommendation; one that can be applied to most patients in most circumstances without reservations. The lowest rating (2C) implies a very weak recommendation; one in which other alternatives may be equally reasonable. For further information see Guyatt G, Schunemann HJ, Cook D, et al, "Applying the Grades of Recommendation for Antithrombotic and Thrombolytic Therapy: The Seventh ACCP Conference on Antithrombotic and Thrombolytic Therapy," *Chest*, 2004, 126(3 Suppl):179S-187S.

TOTAL BLOOD VOLUME

Age	Example Weight (kg) [age]	Approximate Total Blood Volume (mL/kg)[1]	Estimated Total Blood Volume (mL)
Premature infant	1.5	89-105	134-158
Term newborn	3.4	78-86	265-292
1-12 months	7.6 [6 months]	73-78	555-593
1-3 years	12.4 [2 years]	74-82	918-1017
4-6 years	18.2 [5 years]	80-86	1456-1565
7-18 years	45.5 [13 years]	83-90	3777-4095
Adults	70.0	68-88	4760-6160

[1]Approximate total blood volume information compiled from *Nathan and Oski's Hematology of Infancy and Childhood*, 5th ed, Nathan DG and Orkin SH, eds, Philadelphia, PA: WB Saunders, 1998.

ASSESSMENT OF LIVER FUNCTION

Child-Pugh Score

Component	Score Given for Observed Findings		
	1	2	3
Encephalopathy grade[1]	None	1-2	3-4
Ascites	None	Mild or controlled by diuretics	Moderate or refractory despite diuretics
Albumin (g/dL)	>3.5	2.8-3.5	<2.8
Total bilirubin (mg/dL)	<2 (<34 micromoles/L)	2-3 (34-50 micromoles/L)	>3 (>50 micromoles/L)
or Modified total bilirubin[2]	<4	4-7	>7
Prothrombin time (seconds prolonged)	<4	4-6	>6
or INR	<1.7	1.7-2.3	>2.3

[1]**Encephalopathy Grades**

Grade 0: Normal consciousness, personality, neurological examination, electroencephalogram

Grade 1: Restless, sleep disturbed, irritable/agitated, tremor, impaired handwriting, 5 cps waves

Grade 2: Lethargic, time-disoriented, inappropriate, asterixis, ataxia, slow triphasic waves

Grade 3: Somnolent, stuporous, place-disoriented, hyperactive reflexes, rigidity, slower waves

Grade 4: Unrousable coma, no personality/behavior, decerebrate, slow 2-3 cps delta activity

Alternative Encephalopathy Grades

Grade 1: Mild confusion, anxiety, restlessness, fine tremor, slowed coordination

Grade 2: Drowsiness, disorientation, asterixis

Grade 3: Somnolent but rousable, marked confusion, incomprehensible speech, incontinent, hyperventilation

Grade 4: Coma, decerebrate posturing, flaccidity

[2]Modified total bilirubin used to score patients who have Gilbert's syndrome or who are taking indinavir.

Child-Pugh Classification

Class A (mild hepatic impairment): Score 5-6

Class B (moderate hepatic impairment): Score 7-9

Class C (severe hepatic impairment): Score 10-15

References

Centers for Disease Control and Prevention, "Report of the NIH Panel to Define Principles of Therapy of HIV Infection and Guidelines for the Use of Antiretroviral Agents in HIV-Infected Adults and Adolescents," March 23, 2004, located at (URL) http://www.aidsinfo.nih.gov.

U.S. Department of Health and Human Services Food and Drug Administration, "Guidance for Industry, Pharmacokinetics in Patients With Impaired Hepatic Function: Study Design, Data Analysis, and Impact on Dosing and Labeling," May 2003, located at (URL) http://www.fda.gov/cder/guidance/3625fnl.pdf.

HOTLINE PHONE NUMBERS

AIDS Hotline	800-342-2437
American Association of Poison Control Centers (AAPCC)	
Poison Prevention	202-362-7217
Emergency	800-222-1222
American College of Clinical Pharmacy (ACCP)	816-531-2177
American Dental Association (ADA)	312-440-2500
American Medical Association (AMA)	800-621-8335
American Pharmacists Association (APhA)	202-628-4410
American Society of Health-System Pharmacists	866-270-0681
Animal Poison Control Center (24-hours)	888-426-4435
Canadian Pharmacists Association	613-523-7877
Center for Disease Control	1-800-CDC-INFO
FDA (Rare Diseases/Orphan Drugs)	800-300-7469
National Cancer Institute	1-800-4-CANCER
Asthma and Allergy Foundation of America	1-800-7-ASTHMA
Epilepsy Foundation	800-332-1000
National Council on Patient Information & Education	301-656-8565
National Institute of Health	301-496-4000
National Capital Poison Center	202-362-3867
Emergency	800-222-1222
Pediatric Pharmacy Advocacy Group (PPAG) Membership Information	901-380-3617
National Pesticide Information Center	800-858-7378
Rocky Mountain Poison Control Information	800-222-1222

ENDOCARDITIS PROPHYLAXIS

Recommendations by the American Heart Association (*Circulation*, 2007, 115:1-20)

Consensus Process – The recommendations were formulated by the writing group after analyses of relevant literature regarding procedure-related bacteremia and infective endocarditis *in vitro* susceptibility data of the most common microorganisms that cause infective endocarditis, results of prophylactic studies in animal models of experimental endocarditis, and retrospective and prospective studies of prevention of infective endocarditis. The consensus statement was subsequently reviewed by outside experts not affiliated with the writing group and by the Science Advisory and Coordinating Committee of the American Heart Association. These guidelines are meant to aid practitioners but are not intended as the standard of care or as a substitute for clinical judgment.

Table 1. Cardiac Conditions Associated With the Highest Risk of Adverse Outcome From Endocarditis[1]

Prophylaxis With Dental Procedures Is Recommended

- Prosthetic cardiac valves
- Previous infective endocarditis
- Congenital heart disease (CHD)
  - Unrepaired cyanotic CHD, including palliative stunts and conduits
  - Completely repaired congenital heart defect with prosthetic material or device, whether placed by surgery or by catheter intervention, during the first 6 months after the procedure[1]
  - Repaired CHD with residual defects at the site or adjacent to the site of a prosthetic patch or prosthetic device (which inhibit endothelialization)
  - Cardiac transplantation recipients who develop cardiac valvulopathy

Endocarditis Prophylaxis Not Recommended

- Negligible-Risk Category (no greater risk than the general population)
  - Isolated secundum atrial septal defect
  - Surgical repair of atrial septal defect, ventricular septal defect, or patent ductus arteriosus (without residua beyond 6 months)
  - Previous coronary artery bypass graft surgery
  - Mitral valve prolapse without valvar regurgitation
  - Physiologic, functional, or innocent heart murmurs
  - Previous Kawasaki disease without valvar dysfunction
  - Previous rheumatic fever without valvar dysfunction
  - Cardiac pacemakers (intravascular and epicardial) and implanted defibrillators

[1]Prophylaxis is recommended because endothelialization of prosthetic material occurs within 6 months after the procedure.

Table 2. Dental Procedures and Endocarditis Prophylaxis

Dental Procedures for Which Endocarditis Prophylaxis Is Recommended for Patients in Table 1
All dental procedures that involve manipulation of gingival tissue or the periapical region of teeth or perforation of the oral mucosa
Endocarditis Prophylaxis Not Recommended
Restorative dentistry[1] (operative and prosthodontic) with or without retraction cord
Local anesthetic injections through noninfected tissues
Intracanal endodontic treatment; post placement and buildup
Placement of rubber dams
Postoperative suture removal
Placement of removable prosthodontic or orthodontic appliances
Taking of oral impressions
Fluoride treatments
Taking of oral radiographs
Orthodontic appliance adjustment
Bleeding from trauma to the lips or oral mucosa
Shedding of primary teeth

[1]This includes restoration of decayed teeth (filling cavities) and replacement of missing teeth.

ENDOCARDITIS PROPHYLAXIS *(Continued)*

Table 3. Recommended Standard Prophylactic Regimen for Procedures on Respiratory Tract or Infected Skin, Skin Structures, or Musculoskeletal Tissue

Endocarditis Prophylaxis Recommended

Only for patients with underlying cardiac conditions associated with the highest risk of adverse outcome from Table 1 (use antibiotic prophylaxis with a regimen listed in Table 5)

Respiratory tract invasive procedure that involves incision or biopsy of respiratory mucosa

Tonsillectomy or adenoidectomy

For patients who undergo an invasive respiratory tract, procedure to treat an established infection (ie, drainage of an abscess or empyema), antibiotic regimen should contain an agent active against *Streptococcus* viridans group (see medications in Table 5)

If infection is caused by *Staphylococcus aureus*, the antibiotic regimen should contain an antistaphylococcal penicillin or cephalosporin, or vancomycin in patients unable to tolerate a β-lactam

If infection is caused by MRSA, administer vancomycin

Endocarditis Prophylaxis Not Recommended

Respiratory Tract
- Endotracheal intubation
- Bronchoscopy with a flexible bronchoscope, with or without biopsy
- Tympanostomy tube insertion

Gastrointestinal Tract
- Transesophageal echocardiography
- Endoscopy with or without gastrointestinal biopsy

Genitourinary Tract
- Vaginal hysterectomy
- Vaginal delivery
- Cesarean section
- In uninfected tissues:
  - Urethral catheterization
  - Uterine dilatation and curettage
  - Therapeutic abortion
  - Sterilization procedures
  - Insertion or removal of intrauterine devices

Other
- Cardiac catheterization, including balloon angioplasty
- Implanted cardiac pacemakers, implanted defibrillators, and coronary stents
- Incision or biopsy or surgically scrubbed skin
- Circumcision
- Ear and body piercing
- Tattooing

Table 4. Recommended Standard Prophylactic Regimen for Antibiotic Prophylaxis Solely to Prevent Infective Endocarditis (Note: NOT Recommended for GU or GI Tract Procedures)

For patients with underlying cardiac conditions associated with the highest risk of adverse outcome from Table 1 who are scheduled for an elective cystoscopy or other urinary tract manipulation and who have an enterococcal UTI or colonization, antibiotic therapy to eradicate enterococci from the urine before the procedure may be reasonable.

If the urinary tract procedure is not elective, it may be reasonable to administer an active agent against enterococci as part of the empiric antimicrobial regimen.

Preferred agent: Amoxicillin or ampicillin

If patient is unable to tolerate ampicillin: Vancomycin

	Dosage for Adults	Dosage for Children[1]
Vancomycin	1 g I.V. infused **slowly over 1 h**; complete infusion within 30 minutes before procedure	20 mg/kg I.V. infused **slowly over 1 h**; complete infusion within 30 minutes before procedure

[1]Children's dose should not exceed adult dosage.

If infection is caused by known or suspected strain of resistant Enterococcus: Consult with an infectious diseases expert.

Table 5. Endocarditis Prophylaxis for a Dental Procedure

	Dosage for Adults	Dosage for Children[1]
Oral		
Amoxicillin[2]	2 g 30-60 min before procedure	50 mg/kg 30-60 min before procedure
Penicillin or ampicillin allergy:		
Clindamycin **or**	600 mg 30-60 min before procedure	20 mg/kg 30-60 min before procedure
Cephalexin (not to be used in individuals with immediate-type hypersensitivity reaction to penicillins) **or**	2 g 30-60 min before procedure	50 mg/kg 30-60 min before procedure
Azithromycin or Clarithromycin	500 mg 30-60 min before procedure	15 mg/kg 30-60 min before procedure
Parenteral		
Ampicillin	2 g I.M. or I.V. 30-60 min before procedure	50 mg/kg I.M. or I.V. 30-60 min before procedure
Penicillin allergy:		
Clindamycin **or**	600 mg I.V. 30-60 min before procedure	20 mg/kg I.V. 30-60 min before procedure
Cefazolin or ceftriaxone (not to be used in individuals with immediate-type hypersensitivity reaction to penicillins)	1 g I.M. or I.V. 30-60 min before procedure	50 mg/kg I.M. or I.V. 30-60 min before procedure

[1]Children's dose should not exceed adult dosage.

[2]Amoxicillin is recommended because of its excellent bioavailability and good activity against streptococci and enterococci.

References

Wilson W, Taubert KA, Gewitz M, et al, "Prevention of Infective Endocarditis. Guidelines From the American Heart Association," *Circulation*, 2007, 115:1-20.

PEDIATRIC HIV

Selected tables from the Centers for Disease Control and Prevention, "Guidelines for the Use of Antiretroviral Agents in Pediatric HIV Infection," first published in *MMWR*, 1998:47(No.RR-4), April 17, 1998, updated as a "Living Document", October 26, 2006, located at (URL) http://www.aidsinfo.nih.gov.

1994 Revised Human Immunodeficiency Virus Pediatric Classification System: Immune Categories Based on Age-specific CD4+ T cell and Percentage[1]

Immune Category	<12 mo		1-5 y		6-12 y	
	No./mm³	%	No./mm³	%	No./mm³	%
Category 1 no suppression	≥1500	≥25	≥1000	≥25	≥500	≥25
Category 2 moderate suppression	750-1499	15-24	500-999	15-24	200-499	15-24
Category 3 severe suppression	<750	<15	<500	<15	<200	<15

[1]Modified from: CDC,"1994 Revised Classification System for Human Immunodeficiency Virus Infection in Children Less Than 13 Years of Age," *MMWR*, 1994, 43(RR-12):1-10.

1994 Revised Human Immunodeficiency Virus Pediatric Classification System: Clinical Categories[1]

Category N: Not Symptomatic
Children who have no signs or symptoms considered to be the result of HIV infection or who have only **one** of the conditions listed in category A

Category A: Mildly Symptomatic
Children with **two** or more of the following conditions, but none of the conditions listed in categories B and C:

- Lymphadenopathy (≥0.5 cm at more than 2 sites; bilateral = 1 site)
- Hepatomegaly
- Splenomegaly
- Dermatitis
- Parotitis
- Recurrent or persistent upper respiratory infection, sinusitis, or otitis media

Category B: Moderately Symptomatic
Children who have symptomatic conditions attributed to HIV infection, other than those listed for category A or category C. Examples of conditions in clinical category B include but are not limited to the following:

- Anemia (<8 g/dL), neutropenia (<1000/mm³), or thrombocytopenia (<100,000/mm³) persisting ≥30 days
- Bacterial meningitis, pneumonia, or sepsis (single episode)
- Candidiasis, oropharyngeal (ie, thrush) persisting for >2 months in children aged >6 months
- Cardiomyopathy
- Cytomegalovirus infection with onset before age 1 month
- Diarrhea, recurrent or chronic
- Hepatitis
- Herpes simplex virus (HSV) stomatitis, recurrent (ie, more than two episodes within 1 year)
- HSV bronchitis, pneumonitis, or esophagitis with onset before age 1 month
- Herpes zoster (ie, shingles) involving at least two distinct episodes or more than one dermatome
- Leiomyosarcoma
- Lymphoid interstitial pneumonia (LIP) or pulmonary lymphoid hyperplasia complex
- Nephropathy
- Nocardiosis
- Fever lasting >1 month
- Toxoplasmosis with onset before age 1 month
- Varicella, disseminated (ie, complicated chickenpox)

Category C: Severely Symptomatic
Children who have any condition listed in the 1987 surveillance case definition for acquired immunodeficiency syndrome, with the exception of LIP (which is a category B condition).

[1]Centers for Disease Control and Prevention, "1994 Revised Classification System for Human Immunodeficiency Virus Infection in Children Less Than 13 Years of Age," *MMWR*, 1994, 43(RR-12):1-10.

Indications for Initiation of Antiretroviral Therapy in Children Infected With Human Immunodeficiency Virus

This table provides general guidance rather than absolute recommendations for an individual patient. Factors to be considered in decisions about initiation of therapy include the risk of disease progression as determined by CD4+ percentage or count and plasma HIV RNA copy number, the potential benefits and risks of therapy, and the ability of the caregiver and child to adhere to administration of the therapeutic regimen. Issues associated with adherence should be fully assessed, discussed, and addressed with the caregiver and child, if age-appropriate, before the decision to initiate therapy is made.

Age	Criteria	Recommendation
<12 mo	• HIV-related symptoms[1] **or**	Treat
	• Asymptomatic[2] **and** CD4 <25%	Treat
	• Asymptomatic[2] **and** CD4 ≥25%	Consider[3]
1-<4 y	• AIDS or significant HIV-related symptoms[4] **or**	Treat
	• Asymptomatic or mild symptoms[5] **and** CD4 <20%	Treat
	• Asymptomatic or mild symptoms[5] **and** – CD4 20% to 24% **or** – HIV RNA ≥100,000 copies/mL	Consider
	• Asymptomatic[2] **and** – CD4 ≥25% **and** – HIV RNA <100,000 copies/mL	Defer[6]
≥4-12 y	• AIDS or significant HIV-related symptoms[4] **or**	Treat
	• Asymptomatic or mild symptoms[5] **and** CD4 <15%[7]	Treat
	• Asymptomatic or mild symptoms[5] **and** – CD4 15% to 24% **or** – HIV RNA ≥100,000 copies/mL	Consider
	• Asymptomatic[2] **and** – CD4 ≥25% **and** – HIV RNA <100,000 copies/mL	Defer[6]
≥13 y	• AIDS or significant HIV-related symptoms[4] **or**	Treat
	• Asymptomatic or mild symptoms[5] **and** CD4 <200 cells/mm^3	Treat
	• Asymptomatic or mild symptoms[5] **and** – CD4 201-350 cells/mm^3 **or** – HIV RNA ≥100,000 copies/mL	Consider
	• Asymptomatic[2] **and** – CD4 >350 cells/mm^3 **and** – HIV RNA <100,000 copies/mL	Defer[6]

[1]CDC clinical category A, B, C.

[2]CDC clinical category N.

[3]Because HIV infection progresses more rapidly in infants than older children or adults, some experts would treat all HIV-infected infants age <6 months or <12 months, regardless of clinical, immunologic, or virologic parameters.

[4]CDC clinical category C and B (except for the following category B condition: Single episode of serious bacterial infection or lymphoid interstitial pneumonitis).

[5]CDC clinical category A or N or the following category B conditions: Single episode of serious bacterial infection or lymphoid interstitial pneumonitis.

[6]Clinical and laboratory data should be re-evaluated every 3-4 months.

[7]Or for children in upper end of this age category, absolute CD4 cell count is <200-300 cells/mm^3.

PEDIATRIC HIV *(Continued)*

Recommended Antiretroviral Regimens for Initial Therapy for Human Immunodeficiency Virus (HIV) Infection in Children

A combination antiretroviral regimen in treatment-naive children generally contains 1 NNRTI or 1 PI combined with a 2-drug NRTI backbone. A 3-drug NRTI regimen consisting of zidovudine, abacavir, and lamivudine is recommended only if a PI or NNRTI-based regimen can't be used. Regimens should be individualized based on advantages and disadvantages of each combination.

Non-nucleoside Reverse Transcriptase Inhibitor-Based Regimens	
Preferred regimen	Children ≥3 years: 2 NRTIs **plus** efavirenz[1]
	Children <3 years or who can't swallow capsules: 2 NRTIs **plus** nevirapine[1]
Alternative	2 NRTIs **plus** nevirapine (children ≥3 years)
Protease Inhibitor-Based Regimens	
Preferred regimen	2 NRTIs **plus** lopinavir/ritonavir
Alternative	2 NRTIs **plus** nelfinavir (children >2 years)
Use in Special Circumstances	
	1 or 2 NRTIs **plus** nelfinavir **plus** (efavirenz [children ≥3 years] **or** nevirapine)
	2 NRTIs **plus** (ritonavir **or** indinavir **or** amprenavir [children ≥4 years])[2]
	Zidovudine **plus** lamivudine **plus** abacavir
	2 NRTIs **plus** low-dose ritonavir **plus** (indinavir **or** fosamprenavir **or** saquinavir), only in adolescents who can receive adult doses
2-Drug NRTI Backbone Options (for use in combination with additional drugs)	
Preferred	Zidovudine **plus** (lamivudine **or** didanosine **or** emtricitabine)
	Didanosine **plus** (lamivudine **or** emtricitabine)
Alternative	Abacavir **plus** (zidovudine **or** lamivudine **or** emtricitabine **or** stavudine)
	Stavudine **plus** (lamivudine **or** emtricitabine)
Use in special circumstances	Stavudine **plus** didanosine
Insufficient Data to Recommend	
	Dual PIs with the exception of lopinavir/ritonavir[3]
	NRTI **plus** NNRTI **plus** PI[4]
	Tenofovir-containing regimens
	Enfuvirtide (T-20)-containing regimens
	Atazanavir-containing regimens
	Darunavir-containing regimens
	Fosamprenavir-containing regimens[5]
	Tipranavir-containing regimens

NRTI = nucleoside analogue reverse transcriptase inhibitor.

NNRTI = non-nucleoside analogue reverse transcriptase inhibitor.

PI = protease inhibitor.

[1]Efavirenz is currently available only in capsule form; nevirapine would be preferred NNRTI for children <3 years of age or who require a liquid formulation.

[2]Amprenavir should not be administered to children <4 years of age due to the propylene glycol and vitamin E content of the oral liquid preparation and lack or pharmacokinetic data in this age group.

[3]With the exception of lopinavir/ritonavir, data on the pharmacokinetics and safety of dual PI combinations are limited; use of dual PIs other than lopinavir/ritonavir as components of initial therapy is not recommended, although such regimens may have utility as secondary treatment regimens for children who have failed initial therapy. The use of low-dose ritonavir-boosted indinavir, fosamprenavir, or saquinavir can be considered in special circumstances for adolescents who can receive standard adult doses.

[4]With the exception of efavirenz plus nelfinavir plus 1 or 2 NRTIs, which has been studied in HIV-infected children and shown to have virologic and immunologic efficacy in a clinical trial.

[5]Use of low-dose ritonavir-boosted fosamprenavir can be considered as initial therapy in special circumstances for adolescents who can receive standard adult doses.

Considerations for Changing Antiretroviral Therapy for Human Immunodeficiency Virus (HIV)-Infected Children

Virologic Considerations[1]

- **Incomplete viral response to therapy:**
  - *For previously antiretroviral-naive or children with limited antiretroviral experience:* <1.0 $\log_{10}$ decrease in HIV RNA copy number from baseline after 8-12 weeks of therapy, or repeated HIV RNA >400 copies/mL after 6 months of therapy.[2]
  - *For children with more extensive antiretroviral experience:* <1 $\log_{10}$ decrease in HIV RNA after 6 months of treatment with a new therapeutic regimen.
- **Viral rebound:**
  - *For children who have previously suppressed viral replication to undetectable levels:* Repeated detection of HIV RNA >400 copies/mL.[3]
  - *For children who demonstrated an initial HIV RNA response but still had low levels of detectable HIV RNA:* Confirmed >0.5 $\log_{10}$ (>3-fold) increase in HIV RNA copy number for children age ≥2 years or >0.7 $\log_{10}$ (>5-fold) increase for children age <2 years.

Immunologic Considerations[1]

- **Incomplete immunologic response to therapy:** Failure of a child with severe immune suppression (CD4 percentage or cell count in CDC immune class 3) to improve CD4 percentage by at least 5 percentage points above baseline or, for children age 4-6 years, to increase their CD4 cell count by at least 50 cells/mm^3 above baseline over the first year of therapy.
- **Immunologic decline:** Persistent decline of 5 percentage points in CD4 percentage or decline to below pretherapy baseline in CD4 absolute cell count in children who are age 4-6 years at baseline.

Clinical Considerations

- **Progressive neurodevelopmental deterioration**
- **Growth failure:** Persistent decline in weight-growth velocity despite adequate nutritional support and without other explanation
- **Severe or recurrent infection or illness:** Recurrence or persistence of AIDS-defining conditions or other serious infections

[1]At least two measurements (taken 1 week apart) should be performed before considering a change in therapy.

[2]The initial HIV RNA level of the child at the start of therapy and the level achieved with therapy should be considered when contemplating potential drug changes. For example, an immediate change in therapy may not be warranted if there is a sustained 1.5-2.0 $\log_{10}$ decrease in HIV RNA copy number, even if RNA remains detectable at low levels.

[3]Continued observation with more frequent evaluation of HIV RNA levels should be considered if the HIV RNA increase is limited (ie, <5000 copies/mL). The presence of repeatedly detectable or increasing RNA levels suggests the development of resistance mutations.

PEDIATRIC HIV *(Continued)*

Strategies to Improve Adherence to Antiretroviral Medication Regimens in Children

Initial Intervention Strategies

- Establish trust and identify mutually acceptable goals for care.
- Obtain explicit agreement on need for treatment and adherence.
- Identify depression, low self-esteem, or drug use, or other mental health issues for the child/adolescent and/or caregiver that may decrease adherence. Treat prior to starting therapy, if possible.
- Identify family, friends, health team members, or others who can help with adherence support.
- Educate patient and family about the critical role of adherence in therapy outcome.
- Specify the adherence target: 95% of prescribed doses.
- Educate patient and family about the relationship between partial adherence and resistance.
- Educate patient and family about resistance and constraint of later choices of antiretroviral drug; explain that while a failure of adherence may be temporary, the effects on treatment choice may be permanent.
- Develop a treatment plan that the patient and family understand and to which they feel committed.
- Establish readiness to take medication by practice sessions or other means.
- For patient education and to assess tolerability of medications chosen, consider a brief period of hospitalization at start of therapy in selected circumstances,

Medication Strategies

- Choose the simplest regimen possible, reducing dosing frequency and number of pills.
- Choose a regimen with dosing requirements that best conform to daily and weekly routines and variations in patient and family activities.
- Choose the most palatable medicine possible (pharmacists may be able to add syrups or flavoring agents to increase palatability).
- Choose drugs with the fewest side effects; provide anticipatory guidance for management of side effects.
- Simplify food requirements for medication administration.
- Prescribe drugs carefully to avoid adverse drug-drug interactions.

Follow-up Intervention Strategies

- Monitor adherence at each visit, as well as in between visits by telephone or letter as needed.
- Provide ongoing support, encouragement, and understanding of the difficulties of the demands of attaining >95% adherence with medication doses.
- Use patient education aids including pictures, calendars, and stickers.
- Use pillboxes, reminders, alarms, pagers, and timers.
- Provide nurse, social worker, or other practitioner adherence clinic visits or telephone calls.
- Provide access to support groups, peer groups, or one-on-one counseling for caregivers and patients, especially for those with known depression or drug use issues which are known to decrease adherence.
- Provide pharmacist-based adherence support.
- Consider gastrostomy tube use in selected circumstances.
- For selected circumstances of apparent virologic failure, consider a brief period of hospitalization to assess adherence and reinforce that medication adherence is fundamental to successful antiretroviral therapy.
- Consider directly observed therapy at home, in the clinic, or during a brief inpatient hospitalization.

ADULT AND ADOLESCENT HIV

Selected tables from the Centers for Disease Control and Prevention, "Report of the NIH Panel to Define Principles of Therapy of HIV Infection and Guidelines for the Use of Antiretroviral Agents in HIV-Infected Adults and Adolescents," first published in *MMWR*, 1998:47(No. RR-5), April 24, 1998, updated as a "Living Document," October 10, 2006, located at (URL) http://www.aidsinfo.nih.gov.

Goals of HIV Therapy and Strategies to Achieve Them

Goals of Therapy

- Maximal and durable suppression of viral load
- Restoration and/or preservation of immunologic function
- Improvement of quality of life
- Reduction of HIV-related morbidity and mortality

Strategies to Achieve Goals of Therapy

- Maximize adherence to the antiretroviral regimen
- Rational sequencing of drugs
- Preservation of future treatment options
- Selection of appropriate combination therapy
- Optimize initial regimen with use of pretreatment genotypic drug resistance testing
- Optimize antiretroviral regimen with use of therapeutic drug monitoring in selected clinical settings

Indications for Plasma HIV RNA Testing[1]

Clinical Indication	Information	Use
Syndrome consistent with acute HIV infection	Establishes diagnosis when HIV antibody test is negative or indeterminate	Diagnosis[2]
Initial evaluation of newly diagnosed HIV infection	Baseline viral load "set point"	Use in conjunction with CD4$^+$ T-cell count for decision to start or defer therapy
Every 3-4 months in patients not on therapy	Changes in viral load	Use in conjunction with CD4$^+$ T-cell count for decision to start therapy
2-8 weeks after initiation of or change in antiretroviral therapy	Initial assessment of drug efficacy	Decision to continue or change therapy
3-4 months after start of therapy	Assessment of virologic effect of therapy	Decision to continue or change therapy
Every 3-4 months in patients on therapy	Durability of antiretroviral effect	Decision to continue or change therapy
Clinical event or significant decline in CD4$^+$ T cells	Association with changing or stable viral load	Decision to continue, initiate, or change therapy

[1]Acute illness (eg, bacterial pneumonia, tuberculosis, herpes simplex virus, *Pneumocystis jiroveci* pneumonia), and vaccinations can cause an increase in plasma HIV RNA for 2-4 weeks; viral load testing should not be performed during this time. Plasma HIV RNA results should usually be verified with a repeat determination before starting or making changes in therapy.

[2]Diagnosis of HIV infection made by HIV RNA testing should be confirmed by standard methods (ie, ELISA and Western blot testing) performed 2-4 months after the initial indeterminate or negative test.

ADULT AND ADOLESCENT HIV *(Continued)*

Indications for Initiating Antiretroviral Therapy for the Chronically HIV-1-Infected Patient

The optimal time to initiate therapy is unknown among persons with asymptomatic disease and CD4⁺ T-cell count of >200 cells/mm³. This table provides general guidance rather than absolute recommendations for an individual patient. All decisions regarding initiating therapy should be made on the basis of prognosis as determined by the CD4⁺ T-cell count and level of plasma HIV RNA, the potential benefits and risks of therapy, and the willingness of the patient to accept therapy.

Clinical Category	CD4⁺ T-Cell Count	Plasma HIV RNA	Recommendation
AIDS-defining illness or severe symptoms[1]	Any value	Any value	Treat
Asymptomatic[2]	<200/mm³	Any value	Treat
Asymptomatic	>200/mm³ but ≤350/mm³	Any value	Treatment should be offered following full discussion of pros and cons with each patient
Asymptomatic	>350/mm³	≥100,000	Most clinicians recommend deferring therapy, but some clinicians will treat
Asymptomatic	>350/mm³	<100,000	Defer therapy

[1]AIDS-defining illness per Centers for Disease Control, 1993. Severe symptoms include unexplained fever or diarrhea >2-4 weeks, oral candidiasis, or >10% unexplained weight loss.

[2]Clinical benefit has been demonstrated in controlled trials only for patients with CD4⁺ T cells <200/mm³; however, the majority of clinicians would offer therapy at a CD4⁺ T-cell threshold <350/mm³. A collaborative analysis of data from 13 cohort studies from Europe and North America found that lower CD4 count, higher HIV viral load, injection drug use, and age >50 were all predictors of progression to AIDS or death in antiretroviral naive patients beginning combination antiretroviral therapy. These data indicate that the prognosis is better for patients who initiate therapy at >200 cells/mm³, but risk after initiation of therapy does not vary considerably at >200 cells/mm³.

Early vs Delayed Treatment

Benefits and Risks of Delayed Initiation of Therapy in the Asymptomatic HIV-Infected Patient[1]

Benefits	Risks
• Avoid treatment-related negative quality of life effects (ie, inconvenience) • Avoid drug-related adverse events • Delay development of drug resistance • Preserve maximum number of available and future drug options • More time for patient to understand treatment demands • Decreased total time on medications with reduced chance of treatment fatigue • More time for development of more potent, less toxic, and better studied combination regimens	• Possibly irreversible immune system depletion • Possibly greater difficulty in suppressing viral replication • Possibly increased risk of progression to AIDS • Possibly increased risk of HIV transmission[2] • Control of viral replication more difficult to achieve and maintain

[1]See table, "Indications for the Initiating Antiretroviral Therapy for the Chronically HIV-1-Infected Patient," for consensus recommendations regarding when to initiate therapy.

[2]Antiretroviral therapy cannot substitute for primary HIV prevention measures (eg, use of condoms and safer sex practices).

Antiretroviral Components Recommended for Treatment of HIV-1 Infection in Treatment-Naive Patients

A combination antiretroviral regimen in treatment-naive patients generally contains 1 NNRTI + 2 NRTIs or a single or ritonavir-boosted PI + 2 NRTIs. Selection of a regimen for an antiretroviral-naive patient should be individualized based on virologic efficacy, toxicities, pill burden, dosing frequency, drug-drug interaction potential, and comorbid conditions. Components listed below are designated as preferred when clinical trial data suggest optimal and durable efficacy with acceptable tolerability and ease of use. Alternative components are those that clinical trial data show efficacy but that have disadvantages, such as antiviral activity or toxicities, compared with the preferred agent. In some cases, for an individual patient, a component listed as alternative may actually be the preferred component. Clinicians initiating antiretroviral regimens in the HIV-1-infected pregnant patient should refer to **"Recommendations for Use of Antiretroviral Drugs in Pregnant HIV-1-Infected Women for Maternal Health and Intervention to Reduce Perinatal HIV-1 Transmission in the United States"** at **http://aidsinfo.nih.gov/guidelines.**

To construct an antiretroviral regimen, select 1 component from Column A + 1 from Column B.					
	Column A (NNRTI or PI Options – in alphabetical order)				Column B (Dual-NRTI Options – in alphabetical order)
Preferred Components	**NNRTI-** efavirenz[1]	**or**	**PI-** atazanavir + ritonavir fosamprenavir + ritonavir (2x/day) lopinavir/ritonavir[2] (2x/day) (coformulated)	+	tenofovir/emtricitabine[3] (coformulated); **or** zidovudine/lamivudine[3] (coformulated)
Alternative to Preferred Components	**NNRTI-** nevirapine[4]	**or**	**PI-** atazanavir[5] fosamprenavir fosamprenavir + ritonavir (1x/day) lopinavir/ritonavir (1x/day) (coformulated)		abacavir/lamivudine[3] (coformulated) didanosine + (emtricitabine or lamivudine)
Other Possible Options			See next table		See next table

[1]Efavirenz is not recommended for use in the first trimester of pregnancy or in sexually active women with child-bearing potential who are not using effective contraception.

[2]The pivotal study that led to the recommendation of lopinavir/ritonavir as a preferred PI component was based on twice-daily dosing. A smaller study has shown similar efficacy with once-daily dosing but also showed a higher incidence of moderate to severe diarrhea with the once-daily regimen (16% vs 5%).

[3]Emtricitabine may be used in place of lamivudine and vice versa.

[4]Nevirapine should not be initiated in women with $CD4^+$ T-cell count >250 cells/mm^3 or in men with $CD4^+$ T-cell count >400 cells/mm^3 because of increased risk of symptomatic hepatic events in these patients.

[5]Atazanavir must be boosted with ritonavir if used in combination with tenofovir.

ADULT AND ADOLESCENT HIV *(Continued)*

Antiretroviral Components That Are Acceptable as Initial Antiretroviral Components but Are Inferior to Preferred or Alternative Components

Antiretroviral Drugs or Regimens (in alphabetical order)	Reasons for Generally Not Recommending the Drugs or Regimens as Initial Therapy	Special Circumstances in Which the Drugs or Regimens May Be Used
Abacavir/lamivudine/ zidovudine (coformulated) as triple-NRTI combination regimen	Inferior virologic efficacy	When PI or NNRTI-based regimens cannot be used based on toxicities or concerns of significant drug-drug interactions
Nelfinavir	Inferior virologic efficacy	Most experience with pregnant patients with good tolerability and adequate pharmacokinetic data
Saquinavir (ritonavir-boosted)	• Inferior to lopinavir/ ritonavir • Minimal efficacy data in treatment-naive patients	When preferred or alternative PI components cannot be used based on toxicities or concerns of significant drug-drug interactions
Stavudine + lamivudine	Significant toxicities including lipoatrophy, peripheral neuropathy, hyperlactatemia including symptomatic and life-threatening lactic acidosis, hepatic steatosis, and pancreatitis	When preferred or alternative dual-NRTI combination cannot be used

Antiretroviral Components Not Recommended as Initial Therapy

Antiretroviral Drugs or Components (in alphabetical order)	Reasons for Not Recommending as Initial Therapy
Darunovir (ritonavir-boosted)	• Lack of data in treatment-naive patients
Delavirdine	• Inferior virologic efficacy • Inconvenient dosing (3 times/day)
Didanosine + tenofovir	• High rate of early virologic failure • Rapid selection of resistant mutations • Potential for immunologic nonresponse/CD4+ decline
Enfuvirtide	• No clinical trial experience in treatment-naive patients • Requires twice daily subcutaneous injections
Indinavir (unboosted)	• Inconvenient dosing (3 times/day with meal restrictions) • Fluid requirement
Indinavir (ritonavir-boosted)	• High incidence of nephrolithiasis
Ritonavir as sole PI	• High pill burden • Gastrointestinal intolerance
Saquinavir (unboosted)	• High pill burden • Inferior virologic efficacy
Tipranavir (ritonavir boosted)	• Lack of data in treatment-naive patients
Zalcitabine + zidovudine	• Inferior virologic efficacy • Higher rate of adverse effects than other dual-NRTI alternatives

Antiretroviral Regimens or Components That Should Not Be Offered at Any Time

	Rationale	Exception
	Antiretroviral Regimens Not Recommended	
Monotherapy with NRTI or NNRTI	• Rapid development of resistance • Inferior antiretroviral activity when compared to combination with three or more antiretrovirals	Pregnant women with pretreatment HIV-RNA <1000 copies/mL using zidovudine monotherapy for prevention of perinatal HIV transmission and not for HIV treatment for the mother[1]; however, combination therapy is generally preferred
Dual-NRTI regimens	• Rapid development of resistance • Inferior antiretroviral activity when compared to combination with three or more antiretrovirals	
Triple-NRTI regimens except for abacavir/zidovudine/lamivudine or possibly tenofovir + zidovudine/lamivudine	• High rate of early virologic nonresponse seen when this triple NRTI combination including ABC/TDF/3TC or TDF/ddI/3TC were used as initial regimen in treatment-naive patients • Other 3-NRTI regimens have not been evaluated	Abacavir/zidovudine/lamivudine; and possibly tenofovir + zidovudine/lamivudine

ADULT AND ADOLESCENT HIV *(Continued)*

Antiretroviral Regimens or Components That Should Not Be Offered at Any Time *(continued)*

	Rationale	Exception
Antiretroviral Components Not Recommended as Part of Antiretroviral Regimen		
Amprenavir oral solution in: • pregnant women • children <4 y • patients with renal or hepatic failure • patients on metronidazole or disulfiram	Oral liquid contains large amount of the excipient propylene glycol, which may be toxic in the patients at risk	No exception
Amprenavir + fosamprenavir	Amprenavir is the active antiviral for both drugs, combined use have no benefit and may increase toxicities	No exception
Amprenavir oral solution + ritonavir oral solution	The large amount of propylene glycol used as a vehicle in amprenavir oral solution may compete with ethanol (the vehicle in oral ritonavir solution) for the same metabolic pathway for elimination. This may lead to accumulation of either one of the vehicles.	No exception
Atazanavir + indinavir	Potential additive hyperbilirubinemia	No exception
Didanosine + stavudine	• High incidence of toxicities – peripheral neuropathy, pancreatitis, and hyperlactatemia • Reports of serious, even fatal, cases of lactic acidosis with hepatic steatosis with or without pancreatitis in pregnant women[1]	When no other antiretroviral options are available and potential benefits outweigh the risks[1]
Didanosine + zalcitabine	Additive peripheral neuropathy	No exception
Efavirenz in first trimester of pregnancy or in women with significant childbearing potential[1]	Teratogenic in nonhuman primates	When no other antiretroviral options are available and potential benefits outweigh the risks[1]
Emtricitabine + lamivudine	• Similar resistance profile • No potential benefit	No exception
Lamivudine + zalcitabine	*In vitro* antagonism	No exception
Nevirapine initiation in treatment-naive women with CD4 >250 cells/mm^3 or in treatment-naive men with CD4 >400 cells/mm^3	Higher incidence of symptomatic (including serious and even fatal) hepatic events in these patient groups	Only if the benefit clearly outweighs the risk
Saquinavir as **single** protease inhibitor	• Poor oral bioavailability (4%) • Inferior antiretroviral activity when compared to other protease inhibitors	No exception
Stavudine + zalcitabine	Additive peripheral neuropathy	No exception
Stavudine + zidovudine	Antagonistic effect on HIV-1	No exception

[1]When constructing an antiretroviral regimen for an HIV-infected pregnant woman, please consult "Public Health Service Task Force Recommendations for the Use of Antiretroviral Drugs in Pregnant HIV-1-Infected Women for Maternal Health and Interventions to Reduce Perinatal HIV-1 Transmission in the United States" in **http://www.aidsinfo.nih.gov/guidelines**.

Summary of Guidelines for Changing an Antiretroviral Regimen for Suspected Treatment Regimen Failure

Patient Assessment

- Review antiretroviral treatment history.
- Assess for evidence of clinical progression (eg, physical exam, laboratory and/or radiologic tests).
- Assess adherence, tolerability, and pharmacokinetic issues.
- Distinguish between limited, intermediate, and extensive prior therapy and drug resistance.
- Perform resistance testing while patient is taking therapy (or within 4 weeks after regimen discontinuation).
- Identify active drugs and drug classes to use in designing new regimen.

Patient Management: Specific Clinical Scenarios

- **Limited or intermediate prior treatment with low (but not suppressed) HIV RNA level (eg, up to 5000 copies/mL):** The goal of treatment is to resuppress HIV RNA to below level of assay detection. Consider intensifying with one drug (eg, tenofovir) or pharmacokinetic enhancement (use of ritonavir boosting of a protease inhibitor), perform resistance testing if possible, or most aggressively, change two or more drugs in the regimen. If continuing the same treatment regimen, HIV RNA levels should be followed closely because ongoing viral replication will lead to accumulation of additional resistance mutations.
- **Limited or intermediate prior treatment with resistance to one drug:** Consider changing the one drug, pharmacokinetic enhancement (few data available), or, most aggressively, change two or more drugs in the regimen.
- **Limited or intermediate prior treatment with resistance to more than one drug:** The goal of treatment is to suppress viremia to prevent further selection of resistance mutations. Consider optimizing the regimen by changing classes (eg, PI-based to NNRTI-based and vice versa) and/or adding new active drugs. (See table **Treatment Options Following Virologic Failure on Antiretroviral Therapy Regimens**.)
- **Prior treatment with no resistance identified:** Consider the timing of the drug resistance test (eg, was the patient off antiretroviral medications?) and/or nonadherence. Consider resuming the same regimen or starting a new regimen and then repeating genotypic testing early (eg, 2-4 weeks) to determine if a resistant viral strain emerges on treatment.
- **Extensive prior treatment and drug resistance:** In patients with active antiretroviral agents available (eg, an active ritonavir-boosted PI and enfuvirtide), the goal of therapy is suppression of viremia. In patients without active antiretroviral agent available and with ongoing viremia, the goal of therapy is preservation of immune responses and delay of clinical progression. It is reasonable to continue the same antiretroviral regimen if there are few or no treatment options. In general, avoid adding a single active drug because of the risk for the rapid development of resistance to that drug. In advanced HIV disease with a high likelihood of clinical progression (eg, $CD4^+$ cell count <100 cells/mm^3), adding a single drug may reduce the risk of immediate clinical progression. In this complicated scenario, expert advise should be sought.
- **Immunologic failure (or blunted CD4 response) with virologic suppression:** Immunologic failure (or blunted $CD4^+$ cell response) may not warrant a change in therapy in the setting of suppressed viremia. Assess for other causes of immunosuppression (eg, HIV-2, HTLV-1, drug toxicity). The combination of didanosine and tenofovir has been associated with $CD4^+$ cell declines or blunted $CD4^+$ cell responses. In the setting of immunologic failure (or blunted $CD4^+$ response), it would be reasonable to change one of these drugs. Intensifying with additional antiretroviral drugs or the use of immune-based therapies (eg, interleukin-2) to improve immunologic responses remain unproven strategies and generally should not be offered.

ADULT AND ADOLESCENT HIV *(Continued)*

Treatment Options Following Virologic Failure on Antiretroviral Therapy Regimens

First Virologic Failure

Regimen Class	Initial Regimen	Recommended Change[1]
NNRTI	2 NRTIs + NNRTI	• 2 NRTIs (based on resistance testing) + PI (with or without low-dose ritonavir)
PI	2 NRTIs + PI (with or without low-dose ritonavir)	• 2 NRTIs (based on resistance testing) + NNRTI • 2 NRTIs (based on resistance testing) + alternative PI (with low-dose ritonavir; based on resistance testing) • NRTI(s) (based on resistance testing) + NNRTI + alternative PI (with low-dose ritonavir; based on resistance testing)
Triple-NRTI	3 nucleosides	• 2 NRTIs (based on resistance testing) + NNRTI or PI (with or without low-dose ritonavir) • NNRTI + PI (with or without low-dose ritonavir) • NRTI(s) (based on resistance testing) + NNRTI + PI (with or without low-dose ritonavir)
Three-class	NRTI + NNRTI + PI	• >1 NRTIs (based on resistance testing) + a newer PI (with low-dose ritonavir; based on resistance testing) ± enfuvirtide

[1]Antiretroviral therapy regimens should be selected on the basis of treatment history and drug-resistance testing to optimize antiretroviral potency in the second regimen. This is particularly important in selecting NRTIs for an NNRTI-based regimen where drug resistance may occur rapidly to the NNRTI if the NRTIs are not sufficiently potent. **Note:** NNRTIs generally should not be used following the development of NNRTI-resistance because of the risk for selection of additional NNRTI-associated mutations.

Recommendations for Using Drug-Resistance Assays

Clinical Setting / Recommendation	Rationale
Drug-Resistance Assay Recommended	
In acute HIV infection: If the decision is made to initiate therapy at this time, testing is recommended prior to initiation of treatment. A genotypic assay is generally preferred.	Drug resistance testing will determine if drug-resistant virus was transmitted and will help to design initial or changed (if therapy was initiated prior to test results) regimens accordingly.
If treatment is deferred, resistance testing at this time should still be considered	Earlier testing may be considered because of the potentially greater likelihood that transmitted resistance-associated mutations will be detected earlier in the course of HIV infection.
In chronic HIV infection: Drug resistance testing is recommended prior to initiation of therapy. A genotypic assay is generally preferred.	Transmitted HIV with baseline resistance to at least one drug may be seen in 6% to 16% of patients. Suboptimal virologic responses may be seen in patients with baseline resistant mutations.
Resistance testing earlier in the course of HIV infection may be considered.	Earlier testing may be considered because of the potentially greater likelihood that transmitted resistance-associated mutations will be detected earlier in the course of HIV infection.
With virologic failure during combination antiretroviral therapy	Determine the role of resistance in drug failure and maximize the number of active drugs in the new regimen, if indicated.
With suboptimal suppression of viral load after antiretroviral therapy initiation	Determine the role of resistance and maximize the number of active drugs in the new regimen, if indicated.
Drug-Resistance Assay Not Usually Recommended	
After discontinuation of drugs	Drug-resistance mutations may become minor species in the absence of selective drug pressure, and available assays may not detect minor drug-resistant species. If testing is performed in this setting, the detection of drug resistance may be of value, but its absence does not rule out the presence of minor drug-resistant species.
When plasma viral load <1000 copies/mL	Resistance assays cannot be consistently performed because of low HIV RNA levels; patients/providers may incur charges and not receive results.

Therapeutic Drug Monitoring

As with other notable drug classes (eg, antibiotics, anticonvulsants), the goal of therapeutic drug monitoring (TDM) is to maximize therapeutic efficacy and minimize drug-related toxicities. The utility of TDM in the setting of antiretroviral drug therapy is supported by data showing considerable interpatient variability with respect to drug concentrations among patients taking similar doses, as well as data demonstrating concentration/effect and concentration/toxicity correlations. The optimal plasma concentrations of many antiretroviral drugs have yet to be determined (eg, NRTIs). Those drugs for which target trough levels are defined are shown in the following table.

ADULT AND ADOLESCENT HIV *(Continued)*

Suggested Minimum Target Trough Concentrations for Persons With Wild-Type HIV-1

Drug	Concentration (ng/mL)
Amprenavir or Fosamprenavir	400 (concentration assayed as amprenavir)
Atazanavir	150
Indinavir	100
Lopinavir / ritonavir (Kaletra®)	1000
Nelfinavir[1]	800
Ritonavir[2]	2100
Saquinavir	100-250
Efavirenz	1000
Nevirapine	3400

[1]Measurable active M8 metabolite.
[2]Ritonavir given as a single PI.

Associated Signs and Symptoms of Acute Retroviral Syndrome and Percentage of Expected Frequency

- Fever (96%)
- Lymphadenopathy (74%)
- Pharyngitis (70%)
- Rash (70%)
  - Erythematous maculopapular with lesions on face and trunk and sometimes extremities, including palms and soles
  - Mucocutaneous ulceration involving mouth, esophagus, or genitals
- Myalgia or arthralgia (54%)
- Diarrhea (32%)
- Headache (32%)
- Nausea and vomiting (27%)
- Hepatosplenomegaly (14%)
- Weight loss (13%)
- Thrush (12%)
- Neurologic symptoms (12%)
  - Meningoencephalitis or aseptic meningitis
  - Peripheral neuropathy or radiculopathy
  - Facial palsy
  - Guillain-Barré syndrome
  - Brachial neuritis
  - Cognitive impairment or psychosis

Reference

Niu MT, Stein DS, and Schnittman SM, "Primary Human Immunodeficiency Virus Type 1 Infection: Review of Pathogenesis and Early Treatment Intervention in Humans and Animal Retrovirus Infections," *J Infect Dis*, 1993, 168(6):1490-501.

PERINATAL HIV

Selected tables from the Perinatal HIV Guidelines Working Group, Public Health Service Task Force, "Recommendations for Use of Antiretroviral Drugs in Pregnant HIV-1-Infected Women for Maternal Health and Interventions to Reduce Perinatal HIV-1 Transmission in the United States," October 12, 2006, located at (URL) http://www.aidsinfo.nih.gov.

Pediatric AIDS Clinical Trials Group (PACTG) 076 Zidovudine (ZDV) Regimen

ZDV Perinatal Transmission Prophylaxis Regimen

Time of ZDV Administration	Regimen
Antepartum	Oral administration (to the pregnant woman) of 100 mg ZDV 5 times daily,[1] initiated at 14-34 weeks gestation and continued throughout the pregnancy.
Intrapartum	During labor, intravenous administration (to the pregnant women) of ZDV in a 1-hour initial dose of 2 mg/kg body weight, followed by a continuous infusion of 1 mg/kg body weight/hour until delivery.
Postpartum	Oral administration of ZDV to the newborn infant (ZDV syrup at 2 mg/kg body weight/dose every 6 hours) for the first 6 weeks of life, beginning at 8-12 hours after birth.[2]

[1]Oral ZDV administered as 200 mg 3 times daily or 300 mg twice daily is currently used in general clinical practice and is an acceptable alternative regimen to 100 mg orally 5 times daily.

[2]Intravenous dosage for full-term infants who cannot tolerate oral intake is 1.5 mg/kg body weight intravenously every 6 hours. ZDV dosing for infants <35 weeks gestation at birth is 1.5 mg/kg/dose intravenously, or 2 mg/kg/dose orally, every 12 hours, advancing to every 8 hours at 2 weeks of age if >30 weeks gestation at birth or at 4 weeks of age if <30 weeks gestation at birth.

Clinical Scenarios and Recommendations for the Use of Antiretroviral Drugs to Reduce Perinatal Human Immunodeficiency Virus Type (HIV-1) Transmission

SCENARIO #1
HIV-1-infected pregnant women who have not received prior antiretroviral therapy

- Pregnant women with HIV-1 infection must receive standard clinical, immunologic, and virologic evaluation. Recommendations for initiation and choice of antiretroviral therapy should be based on the same parameters used for persons who are not pregnant, although the known and unknown risks and benefits of such therapy during pregnancy must be considered and discussed.
- The three-part ZDV chemoprophylaxis regimen, initiated after the first trimester, is recommended for all pregnant women with HIV-1 infection regardless of antenatal HIV RNA copy number to reduce the risk for perinatal transmission.
- The combination of ZDV chemoprophylaxis with additional antiretroviral drugs for treatment of HIV-1 infection is recommended for infected women whose clinical, immunologic, or virologic status requires treatment or who have HIV-1 RNA over 1000 copies/mL regardless of clinical or immunologic status, and can be considered for women with HIV-1 RNA <1000 copies/mL.
- Women who are in the first trimester of pregnancy may consider delaying initiation of therapy until after 10-12 weeks' gestation.

PERINATAL HIV *(Continued)*

SCENARIO #2
HIV-1-infected women receiving antiretroviral therapy during the current pregnancy

- HIV-1-infected women receiving antiretroviral therapy in whom pregnancy is identified after the first trimester should continue therapy. ZDV should be a component of the antenatal antiretroviral treatment regimen after the first trimester whenever possible, although this may not always be feasible.
- For women receiving antiretroviral therapy in whom pregnancy is recognized during the first trimester, the woman should be counseled regarding the benefits and potential risks of antiretroviral administration during this period, and continuation of therapy should be considered. If therapy is discontinued during the first trimester, all drugs should be stopped and reintroduced simultaneously to avoid the development of drug resistance.
- Regardless of the antepartum antiretroviral regimen, ZDV administration is recommended during the intrapartum period and for the newborn.

SCENARIO #3
HIV-1-infected women in labor who have had no prior therapy

Several effective regimens are available (see Comparison of Intrapartum / Postpartum Regimens). These include:

- intrapartum intravenous ZDV followed by 6 weeks of ZDV for the newborn
- oral ZDV and 3TC during labor, followed by 1 week of oral ZDV-3TC for the newborn
- a single-dose nevirapine at the onset of labor followed by a single dose of nevirapine for the newborn at age 48 hours, and
- the single-dose maternal/infant nevirapine regimen combined with intrapartum intravenous ZDV and 6-week ZDV for the newborn

If single-dose nevirapine is given to the mother, alone or in combination with ZDV, consideration should be given to adding maternal ZDV/3TC starting as soon as possible (intrapartum or immediately postpartum) and continuing for 3-7 days, which may reduce development of nevirapine resistance.

In the immediate postpartum period, the woman should have appropriate assessments (eg, CD4+ count and HIV-1 RNA copy number) to determine whether antiretroviral therapy is recommended for her own health.

SCENARIO #4
Infants born to mothers who have received no antiretroviral therapy during pregnancy or intrapartum

- The 6-week neonatal ZDV component of the ZDV chemoprophylactic regimen should be discussed with the mother and offered for the newborn.
- ZDV should be initiated as soon as possible after delivery – preferably within 6-12 hours of birth.
- Some clinicians may choose to use ZDV in combination with other antiretroviral drugs, particularly if the mother is known or suspected to have ZDV-resistant virus. However, the efficacy of this approach for prevention of transmission has not been proven in clinical trials, and appropriate dosing regimens for neonates are incompletely defined for many drugs.
- In the immediate postpartum period, the woman should undergo appropriate assessments (eg, CD4+ count and HIV-1 RNA copy number) to determine if antiretroviral therapy is required for her own health. The infant should undergo early diagnostic testing so that if HIV-1-infected, treatment can be initiated as soon as possible.

Note: Discussion of treatment options and recommendations should be noncoercive, and the final decision regarding the use of antiretroviral drugs is the responsibility of the woman. A decision to not accept treatment with ZDV or other drugs should not result in punitive action or denial of care. Use of ZDV should not be denied to a woman who wishes to minimize exposure of the fetus to other antiretroviral drugs and who, therefore, chooses to receive only ZDV during pregnancy to reduce the risk for perinatal transmission.

Comparison of Intrapartum / Postpartum Regimens for HIV-1-Infected Women in Labor Who Have Had No Prior Antiretroviral Therapy (Scenario #3)

ZDV

Source of Evidence: Epidemiologic data, U.S.; compared to no ZDV treatment

Maternal Intrapartum: 2 mg/kg intravenous bolus, followed by continuous infusion of 1 mg/kg/h until delivery

Infant Postpartum: 2 mg/kg orally every 6 hours for 6 weeks[1]

Data on Transmission: Transmission 10% with ZDV compared to 27% with no ZDV treatment, a 62% reduction (95% CI, 19% to 82%)

Advantages: Has been standard recommendation

Disadvantages:

- Requires intravenous administration and availability of ZDV intravenous formulation
- Adherence to 6-week infant regimen
- Reversible, mild anemia with 6-week infant ZDV regimen

ZDV / 3TC

Source of Evidence: Clinical trial, Africa; compared to placebo

Maternal Intrapartum: ZDV 600 mg orally at onset of labor, followed by 300 mg orally every 3 hours until delivery **and** 3TC 150 mg orally at onset of labor, followed by 150 mg orally every 12 hours until delivery

Infant Postpartum: ZDV 4 mg/kg orally every 12 hours **and** 3TC 2 mg/kg orally every 12 hours for 7 days

Data on Transmission: Transmission at 6 weeks 9% with ZDV-3TC vs 15% with placebo, a 42% reduction

Advantages: Oral regimen; adherence easier than 6 weeks of ZDV

Disadvantages: Requires administration of two drugs

Nevirapine

Source of Evidence: Clinical trial, Africa; compared to oral ZDV given intrapartum and for 1 week to the infant

Maternal Intrapartum: Single 200 mg oral dose at onset of labor; consider adding intrapartum ZDV/3TC and 3-7 days of ZDV/3TC postpartum to reduce nevirapine resistance

Infant Postpartum: Single 2 mg/kg oral dose at age 48-72 hours[2]

Data on Transmission: Transmission at 6 weeks 12% with nevirapine compared to 21% with ZDV, a 47% reduction (95% CI,[1] 20% to 64%)

Advantages: Inexpensive; oral regimen; simple, easy to administer; can give directly observed treatment

Disadvantages:

- Unknown efficacy if mother has nevirapine-resistant virus
- Nevirapine resistance mutations have been detected postpartum in some women and in infants who became infected despite prophylaxis

PERINATAL HIV *(Continued)*

ZDV-Nevirapine

Source of Evidence: Theoretical

Maternal Intrapartum: ZDV 2 mg/kg intravenous bolus, followed by continuous infusion of 1 mg/kg/h until delivery **and** nevirapine single 200 mg oral dose at onset of labor; consider adding intrapartum ZDV/3TC and 3-7 days of ZDV/3TC postpartum to reduce nevirapine resistance

Infant Postpartum: ZDV 2 mg/kg orally every 6 hours for 6 weeks **and** nevirapine single 2 mg/kg oral dose at age 48-72 hours[2]

Data on Transmission: No data

Advantages: Potential benefit if maternal virus is resistant to either nevirapine or ZDV; synergistic inhibition of HIV replication with combination *in vitro*

Disadvantages:

- Requires intravenous administration and availability of ZDV intravenous formulation
- Adherence to 6-week infant ZDV regimen
- Unknown if additive efficacy with combination
- Nevirapine resistance mutations have been detected postpartum in some women and in infants who became infected despite prophylaxis

ZDV = zidovudine, CI = confidence interval, 3TC = lamivudine.

Footnotes

[1]ZDV dosing for infants <35 weeks gestation at birth is 1.5 mg/kg/dose intravenously, or 2 mg/kg/dose orally, every 12 hours, advancing to every 8 hours at 2 weeks of age if ≥30 weeks gestation at birth or at 4 weeks of age if <30 weeks gestation at birth.

[2]If the mother received nevirapine <1 hour prior to delivery, the infant should be given 2 mg/kg oral nevirapine as soon as possible after birth and again at 48-72 hours.

Antiretroviral Drug Resistance and Resistance Testing in Pregnancy

- HIV drug resistance testing is recommended for:
  a. All pregnant women not currently receiving antiretrovirals, before starting treatment or prophylaxis.
  b. All pregnant women receiving antenatal antiretroviral therapy who have virologic failure with persistently detectable HIV RNA levels or who have suboptimal viral suppression after initiation of antiretroviral therapy.
- For optimal prevention of perinatal transmission, empiric initiation of antiretroviral therapy before results of resistance testing are available may be warranted, with adjustment as needed after the results are available.
- The use of highly active antiretroviral combination therapy to maximally suppress viral replication during pregnancy is the most effective strategy to prevent the development of resistance and to minimize the risk of perinatal transmission.
- All pregnant women should be counseled about the importance of adherence to prescribed antiretroviral medications to reduce the potential for development of resistance.
- The addition of single-dose maternal/infant NVP to an ongoing highly active combination antiretroviral therapy regimen does not provide additional efficacy in reducing perinatal transmission and may result in NVP drug resistance in the mother, and is therefore not recommended.
- NVP-based combination therapy should not be initiated in women with CD4 count >250 cells/mm^3 unless the benefit clearly outweighs the risk due to concern about increased risk of hepatic toxicity. However, some pregnant women may receive an NVP-based combination antiretroviral therapy regimen for prophylaxis only, with plans to discontinue therapy after delivery. In this situation, consideration should be given to continuing the nucleoside analogue agents for 3-7 days after stopping NVP to minimize the risk of NVP resistance.
- Women who have documented ZDV resistance and are on regimens that do not include ZDV for their own health should still receive intravenous ZDV during labor whenever possible, along with their established antiretroviral regimens, and oral ZDV for their infants according to the PACTG 076 protocol. For women who are receiving a stavudine-containing regimen, stavudine should be discontinued during labor while intravenous ZDV is being administered.
- The optimal prophylactic regimen for newborns of women with ARV resistance is unknown. Therefore, ARV prophylaxis for an infant born to a woman with known or suspected drug resistance should be determined in consultation with a pediatric HIV specialist, preferably before delivery.

Clinical Scenarios and Recommendations Regarding Mode of Delivery to Reduce Perinatal Human Immunodeficiency Virus Type (HIV-1) Transmission

SCENARIO A

HIV-1-infected women presenting in late pregnancy (after about 36 weeks of gestation), known to be HIV-1-infected but not receiving antiretroviral therapy, and who have HIV-1 RNA level and lymphocyte subsets pending but unlikely to be available before delivery.

Recommendations

Therapy options should be discussed in detail. The woman should be started on antiretroviral therapy including at least the PACTG 076 ZDV regimen. The woman should be counseled that scheduled cesarean section is likely to reduce the risk of transmission to her infant. She should also be informed of the increased risks to her of cesarean section, including increased rates of postoperative infection, anesthesia risks, and other surgical risks.

If cesarean section is chosen, the procedure should be scheduled at 38 weeks of gestation based on the best available clinical information. When scheduled cesarean section is performed, the woman should receive continuous intravenous ZDV infusion beginning 3 hours before surgery and her infant should receive 6 weeks of ZDV therapy after birth. Options for continuing or initiating combination antiretroviral therapy after delivery should be discussed with the woman as soon as her viral load and lymphocyte subset results are available.

SCENARIO B

HIV-1-infected women who initiated prenatal care early in the third trimester, are receiving highly active combination antiretroviral therapy, and have an initial virologic response, but have HIV-1 RNA levels that remain substantially over 1000 copies/mL at 36 weeks of gestation.

Recommendations

The current combination antiretroviral regimen should be continued as the HIV-1 RNA level is dropping appropriately. The woman should be counseled that although she is responding to the antiretroviral therapy, it is unlikely that her HIV-1 RNA level will fall below 1000 copies/mL before delivery. Therefore, scheduled cesarean section may provide additional benefit in preventing intrapartum transmission of HIV-1. She should also be informed of the increased risks to her of cesarean section, including increased rates of postoperative infection, anesthesia risks, and surgical risks.

If she chooses scheduled cesarean section, it should be performed at 38 weeks' gestation according to the best available dating parameters, and intravenous ZDV should be begun at least 3 hours before surgery. Other antiretroviral medications should be continued on schedule as much as possible before and after surgery. The infant should receive oral ZDV for 6 weeks after birth. The importance of adhering to therapy after delivery for her own health should be emphasized.

SCENARIO C

HIV-1-infected women on highly active combination antiretroviral therapy with an undetectable HIV-1 RNA level at 36 weeks of gestation.

Recommendations

The woman should be counseled that her risk of perinatal transmission of HIV-1 with a persistently undetectable HIV-1 RNA level is low, probably 2% or less, even with vaginal delivery. There is currently no information to evaluate whether performing a scheduled cesarean section will lower her risk further.

Cesarean section has an increased risk of complications for the woman compared to vaginal delivery, and these risks must be balanced against the uncertain benefit of cesarean section in this case.

PERINATAL HIV *(Continued)*

SCENARIO D

HIV-1-infected women who have elected scheduled cesarean section but present in early labor or shortly after rupture of membranes.

Recommendations

Intravenous ZDV should be started immediately since the woman is in labor or has ruptured membranes.

If labor is progressing rapidly, the woman should be allowed to deliver vaginally. If cervical dilatation is minimal and a long period of labor is anticipated, some clinicians may choose to administer the loading dose of intravenous ZDV and proceed with cesarean section to minimize the duration of membrane rupture and avoid vaginal delivery. Others might begin Pitocin® augmentation to enhance contractions and potentially expedite delivery.

If the woman is allowed to labor, scalp electrodes and other invasive monitoring and operative delivery should be avoided if possible. The infant should be treated with 6 weeks of ZDV therapy after birth.

IMMUNIZATION GUIDELINES

Standards for Pediatric Immunization Practices

Standard 1.	Immunization services are readily available.
Standard 2.	There are no barriers or unnecessary prerequisites to the receipt of vaccines.
Standard 3.	Immunization services are available free or for a minimal fee.
Standard 4.	Providers utilize all clinical encounters to screen and, when indicated, immunize children.
Standard 5.	Providers educate parents and guardians about immunizations in general terms.
Standard 6.	Providers question parents or guardians about contraindications and, before immunizing a child, inform them in specific terms about the risks and benefits of the immunizations their child is to receive.
Standard 7.	Providers follow only true contraindications.
Standard 8.	Providers administer simultaneously all vaccine doses for which a child is eligible at the time of each visit.
Standard 9.	Providers use accurate and complete recording procedures.
Standard 10.	Providers co-schedule immunization appointments in conjunction with appointments for other child health services.
Standard 11.	Providers report adverse events following immunization promptly, accurately, and completely.
Standard 12.	Providers operate a tracking system.
Standard 13.	Providers adhere to appropriate procedures for vaccine management.
Standard 14.	Providers conduct semiannual audits to assess immunization coverage levels and to review immunization records in the patient populations they serve.
Standard 15.	Providers maintain up-to-date, easily retrievable medical protocols at all locations where vaccines are administered.
Standard 16.	Providers operate with patient-oriented and community-based approaches.
Standard 17.	Vaccines are administered by properly trained individuals.
Standard 18.	Providers receive ongoing education and training on current immunization recommendations.

Recommended by the National Vaccine Advisory Committee, April 1992.
Modified by the United States Public Health Service, 1993.
Endorsed by the American Academy of Pediatrics, May 1992.

The Standards represent the consensus of the National Vaccine Advisory Committee (NVAC) and of a broad group of medical and public health experts about what constitutes the most desirable immunization practices. It is recognized by the NVAC that not all of the current immunization practices of public and private providers are in compliance with the Standards. Nevertheless, the Standards are expected to be useful as a means of helping providers to identify needed changes, to obtain resources if necessary, and to actually implement the desirable immunization practices in the future.

IMMUNIZATION GUIDELINES *(Continued)*

Dosage and Administration Guidelines for Vaccines Available in the United States

Vaccine	Dosage	Route of Administration	Type
DT[1]	0.5 mL	I.M.; do not give SubQ	Toxoids
Td[1]	0.5 mL	I.M.; do not give SubQ	Toxoids
DTaP (Tripedia®, Infanrix®, Daptacel®)[2]	0.5 mL	I.M.; do not give SubQ	Diphtheria and tetanus toxoids with inactivated acellular pertussis
Tdap (Adacel™, Boostrix®)[3]	0.5 mL	I.M.; do not give SubQ	Tetanus toxoid, reduced diphtheria toxoid, and acellular pertussis
DTaP-PRP-T (Tripedia®/ ActHIB®, TriHIBit®)	0.5 mL	I.M.; do not give SubQ	Polysaccharide-protein conjugate with toxoids and inactivated bacteria
DTaP and hepatitis B (recombinant) and inactivated poliovirus vaccine combined (Pediarix™)	0.5 mL	I.M.; do not give SubQ	Diphtheria and tetanus toxoids with inactivated acellular pertussis, recombinant – derived inactivated viral antigen and inactivated virus
Haemophilus B conjugate vaccine	0.5 mL	I.M. PRP-D, HbOC, or PRP-T can be given SubQ in individuals at risk of hemorrhage	Polysaccharide protein conjugate
HibTITER® (HbOC),[4] manufactured by Lederle Laboratories	0.5 mL	I.M.	Oligosaccharide (diphtheria CRM_{197} protein conjugate)
PedvaxHIB® (PRP-OMP),[5] manufactured by MSD	0.5 mL	I.M.; do not give SubQ	Polysaccharide (meningococcal protein conjugate)
ActHIB® (PRP-T), manufactured by Pasteur Merieux Serums & Vaccines	0.5 mL	I.M.	Tetanus toxoid protein conjugate
Haemophilus b conjugate – PRP-OMP and hepatitis B (recombinant) (Comvax®)	0.5 mL	I.M.; do not give SubQ	Polysaccharide-protein conjugate with inactivated virus
Hepatitis A vaccine, inactivated		I.M.; do not give SubQ	Inactivated virus
Havrix®			
Children 1-18 y	0.5 mL (720 ELISA units) with 2nd dose given 6-12 mo later		
Children >18 y and adults	1 mL (1440 ELISA units) with 2nd dose given 6-12 mo later		
VAQTA®			
Children 1-17 y	0.5 mL (25 units) with 2nd dose given 6-18 mo later		
Children >17 y and adults	1 mL (50 units) with 2nd dose given 6 mo later		
Hepatitis B[6]		I.M. in the anterolateral thigh or in the deltoid muscle[8]	Yeast recombinant-derived inactivated viral antigen
Infants born to HB_sAg-negative mothers, children, and adolescents <20 y[7]			
Recombivax HB® (MSD)	5 mcg (0.5 mL)		
Engerix-B® (SKF)	10 mcg (0.5 mL)		
Infants born to HB_sAg-positive mothers (both immunization with hepatitis B and administration of 0.5 mL hepatitis B immune globulin is recommended for **infants** born to HB_sAg-positive mothers using different administration sites) within 12 hours of birth; administer vaccine at birth; repeat vaccine dose at 1 and 6 months following the initial dose			
Recombivax HB® (MSD)	5 mcg (0.5 mL)		
Engerix-B® (SKF)	10 mcg (0.5 mL)		

Dosage and Administration Guidelines for Vaccines Available in the United States *(continued)*

Vaccine	Dosage	Route of Administration	Type
Adolescents 11-15 y			
Recombivax HB® (MSD)	10 mcg (1 mL) 2nd dose given 4-6 mo after the first dose (alternate two-dose hepatitis B vaccination schedule)		
Adults ≥20 y			
Recombivax HB® (MSD)	10 mcg (1 mL)		
Engerix-B® (SKF)	20 mcg (1 mL)		
Dialysis patients and immunosuppressed patients			
Recombivax HB® (MSD)	<20 y: 20 mcg (0.5 mL); ≥20 y, 40 mcg (1 mL) using special dialysis formulation		
Engerix-B® (SKF)[9]	<20 y, 20 mcg (1 mL); ≥20 y, 40 mcg (2 mL), give as two 1 mL doses at different sites		
Influenza		I.M. (2 doses 4+ weeks apart in children <9 years of age not previously immunized; only 1 dose needed for annual updates)	Inactivated virus subvirion (split) (contraindicated in patients allergic to chicken eggs)
Split virus only in pediatric patients			
6-35 mo	0.25 mL (1 or 2 doses)		
3-8 y	0.5 mL (1 or 2 doses)		
≥9 y	0.5 mL (1 dose)		
Measles	0.5 mL	SubQ	Live virus (contraindicated in patients with anaphylactic allergy to neomycin)

Most areas: Two doses (1st dose at 15 months with MMR; 2nd dose at 4-6 years or 11-12 years, depending on local school entry requirements)

High-risk area: Two doses (1st dose at 12 months with MMR; 2nd dose as above)

Children 6-15 months in epidemic situations: Dose is given at the time of first contact with a health care provider; children <1 year of age should receive single antigen measles vaccine. If vaccinated before 1 year, revaccinate at 15 months with MMR. A 3rd dose is administered at 4-6 years or 11-12 years, depending on local school entry requirements.

Vaccine	Dosage	Route of Administration	Type
Meningococcal			
Menactra™			Polysaccharide diphtheria toxoid conjugate
Adolescents and adults (11-55 y)	0.5 mL	I.M.	
Menomune®-A/C/Y/W-135			
Children ≥2 y and adults	0.5 mL[10]	SubQ	Polysaccharide
MMR[11]	0.5 mL	SubQ	Live virus
MR	0.5 mL	SubQ	Live virus
Mumps	0.5 mL	SubQ	Live virus
Pneumococcal heptavalent (Prevnar®)[12]	0.5 mL	I.M.	Protein-conjugated polysaccharide
Pneumococcal polyvalent[13]	0.5 mL (≥2 y)	I.M. or SubQ (I.M. preferred)	Polysaccharide
Poliovirus (OPV) trivalent	0.5 mL	Oral	Live virus
Poliovirus (IPV)[14] trivalent	0.5 mL	SubQ or I.M.	Inactivated virus

IMMUNIZATION GUIDELINES *(Continued)*

Dosage and Administration Guidelines for Vaccines Available in the United States *(continued)*

Vaccine	Dosage	Route of Administration	Type
Rabies			
Human diploid cell vaccine (Imovax®)	1 mL	I.M.[15] or	Inactivated virus
(HDCV)	0.1 mL	I.D.[16]	
Rabies vaccine adsorbed (RVA)	1 mL	I.M.[15]	Inactivated virus
Purified chick embryo cell (PCEC) (RabAvert™)	1 mL	I.M.[15]	Inactivated virus
Rubella	0.5 mL (≥12 mo)[17]	SubQ	Live virus
Tetanus (adsorbed)[18]	0.5 mL	I.M.	Toxoid
Tetanus (fluid)	0.5 mL	I.M., SubQ	Toxoid
Typhoid			
Injection, solution (Typhim Vi®)		I.M.	Polysaccharide
Children ≥2 y and adults: Primary immunization: 0.5 mL; Booster: 0.5 mL every 2 years			
Oral (Vivotif® Berna)		P.O.	Live bacteria
Children ≥6 y and adults: Primary immunization: 1 capsule qod (days 1, 3, 5, and 7); Booster: Repeat primary immunization series every 5 years.			
Varicella (Varivax®)	0.5 mL	SubQ	Live virus
Children 12 mo:Initial dose: 0.5 mL dose; Booster: 0.5 mL at 4-6 y			
Children 7-13 years: Initial: 0.5 mL; Booster: 0.5 mL at least 3 months following initial dose			
Adolescents ≥13 y and adults: 0.5 mL dose x 2 (second 0.5 mL dose is administered 4 to 8 weeks later)			
Yellow fever	0.5 mL[19]	SubQ	Live attenuated virus
Children ≥9 mo and adults: Initial dose: 0.5 mL; Booster: 0.5 mL every 10 years			

[1]DT for use in children <7 years of age. Td contains same amount of tetanus toxoid as DT & DTP, but a reduced dose of diphtheria toxoid. Td for use in children ≥7 years of age.

[2]DTaP is the recommended vaccine for primary vaccination against diphtheria, tetanus, and pertussis; including completion of the series in children who have received 1 or more doses of whole-cell DTP. The occurrence of fever and local reactions is lower with acellular pertussis vaccine than with whole-cell DTP.

[3]A single dose of Tdap should be given instead of Td in adolescents who have completed the recommended childhood DTP/DTaP series and have not received Td or Tdap; preferred age of vaccination with Tdap is 11-12 years of age. Adolescents who received Td but not Tdap and who have completed the recommended childhood DTP/DTaP series are encouraged to receive Tdap; an interval of at least 5 years between Td and Tdap is recommended, but lesser intervals may be used if the benefit outweighs the risk.

[4]The conjugate (HbCV) vaccine is preferred over the polysaccharide (HbPV) vaccine. In children with a high risk for *Haemophilus influenzae* type b disease and HbCV is unavailable, an acceptable alternate is to give HbPV at 18 months of age with a 2nd dose at 24 months of age. Children <5 years of age who were previously vaccinated with HbPV between 18-23 months of age should be revaccinated with a single dose of HbCV at least 2 months after the initial dose of HbPV. Either HbCV or HbPV can be administered up to the 5th birthday. However, they are generally not recommended for children >5 years of age.

[5]PRP-OMP (PedvaxHIB®) manufactured by Merck, Sharp & Dohme is initiated at 2 months of age for 3 doses (2 months, 4 months and 12 months). If initiated at 7-11 months of age, 3 doses are administered (initial 2 doses at 2-month intervals, 3rd dose at 15-18 months of age); if initiated at 12-14 months of age, 2 doses are administered at 2- to 3-month intervals between doses; if initiated at 15-59 months of age, 1 dose is administered.

[6]Hepatitis B vaccine can be given at the same time with DTP, HbOC, polio, and/or MMR; administer 3 doses at 0, 1, and 6 months).

[7]Administer to newborns at 0-2 days of age before hospital discharge; repeat at 1-2 months and 6-18 months following the initial dose. If not vaccinated at birth, administer at 2, 4, and 6-18 months of age.

[8]Aluminum-absorbed vaccines must be injected deep in the muscle mass and not SubQ because they can cause local irritation, inflammation, granuloma formation, and necrosis. Only patients (ie, hemophiliacs) who are at risk of hemorrhage following I.M. injections should receive hepatitis B vaccine SubQ

[9]Engerix-B® — an alternate schedule for postexposure prophylaxis or more rapid induction using 4 doses at 0, 1, 2, and 12 months of age is recommended.

[10]Indicated in children ≥2 years of age at risk (anatomic or functional asplenia, those with terminal complement component or properdin deficiencies), in epidemic or highly endemic areas. The American College Health Association recommends immunization of college students.

[11]See measles.

[12]Routine administration to all children ≤23 months at 2, 4, 6, and 12-15 months. Initial dose should be given no earlier than at 6 weeks of age. Recommended for children 24-59 months who are at high risk for invasive pneumococcal infection.

[13]Indicated for children with sickle cell disease; asplenia; nephrotic syndrome or chronic renal failure; conditions associated with immunosuppression; CSF leaks; HIV infection. Advisory Committee on Immunization Practices (ACIP) also recommends that patients ≥2 years of age with chronic cardiovascular disease, chronic pulmonary disease, diabetes mellitus, or chronic liver disease receive pneumococcal immunization. Patients ≥2 years of age living in special environments in which the risk of invasive pneumococcal disease is high (ie, Alaskan native and certain American Indian populations) should receive pneumococcal immunization.

[14]The primary series consists of 3 doses. The first 2 doses should be administered at an interval of 8 weeks beginning at 2 months of age (minimum age of 6 weeks). The 3rd dose should be given at 6-18 months of age. A booster dose of 0.5 mL should be given to all children who have completed the primary series, before entering school. However, if the 3rd dose of the primary series is given on or after the 4th birthday, a 4th dose is not required before entering school. When polio vaccine is given to persons >18 years of age, IPV should be given.

[15]In infants and small children, I.M. injection can be given into the midlateral aspect of the thigh; in older children and adults, I.M. injection can be given into the deltoid muscle. For postexposure prophylaxis, repeat doses are given on days 3, 7, 14, and 28 after the first dose. Initiate and complete immunization series with one vaccine product. Intradermal vaccine is not advised for postexposure prophylaxis.

[16]For pre-exposure prophylaxis against rabies for high-risk individuals, 1 mL I.M. or 0.1 mL intradermal is administered on days 0, 7, and 21 (or 28). Both I.M. and I.D. dosage forms are available. Preferred site for intradermal administration is the skin in the deltoid area. Patients taking chloroquine or mefloquine should only receive rabies vaccine by the I.M. route. Do **not** administer intradermally to minimize potential for vaccine failure.

[17]As MMR in a 2-dose schedule.

[18]Adsorbed preferred to fluid toxoid because of longer lasting immunity.

[19]≥9 months of age living in or traveling to endemic areas. Contraindicated in infants <4 months of age and in patients who have had an anaphylactic reaction to eggs. Increased risk of encephalitis associated with use of yellow fever vaccine in infants <9 months of age.

Note: For each vaccine, check the manufacturer's package insert for specific product information since preparations may change from time to time.

References

Advisory Committee on Immunization Practices, Measles Prevention, Recommendations of the Immunization Practices Advisory Committee, *MMWR Morb Mortal Wkly Rep*, 1989, 38(5-9):1-18.

American Academy of Pediatrics, "Report of the Committee on Infectious Diseases," Red Book®, 26th ed, 2003.

American Academy of Pediatrics, Committee on Infectious Diseases, "Acellular Pertussis Vaccines: Recommendations for Use as the Fourth and Fifth Doses," *Pediatrics*, 1992, 90:121-3.

American Academy of Pediatrics, Committee on Infectious Diseases, "Universal Hepatitis B Immunization," *Pediatrics*, 1992, 89(4 Pt 2):795-800.

American Academy of Pediatrics, Committee on Infectious Diseases, "Recommendations for the Use of Live Attenuated Varicella Vaccine," *Pediatrics*, 1995, 95(5):791-6.

American Academy of Pediatrics, Committee on Infectious Diseases, "Policy Statement: Recommendations for the Prevention of Pneumococcal Infections, Including the Use of Pneumococcal Conjugate Vaccine (Prevnar®), Pneumococcal Polysaccharide Vaccine, and Antibiotic Prophylaxis," *Pediatrics*, 2000, 106(2 Pt 1): 362-6.

American Academy of Pediatrics, Committee on Infectious Diseases, "Recommended Childhood and Adolescent Immunization Schedule – United States, 2006," *Pediatrics*, 2006, 117:239-40.

CDC, "Notice to Readers: Alternate Two-Dose Hepatitis B Vaccination Schedule for Adolescents Aged 11-15 Years," *MMWR Morb Mortal Wkly Rep*, 2000, 49(12):261.

CDC, "Recommended Childhood and Adolescent Immunization Schedule – United States, 2006," *MMWR*, 2005, 54(51 & 52):Q1-4.

IMMUNIZATION GUIDELINES *(Continued)*

Currently Recommended Regimens for Routine *Haemophilus influenzae* Type b Conjugate Immunization for Children Immunized Beginning at 2-6 Months of Age[1]

Vaccine Product at Initiation	Total No. of Doses to Be Administered	Recommended Regimens
HbOC or PRP-T	4	3 doses at 2-month intervals initially; fourth dose at 12-15 months of age; any conjugate vaccine for dose 4[2]
PRP-OMP	3	2 doses at 2-month intervals initially; when feasible, same vaccine for doses 1 and 2; third dose at 12-15 months of age; any conjugate vaccine for dose 3[2]

[1]These vaccines may be given in combination products or as reconstituted products with DTaP or DTP, provided the combination or reconstituted vaccine is approved by the U.S. Food and Drug Administration for the child's age and the administration of the other vaccine component(s) also is justified.

[2]The safety and efficacy of PRP-OMP, PRP-T, HbOC, and PRP-D are likely to be equivalent for children ≥12 months of age. If a different product is given for dose 2, then the recommendations for that product (eg, HbOC or PRP-T) apply.

Adapted from "Report of the Committee on Infectious Diseases," *2000 Red Book®*, 25th ed, 268.

Recommendations for Pneumococcal Conjugate Vaccine Use Among Healthy Children During Moderate and Severe Shortages

Age at First Vaccination (mo)	No Shortage[1]	Moderate Shortage	Severe Shortage
<6	2, 4, 6, and 12-15 months	2, 4, and 6 months (defer fourth dose)	2 doses at 2-month interval in first 6 months of life (defer third and fourth doses)
7-11	2 doses at 2-month interval; 12-15 month dose	2 doses at 2-month interval; 12-15-month dose	2 doses at 2-month interval (defer third dose)
12-23	2 doses at 2-month interval	2 doses at 2-month interval	1 dose (defer second dose)
>24	1 dose should be considered	No vaccination	No vaccination
Reduction in vaccine doses used[2]		21%	46%

[1]The vaccine schedule for no shortage is included as a reference. Providers should not use the no shortage schedule regardless of their vaccine supply until the national shortage is resolved.

[2]Assumes that approximately 85% of vaccine is administered to healthy infants beginning at age <7 months; approximately 5% is administered to high-risk infants beginning at age <7 months; and approximately 10% is administered to healthy children beginning at age 7-24 months. Actual vaccine savings will depend on a provider's vaccine use.

Adapted from the Advisory Committee on Immunization Practices, "Updated Recommendations on Use of Pneumococcal Conjugate Vaccine in a Setting of Vaccine Shortage," *MMWR Morb Mortal Wkly Rep*, 2001, 50(50):1140-2.

Recommended Regimens for Pneumococcal Conjugate Vaccine Among Children With a Late Start or Lapse in Vaccine Administration

Age at Examination (mo)	Previous Pneumococcal Conjugate Vaccination History	Recommended Regimen[1]
2-6	0 doses	3 doses 2 months apart, 4th dose at 12-15 months
	1 dose	2 doses 2 months apart, 4th dose at 12-15 months
	2 doses	1 dose, 4th dose at 12-15 months
7-11	0 doses	2 doses 2 months apart, 3rd dose at 12-15 months
	1 or 2 doses before age 7 months	1 dose at 7-11 months, with another dose at 12-15 months (≥2 months later)
12-23	0 doses	2 doses ≥2 months apart
	1 dose before age 12 months	2 doses ≥2 months apart
	1 dose at ≥12 months	1 dose ≥2 months after the most recent dose
	2 or 3 doses before age 12 months	1 dose ≥2 months after the most recent dose
24-59		
Healthy children[2]	Any incomplete schedule	Consider 1 dose ≥2 months after the most recent dose
High risk[3]	<3 doses	1 dose ≥2 months after the most recent dose and another dose ≥2 months later
	3 doses	1 dose ≥2 months after the most recent dose

[1]For children vaccinated at age <1 year, the minimum interval between doses is 4 weeks. Doses administered at ≥12 months should be at least 8 weeks apart.

[2]Providers should consider 1 dose for healthy children 24-59 months, with priority to children 24-35 months, American Indian/Alaska native and black children, and those who attend group child care centers.

[3]Children with sickle cell disease, asplenia, human immunodeficiency virus infection, chronic illness, cochlear implant, or immunocompromising condition.

Adapted from "CDC. Notice to Readers: Pneumococcal Conjugate Vaccine Shortage Resolved," *MMWR Morb Mortal Wkly Rep*, 2003, 52(19):446-7.

IMMUNIZATION GUIDELINES *(Continued)*

Persons Who Should Receive Pre-exposure Hepatitis B Immunization

- All infants
- Children at high risk for early childhood HBV infection
- Adolescents: Hepatitis B vaccination should be given by or before 11-12 years of age. Special efforts should be made to vaccinate all adolescents, not only those at high risk
- Hemophiliac patients and other recipients of certain blood products
- Intravenous drug abusers
- Heterosexual persons who have had more than one sex partner in the previous 6 months and/or those with a recent episode of a sexually transmitted disease
- Sexually active men who have sex with men
- Household and sexual contacts of HB_sAg-positive persons
- Members of households with adoptees who are hepatitis B surface antigen-positive
- Children and other household contacts in populations of high HBV endemicity
- Staff and residents of institutions for the developmentally disabled
- Staff of nonresidential day care and school programs for developmentally disabled if attended by known HB_sAg-positive persons
- Hemodialysis patients
- Healthcare workers and others with occupational risk of exposure to blood or blood-contaminated body fluid
- International travelers to areas of high or intermediate HBV endemicity
- Inmates of long-term correctional facilities

Adapted from American Academy of Pediatrics, Report of the Committee on Infectious Diseases, *Red Book*, 25th ed, 2000, 296.

See Recommended Immunization Schedule for Ages 0-6 Years and 7-18 Years charts for recommended Hepatitis B immunization schedule.

Recommended Immunization Schedule for Ages 0-6 Years United States, 2007

Vaccine ▼ / Age ▶	Birth	1 mo	2 mo	4 mo	6 mo	12 mo	15 mo	18 mo	19-23 mo	2-3 y	4-6 y
Hepatitis B[1]	HepB	HepB		*See footnote 1*	HepB				HepB series		
Rotavirus[2]			Rota	Rota	Rota						
Diphtheria, tetanus, pertussis[3]			DTaP	DTaP	DTaP		DTaP				DTaP
Haemophilus influenzae type b[4]			Hib	Hib	*Hib*[4]	Hib		Hib			
Pneumococcal[5]			PCV	PCV	PCV	PCV				PCV / PPV	
Inactivated poliovirus			IPV	IPV	IPV						IPV
Influenza[6]					Influenza (yearly)						
Measles, mumps, rubella[7]						MMR					MMR
Varicella[8]						Varicella					Varicella
Hepatitis A[9]						HepA (2 doses)				HepA series	
Meningococcal[10]										MPSV4	

Range of recommended ages | Catch-up immunization | Certain high-risk groups

This schedule indicates the recommended ages for routine administration of currently licensed childhood vaccines, as of December 1, 2006, for children through age 6 years. For additional information see **www.cdc.gov/nip/recs/child-schedule.htm**. Any dose not administered at the recommended age should be administered at any subsequent visit when indicated and feasible. Additional vaccines may be licensed and recommended during the year. Licensed combination vaccines may be used whenever any components of the combination are indicated and other components of the vaccine are not contraindicated and if approved by the Food and Drug Administration for that dose of the series. Providers should consult the respective Advisory Committee on Immunization Practices (ACIP) statement for detailed recommendations. Clinically significant adverse events that follow immunization should be reported to the Vaccine Adverse Event Reporting System (VAERS). Guidance about how to obtain and complete a VAERS form is available at **http://www.vaers.hhs.gov** or by telephone, **800-822-7967**.

[1]**Hepatitis B vaccine (HepB).** *(Minimum age: birth)*

At birth:
- Administer monovalent HepB to all newborns prior to hospital discharge.
- If mother is HB_sAg-positive, administer HepB and 0.5 mL of hepatitis B immune globulin (HBIG) within 12 hours of birth.
- If mother's HB_sAg status is unknown, administer HepB within 12 hours of birth. Determine the HB_sAg status as soon as possible and if HB_sAg-positive, administer HBIG (no later than age 1 week).
- If mother is HB_sAg-negative, the birth dose can only be delayed with physician's order and mothers' negative HB_sAg laboratory report documented in the infant's medical record.

Following the birth dose:
- The HepB series should be completed with either monovalent HepB or a combination vaccine containing HepB. The second dose should be administered at age 1–2 months. The final dose should be administered at age ≥24 weeks. Infants born to HB_sAg-positive mothers should be tested for HB_sAg and antibody to HB_sAg after completion of 3 or more doses in a licensed HepB series, at age 9–18 months (generally at the next well-child visit).

4-month dose of HepB:
- It is permissible to administer 4 doses of HepB when combination vaccines are given after the birth dose. If monovalent HepB is used for doses after the birth dose, a dose at age 4 months is not needed.

[2]**Rotavirus vaccine (Rota).** *(Minimum age: 6 weeks)*
- Administer the first dose between 6 and 12 weeks of age. Do not start the series later than age 12 weeks.
- Administer the final dose in the series by 32 weeks of age. Do not administer a dose later than age 32 weeks.
- There are insufficient data on safety and efficacy outside of these age ranges.

[3]**Diphtheria, tetanus toxoids, and acellular pertussis vaccine (DTaP).** *(Minimum age: 6 weeks)*
- The fourth dose of DTaP may be administered as early as age 12 months, provided 6 months have elapsed since the third dose.
- Administer the final dose in the series at age 4-6 years.

[4]***Haemophilus influenzae* type b conjugate vaccine (Hib).** *(Minimum age: 6 weeks)*
- If PRP-OMP (PedvaxHIB® or ComVax® [Merck]) is administered at ages 2 and 4 months, a dose at age 6 months is not required.
- TriHiBit® DTaP/Hib combination products should not be used for primary immunization but can be used as boosters following any Hib vaccine in ≥12 months olds.

[5]**Pneumococcal vaccine.** *(Minimum age: 6 weeks for Pneumococcal Conjugate Vaccine (PCV); 2 years for Pneumococcal Polysaccharide Vaccine (PPV))*
- Administer PCV at ages 24-59 months in certain high-risk groups. Administer PPV to certain high-risk groups aged ≥2 years. See *MMWR*, 2000, 49(RR-9):1-35.

[6]**Influenza vaccine.** *(Minimum age: 6 months for trivalent inactivated influenza vaccine (TIV); 5 years for live, attenuated influenza vaccine (LAIV)*
- All children aged 6–59 months and close contacts of all children aged 0–59 months are recommended to receive influenza vaccine.
- Influenza vaccine is recommended annually for children aged ≥59 months with certain risk factors, healthcare workers, and other persons (including household members) in close contact with persons in groups at high risk. See *MMWR*, 2006, 55(RR-10):1-41.
- For healthy persons aged 5–49 years, LAIV may be used as an alternative to TIV.
- Children receiving TIV should receive 0.25 mL if aged 6–35 months or 0.5 mL if aged ≥3 years.
- Children aged <9 years who are receiving influenza vaccine for the first time should receive 2 doses (separated by ≥4 weeks for TIV and ≥6 weeks for LAIV).

[7]**Measles, mumps, and rubella vaccine (MMR).** *(Minimum age: 12 months)*
- Administer the second dose of MMR at age 4-6 years. MMR may be administered prior to age 4-6 years, provided ≥4 weeks have elapsed since the first dose and both doses are administered at age ≥12 months.

[8]**Varicella vaccine.** *(Minimum age: 12 months)*
- Administer the second dose of varicella vaccine at age 4-6 years. Varicella vaccine may be administered prior to age 4-6 years, provided that ≥3 months have elapsed since the first dose and both doses are administered at age ≥12 months. If second dose was administered ≥28 days following the first dose, the second dose does not need to be repeated.

[9]**Hepatitis A vaccine (HepA).** *(Minimum age: 12 months)*
- HepA is recommended for all children at 1 year of age (ie, 12-23 months). The 2 doses in the series should be administered at least 6 months apart.
- Children not fully vaccinated by age 2 years can be vaccinataed at subsequent visits.
- HepA is recommended for certain other groups of children including in areas where vaccination programs target older children. See *MMWR*, 2006, 55(RR-7):1:23.

[10]**Meningococcal polysaccharide vaccine (MPSV4).** *(Minimum age: 2 years)*
- Administer MPSV4 to children age 2-10 years with terminal complement deficiencies or anatomic or functional asplenia and certain other high risk groups. See *MMWR*, 2005, 54(RR-7):1:21.

Approved by the Advisory Committee on Immunization Practices (**www.cdc.gov/nip/acip**), the American Academy of Pediatrics (**www.aap.org**), and the American Academy of Family Physicians (**www.aafp.org**).

Reference:

"Recommended Immunization Schedules for Persons Aged 0-18 Years — United States, 2007," *MMWR* , 2007, 55(51):Q1-4.

IMMUNIZATION GUIDELINES *(Continued)*

Recommended Immunization Schedule for Ages 7-18 Years United States, 2007

Vaccine ▼ / Age ▶	7-10 y	11-12 y	13-14 y	15 y	16-18 y
Tetanus, diphtheria, pertussis[1]	*See footnote 1*	Tdap	Tdap		
Human papillomavirus[2]	*See footnote 2*	HPV (3 doses)	HPV series		
Meningococcal[3]	MPSV4	MCV4	MCV4[3] / MCV4		
Pneumococcal[4]	PPV				
Influenza[5]	Influenza (yearly)				
Hepatitis A[6]	HepA series				
Hepatitis B[7]	HepB series				
Inactivated poliovirus[8]	IPV series				
Measles, mumps, rubella[9]	MMR series				
Varicella[10]	Varicella series				

Range of recommended ages — Catch-up immunization — Certain high-risk groups

This schedule indicates the recommended ages for routine administration of currently licensed childhood vaccines, as of December 1, 2006, for children aged 7-18 years. For additional information see **www.cdc.gov/nip/recs/child-schedule.htm**. Any dose not administered at the recommended earlier age should be administered at any subsequent visit when indicated and feasible. Additional vaccines may be licensed and recommended during the year. Licensed combination vaccines may be used whenever any components of the combination are indicated and other components of the vaccine are not contraindicated and if approved by the Food and Drug Administration for that dose of the series. Providers should consult the respective Advisory Committee on Immunization Practices (ACIP) statement for detailed recommendations. Clinically significant adverse events that follow immunization should be reported to the Vaccine Adverse Event Reporting System (VAERS). Guidance about how to obtain and complete a VAERS form is available at **www.vaers.hhs.org** or by telephone, **800-822-7967**.

[1]**Tetanus and diphtheria toxoids and acellular pertussis vaccine (Tdap).** *(Minimum age: 10 years for BOOSTRIX® and 11 years for ADACEL™)*
- Administer at age 11-12 years for those who have completed the recommended childhood DTP/DTaP vaccination series and have not received a Td booster dose.
- Adolescents 13-18 years who missed the 11-12 year Td/Tdap booster dose should also receive a single dose of Tdap if they have completed the recommended childhood DTP/DTaP vaccination series.

[2]**Human papillomavirus vaccine (HPV).** *(Minimum age: 9 years)*
- Administer the first dose of the HPV vaccine series to females at age 11-12 years.
- Administer the second dose 2 months after the first dose and the third dose 6 months after the first dose.
- Administer the HPV vaccine series to females at age 13-18 years if not previously vaccinated.

[3]**Meningococcal vaccine.** *(Minimum age: 11 years for meningococcal conjugate vaccine (MCV4); 2 years for meningococcal polysaccharide vaccine (MPSV4))*
- Administer MCV4 at age 11-12 years and to previously unvaccinated adolescents at high school entry (~15 years of age).
- Administer MCV4 to previously unvaccinated college freshmen living in dormitories; MPSV4 is an acceptable alternative.
- Vaccination against invasive meningococcal disease is recommended for children and adolescents aged ≥2 years with terminal complement deficiencies or anatomic or functional asplenia and certain other high-risk groups. See *MMWR*, 2005, 54(RR-7):1:21. Use MPSV4 for children aged 2-10 years and MCV4 or MPSV4 for older children.

[4]**Pneumococcal polysaccharide vaccine (PPV).** *(Minimum age: 2 years)*
- Administer for certain high-risk groups. See *MMWR*, 1997, 46(RR-08), 1-24 and *MMWR*, 2000, 49(RR-9):1-35.

[5]**Influenza vaccine.** *(Minimum age: 6 months for trivalent inactivated influenza vaccine (TIV); 5 years for live, attenuated influenza vaccine (LAIV)*
- Influenza vaccine is recommended annually for persons with certain risk factors, healthcare workers, and other persons (including household members) in close contact with persons in groups at high risk. See *MMWR*, 2006, 55(RR-10);1-41.
- For healthy persons aged 5–49 years, LAIV may be used as an alternative to TIV.
- Children aged <9 years who are receiving influenza vaccine for the first time should receive 2 doses (separated by ≥4 weeks for TIV and ≥6 weeks for LAIV).

[6]**Hepatitis A vaccine (HepA).** *(Minimum age: 12 months)*
- The 2 doses in the series should be administered at least 6 months apart.
- HepA is recommended for certain other groups of children including in areas where vaccination programs target older children. See *MMWR*, 2006, 55(RR-7):1:23.

[7]**Hepatitis B vaccine (HepB).** *(Minimum age: birth)*
- Administer the 3-dose series to those who were not previously vaccinated.
- A 2-dose series of Recombivax HB® is licensed for 11-15 year olds.

[8]**Inactivated poliovirus vaccine (IPV).** *(Minimum age: 6 weeks)*
- For children who received an all-IPV or all-oral poliovirus (OPV) series, a fourth dose is not necessary if third dose was administered at age ≥4 years.
- If both OPV and IPV were administered as part of a series, a total of 4 doses should be given, regardless of the child's current age.

[9]**Measles, mumps, and rubella vaccine (MMR).** *(Minimum age: 12 months)*
- If not previously vaccinated, administer 2 doses of MMR during any visit with ≥4 weeks between the doses.

[10]**Varicella vaccine.** *(Minimum age: 12 months)*
- Administer 2 doses of varicella vaccine to persons without evidence of immunity.
- Administer 2 doses of varicella vaccine to persons aged ≤13 years at least 3 month apart. Do not repeat the second dose, if administered ≥28 days following the first dose.
- Administer 2 doses of varicella vaccine to persons aged ≥13 years at least 4 weeks apart.

Approved by the Advisory Committee on Immunization Practices (**www.cdc.gov/nip/acip**), the American Academy of Pediatrics (**www.aap.org**), and the American Academy of Family Physicians (**www.aafp.org**).

Reference:

"Recommended Immunization Schedules for Persons Aged 0-18 Years — United States, 2007," *MMWR* , 2007, 55(51):Q1-4.

Recommended Immunization Schedule for Children and Adolescents Who Start Late or Who Are >1 Month Behind – United States, 2007

Tables 1 and 2 give catch-up schedules and minimum intervals between doses for children who have delayed immunizations. There is no need to restart a vaccine series regardless of the time that has elapsed between doses. Use the table appropriate for the child's age.

Table 1. Catch-up Schedule for Ages 4 Months - 6 Years

Vaccine (Minimum Age for Dose 1)	Minimum Interval Between Doses			
	Dose 1 to Dose 2	**Dose 2 to Dose 3**	**Dose 3 to Dose 4**	**Dose 4 to Dose 5**
HepB[1] (birth)	4 weeks	8 weeks (and 16 weeks after 1st dose)		
Rotavirus[2] (6 wk)	4 weeks	4 weeks		
DTaP[3] (6 wk)	4 weeks	4 weeks	6 months	6 months[3]
Hib[4] (6 wk)	**4 weeks** if 1st dose given at age <12 months **8 weeks (as final dose)** if 1st dose given at age 12-14 months **No further doses needed** if 1st dose given at age ≥15 months	**4 weeks[4]** if current age <12 months **8 weeks (as final dose)[4]** if current age ≥12 months and 2nd dose given at age <15 months **No further doses needed** if previous dose given at age ≥15 months	**8 weeks (as final dose)** This dose only necessary for children age 12 months - 5 years who received 3 doses before age 12 months	
PCV[5] (6 wk)	**4 weeks** if 1st dose given at age <12 months and current age <24 months **8 weeks (as final dose)** if 1st dose given at age ≥12 months or current age 24-59 months **No further doses needed** for healthy children if 1st dose given at age ≥24 months	**4 weeks** if current age <12 months **8 weeks (as final dose)** if current age ≥12 months **No further doses needed** for healthy children if previous dose given at age ≥24 months	**8 weeks (as final dose)** This dose only necessary for children age 12 months - 5 years who received 3 doses before age 12 months	
IPV[6] (6 wk)	4 weeks	4 weeks	4 weeks[6]	
MMR[7] (12 mo)	4 weeks			
Varicella[8] (12 mo)	3 months			
HepA[9] (12 mo)	6 months			

IMMUNIZATION GUIDELINES *(Continued)*

Table 2. Catch-up Schedule for Ages 7-18 Years

Vaccine (Minimum Age for Dose 1)	Minimum Interval Between Doses			
	Dose 1 to Dose 2	Dose 2 to Dose 3	Dose 3 to Dose 4	Dose 4 to Dose 5
Td/TdaP[10] (7 y[10])	4 weeks	**8 months** if first dose given at age <12 months **6 months** if first dose given at age ≥12 months	**6 months** if first dose given at age <12 months	
HPV[11] (9 y)	4 weeks	12 weeks		
HepA[9] (12 mo)	6 months			
HepB[1] (birth)	4 weeks	8 weeks (and 16 weeks after first dose)		
IPV[6] (6 wk)	4 weeks	4 weeks	4 weeks[6]	
MMR[7] (12 mo)	4 weeks			
Varicella[8] (12 mo)	**4 weeks** if first dose given at age ≥13 years **3 months** if first dose given at age <13 years			

Footnotes to Table 1 and Table 2

[1]**HepB (hepatitis B).** *(Minimum age: birth)*
- Administer the 3-dose series to those who were not previously vaccinated.
- A 2-dose series of Recombivax HB® is licensed for 11-15 year olds.

[2]**Rotavirus (Rota).** *(Minimum age: 6 weeks)*
- Do not start the series later than age 12 weeks.
- Administer the final dose in the series by 32 weeks of age. Do not administer a dose later than age 32 weeks.
- There are insufficient data on safety and efficacy outside of these age ranges.

[3]**DTaP (diphtheria and tetanus toxoids and acellular pertussis).** *(Minimum age: 6 weeks)*
- The fifth dose is not necessary if the fourth dose was administered at age ≥4 years.
- DTaP is not indicated for persons age ≥7 years.

[4]**Hib *(Haemophilus influenzae* type b conjugate).** *(Minimum age: 6 weeks)*
- Vaccine is not generally recommended for children age ≥5 years.
- If current age <12 months and the first 2 doses were PRP-OMP (PedvaxHIB® or ComVax® [Merck]), the third (and final) dose should be administered at age 12-15 months and at least 8 weeks after the second dose.
- If first dose given at age 7-11 months, give 2 doses separated by 4 weeks plus a booster at age 12-15 months.

[5]**PCV (pneumococcal conjugate vaccine).** *(Minimum age: 6 weeks)*
- Vaccine is not generally recommended for children age ≥5 years.

[6]**IPV (inactivated poliovirus).** *(Minimum age: 6 weeks)*
- For children who received an all-IPV or all-oral poliovirus (OPV) series, a fourth dose is not necessary if third dose was administered at age ≥4 years.
- If both OPV and IPV were administered as part of a series, a total of 4 doses should be given, regardless of the child's current age.

[7]**MMR (measles, mumps, and rubella).** *(Minimum age: 12 months)*
- The second dose of MMR is recommended routinely at age 4-6 years, but may be administered earlier if desired.
- If not previously vaccinated, administer 2 doses of MMR during any visit with ≥4 weeks between the doses.

[8]**Varicella.** *(Minimum age: 12 months)*
- The second dose of varicella vaccine is recommended routinely at age 4-6 years but may be administered earlier if desired.
- Do not repeat the second dose in persons age <13 years, if administered ≥28 days following the first dose.

[9]**HepA (hepatitis A).** *(Minimum age: 12 months)*

- HepA is recommended for certain groups of children including in areas where vaccination programs target older children. See *MMWR*, 2006, SS(RR-7):1-23.

[10]**Td (tetanus and diphtheria toxoids) and Tdap (tetanus and diphtheria toxoids and acellular pertussis).** *(Minimum ages: 7 years for Td, 10 years for BOOSTRIX®, and 11 years for ADACEL™)*

- Tdap should be substituted for a single dose of Td in the primary catch-up series or as a booster if age-appropriate; use Td for other doses.
- A 5-year interval from the last Td dose is encouraged when Tdap is used as a booster dose. A booster (fourth) dose is needed if any of the previous doses were administered at age <12 months. Refer to ACIP recommendations for further information. See *MMWR*, 2006, SS(RR-3):L34.

[11] **HPV (human papillomavirus).** *(Minimum age: 9 years)*

- Administer the HPV vaccine series to females at age 13-18 years if not previously vaccinated.

Reporting Adverse Reactions

For information on reporting reactions following immunization, visit **www.vaers.hhs.gov** or call the 24-hour national toll-free information line **800-822-7967**. Report suspected cases of vaccine-preventable diseases to your state or local health department. For additional information including precautions and contraindications for immunization, visit the National Center for Immunization and Respiratory Diseases at **www.cdc.gov/ncird** or contact **800-CDC-INFO (800-232-4636)**.

IMMUNIZATION GUIDELINES *(Continued)*

Recommended Immunization Schedules for Children Not Immunized in the First Year of Life

Recommended Time/Age	Immunization(s)[1]	Comments
Younger Than 7 Years		
First visit	DTaP, Hib, HBV, MMR	If indicated, tuberculin testing may be done at same visit. If child is ≥5 y of age, Hib is not indicated in most circumstances.
Interval after first visit		
1 mo (4 wk)	DTaP, IPV, HBV, Var[2]	The second dose of IPV may be given if accelerated poliomyelitis immunization is necessary, such as for travelers to areas where polio is endemic.
2 mo	DTaP, Hib, IPV	Second dose of Hib is indicated only if the first dose was received when <15 mo.
≥8 mo	DTaP, HBV, IPV	IPV and HBV are not given if the third doses were given earlier.
Age 4-6 y (at or before school entry)	DTaP, IPV, MMR[3]	DTaP is not necessary if the fourth dose was given after the fourth birthday; IPV is not necessary if the third dose was given after the fourth birthday.
Age 11-12 y	See footnote 4	
7-12 Years		
First visit	HBV, MMR, dT, IPV	
Interval after first visit		
2 mo (8 wk)	HBV,[5] MMR,[3] Var, dT, IPV	IPV also may be given 1 mo after the first visit if accelerated poliomyelitis immunization is necessary.
8-14 mo	HBV,[5] dT, IPV	IPV is not given if the third dose was given earlier.
Age 11-12 y	See footnote 4	

[1] If all needed vaccines cannot be administered simultaneously, priority should be given to protecting the child against those diseases that pose the greatest immediate risk. In the United States, these diseases for children <2 years usually are measles and *Haemophilus influenzae* type b infection; for children >7 years, they are measles, mumps, and rubella. Before 13 years of age, immunity against hepatitis B and varicella should be ensured. DTaP, HBV, Hib, MMR, and Var can be given simultaneously at separate sites if failure of the patient to return for future immunizations is a concern.

[2] Varicella vaccine can be administered to susceptible children any time after 12 months of age. Unimmunized children who lack a reliable history of varicella should be immunized before their 13th birthday.

[3] Minimal interval between doses of MMR is 1 month (4 weeks).

[4] See Recommended Immunization Schedule for Ages 0-6 Years and 7-18 Years charts for recommended Hepatitis B immunization schedule.

[5] HBV may be given earlier in a 0-, 2-, and 4-month schedule.

Adapted from American Academy of Pediatrics, Report of the Committee on Infectious Diseases, *Red Book*, 25th ed, 2000.

Spacing Live and Killed Antigen Administration Guidelines

Antigen Combinations	Recommended Minimum Interval Between Doses
≥2 killed antigens	None. May be given simultaneously or at any interval between doses. Vaccines associated with systemic reactions (cholera, plague, and parenteral typhoid) should be given on separate occasions.
Killed and live antigens	None. May be given simultaneously or at any interval between doses. (**Exception:** Concurrent administration of cholera and yellow fever vaccines should be avoided. Separate these vaccines by at least 3 weeks.)
≥2 live antigens parenteral	4-week minimum interval if not administered simultaneously. Live oral vaccines (eg, Ty21a typhoid vaccine, oral polio vaccine) can be administered simultaneously or at any interval before or after inactivated or live parenteral vaccines.

Passive Immunization Agents — Immune Globulins

Immune Globulin		Dosage	Route
Hepatitis B (H-BIG®)			I.M.
percutaneous inoculation		0.06 mL/kg/dose (within 24 hours) (5 mL max)	
perinatal		0.5 mL/dose (within 12 hours of birth)	
sexual exposure		0.06 mL/kg/dose (within 14 days of contact) (5 mL max)	
Immune globulin (IG)			I.M.[1]
hepatitis A prophylaxis		0.02 mL/kg/dose (as soon as possible or within 2 weeks after exposure) (postexposure prophylaxis)	
	<2 y:	0.06 mL/kg/dose (≥3 months or long-term exposure) repeat every 5 months with continuous exposure	
	≥2 y:	0.02 mL/kg (3- to 5-month exposure) may be given to travelers whose departure is imminent with hepatitis A vaccine 0.06 mL/kg (long-term exposure) and hepatitis A vaccine	
hepatitis B		0.06 mL/kg/dose (H-BIG® should be used)	
hepatitis C		0.06 mL/kg/dose (percutaneous exposure)	
measles[2]		0.25 mL/kg/dose (max: 15 mL/dose) (within 6 days of exposure) 0.5 mL/kg/dose (max: 15 mL/dose) (immunocompromised children)	
Rabies[3]		20 IU/kg/dose (within 3 days)	
Tetanus (serious, contaminated, wounds; <3 previous tetanus vaccine doses)		250-500 units/dose	I.M.
Varicella-zoster[4] (VZIG)		Within 48 hours but not later than 96 hours after exposure	I.M.[5]
		0-10 kg: 125 units = 1 vial	
		10.1-20 kg: 250 units = 2 vials	
		20.1-30 kg: 375 units = 3 vials	
		30.1-40 kg: 500 units = 4 vials	
		>40 kg: 625 units = 5 vials	

[1]Deep I.M. in the gluteal region for large doses only. Deltoid muscle or the anterolateral aspect of the thigh are preferred sites for injection. No greater than 5 mL/site in adults or large children; 1-3 mL/site in small children and infants. Max: 20 mL at one time. Pregnant women and infants should receive a thimerosol-free preparation.

[2]IG prophylaxis may not be indicated in a patient who has received IGIV within 3 weeks of exposure.

[3]½ of dose used to infiltrate the wound with the remaining ½ of dose given I.M. Rabies immune globulin is not recommended in previously HDCV immunized patients.

[4]Infants born to women who develop varicella within 5 days before or 48 hours after delivery should receive 125 units I.M. as a single dose.

[5]No greater than 2.5 mL of VZIG/one injection site. Doses >2.5 mL should be divided and administered at different sites.

IMMUNIZATION GUIDELINES *(Continued)*

Suggested Intervals Between Administration of Immune Globulin Preparations for Various Indications and Measles Immunization[1]

Indication	Dose (including mg IgG/kg)	Time Interval (mo) Before Measles or Varicella Vaccination
Tetanus (TIG) prophylaxis	I.M.: 250 units (10 mg IgG/kg)	3
Hepatitis A (IG) prophylaxis		
Contact prophylaxis	I.M.: 0.02 mL/kg (3.3 mg IgG/kg)	3
International travel	I.M.: 0.06 mL/kg (10 mg IgG/kg)	3
Hepatitis B prophylaxis (HBIG)	I.M.: 0.06 mL/kg (10 mg IgG/kg)	3
Rabies immune globulin (RIG)	I.M.: 20 IU/kg (22 mg IgG/kg)	4
Varicella prophylaxis (VZIG)	I.M.: 125 units/10 kg (20-40 mg IgG/kg) (max: 625 units)	5
Measles prophylaxis (IG)		
Standard (ie, nonimmunocompromised contact)	I.M.: 0.25 mL/kg (40 mg IgG/kg)	5
Immunocompromised contact	I.M.: 0.50 mL/kg (80 mg IgG/kg)	6
Blood transfusion		
RBCs, washed	I.V.: 10 mL/kg (negligible IgG/kg)	0
RBCs, adenine-saline added	I.V.: 10 mL/kg (10 mg IgG/kg)	3
Packed RBCs	I.V.: 10 mL/kg (20-60 mg IgG/kg)	5
Whole blood cells	I.V.: 10 mL/kg (80-100 mg IgG/kg)	6
Plasma/platelet products	I.V.: 10 mL/kg (160 mg IgG/kg)	7
Replacement therapy for immune deficiencies	I.V.: 300-400 mg/kg (as IGIV)[2]	8
Immune thrombocytopenic purpura[3]	I.V.: 400 mg/kg (as IGIV) I.V.: 1000 mg/kg (as IGIV)	8 10
Kawasaki disease	I.V.: 2 g/kg (as IGIV)	11
RSV prophylaxis	I.V.: 750 mg/kg (as RSV-IVIG)	9
RSVIG monoclonal antibody (Synagis™)	I.M.: 15 mg/kg	None

[1]This table is not intended for determining the correct indications and dosage for the use of immune globulin preparations. Unvaccinated persons may not be fully protected against measles during the entire suggested time interval, and additional doses of immune globulin and/or measles vaccine may be indicated after measles exposure. The concentration of measles antibody in a particular immune globulin preparation can vary by lot. The rate of antibody clearance after receipt of an immune globulin preparation also can vary. The recommended time intervals are extrapolated from an estimated half-life of 30 days of passively acquired antibody and an observed interference with the immune response to measles vaccine for 5 months after a dose of 80 mg IgG/kg.

[2]Measles vaccination is recommended for most HIV-infected children who do not have evidence of severe immunosuppression, but it is contraindicated for patients who have congenital disorders of the immune system.

[3]Formerly referred to as idiopathic thrombocytopenic purpura.

Modified from *Red Book 2000: Report of the Committee on Infectious Diseases*, 25th ed, Elk Grove Village, IL: American Academy of Pediatrics, 390; Recommendations of the Advisory Committee on Immunization Practices (ACIP) and the American Academy of Family Physicians (AAFP), "General Recommendations on Immunization," *MMWR Morb Mortal Wkly Rep*, 2002, 51(RR-2), 1-36.

Recommended for Routine Immunization of HIV-Infected Children — United States

Vaccine	Known HIV Infection: Asymptomatic	Known HIV Infection: Symptomatic
DTaP	Yes	Yes
OPV	No	No
IPV	Yes	Yes
MMR	Yes	Yes[1]
Hib	Yes	Yes
Pneumococcal	Yes	Yes
Influenza[2]	Yes	Yes
Varicella	Consider	Consider
BCG	No	No
Hepatitis A	[3]	[3]
Hepatitis B	Yes	Yes

[1]Severely immunocompromised HIV-infected children should not receive MMR.

[2]Administer influenza vaccine each autumn and repeat annually for HIV-exposed infants ≥6 months of age, HIV-infected children and adolescents, and household contacts of HIV-infected persons.

[3]The immune response in immunocompromised persons, including persons with HIV, may be suboptimal.

RECOMMENDATIONS FOR TRAVELERS

Recommended Immunizations for Travelers to Developing Countries[1]

Immunizations	Length of Travel: Brief, <2 wk	Length of Travel: Intermediate, 2 wk - 3 mo	Length of Travel: Long-term Residential, >3 mo
Review and complete age-appropriate childhood schedule • DTaP; poliovirus vaccine, and *H. influenzae* type b vaccine may be given at 4 wk intervals if necessary to complete the recommended schedule before departure • Measles: 2 additional doses given if younger than 12 mo of age at first dose • Varicella • Hepatitis B[2]	+	+	+
Yellow fever[3]	+	+	+
Hepatitis A[4]	+	+	+
Typhoid fever[4]	±	+	+
Meningococcal disease[5]	±	±	±
Rabies[6]	±	+	+
Japanese encephalitis[3]	±	±	+

[1]+ = recommended; ± = consider.

[2]If insufficient time to complete 6-month primary series, accelerated series can be given.

[3]For endemic regions, see *Health Information for International Travel* in *Red Book®*. For high-risk activities in areas experiencing outbreaks, vaccine is recommended even for brief travel.

[4]Indicated for travelers who will consume food and liquids in areas of poor sanitation.

[5]For endemic regions of Africa, during local epidemics, and travel to Saudi Arabia for the Hajj.

[6]Indicated for person with high risk of animal exposure, and for travelers to endemic countries.

Adapted from "Report of the Committee on Infectious Diseases," *2000 Red Book®*, 25th ed, 78.

IMMUNIZATION GUIDELINES *(Continued)*

Recommendations for Pre-exposure Immunoprophylaxis of Hepatitis A Virus Infection for Travelers[1]

Age (y)	Likely Exposure (mo)	Recommended Prophylaxis
<2	<3	IG 0.02 mL/kg[2]
	3-5	IG 0.06 mL/kg[2]
	Long-term	IG 0.06 mL/kg at departure and every 5 mo if exposure to HAV continues[2]
≥2	<3[3]	HAV vaccine[4,5] or
	3-5[3]	HAV vaccine[4,5] or IG 0.06 mL/kg[2]
	Long-term	HAV vaccine[4,5]

[1] IG = immune globulin; HAV= hepatitis A virus.
[2]IG should be administered deep into a large muscle mass. Ordinarily, no more than 5 mL should be administered in one site in an adult or large child; lesser amounts (maximum 3 mL) should be given to small children and infants.
[3]Vaccine is preferable, but IG is an acceptable alternative.
[4]To ensure protection in travelers whose departure is imminent, IG also may be given.
[5]Dose and schedule of hepatitis A vaccine as recommended according to age.
Adapted from "Report of the Committee on Infectious Diseases," *2000 Red Book®*, 25th ed, 282.

MALARIA

Prevention of Malaria

Drug[1]	Adult Dosage	Pediatric Dosage
	Chloroquine-Sensitive Areas[2]	
Chloroquine phosphate[3,4]	500 mg (300 mg base), once/ week[5]	5 mg/kg base once/week, up to adult dose of 300 mg base[5]
	Chloroquine-Resistant Areas[2]	
Mefloquine[4,6,7]	250 mg once/week[5]	<15 kg: 5 mg/kg[5] 15-19 kg: 1/4 tablet[5] 20-30 kg: 1/2 tablet[5] 31-45 kg: 3/4 tablet[5] >45 kg: 1 tablet[5]
or		
Doxycycline[4,8]	100 mg/d[9]	2 mg/kg/d, up to 100 mg/d[9]
or		
Atovaquone/ proguanil[4,10]	250 mg/100 mg (1 tablet) daily[11]	11-20 kg: 62.5 mg/25 mg[10,11] 21-30 kg: 125 mg/50 mg[10,11] 31-40 kg: 187.5 mg/75 mg[10,11] >40 kg: 250 mg/100 mg[10,11]
Alternative:		
Primaquine[8,12,13]	30 mg base daily	0.5 mg/kg base daily
Chloroquine phosphate[3]	500 mg (300 mg base) once/ week[5]	5 mg/kg base once/week, up to adult dose of 300 mg base[5]
plus		
Proguanil[14]	200 mg once/day	<2 y: 50 mg once/day 2-6 y: 100 mg once/day 7-10 y: 150 mg once/day >10 y: 200 mg once/day

[1]No drug regimen guarantees protection against malaria. If fever develops within a year (particularly within the first 2 months) after travel to malarious areas, travelers should be advised to seek medical attention. Insect repellents, insecticide-impregnated bed nets, and proper clothing are important adjuncts for malaria prophylaxis.

[2]Chloroquine-resistant *P. falciparum* occurs in all malarious areas except Central America west of the Panama Canal Zone, Mexico, Haiti, the Dominican Republic, and most of the Middle East (chloroquine resistance has been reported in Yemen, Oman, Saudi Arabia, and Iran).

[3]In pregnancy, chloroquine prophylaxis has been used extensively and safely.

[4]For prevention of attack after departure from areas where *P. vivax* and *P. ovale* are endemic, which includes almost all areas where malaria is found (except Haiti), some experts prescribe in addition primaquine phosphate 26.3 mg (15 mg base)/day or, for children, 0.3 mg base/kg/day during the last 2 weeks of prophylaxis. Others prefer to avoid the toxicity of primaquine and rely on surveillance to detect cases when they occur; particularly when exposure was limited or doubtful.

[5]Beginning 1-2 weeks before travel and continuing weekly for the duration of stay and for 4 weeks after leaving.

[6]In the U.S., a 250 mg tablet of mefloquine contains 228 mg mefloquine base. Outside the U.S., each 275 mg tablet contains 250 mg base.

[7]The pediatric dosage has not been approved by the FDA, and the drug has not been approved for use during pregnancy. However, it has been reported to be safe for prophylactic use during the second or third trimester of pregnancy and possibly during early pregnancy as well (CDC Health Information for International Travel, 2001-2003, 113; BL Smoak, Writer JV, Keep LW, et al, "The Effects of Inadvertent Exposure of Mefloquine Chemoprophylaxis on Pregnancy Outcomes and Infants of US Army Servicewomen," *J Infect Dis*, 1997, 176(3):831-3). Mefloquine is not recommended for patients with cardiac conduction abnormalities. Patients with a history of seizures or psychiatric disorders should avoid mefloquine (*Medical Letter*, 1990, 32:13). Resistance to mefloquine has been reported in some areas, such as Thailand; in these areas, doxycycline should be used for prophylaxis. In children <8 years of age, proguanil plus sulfisoxazole has been used (KN Suh and JS Keystone, *Infect Dis Clin Pract*, 1996, 5:541).

[8]An approved drug, but considered investigational for this condition by the U.S. Food and Drug Administration.

[9]Beginning 1-2 days before travel and continuing for the duration of stay and for 4 weeks after leaving. Use of tetracyclines is contraindicated in pregnancy and in children <8 years of age. Doxycycline can cause gastrointestinal disturbances, vaginal moniliasis, and photosensitivity reactions.

[10]Atovaquone plus proguanil is available as a fixed-dose combination tablet: adult tablets (250 mg atovaquone/100 mg proguanil, *Malarone*) and pediatric tablets (62.5 mg atovaquone/25 mg proguanil, *Malarone Pediatric*). To enhance absorption, it should be taken within 45 minutes after eating (Looareesuwan S, Chulay JD, Canfield CJ, et al, "Malarone (Atovaquone and Proguanil

MALARIA *(Continued)*

Hydrochloride): A Review of Its Clinical Development for Treatment of Malaria. Malarone Clinical Trials Study Group," *Am J Trop Med Hyg*, 1999, 60(4):533-41). Although approved for once daily dosing, to decrease nausea and vomiting the dose for treatment is usually divided in two.

[11]Shanks GE et al, *Clin Infect Dis*, 1998, 27:494; Lell B, Luckner D, Ndjave M, et al, "Randomised Placebo-Controlled Study of Atovaquone Plus Proguanil for Malaria Prophylaxis in Children," *Lancet*, 1998, 351(9104):709-13. Beginning 1-2 days before travel and continuing for the duration of stay and for 1 week after leaving. In one study of malaria prophylaxis, atovaquone/proguanil was better tolerated than mefloquine in nonimmune travelers (Overbosch D, Schilthuis H, Bienzle U, et al, "Atovaquone-Proguanil Versus Mefloquine for Malaria Prophylaxis in Nonimmune Travelers: Results From a Randomized, Double-Blind Study," *Clin Infect Dis*, 2001, 33(7):1015-21).

[12]Primaquine phosphate can cause hemolytic anemia, especially in patients whose red cells are deficient in glucose-6-phosphate dehydrogenase. This deficiency is most common in African, Asian, and Mediterranean peoples. Patients should be screened for G6PD deficiency before treatment. Primaquine should not be used during pregnancy.

[13]Several studies have shown that daily primaquine, beginning 1 day before departure and continued until 7 days after leaving the malaria area, provides effective prophylaxis against chloroquine-resistant *P. falciparum* (Baird JK, Lacy MD, Basri H, et al, "Randomized, Parallel Placebo-Controlled Trial of Primaquine for Malaria Prophylaxis in Papua, Indonesia," *Clin Infect Dis*, 2001, 33(12):1990-7). Some studies have shown less efficacy against *P. vivax*. Nausea and abdominal pain can be diminished by taking with food.

[14]Proguanil (Paludrine – Wyeth Ayerst, Canada; AstraZeneca, United Kingdom), which is not available alone in the U.S.A. but is widely available in Canada and Europe, is recommended mainly for use in Africa south of the Sahara. Prophylaxis is recommended during exposure and for 4 weeks afterwards. Proguanil has been used in pregnancy without evidence of toxicity (Phillips-Howard PA and Wood D, "The Safety of Antimalarial Drugs in Pregnancy," *Drug Saf*, 1996, 14(3):131-45).

Adapted from "Report of the Committee on Infectious Diseases," *2003 Red Book®*, 26th ed, 760-1.

Malaria Treatment

Recommended Drug	Adult Dose[1,8]	Pediatric Dose[1,8] *(Pediatric dose should NEVER exceed adult dose)*	Region Infection Acquired
Uncomplicated Malaria / *P. falciparum* **or** Species Not Identified (If "species not identified" is subsequently diagnosed as *P. vivax* or *P. ovale*, see *P. vivax* and *P. ovale* (below) regarding treatment with primaquine)			
Chloroquine phosphate (Aralen® and generics)	600 mg base (= 1000 mg salt) P.O. immediately, followed by 300 mg base (= 500 mg salt) P.O. at 6, 24, and 48 hours Total dose: 1500 mg base (= 2500 mg salt)	10 mg base/kg P.O. immediately, followed by 5 mg base/kg P.O. at 6, 24, and 48 hours Total dose: 25 mg base/kg	**Chloroquine-sensitive** (Central America west of Panama Canal; Haiti; the Dominican Republic; and most of the Middle East)
2nd line alternative for treatment: Hydroxychloroquine (Plaquenil® and generics)	620 mg base (= 800 mg salt) P.O. immediately, followed by 310 mg base (= 400 mg salt) P.O. at 6, 24, and 48 hours Total dose: 1550 mg base (= 2000 mg salt)	10 mg base/kg P.O. immediately, followed by 5 mg base/kg P.O. at 6, 24, and 48 hours Total dose: 25 mg base/kg	
A. Quinine sulfate[2] plus one of the following: Doxycycline, tetracycline, or clindamycin	**Quinine sulfate:** 542 mg base (= 650 mg salt)[3] P.O. tid x 3-7 days **Doxycycline:** 100 mg P.O. bid x 7 days **Tetracycline:** 250 mg P.O. qid x 7 days **Clindamycin:** 20 mg base/kg/day P.O. divided tid x 7 days	**Quinine sulfate:** 8.3 mg base/kg (= 10 mg salt/kg) P.O. tid x 3-7 days **Doxycycline**[4]: 2.2 mg/kg P.O. every 12 hours x 7 days **Tetracycline**[4]: 25 mg/kg/day P.O. divided qid x 7 days **Clindamycin:** 20 mg base/kg/day P.O. divided tid x 7 days	**Chloroquine-resistant or unknown resistance**[1](All malarious regions except those specified as chloroquine-sensitive listed in the box above. Middle Eastern countries with chloroquine-resistant *P. falciparum* include Iran, Oman, Saudi Arabia, and Yemen. Of note, infections acquired in the Newly Independent States of the former Soviet Union and Korea to date have been uniformly caused by *P. vivax* and should therefore be treated as chloroquine-sensitive infections.)

MALARIA *(Continued)*

Malaria Treatment *(continued)*

Recommended Drug	Adult Dose[1,8]	Pediatric Dose[1,8] *(Pediatric dose should NEVER exceed adult dose)*	Region Infection Acquired
B. Atovaquone-proguanil (Malarone®)[5]	**Adult tab = 250 mg atovaquone/100 mg proguanil** 4 adult tabs P.O. qd x 3 days	**Adult tab = 250 mg atovaquone/100 mg proguanil** **Peds tab = 62.5 mg atovaquone/25 mg proguanil** 5-8 kg: 2 peds tabs P.O. qd x 3 d 9-10 kg: 3 peds tabs P.O. qd x 3 d 11-20 kg: 1 adult tab P.O. qd x 3 d 21-30 kg: 2 adult tabs P.O. qd x 3 d 31-40 kg: 3 adult tabs P.O. qd x 3 d >40 kg: 4 adult tabs P.O. qd x 3 d	
C. Mefloquine (Lariam® and generics)[6]	684 mg base (= 750 mg salt) P.O. as initial dose, followed by 456 mg base (= 500 mg salt) P.O. given 6-12 hours after initial dose Total dose = 1250 mg salt	13.7 mg base/kg (= 15 mg salt/kg) P.O. as initial dose, followed by 9.1 mg base/kg (= 10 mg salt/kg) P.O. given 6-12 hours after initial dose Total dose = 25 mg salt/kg	
Uncomplicated Malaria / *P. malariae*			
Chloroquine phosphate	Treatment as above	Treatment as above	**All regions**
2nd line alternative for treatment: Hydroxychloroquine	Treatment as above	Treatment as above	
Uncomplicated Malaria / *P. vivax* **or** *P. ovale*			
Chloroquine phosphate plus primaquine phosphate[7]	**Chloroquine phosphate:** Treatment as above **Primaquine phosphate:** 30 mg base P.O. qd x 14 days	**Chloroquine phosphate:** Treatment as above **Primaquine phosphate:** 0.5 mg base/kg P.O. qd x 14 days	**All regions[8] Note:** For suspected chloroquine-resistant *P. vivax*, see row below
2nd line alternative for treatment: Hydroxychloroquine plus primaquine phosphate[7]	**Hydroxychloroquine:** Treatment as above **Primaquine phosphate:** 30 mg base P.O. qd x 14 days	**Hydroxychloroquine:** Treatment as above **Primaquine phosphate:** 30 mg base P.O. qd x 14 days	

Malaria Treatment *(continued)*

Recommended Drug	Adult Dose[1,8]	Pediatric Dose[1,8] *(Pediatric dose should NEVER exceed adult dose)*	Region Infection Acquired
Uncomplicated Malaria / *P. vivax*			
A. Quinine sulfate[2] plus either doxycycline or tetracycline plus primaquine phosphate[7]	**Quinine sulfate:** Treatment as above **Doxycycline or tetracycline:** Treatment as above **Primaquine phosphate:** Treatment as above	**Quinine sulfate:** Treatment as above **Doxycycline or tetracycline[4]:** Treatment as above **Primaquine phosphate:** Treatment as above	**Chloroquine-resistant[8]** (Papua New Guinea and Indonesia)
B. Mefloquine plus primaquine phosphate[7]	**Mefloquine:** Treatment as above **Primaquine phosphate:** Treatment as above	**Mefloquine:** Treatment as above **Primaquine phosphate:** Treatment as above	
Uncomplicated Malaria: Alternatives for Pregnant Women[9,10,11,12]			
Chloroquine phosphate	Treatment as above	Not applicable	**Chloroquine-sensitive[12]** (See uncomplicated malaria sections above for chloroquine-sensitive *Plasmodium* species by region)
2nd line alternative for treatment: Hydroxychloroquine	Treatment as above	Not applicable	
Quinine sulfate[2] plus clindamycin	**Quinine sulfate:** Treatment as above **Clindamycin:** Treatment as above	Not applicable	**Chloroquine-resistant *P. falciparum*[9,10,11]** (See uncomplicated malaria sections above for regions with known chloroquine resistant *P. falciparum*)
Quinine sulfate	650 mg[3] salt P.O. tid x 7 days	Not applicable	**Chloroquine-resistant *P. vivax*[9,10,11,12]** (See uncomplicated malaria sections above for regions with chloroquine-resistant *P. vivax*)

Malaria Treatment *(continued)*

Recommended Drug	Adult Dose[1,8]	Pediatric Dose[1,8] ***(Pediatric dose should NEVER exceed adult dose)***	Region Infection Acquired
Severe Malaria[13,14,15,16]			
Quinidine gluconate[14] plus one of the following: Doxycycline, tetracycline, or clindamycin	**Quinidine gluconate:** 6.25 mg base/kg (= 10 mg salt/kg) loading dose I.V. over 1-2 hours, then 0.0125 mg base/kg/min (= 0.02 mg salt/kg/min) continuous infusion for at least 24 hours. An alternative regimen is 15 mg base/kg (= 24 mg salt/kg) loading dose I.V. infused over 4 hours, followed by 7.5 mg base/kg (= 12 mg salt/kg) infused over 4 hours every 8 hours, starting 8 hours after the loading dose (see package insert). Once parasite density <1% and patient can take oral medication, complete treatment with oral quinine, dose as above. Quinidine/quinine course = 7 days in Southeast Asia; = 3 days in Africa or South America. **Doxycycline:** Treatment as above. If patient not able to take oral medication, give 100 mg I.V. every 12 hours and then switch to oral doxycycline (as above) as soon as patient can take oral medication. For I.V. use, avoid rapid administration. Treatment course = 7 days. **Tetracycline:** Treatment as above **Clindamycin:** Treatment as above. If patient not able to take oral medication, give 10 mg base/kg loading dose I.V. followed by 5 mg base/kg I.V. every 8 hours. Switch to oral clindamycin (oral dose as above) as soon as patient can take oral medication. For I.V. use, avoid rapid administration. Treatment course = 7 days.	**Quinidine gluconate:** Same mg/kg dosing and recommendations as for adults. **Doxycycline[4]:** Treatment as above. If patient not able to take oral medication, may give I.V. For children <45 kg, give 2.2 mg/kg I.V. every 12 hours and then switch to oral doxycycline (dose as above) as soon as patient can take oral medication. For children ≥45 kg, use same dosing as for adults. For I.V. use, avoid rapid administration. Treatment course = 7 days. **Tetracycline[4]:** Treatment as above **Clindamycin:** Treatment as above. If patient not able to take oral medication, give 10 mg base/kg loading dose I.V. followed by 5 mg base/kg I.V. every 8 hours. Switch to oral clindamycin (oral dose as above) as soon as patient can take oral medication. For I.V. use, avoid rapid administration. Treatment course = 7 days.	**All regions**

Source: http://www.cdc.gov/malaria/diagnosis_treatment/tx_clinicians.htm

[1]**Note:** There are three options (A, B, or C) available for treatment of uncomplicated malaria caused by chloroquine-resistant *P. falciparum.* Options A and B are equally recommended. Because of a higher rate of severe neuropsychiatric reactions seen at treatment doses, we do not recommend option C (mefloquine) unless options A and B cannot be used. For

option A, because there is more data on the efficacy of quinine in combination with doxycycline or tetracycline, these treatment combinations are generally preferred to quinine in combination with clindamycin.

[2]For infections acquired in Southeast Asia, quinine treatment should continue for 7 days. For infections acquired in Africa and South America, quinine treatment should continue for 3 days.

[3]U.S. manufactured quinine sulfate capsule is in a 324 mg dosage; therefore 2 capsules should be sufficient for adult dosing.

[4]Doxycycline and tetracycline are not indicated for use in children <8 years old. For children <8 years old with chloroquine-resistant *P. falciparum*, quinine (given alone for 7 days or given in combination with clindamycin) and atovaquone-proguanil are recommended treatment options; mefloquine can be considered if no other options are available. For children <8 years old with chloroquine-resistant *P. vivax*, quinine (given alone for 7 days) or mefloquine are recommended treatment options. If none of these treatment options are available or are not being tolerated and if the treatment benefits outweigh the risks, doxycycline or tetracycline may be given to children <8 years old.

[5]Give atovaquone-proguanil with food. If patient vomits within 30 minutes of taking a dose, then they should repeat the dose.

[6]Treatment with mefloquine is not recommended in persons who have acquired infections from the Southeast Asian region of Burma, Thailand, and Cambodia due to resistant strains.

[7]Primaquine is used to eradicate any hypnozoite forms that may remain dormant in the liver, and thus prevent relapses, in *P. vivax* and *P. ovale* infections. Because primaquine can cause hemolytic anemia in persons with G6PD deficiency, patients must be screened for G6PD deficiency prior to starting treatment with primaquine. For persons with borderline G6PD deficiency or as an alternate to the above regimen, primaquine may be given 45 mg orally one time per week for 8 weeks; consultation with an expert in infectious disease and/or tropical medicine is advised if this alternative regimen is considered in G6PD-deficient persons. Primaquine must not be used during pregnancy.

[8]**Note:** There are two options (A or B) available for treatment of uncomplicated malaria caused by chloroquine-resistant *P. vivax*. High treatment failure rates due to chloroquine-resistant *P. vivax* have been well documented in Papua New Guinea and Indonesia. Rare case reports of chloroquine-resistant *P. vivax* have also been documented in Burma (Myanmar), India, and Central and South America. Persons acquiring *P. vivax* infections outside of Papua New Guinea or Indonesia should be started on chloroquine. If the patient does not respond, the treatment should be changed to a chloroquine-resistant *P. vivax* regimen and CDC should be notified (Malaria Hotline number: (770) 488-7788 Monday-Friday, 8 AM to 4:30 PM EST or (770) 488-7100 after hours, weekends, and holidays). For treatment of chloroquine-resistant *P. vivax* infections, options A and B are equally recommended.

[9]For pregnant women diagnosed with uncomplicated malaria caused by chloroquine-resistant *P. falciparum* or chloroquine-resistant *P. vivax* infection, treatment with doxycycline or tetracycline is generally not indicated. However, doxycycline or tetracycline may be used in combination with quinine (as recommended for nonpregnant adults) if other treatment options are not available or are not being tolerated, and the benefit is judged to outweigh the risks.

[10]Because there are no adequate, well-controlled studies of atovaquone and/or proguanil hydrochloride in pregnant women, atovaquone-proguanil is generally not recommended for use in pregnant women. For pregnant women diagnosed with uncomplicated malaria caused by chloroquine-resistant *P. falciparum* infection, atovaquone-proguanil may be used if other treatment options are not available or are not being tolerated, and if the potential benefit is judged to outweigh the potential risks. There are no data on the efficacy of atovaquone-proguanil in the treatment of chloroquine-resistant *P. vivax* infections.

[11]Because of a possible association with mefloquine treatment during pregnancy and an increase in stillbirths, mefloquine is generally not recommended for treatment in pregnant women. However, mefloquine may be used if it is the only treatment option available and if the potential benefit is judged to outweigh the potential risks.

[12]For *P. vivax* and *P. ovale* infections, primaquine phosphate for radical treatment of hypnozoites should not be given during pregnancy. Pregnant patients with *P. vivax* and *P. ovale* infections should be maintained on chloroquine prophylaxis for the duration of their pregnancy. The chemoprophylactic dose of chloroquine phosphate is 300 mg base (= 500 mg salt) orally once per week. After delivery, pregnant patients who do not have G6PD deficiency should be treated with primaquine.

[13]Persons with a positive blood smear **or** history of recent possible exposure and no other recognized pathology who have one or more of the following clinical criteria (impaired consciousness/coma, severe normocytic anemia, renal failure, pulmonary edema, acute respiratory distress syndrome, circulatory shock, disseminated intravascular coagulation, spontaneous bleeding, acidosis, hemoglobinuria, jaundice, repeated generalized convulsions, and/or parasitemia of >5%) are considered to have manifestations of more severe disease. Severe malaria is practically always due to *P. falciparum*.

MALARIA *(Continued)*

[14]Patients diagnosed with severe malaria should be treated aggressively with parenteral antimalarial therapy. Treatment with I.V. quinidine should be initiated as soon as possible after the diagnosis has been made. Patients with severe malaria should be given an intravenous loading dose of quinidine unless they have received >40 mg/kg of quinine in the preceding 48 hours or if they have received mefloquine within the preceding 12 hours. Consultation with a cardiologist and a physician with experience treating malaria is advised when treating malaria patients with quinidine. During administration of quinidine, blood pressure monitoring (for hypotension) and cardiac monitoring (for widening of the QRS complex and/or lengthening of the QT_c interval) should be monitored continuously and blood glucose (for hypoglycemia) should be monitored periodically. Cardiac complications, if severe, may warrant temporary discontinuation of the drug or slowing of the intravenous infusion.

[15]Consider exchange transfusion if the parasite density (ie, parasitemia) is >10% **or** if the patient has altered mental status, nonvolume overload pulmonary edema, or renal complications. The parasite density can be estimated by examining a monolayer of red blood cells (RBCs) on the thin smear under oil immersion magnification. The slide should be examined where the RBCs are more or less touching (approximately 400 RBCs per field). The parasite density can then be estimated from the percentage of infected RBCs and should be monitored every 12 hours. Exchange transfusion should be continued until the parasite density is <1% (usually requires 8-10 units). I.V. quinidine administration should not be delayed for an exchange transfusion and can be given concurrently throughout the exchange transfusion.

[16]Pregnant women diagnosed with severe malaria should be treated aggressively with parenteral antimalarial therapy.

CONTRAINDICATIONS AND PRECAUTIONS TO COMMONLY USED VACCINES

Vaccine	Contraindications	Precautions[1]	Vaccines Can Be Administered
General for all vaccines, including diphtheria and tetanus toxoids and acellular pertussis vaccine (DTaP); pediatric diphtheria-tetanus toxoid (DT); adult tetanus-diphtheria toxoid (Td); inactivated poliovirus vaccine (IPV); measles-mumps-rubella vaccine (MMR); *Haemophilus influenzae* type b vaccine (Hib); hepatitis A vaccine; hepatitis B vaccine; varicella vaccine; pneumococcal conjugate vaccine (PCV); influenza vaccine; and pneumococcal polysaccharide vaccine (PPV)	• Serious allergic reaction (eg, anaphylaxis) after a previous vaccine dose • Serious allergic reaction (eg, anaphylaxis) to a vaccine component	• Moderate or severe acute illnesses with or without a fever	• Mild acute illness with or without fever • Mild to moderate local reaction (ie, swelling, redness, soreness); low-grade or moderate fever after previous dose • Lack of previous physical examination in well-appearing person • Current antimicrobial therapy • Convalescent phase of illnesses • Premature birth (hepatitis B vaccine is an exception in certain circumstances)[2] • Recent exposure to an infectious disease • History of penicillin allergy, other nonvaccine allergies, receiving allergen extract immunotherapy • Temperature <40.5°C, fussiness or mild drowsiness after a previous dose of diphtheria toxoid-tetanus toxoid-pertussis vaccine (DTP)/DTaP • Family history of seizures[3] • Family history of sudden infant death syndrome • Family history of an adverse event after DTP or DTaP administration • Stable neurologic conditions (eg, cerebral palsy, well-controlled convulsions, developmental delay)
DTaP	• Severe allergic reaction after a previous dose or to a vaccine component • Encephalopathy (eg, coma, decreased level of consciousness, prolonged seizures) within 7 days of administration of previous dose of DTP or DTaP • Progressive neurologic disorder, including infantile spasms, uncontrolled epilepsy, progressive encephalopathy; defer DTaP until neurologic status clarified and stabilized	• Fever >40.5°C ≤48 hours after vaccination with a previous dose of DTP or DTaP • Collapse or shock-like state (ie, hypotonic hyporesponsive episode) ≤48 hours after receiving a previous dose of DTP/DTaP • Seizure ≤3 days of receiving a previous dose of DTP/DTaP[3] • Persistent, inconsolable crying lasting ≥3 hours, ≤48 hours after receiving a previous dose of DTP/DTaP • Moderate or severe acute illness with or without fever	Same as above

CONTRAINDICATIONS AND PRECAUTIONS TO COMMONLY USED VACCINES *(Continued)*

Vaccine	Contraindications	Precautions[1]	Vaccines Can Be Administered
DT, Td	• Severe allergic reaction after a previous dose or to a vaccine component	• Guillain-Barré syndrome ≤6 weeks after previous dose of tetanus toxoid-containing vaccine • Moderate or severe acute illness with or without fever	Same as above
IPV	• Severe allergic reaction to previous dose or vaccine component	• Pregnancy • Moderate or severe acute illness with or without fever	—
MMR[4]	• Severe allergic reaction after a previous dose or to a vaccine component • Pregnancy • Known severe immunodeficiency (eg, hematologic and solid tumors; congenital immunodeficiency; long-term immunosuppressive therapy,[5] or severely symptomatic human immunodeficiency virus [HIV] infection)	• Recent (≤11 months) receipt of antibody-containing blood product (specific interval depends on product) • History of thrombocytopenia or thrombocytopenic purpura • Moderate or severe acute illness with or without fever	• Positive tuberculin skin test • Simultaneous TB skin testing[6] • Breast-feeding • Pregnancy of recipient's mother or other close or household contact • Recipient is child-bearing-age female • Immunodeficient family member or household contact • Asymptomatic or mildly symptomatic HIV infection • Allergy to eggs
Hib	• Severe allergic reaction after a previous dose or to a vaccine component • Age <6 weeks	• Moderate or severe acute illness with or without fever	—
Hepatitis B	• Severe allergic reaction after a previous dose or to a vaccine component	• Infant weighing <2000 g[2] • Moderate or severe acute illness with or without fever	• Pregnancy • Autoimmune disease (eg, systemic lupus erythematosis or rheumatoid arthritis)
Hepatitis A	• Severe allergic reaction after a previous dose or to a vaccine component	• Pregnancy • Moderate or severe acute illness with or without fever	—
Varicella	• Severe allergic reaction after a previous dose or to a vaccine component • Substantial suppression of cellular immunity • Pregnancy	• Recent (≤11 months) receipt of antibody containing blood product (specific interval depends on product) • Moderate or severe acute illness with or without fever	• Pregnancy of recipient's mother or other close or household contact • Immunodeficient family member or household contact[7] • Asymptomatic or mildly symptomatic HIV infection • Humoral immunodeficiency (eg, agammaglobulinemia)
PCV	• Severe allergic reaction after a previous dose or to a vaccine component	• Moderate or severe acute illness with or without fever	—

Vaccine	Contraindications	Precautions[1]	Vaccines Can Be Administered
Influenza	• Severe allergic reaction to previous dose or vaccine component, including egg protein	• Moderate or severe acute illness with or without fever	• Nonsevere (eg, contact) allergy to latex or thimerosal • Concurrent administration of Coumadin® or aminophylline
PPV	• Severe allergic reaction after a previous dose or to a vaccine component	• Moderate or severe acute illness with or without fever	—

[1]Events or conditions listed as precautions should be reviewed carefully. Benefits and risks of administering a specific vaccine to a person under these circumstances should be considered. If the risk from the vaccine is believed to outweigh the benefit, the vaccine should not be administered. If the benefit of vaccination is believed to outweigh the risk, the vaccine should be administered. Whether and when to administer DTaP to children with proven or suspected underlying neurologic disorders should be decided on a case-by-case basis.

[2]Hepatitis B vaccination should be deferred for infants weighing <2000 g if the mother is documented to be hepatitis B surface antigen (Hb_sAg)-negative at the time of the infant's birth. Vaccination can commence at chronological age 1 month. For infants born to Hb_sAg)-positive women, hepatitis B immunoglobulin and hepatitis B vaccine should be administered at or soon after birth regardless of weight.

[3]Acetaminophen or other appropriate antipyretic can be administered to children with a personal or family history of seizures at the time of DTaP vaccination and every 4-6 hours for 24 hours thereafter to reduce the possibility of postvaccination fever (source: American Academy of Pediatrics, Pickering LK, ed, "Active Immunization," *2000 Red Book®*, Report of the Committee on Infectious Diseases, 25th ed, Elk Grove Village, IL: American Academy of Pediatrics, 2000).

[4]MMR and varicella vaccines can be administered on the same day. If not administered on the same day, these vaccines should be separated by ≥28 days.

[5]Substantially immunosuppressive steroid dose is considered to be ≥2 weeks of daily receipt of 20 mg or 2 mg/kg body weight of prednisone or equivalent.

[6]Measles vaccination can suppress tuberculin reactivity temporarily. Measles-containing vaccine can be administered on the same day as tuberculin skin testing. If testing cannot be performed until after the day of MMR vaccination, the test should be postponed for ≥4 weeks after the vaccination. If an urgent need exists to skin test, do so with the understanding that reactivity might be reduced by the vaccine.

[7]If a vaccine experiences a presumed vaccine-related rash 7-25 days after vaccination, avoid direct contact with immunocompromised persons for the duration of the rash.

Adapted from "Recommendations and Reports," *MMWR Morb Mortal Wkly Rep*, 2002, 51(RR-2):9-10.

SKIN TESTS FOR DELAYED HYPERSENSITIVITY

Skin tests for delayed hypersensitivity are used diagnostically to assess previous infection (ie, PPD, histoplasmin, and coccidioidin) or used to evaluate cellular immune function by testing for anergy (ie, mumps, *Candida*, tetanus toxoid, trichophyton, PPD). Anergy, a defect in cell-mediated immunity, is characterized by a depressed response or lack of response to skin testing with injected antigens. Anergy has been associated with congenital and acquired immunodeficiencies, and malnutrition.

***Candida* 1:100**

Dose = 0.1 mL intradermally (30% of children younger than 18 months of age and 50% older than 18 months of age respond)

Can be used as a control antigen

Histoplasmin 1:100

Dose = 0.1 mL intradermally (yeast derived)

Mumps 40 cfu per mL

Dose = 0.1 mL intradermally (contraindicated in patients allergic to eggs, egg products, or thimerosal)

Purified Protein Derivative 5 TU (PPD[1] Mantoux Tuberculin)

Screening for tuberculosis:

Children who have no risk factors but who reside in high-prevalence regions: skin test at 4-6 years and 11-16 years of age

Children exposed to HIV-infected individuals, homeless, residents of nursing homes, institutionalized adolescents, users of illicit drugs, incarcerated adolescents, and migrant farm workers: skin test every 2-3 years

Children at high risk (children infected with HIV, incarcerated adolescents): annual skin testing

Dose = 0.1 mL intradermally

Definition of positive Mantoux skin test (regardless of previous BCG administration):

Reaction ≥5 mm for high-risk group (children in close contact with known or suspected infectious cases of tuberculosis; children suspected to have disease based on clinical and/or roentgenographic evidence; and children with underlying host factors (immunosuppressive conditions, receiving immunosuppressive therapy, and HIV infection).

Reaction ≥10 mm for children <4 years; those with medical diseases who are at increased risk for dissemination or for those at increased risk because of environmental exposure.

Reaction ≥15 mm for children ≥4 years of age including those with no risk factors.

[1]PPD 1 TU (first strength) is only used in individuals suspected of being highly sensitive. PPD 250 TU (second strength) is used only for individuals who fail to respond to a previous injection of 5 TU, or anergic patients in whom TB is suspected.

Tetanus Toxoid 1:5

Dose = 0.1 mL intradermally (29% of children younger than 2 years of age and 78% older than 2 years of age respond if they have received 3 immunizing doses)

Can be used as a control antigen.

Tine Test

Indication: survey and screen for exposure to tuberculosis (grasp forearm firmly; stretch the skin of the volar surface tightly; apply the tines to the selected site; press for at least one second so that a circular halo impression is left on the skin)

General Information

1. Intradermal skin tests should be injected in the flexor surface of the forearm.
2. A pale wheal 6-10 mm in diameter should form over the needle tip as soon as the injection is administered. If no bleb forms, the injection must be repeated.
3. Space skin tests at least 2 inches apart to prevent reactions from overlapping.
4. Read skin tests for diameter of induration and presence of erythema at 24, 48, and 72 hours. Reactions occurring before 24 hours are indicative of an immediate rather than a delayed hypersensitivity reaction.
5. False-negative results may occur in patients with malnutrition, viral infections, febrile illnesses, immunodeficiency disorders, severe disseminated infections, uremia, patients who have received immunosuppressive therapy (steroids, antineoplastic agents), patients who have received a recent live attenuated virus vaccine (MMR, measles).
6. False-positive results may occur in patients sensitive to ingredients in the skin test solution such as thimerosal; cross-sensitivity between similar antigens; or with improper interpretation of skin test.
7. Side effects are pain, blisters, extensive erythema, and necrosis at the injection site.

   Emergency equipment and epinephrine should be readily available to treat severe allergic reactions that may occur.

Recommended Interpretation of Skin Test Reactions

Reaction	Local Reaction	
	After Intradermal Injections of Antigens	After Dinitrochlorobenzene
1+	Erythema >10 mm and/or induration >1-5 mm	Erythema and/or induration covering <1/2 area of dosing site
2+	Induration 6-10 mm	Induration covering >1/2 area of dose site
3+	Induration 11-20 mm	Vesiculation and induration at dose site or spontaneous flare at days 7-14 at the site
4+	Induration >20 mm	Bulla or ulceration at dose site or spontaneous flare at days 7-14 at the site

References

American Academy of Pediatrics Committee on Infectious Diseases, "Screening for Tuberculosis in Infants and Children," *Pediatrics*, 1994, 93(1):131-4.

American Academy of Pediatrics Committee on Infectious Diseases, "Update on Tuberculosis Skin Testing of Children," *Pediatrics*, 1996, 97(2):282-4.

MANAGEMENT OF HEALTHCARE WORKER EXPOSURES TO HBV, HCV, AND HIV

Adapted from Updated U.S. Public Health Service Guidelines for the Management of Occupational Exposures to HIV and Recommendations for Postexposure Prophylaxis, "Recommended HIV Postexposure Prophylaxis (PEP) for Percutaneous Injuries," *MMWR Recomm Rep*, 2005, 54(RR-9):3-17.

Factors to Consider in Assessing the Need for Follow-up of Occupational Exposures

- **Type of exposure**
  - Percutaneous injury
  - Mucous membrane exposure
  - Nonintact skin exposure
  - Bites resulting in blood exposure to either person involved
- **Type and amount of fluid/tissue**
  - Blood
  - Fluids containing blood
  - Potentially infectious fluid or tissue (semen; vaginal secretions; and cerebrospinal, synovial, pleural, peritoneal, pericardial, and amniotic fluids)
  - Direct contact with concentrated virus
- **Infectious status of source**
  - Presence of HB_sAg
  - Presence of HCV antibody
  - Presence of HIV antibody
- **Susceptibility of exposed person**
  - Hepatitis B vaccine and vaccine response status
  - HBV, HCV, HIV immune status

Evaluation of Occupational Exposure Sources

Known sources

- Test known sources for HB_sAg, anti-HCV, and HIV antibody
  - Direct virus assays for routine screening of source patients are **not** recommended
  - Consider using a rapid HIV-antibody test
  - If the source person is **not** infected with a blood-borne pathogen, baseline testing or further follow-up of the exposed person is **not** necessary
- For sources whose infection status remains unknown (eg, the source person refuses testing), consider medical diagnoses, clinical symptoms, and history of risk behaviors
- Do not test discarded needles for blood-borne pathogens

Unknown sources

- For unknown sources, evaluate the likelihood of exposure to a source at high risk for infection
  - Consider the likelihood of blood-borne pathogen infection among patients in the exposure setting

Recommended Postexposure Prophylaxis for Exposure to Hepatitis B Virus

Vaccination and Antibody Response Status of Exposed Workers[1]	Treatment		
	Source HB_sAg[2]-Positive	Source HB_sAg[2] -Negative	Source Unknown or Not Available for Testing
Unvaccinated	HBIG[3] x 1 and initiate HB vaccine series[4]	Initiate HB vaccine series	Initiate HB vaccine series
Previously vaccinated			
Known responder[5]	No treatment	No treatment	No treatment
Known nonresponder[6]	HBIG[3] x 1 and initiate revaccination or HBIG x 2[7]	No treatment	If known high risk source, treat as if source was HB_sAg-positive
Antibody response unknown	Test exposed person for anti-HB_s[8] 1. If adequate,[5] no treatment is necessary 2. If inadequate,[6] administer HBIG[3] x 1 and vaccine booster	No treatment	Test exposed person for anti-HB_s 1. If adequate,[4] no treatment is necessary 2. If inadequate,[4] administer vaccine booster and recheck titer in 1-2 months

[1]Persons who have previously been infected with HBV are immune to reinfection and do not require postexposure prophylaxis.

[2]Hepatitis B surface antigen.

[3]Hepatitis B immune globulin; dose is 0.06 mL/kg intramuscularly.

[4]Hepatitis B vaccine.

[5]A responder is a person with adequate levels of serum antibody to HB_sAg (ie, anti-HB_s $\geq$10 mIU/mL).

[6]A nonresponder is a person with inadequate response to vaccination (ie, serum anti-HB_s <10 mIU/mL).

[7]The option of giving one dose of HBIG and reinitiating the vaccine series is preferred for nonresponders who have not completed a second 3-dose vaccine series. For persons who previously completed a second vaccine series but failed to respond, two doses of HBIG are preferred.

[8]Antibody to HB_sAg.

MANAGEMENT OF HEALTHCARE WORKER EXPOSURES TO HBV, HCV, AND HIV *(Continued)*

Recommended HIV Postexposure Prophylaxis (PEP) for Percutaneous Injuries

Exposure Type	Infection Status of Source				
	HIV-Positive, Class 1[1]	HIV-Positive, Class 2[1]	Source of Unknown HIV Status[2]	Unknown Source[3]	HIV-Negative
Less severe[4]	Recommend basic 2-drug PEP	Recommend expanded ≥3-drug PEP	Generally, no PEP warranted; however, consider basic 2-drug PEP[5] for source with HIV risk factors[6]	Generally, no PEP warranted; however, consider basic 2-drug PEP[5] in settings in which exposure to HIV-infected persons is likely	No PEP warranted
More severe[7]	Recommend expanded 3-drug PEP	Recommend expanded ≥3-drug PEP	Generally, no PEP warranted; however consider basic 2-drug PEP[5] for source with HIV risk factors[6]	Generally, no PEP warranted; however, consider basic 2-drug PEP[5] in settings in which exposure to HIV-infected persons is likely	No PEP warranted

[1]HIV-positive, class 1 – asymptomatic HIV infection or known low viral load (eg, <1500 ribonucleic acid copies/mL). HIV-positive, class 2 – symptomatic HIV infection, AIDS, acute seroconversion, or known high viral load. If drug resistance is a concern, obtain expert consultation. Initiation of PEP should not be delayed pending expert consultation, and, because expert consultation alone cannot substitute for face-to-face counseling, resources should be available to provide immediate evaluation and follow-up care for all exposures.

[2]For example, deceased source person with no samples available for HIV testing.

[3]For example, a needle from a sharps disposal container.

[4]For example, solid needle or superficial injury.

[5]The recommendation "consider PEP" indicates that PEP is optional; a decision to initiate PEP should be based on a discussion between the exposed person and the treating clinician regarding the risks versus benefits of PEP.

[6]If PEP is offered and administered and the source is later determined to be HIV-negative, PEP should be discontinued.

[7]For example, large-bore hollow needle, deep puncture, visible blood on device, or needle used in patient's artery or vein.

Recommended HIV Postexposure Prophylaxis (PEP) for Mucous Membrane Exposures and Nonintact Skin[1] Exposures

Exposure Type	Infection Status of Source				
	HIV-Positive, Class 1[2]	HIV-Positive, Class 2[2]	Source of Unknown HIV Status[3]	Unknown Source[4]	HIV-Negative
Small volume[5]	Consider basic 2-drug PEP[6]	Recommend basic 2-drug PEP	Generally, no PEP warranted[7]	Generally, no PEP warranted	No PEP warranted
Large volume[8]	Recommend basic 2-drug PEP	Recommend expanded ≥3-drug PEP	Generally, no PEP warranted; however consider basic 2-drug PEP[6] for source with HIV risk factors[7]	Generally, no PEP warranted; however, consider basic 2-drug PEP[6] in settings in which exposure to HIV-infected persons is likely	No PEP warranted

[1]For skin exposures, follow-up is indicated only if evidence exists of compromised skin integrity (eg, dermatitis, abrasion, or open wound).

[2]HIV-positive, class 1 – asymptomatic HIV infection or known low viral load (eg, <1500 ribonucleic acid copies/mL). HIV-positive, class 2 – symptomatic HIV infection, AIDS, acute seroconversion, or known high viral load. If drug resistance is a concern, obtain expert consultation. Initiation of PEP should not be delayed pending expert consultation, and, because expert consultation alone cannot substitute for face-to-face counseling, resources should be available to provide immediate evaluation and follow-up care for all exposures.

[3]For example, deceased source person with no samples available for HIV testing.

[4]For example, splash from inappropriately disposed blood.

[5]For example, a few drops.

[6]The recommendation "consider PEP" indicates that PEP is optional; a decision to initiate PEP should be based on a discussion between the exposed person and the treating clinician regarding the risks versus benefits of PEP.

[7]If PEP is offered and administered and the source is later determined to be HIV-negative, PEP should be discontinued.

[8]For example, a major blood splash.

MANAGEMENT OF HEALTHCARE WORKER EXPOSURES TO HBV, HCV, AND HIV *(Continued)*

Situations for Which Expert[1] Consultation for HIV Postexposure Prophylaxis Is Advised

- **Delayed (ie, later than 24-36 hours) exposure report**
  - The interval after which there is no benefit from postexposure prophylaxis (PEP) is undefined
- **Unknown source (eg, needle in sharps disposal container or laundry)**
  - Decide use of PEP on a case-by-case basis
  - Consider the severity of the exposure and the epidemiologic likelihood of HIV exposure
  - Do not test needles or sharp instruments for HIV
- **Known or suspected pregnancy in the exposed person**
  - Does not preclude the use of optimal PEP regimens
  - Do not deny PEP solely on the basis of pregnancy
- **Breast-feeding in the exposed person**
  - Use of optimal PEP regimen not precluded
  - PEP should not be denied solely on the basis of breast-feeding
- **Resistance of the source virus to antiretroviral agents**
  - Influence of drug resistance on transmission risk is unknown
  - Selection of drugs to which the source person's virus is unlikely to be resistant is recommended, if the source person's virus is unknown or suspected to be resistant to ≥1 of the drugs considered for the PEP regimen
  - Resistance testing of the source person's virus at the time of the exposure is not recommended
  - Initiation of PEP not to be delayed while awaiting results of resistance testing
- **Toxicity of the initial PEP regimen**
  - Adverse symptoms, such as nausea and diarrhea, are common with PEP
  - Symptoms can often be managed without changing the PEP regimen by prescribing antimotility and/or antiemetic agents
  - Modification of dose intervals (ie, administering a lower dose of drug more frequently throughout the day, as recommended by the manufacturer), in other situations, might help alleviate symptoms

[1]Local experts and/or the National Clinicians' Postexposure Prophylaxis Hotline (PEPline 1-888-448-4911).

Occupational Exposure Management Resources

National Clinicians' Postexposure Prophylaxis Hotline (PEPline) Run by University of California-San Francisco/San Francisco General Hospital staff; supported by the Health Resources and Services Administration Ryan White CARE Act, HIV/AIDS Bureau, AIDS Education and Training Centers, and CDC	Phone: (888) 448-4911 Internet: http://www.ucsf.edu/hivcntr
Needlestick! A website to help clinicians manage and document occupational blood and body fluid exposures. Developed and maintained by the University of California, Los Angeles (UCLA), Emergency Medicine Center, UCLA School of Medicine, and funded in part by CDC and the Agency for Healthcare Research and Quality.	Internet: http:// www.needlestick.mednet.ucla.edu
Hepatitis Hotline	Phone: (888) 443-7232 Internet: http://www.cdc.gov/hepatitis
Reporting to CDC: Occupationally acquired HIV infections and failures of PEP	Phone: (800) 893-0485
HIV Antiretroviral Pregnancy Registry	Phone: (800) 258-4263 Fax: (800) 800-1052 Address: 1410 Commonwealth Drive, Suite 215 Wilmington, NC 28405 Internet: http://www.glaxowellcome.com/preg_reg/antiretroviral
Food and Drug Administration Report unusual or severe toxicity to antiretroviral agents	Phone: (800) 332-1088 Address: MedWatch HF-2, FDA 5600 Fishers Lane Rockville, MD 20857 Internet: http://www.fda.gov/medwatch
HIV / AIDS Treatment Information Service	Internet: http://www.aidsinfo.nih.gov

MANAGEMENT OF HEALTHCARE WORKER EXPOSURES TO HBV, HCV, AND HIV *(Continued)*

Management of Occupational Blood Exposures

Provide immediate care to the exposure site

- Wash wounds and skin with soap and water
- Flush mucous membranes with water

Determine risk associated with exposure by:

- Type of fluid (eg, blood, visibly bloody fluid, other potentially infectious fluid or tissue, and concentrated virus)
- Type of exposure (ie, percutaneous injury, mucous membrane or nonintact skin exposure, and bites resulting in blood exposure)

Evaluate exposure source

- Assess the risk of infection using available information
- Test known sources for HB_sAg, anti-HCV, and HIV antibody (consider using rapid testing)
- For unknown sources, assess risk of exposure to HBV, HCV, or HIV infection
- Do not test discarded needle or syringes for virus contamination

Evaluate the exposed person

- Assess immune status for HBV infection (ie, by history of hepatitis B vaccination and vaccine response)

Give PEP for exposures posing risk of infection transmission

- HBV: See Recommended Postexposure Prophylaxis for Exposure to Hepatitis B Virus Table
- HCV: PEP not recommended
- HIV: See Recommended HIV Postexposure Prophylaxis for Percutaneous Injuries Table and Recommended HIV Postexposure Prophylaxis for Mucous Membrane Exposures and Nonintact Skin Exposures Table
  - Initiate PEP as soon as possible, preferably within hours of exposure
  - Offer pregnancy testing to all women of childbearing age not known to be pregnant
  - Seek expert consultation if viral resistance is suspected
  - Administer PEP for 4 weeks if tolerated

Perform follow-up testing and provide counseling

- Advise exposed persons to seek medical evaluation for any acute illness occurring during follow-up

HBV exposures

- Perform follow-up anti-HB_s testing in persons who receive hepatitis B vaccine
  - Test for anti-HB_s 1-2 months after last dose of vaccine
  - Anti-HB_s response to vaccine cannot be ascertained if HBIG was received in the previous 3-4 months

HCV exposures

- Perform baseline and follow-up testing for anti-HCV and alanine amino-transferase (ALT) 4-6 months after exposures
- Perform HCV RNA at 4-6 months if earlier diagnosis of HCV infection is desired
- Confirm repeatedly reactive anti-HCV enzyme immunoassays (EIAs) with supplemental tests

HIV exposures

- Perform HIV antibody testing for at least 6 months postexposure (eg, at baseline, 6 weeks, 3 months, and 6 months)
- Perform HIV antibody testing if illness compatible with an acute retroviral syndrome occurs
- Advise exposed persons to use precautions to prevent secondary transmission during the follow-up period
- Evaluate exposed persons taking PEP within 72 hours after exposure and monitor for drug toxicity for at least 2 weeks

Basic and Expanded HIV Postexposure Prophylaxis Regimens

BASIC REGIMENS

Zidovudine (Retrovir®; ZDV; AZT) + lamivudine (Epivir®; 3TC); available as Combivir®

Preferred dosing

- ZDV: 300 mg twice daily or 200 mg three times daily, with food; total: 600 mg daily
- 3TC: 300 mg once daily or 150 mg twice daily
- Combivir®: One tablet twice daily

Advantages

- ZDV associated with decreased risk for HIV transmission
- ZDV used more often than other drugs for PEP for healthcare personnel (HCP)
- Serious toxicity rare when used for PEP
- Side effects predictable and manageable with antimotility and anti-emetic agents
- Can be used by pregnant HCP
- Can be given as a single tablet (Combivir®) twice daily

Disadvantages

- Side effects (especially nausea and fatigue) common and might result in low adherence
- Source-patient virus resistance to this regimen possible
- Potential for delayed toxicity (oncogenic/teratogenic) unknown

Zidovudine (Retrovir®; ZDV; AZT) + emtricitabine (Emtriva®; FTC)

Preferred dosing

- ZDV: 300 mg twice daily or 200 mg three times daily, with food; total: 600 mg/day, in 2-3 divided doses
- FTC: 200 mg (one capsule) once daily

Advantages

- ZDV: See above
- FTC
  - Convenient (once daily)
  - Well tolerated
  - Long intracellular half-life (~40 hours)

Disadvantages

- ZDV: See above
- FTC
  - Rash perhaps more frequent than with 3TC
  - No long-term experience with this drug
  - Cross resistance to 3TC
  - Hyperpigmentation among non-Caucasians with long-term use: 3%

Tenofovir DF (Viread®; TDF) + lamivudine (Epivir®; 3TC)

Preferred dosing

- TDF: 300 mg once daily
- 3TC: 300 mg once daily or 150 mg twice daily

Advantages

- 3TC: See above
- TDF
  - Convenient dosing (single pill once daily)
  - Resistance profile activity against certain thymidine analogue mutations
  - Well tolerated

Disadvantages

- TDF
  - Same class warnings as nucleoside reverse transcriptase inhibitors (NRTIs)
  - Drug interactions

MANAGEMENT OF HEALTHCARE WORKER EXPOSURES TO HBV, HCV, AND HIV *(Continued)*

- Increased TDF concentrations among persons taking atazanavir and lopinavir/ritonavir; need to monitor patients for TDF-associated toxicities

– Preferred dosage of atazanavir if used with TDF: 300 mg + ritonavir 100 mg once daily + TDF 300 mg once daily

Tenofovir DF (Viread®; TDF) + emtricitabine (Emtriva®; FTC); available as Truvada®

Preferred dosing

– TDF: 300 mg once daily
– FTC: 200 mg once daily
– As Truvada®: One tablet daily

Advantages

– FTC: See above
– TDF
  - Convenient dosing (single pill once daily)
  - Resistance profile activity against certain thymidine analogue mutations
  - Well tolerated

Disadvantages

– TDF
  - Same class warnings as NRTIs
  - Drug interactions
  - Increased TDF concentrations among persons taking atazanavir and lopinavir/ritonavir; need to monitor patients for TDF-associated toxicities
  - Preferred dosing of atazanavir if used with TDF: 300 mg + ritonavir 100 mg once daily + TDF 300 mg once daily

ALTERNATE BASIC REGIMENS

Lamivudine (Epivir®; 3TC) + stavudine (Zerit®; d4T)

Preferred dosing

– 3TC: 300 mg once daily or 150 mg twice daily
– d4T: 40 mg twice daily (can use lower doses of 20-30 mg twice daily if toxicity occurs; equally effective but less toxic among HIV-infected patients with peripheral neuropathy); 30 mg twice daily if body weight is <60 kg

Advantages

– 3TC: See above
– d4T: Gastrointestinal (GI) side effects rare

Disadvantages

– Possibility that source-patient virus is resistant to this regimen
– Potential for delayed toxicity (oncogenic/teratogenic) unknown

Emtricitabine (Emtriva®; FTC) + stavudine (Zerit®; d4T)

Preferred dosing

– FTC: 200 mg daily
– d4T: 40 mg twice daily (can use lower doses of 20-30 mg twice daily if toxicity occurs; equally effective but less toxic among HIV-infected patients who developed peripheral neuropathy); if body weight is <60 kg, 30 mg twice daily

Advantages

– 3TC and FTC: See above; d4T's GI side effects rare

Disadvantages

– Potential that source-patient virus is resistant to this regimen
– Unknown potential for delayed toxicity (oncogenic/teratogenic) unknown

Lamivudine (Epivir®; 3TC) + didanosine (Videx®; ddI)

Preferred dosing

– 3TC: 300 mg once daily or 150 mg twice daily

- ddI: Videx® chewable/dispersible buffered tablets can be administered on an empty stomach as either 200 mg twice daily or 400 mg once daily. Patients must take at least two of the appropriate strength tablets at each dose to provide adequate buffering and prevent gastric acid degradation of ddI. Because of the need for adequate buffering, the 200 mg strength tablet should be used only as a component of a once-daily regimen. The dose is either 200 mg twice daily or 400 mg once daily for patients weighing >60 kg and 125 mg twice daily or 250 mg once daily for patients weighing >60 KG.

Advantages

- ddI: Once-daily dosing option
- 3TC: See above

Disadvantages

- Tolerability: Diarrhea more common with buffered preparation than with enteric-coated preparation
- Associated with toxicity: Peripheral neuropathy, pancreatitis, and lactic acidosis
- Must be taken on empty stomach except with TDF
- Drug interactions
- 3TC: See above

Emtricitabine (Emtriva®; FTC) + didanosine (Videx®; ddI)

Preferred dosing

- FTC: 200 mg once daily
- ddI: See above

Advantages

- ddI: See above
- FTC: See above

Disadvantages

- Tolerability: Diarrhea more common with buffered than with enteric-coated preparation
- Associated with toxicity: Peripheral neuropathy, pancreatitis, and lactic acidosis
- Must be taken on empty stomach except with TDF
- Drug interactions
- FTC: See above

PREFERRED EXPANDED REGIMEN

Basic regimen plus:

Lopinavir / Ritonavir (Kaletra®; LPV/RTV)

Preferred dosing

- LPV/RTV: 400 mg/100 mg = twice daily with food

Advantages

- Potent HIV protease inhibitor
- Generally well-tolerated

Disadvantages

- Potential for serious or life-threatening drug interactions
- Might accelerate clearance of certain drugs, including oral contraceptives (requiring alternative or additional contraceptive measures for women taking these drugs)
- Can cause severe hyperlipidemia, especially hypertriglyceridemia
- GI (eg, diarrhea) events common

ALTERNATE EXPANDED REGIMEN

Basic regimen plus one of the following:

Atazanavir (Reyataz®; ATV) ± ritonavir (Norvir®; RTV)

Preferred dosing

- ATV: 400 mg once daily, unless used in combination with TDF, in which case ATV should be boosted with RTV, preferred dosing of ATV 300 mg + RTV: 100 mg once daily

MANAGEMENT OF HEALTHCARE WORKER EXPOSURES TO HBV, HCV, AND HIV *(Continued)*

Advantages

- Potent HIV protease inhibitor
- Convenient dosing – once daily
- Generally well tolerated

Disadvantages

- Hyperbilirubinemia and jaundice common
- Potential for serious or life-threatening drug interactions
- Avoid coadministration with proton pump inhibitors
- Separate antacids and buffered medications by 2 hours and H_2-receptor antagonists by 12 hours to avoid decreasing ATV levels
- Caution should be used with ATV and products known to induce PR prolongation (eg, diltiazem)

Fosamprenavir (Lexiva™; FOSAPV) ± ritonavir (Norvir®; RTV)

Preferred dosing

- FOSAPV: 1400 mg twice daily (without RTV)
- FOSAPV: 1400 mg once daily + RTV 200 mg once daily
- FOSAPV: 700 mg twice daily + RTV 100 mg twice daily

Advantages

- Once daily dosing when given with ritonavir

Disadvantages

- Tolerability: GI side effects common
- Multiple drug interactions. Oral contraceptives decrease fosamprenavir concentrations.
- Incidence of rash in healthy volunteers, especially when used with low doses of ritonavir. Differentiating between early drug-associated rash and acute seroconversion can be difficult and cause extraordinary concern for the exposed person.

Indinavir (Crixivan®; IDV) ± ritonavir (Norvir®; RTV)

Preferred dosing

- IDV 800 mg + RTV 100 mg twice daily without regard to food

Alternative dosing

- IDV: 800 mg every 8 hours, on an empty stomach

Advantages

- Potent HIV inhibitor

Disadvantages

- Potential for serious or life-threatening drug interactions
- Serious toxicity (eg, nephrolithiasis) possible; consumption of 8 glasses of fluid/day required
- Hyperbilirubinemia common; must avoid this drug during late pregnancy
- Requires acid for absorption and cannot be taken simultaneously with ddI, chewable/dispersible buffered tablet formulation (doses must be separated by ≥1 hour)

Saquinavir (Invirase®; SQV) + ritonavir (Norvir®; RTV)

Preferred dosing

- SQV: 1000 mg (given as Invirase®) + RTV 100 mg, twice daily
- SQV: Five capsules twice daily + RTV: One capsule twice daily

Advantages

- Generally well-tolerated, although GI events common

Disadvantages

- Potential for serious or life-threatening drug interactions
- Substantial pill burden

Nelfinavir (Viracept®; NFV)

Preferred dosing

- NFV: 1250 mg (2 x 625 mg or 5 x 250 mg tablets), twice daily with a meal

Advantages

- Generally well-tolerated

Disadvantages

- Diarrhea or other GI events common
- Potential for serious and/or life-threatening drug interactions

Efavirenz (Sustiva®; EFV)

Preferred dosing

- EFV: 600 mg daily, at bedtime

Advantages

- Does not require phosphorylation before activation and might be active earlier than other antiretroviral agents (a theoretic advantage of no demonstrated clinical benefit)
- Once daily dosing

Disadvantages

- Drug associated with rash (early onset) that can be severe and might rarely progress to Stevens-Johnson syndrome
- Differentiating between early drug-associated rash and acute seroconversion can be difficult and cause extraordinary concern for the exposed person
- Central nervous system side effects (eg, dizziness, somnolence, insomnia, or abnormal dreaming) common; severe psychiatric symptoms possible (dosing before bedtime might minimize these side effects)
- Teratogen; should not be used during pregnancy
- Potential for serious or life-threatening drug interactions

ANTIRETROVIRAL AGENTS GENERALLY NOT RECOMMENDED FOR USE AS PEP

Nevirapine (Viramune®; NVP)

Disadvantages

- Associated with severe hepatotoxicity (including at least one case of liver failure requiring liver transplantation in an exposed person taking PEP)
- Associated with rash (early onset) that can be severe and progress to Stevens-Johnson syndrome
- Differentiating between early drug-associated rash and acute seroconversion can be difficult and cause extraordinary concern for the exposed person
- Drug interactions: Can lower effectiveness of certain antiretroviral agents and other commonly used medicines

Delavirdine (Rescriptor®; DLV)

Disadvantages

- Drug associated with rash (early onset) that can be severe and progress to Stevens-Johnson syndrome
- Multiple drug interactions

Abacavir (Ziagen®; ABC)

Disadvantages

- Severe hypersensitivity reactions can occur, usually within the first 6 weeks
- Differentiating between early drug-associated rash/hypersensitivity and acute seroconversion can be difficult

MANAGEMENT OF HEALTHCARE WORKER EXPOSURES TO HBV, HCV, AND HIV *(Continued)*

Zalcitabine (Hivid®; ddC)

Disadvantages

- Three times a day dosing
- Tolerability
- Weakest antiretroviral agent

ANTIRETROVIRAL AGENT FOR USE AS PEP ONLY WITH EXPERT CONSULTATION

Enfuvirtide (Fuzeon™; T20)

Preferred dosing

- T20: 90 mg (1 mL) twice daily by subcutaneous injection

Advantages

- New class
- Unique viral target; to block cell entry
- Prevalence of resistance low

Disadvantages

- Twice-daily injection
- Safety profile: Local injection site reactions
- Never studied among antiretroviral-naive or HIV-negative patients
- False-positive EIA HIV antibody tests might result from formation of anti-T20 antibodies that cross-react with anti-gp41 antibodies

NORMAL LABORATORY VALUES FOR CHILDREN

		Normal Values
CHEMISTRY		
Albumin	0-1 y	2.0-4.0 g/dL
	1 y to adult	3.5-5.5 g/dL
Ammonia	Newborns	90-150 mcg/dL
	Children	40-120 mcg/dL
	Adults	18-54 mcg/dL
Amylase	Newborns	0-60 units/L
	Adults	30-110 units/L
Bilirubin, conjugated, direct	Newborns	<1.5 mg/dL
	1 mo to adult	0-0.5 mg/dL
Bilirubin, total	0-3 d	2.0-10.0 mg/dL
	1 mo to adult	0-1.5 mg/dL
Bilirubin, unconjugated, indirect		0.6-10.5 mg/dL
Calcium	Newborns	7.0-12.0 mg/dL
	0-2 y	8.8-11.2 mg/dL
	2 y to adult	9.0-11.0 mg/dL
Calcium, ionized, whole blood		4.4-5.4 mg/dL
Carbon dioxide, total		23-33 mEq/L
Chloride		95-105 mEq/L
Cholesterol	Newborns	45-170 mg/dL
	0-1 y	65-175 mg/dL
	1-20 y	120-230 mg/dL
Creatinine	0-1 y	≤0.6 mg/dL
	1 y to adult	0.5-1.5 mg/dL
Glucose	Newborns	30-90 mg/dL
	0-2 y	60-105 mg/dL
	Children to Adults	70-110 mg/dL
Iron	Newborns	110-270 mcg/dL
	Infants	30-70 mcg/dL
	Children	55-120 mcg/dL
	Adults	70-180 mcg/dL
Iron binding	Newborns	59-175 mcg/dL
	Infants	100-400 mcg/dL
	Adults	250-400 mcg/dL
Lactic acid, lactate		2-20 mg/dL
Lead, whole blood		<10 mcg/dL
Lipase	Children	20-140 units/L
	Adults	0-190 units/L
Magnesium		1.5-2.5 mEq/L
Osmolality, serum		275-296 mOsm/kg
Osmolality, urine		50-1400 mOsm/kg
Phosphorus	Newborns	4.2-9.0 mg/dL
	6 wk to 19 mo	3.8-6.7 mg/dL
	19 mo to 3 y	2.9-5.9 mg/dL
	3-15 y	3.6-5.6 mg/dL
	>15 y	2.5-5.0 mg/dL

NORMAL LABORATORY VALUES FOR CHILDREN *(Continued)*

		Normal Values
CHEMISTRY		
Potassium, plasma	Newborns	4.5-7.2 mEq/L
	2 d to 3 mo	4.0-6.2 mEq/L
	3 mo to 1 y	3.7-5.6 mEq/L
	1-16 y	3.5-5.0 mEq/L
Protein, total	0-2 y	4.2-7.4 g/dL
	>2 y	6.0-8.0 g/dL
Sodium		136-145 mEq/L
Triglycerides	Infants	0-171 mg/dL
	Children	20-130 mg/dL
	Adults	30-200 mg/dL
Urea nitrogen, blood	0-2 y	4-15 mg/dL
	2 y to Adult	5-20 mg/dL
Uric acid	Male	3.0-7.0 mg/dL
	Female	2.0-6.0 mg/dL
ENZYMES		
Alanine aminotransferase (ALT) (SGPT)	0-2 mo	8-78 units/L
	>2 mo	8-36 units/L
Alkaline phosphatase (ALKP)	Newborns	60-130 units/L
	0-16 y	85-400 units/L
	>16 y	30-115 units/L
Aspartate aminotransferase (AST) (SGOT)	Infants	18-74 units/L
	Children	15-46 units/L
	Adults	5-35 units/L
Creatine kinase (CK)	Infants	20-200 units/L
	Children	10-90 units/L
	Adult male	0-206 units/L
	Adult female	0-175 units/L
Lactate dehydrogenase (LDH)	Newborns	290-501 units/L
	1 mo to 2 y	110-144 units/L
	>16 y	60-170 units/L

Blood Gases

	Arterial	Capillary	Venous
pH	7.35-7.45	7.35-7.45	7.32-7.42
pCO_2 (mm Hg)	35-45	35-45	38-52
pO_2 (mm Hg)	70-100	60-80	24-48
HCO_3 (mEq/L)	19-25	19-25	19-25
TCO_2 (mEq/L)	19-29	19-29	23-33
O_2 saturation (%)	90-95	90-95	40-70
Base excess (mEq/L)	-5 to +5	-5 to +5	-5 to +5

Thyroid Function Tests

T_4 (thyroxine)	1-7 d	10.1-20.9 mcg/dL
	8-14 d	9.8-16.6 mcg/dL
	1 mo to 1 y	5.5-16.0 mcg/dL
	>1 y	4.0-12.0 mcg/dL
FTI	1-3 d	9.3-26.6
	1-4 wk	7.6-20.8
	1-4 mo	7.4-17.9
	4-12 mo	5.1-14.5
	1-6 y	5.7-13.3
	>6 y	4.8-14.0
T_3	Newborns	100-470 ng/dL
	1-5 y	100-260 ng/dL
	5-10 y	90-240 ng/dL
	10 y to Adult	70-210 ng/dL
T_3 uptake		35%-45%
TSH	Cord	3-22 micro international units/mL
	1-3 d	<40 micro international units/mL
	3-7 d	<25 micro international units/mL
	>7 d	0-10 micro international units/mL

NORMAL LABORATORY VALUES FOR CHILDREN
(Continued)

Hematology Values

Age	Hgb (g/dL)	Hct (%)	RBC (mill/mm^3)	RDW	MCV (fL)	MCH (pg)	MCHC (%)	PLTS (x 10^3/mm^3)
0-3 d	15.0-20.0	45-61	4.0-5.9	<18	95-115	31-37	29-37	250-450
1-2 wk	12.5-18.5	39-57	3.6-5.5	<17	86-110	28-36	28-38	250-450
1-6 mo	10.0-13.0	29-42	3.1-4.3	<16.5	74-96	25-35	30-36	300-700
7 mo to 2 y	10.5-13.0	33-38	3.7-4.9	<16	70-84	23-30	31-37	250-600
2-5 y	11.5-13.0	34-39	3.9-5.0	<15	75-87	24-30	31-37	250-550
5-8 y	11.5-14.5	35-42	4.0-4.9	<15	77-95	25-33	31-37	250-550
13-18 y	12.0-15.2	36-47	4.5-5.1	<14.5	78-96	25-35	31-37	150-450
Adult male	13.5-16.5	41-50	4.5-5.5	<14.5	80-100	26-34	31-37	150-450
Adult female	12.0-15.0	36-44	4.0-4.9	<14.5	80-100	26-34	31-37	150-450

WBC and Diff

Age	WBC (x $10^3/mm^3$)	Segs	Bands	Lymphs	Monos	Eosinophils	Basophils	Atypical Lymphs	No. of NRBCs
0-3 d	9.0-35.0	32-62	10-18	19-29	5-7	0-2	0-1	0-8	0-2
1-2 wk	5.0-20.0	14-34	6-14	36-45	6-10	0-2	0-1	0-8	0
1-6 mo	6.0-17.5	13-33	4-12	41-71	4-7	0-3	0-1	0-8	0
7 mo to 2 y	6.0-17.0	15-35	5-11	45-76	3-6	0-3	0-1	0-8	0
2-5 y	5.5-15.5	23-45	5-11	35-65	3-6	0-3	0-1	0-8	0
5-8 y	5.0-14.5	32-54	5-11	28-48	3-6	0-3	0-1	0-8	0
13-18 y	4.5-13.0	34-64	5-11	25-45	3-6	0-3	0-1	0-8	0
Adults	4.5-11.0	35-66	5-11	24-44	3-6	0-3	0-1	0-8	0

Segs = segmented neutrophils.
Bands = band neutrophils.
Lymphs = lymphocytes.
Monos = monocytes.

NORMAL LABORATORY VALUES FOR CHILDREN
(Continued)

Erythrocyte Sedimentation Rates and Reticulocyte Counts

Sedimentation rate, Westergren	Children	0-20 mm/hour
	Adult male	0-15 mm/hour
	Adult female	0-20 mm/hour
Sedimentation rate, Wintrobe	Children	0-13 mm/hour
	Adult male	0-10 mm/hour
	Adult female	0-15 mm/hour
Reticulocyte count	Newborns	2%-6%
	1-6 mo	0%-2.8%
	Adults	0.5%-1.5%

Cerebrospinal Fluid Values, Normal

Cell count		% PMNs
Preterm mean	9 (0-25.4 WBC/mm^3)	57%
Term mean	8.2 (0-22.4 WBC/mm^3)	61%
>1 mo	0.7	0
Glucose		
Preterm	24-63 mg/dL	mean 50
Term	34-119 mg/dL	mean 52
Children	40-80 mg/dL	
CSF glucose/blood glucose		
Preterm	55-105%	
Term	44-128%	
Children	50%	
Lactic acid dehydrogenase	5-30 units/mL	mean 20 units/mL
Myelin basic protein	<4 ng/mL	
Pressure: Initial LP (mm H_2O)		
Newborns	80-110 (<110)	
Infants/children	<200 (lateral recumbent position)	
Respiratory movements	5-10	
Protein		
Preterm	65-150 mg/dL	mean 115
Term	20-170 mg/dL	mean 90
Children		
Ventricular	5-15 mg/dL	
Cisternal	5-25 mg/dL	
Lumbar	5-40 mg/dL	

APGAR SCORING SYSTEM

	Score		
Sign	**0**	**1**	**2**
Heart rate	Absent	Under 100 beats per minute	Over 100 beats per minute
Respiratory effort	Absent	Slow (irregular)	Good crying
Muscle tone	Limp	Some flexion of extremities	Active motion
Reflex irritability	No response	Grimace	Cough or sneeze
Color	Blue, pale	Pink body, blue extremities	All pink

From Apgar V, "A Proposal for a New Method of Evaluation of the Newborn Infant," *Anesth Analg*, 1953, 32:260.

FETAL HEART RATE MONITORING

Normal Heart Rates

Fetal heart rate (FHR) 120-160 bpm. Isolated accelerations are normal and considered reassuring. Mild (100-120 bpm) and transient bradycardias may be normal. Normal fetal heart rate tracings show beat-to-beat variability of 5-10 bpm (poor beat-to-beat variability suggests fetal hypoxia).

Abnormal Heart Rates

Bradycardia (FHR <120 bpm): Potential causes include fetal distress, drugs, congenital heart block (associated with maternal SLE, congenital cardiac defects).

Tachycardia (FHR >160 bpm): Potential causes include maternal fever, chorioamnionitis, drugs, fetal dysrhythmias, eg, SVT (with or without fetal CHF).

Decreased Beat-to-Beat Variability

Results from fetal CNS depression. Potential causes include fetal hypoxia, fetal sleep, fetal immaturity, and maternal narcotic/sedative administration.

Fetal Heart Rate Decelerations

Type 1 (early decelerations)

- Seen most commonly in late labor
- Mirror uterine contractions in time of onset, duration, and resolution
- Uniform shape
- Usually associated with good beat-to-beat variability
- Heart rate may dip to 60-80 bpm
- Associated with fetal head compression (increases vagal tone)
- Considered benign, and not representative of fetal hypoxia

APGAR SCORING SYSTEM *(Continued)*

Type 2 (late decelerations)

- Deceleration 10-30 seconds after onset of uterine contraction
- Heart rate fails to return to baseline after contraction is completed
- Asymmetrical shape (longer deceleration, shorter acceleration)
- Late decelerations of 10-20 bpm may be significant
- Probably associated with fetal CNS and myocardial depression

Type 3 (variable decelerations)

- Heart rate variations do not correlate with uterine contractions
- Variable shape and duration
- Occur occasionally in many normal labors
- Concerning if severe (HR <60 bpm), prolonged (duration >60 seconds), associated with poor beat-to-beat variability, or combined with late decelerations
- Associated with cord compression (including nuchal cord)

Reference

Manual of Neonatal Care, Joint Program in Neonatology, 1991.

CREATININE CLEARANCE ESTIMATING METHODS IN PATIENTS WITH STABLE RENAL FUNCTION

The following formulas provide an acceptable estimate of the patient's creatinine clearance except when:

a. The patient's serum creatinine is changing rapidly (either up or down).

b. Patients are markedly emaciated.

In these situations (a and b above), certain assumptions have to be made:

a. In patients with rapidly rising serum creatinines (ie, increasing by >0.5-0.7 mg/dL/day), it is best to assume that the patient's creatinine clearance is probably less than 10 mL/minute.

b. In emaciated patients, although their actual creatinine clearance is less than their calculated creatinine clearance (because of decreased creatinine production), it is not possible to predict easily how much less.

Estimation of creatinine clearance using serum creatinine and body length (to be used when an adequate timed specimen cannot be obtained). **Note:** This formula may not provide an accurate estimation of creatinine clearance for infants <6 months of age or for patients with severe starvation or muscle wasting.

$CL_{cr} = K \times L/S_{cr}$

where:

Cl_{cr} = creatinine clearance in mL/minute/1.73 m^2

K = constant of proportionality that is age specific

Age	K
Low birth weight ≤1 y	0.33
Full-term ≤1 y	0.45
2-12 y	0.55
13-21 y female	0.55
13-21 y male	0.70

L = length in cm

S_{Cr} = serum creatinine concentration in mg/dL

Reference

Schwartz GJ, Brion LP, and Spitzer A, "The Use of Plasma Creatinine Concentration for Estimating Glomerular Filtration Rate in Infants, Children and Adolescents," *Ped Clin N Amer*, 1987, 34:571-90.

Children 1-18 years

Method 1: (Traub SL, Johnson CE, *Am J Hosp Pharm*, 1980, 37:195-201)

Equation:

$$Cl_{cr} = \frac{0.48 \times (\text{height})}{S_{cr}}$$

where

Cl_{cr} = creatinine clearance in mL/min/1.73 m^2

S_{cr} = serum creatinine in mg/dL

Height = height in cm

Method 2: See nomogram.

CREATININE CLEARANCE ESTIMATING METHODS IN PATIENTS WITH STABLE RENAL FUNCTION *(Continued)*

Children 1-18 Years

The nomogram below is for rapid evaluation of endogenous creatinine clearance (Cl_{cr}) in pediatric patients.

To predict Cl_{cr}, connect the child's S_{cr} (serum creatinine) and Ht (height) with a ruler and read the Cl_{cr} where the ruler intersects the center line.

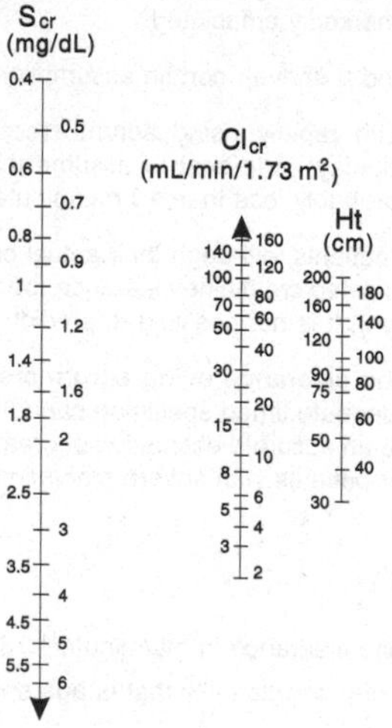

Adults 18 years and older

Method 1: (Cockroft DW and Gault MH, *Nephron*, 1976, 16:31-41)

Estimated creatinine clearance (Cl_{cr}) (mL/min):

$$\text{Male} = \frac{(140 - \text{age})\ \text{IBW (kg)}}{72 \times \text{serum creatinine}}$$

$$\text{Female} = \text{Estimated } Cl_{cr} \text{ male} \times 0.85$$

Note: The use of the patient's ideal body weight (IBW) is recommended for the above formula except when the patient's actual body weight is less than ideal. Use of the IBW is especially important in obese patients. See appendix Growth & Development section for Ideal Body Weight Calculation.

Method 2: (Jelliffe RW, *Ann Intern Med*, 1973, 79:604)

Estimated creatinine clearance (Cl_{cr}) (mL/min/1.73 m^2):

$$\text{Male} = \frac{98 - 0.8\ (\text{age} - 20)}{\text{serum creatinine}}$$

$$\text{Female} = \text{Estimated } Cl_{cr} \text{ male} \times 0.90$$

RENAL FUNCTION TESTS

Endogenous creatinine clearance vs age (timed collection)

Creatinine clearance (mL/min/1.73 m²) = $(Cr_uV/S_{Cr}T)$ (1.73/A)

where:

Cr_u	=	Urine creatinine concentration (mg/dL)
V	=	Total urine volume collected during sampling period (mL)
S_{Cr}	=	Serum creatinine concentration (mg/dL)
T	=	Duration of sampling period (min) (24 h = 1440 min)
A	=	Body surface area (m²)

Age-specific normal values

5-7 d	50.6±5.8 mL/min/1.73 m²
1-2 mo	64.6±5.8 mL/min/1.73 m²
5-8 mo	87.7±11.9 mL/min/1.73 m²
9-12 mo	86.9±8.4 mL/min/1.73 m²
≥18 mo	
male	124±26 mL/min/1.73 m²
female	109±13.5 mL/min/1.73 m²
Adults	
male	105±14 mL/min/1.73 m²
female	95±18 mL/min/1.73 m²

Note: In patients with renal failure (creatinine clearance <25 mL/min), creatinine clearance may be elevated over GFR because of tubular secretion of creatinine.

Serum BUN:Serum Creatinine Ratio

Serum BUN (mg/dL):serum creatinine (mg/dL)

Normal BUN:creatinine ratio is 10-15.

BUN:creatinine ratio >20 suggests prerenal azotemia (also seen with high urea-generation states such as GI bleeding).

BUN:creatinine ratio <5 may be seen with disorders affecting urea biosynthesis such as urea cycle enzyme deficiencies and with hepatitis.

Fractional Sodium Excretion

Fractional sodium secretion (FENa) = Na_uS_{cr} / Na_sCr_u x 100%

where:

Na_u	=	Urine sodium (mEq/L)
Na_s	=	Serum sodium (mEq/L)
Cr_u	=	Urine creatinine (mg/dL)
S_{Cr}	=	Serum creatinine (mg/dL)

FENa <1% suggests prerenal failure
FENa >2% suggest intrinsic renal failure
(for newborns, normal FENa is approximately 2.5%)

Note: Disease states associated with a falsely elevated FENa include severe volume depletion (>10%), early acute tubular necrosis and volume depletion in chronic renal disease. Disorders associated with a lowered FENa include acute glomerulonephritis, hemoglobinuric or myoglobinuric renal failure, nonoliguric acute tubular necrosis, and acute urinary tract obstruction. In addition, FENa may be <1% in patients with acute renal failure **and** a second condition predisposing to sodium retention (eg, burns, congestive heart failure, nephrotic syndrome).

RENAL FUNCTION TESTS *(Continued)*

Urine Calcium:Urine Creatinine Ratio (spot sample)

Urine calcium (mg/dL): urine creatinine (mg/dL)

Normal values <0.21 (mean values 0.08 males, 0.06 females)

Premature infants show wide variability of calcium:creatinine ratio, and tend to have lower thresholds for calcium loss than older children. Prematures without nephrolithiasis had mean Ca:Cr ratio of 0.75±0.76. Infants with nephrolithiasis had mean Ca:Cr ratio of 1.32±1.03 (Jacinto, et al, *Pediatrics*, vol 81, p 31).

Urine Protein:Urine Creatinine Ratio (spot sample)

P_u/Cr_u	Total Protein Excretion (mg/m²/day)
0.1	80
1	800
10	8000

where:

P_u = Urine protein concentration (mg/dL)

Cr_u = Urine creatinine concentration (mg/dL)

Serum Osmolality

Predicted serum osmolality =

2 x Na (mEq/L) + BUN (mg/dL) / 2.8 + glucose (mg/dL) / 18

High Anion Gap (see Toxicology section)

ACID / BASE ASSESSMENT

Henderson-Hasselbalch Equation

$pH = 6.1 + \log (HCO_3^- / (0.03) (pCO_2))$

Alveolar Gas Equation

P_iO_2	=	f_iO_2 x (total atmospheric pressure – vapor pressure of H_2O at 37°C)
	=	f_iO_2 x (760 mm Hg – 47 mm Hg)
PAO_2	=	$P_iO_2 - PACO_2 / R$

Alveolar/arterial oxygen gradient = $PAO_2 - PaO_2$

Normal ranges:

Children	15-20 mm Hg
Adults	20-25 mm Hg

Where:

P_iO_2	=	Oxygen partial pressure of inspired gas (mm Hg) (150 mm Hg in room air at sea level)
f_iO_2	=	Fractional pressure of oxygen in inspired gas (0.21 in room air)
PAO_2	=	Alveolar oxygen partial pressure
$PACO_2$	=	Alveolar carbon dioxide partial pressure
PaO_2	=	Arterial oxygen partial pressure
R	=	Respiratory exchange quotient (typically 0.8, increases with high carbohydrate diet, decreases with high fat diet)

Acid / Base Disorders

Acute metabolic acidosis (<12 h duration)

$PaCO_2$ expected = $1.5 (HCO_3^-) + 8 \pm 2$

or

expected change in pCO = (1-1.5) x change in HCO_3^-

Acute metabolic alkalosis (<12 h duration)

expected change in pCO_2 = (0.5-1) x change in HCO_3^-

Acute respiratory acidosis (<6 h duration)

expected change in HCO_3^- = 0.1 x pCO_2

Acute respiratory acidosis (>6 h duration)

expected change in HCO_3^- = 0.4 x change in pCO_2

Acute respiratory alkalosis (<6 h duration)

expected change in HCO_3^- = 0.2 x change in pCO_2

Acute respiratory alkalosis (>6 h duration)

expected change in HCO_3^- = 0.5 x change in pCO_2

ACUTE DYSTONIC REACTIONS, MANAGEMENT

1. **Confirm that patient has stable airway and adequate respiratory activity.**

2. Administer **one** of the following:

   Diphenhydramine 0.7-1 mg/kg/dose I.V./P.O. q4-6h prn **or**

   Hydroxyzine 0.5-1 mg/kg/dose I.M./P.O. q4-6h prn (adult dose: 25-100 mg I.M./P.O. q6h) **or**

   Children >3 years: Benztropine 0.02-0.05 mg/kg/dose or maximum of 1-2 mg I.V./P.O. (avoid use in children <3 years of age except in cases of extreme emergency)

Agents which predispose patients to acute dystonic reactions, such as phenothiazine neuroleptics or antiemetics, often have long therapeutic half-lives. Anticholinergic administration should therefore be continued for 6-24 hours after discontinuation of phenothiazine therapy.

PREPROCEDURE SEDATIVES IN CHILDREN

Purpose: The following table is a guide to aid the clinician in the selection of the most appropriate sedative to sedate a child for a procedure. One must also consider:

- Not all patients require sedation. It is dependent on the procedure and age of the child.
- When sedation is desired, one must consider the time of onset, the duration of action, and the route of administration.
- Each of the following drugs is well absorbed when given by the suggested routes and doses.
- Each drug was assigned an "intensity" based upon the class of drug, dose, and route.[1]
  - Conscious sedation: A medically controlled state of depressed consciousness that retains the patient's ability to independently and continuously maintain a patent airway, respond appropriately to physical stimulation and/or verbal commands. The protective reflexes are maintained.
  - Deep sedation: A medically controlled state of depressed consciousness associated with partial or complete loss of protective reflexes and inability to respond appropriately to physical stimulation and/or verbal commands.
- Those drugs classified as producing deep sedation require more frequent monitoring postprocedure.
- For painful procedures, an analgesic agent needs to be administered.

Sedatives Used to Produce Conscious Sedation

Drug	Route	Dose (mg/kg)	Onset (min)	Duration (h)	Comments
Chloral hydrate	P.O./P.R.	25-100	10-20	4-8	May cause hepatic neoplasms in rats; maximum single dose: infants: 1 g; children: 2 g
Diazepam[2,3] (Valium®)	P.O.	0.2-0.3 90 min prior	60-90	6-8	Maximum oral dose: 10 mg
	I.V.	0.1-0.2	1-3	6-8	Maximum dose I.V.: 5 mg; due to poor absorption and tissue irritation, I.M. route **not** recommended
	P.R.	0.2-0.4	2-10	6-8	May use I.V. solution rectally
"DPT" cocktail[4] (Demerol®, Phenergan®, Thorazine®)	I.M.	Demerol® 1-2, Phenergan® 0.5-1, Thorazine® 0.5-1	30	2-14	May be mixed in single syringe; I.M. only. This combination of agents may have a higher rate of adverse effects compared with alternative sedative/analgesics.
Fentanyl	Trans-mucosal	5-15 mcg/kg	5-15	1-2	Maximum transmucosal dose: 400 mcg
	I.M.	1-3 mcg/kg	7-15	1-2	
	I.V.	1-3 mcg/kg	Immediate	30-60 min	
Lorazepam[5] (Ativan®)	P.O.	0.05; 90-120 min prior	60	8-12	
	Deep I.M.	0.05; 90-120 min prior	30-60	8-12	
	I.V.	0.05; over 5-10 min	15-30	8-12	

PREPROCEDURE SEDATIVES IN CHILDREN *(Continued)*

Sedatives Used to Produce Conscious Sedation *(continued)*

Drug	Route	Dose (mg/kg)	Onset (min)	Duration (h)	Comments
Meperidine (Demerol®)	P.O.	2-4	10-15	2-4	Doses I.M./I.V. >2 mg/kg are considered deep sedation
	I.M.	0.5-2	10-15	2-4	
	I.V.	0.5-2	5	2-3	
Midazolam[6,7] (Versed®)	P.O.	0.2-0.4; 30-45 min prior	20-30	1-2	Maximum oral dose: 15 mg
	Deep I.M.	0.1-0.15; 30-60 min prior	15	1-2	Maximum total dose: 10 mg
	I.V.	**6 mo - 5 y:** 0.05-0.1; **6-12 y:** 0.025-0.05; **>12 y - Adult:** 2.5-5 mg (total dose); give over 10-20 min	1-5	1-2	Maximum concentration: 1 mg/mL; maximum I.M./I.V. dose: 6 mo - 5 y: 6 mg 6 y - Adult: 10 mg
	P.R.	0.3	20-30	1-2	Dilute injection in 5 mL NS; administer rectally
	Intranasal	0.2-0.3	5	30-60 min	Administer nasally: Use a 1 mL needleless syringe into the nares over 15 seconds; use 5 mg/mL concentration; $\frac{1}{2}$ dose may be administered into each nare
Morphine	P.O.	0.2-0.5	20-30	3-5	
	I.M.	0.05-0.2	20-30	3-5	
	I.V.	0.05-0.2	10-15	2-5	

Note: See individual drug monographs for further information.

Sedatives Used to Produce Deep Sedation

Drug	Route	Dose (mg/kg)	Onset (min)	Duration (h)	Comments
Methohexital[8,9] (Brevital®)	I.M.	5-10	5	1-1.5	Maximum concentration for I.M./I.V.: 50 mg/mL; maximum I.M./I.V. dose: 200 mg. Greater incidence of adverse effects with I.V. use.
	I.V.	0.75-2	1	7-10 min	
	P.R.	20-35	5-10	1-1.5	Shorter duration of action than thiopental; rectal given as a 10% solution in sterile water; maximum dose rectal: 500 mg
Pentobarbital	P.O./I.M./P.R.	2-6	10-25	1-4	Maximum I.M./I.V./P.O./P.R. dose: 100 mg
	I.V.	1-3	1	15 min	
Thiopental[10,4] (Pentothal)	I.V.	4-6	0.5-1	5-10 min	
	P.R.	25; immediately prior to procedure	10	1-5	Variable rectal absorption; may use additional 12.5 mg/kg if necessary; maximum rectal dose: 1-1.5 g

Note: See individual drug monographs for further information.

Sedatives Used to Produce Dissociative Anesthesia (Monitor as if deep sedation)

Drug	Route	Dose (mg/kg)	Onset (min)	Duration	Comments
Ketamine	P.O.	6-10; 30 min prior	30-45	10-30	Use only under direct supervision of physicians experienced in administering general anesthetics; has analgesic effects; may use injectable product orally diluted in a beverage of the patient's choice
	I.M.	3-7	7	12-25	
	I.V.	0.5-2	1	5-10	

Note: See individual drug monographs for further information.

Footnotes

1. Committee on Drugs, Section of Anesthesiology, American Academy of Pediatrics, "Guidelines for Monitoring and Management of Pediatric Patient During and After Sedation for Diagnostic and Therapeutic Procedures," *Pediatrics*, 1992, 89:1110-5.
2. Yager JY and Seshia SS, "Sublingual Lorazepam in Childhood Serial Seizures," *Am J Dis Child*, 1988, 142(9):931-2.
3. Fell D, Gough MB, Northan AA, et al, "Diazepam Premedication in Children," *Anaesthesia*, 1985, 40:12-7.
4. Burckart GJ, White III TJ, Siegle RL, et al, "Rectal Thiopental Versus an Intramuscular Cocktail for Sedating Children Before Computer Tomography," *Am J Hosp Pharm*, 1980, 37:222-4.
5. Burtles R and Astley B, "Lorazepam in Children," *Br J Anaesth*, 1983, 55:275-9.
6. Roelofse JA, van der Bijl P, Stegmann DH, et al, "Preanesthetic Medication With Rectal Midazolam in Children Undergoing Dental Extractions," *J Oral Maxillofac Surg*, 1990, 48(8):791-7.
7. Wilton NC, Leigh J, Rosen DR, et al, "Preanesthetic Sedation of Preschool Children Using Intranasal Midazolam," *Anesthesiology*, 1988, 60(6):972-5.
8. Elman DS and Denson JS, "Preanesthetic Sedation of Children With Intramuscular Methohexital Sodium," *Anesth Analg*, 1965, 44(5):494-8.
9. Miller JR, Grayson M, and Stoelting VK, "Sedation With Intramuscular Methohexital Sodium," *Am J Ophthalmol*, 1966, 62(1):38-43.
10. "Drug Evaluations," *AMA*, 1980.

FEBRILE SEIZURES

A febrile seizure is defined as a seizure occurring for no reason other than an elevated temperature. It does not have an infectious or metabolic origin within the CNS (ie, it is not caused by meningitis, encephalitis, or acute electrolyte imbalance). Fever is usually >102°F rectally. Febrile seizures are the most common form of childhood seizures, occurring in 2% to 5% of children. Most febrile seizures occur between 6 months and 5 years of age, with a peak incidence at 18 months of age. There are three types of febrile seizures:

1. **Simple** febrile seizures are generalized (ie, nonfocal) febrile seizures of less than 15 minutes duration. They do not occur in multiples (ie, they occur only once during a 24-hour period).
2. **Complex** febrile seizures are febrile seizures that are either focal, have a focal component, are longer than 15 minutes in duration, are multiple febrile seizures that occur within 30 minutes, or recur in 24 hours.
3. **Febrile status epilepticus** is a febrile seizure lasting longer than 30 minutes.

Note: Febrile seizures should not be confused with true epileptic seizures associated with fever or "seizure with fever." "Seizure with fever" includes seizures associated with acute neurologic illnesses (ie, meningitis, encephalitis). Infants and children who present with fever and seizures need to be appropriately diagnosed, as there are other conditions which may precipitate seizures in a child with fever (see Srinivasan, 2005).

Acute treatment of an ongoing febrile seizure: Since most febrile seizures are brief in duration, the primary acute treatment of an ongoing febrile seizure is basic first aid seizure management. No other intervention is usually needed. For febrile seizures that last longer than 10 minutes, rectal diazepam is effective in terminating the seizure and is considered the treatment of choice for intervention outside the hospital (Shinnar, 2002). Intravenous diazepam is alse effective and is usually used in the emergency department or hospital setting. Antipyretics are indicated to treat the child's temperature, but do not prevent the recurrence of a febrile seizure.

Long-term treatment to prevent recurrence of febrile seizures: Long-term prophylaxis with daily administration of phenobarbital or valproic acid has been shown to be effective in reducing the risk of subsequent febrile seizures. The intermittent administration of oral or rectal diazepam at the time of febrile illness has also been shown to be effective. **Note:** Daily administration of carbamazepine or phenytoin and use of antipyretic agents alone, are **not** effective in preventing recurrent febrile seizures.

The 1980 NIH Consensus paper stated that after the first febrile seizure, long-term prophylaxis should be considered under any of the following:

1. Presence of abnormal neurological development or abnormal neurological exam
2. Febrile seizure was complex in nature:
   - duration >15 minutes
   - focal febrile seizure
   - followed by transient or persistent neurological abnormalities
3. Positive family history of afebrile seizures (epilepsy)

Also consider long-term prophylaxis in certain cases if:

1. the child has multiple febrile seizures
2. the child is <12 months of age

However, long-term daily administration of phenobarbital or valproic acid and intermittent administration of diazepam is not without risks. Phenobarbital may cause behavioral problems (eg, hyperactivity, irritability), sleep disorders, or hypersensitivity reactions (such as rash or rarely, Stevens-Johnson syndrome). Several studies have also identified a negative effect on learning and cognitive performance in children receiving phenobarbital. Valproic acid has the potential to cause life-threatening hepatotoxicity. It may also cause thrombocytopenia, pancreatitis, GI disturbances, and weight gain or loss. Adverse reactions of diazepam include drowsiness, sedation, lethargy, and ataxia. These adverse effects could mask signs of an evolving CNS infection or process. Thus, these potential risks of long-term treatment need to be weighed against the benefits of preventing the recurrence of febrile seizures.

It is important to note that the risk of recurrent febrile seizures is low for children with **simple** febrile seizures. In 1999, the American Academy of Pediatrics assessed the benefits and risks of long-term anticonvulsant treatment and developed a practice parameter with recommendations. Although daily use of phenobarbital or valproic acid and intermittent administration of diazepam were found to be effective in reducing the risk of recurrent febrile seizures, the potential toxicities associated with these treatments outweigh the relatively minor risks associated with simple febrile seizures. **Therefore, neither continuous (ie, daily administration) nor intermittent anticonvulsant treatment is recommended for neurologically healthy infants and children, 6 months to 5 years of age, who have had one or more simple febrile seizures.** In certain cases (eg, when parental anxiety over febrile seizures is severe), intermittent oral diazepam, administered at the onset of a febrile illness, may be effective in preventing febrile seizure recurrence.

In cases where long-term anticonvulsant prophylaxis is used, it is usually continued for 2 years or 1 year after the last seizure, whichever is longer. Daily administration of phenobarbital requires therapeutic serum concentrations ≥15 mcg/mL to be effective. Due to the potential risk of hepatotoxicity, valproic acid is usually reserved for patients who have significant adverse effects to phenobarbital. The administration of rectal diazepam (as a solution or suppository) at the time of the febrile illness has been shown to be as effective as daily phenobarbital in preventing recurrences of febrile seizures. A rectal diazepam dosage form is available in the United States; however, some centers are still using the injectable form of diazepam rectally. The solution for injection must be filtered prior to use if drawn from an ampul. Like other agents, oral diazepam must be dosed appropriately to be effective. A double-blind, controlled trial found that oral diazepam administered in doses of 0.33 mg/kg/dose given every 8 hours when the child has a fever, reduced the risk of recurrent febrile seizures (see Rosman, 1993). However, a study by Uhari (1995) showed that lower doses of diazepam, 0.2 mg/kg/dose, were not effective.)

References

American Academy of Pediatrics, Committee on Quality Improvement, Subcommittee on Febrile Seizures, "Practice Parameter: Long-Term Treatment of the Child With Simple Febrile Seizures," *Pediatrics*, 1999, 103(6):1307-9.

Baumann RJ, "Prevention and Management of Febrile Seizures," *Paediatr Drugs*, 2001, 3(8):585-92.

Baumann RJ and Duffner PK, "Treatment of Children With Simple Febrile Seizures: The AAP Practice Parameter," *Pediatr Neurol*, 2000, 23:11-7.

Berg AT, Shinnar S, Hauser WA, et al, "Predictors of Recurrent Febrile Seizures: A Meta-Analytic Review," *J Pediatr*, 1990, 116(3):329-37.

Camfield PR, Camfield CS, Gordon K, et al, "Prevention of Recurrent Febrile Seizures," *J Pediatr*, 1995, 126(6):929-30.

NIH Consensus Statement, "Febrile Seizures: A Consensus of Their Significance, Evaluation and Treatment," *Pediatrics*, 1980, 66(6):1009-12.

Rosman NP, Colton T, Labazzo J, et al, "A Controlled Trial of Diazepam Administration During Febrile Illnesses to Prevent Recurrence of Febrile Seizures," *N Engl J Med*, 1993, 329(2):79-84.

Shinnar S and Glauser TA, "Febrile Seizures," *J Child Neurol*, 2002, 17:S44-52.

Srinivasan J Wallace KA, and Scheffer IE, "Febrile Seizures" *Australian Family Physician*, 2005, 34(12):1021-5.

Uhari M, Rantala H, Vainionpää L, et al, "Effect of Acetaminophen and of Low Intermittent Doses of Diazepam on Prevention of Recurrences of Febrile Seizures," *J Pediatr*, 1995, 126(6):991-5.

CAUSES OF NEONATAL SEIZURES

1. Trauma
   a. subdural hematoma
   b. intracortical hemorrhage
   c. cortical vein thrombosis
2. Asphyxia — subependymal hemorrhage
3. Congenital abnormalities (cerebral dysgenesis)
   a. lissencephaly
   b. schizencephaly
4. Hypertension
5. Metabolic
   a. hypocalcemia
      - hypomagnesemia
      - high phosphate load
      - IDM (infants of diabetic mothers)
      - hypoparathyroidism
      - maternal hyperparathyroidism
      - idiopathic
      - DiGeorge's syndrome
   b. hypoglycemia
      - galactosemia
      - IUGR (intrauterine growth retardation)
      - IDM (infants of diabetic mothers)
      - glycogen storage disease
      - idiopathic
      - methylmalonic acidemia
      - propionic acidemia
      - maple syrup urine disease
      - asphyxia
   c. electrolyte imbalance
      - hypernatremia
      - hypomagnesemia
      - hyponatremia
6. Infections
   a. bacterial meningitis
   b. cerebral abscess
   c. herpes encephalitis
   d. Coxsackie meningoencephalitis
   e. cytomegalovirus
   f. toxoplasmosis
   g. syphilis

7. Drug withdrawal
    a. methadone
    b. heroin
    c. barbiturate (short-acting, such as secobarbital and butalbital)
    d. propoxyphene
    e. benzodiazepines (chlordiazepoxide, diazepam)
    f. cocaine
    g. ethanol
    h. codeine
8. Pyridoxine dependency
9. Amino acid disturbances
    a. maple syrup urine disease
    b. urea cycle abnormalities
    c. nonketotic hyperglycinemia
    d. ketotic hyperglycinemia
    e. Leigh disease
    f. isovaleric acidemia
10. Toxins
    a. local anesthetics
    b. isoniazid
    c. lead
    d. indomethacin (from breast feeding)
    e. fentanyl
11. Familial seizures
    a. neurocutaneous syndromes
        - tuberous sclerosis
        - incontinentia pigmenti
    b. genetic syndromes
        - Zellweger's
        - Smith Lemli Opitz
        - neonatal adrenoleukodystrophy
    c. benign familial epilepsy
12. Cerebral hemorrhage
    a. intraventricular
    b. subarachnoid
    c. subdural

Adapted from Painter MJ, Bergman I, and Crumrie P, "Neonatal Seizures," *Pediatr Clin North Am*, 1986, 33:91-107.

ANTIEPILEPTIC DRUGS

Antiepileptic Drugs for Children and Adolescents by Seizure Type and Epilepsy Syndrome

Seizure Type or Epilepsy Syndrome	First Line Therapy	Alternatives
Partial seizures (with or without secondary generalization)	Carbamazepine, oxcarbazepine, or phenytoin	**Second choice:** Gabapentin, lamotrigine, topiramate, or valproate **Third choice:** Tiagabine, zonisamide, phenobarbital, or primidone **Consider:** Benzodiazepine, acetazolamide, vigabatrin, or felbamate
Generalized tonic-clonic seizures	Valproate, carbamazepine, or phenytoin	**Second choice:** Topiramate or lamotrigine **Third choice:** Phenobarbital or primidone **Consider:** Zonisamide
Childhood absence epilepsy		
Before 10 years of age	Ethosuximide (only if no convulsive seizures) or valproate	**Second choice:** Lamotrigine **Third choice:** Methsuximide, acetazolamide, benzodiazepine, topiramate, or zonisamide
After 10 years of age	Valproate	**Second choice:** Lamotrigine **Third choice:** Ethosuximide, methsuximide, acetazolamide, benzodiazepine, topiramate or zonisamide
Juvenile myoclonic epilepsy	Valproate	**Second choice:** Lamotrigine, topiramate, or clonazepam **Third choice:** Phenobarbital, primidone, carbamazepine, or phenytoin **Consider:** Felbamate
Progressive myoclonic epilepsy	Valproate	**Second choice:** Valproate plus clonazepam, or phenobarbital
Lennox-Gastaut and related syndromes	Valproate	**Second choice:** Topiramate, lamotrigine **Third choice:** Ketogenic diet, vagal nerve stimulation, felbamate, benzodiazepine, or phenobarbital **Consider:** Ethosuximide, methsuximide, ACTH or steroids, pyridoxine or vigabatrin
Infantile spasms	ACTH (or steroids), vigabatrin, or valproate	**Second choice:** Topiramate **Third choice:** Lamotrigine, tiagabine, or benzodiazepine **Consider:** Pyridoxine, felbamate, or zonisamide
Benign epilepsy of childhood with centrotemporal spikes	Gabapentin or valproate	**Second choice:** Carbamazepine or phenytoin **Third choice:** Phenobarbital, primidone, or benzodiazepine **Consider:** Lamotrigine or topiramate
Neonatal seizures	Phenobarbital	**Second choice:** Phenytoin **Consider:** Clonazepam, primidone, valproate, or pyridoxine

Adapted from Bourgeois BF, "Antiepileptic Drugs in Pediatric Practice," *Epilepsia*, 1995, 36(Suppl 2):S34-S45 and Bourgeois BF, "New Antiepileptic Drugs in Children: Which Ones for Which Seizures?" *Clin Neuropharmacol*, 2000, 23(3):119-32.

COMA SCALES

Glasgow Coma Scale

Activity	Best Response	Score
Eye opening	Spontaneous	4
	Responds to voice	3
	Responds to pain	2
	No response	1
Verbal response	Oriented and appropriate	5
	Confused / disoriented conversation	4
	Inappropriate words	3
	Nonspecific sounds (incomprehensible)	2
	No response	1
Motor response	Follows commands	6
	Localizes pain	5
	Withdraws to pain	4
	Abnormal flexion (decorticate posturing)	3
	Abnormal extension (decerebrate posturing)	2
	No response	1

Modified Coma Scale for Infants

Activity	Best Response	Score
Eye opening	Spontaneous	4
	Responds to voice	3
	Responds to pain	2
	No response	1
Verbal response	Coos, babbles	5
	Irritable	4
	Cries to pain	3
	Moans to pain	2
	No response	1
Motor response	Normal spontaneous movements	6
	Withdraws to touch	5
	Withdraws to pain	4
	Abnormal flexion (decorticate posturing)	3
	Abnormal extension (decerebrate posturing)	2
	No response	1

Interpretation of Coma Scale Scores
Maximum Score: 15; Minimum Score: 3
(low score indicates greater severity of coma)

Range of Score	Interpretation
3- 8	Coma. Severe brain injury. Immediate action needed. Notify ICU staff STAT. Will require intubation regardless of respiratory status.
9-12	Lethargic. Needs close observation in special care unit. Frequent neuro checks. Notify ICU staff.
13-14	Needs observation
15	Normal

References

James HE, "Neurologic Evaluation and Support in the Child With an Acute Brain Insult," *Pediatr Ann*, 1986, 15(1):16-22.

Jennett B and Teasdale G, "Aspects of Coma After Severe Head Injury," *Lancet*, 1977, 1(8017): 878-81.

ASTHMA

Adapted from National Asthma Education and Prevention Program (NAEPP) Expert Panel Report, "Guidelines for the Diagnosis and Management of Asthma – Update on Selected Topics 2002," NIH Publication No. 02-5075 (www.nhlbi.nih.gov/guidelines/asthma/index.html)

MANAGEMENT OF ASTHMA IN INFANTS, CHILDREN, AND ADULTS

Goals of Asthma Treatment

- Minimal or no chronic symptoms day or night
- Minimal or no exacerbations
- No limitations on activities; no school/work missed
- Minimal use of inhaled short-acting beta$_2$-agonist (<1 time/day, <1 canister/month)
- Minimal or no adverse effects from medications
- Children >5 years of age and adults only: PEF >80% of personal best

Education

- Teach self-management.
- Teach about controlling environmental factors (avoidance of allergens or other factors that contribute to asthma severity).
- Review administration technique and compliance with patient.
- May use a written action plan to help educate.

Stepwise Approach for Managing Infants and Young Children (≤5 Years of Age) With Acute or Chronic Asthma[1]

Symptoms[2]	Long-Term Control (Daily Medications)
STEP 4: Severe Persistent	
Day: Continual Night: Frequent	• **Preferred treatment:** **– High dose inhaled corticosteroid** **AND** **– Long-acting inhaled beta$_2$-agonist** **AND**, if needed – Long-term oral corticosteroids (2 mg/kg/day, generally do not exceed 60 mg/day). (Make repeated attempts to reduce systemic corticosteroids and maintain control with high-dose inhaled corticosteroids.)
STEP 3: Moderate Persistent	
Day: Every day Night: >1 night/week	• **Preferred treatment:** **– Low-dose inhaled corticosteroid** **AND** **Long-acting inhaled beta$_2$-agonist** **OR** **Medium-dose inhaled corticosteroid** • Alternatives: – Low-dose inhaled corticosteroid and either leukotriene receptor antagonist or theophylline
	If needed (especially with recurring severe exacerbations): • **Preferred treatment:** **– Medium-dose inhaled corticosteroid and long-acting inhaled beta$_2$-agonist** • Alternatives: – Medium-dose inhaled corticosteroid and either leukotriene receptor antagonist or theophylline
STEP 2: Mild Persistent	
Day: >2 days/week but <1 time/day Night: >2 nights/month	• **Preferred treatment:** **– Low-dose inhaled corticosteroid (with nebulizer or MDI with holding chamber with or without face mask or DPI)** • Alternatives: Cromolyn (nebulizer is preferred or MDI with holding chamber) **OR** Leukotriene receptor antagonist

Stepwise Approach for Managing Infants and Young Children (≤5 Years of Age) With Acute or Chronic Asthma[1]

Symptoms[2]	Long-Term Control (Daily Medications)
	STEP 1: Mild Intermittent
Day: ≤2 days/week Night: ≤2 nights/month	No daily medication needed

[1]Classify severity. The presence of one of the features of severity is sufficient to place a patient in that category. An individual should be assigned to the most severe grade in which any feature occurs. The characteristics noted in this figure are general and may overlap because asthma is highly variable. Furthermore, an individual's classification may change over time.

[2]Patients at any level of severity can have mild, moderate, or severe exacerbations. Some patients with intermittent asthma experience severe and life-threatening exacerbations separated by long periods of normal lung function and no symptoms.

↓ Step Down
Review treatment every 1-6 month; a gradual stepwise reduction in treatment may be possible.

↑ Step Up
If control is not achieved, consider step up. But first: review patient medication technique, adherence, and environmental control (avoidance of allergens or other precipitant factors)

Quick Relief – All Patients

- Bronchodilator as needed for symptoms ≤2 times/week. Intensity of treatment will depend upon severity of exacerbation (see "Management of Asthma Exacerbations"). Either:
  - Preferred treatment: Inhaled short-acting beta$_2$-agonist by nebulizer or face mask and spacer/holding chamber

    or
  - Alternative treatment: Oral beta$_2$-agonist
- With viral respiratory infection:
  - Bronchodilator q4-6h up to 24 hours (longer with physician consult) but, in general, repeat no more than once every 6 weeks.
  - Consider systemic corticosteroid if current exacerbation is severe or patient has history of severe exacerbations.
- Use of short-acting inhaled beta$_2$-agonist on a daily basis, or increasing use, indicates the need to initiate or titrate long-term control therapy.

Notes:

- **The stepwise approach presents guidelines to assist clinical decision making. Asthma is highly variable; clinicians should tailor specific medication plans to the needs and circumstances of individual patients.**
- Gain control as quickly as possible; then decrease treatment to the least medication necessary to maintain control.
- A rescue course of systemic corticosteroid may be needed at any time and step.
- In general, use of short-acting beta$_2$-agonist on a daily basis indicates the need for additional long-term control therapy.
- There are very few studies on asthma therapy for infants.
- Studies comparing medications in children <5 years of age are not available.
- Consultation with an asthma specialist is recommended for moderate or severe persistent asthma. Consider consultation for patient with mild persistent asthma.
- Initiation of long-term control therapy should be considered in infants and young children who have had >3 episodes of wheezing in the past year that lasted >1 day and affected sleep and who have risk factors for asthma.
- Inhaled corticosteroids improve health outcomes for children with mild-moderate persistent asthma. Monitor growth of children taking corticosteroids by any route. If growth appears slowed, weigh the benefits against the risks.
- Antibiotics are not recommended for treatment of acute asthma exacerbations except where there is evidence or suspicion of bacterial infection.

ASTHMA *(Continued)*

Stepwise Approach for Managing Asthma in Children >5 Years of Age, Adolescents, and Adults: Treatment[1]

Symptoms[2]	Lung Function[3]	Long-Term Control (Daily Medications)
STEP 4: Severe Persistent		
Day: Continual Night: Frequent	PEF/FEV$_1$ ≤60% PEF variability >30%	• **Preferred treatment:** **– High dose inhaled corticosteroid** **AND** **– Long-acting inhaled beta$_2$-agonist** **AND,** if needed – Long-term oral corticosteroids (2 mg/kg/day, generally do not exceed 60 mg/day). (Make repeated attempts to reduce systemic corticosteroids and maintain control with high-dose inhaled corticosteroids.)
STEP 3: Moderate Persistent		
Day: Every day Night: >1 night/week	PEF/FEV$_1$ >60% - <80% PEF variability >30%	• **Preferred treatment:** **– Low-medium dose inhaled corticosteroid** **AND** **– Long-acting inhaled beta$_2$-agonist** • Alternatives: – Increase inhaled corticosteroids within medium-dose range **OR** – Low-medium dose inhaled corticosteroids and either leukotriene receptor antagonist or theophylline
		If needed (especially with recurring severe exacerbations): • **Preferred treatment:** – Increase inhaled corticosteroids within medium-dose range, and add long-acting inhaled beta$_2$-agonist • Alternatives: – Increase inhaled corticosteroids in medium-dose range, and add either leukotriene receptor antagonist or theophylline
STEP 2: Mild Persistent		
Day: >2 days/week but <1 time/day Night: >2 nights/month	PEF/FEV$_1$ ≥80% PEF variability 20%-30%	• **Preferred treatment:** **– Low-dose inhaled corticosteroid** • Alternatives: Cromolyn, leukotriene receptor antagonist, nedocromil, or sustained release theophylline (serum concentration 5-15 mcg/mL)
STEP 1: Mild Intermittent		
Day: ≤2 days/week Night: ≤2 nights/month	PEF/FEV$_1$ ≥80% PEF variability <20%	No daily medication needed. A course of systemic corticosteroids is recommended for severe exacerbations.

[1]Classify severity. The presence of one of the features of severity is sufficient to place a patient in that category. An individual should be assigned to the most severe grade in which any feature occurs. The characteristics noted are general and may overlap because asthma is highly variable. Furthermore, an individual's classification may change over time.

[2]Patients at any level of severity can have mild, moderate, or severe exacerbations. Some patients with intermittent asthma experience severe and life-threatening exacerbations separated by long periods of normal lung function and no symptoms.

[3]PEF is % of personal best and FEV$_1$ is % predicted.

↓ Step down
Review treatment every 1-6 months; a gradual stepwise reduction in treatment may be possible.

↑Step up
If control is not maintained, consider step up. First, review patient medication technique, adherence, and environmental control.

Quick Relief – All Patients

- Short-acting bronchodilator: **Inhaled beta$_2$-agonists** as needed for symptoms.
- Intensity of treatment will depend on severity of exacerbation; see "Management of Asthma Exacerbations".
- Use of short-acting inhaled beta$_2$-agonists on a daily basis, or increasing use, indicates the need to initiate or titrate long-term control therapy.

Notes:

- **The stepwise approach presents general guidelines to assist clinical decision making; it is not intended to be a specific prescription. Asthma is highly variable; clinicians should tailor specific medication plans to the needs and circumstances of individual patients.**
- Gain control as quickly as possible; then decrease treatment to the least medication necessary to maintain control.
- A rescue course of systemic corticosteroids may be needed at any time and at any step.
- Some patients with intermittent asthma experience severe and life-threatening exacerbations separated by long periods of normal lung function and no symptoms. This may be especially common with exacerbations provoked by respiratory infections. A short course of systemic corticosteroids is recommended.
- At each step, patients should control their environment to avoid or control factors that make their asthma worse.
- Antibiotics are not recommended for treatment of acute asthma exacerbations except where there is evidence or suspicion of bacterial infection.
- Consultation with an asthma specialist is recommended for moderate or severe persistent asthma.
- Peak flow monitoring for patients with moderate-severe asthma should be considered.

ASTHMA *(Continued)*

Management of Asthma Exacerbations: Home Treatment[1]

Assess Severity

Measure PEF: Value <50% personal best or predicted suggests severe exacerbation.

Note signs and symptoms: Degrees of cough, breathlessness, wheezing, and chest tightness correlate imperfectly with severity of exacerbation. Accessory muscle use and suprasternal retractions suggest severe exacerbation.

Initial Treatment

Inhaled short-acting $beta_2$-agonist: Up to three treatments of 2-4 puffs by MDI at 20-minute intervals or single nebulizer treatment.

Good Response

Mild Exacerbation

PEF >80% predicted or personal best

No wheezing or shortness of breath

Response to $beta_2$-agonist sustained for 4 hours

- May continue $beta_2$-agonist every 3-4 hours for 24-48 hours
- For patients on inhaled corticosteroids, double dose for 7-10 days.

Then:

- Contact clinician for follow-up instructions.

Incomplete Response

Moderate Exacerbation

PEF 50%-80% predicted or personal best

Persistent wheezing and shortness of breath

- Add oral corticosteroid
- Continue $beta_2$-agonist

Then:

- Contact clinician urgently (this day) for instructions.

Poor Response

Severe Exacerbation

PEF <50% predicted or personal best

Marked wheezing and shortness of breath

- Add oral corticosteroid
- Repeat $beta_2$-agonist immediately
- If distress is severe and nonresponsive, call your physician and proceed to emergency department; consider calling ambulance or 9-1-1.

Then:

- Proceed to emergency department.

[1]Patients at high risk of asthma-related death should receive immediate clinical attention after initial treatment. Additional therapy may be required.

Management of Asthma Exacerbations: Emergency Department and Hospital-Based Care

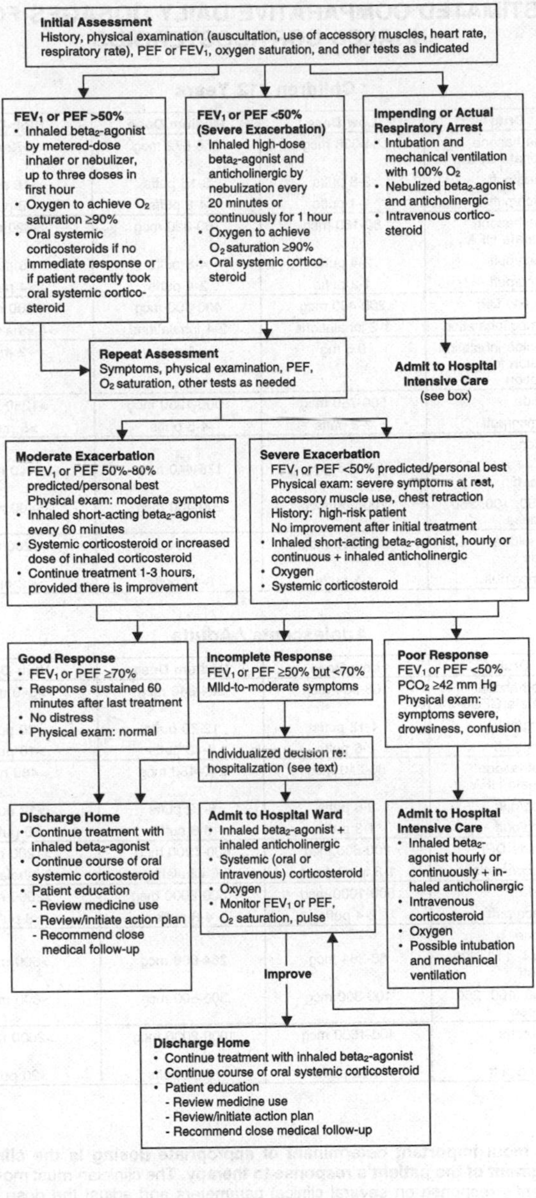

ASTHMA *(Continued)*

ESTIMATED COMPARATIVE DAILY DOSAGES FOR INHALED CORTICOSTEROIDS

Children ≤12 Years

Drug	Low Dose	Medium Dose	High Dose
Beclomethasone dipropionate CFC	84-336 mcg	336-672 mcg	>672 mcg
42 mcg/puff	2-8 puffs	8-16 puffs	>16 puffs
84 mcg/puff	1-4 puffs	4-8 puffs	>8 puffs
Beclomethasone dipropionate HFA	80-160 mcg	160-320 mcg	>320 mcg
40 mcg/puff	2-4 puffs	4-8 puffs	>8 puffs
80 mcg/puff	1-2 puffs	2-4 puffs	>4 puffs
Budesonide DPI	200-400 mcg	400-800 mcg	>800 mcg
200 mcg/inhalation	1-2 inhalations	2-4 inhalations	>4 inhalations
Budesonide inhalation suspension for nebulization	0.5 mg	1 mg	2 mg
Flunisolide	500-750 mcg	1000-1250 mcg	>1250 mcg
250 mcg/puff	2-3 puffs	4-5 puffs	>5 puffs
Fluticasone			
MDI: 44, 110, 220 mcg/puff	88-176 mcg	176-440 mcg	>440 mcg
DPI: 50, 100, 250 mcg/dose	100-200 mcg	200-400 mcg	>400 mcg
Triamcinolone acetonide	400-800 mcg	800-1200 mcg	>1200 mcg
100 mcg/puff	4-8 puffs	8-12 puffs	>12 puffs

Adolescents / Adults

Drug	Low Dose	Medium Dose	High Dose
Beclomethasone dipropionate CFC	168-504 mcg	504-840 mcg	>840 mcg
42 mcg/puff	4-12 puffs	12-20 puffs	>20 puffs
84 mcg/puff	2-6 puffs	6-10 puffs	>10 puffs
Beclomethasone dipropionate HFA	80-240 mcg	240-480 mcg	>480 mcg
40 mcg/puff	2-6 puffs	6-12 puffs	>12 puffs
80 mcg/puff	1-3 puffs	3-6 puffs	>6 puffs
Budesonide DPI	200-600 mcg	600-1200 mcg	>1200 mcg
200 mcg/inhalation	1-3 inhalations	3-6 inhalations	>6 inhalations
Flunisolide	500-1000 mcg	1000-2000 mcg	>2000 mcg
250 mcg/puff	2-4 puffs	4-8 puffs	>8 puffs
Fluticasone			
MDI: 44, 110, 220 mcg/puff	88-264 mcg	264-660 mcg	>660 mcg
DPI: 50, 100, 250 mcg/dose	100-300 mcg	300-600 mcg	>600 mcg
Triamcinolone acetonide	400-1000 mcg	1000-2000 mcg	>2000 mcg
100 mcg/puff	4-10 puffs	10-20 puffs	>20 puffs

Notes:

- **The most important determinant of appropriate dosing is the clinician's judgment of the patient's response to therapy.** The clinician must monitor the patient's response on several clinical parameters and adjust the dose accordingly. The stepwise approach to therapy emphasizes that once control of asthma is achieved, the dose of mediation should be carefully titrated to the minimum dose required to maintain control, thus reducing the potential for adverse effect.
- The reference point for the range in the dosages for children is data on the safety on inhaled corticosteroids in children, which, in general, suggest that the dose

ranges are equivalent to beclomethasone dipropionate 200-400 mcg/day (low dose), 400-800 mcg/day (medium dose), and >800 mcg/day (high dose).

- Some dosages may be outside package labeling.
- Metered-dose inhaler (MDI) dosages are expressed as the actuator dose (the amount of drug leaving the actuator and delivered to the patient), which is the labeling required in the United States. This is different from the dosage expressed as the valve dose (the amount of drug leaving the valve, all of which is not available to the patient), which is used in many European countries and in some of the scientific literature. Dry powder inhaler (DPI) doses (eg, Turbuhaler) are expressed as the amount of drug in the inhaler following activation.

ESTIMATED CLINICAL COMPARABILITY OF DOSES FOR INHALED CORTICOSTEROIDS

Data from *in vitro* and in clinical trials suggest that the different inhaled corticosteroid preparations are not equivalent on a per puff or microgram basis. However, it is not entirely clear what implications these differences have for dosing recommendations in clinical practice because there are few data directly comparing the preparations. Relative dosing for clinical comparability is affected by differences in topical potency, clinical effects at different doses, delivery device, and bioavailability. The Expert Panel developed recommended dose ranges for different preparations based on available data and the following assumptions and cautions about estimating relative doses needed to achieve comparable clinical effect.

Relative Topical Potency Using Human Skin Blanching

- The standard test for determining relative topical anti-inflammatory potency is the topical vasoconstriction (MacKenzie skin blanching) test.
- The MacKenzie topical skin blanching test correlates with binding affinities and binding half-lives for human lung corticosteroid receptors (see following table) (Dahlberg, et al, 1984; Hogger and Rohdewald 1994).
- The relationship between relative topical anti-inflammatory effect and clinical comparability in asthma management is not certain. However, recent clinical trials suggest that different *in vitro* measures of anti-inflammatory effect is not certain. However, recent clinical trials suggest that different *in vitro* measures of anti-inflammatory effect correlate with clinical efficacy (Barnes and Pedersen 1993; Johnson 1996; Kamada, et al, 1996; Ebden, et al, 1986; Leblanc, et al, 1994; Gustaffson, et al, 1993; Lundback, et al, 1993; Barnes, et al, 1993; Fabbri, et al, 1993; Langdon and Capsey, 1994; Ayres, et al, 1995; Rafferty, et al, 1985; Bjorkander, et al, 1982, Stiksa, et al, 1982; Willey, et al, 1982.)

Medication	Topical Potency (Skin Blanching)[1]	Corticosteroid Receptor Binding Half-Life	Receptor Binding Affinity
Beclomethasone dipropionate (BDP)	600	7.5 hours	13.5
Budesonide (BUD)	980	5.1 hours	9.4
Flunisolide (FLU)	330	3.5 hours	1.8
Fluticasone propionate (FP)	1200	10.5 hours	18.0
Triamcinolone acetonide (TAA)	330	3.9 hours	3.6

[1]Numbers are assigned in reference to dexamethasone, which has a value of "1" in the MacKenzie test.

ASTHMA *(Continued)*

Relative Doses to Achieve Similar Clinical Effects

- Clinical effects are evaluated by a number of outcome parameters (eg, changes in spirometry, peak flow rates, symptom scores, quick-relief beta$_2$-agonist use, frequency of exacerbations, airway responsiveness).
- The daily dose and duration of treatment may affect these outcome parameters differently (eg, symptoms and peak flow may improve at lower doses and over a shorter treatment time than bronchial reactivity) (van Essen-Zandvliet, et al, 1992; Haahtela, et al, 1991)
- Delivery systems influence comparability. For example, the delivery device for budesonide (Turbuhaler) delivers approximately twice the amount of drug to the airway as the MDI, thus enhancing the clinical effect (Thorsson, et al, 1994; Agertoft and Pedersen, 1993).
- Individual patients may respond differently to different preparations, as noted by clinical experience.
- Clinical trials comparing effects in reducing symptoms and improving peak expiratory flow demonstrate:
  - BDP and BUD achieved comparable effects at similar microgram doses by MDI (Bjorkander, et al, 1982; Ebden, et al, 1986; Rafferty, et al, 1985).
  - BDP achieved effects similar to twice the dose of TAA on a microgram basis.

Reference

National Asthma Education and Prevention Program (NAEPP), Clinical Practice Guidelines, Expert Panel Report 2, "Guidelines for the Diagnosis and Management of Asthma," NIH Publication No. 97-4051, July 1997.

NORMAL RESPIRATORY RATES

Hour After Birth	Average Respiratory Rate	Range
1st hour	60 breaths/minute	20-100
2-6 hours	50 breaths/minute	20-80
>6 hours	30-40 breaths/minute	20-60

Age (years)	Mean RR (breaths/minute)
0-2	25-30
3-9	20-25
10-18	16-20

BLOOD LEVEL SAMPLING TIME GUIDELINES

Drug	Infusion Time	Therapeutic Range	When to Draw Levels
Amikacin sulfate			
I.V.	30 min	Peak: 20-30 mcg/mL	Peak: 30 min after end of 30 min infusion
		Trough: <10 mcg/mL	Trough: Within 30 min before next dose
I.M.			Peak: 1 h after I.M. injection
			Trough: Within 30 min before next dose
Carbamazepine		4-12 mcg/mL	Just before next dose
Chloramphenicol			
I.V.	30 min	Peak: 15-25 mcg/mL	Peak: 90 min after end of 30 min infusion
			Trough: Just before next dose
P.O.			Peak: 2 h post-P.O. dose
Cyclosporine			
I.V./P.O.		BMT 100-200 ng/mL	Just before next dose
		Liver transplant 200-300 ng/mL	
		Renal transplant 100-200 ng/mL	
Digoxin			
I.V./P.O.		Age and disease related: 0.8-2 ng/mL	6 h postdose to just before next dose
Ethosuximide			
P.O.		40-100 mcg/mL	Just before next dose
Flucytosine			
P.O.		25-100 mcg/mL	Peak: 2 h postdose after at least 4 d of therapy
Fosphenytoin (measure phenytoin levels)			
I.V.		Phenytoin: 10-20 mcg/mL	Peak: 2 h after end of an infusion
I.M.			Peak: 4 h after I.M. injection
Gentamicin			
I.V.	30 min	Peak: 4-10 mcg/mL	Peak: 30 min after end of 30 min infusion
		Trough: 0.5-2 mcg/mL	Trough: Within 30 min before next dose
I.M.			Peak: 1 h after I.M. injection
			Trough: Within 30 min before next dose
Phenobarbital		15-40 mcg/mL	Trough: Just before next dose
Phenytoin			
P.O., I.V.		10-20 mcg/mL	Trough: Just before next dose
I.V.			Post-load/Peak: 1 h after end of infusion
Theophylline			
I.V. bolus	30 min	10-20 mcg/mL	Peak: 30 min after end of 30 min infusion
Continuous infusion			16-24 h after the start or change in a constant I.V. infusion
P.O. liquid, fast-release tablet (Somophyllin®, Slo-Phyllin® liquid & tablet)			Peak: 1 h postdose Trough: Just before next dose

(continued)

Drug	Infusion Time	Therapeutic Range	When to Draw Levels
P.O. slow-release (Theo-Dur®, Slo-Phyllin® GC, Slo-bid®)			Peak: 4 h postdose Trough: Just before next dose
Tobramycin			
I.V.	30 min	Peak: 4-10 mcg/mL	Peak: 30 min after end of 30 min infusion
		Trough: 0.5-2 mcg/mL	Trough: Within 30 min before next dose
I.M.			Peak: 1 h post-I.M. injection
			Trough: Within 30 min before next dose
Trimethoprim			
I.V., dose 20 mg/kg	60 min	Peak: 5-10 mcg/mL	Peak: 30 min after end of 60 min infusion
I.V., dose 8-10 mg/kg		Peak 1-3 mcg/mL	
P.O.			Peak: 1 h postdose
Valproic acid			
P.O.		50-100 mcg/mL	Trough: Just before next dose
Vancomycin	60 min	Peak: 25-40 mcg/mL	Peak: 20-30 min after end of 60 min infusion[1]
		Trough: 5-15 mcg/mL	Trough: Within 30 min before next dose

[1]Some institutions may draw vancomycin peak 1 hour after 1-hour infusion and accept the lower range of therapeutic.

OVERDOSE AND TOXICOLOGY[1]

Drug or Drug Class	Signs / Symptoms	Treatment/Comments
Acetaminophen	Nausea, vomiting, diaphoresis, delirium, fever, coma, vascular collapse, hepatic necrosis, transient azotemia, renal tubular necrosis	Assess severity of ingestion; doses ≥150 mg/kg for children and 7.5 g for adults are thought to be toxic. Obtain serum concentration ≥4 hours postingestion and use acetaminophen nomogram to evaluate need for acetylcysteine. Empty stomach with ipecac (if <1 hour postingestion) or gastric lavage. May administer activated charcoal for one dose, this may decrease absorption of acetylcysteine if given within 1 hour of orally administered acetylcysteine. For unknown ingested quantities and for significant ingestion, give acetylcysteine orally (diluted 1:4 with juice or carbonated beverage); initial: 140 mg/kg then give 70 mg/kg every 4 hours for 17 doses. An I.V. formulation is also available. For I.V. treatment, administer 150 mg/kg (over 15 minutes) followed by 50 mg/kg (over 4 hours), followed by 100 mg/kg (over 16 hours). See acetylcysteine monograph *on page 51*.
Alpha-adrenergic blocking agents	Hypotension, drowsiness	Induce emesis, give activated charcoal, additional treatment is symptomatic; use I.V. fluids, dopamine, or ephedrine to treat hypotension. Epinephrine may worsen hypotension due to beta effects.
Aminoglycosides	Ototoxicity, nephrotoxicity, neuromuscular toxicity	Hemodialysis or peritoneal dialysis may be useful in patients with decreased renal function.
Anticholinergics, antihistamines	Coma, hallucinations, delirium, tachycardia, dry skin, urinary retention, dilated pupils	For life-threatening arrhythmias or seizures physostigmine may be used.
Anticholinesterase agents	Nausea, vomiting, diarrhea, miosis, CNS depression, excessive salivation, excessive sweating, muscle weakness	Suction oral secretions, decontaminate skin, atropinize patient; atropine dose must be individualized. Infants and children: Initial dose: 0.01-0.02 mg/kg/dose; may need to increase as high as 0.05 mg/kg. Adults: Initial atropine dose: 1 mg; may need to increase to 2-5 mg/dose; pralidoxime (2-PAM) may need to be added for severe intoxications.
Barbiturates	Respiratory depression, circulatory collapse, bradycardia, hypotension, hypothermia, slurred speech, confusion	Repeated oral doses of activated charcoal given every 3-6 hours will increase clearance: Children: 1-2 g/kg/dose; adults: 30-60 g. Assure GI motility, adequate hydration, and renal function. Urinary alkalinization with I.V. sodium bicarbonate will increase renal elimination of longer-acting barbiturates (eg, phenobarbital).
Benzodiazepines	Respiratory depression, apnea, hypoactive reflexes, hypotension, slurred speech, unsteady gait, coma	For comatose patient, use gastric lavage with endotracheal tube in place to prevent aspiration; flumazenil, a benzodiazepine antagonist, can be used to reverse the effects of benzodiazepines. See Flumazenil monograph *on page 667* for dose. Action of flumazenil may be shorter than duration of benzodiazepine; repeat doses as needed. Norepinephrine, phenylephrine, or dopamine may be used to treat hypotension; dialysis is of limited value; support blood pressure and respiration.

Drug or Drug Class	Signs / Symptoms	Treatment/Comments
Beta-adrenergic blockers	Hypotension, bronchospasm, bradycardia, hyperglycemia, or hypoglycemia	Induce emesis, followed by activated charcoal; treat symptomatically; glucagon, atropine, isoproterenol, or cardiac pacing may be needed to treat bradycardia, conduction defects, or hypotension
Carbamazepine	Dizziness, drowsiness, ataxia, involuntary movements, opisthotonos, seizures, nausea, vomiting, agitation, nystagmus, coma, urinary retention, respiratory depression, tachycardia	Use supportive therapy, general poisoning management as needed; use repeated oral doses of activated charcoal given every 3-6 hours to decrease serum concentrations; children 1-2 g/kg/dose, adults: 30-60 g/dose; charcoal hemoperfusion may be needed; treat hypotension with I.V. fluids, dopamine, or norepinephrine; monitor EKG; diazepam may control convulsions but may exacerbate respiratory depression
Cardiac glycosides	Hyperkalemia may develop rapidly and result in life-threatening cardiac arrhythmias, progressive bradyarrhythmias, 2nd or 3rd degree heart block unresponsive to atropine, ventricular fibrillation, asystole	Obtain serum drug level, induce emesis or perform gastric lavage; give activated charcoal to reduce further absorption; atropine may reverse heart block, phenytoin will improve A-V conduction; digoxin immune Fab (digoxin specific antibody fragments) is used in life-threatening cases, each 38 mg of digoxin immune Fab binds with 0.5 mg of digoxin or digitoxin; see Digoxin Immune Fab monograph *on page 498* for dosing recommendations
Heparin	Severe hemorrhage	1 mg of protamine sulfate will neutralize approximately 90 units of heparin sodium (bovine) or 115 units of heparin sodium (porcine) or 100 units of heparin calcium (porcine)
Hydantoin derivatives	Nausea, vomiting, nystagmus, slurred speech, ataxia, coma	Gastric lavage or emesis; repeated oral doses of activated charcoal may increase clearance of phenytoin. Children: 1-2 g/kg/dose, adults: 30-60 g/dose activated charcoal every 3-6 hours until nontoxic serum concentration is obtained; assure adequate GI motility, supportive therapy; dialysis may be helpful.
Iron	Lethargy, nausea, vomiting, green or tarry stools, hypotension, weak rapid pulse, metabolic acidosis, shock, coma, hepatic necrosis, renal failure, local GI erosions	Induce emesis if awake or lavage with saline solution; give deferoxamine mesylate I.V. at 15 mg/kg/hour in cases of severe poisoning (serum Fe >350 mcg/mL) and continue chelation therapy for 24 hours after child is excreting normal color urine; urine output should be maintained at >2 mL/kg/hour to avoid hypovolemic shock
Isoniazid	Nausea, vomiting, blurred vision, CNS depression, intractable seizures, coma, metabolic acidosis	Control seizures with diazepam; if suspected ingestion of >80 mg/kg, give pyridoxine I.V. equal dose to the suspected overdose of isoniazid; lavage after seizure control is reached; force diuresis with I.V. fluids; hemo- or peritoneal dialysis may be beneficial in severe cases
Nonsteroidal anti-inflammatory drugs	Dizziness, abdominal pain, sweating, apnea, nystagmus, cyanosis, hypotension, coma	Induce emesis; give activated charcoal via NG tube; provide symptomatic and supportive care.

OVERDOSE AND TOXICOLOGY[1] *(Continued)*

Drug or Drug Class	Signs / Symptoms	Treatment/Comments
Opiates and morphine analogs	Respiratory depression, miosis, hypothermia, bradycardia, circulatory collapse, pulmonary edema, apnea	Establish airway and adequate ventilation; give naloxone 0.1 mg/kg for children up to 5 years of age or 20 kg; for those >5 years or 20 kg give 2 mg naloxone; repeat doses every 2-3 minutes if needed; additional doses may be needed every 20-60 minutes. May need to institute continuous infusion, as duration of action of opiates can be longer than duration of action of naloxone.
Phenothiazines	Deep, unarousable sleep, anticholinergic symptoms, extrapyramidal signs, diaphoresis, rigidity, tachycardia, cardiac dysrhythmias, hypotension, or hypertension	Emesis or gastric lavage; do **not** dialyze; use I.V. benztropine mesylate 0.02-0.05 mg/kg/dose or for adults 1-2 mg/dose slowly over 3-6 minutes for extrapyramidal signs; use loading dose of phenytoin 10-15 mg/kg slow I.V. push for ventricular dysrhythmias; use I.V. fluids and norepinephrine or phenylephrine to treat hypotension; avoid epinephrine which may cause hypotension due to phenothiazine-induced alpha-adrenergic blockade and unopposed epinephrine B_2 action; dantrolene orally 0.5 mg/kg/dose every 12 hours may help with the rigidity
Salicylates	Nausea, vomiting, respiratory alkalosis, hyperthermia, dehydration, hyperapnea, tinnitus, headache, dizziness, metabolic acidosis, coma	Induce emesis or gastric lavage immediately; give charcoal with cathartic via NG tube; correct fluid imbalance by giving D_5LR at 10-20 mL/kg/hour for 1-2 hours, more rapid fluid resuscitation may be needed for patients in shock; use sodium bicarbonate to correct metabolic acidosis and enhance renal elimination by alkalinizing the urine; give supplemental potassium after renal function has been determined to be adequate. Monitor electrolytes; obtain serum salicylate level ≥6 hours postingestion; use poisoning nomogram to assess the significance of the ingestion and the need for more aggressive measures.
Tricyclic antidepressants	Agitation, confusion, hallucinations, urinary retention, hypothermia, hypotension, tachycardia, arrhythmias, widened QRS complex, prolonged PR intervals	Maintain normal temperature; correct acidosis with sodium bicarbonate to increase protein binding and decrease free fraction; correction of acidosis may decrease cardiovascular toxicities; avoid disopyramide, procainamide, and quinidine; lidocaine, phenytoin or propranolol may be necessary; reserve physostigmine for refractory life-treating anticholinergic toxicities. For life-threatening arrhythmias or seizures: Children: I.V., slow: Physostigmine 0.01-0.03 mg/kg/dose up to 0.5 mg/dose over 2-3 minutes, repeat in 5 minutes (maximum total dose is 2 mg). Adolescents and adults: 2 mg/dose physostigmine, may repeat 1-2 mg in 20 minutes and give 1-4 mg slow I.V. over 5-10 minutes if signs and symptoms recur.
Warfarin	Internal or external hemorrhage, hematuria	For moderate overdoses, give oral or I.V. phytonadione; for severe hemorrhage, give fresh frozen plasma or whole blood

Drug or Drug Class	Signs / Symptoms	Treatment/Comments
Xanthine derivatives	Vomiting, abdominal pain, bloody diarrhea, tachycardia, extrasystoles, tachypnea, tonic/clonic seizures	Induce emesis, except in a convulsive patient; give activated charcoal orally; repeated oral doses of activated charcoal may increase clearance; children: 1-2 g/kg/dose, adults: 30-60 g/ dose of activated charcoal every 3-6 hours until nontoxic serum concentrations are obtained. Assure adequate GI motility, supportive therapy; charcoal hemoperfusion can also be effective in decreasing serum concentrations.

[1]As for all overdoses and toxic ingestions, provide airway, breathing, and cardiac support; use appropriate general poisoning management and give general supportive therapy when needed (eg, I.V. fluids, blood pressure support, control seizures, etc). Consult more specific toxicology references (eg, Leikin JB and Paloucek FP, *Poisoning & Toxicology Handbook*, Hudson, OH: Lexi-Comp Inc, 1998, and Poisondex®) for further information.

COMMONLY USED ANTIDOTES FOR ACUTE OVERDOSES

While certain drugs may modify symptoms produced by a toxin, only a relatively few toxins have specific antidotes. The purpose of this chart is to identify those drugs, non-medicinal chemicals, plants, snakes, and spiders to which specific antidotes exist. Please refer to the specific monograph for dosing information. This information does not preclude the use of "conventional" therapeutic modalities for the treatment of intoxication (eg, emesis, lavage, charcoal, etc).

Poisoning Agent	Antidote(s)	Indications	Comments
Chemicals, Nonmedicinal			
Arsenic	Dimercaprol (BAL in Oil®)	• Symptomatic arsenic exposure	• Monitor for hypertension, tachycardia, hyperpyrexia, and urticaria • Pretreatment with diphenhydramine may diminish side effects
Calcium oxide	Edetate calcium disodium (EDTA) (Calcium Disodium Versenate®)	• Eye exposure from calcium oxide	• Immediate irrigation with saline followed by an irrigation with 0.01-0.05 M EDTA solution for at least 15 minutes
Carbon monoxide	Oxygen	• Any suspected carbon monoxide intoxication • Hyperbaric oxygen for any patient with signs and symptoms of severe intoxication regardless of the carboxyhemoglobin concentration • Patients with ischemic heart disease, acute ECG changes, anemia, seizure history, or pregnancy should receive hyperbaric oxygen if the carboxy hemoglobin (COHB) >20% or if any acute symptoms are present	
Carbamate insecticides	Atropine	• Symptomatic bradycardia • Myoclonic seizures, severe hallucinations, weakness, arrhythmias, excessive salivation, involuntary urination and defecation	• Caution should be used in patients with narrow-angle glaucoma, cardiovascular disease, or pregnancy • Plasma and/or erythrocyte cholinesterase levels will be depressed from normal
Copper	Penicillamine (Cuprimine®, Depen®)	• Symptomatic copper intoxication	• Little experience with chelation therapy in the setting of acute ingestion
Cyanide	Amyl nitrite, sodium nitrite, sodium thiosulfate (cyanide antidote kit)	• Begin treatment at the first sign of toxicity if exposure is known or strongly expected	• Do not use methylene blue to reduce elevated methemoglobin levels • Oxygen therapy may be useful when combined with sodium thiosulfate therapy

Poisoning Agent	Antidote(s)	Indications	Comments
Ethylene glycol	Ethanol **OR** Fomepizole (Antizol®)	• Ingestion of >0.25 mL/kg ethylene glycol • Ethylene glycol serum level >20 mg/dL • History or strong clinical suspicion of ingestion and at least two of the following criteria: Arterial pH <7.3 Serum bicarbonate <20 mEq/L Osmolality gap >10 mOsm/L Urinary oxalate crystals present	• Goal: Blood ethanol concentration at least 100 mg/dL (22 mmol/L) • Indications for use of fomepizole over ethanol: Ingestion of multiple substances resulting in depressed level of consciousness, altered consciousness, lack of adequate intensive care staffing or laboratory support to monitor ethanol, critically-ill patient with anion gap metabolic acidosis of unknown origin and potential exposure to ethylene glycol, or patients with active hepatic disease • Continue therapy until ethylene glycol level <10 mg/dL • Monitor blood glucose especially in children as ethanol may cause hypoglycemia
Hydrazine	Pyridoxine (vitamin B_6)	• Antidote for seizures and coma	
Hydrofluoric acid (HF)	Calcium gluconate	• Dermal burns (topical treatment with calcium gluconate gel for dermal exposures of HF <20% concentration) •SubQ injections of calcium gluconate for dermal exposures of HF >20% concentration or failure to respond to calcium gluconate gel	• Oral calcium also used as fluoride-binding agent following oral ingestion • Hypocalcemia occurs frequently following oral ingestion and dermal exposure • Topical calcium gels are not available commercially in U.S.; may be compounded; see Extemporaneous Preparations, Calcium Supplements *on page 272* •Injections of calcium gluconate should not be used in digital area
Hydrogen sulfide	Amyl nitrite **AND** Sodium nitrite	• Severe anoxia, if therapy can be started early – within one hour of exposure	• Do **NOT** use sodium thiosulfate
Lead	Edetate calcium disodium (EDTA) (Calcium Disodium Versenate®) **with or without** Dimercaprol (BAL in Oil®)	Use both calcium EDTA and BAL: • Symptoms of lead encephalopathy and/or blood lead level >70 mcg/dL • Symptomatic without encephalopathy or asymptomatic with blood lead level >70 mcg/dL Use only EDTA for: • Asymptomatic with blood lead level 45-69 mcg/dL	• Do not confuse or interchange therapy of **calcium** disodium edetate with disodium edetate (Chealamide®, Disotate®, Endrate®) – tetany and possibly fatal hypocalcemia may occur • Calcium EDTA should only be administered after adequate urine flow is established • If urine flow is not established, hemodialysis must accompany calcium EDTA dosing
	Succimer (Chemet®)	• Lead level >45 mcg/dL in patients without encephalopathy or protracted vomiting	• Do not use with calcium disodium edetate or BAL

COMMONLY USED ANTIDOTES FOR ACUTE OVERDOSES *(Continued)*

Poisoning Agent	Antidote(s)	Indications	Comments
Manganese	Edetate calcium disodium (EDTA) (Calcium Disodium Versenate®)		• Do not confuse or interchange therapy of **calcium** disodium edetate with disodium edetate (Chealamide®, Disotate®, Endrate®) – tetany and possibly fatal hypocalcemia may occur • Calcium EDTA should only be administered after adequate urine flow is established
Methanol	Ethanol **OR** Fomepizole (Antizol®)	• Anion gap metabolic acidosis associated with a history of methanol ingestion • Methanol blood level >20 mg/dL (6.2 mmoles/L) • Any symptomatic patient with a history of methanol ingestion	• Goal: Ethanol blood level 100-130 mg/dL (22-28 mmoles/L) • Continue therapy until methanol blood level <10 mg/dL • Fomepizole therapy is considered investigational
Organophosphate insecticides	Atropine Pralidoxime (2-PAM, Protopam®)	• Symptomatic bradycardia • Myoclonic seizures, severe hallucinations, weakness, arrhythmias, excessive salivation, involuntary urination and defecation	• Caution should be used in patients with narrow-angle glaucoma, cardiovascular disease, or pregnancy •Most effective when used in initial 24-36 hours after exposure • Plasma and/or erythrocyte cholinesterase levels will be depressed from normal
		Drug / Drug Class	
Acetaminophen	Acetylcysteine (Mucomyst®)	• Serum acetaminophen level >150 mcg/mL at 4 hours postingestion (see Acetaminophen *on page 42*) • Acute ingestion with dose ≥150 mg/kg (child) or 7.5 g (adolescent/adult) within 24 hours of presentation if results of plasma levels cannot be obtained within 8-10 hours of ingestion • Unknown quantity ingested and <24 hours have elapsed since the time of ingestion or unable to obtain serum acetaminophen levels within 12 hours of ingestion • Consider repeating an acetaminophen level 4-6 hours after an initial 4-hour level that is under the treatment range if extended release acetaminophen was ingested • Patients presenting >24 hours postacute ingestion who have measurable levels or biochemical evidence of hepatic injury	• Activated charcoal has been shown to adsorb acetylcysteine; therefore, administer activated charcoal before 4-hour acetaminophen level is drawn • If patient vomits within 1 hour of an oral acetylcysteine dose, readminister the dose • I.V. N-acetylcysteine is now available in the U.S. (see acetylcysteine monograph *on page 51*).

Poisoning Agent	Antidote(s)	Indications	Comments
Anticholinergics	Physostigmine (Antilirium®)	• Refractory seizures or arrhythmias unresponsive to conventional therapy • Symptoms should be life-threatening	• Due to potential for producing severe adverse effects, (eg, seizures, bradycardia) routine use of physostigmine is controversial • Atropine should be available to reverse life-threatening cholinergic effects of physostigmine
Baclofen	Physostigmine (Antilirium®)	• Distinguish anticholinergic delirium from other causes of altered mental status	• Long-lasting reversal of anticholinergic signs and symptoms is generally not achieved due to the relatively short duration of action of physostigmine • Atropine should be available to reverse life-threatening cholinergic effects of physostigmine
Benzodiazepines	Flumazenil (Romazicon®)	• Reverses sedative effects of benzodiazepines	• May procipitate benzodiazepine withdrawal in dependent patients • Not indicated for ethanol, barbiturate, general anesthetic, or narcotic overdose • Mixed drug overdose patients who have ingested drugs that increase the likelihood of seizures (eg, cocaine, lithium, cyclic antidepressants) are at extremely high risk for seizures when flumazenil is used • Action of flumazenil may be shorter than duration of benzodiazepines; repeat doses of flumazenil may be needed • Contraindicated in patients given benzodiazepines for potentially life-threatening conditions (eg, increased intracranial pressure, seizures) and patients with signs of serious cyclic-antidepressant overdosage
Beta-blockers	Isoproterenol (Isuprel®)	• Reversal of bradycardia and hypotension	
	Glucagon	• Reversal of bradycardia unresponsive to isoproterenol	• Glucagon activates adenyl cyclase system at a different site than isoproterenol • Requires liver glycogen stores for hyperglycemic response • I.V. glucose must also be given in treatment of hypoglycemia

COMMONLY USED ANTIDOTES FOR ACUTE OVERDOSES *(Continued)*

Poisoning Agent	Antidote(s)	Indications	Comments
Calcium channel blockers	Calcium chloride **OR** Calcium gluconate	• Reversal of cardiovascular effects of calcium channel blockers (calcium antagonists)	• Monitor serum calcium levels • Calcium is most effective in mild to moderate intoxications • May not be effective in correcting symptomatic bradyarrhythmias
Digitalis glycosides	Digoxin immune Fab (Digibind®)	• Treatment of potentially life-threatening digoxin or digitoxin intoxication in carefully selected patients [serum digoxin level >10 ng/mL or ingestion of >4 mg (child) or >10 mg (adult)] • Life-threatening ventricular arrhythmias secondary to digoxin or digitoxin • Hyperkalemia (K^+ >5 mEq/L) in the setting of digitalis toxicity • Life-threatening cardiac arrhythmias, progressive bradyarrhythmias, second or third degree heart block unresponsive to atropine	• Monitor potassium levels and continuous EKG • Digibind® interferes with the interpretation of serum digoxin/digitoxin levels
Heparin, Enoxaparin, Dalteparin	Protamine	• Severe hemorrhage	• Effect can be immediate and last for 2 hours • Protamine dosage related to anticoagulant dosage and time of anticoagulant administration • Monitor PTT • Monitor for hypotension
Insulin	Dextrose (25%-50%)	• Severe, symptomatic hypoglycemia	• Very hypertonic solutions; dilute with sterile water prior to I.V. administration
Iron	Deferoxamine (Desferal®)	• Serum iron level >350 mcg/mL • Inability to obtain serum iron level within a reasonable time and patient is symptomatic	• Passing of vin rose colored urine indicates free iron was present • Discontinue therapy when urine returns to normal color • Monitor for hypotension during treatment
Isoniazid	Pyridoxine (vitamin B_6)	• Ingestion of >80 mg/kg isoniazid	
Neuromuscular blocking agents, nondepolarizing (eg, pancuronium)	Edrophonium **OR** Neostigmine **OR** Pyridostigmine	• Reversal of neuromuscular blockade	• Atropine should be available to treat acute cholinergic crisis • Not effective for reversal of **depolarizing** neuromuscular blocking agents (eg, succinylcholine)

Poisoning Agent	Antidote(s)	Indications	Comments
Opiates	Naloxone (Narcan®)	• Reversal of symptoms associated with severe toxicity	• May precipitate withdrawal symptoms in patients with physical dependence to opiates • For prolonged intoxication, a continuous infusion may be used
Phenothiazines	Diphenhydramine (Benadryl®) **OR** Benztropine (Cogentin®)	• Reversal of phenothiazine-induced dystonic reactions	
	Sodium bicarbonate	• Reversal of "quinidine-like" cardiovascular effects (eg, prolonged QRS complex) – QRS duration >100 msec – Ventricular dysrhythmias and hypotension	• Goal is arterial pH of 7.45-7.55 and urine pH of 7.5-8 • Attempts at urine alkalinization may be dangerous in patients with renal dysfunction or where sodium and fluid overload may compromise respiratory or cardiac status
Tricyclic antidepressants	Sodium bicarbonate	• Reversal of "quinidine-like" cardiovascular effects (eg, prolonged QRS complex) – QRS duration >100 msec – Ventricular dysrhythmias and hypotension	• Goal is arterial pH of 7.45-7.55 and urine pH of 7.5-8 • Attempts at urine alkalinization may be dangerous in patients with renal dysfunction or where sodium and fluid overload may compromise respiratory or cardiac status
Warfarin	Phytonadione (vitamin K_1)	• Large, acute ingestion • Prothrombin time greater than normal	• Vitamin K is relatively contraindicated in patients with prosthetic heart valves unless toxicity is life-threatening
Zinc	Edetate calcium disodium (EDTA) **and/or** Dimercaprol (BAL in Oil®)	• Symptomatic zinc ingestion	• Few case reports • Monitor zinc levels
		Plants	
Foxglove Oleander	Digoxin immune Fab (Digibind®)	• Severely intoxicated patients who fail to respond to conventional therapy • Life-threatening ventricular arrhythmias, progressive bradyarrhythmias, or second- or third degree heart block not responsive to atropine • Hyperkalemia (K^+ >5 mEq/L) in the setting of digitalis toxicity	• Monitor potassium levels and continuous EKG
Mushroom (genus *Gyomitra*)	Pyridoxine (vitamin B_6)		
Mushrooms containing muscarine (inocybe or clitocybe)	Atropine	•Myoclonic seizures, severe hallucinations, weakness, arrhythmias, excessive salivation, involuntary urination and defecation	•Atropine should only be used when indicated; otherwise use may result in anticholinergic poisoning

COMMONLY USED ANTIDOTES FOR ACUTE OVERDOSES *(Continued)*

Poisoning Agent	Antidote(s)	Indications	Comments
Snake Bites			
Coral snakes (Eastern and Texas coral snakes only)	Antivenin *(Micrurus fulvius)*		• Not effective for Arizona or Sonoran coral snakes • Skin testing is recommended • Treatment for hypersensitivity reactions, including anaphylaxis, should be available
Pit vipers (Rattlesnakes, cottonmouths, copperheads)	Antivenin *(Crotalidae)* Polyvalent (equine origin)	• Administration within 4 hours of envenomation is ideal; however, administer within 30 hours in all severe cases of poisoning	• Skin testing is recommended • Treatment for hypersensitivity reactions, including anaphylaxis, should be available
Spiders, Scorpions			
Black widow spider	Antivenin *(Lactrodectus mactans)*	• Severe symptoms including respiratory failure, seizures, or pain and spasms not relieved by calcium, muscle relaxants, or analgesics • Symptomatic pregnant patients • Children <5 years or adults >60 years (at greatest risk for severe toxicity)	• Either dermal or conjunctival sensitivity testing should be done prior to administration of antivenin
Scorpion	Antivenin *(Centruroides)*		• No FDA-approved *Centruroides* antivenin in U.S.; only a *Centruroides exilicauda (sculpturatus)*-specific antivenin is available in Arizona (for intrastate use only)

Leikin JR and Paloucek FP, "Poisoning & Toxicology Compendium," Hudson, OH: Lexi-Comp, Inc, 1998.

Mowry JB, Furbee RB, and Chyka PA, "Poisoning," *Essentials of Critical Care Pharmacology,* 3rd ed, Baltimore, MD: Williams & Wilkens, 1994, 501-29.

Zed PJ and Krenzelok EP, "Treatment of Acetaminophen Overdose," *Am J Health Syst Pharm,* 1999, 56(11):1081-91.

ANION GAP

Definition: The difference in concentration between unmeasured cation and anion equivalents in serum.

Anion gap = Na^+ - Cl^- - HCO_3^-
(The normal anion gap is 10-14 mEq/L.)

Differential diagnosis of increased anion gap

- Organic anions
  - Lactate (sepsis, hypovolemia, large tumor burden)
  - Pyruvate
  - Uremia
  - Ketoacidosis (β-hydroxybutyrate and acetoacetate)
  - Amino acids and their metabolites
  - Other organic acids (eg, formate from methanol, glycolate from ethylene glycol)
- Inorganic anions
  - Hyperphosphatemia
  - Sulfates
  - Nitrates
- Medications and toxins
  - Penicillins and cephalosporins
  - Salicylates (including aspirin)
  - Cyanide
  - Carbon monoxide

Differential diagnosis of decreased anion gap

- Organic cations
  - Hypergammaglobulinemia
- Inorganic cations
  - Hyperkalemia
  - Hypercalcemia
  - Hypermagnesemia
- Medications and toxins
  - Lithium
- Hypoalbuminemia

LABORATORY DETECTION OF DRUGS IN URINE

Agent	Time Detectable in Urine[1]
Alcohol	12-24 h
Amobarbital	2-4 d
Amphetamine	2-4 d
Butalbital	2-4 d
Cannabinoids	
Occasional use	2-7 d
Regular use	30 d
Cocaine (benzoylecgonine)	12-72 h
Codeine	2-4 d
Chlordiazepoxide	30 d
Diazepam	30 d
Ethanol	12-24 h
Heroin (morphine)	2-4 d
Hydromorphone	2-4 d
Marijuana	
Occasional use	2-7 d
Regular use	30 d
Methamphetamine	2-4 d
Methaqualone	2-4 d
Morphine	2-4 d
Pentobarbital	2-4 d
Phencyclidine (PCP)	
Occasional use	2-7 d
Regular use	30 d
Phenobarbital	30 d
Secobarbital	2-4 d

[1]The periods of detection for the various abused drugs listed above should be taken as estimates since the actual figures will vary due to metabolism, user, laboratory, and excretion.

Adapted from Chang JY, "Drug Testing and Interpretation of Results," *Pharmchem Newsletter*, 1989, 17:1.

OSMOLALITY

Definition: The summed concentrations of all osmotically active solute particles.

Predicted serum osmolality =

2 Na^+ (mEq/L) + glucose (mg/dL) / 18 + BUN (mg/dL) / 2.8

The normal range of serum osmolality is 285-295 mOsm/L.

Differential diagnosis of increased serum osmolal gap (increased by >10 mOsm/L)

Medications and toxins

- Alcohols (ethanol, methanol, isopropanol, glycerol, ethylene glycol)
- Mannitol
- Paraldehyde

SALICYLATE INTOXICATION

Serum Salicylate Level and Severity of Intoxication Single Dose Acute Ingestion Nomogram

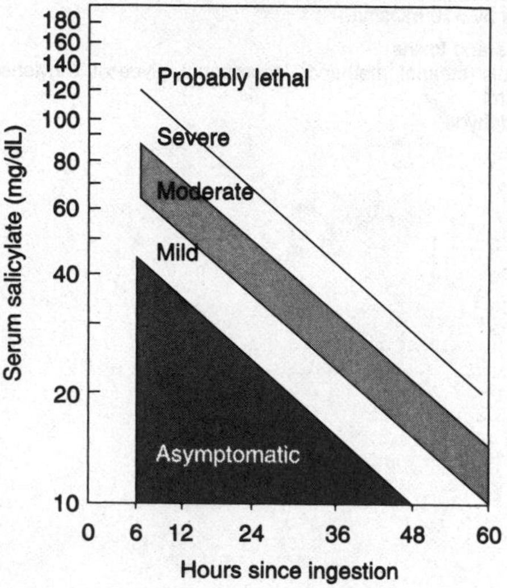

Nomogram relating serum salicylate concentration and expected severity of intoxication at varying intervals following the ingestion of a single dose of salicylate.
From Done AK, "Aspirin Overdosage: Incidence, Diagnosis, and Management," *Pediatrics*, 1978, 62:890-7 with permission.

ACETAMINOPHEN

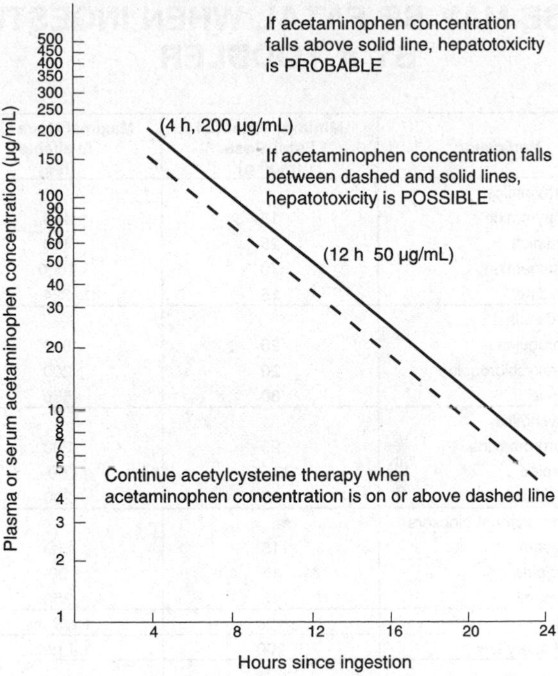

Nomogram relating plasma or serum acetaminophen concentration and probability of hepatotoxicity at varying intervals following ingestion of a single toxic dose of acetaminophen. Modified from Rumack BH, Matthew H, "Acetaminophen Poisoning and Toxicity", Pediatrics, 1975, 55:871-6,
© American Academy of Pediatrics, 1975, and from Rumack BH, et al, "Acetaminophen Overdose", *Arch Intern Med*, 1981, 141:380-5, © American Medical Association.

MEDICATIONS FOR WHICH A SINGLE DOSE MAY BE FATAL WHEN INGESTED BY A TODDLER

Medication[1]	Minimal Potential Fatal Dose (mg/kg)	Maximal Dose Unit Available (mg)
Antiarrhythmics		
Disopyramide	15	150
Flecainide	25	150
Procainamide	70	1000
Quinidine	15	324
Antimalarials		
Chloroquine	20	500
Hydroxychloroquine	20	200
Quinine	80	650
Antipsychotics		
Chlorpromazine	25	200
Loxapine	30-70	50
Thioridazine	15	200
Calcium channel blockers		
Diltiazem	15	360
Nifedipine	15	90
Verapamil	15	360
Camphor	100	1 g/5 mL
Methyl salicylate	200	1.4 g/mL
Narcotics		
Codeine	7-14	60
Hydrocodone	1.5	60 mg/5 mL
Methadone	1-2	40
Morphine		200
Oral hypoglycemics		
Chlorpropamide	5	25
Glibenclamide	0.1	2.5
Glipizide	0.1	5
Podophyllin 25%	15-20	1.25 g/5 mL
Theophylline	8.4	500
Tricyclic antidepressants		
Amitriptyline	15	100
Desipramine	15	150
Imipramine	15	75

[1]Assumptions: Toddler would weigh 10 kg; the lowest described or estimated fatal dose (adjusted for body weight) was used; the toddler is healthy, with normal drug metabolism.

Adapted from Bar-Oz B, Levichek Z, and Koren G, "Medications That Can Be Fatal for a Toddler With One Tablet or Teaspoonful: A 2004 Update," *Paediatr Drugs*, 2004, 6(2):123-6.

BREAST-FEEDING AND DRUGS

Prior to recommending or prescribing medications to a lactating woman, the following should be considered:

- Is drug therapy necessary?
- Can drug exposure to the infant be minimized? (Using a different route of administration, timing of the dose in relation to breast-feeding, length of therapy, using breast milk stored prior to treatment, etc)
- The infants age and health status (their own ability to metabolize the medication)
- The pharmacokinetics of the drug
- Will the drug interact with a medication the infant is prescribed?
- If medications must be used, pick the safest drug possible.
- In situations where the only drug available may have adverse effects in the nursing infant, consider measuring the infants blood levels.

The tables presented below have been adapted from the American Academy of Pediatrics Committee on Drugs report "Transfer of Drugs and Other Chemicals Into Human Milk," September 2001. It should not be inferred that if a medication is not in the tables it is considered safe for administration to a lactating woman; only that published reports concerning their use were not available at the time the report was published.

Table 1. Cytotoxic Drugs

Cyclophosphamide	Doxorubicin
Cyclosporine	Methotrexate

These are medications thought to interfere with cellular metabolism in the nursing infant. Immune suppression may be possible; effects on growth or carcinogenesis are not known. In addition, doxorubicin is concentrated in human milk; methotrexate is associated with neutropenia in the nursing infant.

Table 2. Drugs of Abuse

Amphetamine	Marijuana
Cocaine	Phencyclidine
Heroin	

Drugs of abuse are not only dangerous to the nursing infant, but also to the mother. Women should be encouraged to avoid their use completely. Effects to the infant reported with amphetamine use in the mother include irritability and poor sleeping; it is also a substance that is concentrated in human milk. Cocaine may cause irritability, vomiting, diarrhea, tremors, or seizures in the infant. Heroin may also cause tremors as well as restlessness, vomiting, and poor feeding.

Nicotine, which was previously on this list, is associated with decreased milk production, decreased weight gain in the infant, and possible increased respiratory illness in the infant. Although there are still questions outstanding regarding smoking and breast-feeding, women should be counseled on the possible effects to their infants and offered aid to smoking cessation if appropriate.

BREAST-FEEDING AND DRUGS *(Continued)*

Table 3. Radioactive Compounds That Require Temporary Cessation of Breast-Feeding

Drug	Recommended Time for Cessation of Breast-Feeding
Copper 64 (^{64}Cu)	Radioactivity in milk present at 50 h
Gallium 67 (^{67}Ga)	Radioactivity in milk present for 2 wk
Indium 111 (^{111}In)	Very small amount present at 20 h
Iodine 123 (^{123}I)	Radioactivity in milk present up to 36 h
Iodine 125 (^{125}I)	Radioactivity in milk present for 12 d
Iodine 131 (^{131}I)	Radioactivity in milk present 2-14 d, depending on study
Iodine^{131}	If used for thyroid cancer, high radioactivity may prolong exposure to infant
Radioactive sodium	Radioactivity in milk present 96 h
Technetium-99m (^{99m}Tc), ^{99m}Tc macroaggregates, ^{99m}Tc O4	Radioactivity in milk present 15 h to 3 d

Consider pumping and storing milk prior to study for use during the radioactive period. Pumping should continue after the study to maintain milk production; however, this milk should be discarded until radioactivity is gone. Notify nuclear medicine physician prior to study that the mother is breast-feeding; a short-acting radionuclide may be appropriate. Contact Radiology Department after testing is complete to screen milk samples before resuming feeding.

Table 4a. Psychotropic Drugs Whose Effect on Nursing Infants Is Unknown But May Be of Concern

Antianxiety	Antidepressant	Antipsychotic
Alprazolam	Amitriptyline	Chlorpromazine
Diazepam	Amoxapine	Chlorprothixene
Lorazepam	Bupropion	Clozapine[1]
Midazolam	Clomipramine	Haloperidol
Perphenazine	Desipramine	Mesoridazine
Prazepam[1]	Dothiepin	Trifluoperazine
Quazepam	Doxepin	
Temazepam	Fluoxetine	
	Fluvoxamine	
	Imipramine	
	Nortriptyline	
	Paroxetine	
	Sertraline[1]	
	Trazodone	

[1]Drug is concentrated in human milk.

Psychotropic medications usually appear in the breast milk in low concentrations. Although adverse effects in the infant may be limited to a few case reports, the long half-life of these medications and their metabolites should be considered. In addition, measurable amounts may be found in the infants plasma and also brain tissue. Long-term effects are not known. Colic, irritability, feeding and sleep disorders, and slow weight gain are effects reported with fluoxetine. Chlorpromazine may cause galactorrhea in the mother, while drowsiness and lethargy have been reported in the nursing infant. A decline in developmental scores has been reported with chlorpromazine and haloperidol.

Table 4b. Additional Drugs Whose Effect on Nursing Infants Is Unknown But May Be of Concern

Drug	Reported Effect In Nursing Infant
Amiodarone	Hypothyroidism
Chloramphenicol	Idiosyncratic bone marrow suppression
Clofazimine	Increase in skin pigmentation; high transfer of mothers dose to infant is possible
Lamotrigine	Therapeutic serum concentrations in infant
Metoclopramide[1]	
Metronidazole	
Tinidazole	

[1]Drug is concentrated in human milk.

No adverse effects to the infant have been reported for metoclopramide; however, it should be recognized that it is a dopaminergic agent. Metronidazole and tinidazole are *in vitro* mutagenic agents. In cases where single dose therapy is appropriate for the mother, breast-feeding may be discontinued for 12-24 hours to allow excretion of the medication.

Table 5. Drugs That Have Been Associated With Significant Effects on Some Nursing Infants and Should Be Given to Nursing Mothers With Caution[1]

Drug	Reported Effect
Acebutolol	Hypotension, bradycardia, tachypnea
5-Aminosalicylic acid	Diarrhea (one case)
Atenolol	Cyanosis, bradycardia
Bromocriptine	Suppresses lactation; may be hazardous to the mother
Aspirin (salicylates)	Metabolic acidosis (one case)
Clemastine	Drowsiness, irritability, refusal to feed, high-pitched cry, neck stiffness (one case)
Ergotamine	Vomiting, diarrhea, convulsions (doses used in migraine medications
Lithium	One-third to one-half therapeutic blood concentration in infants
Phenindone	Anticoagulant: increased prothrombin and partial thromboplastin time in one infant; not used in the United States
Phenobarbital	Sedation; infantile spasms after weaning from milk-containing phenobarbital, methemoglobinemia (one case)
Primidone	Sedation, feeding problems
Sulfasalazine (salicylazosulfapyridine)	Bloody diarrhea (one case)

[1]Blood concentration in the infant may be of clinical importance; measure when possible.

BREAST-FEEDING AND DRUGS *(Continued)*

Table 6. Maternal Medication Usually Compatible With Breast-Feeding

Drug	Reported Effect
Acetaminophen	
Acetazolamide	
Acitretin	
Acyclovir[1]	
Alcohol (ethanol)	Large amounts may lead to drowsiness, diaphoresis, deep sleep, weakness, decreased linear growth, and/or abnormal weight gain. Ingestion of 1 g/kg/d decreases mothers milk ejection reflex.
Allopurinol	
Amoxicillin	
Antimony	
Atropine	
Azapropazone (apazone)	
Aztreonam	
B_1 (thiamine)	
B_6 (pyridoxine)	
B_{12}	
Baclofen	
Barbiturate	Refer to Table 5
Bendroflumethiazide	Lactation suppressed
Bishydroxycoumarin (Dicumarol®)	
Bromide	Rash, weakness, absence of cry with maternal intake of 5.4 g/d
Butorphanol	
Caffeine	Irritability and poor sleep may be seen with >2-3 cups/d; excreted slowly
Captopril	
Carbamazepine	
Carbetocin	
Carbimazole	Goiter
Cascara	
Cefadroxil	
Cefazolin	
Cefotaxime	
Cefoxitin	
Cefprozil	
Ceftazidime	
Ceftriaxone	
Chloral hydrate	Sleepiness
Chloroform	
Chloroquine	
Chlorothiazide	
Chlorthalidone	Slow excretion
Cimetidine[1]	
Ciprofloxacin	Theoretically, may affect cartilage in weight-bearing joints; pseudomembranous colitis reported in one infant
Cisapride	
Cisplatin	Not found in milk
Clindamycin	

Table 6. Maternal Medication Usually Compatible With Breast-Feeding *(continued)*

Drug	Reported Effect
Clogestone	
Codeine	
Colchicine	
Contraceptive pill with estrogen and progesterone	Breast enlargement (rare), decreased milk production and protein count (unconfirmed)
Cycloserine	
D (vitamin)	Infant calcium levels should be monitored if mother receives pharmacologic doses
Danthron	Bowel activity increased
Dapsone	No effects reported, but sulfonamide detected in infants urine
Dexbrompheniramine maleate with d-isoephedrine	Crying, poor sleeping patterns, irritability
Diatrizoate	
Digoxin	
Diltiazem	
Dipyrone	
Disopyramide	
Domperidone	
Dyphylline[1]	
Enalapril	
Erythromycin[1]	
Estradiol	Withdrawal, vaginal bleeding
Ethambutol	
Ethanol	See alcohol
Ethosuximide	No effects reported, but detected in infants urine
Fentanyl	
Fexofenadine	
Flecainide	
Fleroxacin	In one report, a single 400 mg dose was administered to the mother and breast milk not given to infant for 48 hours
Fluconazole	
Flufenamic acid	
Fluorescein	
Folic acid	
Gadopentetic (Gadolinium)	
Gentamicin	
Gold salts	
Halothane	
Hydralazine	
Hydrochlorothiazide	
Hydroxychloroquine[1]	
Ibuprofen	
Indomethacin	Seizure (one case)
Iodides	May affect thyroid activity; see Iodine
Iodine	Goiter
Iodine (povidone-iodine/ vaginal douche)	Increased iodine levels in breast milk; iodine odor on infants skin
Iohexol	
Iopanoic acid	
Isoniazid	Metabolite secreted in breast milk; no hepatotoxicity reported in infant

BREAST-FEEDING AND DRUGS *(Continued)*

Table 6. Maternal Medication Usually Compatible With Breast-Feeding *(continued)*

Drug	Reported Effect
Interferon alfa	
Ivermectin	
K_1 (vitamin)	
Kanamycin	
Ketoconazole	
Ketorolac	
Labetalol	
Levonorgestrel	
Levothyroxine	
Lidocaine	
Loperamide	
Loratadine	
Magnesium sulfate	
Medroxyprogesterone	
Mefenamic acid	
Meperidine	
Methadone	
Methimazole (active metabolite of carbimazole)	
Methyldopa	
Methprylon	Drowsiness
Metoprolol[1]	
Metrizamide	
Metrizoate	
Mexiletine	
Minoxidil	
Morphine	No effects reported but found in infants serum
Moxalactam	
Nadolol[1]	
Nalidixic acid	Hemolysis reported in infant with glucose-g-phosphate dehydrogenase deficiency
Naproxen	
Nefopam	
Nifedipine	
Nitrofurantoin	Hemolysis reported in infant with G6PD deficiency
Norethynodrel	
Norsteroids	
Noscapine	
Ofloxacin	Theoretically, may affect cartilage in weight-bearing joints
Oxprenolol	
Phenylbutazone	
Phenytoin	
Piroxicam	
Prednisolone	
Prednisone	
Procainamide	
Progesterone	
Propoxyphene	
Propranolol	

Table 6. Maternal Medication Usually Compatible With Breast-Feeding *(continued)*

Drug	Reported Effect
Propylthiouracil	
Pseudoephedrine[1]	
Pyridostigmine	
Pyrimethamine	
Quinidine	
Quinine	
Riboflavin	
Rifampin	
Scopolamine	
Secobarbital	
Senna	
Sotalol	
Spironolactone	
Streptomycin	
Sulbactam	
Sulfapyridine	Use with caution in infants with G6PD deficiency and in ill, stressed, or premature infants
Sulfisoxazole	Use with caution in infants with G6PD deficiency and in ill, stressed, or premature infants
Sumatriptan	
Suprofen	
Terbutaline	
Terfenadine	
Tetracycline	Negligible absorption by infant; potential to stain infants unerupted teeth
Theophylline	Irritability
Thiopental	
Thiouracil	
Ticarcillin	
Timolol	
Tolbutamide	Jaundice is possible
Tolmetin	
Trimethoprim and sulfamethoxazole	
Triprolidine	
Valproic acid	
Verapamil	
Vitamin (see individual entries, eg, B_1, B_6, B_{12}, D, K)	
Warfarin	
Zolpidem	

[1]Drug is concentrated in human milk.

BREAST-FEEDING AND DRUGS *(Continued)*

Table 7. Selected Food and Environmental Agents

Agent	Effect Related to Breast-Feeding
Aspartame	Use with caution if mother or infant has phenylketonuria
Chocolate	Irritability or increased bowel activity observed in infant when >16 oz/d consumed by mother
Fava beans	Hemolysis reported in infant with G6PD deficiency
Hexachlorobenzene	Skin rash, diarrhea, vomiting, dark urine, neurotoxicity, death
Hexachlorophene	No effects reported; however, possibility of milk contamination following nipple washing
Lead	Neurotoxicity possible
Mercury, methylmercury	Possible effects on neurodevelopment
Silicone breast implants	Breast-feeding not contraindicated
Vegetarian diet	B_{12} deficiency

References

American Academy of Pediatrics Committee on Drugs, "Transfer of Drugs and Other Chemicals Into Human Milk," *Pediatrics*, 2001, 108(3): 776-89.

2000 Red Book: Report of the Committee on Infectious Diseases, 25th ed, Elk Grove Village, IL: American Academy of Pediatrics, 2000, 98-104.

COMPATIBILITY OF MEDICATIONS MIXED IN A SYRINGE

	Atropine	Chlorpromazine	Codeine	Diphenhydramine	Droperidol	Fentanyl	Glycopyrrolate	Hydroxyzine	Meperidine	Metoclopramide	Midazolam	Morphine	Pentazocine	Pentobarbital†	Prochlorperazine	Promazine	Promethazine	Trimethobenzamide
Atropine		C	•	C	C	C	C	C	C	C	C	C	C	C	C	C	C	•
Chlorpromazine	C		•	C	C	C	C	C	C	C	C	C	C	X	C	C	C	•
Codeine	•	•		•	•	•	C	C	•	•	•	•	•	X	•	•	•	•
Diphenhydramine	C	C	•		C	C	C	C	C	C	C	C	C	X	C	C	C	•
Droperidol	C	C	•	C		C	C	C	C	C	C	C	C	X	C	C	C	•
Fentanyl	C	C	•	C	C		C	C	C	C	C	C	C	X	C	C	C	•
Glycopyrrolate	C	C	C	C	C	C		C	C	•	C	C	X	X	C	C	C	C
Hydroxyzine	C	C	C	C	C	C	C		C	C	C	C	C	X	C	C	C	•
Meperidine	C	C	•	C	C	C	C	C		C	C	X	C	X	C	C	C	•
Metoclopramide	C	C	•	C	C	C	•	C	C		C	C	C	•	C	C	C	•
Midazolam	C	C	•	C	C	C	C	C	C	C		C	•	X	X	C	C	C
Morphine	C	C	•	C	C	C	C	C	C	C	C		C	X	C*	C	C	•
Pentazocine	C	C	•	C	C	C	C	C	C	C	•	C		X	C	C	C	C
Pentobarbital†	C	X	X	X	X	X	X	X	X	•	X	X	X		X	X	X	•
Prochlorperazine	C	C	•	C	C	C	C	C	C	C	X	C*	C	X		C	C	•
Promazine	C	C	•	C	C	C	C	C	C	C	C	C	C	X	C		C	•
Promethazine	C	C	•	C	C	C	C	C	C	C	C	C	C	X	C	C		•
Trimethobenzamide	•	•	•	•	•	•	C	•	•	•	C	•	C	•	•	•	•	

C = physically compatible if used within 15 minutes after mixing in a syringe.
X = incompatible.
• = no documented information.
C* = potential incompatibility produced by certain manufacturers.
† = compatibility profile is characteristic of most barbiturate salts, such as phenobarbital and secobarbital.

The following combinations have been found to be compatible:

atropine / meperidine / promethazine
atropine / meperidine / hydroxyzine
meperidine / promethazine / chlorpromazine

The following drugs should not be mixed with any other drugs in the same syringe:

diazepam, chlordiazepoxide

References

Forman JK and Sourney PF, "Visual Compatibility of Midazolam Hydrochloride With Common Preoperative Injectable Medications," *Am J Hosp Pharm*, 1987, 44(10):2298-9.

King JC, "Guide to Parenteral Admixtures," St Louis, MO: Cutter Laboratories, 1986.

Parker WA, *Hosp Pharm*, 1984, 19:475-8.

Trissel LA, "Handbook on Injectable Drugs," 5th ed, Bethesda, MD: American Society of Health-System Pharmacists, Inc, 1988.

Stevenson JG and Patriarca C, "Incompatibility of Morphine Sulfate and Prochlorperazine Edisylate in Syringes," *Am J Hosp Pharm*, 1985, 42:2651.

CONTROLLED SUBSTANCES

Note: These are federal classifications. Your individual state may place a substance into a more restricted category. When this occurs, the more restricted category applies. Consult your state law.

Schedule I = C-I

The drugs and other substances in this schedule have no legal medical uses except research. They have a **high** potential for abuse. They include opiates, opium derivatives, and hallucinogens.

Schedule II = C-II

The drugs and other substances in this schedule have legal medical uses and a **high** abuse potential which may lead to severe dependence. They include former "Class A" narcotics, amphetamines, barbiturates, and other drugs.

Schedule III = C-III

The drugs and other substances in this schedule have legal medical uses and a **lesser** degree of abuse potential which may lead to **moderate** dependence. They include former "Class B" narcotics and other drugs.

Schedule IV = C-IV

The drugs and other substances in this schedule have legal medical uses and **low** abuse potential which may lead to **moderate** dependence. They include barbiturates, benzodiazepines, propoxyphenes, and other drugs.

Schedule V = C-V

The drugs and other substances in this schedule have legal medical uses and **low** abuse potential which may lead to **moderate** dependence. They include narcotic cough preparations, diarrhea preparations, and other drugs.

FEVER DUE TO DRUGS

Most Common

Atropine
Amphotericin B
Asparaginase
Barbiturates
Bleomycin
Cephalosporins
Interferon
Methyldopa
Penicillins
Phenytoin
Procainamide
Quinidine
Salicylates (high doses)
Streptomycin
Sulfonamides

Less Common

Allopurinol
Antihistamines
Azathioprine
Carbamazepine
Cimetidine
Cisplatin
Colistimethate
Diazoxide
Folic acid
Hydralazine
Hydroxyurea
Imipenem
Iodides
Isoniazid
Mercaptopurine
Metoclopramide
Nifedipine
NSAIDs
Nitrofurantoin
Pentazocine
Procarbazine
Propylthiouracil
Rifampin
Streptokinase
Triamterene
Vancomycin

References

Cunha BA, "Antibiotic Side Effects," *Med Clin North Am*, 2001, 85(1):149-85.
Mackowiak PA and LeMaistre CF, "Drug Fever: A Critical Appraisal of Conventional Concepts. An Analysis of 51 Episodes in Two Dallas Hospitals and 97 Episodes Reported in the English Literature," *Ann Intern Med*, 1987, 106(5):728-33.
Tabor PA, "Drug-Induced Fever," Table 2, "Drugs Implicated in Causing a Fever," *Drug Intell Clin Pharm*, 1986, 20(6):416.

DISCOLORATION OF FECES DUE TO DRUGS

Black
Acetazolamide
Alcohols
Alkalies
Aluminum hydroxide
Aminophylline
Aminosalicylic acid
Amphetamine
Amphotericin
Antacids
Anticoagulants
Aspirin
Betamethasone
Bismuth
Charcoal
Chloramphenicol
Chlorpropamide
Clindamycin
Corticosteroids
Cortisone
Cyclophosphamide
Cytarabine
Dicumarol
Digitalis
Ethacrynic acid
Ferrous salts
Floxuridine
Fluorides
Fluorouracil
Halothane
Heparin
Hydralazine
Hydrocortisone
Ibuprofen
Indomethacin
Iodine drugs
Iron salts
Levarterenol
Levodopa
Manganese
Melphalan
Methylprednisolone
Methotrexate
Methylene blue
Oxyphenbutazone
Paraldehyde
Phenacetin
Phenolphthalein
Phenylbutazone
Phenylephrine
Phosphorous
Potassium salts
Prednisolone
Procarbazine
Pyrvinium
Reserpine
Salicylates
Sulfonamides
Tetracycline
Theophylline
Thiotepa
Triamcinolone
Warfarin

Blue
Chloramphenicol
Methylene blue

Dark Brown
Dexamethasone

Gray
Colchicine

Green
Indomethacin
Iron
Medroxyprogesterone

Greenish Gray
Oral antibiotics
Oxyphenbutazone
Phenylbutazone

Light Brown
Anticoagulants

Orange-Red
Phenazopyridine
Rifampin

Pink
Anticoagulants
Aspirin
Heparin
Oxyphenbutazone
Phenylbutazone
Salicylates

Red
Anticoagulants
Aspirin
Heparin
Oxyphenbutazone
Phenolphthalein
Phenylbutazone
Pyrvinium
Salicylates
Tetracycline syrup

Red-Brown
Oxyphenbutazone
Phenylbutazone
Rifampin

Tarry
Ergot preparations
Ibuprofen
Salicylates
Warfarin

White/Speckling
Aluminum hydroxide
Antibiotics (oral)
Indocyanine green

Yellow
Senna

Yellow-Green
Senna

Adapted from Drugdex® — Drug Consults, Micromedex, Vol 62, Denver, CO: Rocky Mountain Drug Consultation Center, 1998.

DISCOLORATION OF URINE DUE TO DRUGS

Black
Cascara
Cotrimoxazole
Ferrous salts
Iron dextran
Levodopa
Methocarbamol
Methyldopa
Naphthalene
Pamaquine
Phenacetin
Phenols
Quinine
Sulfonamides

Blue
Anthraquinone
DeWitt's pills
Indigo blue
Indigo carmine
Methocarbamol
Methylene blue
Mitoxantrone
Nitrofurans
Resorcinol
Triamterene

Blue-Green
Amitriptyline
Anthraquinone
DeWitt's pills
Doan's® pills
Indigo blue
Indigo carmine
Magnesium salicylate
Methylene blue
Resorcinol

Brown
Anthraquinone dyes
Cascara
Chloroquine
Hydroquinone
Levodopa
Methocarbamol
Methyldopa
Methocarbamol
Metronidazole
Nitrofurans
Nitrofurantoin
Pamaquine
Phenacetin
Phenols
Primaquine
Quinine
Rifabutin
Rifampin
Senna
Sodium diatrizoate
Sulfonamides

Brown-Black
Isosorbide mono- or dinitrate
Methyldopa
Metronidazole
Nitrates
Nitrofurans
Phenacetin
Povidone iodine
Quinine
Senna

Dark
p-Aminosalicylic acid
Cascara
Levodopa
Metronidazole
Nitrites
Phenacetin
Phenol
Primaquine
Quinine
Resorcinol
Riboflavin
Senna

Green
Amitriptyline
Anthraquinone
DeWitt's pills
Indigo blue
Indigo carmine
Indomethacin
Methocarbamol
Methylene blue
Nitrofurans
Phenols
Propofol
Resorcinol
Suprofen

Green-Yellow
DeWitt's pills
Methylene blue

Milky
Phosphates

Orange
Chlorzoxazone
Dihydroergotamine mesylate
Heparin sodium
Phenazopyridine
Phenindione
Rifabutin
Rifampin
Sulfasalazine
Warfarin

Orange-Red-Brown
Chlorzoxazone
Doxidan
Phenazopyridine
Rifampin
Warfarin

Orange-Yellow
Fluorescein sodium
Rifampin
Sulfasalazine

Pink
Aminopyrine
Anthraquinone dyes
Aspirin
Cascara
Danthron
Deferoxamine
Merbromin
Methyldopa
Phenazopyridone
Phenolphthalein
Phenothiazines
Phenytoin
Salicylates
Senna

Purple
Phenolphthalein

Red
Anthraquinone
Cascara
Chlorpromazine
Daunorubicin
Deferoxamine
Dihydroergotamine mesylate
Dimethyl sulfoxide
DMSO
Doxorubicin
Heparin
Ibuprofen
Methyldopa
Oxyphenbutazone
Phenacetin
Phenazopyridine
Phenolphthalein
Phenothiazines
Phensuximide
Phenylbutazone
Phenytoin
Rifampin
Senna

Red-Brown
Cascara
Deferoxamine
Methyldopa
Oxyphenbutazone
Pamaquine
Phenacetin
Phenazopyridine
Phenolphthalein
Phenothiazines
Phenylbutazone
Phenytoin
Quinine
Senna

Red-Purple
Chlorzoxazone
Ibuprofen
Phenacetin
Senna

DISCOLORATION OF URINE DUE TO DRUGS *(Continued)*

Rust
Cascara
Chloroquine
Metronidazole
Nitrofurantoin
Pamaquine
Phenacetin
Quinacrine
Riboflavin
Senna
Sulfonamides

Yellow
Nitrofurantoin
Phenacetin
Quinacrine
Riboflavin
Sulfasalazine

Yellow-Brown
Aminosalicylate acid
Bismuth
Cascara
Chloroquine
DeWitt's pills
Methylene blue
Metronidazole
Nitrofurantoin
Pamaquine
Primaquine
Quinacrine
Senna
Sulfonamides

Yellow-Pink
Cascara
Senna

Adapted from Drugdex® — Drug Consults, Micromedex, Vol 62, Denver, CO: Rocky Mountain Drug Consultation Center, 1998.

DRUGS IN PREGNANCY

Medications Known to Be Teratogens

- Alcohol
- Androgens
- Anticonvulsants
- Antineoplastics
- Cocaine
- Diethylstilbestrol
- Etretinate
- Iodides (including radioactive iodine)
- Isotretinoin
- Lithium
- Live vaccines
- Methimazole
- Penicillamine
- Tetracyclines
- Warfarin

Medications Suspected to Be Teratogens

- ACE inhibitors
- Benzodiazepines
- Estrogens
- Oral hypoglycemic drugs
- Progestogens
- Quinolones

Medications With No Known Teratogenic Effects[1]

- Acetaminophen
- Cephalosporins
- Corticosteroids
- Docusate sodium
- Erythromycin
- Multiple vitamins
- Narcotic analgesics
- Penicillins
- Phenothiazines
- Thyroid hormones
- Tricyclic antidepressants

[1]No drug is absolutely without risk during pregnancy. These drugs appear to have a minimal risk when used judiciously in usual doses under the supervision of a medical professional.

Medications With Nonteratogenic Adverse Effects in Pregnancy

- Antithyroid drugs
- Aminoglycosides
- Aspirin
- Barbiturates (chronic use)
- Benzodiazepines
- Beta-blockers
- Caffeine
- Chloramphenicol
- Cocaine
- Diuretics
- Isoniazid
- Narcotic analgesics (chronic use)
- Nicotine
- Nonsteroidal anti-inflammatory agents
- Oral hypoglycemic agents
- Propylthiouracil
- Sulfonamides

Adapted from DiPiro JT, Talbert RL, Hayes PE, et al, "Therapeutic Considerations During Pregnancy and Lactation," *Pharmacotherapy: A Pathophysiologic Approach*, 4th ed, Stamford, CT: Appleton & Lange, 1999.

MILLIEQUIVALENT FOR SELECTED IONS

Approximate Milliequivalents — Weights of Selected Ions

Salt	mEq/g Salt	mg Salt/mEq
Calcium carbonate ($CaCO_3$)	20	50
Calcium chloride ($CaCl_2•2H_2O$)	14	73
Calcium gluconate (Ca $gluconate_2•1H_2O$)	4	224
Calcium lactate (Ca $lactate_2•5H_2O$)	6	154
Magnesium sulfate ($MgSO_4$)	16	60
Magnesium sulfate ($MgSO_4•7H_2O$)	8	123
Potassium acetate (K acetate)	10	98
Potassium chloride (KCl)	13	75
Potassium citrate (K_3 citrate$•1H_2O$)	9	108
Potassium iodide (KI)	6	166
Sodium bicarbonate ($NaHCO_3$)	12	84
Sodium chloride (NaCl)	17	58
Sodium citrate (Na_3 citrate$•2H_2O$)	10	98
Sodium iodide (NaI)	7	150
Sodium lactate (Na lactate)	9	112
Zinc sulfate ($ZnSO_4•7H_2O$)	7	144

Valences and Approximate Weights of Selected Ions

Substance	Electrolyte	Valence	Ionic Wt
Calcium	Ca^{++}	2	40
Chloride	Cl^-	1	35.5
Magnesium	Mg^{++}	2	24
Phosphate	PO_4^{3-}	3	95[1]
	HPO_4^{2-}	2	96
	$H_2PO_4^-$	1	97
Potassium	K^+	1	39
Sodium	Na^+	1	23
Sulfate	SO_4^{2-}	2	96[1]

[1]The atomic weight of phosphorus is 31, and of sulfur is 32.

PEDIATRIC MEDICATION ADMINISTRATION

Adapted from *Giving Your Child Medicine – Ways to Ensure Your Child Receives the Correct Dose of Medicine*, patient booklet, Lexi-Comp, Inc, 2002.

General Advice

Administering medicine to a sick child can be extremely challenging for parents and caregivers. Dosages are calculated by taking the child's age and/or weight into consideration. Infants and young children require very small doses of medicines, thus making accurate measurement very important.

Special measuring devices are available to accurately and easily provide the prescribed dosage. Measuring out a dose with common household utensils can lead to unacceptable inaccuracies. Improper measurement can also cause increased side effects, and over- or under-dosing.

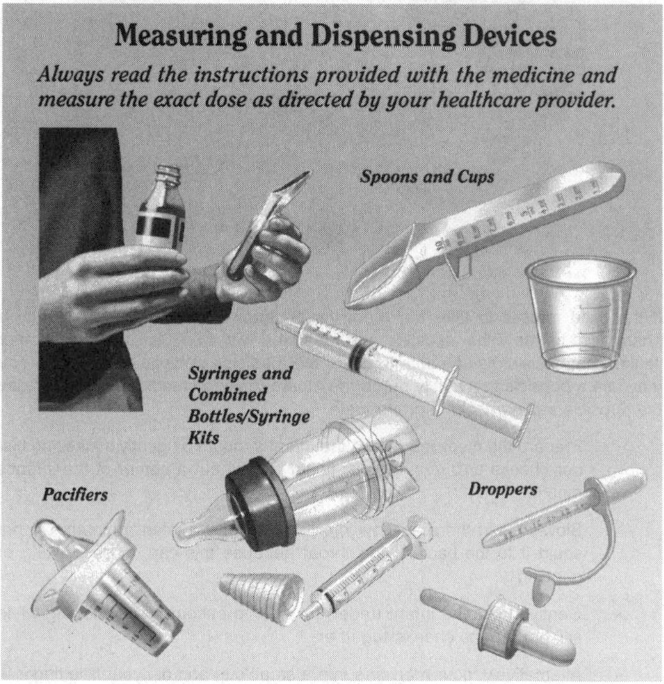

PEDIATRIC MEDICATION ADMINISTRATION *(Continued)*

Liquids

Use either an oral syringe, a medicine dropper, a medicine spoon, or a medicine cup (only for older children) when giving your child oral liquids. You can purchase any of these at a local pharmacy if not provided with your child's medicine. There are specialized pacifiers and bottles designed as medicine delivery aids for children <2 years of age.

- If the medicine can be given on an empty stomach, give right before a feeding.
- Hold an infant in the normal feeding position, or put in a highchair or car seat.

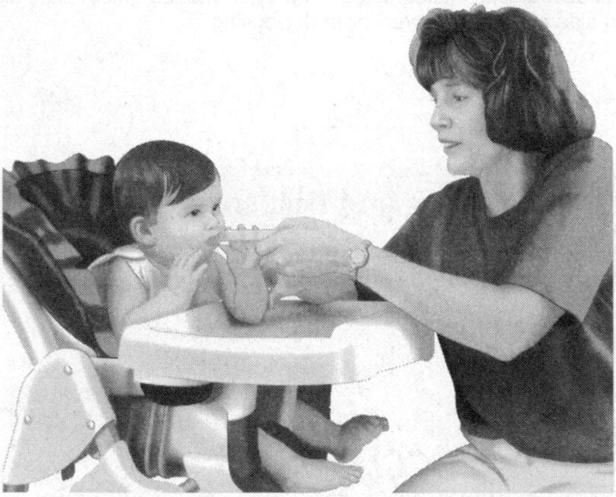

If the child refuses to take the medicine because of bad taste, check with a pharmacist to see if the medicine can be mixed with fruit juice, milk, or another liquid. Pharmacists may be able to flavor the medicine to disguise the taste. You may use a popsicle to partially numb the mouth, give the medicine, and then use the popsicle again to help improve taste.

- Prepare the medicine. Open the infant's mouth by gently squeezing his/her cheeks or by using your finger to pull out a corner of the infant's mouth.
- Slowly squirt the medicine into the side of the infant's mouth. Do not squirt it to the back of the throat because this can cause choking or gagging.
- Gently stroke the infant under the chin to encourage swallowing while still holding the cheeks together.
- Alternatively, pour medicine into a small cup and dip your little finger in it. Let the infant suck it off your finger.
- Young children may want to be in control of taking the medicine by guiding the dropper or spoon into their mouth.
- Rinse measuring device with warm water after each use.

Droppers or cups which come with specific medicines should not be used to administer other medicine.

Eye Drops and Ointments

- Wash your hands before and after use.
- Hold container between hands to bring eye drops or ointment to room temperature before using.
- Clean child's eye of secretions and old medicine if necessary.
- Gently wipe the eye with a damp gauze or cotton pad.
- Tilt child's head back and to the side of the affected eye.
- Do not touch the container tip to eye, lid, or other skin.

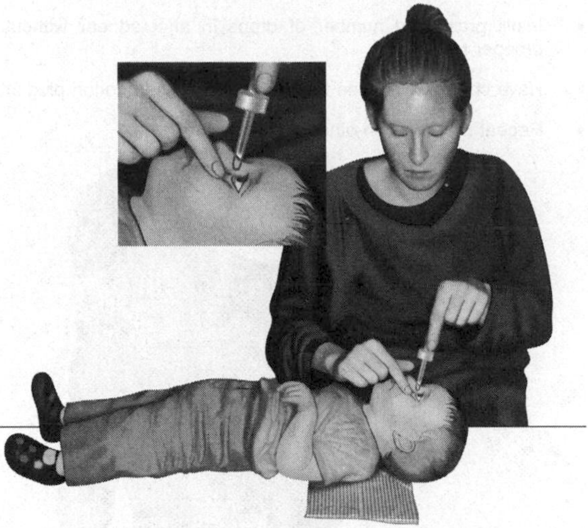

Drops

- If the drops are a suspension, shake the bottle well.
- Gently press the skin under the lower eyelid and pull the lower eyelid away from the eye slightly until you can see a small pouch.
- Insert 1 drop. Wait 1 minute between drops if more than one eye medicine is prescribed.
- After using medicine, ask the child to keep eyes closed. Apply light pressure to the inside corner of the eye.
- Do this for 3-5 minutes. This keeps the medicine in the eye.

Ointment

- If you are using an ointment, gently pull down the lower lid and squeeze in the prescribed amount.
- Release the lower eyelid and instruct the child to keep eyes closed for 1-2 minutes. This will put the medicine in contact with the eye.

PEDIATRIC MEDICATION ADMINISTRATION *(Continued)*

Ear Drops

- Wash your hands before and after use.
- Warm the medicine by holding the bottle between your hands.
- If the drops are a suspension, shake the bottle well.
- For children <3 years of age, pull the outer ear outward and downward.
- For children ≥3 years of age, pull the outer ear outward and upward.
- Instill prescribed number of drops in affected ear without touching dropper to ear.
- Have child stay on side for 2 minutes or insert cotton plug into ear.
- Repeat procedure in other ear if necessary.

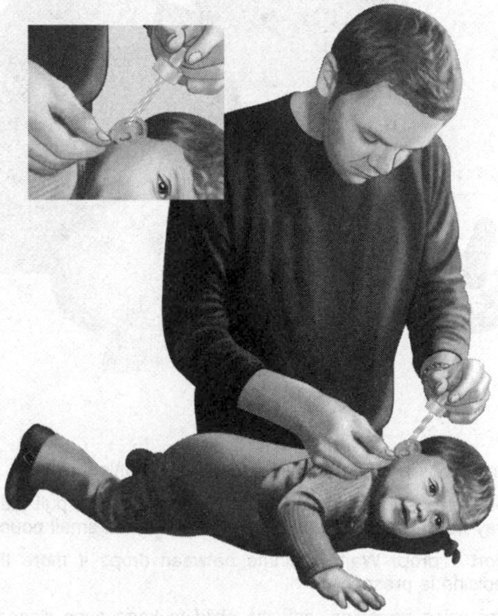

Topical Creams and Ointments

If no specific directions have been given, follow these general guidelines:

- For use on skin only. Keep out of mouth, nose, and eyes (may burn).
- Wash your hands before and after use.
- Clean affected area and dry well before use.
- Apply a thin layer of medicine to the affected skin and rub in gently. Some medicines can be poured or squeezed onto a gauze pad, cotton swab, or cotton ball to apply.
- Do not put coverings (bandages, dressings) over the area unless told to do so by a healthcare provider.

Nose Drops

- Wash your hands before and after use.
- Warm the medicine by holding the bottle between your hands.
- If the drops are a suspension, shake the bottle well.
- Try to clear mucus out of nose. For infants and small children, you can use a nasal aspirator (bulb syringe) or gently twirl a moist cotton swab inside each nostril.

  Do not reach too far into the nostril with the swab or bulb syringe.

  For older children, have the child blow nose.
- Infants can be cradled in your arms in a lying position with head tilted back slightly.

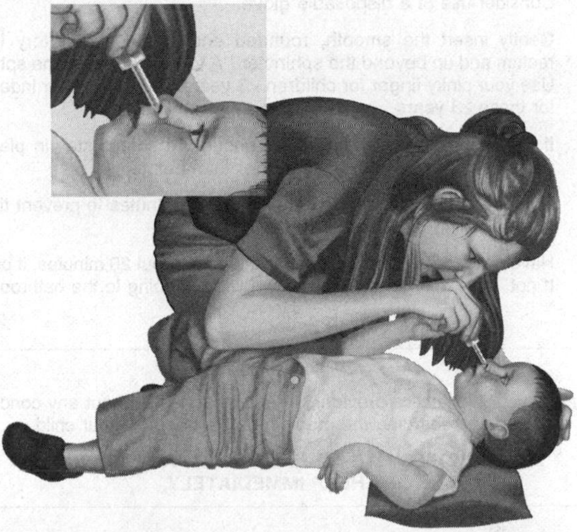

- Young children should lie on their back with a small pillow between their shoulders.
- Have them tilt head back over top of pillow. Older children can sit up with the head tilted back.
- Tell older children they may be able to taste the medicine.
- Draw the correct amount of medicine into the dropper, insert the dropper slightly into the nostril, and squeeze the medicine in without touching dropper to the nose.
- Repeat procedure in other nostril if necessary.
- Keep the child's head tilted back for 2 minutes.
- If child coughs, sit him/her upright.

PEDIATRIC MEDICATION ADMINISTRATION *(Continued)*

Rectal Suppositories

- Wash your hands before and after use.
- If appropriate, store suppository in refrigerator or run it under cold water with the wrapper still on to make it firm enough to place in rectum. Ask pharmacist if you are able to safely store medicine in a refrigerator.
- Infants should be facedown across your knees. An older child can lie on his/her side with knees drawn to chest.
- Remove the wrapper.
- Moisten suppository with water or place a small amount of petroleum jelly on the tip.
- Consider use of a disposable glove.
- Gently insert the smooth, rounded end of the suppository into the rectum and up beyond the sphincter ($^1/_2$ to 1 inch beyond the sphincter). Use your pinky finger for children <3 years of age and your index finger for those ≥3 years.
- If the suppository is inserted far enough, it should stay in place. If it comes out, reinsert it slightly farther than before.
- Hold the buttocks together for a couple of minutes to prevent the child from expelling the suppository.
- Have child remain in the same position for about 20 minutes, if possible. If not, have him/her sit or lie down without going to the bathroom.

If in doubt...

Speak to your healthcare provider or your pharmacist about any concerns you have regarding the medicine prescribed for your child.

IF YOUR CHILD HAS A REACTION TO ANY MEDICINE, GET HELP IMMEDIATELY.

Do's and Don'ts

DO wash your child's hands immediately if medicine gets on them.

DO use distractions such as toys, songs, stories, or rhymes to keep your child busy while trying to give medicine.

DO get another adult to help hold the infant while you give the medicine, or use a car seat to hold the infant or child still.

DO try a different form of the medicine. A child might prefer a chewable tablet or a form that can be sprinkled on food.

DO teach your child about the illness and why he/she has to take medicine. Your healthcare provider or librarian may have books about children who are sick or need to take medicine.

DO help your child gain some control by letting him/her make age-appropriate decisions about care.

DO use prescription as directed, even if your child is feeling better.

DO store medicine out of the reach of children and pets.

DO NOT measure medicine for an infant with a medicine cup (use an oral syringe, a medicine dropper, or a medicine spoon).

DO NOT use a teaspoon or tablespoon from your silverware to measure medicine for your child.

SEROTONIN SYNDROME

Diagnostic Criteria for Serotonin Syndrome

- Recent addition or dosage increase of any agent increasing serotonin activity or availability (usually within 1 day)
- Absence of abused substances, metabolic infectious etiology, or withdrawal
- No recent addition or dosage increase of a neuroleptic agent prior to onset of signs and symptoms
- Presence of three or more of the following: (% incidence)

Agitation (34%)
Abdominal pain (4%)
Ataxia/incoordination (40%)
Diaphoresis (45%)
Diarrhea (8%)
Hyperpyrexia (45%)
Hypertension/hypotension (35%)
Hyperthermia
Hyperreflexia (52%)
Mental status change – cognitive behavioral changes:
- Anxiety (15%)
- Euphoria/hypomania (21%)
- Confusion (51%)
- Agitation (34%)
- Disorientation
- Coma/unresponsiveness (29%)

Muscle rigidity (51%)
Mydriasis
Myoclonus (58%)
Nausea (23%)
Nystagmus (15%)
Restlessness/hyperactivity (48%)
Salivation (2%)
Seizures (12%)
Shivering (26%)
Sinus tachycardia (36%)
Tachypnea (26%)
Tremor (43%)
Unreactive pupils (20%)

Drugs (as Single Causative Agent) Which Can Induce Serotonin Syndrome

Specific serotonin reuptake inhibitors (SSRI)
MDMA (Ecstasy)
Clomipramine

Drug Combinations Which Can Induce Serotonin Syndrome[1]

Alprazolam – Clomipramine
Amphetamines – MAO inhibitors
Amphetamines – SSRIs (Citalopram, Fluoxetine, Fluvoxamine, Paroxetine, Sertraline)
Amphetamines – Tricyclic antidepressants
Amitriptyline – Dihydroergotamine
Amitriptyline – Lithium – Trazodone
Amitriptyline – Sertraline
Anorexiants – MAO inhibitors
Bromocriptine – Levodopa/Carbidopa
Buspirone – Nefazodone
Buspirone – SSRIs (Citalopram, Fluoxetine, Fluvoxamine, Paroxetine, Sertraline)
Buspirone – Trazodone
Buspirone – Tricyclic antidepressants
Carbamazepine – Fluoxetine
Citalopram – Moclobemide
Clomipramine – Alprazolam
Clomipramine – Clorgiline
Clomipramine – Lithium
Clomipramine – MAO inhibitors
Clomipramine – Moclobemide
Clomipramine – S-adenosylmethionine
Clomipramine – Tranylcypromine
Clorgiline – Clomipramine
Dextromethorphan – MAO inhibitors
Dextromethorphan – SSRIs (Citalopram, Fluoxetine, Fluvoxamine, Paroxetine, Sertraline)
Dextropropoxyphene – Phenelzine – Trazodone
Dihydroergotamine – Amitriptyline
Dihydroergotamine – Paroxetine
Dihydroergotamine – SSRIs (Citalopram, Fluoxetine, Fluvoxamine, Paroxetine, Sertraline)
Dihydroergotamine – Tricyclic antidepressants
Fentanyl – SSRIs (Citalopram, Fluoxetine, Fluvoxamine, Paroxetine, Sertraline)
Fluoxetine – Carbamazepine
Fluoxetine – Remoxipride
Fluoxetine – Tryptophan
Levodopa/Carbidopa – Bromocriptine

SEROTONIN SYNDROME *(Continued)*

Linezolid - SSRIs (Citalopram, Fluoxetine, Fluvoxamine, Paroxetine, Sertraline)
Linezolid – Tramadol
Linezolid – Tricyclic antidepressants
Lithium – Amitriptyline – Trazodone
Lithium – Clomipramine
Lithium – SSRIs (Citalopram, Fluoxetine, Fluvoxamine, Paroxetine, Sertraline)
Lithium – Tricyclic antidepressants
Lithium – Venlafaxine
Lysergic acid diethylamide (LSD) – SSRIs (Citalopram, Fluoxetine, Fluvoxamine, Paroxetine, Sertraline)
Metoclopramide – Sertraline
Metoclopramide – Venlafaxine
MAO inhibitors – Amphetamines
MAO inhibitors – Anorexiants
MAO inhibitors – Clomipramine
MAO inhibitors – Dextromethorphan
MAO inhibitors – Meperidine
MAO inhibitors – Nefazodone
MAO inhibitors – Serotonin agonists
MAO inhibitors – S-adenosylmethionine
MAO inhibitors – SSRIs (Citalopram, Fluoxetine, Fluvoxamine, Paroxetine, Sertraline)
MAO inhibitors – St John's Wort
MAO inhibitors – Tramadol
MAO inhibitors – Trazodone
MAO inhibitors – Tricyclic antidepressants
MAO inhibitors – Tryptophan
MAO inhibitors – Venlafaxine
Meperidine – MAO inhibitors
Meperidine – Moclobemide
Meperidine – Nefazodone
Meperidine – SSRIs (Citalopram, Fluoxetine, Fluvoxamine, Paroxetine, Sertraline)
Moclobemide – Citalopram
Moclobemide – Clomipramine
Moclobemide – Meperidine
Moclobemide – Pethidine
Moclobemide – SSRIs (Citalopram, Fluoxetine, Fluvoxamine, Paroxetine, Sertraline)
Moclobemide – Tricyclic antidepressants
Nefazodone – Buspirone
Nefazodone – MAO inhibitors
Nefazodone – Meperidine
Nefazodone – Serotonin agonists
Nefazodone – SSRIs (Citalopram, Fluoxetine, Fluvoxamine, Paroxetine, Sertraline)
Nefazodone – Trazodone
Nefazodone – Tramadol
Nefazodone – Valproic Acid
Nortriptyline – Trazodone
Paroxetine – Dihydroergotamine
Paroxetine – Trazodone
Pethidine – Moclobemide
Phenelzine – Trazodone – Dextropropoxyphene
Remoxipride – Fluoxetine
S-adenosylmethionine – Clomipramine
S-adenosylmethionine – MAO inhibitors
S-adenosylmethionine – SSRIs (Citalopram, Fluoxetine, Fluvoxamine, Paroxetine, Sertraline)
S-adenosylmethionine – Tricyclic antidepressants
Selegiline (high-dose) – SSRIs (Citalopram, Fluoxetine, Fluvoxamine, Paroxetine, Sertraline)
Selegiline (high-dose) – Tricyclic antidepressants
Selegiline (high-dose) – Venlafaxine
Serotonin agonists (Sumatriptan, others) – MAO inhibitors
Serotonin agonists (Sumatriptan, others) – Nefazodone
Serotonin agonists (Sumatriptan, others) – SSRIs (Citalopram, Fluoxetine, Fluvoxamine, Paroxetine, Sertraline)
Serotonin agonists (Sumatriptan, others) – TCAs
Serotonin agonists (Sumatriptan, others) – Tramadol
Sertraline – Amitriptyline
Sibutramine – SSRIs (Citalopram, Fluoxetine, Fluvoxamine, Paroxetine, Sertraline)
SSRIs – Amphetamines
SSRIs – Buspirone
SSRIs – Dextromethorphan
SSRIs – Dihydroergotamine
SSRIs – Fentanyl
SSRIs – Linezolid
SSRIs – Lithium
SSRIs – Lysergic acid diethylamide (LSD)
SSRIs – MAO inhibitors
SSRIs – Meperidine
SSRIs – Moclobemide
SSRIs – Nefazodone
SSRIs – S-adenosylmethionine
SSRIs – Selegiline (high-dose)
SSRIs – Serotonin agonists
SSRIs – Sibutramine
SSRIs – St John's Wort
SSRIs – Tramadol
SSRIs – Trazodone

SSRIs – Tricyclic antidepressants
SSRIs – Tryptophan
St John's Wort – MAO inhibitors
St John's Wort – SSRIs (Citalopram, Fluoxetine, Fluvoxamine, Paroxetine, Sertraline)
St John's Wort – Tricyclic antidepressants
Sympathomimetics – Tricyclic antidepressants
Tramadol – Linezolid
Tramadol – MAO inhibitors
Tramadol – Nefazodone
Tramadol – Serotonin agonists
Tramadol – SSRIs (Citalopram, Fluoxetine, Fluvoxamine, Paroxetine, Sertraline)
Tramadol – TCAs
Tranylcypromine – Clomipramine
Trazodone – Buspirone
Trazodone – Lithium – Amitriptyline
Trazodone – MAO inhibitors
Trazodone – Nefazodone
Trazodone – Nortriptyline
Trazodone – Paroxetine
Trazodone – SSRIs (Citalopram, Fluoxetine, Fluvoxamine, Paroxetine, Sertraline) (theoretical)
Tricyclic antidepressants – Amphetamines
Tricyclic antidepressants – Buspirone
Tricyclic antidepressants – Dihydroergotamine
Tricyclic antidepressants – Linezolid
Tricyclic antidepressants – Lithium
Tricyclic antidepressants – MAO inhibitors
Tricyclic antidepressants – Moclobemide
Tricyclic antidepressants – S-adenosylmethionine
Tricyclic antidepressants – Serotonin agonists
Tricyclic antidepressants – SSRIs (Citalopram, Fluoxetine, Fluvoxamine, Paroxetine, Sertraline)
Tricyclic antidepressants – St John's Wort
Tricyclic antidepressants – Sympathomimetics
Tricyclic antidepressants – Tramadol
Tryptophan – Fluoxetine
Tryptophan – MAO inhibitors
Tryptophan – SSRIs (Citalopram, Fluoxetine, Fluvoxamine, Paroxetine, Sertraline)
Valproic acid – Nefazodone
Venlafaxine – Lithium
Venlafaxine – MAO inhibitors
Venlafaxine – Selegiline (high-dose)

[1]When administered within 2 weeks of each other.

Guidelines for Treatment of Serotonin Syndrome

Therapy is primarily supportive with intravenous crystalloid solutions utilized for hypotension and cooling blankets for mild hyperthermia. Norepinephrine is the preferred vasopressor. Chlorpromazine or dantrolene sodium may have a role in controlling fevers, although there is no proven benefit. Benzodiazepines are the first-line treatment in controlling rigors and thus, limiting fever and rhabdomyolysis, while clonazepam may be specifically useful in treating myoclonus. Endotracheal intubation and paralysis may be required to treat refractory muscular contractions. Tachycardia or tremor can be treated with beta-blocking agents; although due to its blockade of 5-HTIA receptors, the syndrome may worsen. Serotonin blockers such as diphenhydramine, cyproheptadine, or chlorpromazine have been used with variable efficacy. Methysergide and nitroglycerin (I.V. infusion with lorazepam) also has been utilized with variable efficacy in case reports. It appears that cyproheptadine is most consistently beneficial.

Recovery seen within 1 day in 70% of cases; mortality rate is about 11%.

References

Gardner DM and Lynd LD, "Sumatriptan Contraindications and the Serotonin Syndrome," *Ann Pharmacother*, 1998, 32(1):33-8

Gitlin MJ, "Venlafaxine, Monoamine Oxidase Inhibitors, and the Serotonin Syndrome," *J Clin Psychopharmacol*, 1997, 17:66-7.

Heisler MA, Guidery JR, and Arnecke B, "Serotonin Syndrome Induced by Administration of Venlafaxine and Phenelzine," *Ann Pharmacother*, 1996, 30:84.

Hodgman MJ, Martin TG, and Krenzelok EP, "Serotonin Syndrome Due to Venlafaxine and Maintenance Tranylcypromine Therapy," *Hum Exp Toxicol*, 1997, 16:14-7.

John L, Perreault MM, Tao T, et al, "Serotonin Syndrome Associated With Nefazodone and Paroxetine," *Ann Emerg Med*, 1997, 29:287-9.

LoCurto MJ, "The Serotonin Syndrome," *Emerg Clin North Am*, 1997, 15(3):665-75.

Martin TG, "Serotonin Syndrome," *Ann Emerg Med*, 1996, 28:520-6.

Mills K, "Serotonin Toxicity: A Comprehensive Review for Emergency Medicine," *Top Emerg Med*, 1993, 15:54-73.

SEROTONIN SYNDROME *(Continued)*

Mills KC, "Serotonin Syndrome: A Clinical Update," *Crit Care Clin*, 1997, 13(4):763-83.
Nisijima K, Shimizu M, Abe T, et al, "A Case of Serotonin Syndrome Induced by Concomitant Treatment With Low-Dose Trazodone, and Amitriptyline and Lithium," *Int Clin Psychopharmacol*, 1996, 11:289-90.
Sobanski T, Bagli M, Laux G, et al, "Serotonin Syndrome After Lithium Add-On Medication to Paroxetine," *Pharmacopsychiatry*, 1997, 30:106-7.
Sporer, "The Serotonin Syndrome: Implicated Drugs, Pathophysiology and Management," *Drug Safety*, 1995, 13(2):94-104.
Sternbach H, "The Serotonin Syndrome," *Am J Psychiatry*, 1991, 146:705-7.
Van Berkum MM, Thiel J, Leikin JB, et al, "A Fatality Due to Serotonin Syndrome," *Medical Update for Psychiatrists*, 1997, 2:55-7.

SODIUM CONTENT OF SELECTED MEDICINALS

Name and Dosage Unit[1]	Sodium mg	Sodium mEq
Antibiotics		
Amikacin sulfate, 1 g	29.9	1.3
Aminosalicylate sodium, 1 g	109	4.7
Ampicillin, suspension, 250 mg/5 mL, 5 mL	10	0.4
Ampicillin sodium, 1 g	66.7	3
Carbenicillin disodium, 382 mg (tablet)	23	1
Cefazolin sodium, 1 g	47	2
Cefotaxime sodium, 1 g	50.6	2.2
Cefoxitin sodium, 1 g	53	2.3
Ceftriaxone sodium, 1 g	60	2.6
Cefuroxime, 1 g	54.2	2.4
Chloramphenicol sodium succinate, 1 g	51.8	2.3
Dicloxacillin, 250 mg (capsule)	13	0.6
Erythromycin ethyl succinate, suspension 200 mg/5 mL	29	1.3
Erythromycin Base Filmtab®, 250 mg	70	3
Metronidazole, 500 mg I.V.	322	14
Nafcillin sodium, 1 g	66.7	2.9
Nitrofurantoin, suspension, 25 mg/5 mL	7	0.3
Penicillin G potassium, 1,000,000 units I.V.	7.6	0.3
Penicillin G sodium, 1,000,000 units I.V.	46	2
Penicillin V potassium, suspension, 250 mg/5 mL	38	1.7
Piperacillin sodium, 1 g	42.6	1.8
Ticarcillin disodium, 1 g	119.6	5.2
Antacids, Liquid (content per 5 mL)		
ALternaGEL®	2	0.1
Gaviscon®	13	0.57
Maalox®	1.3	0.06
Tums E-X™	<4.8	<0.2
Sodium Content of Miscellaneous Medicinals		
Acetazolamide sodium, 500 mg	47.2	2.05
Chlorothiazide sodium, 500 mg	57.5	2
Cisplatin, 10 mg	35.4	1.54
Edetate calcium disodium, 1 g	122	5.3
Fleet® Enema, 4.5 oz	5000[2]	218
Fleet® Phospho®-Soda, 20 mL	2217	96.4
Hydrocortisone sodium succinate, 1 g	47.5	2.07
Hypaque® M 75%, injection, 20 mL	200	8.7
Hypaque® M 90%, injection, 20 mL	220	9.6
Metamucil® Instant Mix (orange)	6	0.27
Methotrexate sodium, 100 mg vial	20	0.86
Methotrexate sodium, 100 mg vial (low sodium)	15	0.65
Naproxen sodium, 250 mg (tablet)	23	1
Neutra-Phos®, capsule and 75 mL reconstituted solution	164	7.13
Pentobarbital sodium, 50 mg/mL	5	0.2

SODIUM CONTENT OF SELECTED MEDICINALS *(Continued)*

Name and Dosage Unit[1]	Sodium	
	mg	mEq
Phenobarbital sodium, 65 mg, 1 mL vial	6	0.3
Phenytoin sodium, 1 g	88	3.8
Promethazine expectorant, 5 mL	53	2.3
Shohl's solution modified, 1 mL	23	1
Sodium ascorbate, 500 mg acid equivalent	65.3	2.84
Sodium bicarbonate, 50 mL 8.4%	1150	50
Sodium nitroprusside, 50 mg	7.8	0.34
Sodium polystyrene sulfonate, 1 g	94.3[3]	4.1
Thiopental sodium, 1 g	86.8	3.8
Valproate sodium, 250 mg/5 mL, 5 mL	23	1

[1]Product formulations and hence sodium content are subject to change by the manufacturer.

[2]Average systemic absorption 250-300 mg.

[3]Total sodium content. Only about 33% is liberated in clinical use.

SUGAR-FREE LIQUID PHARMACEUTICALS

The following sugar-free liquid preparations are listed by therapeutic category and alphabetically within each category. Please note that product formulations are subject to change by the manufacturer. Some of these products may contain sorbitol, alcohol, xylitol, or other sweeteners which may be partially metabolized to provide calories.

Analgesics

- Acetaminophen Elixir (various)
- APAP/APAP Plus
- Febrol® and Febrol® EX
- Mapap® Drops
- Methadone Hydrochloride Intensol
- Paregoric USP (Abbott)
- Silapap®
- Tylenol® Drops

Antacids / Antiflatulents

- Alcalak®
- Aldroxicon®
- Aluminum Hydroxide Suspension
- Baby Gasz Drops
- Citrocarbonate® Granules
- Gaviscon® Liquid
- Maalox® Plus Suspension
- Maalox® Suspension
- Maalox® Therapeutic Concentrate
- Magnesia and Alumina Oral Suspension USP (Abbott, Phillips Roxane)
- Milk of Bismuth
- Milk of Magnesia USP
- Mylanta® Liquid
- Mylicon® Drops
- Pepto-Bismol® Liquid and Tablets
- Riopan Plus®
- Riopan® Suspension

Antiasthmatics

- Alupent® Syrup
- Elixophyllin® Elixir
- Organidin® NR

Antidepressants

- Celexa™ Solution
- Prozac® Solution
- Sinequan® Oral Concentrate

Antidiarrheals

- Corrective Mixture With Paregoric
- Diotame®
- Kaolin Mixture With Pectin NF (Abbott)
- Kaolin-Pectin Suspension (Phillips Roxane)
- Konsyl® Powder
- Lomanate®
- Lomotil® Liquid
- Paregoric USP (various)
- Parepectolin® (various)
- Pepto-Bismol®
- St Joseph® Antidiarrheal

SUGAR-FREE LIQUID PHARMACEUTICALS *(Continued)*

Antiepileptics
- Mysoline® Suspension

Antihistamine-Decongestants
- Bromphen® Elixir
- Dimetapp® Elixir
- Isoclor® Liquid and Capsules
- Naldecon® Pediatric Drops and Syrup
- Naldecon® Syrup
- Phenergan® Syrup
- Rondec® DM Drops
- S-T® Forte® Liquid
- Tavist® Syrup
- Vistaril® Oral Suspension
- Zyrtec® Syrup

Anti-infectives
- Augmentin® Suspension
- Furadantin® Oral Suspension
- Sulfamethoxazole and Trimethoprim Suspension (Biocraft, Beecham, Burroughs Wellcome)
- Vibramycin® Syrup
- Zovirax® Suspension

Corticosteroids
- Decadron® Elixir
- Dexamethasone Solution (Roxane)
- Dexamethasone Intensol Solution
- Pediapred® Oral Liquid
- Prelone® Syrup

Cough Medicines
- Chlorgest-HD®
- Codiclear® DH Syrup
- Codimal® DM
- Contac Jr® Liquid
- Dimetane®-DC Cough Syrup
- Dimetane®-DX Cough Syrup
- Entuss® Expectorant Liquid
- Histafed® Pediatric Liquid
- Hycomine® Syrup and Pediatric Syrup
- Medicon® D
- Medi-Synal®
- Naldecon-DX® Pediatric Drops and Syrup
- Naldecon-DX® Adult Liquid
- Non-Drowsy Comtrex®
- Organidin® NR
- Potassium Iodide Solution (various)
- Robitussin-CF® Liquid
- Robitussin® Night Relief Liquid
- Rondec®-DM Drops
- Rondec®-DM Syrup
- Ryna® Liquid
- Ryna-C® Liquid
- Ryna-CX® Liquid
- Scot-Tussin® DM Syrup
- Scot-Tussin® Expectorant
- Scot-Tussin® DM Cough Chasers
- Silexin® Cough Syrup
- Sudodrin®/Sudodrin® Forte®
- Terpin® Hydrate With Codeine Elixir (various)
- Tolu-Sed® Cough Syrup
- Tolu-Sed® DM
- Tricodene® Liquid
- Tussirex® Sugar-Free

Dental Preparations and Fluoride Preparations

Cepacol® Mouthwash
Cepastat® Mouthwash and Gargle
Chloraseptic® Mouthwash and Gargle
Fluorigard® Mouthrinse
Fluorinse®
Flura-Drops®
Flura-Loz®
Flura® Tablets
Gel-Kam®
Karigel®
Karigel® N
Luride® Drops
Luride® SF Lozi-Tabs
Luride® 0.25 and 0.5 Lozi-Tabs
Luride® Lozi-Tabs
Pediaflor® Drops
Phos-Flur® Rinse/Supplement
Point-Two® Mouthrinse
Prevident® Disclosing Drops
Thera-Flur® Gel and Drops

Diagnostic Agents

Gastrografin®

Dietary Substitutes

Co-Salt®

Iron Preparations / Blood Modifiers

Amicar® Syrup
Geritol® Complete Tablets
Geritonic™ Liquid
Hemo-Vite® Liquid
Iberet® Liquid
Iberet®-500 Liquid
Niferex®
Nu-Iron® Elixir
Vita-Plus H® Half Strength, Sugar-Free
Vita-Plus H®, Sugar-Free

Laxatives

Aromatic Cascara Fluidextract USP
Castor Oil
Castor Oil (flavored)
Castor Oil USP
Colace®, Liquid
Emulsoil®
Fiberall® Powder
Hydrocil® Instant Powder
Hypaque® Oral Powder
Kondremul®
Kondremul® With Cascara
Kondremul® With Phenolphthalein
Konsyl® Powder
Liqui-Doss®
Magnesium Citrate Solution NF
Metamucil® Instant Mix (lemon-lime or orange)
Metamucil® SF Powder
Milk of Magnesia
Milk of Magnesia/Cascara Suspension
Milk of Magnesia/Mineral Oil Emulsion (various)
Mineral Oil (various)
Neoloid® Liquid
NuLYTELY®
Sodium Phosphate & Biphosphate Oral Solution USP (Phillips Roxane)

SUGAR-FREE LIQUID PHARMACEUTICALS *(Continued)*

Potassium Products

- Cena-K® Solution
- Kaon® Elixir (grape and lemon-lime flavor)
- Kaon-Cl® 20% Liquid
- Kay Ciel® Elixir
- Kay Ciel® Powder
- Klor-Con®/25 Powder
- Klor-Con® EF Tablets
- Klor-Con® Liquid 20%
- Klor-Con® Powder
- Potassium Chloride Oral Solution USP 5%, 10%, and 20% (various)
- Potassium Gluconate Elixir NF
- Rum-K® Solution
- Tri-K® Liquid

Sedatives-Tranquilizers-Antipsychotics

- Butabarbital Sodium Elixir
- Butisol Sodium® Elixir
- Haldol® Concentrate
- Loxitane® C Drops
- Mellaril® Concentrate
- Serentil® Concentrate
- Thorazine® Concentrate

Vitamin Preparations-Nutritionals

- Bugs Bunny™ Chewable Tablets
- Bugs Bunny™ Plus Iron Chewable Tablets
- Bugs Bunny™ With Extra C Chewable Tablets
- Bugs Bunny™ Plus Minerals Chewable Tablets
- Calciferol™ Drops
- Caltrate® 600 Tablets
- Cod Liver Oil (various)
- DHT™ Intensol Solution (Roxane)
- Drisdol® in Propylene Glycol
- Flintstones™ Complete Chewable Tablets
- Flintstones™ With Extra C Chewable Tablets
- Flintstones™ Plus Iron Chewable Tablets
- Oyst-Cal® 500 Tablets
- Pediaflor®
- PMS® Relief
- Poly-Vi-Flor® Drops
- Poly-Vi-Flor®/Iron Drops
- Poly-Vi-Sol® Drops
- Poly-Vi-Sol®/Iron Drops
- Posture® Tablets
- Spiderman™ Children's Chewable Vitamin Tablets
- Spiderman™ Children's Plus Iron Tablets
- Theragran® Jr Children's Chewable Tablets
- Tri-Vi-Flor® Drops
- Tri-Vi-Sol® Drops
- Tri-Vi-Sol®/Iron Drops
- Vi-Daylin® ADC Drops
- Vi-Daylin® ADC/Fluoride Drops
- Vi-Daylin® ADC Plus Iron Drops
- Vi-Daylin® Drops
- Vi-Daylin®/Fluoride Drops
- Vi-Daylin® Plus Iron Drops
- Vitalize®

Miscellaneous

- Altace™ Capsules
- Bicitra® Solution
- Colestid® Granules
- Digoxin® Elixir (Roxane)
- Lipomul®
- Lithium Citrate Syrup
- Neutra-Phos® Powder
- Neutra-Phos®-K Powder
- Nicorette® Chewing Gum
- Polycitra®-K Solution
- Polycitra®-LC Solution
- Tagamet® Liquid

References

Hill EM, Flaitz CM, and Frost GR, "Sweetener Content of Common Pediatric Oral Liquid Medications," *Am J Hosp Pharm*, 1988, 45:135-42.

Kumar A, Rawlings RD, and Beaman DC, "The Mystery Ingredients: Sweeteners, Flavorings, Dyes, and Preservatives in Analgesic/Antipyretic, Antihistamine/Decongestant, Cough and Cold, Antidiarrheal, and Liquid Theophylline Preparations," *Pediatrics*, 1993, 91:927-33.

"Sugar Free Products," *Drug Topics Red Book*, 2005, 29-33.

CARBOHYDRATE CONTENT OF MEDICATIONS

Description (Brand Name)	Dosage Unit	Grams Carbohydrate per Dosage Unit
Analgesics / Antipyretics		
Acetaminophen extended release caplets (Tylenol®)	650 mg	<0.03
Acetaminophen extra strength caplets (Tylenol®)	500 mg	<0.05
Acetaminophen extra strength gel caps (Tylenol®)	500 mg	<0.05
Acetaminophen infant drops (grape and cherry) (Tylenol®)	0.8 mL	<0.71
Acetaminophen liquid suspension cherry) (Tylenol®)	160 mg/5 mL	<5
Acetaminophen regular strength caplets (Tylenol®)	325 mg	<0.04
Acetaminophen elixir (Tylenol®)	160 mg/5 mL	<1.6
Acetaminophen extra strength liquid (Tylenol®)	1000 mg/30 mL	<5.7
Acetaminophen junior strength swallowable caplets (Tylenol®)	160 mg	<0.4
Acetaminophen grape flavored suspension (Tylenol®)	160 mg/5 mL	<4.8
Acetaminophen elixir with codeine (Tylenol® With Codeine) *0.35 g ethyl alcohol/5 mL	120 mg/5 mL	3
Acetaminophen with codeine tablets (Tylenol® With Codeine)	All strengths	0.05
Acetaminophen chewable tablets (Tylenol®)	80 mg	0.25
Effervescent flavored antacid and pain reliever (Alka-Selzer®)	325 mg	0.01
Ibuprofen tablets (Advil®)	200 mg	0.23
Ibuprofen drops (Motrin®)	40 mg/mL	<0.41
Ibuprofen suspension (Motrin®)	100 mg/5 mL	<0.63
Ibuprofen chewable tablets (Motrin®)	50 mg	<0.28
Ibuprofen chewable tablets (Motrin®)	100 mg	<0.54
Antibiotics		
Amoxicillin pediatric drops (Amoxil®)	50 mg/mL	1.6
Amoxicillin oral suspension (Amoxil®)	125 mg/5 mL	1.7
Amoxicillin oral suspension (Amoxil®)	250 mg/5 mL	1.85
Amoxicillin chewable tablets (Amoxil®)	125 mg	0.05
Amoxicillin chewable tablets (Amoxil®)	250 mg	0.34
Amoxicillin capsules (Amoxil®)	250 mg	0
Amoxicillin capsules (Amoxil®)	500 mg	0
Amoxicillin oral suspension (Trimox®)	125 mg/5 mL	3.3

Description (Brand Name)	Dosage Unit	Grams Carbohydrate per Dosage Unit
Amoxicillin oral suspension (Trimox®)	250 mg/5 mL	3.3
Amoxicillin capsules (Trimox®)	250 mg	0
Amoxicillin capsules (Trimox®)	500 mg	0
Amoxicillin/clavulanate potassium oral suspension (Augmentin®)	125 mg/5 mL	0.52
Amoxicillin/clavulanate potassium oral suspension (Augmentin®)	200 mg/5 mL	0.06
Amoxicillin/clavulanate potassium oral suspension (Augmentin®)	250 mg/5 mL	0.6
Amoxicillin/clavulanate potassium oral suspension (Augmentin®)	400 mg/5 mL	0.06
Amoxicillin/clavulanate potassium chewable tablets (Augmentin®)	125 mg	0.08
Amoxicillin/clavulanate potassium chewable tablets (Augmentin®)	250 mg	0.34
Amoxicillin/clavulanate potassium chewable tablets (Augmentin®)	400 mg	0.36
Amoxicillin/clavulanate potassium tablets (Augmentin®)	250 mg	0.02
Amoxicillin/clavulanate potassium tablets (Augmentin®)	500 mg	0.02
Amoxicillin/clavulanate potassium tablets (Augmentin®)	875 mg	0.03
Ampicillin oral suspension (Omnipen®)	125 mg/5 mL	4
Ampicillin oral suspension (Omnipen®)	250 mg/5 mL	4
Azithromycin oral suspension (Zithromax®)	100 mg/5 mL	3.86
Azithromycin tablets (Zithromax®)	250 mg	0.06
Cefaclor oral suspension (Ceclor®)	125 mg/5 mL	2.95
Cefaclor oral suspension (Ceclor®)	187 mg/5 mL	2.83
Cefaclor oral suspension (Ceclor®)	250 mg/5 mL	2.83
Cefaclor oral suspension (Ceclor®)	375 mg/5 mL	2.6
Cefaclor pulvules (Ceclor®)	250 mg	0.04
Cefaclor pulvules (Ceclor®)	500 mg	0.07
Cefadroxil oral suspension (Duricef®)	250 mg/5 mL	3
Cefadroxil oral suspension (Duricef®)	125 mg/5 mL	3.1
Cefadroxil capsules (Duricef®)	500 mg	0.13
Cefadroxil film-coated tablets (Duricef®)	1 g	0.13
Cefixime oral suspension (Suprax®)	100 mg/5 mL	2.7
Cefixime tablets (Suprax®)	200 mg	0.06
Cefixime tablets (Suprax®)	400 mg	0.12
Cefpodoxime proxetil oral suspension (Vantin®)	50 mg/5 mL	3
Cefpodoxime proxetil oral suspension (Vantin®)	100 mg/5 mL	3.05
Cefpodoxime proxetil tablets (Vantin®)	100 mg	0.04

CARBOHYDRATE CONTENT OF MEDICATIONS
(Continued)

Description (Brand Name)	Dosage Unit	Grams Carbohydrate per Dosage Unit
Cefpodoxime proxetil tablets (Vantin®)	200 mg	0.08
Cefprozil oral suspension (Cefzil®)	125 mg/5 mL	2
Cefprozil oral suspension (Cefzil®)	250 mg/5 mL	1.9
Cefprozil tablets (Cefzil®)	250 mg	0.02
Cefprozil tablets (Cefzil®)	500 mg	0.03
Cefuroxime axetil suspension (Ceftin®)	125 mg/5 mL	3.23
Cefuroxime axetil tablets (Ceftin®)	125 mg	0
Cefuroxime axetil tablets (Ceftin®)	250 mg	0
Cefuroxime axetil tablets (Ceftin®)	500 mg	0
Cephalexin oral suspension (Keflex®)	125 mg/5 mL	3.13
Cephalexin oral suspension (Keflex®)	250 mg/5 mL	3.03
Cephalexin pulvules (Keflex®)	250 mg	0.13
Cephalexin pulvules (Keflex®)	500 mg	0.13
Ciprofloxacin tablets (Cipro®)	250 mg	0.04
Ciprofloxacin tablets (Cipro®)	500 mg	0.07
Ciprofloxacin tablets (Cipro®)	750 mg	0.11
Ciprofloxacin oral suspension (Cipro®)	250 mg/5 mL	1.4
Ciprofloxacin oral suspension (Cipro®)	500 mg/5 mL	1.3
Clarithromycin suspension (Biaxin®)	125 mg/5 mL	3
Clarithromycin suspension (Biaxin®)	250 mg/5 mL	2.3
Clarithromycin tablets (Biaxin®)	250 mg	0.07
Clarithromycin tablets (Biaxin®)	500 mg	0
Erythromycin base tablets (Ery-Tab®)	333 mg	0
Erythromycin base tablets (Ery-Tab®)	500 mg	0
Erythromycin estolate oral suspension (Ilosone®)	125 mg/5 mL	1.85
Erythromycin estolate oral suspension (Ilosone®)	250 mg/5 mL	1.8
Erythromycin estolate pulvules (Ilosone®)	250 mg	0
Erythromycin estolate tablets (Ilosone®)	500 mg	0.11
Erythromycin ethylsuccinate drops (EryPed®)	10 mg/2.5 mL	1.5
Erythromycin ethylsuccinate chewable tablets (EryPed®)	200 mg	1.44
Erythromycin ethylsuccinate suspension (E.E.S.®)	200 mg/5 mL	3.5
Erythromycin ethylsuccinate suspension (E.E.S.®)	400 mg/5 mL	3.5

Description (Brand Name)	Dosage Unit	Grams Carbohydrate per Dosage Unit
Erythromycin ethylsuccinate granules (E.E.S.®)	200 mg/5 mL	1.5
Erythromycin ethylsuccinate filmtabs (E.E.S.®)	400 mg	0.2
Erythromycin ethyl + sulfisoxazole acetyl suspension (Pediazole®)	200 mg/5 mL	1.9
Erythromycin ethyl + sulfisoxazole acetyl suspension (Pediazole®)	600 mg/5 mL	1.9
Loracarbef oral suspension (Lorabid®)	100 mg/5 mL	3.15
Loracarbef oral suspension (Lorabid®)	200 mg/5 mL	3.03
Loracarbef pulvules (Lorabid®)	200 mg	0.22
Loracarbef pulvules (Lorabid®)	400 mg	0.11
Nitrofurantoin oral suspension (Furadantin®)	25 mg/5 mL	0.7
Penicillin V potassium oral suspension	125 mg/5 mL	2.53
Penicillin V potassium oral suspension	250 mg/5 mL	3.28
Penicillin V potassium tablets	250 mg	0.09
Penicillin V potassium tablets	500 mg	0
Trimethoprim (TMP) and sulfamethoxazole (SMX) suspension (Septra®)	40 mg TMP/200 mg SMX/5 mL	2.35
Trimethoprim (TMP) and sulfamethoxazole (SMX) grape suspension (Septra®)	40 mg TMP/200 mg SMX/5 mL	2.35
Trimethoprim (TMP) and sulfamethoxazole (SMX) tablets (Septra®)	80 mg TMP/400 mg SMX/5 mL	0
Trimethoprim (TMP) and sulfamethoxazole (SMX) double strength tablets (Septra®)	160 mg TMP/800 mg SMX/5 mL	0
Antiepileptic Drugs		
Carbamazepine suspension (Tegretol®)	100 mg/5 mL	2.65
Carbamazepine chewable tablets (Tegretol®)	100 mg	0.28
Carbamazepine tablets (Tegretol®)	200 mg	0.06
Clonazepam tablets (Klonopin®)	0.5 mg	0.14
Clonazepam tablets (Klonopin®)	1 mg	0.14
Clonazepam tablets (Klonopin®)	2 mg	0.14
Ethosuximide syrup (Zarontin®)	250 mg/5 mL	3.63
Ethosuximide capsules (Zarontin®)	250 mg	0.13
Felbamate solution (Felbatol®)	600 mg/5 mL	1.5
Felbamate tablets (Felbatol®)	400 mg	0.13
Felbamate tablets (Felbatol®)	600 mg	0.19
Gabapentin tablets (Neurontin®)	100 mg	0.03
Gabapentin tablets (Neurontin®)	300 mg	0.07
Gabapentin tablets (Neurontin®)	400 mg	0.1
Lamotrigine tablets (Lamictal®)	25 mg	0.03

CARBOHYDRATE CONTENT OF MEDICATIONS *(Continued)*

Description (Brand Name)	Dosage Unit	Grams Carbohydrate per Dosage Unit
Lamotrigine tablets (Lamictal®)	100 mg	0.11
Lamotrigine tablets (Lamictal®)	150 mg	0.16
Lamotrigine tablets (Lamictal®)	200 mg	0.14
Lamotrigine chewable/dispersible tablets (Lamictal®)	5 mg	0
Lamotrigine chewable/dispersible tablets (Lamictal®)	25 mg	0
Phenobarbital elixir *0.71 g ethyl alcohol/5 mL	20 mg/5 mL	3.4
Phenobarbital tablets	15 mg	0.06
Phenobarbital tablets	30 mg	0.07
Phenobarbital tablets	60 mg	0.1
Phenytoin suspension (Dilantin®)	125 mg/5 mL	1.39
Phenytoin infatabs (Dilantin®)	50 mg	0.48
Phenytoin kapseal (Dilantin®)	30 mg	0.15
Phenytoin kapseal (Dilantin®)	100 mg	0.11
Primidone oral suspension (Mysoline®)	250 mg/5 mL	0
Primidone tablets (Mysoline®)	50 mg	0.03
Primidone tablets (Mysoline®)	250 mg	0.03
Sodium divalproex sprinkle capsules (Depakote®)	125 mg	0.05
Sodium divalproex tablets (Depakote®)	125 mg	0.03
Sodium divalproex tablets (Depakote®)	250 mg	0.05
Sodium divalproex tablets (Depakote®)	500 mg	0.1
Tiagabine tablets (Gabitril®)	4 mg	0.05
Tiagabine tablets (Gabitril®)	12 mg	0.14
Tiagabine tablets (Gabitril®)	16 mg	0.19
Tiagabine tablets (Gabitril®)	20 mg	0.23
Topiramate tablets (Topamax®)	25 mg	0.04
Topiramate tablets (Topamax®)	100 mg	0.17
Topiramate tablets (Topamax®)	200 mg	0.09
Valproic acid syrup (Depakene®)	250 mg/5 mL	4.5
Valproic acid capsules (Depakene®)	250 mg	0
Antifungals		
Fluconazole oral suspension (Diflucan®)	10 mg/mL	2.88
Fluconazole oral suspension (Diflucan®)	40 mg/mL	2.73
Fluconazole tablets (Diflucan®)	50 mg and 100 mg	0
Nystatin oral suspension	100,000 units/mL	0.61
Nystatin oral suspension (Mycostatin®)	100,000 units/mL	0.60
Nystatin tablets (Mycostatin®)	500,000 units	0.11

Description (Brand Name)	Dosage Unit	Grams Carbohydrate per Dosage Unit
Antihistamines		
Cetirizine syrup (Zyrtec®)	5 mg/5 mL	3
Cetirizine tablets (Zyrtec®)	5 mg	0.08
Cetirizine tablets (Zyrtec®)	10 mg	0.16
Diphenhydramine elixir (Benadryl®)	5 mL	1.5
Hydroxyzine syrup (Atarax®)	10 mg/5 mL	5.88
Hydroxyzine tablets (Atarax®)	10 mg	0.04
Hydroxyzine tablets (Atarax®)	25 mg	0.05
Hydroxyzine tablets (Atarax®)	50 mg	0.07
Hydroxyzine tablets (Atarax®)	100 mg	0.1
Hydroxyzine suspension (Vistaril®)	25 mg/5 mL	5.83
Hydroxyzine capsules (Vistaril®)	25 mg	0.03
Hydroxyzine capsules (Vistaril®)	50 mg	0.07
Hydroxyzine capsules (Vistaril®)	100 mg	0.11
Antinausea Medications		
Dimenhydrinate chewable tablets (Dramamine®)	50 mg	<0.5
Meclizine tablets (Dramamine II®)	25 mg	<0.25
Antivirals		
Acyclovir suspension (Zovirax®) *1.75 g of sorbitol	200 mg/5 mL	0
Acyclovir tablets (Zovirax®)	400 mg	0.02
Acyclovir capsules (Zovirax®)	200 mg	0.21
Zidovudine syrup (Retrovir®)	50 mg/5 mL	2.15
Zidovudine tablets (Retrovir®)	300 mg	0.02
Zidovudine capsules (Retrovir®)	100 mg	0.09
Cough and Cold Preparations		
Brompheniramine pseudoephedrine tablets (Dristan® Allergy)	4 mg 60 mg	0
Chlorpheniramine phenylpropanolamine chewable tablets (Allerest® Children's)	1 mg 9.4 mg	0.25
Chlorpheniramine phenylpropanolamine dextromethorphan aspirin effervescent tablets (Alka-Selzer Plus® Cold and Cough)	2 mg 10 mg 20 mg 325 mg	0.01
Chlorpheniramine phenylephrine dextromethorphan syrup	4 mg/5 mL 10 mg/5 mL 15 mg/5 mL	3.6
Dextromethorphan guaifenesin syrup (Robitussin® DM) *2.24 g sorbitol/5 mL	10 mg/5 mL 100 mg/5 mL	0
Dextromethorphan pseudoephedrine syrup (Robitussin® Pediatric Cough and Cold)	7.5 mg/5 mL 15 mg/5 mL	1.35
Triprolidine pseudoephedrine syrup (Actifed®)	1.25 mg/5 mL 30 mg/5 mL	5

CARBOHYDRATE CONTENT OF MEDICATIONS
(Continued)

Description (Brand Name)	Dosage Unit	Grams Carbohydrate per Dosage Unit
Decongestant / Nasal Preparations		
Oxymetazoline nasal spray	0.05%	0
Phenylephrine (Neo-Synephrine® Pediatric Formula Nasal Drops)	0.125%	0
Xylometazoline (Otrivin® Pediatric Nasal Drops)	0.05%	0
Fluoride		
Sodium fluoride (Luride® Drops (peach flavor)	0.5 mg/mL (fluoride ion)	0.7
Laxatives		
Docusate sodium sorbitol glycerin capsules (Correctol® Extra Gentle Stool Softener)	100 mg	0.13
Docusate sodium liquigels (Surfak®)	240 mg	0.37
Docusate sodium syrup	20 mg/5 mL	1.4
Glycerin suppositories	82.5% glycerin/1.35 g	1.11
Magnesium hydroxide in purified water and mineral oil	300 mg/5 mL	0
Magnesium hydroxide (Phillips'® MOM Mint)	40 mEq elem mg/15 mL	0
Mono and dibesic sodium phosphate enema (Fleets®)	Enema	0
Senna children's syrup (Senokot® Children's)	5 mL	3.3
Senna syrup (Senokot®)	5 mL	3.3
Senna granules (Senokot®)	Teaspoonful	2
Senna tablets (Senokot®)	Tablet	0.03
Senna tablets (Senokot-S®)	Tablet	0.05
Senna tablets (SenokotXTRA®)	Tablet	0.08
Multiple Vitamin and Mineral Supplements		
Multiple vitamin and mineral supplement (Bugs Bunny Complete)	Chewable tablet (sugar free)	0.37
Multiple vitamin and mineral supplement (Bugs Bunny Plus Iron)	Chewable tablet	0.47
Multiple vitamin and mineral supplement (Bugs Bunny With Extra C)	Chewable tablet	0.32
Multiple vitamin and mineral supplement (Centrum® Advanced Formula Liquid)	15 mL	6.25
Multiple vitamin and mineral supplement (Centrum® Advanced Formula Tablets)	Tablet	0.25
Multiple vitamin and mineral supplement (Centrum® Kids Rugrats™ Extra Calcium)	Chewable tablet	<0.5
Multiple vitamin and mineral supplement (Centrum® Kids Rugrats™ Extra C)	Chewable tablet	<0.5

Description (Brand Name)	Dosage Unit	Grams Carbohydrate per Dosage Unit
Multiple vitamin and mineral supplement (Centrum® Kids Rugrats™ Complete)	Chewable tablet	<0.5
Multiple vitamin and mineral supplement (Flinstones® Plus Extra C)	Chewable tablet	<0.6
Multiple vitamin and mineral supplement (Flinstones® Plus Iron)	Chewable tablet	0.65
Multiple vitamin and mineral supplement (Flinstones® Plus Calcium)	Chewable tablet	0.11
Multiple vitamin and mineral supplement (Flinstones® Original)	Chewable tablet	0.70
Multiple vitamin and mineral supplement (Flinstones® Complete)	Chewable tablet (sugar free)	0.37
Multiple vitamin and mineral supplement (Unicap®)	Tablet	0.25
Multiple vitamin and mineral supplement (Unicap®)	Capsule	0.25
Calcium Containing Vitamin Products		
Calcium carbonate capsules (Calci-Mix®)	1250 mg	0
Calcium carbonate tablets (Caltrate® 600)	1500 mg	0.25
Calcium citrate capsules (Citracal®)	2,376 mg	0
Calcium carbonate tablets	640 mg	0.05
Calcium carbonate, iron, vitamin D tablets (Caltrate® 600 + Iron and Vitamin D)	1500 mg	0.25
Calcium carbonate gelcap (Liqui-Cal®)	600 mg	0.16
Calcium carbonate suspension	1250 mg/5 mL	1.75
Calcium citrate + magnesium gelcap	Gelcap	0.15
Calcium citrate, vitamin D, vitamin A tablets (Nutravescent®)	250 mg	0.07
Calcium, elemental (Calcet®)	Tablet	0.07
Calcium-iron multivitamin (Calcet® Plus)	Tablet	0.07
Calcium citrate (Citracal®)	950 mg	0
Iron-Containing Vitamin Products		
Ferrous fumarate (Ferro-Sequels®)	Capsule	0.5
Ferrous sulfate drops (Fer-In-Sol®)	75 mg/0.6 mL	0.7
Ferrous sulfate syrup (Fer-In-Sol®)	90 mg/5 mL	6.25
Iron, vitamin B, vitamin D drops (Poly-Vi-Sol® With Iron)	10 mg/mL	0.63
Iron, vitamins A, D, E, C drops (Vi-Daylin® + Iron Drops)	20 mg/mL	0.75
Iron, vitamins A, D, E, C liquid (Vi-Daylin® Liquid With Iron)	10 mg/5 mL	5
Iron, vitamins A, D, E, C, folic acid chewable tablets (Vi-Daylin® Chewable With Iron)	12 mg 0.3 mg	0.43

CARBOHYDRATE CONTENT OF MEDICATIONS
(Continued)

Description (Brand Name)	Dosage Unit	Grams Carbohydrate per Dosage Unit
Miscellaneous		
Aminocaproic acid syrup (Amicar®)	250 mg/mL	0.26
Calcium carbonate tablets (Mylanta® Children's Chewables)	400 mg	0.93
Calcium carbonate suspension (Mylanta® Children's Suspension)	400 mg/5 mL	1.5
Calcium carbonate tablets (Tums® Regular)	500 mg	0.75
Calcium carbonate tablets (Tums® 500)	1250 mg	1.9
Calcium carbonate extra strength tablets (Tums® E-X)	750 mg	1.1
Calcium carbonate ultra tablets (Tums® Ultra)	1000 mg	1.5
Calcium carbonate sugar free extra strength tablets (Tums® Extra Strength Sugar Free)	750 mg	0.5
Carnitine solution (Carnitor®)	1 g/10 mL	0.48
Chloral hydrate	500 mg/5 mL	3
Chlorothiazide suspension (Diuril®) *0.025 ethyl alcohol/5 mL	250 mg/5 mL	2
Cimetidine tablets (Tagamet®)	200 mg	0.01
Cimetidine tablets (Tagamet®)	300 mg	0.01
Cimetidine tablets (Tagamet®)	400 mg	0.01
Cimetidine tablets (Tagamet®)	800 mg	0.02
Cimetidine liquid (Tagamet®) *0.5 ethyl alcohol/5 mL	300 mg/5 mL	2.8
Citalopram solution (Celexa™)	10 mg/5 mL	2.5
Clindamycin solution (Cleocin®)	75 mg/5 mL	1.89
Clonidine tablets (Catapres®)	0.1 mg	0.12
Clonidine tablets (Catapres®)	0.2 mg	0.11
Clonidine tablets (Catapres®)	0.3 mg	0.16
Cyclosporine oral suspension (Neoral®)	100 mg/mL	0
Cyclosporine capsules (Neoral®)	25 mg	0.01
Cyclosporine capsules (Neoral®)	100 mg	0.04
Cyclosporine oral suspension (Sandimmune®) *0.12 ethyl alcohol/mL	100 mg/mL	0
Cyclosporine capsules (Sandimmune®)	25 mg	0
Cyclosporine capsules (Sandimmune®)	50 mg	0.01
Cyclosporine capsules (Sandimmune®)	100 mg	0
Dexamethasone oral solution (Dexamethasone Intensol®) *0.3 ethyl alcohol/mL	0.5 mg/5 mL 1 mg/mL	1.7 0

Description (Brand Name)	Dosage Unit	Grams Carbohydrate per Dosage Unit
Diazepam oral solution	5 mg/5 mL	1
Digoxin pediatric elixir (Lanoxin®) *0.1 ethyl alcohol/mL	0.05 mg/mL	0.3
Digoxin tablets (Lanoxin®)	0.25 mg	0.10
Digoxin tablets (Lanoxin®)	0.125 mg	0.09
Famotidine oral suspension (Pepcid®)	40 mg/5 mL	1.19
Famotidine tablets (Pepcid®)	20 mg	0.09
Famotidine tablets (Pepcid®)	40 mg	0.08
Fluoxetine liquid (Prozac®)	20 mg/5 mL	1
Fluoxetine capsules (Prozac®)	10 mg	0.22
Fluoxetine capsules (Prozac®)	20 mg	0.21
Furosemide tablets (Lasix®)	20 mg	0.06
Furosemide tablets (Lasix®)	40 mg	0.11
Furosemide tablets (Lasix®)	80 mg	0.22
Furosemide elixir (Lasix®)	10 mg/mL	0.8
Glycopyrrolate tablets (Robinul®)	1 mg	0.1
Glycopyrrolate tablets (Robinul®)	2 mg	0.18
Loperamide (Imodium® A-D) *0.26 ethyl alcohol/5 mL	1 mg/5 mL	4.13
Megaldrate, simethicone suspension (Riopan Plus®)	5 mL	0.37
Magnesium hydroxide, aluminum hydroxide, simethicone (Mylanta®)	Tablet – regular strength	0.49
Magnesium hydroxide, aluminum hydroxide, simethicone (Mylanta®)	Tablet – double strength	0.83
Magnesium carbonate, calcium carbonate (Mylanta®)	Gel capsule	0
Magnesium hydroxide, aluminum hydroxide, simethicone (different flavors available) (Mylanta®)	Liquid – regular strength, 5 mL	0.67
Magnesium hydroxide, aluminum hydroxide, simethicone (Mylanta®)	Liquid – double strength, 5 mL	0.67
Mesalamine capsules (Pentasa®)	250 mg	0.23
Metoclopramide syrup (Reglan®)	5 mg/5 mL	1.75
Metoclopramide tablets (Reglan®)	5 mg	0.11
Metoclopramide tablets (Reglan®)	10 mg	0.10
Nifedipine capsules (Procardia®)	10 mg	0.10
Nifedipine capsules (Procardia®)	20 mg	0.12
Potassium chloride (Rum-K®)	10 mEq/5 mL	2.26
Potassium chloride 10% *0.25 ethyl alcohol/5 mL	6.67 mEq/5 mL	0.25
Potassium chloride (Kaochlor® SF) *0.25 ethyl alcohol/5 mL	6.67 mEq/5 mL	0
Potassium citrate/sodium citrate (Polycitra®)		0
Prednisolone syrup (Prelone®)	5 mg/5 mL	2.01
Prednisolone syrup (Prelone®)	15 mg/5 mL	3.55
Prednisolone oral solution (Pediapred®)	5 mg/5 mL	1.53

CARBOHYDRATE CONTENT OF MEDICATIONS
(Continued)

Description (Brand Name)	Dosage Unit	Grams Carbohydrate per Dosage Unit
Prednisone oral solution *0.25 ethyl alcohol/5 mL	5 mg/5 mL	1.8
Ranitidine syrup (Zantac®)	150 mg/10 mL	1
Ranitidine efferdose granules (Zantac®)	150 mg/packet	0
Ranitidine efferdose tablets (Zantac®)	150 mg	0
Ranitidine tablets (Zantac®)	All strengths	0
Simethicone drops (Mylicon®)	40 mg/0.6 mL	<0.071
Theophylline elixir (Elixophyllin®) *0.86 ethyl alcohol/5 mL	26.67 mg/5 mL	0.31
Vitamin D drops (Drisdol®)	8000 units/mL	0
Vitamin E drops (Aquasol E®)	15 units/0.3 mL	0.06

References

Adapted from Feldstein TJ, "Carbohydrate and Alcohol Content of 200 Oral Liquid Medications for Use in Patients Receiving Ketogenic Diets," *Pediatrics*, 1996, 97:506-11.

Adapted from McGhee B and Katyal N, "Avoid Unnecessary Drug-Related Carbohydrates for Patients Consuming the Ketogenic Diet," *J Am Diet Assoc*, 2001, 101(1):87-101.

ORAL MEDICATIONS THAT SHOULD NOT BE CRUSHED OR ALTERED

There are a variety of reasons for crushing tablets or capsule contents prior to administering to the patient. Patients may have nasogastric tubes which do not permit the administration of tablets or capsules; an oral solution for a particular medication may not be available from the manufacturer or readily prepared by pharmacy; patients may have difficulty swallowing capsules or tablets; or mixing of powdered medication with food or drink may make the drug more palatable.

Generally, medications which should not be crushed fall into one of the following categories.

- **Extended-Release Products**. The formulation of some tablets is specialized as to allow the medication within it to be slowly released into the body. This is sometimes accomplished by centering the drug within the core of the tablet, with a subsequent shedding of multiple layers around the core. Wax melts in the GI tract. Slow-K® is an example of this. Capsules may contain beads which have multiple layers which are slowly dissolved with time.

  Common Abbreviations for Extended-Release Products

CD	Controlled dose
CR	Controlled release
CRT	Controlled-release tablet
LA	Long-acting
SR	Sustained release
TR	Timed release
TD	Time delay
SA	Sustained action
XL	Extended release
XR	Extended release

- **Medications Which Are Irritating to the Stomach**. Tablets which are irritating to the stomach may be enteric-coated which delays release of the drug until the time when it reaches the small intestine. Enteric-coated aspirin is an example of this.

- **Foul-Tasting Medication**. Some drugs are quite unpleasant to taste so the manufacturer coats the tablet in a sugar coating to increase its palatability. By crushing the tablet, this sugar coating is lost and the patient tastes the unpleasant tasting medication.

- **Sublingual Medication**. Medication intended for use under the tongue should not be crushed. While it appears to be obvious, it is not always easy to determine if a medication is to be used sublingually. Sublingual medications should indicate on the package that they are intended for sublingual use.

- **Effervescent Tablets**. These are tablets which, when dropped into a liquid, quickly dissolve to yield a solution. Many effervescent tablets, when crushed, lose their ability to quickly dissolve.

Recommendations

1. It is not advisable to crush certain medications.
2. Consult individual monographs prior to crushing capsule or tablet.
3. If crushing a tablet or capsule is contraindicated, consult with your pharmacist to determine whether an oral solution exists or can be compounded.

ORAL MEDICATIONS THAT SHOULD NOT BE CRUSHED OR ALTERED *(Continued)*

Drug Product	Dosage Form	Dosage Reasons / Comments
Accuhist®	Tablet	Slow release[8]
Accutane®	Capsule	Mucous membrane irritant
Aciphex™	Tablet	Slow release
Adalat® CC	Tablet	Slow release
Adderall XR™	Capsule	Slow release[1]
Advicor®	Tablet	Slow release
Aerohist®	Tablet	Slow release
Afeditab™ CR	Tablet	Slow release
Aggrenox®	Capsule	Slow release **Note:** Capsule may be opened; contents include an aspirin tablet that may be chewed and dipyridamole pellets that may be sprinkled on applesauce
Alavert™ Allergy Sinus 12 Hour	Tablet	Slow release
Aldex™	Tablet	Slow release
Allegra-D®	Tablet	Slow release
Altocor™	Tablet	Slow release
Arthritis Bayer® Time Release	Capsule	Slow release
Arthrotec®	Tablet	Enteric-coated
A.S.A.® Enseals®	Tablet	Enteric-coated
Asacol®	Tablet	Slow release
Ascriptin® A/D	Tablet	Enteric-coated
Ascriptin® Extra Strength	Tablet	Enteric-coated
Augmentin XR™	Tablet	Slow release[2, 8]
Avinza™	Capsule	Slow release[1] (not pudding)
Avodart™	Capsule	Teratogenic potential[9]
Azulfidine® EN-tabs®	Tablet	Enteric-coated
Bayer® Aspirin EC	Caplet	Enteric-coated
Bayer® Aspirin, Low Adult 81 mg	Tablet	Enteric-coated
Bayer® Aspirin, Regular Strength 325 mg	Caplet	Enteric-coated
Biaxin® XL	Tablet	Slow release
Biltricide®	Tablet	Taste[8]
Bisacodyl	Tablet	Enteric-coated[3]
Bontril® Slow-Release	Capsule	Slow release
Bromfenex® PD	Tablet	Slow release
Calan® SR	Tablet	Slow release[8]
Carbatrol®	Capsule	Slow release[1]
Cardene® SR	Capsule	Slow release
Cardizem®	Tablet	Slow release
Cardizem® CD	Capsule	Slow release[1]
Cardizem® LA	Tablet	Slow release
Cardizem® SR	Capsule	Slow release[1]
Carter's Little Pills®	Tablet	Enteric-coated
Cartia® XT	Capsule	Slow release
Ceftin®	Tablet	Taste[2] **Note:** Use suspension for children
CellCept®	Capsule, tablet	Teratogenic potential[9]
Charcoal Plus®	Tablet	Enteric-coated
Chloral Hydrate	Capsule	**Note:** Product is in liquid form within a special capsule[2]
Chlor-Trimeton® 12-Hour	Tablet	Slow release[2]

Drug Product	Dosage Form	Dosage Reasons / Comments
Cipro™	Tablet	Taste[5]
Cipro® XR	Tablet	Slow release
Claritin-D® 12-Hour	Tablet	Slow release
Claritin-D® 24-Hour	Tablet	Slow release
Colace®	Capsule	Taste[5]
Colestid®	Tablet	Slow release
Comhist® LA	Capsule	Slow release[1]
Commit™	Lozenge	**Note:** Integrity compromised by chewing or crushing
Compazine® Spansule®	Capsule	Slow release[2]
Concerta®	Tablet	Slow release
Contac® 12-Hour	Tablet	Slow release
Cotazym-S®	Capsule	Enteric-coated[1]
Covera-HS™	Tablet	Slow release
Creon® 5, 10, 20	Capsule	Slow release[1]
Crixivan®	Capsule	Taste **Note:** Capsule may be opened and mixed with fruit puree (eg, banana)
Cymbalta®	Capsule	Enteric-coated
Cytovene®	Capsule	Skin irritant
Cytoxan®	Tablet	**Note:** Drug may be crushed, but maker recommends using injection
Dallergy®	Capsule	Slow release
Dallergy-JR®	Capsule	Slow release
Deconamine® SR	Capsule	Slow release[2]
Defen L.A.®	Tablet	Slow release[8]
Depakene®	Capsule	Slow release mucous membrane irritant[2]
Depakote®	Tablet	Slow release
Depakote® ER	Tablet	Slow release
Desoxyn®	Tablet	Slow release
Desyrel®	Tablet	Taste[5]
Detrol® LA	Capsule	Slow release
Dexedrine® Spansule®	Capsule	Slow release
Diamox® Sequels®	Capsule	Slow release
Dilacor® XR	Capsule	Slow release
Dilatrate-SR®	Capsule	Slow release
Diltia XT®	Capsule	Slow release
Ditropan® XL	Tablet	Slow release
Dolobid®	Tablet	Irritant
Donnatal® Extentab®	Tablet	Slow release[2]
Doryx®	Capsule	Enteric-coated
Drisdol®	Capsule	Liquid filled[4]
Drixoral®	Tablet	Slow release[2]
Drixoral® Plus	Tablet	Slow release
Drixoral® Sinus	Tablet	Slow release
Dulcolax®	Capsule	Liquid-filled
Dulcolax®	Tablet	Enteric-coated[3]
Duratuss® G	Tablet	Slow release[9]
Duratuss® GP	Tablet	Slow release[8]
Dynabac®	Tablet	Enteric-coated
DynaCirc® CR	Tablet	Slow release
Easprin®	Tablet	Enteric-coated
EC-Naprosyn®	Tablet	Enteric-coated
Ecotrin® Adult Low Strength	Tablet	Enteric-coated

ORAL MEDICATIONS THAT SHOULD NOT BE CRUSHED OR ALTERED *(Continued)*

Drug Product	Dosage Form	Dosage Reasons / Comments
Ecotrin® Maximum Strength	Tablet	Enteric-coated
Ecotrin® Regular Strength	Tablet	Enteric-coated
E.E.S.® 400	Tablet	Enteric-coated[2]
Effexor® XR	Capsule	Slow release
Efidac/24® Pseudoephedrine	Tablet	Slow release
Efidac® 24	Tablet	Slow release
E-Mycin®	Tablet	Enteric-coated
Entex® LA	Capsule	Slow release[2]
Entex® PSE	Capsule	Slow release
Entocort™ EC	Capsule	Enteric-coated[1]
Ergomar®	Tablet	Sublingual form[7]
Eryc®	Capsule	Enteric-coated[1]
Ery-Tab®	Tablet	Enteric-coated
Erythrocin Stearate	Tablet	Enteric-coated
Erythromycin Base	Tablet	Enteric-coated
Eskalith CR®	Tablet	Slow release
Evista®	Tablet	Taste; teratogenic potential[9]
Extendryl JR	Capsule	Slow release
Extendryl SR	Capsule	Slow release[2]
Feldene®	Capsule	Mucous membrane irritant
Feosol®	Tablet	Enteric-coated[2]
Feratab®	Tablet	Enteric-coated[2]
Fergon®	Tablet	Enteric-coated
Fero-Grad 500®	Tablet	Slow release
Ferro-Sequels®	Tablet	Slow release
Flagyl ER®	Tablet	Slow release
Flomax®	Capsule	Enteric-coated[1]
Fosamax®	Tablet	Mucous membrane irritant
Fumatinic®	Capsule	Slow release
Geocillin®	Tablet	Taste
Gleevec®	Tablet	Taste[8] **Note:** May be dissolved in mineral oil or apple juice
Glucophage® XR	Tablet	Slow release
Glucotrol® XL	Tablet	Slow release
Gris-PEG®	Tablet	**Note:** Crushing may result in precipitation of larger particles.
Guaifed®	Capsule	Slow release
Guaifed®-PD	Capsule	Slow release
Guaifenex® DM	Tablet	Slow release[8]
Guaifenex® LA	Tablet	Slow release[8]
Guaifenex® PSE	Tablet	Slow release[8]
Guaimax-D®	Tablet	Slow release
Hista-Vent® DA	Tablet	Slow release[8]
Humibid® DM	Tablet	Slow release
Humibid® LA	Tablet	Slow release
Iberet® Filmtab	Tablet	Slow release[2]
Iberet®-500	Tablet	Slow release[2]
Iberet-Folic-500®	Tablet	Slow release
ICAPS® Time Release	Tablet	Slow release
Imdur™	Tablet	Slow release[8]
Inderal® LA	Capsule	Slow release
Inderide® LA	Capsule	Slow release

Drug Product	Dosage Form	Dosage Reasons / Comments
Indocin® SR	Capsule	Slow release[1,2]
InnoPran XL™	Capsule	Slow release
Ionamin®	Capsule	Slow release
Isoptin® SR	Tablet	Slow release
Isordil® Sublingual	Tablet	Sublingual form[7]
Isosorbide Dinitrate Sublingual	Tablet	Sublingual form[7]
Isosorbide SR	Tablet	Slow release
K+ 8®	Tablet	Slow release[2]
K+ 10®	Tablet	Slow release[2]
Kadian®	Capsule	Slow release[1] **Note:** Do not give via N/G tubes
Kaon-Cl®	Tablet	Slow release[2]
K-Dur®	Tablet	Slow release
Klor-Con®	Tablet	Slow release[2]
Klor-Con® M	Tablet	Slow release[2]
Klotrix®	Tablet	Slow release[2]
K-Lyte®	Tablet	Effervescent tablet[6]
K-Lyte/Cl®	Tablet	Effervescent tablet[6]
K-Lyte DS®	Tablet	Effervescent tablet[6]
K-Tab®	Tablet	Slow release[2]
Lescol® XL	Tablet	Slow release
Levbid®	Tablet	Slow release[8]
Levsinex® Timecaps®	Capsule	Slow release
Lexxel®	Tablet	Slow release
Lipram 4500	Capsule	Enteric-coated[1]
Lipram-CR	Capsule	Enteric-coated[1]
Lipram-PN	Capsule	Enteric-coated[1]
Lipram-UL	Capsule	Enteric-coated[1]
Lipram (all products)	Capsule	Slow release[1]
Liquibid-PD	Tablet	Slow release[8]
Lithobid®	Tablet	Slow release
Lodine® XL	Tablet	Slow release
Lodrane® LD	Capsule	Slow release[1]
Mag-Tab® SR	Tablet	Slow release
Maxifed®	Tablet	Slow release
Maxifed® DM	Tablet	Slow release
Maxifed-G®	Tablet	Slow release
Mestinon® Timespan®	Tablet	Slow release[2]
Metadate® CD	Capsule	Slow release[1]
Metadate™ ER	Tablet	Slow release
Methylin™ ER	Tablet	Slow release
Micro-K®	Capsule	Slow release
Modane®	Tablet	Enteric-coated
Motrin®	Tablet	Taste[5]
MS Contin®	Tablet	Slow release[2]
Mucinex®	Tablet	Slow release
Myfortic®	Tablet	Slow release
Naprelan®	Tablet	Slow release
Nasatab® LA	Tablet	Slow release[8]
Nexium®	Capsule	Slow release[1]
Niaspan®	Tablet	Slow release
Nicotinic Acid	Capsule, tablet	Slow release
Nifediac™ CC	Tablet	Slow release
Nitrostat®	Tablet	Sublingual route[7]
Norflex™	Tablet	Slow release

ORAL MEDICATIONS THAT SHOULD NOT BE CRUSHED OR ALTERED *(Continued)*

Drug Product	Dosage Form	Dosage Reasons / Comments
Norpace® CR	Capsule	Slow release form within a special capsule
Oramorph SR®	Tablet	Slow release[2]
Oruvail®	Capsule	Slow release
OxyContin®	Tablet	Slow release
Palgic®-D	Tablet	Slow release[8]
Pancrease®	Capsule	Enteric-coated[1]
Pancrease® MT	Capsule	Enteric-coated[1]
Pancrecarb MS®	Capsule	Enteric-coated[1]
Pangestyme™ CN 10	Capsule	Enteric-coated
Pangestyme™ CN 20	Capsule	Enteric-coated
Pangestyme™ EC	Capsule	Enteric-coated
Pangestyme™ MT 16	Capsule	Enteric-coated
Pangestyme™ UL 12	Capsule	Enteric-coated
Pangestyme™ UL 18	Capsule	Enteric-coated
Pangestyme™ UL 20	Capsule	Enteric-coated
PanMist®-DM	Tablet	Slow release[8]
PanMist®-Jr	Tablet	Slow release[8]
PanMist®-LA	Tablet	Slow release[8]
Pannaz®	Tablet	Slow release[8]
Papaverine Sustained Action	Capsule	Slow release
Paxil CR™	Tablet	Slow release
Pentasa®	Capsule	Slow release
Perdiem® Fiber Therapy	Granules	Wax coated
PhenaVent™ D	Tablet	Slow release
Plendil®	Tablet	Slow release
Prelu-2®	Capsule	Slow release
Prevacid®	Capsule	Slow release
Prevacid®	Suspension	Slow release **Note:** Contains enteric-coated granules
Prilosec®	Capsule	Slow release
Procainamide HCl SR	Tablet	Slow release
Procanbid®	Tablet	Slow release
Procardia®	Capsule	Delays absorption[2, 5]
Procardia XL®	Tablet	Slow release **Note:** AUC is unaffected.
Profen II®	Tablet	Slow release[8]
Profen II DM®	Tablet	Slow release[8]
Profen Forte™ DM	Tablet	Slow release
Pronestyl®-SR	Tablet	Slow release
Propecia®	Tablet	**Note:** Women who are, or may become, pregnant, should not handle crushed or broken tablets
Proscar®	Tablet	**Note:** Women who are, or may become, pregnant, should not handle crushed or broken tablets
Protonix®	Tablet	Slow release
Quibron-T/SR®	Tablet	Slow release[2]
Rescon-Jr	Tablet	Slow release
Respa-DM®	Tablet	Slow release[8]
Respaire®-120 SR	Capsule	Slow release
Ritalin® LA	Capsule	Slow release

Drug Product	Dosage Form	Dosage Reasons / Comments
Ritalin-SR®	Tablet	Slow release
Rondec-TR®	Tablet	Slow release[2]
Rythmol® SR	Capsule	Slow release
Sinemet® CR	Tablet	Slow release
SINUvent® PE	Tablet	Slow release[8]
Slo-Niacin®	Tablet	Slow release[8]
Slow Fe®	Tablet	Slow release
Slow-Mag®	Tablet	Slow release
Somnote™	Capsule	Liquid filled
Sudafed® 12-Hour	Capsule	Slow release[2]
Sular®	Tablet	Slow release
Sulfazine EC	Tablet	Enteric-coated
Symax SR	Tablet	Slow release
Taztia XT™	Capsule	Slow release
Tegretol®-XR	Tablet	Slow release
Temodar®	Capsule	**Note:** If capsules are accidentally opened or damaged, rigorous precautions should be taken to avoid inhalation or contact of contents with the skin or mucous membranes[9]
Tessalon®	Capsule	Slow release
Theo-24®	Tablet	Slow release[2]
Theochron®	Tablet	Slow release
Tiazac®	Capsule	Slow release
Topamax®	Capsule	Taste[1]
Topamax®	Tablet	Taste
Toprol-XL®	Tablet	Slow release
Touro™ CC	Tablet	Slow release
Touro EX®	Tablet	Slow release
Touro LA®	Tablet	Slow release
Tranxene® SD™	Tablet	Slow release
Trental®	Tablet	Slow release
TripTone®	Tablet	Slow release
Tylenol® Arthritis Pain	Tablet	Slow release
Tylenol® 8 Hour	Tablet	Slow release
Ultrase®	Capsule	Enteric-coated[1]
Ultrase® MT	Capsule	Enteric-coated[1]
Uniphyl®	Tablet	Slow release
Urocit®-K	Tablet	Wax-coated
Verelan®	Capsule	Slow release[1]
Videx® EC	Capsule	Slow release
Voltaren®-XR	Tablet	Slow release
VoSpire ER™	Tablet	Slow release
Wellbutrin SR®	Tablet	Slow release
Wellbutrin XL™	Tablet	Slow release
Xanax XR®	Tablet	Slow release
Z-Cof LA	Tablet	Slow release[8]
Zephrex LA®	Tablet	Slow release
ZORprin®	Tablet	Slow release
Zyban®	Tablet	Slow release

ORAL MEDICATIONS THAT SHOULD NOT BE CRUSHED OR ALTERED *(Continued)*

[1]Capsule may be opened and the contents taken without crushing or chewing; soft food such as applesauce or pudding may facilitate administration; contents may generally be administered via nasogastric tube using an appropriate fluid, provided entire contents are washed down the tube.

[2]Liquid dosage forms of the product are available; however, dose, frequency of administration, and manufacturers may differ from that of the solid dosage form.

[3]Antacids and/or milk may prematurely dissolve the coating of the tablet.

[4]Capsule may be opened and the liquid contents removed for administration.

[5]The taste of this product in a liquid form would likely be unacceptable to the patient; administration via nasogastric tube should be acceptable.

[6]Effervescent tablets must be dissolved in the amount of diluent recommended by the manufacturer.

[7]Tablets are made to disintegrate under the tongue.

[8]Tablet is scored and may be broken in half without affecting release characteristics.

[9]Skin contact may enhance tumor production; avoid direct contact.

Adapted from Mitchell JF, "Oral Dosage Forms That Should Not Be Crushed-2004," available at: www.hospitalpharmacyjournal.com.

THERAPEUTIC CATEGORY & KEY WORD INDEX

INTERNATIONAL TRADE NAMES INDEX

The following countries are included in this index and are abbreviated as follows:

Antilles (Netherlands) (AN)
Argentina (AR)
Australia (AU)
Austria (AT)
Bahamas (BS)
Bahrain (BH)
Bangladesh (BD)
Barbados (BB)
Belgium (BE)
Belize (BZ)
Benin (BJ)
Bermuda (BM)
Bolivia (BO)
Brazil (BR)
Bulgaria (BG)
Burkina Faso (BF)
Canada (CA)
Chile (CL)
China (CN)
Colombia (CO)
Costa Rica (CR)
Croatia (HR)
Cuba (CU)
Cyprus (CY)
Czech Republic (CZ)
Denmark (DK)
Dominican Republic (DO)
Ecuador (EC)
Egypt (EG)
El Salvador (SV)
Estonia (EE)
Ethiopia (ET)
Finland (FI)
France (FR)
Gambia (GM)
Germany (DE)
Ghana (GH)
Great Britain [UK] (GB)
Greece (GR)
Guatemala (GT)
Guinea (GN)
Guyana (GY)
Honduras (HN)
Hong Kong (HK)
Hungary (HU)
Iceland (IS)
India (IN)
Indonesia (ID)
Iran (IR)
Iraq (IQ)
Ireland (IE)
Israel (IL)
Italy (IT)
Ivory Coast (CI)
Jamaica (JM)
Japan (JP)
Jordan (JO)
Kenya (KE)
Korea (KR)
Kuwait (KW)
Latvia (LV)
Lebanon (LB)
Liberia (LR)
Libya (LY)
Liechtenstein (LI)
Lithuania (LT)
Luxembourg (LU)
Malawi (MW)
Malaysia (MY)
Mali (ML)
Malta (MT)
Mauritania (MR)
Mauritius (MU)
Mexico (MX)
Monaco (MC)
Morocco (MA)
Netherlands (NL)
New Zealand (NZ)
Nicaragua (NI)
Niger (NE)
Nigeria (NG)
Norway (NO)
Oman (OM)
Pakistan (PK)
Panama (PA)
Paraguay (PY)
Peru (PE)
Philippines (PH)
Poland (PL)
Portugal (PT)
Puerto Rico (PR)
Qatar (QA)
Republic of Yemen (YE)
Romania (RO)
Russia (RU)
Saudi Arabia (SA)
Senegal (SN)
Seychelles (SC)
Sierra Leone (SL)
Singapore (SG)
Slovakia (SK)
Slovenia (SI)
South Africa (ZA)
Spain (ES)
Sri Lanka (LK)
Sudan (SD)
Surinam (SR)
Sweden (SE)
Switzerland (CH)
Syria (SY)
Taiwan (TW)
Tanzania (TZ)
Thailand (TH)
Trinidad (TT)
Turkey (TR)
Uganda (UG)
Ukraine (UA)
United Arab Emirates (AE)
Uruguay (UY)
Venezuela (VE)
Vietnam (VN)
Yugoslavia (YU)
Zambia (ZM)
Zimbabwe (ZW)

NOTES

NOTES

NOTES

NOTES

NOTES

NOTES

NOTES

NOTES

NOTES

NOTES

NOTES

NOTES

NOTES

Other Products Offered by Lexi-Comp®

Anesthesiology & Critical Care Drug Handbook

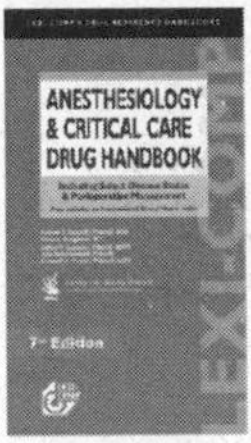

Designed for anesthesiologists, critical care practitioners, and all healthcare professionals involved in the care of surgical or ICU patients.

Includes: Comprehensive drug information to ensure the appropriate clinical management of patients; Intensivist and Anesthesiologist perspective; Over 2000 medications most commonly used in the preoperative and critical care setting; and Special Topics/Issues section with frequently encountered patient conditions

Clinician's Guide to Diagnosis

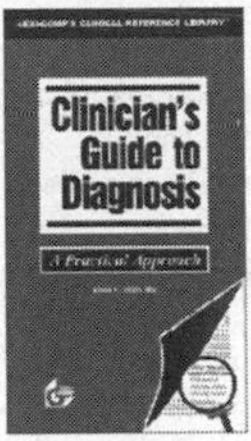

A reference with a practical approach to commonly-encountered symptoms, designed to follow the logical thought process of a seasoned clinician.

Includes: Evidence-based, easy-to-find answers to the questions that commonly arise in the symptom evaluation process; Over 35 algorithms that provide parallel references to the information in each chapter

Clinician's Guide to Internal Medicine

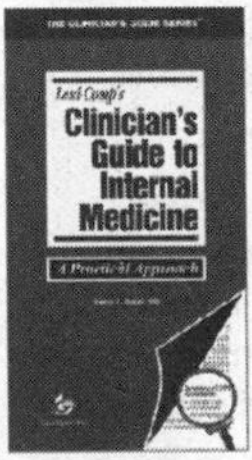

Quick access to essential information covering diagnosis, treatment, and management of commonly-encountered patient conditions in Internal Medicine.

Includes: Practical approaches ideal for point-of-care use; Algorithms to establish a diagnosis and select the appropriate therapy; and Tables to summarize diagnostic and therapeutic strategies

Clinician's Guide to Laboratory Medicine

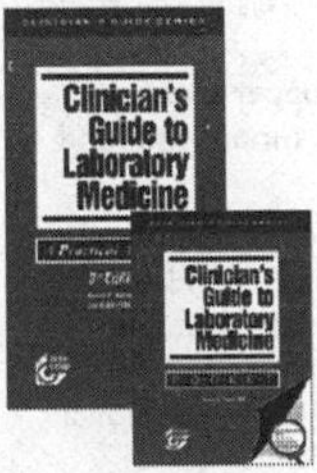

A resource providing a logical step-by-step process from an abnormal lab test to diagnosis. This two-book set provides you with a full size guide and a portable pocket version for convenient referencing.

Includes: 137 chapters; 700 charts, tables, and algorithms; and sections such as neurology, infectious diseases, and obstetrics/gynecology

To order call Customer Service at 1-866-397-3433 or go to www.lexi.com.

Outside of the U.S. call: 330-650-6506 or www.lexi.com

Other Products Offered by Lexi-Comp®

Drug Information Handbook for Oncology

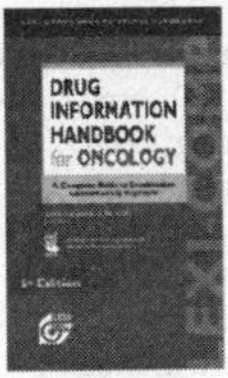

Designed for oncology professionals requiring information on combination chemotherapy regimens and dosing protocols.

Includes: Monographs containing warnings, adverse reaction profiles, drug interactions, dosing for specific indications, vesicant, emetic potential, combination regimens, and more; Where applicable, a special Combination Chemotherapy field that will link you to specific oncology monographs; Special Topics such as Cancer Treatment Related Complications, Bone Marrow Transplantation, and Drug Development

Drug Information Handbook for Perioperative Nursing

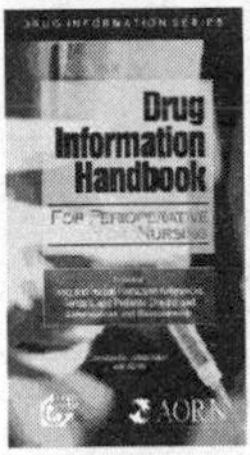

Designed especially for perioperative nurses, Registered Nurses practicing in operative and interventional procedure settings, and upper-division nursing students seeking a distinctive reference for dosing, administration, monitoring, and patient education criteria for perioperative patient care environments. Includes: Up to 40 fields per monograph including Medication Safety data; Adult, Pediatric, and Geriatric Dosing guidelines; and information on each phase of the perioperative encounter, with emphasis on special situations central to perioperative patient care.

Drug Information Handbook for Psychiatry

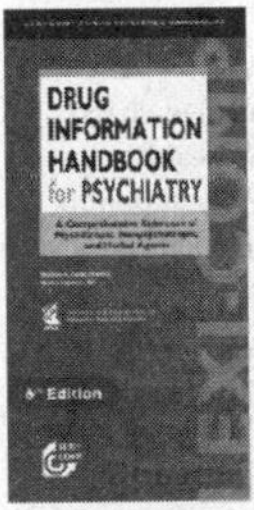

Designed for any healthcare professional requiring quick access to comprehensive drug information as it relates to mental health issues.

Includes: Detailed drug monographs for psychotropic, nonpsychotropic, and herbal medications; Special fields such as Mental Health Comment (useful clinical pearls), Medication Safety Issues, Effects on Mental Status, and Effects on Psychiatric Treatment.

Geriatric Dosage Handbook

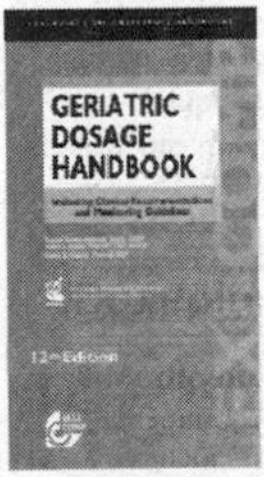

Designed for any healthcare professional managing geriatric patients.

Includes: Complete adult and geriatric dosing; Special geriatric considerations; Up to 36 key fields of information in each monograph including Medication Safety Issues; and Extensive information on drug interactions as well as dosing for patients with renal/hepatic impairment.

To order call Customer Service at 1-866-397-3433 or go to www.lexi.com.
Outside of the U.S. call: 330-650-6506 or www.lexi.com

Other Products Offered by Lexi-Comp®

Laboratory Test Handbook

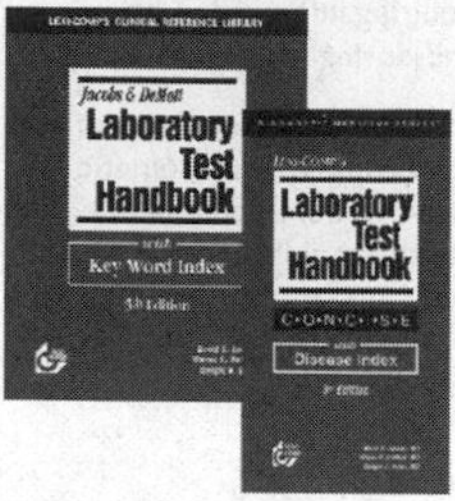

An invaluable source of information for anyone interested in diagnostic laboratory testing. Includes: 960 tests; Up to 25 fields per test; Extensive cross-referencing; Over 12,000 references; and Key Word Index: test result, disease, organ system and syndrome.
Clinicians, nurse practitioners, residents, nurses, and students will appreciate the Concise version of the *Laboratory Test Handbook* for its convenience as a quick reference. This abridged version includes 876 tests.

Pharmacogenomics Handbook

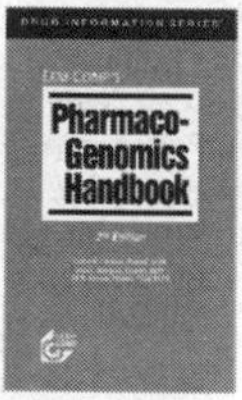

Ideal for any healthcare professional or student wishing to gain insight into the emerging field of pharmacogenomics.
Includes: Information concerning key genetic variations that may influence drug disposition and/or sensitivity; brief introductions to fundamental concepts in genetics and genomics. A foundation for all clinicians who will be called on to integrate rapidly-expanding genomic knowledge into the management of drug therapy.

Pharmacology Companion Guide

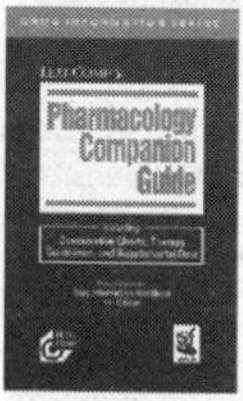

This guide supplies the best of Lexi-Comp's comparative charts, therapy guidelines, and supplemental data. Ideal for healthcare providers who require a quick reference to all the key appendix information found in our popular *Drug Information Handbook* or as a companion to our PDA software.

Includes: Abbreviations and measurements; ACLS Algorithms; Cytochrome P450 and Drug Interactions; and Laboratory Values

Pediatric Pharmacology Companion Guide

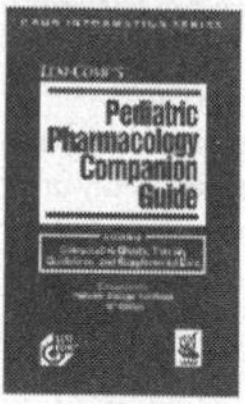

This guide supplies the best of Lexi-Comp's comparative charts, therapy guidelines, and supplemental data. Ideal as a quick reference to all the key appendix information found in our popular *Pediatric Dosage Handbook* or as a companion to our PDA software.

Includes: Apgar Scoring System; CPR Pediatric Drug Dosages; Immunization Guidelines; and Pediatric ALS Algorithms

To order call Customer Service at 1-866-397-3433 or go to www.lexi.com.
Outside of the U.S. call: 330-650-6506 or www.lexi.com